Meyler's Side Effects of Drugs

Complementary to this volume:

SIDE EFFECTS OF DRUGS ANNUALS 1–19 (1977–1995)
Edited by M.N.G. Dukes (Annuals 1–15) and J.K. Aronson (Annuals 16–18)

SEDBASE – The Side Effects of Drugs Database

DRUG-INDUCED DISORDERS
Edited by M.N.G. Dukes

Vol. 1 Drug-Induced Hepatic Injury, 2nd Edition (1992)
B.H.Ch. Stricker and P. Spoelstra

Vol. 2 Drug-Induced Diseases in the Elderly (1986)
F.I. Caird and P.J.W. Scott

Vol. 3 Treatment-Induced Respiratory Disorders (1989)
G.M. Akoun and J.P. White

Vol. 4 Drug-induced Immune Disease (1990)
J. Descotes

UNWANTED EFFECTS OF COSMETICS AND DRUGS USED IN DERMATOLOGY
3rd EDITION (1994)
A.C. de Groot, J.W. Weyland and J.P. Nater

IMMUNOTOXICOLOGY OF DRUGS AND CHEMICALS, 2nd EDITION (1986)
J. Descotes

DRUGS AND HUMAN LACTATION, Second Edition (1996)
P.N. Bennett

RESPONSIBILITY FOR DRUG-INDUCED INJURY (1988)
M.N.G. Dukes and B. Swartz

DRUG SAFETY IN PREGNANCY (1990)
P.I. Folb

The International Journal of RISK AND SAFETY IN MEDICINE
Edited by M.N.G. Dukes

Publishing history of Meyler's Side Effects of Drugs

1951	*First published in Dutch*	L. Meyler
1952	*First published in English*	L. Meyler
1957	*First updating volume*	Edited by L. Meyler
1958	*Second edition*	Edited by L. Meyler
1960	*Third edition*	Edited by L. Meyler
1964	*Fourth edition*	Edited by L. Meyler
1966	*Fifth edition*	Edited by L. Meyler, C. Dalderup, W. van Dijl and H.G.D. Bouma
1968	*Sixth edition*	Edited by L. Meyler and A. Herxheimer
1972	*Seventh edition*	Edited by L. Meyler and A. Herxheimer
1975	*Eighth edition*	Edited by M.N.G. Dukes
1980	*Ninth edition*	Edited by M.N.G. Dukes
1984	*Tenth edition*	Edited by M.N.G. Dukes
1988	*Eleventh edition*	Edited by M.N.G. Dukes
1992	*Twelfth edition*	Edited by M.N.G. Dukes
1996	*Thirteenth edition*	Edited by M.N.G. Dukes

Meyler's Side Effects of Drugs

An Encyclopedia of Adverse Reactions and Interactions

Thirteenth Edition

Editor

M.N.G. DUKES, M.D., M.A., LL.M.

Professor of Drug Policy Science
University of Groningen, The Netherlands

Co-Editors

J.K. Aronson, M.A., D.PHIL., M.B., F.R.C.P., Oxford
P.I. Folb, M.D., F.R.C.P., Cape Town
R. Hoigné, M.D., Berne
P.K.M. Lunde, Ph.D., Oslo
C.B.M. Tester-Dalderup, M.D., Edmonton
C.J. Van Boxtel, Ph.D., Amsterdam
B. Vrhovac, Ph.D., Zagreb

1996

ELSEVIER Amsterdam—Lausanne—New York—Oxford—Shannon—Tokyo

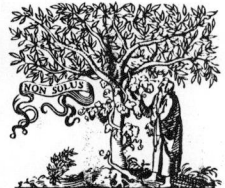

This book is printed on acid free paper.

ISBN 0 444 82405 7

Library of Congress Cataloging in Publication Data
Please refer to Card No. 80-647056

Published by:
Elsevier Science B.V.
P.O. Box 211
1000 AE Amsterdam
The Netherlands

Printed in The Netherlands

Editor

Responsibility for Chapters:

M.N.G. DUKES, M.A., D. PHIL., M.B., F.R.C.P.
Trosterudveien 19
0386 Oslo
Norway

Neuroleptics and antipsychotics
Anticonvulsants
Antipyretic analgesics
Antihistamines (H_1-receptor antagonists)
Antiallergic drugs and antitussives
Anthelminthic drugs
Blood, blood components, plasma and plasma products
Gastrointestinal drugs
Vitamins
Corticotrophins and corticosteroids
Thyroid and antithyroid drugs
Insulin, glucagon and oral hypoglycemic drugs
Drugs affecting lipid metabolism
Radiological contrast media and radiopharmaceuticals
Risks associated with complementary therapies

Co-editors

Responsibility for Chapters:

J.K. ARONSON, M.A., D. PHIL., M.B., F.R.C.P.
Department of Clinical Pharmacology
Radcliffe Infirmary
University of Oxford
Woodstock Road
Oxford, OX2 6HE
United Kingdom

Positive inotropic drugs and drugs used in dysrhythmias
Antianginal and β-adrenoceptor blocking drugs
Drugs acting on the cerebral and peripheral circulations and drugs used in the treatment of migraine
Antihypertensive drugs
Diuretics

P.I. FOLB, M.D., F.R.C.P.
Professor of Pharmacology
University of Cape Town Medical School
Groote Schuur Hospital
Observatory
7925 South Africa

Dermatological drugs, topical agents and cosmetics
Metals
Metal antagonists
Cytostatic and immunosuppressive drugs
Drugs used in ocular treatment
Miscellaneous drugs and materials

R. HOIGNÉ, M.D.
Scientific Secretariat CHDM
Zieglerspital
CH-3007 Bern
Switzerland

β-Lactam antibiotics
Reactions typically shared by more than one class of β-lactam antibiotics
Penicillins
Cephalosporins
β-Lactam antibiotics other than penicillins and cephalosporins
Miscellaneous antibiotics
Sulfonamides, other folic acid antagonists and miscellaneous antibacterial drugs
Antiviral drugs
Drugs used in tuberculosis and leprosy

Co-editors	*Responsibility for Chapters:*
P.K.M. LUNDE, PH.D. Director, Institute for Pharmacotherapy P.O. Box 1065, Blindern 0316 Oslo Denmark	Central nervous system stimulants and anorectic agents Drugs of abuse Hypnotics and sedatives Opioid analgesics and narcotic antagonists Antifungal drugs Antiprotozoal drugs
C.B.M. TESTER-DALDERUP, M.D. P.O. Box 11291 Edmonton, Alberta T5J 3JK5 Canada	Antiseptic drugs and disinfectants Intravenous infusions—solutions and emulsions Drugs acting on the immune system Miscellaneous hormones Prostaglandins
C.J. VAN BOXTEL, PH.D. Department of Internal Medicine Academic Medical Center Meibergdreef 9 1105 AZ Amsterdam	Antidepressant drugs Lithium Neuromuscular blocking agents and skeletal muscle relaxants Drugs affecting autonomic functions or the extrapyramidal system Immunobiological preparations
B. VRHOVAC, PH.D. Department of Medicine University Hospital Medical School Kispaticeva 12 41000 Zagreb Croatia	Anti-inflammatory analgesics and drugs used in gout General anesthetics and therapeutic gases Local anesthetics Drugs affecting blood clotting, fibrinolysis, and hemostasis Hemostatic agents Hormonal contraceptives Sex hormones

Contributors

J.K. ARONSON, M.A., D. PHIL., M.B., F.R.C.P.
Department of Clinical Pharmacology, Radcliffe Infirmary, University of Oxford, Woodstock Road, Oxford, OX2 6HE, United Kingdom

I. AURSNES, M.D.
Department of Pharmacotherapeutics, University of Oslo, P.O. Box 1065, Blindern, 0316 Oslo 3, Norway

Z. BAUDOIN, M.D.
Section of Anaesthesiology, Department of Surgery, Clinical Hospital Centre, Zagreb 12 Kispaticeva, 10000 Zagreb, Croatia

C. BINDSLEV-JENSEN, M.D., PH.D
Department of Dermatology, Odense University Hospital, 5000 Odense C, Denmark

LUCIANO BISCARINI, M.D.
IMISO, University Degli Studi Di Perugia, 06122 Perugia, Italy

J. BLASER, PH.D.
Division of Infectious Diseases, University Hospital of Zürich, Department of Internal Medicine, Zürich, Switzerland

S. BORG, M.D., PH.D.
Department of Clinical Neurosciences, St. Göran Clinic, Karolinska Institute, P.O. Box 12 557, 102 29 Stockholm, Sweden

C.C.E. BRODIE MEIJER
M.v.R. Altenahof 5, 1183 BT Amstelveen, The Netherlands

K. BRODIN
Department of Clinical Neurosciences, St. Göran Clinic, Karolinska Institute, P.O. Box 12 557, 102 29 Stockholm, Sweden

J. CARON, M.D.
Pharmacovigilance, Pharmacologie – CHRU, 1, Place de Verdun, 59045 Lille Cedex, France

A. CASTOT, M.D.
Centre de Pharmacovigilance, Hôpital Fernand Widal, 200, rue du Faubourg Saint-Denis, 75475 Paris Cedex 10, France

A. CERNY, M.D.
Medical Clinic, Zieglerspital, Postfach 2600, 3001 Bern, Switzerland

L.G. CLELAND
Rheumatology Unit, Royal Adelaide Hospital, North Terrace, Adelaide SA 5000, Australia

P. COATES, M.D.
Department of Medicine, The Endocrine and Metabolic Unit, Royal Adelaide Hospital, North Terrace, Adelaide, South Australia 500

P. COTTAGNOUD, M.D.
Department of Internal Medicine, Inselspital, 3010 Bern, Switzerland

A.C. DE GROOT, M.D., PH.D.
Department of Dermatology, Carolus-Liduina Hospital, P.O. Box 1101, 5200 BD Den Bosch, The Netherlands

P.A.G.M. DE SMET, PH.D.
Drug Information Center, Royal Dutch Association for the Advancement of Pharmacy, The Hague, The Netherlands

T.G.B.M. DE VRIES
Department of Clinical Pharmacology, Rijksuniversiteit, Bloemsingel 1, 9713 BZ Groningen, The Netherlands

J. DESCOTES, M.D., PHARM. D., PH.D.
Department of Pharmacology & Med. Toxicology, Fac. de Médecine Alexis Carrel, INSERM U80, F 69008 Lyon, France

S. DITTMANN, M.D., D.SC.MED.
a.i. Integrated Programme on Communicable Diseases, World Health Organization, 8 Scherfigsvej, 2100 Copenhagen O, Denmark

M.N.G. DUKES, M.D., M.A., LL.M.
Trosterudveien 19, 0386 Oslo, Norway

I.R. EDWARDS
WHO Collaborating Centre for International Drug Monitoring, P.O. Box 26, SE-751 03 Uppsala, Sweden

E.H. ELLINWOOD, JR., M.D.
Department of Psychiatry, Behavioral Neuropharmacology Section, Duke University Medical Center, Box 3870, Durham NC 27710, U.S.A.

H.L. ELLIOTT, M.D.
Department of Medicine and Therapeutics, Gardiner Institute, Western Infirmary, 46 Church Street, Glasgow G11 6NT, United Kingdom

E. ERNST
Center for Complementary Health Studies, University of Exeter, 25 Victoria Park Road, Exeter EX2 4NT, United Kingdom

P.I. FOLB, M.D., F.R.C.P.
Department of Pharmacology, Groote Schuur Hospital, K45 Old Main Building, Observatory, Cape Town, 7925 South Africa

F. FOLLATH, M.D.
Department of Internal Medicine, Universitätsspital Zürich, Rämistrasse 100, 8091 Zürich, Switzerland

H.M.P. FREIE
Rijksweg 68, 6247 AK Gronsveld, The Netherlands

P.J. GEERLINGS
Jellinek Kliniek, Postbus 3907, 1001 AS Amsterdam, The Netherlands

D. GERMANN, M.D.
Fachbereich für Diagnostische Virologie und Immunologischer Infektnachweis, Institut für Medizinische Mikrobiologie, Friedbühlstrasse 51, 3010 Bern, Switzerland

H. HAAK
Herbenusstraat 99A, 6211 RC Maastricht, The Netherlands

F. HACKENBERGER, M.D.
Bundesinstitut für Arzneimittel, Seestrasse 10, 13353 Berlin, Germany

E. HELSING, PH.D.
Trosterudveien 19, 0386 Oslo, Norway

C.L. HILL, M.D.
Rheumatology Registrar, Rheumatology Unit, Royal Adelaide Hospital, North Terrace, Adelaide, South Australia 5000

R. HOIGNÉ, M.D.
Scientific Secretariat CHDM, Zieglerspital, 3007 Bern, Switzerland

A.M.M. KADDU, M.D.
The National Drug Authority, c/o National Medical Stores, Entebbe, Uganda

H. KELLER, M.D.
Medical Clinic, Tiefenauspital, 3004 Bern, Switzerland

C. KOCH, M.D.
Division of Immunology, State Serum Institute, Artillerivej 5, DK-2300 Copenhagen 5, Denmark

H.M.J. KRANS, M.D.
Stofwisselingsziekten en Endocrinologie, Gebouw 1, C4-R, Academisch Ziekenhuis Leiden, Postbus 9600, 2300 RC Leiden, The Netherlands

R. LAVERTY, M.SC., PH.D.
Department of Pharmacology, Medical School, University of Otago, P.O. Box 913, Dunedin, New Zealand

T.H. LEE
Department of Psychiatry, Behavioral Neuropharmacology Section, Duke University Medical Center, Box 3870, Durham NC 27710, U.S.A.

P. LEUENBERGER, M.D.
Département de Médecine Interne, Division de Pneumologie, CHUV, 1011 Lausanne, Switzerland

M. LEUWER
Abteilung Anästhesiologie II, Zentrum Anästhesiologie, Medizinische Hochschule, Konstanty Gutschow Str. 8, 30625 Hannover, Germany

C. LIBERSA, M.D.
Centre Hospitalier Régional et Universitaire de Lille, Place de Verdun, F 59045 Lille Cedex, France

P.O. LIM, M.D.
Department of Pharmacology and Clinical Pharmacology, Ninewells Hospital and Medical School, University of Dundee, Dundee DD1 9SY, United Kingdom

K.M. LULICH, M.D.
Department of Pharmacology, Queen Elizabeth II Medical Center, University of Western Australia, Nedlands WA 6907, Australia

T.M. MACDONALD, M.D., F.R.C.P.
Department of Pharmacology & Clinical Pharmacology, Ninewells Hospital and Medical School, University of Dundee, Dundee DD1 9SY, United Kingdom

R. MALINVERNI, M.D.
Oberarzt Medizinische Poliklinik, Inselspital, 3010 Bern, Switzerland

P. MAURER, M.D.
Medical Clinic, Zieglerspital, Postfach 2600, 3001 Bern, Switzerland

M.F. McCANN, M.D.
Chapel Hill, NC 27514, U.S.A.

G.T. McINNES, B.SC., M.D., F.R.C.P.
Department of Medicine and Therapeutics, Gardiner Institute, Western Infirmary, University of Glasgow, Glasgow G11 6NT, United Kingdom

D. MENKES
University of Otago, P.O. Box 913, Dunedin, New Zealand

R.H.B. MEYBOOM, M.D.
Bremhoeven 1, 5244 GV Rosmalen, The Netherlands

J. MOTSCH, M.D.
Klinik für Anästhesiologie, Im Neuenheimer Feld 110, G-69120 Heidelberg, Germany

K.A. NEFTEL, M.D.
Chefarzt Medizinische Klinik, Zieglerspital, 3007 Bern, Switzerland

H. OLSEN
Psychiatrisk Klinikk, Vinderen, Postboks 85, 0319 Oslo, Norway

J.W. PATERSON, M.D.
Department of Pharmacology, Queen Elizabeth II Medical Centre, University of Western Australia, Nedlands WA 6907, Australia

B.C.P. POLAK, M.D.
The Rotterdam Eye Hospital, P.O. Box 70030, 3000 LM Rotterdam, The Netherlands

Ch. RUEF, M.D.
Leiter der Spitalhygiene, Department of Internal Medicine, Universitätsspital, Rämistrasse 100, 8091 Zürich, Switzerland

A. SCHAFFNER, M.D.
Direktor Medizinische Klinik B, Department of Internal Medicine, Universitätsspital, Rämistrasse 100, 8091 Zürich, Switzerland

K. SCHOPFER, M.D.
Direktor, Institut für Medizinische Mikrobiologie, Friedbühlstrasse 51, 3010 Bern, Switzerland

M. SCHOU, M.D.
Psychiatric Hospital, 2 Skovagervej, 8240 Risskov, Denmark

P. SENANAYAKE
International Planned Parenthood Federation, Regent's College, Inner Circle, Regent's Park, London NW1 4NS, United Kingdom

G.M. SIMPSON, M.D.
Department of Psychiatry, Division of Clinical Psychopharmacology, Medical College of Pennsylvania, 3200 Henry Avenue, Philadelphia, PA 19129, U.S.A.

R. SONNTAG, M.D.
Institute of Medical Oncology, Inselspital, 3010 Bern, Switzerland

J.J. SRAMEK Jr
Department of Psychiatry, Division of Clinical Psychopharmacology, Medical College of Pennsylvania, 3200 Henry Avenue, Philadelphia, PA 19129, U.S.A.

C.B.M. TESTER-DALDERUP, M.D.
P.O. Box 11291, Edmonton, Alberta T5J 3K5, Canada

C. THOMAS, M.D.
Centre Hospitalier Régional et Universitaire de Lille, Place de Verdun, F 59045 Lille Cedex, France

R. VERHAEGHE, M.D.
Department of Internal Medicine, University Hospital Gasthuisberg, Herestraat 49, 3000 Leuven, Belgium

T. VIAL
Centre Regional de Pharmacogivilance, Hôpital Edouard Herriot, Place d'Arsonval, 69437 Lyon Cedex 03, France

B. VRHOVAC
Department of Medicine, University Hospital Medical School, Kispaticeva 12, 41000 Zagreb, Croatia

J. WEEKE
Department M, Endocrinology and Diabetes, University Hospital in Aarhus, 8000 Aarhus C, Denmark

M. ZOPPI, M.D.
Medical Clinic, Zieglerspital, Postfach 2600, 3001 Bern, Switzerland

Preface

Meyler and adverse reactions: today and tomorrow

When Leo Meyler of the University of Groningen published his first edition of *Side Effects of Drugs* in 1952 it was unique in the world. Remarkably, despite the vast worldwide increase in interest in drug adverse reactions, his book has remained unique throughout thirteen editions. Other books have come and gone, most of them looking at adverse reactions in other ways or from a particular angle; they have ranged from the splendid to the merely sensational. Yet Meyler has continued to serve the goal which its founder set for it: to provide the clinician and medical investigator with a reliable and critical overview of all that is known—and much that is merely suspected but unproven—with respect to the adverse reactions and interactions of drugs.

The published literature is obviously not the only source of information on suspected adverse reactions. National monitoring systems, based on spontaneous reports from physicians on their experience with drugs, complement what is published in the journals; they sometimes provide the first tentative signal of the existence of a possible problem, a signal which will have to be confirmed or disproven by formal studies or much wider experience, and thus through the medium of the literature. Yet even today a substantial proportion of early warning signals appear first in the medical literature. It is the task of the expert authors of Meyler to consider them and advise the practitioner as to whether and how they might be of relevance to his or her practice.

The examination of new evidence inevitably goes hand in hand with re-examination of older material; where a report of a possible adverse reaction appeared five years ago yet has remained unconfirmed, is it not time to regard it as a false trail and set it aside? Oddly, Meyler has occasionally been taken to task by authors whose favourite adverse effects (sometimes first described by themselves) have been deleted from its pages, but wherever this has happened it has been the result of meticulous reassessment. As the book has expanded it has sometimes been tempting, too, to delete reference to old drugs; but often one finds that in certain parts of the world these are still widely used (amidopyrine is a discreditable example) and even where they have disappeared their past use may still result in adverse effects, as the long history of diethylstilbestrol shows.

In the course of a generation several basic changes have been made to the Meyler volumes in order to meet changing conditions. The enormous expansion in published data has led to the creation of a team of editors and contributors many times larger than that engaged in the work during its early years. The group, originally based largely in The Netherlands and the United Kingdom, now includes experts from a wide range of countries on different continents. The most important change came in 1977 when the newly created *Side Effects of Drugs Annual* took over the vast task of dealing critically and in detail with individual case-reports, serving at the same time to provide a yearly update to the main volume. A further step was the institution of an experimental database in 1987 which brought *Meyler* firmly into the electronic age. With the present volume we proceed a step further: this thirteenth edition will provide the basis for a compact disk to endow the user with the possibility of searching rapidly and reliably for current facts and opinions relating to drug side effects.

Despite all that has been done in the last four decades to promote drug safety, the absolute number of supposed drug injuries recorded annually has gone on growing, in part because of the more intensive use of medicaments (overconsumption all too often having replaced underconsumption) and the multiplication of new compounds, as well as the commercialization of remedies derived from traditional medicine. An informed view of side effects is a vital tool, not only in assessing these problems when they do occur, but in learning from them so that they can be rendered as rare as is humanly possible. Above all, the analyses provided in these volumes often make it possible to relate risk to benefit; drugs will rarely be entirely free of problems, and it is of the greatest importance to practitioner and patient, where risks are present, to decide whether they can be fairly accepted or not, in view of the benefits which the drug may provide.

I would like to express my sincere thanks to the many Contributors and to the Co-editors who have rendered possible the compilation of this Thirteenth Edition of *Meyler*, as well as the editorial staff of Elsevier Science B.V. for their constant encouragement and support.

M.N.G. DUKES
Oslo
Norway

October 1996

Contents

How to use this book

THE SCOPE OF *MEYLER'S SIDE EFFECTS OF DRUGS*

This book is designed as a general reference work on the adverse reactions to (and interactions of) medicinal substances. It can be used independently or alongside the companion *Side Effects of Drugs Annual* which is published each year and provides a critical survey of the latest developments in this field, with extensive references to the literature.

PRESENTATION OF DATA

The great majority of drugs used in medicine at the present day belong to well-defined families of substances with a close pharmacological and/or chemical relationship to one another, e.g. the phenothiazines, the cephalosporin antibiotics and the β-adrenoceptor blockers. In considering adverse reactions it is generally expedient to review such a group as a whole, since the undesired effects of one member of the group are likely to occur with others as well. Each chapter therefore presents one or more *Side Effects Monographs*; a monograph may discuss a group of related drugs or the best-known representative of the group; it is followed by shorter accounts of the individual drugs, pointing to matters in which these differ from the general pattern. Monographs are presented according to a standard format so that information can be readily located without constant reference to the indexes. The format, as well as a list of the monographs to be found in this volume, will be found on pages xxi–xxiii.

SPECIAL CHAPTERS

In a small number of chapters, particularly those where large numbers of substances are in use (e.g. 'Dermatological Drugs, Topical Agents and Cosmetics'), the material has been differently presented, extensive use being made of tables.

CLASSIFICATION

Drugs are classified according to their main field of application or to the properties for which they are most generally recognized. In borderline cases, however, some supplementary discussion has been included in other chapters relating to secondary fields of application. Fixed combinations of drugs are dealt with according to their most characteristic compound.

DRUG NAMES

Drug products are in general dealt with in the text under their most usual non-proprietary name; where these are not available, chemical names have been used; fixed combinations usually do not have a non-proprietary connotation and here trade names have been used as necessary.

SYSTEM OF REFERENCES

References in the text are coded as follows:

R: In the original paper, the point is *reviewed* in some detail with reference to other literature.
r: The original paper *refers* only briefly to the point, on the basis of evidence adduced by other writers.
C: The original paper presents *detailed original clinical evidence* on this point.
c: The original paper provides *clinical evidence*, but only *briefly*.

The code has not been applied to animal pharmacological papers or statements by administrative or regulatory bodies. The various editions of *Meyler's Side Effects of Drugs* are cited in the text as SED-9, SED-10 etc.; *Side Effects of Drugs Annuals 1—19* are cited as SEDA-1, SEDA-2 etc.

In the interests of clarity, this volume provides only salient references. For facts which are widely known and beyond dispute, references are generally omitted, or the reader is referred to documented reviews in the early volumes of *Meyler*. For those facts which have emerged since 1977, selected references are complemented by cross-references to the full reviews in the *Side Effects of Drugs Annuals*.

Readers anxious to trace all references on a particular topic, including those which duplicate earlier work, are advised to consult *Adverse Reactions Titles*, a monthly bibliography of titles from leading biomedical journals published throughout the world, compiled by the Excerpta Medica International Medical Abstracting Service. *Adverse Reactions Titles*, now in its twenty-eighth year, is available in most medical libraries throughout the world.

INDEXES

Index of Drugs: This index provides a complete listing of all mentions of a drug in this volume.

Index of Side Effects: This index is necessarily selective, since a particular side effect may be caused by very large numbers of compounds; the index is therefore mainly directed to those side effects which are acute or life-threatening or are discussed in special detail. Before assuming that a given drug does not have a particular side effect, one should consult the relevant chapters.

To help the clinical reader, side effects are classified according to the system or phenomenon involved, the grouping being very similar to that of the monographs. All adverse reactions involving the skin will for example be found together, listed under both general and specific headings; in looking for drugs causing 'erythema' or 'pruritus', one will thus also be able to check rapidly whether these drugs also affect the skin or hair in other ways.

For *interactions*, the reader should refer to the Index of Drugs where all interactions are listed under the drugs concerned, irrespective of the chapter in which they appear.

It should be borne in mind that American spelling has been used throughout, e.g. anemia, estrogen etc. (instead of anaemia, oestrogen etc.).

The indexes have been compiled by M. Kettner and M. Hulsman, The Netherlands.

Side effects monographs

Monographs are presented according to the standard format given below so that information can be readily located without constant reference to the indexes.

Drug

ADVERSE REACTION PATTERN

A summary of the principal characteristics with special reference to:
General and toxic reactions
Hypersensitivity reactions
Tumor-inducing effects

EFFECTS ON ORGANS AND SYSTEMS

Cardiovascular
Respiratory
Nervous system
Endocrine, metabolic
Mineral and fluid balance
Hematological
Liver
Gastrointestinal
Urinary system
Skin and appendages
Special senses
Musculoskeletal system
Sexual function
Miscellaneous

Hypersensitivity reactions

Risk situations An outline of situations in which use of the drug involves special risks and may be contraindicated

Withdrawal effects

Second-generation effects
Use in pregnancy
Use in lactation
Effects on fertility
Genetic effects

Overdosage

Interactions

Interference with diagnostic routines

Where there is no information on particular topics, the section in question is omitted; if adverse reactions have been proven to be absent, this will be stated.

The following monographs are to be found in this volume (numbers refer to pages):

Meyler's Side Effects of Drugs, 13th Edition
M.N.G. Dukes, editor

SECTION EDITOR: P.K.M. LUNDE

Everett H. Ellinwood and Tong H. Lee

1 Central nervous system stimulants and anorectic agents

CENTRAL NERVOUS SYSTEM STIMULANTS

XANTHINES

The methylated xanthines (caffeine, theophylline and theobromine) excite the central nervous system at all levels. First, the cortex is affected, then the medulla, and finally the cord is stimulated by very large amounts. Simultaneously, augmented appreciation of sensory stimuli occurs which leads to hyperesthesia. The cardiovascular system is also affected, since xanthines directly stimulate both the myocardium and medullary vagal nuclei. Consequently, two opposing actions result, leading either to bradycardia or to tachycardia and/or arrhythmias. The effects on blood pressure are also impossible to predict: central vasomotor and direct myocardial stimulation favor an increase, whereas central vagal stimulation and peripheral vasodilation favor a decrease in blood pressure. Combinations of these pharmacological effects may produce unpredictable adverse reactions according to the pre-existing pathophysiological conditions. In addition, prevalent combined use in the general population of caffeine with other substances (e.g. nicotine) makes it difficult to attribute some of the adverse caffeine reactions directly to the drug itself, rather than the other substance or drug interactions.

Caffeine

Caffeine is the xanthine most often used to stimulate the central nervous system to combat fatigue and drowsiness.

ADVERSE REACTION PATTERN

General and toxic reactions In addition to the central nervous system, caffeine stimulates the respiratory center, skeletal muscles and gastric secretion and, to a lesser extent, will act on the kidney to produce diuresis. Most adverse reactions to it will be the result of accentuated pharmacological actions including those described above under 'Xanthines' and they may become especially evident in pathologically or genetically predisposed individuals. It is well known that differences in the levels of N-acetylation metabolic enzymes in the liver secondary to genetic polymorphism may lead to differential susceptibility to caffeine (xanthine) toxicity (1^C). A certain degree of tolerance may develop to some of the pharmacological actions of caffeine, but little or no tolerance has been observed to its central stimulatory effects; however, some kind of psychic habituation may develop on prolonged consumption. The term 'caffeinism' refers to a state of acute or chronic toxicity resulting from the ingestion of high doses of caffeine. In general, an intake of 500–600 mg of caffeine per day (approx. 7–9 cups of tea or 4–7 cups of coffee) is currently regarded as representing a significant health risk. The symptoms of caffeinism include behavioral, psychophysiological and affective manifestations. They include restlessness, anxiety, irritability, agitation, muscle tremor, insomnia, headache, sensory disturbances, diuresis, cardiovascular symptoms and gastrointestinal complaints (SEDA-10, 5). With very high, exaggerated doses, caffeine may even produce epileptiform convulsions. Acute overdosage of caffeine may occur and produce severe CNS excitation in sensitive individuals and small children (SEDA-15, 1). A case of self-limited, tonic/clonic seizure has been reported in a postpartum patient after receiving 500 mg of caffeine sodium benzoate for treatment of post-lumbar puncture headache; prolonged half-life of the drug has been implicated (SEDA-17, 1). Caffeine may also be responsible for arrhythmias in neonates, following maternal usage in pregnancy (SEDA-14, 1). Because of a significant abuse potential and their potential toxicity, preparations containing a high content of caffeine have been made available by prescription only in some European countries.

Hypersensitivity reactions Workers in the coffee industry rather frequently develop allergic reactions in the form of dermatitis, rhinitis and bronchial asthma on exposure to dust in the process of stripping the chaff from raw beans prior to roasting (SED-9, 1). This may or may not be a reaction to caffeine itself.

Tumor-inducing effects The ability of caffeine to catalyze the formation of *N*-nitrosamine in the digestive tract has raised the question of its being carcinogenic (see 'Gastrointestinal' below). A possible association between the use of caffeine and the occurrence of fibrocystic breast disease has been suggested (2[C]). A study on benign proliferative endothelial disorder of the breast did not show any association between this disorder and methylxanthine consumption (SEDA-15, 1).

ORGANS AND SYSTEMS

Cardiovascular The debate continues over the association between caffeine intake and cardiovascular disease. An increase in mean blood pressure, glucose, and free fatty acid levels, as well as urinary catecholamine excretion has been found after acute ingestion of 150 mg of caffeine (SEDA-4, 4). In patients with pre-existing heart disease, caffeine intake has been noted to lower the effective and functional refractory period of the atrioventricular node (SEDA-4, 5). A two-fold increased risk of myocardial infarction has been suggested for women drinking 6 or more cups of coffee a day (3[C]), and two studies have documented that men drinking 5 or more cups of coffee a day had an approximately 2-fold increase in risk of myocardial infarction (4[C]) or coronary artery disease (5[C]). However, prospective studies of the relationship between caffeine consumption and increased risk of coronary artery disease (or stroke) have been negative (SEDA-15, 1) or inconclusive (6[C], 7[C]), as has been the association between the consumption of coffee and serum cholesterol concentration assessed in 24 cross-sectional epidemiological studies (SEDA-15, 1). However, a Finnish study did show a positive dose relationship with serum cholesterol after adjustment for confounding variables, which was not seen in women. There is also a suggestion that the relationship is only seen with boiled and not instant or filter coffee (SEDA-15, 1).

Nervous system *Insomnia*, *anxiety*, *tachycardia* and *tremor* are among the symptoms most commonly reported with use of caffeine. *Tenseness* and *irritability* also occur and, with high intake, symptoms resembling those of anxiety neurosis have occurred (8[C]). A case of 'caffeine psychosis' has also been reported (SED-8, 4). Dose-response associations have not been particularly well studied, but some are known to exist (SEDA-7, 6). Paradoxically, six cases have been reported of pathological sleepiness induced by caffeine (9[C]).

Endocrine, metabolic The major metabolic effect of caffeine is to produce an *increase in free fatty acids* and *hyperglycemia* (SED-8, 3, 4).

Gastrointestinal Large doses of caffeine may cause *nausea* and *vomiting*. Caffeine is a strong stimulant of hydrochloric acid secretion (10[C]) and has been incriminated in exacerbating duodenal ulcers. However, decaffeinated coffee has been also reported to be as potent as instant coffee in stimulating gastric acid secretion 10[C]).

Caffeine (and theophylline) and pancreatic cancer A relationship between coffee consumption and pancreatic cancer has been reported in a case control study by MacMahon et al. (SEDA-7, 8). These authors observed an unexpected increase in pancreatic cancer associated with an increase in coffee drinking (relative risk, 2.6 for males). These same workers studied changes in mortality for pancreas cancer in different countries in relation to changes in coffee consumption and found a significant relationship between increases in coffee consumption and increases in mortality from pancreatic cancer. However, the data on which the findings were based were crude. An excess in mortality from pancreatic cancer has been noted among US male veterans admitted to hospitals for bronchial asthma and discharged on various bronchodilators, pointing to a possible connection with theophylline (SEDA-7, 8).

Urinary system Large doses of caffeine may cause diuresis. Administration of caffeine citrate daily increased the mean urinary excretion rate of tubular cells and red blood cells in volunteers (SED-8, 1). The nephrotoxicity of analgesic/antipyretic drug combinations may be the result of a combined effect in which aspirin, phenacetin and caffeine all play a role (SEDA-4, 5). In a study of 20 women with confirmed detrusor instability and 10 asymptomatic women, caffeine administration in the former was associated with a significant increase in detrusor pressure on bladder filling, but no difference in volume at first contraction, height of contraction, or bladder capacity (11[C]).

Skin and appendages *Urticaria* as an allergic response to caffeine has been reported (SEDA-4, 5).

Risk situations In patients who have an irritable myocardium subject to *dysrhythmia*, restriction of caffeine may be indicated. The drug may also add to the rise in renin and noradrenaline seen in cirrhotic patients and may also considerably aggravate the diarrhea in patients with irritable colon (SEDA-15, 1).

Use in infants Xanthines have been prescribed to infants at risk for sudden infant death syndrome or idiopathic apnea of prematurity (see 'Theophylline and related substances' below, under 'Risk situations'. About 50% of 30 infants treated with caffeine (and two/three of 18 infants treated with theophylline) exhibited significant increases in episodes of gastroesophageal reflux (12[C]). The authors stress that screening for gastrointestinal reflux should precede the administration of caffeine (and theophylline) to infants at risk for sudden infant death syndrome. As expected, the frequency of side effects such as tachycardia and gastrointestinal reflux appears to be lower with lower doses of caffeine (e.g. 2.5 mg/kg, q.d., SEDA-17, 1).

Use in children In an experimental study of normal boys, increases in subjective anxiety were found in 'chronic' low-caffeine users and withdrawal symptoms in high-caffeine users. No 'beneficial' effects of caffeine use were found (SEDA-7, 22). The UK Committee on Review of Medicine recommends that children should take caffeine only in analgesic products and in a dose related to their age (SEDA-5, 6).

Withdrawal effects Restlessness, irritability and headache are withdrawal effects attributable to caffeine. These and other symptoms may occur with lower dose caffeine use than generally supposed (13[C]). The caffeine withdrawal headache may be responsible for the widespread practice of taking caffeine containing analgesics habitually since a withdrawal headache could create a vicious cycle of drug use (SEDA-5, 6).

Second-generation effects *Pre-pregnancy effects* One review (SEDA-5, 32) suggests that the use of caffeine to improve the mobility of human sperm used in artificial insemination may be very risky due to the potential for chromosomal damage and also possible damage to the fertilized ovum.

Another study (SEDA-9, 2) suggested that a high daily intake of caffeine may predispose a woman to reproductive difficulties. Although delayed mitosis and excessive chromatic breaks have been noted in human lymphocytic cultures in which caffeine was added (14[R]), the rapid and almost complete metabolism of caffeine in man may be a factor which protects against the various deleterious effects found in in vitro human cell-culture studies and in animal studies.

Epidemiological studies requiring further verification have suggested a relationship between caffeine intake and reduced fertility, even at a consumption level as little as the caffeine equivalent of more than 1 cup of brewed coffee per day (SEDA-14, 1).

Use in pregnancy In two studies (SEDA-6, 9) a relationship was found between caffeine consumption and embryo toxicity. In one, a high rate of spontaneous abortions, stillbirth, and prematurity at birth was associated with ingestion of more than 600 mg of caffeine per day by either the mother or father. In the other, it was found that a daily intake of more than 8 cups of coffee (by the mother) increased the frequency of congenital malformations.

Concern about the possible harmful effects of caffeine on the outcome of pregnancy has evolved mainly from studies of animals which have indicated a decrease in intrauterine fetal growth. However, the implications of these data for man are unclear because of the differences in mode of exposure to caffeine, the amounts consumed, and the metabolism of the drug. Morris and Weinstein (SEDA-7, 8) reviewed the current data on the possible effects of caffeine intake on the human fetus and concluded that the scientific data available at the present time could not answer the question. Linn et al. (SEDA-7, 8) analyzed interview and medical record data of 12 205 non-asthmatic women to evaluate the relationship between coffee consumption and adverse outcome of pregnancy. Their findings were negative.

In a study of eight pregnant women at 32—36 weeks of gestation, 2 cups of caffeinated or decaffeinated coffee were associated with an increase in the incidence of fetal breathing activity and the caffeinated coffee was associated with a significant fall in baseline fetal heart rate (15[C]). Three cases of fetal arrhythmia resulting from excessive intake of caffeine by the mother during pregnancy have been reported (SEDA-14, 1).

Use during lactation The relationship between serum and breast milk concentrations of caffeine has been studied (SEDA-6, 8). The caffeine accumulated in the infant would depend on the average concentration in maternal serum and breast milk over time, the volume of milk ingested, and particularly the infant's clearance rate for caffeine. The relationship between methylxanthine consumption and fibrocystic breast disease has also been studied (SEDA-6, 8). It was concluded that in women who are predisposed to fibrocystic disease, methylxanthines are factors in the development of the disease. The mechanism of this effect of methylxanthines might be connected with an inhibitory action on the activity of cyclic AMP and cyclic GMP phosphodiesterases.

Overdosage Excessive amounts (1 gram or more) of

caffeine may cause untoward central nervous effects including psychotic organic brain syndrome (SEDA-5, 6).

Oral route Oral doses causing fatalities are stated to range from 3 to 50 grams of caffeine, but death from excessive caffeine ingestion is rare, perhaps due to the emetic effect of the drug. Death may be due to cardiovascular shock, but chronic potentially lethal toxicity, even for heavy coffee- or tea-drinkers, is very unlikely to occur since 60—100 cups per day would be required if an average of 100 mg of caffeine is present in a cup of coffee or tea (50—100 mg).

Percutaneous Caffeine is well absorbed when applied in a vehicle such as anhydrous eucerine.

Intravenous route In two instances in which caffeine was given intravenously, convulsions and death were recorded at doses of 400 mg and 3.2 grams, respectively (SED-9, 2, 3).

Interactions A recent comprehensive textbook lists more than 40 drugs which interact with caffeine (16^C). These drugs include antiarrhythmics (e.g. mexiletine; reduced caffeine clearance), benzodiazepines (e.g. diazepam; counteracted sedative effect), β-blockers (e.g. propranolol; raised blood pressure), disulfiram (reduced caffeine clearance). Caffeine may alter blood levels of *neuroleptics* (SEDA-5, 6). The pharmacokinetics of caffeine are greatly altered by concomitant administration of the myorelaxant, *idrocilamide*, which has been shown to inhibit the biotransformation of caffeine and increase its half-life 9 times (SEDA-5, 7). Consequently, when idrocilamide is prescribed, partial or total abstinence from caffeine-containing products should be enforced. Phenylpropanolamine, which is available as an over-the-counter preparation for weight loss, also inhibits caffeine metabolism leading to excessive stimulation (e.g. manic psychosis, SEDA 17, 1). In addition to the above list, many of the interactions discussed for 'Theophylline and related substances' also apply to caffeine.

Caffeine has been included in a wide variety of fixed drug combinations (e.g. non-steroid anti-inflammatory agents or antihistamines). The inclusion is aimed at increasing bioavailability (e.g. antipyrine), counteracting side effects of the other drug (e.g. sedation induced by antihistamines), or providing additional therapeutic efficacy (aspirin?). The use of combination drugs complicates the evaluation of caffeine side effects (see "Interactions" for "Theophyllines and related substances").

Interference with diagnostic routines The association of caffeine intake with a rise in serum free fatty acids, hyperglycemia and increased catecholamine levels suggests that caffeine may alter the results of a wide variety of metabolic studies. False-positive dexamethasone suppression test has been associated with ingestion of caffeine equivalent to 4—5 cups of coffee.

Theophylline and related substances

Due to their ability to relax bronchial muscles, theophylline and related compounds are used chiefly in the maintenance treatment of asthma and chronic obstructive pulmonary disease. Theophylline has also been used in the treatment of prolonged apnea of pre-term infants. In terms of treating acute asthmatic exacerbations (status asthmaticus) in emergency rooms, the controversy concerning a possible benefit of including theophylline (aminophylline) in the treatment regimen has not been resolved (2^C, 3^C; see below under 'Interactions'). The bronchodilator effect of theophylline is related to serum concentrations with the effect beginning at 5—8 μg/ml and virtually no additional effects occurring beyond 20 μg/ml. The relationship of relatively minor side effects to serum concentration is idiosyncratic below 15 μg/ml; above that level, the relationship becomes more consistent and more serious side effects also are increasingly likely, i.e. toxic effects; the latter are frequent at about 20 μg/ml. Therefore, the therapeutic range is usually considered to be 10—20 μg/ml with titration of dose to achieve levels within the range of 10—15 μg/ml being optimal. Controversy remains in this area, however, with, for example, the authors of one study finding that the clinical response to theophylline correlated significantly with the log plasma theophylline concentration and other authors claiming that clinical aspects are more relevant for dose correction during therapy than the determination of actual serum concentrations (SEDA-12, 3). A variety of factors influences the metabolism of these compounds, including the pronounced inter-individual differences in metabolism, illnesses for which these drugs are prescribed, other pathological conditions, and factors such as smoking, age and weight. the use of these drugs requires extremely close attention and a host of authors have stressed the importance of monitoring serum levels as well as the clinical condition of the patient and side effects.

An example of some of the complexity encountered is the initiation of chronic bronchodilator therapy using oral theophylline. Approximate initial daily doses are as follows: 6 mg/kg for adult non-smokers; 10 mg/kg for adult smokers; 12 mg/kg for children under 12.

Increases in dose, if any, are made in small increments after about 3 days depending on clinical response and serum theophylline concentration. Proper dosing in itself is complicated by two factors: variable bioavailability among the different products used and elimination kinetics in which blood concentration-dependent kinetics are probable but poorly defined.

Theophylline has been combined chemically to produce aminophylline (the ethylenediamine salt), choline theophyllinate, and other compounds. Several sustained-release forms are available. Absorption of most of the standard forms results in maximum serum levels at 1—3 hours and with sustained-release forms at up to 6 hours. Aminophylline is the most widely used theophylline compound; theophylline is here combined with ethylenediamine to enhance its solubility. Since ethylenediamine is considered to be therapeutically inert, all effects of aminophylline, except for allergic reactions, are considered to stem from the theophylline component.

Among the methylated xanthines, theophylline is the least active cerebral stimulant, its most pronounced feature being stimulation of the medullary respiratory center, circulatory system and smooth muscles of the bronchi. Therapeutic use and untoward responses will derive from these basic pharmacological features which, apart from the desired actions, may produce the untoward effects reviewed. Serious adverse reactions are rare with appropriate blood concentrations; however, it is difficult to control theophylline levels, especially when given by mouth, absorption being erratic. When given intravenously, slow administration is advised. With both oral and parenteral administration, monitoring of serum theophylline levels with individual adjustment of dosage is necessary.

ADVERSE REACTION PATTERN

General and toxic reactions Nausea, vomiting, headache, dizziness, tachycardia, dysrhythmia, vascular collapse, tremor, agitation and convulsions have been described. Although 1% of children and 4% of adults are unable to tolerate even low serum levels, the incidence of adverse effects during therapeutic use is generally related to the logarithm of the serum concentration. However, the relationship between the severity of the symptoms of theophylline poisoning and serum drug concentration is less clear and may well depend on the chronicity of the overdose (SEDA-9, 7—8) (see 'Overdosage').

Hypersensitivity reactions True allergy to theophylline may occur but is probably rare. Hypersensitivity to aminophylline is most likely due to the ethylenediamine component. Two immunogenic types of reactions have been described, one of urticaria and general pruritus and the other involving thrombocytopenia and hemorrhagic diathesis (SED-8, 1). Also reported have been contact dermatitis, exfoliative erythroderma accompanied by bronchospasm and pruritus, generalized dermal reactions (SED-10, 4), severe generalized symptoms with high fever (17), and aggressive behavior in a child (18^C).

Tumor-inducing effects The observation of excess mortality from cancer in the pancreas among US male veterans admitted to hospital for bronchial asthma and discharged on various bronchodilators has raised the question of a possible connection the theophylline. See under 'Caffeine' above.

ORGANS AND SYSTEMS

Cardiovascular The relationship between toxicity and excessive theophylline serum concentrations has been confirmed, tachycardia being a frequent indication of toxic symptoms (SED-9, 3). It appears that the cardiac and metabolic effects of theophylline are at least partly related to catecholamine release (SEDA-13, 1). The importance of appropriate dosage has been stressed in several papers, all indicating the particular risk of ventricular fibrillation in subjects with respiratory distress (19). The authors point to the potentially lethal effect of serum theophylline levels in excess of 20 μg/ml. One can conclude from another study that half the patients with serum concentrations greater than 35 μ/ml experienced life-threatening *arrhythmias* (SEDA-7, 7). In one study of the effect of orally administered aminophylline on cardiac arrhythmias in 15 patients with chronic obstructive pulmonary disease, it was concluded that aminophylline had both arrhythmogenic and chronotropic effects but did not change the grade of arrhythmia (SEDA-7, 7). Another study of 16 patients demonstrated a relationship between use of theophylline and the precipitation of *multifocal atrial tachycardia* (20^C). Whereas elevated blood theophylline concentrations are likely in themselves to produce cardiovascular complications, patients with pre-existing cardiac disease are at greater risk for toxic effects.

Respiratory Aggravation of bronchial asthma is sometimes experienced with the use of aminophylline. Sensitization to the ethylenediamine component is considered to be responsible (SEDA-6, 5).

Nervous system In addition to the more commonly experienced side effects of *tremor*, *dizziness*, *anxiety*, *agitation*, *insomnia*, *visual disturbances* and *seizures*, *depression*, *confusion* (SEDA-6, 1) *acute dyskinesias* (SEDA-17, 1), and *toxic psychosis* have also been reported (SED-10, 5). Seizures with focal onset have been described during treatment with aminophylline of status asthmaticus in adult patients with no previous history of epilepsy (21[C]). Although serum theophylline concentrations are an unreliable predictor of seizures, seizures occur most commonly at serum concentrations >40—50 μg/ml (22[C]). Older patients may be more likely to experience seizures than younger ones at similar theophylline concentrations (23[C]). Patients with pre-existing central nervous system abnormalities (24[C]) or severe pulmonary diseases may also be at increased risk (SEDA-17, 1). Theophylline-induced seizures were reported in two neonates (SEDA-6, 2); the serum theophylline concentration during seizures was 51 μg/ml. A 3.5-month-old girl treated with theophylline had a seizure while hospitalized; in the following months, she manifested a mixed seizure disorder and subsequently exhibited symptoms of moderately severe right brain damage (25[C]). Because toxic symptoms prior to seizures may be absent or undetected, such events underline the need for blood level monitoring during theophylline therapy. Theophylline may disturb sleep more profoundly in caffeine-sensitive subjects (SEDA-15, 1). The concern that cognitive function may be impaired in children on theophylline is still not resolved (SEDA-14, 1; SEDA-15, 1); a recent review suggests that detrimental effects of theophylline on various measures of cognitive function might be measure specific (4[R]).

Endocrine, metabolic The endocrine and metabolic effects of intravenous infusions of aminophylline have been studied in a series of healthy young subjects with regard to serum glucose, insulin, glucagon, cortisol and free fatty acid levels. Infusion of aminophylline which produced theophylline levels in the usual therapeutic range (10—20 μg/ml) caused only small increases in plasma glucose levels but rapid, pronounced and prolonged rises in *free fatty acids*. Increases in free fatty acid concentrations paralleled the rise in theophylline levels (SEDA-6, 6).

Liver Since about 90% of theophylline is eliminated via metabolism in the liver, the functional competency of that organ is intimately interrelated with toxic effects on other systems (see 'Risk situations' below). *Hepatitis* has been reported in two patients with strong evidence of causality (SEDA-15, 1).

Gastrointestinal The commonest gastrointestinal side effects of aminophylline administration in adults are *nausea* and *gastrointestinal irritation*, which are primarily a function of serum theophylline concentrations, although some additional local irritation may be produced by oral administration. Nausea was reported in six (and a seizure in one) of 20 asthmatic patients with serum concentrations of 20 μg/ml of theophylline (SED-9, 4). In a survey of 2766 theophylline-treated patients suffering from cardiac or pulmonary diseases, 10.8% experienced side effects, most of which were gastrointestinal disturbances (7.8%) (SED-9, 4). In a report of two cases of hematemesis (SEDA-5, 5) it was concluded that both a local irritant action of aminophylline and a susceptibility to systemic toxic effects at lower serum theophylline concentrations were responsible in the two elderly patients studied. A pediatric case of non-allergic proctitis associated with aminophylline suppository has also been reported (SEDA-17, 1). For a discussion of the relationship between theophylline and pancreatic cancer, see 'Caffeine' above, under 'Gastrointestinal'.

Skin and appendages See 'Adverse reaction pattern' above. In addition, three new cases of cutaneous eruptions have been reported as due to aminophylline, these patients having probably been sensitized by the use of a multi-antibiotic cream preparation also containing ethylenediamine (SEDA-12, 4). A case of severe Stevens-Johnson syndrome after administration of slow-release theophylline has been reported (26[C]).

Immune processes Salivary IgA was significantly reduced in asthmatic children treated with theophylline as compared to healthy controls or unmedicated asthmatic patients (27[R]). The finding is in harmony with earlier statements that theophylline decreases the bactericidal capacity of leukocytes and affects suppressor T-cells (SEDA-11, 6).

Miscellaneous The following have been reported: exacerbation of spasticity in a post-CVA hemiplegic patient (28[C]); unexpected dangers of theophylline toxicity in a patient found to have hypothyroidism (29[C]); and *esophageal ulceration* resulting from pills which have been taken with insufficient fluid and/or while in a recumbent posture (30[CR], 31[C]).

Risk situations The two greatest risks are inherent: the narrow therapeutic range, and the significant differences in individual response to drug administration, even in healthy controls (SEDA-4, 3). Relative high-risk situations can be identified in relation to patient age and certain illnesses.

The young: (*a*) *prematurity* Serious difficulties arise with respect to the administration of theophylline to premature newborns. These are explained by peculiarities in the biotransformation of the drug in prematurity. Transformation of theophylline to caffeine in premature newborns is explained by the lack of enzymes providing desmethylation and C-hydroxylation and by the predominant *N*-methylase activity. High serum caffeine concentrations have been found in two studies (SEDA-4, 3) of premature newborns with respiratory disturbances who had received theophylline. Caffeine and theophylline synergism was incriminated in the development of toxic reactions in these children. In another study, clinically significant hyperglycemia was found in 13% of pre-term infants undergoing theophylline therapy (32[C]). Plasma glucose should be monitored in pre-term infants receiving theophylline. There is some evidence (SED-10, 5) that administration of a basic 4.5 mg/kg dose of theophylline followed by a maintenance dose (1.2—1.52 mg/kg every 8—12 hours) is most likely to correct respiratory disturbances in premature newborns while avoiding the occurrence of side effects. Because of simpler dosing regimens, some pediatricians prefer caffeine as the drug of choice for treating premature neonates (5[r], 33[C]).

(*b*) *Term infants* Another study (SEDA-4, 3) urged caution in using theophylline for wheezing in very young infants until its pharmacokinetics have been further studied in full-term infants younger than 3 months of age. A further study measured cerebral blood flow velocity in infants treated with an intravenous bolus dose of aminophylline (34[CR]). The reduction in cerebral blood flow velocity which occurred may have been the result of a reduction in P_{CO_2}, due to the administration of aminophylline.

Children In another report (SEDA-5, 4), convulsions were attributed to theophylline given for bronchial asthma in the usual recommended dosage with serum levels within the accepted non-toxic range of 10—20 μg/ml. Young children may be more prone to develop excitement and dehydration due to diuresis and vomiting. Two afebrile children have reported visual hallucinations during theophylline toxicity (SEDA-13, 2).

It is concluded that despite the recommendation for higher initial doses in young children, dosage management is more difficult due to the greater likelihood of toxicity, which is probably a reflection of more erratic and less well-studied pharmacodynamics.

The elderly It is not entirely clear whether the risk of toxicity in the elderly is a function of an age-related difference in metabolism, i.e. slower, a tendency for systemic toxic effects to develop at relatively lower serum concentrations, or whether the elderly are more likely to have conditions which influence the pharmacokinetics of theophylline, e.g. cardiac failure, liver disease, chronic obstructive pulmonary disease. In a review of 72 consecutive patients referred to a regional poison center with chronic theophylline intoxication, stratification of data by chronological age revealed a stepwise increase in the frequency of life-threatening events with advancing years causing the authors to suggest that elderly patients have an inordinately greater risk of such events than younger patients (35[C]).

In an investigation of 510 episodes of elevated theophylline levels in 214 hospitalized patients, the authors concluded that life-threatening events may occur in critically ill patients or patients with past seizures or arrhythmias with mildly elevated (21—40 μg/ml) theophylline levels (36[C]).

One study (SEDA-5, 1) indicated that maintenance dosage should be reduced by approximately 25% in the elderly to maintain plasma levels in the therapeutic range. Other reports (SEDA-7, 6; SEDA-8, 1) have implicated chronic obstructive pulmonary disease and cardiac failure in elderly patients whose reduced theophylline clearances led to toxic reactions or potentially toxic plasma concentrations. In the latter study, it was suggested that aminophylline doses be reduced by 50% when clinical signs of cardiac failure are present in order to avoid excessive drug accumulation.

Illnesses As pointed out above, patients with cardiac disorders may be at greater risk. Erratically altered serum theophylline concentrations have been found in patients with bronchial asthma and severe or chronic obstructive pulmonary diseases (SEDA-4, 2), but in intercurrent respiratory diseases, theophylline clearance is characteristically reduced (SED-10, 6; SEDA-8, 12; SEDA-10, 11). A great variation in tolerance to theophylline was found in children with cystic fibrosis who were given high doses of 10 mg/kg 3 times a day for a period of 3—4 weeks. Some children tolerated high blood levels of theophylline, but most experienced nausea and vomiting or headache even when their plasma levels were appropriate. The decreased tolerance in this group of patients may stem from liver dysfunction which is present in a high percentage of cystic fibrosis sufferers and/or may indicate development of a certain degree of drug tolerance with long-term usage (SED-9, 4). In cirrhosis of the liver, the half-life of theophylline increases approximately 3-fold, drug clearance diminishes, and the incidence of side effects increases simultaneously (SED-10, 6).

Patients receiving electroconvulsive therapy (*ECT*) Three cases are known to have occurred in which patients being treated with theophylline developed status epilepticus after an ECT treatment and subsequently died. Serum theophylline levels at the time of ECT were estimated, from *proximal* samples, to be 20—25 μg/ml. For patients receiving concomitant theophylline treatment and ECT, a suggested procedure is to withhold the theophylline dose and obtain a serum level in the morning prior to ECT. ECT probably should not be administered at serum theophylline levels above 20 μg/ml.

Second-generation effects *Pregnancy* Arwood et al. (SEDA-5, 3) demonstrated the ability of theophylline to cross the placenta, resulting in potentially dangerous serum theophylline concentrations in the neonate. This is of practical importance since 1.3% of pregnant women are asthmatics. In one neonate they studied the serum theophylline concentration of 14 μg/ml was 3 μg/ml higher than cord or maternal serum concentrations. They concluded that neonates of mothers receiving theophylline products should be monitored for pharmacological effects of theophylline. Another study has pointed out that asthmatics receiving theophylline therapy had a longer average duration of labor than did untreated women, since theophylline inhibited uterine contractions (SEDA-5, 3). Symptoms have been described of irritability, vomiting and jitteriness in an infant, possibly related to ingestion of aminophylline during pregnancy by an asthmatic mother (37[R]).

Lactation The kinetics of theophylline transfer into breast milk have been studied in three lactating women given theophylline intravenously (SEDA-6, 2). The data indicated that theophylline accumulation to toxic concentrations should not occur in most breast-fed infants, but that serum theophylline concentrations in the mother should be kept as low as possible and transfer will be minimal if infants are nursed just before the mother takes her theophylline dose.

Fertility Effects on fertility are not known.

Genetic effects These are not well known. The ability of theophylline to suppress phosphodiesterase and cyclic AMP activity, and to increase calcium transport in animal experimentation studies (SEDA-4, 25) indicates a potential for teratogenic action. An increased rate of sister chromatic exchange rate, an indication of mutagenicity, has been also reported (SEDA-17, 1).

Overdosage The effect of theophylline is cumulative and a real danger of overdosage may be compounded if the drug is given repeatedly. Indications of intoxication, however, have been described in young children after a single suppository (SED-9, 4). Symptoms of overdosage have been described above (see 'General and toxic reactions') and elsewhere. The highly variable interindividual differences in metabolism and disease-related alterations in metabolism of the various medicinal preparations result in iatrogenically induced overdosage. The tendency of patients to increase their medication as their condition deteriorates is a second major source of overdosing.

Amount of drug administered, per se, whether putative or known, is less likely to correlate with untoward reactions than is serum concentration. Likewise, the correlation of serum concentration with relatively minor side effects is unreliable. More reliable is the escalating correlation of serious toxic effects with serum concentrations rising above 15 μg/ml.

The use of hemodialysis or hemoperfusion in the management of theophylline toxicity remains controversial (SEDA-8, 11—12; SEDA-9, 10; SEDA-11, 5—6). The recommendation that these treatments be considered for patients who fail to respond to supportive care is complicated by findings that, once major complications have occurred, the benefits from these risky procedures are greatly reduced. Furthermore, the relationship between the severity of clinical manifestations of theophylline poisoning and serum drug concentrations is unclear. A beginning has been made in clarifying this relationship, however, with the finding that patients with theophylline overdose caused by chronic repeated over-medication frequently develop seizures and arrhythmias with serum concentrations of 40—70 μg/ml, while those with acute single ingestion are highly unlikely to suffer serious complications unless serum concentrations exceed 100 μg/ml. According to this study, single-overdose patients were easily recognized by the presence of hypotension, hypokalemia, and low serum bicarbonate, features not present in patients with chronic overdose (SEDA-11, 5—6; 38[R]). These findings warrant further study and could lead to better indicators for more aggressive treatment prior to the advent of major complications.

In a clinical trial on normal volunteers theophylline was shown to decrease circulating pyridoxal-5′-phosphate (Vitamin B_6) levels, presumably via noncompetitive inhibition of pyridoxal kinase. Theophylline levels of approximately 10 μg/ml produced only partial inhibition, plasma pyridoxal kinase and pyridoxal levels being unaffected. The authors speculated that with theophylline overdose and greater inhibition, vitamin B_6 deficiency might contribute to seizures (SEDA-14, 2).

Interactions Both positive and negative drug interactions have been reported for theophylline. A recent debate was triggered by the suggestion of increased mortality due to greater use of theophylline and additive toxicity between oral theophylline and inhaled β-agonists (SEDA-7, 1). The issue continues in debate. Some authors conclude that a combination of theophylline and β-agonists in low doses will give equal and possibly superior results over full doses of either agent and may produce fewer adverse effects (SEDA-7, 2;

SEDA-8, 13). No one has yet documented any serious synergistic toxicity from a combination of theophylline and a β-agonist in appropriate doses, and it seems clear that the patient with severe asthma who is undertreated is much more at risk of death than one who receives concomitant theophylline and adrenergic drug treatment in appropriate doses and sequence (SEDA-9, 10–11).

The effect of *combination products* has been discussed (SEDA-6, 2; SEDA-11, 7). The use of combination drugs complicates the evaluation of side effects, particularly theophylline and *ephedrine*. The likelihood of side effects of each component and synergistic effects between components must be evaluated in relation to the clinical condition of the patient A positive feature is the likelihood of greater compliance with an effective combination product.

Adverse reactions to theophylline have been found to be more common in patients concurrently receiving tetracycline (SED-9, 4).

Pharmacokinetic interactions The concomitant use of drugs which decrease theophylline clearance can produce toxic serum concentrations with therapeutic doses of theophylline. The majority of these drugs are believed to exert this effect by inhibiting the hepatic microsomal P450-metabolizing enzymes which are responsible for the biotransformation of theophylline. Such drugs include the xanthine oxidase inhibitor allopurinol, histamine-2 receptor antagonists (cimetidine in particular), some of the new antidepressants (fluvoxamine), and oral contraceptives. Also included are a variety of antimicrobials, e.g. tetracycline, the macrolide (erythromycin and troleandomycin) and fluoroquinolone (ciprofloxacin, norfloxacin) antibiotics, possibly cephalosporin, the antitubercular isoniazid, anthelmintics (thiabendazole; possibly pyrantel), and antiviral agents (influenza vaccine and vidarabine). Antacids act by increasing theophylline absorption.

Other drugs decreasing theophylline clearance, but via unknown mechanisms, are cardiac medications (the β-blocker propranolol and the calcium channel blockers, nifedipine and verapamil) and an antiarrhythmic, mexiletine. Considering increased theophylline levels can lead to increased propensity toward central and, in particular, cardiac stimulation (e.g. arrhythmia, see above), it may be prudent to avoid using a combination of a theophylline preparation and cardiac medications, especially antiarrhythmics.

Conversely, drugs which have been shown to induce P450 enzymes increase theophylline clearance and lower blood concentrations. These include the barbiturates, phenytoin, and carbamazepine, and the RNA polymerase antibiotic, rifampicin. Increased clearance also occurs with use of high-protein diets, marijuana, and tobacco either smoked, chewed, or dipped. With phenytoin the interaction is two-sided: in combined use, the plasma concentrations of both drugs may fall. This can result in poor seizure and respiratory control on the one hand, and in a toxic drug concentration of one drug given in unchanged doses when the other is withdrawn, on the other hand.

The *quinine* component of Quinamm has been implicated in elevated serum theophylline levels in an elderly patient (39[CR]).

In a case report of theophylline–lithium interaction, renal lithium clearance increased with resultant lowering of the serum *lithium* concentration (40[C]).

In a study of a single-dose interaction of theophylline and *prednisolone*, the plasma concentrations of both drugs were slightly lower when they were given in combination than when given alone (41[C]).

Recommendations have been presented for correction of theophylline doses during concomitant medication with some of the above drugs (SEDA-8, 13; 42[R]). Co-medication with phenobarbital may require an increase in the theophylline dose by about 30%; concurrent use with phenytoin may require an increase in theophylline by as much as 75%. Concomitant therapy with allopurinol, cimetidine, erythromycin, furosemide, isoprenaline or propranolol may, on the other hand, require a decrease of the theophylline dose by about 20–30%; for oleandomycin the decrease should be about 50%.

Despite the ability of theophylline to reduce blood levels of digitalis in digitalis intoxication (43[C]), therapeutic doses of theophylline can evoke arrhythmias in the presence of high normal levels of *digoxin* (44[C]).

Caffeine may accumulate to toxic levels during treatment with theophylline (45[C]). Likewise concomitant administration of caffeine and theophylline may significantly increase plasma theophylline concentrations as well as reduce the clearance rate of theophylline and its metabolites (46[C]).

The interaction between certain new *cephalosporins* (including moxalactam) and the alcohol in theophylline elixir may produce a 'disulfiram-like' reaction (47[C]).

Antagonism to *pancurorium* has been found with theophylline levels in excess of the recommended therapeutic range (SEDA-5, 4).

Finally, food intake may influence both the absorption and clearance rates of theophylline. One study documented that the absorption of a retard preparation of theophylline was very slow after an overnight fast in contrast to absorption, reflected by serum peak drug levels, after a test meal. The effect may be dosage-related, but concern about the potential for inducing toxic drug levels arises because product approval studies of bioavailability have been performed only in fasting subjects (SEDA-11, 7). More specifically, dietary protein has been found to significantly influence theophylline clearance, with a low-protein diet decreasing theophylline clearance and a high-protein diet increasing it. The implications for clinical practice have not been elaborated, but dietary extremes are contraindicated for patients undergoing theophylline therapy (47[C]).

Newer theophyllines and combination with β-agonists The use of intravenous aminophylline and salbutamol together seems to give no additional benefit and an additive chronotropic effect on the heart. In contrast, the addition of inhaled terbutaline or salbutamol to a well-controlled oral theophylline regimen might give additive benefits, which may in turn allow for rather lower doses of theophylline to be used; conversely theophylline may be added with useful effect to inhaled β-agonists without increasing the risk of dysrrhythmias (SEDA-15, 1).

Interference with diagnostic routines *Sulfamethoxazole* distorts the results of high-pressure liquid chromatography used for detection of theophylline plasma concentrations and the antibiotic should be withdrawn 24 hours before the procedure (SEDA-6, 7).

INDIVIDUAL COMPOUNDS

Enprofylline *(SEDA-8, 15; SEDA-9, 12)*

Pauwels (48[C]) has reported briefly on the efficacy and tolerance of enprofylline (3-propylxanthine), a recently developed xanthine derivative which weight-for-weight is about 5 times more active than theophylline as a bronchodilator. The therapeutic plasma concentration is about 3 μg/ml. Enprofylline seems to be practically devoid of adenosine-antagonistic activity in the systems studied, namely the trachea, brain, kidney and smooth muscle.

The most severe side effects of theophylline, namely seizures, are claimed to be absent even at high doses of enprofylline, although other disadvantages such as cardiovascular effects, nausea, vomiting and headache are observed.

Enprofylline looks promising as a new bronchodilating drug, although it has a short half-life (about 2 hours). However, much more information is needed before the claim of greater safety can be taken seriously.

One other report throws a little more light on the drug. Laursen et al. (49[C]) evaluated the drug for intravenous use. In six asthmatic patients, the possibility of obtaining a steady-state plasma level of 5 mg/l of enprofylline by administration of two constant rate infusions was examined. The side effects and bronchodilatation produced by the drug were compared with those obtained with theophylline at a steady-state level of 15 μg/ml. Headache, nausea and vomiting became pronounced in two patients in whom the plasma enprofylline level was about 6 μg/ml.

The authors concluded that by varying the infusion rate the plasma level of enprofylline can be controlled like that of theophylline, but they too stress the need for further study of efficacy versus side effects.

Proxyphylline *(SEDA-10, 12)*

In a short-term study, a new sustained-release formulation of proxyphylline (2400 mg/day) was compared with theophylline (800 mg/day) and placebo (50[C]). A double-blind cross-over design was used; 10 adult asthmatics participated. No significant differences were found between the treatments with regard to relief of asthma symptoms, need for additional medication or the incidence and intensity of side effects.

The adverse reactions noted included loss of appetite, palpitations, headache, nausea, stomach ache, muscle tremor and sleep disturbances.

Other theophylline derivatives

Side effects of other newer theophylline-derived compounds have been recently reviewed (SEDA-17, 1). Whether or not newer drugs possess similar efficacy and/or better tolerability than the 'classic' theophylline preparations is still controversial.

NON-SPECIFIC ANALEPTICS

Non-specific analeptics are capable of producing wide-spread stimulation of the central nervous system. The use of stimulants for depressed respiration is of doubtful value, particularly since most analeptics cannot act selectively without affecting motor centers in the central nervous system. They stimulate all levels of the cerebrospinal axis and in sufficient doses produce tonic-clonic convulsions (51[R], 52[R]). Moreover, with analeptics, side effects indicative of subconvulsive central nervous stimulation are common, i.e. tachycardia, hypertension, coughing, sneezing, vomiting, itching, tremors and muscle rigidity. At low doses, doxapram, ethamivan and nikethamide stimulate respiration with little generalized excitation, but only doxapram seems to act specifically on carotid chemoreceptors

(53[C]). The margin of safety for doses that stimulate the central nervous system is generally very narrow and unpredictable. In deeply comatose patients, analeptics might be effective when given in doses which normally would produce convulsions.

Aminophenazole

The adverse reactions reported with aminophenazole comprise restlessness, prolonged and forced expiration, nausea and vomiting, sweating, and skin reactions including rashes, occasionally oral lichenoid eruptions and ulceration (SED-9, 5). Muscle twitching and mental disorientation also may occur in the elderly. With large doses of aminophenazole, convulsions may occur (SED-9, 5).

Doxapram

Generalized stimulation of the nervous system has been observed with this drug, particularly in large doses. Adverse reactions recorded have been hyperactivity, tachycardia, increased deep tendon reflexes and muscle twitching, and laryngospasm. Elevation of blood pressure may also occur. Doxapram is contraindicated in epilepsy or other convulsive disorders and in hypertension.

Side effects of doxapram are not long-lasting because of its short half-life in plasma. Of 20 patients aged 72 treated by infusion with low doses of doxapram, four developed violent restlessness, confusion and hallucinations. Of these, three patients were known to have excessive alcohol intake and two patients abnormal liver function. The reactions were relatively brief and were related to the beginning and ending of doxapram administration.

In seven post-anesthetic patients treated with doxapram, the side effects were not serious and comprised excessive coughing, weeping, muscle tremor, nausea and hysterical reactions to dreaming. Sweating, excessive salivation and vomiting, however, were noted in the control patients, and the authors concluded that, all in all, recovery was smoother with doxapram (SED-9, 5).

A very high incidence of adverse reactions such as hot flushes, sweating, hyperventilation, tremor, nausea and vertigo has been described in postoperative analgesia combined with doxapram 1 mg/kg (SED-9, 5).

Arrhythmias consisting of self-limited ventricular extrasystoles or single premature ventricular contractions were observed after doxapram had been given by injection (SED-9, 5). The possibility was raised that electrocardiographic arrhythmias occurring in anesthesia could be associated with analeptic administration (SED-9, 5). However, in a study of 285 surgical patients, respiratory stimulation could safely be performed with doxapram, especially with small, frequently repeated doses. Side effects that occurred included neuromuscular signs of excessive central nervous system stimulation in a very few patients on a 1 mg/kg dose. Seven patients exhibited excitement, tremor was evident in three and rigidity in two. Coughing, laryngospasm and salivation are probably physiological manifestations of the return of protective reflexes secondary to arousal (SED-9, 5).

The mean pulmonary arterial pressure was significantly, but not severely, increased in 10 patients receiving intravenous infusions of doxapram (SED-8, 5).

A case of reversible hepatotoxicity has been attributed to doxapram (54[C]).

Ethamivan

The incidence of side effects from intravenous administration of ethamivan has been stated to be fairly high. Laryngospasm, sneezing and substernal chest pain have been among the reactions recorded after intravenous infusion; when given too rapidly or in too high a dose, generalized convulsions may sometimes occur (SED-9, 6). Epilepsy and monoamine oxidase inhibitors are contraindications to ethamivan medication.

Flurotyl

Flurotyl, a hexafluorinated ether, has been used as a therapeutic inhalation convulsant in psychiatry. Its use intravenously as a polyethylene glycol solution has been discontinued because of possible renal damage. In most Western and North American countries, flurotyl is not recommended because of variations in response and dosing difficulties. Electroconvulsive therapy (ECT) remains the preferred treatment.

A study of depressive patients treated alternately with flurotyl and ECT indicated that the main adverse reactions are restlessness, confusion, dysphasia, headache and dysmelia (SED-8, 5). Some patients on low doses of flurotyl have shown prolonged muscle twitching, occasionally intermittent jerky movements of the limbs (SED-9, 2), and sore throat (SED-9, 2). Other serious unwanted effects were seen in the same study: three patients required thiopentone to control restlessness, one patient had several runs of jerky movements, and four patients were severely confused, disoriented and dysphasic, violently resisting any attempts at interference. One of them also experienced a 5-minute fit following 3 ml of flurotyl and developed, in addition to the described syndrome, neck stiffness and epigastric tenderness. Lumbar puncture was normal and after 24 hours the patient had recovered. The authors believed this not to be a dose-dependent reaction and concluded that flurotyl, because of its high incidence of adverse reactions, is unlikely to become an alternative to ECT. Other investigators believe the convulsions produced by flurotyl differ qualitatively from those of ECT. Unpredictable effects were noted in a large survey of 2000 flurotyl convulsive treatments (55[C]).

In a series of 135 treated schizophrenic patients, two developed states resembling toxic delirium in which they became hyperactive, delusional and hostile. This reaction was not observed in depressed patients. The authors noted that prolonged and multiple seizures may result from overdosage or interaction with other drugs, e.g. phenothiazines. Spinal fluid pressure was found to be more elevated by flurotyl treatment than by ECT (SED-8, 6).

Flurotyl is excreted by the lungs and a hypothetical possibility that apnea, cardiac arrest or vascular collapse will occur exists. Recommendations have therefore been made that resuscitation measures be available whenever convulsant therapy is given (56[R]).

Upper respiratory tract infection has been considered a contraindication to flurotyl therapy, but this has been disregarded by others who have not observed ill effects in such cases.

Use in pregnancy The general indications are similar to those for ECT and the bar to its being given to pregnant women is due to the fact that no clinical or animal teratogenic studies are available. There is a report of one patient who received treatment in her first trimester and subsequently delivered a healthy baby (57[C]).

Interactions Flurotyl is not recommended for use *together with monoamine oxidase inhibitors*, *phenothiazines* or Rauwolfia preparation, since these all lower the seizure threshold.

Lobeline

Nausea, vomiting, coughing, tremor and dizziness have been noted with an average dose of lobeline. In addition, profuse diaphoresis, paresis, tachycardia, hypotension, hypothermia, coma and death may occur with overdosage. Lobeline taken as a 'smoking cure' may cause nausea, sweating and palpitations when a cigarette is smoked.

Nikethamide

In addition to generalized restlessness, the side effects resulting from nikethamide are itching, flushing, sweating, coughing, nausea, vomiting and muscle twitching, especially of the face. These are actually toxic effects of overdosage, the margin between the clinically effective dose and that producing toxicity being very narrow.

Pentetrazole (metrazole, pentylenetetrazole, senilex)

Adverse reactions were mild in a controlled clinical study on the efficacy of pentetrazole, alone and in combination with nicotinic acid, in 30 chronic hospitalized geriatric patients. Improvement was better with the combined treatment and only one subject, a 71-year-old woman, developed restlessness, anorexia and weight loss (SED-8, 6). Irritability, altered consciousness and autonomic reactions together with improvement in thought content and in the memory test were noted in a double-blind placebo-controlled study using pentylenetetrazole 200 mg daily in 20 geriatric patients. Nine of the 10 patients lost weight (SED-9, 6). The general consensus is that pentetrazole does not have a place in the current treatment of senility or respiratory depression (53[C]).

Picrotoxin

This non-nitrogenous plant derivative is a powerful stimulant of all parts of the central nervous system, acting on the chloride iontophore—γ-aminobutyric acid complex in a manner opposite to that of barbiturates. Larger doses are required to produce convulsions in a 'spinal' than in an intact animal. The adverse effects resemble those of nikethamide; 20 mg can cause severe poisoning.

Prethcamide

Flushing, paresthesia, headache, restlessness, muscle twitching, tremor and dyspnea have been ascribed to prethcamide. Convulsions, too, have been reported but are rare. When the drug was given intravenously, the incidence of side effects was assessed at 25% (SED-8, 7).

Strychnine

Excitation in all parts of the central nervous system is brought about by strychnine which is a powerful convulsant with a characteristic motor pattern. Since strychnine convulsions also occur in 'spinal' animals, the convulsion is termed a 'spinal convulsion', but other parts of the central nervous system also are excited by doses that produce motor manifestations in a spinal animal. Strychnine does not selectively stimulate the medulla and therefore cannot be regarded as a useful respiratory analeptic (58[R])

Strychnine poisoning In cases of poisoning the first effect produced is stiffness of the face and neck muscles; death results from medullary paralysis.

STIMULANT AND ANORECTIC AGENTS

Discussion of stimulant and anorectic side effects is best understood from the perspective of therapeutic indications, target populations, and the potential for abuse of many of the compounds. A reduction in toxic morbidity indices for those stimulants used in medical practice has come in recent years from physician and patient education, along with a narrowing of the range of therapeutic indications for use of this group of drugs. Moreover, legal sanctions have decreased drug supplies and constricted non-medical use. The development of anorectics with less stimulating, euphoriant properties has also helped to reduce abuse. As with all drugs with the potential for abuse and dose escalation, the main toxic side effects are secondary to either: (a) overdose, (b) chronic high-dose utilization or (c) intravenous administration of unfiltered or unknown drugs as well as infectious agents including HIV and hepatitis B. Toxic effects from anorectics with less euphoriant properties are known and in part reflect both the recreational user's naivety and unscrupulous 'look-alike' drug packaging. The amphetamine epidemic of the 1960s and early 1970s has now been replaced in the United States and many Western nations by cocaine abuse. Methamphetamine abuse has increased in several locales including the Pacific Basin.

Side effects of 'catecholaminergic stimulants' fall into several categories based on doses, time after dose, chronicity of use, and pattern of use-abuse, e.g. 4—5-day bingeing episodes. Adverse effects not only include responses during the period of use but also the intermediate and long-term residual effects following withdrawal. For example, it is well known that once a stimulant psychosis has developed with chronic abuse, that long after withdrawal only one or two moderate doses of stimulant are required to induce the full-blown psychosis in its original form (59[CR]). Similarly the precipitous slide to severe re-addiction in former abusers re-introduced to stimulants illustrates this adverse residual propensity that exists even in the long-term withdrawal state.

Rapid administration by intravenous or inhalation route of administration can induce very high concentrations in areas of high vascular perfusion, heart and brain before eventual distribution to other tissues. Under these conditions in the heart not only does a catecholaminergic storm take place, but also local anesthetic conduction prolongation has the potential for toxic interaction, with the catechol reduction of refractory period increasing the potential re-entrant arrhythmias in addition to any anoxic overload from CNS seizures. Once beyond the immediate vulnerability period, accumulation of stimulant on board (e.g. frequent overdosing, accidents from body packing of condom-filled stimulants to avoid detection) leads to a different cascade of events precipitating death. Catecholaminergic hypermetabolism, states with hyperpyrexia acidosis, and anorexia aggravated by repeated seizure usually is an outcome taking place over a period of hours, usually ending in cardiac collapse (60[C], 61[R]). On the other hand, chronic dosing can induce catecholaminergic cardiomyopathy, e.g. contraction bands, cardiomegaly (62[C]—64[R]), repeated vasospastic insults to cerebral and coronary arteries (63[C]). Whether these chronic effects predispose to increased sensitivity to acute dosing toxicity has not been systematically explored.

In addition to other chronic changes noted in abusers, personality deterioration under the effects of the drug carries a significant association with high-risk behaviors which are a source of physical and psychiatric morbidity and mortality. These include: (a) suicide, (b) violent trauma and aggressive behavior and, (c) high-risk methods of drug use (e.g. needle sharing) and high-risk sexual behavior with increased morbidity for HIV, hepatitis B and other infections.

The stimulant properties of cocaine are similar to those of amphetamines, though differences are notable, in part, because of the very short plasma half-life of cocaine. These differences are highlighted below under 'Amphetamines' and 'Cocaine'. However, cocaine has the same problems of abuse potential as other stimulants and at high doses causes stimulant psychosis (65[R]). In addition, even used as a local nasopharyngeal anesthetic, it has toxic effects in high doses.

Stimulants of the amphetamine and methylphenidate type have specific indications for narcolepsy and the hyperactivity syndrome in children. With the use of stimulants for these therapeutic indications usually at moderate dose levels, careful monitoring for emergent psychosis, agitation and abuse is important. Even periodic checks for monodelusional syndromes are important at doses in the mid-to-high range (66[R]).

The use of amphetamine-type stimulants for depression, fatigue and psychasthenia since the early 1970s fell into disfavor because of the potential for abuse and the low rates of success, especially after tolerance is established. Recently, there have been reports and reviews on the successes in carefully selected groups of patients (67[R], 68[C], 69[R]). The underlying symptom profile that appears to characterize patients responding to stimulants is that of mild anhedonia, lack of mental and physical energy, easy fatiguability, and low self-esteem yet in the absence of the marked depressed mood disturbance, guilt and hopelessness associated with major depression. Examples include dysthymia disorders, medically ill patients (especially post-stroke), depression patients, hospitalized cancer patients, significant cardiovascular disorders all associated with anergia and fast fatiguability. More recently, HIV-related neuropsychiatric symptoms including depression are reported to respond to psychostimulants (68[C], 69[R], 70[C]). Withdrawn apathetic geriatric patients without major dementia are reported to have positive responses (71[R]). General adverse effects are stated to be relatively mild, such as tachycardia, agitation, and all reversed on withdrawal (SEDA-17, 1). The combination of stimulants with monoamine oxidase inhibitors in treatment-resistant depressed patients has been recently reported (72[C]) (SEDA-17). However, this use should be restricted to patients where careful monitoring by specialists is involved because of the potential for hypertensive crisis.

The use of stimulants in hyperactive attentional disorder children remains a major part of treatment. Specific problems with reduced growth are of concern even though growth accelerates during drug holidays (SEDA-6, 4). Drug levels in children on a mg/kg basis are sometimes as high as those reported to produce chronic central nervous system changes in animal studies.

In older patients, a variety of milder stimulants including pemoline, hydergine and piracetam have been used for their mental energizing and alerting properties and successes have been reported; the acute and chronic toxic effects of stimulants in older persons or even older lab animals has not been systematically examined. The greater toxicity of stimulants under high ambient temperatures could prove toxic to geriatric patients vulnerable to heat exhaustion.

The prototype for anoretic drugs is amphetamine. Methamphetamine, benzphetamine, phenmetrazine, phendimetrazine, phentermine, chlorphentermine, chlorterimine, mazindol, diethylpropion and fenfluramine are the more commonly used anorectics. The relative reinforcing effects or abuse potential of these drugs is thought to be related to their potency in releasing dopamine from nerve terminals as compared to serotonin release. Amphetamine, methamphetamine and phenmetrazine are potent dopamine releasers with high euphoriant and stimulant properties, whereas the compounds with halide substitution in the phenol ring, i.e. fenfluramine and chlorphentermine, are more potent releasers of serotonin and have greater sedative action at anorectic doses. Thus, in summary, those drugs with relatively strong serotoninergic to dopaminergic releasing properties seem to provide anorectic effects without euphoria except at high doses, and should be considered first in any patient who has potential for abuse (66[R]) (73[R] and 74[CR] from SEDA-17).

The combination of cocaine and ethanol leads to the formation of coc-ethanol, the adverse effects of which has not been systematically assessed.

Cocaine

An epidemic of abuse continues in many countries for the local anesthetic-stimulant drug, cocaine. There may be about 5 million regular cocaine users in the United States; the number of users who experience significant difficulties including serious as well as fatal medical complications continues to be reported frequently (61[R], 75). The smoking of free-base cocaine, sometimes sold as 'crack' or 'rock' on the streets, is common. The inexpensive widely available 'crack' formulation is prepared by alkalinizing cocaine hydrochloride and precipitating the resultant alkaloidal free-base cocaine which, unlike the hydrochloride, is not destroyed by heat when smoked. Smoking provides a rapid effect, comparable to that of intravenous injection. The intense euphoria, followed within minutes by a let down dysphoria, leads to frequent dosing and greater potential for rapid addiction (76[R]). As with amphetamines, the euphoric effect may enhance craving and the repeated reinforcement may lead to conditioned drug responses which facilitate dependence. Facilitated conditioned effects with cocaine may be due to cocaine's rapid elimination and the development of acute tolerance. Frequent repeated dosing becomes necessary to sustain euphoria, thereby promoting a tight temporal juxtaposition of euphoria with the recent antecedent drug-taking events (75[R]).

ADVERSE REACTION PATTERN

General and toxic reactions Cocaine has a spectrum of pharmacological effects. Initial action induces excitement and euphoria; later, with higher doses, lower centers become involved, producing decreased coordination, tremors, hyperreflexia, increased respiratory rate and, at times, nausea, vomiting and convulsions. The symptoms are eventually followed by CNS depression. Cardiovascular effects include tachycardia, hypertension and increased cardiac irritability; large intravenous doses may produce cardiac failure. If applied to mucous membranes, it causes local vasoconstriction and, with chronic use, necrosis. As a general rule, the mortality is higher when cocaine is used intravenously or as smoked free base than if taken nasally or orally (77[R]). The symptoms of acute cocaine poisoning include agitation, diaphoresis, tachycardia, grand mal seizures, severe respiratory and metabolic acidosis, apnea and ventricular arrhythmias. Seizures ensue at high doses and their control with sedatives is important to reduce lethality (73[C]). The idiopathic cardiac rhythms have been ascribed to a direct toxic effect of cocaine and a secondary sensitization of ventricular tissue for catecholamines (78[C]) along with slowed cardiac conduction secondary to local anesthetic effects.

Cocaine fatal toxicity Death from cocaine often occurs within 2—3 minutes, suggesting direct cardiac toxicity, fatal arrhythmia, and depression of medullary respiratory centers as common causes of death (74[r], 79[r]). Thus, cocaine's local anesthetic properties may contribute additional hazards when high doses are used, reminiscent of cocaine fatal toxicities reported in the era when it was used as a mucous membrane paste for nasopharyngeal surgery (80[r]).

Periods of increased cocaine use, especially intravenous, free-base inhalation and high-dose use, as expected were associated with cocaine-related deaths. For example, according to the Drug Abuse Warning Network, a 3-fold increase in such deaths from 195 to 580 per year occurred in the United States between 1981 and 1985. Despite the importance of these mortality data, relatively little is known of the types of pathophysiological sequences involved in the cascade of events leading to death. More importantly, there is a paucity of guidelines to the appropriate diagnostic and treatment strategies for the various pre-fatal conditions.

Myocardial infarction has increased as a complication of cocaine abuse (62[C], 63[C]). Dilated cardiomyopathies, with subsequent recurrent myocardial infarction, have been associated with long-term use of cocaine, raising the possibility of chronic effects on the heart (81[CR]). Many victims have evidence of pre-existent fixed coronary artery disease precipitated by cocaine use (SEDA-9, 35; 82[CR], 83[R], 84[R]). However, myocardial infarction has been noted even in young intranasal users with no evidence of coronary disease (85[CR]) defined either by autopsy or angiography (86[CR], 87[R]). Some studies suggest that seizures may be a major determinant of fatal outcomes. Associated hyperthermia may contribute as a primary cause in cases of fatal hyperpyrexia, as well as potentiate the hypoxic cardiovascular events in cardiac deaths in those that survive the initial acute dose (88[R], 89[R]). The final agonal events in cocaine toxic deaths involve the combination of sympathomimetic myocardial responses and/or cardiac conduction slowing, secondary to cocaine's local anesthetic effect, leading to arrhythmias (90[R]). In reported fatal overdoses, convulsions and death have usually occurred within minutes. Most patients who have survived for the first 3 hours after an initial acute overdose have been likely to recover. Treatment of the toxicity reaction includes respiratory and cardiovascular resuscitative measures. Short-acting barbiturates, benzodiazepines, propranolol and phentolamine have all been used with some success (86[R], 91[C]). In one study of 60 cocaine-related deaths, autopsy findings were non-specific, but typical of those found in respiratory depression of central origin (92[R]).

ORGANS AND SYSTEMS

Cardiovascular The *tachycardia* and *vasoconstriction* from cocaine can exacerbate coronary insufficiency, complicated by arrhythmias and hypertensive and vascular hemorrhage (61[R]). Sudden deaths have been reported in patients with angina (93[R]). Chronic dosing includes cardiomyopathy and cardiomegaly; other chronic conditions include endocarditis thrombophlebitis. Crack smoking has led to pneumo-pericardium (94[R]).

Nervous system Cocaine *lowers the seizure threshold* and may therefore be dangerous to patients already at risk of seizures (94[R]). As with several other drugs, e.g. marijuana, PCP, and LSD, cocaine use is being reported as a precipitant of panic disorder which continues autonomously long after drug withdrawal (95[C]). Cerebrovascular local vasoconstriction and sudden increase in blood pressure probably underlie the many reports of cocaine-induced strokes, CNS hemorrhage, and migraine (96[R]) (SEDA-17, 4).

Metabolic *Blood sugar* levels may become labile in diabetics using cocaine, not only because their diet changes, but also because adrenaline levels affect the mobilization of glucose (97[R]).

Gastrointestinal Gastrointestinal symptoms, especially *diarrhea*, are known to occur following cocaine use. Cases of more severe *abdominal distress* have required surgical intervention and may be due to bowel infarctions or pneumo-peritoneum (61^R, 97^C, 98^C).

Miscellaneous Other complications include a report of fatal *pulmonary edema* that developed in a 36-year-old man shortly after injecting free-base cocaine intravenously (99^C); three cases of *generalized seizures* occurring shortly after the intravenous use of cocaine (100^R); two cases of *connective tissue disease* (101^R); spontaneous *pneumomediastinum* reported with the inhalation of free-base cocaine (102^C); and exacerbation of *Gilles de la Tourette syndrome* (103^C).

Second-generation effects Neonatal effects are evident in several organ systems when exposure has been in utero. These complications have effects both on the outcome of the pregnancy and the behavior of the neonate. The increased incidence of genital malformations has been noted frequently (104^R). Gastrointestinal disorders include cases of necrotizing enterocolitis and intestinal atresia (105^C). Ankyloglossia is noted to be 3.5 times more common in cocaine neonates. Other facial, vertebral, and cardiovascular defects have been described (SEDA-17, 4). In general, these defects have been ascribed to the interruption of intrauterine blood supply with subsequent destruction of the fetal structure, but the mechanism remains unclear. The data suggested that cocaine-exposed infants may be at increased risk for congenital malformations (106^R). There are increasing reports of intrauterine growth retardation, neurobehavioral abnormalities, cerebral injury, and cardiac anomalies in 'coke babies' (SEDA-14, 15).

The amphetamines

Amphetamine itself is a sympathomimetic compound derived from phenylethylamine; however, the name has tended to become generic for the entire group of related substances, three of the best known being dexamphetamine, methamphetamine and benzamphetamine.

The amphetamines have marked psychomotor stimulant activity in addition to their peripheral sympathomimetic actions. When an amphetamine is taken, even in a therapeutic dose, most people experience a sensation of enhanced energy or vitality. This feeling may, with repetitive intake of the drug, follow different patterns. Most often, euphoria will develop, usually with a sense of heightened function or perception, and occasionally compulsive behavior as well as hallucinogenic delusions. It may also induce dysphoria in certain (especially older) individuals. The euphoric effect may enhance craving for amphetamine and the repeated reinforcement may lead to conditioned drug responses which may facilitate dependence. Progression to severe dependence is highly dependent upon individual vulnerability, the circumstances, the setting, the pattern of use and especially the escalation to high-dose patterns of use. Although most people probably use amphetamines for the original reason they were prescribed and do not escalate the dosage, a significant proportion do, highlighting the abuse potential. The amphetamines sometimes are used recreationally for years at moderate levels. Once inhalation and intravenous routes of administration or higher doses are used, a 'high-dose transition' into abuse usually occurs, and the capacity for low-dose occasional use is lost, presumably, forever (see 'Abuse and dependence' below).

Realization of the risk of abuse and of dependence has led to the present attitude that there may be only a restricted place for amphetamines in medicine. Perhaps low-dose, short-term use in combating fatigue and altering depressed mood could be justified, but only for specific indications and under continuous medical supervision.

The following monograph will deal primarily with the adverse reactions to amphetamine itself and its three close congeners.

ADVERSE REACTION PATTERN

General and toxic reactions By releasing monoamines from the brain and thereby stimulating noradrenergic, serotonergic and particularly dopaminergic receptors, the amphetamines may, under certain circumstances, induce psychosis and compulsive behavior, as well as hallucinogenic auditory delusions of vague noises similar to those experienced in paranoid schizophrenia. In addition, amphetamines give rise to an acute 'toxic psychosis' with visual hallucinations, usually after one or two extremely large doses (107^r).

The multiplicity of action from overdosage of amphetamines can result in restlessness, dizziness, tremor, hyperactive reflexes, talkativeness, tenseness, irritability and insomnia; less commonly, one sees euphoria, confusion, anxiety, delirium, hallucinations, panic states, suicidal and homicidal tendencies, excessive sweating, dry mouth, metallic taste, anorexia, nausea, vomiting, diarrhea and abdominal cramps. Fatal poisoning is usually associated with hyperpyrexia, convulsions, coma or cerebral hemorrhage. In addition, peripheral excitation of smooth muscles or blood vessels supplying skeletal muscles, as well as those of gut and bronchi, have been described among the pharmacological responses observed with the use of amphetamines. Other effects have been excitatory actions, including increased heart rate, causing palpitations and arrhythmias, and metabolic effects such as glycogenolysis in liver and adipose tissue.

Hypersensitivity reactions An anaphylactic reaction following injection of crushed tablets equivalent to 45 mg of amphetamine occurred in a young woman; in others, injected with the same solution and at the same time, no adverse effects were experienced (SED-9, 8). The reaction may have involved amphetamine or excipients. A recent report indicates scleroderma is a potential consequence of various stimulants used for appetite control (108[C]).

Tumor-inducing effects These have not been reported.

ORGANS AND SYSTEMS

Cardiovascular *Tachycardia*, *arrhythmias* and a *rise in blood pressure* have been described following the administration of centrally acting sympathomimetic amines. Acutely administered amphetamine to men with a history of amphetamine abuse enhanced the pressor effect of tyramine and noradrenaline, while continuous amphetamine led to a tolerance of the pressor response to tyramine. As was found with intravenous amphetamines, cardiomyopathy, cardiomegaly, and pulmonary edema have been reported with smoking of crystal methamphetamine (63[C], 129[R], 130[C]).

Of the other central stimulants, aminorex and doxapram have been observed to induce chronic pulmonary hypertension; chlorphentermine, phentermine, phenmetrazine and D-norpseudoephedrine might also have this effect (SED-9, 8). It is not a common complication of treatment with any anorectic agent, however, and may involve a genetic predisposition (SED-9, 8). Pulmonary hypertension may develop or be diagnosed a long time after an anorectic agent has been taken.

Nervous system *Psychoses* in persons taking amphetamines were first reported many years ago and the question was posed whether these states were due to the amphetamines or to co-existing and exacerbated paranoid-schizophrenic illness. It was demonstrated in one study that most psychotic symptoms remitted before the excretion of amines had fallen to its normal base level (SED-9, 8). The psychotic syndrome was indistinguishable from paranoid schizophrenia with short periods of disorientation and could appear after a single dose (many had taken the equivalent of some 100×5 mg tablets (orally) of amphetamine or methamphetamine) without, or with, simultaneous ingestion of alcohol, and was most accentuated in addicts (SED-9, 9). A picture of amphetamine psychosis was also demonstrated in 14 people in Australia (59[CR]); here, the hallucinations predominating were visual, which is unusual for schizophrenia (SED-8, 11). Similarly, in contrast to schizophrenia, vision was noted to be the primary sensory mode in hallucinations, thinking disorders and body schema distortions of amphetamine addicts, according to a study in 25 patients (131[C]).

Other studies were carried out in human volunteers previously dependent on amphetamines, dosing to a level at which amphetamine psychosis was produced in order to examine the mechanism of action and the pharmacokinetics of amphetamine and a possible relationship to schizophrenia (132[R], 133[C]). Psychosis was induced by moderately high doses of amphetamine and the psychotic symptoms were often a replication of the chronic amphetamine psychosis (Australian study), raising the question of whether establishment of chronic stimulant psychosis leaves a residual vulnerability to psychosis precipitated by stimulants. The mechanism might be similar to the one operating in reverse tolerance noted in experimental animals (112). Underlying psychosis can be precipitated; an increase in schizophrenic symptoms (SED-8, 12) was observed in 17 actively ill schizophrenic patients after a single injection of amphetamine.

Amphetamine psychosis is relatively rare in children, even in hyperactive children on large amphetamine doses; amphetamine psychosis was reported in an 8-year-old child with a hyperkinetic syndrome (SED-8, 12). Large doses of amphetamine can cause disruption of thinking, but amphetamine psychosis as generally observed is not accompanied by the degree of disorganization normally seen in schizophrenia (SED-9, 8).

Stereotyped behavior A type of automatic behavior which can continue for hours has been observed in addicts who inject large doses of central nervous system stimulants. Dyskinetic symptoms may appear as strange facial and tongue movements or jerky motions of the arms and legs with a never-ceasing repetition of certain actions. Such stereotyped activity are induced in laboratory animals with high doses of amphetamine.

Fatal toxicity The problem of fatal overdose is central to the problem of frequently repeated intravenous high-dose abuse of stimulants of unknown quality and quantity. Fatal overdose is less frequent among experienced chronic users than in naive or episodic high-dose users (109[r], 110[r], 111[CR]), in part due to the establishment with chronic use of tolerance to the induced hyperpyrexia and hypertension. Rare individuals have used up to 1—3 g of oral amphetamine per day for many years without problems of overdosing, yet toxic overdoses are reported on an acute basis at 100—200 mg (112[R]). Among the stimulants, toxic overdosing has been best documented for amphetamines and there is little evidence of differential overdose toxicity among the group, with the possible exception of cocaine. Hyperpyrexia, seizures, hypertensive cerebrovascular hemorrhage, ventricular fibrillation, left ventricular failure and complications of intravenous drug abuse have all been reported as causes of deaths (110[R], 111[CR], 113[R], 114[R]).

Amphetamine and brain damage The question of permanent brain damage being caused by amphetamine in large doses has been repeatedly raised in the past from animal studies (115[r], 116[r]), yet definitive studies in man have not been accomplished. The vasculitis of large elastic vessels found in chronic animal studies has been reported to involve the internal carotid artery in man (117[r]); intravenous administration is secondarily implicated. In man and animals, behavioral changes continue for several months after withdrawal of amphetamine; chronic residual changes have been reported mainly in monoaminergic neurons or terminals either as structural changes or as residual depletion of monoamines and synthesizing enzymes (112[R]).

Dyskinesias Although controversial, there is a growing consensus that stimulants provoke, cause or exacerbate Gilles de la Tourette syndrome (GTS) (SEDA-7, 10). It is based on the observation that stimulants such as the amphetamines, methylphenidate, pemoline, etc., facilitate dopamine retention at the synaptic cleft. On one side, there are many case reports and studies (118[CR]) reporting that stimulants prescribed for attention deficit disorder in children vulnerable for GTS develop exacerbated motor and phonic tics. These studies suggest: (a) that GTS should be a contraindication for stimulant use for hyperactive syndromes; and (b) that a family history of dyskinesias should be considered as a contraindication. Shapiro and Shapiro (119[CR]) in their critical review of the literature and their own studies conclude that there is virtually no evidence that stimulants in clinically appropriate doses provoke GTS; they believe that dyskinesias are a function of elevated doses. The caution remains that assiduously careful periodic examination for dyskinesia should be performed in patients on stimulants. It is not known whether structural changes in the central nervous system accompany stimulant-induced dyskinesias.

Personality degeneration A report on a double-blind, placebo-controlled, short-term study describes significant personality deterioration in five of 26 children treated with dextroamphetamine (SED-9, 9; 120[r]).

Hematological An isolated case of acute myeloblastic leukemia has been reported in a 24-year-old man who had taken massive doses of amphetamine over more than 2 years (SED-8, 13).

Endocrine, metabolic See discussion of retardation of growth (height and weight) in hyperactive children treated with amphetamine (SED-9, 9) in section on 'Methylphenidate'.

Sexual behavior Reports of effects of amphetamine on sexual behavior refer variously to unchanged, decreased, mixed and heightened sexual performance (SED-9, 9).

Risk situations Special caution should be applied to the use of amphetamines in *geriatric patients*, in view of the likelihood of stimulation of adrenergic receptors and, in particular, of cardiovascular and respiratory functions. Periodic users especially need to be wary of acute use under circumstances of *exercise* and *environmental heat*, due to the potential of heat stroke.

Second-generation effects *Use in pregnancy* Studies were carried out in pregnant women who reported for prenatal care between 1959 and 1966. The severe congenital defect rate per 100 liveborn was compared up to the fifth year of life in children whose mothers had, or had not, taken amphetamines (and similar drugs) during pregnancy. An excess of oral clefts was noted in the offspring of mothers who had taken amphetamines in the first 56 days from their last menstrual period, but this was considered to be either a chance finding or one element in a multifactorial situation (SED-9, 9).

Interactions Amphetamines and other stimulatory anorectic agents, apart from fenfluramine (see below), would be expected to impair the hypotensive effects of *adrenergic neuron-blocking drugs* such as guanethidine. Not only do they release noradrenaline from stores in adrenergic neurons, and block the re-uptake of released noradrenaline into the neuron, but they also impair re-entry of the antihypertensive drugs.

This group of stimulatory drugs should not be used together with or within 14 days of taking any *monoamine oxidase inhibitor*. Severe hypertensive reactions and, on occasion, confusional states (e.g. with fenfluramine) may be produced (SED-9, 9).

Tricyclic antidepressants increase blood levels of amphetamine; *barbiturates* and *benzodiazepines* may enhance amphetamine hypermotility. A point which should be taken into consideration when treating amphetamine psychosis is that chlorpromazine increases the half-life of amphetamine. Prior chronic treatment with *narcotics* may have a residual effect of enhancing subsequent behavioral response to stimulants. *Alcohol* increases blood levels of amphetamines.

Abuse and dependence The most important problem encountered with amphetamines has been their abuse and the development of dependence on them. The most rapid onset of an amphetamine epidemic occurred in Japan where previously little or no abuse has been present (104[R]). Although a high proportion of amphetamine users probably already have emotional and social difficulties, sustained abuse may result in serious psychiatric complications ranging from severe personality disorders to chronic psychoses (121[R], 122[C]). Whereas signs of intense physical dependence are not considered to occur (SED-9, 9), withdrawal may be associated with intense depression (SED-9, 9; 80[R]), and relapses in psychiatric disorders have been frequently noted. A number of countries where the problem became widespread have banned amphetamines from their therapeutic armamentaria and Australia has restricted their use to narcolepsy and behavioral disorders of children. Amphetamine dependence developed into a serious problem in the USA (and to a lesser extent in the UK) where it followed the typical pattern of drug dependence (SED-9, 7, 10).

Continuing critical re-assessment of the usefulness versus the harmfulness of amphetamines has led to further restrictions in their use (SED-9, 10). They have been placed under rigid control in many countries by new legislation and at the same time recommendations to cease prescribing them have been made. The World Health Organization and United Nations have also stressed the need for strict control of amphetamines (SED-9, 10; 123[R]).

INDIVIDUAL COMPOUNDS

Benzphetamine

Euphoria and other stimulatory effects on the central nervous system causing restlessness, sleeplessness and dizziness, gastrointestinal disturbances (including dry mouth and loss of appetite) and cardiovascular changes were observed with this appetite depressant.

Dexamphetamine ((+)-amphetamine)

(+)-Amphetamine is significantly more powerful than (−)-amphetamine, the use of the former as an anorectic having rapidly declined because of realization of its abuse and addiction potentials. These arise mainly from euphoria which may be followed by depression as the effect of the drug wears off. Stimulant effects were reported in 23% of 347 patients using dextroamphetamine as an anorectic (SED-9, 10).

Dexamphetamine is extremely variable in its effect on the individual, even producing drowsiness in a small proportion of subjects. Postmenopausal women are more prone to develop drowsiness, anger and sadness than euphoria (124[C]). Side effects due to sympathetic overactivity are fairly common but not usually serious. However, in view of dexamphetamine's addiction potential, other anorectics should be considered first.

Hyperinsulinemia secondary to chronic administration of D-amphetamine with a decrease in fasting blood sugar after a few weeks of application has been described (SED-9,10).

Methylenedioxymethamphetamine (MDMA)

MDMA, a recreational drug often known as 'ecstasy' is gaining popularity in many areas. MDMA which, at lower doses, is described as a pleasant altered state of mind during which emotional closeness is enhanced, is being used in high doses and settings where toxicity is frequently reported. The British literature has reported considerable adverse effects from its use at rave dances. Associated with increased physical activity and alteration in thermoregulation, MDMA is reported to cause unconsciousness, seizures, hyperthermia, tachycardia, hypotension, disseminated intravascular coagulation, and acute renal failure as well as death.

Methylphenidate (Ritalin)

Methylphenidate is a piperidine derivative structurally related to amphetamine. It is a milder central nervous system stimulant than amphetamine. Large doses, however, will produce symptoms of generalized central nervous system stimulation and lead to convulsions. It is more active than amphetamine as an antidepressant, as treatment for overdosage of depressant drugs, and in exacerbating schizophrenic symptoms. Occasionally anorexia, nausea, dry mouth, nervousness, insomnia, dizziness and palpitations have been recorded in patients on methylphenidate.

Considerable concern surrounds the use of methylphenidate and, to a lesser extent, amphetamine and pemoline in hyperactive or attention deficit syndrome in children and possible detrimental effects on general physical and emotional growth and central nervous system development. The US FDA Psychopharmacology Pediatric Subcommittee reviewed the literature relevant to growth suppression by stimulants in the treatment of hyperkinetic syndrome. There is clear evidence of temporary retardation in growth in weight and suggestion of temporary slowing of stature growth related to drug dose and absence of drug holidays during the prepubertal period (125[CR]–127[CR]). To allow for growth rebound, the importance of drug holidays is evident in children requiring higher doses and manifesting drug plateaus.

Abuse and psychosis Methylphenidate shares the pharmacological properties and the abuse potential of the amphetamines. When given intravenously, it has been found to activate psychotic symptoms in schizophrenic patients if administered during the active phase of their illness but not after remission. It failed to produce a psychotic reaction in most manic or depressed patients or in normal subjects (128[C]).

In hyperactive children, gross behavioral changes with hallucinations were encountered after brief administration of modest doses of methylphenidate. The reaction subsided after withdrawal of the drug (127[CR]).

In one double-blind study, undesirable personality changes consisting of lethargic and apathetic behavior occurred in six out of 98 hyperactive children aged 6–12 years and treated with methylphenidate for 16 weeks. Withdrawal of medication resulted in a prompt switch from the characteristic mental depression to usual behavior (SED-9, 11).

There appears to be a large variation in individual responses to methylphenidate among hyperactive children with minimal brain dysfunction. It is therefore advisable to start with small divided doses since some symptoms (extrapyramidal and seizure-like) could be dose-related.

As with use of other stimulants, chorea (134[C]) and choreoathetosis (135[C]) can be precipitated in children as well as adults at methylphenidate doses ranging from therapeutic to abuse levels. These symptoms respond to drug cessation or neuroleptics.

Cardiovascular and visceral Significant increases in blood pressure and/or pulse rate following oral administration of methylphenidate are more frequent when it is given parenterally (SED-9, 11; SEDA-4, 9).

Arrhythmias, shock, cardiac muscle pathology, and liver pathology have all been cited in specific case reports (SED-8, 21; SED-9, 11).

Increased blood levels of SGPT, SGOT and alkaline phosphatase were reported in a 67-year-old woman with a cerebrovascular accident who had taken methylphenidate 10 mg thrice daily. Nausea, vomiting and dizzy spells occurred. The drug was discontinued and liver enzymes returned to normal levels, but when the patient was rechallenged with a small dose of 2.5 mg methylphenidate, the pathological changes recurred (SED-9, 11).

The abdominal distress occasionally observed can be alleviated either by reduction of the dose or by administering the drug immediately after meals.

Complications of abuse Chronic parenteral injection of (resolved methylphenidate hydrochloride tablets intended for oral use has led to cutaneous reactions. Pulmonary granulomata were seen in two patients who died as a consequence of drug abuse (SED-8, 22). In one case bullous erythema multiforme was described and considered unlikely to be due to the excipients in the tablets. Cornstarch, talc and binders do, however, cause significant microemboli noticeable on retinoscopic examination and may cause pulmonary hypertension (SEDA-4, 9).

Five patients suffered skin abscesses or cellulitis following parenteral methylphenidate abuse (SED-9, 11). Such lesions may arise from local vasospasm and chemical irritation and be susceptible to secondary infection.

Interactions Methylphenidate raises the levels of *phenobarbital*, *phenytoin*, *imipramine* and *desipramine* in serum, and slows the rate of disappearance from the serum of *ethylbiscoumacetate*. Enhanced *anticoagulant* action may therefore occur in the presence of methylphenidate (SED-9, 11).

Hypertensive episodes occurred in three adults after combining methylphenidate with *tricyclic antidepressants* (SED-9, 11).

ANORECTICS

When it was first introduced, one of the most frequent uses of amphetamine was as an anorexigenic agent in the treatment of obesity. A number of anorectic agents, many of them related to amphetamine, have since been manufactured. The majority of these are stimulants of the central nervous system; in descending order of approximate stimulatory potency, they are dexamphetamine, phentermine, chlorphentermine, mazindol, diethylpropion and fenfluramine. The last of these has a stimulatory effect only with overdosage. One of the problems that has concerned clinicians over the use of anorectics for the treatment of weight reduction is that despite the 6 weeks to 3 months of weight reduction efficacy the effects begins to wear off and, on cessation of use, weight gain rebounds. More recently, the comprehensive study examine the long-term efficacy and safety of fenfluramine plus phentermine in combination in a weight reduction program in 121 obese sub-

jects (*SEDA*-17; *and* 75[r], 76[R], 136[C], 137[C] from SEDA-17). The combination of drugs along with group therapy, individual dietary counseling and exercise resulted in weight loss during treatment occurring for up to 2 years; between 2 and 3 years, and beyond 3 years, treatment helped the participants to maintain weight loss. The most commonly used doses were 50 mg of fenfluramine plus 15 mg of phentermine given either continuously or intermittently. Remarkably, the drug related dropouts during the four studies (because of adverse drug effects, lack of efficacy, or fear of medication) were 22 of the 121 subjects. Must of the dropouts occurring after week 34. Most common adverse effects in descending order of frequency were dry mouth, insomnia, constipation, and cardiovascular effects. Thus, this study clearly shows that extensive weight reduction is possible with this combination of anorectics and it has a relatively low adverse effect profile.

Fenfluramine (Ponderal, Ponderax)

ADVERSE REACTION PATTERN

General and toxic reactions Although structurally resembling amphetamine, fenfluramine does not in normal therapeutic doses produce central nervous system-stimulating effects. The main adverse effects encountered with fenfluramine in two double-blind studies were sedation and drowsiness in addition to abdominal discomfort and dry mouth (SED-9, 12; 138[C]). Very rarely were these severe enough to justify withdrawal from trial. With fairly high doses, the above-mentioned adverse effects became more severe and frequent. Drowsiness and gastrointestinal disturbances consisting of colicky abdominal pain were among the most outstanding adverse effects in several other studies, most of them double-blind; dizziness, light-headedness and headaches were less frequent but occasionally quite marked (SED-9, 12).

Dexfenfluramine, the dextro-rotatory isomer is now being widely marked as an appetite suppressant adjunct in the management of obesity. It appears to be a pure serotonin agonist without the dopaminergic and sympathetic activity of the racemic weight both short- and long-term, and the adverse effects seen with greater frequency than in the placebo controls, over a 12-month period, were tiredness, nausea, diarrhea, and dry mouth (139[R], 140[C]). Mydriasis, depression, withdrawal depression, insomnia, nervousness, headache and urinary frequency have also been reported. Most symptoms were mild and disappeared with continuing treatment. Pulmonary hypertension has also been reported in the literature on four patients so far (141[C], 142[C]) (see also 177[C]).

So far published clinical experience indicates that the greater selectivity of the dextro-rotatory isomer leads to good tolerability. There has been only one long-term, i.e. greater than 6 months, trial on which to base this opinion (140[C]). Since weight increase is common after cessation of treatment, long-term treatment is likely to be sought and given. It is recommended that other support and treatment should be offered, since long-term safety over 6 months requires confirmation. Because studies on laboratory animals, including squirrel monkeys, indicate there is a dose-dependent depletion of serotonin and metabolites along with a reduced number of uptake sites that has a persistent time-course, concern has always been that humans may have a potential neurotoxic response. The same case applies to dexfenfluramine. However, it has also been pointed out that dexfenfluramine has been used by more than 5 million patients for 6 years, and the parent compound by more than 20 million patients for 26 years, and yet it has not been associated with any serotonergic-mediated functional CNS pathology in man (SEDA-17, 1).

Hypersensitivity reactions These have not been reported.

Tumor-inducing effects These have not been described.

ORGANS AND SYSTEMS

Cardiovascular In a few patients, *hypertension* was induced or aggravated by fenfluramine. The hypertension disappeared on discontinuing the drug but could not in all instances be re-induced by rechallenge (SED-9, 12).

Respiratory Progressive *pulmonary hypertension* has been seen in two patients taking fenfluramine for only 8 months (SEDA-6, 9). Symptoms decreased on withdrawal but returned in one patient when rechallenged. In the US there is specific warning labeling for pulmonary hypertension. Because of the foregoing pulmonary problems with aminorex, these case reports must be taken seriously and patients on fenfluramine should be periodically evaluated.

Nervous system The frequent occurrence of *sedation*, *drowsiness*, *light-headedness* and *headaches* has been referred to in the general section above.

Impaired power of concentration during the first

week, insomnia, apathy tiredness, *general memory decrease* and a *feeling of derealization* but not mood elevation were noted in healthy persons given fenfluramine (SEDA-13; 143[R]). *Depression* can occur during treatment but is more common during the first few days following sudden discontinuation of treatment (SED-9, 12). Moreover, abrupt cessation of fenfluramine treatment has also led to *feelings* of dizziness, nausea and restlessness in about 20% of patients. An explanation for the depression and irritability encountered after sudden withdrawal of treatment may be a rapid reduction in 5-hydroxytryptamine, since it has been shown that the central effect of fenfluramine is mediated by 5-hydroxytryptamine.

Of special interest are studies on the interrelationship between fenfluramine and *sleep*. In chronic psychiatric cases, following the intake of 40 or 80 mg of fenfluramine, patients fell asleep in a normal way but a few hours later they were troubled with a peculiar feeling of uneasiness which kept them awake for the rest of the night. The following night, however, patients fell asleep more quickly, regardless of the medication. Moreover, one patient experienced nightmares following daily intake of two tablets; when the dosage was reduced to a single morning tablet, the nightmares ceased (SED-8, 19). About half of a group of 50 obese women treated over a period of 20 weeks with various doses increasing gradually up to the maximum tolerated level of 160 mg per day, and then decreasing again, reported increased dreaming (144[C]). In another study, increased dreaming was reported in patients receiving relatively small doses of fenfluramine (SED-9, 12).

Psychosis The clinical picture of fenfluramine-treated subjects is usually not one of stimulation but of calmness or drowsiness. However, in the predisposed, the drug may precipitate psychotic illness. Several published cases illustrate this (SED-8, 19).

Dyskinesia A 43-year-old woman experienced tightening retrocollic movements of the head and neck with tongue and throat muscle spasm following a single fenfluramine tablet (SED-8, 19).

Impotence There have been occasional reports of male impotence which disappeared upon discontinuation of the drug. Very-high-dose regimens of 240 mg daily seem to produce a fairly high incidence of libido loss, especially in women (145[R]).

Endocrine, metabolic Fenfluramine tends to improve glucose tolerance and to cause small but significant reductions in fasting blood cholesterol and β-lipoprotein concentrations. Although it has been suggested that metabolic effects may play a role in the weight reduction attained when fenfluramine is used as an anorectic agent, and that the drug might even be used to reduce blood lipids, the metabolic effects observed are slight and of dubious clinical importance.

Hematological A hemoglobin concentration of 5.1 g/100 ml and a positive direct Coombs test with antibodies of Type 1g were described in a 46-year-old woman treated for obesity with fenfluramine. The Coombs test became negative and the patient recovered following prednisolone infusion. Two other cases are known of *anemia* in patients who received fenfluramine and propranolol (SED-9, 13).

Gastrointestinal *Diarrhea*, *dry mouth* and *nausea* have been reported.

Other organs and systems *Shivering*, *teeth grinding* and *alopecia* have occasionally been reported as adverse effects of fenfluramine (SED-9, 12).

Sustained-release preparations Patients given extended-action fenfluramine tablets 60 mg once a day experienced side effects similar to those on the regular preparation 20 mg t.i.d. Weight loss was greater with the sustained-release form, probably due to better patient compliance in taking the drug.

Risk situations In view of possible interactions with general anesthetics (see below), the drug should be discontinued some time before *surgery* is undertaken. In *liver disease*, metabolism of the drug will be impaired. It would seem wise to avoid the drug in patients prone to endogenous *depression* or to *psychosis*.

Overdosage A systematic study of fenfluramine poisoning in 96 (38 in detail) human subjects is reported by Von Muhlendahl and Krienke (146[CR]). Seventy-five percent of patients taking more than 15 mg/kg had convulsions and coma. Increased muscle tonus, hyperreflexia, or clonus were common; one-third had hyperthermia, but less than 10% died of hyperthermia; symptoms could last for days. Blood levels of 240—850 ng/ml were associated with tachycardia, mydriasis and confusion. Deaths occurred beginning at 650 ng/ml. Early gastric lavage, use of activated charcoal, diazepam for seizures, chlorpromazine and cold blanket for malignant hyperthermia, and lidocaine and constant electrocardiographic monitoring for extrasystoles were recommended by the authors.

Interactions Following a case report on death after an anesthetic that occurred in a 23-year-old woman who had been taking fenfluramine, a study was undertaken in rabbits to investigate the possibility of interaction between fenfluramine and halothane. ECG and phonocardiographic changes were recorded in rabbits on the combined treatment which could not readily be reversed with β-blockers and resuscitative drugs. It was recommended that fenfluramine be discontinued a week prior to anesthesia (SED-9, 13).

Fenfluramine can produce an acute confusional state if given together with *monoamine oxidase inhibitors* (SED-9, 9).

Abuse Fenfluramine has the potential to become a drug of *abuse* when used in high dosage. Sixty of 438 drug-dependent subjects gave a history of fenfluramine abuse and experienced euphoria, depersonalization and perceptual changes following ingestion of up to 400 mg (SED-9, 13). In another report, three of eight subjects receiving 240 mg fenfluramine daily experienced psychedelic states (SED-9, 13). A case of dependence on fenfluramine at an average daily dose of 240 mg was described in a 28-year-old woman (SEDA-1, 5). Overdosage of fenfluramine will therefore result in amphetamine-like adverse effects. However, while tolerance to the anorectic effects of fenfluramine appears to set in after 6—12 months, tolerance to adverse effects is much more rapid in onset. In addition, although cases of fenfluramine abuse were noted, they were rare and it was not the drug of first choice.

INDIVIDUAL COMPOUNDS

Aminorex

Aminorex has been identified as a cause of primary pulmonary hypertension and consequent death (147[C], 148[C]). The fulminant character and rapid development of the disease characterized by dyspnea, arrhythmias, peripheral edema, dizziness, cyanosis, chest pain and syncope, in the absence of usual causes of pulmonary vascular disease, suggested the possibility of its being drug-induced. Long-term follow-up of aminorex-induced primary pulmonary hypertension indicated that the syndrome has a chronic course with long-term survival possible (149[CR]). Aminorex was therefore withdrawn from the market some 20 years ago. However, work to identify the mechanism of the pathogenic effect has continued in view of the risk that other agents might behave similarly. Long-term administration of aminorex fumarate in rats failed to induce hypertensive pulmonary vascular disease, but in dogs an increase in pulmonary pressure did occur. Other appetite depressants too have been implicated in primary pulmonary hypertension (SEDA-3, 3).

Two interesting cases of supposedly delayed reactions to aminorex have been described (150[C]). Both concerned pulmonary hypertension, one in a subject who had taken aminorex 6 years previously. In the other a reaction of limited duration was experienced 8 years after aminorex treatment.

Chlofex

This anorectic compound is similar in structure to chlorphentermine. It has produced adverse effects similar to those of other appetite depressants. Outstanding among them were sleeplessness, headache, increased sweating, and dryness of the mouth.

Chlorphentermine

Chlorphentermine has a long plasma half-life of about 5 days, so there is a clear risk of accumulation in the blood with continued administration (SED-9, 14).

Much less stimulation of the central nervous system has been reported in patients on chlorphentermine than in those on dexamphetamine. Less frequent, too, were complaints of light-headedness, tremors, *restlessness*, nervousness and insomnia. Patients on chlorphentermine have experienced drowsiness.

Considerable animal research has been accomplished on possible anorectic-induced lipoidosis and pulmonary hypertension. Chlorphentermine, along with the extensively used imipramine and other cationic drugs, induces a generalized lipoidosis especially in chronic very high doses which can lead to toxic cellular changes in lung, muscle, neurohypophysis and retina, and can induce anterior polar cataracts in the eye (151[cR]—155[cR]). Those drugs causing lipoidosis also have a marked tendency to accumulate in lung (156[cR]). The clinical relevance of these findings in animals is not established, especially since imipramine has been used chronically in high doses for years in depressed patients. The focus of toxic research has been with anorectics with potent serotonergic effects similar to aminorex. In summary, pathological changes of the lungs were produced with chlorphentermine in laboratory animals (SED-9, 14). Pulmonary complications might therefore be brought about in human subjects, which puts in doubt the wisdom of continuing to recommend this drug as an anorectic until more definitive studies are available.

Chlorphentermine has been found to reduce systolic blood pressure.

In a study of 25 patients who had taken chlorphentermine 3×25 mg daily, constipation and dryness of the mouth were found to be more frequent than with other appetite depressants. In another comparative study with phenmetrazine in volunteers, constipation and dry mouth were again among the more frequent adverse reactions, along with sleepiness and increases in motor activity and micturition (SED-8, 16).

Diethylpropion, Syn. amfepramone (Dospan, Tenuate)

Reports on the frequency of adverse reactions to diethylpropion are not entirely consistent. The number of side effects reported by patients taking diethylpropion closely paralleled that with placebo in one study involving 90 obese individuals. In another 16-week controlled study comprising 95 subjects who received 25 mg of diethylpropion t.i.d., the main adverse effect reported was nervousness. Follow-up over 3 years of 121 obese patients, using a shorter-acting form of diethylpropion with an average treatment of 4.4 months, indicated that adverse effects occurred in less than 9%. They comprised nausea, vertigo in two patients, and nervousness and palpitation in another two; treatment was discontinued in three cases because of nausea, insomnia and paresthesia (157[C]). With long-acting diethylpropion in a double-blind 16-week crossover study carried out in 102 Austrian patients, adverse effects listed included nervousness, tension, nausea, dizziness, light-headedness and dry mouth (SED-9, 14). The main unwanted effects noted in a double-blind trial of sustained-release diethylpropion (tenuate, Dospan) in 50 pregnant women were euphoria, sweating, irritability and palpitations. Nervousness and insomnia were reported in another controlled study in 75 pregnant women (SEDA-8, 17). In neither of the last two studies were the adverse reactions serious enough to justify discontinuation of treatment.

There are some reports of addiction and psychotic manifestations with diethylpropion (158[cR]), but these are much less frequent than in association with amphetamine or phenmetrazole.

Altogether the effects of diethylpropion on the central nervous system are much less common than those of dexamphetamine. Seventy-eight patients who had to stop treatment with amphetamine and benzphetamine were able to continue therapy with diethylpropion. Even insomnia is uncommon if the drug is taken early in the day.

A comparative study using a fixed combination of 75 mg of diethylpropion plus 10 mg of diazepam showed that the side effects were mild and less than those found with other anorexigenic preparations (SED-9, 14). Adverse effects, however, were observed in about 50% of the patients and constituted dry mouth, nervousness and mild depression.

Fenproporex (Perphoxene, Teqisec)

One of the lesser known anorectics, fenproporex, is structurally related to amphetamine to which it is rapidly broken down after oral ingestion. Stimulating effects, as well as somnolence, and electroencephalographic abnormalities are reported to be the major undesired reactions (SED-9, 16).

Mazindol (AN-448, Sanorex, Teronac, SAH-42-548)

Mazindol is a tricyclic compound with central nervous system stimulant properties similar to amphetamine. It releases and blocks re-uptake of dopamine as well as noradrenaline (159[cR]) and the action of these catechols, not serotonin, is responsible for its anorectic activity. With fairly high doses (6 mg/day) central nervous system effects were reported in 30% of 23 patients (160[C]). No euphoria seems to be present with therapeutic doses of mazindol, but higher doses may produce euphoria. It has a much lower addiction potential than the amphetamines and practically no cases have been reported of physical withdrawal syndrome on discontinuation of the drug.

The most frequently occurring adverse effects in a multicenter open study in 274 subjects in Ireland were dry mouth, nausea, insomnia, constipation, headache and dizziness. Restlessness and drowsiness were each complained of by four patients. The incidence of side effects was higher at the beginning of the study but dropped progressively throughout the 12-week treatment period (SEDA-1, 6).

In a double-blind 12-week study of 50 obese patients adverse effects consisted of dry mouth and a tendency to constipation, except for one case of angioneurotic edema and another of peripheral edema and vomiting (SEDA-1, 6).

Another double-blind study over a 12-week period of 60 obese patients on mazindol also rendered minimal adverse effects. In this instance, the complaints were of insomnia and nausea (SED-9, 15).

It should be pointed out that side effects to mazindol will appear in higher frequency and intensity in patients treated for longer periods of time and when combined with a hypocaloric diet (SED-9, 15).

A double-blind study was also carried out in 40 obese subjects with stabilized controlled diabetes mellitus and without any history of emotional instability, drug dependence, or cardiovascular disease. Single cases of mild dry mouth and vertigo were reported (SED-9, 15).

Impaired power of concentration but not mood-elevating properties were noted in healthy subjects who had taken the drug for 3 weeks. Other reported adverse effects were considered to be more of a peripheral than of a central nature. No effect on standing blood pressure and pulse was seen. In another study, however, a drug-dependent increase in heart rate, probably due to an amphetamine-like stimulatory effect, was ascribed to mazindol (SED-9, 15).

Phendimetrazine (see also 'Phenmetrazine)

Glossitis, stomatitis, dry mouth, nausea, abdominal pain, cramps, constipation, difficulty in micturition and headache are the reported adverse reactions to this drug. Phendimetrazine, of which approximately 30% is rapidly metabolized to phenmetrazine in the human body (147[cR]), has been abused in Sweden.

Phenmetrazine (Preludin)

The main adverse effects reflect central nervous system stimulation and resemble those of other stimulants (see above).

Abuse There are many reports of abuse of this drug. Nervousness, hyperexcitability, euphoria and insomnia, although less frequent than with amphetamines, have been observed with average doses of phenmetrazine. Dizziness, headache, nausea, dryness of the mouth and urticaria have also been recorded. With large doses of phenmetrazine, these adverse reactions were more pronounced. Paranoid psychosis was produced in addicts, and with chronic ingestion psychotic manifestations were evident as with amphetamine.

In Sweden, phenmetrazine has been extensively abused and misused, sometimes with intravenous application. Addicts who had previously been taking morphine stated that phenmetrazine gave them a sense of well-being and overconfidence. A high incidence of criminal activity was noted in phenmetrazine users whose primary objective was obtaining money for the drug. Their average doses were 30—60 tablets at a time, repeated 4—5 times a day (SED-9, 15).

Long-term effects Some incidents have been reported of encephalopathy as a result of phenmetrazine toxicity. There were also two cases in which damage to the central nervous system was found following long-term treatment with phenmetrazine; in one, disseminated lesions were described and, in the other, hemiparesis and sensory motor aphasia (SED-9, 15).

Teratogenic effects On very rare occasions, congenital defects in the newborn have been associated with phenmetrazine consumption by the expectant mother.

Phentermine (Mirapront)

With phentermine, adverse effects due to stimulation of the central nervous system are less than with dexamphetamine, although in one study withdrawal from medication use was as high as 16 out of 177 patients (9%) because of adverse effects, and two out of 13 healthy young volunteers withdrew because of unacceptable stimulation (161[C]).

Insomnia is one of the most common side effects of phentermine. In a survey carried out in Edinburgh, 19.9% of the subjects on the test drug reported insomnia as against 62% of those on the placebo (SED-9, 13).

Some cases of toxic psychosis are reported for abused doses of phentermine (162[cR]).

A well-documented case was described of fatal pulmonary hypertension in a 32-year-old man who had been taking phentermine in unknown doses for 4 months (SED-9, 16).

SK&F-70948

A low incidence of side effects was reported with SK&F-70948 (4'-chloro-2-(ethylamino)propiophenone) used as a sustained-release anorectic (SED-9, 17).

Clortermine (voramil)

An α-dimethylphenethylamine chlorine derivative, voramil appears to suppress food-reinforced behavior without concomitant stimulation or depression of the central nervous system. Headache, in four subjects severe enough to stop treatment, was the main characteristic complaint in 49 obese people taking voramil 50 mg daily. In all cases, the complaints were drug- and not placebo-related (SED-9, 17).

CONCLUDING REMARKS

The group of drugs dealt with in this last section are mostly used as anorectic agents and produce side effects mainly of the central nervous system sympathomimetic type. Therapy, employing the use of these drugs, should therefore be allowed only under strict medical supervision to ensure the earliest possible detection of any signs of drug abuse. Long-term drug treatment of obesity should be avoided altogether.

Introduction of long-acting preparations has provided some improvement in the mode of application of anorectics. Steady release of the drug permits a constant level in the blood throughout the entire day. Thus, a sudden excess of physiological hunger is prevented, and side effects involving the central nervous system are diminished.

OTHER CENTRALLY ACTING DRUGS

Hydergine (co-dergocrine) *(for main review, see Chapter 19)*

Hydergine, a preparation of dihydrogenated ergot alkaloids, is usually mentioned for its therapeutic effects on mood depression, confusion, and lack of self-care in the elderly. It acts purportedly through improvement of cerebral blood flow. The basis of these indications has been reviewed and can only be partially validated (163[cR]). Surprisingly few adverse effects have been reported and include sinus bradycardia, nausea and a single case report of vasospastic angiitis (164[cR]). Due to its current popularity in some countries, more careful assessment of therapeutic and side effects is needed.

Norephedrine (phenylpropanolamine)

In contrast to its usual formulation in decongestant preparations, norephedrine has recently been introduced as an anorectic agent administered in doses of 3×25 mg daily. Adverse effects from therapeutic and toxic doses of phenylpropanolamine (PPA) continue to be reported (SEDA-9, 2; SEDA-10, 3; SEDA-11, 1). At single doses (50 mg), PPA increased diastolic blood pressure to over 100 mmHg in 12% of adults. A warning was issued by the Swiss Pharmaceutical Association that norephedrine may induce severe sympathomimetic side effects, including hypertensive crises, arrhythmias and tachycardia (SED-9, 16; SEDA-5, 11; SEDA-7, 12; see also Chapter 13). Psychosis has also been reported. Although irritability and insomnia are frequent in adults, behavioral disturbances (restlessness, irritability, aggressiveness and sleep disturbances) as well as seizures and delirium with hallucinations have been most frequently observed in children (SEDA-11, 1; 165[R]).

As with several other sympathomimetics, norephedrine is often sold illegally in special packages as a look-alike for more euphoriant/alerting stimulants. Both the absolute increase in utilization and the changes in the type of user have been associated with many reports of overdose consequences, including hypertension, cardiac arrhythmias (SEDA-9, 10, 11), cerebral hemorrhage (166[C], 167[C]; SEDA-11, 2), neuropsychiatric symptoms, including agitation and acute psychosis, and seizures (SED-9, 4; 156[C]). A neuroleptic malignant-like syndrome has been reported when PPA was combined with neuroleptic medication (168[C]).

Some consider that adverse reports need to be tempered against the large number of clinical trials reporting safety and the extensive prescription and non-prescription base from which adverse effects are reported (169[C], 170[C]). Similar consideration of the extensive use relative to the toxic consequences of overdose, e.g. paranoid psychosis or hallucinosis (SEDA-8, 10), could be given to pseudoephedrine. Children appear to be sensitive to therapeutic doses of pseudoephedrine in the development of hallucinosis as well as irritability and insomnia syndromes (171[C], 172[C]).

Nootropic drugs

With the advent of an increasing geriatric population the active search for drugs that activate cognitive psychomotor responsivity continues. In contrast to the utilization of milder stimulants such as pemoline in geriatric patients, neurotropic drugs are sought to act more selectively at cortical levels to stimulate without producing sedation or behavioral effects.

Sydnocarb is a Soviet psychostimulant derivative of the sydnonine series which has a more gradual onset and longer duration of action that amphetamine. Therapeutic doses are stated not to induce euphoria or motor activation and withdrawal from medication not to be associated with depression. The most notable adverse effects are insomnia, anorexia and activation of neurotic and psychotic symptoms in predisposed individuals (SEDA-4, 11); the presence of these psychopathological states has been considered a contraindication to using the drug. Insomnia is avoided by eliminating the evening dose.

REFERENCES

1. Benet LZ, Kroetz DL, Sheiner LB. Pharmacokinetic: the dynamics of drug absorption, distribution, and elimination. In: Hardman, JG, Limbird, LE, Molinoff, PB, Ruddon, RW, Gilman AG, eds. Goodman and Gilman's The Pharmacological Basis of Therapeutics, 9th edn. New York: McGraw Hill, 1996;28.
2. Boyle CA, Berkowitz GS, LiVolsi VA et al. Caffeine consumption and fibrocystic breast disease: a case-control epidemiologic study. J Natl Cancer Inst 1984;72:1015.
3. Mann JI, Thorogood M. Coffee drinking and myocardial infarction. Lancet 1975;i:1215.
4. International Coffee Organization. United States of

America: coffee drinking study. London: International Coffee Organization, 1989.
5. LeGrady D, Dyer AR, Shekelle RB, et al. Coffee consumption and mortality in the Chicago Western Electric Company Study. Am J Epidemiol 1987;87:586.
6. Hemminki E, Pesonen T. Regional coffee consumption and mortality from ischemic heart disease in Finland. Acta Med Scand 1977;201:127.
7. Yano K, Rhoads GG, Kagan A. Coffee, alcohol, and risk of coronary heart disease among Japanese men living in Hawaii. N Engl J Med 1977;297:405.
8. Greden JF. Anxiety or caffeinism: a diagnostic dilemma. Am. J. Psychiatry 1974;131:1089.
9. Regestein OR. Pathologic sleepiness induced by caffeine. Am J Med 1989;87:586.
10. Cohen S, Booth GH Jr. Gastric acid secretion and lower esophageal sphincter pressure in response to coffee and caffeine. N Engl J Med 1975;293:897.
11. Creighton SM, Stanton SL. Caffeine: does it affect your bladder? Br J Urol 1990;66:613.
12. Vandenplas Y, DeWolf P, Sacre L. Influence of xanthines on gastroesophageal reflux in infants at risk for sudden infant death syndrome. Pediatrics 1986;77:807.
13. Griffiths RR, Evans SM, Heishman SJ et al. Low-dose caffeine physical dependence in humans. J Pharmacol Exp Therap 1990;255:1123.
14. Mulvihill JJ. Caffeine as teratogen and mutagen. Teratology 1973;8:69.
15. Salvador HS, Koos BJ. Effects of regular and decaffeinated coffee on fetal breathing and heart rate. Am J Obstet Gynecol 1989;160:1043.
16. Stockley, IH. Drug interactions: A Source Book of Adverse Interactions. Their Mechanisms, Clinical Importance and Management, 3rd edn. London: Blackwell Scientific, 1994.
17. Thompson PJ, Gibb W, Cole P, Citron KM. Generalized allergic reactions to aminophylline. Thorax 1984;39:600.
18. Niggemann B. Aggressives Verhalten als Nebenwirkung des Athylendiamins (nicht aber des Theophyllins). Monatsschr Kinderheilkd 1985;133:487.
19. Chaithiraphan S. Fatal complication associated with intravenous use of aminophylline. J Med Assoc Thailand 1976;59:507.
20. Levine JH, Michael JR, Guarnieri T. Multifocal atrial tachycardia: a toxic effect of theophylline. Lancet 1985;i:12.
21. Schwartz MS, Scott DC. Aminophylline-induced seizure. Epilepsia 1974;15:601.
22. Burkle WS, Gwizdala CJ. Evaluation of 'toxic' serum theophylline concentrations. Am J Hosp Pharmacy 1981; 38:1164.
23. Aitken ML, Martin TR. Life-threatening theophylline toxicity is not predictable in serum levels. Chest 1987;91:10.
24. Covelli HD, Knodel AR, Heppner BT. Predisposing factor to apparent theophylline-induced seizures. Ann Allergy 1985;54:411.
25. Noetzel MJ. Theophylline neurotoxicity resulting in significant unilateral brain-damage. Dev Med Child Neurol 1985;27:242.
26. Brook U, Singer L, Fried D. Development of severe Stevens-Johnson Syndrome after administration of slow-release theophylline. Ped Dermatol 1989;6:126.
27. Ben-Aryeh H, Colin A. Salivary composition asthmatic children on theophylline. Isr J Med Sci 1985;21:460.
28. Clark JE, Devenport JK. Theophylline exacerbating spasticity. J Am Med Assoc 1983;250:485.
29. Aderka D, Shavit G, Garfinkel D et al. Life-threatening theophylline intoxication in a hypothyroid patient. Respiration 1983;44:77.
30. D'Arcy PF. Drug reactions and interactions. Pharm Int 1984;5:117.
31. Stoller JL. Oesophageal ulceration and theophylline. Lancet 1985;ii:328.
32. Srinivasan G, Singh J, Cattamanchi G et al. Plasma glucose changes in preterm infants during oral theophylline therapy. J Pediatr 1983;103:473.
33. Serafin WE. Drugs used in the treatment of asthma. In: Hardman JG, Limbird LE, Molinoff PB, Ruddon RW, Gilman AG, eds. Goodman and Gilman's The Pharmacological Basis of Therapeutics, 9th edn. New York: McGraw Hill, 1996;659–682.
34. Rosenkrantz TS, Oh W. Aminophylline reduces cerebral blood flow velocity in low-birth-weight infants. Am J Dis Child 1984;138:489.
35. Shannon M, Lovejoy FH. The influence of age vs peak serum concentration on life-threatening events after chronic theophylline intoxication. Arch Intern Med 1990;150:2045.
36. Emerman CL, Devlin C, Connors AF. Risk of toxicity in patients with elevated theophylline levels. Ann Emergency Med 1990;19:643.
37. Khadem B. Aminophylline poisoning in children: report of two cases. Harper Hosp Bull 1982;20:179.
38. Olson KR, Benowitz NL, Woo OF et al. Theophylline overdose: acute single ingestion versus chronic repeated medication. Am J Emerg Med 1985;3:386.
39. Shane R. Potential toxicity of theophylline in combination with Quinamm (Letter to Editor). Am J Hosp Pharm 1982;39:40.
40. Cook BL, Smith RE, Perry PJ et al. Theophylline–lithium interaction. J Clin Psychiatry 1985;46:278.
41. Anderson JL, Ayres JW, Hall CA. Potential pharmacokinetic interaction between theophylline and prednisone. Clin Pharmacol 1984;3:187.
42. Jonkman JHG, Koeter GH, Berg WC. Geneesmiddelen met een therapeutisch belangrijke invloved op de farmacokinetiek van theofylline. Pharm Weekbl 1983;118:185.
43. Tamburrini LR, Curri G, Mian G et al. Digitale-teofillina antagonismo della tecfillina nella farmacocinctica della digcssina in alcuni soggetti vecchi intossicati: implicazioni clinicobiometriche. Prog Med 1984;40:295.
44. Marchlinski FE, Miller JM. Atrial arrhythmias exacerbated by theophylline. Chest 1985;88:931.
45. Iversen SA, Murphy PG, Leakey TEB et al. Unsuspected caffeine toxicity complicating theophylline therapy. Hum Toxicol 1984;3:509.
46. Jonkman JH, Sollie FA, Sauter R, et al. The influence of caffeine on the steady-state pharmacokinetics of theophylline Clin Pharmacol Ther 1990;49:248.
47. Brown KR, Guglielmo BJ, Pons VG, Jacobs RA. Theophylline elixir, moxalactam, and a disulfiram reaction. Ann Intern Med 1982;97:621.
48. Pauwels R. Enprofylline: a new a bronchodilating xanthine derivative. Eur J Respir Dis 1983;64:331.
49. Laursen LC, Johannesson N, Fagerstrom P-Q, Weeke B. intravenous administration of enprofylline to asthmatic patients. Eur J Clin Pharmacol 1983;24:323.
50. Mosbech H, Paulsen H, Sobord M. Controlled-release

theophylline and proxyphylline in asthmatics: a comparative study. Pharmatherpeutica 1984;3:626.
51. Hahn F. Analeptics. Pharmacol Rev 1960;12:447.
52. Esplin DW, Zablocka-Esplin B. Mechanism action of convulsants. In: Jasper HH, Ward AA, Pope, eds. Basic Mechanisms of The Epilepsies. Boston: Little, Brown and Company, 1969;167.
53. Hirsh K, Wang SC. Selective respiratory action of doxapram compared to pentylenetetrazol. J Pharmacol Exp Ther 1974;189:1.
54. Fancourt GJ, Ashton RJ, Talbot IC et al. Hepatic necrosis with doxapram hydrochloride. Postgrad Med J 1985;61:833.
55. Dolenz B. Flurothyl (Indoklon) side effect. J Psychiatry 1967;123:11.
56. Council on Drugs. A convulsant agent for psychiatric use. J Am Med Assoc 1966;196:29.
57. Hirsh K, Want SC. Selective respiratory action of doxapram compared to pentylenetetrazol. J Pharmacol Exp Ther 1974;189:1.
58. Curtis DR. The pharmacology of post-synaptic inhibition. Prog Prain Res 1969;31:179.
59. Bell ES. The experimental reproduction of amphetamine psychosis. Arch Gen Psychiatry 1973;29:35.
60. Lathers CM, Tyau LSY, Spino MM et al. Cocaine-induced seizures, arrythmias and sudden death. J Clin Pharmacol 1988;28:584.
61. Stein R, Ellinwood EH Jr. Medical complication of cocaine abuse. Drug Ther 1990;10:40.
62. Jiang JP, Downing SE. Catecholamine cardiomyopathy: review and analysis of pathogenic mechanisms. J Biol Med 1990;63:581.
63. Hong R, Matsuyama E, Nur K. Cardiomyopathy associated with the smoking of crystal methamphetamine. J Am Med Assoc 1991;265:1152.
64. Karch SB, Billingham E. The pathology and etiology of cocaine-induced heart disease. Arch Pathol Lab Med 1988;112:225.
65. Ellinwood EH Jr, Petrie WM. Dependence on amphetamine, cocaine, and other stimulants. In: Pradhan SN, ed. Drug Abuse: Clinical and Basic Aspects. New York: C.V. Mosby, 1977;248.
66. Ellinwood EH Jr. Emergency treatment of acute adverse reactions to CNS stimulants. In: Bourne P, ed. Acute Drug Abuse Emergencies: A Treatment Manual. New York: Academic Press, 1976;115.
67. Fawcett JF, Busch KA. Stimulants in psychiatry. In: Schatzberg AF, Nemeroff CB, eds. The American Psychiatric Press Textbook of Psychopharmacology. Washington, DC: American Psychiatric Press, Inc, 1995;417.
68. Angrist B, D'Hollosy M, Sanfilipo M, et al. Central nervous system stimulants as symptomatic treatments for AIDS-related neuropsychiatric impairment. J Clin Psychopharmacol 1992;12:268–272.
69. Satel SL, Nelson JC. Stimulants in the treatment of depression: a critical review. J Clin Psychiatry. 1989;50:241–249.
70. Holmes VF, Fernandez F, Levy JK. Psychostimulant response in AIDS-related complex patients. J Clin Psychiatry 1989;50:5–8.
71. Chiarello RJ, Cole JO. The use of psychostimulants in general psychiatry. Arch Gen Psychiatry 1987;44:286-295.
72. Fawcett J, Ktavitz HM, Zajeck A, Schall MR. CNS stimulant potentiation of monoamine oxidase inhibitors. J Clin Psychopharmacol 1991;11:127.
73. Jonsson S, O'Meara M, Young JB. Acute cocaine poisoning. Am J Med 1983;75:1061.
74. Barinerd H, Krupp M, Chatton J et al, eds. Current Medical Diagnosis and Treatment. Los Altos, CA: Lange Medical Publishers, 1970.
75. Clayton RR. Cocaine use in the United states: in a blizzard or just being snowed? NIDA Res Monogr 1985;61:8.
76. Gawin JH, Ellinwood EH. Cocaine and other stimulants: actions, abuse and treatment. N Eng J Med 1986;318:1173.
77. Stark TW, Pruet CW, Stark DU. Cocaine toxicity. Ear Nose Throat J 1983;62:155.
78. Nanji AA, Eilipenko JD. Asystole and ventricular fibrillation associated with cocaine intoxication. Chest 1984; 85:132.
79. Moe GK, Akildskov JA. Antiarrhythmic drugs. In: Gilman AG, Goodman LS, eds. The Pharmacological Basis of Therapeutics. New York: MacMillan, 1970.
80. Ellinwood EH Jr, Petrie WM. Drug induced psychoses. In: Pickens RW, Heston LL, eds. Psychiatric Factors in Drug Abuse. New York: Grune and Stratton, 1979;301.
81. Weiner RS, Lockhart JT, Schwartz RG. Dilated cardiomyopathy and cocaine abuse: report of two cases. Am J Med 1986;81:699.
82. Mathias DW. Cocaine-associated myocardial ischemia: review of clinical and angiographic findings. Am J Med 1986;81:675.
83. Anonymous. Adverse effects of cocaine abuse. Med Lett Drugs Ther 1984;26:51.
84. Caruana DS, Weinbach B, Goerg D et al. Cocaine-packet ingestion: diagnosis, management and natural history. Ann Intern Med 1984;100:73.
85 Isner JM, Estes NA, Tompson PD et al. Acute cardiovascular events temporally related to cocaine abuse. N Engl J Med 1985;315:1438.
86. Minor RL, Scott BD, Brown DD. Cocaine-induced myocardial infarction in patients with normal coronary arteries. Ann Intern Med 1991;115:797-806.
87. Virmani R. Cocaine-associated cardiovascular disease: clinical and pathological aspects. In: Thadani P, ed. NIDA Research Monograph, 106. Rockville, MD: US HHS, 1991;220–229.
88. Catraras D, Waters IW. Acute cocaine intoxication in the conscious dog: studies on the mechanism of lethalily. J Pharmacol Exp Ther 1981;217:350.
89. Covino BG, Vasalla HG. Local Anesthetics: Mechanism of Action and Clinical Use. New York: Grune and Stratton, 1976;127.
90. Jaffe JH. Drug addiction and drug abuse. In: Gilman AG, Goodman LS, Rall TW, Murad F, eds. The Pharmacological Basis of Therapeutics, 7th edn. New York: McMillan, 1985;54.
91. Hollander JE, Carter WA, Hoffman RS. Use of phentolamine for cocaine-induced myocardial ischemia. New Engl J Med 1992;327:361.
92. Mittleman RE, Weth CV. Death caused by recreational cocaine use. J Am Med Assoc 1984;252:1889.
93. Cohen S. Reinforcement and rapid delivery systems: understanding adverse consequences of cocaine. NIDA Res Monogr 1985;61:151.
94. Gregler LL, Mark H. Medical complications of cocaine abuse. N Engl J Med 1986;315:1495.
95. Aronson TA, Criag TJ. Cocaine precipitation of panic disorder. Am J Psychiatry 1986;143:643.
96. Rowbotham MC. Neurologic aspects of cocaine use. West J Med 1988;149:442.

97. Nalbandian LL, Sheth N, Dietrich R et al. Intestinal ischemia caused by cocaine ingestion: report of two cases. Surgery 1985;97:374.
98. Fishel R, Hamamoto G, Barbul A et al. Cocaine colitis: is this a new syndrome? Dis Colon Rectum 1985;28:264.
99. Allred RJ, Ewer S. Fatal pulmonary edema following intravenous 'free-base' cocaine use. Ann Emerg Med 1981;10:441.
100. Myers JA, Earnest MP. Generalized seizures and cocaine abuse. Neurology 1984;34:675.
101. Trozak DJ, Gould WM. Cocaine abuse and connective tissue disease. J Am Acad Dermatol 1984;10:525.
102. Hunter JG, Loy HC, Markovitz L, Kim US. Spontaneous pneumomediastinum following inhalation of alkaloidal cocaine and emesis. Mt Sinai J Med 1986;53:491.
103. Mesulam MM. Cocaine and Tourette's syndrome. N Engl J Med 1986;315:398.
104. Masaki T. The amphetamine problem in Japan: annex to Sixth Report of Expert Committee on Drugs Liable to Produce Addiction. WHO Techn Rep Ser 1956;102:14.
105. Downing GJ, Horner SR, Kilbride HW. Characteristics of perimatal cocaine-exposed infants with necrotizing entercolitis (Letter to the Editor). Am J Dis Child 1991;145:26-27.
106. Chasnoffi J, Burns WJ, Schnoll SH et al. Cocaine use in pregnancy. N Engl J Med 1985;313:666.
107. Kramer JC, Fischmim VS, Littlefield DC. Amphetamine abuse: pattern and effects of high doses taken intravenously. J Am Med Assoc 1967;201:89.
108. Aeschlimann A, de Truchis P, Kahn MF. Scleroderma after therapy with appetite suppressants: report on four cases. Scand J Rheumatology 1990;19:87.
109. Ellinwood EH Jr. Emergency treatment of acute reactions to CNS stimulants. J Psychedelic Drugs 1972;5:147.
110. Kalant H, Kalant OJ. Death in amphetamine users: causes and rates. Can Med Assoc J 1975;112:299.
111. Nausieda PA. Central stimulant toxicity. In: Vinken PJ, Bruyn GW, eds. Handbook of Clinical Neurology. Intoxications of the Nervous System, Part 11, Amsterdam: Elsevier/North-Holland Biomedical Press, 1979;223.
112. Ellinwood EH Jr, Kilbey MM. Fundamental mechanisms underlying altered behavior following chronic administration of psychomotor stimulants. Biol Psychiatry 1980; 15:749.
113. Delaney P, Estes M. Intracranial hemorrhage with amphetamine abuse. Neurology 1980;30:1125.
114. Olsen ER. Intracranial hemorrhage and amphetamine usage. Angiology 1977;38:464.
115. Ellinwood EH Jr, Duarte-Escalante O. Central nervous system cytopathological changes in cat with chronic methedrine intoxication. Brain Res 1970;21:151.
116. Wagner GC, Ricaurte GA, Seiden LS et al. Longlasting depletions of striatal dopamine and loss of dopamine uptake sites following repeated administration of methamphetamine. Brain Res 1980;181:151.
117. Bostwick D. Amphetamine induced cerebral vasculitis. Hum Pathol 1981;12:1031.
118. Lowe TL, Cohen DG, Detlor J et al. Stimulant medications precipitate Tourette's syndrome. J Am Med Assoc 1982;247:1929.
119. Shapiro AK, Shapiro E. Do stimulants provoke, cause or exacerbate tics and Tourette's syndrome? Compr Psychiatry 1981;22:265.
120. Greenberg LM, McMahon SA, Deem MA. Side effects of dextroamphetamine therapy of hyperactive children. West J Med 1974;120:105.
121. Unwin JR. Illicit drug use among Canadian youth. Can Med Assoc J 1968;98:402.
122. Korman ME, Unna KR. Effects of chronic administration of the amphetamines and other stimulants on behaviour. Clin Pharmacol Ther 1968;9:240.
123. Ellinwood EH Jr. Assault and homicide associated with amphetamine abuse. Am J Psychiatry 1979;3:25.
124. Halbach U, Asnis G, Ross D et al. Amphetamine induced dysphoria in post-menopausal women. Br J Psychiatry 1981;138:470.
125. Roche AF, Lipman RS, Overall JE et al. The effects of stimulant medication of growth of hyperkinetic children. Pediatrics 1979;63:847.
126. Dickinson LD, Lee J, Ringdah IC et al. Impaired growth in hyperkinetic children receiving pemoline. J Pediatr 1979;94:538.
127. Safer JJ, Allen RP, Barr E. Growth rebound after termination of stimulant drugs. J Pediatr 1975;86:709.
128. Janowsky DS, Yousef MK, Davis JM et al. Provocation of schizophrenic symptoms by intravenous administration of methylphenidate. Arch Gen Psychiatry 1973;28:185.
129. Ellenhorn DJ, Barceloux DG. Amphetamines. In: Medical Toxicology: Diagnosis and Treatment of Human Poisoning. New York: Elsevier Science Publishers, 1988;625.
130. Call T, Hartneck J, Dickenson W et al. Acute cardiomyopathy secondary to intravenous amphetamine abuse. Ann Intern Med 1982;97:559.
131. Ellinwood EH Jr. Amphetamine psychosis. 1. Description of the individuals and process. J Nerv Ment Dis 1967;144:273.
132. Griffith JD, Cavanaugh JH, Held J et al. Experimental psychosis induced by the administration of D-amphetamine. In: Costa E, Garattini S, eds. Amphetamines and Related Compounds. New York: Raven Press, 1970;897.
133. Griffith JD, Cavanaugh JH, Held J et al. Dextroamphetamine: evaluation of psychomimetic properties in man. Arch Gen Psychiatry 1972;26:79.
134. Extein I. Methylphenidate induced choreoathetosis. Am J Psychiatry 1973;136:252.
135. Weiner WJ, Nausieda PA, Klawans HL. Methylphenidate-induced chorea: case report and pharmacologic implications. Neurology 1973;28:1041.
136. Campbell DB. Absorption, distribution, and metabolism of fenfluramine. Vie Med Can Fr 1973;2:34.
137. Kruk ZL, Zarrindast MR. The effect of anorectic drugs on uptake and release of brain monoamines. Br J Pharmacol 1976;58:365.
138. Owen HJ. Acceptability of prolonged release fenfluramine capsules in obese patients in general practice. Postgrad Med J 1975;51:176.
139. Guy-Grand B. Therapeutic use of dexfenfluramine in obesity. In: Bender et al, eds. Body Weight Control. The Physiology, Clinical Treatment and Prevention of Obesity. London: Churchill Livingstone, 1987;280.
140. Guy-Grand B, Apfelbaum M, Crepaldi G et al. International trial of long-term dexfenfluramine in obesity. Lancet 1989;2:1142.
141. Atanassoff PG, Weiss BM, Schmid ER, Tornia M. Pulmonary hypertension and dexfenfluramine (Correspondence). Lancet 1992;339:436.
142. Roche N, Labrune S, Braun J-M, Huchon GJ. Pulmonary hypertension and dexfenfluramine (Correspondence). Lancet 1992;339:436.

143. Holmstrand J, Jonsson J. Subjective effects of two anorexigenic agents, fenfluramine and AN 488, in normal subjects. Postgrad Med 1975;51(Suppl 1):183.
144. Innes JA, Watson ML, Ford MJ et al. Plasma fenfluramine and imipramine. Br Med J 1977;3:70.
145. Pinder RM, Brogden RN, Sawyer PR et al. Fenfluramine: a review of its pharmacological properties and therapeutic efficacy in obesity. Drugs 1975;10:241.
146. Von Muhlendahl DE, Krienke EG. Fenfluramine poisoning. Clin Toxicol 1979;4:97.
147. Hager W, Thiede D, Wink K. Primar vaskulare pulmonale Hypertonie und Appetitzugler. Med Klin (Munich) 1971;66:386.
148. Follath F, Burkart F, Schweizer W. Drug-induced pulmonary hypertension. Br Med J 1971;1:265.
149. Mlczoch J, Probst P, Szeless S et al. Primary pulmonary hypertension: follow-up of patients with and without anorectic drug intake. Cor Vasa 1980;22:251.
150. Simon H, Felix R. Reversibele pulmonalarterielle Hypertonie nach Einnahme von Menocil. Med Klin (Munich) 1977;72:1685.
151. Schmalbruch H. The early changes in experimental myopathy induced by chlorphentermine. J Neuropathol Exp Neurol 1980;39(1):65.
152. Grabner R, Meerbach W. Monphological and biochemical alterations of the lung after application of chlorphentermine. Exp Pathol 1979;17(6):303.
153. Bucheim W, Drenckhahn D, Lullman-Rauch R. Freeze-fracture studies of cytoplasmic inclusions occurring in experimental lipidosis as induced by amphilic catatonic drugs. Biochim Biophys Acta 1979;575:71.
154. Kacew W, Nanbaitz R. A comparative ultrastructural and biochemical study between the effects of chlorphentermine and phentermine on rat lung. Exp Mol Pathol 1977; 27(1):106.
155. Krenckhah D. Anterior polar cataract and lysosomal alterations in the lens of rats treated with the amphiphilic lipidosis—including chloroquine and chlorphentermine. Virchows Arch B 1973;27(3):255.
156. Wilson AG, Pickett RD, Eling TE et al. Studies on the persistence of basic amines in the rabbit lung. Drug Metab Dispos 1979;7(6):420.
157. Matthews PA. Diethylpropion in the treatment of obese patients seen in general practice. Curr Ther Res Clin Exp 1975;17:340.
158. Willis JHP. The natural history of anorectic drug abuse. In: Garattini S, Samanin R, eds. Central Mechanisms of Anorectic Drugs. New York: Raven Press, 1978;367.
159. Garattini S, Borroni E, Mennini T et al. Differences and similarities among anorectic agents. In: Garattini S, Samanin R, eds. Central Mechanisms of Anorectic Drugs. New York: Raven Press, 1978;131.
160. De Felice EA, Bronstein S, Cohen A. Double blind comparison of placebo and 42 548, a new appetite depressant in obese volunteers. Curr Ther Res Clin Exp 1969;11:256.
161. Malcolm AD, Mace PM, Outar KP, Pawan GIS. Experimental evaluation of anorexigenic agents in man: a pilot study. Proc Nutr Soc 1972;31:12A.
162. Munro JF. Clinical aspects of treatment of obesity by drugs: a review. Int J Obesity 1979;3:171.
163. Medical Letter (on Drugs and Therapies). Deapril-ST for senile dementia. Med Letter 1977;19(15):61.
164. O'Cayley AC, MacPherson A, Wedgewood J. Sinus bradycardia following treatment with hydergine for cerebrovascular insufficiency. Br Med J 1975;4(599S):384.
165. Dupuis L, Spielberg S. Oral decongestants—facts and fiction. On Contin Pract 1985;12:22.
166. McDowell JR, LeBlanc HJ. Phenylpropanolamine and cerebral hemorrhage. West J Med 1985;142:688.
167. Kikta DG, Devereaux MW, Chandar K. Intracranial hemorrhages due to phenylpropanolamine. Stoke 1985;16: 510.
168. Castellani S. Catatonia associated with phenylproreport. J Clin Psychiatry 1985;46:288.
169. Clark JF, Simon WA. Cardiac arrhythmias after phenylpropanolamine ingestion. Drug Intell Clin Pharm 1983; 17:737.
170. Jick H, Aselton P, Hunter JR. Phenylpropanolamine and cerebral hemorrhage. Lancet 1984;i:1017.
171. Sankey R, Nunh AJ, Silis JA. Visual hallucinations in children receiving decongestants. Br Med J 1984;288:1369.
172. Bain J. Visual hallucinations in children receiving decongestants. Br Med J 1984;288:1688.
173. Hakkarainen H, Hakamies L. Piracetam in the treatment of post-concussional syndrome a double blind study. Eur Neurol 1978;15:50.
174. Parnetti L, Bartorelli L, Bonaiuto S et al. Aniracetam (Ro-13-5057) for the treatment of senile dementia of Alzheimer type: results of a multicentric clinical study. Dementia 1991;2:262—267.
175. Tolman KG, Freston JW, Berenson MM, Sannella JJ. Hepatotoxicity due to pemoline. Digestion 1973;9:532.
176. Pratt DS, Dubois RS. Hepatotoxicity due to pemoline (Cylert): a report of two cases. J Pediatr Gastroenterol Nutr 1990;10:239.
177. Brenot F, Herve P, Petitpretz P, Duroux P, Simmoneau G. Primary pulmonary hypertension and fenfluramine. Br Heart J 1993;70:537—541.

Meyler's Side Effects of Drugs, 13th Edition
M.N.G. Dukes, editor

SECTION EDITOR: C. VAN BOXTEL

Stefan Borg and Kerstin Brodin

2 Antidepressant drugs

HISTORICAL OVERVIEW

Effective antidepressant drugs have now been available for 40 years. In the last two decades, a single theory of drug action (the catecholamine hypothesis) involving relatively few drugs, a clear-cut classification system and restricted indications have been replaced by multiple mechanisms of action, many new drugs that cut across the traditional chemical categories and novel indications in addition to antidepressant actions.

Side effects have played a significant part in shaping this evolutionary process. Fear of electroshock therapy coupled with the adverse effects and addictive potential of amphetamines created a climate of ready acceptance when it was discovered in 1956 that iproniazid produced both mood elevation and possessed the property of inhibiting monoamine-oxidase (MAO) (1[R]).

Early reports of liver damage with iproniazid led in turn to the introduction of newer, structurally different compounds that also inhibited MAO. Simultaneously, the same unwanted adverse effect of liver damage due to chlorpromazine led to the synthesis of safer phenothiazine analogs and to the discovery that among them imipramine benefited the more depressed schizophrenic patients (2[R]).

By 1962, both the MAO inhibitors and imipramine congeners (or tricyclic compounds) were in extensive and about equal use as antidepressants. It was then discovered that inhibition of the ubiquitous enzyme, MAO, occurred in the liver and gut as well as the brain, allowing access of tyramine from foods to the general circulation and provoking hypertensive crises with occasional fatalities (3[R]). As a result, the MAO inhibitors fell into relative disuse. Coupled with a renaissance of interest in the MAO inhibitors there have been attempts to find 'selective' enzyme inhibitors (Type 'A' or Type 'B' inhibitors) which would affect particular substrates and hence be free of the more serious adverse interactions. Moclobemide, was the first Type 'A' inhibitor, that became commercially available as an antidepressant, and selegeline, a Type 'B' inhibitor, is used in the treatment of Parkinson's disease. (Developmental MAO inhibitors have been discussed in more detail in SEDA-12, 8.) Table 1 lists the available and experimental MAO inhibitors.

Meanwhile, tricyclic antidepressants have proliferated: at least 22 compounds have been widely clinically tested and most are commercially available in at least one country (Table 2). The prototype tricyclic structure of imipramine consists of a 7-membered (imino) 'sandwiched' between two 6-membered benzene rings. This structure has been altered in three different ways: modification in the aliphatic side chain, insertions into the central 7-membered ring and deletions or additions to one of the 6-membered benzene side rings. These chemical manipulations have produced some changes in the biomedical and pharmacological profiles of the compounds in animals. At first, this created hopes for specificity or relative safety over the prototype compounds in man. However, none of these changes has produced an antidepressant that is more effective; approximately 80% of a heterogeneous population will respond to adequate treatment with any tricyclic compound. The differential effects of some of these drugs on one or other neurotransmitter substance have given rise to claims for biochemical specificity in the treatment of selected subtypes of affective disorder, but this also is uncorroborated by well-controlled studies. However, these structural and biochemical distinctions do translate into differences in side-effect profiles that have occasional significance in clinical management and use.

The fact that the basic tricyclic configuration has been so extensively manipulated to such little effect, and the rising concern over cardiotoxicity and fatalities due to overdose with tricyclic drugs, led to a search for more novel and safer chemical compounds. Because it is over 20 years since the early antidepressant prototypes were developed, these compounds are often considered to be 'second generation' drugs. Table 3 lists the compounds in this category that are currently available or are in advanced stages of clinical testing. These drugs have a variety of chemical structures and differ in their actions on the various neurotransmitter systems but appear to be equally effective as antidepressants. The clinical claims for these new compounds often reflect the deficiencies and drawbacks to existing drugs. It is

Table 1. *Monoamine-oxidase (MAO) inhibitors which have been studied or are presently commercially available for treating depression or for other purposes*

Compound	Structure	Comments
Fenoxypropazine	Hydrazine	The first 6 drugs are earlier compounds which produced liver damage; obsolete in many countries
Iproniazid*	Hydrazine	
Isocarboxazid*	Hydrazine	
Mebanazine	Hydrazine	
Pheniprazine	Hydrazine	
Pivhydrazine	Hydrazine	
Nialamide*	Hydrazine	Little used today
Phenelzine*	Hydrazine	Widely used
Tranylcypromine*	Cyclopropylamine	Most 'amphetamine-like'; high propensity for food and drug interactions
Pargyline*	Propinylbenzylamine	Indicated for hypertension
Furazolidone*	Nitrofuran	Antimicrobial agent (giardiasis)
Procarbazine*	Methylhydrazine	Antineoplastic agent
Clorgiline	Propylamine	Experimental Type A MAO inhibitor (serotonin/noradrenaline)
Selegiline*	Propinylamine	Type B MAO inhibitor (phenylethylamine)
Moclobemide*	Benzamide	Type A MAO inhibitor
Toloxatone*		Type A MAO inhibitor
Brofaromine*		Type A MAO inhibitor

* Compounds that are commercially available at present.

Table 2. *Tricyclic antidepressant compounds which have been widely studied or are presently available for treating depression*

Compound	Structure	Comments
Imipramine*	Dibenzapine; tertiary amine	Prototype compound
Desipramine*	Secondary amine	First metabolite of imipramine
Amitriptyline*	Dibenzocycloheptene; tertiary amine	
Nortriptyline*	Secondary amine	First metabolite of amitriptyline
Protriptyline*	Secondary amine	Most potent; least sedative
Doxepin*	Dibenzoxepine ring	Sedative
Clomipramine*	Halogenated ring	Available for intravenous use
Dimetacrin*	Acridine ring	
Lofepramine*	Propylamine side chain	
Noxiptiline*	Oxyimino side chain	
Butriptyline*	Isobutyl side chain	More potent dopamine effects
Pizotifen*	Piperidine side chain	
Imipraminoxide	Oxygenated ring	Metabolite of imipramine
Amitriptylinoxide	Oxygenated ring	Metabolite of amitriptyline
Dibenzepin*	Dibenzodiazepine ring	
Melitracen*	Anthracene ring	
Amoxapine*	Dibenzoxazepine ring; piperazine side chain	Less potent than other TCA
Iprindole*	6—5—8 ring structure, indole nucleus	Weak action on amine pump mechanism
Dosulepin*	Dibenzothiepine ring	
Trimipramine*	Propyl side chain	
Amineptine*	7-Carbon side chain	Less sedative profile than other TCA
Opipramol*	Piperidine side chain	

* Compounds that are commercially available at present.

hoped that each new compound will act more quickly, have fewer anticholinergic effects, be safer in overdose, and be relatively free from serious adverse effects such as alterations in cardiac function or seizure threshold. While there is an element of reality to some of these claims, they must be interpreted cautiously. Few biological or pathophysiological derangements are restored to normal by drugs in less than a week. Few chemically active compounds are so selective that they work at a single site or are so specific that they bind to only one receptor. Delayed responses, unwanted effects and multiple actions are to be expected, especially when drugs are directed at a finely tuned and well-protected organ like the brain.

Table 3. *'Second generation' antidepressant drugs (including selective serotonin re-uptake inhibitors (SSRIs))*

Compound	Structure	Comments
Buproprion	Aminoketone	Modulate dopaminergic function, increased risk of seizures in high doses
Maprotiline	Tetracyclic	Strong inhibitory effect on noradrenaline uptake; Skin rashes (3%); increased incidence of seizures in overdose; similar side-effect profile to tricyclic compounds
Mianserin	Tetracyclic	Sedative profile, increased incidence of agranulocytosis; possibly safer in overdose; fewer cardiac effects
Nefazodone	Fenylpiperazine	Weak serotonin uptake inhibitor; blocks 5-HT_2-receptors; chemically related to trazodone
Trazodone	Triazolopyridine	Weak effect on serotonin uptake; blocks 5-HT_2-receptors; fewer peripheral anticholinergic properties; sedative profile
Tryptophan	Amino acid	Precursor to serotonin; withdrawn in many countries due to EMS-syndrome
Venlafaxine	Bicyclic; cyclohexanol	Serotonin- and noradrenaline-uptake inhibitor; nausea, sexual dysfunction and cardiovascular side effects; activating
Viloxazine	Bicyclic	Fewer anticholinergic or sedative effects and weight gain; causes nausea and vomiting and weight loss; may precipitate migraine
Citalopram	Bicyclic	SSRI; fewer anticholinergic and cardiovascular effects; gastrointestinal disturbances early in treatment.
Fluoxetine	Bicyclic	
Fluvoxamine	Monocyclic	
Paroxetine	Bicyclic; fluorophenyl, piperidine derivative	
Sertraline	Bicyclic	

A CONTEMPORARY PERSPECTIVE

Certain general principles may prove helpful in gaining a perspective on the field of antidepressant drug therapy and its safety.

Research in receptor-binding assays has revealed the variable degree to which antidepressant compounds affect different neurotransmitter mechanisms within both the peripheral and central nervous system, as well as the extent to which chemical structure influences such activity (4[R]). The significance of such differences remains in doubt with regard to both beneficial and adverse effects, as well as calling into question the validity of the catecholamine hypothesis and its underlying assumption that the action of all effective antidepressants is mediated via an increase in turnover of catecholamines at central synapses (5[R]). Some idea of the growing complexity and uncertainty in this area can be gained by considering the following factors:

(1) Much of the research is conducted in animals, often on isolated tissues. However, newer drugs have appeared (such as mianserin) that were largely inert in traditional animal models, but were selected on the basis of novel techniques such as computerized EEG profiles in man (6[C]).

(2) The same drug often affects several neurotransmitter systems to differing degrees (serotonin, acetylcholine, noradrenaline, histamine, dopamine). Table 4 (4[R]) illustrates the complexity of the relationship between the pharmacological properties of compounds and their wanted and unwanted clinical consequences.

(3) The same drug may influence central and peripheral receptors within the same neurotransmitter system to a variable degree, e.g. acetylcholine, α-adrenergic receptors.

(4) Drugs which differ profoundly in their actions on different neurotransmitters appear to be equally effective antidepressants when given to heterogeneous patient groups, perhaps because the same end-result may occur irrespective of whether the drug affects an excitatory or inhibitory system.

(5) The effects of the same drug on separate neurotransmitter systems show a different time and dose relationship. For example, the effect of tricyclic antidepressant drugs on the acetylcholine system is maximal within 5 hours of the first dose, after which time tolerance develops slowly over several weeks (7[C]). The effects of these compounds on the peripheral cholinergic system display a linear dose—response relationship, but their central sedative effects appear to be maximal at low dosages and do not increase further (8[Cr]).

(6) Drug effects may alter over time due to the develop-

Table 4. *Pharmacological properties of antidepressants and clinical consequences**

Property	Possible clinical consequences
Blockade of noradrenaline uptake	Alleviation of depression Blockade of the antihypertensive effects of guanethidine, clonidine and α-methyldopa Augmentation of sympathomimetic amines
Blockade of serotonin uptake	Alleviation of depression Postural hypotension
Blockade of histamine H_1-receptors	Potentiation of central depressant drugs Sedation, drowsiness Weight gain Hypotension
Blockade of muscarinic receptors	Blurred vision Dry mouth Sinus tachycardia Constipation Urinary retention Memory dysfunction
Blockade of α_1-adrenergic receptors	Potentiation of the antihypertensive effect of prazosin Postural hypotension, dizziness Reflex tachycardia
Blockade of α_2-adrenergic receptors	Blockade of the antihypertensive effects of clonidine and α-methyldopa

* Reprinted from Richelson (4[R]) by courtesy of the Editors of the *Journal of Clinical Psychiatry*.

ment of increased or decreased receptor sensitivity. The outcome of these temporal actions may depend on whether an excitatory or inhibitory feedback system is implicated. For instance, α_2-adrenergic fibers are desensitized by chronic antidepressant administration, reducing inhibitory feedback and enhancing release of neurotransmitters in a manner that may account for the delayed onset of clinical activity (9[Cr]).

(7) Irrespective of which neurotransmitter they act upon, drugs may do so by one or more of at least three mechanisms. These are a direct action at the receptor site (agonist or antagonist), the blockade of re-uptake from the synaptic cleft into storage sites or an alteration in the sensitivity or density of receptors over time (up- or down-regulation).

(8) Drugs that were once neatly placed in a particular category of drug action appear less selective than their chemical structure once suggested. Examples include thioridazine (classified as both an antidepressant and major tranquilizer) and alprazolam (classified as an antidepressant and minor tranquilizer). This may change now that developments in molecular biology are making it feasible to design compounds that appear to be acting on a single neurotransmitter by only one mechanism (such as the re-uptake of serotonin or noradrenaline). However, there are both theoretical and clinical reasons for doubting if specificity is attainable. One study (10[C]) found that depressed outpatients did equally well on a predominant serotonin re-uptake inhibitor (zimeldine 200 mg/day) as on a noradrenaline uptake inhibitor (maprotiline 150 mg/day). A review of both clinical and animal research (11[R]) on serotonin re-uptake inhibitors concluded that antidepressants were not likely to be specific from a nosological viewpoint and that alterations in both serotonin and noradrenaline availability were requisites for an optimal antidepressant response.

In a recent review the evidence regarding the relationship between the specificity of antidepressants in modulating neurotransmitter systems and their therapeutic activity has been assessed (12[r]) and the question of a common mode of action of all antidepressants irrespective of presumed differences in specificity for transmitter systems is discussed.

(9) The concentration of drug in plasma (and presumably at central receptor sites) varies 20-fold between individuals given identical amounts. Any relationship between plasma level and clinical response appears to differ within compounds of the same class (for imipramine it is linear and for nortriptyline parabolic). For a majority of compounds, such data are inconclusive or lacking.

Additional complexity to the understanding and interpretation of antidepressant drug action is contributed to by the ability to measure changes in neuroendocrine function with regard to both hypothalamic dysfunction as evidenced by the dexamethasone suppression test (13[Cr]) and alterations in the pituitary—thyroid axis as evidenced by a blunted response to thyrotrophin-releasing hormone (14[Cr]). To date, these tests have not fulfilled hopes of providing specific indications for drug selection or explanations of side-effect susceptibility.

Finally, antidepressant drugs are today used in variety of conditions including chronic pain management (15[C]), panic disorders (16[R]), sleep disturbance (17[R]) and obsessive compulsive disorder (18[r]).

All of the above factors have added immeasurably to the complexity of selection among the antidepressant drugs for the practicing clinician. In seeking a rational basis for action, safety remains a prime consideration. A consistent feature of the literature on all psychotropic drugs is the extended time periods that occur between the introduction of a new compound and the discovery of its full range of adverse effects. For example, the paranoid psychoses due to amphetamine and its congeners were first accurately described in 1958 (19[Cr]), over 20 years after their introduction into clinical medicine. The interactions between foodstuffs and MAO inhibitors were described in detail in 1963 (3[R]) after these drugs had been available as antidepressants for more than 5 years. New side effects have been attributed to the tricyclic antidepressants after decades of extensive use.

Physicians who use the newer second-generation compounds as 'first choice' drugs should remain alert to the possibility of novel previously undetected adverse effects and, when possible, should communicate their observations to the appropriate drug-regulatory agency. A tendency to dismiss the somatic complaints of psychiatric patients contributes to delayed recognition of drug complications. Lack of communication concerning such observations delays the development of consensus about potential new adverse effects. This problem is highlighted by the withdrawal of zimeldine and nomifensine due to side effects which were first detected or became problematical long after they were first marketed, as well as by the decision to withhold buproprion on the eve of its distribution in the United States. For pharmaceuticals as a whole it is estimated that approximately one in ten newly introduced drugs will be withdrawn within 2 years due to unexpected toxicity.

The common shortcomings of all currently available antidepressants require careful management. For instance, the risk of suicide when inertia is overcome early in treatment, but before mood is elevated, is an example that requires frequent enquiry and stringent prescribing to avoid a potentially lethal overdose with medication.

A final practical question that relates to the use of any antidepressant is the degree to which side effects or fear of them reduce patient compliance. This is especially important with antidepressants, because side effects occur early in treatment while improvement is often delayed. A review (20[R]) concludes that despite the poor quality of research on compliance there is a consensus that side effects do interfere with effective management. About a fifth of depressed patients refuse drug therapy and half of those in treatment drop out before complete recovery. Although side effects contribute, so do the patient's attitudes and beliefs about the appropriateness and safety of medication. Strategies to decrease side effects and improve compliance include plasma monitoring, once-a-day regimens, educational techniques and selection of particular drugs based on individual patient needs.

In the sections that follow, the MAO inhibitors, tricyclic antidepressants and selective serotonin re-uptake inhibitors are discussed in relation to both drug class-related and compound-specific side effects. The other second-generation drugs are each considered separately

Monoamine-oxidase inhibitors

All of the available monoamine-oxidase (MAO) inhibitors (with the exception of moclobemide, toloxatone, brofaromine and selegeline) act via a 'suicide' mechanism by forming a long-lasting, irreversible, competitive inhibition of the mitochondrial enzyme which persists until new enzyme is manufactured (21[R]). Most of these drugs have also been shown to produce a non-specific decrease in the activity of hepatic drug-metabolizing enzymes.

Table 1 lists the MAO inhibitors that are already available or under investigation. These compounds fall into different chemical categories which include compounds that have antidepressant, antihypertensive (pargyline), antineoplastic (procarbazine) and antimicrobial (furazolidone) properties as well as beneficial effects in the treatment of Parkinson's disease (selegeline).

The MAO inhibitors epitomize cyclical fashions in drug use and the impact of side effects on this process. They were the first psychotropic drugs for which a clear biochemical action was defined. Early excitement was quickly tempered by the reports of liver toxicity in the hydrazine derivatives, leading to synthesis of the cyclopropylamine drug, tranylcypromine. This compound was the most implicated in the food and drug interaction that led to an overall decline in the popularity of this category of antidepressant agents.

Ten to 15 years ago there was a re-appraisal of the risk/benefit ratios of the MAO inhibitors. This included both the search for 'safer' and more selective or rapidly reversible enzyme inhibitors (moclobemide, toloxatone and brofaromine now available), as well as a review and retrial of the older compounds.

The scientific underpinnings of this renaissance are discussed in a review (22[R]). As previously noted (SED-10, 28), much of the earlier work was conducted using inadequate doses of phenelzine. Later investigations using adequate drug levels (to produce 85% or more enzyme inhibition) have validated the efficacy of this MAO inhibitor. A review (23[CR]) of 11 studies conducted in 1963—1982 that compared MAO inhibitors and tricyclic compounds showed that three found no difference, four showed the tricyclics to be superior and three showed the MAO inhibitors to be better. The three studies which favoured the MAO inhibitors were among the four most recently conducted (all since 1979). An article in 1985 entitled 'Should the use of the

MAO inhibitors be abandoned?' (24[R]) was accompanied by commentaries from six British and US experts in psychopharmacology. The consensus was clearly in favour of continued use, with the recognition that even if a specific responder is difficult to define, there are individuals who respond when all other drugs have failed. No clear-cut clinical or metabolic features distinguish such individuals; an earlier claim that clinical response and side-effect susceptibility might be influenced by genetically determined rapid or slow acetylation of phenelzine was not confirmed in a review of seven studies (25[R]).

During recent years there has been a large number of studies on the efficacy and toxicity of the selective Type A MAO-inhibitors (SEDA-16, 7–8; SEDA-17, 16; SEDA-18, 16)

ADVERSE REACTION SUMMARY

General and toxic reactions Problems with the non-selective irreversible MAO inhibitors arise for two reasons: the large number of amines that are substrates for the enzyme and the fact that these drugs also inhibit non-specific drug-metabolizing enzymes in the liver. Together, these two actions produce a lengthy list of interactions with substances, the effects of which may be enhanced or prolonged both during treatment with an MAO inhibitor and for up to 2 weeks afterwards due to the irreversible nature of the enzyme inhibition (see Table 5).

Amines that serve as substrates include both the real and synthetic ephedrine congeners contained in prescribed and proprietary preparations as well as amines such as tyramine that occur naturally in a variety of protein-containing foods in which amines are produced by the bacterial decarboxylation of the amino acids. When these 'indirectly acting' amines are ingested, they are normally destroyed by MAO activity in the intestine or liver; after treatment with an MAO inhibitor, they gain access to the systemic circulation, resulting in a release of noradrenaline from the sympathetic nerve terminals. If the amount ingested is sufficient, this produces symptoms similar to those of a pheochromocytoma with a paroxysmal increase in blood pressure, sudden severe occipital headache and cardiac irregularities. In rare instances, death may result due to cerebral hemorrhage or cardiac failure.

The MAO inhibitors' actions on non-specific hepatic drug-metabolizing enzymes result in the potentiation of effects due to a large number of drugs including narcotic analgesics, barbiturates and anesthetics. This fact may complicate elective or emergency surgery in patients taking these antidepressants, with occasionally fatal results.

In addition to the lengthy list of potential drug interactions, MAO inhibitors produce some toxic effects of their own including the hepatocellular damage that led to withdrawal of the earlier hydrazine derivatives. Hypotension is often a pronounced side effect (possibly due to the accumulation of a pseudotransmitter normally metabolized by MAO) and other autonomic disturbances such as dry mouth, sweating, constipation and weight gain are quite common.

Differences between MAO inhibitors in side-effect profiles are poorly substantiated and confounded by different usage patterns and drug po-

Table 5. *Interactions with monoamine-oxidase inhibitors*

Hypertensive crises: Potentiation of central effects of drugs or food components due to MAO inhibition
Amphetamine and congeners
Ephedrine and congeners
Levodopa
Prescribed or proprietary amines (or precursors)
Reserpine
Tryptophan
Alcohol (wine, beer)
Amine-containing foodstuffs
Banana (peel)
Broad beans (including pods)
Caviar
Cheese
Chicken livers
Chocolate
Pickled herring
Yeast extracts (marmite, packeted soups)
Serotonin syndrome
Pethidine, meperidine
Dextromethorphan
Tryptophan
Tricyclic antidepressants
Selective serotonin re-uptake inhibitors
Trazodone and dextropropoxyphen (combined with phenelzine)
Potentiation or prolongation of other drug effects due to hepatic drug-metabolizing enzyme inhibition
Alcohol (all types)
Anesthetics
Antihistamines
Antiparkinsonian agents
Barbiturates
Benzodiazepines
Chloral hydrate
Hypoglycemic agents
Opiate analgesics
Thyroid extract
Tricyclic antidepressants

tencies. The selective MAO inhibitors are considered separately below.

Hypersensitivity reactions Drug rashes have been reported, but their relationship to drug ingestion is poorly substantiated. The hepatocellular damage caused by hydrazine derivatives probably belongs in this category.

Tumor-inducing effects A single case of angiosarcoma in the liver has been reported in a patient taking phenelzine (26[C]) and similar tumors have occurred in mice treated with the same MAO inhibitor.

ORGANS AND SYSTEMS

Cardiovascular During the period of MAO inhibition, the concentration of noradrenaline, dopamine and serotonin rises in the central nervous system and heart because their breakdown is slowed. The activity of the precursors of these amines—dopa and 5-hydroxytryptophan—is greatly augmented. The effects are similar to those of the postganglionic blocking amines; *postural hypotension* occurs and *cardiac output is reduced*, possibly due to the accumulation of a pseudotransmitter. The hypotensive effects of the MAO inhibitors differ from those of the tricyclic antidepressants because they affect supine blood pressure as well as postural changes. This fact was confirmed both in a study (27[CR]) involving tranylcypromine and in an evaluation (28[CR]) of blood pressure changes in 14 patients treated with phenelzine averaging 65 mg/day for at least 3 weeks. The drug-free mean lying systolic blood pressure was 127 mmHg. It decreased significantly (mean drop 5 mmHg) by the end of the first week. By contrast, the mean baseline orthostatic drop of 2 mmHg did not increase significantly until the end of the second week of treatment and it continued to increase. Two patients developed profound orthostatic drops of up to 50 mmHg after more than 2 weeks of treatment. One patient's hypotension and symptoms (light-headedness and ataxia) improved on treatment with fludrocortisone (a mineralocorticoid), but the other did not and required drug discontinuation. The authors comment that the delayed development of orthostatic hypotension requires cautious long-term monitoring.

Hypertensive crises usually occur when MAO inhibitors are combined with other drugs or foodstuffs which give rise to interactions (see below).

Autopotentiation of hypertensive effects A small proportion of hypertensive crises appears not to be provoked by known drug or dietary precipitants (29[C]). In a recent review, 12 reports of spontaneous hypertension in patients treated with tranylcypromine or phenelzine are described. A family history of hypertension may be a risk factor (SEDA-18, 14). A significant increase in supine blood pressure without similar changes in standing blood pressure following administration of tranylcypromine has also been described (SEDA-17, 17).

Bradycardia also occurs; a report of two cases of 'interaction' with β-blockers (nadolol and metoprolol) is of interest and several possible mechanisms are discussed (30[C]).

Nervous system *Autonomic side effects* A carefully controlled comparison (31[Cr]) of treatment with phenelzine (up to 90 mg/day, mean dose 77 mg) and imipramine (up to 150 mg/day, mean dose 139 mg) found no significant difference between drugs, during a 3-week course of treatment, in the incidence of dry mouth, blurred vision, constipation and urinary difficulty.

Central nervous system Day-time somnolence and fatigue have been reported following tranylcypromine, phenelzine or isocarboxazide (SEDA-16, 8; SEDA-17, 16). In the study comparing phenelzine and imipramine reported above (31[Cr]) there were important and significant differences between drugs: 19% of the phenelzine patients reported drowsiness compared to none on imipramine, moreover, 18 patients taking phenelzine had to be discontinued compared to one on imipramine (who developed urinary retention); four patients developed antisocial behavior, three showed an overt paranoid psychosis, and one experienced a hypertensive crisis despite all precautions to avoid interacting foods and drugs. There has also been a case report of a delusional parasitosis following administration of phenelzine. Hyperthermia and labile blood pressure, perhaps due to drug interaction between clomipramine, phenelzine and chlorpromazine has been described in one patient and central nervous system toxicity was also reported after abrupt switch from phenelzine to isocarboxazide (SEDA-17, 17). A case of dose-related visual hallucinations in a patient with macular degeneration receiving phenelzine has been reported (32[C]). The authors discuss the possibility of deprivation-induced visual phenomena intensified by increased central monoamine levels.

The authors who had previously reported a case of carpal tunnel syndrome due to *pyridoxine deficiency* in a patient on tranylcypromine (SEDA-9, 21) have since collected data (33[C]) on six patients treated with phenelzine (up to 75 mg/day for up to 4 months). All of these developed low levels of pyridoxine and a variety of symptoms including numbness, paresthesias, and edema of the hands as well as 'electric shock' sensation in the head, neck and arms. The symptoms resolved completely following the addition of pyridoxine 150—300 mg/day to the treatment regimen.

Neuromuscular effects The propensity for MAO inhibitors to produce symptoms related to neuromuscular excitability has been recognized in cases of overdose (SEDA-10, 18) and in interactions with other antidepressants or tryptophan (SEDA-10, 16, 17) when it has often been described as the 'serotonin syndrome' (34[C]). A thorough review (35[R]) of the preclinical and clinical literature draws attention to these phenomena occurring at clinical dose levels with an MAO inhibitor alone and speculates that the mechanism is related to a combination of increased serotonergic tone and central disinhibition of α-motorneuron-mediated spinal activity. The authors tabulate and discuss 10 previous reports of myoclonus, hyperreflexia, muscle twitching, and increased muscle tone, in patients treated with all the available MAO inhibitors. These neuromuscular effects appear to occur in up to 15% or more of patients and are more likely when tryptophan is given in combination. Their appearance is usually after 10–14 days treatment; tolerance does not occur, but they may decrease or disappear with dose reduction. The symptoms predominate during sleep but occur less often in a waking state and are often associated with muscle or joint pain.

The MAO inhibitors may be used in patients who have *Parkinson's disease* for two reasons. Firstly, this is a disorder in which depression is common. Secondly, the selective Type B inhibitor, selegiline (deprenyl), may benefit patients with parkinsonism, possibly due to a relative increase in brain dopamine levels (36[C]) and this drug is now commercially available for this indication.

A possible hypertensive interaction between phenelzine and amantadine in Parkinson's disease has previously been reviewed (SEDA-10, 17).

A further potential risk of using a non-selective inhibitor in such patients is illustrated by separate reports of the appearance of *parkinsonism* in patients treated with phenelzine (37[C], 38[C]).

Pande and Max (39[C]) have described the occurrence of *dystonia* in a woman of 65 who had been receiving tranylcypromine 10 mg twice daily for 3 days in an attempt to control major long-term depression which had failed to respond to other agents. The condition receded 48 hours after drug withdrawal but returned on rechallenge with the original dose.

Speech blockage has previously occurred due to a number of tricyclic compounds, to maprotiline and to alprazolam. A case has now been reported due to an MAO inhibitor (40[C]) in a 34-year-old woman who developed difficulty in finding words 2 months after starting treatment with phenelzine 45 mg/day. Because of associated insomnia no attempt at dose adjustment was made and the drug was discontinued. The side effect disappeared and did not recur when the patient's depression was successfully treated with maprotiline 175 mg/day.

Mineral and fluid balance *Inappropriate secretion of antidiuretic hormone* (41[C]) may be the mechanism of action underlying the cases of peripheral edema described previously (SED-6, 28; SEDA-2, 12). Diuretics are not helpful, but dose reduction produces relief (42[C]).

Hematological *Leukopenia* and *agranulocytosis* are well-recognized complications of treatment with tricyclic antidepressants and have been reported with some second-generation compounds. A report (43[Cr]) of leukopenia in a patient treated with phenelzine draws attention to five other unpublished cases and to previous published reports involving isocarboxazid, tranylcypromine and etryptamine.

Liver The early reports of hepatotoxicity with iproniazid led to the synthesis of non-hydrazine inhibitors and a report from France (44[CR]) reaffirms the frequency and severity of this side effect. Nineteen drug surveillance centers reported 91 cases of *hepatitis* due to all antidepressants (11 on iproniazid) in a 5-year period. *Cytolytic reactions* occurred in 11 patients treated with iproniazid and five died. A high level of antimitochondrial antibody (M6) was found in five patients.

A carefully controlled study showed that patients with impaired liver function are especially sensitive to tranylcypromine, sometimes developing obtunded consciousness and slow EEGs similar to those found in hepatic encephalopathy (45[CR]).

Skin *Photosensitivity* to MAO inhibitors must be most unusual, but a well-authenticated report has been published (46[C]).

Sexual function Relative *impotence* and *delayed ejaculation* in men and *difficulty in achieving orgasm* in two women have been reported due to a variety of MAO inhibitors used to treat narcolepsy (47[C]), phobic anxiety (48[C]) and depression (49[C]–51[C]).

Sexual symptoms often display a dose relationship with increased incidence at higher doses. As always with sexual disorders, there is a delicate interplay between psychic and pathophysiological influences. In male patients with premature ejaculation this 'side effect' may even be considered therapeutic.

Risk situations It is inadvisable to administer MAO inhibitors to *schizophrenic* patients, even when they seem to be in an anergic or depressive state, since they may precipitate psychotic crises; in addition, it is difficult to ensure that such patients respect the necessary dietary restrictions, i.e. avoidance of tyramine-containing foods.

Because of the concern expressed about the use of tricyclic antidepressants in the *elderly*, MAO inhibitors have been studied in this population (52[C]). Patients with dementia benefited in mood (but not cognition) and some non-demented patients also improved. Side effects were considered less frequent or troublesome than those due to tricyclic compounds, although one patient on tranylcypromine became paranoid and another on phenelzine developed a choreiform movement disorder. The fact that MAO levels increase with age provides logic to support the use of these drugs in the elderly, but their hypotensive effects and interactions with other drugs and foods suggest that they should be used with extreme caution in a population exposed to polypharmacy whose comprehension and compliance with warnings may be impaired.

Withdrawal effects (*see also 'Abuse potential' below*) Increasing use of any drug for a chronic condition is associated with an increase in the number of individuals treated for prolonged periods and with potential problems relating to dependency and drug withdrawal. A study (53[C]) of the use of phenelzine in continuation therapy after recovery from an acute episode of depression found that relapse rates were higher in patients subjected to tapered withdrawal than in those continued on the therapeutic dose.

Another study (54[Cr]) looked at the effects of sudden drug withdrawal in 34 patients on phenelzine and 17 on tricyclic antidepressants who had been treated for a mean duration of over 9 months. Depressed patients on phenelzine showed significantly more symptoms than depressed patients taking tricyclic antidepressants, and a third of them relapsed compared with a quarter on the tricyclic. At 3 months follow-up 47% of the patients on phenelzine had resumed treatment compared with 23% on the tricyclic.

An attempt to distinguish between withdrawal and relapse on the basis of rapidity and severity of symptoms did not differentiate, but about a third of patients in both groups developed new symptoms of adrenergic hyperactivity including anxiety and perceptual disturbances. Another study (55[C]) reports the occurrence of acute psychotic symptoms in two young women shortly after cessation of treatment with phenelzine 90 mg/day for a month.

The literature on a withdrawal syndrome (SEDA-10, 17) has been expanded by further reports. One of these (56[C]) involved the development of an acute toxic delirious state 3 days after cessation of phenelzine and another (57[C]) concerned patients who became manic following discontinuation of isocarboxazid. A withdrawal state similar to that caused by withdrawal of amphetamines has been described following discontinuation of tranylcypromine (SEDA-16, 8; SEDA-18, 14).

Overdosage The fatal toxicities of antidepressants in England, Scotland and Wales during the periods 1975—1984 and 1985—1989 have been compared in epidemiological retrospective studies (58[C], 59[C]). The fatal toxicity index (deaths per million prescriptions) for individual drugs or groups of drugs was used to give an indication of the relative toxicities of the different drugs. During the two periods there were a total of 24 deaths due to tranylcypromine, 33 due to phenelzine and three to isocarboxazid. The fatal toxicity index for tranylcypromine was significantly higher than the mean of all antidepressants, while that for the other MAO-inhibitors was lower. The majority of all deaths from antidepressant poisoning was due to two tricyclic drugs (amitriptyline and dothiepin) and they as well as the whole group of older tricyclics had a fatal toxicity index significantly higher than the mean (59[C]). It must of course be kept in mind that the fatal toxicity index of a drug is influenced by many other factors than the inherent toxicity of the drug. Such factors are the patient population to whom the drug is prescribed, including differences in severity of illness and suicidality, prescription for other indications than depression and doses prescribed.

The minimum fatal dose of non-selective MAO-inhibitors is of the order of 5—10-times the maximum daily dose, although individuals have been reported to survive such amounts. The symptoms of overdose may be initially mild and deceptive, but progress over 24 hours to include agitation, tremor, alternating low and high blood pressure, severe muscle spasms, hyperpyrexia and convulsions. Symptomatic treatment has been the use of the β-blocker practolol (10 mg i.v., repeated after 2 hours) and the use of muscle relaxants with assisted respiration (60[Cr]) which may help reduce pyrexia by abolishing excessive muscle activity. Active elimination techniques are unhelpful (61[R]) according to a comprehensive review of antidepressant overdosage.

In one case (62[Cr]) in which the patient took 900 mg of phenelzine the authors recorded the marked excess of urinary and plasma catecholamines analogous to pheochromocytoma and successfully managed the patient with α-adrenergic antagonists. In another patient (63[Cr]), who probably took a larger dose of around 2000 mg of phenelzine, hyperpyrexia was a prominent feature (this was atypically absent in the first case). The authors noted the clinical similarities to malignant hyperthermia and neuroleptic malignant syndrome and the patient recovered dramatically with the use of dantrolene sodium, a lipid-soluble hydantoin analog that relaxes skeletal muscle directly.

Abuse potential Griffin et al. (64[Cr]) have described four more cases of addiction to tranylcypromine in addition to the three reported in the literature since 1965. The dose of tranylcypromine taken varied between 150 and 300 mg daily. The mild euphoriant properties of tranylcypromine reflect its structural resemblance to amphetamine and probably account for the tolerance and addiction potential in predisposed individuals. In a recent review (65[CR]) the authors had found a total of 18 cases of tranylcypromine abuse. Thereafter, two additional reports have appeared (SEDA-17, 17; 66[C]). In one of these cases (66[C]) the patient ingested 440 mg tranylcypromine daily without any side-effects. The patient has reported that she was longing for the 'energising' effect of the drug and for the feeling of 'freedom and power'. Withdrawal of the drug resulted in repeated generalized seizures and status epilepticus. Abuse of phenelzine has not been observed.

Interactions A cause-and-effect relationship for interactions between non-selective MAO inhibitors and other substances is often difficult to establish, for two reasons (67[CR]). Firstly, MAO inhibitors act by forming an irreversible combination with the enzyme which is continuously being resynthesized in the body. The level of enzyme inhibition therefore varies with the dose and duration of treatment, and may persist to some degree for up to 2 weeks after treatment ceases. Secondly, the amine composition of foodstuffs is also variable and unpredictable; any protein food which contains decarboxylating bacteria may produce amines by conversion of amino acids to amines such as tyramine, phenylethylamine and histamine. For example, identically appearing pieces of cheese may vary 100-fold in tyramine content. It is the diversity and number of substances listed in Table 5, as well as the unpredictability in the occurrence of adverse effects, that has contributed to the unpopularity of the MAO inhibitors as therapeutic agents.

There are two facts that simplify the understanding and use of these drugs.

(1) The interactions listed in Table 5 fall into three categories: either a *hypertensive crisis* due to the release and potentiation of catecholamines similar to that experienced in pheochromocytoma, a *serotonin syndrome* caused by excess serotonin availability in the CNS or an *exacerbation or prolongation of the normally occurring actions of the drug* (sedation or coma due to alcohol, anesthetics or opiate analgesics; atropine-like central toxicity due to tricyclic antidepressants). The consequences of the hypertensive interaction are in fact variable; many individuals remain unaware of relatively minor increases in blood pressure. However, if the rise is large and rapid (an increase of 30 mmHg or more in systolic pressure within 20 min), the patient experiences a sudden severe occipital headache and palpitations, which may be associated in rare instances with subarachnoid hemorrhage or cardiac failure if the cerebral vasculature or cardiac musculature are already weakened. The serotonin syndrome is characterised by three or more of the following symptoms: confusion, hypomania, agitation, myoclonus, hyperreflexia, hyperthermia, shivering, diaphoresis, ataxia and diarrhoea (68[R]). It is most commonly seen in patients treated with a combination of drugs which increase serotonin availability by different mechanisms. In a recent review by Sporer (69[R]) drug combinations that have been reported to cause the serotonin syndrome are listed and pathophysiology of the syndrome is discussed. It is probably mediated through stimulation of the 5-HT_{1A} receptor, but interaction with dopamine and with 5-HT_2 receptors are also discussed. In the majority of the reported cases the drug combination associated with the syndrome includes a MAO inhibitor (see Table 5). Occurrence of the syndrome seems to be rare, although it has been reported more frequently during the last years often due to a combination of MAO-inhibitor and selective serotonin re-uptake inhibitor. In most cases the symptoms are mild and resolve rapidly after drug withdrawal and supportive therapy. It must, though, be borne in mind that this syndrome may be fatal and if combinations of serotonergic drugs are used it should be with great caution. The interactions of MAO inhibitors with opiates, which may lead to sudden and fatal reactions are discussed in SEDA 18 (pp. 14—15). A flushing reaction has been associated with interaction between phenelzine and clonazepam (SEDA-17, 17).

(2) A second factor that can add to the safer use of these drugs is to recognize that adequate patient education is essential. The patients must be aware of the name and nature of the drug they are taking and its potential to interact with both proscribed foods as well as any other prescribed or proprietary medication. Additionally, the patients should understand what symptoms may indicate an interaction, such as unexpected drowsiness (after alcohol or other drugs) or sudden severe headache (within 2 hours of a meal or medication). Because of the many variables involved, foods or medications that are taken with impunity on one occasion may interact dangerously on another. The director of a British

counselling service has reported that of 119 patients treated with MAO inhibitors who experienced problems, 35 reported hypertensive crises. Four of these were fatal (70[C]). Despite warnings, these patients had eaten amine-containing foodstuffs or taken over-the-counter cold remedies. The MAO inhibitors should not be prescribed unless the patient is able to understand such instructions, repeat them back after explanation, and compliance can be confirmed at subsequent inquiry. Those who take multiple medications, who have difficulty with comprehension or compliance (such as the elderly) or who become overly fearful following such explanations should not be prescribed these drugs.

The management of a patient experiencing these drug interactions depends on their nature. In the case of symptoms due to exacerbation or prolongation of drug effects, specific (if available) or supportive measures (cardiovascular or respiratory) may be indicated. In the case of a hypertensive crisis, symptoms usually abate in 1—2 hours as the blood pressure falls. If seen early, or if hypertension persists or recurs, the high blood pressure can be treated with phentolamine or chlorpromazine given parenterally, but the dangers of invoking rebound hypotension should be weighed carefully.

Comparative risks of MAO inhibitors compared with tricyclic compounds As pointed out above, the MAO inhibitors suffered a long period of disgrace largely because of their troublesome interactions. Their risks still exceed those of the tricyclic compounds, but some experienced clinicians feel that they can be safely used, provided appropriate precautions are taken.

Of particular interest is a chart review (71[C]) of 198 patients aged 19—64 treated in a university research clinic by psychiatrists who 'specialized in pharmacologic treatment of affective disorders'. The majority of the patients (130) were atypical depressives who participated in a 6- or 12-week double-blind study comparing phenelzine, imipramine or placebo. Patients were treated after conclusion of the trial and the sample was expanded to include other patients attending the clinic.

Based on clinical experience and literature review, the authors selected 14 side effects generally considered to cause 'serious medical risk or subjective discomfort great enough to require drug discontinuation'.

The results show that 14% of patients on placebo, 27% on imipramine, 43% on tranylcypromine and 64% on phenelzine had serious side effects; 38% of patients had two or more serious side effects and all except one of them was taking phenelzine. The differences between imipramine and phenelzine were highly significant. Treatment over time revealed that by 33 weeks less than half the imipramine patients suffered a serious side effect compared with over 90% of phenelzine-treated patients. Side effects were sufficiently severe to cause discontinuation of drug in 45% of patients.

None of the 14 selected side effects was more common in patients treated with imipramine. The serious side effects that were clearly more common on phenelzine included hypomania (10% of patients), hypertensive crises (8%), weight gain over 15 pounds (8%), and anorgasmia and impotence (22%).

In a second article (72[C]) the authors discuss details of the side effects and state their conclusions. Of the 11 patients who suffered a hypertensive crisis, six ate tyramine-containing foods 'despite meticulous dietary review and cautioning' and three took ephedrine-containing medications. Four of the 11 patients with hypertensive crises obtained emergency medical treatment in local hospitals and a fifth patient was hospitalized in coma with intracranial bleeding due to an unsuspected aneurysm.

Brofaromine

Brofaromine is a new selective Type A MAO inhibitor. In an open study of brofaromine in endogenous depression side effects were reported in nine out of 51 patients. These included dry mouth, dizziness, tremor, hypomania, anxiety and memory problems (SEDA-17, 16).

Moclobemide

Moclobemide was the first selective Type A MAO inhibitor that became commercially available. It is also reversibly bound to the enzyme, considerably shortening its effect. Both of these characteristics reduce the risk of hypertensive crises (73[R], 74[C]).

A number of studies have been published in which adverse effects are well reported, mainly comparing moclobemide with 'standard' antidepressants. The consensus has been that the new drug produces fewer anticholinergic effects than clomipramine or imipramine, and less orthostatic hypotension and dizziness than either of those drugs. Main problems reported early were insomnia, agitation and paresthesias (75[c]—81[c]). The most common side effects reported in controlled trials have been insomnia and nausea (SEDA-18, 15). In a multicenter trial comparing moclobemide, amitriptyline and placebo, gastrointestinal discomfort, headache and dizziness occurred in over 20% of moclobemide-treated patients and insomnia was also a common complaint (82[C]). In a study in healthy volunteers there was no effects of moclobemide on psychomotor performance. Acute confusion and agitation has been reported in one patient who dropped out of a clinical trial due to this adverse effect (SEDA-16, 7). In a recent report hypomania has been attributed to moclobemide in two cases (SEDA-17, 16). Cases of aggressive behaviour and mild manic symptoms have been described in severely depressed patients, refractory to other treatments, who received moclobemide therapy (SEDA-18, 15). In a controlled multicenter study of 115 inpatients with relatively severe depression, moclobemide was found to be better tolerated but showed a weaker therapeutic effect than clomipramine. Nine of the patients in the moclobemide group dropped out of the study due to worsening of depression and suicidality, though it is possible that the moclobemide dose used (400 mg/day) was insufficient (SEDA-18, 15).

Patients taking moclobemide can follow a normal diet since there is no significant potentiation of tyramine. Two studies reported single cases of rise in blood pressure following moclobemide: in one this was a 40 mmHg increase in systolic pressure after one dose on only 1 day of treatment in 4 weeks (80[c]), while the other report only refers to 'episodes of hypertension' without further comment (76[c]). Interactions were not suggested in either paper as a possible etiological factor. Moclobemide increased the pressor effect of ephedrine in a study in healthy volunteers (SEDA-18, 16) and the subjects also experienced increased side effects as lightheadedness and palpitations. Thus, this reversible MAO inhibitor may potentiate the effect of indirect sympathomimetics, while the combination should be used with caution. L-Dopa and benserazide was given together with moclobemide to normal volunteers. No hypertension was noted but the combination was poorly tolerated with headache and insomnia commonly reported (SEDA-18, 16).

Five fatal cases of serotonin syndrome following combined overdoses of moclobemide and citalopram and moclobemide and clomipramine have been reported (SEDA-18, 16). Two additional cases of this syndrome following the combined treatment of moclobemide and tricyclic antidepressants has been reported in the literature (69[R]).

Cases with overdoses of moclobemide (950 mg, and 1.55 and 1.50—2 grams) showed symptoms of drowsiness, disorientation and hyporeflexia (83[c], 84[c]).

Toloxatone

Like moclobemide, the selective and reversible Type A MAO inhibitor toloxatone is thought to be relatively safe in combination with sympathomimetics (SEDA-18, 16). However, sweating, tachycardia and headache have been reported in a case where terbutaline was added to toloxatone and phenylephrine treatment (SEDA-18, 16). In healthy volunteers doses up to 600 mg/day did not produce hypertensive reactions with oral tyramine (SEDA 17, 17). Two fatal cases of fulminant hepatitis have been reported in patients treated with toloxatone (SEDA-16, 7).

Tricyclic antidepressants

No accurate data exist on the worldwide relative use of the many tricyclic compounds listed in Table 2 and availability of particular drugs differs between countries. The dosage range for all of these compounds is 50—300 mg/day with the exception of nortriptyline, which has an upper limit of 200 mg, and protriptyline, which is a more potent compound with a range of 10—60 mg/day. Well-controlled comparative studies are relatively few, but it is clear that these drugs resemble each other more than they differ. Their adverse effects will be discussed as a class with distinguishing features mentioned when relevant.

ADVERSE REACTION PATTERN

General and toxic reactions The tricyclic antidepressants have been shown to interfere with the activity of at least five putative neurotransmitters by several different potential mechanisms at both central and peripheral sites. This gives rise to uncertainty in understanding the mechanisms that underlie a bewildering variety of unwanted effects that are further modified by temporal factors probably related to changes in receptor sensitivity. Differences between drugs are often inferred on the basis of selective effects on isolated organs in specific species, but their relevance to actions in man is largely unsubstantiated due to a relative absence of early clinical-pharmacology studies in this category of compounds. There is also a high base rate for spontaneously occurring complaints or placebo-induced side effects in psychiatric populations that complicates interpretation even in controlled studies.

There is a wide range of interindividual sensitivity and susceptibility between patients and very little consistent correlation between plasma levels and particular side effects.

All tricyclic compounds (with the possible exception of protriptyline) have sedative effects, but to a variable degree that may be wanted or unwanted depending on a particular patient's apathy or agitation. A spectrum of anticholinergic activity is also observable in clinical-pharmacology studies which may give rise to troublesome side effects such as dry mouth, sweating, confusion, constipation, blurred vision and urinary hesitancy depending on individual patient susceptibility. Weight gain is a common and troublesome side effect of unknown cause.

The side effects of most serious concern relate to the cardiovascular system and seizure threshold. Actions on the adrenergic and cholinergic systems probably contribute to both hypotensive effects and direct cardiac actions that include alterations in heart rate, quinidine-like delays in conduction and decreases in myocardial contractility. The seizure threshold is lowered, increasing the frequency of epileptic convulsions. All these side effects can occur in therapeutic dosages in susceptible populations such as the elderly, children, and cardiac or epileptic patients, but are also a major cause of morbidity and mortality in accidental or intended overdose. Doses in excess of 0.5 grams can be seriously toxic and fatalities are fairly common when 2 grams or more are ingested.

Hypersensitivity reactions Tricyclic antidepressants have been reported rarely to produce cholestatic jaundice and agranulocytosis. The rare liver necrosis may reflect severe hypersensitivity. Two fatal cases of hypersensitivity myocarditis and hepatitis have been described (85[c]). A variety of dermatological manifestations are alleged (rash, urticaria, vasculitis), but their relationship to drug ingestion is often uncertain. A single case of pulmonary hypersensitivity with pleural effusions and eosinophilia has been reported with desipramine (86[C]).

Tumor-inducing effects These have not been reported.

GENERAL TOPICS

Plasma levels and side effects Plasma levels of antidepressants are influenced by pharmacogenetic factors and age, as well as interactions due to concomitant treatment with other drugs. A number of studies have attempted to define the relationship between the plasma levels of tricyclic antidepressants and their side effects. Like the data relating therapeutic outcome to plasma levels (87[R]) the results are conflicting (SEDA-3, 12; SEDA-5, 15). Sometimes there is a clear relationship between cardiac toxicity and elevated plasma levels (88[C], 89[CR], 90[C]) but in some individuals cardiotoxic effects occur at presumed therapeutic levels. Sporadic reports of severe side effects, mostly of the anticholinergic type, have often been associated with high plasma levels of amitriptyline or nortriptyline (91[C], 92[C]), although these vary with each drug and from patient to patient. Preskorn and Jerkovich found that the risk of central nervous system toxicity in patients treated with tricyclic antidepressants was correlated with plasma concentrations, age and gender (SEDA-16, 8; SEDA-17, 17). It may be concluded that routine plasma level monitoring is generally of little practical value in management of patients with side effects but, in view of the great interindividual variability in pharmacokinetics of the tricyclic antidepressants, it may be useful in those patients who report side effects at low doses.

Side effects in the elderly The elderly are often taking other drugs that may cause depression or interact with its treatment (93[R]). These potential sources of variance are superimposed on the wide range of plasma levels reported among individuals and the differences between drugs in dose—response profiles. The dictates of safe practice are that treatment in the elderly be initiated at lower dosages (50 mg imipramine or equivalent daily) in divided amounts with smaller increments (50 mg imipramine per week) and reduced total dose range (75—150 mg/day except in exceptional circumstances) (94[R]). Close attention should be paid to the potential anticholinergic, neurological or cardiovascular complications to which the elderly are especially vulnerable (95[R]). The greater risk of elderly to develop side effects has been discussed in SEDA-18 (p. 17).

Once-daily dosage Most studies that compare once-daily with divided regimens for a variety of tricyclic compounds have reported equal efficacy and reduced side effects on the once-daily regimens (SEDA-3, 10).

The significance of such regimens on compliance may have been exaggerated somewhat. Multiple drugs have a much clearer impact on compliance than do multiple dosages of a single drug. Compliance is not usually impaired until more than three tablets daily are prescribed (96[R]). A patient who forgets to take a single dose on a once-daily regimen loses more therapeutic effect than a patient who is equally forgetful on a divided regimen. Divided regimens may also be useful for patients who benefit from the short-term sedative action of these drugs during the daytime.

Some side effects may be more marked in single large doses, particularly in vulnerable patients. One study reported an increased frequency of frightening dreams when tricyclic antidepressants were given in a single bedtime dose (97[C]). Elderly patients given large single doses at bedtime may be at risk of dizziness, ataxia and confusion caused by postural hypotension when they attempt to get out of bed in the dark (98[C]).

Compatibility with electroconvulsive therapy An important practical question concerns the compatibility of tricyclic antidepressants and electroconvulsive therapy (ECT). This has been studied in 15 patients receiving 150—250 mg/day of imipramine or amitriptyline who received four to 16 ECT treatments (99[CR]). Continuous monitoring of cardiac function by oscilloscopy revealed arrhythmias in 40% of the ECT sessions. Single premature atrial contractions were noted in 46 out of 151 sessions and one to three premature ventricular beats occurred in 12 sessions. Transient ventricular tachycardia occurred in one 32-year-old woman taking 250 mg amitriptyline, who received 12 ECT treatments. The authors conclude that the cardiac effects are similar to those observed in previous studies of ECG changes during ECT in patients not taking antidepressants, and express the opinion that combined therapy does not involve any increased risk of serious cardiac arrhythmia. A controlled comparison (100[C]) of ECT given to 19 patients receiving tricyclic antidepressants and 27 control patients revealed no difference in heart rate, blood pressure or ectopic heart beats.

Tricyclic antidepressants and enuresis Although pediatric psychopharmacology is a much-neglected science, nocturnal enuresis is an area of extensive research. An earlier review (101[R]) catalogued almost 100 publications on the topic. The tricyclic antidepressants have shown efficacy in adequate and well-controlled trials and over 40 publications had appeared before 1970. At that time, the side effects appeared minimal and comparable to those encountered in adults. Since then, considerable concern has developed over the cardiotoxic effects and risks due to accidental overdose in children. The earlier reports were summarized in SEDA-1 (p. 10). SEDA-2 (p. 10) reviewed a method of managing overdose in children, and SEDA-3 (p. 9) reported an additional death in a 16-month-old infant.

Sudden death, possibly related to cardiac effects in children and adolescents, has been discussed in the SED Annuals 15, 16 and 18, and it is concluded that children receiving tricyclic antidepressants require careful monitoring of the ECG even when relatively low doses are used (SEDA-18, 18).

The symptoms of intoxication in children being treated with tricyclic antidepressants may fail to be recognized in time, as demonstrated in a number of cases published in the former German Democratic Republic (102[CR]) which led to serious consideration of the abandonment of such treatment in that country.

The British Committee on Review of Medicines has recommended that these drugs should not be used in children under 6 years of age and be given for periods not to exceed 3 months and then only after full examination (including ECG) and consideration of other treatment.

ORGANS AND SYSTEMS

Cardiovascular The cardiac toxicity of tricyclic antidepressants has been a source of continued concern in 'at risk' populations as well as in adults and children due to intended or accidental overdose. Unwanted cardiovascular effects represent a major therapeutic limitation for this category of drugs and a potential area of advantage among tricyclic compounds of differing structure as well as between these compounds and the newer, second-generation antidepressant drugs. The cardiovascular effects of tricyclic and the new generation of antidepressants have recently been reviewed (SEDA-18, 16—17; 103[R]).

Since the inception of the SED Annuals in 1977, each volume has reported the evolving literature and focused on the specific aspects including direct myocardial actions (SEDA-12, 13), hypotension (SEDA-12, 13) and the incidence, severity and management of overdose in adults and children (SEDA-10, 19; SEDA-11, 16) (88[C], 104[C]—105[C], 106[CR], 107[c], 108[c]).

Direct myocardial actions Tricyclic antidepressants are highly concentrated in the myocardium; this may account for the vulnerability of the heart as a target organ as well as for the inconsistent and inconclusive relationships reported between plasma levels of a drug and specific manifestations of cardiac toxicity. The drugs interfere with the normal rate, rhythm and contractility of the heart through actions on both nerve and muscle that are mediated by at least four different mechanisms (singly, in combination or due to imbalance) including an anticholinergic action, interference with re-uptake of adrenergic amines, direct myocardial depression, and alterations in membrane permeability due to lipophilic and surfactant properties.

Acute experiments in animals have shown a negative inotropic effect sufficient to induce congestive cardiac failure in dogs, but a carefully conducted chronic study in man did not show impaired left ventricular function in depressed patients with concurrent congestive failure (SEDA-9, 18). In a further study (109[C]) nortriptyline (mean daily dosage 76 mg, mean plasma level 107 ng/ml) was given to 21 depressed patients with either congestive cardiac failure or enlarged hearts. In this study nortriptyline was effective and well tolerated, producing only one episode of intolerable hypotension.

The most readily observable change in cardiac function is the *sinus tachycardia* which occurs in a majority of treated patients, but to a variable degree, and which is correlated to a weak or inconsistent degree with plasma levels (88[C], 104[C]—105[C]). The mechanism may be related to both central and peripheral effects on cholinergic and adrenergic systems, but is not simply a reflex response to hypotension (88[CR]). The presence of tachycardia can serve as an indirect measure of compliance (88[C]), but it is seldom a cause for concern, except in individuals who anxiously monitor their own physiological function.

The complex changes that occur in *cardiac rhythm* have been intensively studied using 24-hour high-speed and fidelity ECG tracings, and the technique of His bundle electrocardiography (110[CR], 111[C]) as well as cardiac catheterization (112[C], 113[C]). The changes in *conduction* and *repolarization* are manifested as prolongation of the PR, QRS and QT intervals and flattening or inversion of the T-waves on routine ECGs; the conduction delay occurs distal to the atrioventricular node and is apparent as a prolonged H-V interval (time from activation of the bundle of His to contraction of ventricular muscle). This effect resembles that due to Type I cardiac antiarrhythmic drugs such as quinidine and procainamide. These conduction changes may result in *atrioventricular or bundle branch blockage* and may predispose to re-entrant excitation currents with *ventricular ectopic beats, tachycardia or fibrillation*.

The implications and complications of these changes in cardiac function and rhythm are less clear; knowledge of their existence provoked concern about the incidence of *sudden death* in patients with cardiovascular disease, but the evidence from epidemiological sources remains equivocal (106[CR]). General guidelines for the use of these drugs in the elderly have been discussed above and a review of studies on the cardiovascular effects of therapeutic doses of tricyclics supports their use in elderly patients and those with pre-existing cardiovascular disease, provided due precautions are taken. Recently atrial fibrillation was reported in predisposed elderly subjects (SEDA-18, 19). In children treated with desipramine there are reports on sudden death (114[C], 115[C]) and tachycardia and ECG evidence of an intraventricular conduction defect (SEDA-18, 18; 116[C]).

The antiarrhythmic effect of imipramine was first reported in 1977 during treatment of two depressed patients whose ventricular premature depolarizations improved during treatment (117[C]). While it is reassuring to note these antiarrhythmic effects, it is also important to recognize that tricyclic compounds may still trigger serious arrhythmias at higher dose levels and perhaps also in situations where the myocardium is sensitized.

Caution should be exercised in patients after a recent myocardial infarction who have evidence of impaired conduction (first-degree heart block, bundle-branch block or prolonged QTc interval) since tricyclic antidepressants might theoretically add to the already increased risk of ventricular fibrillation in such patients (95[CR]). Earlier reviews in these volumes have discussed these effects and given practical guidelines for the use of tricyclic antidepressants in patients with heart disease (118[R]).

There is sometimes a clear-cut relationship between cardiac toxicity and elevated plasma levels (SEDA-18, 18; 88[C], 89[CR], 90[C]), but this may not always be so in individuals who are highly sensitive to the drug or in whom prolonged treatment may have led to accumulation of drug in the myocardium despite normal plasma levels. Routine plasma level monitoring does not seem indicated since plasma levels account for only a small part of the variance in cardiac effects (104[C]). If an individual patient shows significant changes clinically or on repeat ECG, then a spot measurement may reveal an elevated plasma level requiring dose reduction.

To date, there have been no prospective studies that clearly demonstrated increased mortality in cardiac patients following use of a tricyclic antidepressant. It has been suggested that the overall mortality due to cardiac disease may be higher in depressed patients who remain untreated than in those who receive either an antidepressant or ECT (119[CR]). Even in patients who have chronic heart disease, the risks of effective treatment with a tricyclic appear minimal (120[C]).

Hypotension As many as 20% of patients treated with adequate doses of a tricyclic may experience marked postural hypotension; this effect does not appear to be consistently correlated with plasma levels of drug and tolerance does not develop during treatment (121[c], 122[C], 123[CR]). The mechanism for this effect remains uncertain; it has been attributed to a peripheral antiadrenergic action, a myocardial depressant effect and to an action mediated by α-adrenergic receptors in the central nervous system (124[CR]). Studies of left ventricular function in human subjects are conflicting. One study using systolic time intervals (125[C]) found a decrement in left ventricular function with therapeutic doses, while two that have observed cardiac function directly with cardiac catheterization following overdose (126[Cr], 127[C]) have found no evidence of impaired myocardial efficiency and the hypotension persisted after left ventricular filling pressures and cardiac output were normal.

Postural hypotension can lead to significant problems in some patients, including severe falls and lacerations. Its occurrence may be predictable, since patients who have elevated systolic pressures and who show a pronounced postural drop before treatment are most likely to experience drug-induced hypotension (124[CR]). Such patients should be cautioned to rise slowly from sedentary positions and, since the elderly may be especially at risk for falls at night, single large bedtime doses of sedative tricyclic drugs should be avoided. These preventive measures are the most helpful, since the hypotensive effect is not directly related to plasma levels of drug, may not improve with dose reduction, and the wisdom of using sympathomimetic drugs to counter this unwanted effect is questionable (128[C]).

Cardiovascular complications of overdose The relationship between dose of tricyclic antidepressant ingested and development of life-threatening cardiovascular complications is inexact and individually variable (129[C], 130[C]), although plasma levels above 1000 ng/ml are cause for serious concern. Plasma levels vary widely and absorption can be delayed or deceptive due to gastric stasis and enterohepatic recycling (131[Cr]). Dysrhythmias may occur for the first time for up to 36 hours after drug ingestion or admission to hospital (131[Cr]). The frequency of serious cardiac conditions in one series of 68 cases (132[C]) was almost double (46%) in patients who took over 2000 mg of imipramine or its equivalent as compared to those who took less (only 25%). The cardiovascular complications reported in an intensive study of 35 overdose patients (126[Cr]) found that about half (51%) had significant hypotension and four-fifths (80%) had abnormal ECGs. The latter consisted of sinus tachycardia (71%) and various abnormalities reflective of impaired conduction including prolongation of QT_c interval (86%), prolongation of QRS complex (29%) and prolonged PR interval (11%). Abnormal ST and T-wave segments were found in about a quarter of patients (28%). Despite these manifestations of disturbed conduction and repolarization, there were relatively few arrhythmias; 13 patients (37%) had ventricular ectopic beats lasting up to 72 hours after admission which subsided within 36 hours in most (10) cases. No patients developed sustained repetitive ventricular tachyarrhythmias and the authors speculate that bizarre wide QRS complexes reflective of aberrantly conducted supraventricular tachycardia (present in cases) may sometimes be misinterpreted as ventricular tachycardia.

The basic principles of intensive supportive care should be applied early and artificial ventilation may often be necessary, since respiratory depression is more frequent than commonly supposed (133[C], 134[C]). Patients whose initial (or subsequent) ECG shows a dysrhythmia should be placed on a cardiac monitor for 24 hours. A discussion (135[R]) of monitoring policy for cardiac complications found that among 75 patients with overdose nobody with a normal ECG and level of consciousness for 24 hours went on to develop any significant arrhythmia. However, a case was subsequently reported (136[C]) of a patient who died an acute cardiac death 57 hours after admission and 33 hours after normalization of the ECG. The authors suggest that prolonged monitoring may be justified in individuals who have taken antidepressants for prolonged periods compared to those who overdose early in treatment.

More specific treatment to combat cardiotoxic effects is usually necessary in only a minority of instances; in the series reported above (126[Cr]), five patients (14%) experienced marked hypotension. Initial low left ventricular filling pressures were corrected within 3 hours by infusion of normal saline (1.5 ± 0.7 liters). Systemic hypotension persisted and was corrected by infusion of sympathomimetic amines. Langou et al. (126[Cr]) recommend routine insertion of a pulmonary artery catheter, with continuous monitoring of blood gases, pulmonary arterial pressure, left atrial wedge pressure and cardiac output. Volume expansion is suggested for low left atrial pressure with dopamine infusion to improve myocardial contractility if cardiac output remains low.

The management of ventricular ectopic activity is based on recognition of the quinidine-like basis of the conduction defect; in the series reported above (126[Cr]), all 13 patients with ventricular arrhythmias responded to intravenous infusion of lidocaine (2.0 ± 0.5 mg/min). This fact alone might account for the absence of any fatalities in this series.

Another indirect method of benefiting the patient with cardiotoxic effects has been the alkalinization of the plasma to pHs of 7.50—7.55 using sodium bicarbonate infusions (137[C]). This technique enhances plasma protein binding, thus making the drug less available to the tissues. It is claimed that this technique may result in a reversal of both hypotension and cardiac dysrhythmias without the risk of unwanted effects due to more specific pharmacological agents (131[Cr]). Recommendations for the management of poisoning with tricyclics given in a recently published review of the literature are summarized in SEDA-16 (p. 8).

Differences between tricyclic compounds Among the tricyclic antidepressants, there has been evidence to suggest that doxepin may have significantly less of a direct cardiotoxic effect (138[R]). However, a complete review of all the animal and clinical data cautions that doxepin overdose may still cause lethal arrhythmias in man, probably by producing more marked respiratory depression.

Three different studies conclude that there is less relative risk of hypotension in patients treated with nortriptyline (139[C]—141[C]) than with other tricyclic compounds. A similar claim has been made for doxepin (142[C]).

Increased pulse rate and blood pressure have been associated with desipramine in the treatment of bulimia nervosa (SEDA-17, 18).

Respiratory There is one case report of decreased ventilatory response to hypercapnia following nortriptyline in a woman with chronic obstructive pulmonary disease (SEDA-18, 19).

Nervous system Miscellaneous symptoms which have been attributed to the tricyclic antidepressants include fatigue, weakness, dizziness, headache and tremor; patients may be prone to fall because of these disturbances.

Seizures are serious adverse events associated with the use of antidepressants and the relative frequency of this side effect for different antidepressants has for a long time been a matter of controversy. A recent review (143[R]) critically evaluated the literature taking into account predisposing factors for seizures, drug doses, plasma drug level and duration of drug treatment. They found that a significant proportion of seizures occur in predisposed individuals, and that seizure risk for most antidepressants increases with dose or blood level. Following overdose the seizure risk seems to be higher for amoxapine and the tetracyclic drug maprotiline than for other antidepressants, but for several drugs there are not enough data to estimate that risk. Imipramine was found to be the most frequently studied tricyclic and the literature indicates a seizure risk of 0.3–0.6% at effective doses. For several of the second generation antidepressants a lower seizure risk has been reported in large clinical trials. Caution with all antidepressants should certainly be exercised in people predisposed to seizure activity by brain damage or alcohol and drug abuse.

A potential risk factor may be the concurrent use of lithium. A well-documented case report (144[C]) describes a 34-year-old woman treated with amitriptyline 300 mg each night for several years. Six days after starting lithium 300 mg t.i.d. the patient experienced several grand-mal seizures. A second episode occurred on re-exposure to lithium.

Patients with phobias or panic disorders display extreme sensitivity to side effects of tricyclic drugs early in treatment. They often manifest a syndrome of fine tremors, insomnia and anxiety that can be characterized as '*jitteriness*' and which is sometimes attributed to adrenergic hypersensitivity (SEDA-13, 9). Yeragani et al. (SEDA-17, 19; 145[C]) found significantly lower *serum iron levels* in jittery patients than those who were not affected. The authors suggest this may be related to the role of iron as a co-factor for tyrosine hydroxylase. This deserves further research.

Because the tricyclic antidepressants suppress REM sleep, they have been used in the management of narcolepsy and cataplexy when amphetamines fail or abuse potential is high. Clomipramine has been reported most effective, possibly due to more pronounced actions on serotonergic mechanisms (146[C]).

Three separate reports in the literature (147[C]–149[C]) refer to a type of *difficulty in articulation* described as 'speech blockade' or 'dysarthria'. The disturbance is described as a delay in thinking and speech, in which the patient has difficulty conceiving or transferring the next logical thought into words. The effect resembles a stammer.

Cognitive impairment has been associated with nortriptyline in elderly subjects (SEDA-17, 19).

There have been sporadic reports of *bilateral foot-drop* with peroneal nerve involvement (150[C]).

A *major neuropathy*, with high stepping gait, and inability to dorsiflex the foot, occurred in an 84-year-old woman. This presumed adverse effect remitted 8 weeks after stopping treatment (151[C]).

Unusual psychiatric or neurological reactions have several times been observed, generally where mixtures of drugs (often including maprotiline) have been given (152[C]). The symptoms comprised ataxia, akathisia, hypokinetic disorders of speech and motion, a 'dream state' and transient derangement of memory.

Confusional reactions were observed in 13% of 150 patients being treated with tricyclic drugs, occurring in as many as 35% of patients over 40 years of age. All responded rapidly to withdrawal of the drug (SEDA-9, 26).

Older persons are supposedly sensitive to the provocation of delirium by centrally acting anticholinergic drugs. Such side effects variously take the form of anxiety, agitation or frank hypomania. The situation may be rendered more likely if the patient is also receiving antipsychotic drugs, most of which also have a weak anticholinergic effect, and/or antiparkinson drugs of the anticholinergic type. Although long recognized as a risk associated with the anticholinergic properties of these drugs, one report (153[CR]) suggests the incidence may be lower than is often assumed. An epidemiological study from a (West) German multicenter drug surveillance system (154[C]) studied this side effect in almost 14 000 patients during a 5-year time period. Exposure-related incidence rates were 1.2% for tricyclic antidepressants compared to 0.8% for both tranylcypromine and neuroleptics. The risk increased steadily with age in both sexes and all diagnostic subgroups and was 6-

fold higher in those over age 60 (3.4%). Also at higher risk were women and patients with affective psychosis.

The neuroleptic malignant syndrome has been reported in association with the antidepressants amoxapine (SEDA-16, 9; SEDA-17, 18; 155[C]), trimipramine (156[C]) and desipramine (SEDA-17, 18). In most cases reported the patients were being treated with several other drugs, but there are reports of this syndrome in association with amoxapine or desipramine alone.

Aggressiveness during treatment in patients taking imipramine and amitriptyline in relatively low doses has been described (157[C]). *Violent behaviour* has also been attributed to amitriptyline (SEDA-17, 18).

A *serotonin syndrome* has been reported in a man taking clomipramine alone. This syndrome has been associated with several tricyclic antidepressants when they are used in combination with MAO-inhibitors (69[R]).

Extrapyramidal symptoms Tricyclic antidepressants are often listed among the manifold drugs capable of producing bucco-facio-lingual or choreoathetoid movements, and there are documented cases reported (158[Cr]). A putative mechanism is the central anticholinergic action of the antidepressant upsetting the balance between dopaminergic and cholinergic systems. The spontaneous occurrence of this syndrome makes it difficult to establish a cause-and-effect relationship, although both the patients described in the above report experienced symptoms again when rechallenged with the drug (amitriptyline in normal dosages for several weeks).

A more clear-cut cause-and-effect relationship seems to be present in the parkinsonian symptoms that occasionally occur on high-dosage tricyclic therapy in susceptible individuals (particularly elderly females). Because of its piperazine side chain and structural resemblance to phenothiazines, amoxapine has antidopaminergic properties that appear to produce typical dystonic reactions (159[C]), but other tricyclic antidepressants may also be implicated in producing the full range of so-called extrapyramidal syndromes including akathisia, dystonic reactions, parkinsonism and tardive dyskinesia. Case reports are described in SEDA-16 (p. 9), SEDA-17 (p. 18) and SEDA 18 (p. 18).

We have previously reported (SED-11, 40) the widely held belief that there is a significant risk that tricyclic antidepressants may precipitate *mania* or *rapid cycling* in up to 10% of patients and that various clinical features may increase this possibility, including being female, younger, having an earlier onset of illness and a positive first-degree family history. Biochemical risk factors have been alleged to include patients who have a low urinary excretion of MHPG; the risk is possibly greater in patients treated with tricyclic antidepressants rather than MAO inhibitors and particularly clomipramine.

The data on which these conclusions were based have now been rigorously analyzed (160[R]) in an article which reviews the controversy around the alternative suggestion that the so-called switch effect is a random manifestation of bipolar illness. There is an absence of both prospective or long-term placebo-controlled studies and the existing research has suffered from unrepresentative samples and poor definition of manic outcomes. The conclusion of this review was that '. . . some bipolar patients and few if any unipolar patients become manic when they are treated with antidepressants. A small number of patients develop rapid cycling.'

This more cautious conclusion is supported by a prospective study (161[CR]) of 230 carefully selected patients with recurrent depression (at least two episodes, with an average of six) treated with imipramine (200 mg daily) for an average of over 46 weeks. Mania and hypomania were defined and measured by the Raskin rating scale. Only six patients (2.6%) developed hypomania and four of these did so after discontinuation of treatment, suggesting a withdrawal effect. Younger patients, women and those with a previous history of hypomania (Bipolar II) were no more likely to switch than unipolar patients.

These results suggest that the risk of mania or hypomania in long-term treatment of recurrent unipolar depressed patients is relatively small. The 12 placebo-controlled studies of acute treatment in less carefully defined samples support a higher incidence rate of around 6–7% for hypomania and 1–2% for mania but may be inflated by the inclusion of bipolar patients with a high risk of a spontaneous switch (160[R]).

Endocrine, metabolic *Weight gain* has long been known as a concomitant of antidepressant and antipsychotic therapy. It may be part of the improved mental state but, aside from that, there appears to be a physiological component with an increased craving for sweets (162[CR]). No abnormalities have been found in fasting glucose and insulin levels or in intravenous insulin tolerance tests (162[CR], 163[CR]). Another possible suggestion for weight gain was that taste perception in depressed people improves after therapy with tricyclic antidepressants (164[C]). A study on 50 depressed patients attempted to address some of these issues (165[C]). An increased energy efficiency during antidepressive treatment has also been suggested to be the reason for weight gain (SEDA-17, 8). A warning to diabetic patients that masking of hypoglycemia can occur seems appropriate (166[C]).

Inappropriate antidiuretic hormone secretion The US Department of Health and Welfare's 'Division of Drug Experience' issued a note on five cases of the 'syndrome of inappropriate antidiuretic hormone secretion' and drugs which have been ascribed to it (167[Cr]). All involved drugs possessed a tricyclic structure; one patient was being treated with the antidepressant, imipramine, others with the closely related muscle relaxant, cyclobenzaprine, and the remaining three with the antiepileptic drug, carbamazepine. The imipramine dose was 50 mg/day for 3 weeks and the patient was a woman of 72. Other cases have been reported, involving amitriptyline (168[C]), imipramine and protriptyline (SEDA-17, 17).

Prolactin levels are very rarely altered during treatment with tricyclic antidepressants, but this is more likely to occur and to produce symptoms of galactorrhea or amenorrhea with clomipramine and amoxapine and when there are other contributory factors that may stimulate prolactin secretion, such as stress or treatment with ECT (169[Cr]).

Hematological *Agranulocytosis* has been associated with tricyclics (170[CR]). Of 21 cases, eight were fatal and 12 recovered after 3—20 days.

Two cases of *non-thrombocytopenic purpura* were observed in patients treated with tricyclics. Both responded to discontinuation of treatment (171[C]). True thrombocytopenia with counts as low as 12 000 platelets per microliter was observed in a 79-year-old woman treated with doxepin. During a later course of treatment with amitriptyline, thrombocytopenia recurred, but it did not appear when she was treated with imipramine (172[C]). Cross-sensitivity must be highly specific to the chemical structure, doxepin and amitriptyline being more like each other than imipramine. Occasional cases of blood dyscrasias with tricyclics continue to be reported (SEDA-12, 46; SEDA-18, 18). Antidepressant-induced blood dyscrasias have recently been reviewed (173[R]).

Liver *Jaundice* associated with *cholestasis* was among the first side effects reported with phenothiazines, tricyclic antidepressants and monoamine-oxidase inhibitors. Its incidence appears to have declined for reasons that are not understood, but under-reporting may be a factor. Elevation of liver enzymes, especially transaminases and alkaline phosphatases, is quite common during treatment with both phenothiazines and tricyclic antidepressants. Such findings are usually benign, but one careful study (174[C]) of a patient taking amitriptyline revealed biopsy findings of mononuclear and eosinophilic infiltration; cholestasis and clinical jaundice were absent. In a controlled study comparing lofepramine and the selective serotonin re-uptake inhibitor fluoxetine, significant increase in alkaline phosphatase, ALT and GT were seen in lofepramine- but not in fluoxetine-treated patients (175[C]).

More serious and sometimes fatal *liver necrosis* has been reported with a number of different tricyclic structures and probably represents an extreme form of allergic hypersensitivity (176[CR], 177[C]).

A case (178[C]) involving a 33-year-old woman treated with imipramine 300 mg daily for over a month led the authors to suggest that once-daily dosage may pose a special hazard because peak levels may exceed the toxic level even though steady-state plasma levels are in the normal range.

A particular hazard appears to be posed by amineptine. French authors reported over 26 cases of toxic hepatitis (179[Cr]). In most instances, hepatitis occurred within the normal dose range and recurred on rechallenge with drug, but in several instances it was reported after an overdose.

There is no indication for routine liver-function tests in patients receiving tricyclic antidepressants; elevated transaminases and alkaline phosphatases within the upper ranges of normal are not a cause for serious concern unless accompanied by clinical signs or symptoms indicative of liver dysfunction.

Anticholinergic activity Several organ systems are the target for the anticholinergic (antimuscarinic) activity of these compounds. They constitute the most common and troublesome adverse effects of the tricyclic antidepressants, but the peripheral anticholinergic actions may also be put to therapeutic use in such conditions as irritable bowel syndrome, premature ejaculation and nocturnal enuresis.

Experiments on receptor binding in the rat brain and guinea-pig ileum have shown a spectrum of activity at the muscarinic acetylcholine receptor for different tricyclic antidepressants (180[C]). Comparison of five compounds revealed that amitriptyline and doxepin were the most potent and desipramine the least active, with imipramine and nortriptyline being intermediate. Single-dose experiments in human volunteers (given up to 100 mg of each drug) have confirmed the same rank ordering of effect for both the peripheral anticholinergic actions (on salivary flow) and the central effects (sedation and other measures on a mood scale) (181[C]). The significance of these differences between relatively low single doses of these drugs in healthy volunteers should not be uncritically extended to clinical practice. However, they do provide a rationale for selecting among the different drugs for patients in whom either a high degree of sedation is desirable or anticholinergic effects are likely to be especially troublesome. No tricyclic compound is entirely free of anticholinergic action and individual differences in susceptibility or metabolism can still give rise to serious problems in some patients. It is also difficult to predict which particular organ system will become the major target for anticholinergic activity; some patients complain bitterly of *dry mouth*, others report *blurred vision* and some develop *bowel or bladder symptoms*. Careful history taking and physical examination will often reveal a possible cause for concern, based on the patient's previous response to similar drugs, existing disease (such as narrow-angle glaucoma, enlarged prostate, constipation) or advancing age.

Two unusual and seldom considered consequences of the anticholinergic actions of tricyclic compounds have been mentioned. The first (182[C]) concerns the *potential damage to the corneal epithelium* in patients who wear contact lenses due to decreased lacrimation and relative accumulation of mucoid secretions. The second (183[C]) reported the development of *rampant dental caries* due to *xerostomia* in a patient treated for over 2 years with up to 300 mg/day of doxepin. The author of this article warned of the need to counsel patients to carry out rigorous and regular dental hygiene as well as simple measures to promote increased salivation such as sugarless lemon drops or chewing gum. In another study there was an increase in the number of decayed teeth in a group of 35 children treated with amitriptyline or nortriptyline for enuresis compared to a smaller group of untreated enuretic children and to a larger matched population control group (184[C]).

It is valuable to know that adverse anticholinergic effects may occur immediately following the first dose of a tricyclic antidepressant. They are a major cause of poor compliance in patients who expect immediate relief, but who are not properly prepared for the delay that can occur in the beneficial effects of these drugs on mood and energy which are probably related to their effects on catecholamines and are dependent on higher plasma levels.

Gastrointestinal system Simple dietary advice concerning bulk foods may diminish the significance of minor bowel disturbances. More serious complications that can arise include paralytic ileus which may be life-threatening, especially in the elderly (185[c]). A less well-known adverse effect is the potential for aggravating or even possibly inducing a hiatus hernia, presumably due to the anticholinergic action of these drugs on the cardiac sphincter (186[C]).

Genitourinary system Clinical experiments have shown that the tricyclic antidepressants increase bladder sphincter tone and the volume of fluid necessary to trigger detrusor contraction (187[CR]). Such effects may account for the efficacy of tricyclic antidepressants in nocturnal enuresis, where the benefit occurs early and at a low dosage consistent with anticholinergic activity. This pharmacological action may produce hesitancy and more serious problems with urinary retention can occur, especially in predisposed males who have an enlarged prostate gland.

Renal damage from tricyclics has been suggested on only one occasion. A 65-year-old man receiving 300 mg/day developed toxic psychosis, anorexia and nausea following 24 days of treatment. He was mildly azotemic, but these changes quickly reverted following discontinuation of the drug. No biopsy or kidney function tests were reported. The findings are entirely compatible with prerenal azotemia associated with diminished fluid intake during a drug-induced psychosis (188[C]).

The eye Loss of accommodation and blurred vision are common inconveniences that can usually be tolerated in the knowledge that they lessen with the duration of treatment. Exacerbation of narrow-angle glaucoma in the elderly can occur, but is not an absolute contraindication to treatment with a tricyclic antidepressant since the anticholinergic effects can be balanced by judicious use of pilocarpine (189[c], 190[R]).

Sexual function A review of the literature (191[R]) regarding sexual dysfunction due to antidepressant drugs in men draws a distinction between erectile dysfunction, ejaculatory problems and changes in libido. A complicating factor is the lack of information concerning the base rate of these problems due to depression itself. The review draws on both published findings and reports provided by the pharmaceutical manufacturers. *Impotence* due to loss of erectile function has been reported involving all of the commonly used tricyclic compounds in the low normal dose ranges. *Delayed and occasionally painful ejaculation* occur and recently four cases of painful ejaculation in association with imipramine and clomipramine were reported (SEDA-17, 18). Both *increased and decreased libido* have been reported, but it is virtually impossible to distinguish drug relatedness from the natural history of the condition. A small number of uncontrolled studies have reported therapeutic benefits in patients with premature ejaculation or disturbed sexual function accompanied by clinical depression (192[C]).

The mechanism of action mediating the sexual dysfunction is assumed to be anticholinergic and one author has suggested (193[C]) taking prostigmine 15 mg 1 hour before intercourse to reverse ejaculatory dysfunction.

In addition to these reports of sexual dysfunction in men, *delay of orgasm* or *lost ability to obtain orgasm* has also been reported in women (194[C]).

Skin Skin *rashes* are so common that it is difficult to determine a cause-and-effect relationship to drug treatment. A choice must be made between waiting to see if the rash clears despite continued treatment or switching to a different compound and, if necessary, rechallenging the patient at a later date. Other skin reactions reported include *cutaneous vasculitis, urticaria and photosensitivity*. A *grey discoloration of the skin* in photo-exposed areas have been associated with long-term therapy with imipramine and desipramine (SEDA-17, 19; SEDA-18, 18). Pigmentary changes in the iris were also reported in one of the cases. Amineptine has been reported (195[C]) to cause a particularly active *acne*, occurring beyond the usual distribution on the body and beyond the usual age, especially in women. The action recommended is cessation of amineptine. A single case of a *rosacea-like eruption* on the face of a 76-year-old woman was also caused by this drug, and the association was confirmed by re-challenge (196[C]).

Special senses *Vision* (*see also 'Anticholinergic activity' above*) Bright light treatment is used for mood disorders and it has been suggested that antidepressants which may act as photosensitisers could enhance the effect of bright light on the eye giving rise to adverse effects (SEDA-18, 17).

Hearing An example of an unwanted effect to appear after prolonged availability of a particular type of drug is the *tinnitus* reported to occur during treatment with tricyclic antidepressants. An early trial of imipramine (197[C]) reported two cases of transient *deafness*, but in the subsequent 20 years no auditory manifestations were recorded. In 1980, a report appeared (198[Cr]) concerning four patients all treated with imipramine in daily dosages below 150 mg. Each patient complained of buzzing or ringing in the ears. In each case the symptoms improved or disappeared on dose reduction with maintenance of therapeutic benefit and in one instance the patient was switched to an equivalent dosage of desipramine without a recurrence.

A further case report (199[C]) concerned a patient treated with protriptyline 45 mg daily who developed ringing in both ears after 12 days of treatment. The symptom severity decreased with dosage reduction and disappeared entirely after desipramine (100 mg daily) was substituted. The authors of this report speculate on the possible mechanism and postulate a non-vibratory tinnitus originating from either neurological factors or changes in blood flow. A chart review of 475 patients treated with tricyclic antidepressants (200[CR]) found five patients with tinnitus. Each developed the symptom in the second or third week of treatment at daily dosages of imipramine between 150 and 250 mg with plasma levels between 200 and 400 ng/ml. In every case tinnitus subsided spontaneously within a further 2—4 weeks of its onset even though dosage and plasma levels remained constant.

Another unusual disturbance of hearing has been reported in a child being treated with tricyclics. Auditory acuity was normal, but discriminative ability for both clear and distorted speech was depressed. The disorder cleared within some days of the withdrawal of the drug (201[C]).

Musical hallucinations have been reported in association with clomipramine (SEDA-17, 18).

Risk situations A variety of high-risk situations have been described throughout this Chapter, including children, the elderly, physically impaired and suicidal patients.

Withdrawal effects There is compelling evidence for a withdrawal syndrome due to abrupt discontinuation of tricyclic antidepressants (SEDA-5, 16) and the literature has recently been reviewed (202[R]). Many of the symptoms seen after acute withdrawal have been attributed to rebound cholinergic activation.

Reports have involved both imipramine and doxepin (203[CR]). Symptoms occur as early as the morning following a missed dose (204[C]), but more often after 48 hours and up to 2 weeks following discontinuation. They include anxiety, restlessness, diaphoresis, diarrhea, hot or cold flushes and piloerection. Amitriptyline withdrawal was followed by similar kinds of physical symptoms 36 hours after the last dose followed by severe depressive illness (SEDA-17, 18). A case of delirium following discontinuation of doxepine has been reported (205[C]) as well as instances of mania (206[CR]). A case with pronounced neurological symptoms following sudden cessation of amitriptyline has been described (SEDA-18, 18).

The existence of a withdrawal syndrome was subjected to a controlled test (203[CR]) in seven patients who had been maintained on chronic administration of amitriptyline (up to 250 mg daily), imipramine (200 mg daily) or desipramine (250 mg daily). After 4 weeks of supervised drug-taking, a placebo was substituted under double-blind conditions for 10—21 days. There were increases in both plasma and urine MHPG levels beginning within 36 hours and reaching a peak 3 weeks after discontinuation which averaged 74% above the baseline. Despite this pronounced neurochemical change there were no alterations in pulse rate or heart beat and only two patients experienced clear increases in anxiety.

There is clearly a need for larger controlled studies to determine the incidence and severity of withdrawal effects following cessation of tricyclic treatment. Based on uncontrolled observation, it has been suggested that the incidence varies from under a quarter to over a half of patients.

A report of three cases (207[Cr]) has suggested that central cholinergic overactivity is implicated and atropine sulfate (3 mg daily) or synthetic anticholinergic agents (benztropine mesylate 4 mg daily) were reported to successfully ameliorate withdrawal symptoms within a few hours. The authors suggest that this technique may be especially useful in patients who must be abruptly discontinued from tricyclics because the patient develops an allergic or idiosyncratic reaction to drug.

Second-generation effects An experimental study in chick embryos revealed a high prevalence of abnormalities, but the doses of imipramine used were close to lethal levels. *Microphthalmia*, *micromelia* and *reduced body size* were among several abnormalities noted (208[R]).

Clinically, the issue of dysmorphogenesis due to these drugs was first seriously discussed after a report on three possible cases by McBride from Australia in 1972 (209[c]). Although the data underlying this report were later discredited, it led to a careful study of the case records of women who had taken tricyclic antidepressants in pregnancy and more than 300 cases were rapidly identified in which such treatment had been followed by the birth of a normal infant. Other negative reports exonerating the drugs have appeared since (210[R]–213[R]), although sporadic case-reports continue to occur (214[CR]).

In spite of these reports negating a possible association between tricyclics and teratogenicity, it might be advisable to avoid these drugs during pregnancy, especially in the early stages, unless there is a compelling need for them. In many of the reports the drugs were used in low doses or for indications not justifying their application.

Effects on the neonate There are few reports concerning the excretion of antidepressant drugs in breast milk even though postpartum depression is a relatively common occurrence. A 32-year-old woman was treated with imipramine 200 mg daily from 1 month post partum (215[CR]). Detectable levels of both imipramine and desipramine were present in breast milk. Although the infant suffered no adverse effects, the authors advise caution because of the known hypersensitivity of young children to tricyclic antidepressants.

In two investigations simultaneous measurements of levels of antidepressant in the mother's plasma and milk revealed almost identical amounts of amitriptyline (216[C]) and desipramine (217[C]).

There is also a report (218[C]) of an 8-week-old breast-fed infant whose mother was treated with doxepin. Four days after an increase in the daily dosage from 10 to 75 mg the infant developed *respiratory depression* accompanied by an accumulation of the desmethylated derivative of doxepin in the baby's plasma.

Instances of *distress* in the newborn have been reported following treatment of the mothers with tricyclics in the period prior to delivery (219[CR]). In one case, an infant demonstrated signs of congestive heart failure without cardiac abnormality; in another, tachycardia and myoclonus were observed; a third infant showed respiratory distress and neuromuscular spasms. These clinical manifestations were thought to result from both the adrenergic and anticholinergic effects of the drug which readily passes the placenta and should be avoided during the perinatal period.

Another interesting observation (220[C]) has included the suggestion that effects noted in the neonate may be due to withdrawal from maternal antidepressants following birth. Two cases of *neonatal convulsions* are reported in infants whose mothers had been treated with clomipramine. In both cases the seizures occurred on the first day of life coincident with decline in plasma clomipramine levels. In one case the convulsions were controlled by administration of clomipramine followed by a tapered withdrawal. *Hypotonia* has been described in four cases where one of the children also developed jitteriness (SEDA-17, 18).

Overdosage Both accidental and intended overdose are relatively frequent problems which pose difficult management problems. Particular concern has been expressed for children either because they gain access to parents' tablets or have been treated for enuresis. During 1 year a Melbourne hospital admitted 35 children poisoned with tricyclics (221[R]). In 1979 it was reported that tricyclics had replaced salicylates as the commonest cause of accidental death in English children under the age of 5 which illustrates the risk with these drugs. An editorial in The Lancet (222[R]) expresses concern about this and Swiss federal statistics raise similar concerns (223[C]).

The majority of all deaths from antidepressant poisoning in England, Scotland and Wales during the periods 1975–1984 and 1985–1989 was due to two tricyclic drugs, amitriptyline and dothiepin, and they, as well as the whole group of older tricyclics, had a fatal toxicity index (deaths per million prescriptions) significantly higher than the mean (59[C]).

A major problem in evaluating the incidence and severity of the complications due to overdose in adults has been the reporting of individual cases or selected samples, often with the inclusion of patients who have taken multiple drugs or who suffer from concurrent physical disease. More reliable epidemiological surveys from a number of different countries (224[CR], 225[R], 226[CR]) indicate that the mean ingested overdose of a tricyclic antidepressant in adults is around 1000 mg, and that only about 3% of patients ingest a sufficient amount to cause fatal complications. There is considerable individual variability in response to overdose and there are conflicting reports on the degree to which there is a relationship between plasma levels and complications. One large study (227[C]) found that plasma levels in excess of 1000 ng/ml were associated with coma, convulsions, cardiac arrhythmias and a need for supportive measures. In other studies there has been no clear-cut correlation between the plasma concentration and the incidence of toxic complications (228[C]). The cardiac complications have been reviewed above and are serious, but should not detract from other serious effects. A review of all deaths due to these drugs in Britain during 1976 (229[CR]) found that dysrhythmias were less common than supposed (11 of 113 patients who died in hospitals), but that respiratory depression was more frequent (54 of 113 patients). Some such deaths might have been avoided by more frequent artificial ventilation and better attention to the principles of supportive care.

Management of overdose Dziukas and Vohra (230[R]) have in a recent review analyzed the literature on poisoning with tricyclic antidepressants. Their recommendations for the management of overdose are summarized in SEDA-16 (p. 8).

Interactions The large number of drugs with which tricyclic antidepressants may interact are summarized in Table 6 and those of major concern are discussed in more detail below.

Monoamine-oxidase (MAO) inhibitors The interactions of tricyclics and MAO inhibitors are so well known and so dangerous that they have constituted a formidable barrier to their combined clinical use. The temptation to treat refractory patients with this combination is great, but considerable caution should be applied (231[R], 232[R]) and it should be remembered that there is no firm proof of the superiority of such combinations. Several reviews (233[R]—235[R]) have arrived at the conclusion that the dangers of these interactions have been overstated and potential therapeutic advantages underestimated. On the other hand, reports of serious and fatal complications continue to appear (236[C], 237[C]).

Benzodiazepines A report (238[C]) describes four patients who developed adverse effects attributable to the combination with tricyclics including exacerbations of delusional thought disorder.

Phenothiazines A report in the Scandinavian literature (239[C]) concerns two patients on combinations of neuroleptics and tricyclic antidepressants who developed epileptic seizures. Risk of seizures is greater in patients with existing brain damage or epilepsy and in cases of high dosage, sudden increase in dosage or shortly after introduction of a second preparation.

The possible mechanism for these interactions with phenothiazines consists of elevated plasma levels of the tricyclic compounds due to competition for the hepatic cytochrome P-450 system that metabolizes both types of compounds (SEDA-9, 30; 240[C]). Antidepressant plasma levels may increase by up to 70% (241[C]).

A particularly dangerous combination is that of thioridazine with a tricyclic antidepressant since both are known to produce cardiac toxicity. One report (242[C]) concerns two young patients who developed ventricular arrhythmias from which they were fortunate to recover.

Other psychotropic drugs The evidence for interactions with other commonly prescribed psychotropic drugs is reviewed more extensively in SEDA-8 (p. 25).

SSRI Fluoxetine may raise blood levels of desipramine as well as nortriptyline if both drugs are given concurrently (243[C], 244[C], 245[R], 246[C]).

Cardiovascular drugs The safe management of either depressed patients with pre-existing cardiovascular disease or patients with cardiac complications of overdose depends on a knowledge of potential interactions among the different drugs used. The tricyclic antidepressants interact with directly and indirectly acting pressor amines, anticoagulants, antihypertensive agents and antiarrhythmic drugs, all of which may be prescribed in cardiovascular conditions.

Tricyclic antidepressants act on both pre- and postsynaptic neurons as well as on both α- and β-adrenergic receptors. Because their principal action is to block the re-uptake of noradrenaline at the presynaptic neuron, they potentiate the hypertensive effects of both directly and indirectly acting amines (247[C]—250[C]). The hypertensive effects of phenylephrine are increased by 2—3-fold and of noradrenaline by 4—8-fold. Even the administration of local anesthetics containing noradrenaline as a vasoconstrictor has proved fatal. The types of compounds that may produce this interaction and the symptoms that result have been previously reviewed in more detail (SEDA-1, 11).

The interaction with methylphenidate (250[C]) may be of particular significance because of claims that tricyclic antidepressants and methylphenidate have a synergistic effect on mood due to interference by methylphenidate with the metabolism of imipramine, resulting in increased blood levels of the tricyclic antidepressant. The occurrence of this hypertensive interaction calls for cau-

Table 6. *Interactions between tricyclic antidepressants and other substances*

Interacting substances	Type of interaction(s)	Comments
MAO inhibitors	Increased incidence of weight gain Increased anticholinergic effects Hyperthermia, hyperflexia, convulsions, death (very rare)	See text; see also monograph on MAO inhibitors earlier in this Chapter
Sympathomimetic agents	Potentiation of hypertensive effects with phenylephrine, noradrenaline, methylphenidate	Similar potentiation of effects with pheochromocytoma
Steroids	Metabolic interference Receptor interaction	Altered bioavailability of tricyclic drug Akathisia, exacerbation of psychosis
Alcohol	Additive sedative effects	May be more pronounced with more sedative tricyclic compounds
Morphine	Potentiation of analgesic effect of morphine	May partly be due to increased bioavailability of morphine
Phenothiazines	Increased plasma levels of tricyclic drug Possible potentiation and/or increased speed of onset of antidepressant effect Enhanced cardiotoxic effects with thioridazine	Due to impaired metabolism Presynaptic α_2-adrenergic blockade (animal studies) Ventricular arrhythmias may occur
Barbiturates	Decreased plasma levels of tricyclic drug	Hepatic microsomal induction
SSRI	Increased plasma level of tricyclic drug	Due to impaired metabolism
Cigarette-smoking	Decreased plasma levels of tricyclic drug	Probably increased metabolism
Disulfiram	Increased plasma levels of tricyclic drug	Probably impaired metabolism
Methylphenidate	Increased plasma levels of tricyclic drug	Probably impaired metabolism
Thyroid hormone	Increased receptor sensitivity to catecholamines	May manifest as spurious hyperthyroidism, increased cardiac irregularity, or enhanced therapeutic action of tricyclic in some cases
Anticholinergic agents	Additive effects on pupil, CNS, bowel and bladder	Particularly likely to occur when a tricyclic drug, phenothiazine and antiparkinsonian agent are prescribed concurrently
Antihypertensive agents	Reversal of hypotensive effects of clonidine, reserpine, α-methyldopa and guanethidine	Hypertension should be controlled with diuretics, β-blocking agents or vasodilators before treatment of depression
Membrane-stabilizing drugs (quinidine type)	Dose-related synergism	Digitalis preferred; free of interactions
Minocycline	Hyperpigmentation	Increased hemosiderosis
Cimetidine	Increased bioavailability of tricyclic drug	Due to impaired hepatic extraction

tion in the use of such combinations for which there is no established evidence.

Tricyclic antidepressants also reverse the hypotensive effects of postganglionic blocking agents, guanethidine, reserpine, clonidine and α-methyldopa, so that the addition of a tricyclic drug can result in loss of blood pressure control (251[R], 252[R]). Sudden withdrawal of a tricyclic compound from a patient stabilized with these compounds can also result in serious hypotension. An additional reason for avoiding drugs such as reserpine, methyldopa and propranolol in depressed cardiovascular patients is that these drugs may also cause or aggravate depression. Because of their similar lipophilic and surfactant properties, tricyclic antidepressants interact with membrane-stabilizing drugs of the quinidine type to interfere with the voltage-dependent stimulus and produce a dose-related synergism (253[R]). Digitalis preparations and β-blocking agents are free of this interaction, although animal studies have suggested an increased lethality of digoxin in rats pretreated with tricyclic antidepressants (254[C]) and propanolol may potentiate direct depression of myocardial contractility due to the tricyclic antidepressants. For all of the above reasons, the preferred treatment for tricyclic-induced arrhythmias is lidocaine. Even this is reported to be only variably effective and possibly to potentiate the hypotensive effects of tricyclic drugs (131[Cr]).

Overall, the multiple sites and mechanisms of action of the tricyclic compounds create at least the potential for an interaction with a variety of cardiovascular agents; exceptions occur only when another agent acts at a site unaffected by the tricyclic compound (such as diuretics on the kidney) or through a mechanism not directly related to adrenergic or cholinergic receptor activity. This suggests that each patient should be managed individually and conservatively; when more than one drug is prescribed, a knowledge of basic pharmacological mechanisms can enhance interpretation of the results obtained or the interactions that may (or may not) occur.

Anticoagulants Tricyclic antidepressants may interfere with the metabolism of oral anticoagulants and may increase their serum levels and prolong their pharmacological half-lives by as much as 300% (255[C]). Prothrombin levels should be carefully monitored in patients receiving oral anticoagulants.

Sex hormones Oral contraceptives have a complex effect on the metabolism of tricyclic drugs, resulting in decreased bioavailability (256[C]). Conjugated estrogens have also been reported to cause akathisia in some patients (257[C]) treated with tricyclic drugs.

Corticosteroids Patients treated with prednisone have experienced psychosis (258[C], 259[C]). Both this and the above-mentioned reaction with estrogens may be due to an interaction at dopamine receptor sites.

Alcohol Alcohol in combination with tricyclics impairs performance and it is customary to caution patients about this possibility when driving or handling machinery. Not only may additive impairment occur (mediated at the receptor level), but alcohol may modify the metabolism of the antidepressant (SEDA-8, 24).

Levodopa The anticholinergic effects of imipramine and other tricyclics may delay gastrointestinal motility enough to interfere with the absorption of various other drugs. Such was the case in an experimental study of the absorption of levodopa in four normal subjects (260[C]). It is likely that this action of the drug may interfere with absorption of other drugs as well, especially those, such as chlorpromazine, which are extensively metabolized during their stay in the gut.

Thyroid hormone Spurious hyperthyroidism was observed in a child receiving thyroid hormone and imipramine for enuresis (261[C]). The ability of thyroid hormone to increase receptor sensitivity to catecholamines has long been known and has been used to enhance clinical response in some refractory patients, especially women.

Anesthetic agents A brief report (262[CR]) from France concerns patients on tricyclic antidepressants which could not be discontinued before surgery. A total of 190 such patients underwent general and 61 local or regional anesthesia. There was no change in the cardiovascular effect of halothane, induction time with pentobarbital, propanidid or ketamine, and duration of depolarization or recovery time. The general conclusion was that it is safer to continue treatment with tricyclics than to risk potential disruption due to discontinuation of the drugs before surgery.

Electroconvulsive therapy The question of an interaction between tricyclics and ECT is discussed separately above.

INDIVIDUAL TRICYCLIC ANTIDEPRESSANTS

Amineptine

Amineptine has a 7-membered carbon side chain and is reported to have more stimulant and fewer sedative effects than other tricyclic compounds, possibly due to differential actions on dopaminergic rather than serotonergic mechanisms. As noted above, the compound appears to have an unusual propensity for causing hepatocellular damage that may limit its clinical utility (44[CE]).

Amineptine increases the release and reduces the reuptake of dopamine and it is therefore not surprising that an amphetamine-like drug dependence has been reported to occur for this antidepressant (263[C], 264[C], 265[C]). A withdrawal state occurs which may be improved by clonidine treatment (SEDA-16, 8).

Amitriptyline *N*-oxide

This metabolite of amitriptyline was compared with the parent drug. The antidepressant effects were comparable, but the metabolite was thought to have fewer side effects, especially cardiotoxic ones. The latter conclusion was based on the absence of ECG abnormalities among 15 patients treated (266[C]), but this is a very limited series on which to base such a conclusion.

Amoxapine

A major review (267[R]) of amoxapine and its pharmacology concludes that it is similar in clinical efficacy and potency to standard tricyclic compounds with a sedative action intermediate between amitriptyline and imipramine.

As previously noted (SEDA-4, 21; SEDA-5, 17), amoxapine has a tricyclic nucleus with a modified piperazine side chain and is closely related to the neuroleptic, loxapine. In animal studies, amoxapine has no antiserotinergic properties and less anticholinergic activity than prototype drugs. Peak plasma levels are achieved in less than 2 hours and the half-lives of the parent drug and its two active metabolites are 8, 6 and 30 hours.

Amoxapine is less potent than other tricyclic antidepressants with a therapeutic dose range of 75—600 mg daily (usual doses 200—400 mg daily). Clinical effects have not been consistently correlated with plasma levels, but the compound shows comparable efficacy to other tricyclics in heterogeneous populations of depressed patients. Controlled comparisons show its clinical profile to be very similar to imipramine (268[C]) and somewhat less sedative than amitriptyline (269[C]—271[C]). In two of these studies (269[C], 271[C]) results confirmed the suggestion of a somewhat earlier onset of action.

Amoxapine appears to share the same commonly occurring side effects as other tricyclic compounds including those attributable to anticholinergic activity. Its structural similarity to the neuroleptic compounds appears to confer an additional hazard of side effects usually found in that category of drugs, such as galactorrhea and extrapyramidal disorders (SEDA-9, 20). In a study of its potential neuroleptic properties (272[Cr]), amoxapine and its metabolite, 7-hydroxyamoxapine, were found to show potent neuroleptic activity using a radioreceptor assay both in vivo and using plasma drawn from patients receiving treatment with neuroleptics or antidepressants. Patients receiving amoxapine had comparable neuroleptic activity to those receiving loxapine while none of the other tricyclic antidepressants showed this property (amitriptyline, nortriptyline, imipramine and desipramine). Additional reports of side effects attributable to its neuroleptic profile continue to appear including tardive dyskinesia (273[C], 274[C]), acute torticollis (275[C]) and malignant neuroleptic syndrome (SEDA-16, 9; SEDA-17, 18; 276[C]).

A bleak picture has rapidly evolved for amoxapine with regard to its toxicity in overdose. Thirty-three cases were reported (277[Cr]) over an 18-month period from Washington DC and New Mexico Poison Centers. These cases included five patients who died and 12 who developed seizures. Thus, the mortality rate of 15.2% greatly exceeds that of 0.7% for other antidepressants in the same centers and the seizure rate is 36.4 compared to 4.3%. The authors express concern that 'the striking CNS toxicity of amoxapine overdose with frequent, persistent, and poorly controlled seizure activity is disconcerting'. In a retrospective study comparing the fatal toxicities of antidepressants in England, Scotland and Wales in 1987—1992 it was found that the number of deaths per million prescriptions of amoxapine was significantly higher than expected (278[C]).

Renal damage have occurred in cases of amoxapine overdose. Acute renal failure and rhabdomyolysis were reported (279[Cr]) in a 27-year-old man who took 1—2 grams of amoxapine. The authors recommend aggressive volume expansion and diuresis with loop diuretics because of the futility of hemodialysis. Another case (280[C]) involved a 24-year-old man who took 4 grams of amoxapine and developed gross hematuria and serum uric acid elevations on the second day of hospitalization. As in previously reported cases, the serum creatinine phosphokinase was grossly elevated. The patient remained obtunded and stuporous for 7 days but eventually recovered.

A further interesting reminder of the structural resemblance of amoxapine to the neuroleptics is provided by a side effect reported both with amoxapine and its close congener, loxapine (281[C]). A 49-year-old woman with no history of diabetes was admitted in unexplained hyperglycemic coma (blood glucose 942 mg/100 ml) while taking lithium 1500 mg/day and loxapine 150 mg/day. The patient responded to insulin infusion, but insulin responses on testing were not delayed and suggested an iatrogenic rather than a diabetic cause. The fasting glucose fell to 150 mg/100 ml after discontinuing loxapine but remaining on lithium. Two weeks later amoxapine 150 mg was started and the patient became acutely confused with a serum glucose of 205 mg/100 ml. Two weeks after stopping amoxapine the serum glucose returned to normal. The authors speculate that a common metabolite of both drugs, 7-hydroxyamoxapine, was responsible for the hyperglycemic response due to its antidopaminergic properties.

Overall, amoxapine appears to have an advantage over other tricyclic compounds of possible earlier onset of action and relative freedom from serious cardiotoxic effects. Its major drawbacks are its potential for inducing neuroleptic side effects, a high incidence of seizures and fatalities in overdose (277[Cr]) and the possibility of long-term neurological damage.

Butriptyline

Butriptyline is the isobutyl side-chain homolog of amitriptyline. Side effects reported in two open studies (282[C], 283[C]) are no different from those of other tricyclics.

Clomipramine

Clomipramine is the imipramine analog of chlorpromazine. Adding a chloride atom does little for imipramine, while the difference between chlorpromazine and promazine is great. Most clinical trials fail to show any superiority of the chlorinated compound over imipramine; the side-effect profile is similar (284[R]), but drowsiness, confusion and 'feeling awful' are commonly reported (285[C]). In a controlled comparison between clomipramine and amitriptyline the former drug produced a greater frequency of side effects, especially drowsiness (286[c]). Overdose toxicity is the same as with other tricyclics (287[CR]) fatal interactions with MAO inhibitors have been reported (SEDA-18, 16; 288[C]). Altogether, toxic effects are not substantially different.

The intravenous route seems fraught with danger and without any demonstrable advantages. A 31-year-old woman who received 300 mg by this route developed seizures and cardiac arrest on the 15th day; she was successfully resuscitated (289[c]). Seizures were also encountered in four of 50 patients undergoing a course of intravenous treatment. Those vulnerable to this complication were not identified in advance by prescreening EEGs (290[C]). Intravenous administration invariably produced ECG changes in a group of geriatric patients. Sometimes the changes were slow to reverse (291[C]). Venous thrombosis is a recognized complication of tricyclic antidepressants. A case of thrombosis of the cerebral veins occurred in a 61-year-old woman following intravenous clomipramine and the authors (292[C]) suggest that the risk may be greater when the intravenous route is used.

Four patients taking up to 100 mg/day developed uncontrollable episodes of yawning. In three cases (two males and one female) this was associated with sexual arousal, in two instances by spontaneous orgasm. In all four patients the symptoms disappeared after drug discontinuation (293[C]).

Delay or complete abolition of ejaculation is attributed to fairly strong peripheral α-adrenoceptor blocking activity (294[CR]). Impotence may be due to a ganglionic blocking action.

This drug has also aroused interest because of an action on prolactin release, which occurs with major tranquilizers but not with other tricyclics (295[CR]). This action of clomipramine is related to its chemical structure and reflects a greater effect on dopamine metabolism and serotonin uptake compared with other antidepressants.

Clomipramine is also widely used in the treatment of phobic and obsessive-compulsive disorders (296[C], 297[C], 298[R]) as well as in panic disorders (299[C]).

Dibenzepin

This compound is a 6—7—6 tricyclic of the dibenzodiazepine type. A comparison with imipramine was said to show equal efficacy. Side effects were comparable in type and degree (300[CR]).

Dimethacrine

This 6—6—6 tricyclic drug, an acridine derivative, was found to be less effective than imipramine, while producing more weight loss and more abnormal liver function tests (301[CR]).

Dosulepin (dothiepin)

This compound has been available in Europe for over 30 years and is particularly popular in Britain. An extensive review (302[R]) catalogs its structure, animal and clinical pharmacology. The compound appears to be equivalent to amitriptyline although few studies report dosages above 225 mg.

Compared to amitriptyline the compound is equally effective and sedative with somewhat fewer anticholinergic side effects reported in several studies. However, it does not appear to have been compared to other less sedative or anticholinergic tricyclic compounds or to second generation drugs. Although claimed to have fewer cardiovascular effects, this is not well substantiated in controlled comparative studies and the cardiovascular and other effects of overdose appear to be identical for all tricyclic compounds. Fetal tachyarrhythmia was believed to be caused by maternal ingestion of dothiepin (303[C]).

Imipramine *N*-oxide

This imipramine metabolite was compared with the parent drug. Efficacy was identical; side effects were the same, but possibly less frequent (304[CR]).

Iprindole

Iprindole is a 6—5—8 tricyclic compound with the first two rings forming an indole nucleus (SED-7, 27). It is of some theoretical interest in that it is weak in its action on the amine pump mechanism. Side effects are reported as being similar to those of other tricyclics (305[CR], 306[CR]).

The major side effect of serious concern has been jaundice. A review of 21 cases of liver damage during iprindole treatment revealed onset between 4 and 21 days after starting treatment (307[C]). Recovery was rapid when the drug was withdrawn. Liver biopsy showed predominantly cholestasis. This complication seems to be similar to that seen after chlorpromazine. In one instance (308[C]) jaundice was accompanied by a marked eosinophilia of 30% and laboratory signs suggesting some hepatocellular damage as well. Jaundice promptly recurred when the drug was re-administered. All signs point to the reaction being allergic in nature.

Lofepramine

Lofepramine is an imipramine analog with animal pharmacology suggestive of low toxicity (309[CR]). Clinical efficacy is similar to that of imipramine and amitriptyline. Patients on lofepramine report less dry mouth and fewer disturbances of accommodation as well as drowsiness, but a greater incidence of tremor (310[CR]).

Lofepramine has apparently not been compared clinically with desipramine to which it is mainly metabolized. The claim that lofepramine has fewer side effects than traditional tricyclic compounds must be viewed with scepticism (SEDA-11, 14).

Melitracen

Melitracen is structurally and pharmacologically related to imipramine with two methyl groups attached to the central ring. It has shown comparable efficacy to amitriptyline, with a somewhat more rapid effect and similar side effects (311[C]).

Noxiptiline

Noxiptiline is another tricyclic compound in which the main change from amitriptyline is the longer side chain, containing an oxyimino-grouping (see SED-7, 20). A comparison with imipramine revealed no difference in therapeutic efficacy. As regards side effects, there seemed to be more mental symptoms, such as delirium (312[CR]).

Pizotifen

This modification of the conventional tricyclics has a 5-membered third ring containing a sulfur atom. One clinical report suggests that it has effects and side effects resembling those of amitriptyline (313[C]), but it is also closely related to cyproheptadine and generally more prone to cause drowsiness and increased appetite, as cyproheptadine does; it is discussed in Chapter 13.

'SECOND-GENERATION' ANTIDEPRESSANT DRUGS

The newer antidepressants that have followed the monoamine-oxidase inhibitors and tricyclic antidepressants are listed in Table 3. They have a wide variety of chemical structures and pharmacological profiles and are categorized as 'second generation' antidepressants solely for convenience. Although they are widely considered to be equally effective with one another and with the older compounds, they each have differing side-effect profiles. No new antidepressant has proven sufficiently free of adverse effects to establish itself as a routine 'first choice' compound over the older remedies; some share a similar side-effect profile to the tricyclic compounds and others have been found to produce novel or unexpected side effects. The complete categorization of each compound depends on wide-scale general use beyond the artificial confines of clinical trials. This also includes the experience that accumulates from the victims of overdose which cannot be anticipated before a new drug is released. The second generation drugs are discussed separately below. The selective serotonin uptake inhibitors are dealt with as a group since they have many class specific side effects.

Bupropion (mefebutamone)

Bupropion has previously been reviewed in SED Annuals (SEDA-8, 18; SEDA-10, 20). Early in 1986 advertising began to appear in advance of the drug's expected release in the United States. Abruptly, in March, distribution was halted due to reports of seizures in patients with bulimia treated with buproprion. However, data have suggested that bupropion has approximately the same seizure potential as the tricyclic compounds (SEDA-8, 30), although the manufacturers have previously noted an increased risk of seizures in patients receiving over 600 mg of bupropion daily in combination with lithium or antipsychotic medication (SEDA-10, 20). In a recent report a higher seizure risk for bupropion than for tricyclics was reported in patients taking bupropion in doses over 450 mg/day (SEDA 17, 21).

Another concern about this compound relates to its activating properties and the risk of provoking psychotic symptoms (SEDA-8, 31). In an open clinical trial, two of 16 patients became psychotic and were dropped from the study (314[c]). A more detailed report of this side effect (315[C]) concerns four of 13 patients who became psychotic on a trial of bupropion. Three of the patients had a history of psychosis, but none had previously shown this response to other antidepressants. The dose range of bupropion is considered to be 300—750 mg daily and the psychotic symptoms occurred at daily dosages of 300—500 mg daily. In two cases symptoms did not occur at lower dosages, but in one instance this was therapeutically inadequate.

Additional reports of psychotic reactions and a manic syndrome associated with bupropion have appeared (SEDA-16, 10; SEDA-17, 21). In two of these cases a drug interaction with fluoxetine, reducing the metabolism of bupropion, could not be excluded. Cases of visual hallucinations and tinnitus have also been reported (SEDA-17, 21).

Maprotiline

Maprotiline has a tetracyclic structure in which the tricyclic nucleus contains a fourth ring formed by an ethylene bridge vertical to the major plane of the molecule (SEDA-5, 34). It exhibits a strong inhibitory effect on noradrenaline uptake across cell membranes and relatively weak effects on serotonergic mechanisms. The biological half-life averages 43 hours (316[R]), allowing once-daily dosing.

Following the release of the drug in Britain, information was collected from 10 000 patients treated in general practice during a 9-month period (317[CR]). Patients were given 75 mg daily, preferably at night, and were followed for 3 weeks. By the end of that time, 1343 patients had dropped out due to side effects. Drowsiness was the commonest of these, followed by dizziness and headache. Skin rashes reached a constant peak incidence of about 3% after 2 weeks treatment; this same side effect was found in some earlier clinical trials (SEDA-2, 12).

Blood levels were measured in two trials conducted in general practice (318[CR]). On both regimens (single and divided doses), a steady state was reached after 1 week, but there was considerable individual variability (up to 10-fold) in plasma levels. A multicenter study of over 2000 records from more than 500 general practitioners (319[CR]) showed that the onset of action usually occurs within the first week of treatment and that the effect is complete after 3—4 weeks with roughly half of the total improvement occurring by the end of the first week.

A number of studies have compared maprotiline with other antidepressants. There was no significant difference in side effects when compared with doxepin (320[CR]), amitriptyline (321[CR]) or imipramine (322[CR]). Maprotiline is among the antidepressants with the lowest-reported incidence of tachycardia and postural hypotension.

Reports of overdosage relate to doses ranging from 750 to 3200 mg (323[C], 324[C]); symptoms comprised lowered consciousness, convulsions, confusion, disorientation, visual hallucinations and ECG changes similar to tricyclic compounds. A report (325[C]) of 41 patients with overdose due to maprotiline notes that cardiotoxicity was equal to or greater than tricyclic drugs. In one case of maprotiline overdose the patient developed mania (SEDA-17, 22).

Information released by the UK Committee on Safety of Medicines (326[r]) revealed that maprotiline appeared to carry a disproportionate risk of inducing seizures. This was supported by a study (327[C]) of 186 patients admitted to a medical center over 1 year and treated with antidepressants. Only one of 45 patients given tricyclic compounds and none of the 109 patients not receiving antidepressants had a seizure. In contrast, five of 32 patients on maprotiline had seizures, and this was a significant difference. Those patients who developed seizures were aged 20—66 and none had a previous history. Daily doses of maprotiline ranged from 75 to 300 mg, and each patient had undergone a dose increase in the week before the seizure. A report based on experience in one hospital, in addition to a review of 87 cases reported to the manufacturer, revealed that seizures tended to occur at high doses (irrespective of dose escalation or plasma levels), and that seizures presented after patients had been on maprotiline for several weeks (328[C]). Post-marketing surveillance has also shown a higher seizure risk with maprotiline than with tricyclics, but since the maximum dose of maprotiline was reduced from 300 to 225 mg few seizures have been reported (SEDA-17, 22).

Another side effect that has been reported with other antidepressants is speech blockage, and a case is described of a 54-year-old man who developed a stammering speech and speech blockade while taking maprotiline 75 mg/day that responded to a decrease in dose to 50 mg/day, re-appeared with another challenge of 75 mg/day, and did not respond to physostigmine intramuscularly on two occasions. This side effect also did not occur when the patient was taking desipramine 50 mg/day (329[C]).

A case of myoclonus due to maprotiline has been reported (330[C]). Further neuromuscular symptoms that have been reported with maprotiline include cerebellar ataxia in a 54-year-old man with a history of unipolar depression and chronic alcohol abuse who was taking maprotiline 200 mg/day (331[C]). The question of whether his history of alcohol abuse contributed to sensitizing his cerebellum to maprotiline-induced ataxia was unresolved.

A fatal overdose has also been reported in detail (332[C]): a 13-year-old girl took 3000 mg of maprotiline and subsequently developed a lactic acidosis which the authors believe responsible for her death. Another death due to maprotiline has been reported in the United States (333[c]) in a 23-year-old woman who ingested 4.5—6.0 grams of drug.

An unexpected side effect reported is the occurrence of galactorrhea (334[C]) in a 23-year-old woman 2 weeks after starting treatment with maprotiline 50 mg/day (increased to 75 mg after 10 days). The condition subsided after the drug was discontinued.

An often troublesome side effect of antidepressant medication is weight gain. Two cases of this side effect in association with maprotiline have now been reported by the same author (335[C]). Both patients were being treated with relatively low doses of maprotiline.

One case of neutropenia has also been reported (336[c]) in a 51-year-old woman who took 150 mg daily for several months and developed a myeloid hyperplasia with a virtual absence of mature granulocytes. The patient recovered fully with conservative management.

As noted previously (SEDA-10, 21), hepatotoxicity has been reported with maprotiline, and another report in a 54-year-old man who was being treated for a chronic head and neck pain has been published (337[C]).

A case of exercise-induced bronchospasm has been reported in a patient treated with maprotiline (338[C]).

Ichthyosiform desquamation of the skin and alopecia have been reported in a woman treated with maprotiline (SEDA-17, 22).

Overall, maprotiline has not been shown to have any significant benefits over traditional tricyclic compounds, but it suffers from additional hazards such as skin rashes and seizures in overdose.

Mianserin

This tetracyclic compound, somewhat related to cyproheptadine (SEDA-5, 18, 19), is an effective antidepressant with anti-serotonin properties and a sedative profile (339[R]). The freedom from anticholinergic effects reported in clinical studies is supported by a double-blind comparative study in normal volunteers (340[C]) comparing mianserin (10—60 mg daily), amitriptyline (25—150 mg daily) and placebo. Mianserin tended to increase saliva flow, while amitriptyline significantly decreased it. However, a further experiment (341[C]) in normal volunteers found that single doses of mianserin (50—70 mg) produced a significant 29% reduction of salivation compared to placebo. This may account for the glossitis previously reported (SEDA-9, 23).

The putative benefits of this compound are its alleged safety in overdose, which may be related to a reduced risk of cardiovascular side effects and convulsions. Data from the UK Committee on Safety of Medicines (326[r]) indicates that mianserin accounts for 11% of reported convulsions and 5.8% of use, placing it intermediate between amitriptyline and maprotiline. On the other hand, the London Poisons Unit survey, involving 84 patients who took mianserin alone (up to 1000 mg), revealed no deaths and no patients with convulsions (342[C]). A survey (343[Cr]) of 100 cases of overdose with mianserin reported to the London Centre of the UK Poisons Information Service included 54 patients who took mianserin alone in amounts up to and in excess of 1000 mg (three cases). Plasma mianserin concentrations ranged from 70—665 ng/l (mean therapeutic concentration is 50 ng/l). There were no reports of convulsions, cardiac arrhythmias or deep coma in any patient taking mianserin alone, but two deaths occurred in patients who took multiple drugs. The authors conclude that in acute overdose mianserin is less toxic than tricyclic antidepressants.

A study (344[CR]) of 40 cases reported to the UK Committee on Safety of Medicines concerned patients who experienced seizures during treatment with therapeutic dosages of mianserin. Its final conclusion is that mianserin is probably no more likely to produce convulsions in therapeutic dosages than tricyclic compounds. When it does so, seizures are more likely to occur in the first 2 weeks of treatment in patients with a family or personal history indicative of risk, and following a dose increment.

A two-part clinical pharmacology study (345[C]) also reports the relative freedom from cardiotoxic effects. Fifty patients with a variety of cardiac conditions who were taking anticoagulants were given either mianserin (up to 30 or 60 mg at two dose levels) or placebo. There were no differences in ECGs, blood pressure or pulse rate either within or between treatment conditions after 3 weeks of treatment. In a second part to the experiment, mianserin (up to 60 mg daily) was compared to amitriptyline (up to 150 mg daily) and placebo in 18 normal volunteers. Measurements included systolic time intervals, ECGs at rest and during exercise, echocardiography and blood pressure monitoring. The results showed a negative inotropic effect due to amitriptyline consistent with a decrease in myocardial contractility. No such effects were noted with mianserin; if anything, there was a favorable effect on cardiac function due to an increase in ejection fraction. The results of both these experiments led the authors to conclude that mianserin is an antidepressant with very low cardiac toxicity.

Another study (346[Cr]) of the ECG effects and a review of previous experiments on doses of mianserin up to 120 mg/day showed no consistent cardiovascular effects, although four patients who received 40 mg/day for 13 months did experience significant increases in pulse rate with prolonged PR intervals and decreased T-wave amplitude. Fainting and persistent bradycardia were noted in a woman following a single dose of 60 mg mianserin and the same symptoms occurred at rechallange (SEDA-17, 21).

Another report (347[C]) documents two instances of possible cardiac effects due to mianserin in elderly patients with pre-existing cardiovascular disorders. A 71-year-old man with hypertension treated with 30 mg/day developed cardiac failure and a 66-year-old woman with mitral regurgitation and atrial fibrillation developed hypokalemia and a variety of rhythm disturbances on dosages of 40 mg or above.

These reports emphasize that the benefits of mianserin with regard to reduced anticholinergic and cardiotoxic effects are relative and not absolute.

Mianserin has already been shown to lack potential for peripheral adrenergic interactions, but because it does have α-adrenoceptor activity the purpose of another study (348[C]) was to investigate the interaction with the centrally acting drugs, clonidine and methyldopa. In normal volunteers, pretreatment with mianserin 60 mg/day for 3 days did not modify the hypotensive effects of a single dose of clonidine 300 mg. In 11 patients with essential hypertension the addition of mianserin 60 mg/day (in divided doses) for 2 weeks did not produce any loss of existing hypotensive effect in patients already treated with clonidine or methyldopa. In the patients treated with methyldopa, some additive hypotensive effects were apparent after the first dose of mianserin, but these were not significant after 1 or 2 weeks of combined treatment.

The results of this study appear to justify the authors' conclusion that adding mianserin to existing treatment with centrally acting hypotensive agents will not result in loss of blood pressure control.

In 1979 a first case of leukopenia due to mianserin was reported (349[C]) followed by another instance (350[C]). In July, 1980, the Australian Drug Evaluation Committee issued a preliminary caution concerning further cases reported to its National Monitoring Centers. Six months later, it published detailed reports of four further cases (351[Cr]), all of which had occurred within 1 year of the compound being marketed in Australia despite 6 years of use in Europe. Inquiries revealed reports of seven similar episodes held by drug surveillance organizations in other countries and the Committee expressed its concern that: 'If a causal relationship between mianserin and these blood disorders is subsequently confirmed, the incidence of disorders due to mianserin may be significantly greater than that of disorders due either to the phenothiazines or the tricyclic antidepressants' (351[Cr]).

The UK Committee on Safety of Medicines (351[r]) also issued a statement concerning 15 reports which the Committee received in 5 years. Three of the patients subsequently died as a result, one with aplastic anemia, one with granulocytopenia and a third with both red and white cell hypoplasia.

The New Zealand Department of Health's Clinical Services Letter makes mention of three cases of agranulocytosis which occurred in New Zealand in 1982 (352[r]). Another report (353[C]) described thrombocytopenia and leukopenia based on an immune mechanism without generalized marrow depression.

Recently Coulter and Edwards reported a high incidence rate of agranulocytosis from the IMMP in New Zealand—one case out of 1822 and one fatal case out of 11 537 (354[C]).

Other side effects reported with mianserin are cases of restless legs (SEDA-14, 15; SEDA-17, 21) and joint symptoms and arthritis (SEDA-16, 11). Hepatotoxicity due to mianserin have been reported in eight cases (SEDA-17, 22).

Despite the safety of mianserin in overdose and its freedom from cardiotoxic effects it suffers from the hazard of blood disorders with relatively high risk of agranulocytosis.

Nefazodone

This recently marketed compound is related chemically to trazodone. It is a potent 5-HT_2 receptor antagonist at the postsynaptic receptor and a weak serotonin re-uptake inhibitor. In clinical trials it has been shown to be more effective than placebo and comparable to imipramine. Reported side-effects are somnolence, dizziness, asthenia, dry mouth, nausea, constipation, headache and amblyopia (355[C], 356[r]).

Nomifensine (*withdrawn*)

Nomifensine was first introduced in 1977 and eventually became available in over 70 countries. Its career lasted for 9 years. There has been increasing evidence of problems with its side effects since 1981 (SEDA-5, 19) when cases of 'drug fever' were already recorded. As noted in detail in SEDA-10 (pp. 22, 23), this vague term covers a multitude of sins, the origins of which were finally elucidated at almost the exact moment when nomifensine was approved for release in the United States. Finally, in January 1986, the manufacturers withdrew nomifensine worldwide, citing the grave concern created particularly by cases of rapid acute hemolytic anemia with intravascular hemolysis (SEDA-10, 22).

Trazodone

Trazodone was first reviewed in this series in SEDA-7 in 1983 (pp. 19—21), but views on the profile of the drug have continued to change since that time. It is a triazolopyridine derivative of novel chemical structure developed from innovative animal models constructed around the hypothesis that depression in man is a disturbance in the emotional integration of unpleasant experiences analogous to noxious stimuli in animals. Not surprisingly, this approach has yielded a compound that differs pharmacologically from the tricyclic antidepressants by being inactive in most traditional test systems, relatively impotent as regards inhibition of brain uptake of noradrenaline, and weak in antimuscarinic properties. Instead, the compound shows selective inhibition of 5-hydroxytryptamine uptake and interaction with binding sites as well as α-adrenergic blocking effects (at both pre- and post-synaptic receptors) (357[R]). It also shows some activity in anti-anxiety test systems.

The compound is rapidly absorbed with peak plasma levels 0.5—2 hours after ingestion. It is extensively metabolized and eliminated mainly via the kidneys with a relatively short half-life of 13 hours for total drug and metabolites.

In human pharmacology (358[R]), trazodone produces marked sedation and lethargy within an hour, lasting up to 6 hours, and is about half as potent as imipramine.

A review (359[R]) of controlled clinical studies in depressed patients in Europe and America shows that the drug is superior to placebo; comparisons with standard antidepressants show that it can be equally effective when compared with imipramine, amitriptyline or placebo (358[R], 359[R]). The doses of trazodone needed to secure an equivalent effect were generally double those of the tricyclic compound and ranged from 150 to 800 mg daily.

One study compared the therapeutic response to plasma levels (360[C]) in 28 depressed inpatients treated with up to 600 mg daily for 4 weeks. Plasma levels showed an 8-fold variation between individuals and while there was a significant relationship between dosage and plasma level overall, there was no relationship to outcome and no significant difference between the mean plasma level of responders (1.51 ± 0.29 μg/ml) and non-responders (1.64 ± 0.168 μg/ml).

The short half-life of this compound gives rise naturally to questions concerning the optimal frequency of dosing. The general practitioner research group in Britain (361[C]) has conducted a series of trials comparing trazodone given once, twice and thrice daily to anxious and depressed outpatients treated with up to 200 mg daily. Efficacy was the same with all three regimens, although there were more complaints of dizziness and fewer of drowsiness on the thrice daily regimen.

In a review in 1980 (362[r]), there were 68 cases of trazodone overdosage in amounts ranging up to 5 grams (12 times the maximum therapeutic dose). The predominant symptom was drowsiness, and rarely coma. Patients also complained of dizziness. There were no deaths in patients who took trazodone alone and only two in those who took it in combination with other potentially lethal drugs. A brief review of data obtained from 46 cases of trazodone overdose reported to the National Poison Information Service in London revealed that 25 of the patients were overdosed with trazodone alone and 21 took trazodone in combination with other drugs (363[R]).

The mean dose in 23 adult patients who took trazodone alone was 1.4 grams with the most commonly reported symptoms being drowsiness, dizziness and vomiting. Two patients were unconscious but responded to minimal stimuli. This group of patients responded to gastric lavage or emesis, and each made an uneventful recovery. A 6-year-old child who took 200 mg trazodone had no symptoms and a 10-year-old who took an unstated amount of the drug had abdominal pains only. In the 21 patients who ingested other drugs, the mean trazodone ingestion was 3.4 grams with three of the patients being in 'moderately severe comas' but responding to painful stimuli, and 13 being drowsy. All of these patients also made a satisfactory recovery.

This retrospective questionnaire study has inherent methodological flaws, but it does tend to lend credence to trazodone's reported safety in overdose.

Early attempts to differentiate this compound from tricyclic antidepressants suggested that it might be relatively free from cardiotoxic effects based on animal research and restricted experience with overdose

(SEDA-7, 19–21). This no longer appears to be the case. Investigators conducting a special study of the effects of trazodone on the cardiovascular system published a preliminary communication (364[C]) concerning two patients who experienced ventricular arrhythmias out of a total of 20 subjects studied. Others have reported ventricular tachycardia (365[C]–367[C]), atrial fibrillation (368[C]) and complete heart block (369[C]) with trazodone.

Additive hypotensive effects of trazodone and phenothiazines has also been reported (370[C]). Another cardiovascular side effect that has been noted with trazodone is peripheral edema as outlined in a recent report of 10 cases (371[C]).

Conversion to mania has been reported in unipolar (372[C], 373[C]) and bipolar (373[C]) depressed patients treated with trazodone.

The manufacturers of trazodone received 30 unpublished reports of seizures in patients, the majority of whom had evidence of seizure predisposition or concurrent contributory conditions. The first published report (374[C]) involved a 50-year-old woman with an EEG abnormality but no history of epilepsy, who had been uneventfully treated for years with amitriptyline and perphenazine but who suffered two seizures 18 days after switching to trazodone 50 mg. Another report was of a 47-year-old man who developed 30-second episodes of facial contortions, aphasia, garbled speech, neologism, nocturnal episodes of deep breathing, swallowing and incomprehensible speech after 3 weeks of treatment with trazodone 150 mg/day. With discontinuation of trazodone, his symptoms remitted but an EEG revealed a left anterior lobe spike. The patient was treated with carbamazepine and within 6 months was neither depressed nor had any further convulsive symptoms (375[C]).

An instance of inhibition of ejaculation was reported (376[Cr]) in a middle-aged man 1 week after treatment with trazodone 100 mg at night. The symptoms remitted 3 days after discontinuing trazodone and did not return when treatment was changed to doxepin 50 mg/day. Because of this selectivity and the fact that trazodone has relatively more α-adrenergic blocking action and less anticholinergic activity than doxepin, the author speculates that this is the possible mechanism

An unusual and potentially tragic new side effect of trazodone is the occurrence of severe and persistent priapism. In a communication from the manufacturers (February, 1987), it was noted that there had been 136 reports of 'increased penile tumescence' in patients taking trazodone. These included all reports of abnormal erectile activity (including inappropriate erections of a few minutes' duration, increased nocturnal tumescence, and the return of erectile activity to a previously impotent patient). The company reported that the incidence of all abnormal erectile activity was approximately one in 6000 male patients, that in 36 of these 136 patients surgical intervention had been performed, and that at least nine of these patients were impotent. They also reported that in addition to the 136 United States cases, there were five case reports from other countries, with one requiring surgery. Additionally, there was one 'unsubstantiated report' of the occurrence of clitoral tumescence in a female patient. The company suggests that early intervention is the treatment of choice, and that the drug should be discontinued immediately upon signs of prolonged erections. If conservative measures fail, they recommend considering intracavernosal irrigation with a weak solution of adrenaline (377[Cr]). This rare side effect has been reported previously with a number of psychoactive and antihypertensive drugs (phenothiazines, guanethidine, prazosin, hydralazine) and has been ascribed to their α-adrenoceptor antagonist activity. The same mechanism probably explains the cases due to trazodone and the frequency with which it has been reported with this relatively recently introduced antidepressant raises serious concerns. Increased libido (378[C]) as well as anorgasmia (379[C]) has also been reported in patients treated with trazodone.

Another side effect reported with trazodone which also occurs with tricyclic antidepressants is delirium (380[C]).

Three cases of palinopsia (the persistence or reappearance of an image of a recently viewed object) have been reported (SEDA-17, 22) and the authors speculate that this effect may be due to some pharmacological effects resembling LSD and mescaline.

Liver toxicity, a known hazard with tricyclic compounds, has reported (381[C], 382[C]).

Trazodone has been reported to cause generalized erythematous maculopapular eruptions (383[C]), erythema multiforme (although the patient was also on lithium) (384[C]) and provocation of generalized pustular psoriasis in a patient who had stable plaque psoriasis for 19 years (385[C]).

In general, trazodone is a markedly sedative drug, very similar in profile to amitriptyline. Although claimed to be relatively free of effects usually attributed to anticholinergic activity, it does cause complaints of dry mouth and blurred vision which may be mediated through its actions on α-adrenergic mechanisms. Urinary retention has been reported in 69-year-old woman treated with the combination of trazodone and an anticholinergic drug (isopropramide iodide) (386[C]). Cholinergic overactivity syndrome has also been described in two patients upon discontinuation of trazodone (387[C]). Current experience in therapeutic and toxic dose ranges throws much doubt on earlier claims for its greater safety and indicates that it raises some unanticipated problems.

Tryptophan

The possibility that mental illness may be alleviated by biogenic amine precursors appeals to scientists and public alike (SEDA-4, 18). The availability of amino acids in health food stores and a contemporary interest in natural remedies led to reported widespread use of tryptophan to treat depression. It was estimated in 1976 that, up to that time, several hundred patients with affective disorders had been studied and results reported in at least 21 papers (388[CR]). Results of clinical trials with L-tryptophan in the treatment of depressive disorders are inconsistent (389[CR]).

It has been suggested in a survey (390[R]) that there may be some benefit in selected patients, particularly those with psychomotor retardation. Unfortunately, most of these reports have appeared as letters to the editors of journals (391[c]—393[c]) or as preliminary communications (394[C]). In addition to the possible absence of any consistent effect, there are many plausible reasons to explain the variability in response. Tryptophan has been given in both the racemic and isomeric (L) form, both alone and with a number of substances intended to increase synthesis or availability of serotonin, including MAO inhibitors (395[C]), potassium or carbohydrate supplements (396[C]) and coenzymes such as pyridoxine or ascorbic acid (397[C]). It has also been suggested that tryptophan plasma levels show a 'therapeutic window' (391[c]) and that repeated administration induces hepatic tryptophan pyrrolase, resulting in lowered plasma levels and loss of therapeutic effect after 2 weeks of treatment (394[C]). Attempts have been made to reduce this by administration of nicotinamide (391[c]).

Added to the difficulty of interpreting possible benefits due to tryptophan has been the scarce information on adverse effects. This may be partly accounted for by the assumed safety of a natural substance, but it is also contributed to by the preliminary nature of many communications. In at least two studies (392[c], 394[C]) in which tryptophan was compared with a tricyclic antidepressant, inquiry was deliberately avoided to protect the double blind integrity of the study. Two studies do report the absence of any consistent or definite changes in hematological values, serum electrolytes, plasma proteins or liver function after 4 weeks of treatment with up to 8 grams of L-tryptophan daily (394[C], 397[C]). Nausea early in treatment (398[c]), 'light-headedness', which does not appear to be related to postural hypotension (399[c]) and deterioration in mental status (400[C], 401[c]) has been reported. Hypomania following the combination of tryptophan and a MAO-inhibitor has been reported (401[c]) and toxic effects including muscle tremors, hypomanic mood, hyperreflexia and bilateral Babinski signs were seen in a patient treated with phenelzine and tryptophan. No severe or irreversible side effects had been reported until 1989 when an eosinophilia-myalgia (EMS) syndrome associated with the ingestion of L-tryptophan was reported and L-tryptophan-containing products were withdrawn from the market. It is suspected to be due to an impurity in the L-tryptophan-containing products from one manufacturer (SEDA-18, 22). The EMS syndrome includes intense circulating eosinophilia, myalgia, neuropathy, scleroderma and pulmonary symptoms. Mortality data has recently been reviewed. L-Tryptophan has been withdrawn from therapeutic use in many countries. It has, however, recently become available again in the UK for the combination treatment of patients with long-standing refractory depression provided careful precautions are taken (SEDA-18, 22).

Venlafaxine

This newly approved antidepressant is a serotonin- and NA-uptake inhibitor.

Clinical trials have shown efficacy comparable to tricyclic antidepressants. Venlafaxine may cause troublesome side effects such as nausea, sexual dysfunction and cardiovascular side effects with a dose-dependent increase in blood pressure.

Venlafaxine is activating and other adverse effects noted are insomnia, nervousness, and loss of body weight. Data from clinical trials have shown that venlafaxine may be a particularly effective drug for treatment-resistant depression (356[r], 402[c]).

Viloxazine

This bicyclic compound is related structurally (but not pharmacologically) to the β-adrenergic blocking agents. In animal tests, its profile shows properties of both the imipramine-like compounds (reversal of reserpine-induced hypothermia) and amphetamine (stimulation of the EEG). A review (403[R]) of animal and clinical data confirmed the impression of a compound with efficacy comparable to imipramine but with a different side-effect profile. There is a reduced frequency of anticholinergic and sedative effects as well as a tendency to lose weight rather than to gain. However, the compound has some limiting side effects of its own. These include nausea, vomiting and gastrointestinal distress which may be reduced by the use of an enteric-coated preparation. Viloxazine has also been implicated in the production of migraine headaches, even in patients with no previous history (404[C]).

It is claimed that viloxazine is relatively free of cardiotoxic effects and therefore safest in patients who overdose. Twelve cases of overdose have been reported with complete recovery and no detectable ECG alterations (SEDA-1, 9). An authoritative review (405[R]) concludes that although coma, hypotension and loss of tendon reflexes have been reported, most cases do not develop serious complications.

Viloxazine has previously been reported free of epileptogenic properties (SEDA-10, 52). A case review (406[CR]) of eight patients (six reported to the UK Committee on Safety of Medicines and two from Japan) concluded that a possible causal connection with seizures existed in only two cases and that such an action was inconsistent with animal studies and a worldwide review of clinical trials. This review concludes that if a risk of inducing epilepsy exists with viloxazine, it is probably only one tenth that of tricyclic compounds.

Another study (407[C]) in seven epileptic patients taking carbamazepine found that the addition of viloxazine (300 mg/day) resulted in a pronounced increase in plasma levels of the anticonvulsant (8.1 ± 2.5 to 12.1 ± 2.5 ng/ml) with symptoms of intoxication (dizziness, fatigue, ataxia and drowsiness) which disappeared when viloxazine was stopped. The mechanism is unclear, but serum levels of phenytoin in two patients were unchanged.

Although hypotension and tachycardia can occur with this bicyclic compound, an extensive review of its animal and clinical pharmacology suggests that it is relatively free of direct cardiotoxic effects (403[R]). In a controlled clinical comparison (408[C]) between doxepin and viloxazine (150–450 mg daily), one patient receiving viloxazine developed chest pains after 26 days of treatment; an ECG confirmed changes compatible with ischemia, but there were no progressive ECG or enzyme changes and the patient recovered fully after being dropped from the study.

Overall, viloxazine appears to be an effective antidepressant with a profile that clearly distinguishes it from tricyclic antidepressants. Although it has unique side effects of its own, these are not life-threatening and the compound appears relatively safe in overdose.

Zimeldine *(withdrawn)*

Zimeldine was withdrawn worldwide because of induction of Guillain-Barré syndrome as part of a serum sickness-like complication. For those who are interested in the instructive history of the drug, zimeldine was reviewed in SEDA-8 (Chapter 21).

Selective serotonin re-uptake inhibitors (SSRI)

This newly developed class of antidepressants at present includes five drugs that are commercially available—citalopram, fluoxetine, fluvoxamine, paroxetine and sertraline. They are now widely marketed and in many countries are a main alternative to TCA in the treatment of depression. The five SSRIs are structurally diverse but have in common that they are all inhibitors of serotonin-uptake with much less effect on NA-uptake. In addition they have slight or no inhibitory effect on histaminergic, adrenergic, serotonergic, dopaminergic or cholinergic receptors (409[R]). The SSRIs are eliminated mainly through hepatic metabolism. Half-lives are variable being about 1 day for fluvoxamine, paroxetine and sertraline (12[r], 410[r], 411[C], 412[C]), 1.5 days for citalopram (413[C]) while that of fluoxetine is about 2–3 days (414[C]). Norfluoxetine, the main metabolite of fluoxetine, is a potent and selective serotonin uptake inhibitor and since this metabolite also has a very long plasma half-life (7–15 days) it contributes significantly to the clinical effect. Norsertraline, the desmethyl metabolite of sertraline, is also an inhibitor of serotonin re-uptake but with much lower potency than sertraline and although its elimination half-life is approximately 2.5-times longer than sertraline it is not considered to contribute to the clinical effect (410[r]). The main metabolite of citalopram, desmethylcitalopram, is pharmacologically active but has much lower potency than the parent compound (409[R]). Fluvoxamine and paroxetine metabolites are inactive with respect to monoamine uptake (12[r]). The major advantage of SSRIs over classic tricyclic antidepressants are less anticholinergic side effects and no severe cardiotoxicity. There seem to be little difference between the SSRIs with respect to frequency and severity of adverse effects. The adverse effects occurring most frequently are gastrointestinal disturbances (nausea, diarrhea/loose stools, constipation), with an incidence of 6–37%, CNS-effects (insomnia, somnolence, tremor, dizziness and headache) 11–26%, and effects on autonomic nervous system (dry mouth and sweating) 9–30% (12[r], 415[C]). Weight gain or weight loss have been documented in low frequency (12[r]). The side effects will be discussed for the class of drugs with compound specific side effects mentioned when relevant.

ADVERSE REACTION PATTERN

General and toxic reactions There seem to be little difference between the SSRIs with respect to frequency and severity of adverse effects. Compared to the tricyclic drugs they have less anticholinergic effects and they have no severe cardiotoxicity. The adverse effects occurring most frequently are gastrointestinal disturbances (such as nausea, diarrhea/loose stools or constipation), CNS-effects (including insomnia, somnolence, tremor, dizziness and headache) and effects on the autonomic nervous system (such as dry mouth and sweating). A rather high frequency of sexual disturbances have also been reported. SSRIs may selectively inhibit hepatic enzymes giving rise to a pharmacokinetic interaction with other drugs metabolized by these enzymes and a pharmacodynamic interaction may occur when SSRIs are given in combination with other serotonergic drugs which may cause serotonergic hyperstimulation, a 'serotonin syndrome'. The SSRIs are considered to be safe in overdose.

Hypersensitivity reactions Skin reactions to SSRIs have been reported.

ORGANS AND SYSTEMS

Cardiovascular SSRIs seem to be safe drugs which, unlike the TCA, are not associated with severe cardiotoxicity. It must, though, be kept in mind that there are no systematic studies yet that evaluate the occurrence of cardiovascular side effects of these drugs in depressed patients with concomitant heart disease. A few case reports on cardiac side effects have appeared in the literature. An elderly man developed *atrial fibrillation* and *bradycardia* shortly after starting fluoxetine treatment, and again on re-challenge of the drug (SEDA-16, 9). Dose-dependent bradycardia with dizziness and syncope has also been described in a few patients on fluoxetine therapy (SEDA-16, 9). A slight but clinically irrelevant reduction of heart rate has been reported for fluvoxamine in two studies on cardiac effects of this drug (416[C], 417[C]). There is one case report of *supraventricular tachycardia* in a woman with no previous cardiovascular disease, but the association to the fluoxetine treatment is unclear since there was no re-challenge (SEDA-16, 9). *Sudden death* in three elderly women with pulmonary disease and atrial fibrillation who had recently started fluoxetine treatment has been reported. The authors recommended caution in this group of patients even though no causal link with fluoxetine was established (SEDA-17, 19).

Nervous system *Extrapyramidal symptoms* (including Parkinsonism, akathisia, acute dystonia and dyskinesia) have been reported in association with the SSRIs. Precipitation of extrapyramidal disorder in fluoxetine-treated patients, especially in the presence of predisposing factors, has been previously reported (SEDA-14, 14). Several cases where fluoxetine treatment worsened Parkinsonian disability have been described and the problem of exacerbation of Parkinson's disease by fluoxetine has recently been reviewed (SEDA-18, 19). Thus, current data suggest that SSRIs should be used with caution in patients with Parkinsonian disease.

Lipinski et al. (418[C]) reported five patients on fluoxetine who developed *akathisia* and hypothesized an enhanced serotonergic inhibition of dopamine neurons as the explanation. A causal link between fluoxetine-induced akathisia and suicidal behaviour has been suggested (SEDA-17, 19; SEDA-18, 19) and akathisia has also been associated with 'indifference' (SEDA-18, 19). Two cases of sertraline-induced akathisia have also been reported (SEDA-18, 19).

Acute dystonia has been described during the first days of paroxetine treatment (SEDA-17, 19) and there is also one case report on dystonic reaction associated with fluvoxamine (SEDA-18, 20).

One case of *neuroleptic malignant syndrome* during fluoxetine treatment has also been described (419[C]).

Psychomotor retardation with semi-stupor has been reported in one patient following paroxetine, however she had concomitant treatment with antipsychotic drugs which may have contributed to the symptoms (SEDA-18, 20).

Cognitive function may be impaired, a negative effect on learning and memory has been described for fluoxetine (SEDA-17, 20)

Reports of acute *mania* and manic-like behaviour after treatment with fluoxetine or fluvoxamine have appeared (SEDA-13, 12; SEDA-17, 20; SEDA-18, 20), but there is not enough data to evaluate the incidence of this reaction. The literature and controversies concerning precipitation of mania in association with classic TCAs are discussed above.

One case of *tics* following long-term fluoxetine therapy has been described, the symptoms subsided several months after discontinuation of the drug (SEDA-18, 19). One case of migraine associated with fluoxetine has also been reported with no further attacks when the drug was discontinued (SEDA-18, 20).

Five years ago Teicher et al. (420[C]) reported a group of patients who developed intense *suicidal preoccupation* after 2—7 weeks of fluoxetine. However, the causal link between the drug and the suicidal ideas in Teichers report has been questioned (SED-12, 57; SEDA-15, 15; SEDA-17, 19). There have been further case reports of suicidal ideation associated with fluoxetine (SEDA-16, 9; SEDA-17, 19) while in other reports, including one controlled trial, no increase was seen (SEDA-16, 9—10). Although a meta-analysis of controlled trials did not point to a greater risk of suicide attempts or suicidal ideation with fluoxetine than with TCA (421[R]) more data is needed to answer this question.

Seizures have been reported in a predisposed subject given fluvoxamine (SEDA-17, 20). Fluoextine has been associated with seizures both in therapeutic doses (422[R], 423[C]) and in overdose (422[R], 424[C]). It has also been shown to lengthen seizure duration during ECT (SEDA-17, 20).

An unusual case of *stuttering* was reported by Guthrie et al. (425[c])

Three cases of fluvoxamine-induced *polydipsia* have been reported (SEDA-18, 20).

Endocrine, metabolic The *syndrome of inappropriate secretion of antidiuretic hormone* (SIADH) was mentioned as a possible side effect of fluoxetine in SEDA-14. Now there are case reports of this syndrome in association with both fluoxetine, paroxetine and fluvoxamine (SEDA-18, 20; 426[C]). The mechanism of this effect is not known. In several of the case reports the patients are elderly persons and it must be considered that this group of patients may be at a greater risk to develop this rare side effect.

Serotonin pathways are involved in the regulation of prolactin secretion and *amenorrhea, galactorrhea and hyperprolactinemia* have been reported in a patient, already taking an antipsychotic drug, after starting treatment with fluvoxamine (SEDA-17, 20). Galactorrhea has also been reported in a patient treated with sertraline, lactation ceased after discontinuation of the drug (SEDA-18, 20).

Hematological There are case reports on *petechiae* and *prolongation of bleeding time* associated with fluoxetine (SEDA-16, 10).

Gastrointestinal Gastrointestinal side effects are one of the major disadvantages of SSRIs. The most common one is *nausea* and in reports that summarize information from clinical trials with the SSRIs the incidence of this side effect is said to be 20% or more for paroxetine (427[R], 428[C]), sertraline (429[R]), fluvoxamine (430[R]) and fluoxetine (431[R]). A frequency of about 20% has also been reported for citalopram in controlled trials (432[C], 415[C]). Though nausea may lead to drug discontinuation it usually disappears after a few weeks treatment. Other gastrointestinal symptoms that occur rather frequently with fluoxetine and sertraline are *loose stools* and *diarrhea* (356[r], 429[R], 431[R]) while *constipation* has been more frequently reported with fluvoxamine (430[R]) and paroxetine (427[R], 428[C]).

Skin and appendages Skin reactions to SSRIs have been reported (SEDA-17, 20; SEDA-18, 20), and rash due to fluoxetine occurs in a few percent of treated patients (433[r]). One case of *toxic epidermal necrolysis* after fluvoxamine has been described. Although the patient received concomitant medication, the authors concluded that the skin reaction probably was due to fluvoxamine (SEDA-18, 20). Fluoxetine has also been implicated in two cases of *psoriasis* (SEDA-17, 20). Remission of Raynaud's phenomenon was seen in a woman prescribed fluoxetine as a part of a study to assess the effect of the SSRI on nicotine withdrawal (SEDA-18, 20).

Reversible *hair loss* has been reported in patients taking fluoxetine (SEDA-16, 10; SEDA-17, 20).

Sexual function Fluoextine may cause impairment of sexual function in both sexes, particularly *anorgasmia* (SEDA-14, 14; SEDA-17, 21; SEDA-18, 21). Sexual dysfunction as delayed orgasm or anorgasmia has been reported to occur in 5—10% of fluoxetine-treated patients (434[C], 435[C]). Sexual disturbance has also been associated with sertraline (436[r]). A high frequency has been reported in studies where high doses were used. In a double-blind, placebo-controlled study of sertraline and amitriptyline in outpatients with major depression, male sexual dysfunction, mainly *ejaculatory disturbance*, was reported significantly more often in the sertraline-treated group, i.e. in 21% of the patients (437[C]). Male sexual dysfunction in 15% of sertraline-treated patients has also been reported by Doogan (438[C]). Delayed ejaculation associated with paroxetine has been reported (SEDA-18, 21). Fluoxetine has also been implicated in a case of *prolonged erection* (SEDA-18, 21). An unusual case of yawning, *clitoral engorgement* and *spontaneous orgasm* associated with fluoxetine has been described (439[C]). *Penile anesthesia* has been reported to occur in association with fluoxetine and sertraline (SEDA-17, 20). The overall frequency of sexual disturbances with the different SSRIs is difficult to estimate. It must be borne in mind that many patients would hesitate to mention these types of adverse effects unless questioned by the doctor and it could be questioned if they are properly evaluated in many studies.

Immunological Three cases of *herpes simplex reactivation* associated with fluoxetine therapy have been described (SEDA-16, 10).

Hypersensitivity reactions Skin reactions have been reported (see above).

Risk situations Severe interactions with MAO-inhibitors are discussed below.

Withdrawal effects Sudden withdrawal of paroxetine has been associated with nausea, dizziness, tremor, insomnia and agitation (SEDA-17, 20). There is a recent report of an additional three cases of withdrawal reaction after paroxetine, despite tapering of the dose during 7—14 days prior to discontinuation. Symptoms are the same as in earlier reports but also included myalgia in one of the cases and rhinorrhea and visual phenomena similar to those associated with migraine in another. The authors suggest that cholinergic mechanisms as well as functional changes in the 5-HT system may play a role in the mediation of the withdrawal symptoms (440[C]). Withdrawal symptoms have also been reported for fluvoxamine (SEDA-17, 20; SEDA-18, 21) and recently for sertraline (441[C]). In the latter case all symptoms, which included gastrointestinal discomfort, insomnia and influenza-like symptoms, remitted when sertraline was restarted. Fluoxetine-related withdrawal effects have been reported in a neonate whose mother had received fluoxetine during pregnancy (SEDA-18, 21).

Overdosage The SSRIs are considered to be much safer in overdose than the tricyclic antidepressants. Fatal cases are rare. Two deaths involving fluoxetine overdose have been reported during clinical trials, but in both cases other drugs were also involved. One patient who ingested 3000 mg recovered completely (433[r]). In seven patients who ingested up to 2.6 grams of sertraline there were no serious sequelae (429[R]). Gastrointestinal symptoms and CNS disturbances were seen in patients taking overdoses of paroxetine, the largest amount being 850 mg (436[R]). There are four reported cases of overdose with fluvoxamine (442[R]) in amounts ranging from 600 to 2500 mg. Details of these overdoses are sparse, but the patient who took 2.5 grams (along with 100 brompheniramine tablets and six flurazepam tablets) exhibited mildly 'hypomanic' and 'aggressive' behavior which resolved in 8 hours.

Interactions For the SSRIs there are two types of interactions that are of major concern: SSRIs may selectively inhibit hepatic enzymes giving rise to a pharmacokinetic interaction with other drugs metabolized by these enzymes and a pharmacodynamic interaction may occur when SSRIs are given in combination with other serotonergic drugs which may cause serotonergic hyperstimulation: a 'serotonin syndrome'. Fluoxetine gives reason for special concern since reactions may occur weeks after discontinuation of fluoxetine due to the long half-life of both parent compound and metabolite.

Paroxetine and fluoxetine are potent inhibitors of cytochrome P450 2D6 which may cause interactions with tricyclics, neuroleptics and some antiarrhythmics that are metabolized by this enzyme. Fluvoxamine has been shown to be a potent inhibitor of cytochrome P450 1A2 which may lead to interactions with several tricyclics as well as theophylline (443[R]). A number of cases of interactions between these SSRIs and tricyclics (444[C], 445[C]) and SSRIs and neuroleptics have been reported, and increased plasma level of carbamazepine in combination with fluoxetine has also been described (SEDA-17, 21; SEDA-18, 21). An interaction between metoprolol and fluoxetine with severe bradycardia has been described (SEDA-18, 21).

Agents that have been reported to cause a serotonin syndrome with SSRIs are MAO-inhibitors, including reversible MAO-A and MAO-B inhibitors, dextromethorphan, tryptophan, lithium, pentazocine and carbamazepine (SEDA-17, 21; SEDA-18, 22; 69[R]).

Pseudo-pheochromocytoma with hypertension, palpitations and headache have been reported in a patient treated with fluoxetine and selegeline (SEDA-18, 21).

Fluoxetine

The manufacturers of fluoxetine have published (422[R]) a review of side effects noted in 1378 patients treated for up to 2 years.

The major side effects confirm the stimulant profile of the compound and relative lack of anticholinergic actions. The most frequent side effects, occurring in 10—25% of the patients, were nausea (25%), nervousness, insomnia, headache, tremor, anxiety, drowsiness, dry mouth, sweating and diarrhea (10%). Most of these side effects occurred early in treatment and seldom led to drug discontinuation.

Analysis of severe side effects that caused drug discontinuation showed that psychotic reactions occurred in nine of 1378 patients. In four instances this appeared to be a stimulant psychosis and in three a conversion to mania.

Fluoxetine appears not to have the cardiovascular effects associated with tricyclic compounds, but 10 patients did discontinue treatment because of tachycardia, palpitations and dyspnea. Two older women suffered myocardial infarctions and subsequently died, although these events may not have been drug-related.

Another 16 patients discontinued treatment because of various skin rashes and eight because of blurred vision.

Altogether, nine patients took overdoses in amounts up to 3000 mg (37 times the recommended dose). One patient, who also took several other drugs including amitriptyline, died, but the other eight all recovered with relatively minor symptoms in most cases.

Four patients had suspected seizures during studies

and one who took a 3000 mg overdose had unequivocal convulsions but recovered.

Two particular side effects which led to the withdrawal of zimeldine are of special concern and have provoked close scrutiny of this combined data base. The first is the flu-like syndrome which occurred in up to 10% of patients taking zimeldine and in a few instances led to a peripheral neuropathy. Only three of the 1378 patients were found to have 'flu-like' symptoms and all recovered fully. Only one had a clinically insignificant elevation of liver enzymes. The specificity of this particular side effect to zimeldine is supported by noting that two patients who took both drugs experienced the flu-like syndrome on zimeldine but not on fluoxetine.

Fluoxetine causes weight loss in contrast to tricyclics. Fawcett et al. (446[c]) found a mean drop in weight of 3.88 pounds over 6 weeks compared to a gain of 4.6 pounds on amitriptyline. The subject is reviewed in a paper by Kinner-Parker et al. (447[R]), the effect clearly being advantageous in some patients and not in others.

The problem of the long half-life of fluoxetine leading to interactions with MAO inhibitors even after withdrawal has been discussed previously (SEDA-14) and made the manufacturer circulate a warning to that effect. A report has also been published of lithium toxicity induced by combined treatment (448[C]).

Fluvoxamine

Fluvoxamine has a plasma half-life of 15 hours and shows peak plasma levels between 1 and 8 hours after oral dosing (449[r]). It is metabolized by oxidation, oxidative deamination, and hydrolysis into nine metabolites, none of which is pharmacologically active (450[R]). Studies of single versus multiple dosing have revealed no significant differences between them (451[C], 452[C]). Treatment doses are in the 150—300 mg daily range, and once-a-day dosing is possible.

Fluvoxamine is a non-sedating antidepressant with fewer anticholinergic side effects than imipramine or clomipramine (453[C], 454[C]). Its major side effects like other serotonergic antidepressants, include nausea and vomiting. A 1-year study in 31 patients reported agitation, which required discontinuation in two of the patients early in treatment (455[C]), along with dry mouth, tremor, and insomnia. The increased agitation and insomnia may require the addition of a sedative or hypnotic.

There appear to be no specific changes in laboratory values with fluvoxamine in many of the reports (449[r], 456[r], 457[c]), and although others (458[C]) have reported a significant decrease in platelet count and an increase in serum creatinine, most of these values remained well within the normal range.

RATIONAL DECISION-MAKING AND CHOICE AMONG ANTIDEPRESSANTS

An increase in the number of new compounds raises the question of how to choose between them (SEDA-10, 53). Traditionally this issue is determined by comparisons in controlled clinical trials but, as discussed above (see lofepramine), most of the effort in new drug development is directed toward comparisons with the tertiary amine tricyclic derivatives. The question of choice between MAO inhibitors and tricyclics has been discussed earlier in this Chapter, but there are very few direct comparisons between different second-generation compounds.

Another potential source of guidance is information derived from systematic collection of data on side effects after a drug is marketed. A report from Germany (459[C]) describes two methods of drug surveillance and discusses the information obtained and its shortcomings. Two university psychiatric hospitals collaborated in the systematic recording of all psychotropic drug use and the occurrence of side effects evaluated for both causal relationship and severity. The data reviewed were adverse reactions considered to be probably or definitely drug-related and severe enough to warrant discontinuation. Drugs studied were amitriptyline, clomipramine, dibenzepin and doxepin as well as four second-generation compounds: nomifensine, mianserin, maprotiline and zimeldine. Unfortunately the data were collected from 1979 to 1982 and two of the latter compounds have since been withdrawn. In general, adverse reactions were less common with second-generation drugs (3.1%), although maprotiline (9.1%) did not differ from the tricyclic compounds (7.4%). Within the latter group, doxepin had a surprisingly low incidence (1.3%). This was attributed to the fact that the compound is used in Germany in low dosage to treat drug-withdrawal syndromes. This emphasizes a weakness in this type of surveillance system which cannot control for differences in use based on dosage, indications or patient variables.

The second type of surveillance system was the voluntary reporting of adverse reactions to the German Medicines Commission. The information obtained was compared to similar data collected by the World Health Organization (WHO). The limitation of this type of reporting is that it does not control for extent of drug use and is subject to seasonal and temporal fluctuations.

Analysis of these data revealed the typical side effects associated with tricyclic compounds with no difference among them. Each second-generation drug had a unique profile and the severe side effects which led to the withdrawal of nomifensine and zimeldine showed up clearly. In the WHO data set, mianserin was associated with a disproportionate number of blood dyscrasias (SEDA-10, 21). This risk was confirmed by information from the UK Committee on Safety of Medicines showing an excess of hematological reactions (12 fatal). These have predominantly been leukopenia or agranulocytosis and the elderly appear particularly susceptible. As a result, the manufacturers have modified their labeling and now recommend a routine blood count every 4 weeks during the first 3 months of treatment.

The treating psychiatrist is confronted both with a dearth of comparative information and with the knowledge that new and sometimes severe or fatal side effects continue to appear long after a compound has been tested or approved for marketing. For these reasons the second-generation drugs are more likely to be used only after a tricyclic antidepressant has already failed or is contraindicated. It is important to recognize that this alone has a powerful impact on prescribing preferences and practice. Drugs that are used as 'first choice' agents obtain better results because placebo responses and spontaneous remission are attributed to them whilst 'second choice' compounds are given more often to treatment-refractory or side-effect-sensitive individuals who fail to benefit from traditional drugs (460[C]). Another bias may operate if treatment with a tricyclic compound or MAO inhibitor is abruptly terminated and withdrawal symptoms are attributed as side effects to the newly prescribed drug. It is important to be aware of these built-in biases that operate against new compounds since the treating psychiatrist is liable to become disillusioned when the newer drugs fail to produce the results reported in clinical trials.

All the second-generation drugs have been shown to be more effective than placebo and not significantly different from other active treatment in short-term clinical trials. In most studies they have been compared with tricyclic compounds.

At present, choice between newer compounds is based neither on differences in efficacy, alleged biochemical mechanisms nor clinical subtypes of depression. The criteria are therefore the same as exist for the older antidepressant drugs. These are:

Desired degree of sedative or stimulant action The degree of agitation or apathy will influence the choice between sedative agents like trazodone, mianserin or maprotiline and compounds which have a more stimulant profile. In general, sedative antidepressants are much more widely prescribed (particularly in primary-care settings) partly because they can be given at night-time with the benefit that they alleviate insomnia and avoid the need for additional hypnotic medications. All of the newer sedative compounds can be given once daily, whereas some of the more stimulant compounds have shorter half-lives and require divided regimens. This means that use of the more stimulant compounds may produce the double disadvantage of increased frequency of medication with the possible need for adjunctive sedative-hypnotic drugs and the risk of poorer patient compliance. This is a factor that is not well tested within the artificial confines of a drug trial where compliance is assured.

Patient susceptibility and side-effect profile Many of the newer drugs are particularly useful for individuals with pre-existing physical conditions or idiosyncratic responses that make them susceptible to the side effects of tricyclic antidepressants or MAO inhibitors.

Most of the newer compounds have been routinely tested in geriatric subpopulations and found to be relatively safe, with the same common-sense recommendations to use about half the normal adult dose and titrate upwards slowly.

Several of the newer drugs have been reported to lower seizure thresholds in some individuals. Since the relative risk of seizures due to different antidepressants is difficult to estimate, there is no compound that can be declared unequivocally safe. There is evidence that maprotiline induces seizures more commonly than other antidepressants in overdose.

An obvious area of need is for drugs without the cardiotoxic actions of the tricyclic compounds. Although trazodone held early promise and does not cause conduction defects, there is some evidence of direct myocardial actions. This leaves mianserin as the only sedative compound that has a clean cardiac profile, and with the added advantage that it does not interact with antihypertensive agents. All of the more stimulant drugs appear to be relatively non-cardiotoxic.

Freedom from the commoner but troublesome anticholinergic and autonomic side effects of the tertiary amine tricyclic antidepressants is a fairly clear-cut advantage to most of the newer compounds. Absence of weight gain with the more stimulant drugs is particularly valuable.

Finally, with the exception of maprotiline, the newer drugs appear much safer when taken in overdose than are either the tricyclic compounds or MAO inhibitors.

Compatibility with concurrent medications Knowledge about interactions is another area that waits upon widespread use of a compound and its administration to individuals taking other medications.

REFERENCES

1. Kline N. Monoamine oxidase inhibitors: an unfinished picaresque tale. In: Ayd F, Blackwell B, eds. Discoveries in Biological Psychiatry. Philadelphia-Toronto: Lippincott, 1970;194.
2. Kuhn R. The imipramine story. In: Ayd F, Blackwell B, eds. Discoveries in Biological Psychiatry. Philadelphia-Toronto: Lippincott, 1970;205.
3. Blackwell B. The process of discovery. In: Ayd F, Blackwell B, eds. Discoveries in Biological Psychiatry. Philadelphia-Toronto: Lippincott, 1970;11.
4. Richelson E. Pharmacology of antidepressants in the United States. J Clin Psychiatry 1982;43/11(Sect 20):4.
5. Zis AP, Goodwin FK. Novel antidepressants and the biogenic amine hypothesis of depression. Arch Gen Psychiatry 1979;36:1097.
6. Fink M. Predictions of clinical activity of psychoactive drugs: application of cerebral electrometry in Phase I studies. In: Sudilofsky A, Gershon S, Beer B, eds. Predictability in Psychopharmacology. New York: Raven Press, 1975;65
7. Palmai CT, Blackwell B, Maxwell AE, Morgenstern F. Patterns of salivary flow in depressive illness and during treatment. Br J Psychiatry 1967;113:1297.
8. Blackwell B, Stepfopoulos A, Enders Petal. The anticholinergic activity of two tricyclic antidepressants. Am J Psychiatry 1978;135:722.
9. Charney DS, Heninger GR, Sternberg DE et al. Presynaptic adrenergic receptor sensitivity in depression. Arch Gen Psychiatry 1981;38:1334.
10. Nyström C, Hällström T. Double-blind comparison between a serotonin and a noradrenaline reuptake blocker in the treatment of depressed outpatients. Acta Psychiatr Scand 1985;72:6.
11. Van Praag HM, Kahn R, Asnis GM et al. Therapeutic indications for serotonin-potentiating compounds: a hypothesis. Biol Psychiatry 1987;22:205.
12. Leonard BE. The comparative pharmacology of new antidepressants. J Clin Psychiatry 1993;54(Suppl 8):3.
13. Carroll BJ, Feinberg M, Greden JF et al. A specific laboratory test for the diagnosis of melancholia. Arch Gen Psychiatry 1981;38:15.
14. Loosen PT, Prange AJ. Serum thyrotrophin response to thyrotrophin-releasing hormone in psychiatric patients: a review. Am J Psychiatry 1982;139:405.
15. Hendler N. The anatomy and pharmacology of chronic pain. J Clin Psychiatry 1982;43:15.
16. Pohl R, Berchow R, Rainey JM. Tricyclic antidepressants and monoamine oxidase inhibitors in the treatment of agoraphobia. J Clin Psychopharmacol 1982;2:399.
17. Kupfer D. Sleep, antidepressants and affective disease. J Clin Psychiatry 1982;43/11(Sect 2):30.
18. Åberg-Wistedt A. The antidepressant effects of 5-HT uptake inhibitors. Br J Psychiatry 1989;155(Suppl 8):32.
19. Connell PH. Amphetamine psychosis. Maudsley Monogr 1958;5.
20. Blackwell B. Antidepressant drugs: side effects and compliance. J Clin Psychiatry 1982;43/11(Sect 2):14.
21. Youdim MBH, Finberg JPM. Monoamine oxidase inhibitor antidepressants. In: Grahame-Smith DG, Cohen PJ, eds. Preclinical Psychopharmacology. Amsterdam: Excerpta Medica, 1983;38.
22. Murphy DL, Sunderland T, Cohen RM. Monoamine-oxidase-inhibiting antidepressants: a clinical update. Psychiatr Clin North Am 1984;7:549.
23. Liebowitz MR, Quitkin FM, Steward JW et al. Phenelzine vs imipramine in atypical depression: a preliminary report. Arch Gen Psychiatry 1984;41:669.
24. White K, Simpson G. Should the use of MAO inhibitors be abandoned? Integrat Psychiatry 1985;3:34.
25. Rose S. The relationship of acetylation phenotype to treatment with MAOIs: a review. J Clin Psychopharmacol 1982;2:161.
26. Daneshmend TK, Scott GL, Bradfield JMB. Angiosarcoma of liver associated with phenelzine. Br Med J 1979;1:6179.
27. Razani J, White KL, White J et al. The safety and efficacy of combined amitriptyline and tranylcypromine antidepressant treatment: a controlled trial. Arch Gen Psychiatry 1983;40:657.
28. Kronig MH, Roose SP, Walsh BT et al. Blood pressure effects of phenelzine. J Clin Psychopharmacol 1983;3:307.
29. Linet LS. Mysterious MAOI hypertensive episodes. J Clin Psychiatry 1986;47:563.
30. Blackwell B. Clinical and Pharmacological Observations of the Interactions of Monoamine Oxidase Inhibitors, Amines and Foodstuffs. Cambridge University: M.D. Thesis, 1966.
31. Evans DL, Davidson J, Raft D. Early and late side effects of phenelzine. J Clin Psychopharmacol 1982;2:208.
32. Galynker I, Kampf R, Rosenthal R. Dose-related visual hallucinations in macular degeneration patients receiving phenelzine. Am J Psychiatry 1994;151(3):450.
33. Stewart JW, Harrison W, Quitkin F et al. Phenelzine-induced pyridoxine deficiency. J Clin Psychopharmacol 1984;4:225.
34. Jack RA. Myoclonus, hyperreflexia, and diaphoresis. Can J Psychiatry 1986;31:178.
35. Lieberman JA, Kane JM, Reife R. Neuromuscular effects of monoamine oxidase inhibitors. J Clin Psychopharmacol 1985;5:221.
36. Riederer P, Reinolds GP. Deprenyl is a selective inhibitor of brain MAO-B in the long-term treatment of Parkinson's disease. Br J Clin Pharmacol 1980;9:88.
37. Teusink JP, Alexopoulos GS, Shamoian CA. Parkinsonian side effects induced by a monoamine oxidase inhibitor. Am J Psychiatry 1984;141:118.
38. Gillman MA, Sandyk R. Parkinsonism induced by a monoamine oxidase inhibitor. Postgrad Med J 1986;62:235.
39. Pande AC, Max PA. A dystonic reaction occurring during treatment with tranylcypromine. J Clin Psychopharmacol 1989;9:229.
40. Goldstein DM, Goldberg RL. Monoamine oxidase inhibitor-induced speech blockage. J Clin Psychiatry 1986; 47:604.
41. Peterson JC, Pollback RW, Mahoney JJ, Fuller TJ. Inappropriate antidiuretic hormone secondary to a monoamine oxidase inhibitor. J Am Med Assoc 1978;239:1422.
42. Dunleavy DLF. Phenelzine and oedema. Br Med J 1977;1:1353.
43. Tipermas A, Gilman HE, Russakoff M. A case report of leukopenia associated with phenelzine. Am J Psychiatry 1984;141:806.
44. Lefebvre B, Castot A, Danan G et al. Hépatites aux antidépresseurs. Thérapie 1984;39:509.

45. Morgan MH, Read AE. Antidepressants and liver disease. Gut 1972;13:697.
46. Bonkovsky HL, Blanchette PL, Schned AR. Severe liver injury due to phenelzine with unique hepatic deposition of extracellular material. Am J Med 1986;80:689.
47. Wyatt RJ, Fram DH, Buchbinder R, Snyder F. Treatment of intractable narcolepsy with a monoamine oxidase inhibitor. N. Engl J Med 1971;285:987.
48. Hollender MH, Ban TA. Ejaculatio retarda due to phenelzine. Psychiatr J Univ Ottawa 1979;IV:233.
49. Rapp MS. Two cases of ejaculatory impairment related to phenelzine. Am J Psychiatry 1979;136:1200.
50. Barton JL. Orgasmic inhibition by phenelzine. Am J Psychiatry 1979;136:1616.
51. Lesko LM, Stotland NL, Segraves RI. Three cases of female anorgasmia associated with MAOIs. Am J Psychiatry 1982;139:1353.
52. Ashford JW, Ford CV. Use of MAO inhibitors in elderly patients. Am J Psychiatry 1979;136:1466.
53. Davidson J, Raft D. Use of phenelzine in continuation therapy. Neuropsychobiology 1984;11:191.
54. Tyrer P. Clinical effects of abrupt withdrawal from tricyclic antidepressants and monoamine oxidase inhibitors after long-term treatment. J Affect Disord 1984;6:1.
55. Liskin B, Roose SP, Walsh T et al. Acute psychosis following phenelzine discontinuation. J Clin Psychopharmacol 1985;5:46.
56. Modai I, Beigel Y, Cygielman G. Urinary amine metabolite excretion in a patient with adrenergic hyperactivity state: reaction to phenelzine withdrawal and combined treatment. J Clin Psychiatry 1986;47:92.
57. Rothschild AJ. Mania after withdrawal of isocarboxazid. J Clin Psychopharmacol 1985;5:340.
58. Cassidy S, Henry JA. Fatal toxicity of antidepressant drugs in overdose. Br Med J 1987;295:1021.
59. Henry JA, Antao CA. Suicide and fatal antidepressant poisoning. Eur J Med 1992;1:343.
60. Shepherd JT, Whiting B. Beta-adrenergic blockage in the treatment of MAOI self-poisoning. Lancet 1974;ii:1021.
61. Crome P. Antidepressant overdose. Drugs 1982;23:431.
62. Breheny FX, Dobb GJ, Clarke GM. Phenelzine poisoning. Anaesthesia 1986;41:53.
63. Kaplan RF, Feinglass NG, Webster W et al. Phenelzine overdose treated with dantrolene sodium. J Am Med Assoc 1986;255:642.
64. Griffin N, Draper RJ, Webb MGT. Addiction to tranylcypromine. Br Med J 1981;283:346.
65. Briggs NC, Jefferson JW, Koenecke FH. Tranylcypromine addiction: a case report and review. J Clin Psychiatry 1990;51:426.
66. Vartzopoulus D, Krull F. Dependence on monoamine oxidase inhibitors in high dose. Br J Psychiatry 1991;158:856.
67. Blackwell B, Marley E, Price J, Taylor D. Hypertensive interactions between monoamine oxidase inhibitors and food stuffs. Br J Psychiatry 1967;113:349.
68. Sternbach H. The serotonin syndrome. Am J Psychiatry 1991;148(6):705.
69. Sporer KA. The serotonin syndrome. Implicated drugs, pathophysiology and management. Drug Safety 1995; 13(2):94.
70. Wright SP. Hazards with monoamine oxidase inhibitors: a persistent problem. Lancet 1978;i:284.
71. Rabkin J, Quitkin F, Harrison W et al. Adverse reactions to monoamine oxidase inhibitors. I. A comparative study. J Clin Psychopharmacol 1984;4:270.
72. Rabkin J, Quitkin FM, McGrath P et al. Adverse reactions to monoamine oxidase inhibitors. II. Treatment correlates and clinical management. J Clin Psychopharmacol 1984;5:2.
73. Amrein R, Allen SR, Guentert TW et al. The pharmacology of reversible monoamine oxidase inhibitors. Br J Psychiatry 1989;155(Suppl 6):66.
74. Simpson GM, De Leon J. Tyramine and new monoamine oxidase inhibitor drugs. Br J Psychiatry 1989;155(Suppl 6):32.
75. Versiani M, Oggero U, Alterwain Petal. A doubleblind comparative trial of moclobemide v. imipramine and placebo in major depressive episodes. Br J Psychiatry 1989;155(Suppl 6):72.
76. Realini R, Mascetti R, Calanchini C. Efficacité et tolerance du moclobemide (Ro 11-1163 Aurorix) en comparaison avec la maprotiline chez des patients ambulatoires présentant un épisode dépressif majeur. Psychol Méd 1989;21:1689.
77. Laux G. Moclobemid in der Depressionsbehandlung—eine Übersicht Psychiatr Prax 1989;16:37.
78. Koczkas C, Holm P, Karlsson A et al. Moclobemide and clomipramine in endogenous depression: a randomized clinical trial. Acta Psychiatr Scand 1989;79:523.
79. Larsen JK, Holm P, Hoyer E et al. Moclobemide and clomipramine in reactive depression. Acta Psychiatr Scand 1989;79:530.
80. Baumhackl U, Bizière K, Fischbach Ret al. Efficacy and tolerability of moclobemide compared with imipramine in depressive disorder (DSM-III): an Austrian double-blind, multicentre study. Br J Psychiatry 1989;155(Suppl 6):78.
81. Burner M. Antidépresseur inhibiteur reversible et sélectif de la MAO-A. Méd Hyg 1990;48:2245.
82. Bakish D, Bradwejn J, Nair N, McClure J, Remick R, Bulger B. A comparison of moclobemide, amitriptyline and placebo in depression: a Canadian multicentre study. Psychopharmacology 1992;106:S98. Erratum in Psychophaarmacology 1993;111:389.
83. Vine R et al. A case of moclobemide overdose. Int Clin Psychopharmacol 1988;3:325.
84. Heinz G et al. Overdose with moclobemide (Letter to Editor). J Clin Psychiatry 1986;47:8.
85. Morrow PL, Hardin NJ, Bonadies J. Hypersensitivity myocarditis and hepatitis associated with imipramine and its metabolite, desipramine. J Forensic Sci 1989;34:1016.
86. Carlson DH, Healy J. Pulmonary hypersensitivity to desipramine. South Med J 1982;75:514.
87. Task Force on the Use of Laboratory Tests in Psychiatry. Tricyclic antidepressants—blood level measurements and clinical outcome: an APA task force report. Am J Psychiatry 1985;142:155.
88. Ziegler VE, Co BT, Biggs JT. Plasma nortriptyline levels and ECG findings. Am J Psychiatry 1977;134:441.
89. Kantor SJ, Glassman AH, Bigger JT et al. The cardiac effects of therapeutic plasma concentration of imipramine. Am J Psychiatry 1978;135:534.
90. Kantor SJ, Bigger JT, Glassman AH et al. Imipramine-induced heart block: a longitudinal case study. J Am Med Assoc 1975;231:1364.
91. Preskorn SH, Biggs JT. Use of tricyclic antidepressant blood levels. N Engl J Med 1978;298:166.
92. Carr AC, Hobson RP. High serum concentrations of antidepressants in elderly patients. Br Med J 1978;2:1151.
93. Salzman C, Shader RI. Drugs that may contribute to depression in the elderly. In: Raskin A, Jarvik LF, eds.

Psychiatric Symptoms and Cognitive Loss in the Elderly. New York: Wiley and Sons, 1979;57.
94. Gulevich G. Psychopharmacological treatment of the aged. In: Barelos ID et al., eds. Psychopharmacology. Oxford-London-New York: Oxford University Press, 1977;448.
95. Wasylenki D. Depression in the elderly. Can Med Assoc J 1980;122:525.
96. Blackwell B. The drug regimen and treatment compliance. In: Haynes RB, Taylor DW, Sacket DL, eds. Compliance in Health Care. Baltimore: Johns Hopkins University Press, 1979;144.
97. Flemenbaum A. Pavor nocturnus: a complication of single daily tricyclic or neuroleptic dosage. Am J Psychiatry 1976;133:570.
98. Carr AC, Hobson RP. High serum concentration of antidepressants in elderly patients. Br Med J 1978;2:1151.
99. Hoppe E, Kramp P, Sandoe E, Bolwig TG. Elektrokonvulsiv behandling og tricykliske antidepressiva: risiko for udvikling af hjertearitmi. Ugeskr Laeg 1977;139:2636.
100. Azar I, Lear E. Cardiovascular effects of electroconvulsive therapy in patients taking tricyclic antidepressants. Anesth Analg 1984;63:1139.
101. Blackwell B, Currah J. The psychopharmacology of nocturnal enuresis. In: Kolvin IL, MacKeith RC, Meadow SR, eds. Bladder Control and Enuresis. London: William Heinemann Medical Books, Ltd., 1973;231.
102. Ratzman GW, Seer OR. Zur Symptomatologie toxischer Nebenwirkungen bei der Therapie der Enuresis im Kindesalter mit Imipramin (Pryleugan). Dtsch Gesundheitswes 1978;33:XII.
103. Glassman AH, Preud'homme XA. Review of the cardiovascular effects of heterocyclic antidepressants. J Clin Psychiatry 1993;54(Suppl 2):16.
104. Veith RC, Friedel RO, Bloom V, Bielski R. Electrocardiogram changes and plasma desipramine levels during treatment of depression. Clin Pharmacol Ther 1980;27 796.
105. Spiker DG, Weiss AN, Chang JS et al. Tricyclic antidepressant overdose: clinical presentation and plasma levels. Clin Pharmacol Ther 1975;18:539.
106. Burrows GD, Vohra J, Hunt D et al. Cardiac effects of different tricyclic antidepressant drugs. Br J Psychiatry 1976;129:335.
107. Hallstrom C, Gifford L. Antidepressant blood levels in acute overdose. Postgrad Med 1976;52:687.
108. Petit JM, Spiker DG, Ruwitch JF et al. Tricyclic antidepressant plasma levels and adverse effects after overdose. Clin Pharmacol Ther 1977;21:47.
109. Roose SP, Glassman AH, Giardina EGV et al. Nortriptyline in depressed patients with left ventricular impairment. J Am Med Assoc 1986;256:3253.
110. Bigger JT, Kantor SJ, Glassman AH et al. Cardiovascular effects of tricyclic antidepressant drugs. In: Lipton MA, Dimascio A, Killam KF, eds. Psychopharmacology: A Generation of Progress. New York: Raven Press, 1978;1033.
111. Burrows GD, Vohra J, Dumovic P et al. Tricyclic antidepressant drugs and cardiac conduction. Prog Neuro-Psychopharmacol 1977;1:329.
112. Brorson L, Wennerblom B. Electrophysiological methods in assessing cardiac effects of the tricyclic antidepressant imipramine. Acta Med Scand 1978;203:429.
113. Schlery BJ, Lau SH, Helfert RH et al. Catheter technique for recording His bundle activity in man. Circulation 1969;39:13.
114. Anon. Sudden death in children treated with a tricyclic antidepressant. Med Lett Drugs Ther 1990;32:53.
115. Riddle MA, Nelson JC, Kleinman CS et al. Sudden death in children receiving Norpramin: a review of three reported cases and commentary. J Am Acad Child Adolescent Psychiatry 1991;30:104.
116. Biederman J, Baldessarini RJ, Wright V et al. A double-blind placebo controlled study of desipramine in the treatment of ADD:II. Serum drug levels and cardiovascular findings. J Am Acad Child Adolesc Psychiatry 1989;28:903.
117. Bigger JT Jr, Giardina EGV, Perel JM et al. Cardiac antiarrhythmic effect of imipramine hydrochloride. N. Engl J Med 1977;296:206.
118. Todd RD, Faber R. Ventricular arrhythmias induced by doxepin and amitriptyline: case report. J Clin Psychiatry 1983;44:423.
119. Avery D, Winokur G. Mortality in depressed patients treated with electroconvulsive therapy and antidepressants. Arch Gen Psychiatry 1976;33:1029.
120. Veith RC, Raskind M, Caldwell JH et al. Cardiovascular effects of tricyclic antidepressants in depressed patients with chronic heart disease. N Engl J Med 1982;306:954.
121. Ziegler VE, Taylor JR, Wetzel RD, Biggs JT. Nortriptyline plasma levels and subjective side effects. Br J Psychiatry 1978;132:55.
122. Resiby N, Gram LF, Bech P et al. Imipramine: clinical effects and pharmacokinetic variability. Psychopharmacology 1977;54:263.
123. Glassman AH, Giardina EV, Perel JM et al. An important side effect of imipramine: postural hypotension. Lancet 1979;i:468–472.
124. Van Zwieten PA. The central action of antihypertensive drugs, mediated via central alpha receptors. J Pharm Pharmacol 1973;25:89.
125. Taylor DJE, Braithwaite RA. Cardiac effects of tricyclic medication: a preliminary study of nortriptyline. Br Heart J 1978;40:1005.
126. Langou RA, Dyke CV, Tahan SR, Cohen LS. Cardiovascular manifestations of tricyclic antidepressant overdose. Am Heart J 1980;100:458.
127. Thorstrand C. Cardiovascular effects of poisoning with tricyclic antidepressants. Acta Med Scand 1974;194:505.
128. Sternon J, Owieczka J. La prophylaxie de l'hypotension orthostatique induite par les antidepresseurs tricycliques. Ars Med (Bruxelles) 1979;34:641.
129. Siddiqui JH, Vakassi MM, Ghani MF. Cardiac effects of amitriptyline overdose. Curr Ther Res Clin Exp 1977;22:321.
130. O'Brien JP. A study of low-dose amitriptyline overdose. Am J Psychiatry 1977;134:66.
131. Hoffman JR, McElroy CR. Bicarbonate therapy for dysrhythmia and hypotension in tricyclic antidepressant overdose. West J Med 1981;134:60.
132. Serafimouski N, Thorball N, Asmussen I, Lunding M. Tricyclic antidepressive poisoning with special reference to cardiac complications. Acta Anaesthesiol Scand 1975; 19(Suppl 57):55.
133. Crome P, Newman B. Fatal tricyclic antidepressant poisoning. J R Soc Med 1979;72:649.
134. Xarau SN, Trias PN, Georges AG et al. Severe acute poisoning following the ingestion of tricyclic antidepressants. Med Clin (Barcelona) 1980;74:257.
135. Goldberg RJ, Capone RJ, Hunt JD. Cardiac complications following tricyclic antidepressant overdose. J Am Med Assoc 1985;254:1772.
136. McAlpine SB, Calabro JJ, Robinson MD et al. Late death in tricyclic antidepressant overdose revisited. Ann Emerg Med 1986;15:1349.

137. Brown TCK, Barker GA, Dunlop ME et al. The use of sodium bicarbonate in the treatment of TCA-induced arrhythmias. Anaesth Intensive Care 1976;1:203.
138. Pinder RM, Brogden RN, Speight TM, Avery GS. Doxepin up-to-date: a review of its pharmacological properties and therapeutic efficacy with particular reference to depression. Drugs 1977;13:161.
139. Reed K, Smith RC, Schoolar JC et al. Cardiovascular effects of nortriptyline in geriatric patients. Am J Psychiatry 1980;137:986.
140. Roose SP, Glassman AH, Siris SG et a]. Comparison of imipramine- and nortriptyline-induced orthostatic hypotension: a meaningful difference. Brief Reports 1981;I:316.
141. Thayssen P, Bjerre M, Kragh-Sorensen P et al. Cardiovascular effects of imipramine and nortriptyline in elderly patients. Psychopharmacology 1981;74:360.
142. Neshkes RF, Gerner R, Jarvik LF et al. Orthostatic effect of imipramine and doxepin in depressed geriatric outpatients. J Clin Pharmacol 1985;5:102.
143. Rosenstein DL, Nelson JC, Jacobs SC. Seizures associated with antidepressants: a rewiev. J Clin Psychiatry 1993;54:289.
144. Solomon JG. Seizures during lithium amitriptyline therapy. Postgrad Med 1979;66:145.
145. Yeragahi VK, Pohl R, Balon R et al. Low serum iron levels and tricyclic antidepressant-induced jitteriness. J Clin Psychopharmacol 1989;9:447.
146. Bental E, Lavie P, Sharf B. Severe hypermotility during sleep in treatment of cataplexy with clomipramine. Isr J Med Sci 1979;15:607.
147. Schatzberg AF, Cole JO, Blumer DP. Speech blockage: a tricyclic side effect. Am J Psychiatry 1978;135:600.
148. Quader SE. Dysarthria: an unusual side effect of tricyclic antidepressants. Br Med J 1977;2:97.
149. Saunders M. Dysarthria: an unusual side effect of tricyclic antidepressants. Br Med J 1977;2:317.
150. Casarino JP. Neuropathy associated with amitriptyline: bilateral footdrop. NY State J Med 1977;77:2124.
151. Yeragani VK, Meiri P, Balon Retal. Effect of imipramine treatment on changes in heart rate and blood pressure during postural and isometric handgrip tests. Eur J Clin Pharmacol 1990;38:139.
152. Davies RK, Tucker GJ, Harrow M, Detre TP. Confusional episodes and antidepressant medication. Am J Psychiatry 1971;128:127.
153. Meyers BS, Mei-Tal V. Psychiatric reactions during tricyclic treatment of the elderly reconsidered. J Clin Psychopharmacol 1983;3:2.
154. Schmidt LG, Grohmann R, Strauss A et al. Epidemiology of toxic delirium due to psychotropic drugs in psychiatric hospitals. Compr Psychiatry 1987;28:242.
155. Washington C, Haines HA, Tam CW. Amoxapine-induced neuroleptic malignant syndrome. DICP (Ann Pharmacother) 1989;23:713.
156. Langlow JR, Alarcon RD. Trimipramine-induced neuroleptic malignant syndrome after transient psychogenic polydipsia in one patient. J Clin Psychiatry 1989;50:144.
157. Rampling D. Aggression: a paradoxical response to tricyclic antidepressants. Am J Psychiatry 1978;135:117.
158. Fann WE, Sullivan J, Richman BW. Dyskinesias associated with tricyclic antidepressants. Br J Psychiatry 1976;128:490.
159. Steele TE. Adverse reactions suggesting amoxapine induced dopamine blockade. Am J Psychiatry 1982;139:1500.
160. Wehr TA, Goodwin FK. Can antidepressants cause mania and worsen the course of affective illness? Am J Psychiatry 1987;144:1403.
161. Kupfer DJ, Carpenter LL, Frank E. Possible role of antidepressants in precipitating mania and hypomania in recurrent depression. Am J Psychiatry 1988;145:804.
162. Paykel ES, Meuller PS, De la Vergne PM. Amitriptyline, weight gain and carbohydrate craving: a side effect. Br J Psychiatry 1973;123:501.
163. Nakra BR, Rutland P, Verma S, Gaind R. Amitriptyline and weight gain: a biochemical and endocrinological study. Curr Med Res Opin 1977;4:602.
164. Steiner JE, Rosenthal-Zifroni C, Edelstein EL. Taste perception in depressive illness. Isr Ann Psychiatry 1969;7(2):223.
165. Fernstrom MH, Krowinski RL, Kupfer DJ. Appetite and food preference in depression: effects of imipramine treatment. Biol Psychiatry 1987;22:529.
166. Sherman KE, Bornemann M. Amitriptyline and asymptomatic hypoglycemia. Ann Intern Med 1988;109:683.
167. Anonymous. SIADH and drugs possessing the tricyclic structure. In: ADR Highlights, 81-19, June 17. Rockville, MD: FDA Division of Drug Experience, 1981;1.
168. Luzecky MH, Burman KD, Schultz ER. The syndrome of inappropriate secretion of antidiuretic hormone associated with amitriptyline administration. South Med J 1974;67:495.
169. Anand VS. Clomipramine induced galactorrhoea and amenorrhoea. Br J Psychiatry 1985;147:87.
170. Albertine RS, Penders TM. Agranulocytosis associated with tricyclics. J Clin Psychiatry 1978;39:483.
171. Kozakoya M. Liekova purpura po antidepresivach. Cesk Dermatol 1971;46:158.
172. Nixon DD. Thrombocytopenia following doxepin treatment. J Am Med Assoc 1972;220:418.
173. Levin GM, DeVane CL. A review of cyclic antidepressant-induced blood dyscrasias. Ann Pharmacother 1992;26:378.
174. Yon J, Anuras S. Hepatitis caused by amitriptyline therapy. J Am Med Assoc 1975;232:833.
175. Robertson MM, Abou Saleh MR, Harrison DA et al. A double blind controlled comparison of fluoxetine and lofepramine in major depressive illness. J Psychopharmacol 1994;8(2):98—103.
176. Schiff L, ed. Diseases of the Liver. Philadelphia: Lippincott, 1982;604.
177. Van Vliet ACM, Frenkel M, Wilson JHP. Acute leverinsufficientie na Opipramolgebruik. Ned T Geneesk 1977;121:1325.
178. Moskovitz R, DeVane L, Harris R, Stewart RB. Toxic hepatitis and single daily dosage imipramine therapy. J Clin Psychiatry 1982;43:165.
179. Andrew J, Doll J, Coffimer C. Hepatitis due a l'amineptine: quatre observations. Gasteroenterol Clin Biol 1982; 6:915.
180. Snyder SH, Yamanura HI. Antidepressants and the muscarinic acetylcholine receptor. Arch Gen Psychiatry 1977; 34:236.
181. Blackwell B, Peterson GR, Kuzma RJ, Adolphe A. The effect of five tricyclic antidepressants on salivary flow and mood in healthy volunteers. Commun Psychopharmacol 1980;4:255.
182. Litovitz GL. Amitriptyline and contact lenses. J Clin Psychiatry 1984;45:188.
183. Slome BA. Rampant caries: a side effect of tricyclic

antidepressant therapy. Gen Dent 1984;November–December;494.
184. Von Knorring A, Wahlin Y. Tricyclic antidepressants and dental caries in children. Neuropsychobiology 1986; 15:143.
185. Clarke IMC. Adynamic ileus and amitriptyline. Br Med J 1971;2:531.
186. Tyber MA. The relationship between hiatus hernia and tricyclic antidepressants: a report of five cases. Am J Psychiatry 1975;132:652.
187. Appel P, Eckel H, Harrer G. Veranderungen des Blasen- und Blasensphinktertonus durch Thymoleptika. Int Pharmacopsychiatry 1971;6:15.
188. Sathananthan G, Gershon S. Renal damage due to imipramine. Lancet 1973;i:833.
189. Nouri A, Cuendet JF. Atteintes oculaires au cours des traitements aux thymoleptiques. Schweiz Med Wochenschr 1971;101:1178.
190. Reid WH, Biouin P, Schermer M. A review of psychotropic medications and the glaucomas. Int Pharmacopsychiatry 1976;11:163.
191. Mitchell JE, Popkin MK. Antidepressant drug therapy and sexual dysfunction in men: a review. J Clin Psychopharmacol 1983;3:76.
192. Renshaw DC. Doxepin treatment of sexual dysfunction associated with depression. In: Sinequan: A Monograph of Clinical Studies. Amsterdam: Excerpta Medica, 1975.
193. Kraupel Taylor F. Loss of libido in depression. Br Med J 1972;1:305.
194. Yeragani VK. Anorgasmia associated with desipramine. Can J Psychiatry 1988;33:76.
195. Thioly-Bensoussan D, Charpentier A, Triller R et al. Acne iatrogène à l'amineptine (Survector): à propos de 8 cas. Ann Dermatol Vénéréol 1988;115:1177.
196. Jeanmougin M, Civatte J, Cavelier-Balloy B. Toxidermie rosacéiforme à l'amineptine (Survector). Ann Dermatol Vénéréol 1988;115:1185.
197. Barker PA, Ashcroft GW, Binns JK. Imipramine in chronic depression. J Ment Sci 1960;106:1447.
198. Racy J, Ward-Racy EA. Tinnitus in imipramine therapy. Am J Psychiatry 1980;137:854.
199. Evans DL, Golden RN. Protriptyline and tinnitus. J Clin Psychopharmacol 1981;1:404.
200. Tandon R, Grunhaus L, Greden JF. Imipramine and tinnitus. J Clin Psychiatry 1987;48:109.
201. Smith KE, Reece CA, Kauffman R. Ototoxic reaction associated with use of nortriptyline hydrochloride: case report. J Pediatr 1972;80:1046.
202. Dilsaver SC. Antidepressant withdrawal syndromes: phenomenology and pathophysiology. Acta Psychiatr Scand 1989;79:113.
203. Charney DS, Heninger GH, Steinberg HL. Abrupt discontinuation of tricyclic antidepressant drugs: evidence for noradrenergic activity. Br J Psychiatry 1982;141:377.
204. Stern SL, Mendels J. Withdrawal symptoms during the course of imipramine therapy. J Clin Psychiatry 1980;41:66.
205. Santos AB, McCurdy L. Delirium after abrupt withdrawal from doxepin: case report. Am J Psychiatry 1980;137:239.
206. Mirin SM, Schatzberg AF, Creasey DE. Hypomania and mania after withdrawal of tricyclic antidepressants. Am J Psychiatry 1981;138:87.
207. DiSalver SC, Feinberg M, Greden JF. Antidepressant withdrawal symptoms treated with anticholinergic drugs. Am J Psychiatry 1983;140:249.
208. Gilani SH. Imipramine and congenital abnormalities. Pathol Microbiol (Basel) 1974;40:37.
209. McBride NG. Limb deformities associated with iminodibenzyl hydrochloride. Med J Aust 1972;1:492.
210. Crombie DL, Pinsent RJ, Fleming D. Imipramine in pregnancy. Br Med J 1972;1:745.
211. Kuenssberg EV, Knox JDE. Imipramine in pregnancy. Br Med J 1972:2:292.
212. Idanpään-Heikkilä J, Saxen L. Possible teratogenicity of imipramine/chloropyramine. Lancet 1973;ii:282.
213. Fu Tsu-Her, Jarvik LF, Yen Fu-Sun et al. Effects of imipramine on chromosomes in psychiatric patients. Neuropsychobiology 1978;4:113.
214. Anonymous. Report on clomipramine H. Kuwait Univ Drug Adverse React Ser 1983;2:14.
215. Sovner R, Orsulak PJ. Excretion of imipramine and desipramine in human breast milk. Am J Psychiatry 1979;136:451.
216. Pittard WB, O'Neal W. Amitriptytine excretion in human milk. J Clin Psychopharmacol 1986;6:383.
217. Stancer HC, Reed KL. Desipramine and 2-hydroxydesipramine in human breast milk and the nursing infant's serum. Am J Psychiatry 1986;143:1597.
218. Matheson I, Pande H, Alertsen AR. Respiratory depression caused by N-desmethyldoxepin in breast milk (Letter to Editor). Lancet 1985;ii:1124.
219. Eggermont E, Raveschot J, Deneve V, Casteels-Van Daele M. The adverse influence of imipramine on the adaptation of the newborn infant to extrauterine life. Acta Paediatr Belg 1972;26:197.
220. Cowe L, Lloyd DJ, Dowling S. Neonatal convulsions caused by withdrawal from maternal clomipramine. Br Med J 1982;284:1837.
221. Brown TCH, Dwyer ME, Stocks JG. Antidepressant overdosage in children: a new menace. Med J Aust 1971; 2:848.
222. Editorial. Tricyclic antidepressant poisoning in children. Lancet 1979;ii:1116.
223. Haner H, Brandenberger H, Pasi A et al. Tricyclic antidepressants as a cause of unexpected death. Z Rechtsmed 1980;84:255.
224. Biggs JT. Clinical pharmacology and toxicology of antidepressants. Hosp Pract 1978;13:79.
225. O'Brien JP. A study of low-dose amitriptyline overdose. Am J Psychiatry 1977;134:66.
226. Van de Ree JK, Zimmerman ANE, Van Heijst ANP. Intoxication by tricyclic antidepressant drugs. Neth J Med 1977;20:149.
227. Petit JM, Spiker DG, Ruwitch JF et al. Tricyclic antidepressant plasma levels and adverse effects after overdose. Clin Pharmacol Ther 1977;21:47.
228. Hultén BÅ, Adams R, Askenasi R et al. Predicting severity of tricyclic antidepressant overdose. Clin Toxicol 1992;30(2):161.
229. Crome P, Newman B. Fatal tricyclic antidepressant poisoning. J R Soc Med 1979;72:649.
230. Dziukas LJ, Vohra J. Tricyclic antidepressant poisoning. Med J Aust 1991;154:344–350.
231. Fréjaville JP. De mauvais mélanges d'antidépresseurs. Concours Méd 1972;94:8543.
232. Ponto LB, Berry PJ, Liskow BI, Seaba HH. Drug therapy review: tricyclic antidepressant and monoamine oxidase inhibitor combination therapy. Am. J Hosp Pharm 1977; 34:954.

233. Goldberg RS, Thornton WE. Combined tricyclic-MAO therapy for refractory depression: a review, with guidelines for appropriate usage. J Clin Pharmacol 1978;18:143.
234. Anath J, Luchins DJ. Combined MAOI-tricyclic therapy (a critical review). Indian J Psychiatry 1976;18:26.
235. White K, Simpson G. Combined MAOI-tricyclic antidepressant treatment: a re-evaluation. J Clin Psychopharmacol 1981;1:264.
236. Anonymous. Antidepressant interaction led to death. Pharmaceut J (February) 1982;13:191.
237. Graham PM, Potter JM, Paterson JW. Combination MAO inhibitor tricyctic interaction. Lancet 1982;ii:440.
238. Beresford TP, Feinsilver DL, Hall RCW. Adverse reactions to a benzodiazepine tricyclic antidepressant compound. J Clin Psychopharmacol 1981;1:392.
239. Waehrens AJ. Krampeanfald ved samtidig behandling med neuroleptika og antidepressiva. Ugeskr Laeger 1982; 144:106.
240. Siris SG, Cooper TB, Rifkin AR et al. Plasma imipramine concentrations in patients receiving concomitant fluphenazine decanoate. Am J Psychiatry 1982;139:104.
241. Linnoila M, George L, Guthrie S. Interaction between antidepressants and perphenazine in psychiatric patients. Am J Psychiatry 1982;139:1329.
242. Heiman EM. Cardiac toxicity with thioridazire-tricyclic antidepressant combination. J Nerv Ment Dis 1977;135:139.
243. Goodluck PJ. Influence of fluoxetine on plasma levels of desipramine. Am J Psychiatry 1989;146:552.
244. Bell IR, Cole JO. Fluoxetine induces elevation of desipramine level and exacerbation of geriatric nonpsychotic depression. J Clin Psychopharmacol 1988;8:447.
245. von Ammon Cavanaugh S. Drug-drug interactions of fluoxetine with tricyclics. Psychosomatics 1990;31:273.
246. Vaughan DA. Interaction of fluoxetine with tricyclic antidepressants (letter). Am J Psychiatry 1988;45:1478.
247. Rumack BH, Anderson RJ, Wolfe R et al. Ornade and anticholinergic toxicity: hypertension, hallucinations and arrhythmias. Clin Toxicol 1974;7:573.
248. Chamberts T, Kindley AD. Amitriptyline poisoning in childhood. Br Med J 1974;2:687.
249. Kadar D. Amitriptyline and isoproterenol: fatal drug combination. Can Med Assoc J 1975;112:556.
250. Flemenbaum A. Hypertensive episodes after adding methylphenidate (Ritalin) to tricyclic antidepressants. Psychosomatics 1972;8:265.
251. Cocco G, Ague C. Interactions between cardioactive drugs and antidepressants. Eur J Clin Pharmacol 1977; 11:389.
252. Reda G, Lacerna F, Reda M, Lauro R. Interazioni tra farmaci antidepressi ed antipertensivi. Riv Psichiatr 1977; XII:309.
253. Cocco G, Ague C. Interactions between cardioactive drugs and antidepressants. Eur J Clin Pharmacol 1977; 11:389.
254. Attree T, Sawyer P, Turnbull MJ. Interaction between digoxin and tricyclic antidepressants in the rat. Eur J Pharmacol 1972;19:294.
255. Vessell ES, Passananti T, Greene FE. Impairment of drug metabolism in man by allopurinol and nortriptyline. N Engl J Med 1976;283:1484.
256. Abernethy DR, Greenblatt DJ, Shader RI. Imipramine disposition in users of oral contraceptive steroids. Clin Pharmacol Ther 1984;35:792.
257. Krishnan KRR, France RD, Ellinwood EH Jr. Tricyclic-induced akathisia in patients taking conjugated estrogens. Am J Psychiatry 1984;141:696.
258. Hall RCW, Popkin MK, Kirkpatrick B. Tricyclic exacerbation of steroid psychosis. J Nerv Ment Dis 1978; 166:738.
259. Malinow KL, Dorsch C. Tricyclic precipitation of steroid psychosis. Pscyhiatr Med 1985;2:351.
260. Messiha FS, Morgan JP. Imipramine-mediated effects on levodopa metabolism in man. Biochem Pharmacol 1974;23:1503.
261. Colantonio L, Orson J. Hyperthyroidism with normal T4-induction by imipramine. Clin Pharmacol Ther 1975; 15:203.
262. Meignan L. Anesthésie et anti-dépresseurs tricycliques. Cah Anesthesiol 1977;25:735.
263. Ginestet D, Cazas O, Branciard M. Deux cas de dependance à l'amineptine. Encéphale 1984;10:189.
264. Castot A, Benzaken C, Wagniart F et al. Surconsommation d'amineptine. Thérapie 1990;45:399.
265. Bertschy G, Luxembourger I, Bizouard P et al. Dépendance à l'amineptine. Encéphale 1990;16:405.
266. Godt HH, Fredslund-Andersen K, Edlund AH. Amitriptyline N-oxid, et nyt antidepressivum: sammenlignende klinisk vurdering i forhold til amitriptylin. Nord Psykiatr T 1971;25:237.
267. Jue SG, Dawson GW, Brogden RN. Amoxapine: a review of its pharmacology and efficacy in depressed states. Drug 1982;24:1.
268. Bagodia VN, Shah LP, Pradan PV, Gada MT. A double-blind controlled study of amoxapine and imipramine in cases of depression. Curr Ther Res Clin Exp 1979;26:417.
269. Sethi BB, Sharma I, Singh H, Metha VK. Amoxapine and amitriptyline: a double-blind study in depressed patients. Curr Ther Res Clin Exp 1979;25:726.
270. Fruensgaard K, Hansen CE, Korsgaard S et al. Amoxapine vs. amitriptyline in endogenous depression. Acta Psychiatr Scand 1979;59:502.
271. Kaumeier HS, Haase HJ. A double-blind comparison between amoxapine and amitriptyline in depressed inpatients. Int J Clin Pharmacol 1980;18:177.
272. Cohen BM, Harris PQ, Alterman RI, Cole JO. Amoxapine: neuroleptic as well as antidepressant? Am J Psychiatry 1982;139:1165.
273. Huang CC. Persistent tardive dyskinesia associated with amoxapine therapy. Am J Psychiatry 1986;143:1069.
274. Price WA, Giannini AJ. Withdrawal dyskinesia following amoxapine therapy. J Clin Psychiatry 1986;47:329.
275. Matot JP, Ziegler M, Olie JP et al. Amoxapine: an antidepressant which can cause extrapyramidal side-effects? Thérapie 1985;40:187.
276. Burch EA Jr, Downs J. Development of neuroleptic malignant syndrome during simultaneous amoxapine treatment and alprazolam discontinuation (Letter to Editor). J Clin Psychopharmacol 1987;7:55.
277. Litovitz TL, Troutman WG. Amoxapine overdose: seizures and fatalities. J Am Med Assoc 1983;250:1069.
278. Henry JA, Alexander CA, Sener EK. Relative mortality from overdose of antidepressants. Br Med J 1995; 310:221.
279. Jennings AE, Levey AS, Harrington JT. Amoxapine-associated acute renal failure. Arch Intern Med 1983; 143:1525.
280. Thompson M, Dempsey W. Hyperuricemia, renal failure, and elevated creatine phosphokinase after amoxapine overdose. Clin Pharm 1983;2:579.

281. Tollefson G, Lesar T. Nonketotic hyperglycemia associated with loxapine and amoxapine: case report. J Clin Psychiatry 1983;44:347.
282. Madalena JC, De Matos HG. Preliminary clinical observations with butriptyline. J Med (Basel) 1971;2:322.
283. Grivois H. Butriptyline: a new antidepressant compound. J Med (Basel) 1971;2:276.
284. Collins GH. The use of parenteral and oral chlorimipramine (Anafranil) in the treatment of depressive states. Br J Psychiatry 1973;122:189.
285. Capstick N. Psychiatric side-effects of clomipramine (Anafranil). J Int Med Res 1973;1:444.
286. Rickels K, Weise CC, Csanalosi I et al. Clomipramine and amitriptyline in depressed outpatients: a controlled study. Psychopharmacologia 1974;34:361.
287. Haqqani MT, Gutteridge DR. Two cases of clomipramine hydrochloride (Anafranil) poisoning. Forensic Sci 1974;3:83.
288. Beaumont G. Drug interactions with clomipramine (Anafranil). J Int Med Res 1973;1:480.
289. Singh G. Cardiac arrest with clomipramine. Br Med J 1972;3:698.
290. Dickson J. Neurological and EEG effects of clomipramine (Anafranil). J Int Med Res 1973;1:449.
291. Symes MH. Cardiovascular effects of clomipramine (Anafranil). J Int Med Res 1973;1:460.
292. Eikmeier G, Kuhlmann R, Gastpar M. Thrombosis of cerebral veins following intravenous application of clomipramine. J Neurol Neurosurg Psychiatry 1988;51:1461.
293. McClean JD, Forsythe RG, Kapkin IA. Unusual side effects of clomipramine associated with yawning. Can J Psychiatry 1983;28:569.
294. Beaumont G. Sexual side-effects of clomipramine (Anafranil). J Int Med Res 1973;1:469.
295. Jones RB, Luscombe DK, Groom GV. Plasma prolactin concentrations in normal subjects and and depressive patients following oral clomipramine. Postgrad Med J 1977;53(Suppl 4):166.
296. Yaryura-Tobias JA, Neziroglu F, Bergman L. Chlorimipramine for obsessive-compulsive neurosis: an organic approach. Curr Ther Res 1976;20:541.
297. De Silva FR, Wijewickrama HS. Clomipramine in phobic and obsessional states: preliminary report. NZ Med J 1976;84:4.
298. Kelly MW, Myers CW. Clomipramine: a tricyclic antidepressant effective in obsessive compulsive disorder. Ann Pharmacother 1990;24:739.
299. Modigh K, Westberg P, Eriksson E. Superiority of clomipramine over imipramine in the treatment of panic disorder: a placebo controlled trial. J Clin Psychopharmacol 1992;12:251.
300. Sim M, Armitage GH, Davies WH, Gordon EB. The treatment of depressive states: a comparative trial of dibenzepin (Noveril) with imipramine (Tofranil). Clin Trial J 1971;1:29.
301. Abuzzahab FS Sr. A double-blind investigation of dimethacrine versus imipramine in hospitalized depressive states. Int J Clin Pharmacol 1973;8:244.
302. Goldstein BJ, Claghorn JL. An overview of seventeen years of experience with dothiepin in the treatment of depression in Europe. J Clin Psychiatry 1980;41:64.
303. Prentice A, Brown R. Fetal tachyarrhythmia and maternal antidepressant treatment. Br Med J 1989;298:190.
304. Rapp W, Noren MB, Pedersen F. Comparative trial of imipramine N-oxide and imipramine in the treatment of outpatients with depressive syndromes. Acta Psychiatr Scand 1973;49:77.
305. Martin ICA, Hossain M, Hart J. Treatment of marked, persistent mood depression: a double-blind comparison of iprindole (Prondol) with nortriptyline. Clin Trials J 1972; 3:39.
306. Narayanan HS, Reddy CNN, Rao BSSR. A comparative double-blind evaluation of iprindole and imipramine in the treatment of depressive states. Indian J Med Sci 1973;27:1.
307. Adjukiewicz AB, Grainger J, Scheuer PJ, Sherlock S. Jaundice due to iprindole. Gut 1971;12:705.
308. Aylett MJ. Allergy to iprindole (Prondol) with hepatotoxicity. Br Med J 1971;1:112.
309. D'Elia G, Borg S, Hermann L et al. Comparative clinical evaluation of lofepramine and imipramine. Acta Psychiatr Scand 1977;55:10.
310. Bernik V, Maia E. Therapeutical and clinical evaluation of a new antidepressant drug, lofepramin (EMD 31. 802), in comparison to amitriptyline in the treatment of depression. Rev Bras Clin Ter 1978;7:43.
311. Francesconi G, LoCascio A, Mellina S et al. Controlled comparison of melitracen and amitriptyline in depressed patients. Curr Ther Res Clin Exp 1976;20:529.
312. Berner P, Guss H, Hofmann G et al. Doppelblindpr—fung von Antidepressiva (Noxiptilin—Imipramin). Arzneim. Forsch 1971;21:638.
313. Olgiati S, Calobrisi A. Clinical results with pizotyline in depression. Dis Nerv Syst 1974;35:35.
314. Dufrensne R, Becker R, Blitzer R et al. Safety and efficacy of bupropion. Drug Dev Res 1985;6:39.
315. Golden R, James S, Sherer M et al. Psychoses associated with bupropion treatment. Am J Psychiatry 1985; 142:1459.
316. Wells BG, Gelenberg AJ. Chemistry, pharmacology, pharmacokinetics, adverse effects and efficacy of the antidepressant maprotiline hydrochloride. Pharmacotherapy 1981; 1:121.
317. Forrest WA. Maprotiline (Ludiomil) in depression: a report of a monitored release study in general practice. J Int Med Res 1977;5(Suppl 4):112.
318. Miller PI, Beaumont G, Seldrup J et al. Efficacy, side effects, plasma and blood levels of maprotiline (Ludiomil). J Int Med Res 1977;5(Suppl 4):101.
319. Forrest WA. Maprotiline (Ludiomil) in depression: a multicenter assessment of onset of action, efficacy and tolerability. J Int Med Res 1977;5(Suppl 4):116.
320. Väisänen E, Naarala M, Kontianen H et al. Maprotiline and doxepin in the treatment of depression. Acta Psychiatr Scand 1978;57:193.
321. Dell AJ. A comparison of maprotiline (Ludiomil) and amitriptyline (1). J Int Med Res 1977;5(Suppl 4):22.
322. Claghorn JL. A double-blind study of maprotiline (Ludiomil) and imipramine in depressed outpatients. Curr Ther Res Clin Exp 1977;22:446.
323. Lutier F, Lefebvre JP, Stephan E. Intoxication aiguë par le Ludiomil. Arch Méd Normandie 1977;8:539.
324. Park J, Proudfoot AT. Acute poisoning with maprotiline hydrochloride. Br Med J 1977;1:1573.
325. Knudsen K, Heath A. Effects of self poisoning with maprotiline. Br Med J 1984;288:601.
326. Edwards JG. Antidepressants and convulsions. Lancet 1979;ii:1368.

327. Jabbari B, Bryan GE, Mars LEE, Gunderson CH. Incidence of seizures with tricyclic and tetracyclic antidepressants. Arch Neurol 1985;42:480.
328. Syssain EC, Schatzberg AF, Woods BT et al. Maprotiline treatment in depression. Arch Gen Psychiatry 1986; 43:86.
329. Sandyk R. Speech blockage induced by maprotiline. Am J Psychiatry 1986;143:391.
330. Decastri RN. Antidepressants and myoclonus: case report. J Clin Psychiatry 1985;46:7.
331. Buckler RA, Friedman JH. Maprotiline-induced ataxia. J Clin Psychopharmacol 1986;6:382.
332. Alten HE, Koppel C, Ibe K. Akute Vergiftung mit Maprotiline mit lethalem Ausgang. Intensivmedizin 1980; 17:71.
333. Rejent TA, Doyle RE. Maprotiline fatality: case report and analytical determination. J Analyt Toxicity 1982;6:199.
334. Perez OE, Henriquez N. Galactorrhea associated with maprotiline HCI. Am J Psychiatry 1983;140:641.
335. Nakra BRS, Grossberg GT. Carbohydrate craving and weight gain with maprotiline. Psychosomatics 1986;27:376.
336. Ream CS, Kerr RO. Neutropenia associated with maprotiline. J Am Med Assoc 1982;248:871.
337. Aleem A, Lingam V. Hepatotoxicity following treatment with maprotiline. J Clin Psychopharmacol 1987;7:54.
338. Dubovsky SL, Freed C. Exercise-induced bronchospasm caused by maprotiline. Psychosomatics 1988;29:104.
339. Brogden RN, Heel RC, Speight TM, Avery GS. Mianserin: a review of its pharmacological properties and therapeutic efficacy in depressive illness. Drugs 1978;16:273.
340. Kopera H. Anticholinergic effects of mianserin. Curr. Med Res Opin 1980;6(Suppl 7):132.
341. Clemmesen L, Jensen E, Min SK et al. Salivation after single-doses of the new antidepressants femoxetine, mianserin and citalipram: a cross-over study. Pharmacopsychiatry 1984;17:126.
342. Shaw WL. The comparative safety of mianserin in overdose. Curr Med Res Opin 1980;6(Suppl 7):44.
343. Chand S, Crome P. One hundred cases of acute intoxication with mianserin hydrochloride. Pharmakopsychiatrie 1981;14:15.
344. Edwards JG, Glen-Bott M. Mianserin and convulsive seizures. Br J Clin Pharmacol 1983;15:229S.
345. Kopera H, Klein W, Schenk H. Psychotropic drugs and the heart: clinical implications. Prog Neuro-Psychopharmacol 1980;4:527.
346. Goldie A, Edwards JG. Electrocardiographic changes during treatment with maprotiline and mianserin. Neuropharmacology 1984;23:273.
347. Whiteford H, Klug P, Evans L. Disturbed cardiac function possibly associated with mianserin therapy. Med J Aust 1984;140:166.
348. Elliott HL, Whiting B, Reid JL. Assessment of the interaction between mianserin and centrally-acting antihypertensive drugs. Br J Clin Pharmacol 1983;15:323S.
349. Curson DA, Hale AS. Mianserin and agranulocytosis. Br Med J 1979;1:378.
350. McHarg AM, McHarg JF. Leucopenia in association with mianserin treatment. Br Med J 1979;1:623.
351. Australian Adverse Drug Reactions Advisory Committee. Mianserin: a possible cause of neutropenia and agranulocytosis. Med J Aust 1980;2:673.
352. Anonymous. Side effects associated with mianserin. Scrip 1982;707:11.
353. Stricker BHC, Barendregt JNM, Claas FHJ. Thrombocytopenia and leucopenia with mianserin-dependent antibodies. Br J Pharmacol 1985;19:102.
354. Coulter DM, Edwards IR. Mianserin and agranulocytosis in New Zealand. Lancet 1990;336:785.
355. Fontaine R. Novel serotonergic mechanismsand clinical experience with nefazodone. Clin Neuropharmacol 1992; 15(Suppl 1, part A):99A.
356. Nemeroff CB. Evolutionary trends in the pharmacotherapeutic management of depression. J Clin Psychiatry 1994;55(Suppl 12):3.
357. Riblet LA, Taylor DP. Pharmacology and neurochemistry of trazodone. J Clin Psychopharmacol 1981;1(Suppl):175.
358. Brogden RN, Heel RC, Speight TM, Avery GS. Trazodone: a review of its pharmacological properties and therapeutic use in depression and anxiety. Drugs 1981;21:401.
359. Davis JM, Vogel C. Efficacy of trazodone: data from European and United States studies. J Clin Psychopharmacol 1981;1(Suppl):275.
360. Mann JJ, Georgotas A, Newton R, Gershon S. A controlled study of trazodone, imipramine and placebo in outpatients with endogenous depression. J Clin Psychopharmacol 1981;1:75.
361. Wheatley D. Trazodone in depression Int Pharmacopsychiatry 1980;15:240.
362. Faillace LA. Antidepressant therapy: risks and alternatives Emerg Med Spec 1983;Suppl, January):20.
363. Ali CJ, Henry JA. Trazodone overdosage: experience over five years. Neuropsychobiology 1986;15(Suppl 1):44.
364. Janowsky D, Curtis G, Zisook Set al. Trazodone-aggravated ventricular arrhythmias. J Clin Psychopharmacol 1983;3:372.
365. Vlay SC, Friedling S. Trazodone-exacerbation of VT (Letter to Editor). Am Heart J 1983;106:604.
366. Vitulo R, Wharton M, Allen N, Pritchett E. Trazodone-related exercise-induced non-sustained ventricular tachycardia. Chest 1990;98:247.
367. Aronson MD, Hafez H. A case of trazodone-induced ventricular tachycardia. J Clin Psychiatry 1986;47:388.
368. White WB, Wong SHY. Rapid atypical fibrillation associated with trazodone hydrochloride. Arch Gen Psychiatry 1985;42:424.
369. Rausch JL, Pavlinac DM, Newman PE. Complete heart block following a single dose of trazodone. Am J Psychiatry 1984;141:1472.
370. Asayesh K. Combination of trazodone and phenothiazines: a possible additive hypotensive effect. Can J Psychiatry 1986;31:857.
371. Barrnett J, Frances A, Kocsis J et al. Peripheral edema associated with trazodone: a report of ten cases. J Clin Psychopharmacol 1985;5:161.
372. Warren M, Bick PA. Two case reports of trazodone-induced mania. Am J Psychiatry 1984;141:1103.
373. Knobler HY, Itzchaky S, Emanuel D et al. Trazodone-induced mania. Br J Psychiatry 1986;149:787.
374. Lefkowitz D, Kilgo G, Lee S. Seizures and trazodone therapy. Arch Gen Psychiatry 1985;42:523.
375. Tasini M. Complex partial seizures in a patient receiving trazodone. J Clin Psychiatry 1986;47:318.
376. Jones SD. Ejaculatory inhibition with trazodone. J Clin Psychopharmacol 1984;4:279.
377. Goldstein I, Payton TR. Pharmacologic detumescence—the alternative to surgical shunting J Urol 1986;135:308A.

378. Gartrell N. Increased libido in women receiving trazodone. Am J Psychiatry 1986;143:781.
379. Garvey MJ. Occurrence of myoclonus in patients treated with cyclic antidepressants. Arch Gen Psychiatry 1987;44:269.
380. Damlouji NF, Ferguson JM. Trazodone-induced delirium in bulimic patients. Am J Psychiatry 1984;143:434.
381. Sheikh KH, Nies AS. Trazodone and intrahepatic cholestasis. Ann Intern Med 1983;99:572.
382. Chu AG, Gunsolly BL, Summers RW et al. Trazodone and liver toxicity. Ann Intern Med 1983;99:128.
383. Rongioletti F et al. Drug eruption for trazodone (Letter to Editor). J Am Acad Dermatol 1986;14:274.
384. Ford HE, Jenike MA. Erythema multiforme associated with trazodone therapy: case report. J Clin Psychiatry 1985;46:294.
385. Barth JH, Baker H. Generalized pustular psoriasis precipitated by trazodone in the treatment of depression. Br J Dermatol 1986;115:629.
386. Chan CH, Ruskiewicz RJ. Anticholinergic side effects of trazodone combined with another pharmacologic agent. Am J Psychiatry 1990;147:533.
387. Montalbetti DJ, Zis AP. Anticholinergics for trazodone withdrawal. J Clin Psychopharmacol 1988;8:73.
388. Farkas F, Dunner DL, Fieve RR. L-Tryptophan in depression. Biol Psychiatry 1976;11:295.
389. Mendels J, Stinhett JL, Burns D, Frazer A. Amine precursors and depression. Arch Gen Psychiatry 1975;32:22.
390. Cooper AJ. Tryptophan antidepressant 'physiological sedative': fact or fancy? Psychopharmacology 1979;61:97.
391. Chouinard G, Young SN, Annable L, Sourkes TL. Tryptophan dosage critical for its antidepressant effect (Letter to Editor). Br Med J 1978;1:1422.
392. Rao B, Broadhurst AD. Tryptophan and depression (Letter to Editor). Br Med J 1976;1:460.
393. Jensen K, Freunsgaard K, Ahlfors UG et al. Tryptophan/imipramine in depression (Letter to Editor). Lancet 1975;ii:920.
394. Herrington RN, Bruce A, Johnstone EG, Lader MH. Comparative trial of L-tryptophan and amitriptyline in depressive illness. Psychol Med 1976;6:673.
395. Coppen A, Shaw DM, Farrell JP. Potentiation of the antidepressant effect of a monoamine oxidase inhibitor by tryptophan. Lancet 1963;i:79.
396. Coppen A, Shaw DM, Herzberg B, Maggs R. Tryptophan in the treatment of depression. Lancet 1967;ii:1178.
397. Herrington RN, Bruce A, Johnstone EC. Comparative trial of L-tryptophan and ECT in severe depressive illness. Lancet 1974;ii:751.
398. Broadhurst AD. L-Tryptophan versus E.C.T. (Letter to Editor) Lancet 1970;i:1392.
399. Carroll BJ, Mowbray RM, Davies B. Sequential comparison of L-tryptophan with ECT in severe depression. Lancet 1970;ii:967.
400. Murphy DL, Baker M, Goodwin RK et al. L-Tryptophan in affective disorders: indolamine changes and differential clinical effects. Psychopharmacology 1974;34:11.
401. Gayford JJ, Parker AL, Philips EM, Roswell AR. Whole blood 5-hydroxytryptophan during treatment of endogenous depressive illness. Br J Psychiatry 1973 122:597.
402. Montgomery SA. Venlafaxine: a new dimension in antidepressant pharmacotherapy (Academic highlights). J Clin Psychiatry 1993;54:119.
403. Pinder RM, Brogden RN, Speight TM, Avery GS. Viloxazine: a review of its pharmacological properties and therapeutic efficacy in depressive illness. Drugs 1977;13:401.
404. Barnes TRE, Greenwood DT. Viloxazine and migraine. Lancet 1979;ii:1368.
405. Crome P. Antidepressant overdosage. Drugs 1982; 23:431.
406. Edwards JG, Glen-Bott M. Does viloxazine have epileptogenic properties? J Neurol Neurosurg Psychiatry 1984;47:960.
407. Pisani F, Narbone M, Fazio A et al. Effect of viloxazine on serum carbamazepine levels in epileptic patients. Epilepsia 1984;25:482.
408. Pinder RM, Brogden RN, Speight TM, Avery GS. Doxepin up-to-date: a review of its pharmacological properties and therapeutic efficacy with particular reference to depression. Drugs 1977;13:161.
409. Hyttel J. Pharmacological charaterization of selective serotonin reuptake inhibitors (SSRIs) Int Clin Psychopharmacol 1994;9(Suppl 1):19—26.
410. Doogan DP, Caillard V. Sertraline: a new antidepressant. J Clin Psychiatry 1988;49(Suppl):46—51.
411. Kaye CM, Haddock RE, Langley PF et al. A review of the metabolism and pharmacokinetics of paroxetine in man. Acta Psychiatr Scand 1989;80(Suppl 350):60.
412. Benfield P, Ward A. Fluvoxamine. A review of its pharmacodynamic and pharmacokinetic properties, and therapeutic efficacy in depressive illness. Drugs 1986;32(Suppl 4):313.
413. Kragh-Sörensen P, Fredricson Overö K, Lindegaard Petersen O, Jensen K, Parnas W. The kinetics of citalopram: Single and multiple dose studies in man. Acta Pharmacol Toxicol 1981;48:53.
414. Bergstrom RF, Lemberger L, Farid NA. Clinical pharmacology and pharmacokinetics of fluoxetine: a review. Br J Psychiatry 1988;153(Suppl 3):47.
415. Dencker SJ, Hopfner Petersen HE. Side effect profile of citalopram and and reference antidepressants in depression. In: Montgomery SA, ed. Citalopram—The New Antidepressant From Lundbeck Research. Amsterdam: Excerpta Medica, 1989;31.
416. Roos C. Cardiac effects of antidepressant drugs: a comparison of the tricyclic antidepressants and fluvoxamine. Br J Clin Pharmacol 1983;15:439S.
417. Robinson JF, Doogan DP. A placebo controlled study of the cardiovascular effects of fluvoxamine and clovoxamine in human volunteers. Br J Clin Pharmacol 1982;14:805.
418. Lipinski JF, Mallya G, Zimmerman P et al. Fluoxetine-induced akathisia: clinical and theoretical implications. J Clin Psychiatry 1989;50:339.
419. Halman M, Goldbloom DS. Fluoxetine and neuroleptic malignant syndrome. Biol Psychiatry 1990;28:518.
420. Teicher MH, Glod C, Cole JO. Emergence of intense suicidal preoccupation during fluoxetine treatment. Am J Psychiatry 1990;147:2.
421. Beasley CM Jr, Dorniseif BE, Bosomworth JC et al. Fluoxetine and sucide: a meta-analysis of controlled trials of treatment for depression Br Med J 1991;303:685 (erratum 968).
422. Wernicke JF. The side effect profile and safety of fluoxetine. J Clin Psychiatry 1985;46:59.
423. Weber JJ. Seizure activity associated with fluoxetine therapy Clin Pharm 1989;8:296.
424. Riddle MA, Brown N, Dzubinski D et al. Fluoxetine overdose in an adolescent. J Am Acad Child Adolesc Psychiatry 1989;28:587.

425. Guthrie S, Grunhaus L. Fluoxetine-induced stuttering. J Clin Psychiatty 1990;51:85.
426. Staab J et al. Transient SIADH associated with fluoxetine. Am J Psychiatry 1990;147:1569.
427. Dunbar GC. An interim overview of the safety and tolerability of paroxetine. Acta Psychiatr Scand 1989; 80(Suppl 350):135.
428. Boyer WF, Blumhardt CL. The safety profile of paroxetine. J Clin Psychiatry 1992;53(Suppl 2):61.
429. Murdoch D, McTavish D. Sertraline: A review of its pharmacodynamic and pharmacokinetic properties and therapeutic potential in depression and obsessive-compulsive disorder. Drugs 1992;44:604.
430. Benfield P, Ward A. Fluvoxamine: a review of its pharmacodynamic and pharmacokinetic properties, and therapeutic efficacy in depressive illness. Drugs 1986;32:313.
431. Stokes PE. Fluoxetine: A five year review. Clin Ther 1993;15(2):216.
432. Shaw DM, Crimmins R. A multicenter trial of citalopram and amitriptyline in major depressive illness. In: Montgomery SA, ed. Citalopram—The New Antidepressant From Lundbeck Research. Amsterdam: Excerpta Medica, 1989;43.
433. Cooper GL. The safety of fluoxetine—an update. Br J Psychiatry 1988;153:77.
434. Stark P, Hardison CD. A review of multicenter controlled studies of fluoxetine vs. imipramine and placebo in outpatients with major depressive disorder. J Clin Psychiatry 1985;46:53.
435. Herman JB, Brotman AW, Pollack MH et al. Fluoxetine-induced sexual dysfunction. J Clin Psychiatry 1990;51:25.
436. Grimsley AR, Jann MW. Paroxetine, sertraline and fluvoxamine: new selective serotonin reuptake inhibitors. Clin Pharmacy 1992;11:930—957.
437. Reimherr FW, Chouinard G, Cohn CK et al. Antidepressant efficacy of sertraline: a double-blind placebo- and amitriptyline-controlled, multicenter comparison study in outpatients with major depression. J Clin Psychiatry 1990;51(12, Suppl B):18.
438. Doogan DP. Tolerability and safety of sertraline: experience world-wide. Int Clin Psychopharmacol 1991; 6(Suppl 2):47.
439. Modell JG. Repeated observations of yawning, clitoral engorgement and orgasm associated with fluoxetine administration. J Clin Psychopharmacol 1989;9:63.
440. Barr LC, Goodman WK, Price LH. Physical symptoms associated with paroxetine discontinuation. Am J Psychiatry 1994;151:289.
441. Louie AK, Lannon RA, Ajari, LJ. Withdrawal reaction after sertraline discontinuation. Am J Psychiatry 1994; 151:450.
442. Bradford LD, Coleman BS, Hoeve L et al. Summary of fluvoxamine maleate. Duphar Report No. H114.058, 1984.
443. Brosen K. The pharmacogenetics of the selective serotonin reuptake inhibitors. Clin Invest 1993;71:1002—1009.
444. Aranow RB, Hudson JI, Pope HG et al. Elevated antidepressant plasma levels after addition of fluoxetine. Am J Psychiatry 1989;146:911.
445. Preskorn SH, Beber JH, Faul JC et al. Serious adverse effects of combining fluoxetine and tricyclic antidepressants. Am J Psychiatry 1990;147:532.
446. Fawcett J, Zajecka JM, Kravitz HM et al. Fluoxetine versus amitriptyline in adult outpatients with major depression. Psychiatry Res 1989;45:821.
447. Kinner-Parker JL, Smith D, Ingle SF. Fluoxetine and weight: something lost and something gained? Clin Pharmacology 1989;8:727.
448. Salama AA, Shafey M. A case of severe lithium toxicity induced by combined fluoxetine and lithium carbonate. Am J Psychiatry 1989;146:278.
449. Doogan DP. Fluvoxamine as an antidepressant drug. Neuropharmacology, 1980;19:1215.
450. Claassen V. Review of the animal pharmacology and pharmacokinetics of fluvoxamine. Br J Clin Pharmacol 1983;15:349S.
451. Siddiqui UA, Chakravarti SK, Jesinger DK. The tolerance and antidepressive activity of fluvoxamine as a single dose compared to a twice daily dose. Curr Med Res Opin 1985;9:681.
452. De Wilde JEM, Mertens C, Wakelin JS. Clinical trials of fluvoxamine vs chlorimipramine with single and three times daily dosing. Br J Clin Pharmacol 1983;15:427S.
453. Itil TM, Shrivastava RK, Mukherjee S et al. A double-blind placebo-controlled study of fluvoxamine and imipramine in outpatients with primary depression. Br J Clin Pharmacol 1983;15:433S.
454. Klok CJ, Brouwer GJ, Van Praag HM et al. Fluvoxamine and clomipramine in depressed patients. Acta Psychiatr Scand 1981;64:1.
455. Feldman HS, Denber HCB. Long-term study of fluvoxamine: a new rapid-acting antidepressant. Int Pharmacopsychiatry 1982;17:114.
456. Coleman BS, Block BA. Fluvoxamine maleate, a serotonergic antidepressant: a comparison with clorimipramine. Prog Neuro-Psychopharmacol Biol Psychiatry 1982;6:475.
457. De Wilde JEM, Doogan DP. Fluvoxamine and chlorimipramine in endogenous depression. J Affect Disorders 1982;4:249.
458. Guelfi JD, Dreyfus JF, Pichot P et al. A double-blind controlled clihical trial comparing fluvoxamine and imipramine. Br J Clin Pharmacol 1983;14:411S.
459. Schmidt LG, Grohmann B, Muller-Oerlinghausen H et al. Adverse drug reactions to first and second generation antidepressants: a critical evaluation of drug surveillance data. Br J Psychiatry 1986;148:38.
460. Blackwell B, Taylor D. An operational evaluation of MAOI. Proc R Soc Med 1967;60:830.

Meyler's Side Effects of Drugs, 13th Edition
M.N.G. Dukes, editor

SECTION EDITOR: C.J. VAN BOXTEL

M. Schou

3 Lithium

GENERAL CONSIDERATIONS *(SED-12, 79; SEDA-15, 20; SEDA-16, 13; SEDA-17, 26; SEDA-18, 25)*

Treatment with lithium (or rather with lithium salts) is used to some extent for somatic diseases (cluster headache, the on-off phenomenon in the treatment of Parkinson's disease, neutropenia caused by cancer chemotherapy, recurrent herpes simplex virus infections, seborrheic dermatitis), but it is used most widely in psychiatry, and for many severely ill manic-depressive patients it offers unique benefits. One has estimated that in industrialized countries about one person out of every 1000 in the population is on lithium treatment at any given time.

The main use of lithium is prophylactic, i.e. to ameliorate or prevent further recurrences in manic-depressive illness of the bipolar type (manias and depressions) and the unipolar type (depressions only, major affective disorder). Although manifest depression is not a primary indication for lithium treatment, lithium can augment the effect of antidepressants in patients resistant to these drugs given alone. In the prevention of recurrent unipolar illness, lithium is as effective as maintenance treatment with antidepressant drugs. In recurrent bipolar illness, carbamazepine or valproate may be tried as prophylactic alternatives in patients who do not respond to or do not tolerate lithium. In the treatment of manifest mania, lithium is clearly effective, although the effect sets in rather slowly. There is evidence of favorable effects of lithium in schizoaffective illness, in cases of emotional instability in children and adolescents, and in pathological impulsive aggressiveness. While manic-depressive patients in general have a markedly increased mortality, mostly from suicide, patients in long-term lithium treatment have a mortality that is the same as or only slightly higher than that of the general population. In patients who have discontinued lithium, the mortality is significantly higher.

As appears from the present review, lithium treatment may produce side effects, but usually the benefits of the therapy outweigh the drawbacks, provided the treatment is given in proper dosage and on appropriate clinical indications. If they do not, the treatment can be discontinued and the side effects disappear.

PHARMACOKINETICS

Lithium (or rather the lithium ion) is readily absorbed in the gastrointestinal tract. It is eliminated almost exclusively through the kidneys, and renal lithium clearance is under ordinary circumstances about one-fourth of creatinine clearance. It falls when the glomerular filtration rate falls, for example in kidney disease, but it may also fall independently of or disproportionately more than the creatinine clearance if fluid or sodium balance are negative.

Monitoring of the serum lithium concentration helps to maintain therapeutic and prophylactic efficacy and to avoid toxicity. The serum concentration of lithium rises during absorption of the drug, and it is therefore important for monitoring purposes that blood samples are drawn under standardized conditions, about 12 hours after the last intake of lithium and after achievement of steady-state, i.e. not less than 4—5 days after initiation of treatment and after change of dosage. The standardized serum lithium concentration is proportional to the lithium maintenance dosage. Recommenced serum lithium concentrations are within the range 0.5—0.8 mmol/l; this is the level to aim for when patients are started on lithium treatment, and for most patients it provides ample protection against further manic and depressive recurrences with a minimum of side effects. In some patients subsequent adjustment to serum levels below or above the standard range may be necessary, namely if patients do not tolerate lithium or if they do not respond to it, but lithium concentrations lower than 0.3 mmol/l are usually ineffective, and concentrations higher than 1.0 mmol/l are often associated with troublesome side effects. Elderly persons should not be deprived of well-indicated lithium treatment, but doses must generally be lower. A consistent rise in serum lithium concentration with unaltered lithium dose or a disproportionate rise after an increase of dose may indicate a fall of renal lithium clearance and should lead to further examination.

Lithium is administered in one or more daily doses and as conventional or slow-release tablets. The treatment regimen may influence some side effects, but it is of more importance to keep the lithium dosage and the serum lithium concentration as low as is compatible with prophylactic efficacy.

SIDE EFFECTS AND DURATION OF TREATMENT

Initial side effects, seen frequently during the first 1–2 weeks of lithium treatment, resemble to some extent those seen in mild intoxication: apathy, drowsiness, muscular weakness, unsteady gait, and indistinct speech, except that nausea and loose stools are more frequent.

Side effects of lithium are usually more pronounced at higher doses and serum concentrations (SEDA-17, 28 (special review)) and can usually be prevented, ameliorated (SEDA-18, 25), or treated through use of the lowest effective dose, clinical and laboratory monitoring, or appropriate adjunctive medication.

Some patients have by now received prophylactic lithium treatment more or less continuously for 30–35 years. The question of special late side effects has naturally arisen, but none has so far been detected.

INSTRUCTION AND INFORMATION

Safe and effective lithium treatment requires close cooperation between physician, patient, and relatives, and it is imperative that all three groups are well informed about treatment guidelines, benefits, side effects, risks, and precautions. Verbal instruction should be supplemented with appropriate written information (1^R–10^R).

ADVERSE REACTION PATTERN

General and toxic reactions Side effects may be seen at the higher end of the therapeutic serum lithium range. They include hand tremor, weight gain, goiter, hypothyroidism, edema, acne, and psoriasis. Polyuria and polydipsia are infrequent with the doses and serum concentrations used today. Cardiac side effects are rare and reversible. Transient impairment of memory can occur. Lithium does not produce dependence. Mild lithium poisoning is characterized by apathy, drowsiness, muscle weakness, unsteady gait, and dysarthria. Severe intoxication may resemble cerebral hemorrhage with impaired consciousness or coma, increased muscle tone, and occasionally generalized seizures.

Hypersensitivity reactions Lithium does not act as an allergen.

Tumor-inducing effects Development of leukemia and thyroid carcinoma has occasionally been observed during lithium treatment, but a causative role for lithium has not been demonstrated.

Second generation effects See p. 85.

ORGANS AND SYSTEMS *(SEDA-17, 26; SEDA-18, 26)*

Cardiovascular Cardiac abnormalities during lithium treatment may include *reversible changes of sinus node activity*, *atrioventricular block*, *arrhythmia*, *paroxysmal bundle branch block*, *T-wave changes*, and variations of *repolarization*.

Cardiovascular side effects of lithium are rare, benign, and reversible, and heart disease is not an absolute contraindication against lithium treatment; prophylactic alternatives such as tricyclic antidepressants are likely to be more cardiotoxic. Electrocardiographic monitoring is advisable when lithium is administered to patients with known arrhythmias or conduction disorders.

Lithium does not affect arterial *blood pressure*. Before treatment the manic-depressive patients' blood pressure is slightly lower in spring and fall than in summer and winter; during lithium treatment these seasonal variations disappear.

Nervous system For some patients *hand tremor* remains one of the most troublesome side effects of lithium treatment; the persons affected are often those with pre-existing tremor or a family history of tremor. The tremorigenic effects of lithium and antidepressants potentiate each other. The prevalence of tremor falls with increasing duration of treatment. Like essential tremor, lithium-induced tremor may be aggravated by smoking and the consumption of caffeine-containing drinks. Reduction of the lithium dose is often sufficient to relieve the tremor, but this is not always possible without loss of prophylactic effect. The tremor usually responds to β-blockers in low dosage, for example 10–20 mg of propranolol taken 30 minutes before a meeting or party where tremor might be embarrassing.

Cogwheel rigidity not subjectively apparent to the patients, reversible *Parkinson-like effects*, *muscular fatigue*, and *restless legs* have been reported. Rare instances of reversible *pseudotumor cerebri* (benign intracranial hypertension, papilledema, headache, downbeat nystagmus, ophthalmoplegia) may be seen. Pre-existing vestibulo-cerebellar abnormalities are present in some of these patients; others may suffer from undetected hypothyroidism.

In association with lithium treatment (occasionally lithium intoxication) there have been scattered reports of *paresthesia*, *alexithymia*, *myasthenia gravis*, *chorea*, *parkinsonism*, and *aggravation of petit-mal epilepsy*, as well as *ataxia*, *dysarthria*, *tardive dyskinesia*, and *electroencephalographic abnormalities*. In some cases there were predisposing factors such as organic brain damage or alcoholic encephalopathy. *Creutzfeldt-Jakob-like syndromes* with dementia, myoclonus, and EEG abnormalities have been seen; whereas the spontaneous Creutzfeldt-Jakob-like syndrome has a poor prognosis, the drug-induced states usually resolve shortly after drug withdrawal.

Psychological In view of its pronounced effect on episodes of abnormal mood and activity it is striking how little lithium treatment affects normal mental processes. Most patients on lithium feel normal and function normally. When lithium-treated patients spontaneously complain of, or reply to questions about, mental trouble, it is often difficult to distinguish between side effects of the drug, the result of disappearance of subjectively pleasant mild manias, and manifestation of possible remnants of depression. Complaints of '*a certain lack of emotional color*' are, for example, difficult to place. *Changes in personality characteristics* have been ascribed partly to improvement induced by lithium and partly to effects of lithium on characteristic individual features.

In sensitive patients lithium may induce *memory impairment* and *prolonged reaction time*, but it is often difficult to assess the contribution of other factors, for example depression, previous electroconvulsive therapy, or concurrently administered drugs. Psychological side effects of lithium are dose-dependent and reversible; they can often be alleviated or removed through a reduction of the dose and serum concentration.

Psychological tests performed on patients taking lithium have not given consistent or reliable results. Short-term studies on healthy volunteers have shown effects on mood stability, interest, achievement, and personality, but no clear impairment of cognitive functions (SED-12, 18; SEDA-18, 26).

Assessment of *car-driving ability*, carried out in simulators, has given variable results. Presumably most of the many thousands of manic-depressive patients maintained on lithium drive a car or operate a machine, and yet the author of the present review has never heard of a car or machine accident where lithium treatment was implicated. He nevertheless makes it his habit to advise patients starting lithium treatment to abstain from car driving until they have found out whether the treatment affects their motor coordination.

There is an association between manic-depressive illness and the artistic temperament (11), and the patients' *creative ability* may decrease during lithium treatment. But equally often it remains unaffected, and more often it is increased because prevention of manic and depressive episodes facilitates a more steady work rhythm and better artistic discipline (12[C]).

Dependence on lithium has never been demonstrated, although like most drugs lithium has occasionally been used by multi-drug addicts in the hope of experiencing exotic effects, sometimes with the result that they felt their 'highs' becoming less high.

Endocrine, metabolic (*SED*-12, 81; *SEDA*-18, 27) Lithium inhibits release of thyroid hormone from the gland and may enhance its peripheral degradation. *Hypothyroidism* and *goiter* are reported with widely varying frequencies; unfortunately most such reports do not distinguish between prevalence and incidence. Prospective studies from Sweden and Denmark have shown the incidence of hypothyroidism requiring thyroxine treatment to be 2 per 100 patient-years of lithium exposure. Serum thyrotropin (TSH) may rise and serum thyroxine fall transitorily within the first 6—12 months of lithium treatment, most pronounced in patients with a past history of thyroid illness. Single abnormal values of serum TSH and serum thyroxine may occur, followed shortly by normal values. Patients with aberrant values should therefore be re-examined rather than started on thyroxine treatment on the basis of a single abnormal laboratory finding. Lithium-induced goiter is significantly correlated with smoking. Elevated titers of thyroid antibodies have been seen but do not necessarily indicate development of hypothyroidism. *Hyperthyroidism* may develop during lithium treatment, but it is much rarer than hypothyroidism.

Lithium-induced goiter and myxedema are not serious clinical problems once they are diagnosed; it is important to avoid mistaking mild myxedema for a depressive recurrence. Addition of thyroxine to the regimen invariably leads to normalization of thyroid size and function. Such treatment may be considered even in the absence of overt clinical hypothyroidism if serum TSH is consistently elevated and there are psychological complaints that might be of hypothyroid origin. Concurrent thyroxine treatment has occasionally improved lithium-treated patients' life quality to a marked degree.

Although lithium-induced *hyperparathyroidism with hypercalcemia* (13[R], 14[C]) usually disappears when lithium administration is stopped, continuation of treatment can be necessary for the patient's mental health, and surgical intervention may be indicated.

Weight gain during the first 1—2 years of lithium treatment may have several causes. In one study, appetite was increased in only one third of the patients, but nearly all patients experienced increased thirst and drank much because of their lithium-induced polydipsia. Weight gain during lithium treatment occurs especially in patients already overweight before the treatment, in bipolar patients, and in patients given lithium and antidepressant drugs together. Patients with lithium-induced weight gain must exercise and cut down on calories. The possibility of hypothyroidism should not be forgotten.

Development of *diabetes mellitus* during lithium treatment is so rare that coincidence is the most likely explanation.

Mineral and fluid balance Transitory edema is usually a lithium side effect without great importance in itself, but it may lead to increased risk of lithium poisoning if treated incautiously with diuretic drugs.

Renal lithium clearance falls when sodium or water balance become negative.

Hematological Lithium often induces *leukocytosis*, and *increased platelet counts* have also been observed. *Leukemia* has infrequently developed during lithium treatment, but a causal relationship is not established. Determinations of *blood folate* during lithium treatment have shown decrease in plasma and increase in erythrocyte levels.

Gastrointestinal Both *hypersalivation* and *hyposalivation* have been seen in lithium-treated patients, but complaints of *dry mouth* are rare. Lithium-induced *diarrhea* (*loose stools*, *defecation urge*) is significantly more frequent when serum lithium is over rather than when it is under 0.8 mmol/l.

Urinary system (*SEDA*-14, 18 (*special review*)) Observation of *morphological changes* in the kidneys of lithium-treated patients about 25 years ago created fear that long-term lithium treatment might lead to deterioration of glomerular function and eventually to renal failure. However, similar structural changes have been seen in manic-depressive patients before lithium treatment, and extensive cross-sectional and longitudinal studies on kidney function in patients given lithium for many years have shown that the risk of lithium-induced lowering of the *glomerular filtration rate* is very small (14[C], 15[R], 16[R]). It is not possible to decide whether the few cases of renal insufficiency that have been reported (17[C], 18[C], 19[C]) are rare and late side effects of the lithium treatment or coincidences. Renal insufficiency without known cause does develop in the general population; the incidence of renal failure among manic-depressive patients not given lithium is unknown.

Impairment of renal concentrating ability may develop as a result of lithium-induced reduction of the sensitivity of the distal tubules to the action of the antidiuretic hormone. This may or may not be associated with *polyuria* and *polydipsia*. These side effects are significantly less frequent with low than with high lithium doses and serum levels. Treatment with thiazide diuretics or amiloride may be effective but is potentially dangerous, because it tends to lower the renal lithium clearance. Treatment with furosemide seems safer (20[C]). The hypothesis that polyuria is lowered by administration of lithium in one rather than two or three daily doses (21[C]) has not been confirmed in properly conducted trials (22[C], 23[C], 24[C]). Supplementation with potassium (25[C]) or inositol (26[C]) is still at an experimental stage. Even a marked lowering of the renal concentrating ability does not constitute grounds for discontinuing prophylactically effective and otherwise well-tolerated lithium treatment.

There have been reports about development of a *nephrotic syndrome* with proteinuria and edema formation during lithium treatment or treatment with lithium in combination with other psychotropic drugs. The frequency is so low that one might consider coincidence the most likely explanation, but in some instances the proteinuria disappeared when lithium treatment was discontinued and reappeared when it was resumed. One is presumably dealing with an idiosyncratic reaction in particularly sensitive patients.

Skin and appendages (27[R]) Acne and treatment-resistant psoriasis may develop or become exacerbated during lithium treatment. *Hair loss*, *change of hair texture*, and *nail dystrophy* can also occur, the first sometimes associated with hypothyroidism. There have been reports of *maculopapular eruptions*, *exfoliative dermatitis*, *subcorneal pustular dermatosis*, *erythema multiforme*, *hydradenitis suppurativa* and *keratosis follicularis*. Exacerbation of *Darier's disease* has been seen.

Special senses Lithium may affect *foveal dark-adaptation*, but this apparently has little functional importance, for example for car driving. Lithium may further cause *visual field changes*, usually unnoticed by the patients, and *increased sensitivity to acute light effects*. It is possible that patients in lithium treatment are at extra risk of retinal affection when exposed to bright light, for example during light therapy for seasonal affective disorder.

Musculoskeletal system Although some older studies of bone density and bone mineral content appeared to show that lithium induces *osteopenia*, later results have been equivocal. In a recent study of 26 manic-depressive patients treated with lithium for 10 years or longer bone mineral densities did not differ significantly from those of matched normal controls

(28[C]). Bone fractures have not been reported to occur with increased frequency during lithium therapy.

Sexual function *Lowering of libido and potency* do not occur more frequently in lithium-treated patients than among mentally healthy controls.

Second-generation effects The question of possible *teratogenic effects* of first-trimester in utero exposure to lithium continues to attract attention. Evidence obtained previously from retrospective, and hence unavoidably biased, studies (29[R]) has in recent years been supplemented by cohort and case-control studies without such bias (30[C], 31[R]). They have shown that the risk of lithium-induced teratogenesis is markedly lower than previously assumed. The last-mentioned review gives detailed, and in my opinion excellent, advice about lithium treatment in women of childbearing potential.

A questionnaire study of the later development of children exposed to lithium during pregnancy and born without malformations failed to provide evidence of a higher risk of somatic or mental developmental anomalies than in a control group consisting of the lithium children's siblings.

Lithium treatment during lactation Lithium passes from blood into milk, and the nursing infant's serum concentration is one-tenth to one-half that of the mother's. It is, however, a moot question whether this is sufficient reason for women in lithium treatment to bottle-feed rather than breast-feed their children.

Risk situations Risk situations include intercurrent physical disease with fever, use of a low-salt diet, rigorous slimming regimens, treatment with diuretics (except perhaps furosemide), treatment with non-steroidal anti-inflammatory agents and with antihypertensive ACE-inhibitors, profuse sweating, major surgery, and manic and depressive recurrence with reduced intake of food and fluid. In risk situations it is wise to stop lithium temporarily or to reduce the dosage. Patients with lithium-induced polyuria are at extra risk of dehydration if they vomit massively or do not drink amply, for example if they are unconscious for a long time or are deprived of fluid prior to surgery with narcosis. Under these circumstances parenteral fluid administration may be required.

Withdrawal effects When prophylactic lithium treatment is stopped, there is risk of recurrence of the disease, because the protection of the treatment is brought to an end. It has been claimed that discontinuation of lithium, especially abrupt discontinuation, produces a '*lithium withdrawal syndrome*', but a critical analysis of the literature failed to disclose evidence of either *abstinence symptoms* or *rebound phenomena* (32[R]).

Intoxication (33[R]) In the present series of reviews this section is customarily entitled 'Overdosage', but I have asked the editor's permission to use instead the title shown above. The reason is that lithium poisoning may develop not only as a result of overdosage, for example by mistake or with suicidal intent. It may also be caused by a fall in the lithium clearance during kidney disease or as a result of negative sodium or water balance (see under 'Risk situations' above).

Signs of incipient intoxication may include apathy, drowsiness, muscular weakness, unsteady gait, and indistinct speech. In fully developed intoxication there is impaired consciousness or coma, possibly seizures, and increased or decreased deep reflexes. The patients look ill, pinched, grey, and cold. The condition may deteriorate for some days in spite of falling serum lithium concentration.

Treatment of lithium intoxication (34[R], 35[C], 36[C]) involves careful monitoring and, if necessary, correction, of renal function and fluid and electrolyte balance. Hemodialysis effectively removes lithium from the body, and it should be repeated if there is pronounced rebound of serum lithium. Bicarbonate dialysis seems more effective than acetate dialysis (37[C]). Continuous hemodiafiltration or hemodia-diffusion-filtration may be better than intermittent hemodialysis because rebound is avoided (38[C], 39[C]), but so far few patients have been given these treatments.

Lithium intoxication may lead to death or permanent *cerebellar damage* (40[R], 41[C]); it should always be regarded as potentially dangerous. The best precaution is avoidance of risk situations and alertness to danger signs. Patients, relatives, and physicians must be properly instructed.

Interactions *(SED-12, 83; SEDA-18, 30 (special review))* Interaction with *neuroleptics* has attracted a good deal of attention, partly due to a sensational but hardly representative report 20 years ago. Extensive studies show that permanent brain damage is not a characteristic of such interaction, which is rare if neuroleptic doses are kept low or moderate, for example lower than 20 mg of haloperidol daily (42[R]). Elderly persons are, not surprisingly, especially vulnerable, and yet one cannot avoid the impression that they are all too often subjected to polypharmacy and large doses.

There is evidence that the combination of lithium with *antidepressant drugs* offers prophylactic advantage in unipolar patients, and addition of lithium to antidepressants may produce therapeutic response in patients who have proven refractory to the latter drugs given alone. Combined administration of antidepressants and lithium increases their potential for inducing tremor and weight gain. When lithium and antidepressants are given together over a long period, some bipolar patients become 'rapid cyclers', i.e. prone to frequent recurrences. This may, however, be an effect of the antidepressant treatment as such rather than of the combination.

A number of reports have dealt with interaction of lithium and *specific serotonin re-uptake inhibitors*, such as *fluoxetine* and *fluvoxamine*, but since we do not know how often lithium has been used in combination with these drugs, it is not possible to decide whether interactions are frequent or rare or perhaps merely coincidental. The majority of studies on lithium augmentation with fluoxetine or fluvoxamine in treatment-resistant depression do not mention adverse interactions (SEDA-18, 30 (special review)).

In patients who do not respond to prophylactic lithium alone, combined treatment with *carbamazepine* may, according to anecdotal evidence, have a good chance of providing help. Adverse effects of the combination may involve ataxia, dizziness, and feelings of unreality, but this is rare. When lithium is combined with carbamazepine, it reverses the leukopenia induced by the latter drug; the antithyroid effects of the two are additive.

Although *electroconvulsive therapy* (*ECT*) does not seem to affect lithium clearance or serum lithium values (and lithium has not been shown to alter the seizure threshold), there may occasionally be interaction between the two therapies with production of confusion, disorientation, restlessness, memory impairment, and electroencephalographic seizure activity. Under appropriate safeguards, combining lithium and ECT may nevertheless be justified in patients unresponsive to either treatment given alone, for example patients who show manic or depressive aggravation immediately after discontinuation of lithium (43[R], 44[R]).

The clinically most important drug interaction of lithium is with *diuretics*, even though reports of such interactions have been rare in recent years. Perhaps warnings are beginning to have an effect. Furosemide may be the safest choice if diuretic treatment is required (20[C], 45[C]).

Interaction between lithium and *non-steroidal anti-inflammatory drugs* (*NSAIDs*) has been reported sufficiently often to be regarded as established. The interaction is clearly at the renal level; lithium clearance falls and the serum lithium concentration rises. An action via inhibition of prostaglandin synthesis seems likely. Aspirin and sulindac may be the safest choices for patients in lithium treatment (46[R]).

Problems can arise with *antihypertensive treatment*. Therapy with thiazides in inadvisable; furosemide may be the least dangerous. Interaction with *ACE inhibitors* (inhibitors of the enzyme that converts angiotensin I to angiotensin II) such as *enalapril*, *captopril*, *lisinopril*, *ramipril* and *quinapril* can lead to impaired glomerular filtration and elevation of serum creatinine and serum lithium. β-Receptor blocking agents may be the best choice in treatment of hypertension in lithium-treated patients.

There is no evidence that lithium and anesthetics interact, but surgeons and anesthesiologists should be aware of the risk of lithium accumulation when fluid and electrolyte balance is deranged in connection with surgery. Administration of *depolarizing agents* to patients on lithium has occasionally led to prolonged neuromuscular blockade.

Alcohol may accelerate lithium excretion in women but hardly to a clinically significant degree. Serum lithium may rise and hand tremor develop when patients change from a hospital regime with high intake of coffee to a home environment with low intake. Laxatives such as ispaghula husk and psyllium may inhibit absorption of lithium from the gastrointestinal tract.

REFERENCES

1. Schou M. Le Lithium: Guide pratique pour les medécins et les patients. Paris: Presses Universitaires de France, 1984.
2. Schou M. Lithium Treatment of Manic-Depressive Illness: A Practical Guide (title in Japanese). Tokyo: Igakushup-pan-Sha, 1984.
3. Schou M. Il trattamento con litio della malattia maniacodepressiva. Roma: Athena Editrice, 1986.
4. Schou M. Lithium v léčbě maniodepresivniho onemocněni. Praha: Avicenum, 1987.
5. Schou M. Litiumbehandling av manodepressiv siukdom: En vägledning, 2nd edn. Södertälje: Astra, 1990.
6. Schou M. Lithium treatment of manic-depressive illness: a practical quide (title in Greek). Athens: Zymel, 1990.
7. Schou M. Lithiumbogen: Lithiumbehandling af maniodepressiv sygdom, 3rd edn. Copenhagen: Rygaard and Welner, 1991.
8. Schou M. Lithium-Behandlung der manisch-depressiven Krankheit: Informationen für Arzt, Patient und Angehöriqe, 3rd revised edn. Stuttgart: Thieme, 1991.
9. Schou M. Treatment of Manic-Depressive Illness: A Practical Guide, 5th revised edn. Basel—Freiburg—Paris—London—New York—New Delhi—Singapore—Tokyo—Sydney: Karger, 1993.
10. Schou M. Lit w leczeniu chorób afektywnych: Przewodnik praktyczny. Warshawa: Fundacja IPN, 1994.
11. Jamison KR. Touched with fire: Manic-depressive illness

and the artistic temperament. New York: Free Press (MacMillan), 1993.
12. Schou M. Artistic productivity and lithium prophylaxis in manic-depressive illness. Br J Psychiatry 1979;135:97.
13. Brochier T, Adnet-Kessous J, Barillot M, Pascalis JG. Hyperparathyroidie sous lithium. Encephale 1994;20:339.
14. Kallner G, Petterson U. Renal, thyroid and parathyroid function during lithium treatment: laboratory tests in 207 people treated for 1—30 years. Acta Psychiatr Scand 1995;91:48.
15. Schou M. Effects of long-term lithium treatment on kidney function: an overview. J Psychiatr Res 1988;22:287.
16. Waller DG, Edwards JG. Lithium and the kidney: an update. Psychol Med 1989;19:825.
17. von Knorring L, Wahlin A, Nyström K, Bohman SO. Uraemia induced by long-term lithium treatment. Lithium 1990;1:251.
18. Gitlin MJ. Lithium-induced renal insufficiency. J Clin Psychopharmacol 1993;13:276.
19. Schou M. Personal observation, 1994.
20. Shalmi M, Thomsen K. Renal elimination of lithium. In: Birch NJ, ed. Lithium and the Cell: Pharmacology and Biochemistry. London: Academic Press, 1991;249.
21. Mellerup ET, Plenge P. The side effects of lithium. Biol Psychiatry 1990;28:464.
22. Muir A, Davidson R, Silverstone T, Dawnay A, Forsling ML. Two regimens of lithium prophylaxis and renal function. Acta Psychiatr Scand 1989;80:579.
23. Abraham G, Delva N, Waldron J, Lawson JS Owen J. Lithium treatment: a comparison of once- and twice-daily dosing. Acta Psychiatr Scand 1992;85:65.
24. O'Donovan C, Hawkes J, Bowen R. Effect of lithium dosing schedule on urinary output. Acta Psychiatr Scand 1993;87:92.
25. Musa MN, Tripuraneni BR. Lithium-induced polyuria ameliorated by potassium supplementation. Lithium 1993;4:199.
26. Bersudsky Y, Vinnitsky I, Grisaru N, Yaroslavsky U, Gheorghiu S, Igvi D, Kofman 0, Belmaker RH. The effect of inositol on lithium-induced polyuria-polydipsia in rats and humans. Hum Psychopharmacol 1993;7:403.
27. Krahn LE, Goldberg RL. Psychotropic medications and the skin. Adv Psychosom Med 1994;21:90.
28. Nordenström J, Elvius M, Bågedahl-Strindlund M, Zhao B, Törring 0. Biochemical hyperparathyroidism and bone mineral status in patients treated long-term with lithium. Metabolism 1994;43:1563.
29. Schou M. Lithium treatment during pregnancy, delivery, and lactation: an update. J Clin Psychiatry 1990;51:410.
30. Jacobson SJ, Jones K, Johnson K, Ceolin L, Kaur P, Sahn D, Donnenfeld AE, Rieder M, Santelli R, Smythe J, Pastuszak A, Einarson T, Koren G. Prospective multicentre study of pregnancy outcome after lithium exposure during first trimester. Lancet 1992;339:530.
31. Cohen LS, Friedman JM, Jefferson JW, Johnson EM, Weiner ML. A reevaluation of risk of in utero exposure to lithium. J Am Med Assoc 1993;271:146.
32. Schou M. Is there a lithium withdrawal syndrome? An examination of the evidence. Br J Psychiatry 1993;163:514.
33. Bell AJ, Ferrier IN. Lithium induced neurotoxicity at therapeutic levels: an aetiological review. Lithium 1994;5:181.
34. Groleau G. Lithium toxicity. Emerg Med Clin N Am 1994;12:511.
35. Kasahara H, Shinozaki T, Nukariya K, Nishimura H, Nakano H, Nakagawa T, Ushijima S. Hemodialysis for lithium intoxication: preliminary guidelines for emergency. Jpn J Psychiatr Neurol 1994;48:1.
36. Okusa MD, Crystal LJT. Clinical manifestations and management of acute lithium intoxication. Am. J. Med 1994;97:383.
37. Szerlip HM, Heeger P, Feldman GM. Comparison between acetate and bicarbonate dialysis for the treatment of lithium intoxication. Am J Nephrol 1992;12:116—120.
38. Bellomo R, Boyce N. Current approaches to the treatment of severe lithium intoxication. Lithium 1992;3:245—248
39. Leblanc M, Raymond M, Pichette V, Isenring P, Bonnardeaux A, Geadah D, Boucher A, Cardinal J. High dialysate flow rate continuous arteriovenous haemodialysis: an effective approach to treat lithium intoxication. Nephrol Dialys Transplant 1994;9:1011.
40. Schou M. Long-lasting neurological sequelae after lithium intoxication. Acta Psychiatr Scand 1984;70:594.
41. Schneider JA, Mirra SS. Neuropathologic correlates of persistent neurologic deficit in lithium intoxication. Ann Neurol 1994;36:928.
42. Schou M. Adverse lithium-neuroleptic interactions: are there permanent effects? Hum Psychopharmacol 1990;5:263.
43. Schou M. Lithium and electroconvulsive therapy: adversaries, competitors, allies? Acta Psychiatr Scand 1991; 84:435.
44. Lippmann SB, El-Mallakh R. Can electroconvulsive therapy be given during lithium treatment? Lithium 1994; 5:205.
45. Crabtree BL, Mack JE, Johnson CD, Amyx BC. Comparison of the effects of hydrochlorothiazide and furosemide on lithium disposition. Am J Psychiatry 1991;148:1060.
46. Johnson AG, Seideman P, Day RO. Adverse drug interactions with nonsteroidal anti-inflammatory drugs (NSAIDs): recognition, management and avoidance. Drug Safety 1993;8:99.

Meyler's Side Effects of Drugs, 13th Edition
M.N.G. Dukes, editor

SECTION EDITOR: P.K.M. LUNDE

Peter J. Geerlings

4 Drugs of abuse

The range of drugs dealt with in this chapter will, as in earlier volumes, continue to be limited to those psychoactive substances which are mainly used for non-medical purposes, generally in order to produce pleasurable, stimulating or desirable effects. These psychoactive substances comprise the cannabinoids, hallucinogens, stimulant-hallucinogens ('designer' drugs), cocaine, phencyclidine and a number of volatile solvents. Although cannabinoids (tetrahydrocannabinol) and phencyclidine are hallucinogenic, their pharmacology, patterns of use and clinical presentations set them apart. Tobacco and alcohol were not included in earlier editions and are again left out of consideration in this volume, since each of them is the subject of a massive and specialized literature which is reviewed in other publications. Drugs which are primarily used for legitimate purposes but which are also the subject of abuse—such as certain opioids, stimulants and sedative/tranquilizers—are dealt with primarily in their own chapters of this volume.

GENERAL CONSIDERATIONS

Many of the psychic manifestations associated with taking a drug depend to a significant extent on the characteristics of the user, his or her experience with this and other drugs, the pharmacological actions of the drug and the environment in which the drug is taken. The effects of a drug are not always predictable, even in the same individual and in the same environment; they also vary with the emotional state of the user prior to administration. The drug user himself (or herself) may also be entirely uncertain as to what drug has been taken, since it is likely to have been bought on the illegal market which is a highly undependable source of supply, and where substitution and contamination are likely to be common.

It is possible to classify users of psychoactive substances for non-medical purposes into a number of different groups. Most users of psychoactive substances, for example cannabis and methylenedioxymethamphetamine (MDMA, also known as 'ecstasy') probably use them only on one occasion, or a very few times, with groups of friends. Others users take psychoactive substances repeatedly though irregularly, as a rule with groups of friends at parties; 'ecstasy' in particular has proved to be a popular drug for house parties.

The route of administration for drugs of abuse may itself be such as to lead to physical damage and disease. Intravenous administration (or indeed any parenteral route of use) carries with it the possibility of inducing thrombophlebitis, chronic abscesses, tissue necrosis, scarring, local and systemic infections. The risks attendant on the use of non-sterile (and hence often contaminated) syringes and needles have been increased in the last decades with the possible transmission of viral infections, including HIV, hepatitis B and hepatitis C. In addition, effects on the immune system have been reported leading to hypersensitivity reactions and systematic vasculitis or glomerulonephritis. The use of illicit injectables, which may well have been prepared from what were originally tablets, often leads to systematic and particularly pulmonary embolism because of contamination with such excipients as starch, talc or synthetic materials. Inhalation of certain substances may promote mechanical damage to the nose and the respiratory system. All psychoactive substances influence various forms of psychomotor performance during the phase of intoxication, and this can naturally include impairment of the ability to drive.

Cannabis and related agents

Cannabis is the abbreviated name for the hemp plant *Cannabis sativa*. The common names for cannabis include: marijuana, grass and weed. Other names for cannabis refer to particular strains; they include bhang and ganja. The most potent forms of cannabis come from the flowering tops of the plants or from the dried resinous exudate of the leaves, and are referred to as hashish or hash. Cannabis is one of the oldest and most widely used drugs in the world.

PHARMACOLOGY

The primary active component of cannabis is δ^9-tetrahydrocannabinol (THC). Δ^9-THC is responsible for the greater part of the pharmacological effects of the cannabis complex. Δ^8-THC is also active. However the cannabis plant contains more than 400 chemicals, of which some sixty are chemically related to Δ^9-THC, and it is evident that the exact proportions in which these are present may vary considerable with the way in which the material has been harvested and prepared. In man, Δ^9-THC is rapidly converted to 11-hydroxy Δ^9-THC (1), the metabolite which is active in the central nervous system. A specific receptor for the cannabinols has been identified; it is a member of the G-protein linked family of receptors (2). The cannabinoid receptor is linked to the inhibitory G-protein which is linked to adenyl cyclase in an inhibitory fashion (3). The cannabinoid receptor is found in the highest concentrations in the basal ganglia, the hippocampus and the cerebellum with lower concentrations in the cerebral cortex.

When cannabis is smoked, the euphoric effects appear within minutes, reaching a maximum in about 30 minutes and lasting up to 4 hours. Some of the motor and cognitive effects may persist for 5—12 hours. Cannabis can also be taken orally, being used to prepare food, such as cakes.

Many variables affect the psychoactive properties of cannabis including the potency of the cannabis used, the route of administration, the smoking technique, the dose, the setting, the user's past experience, the user's expectations and the user's biological vulnerability to the effects of the drug.

The effects may be considered under two main headings, reflecting the psychoactive and the autonomic activity, respectively, in addition to which there are direct toxic effects.

The *autonomic* activity leads to tachycardia, peripheral vasodilation, conjunctival congestion, hyperthermia, bronchodilation, dry mouth, nystagmus, tremors, ataxia, hypotension, nausea and vomiting, i.e. a spectrum of effects which resembles closely the consequences of overdosage with anticholinergic agents. In some individuals sleep disturbances are seen. Increased appetite and dry mouth are other common effects of cannabis intoxication.

The most frequently reported *psychoactive* effects include enhanced sensory perception (e.g. a heightened appreciation of colour and sound). Cannabis intoxication commonly heightens the user's sensitivity to other external stimuli as well but subjectively slows down the appreciation of time. In high doses the user may also experience depersonalization and derealization. Various forms of psychomotor performances including driving are significantly impaired for 8—12 hours after using cannabis.

The most serious potential *toxic* effects of cannabis use on physique are those which result from of the inhalation of the same carcinogenic hydrocarbons that are present in tobacco, and some data indicate that heavy cannabis users are at risk for chronic respiratory diseases and lung cancer.

ADVERSE REACTION PATTERN

General and toxic reactions These reactions have been reported at relatively low doses and principally affect the psyche, leading to anxiety states, panic reactions, restlessness, hallucinations, fear, confusion and, rarely, toxic psychosis. These effects appear to be reversible (4^R).

Hypersensitivity reactions These are rare, but a few have been reported following inhalation. Delayed hypersensitivity reactions, particularly affecting vascular tissue, have been recorded with chronic systemic administration.

Tumour-inducing effects These are difficult to attribute to cannabis alone. Animal studies have demonstrated neoplastic pulmonary lesions superimposed on chronic inflammation, but such pathology may be associated primarily with the 'tar' produced by burning marijuana. The most serious potential adverse effects of cannabis use come from of the inhalation of the same carcinogenic hydrocarbons that are present in tobacco, and some data indicate that heavy cannabis users are at risk for chronic respiratory diseases and lung cancer.

ORGANS AND SYSTEMS

Cardiovascular *Peripheral vasodilatation* with increased blood flow, orthostatic hypotension, and tachycardia may occur with normal doses of recreational cannabis use. High doses of THC taken intravenously have been frequently associated with *premature ventricular beats* with decreased PR intervals and T-wave amplitude, to which tolerance readily develops and which are reversible on drug withdrawal. While the other cardiovascular effects tend to decrease in chronic smokers, the degree of tachycardia continues to be exaggerated with exercise as shown with bicycle ergometry.

The cardiovascular effects may possibly present a risk to persons with existing cardiovascular disorders, but otherwise in adults with normal cardiovascular functions there is no evidence of any permanent damage associated with marijuana (4^R, 5^C, 6^r).

Respiratory Acute inhalation of marijuana or THC induces bronchodilatation, but with chronic use resistance in the bronchioles increases (7^C, 8^C). Prolonged use of cannabis by inhalation may induce chronic *inflammatory changes* in the bronchial tree, in part related to the inhalants accompanying the smoke. In some cases *asthmatic attacks* and *glottal and uvular angio-edema* may occur. *Decreased respiratory gas exchange* has been reported in long-term smokers, and under experimental conditions THC can *depress respiratory function* slightly and act as a *respiratory irritant*. In fact, chronic marijuana cigarette smoking and chronic tobacco cigarette smoking produce very similar changes but these manifest themselves after smoking fewer cigarettes when marijuana is smoked instead of tobacco. Tashkin and colleagues in a series of studies have shown that with marijuana cigarette inhalation, where there is never the interposition of a filter, inhalation is deeper and the smoke is held in the lungs for a longer period than when smoking commercially produced tobacco-based cigarettes (9^C). As a consequence there is greater build-up of carbon monoxide, reduction in carboxyhemoglobin saturation, and alveolar cellular irritation with depression of macrophages (SEDA-13, 25). *Pneumothorax*, *pneumopericardium* and *pneumomediastinum* have been reported when positive pulmonary pressure is applied or a Valsalva manoeuvre used, as often happens (10^C, 11^C).

Nervous system As discussed in the introduction to this chapter, the effects of cannabis on the user's nervous system vary with a number of personal and social factors. However some guidance as to the essential effects of the drug can be derived from investigations with THC and marijuana in non-user volunteer subjects. Blood levels of THC greater than 75 mg/ml prove under these conditions to be associated with euphoria, and somewhat higher levels with dissociation of events and memory and impairment of psychomotor tasks lasting over 24 hours (4^R).

Tolerance develops with repeated use, and withdrawal symptoms occur after regular prolonged use. Occasional use does not appear to be associated with major consequences. Long-term heavy use of cannabis impairs mental performance, induces memory defects (especially for short-term memory), leads to disorganization of thinking and interferes with social integration. Both occasional and regular users have been reported to suffer inexplicably from sudden panic attacks, paranoia, hallucinations or feelings of unreality (depersonalization and derealization). A number of psychologists (12^C) have shown that adolescents with pre-existing disabilities in learning and cognition have experienced serious aggravation of their problem from regular use of cannabis. In young children accidental ingestion leads to the rapid onset of drowsiness, hypotonia, dilated pupils and coma. Fortunately, gradual recovery occurs spontaneously, barring accidents. While chronic adult users may display apathy and impaired concentration, these effects are possibly in part associated with other factors. No permanent organic brain damage has been demonstrated (13^C, 14^C).

Abrupt withdrawal of high-level use of cannabinoids induces irritability, restlessness and insomnia, with a rebound increase in REM sleep, tremor and anorexia lasting up to a week (15^r, 16^R, 17^C, 18^C).

Endocrine, metabolic It has been demonstrated in animals (particularly monkeys) that cannabis will depress ovarian and testicular function. In man chronic use has been associated with decreased serum FSH and LH levels in a few persons, often accompanied by decreases in serum testosterone, oligospermia, decreased sperm mobility and gynecomastia (19^C). There is no evidence of impairment of male fertility; no studies have been carried out on female fertility. There is evidence of slightly shortened gestation periods in chronic users (20^C). There are variable non-specific effects on serum prolactin and growth hormone and a rise in plasma cortisol levels has been recorded in one study.

Hematological The hematological changes very occasionally noted, polycythemia, appear to be secondary to reduced pulmonary oxygen exchange (see 'Respiratory' above).

Special senses No consistent changes have been reported apart from a decrease in intraocular pressure. The initial decrease in intraocular pressure has been shown to be followed by a rebound increase associated with increased prostaglandin levels.

Immune function In vitro studies have shown that THC depresses lymphocyte and macrophage activity in cell cultures, while in vivo studies in rats have shown a direct suppression of natural killer (NK) cell activity and an impairment of T-lymphocyte transformation with phytohemagglutinin (PHA) by concentrations of cannabinoids achievable with the usual doses (21). Variable results have been obtained in man in tests of circulating T-cells and hormonal immunity (23^c).

Various studies in animals and in man have shown that chronic dosage often suppresses the immune system's response to inhaled bacterial or fungal material. In this connection it is highly relevant to note that a contaminant mould (*Aspergillus*) found in cannabis may predispose immunocompromised cannabis smokers to infection. It has been suggested that baking the cannabis (at 300°F for 15 minutes) before smoking it will kill the fungus and reduce the potential risk of smoking (22[c]).

Risk situations Persons with pre-existent coronary artery disease may experience an increased incidence of anginal attacks. In individuals with some degree of mental disorder or instability, toxic psychoses or aggravation of schizophrenia may occur. The control of epilepsy may be deranged. Users undergoing anesthesia may react in an unexpected way and may exhibit a greater degree of CNS depression than expected. Because of impairment of judgment and psychomotor performance, users should not drive or operate machinery for at least 24 hours after administration.

Withdrawal effects While a withdrawal syndrome similar to that generally described with opiates is not seen, abrupt withdrawal after habitual use leads to tremor, anorexia, restlessness, irritability and insomnia.

Second-generation effects In animals, THC has been shown to cross the placenta and to be excreted in breast milk. There is conflicting evidence concerning teratogenicity in animals but no definitive evidence of this in man. However, there have been many anecdotal reports of abnormalities. Although these were without any consistent characteristics, the descriptions would fit more easily into the fetal alcohol syndrome (24[c], 25[R], 26[Cr], 27[cR]). Clinical evaluation of the use of cannabis during pregnancy is indeed complicated by the frequent concomitant use of tobacco and alcohol.

In monkeys as well as in man, behavioral anomalies have been identified in the offspring of women exposed to cannabis during pregnancy. These include decreased visual responses, increased auditory responses and decreased quietude. Most of the effects were gone within 4—5 weeks post partum and no abnormalities were noted at 1 year.

Interactions Additive psychoactive effects sought by users may be achieved by combinations of cannabis and short-acting *barbiturates* and *alcohol*, but at the same time the ability of THC to induce microsomal enzymes will increase the rate of metabolism of barbiturates and alcohol and thus diminish the additive effects (15[r]).

Cannabis has been reported as influencing the effects of psychotropic drugs such as *opioids*, *anticholinergics* and *antidepressants*, though in a variable manner.

Concurrent administration with *disulfiram* is associated with hypomania (28[c]).

The anticholinergic effects of cannabis may result in interactions with *antiarrhythmic agents* and *antihypertensive drugs*.

Hallucinogens

Hallucinogens or psychedelics, of which LSD is the best known example, are drugs characterized by their capacity to induce hallucinations and disturbances of perception, feeling and thought at relatively low doses. The substances are also associated with the phenomenon of 'persisting perception disorder' or 'flashbacks'—spontaneous, transitory recurrences of the substance-induced experience even weeks after the last dose of drug. Earlier editions of this volume used the older term 'psychedelics'; its replacement by the term 'hallucinogens' is in accordance with the current nomenclature of the American Classification of Mental Disorders, the Diagnostic and Statistical Manual of Mental Disorders (DSM-IV) (29), and the latest WHO International Classification of Diseases (ICD-10) (30).

The hallucinogens are thought to act at multiple levels of the central nervous system, often as partial agonists at presynaptic receptors, and for 5-HT, inhibiting release and reducing the rate of firing (31).

The most potent of the group is lysergic acid diethylamide (LSD). The substance is generally consumed orally; its initial effects, anticholinergic-sympathomimetic in type, appear within about half an hour of ingestion and include tachycardia, hyperthermia, mydriasis, piloerection, hypertension and occasionally nausea and vomiting. The more important psychoactive effects develop 1—2 hours later and may last in some instances from 24 to 48 hours. Perception may be strikingly heightened and distorted, and initial perceptions may mask and overshadow later sensory perception. The user often grossly exaggerates his mental and emotional capacities, attributing to himself extraordinary powers. Visual hallucinations, loss of appreciation of time and space, and instability of mood are common. Meaningfullness and a sense of universal union often predominate. A significant problem in 'street purchase' is the uncertain quality and likely impurity of the material obtained. Doses of 25 μg LSD and more are sufficient to induce the psychophysiological effects, which are generally dose-related up to a level of 500 μg. The actual half-life of the drug in man is about 3 hours; its effects last considerably longer (32[R]).

Acute panic attacks and hallucinogen-induced psycho-tic disorder are frequently the consequence of use of hallucinogens in persons with pre-existing personality disorder or pre-psychotic personalities. Suicide and self-injury have been reported after the use of hallucinogens. Prolonged psychotic disorders may occur, but psychiatric opinion is divided as to whether these occur only in persons with pre-existent disorders or in 'normal' individuals as well. 'Flashbacks' occur particularly where there has been prolonged heavy use, but eventually disappear (SED-11, 83; 32[R], 33[cR]).

ADVERSE REACTION PATTERN

General and toxic reactions These include, principally, changes in perception, mood and behaviour, leading in many instances to acute panic, hallucinations, delusion and in some cases to a classical psychosis. Repeated use leads to persistence of these effects with 'flashbacks' occurring even after use has been discontinued. Self-injury and suicides may result (34[R]).

Hypersensitivity reactions These seem to be exceedingly rare and no reports have been validated.

Tumor-inducing effects These remain a possibility as a consequence of various reports from animal and human studies showing that chromosomal abnormalities may be associated with exposure to LSD. However, its ability to exert mutagenic effects in practice is questionable, and no useful evidence for or against its potential for carcinogenicity has been produced for LSD (35[R]).

ORGANS AND SYSTEMS

Cardiovascular Vasoconstriction has been associated with LSD, affecting both cerebral and peripheral circulation, but it is not usually significant at ordinary doses in persons with a normal circulatory system.

Nervous system The effects of LSD on the central nervous system were usefully categorized in earlier volumes and recent work gives little reason to modify the assessment presented at that time. There is no progression from one type to another, but the various features tend to merge, particularly with continuing use.

Hallucinogen-induced mood disorder is associated with changes in affect varying from euphoria to manic-like symptoms, panic/fear, and depression, often occurring within minutes and often varying in the same individual on different occasions. Changes in sensory perception, with a loss of ability to distinguish temporal or spatial reality and sensory hallucinations, particularly visual and tactile, are frequent, with a tendency to assume god-like attributes. These features often merge in a psychosis, particularly with repeated use. Whether a chronic psychosis after LSD is the result of the drug ingestion or of a combination of both the drug ingestion and predisposing factors is currently an unanswerable question.

The repeated use of LSD is associated not only with psychoses but also with *more specific neurological signs and symptoms* including ataxia, incoordination, dysphasia, paresthesia and tremor. Convulsions have been reported. 'Flashbacks' or the return of hallucinogenic effects, occur in almost a quarter of persons who have been using LSD, particularly if they are using other CNS stimulants such as alcohol or marijuana. The individuals may experience distortions of perception of objects, space or time, which intrude without warning into reality, resulting in delusions, panic and unusual images. A 'trailing phenomenon' has also been reported, in which the visual perception of objects is reduced to a series of interrupted pictures rather than a constant view. The frequency of these events may slowly decrease over several years but in a significant number their incidence later increases (32[R], 34[R]).

Hematological The only hematological effect reported has been an increased rate of blood clotting associated with severe hyperthermia (see below).

Gastrointestinal Evidence of increased gastrointestinal irritability is often encountered, with nausea, vomiting and diarrhoea.

Special senses Apart from the visual hallucinations already discussed, diplopia, blurred vision, mydriasis and other visual disturbances occur (36[R]). The pupillary dilatation, combined with a disturbance in sensory appreciation, has led to a number of instances of retinal damage following continued exposure to direct sun.

Other organs and systems A number of cases of *retroperitoneal fibrosis* have been reported—not unexpectedly in view of the similarity in chemical structure between LSD and methysergide (34[r]).

Hyperthermia may occur but does so very seldom with the usual doses. It has been produced experimentally with high doses.

Risk situations Persons with mental instability, schizophrenia or a family history thereof may be at considerable risk of developing LSD psychoses. Persons with epilepsy may be more prone to convulsions with a reduction in convulsant threshold.

Second-generation effects Animal studies have not indicated a teratogenic effect with LSD. Various publications have referred to a high incidence of abortions and of congenital abnormalities associated with LSD. However none of these gives any consistent pattern of abnormality, nor has there been an acceptable control group (35).

Interactions *Phenothiazines* and *butyrophenones* can counteract the psychoactive effects of LSD and *benzodiazepines* may depress the effects (37[r]). *Reserpine* will aggravate the effects of LSD, as will *MAO inhibitors*, *cannabis* and *amphetamines* will also accentuate its effects.

OTHER HALLUCINOGENIC DRUGS

Dimethyltryptamine

Dimethyltryptamine (DMT) is inactive by mouth and is only used by inhalation or injection. Its effects are similar to those of LSD.

Mescaline

The effects of the hallucinogen mescaline, which is derived from the peyote cactus, were investigated in a psychiatric research study (38[C]). Psychosis induced during the experiment was measured with the Brief Psychiatric Rating Scale and the Paranoid Depression Scale. Neuropsychological measures detected decreased functioning of the right hemisphere after use of the drug. Single photon emission computed tomography (SPECT) studies demonstrated a hyperfrontal pattern with an emphasis on the right hemisphere during mescaline use. The authors discussed the possible educational value of experimentally induced psychosis toward understanding the psychotic state.

Prolongation of psychoactive effects for about 12 hours has been reported, the effects being similar to those of LSD.

Psilocin
Psilocybin

These substances, both derived from certain mushrooms, have very short periods of activity, usually 6–8 hours. The effects resemble those of LSD.

'STIMULANT-HALLUCINOGENS'

During the last few years, use of the group of 'stimulant-hallucinogens' or 'designer drugs'—created explicitly to meet illicit demand—has increased. Methylenedioxymethamphetamine (MDMA) is the best known example of these drugs.

There have been several recent reports about the use and effects of MDMA, a recreational drug often known as 'ecstasy' that appears to be gaining in popularity world-wide. MDMA reportedly has the ability to produce a pleasant altered state of mind, during which feelings of emotional closeness can be enhanced (39[R]). In the 1970s and 1980s this effect of the drug caused some clinicians to advocate its use as an adjunct to psychotherapy (40[R]).

MDMA has a mild stimulant effect and a modest hallucinogenic potential. The results of a recent study in Australia suggested that tolerance may develop to its effects, but that adverse effects can increase with continued use (41[R]). Recent reports in the British literature have highlighted some disturbing effects associated with its use, particularly when it is used while dancing vigorously at 'rave' parties (42[R]).

In this setting, with increased physical activity, MDMA can cause *unconsciousness, seizures, hyperthermia, tachycardia, hypotension, disseminated intravascular coagulation, rhabdomyolysis, and acute renal failure* (43[R]). Severe complications of MDMA are also linked to uncontrolled fluid intake, hemodilution and salt losing syndromes. Deaths after the use of MDMA in such settings have been described in the British literature (44[r]). It has been suggested that severe toxicity from MDMA may result from an alteration in the thermoregulation induced by the drug in the face of excessive activity in warm environments (45[R]).

It has also been noted that case reports have suggested that repeated use of MDMA may be associated with jaundice or hepatomegaly, but that there is no way of knowing whether this apparent hepatotoxicity with MDMA is due to the drug or to an additive or contaminant in the available formulations (45[R]).

Further reports on MDMA or 'ecstasy' have appeared in the literature. These reports suggest that the relationship between the dose of 'ecstasy' and the possible development of complications from it may not be straightforward. Some people have problems with very small amounts. For example, a 21-year-old woman developed a protracted psychotic depersonalization disorder with suicidal tendency after taking two tablets of ecstasy for the first time (46[c]). In another case, a 23-year-old man with no prior psychiatric history developed panic disorder after ingesting a single dose (47[c]). In a third case, psychosis occurred in an 18-year-old male who had used the drug on an occasional recreational basis (48[c]).

The number of deaths associated with 'ecstasy' appears to be increasing. In one reported case, death occurred in an 18-year-old man after ingesting three tablets of the drug (49[c]); in another case, a single tablet and a quantity of amphetamine had been ingested (50[c]). Review of the death of six patients following 'ecstasy' use noted common effects—uncontrollable bleeding due to disseminated intravascular coagulation (DIC), progressive acidosis and multiple organ failure (51[c]). In all six cases, DIC or rhabdomyolysis was the prominent feature.

With MDMA's use becoming more widespread, other effects are also being reported. Spontaneous *pneumomediastinum* was noted in a 17-year-old man who presented to an emergency room with chest pain and vomiting after ingesting two tablets of 'ecstasy' (52[c]). *Dryness of the mouth* with possible increased risk of enamel erosion and dental caries has also been described in MDMA users (53[cR]). Since the toxic effects of MDMA resemble certain features of both the 'serotonin' syndrome and the neuroleptic malignant syndrome (NMS), some have suggested that MDMA may have combined actions on both the dopamine and serotonin systems (54[R]). Treatment of MDMA overdose with dantrolene (which may be helpful in cases of NMS) does not however appear useful in dealing with MDMA toxicity (55[c]).

Tolerance and dependence There are few pre-clinical or clinical data to suggest that repeated use of MDMA is associated with increased tolerance or dependence. However, anecdotal reports suggest that, in some individuals, increasing amounts of MDMA are used in order to achieve the same reinforcing psychoactive effects (56, 57).

Neuropsychiatric side-effects Reports of adverse neuropsychiatric manifestations associated with MDMA use have included descriptions of *flashbacks*, *anxiety*, *insomnia* (58), *panic attacks* (59, 60) and *psychosis* (61). Sub-acute adverse effects which have been reported following MDMA use have included *drowsiness*, *depression*, *anxiety* and *irritability* (62). Many other workers have contributed to the literature with cases of prolonged or chronic effects including panic disorder (63, 47), psychosis (57, 61, 64), flashbacks (61), major depressive disorder (60, 65) and memory disturbance (60). The observation that only certain individuals develop neuropsychiatric disturbances following MDMA use suggests that certain predisposing psychiatric factors (or high dose regimens) may make some individuals more vulnerable to these untoward effects.

Stimulants

The best known stimulants are amphetamine and cocaine.

Amphetamines are considered in another chapter of this book.

Cocaine has in recent decades become a very widely abused substance in many parts of the world.

A range of health problems result from of cocaine use. The mental consequences most commonly described include paranoia, memory loss, depression, anxiety reactions, loss of cognitive skills, apathy, mood swings, aggression, psychotic reactions with paranoid delusions and hallucinations are reported. Deaths occur not only from overdose but also from drug-induced mental states that may lead to serious injuries (66).

ORGANS AND SYSTEMS

Cardiovascular The toxic effects of cocaine on cardiac function continue to be meticulously documented. Cocaine abuse is a risk factor for *myocardial ischemia*, *infarction* and *dysrhythmias*, as well as *pulmonary edema*, *ruptured aortic aneurysm*, *infectious endocarditis*, *vascular thrombosis*, *myocarditis* and *dilated cardiomyopathy* (67[R]). Acute doses of cocaine suppress myocardial contractility, reduce coronary caliber and coronary blood flow, induce electrical abnormalities in the heart, and increase heart rate and blood pressure. These effects can lead to *myocardial ischemia* (68[R], 69[r]). However, intranasal cocaine in doses used medicinally or recreationally does not have a deleterious effect on intracardiac pressures and left ventricular performance (70[c]).

Cocaine-induced *infarction* as a consequence of ischemia has been one of the most frequent toxic complications reported after cocaine use. In one review of 114 cases, coronary anatomy, defined either by angiography or autopsy, was normal in 38% of chronic cocaine users who developed a myocardial infarction (71[CR]). In another recent review it has been concluded that "the vast majority of patients dying with cocaine toxicity, either have no pathologic changes in the heart, or only minimal changes" (72[R]). There may be a delay between the use of cocaine and the development of chest pain (73[c]). The results of a study of 101 consecutive patients admitted with acute chest pain related to cocaine use suggested that cocaine commonly causes chest pain that may not be secondary to myocardial ischemia (74[c]). The use of intranasal cocaine for therapeutic purposes (to treat epistaxis) has been associated with myocardial infarction in a 57-year-old man with hypertension and stable angina (75[c]).

In a review of the literature, 91 patients with cocaine-induced myocardial infarction (MI), were identified (76[R]). Myocardial infarction occurred in 44 patients after intranasal use, in 27 after smoking and in 19 after intravenous use. Almost half had a prior episode of chest pain. Two thirds had their myocardial infarction within 3 hours of cocaine use. Acute complications related to the myocardial infarction occurred in 18 patients. Of 24 patients followed up, 58% had subsequent cardiac complications. A recent report suggests that two phase myocardial imaging with ^{99m}Tc-sestamibi (symptomatic and asymptomatic) can be a helpful tool for definitive diagnosis of cocaine-induced myocardial infarction in patients with a history of cocaine use, chest pain and a non-diagnostic electrocardiogram (ECG) (77[C]). Interestingly, damage to the myocardium associated with cocaine use may be unrecognized by the abuser (78[C]). Major electrocardiographic findings (including myocardial infarction, myocardial ischemia and bundle branch block) were recorded during a review of 99 ECGs of known cocaine abusers. None of the 11 patients with major ECG changes had reported a past history of cardiac disease or had complained of chest pain. The mechanism by which cocaine induces acute myocardial damage remains unclear and is under investigation. A recent study involved the administration of intravenous cocaine (in dosages commonly self-administered) and placebo to 20 healthy cocaine abusers. None of the subjects developed myocardial ischemia or ventricular dysfunction on 2-dimensional echocardiogram during the test (79[C]).

There are two new case reports of the occurrence of *dissection of the aorta* during cocaine use. In a 35-year-old man, who used free base cocaine, a non-rupturing lesion extending to and involving the coronary arteries resulted in sudden death (80[c]). In a second case, a 58-year-old man developed acute abdominal pain within 5 minutes of subcutaneous cocaine injection (81[c]). The dissection was distal to the subclavian artery and extended into the left iliac artery. The authors of these two reports note that of the six cases of this rare complication reported in the past 5 years, all involved men with pre-existing essential hypertension.

Respiratory Recent literature has contributed to existing knowledge of the well-recognized respiratory effects of cocaine (82[c]). In a study of 177 heavy cocaine users (compared to 75 non-cocaine users), some of whom were also tobacco or marijuana users, cocaine use was associated with a high prevalence of acute respiratory symptoms, including coughing up black sputum, chest pain, and palpitations as compared with the non-cocaine using controls. However, chronic respiratory symptoms occurred at similar frequencies in both groups. In cocaine-only smokers, mild impairments in DLCO (diffusing capacity of the lung for carbon monoxide—suggesting pulmonary capillary membrane damage) and abnormalities in specific airway conductance (suggesting injury to the upper airway or the large intrathoracic bronchi) were noted.

As reported in earlier volumes in this series, passive inhalation of free-base cocaine in small children may lead to serious consequences. A previously healthy 3-week-old male infant developed pulmonary edema and other autonomic manifestations of cocaine exposure from such passive use (83[c]). The urinary drug screen was positive for benzoylecgonine, a cocaine metabolite.

Reports of *acute pulmonary syndromes* after the inhalation of cocaine have long been familiar and they continue to appear. In one case, a 32-year-old woman rapidly developed progressive deterioration of respiratory function leading to end-stage lung disease (84[c]). An open lung biopsy showed an inflammatory process with extensive accumulation of free silica. The authors cautioned that some cocaine may contain silica, which could lead to severe pulmonary complications after smoking. In a second report, a 27-year-old man was described who twice developed inflammatory lung disease (with a predominance of eosinophils) after inhaling 'crack' cocaine (85[c]). Corticosteroid treatment led to prompt resolution on both occasions. In a third case, a 23-year-old woman developed pulmonary infarction associated with the use of 'crack' cocaine (86[c]).

Otolaryngological Intranasal use, a common method of cocaine abuse, has been associated with *chronic sinusitis*, *septal perforation*, and *saddle nose*. *Pott's puffy tumor*, a subperiosteal infection of the frontal bone, has recently been described in a 34-year-old man with a history of chronic intranasal cocaine use (87[c]). This condition, which is a rare complication of frontal sinusitis, appeared to develop secondary to the insertion of foreign bodies into the nose to facilitate inhalation of cocaine. The local trauma and the cocaine-induced vasoconstriction may have led to the complication.

Nervous system The literature on the adverse effects of cocaine on the nervous system continues to expand. In a recent review, *subarachnoid hemorrhage* was temporally related to cocaine abuse in cases studied (88[CR]). All 12 cases involved young adult abusers who had underlying cerebral aneurysms that had ruptured. Hypertension was a probable contributing factor.

Another less common complication of cocaine use is *cerebral vasculitis* (89[Cr]); it is known that during cocaine use, a hypersensitivity drug-induced vasculitis can develop.

Cocaine's effects and/or the effects of cocaine withdrawal on *neurotransmitter activity* have been evaluated in several studies. Although changes in dopaminergic activity appear to be associated with early cocaine abstinence, *extrapyramidal symptoms* (due to alterations in dopamine functioning) have only infrequently been reported in cocaine users. In a recent report, however, extrapyramidal symptoms of classic muscle stiffness and cogwheeling at the elbow occurred during the 'crash' phase of a 40-year-old man's cocaine withdrawal (90[c]). In a second report, cocaine-associated movement disorders were described (91[c]). Motor and vocal tics, preexisting tremors and generalized dystonia were induced or exacerbated by drug use, and continued even after cocaine use ended. Lastly, dopamine dysregulation (i.e. decreased dopamine DC receptor availability in association with reduced frontal metabolism), was demonstrated by positive emission tomography in 20 chronic cocaine abusers (92[c]). Findings were prominent in the orbito-frontal, cingulate and prefrontal cortices 3—4 months after detoxification. The author offered the hypothesis that dysregulation of these brain areas may result in compulsive drug-taking behavior.

The *disruption of normal sleeping patterns* during cocaine withdrawal may be related to effects on the cholinergic system. In a recent study of nine patients undergoing cocaine withdrawal (93[c]), REM (rapid eye movement) latency was markedly shortened, REM sleep percentage was increased, REM density was very high and the total sleep period was long during the first week. Such REM changes are thought to be related to changes in cholinergic activity. At week 3, characteristic chronic insomnia was observed.

Reports on effects of cocaine withdrawal on *cognition* have also appeared. Impairments in memory, visuospatial abilities and concentration were present in 16 cocaine abusers during the first 2 weeks of abstinence (94[c]). Measured deficits were independent of withdrawal-related depression. The effects of cocaine on cognitive functions are beginning to be measured in controlled studies. The preliminary results of a study of 20 heavy cocaine abusers and a group of matched controls have shown impaired function on neuropsychological tests in 50% of the abusers compared with 15% of the controls. Problems with concentration, memory, problem solving, and abstracting were noted in the cocaine users. The greatest loss of memory was found in the heavy users; recent cocaine use was associated with poorer oral fluency and arithmetic scores (105[c]).

Cocaine also has important effects on the physical processes controlled by the central nervous system, e.g. *seizures* occur in chronic cocaine abusers. A case of aggravation of generalized tonic-clonic seizures (which occurred initially during the use of crack but later continued independently of the drug) has recently been described, with progressive EEG abnormalities (95[c]). In this case, the development of the seizures suggested that cocaine may stimulate kindling, with progressive intensification of after-discharges and the eventual emergence of seizure activity.

Cocaine may cause a variety of intracranial effects, ranging from *headache* to *stroke*. Approximately 60—75% of chronic cocaine abusers report severe headaches (97[R]), and these can resemble migraine; migraine-like symptoms may include auras, visual field changes, and paraphasias (96[c]). *Hypertensive encephalopathy* may follow the use of cocaine (98[c]), as may *cerebral hemorrhage* (99[c], 100[c]) or *rupture of a cerebral aneurysm* (101[c]). *Cerebral infarction* is significantly more common among users of cocaine alkaloid (crack) than cocaine hydrochloride (102[c]).

A case of *dystonia* developing shortly after the use of cocaine was described in SEDA-16 (p. 24). In a recent retrospective study of 116 patients treated with neuroleptic drugs, 42% of cocaine users versus 14% of non-users developed this neurological complication (103[c]). This suggests that the use of cocaine may be a major risk factor for acute dystonic reactions secondary to the use of neuroleptic drugs.

Sniffing cocaine may unmask and then exacerbate *myasthenia gravis*. A 24-year-old woman who developed myasthenia gravis during cocaine use has recently been described (104[c]). The authors speculated that while cocaine did not cause impairment of motor neuron axons for neuromuscular transmission, a reduction in the number of acetylcholine receptors per neuromuscular junction (as occurs in myasthenia gravis) may have increased the susceptibility to an effect of cocaine.

Frankly *psychiatric symptoms* induced by cocaine use have been in reported in earlier volumes in this series, and two recent reports illustrate the problem. In one report, a positive association between panic disorder and cocaine use is noted (106[cR]). Among 280 patients in a methadone maintenance clinic, prevalence of panic disorder increased from 1 to 6% over a decade. A marked rise in the frequency of cocaine abuse coincided in time with this outbreak. The authors suggest that episodes of panic occurring in cocaine users may result in hospitalizations for either psychiatric or medical illness. The second report, a prospective epidemiological study using data from the Epidemiologic Catchment Area (ECA) surveys (1980—1984), evaluated suspected risk factors for obsessive compulsive disorder (OCD) (107[c]). The authors found that users of both cocaine and marijuana were at increased risk of OCD as compared to non-users of illicit drugs, but cocaine use alone was not associated with an increased risk of OCD, within the limited sample size.

In another study psychiatric effects were evaluated in 55 individuals with cocaine dependence (108[R]). Of these cocaine abusers, 53% reported transient cocaine-induced psychotic symptoms. Paranoid delusions (related to drug use) and auditory hallucinations were often reported. In addition, almost one-third (all of whom also described psychotic symptoms) reported transient behavioral stereotypes. A case of paranoid psychosis has been described in a 64-year-old man who had first begun to use crack cocaine 6 months previously. The paranoid symptoms continued for 3 weeks after he stopped using 'crack'. The author suggested that the man's age may have made him particularly sensitive to the psychiatric effects of cocaine (109[c]).

Recent work with single-photon emission computerized tomography (SPECT) suggests that some psychiatric symptoms in cocaine users may be associated with changes in blood flow (110[C]). Multiple scalloped areas of diminished cerebral blood flow (especially periventricular regions and deep portions of the brain) have been seen. Hypoperfusion has also been noted in the frontal lobes of cocaine users with mania.

Gastrointestinal Five cases of *gastric perforation* (rather than the more common duodenal perforation) have been reported in young male smokers of 'crack', all of whom had only brief histories of prodromal symptoms (111[r]). The authors postulated that crack, by an uncertain mechanism, may have accounted for the gastric perforation in these individuals, none of whom had long-standing peptic ulcer disease.

Liver Cocaine has been associated with liver toxicity, as discussed in various Annuals in this series. A 23-year-old man became unresponsive and had a seizure after ingesting cocaine and alcohol (112[c]). Severe liver necrosis developed and radio-imaging with ^{99m}Tc-PYP clearly documented the hepatocellular damage.

Urinary system *Acute renal failure* with malignant hypertension, apparently precipitated by cocaine-induced vasoconstriction, has been described in a 33-year-old woman who had pre-existing scleroderma and normal renal function (113[c]). She was successfully treated with hemodialysis.

Special senses *Ophthalmic effects* associated with cocaine may occur both during active drug use and during early abstinence. Corneal ulcer secondary to smoking crack cocaine has been reported in a 27-year-old woman (114[c]). A case of acute iritis has been reported after the intranasal use of cocaine (115[c]).

New cases of the clinical entity known as 'crack eye syndrome' continue to be reported, for example in a paper in which 14 crack cocaine users presented with corneal problems (137[C]): 10 had corneal ulcers infected with both bacterial and fungal organisms; four had corneal epithelial defects. All 14 patients in the group were actively smoking crack on a daily basis. The authors suggest that crack smoking appears to predispose users, through some unclear mechanism, to corneal epithelial changes, infection and perforation. Typical presentations include the loss of vision associated with or without pain. In another report, a 29-year-old woman with a painful corneal ulcer related to cocaine abuse, was found to be placing cocaine powder directly in the affected eye to reduce the pain (138[c]). Her history included prior corneal perforations. Such topical use of cocaine may aggravate the condition.

Immunological and hypersensitivity reactions The prevalence of infection with the human immunodeficiency virus (HIV) among drug abusers, including cocaine users, is increasing, as is research interest in the effects of cocaine on the immune system. Two separate reports have suggested that cocaine may compromise immunological function. In one study, human mononuclear cells were stimulated in vitro with mitogens in the presence and absence of cocaine (116). In this study, cocaine inhibited the proliferation of the mononuclear cells. In a second study, cocaine amplified HIV-1 replication in co-cultures containing cytomegalovirus-activated peripheral blood mononuclear cells (117[r]).

Second generation effects *Use in pregnancy* Some of the risks run by the pregnant cocaine-using mother and her child (such as pre-term labor and premature delivery) have been previously reported (118[R]).

A recent retrospective study with data from a large perinatal registry showed that there was an increased risk of intrapartum placenta previa among women who used cocaine, compared with those who did not use drugs or alcohol (119[R]). Another apparent obstetric risk of cocaine use, as described in a case report, is rupture of a uterine scar (from a previous cesarian section); extensive laceration of the maternal urinary bladder was seen after a vaginal birth in a 34-year-old woman whose urine tested positive for cocaine (120[c]). The authors postulated that the injury may have resulted from a cocaine-augmented contractile response of the pregnant uterus. Lastly a 'pre-eclampsia-like' syndrome has recently been described, characterized by acute hypertension and a low platelet count, in a 33-year-old female cocaine user; her 20-week-old fetus died (121[c]).

Neonatal effects Cocaine exposure in utero may cause effects on various fetal organ systems. Gastrointestinal disorders, including 10 cases of necrotizing enterocolitis (122[C]), one case of intestinal atresia, and one case of spontaneous colonic perforation, have been reported (123[c]).

The effects of cocaine exposure on the fetal respiratory system are under investigation. In one recent study, respiratory rates in the 3-week-old babies of mothers who had used cocaine during pregnancy were found to be higher than expected; in addition newborn babies who had been exposed prenatally to both cocaine and narcotics exhibited abnormal control of breathing (following hypercapnia challenge) during the first few months of life (124[C]). The preliminary results of another study are also of some interest; this prospective study of maternal drug abuse showed a reduced incidence of respiratory distress syndrome among premature infants prenatally exposed to cocaine (125[C]). The authors noted that while this finding needs to be confirmed, it may suggest that fetal lung maturation can be accelerated by exposure to cocaine.

A study of 500 neonates showed that ankyloglossia, a defect in the attachment of the tongue within the mouth, was 3.5 times more common in cocaine-exposed neonates than in others (126[C]). Two other clinical syndromes involving anomalies of multiple fetal organ systems in fetuses of cocaine-abusing women have also recently been described. In one case, an infant with Pena-Shokeir phenotype (including facial, musculoskeletal, pulmonary, and cardiac malformations accompanied by extensive brain damage) was born to a cocaine-abusing mother (127[c]). The infant died shortly after birth. Another infant exposed to cocaine in utero had a combination of facial, ear, eye, and vertebral anomalies, accompanied by cardiac, central nervous system, and other malformations (41[c]).

The potential effect of cocaine on the developing central nervous system continues to be an area of great importance. In two recent reports, it has been suggested that brain hemorrhages (128[c]) and asymmetrical growth retardation may occur (129[c]). A review of the recent literature (130[R]) has emphasized the importance of further in-depth analysis and the need for longitudinal follow-up of the exposed population.

It is unclear by what mechanism cocaine may affect the fetus. Recent evidence suggests that interruption of the intrauterine blood supply with subsequent destruction of the fetal structure may account for some of the drug's effects (131[R]). In a recent report on the autopsy of a 6-month-old fetus who had been exposed to cocaine and who had a single-ventricle heart, the authors suggested that coronary spasms, resulting in infarction, may have destroyed the right ventricle (132[c]).

By contrast, in light-to-moderate cocaine users, pronounced untoward effects on the fetus were reportedly less than in other studies (133[C]). In this report, 34 light-to-moderate cocaine abusers and 600 non-users from a public prenatal care clinic were studied during the course of pregnancy. In all cases the cocaine had been taken intranasally and the majority of users reduced their intake during pregnancy; none had been referred for drug abuse counseling and none was taking drug treatment. The authors concluded that there was no significant difference in obstetric complications among these mild cocaine users compared with non-users, and no significant differences in infant growth, morphology, or behavior. However, the cocaine users had histories of more fetal losses. Also, during pregnancy they suffered more infectious diseases, such as hepatitis, herpes simplex, infections, and gonorrhea.

As noted in previous Annuals, the literature on maternal cocaine use and its possible outcomes is problematic, because many of the studies have been flawed methodologically (134[R]).

Interactions Cocaine is often used in conjunction with other drugs, primarily in the context of multi-substance abuse. When used with *alcohol*, there may be enhanced hepatotoxicity, and the possibility of enhanced cardiotoxicity (135[R]). Taking of *MAO inhibitors* together with cocaine may in theory result in serious hypertension, although case reports have been relatively few in number (135[R]).

Cocaine combined with *indomethacin* (in a 23-year-old pregnant woman at 34 weeks gestation) may have been the cause of fetal anuria and neonatal gastric hemorrhage (136[c]).

Phencyclidine

Phencyclidine or 1-(1-phenylcyclohexy-1)piperidine (known as PCP or 'angel dust') was originally developed as an anesthetic but it was abused as a illicit drug from the late 1960s onwards. The psychoactive effects of phencyclidine are stimulant and similar to the effects of hallucinogens. Hallucinations are often bizarre, frightening and self-challenging. Aggressive behavior, usually with amnesia, is common. Self-destructive actions are also seen. Overdosage is associated with paresthesia, slurred speech, ataxia and later catatonia, dilated pupils and coma with tachycardia, hypertension and arrhythmias. Seizures and deaths have occurred (SED-11, 86; 59[c]).

Phencyclidine is an antagonist of the *N*-methyl-D-aspartate (NMDA) subtype of glutamate receptors and a dopamine agonist, and has anticholinergic properties through blockade of ion channels in acetylcholine receptors. It is still used in some countries as an anti-Parkinson agent (SED-11, 86; 139[R], 140[c], 141[R]).

Organic solvents

Lighter fuels, benzene, toluene, cleaning fluids (carbon tetrachloride), petrol and paraffin and even the fluorocarbon propellants found in various household sprays and medications have all been used, particularly by children, to produce changes in consciousness. They are all inhaled, often with the aid of a plastic bag, and since they are lipid soluble they are readily concentrated in brain tissue. As with many anesthetics there is an early period of hyperactivity, excitement and intoxication followed by sedation and confusion. Prolonged or regular use can induce serious toxicity with bone marrow depression, cardiac arrhythmias, peripheral neuropathy, cerebral damage, and liver and kidney disorders (SED-12, 37; 142[R]).

REFERENCES

1. Woody GE, MacFadden W. Cannabis-related disorders. In: Comprehensive Textbook of Psychiatry/vi. Vol 1, 6th edn. 1995;810—817.
2. Herkenham M. Cannabinoid receptor localization in brain: relationship to motor and reward systems. In: The Neurobiology of Drug and Alcohol Addiction. Ann NY Acad Sci 1992;654:19—33.
3. Childers SR, Fleming L, Konkoy Ch, Marckel D, Pacheco M, Sexton T, Ward S. Opioid and cannabinoid receptor inhibition of adenylyl cyclase in brain. In: The Neurobiology of Drug and Alcohol Addiction. Ann NY Acad Sci 1992;654:33—52.
4. Institute of Medicine. Marijuana and Health. Washington, DC: National Academy Press, 1982.
5. Avakian EV, Horvath SM, Michaeal ED et al. Effect of marijuana on cardiorespiratory responses to submaximal exercise. Clin Pharmacol Ther 1979;26:777–781.
6. Reiman AS. Marijuana and health. N Engl J Med 1982;306:604.
7. Wu TC, Tashkin DP, Djahed B, Rose JE. Pulmonary hazards of smoking marijuana as compared with tobacco. N Engl J Med 1988;318:347.
8. Taskin PP, Calvarese BM, Simmons MS et al. Respiratory status of seventy-four habitual marijuana smokers. Chest 1980;78:699.
9. Tashkin DP. Pulmonary complications of smoked substance abuse. West J Med 1990;152:525.
10. Douglass RE, Levison MA. Pneumothorax in drug abusers: an urban epidemic? Ann Surg 1986;52:377.
11. Tashkin DP, Coulson AH, Clark VA et al. Respiratory symptoms and lung function in habitual heavy smokers of marijuana and tobacco, smokers of tobacco alone, and nonsmokers. Am Rev Respir Dis 1987;135:209.
12. Schwartz RH, Groenewald PJ, Klitzner M, Fedic P. Short-term memory impairment in cannabis dependent adolescents. Am J Dis Child 1989;143:1214.
13. Wert RC, Raulin ML. The chronic cerebral effects of cannabis use. I. Methodological issues and neurological findings. Int J Addict 1986;21:605.
14. Wert RC, Raulin ML. The chronic cerebral effects of cannabis use. II. Psychological findings and conclusions. Int J Addict 1986;21:629.
15. Jones RT. Cannabis and health. Annu Rev Med 1983;34:247.
16. World Health Organization. Report of an ARF/WHO Scientific Meeting on Adverse Health and Behavior Consequences of Cannabis Use, Toronto, Ont: WHO Addiction Research Foundation, 1981.
17. Carney MWP, Bacelle L, Robinson B. Psychosis after cannabis abuse. Br Med J 1984;288:1047.
18. Liakos, A, Boulougouris JC, Stefanis C. Psycho-physiologic effects of acute cannabis smoking in longterm users. Ann NY Acad Sci 1976;282:375.
19. Kolodny RC, Masters WH, Kolodner RM, Toro G. Depression of plasma testosterone levels after chronic intensive marijuana use. N Engl J Med 1974;290:872.
20. Fried PA, Watkinson B, Willan A. Marijuana use during pregnancy and decreased length of gestation. Am J Obstet Gynecol 1984;150:23.
21. Klein TW, Newton C, Friedman H. Inhibition of natural killer cell function by marijuana components. J Toxicol Environ Health 1987;20:321.
22. Levitz SM, Diamond RD. Aspergillosis and marijuana (Letter to the Editor). Ann Intern Med 1991;115:578—579.
23. Pillai Radhakrishna Nair, Bindu S, Watson RR. Aids, drugs of abuse and the immune system. Arch Toxicol 1991;65:609.
24. Quazi QH, Mariano E, Milman DH et al. Abnormal fetal development linked to intrauterine exposure to marijuana. Dev Pharmacol Ther 1985;8:141.
25. Fried PA. Marijuana use by pregnant women and effects on offspring: an update. Neurobehav Toxicol Teratol 1982;4:451.
26. Greenland S, Staisch KJ, Brown N et al. Effects of marijuana on human pregnancy, labor, and delivery. Neurobehav Toxicol Teratol 1982;4:447.
27. Nahas G, Frick HG. Developmental effects of cannabis. Neurotoxicology 1986;7:381.
28. Lacoursiere RB, Swatek R. Adverse interaction between disulfiram and marijuana: a case report. Am J Psychiatry 1983;140:243.
29. American Psychiatric Association. Diagnostic and Statistical Manual of Mental Disorders, Fourth Edition, Washington DC, American Psychiatric Association, 1994.
30. World Health Organization. The ICD-10 Classification of Mental and Behavioral Disorders: Clinical Descriptions and Diagnostic Guidelines. Geneva: WHO, 1992.
31. Haigler, HJ, Aghajanian GK. Serotonin receptors in the brain. Fed Proc 1977;36:2159.
32. Watson SJ. Hallucinogens and other psychotomimetics: biological mechanisms. In: Barchas JD, Berger PA, Ciorenello RD, Elliot GR, eds. Psychopharmacology from Theory to Practise. New York: Oxford University Press, 1977.
33. Alarcon RD, Dickinson WA, Dohn HH. Flashback phenomena: clinical and diagnostic dilemmas. J Nerv Ment Dis 1982;217.
34. Strassman RJ. Adverse reactions to psychodelic drugs. J Nerv Ment Dis 1984;172:577.
35. Tuchmann-Duplessis H. In: Avery GS, ed. Monographs on Drugs, Vol 2, Drug Effects on the Fetus. London: ADIS, 1975;158.
36. Abraham HD. Visual phenomenology of the LSD flash. Arch Gen Psychiatry 1983;40:884.
37. Vardy MM, Kay SR. LSD psychosis or LSD-induced schizophrenia. Arch Gen Psychiatry 1983;40:877.

38. Hermle L, Fünfgeld M, Oepen G, Botsch H, Borchardt D, Gouzoulis E, Ferhrenback RA, Spitzer M. Mescaline-induced psychopathological, neuropsychological, and neurometabolic effects in normal subjects: Experimental psychosis as a tool for psychiatric research. Biol Psychiatry 1992; 32:976–991.
39. Solowij N, Hall W, Lee N. Recreational MDMA use in Sydney: a profile of 'ecstasy' users and their experiences with the drug. Br J Addict 1992;87:1161–1172.
40. Liester MB, Grob CS, Bravo GL, Walsh RN. Phenomenology and sequelae of 3,4-methylenedioxymethamphetamine use. J Nerv Ment Dis 1992;180:345–352.
41. Lessick M, Vasa R, Israel J. Severe manifestations of oculoauriculovertebral spectrum in a cocaine exposed infant. J Med Genet 1991;28:803–804.
42. Henry JA. Ecstasy and the dance of death: severe reactions are unpredictable. Br Med J 1992;305:5–6.
43. Gelenberg AJ. One man's ecstasy. Biol Ther Psychiatry Newsletter 1992;15:45, 47.
44. Screaton GR, Cairns HS, Sarner M, Singer M, Trasher A, Cohen SL. Hyperpyrexia and rhabdomyolysis after MDMA ('ecstasy') abuse (Letter to the Editor). Lancet 1992;339:677–678.
45. Henry JA, Jeffreys KJ, Dawling S. Toxicity and deaths from 3,4-methylenedioxymethamphetamine ('ecstasy'). Lancet 1992;340:384–387.
46. Wodarz N, Böning J. 'Ecstasy'—induziertes psychotisches Depersonalisationssyndrom. Nervenarzt 1993;64: 478–480.
47. McCann UD, Ricaurte GA. MDMA ('Ecstasy') and panic disorder: induction by a single dose. Biol Psychiatry 1992;32:950–953.
48. Williams H, Meagher D, Galligan P, McCann UD, Ricaurte GA. MDMA ('Ecstasy'); a case of possible drug-induced psychosis. IJMS 1992;162:43–44.
49. Campkin NTA, Davies UM. Another death from Ecstasy. JR Soc Med 1992;85:61.
50. Barrett JP, Taylor GT. 'Ecstasy' ingestion: a case report of severe complications. JR Soc Med 1993;86:233–234.
51. Barrett JP. 'Ecstasy' misuse—overdose or normal use? Anesthesia 1993;48:83.
52. Levine AJ, Rees GM. 'Ecstasy' induced pneumomediastinum. JR Soc Med 1993;86:232–233.
53. Duxbury AJ. Ecstasy—dental implications. Br Dental J 1993;175:38.
54. Ames D, Wirshing WC. Ecstasy, the serotonin syndrome, and neuroleptic malignant syndrome—a possible link? J Am Med Assoc 1993;269:869.
55. Campkin NTA, Davies UM. Treatment of 'ecstasy' overdose with dantrolene. Anesthesia 1993;48:82–83.
56. McCann UD, Ricaurte GA. Major metabolites of 3,4-methylene-dioxyamphetamine not mediate its toxic effects on brain serotonin neurons. Brain Res 1991;545:270–282.
57. McGuire P, Fahy T. Chronic paranoid psychosis after misuse of MDMA ('ecstasy'). Br Med J 1991;302:697.
58. Greer G, Strassman RJ. Information on Ecstasy. Am J Psychiatry 1985;142:1391.
59. Whitaker-Azmitia PM, Aronson TA. 'Ecstasy' (MDMA)-induced panic. Am J Psychiatry 1989;146:119.
60. McCann UD, Ricaurte GA. Lasting neuropsychiatric sequelae of (±)-methylenedioxymethamphetamine ('ecstasy') in recreational users. J Clin Psychopharmacol 1991;11:302–305.
61. Creighton FJ, Black DL, Hyde CE. Ecstasy psychosis and flashbacks. Br J Psychiatry 1991;159:713–715.
62. Peroutka SJ, Newman H, Harris H. Subjective effects of 3,4-methylenedioxymethamphetamine in recreational users. Neuropsychopharmacology 1988;1:273–277.
63. Pallanti S, Mazzi D. MDMA (Ecstasy) precipitation of panic disorder. Biol Psychiatry 1992;32:91–94.
64. Schifano F. Chronic atypical psychosis associated with MDMA ('ecstasy') abuse. Lancet 1991;338:1335.
65. Benazzi F, Mazzoli M. Psychiatric illness associated with 'ecstasy'. Lancet 1991;338:1520.
66. Marzuk PM, Tardiff K, Leon AC et al. Fatal injuries after cocaine use as a leading cause of death among young adults in New York City. 1995;332:1753–1757.
67. Cregler LL. Cocaine: the newest risk factor for cardiovascular disease. Clin Cardiol 1991;14:449–456.
68. Kloner RA, Hale S, Alker K, Rezkalla S. The effects of acute and chronic cocaine use on the heart. Circulation 1992;85:407–409.
69. Thadani P. Cardiovascular toxicity of cocaine: underlying mechanisms. US Department of Health and Human Services, Public Health Serv. Res. Monograph, 1991;108.
70. Boehrer JD, Moliterno DJ, Willard JE. Hemodynamic effects of intranasal cocaine in humans. J Am Coll Cardiol 1992;20:90–93.
71. Minor RL, Scott BD, Brown DD. Cocaine-induced myocardial infarction in patients with normal coronary arteries. Ann Intern Med 1991;115:797–806.
72. Virmani R. Cocaine-associated cardiovascular disease: clinical and pathological aspects. In: Thadani P, ed. NIDA Research Monograph 108. Rockville, MD: US HHS, 1991; 220–229.
73. Amin M, Gabelman G, Karpel J, Buttrick P. Acute myocardial infarction and chest pain syndromes after cocaine use. Am J Cardiol 1990;66:1434–1437.
74. Sharkey SW, Glitter MJ, Goldsmith SR. How serious is cocaine-associated acute chest pain syndromes after cocaine use. Cardiol Board Rev 1992;9:58–66.
75. Ross GS, Bell J. Myocardial infarction associated with inappropriate use of topical cocaine as treatment for epistaxis. Am J Emerg Med 1992;10:219–222.
76. Hollander JE, Hoffman RS. Cocaine-induced myocardial infarction: an analysis and review of the literature. J Emerg Med 1992;10:169–177.
77. Yuen-Green MS, Yen C-K, Lim AD, Lull RJ. Tc-99m sestamibi myocardial imaging at rest for evaluation of cocaine-induced myocardial ischemia and infarction. Clin Nucl Med 1992;17:923–925.
78. Tanenbaum JH, Miller F. Electrocardiographic evidence of myocardial injury in psychiatrically hospitalized cocaine abusers. Gen Hosp Psychiatry 1992;14:201–203.
79. Eisenberg MJ, Mendelson J, Evans GT, Jue J, Jones RT, Schiller NB. Left ventricular function immediately after intravenous cocaine: a quantitative two-dimensional echocardiographic study. J Am Coll Cardiol 1993;22:1581–1586.
80. Cohle SD, Lie JT. Dissection of the aorta and coronary arteries associated with acute cocaine intoxication. Arch Pathol Lab Med 1992;116:1239–1241.
81. Fisher A, Holroyd BR. Cocaine-associated dissection of the thoracic aorta. J Emerg Med 1992;10:723–727.
82. Tashkin DP, Gorelick D, Khalsa M-E, Simmons M, Chang P. Respiratory effects of cocaine freebasing among habitual cocaine users. In: Cocaine: Physiological and Physiopathological Effects. New York: The Haworth Press, 1992;59–70.
83. Battle MA, Wilcox WD. Pulmonary edema in an infant

following inhalation of free-base ('crack') cocaine. Clin Pediatr 1992;32:105–106.
84. O'Donnel AE, Mappin G, Sebo TJ, Tazelaar H. Interstitial pneumonitis associated with 'crack' cocaine abuse. Chest 1991;100:1155–1157.
85. Oh PI, Balter MS. Cocaine induced eosinophilic lung disease. Thorax 1992;47:478–479.
86. Delaney K, Hoffman RS. Pulmonary infarction associated with crack cocaine use in a previously healthy 23-year-old woman. Am J Med 1991;91:92–94.
87. Noskin GA, Kalish SB. Pott's puffy tumor: a complication of intranasal cocaine abuse. Rev Infect Dis 1991; 13:606–608.
88. Oyesiku NM, Colohan ART, Barrow DL, Reisner A. Cocaine-induced aneurysmal rupture: An emergency negative factor in the natural history of intracranial aneurysms? Neurosurgery 1993;32:518–526.
89. Morrow PL, McQuillen JB. Cerebral vasculitis associated with cocaine abuse. J Forensic Sci 1993;38:732–738.
90. Satel Sl, Swann AC. Extrapyramidal symptoms and cocaine abuse. Am J Psychiatry 1993;150:347.
91. Cardoso FEC, Jankovic J. Cocaine-related movement disorders. Mov Disord 1993;8:175–178.
92. Volkow ND, Fowler JS, Wang G-J, Hitzemann R, Logan J, Schlyer DJ, Dewey SL, Wolf AP. Decreased dopamine D2 receptor availability is associated with reduced frontal metabolism in cocaine abusers. Synapse 1993;14:169–177.
93. Kowatch RA, Schnoll SS, Knisely JS, Green D, Elswick RK. Electroencephalographic sleep and mood during cocaine-withdrawal. In: Cocaine: Physiological and Physiopathological Effects. New York: The Haworth Press, 1992;21–45.
94. Berry J, van Gorp WG, Herzberg DS, Hinkin C, Boone K, Steinman L, Wilkins JN. Neuropsychological deficits in abstinent cocaine abusers: preliminary findings after two weeks of abstinence. Drug Alcohol Depend 1993;32:231–237.
95. Dhuna A, Pascual-Leone A, Langendorf F. Chronic, habitual cocaine abuse and kindling-induced epilepsy: a case report. Epilepsia 1991;32:890–894.
96. Mossman SS, Goadsby PJ. Cocaine abuse simulating the aura of migraine. J Neurol Neurosurg Psychiatry 1992;55:628.
97. Dhuna A, Pascual-Leone A, Belgrade M. Cocaine-related vascular headaches. J Neurol Neurosurg Psychiatry 1991;54:803–806.
98. Grewal RP, Miller BL. Cocaine induced hypertensive encephalopathy. Acta Neurol 1991;13:279.
99. Yapor WY, Gutierrez FA. Cocaine-induced intratumoral hemorrhage: Case report and review of the literature. Neurosurgery 1992;30:288–291.
100. Ramadan NM, Levine SR, Welch KMA. Pontine hemorrhage following 'crack' cocaine use. Neurology 1991;41:946–947.
101. Chadan N, Thierry A, Sautreaux JL. Rupture anévrysmale et toxicomanie á la cocaïne. Neurochirurgie 1991; 37:403–405.
102. Levine SR, Brust JCM, Futrell N, Brass LM, Blake D, Fayad P, Schultz LR, Millikan CH, Ho K-L, Welch KMA. A comparative study of the cerebrovascular complications of cocaine. Neurology 1991;41:1173–1177.
103. Hegarty AM, Lipton RG, Merriam AE, Freeman K. Cocaine as a risk factor for acute dystonic reactions. Neurology 1991;41:1670–1672.
104. Berciano J. Oterino A, Rebollo M, Pascal J. Myasthenia gravis unmasked by cocaine abuse (Letter to the Editor). New Engl J Med 1991;169:892.
105. O'Malley S, Adamse M, Heaton RK, Gawin FH. Neuropsychological impairment in chronic cocaine abusers. Am J Drug Alcohol Abuse 1992;18:131–144.
106. Rosen MI, Kosten T. Cocaine-associated panic attacks in methadone-maintained patients. Am J Drug Alcohol Abuse 1992;18:57–62.
107. Crum RM, Anthony JC. Cocaine use and other suspected risk factors for obsessive-compulsive disorder: a prospective study with data from the Epidemiologic Catchment Area surveys. Drug Alcohol Depend 1993;31:281–295.
108. Brady KT, Lydiard RB, Malcolm R, Ballenger JC. Cocaine-induced psychosis. J Clin Psychiatry 1991;52:509–512.
109. Nambudiri DE, Young RC. A case of late-onset crack dependence and subsequent psychosis in the elderly. J Subst Abuse Treat 1991;8:253–255.
110. Miller BL, Mena I, Biombetti R, Villanueva-Meyer J, Djenderedjian AH. Neuropsychiatric effects of cocaine: SPECT measurements. In: Cocaine: Physiological and Physiopathological Effects. New York: The Haworth Press, 1992;47–58.
111. Abramson DL, Gertler JP, Lewis T, Kral JG. Crack-related perforated gastropyloric ulcer. J Clin Gastroenterol 1991;13:17–19.
112. Whitten CG, Luke BA. Liver uptake to Tc-99m PYP. Clin Nucl Med 1991;16:492–494.
113. Lam M, Ballou SP. Reversible scleroderma renal crisis after cocaine use. New Engl J Med 1992;36:1435.
114. Zagelbaum BM, Tannenbaum MH, Hersh PS. Candida albicans corneal ulcer associated with crack cocaine. Am J Ophthalmol 1991;111:248–249.
115. Wang ESJ. Cocaine-induced iritis. Ann Emerg Med 1991;20:192.
116. Delafuente JC, DeVane L. Immunologic effects of cocaine and related alkaloids. Immunopharmacol Immunotoxicol 1991;13:11–23.
117. Peterson PK, Gekker G, Chao CC, Schut R, Verhoef J, Edel man CK, Erice A, Balfour HH Jr. Cocaine amplifies HIV-1 replication in cytomegalovirus-stimulated peripheral blood mononuclear cell cocultures. J Immunol 1992; 149:676–680.
118. Spence MR, Williams R, DiGregorio GJ, Kirby-McDonnell A, Polansky M. The relationship between recent cocaine use and pregnancy outcome. Obstet Gynecol 1991;78:326–329.
119. Handler A, Kistin N, Davis F, Ferre C. Cocaine use during pregnancy: perinatal outcomes. Am J Epidemiol 1991;133:818–825.
120. Hsu C-D, Chen S, Feng TI, Johnson TRB. Rupture of uterine scar with extensive maternal bladder laceration after cocaine abuse. Am J Obstet Gynecol 1992;167:129–130.
121. Abramowicz JS, Sherer DM, Woods JR Jr. Acute transient thrombocytopenia associated with cocaine abuse in pregnancy. Obstet Gynecol 1991;78:499–501.
122. Downing GJ, Horner SR, Kilbride HW. Characteristics of perinatal cocaine-exposed infants with necrotizing enterocolitis (Letter to the Editor). Am J Dis Child 1991;145:26–27.
123. Spinazzola R, Kenigsberg K, Usmani SS, Harper RG. Neonatal gastrointestinal complications of maternal cocaine abuse. NY State J Med 1992;92:22–23.
124. McCann EM, Lewis K. Control of breathing in babies

of narcotic-and cocaine-abusing mothers. Early Hum Dev 1991;27:175–186.

125. Zuckerman B, Maynard EC, Cabral H. A preliminary report of prenatal cocaine exposure and respiratory distress syndrome in premature infants. Am J Dis Child 1991;145:696–698.

126. Harris EF, Friend GW, Tolley EA. Enhanced prevalence of ankyloglossia with maternal cocaine use. Cleft Palate-Craniofacial J 1992;29:72–76.

127. Lavi E, Monotone KT, Rorke LB, Kliman HJ. Fetal akinesia deformation sequence (Pena-Shokeir phenotype) associated with acquired intra-uterine brain damage. Neurology 1991;41:1467–1468.

128. Kapur RP, Shaw CM, Shepard TH. Brain hemorrhages in cocaine-exposed human fetuses. Teratology 1991;44:11–18.

129. Little BB, Snel LM. Brain growth among fetuses exposed to cocaine in utero: asymmetrical growth retardation. Obstet Gynecol 1991;77:361–364.

130. Kosofsky BE. The effect of cocaine on developing human brain. NIDA Res Monogr 1991;114:128–143.

131. Jones KL. Developmental pathogenesis of defects associated with prenatal cocaine exposure: fetal vascular disruption. Clin Perinatol 1991;18:139–146.

132. Shephard TH, Fantel AG, Kapur RP. Fetal coronary thrombosis as a cause of single ventricular heart. Teratology 1991;43:113–117.

133. Richardson GA, Day NL. Maternal and neonatal effects of moderate cocaine use during pregnancy. Neurotoxicol Teratol 1991;13:455–460.

134. Chasnoff IJ. Methodological issues in studying cocaine use in pregnancy: a problem of definitions. NIDA Res Monogr 1991;108:55–65.

135. Sands BF, Ciraulo DA. Cocaine drug-drug interactions. J Clin Psychopharmacol 1992;12:49–55.

136. Carlan SJ, Stromquist C, Angel JL, Harris M, O'Brien WF. Cocaine and indomethacin: fetal anuria, neonatal edema, and gastrointestinal bleeding. Obstet Gynecol 1990;78:501–503.

137. Sachs R, Zagelbaum BM, Hersh PS. Corneal complications associated with the use of crack cocaine. Ophthalmology 1993;116:241–242.

138. Zagelbaum BM, Donnenfield ED, Perry HD, Buxton J, Buxton D, Hersh PS. Corneal ulcer caused by combined intravenous and anesthetic abuse of cocaine-induced bilateral amblyopia. Am J Emerg Med 1993;11:35–37.

139. Balster RL, Wessinger WD. Central nervous system depressant effects of phencyclidine. In: Kameka JM et al, eds. Phencyclidine and Related Amylcyclohexylamine. Ann Arbor, MI: NPP Books, 1983;299.

140. McCarnon MM, Schulze BW, Thompson GA et al. Acute phencyclidine intoxication. Ann Emerg Med 1981; 10:237.

141. Peterson RC, Stillman RC. Phencyclidine. A Review. Rockville, MD: National Institute on Drug Abuse, 1978.

142. Westermeyer J. The psychiatrist and solvent-inhalant abuse. recognition, assessment and treatment. Am J Psychiatry 1987;144:903.

Meyler's Side Effects of Drugs, 13th Edition
M.N.G. Dukes, editor

SECTION EDITOR: P.K.M. LUNDE

David B. Menkes and Richard Laverty

5 Hypnotics and sedatives

The use of hypnotics and sedatives continues to be common in most industrialized societies and new agents with greater selectivity or safety are being introduced or sought. The elderly, in particular, commonly use pharmacological assistance to induce or maintain sleep, although many more individuals complain of insomnia than actually get any advice or medication for this problem. Similarly anxiety disorders, while common and debilitating, are often untreated.

The elderly are at particular risk from the behavioural and cognitive toxicity of hypnotics in part due to pharmacokinetic changes with age. It is not surprising that the side-effects of hypnotics are of particular concern in this large and increasing proportion of the population. Sedative drugs are similar agents pharmacologically which are aimed at dealing with problems during the waking hours, particularly excessive anxiety. Anxiolytics (which may be a better term for these agents) seem to cause somewhat different problems, perhaps because they generally have slower absorption and elimination, are taken at lower doses, and have consumers who are better motivated and of a more mixed age distribution. However, some users of hypnosedatives inevitably find in their pharmacological properties some aspect that is rewarding, either by relief of symptoms, selective amnesia or mood elevation, which leads to continued use and the creation of a dependent state. It should be remembered that non-drug therapies are often appropriate for patients with anxiety or insomnia, and that such individuals often need education, and encouragement to persist with such treatment (1[r]). Unfortunately, many practitioners find it easier to prescribe a chemical remedy and thereby collude with industry in promoting drug treatment of what are often social or life-style problems. History has taught how many 'safe' remedies have turned out to have serious problems associated with their use, and the benzodiazepines are no exception.

Despite a recent tendency to decreasing use in Western countries, in both relative and absolute terms, the benzodiazepines are still predominant, particularly as hypnotics (SEDA-18, 43; 2[R]). This class name is somewhat misleading as there are newer agents, such as zopiclone and zolpidem, which are chemically distinct from the benzodiazepines, but which act on the same γ-aminobutyrate (GABA) receptor complex and therefore can be included in a common category. Conversely other agents, such as clobazam, have a chemically different benzodiazepine ring structure, and slightly different pharmacological properties, which make their classification difficult. The other large group, now only of historic importance as far as hypnotic and sedative properties are concerned, is the barbiturates; the reader should consult earlier editions of this book for details of these agents (SED-11, 97; SEDA-14, 41). There is little justification for their continued use as hypnotics or sedatives due to their much greater toxicity and dependence-inducing properties.

Other GABA enhancers are still used, especially as hypnotics, despite being arguably more toxic than the benzodiazepines. Chloral hydrate, in its many pharmaceutical forms, is still widely used; chlormethiazole continues to be used as a hypnotic in the elderly as well as for alcohol withdrawal; meprobamate likewise is still used as an anxiolytic despite greater abuse potential and suicide risk than benzodiazepines. Acting through an entirely different mechanism, sedating histamine antagonists have been used extensively in the past, particularly in children, and this use continues because of their ready availability in over-the-counter preparations and their relative advantages in dependence- and abuse-prone insomniacs. The use of over-the-counter hypnotics (e.g. promethazine), which may exceed that of the benzodiazepines, has not been systematically studied (3[R]) but can be problematic as many of the older antihistamines are quite non-specific in their actions and have strong antimuscarinic and/or α_1-adrenolytic activity. They are also toxic in overdose (a problem compounded by concomitant alcohol) and may cause prolonged 'hangover' sedation.

Strong antihistaminic activity also confers sedative properties on some of the tricyclic antidepressants, especially doxepin, amitriptyline and trimipramine, which are used for this purpose particularly in the elderly; fortunately, they are usually prescribed in low dose and used by the patients on an 'as required' basis, rather than as continuous therapy, and so they remain generally safe and effective as hypnotics. Similarly some sedating phenothiazines, such as chlorpromazine, methotrimeprazine (levomepromazine) or thioridazine, are used in aged patients with insomnia and agitation. As with over-the-counter hypnotic antihistamines, tricyclic antidepressants and antipsychotics also typically exhibit antimuscarinic and α_1-adrenolytic activity. These properties lead to side-effects which limit their use, particularly in the elderly, to the extent that such drugs are sometimes called 'sedative-autonomic' instead of sedative-hypnotic.

In recent years, a number of new drugs with anxiolytic or hypnotic effects have been introduced, often with pharmacological properties that suggest a further distinct mechanism of action. Of interest in this category are buspirone and ritanserin, which are thought to act through effects on the receptors for 5-hydroxytryptamine, rather than on GABA or histamine receptors. Other drugs, e.g. clonidine, acting on α_2-adrenoceptors, also have sedative effects. It is obvious that much more needs to be known about neurotransmission in the brain and the relation between various transmitters and the complex processes of sleep and arousal. In this chapter, the main group of drugs, the benzodiazepines, will be discussed at first in general and then in terms of the specific, usually the newer, agents; the other classes of hypnotic and sedative drugs will be discussed towards the latter part of the chapter.

The benzodiazepines

GENERAL CONSIDERATIONS

The benzodiazepines typically share hypnotic, anxiolytic, myorelaxant and anticonvulsant activity. Because their efficacy and tolerability are generally good, especially in the short term, these drugs have been used extensively and are likely to continue to be used for many years to come. However, their less specific use in the medically or psychiatrically ill, and in healthy individuals experiencing life-change stress or non-specific symptoms, has often been inappropriate, sometimes dangerous (SEDA-18, 43). The pharmacoepidemiology of benzodiazepine use has been carefully studied in the USA (2[R]) and in France, where 7% of the adult population (17% of those over 65 years) are regular users (4[Cr]). The need to reduce spending on pharmaceutical products, as well as the very real likelihood of inducing iatrogenic disease (e.g. cognitive impairment, drug dependence, withdrawal syndromes), has prompted many reviews aimed at discouraging indiscriminate use.

Authorities differ in their appraisal of the extent of the problem. A comprehensive review of benzodiazepine-induced adverse effects and liability to abuse and dependence which concludes that most benzodiazepine use is both appropriate and helpful (2[R]) has been challenged in commentary in the same journal (5[r], 6[r]). A balanced clinical overview of benzodiazepine use (7[R]) includes a set of recommendations on appropriate prescribing and avoiding adverse effects, including tolerance/dependence. Similarly, guidelines for management of insomnia, and the judicious use of hypnotics, are included in a recent review (8[R]). Recently, a number of new indications for benzodiazepines have been proposed, most notably catatonia (in conjunction with antipsychotics) and panic disorder (9[r]). (Antidepressants, especially the SSRIs, are tending to replace the use of benzodiazepines in anxiety disorders generally.)

There is little question that benzodiazepines are frequently over-prescribed to hospital patients (SEDA-17, 42), and their continuation after discharge constitutes a significant source of long-term users. Anxiety symptoms and insomnia occur commonly in the medically ill population, and are often due to specific physical causes, as a reaction to the illness, or to intercurrent psychiatric illness such as depression. Accordingly, the systematic assessment of such patients allows remediable causes to be identified, and use of hypnosedatives to be minimized. As in the elderly, the medically ill are prone to adverse effects of benzodiazepines, and alternatives are worth considering (10[R]). Benzodiazepines are particularly likely to cause adverse effects in patients with HIV infection and other causes of organic brain syndrome (11[cr]).

The important advantages of the benzodiazepines over their predecessors are their relatively reduced level of psychomotor impairment, drowsiness and respiratory inhibition, and consequently their relative safety in overdose. However, it must be emphasized that these advantages are relative and that the low toxicity potential does not apply when other agents are also present; in particular the combination of benzodiazepines with alcohol can be dangerous (12[R]). In addition to the cotoxicity seen with other CNS depressants, benzodiazepines contribute to suicide risk (13[cr]); they may facilitate self-injurious behaviour by disinhibiting reckless or suicidal impulses. In accord with earlier findings, a recent study indicates that benzodiazepines are the most commonly represented drug class in both attempted and completed suicide (14[Cr]). Before prescribing any drugs of this class, clinicians are exhorted to assess both sui-

Table 1. *Benzodiazepines having long half-life, active metabolites: route of metabolism and predominant metabolite half-times*

To desmethyldiazepam	$t_{1/2}$ β(h)	To other metabolites	$t_{1/2}$ β(h)
Clorazepate	40–100	Chlordiazepoxide	40–100
Diazepam		Clobazam	30–150
Halazepam		Flurazepam	40–120
Medazepam		Quazepam	25–120
Prazepam			

cidality and alcohol problems; a quick and valid screen for the latter is readily available (15[R]).

As far as is presently known, benzodiazepines and similar drugs (zopiclone, zolpidem) act by a single mechanism, interacting at the GABA receptor complex to enhance the ability of GABA to open the chloride ion channel and thereby hyperpolarize the neuronal membrane. It is usual, therefore, to classify benzodiazepines, and recommend their clinical use, on the basis of their duration of action or their half-life in the body. While this is without doubt a useful and scientifically satisfying means of classification it is over-simplistic and may fail to recognize other important pharmacokinetic factors.

The first factor that is considered significant is the metabolism of benzodiazepines to pharmacologically active metabolites. Many newer benzodiazepines intended for use as long-acting anxiolytic or sedative agents were in fact intended to be so metabolized to ensure stable blood and therapeutic levels over prolonged periods. Drugs with long durations of effect due at least in part to the formation of active metabolites are listed in Table 1.

Another, often neglected, aspect of the pharmacokinetics of benzodiazepines is their rate of onset of action. The barbiturates, even more than the benzodiazepines, could have been categorized as quick, medium or slow in onset and used accordingly. Similarly the properties and therapeutic benefits of the benzodiazepines depend to a considerable degree on the rapidity of onset of a perceived effect. This is true particularly of a hypnotic, in that the sufferer wishes to feel the effect coming on quickly; unfortunately this property also determines significantly the abuse potential. For most drugs of abuse, it is the behavioural changes associated with a rapid rise of drug blood level that is sought, whether the drug is abused by intravenous injection, nasal or bronchial absorption or, as with alcohol, rapid oral absorption from an empty stomach (16[R]). Rapid absorption and quick rise in blood levels explains why diazepam and flunitrazepam are effective hypnotics, even though after tissue redistribution and loss of immediate effect they have long terminal half-lives of elimination. It also explains the preference and so the increased liability for abuse of drugs like diazepam (16[R]) and flunitrazepam, especially when the latter is snorted (17[cr]). Since temazepam, as a soft gelatine liquid-containing capsule, is much more quickly absorbed than the hard capsule or tablet, it is the preferred form for hypnotic (Table 2) and 'recreational' use (and for this reason is restricted in some countries). Kinetic differences between drugs and between formulations partially explain why comparing 'equipotent'

Table 2. *Approximate times for maximum blood levels and half-times for elimination of benzodiazepines*

	Approx t_{max} (h)	Approx $t_{1/2}$ β(h)
Slow absorption		
Clonazepam	2–4	20–40
Loprazolam	2–5	5–15
Lorazepam	2	10–20
Oxazepam	2	5–15
Temazepam (hard capsules)	3	8–20
Intermediate absorption and elimination		
Alprazolam	1–2	12–15
Bromazepam	1–4	10–25
Chlordiazepoxide	1–2	10–25
Slow elimination (with active metabolites)		
Flurazepam	1.5	40–120
Clobazam	1–2	20–40
Clorazepate	1	40–100
Quazepam	1.5	15–35
Slow elimination *but* rapid redistribution		
Diazepam	1	20–70
Flunitrazepam	1	10–40
Nitrazepam	1	20–30
Rapid elimination *and* redistribution		
Lormetazepam (soft capsule)	1	8–20
Temazepam (soft capsule)	1	8–20
Rapid elimination		
Brotizolam	1	4–7
Zolpidem	1.5	2–5
Zopiclone	1.5	5–8
Very rapid elimination		
Midazolam	0.3	1–4
Triazolam	1	2–5

doses of benzodiazepines is difficult (see *Effects on Cognition*, below).

The route of metabolism can also be significant, particularly in those with liver disease. The complex interaction between hepatic dysfunction and benzodiazepines has been reviewed (18[R]); these drugs affect liver function in such individuals more readily than in normals, and also may directly contribute to hepatic coma, as shown by the ability of benzodiazepine antagonists to transiently reverse the coma (18[R]). The elderly appear to be at increased risk only if physically unwell, and particularly if taking multiple medications.

Rapid absorption, often followed by rapid redistribution to tissue stores with consequent falls in brain and blood drug levels, play a significant role in the quick onset and cessation of perceived effects, but long-term actions, e.g. mild sedative and anti-anxiety effects, are a consequence of slow hepatic clearance either by hydroxylation with subsequent conjugation to a glucuronide, or by microsomal metabolism to other possibly pharmacologically active metabolites. Agents subject to microsomal metabolism and/or oxidation may accumulate more rapidly in elderly patients with reduced liver function; only the metabolism of drugs such as oxazepam, lorazepam and temazepam that predominantly undergo glucuronidation are not affected by liver function, nor suffer from interference by drugs such as cimetidine, estrogens or erythromycin, which may compete for the enzyme pathways (see *Interactions*, below).

The mechanism of action of benzodiazepines remains a topic of research interest and of considerable progress, more marked at the bench than in the clinic. The use of techniques of molecular biology to clone the benzodiazepine receptor and the other components of the GABA receptor/chloride channel complex has indicated that there are likely to be many variant forms of the receptor, due to the multiplicity of protein subunits that constitute the receptor. This has given rise to the hope that more selective agonist drugs, for example zolpidem, may produce fewer adverse effects, particularly withdrawal phenomena (19[R]). In addition to multiple receptor subtypes, there are also developments, possibly inter-linked, in our views on how drugs may interact with their receptor sites to produce effects. The concepts of agonists, partial agonists and antagonists have been around for a sufficient period to have achieved respectability; classifying drugs as inverse agonists, and even partial inverse agonists, increases the complexity considerably, and the relationships between these mechanistic classifications, and their effect at cellular or whole organism levels, remain to be clarified. The suggestion that partial agonists (such as alpidem) have greater anxiolytic potency for given sedative properties (20[R]) or that they will be less prone to abuse (19[R]) will stimulate much further research.

ADVERSE REACTION PATTERN

General and toxic reactions The most frequent side-effect is drowsiness, which may be accompanied by in-coordination or ataxia. Problems with driving or falls may result. Memory impairment, loss of insight and transient euphoria are common; paradoxical reactions of irritability, abnormal or aggressive behaviour, and excitement have been documented. Tolerance to sedation typically occurs with continued use.

Physical dependence on benzodiazepines is now recognized as a major problem, and can be shown after relatively short periods of treatment (21[R]; 22[R]). Abrupt withdrawal can induce severe anxiety, perceptual changes, convulsions or delirium. It may masquerade as a return of the original symptoms in a more severe form (rebound), or present with additional features (SEDA-17, 42). Up to 90% of regular benzodiazepine users experience adverse symptoms on discontinuation; the distinction of rebound, withdrawal syndrome and recurrence is presented in detail (4[Cr]).

Rebound insomnia or heightened day-time anxiety can occur, particularly after short-acting benzodiazepine hypnotics (7[R], 23[C]; 24[C]).

Benzodiazepines have a very high therapeutic index of safety, with little effect on most systems (other than the CNS) in high dose. However, their toxicity increases markedly when combined with other CNS depressant drugs, such as alcohol. Brain injured patients may be particularly susceptible to adverse neurological or behavioral effects (SEDA-18, 43; 11[cr]).

Hypersensitivity reactions These remain rare. A few cases of anaphylaxis have been described, though usually these have been with the injectable forms and may involve the stabilizing agents (25[c]). Lesser reactions are also reported (SEDA-17, 44–45).

Tumor-inducing effects These have been observed in animals (SEDA-6, 39) but inconsistently; human reports are essentially negative.

Second generation effects These are infrequent and usually reversible; transfer from the mother may affect the fetus, newborn or lactating infant (26[R]).

ORGANS AND SYSTEMS

Cardiovascular *Hypotension* follows the intravenous injection of benzodiazepines, but is usually mild and transient (SED-11, 92; 27[C]). Acute rhabdomyolysis, usually associated with intravascular injection, has also been seen after an oral overdose of temazepam (SEDA-17, 45).

Local reactions to injected diazepam occur quite frequently, and may progress to compartment syndrome (SEDA-17, 44). In one study (28[C]), two-thirds of patients experienced some problem, the majority eventually progressing to thrombophlebitis. Flunitrazepam is similar to diazepam in this regard (29[C]). Altering the formulation by changing the solvent or using an emulsion did not affect the outcome greatly (30[C]). Midazolam being water-soluble might be expected to produce fewer problems; in five separate studies the incidence of thrombophlebitis was nil, in two others the incidence was 8—0%, less than with diazepam but similar to thiopentone and saline (31[r]).

Respiratory *Respiratory depression* has been reported as the commonest adverse effect on intravenous diazepam (27[C]), especially at the extremes of age. Midazolam has similar effects (32[C]). It must be accepted that all benzodiazepines have the potential to cause respiratory depression, particularly in bronchitic patients, through drowsiness and reduction in exercise tolerance (33[C]). Rectal administration of, for example, diazepam may offer advantages in unconscious or uncooperative patients, and is notably less prone than parenteral dosing to produce respiratory depression.

Nervous system *Effects on performance* Since all benzodiazepines have the potential to cause drowsiness and sedation, it must be accepted that motor and mental performance will be affected. Driving is one motor and mental task that is particularly likely to be impaired (SEDA-7, 46); it has been shown that hypnotics, like alcohol, impair actual driving performance (34[CR]) as well as psychomotor tests undertaken in laboratory situations (19[R]). As with alcohol, the maximal impairment occurs while the drug blood levels are rising (35[C]), rather than when they have peaked, are stable or are falling. The motor and mental performance decrements induced by hypnotics, especially in the elderly (36[R]) are evident in increased incidence of falls, often resulting in fracture of the hip (37[CR]). Non-benzodiazepine drugs with short elimination half-lives (less than 24 hours) caused no increased risk, but benzodiazepines with longer half-lives, as with tricyclic antidepressants and antipsychotic drugs, almost doubled the risk ratio.

Fit young subjects had no impairment of their exercise ability after temazepam or nitrazepam, although nitrazepam caused a subjective feeling of 'hang-over' (38[C]).

Effects on cognition The amnestic effects of benzodiazepines (SEDA-17, 42) have been used as an advantage in minor surgery (male doctors and dentists are advised to have a chaperone present when using this procedure with female patients) particularly with the use of midazolam and other short-acting compounds. However, an unwanted amnesia has been found in many instances, particularly associated with the use of triazolam as a hypnotic or as an aid for travellers (39[CR], 40[R]). The combination of a short half-life with a powerful agent, especially when used in the higher doses available when the drug was initially launched, makes triazolam particularly prone to this problem. Flurazepam and temazepam use initiated very few reports of adverse effects on memory, though flurazepam did cause daytime sedation. Temazepam was low in adverse reactions reports, but was also reported more often as being without adequate hypnotic effect. Ironically, temazepam produces more, and oxazepam less, sedation than other benzodiazepines in overdose (41[cr]).

The role of benzodiazepines in brain damage has been reviewed (SEDA-14, 36). Cognitive impairments in long-term users may be detected in up to half the subjects compared with 16% of controls. Cognitive toxicity is more common with benzodiazepines than other anticonvulsants, with the possible exception of phenobarbitone (42[R]).

Excessive anxiety and tremulousness, hyperexcitability, confusion and hallucinations were all reported more frequently with triazolam than with temazepam or flurazepam, when spontaneous reporting was analysed (39[CR]). Whether this is dose-related, and perhaps related to the rapid changes in blood level with triazolam, is not clear. Confusion is common, particularly in the elderly who may have impaired clearance of drugs, and must always be regarded as possibly drug-induced. Dose- and age-related increases in adverse central nervous effects from benzodiazepines (40[R]) are well documented. The use of these drugs in the elderly has been reviewed, with recommendations about maximizing the benefit-to-risk ratio in this group prone to cognitive and other adverse effects (43[R]).

Sleep The use of benzodiazepines, particularly the short-acting compounds such as triazolam, for the induction of sleep has provoked much scientific discussion over the past few years (SEDA-17, 42). The debate rages over the risks and benefits of a short-acting compound, in inducing bizarre behaviour or rapid withdrawal with daytime anxiety, compared with the possibility of 'hang-over' sedation and performance deficits with longer-acting compounds (44[C]). The treatment of sleep disorders is complex because of the complex nature of sleep and the variety of factors that may give rise to sleep disorders (40[R]). Consequently such treatment should be selected and proferred carefully, with due regard for all the factors, not treated cavalierly with the latest 'flavour-of-the-month' benzodiazepine. Non-drug treatments should be considered first; pharmacological treatment should take into consideration any pre-existing factors, e.g. anxiety, depression, duration and nature of medical problems, pain, etc. (8[R]).

Paradoxical effects Depression is commonly seen, either during benzodiazepine treatment, or as a complication of withdrawal (SEDA-17, 42). Benzodiazepines used as anxiolytics or hypnotics may increase irritability and depression and, less commonly, lead to manic episodes (45[C], 46[C]). They typically suppress REM sleep, with consequent rebound dreaming and restlessness on withdrawal, leading to poorer sleep patterns (SEDA-12, 42; 47[R]). While they are generally regarded as tranquillizing, benzodiazepines, in some individuals and particularly in combination with alcohol, may release aggression and induce anti-social behaviour (48[C]). The combination of abnormal behaviour and amnesia produced by benzodiazepines can be particularly dangerous. Non-medical use of flunitrazepam (49[C]) seems particularly prone to reveal paradoxical rage and aggression, with consequent forensic problems. A controlled study indicated that lorazepam was more likely to provoke aggression than oxazepam (50[Cr]).

Review of a Canadian ADR database showed several cases of previously unreported benzodiazepine-induced adverse effects, including hallucinations and encephalopathy (51[c]), although whether benzodiazepines alone were responsible is difficult to confirm. An earlier report showed that schizophreniform auditory hallucinations could follow benzodiazepine withdrawal (52[c]).

Endocrine and other effects Benzodiazepines appear free of effects on most endocrine systems. Gynaecomastia, with raised oestradiol, in men on diazepam treatment has been reported (53[C]).

Jaundice following benzodiazepines has been reported, though only in few cases have they been the only drugs involved; (SED-12, 97).

Nausea has been reported as commoner in children, but the incidence usually does not greatly exceed that found following placebo treatment. Gastrointestinal disturbances have been found more frequently with the newer, non-benzodiazepine agents, e.g. zopiclone, buspirone (54[R], 55[R]).

Skin rashes have been reported; an incidence of 0.4 per 1000 was found for diazepam in the Boston Collaborative Surveillance Program (56[R]).

Sexual effects *Female orgasm* is inhibited by a number of central depressant and psychotropic drugs including antipsychotics, antidepressants and anxiolytic benzodiazepines (57[r]). A clinical survey of bipolar patients on lithium showed that the co-administration of benzodiazepines was associated with a significantly increased risk (49%) of sexual dysfunction in both men and women (58[Cr]).

Dependence and withdrawal *(SEDA-12, 40; SEDA-13, 33; SEDA-14, 35; SEDA-17, 43)* The likelihood and possible severity of dependence on, and withdrawal from, benzodiazepines remains a matter for considerable publicity, especially with regard to the newer, short-acting compounds (21[R]).

Withdrawal symptoms occur in at least one-third of long-term users (over 1 year) even if the dose is gradually tapered (59[R]). Symptoms come on within 2—3 days of finally stopping a short- or medium-acting benzodiazepine, or 7—10 days after a long-acting drug; the former tend to produce a more marked withdrawal syndrome (19[R]). Lorazepam and alprazolam appear particularly difficult to quit. Symptoms usually last 1—6 weeks but may persist for many months, leaving the patient in a vulnerable state with likely recurrence of the original disorder and of self-medication. Withdrawal symptoms may occur within 4—6 weeks of daily benzodiazepine use (60[R]), quite possibly earlier in susceptible individuals.

Symptoms on withdrawal are variable in nature and degree. Rebound insomnia may be observed one or two nights after discontinuation of short-acting drugs. Anxiety is common, with both psychological and physical manifestations including apprehension, panic, insomnia, palpitations, sweating, tremor and gastrointestinal disturbances. Depression has also been seen after withdrawal (61[C]). Increased or distorted sensory perceptions may be experienced, such as photophobia, altered (metallic) taste, hypersensitivity to touch and pain. Flu-like muscle aches and spasms, unsteadiness and clumsiness are common. Perceptual distortions include burning or creeping of the skin and apparent movement or changes in objects or self (59[R]). General malaise with loss of appetite may occur. As with alcohol, paranoid psychosis, delirium, and epileptic fits are possible on withdrawal (SED-12, 97). With careful handling, often involving psychological and sometimes adjunctive pharmacological support, motivated patients dependent on benzodiazepines can usually be successfully withdrawn. Guidelines to management of such patients have been concisely presented (22[R]).

Second-generation effects Benzodiazepines readily

pass from the mother to fetus through the placenta (62[R]), and are also secreted in milk in relatively small amounts (26[R]). Pregnant women may have some risk of congenital malformation if given benzodiazepines during the 1st trimester, but data are contradictory and any real effect would appear to be small (26[R]). The risk of benzodiazepine-induced birth defects thus remains uncertain (63[R]), despite two cases of fetal-alcohol syndrome abnormalities reported after benzodiazepine exposure alone (64[C]).

A further concern exists regarding cognitive development after in utero exposure to benzodiazepines. It now appears that the slowed intellectual progress seen in some children exposed in utero will 'catch up' in most cases by age 4 (26[R]). Unfortunately, the impact of sedative-hypnotic use during pregnancy is often complicated by the abuse of multiple agents, poor maternal nutrition and antenatal care, and may be further confounded by social and environmental deprivation which the infant often faces after birth (26[R], 65[R]). More definite, but short-lived problems occur with benzodiazepines given in late pregnancy and during labour—here floppiness, apnea and withdrawal in the infant can pose clear clinical problems (26[R], 66[cR]). Thus pregnant women should avoid benzodiazepines if possible, especially during late pregnancy and labour.

During lactation, longer acting agents are relatively contraindicated, particularly with continued administration beyond 3—5 days, owing to the likelihood of infant sedation (66[cR], 67[R]). Short acting benzodiazepines and zopiclone are probably safe, especially if restricted to single doses or for short courses of therapy (26[R], 68[R]). Zopiclone and midazolam, for example, become undetectable in breast milk 4—5 hours after a dose (69[cr]).

Interactions *Pharmacodynamic* The interactions of benzodiazepines with other CNS depressants, especially alcohol and other GABA-enhancers, has been reviewed (70[R]). The unwitting potentiation of sedative effects from benzodiazepines with sedating antihistaminics (e.g. tricyclic antidepressants or antipsychotics, over-the-counter remedies) can also pose problems. Other drugs with CNS depressant effects (opioids, anticonvulsants, general anaesthetics) also can add to, and complicate, the depressant action of benzodiazepines.

Caffeine and other central stimulants have an obvious potential to reverse any daytime sedation from benzodiazepine hypnotic use. A positive effect of caffeine (250 mg) on early-morning performance was seen following placebo and flurazepam (30 mg) given the night before (71[C], 72[C]) particularly in terms of subjective assessment of mood and sleepiness. One cannot assume, however, that the alerting effect of caffeine necessarily reverses the amnestic or disinhibiting effects of benzodiazepines. Other drugs with direct or indirect CNS stimulant activity (theophylline, ephedrine, amphetamine and analogues) have similar effects and may counteract, or increase the perceived 'need' for hypnosedatives.

Pharmacokinetic Omeprazole may, like cimetidine, impair benzodiazepine metabolism and lead to side-effects (SEDA-18, 43). Other drugs, including antibiotics (erythromycin, chloramphenicol, isoniazid), antifungals (ketoconazole and analogues), some SSRIs (fluoxetine, paroxetine) and calcium antagonists (diltiazem, verapamil) may also compete for hepatic metabolic pathways. Dietary influences (e.g. grapefruit juice, which contains extremely potent enzyme inhibitors) should not be ignored.

Enzyme induction may become problematic with co-administration of benzodiazepines and rifampicin or certain anticonvulsants (phenobarbitone, phenytoin, carbamazepine). Despite enzyme stimulation, the net effect of adding these anticonvulsants may still be to augment benzodiazepine-induced sedation.

Medico-legal Medico-legal problems especially with the use of triazolam have been discussed previously (SEDA-13, 33); debate continues on the interpretation of evidence pointing to an increased incidence of adverse behavioural effects with triazolam (73[R]) and other short-acting high-potency agents (7[R]). Efforts to restrict benzodiazepines in New York State (2[R]) and to ban triazolam in the United Kingdom (74[r]) have likewise been fraught with controversy.

INDIVIDUAL BENZODIAZEPINES OR RELATED DRUGS

Since many of the properties of the benzodiazepines and related compounds such as zopiclone and zolpidem appear to be very similar, it would be useless to repeat the general effects for all compounds. In this section, only the newer compounds, or unusual observations on the older compounds, will be reviewed.

Alprazolam *(SEDA-12, 43; SEDA-13, 35; SEDA-14, 38)*

This triazolobenzodiazepine has been marketed as an anxiolytic with additional antidepressant properties; its analogue adinazolam also exhibits partial antidepressant activity (75[cr]). Like other benzodiazepines, alprazolam is effective in acute and generalised anxiety; its further efficacy in panic disorder (76[C], 77[Cr]), premenstrual syndrome (78[R]) and chronic pain (79[R]) is complicated by high rates of adverse effects in the treatment of each of those conditions. Alprazolam shows the expected range of benzodiazepine-like side-effects, although dependence and withdrawal from dependence appear to present greater problems than with other benzodiazepines or related compounds (SED-12, 98). Pharmacological strategies for discontinuing alprazolam, by switching to a longer-acting agent, have been proposed (80[c]). Serious mood swings to mania or depression can be seen in panic disorder patients treated with alprazolam (SED-12, 98), and disinhibition can be a major problem in patients with borderline personality disorder (81[c]). In common with other benzodiazepines, alprazolam produces additional performance impairments when taken together with alcohol (82[C]).

Bromazepam

This moderately short-acting benzodiazepine (half-time of elimination about 12 hours) has been used in the treatment of anxiety states and has the usual effects, e.g. amnesia and depressed psychomotor performance, though less depression than with lorazepam has been reported (SED-12, 98). The basis of rare extrapyramidal effects with bromazepam and diazepam are unexplained (SEDA-18, 44).

Clobazam (*see also Chapter 7*)

This 1,5-benzodiazepine differs in its chemical structure from most other benzodiazepines, and it has been claimed to have less sedative effects for its effective anti-convulsant and anti-anxiety effects (SED-12, 98). A number of metabolic interactions between clobazam and other anti-epileptic drugs have been reported, in particular phenytoin intoxication after the addition of clobazam (SED-12, 98). Clobazam has similar effects on anxiety as other benzodiazepines. Used as an anticonvulsant, clobazam has been shown in a review to be generally well tolerated in epileptic patients, many showing little evidence of tolerance (83[R]). Whether due to tolerance or not, clobazam tends to be less sedating than clonazepam.

Clonazepam *(SEDA-13, 35; SEDA-18, 44)*

This is another benzodiazepine used predominantly for epilepsy, particularly status epilepticus and, more recently, for panic disorder (SED-12, 98). Although commonly used in the adjunctive management of chronic pain, benzodiazepines generally do not possess analgesic activity per se. One exception may be stabbing/-lancinating neuropathic pain which often responds to anticonvulsant benzodiazepines, particularly clonazepam. Nevertheless, the use of these drugs in pain syndromes is generally contraindicated (SEDA-17, 42), due both to the availability of alternative agents with comparable or superior efficacy, and the significant incidence of adverse effects in this population, including depression, self-poisoning, cognitive impairment, and dependence (79[R]).

Diazepam *(SEDA-16, 32; SEDA-17, 44)*

Due in part to its continued widespread use, number of unusual side-effects of diazepam continue to be reported. These include cases of urinary retention and compartment syndrome, which are not explicable based on the known pharmacology. On the other hand, accumulation of diazepam, and attendant complications of obtundation and respiratory depression, may be understood in terms of its long half-life, particularly in the elderly and medically ill.

Flunitrazepam *(SEDA-12, 44; SEDA-18, 44)*

This drug has acquired a reputation for toxicity and abuse potential (17[cr]). It has a rapid onset of action but a long half-time of elimination; the previously recommended hypnotic dose (1—2 mg) is excessive and like some other benzodiazepines, e.g. triazolam, is safer in a smaller dose (84[C]). Although its outpatient use in abuse-prone individuals is hazardous, intravenous flunitrazepam has been found useful for alcohol withdrawal delirium.

Lorazepam *(SEDA-14, 39)*

Being a widely used drug it has already been reported to cause a number of rare side-effects; including a manic-like reaction on withdrawal, delirium in a burn patient (SED-12, 99), and a paradoxical precipitation of tonic seizures in a child. Lorazepam has been shown to disinhibit aggression (50[Cr]) and impair memory more than its chemically and kinetically similar analogue, oxazepam (85[C]). It has also been shown to have a considerable abuse potential, and to pose particular difficulties in withdrawal (19[R]). On the other hand, a sizeable sample (n=97) of chronic users wishing to discontinue were found to generally use stable or decreasing doses on an 'as needed' basis (86[Cr]).

Midazolam *(SEDA-13, 35; SEDA-14, 39; SEDA-17, 44; SEDA-18, 44)*

This is used mainly in parenteral form in anaesthesia, and more recently in status epilepticus (87[cr]). Its pharmacology and therapeutics have been extensively reviewed (88[R]). It produces greater amnesia than diazepam, useful in terms of its anaesthetic use, but carries a risk of cardiorespiratory depression and death (SED-12, 99). Behavioural disinhibition (SEDA-18, 44) and acute withdrawal appear relatively common; hallucinations, flumazenil-reversible dystonia, and hypersensitivity have all been observed (SED-12, 99; SEDA-17, 44). Midazolam has been carefully evaluated for adverse effects when used with critically ill infants and children; only the latter showed difficulties; particularly prolonged obtundation and withdrawal were noted (89[Cr]). The availability of the specific benzodiazepine antagonist, flumazenil, to correct any adverse or overdose effects from injected midazolam should not encourage laxity in its use. A number of recent reports highlight the kinetic interactions between midazolam and other drugs (see *Interactions*, above).

Temazepam *(SEDA-17, 45; SEDA-18, 44)*

Temazepam has favourable kinetics for use as a hypnotic (7[R]), and is widely prescribed for this purpose. As mentioned above, the soft capsules are more rapidly absorbed and are also liable to intravenous abuse, often together with other substances. The resulting medical problems are varied, often serious, as reviewed in the Annuals.

Triazolam *(SEDA-13, 36; SEDA-14, 40; SEDA-17, 45; SEDA-18, 44)*

Triazolam continues to dominate the controversial literature (73[r]). Much of this has already been referred to above and has been reviewed (7[R], 90[R]). Much of the adverse effect literature is based on doses of 0.25 mg and above; the reduction in recommended dose to 0.125 mg may improve therapeutic safety at the cost of compromising hypnotic efficacy in most patients. A low therapeutic index is also suggested by the possibility of amnesia even after a single dose (91[CR]) and triazolam does appear associated with a greater incidence of behavioural disturbance than other hypnotics, such as temazepam. A case of recurrent, iatrogenic Kleine-Levin syndrome with irritability, hyperphagia and amnesia (92[cr]) provides a further example of the bizarre behaviour not infrequently seen with triazolam at high dose (0.5 mg). At this dose, triazolam produces too many adverse effects on sleep and memory to be useful to the military; elderly patients are particularly sensitive even to lower doses due in part to reduced clearance of the drug (SED-12, 99). Amnesia and confusion, which can occur even after single-dose use of triazolam, are accentuated by continued use, with frank psychopathology being observed in psychiatric patients during 2 weeks use and during withdrawal (93[C]).

BENZODIAZEPINE-LIKE DRUGS

Zolpidem and Alpidem *(SEDA-17, 46; SEDA-18, 45)*

These drugs are chemically quite different from the benzodiazepines and appear to bind selectively to a subset of benzodiazepine receptors (19[R]). This property may account for their apparently milder withdrawal effects and, in the case of alpidem, a relative dominance of anxiolytic over sedative and cognitive effects (19[R]). Zolpidem has hypnotic efficacy comparable to short/-medium-acting benzodiazepines, and has similar or possibly fewer adverse effects at therapeutic doses (94[R], 95[R], 96[Cr]) except for gastrointestinal disturbances, which appear more common, and recent reports of visual hallucinations (SEDA-17, 46; SEDA-18, 45). Zolpidem also appears relatively toxic in overdose due to respiratory depression, based on one case report (97[cr]). Alpidem has now been withdrawn due to hepatotoxicity but other, similar, drugs are expected to follow. The effects of both drugs are reversed by flumazenil (98[R]).

Zopiclone and Suriclone *(SEDA-12, 46; SEDA-13, 37; SEDA-15, 40; SEDA-17, 47)*

These also have similarities to the benzodiazepines in their pharmacology (binding close to the same site), but not in their chemistry. They are cyclopyrrolones; this may be compared with zolpidem which is an imidazopyridine and with the benzodiazepine ring structure present in most other class members. Zopiclone has been widely used as a hypnotic, comparable to estazolam (99[cr]). It appears to have no notable side-effects which would not to be expected from its pharmacological and pharmacokinetic properties, with the exception (like zolpidem) of increased gastrointestinal disturbances and visual hallucinations (100[R], 101[cr]). Of interest, subchronic zopiclone has been found to produce minimal changes in the sleep EEG (102[cr]), but direct comparison with the benzodiazepines is lacking. Its liability for abuse appears similar to that of the benzodiazepines (SEDA-17, 47). Suriclone has been found efficacious as an anxiolytic, and had the notable advantages of minimal sedation and cognitive toxicity, and withdrawal effects mild in comparison with diazepam or lorazepam (19[R]). Its withdrawal from further development is a mystery.

BENZODIAZEPINE ANTAGONISTS

Flumazenil *(SEDA-12, 45; SEDA-13, 36; SEDA-14, 40; SEDA-15, 39)*

This drug is increasingly in use as an antagonist in the treatment of benzodiazepine poisoning or reversal of benzodiazepine effects in anaesthesia (12[R], 103[R]) or in the neonate (104[C]). Guidelines for use of flumazenil have been summarised (105[R]). The problems in its use are those of dose adjustment, to avoid panic anxiety or other signs of excessively rapid benzodiazepine withdrawal, or pharmacokinetic problems due to the short half-life of flumazenil (about 1 hour) compared with the longer half-time of elimination of most benzodiazepines (106[R]). Its use is also commonly associated with emesis and headache, and rarely with psychosis or sudden cardiac death (SEDA-17, 46), especially in mixed overdoses. Flumazenil was not effective in reversing the amnesic effects of midazolam (107[C]), but interestingly may be useful in hepatic coma, regardless of aetiology (18[R]). In chronic benzodiazepine dependence or in mixed drug overdose, flumazenil may trigger convulsions. Benzodiazepine plasma levels are not generally useful, but may assist in the diagnosis of overdose and thus guide use of antagonists (108[C]).

NON-BENZODIAZEPINES AS ANXIOLYTICS AND HYPNOTICS

Buspirone *(SEDA-12, 45; SEDA-13, 37; SEDA-14, 41; SEDA-15, 39; SEDA-17, 46; SEDA-18, 45)*

This azapirone drug, similar to its analogue ipsaperone, is chemically and pharmacologically dissimilar to the benzodiazepines and appears useful in generalised anxiety *and* in depression (109[CR]). In contrast to benzodiazepines, buspirone shows an antidepressant-like therapeutic latency (19[R]) and for this reason needs to be given with considerable education and encouragement. Recent studies have also shown it to be efficacious as an antidepressant adjuvant in refractory depression with (110[c]) and without obsessive-compulsive symptoms (111[cr]). Buspirone has also shown surprising efficacy in treating agitation or aggression associated with organic brain disease (112[cR]). Originally thought to act through a dopaminergic mechanism, it is now regarded as acting therapeutically as a serotonin ($5HT^{1A}$) (partial) agonist and produces dose-related side-effects similar to the serotonin uptake inhibitors (nausea, headache, insomnia, dizziness) (19[R]) and, like them, may interact with MAOIs in producing a serotonin syndrome (113[R]). An uncommon association with extrapyramidal movement disorders (SEDA-17, 46; SEDA-18, 45) may reflect its structural relation to neuroleptics.

Compared with benzodiazepines, buspirone causes less sedation and memory impairment (114[CR]), has little interaction with alcohol (19[R], 115[CR]), and is essentially devoid of problems of tolerance and dependence. Despite continuing scrutiny, buspirone has shown little, if any, abuse potential (19[R]). These advantages are important in treating particular groups of patients, particularly the elderly and medically ill (116[R], 117[R]). Because of its virtual absence of respiratory depressant effects compared to benzodiazepines (118[C]), buspirone may be especially useful in treating anxious patients with lung disease (119[cr]). It may also have advantages in treating individuals prone to alcohol problems (115[R]), although habitual users of benzodiazepines are often unwilling to persist with buspirone treatment (19[R]), necessary due to its antidepressant-like therapeutic latency. Unlike carbamazepine or tricyclic antidepressants, buspirone does not appear helpful in the management of benzodiazepine withdrawal (4[Cr]).

Chloral hydrate *(SEDA-12, 46)*

Chloral hydrate, in its various pharmaceutical formulations, continues to be used for sleep disorder and for pre-operative sedation, especially in children (120[CR]). As an alternative to the hypnotic benzodiazepines, it has essentially similar properties and problems. Its reputation for safety, however, has been challenged by recent data which indicate that chloral hydrate and short-acting barbiturates are particularly lethal when taken in overdose (121[Cr]). Liver damage and cardiac toxicity, consistent with the chemical similarities between trichlorethanol, chloroform and alcohol, can occur; allergic skin reactions continue to be reported. Concern about carcinogenicity is not supported by its prolonged successful therapeutic use. Hyperbilirubinemia in neonates associated with chloral hydrate use (122[CR]) may be due to the more prolonged half-life of trichlorethanol in newborns compared with adults (37 vs. 14 hours).

Clomethiazole (Chlormethiazole) *(SEDA-12, 46; SEDA-14, 41)*

This sedative-hypnotic has been used extensively in the treatment of alcohol withdrawal, as well as for sedation and sleep induction in the elderly. In addition to GABA-enhancement which it shares with the benzodiazepines, clomethiazole also enhances the activity of another inhibitory amino acid, glycine. Whether this property is clinically important is uncertain. As well as the expected effects of sedation and memory impairment, it produces nasal irritation especially in younger patients, in whom the drug has a shorter half-life. Its use in alcohol withdrawal is becoming less common, possibly due to the demonstrated safety and efficacy of longer acting benzodiazepines, and alternatives such as carbamazepine. As with other GABA enhancers, clomethiazole is highly abusable in susceptible individuals and should not be used for outpatient detoxication. On the other hand, clomethiazole has been reported to maintain efficacy with apparently less dependence than temazepam during prolonged use (123[C]). Hypotension, phlebitis, and respiratory depression can occur after intravenous use. While effects in the elderly may be generally increased, the incidence of side-effects remains similar to that seen in younger subjects (124[C]). Clomethiazole, like the benzodiazepines, has an additive effect with other CNS depressants, and may result in profound bradycardia when combined with β-adrenoceptor antagonists. A notable kinetic interaction occurs with cimetidine, which can reduce clomethiazole clearance by 60—70%.

Ritanserin *(SEDA-12, 46)*

This selective $5HT_2$-receptor antagonist has been shown to increase slow-wave sleep in normal volunteers (125[C]); it improved sleep in middle-aged poor sleepers (126[C]), but on withdrawal after 20 days treatment showed rebound sleep impairment, worst three nights after withdrawal, consistent with its long half-time of elimination (40 hours). Ritanserin is thus unlikely to be useful as a hypnotic, but analogs with more appropriate kinetics will be of interest.

Tiapride

Tiapride, an atypical antipsychotic with anxiolytic activity, appears useful in alcohol withdrawal as an alternative to the benzodiazepines (127[cr]). It is unlikely to show problems of dependence or abuse. Its use may be limited by its lack of anticonvulsant activity, and by the risk of tardive dyskinesia with long-term use.

Trimipramine

This sedating tricyclic antidepressant has been used as a hypnotic (128[CR]), an activity it shares with other drugs of its class, notably amitriptyline and doxepin, and with the tetracyclic mianserin. Trimipramine may be preferred for this purpose, since it has less effect on sleep architecture, including REM (129[C]), and has only a modest propensity to produce rebound insomnia in a subset of patients (130[Cr]). It may be particularly appropriate for individuals at risk of benzodiazepine abuse. The usual pattern of tricyclic side-effects, especially antimuscarinic and hypotensive, may be expected. Some authors, enthusiastic about GABA enhancers, contend that antidepressants are not useful hypnotic alternatives (9[R]).

Antidepressant drugs of various classes (tricyclics, MAOIs, SSRIs) are now appreciated to have broad efficacy in generalised anxiety and in panic disorder, for which they are now the treatment of choice (131[r]). While not prone to benzodiazepine-like dependence or abuse, they do have a significant therapeutic latency and the older drugs are very toxic in overdose.

Vigabatrin

Vigabatrin (γ-vinyl-GABA), a recently introduced GABA-transaminase inhibitor, is effective in certain epilepsies and may also be useful in relieving the excessive startle response characteristic of post-traumatic stress disorder (132[cr]). Benzodiazepine use has been discouraged in this disorder (133[R]), and whether vigabatrin will have less problems in terms of dependence and abuse remains to be seen. Vigabatrin appears similar to conventional anticonvulsants in terms of its side-effect profile, and is said to have prominent behavioural toxicity in some patients (134[r]). In certain settings, vigabatrin has been reported to have subtantially fewer adverse effects than the benzodiazepines (135[c]).

REFERENCES

1. Byrne A. Benzodiazepines: the end of a dream. Aust Family Phys 1994;23:1584.
2. Woods JH, Winger G. Current benzodiazepine issues. Psychopharmacology 1995;118:107.
3. Pillitteri JL, Kozlowski LT, Person DC, Spear ME. Over-the-counter sleep aids: widely used but rarely studied. J Substance Abuse 1994;6:315.
4. Pelissolo A, Bisserbe JC. (Dependence on benzodiazepines. Clinical and biological aspects). Encephale 1994;20: 147.
5. Lader M. Commentary on review by Woods and Winger. Psychopharmacology 1995;118:118.
6. Griffiths RR. Commentary on review by Woods and Winger. Psychopharmacology 1995;118:116.
7. Ashton H. Guidelines for the rational use of benzodiazepines. When and what to use. Drugs 1994;48:25.
8. Pagel JF. Treatment of insomnia. Am Family Phys 1994;49:1417.
9. Laux G. (Current status of treatment with benzodiazepines). Nervenarzt 1995;66:311.
10. Wise MG, Griffies WS. A combined treatment approach to anxiety in the medically ill. J Clin Psychiatry 1995; 56(Suppl 2):14.
11. Ayuso JL. Use of psychotropic drugs in patients with HIV infection. Drugs 1994;47:599.
12. Gaudreault P, Guay J, Thivierge RL et al. Benzodiazepine poisoning: clinical and pharmacological considerations. Drug Safety 1991;6:247.
13. Taiminen TJ. Effect of psychopharmacotherapy on suicide risk in psychiatric inpatients. Acta Psychiatr Scand 1993;87:45.
14. Michel K, Waeber V, Valach L, Arestegui G, Spuhler T. A comparison of the drugs taken in fatal and nonfatal self-poisoning. Acta Psychiatr Scand 1994;90:184.
15. Bohn MJ, Babor TF, Kranzler HR. The Alcohol Use Disorders Identification Test (AUDIT): Validation of a screening instrument for use in medical settings. J Studies Alcohol 1995;56:423.
16. Griffiths RR, McLeod DR, Bigelow GE et al. Comparison of diazepam and oxazepam: preference, liking and extent of abuse. J Pharmacol Exp Ther 1984;229:501.
17. Bond A, Seijas D, Dawling S, Lader M. Systemic absorption and abuse liability of snorted flunitrazepam. Addiction 1994;89:821.
18. Ananth J, Swartz R, Burgoyne K, Gadasally R. Hepatic disease and psychiatric illness: relationships and treatment. Psychother Psychosom 1994;62:146.
19. Lader M. Clinical pharmacology of anxiolytic drugs: Past, present and future. In: Biggio G, Sanna E, Costa E, eds. GABA-A Receptors and Anxiety: From Neurobiology to Treatment. New York: Raven Press, 1995;135.
20. Haefely W, Martin JR, Schoch P. Novel anxiolytics that act as partial agonists at benzodiazepine receptors. Trends Pharmacol Sci 1990;11:452.
21. Woods JH, Katz JL, Winger G. Abuse liability of benzodiazepines. Pharmacol Rev 1987;39:251.
22. Ashton H. The treatment of benzodiazepine dependence. Addiction 1994;89:1535.
23. Adam K, Oswald I. Can a rapidly-eliminated hypnolic cause daytime anxiety? Pharmacopsychiatry 1989;22:115.
24. Kales A, Manfredi RL, Vgontzas AN et al. Rebound insomnia after only brief and intermittent use of rapidly eliminated benzodiazepines. Clin Pharmacol Ther 1991;49;468.
25. Deardon DJ, Bird GLA. Acute (Type 1) hypersensitivity to I.V. Diazemuls Br J Anaesth 1987;59:391.
26. McElhatton PR. The effects of benzodiazepine use during pregnancy and lactation. Reproduct Toxicol 1994;8:461.
27. Donaldson D, Gibson G. Systemic complications with intravenous diazepam. Oral Surg 1980;49:126.
28. Glaser JW, Blanton PL, Thrush WJ. Incidence and extent of venous sequelae with intravenous diazepam utilizing a standardized conscious sedation technique. J Periodontol 1982;53:700
29. Mikkelson H. Hoel TM, Bryne H. Local reactions to i.v. injections of diazepam, flunitrazepam and isotonic saline. Br J Anaesth 1981;52;817.
30. Jensen S. Huttel MS, Olesen AS. Venous complications after i.v. administration of Diazemuls(diazepam) and Dormicum(midazolam). Br J Anaesth 1981;53,1083.
31. Reves JG, Fragen RJ, Vinik HR et al. Midazolam: pharmacology and uses. Anesthesiology 1985;62:310.
32. Dundee JW. Halliday MJ, Harper KW. Midazolam: a review of its pharmacological properties and therapcutic use. Drugs 1984;28:519.
33. Woodcock AA, Gross ER, Geddes DM. Drug treatment of breathlessness: contrasting effects of diazepam and promethazine in pink puffers. Br Med J 1981;2:343.
34. O'Hanlon JF, Volkerts ER. Hypnotics and actual driving performance. Acta Psychiatr Scand Suppl 1986;332:95.
35. Ellinwood EH, Linnoila M, Easler ME et al. Onset of peak impairment after diazepam and after alcohol. Clin Pharmacol Ther 1981;30:534.
36. Kruse WH-H. Problems and pitfalls in the use of benzodiazepines in the elderly. Drug Safety 1990;5:328.
37. Ray WA, Griffin MR, Schaffner W et al. Psychotropic drug use and the risk of hip fracture. N Engl J Med 1987;316:363.
38. Charles RB, Kirkham AJ, Guyatt AR et al. Psychomotor, pulmonary and exercise responses to sleep medication. Br J Clin Pharmacol 1987;24:191.
39. Bixler EO, Kales A, Brubaker BH et al. Adverse reactions to benzodiazepine hypnotics: spontaneous reporting system. Pharmacology 1987;35:286.
40. Gillin JC, Byerley WF. The diagnosis and management of insomnia. N Engl J Med 1990;322:239.
41. Buckley NA, Dawson AH, Whyte IM, O'Connell DL. Relative toxicity of benzodiazepines in overdose. Br Med J 1995;310:219.
42. Meador KJ. Cognitive side effects of antiepileptic drugs. Can J Neurol Sci 1994;21:S12.
43. Shorr RI, Robin DW. Rational use of benzodiazepines in the elderly. Drugs Aging 1994;4:9.
44. McClure DJ, Walsh J, Chang H et al. Relative abuse liability of lorazepam and diazepam: an evaluation in 'recreational' drug users. J Clin Pharmacol 1988;28:52.
45. Strahan A, Rosenthal J, Kaswan M et al. Three case reports of acute paroxysmal excitement associated with alprazolam treatment. Am J Psychiatry 1985;142:859.

46. Rigby J, Harvey M, Davies DR. Mania precipitated by benzodiazepine withdrawal. Acta Psychiatr. Scand., 1989;79:406.
47. Gillin JC, Spinweber CL, Johnson LC. Rebound insomnia: a critical review. J. Clin. Psychopharmacol., 1989;9:161.
48. Brahams D. Iatrogenic crime: criminal behaviour in patients receiving drug treatment. Lancet 1987;1:874.
49. Dobson J Sedatives/hypnotics for abuse. NZ Med J 1989;102:651.
50. Bond A, Lader M. Differential effects of oxazepam and lorazepam on aggressive responding. Psychopharmacology 1988;95:369.
51. Patten SB, Love EJ. Neuropsychiatric adverse drug reactions: passive reports to Health and Welfare Canada's adverse drug reaction database (1965—present). Int J Psychiatry Med 1994;24:45.
52. Roberts K, Vass N. Schneiderian first-rank symptoms caused by benzodiazepine withdrawal. Br J Psychiatry 1986;148:593.
53. Bergman D. Futterweit W, Segal R et al. Increased oestradiol in diazepam-related gynaecomastia. Lancet 1981;2:1225.
54. Monchesky TC, Billings BJ, Phillips R. Zopiclone: a new nonbenzodiazepine hypnotic used in general practice. Clin Ther 1986;8:283.
55. Newton RE, Marunycz JD, Alderdice MT et al. Review of the side-effect profile of buspirone. Am J Med 1986;80:17.
56. Bigby M, Jick S, Jick H et al. Drug-induced cutaneous reactions. J Am Med Assoc 1986;256:3358.
57. Shen WW, Sata LS. Inhibited female orgasm resulting from psychotropic drugs. A five-year, updated, clinical review. J Reprod Med 1990;35:11.
58. Ghadirian A-M, Annable L, Belanger M-C. Lithium, benzodiazepines and sexual function in bipolar patients. Am J Psychiatry 1992;149:801.
59. Lader M, Morton S. Benzodiazepine problems. Br J Addict 1991;86:823.
60. Miller NS, Gold MS. Benzodiazepines: tolerance, dependence, abuse, and addiction. J Psychoact Drugs 1990;22:23.
61. Olajide D, Lader M. Depression following withdrawal from long-term benzodiazepine use: a report of four cases Psychol Med 1984;14:937.
62. Ashton H. Disorders of the foetus and infant In: Davies D.M. (Ed.), Textbook of Adverse Drug Reactions, 3rd ed. Oxford: Oxford University Press, 1985;77.
63. Rosenberg L, Mitchell AA, Parsells JL et al. Lack of relation of oral clefts to diazepam use during pregnancy. N Engl J Med 1983;309:1282.
64. Laegreid L, Olegard R, Wahlstrom J et al. Abnormalities in children exposed to benzodiazepines in utero. Lancet 1987;1:108.
65. Thadani PV. Biological mechanisms and perinatal exposure to abused drugs. Synapse 1995;19:228.
66. Boutroy MJ. Drug-induced apnea. Biol Neonate 1994;65:252.
67. Spigset O. Anaesthetic agents and excretion in breast milk. Acta Anaesthesiol Scand 1994;38:94.
68. Pons G, Rey E, Matheson I. Excretion of psychoactive drugs into breast milk. Pharmacokinetic principles and recommendations. Clin Pharmacokinet 1994;27:270.
69. Matheson I, Lunde PKM, Bredesen JE. Midazolam and nitrazepam in the maternity ward: milk concentrations and clinical effects. Br J Clin Pharmacol 1990;30:787.
70. Hollister LE. Interactions between alcohol and benzodiazepines. Recent Dev Alcohol 1990;8:233.
71. Johnson LC, Spinweber CL, Gomez SA et al. Daytime sleepiness, performance, mood, nocturnal sleep: the effect of benzodiazepine and caffeine on their relationship. Sleep 1990;13:121.
72. Johnson LC, Spinweber CL, Gomez SA. Benzodiazepines and caffeine: effect on daytime sleepiness, performance, and mood Psychopharmacology, 1990;101:160.
73. O'Donovan MC, McGuffin P. Short acting benzodiazepines—dream drugs or nightmare? Br Med J 1993;306:945.
74. Dyer C. Halcion edges its way back into Britain in low doses. Br Med J 1993;306:1085.
75. Ansseau M, Devoitille J-M, Papart P, Vanbrabant E, Mantanus H. Comparison of adinazolam, amitriptyline and diazepam. J Clin Psychopharmacol 1991;11:160.
76. Andersch S, Rosenburg NK, Kullingsjo H et al. Efficacy and safety of alprazolam, imipramine and placebo in treating panic disorder. A Scandinavian multicenter study. Acta Psychiatr Scand 1991; Suppl. 365:18.
77. O'Sullivan GH, Noshivani H, Basoglu M, Marks IM, Swinson R et al. Safety and side-effects of alprazolam. Controlled study in agoraphobia with panic disorder. Br J Psychiatry 1994;165:79.
78. Mortola JF. A risk-benefit appraisal of drugs used in the management of premenstrual syndrome. Drug Safety 1994;10:160.
79. Reddy S, Patt RB. The benzodiazepines as adjuvant analgesics. J Pain Symptom Management 1994;9:510.
80. Rosenbaum JF. Switching patients from alprazolam to clonazepam. Hosp Community Psychiatry 1990;41:1302.
81. Gardner DL, Cowdry RW. Alprazolam-induced dyscontrol in borderline personality disorder. Am J Psychiatry 1985;142:98.
82. Linnoila M, Stapleton JM, Lister R et al. Effects of single doses of alprazolam and diazepam, alone and in combination with ethanol, on psychomotor and cognitive performance and on autonomic nervous system reactivity in healthy volunteers. Eur J Clin Pharmacol 1990;39:21.
83. Remy C. Clobazam in the treatment of epilepsy: a review of the literature. Epilepsia 1994;35(Suppl 5):S88.
84. Grahnen A, Wennerlund P, Dahlstrom B et al. Inter- and intraindividual variability in the concentration — effect (sedation) relationship of flunitrazepam. Br J Clin Pharmacol 1991;31:89.
85. Curran HV, Schiwy W, Lader M. Differential amnesic properties of benzodiazepines: a dose-response com- parison of two drugs with similar elimination half-lives. Psychopharmacology 1987;92:358.
86. Romach M, Busto U, Somer G, Kaplan HL, Sellers E. Clinical aspects of chronic use of alprazolam and lorazepam. Am J Psychiatry 1995;152:1161.
87. Parent JM, Lowenstein DH. Treatment of refractory generalized status epilepticus with continuous infusion of midazolam. Neurology 1994;44:1837.
88. Lauven PM. Pharmacology of drugs for conscious sedation. Scand J Gastroenterol Suppl 1990;179:1.
89. Hughes J, Gill A, Leach HJ, Nunn AJ, Billingham I et al. A prospective study of the adverse effects of midazolam on withdrawal in critically ill children. Acta Paediatr 83, (1994)1194.
90. Schneider PJ, Perry PJ. Triazolam — an 'abused drug' by the lay press? Drug Intell Clin Pharm 1990;24:389.

91. Bixler EO, Kales A, Manfredi RL et al. Next-day memory inpairment with triazolam use. Lancet 1991;337:827.
92. Menkes DB. Triazolam-induced nocturnal bingeing with amnesia. Aust NZ J Psychiatry 1992;26:320.
93. Soldatos CR, Sakkas PN, Bergiannaki JD et al. Behavioral side effects of triazolam in psychiatric inpatients: report of five cases. Drug Intell Clin Pharm 1986;20:294.
94. Langtry HD, Benfield P. Zolpidem. A review of its pharmacodynamic and pharmacokinetic properties and therapeutic potential. Drugs 1990;40:291.
95. Declerck AC. Is 'poor sleep' too vague a concept for rational treatment? J Int Med Res 1994;22:1.
96. Rosenberg J, Ahlstrom F. Randomized, double blind trial of zolpidem 10 mg versus triazolam 0.25 mg for treatment of insomnia in general practice. Scand J Primary Health Care 1994;12:88.
97. Lheureux P, Debailleul G, DeWitte O, Askenasi R. Zolpidem intoxication mimicking narcotic overdose: Response to flumazenil. Hum Exp Toxicol 1990;9:105.
98. Zivkovic B, Morel E, Joly D et al. Pharmacological and behavioral profile of alpidem as an anxiolytic. Pharmacopsychiatry 1990;3:108.
99. Li S, Wang C. A comparative study of imovane and estazolam treatment on sleep disturbances. Chinese Med Sci J 1995;10:56.
100. Goa KL, Heel RC. Zopiclone. A review of its pharmacodynamic and pharmacokinetic properties and therapeutic efficacy as an hypnotic. Drugs 1986;32:48.
101. Mahendran R, Chee KT, Peh LH, Wong KE, Lin L. A postmarketing surveillance study of zopiclone in insomnia. Singapore Med J 1994;35:390.
102. Roschke J, Mann K, Aldenhoff JB, Benkert O. Functional properties of the brain during sleep under subchronic zopiclone administration in man. Eur Neuropsychopharmacol 1994;4:21.
103. Brogden RN, Goa KL. Flumazenil: a reappraisal of its pharmacological properties and therapeutic efficacy as a benzodiazepine antagonist. Drugs 1991;42:1061.
104. Richard P, Autret E, Bardol J et al. The use of flumazenil in a neonate. J Toxicol Clin Toxicol 1991;29:137.
105. Cone AM, Stott SA. Flumazenil. Br J Hosp Med 1994; 51:346.
106. Geller E. Halpern P. Benzodiazepine antagonists and inverse agonists. Curr Opin Anaesthesiol 1990;3:568.
107. Curran HV, Birch B. Differentiating the sedative, psychomotor and amnesic effects of benzodiazepines: a study with midazolam and the benzodiazepine antagonist, flumazenil. Psychopharmacology 1991;103:519.
108. Nishikawa T, Suzuki S, Ohtani H, Eizawa NW, Sugiyama T et al. Benzodiazepine concentrations in sera determined by radioreceptor assay for therapeutic-dose recipients (published erratum appears in Am J Clin Pathol 1995;103(3):376). Am J Clin Pathol 1994;102:605.
109. Rickels K, Amsterdam J, Clary C et al. Buspirone in depressed outpatients: a controlled study. Psychopharmacol Bull 1990;26:163.
110. Menkes DB. Buspirone augmentation of sertraline. Br J Psychiatry 1995;166:823.
111. Joffe RT, Schuller DR. An open study of buspirone augmentation of serotonin reuptake inhibitors in refractory depression. J Clin Psychiatry 1993;54:269.
112. Stanislav SS, Fabre T, Crimson ML, Childs A. Buspirone's efficacy in organic-induced aggression. J Clin Psychopharmacol 1994;14:126.
113. Napoliello MJ, Domantay AG. Buspirone: a worldwide update. Br J Psychiatry 1991;159(Suppl 12):40.
114. Alford C, Bhatti JZ, Curran S et al. Pharmacodynamic effects of buspirone and clobazam. Br J Clin Pharmacol 1991;32:91.
115. Escande M, Frexinos M, Fabre S. (A new generation of tranquilizing agents). Rev Praticien 1994;44:2316.
116. Steinberg JR. Anxiety in elderly patients. A comparison of azapirones and benzodiazepines. Drugs Aging 1994;5:335.
117. Weiss KJ. Management of anxiety and depression syndromes in the elderly. J Clin Psychiatry 1994;55(Suppl):5.
118. Rapoport DM, Greenberg HE, Goldring RM. Differing effects of the anxiolytic agents buspirone and diazepam on control of breathing. Clin Pharmacol Ther 1991;49:394.
119. Craven J, Sutherland A. Buspirone for anxiety disorders in patients with severe lung disease. Lancet 1991;338:249.
120. Fox BE, O'Brien CO, Kangas KJ et al. Use of high dose chloral hydrate for ophthalmic exams in children: a retrospective review of 302 cases. J Pediatr Ophthalmol Strabismus 1990;27:242.
121. Buckley NA, Whyte IM, Dawson AH, McManus PR, Ferguson NW. Correlations between prescriptions and drugs taken in self-poisoning. Implications for prescribers and drug regulation (see comments). Med J Aust 1995;162:194.
122. Lambert GH, Muraskas J, Anderson CL et al. Direct hyperbilirubinemia associated with chloral hydrate administration in the newborn. Pediatrics 1990;86:277.
123. Bayer AJ, Bayer EM, Pathy MS et al. A doubleblind controlled study of chlormethiazole and triazolam as hypnotics in the elderly. Acta Psychiatr Scand Suppl 1986;329:104.
124. Fagan D, Lamount M, Jostell KG et al. A study of the psychometric effects of chlormethiazole in healthy young and elderly subjects. Age Ageing 1990;19:395.
125. Idzikowski C, Mills FJ, James RJ. A dose-response study examining the effects of ritanserin on human slow wave sleep. Br J Clin Pharmacol 1991;31:193.
126. Adam K, Oswald I. Effects of repeated ritanserin on middle-aged poor sleepers. Psychopharmacology 1989;99:219.
127. Peters DH, Faulds D. Tiapride. A review of its pharmacology and therapeutic potential in the management of alcohol dependence syndrome. Drugs 1994;47:1010.
128. Settle EC, Ayd FJ. Trimipramine: twenty years' worldwide clinical experience. J Clin Psychiatry 1980;41:266.
129. Dunleavy DLF, Brezinova V, Oswald I et al. Changes during weeks in effects of tricyclic drugs on the human sleeping brain. Br J Psychiatry 1972;120:663.
130. Hohagen F, Montero RF, Weiss E, Lis S, Schonbrunn E et al. Treatment of primary insomnia with trimipramine: an alternative to benzodiazepine hypnotics? Eur Arch Psychiatry Clin Neurosci 1994;244:65.
131. Menkes DB. Antidepressant drugs. New Ethicals 1994;31:101.
132. Macleod AD. Vigabatrin and post-traumatic stress disorder. J Clin Psychopharmacol 1995;in press.
133. McIvor RJ, Turner SW. Drug treatment in post-traumatic stress disorder. Br J Hosp Med 1995;53:501.
134. British National Formulary, 30th edition. London: British Medical Association, 1995;204.
135. Feucht M, Brantner-Inthaler S. Gamma-vinyl-GABA (vigabatrin) in the therapy of Lennox-Gastaut syndrome: an open study. Epilepsia 1994;35:993.

Meyler's Side Effects of Drugs, 13th Edition
M.N.G. Dukes, editor

SECTION EDITOR: M.N.G. DUKES

George M. Simpson, Edmond H. Pi and John J. Sramek, Jr.

6 Neuroleptics and antipsychotics

INTRODUCTION

Since the introduction of chlorpromazine in the early 1950s, a large number of phenothiazines with antipsychotic properties have been discovered. A variety of other chemical structures with similar therapeutic properties have also been introduced. All these drugs have the capacity to relieve psychotic symptoms and they have profoundly benefitted psychiatry. The range of usefulness of these agents includes the treatment of schizophrenia, mania, certain organic psychoses, certain depressive states, and a variety of lesser indications. In schizophrenia, they are used not only to treat acute episodes, but also for long-term maintenance treatment.

These drugs also have a distinct pattern of side effects, some of them severe; the latter are, in part, due to the effect which these drugs—with the partial exception of 'atypical' neuroleptics such as clozapine—have on the extrapyramidal system. No systematic reporting and evaluating system for documenting their side effects has evolved. Even the recognition of a side effect may be difficult in an individual case: e.g., akathisia may be difficult to differentiate from an exacerbation of the illness and often has a deleterious effect on compliance (1[R]), Thus, the true incidence of side effects or unwanted effects is not available, and it is often uncertain to what extent one drug differs from another in this respect.

There have been many shifts of view on the correct dosage to be employed, and no simple rules can be given. For example, some adverse reactions are more prone to occur at high or more prolonged doses, yet once they have been established, certain of them may, within limits, be aggravated by lowering the dose and alleviated by raising it. In one double-blind study, newly admitted schizophrenic patients were randomly given 10, 30 or 80 mg/day of oral haloperidol. Survival analysis showed no differences among the three groups, nor were there any differences in the extrapyramidal syndrome (EPS) between the groups. Another study comparing 10, 20 and 30 mg of oral fluphenazine found no differences in outcome, but a dose-related EPS effect (154). These findings throw into profile the very important clinical issue of whether higher dosages of antipsychotics provide any additional beneficial effect in the treatment of acute or exacerbated schizophrenia, and whether such doses are really more prone to produce EPS (as commonly believed) or not. More recent opinion would be that high doses are no more beneficial and cause more side effects (2[Cr]).

The wide range of dosage used, not only in different conditions, but also within the same condition, may be related to the large inter-individual differences in plasma levels. Despite much research in the last decade, consistent relationships between plasma levels of neuroleptics (including their metabolites) and therapeutic effects have not been demonstrated. The relationship between unwanted effects and plasma levels remains indistinct. A relationship between plasma and CSF levels and extrapyramidal side effects has been claimed (SED-11, 105). Behavioral worsening on high-dose neuroleptics is a well-recognized clinical phenomenon (3[c], 4[c]). This has also been described in patients with very high plasma levels of neuroleptics (5[C]), Convulsions have also been described in association with very high circulating levels of clozapine (6[c]), While there are no clear indications at the present time for routine monitoring of plasma levels, such measurement may be helpful in evaluating and managing treatment failures or dealing with unusual or severe side effects. The entire problem of finding for the individual patient a dosage which balances safety against efficacy is likely in this field to center on the issue of avoiding severe neurological problems such as tardive dyskinesia; the dosage question is therefore further discussed in the neurological section of the monograph which follows.

CHOICE OF NEUROLEPTIC

In controlled studies, all current neuroleptics have been shown to be similar in therapeutic efficacy, provided they are used in truly equivalent doses. Occasional differences may relate to the methodology of the studies, e.g. diagnoses, difficulties of arriving at equivalent dosages in early studies of new drugs, etc. Drugs such as promazine are much less potent on a milligram basis and less efficacious perhaps because of side effects which may well prevent the prescription of equivalent therapeutic dosages. The choice of a drug, therefore, depends on other factors, namely the side-effect profile of the drug, the clinical characteristics of the patients, and perhaps the desired route of administration. If rapid treatment is necessary, a drug which has a parenteral form will be required. In other situations, an oral liquid may be deemed necessary; in situations where compliance is a problem, oral long-acting agents such as penfluridol can be given at weekly intervals under appropriate supervision. Otherwise, parenteral long-acting agents such as fluphenazine decanoate may be given at more extended intervals.

From a therapeutic point of view, all neuroleptics are equal; no single drug or chemical class appears to be superior to another. While there is a good rationale for using 'more sedative' drugs for treating excited patients, there has nonetheless been a tendency of late to use more potent drugs which can be administered parenterally in higher dosages. A rationale for using more than one neuroleptic in certain situations perhaps exists, but data to support this are lacking. In younger excited males who are vulnerable to acute dystonic reactions, the use of more sedative agents such as chlorpromazine or thioridazine that are less likely to produce extrapyramidal side effects (particularly acute dystonic reactions) may have merit. At the other end of the scale, patients who are elderly or vulnerable to cardiac arrhythmias may do better on low dosages of more potent neuroleptics such as haloperidol, fluphenazine and thiothixene. Low-potency agents have a side-effect profile characterized by sedation and multiple peripheral effects, most notably anticholinergic (blurred vision, constipation, ejaculatory disturbance), cardiovascular (hypotension, arrhythmias) and endocrine (weight gain, sexual dysfunction). In a hot, sunny climate, one might recommend not to use chlorpromazine because of increased problems of photosensitivity. While high-potency drugs have minimal peripheral effects, they cause more CNS effects such as extrapyramidal side effects and behavioral changes.

In general, one selects an agent according to the clinical condition of the patient, prior response to a specific agent (if known), compliance, the patient's age and physical status and the side effects that would be more or less acceptable in individual subjects. The adage that one should not dismiss older drugs simply because they are old is very applicable here; neuroleptics, which have been available for a long time, may be a better choice for routine use because their properties and risks are best defined. They may also be preferable for use in specialized cases, e.g. pregnancy, than drugs about which we still know less. Every clinician using drugs of this type should be familiar with several different neuroleptics that have between them a spectrum of side effects and potencies, so that he can select and modify his treatment. Even if 'atypical' neuroleptics like clozapine become widely available and practical to use, it is unlikely that this spectrum of variation will expand very much, or that one new drug will become dominant; alternative drugs will continue to be necessary. An awareness of the side effect profile of individual neuroleptics will continue to be a major determining factor in the choice of an antipsychotic agent. Clozapine possesses certain advantages over typical neuroleptics. It has been found to be particularly efficacious in the treatment of negative symptoms of schizophrenia and has significant therapeutic effects in treatment-resistant patients, both on positive and negative symptoms. Clozapine does not produce extrapyramidal side effects and improves and may prevent tardive dyskinesia (155[R]).

Risperidone has been found efficacious on both positive and negative symptoms and has a reduced risk for extrapyramidal side effects (156[C]). A clear relationship between dose and extrapyramidal side effects was reported (157[C]). Comprehensive reviews of specific antipsychotics including clozapine, raclopride, remoxipride, risperidone and zotepine have been provided in earlier volumes (SEDA-16, 55; SEDA-17, 58; SEDA-18, 52). If the superiority of atypical neuroleptics is persistently demonstrated and the side effect profile is advantageous, then it is possible that in the future, choice of agents will be between one atypical and another.

The neuroleptics and antipsychotics

In the present Chapter, information on all neuroleptic drugs will be dealt with in a single monograph; the limited variations between the alternative drugs in the class will be dealt with in the appropriate subsections of the monograph.

ADVERSE REACTION PATTERN

General and toxic reactions Neuroleptics can produce a variety of adverse effects in several organ systems. Extrapyramidal reactions and sedation are routinely encountered nervous system side effects; less frequently observed are seizures, unwanted behavioral effects, and tardive dyskinesia. Most neuroleptics exert anticholinergic effects and commonly produce dry mouth, blurred vision and constipation. Postural hypotension is described as a common side effect. These effects usually disappear when a neuroleptic is stopped or dosage is reduced.

Non-specific, usually reversible, ECG changes have been reported, but their relationship to myocardial toxicity has not been confirmed. Sudden death related to cardiac arrest cannot be fully explained on the basis of the administration of neuroleptics. Weight gain is a common side effect of neuroleptics. Breast engorgement and galactorrhea may occur in females and even in males on neuroleptics. Amenorrhea, gynecomastia, hyperglycemia, hypoglycemia, elevation of growth hormone, inappropriate ADH secretion and disturbance of sex hormones have been reliably documented although they remain unusual.

Hypersensitivity reactions Neuroleptics infrequently produce allergic reactions. There are no known reports of anaphylactic reactions with these agents, but various skin reactions, e.g. rashes, photosensitivity and dermatitis, may be viewed as delayed forms of hypersensitivity. Jaundice and blood dyscrasias hemolytic anemia, agranulocytosis) are rare and may represent types allergic reactions.

Tumor-inducing effects Since neuroleptics elevate prolactin levels, there is concern that this may increase the risk of development of breast cancer. Although studies have failed to implicate an association, it would be best to avoid neuroleptics in a patient with a hormone-dependent breast tumor.

ORGANS AND SYSTEMS

Cardiovascular *Hypotension* is the most commonly observed cardiovascular side effect of antipsychotics, particularly following administration of those which are also potent α-adrenergic receptor blockers such as chlorpromazine, thioridazine and clozapine. A central mechanism involving the vasomotor regulatory center may also contribute to the lowering of blood pressure. Antipsychotics of high and intermediate potency such as haloperidol and loxitane have minimal alpha-blocking effects and would be less apt to cause such changes, although in one report, orthostatic changes (30 mmHg decrease) were reported with these drugs in 27 and 22% of cases, respectively (SED-11, 106). An exception to the relatively safe use of high-potency agents has been noted in the combination of droperidol with the narcotic fentanyl which may cause marked hypotension (7[C]). Orthostatic hypotension and syncope have been reported following initiation of clozapine therapy (158[C]).

Hypotensive episodes often arise following postural changes and may, therefore, be particularly hazardous in susceptible patients such as the elderly and in those with depleted intravascular volume or compromised cardiovascular output. The risk of orthostatic hypotension is markedly increased following parenteral administration. The combination of α-adrenergic receptor blockade and sedative effects may explain the increased risk of falling and suffering hip fractures when taking antipsychotics (SEDA-12, 52).

Antipsychotics may *increase resting and exercise heart rates* as a consequence of their vagolytic activity, but bradycardia is unusual. Reduction in exercise-induced cardiac output may be seen as a result of drug-induced increases in plasma levels of catecholamines and concurrent α-adrenergic receptor blockade (8[C]).

ECG changes are relatively common during treatment with antipsychotics, but there is a lack of unanimity regarding the clinical significance of these findings. Those ECG changes generally considered benign and non-specific are reversible after discontinuation of treatment. Potentially more serious changes include increased QT intervals, depressed ST segments, flattened T-waves and appearance of U-waves. Non-specific T-wave changes may be more commonly seen during the mid-afternoon, and may be related to the potassium shift and other changes which result after food and glucose ingestion, so that a pre-breakfast ECG may be more desirable. Two types of T-wave changes have been characterized following treatment with thioridazine: Type I (with rounded, levelled or notched T-waves), and Type II (with diphasic waves) (9[C]), Increases in the QT interval are most commonly seen with thioridazine and represent delayed ventricular repolarization (quinidine-like effects) and have spurred the investigation of these agents for their antiarrhythmic activity (SEDA-5, 42). However, *cardiac arrhythmias* have been reported and include atrial arrhythmias, ventricular tachycardia and fibrillation. Several cases of torsade de pointes arrhythmia have been reported in association with thioridazine (10[C], 11[C]). While the risk of cardiac arrhythmias appears to be dose-related, one should remember that the risk may be increased by pre-existing cardiovascular pathology (SEDA-2, 48), interactions with other cardiovascular or psychotropic medications (particularly the highly anticholinergic tricyclic antidepressants), the increased cardiac sensitivity of the elderly, hypokalemic states and vigorous exercise. In the elderly, it may be advisable to avoid low-potency neuroleptics such as thioridazine which produce significantly more ECG changes than do high-potency agents such as fluphenazine (12[C]). In any patient with pre-existing heart disease, a pre-treatment ECG with routine ECG follow-up is to be recommended.

The possibility that some of the cardiac effects of thioridazine and chlorpromazine may be related to metabolites as well as the parent compound has been explored (9[C], 13[r]) but needs further investigation.

The role of neuroleptics in the etiology of *sudden death* is controversial (SEDA-18, 47; 159[C]R). There may be multiple non-cardiac etiologies including asphyxia, convulsions or hyperpyrexia. However, some cases of sudden death in apparently young healthy individuals may be directly attributable to cardiac arrhythmias following treatment with thioridazine or chlorpromazine (14[R]); there have also been reports on parenteral and high-dose haloperidol which implicate a cardiotoxic mechanism (SED-11, 107) and this may also hold true for any other neuroleptic used in a similar manner. One case of asystolic cardiac arrest was reported following intravenous administration of haloperidol (15[c]). Also, four cases of torsade de pointes have been reported with intravenous haloperidol used with lorazepam to treat delirium (SEDA-18, 47; 160[c]). One report reviews the possibility of acid mucopolysaccharide deposition associated with antipsychotic treatment as a possible mechanism contributing to rare cardiovascular adverse events (SED-11, 107).

Respiratory The *gag and cough reflexes* may be suppressed by neuroleptics (SED-11, 107). Periodic examination of the gag reflex, particularly in patients with tardive dyskinesia has been recommended. Acute *respiratory failure* which may be complicated by pneumonia has been reported in psychiatric patients receiving long-term neuroleptic treatment (SED-11, 107). In addition, *pulmonary embolism* without a primary focus was surprisingly frequent among cases of sudden death. *Aspiration asphyxia* in patients treated with neuroleptics has been described (SED-11, 107) and it has been suggested that this could have been due to laryngeal-pharyngeal dystonia (16[c]).

A single case of fatal *pulmonary edema* was reported in 1982 in association with haloperidol use (17[c]). Diaphragmatic, laryngeal and glottal dyskinesias have been described as part of the tardive dyskinesia syndrome and may cause respiratory complications (18[c], 19[c]).

Nervous system *Behavioral side effects* Oversedation and/or drowsiness is the most common side effect of neuroleptic administration. Most patients develop tolerance to this effect. In addition, neuroleptics may cause a depression-like syndrome. This should be differentiated from neuroleptic-induced akinesia. Long-acting drugs have been particularly implicated (SED-11, 107; 20[R]). However, double-blind randomized investigation comparing depressive symptoms related to the use of a placebo with the continued use of long-acting neuroleptics did not support this conclusion (21[C]).

Toxic delirium caused by neuroleptics with potent anticholinergic properties has been widely reported (SED-11, 107). Physostigmine can alleviate these toxic symptoms and is a useful diagnostic procedure. Other uncommon behavioral effects include psychotic exacerbation, catatonia-like states and Klüver-Bucy-like syndrome (SED-9, 81; SEDA-7, 67; 20[R]).

The extent to which neuroleptics *impair mental activity* is disputed. A recent study showed that the more anticholinergic antipsychotic agents impaired short-term verbal memory (SEDA-18, 48; 161[CR]). One study actually reported that schizophrenic patients who ingested neuroleptics showed superior information-processing as compared with unmedicated schizophrenic patients; the authors claimed that neuroleptics probably do not cause, and may actually reverse, slowness of information-processing in schizophrenic patients (22[c]). However, a substantial number of schizophrenic patients declare that neuroleptics slow their thinking, cause them to forget, and take away interest and motivation. These responses to neuroleptics are claimed to be dysphoric and often are associated with drug-induced extrapyramidal symptoms, particularly akathisia (23[C]). Akinesia may also contribute to feelings of apathy and diminished spontaneity, and can be difficult to distinguish from the negative symptoms of schizophrenia or the psychomotor retardation of post-psychotic depression (24[C]).

Effects on the convulsive threshold Neuroleptics cause slowing of alpha-rhythm, increased synchronization and amplitude with superimposed sharp fast activity. They also induce discharge patterns in the EEG similar to those associated with epileptic seizure disorders, of the grand mal or focal types (SED-11, 108). The incidence of convulsion associated with typical neuroleptic administration is relatively rare (probably less than 1%) (SED-9, 81).

Predisposing factors to neuroleptic-induced seizures include abnormal EEG, pre-existing CNS abnormalities, parenteral administration of high doses of neuroleptics, and a family history of seizure or febrile convulsions (25[r]).

It has been suggested that the less potent sedative neuroleptics (aliphatic or piperidine phenothiazines) lower the convulsive threshold more than do the potent neuroleptics (piperazine phenothiazines) (26[C]). However, variable and unpredictable effects on seizure activity related to butyrophenone usage in man have been reported recently (27[c]). The reported prevalence of seizures with clozapine is apparently higher than the average, approximately 5%, and is dose-dependent. A recent report described four patients who developed seizure activity while taking therapeutic or subtherapeutic doses of this drug (28[Cr]). An in vitro technique, claimed to assess the relative risks for neuroleptic-induced seizures, was reported to produce striking differences between neuroleptics in spike activity in hippocampal slices. Tentatively, molindone, pimozide and butaclamol appeared to be the safest compounds in vitro (29[C]). Data generated from a well-designed in vivo study are needed before any conclusion can be drawn.

Extrapyramidal side effects can be classified into four main groups, i.e. acute dystonic reactions, akathisia, (pseudo)parkinsonism and tardive dyskinesia. In addition, there are a series of less common tardive conditions which will be discussed later in this section. Except for tardive dyskinesia the extrapyramidal side effects are, in large part, reversible by prescribing anticholinergic agents and discontinuing or lowering the dose of the neuroleptics. These effects have been well reviewed much earlier in this series and elsewhere (SED-9, 78; SEDA-7, 61; SEDA-16, 40; SEDA-18, 48; 20[R]). Several studies have found a relationship between the neuroleptic dosages, extrapyramidal side effects, and the degree of D_2 receptor occupancy (SEDA-18, 48; 162[Cr], 163[CR]).

(*a*) *Acute dystonic reactions* These are dramatic, acute-onset muscular spasms that take place within the first 24—48 hours after starting therapy, or in a few cases when the dosage is increased. The muscles of the head and neck are mainly affected: opisthotonos, torticollis, oculogyric crisis and macroglossia (all of which may be seen together) are dramatic effects relieved by the use of intramuscular antiparkinsonian or antihistaminic drugs. Acute laryngeal dystonia is probably an under-reported yet potentially lethal side effect. A recent comprehensive review strongly advocates immediate intravenous administration of anticholinergic drugs to relieve acute dystonia. Males are more prone than females to this reaction, and the young more so than the elderly (30[R]). Drug-induced dystonia can also be precipitated by emotional arousal (31[C], 164[C]).

(*b*) *Akathisia* This is a variant of the restless legs syndrome associated with anxiety and/or dysphoria; it may be confused with an exacerbation of the disorder undergoing treatment. Subjects show various degrees of restlessness, inability to sit or stand still; in severe cases, it may merge with behavioral disorders. Antiparkinsonian agents are sometimes helpful, beta-blockers are often more helpful.

(*c*) (*'Pseudo')parkinsonism* induced by these drugs is clinically indistinguishable from postencephalitic or classical parkinsonism. It begins in the head and neck region and produces a loss of movement in the muscles which spreads to the arms, producing varying degrees of akinesia and rigidity.

(*d*) *Tardive dyskinesia* Originally, tardive dyskinesia was described as comprising spontaneous irregular movements, mainly affecting the mouth and tongue; chewing, licking, smacking movements of the tongue and lips were involved including protrusion of the tongue outside the buccal cavity and various abnormal movements of the tongue within the buccal cavity. In addition to the above, this condition is now known to include choreoathetoid movements of the fingers and toes, sometimes associated with rocking movements, akathisia and, in other individuals, truncal muscles and respiratory muscles may be involved.

Tardive dyskinesia usually occurs after long-term usage of neuroleptics, but some cases of early onset (less than 1 year) have been reported (SED-11, 108). A prospective study reported that the cumulated incidence of tardive dyskinesia was 5% after 1 year, 10% after 2 years, 15% after 3 years, and 19% after 4 years. The authors suggested that the prevalence increases with increasing duration of neuroleptic exposure and that the increase is linear at least for the first 4—5 years of such exposure (32[Cr]). Recently, in one study, the average incidence rate of tardive dyskinesia was 0.053 per year and the 5-year risk was 20% (SEDA-18, 49; 165[CR]). In another study, cumulative incidence of tardive dyskinesia was 26, 52 and 60% after 1, 2 and 3 years, respectively, in patients over age 45 (166[CR]). The figures are nevertheless variable from center to center. A prevalence ranging from 0.5 to 65% has been reported in patients receiving neuroleptics (33[R]). One review goes so far as to suggest that the prevalence of tardive dyskinesia among all patients taking neuroleptics is so low as not to justify any alarm (34[r]). No cases of the severe form were found in a 12-year follow-up study of 99 chronically hospitalized patients who had received extensive neuroleptic treatment (35[c]). Absence of severe tardive dyskinesia was reported in a group of Hungarian schizophrenic outpatients (36[c]). Prevalence ranges from 8.4 to 20.6% were reported in other cross-cultural studies comparing different ethnic groups (37[R], 38[C], 39[c], 40[C]). This wide variation in prevalence is perhaps due to a lack of precise objective definition of the syndrome. The availability of standardized rating scales (41[CR]) and research diagnostic criteria represents a significant advance in resolving these problems (42[Cr]). A multinational study of tardive dyskinesia in Asians (N=982) found the overall prevalence of tardive dyskinesia was 17% (ranging from 8.2 to 22.1%). There was a significant difference in tardive dyskinesia prevalence among different sites with the same ethnic group. Reasons for such a difference remains unclear. At present there is little convincing evidence that interethnic differences in the prevalence of tardive dyskinesia truly exist (167[c], 168[CR]). The tongue protrusion test, i.e. inability to maintain tongue protrusion, was found to be a measure of severity, present mainly when tardive dyskinesia occurred in an advanced form; abnormal movements within the buccal cavity occurred over a much wider range of severity, suggesting that abnormal tongue movements may prove a more helpful sign for early detection of tardive dyskinesia (43[c]).

Considerable information, although not entirely consistent, is available regarding *predisposing factors* (SED-11, 108; 33[R], 44[R], 45[cr]). The condition is apparently more common in women and in the elderly; elderly females in particular seem prone to develop the condition in a relatively severe form (SED-11, 108; 33[R], 46[c]). It has been suggested that estrogen may play a role in the higher prevalence of tardive dyskinesia among females (47[c], 48[cr]). Here too, however, the epidemiology is challenged; not all studies confirm that females are more vulnerable to tardive dyskinesia (49[cr]), though the consensus would support this conclusion. The tardive dyskinesia incidence among patients with extrapyramidal syndromes (EPS) has been found markedly higher than that of a comparison group without EPS. Overall, the hazard rate for the EPS patients is 2.32-times that of the others, and the risk ratio could be even higher during the first 2 years of exposure (32[R]).

Whether certain neuroleptics are more prone than others to cause tardive dyskinesia remains unknown (44[R]), but virtually all currently prescribed neuroleptics, with possible exception of 'atypical' neuroleptics such as clozapine (169[Cr]) have been associated with it. A review of the literature did not support the notion that medications with central anticholinergic properties constitute a particular risk factor in tardive dyskinesia. However, antiparkinsonian medications of the anticholinergic type tend to produce reversible increases in the severity of dyskinetic movements and authors suggest that antiparkinsonian agents can be used as pharmacological probes in the evaluation of neuroleptic-induced movement disorders (36[C], 50[R], 51[c]); a history of drug-induced parkinsonism and tardive dyskinesia is sometimes strongly associated.

Prolonged treatment with neuroleptic drugs was found to increase the risk of tardive dyskinesia (49[cr]); this finding has been supported by the preliminary results of a prospective study of the condition but again one encounters inconsistent results (44[R], 45[cr]). One particular outpatient study reported that the duration of treatment with neuroleptics did not seem to explain the differences in severity of tardive dyskinesia (46[c]). A positive correlation between tardive dyskinesia and circulating neuroleptic concentrations has been reported (52[c]); however, in one study no significant difference in serum levels of thioridazine, its metabolites, or radio-receptor activity values was found between patients with and without tardive dyskinesia (53[c]). Histories of more and longer drug-free periods were found more commonly in moderate and severe tardive dyskinesia than in mild forms (54[C]). A positive association between neuroleptic-free periods and persistent tardive dyskinesia (55[r]) has been reported. Some studies have suggested that diabetes mellitus may be a risk factor for tardive dyskinesia (SEDA-16, 47; 170[CR]).

There are various other possible risk factors, e.g. organicity, affective disorder, history of electroconvulsive therapy or alcohol abuse, and individual susceptibility (56[R]).

There are insufficient data to support the use of drug holidays in detecting the risk of tardive dyskinesia, but they may help to diagnose the covert type by unmasking dyskinesia (44[R]).

The rate of *reversibility* of tardive dyskinesia following drug termination has been reported to range from 0 to 90% (33[R]). Since subjective complaints are rarely made by patients with tardive dyskinesia (57[C]), periodic assessment of dyskinetic movements is essential to make an early diagnosis and, furthermore, it may increase the opportunity to reverse the disorder. Some reports are relatively encouraging regarding reversibility (58[C], 59[C]); characteristics and both reversible and irreversible forms have been reviewed, but no firm conclusion can be drawn (60[R]). However, the prognosis of tardive dyskinesia was better for those patients treated for a smaller proportion of time during the follow-up period and for those treated with lower modal doses during follow-up (37[C]).

In dealing with the whole problem of dyskinesia the pre-eminent role of prevention must be emphasized (56[R]), particularly because the *treatment* is so unrewarding. Various agents for the treatment of tardive dyskinesia have been studied; they include agonists and antagonists of various CNS neurotransmitter systems, as well as a group of newer dopamine antagonists which supposedly act only at D_2-receptors (dopamine receptor sites not linked to adenylcyclase). The few supposedly-positive results which have been claimed for a number of drugs must be interpreted with great caution (SEDA-18, 49; 61[R]). Reserpine has been used with apparent improvement in symptoms, but deterioration followed withdrawal of the drug (62[C]), and reserpine has indeed also been reported to cause the condition. A double-blind study dating back to 1982 using propranolol in treating tardive dyskinesia showed short-term improvement and two of four subjects responded to long-term propranolol use (63[c]), but unfortunately this study has not been replicated. Tetrahydroisoxazolpyridinol (THIP), a new and less toxic analogue of γ-aminobutyric acid (GABA) which acts as a GABA antagonist, produced no change in tardive dyskinesia either in a dose-finding study or a 4-week placebo-controlled study, but pre-existing parkinsonism increased significantly and eye-blinking rates decreased (64[C]); again, these are preliminary findings more than a decade old and hard to interpret. More recently, vitamin E (α-tocopherol), with its antioxidant properties, has been reported efficacious in the treatment of tardive dyskinesia (65[Cr], 66[C]; SEDA-17, 56).

Many other *differential diagnoses* must be considered in evaluating tardive dyskinesia. Spontaneous dyskinesias are, for example, not rare; they were found in 5.8±1.0% of individuals in 18 population studies (SED-11, 109). Especially among elderly patients, even higher rates have been recorded; senile dyskinesias were reported in two studies of drug-free elderly subjects and found to be present in 9 and 37% of individuals, respectively (67[C], 68[C]). There is also evidence that dyskinetic movements can be a feature of severe chronic schizophrenia unmodified by neuroleptics (SED-11, 109; 69[C]), which could mean that neuroleptics may merely be triggering already latent dyskinesias in schizophrenic patients.

Tardive akathisia Akathisia, where it occurs, can be an early problem, appearing within days or weeks of initiation of therapy, but this is not necessarily the case. A 1986 review (70[R]) considered 24 cases of tardive akathisia seen over a long period; in three of these the condition had appeared after only 1 or 2 months of neuroleptic therapy but the remainder had been treated for at least 1 year; seven had been treated with neuroleptics for at least 5 years. Whereas tardive dyskinesia most often starts in the bucco-oral region, then extends to the fingers and occasionally to the lower limbs and trunk, tardive akathisia most often affects the lower extremities or is described as a generalized sensation throughout limbs and trunk. Moreover, while a decrease in medication will induce a temporary worsening of masked tardive dyskinesia and an increased dose an improvement, the effects of dose changes on akathisia are less certain.

Tardive Tourette's syndrome There have been at least seven published cases of Tourette's syndrome ascribed to antipsychotic drugs and emerging either during treatment or following cessation of therapy. Some authors believe that the tardive Tourette-like syndrome may be a subtype of the more frequent tardive dyskinesia, because it can be masked by an increase in neuroleptic administration and exacerbated by neuroleptic withdrawal. However, the type of symptoms described can readily be confused with exacerbation of the underlying psychosis; misdiagnosis of the condition, at least in some of the published case-reports, cannot be completely ruled out.

Tardive dystonia This is a rare, late-onset, persistent dystonia associated with neuroleptic treatment. Prevalence of this condition, which usually affects younger and male patients, is reported at 1—2% (71[C]). It tends to affect the muscles of the neck, shoulder girdle, and trunk causing opisthotonos. *Pisa syndrome* is a special form involving tonic flexion of the trunk to one side accompanied by slight backward rotation in the absence of other dystonic symptoms. Sometimes, patients with tardive dystonia can become incapacitated (72[r], 73[C]). Differential diagnoses include idiopathic torsion dystonia, parkinsonism idiopathic torticollis, Huntington's disease, Wilson's disease, and Meige's syndrome (blepharospasm, oro-mandibular dystonia). Anticholinergics, cholinergics, dopamine agonists, dopamine-depleting agents, dopamine blockers, beta-blockers, GABA agonists, benzodiazepines, carbamazepine, electroconvulsive therapy and thalamotomy have been used to treat this condition, but none has shown any definitive, consistent therapeutic effects (71,74). Clozapine would be particularly indicated for subjects who remain psychotic.

'Rabbit syndrome' is considered as a late-onset extrapyramidal side effect associated with antipsychotics. This syndrome is characterized by a rapid tremor of the lips and occasionally the jaw. The movements usually respond well to antiparkinsonian agents and discontinuation of antipsychotics. It has been suggested that the rabbit syndrome is the clinical 'opposite' of tardive dyskinesia (75[R]).

Low-dose maintenance treatment for schizophrenia The acceptability of neuroleptic medication, by both patient and doctor, may be limited by extrapyramidal and other side effects. If these are dose-related, using the lowest effective dose for maintenance treatment may minimize their risk (SEDA-17, 49). Unfortunately, there is little evidence available on how low a dose should be to prevent relapse. As a result, there may be a general tendency to administer higher doses than necessary. Kane et al. (76[c]) carried out a double-blind study comparing a group of stabilized outpatients taking a low dose of fluphenazine enanthate (1.25—5 mg every 2 weeks) with a group taking a standard dose (12.5—50 mg every 2 weeks). Relapse rates were higher in the low-dose group (56%) than in the standard-dose group

(7%). However, patients in the low-dose group had a better outcome in terms of some measures of psychosocial adjustment and family satisfaction. Patients in the low-dose group showed fewer signs of tardive dyskinesia, and relapses led less frequently to re-admission to hospital; they also responded more readily to treatment with temporary increases in medication than patients treated with standard doses. Later, Marder et al. (77[C]) compared a low (5 mg) with a standard (25 mg) dose of fluphenazine decanoate given every 2 weeks. One-year survival analysis disclosed that there were no statistically significant differences between the two doses in their ability to prevent relapse. Evaluation of the survival with each dose revealed no significant difference at one year, but significantly better survival was seen with the 25-mg dose (64%) than with the 5-mg dose (31%) at 2 years (171[CR]).

Kane (78[R]) has reviewed the dose-response relationships for a variety of side effects of antipsychotic drugs. Although the dose-response relationships for extrapyramidal effects are not fully understood, the available evidence does support, according to Kane, a dose effect. This relationship is probably not linear and may be influenced by a variety of factors, but it is reasonable to conclude that systematic attempts to use the lowest possible clinically effective dosage should be strongly encouraged. Kane speculates that it is possible that for patients vulnerable to the development of tardive dyskinesia, a dose-response relationship occurs at a relatively low cumulative or average daily dose, whereas for patients without underlying vulnerability, increasing doses beyond this range may not lead to substantial increases in the risk of tardive dyskinesia. Hyperprolactinemia is dose-related, but there is wide interindividual variability in the magnitude of this effect. The same applies to peripheral autonomic effects.

Since, in most patients, high doses do not lead to better therapeutic effects but are associated with more frequent and severe side effects, the use of the least amount of medication necessary to produce antipsychotic benefits is recommended. When sedation is required, the concurrent use of moderate doses of a neuroleptic with a benzodiazepine may be preferable to the use of high doses of a neuroleptic.

Myasthenia gravis induced by neuroleptics has been reported (SED-11, 110). such cases may be due to impairment of neuromuscular transmission induced by neuroleptics. Three cases of radial nerve palsy were reported in demented elderly patients confined to wheelchairs who were treated with haloperidol. The combination of extrapyramidal and sedative side effects, added to wheelchair confinement, may have resulted in pressure on the upper arm with subsequent neuropathy (79[C]).

Neuroleptic malignant syndrome (*'syndrome malin'*) The neuroleptic malignant syndrome is a rare but potentially fatal disorder characterized by muscular rigidity, hyperthermia, altered consciousness and autonomic dysfunction (80[R]). This description applies to most of the approximately 70 cases reported to date since 1960, but the syndrome is still poorly defined and overlaps to some extent with lethal catatonia, neuroleptic-induced hyperpyrexia and sudden death due to cardiac arrhythmias. Similar symptoms have also been reported in non-schizophrenic patients following exposure to dopamine-depleting drugs (81[C]) and after withdrawal of indirect dopamine agonists (82[C]), and no consensus has been attained as to the boundaries, etiology or management of the syndrome (SEDA-18, 50). The prevalence has been suggested as less than 1% (83[C]), but the precise frequency is unknown and a trend towards fewer reports in recent years suggests that other factors (such as the use of lower neuroleptic dosages) may come into play. There is no consistent evidence that one neuroleptic drug or class is more or less likely to produce neuroleptic malignant syndrome, and the disorder has been reported with clozapine (SEDA-12, 52; 84[C], 85[C], 172[C]). The highest risk of developing the syndrome appears to exist when neuroleptic treatment is initiated or when the dose is increased. The appearance of severe extrapyramidal dysfunctions, primarily rigidity, underlies the majority of case-reports, and may provide the key to understanding and preventing the syndrome. The appearance of severe rigidity may well explain the increased body temperature because of heat build-up by the muscles and it may well contribute to the elevation of serum CPK, reflecting a risk of myoglobinuria and acute renal failure. Increased temperature (hyperthermia) can lead to dehydration and electrolyte imbalance, leaving the patient at risk for infections and other medical consequences. Laboratory abnormalities may include elevated CPK and electrolyte abnormalities, but these are generally not diagnostic since they can be significantly elevated in other hyperthermic conditions. A 1986 review by Levinson and Simpson (86[R]) argues strongly that the neuroleptic malignant syndrome may represent a heterogeneous group of neuroleptic-induced extrapyramidal syndromes with concurrent fever, and it questions the existence of neuroleptic malignant syndrome as a unitary syndrome. The syndrome shares clinical features with the genetic-acquired malignant hyperthermia, but there does not appear to be a common peripheral pathophysiological link between the two (SED-11, 111). The neuroleptic-induced syndrome is reported most often in young males, may appear suddenly days to weeks after initiating or intensifying drug therapy, and usually lasts 5—10 days after its discontinuation. Relatively more cases have been associated with high-potency antipsychotics, and the course of the syndrome may be particularly prolonged and difficult to treat when depot forms of these drugs have been used.

Early recognition and prompt treatment of this severe extrapyramidal syndrome, in particular an immediate recognition of new rigidity, may be the best means of arresting its progress and preventing further complications. If the condition is accompanied by fever, the clinician must naturally evaluate the patient for other possible causes of fever such as viral infection and for associated symptoms suggesting such alternatives; there should, however, be no delay in instituting appropriate treatment of severe extrapyramidal syndrome and in particular anticholinergic treatment of severe parkinsonian rigidity. There is no proven, specific treatment at the present time, but immediate discontinuation of antipsychotics is essential, followed by supportive therapy and intensive monitoring of respiratory, renal and cardiac function. Anticholinergic agents are often used, but where fever exceeds a temperature of 101°F, anticholinergics may exacerbate fever and other treatments might then be preferred. It should be remembered that the simultaneous withdrawal of antipsychotic and anticholinergic agents can produce a worsening of EPS and that anticholinergics, if possible, should be continued for one week after the cessation of the antipsychotic. Amantadine (87[c]), dantrolene sodium (88[C], 89[C]) and bromocriptine (90[C]) have been successful as empiric therapy in isolated case-reports, but need further experience and investigation before their effectiveness can be properly assessed. In the present view, dopamine agonists are preferred when the temperature exceeds 101—103°F, and muscle contraction can be further alleviated with dantrolene or benzodiazepines. Following resolution of symptoms, neuroleptics can be reintroduced safely in a majority of patients (91[C]). In all cases the lowest effective dose of neuroleptic should be used, along with anticholinergic therapy or the use of thioridazine with its inherent anticholinergic effects. Comprehensive reviews of neuroleptic malignant syndrome have been provided earlier in these volumes (SEDA-11, 47; SEDA-14, 50).

Endocrine, metabolic *Weight gain* is a common side effect of neuroleptics, produced more frequently by low-potency agents, e.g. chlorpromazine, thioridazine and clozapine, than by those of high potency, e.g. haloperidol and fluphenazine. The mechanism involved is poorly understood (SED-11, 111). Reduction of weight has been observed after discontinuation of neuroleptic treatment (92[C]).

Temperature regulation Antipsychotics interfere with the temperature regulatory function of the hypothalamus, and also peripherally with the sweating mechanism, resulting in poikilothermy. This can result in either hyperthermia or hypothermia, depending on environmental temperature. Clozapine often causes a benign and transient increase in body temperature early in treatment.

Neuroendocrine effects of neuroleptics include elevated growth hormone, inappropriate ADH and prolactin secretion, and disturbance of sex hormones (SED-11, 111). Galactorrhea and gynecomastia may be caused by the elevation of prolactin induced by neuroleptics. A correlation between serum levels of neuroleptics and prolactin has been claimed (93[c], 94[c]), but this is not linear at all ranges. No further elevation of plasma prolactin level could be observed with higher dosages of haloperidol (>100 mg/day). This was explained as being related to saturation of the pituitary dopamine receptors by a modest amount of haloperidol (94[c]). A low prolactin level during maintenance neuroleptic treatment predicted relapse after neuroleptic withdrawal and it was suggested that serum prolactin level may be helpful in monitoring drug treatment (95[c]). Hirsutism, amenorrhea and a false-positive pregnancy test associated with neuroleptic treatment were also reported (SED-11, 111; 173[C]).

There is concern that neuroleptics may increase the risk of breast cancer because of elevated prolactin levels. For a long period, findings did not confirm this association (96[C]), but a recent Danish cohort study of 6152 patients found a slight increase in the risk of breast cancer among schizophrenic women (97[C]).

Sexual dysfunction Neuroleptic-induced sexual dysfunctions including erectile and ejaculatory dysfunctions as well as changes in the quality of orgasm and in libido appear to be benign and reversible with cessation of neuroleptic therapy. Priapism, although infrequent, necessitates prompt urological consultation and sometimes even surgical intervention (98[r]). Although the mechanism involved in neuroleptic-induced male sexual dysfunction is not entirely understood, it may be at several different levels including the cortex, hypothalamus, pituitary gland and the gonads, e.g. gonadotrophins and testosterone. An additional mechanism involves the sympathetic and parasympathetic nervous systems and may explain why thioridazine and other highly anticholinergic agents are mainly responsible for sexual dysfunction in men including impotence and retrograde ejaculation (98[r], 99[r]). A case of thioridazine-induced inhibition of female orgasm has also been reported (100[c]). The first report of spontaneous ejaculation associated with the therapeutic use of antipsychotic drugs was described in 1983 by Keitner and Selub (101[C]).

Mineral and fluid balance *Water retention* and *edema* occur very rarely during treatment with antipsychotics. Water intoxication has been reported following treatment with thioridazine and may be due to the pronounced anticholinergic properties of this agent and/or direct stimulation of the hypothalamic thirst center (102[C]).

Polyuria and polydipsia have long been associated with schizophrenia, and neuroleptics appear to aggravate these symptoms, sometimes with a concomitant syndrome of inappropriate antidiuretic hormone. Therefore, at present, care should be taken when treating hyponatremic patients with neuroleptic medication (103[C]).

In one controlled study, 12 patients who were receiving various antipsychotics had significantly *increased urinary calcium and hydroxyproline levels* and *decreased urinary alkaline phosphatase* as compared to five normal controls (104[C]). The possibility of reduction in bone mineralization may contribute to the increased risk of hip fracture associated with antipsychotic treatment in the elderly.

Hematological Rarely-reported hematological reactions to various antipsychotics include *agranulocytosis, thrombocytopenic purpura, hemolytic anemia, and leukopenia*. These are thought to represent a form of allergic or hypersensitivity reaction since they are apparently not dose related, although this has been questioned in one detailed case report involving chlorpromazine-induced agranulocytosis (105[c]). Neutropenia has been reported after accidental acute ingestion of approximately 1.53 g of chlorpromazine in a 5-year-old girl (106[C]), implicating a direct toxic effect on the bone marrow. The reported incidence of agranulocytosis is variable, ranging from 1 in 3000—4000 to 1 in 250 000. Most cases are seen within the first 2 months after beginning treatment, but there have been a few reports in which this occurred only after many years. Frequent white cell counts may be of limited value in monitoring for development of this rare but potentially fatal reaction, since counts fall rapidly and abruptly. Careful attention should be given to possible early warning signs such as fever, sore throat and adenopathy. Treatment requires discontinuing the antipsychotic immediately and instituting preventive measures against infection. Granulocyte colony-stimulating factor (GCSF) has been used to treat antipsychotic-induced agranulocytosis (174[C]).

The estimated incidence of clozapine agranulocytosis, originally determined to be 2.1 per 1000 in a selected Finnish population (SED-9, 83), led to the drug's prolonged withdrawal, followed a decade later in certain countries by a cautious reintroduction with hematological monitoring. With madatory hematological monitoring prescribed by the Clozaril Patient Management System in the U.S., the cumulative incidence of agranulocytosis was 0.8% at 1 year, and 0.9% at 1.5 years of treatment, and the risk was not found to be related to dosage (SEDA-18, 54; 175[R]). Because of the unusually high incidence of agranulocytosis in Finnish and Jewish patients, an ethnic risk factor for agranulocytosis has been suggested. Human leukocyte antigen (HLA)-B38 phenotype was found in 83% of patients who developed agranulocytosis and in 20% of clozapine-treated patients who did not develop agranulocytosis (107[C]). Gene products contained in the haplotype may thus be involved in mediating drug toxicity.

Liver *Hepatotoxicity* associated with chlorpromazine therapy was noted soon after its introduction, but is considered to be a rare side effect today. Occasional reports of *cholestatic jaundice* with thioxanthenes, and haloperidol have also been published (SED-9, 83; 108[C]). Jaundice generally occurs within 24 weeks after the drug is started and has many characteristics of an allergic reaction, i.e. non-dose-related, and accompanied by fever, rashes and eosinophilia, although a direct toxic mechanism has also been implicated. Symptoms generally subside rapidly upon discontinuation of the agent, but cholestasis may be prolonged. Hepatotoxicity may be as frequent with piperidine and piperazine phenothiazine compounds as with chlorpromazine, despite previous literature suggestions that the toxicity of these compounds is less. Jones et al. (109[CR]) found evidence of a significant hepatotoxic effect for the phenothiazines and for persons under age 50, but not over 50, relative to comparable population control.

More commonly seen are minor abnormalities in liver function tests following treatment with various antipsychotics, and these appear to be dose-related.

Gastrointestinal *Dry mouth* is a commonly reported autonomic side effect of antipsychotics and is seen more frequently with agents having prominent anticholinergic properties such as thioridazine and chlorpromazine, although the highly muscarinic clozapine has been associated with nocturnal hypersalivation. Dry mouth is mainly a nuisance, but its persistence may promote the development of dental caries, oral motuliasis and infective parotitis. When feasible, once daily administration of antipsychotics at bedtime often helps to alleviate the problem of dry mouth. One should also avoid concurrent administration of multiple drugs with additive anticholinergic effects. Sugarless gum or candy, frequent sips of water and/or ice chips, may help relieve dry mouth.

Constipation is also common with the highly anticholinergic antipsychotics, but is easily remedied by administration of laxatives. Nevertheless, the possibility of *fatal intestinal dilatation*, although very rare, warrants careful evaluation of persistent complaints of constipation, particularly when vomiting, abdominal pain, distension or tenderness are present (110[CR]). By promoting intestinal stasis, antipsychotics may very rarely cause increased intra-abdominal pressure and disrupt the vascular supply to the gut, leading to necrotizing enterocolitis (SED-11, 112). Acute colitis is a rare gastrointestinal effect of antipsychotics (176[C]).

Urinary system *Urinary retention, incontinence or dysuria* may be encountered occasionally with antipsychotics having more marked anticholinergic properties. A case of retroperitoneal fibrosis attributable to haloperidol was reported; since this condition affects the kidney, it should be differentiated from other causes of obstructive uropathy (111[c]).

Skin and appendages Many cutaneous reactions have been reported with the use of antipsychotics, including *urticaria, abscesses* following intramuscular administration, *rashes, photosensitivity or exaggerated sunburn, contact dermatitis, and melanosis or blue-gray skin discoloration*. Skin rashes are usually benign and are perhaps the most common type of cutaneous reaction encountered. Chlorpromazine is most often implicated (incidence 5—10%). Cutaneous lesions consisting of telangiectatic macules have been reported with thiothixene (112[C]). Non-phenothiazines such as haloperidol and loxitane may cause fewer urticarial reactions. As with any other class of drug, patients may be allergic to excipients in various tablet or capsule forms, or to preservatives, e.g. methylparaben, in liquid dosage forms (113[Cr]). Chlorpromazine most often causes photosensitivity reactions (incidence around 3%) which may result from formation of a cytotoxic by-product after exposure to ultraviolet light. Patients can be advised to avoid prolonged exposure to strong indoor light, as well as to wear protective clothing and to use a combination of *p*-aminobenzoic acid and benzophenone sunscreen when exposure to strong sunlight is unavoidable.

Potentially serious skin reactions are best treated by discontinuing the offending agent and switching to a structurally unrelated antipsychotic. When the offending agent is a phenothiazine, replacement by nonphenothiazines such as haloperidol or molindone may be preferable to use of the more closely related thioxanthenes.

Skin discoloration is more common in females and generally occurs over the exposed parts of the body. This reaction may be caused by deposition of melanin—drug complexes and was more commonly observed in the decade following the introduction of the phenothiazines into clinical practice, but it is rarely seen today (114[c]).

Seborrheic dermatitis has been observed in patients chronically treated with antipsychotic drugs (SEDA-17, 57), and this side effect appears to be highly associated with drug-induced parkinsonism.

More serious types of cutaneous reactions are rare, but angioneurotic edema, non-thrombocytopenic purpura, exfoliative dermatitis and Stevens-Johnson syndrome have been reported, as well as rare disorders of connective tissue resembling systemic lupus erythematosus reported with chlorpromazine, perphenazine and chlorprothixene (115[c]).

Special senses Various antipsychotics, particularly low-dose phenothiazines and thioxanthenes, commonly produce blurred vision (*mydriasis*) secondary to their anticholinergic activity. This is primarily a nuisance except in the rare patient with narrow-angle glaucoma.

Of more concern are two distinct types of adverse effects in the eye which may be produced by various antipsychotics: *lenticular and corneal deposits* and *pigmentary retinopathy*. Deposits in the lens or cornea are probably the results of melanin—drug complex deposition and are best detected by slit-lamp examination. These deposits are probably dose-related since they generally occur only after years of treatment. Fortunately, they are in large part benign and reversible, but if undetected they may progress to interfere with vision. They are most often reported with chlorpromazine or thioridazine and may occur in association with pigmentary changes in the skin. Non-phenothiazines appear to have minimal propensity to cause oculocutaneous reactions and may be preferred in cases where these problems have occurred during treatment with phenothiazines (SED-11, 113), although the patient should still be closely monitored.

Pigmentary retinopathy, which can seriously impair vision, is specifically associated with thioridazine and has occurred more frequently on high and prolonged dosage (e.g. 1200—1800 mg/day for weeks to months), although one case is on record where the daily dose was only 700 mg (SED-11, 113). Large-scale surveys have confirmed the relative safety of doses up to 800 mg/day (20[r]); at any dose, however, any complaint by the patient of brownish discoloration of vision or impaired dark adaptation requires immediate evaluation.

A variety of *rarer ocular effects* have been reported, including oculomotor palsies, transient myopias, optic atrophy, blue-green blindness and night-blindness. For a long time, there has been some suspicion that neuroleptics might increase the risk of cataract (116[R]).

Miscellaneous *Epistaxis* has been reported in three patients with hypertension while receiving thioridazine (117[C]).

Risk situations The contraindications to neuroleptic therapy include *comatose states*, the presence or withdrawal of high doses of *other CNS depressants* (alcohol, barbiturates, narcotics etc.), serious *hematological conditions* (e.g. bone marrow suppression) and a previous history of *hypersensitivity* reactions, e.g. jaundice or severe photosensitivity. Since neuroleptics cause sedation, they may impair mental or physical abilities (including reaction times), especially during the first few days of therapy. Use of neuroleptics in *pregnancy* and by *nursing mothers* is not advised, but if they are indeed needed, chlorpromazine or trifluoperazine may be the drugs of choice.

Neuroleptics have been prescribed to children for the treatment of psychotic disorders, Tourette's syndrome, attention deficit disorder, hyperactivity, behavioral and psychiatric complications of mental retardation, and pervasive developmental disorders, e.g. infantile autism (118[r]). Side effects of neuroleptics in children may be unpredictable and a suggestion that they could be a cause of sudden infant death remains a hypothesis (119[r]). Significant weight gain has been reported to occur in almost 100% of neuroleptic-treated children, and there seems to be a relatively high incidence of extrapyramidal side effects in these young patients (120[r]). Since there is little information regarding the pharmacokinetics and pharmacodynamics of neuroleptics in pediatric populations, careful supervision of treatment is vital; the use of high-dose treatment is inadvisable.

Similar principles apply when treating the geriatric population, primarily because there is wide individual variation in the extent to which *older people* tolerate these drugs.

Withdrawal effects A variety of somatic complaints has been reported in patients abruptly withdrawn from neuroleptics. The incidence of these complaints varies widely in different reports, from 0 to 75%. Common complaints include headache, vomiting, nausea, diarrhea, insomnia, abdominal pain, rhinorrhea and muscle aches. On rare occasions, the symptoms resemble those of benzodiazepine withdrawal (appetite change, dizziness, tremulousness, numbness, nightmares, a bad taste in the mouth, fever, perspiration, vertigo, tachycardia and anxiety), but it is quite possible that in some of the reported cases, there actually has been benzodiazepine withdrawal. Some of these symptoms may also have been linked to the simultaneous withdrawal of anticholinergic agents (SED-11, 113; 121[c]). Parkinsonism, not explained by discontinuation of anticholinergics, has also been reported as an unusual withdrawal effect of neuroleptic drugs (122[C]).

Worsening of psychotic symptoms and/or dyskinetic movements may be seen when dosages are lowered or the neuroleptic is discontinued. A functional increase in mesolimbic and striatal dopaminergic sensitivity has been suggested as an explanation for these phenomena (123[R]). Psychotic relapse is rarely seen in the first 2 weeks after discontinuing neuroleptics, but physical withdrawal symptoms generally have their onset within 48 hours of the last dose (SEDA-14, 54).

Abrupt clozapine withdrawal, or even dosage reduction can result in psychosis and/or delirium (177[C], 178[C], 179[C]). Clozapine withdrawal has also been associated with nausea, vomiting, diarrhea, headache, restlessness, agitation and sweating (155[r], 180[r]), which occur as the result of cholinergic rebound and which may respond to anticholinergics (181[C]). Appearance of delirium and return of dyskinetic movements can take place in days after clozapine withdrawal.

Withdrawal emergent syndrome has been described in children (119[r], 120[r]) and consists of nausea, vomiting, ataxia and choreiform dyskinesia primarily affecting the extremities, trunk and head following sudden stoppage of neuroleptic treatment (124[c]). In one study, withdrawal symptoms were observed in 51% of children, twice as many children being affected by the withdrawal of low-dose, high-potency compounds compared with others. Symptoms usually appear within a few days to 2 weeks after drug withdrawal; spontaneous remission is likely within the next 8–12 weeks. The syndrome is still not well understood.

Second-generation effects *Use in pregnancy* All antipsychotic agents cross the placenta and reach the fetus in potentially significant amounts. However, most large-scale controlled studies conclude that these agents can be used safely during pregnancy (20[R]). There are nevertheless, as one would expect with such widely used drugs, isolated case-reports of malformations (SED-11, 114). Several instances of limb reduction following use of haloperidol during pregnancy suggest that it would be prudent not to administer this agent during the first trimester, the period of limb development (125[C]). There is also reason to argue that prenatally administered drugs of this class influence the offspring after the drug has been eliminated, and can produce 'behavioral teratogenicity'; since neurotransmitter systems continue to develop long after birth, such drugs might influence behavior in an adverse way over a very long period

(126[R]). In general, the best recommendation is to avoid any drug during the first trimester and only to employ drugs thereafter if the benefits to the mother and fetus outweigh any possibility of risk. Should an antipsychotic be required during pregnancy, one would prefer to use an agent such as chlorpromazine or trifluoperazine, as there is considerably more worldwide experience with these drugs than with newer antipsychotics (20[R]).

A variety of pharmacological effects may be seen in the infant after birth, particularly when the mother has received these agents in the weeks prior to delivery. These include postnatal depression and acute dystonic reactions (which may interfere with normal delivery). Hypotonia may persist for months (127[C]) and may respond to diphenhydramine, 5 mg/kg per day. Neonatal jaundice, hyperbilirubinemia and melanin deposits in the eyes may be seen when antipsychotics have been given during the last trimester or longer during pregnancy.

Lactation Neuroleptics appear in breast milk at concentrations that are very low but probably related to the amount of maternal dose ingested per day. Typical regimens of antipsychotics yield low or negligible levels (20[R], 128[C]). Until these issues are further clarified, it would be best to avoid breast-feeding while receiving antipsychotics.

Effects on fertility The effects of antipsychotics on fertility are not well known; present data are controversial, being often based on animal studies, e.g. reduction in male rat copulation by chlorpromazine. However, oligospermia, polyspermia, necrospermia and decreased sperm motility have been reported with various phenothiazines and butyrophenones; these are likely to improve when the drug is discontinued (129[R]).

Overdosage Antipsychotics are often ingested in accidental overdosage or suicide attempts, but mortality from this group of drugs is generally low and infrequently associated with residual impairment. However, an important exception to this would be concomitant drug ingestion with alcohol, tricyclic antidepressants or antiparkinsonian agents. In acute overdosage of antipsychotics alone, the most serious complications include shock, seizures and cardiac arrhythmias. These can be more problematic when the ingested antipsychotics are of the low-potency type, e.g. thioridazine and chlorpromazine, taken in high dosages. However, a review of acute loxapine overdosage also indicates a high potential for serious neurological problems and cardiotoxicity with this high-potency agent (130[C]). Acute extrapyramidal reactions occur more often after ingestion of high-potency drugs such as haloperidol and fluphenazine; these respond to parenteral administration of benztropine, but anticholinergics should be used judiciously so as not to worsen peripheral or central autonomic toxicity. Other serious, but less frequent, complications include paralytic ileus and hypothermia. Acute renal failure has been very rarely reported, but is apparently reversible and may occur secondary to severe hypotension or other etiology following an acute ingestion (131[C]).

Interactions *Adrenolytics* Antipsychotics may intensify the effects of α-adrenoceptor blocking agents, e.g. phentolamine, causing severe hypotension (120[r]).

Alcohol Alcohol-induced CNS and respiratory depression is enhanced by antipsychotics (132[r]), but enhancement may be slight if both are used at reasonable levels (133[R]). Haloperidol (but not chlorpromazine) was found to increase blood alcohol levels (134[C]).

Antacids Antacids containing aluminium and magnesium ions may reduce the gastrointestinal absorption of chlorpromazine and other phenothiazines by forming complexes (135[r]). The clinical significance of this is unknown.

Anticoagulants Concurrent administration with phenothiazines may cause an increased hypoprothrombinemic effect, presumably due to enzyme competition. However, haloperidol has been reported to lower anticoagulant effectiveness through enzyme induction (136[r]).

Antidepressants Various antipsychotics have been reported to inhibit the metabolism of imipramine, nortriptyline and amitriptyline (SED-11, 114). In one study, patients receiving amitriptyline or nortriptyline in combination with perphenazine had up to 70% higher antidepressant levels than patients receiving antidepressants alone (137[r]). While of less clinical significance, the levels of neuroleptics may also be raised.

Antidiabetics Because phenothiazines affect carbohydrate metabolism, they may interfere with control of diabetic patients (132[r]).

Antihypertensives Antipsychotics may enhance the hypotensive action of antihypertensive drugs due to their ability to produce α-adrenoceptor blockade. However, phenothiazines may inhibit the hypotensive action of guanethidine (133[R]). This antagonism may not occur with molindone (136[r]). Combined use of antipsychotics and thiazide diuretics has rarely resulted in severe hypotension and diuretic-induced hypokalemia may potentiate thioridazine-induced cardiotoxicity (136[r]). Phenothiazines decrease hepatic metabolism and thereby increase plasma levels of propranolol (136[r]). In addition, in one report, a schizophrenic patient experienced delirium, grand mal seizures and photosensitivity after addition of propranolol to a chlorpromazine regimen, suggesting that neuroleptic levels are increased by propranolol (138[C]). Nevertheless, high dosages of propranolol (up to 2 g) have been used in combination with chlorpromazine to treat schizophrenia. The cardiac effects of neuroleptics can be potentiated by propranolol (139[r]).

Benzodiazepines Several reports of synergistic reactions, resulting in increased sedation and ataxia, have been reported when lorazepam was initiated in patients already receiving clozapine (182[C]).

Bromocriptine The dopamine-blocking activity of antipsychotics may antagonize the effects of bromocriptine. Conversely, bromocriptine has been reported to cause exacerbation of schizophrenic symptoms (140[C]).

Caffeine Excessive intake of caffeine may cause CNS stimulant effects which can worsen psychosis and thus interfere with the results of neuroleptic treatment (141[R]). Neuroleptics may precipitate from solution when mixed with coffee or tea (142[C]), but the clinical significance of this interaction is unknown (143[C]).

Carbamazepine Neuroleptic plasma levels can be lowered by carbamazepine, and patients should be monitored for reduced antipsychotic clinical efficacy (144[C]).

Corticosteroids By reducing gastrointestinal motility, antipsychotics may enhance the absorption of corticosteroids (132[r]).

Digoxin By reducing gastrointestinal motility, antipsychotics may increase the bioavailability of digoxin and other ionotropic agents and thereby increase the potential for toxicity (133[R]).

Levodopa Levodopa and an antipsychotic may interfere with the effects of each other when administered concurrently; the patient should be monitored for deterioration in both parkinsonism and mental state.

Lithium Neurotoxicity has been reported in around 20 patients treated with the combination of lithium and haloperidol; several cases of lithium—thioridazine neurotoxicity have also been reported. The etiology of this interaction has not been resolved and, in general, lithium seems compatible with all antipsychotics, although patients should be carefully monitored (145[R], 183[R], 184[R]). Persistent dysarthria with apraxia associated with a combination of lithium carbonate and haloperidol was reported (146[C]).

Methyldopa Dementia has been reported when methyldopa was combined with haloperidol (147[C]).

Monoamine oxidase inhibitors There may be additive hypotensive effects when these drugs are combined with antipsychotics.

Narcotic analgesics CNS and respiratory depression due to narcotic analgesics can be enhanced by antipsychotics (132[r]).

Oral contraceptives Estrogen-containing preparations may further promote neuroleptic-induced prolactin stimulation (132[r]).

Phenytoin Antipsychotics may decrease phenytoin levels by inducing liver enzymes (148[r]) but occasionally serum levels are increased (149[r]). Phenytoin may also decrease antipsychotic levels (150[c]).

Propranolol see under 'Antihypertensives'.

Quinidine Concurrent administration with antipsychotics, particularly thioridazine, can lead to additive myocardial depression (136[r]).

Sedatives and hypnotics Neuroleptics increase barbiturate and sedative-hypnotic sleep time and respiratory depression. Lower doses of barbiturates or other hypnotics may be indicated in patients receiving antipsychotics (136[r]).

Cigarette smoking Smoking appears to have important effects on plasma concentrations. Pantuck and colleagues found that chlorpromazine levels are reduced by 36% in smokers (151[C]), and in an analysis of a number of factors that potentially influence chlorpromazine levels, smoking may be second in importance only to dosage (152[C]).

Sympathomimetics Antipsychotics may reduce or block the pressor effects of α-adrenoceptor agonists. When using sympathomimetics having both α- and β-activity, antipsychotic blockade of α-adrenoceptors may lead to unopposed β-predominance, resulting in severe hypotension (136[r]). Levarterenol or phenylephrine may be safer to use when the patient is receiving chlorpromazine or other antipsychotic agents (133[r]).

Interference with diagnostic routines Alterations in various laboratory values may be the result of pharmacological actions, such as elevated glucose or decreased serum urate (2—3 days delay). One must also keep in mind those alterations which indicate end-organ toxicity, including elevated serum transaminases, alkaline phosphatase or bilirubin (due to hepatic necrosis, hypersensitivity or jaundice), or increased prothrombin time or serum cholesterol (by cholestasis, hepatic toxicity).

Methodological interference has been reported between chlorpromazine and various laboratory tests, resulting in overestimation of cholesterol (Zlatkis-Zak reaction), false findings of increased CSF protein (Folin-Ciocalteau method) or decreased readings for haptoglobin (153[R]). Phenothiazines can also cause a false-positive pregnancy test (but only when using the virtually obsolete Ascheim-Zondek animal test method) or increased urinary ketones (ferric chloride test), urinary steroids (colorimetry) or oxosteroids (Porter-Silber test) (SED-11, 115).

REFERENCES

1. van Putten T. Why do schizophrenic patients refuse to take their drugs? Arch Gen Psychiatry 1974;31:67.
2. Rifkin A, Doddi S, Karajgi B et al. Dosage of haloperidol for schizophrenia. Arch Gen Psychiatry 1991;48:166.
3. Simpson GM, Varga E, Haher EJ. Psychotic exacerbations produced by neuroleptics. Dis Nerv Syst 1976;37:367.
4. van Putten T, Mutalipassi LR. Fluphenazine enanthate induced decompensations. Psychosomatics 1975;16:37.
5. Curry SH, Davis JM, Ianowsky DS, Marshall JHL. Factors affecting chlorpromazine plasma levels in psychiatric patients. Arch Gen Psychiatry 1970;22:209.
6. Simpson GM, Cooper TB. Clozapine plasma levels and convulsions. Am J Psychiatry 1978;135:99.
7. Mandelstam JP. An inquiry into the use of Innovar for pediatric premedication. Anesth Analg 1970;49:746.
8. Carlsson C, Dencker SJ, Gramby G et al. Norepinephrine in blood, plasma and urine during chlorpromazine treatment. Lancet 1966;i:1208.
9. Axelsson R, Aspenstrom G. Electrocardiographic changes and serum concentrations in thioridazine-treated patients. J Clin Psychiatry 1982;43:332.
10. Kiriike N, Maeda Y, Nishinaki S et al. Iatrogenic torsade de pointes induced by thioridazine. Biol Psychiatry 1987; 22:99.
11. Connolly MJ, Evemy KL, Snow MH. Torsade de pointes ventricular tachycardia in association with thioridazine therapy: report of two cases. New Trends Arrhythmias 1985; 1:157.
12. Branchey MH, Lee JH, Amin R et al. High and low potency neuroleptics in elderly psychiatric patients. J Am Med Assoc 1978;239:1860.
13. Dahl S. Active metabolites of neuroleptic drugs: possible contribution to therapeutic and toxic effects. Ther Drug Monit 1982;4:33.
14. Risch SC, Groom GP, Janowsky DS. The effects of psychotropic drugs on the cardiovascular system. J Clin Psychiatry 1982;43:16.
15. Nuyse F, van Schijndel RD. Naloperidol and cardiac arrest. Lancet 1988;ii:568.
16. Flaherty JA, Lahmeyer HW. Laryngeal-pharyngeal dystonia as a possible cause of asphyxia with haloperidol treatment. Am J Psychiatry 1978;135:1414.
17. Mahutte CK. Naloperidol and sudden death due to pulmonary edema. Arch Intern Med 1982;142:1952.
18. Faheem AD, Brightwell DR, Burton GC, Struss A. Respiratory dyskinesia and dysarthria from prolonged neuroleptic use: tardive dyskinesia? Am J Psychiatry 1982;139:517.
19. Portnoy RA. Hyperkinetic dysarthria as an early indication of impending tardive dyskinesia. J Speech Hear Disord 1979;44:214.
20. Simpson GM, Pi EH, Sramek JJ. Adverse effects of antipsychotic agents. Drugs 1981;2:128.
21. Wistedt B. Neuroleptics and depression. Arch Gen Psychiatry 1982;39:745.
22. Braff DL, Saccuzzo DP. Effect of antipsychotic medication on speed of information processing in schizophrenic patients. Am J Psychiatry 1982;139:1127.
23. van Putten T, May PRA, Marder SR et al. Subjective response to antipsychotic drugs. Arch Gen Psychiatry 1981; 38:187.
24. Rifkin A, Quitkin F, Klein DF. Akinesia: a poorly recognized drug-induced extrapyramidal behavior disorder. Arch Gen Psychiatry 1975;32:672.
25. Sriwatanakul K. Minimizing the risk of antipsychotic-associated seizures. Drug Ther 1982;12:65.
26. Itil TM. Comparison of the clinical and EEG effects of molindone and trifluoperazine in acute schizophrenic patients. Behav Neuropsychiatry 1971;3:25.
27. Baldessarini RJ. Drugs and the treatment of psychiatric disorders. In: Goodman LS, Gilman A, eds. The Pharmacological Basis of Therapeutics. New York: MacMillan, 1980;391.
28. Heller E, Binder RL. Clozapine and seizures. Am J Psychiatry 1990;147:1069.
29. Oliver AP, Luchins DJ, Wyatt RJ. Neuroleptic induced seizures: an in vitro technique for assessing relative risk. Arch Gen Psychiatry 1982;39:206.
30. Koek RJ, Pi EH. Acute laryngeal dystonic reactions to neuroleptics. Psychosomatics 1989;30:359.
31. Sovner R, McGorrill S. Stress as a precipitant of neuroleptic-induced dyskinesia. Psychosomatics 1982;23:707.
32. Kane JM, Woerner M, Borenstein M et al. Integrating incidence and prevalence of tardive dyskinesia. Psychopharmacol Bull 1986;22:254.
33. Simpson GM, Pi EH, Sramek JJ. Management of tardive dyskinesia: current update. Drugs 1982;23:382.
34. Ananth J. Tardive dyskinesia: myth and reality. Psychosomatics 1980;21:389.
35. Gardos G, Cole JO. Overview: public health issues in tardive dyskinesia. Am J Psychiatry 1980;137:776.
36. Gardos G, Samu I, Kallos M. Absence of severe tardive dyskinesia in Hungarian schizophrenic outpatients. Psychopharmacology 1980;71:29.
37. Pi EH, Kusuda M, Gray GE et al. Cross-cultural psychopharmacology: neuroleptic-induced movement disorders. In: Eckert GM, Forrest IT, Gupta RR et al, eds. Thiazines and Related Compounds. Melbourne, Florida: Krieger Publishing Company, 1991.
38. Ko GN, Zhang LD, Yan WW et al. The Shanghai 800: prevalence of tardive dyskinesia in a Chinese psychiatric hospital. Am J Psychiatry 1989;146:387.
39. Binder RL, Kazamatsuri H, Nishimura T et al. Tardive dyskinesia and neuroleptic-induced parkinsonism in Japan. Am J Psychiatry 1987;144:1494.
40. Sramek J, Roy S, Ahrens T et al. Prevalence of tardive dyskinesia in three ethnic groups of chronic psychiatric patients. J Hosp Community Psychiatry 1991;42:590.
41. Simpson GM, Lee JH, Zoubok B, Gardos G. A rating scale for tardive dyskinesia. Psychopharmacology (1979) 64, 171.
42. Schoolar NR, Kane JM. Research diagnosis for tardive dyskinesia. Arch Gen Psychiatry 1982;39:486.
43. Pi EH, Simpson GM. Tardive dyskinesia and abnormal tongue movements. Br J Psychiatry 1981;139:526.
44. Kane, JM, Smith JM. Tardive dyskinesia, prevalence and risk factors, 1959 to 1979. Arch Gen Psychiatry 1982;39:473.
45. Kane JM, Woerner M, Wernhold P, Wegner J Results from a prospective study of tardive dyskinesia over a 2-year period development: preliminary findings. Psychopharmacol Bull 1982;18:82.
46. Johnson GFS, Hunt GE, Rey JM. Incidence and severity of T.D.-increase with age. Arch Gen Psychiatry 1982;39:486.
47. Chouinard G, Jones P, Annable L, Ross-Chouinard A.

Sex differences and tardive dyskinesia. Am J Psychiatry 1980;137:507.
48. Gordon J, Borison R, Diamond B. Modulation of dopamine receptor sensitivity by estrogen. Biol Psychiatry 1980;15:389.
49. Perenji A, Arato M. Tardive dyskinesia on Hungarian psychiatric wards. Psychosomatics 1980;21:904.
50. Gardos G, Cole JO. Tardive dyskinesia and anticholinergic drugs. Am J Psychiatry 1983;140:200.
51. Chouinard G, Bradwejn J. Reversible and irreversible tardive dyskinesia: a case report. Am J Psychiatry 1982; 139:360.
52. Jeste DV, Linnoila M, Wagner RL, Wyatt RJ. Serum neuroleptic concentrations and T.D. Psychopharmacology 1982;76:377.
53. Widerlöv EW, Häggström J-E, Kilts CD et al. Serum concentrations of thioridazine, its major metabolites and serum neuroleptic-like activities in schizophrenics with and without tardive dyskinesia. Acta Psychiatr Scand 1982; 66:294.
54. Yassa R, Nair NPV, Iskandar H et al. Factors in the development of severe forms of tardive dyskinesia. Am J Psychiatry 1990;147:1156.
55. Jeste DV, Potkin SG, Sirha S et al. Tardive dyskinesia-reversible and persistent. Arch Gen Psychiatry 1979;36:585.
56. Pi EH, Simpson GM. Prevention of tardive dyskinesia. In: Shah NS, Donald AG, eds. Neurobehavioral Dysfunction Induced by Psychotherapeutic Agents. Neurophysiological, Neuropharmacological Bases and Clinical Implications. New York: Plenum Publishing Corp, 1983.
57. Rosen AM, Mukherjee S, Olarte S et al. Perception of tardive dyskinesia in outpatients receiving maintenance neuroleptics. Am J Psychiatry 1982;139:372.
58. Wegner JT, Kane JM. Follow-up study on the reversibility of tardive dyskinesia. Am J Psychiatry 1982;139:368.
59. Seeman M. Tardive dyskinesia: two year recovery. Comp. Psychiatry 1981;22:189.
60. Jeste DV, Wyatt RT. Changing epidemiology of tardive dyskinesia: an overview. Am J Psychiatry 1981;138:297.
61. Jeste DV, Wyatt RJ Therapeutic strategies against tardive dyskinesia: two decades of experience. Arch Gen Psychiatry 1982;39:803.
62. Donatelli A, Geisen L, Feuer E. Case report of adverse effect of reserpine on tardive dyskinesia. Am J Psychiatry 1983;140:239.
63. Schrodt GR, Wright JH, Simpson R et al. Treatment of tardive dyskinesia with propranolol. J Clin Psychiatry 1982;43:328.
64. Korsgaard S, Casey DE, Gerlach J et al. The effect of tetrahydroisoxazolo-pyridinol (THIP) in tardive dyskinesia: a new γ-amino butyric acid agonist. Arch Gen Psychiatry 1982;39:1017.
65. Elkashef AM, Ruskin E, Bacher N et al. Vitamin E in the treatment of tardive dyskinesia. Am J Psychiatry 1990; 147:505.
66. Lohr JB, Cadet JL, Lohr MA et al. Alphatocopherol in tardive dyskinesia. Lancet 1987;i:913.
67. Delwaide PJ, Desseilles M. Spontaneous buccolinguofacial dyskinesia in the elderly. Acta Neurol Scand 1977; 56:256.
68. Varga E, Sugerman AA, Varga V, Zomorodi A et al. Prevalence of spontaneous oral dyskinesia in elderly persons. Paper presented at: 12th CINP Congress, Gothenburg, 1980.
69. Owens DGC, Johnstone EC, Frith CD. Spontaneous involuntary disorders of movement: their prevalence, severity, and distribution in chronic schizophrenics with and without treatment with neuroleptics. Arch Gen Psychiatry 1982;39:452.
70. Jeste DV, Wisniewski AA, Wyatt RJ Neuroleptic-associated tardive syndromes. Psychiatr Clin North Am 1986; 9:183.
71. Yassa R, Nair V, Dimity R. Prevalence of tardive dystonia. Acta Psychiatr Scand 1986;73:629.
72. Simpson GM, Pi EH, Sramek JJ An update on tardive dyskinesia. Hosp Community Psychiatry 1986;37:362.
73. Yadalam KG, Korn ML, Simpson GM. Tardive dystonia: four case histories. J Clin Psychiatry 1990;51:17.
74. Burke RE, Fahn S, Jankovic L et al. Tardive dystonia: late-onset and persistent dystonia caused by antipsychotic drugs. Neurology 1982;32:1335.
75. Deshmukh DH, Joshi VS, Agarwal MR. Rabbit syndrome a rare complication of long-term neuroleptic medication. Br J Psychiatry 1990;157:293.
76. Kane JM, Rifkin A, Woerner M et al. Low-dose neuroleptic treatment of outpatient schizophrenics. 1. Preliminary results from relapse rates. Arch Gen Psychiatry 1983;40:893.
77. Marder SR, van Putten T, Mintz I et al. Costs and benefits of two doses of fluphenazine. Arch Gen Psychiatry 1984;41:1025.
78. Kane JM. Antipsychotic drug side effects: their relationship to dose. J Clin Psychiatry 1985;46:16.
79. Sloane PD, McLeod MM. Radial nerve palsy in nursing home patients: association with immobility and haloperidol. J Am Geriatr Soc 1987;35:465.
80. Caroff SN. The neuroleptic malignant syndrome. J Clin Psychiatry 1980;41:79.
81. Burke RE, Fahn S, Mayeux R et al. Neuroleptic malignant syndrome caused by dopamine-depleting drugs in a patient with Huntingdon's disease. Neurology 1981;31:1022.
82. Keyser DL, Rodnitzky RL. Neuroleptic malignant syndrome in Parkinson's disease after withdrawal or alteration of dopaminergic therapy. Arch Intern Med 1991;151:794.
83. Keck PE, Pope HG, McElroy SL. Frequency and presentation of neuroleptic malignant syndrome: a prospective study. Am J Psychiatry 1987;144:1344.
84. Anderson ES, Powers PS. Neuroleptic malignant syndrome associated with clozapine use. J Clin Psychiatry 1991;52:102.
85. Das Gupta H, Young A. Clozapine-induced neuroleptic malignant syndrome. J Clin Psychiatry 1991;52:105.
86. Levinson DF, Simpson GM. Neuroleptic-induced extrapyramidal symptoms with fever. Arch Gen Psychiatry 1986;43:839.
87. Mccarron MM, Boettger ML, Peck JJ A case of neuroleptic malignant syndrome successfully treated with amantadine. J Clin Psychiatry 1982;43:381.
88. Coons DJ, Hillman FJ, Marshall RW. Treatment of neuroleptic malignant syndrome with dantrolene sodium: a case report. Am J Psychiatry 1982;139:944.
89. Goekoop JG, Carbaat PA. Treatment of neuroleptic malignant syndrome with dantrolene. Lancet 1982;ii:49.
90. Mueller PS, Vester JW, Fermaglich J Neuroleptic malignant syndrome: successful treatment with bromocriptine. J Am Med Assoc 1983;249:386.
91. Rosebush PI, Stewart TD, Gelenberg AJ Twenty neuroleptic rechallenges after neuroleptic malignant syndrome in 15 patients. J Clin Psychiatry 1989;50:295.
92. Wistedt B. A depot neuroleptic withdrawal study: a

controlled study with the withdrawal of depot fluphenazine decanoate and depot flupenthixol decanoate in chronic schizophrenic patients. Acta Psychiatr Scand 1981;64:65.
93. Moller HJ, Kissling W, Maurach R. Beziehungen zwischen Haloperidol-Serumspiegel, Prolactin-Setumspiegel, antipsychotischem Effekt und extrapyramidalen Begleitwirkungen. Pharmacopsychiatrica 1981;14:27.
94. Zarifian E, Scotton B, Bianchetti G et al. High doses of haloperidol in schizophrenia: a clinical, biochemical, and pharmacokinetic study. Arch Gen Psychiatry 1982;39:212.
95. Brown WA, Laughren T. Low serum prolactin and early relapse following neuroleptic withdrawal. Am J Psychiatry 1981;138:237.
96. Schyve PM, Smithline F, Meltzer H. Neuroleptic-induced prolactin level elevation and breast cancer. Arch Gen Psychiatry 1978;35:1291.
97. Mortensen PB. The incidence of cancer in schizophrenic patients. J Epidemiol Community Health 1989;43:43.
98. Mitchell JE, Popkin MH. Antipsychotic drug therapy and sexual dysfunction in men. Am J Psychiatry 1982; 139:633.
99. Siris SG, Siris ES, Vankammen DP et al. Effects of dopamine blockage on gonadotropins and testosterone in men. Am J Psychiatry 1980;137:211.
100. Shen WW, Park S. Thioridazine-induced inhibition of female orgasm. Psychiatr J Univ Ottawa 1982;7:249.
101. Heitner GI, Selub S. Spontaneous ejaculations and neuroleptics. J Clin Psychopharmacol 1983;3:34.
102. Rao KJ, Miller M, Moses A. Water intoxication and thioridazine (Me11ari1). Ann Intern Med 1975.82:61.
103. Lawson WB, Karson CN, Bigelow LB. Increased urine volume in chronic schizophrenic patients. Psychiatry Res 1985;14:323.
104. Higuchi T, Komoda T, Sugishita M et al. Certain neuroleptics reduce bone mineralization in schizophrenic patients. Neuropsychobiology 1987;18:185.
105. Marcus J, Mulvihill F. Agranulocytosis and chlorpromazine. J Clin Psychiatry 1978;39:784.
106. Burckart GJ Neutropenia following acute chlorpromazine ingestion. Clin Toxicol 1981;18:797.
107. Lieberman JA, Yunis J, Egea E et al. HLA-B38, and clozapine-induced agranulocytosis in Jewish patients with schizophrenia. Arch Gen Psychiatry 1990;47:945.
108. Dincsoy HP, Saelinger DA. Haloperidol-induced chronic cholestatic liver disease. Gastroenterology 1982; 83:694.
109. Jones JK, van de Carr SW, Zimmerman H, Leroy A. Hepatotoxicity associated with phenothiazines. Psychopharmacol Bull 1983;19:24.
110. Evans D, Rogers J, Peiper S. Intestinal dilatation associated with phenothiazine therapy: a case report and literature review. Am J Psychiatry 1979;136:970.
111. Jeffries JJ, Lyall WA, Bezchlibnyk K et al. Retroperitoneal fibrosis and haloperidol. Am J Psychiatry 1982; 139:1524.
112. Matsuoka LY. Thlothixene drug sensitivity. J Am Acad Dermatol 1982;7:405.
113. Kaminer Y, Apter A, Tyano S et al. Use of macrophage migration inhibition factor test to determine the cause of delayed hypersensitivity reaction to haloperidol syrup. Am J Psychiatry 1982;139:1503.
114. Ananth J, Yassa R. Tardive dyskinesia and skin pigmentation. Br J Psychiatry 1982;141:194.
115. McNevin S, Mackay M. Chlorprothixene-induced systemic lupus erythematosus. J Clin Psychopharmacol 1982; 2:411.
116. Editorial. Epidemiology of cataract. Lancet 1982;i:1392.
117. Idupuganti S. Epistaxis in hypertensive patients taking thioridazine. Am J Psychiatiy 1982;139:1083.
118. Biederman J New directions in pediatric psychopharmacology. Drug Ther 1982;12:33.
119. Polizos P, Engelhardt DM. Dyskinetic phenomena in children treated with psychotropic medication. Psychopharmacol Bull 1978;14:65.
120. Polizos P, Gualtieri DT, Barnhill J, McGimsey J Tardive dyskinesia and other movement disorders in children treated with psychotropic drugs. J Am Acad Child Psychiatry 1980;19:491.
121. Mitchell JE. Discontinuation of antipsychotic drug therapy. Psychosomatics 1981;22:241.
122. Ceccherini HA, Yarden PE, Guazzelli M et al. Parkinsonism following neuroleptic withdrawal. Arch Gen Psychiatry 1989;46:383.
123. Chouinard G, Jones BD. Neuroleptic-induced supersensitivity psychosis: clinical and pharmacologic characteristics. Am J Psychiatry 1980;137:16.
124. Polizos P, Engelhardt DM, Hoffman SP. Neurological consequences of psychotropic drug withdrawal in schizophrenic children. J Autism Child Schizophr 1973;3:247.
125. Kopelman AE, McCullan FW, Heggeness L. Limb malformations following maternal use of haloperidol. J Am Med Assoc 1975;231:62.
126. Coyle I, Wayner MJ, Singer G. Behavioral teratogenesis: a critical evaluation. Pharmacol Biochem Behav 1976;4:191.
127. O'Connor M, Johnson GH, James DI. Interuterine effect of phenothiazines. Med. J Aust 1981;1;416.
128. Stewart KB, Karas B, Springer PK. Haloperidol excretion in human milk. Am J Psychiatry 1980;137:849.
129. Blair JH, Simpson GM. Effect of antipsychotic drugs on reproductive functions. Dis Nerv Syst 1966;27:645.
130. Peterson CD. Seizures induced by acute loxapine overdosage. Vet. Hum. Toxicol 1980;22(Suppl 2):52.
131. Rossen B, Sterness I. The pathophysiology of acute renal failure after chlorprothlxene overdosage. Acta Med Scand 1981;209:525.
132. Griffin JP, D'Arcy PF. A Manual of Adverse Drug Interactions. Bristol: John Wright and Sons Ltd, 1979.
133. Shopsin B, Kline NS, Ayd F et al. In: Evaluation of Drug Interactions, 2nd edn. Washington, DC: American Pharmaceutical Association, 1976;25,81,122,397.
134. Morselli PL. Further observations on the interaction between ethanol and psychotropic drugs. Arzneim-Forsch 1971;2:20.
135. Shader RI, Ciraulo DA, Greenblatt DJ Drug interactions involving psychotropic drugs. Psychosomatics 1978; 19:671.
136. Risch SC, Groom GP, Janowsky DS. The effects of psychotropic drugs on the cardiovascular system. J Clin Psychiatry 1982;43:16.
137. Linnoila M, George L, Guthrie S. Interaction between antidepressants and perphenazine in psychiatric inpatients. Am J Psychiatry 1982;139:1329.
138. Miller FA, Rampling D. Adverse effects of combined propranolol and chlorpromazine therapy. Am J Psychiatry 1982;139:1198.
139. Ayd FJ Loxapine update 1966–1977. Dis Nerv Syst 1977;38:883.

140. Frye PE, Pasiser SF, Kim MH et al. Bromocriptine associated with symptom exacerbation during neuroleptic treatment of schizoaffective schizophrenia. J Clin Psychiatry 1982;43:252.
141. Bezchlinbnyk KZ, Jeffries JJ Should psychiatric patients drink coffee? Can Med Assoc 1981;124:357.
142. Kulhanek F, Linde OK, Meisenberg G. Precipitation of antipsychotic drugs in interaction with coffee or tea (Letter to Editor). Lancet 1979;ii:1130.
143. Bowen S, Taylor KM, Gibb IA. Effect of coffee and tea on blood levels and efficacy of antipsychotic drugs. Lancet 1981;i:1217.
144. Fast DK, Jones BD, Kusalic M et al. Effect of carbamazepine on neuroleptic plasma levels and efficacy. Am J Psychiatry 1986;143:117.
145. Jefferson JW, Greist JH, Baudhuin M. Lithium: interactions with other drugs. J Clin Psychopharmacol 1981;1:124.
146. Bond WS, Carvalho M, Foulks EF. Persistent dysarthria with apraxia associated with a combination of lithium carbonate and haloperidol. J Clin Psychiatry 1982;43:256.
147. Thornton WE. Dementia induced by methyldopa with haloperidol. N Engl J Med 1976;27:1222.
148. Gram LF, Christiansen J, Overo KF. Interaction between neuroleptics and tricyclic antidepressants In: Morselli PL, Garranttini S, Cohen SN, eds. Drug Interaction. New York: Raven Press, 1974;271.
149. Kutt H, McDowell F. Management of epilepsy with diphenylhydantoin sodium. J Am Med Assoc 1968;203:969.
150. Linnoila M, Viukari M, Vaisanen K et al. Effect of anticonvulsants on plasma haloperidol and thioridazine levels. Am J Psychiatry 1980;137:819.
151. Pantuck EJ, Pantuck CB, Anderson KE et al. Cigarette smoking and chlorpromazine disposition and actions. Clin Pharmacol Ther 1982;31:533.
152. Sramek J, Herrera J, Roy S et al. An analysis of steady-state chlorpromazine plasma levels in the clinical setting. J Clin Psychopharmacol 1987;7:117.
153. Sher PP. Drug interferences with clinical laboratory tests. Drugs 1982;24:24.
154. Levinson DF, Simpson GM, Singh H. Fluphenazine dose, clinical response and extrapyramidal symptoms. Arch Gen Psychiatry 1990;47:761.
155. Simpson GM, Varga E. Clozapine—a new antipsychotic agent. Curr Ther Res 1974;16:679—686.
156. Marder SR, Meibach RC. Risperidone in the treatment of schizophrenia. Am J Psychiatry 1994;151:825—835.
157. Jansen PAJ, Niemegeers CJE, Awouters F et al. Pharmacology of risperidone (R64766), a new antipsychotic with serotonin S2 and dopamine D2 antagonistic properties. J Pharmacol Exp Ther 1988;244:685—693.
158. Bredbacka PE, Paukkala E, Kinnunen E, Koponen H. Can cardiorespiratory dysregulation induced by clozapine monotherapy be predicted? Int Clin Psychopharmacol 1993;8:205—206.
159. Mehtonen O-P, Aranko, K, Malkonen L, Vapaatalo H. A survey of sudden death associated with the use of antipsychotic or antidepressnat drugs. Acta Psychiat Scand 1991;84:58—64.
160. Wilt JL, Minnema AM, Johnsons RF, Rosenblum AM. Torsades de pointes associated with the use of intravenous haloperidol. Ann Intern Med 1993;119:391—394.
161. Eitan N, Levin Y, Ben-Artzi E, Levy A, Neumann M. Effects of antipsychotic drugs on memory functions of schizophrenic patients. Acta Psychiat Scand 1992;85:74—76.
162. Farde L, Nordstrom A-L, Wiesel F-A, Pauli S, Halldin C, Sedvall G. Positron emission tomographic analysis of central D1 and D2 dopamine receptor occupancy in patients treated with classical neuroleptics and clozapine. Relation to extrapyramidal side effects. Arch Gen Psychiatry 1992; 49:538—544.
163. Nordstrom A-L, Farde L, Wiesel F-A, Forslund K, Pauli, S, Halldin, C, Uppfeldt G. Central D2 dopamine receptor occupancy in relation to antipsychotic drug effects: a double-blind PET study of schizophrenic patients. Biol Psychiat 1992;33:227—235.
164. Angust JW, Simpson, GM. Hysteria and drug-induced dystonia. Acta Psychiat Scand (Suppl) 1970;212:52—58.
165. Morgenestern H, Glazer WM. Identifying risk factors for tardive dyskinesia among long-term outpatients maintained with neuroleptic medications. Results of the Yale Tardive Dyskinesia Study. Arch Gen Psychiatry 1993; 50:723—733.
166. Jeste DV, Caliguri MP, Paulsen JS, Heaton RK, Lacro JP, Harris MJ, Bailey A, Fell RL, McAdams LA. Risk of tardive dyskinesia in older patients: A prospective longitudinal study of 266 outpatients. Arch Gen Psychiatry 1995;52:756—765.
167. Pi EH, Gutierrez MA, Gray GE. Cross-cultural studies in tardive dyskinesia. Am J Psychiatry 1993;150:991.
168. Pi EH, Gutierrez, MA, Gray GE. Tardive dyskinesia: cross-cultural perspective. In: Lin KM et al, eds. Psychopharmacology and Psychobiology of Ethnicity. American Psychiatric Press Inc, 1993;153—167.
169. Kane JM, Woerner MG, Pollack S, Safferman AZ, Lieberman JA. Does clozapine cause tardive dyskinesia? J Clin Psychiatry 1993;54:327—330.
170. Woerner MG, Saltzl BL, Kane JM, Lieberman JA, Alvir JMJ Diabetes and development of tardive dyskinesia. Am J Psychiatry 1993;150:966—968.
171. Marder SR, Van Putten T, Mintz J, Lebell M, McKenzie J, May PRA. Low- and conventional dose maintainance therapy with fluphenazine decanoate. Two-year outcome. Arch Gen Psychiatry 1987;44:518—521.
172. Reddig S, Minnema AM, Tandon R. Neuroleptic malignant syndrome and clozapine. Ann Clin Psychiatry 1993;5:25—27.
173. Phillips P, Shraberg D, Weitzel WD. Hirsutism associated with long-term phenothiazine neuroleptic therapy. J Am Med Assoc 1979;241:920—921.
174. Kendra JR, Rugman FP, Flaherty TA, Myers A, Horsfield N, Barton A, Russell L. First use of G-CSF in chlorpromazine-induced agranulocytosis: report of two cases. Postgrad Med J 1993;69:885—887.
175. Alvir, JM, Lieberman JA, Safferman AZ, Schwimmer JL, Schaaf JA. Clozapine induced agranulocytosis. Incidence and risk factors in the United States. New Engl J Med 1993;329:162—167.
176. Larrey D, Lainey E, Blanc P, Diaz D, David R, Biaggi A, Barneon G, Bottai T, Potet F, Michel H. Acute colitis associated with prolonged administration of neuroleptics. J Clin Gastroenterol 1992;14:64—67.
177. Ekblom B, Eriksson K, Lindstrom LH. Supersensitivity psychosis in schizophrenic patients after sudden clozapine withdrawal. Psychopharmacology 1984;83:293—294.
178. Perenyi A, Kuncz E, Bagdy G. Early relapse after sudden withdrawal or dose reduction of clozapine. Psychopharmacology 1985;86:244.
179. Eklund K. Supersensitivity and clozapine withdrawal. Psychopharmacology 1987;91:135.

180. Liebermnan JA, Kane JM, Johns CA. Clozapine: guidelines for clinical management. J Clin Psychiatry 1989; 50:329–338.
181. DeLeon J, Stanilla JK, White AO, Simpson GM. Anticholinergics to treat clozapine withdrawal. J Clin Psychiatry 1994;55:3.
182. Cobb CD, Anderson CB, Seidel, DR. Possible interaction between clozapine and lorazepam. Am J Psychiatry 1991;148:1606–1607.
183. Waddington JL. Some pharmacological aspects relating to the issue of possible neurotoxic interactions during combined lithium-neuroleptic therapy. Hum Psychopharmacol 1990;5:293–297.
184. Batchelor DH, Lowe MR. Reported neurotoxicity with the lithium/haloperidol combination and other neuroleptics. A literature review. Hum Psychopharmacol 1990;5:275–280.

Meyler's Side Effects of Drugs, 13th Edition
M.N.G. Dukes, editor

SECTION EDITOR: M.N.G. DUKES

M.N.G. Dukes

7 Anticonvulsants

COMPLICATIONS OF ANTICONVULSANT THERAPY AS SUCH

Complications during treatment with anticonvulsants or antiepileptic drugs may be specific to particular drugs (such as gingival hyperplasia induced by phenytoin or connective tissue disorders induced by barbiturates). More commonly, however, identical or similar side effects are shared by several antiepileptic drugs, e.g. hypersensitivity reactions. In addition, complications during treatment may be an expression of an interaction between an antiepileptic drug and the epilepsy itself or underlying conditions; this may well apply to second-generation effects and cognitive dysfunction; sometimes such a supposed 'adverse effect' may be *entirely* due to the pathological condition and not to the drug at all.

The problems most commonly seen during treatment with antiepileptic drugs as a group are dose-related, mild and transient neurological side effects, such as cerebello-vestibular or oculomotor dysfunction, but systemic toxicity can affect any organ or system.

Second-generation effects The conclusions advanced in many earlier volumes in this series still apply; the incidence of congenital anomalies among babies born to epileptic women is 2—3 times higher than in the healthy population. The disease itself, either in the mother or the father is partly to blame (a point to which we return below) but the incidence is nevertheless somewhat higher in epileptic mothers who have received anticonvulsants during pregnancy than in those untreated.

None of the major anticonvulsants—phenytoin, carbamazepine, valproate and phenobarbital—is to be regarded as free from teratogenic effects, and no one drug is clearly safer than any other in this regard. For a time it was believed that sodium valproate might be relatively safe, but it proves to be associated with congenital malformations similar to those ascribed to the other anticonvulsants, namely *neural tube defects* (1[c]), *congenital heart lesions*, *digital anomalies* and *oral clefts*; the incidence of spina bifida with carbamazepine has been estimated at 1% (SEDA-16, 72). Incidentally, a congenital rib anomaly and an optic nerve hyperplasia have been described with this drug (ibid). Phenytoin has been found to produce a high incidence of hypoplastic nails in the infant, especially if serum phenytoin concentrations in the mother have been high (1a[C]) (Table 1).

Pregnant epileptic women having anticonvulsant treatment should be told that there is a 90% chance of having a normal child and that maternal serum α-fetoprotein, uterine ultrasonography and diagnostic amniocentesis may be used to help in detecting any fetal abnormalities.

In addition to major structural malformations a number of mostly craniofacial dysmorphic features, notably *growth retardation*, *microcephaly*, *and mental retardation* have been described as comprising a '*fetal antiepileptic drug syndrome*' (Table 1). This syndrome, originally attributed only to hydantoin, and at one time indeed known as the 'fetal hydantoin syndrome', has since been observed in children exposed to phenytoin, carbamazepine, primidone and valproate. A broad range of signs is observed in at most 5—10% of children exposed to these drugs in utero, but individual signs noted in Table 1, e.g. hypertelorism, are observed in as many as 52%, and digital hypoplasia in 23% of exposed children. Few results from controlled studies are available, and the selection criteria and methods of ascertainment are normally not fully agreed (2[R]); one regularly encounters new phenomena which tend to be grouped under this heading with little justification, e.g. rare case of holoprosencephaly described in 1993 (SEDA-18, 60). Certainly there seem to be differences between the various anticonvulsant drugs as regards the pattern of defects induced, but since these vary from case to case, even with the same drug, exact comparisons are not possible. In one prospective study the association between prenatal phenytoin exposure and digital hypoplasia or hypertelorism was confirmed, but in fact none of the exposed children exhibited, at the age of 5.5 years, all of the main characteristics of the hydantoin syndrome. The risk of developmental disturbances seemed to be lower than the 7—11% risk of fetal hydantoin syndrome reported earlier (3[CR]).

Table 1. *Anomalies in the fetal anticonvulsant syndrome*

Growth and performance
Motor or mental deficiency
Microcephaly
Prenatal growth deficiency
Postnatal growth deficiency
Craniofacial
Short nose with low nasal bridge
Hypertelorism
Epicanthic folds
Ptosis of eyelid
Strabismus
Low-set and/or abnormal ears
Wide mouth
Prominent lips
Cleft palate
Metopic sutural ridging
Wide fontanelles
Limbs
Hypoplasia of nails and distal phalanges
Fingerlike thumb
Abnormal palmar creases
Five or more digital arches
Other
Short or webbed neck, low hairline
Coarse hair
Widely spaced, hypoplastic nipples
Rib, sternal or spinal anomalies
Hernias
Undescended testes

A further factor complicating comparisons is dosage and the common use of multiple drug regimes. It has been suggested that high doses of antiepileptic drugs, especially as part of multiple drug therapy (and particularly if this includes valproate) may carry particular risks for the fetus (SED-12, 123). In one small series of meningomyoceles and dysmorphic features associated with valproate, the risk and severity seemed to be greater where a benzodiazepine had also been taken (4^{C}).

Neither epilepsy nor prenatal exposure to antiepileptic drugs have been found to be associated with an increased risk of *spontaneous abortion* (5^{R}).

Based on a case history of *fetal hemorrhage* attributed to maternal antiepileptic drug treatment, and a review of other relevant papers, it has been authoritatively recommended that epileptic mothers receive vitamin K tablets throughout the month before delivery and intravenously during labour (6^{R}). Blood specimens should be taken for immediate clotting tests and if a diminution is found in vitamin K-dependent factors, fresh frozen plasma should be administered. The right approach may need yet further evaluation, since a recent controlled study shows that while vitamin K deficiency is common in newborn infants exposed to these drugs in utero their mothers rarely show such a deficiency (SEDA-18, 60—61).

Mechanisms, risk factors and prophylaxis It has long been suspected that anticonvulsants exert their teratogenic effect by inducing folate deficiency, and there is some retrospective and prospective work which supports this belief. Any folate deficiency found in the mother should certainly be corrected. A further theory has attributed the teratogenicity of hydantoin to epoxide metabolites of the drugs; this now seems unlikely, though there is evidence that a genetic defect in arene oxide detoxification can increase the risk of major birth defects (SED-12, 123). An enzymatic marker (epoxide hydroxylase) may perhaps prove useful in identifying infants who are at greater risk than others of teratogenic effects from anticonvulsants (7^{c}).

Although one repeatedly encounters convincing evidence, touched on above, that epilepsy itself is responsible for some congenital defects irrespective of whether drugs have been taken or not, there is much difficulty in arriving at the absolute truth. No physician will, after all, deliberately withhold drugs from women who need them in order to conduct a perfectly designed comparative study. If one relies on retrospective experience, it is clear that those epileptic women who did not receive drugs are likely to have been those in whom the condition is relatively mild, thus distorting the findings. Work continues in the hope of solving these puzzles.

The possible influence of epilepsy-related factors on the rate of facial clefts and congenital malformations in children of epileptic parents has several times been evaluated. The data suggest a joint effect of the disease and the drugs, the latter eliciting a latent tendency in epileptic populations to this type of defect. On the other hand, no genetic element was found as regards the occurrence of congenital heart defects in the children of epileptic families. A further complicating factor could be exerted by the occurrence of seizures during pregnancy, e.g. interfering with fetal blood supply; although this has been contested (8^{c}). One, a prospective study published in 1990, does seem to show that seizures during pregnancy impair the subsequent cognitive ability and psychomotor function of the child (SEDA-16, 70).

Physical and mental development Quite apart from evident physical congenital defects, the possibility has been raised that a child seemingly normal at birth might as a result of exposure to anticonvulsants later show impaired physical or mental development. Postnatal growth and the appearance of mental deficiency have been compared in children of epileptic mothers not exposed to antiepileptic drugs and in non-epileptic controls. Delays in height and weight gain were detected in the epileptic series after the first postnatal month, but weight at 5.5 years of age was not affected. A reduced mean head circumference without obvious intellectual impairment was found in children exposed to single drug therapy with carbamazepine and barbiturates. A lesser parental mean head circumference in the epileptic series as a whole was however a major confounding factor (9[C]). This type of prospective work on mental development however continues to show how difficult it can be to draw meaningful conclusions; in all probability, the incidence of mental deficiency in children of epileptic mothers is similar to that in the general population, though general intelligence may be lower and specific forms of cognitive dysfunction somewhat more frequent, irrespective of whether drugs have been used or not.

Hepatotoxicity Virtually all of the major antiepileptic drugs can cause hepatotoxicity, although a fatal outcome is rare. Liver enzymes are increased up to 3 times the normal limit in up to 40% of patients treated with major antiepileptic drugs without any additional laboratory or clinical evidence for overt hepatic disease. Hepatic disease may occur as part of a hypersensitivity reaction with skin rashes and fever in the early weeks of treatment with phenytoin, carbamazepine, phenobarbital and primidone. For valproate a hepatic hypersensitivity reaction has not been described. In addition, hepatic disease may rarely develop after many years of treatment with phenytoin, carbamazepine, phenobarbital or primidone without any signs of hypersensitivity. Once hepatotoxicity develops, mortality rates are 10–38% with phenytoin and some 25% for carbamazepine (10[C]). Histological examination often reveals granulomatous hepatitis. Elderly patients may be at a higher risk (11[CR]), although risk factors are not firmly established. The factors determining a fatal outcome have been more clearly defined; it is most likely to ensue in children under the age of 2 years who are receiving several antiepileptic drugs and have additional handicaps. As compared with other antiepileptic drugs, valproate given alone seems least likely to lead to fatal liver damage, at least in adults (12[R]). However, as noted later in this chapter, valproate can induce carnitine deficiency, and this has been suggested as a reason for the (usually mild) hepatic effects which it does exert.

Endocrine, metabolic Most anticonvulsant drugs interfere to some extent with endocrine function, but actual clinical symptoms of endocrine dysfunction seldom result. Phenytoin inhibits the release of *antidiuretic hormone* (*ADH*) (13[C]), but this does not result in any clinical derangement. However, hyponatremia, reduced plasma osmolality and water intoxication due to inappropriate secretion of ADH are well-known dose-related effects of carbamazepine and its keto-analog, oxcarbazepine.

Franceschi et al. (14[CR]) evaluated the effects of long-term anticonvulsant treatment on hypothalamic-pituitary function in patients with epilepsy of mild to moderate severity. The *growth hormone* secretion response to levodopa stimulation was not affected by carbamazepine or phenobarbital, whereas phenytoin and anticonvulsant polytherapy induced an increase in the GH level and valproate a decrease at varying times after the administration of levodopa. In epileptic men, carbamazepine, phenobarbital, phenytoin and anticonvulsant polytherapy increased both basal and stimulated levels of *prolactin*, whereas valproate did not.

Masala et al. (15[C]) found that in boys treated with phenobarbital the baseline concentrations of *luteinizing hormone* and *follicle-stimulating hormone* were reduced as well as their response to stimulation with the releasing hormone. Baseline prolactin concentration was raised in comparison with normal children and the response of prolactin levels to stimulation was impaired.

Franceschi's work, cited above, concluded that neither phenytoin, valproate, carbamazepine or phenobarbital alone nor anticonvulsant multi-drug therapy significantly changed the circadian *ACTH/cortisol* rhythm in epileptic patients. However, γ-aminobutyric acid (GABA) and valproate do inhibit corticotrophin-releasing factor and thus depress corticotrophin levels, and valproate has actually been used in the treatment of Nelson's syndrome (16[C]). Kritzler et al. (17[C]) found reduced basal ACTH levels in seven children on long-term treatment with valproate, while Ostrowska et al. found that serum concentrations of progesterone and cortisol and the excretion of 17-hydroxycorticosteroid were lower in untreated patients with epilepsy, and further decreased during treatment with phenytoin (18[C]).

Total and free *thyroxine* as well as *tri-iodothyronine* decrease during treatment with phenytoin and carbamazepine, but thyroid-stimulating hormone remains normal or slightly increased (19[C]). The normal level of the latter could indicate some pituitary dysfunction; however, the main reason for the reduction in the thyroid hormone levels is their increased hepatic metabolism due to liver enzyme induction. Hypothyroidism has been described in some patients who may actually require thyroxine replacement therapy as a result of treatment with phenytoin or carbamazepine (20[C]). In contrast to earlier reports Isojärvi (21[C]) found no changes in thyroid hormones during treatment with valproate.

Effects on sex hormones are several and somewhat contradictory. Bound serum *testosterone* increases during treatment with phenytoin, carbamazepine, phenobarbital and primidone due to the increased synthesis of the specific transport protein, sex hormone-binding globulin (SED-12, 124). The metabolic clearance of testosterone is also reduced (SEDA-16, 70). Clinically, Toone et al. (22[C]) found that sexual activity appeared to be reduced, while mean plasma levels of LH, FSH, PRL and SHBG were elevated in 27 epileptic patients on anticonvulsant therapy (phenytoin, primidone, phenobarbital or combinations of these) as compared with controls. The decreased sexual activity often complained of (and possibly impotence, as reported anecdotally) may be related to the decrease in free testosterone or its increased breakdown under the influence of these enzyme-inducing anticonvulsants. Since then, MacPhee's group have recommended choosing valproate for epileptic patients with dysfunctional libido or impotence because it apparently does not reduce free hormone concentrations in the blood (23[R]).

Effects on *sex hormones in women* of fertile age run somewhat parallel to those in men, at least if a study of carbamazepine is representative. The concentration of sex hormone-binding globulin increases while those of dihydroepiandrosterone and the free androgen index fall. These changes persist. In contrast, the reduction observed in pituitary responsiveness and in serum basal LH concentration are transitory. The serum progesterone concentrations fall only after long-term treatment (23a[C]).

Phenytoin and carbamazepine increase free serum *cortisol* (24[c]), but no cases with the clinical features of Cushing's syndrome have been described. As noted above, valproate inhibits corticotrophin-releasing factor and this can reduce serum cortisol.

Valproate therapy is often associated with decreased *carnitine* concentration and occasionally with true carnitine deficiency, especially in young children with neurological disabilities taking several antiepileptic drugs. Carnitine measurement and supplementation may be useful in patients with symptoms and signs suggestive of carnitine deficiency.

Phenytoin intoxication may produce *hyperglycemia* (SED-10, 112). A decrease in the insulin response to glucose has been noted during long-term treatment with therapeutic doses of phenytoin, but glucose intolerance does not arise, probably due to a concomitant increase in sensitivity to the effect of insulin.

Effects on calcium and bone Significant reductions in serum calcium and phosphate and an increase in serum alkaline phosphatase may be found in up to 50% of adult patients treated for epilepsy. It has been suggested that these changes are caused by a disturbance of hepatic hydroxylation of vitamin D_3 to 25-hydroxycholecalciferol (25-OH-D), which is the immediate precursor of 1,25-dihydroxycholecalciferol, the active form of vitamin D on bone and intestine. Increased excretion of both 25-OH-D and 1,25-$(OH)_2$D has also been incriminated, and it has also been suggested with some evidence that these drugs interfere with the action of 1,25-$(OH)_2$D on bone and/or that induction of hepatic enzymes is involved (SEDA-16, 71). Whatever the mechanism, a periodic check on serum calcium, phosphate and alkaline phosphatase levels should be kept on patients at increased risk for anticonvulsant osteomalacia, e.g. as a result of low vitamin D intake, inactivity, or lack of exposure to sunlight in institutionalized handicapped children (25[R]). The risk of age-related fractures in patients with epilepsy is not greatly increased by long-term use of antiepileptic drugs (26[C]). There is now evidence that treatment with cholecalciferol may be useful (SEDA-16, 70).

Mineral, fluid balance Immunoreactive *parathyroid hormone* concentrations were found to be increased during anticonvulsant treatment while bone mineral content was reduced. Hypocalcemia and osteopenia occurred in spite of normal mean levels of serum 25-OH-D and 1,25-$(OH)_2$D, suggesting that the hypocalcemia was independent of the effect of the drugs on vitamin D metabolism. Bone biopsies showed increased osteoid but normal calcification front formation, an accelerated rate of mineralization and a decreased mineralization lag time, suggesting increased skeletal turnover rather than osteomalacia (27[R]).

Cholesterol and lipids Anticonvulsant treatment, perhaps of any type, produces changes in blood lipids (SEDA-5, 59), but like many other metabolic effects it is not at all clear that these are clinically of significance. The effect of three drugs were compared in 1991 by Calandre et al. in 101 epileptic patients with matched controls. Patients on valproate had lower total and LDL cholesterol than controls; with carbamazepine there were higher levels of HDL cholesterol and apolipoprotein A; patients on phenobarbital had higher concentrations of total and HDL cholesterol and of apolipoproteins A and B. The total/HDL cholesterol ratio was significantly lower than control values with valproate and carbamazepine but not with phenobarbital. Remarkably, the changes did not correlate with drug concentrations or the duration of treatment (27a[Cr]). It is not clear that all these effects persist as treatment continues (*see carbamazepine monograph below*).

Nervous system (*see Table* 2) Most major anticonvulsants, including valproate, can produce, albeit rarely, a reversible subacute or chronic *encephalopathy* consisting of neurological dysfunction, mostly cerebellove-

Table 2. *'Neuropsychiatric toxicity' of anticonvulsant drugs*

Toxicity	Drug
Peripheral neuropathy	Carbamazepine
	Phenobarbital
	Phenytoin
	Primidone
Cerebellar ataxia	Barbiturates (?)
	Phenytoin
Involuntary movements	
Dystonia	Carbamazepine
	Phenytoin
Asterixis	Carbamazepine
	Barbiturates
	Phenytoin
Parkinsonism	Phenytoin
	Valproate
Tremor	Valproate
Behavioral disorders	Barbiturates
	Benzodiazepines
	Carbamazepine (?)
	Ethosuximide
	Phenytoin
	Valproate
Impaired cognitive function	Barbiturates
	Benzodiazepines (clobazam < clonazepam)
	Carbamazepine
	Phenytoin
	Valproate

stibular and oculomotor disturbances with diplopia, nystagmus and oscillopsia; much less commonly one observes dyskinesia, parkinsonism, monoplegia, Babinski reflexes, exacerbation of seizures, CSF protein and slowing of EEC activity. In addition, cognitive function and mood are usually impaired and may even be the predominant finding. Uncommon neurological side effects include dysfunction of the optic nerve and retinal disorders induced by phenytoin and carbamazepine, as revealed by color vision defects and increased glare sensitivity (28[C]). Carbamazepine has induced non-epileptic *myoclonus* in a body with benign occipital epilepsy (29[C]).

Restless legs were observed in patients with epilepsy taking phenytoin and methsuximide and subsided with a change of antiepileptic treatment or reduction in the dose (SED-12, 125). Experimental or clinical evidence of *polyneuropathy*, commonly with paresthesia, was found in 53% of a series of patients treated for at least 6 months with carbamazepine, phenytoin, phenobarbital and/or valproate (SEDA-18, 60), and a more specific study has provided evidence that both carbamazepine and phenobarbital are toxic to peripheral nerve fibres (SEDA-17, 72).

Patients with existing movement disorders may develop *tics* (30[C]) when treated with anticonvulsant drugs and in rare cases *parkinsonism* may develop. Four cases of reversible parkinsonism have been described during treatment with valproate (31[C]). Reversible *pseudoatrophy of the brain* has been observed with valproate monotherapy (32[C]).

Phenytoin even, at plasma concentrations below 20 μg/ml, has been associated with *worsening of cerebellar ataxia* and *exacerbation of seizures* in patients with Baltic myoclonic epilepsy (33[C]), and the drug should be avoided in patients with this condition.

Effects on cognitive function Cognitive dysfunction in patients with epilepsy may be influenced by many factors other than drugs; they include the duration, frequency and etiology of the disease, the type of seizure, hereditary factors and psychosocial influences. The cognitive effects of antiepileptic drugs will naturally be less if doses are kept as low as possible (e.g. with valproate less than 20 mg/day) and if a single drug is used rather than multiple drug treatment.

Carbamazepine and phenytoin have similar neuropsychological effects, with impairment of memory and of psychomotor performance (SEDA-16, 70). Increasing concentrations of carbamazepine and its active metabolite, carbamazepine-10,11-epoxide, were found to be correlated with decreasing psychomotor and cognitive function in epileptic patients (34[C]).

Cognitive side effects, especially impairment of memory and visual information processing, improve when patients are transferred from conventional to controlled-release preparations of carbamazepine (35[C]).

Subtle differences may exist in this respect between phenytoin, carbamazepine, phenobarbital and primidone, but controlled trials however, found no major differences between them. It is possible that valproate does have less effect on cognitive function, but this needs confirming in work on a larger scale (36[C]).

Phenytoin, phenobarbital and possibly carbamazepine may produce a usually mild, distal motor-sensory *peripheral neuropathy* (37[C]). Folate therapy seemed to reverse the abnormalities in sensory and motor nerve distal latencies. It is not known whether the neuropathy is progressive, but isolated case reports have claimed resolution after stopping treatment. Permanent neuropathy due to phenytoin (and perhaps barbiturates) may result from prolonged or repeated episodes of intoxication or folate deficiency. The predominant electrophysiological change in patients taking phenytoin in therapeutic doses has been found to be a reduction in the amplitude of sensory nerve action potential with

Table 3. *Adverse dermatological effects of individual anticonvulsants (115[R])*

	Pheny-toin	Mepheny-toin	Phenobar-bital	Primidone	Carbama-zepine	Valproic acid	Ethosuxi-mide	Lamo-trigine
Exanthemas	+		+		+	+	+	+
Exfoliative dermatitis	+		+	+	+		+	+
Stevens-Johnson syndrome	+	+	+	+	+		+	+
Lyell syndrome	+	+	+	+	+			
Dermatomyositis	+		+	+	+		+	
Erythema nodosum			+					
Pigmentation	+	+						
Hair alterations	+	+				+		
Acne	+		+	+				

relative preservation of the conduction velocity. This contrasts with the moderate slowing of sensory nerve conduction velocity among patients with phenytoin toxicity.

Mechanisms It is possible, according to experimental work from Japan, that some of the effects of anticonvulsants on the nervous system result from an impaired blood flow to the brain (37a[r]).

Urinary system There is laboratory test evidence that valproate (and to a lesser degree carbamazepine) increases excretion of NAG (*N*-acetyl-β-glucosaminidase) which is a marker of renal tubular integrity. This could be a harmless physiological response to the drugs without clinical significance (SEDA-18, 60).

Skin and appendages *All* major anticonvulsants have adverse effects on the skin (Table 3). Valproic acid has not been reported to induce exfoliative dermatitis, Stevens-Johnson syndrome or Lyell syndrome. Plasmapheresis has recently been recommended for the emergency treatment of patients with Lyell syndrome as a side effect of these drugs (38[C]). Patients receiving cranial irradiation and phenytoin may be at increased risk for developing Stevens-Johnson syndrome and Lyell syndrome.

Withdrawal effects Recent data argue against the occurrence of withdrawal seizures and suggest that worsening of seizures following discontinuation of phenytoin, carbamazepine, phenobarbital or valproic acid in patients with persistent seizures receiving several antiepileptic drugs more probably reflects loss of therapeutic drug effects than a true abstinence phenomenon (39[C]).

Antiepileptic drug intoxication Antiepileptic drug intoxication in epileptic patients may be entirely unexpected and unexplained (41%) but some cases are due to inappropriate self-adjustment of dosage (34%), suicide attempts (18%), inappropriate caretaker dose adjustment (9%), accidental ingestion (8%), drug interaction (6%), or intercurrent illness (2%) (40[C]). Most patients exhibit oculomotor and vestibulocerebellar dysfunction.

Drug interactions Tables 4 and 5 list the drugs which are currently known to increase or reduce the effects of anticonvulsants by affecting their blood levels. In addition, some of their effects (notably sedation) may be increased by other drugs having similar properties, and in various respects (see monographs) the various anticonvulsants can potentiate one another's effects. Table 6 lists those drugs the effects of which can be reduced by anticonvulsants.

HYDANTOIN DERIVATIVES

Phenytoin

ADVERSE REACTION PATTERN

General and toxic reactions Phenytoin induces vestibulo-cerebellar, oculomotor and cognitive dysfunction. Gingival hyperplasia and hirsutism are frequent. Retinal, movement and peripheral nerve disorders and endocrine changes are uncommon. Interstitial nephritis, interstitial pneumonia or hepatic injury are rarely observed. High intravenous doses are cardiotoxic.

Hypersensitivity reactions Phenytoin produces a hypersensitivity syndrome which ranges from exanthema and fever to life-threatening Stevens-Johnson syndrome and Lyell syndrome with mucosal involvement and bullous exanthema. Hepatic, cardiac, muscular, pulmonary, hematological, reticuloendothelial and renal involvement may occur. Systemic lupus erythematosus may be in-

Table 4. *Drugs which increase the blood levels of anticonvulsants*

Anticonvulsant affected	Drugs responsible
Phenytoin	Acetazolamide
	Azapropazone
	Chloramphenicol
	Chlorpheniramine
	Cimetidine
	Clobazam
	Co-trimoxazole
	Dextropropoxyphene
	Dicoumarol
	Disulfiram
	Isoniazid
	Miconazole
	Metronidazole
	Phenylbutazone
	Phenothiazines
	Sulfaphenazole
	Sulfinpyrazone
	Sultiame
	Viloxazine
Phenobarbital	Phenytoin
Primidone	Valproate
Ethosuximide	Phenytoin
	Valproate
Lamotrigine	Valproate
Clonazepam	Cimetidine
Carbamazepine	Cimetidine
	Danazol
	Erythromycin
	Denzimole
	Dextropropoxyphene
	Diltiazem
	Fluvoxamine
	Isoniazid
	Lamotrigine
	Triacetyloleandomycin
	Valnactamide
	Valpromide
	Verapamil

duced. In children, serum IgA concentrations often fall.

Tumor-inducing effects Neuroblastoma has been reported in single cases in possible association with the fetal hydantoin syndrome. Phenytoin can induce pseudolymphoma and, very exceptionally, a condition closely resembling malignant lymphoma. The finding of (reversible) spleen enlargement containing solid lesions in one elderly patient has led to the suggestion that this may have occurred in other cases as well but have been missed before the advent of computed tomography (40a[C]).

Table 5. *Drugs which reduce the blood levels of anticonvulsants*

Anticonvulsant affected	Drugs responsible
Phenytoin	Carbamazepine
	Dichloralphenazone
	Folic acid
	Phenobarbital
	Primidone
	Vigabatrin
	Viloxazine
Carbamazepine	Phenobarbital
	Phenytoin
	Primidone
Ethosuximide	Carbamazepine
Clonazepam	Carbamazepine
	Phenobarbital
	Phenytoin
	Primidone
Lamotrigine	Carbamazepine
	Phenobarbital
	Phenytoin
Valproate	Carbamazepine
	Phenobarbital
	Phenytoin

ORGANS AND SYSTEMS

General It should be borne in mind that laboratory findings regarding total serum concentrations may be misleading in cases where plasma protein binding is impaired; despite a 'normal' total figure, the free phenytoin may be in the toxic range (SEDA-18, 67–68; 40b[c]).

Cardiovascular Intravenous phenytoin can be cardiotoxic, but oral phenytoin, by elevating serum high density lipoprotein, may in the long run be cardioprotective since high-density lipoprotein is inversely related to the risk of coronary artery disease (41[R]). Fatal *cardiovascular collapse* has been reported in two cases after manual infusion of phenytoin in total doses of 500 and 880 mg, respectively, at a rate of 35 mg/min. The authors concluded that the phenytoin concentration was too high (42[C]).

Taliercio et al. (43[C]) described a case of *hypersensitivity myocarditis* which was probably initiated by phenytoin. Carbamazepine may also have been a contributing factor in this case. The mechanism of the reaction was postulated to be delayed hypersensitivity.

Extravasation of intravenously injected phenytoin can cause serious damage, including tissue necrosis, even demanding amputation (43a[C]).

Table 6. *Drugs affected by anticonvulsants*

Anticonvulsant responsible	Drug whose effect is reduced
Phenytoin	Busulfan Corticosteroids Cyclosporin Digitoxin Doxycycline Metronidazole Metyrapone Mexiletine Oral contraceptives Quinidine Thyroxine Warfarin (may be increased or reduced)
Phenobarbital	Chenodeoxycholic acid Cyclosporin Theophylline
Primidone	Corticosteroids Coumarin anticoagulants Digitoxin Doxycycline Griseofulvin Metronidazole Oral contraceptives Phenothiazines Quinidine Tricyclic antidepressants
Carbamazepine	Corticosteroids Cyclosporin Coumarin anticoagulants Doxycycline Haloperidol Oral contraceptives Vecuronium
Oxcarbazepine	Oral contraceptives Felodipine
Phenytoin + carbamazepine or phenobarbital	Mianserin

Respiratory *Interstitial pneumonitis* is extremely rare. This hypersensitivity syndrome responds to stopping phenytoin treatment and to use of corticosteroids.

Nervous system As noted in the introductory section and Table 2, phenytoin can induce a range of psychiatric and neurological disorders. A common effect is horizontal *nystagmus* on lateral gaze, but severe intoxication may occasionally produce upbeat, downbeat nystagmus or periodic alternating forms of nystagmus. Uncommon are reversible *mono- or hemiplegia*, *reversible spastic rigidity*, *hyperreflexia* and *clonus*, *hyperkinetic disorders*, *choreoathetosis*, *hemiballism*, *hemichoreiform movements*, *local dystonia in the foot*, *generalized myoclonus*, and reversible *parkinsonism*.

Phenytoin *encephalopathy* may occur with or without dyskinesia or focal neurological deficit, nystagmus or ataxia; the frequency of seizures may increase progressively, and the electroencephalogram may show paroxysmal activity and slowing. Phenytoin may rarely induce *cerebellar degeneration* (44[C]). Patients at risk are those with uncorrected prolonged oculo-cerebellar toxic signs, with prolonged status epilepticus, a history of multiple electroshock treatment or suffering from a hypoxic-ischemic encephalopathy. In one study, cerebellar atrophy, which does not necessarily produce clinical cerebellar symptoms, was found to be significantly correlated with both the duration of the epilepsy and the total amount of phenytoin ingested during the patient's lifetime (45[C]).

Pre-existing *myasthenia gravis* may be aggravated by phenytoin. possibly because of its neuropathogenic effects (SEDA-7, 78).

It is important to realize that the susceptibility to neurological complications of the type described above and in Table 2 may be much greater if the patient has an organic brain disorder. Haider and Abbott (45a[C]) described in 1990 a woman of 54 with a frontal glioma who received a normal loading dose; at phenytoin serum levels of only 12 mg/l she developed choreoathetoid movements, bizarre speech and mental confusion, resolving within 24 hours of withdrawing the drug.

Endocrine, metabolic Reduced blood *thiamine* levels and very occasional *hyperglycemia* have been reported.

Serum high-density lipoprotein *cholesterol* levels are raised by phenytoin treatment (46[C]), probably through changes in endogenous triglyceride metabolism. Phenytoin also produces an increase in serum triglyceride and cholesterol levels via its effect on hepatic lipid metabolism (47[C]).

It was known as early as 1971 that phenytoin could cause hyperglycemia, and at that time evidence was advanced that this might involve inhibition of insulin release. Occasional cases are still being reported, alongside evidence from cell cultures that the drug might induce a post-binding defect in the action of insulin (47[a]).

Hematological Combined use of cimetidine and phenytoin led to severe *thrombocytopenia* in just four of 1512 neurosurgical patients; there was severe megakaryocyte depression in the bone marrow (48[C]). Phenytoin-induced *IgA depression* was observed in 9% of treated children (49[C]); there was no relationship to the type of epilepsy or the plasma concentration of phenytoin. A single case has been reported in which deficiencies of IgG2 and IgG4 were also found (SEDA-17, 73). In one reported case a panhypogammaglobulinemia was observed, fully reversible though liver function abnormalities tended to persist (SEDA-16, 73).

No detectable cytogenetic effects of phenytoin or carbamazepine were found in peripheral *leukocytes* of patients with epilepsy (50[C]). O'Reilly and Hamilton (51[C]) described a patient who developed spontaneous *hemophilia* due to a neutralizing inhibitor to Factor VIII thought to be an antibody induced by long-term phenytoin therapy. A single case of *hemolytic anemia* due to diphenylhydantoin and associated with *renal failure* and a case of *pure red cell aplasia* were reported in 1980 (SED-12, 129).

A dose-related *reduction in the production of vitamin K-dependent clotting factors* has been found in animals.

Megaloblastic anemias, *pancytopenias* and *disseminated lupus erythematosus* have very rarely been attributed to phenytoin, but *aplastic anemia* has been observed with mephenytoin.

Liver The association of diphenylhydantoin therapy with acute *hepatic injury* has been recognized for about 30 years, and by 1980 Mullick and Ishak (52[R]) were able to collect 20 relevant case reports. The interval between the beginning of treatment and the development of signs and symptoms ranged from 1 to 8 weeks in the acute cases, and from 4 months to several years in the chronic cases. Of the 16 patients with acute hepatic complications, 75% had fever and 62.5% had a rash in addition to the symptoms and signs of liver disease. Jaundice occurred in 44% of cases, hepatomegaly in 12.5% and lymphadenopathy and splenomegaly in 60%. Less common signs and symptoms included sore throat, malaise, chills, myalgia and pruritus. Of these 20 patients, 14 recovered after phenytoin was discontinued, but six died (Table 7). *Chronic hepatitis* is rare, but in one recent adult case causal association with phenytoin was demonstrated by withdrawal and rechallenge (52a[c]).

It has been suggested that an inherited defect in response to arene oxide metabolites of phenytoin may predispose some patients to the hepatotoxic effects of the drug.

Gastrointestinal *Gingival hyperplasia* has classically been observed in at least one-third of all epileptic patients treated with phenytoin. With improved oral hygiene and changes in the spectrum of antiepileptic drugs, this reversible complication seems to be diminishing in importance (SED-12, 129), but there is clear evidence that many patients do experience a tissue overgrowth effect with phenytoin which is at the root of the problem (SEDA-16, 72). Inoue and Harrison (53[r]) suggested some years ago that supplements of folic acid may also help to overcome this troublesome complication.

A possibly unique case of reversible *hypertrophy of the submandibular salivary gland* in a boy of 16 with high serum phenytoin concentrations has been described; no cause other than the drug could be identified (SEDA-18, 67).

Urinary system Hyman et al. (54[C]) described a child with diphenylhydantoin sensitivity who developed *autoimmune interstitial nephritis* associated with tubular deposits of diphenylhydantoin and circulating antitubular basement-membrane antibodies.

Skin and appendages *Diffuse fasciitis with eosinophilia* (a variant of scleroderma), hypertrophic *retroauricular folds*, and *local skin and soft tissue reactions* to intravenous phenytoin have been noted.

In one highly unusual case reported in 1984, a 10-year-old black girl developed *toxic epidermal necrolysis* as part of a severe hypersensitivity reaction to phenytoin, followed remarkably by *universal cutaneous depigmentation*. Skin biopsy and electron microscopy revealed no detectable melanocytes (55[C]). Toxic epidermal necrolysis without this sequel has been described by others, and a fatal case has been described by Schmidt and Kluge (56[C]); more recently there has been a case of *Stevens-Johnson syndrome* which remarkably did not recur when ethytoin was substituted for phenytoin (SEDA-18, 67).

Equally unusual was a case of generalized *nodular cutaneous pseudolymphoma* without any evidence of phenytoin hypersensitivity. Although the histology suggested malignant change, the condition resolved entirely within a fortnight of withdrawing the drug (56a[C]).

One 3-year prospective study of patients taking phenytoin, recorded an *erythematous morbilliform rash* in 8.5% of cases, starting within 3 weeks of initiation of treatment and with a marked seasonal association (57[R]).

Reticuloendothelial system *Pseudolymphomatous reactions*, *malignant lymphoma*, *angioimmunoblastic lymphadenopathy* (with clinical features overlapping with systemic lupus erythematosus) and phenytoin-induced *serum sickness* have been noted in individual cases. A remarkable report relates to a boy in whom a condition indistinguishable from malignant *histiocytosis* appeared yet resolved after drug treatment (SEDA-16, 73).

The phenytoin *hypersensitivity syndrome* is well recognized and ranges from a simple rash with fever to a fulminant fatal illness with *exfoliative dermatitis*, *vasculitis* and *disseminated intravascular coagulation*. The most common features are variable combinations of fever, eosinophilia, lymphadenopathy, hepatosplenomegaly, atypical lymphocytes, blood dyscrasias, serum sickness, hepatitis and renal failure. Polymyositis may occur and the pseudolymphoma syndrome is another variant.

Wolf et al. (58[C]) have described a skin reaction resembling *mycosis fungoides* and accompanied by lymphadenopathy and hepatosplenomegaly which occurred during treatment with phenytoin and resolved completely after stopping it.

Second-generation effects See introductory section of this Chapter.

Overdosage A case of severe phenytoin poisoning in a neonate very rapidly responded to peritoneal dialysis, suggesting that much of the phenytoin was unbound; which, in this particular case, may have resulted from hypoalbuminemia in the child (SEDA-16, 73).

Risk situations It has been suggested that patients receiving *cranial irradiation* may be at particular risk of developing the more severe type of skin reaction to phenytoin (SEDA-18, 67).

Interactions A large number of interactions between phenytoin and other drugs are summarized in Tables 4—6 and only selected interactions are listed below.

Phenytoin reduces the effectiveness of *oral contraceptives* probably by inducing the hepatic enzymes which break them down; it has been suggested that the risk of pregnancy may therefore be raised by a factor of 25 (59[R]).

Isoniazid may promote the neurotoxicity of phenytoin by interfering with the clearance of the drug.

Large doses of *aspirin* (975 mg 4-hourly) may cause a small rise in the free concentration of phenytoin and a fall in mean total concentration of phenytoin.

Phenytoin decreases the blood concentration of *dexamethasone*; conversely, phenytoin blood concentration may increase as a result of concurrent administration of dexamethasone (60[R]), and it has been suggested that particular risks attach to the triple combination of phenytoin with cimetidine and dexamethasone (SEDA-18, 67). It is possible that downregulation of epoxide hydrolase by glucocorticoids is involved.

Miconazole elevates serum phenytoin concentration.

Carbamazepine

Most side effects of carbamazepine are mild, transient, and reversible upon dose adjustment, though this may entail reducing the dose below the effective level. The rate of withdrawal because of adverse effects has been found to be about 6% (SEDA-16, 71). Direct reports to the manufacturer in the United States from 1975 to 1986 totalled 371 hematological, 396 dermatological, and 156 hepatic and pancreatic occurrences out of more than 4 million patients treated. Hematological side effects included 27 cases of aplastic anemia and 10 cases of agranulocytosis. Overall, 50—70% of children and adults reported side effects during treatment with carbamazepine (61[R]). Virtually all hepatic disorders and severe skin reactions, as well as the majority (60%) of the hematological reactions, occurred within the first 2 months of treatment. In view of the very low incidence of reported serious blood dyscrasias, such as pancytopenia (0.04 per million prescribed daily doses) and agranulocytosis (0.06 per million prescribed daily doses), continuous hematological monitoring seems to be of little value. The elderly appear to be at increased risk of developing blood dyscrasias and liver reactions, and alcohol abusers appear to represent a high-risk group for developing serious skin reactions (62[R]).

ADVERSE REACTION PATTERN

General and toxic reactions Cerebellovestibular and oculomotor dysfunction with diplopia, nystagmus, ataxia and gastrointestinal dysfunction with nausea are common with carbamazepine. Uncommon are involuntary movements, myoclonus, exacerbation of seizures and movement disorders, hyponatremia, water retention, hepatic damage and cardiac conduction dysfunction.

Hypersensitivity reactions Skin rashes with fever occur in about 8% of cases with an occasional Stevens-Johnson syndrome and Lyell syndrome. Lymphadenopathy tends to be prominent and the condition can resemble infectious mononucleosis. Carbamazepine induces systemic lupus erythematosus. Desensitization to carbamazepine seems to be feasible.

Tumor-inducing effects These have not been described.

ORGANS AND SYSTEMS

Cardiovascular Carbamazepine may exert negative chronotropic and dromotropic effects on the cardiac conduction system; there is evidence of a drug-induced defect in His-Purkinje conduction (SEDA-16, 71). A small number of case reports have described reversible *atrioventricular block* during carbamazepine intoxication among young persons between 10 and 48 years old (SED-12, 130), while *asystole* has been described in an older patient with pre-existent Guillain-Barré syndrome (SEDA-18, 61). *Bradyarrhythmias* of different types and severity have been reported, especially in the elderly, but were completely reversible on withdrawal or reduction of the dose level. When the prevalence of bradyarrhythmias was compared in 48 patients, all 40 years or older, on continuous carbamazepine treatment for various neurological disorders, with that in an age-stratified reference group, there were no differences between the two age groups. The authors concluded that carbamazepine did not increase the risk for bradyarrhythmias in the vast majority of patients (63[C]).

In one published case in 1980, *congestive heart failure* occurred in a young man and was considered possibly attributable to carbamazepine (SED-12, 130); there appear to have been no subsequent reports. Boesen et al. (64[C]) described three cases of carbamazepine-induced *Stokes-Adams attacks* caused by intermittent total atrioventricular block, sinoatrial block with functional escape rhythm and intermittent asystole. They recommended that if syncope or changes in seizure type occur in patients taking carbamazepine, cardiac conduction be assessed.

Respiratory Acute *pulmonary hypersensitivity* with acute dyspnea, crackling rales, rash, eosinophilia and a reticular pattern on chest X-ray may arise during carbamazepine therapy but is rare, though cases continue to be reported (SEDA-18, 61; 65[C]). Lewis and Rosenbloom (66[C]) described an 8-year-old boy who developed a hypersensitivity reaction to carbamazepine, manifested by fever, maculopapular erythematous rash, lymphadenopathy, hepatosplenomegaly, and asthma with eosinophilia. This resolved rapidly on stopping the drug. Sometimes the picture is not at all clear; one report describes generalized radiological changes in the lung accompanied by pleuritic pain and dyspnea; the condition resolved within a month of drug withdrawal (SEDA-16, 71).

Nervous system (*see also the introductory section to this Chapter and Table* 2) *Asterixis*, *dystonic movements* and *tremor* have been ascribed to carbamazepine therapy, as have *orofacial and lingual dyskinesia* (67[C]) and oculogyric crises (68[C]). *Dystonia* progressing to *ophisthotonus* was seen (69[C]) on four occasions in three brain-damaged children taking a total daily dose of 25 mg/kg orally.

Neglia et al. (70[C]) described three patients who either experienced the onset (one case) or exacerbation of *multiple motor tics and vocalizations* 2–4 weeks after starting carbamazepine treatment in normal doses for control of suspected seizures. In two of these patients, in whom these complications were present during the EEG recordings, they proved not to be associated with paroxysmal discharges. The motor tics did not resolve or return to pre-treatment frequency after stopping the carbamazepine. On the other hand, Robertson et al. has reported on pediatric cases without pre-existing movement disorders in whom facial tics appeared and were fully reversible, sometimes even during continuing treatment (70[a]C).

Carbamazepine-induced myoclonic, atonic and absence *seizures* have been described even in the early literature; the problem seems to be common in children and adolescents; both generalized and partial seizures can sometimes be worsened by the drug (SEDA-18, 62). A recent clinical paper (71[C]) notes that the type of symptom most commonly aggravated was the generalized atypical absence. An EEG bilaterally synchronous spike and wave discharge of 2.5 and 3 cycles per second was found to be predictive of increased atypical absence seizures with carbamazepine, whereas generalized bursts of spikes and slow waves of 1–2 cycles per second suggested an increased risk of generalized convulsive seizures.

Carbamazepine and phenytoin seem to produce fewer serious neurological side effects than primidone or phenobarbital, but their *behavioral* side effects are similar. Carbamazepine has been found to cause less impairment of attention and concentration and of motor performance than the other three drugs (72[C]). However, a study of psychomotor activity in 13 patients given 200 mg twice daily did demonstrate acute initial impairment (e.g. of movement time and finger tapping rate) with a maximum after a week of treatment and a return to normal by the fourth week (72a[C]).

The *neuroleptic malignant syndrome* has been observed with carbamazepine in a middle-aged man who had earlier experienced the same reaction to thiothixine (SEDA-17, 72).

Aseptic meningitis has been described three times in the published literature in patients taking carbamazepine; it is fully reversible if the drug is stopped (72b[cr]).

Traccis et al. (73[R]) evaluated *peripheral nerve function* in 30 epileptic patients on chronic carbamazepine therapy and 20 healthy controls. A mild progressive reduction of motor and sensory conduction velocities was found in patients on long-term treatment with the drug. Carbamazepine plasma levels were constantly within the therapeutic range. Folic acid levels were below normal in 50%, and they suggested that this might have played a part in the development of peripheral nerve dysfunction.

Endocrine, metabolic (*see also introductory section*) *Hyponatremia, reduced plasma osmolality* and *water intoxication*, probably ascribable to inappropriate secretion of antidiuretic hormone are well-known effects of carbamazepine. It has been shown that this effect can be blocked by phenytoin (SED-12, 131). It has been assumed that this effect of phenytoin could be due to inhibition of antidiuretic hormone release, but later it was shown that phenytoin simply reduced the serum level of carbamazepine.

Biochemical, but not clinical, evidence of *osteomalacia* due to carbamazepine was described for the first time in 1980. Later, Hoikka et al. (74[CR]) found features of histological osteomalacia in two of 18 biopsies. Rajantie et al. found reduced levels of serum calcium and 25-hydroxyvitamin D and higher alkaline phosphatase in 20 institutionalized mentally retarded children taking carbamazepine as compared with controls (75[E]).

Carbamazepine (like clonazepam and valproate) increased the production of *porphyrin* in a chick-embryo hepatocyte culture (SED-12, 131) and none of these drugs should if possible be used in porphyric patients. There are clinical grounds for this view; Laiwah et al. (76[c]) described a case of acute porphyria following treatment of epilepsy with carbamazepine; they suggest that carbamazepine exerts a direct suppressant effect on uroporphyrin-1-synthase in addition to its indirect enzyme-inducing properties. It has since been argued that this effect could be due to depression of 5-aminolevulinic acid dehydrase levels (SED-12, 131).

As noted in the introductory section to this chapter, it is not clear that the effects of anticonvulsants on *high-density lipoprotein cholesterol* are of clinical importance but, if anything, some of them may be favourable as regards the risk of atherosclerosis and coronary heart disease (SEDA-18, 62). A 5-year prospective study with carbamazepine showed that during treatment serum total cholesterol and high-density lipoprotein remained consistently elevated, whereas an associated increase in serum triglycerides and low-density lipoprotein was transient (76a[C]).

Mineral and fluid balance (*see also 'Endocrine, metabolic' in introductory section*). In one case of hyponatremia in a boy of 13 the drug seems to have induced both *fluid retention* and *cardiomegaly* (SEDA-18, 61).

Hematological *Leukopenia* occurs in approximately 12% of children and 7% of adults, usually during the first 3 months of treatment, with a higher risk in those with a low or low-normal pre-treatment white blood cell count. The leukopenia often reverses, even if carbamazepine is continued (SED-12, 131). The risk is sufficient to justify careful monitoring of high-risk cases; white cell counts of less than $3000/mm^3$ or neutrophil counts below $1000/mm^3$ warrant a decrease in dose or discontinuation of carbamazepine. In one reported case the patient developed leukopenia with thrombocytopenia and *Henoch-Schönlein purpura* (SEDA-18, 62).

Warren and Steinbook (77[c]) described the occurrence of *reticulocytosis* due to carbamazepine. This was not due to hemolysis or to post-hemorrhagic anemia and blood loss, and probably represented an idiosyncratic reaction.

Some 15 documented cases of *thrombocytopenia*, in at least two instances with the demonstrable presence of antiplatelet antibodies, have been published (SED-12, 131; SEDA-18, 62; 78[c], 79[c]); the manufacturer had, up to 1992, received 47 relevant reports, which is a relatively small number in view of the widespread use of carbamazepine, though the problem of gross underreporting of adverse effects needs to be recognized (SEDA-17, 72). The effect resolves on stopping the drug.

The first reported case of carbamazepine-induced *hemolytic anemia* was described in 1984 (SED-12, 132); the anemia appeared 20 days after starting carbamazepine monotherapy, and resolved after stopping the drug.

A single case of *pure red cell aplasia* in a child of 3 treated for 6 months proved to be reversible when the drug was withdrawn (79a[C]).

There have been several reports (SED-12, 132) of a syndrome resembling *systemic lupus erythematosus* during use of carbamazepine.

Liver Fatal *hepatic failure* in a girl treated with carbamazepine for 6 months was described by Zucker et al. in 1977 (SED-12, 133). Levander (80[C]) observed a granulomatous, non-caseating hepatitis in a 60-year-old woman; it resolved on drug withdrawal. Further cases of granulomatous hepatitis due to carbamazepine have been reported since then (SED-12, 132), the complication appearing within a month of starting the drug; histological appearances included histiocytic, lymphocytic and multinucleated giant-cell infiltration together with some evidence of cholangitis.

Cholestatic hepatitis was seen in a 3-week old infant whose mother had received carbamazepine throughout pregnancy; the condition peaked at 6.5 weeks and then resolved. No other cause could be found, but the association could have been coincidental (SEDA-16, 71).

Gastrointestinal *Gastric intolerance* is uncommon and mild. However there have been several reports of severe but reversible *diarrhea* requiring drug withdrawal, while one other published case from Finland experienced eosinophilic colitis after normal doses, the causal link being confirmed by withdrawal and rechallenge (80a[C]).

Urinary system Some cases of carbamazepine-induced *renal failure* have been published, though they are not firmly documented (SEDA-18, 62). On the other hand, two recent cases of diabetic patients who developed *urinary retention* on low doses (400–600 mg/day) were confirmed by rechallenge; there have been earlier reports, and it seems possible that preexistent autonomic dysfunction predisposes to this adverse effect (80b[cr]).

Skin and appendages The overall incidence of skin reactions has been found in a Japanese pediatric study to be some 10% (SEDA-18, 62), the type of complication varying widely. Erythematous maculopapular *rash* as part of the hypersensitivity syndrome has often been observed as have miliary or diffuse exanthema. The skin rashes can appear alongside other (systemic) manifestations of hypersensitivity. Carbamazepine-associated toxic *epidermal necrolysis* and *exfoliative dermatitis* were reported by Breathnach et al. (81[c]) and Reed et al. (82[C]), respectively. Staughton et al. (83[C]) reported the first case of *toxic pustuloderma* due to carbamazepine. Finger and toe *nail hypoplasia* at birth was found in a child of an epileptic mother after carbamazepine had been started at the 26th week of pregnancy; by the time the infant was aged 3 months, the nails had returned to normal (SED-12, 132).

There is a single report in the published literature of *systemic lupus erythematosus* with skin rash during the use of carbamazepine, the authors believing that there was a causal link (SEDA-18, 63). Again there is a report of severe *serum sickness* in one case, with evidence that an immunoblastic lymphadenopathy was involved; carbamazepine antibodies were present (SEDA-16, 72; SEDA-18, 63). Two cases of *lichenoid eruption* were reported in 1990 from Japan (SEDA-16, 71).

It is important to recognize that even serious skin reactions of the hypersensitivity type to carbamazepine may be temporarily masked by concomitant corticosteroid treatment (84[C]); in mild cases it may be helpful to relieve the condition with antihistamines or corticosteroids.

Patch testing for carbamazepine allergy tends to be positive in some types of case (including exfoliative dermatitis and sometimes maculopapular eruptions) but not in fixed eruptions (84a[Cr]). A successful desensitization procedure, using gradually increasing dosage of carbamzepine over a 6-week period, has been described (SEDA-18, 63).

Risk situations Because of the adverse reactions described above, carbamazepine should only be used with caution in patients with *cardiac, hepatic or renal disorders*. There is one reported case in which carbamazepine caused *pacemaker failure* until the pacemaker was adjusted, no doubt because of the drug's effects on cardiac conduction (SEDA-18, 61).

Second-generation effects (*see also introductory section to this Chapter*) There is specific evidence incriminating carbamazepine, like several other anticonvulsants, as a cause of *neural tube defects*; one recent report on a non-epileptic woman who attempted to commit suicide with carbamazepine (4.8 grams at the third or fourth week) showed that at 20 weeks the fetus had developed a large *myeloschisis* (SEDA-18, 63).

In fact the incidence of congenital defects after valproate use in pregnancy may be very high. In one unselected series of 17 infants exposed in utero, five had major malformations (including heart defects and other abnormalities in four cases and esophageal herniation in the other), four had less serious structural defects and 12 had manifestations of withdrawal (irritability, jitteriness, abnormal tone, seizures, feeding problems) correlated with the dosage of valproate during the last trimester. Four of the affected children also had hypoglycemia (84b[C]).

Overdosage Excessive dosage may result in cardiac arrhythmias and conduction defects, seizures, chorea-like movements, ataxia, fixed dilated pupils, nystagmus, absent reflexes, ophthalmoplegia, liver function disturbances and respiratory depression (SEDA-18, 63; 85[C]). The exact picture is dose-related; a truly massive carbamazepine overdose may result in coma and seizures if plasma concentrations exceed 25 μg/ml; combativeness, hallucinations or choreiform movements can occur at levels of no more than 15–25 μg/ml, and drowsiness and ataxia with levels as low as 11–15 μg/ml. After recovery, relapses can be induced by even mildly excessive plasma levels. Pharmacokinetic studies in cases of intoxication have sometimes shown prolongation of carbamazepine half-life and elevation of the 10,11-epoxide. Repeated gastric lavage, detection and endoscopic elimination of any insoluble tablet coagulum, electrolyte monitoring, and treatment of seizures with diazepam and phenytoin are recommended (SED-12, 132).

Interactions (*See Tables* 4–6) The fact that valproate (and apparently also carbamazepine) reduce the effect of non-depolarizing *muscle relaxants* may not be due exclusively to enzyme induction; it seems likely that these anticonvulsants also interfere with the muscle relaxant effect by up-regulation of acetylcholine receptors (SEDA-18, 63).

Valproate

Both sodium valproate and valproic acid are in use; their effects are similar.

ADVERSE REACTION PATTERN

General and toxic reactions Mild gastrointestinal side effects, weight gain, fine tremor, and drowsiness may occur. Uncommon are hair changes and hematological side effects. Serious side effects include encephalopathy, hepatic injury, pancreatitis and second-generation effects.

Hypersensitivity reactions These are extremely rare.

Tumor-inducing effects These have not been described.

ORGANS AND SYSTEMS

Cardiovascular No adverse effects have been described up to the present.

Respiratory Valproate had long been considered free of adverse respiratory effects, but in 1993 the case of a patient with a bipolar illness was described who, when treated with normal doses of phenytoin, developed *respiratory failure* and truncal weakness; the association appeared to be proven by withdrawal and rechallenge. The authors suggested that the effect could have been due to muscle weakness related to carnitine deficiency or impaired mitochondrial function (85a[C]).

Nervous system (*see also introductory section and Table* 2) Dose-related *tremor* is seen during long-term valproate therapy in about 10% of patients (SED-12, 132). The symptom is reminiscent of adrenergic or essential tremor and responds well to dose reduction or propranolol.

Involuntary movements, twitching of the face and limbs and physiological tremor have been precipitated by sodium valproate, perhaps in patients unduly sensitive to this type of effect. Lautin et al. (86[C]) is one of several workers who have described a *parkinsonian-like* reaction, in their case with tremor of the arms, cogwheel rigidity and circumoral tremor, indistinguishable from the tremor induced by haloperidol and metoclopramide in the same patient (SEDA-18, 68).

Encephalopathy, often associated with hyperammonemia and/or liver failure (see below) has repeatedly been described, with symptoms ranging from stupor to deep coma (SEDA-18, 68; 86a[cR]). Chadwick et al. (87[C]) observed two adults with acute toxic encephalopathy, producing confusion in both of them, hallucinations in one and hyperactive behaviour in the other. Both appeared to experience an increased seizure frequency. All the symptoms resolved with reduction of the valproate dosage.

Psychotic reactions had been reported to the WHO monitoring system on some 16 occasions by 1993, and occasional cases have also been published (87a[C]).

Asterixis has been associated with intoxication by most anticonvulsant drugs; with valproate cases have been seen despite the presence of normal serum levels (SED-12, 133).

As with other anticonvulsant drugs, *drowsiness*, *irritability* and *acute confusional states* may occur. Such effects, sometimes extending to *coma*, have occasionally been seen with valproate, sometimes even in the absence hyperammonemia, increased phenobarbital plasma concentrations or other evidence of possible precipitating causes (SED-12, 133). Valproate-induced stupor tends to be associated with bilaterally synchronous high-voltage, slow-wave EEG activity. One mild but common effect is a *greater depth of sleep* may increase the incidence of enuresis in child patients (see below).

A reversible *dementia* was reported in 1986 (SED-12, 133); it receded within 2 months of discontinuing the drug. Comparative data, examined by the American Academic of Pediatrics Committee on Drugs in 1985, suggest that valproate usually has little effect on *psychological performance* and *cognitive function* as compared with other anticonvulsants (88[R]).

Behavioral problems are infrequent but include *sedation*, *hyperactivity* and *aggression*. Monitoring for such complications in children can require careful questioning of parents, teachers and the patient.

Endocrine, metabolic Asymptomatic *hyperammonemia*, with ammonia levels as high as 140 μmol/l, was found in 29 of a series of 55 patients receiving valproate (89[C]); in these cases the elevated levels were well tolerated. Several explanations for this commonly reported complication have been offered; it may be due to increased renal production of ammonia or inhibition of nitrogen elimination, while carnitine deficiency (see below), nutritional influences and multiple drug therapy have also been thought to play a role. Others have sought an explanation in metabolic abnormalities secondary to increased glycine or propionic acid concentrations (SED-12, 133). Individual metabolic abnormalities are certainly relevant; one fatality in a case of hyperammonemia involved a person suffering from ornithine transcarbamylase deficiency (SED-12, 133; 90[C]), suggesting that if a case of hyperammonemia persists for several months following drug withdrawal one should look for a possible urea cycle enzyme deficiency. There is indeed other evidence pointing to the need for caution in giving valproate to patients with any enzyme disorder; Christmann et al. described an 18-year-old woman with progressive dementia and spastic paraparesis who fell into a coma with hyperammonemia when receiving valproate; moderate hyperammonemia persisted for several months following discontinuation of valproate, a further episode with coma developed without exposure to valproate, and congenital argininemia was diagnosed (91[Cr]). Despite such cases, there is no reason to hesitate in using valproate in an otherwise healthy epileptic patient, even if hyperammonemia develops.

Valproate-induced *carnitine deficiency* (91a[R]) may be due to either reduced production or increased biotransformation and excretion. The effect is usually asymptomatic, but measurement of carnitine levels seems advisable in young children with neurological disabilities who are taking several antiepileptic drugs who appear to be at greatest risk for carnitine deficiency, as well as in patients with symptoms and signs suggesting carnitine deficiency (SED-12, 133). There seems no reason to provide carnitine substitution in asymptomatic cases. All this should not obscure the fact that there seems to be a genuine risk in occasional instances; one case of acute encephalopathy during valproate treatment was found to be associated with biochemical evidence of severe carnitine deficiency, and in turn with a defect of the valproate breakdown process; L-carnitine substitution corrected the biochemical abnormalities but the patient died (91b[c]). In one other reported case, late-onset *lipid storage myopathy* was described, with carnitine deficiency as a secondary phenomenon (91c[c]). Finally one could point to a report of a case in which life-threatening cardiac dysfunction in a boy of 7 required urgent carnitine supplementation (SEDA-17, 74).

Valproate may induce *hyperglycinemia* and *hyperglycinuria* (SED-12, 133) usually without associated clinical symptoms and signs. Elevated spinal fluid glycine levels have been reported in some such patients.

Egger and Brett (92[C]) found that *weight increase* was the commonest side effect in a retrospective study of 100 epileptic children treated with sodium valproate; it occurred in 44 of their cases. It is probably mediated through hypothalamic stimulation or possible changes in fatty acid metabolism (SEDA-17, 74) and seems to be unrelated to dose.

John (94[C]) noted transient *osteosclerosis* of the long bones in a 15-year-old boy taking sodium valproate. His symptoms of severe pain in the extremities as well as positive X-ray findings disappeared after the drug was stopped.

Sodium valproate has been described as causing an attack of acute *porphyria* in a young woman who had epilepsy and acute intermittent porphyria (SED-12, 134). On the other hand, valproate is considered a safe treatment for patients with *porphyria cutanea tarda* (95[R]); this is particularly important since the enzyme-inducing antiepileptic drugs may lead to exacerbation.

Finally, transient *amenorrhea* persisting up to 1 year has more than once been reported in young women following the start of valproate therapy (SEDA-16, 73; 93[C]). From recent work there is reason to think that valproate often causes some form of menstrual disturbance, sometimes with polycystic ovaries and hyperandrogenism; it may inhibit the conversion of testosterone to estradiol (SEDA-18, 68).

Effects on *blood lipids* are reviewed in the general introduction to this Chapter.

Hematological Specific investigation suggests that some form of hematological problem, not necessarily of clinical significance, is present in a third of patients on valproate monotherapy (SEDA-18, 68).

The *thrombocytopenia* associated with valproate treatment may be caused by autoimmune mechanisms (SED-12, 134). Sandler et al. (96[R]) found that among 31 patients on sodium valproate, four had platelet-bound antibodies and one a platelet autoantibody in their sera. Ikeda et al. (97[R]), who studied platelet function in 28 children during treatment with sodium valproate, found that 15 of them showed some platelet dysfunction; abnormalities of clot retraction occurred in two, platelet adhesiveness in nine, ristocetin-induced aggregation in nine, and ADP-induced aggregation in 15. In five of the 15 patients the secondary aggregation was inhibited. No relationship between platelet dysfunction and serum valproate level was recognized. Only two patients showed evidence of bleeding.

Depressed *fibrinogen* serum levels have been found in children receiving valproate alone, but were more marked in those taking valproate together with other anticonvulsants (SED-12, 134). It is unlikely that these effects have any clinical importance except perhaps in patients due to undergo surgery.

A series of other hematological effects have been described incidentally in single patients (SED-12, 134). Those noted earlier in this series of volumes include cases of *bone marrow suppression*, together with *platelet autoantibodies* and a *coagulopathy*, a transient *leukopenia* due to valproate, a case of *lethal bone marrow failure* due to self-poisoning and a case of reversible *intravascular hemolysis and pure marrow red cell aplasia* while being treated with valproate.

A marked reduction in the concentration of von Willebrand factor (and risocetin co-factor) was shown in the majority of pediatric cases taking valproate examined in one study (SEDA-17, 74; 97a) and it does now seem than *hemostasis* may commonly be deranged in patients for this reason, though not always to a clinically serious degree.

Liver The spectrum of hepatotoxicity ranges from transient dose-related and clinically asymptomatic *elevations of liver enzymes* in as many as 40% of the patients to rare, idiosyncratic and often fatal hepatic injury. Elevations of enzyme levels up to 3 times the normal concentration may subside even without a reduction in the daily dose of valproate (98[R]) but the drug should be stopped if enzyme concentrations exceed this level.

Fatal *hepatic failure* is extremely rare; if it occurs at all, it is likely to appear within the first 3 months of treatment. The highest risk level reported (1:500) was found in children under 2 years of age receiving valproate as part of a multiple-drug regimen, and this relatively high rate may have been explained in part by the presence of mental retardation, congenital abnormalities and neurological disorders. In older children and adults the incidence is no more than 1:37 000 for monotherapy and 1:12 000 for multi-drug therapy. Risk factors include familial hepatic disease, and concomitant salicylate intake. The clinical findings are classically those of a severe hepatic disorder; abdominal pains, easy bruising, sudden loss of seizure control and neurological dysfunction, e.g. ataxia, may be early warning signs. Histological features of valproate-induced hepatic injury mainly include microvascular steatosis and necrosis.

The mechanism of valproate-induced fatal hepatotoxicity remains elusive; while valproic acid itself may be the agent responsible for liver damage in susceptible individuals, the acid can undergo biotransformation to its valproate-4-ene metabolite which, both structurally and functionally, resembles 4-pentanoic acid, a known hepatotoxin (SED-12, 135; SEDA-18, 68). The latter irreversibly inhibits the enzymes of the fatty acid β-oxidation complex, causes destruction of cytochrome P450 and generates active metabolites. The recent finding that δ^4-valproate is formed metabolically by the action of hepatic cytochrome P450 enzymes that are induced by phenobarbital and other antiepileptic drugs, offers a plausible explanation for the fact that the latter seem capable of potentiating the hepatotoxicity of valproate both in animal studies and in man. This interaction is the best of reasons for prescribing valproate alone, rather than in combination with other antiepileptic drugs, especially in the youngest children. Similarly, valproate should be avoided in patients with a personal or familial history of liver disorders, and the simultaneous use of salicylates should be avoided.

A *Reye-like syndrome*, as yet occurring only in children, has been described in association with valproate treatment.

Gastrointestinal Sodium valproate may well be associated with the rare development of *acute pancreatitis* (SEDA-18, 69; 99[C]); by 1993 there had been 27 published reports of acute pancreatitis during treatment with the drug (and many unpublished reports as well) and few of these complications seem likely to have been merely coincidental; one patient relapsed on three occasions when rechallenged with the drug, and there have been positive rechallenges in other cases as well. Two deaths have occurred from hemorrhagic pancreatic necrosis. Complications have included *pleural and pericardial effusions*, *coagulopathy*, *pseudocyst*, *ascites*, *wound infection* and *pneumonia*.

Two cases of *stomatitis*, one confirmed by rechallenge, have been described in patients taking normal doses of valproic acid, as has one instance of parotid enlargement (99a[c]). Valproate treatment may also result in *gastritis*, and this should be suspected in children receiving valproate when feeding difficulties arise and persist (SED-12, 135). There have in the course of the years been two published reports of *gingival hyperplasia*, an effect more usually associated with the hydantoins (SEDA-16, 74).

Vomiting, if associated with amnestic episodes, and *feelings of tightness in the throat* and *fear* may be a sign of a partial seizure originating from the insular cortex, rather than a local effect on the gastrointestinal tract.

Urinary system In 1981, Lenoir et al. reported a complete *Fanconi syndrome* in a 9-year-old boy who had taken valproate for a year (100[C]). The proximal renal tubular cells were abnormal on biopsy. Clinical improvement was dramatic after valproate was stopped, and renal function returned to normal within a few months. The case seems to have remained unique, so the causal association with the drug seems dubious.

Enuresis in children can in occasional cases be a problem during treatment with sodium valproate (101[C]). The incidence varies between 1 and 7%. It may be secondary to the polydipsia as a result of the increased thirst due to valproate or perhaps result from the increased depth of sleep associated with valproate.

Skin and appendages Sodium valproate is known to cause transient *loss of hair* and change in *hair texture* (SED-12, 135). Change in *hair color* has also been ascribed to the drug (ibid).

Kinnell (102[c]) reported three cases of *photosensitivity* possibly or probably attributable to valproate. A report of two possible cases of *systemic lupus erythematosus* associated with valproate has so far remained unconfirmed (SEDA-74), but there is a report on two patients who developed *cutaneous vasculitis* during treatment (102a[C]).

Developmental effects A case of valproate-associated *pubertal growth arrest* has been described in a girl of 12 who had been treated for 18 months.

Risk situations Valproic acid should be used only with great caution in patients with *bleeding disorders* and obviously also where there is a personal or family history of *hepatic dysfunction*. Several other problems raised earlier in this Chapter suggest other possible contraindications, e.g. *porphyria* or *carnitine deficiency*. The suggestion has been made that *glutathione peroxidase deficiency* could predispose to severe reactions (such as pancreatic or hepatic failure) in children and that screening for such disorders (whether familial or induced) might render it possible to reduce risk (SEDA-17, 72).

Second-generation effects See introductory section to this Chapter.

Overdosage Accidental overdose of sodium valproate in a 19-month-old boy produced coma and pinpoint pupils which responded to naloxone (103[C]).

Interactions Stupor is an unusual complication following the addition of valproic acid to *other antiepileptic drugs*; when combined with phenobarbital, the serum levels of the latter may rise sufficiently to produce undesirable drowsiness (SED-12, 136). Similarly, valproic acid has been reported to produce a transient increase in *phenytoin* serum levels which later seems to recede despite continuation of treatment (104[C]); it also causes an increase in the serum level of *ethosuximide* (105[C]).

MISCELLANEOUS ANTICONVULSANTS

Acetazolamide

Although better known as a selective diuretic used in glaucoma, acetazolamide is also employed as an anticonvulsant. In a series of 51 adult epileptics taking the drug, six developed *renal calculi* after treatment for 1 or more years. The drug is of course usually regarded as contraindicated in renal disease, and it is important to ensure adequate hydration when it is used (SEDA-16, 71).

Atrium®

Atrium® is a French proprietary mixture containing phenobarbital, febarbamate and diferbarbamate. There have been several cases of *hepatotoxicity*. One recent incident, confirmed by rechallenge, suggests that the components responsible are the carbamates, since the patient had earlier tolerated phenobarbital (105a[cr]).

Clobazam and other barbiturates *(see also Chapter 5)*

Feeley et al. (106[C]) studied this drug in the treatment of catamenial epilepsy. *Sedation* and mild *depression* were the adverse effects most commonly encountered. One patient had transient *galactorrhea* and exhibited *delayed menstruation*; she had no previous history of galactorrhea and had normal prolactin levels. There was some suggestion that the drug became less effective after a period of time. O'Flaherty et al. (107[C]) describe a patient who developed choreoathetosis on completing the slow withdrawal of clonazepam over 9 days.

When one looks at the many open studies conducted with clobazam, the side effects most often reported are mild and transient *drowsiness, dizziness or fatigue*; rather less common are *muscle weakness*, *restlessness*, *aggressiveness*, *weight increase*, *ataxia* and an *unpleasant mood*. Rarely one sees mention of an *atonic state*, *hyperkinetic syndromes*, *delusional state*, *psychotic symptoms*, *behavioral disturbances*, *vertigo*, *hypersalivation* and *edema*. Clobazam appears to have no hematological side effects.

Four episodes of *akathisia* have been described in three patients with a history of brain injury and seizure disorder who were treated with benzodiazepines, perhaps a disinhibitory effect in this type of subject (107a[Cr]).

The development of *tolerance* and exacerbation of seizures following an all too abrupt *withdrawal* are major limitations of clobazam and probably of other benzodiazepines when used in epilepsy (SEDA-18, 61; 108[R]).

Clomethiazole edisilate *(see also Chapter 5)*

Continuous intravenous infusion of clomethiazole edisilate is sometimes used in status epilepticus resistant to intravenous diazepam. When Lingam et al. (109[C]) treated five patients aged between 2 and 8 years with individually adapted infusion rates, using an 8 g/l concentration in 4% dextrose, they experienced problems with *thrombophlebitis* at the site of infusion, especially with infusions lasting longer than 12 hours. *Fever* occurred in all five patients, often severe. Pronounced *headache* occurred in all the children. Clomethiazole edisilate (9 g/l) was given here in an aqueous solution of 4% dextrose, the rate of infusion being adapted as necessary to ensure seizure control.

Clonazepam *(see also Chapter 5)*

A review of side effects reported in seven controlled trials (110[R]) found that adverse effects occurred in 60—90% of cases, and the rate of discontinuation for this reason was as high as 36%. The most common problems were *drowsiness*, *ataxia*, and behavioral and personality changes such as *hyperactivity*, *restlessness*, *reduced attention span*, *irritability*, *disruptiveness* and *aggressiveness*. Major limitations were *hypersalivation* and development of *tolerance*, while upon abrupt withdrawal there tended to be an *exacerbation of the seizures*.

A paradoxical *increase in seizure frequency* may occur in as many as 5—6% of patients treated with this benzodiazepine (111[C]). The mechanism for this is not apparent.

Diazepam *(see also Chapter 5)*

When intravenous diazepam is used in the treatment of status epilepticus, the patient must be assiduously monitored for possible *respiratory depression*, which during intensive treatment may actually demand artificial ventilation.

Ethosuximide

Sodium valproate has generally superseded ethosuximide in the treatment of absence seizures. Side effects include *gastrointestinal disturbances*, *headache*, *drowsiness*, *ataxia*, *granulocytopenia*, *thrombocytopenia*, *systemic lupus erythematosus* and *scleroderma*. Patients may also develop *antinuclear antibodies* and, where this occurs, the patients should be watched carefully for subsequent development of systemic lupus erythematosus which has been seen during use of the drug (111a[C]).

Felbamate

Psychotic reactions, *anxiety* and *nervousness* have been ascribed to felbamate in small placebo-controlled studies (111b[CR]). There is also a fair incidence of *gastrointestinal intolerance*. At present it is difficult to distinguish other possible effects from those ascribable to concurrent medication or to lack of experience with the correct dosage of felbamate. *Interactions* should be anticipated, since felbamate can increase the serum concentrations of the major antiepileptic drugs (SEDA-18, 94).

Gabapentin

There is little published information on the pattern of adverse effects of this drug, other than a review of pre-marketing studies, which do not necessarily correlate well with subsequent field experience (111c[R]); some 10—20% of patients seem to develop *drowsiness*, *fatigue or ataxia* or combinations of these. There was a somewhat lower incidence of *nausea*, *vomiting* and *rhinitis* (SEDA-17, 75; SEDA-18, 64).

In rats used for chronic toxicity studies, acinar cell carcinomas of the pancreas were observed; these are not similar to the primarily ductal carcinoma of the pancreas which occurs in humans, and the significance of the finding is dubious (SEDA-18, 64).

Lamotrigine

Lamotrigine is used as add-on treatment for partial seizures not satisfactorily controlled with other antiepileptic drugs. Since the drug is almost always used as add-on medication it can be difficult to decide which effects are specifically due to lamotrigine. Most of the side-effects are more frequent if carbamazepine is given concurrently.

Nervous system Adverse reactions to lamotrigine are primarily CNS-related and included *dizziness* (in 50% of cases in placebo-controlled trials), *diplopia* (33%), *ataxia* (24%), *blurred vision* (23%) and *somnolence* (14%). Mild or transient side effects include a degree of *irritability* and *aggression* as well as *insomnia* (SEDA-18, 64).

Hematological Lamotrigine is a weak inhibitor of dihydrofolate reductase and may therefore possibly interfere with folate metabolism during long-term therapy. Currently, however, there is no evidence for changes in hemoglobin concentration, mean corpuscular volume, or serum and red blood cell folate concentration in patients treated with lamotrigine for 1 year.

Gastrointestinal *Nausea* and *vomiting* are common but not necessarily long lasting.

Skin and appendages In controlled add-on trials skin *rashes* occurred in up to 10% of patients and led to withdrawal of the drug in 2%. The rash is usually maculopapular. In one trial, two of the children developed *hirsutism*, resolving on drug withdrawal (SEDA-18, 65). Rarely, more severe skin complications including *angio-edema* and *Stevens-Johnson syndrome* have been reported (112[C]). Slow introduction of the drug seems to decrease the risk of the milder skin reactions.

Other reactions Hypersensitivity reactions, though generally affecting the skin, may lead to *pyrexia*. Pharyngitis has been described, but could be coincidental.

There have been occasional reports of fatal multi-organ failure during the treatment of status epilepticus, but such reports are seen from time to time with other antiepileptic drugs and probably represent a complication of the status rather than a drug effect (SEDA-18, 64).

Overdosage There is a case of severe overdosage on record where a dose of 1350 mg had been taken; alongside central nervous system effects there was a striking widening of the QRS complex on the electrocardiogram, which suggests the need for cardiac monitoring in cases of poisoning (112a[c]).

Interactions *Enzyme-inducing anticonvulsants* given simultaneously reduce the effect of lamotrigine by stimulating its breakdown. Conversely, *valproic acid* inhibits its metabolism, as a result of which the dose of lamotrigine can be reduced; use of the two drugs together can result in tremor (SEDA-18, 65). When lamotrigine is given alongside *carbamazepine*, cerebellar dysfunction can occur (ibid).

Loreclezole

When used as add-on therapy for uncontrolled partial seizures, loreclezole produced some *weight loss*, *drowsiness* and *fatigue* (SEDA-16, 74).

Oxcarbazepine

In a comparative trial against carbamazepine, oxcarbazepine produced side effects in 68% of all patients, with a mean of 2.8 side effects per patient (113[C]). As compared with the older drug, oxcarbazepine seems to have a lower allergenic potential, similar or slightly better CNS tolerability and greater antidiuretic activity, but these are only differences of degree. The drug seems to have been withdrawn in about a fifth of patients because of adverse effects.

Hypersensitivity reactions involving the skin (but with only partial cross-reactivity with carbamazepine) have been reported, as have *fever*, *drowsiness*, *fatigue*, *headache*, *dizziness* and *ataxia*. Serum electrolytes were not in all the larger studies, but in some work oxcarbazepine has produced *hyponatremia* (<135 mmol/l) in up to 40% of cases (SED-12, 137). *Diplopia* and *nystagmus* are known from other reports (SEDA-17, 73). Transient *cognitive impairment*, *exacerbation of seizures* and *coma* have been all been reported in single cases, each effect being completely reversed by discontinuation of oxcarbazepine.

Interactions The interactions of oxcarbazepine do not seem to parallel those of carbamazepine (Table 6), though it must be borne in mind that the latter has been used on a much larger scale and data are still accumulating. Interestingly, there is some evidence that oxycarbazepine can be used alongside *carbamazepine* without potentiating the adverse effects of the latter. Volunteer studies have suggested that oxcarbazepine does not interfere with blood levels of the coumarin anticoagulants, and that neither cimetidine nor dextropropoxyphene inhibit the metabolism of oxcarbazepine. However, oxcarbazepine does reduce the availability of *estrogen*, *progestogen* and *felodipine*.

Phenobarbital *(see also Chapter 5)*

Development of *Dupuytren's contracture*, *frozen shoulder*, *Ledderhose syndrome*, *Peyronie's disease*, *fibromas*, and general *joint pain* have all been authoritatively linked at various times to the use of barbiturate antiepileptic drugs (phenobarbital, primidone), especially when these are given long term; the incidence may be some 10% (114[C]). Most of the patients prove to have developed some evidence of connective tissue changes during the first year of treatment, though they only become disabling at a later stage. It is important to recognize these complications early, since in the early phases they seem as a rule to be reversible (SED-12, 137).

Other adverse effects reported in recent years to phenobarbital used in epilepsy have been those familiar through other forms of use of the barbiturates. Incidental reports relate to a *menstrually related mood disorder*, *erythroderma*, and an atypical *lymphocytosis* mimicking cutaneous T-cell lymphoma (SEDA-18, 66).

Primidone

Primidone is in part metabolized to phenobarbital, which is probably responsible for its anticonvulsant effects. The most common side effect is *drowsiness*, but *rashes*, *systemic lupus erythematosus* and a *megaloblastic anemia* reacting to folic acid may occur. A syndrome resembling *diabetes insipidus* as well as *lymphadenopathy*, *toxic epidermal necrolysis*, *thyroid enlargement*, and *edema* have been attributed to primidone. Like barbiturates, the drug should not be given to patients with *acute intermittent porphyria*. The symptoms of acute intoxication are those seen in barbiturate overdosage; massive crystalluria can occur due to the urine being overloaded with hexagonal primidone crystals (115[R]).

Progabide

The most serious adverse effect of progabide is its *hepatotoxicity*. Abnormal liver function tests were reported in 8.4% of a series of 1164 patients; clinical hepatotoxicity occurred in 0.46%; three patients died. Withdrawal of progabide is recommended if liver transaminases exceed twice the normal limit and laboratory monitoring of liver function is always highly advisable (116[R]).

Remacemide

Remacemide hydrochloride is thought to act as a non-competitive antagonist at NMDA receptors; in Phase II trials, the maximum tolerated oral dose is about 600 mg/day in divided doses. The dose-limiting effects have been gastrointestinal and neurological, especially dizziness and light-headedness; elderly subjects with cardiac disorders tolerated the drug well, though some complained of difficulty in concentrating, confusion and mood changes. Enzyme-inducing anticonvulsants given simultaneously markedly reduce the levels of remacemide and its active metabolite, while remacemide seems to raise the levels of concurrently administered carbamazepine (117[cR]).

Stripentol

In 1993, a small open add-on trial of stripentol in doses of 1000—3000 mg/day resulted in occurrence of irritability, lethargy, incoordination, increased sleep, agitation, anorexia, nausea and (sometimes severe) vomiting. The doses used in this study appear to have been excessive; the adverse effects were relieved by dose reduction (118[c]).

Taltrimide

When Taltrimide was used in a controlled trial as add-on therapy, adverse events occurring during its use comprised *headache*, *tiredness*, *insomnia*, *nausea* and *general malaise*. One patient with an allergy to sulfonamides developed *petechiae* and *nasal bleeding* after the first dose (119[C]).

Vigabatrin

Adverse events in patients receiving vigabatrin are usually mild and transient. The most common adverse effects found in a systematic review were *drowsiness*, *fatigue*, *irritability*, *nervousness*, *dizziness*, *weight gain*, *headache*, *confusion* and *depression* (120[R]). The weight gain occurs in as many as 40% of patients during the first 6 months of therapy. Two cases of *akathisia* and *hyperkinesia* have been reported. If the dosage is carefully titrated, there are likely to be no significant psychomotor effects and no changes in laboratory parameters, but the cognitive effects can only be firmly assessed after more experience has been gained.

In a proportion of patients, as with other anticonvulsant drugs, there is *aggravation of the seizure pattern* when vigabatrin is given; one pediatric study has found this effect in 10% of cases, and noted that new seizure types could occur during treatment (SEDA-18, 69—70).

More serious is that *psychotic episodes* and *bipolar disorders* can occur during treatment with vigabatrin or on abrupt withdrawal; the issue was reviewed at length in SEDA-18 (pp. 70—72) to which the reader is referred for a full discussion. It has been claimed that the incidence is much higher than the (already elevated) frequency in an untreated epileptic population where the incidence may be some 2—4%, or as much as 14% in temporal lobe epilepsy. Sander has reported on 14 patients treated with vigabatrin, nine of whom had no previous history of psychosis, who became psychotic after periods of treatment ranging from 5 days to 32 weeks at doses varying from 500 to 4000 mg daily (121[CR]), and in the literature to date it seems that some 5% of patients will show some behavioral change, though it is clear that certain early studies were carried out with relatively high doses. The manufacturer's data present a more optimistic pictures, with figures derived from pre-marketing and adverse reaction-monitoring programmes which are comparable to those described in untreated epileptics (*Marion Merrell Dow, data on file*); the UK Prescription Event Monitoring Centre also shows very low figures (122[R]). However it is not uncommon for adverse reaction figures from these sources to be much lower than those obtained in specific studies. It seems clear that psychosis can be precipitated by vigabatrin, and one's best estimate at present is that some 2—6% of cases will be affected by this or other serious psychiatric complications, the exact incidence will probably be strongly influenced by dosage. One should thus introduce and withdraw the drug cautiously, especially in those with a history of mental disorder (SEDA-16, 74). It is possible that reduced binding of a specific dopamine D_2 receptor ligand in the basal ganglia could explain the psychotic reactions (SEDA-17, 74; SEDA-18, 72).

There have been several published cases of *acute encephalopathy* or conditions pointing to it, associated with vigabatrin treatment. Patients may develop new types of seizures or even status epilepticus, while others may show stupor, dysphoria and slowed EEG background patterns (SEDA-18, 70).

Toxicity studies of long-term administration in mice, rats and dogs have shown dose-related *intramyelinic edema* with microvacuoles in the white matter of the brain. The changes are limited in degree and reversible; it is doubtful whether they have any relevance to the treatment of human subjects, since neither tests in vivo nor post mortem studies have so far given any grounds for concern (SED-12, 137; SEDA-17, 74).

Vigabatrin can produce an *abnormal urinary amino acid pattern* which can be diagnostically confusing (SEDA-16, 74).

Zonisamide

Clinical testing of zonisamide was at one stage discontinued in the United States due to the development of *kidney stones* in several patients after several months of exposure to the drug as an add-on medication. However, the drug apparently continues in use in some countries, notably in Japan and elsewhere in the Far East, and urolithiasis there was reported in only 0.2% of cases studied; trials in western countries have been resumed. In a large Japanese series, the overall incidence of adverse effects was 51%, with 18% withdrawals. The most common problems were *drowsiness*, *ataxia*, *anorexia*, *mental slowing* and *gastrointestinal intolerance* (123).

At excessive serum levels, *acute mania* has been described (SEDA-16, 75). Other side effects have seemed to be most frequent during the initial stages of treatment and comprise *ataxia*, *dizziness*, *nystagmus*, *dysarthria*, *diplopia*, *asterixis*, *tremor*, *confusion*, *nausea*, *vomiting*, *anorexia* and *weight loss*.

REFERENCES

1. Bjerkedal T et al. Valproic acid and spina bifida. Lancet 1982;ii:1096.

1a. D'Souza SW, Robertson IG, Donnal D et al. Fetal phenytoin exposure, hypoplastic nails, and jitteriness. Arch Dis Child 1990;65:320—324.

2. Friis ML. Malformations in children of epileptic patients. In: Comprehensive Epileptology, Vol 24. New York: Raven Press, 1990;309.

3. Gaily E, Granström ML, Hiilesmaa V et al. Minor anomalies in offspring of epileptic mothers. J Pediatr 1988; 112:520.

4. Laegreid L, Kyllerman M, Hedner D et al. Benzodiazepine amplification of valproate teratogenic effects in children of mothers with absence epilepsy. Neuropediatrics 1993;24:88—92.

5. Annegers JF, Baumgartner KB, Hauser WA et al. Epilepsy, antiepileptic drugs, and the risk of spontaneous abortion. Epilepsia 1988;29:451.

6. Moslet U. Hansen ES. A review of vitamin K, epilepsy and pregnancy. Acta Neurol Scand 1992;85:39.

7. Buehler EA, Delimont D, van Waes M et al. Prenatal prediction of risk of the fetal hydantoin syndrome. N Engl J Med 1990;322:1567.

8. Shapiro S, Hark SC, Siskind V. Anticonvulsants and parental epilepsy in the development of birth defects. Lancet 1976;i:272.

9. Gaily E. Development and Growth in Children of Epileptic Mothers. Academic Dissertation, University of Helsinki, 1990.

10. Dreifuss FE, Langer DH, Moline KA et al. Valproic acid hepatic fatalities: II. US experience since 1984. Neurology 1989;39:201.

11. Horowitz S, Patwardhan R, Marcus E. Hepatotoxic reactions associated with carbamazepine therapy. Epilepsia 1988;29:149.

12. Dreifuss FE. Valproate toxicity. In: Levy R, Mattson R, Meldrum B et al, eds. Antiepileptic Drugs, 3rd edn. New York: Raven Press, 1989;643.

13. Fichman MP, Kleeman CR, Bethune JE. Inhibition antidiuretic hormone by diphenylhydantoin. Arch Neurol 1970;55:45.

14. Franceschi M, Perego L, Cavagnini F et al. Effects of long term antiepileptic therapy on the hypothalamic pituitary axis in man. Epilepsia 1984;25:46.

15. Masala A, Meloni T, Alagna S et al. Pituitary responsiveness to gonadotrophin-releasing and thyrotrophin releasing hormones in children receiving phenobarbitone. Br Med J 1980;281:1175.

16. Julesz J, Lis M, Gutkowska J et al. Sodium valproate and Nelson's syndrome. Lancet 1981;i:252.

17. Kritzler RK, Vining EPC, Plotnik LP. Sodium valproate and corticotropin suppression in the child treated for seizures. J Pediatr 1983;102:142.

18. Ostrowska Z, Buntner B, Rosciszewska D et al. Adrenal cortex hormones in male epileptic patients before and during a 2-year phenytoin treatment. J Neurol Neurosurg Psychiatry 1988;51:374.

19. Rootwelt K, Ganes T, Johannesen SJ. Effect of carbamazepine. phenytoin and phenobarbital on serum levels of thyroid hormones and thyrotropin in humans. Scand J Clin Lab Invest 1978;38:731.

20. Aanderud S, Strandjord RE. Hypothyroidism induced by antiepileptic drugs. Acta Neurol Scand 1980;61:330.

21. Isojärvi JIT, Pakarinen AJ, Ylipalosaari PJ et al. Serum

hormones in male epileptic patients receiving anticonvulsant medication. Arch Neurol 1990;47:670.

22. Toone BK, Wheeler M, Fenwick PBC. Sex hormone changes in male epileptics. Clin Endocrinol 1980;12:391.

23. MacPhee GJA, Larkin JC, Butler E et al. Circulating hormones and pituitary responsiveness in young epileptic men receiving long-term anti-epileptic medication. Epilepsia 1988;29:468.

23a. Isojärvi JIT. Serum steroid hormones and pituitary function in female epileptic patients during carbamazepine therapy. Epilepsia 1990;31:438—445.

24. Lühdorf K. Endocrine function and antiepileptic treatment. Acta Neurol Scand Suppl 1983;94:15.

25. Morijiri Y, Sato T. Factors causing rickets in institutionalised handicapped children on anticonvulsant therapy. Arch Dis Child 1981;56:446.

26. Annegers JF, Melton LJ, Sun C et al. Risk of age-related fractures in patients with unprovoked seizures. Epilepsia 1989;30:348.

27. Weinstein RS, Bryce GF, Sappington LJ et al. Decreased serum ionised calcium and normal vitamin D metabolite levels with anticonvulsant drug treatment. J Clin Endocrinol Metab 1984;58:1003.

27a. Calandre EP, Rodruiguez-Lopez C, Blazquez A et al. Serum lipids, lipoproteins and apolipoproteins A and B in epileptic patients treated with valproic acid, carbamazepine or phenobarbital. Acta Neurol Scand 1991;83:250—253.

28. Bayer A, Zrenner E, Thiel HJ et al. Retinal disorders induced by anticonvulsant drugs. In: Abstracts, Second Congress of the International Society of Ocular Toxicology, Deidesheim, May 20—24, 1990.

29. Aguglia U, Zappia M, Quattrone A. Carbamazepine-induced non-epileptic myoclonus in a child with benign epilepsy. Epilepsia 1987;28:515.

30. Kurlan W. Exacerbation of motor ties by phenytoin. Epilepsia 1990;31:468.

31. Power W. Reversible parkinsonism induced by valproate. Neurology 1990;40(Suppl 1):139.

32. McLachlan RS. Pseudoatrophy of the brain with valproic acid monotherapy. Can J Neurol Sci 1987;14:294.

33. Eldridge R, Iivanainen M, Stern R et al. 'Baltic' myoclonus epilepsy: hereditary disorder of childhood made worse by phenytoin. Lancet 1983;ii:838.

34. Gillham RA, Williams N, Wiedmann K et al. Concentration—effect relationships with carbamazepine and its epoxide on psychomotor and cognitive function in epileptic patients. J Neurol Neurosurg Psychiatry 1988;51:929.

35. Aldenkamp AP, Alpherts WCJ, Moerland MC et al. Controlled release carbamazepine: cognitive side effects in patients with epilepsy. Epilepsia 1987;28:507.

36. Gallassi R, Morreale A, Lorusso S et al. Carbamazepine and phenytoin: comparison of cognitive effects in epileptic patients during monotherapy and withdrawal. Arch Neurol 1988;45:892.

37. Eisen AA, Woods JF, Sherwin AL. Peripheral nerve function in long term therapy with diphenylhydantoin. Neurology 1974;54:411.

37a. Jibiki I, Kido H, Yamaguchi N et al. Probable cerebellar abnormality on *N*-isopropyl(iodine-123)-*p*-iodoamphetamine single photon emission computed tomography scans in an epileptic patient receiving long-term high-dose phenytoin therapy. Neuropsychobiology 1993;27:204—209.

38. Kamanabroo D, Schmitz-Landgraf W, Czarnetzki BM. Plasmapheresis in severe drug-induced toxic epidermal necrolysis. Arch Dermatol 1985;121:1548.

39. Duncan JS, Shorvon SD, Trimble MR. Withdrawal symptoms from phenytoin, carbamazepine and sodium valproate. J Neurol Neurosurg Psychiatry 1988;51:924.

40. Manon-Espaillat R, Burnstine FH, Rertder B et al. Antiepileptic drug intoxication: factors and their significance. Epilepsia 1991;32:96.

40a. Rodriguez-Garcia JL, Sánchez-Corral J, Martinez H et al. Phenytoin-induced benign lymphadenopathy with solid spleen lesions mimicking a malignant lymphoma. Ann Oncol 1991;2:443—445.

40b. Phelps SJ, Baldree LA, Boucher BA. Neuropsychiatric toxicity of phenytoin. The importance of monitoring phenytoin levels. Clin Pediatr 1993;32:107—110.

41. Nikkilä EA, Kaste M, Ehnholm C, Vilkari J. Elevation of high density lipoprotein in epileptic patients treated with phenytoin. Acta Med Scand 1978;204:517.

42. York RC, Coleridge ST. Cardiopulmonary arrest following intravenous phenytoin loading. Am J Emerg Med 1988;6:255.

43. Taliercio CP, Olney BA, Lie JT. Myocarditis related to drug hypersensitivity. Mayo Clin Proc 1985;60:463.

43a. Hayes AG, Chesney TM. Necrosis of the hand after extravasation of intravenously administered phenytoin. J Am Acad Dermatol 1993;28:360—363.

44. Koller WC, Sander LG, Fox JH. Phenytoin induced cerebellar degeneration. Ann Neurol 1980;8:203.

45. Botez MI, Attig E, Vezina JL. Cerebellar atrophy in epileptic patients. Can J Neurol Sci 1988;15:299.

45a. Haider Y, Abbott RJ. Phenytoin-induced choreoathetosis. Postgrad Med J 1990;66:1089.

46. Luoma PV, Myllylä VV, Sotaniemi EA, Hokkanen TEJ. Plasma HDL cholesterol in epileptics with elevated triglyceride and cholesterol. Acta Neurol Scand 1979;60:56.

47. Luoma PV, Reunanen MJ, Sotaniemi EA. Changes in serum triglyceride and cholesterol levels during long term phenytoin treatment for epilepsy. Acta Med Scand 1979; 206:229.

47a. Al-Rubeaan K, Ryan EA. Phenytoin-induced insulin insensitivity. Diabetic Med 1991;8:968—970.

48. Yue CP, Mann KS, Chan KH. Severe thrombocytopenia due to combined cimetidine and phenytoin therapy. Case reports. Neurosurgery 1987;20:693.

49. Ruff ME, Pincus LC, Sampson HA. Phenytoin-induced IgA depression. Am J Dis Child 1987;141:858.

50. Flejter WL, Astemhorski JA, Hassel TM et al. Cytogenetic effects of phenytoin and/or carbamazepine on human peripheral leucocytes. Epilepsia 1989;30:374.

51. O'Reilly RA, Hamilton RD. Acquired hemophilia meningioma and diphenylhydantoin therapy. J Neurosurg 1980; 53:600.

52. Mullick FO, Ishak KG. Hepatic injury associated with diphenylhydantoin therapy. A clinicopathologieal study of 20 cases. Am J Clin Pathol 1980;74:442.

52a. Brandenburg AH, Smits MG, Voorbrod BS. Phenytoin-induced chronic hepatitis. Dig Dis Sci 1993;38:740—743.

53. Inoue F, Harrison JV. Folic acid and phenytoin hyperplasia. Lancet 1981;ii:86.

54. Hyman LR, Ballow M, Knieser MR. Diphenylhydantoin interstitial nephritis: role of cellular and humoral immunological injury. J Pediatr 1978;95:915.

55. Schmidt D. Adverse Effects of Antiepileptic Drugs. New York: Raven Press, 1982.

56. Schmidt D, Kluge W. Fatal toxic epidermal necrolysis following reexposure to phenytoin. Epilepsia 1983;54:440.
56a. Braddock SW, Harrington D, Vose J. Generalised nodular cutaneous pseudolyumphoma associated with phenytoin therapy. J Am Acad Dermatol 1992;27:337—340.
57. Leppik IE, Lapora A, Loewenson R. Seasonal incidence of phenytoin allergy unrelated to plasma levels. Arch Neurol 1985;42:120.
58. Wolf R, Kahane E, Sandbank M. Mycosis fungoides-like lesions associated with phenytoin therapy. Arch Dermatol 1985;121:1181.
59. Coulam CB, Annegers JF. Do anticonvulsants reduce the efficacy of oral contraceptives? Epilepsia 1979;20:519.
60. Lawson L, Blouin RA, Smith RB et al. Phenytoin—dexamethasone interaction: a previously unreported observation. Surg Neurol 1981;16:423.
61. Pellock JM. Carbamazepine side effects in children and adults. Epilepsia 1987;28(Suppl 3):564.
62. Askmark H, Wiholm BE. Epidemiology of adverse reactions to carbamazepine as seen in a spontaneous reporting system. Acta Neurol Scand 1990;81:131.
63. Kennebäck C, Bergfeldt L, Tomson T et al. Carhamazepine induced bradycardia—a problem in general or only in susceptible patients? A 24 hour long-term electrocardiogram study. Epilepsy Res 1992.
64. Boesen F, Andersen EB, Jensen EK. Cardiac conduction disturbances during carbamazepine therapy. Acta Neurol Scand 1983;68:49.
65. Mitchell MC, Boitnott K, Arregui A et al. Granulomatous hepatitis associated with carbamazepine. Am J Med 1981;71:733.
66. Lewis IJ, Rosenbloom L. Glandular fever like syndrome, pulmonary eosinophilia, and asthma associated with carhamazepine. Postgrad Med J 1982;58:100.
67. Tridon P, Vidailhet C, Stehlin S. Dyskinésie linguale induite par la carbamazepine. Ann Méd Nancy 1980;19:745.
68. Berchou RC, Rodin A. Carhamazepine induced oculogyric crisis. Arch Neurol 1979;36:522.
69. Crosley CJ, Swender PT. Dystonia associated with carbamazepine administration: experience in brain damaged children. Pediatrics 1979;63:612.
70. Neglia JP, Glaze DG, Zion TE. Ties and vocalizations in children treated with carbamazepine. Pediatrics 1984;73:841.
70a. Robertson PL, Garofalo EA, Silverstein FS. Carbamazepine-induced tics. Epilepsia 1993;34:965—968.
71. Snead OC, Hosey LC. Exacerbation of seizures in children by carbamazepine. N Engl J Med 1985;313:916.
72. Smith DB, Mattson RH, Cramer JA et al. Results of a nation-wide Veterans Administration Cooperative Study comparing the efficacy and toxicity of carbamazepine, phenobarbital, phenytoin, and primidone. Epilepsia 1987;28(Suppl 3):550.
72a. Larkin JG, McKee PJW, Brodie MJ. Rapid tolerance to psychomotor impairment with carbamazepine in epileptic patients. Br J Clin Pharm 1992;33:111—114.
72b. Hemet C, Chassagne P, Levade MH. La carbamazépine, une cause rare de ménigite aseptique. Rev Med Interne 1993;14:607.
73. Traccis S, Monaco F, Sechi GP et al. Long term therapy with carbamazepine: effects on nerve conduction velocity. Eur Neurol 1983;22:410.
74. Hoikka V, Alhava EM, Karjalainen P et al. Carbamazepine and bone mineral metabolism. Acta Neurol Scand 1984;69:77.
75. Rajantie J, Lamberg-Allardt C, Wilska M. Does carbamazepine treatment lead to a need of extra vitamin D in some mentally retarded children? Acta Pediatr Scand 1984;73:325.
76. Laiwah AACY, Thompson GG, Philip M et al. Carbamazepine induced non-hereditary acute porphyria. Lancet 1983;i:790.
76a. Isojarvi JIT, Pakarinen AJ, Myllylä VV. Serum lipid levels during carbamazepine medication: a prospective study. Arch Neurol 1993;50:590—593.
77. Warren JA. Steinbook RM. Case report of carbamazepine induced reticulocytosis. Am J Psychiatry 1983;140:247.
78. Tohen M, Castillo J, Cole JO et al. Thrombocytopenia associated with carbamazepine: a case series. J Clin Psychiatry 1991;52:496—498.
79. Bradley JM, Sagraves R, Kimbrough AC. Carbamazepine induced thrombocytopenia in a young child. Clin Pharm 1985;4:221.
79a. Buitendag DJ. Pure red-cell aplasia associated with carbamazepine. South Afr Med J 1990;78:214—215.
80. Levander HG. Granulomatous hepatitis in a patient receiving carbamazepine. Acta Med Scand 1980;208:333.
80a. Steiner I, Birmanns B. Carbamazepine-induced urinary retention in long-standing diabetes mellitus. Neurology 1993;43:1855—1856.
80b. Anttila V, Valtonen M. Carbamazepine-induced eosinophilic colitis. Epilepsia 1992;33:119—121.
81. Breathnach SM, McGibbon DH, Ive FA et al. Carbamazepine (Tegretol) and toxic epidermal necrolysis: report of three cases with histopathological observations. Clin Dermatol 1982;7:585.
82. Reed MD, Bertino JS, Blumer JL. Carbamazepine associated exfoliative dermatitis. Clin Pharmacol 1982;1:78.
83. Staughton RCD, Harper JI, Rowland Payne CME. Toxic pustuloderma: a new entity? J R Soc Med 1984;77(Suppl 4):6.
84. Lisker-Melman M, Hoofnagle JH. Phenytoin hepatotoxicity masked by corticosteroids. Arch Intern Med 1989; 149:1196.
84a. Alanko K. Patch testing in cutaneous reactions caused by carbamazepine. Contact Dermatitis 1993;29:254—257.
84b. Thisted E, Ebbesen F. Malformations, withdrawal manifestations and hypoglycemia after exposure to valproate in utero. Arch Dis Child 1993;695:288—291.
85. Schmidt D, Rohrer E. Carbamazepine. In: Resor SR Jr, Kutt H, eds. The Medical Treatment of Epilepsy. New York: Marcel Dekker, 1992;293.
85a. Trehan R, Clark CF. Valproic acid-induced truncal weakness and respiratory failure. Am J Psychiatry 1993; 150:1271.
86. Lautin A, Stanley M, Angris TB, Cershon S. Extrapyramidal syndrome with sodium valproate. Br Med J 1979;4:1035.
86a. Duarte J, Macias S, Coria F et al. Valproate-induced coma: case report and literature review. Ann Pharmacother 1993;27:482—583).
87. Chadwick DW, Cumming WJK, Livingstone J, Cartlidge NEP. Acute intoxication with sodium valproate. Ann Neurol 1978;6:552.
87a. Swedish Adverse Drug Reactions Advisory Committee. Valproate-psychosis. Bull SAD-RAC 1990.
88. American Academy of Pediatrics' Committee on Drugs. Behavioral and cognitive effects of anticonvulsant therapy. Pediatrics 1985;76:644.

89. Murphy JV, Marquardt K. Asymptomatic hyperammonaemia in patients receiving valproic acid. Arch Neurol 1982;39:591.
90. Hjelm M, de Silva LV. Seakins JW et al. Evidence of inherited urea cycle defect in a case of fatal valproate toxicity. Br Med J 1986;292:23.
91. Christmann R. Valproate-induced coma in a patient with urea cycle enzyme deficiency. Epilepsia 1990;31:228
91a. Coulter DL. Carnitine, valproate and toxicity. J Child Neurol 1991;6:7–14.
91b. Marukami K, Sugimoto T, Nishida N et al. Abnormal metabolism of carnitine and valproate in case of acute encephalopathy during chronic valproate therapy. Brain Dev 1992;14:178–181.
91c. Papadimitrou A, Servidei S. Late onset lipid storage myopathy due to multiple acylCoA dehydrogenase deficiency triggered by valproate. Neuromusc Disord 1991;1:247–252.
92. Egger J, Brett EM. Effects of sodium valproate in 100 children with special reference to weight. Br Med J 1981;283:577.
93. Margraf JW, Dreifuss FE. Amenorrhea following initiation of therapy with valproic acid. Neurology 1981;31:159.
94. John C. Transient osteosclerosis associated with sodium valproate. Dev Med Child Neurol 1981;23:234.
95. D'Alessandro R, Rocchi E, Cristina E et al. Safety of valproate in porphyria cutanea tarda. Epilepsia 1988;29:159.
96. Sandler RM, Bevan PC, Roberts GE et al. Interaction between sodium valproate and platelets: a further study. Br Med J 1979;4:1476.
97. Ikeda N, Mitsudome A, Ogata H. The platelet dysfunction in children during treatment with sodium valproate. No To Hattaisu 1984;16:27.
97a. Kreuz W, Linde R, Funk M et al. Induction of von Willebrand disease type 1 by valproic acid. Lancet 1990; 335:1350–1351.
98. Dickinson RC, Bassett ML, Searle J et al. Valproate hepatotoxicity: a review and report of two instances in adults. Clin Exp Neurol 1985;21:79.
99. Ng JYK, Disney APS, Jones TE. Acute pancreatitis and sodium valproate. Med J Aust 1982;24:362.
99a. Reisser C, Maier H. Sialadenose durch valproat-dauermedikation. Laryngol Rhinol Otol 1991;70:384–386.
100. Lenoir CR, Perignon JL, Gubler MC. Valproic acid: a possible cause of proximal tubular renal syndrome. J Pediatr 1981;98:503.
101. Choonara IA. Sodium valproate and enuresis. Lancet 1985;i:1276.
102. Kinnell HG. Heated reaction to valproate. Hosp Doctor 1984;C4(23):4.
102a. Kamper AM, Valentijn RM, Stricker BHC et al. Cutaneous vasculitis induced by sodium valproate. Lancet 1991;337:497–498.
103. Steiman GS, Woerpel RW, Sherard ES. Treatment of accidental sodium valproate overdose with an opiate antagonist. Ann Neurol 1979;6:274.
104. Bruni J, Wilder BJ, Willmore LJ, Barbour B. Valproic acid and plasma levels of phenytoin. Neurology 1979;29:904.
105. Mattson RH, Cramer JA. Valproic acid and ethosuximide interaction. Ann Neurol 1980;7:583.
105a. Brocheriou I, Zafrani ES, Navier P. Hepatite aigue sévére imputable à l'Atrium®. Gastroenterol Clin Biol 1993;17:305–306.
106. Feeley M, Calvert R, Gibson J. Clobazam in catamenial epilepsy: a model for evaluating anticonvulsants. Lancet 1982;ii:71.
107. O'Flaherty SO, Evans M, Epps A et al. Choreoathetosis and clonazepam (Letter to Editor). Med J Aust 1985; 142:453.
107a. Joseph AB, Wroblewski BA. Paradoxical akathisia caluses by clonazepam, clorazepate and lorazepam in patients with traumatic encephalopathy and seizure disorders. Behav Neurol 1993;6:221–223.
108. Schmidt D, Rhode M, Wolf Petal. Tolerance to the antiepileptic effect of clobazam. In: Frey HH, Friischer W, Koella WP, Meinardi H, eds. Tolerance to Beneficial and Adverse Effects of Antiepileptic Drugs. New York: Raven Press, 1986.
109. Lingam S, Bertwistle H, Eilisto M, Wilson J. Problems with intravenous chlormethiazole (Heminevrin) in status epilepticus. Br Med J 1980;1:155.
110. Sato S. Clonazepam. In: Levy R, Mattson R, Meldrum B, Penry JK, Dreifuss FE, eds. Antiepileptic Drugs, 3rd edn. New York: Raven Press, 1989;765.
111. Alvarez N, Hartford E, Doubt C. Epileptic seizures induced by clonazepam. Clin EEG 1981;12:57.
111a. Ansell BM. Drug-induced lupus erythematosus in a 9-year-old boy. Lupus 1993;2:193–194.
111b. Wilder B, Campbell KW, Uthman BA et al. Felbamate for intractable epilepsy: a long-term study (Abstract). Epilepsia 1991;32:59.
111c. Goa KL, Sorkin EM. Gabapentin. A review of its pharmacological properties and clinical potential in epilepsy. Drugs 1993;46:402–427.
112. Jawad S, Richens A, Goodwin C et al. Controlled trial of lamotrigine (Lamictal) for refractory partial seizures. Epilepsia 1989;30:356.
112a. Buckley NA, Whyte IM, Dawson AH. Self-poisoning with lamotrigine. Lancet 1993;342:1552–1553.
113. The Scandinavian Oxcarbazepine Study Group. A double-blind study comparing oxcarbazepine and carbamazepine in patients with newly diagnosed, previously untreated epilepsy. Epilepsy Res 1988.
114. Mattson RH, Cramer JA, McCutchen CB et al. Barbiturate-related connective tissue disorders. Arch Intern Med 1989;149:911.
115. Schmidt D, Seldon L. Adverse Effects of Antiepileptic Drugs. New York: Raven Press, 1982.
116. Loiseau P, Duchie B. Progabide. In: Dam M, Gram L, eds. Comprehensive Epileptology. New York: Raven Press, 1990;641.
117. Palmer GC, Clark B, Hutchinson JB. Antiepileptic and neuroprotective potential of remacemide hydrochloride. Drugs Future 1993;18:1021–1942.
118. Farwell JR, Anderson GD, Kerr BM et al. Stripentol in atypical absence seizures in children: an open trial. Epilepsia 1993;34:305–311.
119. Iivainen M, Waltimo O, Parantainen J et al. A controlled study with taltrimide and sodium valproate: valproate effective in partial epilepsy. Acta Neurol Scand 1990; 82:121–125.
120. Richens A. Potential antiepileptic drugs—vigabatrin. In: Levy R, Mattson R, Meldrum B, Penry JK, Dreifuss FE, eds. Antiepileptic Drugs, 3rd edn. New York: Raven Press, 1989;937.
121. Sander JWAS, Hart YM, Trimble MR. Vigabatrin and psychosis. Lancet 1991;335:1279.
122. Mumford JP. Vigabatrin (Sabril). The strategy for preclinical and clinical evaluation. Boll Lega It Epil 1994;in press.
123. Peters DH, Sorkin EM. Zonisamide. A review of its pharmacodynamic and pharmacokinetic properties, and therapeutical potential in epilepsy. Drugs 1992;45:760–787.

Meyler's Side Effects of Drugs, 13th Edition
M.N.G. Dukes, editor

SECTION EDITOR: P.K.M. LUNDE

H. Olsen

8 Opioid analgesics and narcotic antagonists

GENERAL CONSIDERATIONS

INTRODUCTION

Classes of substances Opioids are naturally occurring or synthetic substances which have morphine-like activity. The term *opiate* refers only to substances with morphine-like activity that are derived from opium. Substances which bind to opioid receptors but elicit little agonist activity are known as *opioid antagonists*. Some drugs have both agonist and antagonist effects (*partial agonists*). The opioids and antagonists can be divided into three groups, namely: (a) opioid agonists (morphine and morphine-like opioids); (b) opioid antagonists (e.g. naloxone and naltrexone); and (c) opioid partial agonist = opioid agonists/antagonists (e.g. buprenorphine and nalbuphine).

Three separate categories of *endogenous substances* with morphine-like activity have been identified. These families of neuropeptides are known as 'enkephalins', 'endorphins' and 'dynorphins'. Each family is derived from distinct precursor polypeptide (pro-enkephalin, pro-opiomelanocortin and prodynorfin) and has a characteristic anatomical distribution. The enkephalins and dynorphins are often found to coexist with other neurotransmitters such as serotonin (5-HT) and noradrenaline, but details of how the peptides modulates the activity of co-transmitters await elucidation.

Finally, several molecules with chemical structure similar to morphine have been found in mammalian brain, but it is not certain if these molecules have been derived from dietary sources or if they are synthesized in the brain.

The word *narcotic* was previously used to describe substances with morphine-like activity and is now largely obsolete in the medical literature although it is still used in legal parlance.

Receptors Neurophysiological studies have revealed the existence of a multiplicity of distinct types of receptors that can interact with endogenous peptides or opioid drugs. Three main types of opioid receptor are found, mainly within the central nervous system (CNS), but also in the periphery. These are the mu (μ), kappa (κ), and delta (δ) receptors. Subtypes of each of these have been identified. Opioids interact with these receptors to produce their effects. Primarily by exerting presynaptic inhibition whereby this results in decreased release of excitatory transmitters. Attempts have been made to relate pharmacological effects of opioid drugs to interactions with specific types of receptors. It is thought that analgesia is primarily mediated via activation of μ-receptors at supraspinal sites and κ-receptors within the spinal cord. An opioid drug may interact to a greater or lesser degree with all three types of receptor and act as an agonist, partial agonist, or an antagonist at each one.

The identification of opioid receptors and the discovery of opioid peptides in the mid and late 1970s led to the hope that with greater understanding of fundamental mechanisms, it would be possible to develop new drugs with all the valued properties of known opioids but without their unwanted effects. However, it is probably fair to say that these hopes have remained unrealized, although a synthetic enkephalin (pentapeptide 443C81) which poorly penetrates the blood-brain barrier has been shown to produce a dose-related analgesia without causing significant miosis or reducing minute volume on rebreathing CO_2 in healthy volunteers (SEDA-16, 86).

Differences between individual agents Morphine remains the 'gold standard' against which all others opioids are compared. The majority of opioids are used as analgesics although some are used primarily as antitussives, and others such as loperamide and diphenoxylate are exclusively used in the treatment of diarrhea, whilst fentanyl and its congeners are primarily employed in anesthetic practice. Fentanyl, the oldest of the anesthetic opioid agonists, as well as its derivatives, alfentanil and sufentanil, are used either as anesthetic supplements or in appropriate doses as complete anesthetics. In the field of analgesia, butorphanol and nalbuphine have largely replaced pentazocine because of a lesser tendency to result in dysphoric side effects and, in contrast to the pure agonists, any respiratory depression which may follow their use is not dose-related and reaches a 'ceiling' as the dose increases.

The main characteristics and use of opioid drugs are listed in Table 1. Drugs in widespread clinical use each have a separate monograph.

The clinical use of opioid drugs is continuing to increase, mainly due to development of alternative routes of administration and increasing use in the very young. Pharmacological maneuvers have been made in order to improve analgesic potency and reduce adverse effects. Benzodiazepines have been used to improve analgesic effect (SEDA-17, 78) and methylphenidate has been given to patients in order to reduce drowsiness (SEDA-17, 78). Combination of opioids with non-steroid anti-inflammatory drugs has been used in the provision of analgesia postoperatively with the aim of reducing amounts of opioid required with the consequent reduction in adverse effects (SEDA-18, 79).

Sandler (SEDA-17, 78) has outlined the more novel routes of administration of opioids, including oral, nasal, rectal, transdermal, spinal, and by patient controlled methods.

Degree of risk It is often the side effects of opioids and their dependence-producing properties rather than their beneficial therapeutic effects that are emphasised in medical teaching. World-wide studies in patients with malignant disease have demonstrated the efficacy of these agents in relieving opioid-responsive pain. When used correctly, side effects are usually minimal. However, when used illicitly, opioids are often adulterated with other substances, and therefore some side effects may be due to these adulterants.

Belgrade (1[R]) outlined the strategy to control pain caused by malignant disease and reviewed the classic effects which can be associated with opioid administration. These included constipation, nausea, sedation, pruritus, urinary retention, myoclonus and respiratory depression. The latter is a dose-dependent effect which can be life-threatening. Particular care is needed in opioid-naive individuals, those with compromised respiratory function and in elderly patients.

The use of opioids in very young patients is increasing. In a recent review of pain management in children various routes of administration of opioids and the associated adverse effects have been discussed (SEDA-17, 78).

In a review of pain management in neonates (SEDA-17, 78), attention has been drawn to the adverse effects of i.v. codeine in children and to the risk of convulsions with pethidine in the newborn, because of accumulation of its metabolite, norpethidine. The risk of respiratory depression with morphine was also highlighted and morphine is recommended for use only in neonates who are being ventilated or intensively nursed.

The advent of patient-controlled analgesia (PCA) (SEDA-15, 68) highlights the importance of adequate monitoring in order to avoid potentially catastrophic side effects such as respiratory depression. The experience so far with PCA has been encouraging; patients generally used less morphine than controls but still achieved the same degree of pain control (2[cr]). This supports the view that self-administration of opioids in a medical setting does not put patients at risk of overmedication or drug dependence.

It has been suggested that the risk of producing opioid dependence in the medical setting is greater in those who prescribe and administer them than in those who receive them (3[r]). Several studies have examined the likelihood of producing dependence in patients treated with opioids. In a review of the treatment of cancer pain Foley (4[R]) stated that 'tolerance and physical dependence occur but that psychological dependence (addiction) is rare'. red by others (5[R]). Porter and Jick (6[r]) looked at 11 882 patients who had received at least one opioid preparation and found that addiction was only reasonably well documented in four cases.

In a study of 130 patients with chronic malignant and chronic benign pain attending a pain relief unit over a 3-year period, nine (18%) were considered to be addicted to analgesics on subjective evaluation (7[C]). Coote et al. (8a[c]) reviewed the medication in a series of 71 patients with chronic pain referred to a pain relief centre: 86% were taking analgesics, 58% opioids and 68% psychotropic agents; 49% of those taking opioids were considered to be dependent.

These studies emphasise the need to correctly define the meaning of terms such as 'addiction' and 'dependence' and distinguish between psychological and physical dependence. Failure to do so could lead to the unwitting deprivation of opioids in those patients for whom they provide undisputed benefit with minimal risk.

Finally it must be borne in mind that some of the problems with opiates are treatable: e.g. naloxone can reverse respiratory depression, but care must be taken in opioid-dependent individuals as it may precipitate opioid withdrawal.

OPIOIDS IN PREGNANCY AND LABOR *(SED-11, 137; SEDA-8, 76; SEDA-10, 61; SEDA-17, 85; SEDA-18, 82)*

Reports on the effects of drugs taken by the mother on the fetus and neonate fall into two categories: drugs

Table 1. *Major characteristics and uses of some opioid drugs*

Drug	Typical dose	Route of administration	Pharmacokinetics	Usual indication	Main adverse effects
Agonists					
Morphine	10 mg upwards 3–4 hourly	Oral, injection, intrathecal	$T_{1/2}$ 2–4 h Morphine-6 glucuronide active agonistic metabolite	Severe pain, anesthesia	Sedation, constipation, nausea, vomiting, itching, resp.dep., tolerance and dependence, euphoria
Alfentanil	30–50 μg/kg	Injection, epidural	$T_{1/2}$ 1.6–4 h	Analgesia, anesthesia	As morphine
Codeine	30–60 mg 4-hourly	Oral	$T_{1/2}$ 3–4 h Acts as prodrug, (?) metabolized to morphine by Cyp $2D_6$	Cough, diarrhea, moderate pain	As morphine Lack of effect in poor metab. of Cyp $2D_6$ (?)
Dextromethorphan	10–30 mg 4–8 hourly		$T_{1/2}$ 2.7–3.3 h Gen. reg. metab. by Cyp $2D_6$	Dry, painful cough	
Dextropropoxyphen	65 mg 6–8 hourly	Oral	$T_{1/2}$ 6–32 h Active metabolite (norpropoxyphene) with $T_{1/2}$ 24–42 h	Moderate pain	As morphine Cardiotoxicity, not reversible by naloxone. Convulsions possible due to norpropoxyphene
Fentanyl	50–200 μg	Intravenous, epidural, transdermal patch	$T_{1/2}$ 2–7 h	Acute pain, anesthesia	As morphine
Methadone	10 mg 6–8 hourly	Oral, injection	$T_{1/2}$ 15–60 h	Severe pain, opioid dependence	As morphine
Pethidine (meperidine)	50–150 mg 3-hourly	Oral, intramuscular injection	$T_{1/2}$ 3.2	Moderate/severe pain	As morphine, excitement and convulsions
Sufentanil	up to 8 μg/kg	Intravenous, epidural	$T_{1/2}$ 2.7–6 (12)	Severe pain anesthesia	As morphine
Partial agonists					
Buprenorphine	300–600 μg 6–8 hourly	Sublingual, injection	$T_{1/2}$ 5 (–12)	Moderate/severe pain	As morphine but less pronounced, less reversed by naloxone
Pentazocine	30–60 mg 3–4 hourly	Oral, injection	$T_{1/2}$ 2–4	Acute pain	As morphine, dysphoria
Antagonists					
Naloxone	1.5–3 μg/kg and repeat according to response	Injection	$T_{1/2}$ 1,1	Reversal of opioid-induced respiratory depression	
Naltrexone	25–50 mg daily		$T_{1/2}$ 2,7	Adjunct to prevent relapse in formerly opioid-dependent patients	

given during the course of labor and drugs taken by the drug-dependent mother.

Drugs given during the course of labor In a major review, Fishburne (SEDA-11, 137) described the pharmacokinetics and demonstrated the effects of various systemically administered analgesics on the uterus, fetus and neonate. Ron et al. (SED-11, 137) reported fetal *bradycardia* lasting up to 7 minutes in 53 (2.7%) fetuses out of 1910 following administration of 75 mg pethidine (meperidine) and 25 mg promethazine intravenously to the mothers during labor.

Tajavej et al. (SED-11, 137) carried out a study to examine the relationship between maternal morphine administration during labor and the Apgar score of the baby at birth. The authors concluded that morphine alone did not seem to cause asphyxia at birth but that morphine together with other fetal and/or obstetric factors would definitely be a cause for concern with regard to *birth asphyxia*. Belsey et al. (SED-11, 137) have also assessed the influence of maternal analgesia on *neonatal behavior*. The authors suggest that the newborn infant responds to pethidine in the same way as the adult, but the changes observed were relatively subtle, and comparison of these infants with a control group whose mothers had received no drugs revealed no between-group differences in behavior.

Opioid analgesia may cause prolonged reductions in the baseline variability of the fetus during monitoring in labor (SEDA-17, 85). The mechanism(s) of action is thought to be via a direct effect on the cardiac centers or fetal myocardium. The danger of this is the risk of misinterpretation of the cardiotocogram as being indicative of fetal distress.

Epidural and intrathecal routes for analgesia administration in labor are being increasingly used. When opioids are used as the sole agent, disappointing results due to unwanted adverse effects such as pruritus, nausea, respiratory depression and effects on the neonate, caused by the significant systemic absorption, have been reported and recently commented upon editorially (SEDA-17, 85). Thus combination of opioids (alfentanil, fentanyl, morphine, sufentanil) and local anesthetics (e.g. bupivacaine) is suggested to yield better results (SEDA-18, 83).

The use of alfentanil with bupivacaine via a continuous epidural infusion during labor resulted in a significant reduction in motor blockade compared with a bupivacaine infusion.

No respiratory depression was observed in the mothers although shivering and pruritus were more frequent in the alfentanil group. No difference in the neonatal Apgar scores between the groups were found (SEDA-18, 83).

Cohen et al. (SEDA-18, 83) compared the effects of fentanyl and sufentanil combined with bupivacaine and adrenaline in a PCA-system following cesarean section. The number of requests were greater in the fentanyl group but there was no difference between the groups with regard to sedation, pruritus and nausea. However, the sufentanil group had a significantly higher incidence of vomiting, light-headedness and dizziness.

It is uncertain whether addition of adrenaline to intrathecal sufentanil increases the duration of analgesics during labor. According to Camann et al. (SEDA-18, 83) addition of adrenaline to intrathecal sufentanil did not prolong the duration of analgesia, but reduced incidence and severity of pruritus, whereas Grieco et al. (SEDA-18, 83) reported that addition of adrenaline or morphine to intrathecal sufentanil prolonged the duration of analgesia. However, the morphine group experienced significantly greater nausea and pruritus.

In another study, comparing a single dose of epidural morphine with PCA-epidural fentanyl in patients following cesarean section it was found that the pain relief and the incidence of nausea were similar in both groups, but pruritus was significantly less in the fentanyl group (SEDA-18, 83).

Also, epidural administration of methadone and diamorphine are reported to be useful analgesics during cesarean section, but oxygen desaturation and nausea are more frequent during diamorphine treatment (SEDA-18, 83).

A new variation, combined spinal-epidural administration has been introduced to achieve almost instantaneous analgesia with longer term pain relief (8b). According to a recent publication (9a) this method seems to cause a faster onset of analgesia and less motor blockade compared with standard epidural analgesia.

The administration of intramuscular tramadol (50 or 100 mg) during labor is, according to Viegus et al. (SEDA-18, 83), associated with fewer adverse effects than pethidine (75 mg). Pethidine and the higher dose of tramadol had similar analgesic efficacy, but pethidine was associated with significantly lower neonatal respiratory rate at birth.

Drugs taken by the drug dependent mother A major review of the problems of drug dependence in pregnancy and the clinical management of mother and child was published in 1979 and its findings remain valid today (SED-11, 138).

The adverse consequences for the neonate of drug abuse in pregnancy can be dramatically reduced by comprehensive medical and psychosocial care for the mothers during pregnancy and delivery (SED-11, 138; $9b^{cR}$). Without due care during pregnancy, however, problems are likely.

The long-term consequences of maternal opioid dependency on the child have been examined in detail more recently. Olofsson et al. (SED-11, 138) investigated 89 infants born to mothers addicted to heroin, morphine and methadone. They found that 20% were pre-term and 31% were light for gestational age. Eighty-five percent of the newborns had withdrawal symptoms and 12% had convulsions. Rosen and Johnson (SED-11, 138) reported on the somatic and neurobehavioral findings of children in the first 18 months of life born to methadone-maintained mothers and to a matched drug-free comparison group of mothers. At 18 months the methadone children had: (a) a significantly higher incidence of otitis media; (b) a significant incidence in head circumference below the third percentile; (c) neurological findings in tone discrepancies, developmental delays, poor motor coordination; (d) a high incidence of abnormal eye findings; and (e) significantly lower scores on the Bayley mental and motor developmental indices.

In a study of 72 such children investigated 1—10 years after birth by Olofsson (10^{CR}), only 25% were found to be physically, mentally and behaviorally normal.

Rosen and Johnson (SED-11, 138) evaluated 41 children born to methadone-maintained mothers and 23 children from matched controls at 6 months of age. Their findings showed: delayed motor development in methadone-exposed infants, greater vulnerability of males to adverse environmental conditions, and correlation between early methadone exposure and behavioral abnormalities in adult male rats.

EPIDURAL AND INTRATHECAL ADMINISTRATION OF OPIOIDS *(SEDA-12, 66; SEDA-13, 58; SEDA-14, 66; SEDA-15, 75; SEDA-16, 82; SEDA-17, 85; SEDA-18, 83)*

In comparison with conventional routes, spinal opioid administration carries a potentially greater morbidity. This can only be justified if it results in equal or superior pain relief in comparison with conventional methods with fewer unwanted effects (SED-11, 139).

Although the analgesic effect of spinal opioids is largely due to a spinal effect, the drug may spread rostrally to the brainstem and higher centers with the potential to produce side effects which may be delayed in onset. Lipid solubility influences the rate at which an opioid will be adsorbed into the spinal cord from the cerebrospinal fluid (CSF), and therefore predicts the likelihood of rostral spread. Poorly lipid-soluble drugs such as morphine will linger in the CSF and produce prolonged analgesia which may last 12 hours or more. Such drugs may float rostrally, producing a more widespread but less intense analgesia. However, if the drug reaches opioid receptors in the respiratory center in the fourth ventricle, delayed respiratory depression may occur. In contrast to morphine, fentanyl is very lipid-soluble but short-acting; a single dose will produce highly segmental intense analgesia lasting between 2 and 3 hours. These properties make it suitable for continuous epidural infusion.

Intrathecal route

Technical problems following intrathecal opioids are rare although catheter occlusion and leakage of CSF have been reported (SEDA-17, 85—86; 11^{R}, 12^{Cr}, 13^{Cr}).

In a series of 121 patients with mean follow-up of 68 days (maximum 13 months) Gestin et al. (14^{Cr}) reported an incidence of less than 10%.

Morphine is the opioid chosen most frequently for intrathecal administration. *Central side effects* are as may be expected (see Monograph); with the exception of constipation, urinary retention and respiratory depression, these effects tend to be transient and disappear within a few days of initiation of therapy.

Pruritus is a frequent side effect following intrathecal administration, with an incidence of one-third reported in two studies involving buprenorphine and diamorphine respectively (15^{CR}, 16^{CR}) and over 70% for both diamorphine and morphine in two studies by Jacobson et al. (17^{C}, $18b^{C}$). In the study by Jacobson (17^{C}) the incidence of pruritus was higher with morphine than with methadone; analgesia was also superior. Pruritus has also been reported with intrathecal pethidine (meperidine). Treatment was not reported to be necessary. This effect is not reported to occur following intrathecal β-endorphin (18a, 19). The mechanism of pruritus is not well understood and has been attributed to a disturbance of thiamine metabolism (20^{r}) and to a disturbance of afferent input at supraspinal as well as at spinal receptor sites (21^{C}).

A high incidence of *nausea and vomiting* has been found with intrathecal diamorphine, which may not be dose-related (22). Two studies suggest that the incidence of nausea and vomiting in labor is higher with intrathecal than with epidural opioids (23, 24).

Drowsiness, in addition to *miosis* and *respiratory depression*, is reported by Lazorthes (25^{CR}) after intracerebroventricular administration of morphine in two out of 55 patients who received between 1 and 1.5 mg morphine. A third patient developed *visual hallucinations* and behavioural disorders after 1 mg. All effects were rapidly reversed by systemic administration of naloxone. Swaraj et al. (26[C]) described *urinary retention* in one of a series of patients who had been given 5 mg pentazocine intrathecally whilst others have reported similar findings since.

Respiratory depression occurs more frequently after intrathecal than after epidural opioid administration and may be more of a problem in old age or where there is pre-existent respiratory disease (SED-11, 139). The time of onset is quite variable but usually occurs within 6—10 hours of the opioid injection, although delays of up to 11 hours have been reported (27[CR]). The same authors noted two cases of prolonged respiratory depression lasting 18 hours after single doses of 3 and 5 mg. Repeated doses of naloxone were required, but each incremental dose did not alter the level of analgesia. It has been suggested that opioid-naive patients may be more susceptible to respiratory depression and that posture may also be important (SED-11, 139). Return of normal respiration may take up to 23 hours. Fitzpatrick and Moriarty (28[Cr]) found that peak expiratory flow rate (PEFR) was significantly better in patients who had received intrathecal rather than intravenous morphine following cardiac surgery ($P < 0.01$), but mean $Paco_2$ was significantly higher in patients given 2 mg intrathecal morphine rather than 1 mg intrathecal morphine or intravenous morphine. Yamaguchi (29[CR]) found the effect to be dose dependent.

Intrathecal opioids used in obstetrics seem to be well tolerated by *mother and child* (SED-11, 139, 140).

Glavina and Robertshaw (30[C]) describe a case of *myoclonic spasms* of the legs following intrathecal morphine, which were abolished by intrathecal bupivacaine. *Hyperalgesia* and *myoclonus* was reported after high-dose intrathecal morphine (SEDA-17, 87).

Kleiner et al. (31[C]) reported temporary, totally reversible motor and sensory paralysis following 1.6 mg intrathecal morphine which they attributed not to a direct spinal action of morphine but more probably to cardiovascular changes occurring as a result of pain relief.

Reactivation of herpes simplex following epidural administration of opioids is well known. However there are recent case reports on reactivation of *herpes simplex* following the intrathecal administration of morphine for cesarean section (SEDA-17, 87; SEDA-18, 84).

Knowledge on the use of spinal opioids in *children* is limited, but apparently side effects are similar to those reported in adults (32[R], 33[R], 34[Cr]; SEDA-18, 85). The review by Krane et al. (34[Cr]) also reported a single case of dysphoria but attributed this to systemic absorption.

Epidural route

The nature of the side effects reported following epidural opioids is similar to that reported with the intrathecal route. Again, old age and respiratory disease probably dispose to respiratory depression (SED-11, 138—140). As may be predicted from pharmacokinetic considerations, delayed respiratory depression is more common with epidural morphine than with fentanyl (35).

Pruritus has been noted following epidural morphine, pethidine (meperidine), diamorphine (heroin) and fentanyl with a quoted incidence of 1—100% There appears to be no relationship between dose and incidence of this side effect. Pruritus severe enough to prove troublesome to the patient occurs in only about 1% of cases (SED-11, 139). In one study of postoperative patients who received 10 mg epidural morphine, pruritus was present in 28% of patients (36), but in only 1% of patients in other studies who received 5 and 2 mg morphine (SED-11, 139). With 50 mg epidural pethidine (meperidine) following cesarean section, Brownridge (37) reported a 50% incidence of pruritus but only in one patient was it troublesome.

Ballantyne et al. (38[R], 39[R]) reviewed pruritus in relation to parturition. They found a reported incidence of 42.7% (593 cases) in pregnant women compared with 8.4% (3050 cases) in non-parturients. These findings are borne out in other comparative work (40). Ackerman et al. (41[Cr]) found that pruritus after cesarean section was more common with epidural morphine and fentanyl than with buprenorphine or butorphanol.

Dezeros et al. (42[Cr]) looked at the effect of obstetric epidural administration of a mixture of 8 ml bupivacaine (0.25%) with 50 μg fentanyl on 40 offspring. Fetal distress occurred in 11 babies, five of whom needed resuscitation; there appeared to be no correlation between fetal distress and newborn plasma fentanyl levels.

Suggested mechanisms for the difference in incidence of pruritus in parturients and non-parturients include high plasma levels of maternal endorphins during labour together with more distant spread for morphine within the CSF, competition by estrogen for opioid-binding sites and hormonal modification of endogenous opioid content at opioid receptors. It has also been suggested that the incidence of all side effects following spinal opioids may be higher in pregnant women for the reasons stated above.

A variety of approaches have been used to try and

eliminate the pruritus phenomenon. Substitution of epidural buprenorphine for morphine in combination with bupivacaine relieved severe unremitting pruritus in a single reported case (43[C]). Injection of 10 mg nalbuphine subcutaneously significantly reduced the pruritus induced by epidural fentanyl within 15 minutes in a series of 24 patients (44[CR]). Naltrexone 6 mg by mouth significantly reduced the incidence of pruritus following epidural morphine without affecting analgesia, but a dose of 9 mg was associated with a shorter duration of analgesia (45[R]).

The mechanism whereby spinal opioids cause generalised pruritus is likely to be due to widespread alteration in sensory modulation as it occurs when there is evidence of opioid migration over the entire spinal cord to the brain. The dominant feature of facial pruritus, which is often reported, may be explained by rapid penetration of opioid to the superficially placed caudal portions of the nucleus of the spinal tract of the trigeminal nerve (46). Pruritus is not due to preservatives within the injection, as it occurs with non-preservative-containing opioid solutions (47a). It is unlikely to be due to histamine release, as the effect occurs about 3 hours after spinal or epidural administration (46–49) and occurs with fentanyl which does not cause histamine release in contrast to morphine (50). Intravenous naloxone reverses the pruritus (46).

Whereas a high incidence (50%) of delayed (6 hours) *nausea and vomiting* has been reported in volunteers who received epidural morphine (46), a low incidence has been noted in postoperative patients (51). In another series the incidence of nausea (12%) and vomiting (24%) was similar whether morphine was used intramuscularly or epidurally or saline was injected epidurally (36). In labor the incidence of this side effect has been reported to be low with epidural opioid (37, 52[c]) in comparison with intrathecal opioid (23, 24). The incidence appears to decrease on repeat dosing and is very low in patients with cancer who require long-term opioid administration (27, 53). Nausea and vomiting has also been reported following fentanyl (54[CR], 55[CR]) and pethidine (meperidine) (56[c]). The effects are abolished by intravenous naloxone without diminution of analgesia (57[c]).

Current evidence suggests that the *urodynamic effects* of epidural morphine are not dose-related and the incidence is similar to that reported after intramuscular injections. Urinary retention occurs more frequently following the use of epidural opioids in volunteers as compared with patients (58–61). In one series (46[C]) two patients who had failed to respond to bethanechol 5 mg subcutaneously, responded to intravenous naloxone 400 μg, which suggests that the mechanism involves opioid receptors. Further evidence for involvement of an opioid mechanism is offered in studies by Rawal et al. (59, 62) in which all subjects responded to naloxone 800 μg. The same authors (63) found a 22% incidence of urinary retention in 90 postoperative patients who received epidural morphine. This compares with a rate of 39% reported in another series (36). A dose-response study which used epidural morphine in increments ranging from 0.5 to 8 mg (64) showed a similar incidence of urinary retention with all doses. These results are similar to those in a volunteer study involving 30 subjects who received either 2, 4 or 10 mg epidural morphine (59).

Respiratory depression is reported to occur less frequently after epidural than intrathecal opioid administration (65, 66). It is suggested that older patients and those with increased intrathoracic or intra-abdominal pressure are particularly at risk and require a reduced dosage (67). In Gustafsson's retrospective study (66) in which over 6000 patients received epidural morphine, 220 epidural pethidine (meperidine) and 90 intrathecal morphine, respiratory depression requiring naloxone was reported in approximately 0.33% of patients after epidural morphine and 5.5% of patients after intrathecal morphine. Only two of the patients who received epidural morphine had respiratory depression later than 6 hours after the last dose of opioids. Only three of the 22 patients who had respiratory depression after epidural morphine had not received opioids in addition to the epidural morphine during or after the operation. Ten were more than 70 years old and 10 had thoracic injections. Brownridge (37) reported only one case of respiratory depression in 2000 women who received 9000 doses of epidural pethidine (meperidine) 50 mg. This was due to migration of the catheter into the subarachnoid space.

The time taken for diffusion of poorly lipid-soluble opioids such as morphine from the lumbar subarachnoid space to the fourth ventricle is the most likely explanation for the delayed onset of respiratory depression, which is reported by many authors. Erikson and Jensen (68[CR]) suggest that the frequency of respiratory depression may be influenced by the position of the patient and form of administration, as well as by dosage and volume of the opioid.

Thangathurai et al. (40[c]) used doxapram to treat respiratory depression following administration of epidural morphine; however, the patient still required endotracheal intubation and mechanical ventilation to correct severe hypercapnia.

Markedly lipid-soluble opioids have also been reported to cause respiratory depression. Brockway et al. (69[C]) noted profound respiratory depression 100 minutes after administration of 100 μg of epidural fentanyl, whilst epidural sufentanil caused apnea within a couple of minutes which was successfully reversed with nalbuphine (70^{C}). Epidural buprenorphine in a dose of 150 μg produced prolonged time-dependent biphasic depression of carbon dioxide response in six healthy volunteers. The second maximum occurred between 8 and 10 hours after injection (71^{Cr}). Similar cases have been reported by other authors. *Psychomotor symptoms* have been noted subsequent to epidural buprenorphine (72^{c}). Epidural meptazinol has been described as being well tolerated (73).

A case of respiratory depression occurring 3.5 hours after a 2.5-year-old child had been given a caudal epidural of 100 μg/kg of morphine was reported by Krane (74^{C}). The effects were successfully reversed by intravenous naloxone.

Dougherty et al. (75^{C}) evaluated the efficacy of up to two doses of epidural hydromorphine 1.5 mg in 10 women following cesarean section. The duration of analgesia was 19.3 (±4.2) hours. Adverse effects were pruritus (56—70%), nausea (11—20%), and vomiting in less than 10% There was a significant increase in venous P_{CO_2} 3 hours after the second dose of hydromorphine. No delayed respiratory depression was noted. In a study by Macrae et al. (76^{Cr}) comparing extradural diamorphine 5 mg with extradural phenoperidine 2 mg and intramuscular diamorphine 5 mg, extradural diamorphine produced more prolonged and intense analgesia and no serious side effects were reported. *Maternal pyrexia* had been reported following epidural opioid analgesia during labor. This may be the result of vascular and thermoregulatory modifications induced by the epidural analgesia (77^{Cr}).

A single case of a grand-mal seizure 6 hours after administration of epidural morphine occurred in a 30-year-old known epileptic woman who had undergone cesarean section (78^{cr}). Myoclonic seizures following epidural morphine 25 mg/h and after intrathecal hydromorphone were reported by Parkinson et al. ($79a^{C}$).

Use of epidural opioids in labor may pose a potential risk to the fetus ($79b^{c}$), but Hughes et al. (80^{CR}), in a series of 40 parturients who received either epidural morphine 2—7.5 mg or bupivacaine (10 patients), found that the opioid did not produce respiratory depression in the neonate.

Less frequent reports of adverse reactions associated with the use of epidural opioids include a case of *catatonia* following a continuous infusion of epidural morphine (81^{C}). *Hallucinations* were thought to be an important sign of impending intoxication. An *anaphylactic reaction* to epidural fentanyl has been reported (82^{Cr}). Both severe *hypotension* and severe *hypertension* have occurred following epidural pethidine (meperidine) (83^{Cr}, 84). Two cases of *Meniere-like syndrome* (85; SEDA-16, 83) and *vertical nystagmus* and *blurred vision* (SEDA-16, 83; SEDA-17, 86) have been reported after epidural morphine.

Symptoms of *shock* lasting 2—3 hours occurred in two women with advanced cancer who were commenced on epidural buprenorphine 300 μg following the onset of tolerance to epidural morphine. The buprenorphine was given 12 hours after the last dose of morphine and symptoms started within 2 hours of administration and remitted spontaneously (86^{C}).

Epidural opioids have a much better safety margin in patients who are already tolerant to such drugs (87^{Cr}). Tolerance has also not proven to be a problem ($88a^{CR}$).

Mechanical difficulties in the form of backflow of solution from epidural catheters occurred in 31 out of 32 patients and there were neurological complications in a further two out of eight patients where the catheter had been tunnelled and connected to a subcutaneous access port. Epidural fibrosis with compression of the spinal cord was presumed to be the cause (87^{Cr}). Others have also reported epidural fibrosis to be a complication after long-term epidural morphine administration (SEDA-17, 85).

CURRENT CONCEPTS ON THE TREATMENT OF OPIOID WITHDRAWAL *(SED-11, 140; SEDA-18, 85)*

A variety of treatment regimens were used in the past in an attempt to withdraw patients from opioid addiction ($88b^{R}$). The modern scientific basis for the evaluation of opioid withdrawal regimens was established by Kolb and Himmelsbach (89^{CR}) who concluded that the methods which produced the least discomfort and the best results were either abrupt or rapid withdrawal of the narcotic. Rapid withdrawal consisted of gradually decreasing doses of morphine in 4—10 days. Such methods were in regular use until the advent of methadone as a heroin substitute in the 1950s.

A widely used technique pioneered by Isbell and Vogel (90^{C}) involves the substitution of methadone for the illicit opioid followed by a gradual reduction in the amount of methadone taken. Methadone is used to substitute for a variety of opioid drugs. It is well absorbed after oral ingestion with peak blood concentrations after about 4 hours. Steady-state concentrations are reached about 5 days after initiation of treatment. By virtue of its long duration of action (half-life on regular dosing is about 22 hours), methadone suppresses opioid withdrawal symptoms for 24—36 hours. In the early stages of treatment patients may reports problems such as drowsiness, insomnia, nausea, euphoria, difficulty in micturition, and excessive sweating. With the exception of chronic constipation and excessive sweating these effects do not generally persist.

British studies have shown that, using methadone, about 80% of in-patient subjects but only 17% of outpatients were successfully withdrawn (91, 92). However, the technique is not without its problems, one being that the methadone reduces but does not eliminate withdrawal symptoms. Kleber (93) described the withdrawal response as being akin to a mild case of influenza, objectively mild but subjectively severe. The fear expressed by those dependent on drugs regarding withdrawal symptoms should not be underestimated: these factors are associated with the subsequent severity of withdrawal symptoms, and they are more closely related to symptom severity than drug dosage (94). Methadone substitution can result in a protracted withdrawal response with patients still experiencing significantly more symptoms than controls 2 weeks after discontinuation of drug therapy (95).

A recent study (96[C]) compared the outcomes from a 10-day and 21-day methadone withdrawal programme. Those patients who were withdrawn over 10 days showed a withdrawal syndrome that began to increase in severity from day 3, with peak severity of symptoms on day 13. In the 21-day programme, symptoms began to increase about day 10 with a peak on day 20 and declined thereafter, although some patients were not fully recovered until 40 days after starting withdrawal. Thus the duration of the withdrawal syndrome is much the same for both treatments in terms of symptom severity. It is possible that an exponential rather than linear reduction in the dosage may improve the withdrawal response. Although not scientifically significant, these results may be of clinical significance in that patients may feel it important that they recover from withdrawal as quickly as possible in order to fully participate in other aspects of the drug-withdrawal treatment. However, although there was no difference between the 10-day and 21-day programmes with regard to completion rates for detoxification (70 and 79%, respectively), the drop-out rates after detoxification were significantly different. During the 10 days after the last dose of methadone, the drop-out rate for the 21 day group was 17.5% compared with 30.3% for the 10 day group ($P<0.05$). These results may also have financial implications in respect of the number of subjects who can be admitted to treatment programmes.

Clonidine is a centrally acting α_2-adrenoceptor agonist which decreases sympathetic output from the lower brainstem regions. It appears to ameliorate the opioid withdrawal syndrome by decreasing, central noradrenergic activity. Gold et al. (98[C]) hypothesized that the opioid withdrawal syndrome may be due to increased noradrenergic neuronal activity in areas such as the locus coeruleus (LC) which are regulated by both opioid receptors and α_2-adrenoceptors. Opioids and clonidine both act at the LC to decrease central noradrenergic function. This common pathway hypothesis is supported by the similarity of clonidine and opioid withdrawal with respect to their effect on vital signs, mood and noradrenergic hyperactivity (99[C]). The actions of clonidine are mediated by α-adrenoceptors and are therefore not antagonized by opioid antagonists. Clonidine diminishes noradrenaline release by binding presynaptically to α-adrenoceptors and reverses the increased noradrenaline turnover during withdrawal (100[R]).

There have been many reports on the use of clonidine in the treatment of acute opioid withdrawal (101[C]). A dose of 500 μg daily for 10 days reduced but did not completely abolish withdrawal symptoms in 50 patients dependent on methadone or heroin. Patients still complained of sluggishness, insomnia and bone pain, but there were none of the usual complaints associated with opioid withdrawal such as anxiety, abdominal cramps, chills, muscle spasms, irritability and anger.

Charney et al. (102[cr], 103[cr]) also reported good results from the use of clonidine. Under controlled in-patient conditions, 20 out of 25 patients physically dependent on methadone were able to withdraw completely from methadone at the end of 2 weeks. In most patients, 10—11 days of clonidine administration, with a peak dose of 16 μg/kg per day, resulted in a perceived reduction in symptoms compared with previous attempts to become opioid-free. At these dosages clonidine significantly reduced standing blood pressure without producing clinical problems. Withdrawal symptoms of anxiety, restlessness, insomnia, and muscular aching were still evident.

In a randomised double-blind placebo-controlled trial comparing clonidine with a decreasing dose of methadone there was no difference in success rate, with 42% abstinence reported for clonidine, and 39% for methadone (104[CR]). However, patients receiving clonidine experienced self-rated level of maximum withdrawal symptoms and a higher percentage of days on which self-rated symptoms were high.

Clonidine has been reported to cause decreases of 10—15 mmHg in both diastolic and systolic blood pressure during treatment for opioid withdrawal. Sedation and insomnia have also been noted. It is often difficult to distinguish which symptoms are due to the treatment and which may be caused by the opioid withdrawal syndrome. In a comparison of clonidine and methadone

50% (seven) of patients in the clonidine group were removed from the study because they were rated as experiencing unacceptable side effects compared to one out of 11 in the methadone group. Two of those taking clonidine experienced severe immediate side effects that prevented them from continuing beyond 2 days (105a[C])

One of the limitations of clonidine treatment is that it does not appear to decrease the duration of the opioid withdrawal syndrome. Charney et al. (103[cr]) found that 10 days of clonidine therapy is required to suppress the symptoms of opioid withdrawal from long-acting opioids such as methadone.

Ghodse et al. (105b) have examined the effect of clonidine in the management of opioid-dependent individuals undergoing a 14-day period of gradual methadone detoxification. In those who completed the period, clonidine did not significantly reduce either the symptoms or objective signs of opioid withdrawal. During the trial there was a substantial drop-out rate and several subjects were withdrawn because of hypotension-related symptoms. In those who completed detoxification, clonidine did not reduce either the symptoms or the signs of opioid withdrawal. Due to these results, clonidine seems to have no place as an adjunct to a program of gradual methadone detoxification.

Naltrexone is an orally active long-acting pure opioid antagonist which has no significant actions of its own. It antagonises the actions of morphine-like drugs by preferentially binding to opioid receptors in the brain and other tissues, thereby displacing any opioid present and preventing the binding of any pure opioid agonist subsequently administered.

Charney et al. (106a[Cr]) undertook a large-scale double-blind study using titrated doses of clonidine and naltrexone. Combined clonidine and naltrexone treatment allowed 38 out of 40 patients physically dependent on methadone to withdraw completely in 4–5 days. For most patients naltrexone was gradually increased from 1 to 50 mg/day over 4 days. The dose of clonidine ranged from 200 to 600 μg every 4 hours. After the first 48 hours the dose was rapidly tapered without recurrence of withdrawal symptoms. Flurazepam was used for night sedation. Although clonidine reduced the intensity of naltrexone-induced withdrawal symptoms, it did not eliminate them completely. On the first day after discontinuation of methadone and commencement of naltrexone and clonidine the frequencies of craving, anxiety, restlessness, insomnia, muscular aching, anorexia, hot and cold flushes and diarrhea were significantly higher than whilst taking methadone. However, after 4 days of naltrexone treatment, patients were considerably less symptomatic. In comparison to feelings whilst on methadone, patients complained of significant increases in irritability, 'unpleasantness' and lethargy for the first 3 days of clonidine and naltrexone therapy.

The combined use of clonidine and naltrexone appears to allow successful withdrawal from long-term methadone therapy within 4–5 days of its abrupt discontinuation. Although patient selection may be an important consideration, the apparent success rate compares favorably with other methods and is achieved in a much shorter time (103). Naltrexone may be used on its own in 'detoxified' individuals to discourage relapse.

In some treatment programmes total abstinence is not considered to be a practical objective and treatment may involve the use of drugs such as methadone as maintenance therapy with the expectation of reducing illicit drug consumption (97[C]). Well organized methadone maintenance treatment can reduce the intake of illicit opioids in many injecting drug users (106b, 107a).

The methadone maintenance treatment was established in 1964 in New York City by Vincent Dole and Marie Nyswander.

In the initial studies, heavily heroin addicted subjects were evaluated and stabilized on daily methadone doses in in-patient service before transfer to out-patient clinic for continued treatment. With further experience, it was feasible to drop the in-patient phase, and start with the out-patient clinic.

Outcome studies of methadone maintenance treatment have reported favorable results. High rates of patient retention, reduced criminality and improved social rehabilitation are reported. However, despite its proved effectiveness, it remains a controversial approach among substance abuse treatment providers, public officials, policy makers, the medical profession, and the public at large. Despite the controversy, almost every nation with a significant narcotic addiction problem, has established a methadone maintenance treatment program.

For patients entering treatment from an institution where they have been drug-free, initial daily methadone doses should be no more than 20 mg, otherwise initial daily doses of 30–40 mg should be sufficient to obtain a necessary balance between withdrawal and narcotic symptoms. Thereafter stabilization is achieved by gradually increasing the doses. When methadone is administered in adequate oral doses (usually 60 mg/day or more), a single dose in a stabilized patient lasts between 24 and 36 hours, without creating euphoria and sedation. The tolerance to methadone seems to remain steady, thus patients can be maintained on the same dose, e.g. in some cases more than 20 years.

The methadone dose must be determined indivi-

Table 2 *Interations; opioid analgesics*[a]

Drug	Combined with	Clinical concequences	Proposed mechanism(s)
Codeine	quinidine	decreased analgesic effect (?)	decreased liver metabolism of codeine to morphine
Dextropropoxyphene	carbamazepine	increased effect of carbamazepine	decreased metabolism
	ethanol	increased effect of dextropropoxyphene	decreased metabolism
	fenobarbital	increased effect of phenobarbital	decreased metabolism
	nortriptyline	increased effect of nortriptyline	decreased metabolism
	phenytoin	increased effect of phenytoin	decreased metabolism
Methadone	carbamazepine	decreased effect of methadone	increased metabolism
	cimetidine	increased effect of methadone	decreased metabolism
	phenobarbital	decreased effect of methadone	increased metabolism
	fluvoxamine	increased effect of methadone	decreased metabolism
	phenytoin	decreased effect of methadone	increased metabolism
	rifampicin	decreased effect of methadone	increased metabolism
Morphine	cimetidine	increased effect of morphine (?)	decreased metabolism
	amitriptyline	increased effect of morphine	increased bioavailability
	clomipramine	increased effect of morphine	increased bioavailability
Pethidine	cimetidine	increased effect of pethidine	decreased metabolism
	chlorpromazine	increased toxicity of pethidine	?
	moclobemide	serious CNS-syndrome	?
	selegilin	serious CNS-syndrome	?

[a]See also separate paragraph.

dually, due to individual variability in pharmacokinetics and pharmacodynamics. However, maintenance of appropriate methadone blood levels are recommended.

Tolerance to the narcotic properties of methadone develops within a period of 4—6 weeks, but tolerance to the autonomic effects (e.g. constipation and sweating) develops at a slower rate.

The major side effects during treatment occur during the initial stabilization phase. In addition to constipation and sweating, the most frequent reported side effects are transient skin rash, weight gain and water retention. Drugs reported to interact with methadone are listed in Table 2.

The methadone maintenance treatment is considered to be a medically safe treatment with relatively few and minimal side effects. However, a recent article highlights the danger of serious adverse effects and death with the increasing use of methadone as maintenance therapy in drug addicts. It must be emphasized that the toxicity of a daily maintenance dose of 50—100 mg to a non-tolerant adult and as little as 10 mg to a child can be fatal. There is an increasing number of reports of the death of children of mothers on maintenance therapy due to inadvertent ingestion.

Buprenorphine, a partial opioid agonist has been suggested to be useful for the treatment of cocaine and opiate dependence. A study designed to assess the safety of buprenorphine for this use (SEDA-18, 85) found that there were no adverse effects or serious interactions with a single dose of intravenous morphine or cocaine during daily maintenance on buprenorphine.

Antidepressant, anxiolytic and neuroleptic agents may allow some patients to participate in treatment programmes, especially when drug abuse is associated with a psychiatric disorder such as depression, chronic anxiety or schizophrenia.

Opioids and opioid analgesics *(SEDA-12, 61; SEDA-13, 56; SEDA-14, 62; SEDA-16, 78; SEDA-17, 78; SEDA-18, 79)*

ADVERSE REACTION PATTERN

General and toxic reactions Although opioids share many side effects, qualitative and quantitative differences exist between them. They all cause constipation by virtue of a reduction in gastrointestinal motility. Respiratory depression, cough suppression, nausea, vomiting and urinary retention also occur. With the exception of constipation, tolerance to these effects develops. Physical and psychological dependence is a possibility. Interaction with monoamine oxidase inhibitors leads to central nervous excitation and hypertension.

Hypersensitivity reactions are rare though anaphylactic reactions have occurred following intravenous use and skin phenomena can occur.

Tumor-inducing effects have not been described in man, but recent in vitro work suggested a mutagenic effect for papaveretum in mammalian cell lines apparently related to the noscapine content.

ORGANS AND SYSTEMS

Cardiovascular *Orthostatic hypotension* may occur and is common after intravenous administration. Histamine release sometimes contributes to this phenomenon.

Respiratory Opioids *depress respiration* by virtue of a direct effect on brainstem respiratory centres (107b[cr]). The nadir depends on the route of administration, occurring around 7 minutes after intravenous administration of opioids but not until about 30 minutes following intramuscular use and 90 minutes after subcutaneous injection. Pulmonary *granulomatosis* has occurred (108[R]) and a case of *asthma* after opioid inhalation has been described (109[C]).

Nervous system Opioids produce analgesia without loss of consciousness, although *drowsiness, changes in mood* and *mental clouding* do occur. Responses to painful stimuli are blocked at several locations in the brain resulting in both an alteration in the sensation of pain as well as a change in the affective response. The ability of a patient to perceive pain may remain the same whilst his tolerance to pain is markedly increased (110[R]). Opioids cause *nausea and vomiting* as a result of stimulation of the chemoreceptor trigger zone in the medulla, although tolerance to this effect usually develops within a few days (111[C]).

Morphine and most opioids cause *constriction of the pupil* in man, which may be due to an excitatory action on the autonomic segment of the nucleus of the oculomotor nerve. Tolerance to this miotic effect is not usual.

Single therapeutic doses of opioids produce a shift towards increased voltage and lower frequencies in the *encephalogram* such as occurs in natural sleep or after very low doses of barbiturates. High doses of morphine may cause *sleep disturbances* in some children (SEDA-17, 78). Fentanyl and sufentanil may cause *epileptiform activity* in patients underdoing coronary artery bypass grafting (SEDA-18, 79).

Schnorr and Hempelmann (SEDA-16, 78) mention *catatonia* as a rare complication of prolonged epidural opioid administration in cancer pain.

Bruera et al. (112[cr]) found that patients with advanced cancer who were taking opioids experienced significant but transient *cognitive impairment* when opioid doses were increased. This correlates well with studies of the effect of psychotropic medication on a patient's ability to drive (113[R]).

Endocrine, metabolic Morphine *decreases the response of the hypothalamus* to afferent stimulation. In many species, opioids alter the equilibrium point of the hypothalamic heat-regulatory mechanisms. In patients undergoing surgery, opioids inhibit the stress-induced release of ACTH. Secretion of luteinizing hormone (LH) and thyrothrophin is suppressed, whereas the release of prolactin and, in some cases, growth hormone is enhanced.

Gastrointestinal (*see also 'Nervous system' above*) Opioids *decrease the secretion of hydrochloric acid* and have a marked effect on *gastrointestinal motility*. Gastric emptying is prolonged and the likelihood of esophageal reflux is increased (114). Tone in the antral part of the stomach and first part of the duodenum is increased. Passage of gastric contents through the duodenum may be delayed as much as 12 hours, thus retarding the absorption of orally administered drugs (115). In 260 patients with malignant disease, 23—40% vomited and 8—10% experienced nausea (SEDA-17, 79). Use of transdermal hyoscine (scopolamine) may reduce this problems (SEDA-17, 79). Biliary and pancreatic and intestinal secretions are diminished by morphine and digestion in the small intestine is delayed. Constipation is usual and this complication has been addressed in two recent articles (SEDA-17, 79). Similar effects are seen in the large intestine. Tone of the anal sphincter is increased and the usual reflex relaxation response to rectal distention is reduced. Therapeutic doses of opioids may constrict the sphincter of Oddi such that biliary tract pressure rises 10-fold. Patients with biliary colic may experience an exacerbation of pain after administration of morphine.

Urinary system The urinary voiding reflex is inhibited, with both the tone of the external sphincter and the volume of the bladder increased; therefore *urinary retention* is common.

Skin and appendages *Flushing* of the face, neck and upper thorax may follow therapeutic doses of opioids. These effects may be partly due to release of histamine which is also implicated in the *sweating* and *pruritus* seen after opioid administration. Opioid effects on neurons may partly be involved in the pruritus, as pruritus is provoked by opioids that do not release histamine and is abolished by small doses of naloxone.

Urticaria at the site of injection is due to histamine release. It is seen with pethidine (meperidine) and morphine, but not with oxymorphone, methadone, fentanyl or sufentanil. Levy et al. (116[Cr]) found that wheal and flare responses to various opioids differed.

Risk situations *Renal impairment* can result in clinically significant accumulation of pharmacologically active opioid metabolites and such patients must be monitored for signs of toxicity (SEDA-17, 79; 117[CR], 118[CR]). To date, this effect has been only reported with codeine, morphine and pethidine. Propoxyphene is not recommended in renal failure, as its metabolite norpropoxyphene, which is eliminated via the kidney accumulates causing cardiac depressant effects (SEDA-17, 79).

In patients with a *decreased respiratory reserve*, such as those with emphysema, severe obesity, cor pulmonale and kyphoscoliosis, opioids must be used with caution. The benefits and risks of using opioids in patients taking *mono-amine oxidase inhibitors*, those with a history of *drug abuse*, *asthma*, *hepatic impairment*, *hypotension*, *raised intracranial pressure* or *head injury* as well as during *pregnancy* or *breast feeding* should be carefully considered. *Elderly patients* are particularly at risk as a number of these factors may co-exist in any one individual.

Neonates, *infants* and *children* may also be considered as groups at risk, due to both pharmacokinetic and pharmacodynamic changes. This has recently been reviewed (SEDA-17, 78).

Withdrawal effects Chronic administration of opioids produces physical and psychological dependence. A characteristic withdrawal syndrome occurs when the drug is stopped abruptly or an opioid antagonist is given. In the case of morphine, and other μ-agonists with a similar duration of action, lacrimation, rhinorrhea, yawning and sweating appear about 8—12 hours after the last dose. Symptoms peak about 24—48 hours after cessation of opioid with restlessness, irritability, and insomnia as well as severe sneezing, weakness, anxiety and depression. Other symptoms reported include dilated pupils, anorexia, piloerection, nausea, vomiting, diarrhea, pyrexia, hypertension, muscle cramps, dehydration and weight loss (119[R]).

Second-generation effects Opioids taken in pregnancy by a drug-dependent mother as well as those administered to the parturient can cause *respiratory depression* in the newborn. *Abstinence symptoms* have been reported in infants of mothers who are opioid-dependent at term (120[R]).

Overdosage Acute poisoning involves marked CNS depression with *drowsiness*, *loss of consciousness* and *coma*. Other prominent features are a decreased respiratory rate, hypotension and symmetrical pinpoint pupils (unless the patient has been hypoxic for some time, in which case pupils may be dilated). Decreased urine output, hypothermia, flaccid skeletal muscles and pulmonary edema may also be present. Convulsions have occurred in children.

Rhabdomyolysis in association with myoglobinuric renal failure and cardiac failure has been reported with a variety of agents (SEDA-8, 76; 121[CR]).

Treatment of poisoning Respiratory depression can be rapidly reversed by clearing the airway, ventilating the patient and giving intravenous naloxone. The duration of action of naloxone is generally shorter than that of opioids, necessitating periodic repeated administration.

Interactions Opioids may reduce/prolong the gastrointestinal absorption of other drugs. The partial opioid agonists, e.g. buprenorphine and pentazocine may antagonize the effect of poor opioid agonists.

Clomipramine and amitriptyline enhance the analgesic effect of morphine, probably due to increased biological availability of morphine. Opioid analgesics interact with monoamine oxidase inhibitors causing CNS excitation and hypertension (122). Increased respiratory depression may occur if other respiratory depressant drugs, e.g. *hypnotics*, *sedatives* or *alcohol* are taken concurrently. *Muscle relaxants* and *antihistamines* with sedative properties have a similar effect. Hypotensive effects are increased if opioids and *phenothiazines* are used together (SED-9, 109). The hepatic metabolism of fentanyl and pethidine may be inhibited by *cimetidine*, leading to respiratory depression and sedation (123, 124). *Phenytoin* may enhance the metabolism of pethidine (127[C]) and methadone (128a[C]). There is some evidence that concomitant treatment of pethidine with selegelin or moclobemide may enhance the CNS-toxicity of pethidine. Prolongation of the prothrombin time has been observed in a patient taking warfarin and a compound analgesic containing dextropropoxyphene concurrently (125[C]). Dextropropoxyphene inhibits the oxidative metabolism of *carbamazepine* leading to clinically significant rises in carbamazepine levels (126), also inhibition of the alprazolam and nortriptyline metabolism have been reported.

The enzyme inducing drugs, carbamazepine, phenobarbital, phenytoin and rifampicin enhance the metabolism of methadone, leading to lower serum methadone concentrations (128a[c]).

There is some evidence that fluvoxamine and cimetidine may increase the methadone effects probably due to inhibition of methadone metabolism. Quinidine inhibits the liver metabolism of codeine to morphine. Whether this diminishes or abolishes the analgesic effect of codeine is uncertain (257, 258).

Interference with diagnostic routines Therapeutic doses of morphine may alter the blood levels of *amylase, lipase, lactate dehydrogenase, leucine aminopeptidase, BSP retention, urine glucose* (Benedict's) and *creatine phosphokinase*. Diamorphine has been shown to flatten the *glucose tolerance curve*, increase glycosylation of *HgbA* and depress biological activity of *antithrombin III*.

INDIVIDUAL OPIOIDS

Alfentanil *(SEDA-12, 61; SEDA-14, 62; SEDA-15, 69; SEDA-16, 78; SEDA-17, 79)*

Alfentanil is a potent short-acting opioid used in anesthetic practice. Its rapid onset and short duration of action make alfentanil suitable for use in day care although it is important to treat adverse effects before discharge.

When 30 μg/kg were given to six healthy volunteers no clinical changes in respiratory and cardiovascular function were found (SEDA-16, 78). Bradycardia often occurs with combination of potent short-acting opioid with suxamethonium during induction of anesthesia and alfentanil has been reported to have caused sinus arrest in three patients (SEDA-17, 79).

Nathan (130[R]) found alfentanil particularly prone to cause hemodynamic instability and myocardial ischemia. However, drug interactions or the dosage regimen may have been responsible. Three cases of sinus arrest following alfentanil and succinylcholine have been reported (131[cr]).

Significant *respiratory depression* occurs after alfentanil doses in excess of 1000 μg and delayed-onset respiratory depression has been reported. Used as a general anesthetic for urgent cesarean section, alfentanil may cause marked neonatal respiratory depression, which is reversible with naloxone (SEDA-16, 78).

Increase in intracranial pressure in normal pressure hydrocephalus patients has been described (SEDA-17, 79), and a case of *acute dystonic reaction* in an untreated Parkinson patient has been reported (SEDA-16, 78). Muscular rigidity involving many muscle groups has been described (SEDA-12, 62).

Seizure activity may be less common with alfentanil but certainly does occur.

Alfentanil is associated with a high incidence of nausea and vomiting. It is reported that droperidol may reduce emetic symptoms but moclobemid not (SEDA-17, 79).

A possible *hypersensitivity reaction* to alfentanil was reported in an atopic 13-year-old female who developed life-threatening bronchospasm and confluent urticarial wheals (132[C]).

The incidence of nausea, vomiting, hiccup and tachycardia is comparable to fentanyl. Care is needed when alfentanil is used in the elderly. Elimination of alfentanil is slower in elderly patients 128b[cr]).

There is no significant difference in recovery time between alfentanil and fentanyl. Dechene (129[C]) observed that recovery times were shorter for smokers than for nonsmokers.

Reserpine and alfentanil are reported to cause ventricular dysrythmias (SEDA-17, 79). Powell (SEDA-17, 79) reported the absence of adverse effects when alfentanil was given to a patient taking the monoaminoxidase inhibitor, tranylcypramine.

Alphaprodine *(SEDA-12, 62; SEDA-14, 63)*

Alphaprodine is a synthetic opioid which is rapidly absorbed following oral submucosal injection (133[cR]). It is used in pediatric dentistry, but it has been removed from the market on a number of occasions because of concern about its safety. Problems include *hypoxia, decrease in respiratory rate*, and generalised *venodilatation* with local cyanosis.

Codeine *(SEDA-12, 62; SEDA-15, 69; SEDA-17, 79; SEDA-18, 79)*

In a study comparing side effects following 30, 60 and 90 mg codeine the most frequent side effects of *headache, drowsiness, nausea, thirst* and a feeling of strangeness occurred after 60 and 90 mg doses only. Visuomotor coordination was altered with 60 and 90 mg and dynamic visual acuity with 90 mg only (134[cr]). Decrease in pupil size is related to plasma codeine concentration (135a[C]).

True allergy to opioids is extremely rare. However, codeine allergy resulting in a 'near anaphylactic' reaction has been reported. The management of true codeine allergy was discussed and agents with chemical structure different from the offending drug, such as phenylpiperidines or methadone-like compounds, are recommended (SEDA-17, 80).

Signs of opiate toxicity, reversible with naloxone, were noted in an 80-year-old woman after concomitant treatment with amitriptyline and paracetamol/codeine (Tylex) (SEDA-18, 79).

The metabolism of codeine to morphine is genetically

regulated by the Cyp 2D6 system. Thus, poor metabolizers may lack the analgesic effect of codeine (135b).

Dextromethorphan *(SEDA-12, 62; SEDA - 15, 69; SEDA-16, 79)*

Dextromethorphan is an antitussive morphinan which exerts its action through unknown non-opioid mechanisms. It is sometimes sold without prescription.

In a trial of 11 patients with Huntington's disease side effects were reported in seven patients. These included *eczematoid rash*, *clumsiness*, *dysarthria*, *drowsiness* and worsening *rigidity* (136[CR]).

A possible *interaction* between dextromethorphan and the monoamine-oxidase inhibitor, isocarboxazid, has been described with myoclonic jerks, choreoathetoid movements, and marked urinary retention (137[c]). Dextromethorphan toxicity occurred in a 3-year-old child who ingested possibly up to 270 mg of the drug. Symptoms were reversed by naloxone (138[c]). On two occasions, a *fixed drug eruption* occurred on the arm of a 45-year-old woman after use of dextromethorphan as an antitussive (SEDA-16, 79).

Dextropropoxyphene *(SEDA-12, 62; SEDA-13, 56; SEDA-15, 69; SEDA-17, 80; SEDA-18, 85)*

The most frequently experienced side effects associated with dextropropoxyphene are *dizziness*, *sedation*, *nausea and vomiting*. Other reported effects include *constipation*, *abdominal pain*, *skin rashes*, *light-headedness*, *headache*, *weakness*, *euphoria*, *dysphoria*, minor reversible *visual disturbances* and *liver dysfunction* (139[R]).

Nerve deafness in a 44-year-old woman, co-proxamol (dextropropoxyphene plus paracetamol)-dependent, has been reported (SEDA-17, 80).

Various forms of hepatotoxicity, sometimes involving jaundice or mimicking biliary tract disease have been reported by the UK Committee on Safety of Medicines. In most but not all cases the drug had been taken in conjunction with paracetamol. In some cases, rechallenge was followed by evidence of hepatotoxicity within a few hours, and an immunologically based mechanism is suggested.

Severe *carbamazepine* toxicity can occur if dextropropoxyphene is taken concurrently (140).

Four cases each of *necrotizing anorectitis* and *proctitis* have been reported following long-term (2—24 months) use of suppositories containing dextropropoxyphene and paracetamol (see SEDA-10, 62). *Perineal ulceration* can also occur (141[C]). *Hemolytic anaemia* attributed to the drug has been reported (142[C]) and severe *hypoglycemia* in a patient with chronic renal failure (143[cr]), and in the elderly (SEDA-17, 80).

Recently, the first case report of *fibrous myopathy* after long-term propoxyphene injections have emerged (SEDA-18, 85).

In common with other opioids, dextropropoxyphene has the potential to produce dependence (144[r]). However, the drug has been used to withdraw patients from morphine (145[CR]).

Dextropropoxyphene is widely prescribed in combination with aspirin and in combination with paracetamol. It is particularly dangerous when taken in overdose (146[R]). A mortality rate of 8% was described in a series of 222 self-harm patients (147[CR]). Acute respiratory failure predominated in patients less than 30 years of age whilst cardiotoxic effects predominated in the elderly; cardiorespiratory arrest may occur only 15 minutes after drug ingestion (148[R]).

The cardiac effects are not reversed by naloxone (256[R]), but dopamine may be effective.

Dihydrocodeine *(SEDA-14, 63; SEDA-15, 70; SEDA-16, 79; SEDA-17, 80; SEDA-18, 79)*

Dihydrocodeine is about one-tenth as potent as morphine and similar to codeine in other respects. The most common adverse effects are nausea, vomiting and drowsiness (SEDA-16, 79; SEDA-17, 80; SEDA-18, 79).

Dihydrocodeine was implicated in individual cases of *granulomatous interstitial nephritis* (149[cr]).

Anaphylaxis (150[C]), severe *narcosis* and *acute renal failure* after therapeutic doses (151[cR]), have been reported.

There is a risk in giving dihydrocodeine to the elderly and those with renal impairment.

Fentanyl *(SEDA-12, 62; SEDA-13, 56; SEDA-14, 64; SEDA-15, 70; SEDA-16, 79; SEDA-17, 80; SEDA-18, 80)*

Fentanyl citrate is a synthetic opioid 1000 times more potent than pethidine. It is characterized by a relatively short duration of action, and a rapid reversal of its effects by opioid antagonists (152[R]). The drug is both safe and useful (153[R]), but has typical opioid effects: e.g., even small doses can cause *respiratory depression*. Delayed respiratory depression can be a particular problem in the elderly in whom the elimination half-life is approximately 3 times longer than in younger patients (154[cr]). Respiratory depression has been reversed with nalbuphine; doxapram could only antagonize this effect for 2—5 minutes (155[r]). Chest wall rigidity, sometimes lasting for more than 24 hours and causing hypoxia, may occur postoperatively; it can be attenuated with naloxone or neuromuscular blockers (156[CR]).

Used as a pretreatment for anesthetic induction with etomidate, fentanyl 500 μg produced apnea in 100% of patients and with a 67% incidence of nausea and 47% incidence of vomiting postoperatively (157[Cr]).

Life-threatening complications have included *raised intracranial pressure*, critically reducing cerebral perfusion (158[C]), and *hypertensive crisis* in a patient with previously unknown pheochromocytoma (159[C]).

Fentanyl may also evoke the pulmonary chemoreflex as evidenced by 49.5% of patients in one study and by 28% in another who coughed after administration of fentanyl through a central line (160[Cr]; SEDA-16, 79).

Transdermal fentanyl has a side-effect profile similar to that associated with parenteral administration. Local erythema and rash have been reported (161[CR]) as well as the usual opioid side effects.

Local heating and cutaneous hyperthermia of the patch area may cause lethal problems of overdose due to increased release and absorption (SEDA-18, 80).

Need for prolonged treatment of respiratory depression with naloxone, because of pharmacokinetic variability and/or transdermal drug reservoir has been emphasized by several authors (SEDA-16, 80; SEDA-17, 80).

Fentanyl-induced seizures have been reported (162[CR]).

Movement disorders, without the characteristic autonomic signs of opioid withdrawal, after withdrawal of continuous infusion have been reported to occur in children (SEDA-17, 80).

Several adverse effects have been reported with combined use of fentanyl and midazolam; chest wall rigidity, making ventilation with a bag and mask-system impossible, was reported (SEDA-16, 79). In neonates hypotension may occur (SEDA-16, 80), and a case of respiratory arrest in a child and a case of sudden cardiac arrest were reported (SEDA-16, 80).

However, Laue et al. did not find any cardiac electrophysiological effects of midazolam combined with fentanyl in subjects undergoing cardiac electrophysiological studies (SEDA-18, 80).

Addition of fentanyl to the local anesthetic prilocain does not seem to cause analgesic benefits, but increases the incidence of side effects.

Combining ketorolac with fentanyl for out-patient surgery seems not to offer any advantages over fentanyl alone.

In a situation with decreased concentration of α_1-acid glucoprotein, with decreased binding and increase in the free fraction of highly protein-bound basic drugs like fentanyl, such drugs should be given with caution in order to avoid high concentration and unwanted adverse effects (SEDA-17, 81). Fentanyl may displace bilirubin from albumin in neonates, thus other tried and tested drugs should be used in neonates (SEDA-17, 81).

Heroin (diamorphine) *(SEDA-12, 63; SEDA-14, 64; SEDA-16, 81)*

Diamorphine is a potent opioid which offers no substantial advantages over morphine. Within the United Kingdom it is the preferred parenteral opioid for subcutaneous administration to cachexic cancer patients on the basis of its extreme solubility.

Bilateral *pulmonary edema* associated with heroin abuse has been reported several times (163[cR]) and there is one record of *mixed transcortical aphasia* (164[C]).

Bronchospasm has been noted following use of street heroin, and may be due to contaminants.

A traumatic *skin lesion* with blisters and sweat gland necrosis was described in a 24-year-old male who was comatose as a result of heroin overdose. Immunofluorescence demonstrated deposits of immunoglobulin and C3 in dermal vessels (165[C]).

Heroin was presumed to be the cause of reversible nephrotic syndrome in patients dependent on heroin (166[R]), and renal amyloidosis can be a late effect.

Myoclonic spasm, occurring approximately 24 hours after withdrawal of epidural infusion, has been reported (SEDA-16, 81).

Ketobemidone *(SEDA-16, 81; SEDA-17, 81)*

Ketobemidone is an opioid receptor agonist, with pharmacokinetics and potency similar to morphine. Combined with the antispasmodic drug, *N*,*N*-dimethyl-3,3-diphenyl-1-methylallylamine chloride, ketobemidone (available as Ketogan®) is frequently used in Scandinavia.

In a study of postoperative pain relief, ketobemidone equalled morphine and pethidine with respect to efficacy of analgesia or adverse effects such as *shivering*, *nausea* or *vomiting* (SEDA-16, 81).

Early cough in 40 out of 121 patients given Ketogan for postoperative analgesia has been reported. Four of the patients found it severe and distressing. The lower frequency of cough in patients previously exposed to Ketogan in the premedication may reflect a tachophylaxic reaction (SEDA-17, 81).

Methadone *(SEDA-12, 63; SEDA-14, 64; SEDA-15, 71; SEDA-16, 81; SEDA-17, 81)*

Methadone is a μ-agonist with pharmacological properties similar to morphine.

Methadone-induced *edema* soon after start of treatment is recognized but a case report of distal leg edema after 7 years of treatment was recently published (SEDA-17, 81).

Subcutaneous administration may cause complications like skin *erythema* and *induration* at the injection site (SEDA-16, 81).

Reversible *choreic movements* of the upper limbs, torso and speech mechanism developed in a 25-year-old man taking methadone as a heroin substitute (168[CR]). A variety of complications following parenteral self-administration of oral methadone were noted, including cellulitis abscess formation, necrosis of the skin and deeper tissues, and regional thrombosis, septic and embolic phenomena, often associated with shock and multi-organ failure (169[c]).

Methadone has been used for intrathecal administration. Although this route may provide prolonged analgesia, the adverse effects have been reported to be unacceptable (SEDA-16, 81).

Methadone is extensively used in opioid withdrawal and maintenance programmes (see separate section), and has been safely used for this purpose in pregnancy with only mild effects on the offspring (167[CR]). However, fetal exposure to methadone in utero may cause a *neonatal abstinence syndrome* after delivery.

Rifampicin interaction is thought to have induced acute methadone withdrawal symptoms in two AIDS patients (SEDA-16, 81).

Prolonged therapy with methadone causes increases in thyroxin-binding globulin, triiodothyronine and thyroxine as well as albumin, globulin and prolactin in serum, and these must be monitored (SEDA-15, 71; SEDA-17, 81).

Morphine *(SEDA-12, 63; SEDA-13, 57; SEDA-14, 64; SEDA-15, 71; SEDA-16, 82)*

A similar frequency of adverse effects occurs between buccal and intramuscular morphine, as well as intramuscular and intravenous infusions.

Oral morphine is more effective after repeated rather than single doses. This is probably due to penetration into the central nervous system of morphine-6-glucuronide, the active metabolite (170[R]).

Hallucinations have been described following use of morphine in various dosage forms; one series (171[c]) reported that patients experienced adequate pain relief and no further hallucinations or nightmares when changed to oxycodone. D'Souza (172[C]) reported delusions and hallucinations whilst Jellema (173[C]) observed restlessness, vomiting and disorientation in two male patients over 60 years of age taking slow-release morphine (MST) for relief of pain in advanced cancer. D'Souza's patient was also taking dothiepin.

White et al. (174[C]) showed a clear association between administration of morphine and *dry mouth*.

Other well-documented cases reported in recent years have included non-cardiogenic *pulmonary edema* in three cancer patients, all of whom had received rapidly escalating doses of morphine over a short period (175[C]), evidence of *prolactin release* (176) not antagonised by naloxone, and *purpuric rash* (177[C]).

Adverse cardiac effects due to morphine are rare. They are comprised of inappropriate heart rate responses to hypotension rather than conduction defects. They are not especially associated with inferior cardiac infarction as was previously thought (SED-10, 142).

Bruera et al. (SEDA-16, 82) have commented that some patients developed severe local toxicity during the subcutaneous administration of morphine sulfate (and of hydromorphone) via portable pumps.

Risk situations A higher incidence of adverse effects to morphine has been described in patients with renal impairment who are receiving opioids for some time (118[CR]), and in hemolytic uremic syndrome patients who were given ketamine with subcutaneous morphine postoperatively (178[C]).

A study of patient-controlled analgesia in children suggested that the pharmacokinetics are similar to those in adults, with the exception of young infants (179[Cr]).

Myoclonus may be more likely to occur in patients taking psychotropic or non-steroidal anti-inflammatory drugs as adjunct analgesia (180a[cr]).

Morphine is extensively metabolized. The main metabolite, morphine-3-glucuronide is without analgesic effects, while morphine-6-glucuronide is supposed to be more analgetic/potent than morphine.

Neonates with reduced capacity to morphine-6-glucuronidation may thus have reduced efficacy from the drug, and patients with renal impairment may experience stronger and prolonged effect, due to reduced renal excretion of morphine-6-glucuronides.

Recent studies have indicated that morphine and the two glucuronidated metabolites may have neuroexcitatory effects and affinity with other non-opioid receptors (glycine and/or *N*-methyl-D-aspartate) that is not antagonised by naloxone. Further these 'other opioid' effects may be related to the mechanism of the side effects; hyperalgesia, allodynia and myoclonus which are increasingly reported after high doses of morphine, but that do not seem to occur after methadone, fentanyl, sufentanil and ketobemidone (180b).

Oxycodone *(SEDA-15, 72)*

Oxycodone is an opioid analgesic which is approximately equipotent with morphine. Fishbain et al. (182a[C]) reported a case of atypical oxycodone withdrawal in which the patient experienced restlessness and delusions.

Papaveretum *(SEDA-17, 83)*

Papaveretum (Omnopon, Pantopon) is a mixture of a number of opium alkaloids. There was a 56% incidence of nausea and vomiting with papaveretum in 129 children 24 hours after circumcision using caudal epidural blockade (181[cr]).

Impairment of renal function in a 60-year-old patient after use of papaveretum for perioperative analgesia has been reported (SEDA-17, 83). Because of possible risk of teratogenicity papaveretum is no longer recommended for use in women of child-bearing age (SEDA-17, 83).

Papaverine *(SEDA-12, 64; SEDA-13, 57; SEDA-14, 65; SEDA-15, 72; SEDA-16, 83; SEDA-17, 83)*

Papaverine is a drug closely related to morphine and is also produced by the opium poppy. Pharmacologically it is quite unlike morphine. Its main action being to relax smooth muscle in blood vessels and elsewhere. The mechanism of action is poorly understood, but blockade of calcium channels and phosphodiesterase inhibition seem to be involved.

Papaverine is used for other purposes than morphine; intracavernous injection in diagnosis and treatment of impotence; intracoronary injection for measuring coronary flow reserve.

Intracoronary injection of papaverine has resulted in *ischemic chest pain*, reversed with intracoronary glyceryl trinitrate (184[C]).

Intracoronary papaverine may cause ventricular dysrhythmia lasting less than 1 minute in 1.3% of the patients; women with relatively slow heart rate appear to be predisposed to these adverse effects (SEDA-16, 84). There are case reports of torsades de pointes after 10 mg papaverine intracoronary in a 61-year-old patient and tachycardia deteriorating into ventricular fibrillation in a 49-year-old patient (SEDA-16, 84).

Continuous intravenous infusion of papaverine provided superior pain relief compared to intermittent intramuscular dosing but was associated with potentially life-threatening *respiratory depression* (183[CR]).

Chronic hepatitis, as evidenced by an increase in serum bilirubin and serum glutamic transaminase, has been reported in three cases following long-term papaverine therapy (SEDA-11, 145). Six of 14 patients who were given slow-release papaverine developed abnormal liver function tests. One patient had jaundice and another had abnormal liver function on biopsy (182b[C]).

Intracavernous injection of papaverine is used for treatment of penile erectile failure. Many adverse effects and complications have been reported; mild *discomfort* in the penis during injection, *ecchymosis* at the injection site, *urethral bleeding*, *paresthesia* of the glans, difficulty in reaching *orgasm* and *ejaculation* (SEDA-16, 83).

Priapism may occur in 5—13% of cases if outflow reduction is excessively severe and prolonged, thus maintaining a high concentration of papaverine in the corpus cavernosum. Papaverine is often combined with phentolamine which serves to augment smooth muscle relaxation in addition to blunting adrenergic tone (185[Cr]).

The mechanism of priapism due to papaverine has been investigated by Witt et al. (SEDA-16, 83). Two forms seem to exist, one veno-occlusive priapism with a prolonged painful erection, and one less common form; high-flow priapism with lack of pain and ischemia. The authors emphasize the importance of distinguishing between the two types because they should be treated differently.

Death after papaverine-induced priapism has been reported (SEDA-16, 84).

Smoking diminishes the resulting erection by attenuating intracavernous pressure in response to papaverine (186). *Fibrosis of the corpus cavernosum* may occur on long-term use (187[CR], 188[C]). It may be due to the acidic nature of papaverine which has a pH of 2.7 in comparison with a combination of papaverine and phentolamine which has a pH of 4.5. Stief et al. (189) reported a nil incidence of fibrosis when the less acidic combination with phentolamine was used. Repeated inadvertent injection of the drug superficial to the tunica albuginea may also be a factor (190[c]).

Infective complications of papaverine injection included *inflammation of the corpus cavernosum* (SEDA-16, 84) and *pyogenic granuloma* (SEDA-16, 84). Diabetic patients seem to be more vulnerable to infection of the corpora cavernosum (SEDA-17, 83).

Minor and local complications of intracavernous papaverine include *hematoma*, *ecchymoses*, *severe aching*, and *thickening of the tunica albuginea*. Nodules adjacent to the injection sites but located in the subcutaneous tissue rather than the corpora may be due to incorrect injection technique.

Pentamorphone *(SEDA-15, 74)*

Subjective symptoms in 23 male volunteers who received pentamorphone were *pain on injection*, *headache*, *tiredness*, *euphoria*, *dizziness*, *visual disturbances* and *nausea*. There was no effect on blood pressure or heart rate with doses of 0.015—0.48 μg/kg (191[C]).

Pethidine (meperidine) *(SEDA-12, 65; SEDA-13, 57; SEDA-14, 65; SEDA-15, 74; SEDA-16, 85; SEDA-18, 81)*

Pethidine (meperidine) is about one-tenth as potent as morphine in terms of analgesia. Norpethidine (normeperidine) is an active metabolite of pethidine with a half-life of 15—20 hours which may accumulate in cases of impaired renal function (192) leading to symptoms of overdosage. More common opioid effects associated with pethidine include *myoclonus* and *histamine-releasing activity* (193[cr]). Cases of severe reversible *neurotoxicity* and *parkinsonism* are on record (SED-11, 143; SEDA-18, 82).

Seizures are an uncommon adverse effect of pethidine, although several cases of seizure have been reported, including when pethidine was used in a PCA-system. The metabolite, norpethidine (normeperidine) is considered to be of significant importance in provoking seizure. Risk factors identified are renal failure, sickle-cell anemia, high doses of pethidine, concurrent administration of phenothiazines or drugs that induce hepatic enzymes (SEDA-16, 85; SEDA-18, 82).

Rectal pethidine administration is not advised in children due to enormous variability in bioavailability (SEDA-18, 82). When used for sedation in children undergoing esophagogastroduodenoscopy, *hypoxia with arrhythmia* was more likely to occur with a combination of pethidine and diazepam than with pethidine and midazolam (SEDA-18, 81).

Phenoperidine

Phenoperidine is a potent opioid analgesic often used in neuroleptanalgesia and as a respiratory depressant in ventilated patients. *Intracranial hypertension* occurred within 1 minute in a patient with a severe head injury who received 1 mg phenoperidine intravenously. It was associated with a decrease in arterial blood pressure. A similar reaction occurred when a second 1 mg bolus was given 8 hours later (SED-11, 146).

Sufentanil *(SEDA-12, 66; SEDA-13, 58; SEDA-14, 65; SEDA-15, 74; SEDA-16, 85; SEDA-18, 82)*

Sufentanil, a fentanyl analogue, is a synthetic opioid with high affinity for μ-opioid receptor and high lipid solubility, with a potency some 5—10 times that of the parent drug. Sufentanil is a short acting established analgesic. Frequently side effects are of the opioid-type like; *pruritus*, *sedation*, *nausea* and *vomiting*, as well as *dizziness*, *urinary retention*, *light-headedness*, *miosis* and *shivering* (SEDA-16, 86). *Motor neuron blockade*, *acute hypotension* and *muscle weakness* seem to be rare, affecting less than 1% of patients (SEDA-16, 86).

The incidence of *hypotension* is quoted as 7% and that of *hypertension* 3%. In a double-blind study comparing morphine, pethidine, fentanyl and sufentanil in balanced anesthesia, those patients who received sufentanil showed the least hemodynamic disturbance. In high doses, adverse effects like bradycardia and hypotension may lead to complications in some patients (SEDA-16, 85). Spiess et al. (194[C]) noted sudden hypotension on induction of anesthesia with sufentanil in four patients, in whom the dose varied between 8.4 and 22.7 μg/kg. Other workers noted similar findings at doses of 1 and 1.5 μg/kg.

Clinically significant *bradycardia* or asystole occurred on induction in cases when sufentanil was used in conjunction with vecuronium (195[C], 196[C]).

There are isolated reports of chest wall rigidity following sufentanil (197[c]).

A case report of respiratory arrest 55 minutes following the epidural administration of sufentanil and bupivacaine has been described (SEDA-18, 82). In children when nasally administered sufentanil was used for inducing anesthesia, the ventilatory compliance was mildly or markedly decreased and one required succinylcholine, oxygen and positive pressure ventilation (SEDA-16, 86).

There are case reports on unexpected transient *neurological deficit* after sufentanil in neurosurgical patients (SEDA-16, 85).

Use of epidural sufentanil for labor and delivery, the neonates may suffer subtle neurological signs of drug depression, including mild hypotonia, poor primary reflexes, and poor habituation to repeated stimuli at 1 and 4 hours of life (SEDA-16, 86).

Tramadol *(SEDA-12, 66; SEDA-16, 86; SEDA-17, 84; SEDA-18, 82)*

Tramadol is a new synthetic opioid analgesic with activity at the μ-opioid receptor, but also inhibits neuronal noradrenaline uptake and 5-hydroxytryptamine release. When tramodol 1 mg/kg was given intravenously to 110 adult patients for postoperative shivering, few adverse effects were reported; two had transient *hypotension*, two complained of *nausea* without vomiting. Similarly mild adverse effects were reported in 20% of patients in a trial of tramadol in cancer pain (SEDA-16, 86), and when it was used to relieve severe pain in sports injuries (SEDA-16, 86).

Tramadol is reported not to cause respiratory depression (SEDA-17, 84; SEDA-18, 82), but Vickers et al. (SEDA-17, 84) reported that equipotent doses of tramadol produced less *respiratory depression* with shorter time of duration than morphine.

Adverse effects reported are *nausea*, *vomiting*, *sweating*, *dry mouth*, *dizziness* and *sedation* (SEDA-17, 84).

OPIOID ANTAGONISTS *(SEDA-12, 68; SEDA-13, 60; SEDA-14, 68; SEDA-15, 76; SEDA-16, 87; SEDA-17, 88; SEDA-18, 85)*

The main adverse reactions to the compounds fall into two groups. The first are those caused by a reversal of opioid actions when a drug is used as an antagonist. These include hypotension, pulmonary edema, atrial and ventricular arrhythmias and cardiac arrest. The risk of such effects is increased in patients with pre-existing cardiac abnormalities. The second group of effects results from a direct action of the drug and its actions on the central nervous system, i.e. typical opioid effects, including dependence.

Nalmefene *(SEDA-14, 68; SEDA-15, 76; SEDA-17, 88)*

Nalmefene is a pure opioid antagonist structurally similar to naloxone and naltrexone.

In a trial comparing the efficacy of naloxone and nalmefene in reversing opioid-induced *sedation*, *vertigo and nausea* were observed with nalmefene (199[CR]). Three out of six healthy male volunteers given nalmefene 0.4 mg/70 kg complained of paresthesia in the midthoracic region (200[Cr]).

When nalmefene was given to six men with history of drug abuse, the adverse effects reported were; *agitation*, *irritability*, *muscle tension*, and a *hangover* feeling (SEDA-17, 88).

Naloxone *(SEDA-12, 68; SEDA-15, 76; SEDA-16, 87; SEDA-17, 88)*

Naloxone is generally considered to be an opioid antagonist devoid of pharmacological activity, except for its reversal of opioid effects. Patients with pre-existing cardiac abnormalities are particularly susceptible to effects such as *hypertension*, *pulmonary edema*, *atrial and ventricular arrhythmias*, and *cardiac arrest* which may occur when naloxone is given to reverse opioid effects. As naloxone is widely believed to be innocuous, large maintenance doses of opioids are commonly used in the belief that reversal can be safely achieved at the end of anesthesia. Azar (SED-11, 147) reported severe hypertension and multiple atrial premature contractions following administration of naloxone, especially in patients with coronary heart disease.

Doses of naloxone greater than 1 pg/kg should be given with caution, especially to known hypertensive patients. Massive release of catecholamines in response to pain after administration of naloxone may trigger the typical clinical picture of left ventricular failure.

A fatal case of pulmonary edema in a young man following use of naloxone has been reported (201[C]), although the causal link has been disputed (202[C]).

However release of catecholamines may also be involved in the pathogenesis of pulmonary edema by causing a shift in fluid from the intravascular to the interstitial space. Thus, α-blockers such as phentolamine has been postulated to be beneficial in its management (SEDA-17, 88).

Behavioral effects have been noted after high doses (2 and 4 mg/kg) of naloxone to volunteers. Most subjects experienced an initial 'rush' or 'buzz', tingling or numbness in the extremities, dizziness, a heavy head and reluctance to move or initiate activities, which usually subsided within 15—30 minutes of administration. Transient sweating and yawning occurred later. Nausea and stomach-ache were frequently experienced and in two subjects persisted throughout the day, although in mild form. No pupillary changes or sleepiness were observed. Increasing doses of naloxone were associated with increasingly impaired cognitive performance. *Violent behavior* has been reported to occur after use of naloxone to reverse sedation (SEDA-17, 88).

Mild adverse effects such as dizziness, nausea, coolness of the head, and abdominal pain were reported when moderate doses of naloxone were given to patients with tension headaches (203[CR]).

Convulsions occurred in a baby born to an opioid-dependent mother. This case is unusual as convulsions due to neonatal opioid withdrawal do not usually occur in the first 24 hours after delivery; it suggests that naloxone should be used with great caution in children born to opioid-dependent mothers (204[C]).

Barsan (205a) evaluated the efficacy and toxicity of a naloxone loading dose of 4 mg/kg followed by 2 mg/kg per day in 36 patients with acute stroke. The most common side effect was *nausea and vomiting*, which was easily controlled. The most serious effect was *bradycardia* and *hypotension*, which developed in response to the loading dose. One patient developed hypotension and two developed *focal seizures*, which were ipsilateral to the affected hemisphere; one had *myoclonus*. In another study (SEDA-16, 87), the safety of naloxone in much higher doses was studied in 38 patients suffering from acute ischemic stroke. They were given a loading dose of 160 mg/m^2 over 15 minutes followed by a 24-hour infusion at a rate of 80 mg/m^2 per hour. Twenty-six patients experienced *nausea* and/or *vomiting*, three patients had *behavioural changes* and in seven patients naloxone was discontinued because of adverse effects. The authors concluded that although naloxone is relatively safe in the dosage used, its efficacy in ischemic stroke is unproven.

Marked changes in physiological functions may occur if naloxone is given when the endorphin system has been modified by opioids. Following use of naloxone a decreased plasma prolactin concentration was noted (206[C]) and the abolition of the hypotensive effect of captopril (207[cr]).

Complete resolution of a unilateral neurological deficit associated with anesthesia along with complete resolution of postoperative unilateral EEG evidence of ischemia has occurred when naloxone was given to reverse residual opioid effects (208[cr]).

Naltrexone *(SEDA-12, 68; SEDA-15, 77)*

Reversible hepatocellular injury has been reported with naltrexone in doses of up to 300 mg daily, which is 5 times that usually used for opioid blockade (SED-11, 147). Five of 26 patients treated with naltrexone for obesity developed elevated serum transaminase levels after 3—8 weeks of treatment. In another study in which 60 obese subjects received naltrexone for 8 weeks, abnormal liver function tests were observed in six patients. Three patients failed to complete the course. *Nausea and vomiting* occurred within the first 24 hours of treatment but responded to a reduction in dose. *Changes in mentation* such as *decreased mental acuity*, *depression* and *anxiety* were also noted, all of which resolved when medication was stopped. This is of significance as adverse effects from naltrexone have previously been attributed to mild physical withdrawal syndromes. *Gastrointestinal irritation* and clinically insignificant *increases in blood pressure* are commonly reported effects. *Fatigue*, *irritability* and *decreased food intake* were also reported. One case of *idiopathic thrombocytopenic purpura* is known (209[Cr]).

Behavioral disturbances and aversive effects in particular have been observed when naltrexone has been used for treatment of opioid dependence; symptoms noted were *loss of energy*, *gastrointestinal disturbances* and *mental depression*. When given to a group of clonidine detoxified opioid-dependent subjects, several complained of *anorexia* and *weight loss* (110[C]).

Complaints of *headache* were noted in two children, and an *opioid withdrawal syndrome* in one child during the first 3 days of treatment when naltrexone was given to treat protracted apnea in children with increased β-endorphin concentrations in the cerebrospinal fluid (210[CR]).

PARTIAL OPIOID AGONISTS *(SEDA-12, 68; SEDA-13, 60; SEDA-14, 68; SEDA-15, 77; SEDA-16, 87; SEDA-17, 87; SEDA-18, 85)*

There is some evidence that in the case of partial opioid agonists such as buprenorphine the relative clinical activity of agonist and antagonist actions may differ, depending, among other things, on the dose used.

Buprenorphine *SEDA-12, 68; SEDA-13, 60; SEDA-14, 68; SEDA-15, 77; SEDA-16, 87; SEDA-17, 87)*

Abuse of buprenorphine has been reported in many countries and it is now widely controlled under psychotropic drugs legislation.

Lewis (211[r]) reported that ex-opioid-dependent subjects were clearly able to identify buprenorphine as an opioid in doses ranging from 0.8 to 2 mg.

Although the use of sublingual buprenorphine in management of heroin addiction has been reported (SEDA-16, 88) widespread abuse of buprenorphine by addicts is known (SEDA-16, 88). A new form of buprenorphine abuse has been detected; sublingual tablets being crushed and then snorted (SEDA-16, 88).

Side effects following parenteral, sublingual and rectal use have included *hypotension*, *bradycardia*, *decreased systolic blood pressure*, *decreased stroke volume*, *nausea*, *sweating*, *vomiting*, *vertigo*, *sedation*, and a *reduction in respiratory rate* (212[CR]). In some intravenous studies the incidence of nausea and vomiting has been as high as 20 and 10%, respectively. Hypotension reportedly occurs in 1—5% of patients and hypertension, tachycardia or bradycardia in less than 1%.

Respiratory depression may occur subsequent to buprenorphine. It is often prolonged and may be particularly difficult to reverse (SEDA-16, 87).

Naloxone is of limited use because of its relative inability to displace buprenorphine from opioid receptors. Insignificant effects on circulation and respiration have been reported at lower doses of buprenorphine (4.5—10 μg/kg) (213[CR]).

Gal (214[cr]) reported that naloxone 1 mg had little effect on the respiratory depression caused by buprenorphine 300 μg/70 kg, although both 5 and 10 μg produced consistent reversal, which was more complete with the larger dose. Use of buprenorphine is inadvisable during labor as effects on the fetus cannot be reversed. In clinical practice, respiratory depression is not often a problem except in older and weaker subjects in whom it can be fatal (215[C])

Under some conditions the antagonist action may jeopardise the effect of subsequently administered pure opioid agonists, by blocking μ-opioid receptors so effectively that 'normal' doses of the opioid agonist are ineffective necessitating administration of an increased dose with the attendant risk of respiratory depression. Kints and Stricker in 1987 presented two such cases, one of which was fatal (see SEDA-13, 60). Fortunately such instances appear to be rare. Sedation and nausea are relatively frequent. Used for patient-controlled analgesia, minor *dysphoria* or *euphoria* were reported to occur after buprenorphine (SEDA-16, 88).

In one of three patients receiving epidural buprenorphine for the relief of pain from head and neck cancers, the drug was discontinued because of severe dizziness (SEDA-17, 87). There have been documented cases of *severe pruritus*, *anaphylactic reaction* and *facial and lingual ulcers*, the ulceration following repeated injection of buprenorphine into the left superior cervical ganglion for trigeminal neuralgia (216[C]) of sublingual buprenorphine (217[C]). Ceased gastric emptying and delayed absorption after sublingual buprenorphine is also reported (SEDA-17, 87).

In a double-blind randomised study of three groups of 18 patients having abdominal surgery who received single doses of either intramuscular pethidine (meperidine) 75 mg, with 400 μg sublingual buprenorphine, or 300 μg buprenorphine alone, *sedation* and *nausea* were the most common side effects in all three groups. Patients who received sublingual buprenorphine were significantly less sedated in the immediate postoperative period (218[Cr]).

Butorphanol *(SEDA-13, 60; SEDA-14, 68; SEDA-15, 77; SEDA-16, 88; SEDA-17, 87)*

Butorphanol is a synthetic 14-hydroxymorphinan analogue with a low dependence potential and a low propensity to cause opioid side effects (219[R]). It is a synthetic κ-agonist and μ-antagonist on the opioid receptor system. *Respiratory depression* rises minimally at doses of 2—4 mg. Although cardiovascular toxicity is slight, *elevated pulmonary wedge pressure* has occurred in cardiac catheterisation patients given butorphanol.

In some patient groups, effective doses do cause troublesome effects: e.g. a randomised study involving patients with sickle-cell crisis who received either butorphanol 2 mg intramuscularly or morphine 6 mg intramuscularly, showed an incidence of adverse effects of 23 and 13%, respectively (220a[Cr]). On the other hand, a wide range of doses (4—48 mg/day) over a 1-month period failed to produce scores indicative of euphoric effects, and the withdrawal syndrome resembled a cyclazocine rather than a morphine abstinence effect (219[R]).

Welt (220b[c]) reported two cases of *sinusoidal fetal heart rhythm* where there was a significant temporal relationship between the administration of butorphanol and the onset of the abnormal heart rhythm. In both instances the pattern had reverted to normal when the patient requested further analgesia.

Butorphanol is generally believed to have a much lesser effect on biliary pressure than morphine, fentanyl or pethidine, but 2 mg has caused *biliary spasm*.

A case report of *fibrous myopathy* in a 40-year-old woman who injected butorphanol intramuscularly is on record (SEDA-17, 87).

Butorphanol has been used for epidural anesthesia in obstetric practice without adversely affecting the neonate and no patients suffered pruritus (SEDA-16, 88).

As butorphanol is not orally active, reports of its transnasal administration are of interest. After cesarean section, transnasal butorphanol did not work quite as quickly as intravenous administration. The effect lasted longer but the adverse effects were similar (SEDA-16, 88).

Ciramadol *(SEDA-12, 68)*

Data on the incidence of side effects following normal doses of oral ciramadol are conflicting. Graf et al. (221[Cr]) reported a low incidence of mild side effects, whereas Van Steenberghe et al. (222[C]) found 60 mg ciramadol more effective than 60 mg codeine or placebo, but observed a high incidence of opioid side effects at doses of ciramadol of 15, 30 and 60 mg; some other workers have the same experience.

Conorfone

Conorfone in a 20 mg dose has side effects similar to those of 60 mg codeine, but produces more *drowsiness* (223[C]).

Cyclazocine *(SEDA-12, 69)*

Cyclazocine is an agonist at opioid κ-receptors and it is the drug's affinity for these receptors that is thought to account for *disruption to normal sleep pattern, urination* and sustained *arousal* (224[Cr]). *Visual disturbances* and *racing thoughts* have also be associated with use of cyclazocine. Tolerance to these effects does develop. Abrupt withdrawal of the drug resulted in a classical withdrawal syndrome but without drug-seeking behavior. Adverse effects could be minimized by gradual increments in daily dosage over a period of 3 weeks.

Dezocine *(SEDA-12, 69; SEDA-13, 60; SEDA-16, 88)*

Dezocine is structurally related to pentazocine and reacts primarily with the μ-receptors, but has some affinity for δ- and κ-receptors too. It is a relatively new drug and it is slightly more potent on a weight basis than morphine but with similar side effects at effective levels (2.5—10 mg). According to a recent review (SEDA-16, 88), the most common adverse effects (3—9%) are *nausea and vomiting*, *sedation*, or *local injection site reactions*; *dizziness/vertigo* have also been reported (1—3%). However, in some trials nausea and/or vomiting were reported in 5—22%, while *headache* was the most common CNS complaint (16—35%). Other adverse effects reported in 1% of patients involves the cardiovascular system, respiratory system, urogenital system, CNS, gastrointestinal system and visual senses (SEDA-16, 88).

Meptazinol *(SEDA-12, 69; SEDA-15, 77)*

Meptazinol is a centrally acting opioid analgesic with an affinity for the μ-receptor (226[R]). Common side effects are typically opioid in character; *vomiting* seems to be a problem and *abdominal pain* may occur in some patients. Euphoria and hallucinations are uncommon.

Westcombe and Price (227[C]) found that prophylactic administration of intramuscular prochlorperazine 12.5 mg did not prevent meptazinol-induced emesis; in fact, the incidence of vomiting with this combination was twice the expected frequency; cyclizine was found to be an effective anti-emetic. Prolonged vomiting has followed the use of intravenous meptazinol 50 mg (228[C]).

Clinically and statistically significant *respiratory depression* can occur within 1 minute of the start of a meptazinol infusion at a dose of 1 mg/kg. Respiratory depression was less than seen following pethidine 1 mg/kg but more than observed after 0.5 mg/kg (229[Cr]). Other studies have confirmed these effects. In a study of 49 patients who received either patient-controlled analgesia with meptazinol (20 mg bolus, maximum 120 mg/h) or morphine (2 mg bolus, maximum 12 mg/h) following major orthopedic surgery, there was a tendency for more patients on meptazinol to have obstructive apnea and central apnea.

Nalbuphine *(SEDA-12, 69; SEDA-13, 61; SEDA-14, 68; SEDA-15, 78; SEDA-16, 89; SEDA-17, 87)*

Nalbuphine is a partial opioid agonist structurally similar to naloxone. Like naloxone it has an antagonist action at the μ-receptor, whilst achieving analgesia via an agonist effect at the κ-receptor.

Nalbuphine was shown to be approximately equianalgesic with morphine (230[C]) and hemodynamic and respiratory effects were not statistically significantly different from those seen with morphine (SEDA-14, 69). Other studies show that this also applies to other organ systems.

Cardiac dysrhythmias, hypertension, agitation, nausea and vomiting were recorded when nalbuphine was given to four patients to reverse fentanyl-caused respiratory depression (SEDA-16, 89). A case of fetal sinusoidal rate pattern with nalbuphine is reported (SEDA-17, 87).

Although similar *respiratory depression* occurs with morphine and nalbuphine after single doses, on cumulative dosing there appears to be a ceiling effect with nalbuphine which may also occur with respect to analgesic efficacy (231). Considerable respiratory depression requiring prolonged monitoring has been reported in children (SEDA-16, 89).

The effects of nalbuphine and morphine on *gastrointestinal function* have been compared in 17 volunteers. Nalbuphine 10 mg prolonged gastric emptying to a greater extent than nalbuphine 5 mg or morphine 5 mg, which were about equal in their effects (232[Cr]). However, another study (233[Cr]) found that nalbuphine produced significantly less inhibition of gastrointestinal activity than morphine.

Nalbuphine has been shown to have a similar efficacy

and incidence of side effects when compared with tramadol; paracetamol (acetaminophen) (234[Cr]) and nalbuphine, although when compared with fentanyl arrhythmias and coughing apparently occurred more frequently with nalbuphine (235[CR]).

Transplacental transfer of nalbuphine was measured in eight mothers who underwent cesarean section and were given nalbuphine 200 μg/kg i.v. (±20 μg) along with thiopentone and succinylcholine. The umbilical cord/maternal vein ratio was 1.4:1 at delivery, which occurred between 2 and 10 minutes after nalbuphine injection. Apgar scores at 1 minute were 6.6 (±2.5) and 8.5 (±2.1) at 5 minutes and correlated neither with the serum nalbuphine concentration nor with the time between injection of nalbuphine and delivery (236[cr]). Three cases have been described in which the newborn of mothers who had received nalbuphine during labor developed apnea and cyanosis which required ventilation within 3 minutes of birth (237[C], 238[C]). Additionally, *bradycardia* and *bradypnea* has been reported in babies whose mother were given nalbuphine a few hours before delivery (SEDA-16, 89).

The effect of nalbuphine 20 mg i.v. on *biliary tract pressure* was examined in 10 patients undergoing surgery for symptomatic cholelithiasis and choledocholithiasis. Thirty minutes after administration of nalbuphine there was a statistically significant rise in pressure, but this did not have any apparent deleterious effects (239[C]). Others have suggested nalbuphine to reverse opioid-induced spasm of the sphincter of Oddi (SEDA-17, 88).

The development of dependence is unlikely at doses within the usual analgesic range (240[R]).

Pentazocine *(SEDA-12, 70; SEDA-13, 61; SEDA-15, 78; SEDA-16, 89; SEDA-17, 88)*

The adverse effects of pentazocine in effective doses are again largely typical of its class (241[R], 242[C]), with some quantitative exceptions.

Pentazocine is now controlled under Schedule 3 in the United Kingdom and similar regulations on dependence producing drugs in force elsewhere.

Perceptual disturbances are generally thought to occur more frequently with pentazocine than with other opioids. Objective definition of such phenomena is difficult, but it is interesting to note that in a study of postoperative dreaming following the use of pentazocine and morphine as premedicants there was no statistically significant difference between the two drugs (SED-11, 148).

Pentazocine in a single dose of 30 mg had no effect on motor skills but was found to impair sensory processing and extraocular muscle imbalance. Other effects reported in this study were slight respiratory depression (enhanced by concurrent amitriptyline administration), and feelings of clumsiness, drowsiness, friendliness, contentedness, and a muzzy head (243[Cr]).

Fibrous myopathy and *necrotic ulceration* may occur at the injection site following repeated parenteral administration (241[R]). Also *myocutaneous sclerosis* and extensive *calcinosis* at injection site has been reported (SEDA-17, 88). Pedragosa et al. (244[R]) reported a case of severe renal failure associated with *toxic epidermal necrolysis*. Two distinct types of *skin lesions* were described: scleroderma-like changes, subcutaneous abscesses, cellulitis, ulceration, muscle atrophy and granulomas (all of which are well-recognized consequences of pentazocine abuse), and a generalized erythematous desquamative rash.

Rhabdomyolysis-induced *acute renal necrosis* occurred in a 26-year-old male following concomitant use of pentazocine and alcohol (245[Cr]) and a fatal nephrotic syndrome occurred in a 33-year-old man, with renal glomerular disease, dependent on pentazocine (SEDA-17, 88). Intravenous injection of a mixture of methylphenidate and pentazocine intended for oral use resulted in death due to granulomatosis associated with pulmonary hypertension (246[C]). A further case of large sclerotic and infected areas with multiple depressed atrophic scars at sites of prior ulceration has been described in a 58-year-old nurse who was prescribed parenteral pentazocine. Unsterile injection technique cannot be excluded as a cause (247[c]).

Pentazocine in overdose (248[cr]) can cause generalized tonic-clonic seizures, hypertension, hypotonia, dysphoria, hallucinations, delusions and agitation with a poor response to naloxone. Other authors reported status epilepticus, coma, respiratory depression, acidosis, severe hypotension and ventricular arrhythmias. Increased toxicity is seen in patients who ingest pentazocine with alcohol, antihistamines or CNS depressants; one patient developed opioid pulmonary edema, and one died.

There have been reports of pentazocine-induced *agranulocytosis* in the absence of other predisposing factors (SED-11, 148).

Pentazocine dependence is associated with a mild opioid-like withdrawal syndrome. Abusers sometimes adulterate the pentazocine with tripelennamine ('Ts and blues'). Medical and psychiatric complications can include seizures, abscesses, depression, psychosis, dysphoria, confusion and hallucinations (249[R], 250[cR]). Neonatal withdrawal syndrome has been described with verification by the detection of pentazocine and its metabolites in the urine of both mother and baby.

Within 4 hours of birth the child was irritable, jittery, and hypertonic with a high-pitched cry, voracious appetite and frequent bowel movements. Symptoms improved over 3 days. The mother had been abusing parenteral pentazocine (23—46 mg) for the previous 10 years and injected the last dose of 46 mg some 10 hours prior to delivery (251[c]).

Opioids interact with monamine oxidase inhibitors causing CNS excitation and hypertension. A serious excitatory interaction between fluoxetine and pentazocine has been reported (SEDA-16, 89). The authors commented on the similarity of this syndrome to the reported dangerous interactions between MAO-inhibitors and narcotics, and suggested that increased central 5-HT activity may be the basis of the observed interaction.

Picenadol *(SEDA-14, 69; SEDA-16, 90)*

Picenadol is a racemic mixture of an *N*-methyl-4-phenylpiperidine derivative. It has mixed agonist—antagonist properties which result from the fact that the dextro-isomer is a potent opioid agonist whilst the laevoisomer is an opioid antagonist. Picenadol has also anticholinergic activity. Its adverse effects include *drowsiness*, *dizziness* and *light-headedness* (SEDA-16, 90). In a double-blind study to compare the analgesic potency and side-effect profiles of a single 25 mg oral dose of picenadol with 60 mg codeine and placebo few side effects were reported. *Drowsiness* was the most frequent, with an incidence of 16% (252[CR]).

In a dose of 75 mg, picenadol was reportedly distinguishable from morphine by sedation, dysphoria and hallucinatory activity, probably due to anticholinergic activity; at lower doses it was morphine-like (SEDA-16, 90).

Propiram

Propiram is an orally active analgesic with weak antagonist activity and effects typical of its class (SED-11, 150); recent data seem to be sparse.

Tonazocine *(SEDA-15, 78)*

Tonazocine is a partial opioid agonist which has not been reported to have any adverse effects on the cardiovascular system or to cause clinically significant respiratory depression. Single doses of tonazocine 2, 4 and 8 mg were compared in a postoperative study involving 150 adults. *Drowsiness* was experienced most frequently and *visual hallucinations* occurred in two patients (253[Cr]).

MISCELLANEOUS

Nefopam *(SEDA-15, 79)*

Nefopam is a centrally acting non-opioid analgesic. A variety of side effects has been reported with this drug, namely *nausea*, *vomiting and epigastric pain*, *dizziness*, *drowsiness and mental confusion*, *hypotension*, *tachycardia*, *skin rashes* and *xerostomia* as well as *urinary retention*. Fifty-three cases in which nefopam has been associated with the development of reversible urinary retention, hesitancy, a poor stream, or dribbling have been reported to the UK Committee on Safety of Medicines. The Committee also received 12 reports of *confusion* and 22 of *hallucinations* and has recommended that the drug be used with caution in the elderly, in patients with symptoms of urinary retention or when given concurrently with other medications which have anticholinergic activity (254[r]).

In one study five out of 33 patients (15%) stopped treatment because of the severity of side effects attributed to nefopam (255).

REFERENCES

1. Belgrade MJ. Control of pain in cancer patients. Control Cancer Pain 1989;86:319.
2. Chapman CR, Hill HF. Prolonged morphine selfadministration and addiction liability. Cancer 1989;63:163.
3. Royal College of Surgeons of England. The College of Anaesthetists Commission on the Provision of Surgical Services. Report on the Working Party on Pain after Surgery. London, 1991;12.
4. Foley K. The treatment of cancer pain. N Engl J Med 1985;313:84.
5. Angell M. The quality of mercy. N Engl J Med 1982; 306:99.
6. Porter J, Jick H. Addiction rare in patients treated with narcotics. N Engl J Med 1980;302:123.
7. Evans PJD. Narcotic addiction in patients with chronic pain. Anaesthesia 1981;36:597.

8a. Coote JC, Hughes AM, McKane M et al. Drug consumption in chronic pain patients. Br J Pharm Pract 1986; 9:193.
8b. Bogod D. Advances in epidural analgesia for labour: progress versus prudence. Lancet 1995;345:1129.
9a. Collis RE, Davies DWL, Aveling W. Randomised comparison of combined spinal-epidural and standard epidural analgesia in labour. Lancet 1995;345:1413.
9b. Ghodse AH, Reed JL, Mack JW. The effect of maternal narcotic addiction on the newborn infant. Psychol Med 1977;7:667.
10. Olofsson M, Buckley W, Andersen GE, Friis-Hansen B. Investigation of 89 children born to drug-dependent mothers. II. Follow-up 1—10 years after birth. Acta Paediatr Scand 1983;72:407.
11. Cousins MJ, Mather LE. Intrathecal and epidural administration of opioids. Anesthesiology 1984;61:276.
12. Madrid JI, Fatela LV, Alcorta J et al. Intermittent intrathecal morphine by means of an implantable reservoir. J Pain Symptom Manage 1988;3:67.
13. Dautheribes M, Guérin J. Intrathecal analgesia. A series of 50 cases. Neurochirurgie 1988;33:194.
14. Gestin Y, Pere N, Solasso LC. Long-term intrathecal isobaric morphine treatment. Ann Fr Anésth Réanim 1986;5:346.
15. Lipp M, Daublander M, Lanz E. 0.15 mg intrathecal buprenorphine with spinal anaesthesia: a double-blind study on sensory blockade, postoperative analgesia and side effects. Anaesthesist 1987;36:233.
16. Reay BA, Semple AJ, Macrae WA, Mackenzie N. Low dose intrathecal diamorphine analgesia following major orthopaedic surgery. Br J Anaesth 1989;62:248.
17. Jacobson L, Chapal C, Brody MC et al. Intrathecal methadone and morphine for post-operative analgesia: a comparison of efficacy, duration and side effects. Anesthesiology 1989;70:742.
18a. Oyama T, Matsuki A, Taneichi T et al. Betaendorphin in obstetric analgesia. Am J Obstet Gynecol 1980;137:613.
18b. Jacobson L, Kokri MS, Pridie AK. Intrathecal diamorphine: a dose response study. Ann R Coll Surg Engl 1989; 71:289.
19. Oyama T, Toshiro JIN, Yamaya R. Profound analgesic effects of beta-endorphin in man. Lancet 1980;i:122.
20. Saissy JM. Prurit aprés rachianesthésie à la péthidine. Ann Fr Anesth Réanim 1984;3:402.
21. Shipton EA. Pruritus—a side effect of epidural fentanyl for postoperative analgesia. South Afr Med J 1984;66:61.
22. Barron DW, Strong JE. Safety and efficacy of intrathecal diamorphine. Pain 1984;18:279.
23. Baraka A, Noveihid R, Hajj S. Intrathecal injection of morphine for obstetric analgesia. Anesthesiology 1981; 54:136.
24. Scott PV, Bowen FE, Cartwright P et al. Intrathecal morphine as sole analgesic during labour. Br Med J 1980;281:351.
25. Lazorthes Y. Intracerebroventricular administration of morphine for control of irreducible cancer pain. Ann NY Acad Sci 1988;531:123.
26. Swaraj, Saxena R, Sabzposh SWA, Shakoor A. Effect of intrathecal pentazocine on postoperative pain relief. J Indian Med Assoc 1988;86:93.
27. Glynn CJ, Mather LE, Cousins MJ et al. Spinal narcotics and respiratory depression. Lancet 1979;ii:356.
28. Fitzpatrick GJ, Moriarty DC. Intrathecal morphine in the management of pain following cardiac surgery. Br J Anaesth 1988;60:639.
29. Yamaguchi H, Watanabe S, Motokawa K et al. Intrathecal morphine dose response data for pain relief after cholecystectomy. Anesth Analg 1990;70:168.
30. Glavina MJ, Robertshaw R. Myoclonic spasms following intrathecal morphine. Anaesthesia 1988;43:389.
31. Kleiner LI, Krezeminski J, Rosenwasser RH. Temporary motor and sensory paralysis associated with intrathecal administration of morphine. Neurosurgery 1989;24:756.
32. Tyler DC, Krane EJ. Epidural opioids in children. J Pediatr Surg 1989;24:469.
33. Tobias JD, Deshpande JK, Wetzel RC et al. Care of intrathecal morphine in children. Clin Pediatr 1990;29:44.
34. Krane EJ, Tyler DC, Jacobson LE. The dose-response of caudal morphine in children. Anesthesiology 1989;71:48.
35. Lam AM, Knill RL, Thompson WR et al. Epidural fentanyl does not cause delayed respiratory depression. Can J Anaesth 1983;30:578.
36. Lanz E, Theiss D, Riess W, Sommer V. Epidural morphine for postoperative analgesia. A double-blind study. Anesth Analg 1982;61:236.
37. Brownridge PR. Epidural and intrathecal opiates for postoperative pain relief. Anaesthesia 1983;38:74.
38. Ballantyne JC, Loach AB, Carr DB. Itching after epidural and spinal opiates. Pain 1988;33:149.
39. Ballantyne JC, Loach AB, Carr DB. The incidence of pruritus after epidural morphine. Anaesthesia 1989;44:863.
40. Thangathurai D, Nelson D, Cheung M. Doxapram for respiratory depression after epidural morphine (Letter to Editor). Anaesthesia 1990;45:64.
41. Ackerman WE, Juneja MM, Kaczorowski DM et al. A comparison of the incidence of pruritus following epidural opioid administration in the parturient. Can J Anaesth 1989;36:388.
42. Dezeros G, Levron JC, Simon A et al. Long duration peridural analgesia in Labour by association of bupivacaine and fentanyl. Agressologie 1988;29:33.
43. Keaveny JP, Harper NJN. Treatment of epidural morphine-induced pruritus with buprenorphine (Letter to Editor). Anaesthesia 1989;44:691.
44. Davies GG, From R. A blinded study using nalbuphine for prevention of pruritus induced by epidural fentanyl. Anesthesiology 1988;69:763.
45. Abboud TK, Afrasiabi A, Davidson J et al. Prophylactic oral naltrexone in epidural morphine: effect on adverse reactions and ventilatory responses to CO_2. Anesthesiology 1990;72:233.
46. Bromage PR, Camporesi E, Durant PAC, Neilsen CH. Non-respiratory side effects of epidural morphine. Anesth Analg 1982;61:490.
47a. Sghirlanzoni S, Sala F, Servadio G et al. Epidural morphine and pruritus; the role of sodium metabisulphite. Anesth Reanim 1983;24:177.
47b. Bromage PR, Camporesi E, Durant PAC, Neilsen CH. Rostral spread of epidural morphine. Anesthesiology 1982; 56:431.
48. Bromage PR, Camporesi E, Durant PAC, Neilsen CH. Influence of epinephrine as an adjuvant to epidural morphine. Anesthesiology 1983;58:257.
49. Bromage PR, Camporesi E, Durant PAC, Leslie J. Epi-

dural narcotics in volunteers: sensitivity to pain and to carbon dioxide. Pain 1980;9:145.
50. Rosow CE, Moss J, Philbin DM, Savarese JJ. Histamine release during morphine and fentanyl anaesthesia. Anesthesiology 1982;56:93.
51. Torda TA, Pybus DA. Clinical experience with epidural morphine. Anaesth. Intensive Care 1981;9:129.
52. Perris BW, Malins AF. Pain relief in labour using epidural pethidine with adrenaline. Anaesthesia 1981;36:631.
53. Howard RP, Milne LA, Williams NE. Epidural morphine in terminal care. Anaesthesia 1981;36:51.
54. Lirzin JD, Jacquinot P, Dailland P et al. Controlled trial of extradural bupivacaine with fentanyl, morphine or placebo for pain relief in labour. Br J Anaesth 1989;62:641.
55. Kreitzer JM, Kirshenbaum IP, Eisenkraft JU. Epidural fentanyl by continuous infusion for relief of postoperative pain. Clin J Pain 1989;5:283.
56. Perris BW, Latham BV, Wilson IH. Analgesia following extradural and intramuscular pethidine in postcaesarean section patients. Br J Anaesth 1989;64:355.
57. Rawal N, Wattwil M. Respiratory depression following epidural morphine. An experimental and clinical study. Anesth Analg 1984;63:8.
58. Bromage PR, Camporesi E, Chestnut D. Epidural narcotics for postoperative analgesia. Anesth Analg 1980;59: 473.
59. Rawal N. Mallefors K, Axelsson K et al. An experimental study of urodynamic effects of epidural morphine and of naloxone reversal. Anesth Analg 1983;62:641.
60. Torda TA, Pybus DA, Liberman H et al. Experimental comparison of extradural and intramuscular morphine. Br J Anaesth 1980;52:939.
61. Thompson WR, Smith PT, Hirst M et al. Regional analgesic effect of epidural morphine in volunteers. Can J Anaesth 1981;28:530.
62. Rawal N, Mollefors K, Axelsson K et al. Naloxone reversal of urinary retention after epidural morphine. Lancet 1981;ii:1411.
63. Rawal N, Sjostrand UH, Dahlstrom B. Postoperative pain relief by epidural morphine. Anesth Analg 1981;60:726.
64. Martin R, Salbaing J, Blaise G et al. Epidural morphine for postoperative pain relief. A dose-response curve. Anesthesiology 1982;56:423.
65. Kossmann B, Dick W, Bowdler I et al. The analgesic action and respiratory side effects of epidural morphine. A double-blind trial on patients undergoing vaginal hysterectomy. Reg Anaesth 1984;9:55.
66. Gustafsson LL, Schildt B, Jacobson K. Adverse effects of extradural and intrathecal opiates: report of a nationwide survey in Sweden. Br J Anaesth 1982;54:479.
67. Von Palitzsch J. Respiratory effects of epidural morphine analgesia. Anaesthesiol Reanim 1982;7:335.
68. Eriksen HO, Jensen FM. Side effects of epidural and spinal opiates. Ugeskr Laeg 1982;144:2627.
69. Brockway MS, Noble DW, Sharwood-Smith GH et al. Profound respiratory depression after extradural fentanyl. Br J Anaesth 1990;64:243.
70. Cheng E, May J. Nalbuphine reversal of respiratory depression after epidural sufentanil. Crit Care Med 1989;17:378.
71. Molke Jensen F, Jensen NH, Holk IK, Ravnborg M. Prolonged and biphasic respiratory depression following epidural buprenorphine. Anaesthesia 1987;42:470.
72. MacEvilly M, Carroll CO. Hallucination repression after epidural buprenorphine. Br Med J 1989;298:928.
73. Budd K, Robson PJ, Brown PM. The treatment of chronic pain by the use of meptazinol administration into the epidural space. Postgrad Med J 1983;59(Suppl 1):68.
74. Krane EJ. Delayed respiratory depression in a child after caudal epidural morphine. Anesth Analg 1988;67:79.
75. Dougherty TB, Baysinger CL, Gooding DJ. Epidural hydromorphine for postoperative analgesia after delivery by caesarean section. Reg Anaesth 1986;11:118.
76. Macrae DJ, Munishankrappa S, Burrow LM et al. Double-blind comparison of the efficacy of extradural diamorphine following caesarean section. Br J Anaesth 1987;59:354.
77. Fusi L, Steer PJ, Maresh MJA, Beard RW. Maternal pyrexia associated with the use of epidural analgesia in labour. Lancet 1989;i:1250.
78. Borgeat A, Biollaz J, Depierraz B, Neff R. Grand mal seizure after extradural morphine analgesia. Br J Anaesth 1988;60:733.
79a. Parkinson SK, Bailey SL, Little WL et al. Myoclonic seizure activity in chronic high dose spinal opioid administration. Anesthesiology 1990;72:743.
79b. Nybell-Lindahl G, Carlsson C, Ingemarsson I et al. Maternal and foetal concentrations of morphine after epidural administration during labor. Am J Obstet Gynecol 1981; 139:20.
80. Hughes SC, Rosen MA, Shnider SM et al. Maternal and neonatal effects of epidural morphine for labor and delivery. Anesth Analg 1984;63:319.
81. Engquist A, Jorgensen BC, Andersen HB. Catatonia after epidural morphine. Acta Anaesthesiol Scand 1981; 25:445.
82. Zucker-Pinchoff B, Ramanathan S. Anaphylactic reaction to epidural fentanyl. Anesthesiology 1989;71:599.
83. Balaban M, Slinger P. Severe hypotension from epidural meperidine in a high risk patient after thoracotomy. Can J Anaesth 1989;36:450.
84. Robinson RJS, Metcalf IR. Hypertension after epidural meperidine. Can Anaesth Soc J 1985;32:658.
85. Linder S, Borgeat A, Biollaz J. Meniere-like syndrome following epidural morphine. Anesthesiology 1989;71:782.
86. Christensen FR, Andersen LW. Adverse reaction to extradural buprenorphine. Br J Anaesth 1982;54:476.
87. Driessen JJ, de Mulder PHM, Claessen JJ et al. Epidural administration of morphine for control of cancer pain: Long term efficacy and complications. Clin J Pain 1989;5:217.
88a. Zenz M, Piepenbrock S, Tryba M. Epidural opiates: long-term experiences in cancer pain. Klin Wochenschr 1985;63:225.
88b. Kleber HD, Riordan CF. The treatment of narcotic withdrawal: a historical review. J Clin Psychiatry 1982;43:30.
89. Kolb L, Himmelsbach CK. Clinical studies of drug addiction. III. A clinical review of withdrawal treatment with a method of evaluating abstinence syndromes. Am J Psychiatry 1938;94:759.
90. Isbell H, Vogel VH, Chapman KW. Present status of narcotic addiction with particular reference to medical indications and comparative addiction liability of the newer and older analgesic drugs. J Am Med Assoc 1948;138:1019.
91. Glossop M, Johns A, Green L. Opiate-withdrawal: inpatient vs out-patient programmes and preferred vs random assigment to treatment. Br Med J 1986;293:103.
92. Glossop M, Green L, Phillips G. What happens to opiate addicts immediately after treatment: a prospective follow-up study. Br Med J 1987;294:1377.
93. Kleber HD. Detoxification from narcotics. In: Lowinson

L, Ruiz P, eds. Substance Abuse. Baltimore: Williams and Wilkins, 1981;317.
94. Phillips GT, Glossop M, Bradley B. The influence of psychological factors on the opiate withdrawal syndrome. Br J Psychiatry 1986;149:235.
95. Glossop M, Bradley B, Phillips G. An investigation of withdrawal symptoms shown by opiate addicts during and subsequent to a 21-day in-patient methadone detoxification procedure. Addict Behav 1987;12:1.
96. Glossop M, Griffiths P, Bradley B, Strang S. Opiate withdrawal symptoms in response to a ten day and 21-day methadone withdrawal programme. Br J Psychiatry, 1989; 154:360.
97. Newman RG, Whitehill WB. Double-blind comparison of methadone and placebo maintenance treatments of narcotic addicts in Hong Kong. Lancet 1979;ii:485.
98. Gold MS, Redmond DE, Kleber HD. Noradrenergic hyperactivity in opiate withdrawal supported by clonidine reversal of opiate withdrawal. Am J Psychiatry 1979;136:100.
99. Gold MS, Byck R, Sweeney DR et al. Endorphin locus coeruleus connection mediates opiate action and withdrawal. Biomedicine 1979;30:1.
100. Glossop M. Clonidine and the treatment of the opiate withdrawal syndrome. Drug Alcohol Depend 1988;21:253.
101. Editorial. Clonidine treatment for acute opiate withdrawal. Med Lett 1979;21:100.
102. Charney DS, Kleber HD. Iatrogenic opiate addiction: successful detoxification with clonidine. Am J Psychiatry 1980;137:989.
103. Charney DS, Sternberg DE, Kleber HD et al. The clinical use of clonidine in abrupt withdrawal from methadone, effects on blood pressure and specific signs and symptoms. Arch Gen Psychiatry 1981;38:1273.
104. Rounsaville BJ, Kosten T, Kleber HD. Success and failure of outpatient opioid detoxification: evaluating the process of clonidine and methadone-assisted withdrawal. J Nerv Ment Dis 1985;173:103.
105a. Kleber HD et al. Clonidine in outpatient detoxification from methadone maintenance. Arch Gen Psychiatry 1985;42:391.
105b. Ghodse H, Myles J, Smith SE. Clonidine is not a useful adjunct to methadone gradual detoxification in opioid addiction. Br J Psychiatry 1995;165:370.
106a. Charney DS, Heninger GR, Kleber H. The combined use of clonidine and naltrexone as a rapid safe and effective treatment of abrupt withdrawal from methadone. Am J Psychiatry 1986;143:831.
106b. Lowinson JH, Marion IJ, Joseph H, Dole VP. Methadone maintenance. In: Lowinson JH, Ruiz P, Millman RB, eds. Substance Abuse. A Comprehensive Textbook, second edition. Baltimore: Williams and Wilkins, 1992;550.
107a. Ball JC, Ross A. The Effectiveness of Methadone Maintenance Treatment. New York: Springer-Verlag, 1991; ISBN 0-387-97423-7.
107b. Snir-Mor I, Weinstock M, Davidson JT, Bahar M. Physostigmine antagonises morphine-induced respiratory depression in human subjects. Anesthesiology 1983;59:6.
108. Brashear RE. Effects of heroin, morphine, methadone and propoxyphene on the lung. Semin Respir Med 1980;2:59.
109. Agius R. Opiate inhalation and occupational asthma. Br Med J 1989;298:323.
110. Sternbach HA, Annitto W, Pottash ALC, Gold MS. Anorexic effects of naltrexone in man. Lancet 1982;i:388.
111. Campora E, Merlini L, Pace M et al. The incidence of narcotic-induced emesis. J Pain Symptom Manage 1991;6:428.
112. Bruera E, Macmillan K, Hanson J, Macdonald RN. The cognitive effects of the administration of narcotic analgesics in patients with cancer pain. Pain 1989;39:13.
113. Nielsen SL, Christensen LQ, Neilsen LM. Analgesics, benzodiazepines and traffic. Ugeskr Laeg 1989;151:1822.
114. Duthie DJR, Nimmo WS. Adverse effects of opioidanalgesic drugs. Br J Anaesth 1987;59:61.
115. Goodman A, Gilman A et al. In: Coodman and Gilman's The Pharmacological Basis of Therapeutics, 8th edn. Oxford: Pergamon Press, 1990;494.
116. Levy JH, Brister NW, Shearin A et al. Wheal and flare responses to opioids in humans. Anesthesiology 1989;70:756.
117. McQuay H, Moore RA. Be aware of renal function when prescribing morphine. Lancet 1984;ii:284.
118. Sear JW, Hand CW, Moore RA, McQuay HJ. Studies on morphine disposition: influence of renal failure on the kinetics of morphine and its metabolites. Br J Anaesth 1989;62:28.
119. Eddy NB, Halsbach H, Isbell H, Seevers MH. Drug dependence; its significance and characteristics. Bull WHO 1965;17:569.
120. National Institute on Drug Abuse. Drug Dependence in Pregnancy: Clinical Management of Mother and Child. Services Research Monograph Series, NIDA, DHEW Publication, No. ADM. 1979;79.
121. Scherrer P, Delaloye-Bischof A, Turini G et al. Participation myocardique à la rhabdomyolyse non traumatique après surdosage aux opiates. Schweiz Med Wochenschr 1985;115:1166.
122. British Medical Association and Royal Pharmaceutical Society of Great Britain. British National Formulary, 22nd edn., 1991;458.
123. Knodell RG et al. Drug metabolism by rat and human hepatic microsomes in response to interaction with H_2-receptor antagonists. Gastroenterology 1982:82:84.
124. Lee HR et al. Effect of histamine H_2- receptors on fentanyl metabolism. Pharmacology 1982;24:145.
125. Smith R. Prudden D, Hawkes C. Propoxyphene and warfarin interaction. Drug Intell Clin Pharmacol 1984;18:822.
126. Hansen BS et al. Influence of dextropropoxyphene on steady state serum levels and protein binding of three antiepileptic drugs in man. Acta Neurol Scand 1980;61:357.
127. Pond SM et al. Effect of phenytoin on meperidine clearance and normeperidine formation. Clin Pharmacol Ther 1981;30:680.
128a. Finelli PF. Phenytoin and methadone tolerance (Letter to Editor). N Engl J Med 1976;294:227.
128b. Kent AP, Dodson ME, Bower S. The pharmacokinetics and clinical effects of a low dose of alfentanil in elderly patients. Acta Anaesthesiol Belg 1988;39:25.
129. Dechène JP. Alfentanil as an adjunct to thiopentone and nitrous oxide in short surgical procedures. Can Anaesth Soc J 1985;32:346.
130. Nathan HJ. Narcotics and myocardial performance in patients with coronary artery disease. Can J Anaesth 1988;35:209.
131. Ananthanarayan C. Sinus arrest after alfentanil and suxamethonium. (Letter to Editor). Anaesthesia 1989;44:614.
132. Coventry DM, Stone P. Hypersensitivity reactions to alfentanil. Anaesthesia 1988;43:887.
133. Currie WR, Biery KA, Campbell RL, Mourino AP.

Narcotic sedation: an evaluation of cardiopulmonary parameters and behaviour modification in paediatric dental patients. J Periodont Res 1988;12:230.
134. Bradley CM, Nicholson AN. Effects on an mureceptor agonist (codeine phosphate) on visuomotor coordination and dynamic visual acuity in man. Br J Clin Pharmacol 1986;22:507.
135a. Peacock JE, Henderson PD, Nimmo WS. Changes in pupil diameter after oral administration of codeine. Br J Anaesth 1988;61:598.
135b. Sindrup SH, Brøsen K, Bjerring P, Arendt-Nielsen L, Larsen U, Helle R, Angelo HR, Gram LF. Codeine increases pain thresholds to copper vapor laser stimuli in extensive but not poor metabolizers of sparteine. Clin Pharmacol Ther 1991;49:686.
136. Walker FO, Hunt VP. An open label trial of dextromethorphan in Huntington's disease. Clin Neuropharmacol 1989;12:322.
137. Sovner R, Wolfe V. Interaction between dextromethorphan and monoamine oxidase inhibitor therapy with isocarboxazid (Correspondence). N Engl J Med 1988;319:1671.
138. Katona B, Watson S. Dextromethorphan danger. N Engl J Med 1986;314:993.
139. Grover H. Propoxyphene. J Indian Med Assoc 1988;86:21.
140. Yu YL, Huang CY, Chin D et al. Interaction between carbamazepine and dextropropoxyphene. Postgrad Med 1986;62:231.
141. Bosisio OA, Gonzales AU, Bravard JD et al. Ulcera medicamentosa de ano. Prensa Med Argent 1986;73:437.
142. Fulton JD, McGonigal C. Steroid responsive haemolytic anaemia due to dextropropoxyphene paracetamol combination. J R Soc Med 1989;82:228.
143. Almirall J, Montoliu J, Torras R et al. Propoxyphene-induced hypoglycaemia in a patient with chronic renal failure. Nephron 1989;53:273.
144. Strode SW. Propoxyphene dependence and withdrawal. Am Fam Phys 1985;32:105.
145. Hasday JD, Weintraub M. Propoxyphene in children with iatrogenic morphine dependence. Am J Dis Child 1983;137:745.
146. Proudfoot AT. Clinical features and management of Distalgesic overdose. Hum Toxicol 1984;3(Suppl):855.
147. Sloth Madsen P, Strom J, Reiz S, Bredgaard Sorensen M. Acute propoxyphene self-poisoning in 222 consecutive patients. Acta Anaesthesiol Scand 1984;28:661.
148. Young RJ. Dextropropoxyphene overdose-pharmacological considerations and clinical management. Drugs 1983;26:70.
149. Singer DRJ, Simpson JG, Catto GRD, Johnston AW. Drug hypersensitivity causing granulomatous interstitial nephritis. Am J Kidney Dis 1988;11:357.
150. Panos MZ, Burnett S, Gazzard BG. Use of naloxone in opioid-induced anaphylactoid reaction. Br J Anaesth 1988;61:371.
151. Park GR, Shelly MA, Quinn K et al. Dihydrocodeine—a reversible course of renal failure? Eur. J. Anaesthesiol 1989;6:303.
152. Editorial. High-dose fentanyl. Lancet, 1979;i:81.
153. Chudnofsky CR, Wright SW, Dronen SC et al. The safety of fentanyl use in the emergency department. Ann Emerg Med 1989;18:635.
154. Chung F, Evans D. Low-dose fentanyl: haemodynamic response during induction and intubation in geriatric patients. Can Anaesth Soc J 1985;32:622.
155. Grote B, Kugler J, Gutzeit M, Doenicke A. The influence of doxapram in humans on the respiratory depression by fentanyl. Anaesthesist 1978;27:287.
156. Christian CM, Waller JL, Moldenhauer CC. Postoperative rigidity following fentanyl anaesthesia. Am Soc Anesthesiol 1983;58:275.
157. Stockham RJ, Stanley TH, Pace NL et al. Fentanyl pretreatment modifies anaesthetic induction with etomidate. Anaesth Intensive Care 1988;16:171.
158. Knuttgen D, Doehn M, Eymer D et al. Fentanyl-induced increase in intracranial pressure. Anaesthesist 1989;38:73.
159. Barancik M. Inadvertent diagnosis of phaeochromocytoma after endoscopic premed. Dig Dis Sci 1989;34:136.
160. Bohrer H, Fleischer F, Werning P. Tussive effect of a fentanyl bolus administered through a central venous catheter. Anaesthesia 1990;45:18.
161. Caplan RA, Ready LB, Oden RV et al. Transdermal fentanyl for postoperative pain management, a double blind placebo controlled study. J Am Med Assoc 1989;261:1036.
162. Scott JC, Sarnquist FH. Seizure-like movements during a fentanyl infusion with absence of seizure activity in a simultaneous ECG recording. Anesthesiology 1985;62:812.
163. Reynes AN, Pujol JA, Baixeras RP, Fernandez B. Edema agudo de pulmon unilateral en paciente con sobredosis do heroina y tratado con naloxona intravenosa. Med Clin (Barc) 1990;94:637.
164. Chenery HJ, Murdoch BE. A case of mixed transcortical aphasia following drug overdose. Br J Disord Commun 1986;21:381.
165. Rocamora A, Matarredona J, Sendagorta E, Ledo A. Sweat gland necrosis in drug-induced coma: light and direct immunofluorescence study. J Dermatol 1986;13:49.
166. Llach F, Descoendres C, Massry SG. Heroin associated nephropathy: clinical and histological studies in 19 patients. Clin Nephrol 1979;11:7.
167. Pinto F, Torrioli MG, Casella G et al. Sleep in babies born to chronically heroin-addicted mothers. A follow up study. Drug Alcohol Depend 1988;21:43.
168. Wasserman S, Yahr MD. Choreic movements induced by the use of methadone. Arch Neurol 1980;37:727.
169. Nathan HJ. Narcotics and myocardial performance in patients with coronary artery disease. Can J Anaesth 1988;35:209.
170. Hanks GW, Twycross RG, Bliss JM. Controlled release morphine tablets: a double-blind trial in patients with advanced cancer. Anaesthesia 1987;42:840.
171. Kalso E, Vainio A. Hallucinations during morphine but not during oxycodone treatment. Lancet 1988;ii:912.
172. D'Souza M. Unusual reaction to morphine. Lancet 1987;ii:48.
173. Jellema JG. Hallucination during sustained-release morphine and methadone administration. Lancet 1987;ii:392.
174. White ID, Hoskin PJ, Hanks GW et al. Morphine and dryness of the mouth. Br Med J 1989;298:1222.
175. Bruera E, Miller MJ. Non-cardiogenic pulmonary oedema after narcotic treatment for cancer pain. Pain 1989;39:297.
176. Zis AP, Haskett RF, Albala AA. Prolactin response to morphine in depression. Biol Psychiatry 1986;29:287.
177. Whiston RJ, Griffith CDM, Hopkinson DR. Purpuric rash associated with slow release morphine. Br Med J 1988;296:8.
178. Bristow A, Orlikowski C. Subcutanecous ketamin anal-

gesia post-operative analgesia using subcutaneous infusions of ketamine and morphine. Ann R Coll Surg Engl 1989;71:64.
179. Olkkola KT, Maunuksela E-L, Korpela R, Rosenberg PH. Kinetics and dynamics of postoperative intravenous morphine in children. Clin Pharmacol Ther 1988;44:128.
180a. Potter JM, Reid DB, Shaw RJ et al. Myoclonus associated with treatment with high doses of morphine: the role of supplementary drugs. Br Med J 1989;299:150.
180b. Jacobsen LS, Olsen AK, Sjogren P, Jensen NH. Morfininduseret hyperalgesi, allodyni og myoklonus—nye morfinbivirkninger. Ugeskr Laeger 1995;157:3307.
181. Wilton NCT, Burn JMB. Delayed vomiting after papaveretum in paediatric outpatient surgery. Can Anaesth Soc J 1986;33:741.
182a. Fishbain DA, Goldberg M, Rosomoff RS, Rosomoff H. Atypical oxycodone withdrawal syndrome. Pain Manage March/April, 1989;76.
182b. Pathy MS, Reynolds AJ. Papaverine and hepatotoxicity. Postgrad Med J 1980;56:488.
183. Catling JA, Pinto DM, Jordan C, Jones JG. Respiratory effects of analgesia after cholecystectomy: comparison of continuous and intermittent papaveretum. Br Med J 1980;281:478.
184. Gudipatti CV, Kern MJ, Aguirre FV, Deligonue U. Papaverine-induced chest pain due to coronary vascular steal; demonstration with angiographic and intracoronary flow velocity measurements. Am Heart J 1989;118:404.
185. Lakin MM, Montague DK. Intracavernous injections of papaverine and phentolamine: correlation with penile brachial index. Urology 1989;33:383.
186. Glina S, Reichelt AC, Leao PP et al. Impact of cigarette smoking on papaverine-induced erection. J Urol 1988;140:523.
187. Kirkeby AHJ. Erection resulting from intravenous injection of papaverine. Ugeskr Laeg 1988;150:855.
188. Fuchs ME, Brawer MK. Papaverine-induced fibrosis of the corpus cavernosum. J Urol 1989;141:125.
189. Stief CG, Gall H, Scherb W, Bahren W. Mid term results of autoinjection therapy for erectile dysfunction. Urology 1988;31:483.
190. Desai KM, Gingell JC. Penile corporeal fibrosis complicating papaverine self injection therapy for erectile impotence. Eur J Urol 1988;15:132.
191. Glass PSA, Camporesi EM, Shafron D et al. Evaluation of pentamorphone in humans: a new potent opiate. Anesth Analg 1989;68:302.
192. Kaiko RF, Foley KM, Cirabinski PY et al. Central nervous system excitatory effect of meperidine in cancer patients. Ann Neurol 1983;13:180.
193. Flacke JW, Flacke WE, Boor BC et al. Histamine release by four narcotics: a double-blind study in humans. Anesth Analg 1987;66:723.
194. Spiess BD, Sathoff RH, El-Ganzouri ARS, Ivankovich AD. High-dose sufentanil: four cases of sudden hypotension on induction. Int Anesth Res Soc 1986;65:703.
195. Starr NJ, Sethna DH, Estafanous FG. Bradycardia and asystole following the rapid administration of sufentanil with vecuronium. Anesthesiology 1986;64:521.
196. Dobson JAR, Davies JM, Hodgson GH. Bradycardia after sufentanil and vecuronium. Can J Anaesth 1988;35:S121.
197. Goldberg M, Ishak S, Garcia C et al. Postoperative rigidity following sufentanil administration. Anesthesiology 1985;63:199.
198. Muller H, Stoyanov M, Brahler A, Hempelmann G. Effects of tramadol on haemodynamics and respiration during N_2O-O_2 ventilation and in the postoperative period. Anaesthesist 31:604.
199. Barsan WG, Seger D, Danzl DF et al. Duration of antagonistic effects of nalmefene and naloxone in opiate induced sedation for emergency department procedures. Am J Emerg Med 1989;7:155.
200. Konieczko KM, Jones JG, Barrowcliffe MP et al. Antagonism of morphine-induced respiratory depression with nalmefene. Br J Anaesth 1988;61:318.
201. Wride SRN, Smith RER, Courtney PG. A fatal case of pulmonary oedema in a healthy young male following naloxone administration. Anaesth. Intensive Care 1989; 17:374.
202. Allen T. No adverse reaction. Ann Emerg Med 1989;18:116.
203. Langemark M. Naloxone in moderate dose does not aggravate chronic tension headache. Pain 1989;39:85.
204. Gibbs J, Newson T, Williams J, Davidson DC. Naloxone hazard in infant of opioid abuser. Lancet 1989;ii:159.
205. Barsan WG, Olinger CP, Adams HP et al. Use of high dose naloxone in acute stroke: possible side effects. Crit Care Med 1989;17:762.
206. Rubin P, Swezey S, Blaschke T. Naloxone lowers plasma prolactin in man. Lancet 1979;i:1293.
207. Ajayi AA, Campbell BC, Rubin PC et al. Effect of naloxone on the actions of captopril. Clin Pharmacol Ther 1985;38:560.
208. Krechel SW, Orr RM, Couper NB et al. Naloxone: report of a beneficial side effect. J Neurosurg Anesthesiol 1989;1:346.
209. Atkinson RL, Berke LK, Drake CR et al. Effects of long-term therapy with naltrexone on body weight in obesity. Clin Pharmacol Ther 1985;38:419.
210. Myer EC, Morris DL, Brase DA et al. Naltrexone therapy of apnea in children with elevated cerebrospinal fluid beta-endorphin. Ann Neurol 1990;27:75.
211. Lewis JW. Buprenorphine. Drug Alcohol Depend 1985;14:363.
212. Weiss PL, Ritz R. Analgesic action and side effects of buprenorphine in acute coronary heart disease: a randomised double-blind comparison with morphine. Anaesth Intensivther Notfallmed 1988:23:309.
213. Rifat K, Magnin C, Morel D. L'analgesie per et postopératoire à la buprénorphine: effets cardio-circulatoires et respiratoires. Cah Anesthésiol 1984;32:33.
214. Gal TJ. Naloxone reversal of buprenorphine induced respiratory depression. Clin Pharmacol Ther 1989;45:66.
215. Fincham JE. Cardiopulmonary arrest and subsequent death after administration of buprenorphine in an elderly female: a case report. J Geriatr Drug Ther 1989;3:103.
216. Schleicher G, Lechner W, Muller E. Trophic ulcers after intraganglionic injection of buprenorphine and root canal therapy. Aktuel Dermatol 1985;11:90.
217. Lockhart SP, Baron JH. Tongue ulceration after lingual buprenorphine. Br Med J 1984;288:1346.
218. Carl P, Crawford ME, Madsen NBB et al. Pain relief after major abdominal surgery: a double-blind controlled comparison of sublingual buprenorphine, intramuscular buprenorphine and intramuscular meperidine. Anesth Analg 1987;66:142.
219. Pachter IJ, Evans RP. Butorphanol. Drug Alcohol Depend 1985;14:325.

220a. Gonzalez ER, Ornato JP, Ware D et al. Comparison of intramuscular analgesic activity of butorphanol and morphine in patients with sickle cell disease. Ann Emerg Med 1988;17:788.
220b. Welt SI. Sinusoidal fetal heart rate and butorphanol administration. Am J Obstet Gynecol 1985;152:362.
221. Graf DF, Pandit SK, Kothary SP et al. A double-blind comparison of orally administered ciramadol and codeine for relief of postoperative pain. J Clin Pharmacol 1985;25:590.
222. Van Steenberghe D, Verbist D, Quirynen M et al. Double-blind comparison of the analgesic potency of ciramadol, codeine and placebo against postsurgical pain in ambulant patients. Eur J Clin Pharmacol 1980;31:335.
223. Dionne RA, Wirdezk PR, Butler DP et al. Comparison of conorphone, a mixed agonist-antagonist analgesic, to codeine for postoperative dental pain. Anaesth Prog 1984;31:77.
224. Pickworth WB, Neidert GL, Kay DC. Cyclazocine-induced sleep disruptions in non-dependent addicts. Prog Neuro-Psychopharmacol Biol Psychiatry 1986;1:77.
225. Pandit UA, Kothary SP, Pandit SK. Intravenous dezocine for postoperative pain: a double-blind, placebo controlled comparison with morphine. J Clin Pharmacol 1986;26:275.
226. Holmes B, Ward A. Meptazinol: a review of its pharmacodynamic and pharmacokinetic properties and therapeutic efficacy. Drugs 1985;30:285.
227. Westconbe RE, Price RKJ. Meptazinol in the casualty deparament: a comparison against morphine. Curr Ther Res 1985;37:969.
228. Barnes PRH, Williams CB, Davies RL et al. The use of intravenous meptazinol in colonoscopy. Postgrad Med J 1985;61:221.
229. Kay NH, Allen MC, Bullingham RES et al. Influence of meptazinol on metabolic and hormonal responses following major surgery. Anaesthesia 1985;40:223.
230. Kururattapun SA, Prakanrattana U. Intravenous dezocine for postoperative pain: a double-blind, placebo controlled comparison with morphine. J Clin Pharmacol 1986;26:275.
231. Gannon R. Nalbuphine: (1) 'Adverse effects' and (2) 'Summary and recommendations'. Conn Med 1985;49:681.
232. Yukioka H, Rosen K, Evans KT et al. Gastric emptying and small bowel transit times in volunteers after intravenous morphine and nalbuphine. Anaesthesia 1987;42:704.
233. Shah M, Rosen M, Vickers MD. Effect of premedication with diazepam, morphine, or nalbuphine on gastrointestinal motility after surgery. Br J Anaesth 1984;56:1235.
234. Jain AK, Ryan JR, McMahon FG, Smith G. Comparison of oral nalbuphine, acetaminophen, and their combination in postoperative pain. Clin Pharmacol Ther 1986;39:295.
235. Heintz-Bamberg D, Muller H, Dick W, Reiter G. Comparative studies on haemodynamic parameters under balanced anaesthesia using either nalbuphine or fentanyl. Anaesthesist 1987;36:217.
236. Dadabhoy ZP, Tapia DP, Zsigmond EK. Transplacental transfer of nalbuphine in patients undergoing caesarean section. Acta Anaesthesiol Ital 1988;39:227.
237. Guillonneau M, Jacqz-Aigrain E, De Crepy A, Zeggout H. Perinatal adverse effects of nalbuphine given during parturition. Lancet 1990;i:1588.
238. Sgro C, Escousse A, Tennenbaum D, Couyon JB. Perinatal adverse effects of nalbuphine given during labour. Lancet 1990;ii:1070.
239. Butsch JL, Okoli JA. The effect of nalbuphine on the common bile duct pressure. Am Surg 1988;54:253.
240. Schmidt WK, Tam SW, Shotzberger GS et al. Nalbuphine. Drug Alcohol Depend 1985;14:339.
241. Goldstein G. Pentazocine. Drug Alcohol Depend 1985;14:313.
242. Rudra A. Comparison of buprenorphine, morphine, pethidine, and pentazocine as postoperative analgesic after upper abdominal surgery. Calcutta Med J 1989;86:1.
243. Saarialho-Kere V, Mattila MJ, Seppala T. Parenteral pentazocine: effects on psychomotor skills and respiration and interactions with amitriptyline. Eur J Clin Pharmacol 1988;35:483.
244. Pedragosa R, Vidal J, Fuentes R, Huguet P. Tricotropism by pentazocine. Arch Dermatol 1987;123:297.
245. Tsai J-C, Lai Y-H, Shin S-J et al. Rhabdomyolysis-induced acute tubular necrosis after the concomitant use of alcohol and pentazocine—a case report. Kaohsiung J Med Sci 1987;3:299.
246. Lundquest DE, Winston RY, Edland JF. Maternal death associated with intravenous methylphenidate (Ritalin) and pentazocine (Talwin) abuse. J Forensic Sci 1987;32:798.
247. Furner BB. Parenteral pentazocine: cutaneous complications revisited. J Am Acad Dermatol 1990;22:694.
248. Challoner KR, McCarron MM, Newton EJ. Pentazocine (Talwin) intoxication: report of 57 cases. J Emerg Med 1990;8:67.
249. Showalter CV. T's and blues: abuse of pentazocine and tripelennamine. J Am Med Assoc 1980;244:1224.
250. Lahmeyer HW, Steingold RG. Medical and psychiatric complications of pentazocine and tripelennamine abuse. J Clin Psychiatry 1980;41:275.
251. Wu WH, Teng RJ, Shin HYH. Neonatal pentazocine withdrawal syndrome—a case report with conservative treatment. Clin Med J 1988;42:229.
252. Brunelle RL, George RE, Sunshine A, Hammonds WD. Analgesic effect of picenadol, codeine, and placebo in patients with postoperative pain. Clin Pharmacol Ther 1988;43:663.
253. Lippman M, Mok MS, Farinaci JV et al. Tonazocine mesylate in postoperative pain patients: a double-blind placebo-controlled analgesic study. J Clin Pharmacol 1989;29:373.
254. D'Arcy PF. Drug reactions and interactions. Int Pharm J 1989;3:91.
255. Minotti V, Patoia L, Roila F et al. Double-blind evaluation of analgesic efficacy of orally administered diclofenac, nefopam, and acetylsalicylic acid (ASA) plus codeine in chronic cancer pain. Pain 1989;36:177.
256. Pickar D, Dubois M, Cohen MR. Behavioural change in a cancer patient following intrathecal beta-endorphin administration. Am J Psychiatry 1984;141:103.
257. Desmeules J, Gascon MP, Dayer P, Magistris M. Impact of environmental and genetic factors on codeine analgesia. Eur J Clin Pharmacol 1991;41:23.
258. Sindrup SH, Arendt-Nielsen L, Brøsen K, Bjerring P, Angelo HR, Eriksen B, Gram LF. The effect of quinidine on the analgesic effect of codeine. Eur J Clin Pharmacol 1992;42:587.

Meyler's Side Effects of Drugs, 13th Edition
M.N.G. Dukes, editor

SECTION EDITOR: M.N.G. DUKES

Harm M. Paul Freie

9.1 Antipyretic analgesics

GENERAL CONSIDERATIONS

Although 'over the counter' versions of ibuprofen and naproxen have in recent years been introduced, aspirin and paracetamol remain by far the two most commonly used analgesics, both still being prescribed by physicians and generally used for mild to moderate pain, fever associated with common, everyday illnesses and disorders ranging from head colds and influenza to toothache to headache. Their greatest use is by consumers obtaining them directly at the pharmacy and in many countries outside pharmacies as well. Perhaps this wide availability leads to a lack of appreciation by the lay public that these are medicines with associated adverse effects. Both have at any rate been subject to overuse and excessive use leading to such problems as chronic salicylate intoxication with aspirin, and severe hepatic damage with paracetamol. Both aspirin and paracetamol preparations have also featured in accidental overdosage (particularly in children) as well as intentional overdosage. While it is difficult to treat overdosage with aspirin, it is almost impossible to deal successfully with overdosage with paracetamol unless one is able to commence treatment within 8—12 hours of the mishap.

To offer some protection against misuse of analgesics, many countries have insisted on the use of packs containing total quantities less than the minimum toxic dose, and supplied in child-resistant packaging. Most important, however, is the need to provide education for the lay public to respect such medicines in general for the good they can do, but more especially for the harm that may arise yet which can be avoided.

The antipyretic analgesics share with the non-steroidal anti-inflammatory drugs (NSAIDs) a common mechanism of action, namely the inhibition of prostaglandin synthesis and release. However, aspirin and paracetamol are distinguishable from most of the NSAIDs by their ability to inhibit prostaglandin synthesis in the CNS, and thus the hypothalamic center for body temperature regulation, rather than acting mainly in the periphery.

Endogenous pyrogens (and exogenous pyrogens which exert their effects through the endogenous group) induce the hypothalamic vascular endothelium to produce prostaglandins which activate the thermonuclear neurones via increase in AMP levels. The capacity of the antipyretic analgesics to inhibit hypothalamic prostaglandin synthesis appears to be the basis for their antipyretic action. Neither aspirin nor paracetamol affect synthesis or release of endogenous pyrogens and neither will lower the temperature if it is normal.

While aspirin has a significant inhibitory effect on peripheral prostaglandin synthesis (i.e. inhibition of both cyclo-oxygenase-1 and -2 isoenzymes) as well, paracetamol is less potent as a synthetase inhibitor than the NSAIDs except in the brain, and paracetamol exerts only a weak anti-inflammatory action. It seems relatively simple to ascribe the analgesic activity of aspirin to its capacity to inhibit synthesis with a consequent diminution to inflammatory edema and vasodilatation, since aspirin is most effective in the pain associated with inflammation or injury. However, such a peripheral effect cannot account for the analgesic activity of paracetamol, which is as yet unexplained.

The sale of paracetamol or aspirin in dose forms in which they are combined with other active ingredients, generally for the management of symptoms of upper respiratory tract disorders, offers considerable risk to the consumer since the product as sold may not be clearly identified as containing either of these two analgesics; consequently the patient who is so anxious to allay all his symptoms that he takes several medications concurrently may without knowing it take several doses of aspirin or paracetamol at the same time, perhaps sufficient to induce toxicity. It is essential that product labels clearly state the active ingredients by approved name together with the quantity per dose form (1^c).

Although the various forms of *gastrointestinal damage* (bleeding, ulcer, perforation) are the most common side effects of prostaglandin synthesis inhibitors, and can lead to fatal complications especially in the elderly, the clinically most important side effects involve the kidneys.

ANALGESIC NEPHROPATHY AND URINARY TUMORS

Over the last 40 years there has been a steady evolution in our knowledge of drug-related renal pathology. During the early years (1950s and 1960s) a reasonably well-defined disease was identified comprising interstitial nephritis and renal papillary necrosis. The condition was not uncommon and it was serious. In some cases malignancies also appeared in the urinary system.

Symptoms The analgesic syndrome and the frequency of particular symptoms have been documented in earlier volumes. Diagnoses are usually made in cases of ages 30—70 years, with the peak in the fourth decade, and a familial predisposition. Nocturia resulting from failure to concentrate urine is usually the earliest functional defect.

Epidemiology The prevalence of this complication is variable, but particularly high where there is intensive use of analgesics. The disparity in incidence of nephropathy in various parts of the world is difficult to explain but, despite the general overuse of analgesics, the level of use has varied. There is evidence from animal and clinical work to suggest that hypovolemia plays a part, and that the risk of nephropathy is greatest in females and the elderly. Because of the long latent period which can elapse before the disorder develops, the condition has continued to appear despite the withdrawal of phenacetin, identified as the main culprit. It has been estimated that analgesic-associated nephropathy still accounts for 20% of patients in the United States with interstitial nephritis. In Australia, where phenacetin disappeared before 1975, analgesic nephropathy continued to be a major problem thereafter: 22% of patients newly admitted to the Australian Kidney Foundation's dialysis and transplant registry in 1980 had analgesic nephropathy.

Causation It soon became clear that the major etiological agent was phenacetin, improperly used long-term. This led to the virtual disappearance of this widely-used compound in the mid-1970s, following regulatory action. However, it was well recognised that other analgesics including aspirin could in some way be implicated, as could combinations of aspirin and phenacetin; as the debate developed, the safety of paracetamol and its combination with aspirin—which had only come to the fore on a large scale as phenacetin disappeared—also came to be questioned. The difficulty in assigning specific roles to the various analgesics arises in part from the use of drug combinations—phenacetin was usually combined with aspirin and caffeine—but largely from the prolonged time span (over 10 years) for the development of the disorder. In recent years it has become obvious that many of the NSAIDs are associated with renal disorders arising *de novo* or by aggravation of existent renal dysfunction. The inhibition of PGE_1 synthesis intrarenally leads to a diminution of the vasodilator activity of this prostaglandin which normally contributes to maintenance of renal functional balance and protection against the vasoconstrictive effects of noradrenaline and angiotensin-II and the action of ADH. There is some experimental work suggesting a tendency for phenacetin and its metabolite paracetamol to concentrate in the renal medulla, possibly accounting for the papillary lesions most associated with them.

There is no evidence that short-term use of cyclo-oxygenase inhibitors has any major deleterious effect on renal function in normal individuals.

Associated disorders The incidence of renal carcinomas in analgesic abusers in Switzerland was calculated to be 13-times greater than that in non-abusers (2^R—4^R), while in Australia 47% of tumors were attributed to analgesic abuse and nephropathy (5^r). Patients with analgesic nephropathy have been considered to have a raised risk of atherosclerosis. In a retrospective study their levels of serum cholesterol and triglycerides were significantly higher than in a control group of similar age and having a similar degree of renal insufficiency due to other renal diseases. Some possible mechanisms of hyperlipidemia in analgesic nephropathy have been discussed, as this phenomenon is not sufficiently explained by end-stage renal failure or by protein loss as in the nephrotic syndrome. In the prospective Swiss Analgesic Study, the risk of bacteriuria proved to be about 3 times higher for those who abused analgesics heavily than for matched controls (6^C). The primary causes of mortality in this study were tumors and cardiovascular disease; only 7.5% died from the renal disorder itself.

Clinical evidence suggestive of analgesic nephropathy includes nocturia, renal failure with severe acidosis and persistent urinary tract infection with colic (7^R, 8^r).

Conclusions The history of analgesic nephropathy must not be dismissed as one involving only a drug now obsolete. Phenacetin was unwisely used long-term by a large section of the public, and unless such misuse of analgesics can be avoided, there is much reason to fear that the story will be repeated with other agents and combinations. Also, short-term use of a compound of this class is never a guarantee that nephropathies will not occur.

If analgesics are discontinued in the early phases of nephropathy, there is a reasonable possibility of return to normal renal function. Especially in patients over 65 years of age, who seem to be at particular risk of analgesic nephropathy and who may also have pre-existing renal dysfunction including marginally compensated asymptomatic renal failure, it seems wise to ensure that the dosage of aspirin or paracetamol, or indeed any NSAID is kept as low as possible, that renal function is regularly assessed, and that prolonged use is avoided (7[R]).

ACETYLSALICYLIC ACID AND RELATED COMPOUNDS

Aspirin

ADVERSE REACTION PATTERN

General and toxic reactions As a prostaglandin synthesis inhibitor, aspirin, like other NSAIDs, is associated with irritation of and damage to the gastrointestinal mucosa. In low doses it can also increase bleeding due to inhibition of platelet aggregation; with high doses, prolongation of prothrombin time will contribute to the bleeding tendency. Intensive treatment can also produce unwanted CNS effects (salicylism).

Hypersensitivity reactions Depending on the criteria used, the incidence of aspirin sensitivity is variously estimated as being as low as 1% or as high as 50%, the highest frequency being found in asthmatics. The condition is characterised by bronchospasm (asthma), urticaria, angio-edema, and vasomotor rhinitis, each occurring alone or in combination, often leading to quite severe and even life-threatening reactions. See also 'Allergy or idiosyncrasy' below.

Tumor-inducing effects There have been no clear indications of an association, apart from the possible peripheral contribution of aspirin to the development of urinary tract neoplasms. Indeed, some recent published papers suggest a role for salicylates in decreasing the incidence of colorectal tumors. Such a finding must obviously be investigated in depth.

ALLERGY OR IDIOSYNCRASY

Aspirin has a leading position, next to penicillin, among drugs causing disorders of hypersensitivity. It is perhaps better to refer to idiosyncrasy or sensitivity rather than allergy to aspirin in the absence of identification of a definite antigen—antibody reaction. This topic has been reviewed in length in earlier editions (SEDA-17, 94; SEDA-18, 90—94).

Mechanism The current theory of the mechanism relates to the inhibition of cyclo-oxygenases (9[r]) and a greater degree of interference with PGE_2 synthesis, allowing the bronchoconstricting $PGF_{2\alpha}$ to override in susceptible individuals.

PGE_2 inhibition in the macrophages may also unleash bronchial cytotoxic lymphocytes, generated by chronic viral infection, leading to a destruction of virus-infected cells of the respiratory tract (10[C]). Where urticaria occurs (see below), it may well result from increased SRS-A (leukotrienes LTC_4, D_4 and E_4) release, which also induces bronchoconstriction consequent on the above with a shunt of arachidonic acid toward lipoxygenation in aspirin-sensitive asthmatics (SEDA-18, 93).

Features The features of hypersensitivity include bronchospasm, acute and usually generalized urticaria, angio-edema, severe rhinitis and shock. The reactions may each occur alone or in various combinations, developing within minutes or a few hours of aspirin ingestion and lasting until elimination is complete. They may be life-threatening. The bronchospastic type of reaction is predominant in adults, only the urticarial type being found in children. The frequency of recurrent urticaria is significantly greater in adults (3.8 vs 0.3%).

Epidemiology Aspirin hypersensitivity is relatively common in adults (20%), although often only demonstrable by challenge tests with spirometry; only a fifth of this number may experience problems in practice. Patients with existing asthma and nasal polyps or chronic urticaria have a greater frequency of hypersensitivity (11[R]), and women appear to be more susceptible than men, perhaps particularly during the child-bearing period of life (12[R]). There is considerable cross-reactivity of patients with other NSAIDs or those sensitive to—the now widely banned food colorant—tartrazine (13[C]).

It is notable that acute intolerance to aspirin can develop even in patients who have taken the drug for some years without problems. Cross-sensitization between aspirin and tartrazine is common, e.g. in one series, 24% of aspirin-sensitive patients reacted also to tartrazine (SEDA-9, 76).

Prophylaxis and treatment Avoidance of aspirin and substances to which there is cross-sensitivity is the only satisfactory solution. Desensitization regimens are not usually successful and repeated treatments are needed to maintain any effect which is obtained (14[r], 15[C]).

ORGANS AND SYSTEMS

Cardiovascular Apart from rare reports of variant angina pectoris and vasculitis theoretically related to thromboxane, aspirin is not associated with adverse effects on the cardiovascular system (16[R], 17), except an increase in circulating plasma volume after large doses.

Respiratory The effect of aspirin on bronchial musculature as a sensitivity feature is discussed separately under 'Hypersensitivity' above.

Pulmonary oedema can be induced by salicylates, particularly in the elderly, especially if they are or have been heavy smokers (18[C]).

Nervous system *Salicylism* (see 'Special senses') is a reaction to very high circulating levels of salicylate, characterized by tinnitus, dizziness, confusion and headache. *Encephalopathy* secondary to hyperammonemia has been reported in those rare cases of liver failure associated with high doses of aspirin, and this also forms a major feature of Reye's syndrome (see below).

Endocrine, metabolic Aspirin has been shown to lower plasma glucose levels in C-peptide-positive diabetic subjects and in normoglycemic persons (19[C]). There appears to be little clinical significance for these effects.

Hematological *Thrombocytopenia*, *agranulocytosis*, *neutropenia* and *aplastic anemia* or even *pancytopenia* have been reported in association with aspirin. The prospect for recovery from the latter is poor, mortality approaching 50%. *Hemolytic anemia* may occur in patients with glucose-6-phosphate dehydrogenase or RBC-glutathione peroxidase deficiency (SED-9, 127; 20[C], 21[r]). In how far these reports have anything more than anecdotal value (SEDA-17, 97) remains to be determined. Simple iron deficiency caused by occult blood loss occurs at a frequency of 1% and upper gastrointestinal bleeding resulting from regular aspirin ingestion is the reason for hospitalization in about 15 patients per 100 000 aspirin users per year. Aspirin causes bleeding of sufficient severity to lead to iron deficiency anemia in 10—15% of patients taking it continuously for chronic arthritis. Some individuals are particularly at risk because of pregnancy, age, inadequate diet, menorrhagia, gastrectomy or malabsorption syndromes.

Macrocytic anemia associated with folate deficiency has been described in patients with rheumatoid arthritis and also in patients abusing analgesic mixtures containing aspirin.

Effects on coagulation Aspirin at high doses for several days can decrease prothrombin levels with prolongation of prothrombin time. The effect will contribute to bleeding problems initiated by other factors, including the drug's local irritant effects on epithelial cells. It is therefore very risky to use aspirin in patients with bleeding disorders. The effect will contribute to increased blood loss at parturition, spontaneous abortion or menorrhagia, and may be linked to persistent ocular hemorrhage, particularly in the older age group, with or without associated surgical intervention (22, 23).

By virtue of its effects on both cyclo-oxygenase isoenzymes, aspirin inhibits platelet thromboxane A_2 formation. This effect within the platelet is irreversible and will persist for its lifetime of up to 10 days, since its anucleate state precludes any capacity for *de novo* protein synthesis or new cyclo-oxygenase. It is of clinical significance that the dose of aspirin necessary to inhibit platelet thromboxane A_2 (around 40 mg daily) is much lower than that which is needed to inactivate the subendothelial prostacyclin. Hence, platelet aggregation is inhibited, with some associated dilatation of coronary and cerebral arterioles at doses which do not interfere with prostacyclin inhibition. It is important, in considering the dosage of aspirin for prophylaxis (see below), to appreciate that prostacyclin is a general inhibitor of platelet aggregation while aspirin, as a cyclo-oxygenase inhibitor, affects aggregation from a limited number of stimuli, e.g. ADP, adrenaline, thromboxane A_2. It is also worth recalling that the vascular endothelium can synthesize new cyclo-oxygenase so that any effect on prostacyclin synthesis is of limited duration only (SEDA-12, 74; 24[r]).

A series of long-term studies have been carried out since the 1980s to determine the prophylactic usefulness of these effects on clotting. Many of those have been reviewed earlier in these volumes (SED-11, 160) and the *Side Effects of Drugs Annuals*. The evidence is now clear that aspirin in daily doses of 300 mg may successfully be used for secondary prophylaxis in patients with coronary artery disease in order to reduce the incidence of severe myocardial infarction, and in patients with cerebrovascular disease to decrease the incidence of ischemic attacks and strokes. There is some suggestion that higher doses of aspirin may be required in women. A major drawback has been the high incidence of gastrointestinal side effects and particularly bleeding in aspirin-treated groups (25[C]; 26—28). In view of the age group involved, the latter event can have serious implications. In an attempt to avoid this high proportion of ill-effects and yet retain the benefits of prophylactic antithrombotic treatment, a few trials have been conducted using aspirin at doses of 162 mg (ISIS-2: 29[C]) and 75 mg (RISC: 30[C]) in symptomatic coronary heart disease with good evidence of efficacy. Two studies have been reported in patients with cerebrovascular events, namely the Dutch TIA trial with aspirin 30 vs 283 mg (31[C]) and the SALT study with aspirin 75 mg (32[C]). The former did not show any difference in efficacy between the 30 and 283 mg dose groups, but there was no placebo control. The results in the other study demonstrated a significant reduction in thrombotic stroke. However, hemorrhagic stroke and their increased fatality were evident with aspirin in this study as well as in the Physicians Health Study of 1989 (33[c]). On the other hand, the incidence of serious gastrointestinal events was much lower than previously described.

There is a good prospect that an even lower daily dose of aspirin may offer advantages in antithrombotic prophylaxis without an increased risk of bleeding, but the results of further such studies are still awaited (34[C]).

Liver Aspirin can cause dose-related *focal hepatic necrosis* that is usually asymptomatic or anicteric. Much of the evidence for hepatotoxicity of aspirin and the salicylates has been shown in children (35[cr]), in whom several hundred cases have been described in the literature (36[R]), usually in patients with connective tissue disorders, on relatively high dosage long-term for Still's disease, rheumatoid arthritis or occasionally systemic lupus erythematosus. *Elevations of plasma amino transferases* seem to be the most frequently seen feature—in up to 50% of patients—and are usually reversible when the drug is discontinued, but occasionally may lead to fatal hepatic necrosis. Severe and even fatal *metabolic encephalopathy* may also occur, as in Reye's syndrome (see below). It would seem that one can easily overload the young patient's individual metabolic capacity. The coexistence of hypoalbuminemia may be a particular risk factor; in patients with a hypoalbuminemia of 35 g/l or less, close monitoring of the ASAT (SGOT) is advisable, especially if the level of total serum salicylate is 1.1 mmol/l or higher (37[R]). Plasma salicylate concentrations in serious cases have usually been in excess of 1.4 mmol/l and liver function tests return rapidly to normal when the drug is discontinued. Finally, there are a very small number of cases of *chronic active hepatitis* on record which appeared attributable to aspirin (38[C]).

Reye's syndrome This topic has been dealt with at length in the previous edition of this volume (SED-12, 172); it is repeated here because of its clinical importance and the fact that it is an avoidable risk. First defined as a clinicopathologically distinct syndrome in 1963 by Reye et al., this syndrome came to be regarded some years later as an adverse effect of aspirin. In fact, the position is more complex, and the syndrome still cannot be assigned a specific cause. There is general agreement that the disorder presents a few days after the prodroma of a viral illness. Well over a dozen different viruses have so far been implicated, including influenza A and B, adenovirus, varicella and, most recently, reovirus. Various other factors have also been incriminated including aflatoxins, certain pesticides and such antioxidants as BHT. Only in the case of aspirin have some epidemiological studies been conducted and these appeared to show a close correlation between this compound and cases of Reye's syndrome. It was these studies which led to regulatory action against the promotion of salicylate use in children. Doubt has been thrown on the clarity of the link, and it now seems increasingly likely that while there is some association with aspirin, there is in fact a multifactorial etiology, including some genetic predisposition. Studies in Japan did not support the US findings while studies in Thailand and Canada invoked other factors.

Two characteristic phenomena are present in Reye's syndrome:
1) damage to mitochondrial structures with pleomorphism, disorganization of matrix, proliferation of smooth endoplasmic reticulum and an increase in peroxisomes; mitochondrial enzyme activity is severely diminished but cytoplasmic enzymes are unaffected. The changes appear first in single cells but may spread to all hepatocytes. Recovery may be complete by 5—7 days. While these changes are most evident in liver cells, similar effects have been seen in cerebral neurons and skeletal muscle.

There appears to be a block in β-oxidation of fatty acids (inhibition of oxidation of NAB^+-linked substrates). Aspirin has also been shown in vitro to selectively inhibit mitochondrial oxidation of medium- and long-chain fatty acids.
(2) An acute catabolic state with hypoglycemia, hyperammonemia, elevated serum aspartate aminotransferase and creatine phosphokinase levels, increased urinary nitrogen and serum long chain dicarboxylic acid.

Despite our lack of understanding of the syndrome, the decision taken in many countries to advise against use of salicylates in children already shows an effect in terms of a declining incidence of Reye's syndrome (SEDA-16, 96; SEDA-17, 97).

Gastrointestinal The gastrointestinal side effects of aspirin and the other NSAIDs are the most common and have been discussed in length in earlier volumes (SEDA-16, 96; SEDA-17, 95; SEDA-18, 90—94). As might be expected with an inhibitor of prostaglandin synthesis, the cytoprotective effects of prostaglandin E and prostacyclin (PGI_2) are diminished by aspirin, as is the inhibitory action on gastric acid secretion. This effect may be both direct, as is the case with aspirin released in the stomach (or the lower rectum in the case of aspirin suppositories), and indirect following absorption and distribution via the systemic circulation; attempts to reduce the problems by coating and buffering therefore can have only limited success. The indirect type of effect is demonstrated by the fact that these adverse gastric effects can also be exerted by parenterally administered lysine acetylsalicylate (SEDA-10, 72). The local effects depend in part on the tablet particle size, solubility and rate of gastric absorption, while the most important variable appears to be gastric pH.

While there is a body of opinion which argues against a causative relationship between aspirin ingestion and *chronic gastric ulceration*, the present consensus still favours such a relationship, although admitting that other factors such as *H. pylori* are likely to play a part. Again, patients aged over 65 years and females are more at risk, and those taking aspirin over prolonged periods with a daily dose of about 2 grams or more.

There is no ambiguity about the association of aspirin with *gastritis*, *gastric erosions* or *extensions of existing peptic ulcers*, all of which are demonstrable by endoscopy. Even with one or two doses, superficial erosions have been described in over 50% of normal subjects. This association is now almost universally accepted as the standard basis for comparative testing of NSAIDs and other drugs (39—42). Whether it is of benefit to use other drugs concomitantly to prevent in one way or another the effect of gastric acid on the mucosa, and thus reduce the risk of gastric ulceration, is as yet not clear.

Dyspepsia, nausea and vomiting occur in 2—6% of patients after aspirin ingestion. Rheumatoid patients seem to be more sensitive and the frequency of aspirin-induced dyspepsia in this group is 10—30% (SEDA-9, 129). These symptoms are however generally poor predictors of the incidence of mucosal damage (SEDA-18, 90—92).

The *bleeding* which occurs is usually triggered by erosions and aggravated by the antithrombotic action of aspirin. While reported to occur in up to 100% of regular aspirin takers, bleeding tends to be asymptomatic in young adults, unless associated with peptic ulceration, but is readily detectable by endoscopy and the presence of occult blood in feces. Less commonly, hematemesis and melena are seen. A degree of resultant iron deficiency anemia is common (see 'Hematological'). Such events are more commonly seen in the older age group in whom there is a significant proportion of serious bleeding and even fatalities. Major gastrointestinal bleeding is reported with an incidence of 15 per 100 000 'heavy' aspirin takers. However, the interpretation of 'heavy' and of quantities of aspirin actually taken is to a large extent subjective and very dependent upon the questionable accuracy of patient reporting. The risk appears to be greater in women, smokers, and possibly affected by other factors not yet established (43[C]).

Associated effects Aspirin may also play a role in esophageal bleeding, ulceration or benign stricture and should be considered in patients, particularly the elderly, presenting with any of these features. In addition, there have been reports of rectal stricture in the elderly associated with the use of aspirin suppositories. Effects on both these structures emphasize the significance of a direct local action of aspirin as well as a systemic action and underlines the relevance of the involvement of oxygen-derived free radicals in the pathogenesis of mucosal lesions in the gastrointestinal tract (44[r]—46[r]).

Long-term effects The effects on the stomach of continued exposure to aspirin remain in various respects controversial.

Prophylaxis Intravenous administration, or the use of enteric-coated formulations or products with delayed release all appear to reduce the risk both of bleeding and more particularly of erosions/ulcerations. Because of the indirect effect noted above, such preparations do not, however, eliminate the risk. Use of these forms, or of buffered aspirin, reduces the incidence of gastric or duodenal ulcer to half of that seen with regular aspirin (47, 48).

Considerable attention in recent years has been directed toward the efficacy of using synthetic form of PGE_2, H_2-receptor blockers or proton-pump inhibitors either to heal peptic ulcers associated with use of prostaglandin inhibitors or more significantly to act prophylactically to protect against development of ulceration or bleeding associated with aspirin or the NSAIDs. Since all these agents carry their own potential risks it is more than questionable whether administration to a patient with a normal gastrointestinal mucosa is justified. Generally, use of prostaglandin inhibitors should be limited to the shortest possible duration, thereby minimizing—but not eliminating—the risk of gastrointestinal damage.

Urinary system The possible role of aspirin in analgesic *nephropathy* has been discussed above. Otherwise, effects of aspirin on the kidney are relatively minor, unless there is pre-existent renal disease. When aspirin is used by patients on sodium restriction or with congestive heart failure, there tends to be a decrease in the glomerular filtration rate with preservation of normal renal plasma flow. Some renal tubular epithelial shedding may also occur. In low doses (up to 2 g/day), the drug may cause some decrease in urate excretion and blocks the effects of probenecid and other uricosuric agents. In higher doses (over 5 g/day), the salicylates increase urate excretion and somewhat inhibit the effects of spironolactone, but it is not clear that these phenomena are of importance. At least one study in patients with rheumatoid arthritis on relatively high doses of aspirin alone over prolonged periods has shown evidence of freedom from nephropathy which is reassuring for those using standard therapeutic dosage in patients with rheumatoid arthritis (49[C]). However, even prolonged asymptomatic use is no guarantee for a incidence-free future.

Severe systemic disease involving heart, liver or kidneys seems to predispose the patient to the effects of aspirin and other NSAIDs on renal function (50[C]).

Skin and appendages Hypersensitivity reactions such as *urticaria* and *angio-edema* are relatively common in allergic subjects. *Purpura, hemorrhagic vasculitis, erythema multiforme, Stevens-Johnson Syndrome* and *Lyell's syndrome* have also been reported, fortunately much less frequently in view of their often life-threatening nature. *Fixed drug eruptions*, probably hypersensitive in origin, are periodically described. In some patients they do not recur on rechallenge, i.e. the sensitivity disappears (51[r]).

Special senses With the high levels achieved in attempted suicide, *tinnitus* and *hearing loss* leading to deafness, develop within about 5 hours, usually with regression within 48 hours, but permanent damage may occur. Disturbed balance often with vertigo may develop as well as nausea, usually with maintenance of consciousness, even without treatment. It has been postulated that in this state depolarisation of the cochlear hair cells occurs, similar to the changes induced by pressure.

Myopia A case of acute myopia and increased ocular pressure attributed to aspirin has been described and seems well documented (52[c]).

Musculoskeletal system Increasing evidence is being developed that salicylates together with at least some NSAIDs may suppress proteoglycan biosynthesis independently of effects on prostaglandin synthesis (53[r]). As a consequence, prolonged use of these agents may accentuate deterioration of articular cartilage in weight-bearing arthritic joints. If this is proved, the problem will be of greatest relevance for the elderly with osteoarthritis, a condition in which this use of prostaglandin inhibitors is quite questionable.

Risk situations Aspirin may be considered to be contraindicated in four situations:

(a) In view of the association with Reye's syndrome, use of aspirin in *children* should be avoided unless essential.

(b) Because of the relatively high incidence of aspirin-induced bronchoconstriction, urticaria or anaphylaxis, the drug should not be used in patients with *asthma* or those already believed to be hypersensitive to it, to related agents (NSAIDs) or to tartrazine.

(c) Patients with *peptic ulceration* should not take aspirin.

(d) Aspirin should be avoided in persons with known *coagulopathies* including those induced as part of medical therapeutics.

There are also various situations of relative risk:

(e) Since normal analgesic doses impede excretion of uric acid they are better avoided in *gout*, despite the fact that high (antirheumatic) doses have a uricosuric effect; an additional problem in gout is that salicylates reduce the uricosuric effects of sulphinpyrazone and of probenecid if given to the same patient.

(f) *Children with pyrexia and dehydration* can easily develop salicylate intoxication, and in pyrexial children there may be a remote risk of inducing Reye's syndrome (see above).

(g) Various reports point to a risk of aspirin in *variant angina*. A dose of 4 g/day has been found to provoke attacks both at night time and during the day (27[C], 28[C]), perhaps due to direct triggering of coronary arterial spasm; blockade of the synthesis of PGI_2, which normally protects against vasoconstriction, could be involved.

(h) In *diabetics* aspirin can in theory interfere with insulin and glucagon sufficiently to derange control.

(i) It is wise to withdraw aspirin some days prior to *elective surgery* (even in coronary artery bypass grafting) or *delivery*, especially if extradural anesthesia is performed (54[r]), though recent data seem reassuring (55[R]). The drug increases bleeding at *dental extraction* or perioperatively.

(j) It is wise to avoid *continuous prolonged use in the elderly* who may develop gastrointestinal bleeding. The use of rectal suppositories of aspirin should be avoided in patients with anorectal inflammation.

Because of known or supposed adverse effects discussed elsewhere in this monograph, caution is also indicated in using aspirin in pre-existing *gastrointestinal disease, liver disease, hypoalbuminemia, hypovolemia, in the third trimester of pregnancy* or *perioperatively*, or in *patients with threatening abortion*.

Second-generation effects It is perhaps surprising that aspirin, which itself is teratogenic in rodents, and which by virtue of its capacity to inhibit prostaglandin synthesis would be expected to affect the development of the renal and cardiovascular systems, has as yet shown no clear evidence of teratogenesis when used during pregnancy in human beings. This remains the case despite very widespread use in pregnant women. Possibly the increased production of prostaglandins during pregnancy overrides the effects of aspirin in the usual dosages, and the intervention of placental metabolism protects the human fetus from exposure to aspirin itself. Whatever the explanation, there are very few reports in which aspirin can be implicated as a human teratogen and a few studies (56[C], 57[C]) have provided some positive reassurance.

The role of aspirin as an antithrombotic agent and its ability to promote bleeding mean that it should be avoided in the third trimester of pregnancy and very definitely at parturition. In the latter situation there is a second good reason to avoid aspirin, since the drug's prostaglandin-inhibiting capacity could mean that it will delay parturition and induce early closure of the ductus arteriosus in the near-term fetus, the latter effects being exerted in common with other NSAIDs (58, 59). However, its low-dose use in pregnancy may prevent retardation of fetal growth (EPREDA: 60[C]).

Overdosage *Acute salicylate poisoning* remains a major clinical hazard (61[R]), although associated with low major morbidity and low mortality in contrast to chronic intoxication (SEDA-17, 98). Alkalemia or acidemia, alkaluria or aciduria, hyperglycemia or hypoglycemia, and water and electrolyte imbalances may occur, although the usual picture is one of hypokalemia with metabolic acidosis alongside respiratory alkalosis. Effects on hearing have been referred to above. Nausea, vomiting, tinnitus, hyperpnea, hyperpyrexia, confusion, disorientation, dizziness, coma and/or convulsions are common. They are expressions of the CNS effects of the salicylates. Gastrointestinal hemorrhage is frequent. After ingestion, drug absorption can be prevented by induction of emesis, gastric lavage and the administration of active charcoal; drug excretion is enhanced by forced diuresis with alkalinizing solutions, hemoperfusion and hemodialysis (62[R]). Serum salicylate levels above 3.6 mmol/l are likely to be toxic and levels of 5.4 mmol/l can easily prove fatal. Fluid and electrolyte management is the mainstay of therapy; the immediate aim must be to correct acidosis, hyperpyrexia, hypokalemia and dehydration. In severe cases vitamin K_1 should be given to counteract hypoprothrombinemia.

Chronic salicylate intoxication is commonly associated with chronic daily headaches, lethargy, confusion or coma and, mimicking the symptoms resulting from illness for which the drug was administered, it can easily be misdiagnosed if the physician is not aware that aspirin has been over-used. Depression of mental status is usually present at the time of diagnosis, when the serum salicylate concentration is at a peak. The explanation of depression, manifested by irritability, lethargy and unresponsiveness occurring 1 or 3 days following the initiation of therapy for aspirin intoxication, lies in a persistently high concentration of salicylate within the central nervous system, while the serum salicylate concentration falls to non-toxic values. The delayed unresponsiveness associated with salicylate intoxication appears to be closely associated with the development of cerebral edema of uncertain etiology. The encephalopathy which ensues appears to be directly related to increased intracranial pressure, a known effect of prostaglandin synthesis inhibitors; it has responded to the administration of mannitol (63[CR]).

Interactions It is obvious that the demonstrable effects of aspirin on gastrointestinal mucosa will lead to additive effects if the drug is used concurrently with other drugs having an irritant effect on the stomach, notably *other NSAIDs* or *glucocorticosteroids* (64[r], 65[r]).

Although *ethanol* itself has no effect on bleeding time, it enhances the effect of aspirin when given simultaneously up to at least 36 hours after aspirin ingestion (66[R]). Ethanol also promotes gastric bleeding.

Similarly the effects on coagulation parameters will lead to additive effects if the drug is used concurrently with *anticoagulants*. If the latter are in use, abrupt withdrawal of aspirin will disrupt control of coagulation parameters and require readjustment of anticoagulant dosage. There are also other interactions with anticoagulants: the effect of the *coumarins* is increased by kinetic displacement, and if aspirin causes gastric hemorrhages, the latter may well be more severe when anticoagulants are being given.

Salicylates are strongly protein-bound but can be displaced from binding sites by some *NSAIDs* such as *naproxen*, or in turn displace others such as *piroxicam*. Aspirin will displace *methotrexate* from its binding sites and also inhibit its renal tubular elimination so that dosage of concurrently used methotrexate should be reduced (excluding that of once-a-week low-dose in the treatment of rheumatoid arthritis). Similar displacement by aspirin occurs with *sulfonamides*, *co-trimoxazole* and *sodium valproate* (67[C]).

It is as well to remember that such interactions are reported with normal analgesic dose levels of aspirin, i.e. not with the low dosage being used prophylactically as antithrombotic, and are seldom of clinical significance with a single dose of aspirin.

Aspirin is thought to diminish the antihypertensive effect of *captopril* (68[C]), and it seems to potentiate the effects of *food allergens*, but this is uncertain (SEDA-10, 72).

In two pediatric cases, aspirin has been found to render clinically significant the slight metabolic acidosis commonly induced by *carbonic anhydrase inhibitors* used in glaucoma (SED-9, 79).

Supposed mechanisms of action of plain *intrauterine devices* (IUDs) include a local inflammatory response and increased local production of prostaglandins that prevent sperm from fertilizing ova (69[C], 70[C]). As aspirin has both anti-inflammatory and anti-prostaglandin properties, the contraceptive effectiveness of an IUD may be somewhat reduced by the drug, though the effect on periodic bleeding may prevail.

Risks of enteric-coated aspirin Although use of enteric-coated aspirin can reduce the drug's direct adverse effect on the stomach (SEDA-10, 72), it could in principle transfer these to some extent to the intestine; slow-release NSAIDs have sometimes caused perforations.

Enteric coating slows down absorption of aspirin; in cases of severe overdosage this fact may cause difficulties in diagnosis and treatment since early plasma salicylate measurements are unreliable, the maximum blood levels sometimes not being attained until 60 or 70 hours after the overdose has been taken (71[R], 72[C]). Another complication of the use of enteric-coated aspirin is the risk of gastric outlet obstruction and resulting accumulation of tablets because of subclinical pyloric stenosis.

DRUGS RELATED TO ASPIRIN

Salsalate (salicylsalicylic acid)

Salsalate has been studied from 1969 onwards. Some evidence points to a lesser degree of gastric toxicity than that seen with aspirin, but it is clear that salsalate can produce dyspepsia and occult bleeding when used therapeutically in effective doses.

Diflunisal

This is a salicylic acid derivative, absorbed unchanged from the gastrointestinal tract, reaching peak levels after about 2 hours and metabolized by glucuronidation. Despite an allegedly better tolerance, its side effects and other characteristics are those of aspirin.

Miscellaneous salicylates

Salicylates administered orally have proved in most cases too irritant to the upper gastrointestinal tract and are now usually applied topically. Absorption, though variable, is significant and even by this route the systemic side effects of aspirin are encountered. Pharmaceutical forms of salicylates (mesalazine, sulfasalazine) are available for local release in the lower gastrointestinal tract, intended for the treatment of Crohn's disease and colitis ulcerosa.

Benorilate

The acetylsalicylic ester of paracetamol, benorilate is slowly absorbed unchanged from the gastrointestinal tract but is rapidly hydrolysed to its components—aspirin and paracetamol. Thereafter its effects and kinetics are those of the two moieties. However, the delay in its metabolism reduces the incidence of direct gastric irritation, delays its onset of action, and prolongs its duration of action.

In cases of suspected benorilate overdosage, both salicylate and paracetamol should be assayed; measuring salicylate levels alone will not exclude toxic levels of paracetamol.

ANILINE DERIVATIVES

Paracetamol (acetaminophen)

The use of paracetamol as an antipyretic increased rapidly once phenacetin was no longer available and has received a boost more recently with wide acknowledgement of the role of aspirin as an etiological agent in Reye's syndrome, resulting in the virtual disappearance of children's dose forms of aspirin. While the incidence of adverse effects is reassuringly low, satisfaction must be tempered by the appreciation of the relatively short duration of extensive clinical experience with paracetamol, its low potency as an analgesic and the low public awareness of its potential side effects.

ADVERSE REACTION PATTERN

General and toxic reactions Although acceptably safe in the usual dosage, there have been some reports that in patients with significant hepatic dysfunction or those receiving substances inducing hepatic enzymes (e.g. ethanol, phenobarbital, isoniazid) even these doses may aggravate liver dysfunction, sometimes to the point of inducing hepatic failure. The overdosage problems are substantial, bearing in mind the wide availability and the resistance to treatment.

Hypersensitivity reactions Allergic reactions, including urticaria are seen occasionally. Anaphylactic shock has been reported.

Tumor-inducing effects Animal studies have indicated a carcinogenic effect where paracetamol has been administered for prolonged periods at relatively high dosage. However, no clinical data are so far available to corroborate this finding. The matter cannot be dismissed entirely for the time being in view of a report (73[C]) of the development of chromosomal aberrations in a patient after prolonged use.

ORGANS AND SYSTEMS

Respiratory Paracetamol may *aggravate bronchospasm* in patients sensitive to aspirin and other analgesics. In severe poisoning, paracetamol depresses respiratory function centrally.

Endocrine, metabolic *Hypoglycemia* has been recorded, particularly in children.

Hematological Very occasional but well-documented reports of *thrombocytopenia*, ostensibly associated with circulating antibodies, have appeared in the literature.

Agranulocytosis was recorded in a series in France (74[C]) but does not appear to have been a significant clinical problem elsewhere. A hemolytic crisis has been recorded in a patient with glucose-6-phosphate dehydrogenase deficiency (75).

Liver Paracetamol-induced *hepatic damage* appears with accumulation of cytochrome P450-mediated formation of *N*-acetylimidobenzoquinone, a reactive metabolite normally metabolized by glutathione (76). Saturation of the detoxification path may occur with overdoses of paracetamol (77[R]) or sometimes, as has become evident in recent years, in certain individuals making long-term use of normal dosage (78[C]), in patients with compromised hepatic function or with certain drug combinations.

There is a relatively narrow margin between the maximum recommended daily dose of 4 grams and the minimum toxic dose of 6 grams in healthy patients. As discussed under 'Overdosage', hepatic failure continuing to necrosis occurs early, suddenly, and frequently. If specific treatment is not instituted within a very short interval after ingestion, the mortality rate is high and the changes are irreversible. Children appear to have a relative resistance to paracetamol hepatotoxicity, although they do have some reversible metabolic and enzymatic changes. Recently acute biliary pain with cholestasis has been identified as additional hepatic complication (79[C], 80[C]).

Gastrointestinal In normal doses, paracetamol is, in contradistinction to aspirin and the NSAIDs, well tolerated by the gastrointestinal tract.

Pancreatitis has been reported, but only in association with overdosage.

Urinary system Apart from renal tubular necrosis usually associated with hepatic toxicity, but occasionally seen without hepatic damage, there have been reports of a nephropathy similar to that seen with phenacetin, which has occurred after prolonged use of paracetamol alone, or in combination with other NSAIDs (81[c], 82[r], 83[R]).

Skin *Allergic reactions* are occasionally encountered, as is a *rash*, usually erythematous (84[c], 85[r], 86[c]).

Overdosage *Fulminant hepatic failure* occurs in 1–5% of cases of paracetamol overdosage 3–6 days after ingestion (87[C]), with frequent fatalities in persons ingesting 20–25 grams. There is only a narrow margin between the normal maximum 24-hour dosage and that which is capable of inducing liver damage and acute hepatic failure. Undoubtedly there are certain persons more susceptible than most to paracetamol toxicity, since although a 6-gram dose has been reported as toxic in some cases, it is in the range of 12 grams upwards where most toxicity is seen (77[R], 88[R]). Nomograms have been developed putting paracetamol plasma concentrations over time in relation to possible outcome (SEDA-18, 94–96).

Symptoms and diagnosis While damage to the liver is effected within hours of ingestion, major clinical manifestations are seldom seen until some 24–48 hours have elapsed. Thus early history-taking, a high index of suspicion and prompt and repeated assays of plasma paracetamol levels are essential in dealing with patients in the emergency situation. Primary signs, when they do appear, are those of liver failure, e.g. abdominal pain and tenderness, followed by jaundice, elevated levels of serum transaminases and reduced concentrations of coagulation factors resulting in a prolongation of prothrombin time. It may be up to a week before radical liver failure ensues. Consciousness is not usually lost early on, but resistant cerebral edema may intervene in a few days secondary to the hepatic failure. Acute renal tubular damage occurs in association with the liver damage, together with muscle necrosis and hyperkalemia. The muscle necrosis, as demonstrated at autopsy in fatal cases (89[R]), may itself exacerbate the severe electrolyte derangement seen in liver failure, particularly the marked hyperkalemia. The measuring of serum levels of coagulation factors V (below 10%) and VIII (VIII/V-ratio over 30) may have a predictive value and can thus be helpful in selecting those patients requiring liver transplantation (SEDA-17, 99).

Treatment Gastric lavage, especially in the first 4 hours after ingestion, is highly recommended, whilst the administration of activated charcoal is not vis-a-vis the absorption of the sulfhydryl antidote *N*-acetylcysteine. Since the mechanism of damage appears to be the exhaustion or depletion of sulfhydryl groups as available in glutathione, the treatment consists of early replacement of those groups by administration of an alternative source, either methionine or more readily acetylcysteine, given either orally or intravenously. To be most effective, these should be given within 8—12 hours of ingestion of the overdosage, but even up to 24 hours their administration may improve the outcome (90[R]). The only alternatives are charcoal hemoperfusion and renal dialysis which may be effective up to 18 hours after dosage. However, the longer the time from ingestion to treatment, the less likely the condition is to be reversible and the more certain a fatal outcome. Plasma paracetamol levels of under 1.3 mmol/l usually carry a good prognosis, but single measurements can be misleading because of continuing absorption of the drug. Theoretically, inhibitors of cytochrome P450 like cimetidine may be of value in the treatment of paracetamol overdosage, and preliminary animal data also suggest this (90[R]).

Children of 6 years and under are rarely subject to hepatotoxicity even with accidental overdosage (91[R]), possibly due to age-dependent differences in the paracetamol kinetics (92[C]).

Second-generation effects Paracetamol crosses the placenta readily. However, there has been no published evidence of a teratogenic effect in offspring of mothers taking paracetamol during pregnancy. A case of *fetal death* after a maternal overdose of paracetamol (30 grams) has been described (SEDA-10, 73), but in another similar case where 22.5 grams was taken in the 36th week the fetus survived (SEDA-9, 96).

Risk situations It is generally considered inadvisable to use paracetamol in patients with *active liver disease* or *severe dysfunction*, those with *cachexia*, or in *chronic alcoholics*.

Stable chronic liver disease does not seem to be a contraindication (93[C]).

Interactions *Diflunisal* somewhat increases blood levels of paracetamol while oral contraceptives seem to accelerate its excretion through the kidneys, reducing its effect (SEDA-9, 90). Analgetic 'cocktails' containing paracetamol or concurrent use of potentially hepatotoxic drugs will increase the risk of paracetamol toxicity, while drugs inducing liver microsomal enzymes such as phenobarbital and isoniazid can render paracetamol poisoning more severe (94[c], 95[r]).

A double-blind study on the interaction between *coumarin anticoagulants* and paracetamol revealed a statistically significant lengthening of the thrombotest time during the trial, as compared with placebo (96[c]).

Concomitant administration of paracetamol with *zidovudine* may lead to inhibition of glucuronidation and to potentiation of the toxicity of each drug (97[C], 98[C]).

Interference with diagnostic routines Attention has been drawn to the fact that paracetamol can induce false-positive reactions for *glucose* in serum and blood specimens examined using the YSI glucose analyzer. The effect could be of considerable importance in patients admitted with suspected paracetamol overdosage.

REFERENCES

1. National Drugs Advisory Board. Availability of aspirin and paracetamol. Annual Report 1987;24.
2. Kung LG. Hypernephroid carcinoma and carcinoma of the urinary tract associated with abuse of phenacetin. Schweiz Med Wochenschr 1976;106:47.
3. Gonwa TA, Corbett WT, Schey HM et al. Analgesic associated nephropathy and transitional cell carcinoma of the urinary tract. Ann Intern Med 1980;93:249.
4. Mihatsch MJ, Manz T, Knüsli C et al. Phenacetin abusus. III. Malignant tumors of urinary tract in phenacetin abusers in Basel. Schweiz Med Wochenschr 1980;110:255.
5. Taylor JS. Carcinoma of the urinary tract and analgesic abuse. Med J South Aust (1972) 1, 407.
6. Dubach UC. Die Bedeutung des Analgetikaabusus für chronische Harninfektionen. Therapiewoche 1981;31:7891.
7. Prescott LF. Analgesic nephropathy, a reassessment of the role of phenacetin and other analgesics. Drugs 1982;23:75.
8. Cove-Smith JR, Knapp HR. Analgesic nephropathy: an important cause of chronic renal failure. Q J Med 1978;47:49.
9. Szczeklik A. The cyclooxygenase theory of aspirin-induced asthma. Eur Respir J 1990;3:588.
10. Szczeklik A. Aspirin-induced asthma: pathogenesis and clinical presentation. Allergy Proc 1992;13:163.
11. Oates JA, Fitzgerald GA, Branch RA et al. Clinical implications of prostaglandin and thromboxane formation. N Engl J Med 1988;319:689.
12. Settipane RA, Constantine HP, Settipane GA. Aspirin intolerance and recurrent urticaria in normal adults and children. Allergy 1980;35:149.
13. Farr RS, Spector SL, Wangaard CH. Evaluation of aspirin and tartrazine idiosyncrasy. J Allergy Clin Immunol 1979; 64:667.
14. Editorial. Aspirin sensitivity in asthmatics. Br Med J 1980;281:958.
15. Pleskow WW, Stevenson DD, Mathison DA et al. Aspirin desensitization in aspirin-sensitive asthmatic patients: clinical manifestations and characterization of the refractory period. J Allergy Clin Immunol 1982;69:11.
16. Aspirin Myocardial Infarction Study Research Group. A randomized, controlled trial of aspirin in persons recovered from myocardial infarction. J Am Med Assoc 1980;243:661.
17. Habbad MA, Szwed SA, Haft JI. Is coronary arterial spasm part of the aspirin-induced asthma syndrome? Chest 1986;90:141.
18. Heffner JE, Sahn SA. Salicylate-induced pulmonary oedema. Ann Intern Med 1981;95:405.

19. Prince RL, Larkins RG, Alford FP. The effect of acetylsalicylic acid on plasma glucose and the response of glucose regulatory hormones to intravenous glucose-arginine in insulin treated diabetics and normal subjects. Metabolism 1981;30:293.
20. Meloni T, Forteleoni G, Ogan AP, Franca V. Aspirin-induced acute haemolytic anaemia in glucose-6-phosphate dehydrogenase-deficient children with systemic arthritis. Acta Haematol (Basel) 1989;81:208.
21. Levy M, Heyman A. Hematological adverse effects of analgesic anti-inflammatory drugs. Hematol Rev 1990;4:177.
22. Kingham JD, Chen MC, Levy MH. Macular hemorrhage in the aging: the effects of anticoagulants. N Engl J Med 1988;318:1126.
23. Werblin TP, Pfeiffer RL. Persistent hemorrhage after extracapsular surgery associated with excessive aspirin ingestion. Am J Ophthalmol 1987;104:426.
24. Hanley SP, Bevan J, Cockbill SR et al. Differential inhibition by low-dose aspirin of human venous prostacyclin synthesis and platelet thromboxane synthesis. Lancet 1981;i:969.
25. The Canadian Cooperative Study Group. A randomized trial of aspirin and sulfin-pyrazone in threatened stroke. N Engl J Med 1978;299:53.
26. Peto R, Gray R, Collins R et al. Randomized trial of prophylactic daily aspirin in British male doctors. Br Med J 1988;296:313.
27. Antiplatelet Trialist Collaboration. Secondary prevention of vascular disease by prolonged anti-platelet therapy. Br Med J 1988;296:320.
28. Hennekens CH et al. Aspirin and other antiplatelet agents in the secondary and primary prevention of cardiovascular disease. Circulation 1989;80:749.
29. Second International Study of Infarct Survival Collaborative Group. Randomized trial of intravenous streptokinase, oral aspirin, both, or neither among 17,187 cases of suspected myocardial infarction: ISIS-2. Lancet 1988;ii:349.
30. The RISC Group. Risk of myocardial infarction and death during treatment with low-dose aspirin and intravenous heparin in men with unstable coronary artery disease. Lancet 1991;336:827.
31. The Dutch TIA Trial Study Group. A comparison of two doses of aspirin (30 mg vs 283 mg a day) in patients after a transient ischaemic attack or minor ischaemic stroke. N Engl J Med 1991;325:1261.
32. The SALT Collaborative Group. Swedish Aspirin Low-dose Trial (SALT) of 75 mg aspirin as secondary prophylaxis after cerebrovascular ischaemic events. Lancet 1991;338:1345.
33. Steering Committee of the Physician's Health Study Research Group. Final report on the aspirin component of the ongoing physicians health study. N Engl J Med 1989;321:129.
34. UK-TIA Study Group. The United Kingdom Transient Ischaemic Attack Trial: final results. J Neurol Neurosurg Psychiatry 1991;54:1044.
35. Ivey KJ. Aspirin gastrointestinal toxicity: a review. Arch Ther 1984;1:190.
36. Zimmerman HJ. Effects of aspirin and acetaminophen on the liver. Arch Intern Med 141, l981;141:333.
37. Gitlin N. Salicylate hepatotoxicity: the potential role of hypoalbuminaemia. J Clin Gastroenterol 1980;5:281.
38. Freeland GR, Northington RS, Hedrich DA, Walker BR. Hepatic safety of two analgesics used over the counter: ibuprofen and aspirin. Clin Pharmacol Ther 1988;43:473.
39. Piper DW, McIntosh JH, Ariotti DE et al. Analgesic ingestion and chronic peptic ulcer. Gastroenterology 1981;80:427.
40. Perrault J, Fleming R, Dozoig RR. Surrepetitious use of salicylates: a cause of chronic recurrent gastroduodenal ulcers. Mayo Clin Proc 1988;63:337.
41. Petroski D. Endoscopic comparison of various aspirin preparations—gastric mucosal adaptability to aspirin restudied. Curr Ther Res 1989;45:945.
42. Szabo S. Pathogenesis of gastric mucosal injury. South Afr Med J 1988;2:35.
43. Faulkner G, Prichard P, Sommerville K, Langman MJS. Aspirin and bleeding peptic ulcers in the elderly. Br Med J 1988;297:1311.
44. Bonavina L, De Meester TR, McChesney L et al. Drug-induced esophageal strictures. Ann Surg 1987;206:173.
45. Screiber JB, Covington JP. Aspirin induced esophageal hemorrhage. J Am Med Assoc 1988;259:1647.
46. Barrier CH, Hirshowitz BI. Controversies in the detection and management of NSAID-induced side effects of the upper gastrointestinal tract. Arthritis Rheum 1989;32:926.
47. Mielants H, Veys EM, Verbruggen G et al. Salicylate-induced gastrointestinal bleeding, comparison between soluble buffered, enteric coated and intravenous administration. J Rheumatol 1979;6:210.
48. Malfertheiner P, Stonescu A, Rogatti W, Ditschuneit H. Effects of microencapsulated vs enteric-coated acetylsalicylic acid on gastric and duodenal mucosa: an endoscopic study. J Clin Gastroenterol 1988;10:269.
49. Akyol SM. Thompson M, Kerr DNS. Renal function after prolonged consumption of aspirin. Br Med J 1982;284:631.
50. Plotz PH, Kimberly RP. Acute effects of aspirin and acetaminophen on renal function. Arch Intern Med 1981;141:343.
51. Kanwar AJ, Belhaj MS, Bharija SC et al. Drugs causing fixed eruptions. J Dermatol 1984;11:383.
52. Röhr W-D. Transitorische Myopisierung und Drucksteigerung als Medikamentennebenwirkung. Fortschr Ophthalmol 1984;81:199.
53. Brandt KD, Polmosky MJ. Effects of salicylates and other NSAID on articular cartilage. Am J Med 1984;77:65.
54. Macdonald R. Aspirin and extradural blocks. Br J Anaesth 1991;66:1.
55. De Swiet M, Redman CWG. Aspirin, extradural anaesthesia and the MRC collaborative low-dose aspirin study in pregnancy (CLASP). Br J Anaesth 1992;68:109.
56. Slane D, Siskind V, Heinonen S et al. Aspirin and congenital malformations. Lancet 1976;i:1373.
57. Werler MM, Mitchell AA, Shapiro S. The relation of aspirin use during the first trimester of pregnancy to congenital cardiac defects. N Engl J Med 1989;321:1693.
58. Rumack CM, Guggenheim MA, Rumack BH et al. Neonatal intracranial hemorrhage and maternal use of aspirin. Obstet Gynecol 1980;58:525.
59. Shapiro S, Siskin V, Monson RR et al. Perinatal mortality and birth-weight in relation to aspirin taken during pregnancy. Lancet 1976;i:1375.
60. Uzan S, Beaufils M, Breart G et al. Prevention of fetal growth retardation with low-dose aspirin: findings of the EPREDA trial. Lancet 1991;337:1427.
61. Temple AR. Acute and chronic effects of aspirin toxicity and their treatment. Arch Intern Med 1981;141:364.
62. Meredith TJ, Vale JA. Non-narcotic analgesics. Problems of overdosage. Drugs 1986;32(Suppl 4):177.
63. Dove DJ, Jones T. Delayed coma associated with salicylate intoxication. J Pediatr 1982;100:493.

64. Book PM, Day RO. Non-SAID—Differences and similarities. N Engl J Med 1991;324:1716.
65. Valsecchi RR. Fixed drug eruption to paracetamol. Dermatologica 1989;179:51.
67. Deykin D, Janssen P, McMahon L. Ethanol potentiation of aspirin-induced prolongation of the bleeding time. N Engl J Med 1982;306:852.
68. Farrell K et al. The effect of acetylsalicylic acid on serum free valproate concentrations and valproate clearance in children. Clin Pharmacol Ther 1982;31:642.
69. World Health Organization (WHO). Mechanism of action, safety and efficacy of intrauterine devices. Geneva: WHO,1987;Technical Report Series 753:91
70. Croxatto HB, Ortiz ME, Valdez E. IUD mechanisms of action. In: Bardin CW, Mishell DR (eds): Proceedings from the 4th International Conference on IUDs. Boston: Butterworth-Heinemann, 1994;44.
71. Moore TJ et al. Contribution of prostaglandins to the antihypertensive effect of captopril in essential hypertension. Hypertension 1981;3:168.
72. Poulson AM Jr, Naisbett JP, Chamberlain PhD Jr. Aspirin use in women who become pregnant with an intrauterine device. Fertil Steril 1981;36:421.
73. Editorial. Poisoning with enteric-coated aspirin. Lancet 1981;2:130.
74. Pierce RP, Gazewood J, Blake RL Jr. Salicylate poisoning from enteric-coated aspirin. Delayed absorption may complicate management. Postgrad Med 1991;89:61.
75. Fyfe AI, Wright JM et al. Chronic acetaminophen ingestion associated with (117)(p11:p11)translocation and immune deficiency syndrome. Am J Med 1990;89:443.
76. Duhamel G, Najman A, Gorin NC et al. Aspets actuels de l'agranulocytose. Ann Méd Int 1977;125:303.
77. Heintz B, Bock TA, Kiendorf H, Maurin N. Haemolytic crisis after acetaminophen in glucose-6-phosphate dehydrogenase deficiency. Klin Wochenschr 1989;67:1068.
78. Hinsoin JA, Pohl LR, Monks TJ et al. Acetaminophen-induced hepatotoxicity. Life Sci 1981;29:107.
79. Meredith TJ, Prescott LF, Vale JA. Why do patients still die from paracetamol poisoning? Br Med J 1986;293:345.
80. Itoh S, Matsuo S, Shiomi M et al. Cirrhosis following 12 years of treatment with acetaminophen. Hepato-Gastroenterology 1983;30:58.
81. Waldum HL, Hamre T, Kleveland PM et al. Can NSAIDs cause acute biliary pain with cholestasis? J Clin Gastroenterol 1992;14:328.
82. Wong V, Daly M, Boon A, Heatley V. Paracetamol and acute biliary pain with cholestasis. Lancet 1993;342:869.
83. Schwartz A, Kunzendorf U, Keller F, Offermann G. Progression of renal failure in analgesic-associated nephropathy. Nephron 1989;53:244.
84. McCredie M, Steward JG. Does paracetamol cause urothelial cancer or renal papillary necrosis? Nephron 1988; 49:296.
85. Walker RJ. Paracetamol, nonsteroidal antiinflammatory drugs and nephrotoxicity. NZ Med J 1991;125:182.
86. Meyrick Thomas RH, Munro DD. Fixed drug eruption due to paracetamol. Br J Dermatol 1986;115:357.
87. McInnes GT, Brodie MT. Drug interactions that matter. A critical appraisal. Drugs 1988;36:83.
88. Dussarat GV, Dalger J, Mafort B, Chagnon A. Purpura vasculaire au paracétamol: Une observation. Presse Méd 1988;17:1587.
89. Brotodihardjo AE, Batey RG, Farrell C, Byth K. Hepatotoxicity from paracetamol self-poisoning in Western Sydney: a continuing challenge. Med J Aust 1992;157:385.
90. Stricker BHC, Spoelstra P. Drug-Induced Hepatic Injury. Amsterdam: Elsevier, 1985;51.
91. Ojeda VJ, Shilkin KB, Wright EA et al. Massive hepatic necrosis and focal necrotising myopathy. Lancet 1982;i:172.
92. Lewis RK, Paloucek FP. Assessment and treatment of acetaminophen overdose. Clin Pharm 1991;10:765.
93. Penna A, Buchanan N. Paracetamol poisoning in children and hepatotoxicity. Br J Clin Pharmacol 1991;32:143.
94. Rumore MM, Blaiklock RG. Influence of age-dependent pharmacokinetics and metabolism on acetaminophen hepatotoxicity. J Pharm Sci 1992;81:203.
95. Benson GD. Acetaminophen in chronic liver disease. Clin Pharmacol Ther 1983;33:95.
96. Marsepoils T, Mahassani B, Roudiak N et al. Potentialisation de la toxicité hépatique et rénal du paracétamol par le phénobarbital. Jeur 1989;2:118.
97. Dossing M, Sonne J. Drug-induced hepatic disorders. Incidence, management and avoidance. Drug Safety 1993;9:441.
98. Boeijinga JK, Boerstra EE, Ris P et al. De invloed van paracetamol op antistollingsbehandeling met coumarinederivaten. Pharm Weekbl 1983;118:209.
99. Shriner K, Goetz MB. Severe hepatotoxicity in a patient receiving both acetaminophen and zidovudine. Am J Med 1992;93:94.
100. Ameer B. Acetaminophen hepatotoxicity augmented by zidovudine. Am J Med 1993;95:342.

Meyler's Side Effects of Drugs, 13th Edition
M.N.G. Dukes, editor

SECTION EDITOR: B. VRHOVAC

Luciano Biscarini

9.2 Anti-inflammatory analgesics and drugs used in gout

NON-STEROIDAL ANTI-INFLAMMATORY DRUGS

GENERAL CONSIDERATIONS

Non-steroidal anti-inflammatory drugs (NSAID) are a heterogeneous group of organic acids which exert analgesic, antipyretic, anti-inflammatory and platelet-inhibitory actions.

The number of NSAID is very large. More than 100 are marketed or are at an advanced stage of development worldwide. There are two reasons for the ever-increasing number of NSAID: firstly, their use is constantly expanding and, secondly, the search for new more efficacious and better-tolerated compounds is still being pursued. In fact the search for new less toxic NSAID has received renewed impulse due to recent studies on selective inhibitors of cyclooxygenase 2 (COX-2), nitric oxide-releasing NSAID, peroxidase inhibitors, enantiomers of already known NSAID and cytokine modulating antirheumatic drugs such as tenidap.

Predominantly used in the management of rheumatological conditions, NSAID are considered the drugs of choice in the treatment of the inflammatory arthropathies. However, in recent years, their use has been extended to many non-rheumatological problems (e.g. dysmenorrhea, pain of different origin, neoplastic fever, migraine, thromboembolic disease and patent ductus arteriosus; they are also used for tocolysis and in some neoplastic diseases (see sulindac, below) (1[R]). There are by now several clinical, epidemiological and animal studies indicating that NSAID may reduce the occurrence or progression of colorectal cancer and polyps and perhaps of other gastro-intestinal tumors (2, 3, 4[C]). There are also reports and epidemiological studies on possible protective effect of NSAID on the risk for Alzheimer disease (5, 6). The wide occurrence of these conditions clearly justifies the extensive usage of the drugs employed to treat them, and explains the drug industry's interest in exploiting the potential revenues of such a wide market by commercializing each 'new' NSAID which is developed.

The effort to find new compounds is medically justified by the fact that presently available NSAID are not characterized by a satisfactory risk/benefit ratio. NSAID are the drugs most frequently reported to the various national agencies as being responsible for side effects. In addition, the adverse reaction profile of many NSAID has proved to be completely unacceptable. During the last 15 years, 18 NSAID have been withdrawn from the market or their clinical studies terminated because of unexpected and unacceptable toxicity (7[R]). The large number of NSAID which are available can render selection difficult, since reliable information on their relative efficacy and adverse reactions is usually meagre.

Although the physicochemical features, pharmacokinetics and/or pharmacodynamics of individual NSAID can differ, it is not known to what extent these differences will result in significant differences in the risk/benefit profile in the individual patient (8[R]). Certainly they can influence the adverse reactions and the general pattern of action of a particular subgroup of NSAID or a specific compound within a class, but this still provides no reliable prediction of what the individual patient will experience.

Physicochemically the acidic nature and lipid-solubility of these compounds can be important. The lipid-solubility of an NSAID determines its diffusibility in the central nervous system (CNS) and hence the incidence of CNS-related side effects, as well as, perhaps, adverse skin reactions (9[R], 72[R]). The weak acid nature of these drugs affects their tissue distribution, which explains why they both exert an action at certain sites (e.g. synovial tissue of inflamed joints) and also contribute to the triggering of particular adverse reactions at others (e.g. stomach and renal medulla) (10).

Pharmacodynamic mechanisms may also be crucial. The major mechanism of action of NSAID is generally conceded to be the inhibition of cyclo-oxygenase (COX) activity and consequently of prostaglandin synthesis (11, 12[R], 13[R]). Recently two forms of the COX enzyme have been identified: COX-1, which is constitutively expressed in many cells and tissues, and COX-2, which is selectively induced by proinflammatory cytokines at the site of inflammation. The discovery of a second COX enzyme has led to the hypothesis that toxicity associated with the clinically useful NSAID is caused by the inhibition of COX-1, whereas the anti-inflammatory properties are caused by the inhibition of inducible COX-2 (14). Therefore a selective inhibitor of COX-2 may exert superior anti-inflammatory activity with substantial safety over existing NSAID. The in vitro potency of NSAID as inhibitors of prostaglandin synthesis, which tends to match their anti-inflammatory potency in vivo, varies from one anti-inflammatory agent to another (15[R], 16[R]). Other mechanisms which are poorly understood may be implicated in determining both a drug's activity and its side effects.

Pharmacokinetic aspects may play a critical role in favoring the onset of certain side effects in some patients (17). NSAID have high bioavailability after oral administration, since they are almost entirely absorbed from the gastrointestinal tract (18[R]). The rate and the site of absorption from the gastrointestinal tract may be important; it has been found that formulations designed to spare the stomach from NSAID toxicity instead may damage the intestinal wall; this seems to have been the case with 'Osmosin' (SEDA-8, 103).

NSAID bind avidly to plasma protein. High protein binding theoretically can predispose patients to drug interactions, which occur most frequently with certain NSAID (e.g. butazones) in patients concomitantly treated with such drugs as hypoglycemic agents or oral anticoagulants. The unbound fraction responsible for the pharmacological action of NSAID obviously varies with the plasma albumin concentrations, and the latter may be influenced by active rheumatoid arthritis, genetic factors, sex, age, pregnancy, other drugs, and various disease states, particularly involving the kidney and liver. A correlation between anti-inflammatory action and dose or plasma concentrations has in fact been documented for only a few NSAID, and there is no direct evidence that an increase in free-drug levels is accompanied by greater toxicity. There is however convincing testimony that the dose administered at least contributes to provoking certain side effects (e.g. gastrointestinal and renal). A record-linkage study has revealed an association between NSAID dosage and upper gastrointestinal bleeding (19[R]).

NSAID can be roughly classified into those with a short and those with a long half-life. Although the difference in clinical effects between these two groups is poorly understood, half-lives have served as a rough guide for NSAID dosage regimens, compounds of the latter type being administered only once daily. These NSAID with longer half-lives also may be regarded as having a greater potential to induce side effects, at least in some patients. As the half-lives of NSAID of this type (e.g. piroxicam) may however vary widely in different patients, drug accumulation can occur in some individuals. When using such a long half-life NSAID, loading doses may be given to attain high drug concentrations quickly; such loading doses can however be associated with increased side effects, particularly gastrointestinal intolerance.

NSAID are mainly cleared by the liver; as one would expect, therefore, clearance of a number of NSAID decreases with age (18[R]). The metabolites are generally inactive and excreted in the urine, which as a rule contains very little of the unchanged drug. Conversely, several NSAID which are themselves inactive can be used as 'prodrugs' since they have active metabolites; some of these compounds, such as sulindac, are enterohepatically recycled. Claims that these pro-drugs are less toxic than other compounds are not supported by a firm evidence. Some NSAID, including ketoprofen, fenoprofen, naproxen, carprofen and indometacin are metabolized to acylglucuronide; the metabolites are retained and hydrolyzed to reform the parent compound. This is probably one of the mechanisms of toxicity in patients with renal impairment.

The presented data provide basis for the practical use of NSAID. There can be no doubt that some NSAID are more toxic than others, notably those which exert the greatest inhibitory effect on cyclooxygenase. NSAID which inhibit both cyclooxygenase and lipooxygenase are particularly toxic. The fact that some NSAID are more toxic for single organ systems than others seems to depend on the physicochemical and metabolic characteristics of single drugs or groups of similar drugs. Despite numerous studies, reliable comparison of the adverse effects of the different drugs are scanty. However some data have been produced recently from data bank centers of the Arthritis Rheumatism and Aging Medical Information System (ARAMIS) and are reviewed in SEDA-17, 102. The categories of patients who are at higher risk of adverse reactions when treated with NSAID are well known and can largely be deduced from what has been said above. They comprise the elderly (especially women), pregnant women (including their fetuses), newborn infants, patients with liver, kidney or cardiac disorders and those affected by arterial hypertension, multiple myeloma, peptic disorders or active rheumatoid arthritis. Greater awareness of these risk factors among medical practitioners, limitation of the use of NSAID to those cases where there is a precise indication, development of systems for monitoring unwanted side effects, and performance of adequate well-designed experimental studies would do much to ensure a more correct use of these drugs in clinical practice. Since many NSAID side effects are, with negligible differences, common to the entire NSAID group, these effects will be dealt with below before the various classes of NSAID and individual compounds are discussed.

MAJOR PROBLEMS WITH NON-STEROIDAL ANTI-INFLAMMATORY DRUGS

Gastrointestinal *(SEDA-13, 71; SEDA-14, 79; SEDA-15, 92; SEDA-16, 103; SEDA-17, 108; SEDA-18, 99)* Prostaglandins have a protective effect on the gastrointestinal (GI) mucosa. All NSAID that inhibit nonselectively prostaglandin biosynthesis cause GI mucosal damage. Direct NSAID-mediated acid damage has been identified as a mechanism of GI toxicity (20[R]). Moreover, there are now several in vitro and animal studies that support the role of early vascular changes and highlight the important role of leukocyte adhesion to the endothelium in NSAID gastropathy. The pathogenesis of NSAID-associated gastro-intestinal damage has been re-examined in SEDA-17, 104.

Upper GI toxicity during NSAID therapy is characterized by clinical problems ranging from relatively mild symptoms such as heartburn, dyspepsia and stomach discomfort, to more severe and potentially life-threatening states, e.g. GI erosion or ulceration and GI bleeding or perforation. Although dyspepsia is one of the major factors limiting the use of NSAID in rheumatic disease patients, its presence does not necessarily predict mucosal damage. There is no strict correlation between objective gastroscopy findings and subjective intolerance to medications, or between acute damage and chronic damage or complications. Epigastric pain was the most common symptom in patients admitted to hospital for hematemesis and/or melena in both groups, treated or not with NSAID during the 14 days prior to admission, in a study recently published and reviewed in SEDA-17, 103. 'NSAID gastropathy' is the term proposed by Roth and Bennett to describe upper GI lesions associated with NSAID therapy. It has its own specific features (primarily antral and prepyloric localization, especially in the elderly female NSAID population) which differentiate it from classic peptic ulcer disease (21[R]). Damage to the upper GI tract can also involve the duodenum and, albeit infrequently, the esophagus.

GI damage by NSAID represents a major health problem in current clinical practice and estimates of the absolute risk vary from approximately two cases of serious upper GI adverse effects per 10 000 person-months (22[R]) to a 7-fold increase in the risk of hospitalization in patients with rheumatoid arthritis (23[C]). Estimates of hospitalization for ulcer complications and excess of GI deaths in the United Kingdom have shown that 20—30% of all cases of ulcer complications in subjects aged over 60 which result in hospitalization are directly attributable to the use of NSAID, and that some 10% of these culminate in death (24[C]). For the United Kingdom this would mean that at least 2000 cases of bleeding are induced every year and that about 200 deaths occur (25[C]), in association with approximately 11 million prescriptions. The relative risk reported in various studies has generally been in the range of 3:1—5:1 (26[R]). Fries et al. (27[CR]) have reported a study on 2747 rheumatoid arthritis patients which reveals that those taking NSAID were 5 times more likely (hazard ratio of 5.2) to be hospitalized for an upper GI event than those who were not. The risk of hospitalization for a GI event in these patients was 15.8 per 1000 person-years in individuals taking NSAID, as compared with 3.2 per 1000 person-years for individuals not taking these drugs. Such figures would mean that, on average, of every 100 patients taking NSAID for 1 year, one to two would be hospitalized for a GI event (most commonly an ulcer). A meta-analysis of 16 studies also came to the conclusion that users of NSAID have an approximately 3-times greater relative risk of developing serious adverse GI events than are non-users (28[CR]). This is confirmed by a review of studies published in recent years (29[R]). Case-control and surveillance studies have confirmed previously identified risk factors for peptic ulcer disease, such as age (elderly), history of ulcers and/or gastric bleeding, combination with corticosteroids, combination with other NSAID and, possibly, smoking (SEDA-14, 84). In addition, an interesting new finding has emerged from the data of Fries et al. on rheumatoid arthritis patients taking NSAID (27[Cr]): predisposition to GI events is related to the severity of the rheumatoid arthritis. Other suggested potential risk factors are sex (female), the musculoskeletal diseases for which NSAID are used, the nature of the NSAID itself and dosage. The presence of gastric mucosal erosions at endoscopy was associated with an increased risk of subsequent development of a gastric ulcer irrespective of the prophylactic treatment received (misoprostol vs sucralfate) in chronic NSAID osteoarthritic users evaluated in a large randomized controlled trial (30[C]).

Despite the suggestions made by some authors that some NSAID are more gastrotoxic than others, data on individual drugs have been at best fragmentary (SEDA-14, 85). Two well-conducted studies have recently provided convincing data for clarifying whether some compounds are more likely than others to cause serious adverse gastrointestinal events (31[C], 32[C]). Ibuprofen was associated with the lowest risk of gastrointestinal toxicity; diclofenac, naproxen and possibly indometacin were intermediate, while piroxicam and, in particular azapropazone, had a much higher risk. These results have practical implications: when NSAID treatment is needed the least toxic compound should be selected on the basis of the data provided by these studies and, because of the substantial increase in risk from low-dose to high-dose NSAID therapy, it would be wise, whenever possible, to start treatment with low dosages. Another important finding confirmed by both studies is that risk increased with drug dosage for all drugs combined. The search for less toxic drugs or formulations has been discouraging. Various new formulations may be less gastrotoxic than standard formulations in short-term studies, but their merit has not yet been proven in long-term use. Equally, pro-drugs have not protected users against gastric complications (33[C]). Parenteral and rectal administration of NSAID does not spare the stomach. Other ways of preventing NSAID GI damage that have been investigated are the use of H2-receptor antagonists, the prostaglandin analog misoprostol, or sucralfate. The limited data available indicate that H2-receptor antagonists are unable to prevent NSAID-induced gastric ulcer. Two studies on ranitidine, which report that it reduces the incidence of duodenal ulcers, conflict with others that did not find that it offers protection against gastroduodenal-mucosa lesions (SEDA-14, 86). Studies on misoprostol an oral prostaglandin analog have shown that co-administration of misoprostol and NSAID does significantly reduce the frequency of NSAID-induced gastric ulcer in patients with osteoarthritis (34[C]) and it has been recently demonstrated that misoprostol reduces the occurrence of serious upper gastrointestinal complications (perforation, gastric outlet obstruction, and perhaps bleeding) by 40% compared with placebo in older patients with rheumatoid arthritis treated with NSAID (35, 36). Whether patients who start taking NSAID should routinely have prophylaxis with anti-ulcer drugs is not at all clear; the costs of such co-therapy are obviously high, side-effects of drugs used in prophylaxis must be taken into consideration and it would seem logical to limit it to high-risk cases (see below). Another still unsolved problem is that of the role of *Helicobacter pylori* in NSAID-induced gastroduodenal damage. Current data on the subject suggest that *H. pylori* does not confer increased risk for the development of endoscopically visible gastroduodenal damage or dyspeptic symptoms. It is not clear whether ulcer complications occur with greater frequency in individuals infected with *H. pylori* who are also taking NSAID. For practical purpose, even if reliable data are lacking, it would seem reasonable to eradicate the infection in those patients who need continuous therapy with NSAID (SEDA-17, 105, 37, 38).

As pointed out, NSAID are an important cause of morbidity and mortality in the community, but this is due to their extraordinarily wide use rather than to their intrinsic toxicity. The main way to reduce risks from NSAID in the community should therefore be to limit their use rather than to attempt to lower the relative risk further by widespread co-prescription of other agents, whether these be H2-receptor antagonists, misoprostol, or anticholinergics. 'Protective' co-therapy may have a role but only in a limited number of individuals. When NSAID are thought to be important, as in many cases of rheumatoid arthritis, and the patient is in a high-risk group, consideration should be given to using mucosal-protective agents as well. Fries et al. have proposed an interesting rule that permits the individual risk of rheumatoid arthritis patients to be estimated (27[CR]).

Esophageal damage by NSAID has been considered a rare adverse reaction but it has been underestimated, perhaps because the symptoms of esophagitis can be misinterpreted as being of gastric origin. The clinical pattern is characterized by inflammatory changes (erosive and/or ulcerative esophagitis), ulceration with or without bleeding and/or perforation and strictures. Data (reviewed in SEDA-15) suggest that the frequency of erosive/ulcerative esophagitis in patients taking NSAID is not so low as was previously thought. Semble et al. (39[CR]) found that erosive or ulcerative esophagitis was present in 20% of a consecutive series of 60 arthritic patients who were receiving chronic NSAID therapy: esophageal symptoms were noted in 83% of those with esophagitis. A recent study shows that long-term users of NSAID have fewer esophageal histological abnormalities than patients not receiving NSAID (40). However, more epidemiological and experimental prospective studies are needed to define better the role of NSAID in inducing esophageal injury.

The capacity of NSAID to cause *intestinal damage* has been demonstrated in a case-control study (41[C]) as well as by experience with a special formulation of indometacin ('Osmosin') (SEDA-15, 93). Severe intestinal damage such as perforation and bleeding seems to be a very rare complication of therapy with conventionally formulated NSAID. According to Langman et al. (41[C]) the expected incidence of lower bowel perforations and bleeding is about ten and seven per 100 000 patients respectively. In contrast, uncomplicated intestinal mucosal lesions are more frequent, particularly when NSAID are given long-term (42[R]). Small intestine enteropathy is characterized by inflammation and/or malfunction with an increase in intestinal permeability. The majority of patients are asymptomatic, though a few on long-term treatment present symptoms that mimick the clinical features of Crohn's disease. The fact that NSAID may exacerbate Crohn's disease (SEDA-10, 76) makes differential diagnosis difficult in symptomatic patients. Adverse effects on the small intestine may be more frequent than previously thought and are represented by various pathologies, ranging from asymptomatic enteropathy to severe complications, such as ulceration, bleeding, perforation and stricture (43[R]). An estimate of the prevalence of such lesions associated with the use of NSAID has been provided by a recent prospective autopsy study on 713 patients (44[C]). Nonspecific small-intestinal ulcers were more frequent in the NSAID group than in the control group (8.6 vs 0.6%) and the percentage was slightly higer in long-term than in short-term users. The maiority of the lesions were subclinical, but perforation leading to peritonitis and death was documented in three patients on long-term NSAID therapy. The pathogenesis of NSAID-induced enteropathy is still unknown; the hypotheses are reviewed in SEDA-17, 106. Whether the 'diaphragm disease' (45[R]), found in a few patients, is a new NSAID-related disease or only a variant form of congenital intestinal diaphragm remains to be clarified, even if new reports have been added (46, 47). The causal connection between NSAID administration and large bowel inflammation needs to be substantiated by appropriate epidemiological studies. Many publications have documented an association between NSAID and colonic inflammation (SEDA-10, 77; SEDA-15, 95), but the differential diagnosis between colonic inflammation arising de novo and exacerbation of underlying inflammatory bowel disease can be difficult. However, the role of NSAID in aggravating ulcerative colitis or Crohn's disease or other inflammatory bowel disease is controversial (SEDA-10, 76; SEDA-15, 95).

When administered long-term, the fenamates cause watery diarrhea in a greater proportion of patients than do other NSAID. Colonic ulcerations have been reported following oral ingestion of various NSAID (SEDA-7, 105; SEDA-10, 77; SEDA-15, 95), but the evidence is not entirely convincing. On the other hand, there is firm reason to conclude that there is a direct causal relationship between rectally administered NSAID and rectal ulceration, which seems to occur more frequently when doses are high or treatment prolonged.

Hematological NSAID have been reported to cause potentially severe hematological disorders: *thrombocytopenia*, *agranulocytosis*, *aplastic anemia* and *hemolytic anemia* (48[R]). NSAID as a group do not appear to be particularly prone to cause thrombocytopenia. It is generally mild, reversible and has a low case-fatality rate. However, deaths from *bleeding* have been reported, particularly with phenylbutazone, oxyphenbutazone and indometacin (48[R]).

Pyrazolone derivatives and butazones are most frequently blamed for causing agranulocytosis and aplastic anemia (SEDA-9, 85; SEDA-11, 89). Unfortunately, no reasonably accurate estimate of the overall incidence of either disease or of the risk associated with the use of any particular NSAID is available. The results of the International Agranulocytosis and Aplastic Anemia study published in 1986 (49) have been reviewed in detail in SEDA-11, 89 and in SED-11, 171. This epidemiological study, which is the only one ever performed and was organized by the manufacturer (Hoechst) of the widely incriminated drug dipyrone, revealed an overall annual community agranulocytosis incidence of 4.4 per million (6.2 including hospital cases) with a fatality rate of 10% and an annual mortality rate of 0.4 per million. Analgesics found to be significantly associated with agranulocytosis were dipyrone, indometacin and two butazones (phenylbutazone and oxyphenbutazone). Other pyrazolones such as amidopyrine (which is an acknowledged cause of agranulocytosis) or other NSAID could not be evaluated because of the small number of cases. A population-based case-control study in patients hospitalized with neutropenia has now confirmed the association between NSAID and neutropenia and the differences among various classes of NSAID (50[C]). The data on aplastic anemia are also of interest since this is the first study to provide excess risk estimates of this side effect in NSAID users. The overall annual incidence was found to be 2.2 per million, with a 2-year fatality rate of 40%. An increased risk for aplastic anemia has proved to be significantly associated with any exposure to three drugs: indometacin (multivariate rate ratio 12.7), butazones (8.7) and, unexpectedly, diclofenac (8.8). Whatever the interpretation put upon this study by different manufacturers, the study confirmed that dipyrone can induce agranulocytosis and that indometacin can cause aplastic anemia (51). The high relative risk of diclofenac for aplastic anemia is unexpected and requires confirmation. Hemolytic anemia has occasionally been associated with NSAID; there are a number of reports involving mefenamic acid, ibuprofen and sulindac (52[R]). No evidence has been found that any NSAID, except aspirin, constitutes a particular risk for subjects with glucose-6-phosphate dehydrogenase deficiency.

Urinary system *(SED-11, 172; SEDA-11, 82)* NSAID can produce a whole spectrum of renal diseases: functional renal insufficiency, interstitial nephritis and nephrotic syndrome, nephrotic syndrome without interstitial nephritis, renal papillary necrosis and chronic interstitial nephritis, acute tubular necrosis, vasculitis, glomerulonephritis, and obstructive nephropathy. Moreover, NSAID can interfere with fluid and electrolyte homeostasis, thereby causing edema, hyponatremia, hyperkalemia, and blunting of the natriuretic effects of diuretics.

While misoprostol has been shown to limit NSAID-induced gastric damage, three studies failed to produce evidence that misoprostol prevents NSAID-induced impairment of renal function, but another one indicates that it does prevent cyclosporin nephrotoxicity in renal transplant patients (53[C]). Further studies are, therefore, required to define the value of misoprostol in the protection of renal function (SEDA-16, 106).

Incidence of renal effects and variations in risk Two recent studies suggest that the overall incidence of clinically manifest nephrotoxicity with NSAID is small (54[C], 55[C]). Some particular patient groups, as indicated in the sections which follow, are however at increased risk of particular effects (SEDA-11, 82) and patients with sickle cell anemia can probably be added to the list (SEDA-15, 97).

Although some compound-related variations do occur, the important point to bear in mind is that every type of nephrotoxic effect seems to have been reported with every NSAID at some time; no NSAID is free of nephrotoxic potential. This applies to sulindac as to other NSAID, though there are some disputed claims that this particular compound might have a 'renal function sparing effect' (SEDA-15, 99; 56[R], 57[R]). One study (58[C]) did suggest that renal effects were more likely to occur in patients treated with ibuprofen than those administered piroxicam or sulindac, but it was criticized for flaws in experimental design (59[R]). Erikson et al. have recently provided supporting evidence that sulindac might be relatively safer; they showed that short-term administration of 400 mg/day of sulindac and 750 mg/day of naproxen exerted different effects on the glomerular filtration rate, the renal plasma flow and renal prostaglandin excretion in 10 patients with arthritis and impaired renal function. Whereas no significant changes were documented with sulindac, naproxen provoked a reduction in all three parameters of renal function (60[C]). Such short-term evidence clearly does not rule out the sort of problem in long-term use which constitutes the real challenge.

A recent study that evaluated the risk of *chronic renal disease* associated with the regular use of NSAID revealed that it was twice as high in men over 65 years and that it tended to be even higher in those with heart disease or other disorders which might compromise renal circulation (61[R]). The results of a second investigation, a case control study of 340 patients with end-stage renal disease on hemodialysis maintenance program and 678 hospitalized controls, revealed the same trend (SEDA 16, 105). However, more reliable epidemiological data are needed to demonstrate that regular consumption of NSAID as a single drug can increase the risk of chronic renal disease. NSAID-associate analgesic nephropathy is reviewed in SEDA-18, 100. The actual risk of NSAID-associated acute renal dysfunction also continues to be the subject of controversy. While there is adequate evidence that underlying renal failure, congestive heart failure or cirrhosis are conditions at high risk of NSAID-related renal function impairment, it is still not known whether the old age represent a risk factor, whether the risk of renal impairment varies with different NSAID or whether renal function continues to deteriorate, stabilize or even improve in affected patients with continued use of NSAID. Renal failure caused by use of topical NSAID has been described in three cases until now (SEDA-18, 100).

Types of complication Of the potentially serious side effects of *NSAID functional renal insufficiency*, which is probably the most common, results from the hemodynamic changes secondary to inhibition of prostaglandin synthesis caused by NSAID. The insufficiency and the interference with fluid and electrolyte homeostasis occur in disease states in which prostaglandins have become significant determinants of renal function, such as those characterized by hypovolemic states due to salt depletion or hypoalbuminemia and those where there is pre-existing renal impairment due to age, atherosclerosis, hypertensive renal disease or other intrinsic renal disease. The functional renal insufficiency is usually mild and reversible within a few days after cessation of NSAID therapy, but it can also be severe and irreversible. Early recognition is essential if it is to be reduced. All NSAID can cause this complication.

Symptomatic edema is seen in 2—20% of patients receiving NSAID, hyperkalemia may occur, especially in older patients who often receive potassium-sparing drugs or supplements, and the natriuretic effects of diuretics may be blunted.

Acute interstitial nephritis, which is distinct from the methicillin-like form, is the most important type of organic renal damage resulting from use of NSAID. Its distinguishing feature is a nephrotic syndrome, often with renal failure. The histological picture is one of acute interstitial nephritis combined with a glomerular lesion with fusion of the epithelial foot process. Typically the patients concerned have been taking NSAID over a long period. Acute interstitial nephritis has relatively often been reported in patients on fenoprofen.

Renal papillary necrosis has been repeatedly demonstrated following long-term intake or abuse of aspirin and other NSAID (SEDA-11, 85; SEDA-12, 79).

Acute flank pain syndrome associated with reversible renal failure seems to be very rare and has been described induced mainly by suprofen (SEDA-12, 89), but recently flurbiprofen and ibuprofen have been reported (SEDA-18, 100) as causes of this side effect.

Hypersensitivity reactions *(SEDA-7, 106)* Anaphylactic or anaphylactic-like reactions to NSAID are probably relatively rare events. Even today, the only data available from 1981, when the US Food and Drug Administration's Division of Drug Experience (62[CR]) was notified of 131 cases attributable to various NSAID, tolmetin being the compound most frequently implicated. The figures are distorted by the fact that some of these drugs are much more widely used than others. A retrospective cohort study on 1980—1984 Medicaid billing data from three states in the United States, performed to assess the relative risk of hypersensitivity reactions from different NSAID, failed to confirm previous suggestions that the use of tolmetin is associated with a higher risk of hypersensitivity reactions than administration of other NSAID (63). However, two drugs (glafenine and zomepirac) have been withdrawn from the market because of their propensity to cause severe hypersensitivity reactions. The clinical picture of hypersensitivity reactions may vary from vasomotor rhinitis, urticaria and angio-edema to serious bronchocostriction and, in some cases, anaphylactic shock. Two pathogenic mechanisms have been proposed: the first is an allergic immunological hypersensitivity reaction; the second is a pseudoallergic reaction characterized by mast-cell degranulation by complement components, histamine liberation by drugs and interference with endogenous eicosanoid biosynthesis (64). The former mechanism appears to be responsible for the anaphylactic shock and/or urticaria that may develop after taking amidopyrine or noramidopyrine, the latter for the bronchoconstriction encountered after ingestion of aspirin, noramidopyrine, or of aminophenazone and other pyrazole drugs. It is important to distinguish the two mechanisms since intolerance of the first type is fairly structure-specific and can be avoided by transferring a patient from a drug to which he/she has proved sensitive to NSAID of differing structure, whereas pseudoallergic aspirin-sensitive patients must avoid all NSAID that are effective inhibitors of fatty acid cyclooxygenase.

Skeletal system The suspected but unproven deleterious effects of NSAID on joint, cartilage and bone have been extensively discussed in SEDA-11, 87. Inhibition of glycosaminoglycan synthesis in joint cartilage, inhibition of necrotic bone repair by reduced synthesis of vasodilator prostaglandins which have been demonstrated in both in vitro and animal models, and the deprivation of protective painful stimuli are possible mechanisms of deleterious effects on osteoarthritic joints. As these data derive from experimental models, they cannot however be extrapolated with any degree of certainty to the effects which NSAID exert on the pathophysiological characteristics of the human osteoarthritic joint. Clinical evidence for harmful effects of NSAID on the human hip-joint comes from single case reports or small series of clinical observations, two retrospective studies and a more recent prospective investigation. The last (65[C]) revealed that hip osteoarthritis progressed more rapidly in patients treated with indometacin, a strong prostaglandin-synthesis inhibitor, than in those who received azapropazone, a weak prostaglandin-synthesis inhibitor; this suggests that one should be cautious with the long-term use of the more potent inhibitors of cyclooxygenase in patients with joints severely compromised by osteoarthritis. Other studies have reported that some NSAID have a protective effect on cartilage (66[R]). A recent study on a small group of patients with osteoarthritis of the knee treated with piroxicam supports the hypothesis that, by increasing the load on the joint, the deprivation of painful stimuli puts the patients at risk of more rapid progression of disease (67[C]). More extensive laboratory and clinical research is needed before a consensus can be reached.

Skin and appendages *(SEDA-13, 72)* Skin reactions are reported commonly with NSAID, but the true incidence of effects with the individual NSAID is unknown. There are very few specific epidemiological studies and most information comes from single case reports and data derived from national spontaneous reporting systems. A major study on nearly 20 000 patients by Kaiser et al. found that 0.3% of the 9118 patients being treated with analgesics and NSAID developed skin reactions which were considered to be attributable to these drugs (68[C]).

Although usually mild, skin reactions very often necessitate withdrawal of treatment. At times they may be severe; isoxicam was indeed withdrawn from the market because of the high frequency of severe adverse skin reactions (SEDA-10, 88).

Various types of NSAID-induced *rashes* can be identified. The main morphological patterns are urticarial, maculopapular, vesicular and exfoliative. Cutaneous reactions to NSAID are probably of phototoxic origin and may be associated with systemic hypersensitivity or other allergic reactions. More rarely, NSAID can exacerbate a pre-existing skin disease (e.g. psoriasis, acne). Phototoxic reactions proved to be a considerable problem with benoxaprofen (30—50% of patients treated in the United Kingdom), and were one reason why it did not receive licensing approval in Australia or the Benelux countries, but other NSAID such as azapropazone, piroxicam and fenbufen have been reported to cause higher than average rates of photosensitivity (69[R]). NSAID were among the causal agents of phototoxic reactions most commonly reported to the Australian Adverse Drug Reactions Advisory Committee (70[R], 71[R]).

The wide use of naproxen, sulindac, diclofenac and diflunisal, rather than a greater propensity to cause these side effects, is probably the reason that they were the most frequently implicated. All the same, NSAID do differ in their ability to cause adverse dermatological reactions in terms of both frequency and severity: pyrazolones, butazones and oxicams are most often blamed and, among the arylalkanoic acid derivatives, fenbufen and carprofen are the most frequently incriminated.

The type of cutaneous side-effect observed also varies with different compounds. The most serious life-threatening reactions such as *erythema multiforme* and its variants (Stevens-Johnson syndrome, toxic epidermal necrolysis or Lyell's syndrome, exfoliative erythroderma), are uncommon and probably occur mainly with the butazone derivatives and, to a lesser extent, with piroxicam, sulindac and possibly fenbufen. All NSAID can cause *urticaria*, particularly in aspirin-sensitive patients. However, it is more common with pyrazolone derivatives. *Photosensitivity* is principally a problem with azapropazone, carprofen, tiaprofenic acid and piroxicam (SEDA-9, 84). The reasons for the differences in the cutaneous side-effects of the different NSAID are poorly understood. The only physicochemical characteristic that seems to be important in determining a particular propensity for dermatological adverse reactions is lipophilia (72) since this probably affects the distribution of various NSAID to the skin. In addition, the longer half-life of lipophilic compounds may concomitantly facilitate the persistence of skin reactions. Although no clear relationship has been found between the other pharmacological and kinetic characteristics of NSAID and cutaneous effects, less lipophilic drugs with a short half-life might be preferable.

There are no clearly identifiable predisposing factors for most cutaneous adverse reactions. Urticaria and photosensitivity are exceptions. Many NSAID can provoke urticaria (sometimes associated with angio-edema) in aspirin-sensitive patients. The reaction is probably not immunological in origin, but rather related to prostaglandin inhibition in a patient whose cutaneous mastocytes are more susceptible to the stabilizing effect of prostaglandins. Skin testing in patients with a history of urticarial and/or anaphylactic reactions to analgesics seems of little value in identifying predisposed patients and can be dangerous (73, 74). Skin pigmentation and environmental factors that influence the radiant exposure dose are clearly very important in determining the risk of a phototoxic reaction in a given patient. Since the extreme rarity of life threatening reactions, such as erythema multiforme and toxic epidermal necrolysis, suggests individual susceptibility, efforts have been made to identify predisposed subjects. A study of 25 cases of erythema multiforme and toxic epidermal necrolysis revealed a slight, nonstatistically significant increase in the frequency of the HLA-B12 and DR4 phenotypes, which may mean that genetic factors are involved (75[R]). The possibility of genetic predisposition also seems to be confirmed by the recent finding of a fixed drug eruption in four members of a single family taking feprazone (SEDA-17, 108). From a practical point of view, if a mild reaction occurs, it would seem wise to suggest withdrawal of treatment, even if in some patients the reaction disappears spontaneously despite continuing treatment. Withdrawal of treatment and prompt referral to hospital is imperative if the reaction is severe and/or tends to progress.

Careful clinical monitoring is probably wise in all patients with underlying skin diseases (e.g. acne, psoriasis) receiving NSAID, as some of these compounds can exacerbate their dermatological problems (76[c], 77[c]). Moreover, NSAID should not be used for apparently benign inflammatory cutaneous lesions unless the possibility of infection has been ruled out by appropriate investigations; it is striking that in 11 cases of necrotizing fasciitis (which is usually caused by *Streptococcus pyogenes*) NSAID were suspected to have predisposed to the infection and/or to have caused its fulminant evolution (SEDA-12, 79).

Liver Serious liver reactions to NSAID are rare but unpredictable and this suggests that the majority of reactions are due to hypersensitivity or occasionally idiosyncrasy. The U.S. Food and Drug Administration has, however, recognized liver reactions as a 'class effect' of NSAID. Due to hepatotoxicity, probably dose-related and particularly problematic in the elderly, benoxaprofen was withdrawn from the market in 1982, and ibufenac is not on sale for the same reason. Serious hepatocellular reactions have been well documented with phenylbutazone and the reported case fatality rate is high (78[CR]). Hepatotoxicity has been reported with all of the structural classes of NSAID. The incidence and importance of liver reactions with the commonly used modern NSAID is difficult to assess because there has been little systematic research and, in particular, no large epidemiological studies. Hepatic reactions are more commonly reported with the pyrazolone, indole, and propionic acid groups of compounds than with the fenamate and oxicam classes of NSAID (48[R]). Some national monitoring centers have published their experience on liver toxicity with NSAID and the Swedish and Australian agencies have both drawn attention to an apparently higher frequency of liver reactions with sulindac and diclofenac (79[R], 80[R]). While the reactions to sulindac are characterized by a cholestatic picture, diclofenac is associated with a more acute hepatocellular derangement. Diclofenac is now recognized as a rare cause of acute hepatocellular damage (81[R]).

Three recent epidemiological cohort studies have confirmed that acute liver injury caused by the most frequently used NSAID is rare (SEDA-17, 107, 82).

Second-generation effects *Use in pregnancy and lactation* Many NSAID have provoked teratogenic effects in animals, but there is no evidence from epidemiological studies to suggest that NSAID have an embryotoxic effect in humans. Because of the lack of clinical and epidemiological studies it is impossible to advance any firm recommendations for the correct use of NSAID during the first 6 months of pregnancy. However, the possibility of unrecognized dysmorphogenic effects of NSAID needs to be considered before prescribing, so it would seem wise to use compounds with short elimination half-lives and to administer them at the longest possible dosage intervals. When NSAID are used for dysmenorrhea, it is wise to delay giving them until menstruation has actually started, so as to avoid administration during an unrecognized pregnancy; therapeutically there is no need to give them earlier. There is now no doubt about the ability of NSAID to alter fetal physiology in the last trimester of pregnancy, as well as to prolong gestation and labor, and they should therefore not be used at this time (SEDA-5, 101; SEDA-6, 93; SEDA-7, 108; SEDA-8, 102; SEDA-9, 88; SEDA-11, 88; SEDA-12, 84; SEDA-15, 99).

The ingestion of NSAID during breast feeding seems to present fewer problems. In fact, the newer NSAID are all secreted into milk, but in amounts that are probably too small to affect the breast-fed infant. However, serious side effects in breast-fed children have been described with pyrazolones and indometacin (SEDA-10, 78). Therefore the choice of an NSAID, if its use is strictly indispensable, should be directed to compounds which have a short half-life, and in order to reduce the quantity of drug reaching the child, the drug should be taken by the mother at the time of breast feeding or immediately thereafter, so that the next feed occurs after a time period equivalent to the half-life of the drug.

Cardiovascular *(SEDA-13, 72)* All NSAID, and indometacin in particular, interfere with the control of hypertension in patients receiving diuretics, β-blockers or ACE inhibitors, though no rigorous experimental studies of the effect have been performed (83[R]). Some antihypertensive drugs, particularly diuretics and ACE inhibitors depend, in part, on stimulation of renal prostaglandins for their effect. There is controversy as to whether the relative selectivity of sulindac in normal doses may be an advantage in this situation. A recent meta-analytic trial has shown that certain NSAID (sulindac and aspirin) have a less hypertensive effect than others and that piroxicam exerts the most marked effect (84). Moreover NSAID interact diversely with different antihypertensive drugs; NSAID antagonize the effect of β-blockers and ACE-inhibitors more than that of calcium channel blockers, diuretics and centrally acting α-agonists (85, 86). Among ACE-inhibitors, perindopril has been shown to be efficacious to reduce blood pressure in patients on NSAID-treatment (87).

NSAID may have serious consequences in individuals at risk for cardiovascular insufficiency since they may cause water retention. Hypertension can be aggravated, or the effects of antihypertensive drugs countered, and edema can occur. Van de Ouweland et al. identified 27 cases where there was a possible, or probable, link between NSAID and this condition in 600 elderly patients with documented congestive cardiac failure (88[C]). In some, the mechanism was apparently a decrease in the effect of furosemide treatment, in others it may have been an NSAID-induced imbalance of circulatory homeostasis. Pre-existing renal impairment was not observed in any of the 27 cases identified. This study suggests that *congestive heart failure* may be a complication of NSAID treatment in the elderly.

Respiratory As between 2 and 20% of adult asthmatics exhibit hypersensitivity to aspirin (89[R]), they too must be considered at risk from NSAID. The proposed mechanism is a deficiency in bronchodilator prostaglandins; inhibition of prostaglandins may divert arachidonic acid to produce more leukotrienes, which have bronchoconstrictor activity. Oral challenge to detect aspirin sensitivity in asthmatic patients is an effective but potentially dangerous method for establishing the presence of sensitivity in these patients (90). Occasionally *bronchospasm* may be part of an anaphylactoid reaction to NSAID; zomepirac was withdrawn for this reason. There is an intriguing report that bee-keepers may be at increased risk for severe reactions from bee stings if they are taking NSAID and it has been suggested that the drugs should be prescribed with particular caution for such individuals (91[C]).

Nervous system NSAID cause *headaches* and *confusion* in a relatively small number of recipients. Headache and *dizziness* are reported commonly with indometacin. More severe reactions, including *depersonalization, confusion and paranoia*, have also been reported. It has been suggested that indometacin's chemical similarity to serotonin, an important central neurotransmitter that can cause severe headaches, may be responsible (92[R]).

NSAID should probably be included as one of the many groups of drugs that can cause confusion in elderly subjects. However cognitive function in elderly ambulatory patients was assessed in a recent large retrospective study by a questionnaire and there were no significant differences in the total scores of users and non-users of NSAID (SEDA-17, 106). Moreover another study shows that performance on tests of sensorimotor coordination and short-term memory may improve in healthy elderly volunteers treated with indometacin (93). Some rarer side-effects, such as aseptic meningitis, have been reported with ibuprofen, sulindac and tolmetin (92[R]) in patients with systemic lupus erythematosus.

Interactions The wide use of NSAID, particularly in the elderly, who often take other drugs at the same time, leads to a high risk for clinically significant drug interactions, both pharmacokinetic (already described) and pharmacodynamic. The inhibitory action of phenylbutazone, oxyphenbutazone and azapropazone on the metabolism of other drugs, such as *oral anticoagulants, oral hypoglycemic agents or phenytoin*, is an example of the former mechanism. Other NSAID may inhibit the renal excretion of *lithium* (toxicity is less likely with sulindac, ibuprofen, aspirin) and *methotrexate* (increased toxicity). The second mechanism is exemplified by the interactions between indometacin and other NSAID, except perhaps sulindac, with antihypertensive agents including β-blockers, diuretics and ACE inhibitors. The interactions of NSAID with other drugs recently reviewed by Tonkin and Wing (94[R]) are summarized in Tables 1 and 2.

With respect to interaction between methotrexate and NSAID, a recent paper shows that in contrast to other NSAID such as ibuprofen and salicylates, in clinically relevant doses ketoprofen, flurbiprofen or piroxicam do not appear to affect methotrexate disposition (95).

Two reports that describe neurological adverse effects (dizziness, ambulatory instability and ataxic symptoms) in patients treated with misoprostol and NSAID require confirmation (SEDA-16, 108).

The relevance of interaction between NSAID and cyclosporin is still controversial. An interaction resulting in additive deterioration of renal function has been documented in patients taking cyclosporin together with various NSAID, as reviewed in SEDA-17, 107. The mechanism of this interaction is still uncertain, but may involve the production of prostaglandins and the known effects of NSAID on cyclooxygenase suggests an additive effect in the kidney. The concomitant use of NSAID and cyclosporine requires caution; in fact sulindac, which may be less likely toxic for renal function, may cause an increase of whole blood cyclosporin concentrations by inhibiting hepatic cytochrome P450 (SEDA-17, 107).

INDIVIDUAL NON-STEROIDAL ANTI-INFLAMMATORY DRUGS AND CLASSES

In discussing the extent to which various non-steroidal anti-inflammatory drugs deviate from the general adverse reaction pattern discussed above, it is possible to consider them according to the chemical groups to which they belong. However within these groups some further variations in effect are possible.

In the presentation of the more important anti-inflammatory agents which follows, a grouping according to chemical structure has been adopted. The antipyretic analgesics, including aspirin and its derivatives, are discussed in Chapter 9.1; their segregation from other NSAID is artificial, merely reflecting their primary use in pain relief.

PHENYLBUTAZONE AND RELATED COMPOUNDS

This group of NSAID is characterized by a considerable incidence of side effects which are sometimes very se-

Table 1. *Pharmacokinetic interactions with NSAID*

Drug affected	NSAID implicated	Effect	Approach to management
NSAID affecting other drugs			
Oral anticoagulants	Phenylbutazone Oxyphenbutazone Azapropazone	Inhibition of metabolism of S-warfarin, increasing anticoagulant effect	Avoid NSAID if possible. Careful monitoring where unavoidable (note pharmacodynamic interactions also)
Lithium	Probably all NSAID (? except sulindac, aspirin)	Inhibition of renal excretion of lithium, increasing lithium serum concentrations and increasing risk of toxicity	Use sulindac, aspirin if NSAID unavoidable. Careful monitoring of lithium concentration and appropriate dose reduction
Oral hypoglycemic agents	Phenylbutazone Oxyphenbutazone Azapropazone	Inhibition of metabolism of sulfonylurea drugs, prolonging halflife and increasing risk of hypoglycemia	Avoid this group of NSAID if possible; if not, monitor blood sugar closely
Phenytoin	Phenylbutazone Oxyphenbutazone	Inhibition of metabolism of phenytoin, increasing plasma concentration and risk of toxicity	Avoid this group of NSAIDs if possible; if not, intensive therapeutic drug monitoring
	Other NSAID	Displacement of phenytoin from plasma protein, reducing total concentration for the same unbound (active) concentration	Careful interpretation of phenytoin total concentration; measurement of unbound concentration may be helpful
Methotrexate	Probably all NSAID	Reduced clearance of methotrexate (mechanism unclear) increasing plasma concentration and risk of severe toxicity	Simultaneous dosing is contraindicated. Use of NSAID between cycles of chemotherapy is probably safe
Sodium valproate	Aspirin	Inhibition of valproate metabolism increasing plasma concentration	Avoid aspirin; dose monitoring of plasma concentration if other NSAID used
Digoxin	All NSAID	Potential reduction in renal function (particularly in very young and very old) reducing digoxin clearance and increasing plasma concentration and risk of toxicity. (No interaction if renal function normal)	Avoid NSAID if possible, if not, frequent checks of digoxin plasma concentration and plasma creatinine
Aminoglycosides	All NSAID	Reduction in renal function in susceptible individuals, reducing aminoglycoside clearance and increasing plasma concentration	Close plasma concentration monitoring and dose adjustment
Other drugs affecting NSAID			
Antacids	Indometacin ? Other NSAID	Variable effects of different preparations: —aluminium-containing antacids reduce rate and extent of absorption of indometacin —sodium bicarbonate increases rate and extent of absorption of indometacin	No action required unless marked reduction in absorption results in poor response to NSAID; dose may need to be increased in this case
Probenecid	Probably all NSAID	Reduction in metabolism and renal clearance of NSAID and acyl glucuronide metabolites which are hydrolyzed back to parent drug	May be used therapeutically to increase the response to a given dose of NSAID
Barbiturates	Phenylbutazone ? Other NSAID	Increased metabolic clearance of NSAID	May require higher doses of phenylbutazone
Caffeine	Aspirin	Increased rate of absorption of aspirin	No action required
Cholestyramine	Naproxen and probably other NSAID	Anion exchange resin binds NSAID in gut reducing rate (? and extent) of absorption	Separate dosing times by 4 hours; may need higher than expected dose of NSAID
Metoclopramide	Aspirin	Increased rate and extent of absorption of aspirin in patients with migraine	May be used therapeutically

Reprinted from Tonkin and Wing (94[R]) by courtesy of the Editors of *Clinical Rheumatology*.

Table 2. *Pharmacodynamic interactions with NSAID*

Drug affected	NSAID implicated	Effect	Approach to management
NSAID affecting other drugs			
Antihypertensive agents β-Blockers Diuretics ACE inhibitors Vasodilators	Indometacin Other NSAID (? except sulindac)	Reduction in hypotensive effect, probably related to inhibition of renal prostaglandin synthesis (producing salt and water retention) and vascular prostaglandin synthesis (producing increased vasoconstriction)	Avoid all NSAID in treated hypertensive patients if possible; if not, use sulindac preferentially. May need additional antihypertensive therapy
Diuretics	Indometacin Other NSAID (? except sulindac)	Reduction in natriuretic and diuretic effects; may exacerbate congestive cardiac failure	Avoid NSAID in patients with cardiac failure; use sulindac; monitor clinical signs of fluid retention
Anticoagulants	All NSAID	Gastrointestinal tract mucosal damage, together with inhibition of platelet aggregation, increased risk of GI bleeding in patients on anticoagulants	Avoid all NSAID if possible
Hypoglycemic agents	Salicylate (high dose)	Potentiation of hypoglycemic effects (mechanism unknown)	Monitor blood sugar level
Combination with increased risk of toxicity			
Diuretics General	All NSAID	Combination associated with increased risk of hemodynamic renal failure	Avoid combination if possible
Triamterene	Indometacin	Potentiation of nephrotoxicity, including subjects with normal renal function	Combination contraindicated
Potassium-sparing	All NSAID	Potassium retention and hyperkalemia	Avoid combination; monitor K+

Reprinted from Tonkin and Wing (94[R]) by courtesy of the Editors of *Clinical Rheumatology*.

vere. It is possible that there are differences between the incidence and severity of adverse reactions of the individual compounds.

Phenylbutazone, considered as the founder of the family of modern NSAID and originally employed as a solubilizing agent for aminopyrine, was introduced for the treatment of rheumatoid arthritis and allied disorders in 1949. This group of compounds was used worldwide until the early 1980s when, following increasing expressions of concern as to their safety, Ciba-Geigy published its own international assessment on phenylbutazone (Butazolidine) and oxyphenbutazone (Tanderil), which summarized reports on 1182 deaths associated with the use of these drugs from their introduction up to 1982 (SEDA-9, 85). The report showed that the percentage of serious unwanted effects was high for both phenylbutazone and oxyphenbutazone, and that in both cases the most frequent of these serious problems were dermatological and hematological, closely followed by gastrointestinal disorders. Phenylbutazone and oxyphenbutazone have been removed from the market by regulatory agencies in many countries or limited to prescribing for highly specific purposes since late in 1983. In 1985, Ciba-Geigy decided to stop sales of systemic dosage forms of oxyphenbutazone on a worldwide basis and to reduce further the indications for phenylbutazone (SEDA-9, 85; SEDA-10, 78).

Poisoning *(SEDA-9, 85)* Although the clinical picture of severe poisoning is similar for all these compounds, the intensity of the effect on target organs is different. Aminopyrine, propyphenazone and dipyrone mainly affect the central nervous system (coma, convulsions), followed by the liver. Oxyphenbutazone and phenylbutazone cause liver damage only. Loss of consciousness is rare with dipyrone, but abdominal symptoms are common. Fatal intoxication has occurred in infants after doses of aminopyrine as low as 0.5 g.

Phenylbutazone *(SEDA-10, 78)*

Despite the fact that it has largely been taken out of production, phenylbutazone from various sources is still to be found in many places; it still merits discussion here because of the degree of risk which it presents, for phenylbutazone is a dangerous drug. It should be used only when less toxic alternatives are unavailable.

Phenylbutazone and its congeners are now used only for ankylosing spondylitis and, possibly, for acute gout, psoriatic arthritis, and active rheumatoid arthritis in patients who have not responded to other therapy, including other NSAID. All fixed combinations containing butazone derivatives and a corticosteroid have been removed from the market even in Germany, one of the most lenient countries in the regulation of phenylbutazone use. For other indications, less toxic alternatives suffice (96, 97).

Significant side effects can affect up to 40% of patients (98[r]) and do not often correlate with the dose.

ADVERSE REACTION PATTERN

General and toxic reactions These affect mainly the gastrointestinal system and include symptoms ranging from irritation to ulcer perforation and bleeding. Salt and water retention leads to edema, which is undesirable in older patients, and even to congestive heart failure. Hematological side effects include blood dyscrasias, lymphadenopathy and agranulocytosis. Hepatotoxicity and nephrotoxicity occur (99[C]). Headache is common; other CNS effects are mild. Acute poisoning can be successfully treated by column hemoperfusion (100[C]).

Hypersensitivity reactions can be very severe (101[C]); asthma and systemic lupus erythematosus are recognized problems.

Tumor-inducing effects have not been reported.

ORGANS AND SYSTEMS

Cardiovascular effects due to salt and water retention (see below) are especially dangerous for patients with impaired cardiac function. *Hypertension* due to increased plasma volume readily occurs.

Respiratory Failure of the left ventricle can result in effusions into thoracic cavities. *Asthma* can be provoked. Cross-reactivity with aspirin has been noted (102[C]). A picture resembling allergic alveolitis has been described (103[C])

Nervous system Therapeutic doses can be followed by *headache*, *dizziness* and *vertigo*. Overdoses may cause coma and convulsions. *Psychomotor reactions* related to driving have been reported (104[C]).

Endocrine, metabolic Due to interference with uptake of iodine, *hypothyroidism* and *goitre* can result. The condition is reversible, but an obstructive syndrome due to thyroid enlargement has been observed (105[C]).

Mineral and fluid balance As many as 10% of patients show signs of *salt and fluid retention* and *edema* (101[C]). Increased intravascular fluid volume is responsible for both dilution anemia and increasing cardiac load (SED-8, 216). There is still no explanation for the water retaining effect, which might however reflect increased production of the antidiuretic hormone.

Hematological Phenylbutazone causes many *blood dyscrasias*, some fatal (SED-8, 213; SEDA-2, 92; 101[C], 106[C]). The most serious side effect of phenylbutazone is *aplastic anemia*, which according to Swedish and British sources ends fatally in almost 50% of cases (106[c], 107[R], 108[R]). More than 1100 fatalities from this cause are on record with the principal manufacturer (SEDA-8, Essay).

Specific anti-platelet antibodies can cause *thrombocytopenia* with purpura (109[C]), which can prove fatal. The higher risk of *leukemia* after phenylbutazone administration could be due to the depressed bone marrow acting as a predisposing factor (SED-9, 143; 110[C]).

Liver Phenylbutazone's hepatotoxicity has been clearly documented (111[CR]). The drug probably causes three types of liver damage through three separate pathogenic mechanisms: (a) acute hepatic necrosis, found in overdosage and related to the hepatotoxicity of phenylbutazone and/or its metabolites; (b) mild hepatotoxicity (with or without cholestasis) and granulomas (sometimes also found at extrahepatic sites, with varying degrees of steatosis)—these changes are the result of hypersensitivity, possibly with a certain degree of toxic effect; (c) more pronounced hepatic cellular damage with cholestasis but without granulomas; here the toxic effects play a more important role than hypersensitivity. Concomitant treatment with other hepatotoxic agents may be a predisposing factor for phenylbutazone-induced liver toxicity.

Gastrointestinal Phenylbutazone is a potent gastric and intestinal irritant, which may provoke *ulcers* and *bleeding*. In one study conducted in 1975, at which time the drug was very prominent, 18.7% of 241 cases with acute gastrointestinal bleeding were due to phenylbutazone (112[C]). According to the British Committee on Safety of Medicines, 120 of 1967 adverse reactions attributed to phenylbutazone and its metabolite, oxyphenbutazone, involved gastrointestinal bleeding; of these, 32 ended fatally (113[R]). The risk of developing a peptic ulcer during phenylbutazone therapy is estimated at 1—3% (SED-8, 214). Perforation has also been repeatedly observed (112[C], 114[C]). Other side effects are *nausea*, *vomiting*, *abdominal pain*, *heartburn*, *diarrhea* and *abdominal discomfort*. Even rectal administration and enteric-coated preparations can induce adverse reactions in the upper gastrointestinal tract. In addition, phenylbutazone suppositories can cause *rectal irritation* with mucosal defects, severe *hemorrhagic proctitis* (115[C]), *perforation of the large bowel* and *necrotizing colitis* (116[C]).

Urinary system Although as pointed out in the general section above that renal effects can occur with any NSAID (i.e. also with phenylbutazone), it should be noted that phenylbutazone nephrotoxicity has mainly been reported when the drug was taken in association with other anti-inflammatory drugs (SED-8, 215) or given alone at a high dose (117[R]).

Skin and appendages *Dermal eruptions*, *Quincke's edema* and even *epidermal necrolysis* (SEDA-5, 100; 118[C], 119[R]) can develop during or after phenylbutazone therapy.

Special senses Phenylbutazone can damage the *eyes*. Conjunctivitis, damage to the cornea with vascularization and scarring, adhesion of the lids to the eyeballs, amblyopia, retinal hemorrhage and even blindness have been reported (120[R]).

Local irritation Considerable local irritation and pain at the site of injection are sometimes followed by necrosis. Sterile abscess formation has also been reported (121[C]).

Miscellaneous effects Phenylbutazone infusion for 10 days has induced chromosomal aberrations in rheumatic patients (122[C]), although the significance of this finding is not clear.

Risk situations The risk of adverse drug reactions with phenylbutazone in general increases with *age* (SED-8, 213; 108[R]). The special risks of salt and water retention in *cardiac and renal disease* have already been mentioned. The potential for ulcerogenic activity should be borne in mind if the drug is given to a patient with a *history of ulcer*. Patients *hypersensitive to other drugs* (especially aspirin) should be carefully monitored when taking phenylbutazone.

Second-generation effects There is no evidence that phenylbutazone injures the fetus. If taken during lactation, only small amounts are found in the milk.

Overdosage Acute intoxication with phenylbutazone is dominated by metabolic acidosis, which can progress to coma, seizures, hypotension, shock and oliguria. Kidney and liver reactions, acute bone marrow depression and acute perforation of peptic ulcer have been described (99[C], 122[c], 124[c]).

Interactions What was said in the general section on interactions resulting from protein displacement also applies to phenylbutazone. There is not only a biphasic interaction with *coumarin anticoagulants*; interactions with *sulfonamides*, *oral antidiabetics* and *diphenylhydantoin* have also been described (SED-9, 144; 124[c], 125[c]). Another mechanism of interaction is interference with tubular excretion (*penicillins*, *oral antidiabetics*, *aspirin*) (98[r]). A third mechanism involves the induction of microsomal liver enzymes, resulting in accelerated metabolism of some drugs; which drugs are affected probably depends on their stereochemical structure. Inhibition of the effect of *antihypertensive agents* can probably be explained by the retention of salt and water provoked by phenylbutazone (126[C]). The possibility that an interaction may occur with certain drugs through more than one mechanism must always be borne in mind.

Interference with diagnostic routines Phenylbutazone inhibits the thyroid uptake of iodine and/or competes for protein-binding sites with thyroxine (SED-9, 145), and may thus disrupt the diagnosis of thyroid disorders.

PHENYLBUTAZONE-RELATED COMPOUNDS AND VARIANTS

In some countries many phenylbutazone derivatives are still on the market and until a well-controlled comparative clinical study has proved the opposite, it must be assumed that adverse reactions to all these agents are very similar; numerous individual case-reports also suggest strongly that this is the case. One should be aware of this fact, since a number of these agents have been claimed to be better tolerated, often after only limited experience.

Butacote

Butacote is enteric-coated phenylbutazone, but it produces no less gastrointestinal irritation. One comparative double-blind cross-over trial showed that plain naproxen caused fewer gastrointestinal side effects than Butacote (127[C]).

Oxyphenbutazone

Oxyphenbutazone, already referred to above, is a *p*-hydroxy analog of phenylbutazone and one of the active metabolites of the parent drug. In April 1985, Ciba-Geigy decided to stop sales of systemic dosage forms of oxyphenbutazone on a worldwide basis. The company stated they had reached this decision because a survey had shown that although the recommended limitations on use published for phenylbutazone had been respected to a high degree, this had not been the case with oxyphenbutazone. There was evidence that oxyphenbutazone was more likely to cause death due to bone marrow failure than phenylbutazone (128), as reported on data from the UK Committee on Safety of Medicines. Furthermore, according to Ciba-Geigy's reassessment of phenylbutazone and oxyphenbutazone (January, 1984), oxyphenbutazone with 5.5 (USA) to 12.8 (UK) deaths/million prescriptions appears to be more dangerous than phenylbutazone with 3.8–7.6 deaths/million prescriptions (SEDA-9, 87). Oxyphenbutazone has the same spectrum of activity, therapeutic uses, interactions, dangers and contraindications for clinical use.

Ketophenylbutazone (kebuzone)

Allergic reactions, gastrotoxicity, nephrotoxicity, local reaction with necrosis and liver damage have been reported (SED-11, 176). The Japanese authorities have requested that the package insert should indicate that this drug must be used only as a drug of last resort when other anti-inflammatory agents and uricosurics are ineffective (SEDA-12, 83).

Monophenylbutazone

Adverse reactions similar to those of the parent drug, including dermal reactions (even epidermal necrolysis), gastrotoxicity, hepatotoxicity, nephrotoxicity, edema, headache and hematological side effects (SED-9, 145), have been described.

Azapropazone

Among the drugs of this family, azapropazone deserves particular mention. It is structurally related to phenylbutazone and probably shares the same side effects: gastrotoxicity, skin reactions, headache, vertigo, edema and renal impairment. A review of a very large series described azapropazone side effects in 1724 patients (17.6%) and they were the cause of withdrawal in 3.7%. Surprisingly, however, no phenylbutazone-type blood dyscrasia was observed in this series (SED-11, 176). Hemolytic anemia has been reported in the literature, as well as to the UK Committee on Safety of Medicines (SEDA-10, 79; SEDA-12, 83). More recently, a high percentage of patients taking azapropazone have proved positive to the direct Coombs' test. However, there was no evidence that the positive reaction persisted after treatment had been stopped for several weeks (SEDA-12, 83). Hemolytic anemia has also been described in combination with pulmonary alveolitis, which suggests an allergic or immune reaction to the drug (129[C]). Photosensitivity is a frequently reported side effect of azapropazone; in 1985, 190 reports of photosensitivity were submitted to several national drug-monitoring centres in Europe (SEDA-10, 79; SEDA-12, 83). The reaction is more frequent with azapropazone than with almost any other NSAID.

Azapropazone has the same pattern of interactions with oral anticoagulants (SEDA-2, 98), tolbutamide (130[C]) and phenytoin (131[C], 132[C]) as phenylbutazone. Because of increases in the unbound drug and reduced clearance in renal insufficiency, the dose should be carefully adjusted in patients with liver or renal disease (SEDA-11, 92).

Suxibuzone

Skin reactions, gastrotoxicity, nephrotoxicity, headache and vertigo have been noted. The carcinogenic potential of suxibuzone in animals has attracted attention (133[r]) and has apparently put an end to its career in certain countries.

Feprazone

Skin reactions including severe bullous dermatosis (SEDA-9, 87), gastrotoxicity, nephrotoxicity and edema, as well as headache, tinnitus and depression, have been described (134[C]). Thrombocytopenia and immune complex-mediated hemolytic anemia have been reported (SEDA-7, 108). In an 8-week trial on 2693 patients with rheumatoid arthritis and osteoarthritis, 30% reported side effects and 11% failed to complete the study. Feprazone was withdrawn in the United Kingdom due to its adverse drug reaction resemblance to phenylbutazone and high prescription rates. The fact that two large, but short-term, general practice multicenter studies in Italy on 11 000 patients reported a very low percentage (1.2–9.8%) of side effects (135, 136) casts doubts on the reliability on such studies.

Feprazone has been designated as a last-resort drug by the Japanese Committee on Safety of Drugs (SEDA-12, 83). Contact dermatitis has been recently described with feprazone cream (SEDA-18, 101).

Trimethazone

The usual side effects of this group have been encountered (gastric effects, fluid retention, headache) (SED-9, 145).

Pipebuzone

The curious idea of combining phenylbutazone chemically with piperazine to improve the tolerance of the latter seems to have proved unsuccessful. The frequent occurrence of typical phenylbutazone reactions (abdominal, hematological, renal and allergic, as well as rectal irritation by suppositories) has been reported (SED-9, 145).

Bumadizone

In a study on 647 patients, about 15% experienced side effects (gastrointestinal, fluid retention and hypersensitivity). Treatment was stopped in 7% for this reason (137[C]).

Pyrazine-butazone *(SEDA-12, 83; SEDA-15, 107)*

Gastrointestinal toxicity has been reported in a patient treated short-term with this drug. Although agranulocytosis and liver injury have been associated with pyrazine-butazone, there is no evidence for an immunological mechanism.

PYRAZOLONE DERIVATIVES—ANTIPYRINE AND RELATED COMPOUNDS

Antipyrine (phenazone)

Antipyrine is still employed therapeutically in some countries, though the substance is in fact now used predominantly as a marker of hepatic enzyme drug metabolizing activity. The fact that it is usually taken in combination with other analgesics, and that it is an old compound with little recent investigation makes an exact analysis of its side effects impossible. Antipyrine seems to have a low toxicity index, which corresponds with its weak anti-inflammatory effect. Allergic reactions are very rare (SEDA-6, 92; SEDA-14, 92; SEDA-16, 108), but subjects undergoing the antipyrine test should be informed of the potential risk.

Hematological Until recently, the only hematological side effect known was hemolysis in patients with glucose-6-phosphate dehydrogenase deficiency. An immediate reaction after a single test dose in the form of a latent leukopenic reaction has later been reported (138[C]). Previous sensitization to pyrazolone derivatives was the most probable explanation. More recently agranulocytosis has been reported in six women after the use of a phenazone-containing cream (SEDA-18, 101).

Gastrointestinal Only chronic abuse of antipyrine, probably together with other more aggressive antipyretics, can cause gastric symptoms (139[C]).

Urinary system The nephrotoxicity of antipyrine is well established, but information is limited. Experimental papillary necrosis can easily be provoked; analgesic nephropathy, described earlier, is probably a real danger with antipyrine, especially when it is combined with a stronger prostaglandin inhibitor. The effect is probably toxic since inhibition of prostaglandins is not a marked characteristic of antipyrine. Two reports have suggested a causal link between antipyrine and renal carcinoma such as is well known for phenacetin (140[C], 141[C]), but this has not been confirmed.

Skin Urticarial rashes and erythema are the most common effects, followed by maculopapular eruptions, erythema multiforme, erythema nodosum or even angioneurotic edema (119[R]).

Second-generation effects In spite of the fact that antipyrine easily crosses the placenta, no injury to the fetus has been reported.

Dichloralphenazine

The complexing of antipyrine and chloral hydrate, which dissociates in aqueous solution, is irrational; one must expect the drug to cause the side effects characteristic of its components.

Isopropylantipyrine (propyphenazone)

There are still no indications that isopropylantipyrine really has a lower incidence of side effects than antipyrine as was originally supposed, since neither compound has been widely studied alone. Isopropylantipyrine is one of the most widely used among pyrazolone derivatives, as it is incorporated into numerous over-the-counter analgesics combinations in many countries. Serious generalized urticaria with angioneurotic edema has occurred after ingestion (142[C]). Rechallenge with oral isopropylantipyrine caused a severe anaphylactic reaction in a patient with a negative skin test. Although the case report concerned stresses the importance of oral challenge, it also draws attention to the risk of such a procedure (SEDA-12, 83). Severe hypersensitivity reactions have also been reported more recently (SEDA-16, 108).

Pirazolac *(SEDA-16, 111)*

In basic clinical studies this pyrazoloacetic derivative caused heartburn, upper abdominal pain, and cutaneous side effects (skin eruptions, exacerbation of pre-existing eczema) and eosinophilia in early clinical studies (143[C]). In two comparative studies withdrawal of pirazolac occurred in 15—20% of patients and was more frequent than with the comparative NSAID (indometacin, sulindac) (SEDA-16, 111).

AMIDOPYRINE AND RELATED COMPOUNDS

Amidopyrine (aminophenazone, pyramidone, aminopyrine) *(SEDA-12, 82)*

Amidopyrine is the most toxic and most dangerous of the anti-inflammatory analgesics. Blood dyscrasias not correlated with the dose have been documented beyond any doubt, which suggests a hypersensitivity mechanism.

The hope expressed in an earlier volume that amidopyrine would disappear from the market has yet not been fulfilled. Third World countries are in particular danger (144[C]), and the drug is still very widely produced and used in the Eastern countries; it has however been withdrawn in most developed countries. The Committee on the Safety of Drugs of the Japanese Pharmaceutical Affairs Bureau has recently issued a notification ordering the withdrawal of this drug due to its association with serious side effects, such as hematological disorders (SEDA-12, 82).

Hematological Amidopyrine causes severe bone marrow depression, usually with a fulminant course and high mortality (SED-9, 146). Specific antibodies and leukoagglutinins are sometimes found (145[C]). Agranulocytosis is caused by arrest of maturation at the metamyelocyte stage (146[R]).

Other allergic reactions A variety of allergic skin reactions, acute anaphylactic shock and (in predisposed patients), acute bronchospasm, as well as cross-sensitivity to aspirin, have been reported (147[C]).

Skin Toxic epidermal necrolysis, exfoliative dermatitis and Stevens-Johnson syndrome have been described (SED-8, 210).

Gastrointestinal The gastrotoxicity of amidopyrine is lower than that of other analgesic/anti-inflammatory drugs, probably merely reflecting a lesser anti-inflammatory effect.

Liver Amidopyrine is not hepatotoxic, but liver damage can occur in the course of a general hypersensitivity reaction (148[C]).

Urinary system Since albuminuria, hematuria and acute renal failure have been observed, direct renal damage can follow amidopyrine intake, even in therapeutic doses. A contribution by amidopyrine to analgesic nephropathy is also possible (SED-8, 211).

Tumor-inducing activity Amidopyrine and its derivatives may be metabolized to carcinogenic nitrosamines. The clinical importance of this is not clear (SEDA-2, 389; 149[r]).

Dipyrone (metamizole, noramidopyrine, noraminosulfon, noramidopyrine methanesulfonate) *(SEDA-11, 31; SEDA-12, 83; SEDA-13, 78)*

Phenyldimethylaminophenazone and noramidopyrine are the main derivatives of amidopyrine and it is justifiable to expect that they will provoke the same adverse reactions as amidopyrine itself. Although there is firm evidence to this effect, it has been contested (see 'General Considerations'). Dipyrone, no doubt because of its vast turnover, continues to be attacked and defended with remarkable vigor. One finds on the one hand two extremely critical papers by Offerhaus on the International 'Agranulocytosis Study' (49) and, on the other hand one paper by Levi and Shapiro in which they strongly defend the study (150[R], 151[R]). At the same time, an analysis of all reports on blood disorders attributed to NSAID and submitted to the Finnish National Board of Health during the period 1973—1985 showed that dipyrone was suspected of causing 14 cases of agranulocytosis (three fatal), other pyrazolones four cases, indometacin two cases and ibuprofen one case (152). Dipyrone is still widely prescribed, and commonly also sold as a headache remedy on the open market, in some developing countries, but has been withdrawn from the market in many other parts of the world; in some Western countries it still curiously enjoys a reputation as an injectable product for the relief of renal colic, whereas in other countries it is entirely unknown and apparently not missed. Although the compound is of German origin, the German authorities decided in 1987 to subject all dipyrone products to prescription-only regulations. This measure should be a clear message to the regulatory authorities in other countries where the drug is used without prescription (SEDA-12, 82). According to the Japanese authorities, suppositories and injectable preparations should be used only as last resort drugs, and warnings against shock should be included in the package insert (SEDA-12, 83).

The absolute measure of risk of blood dyscrasias connected with its use is not known (153[R]), but it seems to be unacceptably high. Hemolysis has also been reported (154[Cr]), possibly due to absorption of the drug-antibody immune complexes by the cell membrane. Nephrotoxicity from dipyrone is rare (SEDA-17, 108). Fluid and salt retention have been observed in small children taking dipyrone (155[C]). In an occasional case, intravenous injection of dipyrone seems to cause arterial hypotension (156[C]). Dipyrone was the single most commonly used agent producing adverse drug reaction (mainly hypersensitivity reactions and also anaphylactic shock and two deaths) in a study from India based on reports to an adverse drug reaction monitoring center by general practitioners (SEDA-16, 108).

Sulfenazone

Sulfenazone, a pyrazolone derivative, causes benign intracranial hypertension in children (SEDA-5, 100; 157[C]).

Diftalone

Because of the hepatotoxicity and carcinogenicity (hepatoma) detected in preclinical studies, as well as verified hematotoxicity and gastrointestinal side effects in man, diftalone has been withdrawn by its manufacturer (158).

INDOMETACIN AND RELATED COMPOUNDS

Indometacin (Indocid)

Indometacin is one of the most effective NSAID. As pointed out in the introductory section of this chapter, the majority of its toxic and therapeutic effects are probably due to marked prostaglandin inhibition.

Indometacin is the best known and most thoroughly tested of the indoleacetic acid derivatives. Because of its potency its clinical efficacy is comparable, if not superior, to that of other NSAID, but for precisely the same reason the side effects which attach to this potency—notably involving the gastrointestinal tract and the nervous system—unavoidably limit its use. Patients who do find that they tolerate the drug reasonably well are naturally not anxious to exchange it for any more recent drug with fewer problems but also less potency; a meta-analysis of patients' preference in 37 cross-over trials that compared indometacin with newer NSAID, failed to provide any evidence of a trend for newer NSAID to replace indometacin (159[c]).

ADVERSE REACTION PATTERN

General and toxic reactions Side effects, which involve up to 60% of patients, are closely correlated with the strong anti-inflammatory potency of indometacin. Gastric irritation, including ulcers, bleeding and perforation, predominate. CNS complications are related to cerebral edema. Headache is common. Hematological effects are reported, but are infrequent. Nephrotoxicity is important in pre-existing renal impairment. Ocular toxicity may follow long-term use.

Hypersensitivity reactions Cross-reactivity with aspirin has been reported (160[C]). The hazards of administering topical indometacin to asthmatic patients should be widely known (161[C]).

Tumor-inducing effects have not been demonstrated.

ORGANS AND SYSTEMS

Cardiovascular Clinical experience and the literature provide little evidence that indometacin as a general phenomenon precipitates angina or myocardial infarction. However, an individual angina-provoking effect has been documented (162[C]), and there are reasons to accept that it can happen; certainly, intravenous administration of indometacin increases systemic arterial blood pressure, coronary vascular resistance and myocardial oxygen demands, thereby decreasing coronary flow. A controlled short-term study showed that indometacin increased the blood pressure in patients with mild untreated essential hypertension (SEDA-17, 108). Unlike other NSAID, indometacin also acts as a vasoconstrictor of the cerebral circulation. Cerebral flow is decreased by up to 35% and the cerebral blood flow response to hypercapnia is abolished (SEDA-10, 79). The drug also diminishes blood flow in the splanchnic vascular bed by increasing local vascular resistance, but it does not impair circulation in the forearm and leg muscles. Intravenous administration of indometacin increases systemic arterial blood pressure, especially when given at a high intravenous infusion rate. In view of the increasing use of parenteral administration, the *acute hemodynamic effects* induced by indometacin may now tend to occur more often, especially in the elderly (163[Cr]). The mechanism of indometacin's action on blood flow is poorly understood; it apparently exerts a direct action on the resistance vessels of various regions, which is probably independent of its action on prostaglandin formation. The clinical relevance of this is largely unknown, but it seems wise to prefer other NSAID when treating patients with occlusive vascular diseases that affect the cerebral and/or coronary circulation. Other cardiovascular systemic side effects are due to salt and fluid retention and also to a reduction in the vasodilator action of circulating prostaglandins E_2 and I_2 (164).

Respiratory Prostaglandin inhibition also explains the drug's ability to *provoke or aggravate asthma* in hypersensitive patients (165[R]). There is one entirely credible report that indometacin in ophthalmic solution induced such a degree of deterioration in an asthmatic patient that mechanical ventilation was required (161[C]). Cross-sensitivity between indometacin and aspirin has been observed.

Nervous system Adverse reactions to indometacin involving the central nervous system are frequent and are second in importance only to the drug's gastrointestinal effects. They are attributed to salt and water retention. Up to 60% of patients experience *headache* (often migrainelike), *frontal throbbing* and *vertigo*. *Vomiting*, *tinnitus*, *ataxia*, *tremor*, *dizziness* and *insomnia* follow. *Somnolence*, *confusion* and, especially in the elderly, even *hallucinations* and *psychotic symptoms* have been described. *Coma*, *clonic seizures* and *myoclonic spasms* (SEDA-18, 101) can on occasion develop. Muscle weakness and paresthesias, i.e. *peripheral neuropathy*, may develop in elderly patients, but recede after the drug is withdrawn (166[C], 167[C]). Indometacin is used for non-invasive closure of symptomatic ductus arteriosus in the pre-term infant. Intravenous administration of indometacin causes an instantaneous decrease in cerebral blood flow, thus increasing cerebral vascular resistance. The clinical significance for the nervous system of these hemodynamic changes is unknown (168[C], 169[C]), but they seem to tie up logically with the nervous effects observed (see above). Advantage has been taken of this effect for reducing intracranial hypertension in patients with severe head injury (SEDA-15, 99).

Endocrine, metabolic Indometacin reduces the area under the corticotropin (ACTH) plasma concentration-time curves after insulin in normal males, possibly due to prostaglandin's role in the control of ACTH secretion (170). One report describes low plasma ascorbic acid levels during indometacin treatment, and there is a published case of hyperglycemia (171[c]).

Mineral and fluid balance As mentioned above, *salt and fluid retention* is an adverse effect of indometacin, though it is less important than with the pyrazolone derivatives. The effect can antagonize antihypertensive agents including, β-adrenoreceptor antagonists (172[C], 173[C]). The effect on blood pressure in normotensive patients has not been adequately studied. Severe water intoxication caused by inappropriate ADH secretion has been described in an elderly woman treated with indometacin (SEDA-17, 108).

Hyperkalemia has been reported in patients with preexisting renal disease treated with indometacin (SEDA-4, 65; SEDA-5, 90; SEDA-6, 93) and in a patient with Bartter's syndrome receiving concomitant treatment with oral potassium chloride (SEDA-11, 92). More recently, the use of indometacin caused serum potassium to rise to high levels in a young athlete (SEDA-14, 93).

Hematological *Anemia* due to repetitive gastrointestinal bleeding is a relatively frequent, although indirect, hematological side effect. Blood dyscrasias are seen and *aplastic anemia*, sometimes fatal (174[r]), isolated *granulocytopenia* and *agranulocytosis* have been reported (175[R]). Indometacin was found to be significantly associated with agranulocytosis and aplastic anemia in the International Agranulocytosis and Aplastic Anemia study (49[C]) mentioned earlier in this chapter.

Since indometacin is a platelet-aggregation inhibitor, impairment of thrombocytic function is frequent, but thrombocytopenia is rare. Severe *clotting defects* due to platelet-aggregation inhibition in premature infants has been described (176[C]). Postoperative bleeding is significantly more frequent in indometacin-treated patients than in control subjects. Indometacin should probably not be used postoperatively in patients at increased risk of bleeding (SEDA-8, 103).

Liver In spite of reversible *changes in liver enzyme tests* (177[C]) and a fatal case of acute *hepatocellular necrosis*, which may have been related to indometacin, it is rarely hepatotoxic (178[C]). A recent report describes a case of indometacin-associated primarily *cholestatic* liver injury. The reaction was not severe and recovery was rapid and uneventful (179[C]).

Gastrointestinal *Gastrotoxicity* is the main side effect of indometacin. Gastrointestinal symptoms range from abdominal discomfort to ulcer penetration and perforation (180[C]). Studies by Shorrock et al. tend to support the phenomenon of gastric mucosal adaptation, which has been evoked to explain the relatively low incidence of serious side effects, rather than the acute gastric damage that frequently occurs in short-term studies. In fact, in healthy volunteers, indometacin produced acute gastro-duodenal damage in all cases, but despite continuing administration, endoscopic damage resolved in almost all. The author hypothesized that the severity of the mucosal damage depends on the reduction in mucosal blood flow (SEDA-16, 108; SEDA-17, 108). Perforation of colonic diverticuli has also been described (181[C]). Small bowel ulcerations with thickening of the bowel wall and stricture formation in the terminal ileum and the ileocecal junction have been described in a patient with rheumatoid arthritis on long-term indometacin therapy (SEDA-12, 84). This is one reason why prolonged courses of indometacin treatment should be avoided wherever possible, especially in elderly women.

The use of indometacin suppositories can be associated with rectal irritation, mucosal inflammation or necrosis with bleeding (182[C]). Suppositories do not cause fewer gastric lesions than the oral form of the drug (183). However, the local effect on the gastric mucosa is less important than the systemic one. 'Osmosin', an osmotic pump of indometacin containing potassium bicarbonate, was withdrawn due to a fair number of intestinal irritations, bleeding, perforation and probably even death. These side effects were most likely caused by the much higher local concentrations of indometacin and potassium in the lower part of the gastrointestinal tract produced with this form of administration, which in essence shifted the adverse reactions from the stomach to the intestine (SEDA-8, 103; 184).

Urinary system The most important aspects of the nephrotoxicity of this group of agents have been outlined in the general sections on NSAID above. Indometacin nephrotoxicity is rare in patients with normal renal function, but the drug may aggravate pre-existing renal impairment. Such an effect has been observed in patients with glomerulonephritis, nephrotic syndrome and systemic lupus erythematosus and cirrhosis complicated by ascites (SED-8, 219; SEDA-4, 65; SEDA-7, 108; SEDA-11, 85). The fact that severe but reversible loss of renal function in SLE patients has been reported in the absence of active renal disease suggests that mesangial contraction in the glomerulus could be responsible for a significant reduction in the capillary surface area available for filtration and hence a reduction in the glomerular filtration rate (185, 186). A significant reduction in the glomerular filtration rate and a concomitant drop in renal excretion of sodium and water has recently been demonstrated in patients with compensated cirrhosis without ascites treated with indometacin (SEDA-18, 101).

Two cases of probable indometacin-induced *renal papillary necrosis* have been described in patients with chronic juvenile arthritis (SEDA-8, 103). Reversible *acute renal failure* with eosinophilia has been described (187[C]).

During indometacin therapy, the urinary excretion of *zinc* and *calcium* may increase significantly (188). The clinical relevance of this is not known. Severe *hyperkalemia* was observed in a patient with Bartter's syndrome who was also receiving potassium supplements (189).

The deleterious effect of the drug on renal function has been used as a therapeutic tool to induce medical nephrectomy (SEDA-7, 108).

Skin Skin reactions range from urticaria and pruritus to fixed rashes, purpura and maculopapular, as well as morbilliform, eruptions. Toxic *epidermal necrolysis* has also been described (190[C]). The frequency of skin reactions is lower than that seen with pyrazolone derivatives. There is a cross-sensitivity with aspirin. Whether indometacin *exacerbates psoriasis* is not certain, but one report (191[C]) suggests that it can. Indometacin can also *exacerbate dermatitis herpetiformis* (SEDA-10, 81).

Special senses Prolonged therapy can cause a number of adverse reactions in the *eyes*. Trivial effects are ocular discomfort, conjunctival pain and ocular tension, but mydriasis, photophobia, blurred vision, diplopia, amblyopia and loss of vision may occur. The most serious complications are retinopathy with decreased retinal sensitivity and corneal and retinal pigmentation; they are reversible, but improvement is slow. A recent report on indometacin retinopathy has added more doubt than certainty to the question of the frequency and severity of the retinotoxicity of this drug (SEDA-14, 93). One would be well advised to heed the suggestion that patients undergoing prolonged therapy should be periodically monitored by ophthalmic examination.

Musculoskeletal system *Progressive destruction of large weight-bearing hip joints* was first observed during long-term indometacin therapy more than 20 years ago (SEDA-11, 87; 192[C]). One recent study, which compared the effects of azapropazone and indometacin on osteoarthritis, showed that the osteoarthritic process in the hip progressed more quickly in patients treated with the latter, no doubt a further reflection of its powerful inhibitory effect on prostaglandin synthesis (193[C]). The mechanisms that could be responsible for the deleterious effect of NSAID on osteoarthritic joints have already been noted in the general NSAID section of this chapter and are amply discussed in SEDA-11, 87.

Sexual function Inhibition of prostaglandin synthesis may be involved in the induction of *impotence*. A healthy man was found to be impotent while on short-term treatment with 150 mg indometacin daily (SEDA-5, 101).

Effects on immunoreactivity Masking of infection and alteration of immune reactions have been reported (194[C]). It is not clear whether this finding has any clinical significance.

Parenteral administration Intravenous administration (treatment of ureteral colic) is effective and well tolerated. However, in a trial on 90% of patients receiving slow (5 min) intravenous injection, hypertension, nausea, vertigo, vomiting, and peptic ulcer symptoms were documented (195). Intravenous administration should be avoided in patients with heart failure. Intramuscular indometacin induces few side effects at the site of injection (redness, pain, induration) (SEDA-8, 102) and seems to have better systemic tolerability than intravenous injection: 26% of 388 patients treated with 100 mg/day of indometacin developed a side effect (GI- or CNS-related) and 4.6% interrupted treatment (196[C]).

Risk situations As pointed out above, patients with *asthma* or *allergic rhinitis* can be hypersensitive to indometacin and may develop severe general allergic reactions, especially if they are allergic to aspirin. *Elderly patients* are prone to develop CNS side effects, including psychotic reactions. Gastrotoxicity is also more frequent in this patient group.

Indometacin should probably not be used postoperatively in patients with *increased risk of bleeding* (SEDA-8, 103), because of its anti-platelet activity.

Pharmacokinetic factors (slow metabolism) may underlie the pronounced effect of indometacin on platelet aggregation *in premature infants and small children*. The use of indometacin in children with patent ductus arteriosus (PDA) can be followed by a severe general reaction. Nephrotoxicity, abdominal distension, hemorrhagic enteritis and even necrotizing enterocolitis have been observed (SEDA-10, 81; 176, 197[C]). On the other hand, none of the retrospective studies performed has demonstrated that indometacin-treated infants have a higher incidence of retrolental hyperplasia or visual problems than infants treated otherwise (198[R]). Reopening of the ductus after indometacin-induced occlusion of patent ductus arteriosus has been described (SEDA-18, 101). The dangers of treatment of PDA by intravenous indometacin are few and compared with ligation it is more efficacious and safer.

It has recently been reported that in *athletes* in training for a marathon use of indometacin may prove dangerous since it may provoke hyperkalemia and the risk of serious arrhythmias (SEDA-14, 93).

Pregnant women taking β-blockers should not be prescribed indometacin as it may cause an increase in arterial blood pressure (199).

Second-generation effects It has been suggested that indometacin in pregnancy may be relatively safe provided its use is limited to the first 32 weeks of gestation. A possible teratogenic effect of indometacin has been described to the drug (200[C]).

The situation with respect to use in late pregnancy has been much debated, since by virtue of its ability to inhibit prostaglandin synthesis indometacin can be used to arrest premature labor for a short time, though there is no evidence that it reduces the incidence of premature delivery. The hazards of such use of indometacin as a tocolytic agent seem to outweigh any theoretical advantage, since there are a number of reports on serious adverse neonatal effects following treatment of preterm labor with indometacin; they include premature closure of the ductus arteriosus, pulmonary hypertension with persistent fetal circulation, fetal anuria, severe oligohydramnios, necrotizing enterocolitis, perinatal death, and severe respiratory distress syndrome resulting in oxygen dependence for several days (SED-11, 179; SEDA-5, 101; SEDA-6, 93; SEDA-7, 108; SEDA-8, 102; SEDA-9, 88; SEDA-12, 84; SEDA-15, 99; SEDA-16, 109; SEDA-17, 108). The risks might be linked to the duration of use, but one recent study provides evidence that even when given short-term, indometacin can cause closure of the ductus arteriosus, even if several weeks elapse between treatment and delivery (201[C]). The risks involved in longer-term use are multiple, as various studies show:

The use of indometacin and ibuprofen for longer than 72 hours in 67 women in pre-term labor was significantly associated with more ultrasound-recorded oligohydramnios than either ritodrine or magnesium sulfate treatment. Oligohydramnios developed in 70% of 37 women treated with indometacin, in 27% treated with ibuprofen and in two controls (202).

Cerebral ischemia has also recently been described in premature twins following use of the drug in the mother (203[C]).

The incidence and type of cerebral lesions were studied by ultrasound in 159 pre-term infants: 76 fetuses were exposed to indometacin, used as a tocolytic agent, and for the remaining 83 pregnancies, tocolysis was either not started or was limited to fenoterol. The incidence of periventricular leukomalacia was increased in infants exposed to any tocolytic agent; cystic lesions occurred more commonly in those exposed to indometacin (204[C]).

Oligohydramnios and renal dysgenesis developed in one identical twin exposed to early, prolonged high-dose indometacin. As indometacin has been shown to induce oligohydramnios and renal dysgenesis in fetal monkeys, it may also have induced the abnormalities in this patient (205[C]).

The topic 'Antenatal indometacin therapy' has been extensively reviewed in SEDA-18, 102. New data derived from a recent retrospective cohort study of 57 premature infants, born between the 24th and 30th weeks of gestation, whose mothers had been treated unsuccessfully with indometacin for preterm labor, confirmed several fetal and neonatal complications (206[C]R). However overall data in our possession on the topic give inconclusive or contradictory results on the risk/benefit ratio of the use of indometacin as a tocolytic agent or as treatment for hydramnios (SEDA-18, 102).

The situation regarding use during lactation is uncertain; convulsions occurring in a breast-fed infant have been linked with the fact that indometacin passes into the milk (207[C]).

Genital system Ovulation has been inhibited by indometacin at high doses in women in the preovulatory period (SEDA-16, 109).

Interactions Indometacin decreases the absorption of *aspirin*, potentiates the effect of *anti-platelet drugs and anticoagulants* and decreases the effect of *diuretics* (208[C]). Combination with Moduretic (*amiloride + hydrochlorothiazide*) results in hyperkalemia (209). *Probenecid* inhibits the tubular secretion of indometacin (SEDA-4, 66).

Attenuation of the hypotensive effect of *propranolol* and *thiazide diuretics* by indometacin was demonstrated in a double-blind placebo-controlled comparison of two groups of patients with essential hypertension several years ago (SEDA-6, 94). Two women with pre-eclampsia treated with pindolol and propranolol became profoundly hypertensive when indometacin was added because of premature contractions. Indometacin should not be given to pregnant patients with hypertension being treated with β-blockers (199[C]). The combination with ACE-inhibitors also warrants attention. Although lisinopril and indometacin in association lowered proteinuria in a small group of nephrotic patients, it also caused a decline in renal function and hyperkalemia in a substantial proportion of patients (SEDA-16, 109).

Synergy between indometacin and *cyclophosphamide* has been advanced as the cause of a life-threatening acute water intoxication and severe hyponatremia observed in a patient with multiple myeloma and normal renal function (SEDA-15, 99).

Marked water retention has also been observed during acute administration of *dipyridamole* in combination with indometacin (SEDA-13, 79).

Osmosin (Indosmos)

The fate of this slow-release version of indometacin has been outlined above (see also SEDA-8, Essay and Chapter 10 and SEDA-10, 77).

Indometacin-farnesil The limited initial experience with this lipid-soluble derivative of indometacin esterified with farnesol suggests an adverse effects profile similar to that of indometacin, even if the compound has been synthesized to decrease the gastrotoxicity (SEDA-17, 109).

INDOMETACIN-RELATED SUBSTANCES

Sulindac

There is still no firm evidence that by acting through an active metabolite, sulindac has any distinct advantage over other members of this group. However, its good tolerance in geriatric patients has been stressed (210[C]). The pattern of adverse drug reactions is similar to that of indometacin (211[r]). The incidence of side effects ranges from 16.9% (212[C]) to 50% (213[C]). Compared with other NSAID, sulindac has caused fewer gastrointestinal side effects than aspirin, but in some studies the incidence equalled that of ibuprofen (214[C]), fenoprofen (215[C]) and indometacin itself (216[C]), suggesting that the difference from aspirin simply reflects the absence of the latter's gastroerosive effects.

Cardiovascular Several cardiac abnormalities have been reported (217[R]), including congestive heart failure, arrhythmia and palpitations.

Respiratory Pulmonary infiltrates have been described in a woman with osteoarthritis who had been on sulindac therapy for 6 months (218[C]).

Nervous system Side effects affecting the central nervous system were found in 2.5–6.5% of patients in one study (213[C]). Dizziness, drowsiness and headache, as well as somnolence, vertigo, insomnia and blurred vision, i.e. all side effects described with indometacin, have been observed. Psychiatric symptoms, bizarre behavior and paranoia are possible (219[C]). Acute reversible encephalopathy has been described, accompanied by rash and fever. Like other NSAID, sulindac can cause aseptic meningitis in patients with SLE (SEDA-7, 109). Recurrent aseptic meningitis, described in a patient with no underlying connective tissue disease who had tolerated other NSAID, suggested an immunological hypersensitivity to sulindac (220).

Hematological Agranulocytosis (probably toxicity rather than hypersensitivity) can be caused by sulindac treatment (221[C]), as can bone marrow aplasia (222[C]) and severe thrombocytopenia (223[C], 224[C]). The latter may be the consequence of an autoimmune mechanism which destroys platelets in the presence of sulindac or its metabolite (SEDA-7, 109). Immuno-mediated hemolytic anemia with positive direct antiglobulin test has been reported with sulindac (SEDA-18, 103).

Aplastic anemia which occurred in a woman with osteoarthritis taking sulindac relapsed 3 years later during therapy with fenbufen; the case suggests that extreme caution should be exercised before giving NSAID to a patient who has a previous history of NSAID-related aplastic anemia (225[C]).

Liver Sulindac can cause toxic hepatitis and several cases have been described in the literature, some even with a positive rechallenge (226[C], 227[C]). A retrospective cohort study with secondary case-control analysis suggests that sulindac may cause a higher incidence of acute liver damage than all NSAID together, although the calculated risk is very low (27 per 100 000 prescriptions) (228). The liver function impairment is generally mild and reversible. Analysis of spontaneous reports to Danish Committee on ADR and FDA (SEDA-18, 103) confirms these data. Abdominal pain, nausea, high fever with chills, icterus, raised liver enzyme concentrations and hepatomegaly are characteristic and probably caused by hypersensitivity. Fever, rash and/or eosinophilia reported in 35–55% of patients seems to be a confirmation of an hypersensitivity mechanism (SEDA-18, 103). Cholestatic jaundice has also been described (229[C]) and, more recently, acute cholangitis in combination with acute pancreatitis (SEDA-13, 79).

Gastrointestinal Sulindac can cause all the gastrointestinal side effects associated with indometacin, from dyspepsia to peptic ulcer. Nausea and abdominal pain are the most frequent, followed by constipation (230[R]). Surprisingly, a study in healthy volunteers documented no gastroscopic mucosal damage after 7 days (231[C]), but this recalls other papers published in the past and showing a lack of mucosal damage in short studies even with NSAID known to be gastrotoxic. A giant esophageal ulcer has been described (232[C]).

Sulindac has been reported to be efficacious in reducing the number and size of rectal and colon polyps (233[C]) and it has been demonstrated that colon mucosal synthesis of prostaglandin E_2 and 6-keto-prostaglandin $F_{1\alpha}$ is markedly reduced in patients taking sulindac. The fact that this occurs concomitantly with the regression of the polyps supports the hypothesis that prostaglandins are implicated in the regulation of colonic polyp growth. These observations need to be confirmed in larger series of experiments designed to test the potential antitumor action of NSAID in the intestine.

Urinary system Sulindac may be less likely to induce renal toxicity than other NSAID (234[C]), at least when it is used in low doses, but, as pointed out in the general section of this chapter, there is some disagreement on this point in the literature (235[R], 236[R], 237[C]), and cases of nephrotic syndrome and renal failure have recently been described in five patients (238[C], 239[C]). The risk of severe hyperkalemia is also documented in a series of four cases (240). Data on the supposed ability of sulindac to inhibit the diuretic effect of furosemide are mutually contradictory (241).

Pancreas There are several reports of pancreatitis associated with sulindac (SEDA-4, 66; SEDA-7, 109). Symptoms resembling acute pancreatitis appeared after 3—90 days of sulindac treatment. Rechallenge was positive in one report (242[C]).

Skin Stevens-Johnson syndrome has been reported in females (SEDA-6, 95); all recovered after the drug was withdrawn and corticosteroid treatment initiated. A pernio-like reaction with purple discoloration, swelling, red papules and desquamation of the distal parts of several toes, which resolved after drug discontinuation and recurred after resumption, have been observed (243[C]), as have subcutaneous fat necrosis (SEDA-11, 92), fixed drug reaction (SEDA-12, 84) and toxic epidermal necrolysis (244, 245, 246).

Hypersensitivity reactions Various types of proven or suspected hypersensitivity have already been mentioned, e.g. in connection with the liver, but the exact mechanism of a particular side effect has not always been clear. A case of fever, pharyngitis, cervical lymphadenopathy, leukopenia, liver abnormalities, proteinuria, pulmonary infiltrates and abdominal pain has been described. Another patient who previously took sulindac without problems developed pruritus, dyspnea, perioral edema and lethargy after ingestion of a single 150 mg dose of sulindac. Pneumonitis is probably a part of a general hypersensitivity reaction (SEDA-6, 94; 218, 247[C]).

An anaphylactic reaction has been described (248[C]), while sulindac is also thought to have been responsible for a severe multisystem reaction (possibly again anaphylactic) which involved the cardiovascular, hepatic, pulmonary and hematological systems, in a patient with quiescent SLE (249[C]).

Risk situations Patients with sodium depletion are at risk of developing hyponatremia with all NSAID. Sulindac has also provoked hyponatremia in an elderly patient on a salt-restricted diet (250[C]).

Overdosage Granulocytosis of short duration was described after 12 g of sulindac (251). Eight cases of sulindac overdose have been reported to the UK National Poisons Information Service; all patients remained asymptomatic (SEDA-9, 89).

Interactions Potentiation of warfarin effects by sulindac has been reported (252[C]). Unlike other NSAID, sulindac lacks a potentially toxic interaction with lithium (SEDA-10, 82). Two cases of peripheral neuropathy attributed to a combination of oral sulindac and topical dimethylsulfoxide have been reported (SEDA-9, 89). Like indometacin, sulindac has been observed to interact with propranolol and a thiazide diuretic in a hypertensive patient (SEDA-6, 95).

Glucametacin *(SED-9, 49)*

There is no evidence that this glucosamide derivative of indometacin has any advantage over the parent compound. The same pattern of side effects must be expected. The most common are nausea and heartburn.

Clometacin *(SEDA-10, 82; SEDA-12, 84; SEDA-15, 98)*

Clometacin is another indometacin derivative on the market in a few countries. A retrospective analysis of acute renal failure related to NSAID therapy in France found that clometacin was the most frequently implicated drug. Cases of functional renal insufficiency and interstitial nephritis with nephrotic syndrome were reported (SEDA-12, 84). Thrombocytopenia has also been observed (SEDA-6, 94).

The hepatotoxic potential of clometacin was first reported in France in 1978. Since then many cases of hepatic toxic effects have been described (SEDA-7, 109). Two recently published retrospective studies have detailed the clinical, biochemical, immunological and histopathological features of the condition (253[Cr],

254[Cr]). Patients variously showed jaundice and/or hepatomegaly (90%), weakness (60%), fever (30%) and abdominal pain (20%), with or without diarrhea, nausea and vomiting, usually presenting after long-term use or shortly after a rechallenge. Cutaneous eruptions, generalized pruritus and weight loss were also recorded. The biochemical disorders indicated were hepatocellular hepatitis in the majority and cholestatic hepatitis. High titres of antitissue antibodies and hypergammaglobulinemia were also present in most patients. The histological findings were characteristic of acute hepatitis or chronic active hepatitis. A high prevalence of HLA antigen B8 was found. These immunological features suggest an autoimmune pathogenesis for chronic active hepatitis.

Due to the risk of long-term or repeated use of clometacin, the French authorities have already restricted its use of prescriptions for no more than 8 days. It seems wise to recommend that the drug be no longer used.

Oxametacin

The adverse reaction pattern is similar to that of indometacin. In a recent paper, 17% of 771 patients taking the drug experienced side effects, which led to discontinuation of treatment in 87. Gastrointestinal side effects accounted for 60% and CNS reactions for 31% (headache, dizziness) (255[C]).

Proglumetacin

This indoleacetic acid derivative, again, is particularly prone to cause gastrointestinal side effects: 18–41% of patients in various trials experienced side effects, but not to the extent that they interfered with treatment. Trials that compared proglumetacin with indometacin and oxyphenbutazone concluded that it is equally effective and usually better tolerated (SEDA-5, 103). This finding should not be considered conclusive, since the same claim has commonly been made for other members of this group of analgesics. Then, with the passage of time, the full picture of the usual side effects has emerged.

Acemetacin

Acemetacin is yet another indometacin derivative with the same side effect profile (SEDA-6, 94). In an open multicenter study, 187 of 280 patients experienced side effects (57% gastrointestinal). Treatment had to be stopped in 7% (256[C]). The clinical use of acemetacin is limited and there is no justification for claims that it has advantages over existing NSAID.

Table 3. *Arylalkanoic acid derivatives*

Aceclofenac	Flurbiprofen
Alclofenac	Ibuprofen
Benoxaprofen	Ibuproxam
Bromfenac	Indoprofen
Bucloxic acid	Ketoprofen
Bufexamac	Ketorolac
Butibufen	Lonazolac
Carprofen	Loxoprofen
Clozic	Nabumetone
Dexindoprofen	Naproxen
Diclofenac	Oxaprozin
Diphenpyramide	Pirprofen
Etodolac	Piproxen
Felbinac	Pronoprofen
Fenbufen	Tiaprofenic acid
Fenclofenac	Tolmetin
Fenoprofen	Tropesin
Fentiazac	Suprofen (sutoprofen)
Flunoxaprofen	Zomepirac

Cinmetacin

According to one rather small study, gastrointestinal side effects developed in 13 out of 30 patients (257[C]). It is still too early to make any definitive statements about the efficacy and toxicity of this drug.

Zidometacin

Zidometacin differs from indometacin in having an azido-group in the para-position, whereas indometacin has a benzyl group. It appears to be less ulcerogenic in animals. Epigastric pain, burning and nausea have, however, been experienced by patients treated with this drug (258[C]).

ARYLALKANOIC ACID DERIVATIVES AND RELATED COMPOUNDS

This large group of NSAID is constantly expanding. A great number of agents are now (or have been) on the market in various countries (Table 3). In consequence it is impossible to delineate all the side effects, comparative merits and advantages of any single agent. Nevertheless, some recent developments concerning the apparently specific toxicity of several members of this group deserve attention, especially since similar patterns can be expected in the development of new drugs in the series.

Ibuprofen can be taken as a reference substance. It is a typical member of the group and, because it has been extensively used in many countries for more than two decades and more recently (in lower dosages) as an over-the-counter analgesic, its effects are well known.

Ibuprofen (Brufen, isobutylphenylpropionic acid)

Like other NSAID, ibuprofen is a strong inhibitor of prostaglandin synthesis and many or all of its therapeutic as well as toxic effects may be linked with this characteristic. One gains the general impression that it is less potent and thus less toxic than indometacin in the doses usually employed, but that it has often been used in the past at relatively lower doses than indometacin. In a comparative double-blind cross-over study of ibuprofen, naproxen, fenoprofen and tolmetin in patients with rheumatoid arthritis, ibuprofen in equi-effective doses was the best tolerated drug. However, patients' and physicians' preference ranked naproxen first (259). The controversy over the use of ibuprofen as an antipyretic or analgesic and the question of whether it is safer than paracetamol in children are still opened (SEDA-16, 110; SEDA-17, 110). There are few data on the long-term safety of NSAID in the treatment of juvenile rheumatoid arthritis (JRA). A recent study analyzed the adverse reactions of patients affected by JRA treated long-term with ibuprofen (SEDA-16, 110). Gastrotoxicity was directly correlated with the dose administered and 5% withdrew ibuprofen early because they had gastrointestinal bleeding, vomiting, severe rash, hearing loss and abnormalities in liver function tests.

Sustained-release formulations seem to have the same pattern of adverse effects as conventionally formulated ibuprofen (260[C]), and 4-times-daily treatment is better tolerated than twice-daily administration (SEDA-12, 86).

ADVERSE REACTION PATTERN

General and toxic reactions Gastrointestinal side effects are the most frequent. They occur in up to 30% patients and range from abdominal discomfort to serious bleeding or activation of peptic ulcer. CNS effects with headache and dizziness are very common, but no severe renal impairment has been noted; blood dyscrasias can occur when treatment is prolonged and doses higher. There is no significant general hepatotoxicity, but both liver and central nervous system (meningitis) can be affected as part of a hypersensitivity reaction.

Hypersensitivity reactions The frequency of hypersensitivity reactions is low, but their severity can be considerable. A severe general hypersensitivity reaction, characterized by aseptic meningitis, hypotension, fever, conjunctivitis, arthralgias and leukopenia, has been reported in a woman with SLE (273[C]). Other similar patients have experienced fever with rashes, abdominal pain, headache, nausea and vomiting, signs of liver damage and meningitis. This type of reaction seems to occur especially (but not exclusively) in patients with connective tissue diseases (SEDA-5, 105; SEDA-10, 84) and it can be difficult to differentiate between a hypersensitivity reaction and flaring-up of the disease. Ibuprofen can provoke bronchospasm in asthmatics.

Tumor-inducing effects These have not been reported.

ORGANS AND SYSTEMS

Cardiovascular Apart from the possible consequences of salt and water retention, ibuprofen does not affect myocardial or vascular function. *Congestive heart failure* has rarely been reported.

Respiratory Ibuprofen can provoke *asthmatic attacks* in predisposed individuals, though this is rare. Cross-sensitivity to aspirin probably exists; a fatality has been reported in an asthmatic patient with no history of aspirin sensitivity after taking 2 ibuprofen tablets (SEDA12, 86). Pulmonary infiltrates with eosinophilia have recently been described with ibuprofen (SEDA-18, 104). Two episodes of acute pulmonary edema and progressive pulmonary infiltrates without eosinophilia have been reported in a HIV-infected man after administration of ibuprofen (SEDA-18, 104).

Nervous system CNS effects have already been mentioned. *Headache*, *vertigo*, *tinnitus* and *insomnia* are the most frequent, but are rarely severe. *Depression* and other psychotic reactions have been reported. Some CNS reactions (meningism and meningitis, lethargy and irritability) are thought to be a result of hypersensitivity (261[C]) (SEDA-9, 91; SEDA-18, 104). This data is confirmed by a report of aseptic meningitis with elevated intrathecal IgG synthesis and evidence of immune complexes within the cerebrospinal fluid (SEDA-16, 110).

Endocrine, metabolic An increase in serum levels of *uric acid* has been described (262[C]).

Hematological Ibuprofen *prolongs bleeding time*, although to a lesser extent than aspirin (263). There are reports indicating that a daily dose of less than 1 g does not affect bleeding time (264[C]). *Blood dyscrasias* varying in type and severity have been reported (SED-9, 150; 232[R]). They range from thrombocytopenia and granulocytopenia to agranulocytosis and fatal pancytopenia.

Reversible *pure white-cell aplasia* with bone marrow plasmocytosis and complement-dependent IgG antibody has been observed in one patient (265). Fatal autoimmune *hemolytic anemia* has been attributed to ibuprofen in a patient who was also taking other drugs (266[C]). Reversible hemolytic anemia has been described during ibuprofen treatment, but tartrazine, the orange dye in the coating of the brand used (Motrin 400), may have been responsible (267[C]). Gastrointestinal blood loss can cause *iron deficiency anemia*.

Liver Ibuprofen itself is not hepatotoxic, but the liver can be damaged as part of a generalized hypersensitivity reaction. Toxic hepatitis with Stevens-Johnson syndrome has been described (268[Cr]).

Gastrointestinal When first introduced, the gastrointestinal tolerance of ibuprofen was regarded as better than that of other NSAID, especially aspirin and indometacin. However, when higher doses began to be administered, probably equipotent with the usual doses of these older agents, there seemed to be no significant differences. As with other NSAID there is thus a close correlation between efficacy and side effects. Gastrointestinal side effects include a variety of symptoms such as *irritation*, *nausea*, *anorexia*, *vomiting*, *dyspepsia*, *heartburn*, *abdominal discomfort*, *bleeding*, *hematemesis* and *activation of peptic ulcer*; 10—30% of cases taking prescription doses (e.g. for rheumatic conditions) develop these side effects (SED-9, 150). It is not possible to give a reliable estimate of the frequency when the drug is used as a self-medication analgesic in lower doses, since exact information on complications to self-medication is rarely available and there is always likely to be a proportion of misuse (e.g. ingestion of higher or lower doses than those recommended). *Irritation of the rectal mucosa* after ibuprofen suppositories has also been reported (269[C]). Ulcerative *proctitis* has recently been reported in an SLE patient (SEDA-14, 94). Bleeding from a Meckel's diverticulum has been described with oral ibuprofen (SEDA-17, 110).

Urinary system *Renal function impairment* can follow ibuprofen treatment. It ranges from an insignificant reduction to an acute fall of creatinine clearance to an acute fall associated with a general hypersensitivity reaction, especially in patients with SLE or acute tubular necrosis (270[C]). *Nephrotic syndrome* without renal failure and *acute interstitial nephritis* without nephrotic syndrome have been described after self-administration of over-the-counter ibuprofen (SEDA-12, 86).

Irreversible *renal failure* due to acute cortical necrosis triggered by severe renal hypoperfusion has recently been reported (SEDA-12, 86).

Skin Skin *rashes* are usually present during general hypersensitivity. Urticarial, purpuric and erythematous changes with pruritus have been reported (271[r]); bullous pemphigoid has been described after 6 months of treatment and has been observed in two other patients on ibuprofen (SEDA-14, 94). Photosensitization has also been attributed to ibuprofen (SEDA-17, 110).

Alopecia has been described in black women; normal hair growth returned after therapy was discontinued (SED-11, 183). Ibuprofen can be added to the list of NSAID that can *exacerbate psoriasis* (SEDA-12, 86; SEDA-8, 102; SEDA-7, 108).

Special senses The *ocular reactions* described up to the present are reversible and not severe. They include blurred vision, changes in color perception and toxic amblyopia (272[C]). Use of ibuprofen has been found significantly correlated with high-altitude retinal hemorrhages (SEDA-17, 110)

Risk situations In patients with a history of *peptic ulcer* or *SLE* the risk/benefit ratio must be considered before prescribing ibuprofen. The first group is in danger of ulcer exacerbation and the second of a severe generalized hypersensitivity reaction.

Overdosage In spite of the large number of prescriptions and over-the-counter sale, acute intoxication is rare. Most often the symptoms are limited to nausea and vomiting, but more severe cases, characterized by coma, acidosis, mild hypothermia and non-oliguric renal failure have been described (SEDA-12, 86). Treatment is supportive (SEDA-9, 81).

Interactions A well-documented case of interaction of ibuprofen with *phenytoin*, where the former inhibited degradation of the latter, has been reported (274[C]). Because of its clinical significance, this interaction, which may also occur with other members of the group, should be further studied. Ibuprofen has been reported to interact with *antihypertensive agents* and reduce their efficacy (275[C]). Ibuprofen can increase the serum *lithium* level (SEDA-13, 81) and potentiate methotrexate-induced renal toxicity (276[C]). Acute renal failure has been described in concomitant treatment with ibuprofen and an immunosuppressive drug, tacrolimus, in two liver transplant recipients (SEDA-18, 104).

Ketoprofen *(SEDA-11, 94; SEDA-12, 86; SEDA-15, 101; SEDA-16, 110; SEDA-17, 110; SEDA-18, 104)*

The spectrum of side effects of this NSAID is similar to that of ibuprofen. The overall frequency of adverse reactions has ranged between 15 and 50% in different trials, with gastrotoxicity predominating at a frequency of 6.5—42% (277[R], 278[cr], 279[C]), even when administered rectally. Local symptoms, including rectal bleeding, can accompany treatment with ketoprofen suppositories (8.3% of patients). Studies on a controlled-release formulation revealed a pattern of side effects similar to that found with the usual formulations (SEDA-12, 86). An injectable form of ketoprofen also has acceptable tolerance (277[R], 278[C]). About 4.5% of patients treated with the injectable form have local reactions.

A fatal asthmatic reaction has been described (280[C]), and a case of severe bronchospasm with respiratory and cardiac arrest has been reported in a young man with a history of mild asthma, after the ingestion of ketoprofen (281[C]). Topical application of the drug can also provoke asthma in predisposed subjects (282[C]).

CNS effects are less pronounced than with ibuprofen. A cholinergic crisis was precipitated by a single dose in a myasthenic patient. No hematological toxicity has been reported. Hepatic toxicity has rarely been reported with ketoprofen (SEDA-17, 110). Retention of salt and water, sometimes with a picture of reversible pseudotumor cerebri, can also occur (283[C]). Concurrent administration of aspirin decreases ketoprofen protein binding and increases its plasma clearance. Salicylate also reduces metabolic conversion of ketoprofen to its conjugates and their renal elimination, and also enhances its conversion to nonconjugative metabolites (284[C]).

Like many other NSAID, ketoprofen can cause acute interstitial nephritis (285[C]). Renal failure and nephrotic syndrome due to membranous glomerulonephritis (an unusual cause of NSAID-induced nephrotic syndrome) has been described in an elderly patient on long-term ketoprofen therapy (SEDA-12, 86). Topical application of ketoprofen can cause contact dermatitis like other NSAID (SEDA-18, 104).

Although data from normal subjects indicate no interaction with warfarin, a case of severe gastrointestinal bleeding, and lengthened prothrombin time has been attributed to this drug combination (SEDA-13, 81). Irreversible renal failure has recently been reported in an elderly patient who received ketoprofen in combination with triamterene + hydrochlorothiazide (286[C]). The interaction of triamterene with NSAID is well documented (SEDA-12, 80) and co-administration with ketoprofen has proved dangerous. Ketoprofene use has been followed by red discoloration of the urine (SEDA-16, 110).

Fenoprofen *(SEDA-12, 85; SEDA-13, 81; SEDA-14, 94)*

According to published evidence, fenoprofen causes a rather different spectrum of adverse effects, although gastrotoxicity again predominates, and affects almost 50% of patients. The enteric-coated formulation has also been found to cause gastric and duodenal mucosal damage ranging from minimal submucosal hemorrhage to extensive ulceration (SEDA-13, 81). Blood dyscrasias have been repeatedly reported and include aplastic anemia, pancytopenia, thrombocytopenia, granulocytopenia, agranulocytosis (287[C], 288[C]) and pure red cell aplasia. Thrombocytopenia recedes after withdrawal of the drug; the mechanism is probably peripheral platelet destruction. It is difficult to estimate the frequency of these serious side effects, but it is probably low. Non-oliguric renal failure and hypotension have been observed (SEDA-6, 97), as have acute renal failure and acute interstitial nephritis presenting with nephrotic syndrome (SED-11, 183). In a recent review of acute interstitial nephritis with glomerulopathy due to NSAID, fenoprofen was implicated in 47% of the cases presented (289[R]); fenoprofen nephropathy is immune-mediated, and if drug withdrawal fails to improve renal function, immunosuppressive therapy is indicated (290[C]). Toxic epidermal necrolysis accompanied by high fever has been described in two patients (SEDA-14, 94).

Fenoprofen, like other NSAID, can interfere with some thyroid tests (SEDA-12, 85). There is a report on coma and metabolic acidosis due to an overdose of fenoprofen (291[C]).

Flurbiprofen *(SEDA-10, 83; SEDA-12, 85; SEDA-15, 101; SEDA-17, 109; SEDA-18, 104)*

In one prolonged, open study involving 1200 patients, more than 50% reported adverse reactions and therapy had to be withdrawn in 19% (292[C]). In a short-term multi-center study (293), only 6% patients were withdrawn because of side effects. Elderly patients seem to be particularly sensitive to, and intolerant of, flurbiprofen. One study has reported side effects in 80% of patients (SED-11, 183). There are more gastrointestinal side effects with flurbiprofen treatment than with naproxen or ibuprofen. In a series of controlled double-blind studies, adverse reactions occurred in 27—42% patients and were most commonly gastrointestinal in origin (18—28% patients) (SEDA-12, 85). Local tolerance of suppositories is often satisfactory, but discomfort, irritation, tenesmus and diarrhea have been observed (294[C]). Interstitial nephritis with nephrotic syndrome and one case of renal papillary necrosis have also been recorded (SEDA-12, 86; SEDA-17, 110). CNS effects are fewer than with indometacin (295[C]). Flurbiprofen can be added to the list of NSAID that precipitate, albeit rarely, extrapyramidal reactions

(SEDA-15, 101) and a parkinsonian syndrome has been reported in a predisposed patient (SEDA-15, 101). A leukocytoclastic vasculitis caused by flurbiprofen has been observed in a patient with rheumatoid arthritis (SEDA-15, 101). Two reports of a dermatitis herpetiformis-like drug eruption with flurbiprofen have been published (SEDA-18, 104).

Flurbiprofen can interact with furosemide and decrease its diuretic action (296[C]), and with acenocoumarol to potentiate its anticoagulant effect (SEDA-7, 112). The Japanese regulatory authority has suggested that the data sheet for flurbiprofen include a warning that it can cause convulsions. The reaction has mainly been described in patients taking quinolone antibiotics (SEDA-18, 104). As this interaction has also been described with fenbufen, the concomitant use of these classes of drugs should be avoided (SEDA-18, 104).

Pirprofen *(SEDA-10, 84; SEDA-11, 95; SEDA-12, 88; SEDA-16, 111)*

In an open, non-comparative field trial on 1506 patients, the reported side effects were mainly gastrointestinal and consisted mostly of epigastric pain. As one might expect, the side effects were dose-related. There was one case each of asthmatic attack, iron deficiency anemia, leukopenia and an increase in transaminase to more than 10 times the normal values (297[C]). In a long-term trial, 9.7% of over 3000 patients stopped treatment because of poor tolerability. Laboratory signs of hepatic damage have been documented in 37 patients, including three cases of icteric hepatitis (298[C]); pirprofen can definitely be considered hepatotoxic. The manufacturers decided to discontinue marketing it worldwide, claiming this to be a commercial decision (SEDA-16, 111).

Naproxen *(SEDA-10, 84; SEDA-12, 87; SEDA-14, 95; SEDA-15, 101; SEDA-16, 111; SEDA-17, 112; SEDA-18, 105)*

Side effects of naproxen resemble those of ibuprofen. Possible minor differences in their frequency cannot be assessed with certainty. When long-term naproxen treatment was analyzed in a cohort survey of 881 patients who had been followed for more than 3 years (299[C]), only 8.9% were found to have dropped out because of side effects. In shorter studies, doses of up to 1.5 g/day of naproxen produced no more side effects than lower or standard doses of other NSAID.

The incidence of adverse effects to naproxen in the elderly was found to be comparable to that in younger subjects in an analysis of nine double-blind controlled studies (300[C]).

New formulations (suspension and controlled-release tablets) have been found to have the usual pattern of side effects (SEDA-15, 101).

Respiratory A well-documented eosinophilic interstitial pneumonitis (PIE) and occurrence of pulmonary infiltrates have been reported (301[C]). These data have been confirmed by a more recent review and the incidence of the syndrome PIE seems to be greater in patients taking naproxen than those taking ibuprofen as shown by results fom a survey data of the FDA (SEDA-17, 112).

Nervous system Abnormalities in cognitive capacity and altered behavior have been described in elderly patients taking naproxen (SEDA-8, 107; 302[C]). Peripheral neuropathy has been reported in a patient with psoriatic arthritis while taking naproxen and hydroxychloroquine (SEDA-12, 87). Aseptic meningitis has been attributed to naproxen in a healthy young man taking it for neck pain (SEDA-14, 95).

Hematological Fatal aplastic anemia was reported in a patient taking naproxen as the only drug for 4 months (303[C]). Cases of Coombs-positive, as well as negative, autoimmune hemolytic anemia have been reported (304). Agranulocytosis (SEDA-13, 82) and thrombocytopenia (SEDA-15, 102) have also recently been reported with naproxen.

Liver Pathological liver function tests (SED-9, 152) and hepatic injury have been associated with naproxen therapy (305[Cr]), but no cause-effect relationship has been established with certainty.

Gastrointestinal Naproxen-induced gastrotoxicity has been reported with varying frequency (SED-9, 152; 299[C]). Enteric-coated tablets induced fewer endoscopic lesions in the stomach and duodenal bulb of young volunteers than did enteric-coated granules or plain tablets, but there were no differences in the incidence of middle and distal duodenum lesions (306[C]). An esophageal ulceration with bleeding has been reported in an elderly woman with esophageal dysmotility (SEDA-17, 112). Naproxen did not induce reflux and had no significant effect on motility parameters in normal subjects examined in a recent study (307). Local side effects of naproxen suppositories include edema, erythema and bleeding. They are usually mild. Acute eosinophilic colitis has recently been described associated with naproxen therapy; however, it rapidly resolved when the drug was discontinued (308[C]). An acute pancreatitis has been described in a young woman taking naproxen for dysmenorrhea (SEDA-18, 105).

Urinary system Interstitial nephritis with a rise in serum urea and creatinine, which decreased after withdrawal of naproxen, has been described after 3 months therapy in adults (309[C]) and in a recent report on a young boy (SEDA-16, 111). Oliguric renal failure with nephrotic syndrome and active interstitial nephritis has been described in a young female with SLE on intermittent long-term therapy with naproxen (SEDA-15, 102). A marathon runner, who had taken naproxen until 36 hours before the marathon, developed oliguric acute renal failure that required hemodialysis 2 days after the race (SEDA-12, 87). Edema can also be caused by naproxen. The kidney may be affected in the course of a generalized hypersensitivity reaction. The fact that the serum half-life of naproxen remains unchanged in renal failure can be therapeutically useful (310[C]).

Skin Acne has been reported in a woman treated for primary dysmenorrhea (311). The skin can be affected in the course of generalized allergic reactions (312[C]). Bullous photodermatitis, resembling porphyria cutanea tarda, has been described in patients on long-term treatment (SEDA-12, 87). Hair loss can be also induced by naproxen (SEDA-15, 102). A photodermatitis, defined as pseudoporphyria, has been reported in 21 children with juvenile rheumatoid arthritis and one with SLE after prolonged treatment with naproxen (313[C]) and more recently in another four children with JRA (314). This effect is rare, but since naproxen is a widely used drug in JRA, it is worthy of mention. Some cases of cutaneous necrotizing vasculitis have been described in patients taking naproxen (SEDA-5, 106; SEDA-17, 113).

Special senses Blurred vision and ocular discomfort, as well as lenticular and corneal changes, have been registered in a long-term study (299[C]). Hearing loss and tinnitus (sudden, bilateral and permanent) have also been associated with naproxen (315[Cr]).

Hypersensitivity reactions Generalized reactions have been associated with naproxen therapy (316[C]), including cutaneous vasculitis, nephritis or even paralytic ileus, as well as angiitis with cutaneous, muscular, articular and renal involvement (312[c]). Anaphylactic reactions are also possible. Exacerbation of asthma in sensitive patients seems to be rare.

Genital and sexual function Impotence and failure of ejaculation have been described, the latter with positive rechallenge (317[C]). In women naproxen, like other NSAID, may interfere with the normal course of menstruation; two young women experienced interruption of menstrual blood flow after taking the drug (SEDA-15, 102). Moreover, taken in high doses at mid-cycle, naproxen can inhibit ovulation and cause the so-called luteinized unruptured follicle syndrome (SEDA-16, 111).

Second-generation effects The conclusions presented above regarding the use of indometacin late in pregnancy also hold true for naproxen. Pulmonary hypertension and severe protracted hypoxemia have occurred in babies born to mothers who had been taking naproxen to delay delivery. The babies also had derangement of blood clotting, renal function and bilirubin metabolism. Necroscopy showed subarachnoid hemorrhage, gastric ulcers and constricted ductus arteriosus (318[C]).

Risk situations The safety and the efficacy of NSAID for the relief of the common cold symptoms have been insufficiently studied. Naproxen did not alter virus shedding or the serum neutralizing antibody response in healthy young adults with experimental rhinovirus colds and had some beneficial effect on their symptoms (SEDA-17, 113).

Overdosage Nothing more serious than nausea and indigestion have been reported after 25 g of naproxen (319[C]), whereas 35 g caused an epileptic fit (320[C]R). Metabolic acidosis, loss of consciousness, seizures and apnea have been reported more recently after the ingestion of more than 10 g of naproxen (321[C]).

Interactions Naproxen can interact with diuretics, propranolol and methyldopa (SEDA-8, 107) to decrease their action, and with probenecid to inhibit its metabolism and renal excretion (322[C]) and thus prolong its plasma half-life. A recent study showed that methotrexate can alter naproxen kinetics and vice versa (323).

Diclofenac *(SEDA-11, 82; SEDA-12, 85; SEDA-15, 100; SEDA-16, 109; SEDA-17, 109; SEDA-18, 104)*

The overall incidence of side effects is about 30%. Less than 1% of patients have to be excluded from treatment for this reason. The manufacturer's own analysis of 1966 side effects observed in 987 patients over about 6 years, during which period over 30 million patients had been treated with this drug, provided some interesting quantitative data. Of the total number of adverse reactions, 34.4% were gastrointestinal and 15.6% hematological. The review of data on worldwide safety experience with diclofenac showed that the incidence of serious adverse drug reactions noted in Phase III short-term (1227 patient) and long-term (1173 patient) trials in the United States was as follows: peptic ulcer 0.16 and 0.34%; gastrointestinal bleeding 0.16 and 0.17%; hepatitis 0 and 0.26%; thrombocytopenia 0 and 0.17% (324[R]).

Respiratory Diclofenac has been reported to have caused eosinophilic pneumonitis in a 67-year-old man (SEDA-18, 103).

Nervous system Headache, dizziness, vertigo, insomnia, drowsiness and agitation can be associated with diclofenac treatment. Hallucinatory symptoms and grand mal seizures have also been described (SEDA-16, 109). Toxic encephalitis can be part of a general toxic reaction (325[C]). Diclofenac has provoked aseptic meningitis in patients with SLE (SEDA-17, 109). The frequency of central side effects is 1—9%.

Mineral and fluid balance At least three reports of severe hyponatremia have been described with diclofenac (SEDA-12, 85; SEDA-13, 80; SEDA-18, 103). Interestingly, the last case manifest as the withdrawal of diclofenac and fluid restriction led to normal fluid and electrolyte balance within 10 days, despite concomitant treatment with nabumetone (SEDA-18, 104). It may be that inappropriate ADH secretion does not occur with all NSAID.

Hematological In an analysis of 447 side effects observed in 194 patients from all over the world (326[CR]), 20 patients with blood abnormalities were identified. There were two cases of agranulocytosis and one case of granulocytopenia. One of these patients, who was sensitive to pyrazolone, had taken a pyrazolone compound as well. Immune-mediated agranulocytosis and thrombocytopenia have been reported (SEDA-16, 110). Reversible hemolytic anemia (SEDA-4, 69; 327) and fatal hemolytic anemia have been reported following administration of diclofenac (328). A possibility that this drug causes panmyelopathy has been raised (329[C]). Data from the International Agranulocytosis and Aplastic Anemia Study showed an increased risk of aplastic anemia for diclofenac (multivariate rate-ratio of 8.8) (49). Fatal aplastic anemia has also been described (SEDA-4, 69; 330), as have purpura and thrombocytopenia, although not always with certainty. Spontaneous non-gastrointestinal bleeding (subcutaneous bruises, hematoma, greater wound drainage) has been associated with diclofenac use (SEDA-15, 100).

Liver Liver function may be impaired during diclofenac treatment. It has been suggested that liver damage may be more common than previously thought (SEDA-10, 83; 331[C]) but the risk is in fact closely similar to that recorded with those few other NSAID for which the issue of hepatic injury has been adequately studied. Bioptically proven hepatitis with positive rechallenge and dechallenge has been described (332[C]) and, recently, confirmed (333[C], 334). The usual clinical presentation is that of an acute hepatitis, but chronic active hepatitis has recently been described (333[C], 335[C], 336). Although recovery is usually rapid in the acute form after withdrawal of the drug, fatal cases have occurred (SEDA-11, 93; SEDA-12, 85; SEDA-13, 80; 337). Two patients who developed combined reversible hepatorenal damage have also been reported (338[C], 339[C], 340).

Gastrointestinal Side effects involving this system are particularly frequent (affecting some 13.5—25% of patients) and the incidence of the most serious—peptic ulcer and GI bleeding—has been noted above (324[R]). Rectal administration caused side effects in 15.6% of patients (341[C]); anorectal lesions (erosions, ulcers, stenosis of the anal verge) were observed in patients using suppositories for a relatively short time (342[C]). Perforation of the terminal ileum occurred in a patient who had taken an excessive dose (400 mg/day) of controlled-release diclofenac (343[C]). Colonic stricture, similar to ileum 'diaphragm' disease, described above as an adverse reaction to NSAID, developed in a patient during prolonged intake of a slow-release form of diclofenac (344[C]). Pseudomembranous colitis and colonic ulceration, with or without a diaphragm-like colonic stricture, have been reported recently (SEDA-16, 110; SEDA-17, 109).

Urinary system Renal papillary necrosis and interstitial nephritis with nephrotic syndrome have been documented (345[C], 346[C]). Other cases of nephrotic syndrome, with or without renal failure and apparently due to minimal-change nephropathy (which is relatively more common in NSAID users), have been reported (347[C], 348[C]). Recently the unusual feature of diclofenac-associated renal interstitial mucinosis has been described (SEDA-17, 109). Severe hyponatremia developed in an elderly woman treated with intramuscular diclofenac (SEDA-13, 80).

Skin Allergic skin rashes, serous bullous dermatitis with positive rechallenge and linear IgA deposits along the basal membrane in lesional and perilesional skin have all been reported (349[C]). The death of a patient who developed Stevens-Johnson syndrome must also be mentioned (SEDA-5, 103). Contact dermatitis and a generalized maculopapular eruption caused by delayed hypersensitivity to diclofenac has been reported with topical and oral diclofenac (SEDA-18, 104).

Local reactions Aseptic tissue necrosis after intramuscular injection (Nicolau syndrome) is a serious complication associated with unintentional intra-arterial injection of drugs. Antirheumatic drugs are frequently involved in these reactions and diclofenac has also been implicated (350[c]). Other consequences of the intramuscular administration of diclofenac are the asymptomatic high concentrations of serum CPK or damage to muscle, nerve or blood vessels formerly reported. New reports on these effects continue to appear (SEDA-17, 109), because intramuscular diclofenac is becoming a popular alternative to opioids, especially in post-surgical analgesia. Necrotizing fasciitis has been reported in three patients, two died, as the consequence of severe local reaction associated with intramuscular injection of diclofenac (351). If appropriately diluted and infused intravenously it is usually well tolerated, even if local venous thrombosis has been described (SEDA-17, 109).

Hypersensitivity reactions Acute allergic reactions were reported in 48 patients, and included anaphylactic or anaphylactoid reactions and angioneurotic edema without shock, but no fatalities appeared to have occurred. Two anaphylactic reactions, one fatal, to parenteral diclofenac have recently been reported (SEDA-18, 104). Hepatorenal damage described with the use of diclofenac (SEDA-15, 100), has sometimes been reported with thrombocytopenia and hemolytic anemia, mediated by an immune mechanism (SEDA-16, 110).

Interactions Diclofenac increases plasma levels of lithium by impairing its renal excretion (352[C]). The interaction between diclofenac and triamterene has been reported to be responsible for renal impairment. The nephrotoxicity of cyclosporin may be increased when the drug is used in combination with diclofenac or other NSAID (353[C], 354[C]).

Tolmetin

A large number of patients (32 207 in all) taking part in a short (1—4 weeks) post-marketing study with tolmetin were analyzed (355[C]). Side effects occurred in 12.3% of patients, and led to withdrawal in 3.6%. Tolerability was comparable to that of naproxen, indometacin (SEDA-7, 114), and ibuprofen (SED-9, 152). In another retrospective study of patients treated for a year or more with tolmetin 63.8% reported side effects, generally mild and transitory. In controlled studies, about 10% patients dropped out due to side effects (356[C]). In another study to evaluate the safety of the drug, in which 25 000 prescription records were examined (357[C]), tolmetin induced adverse reactions serious enough to cause hospitalization in only two cases (drug fever and membranous glomerulopathy).

Cardiovascular Increased blood pressure can develop after long-term treatment with tolmetin.

Nervous system The adverse reactions usual for this group have been reported (SEDA-6, 98). An aseptic meningitis similar to that seen with ibuprofen occurred in one female patient (358[C]).

Hematological Acute reversible thrombocytopenic purpura and tolmetin-related antibodies have been reported in a patient with a history of multiple allergies. Rechallenge was positive (359[C]). Eosinophilia in the peripheral blood has also been found (SEDA-6, 98).

Gastrointestinal 31% of patients receiving tolmetin developed gastrointestinal side effects, 2% having a peptic ulcer (356[C]). In older patients, the percentage of peptic ulcer and gastrointestinal bleeding is somewhat higher (360[R]).

Urinary system Reversible renal failure and acute interstitial nephritis have been reported. Another paper attributed a nephrotic syndrome to tolmetin intake, but was unable to establish a firm causal relationship (361[C]). Nephrotic syndrome has also been described in a 16-year-old girl after 6 months of tolmetin treatment (SEDA-16, 122).

Special senses Loss of hearing has been documented (SED-9, 152).

Hypersensitivity reactions From an early phase the high incidence of hypersensitivity reactions with this drug has been striking: e.g. in spontaneous adverse reaction reports, despite a later claim that the high incidence could not be confirmed in a retrospective comparative review (SEDA-6, 98; SEDA-7, 134; 362[C]). Various factors can explain such a discrepancy: e.g. patients covered by such a review may be precisely those who persisted with treatment since they themselves did not experience such reactions. A fatal multisystem toxicity including both renal and hepatic failure with microvesicular fatty change in the liver has been reported with tolmetin ingestion in a young woman (363[C]).

Interactions Combined use of tolmetin with warfarin can markedly increase prothrombin time and cause bleeding (SEDA-13, 82).

Bufexamac

Bufexamac in the form of cream is intended for topical use only (using iontophoresis, ultrasound and massage). Local intolerance is manifested by burning and irritation, attributable to the components of the cream. Urticaria, folliculitis and pyodermia may develop when occlusive dressings are used. The course of contact allergy by bufexamac was particularly protracted and refractory in most of the 24 patients observed in one dermatological hospital between 1983 and 1987 (364[C]). An erythema multiforme-like rash associated with contact dermatitis has been reported recently (SEDA-18, 103).

Fenclofenac

Fenclofenac was withdrawn from the UK market after an official refusal to relicense it because of the unsatisfactory adverse drug reaction profile (365); shortly thereafter, it was withdrawn in all other countries where it had been marketed.

The UK Committee on Safety of Medicines' adverse drug reaction data included records of seven deaths and 895 side effects in patients taking fenclofenac. The majority of the unwanted effects were skin-related. According to Weber (366[R]), who compared the number of reports on adverse reactions to NSAID with the number of prescriptions issued, fenclofenac had the second highest incidence of reported complications and ranked first as regards the number and severity of dermatological reactions.

Fentiazac

This thiazoleacetic acid derivative has the same adverse reaction profile as other NSAID. Side effects affect as many as 56% of patients (5—56%), and are even more frequent than with phenylbutazone (367[C]).

Nervous system Adverse effects involving the central nervous system include headache, dizziness, mental confusion, sedation, giddiness and blurred vision. Dysesthesia and oral paresthesia have also been reported.

Liver In one study seven out of 20 patients with rheumatoid arthritis presented a significant rise in SGOT and alkaline phosphatase levels (368[C]).

Gastrointestinal Pyrosis, epigastric pain, nausea, constipation/diarrhea and occult bleeding are the most frequent gastrointestinal complications. Rectal administration can cause various side effects, both local and systemic.

Tiaprofenic acid *(SEDA-10, 84; SEDA-12, 89; SEDA-18, 106)*

More data are now available on the incidence of side effects caused by this drug (369[R], 370[c], 371[r]). A review of the published studies shows that about 13—15% of patients manifest side effects. The withdrawal rate from therapy because of drug-induced unwanted reactions has ranged from 3.2 to 12% in short-term studies and was 4% in one long-term trial. Side effects have involved the gastrointestinal tract in 8—12% of patients, the central nervous system in 1—10% and the skin (rash, sweating and itching) in 1—4%. Cutaneous photosensitivity and edema have also been reported. The side effect profile does not differ from that of other propionic acid compounds and includes the whole spectrum of gastrointestinal adverse reactions usually found with NSAID (SED-10, 166; SEDA-10, 84). The claim of good tolerance and gastric protection, based on animal data which the company extrapolated to humans, has not been substantiated by appropriate clinical studies (SEDA-12, 89). Although many NSAID have rarely been reported to be responsible for increased urinary frequency and dysuria, and never for severe cystitis, there is now the certainty that tiaprofenic acid can give rise to severe cystitis as described in the review of SEDA-18, 106. The lesson is that careful consideration should be given to symptoms suggestive of chronic cystitis in any patient taking any NSAID.

Butibufen

Experience with butibufen is still limited. Until now only gastrointestinal side effects have been desribed (372[R]).

Fenbufen *(SEDA-15, 100; SEDA-18, 104)*

The profile of fenbufen is similar to that of other NSAID (373[R]). The drop-out rate due to adverse reactions reported in various studies has ranged from 12 to 22%.

Respiratory Fenbufen can cause a pulmonary alveolitis characterized by rash, dry cough, breathlessness, fever, hypoxia, sometimes eosinophilia, and bilateral alveolar shadowing or infiltrates; the condition recedes after withdrawal of the drug (SEDA-12, 85; SEDA-13, 80; SEDA-15, 100).

Nervous system Headache has been reported during treatment with fenbufen.

Hematological Hemolytic anemia, in some cases accompanied by signs of hypersensitivity, has been reported (SEDA-14, 94). Aplastic anemia has been described in two patients taking fenbufen (SEDA-18, 104) but both recovered fully after withdrawal.

Liver The incidence of hepatotoxicity varies greatly. Whereas changes in liver function tests were recorded in 25% patients in an early study (SEDA-4, 68), the finding has not been confirmed by later studies (SEDA-5, 194; SEDA-6, 96). Abnormalities in the liver function of patients with rheumatoid arthritis may be a non-specific reaction to inflammation. However, hepatotoxicity should be watched for in patients on fenbufen treatment.

Skin About 5% of patients experience itching, rashes or erythema multiforme (374[C]). Circulating immunocomplexes have been found (375[C]). The UK Commission on Safety of Medicines issued a warning regarding the high reporting rate of cutaneous adverse reactions with fenbufen and noted that some of them can be followed by a severe illness (SEDA-13, 72; SEDA-14, 94; SEDA-15, 100). A life-threatening reaction (toxic epidermal necrolysis) has also been reported (SEDA-6, 96; SEDA-8, 106) and a 1981—1985 review on the incidence and drug etiology of this condition in France placed fenbufen third among NSAID, after isoxicam and oxyphenbutazone, as a causal factor (376[r]).

Interactions A number of cases of epileptic seizures have been documented in Japan in patients treated with a combination of fenbufen and enoxacin (SEDA-12, 85; SEDA-15, 100).

Carprofen *(SEDA-11, 92; SEDA-13, 79)*

The main side effect problems would seem to be cutaneous and hepatic. Photoreactions to this drug are being increasingly reported and the chemical similarity between carprofen and benoxaprofen is worth noting (SEDA-12, 84). The mechanism of photosensitivity can be either toxic or allergic. Other cutaneous symptoms, such as burning, pruritus, dermatitis and skin redness, have also been reported (377[C]). 14% of 1500 patients enrolled in clinical trials in the United States presented slight transient rises in liver function test indices, but it is difficult to judge the clinical significance of these laboratory abnormalities (SEDA-13, 79). Headache, dizziness, gastrointestinal discomfort, and dysuria have also been described (377[C]). Asthma may be precipitated in aspirin-sensitive persons.

Despite the fact that carprofen is reported to be well tolerated by peptic ulcer patients on ranitidine (378[C]), one should not presume that it can be used without risk in patients with ulcer disease.

Alclofenac *(SED-9, 152; SEDA-3, 94; SEDA-4, 67)*

While the pattern of aclofenac toxicity resembles that of other NSAID, the frequency of various side effects differs widely. Allergic reactions have been reported more frequently and skin rashes have been particularly common. General hypersensitivity reactions, including anaphylactic shock, severe generalized vasculitis, hepatotoxicity and nephrotoxicity, have been observed. For this reason alclofenac has been withdrawn in several countries (379[R]). Blood dyscrasias and neurological symptoms are rare.

Bucloxic acid

Bucloxic acid is not widely used. While the usual symptoms of gastrotoxicity, nephrotoxicity and increased blood pressure have been reported, the most important side effects involve skin and allergic reactions. Quincke's edema has been observed (SED-9, 152; SEDA-1, 93).

Indoprofen

Indoprofen is one of several NSAID withdrawn from the market because of its side effects. Some details are of interest. The UK Licensing Authority suspended the product license for this drug on grounds of safety in 1983, and in 1984 the Italian manufacturer decided to withdraw it from the world market. The UK decision was taken after the discovery of a high level of adverse drug reactions in both a voluntary post-marketing surveillance study and the spontaneous adverse reaction reporting system; the latter noted 217 serious adverse effects, mainly gastrointestinal (bleeding and perforation). According to the manufacturer, the side effect profile seen in the United Kingdom had not emerged in other countries (380[C]). A survey of adverse reactions in 6764 patients, mostly treated for 1 month or less, showed that life threatening events were rare. A post-marketing surveillance study on 3823 osteoarthritic patients found serious adverse reactions to be even less frequent (381[r]). A total of 46 deaths associated with indoprofen has been reported from three countries (Germany 5, UK 34, Italy 7), but only 11 were judged as probably or possibly drug-related. The majority (nine) of these indoprofen-related deaths were caused by gastrointestinal reactions. The ultimate reason advanced by the manufacturer for worldwide withdrawal was claimed to be the finding of carcinogenicity in long-term toxicological animal studies; to what extent the clinical events actually played a role in the decision is not clear.

No interactions have been reported, but the fact that indoprofen prolongs bleeding time and decreases platelet aggregation could be important in this context (382[C]).

Benoxaprofen *(SEDA-12, 84; SEDA-13, 79)*

Since benoxaprofen, like zomepirac, provided an experience from which several lessons can be learnt, it deserves a brief review, even though it was withdrawn 10 years ago; it is after all possible that some newer drugs will prove to share its chemical or pharmacological characteristics and thereby its problems. The compound was originally launched in or about 1980; initial claims had, as is common in this class of agents, been related to a favorable side effect profile and, in this instance, also to what were called 'unique disease-modifying properties' in rheumatoid arthritis. The latter claims appeared to have been based on the fact that the compound had a relatively stronger leukotriene-inhibiting effect (and a somewhat weaker prostaglandin synthetase-inhibiting action) than other NSAID. Having passed all the preclinical and clinical tests and having met the safety requirements set by current drug legislation in many countries (though having been rejected in several on safety grounds), benoxaprofen was suspended by the UK Committee on Safety of Medicines in 1982, about 18 months after marketing; shortly afterwards it was withdrawn worldwide by its manufacturer (383[R]). The end of benoxaprofen reflected a very high incidence of side effects, with skin and nail reactions being prominent as well as liver reactions which (particularly in the elderly) sometimes proved fatal.

Legal aspects The case has led to considerable regulatory and medicolegal discussion in the 10 years since the drug was withdrawn. In the United States, the company was subsequently charged by the Food and Drug Administration with misbranding the drug in a press kit and in associated materials, which contained a false and misleading headline implying that the drug was harmless, despite the fact that the company was aware of a report of fatal cases related to benoxaprofen use. The company's intense marketing campaign has been heavily criticized (384) and it has been noted that the recommendation of the WHO that drugs likely to be used in the elderly should be investigated in the elderly at an early stage had certainly been disregarded in the pre-marketing phase. In the United Kingdom, the manufacturer rejected patient demands to establish a compensation scheme, offering instead a level of financial settlement which patients in turn refused as inadequate. The case shows how poorly suited some legal systems are for dealing with mass personal injury due to drugs.

Liver Fatal liver damage was observed particularly in the United Kingdom and tended to occur in elderly individuals. The complication initially presented as jaundice, or raised liver enzymes (including alkaline phosphatase). Surprisingly, biochemical and histological liver changes were not consistent with major hepatocellular damage. The role of the very long plasma half-life and the significance of the fact that benoxaprofen is excreted in the bile and urine have never been made clear. There were three reports of primary biliary cirrhosis after benoxaprofen, but the causal relationship was not proven (SEDA-12, 84).

Gastrointestinal The hope of improved gastric tolerance with this drug, which as compared with other NSAID is a weaker prostaglandin inhibitor (though probably a stronger leukotriene inhibitor), was not fulfilled. The incidence of this type of reaction, too, was higher in elderly patients.

Urinary system All types of kidney damage were reported, ranging from a transitory fall in glomerular filtration and reversible renal insufficiency (part of multisystem disease with lupus erythematosus cells in the circulation) to nephrotic syndrome.

Skin Cutaneous side effects were perhaps the most frequent problem and (together with hepatic complications) the most serious: 63% of 300 patients treated with this drug for 6 months complained of one or more side effects (total 259 reactions); 69.5% were cutaneous; photosensitivity led to withdrawal in 30.2% of cases. Multiple subepidermal cysts (milia) on sun-exposed skin areas and onycholysis (12.6% of patients) were documented. Other skin reactions included rashes, hypertrichosis, erythema multiforme and Stevens-Johnson syndrome (385[C]). Persistent phototoxicity was reported many months after stopping benoxaprofen (SEDA-12, 84). Although a later study on persistent photosensitivity as a sequel to benoxaprofen administration in 42 subjects failed to confirm the relationship between the photosensitivity and the drug (386), this is contrary to the massive experience in the field.

In retrospect it seems likely that one problem of benoxaprofen was that the drug had largely been studied in clinical work conducted during the winter months, whereas shortly after its launch in the United Kingdom the summer began and patients were exposed to much sunlight.

Diphenpyramide

Diphenpyramide, a phenylacetic derivative, is less efficacious but has fewer side effects than indometacin or phenylbutazone. Gastrointestinal tolerance is, as one would expect, better (387[C]). The most frequent reactions are gastrointestinal and skin (388[R]).

Ibuproxam

Gastrointestinal and skin side effects with this less well-known NSAID have been reported (389[C]).

Zomepirac

Despite the fact that zomepirac is a pyrrole-acetic acid compound closely related to tolmetin, it was claimed to be a new type of analgesic drug. Its history is not unlike that of benoxaprofen. In 1982, due to the severity and frequency of hypersensitivity reactions it was withdrawn voluntarily by the manufacturers worldwide, at least temporarily (390). It has not been relaunched.

The overall incidence of side effects of zomepirac, according to numerous reviews (SEDA-7, 114), is similar to, or somewhat higher than that of other

NSAID. After single oral doses 36% of 496 patients had some side effects. The percentage was even higher (42.5%, 458 out of 1079 patients) for short-term therapy (2 weeks). Due to adverse reactions 3.5% of patients dropped out. Although when given over 2—3 weeks, 65—70% patients experienced adverse effects, the discontinuation rate was comparable to, or lower than, that of other NSAID (391[C], 392[C]). Only the most important side effects will be presented here.

Cardiovascular Weight gain, edema and hypertension have been encountered. The content of sodium (0.34 mmol in 100 mg) could be a risk factor in the long-term treatment of some patients.

Gastrointestinal The side effects of zomepirac on the gastrointestinal tract have been the most frequent reason for interruption of treatment. They are dose-related and, as already mentioned, increase with duration of drug intake. Nausea, vomiting, dyspepsia, discomfort, abdominal pain and diarrhea/constipation have been recorded. Stomatitis and tongue pain have also been reported (393[C]). Zomepirac at a dose of 300 mg increases fecal blood loss, but less than aspirin.

Hypersensitivity reactions Fatal anaphylactic and anaphylactoid reactions have been reported since zomepirac was first used: 10% of all reports on anaphylactic reactions in the United States named zomepirac, making it second only to the much older tolmetin. Hypersensitivity reactions are characterized by hypotension, bronchospasm and serious respiratory distress with or without oropharyngeal edema. Type 3 allergic reactions have also been described. The manufacturer received 1100 reports of allergic reactions in the first 2 years after launching.

Addiction Suspicions based on cluster reports that zomepirac may be addictive have not been confirmed in a comprehensive review (394[r]).

Oxaprozin *(SEDA-11, 94)*

Oxaprozin, according to the controlled studies available, causes side effects in 23—58% of patients. It was considered to be better than aspirin and comparable to other NSAID in long-term studies. However, the treatment had to be interrupted due to side effects in 8—31% of patients.

Nervous system Headache, dizziness, vertigo, and tinnitus are less frequent than with indometacin or aspirin.

Liver Minor rises in transaminase levels have been observed in 10—20% of patients. Liver function should be monitored, especially during the first 6 months of therapy. Now fulminant hepatitis has been reported (395).

Gastrointestinal These are the most frequently reported side effects, though gastroduodenal ulcer or bleeding is rare.

Urinary system Six percent of 847 patients with various rheumatic diseases who took oxaprozin daily for up to 1 year developed significant increases in BUN or creatinine, but there was a serious adverse renal effect in only one patient (SEDA-12, 87).

Skin Less than 5% of patients develop rashes. Some patients have phototoxic reactions (SEDA-12, 87).

Risk situations Older patients are more likely to suffer from gastrointestinal and nephrotoxic reactions. In this respect, oxaprozin differs little from other NSAID.

Interactions The clinical significance of the reduced renal clearance of oxaprozin when it is given concomitantly with cimetidine or ranitidine is not clear (SEDA-12, 87).

Clobuzaril

This methylpropionic acid derivative, thought to have a penicillamine-like effect, was withdrawn from the market because of several reports of Stevens-Johnson syndrome (396[C]).

Dexindoprofen *(SEDA-10, 82; SEDA-11, 93)*

This indoprofen derivative has a similar side-effect pattern to the parent drug. Gastrointestinal, CNS and skin reactions are the most frequent.

Etodolac *(SEDA-10, 83; SEDA-12, 85; SEDA-15, 100; SEDA-18, 104)*

Etodolac, a pyranocarboxylic acid, is a relatively new compound, that was first introduced onto the market in the United Kingdom in 1986. Animal experiments, as well as endoscopic and ^{51}Cr-blood loss studies in man, suggest that its gastroirritancy is low (397[R], 398[R]), but such claims have to be regarded with the reservations expressed earlier in this chapter and those noted with respect to the dose below. Etodolac administered short-term at dosages of 200, 400 and 600 mg b.i.d. caused significantly less damage to both the gastric and the duodenal mucosa than 3.9 g/day aspirin (SEDA-12, 85). It had a less damaging effect on the stomach than naproxen in a short-term endoscopic study in rheumatoid arthritis patients (399[C]). The most frequent side effects among 1379 patients enrolled in various clinical trials were gastrointestinal symptoms: 8.9% of patients experienced nausea, 5.8% epigastric pain, 5.7% heartburn and 5.2% indigestion; 1.9% of patients had to be withdrawn because of these side effects. CNS complaints included dizziness (4.4% patients), headache (6.0%) and tinnitus (2.6%). Skin rashes occurred in 3% of patients (SEDA-12, 85). In 1986 the UK Drug Safety Research Unit at Southampton published a report on its 'prescription event monitoring' study of etodolac (SEDA-13, 80). The drug was rated effective in only 56% of 9109 patients and the Unit was led to the conclusion that the average daily dose used (400 mg) was too low to be effective. In consequence, the adverse reaction figures should be viewed with great caution. Indeed, at an adequate dose level they might actually prove to be unfavorable, since in this study the rate of dyspepsia during the first month was 16 per 1000 as compared to 3 per 1000 for piroxicam. After the first month, rates were similar for etodolac and piroxicam. Few serious events were recorded: exfoliative dermatitis was seen in a patient with psoriatic arthritis and there were 20 cases with hematemesis or melena. By 1988, etodolac had been reported 27 times to the UK Committee on the Safety of Medicines as being suspected of causing serious adverse reactions (400[R]). In a French post-marketing safety study which involved 51 355 patients taking 200—600 mg/day, 10.1% of patients reported a total of 6236 adverse reactions and 9.0% dropped out because of adverse reactions, 21 of which were adjudged severe (401[C]). Another four postmarketing surveillance studies conducted on 8334 patients with rheumatic conditions who received 200—600 mg/day of etodolac for periods ranging from 4 weeks to 1 year revealed that 23% patients reported events and that 9% of all the patients stopped taking the drug because of adverse reactions. Strikingly, gastrointestinal events were the most commonly reported (402[C]). One case of agranulocytosis probably induced by etodolac with the pattern described with other NSAID has been recently reported (403). The long-term treatment safety profile of the new modified-release formulation of etodolac seems to be similar to that of conventional etodolac (SEDA-18, 104).

Flunoxaprofen *(SEDA-10, 83)*

The side effect pattern of this lesser-known NSAID is similar to that of other members of the group. Gastrointestinal disturbances have been described.

Lonazolac

This arylacetic derivative causes side effects comparable to those of other NSAID. Gastrointestinal disturbances are followed in frequency by CNS and skin reactions. Cholestatic hepatitis has also been reported (SEDA-8, 106).

Nabumetone

Nabumetone is a derivative of naproxen. Its effectiveness is related to the formation of the active metabolite, 6-methoxy-2-naphthylacetic acid. After repeated once-daily doses it accumulates in elderly patients but not in others; it would therefore seem prudent to lower the dose in elderly patients. The renal clearance of the active metabolite is very low, but there are still insufficient pharmacokinetic studies to allow the potential renal toxicity of the drug to be assessed. Being a non-acidic compound and a weak inhibitor of prostaglandin synthesis, nabumetone was designed as a pro-drug that could be administered without causing gastric damage; this theoretical advantage is still awaiting clinical confirmation. Though it was found not to exert gastrointestinal toxicity in animals, one has to bear in mind that gastric problems with NSAID are not primarily a local effect but are exerted systemically; a metabolite formed after gastric passage could thus still cause gastric problems. Again, although radiochromium evaluation of GI blood loss in healthy volunteers and endoscopic studies in rheumatoid arthritis patients showed that nabumetone provokes less gastric damage than naproxen, the usual defects of such studies limit their clinical relevance (SEDA-13, 81). The same applies to the preliminary results of an ongoing long-term study on osteoarthritis and rheumatoid arthritis patients which also indicate that nabumetone is less gastrolesive than naproxen, but where the investigation was insufficient to exclude the possibility that the dosage was lower than that needed for optimal efficacy (404[C]). Not unexpectedly, a study in 2000 patients, mostly treated for more than 6 months, elicited an adverse event pattern similar to that of other derivatives of this class of NSAID (SEDA-13, 81). Side effects were reported in 18% of patients and 10% ceased taking the drug due to adverse reactions. Diarrhea was the most common problem (12.8% of patients) followed by abdominal pain (9.9%), dyspepsia (9.3%), nausea (7.8%) and flatulence (4.7%). Ten ulcers were detected. In this and other work, nervous system reactions, cutaneous rashes, edema, unspecified eye disorders and liver function test abnormalities have all been encountered. Findings in another review of clinical trials were similar (405[R]). A post-marketing surveillance study on 10 800 osteoarthritis and rheumatoid arthritis patients, who were followed up at 12 months, noted that 12% of patients discontinued the drug because of adverse events; 11 serious events may have been related to nabumetone therapy and seven of these were gastrointestinal hemorrhage (406[C]).

Suprofen (sutoprofen) *(SEDA-12, Essay, 88; SEDA-15, 102; SEDA-17, 113)*

Suprofen, an α-methyl-4-(2-thienylcarbonyl)-phenylacetic acid, an NSAID specifically studied and promoted as a non-narcotic analgesic for use in many painful conditions, was withdrawn from the market worldwide in 1987. It induced an unusual clinical syndrome of acute flank pain and nephrotoxicity (SEDA-12, 89). A case-control study identified as risk factors male sex, hay fever and asthma, participation in exercise, and alcohol consumption. It has been thought that the pathogenesis of suprofen nephrotoxicity, as studied in young healthy volunteers, involves a transient decrease in renal plasma flow and glomerular filtration rate, possibly due to intratubular precipitation of uric acid (407[C]). Suprofen, which is still available as a 1% ointment in some countries, can cause photodermatitis (SEDA-17, 113).

Ketorolac *(SEDA-12, 86; SEDA-14, 94; SEDA-16, 110; SEDA-17, 112; SEDA-18, 104)*

Ketorolac is a relatively new NSAID which, like several others, is promoted as a non-narcotic analgesic, though this is merely a marketing ploy which does not reflect any special characteristics, unless it be that it is one of (many) NSAID which can be given parenterally when needed. It is a pyrrolizine carboxylic acid derivative, structurally and pharmacologically related to tolmetin, zomepirac and indometacin. The trometamol salt of ketorolac enhances the solubility of the drug and allows its parenteral administration. Preliminary experience shows that single intramuscular injections are better tolerated than morphine. Experience that has matured in the last 4 years (see Review in SEDA-17, 110) confirms that, under the profile of adverse reactions, ketorolac should be considered an NSAID to all effects. Opinions on the safety of ketorolac among the European Community drug regulatory authorities continue to conflict (SEDA-18, 104; 408[C]). The most commonly reported symptoms are stated to be somnolence, headache, dizziness, nausea, dyspepsia and abdominal pain. Edema, hyperkalemia, diarrhea, sweating, self-limited wheezing and itching have also been occasionally reported (SEDA-12, 86; SEDA-16, 110; SEDA-17, 111). There are by now several reports that document the high risk of giving ketorolac to patients with a history of asthma, nasal polyposis and sensitivity to aspirin or any other NSAID (SEDA-18, 105). Gastric lesions (endoscopically demonstrated erosion, ulcers and uncommon giant duodenal or gastric ulcers) have been described in healthy volunteers (SEDA-14, 94) as well as in patients (SEDA-18, 105) parenterally treated with ketorolac (SEDA-14, 94); gastric damage appears to be dose-related (SEDA-17, 112). The drug, like aspirin, is able to prolong bleeding time, but the effect on hemostasis disappears when the drug is eliminated from the body. The clinical significance of the effect of ketorolac on hemostasis in perioperative use is still imperfectly understood. Serious bleeding either at the operative site or in the gastrointestinal tract after the administration of ketorolac has been documented in several reports (SEDA-18, 105). The concomitant use of anticoagulants increases the risk of bleeding (SEDA-18, 105). There are several reports of impairment of renal function by ketorolac (SEDA-17, 112; SEDA-18, 105). The severity of renal impairment can vary from slight to severe forms of renal failure and may also happen after a single administration of 30 mg. Recent major surgery should be considered a risk factor for renal insufficiency, particularly in elderly patients; the use of ketorolac, or other NSAID, for post-operative pain management is therefore warranted only in carefully selected patients. Anaphylaxis and anaphylactoid reactions have been reported (SEDA-17, 112). Because it crosses the placental barrier, it should not be used in pregnant women. When administered to mothers during labor, ketorolac has been shown to inhibit significantly platelet aggregation in neonates (SEDA-14, 94). One case of lithium neurotoxicity resulting from interaction with ketorolac has been reported (409).

Piproxen *(SEDA-12, 88)*

At the time of writing, only preliminary experience with this naproxen derivative seems to have been published, though it is not particularly new. The side-effect profile seems to be similar to that of the parent compound.

Loxoprofen *(SEDA-15, 101; SEDA-17, 112; SEDA-18, 105)*

Data on the safety of loxoprofen are based on an open multicenter trial of about 4000 elderly patients in Japan (SEDA-17, 112). The side effects were mainly gastrointestinal, but other adverse effects, common to every NSAID, have been described: edema, dizziness, skin rashes, pruritus and a case of eosinophilic pneumonia and liver dysfunction (SEDA-17, 112). Two cases of a type I hypersensitivity reaction to this drug, characterized by generalized urticarial rash and dyspnea, have been reported. A fatal asthmatic attack after taking loxoprofen has been described in a young man with a history of asthma and nasal polyps (SEDA-18, 105).

Table 4. *Anthranilic acid derivatives*

Antrafenine	Meclofenamate
Etofenamate	Mefenamic acid
Floctafenine	Niflumic acid
Flufenamic acid	Talinflumate
Glafenine	Tolfenamic acid

Aceclofenac *(SED-11, 186; SEDA-15, 99; SEDA-18, 103)*

A hypersensitivity reaction characterized by multiple purpuric lesions and reduced renal function has been described in an elderly patient (SEDA,18, 103).

Bromfenac

Bromfenac sodium (2-amino-3-(4-bromo-benzoyl)-benzeneacetic acid sodium salt sesquihydrate) is another new NSAID whose reported adverse effects are dizziness, drowsiness, headache, nausea and vomiting (SEDA-17, 109).

Felbinac

Felbinac, an active metabolite of fenbufen, is used as a gel for topical treatment. Itching, rash and eosinophilia can occur (SEDA-16, 110).

Pronoprofen

Mutiple small bowel ulcers and massive bleeding have been described in a patient taking both oral pronoprofen and rectal indometacin (SEDA-17, 113).

Tropesin

Clinical experience with tropesin is still very limited, but, not unexpectedly, its adverse effects profile is similar to that of other compounds of this class (SEDA-17, 113).

ANTHRANILIC ACID DERIVATIVES

Again with this group of anti-inflammatory analgesics (Table 4) the hope of finding a compound with fewer side effects and greater therapeutic potency has not been realized. Some may even cause more side effects than do the older NSAID, but most variations prove to reflect nothing more than differences in dose as related to potency. Several closely related substances in this group—mefenamic, tolfenamic, flufenamic, meclofenamic and niflumic acid—are potentially nephrotoxic and have very similar renal side effects. Three other chemically related members of this group—glafenine, antrafenine and floctafenine (410[R])—similarly have a pattern of side effects in common, with shock in first place; a sensitization mechanism is thought to be responsible for this serious side effect.

Mefenamic acid *(SEDA-12, 90; SEDA-13, 83; SEDA-16, 112)*

It has been argued for more than a decade that, since a wide range of effective and less toxic drugs are available, there seems to be no reason for continuing to prescribe mefenamic acid and related drugs (SEDA-5, 93). All the same, some of the figures have been disputed and, strictly speaking, a comparative controlled study to estimate the incidence of side effects of mefenamic acid is still needed. The main reasons for concern are particular effects which are unexpected for an NSAID, such as hemolytic anemia, and which may therefore take the user by surprise.

Nervous system The occurrence of epileptic seizures in overdosed patients may indicate a degree of CNS toxicity. It has been stated that convulsions in the poisoned patient are more likely to occur with mefenamic acid than with other compounds (411[cr]). Other CNS reactions (headache, etc.) are less frequent than with the arylcarboxylic acid derivatives. Coma has also been described as a consequence of mefenamic acid overdosage (412[C]).

Hematological A number of hematological disturbances have been reported, though their overall incidence is probably moderate. They include hemolytic autoimmune anemia (Coombs-positive), leukopenia, thrombocytopenia and agranulocytosis (SED-8, 223; SEDA-4, 68). Neutropenic reactions have also been described (413[C]); severe neutropenia developed simultaneously with non-oliguric renal failure in two elderly hypothyroid females, and it would therefore seem prudent not to use mefenamic acid in hypothyroid patients (414[C]).

Gastrointestinal The gastrotoxicity of mefenamic acid is pronounced. Other than the common side effects (nausea, anorexia, vomiting, pain, diarrhea), there have been documented reports of acute peptic ulcer, intestinal hemorrhage, hematemesis, abdominal distension and profuse steatorrhea (SEDA-2, 97). Pancreatitis has also been reported. Mefenamic acid, in contrast to other NSAID, can provoke enteritis and colitis in patients with no known predisposing factors (415[C]). The drug has been demonstrated to accelerate bowel transit in healthy volunteers (SEDA-16, 112).

Urinary system The nephrotoxicity of this and anthranilic acid-related derivatives has already been mentioned. A number of renal effects have been demonstrated in animals. Acute renal failure, renal papillary necrosis and non-oliguric renal failure have been reported in man (416[c], 417[c]). Renal biopsies of more recent cases of renal failure have revealed interstitial nephritis, mesangial proliferation and focal pedicel fusion, a previously undescribed finding (418[C]).

Skin Fixed drug eruption has been described in two patients within hours of taking mefenamic acid (SEDA-12, 90). In another case, a multifocal fixed drug eruption mimicked erythema multiforme (419[C]).

Special senses A patient with hyperacusia, vertigo and tinnitus has been described (SEDA-12, 90).

Genital system Although it can be used to relieve dysmenorrhea, mefenamic acid may also delay menstruation for several days (420[C]).

Hypersensitivity reactions Asthma and anaphylactic shock are the most dangerous of the acute hypersensitivity reactions. There is cross-sensitivity with other NSAID (165[R]). Rash, urticaria and pruritus accompany more serious reactions.

Overdosage Mefenamic acid overdose is characterized by CNS symptoms, such as generalized seizures, agitation and confusion sometimes progressing to coma, gastrointestinal problems (bloody diarrhea, abdominal pain and vomiting) and renal impairment (SEDA-13, 83; SEDA-14, 95; 421[r]).

Interactions A possible interaction between mefenamic acid and lithium has been recorded in a patient with reduced renal function (SEDA-13, 83).

Flufenamic acid/Meclofenamic acid *(SEDA-11, 97; SEDA-14, 95)*

These anthranilic acid derivatives are very similar to mefenamic acid. The withdrawal rate attributable to side effects ranges from 7 to 31% and is higher in long-term studies. Flufenamic and meclofenamic acid are not widely prescribed and, in consequence, there is scant evidence to show whether they have any advantage over other NSAID. Both have a high incidence of gastrointestinal side effects (30—60% of patients at recommended doses). Diarrhea, the most important, affects 11—46% of patients (SEDA-4, 68; SEDA-6, 99; SEDA-7, 116; SEDA-14, 95). Thrombocytopenia with positive rechallenge has been described. Rashes appear in less than 10% of patients. Meclofenamic acid has repeatedly exacerbated psoriasis when given for psoriatic arthritis (422[C]).

Niflumic acid *(SEDA-13, 83; SEDA-14, 95)*

The three atoms of fluorine in the niflumic acid molecule may be critically implicated in its side effects. However, bearing in mind that niflumic acid has been on the market in many countries for more than a decade, fluoride-induced side effects (see below) are probably very rare, and they are clinically relevant only if the therapy is very prolonged. There are no adequate prospective studies estimating the comparative advantages and disadvantages of this agent.

Nervous system Headache has been reported as a common side effect of niflumic acid.

Hematological A case of agranulocytosis with a positive lymphocytic stimulation test, which recovered after withdrawal, has been described (423[C]).

Liver Hepatic damage has rarely been reported with this compound (SEDA-1, 90). A fatal case of icteric hepatitis in a patient taking niflumic acid and paracetamol has however been recorded (SEDA-13, 83).

Gastrointestinal Niflumic acid has the same gastrointestinal side effect profile as other anthranilic acids.

Urinary system Nephrotoxic effects have frequently been reported. Whether this really indicates a relatively high renal toxicity potential is an open question. Retention of water with edema, oliguria, proteinuria and an increase in urea and creatinine level have been described (SED-8, 223). Seven cases of acute renal failure in children which had been prescribed a short-term niflumic acid for ear-nose-throat disorders has recently been reported. Signs of hypersensitivity reaction were present in all cases (424).

Musculoskeletal system Niflumic acid has been stated to provoke rhabdomyolysis (SEDA-14, 95). There are several accounts of skeletal fluorosis attributable solely to chronic intoxication with fluoride as a result of long-term use of the drug (up to 11 years) (SEDA-6, 99). As each capsule of niflumic acid contains 50.5 mg fluoride, this could result in a daily intake of up to 0.30 g. The skeletal fluorosis was asymptomatic and discovered only by routine X-ray examination. The homogeneous osteosclerosis was, in all cases, found to be greatest in the axial skeleton. Urinary fluoride was high and associated with hypocalcemia, hypocalciuria and increased serum alkaline phosphatase levels. Bone biopsies disclosed an increase in trabecular bone volume suggestive of bone fluorosis. Persistent ingestion of fluoride leads to a high fluoride content in the bone, where fluorine is trapped, at the site normally occupied by the hydroxyl group in the apatitic mineral lattice (425[r]). Exactly how fluoride causes changes in bone structure and why osteocondensation is unevenly distributed is not known. It is not clear whether osteoid stimulation can increase bone fragility (426). In view of the dangers of fluoride accumulation in renal insufficiency, it seems wise to reccomend that niflumic acid should not be given in this condition. Fluoride osteosis has also been described, again in association with a prolonged flufenamic acid intake (427[C]).

Tolfenamic acid *(SEDA-13, 83; SEDA-18, 107)*

As already pointed out, the main side effects (particularly nephrotoxicity) of tolfenamic acid are similar to those of other anthranilic acids. Dysuria has however been reported more often, and confirmed by positive rechallenge (SEDA-4, 68). A recent report describes fixed drug eruption (SEDA-18, 107). Skin disorders are frequent, as is diarrhea. A rechallenge-positive hepatitis has also been described. Six patients with pulmonary infiltrations, possibly caused by tolfenamic acid, were reported to the Finnish National Centre for Adverse Drug Reaction Monitoring over a 12-year period. The fact that such features as Coombs-positive autoimmune hemolytic anemia and antinuclear antibodies were also present in some patients, suggests an immunological mechanism (SEDA-13, 83).

Glafenine *(SEDA-10, 84; SEDA-12, 90; SEDA-13, 82; SEDA-14, 95; SEDA-15, 102)*

At the time of writing, glafenine appears to have been withdrawn from the market in much of the world (428); up to 1991 it had been on sale in some 70 countries (though never marketed or accepted in others) in spite of a long history of severe reactions (particularly anaphylaxis, fatal hepatotoxicity and nephrotoxicity, seen even in normal doses) adequately documented in these volumes. As late as 1989 the European Community Committee on Proprietary Medicinal Products (CPMP) astonishingly recommended that glafenine be kept on the market, but with stricter control on its distribution and closer side-effect monitoring (429[C]). Firm restrictions or prohibitions nevertheless preceded or followed this recommendation in various European countries, and the CPMP finally condemned the drug in early 1992. Offerhaus has remarked that in view of strikingly poor investigational work and the dangerous adverse effects induced it is difficult to understand the reputation it has enjoyed for the last two decades (SEDA-13, 82).

Cardiovascular A rise in blood pressure coupled with the renal side effects (see below) was reported. Coronary spasm leading to myocardial infarction was described as part of an allergic reaction with Quincke's edema (SED-11, 90).

Hematological Acute hemolytic anemia, probably as part of an allergic reaction, has been reported (SED-9, 154) and leukopenia through an unknown mechanism has occurred. Furthermore, thrombocytopenic purpura with hemorrhage has been documented (430[C]).

Liver Liver injury has repeatedly been described in patients taking glafenine (SEDA-4, 69; SEDA-5, 106). Fatal hepatotoxicity as part of a general toxic reaction has been observed in several cases (431[C]). Glafenine-associated hepatic injury is characterized by a high prevalence of jaundice, a high fatality rate and a predominantly hepatocellular histological pattern of liver lesions, varying from spotty panlobular necrosis, centrilobular and submassive necrosis (acute pattern) to fibrosis and cirrhosis (chronic pattern) (432[C]). Choledocholithiasis composed of glafenic acid has been reported in a patient on long-term therapy with glafenine (SEDA-14, 95).

Gastrointestinal Gastrotoxicity has been reported but, surprisingly, gastrointestinal side effects are not a typical feature of glafenine treatment, perhaps because of its relatively weak effects on prostaglandins.

Urinary system A number of nephrotoxic features of glafenine treatment have been observed in preclinical and clinical studies. Glafenine is nephrotoxic when given in therapeutic doses and more especially in overdose (SEDA-4, 69). Acute oliguria, anuria, increased blood urea and creatinine, proteinuria and the rise of blood pressure already mentioned have been reported repeatedly. Glafenine stones have been documented in five patients (433[C])

Hypersensitivity reactions Although rash has sometimes occurred (434[Cr]), the hypersensitivity reactions giving rise to concern have been much more serious; many acute allergic, anaphylactic reactions have been observed (SEDA-4, 69; SEDA-6, 98; 431[C], 435, 436). Shock was present in more than 50% of these cases, being registered in 24 out of 1517 reports on the drug collected by the Pharmacovigilance Unit in Lyons (434[Cr]). The isolated fever sometimes seen and confirmable by rechallenge (437[C]) is probably also of hypersensitive origin. Interstitial nephritis, hepatitis and pulmonary hypersensitivity have been reported.

Muscle Symptoms of rhabdomyolysis, which started a few hours after glafenine intake and was accompanied by other disorders, were observed in two patients (438[c]).

Interactions Interaction with methotrexate has been described in a patient with rheumatoid arthritis (SEDA-14, 95)

Floctafenine

As already pointed out, floctafenine is very closely related to glafenine and its side-effects profile is similar. As floctafenine has been demonstrated to interact with coumarin anticoagulants, the same may be true for other anthranilic acids (SEDA-7, 116). Since the withdrawal from the market of both antrafenine and glafenine, it is difficult to understand why floctafenine is still used (SEDA-17, 113).

Antrafenine

This anthranilic acid was never widely marketed, but it again closely resembles glafenine and floctafenine (SED-9, 153; SEDA-7, 116; SEDA-11, 96). The same adverse problems must therefore be expected and some have been described, e.g. nephrotoxicity (SEDA-4, 69; 439[c]). Gastrotoxicity has been reported to be less than with aspirin (440[c]), again no doubt merely because it is a weak anti-inflammatory drug.

Etofenamate

Local irritation and contact dermatitis have been described as side effects of this topical agent in 0.8–2% patients (SEDA-11, 97). A large multicenter study of over 4000 patients reported local side effects in 6.4% of patients and they were the reason for treatment being interrupted in 0.3% of them (SEDA-12, 90). When etofenamate is administered intramuscularly it can cause local pain, irritation and sterile abscesses as can happen with other NSAID. Also, general adverse effects are similar with other NSAID: allergic reactions, gastrointestinal disturbances, headache, dizziness and salt and water retention (SEDA-17, 113).

Talinflumate

Talinflumate is a recent addition to the NSAID family. As expected, gastrointestinal side effects are the most frequent (399[R]).

OXICAM DERIVATIVES *(SEDA-10, 85; SEDA-11, 97)*

Drugs belonging to this group, especially isoxicam and piroxicam, have been widely discussed in recent years because of their very high consumption and their still unclear safety profile. Isoxicam has been suspended in several countries (France, Italy) due to a negative benefit/risk ratio. Piroxicam is suspected of pronounced gastrointestinal toxicity, especially in elderly women. The number of adverse reaction reports to this drug is, bearing in mind the vast scale on which it is now used, not disproportionately high.

Piroxicam

Piroxicam was the first of the oxicam compounds and by far the most widely used. It is a prostaglandin- and platelet-aggregation inhibitor. Its long half-life (36–48 hours) allows it to be given in a single daily dose.

Side effect data from 46 trials involving 3827 patients, 2716 of them however treated only short-term (less than 12 weeks), have been reviewed (SEDA-6, 1; 442[R]). In 20 controlled trials that involved 816 patients, side effects occurred in 27.1% of cases and were the reason for discontinuing treatment in 2.2%. However, a non-controlled study registered side effects in only 15.9% of patients. Allowing for all analyses and reviews, it would seem that the overall side-effect profile of piroxicam is qualitatively the same as for other NSAID, with gastrointestinal complaints at the top of the list. Analysis of the side-effect profile of suppository and dispersible tablet formulations shows that it is very like that of the standard capsule (SEDA-13, 83).

A parenteral formulation of piroxicam caused somnolence more frequently than did diclofenac in a double-blind study, whereas diclofenac provoked more gastric discomfort and nausea than piroxicam. Local adverse effects of both drugs were pain, burning and induration at the site of injection (SEDA-15, 103).

In the attempt to reduce gastric toxicity, piroxicam has been complexed with cyclodestrins. Nevertheless studies on healthy volunteers have documented that piroxicam β-cyclodestrin is less toxic than either piroxicam or indometacin. The few clinical data available show that gastrointestinal tract side effects are the most frequent (SEDA-16, 113).

ADVERSE REACTION PATTERN

General and toxic reactions These reactions involve the gastrointestinal system and occur in up to 40% of patients. The incidence of peptic ulcer is about 1% and appears to be dose-related. The incidence rises to 7% in patients who receive doses higher than 20 mg/day for several weeks (443[R]). CNS reactions are the second most frequent type of side effect. Changes in laboratory findings (creatinine, SGOT, SGPT) are frequent, but the clinical relevance of this observation seems to be slight.

Hypersensitivity reactions These do not seem to be a problem with piroxicam treatment, although skin or mucosal reactions have been reported. Shock has been described.

Tumor-inducing effects These have not been reported.

ORGANS AND SYSTEMS

Nervous system Side effects have been described in approximately 11% of patients and include *headache, dizziness, drowsiness, fatigue and sweating* (444[C]).

Mineral and fluid balance Severe *hyponatremia*, clinically characterized by increasing confusion and disorientation, has been reported with piroxicam (SEDA-13, 83).

Hematological Piroxicam can cause *thrombocytopenia*. A well-documented case of thrombocytopenic purpura due to an immunological mechanism has been described (SEDA-13, 83). As a prostaglandin inhibitor, piroxicam also *decreases platelet aggregation* and prolongs bleeding time. *Leukopenia*, with the leukocyte count returning to normal after withdrawal of the drug, has been reported (445). *Agranulocytosis* has been described in a woman who was treated with the drug for 3 days. However, she recovered rapidly after stopping therapy (SEDA-14, 95). Aplastic anemia which completely recovered after withdrawal of piroxicam has been described (SEDA-17, 114). There may be a fall in hemoglobin and hematocrit, unassociated with gastrointestinal blood loss.

Liver A transient *elevation of SGOT and SGPT* can occur. A case of biopsy-proven *hepatitis* has been noted in a patient who was also taking other medication (SEDA-5, 107). Cases of *acute hepatitis* have been described recently. Two elderly women developed acute hepatocellular injury which progressed to fatal *subacute hepatic necrosis* (SEDA-12, 93; 446[C], 447[C]).

Gastrointestinal As indicated above, gastrointestinal side effects are the most frequent. Although *epigastric distress, nausea, abdominal pain, constipation, flatulence and diarrhea* have all been reported, they rarely interfere with treatment. *Esophageal lesions* have been recorded in young healthy volunteers during treatment with piroxicam (448[C]). An unusual case of a *gastrocolic fistula* occurred in an old man treated with piroxicam for 2 months (449[C]). *Peptic ulceration* and *gastrointestinal bleeding* were recorded in 1—1.4% of patients taking 20 mg of piroxicam daily. A dose-response relationship has been found. A daily dose of 40 mg increases the ulcer incidence to 6.9% patients. A comparative trial that studied gastrointestinal blood loss after 972 mg of aspirin taken 4 times a day for 4 days and after various doses of piroxicam (20 mg once, 5 mg 4 times and 10 mg 4 times a day) revealed that piroxicam did not cause an increase in fecal blood loss, whereas aspirin did so. Gastroscopic evidence of irritation was also greater with aspirin (450[C]). The debate on the ulcerogenicity and relative safety of piroxicam continues as new reports are published (SEDA-10, 85, SEDA-11, 97; SEDA-12, 91). No 'perfect' epidemiological study has been carried out to date. Therefore, the only thing that can be said is that piroxicam's ulcerogenicity increases with dose and that in this respect 20 mg/day constitutes 'high-dose' therapy, especially for elderly women patients.

Urinary system Transient and probably insignificant rises in urea or BUN are often associated with piroxicam therapy. Since creatinine levels do not increase, the renal effect of the drug is functional rather than toxic. Renal function should be monitored in long-term therapy and its use avoided in renal insufficiency. An occasional patient develops *edema* and *dysuria*.

Hematuria with purpuric rash and Henoch-Schönlein purpura have been described (451[C]). Fatal *acute renal failure* owing to diffuse interstitial nephritis has recently been described in a young man (SEDA-14, 95). *Hyperkalemia* has been repeatedly described in connection with prolonged piroxicam intake, especially in the elderly (SEDA-8, 110; SEDA-10, 87). Chemotherapy-induced uric acid nephropathy appears to be more frequent when piroxicam is added to cancer chemotherapy.

Skin Minor skin *rashes*, often transient, are a relatively common finding, as is the case with other NSAID. Light-induced skin eruptions have been reported to national ADR monitoring centers in a number of countries and they seem to be particularly frequent with piroxicam. Such *photoreactions* are generally reported to occur only 1—6 days after the start of therapy and are characterized by pruritic, papulovesicular or bullous eruptions, usually restricted to light-exposed areas of the skin. Clinical, histological and provocation studies are not conclusive for distinguishing the eruptions as photoallergic or phototoxic (SEDA-13, 76; SEDA-15, 103; 452[R]). A recent study which revealed a cross-reaction between thiosalicylic acid and piroxicam supports the concept that photosensitive reactions induced by piroxicam have a photoallergic mechanism and can occur soon after the initiation of therapy when patients have previously been sensitized to thiosalicylate (SEDA-16, 113) (453). The wide range of cutaneous side effects is completed by various types of *exanthemas, urticaria, vasculitis* and *life-threatening reactions* (TEN, EM and pemphigus) (SEDA-11, 192; SEDA-8, 110; SEDA-13, 77). Fixed drug eruptions have also been described (SEDA-16, 113). After piroxicam intake and sun exposure a patient with Sjögren's syndrome developed the typical cutaneous lesions and serological markers of SLE, despite drug withdrawal (454[C]).

Special senses *Blurred vision* and *burning eyes*, as well as *tinnitus*, have been reported (SEDA-5, 107). A permanent sensorineural *hearing loss* has been described (455[C]).

Risk situations Clinical and pharmacokinetic data indicate that reduced excretion of piroxicam (impaired renal function in the elderly can lower excretion of the drug by 33%) increases the risk of dose-related gastrointestinal side effects; most reports of such effects indeed relate to *elderly women*. The dose used in this patient group should therefore be as low as possible and certainly not above 20 mg/day. Although the demand from consumers advocates that piroxicam should not be given to the elderly at all attracted worldwide attention, it has not been accepted as valid.

Second-generation effects These have not been reported. See, however, the general section of this chapter.

Interactions Interactions with *lithium* have been reported in the form of increased lithium toxicity, as occurs with some other NSAID (456[C]). Furosemide natriuresis and kaliuresis can be reduced by short-term treatment with piroxicam in hypertensive patients with impaired renal function (SEDA-16, 113). The antipyrine test is used as the index for estimating the ability of a subject to metabolize drugs; the half-life of antipyrine has been reported to be prolonged and metabolic clearance significantly reduced in proportion to the dose of piroxicam administered to healthy young volunteers (SEDA-16, 113).

Isoxicam *(SEDA-11, 97)*

This oxicam derivative has a shorter (30 hours) half-life than piroxicam. However, wide variation in the half-life, plasma clearance values, and mean steady-state plasma levels have been documented. Except for edema, the incidence of other side effects seems to be unrelated to age (457[R]). As already pointed out, serious skin reactions (Stevens-Johnson syndrome and Lyell's disease) have been the cause of temporary withdrawal of isoxicam in several countries, even though analysis of 1800 patients with rheumatoid arthritis or degenerative joint disease failed to confirm any increased risk (458[r]). The main reactions are gastrointestinal (pain, dyspepsia, nausea, vomiting, stomatitis, constipation, occasionally peptic ulcer), which occur in up to 80% of patients, followed by the skin reactions already mentioned. Isoxicam is an example of how reports received by ADR monitoring centers cannot always be quantitatively validated in clinical reviews, though this does not necessarily discount the validity of the former.

Tenoxicam *(SEDA-11, 100; SEDA-14, 95; SEDA-15, 103; SEDA-17, 114; SEDA-18, 107)*

Tenoxicam is a piroxicam analog ($t_{1/2}$, 75 hours) that it is still after some years largely in the clinical evaluation stage. As experience slowly accumulates, it is becoming clear that the pattern of side effects is similar to that of piroxicam. However, tenoxicam seems to cause slightly fewer serious gastrointestinal effects (459[R]). Fecal blood loss is lower than with aspirin (SEDA-8, 111). A large multicenter hospital-based study confirmed that tenoxicam and piroxicam had a similar tolerance rating: 13% of patients suffered severe side effects, most often gastrointestinal (i.e. melena, hematemesis, rectal bleeding, exacerbation of ulcerative colitis) and serious rashes (SEDA-15, 103). Gastrointestinal side effects seem to be more frequent in patients taking higher doses of tenoxicam (460[r]), as one would expect. In an open noncomparative study on 1267 patients performed to examine the safety of tenoxicam in general practice, the commonest adverse reactions were gastrointestinal (11.4%), central and peripheral nervous system disorders (2.8%) and skin reactions (2.5%) (461). Patients treated long-term with tenoxicam seem to be at low risk for nephrotoxic effects; the prevalence of urinary system adverse effects was 0.07% in clinical trials that included 67 000 patients (462). Tenoxicam may provoke severe bronchoconstriction and nasal obstruction in aspirin-sensitive asthmatic patients (SEDA-12, 93). Adverse effects which have been reported also include phototoxic dermatitis, thrombocytopenia, edema of the legs, pruritus and hypersalivation (SEDA-12, 93). More recently three cases of toxic epidermal necrolysis (Lyell's syndrome) have been described (SEDA-17, 114). A fixed drug eruption with cross-sensitivity to droxicam and tenoxicam has been reported (SEDA-18, 107). On the other hand, tenoxicam may not cross-react in patients with photosensitivity to piroxicam (SEDA-18, 107).

Whether the differences in pharmacokinetic parameters found in elderly patients have any clinical significance is unknown (SEDA-12, 93).

Cinnoxicam

The side effects profile of cinnoxicam is similar to that of the other oxicam derivatives. Gastrointestinal (81%), central nervous system and cutaneous effects (4% each) were the most frequent in a multicenter post-marketing surveillance study on 2969 patients; 12% of patients suffered from side effects (SEDA-16, 113).

Droxicam

Droxicam, a pro-drug of piroxicam, has similar side effects to piroxicam in still very limited clinical experience (SEDA-16, 113). Due to numerous Spanish reports of non-fatal liver damage, according to the CPMP the summary of product characteristics should state that serious hepatic damage can occur (SEDA-17, 113).

Lornoxicam

There are insufficient data to indicate whether this drug, chlortenoxicam, is safer for the gastrointestinal tract than other oxicam derivatives (SEDA-16, 113).

MISCELLANEOUS DRUGS

Ademetionine (*S*-adenosylmethionine) *(SEDA-13, 83)*

S-Adenosylmethionine is a physiological product, the anti-inflammatory and analgesic effects of which have been demonstrated in experimental animals. Convincing evidence of these activities in patients is still lacking. Results of clinical trials on the treatment of osteoarthritis, as presented at a recent symposium organized by the manufacturer, and thus open to selection bias, indicated that the drug is well tolerated. In a large uncontrolled short-term Phase IV trial, side effects (moderate or severe) were reported by 21% of the patients and treatment was discontinued because of side effects in 5.2% cases. Side effects were mainly gastrointestinal problems (nausea, stomach ache, heartburn, diarrhea), CNS symptoms (headache, dizziness, sleep disturbances, fatigue) and skin rashes.

Benzydamine (benzindamine) *(SEDA-11, 100; SEDA-12, 94; SEDA-13, 84)*

Skin reactions, including photosensitivity as well as contact dermatitis (when used topically), have been reported.

Cincophen

Only in 1991 did Spanish authorities withdraw cincophen from the market, although it has been known for some time that the drug can cause severe hepatitis (SEDA-17, 114).

Cloximate

This non-steroidal anti-inflammatory drug is approved in a small number of countries, so experience with its use is still limited. A number of the usual side effects have been reported; they include headache, insomnia, drowsiness, anorexia, gastrointestinal symptoms, a transient increase in BUN, leukopenia, thrombocytopenia and exanthema (463[C]).

CPH-8

CPH-8 is composed of two semisynthetic lignam glycosides and, when used in the treatment of rheumatoid arthritis, causes the same gastrointestinal problems as Proresid (see '*Podophyllum derivatives*' below).

Diacerein (diacetylrhein) *(SEDA-14, 96; SEDA-15, 103)*

Very few clinical data are available on rhein, the active metabolite of diacetylrhein, a recently developed anthraquinone derivative, said to be effective in the treatment of osteoarthritis. The drug does not affect arachidonic acid metabolism and might therefore be better tolerated than other NSAID as far as renal and gastric toxicity is concerned. However, epigastric or abdominal pain and diarrhea remain the most frequent side effects; the latter has been confirmed as the most frequent effect (37%) observed in the diacerein group in a recent study on patients with osteoarthritis (464). Skin reactions have also been reported.

Enorfazone

First results of clinical evaluation of this drug indicate sleepiness, dry mouth, rash, and various gastrointestinal disturbances as the most important side effects (465[C]).

Flupirtine

Flupirtine causes predominantly CNS side effects (visual, disorientation, confusion, tremor). About 26% of patients develop minor adverse reactions (466[c]).

Hyaluronate sodium *(SEDA-15, 103)*

Intra-articular sodium hyaluronate injection used for the treatment of osteoarthritis of the knee has been reported to cause hemarthrosis, an increase in joint effusion volume and, possibly, phlebitis. More experience is needed to establish whether this form of treatment is an efficacious and well-tolerated alternative therapy.

Isoxepac

Up to now only gastrointestinal blood loss increases over the pre-treatment levels have been described; evidence for the properties of the drug appears very incomplete (SEDA-8, 110).

IX 207-887

10-Methoxy-4H-benzo-(4,5)cyclohepta-(1,2-6) thiophene-4 yliden acetic acid) is a slow-acting drug for use in rheumatoid arthritis and its mechanism of action involves the inhibition of the release of IL-1. Adverse effects have occurred in 22% of cases. Skin reactions were the most frequent, but hepatitis and gastrointestinal disorders were also reported (SEDA-17, 114).

Lefetamine

Up to the present, sedation, tiredness, gastrointestinal disturbances, headache, sweating and flushing have been observed (467[R]).

MW-2884 *(SEDA-15, 103)*

MW-2884 (10-methoxy-4H-benzo(4,5)-cyclohepto-thiophene-4-glindene-acetic acid) is a monokine-release inhibitor. Twelve patients with rheumatoid arthritis who were so treated presented gastrointestinal disturbances, temporary impairment of liver function and allergic skin reactions; one patient withdrew from the drug because of severe urticaria.

Nefopam *(SEDA-11, 100; SEDA-15, 104)*

Nefopam is an orphenadrine derivative. It is mainly regarded as an analgesic agent. Most of the adverse reactions responsible for the interruption of treatment, the more prominent being nausea, drowsiness and sweating, have been related to the anticholinergic properties of the compound (SEDA-11, 100). The unsatisfactory side-effects profile of this drug has been confirmed in two recent studies carried out on cancer and rheumatoid arthritis (SEDA-15, 104).

Nimesulide

Gastrointestinal symptoms (pyrosis, pain, nausea), cutaneous changes (rash, itching) and CNS side effects (nervousness, vertigo) have been encountered (468[R]). Nimesulide was shown to cause less gastric damage than indometacin in an endoscopic study during short-term treatment (SEDA-15, 104). Thrombocytopenia occurred in a patient with HIV infection treated with nimesulide, but regressed rapidly when the drug was withdrawn (SEDA-14, 96). A fixed drug eruption has been described in the oral cavity of a young woman (SEDA-17, 114). Data from a post-marketing survey of nimesulide in the short-term treatment of osteoarthritis in 22 938 outpatients confirmed that the adverse-effects profile of the drug is similar to that of the other NSAID (SEDA-16, 114). However, the data that nimesulide is well-tolerated in aspirin-sensitive asthmatic patients requires confirmation in more extensive well-conducted studies (SEDA-18, 107).

Orgotein *(SEDA-12, 94; SEDA-14, 96)*

Orgotein is an enzyme (CuZn superoxide dismutase) present in all mammalian cells. It is obtained from bovine liver through various steps including chromatography. Reliable and published clinical experience of its properties is limited. Orgotein can be given parenterally or topically. Local painful subcutaneous reactions, erythema, urticaria and pruritus have been observed (469[R]), as have temperature rise, swelling, redness, heat and pain at the injection site (470[C]).

Two anaphylactic reactions have been reported: one after intra-articular injection, the other after submucosal bladder injection of orgotein. An IgE-mediated mechanism was demonstrated in the former case (SEDA-12, 94; SEDA-14, 96). In Germany, marketing approval for orgotein has been suspended because of severe reactions and deaths most due to hypersensitivity (SEDA-18, 107).

Osmic acid *(SEDA-12, 94)*

Osmic acid is injected into joints for chemical synovectomy. Local pain, fever and effusions are associated with this therapy. Cutaneous necrosis is less frequent. Nerve damage and abnormal urinary findings (hematuria, proteinuria and leukocyturia), possibly related to intraarticular injection of osmic acid, have been reported (SEDA-12, 94). This is a potentially dangerous treatment which certainly should not be given to younger patients.

Oxaceprol

Use of this hydroxyproline derivative has been proposed for treatment of arthrosis. Efficacy and safety have not yet been documented. Gastrointestinal, CNS (headache, dizziness) and skin reactions have been reported (471).

Phenazopyridine *(SEDA-13, 84)*

Phenazopyridine is an azodye introduced as a urinary tract analgesic. Due to its nephrotoxicity (oliguria, cylindruria, decreased creatinine clearance with crystal deposits in renal tubules and interstitial tissue) it should not be used in patients with suspected renal disease and insufficiency or in patients with glucose-6-phosphate dehydrogenase deficiency. Vesical concrements have also been described. Hematological side effects include methemoglobinemia and hemolytic anemia, particularly after overdose (472[C]). Liver and ocular toxicity have been reported (473[R]). Aseptic meningitis has been diagnosed in a patient who had three distinct episodes of fever and confusion after taking the drug (SEDA-13, 84). Because of its toxicity, the traditional use of phenazopyridine as part of a fixed-dose combination no longer seems to be justified and the drug as a whole seems to be ripe for re-assessment.

***Podophyllum* derivatives** *(SEDA-15, 104)*

Proresid (mitopodozide) is a mixture of more than 20 *Podophyllum emodi* derivatives used for many years in some countries for the treatment of rheumatoid arthritis as a disease-modifying agent. It is a microtubulin antagonist that is comparable with colchicine and griseofulvin. Its use, however, has been limited because the treatment is often complicated by severe diarrhea, abdominal pain, nausea and vomiting. Leukopenia and thrombocytopenia have also been reported.

Proquazone/Fluproquazone

These quinazoline derivatives are of minor importance. Gastrointestinal side effects are the most frequent (SEDA-4, 69; SEDA-5, 197; SEDA-10, 88). Because fluproquazone caused hepatic injury in 14% of patients in clinical trials, evaluation was halted (474[C]).

Pyritinol *(SEDA-15, 104)*

This curious old vitamin B_6 derivative was used from 1961 onwards and then largely abandoned as a psychostimulant of doubtful efficacy, but apparently without side effects. When it was re-introduced in some countries for the treatment of rheumatoid arthritis, side effects were registered in 25% of patients. A hypothesis has been advanced that the cross-allergic reaction of pyritinol with D-penicillamine, which is widely used in the treatment of rheumatoid arthritis, is the reason for the apparently higher frequency of problems in rheumatic patients (475[C]R). Side effects include gastrointestinal symptoms (diarrhea, gastralgia, nausea, loss of taste) and skin changes (pemphigus, lichenoid eruption). Thrombocytopenia has also been reported, as has reversible extramembranous glomerulonephritis with a nephrotic syndrome (476[C]), and even a myasthenia-like clinical picture. Acute polymyositis with positive rechallenge has been described (477[C]). An autoimmune hypoglycemic syndrome re-occurred twice in an elderly woman following treatment with pyritinol (SEDA-15, 104).

Rimazolium

In spite of the fact that rimazolium is not a new drug, published experience is very scanty. Vertigo, drowsiness and nausea have been reported (SED-10, 172; SEDA-7, 117).

Romazarit

Romazarit is a slow-acting drug for use in rheumatoid arthritis that was well tolerated in pharmacokinetic studies. It is structurally similar to clobuzarit, which was withdrawn because of four possible cases of Stevens-Johnson syndrome (SEDA-17, 114).

Steopronine *(SEDA-15, 104)*

The side-effect profile of this sulfhydryl compound, which is used in rheumatoid arthritis, seems to be similar to that of penicillamine. In a long-term open study, treatment had to be interrupted in 30% of 36 patients due to severe side effects. Seven patients presented mucocutaneous reactions (dermatitis, pruritus, stomatitis, glossitis, ageusia), three proteinuria and one thrombocytopenia and leukopenia.

Timegadine *(SEDA-15, 104)*

This guanidine derivative inhibits cyclo-oxygenase, lipo-oxygenase and phospholipase activity. Reported side effects are skin rashes, oral lesions, epigastralgia and nausea, dizziness and vertigo, dysuria and sleep disturbances. Liver enzyme changes and pneumonitis have also been described.

DRUGS USED IN THE TREATMENT OF GOUT

Gout and pseudo-gout result from the deposition of uric acid and other crystals in the body due to their

diminished excretion or increased production. The condition may arise in renal failure, be associated with other disease, be induced by drugs (diuretics, cytotoxic drugs, pyrazinamide) or be idiopathic. The latter form is the commonest. These diseases can manifest as an acute condition (starting suddenly or more gradually with acute pain) or as a chronic one with a number of consequences (arthrosis, renal damage, bursitis). Several structurally dissimilar groups of drugs are used in the treatment of acute or chronic gout:
(a) Drugs which decrease the production of uric acid by inhibition of the enzyme xanthine oxidase, e.g. allopurinol.
(b) Drugs which increase uric acid excretion (secretion via the renal tubules) by non-specific inhibition of its tubular reabsorption. Probenecid, sulfinpyrazone and benzbromarone are examples, but many anti-infiammatory drugs also have a uricosuric effect.
(c) Drugs which suppress the symptoms of acute gout, but affect neither the excretion nor production of uric acid. Colchicine, but also anti-inflammatory drugs (except aspirin), belong to this group.

Allopurinol *(SEDA-10, 89; SEDA-12, 94; SEDA-16, 114; SEDA-17, 114; SEDA-18, 107)*

ADVERSE REACTION PATTERN

General and toxic reactions These are rare. Toxic hepatitis, nephrolithiasis and hematological side effects have been described.

Hypersensitivity reactions These are common, sometimes severe, and even fatal. They include generalized vasculitis, a variety of skin eruptions, which can proceed to bullous and toxic exfoliative dermatitis, fever, lymphadenopathy and eosinophilia. If the reaction is severe and generalized, renal, ocular, hematological and hepatic damage, inciuding acute hepatocellular necrosis, may occur. Recovery from such a condition is slow and the prognosis uncertain (SED-10, 172; SEDA-10, 89). There have been attempts at desensitization by slowly increasing the dosage (478[C], 479).

Tumor-inducing effects These have not been reported.

ORGANS AND SYSTEMS

Nervous system Apart from *headache* and *vertigo*, adverse effects involving the nervous system are rare. *Peripheral neuropathy* of a transient nature has been reported (SEDA-18, 107). *Seizures*, which were unresponsive to the customary anticonvulsive therapy but which disappeared when allopurinol was discontinued, have been described in a patient with a primary neurological disorder (480[C]). Occasional reports of a possible anticonvulsive effect of allopurinol have prompted its use in therapy-resistant epileptic patients and withdrawal of the drug in one of these patients precipitated a convulsive status epilepticus (SEDA-16, 114).

Endocrine, metabolic Since allopurinol blocks the conversion of xanthines to uric acid, their excretion in urine is increased; this can create a risk of *xanthine crystal formation* in the urinary system or even in the muscles. It is still an open question whether a predisposition or renal disease must be present in order to precipitate these side effects. It is also not yet known whether increased excretion of *orotic acid* due to interaction of allopurinol with pyrimidine formation has any consequences for the latter's side effects or for its role in reducing glucose tolerance (481[C]).

Hematological *Eosinophilia* and *leukocytosis* are part of a general hypersensitivity reaction. *Leukopenia* and *neutropenia* are sometimes associated with allopurinol treatment. It has been stated that patients on cytostatic therapy are more susceptible to bone marrow depression if they take allopurinol as well (SED-9, 155; 482), but this has not been confirmed by other data (483[C]). *Agranulocytosis* is extremely rare. Cases of *aplastic anemia* have recently been reported (SEDA-13, 84; 484[C], 485[c]), some in patients with renal failure. This confirms the necessity of decreasing the allopurinol dose in patients with renal insufficiency and for monitoring for possible toxicity (SEDA-16, 114).

Liver As pointed out above, hepatitis can be part of a generalized hypersensitivity reaction. *Hepatotoxicity* ranges from mild granulomatous hepatitis to severe hepatocellular necrosis (SED-5, 155; SEDA-4, 70). It seems that renal impairment is a prerequisite for a severe hepatic reaction.

Urinary system Vasculitis due to a general hypersensitivity reaction can cause *renal failure*, *oliguria* and *decreased creatinine clearance*. Histologically, this is due to vasculitis and tubular necrosis with fibrinoid deposits. *Acute renal failure* due to xanthine crystals in the kidney tubules during antineoplastic chemotherapy has been reported (486[C]). Nephrolithiasis as a side effect of allopurinol treatment has also been described. A *granulomatous interstitial nephritis* has been recorded (SEDA-12, 94).

Skin Reactions affecting skin have a general incidence of 10%, being more common in renal patients and in patients receiving thiazide diuretics. Persistently high serum concentrations of oxypurinol correlate well with the development of this syndrome (487[CR]). *Rash, urticaria, erythematous eruptions, papulovesicular reactions* and *pruritus* may be the only sign of hypersensitivity or may be part of a generalized reaction. Such dangerous reactions as *exfoliative dermatitis* and *Lyell's syndrome* can develop but are rarely seen (SEDA-5, 108). Unusual cutaneous lesions characterized by benign lymphocytic infiltration have recently been documented (SEDA-14, 96). Toxic pustuloderma can be added to the list (SEDA-18, 108). The positive association of severe skin reactions with AW33 and B17 in the HLA system suggests a genetic predisposition to these reactions (488).

Other systems *Muscular pain* has been reported. Allopurinol has possible cataractogenic potential, but a recent study found no evidence to confirm this risk (SEDA-15, 104). It has been suggested that allopurinol uncovers *latent lichen planus* (489[C]).

Hypersensitivity reactions Hypersensitivity reaction to allopurinol occurs in about 10—15% of patients. Successful desensitization with both oral and intravenous allopurinol has been reported (SEDA-17, 114). In the 'allopurinol hypersensitivity syndrome' the skin is the organ most prominently involved (490[R]). Symptoms developed after 2—5 weeks of allopurinol treatment. Hepatic involvement was present in 40% and renal involvement in 45% of cases; 25% of patients had combined renal and hepatic lesions. Where such problems occur one can, as pointed out above, discontinue treatment and then start again with smaller but increasing doses, in essence seeking to produce desensitization. The hypersensitivity syndrome has been estimated to occur in 1/1000 hospitalized patients. A major complication of the hypersensitivity syndrome is an extensive cutaneous staphylococcal infection with septicemia and endocarditis. Gastrointestinal hemorrhage, disseminated intravascular coagulation and adult respiratory distress syndrome have also been described. Twenty to 30% of patients with severe hypersensitivity syndrome die. Treatment includes drug withdrawal and use of systemic corticosteroids (prednisone 40—200 mg/dl) for several months.

Risk situations Previous *renal impairment* and *diuretic therapy* predispose to an increased frequency of side effects. The exact mechanism has still to be elucidated. The active metabolite, oxypurinol, accumulates in *renal failure* but also in patients on a *low protein diet*. *Acute gout* can be exacerbated at the beginning of allopurinol treatment unless the drug is combined with colchicine or an anti-inflammatory agent.

Interactions Concomitant treatment of allopurinol with *ampicillin* is stated to increase considerably the incidence of adverse skin reactions: in one study, these occurred in 22.4% of patients taking the combination (491[C]), though the interaction was not confirmed in a later investigation (492[C]). *Thiazides* enhance excretion of orotic acid, which is already increased during allopurinol treatment. The possible implications of this fact for the frequency of side effects are not known. It has been pointed out above that the risk of bone marrow depression by *cytostatics* can be potentiated by allopurinol, but the latter also appears to potentiate the therapeutic effect of cytostatics since it competitively inhibits the metabolic breakdown of these purine derivatives. Recent studies in animals suggest that this reaction only occurs with oral mercaptopurine (493), though there is older evidence that the toxicity of cyclophosphamide and other cytostatics can be increased by allopurinol (SED-9, 156). The dangerous combined use with azathioprine has been confirmed by the occurrence of new cases of bone marrow suppression, particularly in patients with impaired renal function (SEDA-16, 114). When *aluminium hydroxide* is given alongside allopurinol, there can be an increase in serum uric acid, probably because the antacid reduces absorption of allopurinol (SEDA-13, 84). Two well-documented reports described a marked increase of cyclosporin serum concentrations when administered with allopurinol (SEDA-18, 108).

Probenecid *(SED-9, 157)*

This uricosuric agent (ineffective in renal impairment) is generally well tolerated. Soreness of the gums, gastrointestinal irritation, skin rashes and pyrexia as well as nephrotic syndrome have been reported. Interactions of probenecid with contrast media, antibiotics (penicillins, cephalosporins), indometacin and methotrexate (the excretion of which is reduced, leading to an increase in effect) have been documented. Aspirin reduces the effect of probenecid.

Sulfinpyrazone

Sulfinpyrazone, a pyrazolone derivative used both as a uricosuric agent and an anti-platelet drug, has proved to have side effects similar to those produced by phenylbutazone when administered in the long-term (SEDA-6, 104). However, in studies involving a large number of patients and employing the drug for secondary prevention of myocardial infarction (indication which was not accepted) the incidence of side effects (494[C]) has not been considerable.

Respiratory Sulfinpyrazone can precipitate bronchoconstriction in some aspirin-sensitive patients (495[C]). There is no cross-sensitivity with dipyrone.

Hematological Prolonged treatment produces a high incidence of thrombocytopenia and granulocytopenia. After drug withdrawal, these changes are completely reversible (SED-9, 157), but sulfinpyrazone has been involved in the development of myelomonocytic leukemia and multiple myeloma when given together with colchicine (496[C]). Inhibition of platelet aggregation has already been mentioned.

Urinary system Impairment of renal function and even acute renal failure can follow sulfinpyrazone treatment because of various mechanisms, namely immuno-allergic-induced acute interstitial nephritis, inhibition of renal prostaglandins and precipitation of uric acid stones. These changes are probably reversible, since cases in which renal impairment spontaneously normalized upon interruption of treatment have been reported (497[C]). The antinatriuretic effects of sulfinpyrazone could be dangerous in patients with impaired cardiac function (498[C]).

Interactions By reducing the metabolic clearance of warfarin, sulfinpyrazone enhances the hypoprothrombinemic effect of this agent and the consequences can be life-threatening (499[C]). A biphasic interaction (enhancement followed by antagonism) has been described with phenylbutazone therapy. Sulfinpyrazone, like other NSAID, interferes with the antihypertensive action of β-blockers (500[C]).

Benzbromarone

This uricosuric agent causes diarrhea (3—4% of patients), urate and oxylate lithiasis, urinary sand, renal colic and allergy in a small number of patients (501). Hepatic damage, recovered after withdrawal of the drug, has been recently described (SEDA-18, 108). Since it is a coumarin derivative, it may potentiate vitamin K antagonists.

Colchicine *(SED-8, 227; SEDA-12, 94; SEDA-13, 84; SEDA-16, 114)*

This antimitotic agent is highly effective in the treatment of gout but is characterized by considerable toxicity. Diarrhea is indeed used as a criterion for adequate dosage. Accidental overdose occurs relatively often and can be dangerous. For these reasons, NSAID (except aspirin) are often used in acute gout instead of colchicine.

Nervous system Neuropathy, polyneuritis, toxic encephalitis, delirium and coma have been observed in severe colchicine intoxication only. During prolonged treatment, neuritis, muscular weakness and myopathy occur more commonly than previously thought in patients with decreased renal function. In some cases the neuromyopathy was part of a multi-organ system failure, but in others the syndrome was not accompanied by other features of colchicine toxicity. Patients on long-term treatment with colchicine should therefore receive low doses (probably no more than 0.6 mg/day) and have their serum creatine kinase monitored (SEDA-12, 94).

Endocrine, metabolic Transient diabetes and hyperlipidemia have been reported. Metabolic acidosis is probably a consequence of heavy, cholera-like diarrhea. Progressive decrease of libido was attributed to colchicine intake in patients with familial Mediterranean fever (502[C]).

Mineral and fluid balance Ionic imbalance is also associated with diarrhea.

Hematological Bone marrow depression is common after colchicine overdosage and intoxication. It is less common in therapeutic doses. Fatal cases of agranulocytosis are more often associated with bone marrow aplasia (SEDA-4, 70; 503[C]). Bone marrow depression usually occurs between the 3rd and 6th day of acute intoxication. Cytoplasmic inclusions in neutrophils and megaloblastic anemia have been described. Administration of the usual therapeutic doses intravenously and orally to two patients with reduced renal function caused profound and prolonged neutropenia which was complicated by septicemia resulting in death (SEDA-13, 84).

Gastrointestinal GI symptoms commonly develop after therapeutic doses; they are, as indicated above, even used for titration of the dose. Diarrhea is frequent followed by nausea, vomiting and abdominal pain. Long-term therapy may provoke steatorrhea, malabsorption and defects in intestinal enzyme activity.

Urinary system Acute renal failure can be associated with colchicine intoxication.

Skin Blood dyscrasias can be associated with ecchymosis and purpura. Allergic skin changes are rare. Alopecia is common after acute intoxication, but also after prolonged treatment (SEDA-5, 109).

Muscular system Acute rhabdomyolysis with fever, muscle cramps, rises in creatine phosphokinase and lactic acid dehydrogenase, phlebitis at the injection site and transitory leukothrombocytopenia have been reported (504[C]).

Risk situations There is controversy about the long-term toxicity of colchicine. In familial Mediterranean fever, the use of colchicine in low doses (1—2 mg/day) for 15—18 years has been well tolerated even by young patients as reported in a recent study (SEDA-16, 114). Other studies confirm the necessity of adjusting the colchicine dose for creatinine clearance in long-term use to avoid the risk of myoneuropathy (SEDA-16, 114). Moreover colchicine should not be used in patients undergoing hemodialysis since the drug can be removed neither by dialysis nor by exchange transfusion. Parenteral (i.v.) colchicine is, according to published evidence, potentially much more toxic than the oral drug. Because of its very low benefit/toxicity ratio and the availability of less dangerous treatments, colchicine should not be administered intravenously (SEDA-5, 109; SEDA-13, 84; SEDA-16, 115).

Second-generation effects Reversible azoospermia (later not confirmed) was observed after long-term treatment. Due to its antimitotic properties, colchicine should not be given during pregnancy (SED-9, 158).

Overdosage Acute intoxication with colchicine occurs relatively often, because the therapeutic dose is close to the toxic dose. They are characterized by proteiform symptomatology, gastrointestinal, hematological and neurological reactions being the most frequent (SEDA-7, 118). An accidental overdose of colchicine by nasal insufflation has been reported in a young male drug abuser who had mistaken it for methamphetamine. The intoxication picture was one of gastrointestinal distress, myalgia, thrombocytopenia, hypocalcemia and hypophosphatemia (505).

Interactions There is a report of acute reversible cyclosporine toxicity in a renal transplant patient a few days after colchicine was administered for an acute attack of gout (SEDA-16, 115).

REFERENCES

1. Evens RP. Nonrheumatologic uses of NSAIDS. Drug Intell. Clin. Pharm 1984;18:52.
2. Peleg II, Maibach HT, Brown SH, Wilcox CM. Aspirin and nonsteroidal anti-inflammatory drug use and the risk of subsequent colorectal cancer. Arch Intern Med 1994; 154(4):394.
3. Waterhouse DM, Brenner D. Aspirin, NSAIDs, and risk reduction of colorectal cancer. The problem is translation. Arch Intern Med 1994;28(154(4)):366—368.
4. Muscat JE, Stellman SD, Wynder EL. Nonsteroidal anti-inflammatory drugs and colorectal cancer. Cancer 1994; 74(7):1847—1854.
5. Andersen K, Launer LJ, Ott A et al. Do nonsteroidal anti-inflammatory drugs decrease the risk for Alzheimer's disease? The Rotterdam Study. Neurology 1995; 45(8):1441—1445.
6. Rich JB, Rasmusson DX, Folstein-MF et al. Nonsteroidal anti-inflammatory drugs in Alzheimer's disease. Neurology 1995;45(1):51—55.
7. Ransford KD. Introduction and historical aspects of the side-effects of anti-inflammatory analgesic drugs. In: Rainsford KD, Velo JP, eds. Side-effects of Anti-inflammatory Drugs. Part I: Clinical and Epidemiological Aspects. Lancaster: MTP Press 1987;3.
8. Furst DE. The basis for variability of response to anti-rheumatic drugs. Clin Rheumatol 1988;2:395.
9. Brooks PM, Day RO. Non-steroidal anti-inflammatory drugs—differences and similarities. N Engl J Med 1991; 324:1716.
10. Brune K, Graf P. Non-steroid anti-inflammatory drugs: influence of extra-cellular pH on biodistribution and pharmacological effects. Biochem Pharmacol 1978;27:525.
11. Vane JR, Ferreira SH, eds. Anti-inflammatory Drugs. New York: Springer Verlag, 1979.
12. Moncada S, Vane JR. Mode of action of aspirin like drugs. Adv Intern Med 1979;24:1.
13. Abramson SB, Weissmann G. The mechanisms of action of non-steroidal anti-inflammatory drugs. Arthr Rheum 1989;32:1.
14. Vane J Towards a better aspirin. Nature 1994;367:215.
15. Higgs GA, Moncada S, Vane JR. The mode of action of anti-inflammatory drugs which prevent peroxidation of arachidonic acid. Clin Rheum Dis 1980;6:675.
16. Kitchen EA, Dawson W, Rainsford KD, Cawston T. Inflammation and possible modes of action of anti-inflammatory drugs. In: Rainsford KD, ed. Anti-inflammatory and Antirheumatic Drugs, Vol. 1. Boca Raton, FL: CRC Press, 1985;21.
17. Day RO, Graham GG, Williams KM, Champion G, de Jager J Clinical pharmacology of non-steroidal anti-inflammatory drugs. Pharmacol Ther 1987;33:384.
18. Day RO, Graham GG, Williams KM. Pharmacokinetics of non-steroidal anti-inflammatory drugs. Clin Rheumatol 1988;2:363.
19. Carson JL, Strom BL, Morse ML et al. The relative gastrointestinal toxicity of the non-steroidal anti-inflammatory drugs. Arch Intern Med 1987;147:1054.
20. Schoen RT, Vender RJ Mechanism of non-steroidal anti-inflammatory drug-induced gastric damage. Am J Med 1989; 86:449.
21. Roth SH, Bennett RE. Non-steroidal anti-inflammatorydruggastropathy. Arch Intern Med 1987;147:2093.
22. Langman MJS. Epidemiologic evidence on the association between peptic ulceration and anti-inflammatory drug use. Gastroenterology 1989;96(Suppl 2):640.
23. Fries JF, Miller SR, Spitz PW et al. Towards an epidemiology of gastropathy associated with non-steroidal anti-inflammatory drug use. Gastroenterology 1989;96(Suppl 2);647.
24. Henry DA, Johnston A, Dobson A et al. Fatal peptic ulcer complications and the use of non-steroidal anti-inflammatory drugs, aspirin, and corticosteroids. Br Med J 1987;295:1227.
25. Somerville K, Faulkner G, Langman M. Nonsteroidal anti-inflammatory drugs and bleeding peptic ulcer. Lancet 1986;i:462.
26. Pincus T, Griffin M. Gastrointestinal disease associated with non-steroidal anti-inflammatory drugs: new insights

from observational studies and functional status questionnaires. Am J Med 1991;91:209.
27. Fries JF, Williams CA, Bloch DA, Michel BA. Nonsteroidal anti-inflammatory drug-associated gastropathy: incidence and risk factor models. Am J Med 1991;91:213.
28. Gabriel SE, Jakkimainen L, Bombardier C. Risk for serious gastrointestinal complications related to use of nonsteroidal anti-inflammatory drugs. Ann Intern Med 1991; 115:787.
29. Willet LR, Carson TL, Strom BL. Epidemiology of gastrointestinal damage associated with nonsteroidal anti-inflammatory drugs. Drug Safety 1994;10:170.
30. Agrawal NM, Roth S, Graham DY et al. Misoprostol compared with sucralfate in the prevention of non-steroidal anti-inflammatory drug-induced gastric ulcer. Ann Intern Med 1991;115:195.
31. Garcia Rodriguez LA, Jick H. Risk of upper gastrointestinal bleeding and perforation aassociated with individual non-steroidal anti-inflammatory drugs. Lancet 1994;343:769.
32. Langman MJS, Weil J Wainwright P et al. Risk of bleeding peptic ulcer associated with individual non-steroidal anti-inflammatory drugs. Lancet 1994;343:1075.
33. Carson JL, Strom BL, Morse ML et al. The relative gastrointestinal toxicity of the non-steroidal anti-inflammatory drugs. Arch Intern Med 1987;147:1054.
34. Graham DY, Agrawal NM, Roth SH. Prevention of NSAID-induced gastric ulcer with misoprostol: multicentre, double-blind, placebo-controlled trial. Lancet 1988;ii:1277.
35. Levine JS. Misoprostol and nonsteroidal anti-inflammatory drugs: a tale of effects, outcomes, and costs. Ann Intern Med 1995;123:309.
36. Silverstein FE, Graham DY, Senior JR et al. Misoprostol reduces serious gastrointestinal complications in patients with rheumatoid arthritis receiving nonsteroidal anti-inflammatory drugs. A randomized, double-blind, placebo-controlled trial. Ann Intern Med 1995;123(4):241.
37. Laine L, Cominelli F, Sloane R et al. Interaction of NSAIDs and Helicobacter pylori on gastrointestinal injury and prostaglandin production: a controlled double-blind trial. Aliment Pharmacol Ther 1995;9(2):127-135.
38. Kim JG, Graham DY. *Helicobacter pylori* infection and development of gastric or duodenal ulcer in arthritic patients receiving chronic NSAID therapy. The Misoprostol Study Group. Am J Gastroenterol 1994;89(2):203—207.
39. Semble EL, Wu WC, Castell DO. Non-steroidal anti-inflammatory drugs and esophageal injury. Semin Arthr Rheum 1989;19:99.
40. Taha AS, Dahill S, Nakshabendi I et al. Oesophageal histology in long term users of non-steroidal anti-inflammatory drugs. J Clin Pathol 1994;47(8):705—708.
41. Langman MJS, Morgan I, Worral A. Use of anti-inflammatory drugs by patients admitted with small or large bowel perforations and haemorrhage. Br Med J 1985; 290:347.
42. Bjarnason I, Macpherson A. The changing gastrointestinal side effect profile of non-steroidal anti-inflammatory drugs. Scand J Gastroenterol 1989;24:56.
43. Bjarnason I, Hayllar J, Macpherson AJ et al. Side effects of nonsteroidal anti-inflammatory drugs on the small and large intestine in humans. Gastroenterology 1993;104:1832.
44. Allison MC, Howatson AG, Torrance CJ et al. Gastrointestinal damage associated with the use of nonsteroidal anti-inflammatory drugs. New Engl J Med 1992;327:749.
45. Lang J, Price AB, Levi AJ et al. Diaphragm disease: the pathology of NSAID induced small intestinal strictures. J Clin Pathol 1988;41:516.
46. Kwo PY, Tremaine WJ Nonsteroidal anti-inflammatory drug-induced enteropathy: case discussion and review of the literature. Mayo Clin Proc (1995);70(1):55.
47. Speed CA, Bramble MG, Corbett WA, Haslock I. Nonsteroidal anti-inflammatory induced diaphragm disease of the small intestine: complexities of diagnosis and management. Br J Rheumatol 1994;33(8):778.
48. O'Brien WN, Bagby GF. Rare adverse reactions to nonsteroidal anti-inflammatory drugs. Part II. J Rheumatol 1985;12:347.
49. International Agranulocytosis and Aplastic Anemia Study. Risks of agranulocytosis and aplastic anemia: a first report of their relation to drug use with special reference to analgesics. J Am Med Assoc 1986;256:1749.
50. Strom BL, Carson JL, Shinnar R et al. Nonsteroidal anti-inflammatory drugs and neutropenia. Arch Intern Med 1993;153:2119.
51. DeGruchy GC. Drug-Induced Blood Disorders. Melbourne: Blackwell Scientific Publications, 1979.
52. Sanford-Driscoll M, Knodel LC. Induction of hemolytic anemia by non-steroidal anti-inflammatory drugs. Drug Intell Clin Pharm 1986;20:925.
53. Moran M, Mozes MF, Maddux MS et al. Prevention of acute graft rejection by the prostaglandin E1 analogue misoprostol in renal-transplant recipients treated with cyclosporine and prednisone. N Engl J Med 1990;322:1183.
54. Richards IM, Fraser SM, Capell HA et al. A survey of renal function in outpatients with rheumatoid arthritis. Clin Rheumatol 1988;7:267.
55. Allred J, Wong W, Kafetz K. Elderly people taking nonsteroidal anti-inflammatory drugs are unlikely to have excess renal impairment. Postgrad Med J 1989;65:735.
56. Dunn MJ, Simonson M, Davidson EW et al. Nonsteroidal anti-inflammatory drugs and renal function. J Clin Pharmacol 1988;28:524.
57. Stillman MT, Schlesinger PA. Non-steroidal anti-inflammatory drug nephrotoxicity. Should we be concerned? Arch Intern Med 1990;150:268.
58. Whelton A, Stout RL, Spilman PS et al. Renal effects of ibuprofen, piroxicam and sulindac in patients with asymptomatic renal failure. Ann Intern Med 1990;112:568.
59. Murray MD, Brater DC. Adverse effects of nonsteroidal anti-inflammatory drugs on renal function. Ann Intern Med 1990;112:559.
60. Erikson LO, Sturfelt G, Thysell H et al. Effects of sulindac and naproxen on prostaglandin excretion in patients with impaired renal function and rheumatoid arthritis. Am J Med 1990;89:313.
61. Sandler DP, Burr FR, Weinberg CR. Non-steroidal anti-inflammatory drugs and the risk for chronic renal disease. Ann Intern Med 1991;115:165—?.
62. Eaton RA. A comparison of anaphylactoid reactions associated with non-steroidal anti-inflammatory drugs. ADR Highlights 1981;8116.
63. Strom BL, Carson JL, Schinnar R et al. The effect of indication on the risk of hypersensitivity reactions associated with tolmetin sodium vs other non-steroidal anti-inflammatory drugs. J Rheumatol 1988;15:695.
64. Czerniawska-Mysik G, Szczeklik A. Idiosyncrasy to pyrazolone. Drugs Allergy 1981;36:381.
65. Rashad S, Revell P, Hemingway A et al. Effect of nonsteroidal anti-inflammatory drugs on the course of osteoarthritis. Lancet 1989;ii:519.

66. Abdulrhman AA, Davis P. Osteoarthritis 1991. Current drug treatment regimens. Drugs 1991;41:193.
67. Schnitzer TJ, Popovich JM, Andersson GBJ et al. Effect of piroxicam on gait in patients with osteoarthritis of the knee. Arthr Rheum 1993;36:1207.
68. Kaiser U, Sollberger J, Hoigne R et al. Haut-Nebenwirkungen unter nicht-steroidalen Analgetika-Entzundungshemmern und sogenannten leichten Analgetika. Schweiz Med Wochenschr 1987;117:1966.
69. Fowler PD. Aspirin, paracetamol and non-steroidal anti-inflammatory drugs. A comparative review of side-effects. Med Toxicol 1987;2:338.
70. ADRAC. Photosensitivity reactions: a sunburnt country. Aust. Adverse Drug Reactions Bull March, 1983.
71. ADRAC. A sunburnt country revisited. Aust. Adverse Drug Reactions Bull February, (1987).
72. Fenner H. Hautreaktionen durch nicht-steroidale Antirheumatica. Dtsch Apoth Zt 1985;125:2654.
73. Paul E, Hellwich M. Die Wertigkeit des intracutanen Hauttestes bei Analgetika-Unverträglichkeit im Vergleich zur oralen Provokation. Z Hautkrankh 1987;62:705.
74. Maucher OM, Fuchs A. Kontakturtikaria im Epikutantest bei Pyrazolonallergie. Hautartzt 1983;34:383.
75. Roujeau JC, Bracq C, Huyn NT et al. HLA phenotypes and bullous cutaneous reactions to drugs. Tissue Antigens 1986;28:251.
76. Powles AV, Griffiths CEM, Seifert MH et al. Exacerbation of psoriasis by indometacin. Br J Dermatol 1987; 117:799.
77. Sendagorta E, Allegue F, Rocamora A et al. Generalized pustular psoriasis precipitated by diclofenac and indometacin. Dermatologica 1987;175:300.
78. Benjamin SJ, Ishak KG, Zimmerman HJ et al. Phenylbutazone liver injury: a clinical-pathologic survey of 23 cases and review of the literature. Hepatology 1981;1:255.
79. ADRAC. Diclofenac sodium and hepatic injury. Aust Adverse Drug Reactions Bull June, 1986.
80. Wilholm BE, Myrhed M, Ekman E. Trends and patterns in adverse drug reactions to non-steroidal anti-inflammatory drugs reported in Sweden. In: Rainsford KD, Velo JP, eds. Side-effects of Anti-inflammatory Drugs, Part I. Clinical and Epidemiological Aspects. Lancaster: MTP Press, 1987;55.
81. Brooks PM. Side effects of non-steroidal anti-inflammatory drugs. Med J Aust 1988;148:248.
82. Garcia-Rodriguez LA, Williams R, Derby LE, et al. Acute liver injury associated with nonsteroidal anti-inflammatory drugs and the role of risk factors. Arch Intern Med 1994;154(3):311—316.
83. Radack K, Deck C. Do non-steroidal anti-inflammatory drugs interfere with blood pressure control in hypertensive patients? J Cen Intern Med 1987;2:108.
84. Johnson AG, Nguyen TV, Day RO. Do nonsteroidal anti-inflammatory drugs affect blood pressure? A meta-analysis. Ann Intern Med 1994;121(4):289—300.
85. Mene P, Pugliese F, Patrono C. The effects of nonsteroidal anti-inflammatory drugs on human hypertensive vascular disease. Semin Nephrol 1995;15(3):244—252.
86. Klassen DK, Jane LH, Young DY, Peterson CA. Assessment of blood pressure during naproxen therapy in hypertensive patients treated with nicardipine. Am J Hypertens 1995;8(2):146—153.
87. Overlack A, Adamczak M, Bachmann W et al. ACE-inhibition with perindopril in essential hypertensive patients with concomitant diseases. The Perindopril Therapeutic Safety Collaborative Research Group. Am J Med 1994; 97(2):126—134.
88. Van de Ouweland FA, Gribnau FWJ, Meyboom RHB. Congestive heart failure due to non-steroidal anti-inflammatory drugs in the elderly. Age Ageing 1988;17:8.
89. O'Brien WN, Bagby GF. Rare adverse reactions to non-steroidal anti-inflammatory drugs. Part I. J Rheumatol 1985;12:13.
90. Simon RA. Oral challenges to detect aspirin and sulfite sensitivity in asthma. Allerg Immunol Paris 1994;26(6):216—218.
91. Bernard A, Kersley JB. Sensitivity to insect stings in patients taking anti-inflammatory drugs. Br Med J 1986; 292:378.
92. O'Brien WN, Bagby GF. Rare adverse reactions to non-steroidal anti-inflammatory drugs. Part IV. J Rheumatol 1985;12:785.
93. Bruce-Jones PN, Crome P, Kalra L. Indometacin and cognitive function in healthy elderly volunteers. Br J Clin Pharmacol 1994;38(1):45—51.
94. Tonkin AL, Wing LMH. Interactions of nonsteroidal anti-inflammatory drugs. Clin Rheumatol 1988;2:455.
95. Tracy TS, Worster T, Bradley JD et al. Methotrexate disposition following concomitant administration of ketoprofen, piroxicam and flurbiprofen in patients with rheumatoid arthritis. Br J Clin Pharmacol 1994;37(5):453—456.
96. Anonymous. BGA 'loose' butazone Coombs warning. Scrip 1985;974:8.
97. Anonymous. Mofebuzone restriction explained. Scrip 1985;965:1.
98. Martindale: The Extra Pharmacopoeia, 28th ed. London: The Pharmaceutical Press, 1983;273.
99. Prescott LF, Critchley JAJH, Bala-li-Mood M. Phenylbutazone overdosage: abnormal metabolism associated with hepatic and renal damage. Br Med J 1980;281:1106.
100. Berlinger WG, Spector R, Flanigan MJ et al. Hemoperfusion for phenylbutazone poisoning. Ann Intern Med 1982;96:334.
101. Adverse Drug Reactions Advisory Committee. Phenylbutazone. Med J Aust 1979;2:553.
102. Szczeklik A, Gryglewski RJ, Czerniawska-Mysik G. Relationship of inhibition of prostaglandin biosynthesis by analgesics to asthma attack in aspirin sensitive patients. Br Med J 1975;1:67.
103. Thurston JGB, Marks P, Trapnell D. Lung changes associated with phenylbutazone treatment. Br Med J 1976;2:1422.
104. Linnoila M, Seppalla T, Mattila MJ Acute effect of antipyretic analgesics alone or in combination with alcohol on human psychomotor skills related to driving. Br J Clin Pharmacol 1974;1:477.
105. Schwarzmann E, Quest M. Kasuistische Betrachtungen zur Phenylbutazon-Struma. Dtsch Gesundheitswes 1973; 28:1417.
106. Botiger LE, Westerholm B. Drug-induced blood dyscrasias in Sweden. Br Med J 1973;3:339.
107. Botiger LE. Phenylbutazone, oxyphenbutazone and aplastic anemia. Br Med J 1977;2:265.
108. Inman WH. Study of fatal bone marrow depression with special reference to phenylbutazone and oxyphenbutazone. Br Med J 1977;1:1500.
109. Davidson C, Mahohitharajah SM. Drug induced antiplatelet antibodies. Br Med J 1973;1:545.
110. Hartwich G, Lutz H. Occurrence of leukemia. Verh Dtsch Ges Inn Med 1973;79:394.

111. Benjamin SB, Ishak KG, Zimmerman HJ et al. Phenylbutazone liver injuries: a clinical-pathological survey of 23 cases and review of the literature. Hepatology 1981;1:255.
112. Schwenke W, Schwenke G, Willgeroth C. Die grosse obere Gastrointestinalblutung unter besonderer Berucksichtigung der akuten Magenschleimhautlasionen durch Medikamente. Z Gesamte Inn Med Ihre Grenzgeb 1975;30:198.
113. Cuthbert MF. Adverse reactions to non-steroidal antirheumatic drugs. Curr Med Res Opin 1974;2:600.
114. Schwabe H. Magenperforation und Blutung nach langeren Gaben von Antirheumatika. 2. Allgemeinmedizin 1975;51:1097.
115. Cheli T, Chiancamerla G. Proctiti emorragiche da medicamenti locali. Minerva Gastroenterol 1974;20:56.
116. Liaras H, Niedhardt JH, Tairras JP et al. Les enterites et colites aigues necrosantes: essai nosologique et pathogenique-etude clinique: a propos de 8 cas. J Clin (Paris) 1968;96:501.
117. Wigley RAD. The New Zealand experience. Aust NZ J Med 1976;6:37.
118. Eischbeck R, Huhle G, Stiller D, Zucker G. Durch immunologische in vitro Untersuchungen gesicherte hochgradige Phenylbutazon Uberempfindlichkeit bei einem Fall von Morbus Lyell. Dtsch Gesundheitswes 1975;30:2331.
119. Zurcher K, Krebs A. Nebenwirkungen interner Arzneimittel auf die Haut unter besonderer Berücksichtigung neuerer Medikamente. Dermatologica (Basel) 1970;141:119.
120. Willets GS. Ocular side effects of drugs. Br J Ophthalmol 1969;53:252.
121. Hadida A, Groulier P. Necrose de la fesse apres une injection de phenylbutazone. Marseille Chir 1968;20:270.
122. Vormittag W, Kolarz G. Chromosomenuntersuchungen vor und nach Infusionstherapie mit Phenylbutazon. Arzneim-Forsch 1979;29:1163.
123. Farber D, Liel E. Phenylbutazon-Vergiftung in Kindesalter. Tagl Prax 1968;9:231.
124. Anvik T. Acute phenylbutazone poisoning. Tidsskr Nor Laegeforen 1970;90:95.
125. Field JB, Ohta M, Boyle C, Reaner A. Potentiation of acetohexamide hypoglycemia by phenylbutazone. N Engl J Med 1967;277:889.
126. Polak F. Die hemmende Wirkung von Phenylbutazon auf die durch einige Antihypertonika hervorgerufene Blutdrucksenkung bei Hypertonikern. Z Gesamte Inn Med Ihre Grenzgeb 1967;22:375.
127. Ansell BM, Major G, Liyanage SP et al. A comparative study of butacote and naprosyn in ankylosing spondylitis. Eur J Rheumatol Inflam 1980;2:45.
128. Anonymous. Phenylbutazone and oxyphenbutazone: time to call a halt. Drug Ther Bull 1984;22:5.
129. Kalbazzaz MK, Harvey JE, Hoffman JN. Alveolitis and haemolytic anaemia induced by azapropazone. Br Med J 1986;293:1537.
130. Andreasen PB, Simonsen K, Brocks K et al. Hypoglycaemia induced by azapropazone—tolbutamide interaction. Br J Clin Pharmacol 1981;12:581.
131. Geaney DP, Carver JG, Aronson JK et al. Interaction of azapropazone with phenytoin. Br Med J 1982;284:1373.
132. Geaway DP, Carver JG, Davies CL, Aronson JK. Pharmacokinetic investigation of the interaction of azapropazone with phenytoin. Br J Clin Pharmacol 1983;15:727.
133. Anonymous. Other action on suxibuzone. Scrip 1982;669:14.
134. Sturrock R, Isaacs A, Hart FD. Feprazone compared with indometacin in the management of rheumatoid arthritis. Practitioner 1975;215:94.
135. Montanari C et al. Large cooperative multicentric trial with feprazone in the inflammatory process of dental tissues. Curr Ther Res 1975;17:166.
136. Chierichetti S. Esempio di monitoraggio attivo su un farmaco: il feprazone. Emerg Med 1976;500.
137. Du Lac Y. Banc d'essai therapeutique d'un anti-inflammatoire Eumotol. Reumatologie 1979;8:405.
138. Kadar D, Kallow W. Acute and latent leukopenia reaction to antipyrine. Clin Pharmacol Ther 1980;28:820.
139. Drtil J, Sanda Z. Veranderungen der Magenschleimhaut nach Gebrauch einiger Antiasthmatika und Analgetika Antipyretika. Z Gesamte Inn Med 1968;23:236.
140. Johansson S, Angesvall L, Bengtsson U, Wahlquist L. Uroepithelial tumours of the renal pelvis associated with abuse of phenacetin containing analgesics. Cancer 1974; 33:743.
141. Shabert P, Nagel R, Leistenschneider W. Zur Frage der Koinzidenz von Tumoren der oberen Harnwege mit chronischer Einnahme analgetischer Substanzen. In: Haschek H, ed. Internationales Symposium uber Probleme des Phenacetin Abusus. Vienna: Facta Publication, Verlag H, Egerman, 1973;257.
142. Kienlein-Kletschka B, Baurle G. Epicutane Sofort reaktion. Aktuel Dermatol 1981;7:88.
143. Symmons D, Clark B, Panayi G et al. Differentialdosing study of pirazolac, a new non-steroidal anti-inflammatory agent, in patients with rheumatoid arthritis. Curr Med Res Opin 1985;9:542.
144. Epstein P, Judkin JS. Agranulocytosis in Mozambique due to amidopyrine, a drug withdrawn in the West. Lancet 1980;ii:254.
145. Barrett AJ, Weller E, Rozengust N et al. Amidopyrine agranulocytosis: drug inhibition of granulocyte colonies in the presence of patient's serum. Br Med J 1976;2:850.
146. Gondemand M. Acute agranulocytosis induced by amidopyrine or phenothiazine derivatives: report of 31 cases. Semin Hop Paris 1976;52:1513.
147. Bartoli E, Masala RF, Chiandussi L. Drug induced asthma. Lancet 1976;i:1357.
148. Scholz H, Meyer W. Akute Agranulozytose und intrahepatische Cholestase nach Aminophenazon bei einem 12 jahrigen Madchen. Dtsch Gesundheitswes 1972;27:205.
149. World Health Organization. Aminophenazone a possible cancer hazard? WHO Drug Info 1977;July—September:9.
150. Offerhaus L. Metamizol: een honderdjarige treurnis. Ned Tijdschr Geneeskd 1987;131:479.
151. Levy M, Shapiro S. Metamizol: een honderdjarige treurnis. Ned Tijdschr Geneeskd 1987;131:1680.
152. Palva ES, Eranko PO. Dipyrone and agranulocytosis in Finland. Paper presented at: Conference of the International Union of Pharmacology, August, 1987.
153. Heimpel H, Kewitz H. Agranulozytose und Schock nach Metamizol. Dtsch Arztebl 1982;79:48.
154. Ribera A, Monasterio J, Acebedo G et al. Dipyrone induced immune haemolytic anaemia. Vox Sang 1981;41:32.
155. Bajoghli M, Ajudani TS, Gharavi M. Generalized oedema of newborn associated with the administration of dipyrone. Eur J Pediatr 1977;126:271.
156. Zoppi M, Hoigne R, Keller MF et al. Fall in systolic blood pressure due to dipyrone (novaminsulfon): result of the Comprehensive Hospital Drug Monitoring Berne

(CHDMB) (in German). Schweiz Med Wochenschr 1983; 113:1768.
157. Laverda AM, Casara GL, Furlannt M et al. Ipertensione endocranica acuta benigna da sulfafenazone. Riv Ital Pediatr 1981;7:83.
158. Anonymous. Dow Lepetit drops diftalone. Scrip 1977; October 15:22.
159. Gotzsche PC. Patients' preference in indometacin trials: an overview. Lancet 1989;i:88.
160. Smith AP. Response of aspirin allergic patients to challenge by some analgesics in common use. Br Med J 1971;2:494.
161. Sheehan GJ, Kutzner MR, Chin WD. Acute asthma attack due to ophthalmic indometacin. Ann Intern Med 1989;111:337.
162. Golding D. Angina and indometacin. Br Med J 1970; 4:62.
163. Wenmalm A, Carlsson I, Edlund A et al. Central and peripheral haemodynamic effects of non-steroidal anti-inflammatory drugs in man. Arch Toxicol 1984;Suppl 7:350.
164. Dzau VJ, Packer M, Lilly LS et al. Prostaglandins in severe congestive heart failure: relation to activation of the renin-angiotensin system and hyponatremia. N Engl J Med 1984;310:347.
165. Szczeklik A, Grylewski RJ, Czerniawska-Mysik G. Participation of prostaglandins in pathogenesis of aspirinsensitive asthma. Naunyn-Schmiedeberg's Arch Exp Pathol Pharmacol 1977;297:S99.
166. Eade OE, Acheson ED, Cuthbert MF, Hawkes CH. Peripheral neuropathy and indometacin. Br Med J 1975;2:994.
167. Rothermich NO. Deafness and hand tremor with indometacin. J Am Med Assoc 1973;226:1471.
168. Van Bel F, Van de Bor M, Stijnen T et al. Cerebral blood flow velocity changes in preterm infants after a single dose of indometacin: duration of its effect. Pediatrics 1989;84:802.
169. Edwards AD, Wyatt JS, Richardson C et al. Effects of indometacin on cerebral haemodynamics in very preterm infants. Lancet 1990;335:1491.
170. Berine J, Jubiz W. Effect of indometacin on the hypothalamic-pituitary-adrenal axis in man. J Clin Endocrinol 1978;47:713.
171. Thack JR, Bozeman MT. Indometacin induced hyperglycemia. J Am Acad Dermatol 1982;7:502.
172. Durao V, Prata MM, Goncalues LMP. Modification of the antihypertensive effect of beta-adrenoreceptor blocking agents by inhibition of endogenous prostaglandin synthesis. Lancet 1977;ii:1005.
173. Watkins J, Abbott EC, Hensby CN et al. Attenuation of hypotensive effect of propranolol and thiazide diuretics by indometacin. Br Med J 1980;281:702.
174. Menkes E, Kutas GJ Fatal aplastic anemia with indometacin plus acetylsalicylic acid. Can Med Assoc J 1977; 117:118.
175. Cuthbert MF. Adverse reactions to non-steroidal antirheumatic drugs. Curr Med Res Opin 1974;2:600.
176. Friedman Z, Whitman V, Maisels MJ et al. Indometacin disposition and indometacin-induced platelet dysfunction in premature infants. J Clin Pharmacol 1978;18:272.
177. Fenach FF, Bannister WH, Grech JL. Hepatitis with biliverdinaemia in association with indometacin. Br Med J 1967;3:155.
178. De Kraker-Sangster M, Bronkhorst FB, Brandt KH et al. Massale Levercelnecrose na toediening van indometacine in combinatie met aminofenazon. Ned Tijdschr Geneeskd 1981;125:1828.
179. Cappell MS, Kozicky O, Competiello LS. Indometacin-associated cholestasis. J Clin Castroenterol 1988;10:445.
180. MacLaurin BP, Richards DA, Heads D. Indometacin associated peptic ulceration. NZ Med J 1978;88:439.
181. Controt S, Roland D, Barbier J et al. Acute perforation of colonic diverticula associated with short-term indometacin. Lancet 1978;ii:1055.
182. Levy N, Gaspar E. Rectal bleeding and indometacin suppositories. Lancet 1975;i:577.
183. Hansen TM, Matzen P, Madsen P. Endoscopicevaluation of the effect of indometacin capsules and suppositories on the gastric mucosa in rheumatic patients. J Rheumutol 1984;11:484.
184. Anonymous. 'Osmosin' may not reduce indometacin's side effects. Scrip 1983;82:1.
185. ter Borg EJ, de Jong PE, Meijer S et al. Indometacin and ibuprofen induced reversible renal failure in a patient with systemic lupus erythematosus. Neth J Med 1987;30:181.
186. ter Borg EJ, de Jong PE, Meijer S, Kallenberg CGM. Renal effects of indometacin in patients with systemic lupus erythematosus. Nephron 1989;53:238.
187. Fawaz Estrup F, Ho G Jr. Reversible acute renal failure induced by indometacin. Arch Intern Med 1981;141:1670.
188. Ambanelli U, Ferracioli GF, Serventi G et al. Changes in serum urinary zinc induced by ASA and indometacin. Scand J Rheumatol 1982;11:63.
189. Akbarpour F, Afrasiabi A, Vaziri ND. Severe hyperkalemia caused by indometacin and potassium supplementation. South Med J 1985;78:756.
190. O'Sullivan M, Hanly JG, Molloy M. A case of toxic epidermal necrolysis secondary to indometacin. Br J Rheumatol 1983;22:47.
191. Katayma H, Kawada A. Exacerbation of psoriasis induced by indometacin. J Dermatol 1981;8:323.
192. Rubens Duval A, Villiaumey J, Kaplan G, Bailly D. Surmenage et deterioration rapide de coxo-femorales arthrosiques au cours de therapeutiques anti-inflammatoires non corticoides. Rev. Rhum 1970;37:535.
193. Rashad S, Hemingway A, Rainsford K et al. Effect of non-steroidal anti-inflammatory drugs on the course of osteoarthritis. Lancet 1989;ii:519.
194. Romanowska-Gorecka B, Oleszczak B. The masking effect of Indocid on the course of purulent inflammatory processes. Pol Tyg Lek 1969;24:2019.
195. Galassi P, Vicentini C, Scapellato F et al. L'impiego dell'indometacina e del metamizolo per via endovenosa nella colica renale. Minerva Urol 1983;35:295.
196. Vincent G, Vincent H. Indocid 50 mg injectable dans la pathologie disco-vertebrale. Sem Hop 1986;62:2189.
197. Harinck E, Ertbruggen IV, Senders RCh, Moulaert AJ Problems with indometacin for ductus closure. Lancet 1977;ii:245.
198. Merritt TA, Bejar R, Coraza M et al. Clinical trials of intravenous indometacin for closure of the patent ductus arteriosus. Pediatr Cardiol 1983;4:Suppl.2, 71.
199. Schoenfeld A, Freedman S, Hod M et al. Antagonism of antihypertensive drug therapy in pregnancy by indometacin? Am J Obstet Gynecol 1989;161:1204.
200. Di Battista C, Landizi L, Tamborius G. Focomelia et agenesia del pene in neonato. Minerva Pediatr 1975;27:675.
201. Moise Jr KJ, Huhta JC, Sharif DS et al. Indometacin

in the treatment of premature labor: effects on the fetal ductus arteriosus. N Engl J Med 1988;319:327.
202. Hendricks SK, Smith JR, Moore DE et al. Oligohydramnios associated with prostaglandin synthetase inhibitors in preterm labour. Br J Obstet Gynaecol 1990;97:312.
203. Haddad J Indometacin and ischemic brain injury. J Pediatr 1990;116:839.
204. Baerts W, Fetter WP, Hop WC et al. Cerebral lesions in preterm infants after tocolytic indometacin. Dev Med Child Neurol 1990;32:910.
205. Restaino I, Kaplan BS, Kaplan P et al. Renal dysgenesis in a monozygotic twin: association with in utero exposure to indometacin. Am J Med Genet 1991;39:252.
206. Norton ME, Merril J, Cooper BAB, et al. Neonatal complications after the administration of indometacin for preterm labor. New Engl J Med 1993;329:1602.
207. Eeg-Olafsson O, Malmros I, Elwin CE, Sten B. Convulsions in a breast-fed infant after maternal indometacin. Lancet 1978;ii:215.
208. Allan SG, Knox J, Kerr F. Interaction between diuretics and indometacin. Br Med J 1981;283:1611.
209. Mor R, Pitlik S, Rosenfeld JB. Indometacin and Moduretic-induced hyperkalemia. Isr J Med Sci 1983;19:535.
210. Davis P. Comparative efficacy and tolerance of sulindac (Clinoril) in geriatric and nongeriatric patients. Curr Ther Res 1985;37:945.
211. Anonymous. Clinoril adverse reactions. FDA Drug Bull 1979;9:29.
212. Delcambre B. the sulindac profile use of sulindac in hospital and private practice: multicentre study in general practice. Eur J Rheumatol Inflam 1978;1:47.
213. Bordier P, Knutz DD. Sulindac: clinical results of treatment of osteoarthritis. Eur J Rheumatol Inflam 1978;1:27.
214. Andrade L, Fernandez A. Sulindac in the treatment of osteoarthritis: a double blind 8 week study comparing sulindac with ibuprofen and 96 weeks of long term therapy. Eur J Rheumatol Inflam 1978;1:36.
215. Durance RA, Jacobi RK, Thompson M, Whittington JR. A multicentre comparative analgesic study of fenoprofen and sulindac in rheumatoid arthritis. Curr Ther Res 1979;26:79.
216. Calin A, Britton M. Sulindac in ankylosing spondylitis: double blind evaluation of sulindac and indometacin. J Am Med Assoc 1979;242:1885.
217. Anonymous. Clinoril sulindac: cardiac abnormalities. ADR Highlights, 1979;July 3.
218. Takimoto CH, Lynch D, Stulbarg MS. Pulmonary infiltrates associated with sulindac therapy. Chest 1990;97:230.
219. Kruis R, Barger R. Paranoid psychosis with sulindac. J Am Med Assoc 1980;243:1420.
220. Greenberg GN. Recurrent sulindac induced aseptic meningitis in a patient tolerant to other non-steroidal anti-inflammatory drugs. South Med J 1988;81:1463.
221. Romeril KR, Duke DS, Hollings PE. Sulindac induced agranulocytosis and bone marrow culture. Lancet 1981; ii:523.
222. Miller JL. Marrow aplasia and sulindac. Intern. Med 1980;92:129.
223. Stambaugh Jr JE, Gordon RL, Geller R. Leukopenia and thrombocytopenia secondary to clinoril therapy. Lancet 1980;i:594.
224. Rosenbaum JT, O'Connor M. Thrombocytopenia associated with sulindac. Aust Rheum 1981;24:753.
225. Andrews R, Russell N. Aplastic anaemia associated with a non-steroidal anti-inflammatory drug: relapse after exposure to another such drug. Br Med J 1990;301:38.
226. Kaul A, Reddy JC, Fagman E et al. Hepatitis associated with the use of sulindac in a child. J Pediatr 1981;99:652.
227. Smith FE, Lindberg PJ Life threatening hypersensitivity to sulindac. J Am Med Assoc 1980;246:213.
228. Rodriguez LAG, Williams R, Derby LE, Dean A. Acute liver injury associated with nonsteroidal anti-inflammatory drugs and the role of risk factors. Arch Intern Med 1994;154:311.
229. Giroux Y, Moreau M, Kass TG. Cholestatic jaundice caused by sulindac. Can J Surg 1982;25:334.
230. Anonymous. Sulindac (Clinoril) a new drug for arthritis. Med Lett 1979;21:1.
231. Graham DY, Smith L, Holmes GL et al. Nonsteroidal anti-inflammatory effect of sulindac sulfoxide and sulfide on gastric mucosa. Clin Pharmacol Ther 1985;38:65.
232. Levine MS, Rothstein RD, Lanfer I. Giant esophageal ulcer due to Clinoril. Am J Roentgenol 1991;156:955.
233. Rigau J, Pique JM, Rubio E et al. Effects of longterm sulindac therapy on colonic polyposis. Ann Intern Med 1991;115:952.
234. Bunning RD, Barth WF. Sulindac: a potentially renal-sparing non-steroidal anti-inflammatory drug. J Am Med Assoc 1982;248:2864.
235. Dunn MJ, Simonson M, Davidson EW et al. Nonsteroidal anti-inflammatory drugs and renal function. J Clin Pharmacol 1988;28:524.
236. Stillman MT, Schlesinger PA. Non-steroidal anti-inflammatory drug nephrotoxicity. Should we be concerned? Arch Intern Med 1990;150:268.
237. Whelton A, Stout RL, Spilman PS et al. Renal effects of ibuprofen, piroxicam and sulindac in patients with asymptomatic renal failure. Ann Intern Med 1990;112:568.
238. Champion de Crespigny PJ, Becker GJ, Ihle BU et al. Renal failure and nephrotic syndrome associated with sulindac. Clin Nephrol 1988;30:52.
239. Pagniez D, Gosset D, Hardouin P et al. Evolution vers la hyalinose segmentaire et focale d'un syndrome nephrotique a lesions glomerulaires minimes chez une patiente traitee par le sulindac. Nephrologie 1988;9:90.
240. Nesher G, Zimran A, Hershko C. Hyperkalemia associated with sulindac therapy. J Rheumatol 1986;13:1084.
241. Brater DC, Anderson S, Baird B et al. Effects of ibuprofen, naproxen, and sulindac on prostaglandins in men. Kidney Int 1985;27:66.
242. Lilly EL. Pancreatitis after administration of sulindac. J Am Med Assoc 1981;246:2680.
243. Reinertsen JL. Unusual perniolike reaction to sulindac. Arthritis Rheum 1981;24:1215.
244. Breton JC, Pibouin M, Allain H et al. Toxic epidermal necrolysis induced by sulindac. Therapie 1985;40:67.
245. Small RE, Garnett WR. Sulindac-induced toxic epidermal necrolysis. Clin Pharm 1988;7:766.
246. Hovde O. Sulindakindusert toksisk epidermal nekrolyse. Tidsskr. Nor. Laegeforen 1990;110:2537.
247. Fein M. Sulindac and pneumonitis. Ann Intern Med 1981;95:245.
248. Buriish GF, Kalz BL. Sulindac induced anaphylaxis. Ann. Emerg. Med 1981;10:154.
249. Hyson CP, Kazakoff MA. A severe multisystem reaction to sulindac. Arch Intern Med 1991;151:387.
250. Chamontin B, Fille A, Salva P et al. Does selective inhibition of prostaglandins exist? Concerning a case of hyponatremia with sulindac. Presse Med 1988;17:2140.

251. Gross GE. Granulocytosis and a sulindac overdose. Ann Intern Med 1982;96:793.
252. Ross JRY, Beeley L. Sulindac prothrombin time, and anticoagulants. Lancet 1979;ii:1075.
253. Pariente EA, Hamoud, Goldfain D et al. Hepatites a la clometacine (Duperan). Etude retrospective de 30 cas. Un modele d'hepatite autoimmune medicamenteuse? Gastroente'rol. Clin Biol 1989;13:769.
254. Islam S, Mekhloufi F, Paul JM et al. Characteristics of clometacin-induced hepatitis with special reference to the presence of anti-actin cable antibodies. Autoimmunity 1989;2:213.
255. Demay F, De Sy J A new non-steroidal anti-inflammatory drug (NSAID) in current rheumatological practice (oxamethacin). Curr Ther Res 1982;31:113.
256. Heiter A, Tausch G, Eberl R. Ergebnisse einer Langstudie mit Acemetacin bei der Behandlung von Patienten mit chronischer Polyarthritis. Arzneim-Forsch 1980;30:1460.
257. Lucietti MV, Bauchieri G. Studio clinico sulla efficacia e tollerabilita di un nuovo antiflogistico non-steroideo, la cinmetacina. G Clin Med (Bologna) 1980;61:545.
258. Friez L. Preliminary clinical experience with zidometacin. Acta Ther 1985;11:109.
259. Gall EP, Caperton EM, McComb JE et al. Clinical comparison of ibuprofen, fenoprofen calcium, naproxen and tolmetin sodium in rheumatoid arthritis. J Rheumatol 1982;9:402.
260. Fernandez L, Jacoby RK, Smith PJ et al. Comparative trial of standard and sustained release formulations of ibuprofen in patients with osteoarthritis. Curr Med Res Opin 1982;7:610.
261. Samuelson CO Jr, Williams HJ. Ibuprofen associated aseptic meningitis in systemic lupus erythematosus. West J Med 1979;131:57.
262. Chalmers TM. Clinical experience with ibuprofen in rheumatoid arthritis. Schweiz Med Wochenschr 1971; 101:280.
263. McIntyre BA, Philip RB, Inwood MJ. Effect of ibuprofen on platelet function in normal subjects and hemophiliac patients. Clin Pharmacol Ther 1978;24:616.
264. Thilo D, Nyman D, Duckert F. A study of the effect of the antirheumatic drug ibuprofen (Brufen) on patients being treated with the oral anti-coagulant phenprocoumon (Marcoumar). J Int Med Res 1974;2:276.
265. Mamus SW, Burton JD, Groat JD et al. Ibuprofen associated pure white-cell aplasia. N Engl J Med 1986; 314:624.
266. Guidry JB, Ogburn CL, Griffin FM. Fatal autoimmune hemolytic anaemia associated with ibuprofen. J Am Med Assoc 1979;242:68.
267. Law IP, Wickman CJ, Harrison BR. Coombspositive hemolytic anaemia and ibuprofen. South Med J 1979;72:707.
268. Sternlieb P, Robinson ROL. Stevens-Johnson syndrome plus toxic hepatitis due to ibuprofen. NY State J Med 1978;July:1239.
269. Caro H, Conture B, Pethilaz R, Royar JC. Etude clinique sur l'ibuprofen sous forme suppositoires. Gaz Med Fr 1976;83:372.
270. Fong HJ, Cohen AH. Ibuprofen induced acute renal failure with acute tubular necrosis. Am J Nephrol 1982;2:28.
271. Davies EF, Avery GS. Ibuprofen: a review of its pharmacological properties and therapeutic efficacy in rheumatic disorders. Drugs 1971;2:416.
272. Williamson J, Sturrock RD. An ophthalmic study of ibuprofen in rheumatoid conditions. Curr Med Res Opin 1976;4:128.
273. Mandell BF, Raps EC. Severe systemic hypersensitivity reaction to ibuprofen occurring after prolonged therapy. Am J Med 1987;82:817.
274. Sandyk R. Phenytoin toxicity induced by interaction with ibuprofen. South Afr Med J 1982;62:592.
275. Radack KL, Deck CC, Bloomfield SS. Ibuprofen interferes with the efficacy of antihypertensive drugs: a randomized, double blind, placebo-controlled trial of ibuprofen compared with acetaminofen. Ann Intern Med 1987;107:628.
276. Cassano WF. Serious methotrexate toxicity caused by interaction with ibuprofen. Am J Pediatr Hematol Oncol 1989;11:481.
277. Tamisier JN. Ketoprofen. Clin Pharm Dis 1979;5:381.
278. Gougeon J, Mireau-Hottin J, Gailland F. Clinical trial of the injectable form of ketoprofen. Rheumatol Rehabil 1976;15:75.
279. Willans MJ, Digby JW, Topp JR et al. Long term treatment of arthritis disease with ketoprofen (Orudis): a Canadian multicentre evaluation. Curr Ther Res 1979;25:35.
280. Egede F. Fatal asthmatic reaction following ketoprofen (Orudis) (Alreumat). Ugeskr Laeg 1979;141:1151.
281. Schreuder G. Ketoprofen: possible idiosyncratic acute bronchospasm. Med J Aust 1990;152:332.
282. Miyairi A, Ohori K. Aspirin-induced asthma due to rubbing ketoprofen ointment. Kokyu 1990;9:110.
283. Lanzia D, Colombo A, Lorini R, Severi F. Ketoprofen causing pseudotumor cerebri in Bartter's syndrome. N Engl J Med 1979;300:796.
284. Williams RL, Upton EA, Burkin JN, Jones RM. Ketoprofen aspirin interactions. Clin Pharmacol Ther 1981;30:226.
285. Ducret F, Pointet P, Martin D et al. Insuffisance renale aigue reversible induite par le ketoprofene. Nephrologie 1982;3:105.
286. Pazmino PA, Pazmino PB. Ketoprofen induced irreversible renal failure. Nephron 1988;50:70.
287. Simon SD, Kosmin M. Fenoprofen and agranulocytosis. N Engl J Med 1978;299:490.
288. Ashraf M, Pearson RM, Winfield DA. Aplastic anaemia associated with fenoprofen. Br Med J 1982;284:1301.
289. Porile JL, Bakris GL, Garella S. Acute interstitial nephritis with glomerulopathy due to non-steroidal anti-inflammatory agents: a review of its clinical spectrum and effects of steroid therapy. J Clin Pharmacol 1990;30:468.
290. Stachura I, Jayakumar S, Bourke E. T and B lymphocyte subsets in fenoprofen nephropathy. Am J Med 1983;75:9.
291. Kolodzik JM, Eilers MA, Angelos MG. Nonsteroidal anti-inflammatory drugs and coma: a case report of fenoprofen overdose. Ann Emerg Med 1990;19:378.
292. Sheldrake TE, Webber JM, Marsh BD. A long term assessment of flurbiprofen. Curr Med Res Opin 1977;5:64.
293. Benvenuti C, Longoni L. Multicentre study on effectiveness and safety of flurbiprofen versus alternative therapy in 738 rheumatic patients. Curr Ther Res 1983;34:30.
294. Huskisson EC, Woolf DL, Boyle DV, Scott J A trial of naproxen, flurbiprofen, indometacin and placebo in the treatment of osteoarthritis. Eur J Rheumatol Inflam 1980;2:69.
295. De Moor M, Oaghe R. A double blind comparison of flurbiprofen and indometacin suppositories in the treatment of osteoarthritis and rheumatoid diseases. J Int Med Res 1981;9:495.

296. Rawles JM. Antagonism between non-steroidal anti-inflammatory drugs and diuretics. Scot Med J 1982;27:37.
297. Daubresse AJ. Pirprofen for the treatment of rheumatic disorders and post-traumatic lesions. Acta Ther 1984;10:97.
298. Salliere D, Alcalay M. Rangasil en traitement prolonge. Rheumatologie 1986;38:131.
299. Segre E. Long term experience with naproxen: open labeled cohort survey of nearly 900 rheumatoid arthritis and osteoarthritis patients. Curr Ther Res 1980;28:47.
300. Geczy M, Peltier L, Wolbach R. Naproxen tolerability in the elderly—a summary report. J Rheumatol 1987;14:348.
301. Nader DA, Schillaci RF. Pulmonary infiltrates with eosinophilia due to naproxen. Chest 1983;83:280.
302. Wysenbeek AJ, Klein Z, Nakar S, Mane R. Assessment of cognitive function in elderly patients treated with naproxen. A prospective study. Clin Exp Rheumatol 1988; 6:399.
303. Arnold R, Heimpel H. Aplastic anemia after naproxen. Lancet 1980;i:321.
304. Lo TCN, Martin MA. Autoimmune hemolytic anemia associated with naproxen suppositories. Br Med J 1986; 292:1430.
305. Victorino RMM, Baptista A, Silveira JCB et al. Jaundice associated with naproxen. Postgrad Med J 1980;56:368.
306. Aabakken L, Bjornbeth BA, Hofstad B et al. Comparison of the gastrointestinal side effects of naproxen formulated as plain tablets, or enteric-coated granules in capsules. Scand J Gastroenterol 1989;24:Suppl. 163, 65.
307. Scheiman JM, Patel PM, Henson EK et al. Effect of naproxen on gastroesophageal reflux and esophageal function: a randomized, double-blind, placebo-controlled study. Am J Gastroenterol 1995;90(5):754—757.
308. Bridges AJ, Marshall JB, Diaz-Arias AA. Acute eosinophilic colitis and hypersensitivity reaction associated with naproxen therapy. Am J Med 1990;89:526.
309. Cartwright KC, Trotter TL, Cohen ML. Naproxen nephrotoxicity. Ariz Med 1979;36:124.
310. Antilla M, Haataja M, Kasanen S. Pharmacokinetics of naproxen in subjects with normal and impaired renal function. Eur J Clin Pharmacol 1980;18:263.
311. Hamann CO. Severe primary dysmenorrhea treated with naproxen: a prospective double blind, cross-over investigation. Prostaglandins 1980;19:651.
312. Plauvier B, Gosselin B, Hatrou PT et al. Systemic allergic vasculopathy after naproxen. Ann Med Interne 1979;130:173.
313. Levy ML, Barron KS, Eichenfield A, Honig PJ Naproxen-induced pseudoporphyria: a distinctive photodermatitis. J Pediatr 1990;117:660.
314. Girschick HJ, Hamm H, Ganser G, Huppertz HI. Naproxen-induced pseudoporphyria: appearance of new skin lesions after discontinuation of treatment. Scand J Rheumatol 1995;24(2):108—111.
315. Chapman P. Naproxen and sudden hearing loss. J Laryngol Otol 1982;96:163.
316. Grennan DM, Jolly J, Holloway LJ, Palmer DG. Vasculitis in a patient receiving naproxen. NZ Med J 1979;89:48.
317. Wei N, Hood JC. Naproxen and ejaculatory dysfunction. Ann Intern Med 1980;93:933.
318. Wilkinson AR, Aynsley-Green A, Mitchell MD. Persistent pulmonary hypertension and abnormal prostaglandin E levels in premature infants after maternal treatment with naproxen. Arch. Dis. Child 1979;54:942.
319. Fredell EW, Strano LJ Naproxen overdose. J Am Med Assoc 1977;238:938.
320. Court H, Volans GN. Poisoning after overdose with non-steroidal anti-inflammatory drugs. Adverse Drug React Acute Poison Rev 1984;3:1.
321. Martinez R, Smith DW, Frankel LR. Severe metabolic acidosis after acute naproxen sodium ingestion. Ann Emerg Med 1989;18:129.
322. Runkel R, Mroszczak E, Chaplin M et al. Naproxen-probenecid interaction. Clin Pharmacol Ther 1978;24:706.
323. Wallace CA, Smith AL, Sherry DD. Pilot investigation of naproxen/methotrexate interaction in patients with juvenile rheumatoid arthritis. J Rheumatol 1993;20:1764.
324. Catalano MA. Worldwide safety experience with diclofenac. Am J Med 1986;80(Suppl 4B):81.
325. Dandelot JB, Mihout B. Encephalopathie myoclonique au diclofenac. Nouv Presse Med 1978;7:1406.
326. Ciuci AG. A review of spontaneously reported adverse drug reactions with diclofenac sodium. Rheumatol Rehabil 1980;18(Suppl 2):116.
327. Salama A, Gottsche B, Mueller-Eckhardt C. Auto antibodies and drug- or metabolite-dependent antibodies in patients with diclofenac-induced immune haemolysis. Br J Haematol 1991;77:546.
328. Heuft HG, Postels H, Hoppe I et al. Eine todlich verlaufene immunhamolytische Anamie nach Applikation von Diclofenac. Beitr Infusionther 1990;26:412.
329. Porzsolt F, Heit W, Heimpel H, Asheck F. Panmyelopathie nach Einnahme von Diclofenac? Dtsch Med Wochenschr 1979;104:968.
330. Eustace S, O'Neill T, McHale S, Molony J. Fatal aplastic anemia following prolonged diclofenac use in an elderly patient. Ir J Med Sci 1989;158:217.
331. Tanner E, Wachter G, Lasarof J et al. Klinische Erfahrungen mit dem neuen Antirheumatikum Diclofenac. Z Gesamte Inn Med Ihre Grenzgeb 1982;37:8.
332. Dunk AA, Welt RP, Jenkins WJ et al. Diclofenac hepatitis. Br Med J 1982;284:1605.
333. Iveson TJ, Ryley NG, Kelly PMA et al. Diclofenac associated hepatitis. J Hepatol 1990;10:85.
334. Ouellette GS, Slitzky BE, Gates JA et al. Reversible hepatitis associated with diclofenac. J Clin Gastroenterol 1991;13:205.
335. Mazeika PK, Ford MJ. Chronic active hepatitis associated with diclofenac sodium therapy. Br J Clin Pract 1989; 43:125.
336. Sallie RW, McKenzie T, Reed WD et al. Diclofenac hepatitis. Aust NZ J Med 1991;21:251.
337. Helfgott SM, Sandberg-Cook J, Zakim D, Nestler J. Diclofenac-associated hepatotoxicity. J Am Med Assoc 1990;264:2660.
338. Diggory P, Golding RL, Lancaster R. Renal and hepatic impairment in association with diclofenac administration. Postgrad Med J 1989;65:507.
339. Hovette P, Touze JE, Debonne JM et al. Hepatite cholestatique et insuffisance renale aigue au cours d'un traitement par diclofenac. Ann Gastroenterol Hepatol 1989; 25:257.
340. Gray GR. Another side effect of NSAIDs. J Am Med Assoc 1990;264:2677.
341. Baroni L, Comoglio T, Trombetta N et al. Il diclofenac sodico nella terapia ambulatoriale dell'infiammazione o del dolore articolare. Clin Ter 1982;100:383.
342. Gizzi G, Villani V, Brandi G et al. Ano-rectal lesions in patients taking suppositories containing non-steroidal anti-inflammatory drugs. Endoscopy 1990;22:146.

343. Deakin M. Small bowel perforation associated with an excessive dose of slow release diclofenac sodium. Br Med J 1988;297:488.
344. Huber T, Ruchti C, Halter F. Non-steroidal anti-inflammatory drug-induced colonic strictures: a case report. Gastroenterology 1991;100:1119.
345. Wolters J, Van Breda-Vriesman PJC. Minimal change nephropathy and interstitial nephritis associated with diclofenac. Neth J Med 1985;28:311.
346. Campistol JM, Galofre J, Botey A et al. Reversible membranous nepphritis associated with diclofenac. Nephrol Dial Transplant 1989;4:393.
347. Beun GDM, Leunissen KML, Vriesman PJC et al. Isolated minimal change nephropathy associated with diclofenac. Br Med J 1987;295:182.
348. Yinnon AM, Moreb JS, Slotki IN. Nephrotic syndrome associated with diclofenac sodium. Br Med J 1987;295:556.
349. Gabrielson TO, Staerfelt F, Thune PO. Drug induced bullous dermatosis with linear IgA deposits along the basement membrane. Acta Dermatol 1981;61:439.
350. Muller-Vahl H. Aseptische Gewebsnekrose: eine schwerwiegende Komplikation nach intramuskulärer Injektion. Dtsch Med Wochenschr 1984;109:786.
351. Pillans PI, O'Connor N. Tissue necrosis and necrotizing fasciitis after intramuscular administration of diclofenac. Ann Pharmacother 1995;29(3):264—266.
352. Reimann IW, Frolich JC. Effects of diclofenac on lithium kinetics. Clin Pharmacol Ther 1981;30:348.
353. Deray G, Le Hoang P, Aupetit B et al. Enhancement of cyclosporin A nephrotoxicity by diclofenac. Clin Nephrol 1987;27:213.
354. Harris KP, Jenkins D, Walls J Non-steroidal anti-inflammatory drugs and cyclosporin. A potentially serious adverse interaction. Transplantation 1988;46:598.
355. Sarchi C, Cioffi T, Bertelleti D et al. Tolmetin sodium in clinical practice: a survey of 32,007 treated patients. J Int Med Res 1981;9:482.
356. Reid RT, Levin J, Ricca LR et al. Tolmetin sodium in the treatment of osteoarthrtis: an analysis of 725 patients with a year or more of therapy. Curr Ther Res 1982;28:173.
357. Jick H, Jick SS, Hunter JR et al. Follow-up study of tolmetin users. Pharmacotherapy 1989;9:91.
358. Ruppert GB, Barth WF. Tolmetin induced aseptic meningitis. J Am Med Assoc 1981;245:67.
359. Stefanini M, Nassif RI. Acute thrombocytopenic purpura traced to tolmetin-related antibody. Virginia Med 1982;109:171.
360. O'Brien WM. Longterm efficacy and safety of tolmetin sodium in treatment of geriatric patients with rheumatoid arthritis and osteoarthritis: a retrospective study. J Clin Pharmacol 1983;23:309.
361. Chatoyee GP. Nephrotic syndrome induced by tolmetin. J Am Med Assoc 1981;245:1589.
362. Strom BL, Carson JL, Schinnar R et al. The effect of indication on the risk of hypersensitivity reactions associated with tolmetin sodium vs other non-steroidal anti-inflammatory drugs. J Rheumatol 1988;15:695.
363. Shaw GR, Anderson WR. Multisystem failure and hepatic microvescicular fatty metamorphosis have been associated with tolmetin ingestion. Arch Pathol Lab Med 1991; 115:818.
364. Geier J, Fuchs T. Kontaktallergien durch Bufexamac. Med Klin 1989;84:333.
365. Anonymous. Fenclofenac withdrawn. Lancet 1984;ii:56.
366. Weber JCP. Epidemiology of adverse reactions to non-steroidal anti-inflammatory drugs. Adv Inflam Res 1984;6:1.
367. Buerklin EM, Ballard IM. A double blind comparison of fentiazac and phenylbutazone in the treatment of acute tendinitis and bursitis. Curr Med Res Opin 1979;6(Suppl 2):90.
368. Katona G, Boudani A. Efficacy and tolerability of fentiazac in rheumatoid arthritis: double blind study versus indometacine. Curr Med Res Opin 1979;6(Suppl 2):71.
369. Anonymous. The side effects of tiaprofenic acid. Reactions 1985;118:11.
370. Rave O, Penth B. Arzneimittelsicherheit bei Antirheumatika: Ergebnisse einer Breitenprufung mit Tiaprofensaure an 20,947 Patienten. Med Welt 1984;35:1587.
371. Poletto B. Tiaprofenic acid. Clin Rheum Dis 1984; 10:333.
372. Aparicio L. Butibufen. Drugs Today 1979;15:43.
373. Brogden RN, Heel RC, Speight TM et al. Fenbufen: a review of its pharmacological properties and therapeutic use in rheumatic diseases and acute pain. Drugs 1981;21:1.
374. Peacock A, Ledingham J Fenbufen induced erythema multiforme. Br Med J 1981;283:582.
375. Nicolas C, Chouvet B, Cambazard F et al. Accidents cutanes lies a un nouvel anti-inflammatoire: fenbufene. Ann Dermatol Venereol 1983;110:419.
376. Roujeau JC, Guillaume JC, Fabre JP et al. Toxic epidermal necrolysis (Lyell syndrome). Incidence and drug etiology in France, 1981-1985 (1990).
377. Jensen EM, Fossgren J, Kirchheiner B et al. Treatment of rheumatoid arthritis with carprofen (Imadyl) or indometacin: a randomized multicentre trial. Curr Ther Res 1980; 28:882.
378. Czarnobilski Z, Bem S, Czarnobilski K et al. Carprofen and the therapy of gastroduodenal ulcerations by ranitidine. Hepato-Gastroenterology 1985;32:20.
379. Mann RD. Withdrawal of alclofenac (Prinalgin). Br Med J 1979;2:133.
380. Anonymous. Flosin hearing. Scrip 1984;883:14.
381. Emanueli A, Prosperino A, Viaro D. Postmarketing surveillance of indoprofen. In: Proceedings, Scientific Symposium on Indoprofen in Inflammatory and Painful Conditions, Venice. Barnet, Herts: UK. Farmitalia Carlo Erba Ltd, 1982;95.
382. Jacono A, Caso P, Gualtieri S et al. Clinical study of possible interactions between indoprofen and oral anticoagulants. Eur J Rheumatol. Inflam 1981;4:32.
383. Editorial. Benoxaprofen. Br Med J 1982;285:459.
384. Dukes MNG. The seven pillars of foolishness. In: Dukes MNG, ed. Side Effects of Drugs, Annual 8. Amsterdam: Elsevier, 1984:xvii.
385. Halsey JP, Cardoe N. Benoxaprofen: side effect profile in 300 patients. Br Med J 1982;284:1365.
386. Frain-Bell W. A study of persistent photosensitivity as a sequel of the prior administration of the drug benoxaprofen. Br J Dermatol 1989;121:551.
387. Fumagalli M, Montrone F, Vernazza M et al. La difenpiramide nel trattamento dell'artrite reumatoide: studio in doppio cieco a breve termine versus indometacina. Clin Ter 1979;89:581.
388. Jochems OB, Ianbroers IM. Diphenpyramide: a review of its pharmacology and anti-inflammatory effects. Pharmatherapeutica 1986;4:429.
389. Scaranelli M, Delli Gatti I, Menegale G et al. Casi di artrite reumatoide resistent al trattamento con farmaci

antiflogistici non-steroidei: uso di dosi piu elevate di ibuproxam. Gaz Med Ital 1981;140:27.
390. World Health Organization. Zomepirac (United States of America). PHA (DIA), (1983) 83.3.8.
391. Ruoff GE, Andelman SY, Cannella JJ. Long term safety of zomepirac: a double blind comparison with aspirin in patients with osteoarthritis. J Clin Pharmacol 1980;20:377.
392. McMiller JL, Urbamak JR, Boas R. Treatment of chronic orthopedic pain with zomepirac. J Clin Pharmacol 1980;20:392.
393. Bates LH, Triplett WC, Berry ER et al. Stomatitis associated with zomepirac. J Am Med Assoc 1982;247:461.
394. Mendelis PS. Abuse potential associated with nonsteroidal anti-inflammatory drugs. ADR Highlights 1982;82.
395. Purdum PP III, Shelden SL, Boyd JW, Shiffman ML. Oxaprozin-induced fulminant hepatitis. Ann Pharmacother 1994;28(10):1159—1161.
396. Bird HA. Rheumatology and the pharmaceutical industry. J Rheumatol 1983;10:663.
397. Sanda M, Jacob GB, Fliedner L et al. In: Lewis AJ, Furst DE, eds. Non-steroidal Anti-inflammatory Drugs. Mechanisms and Clinical Use. New York, Basel: Marcel Dekker, 1987;349.
398. Lanza FL, Arnold JD. Etodolac, a new nonsteroidal anti-inflammatory drug: gastrointestinal microbleeding and endoscopic studies. Clin Rheumatol 1989;8(Suppl 1):5.
399. Taha AS, McLaughlin S, Sturrock RD, Russell RI. Evaluation of the efficacy and comparative effects on gastric and duodenal mucosa of etodolac and naproxen in patients with rheumatoid arthritis using endoscopy. Br J Rheumatol 1989;28:329.
400. Bem JL, Breckenridge AM, Mann RD, Rawlins MD. Review of yellow cards (1986): report to the Committee on the Safety of Medicines. Br J Clin Pharmacol 1988;26:679.
401. Benhamou CL. Large-scale open trials with etodolac (Lodine) in France: an assessment of safety. Rheumatol Int 1990;10(Suppl):29.
402. Serni U. Global safety of etodolac: reports from worldwide postmarketing surveillance studies. Rheumatol. Int 1990;10(Suppl):23.
403. Cramer RL, Aboko-Cole VC, Gualtieri RJ. Agranulocytosis associated with etodolac. Ann Pharmacother 1994; 28(4):458—460.
404. Roth SH. New understandings of NSAID gastropathy. Scand J Rheumatol 1989;Suppl 78:24.
405. Jenner PN, Johnson ES. Review of the experience with nabumetone in clinical trials outside of the United States. Am J Med 1987;83(Suppl 48):110.
406. Jenner PN. A 12-month postmarketing surveillance study of nabumetone. A preliminary report. Drugs 1990; 40(Suppl 5):80.
407. Abraham PA, Halstenson CE, Opsahl JA et al. Suprofen-induced uricosuria. Am J Nephrol 1988;8:90.
408. Lewis S. Ketorolac in Europe. Lancet 1994;343:784.
409. Iyer V. Ketorolac (Toradol) induced lithium toxicity. Headache 1994;34(7):442—444.
410. Cheymol G, Biour M, Bruneel M et al. Bilan d'une enquete national prospective sur les effets indesirables de la glafenine, de l'antrafenine et de la floctafenine. Therapie 1985;40:45.
411. Prescott LF, Balali-Mood M, Critchely JAJH, Proudfoot AT. Avoidance of mefenamic acid in epilepsy. Lancet 1981;ii:418.
412. Gossinger H, Hruby K, Haubenstock A et al. Coma in mefenamic acid poisoning. Lancet 1982;ii:384.
413. Euber HH, Kleine L, Herrlinger JD. Neutropenie unter Mefenaminsaure. Dtsch Med Wochenschr 1980;22:1192.
414. Handa SI, Freestone S. Mefenamic acid-induced neutropenia and renal failure in elderly females with hypothyroidism. Postgrad Med J 1990;66:557.
415. Phillips MS, Fehilly B, Stewart S et al. Enteritis and colitis associated with mefenamic acid. Br Med J 1983; 287:1626.
416. Robertson CE, Ford MJ, Van Someren V et al. Mefenamic acid nephropathy. Lancet 1980;ii:232.
417. Woods KL. Mefenamic acid nephropathy. Br Med J 1981;282:1471.
418. Jenkins DAS, Harrison DJ, MacDonald MK et al. Mefenamic acid nephropathy: an interstitial and mesangial lesion. Nephrol Dial Transplant 1988;2:217.
419. Sowden JM, Smith AG. Multifocal fixed drug eruption mimicking erytema multiforme. Clin Exp Dermatol 1990; 15:387.
420. Halbert DR. Menstrual delay and dysfuctional uterine bleeding associated with antiprostaglandin therapy for dysmenorrhea. J Reprod Med 1983;28:592.
421. Meredith TJ, Vale JA. Non-narcotic analgesics: problems of overdosage. Drugs 1986;32(Suppl 4):177.
422. Meyerhoff JO. Exacerbation of psoriasis with meclofenamate. N Engl J Med 1983;309:496.
423. Szczeklik A, Gryglewski RJ, Czerniawska Mysik G. Clinical patterns of hypersensitivity to non-steroidal anti-inflammatory drugs and their pathogenesis. J Allergy Clin Immunol 1977;60:276.
424. Lantz B, Cochat P, Bouchet JL, Fischbach M. Short-term niflumic-acid-induced acute renal failure in children. Nephrol Dial Transplant 1994;9(9):1234—1239.
425. Haynes Jr RC, Murad F. Agents affecting calcification, calcium parathyroid hormone, calcitonin, vitamin D and other compounds. In: Goodman LS, Gilman A, eds. The Pharmacological Basis of Therapeutics, 6th ed. New York: MacMillan, 1980;1545.
426. Stevens RM. Chronic fluorosis. Br Med J 1981;282:741.
427. Leroux JL et al. Rev. Med. Ther 1983;17:785.
428. Anonymous. Withdrawal of glafenine. Lancet 1992; 339:357.
429. Herxheimer A. Belgium: withdrawal of glafenine. Lancet 1991;337:102.
430. Bosset JF, Perriguey G, Rozenbaum A. Thrombopenie aigue recidivante apres prise de glafenine: une observation. Nouv Presse Med 1979;8:1606.
431. Ypma RThJM, Festen JJM, DeBruin CD. Hepatotoxicity of glafenine. Lancet 1978;ii:480.
432. Stricker BHC, Blok APR, Bronkhorst FB. Glafenine-associated hepatic injury: analysis of 38 cases and review of the literature. Liver 1986;6:63.
433. Daudon M, Protat MF, Reveillaud RJ Toxicite renale de la glafenine chez l'homme: calculs renaux et insuffisance renale aigue. Ann Biol Clin 1983;41:105.
434. Descotes J, Lery N, Vignean C et al. Bilan des effets secondaires dus a la glafenine au Centre de Pharmacovigilance de Lyon. Therapie 1980;35:405.
435. Stricker BHC, de Groot RRM, Wilson JHP. Anaphylaxis to glafenine. Lancet 1990;336:943.
436. Stricker BHC, de Groot RRM, Wilson JHP. Glafenine-associated anaphylaxis as a cause of hospital admission in The Netherlands. Eur J Clin Pharmacol 1991;40:367.
437. Garre M, Youinou P, Burtin C et al. Fievre isolee: effet secondaire singulier de la glafenine. Therapie 1980;35:752.

438. Rouveix B, Benhamed S, Regnier B. Rhabdomyolyse et glafenine. Therapie 1984;39:53.
439. Leguy Ph, Herve JP, Garre M et al. Nephropathie aigue tubulo-interstitielle apres ingestion d'antrafenine de mecanisme apparemment non immunoallergique. Nouv Presse Med 1981;10:1336.
440. Bressot C, Dechavanne M, Ville D et al. Effet antalgique et pertes sanguines fecales induites par l'antrafenine. Rev Rhum 1981;48:601.
441. Torriani H. Talniflumate. Drugs Today 1983;19:97.
442. Pitts NE. Ubersicht uber die mit Piroxicam in klinischen Untersuchungen gewonnenen Erfahrungen. Aktuel Rheumatol 1980;5:53.
443. Pisko EJ, Rahaman MA, Turner RA et al. Long term efficacy and safety of piroxicam in the treatment of rheumatoid arthritis. Curr Ther Res 1980;27:852.
444. Dessain I, Eistahooks TF, Gordon AI. Piroxicam in the treatment of osteoarthrosis: a multicentre study in general practice involving 1218 patients. J Int Med Res 1979;7:335.
445. Box J, Box P, Turner R, Pisko E. Piroxicam and rheumatoid arthritis: a double blind 16-week study comparing piroxicam and phenylbutazone. In: Piroxicam, International Congress and Symposium Series No. 1, Royal Society of Medicine. London: Academic Press, 1978;40.
446. Planas R, De Leon R, Quer JC et al. Fatal submassive necrosis of the liver associated with piroxicam. Am J Castroenterol 1990;85:468.
447. Honein K, Attali P, Pelletier G, Ink O. Hepatite aigue due au piroxicam: un nouveau cas. Gastroenterol Clin Biol 1988;12:79.
448. Santucci L, Patoia L, Fiorucci S et al. Oesophageal lesions during treatment with piroxicam. Br Med J 1990; 300:1018.
449. Carver N, Wedgwood KR, Ralphs DN. Iatrogenic gastrocolic fistula associated with non-steroidal anti-inflammatory drug administration. Br J Clin Pract 1990;44:759.
450. Bianchine JR, Procter RR, Thomas FB. Piroxicam, aspirin and gastrointestinal blood loss. Clin Pharmacol Ther 1982;32:247.
451. Goebel KM, Muller-Broadmann W. Reversible overt nephropathy with Henoch-Schonlein purpura due to piroxicam. Br Med J 1982;284:311.
452. Ljunggren B. The piroxicam enigma. Photodermatology 1989;6:151.
453. Mammen L, Schmidt CP. Photosensitivity reactions: a case report involving NSAIDs. Am Fam Physician 1995;52(2):575—579.
454. Roura M, Lopez Gil F, Umbert P. Systemic lupus erythematosus exacerbated by piroxicam. Dermatologica 1991; 182:56.
455. Vernick DM, Kelly JH. Sudden hearing loss associated with piroxicam. Am J Otol 1986;7:97.
456. Kerry RJ, Owen G, Michaelson SOG. Possible toxic interaction between lithium and piroxicam. Lancet 1983; i:418.
457. Haslock I. Tolerance of isoxicam with respect to age. In: Amor B, ed. Non-steroidal Anti-inflammatory Agents in the Elderly. Basel: Eular, 1984;114.
458. Burch FX. Evaluation of the safety of isoxicam. Am J Med 1985;79(Suppl 4B):28.
459. Bird HA. International experience with tenoxicam: a review. Scand. J Rheumatol 1988;Suppl 73:22.
460. Gonzalez JP, Todd PA. Tenoxicam—a preliminary review of its pharmacodynamic and pharmacokinetic properties, and therapeutic efficacy. Drugs 1987;34:289.
461. Caughey D, Waterworth RF. A study of the safety of tenoxicam in general practice. NZ Med J 1989;102:582.
462. Heintz RC Tenoxicam and renal function. Drug Safety 1995;12(2):110—119.
463. Kolarz G, Lieni KS, Rcichel H, Scherak O. Doppelblindstudie zwischen Indometacin und Cloximat, einem neuen nichtsteroidalen Anti-rheumatikum. Therapiewoche 1979;29:5898.
464. Nguyen M, Dougados M, Berdah L, Amor B. Diacerhein in the treatment of osteoarthritis of the hip. Arthr Rheum 1994;37(4):529.
465. Anonymous. Emorfazone. Drugs Today 1985;21:63.
466. Galasko CSB, Courtenay PM, Jane M et al. Trial of oral flupirtine maleate in the treatment of pain after orthopaedic surgery. Curr Med Res Opin 1985;9:594.
467. De Angelis L. Lefetamine hydrochloride. Drugs Today 1983;19:82.
468. Biscarini L, Patoia L, Del Favero A. Nimesulide—a new non-steroidal anti-inflammatory agent. Drugs Today 1988;24:23.
469. Huber W, Menander Huber KB. Orgotein. Clin Rheum. Dis 1980;6:465.
470. Lund-Olesen K, Menander-Huber KB. Intraarticular orgotein therapy in osteoarthritis of the knee. Arzneim-Forsch Drug Res 1983;33:1199.
471. Diehl K, Fallot-Burghardt W, Frie A. Die Therapie der Gonarthrose mit Oxaceprol. Therapiewoche 1985;35:51.
472. Jeffery WH, Zelicoff AP, Hardy WR. Acquired methemoglobinemia and hemolytic anemia after usual doses of phenazopyridine. Drug Intell Clin Pharm 1982;16:157.
473. Green ED, Zimmerman RC, Ghurabi WH, Colohan DP. Phenazopyridine hydrochloride toxicity: a cause of drug induced methemoglobinemia. J Am Coll Emerg Phys 1979; 8:426.
474. Lewis JH. Hepatic toxicity of non-steroidal anti-inflammatory drugs. Clin Pharm 1984;3:128.
475. Merand JP, Geniaux M, Tamisier JM et al. Eruption squamocrouteuse a type histologique de lichen plan au cours d'un traitement par le pyritinol. Ann Dermatol Venereol 1980;107:561.
476. Segoud P, Delaas JA, Massias P. Syndrome nephrotique en cours d'une polyarthrite rheumatoide traitee par la pyrithioxine. Rev. Rhum 1979;46:510.
477. Treves R, Tabaraud F, Arnaud M et al. Polymyosite aigue compliquant une polyarthrite rhumatoide traitee a la pyrithioxine. Rev Rhum 1984;51:283.
478. Meyrier A. Desensitization in a patient with renal disease and severe allergy to allopurinol. Br Med J 1976;2:458.
479. Fam AG, Paton TU, Chaiton A. Reinstitution of allopurinol therapy for gouty arthritis after cutaneous reactions. Can Med Assoc J 1980;123:128.
480. Weiss EB, Forman P, Rosenthal IM. Allopurinol induced arteritis in partial HGPRT-ase deficiency: atypical seizure manifestation. Arch Intern Med 1978;138:1743.
481. Schattenkirchner M, Wandrey H. Uber eine Kohlenhydratstoffwechselstorung bei Gichtbehandlung mit Allopurinol. Z Rheumaforsch 1969;28(Suppl 1):410.
482. Boston Collaborative Drug Surveillance Program. Allopurinol and cytotoxic drugs: interaction in relation to bone marrow depression. J Am Med Assoc 1974;227:1036.
483. Stolbach L, Begg C, Bennett JM et al. Evaluation of marrow toxic reaction in patients treated with allopurinol. J Am Med Assoc 1982;247:334.
484. Ohno I, Ishida Y, Hosoya T et al. Allopurinol induced

aplastic anemia in a patient with chronic renal failure. Ryumachi 1990;30:281.
485. Okafuji K, Shinohara K. Aplastic anemia probably induced by allopurinol in a patient with renal insufficiency. Rinsho Ketsueki 1990;31:85.
486. Gomez GA, Stutzman L, Ming Chu R. Xanthine nephropathy during chemotherapy in deficiency of hypoxanthine-guanine phosphoribosyltransferase. Arch Intern Med 1978;138:1017.
487. Hande KR, Noone RM, Stone WJ Severe allopurinol toxicity. Am J Med 1984;76:47.
488. Chan SH, Tan T. HLA and allopurinol drug eruption. Dermatologica 1989;179:32.
489. Chau NY, Reade PC, Rich AM et al. Allopurinol amplified lichenoid reactions of the oral mucosa. Oral Surg 1984;58:397.
490. Lupton GP. Allopurinol hypersensitivity. J Am Acad Dermatol 1979;1:365.
491. Boston Collaborative Drug Surveillance Program. Excess of ampicillin rashes associated with allopurinol of hyperuricemia. N Engl J Med 1972;286:505.
492. Sonntag MR, Zoppi M, Fritschy D et al. Exantheme unter haufig angewandten Antibiotika and antibakteriellen Chemotherapeutika (Penicilline, speziell Aminopenicilline, Cephalosporine und Cotrimoxazol) sowie Allopurinol. Schweiz Med Wochenschr 1986;116:142.
493. Zimm S, Narang PK, Ricardi R et al. The effect of allopurinol on the pharmacokinetics of oral and parenteral (i.v.) 6-mercaptopurine. Proc Am Assoc Cancer Res 1982;23:210 (Abstract).
494. Sherry S. The anturan reinfarction trial. N Engl J Med 1980;303:50.
495. Szczeklik A, Czerniawska-Mysik G, Nizankowska E. Sulfinpyrazone and aspirin-induced asthma. N Engl J Med 1980;303:702.
496. Witwer MU, Schmid FR, Tesar JT. Acute myelomonocytic leukaemia and multiple myeloma after sulphinpyrazone and colchicine treatment of gout. Br Med J 1976;2:89.
497. Durham DS, Ibels LS. Sulphinpyrazone-induced acute renal failure. Br Med J 1981;282:609.
498. Hauselmann HJ, Studer H. Antinatriuretische Wirkung von Sulphinpyrazon. Schweiz Med Wochenschr 1981;111:1030.
499. Bailey RR, Reddy J. Potentiation of warfarin action by sulphinpyrazone. Lancet 1980;i:254.
500. Brater DC. Drug—drug and drug—disease interactions with non-steroidal anti-inflammatory drugs. Am J Med 1986;80(Suppl IA):62.
501. Masbernard A, Giudicelli CP. Ten years experience with benzbromarone in the management of gout and hyperuricemia. South Afr Med J 1981;9:701.
502. Peters RS, Lehman TJA, Schwabe AD. Colchicine use for familial Mediterranean fever. West J Med 1983;138:43.
503. Liu YK, Hymowitz R, Carroll MG. Marrow aplasia induced by colchicine. Arthr Rheum 1978;21:731.
504. Letellier P, Langeard M, Agullo M. Rhabdomyolise secondaire a une serie d'injections intraveineuses de colchicine. J Med Caen 1979;14:157.
505. Baldwin LR, Talbert RL, Samples R. Accidental overdose of insufflated colchicine. Drug Safety 1990;5:305.

Meyler's Side Effects of Drugs, 13th Edition
M.N.G. Dukes, editor

SECTION EDITOR: B. VRHOVAC

Zlatko Baudoin and Bozidar Vrhovac

10 General anesthetics and therapeutic gases

GENERAL TOPICS

RISK FACTORS IN ANESTHESIA

Although a certain number of untoward reactions related to general anesthesia are essentially unpredictable, it is very important for the anesthetist to determine which of his patients are primarily at risk so that safer use of anesthetic agents and better supervision of surgical patients can be achieved.

Underlying disease This is probably one of the most complex risk factors to be dealt with. Although general anesthesia has indeed been shown to be potentially more hazardous in patients with underlying disease in general (1[C]) or specifically suffering from intracardiac conduction disturbances (2[C]), severe hypertension (3[R]), hypothyroidism (4[R]) or cancer (5[R]), it remains extremely difficult to provide clear-cut recommendations because the relative severity of disease in a given patient and his own response to the pathological process needs to be taken into account: while, for instance, thiopental may precipitate cardiovascular collapse, both the pre-existing cardiac status and the dose of the drug are relevant.

Muscular disorders present a special problem. A spectrum of muscle reactions to all the inhalation agents has been described. Masseteric muscle spasm may occur as an isolated phenomenon or it may progress either to rhabdomyolysis with renal failure or to malignant hyperpyrexia (6[C], 7[C], 8[Cr], 9[Cr]). The latter life-threatening condition involves sustained muscle contraction, muscular damage and the production of vast quantities of metabolic heat, carbon dioxide and potassium. Although usually associated with suxamethonium, all the inhalation agents are implicated and will prove to be unsafe if risk factors for this condition are present, e.g. a family history or one of the congenital muscle disorders (10[C]). This must be considered in patients at risk as there are readily acceptable alternatives such as propofol (11[Cr]) and midazolam (12[CR]). Genetic markers for malignant hyperpyrexia may in the near future make identification of risk groups simpler than the currently used muscle biopsy technique (13[C]).

Pre-anesthetic drug therapy This is another risk factor to be considered, the consequences of which are obviously closely related to those of the underlying disease. The problem has attracted considerable attention in recent years and has been extensively reviewed (14[R]). Interactions of drugs with anesthesia are, in this volume, dealt with primarily in reviews of the drugs concerned, i.e. in other chapters. Although many pharmacological interactions with general anesthesia are firmly established, others remain ill-explained or unpredictable. Individual factors are again likely to play a major role. Moreover, pre-anesthetic drug withdrawal in itself may prove more dangerous than continuation of therapy, as exemplified by the case of the antihypertensive agent clonidine (15[C]), or the β-blockers (16[C]).

Factors predisposing to hypersensitivity reactions These have been shown to include atopy, drug allergy, previous exposure to general anesthetics, sex (women) and age (young adults).

Multiple anesthesia The importance of multiple anesthesia should not be overlooked. Patients in whom halothane anesthesia is given twice with an interval of less than 6 weeks are, for example, at major risk of developing jaundice. Some anesthetists avoid any second exposure to this agent.

ANESTHETIC DEATHS

Correct estimates of the incidence of anesthetic deaths are difficult to obtain, since many deaths are multifactorial.

Mortality due to anesthetic drugs is between 1 in

10 000 and 1 in 20 000 (17[R]). The adverse effects of anesthetics have been reviewed (18[R]) and, as is the case of many other classes of drug, two distinct types of problem have been distinguished: *dose related, predictable reactions*, which represent an extension of the normal pharmacological actions of the drug, and *non-dose-related, unpredictable reactions*, which may not appear to be directly related to the pharmacological action of the drug. Dose-related reactions are common and carry a low mortality, while non-dose-related reactions are less common and carry a high mortality.

Inhalation and intravenous anesthetic drugs depress the cardiac, respiratory, and central nervous system in a dose-related manner. In most cases anesthetic drugs are not given alone, and adverse effects may occur as a result of the co-administration of various anesthetic compounds.

A national prospective survey of complications related to anesthesia was carried out in France from 1978 to 1982 (19[C], 20[C]). In a total series of 198 103 anesthesias, only 63 deaths were recorded, of which only 15 were definitely attributed to anesthesia (21[C]). The Confidential Enquiry into Perioperative deaths conducted a decade ago in three British Health Regions (22[R]) and covering a total of 555 248 patients, found that the incidence of death within 30 days following surgery and anesthesia totalled 0.73% (4034 cases). Only about 14 of these deaths were considered to be partly or totally attributable to the anesthesia, and indeed in most of these cases other factors were also involved. Such factors include the surgery itself, the pre-surgical condition and intercurrent illness. In a review of 25 cases of death during anesthesia from 1982 to 1986 (23[R]), only six were considered to be drug-related; of these two were due to overdose and two more were the result of side-effects of non-anesthetic agents.

Finally, except for certain specific effects which have a clear relationship to a particular agent (e.g. liver damage following halothane) it is as a rule difficult to designate one anesthetic as being more risky than another. It has been authoritatively concluded that "the current level of research effort cannot distinguish mortality and serious morbidity between the most common anesthetic agents and the clear differences in hemodynamic patterns among these anesthetic agents have an unknown, perhaps non-existent, relationship with mortality and serious morbidity" (24[R]).

THE SAFETY OF DENTAL ANESTHESIA

Side effects of dental anesthesia represent a special problem. It is commonly difficult to obtain reliable data on the extent to which complications occur during dental anesthesia. Several studies investigating the safety of dental anesthesia have been performed in the US (SEDA-18); unfortunately all of them have their weaknesses. More informative is an American survey in which 47 oral and maxillofacial surgeons were approached directly and all responded. Among the 74 871 patients to whom they had given general anesthesia, there were 250 case of laryngospasm, 51 of phlebitis, 30 of dysrhythmias sufficiently severe to require therapy, 17 of hypotension requiring drug therapy and 13 of bronchospasm. Small numbers of cases suffered allergic reactions requiring drug therapy (four), convulsions (four), hypertension (two), myocardial infarction (two) or vomiting with aspiration (two); in one case an injection was inadvertently given into an artery (25).

ENVIRONMENTAL EXPOSURE

It remains a source of much concern that those working in operating theatres spend their time in such a polluted environment in spite of attempts to introduce scavenging of waste anesthetic gases (26). This is not without its effects. There is for example a relationship between asthma and occupational exposure to various respiratory hazards which include anesthetic gases (27[R]).

Nitrous oxide may be the most serious of the pollutants; female dental assistants exposed to large amounts of nitrous oxide (5 or more hours of exposure per week) are significantly less fertile than women who are not exposed or who are exposed to lower amounts (28[r]). In an epidemiological study anesthetists were found to have significantly greater exposure and perhaps more adverse effects than other operating-room personnel (29[r]). Among women, exposure certainly causes an increased risk of spontaneous abortions in the first trimester, although teratogenicity is a less clear-cut issue. (30[R]).

An impressive French study has examined the risks of occupational exposure of hospital personnel to anesthetics by studying the staff of 18 Paris hospitals (excluding doctors) over a 12-year period (31[CR]): 557 staff exposed to anesthetics were compared to 566 workers less exposed. The most striking finding was that neuropsychological and neurological symptoms (tiredness, nausea, headaches, memory impairment, decrease in reaction time, tingling, numbness, cramps) were reported some 3 times more commonly by workers in less often scavenged theatres than by controls; no difference was found between workers from well-scavenging theaters and controls. It may be noted that neuropsychological symptoms have been reported in several earlier papers over the last three decades (32[C]) and the French findings, though better documented than previous reports, are not surprising.

An interesting paper from Croatia shows significant immunological changes in the peripheral blood film of personnel working in unscavenged operating theatres. Some of the effects persists beyond a 4-week period away from that environment (33[C]).

MALIGNANT HYPERTHERMIA

Although malignant hyperthermia is a rare complication of general anesthesia it remains a topic of considerable interest (34[R]). The incidence of hyperthermia is difficult to determine, but it is currently estimated at 1 in every 10 000–20 000 anesthesias.

Diagnosis Generalized muscle rigidity (found in 70% of the patients involved) and a progressive rise in body temperature (sometimes beyond 43°C) are the main clinical features, frequently associated with excessive tachycardia, hypoxia, metabolic acidosis, cardiac arrhythmias and, less often, disseminated intravascular coagulation, cerebral edema and acute renal failure. Diagnosis essentially relies on clinical signs, i.e. muscle rigidity and hyperpyrexia, and on elevated serum levels of skeletal and cardiac muscle enzymes, e.g. aldolase and creatine phosphokinase.

Prognosis and treatment Around 1970, mortality was as high as 70% but it is now less than 10%. This reduction in mortality has been due to the use of dantrolene, the only specific treatment available, and also to an increased understanding of the condition (34[R]). Doses of dantrolene from 2.5 to 5 mg/kg are usually recommended, given as early as possible to ensure rapid and complete resolution of the hyperthermic response (35[R]). The anesthetic should be withdrawn; one must then commence hyperventilation with 100% oxygen, institute cooling measures immediately, use dantrolene, and maintain hemodynamic and cardiac equilibrium.

Risk factors and prophylaxis Malignant hyperthermia is probably due to the inability of certain individuals to control calcium concentrations within the muscle fiber and may involve a generalized alteration in cellular or subcellular membrane permeability, as suggested from basic research on porcine models. This anomaly is known to be genetically determined but pre-anesthetic evaluation of susceptibility to malignant hyperthermia is a matter of controversy: measurement of blood creatine phosphokinase levels, ATP muscle depletion or myophosphorylase A, histological examination of muscle fibers, and in vitro exposure to caffeine or halothane, have all been proposed. Susceptible patients may, however, require general anesthesia despite the risk.

Prophylactic use of intravenous dantrolene during induction of anesthesia in a dose of 2.4 mg/kg has been recommended (36[R]).

GENERAL ANESTHESIA AND THE IMMUNE RESPONSE

General anesthesia and surgery certainly influence immune responses. However, despite considerable work on the subject, some divergence in interpretation persists (37[R]). In patients with no pre-anesthetic immunological anomaly, general anesthesia is unlikely to affect the immune status significantly (38[C]).

HYPERSENSITIVITY REACTIONS

The issue of hypersensitivity reactions in the course of general anesthesia is a matter of concern for anesthetists. Widespread erythema and edema, the most dangerous form of which is that affecting the glottis, occur in some cases. Hypotension is also seen, together with compensatory tachycardia. Bronchospasm is a common respiratory finding (39[CR]).

Epidemiology Laxenaire et al. (40[CR]) examined 23 444 anesthetic files over a period of 12 months; one patient in 630 presented with generalized erythema and edema, one in 1230 with erythema and hypotension. One patient died of shock. Female patients, patients between the ages of 15 and 25 with a history of allergy, subject with excessive anxiety and those who had previously undergone general anesthesia were confirmed to have a statistically significant higher risk of developing anaphylactoid reactions. The incidence of true anaphylactic reactions (with IgE antibodies being produced) is said to be between one in 4500 and one in 20 000 general anesthetics per year (41). However, the diagnosis is frequently missed (42[R]).

Prediction and mechanism The patient's history is hardly helpful; neither the presence nor the absence of such a reaction to any one drug on a past occasion gives much guidance as to the likelihood of its occurring on future exposure. The mechanisms underlying such reactions may or may not involve histamine release, but the distinction between anaphylactic and anaphylactoid reactions is often unclear for lack of definitive and easily available investigations. Furthermore, because anesthetic drugs are often given rapidly and in combination, it can be impossible to decide which one has been responsible for the reaction. Intradermal injection of a test dose is of limited predictive value (43[R]); false-positive and false-negative results are often obtained, particularly with opiates, tubocurarine and atracurium. What is more, the test is dose-dependent, and it may itself precipitate a hypersensitivity reaction (44[Cr]). Assem (43[R]) concludes that leucocyte histamine release on exposure to drugs can be used in combination with paper radioallergosorbent testing for IgE antibodies, to detect the precise cause of any anaphylactic reaction: these techniques point to neuromuscular blocking drugs as being the most common cause of anaphylaxis.

In a French study, 1585 patients underwent diagnostic investigations after anaphylactic shock during anesthesia; 813 of them were recognized as having had a reaction of immunological origin. The drugs involved were: muscle relaxants 70%, latex 12.6%, anesthetic drugs 5.6%, opioids 1.7%, colloids 4.7%, and antibiotics 2.6% (45[r]). Among the 45 cases in which anesthetics were involved, the agents involved were thiopentone (18 cases), propofol (10), ketamine (one), midazolam (seven), diazepam (five) and flunitrazepam (four). These data did not differ from those reported in the UK (46[r]).

Both authors point to the high proportion of cases in which muscular relaxants are used alongside anesthetics, resulting in a two-fold risk of hypersensitivity.

GENERAL ANESTHESIA AND DRIVING

The actual hazard of driving shortly after general anesthesia is still difficult to evaluate. Although Havard (47[R]) has recommended abstention from driving for 48 hours after general anesthesia, it is still difficult to draw clear-cut conclusions from available data. The matter is also referred to under individual drug headings in this chapter.

HEMOSTASIS AND PLATELET FUNCTIONS

Hemostasis may be deranged both by surgery and general anesthetics (48[R]). Fentanyl, halothane and enflurane have been shown to enhance fibrinolytic activity significantly (49[C]). In addition, a raised plasma β-thromboglobulin level (a good indicator of platelet activation) was found in 61 patients following use of nitrous oxide, oxygen and halothane when they were compared with controls (50[C]).

ANESTHETIC VAPORS

The inhalation agents in common use share similar side-effects, albeit with a differing incidence. Initial hopes of new agents being less problematic have faded as their use increases and familiarity with their adverse effects grows. There is even a report of anaphylaxis with isoflurane (51[c]).

Enflurane

Enflurane is a non-explosive halogenated volatile anesthetic first released for clinical use in 1966. It was developed in the search for agents safer than halothane and methoxyflurane (52[C]). In the course of the years, however, the list of halothane-like side effects has continued to grow.

ADVERSE REACTION PATTERN

General and toxic reactions Enflurane is usually well-tolerated and has no marked toxic effects on organ function. Little cardiovascular or respiratory depression has been noted so far.

Hypersensitivity reactions These are rare. Asthma attacks and bronchospasm have been described.

Tumor-inducing effects These have not been reported.

ORGANS AND SYSTEMS

Cardiovascular Despite somewhat conflicting results, enflurane is generally considered to induce little change in the cardiovascular system. Cardiac output was mildly influenced in healthy men while enflurane's negative inotropic effects (53[C]) were more pronounced in patients with congestive heart failure (54[C]). Myocardial damage was suggested to be an unlikely complication of enflurane anesthesia even in patients with ischemic heart disease (55[C]). *Dysrhythmias* are generally considered to be less frequent or at least less severe with enflurane than with halothane (56[C], 20[C]). However, caution in the use of adrenaline is very advisable, especially in patients with cardiac disease or hyperthyroidism. Isorhythmic atrioventricular dissociation was seen in 16 of 105 patients following use of 1–1.5% enflurane (57[C]).

Respiratory Enflurane is usually not irritant to the respiratory tract, although cases of *bronchospasm* have been reported (58[C]). It is however generally considered a bronchodilator. It causes *respiratory depression* at concentrations greater than 2%.

Nervous system *Cerebral irritability* is a potential consequence of enflurane anesthesia as evidenced by EEG recordings and by reported cases of *convulsions* (SED-11, 208; 59[Cr]). Enflurane should be used with care—though it is probably not entirely contraindicated—in patients with epileptiform tendencies, especially if they are deeply anesthetized and hyperventilated. There are reports of patients having delayed convulsions after light general anesthesia not involving hyperventilation. A patient had a convulsion in a car after being discharged from a day care anesthetic involving enflurane (59[C]).

Bentin et al. (60[C], 61[C]) noted a *decreased capacity for learning and decision-making* in healthy volunteers following exposure to subanesthetic concentrations of enflurane.

Endocrine, metabolic The endocrine effects of enflurane anesthesia are minimal and clinically not significant (62[C]).

Porphyria The effect of enflurane on heme metabolism has been tested in mice (63); in the light of the results the authors decided to add this drug to the list of drugs which can precipitate *acute attacks of porphyria*.

Liver One of enflurane's main advantages over halothane is a reduced rate of liver damage, though such damage can occur. With increasing use since 1980 there has been an increasing number of reports of enflurane-induced *hepatitis* (SED-11, 209), some in patients previously affected by halothane (64[C]), and with some indications that the risk may be higher in obese middle-aged women (65[c]); some fatalities have occurred. All the same, its hepatotoxic potential, though not entirely defined, is probably low, as evidenced by prospective studies of liver function under repeated enflurane anesthesia (66[C]). Indeed, the US Food and Drug Administration decided in May 1982 against incorporating a hepatotoxicity warning on the drug's American labelling, and this policy has been maintained since.

Urinary system *Nephrotoxicity* leading to renal failure, particularly after prolonged anesthesia, is a potential consequence of general anesthesia with enflurane (67[C]). Several cases of renal failure have been described (SED-11, 209) and the mechanism studied. On experimental grounds, it has been suspected that the inorganic fluoride ions to which enflurane is biotransformed may play a role in kidney damage. Despite evidence of the drug's capacity for inducing a significant decrease in maximum urinary osmolarity (tested using vasopressin administration) and in creatinine clearance in healthy volunteers (68[C]), further investigations are warranted. Superimposition of nephrotoxic factors, e.g. drugs or underlying disease, should be avoided (52[C]).

Musculoskeletal system One case of *myoglobinuria*, developing immediately after enflurane anesthesia, has been reported (69[C]).

Risk situations Pre-existing *renal disease* is suspected to increase the risk of enflurane nephrotoxicity.

Second-generation effects Available experimental evidence goes against a teratogenic role of enflurane (52[R]).

Interactions Enflurane was shown to increase the sensitivity of the neuromuscular junction to *d*-tubocurarine in man (70[C]). *Amitriptyline* may potentiate enflurane-induced cerebral irritability (59[C]).

Halothane

Halothane is a non-inflammable hydrocarbon that induces anesthesia with little tendency to excitement. Contrary to earlier assumptions, halothane is biotransformed in the body, a process the consequences of which are discussed below.

Halothane is still the most popular agent for gaseous induction and retains advantages over the other agents in certain situations discussed elsewhere in this chapter; this is the case despite the long debate regarding hepatitis; one may ask what other methods are safer overall (71[R], 72[R]).

ADVERSE REACTION PATTERN

General and toxic reactions Halothane is generally well tolerated. No marked toxic effects on organ function have been described, although the effect on the liver may be toxic rather than allergic. High concentrations can cause some cardiovascular depression. Malignant hyperthermia can occur but is a rarity.

Hypersensitivity reactions The only reaction possibly due to hypersensitivity to halothane, apart from an occasional skin reaction, is hepatitis; the mechanism of the latter is still debated.

Tumor-inducing effects These have not been clearly documented. However, the possible effects of chronic exposure to low concentrations have given rise to some concern (see above).

ORGANS AND SYSTEMS

Cardiovascular Cardiac depressive effects of halothane are frequently referred to in the literature (73[R]). Halothane indeed produces *bradycardia*, but *arrhythmias*, most often ventricular in origin, also occur during maintenance of anesthesia. They were noted in 53% of a series of 679 patients (74[C]). Concomitant administration of cathecholamines may increase the risk of developing such arrhythmias.

Bundle branch block and *aberrant conduction* were noted in children under halothane anesthesia (75[C]).

Halothane, isoflurane, and sevoflurane, are potent coronary vasodilators, able to produce some degree of 'coronary steal' in ischemic regions. Despite this effect, halothane may preferentially dilate large coronary arteries and/or interfere with platelet aggregation. If these experimental effects are confirmed in clinical practise, halothane may be the anesthetic of choice in the non-failing ischemic heart (76[c]).

Halothane has a mild depressive effect on cardiac performance. In the human ventricular myocardium, halothane has been found to interact with L-type calcium channels by interfering with the dihydropyridine binding site. This might, at least in part, explain the negative inotropic effect of halothane (77).

Halothane depressed cardiovascular function significantly more than isoflurane in younger adults, but the falls in systolic and diastolic blood pressure recorded in elderly patients were significantly greater with isoflurane (78[c]).

Halothane can be used as an anesthetic agent during fetal surgery via maternal inhalation and improves surgical exposure by relaxing the uterus. However, the effects of halothane on fetal cardiovascular homeostasis have been evaluated, and the authors concluded that halothane had a significant negative effect on the fetal heart and peripheral vasculature. It was therefore considered a poor anesthetic for this specific purpose (79[C]).

Respiratory Halothane is not irritant to the respiratory tract (see, however, 'Overdosage' below). *Respiratory depression* is a consequence only of high concentrations of halothane. A certain degree of bronchodilatation is observed, and this may explain the fact that a beneficial effect of halothane was described in a 17-year-old woman with status asthmaticus who did not respond to conventional treatment (80[c]). Clearly some caution is needed; the authors point out that the benefits need to be weighed against the seriousness of possible adverse effects such as hypotension, cardiac dysrhythmias, and liver damage, in a patient who is already ill.

Pre-term infants may become apneic during the immediate postoperative period, even if the ventilatory response to CO_2 is not depressed after halothane anesthesia (81[c]). In a prospective study in 167 pre-term infants after inguinal herniorrhaphy with halothane/nitrous oxide anesthesia, only one infant had an episode of apnea up to 2 days postoperatively; however the authors recommend careful monitoring until complete recovery from anesthesia has occurred (82[C]).

Nervous system Halothane can induce *shivering*. It reduces sympathetic activity and increases vagal tone. In contrast to enflurane, cerebral irritability is extremely rare (83[C]). Halothane can cause an *increase in intracranial pressure*, as can other inhalation anesthetics, which can constitute a particular risk if the pressure is already elevated prior to anesthesia and surgery. A slight *depression* of mood lasting up to 30 days along with a non-specific slowing of the EEG for 1—2 weeks was observed after halothane (84[C], 85[C]).

Endocrine, metabolic Halothane in association with suxamethonium is the most frequent cause of *malignant hyperthermia* attributed to general anesthesia.

Mineral and fluid balance An increase in circulating *bromide* and *fluoride* can occur.

Hematological Halothane was shown to produce a parallel *inhibition of in vitro platelet aggregation* and an *increase in bleeding time* (86[C]).

Liver The greatest disadvantage of halothane is its ability to cause liver damage (87[r]). The incidence of death due to this adverse effect was, in a 1993 overview, estimated at one in 35 000 anesthesias (88[R]), which is three times greater than the one in 110 000 incidence reported in 1976 (89[r]). Both immune function and the metabolism of halothane play important roles in the pathophysiology of liver toxicity (90[R]). Human hepatic microsomal carboxylesterase is a target antigen in halothane hepatitis, protein disulfide isomerase is an important factor in the mechanism of liver impairment, and an associated immune response may be involved (SEDA-18, 116). So-called halothane-induced liver antigens are novel antigens found in the livers of some individuals who have been exposed to halothane, but not in the livers of unexposed individuals (91[R]).

It has been suggested that some genetic factor determines the risk of developing of halothane hepatitis (92[Cr]). A report published in 1981 of halothane hepatitis in three pairs of closely related women (98[C]) has raised the possibility of a pharmacogenetic defect in these patients leading to an increased production of hepatotoxic metabolites. Most cases of liver disorders recorded in the literature occurred following either after repeated exposure (93[c]) or prolonged (94[c]) exposure to halothane. In one published case, hepatitis developed 3 weeks after a single halothane anesthesia in a 37-year-old renal transplant recipient who had previously been exposed to isoflurane (95[c]); this report suggests that previous exposure to isoflurane may predispose to subsequent halothane toxicity.

Halothane also reduces liver blood flow during anesthesia and this could increase the release of potentially hepatotoxic halothane metabolites. The role of halothane reductive metabolites and inorganic fluoride which may covalently link to liver macromolecules has been stressed; in keeping with this hypothesis is the observation of halothane hepatitis in patients simultaneously taking enzyme-inducing agents, e.g. barbiturates (96[C]) or rifampicin (97[C]).

It is therefore tempting to suggest that patients with one or several predisposing factors, e.g. a pharmacogenetic trait, hepatic hypoxia or enzymic induction, are likely to produce high amounts of hepatotoxic halothane metabolites which covalently bind to liver macromolecules, rendering them immunogenic. The finding that repeated administration increases the risk of developing halothane jaundice (66[C], 99[C]) supports this hypothesis.

Children as young as 11 months are certainly not exempt from risks of halothane hepatitis, as was once thought to be the case; there are a growing number of case-reports of halothane hepatitis in children (100[CR]).

Gastrointestinal Postoperative nausea and vomiting can occur but are as a rule seldom encountered with halothane.

Urinary system Renal blood flow, glomerular filtration rate and urinary volume are sometimes decreased mildly and reversibly. By contrast, one case of repeated massive *polyuria* has been reported in a 46-year-old man following two operations under halothane (101[C]). Acute renal failure has been described (102[C]) but it is rare.

Skin and appendages A young nurse complained of skin *rash* with edema of the eyelids following repeated professional exposure to halothane (103[C]).

Immunotoxicity Halothane may suppress host defence mechanisms, the clinical consequences of which are again unclear (SED-11, 210).

Risk situations Prior *liver disease* or *recent administration* involves the risk of hepatotoxic effects, as discussed above. *Children* do not always tolerate halothane quite as well as is generally thought; hepatitis and ventricular arrhythmias have been reported.

Second-generation effects Chronic exposure to low concentrations of halothane is a matter of much concern, as discussed above (see 'General' section of this chapter). Furthermore, halothane strongly *reduces uterine contractility* during labor (104[C]) and is readily *excreted in the milk* (105[C]).

Overdosage Suicide attempts with halothane have sometimes succeeded, but in cases which recovered there was no residual damage. A 4-year-old boy was accidentally given halothane intravenously. He fully recovered within a few hours (106[C]). Accidental intravenous injection and illicit inhalation have both caused pulmonary edema.

Interactions The risk of arrhythmias in the case of association with *catecholamines* has already been discussed above. Halothane potentiates *non-depolarizing muscular relaxants* (SED-11, 210).

In one series, postoperative vomiting occurred in 13 of 29 patients who had received halothane in induction, but when *dyxirazine* was added during anesthesia the incidence of postoperative vomiting was significantly reduced (three out of 29 patients) (107[c]).

Chloroform

Chloroform should no longer be used today because of its toxic action on the heart, liver and kidneys, although the exact nature and extent of these complications is still debated (108[R]).

Ether

An *impaired immune response* has been found after diethylether anesthesia and one case of *contact dermatitis* together with a systemic allergic reaction attributed to ether general anesthesia has been described in older literature (SEDA-5, 120).

Isoflurane

Not surprisingly, being an isomer of enflurane, isoflurane has many of the same side effects; it is a potent inhalation anesthetic. Its low level of metabolism (about 0.2%) has encouraged its prolonged use as a sedative agent or bronchodilator in patients in status asthmaticus. However, it may not be as inert in all patients.

A mutagenic effect of isoflurane has been ruled out. A case of *anaphylaxis* was reported in 1988 (51[c]).

Cardiovascular Although atrial *arrhythmia* has

been reported in 3.9% of patients and ventricular arrhythmia reported in 2.5% (109[R]), the arrhythmogenicity of isoflurane has clearly been shown to be less pronounced than that of halothane (110[C]). Indeed, the incidence of dysrhythmias induced by catecholamines in cardiovascular anesthesia and during oral surgery is incontrovertibly reduced by using isoflurane rather than the other agents.

The most controversial side effect of isoflurane is its potential to cause a *coronary steal* in patients with critical stenosis in the coronary circulation. Most recent work suggests that there is no increased risk of myocardial ischemia as long as the hemodynamics, especially the heart rate, are well controlled (111[C]). There are however still isolated reports indicating that the issue is not settled and isoflurane may cause a specific coronary steal even with good hemodynamic control (112[C]).

Respiratory A marked *respiratory depressant effect* has been documented in children (113[C]) and *coughing* associated with nausea and vomiting occurs in roughly 10% of subjects (109[R]).

Like halothane (see above) isoflurane has proved useful in cases of life-threatening acute severe asthma refractory to drug therapy. An 11-year-old girl with acute asthma and severe CO_2 narcosis and ventricular fibrillation induced by hypoxemia was successfully treated with isoflurane in oxygen for 14 hours. Her recovery may have been due to bronchodilatation and the treatment possible because of the low dysrhythmogenic effect of isoflurane (114[c]).

Nervous system *Seizures* are uncommon, but incidental reports continue to appear. Symptoms suggestive of severe sensorimotor *neuropathy* developed in a 40-year-old woman 15 days after admission for severe exacerbation of asthma. During this period she was given isoflurane 0.5—3% in oxygen, vecuronium bromide 4—6 mg/h, and fentanyl 100 μg/h. The neuropathy resolved spontaneously over the next 3 months. The neuromuscular blocking effects of vecuronium bromide can be enhanced by inhalation anesthetics. In this case, isoflurane may have been the triggering drug (115[c]).

Kidney High levels of fluorine ions, potentially damaging to the kidney, may be found after prolonged use (116[c]).

Liver Hepatic damage related to isoflurane anesthesia has very occasionally been described (117[C], 118[C]), the literature including one report of hepatic necrosis and death (119[Cr]).

Endocrine, metabolic Malignant hyperthermia is a possible complication of isoflurane anesthesia (120[C]).

Interactions The infusion requirements of *rocuronium* necessary to maintain twitch depression were reduced by 40% during anesthesia involving isoflurane (121[c]).

Isoflurane in nitrous oxide inhibited *succinylcholine*-induced muscle fasciculation in children (122[c])

Desflurane

Desflurane is a new anesthetic produced by substitution of fluorine for the single chlorine atom in isoflurane. Desflurane is a volatile anesthetic that combines low blood gas solubility with moderate potency and high volatility. Because of these characteristics, desflurane must be used in specific vaporisers, and one must be extremely careful not to interchange the agent or the vaporiser, since serious under- or overdosage will result (123). When using desflurane with the proper equipment, alveolar concentrations can be adjusted more rapidly and precisely during administration, and recovery is quicker in both the short and long term than with other agents (124[R]).

Cardiovascular Desflurane increases the heartrate and reduces both mean arterial pressure and systemic vascular resistance while maintaining cardiac output.

Despite some coronary vasodilatation in dogs, there is no evidence of 'coronary steal' in man. Desflurane may benefit elderly patients by providing a more rapid recovery from anesthesia (125[c]).

Respiratory Desflurane appears to be a mild respiratory irritant (126[R]). Moderate to severe laryngospasm and moderate to severe *coughing* occurred frequently (50% of cases) during induction of anesthesia with desflurane in a series of 206 children aged 1 month to 12 years; the authors concluded that the high incidence of these airway complications during induction limited use of desflurane in pediatric patients, but that anesthesia could be safely maintained with desflurane after induction with another anesthetic (127[cr]).

Nervous system Increasing doses of desflurane produced no demonstrable fall in cerebral blood flow. Consequently, desflurane can be advocated for patients undergoing neurosurgical procedures (128[c]).

Depression of neuromuscular function occurred 10 minutes after the introduction of desflurane 1.3% in a 32-year-old man who had previously received midazolam, fentanyl, and thiopental for induction. On withdrawal his neuromuscular function returned to baseline (129[C]).

Liver and kidney Poorly metabolized gases are generally safer than those which undergo extensive metabolism. Desflurane is poorly metabolized, and appeared to have no toxic effects on the liver and kidneys in 13 young male volunteers (130[c]).

Risk situations In *old people* the MAC of desflurane, with or without nitrous oxide, was less than that reported in patients aged 18—65 years. Doses of desflurane must therefore be reduced in older people, as with all other inhalation agents (131[c]). The question of using deflurane in children is discussed above.

Interaction The MAC of desflurane was found to be significantly reduced 25 minutes after a single dose of *fentanyl* (132[c]).

Adrenalin used during anesthesia may cause ventricular dysrhythmias. The threshold of adrenaline for dysrhythmias is reduced by halothane, but not by desflurane; the dose of adrenalin required to produce dysrhythmias in 50% of patients was 3-fold that needed when anesthesia was with halothane (133[c]).

Sevoflurane

Sevoflurane is an isoflurane-related anesthetic developed more than one decade ago but apparently not widely documented. In Japan, where it came into clinical use in 1990, Ochai et al. (134[C]) have used it in more than 3000 cases. They encountered two incidents of *malignant hypertension*, one of them fatal. In this case, isoflurane had been used early in the anesthesia, and could have been at least in part responsible. There was some reason to consider that the former patient, a girl of 12, had a familiar propensity to malignant hyperthermia as indicated by higher resting P_i/P_{cr} values. It should however be noted that sevoflurane itself can trigger malignant hyperthermia in swine (135).

Sevoflurane can be used both for the induction and maintenance of anesthesia. In a series of 75 patients of ASA grades I or II, recovery from anesthesia after maintenance with sevoflurane/nitrous oxide was significantly faster than with an isoflurane/nitrous oxide combination (136[cr]).

Cardiovascular In a study of 28 subjects given either sevoflurane/nitrous oxide or enflurane/nitrous oxide anesthesia, sevoflurane showed fewer *cardiodepressant* effects than enflurane (137[c]). Nevertheless, in 10 healthy subjects atrial contraction and left ventricular diastolic function, including active relaxation, passive compliance, and elastic recoil, were impaired by sevoflurane (1 MAC) (138[c]).

Nervous system Despite a fall in mean arterial pressure, with a consequent reduction in cerebroperfusion pressure, sevoflurane should be a suitable agent for neuro-anesthesia (139). Even in patients with ischemic cerebrovascular diseases, both the CO_2 response and cerebral autoregulation were well maintained during sevoflurane anesthesia (0.88 MAC) (140[c]).

Liver Sevoflurane can be used to induce hypotension during neurosurgery. Hypotensive anesthesia has a little effect on postoperative liver function (141[c])

A 3-day-old boy underwent inguinal herniorrhaphy under sevoflurane anesthesia, and 2 days later developed vomiting, anorexia, and fever. His AST, ALT, and LDH were increased and peaked 12—16 days after the operation. Viral markers were negative, as was a lymphocyte stimulation test with sevoflurane. Toxic (not allergic) liver damage due to exposure to sevoflurane was considered to be the most probable diagnosis (142[c]).

Urinary system Serum and urinary inorganic fluoride concentrations have been reported to rise after inhalation of sevoflurane (143[c]). The authors concluded that lengthy sevoflurane anesthesia could alter renal function, although there was no other evidence of nephrotoxicity.

Malignant hyperthermia has occurred in people treated with sevoflurane. In the case of a 4-year-old girl, treatment with dantrolene was successful; susceptibility to malignant hyperthermia was later confirmed by muscle biopsy analysis (144[c]). However, a 28-year-old man, who developed malignant hyperthermia after anesthesia induced with isoflurane which was maintained with sevoflurane, died 4 days later despite cooling and intravenous dantrolene (145[C]).

Risk situations A 56-year-old woman with insulinoma operated under sevoflurane anesthesia had an uneventful perioperative course, and the authors suggested that sevoflurane could suppress the spontaneous release of insulin (146[c]). The agent may therefore be useful for anesthesia in patients with insulinoma.

Transplantation A 29-year-old man was anesthetized after renal transplantation with sevoflurane/nitrous oxide/oxygen for replacement of the head of the left femur. His serum fluoride concentration always remained below 40 μmol/l and sevoflurane had little effect on the transplanted kidney. It seems, therefore, that sevoflurane might be suitable for use in such patients (147[C]).

Methoxyflurane

The *nephrotoxicity* of methoxyflurane is well established (148[C]). *Hepatitis* has also been reported (149[C]), with possible cross-allergy between halothane and methoxyflurane.

GASES

Nitrous oxide

Nitrous oxide is a relatively potent analgesic but a weak anesthetic, in use since 1842. At body temperature, its blood/gas partition ratio is only 0.47. It is excreted unchanged via the lungs. Over 120 years of anesthetic use have outlined most of its complications. Because of the large mass of gas delivered to the patient, important physicochemical problems arise. Its ability to diffuse into and expand any air-filled cavities continues to produce new reports. The drug is occasionally abused (150[C]).

ADVERSE REACTION PATTERN

General and toxic reactions Cardiovascular and respiratory depression is the main side effect of nitrous oxide, which is otherwise well tolerated. Peripheral neuropathy and megaloblastic anemia have been reported, generally following chronic exposure. Malignant hyperthermia is extremely rarely encountered. Hypoxia during recovery is a possible complication. Megaloblastic changes herald a depression of immunological competence reflected in an increased postoperative morbidity.

Hypersensitivity reactions Allergy to nitrous oxide does not seem to occur.

Tumor-inducing effects These have been reported in chronic exposure but not substantiated.

ORGANS AND SYSTEMS

Cardiovascular Although *myocardial depression* has been described in normal volunteers following use of 40 or 50% nitrous oxide in oxygen, it is usually mild. It is likely that nitrous oxide can worsen myocardial ischemia in patients with critical coronary stenosis, although this may only be of academic significance (151[C], 152[cr]).

Respiratory While airway conductance may be decreased following nitrous oxide inhalation, respiratory depression is unlikely after short-term exposure (153[C]).

The effects of intraoperative air or nitrous oxide on postoperative oxygen saturation (Sa_{O_2}) in blood have been compared in 40 patients of ASA classes I and II undergoing elective open cholecystectomy. The incidence of hypoxemia was significantly higher in those treated with nitrous oxide than in those given air 48 hours postoperatively (154[c]).

Hypoxemia may also have some mechanical origins: nitrous oxide diffuses into the endotracheal tube cuff, overexpanding it, and can in this way provoke upper airway obstruction, hypoxemia, and trauma in intubated patients during general anesthesia (155[c]).

Nervous system Nitrous oxide is endowed with a potential for abuse (156[R]), one of the major complications of which is *myeloneuropathy*; an alteration of vitamin B_{12} metabolism has been suggested as a mechanism (157[Cr]), and in some cases the patients concerned have been found to have pre-existing subclinical B_{12} deficiency (158[C]). Layzer (159[C]) observed 12 patients heavily exposed to nitrous oxide either deliberately or professionally for periods ranging from 3 month to several years who initially developed numbness in the hands or legs, then the Lhermitte sign, gait ataxia, impotence and sphincter disturbances. Several similar cases have been reported by others (SEDA-11, 110). Numbness and/or muscle weakness were found four times more frequently among exposed than non-exposed dental personnel (160).

Since nitrous oxide does have some effects on the nervous system, it is not entirely surprising to note a further report to the effect that under experimental conditions it can affect *memory*. That memory changes can occur has been known for very long time, but the pattern of the effects now appears to be distinctly odd.

Inhalation of 50 or 70% nitrous oxide in oxygen for 15 minutes was shown to *impair driving skill* (161[C]).

Nitrous oxide can diffuse into any cavity that has air inserted or left in situ. Intraoperative subdural tension pneumocephalus arising during neurosurgery has been described (162[Cr]). Air injected into the epidural space can cause symptomatic pressure effects if nitrous oxide diffuses into the air pocket.

At the very least it now seems that patients receiving the gas should be informed as to the fact that its aftereffects can affect their functioning without their being consciously aware of the fact (163[C]).

Endocrine, metabolic Nitrous oxide inhalation may give false P_{O_2} measurement results and shift the oxyhemoglobin curve to the left (164[C]). Malignant hyperthermia is extremely rare; the possible role of nitrous oxide as a triggering agent has not been confirmed when examined in the porcine model (165).

Hematological The most worrying concern is the effect of nitrous oxide on vitamin B_{12} and folate metabolism. This causes *megaloblastic marrow changes*, the period required depending on the patient's nutritional status (166[Cr]).

Dyshemopoiesis after exposure to nitrous oxide may be mediated through a direct inhibitory effect (167). Although clinical sequelae were not apparent to date, the use of nitrous oxide in bone-marrow transplantation needs to be evaluated further and cannot currently be recommended (168[cr]).

Liver A case of *jaundice* after general anesthesia in which nitrous oxide was the only anesthetic has been described (169[C]). Contamination with halothane was not, however, definitely ruled out.

Gastrointestinal Nausea and vomiting are seldom noted. It had no effect on recovery after laparoscopic cholecystectomy (170[c]).

Urinary system Renal blood flow is moderately reduced. Kidney function disturbances have been described (171).

Special senses Nitrous oxide *increases middle-ear pressure* (172[C]), and spontaneous *tympanic rupture* has been described.

Side effects due to solubility The poor solubility of nitrous oxide may be dangerous for patients with pneumothorax, pneumoperitoneum, ileus or air embolism.

Risk situations Solubility problems lead to risks in patients in whom *air cavities* are present. Chronic exposure of *operating theater personnel* is a matter of concern as pointed out by the US Food and Drug Administration (SEDA-5, 120) (see also introductory section).

Second-generation effects Nitrous oxide has been widely used in pregnancy and generally regarded as safe (173[C]). Some experimental data have suggested a possible teratogenic potential, the clinical relevance of which is still unclear. The interaction with vitamin B_{12} (see above) causes changes in DNA synthesis that could be important in the first trimester of pregnancy. After much analysis of all data concerning women anesthetized in early pregnancy it does not however appear to be of clinical significance (174).

Interactions The uptake of *any other inhalation agent*, given at the same time as nitrous oxide, is accelerated by the rate of uptake of nitrous oxide. This is termed the 'second gas effect' (175). Direct pharmacodynamic interactions do not occur. The addition of nitrous oxide to *halothane* in coronary patients was shown to produce hypotension with a subsequent risk of myocardial damage (176[C]).

Cyclopropane

Cardiac arrhythmias, mainly ventricular in origin, are a frequent complication of high concentrations of cyclopropane; their incidence is further increased by respiratory depression. The risk of explosion in the course of cyclopropane use is important (177[C]).

A certain degree of *liver dysfunction*, as judged by effects on indocyanine green clearance, has been reported.

Nausea and vomiting are fairly frequent after recovery and *delirium* can occur if no narcotic premedication has been given.

Cyclopropane potentiates non-depolarizing neuromuscular blockers.

Oxygen

The duration and extent of hyperoxygenation during anesthesia are generally limited to safe levels. In intensive care, however, a patient's exposure to oxygen may become prolonged and dangerous.

Respiratory Pulmonary toxicity takes the form of an initial exudation of blood and fibrinous fluid into the alveoli, followed by proliferation of fibroblasts and alveolar cells (178). This proliferative phase may be permanent (179). It is reflected in a decreased vital capacity and diffusion capacity (180) and appears to be proportional to the units of pulmonary toxic dose (UPTD) administered; 1 UPTD is equivalent to 1 ATA × 1 minute exposed. If exposure exceeds 1000 UPTD it may be difficult to predict the outcome (181) due to inter-patient differences in susceptibility.

Nervous system CNS toxicity causes convulsant activity resembling 'grand mal' fits (182) and is associated with decreased levels of γ-aminobutyric acid in the brain. Unfortunately, such fits may not be apparent in sedated patients.

Other Other targets of oxygen toxicity include the *eye* (with tunnel vision due an effect on the retina, and in the neonate retrolental fibroplasia), the *red blood cells* (hemolysis) and any *metabolizing cell* because of its susceptibility to chemical toxicity (lipid peroxidation and cell membrane damage) (SED-12, 342).

INTRAVENOUS AGENTS

BARBITURATE ANESTHETICS

Methohexital (methohexitone)

Of a series of 4379 dental patients receiving methohexital, 6.7% experienced *restlessness*, 5.5% *respiratory disorders* (respiratory obstruction, hiccoughing, laryngeal spasm, apnea or sneezing), 1.1% *venous complications*, 1.0% *delayed recovery*, 0.5% *excitation*, 0.27%

nausea and vomiting and 0.2% other mild reactions (183[C]). *Pain* at the site of methohexital injection has been noted in up to 64% of patients; the addition of 10 mg lignocaine significantly decreased the incidence to 22% (184[C]).

Seizures are a possible but rare complication of methohexital administration (185[C]); it is inadvisable to use this drug in a patient with a history of epilepsy.

Vasodilatation and *depressed myocardial contractility* are possible hemodynamic consequences of high-dose methohexital anesthesia.

Rectal administration of methohexital, sometimes used for children with needle-phobia, may cause *apnea*, particularly if there are pre-existent CNS abnormalities (SED-12, 242).

Thiopental sodium

Thiopental sodium, one of the oldest anesthetics, still remains the first choice induction drug for cesarean section (186[r]).

Allergy *Anaphylaxis* has been repeatedly reported following thiopental (SED-10, 190; SED-11, 211) but remains a rare complication with an estimated incidence of one in 30 000. An extreme example reported in 1993 involved a 55-year-old obese man with no history of allergy to penicillin, who had on earlier occasions received sodium thiopentone without reaction; on this occasion he stopped breathing and had severe bronchial constriction and vascular collapse requiring prolonged resuscitation and mechanical ventilation (187[C]).

Fixed drug eruptions after thiopental administration have been reported (188[C]). One case of *immune hemolytic anemia* with acute renal failure has been reported in a 55-year-old patient following induction of anesthesia with 450 mg of thiopental; a specific thiopental antibody was detected. The patient recovered fully (189[C]).

Local complications Inadvertent injection into extravascular tissues will cause pain and swelling, and possibly tissue necrosis. Pain on injection has been noted in 10% of patients (190[C]). Intra-arterial injection causes vascular spasm, and may lead to gangrene of a distal extremity.

Gastrointestinal *Vomiting* is common during many types of anesthesia (191[c]). By reducing upper esophageal sphincter pressure during induction, thiopental may contribute to this complication (192[c]).

Cardiovascular *Cardiovascular depression* is a well-documented complication of thiopental. However, the plasma levels necessary to produce loss of corneal reflex and trapezius muscle tone were found to be only minimally depressant to the heart (193[C]). Problems can in any case be reduced or avoided by proper fluid administration prior to induction of anesthesia, as well as by cautious dosage and administration in patients with uncompensated cardiac failure.

Some cerebral artery aneurysms require cardiopulmonary bypass and deep hypothermic circulatory arrest if they are to be operated upon safely. During such bypass procedures these patients often receive large doses of thiopental in the hope of providing additional cerebral protection. A study in 42 non-cardiac patients has sought to verify the effects of thiopental on hemodynamic parameters; it was concluded that, provided preoperative function is good, thiopental loading to the point of suppressing EEG bursts will cause only negligible cardiac impairment and will not impede separation from the cardiopulmonary bypass. There were no data on patients with cardiac disease (194[c]).

Risk situations In one case, undetected *congenital methemoglobinemia* caused severe cyanosis during anesthesia with 500 mg thiopental and 50% nitrous oxide (195[C]).

The use of thiopental or any other barbiturate is contraindicated in *acute intermittent porphyria*; a progressive neuropathy can occur and may prove to be fatal.

MISCELLANEOUS NON-BARBITURATE ANESTHETICS

Alfadolone (Althesin)
Propanidid

Both these preparations have been withdrawn because of safety considerations regarding the solvent used (Cremophor EL)(SED-11, 211).

Etomidate *(SED-12, 242; SEDA-17, 126)*

Etomidate, a non-barbiturate anesthetic, is considered to be safe, especially in patients with hemodynamic instability. The most common complications of using etomidate are venous sequelae, pain on injection (190[R]) and involuntary muscle movements (SED-11, 211).

Cardiovascular The cardiorespiratory tolerance of etomidate is usually excellent (196[C]), but cardiovascular instability has been described after a bolus dose (197[C]).

Muscular *Involuntary muscle movements* are noted in 20–50% of patients unless fentanyl or a benzodiazepine are given first (SED-11, 211). Myoclonus has been noted, which may be dangerous for open eye surgery (198[c]).

Nervous system Etomidate has been observed to produce activation of *epileptiform activity*, and electrographic seizure during craniotomy in epileptic patients (199[CR]). Generalized seizures have been noted in 20% of 30 patients without a history of epilepsy, following etomidate induction (200[C]). Cerebral excitation may also occur after recovery from etomidate anesthesia, with potential respiratory disturbance (201[Cr], 202[C]).

Caution should be exercised when giving etomidate to patients with a history of seizures (SEDA-18, 113).

Endocrine, metabolic *Cortisol and aldosterone levels* were found to be depressed in adults by etomidate (203[c], 204[c]), but the clinical relevance of the change was minimal after a single bolus (205[c]). A reduction in cortisol has also been reported 2 hours after delivery in 40 infants whose mothers received etomidate for cesarean section. There were also nine cases of severe to moderate hypoglycemia in this study, but the changes in blood glucose concentration were not significantly different from those of the control group (206[C]).

Hematological *Hemolysis* has been reported after the administration of etomidate (207[C]). It may be related to the use of propylene glycol as a solvent (208[C], 209[C]).

Allergy Transient *erythema* has been described, but histamine release does not occur. Etomidate is the induction agent of choice in an atopic patient, in whom etomidate, fentanyl and vecuronium comprise the safest combination of drugs for general anesthesia. However, an anaphylactoid reaction has been observed even after this combination (210[c]) and it can even be life-threatening.

Ketamine

Ketamine is considered to be a safe drug, usable in emergencies. It is widely used by emergency physicians (211[c]) and can be given intravenously, intramuscularly, orally, and even nasally (212[c]).

Cardiovascular *Tachycardia* and *hypertension* are common occurrences after anesthetic induction with ketamine, although the hypertension can be limited by the addition of diazepam (213[C]). Nodal *arrhythmias* may also occur (214[Cr]). Because of possible decreased cardiac and pulmonary performance the use of ketamine should be avoided in critically ill patients (215[C]). Pulmonary vasoconstriction and increased ventricular pre-load secondary to ketamine administration may prove deleterious (216[C]).

Respiratory (see also 'Cardiovascular' above) *Apnea* occurred after the intramuscular injection of ketamine 4 mg/kg to sedate a healthy 4-year-old boy (217[C]). This case illustrates the need for adequate monitoring and preparation for emergency airway management when using ketamine for sedation.

When used in combination with midazolam given by infusion, ketamine provides analgesia and also prevents and relieves bronchospasm (218[c]).

Nervous system Ketamine-induced *hallucinations* have given the drug a bad reputation.

The psychomimetic effects of ketamine, apart from encouraging some illicit use, may lead to distressing psychic disturbances, particularly in children (216[C]); there may be *nightmares, delirium and hallucinations* (219[C]). Prior use of benzodiazepines or opiates limits this effect. Ketamine has been shown to cause a significant elevation of CSF pressure, increased EEG activity and possibly epileptiform discharge. Delayed *acute intracranial hypertension* has been described following ketamine anesthesia (220[C]).

Media reports suggest that in some countries the non-medical (illicit) use of ketamine has greatly increased (221).

Miscellaneous Serum *enzyme levels* (alkaline phosphatase, aspartate aminotransferase, alanine aminotransferase and γ-glutamyltransferase) were found to be elevated in 14 of 34 patients anesthetized with ketamine. The significance of this phenomenon is unknown (222[C]).

Multiple ketamine anesthesias may well prove to be safe (223[C]).

Midazolam

This agent is used for intravenous sedation, rather than for induction of general anesthesia. It can induce an unpleasant state of dysphoria if surgical stimuli are applied to the patient, who may nevertheless appear calm and untroubled. Amnesia is also produced by this drug. Delayed recovery of cognitive function is noted after the use of benzodiazepines as premedication (224).

Cardiorespiratory Midazolam is noted to be *depressant* to both cardiovascular and respiratory function, especially in the elderly (225). As little as 0.01 mg/kg can obtund the response to hypoxia and hypercapnia (226[C]). The simultaneous use of opiates (such as fentanyl) commonly produces *hypoxia* (227[CR]).

Neurological In the presence of acute neurological injuries, midazolam produces a severe risk of raised intracranial pressure (228[Cr]) and the risk of airway obstruction (229[C]) compounds the problem.

Recovery after propofol or midazolam has been compared in two trials (230[c], 231[c]). *Memory* was significantly impaired in the midazolam group, an effect reminiscent of the problems experienced with short-acting oral benzodiazpine hypnotics such as triazolam.

Withdrawal The cessation of an infusion of midazolam, used as sedation in intensive care units, is associated with occasional severe and bizarre behavioral disturbances, particularly in children (232). These again are similar in nature to the withdrawal effects seen with other short-acting benzodiazepines (see Chapter 5).

Interactions *Erythromycin* and midazolam have been previously reported to interact when given orally (SEDA 17; 125), the effect of the latter being potentiated; midazolam should be avoided in patients taking erythromycin or the dose should be reduced by 50—75% (233[c]).

Midazolam produces marked reduction of the *halothane* MAC in humans at lower serum concentrations than are required to cause sleep (234[c]).

Benzodiazepine antagonists

Flumazenil

This topic is primarily dealt with in Chapter 5, but it may be noted here that the antagonist flumazenil is used after midazolam anesthesia or sedation or in the event of overdose (235[c], 236[c]). However, it is not absolutely safe and can cause adverse effects, including nausea, vomiting and a release of catecholamines leading to increases in blood pressure and heart rate; these may be dangerous in patients with cardiovascular diseases (237[r]).

Flumazenil can provoke acute withdrawal reactions and extreme anxiety (238[CR]). Its duration of action (less than 1 hour) may be shorter than the of the original benzodiazepine, which can re-assert its effects while the patient is unobserved.

Propofol

This short-acting intravenous induction agent, now in general use in day-care anesthesia, is being increasingly used in infusions in intensive care units. Recovery from anesthetic doses compares favorably with that following enflurane and isoflurane (239).

Allergy True anaphylaxis to propofol has been observed (240[C]). A fixed drug eruption has also been recorded (241[c]).

Cardiovascular Propofol has a depressant effect, and resets the baroreflex set-point with a tendency to bradycardia (occurring in some 5% of cases), hypotension (16%) or both (1.3%) (242[R]). The hypotension may have been brought about by the effects of propofol in causing peripheral vasodilatation, reduced myocardial contractility, and inhibition of sympathetic nervous system outflow (243[R]).

Respiratory Respiratory depression is well recognized; apnea can be produced, especially with rapid injection (244[C]).

Neurological It has been claimed that propofol produces good recovery after anesthesia. A review of the literature has shown that for operations lasting under 30 minutes, propofol seems to give the best recovery, but for longer operations use of isoflurane gave better quality recovery (245[R]).

Myoclonus and opisthotonos have been noted, especially in children (246[Cr]). Choreoathetosis has also been attributed to propofol (247[c]). However, in experimental studies propofol has been shown to be an effective anticonvulsant against drug-induced seizures (248, 249). It is suggested that the drug inhibits efferent inhibitory neurons in the midbrain and reticular activating system, producing movements which originate subcortically and in the spinal cord (250).

Sexual function Sexual illusions and disinhibition were a problem in two women (aged 20 and 47 years) after sedation with propofol (251[cr]).

Withdrawal Excitation, including 'grand mal' convulsions, has been observed on cessation of a propofol infusion in intensive care (252[C]).

REFERENCES

1. Train M, Lepage JY, Le Forestier K et al. Incidents et accidents observés lors de l'anesthésie-réanimation en chirurgie coronaire. Ann Anesthésiol Fr 1979;5:431.
2. Tachovies D, Poisot D, Erny P et al. Les troubles de la conduction intra-cardiaque en anesthésie-réanimation. Ann Anesthésiol Fr 1979;4:357.
3. Rodriguez PR, Mangans DT. Anesthesia and hypertension. Semin Anaesthesiol 1982;1:226.
4. Murkin JM. Anesthesia and hypothyroidism: a review of thyroxine physiology, pharmacology and anesthetic implications. Anesth Analg 1982;61:371.
5. Chung F. Cancer, chemotherapy and anaesthesia. Can Anaesth Soc J 1982;29:364.
6. McGuire N, Easy WR. Malignant hyperthermia during isoflurane anaesthesia. Anaesthesia 1990;45:124.
7. Rubiano JA, Chang J-L, Carrol J et al. Acute rhabdomy-

olysis following halothane anaesthesia without succinylcholine. Anesthesiology 1987;67:856.
8. Littleford JA, Patel LR, Bosy D et al. Masseter muscle spasm in children, implications of continuing the triggering anesthetic. Anesth Analg 1991;72:151.
9. Lee S-C, Abe T, Sato T. Rhabdomyolysis and accute renal failure following use of succinylcholine and enflurane. J Oral Maxillofac Surg 1987;45:789.
10. Chalkiadis GA, Branch KG. Cardiac arrest after isoflurane anaesthesia in patient with Duchenne's muscular dystrophy. Anaesthesia 1990;45:22.
11. Gallen. Propofol does not trigger malignant hyperthermia (Correspondence). Anaesth Analg 1991;72:406.
12. Brooks JHJ. Midazolam in a malignant hyperthermia-susceptible patients (Correspondence). Anesthesiology 1989;70:167.
13. MacKenzie A, Allen G, Lahey et al. A comparison of the caffeine halothane muscle contrastion test with the molecular genetic diagnosis of malignant hyperthermia. Anesthesiology 1991;75:4.
14. Craig DB, Bose D. Drug interaction in anaesthesia: chronic antihypertensive therapy. Can Anaesth Soc J 1984;31:580.
15. Stevens JE. Rebound hypertension during anesthesia. Anaethesia 1980;35:490.
16. Ponten J, Biber B, Bjurö T et al. Beta-receptor blocker withdrawal: a pre-operative problem in general surgery. Acta Anaesthesiol Scand Suppl. 1982;76:32.
17. Derrington MC, Smith G. A review of studies of anestheetic risk, morbidity and mortality. Br J Anaesth 1987;95:815–833.
18. Berthoud MC, Reilly CS. Adverse effects of general anaesthetics. Drug Safety 1992;7:434–459.
19. Harrison GG. Death attributable to anaesthesia: a 10-year survey (1967–1976). Br J Anaesth 1978;50:1041.
20. Saarnivaara L. Comparison of halothane and enflurane anaesthesia for tonsillectomy in adults. Acta Anaesthesiol Scand 1984;28:319.
21. Vourc'h G, Hatton F, Tiret L, Desmote JM. Étude épidemiologique sur les complications de l'anesthésie en France. Bull Acad Natl Méd 1983;167:939.
22. Buck N, Devlin HB, Lunn JN. The Report of A Confidental Enquiry into Perioperative Deaths. Nuffield Provincial Hospitals Trust and The King's Fund, London. 1987.
23. Gannon K. Mortality associated with anethesia. A case review study. Anaesthesia 1991;46:962.
24. Pace NL. Adverse outcomes and the multicenter study of general anesthesia: II. Anesthesiology 1992;77:394–395.
25. D'Eramo EM. Morbidity and mortality with outpatient anesthesia: the Massachusetts experience. J Oral Maxillofac Surg 1992;50:700–704.
26. Gray WM. Occupational exposure to nitrous oxide in four hospitals. Anaesthesia 1989;44:511.
27. Gold DR. Indoor air polution. Clin Chest Med 1992; 13:215–229.
28. Rowland AS, Baird DD, Weinberg CR, Shore DL, Shy CM, Wilcox AJ. Reduced fertility among women employers as dental assistants to high levels of nitrous oxide. New Engl J Med 1992;327:1026–1027.
29. Sass-Kortsak AM, Purdham JT, Bozek PR, Murphy JH. Exposure of hospital operating room personnel to potentially harmful environmental agents. Am Ind Hyg Assoc J 1992;53:203–209.
30. Eger EI, ed. Nitrous Oxide. Edward Arnold, New York, 1985.
31. Saurel MJ, Estryn-Behar M, Maillard MF et al. Neuropsychological symptoms and occupational exposure to anaesthetics. Br J Ind Med 1992;49:276–281.
32. Vaisman AI. Working conditions in surgery and their effect on the health of anesthesiologists. Eksp Khirurg Anesteziol 1967;12:44–49.
33. Perić M, Vraneš Z, Marušić M. Immunological disturbances in anaesthetic personnel chronically exposed to halothane. Anaesthesia 1991;46:531.
34. Halsall PJ, Ellis FR. Malignant hyperthermia. Bailliere's Clin Anaesthesiol 1993;7:343–356.
35. Harrison GG. Dantrolene—dynamics and kinetics. Br J Anaesth 1988;60:279.
36. Flewellen EH, Nelson TE, Jones WP et al. Dantrolene dose response in awake man: implications for menagement of malignant hyperthermia. Anesthesiology 1983;59:275.
37. Walton B. Anaesthesia, surgery and immunology. Anaesthesia 1978;33:322.
38. Ryhanen P. Effects of anaesthesia and operative surgery on the immune response of patients of different ages. Ann Clin Res 1977;(Suppl 19):9.
39. Clarke RSJ. The clinical presentation of anaphylactoid reactions in anesthesia. Int Anesthesiol Clin 1985;23:1.
40. Laxenaire MC, Manel J, Borgo J, Moneret-Vautrin DA. Facteurs de risque d'histamino-libération: étude prospective dans une population anesthésiée. Ann Fr Anesth Réanim 1985;4:158.
41. Watkins J. Investigation of allergic and hypersensitivity reactions to anesthetic agents. Br J Anaesth 1987;59:104.
42. Youngman PR, Taylor KM, Wilson JD. Anaphylatic reactions to neuromuscular blocking agents: a commonly undiagnosed condition? Lancet 1983;ii:597.
43. Assem ESK. Anaphylactic anaesthetic reactions. Anaesthesia 1990;45:1032.
44. Assem ESK, Symons IE. Anaphylaxis due to suxamethonium in a seven year old child. Anaesthesia 1989;44:121.
45. Laxenaire MC, Moneret-Vautrin DA, Guéant JL et al. Drugs and other agents involved in anaphylactic shock occurring during anaesthesia. A French multicenter epidemiological inquiry. Ann Fr Anesth Réanim 1993;12:91–96.
46. Clarce RSJ, Watkins J. Drugs responsible for anaphylactoid reactions in anaesthesia in the United Kingdom. Ann Fr Anesth Reanim 1993;12:105–108.
47. Havard J. Medical Aspects of Fitness to Drive, 3rd edn. London: A. Rapple, 1976;43.
48. Sparacia A, Mangione S, Sansone A. Alterazioni dell'emostasi in relazione al farmaci anestetici ed all'emostasi ed all'intervento chirurgico. Minerva Anestesiol 1980;46:791.
49. Simpson PJ, Radford SG, Forster SJ et al. The fibrinolytic effects of anesthesia. Anesth Analg 1982;60:319.
50. Zahavi J, Price AJ, Kakkar VV. Enhanced platelet release reaction associated with general anaesthesia. Lancet 1980;i:1132.
51. Slegers-Karsmakers S, Stricker BHCh. Anaphylactic reaction to isoflurane (Correspondence). Anaesthesia 1988; 43:506.
52. Black GW. Enflurane. Br J Anaesth 1979;51:627.
53. Shimosato S, Iwatsuki N, Carter JG. Cardiocirculatory effects of enflurane anaesthesia in health and disease. Acta Anaesthaesiol Scand 1979;71:89.

54. Rifat K. Effets cardiovasculaires de l'enflurane. Med Hyg 1979;37:3602.
55. Reves JG, Samuelson PN, Lell WA et al. Myocardial damage in coronary artery by-pass surgical patients anaesthetized with two anaesthetic techniquee: a random comparison of halothane and enflurane. Can Anaesth Soc J 1980;27:238.
56. Wilatts DG, Harrison AR, Groom JF, Growther A. Cardiac arrhythnias during out-patient dental anaesthesia: comparison of halothane with enflurane. Br J Anaesth 1983;55:399.
57. Chander S. Isorhythmic atrioventricular dissociation during enflurane anaesthesia. South Med J 1982;75:945.
58. Lowry CJ, Fielden BP. Bronchospasm associated with enflurane exposure: three case reports. Anaesth Intensive Care 1976;4:254.
59. Fahy LT. Delayed convulsion after day-care anaesthesia with enflurane. Anaesthesia 1987;42:1327.
60. Bentin S, Collins GI, Adam N. Decision-making behaviour during inhalation of subanaesthetic concentration of enflurane. Br J Anaesth 1978;50:117.
61. Bentin S, Collins GI, Adam N. Effects of low concentrations of enflurane on probability learning. Br J Anaesth 1978;50:1179.
62. Oyama T, Tanigushi K, Whihara A et al. Effects of enflurane anaesthesia and surgery on endocrine function in man. Br J Anaesth 1979;51:141.
63. Buzaleh AM, Enriquez de Salamanca R, Batlle AM. Porphyrinogenic properties of the anesthetic enflurane. Gen Pharmacol 1992;23:665—669.
64. Sigurdsson J, Hreidarsson AB, Thjodleifsson B. Enflurane hepatitis: a report of a case with a previous history of halothane hepatitis. Acta Anaesthesiol Scand 1985;29:495.
65. Paull JD, Fortune DW. Hepatotoxicity and death following two enflurane anaesthetics. Anaesthesia 1987;42:1191.
66. Fee JPJ, Black GW, Dundee JW et al. A prospective study of liver enzymes and other changes following repeat administration of halothane and enflurane. Br J Anaesth 1979;51:1133.
67. Motuz DJ, Watson WA, Barlow JC et al. The increase in urinary alanine aminopeptidase excretion associated with enflurane anesthesia in increased further by aminoglycosides. Anesth Analg 1988;67:770.
68. Mazze RI, Calverley RK, Ty Smith N. Inorganic fluoride nephrotoxicity: Prolonged enflurane and halothane anesthesia in volunteers. Anesthesiology 1977;46:265.
69. Miyagishima T, Takagi N, Oka N et al. Myoglobinuria associated with enflurane anesthesia. Hiroshima J Anesth 1981;16:122.
70. Stanski DR, Ham J, Miller RD, Skeiner LB. Time dependent increase in sensitivity to *d*-tubocurarine during enflurane anesthesia in man. Anesthesiology 1980;52:483.
71. Weis K-H, Engelhardt W. Is halothane obsolete? Two standard judgement. Anesthesia 1989;44:97.
72. Pedersen T, Johansen SH. Serious morbidity attributable to anesthesia. Anaesthesia 1989;44:504.
73. Maze M, Mason DM. Aetiology and treatment of halothane-induced arrhythmias. Clin Anaesthesiol 1983;1:301.
74. Yokoyama K. Arrhythmias due to halothane anesthesia. Jpn J Anesthesiol 1978;27:64.
75. Lindgren L. ECG changes during halothane and enflurane anaesthesia for ENT surgery in children. Br J Anaesth 1981;53:853.
76. Merin RG. Physiology, pathophysiology and pharmacology of the coronary circulation with particular emphasis on anesthetics Anaesthesiol Reanim 1992;17:5—26.
77. Schmidt U, Schwinger RH, Bohm S, Uberfuhr P, Kreuzer E, Reichart B, Meyer L, Erdmann E, Bohm M. Evidence for an interaction of halothane with L-type Ca^{2+} channel in human myocardium. Anesthesiology 1993; 79:332—339.
78. McKinney MS, Fee JP, Clarke RSJ. Cardiovascular effects of isoflurane and halothane in young and elderly adult patients. Br J Anaesth 1993;71:696—701.
79. Sabik JF, Assad RS, Hanley FL. Halothane as an anesthetic for fetal surgery. J Pediatr Surg 1993;28:542—546.
80. Obata T, Masaki T, Nezu T, Iikura Y. Treatment of status asthmaticus with halothane: a case report. Iryo 1992;46:204—210.
81. Palmisano BW, Setlock MA, Doyle MK, Rosner DR, Hoffman GM, Eckert JE. Ventilatory response to carbon dioxide in term infants after halothane and nitrous oxide anesthesia. Anesth Analg 1993;76:1234—1237.
82. Haga S, Shima T, Momose K, Andoch K, Hoshi K, Hashimoto Y. Postoperative apnea in preterm infants after inguinal herniorrhaphy. Masui 1993;42:120—122.
83. Smith PA, McDonald TR, Jones CS. Convulsions associated with halothane anaesthesia: two case reports. Anaesthesia 1966;21:229.
84. Davison LA, Steinhelber JC, Eger IE, Stevens WC. Psychological effects of halothane and isoflurane anesthesia. Anesthesiology 1975;43:313.
85. Burchiel KJ, Stockard JJ, Calverley RK et al. Electroencephalographic abnormalities following halothane anesthesia. Anesth Analg 1978;57:244.
86. Dalsgaard-Nielsen J, Risbo A, Simmelkjarer P, Gormsen J. Impaired platelet aggregation and increased bleeding time during general anaesthesia with halothane. Br J Anaesth 1981;53:1039.
87. Feher J, Vasarhelyi B, Blazovics A. Halothane hepatitis. Orv Hetil 1993;134:1795—1798.
88. Elliot RH, Strunin L. Hepatotoxicity of volatile anaesthetics. Br J Anaesth 1993;70:339—348.
89. Bottiger LE, Dalen E, Hallen B. Halothane-induced liver damage: an analysis of the material reported to the Swedish Adverse Drug Reaction Committee. Acta Anaesthesiol Scand 1976;20:40—46.
90. Smith GC, Kenna JG, Harrison DJ, Tew D, Wolf CR. Autoantibodies to hepatic microsomal carboxylesterase in halothane hepatitis. Lancet 1993;342:963—964.
91. Kenna JG, Knight TL, Van Pelt FN. Immunity to halothane metabolite-modified proteins in halothane hepatitis. Ann NY Acad Sci 1993;685:646—661.
92. Ranek L, Dalhoff K, Enghusen-Poulsen H. Drug metabolite and genetic polymorphism in subjects with previous halothane hepatitis. Scand J Gastroenterol 1993;28:677—680.
93. Dahmash NS, Ayoola EA, Al-Nozha M. Halothane induced hepatotoxicity in a Saudi male. Ann Saudi Med 1993;13:314—316.
94. Shimizu H, Namba H, Ishima T. Liver dysfunction after halothane therapy in two cases with life threatening asthma. KoKyu 1993;12:229—232.
95. Slaytar KL, Sketris IS, Gulanjkar A. Halothane hepatitis in a renal transplant patient previously exposed to isoflurane. Ann Pharmacother 1993;27:101.
96. Bidard JM, Casio N, Gerolami A et al. Deux observations d'hépatite toxique par association d'halothane à un inducteur enzymatique. Nouv Presse Méd 1980;9:883.

97. Steiner F, Pottecher T, Bellocq JP. Ictère grave post opératoire: rôle de l'halothane et des tuberculostatiques. Cah Anesthésiol 1980;23:1019.
98. Hoft RH, Bunker JP, Goodman HI, Gregory PB. Halothane hepatitis in three pairs of closely related women. N Engl J Med 1981;304:1023.
99. Schlippert W, Anuras S. Recurrent hepatitis following halothane exposure. Am J Med 1978;65:25.
100. Kenna JG, Neuberger J, Mieli-Vergani et al. Halothane hepatitis in children. Br Med J 1987;294:1209.
101. Dallera F, Caccialanza E, Segalini A et al. Un caso di poliuria probabilmente da fluotano. Acta Anaesthesiol Ital 1983;34:83.
102. Gelman ML, Lichtenstein NS. Halothane-induced nephrotoxicity. Urology 1981;17:323.
103. Bodman R. Skin sensitivity to halothane vapour. Br J Anaesth 1979;15:1092.
104. Neumark J, Faller T. Halothan, Enfluran und ihr Einfluss auf die Uterusaktivität am Geburts-Termin. Prakt Anaesth 1978;13:7.
105. Coté CJ, Kenepp NB, Reeb SB, Strobel GE. Trace concentrations of halothane in human breastmilk. Br J Anaesth 1976;48:541.
106. Trombini Garcia R, Salomao JB, Benincasa SC et al. Instilagaio acidental de halotano em una criança de quatro anos. J Pediatr 1984;56:323.
107. Karlsson E, Larsson LE, Nilsson K. The effects of prophylactic dixyrazine on postoperative vomiting after two different anaesthetic methods for squint surgery in children. Acta Anaesthesiol Scand 1993;37:45—48.
108. Payne JP. Chloroform in clinical anaesthesia. Br J Anaesth 1981;53:115.
109. Levy WJ. Clinical anaesthesia with isoflurane. Br J Anaesth 1984;56:101S.
110. Rodrigo MCR, Moles TM, Lee PK. Comparison of the incidence and nature of cardiac arrhythmias occurring during isoflurane or halothane anaesthesia. Br J Anaesth 1986; 58:394.
111. Slogoff S, Keats AS. Randomized trial of primary anesthetic agents on outcome of coronary artery bypass operations. Anesthesiology 1989;70:179.
112. Inoue K, Reicheit W, El-Banyosy A et al. Does isoflurane lead to a higher incidence of myocardial infarction and peri-operative death than enflurane in coronary artery surgery? Anesth Analg 1990;71:469.
113. Murat I, Beydon L, Chaussain M et al. Ventilatory changes during nitrous oxide isoflurane anaesthesia in children. Eur J Anaesthesiol 1986;3:403.
114. Shibata Y, Kukita I, Baba T, Goto T, Yoshinaga T. A critical patient relieved from status asthmaticus with isoflurane inhalation therapy. Masui 1993;42:116—119.
115. Du Peloux Menage H, Duffy S, Yates DW, Hughes JA. Reversible sensorimotor impairment following prolonged ventilation with isoflurane and vecuronium for acute severe asthma. Thorax 1992;47:1078—1079.
116. Truog RD, Rice SA. Inorganic fluoride and prolonged isoflurane anesthesia in the intensive care unit. Anesth Analg 1989;69:843.
117. Gregoire S, Kennedy A, Smiley R. Acute hepatitis in a patient with mild factor IX deficiency after anesthesia with isoflurane. Can Med Assoc J 1986;135:645.
118. Scheider DM, Klygis LM, Tsan TK, Caughron MC. Hepatic dysfunction after repeated isoflurane administration. J Clin Gastroenterol 1993;17:168—170.
119. Carrigan TW, Straughen WJ. A report of hepatic necrosis and death following isoflurane anesthesia. Anesthesiology 1987;67:581.
120. Boheler J, Hamrick JC, MacKnight RL, Eger EI. Isoflurane and malignant hyperthermia. Anesth Analg 1982;61:712.
121. Shanks CA, Fragen RJ, Ling D. Continuous infusion of rocuronium in patients receiving balanced enflurane or isoflurane anesthesia. Anesthesiology 1993;78:649—651.
122. Randell T, Yli-Hankala A, Lindgren L. Isoflurane inhibits muscle fasciculations caused by succinylcholine in children. Acta Anaesthesiol Scand 1993;37:262—264.
123. Andrews JJ, Johnston RV, Kramer GC. Consequenses of misfilling contemporary vaporizers with desflurane. Can J Anaesth 1993;40:71—76.
124. Eger EI. Desflurane animal and human pharmacology: aspects of kinetics, safety, and MAC. Anesth Analg 1992;75(Suppl):3—9.
125. Bennett JA, Lingaraju N, Horrow JC, McElrath T, Keykhah MM. Elderly patients recover more rapidly from desflurane than from isoflurane anesthesia. J Clin Anesthesiol 1992;4:378—381.
126. Warltier DC, Pagel PS. Cardiovascular and respiratory actions of desflurane: is desflurane different from isoflurane? Anesth Analg 1992;75(Suppl):17—31.
127. Zwass MS, Fisher DM, Welborn LG, Cote CJ, Davis PJ, Dinner M, Hannallah RS, Liu LM, McGill WA. Induction and maintenance characteristics of anesthesia with desflurane and nitrous oxide in infants and children. Anesthesiology 1992;76:373—378.
128. Ornstein E, Young WL, Fleischer LH, Ostapkovich N. Desflurane and isoflurane have similar effects on cerebral blood flow in patients with intracranial mass lesions. Anesthesiology 1993;79:498—502.
129. Kelly RE, Lien CA, Savarese JJ, Belmont MR, Hartman GS. Depression of neuromuscular function in a patient during desflurane anesthesia. Anesth Analg 1993;76:868—871.
130. Weiskopf RB, Eger EI, Ionescu P, Yasuda N, Cahalan MK, Freire B, Peterson N, Lockhart SH, Rampil IJ, Laster M. Desflurane does not Produce hepatic or renal injury in human volunteers. Anesth Analg 1992;74:570—574.
131. Gold MI, Abello D, Herrington C. Minimum alveolar concentration of desflurane in patients older than 65 yr. Anesthesiology 1993;79:710—714.
132. Sebel PS, Glass PS, Fletcher JE, Murphy MR, Gallagher C, Quill T. Reduction of the MAC of desflurane with fentanyl. Anesthesiology 1992;76:52—59.
133. Moore MA, Weiskopf RB, Eger EI, Wilson C. Arrhythmogenic doses of epinephrine are similar during desflurane or isoflurane anesthesia in humans. Anesthesiology 1993;79:943—947.
134. Ochai R, Toyoda Y, Nishio I et al. Possible association of malignant hyperthermia with sevoflurane anesthesia. Anesth Analg 1992;74:616—618.
135. Shulman M, Braverman B, Ivankovich AD et al. Sevoflurane triggers malignant hyperthermia in swine. Anesthesiology 1981;54:259—260.
136. Smith I, Ding Y, White PF. Comparison of induction, maintenance and recovery characteristics of sevoflurane-N_2O anesthesia. Anesth Analg 1992;74:253—259.
137. Kikura M, Ikeda K. Comparison of effects of sevoflurane/nitrous oxide and enflurane/nitrous oxide on myocardial contractility in humans. Load-independent and noninvasive

assessment with transoesophageal echocardiography. Anesthesiology 1993;79:235–243.
138. Kitahata H, Tanaka K, Kimura H, Saito T. Effects of sevoflurane on left ventricular diastolic function using transesophageal echocardiography. Masui 1993;42:358–364.
139. Takahashi H, Murata K, Ikeda K. Sevoflurane does not increase intracranial pressure in hyperventilated dogs. Br J Anaesth 1993;71:551–555.
140. Kitaguchi K, Ohsumi H, Kuro M, Nakajima T, Hayashi Y. Effects of sevoflurane on cerebral circulation and metabolism in patients with ischemic cerebrovascular disease. Anesthesiology 1993;79:704–709.
141. Hasegawa J, Mitsuhata H, Matsumoto S, Komatsu H, Mizunuma T. The effects of induced hypotension with sevoflurane and PGE 1 on liver function during neurosurgery. Masui 1992;41:772–778.
142. Watanabe K, Hatakena S, Ikemune K, Chigyo Y, Kubozono T, Arai T. A case of suspected liver dysfunction induced by sevoflurane anesthesia. Masui 1993;42:902–905.
143. Kobayashi Y, Ochiai R, Takeda Y, Sekiguchi H, Fukusima K. Serum and urinary fluoride concentrations after prolonged inhalation of sevoflurane in humans. Anesth Analg 1992;74:753–757.
144. Otsuka H, Komura Y, Mayumi T, Yamamura T, Kemmotsu O. Malignant hyperthermia during sevoflurane anesthesia in a child with a central core disease. Anesthesiology 1991;75:699–701.
145. Ochiai R, Toyoda Y, Nishio I, Takeda J, sekiguchi H, Fukushima K, Kohda E. Possible association of malignant hyperthermia with sevoflurane anesthesia. Anesth Analg 1992;74:616–618.
146. Matsumoto M, Sakai H. Sevoflurane anesthesia for a patient with insulinoma. Masui 1992;41:446–449.
147. Saitoh K, Hirabayashi Y, Fukuda H, Shimizu R. Sevoflurane anesthesia in a patient following renal transplantation. Masui 1993;42:746–749.
148. Desmond JW. Methoxyflurane nephrotoxicity. Can Anaesth Soc J 1974;21:294.
149. Sanchez MA, Gonzales-Mirana F, Rodriquez-Harnangez JL. Icteria y metoxiflurano. Rev Esp Anestesiol Reanim 1980;27:481.
150. Li Prema JP, Wellman J, Stern HP. Nitrous oxide abuse: a new case for pneumomediastinum. Radiology 1982; 145:602.
151. Kozmary SV, Lampe GH, Benefield D et al. No finding of increased myocardial ischemia during or after carotid endarterectomy under anesthesia with nitrous oxide. Anesth Analg 1990;71:591.
152. Lampe GH, Donegan GH, Rupp SM et al. Nitrous oxide and epinephrine-induced arrhythmias. Anesth Analg 1990;71:602.
153. Jin T, Ishihara H, Ohshiro Y et al. Effects of nitrous oxide on the circulatory and respiratory functions. Jpn J Anesthesiol 1980;29:458.
154. Maroof M, Khan RM, Siddique M. Ventilation with nitrous oxide during open cholecystectomy increase the incidence of postoperative hypoxemia. Anesth Analg 1993; 76:1091–1094.
155. Komatsu H, Mitsuhata H, Hasegawa J, Matsumoto S. Decreased pressure of endotracheal tube cuff in general anesthesia without nitrous oxide. Masui 1993;42:831–834.
156. Atkinson RM, Moorozumi P, De Wayne-Green J, Kramer JC. Nitrous oxide intoxication: subjective effects in healthy young men. J Psychedelic Drugs 1977;6:317.
157. Nunn JF. Clinical aspects of the interaction between nitrous oxide and vitamin B_{12}. Br J Anaesth 1987;59:3.
158. Holloway KL, Alberico AM. Postoperative myeloneuropathy: a preventable complication in patients with B_{12} deficiency. J Neurosurg 1990;7:732.
159. Layzer PB. Myeloneuropathy after prolonged exposure to nitrous oxide. Lancet 1978;ii:1227.
160. Brodsky JB, Cohen EN, Brown BW et al. Exposure to nitrous oxide and neurologic disease among dental professionals. Anesth Analg 1981;60:297.
161. Moyes D, Cleaton-Jones P, Lelliot J. Evaluation of driving skills after brief exposure to nitrous oxide. South Afr J Med 1979;56:1000.
162. Goodie D, Trail R. Intra-operative subdural tension pneumocephalus arising after opening of the dura. Anesthesiology 1991;74:193.
163. Ramsay DS, Leonesio RJ, Whitney CW et al. Paradoxical effects of nitrous oxide on human memory. Psychopharmacology 1992;106:370–374.
164. Fournier L, Major D. Nitrous oxide effects on pO_2 measurements in the operating room: shift of the oxyhaemoglobin curve. Can Anaesth Soc J 1982;29:498.
165. Gronert CA, Milde JH. Hyperbaric nitrous oxide and malignant hyperthermia. Br J Anaesth 1981;53:1238.
166. Waldman FM, Koblin DD, Lampe GH et al. Hematologic effects of nitrous oxide in surgical patients. Anesth Analg 1990;71:618.
167. Warren DJ, Christensen B, Slordal L. Effects of nitrous oxide on haematopoeses in vitro: biochemical and fuctional features. Pharmacol Toxicol 1993;72:69–72.
168. Carmel R, Rabinowitz AP, Mazumder A. Metabolic evidence of cobalamin deficiency in bone marrow cells harvested for transplantation from donors given nitrous oxide. Eur J Haematol 1993;50:228–233.
169. Hart SM, Fitzgerald PG. Unexplained jaundice following non-halothane anaesthesia. Br J Anaesth 1975;47:1321.
170. Jensen AG, Prevedorors H, Kullman E, Anderberg B, Lennmarken C. Perioperative nitrous oxide does not influence recovery after laparoscopic cholecystectomy. Acta Anaesthesiol Scand 1993;37:683–686.
171. Nuutinen LS. The effect of nitrous oxide on renal function in open heart surgery. Ann Chir Gynaecol 1976;65:200.
172. Casey WF, Drake-Lee AB. Nitrous oxide and middle-ear pressure. Anaesthesia 1982;37:896.
173. Crawford JS, Lewis M. Nitrous oxide in early human pregnancy. Anaesthesia 1986;41:900.
174. Nunn JF. Nitrous oxide and pregnancy. Anaesthesia 1987;42:427.
175. Epstein RM, Rackrow H, Salanitre E, Wolf GL. Influence of the concentration effect on the uptake of anesthetic mixtures—the second gas effect. Anesthesiology 1964; 25:364.
176. Moffitt E, Bussell J, Sethna D et al. Nitrous oxide added to halothane depresses coronary flow and the heart in patients with coronary artery disease. Can Anaesth Soc J 1981;28:497.
177. Jansen U, Moller-Petersen J, Petersen S. An explosion fatality during cyclopropane anaesthesia. Ugeskr. Læg 1979;141:3375.
178. Nash G, Blennerhasset JB, Pontoppidan H. Pulmonary lesions associated with oxygen therapy and artificial ventilation. N Engl J Med 1967;276:368.
179. Kapanci Y, Tosco R, Eggermann J et al. Oxygen pneu-

monitis in man. Light and electron-microscope morphometric studies. Chest 1972;62:162.
180. Clark JM, Lambertsen CJ. Pulmonary oxygen toxicity: a review. Pharm Rev 1971;23:37.
181. Wright WB. Use of the University of Pennsylvania Institute for Environmental Medicine procedure for calculation of pulmonary oxygen toxicity. US Navy Exp Diving Unit Rep 1972;2:72.
182. Donald KW. Oxygen poisoning in man. I and II. Br Med J 1947;1:667, 712.
183. MacDonald D. Methohexitone in dentistry. Aust Dent J 1980;25:335.
184. Millar JM, Barr AM. The prevention of pain on injection. Anaesthesia 1981;36:878.
185. Rockoff MA, Goudsouzian PG. Seizures induced by methohexital. Anaesthesiology 1981;54:333.
186. Celleno D, Capogna G, Emanuelli M, Varrassi G, Muratori F, Costantino P, Sebastiani M. Which drug for cesarean section? A comparison of thiopental sodium, propofol, and midazolam. J Clin Anesth 1993;5:284—288.
187. Seymour DG. Anaphylactic reaction to thiopental. J Am Med Assoc 1993;270:2503.
188. Desmeules H. Nonpigmenting fixed drug eruption after anesthesia. Anesth Analg 1990;70:216.
189. Habibi B, Basty R, Chodez S, Prunat A. Thiopental-related immune hemolytic anemia and renal failure. N Engl J Med 1985;312:353.
190. Kanor P, Dundee JW. Frequency of pain on injection and venous sequelae following the i.v. administration of certain anaesthetics and sedatives. Br J Anaesth 1982;54:935.
191. Vaughan GG, Grycko RJ, Montgomery MT. The prevention and treatment of vomitus during pharmacosedation and general anesthesia. J Oral Maxillofac Surg 1992;50:874—879.
192. Vanner RG, Pryle BJ, O'Dwyer JP, Reynolds F. Upper oesophageal sphincter pressure and the intravenous induction of anaesthesia. Anaesthesia 1992;47:371—375.
193. Becker KE, Tonnesen AS. Cardiovascular effects of plasma levels of thiopental necessary for anesthesia. Anesthesiology 1978;49:197.
194. Stone JG, Young WL, Marans ZS, Khambatta HJ, Solomon RA, Smith CR, Ostapkovich N, Jamdar SC, Diaz J. Cardiac performance preserved despite thiopental loading. Anesthesiology 1993;79:36—41.
195. Festimanni F, Orvieto A, Peduto VA. Metaemoglobinemia congenita come causi di cianosi durante l'anesthesia. Acta Anaesthesiol Ital 1980;31:601.
196. Colvin MP, Savege TM, Newland PE et al. Cardiorespiratory changes following induction of anaesthesia with etomidate in patients with cardiac disease. Br J Anaesth 1979;51:551.
197. Price ML, Millar B, Grounds M, Cashman J. Changes in cardiac index and estimated systemic vascular resistance during induction of anaesthesia with thiopentone, methohexitone, propofol and etomidate. Br J Anaesth 1992;69:172—176.
198. Berry JM, Merin RG. Etomidate myoclonus and the open globe. Anesth Analg 1989;69:256.
199. Krieger W, Koerner M. Generalized grand mal seizure after recovery from uncomplicated fentanyl—etomidate anaesthesia. Anesth Analg 1987;66:283.
200. Nickel B, Schmickaly R. Gesteigerte Anfallsbereitschaft unter Etomidatlangzeitinfusion beim Delirium tremens. Anaesthesist 1985;34:462.
201. Parker CJR. Respiratory disturbance during recovery from etomidate anaesthesia. Anaesthesia 1988;43:16.
202. Hansen HC, Drenck NE. Generalized seizures after etomidate anaesthesia. Anaesthesia 1988;43:805.
203. Weber MM, Lang J, Abedinpour F, Zeilberger K, Adelmann B, Engelhart D. Different inhibitory effect of etomidate and ketoconazole on the human adrenal steroid biosynthesis. Clin Invest 1993;71:933—938.
204. Varga I, Racz K, Kiss R, Futo L, Toth M, Sergev O, Glaz E. Direct inhibitory effect of etomidate od corticosteroid secretion in human pathologic adrenocortical cells. Steroids 1993;58:64—68.
205. Vanacker B, Wiebalck A, Van-Aken H, Sermeus L, Bouillon R, Amery A. Quality of induction and adrenocortical function. A clinical comparison of Etomidate-Lipuro and Hypnomidate. Anaesthesist 1993;42:81—89.
206. Crozier TA, Flamm C, Speer CP, Rath W, Wuttke W, Kuhn W, Kettler D. Effects of etomidate on the adrenocortical and metabolite adaptation of the neonate. Br J Anaesth 1993;70:47—53.
207. Nebauer AE, Doenicke A, Hoernicke R, Angster R, Mayer M. Does etomidate cause haemolysis? Br J Anaesth 1992;60:58—60.
208. Wertz E. Does etomidate cause haemolysis? Br J Anaesth 1993;60:490—491.
209. Doenicke A, Nebauer AE, Hoernecke R, Angster R, Mayer M. Does eomidate cause haemolysis? In response. Br J Anaesth 1993;70:491.
210. Fazerackerley EJ, Martin AJ, Tolhurst-Cleaver CL et al. Anaphylactoid reaction following the use of etomidate. Anaesthesia 1988;43:953.
211. Epstein FB. Ketamine dissociative sedation in pediatric emergency medical practice. Am J Emerg Med 1993; 11:180—182.
212. Weksler N, Ovadia L, Muati G, Stav A. Nasal ketamine for pediatric premedication. Can J Anaesth 1993;40:119—121.
213. Zsigmend EK, Kothary SP, Kumar SM et al. Counteraction of circulatory side effect of ketamine by pretreatment with diazepam. Clin Ther 1980;3:28.
214. Cabbabe EB, Behbahani PM. Cardiovascular reactions associated with the use of ketamine and epinephrine in plastic surgery. Ann Plastic Surg 1985;15:50.
215. Waxman K, Shoemaker WC, Lippmann M. Cardiovascular effects of anesthetic induction with ketamine. Anesth Analg 1980;59:355.
216. Tarnow J, Hess W. Pulmonale Hypertonie und Lungödeem nach Ketamin. Anesthetist 1978;57:486.
217. Smith JA, Santer LJ. Respiratory arrest following intramuscular ketamine injection in a 4-year-old child. Ann Emerg Med 1993;22:613—615.
218. Jahangir SM, Islam F, Aziz L. Ketamine infusion for postoperative analgesia in asthmatics: a comparison with intermittent meperidine. Anesth Analg 1993;76:45—49.
219. Klausen NO, Wiberg-Jorgensen F, Chraemmer-Doigensen B. Psychomimetic reactions following low-dose ketamine infusion. Br J Anaesth 1983;55:297.
220. Fontana M, Mastrostefano R, Pietrangelli A et al. Acute intracranial hypertension syndrome due to ketamine in a patient with delayed radioneurosis simultaning an expanding process. J Neurosurg Sci 1980;24:93.
221. Hall CH, Cassidy J. Young drug users adopt "bad trip" anesthetic. Independent 1992;2:1.
222. Dundee JW, Fee JPH, Moore J et al. Changes in serum

enzyme levels following ketamine infusions. Anaesthesia 1980;35:12.
223. Murray Wilson A. Multiple ketamine anaesthesia. Saudi Med J 1979;1:19.
224. Gast PH, Fisher A, Sear JW. Intensive care sedation now. Lancet 1984;ii:863—864.
225. Editorial. Midazolam—is antagonism justified? Lancet 1988;ii:140.
226. Alexander CM, Gross JB. Sedative doses of midazolam depress hypoxic ventilatory responses in humans. Anesth Analg 1988;67:377.
227. Bailey PL, Pace NL, Ashburn MA et al. Frequent hypoxaemia and apnea after sedation with midazolam and fentanyl. Anesthesiology 1990;73:826.
228. Eldridge FR, Punt JAC. Risks associated with giving benzodiazepines to patients with acute neurological injuries. Br Med J 1990;300:1189.
229. Montravers PH, Dureuil B, Desmonts JM. Effects of midazolam on upper airway resistances. Anesthesiology 1988;69:A824.
230. Atanassoff PG, Alon E, Pasch T. Recovery after propofol, midazolam and methohexitone as an adjunct to epidural anesthesia for lower abdominal surgery. Eur J Anaesthesiol 1993;10:313—318.
231. Crawford M, Pollock J, Anderson K, Glavin RJ, MacIntyre D, Vernon D. Comparison of midazolam with propofol for sedation in outpatient bronchoscopy. Br J Anaesth 1993;70:419—422.
232. Conway EE, Singer LP. Acute benzodiazepine withdrawal after midazolam in children. Crit Care Med 1990;18:461.
233. Olkkola KT, Aranko K, Luurila H, Hiller A, Saarnivaara L, Himberg JJ, Neuvonen PJ. A potentially hazardous interaction between erythromycin and midazolam. Clin Pharmacol Ther 1993;53:298—305.
234. Inagahi Y, Sumikawa K, Yoshiya I. Anesthetic interaction between midazolam and halothane in humans. Anesth Analg 1993;76:613—617.
235. Kitamura N, Sugai T, Hirasawa H, Hayashi S, Kikuchi S. Therapeutic use of flumazenil in mixed overdoses with benzodiazepines. Jpn J Toxicol 1992;5:63—67.
236. Coates W, Evans TC, Jehle D, Harchelroad F, Issacs M. Flumazenil for the reversal of refractory benzodiazepine-induced shock. J Toxicol Clin Toxicol 1991;29:537—542.
237. Kulka PJ, Lauven PM. Benzodiazepine antagonists. An update of their role in the emergency care of overdose patients. Drug Safety 1992;7:381—386.
238. Lopez A, Rebollo J. Benzodiazepine withdrawal syndrome after a benzodiazepine antagonist. Crit Care Med 1990;18:1480.
239. Millar LM, Jewkes CF. Recovery and morbidity after daycase anaesthesia: a comparison of propofol with thiopentone—enflurane without alfentanyl. Anaesthesia 1988;43:738.
240. Laxenaire MC, Gueant JL, Bermejo E et al. Anaphylactic shock due to propofol. Lancet 1988;ii:739.
241. Jamieson V, Mackenzie J. Allergy to propofol? (Correspondence). Anaesthesia 1988;43:70.
242. Hud CC Jr, McLeskey CH, Nahrwold ML, Roizen MF, Stanley TH, Thisted RA, Walawander CA, White PF, Apfelbaum LJ, Grasela TH. Hemodynamic effects of propofol—data from over 25000 patients. Anesth Analg 1993;77(Suppl 4):S21—S29.
243. Searle NR, Sahab P. Propofol in patients with cardiac disease. Can J Anaesth 1993;40:730—747.
244. Gillies GWA, Lees NW. The effects of speed of injection of propofol. A comparison with etomidate. Anaesthesia 1989;44:386.
245. Carpentier JP, Riou O, Petrognani R, Seignot P, Aubert M. Étude comparée du reveil après entretien de l'anesthesie par propofol ou isoflurane. Essai de synthese des clonnées actuelles Cah Anesthesiol 1993;41:327—330.
246. Saunders PRI, Harris ME. Opisthotonus and other neurological sequelae after outpatient anaesthesia. Anaesthesia 1990;45:552.
247. McHugh P. Acute choreoathetoid reaction to propofol. Amaesthesia 1991;46:425.
248. Hassan MM, Hasan ZA, Al Hader AF, Takrouri MS. The anticonvulsant effects of propofol, diazepam and thiopental, against picrotoxin-induced seizure in the rat. Middle East J Anesthesiol 1993;12:113—121.
249. Heavner JE, Arthur J, Zou J, McDaniel K, Tymanszram B, Rosenberg PH. Comparison of propofol with thiopentone for treatment of bupivacaine-induced seizures in rats. Br J Anaesth 1993;71:715—719.
250. Borgeat A, Dessibourg C, Popovic V et al. Propofol and spontaneous movements: an EEG study. Anesthesiology 1991;74:24.
251. Kent EA, Douglas RB, Harrison P, Lema MJ. Sexual illusions and propofol sedation. Anesthesiology 1992;77:1038—1043.
252. Shearer ES. Convulsions and propofol. Anaesthesia 1991;45:255.

Meyler's Side Effects of Drugs, 13th Edition
M.N.G. Dukes, editor

SECTION EDITOR: B. VRHOVAC

M.N.G. Dukes

11 Local anaesthetics

Editorial note *Adverse effects of local anesthetics used in the eye are reviewed primarily in Chapter 47. Lidocaine is used systematically as an antiarrythmic agent, and its adverse effects when so used are discussed in Chapter 17.*

GENERAL

The general pattern of adverse effects to local anesthetics is well established and the literature produces few major surprises from year to year (1^R, 2^R). As in other therapeutic fields, the advantages claimed for newer agents as regards their safety profile have to be regarded with much reserve, since with increasing field experience and adjustment of the dose to optimal levels the tolerability is commonly found to be very similar to that of substances in use for a much longer period.

The adverse effects of local anesthesia fall broadly into three groups. Firstly, there are the effects attributable to the technique itself rather than to the agent used, e.g. needle damage to a vessel or nerve; secondly, there are the local and regional effects of the drug concerned which may be related to its anesthetic activity or a consequence of irritation or allergy. Finally, there are the systemic effects, most usually seen if the agent is inadvertently injected into a vessel in sufficient quantities (3^R).

Some of the effects of local anesthesia are in whole or in part a consequence of using additives, notably vasoconstrictors (added to prolong the local effect) or hyaluronidase to promote penetration (4^C).

As to the frequency of complications, some distinction must also be made between the main groups of local anesthetics, namely the amide-type agents (such as bupivacaine, dibucaine, etidocaine, lidocaine, mepivacaine, and prilocaine) and the non-amides (the remainder); hypersensitivity reactions are for example relatively less common with the amides. However, individual local anesthetics differ as to their systemic toxicity: bupivacaine, dibucaine and tetracaine are considered to be the most toxic derivatives. Furthermore, the individual characteristics of the patient, e.g. age, sex, body weight and the state of cardiac, renal and hepatic function, are known to play an important role (SEDA-17, 134).

SYSTEMIC TOXICITY

As pointed out above, systemic toxicity (5^R) is most likely to be seen if a local anesthetic is by accident injected into a vessel in sufficient quantity. There is, however, also inevitably some diffusion of the local anesthetic into the system from the site where it is used, varying with the degree of vascularization and the technique; intercostal block, for example, produces high plasma concentrations, subcutaneous infiltration much lower levels.

Prophylaxis Such measures as very close monitoring of patients, administration of intravenous fluids before major regional block, immediate availability of drugs and equipment to treat systemic toxicity, pre-oxygenation, injection of a test dose and incremental dosing are important measures if systemic complications from local anesthesia are to be avoided.

Risk groups Cardiotoxicity due to bupivacaine seems to be more likely in *pregnancy*; in the *elderly* some local anesthetics (including lidocaine and bupivacaine) have a longer half-life. *Hyperkalemia*, *acidosis*, *severe hypoxia* and *myocardial ischemia* increase the cardiovascular depressive effects of bupivacaine. Patients with a *pseudocholinesterase defect* may be unable to metabolize a particular local anesthetic and hence be more susceptible to its effects (see 'Chloroprocaine' below). Finally, *infants and young children* are clearly sensitive to the toxic (and especially hematological) effects of local anesthetics which enter the system, even the relatively small amounts which do so after topical use; particularly serious cases have been reported after topical use in children of TAC—a combination of tetracaine, adrenaline and cocaine (6^c, 7^c); a similar problem arises in children when using EMLA cream (2.5% prilocaine and 2.5% lidocaine) (8^c); other cases involving children are discussed throughout this chapter.

Manifestations Although the effects are usually mild, systemic toxicity related to local anesthesia may be fatal. A 1982 paper examined 53 fatalities following the use of local anesthetics in which no evidence pointing to allergy could be obtained (SED-11, 217). The systemic toxicity of local anesthetics mainly involves the central nervous system and the cardiovascular system.

Lidocaine, and probably other local anesthetics, have a convulsant effect at the synaptic junction. They close chloride channels and so depolarize the membrane and facilitate synaptic transmission. Dizziness, tinnitus, muscle twitching, peripheral paresthesias, distorted vision, disorientation and lightheadedness are the most frequently reported neurotoxic side effects. However, as the blood concentrations achieved are sometimes higher than one would anticipate, this dose-dependent neurotoxicity may occasionally prove much more severe than expected, e.g. with frank convulsions. Particular emphasis has been given to adequate oxygenation as a preventive and therapeutic measure with respect to convulsions.

Cardiovascular complications are not uncommonly encountered in the course of local anesthesia; however, most changes are moderate, involving a mild peripheral vasodilatation and depression of cardiac output with a slight increase in the heart rate. Cardiac arrest and marked myocardial depression in which hypoxia again plays a critical role have been rarely reported.

HYPERSENSITIVITY *(see also Chapter 14)*

Contrary to earlier beliefs, systemic hypersensitivity reactions are not a frequent problem in local anesthesia. Systemic toxicity or allergy to hyaluronidase (see above), or to bisulfite or parabens has sometimes been mistakenly classified as hypersensitivity to local anesthetics (SEDA-17, 135). The incidence of true allergy is indeed very low, probably less than 1% of all side effects attributable to these substances. Well-documented case reports are very few, relating particularly to amide-type agents; this appears to be because these agents have the highly antigenic *para*-aminobenzoic acid as a metabolite (SEDA-l3, 98). The use of skin testing to identify a causative drug allergen has been repeatedly advocated by several groups, but the advice has not often been followed. In addition, intradermal testing has, not surprisingly, been found to be very helpful in distinguishing between safe and unsafe agents in patients with a past history of allergy to local anesthesia. For all this, there is a small group of patients who are truly allergic to local anesthetics; careful history taking, e.g. by dentists, remains of importance if they are to be identified and risks avoided.

Both an *anaphylactoid reaction* and *bronchospasm* have been occasionally reported, though the latter could sometimes have been due to a sympathetic nervous blockade allowing unopposed parasympathetic effects (SEDA-18, 143; 9[C]).

Contact hypersensitivity also occurs. Benzocaine is a potent skin sensitizer and several cases of contact dermatitis to lidocaine have been reported. Interestingly enough, some sensitized patients have been found to cross-react with various related local anesthetic agents or chemically similar compounds, including some muscle relaxants (SEDA-15, 117); cross-reactivity between ester-type and amide-type agents, however, seems unlikely and does not appear to be on record.

TERATOGENICITY

The increasing use of in vitro fertilization has raised the question of whether the use of local anesthetics during oocyte removal is innocuous or not. Pharmacological concentrations of anesthetic agents are found in follicular fluid (10[cr]). No clinical effects have been noted, but knowledge of the behavioral effects on the offspring of lidocaine in rats must cause some concern (SEDA-15, 117).

It seems most unlikely that the local anesthetics in current use have any adverse effect on the fetus when employed during pregnancy (11[R]). The influence on the fetus of using local anesthesia in obstetrics is considered in the lidocaine monograph below.

METHEMOGLOBINEMIA

Cases of methemoglobinemia have been reported following the use of benzocaine, cetacaine, lidocaine, novocaine, prilocaine and aniline cocaine, and some are documented in the relevant sections of this chapter. Acquired methemoglobinemia may result from exposure to chemicals containing an aniline group in their chemical structure. Such is the case with benzocaine and procaine while lidocaine and prilocaine are biotransformed to metabolites which contain an aniline group. Toxic blood levels of local anesthetics, aberrant hemoglobin and NADH-methemoglobin reductase deficiency are critical factors favoring the onset of toxic methemoglobinemia. However, methemoglobinemia can occur even in the absence of such risk factors. Young children are most likely to experience clinical effects, but topical use (e.g. of cetacaine) has very occasionally caused severe problems in adults (12[CR]).

Intravenous administration of methylene blue (1–2 mg/kg) and oxygen are the therapeutic measures usually recommended when methemoglobinemia exceeds 30%.

MALIGNANT HYPERTHERMIA

Malignant hyperthermia has occasionally been documented following the use of bupivacaine, lidocaine, procaine and tetracaine, and can presumably occur with related agents as well. The symptoms can include muscular twitching, rigidity, hyperventilation and tachycardia. Even in patients known to be susceptible to this effect, however, local anesthesia is almost always without problems; of a series of 307 susceptible dental patients only one developed the complication after use of amide local anesthesia (13[C]).

EFFECT ON THE IMMUNE RESPONSE

In the very few relevant studies available, local anesthesia was found to *depress* both the immune response and phagocytosis. However, the clinical significance of these findings is highly debatable.

ENDOCRINE AND METABOLIC SIDE EFFECTS

Spinal or epidural analgesia generally exerts only slight effects on endocrine and metabolic parameters and these have no clinical repercussions.

DRUG INTERACTIONS

A positive interaction seems to be the ability of a local anesthetic to potentiate the postoperative analgesic effect of epidural *fentanyl* without an increase in adverse effects; though some earlier work was negative, a 1994 paper showed better analgesia during the first 16—24 hours if 0.1% bupivacaine was added to the opiate (14[C]). However, when fentanyl was added to improve the analgesic effect of bupivacaine in caesarian section, the improvement in analgesic effect was accompanied by an increase in bupivacaine-induced pruritus to as much as 43% (when using 100 μg fentanyl) (15[C]). Similar findings regarding this mutual potentiation of effect have been obtained in several studies with morphine, meperidine or clonidine as the systemic analgesic, lidocaine as the local agent, or when employing the spinal, caudal or suprapubic routes of drug administration; and the benefits have been demonstrated in long-term pain relief as well as in post-operative pain, and in adults as well as children (SEDA-18, 141—142, 146).

In a sense, the addition of *vasoconstrictors* to local anesthetics to prolong their effect involves a deliberate interaction. The addition of *dextran* to a lidocaine—adrenaline solution used for infiltration has been found to reduce the absorption of both agents (16[C]).

As bupivacaine (like some of its congeners) inhibits the inward current of calcium in cardiac tissues, β-blockers and *calcium blockers* may potentiate its cardiotoxicity; such an interaction has been observed clinically between lidocaine and a β-blocking agent (17[c]).

The CNS toxicity of lidocaine was increased in 11 healthy volunteers who simultaneously received *propafenone*; the latter reduced the metabolic breakdown of lidocaine.

EFFECTS RELATED TO THE TECHNIQUE EMPLOYED

Accidents during the administration of local anesthetics are of very many different types, and they are chronicled from year to year in the Side Effects of Drugs Annuals; only a selection of the more serious or frequent types of complication can be presented here. In principle the possibility must always be anticipated that when a local anesthetic is administered some of it will reach organs or tissues for which it is not destined, either because it has been incorrectly administered or because some anatomical or other idiosyncrasy of the patient has resulted in unexpected diffusion or leakage of the agent beyond its intended location. The main problems which result relate either to effects on the *nervous system* or adverse effects resulting from unintended *entry into the general circulation*. Very occasionally, infections are transmitted when injecting local anesthetic agents (SEDA-16, 129).

The early recognition of complications can be very difficult if a local anesthetic is administered during general anesthesia as a means of preventing severe postoperative pain, since the unconscious patient will not recognize the early signs of trouble, such as traumatic paresthesia (18[c]).

Brachial plexus block

The systemic complications of this technique are similar to those seen with others if sufficient drug enters the circulation. Several other complications are more specific to the routine. Local complications include *hematoma* and *infection*. Inadvertent *injection into the subarachnoid space*, occasionally precipitating cerebral or neurological problems, is one life-threatening complication of brachial plexus block. Cases of *pneumothorax* with subsequent recovery have been observed among patients receiving either subaxillary or supraclavicular plexus block. The latter technique is recommended to prevent this complication. Post-block *neuropathies* have been reported. With a good technique, however, brachial plexus block has been successfully used even in treating severe cancer pain, with no problems other than some numbness of the arm (SEDA-18, 142).

Buccal anesthesia

Persistent hiccough, paralysis of cranial nerves and *systemic toxicity* are the main complications of stomatological local anesthesia. *Trismus* has been seldom reported.

Dental anesthesia

Despite the frequent use of local dental anesthesia, adverse effects are uncommon provided the administration is competently performed. A case of *ptosis* is on record (SEDA-15, 118). One group described *acute hypertension* leading to *myocardial infarction* and *pulmonary edema* after use of mepivacaine with levonordefrin (19[c]). *Facial paralysis* is occasionally reported and is not necessarily due to poor technique; in one reported case *vascular spasm* seemed to provide an explanation (SED-12, 252).

Ear, local anesthesia

Transient *vestibular irritation* without hearing loss following infiltration of the auditory canal has been incidentally attributed to diffusion of the local anesthetic from the site of injection.

Extradural analgesia

The consequences of extradural analgesia may prove to vary somewhat with the level at which it is given, though they are not predictable. Thoracic administration was found in a series of patients to produce a degree of hyperglycemia (SED-12, 252). Lumbar extradural analgesia with bupivacaine was found to *increase intracranial pressure* in some patients, apparently those who already have some reduced intracranial compliance, and who may be a risk group (20[C]).

In obstetric patients, extradural analgesia with lidocaine or bupivacaine has been found to produce hypotension in a third of cases, especially where the patient receives the drug in the sitting rather than the lateral position (21[c]).

Hematoma blocks

Like administration onto a mucosal surface, local anesthesia administered directly into a fracture hematoma involves the real likelihood of pronounced systemic absorption and general toxicity (SED-12, 252).

Intercostal nerve block

High spinal anesthesia subsequent to inadvertent injection is again a possible complication of intrathoracic intercostal nerve block (SEDA-12, 252).

Intra-articular anesthesia

This type of anesthesia used in the knee joint has in one case been followed by necrosis of the knee ligament and the skin, apparently due to localized drug-induced embolism (22[c]).

Intradermal anesthesia

Intradermal infusion 70 ml ropivacaine in saline (up to 0.125%) along a proposed abdominal incision line has been found to delay post-operative pain; there was no reduction in the inflammatory response to surgery (23[C]).

Intrapleural anesthesia *(24[CR])*

Intrapleural administration of local anesthetics has been followed by *Horner's syndrome* and *increased skin temperature*, apparently pointing to an influence on the sympathetic nervous system (25[C]); poor technique can result in *pneumothorax* or *infection*.

Intraspinal narcotic analgesia

Following the publication of evidence that small doses of morphine or other narcotics given intrathecally produced long-lasting relief of pain in man, a number of reports dealing with the clinical application of epidural opiates have appeared and many of these relate to the combined use of narcotics with local anesthetics (SED-12, 252; SEDA-18, 145—146; see also 'Drug interactions' above). Side effects are frequently observed, and it is not always clear which of the agents is responsible. Widely distributed *pruritus* is one of the most common problems. *Urinary retention* has also been frequently cited as a side effect, and in one series was encountered early in 33% of cases and late in a further 33% (SEDA-18, 146). In both cases, the underlying mechanism is purely speculative at the present time. Among moderately severe side effects, *sedation*, *nausea*, *hypotension* and bradycardia have been reported less often. Currently, *ventilatory depression* is the only life-threatening complication of intraspinal narcotic analgesia employing morphine. Other aspects of adverse reactions to narcotics (most of which are unrelated to the route of administration) are dealt with in Chapter 8.

Intra-urethral anesthesia

Intra-urethral instillation of anesthetics is most likely to be needed in old people, and these are a risk group when—as can occur—there is marked absorption from the mucosa, especially if it is diseased or damaged. *Seizures* after instillation of lidocaine jelly (e.g. 20 ml of a 2% preparation) have been reported as a consequence (26[c]).

Intravenous regional anesthesia

Systemic toxic reactions (see introductory section) are the commonest complications of intravenous regional anesthesia, occurring soon after the tourniquet is released. One case of a *psychotic reaction* is on record.

Humeral phlebitis seems to have been triggered by this form of anesthesia in a high-risk case, involving a 32-year-old woman smoker using oral contraceptives (27[C]).

Laryngeal anesthesia

Local anesthesia to the larynx, e.g. using 4% lidocaine, is generally entirely safe. *Laryngeal edema* has been reported in a few cases and could be due to a propellant rather than to lidocaine itself (28[c]). An unusual complication is *mydriasis* if part of the spray is accidentally directed to the eye (SEDA-18, 144).

Obstetric local anesthesia

When a local anesthetic is used for episiotomy there is a risk of the needle entering the child's scalp; in two reported cases involving prilocaine this resulted in *cyanosis*, *methemoglobinemia* and *hemolytic anemia* in the child (29[c]).

Ophthalmic local anesthesia

This type of anesthesia is dealt with in Chapter 47.

Paravertebral block

Paravertebral block should be avoided in the cervical and lumbar region due to the possibility of persistent *nerve root damage*. *Postural headache* following thoracic paravertebral nerve block and probably reflecting dural entry has been reported. *Hematuria* due to ureteral or renal injury is an unusual complication of lumbar paravertebral sympathetic block. *Hemidiaphragmatic paralysis* can occur with cervical plexus anesthesia and can be particularly risky in cases of pre-existing airways obstruction (30[Cr]).

Percutaneous analgesia

When administering laser treatment for the correction of vascular defects, it can be necessary to use a topical anesthetic with enhanced absorption. Use of 25% lidocaine in 70% dimethylsulfoxide has proved successful and apart from some transient redness there appear to have been no problems to date.

Perianal anesthesia

Local anesthesia using ointments is very widely applied to relieve the symptoms of hemorrhoids and anal fissures. It should however be realized that absorption through the mucosa can be considerable; one case of *convulsions* as a suspected consequence of such treatment has been cited (SED-12, 253).

Peridural anesthesia and obstetric regional analgesia

Cardiovascular system Abrupt onset of *arterial hypotension* is a possible complication of peridural anesthesia, (31[cr]) particularly in elderly patients. Supplementation with adrenaline in this high-risk group, however, no longer seems defensible; it is better to be cautious with dosage and to monitor the patient closely.

Intracardiac conduction disturbances should not be considered as absolute contraindications to peridural anesthesia: only nine cases of *sinus bradycardia*, easily reversed with atropine sulfate, were noted in a series of 66 patients with such a pathological condition (32[C]).

Use in obstetrics (33[R]) Maternal hypotension and excessive placental transfer of local anesthetics and other drugs, e.g. narcotics or sedatives, given to the mother prior to or during delivery are the main causes of *neonatal death* related to the use of these agents in obstetrics. However, fatalities remain very infrequent.

The question of possible *neurobehavioral effects* in the child as a consequence of obstetric analgesia is still debated; although impairment of visual and neurological performance, decreased alertness and alterations in walking and muscle tone have all been reported, a majority of authors have found normal Apgar scores and psychomotor development following obstetric anesthesia (SED-12, 253), and any functional defects noted at birth are likely to be transient (34[c]).

Currently, the possibility of a *raised maternal mor-*

tality remains a topic of debate, although this is happily a decreasing problem; as recently as 1979, 150 maternal deaths (0.27 per 1000 births) occurred in the Federal Republic of Germany, of which 15—25% were apparently related to regional anesthesia having induced such complications as hypotension, systemic toxicity, total spinal block, hematoma, catheter rupture and uterine injury (SED-12, 253). Clearly, all these things reflect, in part, skills or lack of them; regional anesthesia is probably a safe enough technique for delivery, but it must be competently and carefully performed, whatever the choice of drug.

Peribulbar or retrobulbar block and facial block

Retrobulbar anesthesia, competently administered, is a safe procedure; in one series of 13 000 cases using a curved needle technique, the only serious complication was a single case of *postoperative ischemic neuropathy* (35[C]). Other centers have however experienced recurrent problems with *chemosis* (up to 30%), *sub-conjunctival hemorrhage* and *lid hemorrhage* before perfecting their technique (SEDA-18, 144). Inadvertent injection into the subarachnoid space surrounding the optic nerve has on various occasions led to a bilateral *decrease of vision* and *ophthalmoplegia*, together with varying degrees of *CNS and respiratory depression* (SED-12, 254). However, the work of several groups seems to show that such complications can occur, especially with higher concentrations, independently of any fault in the technique (SED-12, 254). The same seems to apply to *cardiac toxicity*, the anesthetic diffusing readily towards the cerebrospinal fluid (SEDA- 14, 110). *Headache* following bupivacaine-induced block, on the other hand, has been traced to the use of a vasoconstrictor additive, and appears more prone to occur with noradrenaline than with adrenaline (36[c]). Pulmonary edema has several times been described (37[c]). Unwanted *effects on the eye muscles*, occurring in some 1% of retrobulbar blocks, extend to ptosis, horizontal rectus muscle palsy and lagophthalmos; all seem to recover spontaneously within a matter of weeks (38[c]). *Retinal vascular occlusion* is rare, but it can occur in patients with severe vascular disease, without retrobulbar or optic nerve sheath hemorrhage; the mechanism is unclear (SED-12, 254).

Peribulbar anesthesia has incidentally led to *contralateral mydriasis*, *hemiplegic coma* and *damage to the infra-orbital nerve* (SEDA-18, 144). The contralateral eye may exhibit oculomotor weakness (SEDA-16, 130).

Injection of lidocaine and a corticosteroid into the tympanic plexus has been reported to result in taste sense disorders, the mechanism being uncertain (39[c]).

The serious though rare complications seen with ocular block anesthesia have led to alternative approaches, one involving a combination of neuroleptanesthesia with facial nerve block and contact anesthesia on the eye; the complications appear to have been greater rather than less than those with retrobulbar to periocular anesthesia (40[c]).

Regional anesthesia in the arm

After i.v. regional anesthesia one may experience some *systemic effect* once the tourniquet is released, e.g. venous irritation, tachycardia, supraventricular extrasystoles or dizziness.

Regional anesthesia in the neck

With regional anesthesia to the neck there is a risk of inadvertent intra-arterial injection; this could explain one report of *convulsions* in an elderly woman (41[c]).

Spinal and epidural anesthesia

General *Inadvertent intravenous administration*, due to an epidural catheter accidentally being placed in a vein seems particularly easy to detect with lidocaine, since it rapidly leads to tinnitus and a metallic taste in the mouth; it has been suggested that this could be used routinely to check for correct placement of the catheter (42[C]).

The accidental *transformation of epidural to spinal block* may be dramatic, and tracheal intubation may be needed to save the patient's life (43[c]).

Cardiovascular system *Hypotension* is the most frequent side effect of spinal and epidural anesthesia; in one very large series it was found to occur in 11% of the epidural group and 21.6% of the subarachnoid group (44[C]), but the actual figures differ with the anesthetic and concentration used; there may be more problems with tetracaine or lidocaine than with bupivacaine in equivalent doses (SEDA-12, 35; see also 'Lidocaine' below), and the problem is less when the patient is in the lateral rather than the sitting position. One study concluded showed that the use of elastic bandages around the legs would reduce the incidence of hypotension (45[c]). Using bupivacaine and tetracaine together seems to produce a more prolonged analgesic effect without inducing more hypotension than use of these agents separately (SEDA-18, 143). Whether one should attempt to prevent the hypotensive effect by giving adrenaline alongside the anesthetic depends on the patient; in ASA-III patients (those with any type of anesthetic risk) it is wise to do so, whereas in ASA-I- and -

II-type patients the vasoconstrictor risk of the adrenaline outweighs the hypotensive risk of the anesthetic (SED-12, 254). Metaraminol or ephedrine can also be used, the former apparently being more effective (SEDA-18, 143).

In young infants similar problems with blood pressure occur and some changes in heart rate may be found, but they apparently tend to be transient (SEDA-12, 154; 46[c]). In adults *bradycardia* occurs in some 3% of cases.

Myocardial infarction and *heart arrest* preceded by *atrioventricular block* have also been described. Analyzing 900 cases of major anesthetic mishaps giving rise to compensation claims, Caplan et al. (47[CR]) found 14 cases of cardiac arrest of which six were fatal.

Respiratory system *Respiratory depression* was noted in 0.24% of patients from a Chinese series of 10 978 epidural blocks (SED-12, 254). Direct paralysis of respiration probably plays an important role. Respiratory depression with cardiovascular side effects subsequent to miscalculated dose requirements or a misplaced catheter has also been described.

One highly unusual fatality to a mother and her child was described following repeated administration of a local anesthetic for cesarian section; it is believed to have been due to *pulmonary edema* (48[C]).

Nervous system *Headache* is the most common CNS complication (20—40% of patients), but the incidence can be reduced by using smaller needles; premedication with an analgesic does not seem to alleviate the problem. Perhaps similarly common is *pain or cramping in the back or legs* (seen in 30% of a series of cases receiving hyperbaric 5% lidocaine). Both these effects usually decline within 48 hours. However, it should be realized that headache (or psychosis) can be the presenting sign of *subdural hematoma*, which has twice been observed in women given subdural anesthesia for childbirth (SEDA-18, 143).

Peripheral paresthesia (1.13% of patients in the Chinese series already cited) and *paralysis* are the most frequent neurological deficits attributed to spinal and epidural analgesia. These permanent or temporary deficits are caused either by cord ischemia following arterial hypotension or by such damage as production of an epidural or subdural hematoma or injury to the spinal cord and nerve roots as a consequence of needle puncture, introduction of a catheter, infection or chemical irritation. These deficits may be limited to the cranial nerves, resulting for instance in transient *hearing loss* (see also below).

Less frequent neurological complications are *bladder dysfunction* or *sphincter paresis* (49[c]), *cauda equina syndrome*, *intracranial hypertension* and *convulsions*, the latter reflecting systemic toxicity. In cases of preeclampsia, obstetric peridural anesthesia with adrenaline can be used without special risks.

Special senses In some reported series it was striking that transient *hearing loss* after anesthesia with bupivacaine was found with the spinal but not with the epidural method (SEDA-13, 99; SEDA-16, 129; 50[c]). It has been suggested that the etiology could be a decrease in cerebrospinal fluid pressure transmitted through the cochlear aqueduct (51[CR]), a hypothesis which has been both supported and criticized (SEDA-16, 129).

Infection Contamination of catheters, with subsequent clinical infection, is a potential hazard of epidural analgesia. However not every suspected infection is indeed what it seems; an aseptic meningitis has been described following an intradural injection of bupivacaine with methylprednisolone acetate (52[c]).

Endocrine, metabolic Hypoglycemic coma developed in a patient with insulin-dependent diabetes 20 minutes after epidural injection of 6 ml bupivacaine 0.5% (53[CR]), and a smaller reduction in glucose levels is probably more common, perhaps due to the enkephalinergic mechanism (SEDA-16, 130). This effect is in keeping with the finding that the blood sugar response to surgery in women was abolished during epidural analgesia (SED-12, 254).

Sexual organs and function For reasons which are not understood, intraoperative penile erection is sometimes observed, and it may be followed by prolonged *priapism*; the effect is common to spinal, intradural and epidural treatment (SEDA-14, 110).

A long-standing belief that spinal anesthesia in young men reduces sexual potency was not confirmed in a recent retrospective study (SEDA-17, 139).

Obstetric use and second-generation effects In about 10% of cases, obstetric use of epidural anesthesia will cause some bradycardia in the fetus, but this is not a clinical problem (SEDA-15, 119). No increase in bilirubin production as compared with a control group was found in a series of newborn babies whose mothers received an epidural block with bupivacaine during labor (54[c]). On the other hand, in a case where the same method was used but accidental intravenous injection of bupivacaine occurred there were both maternal convulsions and severe fetal bradycardia (55[c]).

Postoperative effects *Postoperative pain* is common and there is evidence that in children simultaneous injection of morphine—despite the opiate's own adverse effects—greatly diminishes this problem (56[C]). Postoperative *shivering* is also common, but it appears to be much lessened if the epidural solutions are warmed to body temperature before injection (SED-12, 255).

Headache and *nausea* occur postoperatively in about half of all cases.

Risk factors *(SEDA-16, 130)* There may be a higher risk of uterine rupture when peridural anesthesia is used in obstetrics in a woman who has earlier undergone a *cesarean section*. The *athletic heart syndrome*, which may be present in professional sportspeople, can result in cardiac complications of epidural anesthesia.

In children who have been born as *premature infants* there is a greater risk that spinal anesthesia will cause apnea. All the same, spinal anesthesia with a sound technique has been used safely in high-risk infants; Sartorelli et al. used tetracaine in 142 such cases; there were only two cases with serious adverse effects, one with (unexplained but treatable) apnea and one in which too high a caudal block resulted in respiratory arrest (57[Cr]).

Stellate ganglion block

Inadvertent spinal anesthesia and subsequent CNS toxicity, e.g. with transient paralysis or apnea, are the main complications of stellate ganglion block. The use of very small test doses and an anterior approach to the stellate ganglion are recommended preventive measures. *Brachial plexus paresis* has also been reported. Accidental *block of the recurrent laryngeal nerve* can cause hoarseness and occasionally aspiration of saliva (58[c]).

In two women with *Raynaud's syndrome* the symptoms were aggravated contralaterally after stellate ganglion block (SEDA-18, 145).

Submucosal and subcutaneous anesthesia

Complications noted at various times with submucosal use include *allergic reactions* to the parabens present in lidocaine, *systemic effects* due to general diffusion (which readily occurs) or *necrosis* (where epinephrine is included in the preparation used) (SEDA-16, 131).

When infiltrating local anesthetics into the skin there is always a potential risk of *intravascular injection* (SEDA-17, 140), but it can be avoided by back-aspiration of the syringe.

Pain following skin infiltration is less likely if the anesthetic is warmed to body temperature before use, and if the pH value is adjusted; if using bicarbonate for the latter purpose its compatibility with the local anesthetic must be considered (SEDA-16, 131).

Subcutaneous fat anesthesia

A weak solution of lidocaine has sometimes been injected into excess fat prior to liposuction, so that the procedure can be carried out without general anesthesia. The technique appears to be without serious complications (59[C]).

EFFECTS ASSOCIATED WITH INDIVIDUAL DRUGS

Lidocaine

Lidocaine is a widely used local anesthetic agent of the amide type with low toxic potential. Its side effects when used as an antiarrhythmic drug are discussed in Chapter 17.

> ADVERSE REACTION PATTERN
>
> **General and toxic reactions** These can occur following inadvertent intravascular injection. CNS toxicity is directly related to blood concentrations, with symptoms ranging from lightheadedness and tinnitus to coma. Cardiovascular depression only occurs at very high blood concentrations. Risks of serious systemic effects do not seem to increase with age. Fatalities have occurred with voluntary intoxication, primarily because of the cardiac effects.
>
> **Hypersensitivity reactions** These are rare, and not all reports are clear, but cases do occur; they are usually mild (SED-12, 255; 60[Cr]). Some patients have been found highly sensitive to lidocaine yet insensitive to other amide-type local anesthetics (61[C]), and the reverse has also been demonstrated (SEDA-14, 109). True anaphylaxis with rechallenge has been documented (62[C]). A few cases of contact dermatitis have been reported.
>
> **Tumor-inducing effects** These have not been described.

ORGANS AND SYSTEMS

Those systemic effects which may occur after accidental intravascular injection are only briefly referred to here; they are as one would expect from the systemic use of the drug (see Chapter 17).

Cardiovascular *Sinus bradycardia* has been seen after a bolus injection of 50 mg, *atrioventricular block* after a dose of 800 mg given in the course of 12 hours, and *left bundle branch block* after a mere subconjunctival injection of lidocaine 2%. One case of high-grade atrioventricular block has been reported in a 14-day-old infant after receiving lidocaine 2 mg/kg i.v. (SED-12, 255). A fatality due to *ventricular fibrillation* after a 50-mg dose and another due to sinus arrest after a 100-mg dose have been reported (SED-12, 255). The degree of *hypotension* occurring after epidural anesthesia with alkalinized lidocaine (with adrenaline) was found to be greater than with a standard commercial solution (SED-12, 255).

Respiratory Life-threatening *bronchospasm* may occur following either spinal or topical use of lidocaine. In one series of patients being treated with lidocaine spray for persistent cough, an increase of airway resistance was found after a 40-mg dose (SED-12, 255). The adult *respiratory distress syndrome* is a possible but rare complication.

Nervous system With increasing blood concentrations following inadvertent intravascular injection, *light-headedness* and *tinnitus*, *visual disturbances*, *muscular twitching*, *convulsions*, *unconsciousness* and finally *coma* have been reported (SED-12, 255).

Hematological One case of severe *thrombocytopenic purpura* with lidocaine-mediated anti-platelet IgM antibody has been reported (SED-12, 255).

Endocrine, metabolic High systemic doses can cause transient hypoglycemia (SED-12, 255).

Skin and appendages Several cases of *contact dermatitis* have been reported. Generalized *exfoliative dermatitis* has also been noted once. Local *inflammation and necrosis*, possibly due to mechanical pressure, are both complications at the injection site.

Special senses *Tinnitus* and *visual disturbances* are early components of a systemic toxic reaction (see above).

Immunotoxicity Various types of *immunodepressant effect* can be detected by laboratory testing though they may have no clinical significance. Lidocaine has been shown to inhibit EA rosetting by human lymphocytes in a dose-dependent manner. Depression in vitro of human leukocyte random motility and phagocytosis has also been reported (SED-12, 256).

Malignant hyperthermia One case of malignant hyperthermia after epidural anesthesia with lidocaine 300 mg and bupivacaine 50 mg combined with adrenaline has been reported (SED-12, 256).

Sexual function Two cases of *impotence* after anesthesia for elective circumcision in adults have been described (SED-12, 256) but it seems very dubious whether this was a pharmacological and not merely a psychological effect.

Risk situations In patients with *heart* and *liver disease* the dose requirement of lidocaine is decreased; the half-life of the compound is substantially longer in patients with liver disease. That *sex* differences may influence lidocaine pharmacokinetics is suggested by one paper reporting higher blood levels in men than in women following administration of the same dose (SED-12, 256).

Second-generation effects Because of rapid transfer across the placenta and prolonged half-life in the newborn, lidocaine may cause *neonatal depression* (SED-12, 256). Fetal *bradycardia* is usually observed only in those fetuses with pre-existing heart rate deceleration. Despite massive intoxication at birth, one child presented a normal behavioral development at 7 months of age (SED-12, 256). The safety of lidocaine in in vitro fertilization is considered in the general section above.

Low concentrations of lidocaine and its metabolite monoethylglycinexylidide have been found in *breast milk* after a dental procedure, but no risk seems to be involved (63[c])

Overdosage Inadvertent intravenous injection of 1 gram of lidocaine resulted in one reported case in *asystole*, *apnea* and grand mal *seizures* with full recovery after 6 hours of intensive resuscitation (SED-12, 256).

Interactions These have been listed in the general section of this Chapter.

Benzocaine

Methemoglobinemia, as discussed in the general section above, is a classical complication of benzocaine and cases continue to occur (SED-12, 256); the problem arises particularly in children (64[c]). Two cases of *photodermatitis* have been described (SED-12, 256).

Benzocaine is in many countries a component of some free-sale preparations for topical use, e.g. in skin creams or throat tablets as well as so-called ‘teething preparations’ for young children. The risk of methemoglobinemia has led to criticism of its free availability. It has among other things been suggested that it should be eliminated from products for use in children, that concentrations in over-the-counter products should be limited and that there should be explicit labelling warnings of the hematological risk (SED-12, 256; SEDA-17, 135; see also reference 64 above).

Bupivacaine

Nervous system Neurological symptoms subsequent to unrecognized intravascular injection are the major complications of bupivacaine: *tinnitus*, *muscle twitching*, *nystagmus* and *convulsions* can occur. The use of vasoconstrictors is probably inadvisable because of their long duration of action. Whether addition of hyperbaric glucose to (0.5%) bupivacaine for spinal anesthesia alters the incidence of *pain* from an orthopedic tourniquet is disputed; some findings suggest that it aggravates the problem (SED-12, 256).

Cardiovascular Bupivacaine-induced cardiotoxicity, notably after epidural use, is a matter of concern and controversy. There is increasing evidence that the risk can be greatly reduced or eliminated by careful dosage and/or the use of lower concentrations (SEDA-12, 108–109; 65[R]). Use of concentrations not exceeding 0.5% has been recommended in order to avoid the risk of *cardiovascular collapse*. *Hypotension*, *fetal bradycardia* and *cardiac rhythm disturbances* have been very occasionally reported (SED-12, 256).

Muscular system A case of *muscular atrophy* after intramuscular injection has been documented (66[C]).

Obstetric risks There is a single study concluding that when local peridural anesthesia is used for cesarian section, bupivacaine (with oxytocin) produces a higher frequency of neonatal jaundice than does similar treatment using lidocaine (SEDA-14, 111).

Risk situations These are noted under the general discussion of systemic reactions to local anesthesia above.

Carticaine

The incidence of *hypotension* and post-anesthetic *headache* after spinal anesthesia was found to be similar to that encountered with lidocaine. *Methemoglobinemia* is a theoretically possible complication, although it has not yet been reported in the published literature. An 11-year-old boy developed severe *dermatomyositis* only a few days after injection of carticaine in the jaw for tooth extraction; cause and effect was not established (SEDA-10, 105).

Centbucridine

Nausea, *vomiting*, *bradycardia*, *backache*, *shivering* and *hypotension* may occur with a similar incidence to that of lidocaine (SED-12, 256).

Chloroprocaine

Local *neural irritation* can occur when large doses are used epidurally or intrathecally, probably because of the low pH and the sodium bisulfite content of some solutions (SEDA-14, 111). Prolonged *neural blocks* have been described, the pathophysiology of which is still controversial (SEDA-10, 105).

Systemic toxicity is low owing to rapid hydrolysis by plasma pseudocholinesterases, but where an atypical pseudocholinesterase is present, complications can occur, notably *convulsions* (67[cr]).

In a series of 25 patients receiving epidural chloroprocaine for various day procedures, 23 had a *fall of arterial blood pressure* by 15%, and in two it fell by 25% (68[c]).

Cocaine *(see also Chapters 1 and 4)*

Because of its rapid absorption by mucous membranes, cocaine applied topically can induce systemic toxic effects. In one woman who (inappropriately) used cocaine on the nasal mucosa to treat epistaxis, myocardial infarction followed (69[c]); another case treated intranasally with nasal cocaine and submucosal lidocaine during general anesthesia developed ventricular fibrillation (SEDA-17, 142).

Dibucaine (2-chloroprocaine)

In in vitro work, dibucaine has been found to affect the platelet membrane, resulting in inhibition of ADP-mediated platelet aggregation (70[C]); it is not known whether this has any clinical significance.

Mepivacaine (Carbocaine)

Mepivacaine may slow the spontaneous *heart rate*. One case of first-degree *atrioventricular block* has been reported. Again, systemic toxicity is the major complication which can prove fatal. Vasoconstrictors are not warranted as they have not been shown to influence the rate of systemic reactions. One case of an *allergic reaction* has been described.

Oxybuprocaine

When used in the eye, some quantities can enter the anterior chamber, and *fibrinous iritis* and moderate *corneal swelling* have incidentally been described (SED-12, 257).

Prilocaine

Methemoglobinemia has been reported after inadvertent intravenous administration, particularly in neonates and children (SEDA-11, 221; 71[C]; see also 'Obstetric local anesthesia' above); in one boy of 6, a 10-ml dose of a 2% solution given for a bilateral percutaneous nephrostomy, produced a degree of cyanosis demanding methylene blue treatment (72[c]). In adults, even those with anemia, the shift in methemoglobin levels, while measurable, is not of clinical significance (SEDA-12, 257; 73[Cr]).

One case of a *hypersensitivity reaction* has been reported (SED-12, 257).

Procaine

Allergic reactions are somewhat more frequent with this ester-type local anesthetic. Today it is most widely used as a component of procaine penicillin, and rare cases of tonic seizures have been reliably attributed to its presence (74[c]).

Ropivacaine

This amide-type local anesthetic has been well studied and many reports have now appeared (SEDA-16, 85). Though the initial clinical reports suggested that there was reduced toxicity to the central nervous system it is now not at all clear that this is the case. The cardiovascular effects seem similar to those of bupivacaine, and it has become clear that hypotension is fairly prominent when ropivacaine is used epidurally, e.g. in one series it was observed in 30% of cases receiving ropivacaine but in only 13% of those given an equivalent dose of bupivacaine (75[C]).

Tetracaine

Tetracaine is 20 times as toxic as procaine and unless great caution is exercised in dosage, marked serious systemic side effects can develop owing to rapid resorption following topical use (e.g. in a 0.5% gargle) (76[c]) or employment in endoscopy. One case of *malignant hyperthermia* has been reported (see above), as well as *anaphylactic shock* following spinal anesthesia (SED-12, 257). When a pneumatic tourniquet is used in spinal anesthesia, *pain* has been found to be twice as frequent with tetracaine (60%) as with bupivacaine (25%) (77[C]).

REFERENCES

1. McCaughey W. Adverse effects of local anesthetics. Drug Safety 1992;7:178—189.
2. Young ER, McKenzie TA. The pharmacology of local anesthetics—a review of the literature. Can Dent Assoc J 1992;58:34—42.
3. Reynolds F. Adverse effects of local anaesthetics. Br J Anaesth 1987;59:78.
4. Muller U, Bircher A, Bischof M. Allergisches Angiödem nach zahnärztlicher Applikation eines Lokalanästhetikum und Hyaluronidase enthaltenden Vorspritzmittels. Schweiz Med Wochenschr 1986;116:1810.
5. Covino BG. Toxicity of local anesthetic agents. Acta Anaesthesiol Belg 1988;39(Suppl 2):159.
6. Mofenson HC, Caraccio TR. Tack up a warning on TAC. Am J Dis Child 1989;143:519.
7. Daya MR, Burton BT, Schleiss MR, DiLiberti JH. Recurrent seizures following mucosal application of TAC. Ann Emerg Med 1988;17:646.
8. Nilsson A, Engberg C, Henneberg S et al. Inverse relationship between age dependent erythrocyte activity of methaemoglobin reductase and prilocaine-induced methaemoglobinaemia during infancy. Br J Anaesth 1990:64:72.
9. McCough E, Cohen JA. Unexpected bronchospasm during spinal anesthesia. J Clin Anesth 1990;2:35—36.
10. Bailey-Pridham DD, Reshef E, Drury K. Follicular fluid lidocaine levels during transvaginal oocyte retrieval. Fertil Steril 1990;53:171.
11. Friedman JM. Teratogen update: anesthetic agents. Teratology 1988;37:69.
12. Ferraro L, Zeichner S, Greenblatt G et al. Cetacaine-induced acute methemoglobinemia. Anesthesiology 1988; 69:614.
13. Minasian A, Yagiela JA. The use of local anestbetics in patients susceptible to malignant hyperthermia. Oral Surg Oral Med Oral Pathol 1988;66:405.
14. Paech MJ, Westmore MD. Postoperative epidural fentanyl infusion—is the addition of 0.1% bupivacaine of benefit? Anaesth Intens Care 1994;22:9—14.
15. Halonen PM, Paatero H, Hovorkl J et al. Comparison of two fentanyl doses to improve epidural anesthesia with 0.5% bupivacaine for caesarian section. Acta Anaesthesiol Scand 1993;37:774—779.
16. Adams HA, Biscoping J, Kafurke H et al. Influence of dextran on the absorption of adrenaline-containing lignocaine solutions: a protective mechanism in local anesthesia. Br J Anaesth 1988;60:645.
17. Wyse DG, Kellen J, Tarn Y et al. Increased efficacy and toxicity of lidocaine in patients on betablockers. Int J Cardiol 1989;21:59.
18. Ecoffey C, Samii K. Complication neurologique après anesthésie péridurale chez un garcon de 15 ans. Ann Fr Anésth Réanim 1990;9:398—400.
19. Pearson AC, Labovitz AJ, Kern MJ. Accelerated hypertension complicated by myocardial infarction after use of a local anesthetic/vasoconstrictor preparation. Am Heart J 1987;114:662.
20. Hilt H, Gramm HJ, Link J. Changes in intracranial pressure associated with extradural anaesthesia. Br J Anaesth 1986;58:676.
21. Reid JA, Thorburn J. Extradural bupivacaine or lignocaine anaesthesia for elective caesarian section: the role of maternal posture. Br J Anaesth 1988;61:149.
22. Wand A, Junger H. Embolia cutis medicamentosa an atypischer Lokalisation. Aktuel Dermatol 1990;16:128—129.
23. Johansson B, Glise H, Hallerbäck B et al. Preoperative local infiltration with ropivacaine for postoperative pain relief after cholecystectomy. Anesth Analg 1994;78:210—214.

24. Escarment J, Leroy P, Baechle JP et al. L'analgésie par administration intrapleurale d'anesthésiques locaux. Cah Anesthésiol 1990;38:411–419.
25. Parkinson SK, Mueller JB, Rich TJ et al. Unilateral Horner's syndrome associated with interpleural catheter injection of local anesthetic. Anesth Analg 1989;68:61.
26. Sundaram MBM. Seizures after intraurethral instillation of lidocaine. Can Med Assoc J 1987;137:219.
27. Laborde Y, Gimenez V, Besset-Lehmann J. Une complication rare de l'anesthésie locorégionale endoveineuse: la phlébite humérale. Presse Méd 1989;18:1527.
28. Ryder W. 'Two cautionary tales'. Anaesthesia 1994; 49:180–181.
29. Menahem S. Neonatal cyanosis, methaemoglobinemia and hemolytic anaemia. Acta Paediatr Scand 1988;77:755.
30. Castresana MR, Masters RD, Castresane EJ et al. Incidence and clinical significance of hemidiaphragmatic paresis in patients undergoing carotid endartercectomy during cervical plexus block anesthesia. J Neurosurg Anesthesiol 1994;6:21–23.
31. Bonnet F, Derosier JP, Pluskwa F et al. Cervical epidural anaesthesia for carotid artery surgery. Can J Anaesth 1990;37:353–358.
32. Tarot JP, Coriat P, Samti K et al. Anesthésie péridurale et trouble de la conduction intracardiaque. Anesth Analg Réanim 1980;37:9.
33. Douglas MJ. Potential complications of spinal and epidural anesthesia for obstetrics. Semin Perinatol 1991; 15:368–374.
34. Morikawa S, Ishikawa J, Kamatsuki H. et al. Neurobehaviour and mental development of newborn infants delivered under epidural analgesia with bupivacaine. Acta Obstet Gynaecol Jpn 1990;42:1495–1502.
35. Teichmann KD, Uthoff D. Retrobulbar (intraconal) anesthesia with a curved needle; technique and results. J Cataract Refract Surg 1994;20:54–60.
36. Pilz J. Kopfschmerz bei ophthalmologischer Lokalanisthesie in Abhängigkeit von der Art des Vasokonstriktorzusatzes. Folia Ophthalmol 1988;13:133.
37. Elk J R. Wood J. Holladay JT. Pulmonary edema, following retrobulbar hlock. J Cataract Refract Surg 1988;14:216.
38. Rao VA, Kawatra VK. Ocular myotoxic effects of local anesthetics. Can J Ophthalmol 1988;23:171.
39. Yamada Y, Tomita H. Influences on taste in the area of chorda tympani nerve after transtympanic injection of local anesthetic (4% Lidocaine). Auris Nasus Larynx 1989; 26(Suppl 1):541.
40. Hodgkins PR, Teye-Botchway L, Morrell AJ et al. Neuroleptanalgesia and extracapsular cataract extraction. Br J Ophthalmol 1992;76:153–156.
41. Brooker CD, Lawson AD. Convulsions following bupivacaine infiltration for excision of carotid body tumour. Anesth Intens Care 1993;21:877–878.
42. Colonna-Romano P, Lingaraju N, Braitman LE. Epidural test dose: lidocaine 100 mg, not chloroprocaine, is a symptomatic market of iv injection in labouring parturients. Can J Anaesth 1993;40:714–717.
43. Becl GN, Griffiths AG. Failed extradural anaeshtesia for Caesarian section. Complications of subsequent spinal block. Anaesthesia 1992;47:690–692.
44. Unzueta Merino MC, Escolan Villen F, Aliaga Font L et al. Revisión de las complicaciones de la anestesia espinal en un periodo de 7 años (1977–1984). Rev Esp Anestesiol Reanim 1986;33:66.
45. Bhagwanjee S, Rocke DA, Rout CC et al. Prevention of hypotension following spinal anaesthesia for elective caesarian section by wrapping of the legs. Br J Anaesth 1990; 65:819–822.
46. Logan MR, Ecoffey C. Spinal anesthesia with isobaric bupivacaine in infants. Anesthesiology 1988;68:601.
47. Caplan PA, Ward RJ, Posner K et al. Unexpected cardiac arrest during spinal anesthesia: a closed claims analysis of predisposing factors. Anesthesiology 1988;68:5.
48. Van Zundert AA, Scott DB. A fatal accident after epidural anesthesia for cesarian section. Acta Anaesthesiol Belg 1989;40:195–199.
49. Schou H, Hole P. Neurologic deficit following spinal anesthesia. Acta Anaesthesiol Belg 1987;38:241.
50. Michel O, Brusis T. Hearing loss as a sequel of lumbar puncture. Ann Otol Rhinol Larygol 1992;101:390–394.
51. Fog J, Wang LP, Sunberg A et al. Hearing loss after spinal anesthesia is related to needle size. Anesth Analg 1990;70:517–522.
52. Thomson SJ, Lomax DM, Collett BJ. Chemical meningism after lumbar facet joint block with local anaesthetic and steroids. Anaesthesia 1991;46:563–564.
53. Romano E, Gullo A. Hypoglycaemic coma following epidural analgesia. Anaesthesia 1980;35:1084.
54. Gale R, Ferguson JE, Stevenson DK. Effect of epidural analgesia with bupivacaine hydrochloride on neonatal bilirubin production. Obstet Gynecol 1987;70:692.
55. Knitza R, Sirl C, Wisser J. Zerebraler Krampfanfall nach Epiduralanästhesie mit Bupivacain zur Sectio caesarea. Geburtsh Frauenheilkd 1988;48:47.
56. Dalens R, Tanguy A, Haberer JP. Lumbar epidural anesthesia for operative and postoperative pain relief in infants and young children. Anesth Analg 1986;5:1069.
57. Sartorelli KH. Abajian JC, Kreutz JM et al. Improved outcome utilizing spinal anesthesia in high-risk infants. J Pediatr Surg 1992;27:1022–1025.
58. Omote K, Kawamata M, Namiki A. Adverse effects of stellate ganglion block on Raynaud's syndrome associated with progressive systemic sclerosis. Anaesth Analg 1993; 77:1056–1060.
59. Klein JA. Tumescent technique for local anesthesia improves safety in large-volume liposuction. Plast Reconstr Surg 1993;92:1085–1098.
60. Adriani J, Coffman VD, Naraghi M. The allergenicity of lidocaine and other amide and related anesthetics. Anesthesiol Rev 1986;13:671.
61. Bonnet MC, Du Cailar G, Deschot J. Anaphylaxie à la lidocaine. Ann Fr Anesth Réanim 1989;8:127.
62. Kennedy KS, Cave RH. Anaphylactic reaction to lidocaine. Arch Otolaryngol Head Neck 1986;112:671.
63. Lebedevs TH, Wojnar-Horton RE, Yapp P et al. Excretion of lignocaine and its metabolite monoethylglycinexylidide in breast milk following itsuse in a dental procedure. A case report. J Clin Periodontol 1993;20:606–608.
64. Gentile DA. Severe methemoglobinemia induced by a topical teething preparation. Pediatr Emerg Care 1987;3:176.
65. Nolte H. Zur Problematik der Cardiotoxizität von Bupivacain 0.75%. Reg Anästh 1986;9:57.
66. Parris WCV, Dettbarn WD. Muscle atrophy following bupivacaine trigger point injection. Anesthesiol Rev 1989; 16:50.
67. Smith AR, Hur D, Resano F. Grand mal seizures after 2-chloroprocaine epidural anesthesia in a patient with plasma cholinesterase deficiency. Anesth Analg 1987;66:677.

68. Allen RW, Fee JPH, Moore J. A preliminary assessment of epidural chloroprocaine for day procedures. Anaesthesia 1993;48:773—775.
69. Ross GS, Bell J. Myocardial infarction associated with inappropriate use of topical cocaine as treatment for epistaxis. Am J Emerg Med 1992;10:219—222.
70. Peerschke EIB. Platelet membrane alteration induced by the local anesthetic dibucaine. Blood 1986;68:463.
71. Menahem S. Neonatal cyanosis, methaemoglobinaemia and haemolytic anaemia. Acta Paediatr Scand 1988;77:755.
72. Kilic I, Kalayci Ö. Methemoglobinemia due to prilocaine local anesthesia. Daga Turk J Med Sci 1993;19:299.
73. Bardoczky GL, Wathieu M, D'Hollander A. Prilocaine-induced methemoglobinemia evidenced by pulse oximetry. Acta Anaesthesiol Scand 1990;14:162.
74. Malone JD, Lebar RD, Hilder R. Procaine-induced seizures after intramuscular procaine penicillin. G Mil Med 1988;153:191.
75. Morrison LMM, Emanuelsson BM, McClure JH et al. Efficacy and kinetics of extradural ropivacaine: comparison with bupivacaine. Br J Anaesth 1994;72:164—169.
76. Patel JHM, Chopra S, Berman MD. Serious systemic toxicity resulting from use of tetracaine for pharyngeal anesthesia in upper endoscopic procedures. Dig Dis Sci 1989; 34:882.
77. Conception MA, Lambert DH, Welch KA et al. Tourniquet pain during spinal anesthesia: a comparison of plain solutions of tetracaine and bupivacaine. Anesth Analg 1988;67:828.

Meyler's Side Effects of Drugs, 13th Edition
M.N.G. Dukes, editor

SECTION EDITOR: C.J. VAN BOXTEL

M. Leuwer and J. Motsch

12 Neuromuscular blocking agents and skeletal muscle relaxants

INTRODUCTION

A great many side effects have been described for muscle relaxants and, as clinicians and pharmacologists examine more critically and monitor more intensively the effects that these drugs produce, it is to be expected that a great many more will be discovered. The more aware the clinician is of the various side effects and interactions of the drugs he uses daily and of the circumstances under which these effects are more likely to appear, the more easily he can avoid 'risk situations' and choose the most suitable, or less dangerous, relaxant for each individual patients

It is difficult to fit muscle relaxants into the form of systematic classification used throughout *Meyler*, but in order to maintain conformity and ease of reference the standard structure is generally adhered to. Under 'Organs and systems', an extra section is inserted at the beginning, namely 'Neuromuscular', and since not only the side effects of relaxants on the various body systems are important but also the effects that the various body systems, in health and disease, have on the actions of relaxants, the headings are used 'two-way' when appropriate. Thus in the 'Cardiovascular' section the effects of a relaxant on that system will be reviewed, whereas in the 'Urinary system' section the adverse effects of the relaxant arising as a consequence of renal dysfunction will be discussed.

Suxamethonium and *d*-tubocurarine are described in greatest detail as principal representatives of the depolarizing and non-depolarizing types of neuromuscular blocking agents, respectively, despite the fact that both drugs are becoming less important in daily practice. The side effects of the other neuromuscular blocking agents are reviewed in relation to these two at greater or shorter length depending on how much has been reported and on the extent to which the relaxation is currently used. Decamethonium, dioxonium, fazadinium and doxacurium which are very seldom, if any used today are dealt with for historical reasons and for matters of completeness.

The centrally acting muscle relaxants such as baclofen or agents with direct musculotropic effects, e.g. dantrolene, are discussed individually. Useful background reading on the side effects and interactions of neuromuscular blocking agents, factors that affect their actions and the possible mechanisms underlying them is to be found in two recently published books (1[R], 2[R]) and several reviews (3[R]—6[R]). Walts (7[R]) has written a relaxed review of the older literature on this subject.

Some general topics which involve both depolarizing and non-depolarizing neuromuscular blocking agents are considered first before the individual relaxants are discussed.

GENERAL CONSIDERATIONS

Hypersensitivity reactions These are known to occur with all neuromuscular blocking agents. The incidence of life-threatening anaphylactic or anaphylactoid reactions occurring during anesthesia is variably reported as being between 1 in 1000 and 1 in 10 000 anesthesias (8, 9[Cr]). The frequency quoted depends on the criteria used. An epidemiological study (10[R]) suggests that the incidence is somewhat greater than 1 in 5000 anesthesias. The mortality from such serious reactions is reported to be in the range of 3.4—6% (9[Cr], 10[R]). Minor systemic reactions attributable to histamine release probably occur in more than 1% of anesthesias (11[R]). Neuromuscular blocking drugs are the triggering agents in 50% or more of these reactions (12[CR], 13[R]), and of them *d*-tubocurarine is the most potent histamine liberator pharmacologically. During the last 15 years, however, several large series of patients have been investigated and these data suggest that suxamethonium and gallamine are nevertheless the relaxants most likely to produce life-threatening reactions, followed by *d*-tubocurarine or alcuronium, if allowances are made for the frequency of usage of the different agents (SEDA-17, 12[R]; 10[R], 12[CR], 14[R], 15[CR], 16[C]). Pancuronium has repeatedly been shown to be the relaxant least often associated with anaphylactoid reactions major or minor.

Anaphylactoid reactions are easily misdiagnosed during anesthesia (17[C]) since circulatory collapse accompanied by sinus tachycardia may be the only signs (11[R]). These are the presenting features in 70—90% of cases. Mucocutaneous manifestations (erythema, urticaria, angioneurotic edema) are reported in 60—80% of reactions, but these are often only noticed much later when the acute phase is over. Bronchospasm is present in about 40% of cases. Reactions are more common in women (up to 80%), in atopic patients and in those who have a history of asthma (who are particularly prone to react with bronchospasm) or allergy, and in patients who have had a previous reaction to anesthetic drugs (12[CR], 14[R]); they also seem to be more common in patients under 40 years of age (15[CR]).

Much controversy surrounds the issue of the possible mechanisms by which a neuromuscular blocking agent produces the clinical picture of an anaphylactoid reaction. Investigations (12[CR], 18[CR], 19[R]) have suggested that IgE are involved in most cases (i.e. the mechanism is a Type I hypersensitivity reaction), although the frequent lack of previous exposure to relaxants would seem to exclude this. Direct histamine release and several other mechanisms have also been postulated (20, 21[R]). Drug-specific IgE antibodies to suxamethonium (22, 23) and other neuromuscular blocking agents (SEDA-17, 149; 24) have been demonstrated. The hypothesis has been put forward that such antibodies are directed against quaternary and tertiary ammonium ion determinants (22, 24). This would help to explain the phenomenon of *cross-reactivity* with different relaxants and also suggests that prior sensitization could occur via other quaternary or tertiary ammonium ion-containing compounds in drugs, cosmetics, disinfectants, etc. (12[CR], 18[CR]). Two quaternary ammonium groups may be necessary for histamine release by neuromuscular blocking agents (20, 19[R]).

The investigation of a reaction during anesthesia requires serial blood samples during the first 24—72 hours and further laboratory tests, such as basophil histamine release, and intradermal skin testing 4—8 weeks later (SEDA-8, 132—133; SEDA-17, 6[C]; 8, 14[R], 21[R], 25[R]). The possibilities of post-mortem diagnosis have now been extended to the use of blood samples taken up to 3 hours after a patient's death and subjected to radioimmunoassays for mast cell tryptase levels and drug-specific IgE-antibodies (SEDA-18, 3[C]).

Opinions differ as to the value and the reliability of intradermal skin testing. The protagonists emphasize that strict criteria must be used in performing and interpreting the tests (26). Radioallergosorbent tests (RAST) which detect IgE antibodies to specific muscle relaxants have been developed (22, 24) and are commercially available for some anesthetic drugs (27[R], 21[R]). The possibility of cross-reactivity with different relaxants should also be investigated and the patient issued with an appropriate 'warning-card'.

Measures for the prevention and treatment of reactions are discussed by Laxenaire et al. (14[R], 15[CR]), Sage (28) and Fisher (29[C]).

Antibiotics Antibiotics in very high concentrations may produce paralysis on their own and have been reported to act additively or synergistically with neuromuscular blocking drugs. The danger of prolonged neuromuscular block is greater with high blood levels, as may occur as a result of absolute overdose, systemic absorption of large quantities from the peritoneal or pleural cavities, or when excretory processes are impaired in renal insufficiency (relative overdose). 'Recurarization' may occur in the recovery period if high blood levels of an antibiotic are achieved in the presence of residual curarization. Myasthenic patients aré particularly at risk, even with normal doses of antibiotics.

The antibiotics known to produce muscle paralysis fall into four main groups. The *aminoglycosides* (streptomycin, neomycin, kanamycin, gentamicin, tetramycin, amikacin, tobramycin, etc.) have a magnesium like effect, acting primarily prejunctionally to diminish transmitter release and also acting postjunctionally to diminish transmitter release and also reducing postjunctional sensitivity to acetylcholine. Their effect can be reversed, partly at least, by calcium or 4-aminopyridine in most cases. Neostigmine may have little effect. Tobramycin is thought also to have a direct effect on muscle. The *polymyxins* (A, B, colistin and colistimethate) probably produce a predominantly postjunctional effect (via ion channel block) and reduce muscle contractility. The block is difficult to reverse, calcium being only partly successful. Neostigmine has been reported to increase blocks produced by polymyxin B and colistin. In such cases 4-aminopyridine might be helpful. The *tetracyclines* produce a small effect partly by calcium chelation, thus reducing transmitter release. Reversal is usually, but inconsistently, obtained with calcium or neostigmine. The *lincosamides* (lincomycin, clindamycin) possess pre- and postjunctional effects, the principal action being probably on the muscle. Their block is difficult to reverse with cholinesterase inhibitors or calcium. *Penicillins* V and G (30[r]) are also reported to produce neuromuscular block in animal preparations, but only at exceptionally high doses. Calcium is effective in reversal. The *acylamino-penicillins* (apalcillin, mezlocillin, piperacillin and azlocillin) have been shown to augment a vecuronium-block (31[C]). A possible 're-curarization' with piperacillin was successfully reversed by neostigmine (32[C]). An unusual high dose of vancomycin has been reported to augment a vecuronium-induced block during recovery, thus delaying the detubation of the patient for about 30 minutes (SEDA 16, 7[C]). In another patient vancomycin prolonged the recovery from a block induced by a suxamethonium infusion for some hours (SEDA-18, 14[C]). If it is suspected that an antibiotic is contributing to a prolonged neuro-muscular block, the patient should be monitored and the effect of calcium (up to 1 gram of calcium chloride slowly) be observed. If this is unsuccessful, neostigmine (max. 5 mg for an adult) or edrophonium (0.5 mg/kg) may be tried, but these agents may intensify a block due to polymyxin B, colistin or lincomycin. 4-Aminopyridine (max. 0.3 mg/kg), if available, may be successful if the other remedies fail. Artificial ventilation should be continued until adequate spontaneous efforts are achieved and other possible factors, such as acidosis or electrolyte disturbances are corrected.

This subject is reviewed in several excellent papers (30[R], 33[R], 34[R]).

Hemodilution Hemodilution (by replacing 1 liter of patient blood by dextran-40 solution) has been reported to increase the potencies and prolong the actions of suxamethonium, pancuronium, *d*-tubocurarine and vecuronium (SEDA-17, 151; 35[C], 36[C]). To avoid this, blood collection should be carried out before the administration of anesthetic drugs.

Age Neonates are said to be more sensitive to non-depolarizing neuromuscular blocking drugs. While it has been suggested that this is only an apparent increase in sensitivity, produced by the lower muscle mass per kilogram body weight of neonates, evidence that maturation of neuromuscular transmission occurs in the 2 months following full-term birth (37[C]), and that the ‘margin of safety’ for neuromuscular transmission is reduced in infants under 12 weeks of age (38[C]), supports the view that smaller doses should be used in the very young. The greater body water content of neonates, however, tends to ‘neutralize’ the increased sensitivity so that several authors recommend similar doses to adults (calculated on a weight basis). Due to a longer elimination half-life, recovery is slower in neonates and maintenance doses are needed at longer intervals (39[C]), certainly where most of the older, long-acting relaxants are concerned. Conflicting data exist as to whether the actions of vecuronium and atracurium (and even pancuronium) are prolonged or not (40[R]). Most investigators concur that neonates and infants require a larger dose per kilogram of suxamethonium (2—4 mg/kg) to achieve an equivalent effect to that seen in adults. In *young* children plasma clearance is quicker (41[C]) and the duration of action of non-depolarizing relaxants is shorter (42[C]) so that doses may have to be given more frequently.

Interindividual variation in dose requirements is even more marked in neonates and infants than in adults, so that monitoring of neuromuscular function is essential. Small dysmature babies, especially with temperatures below 36°C, are notoriously unpredictable in their response to relaxants.

In *the elderly* there is much slower recovery from non-depolarizing relaxants (about 60% in patients over 75 years of age given pancuronium), associated with a decreased rate of elimination (probably through reduced glomerular clearance and, to a lesser extent, decreased hepatic blood flow). The potency of relaxants is not altered. While the initial dose required to produce full relaxation is the same as in young adults, smaller maintenance doses are required at much longer intervals (43[C], 44[C]). The duration of atracurium is not increased since termination of its action is not dependent on renal or hepatic function.

Chapters on the elderly (45[R]) and on pediatric practice (46[R]) in *Clinics in Anaesthesiology* try to reconcile the many conflicting reports on the age-related differences in response to neuromuscular blocking agents. Information on the development of the myoneural junction in infants and animals, together with possible implications for the use of neuromuscular blocking agents, is reviewed by Goudsouzian and Standaert (47[R]).

Temperature In *hypothermia* a decrease in blood flow to muscle increases the time to onset of neuromuscular blockade. The actions (depth of block and duration) of depolarizing relaxants are increased. The potency of non-depolarizing neuromuscular blocking agents is decreased according to some investigators, whereas others maintain that the potency is increased and the duration of action is prolonged (48[C], 49[Cr], 50[Cr]). Hypothermia produces different changes in the twitch (51[C]) and electromyographic (52) responses to nerve stimulation in the absence of relaxants. The excretion and the metabolism of relaxants are decreased by hypothermia.

Acid—base and electrolyte changes Respiratory acidosis tends to potentiate the block produced by non-depolarizing relaxants and respiratory alkalosis produces resistance to their action. A recent laboratory study (SEDA-14, 115—116; 53[r]) suggests that this long-accepted view, while being true for *d*-tubocurarine and vecuronium (possibly via their increased conversion to the bisquaternary form at lower pH), may not hold for metocurine, pancuronium or alcuronium. More clinical research (54[C]) is needed on this subject. There is no consensus on the effects of metabolic acid–base changes. Protein binding of muscle relaxants is maximal between pH 8 and 9 and this may account for larger doses being required in alkalosis. Alkalosis is often associated with hypokalemia. In hypokalemia the actions of non-depolarizing agents may be increased and those of depolarizing agents reduced. Hyperkalemia has the opposite effects, probably via lowering of muscle transmembrane potential. Variations in serum sodium affect neuromuscular blocking agents in a similar manner to potassium changes. However, serum levels of electrolytes do not always reflect intracellular concentrations or, perhaps more important, the intra-/extracellular ion ratios; in addition, changes in pH and the concentrations of potassium, sodium and other electrolytes are linked and have opposing influences at several sites in the processes of neuromuscular function so that the expected effect of a change, taken in isolation, may not be found. Nonetheless, it is of practical importance to note that respiratory acidosis does enhance a non-depolarizing block and makes its reversal by neostigmine more difficult. Such a vicious circle in the recovery room is best broken by ventilating the patient until the cause of the respiratory depression is removed or corrected. Hypermagnesemia enhances the actions of both depolarizing and non-depolarizing neuromuscular blocking agents. Lithium *may* also do this. Hypercalcemia may be associated with prolongation of suxamethonium blockade and reduction in potency of non-depolarizing agents.

DEPOLARIZING NEUROMUSCULAR BLOCKING AGENTS

Suxamethonium (succinylcholine)

Suxamethonium consists of two acetylcholine molecules linked together and, initially, acts like acetylcholine by depolarizing the motor end-plate. Unlike acetylcholine which, on dissociation from the receptor, is immediately destroyed by acetylcholinesterase present in the neuromuscular junction, suxamethonium is hydrolyzed by *plasma* (pseudo-)cholinesterase which is, as the name suggests, present in plasma but not at the neuromuscular junction. Indeed, most of an injected dose of suxamethonium is normally destroyed before it reaches the neuromuscular junction. If the activity of plasma cholinesterase in a particular patient is reduced, more suxamethonium reaches the neuromuscular junction and its action is proportionately prolonged. The molecules of suxamethonium that reach the acetylcholine receptor sites interact repeatedly with them, producing prolonged depolarization of the motor end-plate which becomes surrounded by an electrically inactive zone. The end-result is flaccid paralysis. The action of suxamethonium is terminated by diffusion away from the neuromuscular junction. Hydrolysis results in choline and succinylmonocholine, which has a very weak competitive blocking action and is further slowly hydrolyzed by plasma cholinesterase to choline and succinic acid. Approximately 10% of an intravenous dose is excreted unchanged in the urine. The normal half-life of suxamethonium is 1–2 minutes (55). The usual adult dose of suxamethonium chloride is 0.5–1.5 mg/kg, providing clinical relaxation for some 4–9 minutes. The normal response is highly variable, however, and up to 15 minutes relaxation may result from normal doses. Suxamethonium iodide has about two-thirds the potency of the chloride.

Hypersensitivity reactions Bourne et al. (56[C]), from the results of intradermal injections, concluded that suxamethonium had only 1% of the histamine-releasing activity of *d*-tubocurarine. However, through the years there have been many case-reports of reactions varying from *flushing* and *urticaria* to *bronchospasm* (57[C])–60[C]) and *severe shock* (61[C])–64[C]). That suxamethonium was the agent responsible has been suggested in some cases by the patients reacting on different occasions (65[C], 66[C], 70[C]—with raised plasma histamine and catecholamine levels) and confirmed in others by repeatedly injecting the drug, thereby producing bronchospasm several times in the course of the one anesthesia (67[C], 68[C]). Skin testing has also yielded confirmation, although this can be dangerous (62[C]). More recently, the analysis of large series of patients (12[CR], 14[R], 15[R], 16[C], 17[C], 71[C]) who have suffered severe anaphylactoid reactions during anesthesia, using more sophisticated laboratory and immunological investigations in addition to intradermal skin tests, suggests that suxamethonium may be much more commonly associated with such reactions than was previously believed. In a series of 18 cases (69[Cr]) cardiovascular collapse was the predominant feature in 72% and bronchospasm in 33%; cardiac arrest occurred in five patients. The possible mechanisms involved in anaphylactoid reactions to neuromuscular blocking agents and associated factors are discussed above in the section entitled 'General considerations'. In addition, two new reports (72[C], 73[C]) of anaphylactic reactions involving both thiopental and suxamethonium raise the question of 'aggregate'-induced reactions (72[C]) occurring when drugs are given in such a way that they can interact in the injection system.

ADVERSE REACTION PATTERN

General and toxic reactions Suxamethonium has many unwanted and potentially dangerous side effects. Generalized muscle fasciculations are associated, to a varying degree, with muscle pain, acute elevation of serum potassium which under certain conditions may result in dysrhythmias and cardiac arrest, raised intraocular and intragastric pressures, and rhabdomyolysis and myoglobinuria with, rarely, renal failure. Bradycardia and junctional rhythms are relatively common. Normal doses may result in prolonged paralysis (on rare occasions for several hours) in patients with congenital or acquired plasma cholinesterase abnormality or deficiency.

Hypersensitivity reactions Anaphylactoid reactions have been documented and clinical signs suggestive of histamine release are not uncommon. These are mostly mild such as flushing of the skin, but occasionally bronchospasm and/or hypotension which may lead to circulatory arrest occur. Suxamethonium is the relaxant most commonly associated with the syndrome of malignant hyperthermia.

Tumor-inducing effects These have not been reported.

ORGANS AND SYSTEMS

Neuromuscular The depolarization of the motor endplate receptors produced by suxamethonium (either directly or via repetitive discharge generation by the motor nerve terminals) (74) results in generalized and desynchronized contraction of skeletal muscle fibers. These fasciculations result in aching *muscle pain* (in up to 90% of patients) most commonly in the neck, pectoral region, shoulders and back. The pain is most often experienced the day after operation and is worse in ambulatory patients. It is more common in women than in men. Children, elderly patients, athletes and pregnant women (75[C]) complain less frequently. Africans also seem to be less susceptible (76[C]). The pain appears not to be related to the extent or intensity of the observed fasciculations. The cause of the pain remains unknown, although there are many hypotheses such as damage to muscle (77[Cr], 78[Cr]) resulting from asynchronous contractions of adjacent muscle fibers (79[Cr]), irreversible damage to muscle spindles (80), potassium flux (81[C]), lactic acid (82[Cr]), serotonin (83[C]), calcium influx-associated damage to muscle spindles (84[C]) and prostaglandins (85[C], 86[Cr]). Various measures have been recommended as preventive, but none is effective in all cases. Undoubtedly the most reliable method to date is the injection of a small non-paralyzing dose of a non-depolarizing neuromuscular blocker (gallamine 20 mg, *d*-tubocurarine 3 mg, in adults) 3–4 minutes before the injection of suxamethonium. Gallamine is slightly more effective than *d*-tubocurarine and pancuronium is much less effective than the other two (87[C]–90[C]) in preventing fasciculations. Other measures, much disputed, include the prior injection of diazepam (91[C], 92[C]), procaine or lidocaine (in rather toxic doses), vitamin C, suxamethonium itself (10 mg) and, recently, aspirin (85[C], 86[Cr]). Thiopental, injected immediately beforehand, is also said to reduce myalgia, as is giving the suxamethonium slowly.

Rarely, on injecting suxamethonium, *contracture*, instead of the usual relaxation, of skeletal muscles ensues. This is most often associated with myotonia dystrophica and myotonia congenita. A myotonic reaction has also been reported in a patient with hyperkalemic periodic paralysis (93[C]). Suxamethonium is therefore contraindicated in these conditions, even though normal responses are sometimes seen. Contracture has also been reported as a result of denervation in Pancoast's syndrome and after plexus injuries and, rarely, in patients with amyotrophic lateral sclerosis or multiple sclerosis (94[Cr], 95[C], 96). In denervated muscles the postulated mechanism is direct activation of the contractile mechanism by suxamethonium via the widespread chemosensitivity of the muscle fiber membranes. *Failure of relaxation and generalized muscular rigidity* after suxamethonium is sometimes also seen in patients who develop the syndrome of *malignant hyperthermia* (see under 'Metabolic' effects). *Isolated masseter muscle spasm* is seen more often, being reported particularly in pediatric patients subjected to both suxamethonium and halothane. While some (97[C]) believe that 50% of these patients are susceptible to malignant hyperthermia (MHS), others are not convinced of such a high degree of correlation (98) and hold diverse other factors to be responsible for the majority of cases (99[C], 100[C], 101[Cr]).

Myoglobinuria (110[C]) and *raised serum CPK* (78[C]) have been reported after suxamethonium and would appear to be evidence of muscle damage probably resulting from the fasciculations. Repeated bolus doses of suxamethonium result in higher plasma myoglobin (102[C]) and creatine kinase (78[C]) levels. Myoglobinemia seems to be much more common in children than in adults (SEDA-10, 107; SEDA-11, 121; 103[Cr]) and is more marked when halothane is used (104[C]). On occasion, myoglobinuria results in *renal failure* (105[C], 106[Cr]). An association appears to exist between (latent) *muscular dystrophy* (usually of the *Duchenne* type) and the production of rhabdomyolysis by suxamethonium (SEDA-8, 134—135; 106[Cr], 111[C], 112[C]).

Prolonged paralysis may result from idiosyncrasy, overdose or decreased plasma cholinesterase activity. *Geographical and racial differences* in sensitivity to suxamethonium exist (SEDA-6, 129; 107[R], 113[r]); some of these differences arise from dietary and other environmental factors and others result from variations in plasma cholinesterase genotypes. *Genotypically normal* patients may be clinically paralyzed from a usual (1 mg/kg) dose of suxamethonium for as short as 2 minutes or (rarely) as long as 20 minutes and the duration in general inversely reflects the plasma cholinesterase activity (114[Cr]). *Tachyphylaxis* is associated with repeated doses. Prolonged exposure of the neuromuscular junction to suxamethonium (resulting from repeated bolus injections or during an infusion of the drug or as a consequence of delayed hydrolysis subsequent to genetic or acquired plasma cholinesterase deficiency) is accompanied by the development of a *Phase II block*, with non-depolarizing characteristics and a variably prolonged recovery. This is dependent on both the dose and the duration of exposure to suxamethonium. A cumulative dose of 3—4 mg/kg and an exposure time of 20—30 minutes may be sufficient during halothane anesthesia (108[C]). There is wide variation between patients (109[C]), however, and monitoring of neuromuscular transmission (train-of-four or post-tetanic count) is advisable with cumulative doses greater than 3 mg/kg. *Plasma cholinesterase deficiency* may be hereditary or acquired. The hereditary form is believed to account for two-thirds of suxamethonium-sensitive patients. Genetically determined *plasma cholinesterase variants* hydrolyze suxamethonium much more slowly. About 96% of the population are homozygotes for the normal 'typical' gene, one in 25 are heterozygotes ('typical'/'atypical') and exhibit a slightly prolonged (about 2—4 times normal) response to suxamethonium, and one in 2000—3000 are homozygotes for the 'atypical' gene and exhibit a markedly prolonged response (2—3 hours). The 'silent' gene is much rarer and homozygotes (approximately 0.0006% of the population) have virtually no plasma cholinesterase activity, complete paralysis after suxamethonium lasting many hours. The reviews by Whittaker (115[R]) and Pantuck and Pantuck (116[R]) are recommended for detailed information about the various plasma cholinesterase variants and their relevance. *Acquired plasma cholinesterase deficiency* is clinically less important since paralysis from suxamethonium seldom lasts for more than 20—30 minutes. However, this 'inconvenience' can be avoided by not using suxamethonium in patients known to be at risk. A clinically important prolongation of suxamethonium-paralysis is only to be expected, with the exception of some drug-induced effects (see 'Interactions' section), in patients with more than one cause for reduction in pseudocholinesterase activity. In *malnutrition* and *liver disease* (117[C], 118[C]) synthesis (hepatic) of plasma cholinesterase is reduced. *Neonates* have about 50% of normal adult plasma cholinesterase activity. In pregnancy there is a rapid fall in plasma cholinesterase levels of about 25% in the first trimester, which only returns to normal some 6—8 weeks postpartum (119[Cr]—121[Cr]). Occasionally much greater falls are seen. The lowest average values have been reported (SEDA-5, 135; 122[C], 123[Cr]) in the first week of the puerperium. Similar changes have been reported in gestational trophoblastic disease (hydatidiform mole) (124[C]). *Cancer* is sometimes associated with lower plasma cholinesterase activity (SEDA-5, 136; 125[C]). There is also a case-report of multiple esterase deficiencies in Hodgkin's disease (SEDA-2, 117; 126[C]). Plasma cholinesterase activity has also been reported to be reduced by up to 70—80% in patients with *renal disease and burns*. *Plasmapheresis* (SEDA-5, 135; 127[C], 128[C]) removes cholinesterase, along with other proteins, from the plasma. Numerous drugs, which are described in more detail in the 'Interactions' section, also reduce plasma cholinesterase synthesis or activity, e.g. *estrogens* (and *oral contraceptives*), *glucocorticoids*, *phenelzine*, *organophosphorus compounds* (such as *ecothiopate* eye-drops, insecticides), *carbamates* (insecticides, *bambuterol*), *cytotoxic drugs*, *metoclopramide*, the *ester-type local anesthetic drugs*, and *pancuronium*. The clinically used *anticholinesterases*, such as *neostigmine*, *pyridostigmine*, *hexafluorenium* and *tetrahydroaminoacridine*, will also prolong the action of suxamethonium. A concise update on plasma cholinesterase and its relevance for the anesthetist is provided by Jensen et al. (129[R]).

Neuromuscular disease In *myasthenia gravis* responses to suxamethonium are unpredictable. Resistance has been reported and the development of a phase II block may occur more readily, occasionally leading to prolonged paralysis. The measures used to treat the condition, e.g. plasmapheresis or anticholinesterases, further complicate the picture (see above). Foldes gives an excellent review of this subject (130[R]). Patients with the *Eaton-Lambert syndrome* are very sensitive to all relaxants. Prolonged paralysis after suxamethonium has been reported also in *von Recklinghausen's disease*

(SEDA-2, 117; 131[C]), but resistance to suxamethonium has also been seen (132[C]). *Nemaline myopathy* (133[C]) may be associated with resistance to suxamethonium. The possible association between (latent) *muscular dystrophy of the Duchenne type* and the production of rhabdomyolysis by suxamethonium has already been referred to above. Suxamethonium may cause excessive muscle damage in these patients as manifested not only by severe *myoglobinemia and raised serum creatine kinase levels* but also by an *acute exacerbation of muscle weakness* postoperatively (SEDA-8, 134—135; SEDA-11, 121; 134[Cr], 135[C], 136[Cr], 137[C], 138[Cr]). Such patients may also develop features suggestive of the syndrome of *malignant hyperthermia*. Suxamethonium should not be used in patients who are known to suffer from Duchenne muscular dystrophy or who have a family history suspect for the condition.

The response of patients with neuromuscular disorders to muscle relaxants is reviewed by Azar (139[R]), Martz et al. (140[R]) and Miller and Lee (141[R]).

Cardiovascular *Bradycardia* and other dysrhythmias are common (80% in some series) and occur after the first, and subsequent, injections of suxamethonium in infants and children. In adults, these effects are seen more commonly after second, or later, injections, particularly when the interval between the doses is 2—5 minutes. However, it has been suggested that bradycardia and 'asystole' may now be more frequently seen than previously in adults after a single injection of suxamethonium as a result of the increased use of fentanyl or the omission of atropine beforehand (142[C]). *Nodal rhythm* and '*wandering pacemaker*' are frequent occurrences. The bradycardia is sometimes extreme (asystoles of 15—30 seconds duration have been reported). Usually these minor dysrhythmias revert to normal after a few minutes. Halothane may prolong their presence. The incidence of bradycardic asystole is not known, as atropine (the effective therapy) is usually quickly given.

Serious problems however have been reported in apparently healthy children undergoing minor surgical procedures (SEDA-18, 6[Cr]). The report is dealing with nine children whose cases were collected over a 5-year period by a Malignant Hyperthermia 'Hotline'. Cardiac arrest occurred within 4 minutes after injection of suxamethonium preceded by bradycardia in eight of the children. Resuscitation was difficult and prolonged (up to 70 minutes). Five of the children died. Only one child was known to have muscular dystrophy (Becker) and another muscular hypotonia. But subsequent investigation of the survivors and the children's families revealed that all the others, being apparently healthy before the intervention were suffering from some form of *myopathy*. The authors suppose that hyperkalemia was the cause of cardiac arrest in these children and that when it occurs temporally related to the injection of suxamethonium, as in these cases, intravenous calcium should be the first-line treatment.

This one and other recent reports suggest that the routine use of suxamethonium in pediatric anesthesia should be abandoned. Its use should be reserved for emergency intubation or instances where immediate securing of the airway is necessary.

Tachycardia and *rise in blood pressure* are occasionally seen. Other *supra-ventricular and ventricular dysrhythmias* are much less common. *Ventricular fibrillation* associated with the use of suxamethonium is usually the result of hyperkalemia (see 'Mineral and fluid balance' section), but has been reported also in hypercalcemia (143[C]), and is often seen in the course of malignant hyperthermia. Atropine, especially when given intravenously just before suxamethonium, is the most effective agent for the prevention of dysrhythmias. Hexafluorenium, *d*-tubocurarine, pancuronium and other non-depolarizers have also been reported as being effective in prevention. Severe *hypotension* may occur in patients with anaphylactoid reactions (see 'Hypersensitivity reactions' section above).

On theoretical grounds, suxamethonium, being akin to acetylcholine, may produce effects not only at the neuromuscular junction, but also at autonomic ganglia, at muscarinic receptors and at postganglionic parasympathetic receptors. However, these other cholinoceptors are not so sensitive to its action. Nevertheless, 'stimulation of sympathetic ganglia' has been invoked as possibly responsible for the tachycardia and rise in blood pressure which are sometimes transiently seen after its use. Likewise, stimulation of parasympathetic ganglia or direct stimulation of cardiac muscarinic receptors, may be responsible for the commonly occurring bradycardia. Differences in resting sympathetic and vagal tone have been said to account for the more frequent occurrence of tachycardia in 'vagotonic' adults and bradycardia in 'sympathotonic' children. The transient mild rise in blood pressure is possibly the result of the initial fasciculations inducing an increase in venous return, which may also reflexly result in a slowing of heart rate. Stimulation of afferent receptors in the carotinoid sinus has also been claimed to cause reflex bradycardia. Small doses (20—25 mg) are said to convert nodal to sinus rhythm, and larger doses to depress the sino-auricular node and so cause bradycardia and nodal rhythm. Fasciculations probably produce an increase in afferent discharge from muscle spindles, which may account for the reported arousal pattern on the electroencephalogram and this, in turn, is postulated as a cause of tachycardia and rise in blood pressure. Nigrovic

(144[R]) has proposed a hypothesis involving the modulation of noradrenaline release from postganglionic sympathetic nerve terminals by presynaptic nicotine (+) and muscarinic (−) receptors on these nerve terminals. The refractory period of these presynaptic nicotinic receptors is postulated as being longer than that of the muscarinic receptors which results in a net muscarinic effect (bradycardia) of a second suxamethonium injection within 4—5 minutes of the first dose. To explain the occurrence of bradycardia after an initial injection of suxamethonium in young children, it is postulated that sympathetic nerve terminals mature later, so that muscarinic (bradycardic) effects are unopposed by noradrenaline secretion in the younger patient.

It is to be concluded that while there are innumerable mechanisms whereby cardiovascular changes may be produced, there is no clear indication which are the more relevant, and many of them probably contribute to the final outcome.

Respiratory *Apnea* of variable duration results from muscle paralysis. The return of spontaneous respiration is normally rapid but may be delayed if phase II block develops. This will only be of consequence if it is not detected and spontaneous respiration is permitted before it is adequate (see 'Neuromuscular' section). Exacerbation of muscle weakness in *Duchenne muscular dystrophy* following the injection of suxamethonium may lead to *'delayed' respiratory failure* in the postoperative period (SEDA-11, 121—122; 138[Cr]). Bronchospasm is a feature of approximately one-third of anaphylactoid reactions to suxamethonium (see above) and *laryngeal edema* may also occur, producing intubation problems (145[C]) or respiratory distress and cyanosis after detubation (SEDA-8, 133; 146[C]).

Nervous system (*See also the 'Neuromuscular' and 'Cardiovascular' sections*) An *arousal pattern* may be seen on the electroencephalogram which is possibly the result of increased afferent 'traffic' from muscle spindles. This has been speculated as the cause of *perioperative dreaming* in children in whom an intermittent-suxamethonium technique has been used during light anesthesia (SEDA-13, 102; 147[Cr]). Suxamethonium must be used with caution in *neurological disease* and is better avoided altogether in circumstances where there is a risk of a dangerous rise in serum potassium (see the 'Mineral and fluid balance' section). A transient *rise in intracranial pressure* occurs subsequent to the injection of suxamethonium, probably as a result of an increase in cerebral blood volume. The mean rise of 5—9 mmHg is said to be insignificant. However, the rise is substantial in a number of cases (SEDA-9, 116; 148[C], 149[r]), so that the use of suxamethonium could be catastrophic in patients with reduced intracranial compliance or a cerebral aneurysm.

Endocrine, metabolic (*See also 'Risk situations' section*) The syndrome of *malignant hyperthermia* may be triggered by suxamethonium. The mortality is more than 60% in untreated patients. This syndrome is reported as occurring once in every 15 000—150 000 anesthesias. It may be more common in the Japanese. There are, however, also abortive forms of malignant hyperthermia and many of the typical signs may be produced by other conditions, so that it is difficult to ascertain the precise incidence of the syndrome. Autosomal dominant inheritance, with reduced penetrance and variable expressivity, is the proposed genetic basis for malignant hyperthermia. The etiology is unknown, but is thought to be associated with a rise in free ionized myoplasmic calcium, possibly due to a failure of the sarcoplasmic reticulum to bind calcium. As a result, aerobic and anaerobic metabolism are increased, resulting in the typical features of the syndrome. Halothane and suxamethonium are the most frequent 'triggers', although almost all the inhalational anesthetic agents have been incriminated. While other muscle relaxants (pancuronium, *d*-tubocurarine) have been suggested as triggers in a few cases—and many other drugs used in anesthetized patients also—convincing evidence is lacking at present. It is reasonably suggested that stress plays a role in the development of malignant hyperthermia (150[C]). Several excellent review articles have been written on the subject by Gronert (151[R]), Britt (152[R]) and Schulte-Sasse and Eberlein (153[R]). The last-named authors also discuss apparently related conditions such as rhabdomyolysis and the malignant neuroleptic syndrome, pointing out the many similarities with malignant hyperthermia.

Dantrolene (586[R], 587[R]) is the agent of choice for treatment of malignant hyperthermia and greatly reduces the mortality to under 10% if given in time (SEDA-7, 148; 154[C]), together with general supportive measures. The recommended dose of dantrolene is 1—2.5 mg/kg i.v., repeated at 5—10-minute intervals if necessary to a maximum total dose of 10 mg/kg in 15 minutes. Patients need continuous observation for at least 48 hours after an episode since hyperthermia may recur. Prophylaxis with dantrolene (see the review articles quoted here for details) should be given to patients suspected of being susceptible (155[Cr]) to the syndrome. Dantrolene itself (see later in this Chapter) has side effects which are mostly minor in nature, such as nausea and vomiting, when the drug is used acutely. A case-report has suggested, however, that it may have contributed to *uterine atony* with resulting excessive hemorrhage when given prophylactically after a cesarean section (156[C]), and muscle weakness associated with its oral prophylactic use in a patient with compromised respiratory function is reported to have exacerbated postoperative *respiratory* depression to such an extent that artificial ventilation was required (SEDA-14, 114; 157[Cr]). Intravenous prophylaxis (2.5 mg/kg) just before the induction of anesthesia is currently recommended. The combination with calcium-channel blockers, such as verapamil, may result in severe cardiovascular depression and hyperkalemia (SEDA-9, 122; SEDA-12, 113; 158[r], 159[C]), so that extreme care is required.

Mineral and fluid balance An immediate *rise in serum potassium* occurs. This is probably a result of the repetitive opening of the receptor-linked ion channels and the suxamethonium-induced fasciculations, although it may occur in the absence of visible fasciculations. The rise is normally small, 0.5 mmol/l or less (160). It may be prolonged (SEDA-11, 122; 161[C]) and exaggerated (SEDA-10, 108; 162) in patients taking β-blockers. In *renal insufficiency* the rise after suxamethonium is similar to that in normal cases (163[C]) and is only dangerous if the serum potassium is already high (above 5.5 mmol/l). There are several conditions, however, which may lead to a massive rise in serum potassium, resulting in ventricular fibrillation and cardiac arrest. These include *burns* (164[C], 165[C]), *massive trauma* (166[C], 167[C]), and *neurological diseases or injuries*, especially where denervation is a feature, such as *spinal cord injury* (168[C]), 169), *hemiplegia, multiple sclerosis or muscular dystrophy* (170[R]), *peripheral nerve injuries* (95[C], 171[Cr]) and *polyneuropathy* (172[C], 173[C]). Hyperkalemia has also been reported after suxamethonium in patients with *tetanus* (174[C]), *encephalitis* (175[C]), *Parkinson's disease* (SEDA-6, 129; 176[C]), *muscle wasting* secondary to *chronic arterial insufficiency* (177[C]), *metastatic embryonal rhabdomyosarcoma* (SEDA-14, 114; 178[C]), *ruptured cerebral aneurysms* (SEDA-5, 134; 179[C]), *hyperparathyroidism* (143[C]), and in patients with *severe and long-lasting sepsis* (180[C], 181[C]). Muscle injury with excessive leakage of potassium is postulated as a cause of the hyperkalemia. Re-uptake of potassium into muscle cells may also be hindered. It has been shown that denervation results in a spread of the normally small receptor area of the motor end-plate over the entire muscle fiber membrane, so that eventually the whole membrane surface is directly excitable by depolarizing agents such as acetylcholine or suxamethonium. The immature type of extrajunctional receptor-linked ion channels so formed remain open for a longer time than those at normal motor end-plates. Depolarization by suxamethonium thereby results in an excessive efflux of potassium from ion channels spread over the entire muscle fiber membrane and not just, as normally occurs, from the circumscribed motor end-plate region (182—184). *Prolonged immobilization* may also result in extrajunctional receptor spread (185) and a greater increase in serum potassium than usual after suxamethonium.

There is a *time period* during which patients are at greatest risk from hyperkalemia. In patients suffering from burns or trauma this is generally found to be between 10 and 60 days after the injury, or longer if there is persistent infection and delayed healing. In neurological diseases or injuries the danger period is usually from 3 weeks to 6 months after onset. However, in some cases, such as patients with transverse spinal lesions and tetraplegia, dangerous hyperkalemia has been reported as early as 24—48 hours after the injury, and likewise severe potassium rises have been reported more than 6 months after injury or onset of disease, particularly in patients with progressive lesions (SEDA-6, 128; 170[R]). It has been claimed that non-depolarizing drugs given before suxamethonium attenuate the rise in potassium, but this has been repeatedly shown to be unreliable. It seems advisable to avoid the use of suxamethonium completely in such patients. This subject has been extensively reviewed by Gronert and Theye (186[R]) in the past, and by Yentis (187[R]) more recently.

Liver In severe liver dysfunction the synthesis of plasma cholinesterase may be reduced to such an extent that the action of suxamethonium may be prolonged. This is usually not more than 2 or 3 times the normal duration.

Gastrointestinal Suxamethonium may *increase intragastric pressure*. This is probably a result of the intensity of the fasciculation (188[C]) of the abdominal muscles, although a vagal effect may also contribute. The rise is highly variable, ranging from zero to more than 85 cmH_2O according to many different investigations (189[C]—192[C]). The intragastric pressure at which the lower esophageal sphincter opens is also variable, with a mean of about 28 cmH_2O, depending partly on the angle between the esophagus and the cardia of the stomach (193, 194[C]). There is therefore a danger that the suxamethonium-induced rise in intragastric pressure may produce incompetence of the lower esophageal sphincter and result in *regurgitation*. This risk is likely to be increased in patients with hiatus hernia, gastric and intestinal dilatation, ascites and intra-abdominal tumors. Pregnant patients are especially at risk as the tonus of the lower esophageal sphincter may also be reduced in pregnancy. It has been suggested, however, that suxamethonium causes, either by a direct action on the lower esophageal sphincter or indirectly through a 'pinch action' of the diaphragm, an increase in resistance to opening of the lower esophagus which counteracts the increased intragastric pressure (195[Cr]). Attenuating the fasciculations by giving small doses of non-depolarizing blockers reduces the rise in gastric pressure (191[C], 196[C], 188[C]).

Urinary system In severe renal disease, suxamethonium should only be given if the serum *potassium* is less than 5.5 mmol/l (see 'Mineral and fluid balance' section). The *excretion of neostigmine and pyridostigmine* may be impaired in renal failure and this has been reported (SEDA-9, 117; 197[C]) to have resulted in prolongation of the action of suxamethonium given some hours later. *Myoglobinuria* resulting from suxamethonium administration may cause acute renal failure (105[C], 106[Cr], 198[C]).

Special senses *Intraocular pressure* rises within 20–30 seconds after the injection of suxamethonium. The probable cause is contracture of the extraocular muscles (199[C], 200[C]); a transient dilatation of choroidal blood vessels has also been postulated (201[C]). The extraocular muscles contain fibers which receive multiple innervation and such fibers respond to depolarizers with a sustained contracture, possibly as a result of direct activation of the contractile mechanism by the more extensive area of depolarization (202[R]). The rise in intraocular pressure is about 8 torr on average (203[C]), but can be much greater (204[C]) and usually lasts about 4–6 minutes (205[C]) (up to 15 minutes on occasion). The rise is less during deep anesthesia. If suxamethonium is given when the globe is open, the rise in intraocular pressure results in extrusion of vitreous and other contents such as the lens. Permanent damage and blindness are therefore risks. Suxamethonium is contraindicated in open-eye injuries and during the course of operations when the eyeball is open. In glaucoma the rise is reported to be no greater than in normal patients, although suxamethonium is perhaps better avoided in closed-angle cases on theoretical grounds.

Whilst it has been claimed that the previous injection of small doses of non-depolarizing agents, as used to attenuate fasciculations, and—more open to dispute—prior diazepam, acetazolamide, hexafluorenium, lidocaine and 'self-taming' with suxamethonium itself can prevent or reduce the rise in intraocular pressure, it has repeatedly been demonstrated that these measures are by no means always successful (SEDA-5, 136; 206[C], 207[C], 208[R]), and so suxamethonium remains contraindicated in the above circumstances.

Risk situations In patients with *asthma* or a *history of previous allergy*, suxamethonium should be used with caution in view of its potential for causing allergic reactions and bronchospasm. Where a patient or a relative has had a *previous 'reaction'* to an anesthetic, the possibilities of an atypical cholinesterase genotype or malignant hyperthermia should also be considered. Patients with certain *musculoskeletal and developmental abnormalities*, such as a tendency to joint dislocations, squint, ptosis, hernias, some forms of cryptorchidism, pectus excavatum, kyphosis, foot deformities, and myopathic features, and also those who have reacted to a previous injection of suxamethonium with *generalized muscle rigidity or masseter spasm*, may be more prone to malignant hyperthermia. Dantrolene should be available to every area where anesthetic agents are used.

Suxamethonium fasciculations (or increase in muscle tone) may be dangerous in patients with *fractures* or *dislocations* (especially vertebral, where the drug is relatively contraindicated), in patients with *open-eye injuries* or after the eyeball is opened surgically, in cases where an increase in abdominal pressure must be avoided (*pheochromocytoma, aortic aneurysm, full stomach, ileus*), and in patients where a rise in arterial pressure may be catastrophic (*cerebral aneurysm, raised intracranial pressure*). In *pregnancy* the risk of regurgitation has to be weighed against the advantage of rapid intubation. The use of 'precurarization' with small doses of non-depolarizers may reduce the intensity of the fasciculations, but is by no means reliable. If possible, relaxation is better achieved by using a non-depolarizing agent alone. This is also true of patients prone to develop excessive hyperkalemia (with *burns, massive trauma, denervating injuries and neurological diseases*, etc., during the 6 months or so of the 'danger period' as described in the section on 'Mineral and fluid balance'). Patients with *disease of muscle*—dystrophia myotonica, myotonia congenita, myasthenia gravis, and hyperkalemic periodic paralysis—tend to react unpredictably to suxamethonium. In myasthenia gravis, small doses of suxamethonium may be tried and the resulting effect monitored. In the other diseases listed non-depolarizers, cautiously used, are preferable. Cardiac arrest has been reported in at least two cases of pseudohypertrophic muscular dystrophy (Duchenne type) and excessive muscle damage may be produced by suxamethonium in this condition.

Prolonged paralysis, occasionally lasting hours, is a risk if the patient is, or has been, receiving *certain drugs* (see 'Interactions' section below).

Second-generation effects Maternal doses of suxamethonium up to 200 mg have been reported as not resulting in detectable levels in neonates. Very large bolus doses (300–500 mg) have produced umbilical vein levels up to 2 mg/l, but the neonates showed no adverse effects (209[C], 210[C]). Extreme *reduction in plasma* *cholinesterase activity*, either caused by organophosphorus poisoning (SEDA-8, 136; 211[C]) or genetically determined (SEDA-15, 123; 212[Cr], 213[C]), has resulted in *weakness and respiratory depression in neonates* after normal or small (211[C]) maternal doses.

Interactions *Antibiotics* are discussed in the 'General considerations' section at the beginning of this chapter.

Organophosphorus compounds Ecothiopate eye-drops, used in the treatment of glaucoma, prolong the action of suxamethonium considerably (214[C]). This drug is a long-acting anticholinesterase and inhibits the activity of both acetylcholinesterase and plasma cholinesterase. Plasma cholinesterase activity may be reduced to 5% or less and, on cessation of this therapy, requires 1—2 months for recovery to normal values (215[C], 216[C]). The prolonged anticholinesterase effect is due to the conversion of the enzyme to its stable phosphoryl derivative. If a patient has used ecothiopate eye-drops in the previous 2 months or so, suxamethonium should not be given unless normal plasma cholinesterase activity can be demonstrated.

Various organophosphorus insecticides, such as *parathion and malathion*, may also result in prolonged paralysis after suxamethonium due to reduced free cholinesterase levels (SEDA-8, 136; 211[C], 217[C]), produced in a similar manner to that in the case of ecothiopate (218).

Bambuterol, a drug used to relieve bronchospasm, has been shown to approximately double the duration of action of suxamethonium (SEDA-14, 114; 219[C]). Plasma cholinesterase activity was reduced significantly even 10—12.5 hours after a single 30-mg dose had been given to patients. The interaction is due to carbamate groups binding to plasma cholinesterase.

Phenelzine, a monoamine-oxidase inhibitor, has been reported to cause significant prolongation of suxamethonium paralysis due to depressed plasma cholinesterase levels (to approximately 10% of normal). Recovery of plasma cholinesterase levels took 2 weeks (220[C]).

Metoclopramide, an antiemetic, inhibits the activity of plasma cholinesterase and may prolong the action of suxamethonium (SEDA-14, 115; 221, 222[C]).

Magnesium sulfate is used mostly in the treatment of toxemia of pregnancy. Serum magnesium levels may be raised and, as magnesium inhibits the release of acetylcholine and decreases the sensitivity of the postjunctional membrane, the action of non-depolarizing agents will be prolonged (see 'Interactions' section under '*d*-Tubocurarine'). It is not so clear, however, why the action of suxamethonium is also prolonged (223[C], 224[Cr], 337[C], 338). Suxamethonium fasciculations are reported to be prevented (SEDA-5, 135; 225[C]). It has been suggested that the administration of intravenous magnesium sulfate should be stopped 20—30 minutes before muscle relaxants are given. Monitoring with a nerve stimulator is advisable.

Steroids Estrogens and estrogen-containing contraceptives prolong the action of suxamethonium. Plasma cholinesterase levels are reduced, possibly by the estrogenic depression of hepatic synthesis of plasma cholinesterase, and its isoenzymes are modified (115[R], 226[C], 227[C]). *Stilbestrol*, included in this group, is reported to have caused paralysis for 3 hours in a patient with other aggravating factors (SEDA-4, 89; 228[C]). One would, however, expect little prolongation of suxamethonium paralysis since the decrease in plasma cholinesterase activity (after contraceptives, at least) averages only about 20%. *Prednisone, cortisol and dexamethasone* also reduce plasma cholinesterase activity to a mild or moderate degree (SEDA-15, 122; 229, 230[C], 231[Cr]).

Cytotoxics and immunosuppressive drugs Nitrogen mustards and related agents, such as cyclophosphamide, chlorambucil, triethylmelamine and thiophosphoramide, etc., have produced prolongation of suxamethonium's action (232[C], 233[C]). Plasma cholinesterase activity is reduced, possibly by alkylation of the enzyme by these agents. It is suggested that azathioprine may potentiate suxamethonium via inhibition of phosphodiesterase activity (SEDA-4, 87; 234).

Lithium carbonate, used in psychiatry, delays the onset and prolongs the action of depolarizing relaxants (235[C], 236). The principal mechanism of action is disputed. Factors suggested have been the development of 'dual block', reduced sensitivity of the end-plate for suxamethonium, diminished synthesis or release of acetylcholine, and plasma cholinesterase inhibition (236, 237, 238[r]). The clinical importance is also disputed.

Trimetaphan This ganglion blocker may result in a doubling of the duration of suxamethonium block (239[C], 240, 241[C]). The mechanism is not clear, but may be a competitive effect at the neuromuscular junction. Blockade of end-plate ionic channels has also been suggested (242).

Tacrine (*tetrahydroaminoacridine*) *and hexafluorenium*, both clinically used sometimes to potentiate and prolong the action of suxamethonium (243[C], 244[C]), inhibit plasma cholinesterase. Hexafluorenium also inhibits acetylcholinesterase and has a weak neuromuscular blocking action of the non-depolarizing type; a phase II block develops fairly rapidly when repeated injections of even small doses (0.2—0.3 mg/kg) of suxamethonium are given in combination with hexafluorenium (245[C]); (authors' personal observations). Fasciculations are reportedly reduced and hyperkalemia prevented (SEDA-7, 147; 246[C]), as is an increase in intraocular pressure

(202[C]), when hexafluorenium is given prior to suxamethonium. Because of a lack of consistency of successful results from various investigators, this method is not recommended for patients especially at risk from hyperkalemia or increased intraocular pressure (see previous sections). Simultaneous injection of hexafluorenium and suxamethonium may result in severe bronchospasm.

Aprotinin (*Trasylol*) slightly reduces plasma cholinesterase activity and would only be expected to prolong the action of suxamethonium in combination with other factors. However, re-paralysis has been reported when this agent was used after operations during which suxamethonium had been given alone or in combination with normal doses of *d*-tubocurarine (247[C]).

Antidysrhythmic drugs Quinidine potentiates not only non-depolarizing muscle relaxants but also depolarizing drugs (248). Verapamil may also potentiate the block produced by both types of neuromuscular blocking agent (SEDA-9, 116; 249). Digitalis and suxamethonium may possibly interact and result in a higher frequency of dysrhythmias (250[r]). However, considering the frequency with which digitalized patients receive suxamethonium and the paucity of reports on clinical problems arising, this would seem to be of minor importance. β-Blockers may prolong and possibly exaggerate the rise in serum potassium resulting from the injection of suxamethonium (see 'Mineral and fluid balance' section above).

Local anesthetics Procaine and cocaine are esters hydrolyzed by plasma cholinesterase and may therefore competitively enhance the action of suxamethonium (251). Chloroprocaine may have a similar action. Licocaine also interacts, although the mechanism is not clear unless very high doses are used (252[C]).

Non-depolarizing muscle relaxants and suxamethonium are mutually antagonistic. These agents are often given in small non-paralyzing doses prior to suxamethonium to reduce fasciculations and other adverse effects. Gallium is slightly more effective than *d*-tubocurarine and both these are more effective than pancuronium (see 'Neuromuscular' section above). This 'precurarization' tends to prolong the onset (probably by direct antagonism) and to shorten (*d*-tubocurarine) or lengthen (pancuronium) the duration of action of suxamethonium (253[C]). The latter effect may well be due to inhibition of plasma cholinesterase by pancuronium.

When non-depolarizing agents are given after suxamethonium, even more than 30 minutes later, their action is considerably potentiated and prolonged (SEDA-8, 136; 254[C], 255[C]). This effect (and also the production of a phase II block when suxamethonium is used alone in high or frequently repeated doses) may be the result of an inhibition of transmitter release through a prejunctional action of suxamethonium (6[R]).

Suxamethonium given some time after a paralyzing dose of a non-depolarizing agent (e.g. for peritoneal closure) produces varying effects depending on the depth of residual 'curarization' (256[C]). As it is uncertain what type of block results, this practice cannot be recommended, although few difficulties have been reported in subsequent reversal.

Neostigmine inhibits both plasma cholinesterase and acetylcholinesterase, so that if any suxamethonium is still circulating, its action will be prolonged (by a factor of 2 approximately). This may present problems when neostigmine is administered to antagonize a phase II block (257[C]) (where hypothetical desensitization-block and open channel-block elements may also be intensified) or shortly after suxamethonium is given (as in the example at the end of the previous paragraph). In renal failure both *neostigmine* and *pyridostigmine* administration has resulted in prolongation (by 1—2 hours) of the action of suxamethonium given several hours after renal transplant operations (see 'Urinary system' above).

Other anesthetic agents When mixed, thiopental will hydrolyze suxamethonium due to a pH effect. Ketamine may prolong the action of suxamethonium slightly (258[C], 259[r]); a phase II block might be prolonged more significantly (259[r]), although there is no clinical experience reported. Decreased presynaptic acetylcholine synthesis or release has been postulated as the mechanism (260). Another study (277[C]) found no significant shift in the dose—response curve for suxamethonium with ketamine. *Inhalational agents* potentiate relaxants. Since this is of more clinical importance with regard to non-depolarizing agents, it is discussed later. Tachyphylaxis and phase II block develop earlier and after smaller total doses of suxamethonium when volatile agents such as halothane, enflurane or isoflurane (261[C], 262[C]) are used instead of balanced anesthesia. *Halothane* may increase the incidence of dysrhythmias, especially bradycardia and nodal rhythm, after suxamethonium. *Atropine* and *glycopyrrolate*, particularly when given intravenously just before, afford some protection against suxamethonium dysrhythmias (SEDA-5, 136; 263[C]).

OTHER DEPOLARIZING NEUROMUSCULAR BLOCKING AGENTS

Decamethonium (C 10)

Decamethonium, a depolarizing neuromuscular blocker, is little used nowadays. A dose of 3 mg provides adequate relaxation for intra-abdominal surgery for about 15 minutes, supplements being required at 10–30-minute intervals. It is not so rapid in onset of action as suxamethonium. Fasciculations occur, with similar consequences to those described for suxamethonium. It is not hydrolyzed. Tachyphylaxis occurs and a phase II block develops readily. Decamethonium is *dependent on renal excretion* for the termination of its effects and is therefore contraindicated in renal insufficiency. Its action is also prolonged by hypothermia. Cardiovascular effects are less frequent than with suxamethonium; reduction in heart rate is sometimes seen after a second dose. In high doses, muscarinic actions may be seen and histamine release may occur. The development of myotonia has been precipitated with this relaxant in patients with myotonia congenita and dystrophia myotonica. Hexafluorenium and decamethonium are antagonistic. Potentiation of decamethonium block has been reported with ketamine, and may occur with neostigmine.

Dioxonium
Hexacarbacholine bromide (Imbretil)

These two drugs have been little used and appear to be largely obsolete. Accounts of their adverse reactions will be found in earlier volumes in this series (SED-10, 213; SEDA-6, 131).

NON-DEPOLARIZING NEUROMUSCULAR BLOCKING AGENTS

Non-depolarizing neuromuscular blocking agents compete with acetylcholine for receptors at the neuromuscular junction and clinical relaxation begins when 80–85% of the receptors on the motor end-plate are blocked. They do *not* produce depolarization themselves and, by blocking access to the receptors, prevent the normal acetylcholine-induced depolarization. Flaccid paralysis ensues. Their action terminates when acetylcholine again gains access to the receptors, due to diffusion of the relaxant molecules away from the neuromuscular junction. This may be hastened by greatly increasing the number of acetylcholine molecules at the motor end-plate by giving an anticholinesterase such as neostigmine.

Because all the clinically used relaxants in this group have the same basic mechanism of action, most of their side effects and interactions with other drugs are likely to be very similar, so that what is reported for one may be applicable, to a greater or lesser degree, to others in the group. However, these agents do differ from each other structurally and there are accordingly subtle differences in their modes of action, they have differing affinities for different cholinoceptors at and outwith the neuromuscular junction, their routes of elimination or inactivation also vary and so forth, so that some caution is required when extrapolating findings on one to others in the group.

d-Tubocurarine is the classic non-depolarizing relaxant and will be described in detail. Since pancuronium has been exhaustively investigated too, in some respects even more so, it is accordingly also discussed at length. Major differences from the *d*-tubocurarine and pancuronium patterns of side effects together with effects that have only been described for a specific drug, will be reported in the individual sections on the other non-depolarizing agents. Where a side effect is reported for two or more relaxants, it will—with appropriate referrals—be found in the section pertaining to the relaxant for which it has most clinical relevance. Firstly, some interactions involving non-depolarizing agents in general are described.

INTERACTIONS WITH GENERAL ANESTHETIC AGENTS

The volatile inhalational anesthetic agents and cyclopropane potentiate neuromuscular blocking drugs. The extent depends on the particular relaxant and inhalational agent used and the concentration of the latter. In comparative studies, isoflurane was found to be the most potent in this respect, enflurane was almost as potent and both these were 2–3 times more potent than halothane, which was in turn twice as potent as the standard nitrous oxide (balanced) anesthesia (the volatile agents being administered at concentrations of 1.25 MAC (mean alveolar concentration) and the relaxant studied being *d*-tubocurarine) (264[r]). Concerning the older agents, the relaxant dose can be reduced by half under ether anesthesia and by one-fifth or more when cyclopropane is used. The degrees of potentiation by ether and cyclopropane probably lie between those of enflurane and halothane.

The higher the anesthetic concentration, the greater the degree of potentiation and the smaller the dose of relaxant needed. For example, increasing the alveolar halothane concentration from 0.4 to 1.2% reduces both *d*-tubocurarine and pancuronium requirements by about 60%; an increase in isoflurane concentration from 0.5 to 1.5% reduces the ED_{50} for *d*-tubocurarine by about 40% and that of pancuronium by 70% (265[C]). The full potentiating effect will only be seen when the tissues are saturated by the inhalational agent. Reducing the concentration of the inhalational agent generally reduces the degree of neuromuscular blockade (266[C]), a desirable feature at the end of an operation. However, this maneuver may take some time (perhaps about half-an-hour for enflurane) to be effective and will only diminish the 'volatile' contribution to the total block. Nevertheless, there may be occasions, such as for patients with myasthenia or renal or hepatic disease, where the advantages of using higher inhalational anesthetic concentrations and lower (zero?) doses of relaxants may outweigh the disadvantages (SEDA-7, 141; 267).

The potentiation of *d*-tubocurarine block produced by *enflurane* slowly continues to increase with time, even after the usual equilibration period has passed (SEDA-5, 132; 268[C]). This does not occur with halothane and the discrepancy is said to mean that more *d*-tubocurarine will be required in the first hour of an enflurane anesthesia than during a halothane (equipotent) anesthesia, but that thereafter less will be required under enflurane anesthesia. It is suggested that enflurane, unlike halothane, may produce an effect on muscle which takes time to develop. This may also be part of the mechanism—in addition to the greater potentiating action of enflurane—behind the report (269[C]) of the slower spontaneous recovery from pancuronium and the greatly impaired antagonistic effect of neostigmine in patients anesthetized with enflurane 1.3—1.4% as compared to halothane 0.55—0.65% (end-tidal, in 70% nitrous oxide). The experimental conditions in this last study, however, were somewhat different from usual clinical practice (SEDA-7, 143).

It is unfortunately not possible to come to a categorical conclusion on precisely how great the potentiation of a given relaxant will be by a particular inhalational anesthetic because the effects of inhalational agents here are multifactorial and diverse and the numerous studies done have used different methodologies (265[C], 267[r], 270[r], 271[C]—273[C]). Very approximately, isoflurane and enflurane potentiate the longer-acting relaxants such as *d*-tubocurarine and pancuronium by 50—70% and the shorter-acting agents vecuronium, atracurium and mivacurium by 20—25%. The degree of potentiation reported for the shorter-acting relaxants, however, varies greatly (from 0 to 70% for vecuronium) depending on the duration of exposure of the skeletal muscles to the inhalational agent, the mode of nerve stimulation, whether the relaxant is given as a single bolus or by cumulative bolus doses or by an infusion (steady-state or not), the nature of the circulatory changes produced, etc. The potentiation produced by halothane is much less than for isoflurane and enflurane.

Muscle relaxants may also contribute to anesthesia. Pancuronium 0.1 mg/kg has been reported to *lower the MAC* for halothane by 25% (274[C]). It was conjectured that this could be due to a central effect or peripheral, through reduction of afferent input from muscle spindles to the reticular activating system. Recently, however, a similar though not identical study (SEDA-15, 124; 275[C]) failed to confirm that pancuronium, vecuronium or atracurium lowers the MAC for halothane.

Intravenous anesthetic agents have much less influence on the neuromuscular blocking effects of relaxants and most have no clinically significant effect. However, *ketamine* (SEDA-14, 113) has been reported to significantly potentiate atracurium (276[C]), and also *d*-tubocurarine but not pancuronium (277[C]) in man. Animal studies suggest that all relaxants will be potentiated by ketamine in a dose-dependent manner (259[r], 260). It has been suggested that had Johnston et al. (277[C]) used a higher dose of ketamine (than 75 mg/m^2), then they would have seen potentiation of pancuronium. The main effect of ketamine appears to be a reduction in the sensitivity of the postjunctional membrane to acetylcholine, possibly by ion-channel blockade. *Diisopropylphenol* ('Propofol') has been reported as potentiating vecuronium- and atracurium-induced blocks (SEDA-9, 120; 278[C]). Animal studies suggest that large doses of *pethidine* and *droperidol* may also augment the myoneural effects of neuromuscular blocking agents (SEDA-9, 115; 279). Lastly, laboratory investigations have shown that some *benzodiazepines* may produce biphasic effects (280, 281), higher doses potentiating neuromuscular blocking agents (280, 282); but several human investigations have failed to find a significant effect (283[C]—285[C]); it has been suggested that the agents present in the commercial preparations of some benzodiazepines to render them more water-soluble may mask the benzodiazepine effect (285[C]).

Some time ago Ngai (286[R]) reviewed the topic of general anesthetics and muscle relaxation.

INTERACTIONS BETWEEN NEUROMUSCULAR BLOCKING AGENTS

Interactions between suxamethonium and non-depolarizing agents are discussed in the section on suxamethonium. *Precurarization*, the injection of a small 'non-paralyzing' dose of a non-depolarizer to reduce the fasciculations, etc., from the subsequent injection of suxamethonium, confers many advantages, but the patient must be carefully observed since an unexpected degree of paralysis occasionally ensues (SEDA-6, 130).

This may result from idiosyncrasy, latent myopathy or from one of the other causes of hypersensitivity described later in this chapter (see in particular the 'Neuromuscular' section under '*d*-Tubocurarine').

Interactions between different non-depolarizing neuromuscular blocking agents may result in additive or synergistic effects. When pancuronium is given *together with d*-tubocurarine or metocurine, the resulting block is greater than would be expected if the effects were purely additive. This potentiation is not seen with the metocurine + *d*-tubocurarine combination (287[C]). Synergism resulting from such combinations is suggested as being a postsynaptic effect (288). Advantages of this technique are discussed in the original paper and in SEDA-5 (p. 133). When different non-depolarizing agents are given *consecutively*, the neuromuscular blocking action of the second may be considerably modified by the first; the action of vecuronium, for example, lasts longer than expected if pancuronium has been given initially (SEDA-11, 124; 289[C]). Caution should therefore be exercised when giving a small dose of a normally short-acting non-depolarizer near the end of an operation when another, long-acting, agent has been given earlier. The resulting block may be greater than expected and last much longer than desired. Reversal with anticholinesterases may be difficult at the end of surgery if the block is still greater than 90%.

USE IN THE INTENSIVE CARE UNIT

In the intensive care situation muscle relaxants are sometimes used to keep patients paralyzed for several days, or even weeks. Muscle weakness, causing difficulties in the subsequent weaning of such patients from artificial ventilation has been frequently described (290[C]—295[C]). This problem has been ascribed to a multitude of factors, such as the muscle relaxants themselves and the concomitant use of antibiotics steroids and other drugs, which have effects on neuromuscular functions, dysfunction of liver or kidney leading to impairment of metabolism or elimination of these drugs and their metabolites, respectively, nutritional deficiencies and the effects of sepsis, catabolism and toxins. It has been suggested that prolonged exposure to muscle relaxants and/or prolonged immobilization may result in changes at the neuromuscular junction similar to those seen after denervation (296) or associated with disuse (297). In the last few years evidence has been accumulating for the existence of the specific '*critical illness polyneuropathy*' (SEDA 16, 1[CR]; 2[CR]) which results in weaning difficulties even in patients who have not been given muscle relaxants. The combination of sepsis and multiple organ failure appears to underlie the polyneuropathy which has been diagnosed in more than 50% of such patients who have been septic for more then 2 weeks. Electrophysiological and autopsy findings are consistent with primary axonal degeneration of motor and sensory nerves.

Recently numerous case reports of prolonged weakness in intensive care patients who have received muscle relaxants have been published (SEDA-16, 139—141). Most of these reports have pertained to vecuronium, probably because this relaxant is most commonly used for long-term ventilation in the belief that its relatively short duration of action will result in easy reversal of paralysis when weaning is due. Unfortunately in these reports very large doses have been given for long periods to patients who have dysfunctions of kidney and/or liver, the organs of which elimination and metabolism are dependent. In addition, all to frequently there is little information concerning assessment of neuromuscular function.

Up to now prospective studies on this area are rare (SEDA-16, 8[C]) and further investigations are required urgently. In view of the multitude of causal factors mentioned above it seems advisable to always monitor neuromuscular function and to avoid complete paralysis for any length of time in intensive care patients who are treated with muscle relaxants.

d-Tubocurarine chloride (DT[C])

d-Tubocurarine is the standard non-depolarizing neuromuscular blocking agent against which all the others of the group are compared. The molecule has one quaternary and one tertiary nitrogen, the latter being protonated at body pH in most molecules which therefore function as bisquaternary entities. In addition to its main ('competitive') action at the neuromuscular junction of blocking the access of acetylcholine to the receptor recognition sites, it may also possibly block some ion channels, but only to a small extent and when very high concentrations are present.

About 40—50% of a normal dose of *d*-tubocurarine is bound to plasma proteins, mostly γ-globulins (about 25%). This binding is highly variable, and hence also the amount of non-bound drug available for neuromuscular blockade. Metabolism does not occur. The drug is eliminated principally via glomerular filtration in the urine (about 40—60% in 24 hours), but has an alternative pathway for excretion in the bile (normally only about 12% in 24 hours). The initial dose for healthy patients is 0.2—0.5 mg/kg, dependent on the anesthetic agents used and whether suxamethonium is given beforehand or not. Maintenance doses are about one-third of the initial dose and are required at approximately 30–40-minute intervals.

ADVERSE REACTION PATTERN

Toxic and general reactions A fall in blood pressure occurs almost always with *d*-tubocurarine. This is often mild, but may be marked, particularly if a large dose is given rapidly or if the patient is hypovolemic, or has a diminished cardiac reserve or capacity for vasoconstriction (as is not infrequently the case in old age, in diabetes and in other diseases with sympathetic neuropathy), and is potentiated by other anesthetic agents such as halothane. Myasthenic patients or patients with other neuromuscular pathology are markedly sensitive to non-depolarizing relaxants.

Hypersensitivity reactions Histamine-mediated reactions are common, leading to local weal-and-flare effects near the injection site, frequent hypotension—mostly around a 20% fall—and, occasionally, bronchospasm. Malignant hyperthermia has also been reported after *d*-tubocurarine.

Tumor-inducing effects These have not been reported.

ORGANS AND SYSTEMS

Neuromuscular The blockade of neuromuscular transmission is non-depolarizing in nature and is easily reversed (if twitch height has recovered to at least 10%) by anticholinesterases. *Sensitivity* to *d*-tubocurarine and other non-depolarizing relaxants is *highly variable* even in apparently normal patients, so that the small doses given for precurarization may lead to appreciable paralysis (298, 299[C], 300[C]). More commonly, residual blockade may be detected postoperatively (301[C], 302[C]), long after the expected recovery of neuromuscular transmission.

Racial differences and environmental factors may influence the response to relaxants. Patients in the United States reportedly require less *d*-tubocurarine than in the United Kingdom, and West Indians need more. Difference in cholinesterase activities, perhaps brought about by more organophosphorus insecticides being used in one country than in another, or differences in protein-binding as a result of dietary factors, are possible explanations (303[R]). Recently, vecuronium has been reported to be approximately 30% more potent in Montreal than in Paris (304[C]).

Cumulation may occur and is the more likely if large doses are given too frequently or if excretion is impaired (see 'Urinary system' and 'Liver'). Smaller doses should be given if the patient has received *d*-tubocurarine within the previous 24 hours.

Resistance to the neuromuscular blocking action of *d*-tubocurarine (and other non-depolarizing relaxants) is seen in patients with *burns* (331[C]) (see 'Skin and appendages' section). Also, patients with *upper motor neuron lesions* such as hemiplegia (305[Cr], 306[C]–308[C]) and possibly *multiple sclerosis* (SEDA-13, 105; 309[Cr]) may exhibit a clinically significant resistance to various non-depolarizing blockers. *Lower motor neuron* injury has only been reported to produce this phenomenon in rats (310[r]) or dogs so far. Affected muscles in these conditions are paralyzed to a lesser degree than unaffected muscles and this has to be taken into account when siting the electrodes for monitoring a block and in assessing recovery therefrom. The mechanism is probably a quantitative and/or qualitative change in the acetylcholine receptors. Lastly, resistance is seen too in patients given certain *drugs* such as phenytoin, carbamazepine and, disputedly, azathioprine (see 'Interactions' section).

Greatly *increased sensitivity* occurs in myasthenia (130[R]) and may even be seen in 'premyasthenic' patients with no overt symptoms (311[C]). Increased sensitivity has also been reported in *amyotrophic lateral sclerosis* (312[C]), *von Recklinghausen's disease* (132[C]) and *ocular muscular dystrophy* (313[C]). Patients with *Duchenne muscular dystrophy* have been found to have a prolonged block from the regional curare test (314[C]), but other investigators have disputed whether an altered response to non-depolarizing relaxants occurs in this condition.

The response of patients with neuromuscular disorders to relaxants has been reviewed (139[R]–141[R]).

Cardiovascular *d*-Tubocurarine results commonly in a *fall in blood pressure*, associated with a *slight tachycardia* and a *decrease in total peripheral resistance*; the cardiac output is not affected. The frequency of hypotension is reported as being between 20 and 90%. The wide range probably reflects the methods of measurement, anesthetic agents used and the general condition of the patients in the various studies, as well as the criteria for 'hypotension'. The magnitude of the decrease in blood pressure is generally about 20%, being reached within 5 minutes of the injection. Histamine release is considered to be the principal cause of the hypotension (SEDA-7, 141; 315[C]). It has been suggested recently that prostacyclin, released via histamine acting on H_1-receptors, is the final mediator in the causation of the hypotension; intravenous administration of aspirin or an H_1-antagonist beforehand afforded some protection (SEDA-15, 126; 316[C]). Ganglion blockade may also contribute, particularly if high doses are used (4[R]). Reduction in venous return consequent to muscle relaxation and alterations in intrathoracic and intra-abdominal pressures may also play a role. The fall in blood pressure may be greatly exaggerated in hypovolemic patients, in the elderly and in others with reduced sympathotonicity. *d*-Tubocurarine should be used very cautiously in such patients or, better, another relaxant chosen. Concurrent administration of agents known to produce circulatory depression aggravates the situation. The higher the halothane concentration, for example, the greater the fall in blood pressure after *d*-tubocurarine (317[C]). Since the degree of hypotension seems linked to the dose (315[C]) and rate of injection (318[C]), it seems reasonable to use the smallest dose that produces adequate relaxation (<0.5 mg/kg) and inject it slowly (over at least 180 seconds) (SEDA-7, 141).

Respiratory Apnea is produced. The muscles involved in protecting and maintaining the airway are more sensitive to *d*-tubocurarine than the muscles of ventilation (319[C], 320) so that *aspiration and airway obstruction* are possible in the partially curarized patient at a time when spontaneous ventilation is adequate. Airway obstruction in the presence of vigorous respiratory efforts can eventually (and is rarely reported to) lead to negative pressure *pulmonary edema* (321[Cr], 322[R]). *Hypoventilation* may occur after doses as small as 1.5 mg in exceptionally sensitive patients. Postoperative hypoventilation, or apnea, is a danger in patients given certain antibiotics and antidysrhythmic drugs before or after apparently successful spontaneous reversal or antagonism of a non-depolarizing block (see the 'Interactions' section).

Potentiation of undetected residual curarization may also occur postoperatively from respiratory acidosis.

Histamine release, common with *d*-tubocurarine, may produce *bronchospasm*. *d*-Tubocurarine is relatively contraindicated in asthmatic patients and in those with an allergic diathesis.

Nervous system Minute amounts of *d*-tubocurarine have been detected in cerebrospinal fluid (323[C]). Whilst convulsions have been produced in animals by injection into cerebrospinal fluid and it has been suggested that exceptionally large doses may cause depression of medullary centers, there is insufficient information to draw any conclusions.

Pancuronium is reported to lower the MAC for halothane, but whether this is a central or peripheral action is not known (see page 306).

Autonomic ganglia are partially blocked by *d*-tubocurarine (competition with acetylcholine) and *vasodilatation* is produced. With normal doses, however, these effects are of minor importance.

Both resistance to and increased sensitivity to the action of *d*-tubocurarine and other non-depolarizing relaxants have been reported in various *neurological diseases* (139[R], 140[R]) (see 'Neuromuscular' section above).

Endocrine, metabolic *d*-Tubocurarine (324[C]) has been implicated as a triggering agent, particularly in combination with halothane, for the *malignant hyperthermia* syndrome (see the corresponding 'Suxamethonium' section) although doubts have been expressed (151[R]). Increased muscular tonus is not a feature with *d*-tubocurarine.

Patients with *thyrotoxic myopathy*—as with all forms of myopathy—are exceedingly sensitive to all non-depolarizing agents.

Liver In *liver disease*, increased amounts of *d*-tubocurarine may be required. In the past it has been suggested that this could be due to reduced synthesis of acetylcholinesterase, or to increased levels of γ-globulins binding the relaxant (325[C]), although this is disputed (326[R]). Similar kinetic mechanisms to those suggested for pancuronium (see p. 316) may be involved but there are no studies for *d*-tubocurarine. In primary *liver cancer*, in children, resistance to *d*-tubocurarine (and alcuronium) has been reported (SEDA-13, 104; 327[C]).

Gastrointestinal The motility of the gut may be reduced as a result of ganglion blockade.

Urinary system In *renal insufficiency* the action of *d*-tubocurarine is prolonged. The elimination half-life in the complete absence of renal function is increased by 70% or more. *Hyperkalemia* will tend to diminish the neuromuscular blocking effects. The reduced ability of plasma proteins to bind the drug (328[C]), if this indeed occurs, will result in a greater proportion of 'free' *d*-tubocurarine and, therefore, increased potency.

Increased biliary excretion of *d*-tubocurarine occurs in renal insufficiency and compensates to a varying degree for the reduced renal excretion (329[C]). The slower rate of biliary (as opposed to renal) excretion will result in sharply increasing prolongation of neuromuscular blockade if large single doses are used or if multiple doses are given (330[C]). A single small dose will result in little or no prolongation of effect since redistribution will be mainly responsible for termination of the drug's effect. It has been suggested for several other non-depolarizing relaxants that the initial dose produces less effect in renal insufficiency (SEDA- 13, 103).

Should there be concomitant liver disease, reduction in the capacity of the alternative biliary route for excretion of *d*-tubocurarine will further prolong the action of the drug.

Skin and appendages Patients with *burns* require

more *d*-tubocurarine (and higher plasma levels) for the same depth of block in comparison to non-burned patients (331[C]). The mechanism is not known; it appears not to be altered pharmacokinetics (332[C]). The resistance to non-depolarizing neuromuscular blocking agents (SEDA-8, 136) appears to be influenced by the size of the body surface area burned and by the time which has elapsed since the injury (see 'Atracurium' section). In extensive burns dose requirements are increased approximately by a factor of 2–3.

Special senses *d*-Tubocurarine may, unlike other non-depolarizing relaxants, produce *marked* reduction in intraocular pressure. However, this tends to be associated with undesirable circulatory changes (333[C]). 'Precurarization' is an unreliable technique (207[C]) for preventing suxamethonium-induced increases in intraocular pressure (see further in the 'Suxamethonium' section).

Risk situations In the *elderly*, in *hypovolemic patients*, in patients with *impaired sympathetic autonomic activity*, and in patients operated on in the *anti-Trendelenburg position*, extreme falls in blood pressure may occur with *d*-tubocurarine. Hypotension is aggravated by the use of halothane, in particular, and other drugs which produce circulatory depression. In such cases and in patients with *hypertension*, *coronary artery disease* and *arteriosclerosis*, *d*-tubocurarine is better avoided.

Asthmatic and *atopic* individuals are at special risk from *d*-tubocurarine's histamine-releasing potential, and severe bronchospasm may result.

Myasthenic patients (and possibly also those with *amyotrophic lateral sclerosis* or *von Recklinghausen's disease*) are highly sensitive to non-depolarizing agents and extremely prolonged paralysis will result from normal doses of *d*-tubocurarine.

In *renal failure* the action of *d*-tubocurarine is greatly prolonged if large or repeated doses are used Nevertheless, the elimination of *d*-tubocurarine is less dependent on renal function than gallamine, metocurine or even pancuronium. Concomitant hepatic dysfunction may further delay elimination.

The problem of cumulation, already referred to, may be marked in *intensive care* situations where *d*-tubocurarine is used to maintain long-term paralysis (330[C]). These patients may also have impaired renal and hepatic function, with protein and electrolyte imbalance. The timing of repeat injections of *d*-tubocurarine (and, indeed, all relaxant drugs) in such cases should be guided by monitoring of neuromuscular function (by response to single twitch, train-of-four or, more sensitive but painful, tetanic stimulation) or clinically by observing the return of muscle tone.

Certain drugs may potentiate and prolong the action of *d*-tubocurarine and other relaxants (see further in the 'Interactions' section below).

Second-generation effects *Placental transfer* of *d*-tubocurarine occurs (as with all relaxants) and low levels of the drug have been detected in umbilical blood. Under normal circumstances no untoward effects have been reported in the newborn.

Paralysis of a 28-week fetus whose mother received *d*-tubocurarine for status epilepticus, and joint deformities possibly resulting from 4 weeks' maternal curarization during the first trimester, have been reported (334[C]).

Experiments in animals have shown that *d*-tubocurarine can result in retardation of bone growth in chick embryos (335) and that malformations can be produced by in utero curarization (336). Long-term curarization during pregnancy would seem to be undesirable.

Interactions *Antibiotics* See 'General considerations' at the beginning of this chapter. Interactions with *general anesthetic agents* and with *other neuromuscular blocking agents* are described at the beginning of the 'Non-depolarizing neuromuscular blocking agents' section.

Interactions with various drugs have been reported over many years for the different non-depolarizing neuro-muscular blocking agents. Case-reports often involve only one relaxant. Occasionally studies are done with several agents, but it is rare to have definite evidence of an interaction involving all the members of this relaxant group. The results of animal studies are sometimes difficult to relate to the usual human clinical setting. Nevertheless, it is assumed, perhaps unjustifiably in some instances, that most interactions will be common to all non-depolarizing neuromuscular blocking agents. At any rate, documented evidence of an interaction for one relaxant suggests caution for the others. Most of the drug groups or individual drugs believed to interact with non-depolarizing relaxants are alluded to here, although others are to be found in the interactions sections for other relaxants where they appear to be specifically involved.

Magnesium sulfate is capable of producing neuromuscular transmission failure and enhances the effect of *d*-tubocurarine and other non-depolarizing neuromuscular blocking drugs as well as depolarizing agents (337[C], 338). Not only have potentiation and prolongation of *d*-tubocurarine block been reported, but also respiratory depression when magnesium sulfate was given an hour after reversal of the relaxant. Presumably the muscle weakness resulted from potentiation of residual curarization. Possible mechanisms are discussed in the corresponding 'Interactions' section under 'Suxamethonium'. Whether the effects are additive or synergistic is disputed. Muscle relaxants must be used with caution and in reduced dosage in patients receiving magnesium sulfate. Reversal of the block may be difficult.

Penicillamine See 'Alcuronium' section (p. 320).

Local anesthetic drugs These have diverse effects on the neuromuscular junction. In very large doses they produce paralysis on their own. When the recommended doses are used for local anesthesia, systemic absorption is small and interaction with relaxants is not to be expected. Large doses injected intravascularly (accidentally, or therapeutically for dysrhythmias), however, may potentiate relaxants of both types (251[C], 339[C]) (see also the following section).

Antidysrhythmic drugs Procainamide, lidocaine, propranolol and *diphenylhydantoin* (340[C]), *quinidine* (248), *procaine* and *lidocaine* (341[C]) have all been claimed to enhance the neuromuscular block of *d*-tubocurarine and other non-depolarizing agents. *Bretylium* (342) and *disopyramide* (343) are also reported to have their neuromuscular blocking activities potentiated by low concentrations of *d*-tubocurarine in animal experiments; neostigmine failed to reverse a disopyramide-induced block (SEDA-13, 102: 344). The greatest hazard from these agents is that they may result in 'recurarization' when given postoperatively. With bretylium this may, as a result of its slow kinetics, occur several hours after its administration (SEDA-7, 141; 342). Effects in man have still to be documented for bretylium, but 'recurarization' 15 minutes after adequate reversal of a vecuronium blockade with neostigmine has been described in a patient given disopyramide intravenously (SEDA-14, 116; 345[cr]). *Calcium channel blockers*, such as verapamil and nifedipine, may also potentiate neuromuscular blocking agents (SEDA-9, 116; 249, 346[C]) and it has been suggested that in long-term use they may accumulate in muscle and make block-reversal difficult (347) (see also under 'Vecuronium').

Ganglion-blocking agents Trimetaphan and hexamethonium may potentiate *d*-tubocurarine-induced block, but clinical reports clearly demonstrating this are lacking. *d*-Tubocurarine will increase their hypotensive effect. Neostigmine could theoretically facilitate the postulated end-plate ion channel block of trimetaphan (SEDA-13, 102; 242), which would complicate reversal of neuromuscular block.

Diuretics Furosemide (80—40 mg) has been reported (348[C]) to enhance and prolong *d*-tubocurarine-induced block in anephric patients. In animals (349) low doses have potentiated *d*-tubocurarine (and suxamethonium) probably via presynaptic effects, while high doses (1—40 mg/kg in cats) reversed the neuromuscular actions of these relaxants; the effects of high doses were similar to those of theophylline, and phosphodiesterase inhibition leading to increased acetylcholine release was postulated as one possible mechanism for the antagonism (see also below under 'Pancuronium').

Potassium and magnesium loss as a result of the use of diuretics may affect non-depolarizing relaxants.

Aprotinin (*Trasylol*) Re-paralysis has been reported when this agent was used after suxamethonium and after *d*-tubocurarine reversal (see further in the 'Suxamethonium' section).

Doxapram This drug, used as a respiratory stimulant, has been reported to increase partial *d*-tubocurarine and pancuronium neuromuscular blockade when used in high concentrations in rat experiments (SEDA-14, 113; 350). There are no reports in man so far.

Azathioprine An immunosuppressive agent, this reduces sensitivity to *d*-tubocurarine, gallamine and pancuronium in the cat, possibly as a result of phosphodiesterase inhibition increasing transmitter release (SEDA-4, 87; 234) (in rats, see SEDA-13, 104). In humans with renal failure, azathioprine (3 mg/kg) produced a negligible and transient reduction in the neuromuscular blockade maintained by infusions of atracurium, vecuronium or pancuronium (351[C]).

Aminophylline See Pancuronium, 'Interactions' (p. 318).

Steroids There are several contradictory reports; in general, it seems that the *chronic use* of steroids may reduce sensitivity to non-depolarizing neuromuscular blocking agents while their *acute administration* may lead to potentiation (352[R]). Long-term steroid treatment may be associated with the development of a *myasthenic syndrome* in some patients who will, accordingly, be very sensitive to neuromuscular blocking agents.

OTHER NON-DEPOLARIZING NEUROMUSCULAR BLOCKING AGENTS

Pancuronium bromide

Pancuronium, a non-depolarizing competitive neuromuscular blocking drug, has two quaternary ammonium groups on a steroid (androstane) skeleton. It is about 5—7 times as potent as *d*-tubocurarine. Protein binding occurs to both albumins and globulins, probably only to a relatively slight degree (10—20%), although the extent is disputed, reports varying from 10—90%. In contrast to most other non-depolarizing relaxants, pancuronium is metabolized in the human body (approximately 10—20%). Deacetylation in the liver probably accounts for the greater part of this biotransformation. The major metabolites are mono-(3-OH)-pancuronium, mono-(17-OH)-pancuronium and the (3,17)-dihydroxy derivative; they are active pharmacologically, the dominant (3-OH) metabolite being half as potent and the other two having 2% of the potency of pancuronium. About 40—50% of a dose is normally excreted in the urine and 5—10% in the bile over 24 hours (pancuronium plus metabolites).

Pancuronium is reported to inhibit plasma cholinesterase (353[C]) and this may be part of the explanation why the action of suxamethonium, given after a small dose of pancuronium, is prolonged (see also in the 'Interactions' section under 'Suxamethonium'). It also weakly inhibits acetylcholinesterase. For tracheal intubation the usual dose is 0.1 mg/kg. When given after suxamethonium, 0.05 mg/kg is sufficient for good abdominal relaxation. Further doses of about one-quarter to one-third the size of the initial dose are given at 30—40-minute intervals to maintain relaxation. Reversal is easily achieved with neostigmine, provided there is some spontaneous return of neuromuscular transmission beforehand. If the evoked twitch height is less than 10% of the control value, difficulty may well be experienced in reversing the block; this applies to all non-depolarizing relaxants except, perhaps, vecuronium and atracurium.

The onset time for complete neuromuscular blockade is similar to that for *d*-tubocurarine and other non-depolarizing agents, namely 2—4 minutes. However, this is to some extent dose-dependent, and, because of the relative lack of cardiovascular effects and histamine release, pancuronium can be given safely in higher dosage, thus producing good intubation conditions within 2 minutes. The dose of *d*-tubocurarine required to achieve similar conditions in 2 minutes would result in hypotension. As with *d*-tubocurarine, repeated doses can lead to cumulation and a prolonged block.

Neuromuscular system As with all muscle relaxants, abnormal reactions may be seen in patients with neuromuscular diseases (see '*d*-Tubocurarine' section). In addition, muscle fibrillation has been reported, possibly due to pancuronium, in a patient with metachromatic leukodystrophy (SEDA-3, 113; 354[C]).

Cardiovascular Cardiovascular side effects are minimal with pancuronium. Ganglion blockade does not occur. A slight dose-dependent *rise in heart rate*, *blood pressure and cardiac output* are common (355[C]) but are often masked by the actions of other concomitantly used agents, such as fentanyl or halothane, which produce bradycardia or hypotension. These side effects of pancuronium are thus often beneficial and can be deliberately utilized. Several mechanisms contribute to their inception: vagal blockade via selective blockade of cardiac muscarinic receptors (356), release of noradrenaline from adrenergic nerve endings (357), increase in blood catecholamine levels (358), inhibition of neuronal catecholamine re-uptake (359—361), and direct effects on myocardial contractility (362). These are discussed further by Bowman (1[R], 6[R]) and Marshall (4[R]).

Occasionally *nodal rhythm*, *atrioventricular dissociation and tachydysrhythmias* (such as premature ventricular beats or even bigeminy) develop, but these usually occur in association with halothane. The use of both *halothane* and pancuronium in patients receiving *tricyclic antidepressants* (imipramine), which can also inhibit noradrenaline re-uptake by adrenergic nerve endings, has been reported as resulting in severe tachyarrhythmias. Experiments in dogs have shown this combination to be capable of producing ventricular fibrillation and cardiac arrest (SEDA-4, 88; 363[C]). Enflurane also resulted in tachycardias in dogs given both imipramine and pancuronium acutely, but not when the imipramine was given chronically over 15 days beforehand. Pancuronium should not be used in patients on tricyclic medication.

Supraventricular tachycardia has also been reported after 8 mg pancuronium in a patient receiving *aminophylline* (800 mg/day) (SEDA-7, 143; 364[C]). This drug also has adrenergic effects and halothane anesthesia will increase the risks of tachydysrhythmias when pancuronium is used (365[C]). Severe hypertension together with tachycardia may occur when pancuronium is given to patients with *pheochromocytomas* (SEDA-7, 143; 366[C], 367[C]). It is to be concluded that pancuronium is relatively contraindicated, particularly in combination with halothane, in patients who may have raised catecholamine levels, or who are receiving drugs with sympathomimetic effects. Caution should also be exercised in patients with thyrotoxicosis and with valvular stenoses, coronary artery insufficiency (368[C]) or other conditions where tachycardia is hazardous.

Potentially less dangerous, nodal rhythm may occur after injection of pancuronium. This dysrhythmia and bradycardia appear to be more common when *neostigmine* (and atropine) is given for reversal of a pancuronium-induced neuromuscular blockade than for reversal of a *d*-tubocurarine or alcuronium block (SEDA-7, 143; 369[C]); cholinesterase inhibition by pancuronium may contribute to the bradycardia in these circumstances.

Respiratory See '*d*-Tubocurarine' section (p. 314).

Nervous system Pancuronium has been reported to lower the MAC for halothane by 25% (274[C]), although this has been disputed (SEDA-15, 124; 275[C]) (see 'Interactions with general anesthetic agents', p. 310).

Accidental injection into the cerebrospinal fluid of 4 mg resulted in generalized hypotonia, weakness and hypoventilation (SEDA-15, 126; 370[C]). Neostigmine given intravenously led to prompt recovery.

Metabolic A case of *malignant hyperthermia*, possibly triggered by pancuronium, has been described (SEDA-5, 133; 371[C]), although the relaxant is generally considered to be 'safe' in patients susceptible to the syndrome (151[R]).

Liver In hepatic disease, the use of pancuronium seems to be more problematic than *d*-tubocurarine. Significant prolongation of distribution and elimination half-lives and reduction in plasma clearance have been reported in *cirrhotic* patients, together with a marked increase in apparent volume of distribution (372[C]). This is likely to result in larger initial doses being necessary for adequate relaxation, and prolongation of recovery of neuromuscular function. *Cholestasis* may also prolong the action of pancuronium. Plasma clearance has been reported to be reduced to 50%. This may possibly be a result of elevated bile-salt levels reducing the hepatic uptake (which is an important factor contributing to the total plasma clearance in normal patients) or pancuronium (SEDA-6, 130).

In patients undergoing liver transplantation the dose requirements for pancuronium and vecuronium by intravenous infusion were reduced by 57 and 50%, respectively, during the anhepatic phase (SEDA-17, 28[C]), whereas atracurium requirements were not altered by exclusion of the liver from the circulation. Significant *hyperbilirubinemia* has been reported to occur more frequently in critically ill *neonates* given pancuronium than in a control group (373[C]). The hyperbilirubinemia was increased in the 4 days following cessation of pancuronium treatment whereas during the administration period the hyperbilirubinemia was less in the pancuronium group.

Urinary system Pancuronium appears to be more dependent on renal function for elimination than *d*-tubocurarine. Its action is, in most cases, significantly prolonged in *renal failure* (374[C]) in particular, spontaneous recovery is slow and adequate reversal of the block with neostigmine takes much longer than generally expected (SEDA-7, 144; 375[C]). The response to pancuronium is much more unpredictable in renal failure, with great interindividual variation in duration of blockade. Occasionally resistance to neuromuscular blockade with pancuronium is encountered (SEDA-13, 103; 351[C], 374[C]). This may be because of an increase in the volume of distribution. Pancuronium infusion requirements are greatly reduced in renal failure (SEDA-13, 103; 351[C]) and cumulation with repeated doses will occur. High plasma and tissue levels of the 3-OH metabolite, sufficient to produce significant neuromuscular blockade, have also been measured in anuria (295[C]). Monitoring of neuromuscular function is required in patients with appreciable renal dysfunction.

Skin and appendages In *burned patients* resistance to the neuromuscular blocking action of pancuronium may be encountered (376[C]), as with other non-depolarizing relaxants (see also in '*d*-Tubocurarine' and 'Atracurium' sections).

Hypersensitivity reactions *Histamine release and bronchospasm* are relatively rare with pancuronium but have been reported (SEDA-12, 117; 377[c]–379[c], 380[C])

Second-generation effects Placental transfer occurs, but no untoward effects have been reported in the newborn so far. In an investigation designed to compare the onset and duration of paralysis produced by 0.2 mg/kg pancuronium (n=8) or pipecuronium (n=8) injected into the thighs of fetuses between 30 and 38 weeks gestational age, *tachycardia* occurred in four out of eight fetuses injected with pancuronium. Loss of beat-to-beat variability occurred in two out of the eight fetuses given pancuronium. No such changes were observed in any of the eight fetuses injected with pipecuronium (SEDA-18, 24[C], 25[C]).

Drug interactions Interactions with *tricyclic antidepressants*, *halothane*, *aminophylline*, and *neostigmine* are described in the 'Cardiovascular' section above. Interactions with *suxamethonium* are described in the 'Suxamethonium' section (p. 308) and with *other non-depolarizing relaxants* (p. 312). Further interactions with general anesthetic agents are discussed on page 310 and with *antibiotics* on page 299. Pancuronium-induced neuromuscular blockade may also be affected as a result of interaction with *local anesthetic and antidysrhythmic drugs*, *calcium channel blockers*, *magnesium salts*, *ganglion-blocking agents*, *doxapram*, *azathioprine*, *steroids* and *furosemide*—as listed in the 'Interactions' section under '*d*-Tubocurarine'.

Furosemide Furosemide (1 mg/kg) shortened the recovery time from pancuronium blockade in neurosurgical patients with normal renal function (381[C]). Phosphodiesterase inhibition and increased pancuronium excretion were suggested as possible explanations (cf. *d*-tubocurarine—furosemide interactions, p. 316).

Ciclosporin This immunosuppressive agent has been reported to have been associated with considerable prolongation of neuromuscular paralysis induced by pancuronium (382[C]) in one patient (and also in another given vecuronium). Reversal required both neostigmine and edrophonium. Subsequently, recurarization occurred (SEDA-14, 116). Contributing factors could have been the solvent, cremophor-EL, in the ciclosporin preparation (Sandimmun) and minor renal dysfunction. Potentiation of vecuronium and atracurium in cats has also been described (SEDA-12, 188; 383).

Lithium carbonate Prolonged neuromuscular blockade has been reported in patients on long-term lithium therapy given pancuronium (384[C]). In animal experiments, lithium was found to prolong neuromuscular block due to pancuronium, suxamethonium and decamethonium, but not that due to *d*-tubocurarine and gallamine (236); on the other hand, lithium was reported to have no, or minimal, effects on the blocks produced by pancuronium or *d*-tubocurarine, respectively (SEDA-7, 140; 385). Possible mechanisms of interaction are discussed in the original papers. Caution, and monitoring, would seem advisable.

Aminophylline Aminophylline appears to facilitate neuromuscular transmission, perhaps by increasing neurotransmitter release through raising cyclic AMP levels at the neuromuscular junction via phosphodiesterase inhibition (365[C]). This would account for the antagonism of pancuronium-induced blockade which has been reported to occur in the presence of very high serum levels of theophylline (SEDA-4, 88; 386[C]). A similar effect should theoretically occur with other non-depolarizing relaxants.

Nitroglycerin Experiments in cats have demonstrated a significant prolongation and potentiation of the neuromuscular blockade induced by pancuronium in the presence of a nitroglycerin infusion (1 mg/kg per minute) started before the muscle relaxant was given. No prolongation was seen if suxamethonium, *d*-tubocurarine or gallamine was used in place of pancuronium. Neostigmine reversal of the pancuronium block was not affected nor was the plasma clearance of pancuronium over the 2 hours following the injection (SEDA-4, 88; 387, 388). The cause of this phenomenon and whether it is applicable to man, remains to be elucidated. However, more recent experiments (also in cats), using only moderate doses of pancuronium (and vecuronium), have failed to elicit any potentiation by nitroglycerin (389).

Corticosteroids These have been reported to antagonize neuromuscular blockade due to pancuronium (SEDA-3, 113; 390[C], 391[C]). In vitro studies (rat) have shown a direct facilitating action of prednisolone on neuromuscular transmission (392), so that one would expect some antagonism of non-depolarizing relaxants in general. See also 'Interactions' section under '*d*-Tubocurarine'.

Anticonvulsants The chronic use of diphenylhydantoin (dilantin) has been associated with increased pancuronium requirements during neurosurgical operations (393[C]), although the opposite effect might be expected from its quinine-like membrane-stabilizing activity. Resistance to pancuronium, with a considerable shortening of recovery time, has also been seen in patients on chronic treatment with another anticonvulsant, carbamazepine (SEDA-12, 118; 394[Cr]); an inverse correlation was found between the daily dose and the recovery time. Resistance to metocurine and vecuronium has also been reported in patients on chronic treatment with phenytoin, and resistance to vecuronium has been described in patients taking carbamazepine too.

Interference with diagnostic radiography Complete relaxation in artificially ventilated neonates has resulted in apparent 'gasless abdomens' on radiography and confusion in diagnosis. On discontinuation of paralysis, the normal appearance of gas-filled bowel was restored (395[C]).

Metocurine (dimethyltubocurarine)

This non-depolarizing neuromuscular blocker is a synthetic derivative of *d*-tubocurarine. No metabolites have been detected and the drug depends almost entirely on renal function for its excretion; 40—50% of the drug is excreted in the urine and about 2% (possibly more) in the bile in 24 hours (396[C]). Its potency is approximately twice that of *d*-tubocurarine and a quarter that of pancuronium measured during narcotic—nitrous oxide anesthesia. In onset and duration of action and in speed of recovery it is similar to *d*-tubocurarine and pancuronium (397[C]). The dose for intubation is 0.3 mg/kg; adequate abdominal relaxation is achieved with 0.1—0.2 mg/kg in most patients. As with all neuromuscular blocking agents, there is great individual variation in response so that, if it is desired to give minimal doses, monitoring of the neuromuscular response is advisable. Volatile anesthetics and prior suxamethonium may be expected to reduce dosage requirements, but clinical reports are lacking.

In comparison with *d*-tubocurarine, metocurine has a significantly weaker ganglion-blocking activity (398) and much less tendency to provoke histamine release (399, 400[C]). It does not block cardiac muscarinic receptors (401) at neuromuscular blocking doses. Cardiovascular stability is therefore to be expected with metocurine (402[C]). *Slight tachycardia and fall in blood pressure* have been reported in a third of patients given larger doses (0.4 mg/kg) rapidly, probably as a result of histamine release; but no bronchospasm was seen (397[C]).

Greatly *prolonged duration of paralysis* and a decreased rate of return of neuromuscular function may occur in renal failure, where plasma clearance is significantly reduced and the elimination half-life significantly prolonged (SEDA-7, 142; 403[C]). Metocurine is not the relaxant of choice where renal function is poor.

Patients with *burns* require 2—3 times higher doses of metocurine (SEDA-8, 137; 404[C]) and this phenomenon may persist (in lessening degree) for a year or more (405[C]).

Resistance to metocurine is also described in patients receiving chronic anticonvulsant therapy with *phenytoin* (SEDA-10, 110; 406[C]).

As there are extremely few recent publications on metocurine, it can only be assumed meantime that its side effects and interactions will be similar to those of *d*-tubocurarine and pancuronium, modified by the factors discussed above.

Gallamine triethiodide

For intubation, about 2 mg/kg (some authors say 3—4 mg/kg) are necessary and the duration of effect is then similar to usual (intubating) doses of *d*-tubocurarine or pancuronium. A dose of 1—1.5 mg/kg is usually sufficient for the production of apnea and adequate abdominal relaxation. Such doses are said to be short-acting (20 minutes) but, in the authors' experience, provide clinical relaxation (75% or more depression of twitch height) for some 30—40 minutes. Individual variation is considerable, and complete spontaneous reversal of the block is relatively slow.

Gallamine does not undergo biotransformation and is entirely dependent on glomerular filtration for excretion. In *renal failure* the neuromuscular block is considerably prolonged and the drug is contraindicated.

Histamine release may be associated with its use more often than was previously believed, according to several studies involving large numbers of patients (10[R], 12[CR], 15[CR], 16[C]). Numerous case-reports from the past of reactions involving skin flushing, bronchospasm or cardiovascular collapse possibly due to gallamine are listed in two articles (407[Cr], 408[Cr]), the latter of which describes two anaphylactoid reactions to small pre-curarizing doses of the relaxant.

Tachycardia is an invariable accompaniment to the use of gallamine. It is seen after doses as small as 20 mg and reaches a maximum at around 100 mg in adults (409[C]). It is frequently extreme, rates above 120 per minute being not uncommon. The increase in heart rate outlasts the neuromuscular blocking effect (409[C]). Normal clinical doses also result in a slight increase in mean arterial pressure, a slight decrease in systemic vascular resistance and a marked rise in cardiac index (410[C], 411[C]). These cardiovascular effects are principally accounted for by the strong vagolytic action of gallamine, the cardiac muscarinic receptors (412) being almost as sensitive to its blocking action as the acetylcholine receptors of the neuromuscular junction. Blockade of noradrenaline reuptake and an increased release of noradrenaline from cardiac adrenergic nerve endings (413, 414) may contribute, although an inotropic effect in man is disputed (415[C]). Ganglion-blocking activity is slight and is not seen in the clinical dose range. Marshall (4[R]) and Bowman (6[R], 1[R]) have reviewed the possible mechanisms. Gallamine should therefore not be used when tachycardia has to be avoided.

Placental transfer has been variously reported, usually only small amounts being detected in the umbilical blood, with no clinically obvious effects on the newborn.

Side effects in other disease states and interactions with other drugs are likely to be similar to those reported for *d*-tubocurarine and pancuronium.

Alcuronium (diallyl nortoxiferine)

Alcuronium is a synthetic derivative of toxiferin, an alkaloid of calabash curare, and is a non-depolarizing relaxant with properties and side effects similar to those of *d*-tubocurarine. It is about twice as potent as *d*-tubocurarine, 0.15—0.25 mg/kg usually being adequate for abdominal relaxation, and has a similar onset time and a slightly shorter duration of action.

It is bound to albumin (40%) and requirements for alcuronium are less if the plasma albumin levels are low, as may occur in hepatic disease.

Like *d*-tubocurarine, alcuronium does not undergo biotransformation. Excretion occurs mainly in the urine (80—85%), but, as occurs with *d*-tubocurarine, some is also excreted in the bile (15—20%) (416[C]). Persistent relaxation has been reported in *renal failure* (417[C]) and the drug is relatively contraindicated in this condition.

Histamine release and anaphylactoid reactions occur with alcuronium (418[C]—420[C]). The precise incidence is not clear. Erythema is said to occur much less frequently than after *d*-tubocurarine (421[C]). A retrospective study in Australia (12[CR]) found that 37% of serious anaphylactoid reactions reported there were associated with alcuronium; alcuronium, however, accounted then for almost 50% of the total muscle relaxant consumption in Australia, and if this is taken into account the likelihood of a serious reaction is less than with *d*-tubocurarine, as others have also concluded (16[C]). Clinical features reported range from erythema to severe hypotension and tachycardia (422[C]) and bronchospasm (423[C], 424[C]). A large prospective surveillance study (SEDA-15, 125; 425[C]) involving over 1400 patients given alcuronium (initial dose 0.25+0.09 mg/kg) has reported adverse reactions in almost 18% of the patients, with moderate hypotension (20—50% decrease) in 13%, severe hypotension in 0.8%, and bronchospasm in 0.1%.

Tachycardia, hypotension and a fall in total peripheral resistance occur to an extent similar to that seen with *d*-tubocurarine according to most studies (421[C], 426[C]—428[C]). Others report that these effects are short-lived (429[C]). Doses of 0.2 mg/kg or more may be associated with the more extreme cardiovascular effects. Block of cardiac muscarinic receptors (398), histamine release and, possibly, some ganglionic blockade (although it has a very low ganglion-blocking activity in animals) (398) may all play a role in the production of alcuronium's cardiovascular effects.

In *liver cancer* in children, resistance to alcuronium has been reported (SEDA-13, 104; 327[C]).

In patients with *burns*, dosage requirements are increased (SEDA-8, 137; 430[C]).

Placental transfer (SEDA-6, 130; 431[C]) occurs and is increased if alcuronium is rapidly injected (432[C]). No complications attributable to neuromuscular block were seen in the newborn.

Penicillamine-induced myasthenia gravis (SED-10, 415) was probably the cause of extremely prolonged apnea occurring in two patients given alcuronium (SEDA-12, 111; 433[Cr], 434[Cr]). Patients receiving penicillamine should be treated as myasthenics and, if a muscle relaxant is required, should be given a test dose (of about one-tenth the usual dose), with monitoring of the response, before a full dose is administered.

Other side effects and interactions, though not specifically reported, are probably to be expected as indicated in the '*d*-Tubocurarine' and 'Pancuronium' sections. In two intensive care patients treated with infusion of large amounts of alcuronium *fixed dilated pupils* have been observed. Within 6—24 hours after stopping the infusion of alcuronium the pupils became normally reactive again (SEDA-18, 18[C]). This is a very important and dangerous side effect since the presence of fixed dilated pupils may lead to the mistaken diagnosis of brain death in coma patients if other neurological diagnostic procedures are not carried out.

Fazadinium

Originally claimed, from animal experiments, to be of rapid onset, short duration and free from important side effects, this non-depolarizing relaxant has been found to be less satisfactory in man. Usual doses are 0.5—0.75 mg/kg, although 1 mg/kg is sometimes advocated for fast intubation (within 1—2 min). The duration of action is similar in man to *d*-tubocurarine and pancuronium. Excretion is primarily in the urine (50—80%, mostly in the first 6 hours), although a biliary route is also suggested. Metabolism occurs, probably to a minor extent (1—3% inactive metabolites being detected in the urine).

Histamine release is very uncommon, but hypotension associated with an urticarial rash and two cases of severe bronchospasm and cardiac arrest (in patients who had also received thiopental) have been reported (SEDA-5, 132; 435[C]) as probably being due to fazadinium. Immunological investigations combined with positive intradermal tests have been used to confirm the relaxant as the causative agent in a severe reaction (436[C]).

Cardiovascular effects account for the relative unpopularity of this relaxant. It has some ganglion-blocking activity (398) and blocks cardiac muscarinic receptors in the clinical dose range (437). Its 'vagolytic' potency is about the same as gallamine. Fazadinium, like pancuronium, also blocks the re-uptake of noradrenaline into sympathetic nerve endings. These actions explain its major cardiological side effect, namely *significant tachycardia* (438[C]) which occurs even with small doses and is persistent. It is dose-related (439[C]), the increase in heart rate varying between 30 and 100%, and is associated with a rise in cardiac output and with falls in stroke volume and peripheral resistance. Hypertension or hypotension may occur (440[C], 441[C]). If fazadinium is used injudiciously, extreme and dangerous cardiovascular changes can ensue (SEDA-9, 121; 442[C]).

Placental transfer occurs and, though there may be some fetal uptake, Apgar scores did not appear to be affected (443[C], 444[C]).

As there are extremely few recent publications on fazadinium, it can only be assumed meantime that its side effects and interactions will be similar to those of *d*-tubocurarine and pancuronium, modified by the factors discussed above.

Vecuronium bromide

Much has been published in the last few years over this non-depolarizing relaxant and the early publications are summarized in SEDA-6 (p. 131). Vecuronium is a monoquaternary analog of pancuronium, with a similar speed of onset, a duration of action of 15—30 minutes, rapid spontaneous recovery, and virtually no cumulative effects. Being monoquaternary, it is more lipophilic than pancuronium. About 30% is bound to plasma proteins. It is de-acetylated in the liver, the principal metabolite being the 3-desacetyl derivative, which is believed to have about 50% of the neuromuscular blocking potency of the parent drug in man; small amounts of the 17-desacetyl and the 3,17-didesacetyl derivatives are also formed. In 'balanced' anesthesia it is slightly more potent than pancuronium, but during halothane anesthesia it has been reported to be 1.4 times as potent as the latter drug. Suitable doses during balanced anesthesia are similar to those for pancuronium; *potentiation by volatile agents* (445[C]) permits the reduction of these doses, after equilibration has occurred between the volatile agent and the tissues, by 25 or 45% when halothane or enflurane, respectively, are used, according to older studies (446[C], 447[C]). A more recent investigation (SEDA-13, 105; 448[C]) reports that after 1 hour of constant 90% neuromuscular blockade under nitrous oxide (60%) + isoflurane (1.2% end-tidal) or + enflurane (1.2% end-tidal) anesthesia the vecuronium infusion requirements were reduced by as much as 70% (compared to the nitrous oxide + fentanyl group).

In *animal studies* (449[R], 450, 451[C], 452, 453) histamine release, cholinesterase inhibition and autonomic effects have been found to be minimal and occur only at concentrations of vecuronium considerably greater than those required for neuromuscular block; interactions with antimicrobial agents, analgesics and anesthetic agents were similar to those known for other non-depolarizing relaxants, apart from a possible potentiating effect by metronidazole (451[C]).

These animal findings have been confirmed in man by the relative freedom from side effects reported. In man, the intradermal injection of vecuronium produces a considerably smaller local histamine reaction than does *d*-tubocurarine, metocurine, pancuronium or atracurium (454[C], 455[C]) and plasma histamine is not raised in the clinical dose range (456[C], 457[C]). Nevertheless, minor skin reactions have been reported (458[C], 459[C]), as well as hypotension (460[C]) and severe anaphylactoid reactions with circulatory collapse (461[C], 462[C]) and bronchospasm (463[C], 464[C]). Cross-sensitivity with pancuronium may occur (SEDA-10, 111).

Cardiovascular The expected cardiovascular stability has been confirmed (445[C], 465[C]–467[C]) in man. Even doses as great as 0.28 mg/kg in patients undergoing coronary artery bypass grafting produced negligible effects (468[C]). *Bradycardia* is the only cardiovascular side effect reported, and this is seen in association with opioids such as fentanyl (SEDA-9, 119; 469[C]) and sufentanil (SEDA-11, 125; 470[C]) or other drugs which are themselves capable of producing bradycardia. The lack of vagolytic and sympathomimetic activity on the part of vecuronium means that it does not counteract the bradycardia (or hypotensive) effects of other drugs or surgical manipulations. It is an ideal relaxant for patients with pheochromocytoma (471[C]).

Liver In *liver disease* (cirrhosis and cholestasis) the plasma clearance of vecuronium is reduced, its elimination half-life is increased and its duration of action is prolonged (SEDA-10, 112; 472[C], 473[C]). Rapid uptake in the liver appears to be an important factor in its plasma clearance and in determining its relatively short duration of action; it is estimated that about 40% of the injected drug is excreted via the bile (474[C]). Prolongation of the action of large single doses and cumulation after repeated doses may therefore be expected in liver disease.

Urinary system *Renal dysfunction* has been reported as having no significant effect on the duration of action of vecuronium (SEDA-11, 125; 475[C]–477[C]). Nevertheless, slight resistance to the neuromuscular blocking effect of an initial dose (ED_{50} increased by 20%) and a small reduction (of 23%) in infusion requirements to maintain a 90% block after 1 hour of relaxation have been described in end-stage renal failure (SEDA-13, 103; 351[C]). These findings are in line with those for other non-depolarizing agents, with the exception of atracurium; the changes, however, are minor compared to those for the older relaxants, as is to be expected from vecuronium's kinetics. There is a slight tendency for its action to be prolonged in renal failure, so that monitoring of neuromuscular transmission is advisable if several doses are to be given. About 25–30% of an injected dose is excreted in the urine in normal patients, mostly as unchanged drug.

Risk situations It has been reported (SEDA-17, 29[C]) that spontaneous recovery of neuromuscular function after a bolus dose of vecuronium (0.1 mg/kg) was significantly prolonged in elderly patients in comparison to younger adults. The elimination half-life was significantly prolonged (125 (S.D. 55) versus 78 (21) minutes) and the plasma clearance reduced (2.5 (0.6) versus 5.6 (3.2) ml/kg per minute) in the elderly versus the younger patients.

Second-generation effects Placental transfer occurs (feto-maternal concentration ratio is about 10% less than for pancuronium) and no effects have been detected in the newborn (478[C]). Post-partum, vecuronium has been reported to have an appreciably longer duration of action (SEDA-13, 105; 479[C], 480[C]) when given on a 0.1 mg/kg total body weight basis.

Interactions The interactions of vecuronium are probably similar to those already described for *d*-tubocurarine and pancuronium (see pp. 315 and 318), according to animal studies (451[R]). Interactions which have already been reported specifically for vecuronium are potentiation by the *calcium-channel blockers*, verapamil (SEDA-9, 116; 481[C], 482) and nifedipine (SEDA-11, 126; 483[C]), *dantrolene* (SEDA-11, 126;

484[C]), diisopropylphenol ('Propofol') (SEDA-9, 120; 278[C]), and ketamine and other intravenous anesthetic agents (see p. 311). The effects of *volatile* anesthetic agents are described above.

Ciclosporin has been reported to significantly potentiate vecuronium, prolonging its action considerably and causing difficulties with reversal (SEDA-14, 116; 485[C]) (see also p. 300 above).

Disopyramide has also been associated with impairment of neostigmine-antagonism of a vecuronium-induced neuromuscular block (see p. 312).

Acute administration of *phenytoin* (10 mg/kg i.v.) has been reported to enhance slightly, but statistically significantly, a steady block maintained by an infusion of vecuronium (SEDA-15, 124; 486[C]). This is in contrast to recent reports of resistance to non-depolarizing neuromuscular blocking agents, including vecuronium (SEDA-13, 104; 487[C], 488[C]), associated with the chronic administration of phenytoin and another anticonvulsant drug, *carbamazepine*.

Testosterone enanthate, given over a prolonged (10-year) period to produce virilization, has been claimed to have been responsible for a case of marked resistance to vecuronium (SEDA-14, 116; 489[C]).

Azathioprine has also been reported to reduce the neuromuscular blocking action of vecuronium, but to a clinically insignificant degree (see '*d*-Tubocurarine section').

Antibiotic interactions are described under 'General considerations' (page 298).

The clinical pharmacology of vecuronium and atracurium has been reviewed by Miller et al. (490[R]).

Atracurium dibesilate

Early studies on this new relaxant are reviewed in SEDA-7 (p. 146). In contrast to other non-depolarizing drugs, atracurium is completely broken down at normal blood pH and temperature via Hofmann elimination, principally and, to disputed degrees, by nucleophilic substitution and enzymatic ester hydrolysis (491, 492, 493[R]). Four *metabolites* are known, laudanosine being the main biotransformation product. Atracurium-induced neuromuscular block is easily reversed by neostigmine. It has approximately one-fifth the potency of pancuronium (initial doses of 0.3—0.6 mg/kg and maintenance doses of 0.2 mg/kg being commonly used), an onset of action of 1.2—4 minutes (depending on the dose and the investigator), a medium duration of effect similar to (or slightly longer than) vecuronium, a rapid spontaneous recovery (slightly longer than vecuronium), and a virtual lack of cumulation.

In animal experiments, vagal blockade and changes attributed to histamine release occurred only with large concentrations, many times those providing complete neuromuscular blockade; at high dosage some hypotension was seen, possibly from histamine release; alkalosis diminished the neuromuscular block, and acidosis prolonged it (494). In cats, high doses of some of the breakdown products of atracurium produced dose-dependent neuromuscular blockade, hypotension and autonomic effects (495). However, it was considered that these effects were of no pharmacological significance for man in view of the low potencies of these substances and the quantities likely to be found in man. From interaction studies in cats (496) it was concluded that the action of atracurium is enhanced by *d*-tubocurarine, halothane, gentamicin, neomycin and polymyxin, and antagonized by adrenaline and, transiently, by suxamethonium. Pretreatment with suxamethonium did not affect the subsequent block by atracurium in cats. Ciclosporin has also been reported to potentiate atracurium in cats (SEDA-12, 118; 383).

In man, *histamine* release is common but the clinical significance is disputed. Minor skin reactions lasting 5—30 minutes occur in 10—50% of patients according to various studies (497[C]—500[C]) and are not usually associated with obvious systemic effects. Mirakhur et al. (501[C]) report a 42% incidence in a series comprising 200 patients of cutaneous flushing which was dose-dependent, being 18% at 0.4 mg/kg, 33% at 0.5 and 0.6 mg/kg, and increasing further to 73% at a dose of 1 mg/kg. One patient in their study, in the 1 mg/kg group, developed generalized erythema, hypotension, tachycardia and bronchospasm. Systemic effects (SEDA-10, 109) are, fortunately, much rarer than cutaneous manifestations of histamine release. There are, nevertheless, various reports of hypotension (SEDA-15, 125; 500[C], 5O2[C], 503[C]), angioneurotic edema (500[C]), and bronchospasm (504[C], 502[C]). Extreme sensitivity to an intradermal skin test (0.003 mg), some 24 hours after a severe skin reaction to the intravenous administration of atracurium, has also been described (505[C]). In general, it appears that systemic effects from histamine release are also dose-dependent. Basta et al. (506[C]) have demonstrated that cardiovascular stability is maintained with atracurium up to doses of 0.4 mg/kg. At higher dose levels (0.5 and 0.6 mg/kg), however, these investigators found that arterial pressure decreased by 13 and 20%, and heart rate increased by 5 and 8%, respectively. These effects were maximal at 1—1.5 minutes. Since these cardiovascular effects were associated with facial flushing, it was suggested that they might have resulted from histamine release. In a subsequent study these investigators (507[C]) linked significant cardiovascular changes with increased plasma histamine levels at a dose of 0.6 mg/kg atracurium. Injecting this dose slowly over 75 seconds has been found to reduce the plasma histamine release and the adverse hemodynamic effects (508[C]). A large prospective surveillance study (SEDA-15, 125; 425[C]) involving more than 1800 patients given atracurium found a 10% incidence of adverse reactions, with moderate hypotension (20–50% decrease) in 3.5% and bronchospasm in 0.2% of patients.

Cardiovascular Cardiovascular effects, apart from those resulting from histamine release as discussed above, appear to be almost entirely limited to *bradycardia*. From animal studies, vagolytic (494) and ganglion-blocking (509) effects are very unlikely to occur at neuromuscular blocking doses, and these predictions appear to be borne out by investigations in man in which cardiovascular effects are only reported at high dosage associated with signs suggestive of histamine release (506[C], 507[C], 510[C]). The bradycardia seen (511[C]–513[C]) is occasionally severe but, as with vecuronium, the explanation seems to be that the bradycardic effects of other agents used during anesthesia are not attenuated by atracurium as they are by pancuronium, gallamine or alcuronium which have vagolytic (or sympathomimetic) effects. The possibility that bradycardia may be caused by one of the metabolites, such as laudanosine (SEDA-12, 115) which has a structural similarity to apomorphine, has yet to be excluded. A recent animal study suggests that noradrenaline release from sympathetic nerve terminals may be increased by very large doses of atracurium, probably due to high concentrations of laudanosine (SEDA-14, 117; 514). In the clinical situation cardiovascular effects from this source would only be expected in circumstances leading to much higher than usual laudanosine concentrations. It has been suggested (515[C]) that atracurium is unsuitable for use in patients with a *pheochromocytoma*, increases in catecholamine levels associated with hypertension and other unwanted cardiovascular effects occurring after the (rapid?) injection of relatively large doses (0.6–0.7 mg/kg). However, in an earlier case-report catecholamine levels did not increase and there were no untoward cardiovascular effects following atracurium (516[C]). Nonetheless, considering atracurium's potential for histamine release (which can secondarily lead to increases in circulating catecholamines), vecuronium or pipecuronium would seem to be more logical choices for relaxation in this condition.

An unusual effect, *hypoxemia*, has been reported (SEDA-15, 125; 517[C]) and most probably resulted from an increase in right-to-left cardiac shunting (in a patient with a ventricular septal defect and pulmonary atresia). Atracurium (0.2 mg/kg) may have produced a fall in systemic vascular resistance, perhaps from histamine release; pancuronium was subsequently given without incident.

Metabolism *(see also SEDA-10, 108)* The breakdown of atracurium is *pH- and temperature-dependent*. The effects of pH changes in animal studies are described above. *Hypothermia* (25, 26[C]), during cardiopulmonary by-pass, has been reported as reducing atracurium requirements by half (518[C]); pH changes may also have occurred. It has been recommended that doses also be reduced in small neonates less than 3 days old, particularly if their core temperatures are less than 36°C (519[C]). In elderly patients atracurium infusion requirements appear not to be reduced and its effects are not prolonged (520[C]), probably because the action of atracurium is independent of routes of elimination that are affected by age.

The major metabolite is *laudanosine*. Laudanosine can cross the blood–brain barrier (CSF/plasma ratios of 0.3–0.6 are found in dogs (521)) and produce strychnine-like CNS stimulation which at high plasma levels (around 17 ng/ml) leads to convulsions in dogs (521–523). CSF/plasma ratios of laudanosine in man have been reported to be between 0.01 and 0.14 after a 0.5-mg/kg dose of atracurium in a study in which the highest laudanosine level was 14 ng/ml (524[C]). Much higher CSF laudanosine levels (mean 202 ng/ml, highest level 570 ng/ml) were measured after larger atracurium doses (0.5 mg/kg/hour) during intracranial surgery (SEDA-15, 126; 525[C]). Patients in whom the blood–brain barrier is not intact, such as during neurosurgical procedures, may be at risk from exposure of the brain to unpredictable concentrations of laudanosine (and other drugs). Two patients in the latter study (525[C]) had fits but these were not thought to be related to laudanosine (see also in the 'Interactions' section under 'Isoflurane' below). Under normal circumstances plasma levels in man will be far below those required for significant central nervous stimulation. However, the elimination half-life of laudanosine (521, 526[C]) is considerably longer than that of atracurium (527[C]), so that the possibility of laudanosine cumulation exists if many repeated doses or prolonged infusions of atracurium are given. Laudanosine metabolism may possibly be reduced in liver disease (528), and in renal failure (529[C]) higher plasma levels and an apparently delayed elimination of laudanosine have been reported. The prolonged infusion of atracurium in the intensive care situation (for 38–219 hours) led to slowly increasing plasma laudanosine levels which appeared to level out after 2–3 days (292[C]). The maximum plasma laudanosine concentrations in six patients ranged between 1.9 and 5 μg/ml. There was no evidence of cerebral excitation. Nevertheless, *caution* is urged in patients with *severe hepatic dysfunction* (530[C], 531[r]), *particularly if associated with renal failure*, when repeated bolus doses or an infusion of atracurium are given over a prolonged period. Laudanosine has been reported to increase the MAC for halothane in animals (532).

Of the other metabolites, the acrylate esters might possibly give rise to side effects. Acrylates are highly reactive pharmacologically and are potentially toxic, theoretically having the capacity to form immunogens and to alkylate cellular nucleophils (493[R]), but so far no effects have been reported (533, 534).

Urinary system and liver Renal and liver dysfunction appear to have little effect on the neuromuscular blocking action of atracurium (527[C], 535[C], 536[C]), although resistance has been reported in end-stage renal failure (37% greater ED_{50} values and shorter duration of bolus doses) (SEDA-13, 103; 351[C], 537[C]) The excretion and metabolism of laudanosine is impaired (see above).

Skin and appendages *Burns* are associated with resistance to atracurium (538[C]), as for several other non-depolarizing neuromuscular blocking agents. The EC_{50} is increased and dose requirements may be increased by up to 2—3 times. The resistance varies with the burn area and the time from injury (SEDA-12, 116), being maximal at 15—40 days in patients repeatedly anesthetized.

Miscellaneous Patients with *dystrophia myotonica* may be extremely sensitive to atracurium according to a case-report (SEDA-10, 110; 540[C]) Resistance to atracurium and higher than normal concentrations of acetylcholine receptors in muscle biopsies have been reported in a patient with *multiple sclerosis* (SEDA-13, 105; 309[Cr]).

Second-generation effects Placental transfer occurs (539[C]). A study in 46 patients undergoing cesarean section (SEDA-17, 18[C]) has shown that while the Apgar scores did not differ between neonates whose mothers had received atracurium (0.3 mg/kg) or tubocurarine (0.3 mg/kg), the neurological and adaptive capacity scoring (NACS) values at 15 minutes (but not at 2 and 24 hours) after birth were lower after atracurium. The NACS values were normal in 83% of the babies in the tubocurarine group and in 55% of those in the atracurium group. The difference was primarily due to lower scores for active contraction of the neck extensor and flexor muscles. These results cannot be satisfactorily explained by partial curarization in some neonates of the atracurium group because the placental transfer of atracurium was lower in the atracurium group; the umbilical vein concentrations of atracurium after clamping of the umbilical cord being approximately one-tenth of the EC_{50} for block of neuromuscular transmission in neonates.

Interactions From animal experiments (496), as described at the beginning of this section, it seems likely that drug interactions with atracurium will be similar to those for other non-depolarizing neuromuscular blocking agents. In man, potentiation and prolongation of its action by *halothane* (541[C]—543[C]) has been reported, as has potentiation after 30 minutes of isoflurane anesthesia (544[C]). Whether one should reduce the dose of atracurium (from that used during 'balanced anesthesia') by 20, 30 or 50% if one uses halothane, isoflurane or enflurane, respectively, for an individual patient is probably academic since many other variables, such as the tissue levels of the volatile anesthetic and the response of the individual patient to the neuromuscular blocking agent, will influence the outcome to an equal or even greater extent. If one wishes accurate control of the degree of neuromuscular blockade, then one has to use a monitor. A synergistic interaction between *isoflurane* and atracurium (high doses) has been incriminated in the causation of an increased incidence of grand mal seizures occurring after neurosurgical operations (SEDA-15, 125; 545[Cr]). So far this has not been confirmed. The possible role of a non-intact blood—brain barrier in neurosurgical patients has been alluded to in the section on laudanosine above. The intravenous anesthetic agent, *diisopropylphenol*, is also said to potentiate atracurium (278[C]) and *ketamine* has also been shown to prolong its action slightly (276[C]). Prior administration of *suxamethonium* potentiates the action of atracurium by approximately 30% (546[C]). Small doses of *pancuronium* (0.5 or 1 mg) or *d-tubocurarine* (0.05 or 0.1 mg/kg) administered 3 minutes before atracurium have been shown to synergistically potentiate its action (SEDA-12, 117; 547[C]). *Tamoxifen*, an anti-estrogen, has been associated with a prolonged atracurium block in a patient with breast cancer (SEDA-12, 117; 548[C]). *Azathioprine* (351[C]) has been reported to reduce a constant atracurium blockade transiently and to a clinically insignificant extent (see also 'Interactions' section under '*d*-Tubocurarine' on p. 315).

In contrast to reports on other non-depolarizing neuromuscular blocking agents, resistance to atracurium has not been found in patients on chronic anticonvulsant therapy with *phenytoin* or *carbamazepine* (SEDA-13, 104; 487[C], 488[C]). Another interaction which has been reported not to occur in man is potentiation by the aminoglycoside antibiotics, gentamicin and tobramycin (SEDA-15, 123; 549[Cr]). In animals, however, gentamicin was found to enhance atracurium blockade (496), so further investigation is required to clarify this point.

The clinical pharmacology of vecuronium and atracurium has been reviewed by Miller et al. (490[R]).

Pipecuronium bromide

Pipecuronium bromide is a bisquaternary steroid analog of pancuronium. It was first introduced into clinical use in Eastern Europe several years ago and the early studies are summarized in SEDA-5 (p. 133) and in *Clinics in Anesthesiology* (550[R]). In vitro (551) pipecuronium has been shown to reversibly inhibit both human red cell acetylcholinesterase and human plasma cholinesterase to an extent that might have clinical implications. Its potency is similar to (or slightly greater than) that of pancuronium and its onset and duration are also approximately the same. Cumulation (552[C]) may occur and maintenance doses should be one-quarter to one-sixth of the initial dose to achieve a similar effect, depending on the anesthetic technique used (see below).

No histamine release has been reported and vagolytic or sympathomimetic effects are not seen in the clinical dose range. Rarely, significant *hypotension* has been reported (552[C]), but this was transient and occurred during an unstable phase of anesthesia. *Bradycardia* has also been seen (552[C]) but is usually mild (553[C]), and probably due to the vagotonic effects of concurrently administered drugs as is seen with vecuronium and atracurium (i.e. a minor disadvantage of the relaxant's lack of vagolytic or sympathomimetic effects). Usually, no significant changes in heart rate or blood pressure are seen (554[C]—556[C]), even with doses up to 3 times the ED_{95} (557[C], 558[C]). Cardiovascular stability has also been reported in cardiac patients (559[C]), including ASA class II and III patients about to undergo coronary artery bypass grafting who received doses up to 0.15 mg/kg (560[C]) and those receiving high-dose fentanyl anesthesia (561[C]). The absence of tachycardia in these high-risk cardiac patients, in whom any increase in myocardial O_2 demand is unwanted, was considered an advantage of pipecuronium.

From animal investigations hepatic uptake appears to be a factor in its total plasma clearance, but renal excretion seems to be the main route of elimination. Ligation of renal pedicles in dogs (562) resulted in reduced elimination of the drug with a 4-fold increase in mean residence time and an increase (also 4-fold) of hepatobiliary elimination which, however, did not compensate for the loss of urinary excretion. In humans, approximately 40% of pipecuronium is excreted unchanged in the urine together with another 15% as the 3-OH metabolite in 24 hours (563[Cr]). The elimination half-life is around 135—160 minutes. As expected, *renal dysfunction* is associated with an increase in volume of distribution, a decrease in plasma clearance (1.6 vs. 2.4 ml/kg per minute) and an increase in elimination half-life (263 ± 168 vs. 137 ± 68 minutes) when compared to patients with normal renal function (564[C]). In the latter study there was no statistically significant prolongation of the mean clinical duration of action of pipecuronium, but there was a much greater variation in the renal failure group, with 25% recovery times (after 0.07 mg/kg) ranging from 30 to 267 minutes (controls 55—198 minutes). Also, these patients were undergoing renal transplantation and most of the 'new' kidneys would be expected to show some function and some glomerular excretion of pipecuronium. Prolongation of pipecuronium blockade should be expected in patients with renal failure.

Thiobutobarbital has been noted to prolong the duration of action of pipecuronium in dogs (565), but so far no interaction with (thio-)barbiturates has been reported in man. In patients who have been exposed to *volatile anesthetic agents* for 30 minutes or so there is an increase in potency of pipecuronium to an extent such that doses can be reduced by about a third with isoflurane (566[C]) or enflurane (558[C]) in comparison to those required for balanced anesthesia; halothane appears to be associated with relatively minor changes in potency (566[C]). When the same doses of pipecuronium are given, the duration of blockade (567[C]) is significantly longer during isoflurane anesthesia than during neurolept anesthesia; halothane is also associated with a prolonged action but to a lesser extent.

Doxacurium chloride

Doxacurium chloride is a long-acting non-depolarizing neuromuscular blocking agent. It is a bisquaternary benzylisoquinolinium derivative (a diester). It is subject to minimal hydrolysis by plasma cholinesterase (at about 6% of the rate of hydrolysis of suxamethonium when incubated with purified pooled human plasma cholinesterase) (568[C]). Antagonism with *edrophonium* (1 mg/kg) was considered inadequate in one (EMG) study, whereas no difficulties were experienced with neostigmine (0.05 mg/kg) (569[C]). This requires further investigation before conclusions can be drawn.

No elevation in plasma histamine was found with bolus doses up to 0.08 mg/kg (568[C]), but one case-report (570[C]) in which *transient hypotension* 1 minute after a bolus dose of 0.05 mg/kg via a pulmonary artery cannula, with cutaneous flushing at 2 minutes, suggests that histamine release can occur on occasion. In this case-report, there was no tachycardia and no sign of bronchospasm; the mean arterial pressure fell from 88 to 40 mmHg but, with therapy, recovered within 3 minutes, at which time the skin flushing was fading. In another investigation (571[C]) plasma histamine increased by 200% following doxacurium in 2 patients out of 54, but there were no changes in heart rate or blood pressure. Indeed, cardiovascular stability has been reported in several studies (568[C], 571[C]) and, even in cardiac patients (ASA groups III—IV), only minor clinically insignificant changes have been seen with doses up to 0.08 mg/kg (572[C], 573[C]). *Bradycardia* is occasionally seen, but it is too early to say if this is due to concomitantly given (vagotonic) drugs as is the case with atracurium, vecuronium and pipecuronium or not.

Renal excretion is believed to be the main route of elimination, so that the duration of action of this long-acting relaxant would be expected to be prolonged by renal dysfunction. So far there have been two publications on the use of doxacurium in *chronic renal failure* patients. In the first of these (574[C]) it was reported that the action of doxacurium (0.025 mg/kg bolus dose) was 'markedly but not statistically prolonged'; the mean time to 25% recovery of the twitch height was 121 minutes in the group of patients with renal failure as opposed to 67 minutes in the control group, with great inter-individual variation in both groups. The second paper (575[C]) studied the pharmacokinetics and pharmacodynamics of doxacurium in patients undergoing cadaveric kidney or liver transplantation. These investigators confirmed that the duration of action of doxacurium is more variable and may be greatly prolonged in patients with end-stage renal failure, although once again the results were clinically but not statistically (small numbers of patients and large standard deviations) significant. Plasma clearance was significantly slower and mean residence time significantly greater in the renal transplant group than in control patients. In the patients with *liver disease* there were no significant pharmacokinetic changes detected, but the duration of action of the small (15 μg/kg) dose used here did tend to be somewhat prolonged.

Mivacurium chloride

Mivacurium chloride is a benzylisoquinolinium diester compound with a duration of approximately twice that of suxamethonium. In vitro (576) it is *metabolized to a significant extent by plasma cholinesterase*, and minimally by acetylcholinesterase. The rate of metabolism in vitro is directly related to plasma cholinesterase activity. In pooled human plasma the rate of hydrolysis of mivacurium was 70% that of suxamethonium. It was also estimated, in the same paper, that the half-life for mivacurium ranges from 5 to 10 minutes versus 2 to 5 minutes for suxamethonium. In another study (577[C]) the in vitro hydrolysis of mivacurium, by purified human plasma cholinesterase, occurred at 88% of the rate for suxamethonium. These investigators found a poor correlation between the duration of action of bolus doses of mivacurium and the plasma cholinesterase activity in individual patients, a finding which has also been reported by others (578[C]). However, the average infusion rate to maintain around 95% blockade in individual patients correlated significantly with the patients' plasma cholinesterase activities (579[C]). While metabolites have been detected in both urine and bile, mivacurium seems to depend principally on ester hydrolysis for its plasma clearance so that reduced activity of plasma cholinesterase is likely to result in a prolonged duration of action.

Benzylisoquinolinium compounds have a tendency to evoke *histamine* release and this would seem to be the main source of the cardiovascular changes seen with mivacurium. These have been reported as minimal up to and including twice the ED_{95} dose in several studies (578[C], 580[C], 581[C], 582[C]). At higher dosage (0.2 mg/kg and more) *transient hypotension*, often associated with facial flushing and lasting only some 2—5 minutes, has been described (580[C]) which significantly correlated with increases in plasma histamine; reducing the speed of injection to 30 or 60 seconds reduced the degree of hypotension to insignificant levels. Similar findings in 50% of patients given doses of 0.2 and 0.25 mg/kg are described in another paper (578[C]). In yet another series, mean arterial pressure fell by more than 20% (24—61%) in seven of 15 patients given rapid bolus injections of 0.2—0.25 mg/kg (581[C]).

In patients scheduled for coronary artery bypass grafting or valve replacement (582[C]) significant *hypotension* was seen in two patients (out of 27 given higher doses) even when mivacurium was injected slowly (over 60 seconds); the mean arterial pressure fell by 24 and 50% after the injection of 0.2 and 0.25 mg/kg, respectively. β-Blockers, calcium-channel blockers and nitrates were not discontinued preoperatively in this study. The authors of this paper concluded that 'doses larger than 0.15 mg/kg are probably unnecessary and may contribute to hemodynamic instability at least in cardiac patients'—which seems a fair summing-up.

Inhalation anesthetics appear to have potentiating effect on the neuromuscular blocking action of mivacurium, as with the other non-depolarizing relaxants. With isoflurane (578[C]) and enflurane (583[C]) the ED_{95} is reduced by approximately 25% and the duration of action is somewhat prolonged, although the extent of this is not quite clear yet. Halothane has much less effect (584[C], 585[C]). It has been reported that the duration of mivacurium-induced neuromuscular block is prolonged in patients undergoing renal or liver transplantation (SEDA-17, 25[C]). These results are probably due to the reduced plasma cholinesterase activities in the investigated patients.

SKELETAL MUSCLE RELAXANTS

This group of drugs produces muscle relaxation by depression of interneuronal activity in the spinal cord or by interference with the contractile mechanism of the skeletal muscle. They are used in neurological and musculoskeletal diseases associated with muscular hypertonus and other painful spastic conditions, due mostly to lesions in the central nervous system. Several drugs, including mephenesin, chlorphenesin, carisoprodal, chlorzoxazone, methocarbamol and diazepam, were tried or are still used with varying success for the relief of spasticity. However, the effective treatment of spastic conditions with the above drugs often requires very large doses, which frequently result in over-sedation and depression of voluntary activity. The search continues for more selective agents which relieve the painful muscle spasms without loss of voluntary muscle function and without impairment of CNS function.

Dantrolene sodium

Dantrolene, a hydantoin derivative (see also Chapter 7), is well established in clinical practice, being of greatest value for the reduction of clonus and involuntary muscle spasms (586[R], 587[R]). During the last few years it has been found to be very promising drug for the prophylaxis and treatment of the syndrome of malignant hyperthermia (see the 'Suxamethonium' section). Dantrolene differs from the centrally acting muscle relaxants in that its site of action is beyond the muscle cell membrane. It interferes with the excitation—contraction coupling mechanism of striated muscle, presumably by inhibition of calcium release from the sarcoplasmic reticulum. The recommended clinical doses for the treatment of spastic conditions range between 75 and 400 mg daily per os. The most common adverse reactions, seen in up to 75% of patients, are weakness, fatigue, drowsiness and dizziness. Nausea, vomiting, diarrhea or constipation are also common complaints, but all these adverse reactions tend to disappear as the treatment continues. In general, by adjusting the dose, a satisfactory effect can be achieved with acceptable side effects.

Rare, but occasionally very serious, side effects include hepatotoxicity, respiratory depression, seizures, pleuropericardial reaction and the development of (fatal) lymphocytic lymphoma (SEDA-5, 137). The *hepatotoxicity* consists mainly of minor liver function disturbances (in 1% of patients), with symptoms in 0.35—0.5% and fatal hepatitis in 0.3% (588[C], 589[r]). The risk of severe liver damage is greater with doses above 300—400 mg daily, with prolonged treatment (more than 60 days), in females and in patients older than 35 years. *Respiratory depression* may be seen when the drug is used injudiciously in patients with marginal ventilatory function; the muscle weakness caused by dantrolene can lead to respiratory failure in such patients (SEDA, 114; 157[Cr]). Exacerbation or precipitation of *seizures* has been reported in children with cerebral palsy on long-term treatment with high doses (4—12 mg/kg) (590[C]). Pleuropericardial reactions, with sterile effusions and eosinophilia, have also rarely been reported (in patients taking 225—400 mg/day for 3 months to 4 years) (591[C]). There is no proof of a causal relationship, but the chemically related nitrofurantoin has also been associated with pulmonary reactions, so that patients on dantrolene should be screened periodically. One case of (fatal) *lymphocytic lymphoma* (592[C]) has also been described during high-dose (600 mg/day over 3 years) dantrolene treatment. Again the association is only circumstantial, another hydantoin derivative, phenytoin, being documented as inducing lymphomas. Numbness of hands and feet have also been reported (593[C]); long-term use of the structurally related diphenylhydantoin (phenytoin) has been incriminated in the causation of polyneuropathy. One case of *deafness* after 5 days' treatment (25 mg/day) has been recorded; the patient was on long-term therapy with baclofen and diazepam (594[C]). This may be coincidental. A very tenuous hypothesis, however, is suggested in SEDA-13 (p. 106).

Side effects such as *uterine atony* and a potentially fatal interaction associated with the intravenous use of the drug in the malignant hyperthermia syndrome are discussed in the 'Suxamethonium' section, where the danger of oral dantrolene (4 mg/kg per day) *aggravating pre-existing muscle weakness* to such an extent that artificial ventilation was required is also referenced (a case where the drug was used as prophylaxis against malignant hyperthermia).

Baclofen

Baclofen is a chlorophenyl derivative of γ-aminobutyric acid (GABA), a naturally occurring inhibitory neurotransmitter in the brain and spinal cord. It is of proven therapeutic value in reducing the severity of flexor or extensor spasms resulting from spinal cord injury or disease. The recommended daily (oral) dose is 15 mg (5 mg 3 times daily) which can be carefully increased; however, the total daily dose should not exceed 80 mg (20 mg given 4 times daily).

The most commonly reported side effects include *drowsiness, dizziness, fatigue, confusion, hypotension and nausea. Euphoria or depression* may be produced, and mania has been reported in a schizophrenic patient (SEDA-8, 139; 595[C]). Impairment of speech, memory and mental acuity, associated with an *abnormal electroencephalogram*, has been described in a young patient receiving normal doses (20 mg twice daily); gradual withdrawal restored the patient and electroencephalogram to normal (SEDA-12, 119; 596[C]). Abnormal *EEC changes* have also been reported in a patient with deteriorating multiple sclerosis who developed *encephalopathy* 48 hours after starting baclofen in low dosage (10 mg 3 times daily), but this patient also had renal impairment (see below); withdrawal also led to reversal of symptoms in this case (597[C]). Epilepsy, progressing to status epilepticus, has also been ascribed to baclofen (80 mg/day); the fits stopped on gradual withdrawal of the baclofen (598[C]). In contrast with other reports, this patient had no previous history of seizures. *Sudden withdrawal may cause hallucinations and grand mal convulsions or worsening of pre-existing epilepsy* (SED-9, 206; SEDA-6, 132; 599[C]). The drug should always be withdrawn gradually. Generally, patients with a history of seizures, convulsive disorders, or psychiatric disturbances, and also elderly patients with cerebrovascular disease, should be regarded as patients at risk of developing the more serious side effects (SED-9, 206). Rarely, *deterioration in liver function tests* (increases in SGOT and alkaline phosphatase) may occur (SEDA-6, 132). Toxic reactions characterized by a *psychotic syndrome and myoclonia have been reported due to cumulation of baclofen in patients with impaired renal function* (SEDA-7, 148; 600[C]).

Overdose, which may be absolute or relative (due to impaired renal excretion, or in elderly patients who develop side effects at lower dosage), leads to severe hypotonia, mental confusion and somnolence, respiratory depression and eventually apnea, bradycardia, cardiac conduction abnormalities, hypotension and coma. Convulsions may occur and hypertension has been reported. It is possible that during recovery the picture may be complicated by an acute withdrawal syndrome, with agitation, psychosis, tremor and dystonic movements, convulsions and hallucinations (SEDA-9, 122; SEDA-11, 126; 601[C], 602[Cr], 603[C], 604[CR]).

Intrathecal baclofen has caused *severe hypotonia, respiratory depression and coma*. Primary cardiovascular effects were not a feature here. This picture has been seen not only with high doses (2000 g/day produced flaccid quadriplegia with total areflexia) (SEDA-12, 119; 605[C]) but also following a single bolus dose of 80 g in a patient known to be very sensitive to the action of baclofen (SEDA-15, 128; 606[C]). Drugs injected directly into the cerebrospinal fluid have a tendency to produce unpredictable effects, their spread being influenced not only by the volume administered, but also by the concentration of the drug, its specific gravity in relation to that of cerebrospinal fluid and the positioning of the patient (head-up or -down), and on the speed of injection of bolus doses. Truncal muscle spasms can also increase the spread of drug within the cerebrospinal fluid. All these parameters need to be taken into consideration. Standardization is required as a first step. Rapid bolus injection in particular can produce unexpectedly severe side effects. How does one monitor the spread of baclofen in the cerebrospinal fluid from spinal cord to brain?

Physostigmine has been found to be rapidly effective in reversing not only the respiratory depression but also the coma and hypotonia seen in cases of intrathecal baclofen overdosage (SEDA-15, 128; 606[C]). The doses recommended for physostigmine salicylate were 1—2 mg i.v. over 5—10 minutes, and may have to be repeated after 30—40 minutes as the action of physostigmine is fairly short. Physostigmine may be ineffective, however, where large doses of baclofen are involved (607[C]), and it also has side effects (see Chapter 13), so that the above dosage guidelines should not be exceeded. In particular, *bradycardia and cardiac conduction defects* can be worsened (cardiac arrest has been reported in connection with baclofen) and it should not be used in these circumstances, respiratory support and symptomatic treatment being recommended (608[C]). *Phaclofen* is a more specific baclofen antagonist (609), but more research is required to ascertain if it can be safely used in the treatment of baclofen overdose.

Tricyclic antidepressants may potentiate the muscle relaxant effects of baclofen, resulting in *severe hypotonic weakness* (SEDA-7, 148; 610[C]); the combination has also been incriminated in the causation of *short-term memory impairment* (SEDA-11, 127; 611[C]). An elderly patient with a 4-year history of *Alzheimer's disease* has been reported (SEDA-16, 23[C]) to have developed *chorea* 2 weeks after starting a trial with baclofen. The does had been gradually increased to 15 mg 3 times a day. The chorea ceases within 24 hours after the baclofen was stopped. The authors suggest that the chorea resulted from the combination of the GABA-agonist drug and the deficient cholinergic function of Alzheimer's disease.

Tizanidine

Tizanidine is a centrally acting benzothiadiazol derivative with myotonolytic activity. Although its mechanism of action has not been fully clarified, facilitation of glycine-mediated transmission in the spinal cord might play an important role (612). A total daily dose of 15 mg (5 mg 3 times) is reported to be effective and well tolerated by most patients (613[C]). The documentation of side effects is still fragmentary; tizanidine seems to be a relatively well tolerated and useful antispastic agent.

The most frequently reported side effects include *drowsiness*, *dry mouth* and *muscular weakness* (614[Cr]). Occasionally, *hypotension* may occur. This is usually mild (615[C], 616[C]) but may be more severe in patients on antihypertensive therapy (617[C]—619[C]) in whom the drug should be used with great caution. A small decrease in heart rate has also been reported (620[C]).

Cyclobenzaprine

Cyclobenzaprine is a centrally acting skeletal-muscle relaxant, claimed to be effective in providing relief of muscle spasm, pain and tenderness, and in reducing the limitations imposed thereby on normal daily activities. The recommended total daily dose is 30 mg per os (621[C]). Its chemical structure is similar to the tricyclic antidepressant class of drugs which are known to inhibit neuronal reuptake of noradrenaline. This may occasionally produce marked *arteriolar spasm* due to increased adrenergic tone, precipitating *Raynaud's phenomenon* (SEDA-6, 132). The most common side effects reported so far are *somnolence*, *dry mucous membranes*, *dizziness and confusion*. *Less commonly*, *tachycardia*, *dysarthria*, *disorientation and hallucinations* have been experienced (622[C]). Rarely, *manic psychosis* may be activated in patients with bipolar affective disorders (SEDA-9, 122; 623[C]). Cyclobenzaprine should be looked upon as a tricyclic muscle relaxant and, accordingly, *side effects similar to those seen with the tricyclic antidepressants* (see Chapter 2) are to be expected. Overdose should be treated as for this group of drugs. Noradrenaline reuptake inhibition is a common feature of various drugs. Therefore, severe tachydysrhythmias may occur when such compounds are administered concomitantly (see also in the 'Interactions' section under 'Pancuronium').

Botulinum-A toxin

This is one of several toxins produced by the bacterium *Clostridium botulinum*. The toxin binds irreversibly with nerve endings, preventing the release of the neurotransmitter acetylcholine, so that paralysis of the muscles supplied by the affected nerves ensues. Sprouting of the terminal nerves eventually results in re-innervation of the muscles and return of function.

Originally introduced in the treatment of various ophthalmological disorders to restore the balance of contraction of the extraocular muscles, e.g. in patients with lateral rectus paralysis or strabismus, it is now used mainly in the treatment of blepharospasm. Injections of approximately 12.5—25 units are made into the periocular muscles of each eye. When so used, side effects are seen in 20—51% of treatments and consist of *mild ptosis*, *increased or decreased tear function*, *diplopia*, *and ectropion*. These effects are transient, most lasting about 2 weeks, and generally well-tolerated. Occasionally ptosis is so severe as to be inconvenient for the patient. The blepharospasm is relieved for 2—4 months. Systemic effects have not been reported (624[Cr]).

In the treatment of spastic torticollis, however, there is a tendency to use greater doses (up to 1000 Mouse Units) injected into the neck muscles, and *weakness of the pharyngeal muscles*, *resulting in dysphagia and paralysis of the vocal cords*, has been reported. Difficulty in swallowing and deepening of the voice were found in up to 30% of cases in one series, resolving after 2— 3 weeks (625[C]). A case has been described with severe dysphagia 2 days after an injection, with *unilateral vocal cord paralysis* a week later; swallowing was normal again after 6 weeks (626[C]). The possibility of appreciable effects from this neurotoxin at more distant neuromuscular junctions and the (hypothetical) development of antibodies are theoretical dangers here. Treatment with botulinum toxin of spasmodic torticollis has been reviewed retrospectively in 107 patients (SEDA-17, 45[C]). It was efficacious in 93% but adverse effects occurred in 84%. Initially, 500 mouse units (MU, Porton Down) were injected into each muscle but the incidence of adverse effects led to a reduction in dosage, 200—500 MU being injected depending on the muscle used and on neck thickness. The median dose per treatment was 1000 (range 200—1600) MU on the first visit and 800 MU subsequently. Dysphagia occurred after 44% of the treatments. This was severe in 2% of treatments, allowing only sips of fluid and necessitating hospitalization for two patients because of dehydration. Two patients developed stridor, two experienced substantial weight loss, and one developed pneumonia as a result of aspiration. The risk of dysphagia, according to the authors, is 40% if a sternomastoid is injected and 25% if it is not. The risks of moderate or severe dysphagia are 7 and $<1\%$, respectively. The authors estimated that there is a 3% chance of antibody production with reduced responsiveness during the first 15 months of treatment. They recommended antibody testing for patients who have initial but not subsequent improvement after repeated injections of botulinum toxin.

MISCELLANEOUS

Progabide *(see also Chapter 7)*

Progabide is an anti-spasticity drug which is also being used in the treatment of epilepsy. Together with its metabolites, it acts as an agonist at both GABA-A and GABA-B receptors. A high proportion of patients suffer from transient minor side effects such as *drowsiness, nausea, weakness or dizziness.* Twenty-three percent (seven patients) in one study, given doses up to 45 mg/kg per day, *exhibited significant disturbances in liver function tests* (which returned to normal on withdrawing the drug) (627[C]). If this high incidence of liver toxicity is confirmed, the drug's usefulness will be greatly curtailed.

Chlorzoxazone

Chlorzoxazone is a centrally acting benzoxazole derivative with a weak muscle relaxing effect. It is usually used in combination with acetaminophen for the treatment of painful muscle spasms. The usual dose is 500 mg 3 times a day. *Drowsiness*, *weakness*, *dizziness* and *gastrointestinal complaints* are the most frequent unwanted effects.

The most serious side effect of this older anti-spasticity agent, which fortunately occurs only rarely, is *hepatotoxicity*. An interesting case of jaundice where rechallenge with a single Parafon Forte pill resulted in a dramatic reaction after 5 hours, with fever, chills, nausea, vomiting and recurrence of icterus, has been documented in an article that also reviews some 23 other cases (SEDA-12, 119; 628*Cr*). Acetaminophen (paracetamol) on its own had no adverse effect in this case.

A *spasmodic torticollis*-like syndrome, repeatedly evoked after the ingestion of chlorzoxazone, is an unusual side effect of the drug. Benztropine mesylate, 1 mg i.v., led to resolution of the symptoms within 10 minutes (629[C]).

Chlormezanone

Chlormezanone is a tranquillizer with central muscle relaxant effects. It has been recommended that it should be used in dosages of less than 800 mg orally per day and for relatively short periods (never more than a few weeks). For the most part only minor side effects are seen, such as sedation, dizziness, nausea, and headache, which clear on stopping the drug.

The concomitant use of paracetamol increases the chance of adverse effects, especially erythema and urticaria.

Drug dependence may develop with high dosages or administration for prolonged periods, leading to withdrawal symptoms.

Rarely, cholestatic hepatitis and thombocytopenia occur. One case of fulminant liver necrosis requiring liver transplantation has been reported in a young pregnant woman who had taken chlormezanone (600 mg/day) for 3 weeks (SEDA-17, 47[C]).

REFERENCES

1. Bowman WC. Pharmacology of Neuromuscular Function, 2nd edn. London—Boston—Singapore—Sydney—Toronto—Wellington: Wright, 1990.
2. Agoston S, Bowman WC. eds. Muscle Relaxants, 2nd edn. Monographs in Anaesthesiology, Vol. 19. Amsterdam: Elsevier Science Publishers BV, 1990.
3. Lingle CJ, Steinbach JH. Neuromuscular blocking agents. Int Anesthesiol Clin 1988;26:288.
4. Marshall IG. Pharmacological effects of neuromuscular blocking agents: interaction with cholinoceptors other than nicotinic receptors of the neuromuscular junction. Anest Rianim 1986;27:19 (in English).
5. Standaert FG. Neuromuscular Physiology. In: Miller RD, ed. Anesthesia, 3rd edn. New York: Churchill Livingstone, 1990;659.
6. Bowman WC. Non-relaxant properties of neuro-muscular blocking drugs. Br J Anaesth 1982;54:147.
7. Walts LF. Complications of muscle relaxants. In: Katz RL ed. Muscle Relaxants. Amsterdam: Excerpta Medica, 1975;209.
8. Laxenaire M-C, Moneret-Vautrin DA, Watkins J. Diagnosis of the causes of anaphylactoid anaesthetic reaction. Anaesthesia 1983;38:147.
9. Fisher MMcD, More DG. The epidemiology and clinical features of anaphylactic reactions in anaesthesia. Anaesth Intensive Care 1981;9:226.
10. Hatton F, Tiret L, Maujol L et al. Enquête épidémiologique sur les anesthesies. Ann Fr Anesth Réanim 1983;2:331.
11. Thornton JA, Lorenz W. Histamine and antihistamine in anaesthesia and surgery: report of a symposium. Anaesthesia 1983;38:373.
12. Fisher MMcD, Munro I. Life-threatening anaphylactoid reactions to muscle relaxants. Anesth Analg 1983;62:559.
13. Boileau S, Hammer-Sigiel M, Moeller R, Drouet N. Réévaluation des risques respectifs d'anaphylaxie et d'histaminoblitération avec les substances anesthésiologiques. Ann Fr Anesth Réanim 1985;4:195.
14. Laxenaire MC, Moneret-Vautrin DA, Vervloet D et al. Accidents anaphylactoïdes graves peranesthésiques. Ann Fr Anesth Réanim 1985;4:30.

15. Laxenaire MC, Moneret-Vautrin DA, Vervloet D. The French experience of anaphylactoid reactions. Int Anesthesiol Clin 1985;23:145.
16. Galletly DC, Treuren BC. Anaphylactoid reactions during anaesthesia. Anaesthesia 1985;40:329.
17. Youngman PR, Taylor KM, Wilson JD. Anaphylactoid reactions to neuromuscular blocking agents: a commonly undiagnosed condition? Lancet 1983;ii:597.
18. Vervloet D, Nizankowska E, Arnaud A et al. Adverse reactions to suxamethonium and other muscle relaxants under general anesthesia. J Allergy Clin Immunol 1983; 71:552.
19. Vervloet D. Allergy to muscle relaxants and related compounds. Clin Allergy 1985;15:501.
20. Assem ESK. Characteristics of basophil histamine release by neuromuscular blocking drugs in patients with anaphylactoid reactions. Agents Actions 1984;14:435.
21. Watkins J. Heuristic decision-making in diagnosis and management of adverse drug reactions in anaesthesia and surgery: the case of muscle relaxants. Theor Surg 1989;4:212.
22. Harle DG, Baldo BA, Fisher MMcD. Detection of IgE antibodies to suxamethonium after anaphylactoid reactions during anaesthesia. Lancet 1984;i:930.
23. Vervloet D, Arnaud A, Senlt M et al. Anaphylactic reactions to suxamethonium: prevention of mediator release by choline. J Allergy Clin Immunol 1985;76:222.
24. Baldo BA, Harle DG, Fisher MM. In vitro diagnosis and studies on the mechanism(s) of anaphylactoid reactions to muscle relaxant drugs. Ann Fr Anesth Réanim 1985;4:139.
25. Bird AG. 'Allergic' drug reactions during anaesthesia. Adverse Drug React Bull 1985;110:408.
26. Fisher M. Intradermal testing after anaphylactoid reaction to anaesthetic drugs: practical aspects of performance and interpretation. Anaesth Intensive Care 1984;12:115.
27. Assem ESK. Anaphylactic anaesthetic reactions. The value of paper radioallergosorbent tests for IgE antibodies to muscle relaxants and thiopentone. Anaesthesia 1990; 45:1032.
28. Sage DJ. Management of acute anaphylactoid reactions. Int Anesthesiol Clin 1985;23:175.
29. Fisher MMcD. Clinical observations on the pathophysiology and treatment of anaphylactic cardiovascular collapse. Anaesth Intensive Care 1986;14:17.
30. Sokoll MD, Gergis SD. Antibiotics and neuromuscular function. Anesthesiology 1981;55:148.
31. Tryba M. Wirkungsverstarkung nicht-depolarisierender Muskelrelaxantien durch Acylaminopenicilline. Anaesthesist 1985;34:651.
32. Mackie K, Pavlin EG. Recurrent paralysis following piperacillin administration. Anesthesiology 1990;72:561.
33. Singh YN, Marshall IG, Harvey AL. The mechanisms of the muscle paralysing actions of antibiotics and their interaction with neuromuscular blocking agents. Rev Drug Metab Drug Interact 1980;3:129.
34. Pittinger C, Adamson R. Antibiotic blockade of neuromuscular function. Annu Rev Pharmacol 1972;12:169.
35. Schuh FT. Hämodilution und Wirkungsdauer von Muskelrelaxantien. Anaesthesist 1981;30:44.
36. Schuh FT. Influence of haemodilution on the potency of neuromuscular blocking drugs. Br J Anaesth 1981;53:263.
37. Goudsouzian NG. Maturation of neuromuscular transmission in the infant. Br J Anaesth 1980;52:205.
38. Crumrine RS, Yodlowski EH. Assessment of neuromuscular function in infants. Anesthesiology 1981;54:29.
39. Fisher DM, O'Keeffe CO, Stanski DR et al. Pharmacokinetics of *d*-tubocurarine in infants, children and adults. Anesthesiology 1982;57:203.
40. Goudsouzian NG. Muscle relaxants in paediatric anaesthesia. In: Agoston S, Bowman WC, eds. Muscle Relaxants, 2nd edn. Monographs in Anaesthesiology, Vol 19. Amsterdam: Elsevier, 1990;285.
41. O'Keeffe C, Gregory GA, Stanski DR et al. *d*- Tubocurarine: pharmacodynamics and kinetics in children. Anesthesiology 1979;51:S270.
42. Goudsouzian NG, Liu LMP, Cote CJ. Comparison of equipotent doses of nondepolarizing muscle relaxants in children. Anesth Analg 1981;60:862.
43. Duvaldestin P, Saada J, Berger JL et al. Pharmacokinetics, pharmacodynamics and dose-response relationships of pancuronium in control and elderly subjects. Anesthesiology 1982;56:36.
44. D'Hollander A, Massaux F, Nevelsteen M et al. Age-dependent dose—response relationship of Org NC 45 in anaesthetized patients. Br J Anaesth 1982;54:653.
45. Matteo RS. Use in the elderly. In: Norman J, ed. Clinics in Anaesthesiology, Vol. 3. London—Philadelphia—Toronto: W.B. Saunders Co., 1985;421.
46. Bush GH. Use in paediatric surgery and intensive care. In: Norman J, ed. Clinics in Anaesthesiology, Vol 3. London—Philadelphia—Toronto: W.B. Saunders Co., 1985;405.
47. Goudsouzian NG, Standaert FG. The infant and the myoneural junction. Anesth Analg 1986;65:1208.
48. Ham J, Stanski DR, Newfield P, Miller RD. Pharmacokinetics and dynamics of *d*-tubocurarine during hypothermia in humans. Anesthesiology 1981;55:631.
49. Buzello W, Schlurmann D, Schindler M, Spillner G. Hypothermic cardiopulmonary bypass and neuromuscular blockade by pancuronium and vecuronium. Anesthesiology 1985;62:201.
50. Buzello W, Schlurmann D, Pollmacher T, Spillner G. Unequal effects of cardiopulmonary bypass-induced hypothermia on neuromuscular blockade from constant infusion of alcuronium, *d*-tubocurarine, pancuronium and vecuronium. Anesthesiology 1987;66:842.
51. Heier T, Caldwell JE, Sessler Dl, Miller RD. The effect of local surface and central cooling on adductor pollicis twitch tension during nitrous oxide/isoflurane and nitrous oxide/fentanyl anesthesia in humans. Anesthesiology 1990; 72:807.
52. Engbaek J, Skovgaard LT, Friis B, Kann T. The effect of temperature on the evoked EMG response. Anesthesiology 1989;72:A810.
53. Ono K, Ohta Y, Morita K, Kosaka F. The influence of respiratory-induced acid base changes on the action of nondepolarizing muscle relaxants in rats. Anesthesiology 1988;68:357.
54. Gencarelli PJ, Swen J, Koot HWJ, Miller RD. The effects of hypercarbia and hypocarbia on pancuronium and vecuronium neuromuscular blockades in anesthetized humans. Anesthesiology 1983;59:376.
55. Dal Santo G. Kinetics of distribution on radioactive labelled muscle relaxants. III. Investigations with ^{14}C-succinyldicholine and ^{14}C-succinylmonocholine during controlled conditions. Anesthesiology 1968;29:435.
56. Bourne JG, Collier HOJ, Somers GF. Succinylcholine muscle relaxant of short action. Lancet 1952;i:1225.
57. Smith NL. Histamine release by suxamethonium. Anaesthesia 1957;12:293.

58. Bele-Binda N, Valeri F. A case of bronchospasm induced by succinylcholine. Can Anaesth Soc J 1971;18:116.
59. Dohi S, Ogawa H. The bronchospasm induced by suxamethonium administration. Jpn J Anesth 1973;22:1432.
60. Czekuć E. Bronchospasm following suxamethonium in a 2 year old child. Anesteziol Reanimatol (Warzawa) 1970;2:65.
61. Redderson C, Perkins HM, Adler WH et al. Systemic reaction to succinylcholine: a case report. Anesth Analg 1971;50:49.
62. Sitarz L. Anaphylactic shock following injection of suxamethonium. Anaesth Resusc Intensive Ther 1974;2:83.
63. Mandappa JM, Chandrasekhara PM, Nelvigi RG. Anaphylaxis to suxamethonium. Br J Anaesth 1975;47:523.
64. James OF. Anaphylactoid reaction to suxamethonium. Anaesth intensive Care 1979;7:288.
65. Kepes ER, Haimovici H. Allergic reaction to succinylcholine. J Am Med Assoc 1959;171:548.
66. Jerums G, Whittingham S, Wilson P. Anaphylaxis to suxamethonium. Br J Anaesth 1967;39:73.
67. Fellini AA, Bernstein RL, Zauder HL. Bronchospasm due to suxamethonium. Br J Anaesth 1963;35:657.
68. Katz AM, Mulligan G. Bronchospasm induced by suxamethonium: a case report. Br J Anaesth 1972;44:1097.
69. Laxenaire M-C, Moneret-Vautrin DA, Boileau S. Choc anaphylactique au suxaméthonium: à propos de 18 cas. Ann Fr Anesth Réanim 1982;1:29.
70. Moss J, Fahmy NR, Sunder N, Beaven MA. Hormonal and hemodynamic profile of an anaphylactic reaction in man. Circulation 1981;63:210.
71. Vuitton D, Neidhardt-Audion M, Girardin P et al. Caractéristiques épidemiologiques de 21 accidents anaphylactoïdes peranesthésiques observés dans une population de 12,855 sujets opérés. Ann Fr Anesth Réanim 1985;4:167.
72. Wright PJ, Shortland JR, Stevens JD et al. Fatal haemopathological consequences of general anaesthesia. Br J Anaesth 1989;62:104.
73. Moneret-Vautrin DA, Widner S, Gueant J-L et al. Simultaneous anaphylaxis to thiopentone and a neuromuscular blocker: a study of two cases. Br J Anaesth 1990;64:743.
74. Standaert FG, Adams JE. The actions of succinylcholine on the mammalian motor nerve terminal. J Pharmacol Exp Ther 1965;149:113.
75. Thind GS, Bryson THL. Single dose suxamethonium and muscle pain in pregnancy. Br J Anaesth 1983;55:743.
76. Coxon JD. Muscle pain after suxamethonium. Br J Anaesth 1962;34:750.
77. Paton WDM. The effects of muscle relaxants other than muscular relaxation. Anesthesiology 1959;20:453.
78. Tammisto T, Airaksinen M. Increase of creatine kinase activity in serum as a sign of muscular injury caused by intermittently administered suxamethonium during halothane anaesthesia. Br J Anaesth 1966;38:510.
79 Waters DJ, Mapleson WW. Suxamethonium pains: hypothesis and observation. Anaesthesia 1971;26:127.
80. Rack PMH, Westbury DR. The effects of suxamethonium and acetylcholine on the behaviour of cat muscle spindles during dynamic stretching, and during fusimotor stimulation. J Physiol (London) 1966;186:698.
81. Mayrhofer O. Die Wirksamheit von *d*-Tubocurarin zur Verhutüng der Muskelschmerzen nach Succinylcholin. Anaesthesist 1959;8:313.
82. König W. Über Beschwerden nach Anwendung von Succinylcholin. Anaesthesist 1956;5:50.
83. Kaniaris P, Galanopoulou T, Varnos D. Effects of succinylcholine on plasma 5-HT levels. Anesth Analg 1973; 52:425.
84. Collier CB. Suxamethonium pains and early electrolyte changes. Anaesthesia 1978;33:454.
85. Naguib M, Farag H, Magbagbeola JAO. Effect of pretreatment with lysine acetyl salicylate on suxamethonium-induced myalgia. Br J Anaesth 1987;59:606.
86. McLoughlin C, Nesbitt GA, Howe JP. Suxamethonium induced myalgia and the effect of pre-operative administration of oral aspirin. Anaesthesia 1988;43:565.
87. Cullen DJ. The effect of pretreatment with non-depolarizing muscle relaxants on the neuromuscular blocking action of succinylcholine. Anesthesiology 1971;35:572.
88. Jansen EC, Hansen PH. Objective measurement of succinylcholine-induced fasciculations and the effect of pretreatment with pancuronium or gallamine. Anesthesiology 1979;51:159.
89. Blitt CD, Carlson GL, Rolling G et al. A comparative evaluation of pretreatment with nondepolarizing neuromuscular blockers prior to the administration of succinylcholine. Anesthesiology 1981;55:687.
90. Erkola O, Salmenperä A, Kuoppamäki R. Five nondepolarizing muscle relaxants in precurarization. Acta Anaesthesiol Scand 1983;27:427.
91. Fahmy NR, Malek NS, Lappas DG. Diazepam prevents some adverse effects of succinylcholine. Clin Pharmacol Ther 1979;26:395.
92. Manchikanti L. Diazepam does not prevent succinylcholine-induced fasciculations and myalgia: a comparative evaluation of the effect of diazepam and *d*-tubocurarine pre-treatments. Acta Anaesthesiol Scand 1984;28:523.
93. Flewellen EH, Bodensteiner JB. Anesthetic experience in a patient with hyperkalemic periodic paralysis. Anesthesiol Rev 1980;7:44.
94. Brim VD. Denervation supersensitivity: the response to depolarising muscle relaxants. Br J Anaesth 1973;45:222.
95. Kelly EP. A rise in serum potassium after suxamethonium following brachial plexus injury. Anaesthesia 1982; 37:694.
96. Orndahl G, Stenberg K. Myotonic human musculature: stimulation with depolarizing agents: mechanical registration of the effects of succinyldicholine, succinylmonocholine and decamethonium. Acta Med Scand 1962;172(Suppl 389):3.
97. Rosenberg H, Fletcher JE. Masseter muscle rigidity and malignant hyperthermia susceptibility. Anesth Analg 1986;65:161.
98. Gronert GA. Management of patients in whom trismus occurs following succinylcholine. Anesthesiology 1988;68: 653.
99. Van der Spek AFL, Fang WB, Ashton-Miller JA et al. The effect of succinylcholine on mouth opening. Anesthesiology 1987;67:459.
100. Meakin G, Walker RWM, Dearlove OR. Myotonic and neuromuscular blocking effects of increased doses of suxamethonium in infants and children. Br J Anaesth 1990;65:816.
101. Littleford JA, Patel LR, Bose D et al. Masseter muscle spasm in children: implications of continuing the triggering anesthetic. Anesth Analg 1991;72:151.
102. Plötz J, Braun J. Serummyoglobin nach Wiederholungsgaben von Succinylcholin und der Einfluss von Dantrolen. Anaesthesist 1985;34:513.
103. Plötz J. Nebenwirkungen von Succinylcholin auf die Skelettmuskulatur in Halothannarkose bei Kindern: Prophy-

laxe mit Diallylnortoxiferin, 'self-taming' und Dantrolen. Therapiewoche 1984;34:3168.
104. Harrington JF, Ford DJ, Striker TW. Myoglobinemia after succinylcholine in children undergoing halothane and non-halothane anesthesia. Anesthesiology 1984;61:A431.
105. Hool GJ, Lawrence PJ, Sivaneswaran N. Acute rhabdomyolytic renal failure due to suxamethonium. Anaesth Intensive Care 1984;12:360.
106. McKishnie JD, Muir JM, Girvan DP. Anaesthesia induced rhabdomyolysis—a case report. Can Anaesth Soc J 1983;30:295.
107. Steegmuller H. On the geographical distribution of pseudocholinesterase variants. Humangenetik 1975;26:167.
108. DeCook TH, Goudsouzian NG. Tachyphylaxis and phase-II block development during infusion of succinylcholine in children. Anesth Analg 1980;59:639.
109. Ramsey FM, Lebowitz PW, Savarese JJ, Ali HH. Clinical characteristics of long-term succinylcholine neuromuscular blockade during balanced anesthesia. Anesth Analg 1980;59:110.
110. Airaksinen MM, Tammisto T. Myoglubinuria after intermittent administration of succinylcholine during halothane anaesthesia. Clin Pharmacol Ther 1966;7:583.
111. Ryan JF, Kagen LJ, Hyman AL. Myoglobinemia after a single dose of succinylcholine. N Engl J Med 1971;285:824.
112 Gibbs JM. A case of rhabdomyolysis associated with suxamethonium. Anaesth Intensive Care 1978;6:141.
113. Pantuck EJ, Pantuck CB. Cholinesterases and anticholinesterases. In: Katz RL, ed. Muscle Relaxants. Amsterdam: Excerpta Medica, 1975;155.
114. Viby Mogensen J. Correlation of succinylcholine duration of action with plasma cholinesterase activity in subjects with the genotypically normal enzyme. Anesthesiology 1980;53:517.
115. Whittaker M. Plasma cholinesterase variants and the anaesthetist. Anaesthesia 1980;35:174.
116. Pantuck EJ, Pantuck CB. Cholinesterases and anticholinesterases. In: Katz RL, ed. Muscle Relaxants. Amsterdam: Excerpta Medica, 1975142.
117. Hodges RJH, Harkross J. Suxamethonium sensitivity in health and disease: a clinical evaluation of pseudocholinesterase levels. Br Med J 1954;2:919.
118. Foldes FF, Rendell-Baker L, Birch JH. Causes and prevention of prolonged apnea with succinylcholine. Anesth Analg 1956;35:609.
119. Shnider SM. Serum cholinesterase activity during pregnancy, labor and the puerperium. Anesthesiology 1965; 26:335.
120. Robertson GS. Serum cholinesterase deficiency. II. Pregnancy. Br J Anaesth 1966;38:361.
121. Hazel B, Monier D. Human serum cholinesterase: variations during pregnancy and post-partum. Can Anaesth Soc J 1971;18:272.
122. Evans RT, Wroe JM. Plasma cholinesterase changes in pregnancy. Anaesthesia 1980;35:651.
123 Robson N, Robertson I, Whittaker M. Plasma cholinesterase changes during the puerperium. Anaesthesia 1986; 41:243.
124, Davies JM, Carmichael D, Dymond C. Plasma cholinesterase and trophoblastic disease. Anaesthesia 1983; 38:1071.
125. Kaniaris P, Fassoulaki A, Liarmakopoulou K et al. Serum cholinesterase levels in patients with cancer. Anesth Analg 1979;58:82.
126. Goertz B, Spieckermann B, Leven B et al. Succinylunvertraglichkeit mit achtwochiger Atemlahmung. Intensivmedizin 1977;14:88.
127. Evans RT, MacDonald R, Robinson A. Suxamethonium apnoea associated with plasmapheresis. Anaesthesia 1980;35:198.
128. Paterson JL, Walsh ES, Hall GM. Progressive depletion of plasma cholinesterase during daily plasma exchange. Br Med J 1979;2:580.
129. Jensen FS, Viby Mogensen J, Ostergaard D. Significance of plasma cholinesterase for the anaesthetist. Curr Anaesth Crit Care 1991;2:232.
130. Foldes FF. Myasthenia gravis. In: Katz RL, ed. Muscle Relaxants. Amsterdam: Excerpta Medica, 1975;345.
131. Yamashita M, Matsuki A, Oyama T. Anaesthetic considerations on Von Recklinghausen's disease. Anaesthesist 1977;26:317.
132. Baraka A. Myasthenic response to muscle relaxants in Von Recklinghausen's disease. Br J Anaesth 1974;46:701.
133. Heard SO, Kaplan RF. Neuromuscular blockade in a patient with nemaline myopathy. Anesthesiology 1983; 59:588.
134. McKishnie JD, Muir JM, Girvan DP. Anaesthesia induced rhabdomyolysis—a case report. Can Anaesth Soc J 1983;30:295.
135. Miyamoto K, Sasaki M, Okudo T et al. Four cases suspected of malignant hyperthermia induced by halothane and succinylcholine. Hiroshima J Anesth 1983;18:157.
136. Lewandowski KB. Strabismus as possible sign of subclinical muscular dystrophy predisposing to rhabdomyolysis and myoglobinuria: a study of an affected family. Can Anaesth Soc J 1982;29:372.
137. Linter SPK, Thomas PR, Withington PS et al. Suxamethonium associated hypertonicity and cardiac arrest in unsuspected pseudohypertrophic muscular dystrophy. Br J Anaesth 1982;54:1331.
138. Smith CL, Bush GH. Anaesthesia and progressive muscular dystrophy. Br J Anaesth 1985;57:1113.
139. Azar I. The response of patients with neuromuscular disorders to muscle relaxants: a review. Anesthesiology 1984;61:173.
140. Martz DG, Schreibman DL, Matjasko MJ. Neurological diseases. In: Katz RL, Benumof JL, Kadis LB, eds. Anesthesia and Uncommon Diseases, 3rd edn. Philadelphia: W.B. Saunders, 1990;560.
141. Miller JD, Lee C. Muscle diseases. In: Katz RL, Benumof JL, Kadis LB, eds. Anesthesia and Uncommon Diseases, 3rd edn. Philadelphia: W.B. Saunders, 1990;590.
142. Sorensen M, Engbaek J, Viby-Mogensen J et al. Bradycardia and cardiac asystole following a single injection of suxamethonium. Acta Anaesthesiol Scand 1984;28:232.
143. Smith RB, Petruscak J. Succinylcholine, digitalis and hypercalcemia. Anesth Analg 1972;51:202.
144. Nigrovic V. Succinylcholine, cholinoceptors and catecholamines: proposed mechanism of early adverse haemodynamic reactions. Can Anaesth Soc J 1984;31:382.
145. Ravindran RS, Klemm JE. Anaphylaxis to succinylcholine in a patient allergic to penicillin. Anesth Analg 1980;59:944.
146. Cohen S, Liu KH, Marx GF. Upper airway edema—an anaphylactoid reaction to succinylcholine? Anesthesiology 1982;56:467.
147. O'Sullivan EP, Childs D, Bush GH. Peri-operative dreaming in paediatric patients who receive suxamethonium. Anaesthesia 1988;43:104.

148. Marsh ML, Dunlop BJ, Shapiro HM, Gagnor RL, Rockoff MA. Succinylcholine-intracranial pressure effects in neurosurgical patients. Anesth Analg 1980;59:550.
149. Cottrell JE, Hartung J, Giffin JP, Shwury B. Intracranial and hemodynamic changes after succinylcholine administration in cats. Anesth Analg 1983;62:1006.
150. Gronert GA, Thompson RL, Onofrio BM. Human malignant hyperthermia: awake episodes and correction by dantrolene. Anesth Analg 1980;59:377.
151. Gronert GA. Malignant hyperthermia. Anesthesiology 1980;53:395.
152. Britt BA. Malignant hyperthermia. Can Anaesth Soc J 1985;32:666.
153. Schulte-Sasse U, Eberlein HJ. Neue Erkenntnisse und Erfahrungen auf dem Gebiet der malignen Hyperthermia. Anaesthesist 1986;35:1.
154. Kolb ME, Horne ML, Martz R. Dantrolene in human malignant hyperthermia. Anesthesiology 1982;56:254.
155. Larach MG, Rosenberg H, Larach DR, Broennle AM. Prediction of malignant hyperthermia susceptibility by clinical signs. Anesthesiology 1987;66:547.
156. Weingarten AE, Korsch JL, Neuman GC, Stern SB. Postpartum uterine atony after intravenous dantrolene. Anesth Analg 1987;66:269.
157. Hara Y, Kato A, Horikawa H et al. Post-operative respiratory depression thought to be due to oral dantrolene pretreatment in malignant hyperthermia-susceptible patient. Jpn J Anesth 1988;4:483.
158. Saltzman LS, Kates RA, Corke BC et al. Hyperkalemia and cardiovascular collapse after verapamil and dantrolene administration in swine. Anesth Analg 1984;63:473.
159. Rubin AS, Zablocki AD. Hyperkalemia, verapamil, and dantrolene. Anesthesiology 1987;66:246.
160. Paton WDM. The effects of muscle relaxants other than muscular relaxation. Anesthesiology 1959;20:453.
161. O'Brien DJ, Moriarty DC, Hope CE. The effect of preexisting beta blockade on potassium flux in patients receiving succinylcholine. Can Anaesth Soc J 1986;3:S89.
162. McCammon RL, Stoelting RK. Exaggerated increase in serum potassium following succinylcholine in dogs with beta-blockade. Anesthesiology 1984;61:723.
163. Koide M, Waud BE. Serum potassium concentrations after succinylcholine in patients with renal failure. Anesthesiology 1972;36:142.
164. Schaner PJ, Brown RL, Kirksey TD et al. Succinylcholine-induced hyperkalemia in burned patients. Anesth Analg 1969;48:764.
165. Tolmie JD, Joyce TH, Mitchell GD. Succinylcholine danger in the burned patient. Anesthesiology 1967 28:467.
166. Mazze RL, Escue HM, Houston JB. Hyperkalaemia and cardiovascular collapse following administration of succinylcholine to the traumatized patient. Anesthesiology 1969;31:540.
167. Birch AA, Mitchell OD, Playford GA et al. Changes in serum potassium response to succinylcholine following trauma. J Am Med Assoc 1969;210:490.
168. Stone WA, Beach TP, Hamelberg W. Succinylcholine danger in the spinal-cord-injured patient. Anesthesioloy 1970;32:168.
169. Stone WA, Beach TP, Hamelberg W. Succinylcholine-induced hyperkalemia in dogs with transected sciatic nerves or spinal cords. Anesthesioloy 1970;32:515.
170. Cooprman LH. Succinylcholine-induced hyperkalaemia in neuromuscular disease. J Am Med Assoc 1970;213:1867.
171. Tobey RE, Jacobson PM, Kahle CT et al. The serum potassium response to muscle relaxants in neural injury. Anesthesiology 1972;37:332.
172. Beach TP, Stone WA, Hamelberg W. Circulatory collapse following succinylcholine: report of a patient with diffuse lower motor neurone disease. Anesth Analg 1971;50:431.
173. Fergusson RJ, Wright DJ, Willey RF et al. Suxamethonium is dangerous in polyneuropathy. Br Med J 1981;282:298.
174. Roth F, Wuthrich H. The clinical importance of hyperkalaemia following suxamethonium administration. Br J Anaesth 1969;41:311.
175. Cowgill DB, Mostello LA, Shapiro HM. Encephalitis and a hyperkalemic response to succinylcholine. Anesthesiology 1974;40:409.
176. Gravlee GP. Succinylcholine induced hyperkalemia in a patient with Parkinson's disease. Anesth Analg 1980;59:444.
177. Rao TLK, Shanmugam M. Succinylcholine administration—another contra-indication? Anesth Analg 1979;58:61.
178. Krikken-Hogenberg LG, de Jong JR, Bovill JG. Succinylcholine-induced hyperkalemia in a patient with metastatic rhabdomyosarcoma. Anesthesiology 1989;70:553.
179. Iwatsuki N, Kuroda N, Amaka K et al. Succinylcholine-induced hyperkalemia in patients with ruptured cerebral aneurysms. Anesthesiology 1980;53:64.
180. Kohlschütter B, Baur H, Roth F. Suxamethonium-induced hyperkalaemia in patients with severe intra-abdominal infections. Br J Anaesth 1976;48:557.
181. Kahn TZ, Khan RM. Changes in serum potassium following succinylcholine in patients with infections. Anesth Analg 1983;62:327.
182. Axelsson J, Thesleff S. A study of supersensitivity in denervated mammalian skeletal muscle. J Physiol (London) 1959;149:178.
183. Kendig JJ, Bunker JP, Endow S. Succinylcholine-induced hyperkalemia: effects of succinylcholine on resting potentials and electrolyte distributions in normal and denervated muscle. Anesthesiology 1972;36:132.
184. Cronert CA, Lambert EH, Theye RA. The response of denervated skeletal muscle to succinylcholine. Anesthesiology 1973;53:13.
185. Fischbach CD, Robbins N. Effect of chronic disuse of rat soleus neuromuscular junctions on postsynaptic neuromuscular blockade. J Neurophysiol 1971;34:562.
186. Cronert CA, Theye RA. Pathophysiology of hyperkalemia induced by succinylcholine. Anesthesiology 1975;43:89.
187. Yentis SM. Suxamethonium and hyperkalaemia. Anaesth Intensive Care 1990;18:92.
188. Muravchick S, Burkett L, Cold MI. Succinylcholine-induced fasciculations and intragastric pressure during induction of anesthesia. Anesthesiology 1981;55:180.
189. Salem MR, Wong AY, Lin YH. The effect of suxamethonium on the intragastric pressure in infants and children. Br J Anaesth 1972;44:166.
190. Roe RB. The effect of suxamethonium on intragastric pressure. Anaesthesia 1962;17:179.
191. Miller RD, Way WL. Inhibition of succinylcholine-induced increased intragastric pressure by nondepolarizing muscle relaxants and lidocaine. Anesthesiology 1971;34:185.
192. La Cour D. Rise in intragastric pressure caused by suxamethonium fasciculations. Acta Anaesthesiol Scand 1969,13:255.
193. Marchand P. The gastro-oesophageal 'sphincter' and the mechanism of regurgitation. Br J Surg 1955;42:504.

194. Creenan J. The cardio-oesophageal junction. Br J Anaesth 1961;33:432.
195. Smith C, Dalling R, Williams TIR. Gastro-oesophageal pressure gradient changes produced by induction of anaesthesia and suxamethonium. Br J Anaesth 1978;50:1137.
196. La Cour D. Prevention of rise in intragastric pressure due to suxamethonium fasciculations by prior dose of *d*-tubocurarine. Acta Anaesthesiol. Scand 1970;14:5.
197. Bishop MJ, Hornbein TF. Prolonged effect of succinylcholine after neostigmine and pyridostigmine administration in patients with renal failure. Anesthesiology 1983;58:384.
198. Bennike KA, Jarnum S. Myoglobinuria with acute renal failure possibly induced by suxamethonium: a case report. Br J Anaesth 1964;36:730.
199. Macri FJ, Crimes PA. The effects of succinylcholine on the extraocular striate muscles and on the intraocular pressure. Am J Ophthalmol 1957;44:221.
200. Kornbluth W, Jampolsky A, Tamler E et al. Contraction of the oculorotatory muscles and intraocular pressure. Am J Ophthalmol 1960;49:1381.
201. Adams AK, Barnett KC. Anaesthesia and intraocular pressure. Anaesthesia 1966;21:202.
202. Katz RL, Eakins KE, Lord CO. The effects of hexafluorenium in preventing the increase in intraocular pressure produced by succinylcholine. Anesthesiology 1968;29:70.
203. Taylor TH, Mulcahy M, Nightingale D. Suxamethonium chloride in intraocular surgery. Br J Anaesth 1968;40:113.
204. Lincoff HA, Ellis CH, DeVoe AC et al. The effect of succinylcholine on intraocular pressure. Am J Ophthalmol 1955;40:501.
205. Pandey K, Badola RP, Kumar S. Time course of intraocular hypertension produced by suxamethonium. Br J Anaesth 1972;44:191.
206. Meyers EF, Krupin T, Johnson M et al. Failure of non-depolarizing blockers to inhibit succinylcholine-induced increased intraocular pressure: a controlled study. Anesthesiology 1978;48:149.
207. Cook JH. The effect of suxamethonium on intraocular pressure. Anaesthesia 1981;36:359.
208. Holloway KB. Control of the eye during general anaesthesia for intraocular surgery. Br J Anaesth 1980;52:671.
209. Moya F, Kvisselgaard N. The placental transmission of succinylcholine. Anesthesiology 1961;22:1.
210. Kvisselgaard N, Moya F. Investigation of placental threshold to succinylcholine. Anesthesiology 1961;22:7.
211. Weis OF, Muller FO, Lyell H et al. Materno-fetal cholinesterase inhibitor poisoning. Anesth Analg 1983;62:233.
212. Hoefnagel D, Harris NA, Kim TH. Transient respiratory depression of the newborn. Am J Dis Child 1979;133:825.
213. Cherala SR, Eddie DN, Sechzer PH. Placental transfer of succinylcholine causing transient respiratory depression in the newborn. Anaesth Intensive Care 1989;17:202.
214. Cestzes T. Prolonged apnoea after suxamethonium injection associated with eye-drops containing an anticholinesterase agent. Br J Anaesth 1966;38:408.
215. De Roetth A, Dettbarn WB, Rosenberg P et al. Effect of phospholine iodide on blood cholinesterase levels of normal and glaucoma subjects. Am J Ophthalmol 1965;59:586.
216. McCavin DD. Depressed levels of serum pseudo-cholinesterase with ecothiopate iodide eye drops. Lancet 1965; ii:272.
217. Barnes JM, Davies DR. Blood cholinesterase levels in workers exposed to organophosphorus insecticides. Br Med J 1951;2:816.
218. Little DM. Classical file. Surv Anesth. 1973;17:577.
219. Fisher DM, Caldwell JE, Sharma M, Wiren JE. The influence of bambuterol (carbamylated terbutaline) on the duration of action of succinylcholine-induced paralysis in humans. Anesthesiology 1988;69:757.
220. Bodley PO, Halway K, Potts L. Low serum pseudocholinesterase levels complicating treatment with phenelzine. Br Med J 1969;3:510.
221. Kambam JR, Parris WCV, Franks JJ, Sastry BVR. The inhibitory effect of metoclopramide on plasma cholinesterase activity. Anesth Analg 1988;67:S107.
222. Kao YJ, Turner DR. Prolongation of succinylcholine block by metoclopramide. Anesthesiology 1989;70:905.
223. Morris R, Ciesecke A. Potentiation of muscle relaxants by magnesium sulfate therapy in toxemia in pregnancy. South Med J 1968;61:25.
224. Skaredoff MN, Roaf ER, Datta S. Hyper-magnesaemia and anaesthetic management. Can Anaesth Soc J 1982;29:35.
225. De Vore JS, Asrani R. Magnesium sulfate prevents succinylcholine-induced fasciculations in toxemic parturients. Anesthesiology 1980;52:76.
226. Robertson CS. Serum proteins and cholinesterase changes in association with contraceptive pills. Lancet 1967;i:232.
227. Whittaker M, Charlier AR, Ramaswamy S. Changes in plasma cholinesterase isoenzymes due to oral contraceptives. J Reprod Fertil 1971;26:273.
228. Archer TL, Janowsky EC. Plasma pseudocholinesterase deficiency associated with diethylstilbestrol therapy. Anesth Analg 1978;57:726.
229. Foldes FF, Arai T, Gentsch HH, Zarday Z. The influence of glucocorticoids on plasma cholinesterase. Proc Soc Exp Biol Med 1974;146:918.
230. Verjee ZH, Behal R, Ayim EM. Effect of glucocorticoids on liver and blood cholinesterases. Clin Chim Acta 1977;81:41.
231. Bradamante V, Kunec-Vajic E, Lisic M et al. Plasma cholinesterase activity in patients during therapy with dexamethasone or prednisone. Eur J Clin Pharmacol 1989; 36:253.
232. Zsigmond EK, Robins G. The effect of a series of anticancer drugs on plasmacholinesterase activity. Can Anaesth Soc J 1972;19:75.
233. Gurman GM. Prolonged apnea after succinylcholine in a case treated with cytotoxics for cancer. Anesth Analg 1972;51:761.
234. Dretchen KL, Morgenroth VH, Standaert FG et al. Azathioprine: effects on neuromuscular transmission. Anesthesiology 1976;45:604.
235. Hill GE, Wong KC. Potentiation of succinylcholine neuromuscular blockade by lithium carbonate. Anesthesiology 1976;44:439.
236. Hill GE, Wong KC. Lithium carbonate and neuromuscular blocking agents. Anesthesiology 1977;46:122.
237. Schou M. Possible mechanisms of action of lithium salts: approaches and perspectives. Biochem Soc Trans 1973;1:81.
238. Whittaker M, Spencer R. Plasma cholinesterase variants in patients having lithium therapy. Clin Chim Acta 1977;75:421.
239. Tewfik GI. Trimetaphan, its effect on the pseudocholinesterase level in man. Anaesthesia 1957;12:326.

240. Sklar GS, Lanks KW. Effects of trimetaphan and sodium nitroprusside on hydrolysis of succinylcholine in vitro. Anesthesiology 1977;47:31.
241. Poulon TJ, James FM III, Lockridge O. Prolonged apnea following trimetaphan and succinylcholine. Anesthesiology 1979;50:54.
242. Nakamura K, Hatano Y, Mori K. The site of action of trimetaphan-induced neuromuscular blockade in isolated rat and frog muscle. Acta Anaesthesiol Scand 1988;32:125.
243. Foldes FF, Hilmer NR, Molloy ER et al. Potentiation of the neuromuscular effect of succinylcholine by hexafluorenium. Anesthesiology 1960;21:50.
244. Gordh T, Waklin A. Potentiation of the neuromuscular effect of succinylcholine by tetrahydroamin-acridine. Acta Anaesthesiol Scand 1961;5:55.
245. Walts LF, De Angelis J, Dillon JB. Clinical studies of the interaction of hexafluorenium and succinylcholine in man. Anesthesiology 1970;33:503.
246. Radney PA, El-Gaweet E-S, Novakovic M et al. Prevention of succinylcholine induced hyperkalaemia by neurolept anaesthesia and hexafiuorenium in anephric patients. Anaesthesist 1981;30:334.
247. Chasapakis G, Dimas C. Possible interaction between muscle relaxants and the kallikrein-trypsin inactivator 'Trasylol': report of three cases. Br J Anaesth 1966;38:838.
248. Miller RD, Way WL, Katzung BG. The potentiation of neuromuscular blocking agents by quinidine. Anesthesiology 1967;28:1036.
249. Durant NN, Nguyen N, Katz RL. Potentiation of neuromuscular blockade by verapamil. Anesthesiology 1984; 60:298.
250. Avery GS. Checklist to potential clinically important interactions. Drugs 1973;5:187.
251. Matsuo S, Rao DBS, Chaudry J et al. Interaction of muscle relaxants and local anesthetics at the neuromuscular junction Anesth Analg 1978;57:580.
252. Usubiaga JE, Wikinski JF. Interaction of intravenous administered procaine, lidocaine and succinylcholine in the anesthetized subject. Anesth Analg 1967;46:39.
253. Ivankovich AD, Sidell N, Cairoli JV et al. Dual action of pancuronium on succinylcholine block. Can Anaesth Soc J 1977;24:228.
254. D'Hollander AA, Agoston S, De Ville A et al. Clinical and pharmacological actions of a bolus injection of suxamethonium: two phenomena of distinct duration. Br J Anaesth 1983;55:131.
255. Katz RL. Modification of the action of pancuronium by succinylcholine and halothane. Anesthesiology 1971;35:602.
256. Walts LF, Dillon JB. Clinical studies of the interaction between *d*-tubocurarine and succinylcholine. Anesthesiology 1969;31:39.
257. Gissen AJ, Katz RL, Karis JH et al. Neuromuscular block in man during prolonged arterial infusion with succinylcholine. Anesthesiology 1966;27:242.
258. Bovill JG, Coppel DL, Dundee JW, Moore J. Current status of ketamine anaesthesia. Lancet 1971;ii:1285.
259. Tsai SK, Lee C, Tran B. Ketamine enhances phase I and phase II neuromuscular block of succinylcholine. Can J Anaesth 1989;36:120.
260. Amaki Y, Nagashima H, Radnay PA, Foldes FF. Ketamine interaction with neuromuscular blocking agents in the phrenic nerve—hemidiaphragm preparation of the rat. Anesth Analg 1978;57:238.
261. Hilgenberg JC, Stoelting RK. Characteristics of succinylcholine-produced phase II neuromuscular block during enflurane, halothane, and fentanyl anesthesia. Anesth Analg 1981;60:192.
262. Donati F, Bevan DR. Long-term succinylcholine infusion during isoflurane anesthesia. Anesthesiology 1983; 58:6.
263. Cozanitis DA, Dundee JW, Khan MM. Comparative study of atropine and glycopyrrolate on suxamethonium-induced changes in cardiac rate and rhythm. Br J Anaesth 1980;52:291.
264. Ali HH. Savarese JJ. Monitoring of neuromuscular function. Anesthesiology 1976;45:216.
265. Miller RD, Way WL, Dolan WM et al. The dependence of pancuronium and *d*-tubocurarine induced neuromuscular blockades on alveolar concentrations of halothane and Forane. Anesthesiology 1972;37:573.
266. Gencarelli PJ, Miller RD, Eger EI et al. Decreasing enflurane concentrations and *d*-tubocurarine neuromuscular block. Anesthesiology 1982;56:192.
267. Eger EI. Isoflurane: a review. Anesthesiology 1981;55:559.
268. Stanski DR, Ham J, Miller RD et al. Time-dependent increase in sensitivity *d*-tubocurarine during enflurane anesthesia in man. Anesthesiology 1980;52:483.
269. Delisle S, Bevan DR. Impaired neostigmine antagonism of pancuronium during enflurane anaesthesia in man. Br J Anaesth 1982;54:441.
270. Waud BE. Decrease in dose requirement of *d*-tubocurarine by volatile anesthetics. Anesthesiology 1979;51:298.
271. Rupp SM, Miller RD, Gencarelli PJ. Vecuronium induced neuromuscular blockade during enflurane, isoflurane and halothane anesthesia in humans. Anesthesiology 1984;60:102.
272. Cannon JE, Fahey MR, Castagnoli BA et al. Continuous infusion of vecuronium: the effect of anesthetic agents. Anesthesiology 1987;67:503.
273. Swen J, Rashkovsky OM, Ket JM et al. Interaction between nondepolarizing neuromuscular blocking agents and inhalational anesthetics. Anesth Analg 1989;69:752.
274. Forbes AR, Cohen NH, Eger EI II. Pancuronium reduces halothane requirement in man. Anesth Analg 1979;58:497.
275. Fahey MR, Sessler DI, Cannon JE et al. Atracurium, vecuronium, and pancuronium do not alter the minimum alveolar concentration of halothane in humans. Anesthesiology 1989;71:53.
276. Toft P, Helbo-Hansen S. Interaction of ketamine with atracurium. Br J Anaesth 1989;62:319.
277. Johnston RR, Miller RD, Way WL. The interaction of ketamine with *d*-tubocurarine, pancuronium and succinylcholine in man. Anesth Analg 1974;53:496.
278. Robertson EN, Fragen RJ, Booij LHDJ et al. Some effects of diisopropyl phenol (ICI 35 868) on the pharmacodynamics of atracurium and vecuronium in anaesthetized man. Br J Anaesth 1983;55:723.
279. Boros M, Chaudhry AI, Nagashima H et al. Myoneural effects of pethidine and droperidol. Br J Anaesth 1984; 56:195.
280. Driessen JJ, Vree TB, Van Egmond J et al. In vitro interaction of diazepam and oxazepam with pancuronium and suxamethonium. Br J Anaesth 1984;56:1131.
281. Wali FA. Myorelaxant effect of diazepam: interactions with neuromuscular blocking agents and cholinergic drugs. Acta Anaesthesiol Scand 1985;29:785.

282. Driessen JJ, Vree TB, Van Egmond J et al. Interaction of midazolam with two non-depolarizing neuromuscular blocking drugs in the rat in vivo sciatic nerve tibialis anterior muscle preparation. Br J Anaesth 1985;57:1089.
283. Asbury AJ, Henderson PD, Brown BH et al. Effect of diazepam on pancuronium-induced neuromuscular blockade maintained by a feedback system. Br J Anaesth 1981;53:859.
284. Cronnelly R, Morris RB, Miller RD. Comparison of thiopental and midazolam on the neuromuscular responses to succinylcholine or pancuronium in humans. Anesth Analg 1983;62:75.
285. Driessen JJ, Crul JF, Vree TB et al. Benzodiazepines and neuromuscular blocking drugs in patients. Acta Anaesthesiol Scand 1986;30:642.
286. Ngai SH. Action of general anesthetics in producing muscle relaxation-interaction of anesthetics with relaxants. In: Katz RL, ed. Muscle Relaxants. Amsterdam: Excerpta Medica, 1975;279.
287. Lebowitz PW, Ramsey FM, Savarese JJ et al. Potentiation of neuromuscular blockade in man produced by combinations of pancuronium and metocurine or pancuronium and *d*-tubocurarine, Anesth Analg 1980;59:604.
288. Waud BE, Waud DR. Interaction among agents that block end-plate depolarization competitively. Anesthesiology 1985;63:4.
289. Rashkovsky OM, Agoston S, Ket JM. Interaction between pancuronium bromide and vecuronium bromide. Br J Anaesth 1985;57:1063.
290. Smith CL, Hunter JM, Jones RS. Vecuronium infusions in patients with renal failure in an ITU. Anaesthesia 1987;42:387.
291. Op de Coul AAW, Lambregts PCLA, Koeman J et al. Neuromuscular complications in patients given Pavulon (pancuronium bromide) during artificial ventilation. Clin Neurol Neurosurg 1985;87:17.
292. Yate PM, Flynn PJ, Amold RW et al. Clinical experience and plasma laudanosine concentrations during the infusion of atracurium in the intensive therapy unit. Br J Anaesth 1987;59:211.
293. Rutledge ML, Hawkins EP, Langston C. Skeletal muscle growth failure induced in premature newborn infants by prolonged pancuronium treatment. J Pediatr 1986;109:883.
294. Torres CF, Maniscalco WM, Agostinelli T. Muscle weakness and atrophy following prolonged paralysis with pancuronium bromide in neonates. Ann Neurol 1985;18:403.
295. Vandenbrom RHG, Wierda JMKH. Pancuronium bromide in the intensive care unit: a case of overdose. Anesthesiology 1988;69:996.
296. Berg DK, Hall ZW. Increased extrajunctional acetylcholine sensitivity produced by chronic post-synaptic neuromuscular blockade. J Physiol (London) 1975;244:659.
297. Fischbach GD, Robbins N. Effect of chronic disuse of rat soleus neuromuscular junctions on postsynaptic membrane. J Neurophysiol 1971;34:562.
298. Rao TLK, Jacobs HK. Pulmonary function following 'pretreatment' dose of pancuronium in volunteers. Anesth Analg 1980;59:659.
299. Engbaek J, Viby-Mogensen J. Precurarization—a hazard to the patient? Acta Anaesthesiol Scand 1984;28:61.
300. Musich J, Walts LF. Pulmonary aspiration after a priming dose of vecuronium. Anesthesiology 1986;64:517.
301. Viby-Mogensen J, Chraemmer-Jørgensen B, Ørding H. Residual curarization in the recovery room. Anesthesiology 1979;50:539.
302. Lennmarken C, Löfström JB. Partial curarization in the post operative period. Acta Anaesthesiol Scand 1984;28:260.
303. Stovner J. Clinical Use of Relaxants in Europe. In: Katz RL, ed. Muscle Relaxants. Amsterdam; Excerpta Medica, 1975;268.
304. Fiset P, Donati F, Balendran P et al. Vecuronium is more potent in Montreal than in Paris. Can J Anaesth 1991;39:717.
305. Shayevitz JR, Matteo RS. Decreased sensitivity to metocurine in patients with upper motoneuron disease. Anesth Analg 1985;64:767.
306. Moorthy SS, Hilgenberg JC. Resistance to non-depolarizing muscle relaxants in paretic upper extremities of patients with residual hemiplegia. Anesth Analg 1980;59:624.
307. Graham DH. Monitoring neuromuscular block may be unreliable in patients with upper-motor-neuron lesions. Anesthesiology, 1980;52:74.
308. Laycock JRD, Smith CE, Donati F, Bevan DR. Sensitivity of the adductor pollicis and diaphragm muscles to atracurium in a hemiplegic patient. Anesthesiology 1987;67:851.
309. Brett RS, Schmidt JH, Gage JS et al. Measurement of acetylcholine receptor concentration in skeletal muscle from a patient with multiple sclerosis and resistance to atracurium. Anesthesiology 1987;66:837.
310. Hogue CW, Itani MS, Martyn JAJ. Resistance to *d*-tubocurarine in lower motor neurone injury is dated to increased acetylcholine receptors at the neuromuscular junction. Anesthesiology 1990;73:703.
311. Enoki T, Naito Y, Hirokawa Y et al. Marked sensitivity to pancuronium in a patient without clinical manifestations of myasthenia gravis. Anesth Analg 1989;69:840.
312. Rosenbaum KJ, Neigh JL, Strobd GE. Sensitivity to nondepolarizing muscle relaxants in amyotrophic lateral sclerosis: report of two cases. Anesthesiology 1971;35:638.
313. Robertson JA. Ocular muscular dystrophy. Anaesthesia 1984;39:251.
314. Brown JC, Charlton JE. Study of sensitivity to curare in certain neurological disorders using a regional technique. J Neurol Neurosurg Psychiatry 1975;38:34.
315. Moss J, Roscow CE, Savarese JJ et al. Role of histamine in the hypotensive action of *d*-tubocurarine in humans. Anesthesiology 1981;55:19.
316. Hatano Y, Arai T, Noda J et al. Contribution of prostacyclin to *d*-tubocurarine-induced hypotension in humans. Anesthesiology 1990;72:28.
317. Munger ML, Miller RD, Stevens WC. The dependence of *d*-tubocurarine-induced hypotension on the alveolar concentration of halothane and the presence of nitrous oxide. Anesthesiology 1974;40:442.
318. Stoelting GK, McCammon RL, Hilgenberg JC. Changes in blood pressure with varying rates of administration of *d*-tubocurarine Anesth Analg 1980;59:697.
319. Pavlin EG, Holle RH, Schoene RB. Recovery of airway protection compared with ventilation in humans after paralysis with curare. Anesthesiology 1989;70:381.
320. Knill RL. *d*-Tubocurarine and upper airway obstruction: a historical perspective. Anesthesiology 1989;71:480.
321. Warner LO, Martino JD, Davidson PJ, Beach TP. Negative pressure pulmonary oedema: a potential hazard of muscle relaxants in awake infants. Can J Anaesth 1990; 37:580.
322. Brown RE. Negative pressure pulmonary edema. In: Berry FA ed. Anesthetic Management of Difficult and Routine Pediatric Patients. New York; Churchill Livingstone, 1986;169.

323. Matteo RS, Pua EK, Khambatta HJ et al. Cerebrospinal fluid levels of *d*-tubocurarine in man. Anesthesiology 1977; 46:396.

324. Britt BA, Webb GE, LeDuc C. Malignant hyperthermia induced by curare. Can Anaesth Soc J 1974;21:371.

325. Stovner J, Theodorsen L, Bjelke E. Sensitivity to tubocurarine and alcuronium with special reference to plasma protein pattern. Br J Anaesth 1971;43:385.

326. Duvaldestin P. Common disease states affecting the action of neuromuscular blocking drugs. In: Agoston S, Bowman WC, eds. Muscle Relaxants Monographs in Anaesthesiology, Vol. 19. Amsterdam: Elsevier Science Publishers BV, 1990;253.

327. Brown TCK, Gregory M, Bell B, Campbell PC. Liver tumours and muscle relaxants: electromyographic studies in children. Anaesthesia 1987;42:1284.

328. Miller RD, Eger EI II. Early and late relative potencies of pancuronium and *d*-tubocurarine in man. Anesthesiology 1976;44:297.

329. Cohen EN, Brewer WH, Smith D. The metabolism and elimination of *d*-tubocurarine-H3. Anesthesiology 1967; 28:309.

330. Riordan DD, Gilbertson AA. Prolonged curarization in a patient with renal failure. Br J Anaesth 1971;43:506.

331. Martyn JAJ, Szyfelbein SK, Ali HH et al. Increased *d*-tubocurarine requirement following major thermal injury. Anesthesiology 1980;52:352.

332. Martyn JAJ, Matteo RS, Greenblatt DJ et al. Pharmacokinetics of *d*-tubocurarine in patients with thermal injury. Anesth Analg 1982;61:241.

333. Al-Abrak MH, Samuel JR. Effects of general anaesthesia on the intraocular pressure in man: comparison of tubocurarine and pancuronium in nitrous oxide and oxygen. Br J Ophthalmol 1974;58:806.

334. Older PO, Harris JM. Placental transfer of tubocurarine. Br J Anaesth 1968;40:459.

335. Ahmed W. The effect of relaxant drugs on the growth and development of bone and cartilage in the chick embryo. Ain Shams Med J 1970;21:679.

336. Drachman DB, Coulombre AF. Experimental club-foot and arthrogryposis multiplex congenita. Lancet 1962;ii:523.

337. Ghoneim MM, Long JP. The interaction between magnesium and other neuromuscular blocking agents. Anesthesiology 1970;32:23.

338. Giesecke AH, Morris RE, Dalton MD et al. Of magnesium, muscle relaxants, toxemic parturients, and cats. Anesth Analg 1968;47:689.

339. Telivuo L, Katz RL. The effects of modern intravenous local analgesics on respiration during partial neuromuscular block in man. Anaesthesia 1970;25:30.

340. Harrah MD, Way WL, Katzung BG. The interaction of *d*-tubocurarine with antiarrhythmic drugs. Anesthesiogy 1970;33:406

341. Katz RL, Gissen AJ. Effects of intravenous and intraarterial procaine and Lidocaine on neuromuscular transmission in man. Acta Anaesthesiol Scand Suppl 1969;36:103.

342. Welch GW, Waud BE. Effect of bretylium on neuromuscular transmission. Anaesth Analg 1982;61:442.

343. Healy TEJ, O'Shea M, Massey J. Disopyramide and neuromuscular transmission. Br J Anaesth 1981;52:495.

344. Jones SVP, Marshall IG. Non-competitive effects of disopyramide at the neuromuscular junction: evidence for endplate ion channel block. Br J Anaesth 1987;59:776.

345. Baurain M, Barvais L, d'Hollander A, Hennart D. Impairment of the antagonism of vecuronium-induced paralysis and intraoperative disopyramide administration. Anaesthesia 1989;44:34.

346. Jones RM, Cashman JN, Casson WR, Broadbent MP. Verapamil potentiation of neuromuscular blockade: failure of reversal with neostigmine but prompt reversal with edrophonium. Anesth Analg 1985;64:1021.

347. Bikhazi GB, Leung I, Flores C et al. Potentiation of neuromuscular blocking agents by calcium channel blockers in rats. Anesth Analg 1988;67:1.

348. Miller RD, Sohn YJ, Matteo RS. Enhancement of *d*-tubocurarine neuromuscular blockade by diuretics in man. Anesthesiology 1976;45:442.

349. Scappaticci KA, Ham, JA, Sohn YJ et al. Effects of furosemide on the neuromuscular junction. Anesthesiology 1982;57:381.

350. Pollard BJ, Randall NPC, Pleuvry BF. Doxapram and the neuromuscular junction. Br J Anaesth 1989;62:664.

351. Gramstad L. Atracurium, vecuronium and pancuronium in end-stage renal failure. Br J Anaesth 1987;59:995.

352. Maestrone E. Interaction of neuromuscular blocking agents in surgical patients. In: Agoston S, Bowman WC, eds. Muscle Relaxants. Monographs in Anaesthesiology, Vol 19. Amsterdam: Elsevier, 1990;199.

353. Stovner J, Oftedal N, Holmboe J. The inhibition of cholinesterases by pancuronium. Br J Anaesth 1975;47:949.

354. Quader MA, Healy TEJ. Muscle fibrillation following thiopentone and pancuronium bromide. Anesthesia 1977; 32:644.

355. Coleman AJ, Downing LW, Leary WP et al. The immediate cardiovascular effects of pancuronium, alcuronium and tubocurarine in man. Anaesthesia 1972;27:415.

356. Saxena R, Bonta FL. Mechanism of selective cardiac vagolytic action of pancuronium bromide: specific blockade of cardiac muscarinic receptors. Eur J Pharmacol 1970;11:332.

357. Domenech JS, Garcia RC, Sasian JMR et al. Pancuronium bromide: an indirect sympathomimetic agent. Br J Anaesth 1976;48:1148.

358. Cardan E, Nana A, Domokos M. Blood catecholamine changes after pancuronium bromide administration. In: Abstracts, X Congress of the Scandinavian Society of Anesthesiologists, Lund, 1971;57.

359. Quintana A. Effect of pancuronium bromide on the adrenergic reactivity of the isolated rat vas deferens. Eur J Pharmacol 1977;46:275.

360. Docherty JR, McGrath JC. Potentiation of cardiac sympathetic nerve responses in vivo by pancuronium bromide. Br J Pharmacol 1977;61:472.

361. Docherty JR, McGrath JC. Sympathomimetic effects of pancuronium bromide on the cardiovascular system of the pithed rat: a comparison with the effects of drugs blocking the neuronal uptake of noradrenaline. Br J Pharmacol 1978;64:589.

362. Seed RF, Chamberlain JH. Myocardial stimulation by pancuronium bromide. Br J Anaesth 1977;49:401.

363. Edwards RP, Miller RD, Roizen MF et al. Cardiac responses to imipramine and pancuronium during anesthesia with halothane or enflurane. Anesthesiology 1979;50:421.

364. Belani KG, Anderson WW, Buckley JJ. Adverse drug interaction involving pancuronium and aminophylline. Anesth Analg 1982;61:473.

365. Stirt JA, Sullivan SF. Aminophylline. Anesth Analg 1981;60:587.

366. Hirano S, Ueki O, Misaki T, Hisazumi H. Severe hypertension and tachycardia associated with pancuronium bromide in a patient with asymptomatic pheochromocytoma. Acta Urol Jpn 1984;30:709.
367. Jones RM, Hill AB. Severe hypertension associated with pancuronium in a patient with a phaeochromocytoma. Can Anaesth Soc J 1981;28:394.
368. Thomson IR, Putnius CL. Adverse effects of pancuronium during high-dose fentanyl anesthesia for coronary artery bypass grafting. Anesthesioloy 1985;62:708.
369. Heinonen J, Takkunen O. Bradycardia during antagonism of pancuronium-induced neuromuscular block. Br J Anaesth 1977;49:H09.
370. Peduto VA, Gungui P, DiMartino MR, Napoleone M. Accidental subarachnoid injection of pancuronium. Anesth Analg 1989;69:516.
371 Waterman PM, Albin MS, Smith RB. Malignant hyperthermia; a case report. Anesth Analg 1980;59:220.
372. Duvaldestin P, Agoston S, Henzel D et al. Pancuronium pharmacokinetics in patients with liver cirrhosis. Br J Anaesth 1978;50:H31.
373. Freeman J, Lesko SM, Mitchell AA et al. Hyperbilirubinemia following exposure to pancuronium bromide in newborns. Dev Pharmacol Ther 1990;14:209.
374. Somogyi AA, Shanks CA, Triggs EJ. The effect of renal failure on the disposition and neuromuscular blocking action of pancuronium bromide. Eur J Clin Pharmacol 1977;12:23.
375. Bevan DR, Archer D, Donati F et al. Antagonism of pancuronium in renal failure; no recurarization. Br J Anaesth 1982;54:63.
376. Yamashita M, Shiga T, Matsuki A et al. Unusual resistance to pancuronium in severely burned patients: case reports. Can Anaesth Soc J 1982;29:630.
377. Heath ML. Bronchospasm in an asthmatic patient following pancuronium. Anaesthesia 1973;28:437.
378. Buckland RW, Avery AF. Histamine release following pancuronium. Br J Anaesth 1973;45:518.
379. Mishima S, Yamamura T. Anaphylactoid reaction to pancuronium. Anesth Analg 1984;63:865.
380. Bonnet MC, Julia JM, Chardon P et al. À propos d'un cas d'anaphylaxie au pancuronium. Cah Anesth*siol 1986; 34:253.
381. Azar I, Cottrell J, Gupta B, Turndorf H. Furosemide facilitates recovery of evoked twitch response after pancuronium. Anesth Analg 1980;59:55.
382. Crosby E, Robblee JA. Cyclosporine-pancuronium interaction in a patient with a renal allograft. Can J Anaesth 1988;35:300.
383. Gramstad L, Gjerlow JA, Hysing ES, Rugstad HE. Interaction of cyclosporin and its solvent, cremophor, with atracurium and vecuronium. Br J Anaesth 1986;58:1149.
384. Borden H, Clarke MT, Katz H. The use of pancuronium bromide in patients receiving lithium carbonate. Can Anaesth Soc J 1974;21:79.
385. Waud BE, Farrell L, Waud DR. Lithium and neuromuscular transmission. Anesth Analg 1982;61:399.
386. Doll DC, Rosenberg H. Antagonism of neuromuscular blockade by theophylline. Anesth Analg 1979;58:139.
387. Glisson SN, El-Etr AA, Lim R. Prolongation of pancuronium-induced neuromuscular blockade by intravenous infusion of nitroglycerin. Anesthesiology 1979;51:47.
388. Glisson SN, Sanchez MM, El-Etr AA et al. Nitroglycerin and the neuromuscular blockade produced by gallamine, succinylcholine, *d*-tubocurarine, and pancuronium. Anesth Analg 1980;59:117.
389. Schwarz S, Agoston S, Houwertjes MC. Does intravenous infusion of nitroglycerin potentiate pancuronium- and vecuronium-induced neuromuscular blockade? Anesth Analg 1986;65:156.
390. Meyers EF. Partial recovery from pancuronium neuromuscular blockade following hydrocortisone administration. Anesthesiology 1977;46:148.
391. Laflin MJ. Interaction of pancuronium and corticosteroids. Anesthesiology 1977;47:471.
392. Wilson RW, Ward MD, Johns TR. Corticosteroids: a direct effect at the neuromuscular junction. Neurology 1974;24:1091.
393. Chen J, Kim YD, Dubois M et al. The increased requirement of pancuronium in neurosurgical patients receiving dilantin chronically. Anesthesiology 1983;59:A288.
394. Roth S, Ebrahim ZY. Resistance to pancuronium in patients receiving carbamazepine. Anesthesiology 1987; 66:691.
395. Siegle RL. Neonatal gasless abdomen: another cause. Am J Roentgenol 1980;133:522.
396. Meijer DKF, Weitering JG, Vermeer GA et al. Comparative pharmacokinetics of *d*-tubocurarine and metocurine in man. Anesthesiology 1979;51:402.
397. Savarese JJ, Ali HH, Antonio RP. The clinical pharmacology of metocurine. Anesthesiology 1977;47:277.
398. Hughes R, Chapple DJ. Effects of non-depolarizing neuromuscular blocking agents on peripheral autonomic mechanisms in cats. Br J Anaesth 1976;48:59.
399. McCullough LS, Stone WA, Delaunois AL et al. The effect of dimethyl tubocurarine iodide on cardiovascular parameters, post-ganglionic sympathetic activity and histamine release. Anesth Analg 1972;51:554.
400. Basta SJ, Savarese JJ, Ali HH et al. Histamine-releasing potencies of atracurium, dimethyl tubocurarine and tubocurarine. Br J Anaesth 1983;55:1O5S.
401. Hughes R, Chapple DJ. Cardiovascular and neuromuscular effects of dimethyl tubocurarine in anaesthetized cats and rhesus monkeys. Br J Anaesth 1976;48:847.
402. Hughes R, Ingram GS, Payne JP. Studies on dimethyl tubocurarine in anaesthetized man. Br J Anaesth 1976; 48:969.
403. Brotherton WP, Matteo RS. Pharmacokinetics and pharmacodynammcs of metocurine in humans with and without renal failure. Anesthesiology 1981;55:273.
404. Martyn JAJ, Goudsouzian NG, Matteo RS et al. Metocurine requirements and plasma concentrations in burned paediatric patients. Br J Anaesth 1983;55:263.
405. Martyn JAJ, Matteo RS, Szyfelbein SK et al. Unprecedented resistance to neuromuscular blocking effects of metocurine with persistence after complete recovery in a burned patient. Anesth Analg 1982;61:614.
406. Ornstein E, Matteo RS, Young WL et al. Resistance to metocurine in patients receiving phenytoin. Anesthesiology 1984;61:A314.
407. Harrison GR, Thompson ID. Adverse reaction to methohexitone and gallamine. Anaesthesia 1981;36:40.
408. Harrison JF, Bird AG. Anaphylaxis to precurarising doses of gallamine triethiodide. Anaesthesia 1986;41:600.
409. Eisele JH, Marta JA, Davis HS. Quantitative aspects of the chronotropic and neuromuscular effects of gallamine in anesthetized man. Anesthesiology 1971;35:630.
410. Stoelting RK. Hemodynamic effects of gallamine during halothane-nitrous oxide anesthesia. Anesthesiology 1973; 39:645.

411. Kennedy BR, Farman JV. Cardiovascular effects of gallamine triethiodide in man. Br J Anaesth 1968;40:773.
412. Riker WF, Wescoe WC. The pharmacology of Flaxedil with observations on certain analogs. Ann NY Acad Sci 1951;54:373.
413. Brown BB, Crout JR. The sympathomimetic effect of gallamine on the heart. J Pharmacol Exp Ther 1970;172:266.
414. Vercruysse P, Bossuyt P, Hanegreefs G et al. Gallamine and pancuronium inhibit prejunctional and post-junctional muscarinic receptors in canine saphenous veins. J Pharmacol Exp Ther 1979;209:225.
415. Reitan JA, Fraser AI, Eisele JH. Lack of cardiac inotropic effects of gallamine in anesthetized man. Anesth Analg 1973;52:974.
416. Raaflaub J, Frey P. Zur Pharmakokinetik von Diallylnortoxiferin beim Menschen. Arznzeim-Forsch 1972; 22:73.
417. Havill JH, Mee AD, Wallace MR et al. Prolonged curarisation in the presence of renal impairment. Anaesth Intensive Care 1978;6:234.
418. Chan CS, Yeung ML. Anaphylactic reaction to alcuronium—a case report. Br J Anaesth 1972;44:103.
419. Rowley RW. Hypersensitivity reaction to diallyl nortoxiferine (Alloferine). Anaesth Intensive Care 1975;3:74.
420. Fisher MMcD, Hallowes RC, Wilson RM. Anaphylaxis to alcuronium. Anaesth Intensive Care 1978;6:125.
421. Pandit SK, Dundee JW, Stevenson HM. A clinical comparison of pancuronium with tubocurarine and alcuronium in major cardiothoracic surgery. Anesth Analg 1971;50:926.
422. Panning B, Peest D, Kirchner E, Schedel I. Anaphylactoid Schock mit Alloferin. Anaesthesist 1985;34:211.
423. Fadel R, Herpin-Richard N, Rassemont R et al. Choc anaphylactique à la diallylnortoxiferine: étude clinique et immunologique. Ann Fr Anesth Réanim 1982;1:531.
424. Plötz J, Schreiber W. Vergleichende Untersuchung von Atracurium und Alcuronium zur Intubation älterer Patienten in Halothannarkose. Anaesthesist 1984;33:548.
425. Beemer GH, Dennis WL, Platt PR et al. Adverse reactions to atracurium and alcuronium. A prospective surveillance study. Br J Anaesth 1988;61:680.
426. Baraka A. A comparative study between diallylnortoxiferine and tubocurarine. Br J Anaesth 1967;39:624.
427. Coleman AJ, Downing JW, Leary WP et al. The immediate cardiovascular effects of pancuronium, alcuronium and tubocurarine in man. Anaesthesia 1972;27:415.
428. Brändli FR. Pancuronium and Alcuronium: Ein klinischer Vergleich. Prakt Andsth 1976;11:239.
429. Tammisto T, Welling I. The effect of alcuronium and tubocurarine on blood pressure and heart rate. Br J Anaesth 1969;40:113.
430. Sarubin J. Erhöhter Bedarf an Alloferin bei Verbrennungspatientm Anaesthesist, 1982;31:392.
431. Ho PC, Stephens ID, Triggs EJ. Caesarian section and placental transfer of alcuronium. Anesth Intensive Care 1981;9:113.
432. Thomas J, Climie CR, Mather LE. The placental transfer of alcuronium. Br J Anaesth 1969;41:297.
433. Fried MJ, Protheroe DT. D-Penicillamine induced myasthenia gravis: its relevance for the anaesthetist. Br J Anaesth 1986;58:1191.
434. Blanloeil Y, Baron D, Gazeau MF, Nicolas F. Curarisation prolongée au cours d'un syndrôme myasthénique induit par la D-pénicillamine. Anesth Analg Reanim 1980;37:441.
435. Alexander JP. Adverse reactions following fazadinium—thiopentone induction. Anaesthesia 1979;34:661.
436. Baldassare M, Mastroianni A. Su un grave caso di shock da bromuro di fazadinio. Acta Anaesthesiol Ital 1983;34:91.
437. Marshall IG. The ganglion blocking and vagolytic actions of three short-acting neuromuscular blocking drugs in the cat. J Pharm Pharmacol 1973;25:530.
438. Hughes R, Payne JP, Sugai N. Studies on fazadinium bromide (AH 8165): a new non-depolarizing neuromuscular blocking agent. Can Anaesth Soc J 1976;23:36.
439. Schuh FT. Clinical neuromuscular pharmacology of AH-8165D, an azobisarylimidazo-pyridinium compound. Anaesthesist 1975;24:151.
440. Lyons SM, Clarke RSJ, Young HSA. A clinical comparison of AH 8165 and pancuronium as muscle relaxants in patients undergoing cardiac surgery. Br J Anaesth 1975; 47:725.
441. Lienhart A, Tauvent A, Guggiari M. Effets hémodynamiques des curares. In: Curares et Curarisation, Vol 1. Paris: Librairie Arnette—Amsterdam: Excerpta Medica, 1979;384.
442. Pinaud M, Arnould F, Souron R et al. Influence of cardiac rhythm on the haemodynamic effects of fazadinium in patients with heart failure. Br J Anaesth 1983;55:507.
443. Bertrand JC, Duvaldestin P, Henzel D, Desmonts JM. Quantitative assessment of placental transfer of fazadinium in obstetric anaesthesia. Acta Anaesthesiol Scand 1980; 24:135.
444. Rainaldi MP, Busi T, Melloni C, Boschi S. Pharmacokinetics and placental transmission of fazadinium in elective caesarean sections. Acta Anaesthesiol Scand 1984;28:222.
445. Mirakhur RK, Ferres CJ, Clarke RSJ et al. Clinical evaluation of Org NC 45. Br J Anaesth 1983;55:119.
446. Foldes FF, Bencini A, Newton D. Influence of halothane and enflurane on the neuromuscular effects of Org NC 45 in man. Br J Anaesth 1980;52(Suppl 1):645.
447. Ording H, Viby-Mogensen J. Dose response curves for Org NC 45 and pancuronium. Acta Anaesthesiol Scand 1981;25(Suppl 72):73.
448. Cannon JE, Fahey MR, Castagnoli KP et al. Continuous infusion of vecuronium: the effect of anesthetic agents. Anesthesiology 1987;67:503.
449. Symposium on Org NC 45. Br J Anaesth 1980; 52(Suppl 1).
450. Lee-Son S, Waud BE, Waud DR. A comparison of the neuromuscular blocking and vagolytic effects of Org NC 45 and pancuronium. Anesthesiology 1981;55:12.
451. McIndewar IC, Marshall RJ. Interactions between the neuromuscular blocking drug Org NC 45 and some anaesthetic, analgesic and antimicrobial agents. Br J Anaesth 1981;53:785.
452. Durant NN, Marshall IG, Savage DS et al. The neuromuscular and autonomic blocking activities of pancuronium, Org NC 45, and other pancuronium analogues in the cat. J Pharm Pharmacol 1979;31:831.
453. Marshall RJ, McGrath JC, Miller RD et al. Comparison of the cardiovascular actions of Org NC 45 with those produced by other non-depolarizing neuromuscular blocking agents in experimental animals. Br J Anaesth 1980;52:21S.
454. Booij LHDJ, Krieg N, Crul JF. Intradermal histamine releasing effect caused by Org NC 45: a comparison with pancuronium, metocurine and *d*-tubocurarine. Acta Anaesthesiol Scand 1980;24:393.
455. Robertson EN, Booij LHDJ, Fragen RJ et al. Intradermal histamine release by 3 muscle relaxants. Acta Anaesthesiol Scand 1983;27:203.

456. Basta SJ, Savarese JJ, Ali HH et al. Vecuronium does not alter serum histamine within the clinical dose range. Anesthesiology 1983);59:A273.
457. Goudsouzian NG, Young ET, Moss J, Liu LMP. Histamine release during the administration of atracurium or vecuronium in children. Br J Anaesth 1986;58:1229.
458. Clayton DG, Watkins J. Histamine release with vecuronium (Letter to Editor). Anaesthesia 1984;39:1143.
459. Spence AG, Barnetson R StC. Reaction to vecuronium bromide (Letter to Editor). Lancet 1985;i:979.
460. Lavery GG, Hewitt AJ, Kenny NT. Possible histamine release after vecuronium. (Letter to Editor). Anaesthesia 1985;40:389.
461. Thacker MA, Boon von Ochssee D. Anaphylactoid reaction to vecuronium (Letter to Editor). Anaesth Intensive Care 1988;16:129.
462. Treuren BC, Buckley DHF. Anaphylactoid reaction to vecuronium (Letter to Editor). Br J Anaesth 1990;64:125.
463. Conil C, Bornet JL, Jean-Noël M et al. Choc anaphylactique au pancuronium et au vécuronium. Ann Fr Anesth Réanim 1985;4:241.
464. Holt AW, Vedig AE. Anaphylaxis following vecuronium (Letter to Editor). Anaesth Intensive Care 1988;16:378.
465. Barnes PK, Brindle-Smith G, White WD et al. Comparison of the effects of Org NC 45 and pancuronium bromide on heart rate and arterial pressure in anaesthetized man. Br J Anaesth 1982;54:435.
466. Gregoretti SM, Sohn YJ, Sia RL. Heart rate and blood pressure changes after Org NC 45 (vecuronium) and pancuronium during halothane and enflurane anesthesia. Anesthesiology 1982;56:392.
467. Lienhart A, Desnault H, Guggiari M et al. Vecuronium bromide: dose response curve and haemodynamic effects in anaesthetized man. In: Agoston S, ed. Clinical Experiences with Norcuron. Amsterdam: Excerpta Medica, 1982;46.
468. Morris RB, Cahalan MK, Miller RD et al. The cardiovascular effects of vecuronium (Org NC 45) and pancuronium in patients undergoing coronary artery bypass grafting. Anesthesiology 1983;58:438.
469. Salmenpera M, Peltola K, Takkunen O et al. Cardiovascular effects of pancuronium and vecuronium during high-dose fentanyl anesthesia. Anesth Analg 1983;62:1059.
470. Starr NJ, Sethna DH, Estafanous FG. Bradycardia and asystole following the rapid administration of sufentanil with vecuronium. Anesthesiology 1986;64:521.
471. Gencarelli PJ, Roizen MF, Miller RD et al. Org NC 45 (Norcuron) and phaeochromocytoma: a report of three cases. Anesthesiology 1981;55:690.
472. Lebrault C, Berger JL, d'Hollander AA et al. Pharmacokinetics and pharmacodynamics of vecuronium (Org NC 45) in patients with cirrhosis. Aneshesiology 1985;62:601.
473. Lebrault C, Duvaldestin P, Henzel D et al. Pharmacokinetics and pharmacodynamics of vecuronium in patients with cholestasis. Br J Anaesth 1986;58:983.
474. Bencini AF, Scaf AHJ, Sohn YJ et al. Hepatobiliary disposition of vecuronium bromide in man. Br J Anaesth 1986;58:988.
475. Fahey MR, Morris RB, Miller RD et al. Pharmacokinetics of Org NC 45 (Norcuron) in patients with and without renal failure. Br J Anaesth 1981;53:1049.
476. Bencini AF, Scaf AHJ, Sohn YJ et al. Disposition and urinary excretion of vecuronium bromide in anesthetized patients with normal renal function or renal failure. Anesth Analg 1986;65:245.
477. Bevan DR, Donati F, Gyasi H et al. Vecuronium in renal failure. Can Anaesth Soc J 1984;31:491.
478. Demetriou M, Depoix J-P, Diakite B et al. Placental transfer of Org NC 45 in women undergoing caesarian section. Br J Anaesth 1982;54:643.
479. Hawkins JL, Adenwala J, Camp C, Joyce TH. The effect of H_2-receptor antagonist premedication on the duration of vecuronium-induced neuromuscular blockade in postpartum patients. Anesthesiology 1989;71:175.
480. Camp CE, Tessem J, Adenwala J, Joyce TH. Vecuronium and prolonged neuromuscular blockade in postpartum patients. Anesthesiology 1987;67:1006.
481. Van Poorten JF, Dhasmana KM, Kuypers RSM et al. Verapamil and reversal of vecuronium neuromuscular blockade. Anesth Analg 1984;63:155.
482. Anderson KA, Marshall RJ. The effects of calcium antagonists on the neuromuscular blocking actions of vecuronium bromide in anaesthetized cats. Br J Pharmacol 1983;80:613P.
483. Ilias W, Lackner F, Zekert F. Nifedipin und Vecuronium-bromid: Wie reagiert der mit Ca-Antagonisten behandelte Patient auf nichtdepolarisierende Muskelrelaxantien? Anaesthesist 1985;34:591.
484. Driessen JJ, Wuis EW, Gielen MJM. Prolonged vecuronium neuromuscular blockade in a patient receiving orally administered dantrolene. Anesthesiology 1985;62:523.
485. Wood GG. Cyclosporine—vecuronium interaction. Can J Anaesth 1989;35:358.
486. Gray HStJ, Slater RM, Pollard BJ. The effect of acutely administered phenytoin on vecuronium-induced neuromuscular blockade. Anaesthesia 1989;44:379.
487. Ornstein E, Matteo RS, Schwartz AE et al. The effect of phenytoin on the magnitude and duration of neuromuscular block following atracurium or vecuronium. Anesthesiology 1987;67:191.
488. Ebrahim Z, Bulkley R, Roth S. Carbamazepine therapy and neuromuscular blockade with atracurium and vecuronium. Anesth Analg 1988;67:555.
489. Reddy P, Guzman A, Robalino J, Shevde K. Resistance to muscle relaxants in a patient receiving prolonged testosterone therapy. Anesthesiology 1989;70:871.
490. Miller RD, Rupp SM, Fisher DM et al. Clinical pharmacology of vecuronium and atracurium. Anesthesiology 1984;61:444.
491. Nigrovic V, Auen M, Wajskol A. Enzymatic hydrolysis of atracurium in vivo. Anesthesiology 1985;62:606.
492. Stiller RL, Ryan Cook D, Chakravorti S. In vitro degradation of atracurium in human plasma. Br J Anaesth 1985;57:1085.
493. Nigrovic V. New insights into the toxicity of neuromuscular-blocking drugs and their metabolites. Curr Opin Anaesthesiol 1991;4:603.
494. Hughes R, Chapple DJ. The pharmacology of atracurium: a new competitive neuromuscular blocking agent. Br J Anaesth 1981;53:31.
495. Chapple DJ, Clark JS. Pharmacological action of breakdown products of atracurium and related substances. Br J Anaesth 1983;55(Suppl 1):11S.
496. Chapple DJ, Clark JS, Hughes R. Interaction between atracurium and drugs used in anaesthesia. Br J Anaesth 1983;55(Suppl 1):17S.
497. Lavery GG, Mirakhur RK. Atracurium besylate in paediatric anaesthesia. Anaesthesia 1984;39:1243.
498. Mirakhur RK, Lyons SM, Carson IW et al. Cutaneous

reaction after atracurium (Letter to Editor). Anaesthesia 1983;38:818.
499. Watkins J. Histamine release and atracurium. Br J Anaesth 1986;58:19S.
500. Srivastava S. Angioneurotic oedema following atracurium (Letter to Editor). Br J Anaesth 1984;56:932.
501. Mirakhur RK, Lavery GG, Clarke RSJ et al. Atracurium in clinical anaesthesia: effect of dosage on onset, duration and conditions for tracheal intubation. Anaesthesia 1985;40:801.
502. Siler JN, Mager JG, Wyche MQ. Atracurium: hypotension, tachycardia and bronchospasm. Anesthesiology 1985; 62:645.
503. Lynas AGA, Clarke RSJ, Fee JPH, Reid JE. Factors that influence cutaneous reactions following administration of thiopentone and atracurium. Anaesthesia 1988;43:825.
504. Sale JP. Bronchospasm following the use of atracurium. Anaesthesia 1982;38:511.
505. Aldrete JA. Allergic reaction after atracurium (Letter to Editor). Br J Anaesth 1985;57:929.
506. Basta SJ, Ali HH, Savarese JJ et al. Clinical pharmacology of atracurium besylate (BW33A): a new non-depolarizing muscle relaxant. Anesth Analg 1982;61:723.
507. Basta SJ, Savarese JJ, Ali HH et al. Histamine-releasing potencies of atracurium, dimethyl tubocurarine and tubocurarine. Br J Anaesth 1983;55(Suppl 1):105S.
508. Scott RPF, Savarese JJ, Ali HH et al. Atracurium: clinical strategies for preventing histamine release and attenuating the hemodynamic response. Anesthesiology 1984; 61:A287.
509. Healy TEJ, Palmer JP. In vitro comparison between the neuromuscular and ganglion blocking potency ratios of atracurium and tubocurarine. Br J Anaesth 1982;54:1307.
510. Guggiari M, Gallais S, Bianchi A et al. Effets hémodynamiques de l'atracurium chez l'homme. Ann Fr Anesth Reanim 1985;4:484.
511. Carter ML. Bradycardia after the use of atracurium. Br Med J 1983;287:247.
512. McHutchon A, Lawler PG. Bradycardia following atracurium (Letter to Editor). Anaesthesia 1983;38:597.
513. Woolner DF, Gibbs JM, Smeele PQ. Clinical comparison of atracurium and alcuronium in gynaecological surgery. Anaesth Intensive Care 1984;13:33.
514. Kinjo M, Nagashima H, Vizi ES. Effect of atracurium and laudanosine on the release of ^{3}H-noradrenaline. Br J Anaesth 1989;67:683.
515. Amaranath L, Zanettin GG, Bravo EL et al. Atracurium and pheochromocytoma: a report of three cases. Anesth Analg 1988;67:1127.
516. Stirt JA, Brown RE, Ross WT, Althaus JS. Atracurium in a patient with pheochromocytoma. Anesth Analg 1985; 64:547.
517. Sudhaman DA. Atracurium and hypoxemic episodes (Letter to Editor). Anaesthesia 1990;45:166.
518. Flynn PJ, Hughes R, Walton B. Use of atracurium in cardiac surgery involving cardiopulmonary bypass with induced hypothermia. Br J Anaesth 1984;56:967.
519. Nightingale DA. Use of atracurium in neonatal anaesthesia. Br J Anaesth 1986;58(Suppl 1):32S.
520. D'Hollander AA, Luyckx C, Barvais L et al. Clinical evaluation of atracurium besylate requirement for a stable muscle relaxation during surgery: lack of age-related effects. Anesthesiology 1983;59:237.
521. Hennis PJ, Fahey MR, Miller RD et al. Pharmacology of laudanosine in dogs. Anesthesiology 1984;61:A305.
522. Babel A. Étude comparative de la laudanosine et de la papavérine au point de vue pharmacodynamique. Rev Med Suisse Rom 1899;19:657.
523. Mercier J, Mercier E. Action de quelques alcaloïdes secondaires de l'opium sur l'électrocorticogramme du chien. CR Soc Biol (Paris) 1955;149:760.
524. Fahey MR, Canfell PC, Taboada T et al. Cerebrospinal fluid concentrations of laudanosine after administration of atracurium. Br J Anaesth 1990;64:105.
525. Eddleston JM, Harper NJN, Pollard BJ et al. Concentrations of atracurium and laudanosine in cerebrospinal fluid and plasma during intracranial surgery. Br J Anaesth 1989;63:525.
526. Boheimer N, Ward S, Dopson T et al. Pharmacokinetics of laudanosine and quaternary alcohol after an i.v. bolus dose of atracurium in patients with impaired renal function. Br J Anaesth 1985;57:345P.
527. Fahey MR, Rupp SM, Fisher DM et al. The pharmacokinetics and pharmacodynamics of atracurium in patients with and without renal failure. Anesthesiology 1984;61:699.
528. Sharma M, Fahey MR, Castagnoli K et al. In vitro metabolic studies of atracurium with rabbit liver preparations. Anesthesiology 1984;61:A304.
529. Fahey MR, Rupp SM, Canfell C et al. Effect of renal failure on laudanosine excretion in man. Br J Anaesth 1985;57:1049.
530. Ward S, Weatherley BC. Pharmacokinetics of atracurium and its metabolites. Br J Anaesth 1986;58:6S.
531. Hughes R. Atracurium: an overview. Br J Anaesth 1986;58(Suppl 1):2S.
532. Shi W, Fahey MR, Fisher DM et al. Laudanosine (a metabolite of atracurium) increases the minimum alveolar concentration of halothane in rabbits. Anesthesiology 1985;63:584.
533. Chapple DJ, Clark JS. Pharmacological action of breakdown products of atracurium and related substances. Br J Anaesth 1983;55:11S.
534. Cato AE. Concerning toxicity testing of atracurium (Letter to Editor). Anesthesiology 1985;62:94.
535. Ward S, Neill EAM. Pharmacokinetics of atracurium in acute hepatic failure (with acute renal failure). Br J Anaesth 1983;55:1169.
536. Hunter JM, Jones RS, Utting JE. Use of atracurium in patients with no renal function. Br J Anaesth 1982;54:1251.
537. Vandenbrom RHG, Wierda JMKH, Agoston S. Pharmacokinetics of atracurium and metabolites in normal and renal failure patients. Anesthesiology 1987;67:A606.
538. Dwersteg JF, Pavlin EG, Heimbach DM. Patients with burns are resistant to atracurium. Anesthesiology 1986; 65:517.
539. Flynn PJ, Frank M, Hughes R. Use of atracurium in Caesarean section. Br J Anaesth 1984;56:599.
540. Stirt JA, Stone DJ, Weinberg G et al. Atracurium in a child with myotonic dystrophy. Anesth Analg 1985;64:369.
541. Payne JP, Hughes R. Evaluation of atracurium in anaesthetized man. Br J Anaesth 1981;53:45.
542. Katz RL, Stirt JA, Murray AL et al. Neuromuscular effects of atracurium in man. Anesth Analg 1982;61:730.
543. Stirt JA, Murray AL, Katz RL et al. Atracurium during halothane anesthesia in humans. Anesth Analg 1983;62:207.
544. Rupp SM, Fahey MR, Miller RD. Neuromuscular and cardiovascular effects of atracurium during nitrous oxide fentanyl and nitrous oxide isoflurane anaesthesia. Br J Anaesth 1983;55(Suppl 1):67S

545. Beemer GH, Dawson PJ, Bjorksten AR, Edwards NE. Early postoperative seizures in neurosurgical patients administered atracurium and isoflurane. Anaesth Intensive Care 1989;17:504,
546. Stirt JA, Katz RL, Murray AL et al. Modification of atracurium blockade by halothane and by suxamethonium: a review of clinical experience. Br J Anaesth 1983;55(Suppl 1):715.
547. Gerber HR, Romppainen J, Schwinn W. Potentiation of atracurium by pancuronium and *d*-tubocurarine. Can Anaesth Soc J 1986;33:563.
548. Naguib M, Gyasi HK. Antiestrogenic drugs and atracurium—a possible interaction? Can Anaesth Soc J 1986;33:682.
549. Dupuis JY, Martin R, Tetrault J-P. Atracurium and vecuronium interaction with gentamicin and tobramycin. Can J Anaesth 1989;36:407.
550. Agoston S, Richardson FJ. Pipecuronium bromide (Arduan)—a new long-acting non-depolarizing neuromuscular blocking drug. In: Norman J, ed. Clinics in Anaesthesiology, Vol 3. London—Philadelphia—Toronto: W.B. Saunders, 1985;361.
551. Simon G, Biro K, Karpati E, Tuba Z. The effect of the steroid muscle relaxant pipecurium bromide on the acetylcholinesterase activity of red blood cells in vitro. Arzneim-Forsch/Drug Res 1980;30:360.
552. Wittek L, Gecsényi M, Barna B et al. Report on clinical test of pipecurium bromide. Arzneim-Forsch 1980;30:379.
553. Boros M, Szenohradszky J, Marosi Gy et al. Comparitive clinical study of pipecurium bromide and pancuronium bromide. Arzneim-Forsch 1980;30:389.
554. Alant O, Darvas K, Pulay I et al. First clinical experience with a new neuromuscular blocker pipecurium bromide. Arzneim-Forsch 1980;30:374.
555. Bunjatjan AA, Miheev Vl. Clinical experience with a new steroid muscle relaxant: pipecurium bromide. Arzneim-Forsch 1980;30:383.
556. Newton DEF, Richardson FJ, Agoston S. Preliminary studies in man with pipecurium bromide (Arduan), a new steroid neuromuscular blocking agent. Br J Anaesth 1982;54:789P.
557. Larijani GE, Bartkowski RR, Azad SS et al. Clinical pharmacology of pipecuronium bromide. Anesth Analg 1989;68:734.
558. Foldes FF, Nagashima H, Nguyen HD et al. Neuromuscular and cardiovascular effects of pipecuronium. Can J Anaesth 1990;37:549.
559. Barankay A. Circulatory effects of pipecurium bromide during anaesthesia of patients with severe valvular and ischaemic heart diseases. Arzneim-Forsch 1980;30:386.
560. Tassonyi E, Neidhart P, Pittet J-F et al. Cardiovascular effects of pipecuronium and pancuronium in patients undergoing coronary artery bypass grafting. Anesthesiology 1988;69:793.
561. Stanley JC, Carson IW, Gibson FM et al. Comparison of the haemodynamic effects of pipecuronium and pancuronium during fentanyl anaesthesia. Acta Anaesthesiol Scand 1991;35:262.
562. Khunl-Brady KS, Sharma M, Chung K et al. Pharmacokinetics and disposition of pipecuronium bromide in dogs with and without ligated renal pedicles. Anesthesiology 1989;71:919.
563. Wierda JMKH, Karliczek GF, Vandenbrom RHG et al. Pharmacokinetics and cardiovascular dynamics of pipecuronium bromide during coronary artery surgery. Can J Anaesth 1990;37:183.
564. Caldwell JE, Canfell PC, Castagnoli KP et al. The influence of renal failure on the pharmacokinetics and duration of action of pipecuronium bromide in patients anesthetized with halothane and nitrous oxide. Anesthesiology 1989;70:7.
565. Pulay I, Alant O, Darvas K et al. Respiration paralysing and circulatory effects of a new non-depolarizing relaxant, pipecurium bromide, in anaesthetized dogs. Arzneim-Forsch 1980;30:358.
566. Pittet J-F, Tassonyi E, Morel DR et al. Pipecuronium-induced neuromuscular blockade during nitrous oxide—fentanyl, isoflurane, and halothane anesthesia in adults and children. Anesthesiology 1989;71:210.
567. Wierda JMKH, Richardson FJ, Agoston S. Dose—response relation and time course of action of pipecuronium bromide in humans anesthetized with nitrous oxide and isoflurane, halothane, or droperidol and fentanyl. Anesth Analg 1989;68:208.
568. Basta SJ, Savarffe JJ, Ali HH et al. Clinical pharmacology of doxacurium chloride—a new long-acting nondepolarizing muscle relaxant. Anesthesiology 1988;69:478.
569. Scott RPF, Norman J. Doxacurium chloride: a preliminary clinical trial. Br J Anaesth 1989;62:373.
570. Reich DL. Transient systemic arterial hypotension and cutaneous flushing in response to doxacurium chloride. Anesthesiology 1989;71:783.
571. Murray DJ, Mehta MP, Choi WW et al. The neuromuscular blocking and cardiovascular effects of doxacurium chloride in patients receiving nitrous oxide narcotic anesthesia. Anesthesiology 1988;69:472.
572. Stoops CM, Curtis CA, Kovach DA et al. Hemodynamic effects of doxacurium chloride in patients receiving oxygen sufentanyl anesthesia for coronary artery bypass grafting or valve replacement. Anesthesiology 1988;69:365.
573. Reich DL, Konstadt SN, Thys DM et al. Effects of doxacurium chloride on biventricular cardiac function in patients with cardiac disease. Br J Anaesth 1989;63:675.
574. Cashman JN, Luke JJ, Jones RM. Neuromuscular block with doxacurium (BW A938U) in patients with normal or absent renal function. Br J Anaesth 1990;64:186.
575. Cook DR, Freeman JA, Lai AA et al. Pharmacokinetics and pharmacodynamics of doxacurium in normal patients and in those with hepatic or renal failure. Anesth Analg 1991;72:145.
576. Cook DR, Stiller RL, Weakly JN et al. In vitro metabolism of mivacurium chloride (BW B1090U) and succinylcholine. Anesth Analg 1989;68:452.
577. Savarese JJ, Ali HH, Basta SJ et al. The clinical neuromuscular pharmacology of mivacurium chloride (BW B1090U)—a short-acting nondepolarizing ester neuromuscular blocking drug. Anesthesiology 1988;68:723.
578. Choi WW, Mehta MP, Murray DJ et al. Neuromuscular and cardiovascular effects of mivacurium chloride in surgical patients receiving nitrous oxide—narcotic or nitrous oxide—isoflurane anaesthesia. Can J Anaesth 1989;36:541.
579. Ali HH, Savarese JJ, Embree PB et al. Clinical pharmacology of mivacurium chloride (BW B1090U) infusion: comparison with vecuronium and atracurium. Br J Anaesth 1988;36:641.
580. Savarese JJ, Ali HH, Basta SJ et al. The cardiovascular effects of mivacurium chloride (BW B1090U) in patients receiving nitrous oxide—opiate—barbiturate anesthesia. Anesthesiology 1989;70:386.
581. Caldwell JE, Heier T, Kitts JB et al. Comparison the neuromuscular block induced by mivacurium, suxamethon-

ium or atracurium during nitrous oxide—fentanyl naesthesia. Br J Anaesth 1989;63:393.
582 Stoops CM, Curtis CA, Kovach DA et al. Hemodynamic effects of mivacurium chloride administered to patients during oxygen—sufentanil anesthesia for coronary utery bypass grafting or valve replacement. Anesth Analg 1989; 68:333.
583. Caldwell JE, Kitts JB, Heier T et al. The dose—response relationship of mivacurium chloride in humans using nitrous oxide—fentanyl or nitrous oxide—enflurane anesthesia. Anesthesiology 1989;70:31.
584. Brandom BW, Sarner JB, Woelfel SK et al. Mivacurium infusion requirements in pediatric surgical patients during nitrous oxide—halothane and during nitrous oxide—narcotic anesthesia. Anesth Analg 1990;71:16.
585. From RP, Pearson KS, Choi WW et al. Neuromuscular and cardiovascular effects of mivacurium chloride (BW B1090U) during nitrous oxide—fentanyl—thioentone and nitrous oxide—halothane anaesthesia. Br J Anaesth 1990; 64:193.
586. Britt BA. Dantrolene. Can Anaesth Soc J 1984;31:61.
587. Ward A, Chaffman MO, Sorkin EM. Dantrolene: review of its pharmacodynamic and pharmacokinetic properties and therapeutic uses in malignant hyperthermia, the euroleptic malignant syndrome and an update of its use in muscle spasticity. Drugs 1986;32:130.
588. Utili R, Boitnott JK, Zimmerman HJ. Dantrolene associated hepatic injury. Incidence and character. Gastronterology 1977;72:610.
589. Pinder RM, Brogden RN, Speight TM, Avery GS. Dantrolene sodium: a review of its pharmacological properties and therapeutic efficiency in spasticity. Drugs 1977;13:3.
590. Denhoff E, Feldman S, Smith MG. Treatment of pastic cerebral-palsied children with sodium dantrolene. Dev Med Child Neurol 1975;17:736.
591. Petusevsky ML, Ealing LJ, Rocklin RE et al. Pleuropericardial reaction to treatment with dantrolene. J Am Med Assoc 1979;242:2772.
592. Wan HH, Tucker JS. Dantrolene and lymphocytic lymphoma. Postgrad Med J 1980;56:261.
593. Luisto M, Moller K, Nuutila A et al. Dantrolene sodium in chronic spasticity of varying etiology. Acta Neurol Scand 1982;65:355.
594. Pace-Balzan A, Ramsdan RT. Sudden bilateral senneural hearing loss during treatment with dantrolene sodium (Dantrium). J Laryngol Otol 1988;102:57.
595. Wolf ME. Almy G, Toll M et al. Mania associated with the use of baclofen. Biol Psychiatr 1982;17:757.
596. Wainapel SF, Lee L, Riley TL. Reversible electroencephalogram changes associated with administration of baclofen in a quadriplegic patient: case report. Paraplegia 1986;24:123.
597. Hormes JT, Benarroch EE, Rodriguez M, Klass DW. Periodic sharp waves in baclofen-induced encephalopathy. Arch Neurol 1988;45:814.
598. Rush JM, Gibberd FB. Baclofen-induced epilepsy. J R Soc Med 1990;83:115.
599. Fromm GH, Terrence CF, Chattha AS et al. Baclofen in trigeminal neuralgia. Arch Neurol 1980;37:768.
600. Seyfert S, Kraft D, Wagner K. Baclofen-Dosis bei Haemodialyse und Niereninsuffizienz. Nervenarzt 1981; 52:616.
601. Wimmer C. Über Lioresal®-(Baclofen-) Intoxikationen—Ein kasuistischer Beitrag. Dtsch Gesundheitswes 1982;37:1500.
602. May CR. Baclofen overdose. Ann Emerg Med 1983; 12:171.
603. White WB. Aggravated CNS depression with urinary retention secondary to baclofen administration. Arch Intern Med 1985;145:1717.
604. Nugent S, Katz MD, Little TE. Baclofen overdose with cardiac conduction abnormalities: case report and review of the literature. Clin Toxicol 1986;24:321.
605. Romijn JA, van Lieshout JJ, Velis DN. Reversible coma due to intrathecal baclofen. Lancet 1986;ii:696.
606. Müller-Schwefe G, Penn RD. Physostigmine in the treatment of intrathecal baclofen overdose. Report of three cases. J Neurosurg 1989;71:273.
607. Saltuari L, Baumgartner H, Kofler M et al. Failure of physostigmine in treatment of acute severe intrathecal baclofen intoxication (Letter to Editor). N Engl J Med 1990;322:1533.
608. Penn RD, Kroin JS. Failure of physostigmine in treatment of acute severe intrathecal baclofen intoxication (Letter to Editor). N Engl J Med 1990;322:1533.
609. Kerr DIB, Ong J, Prager RH et al. Phaclofen: a peripheral and central baclofen antagonist. Brain Res 1987; 405:150.
610. Silverglat MJ. Baclofen and tricyclic antidepressants: possible interaction (Letter to Editor). J Am Med Assoc 1981;246:1659.
611. Sandyk R, Gillman MA. Baclofen-induced memory impairment. Clin Neuropharmacol 1985;8:294.
612. Sayers AC, Burki HR, Eichenberger E. The pharmacology of 5-chloro-4-(2-imidazolin-2-yl-amino)-2,1,3,-benzothiadiazole (DS 103—282), a novel myotonolytic agent. Arzneim-Forsch 1980;30:793.
613. Rinne UK. Tizanidine treatment of spasticity in multiple sclerosis and chronic myelopathy. Curr Ther Res 1980; 28:827.
614. Hutchinson DR. Modified release tizanidine: a review. J Int Med Res 1989;17:565.
615. Fryda-Kaurinsky Z, Müller-Fassbender H. Tizanidine (DS103-282) in the treatment of acute paravertebral muscle spasm: a controlled trial comparing tizanidine and diazepam. J Int Med Res 1981;9:501.
616. Goei The HS, Whitehouse IJ. Acomparative trial of tizanidine and diazepam in the treatment of acute cervical muscle spasm. Clin Trials J 1982;19:20.
617. Hennies OL. A new skeletal muscle relaxant (DS 103-282) compared to diazepam in the treatment of muscle spasm of local origin. J Int Med Res 1981;9:62.
618. Hassan N, McLellan DL. Double-blind comparison of single doses of DS 103-282, baclofen and placebo for suppression of spasticity. J Neurol Neurosurg Psychiatry 1980; 43:1132.
619. Stien R, Nordal HJ, Oftedal SI, Slettebo M. The treatment of spasticity in multiple sclerosis: a double-blind clinical trial of a new anti-spastic drug tizanidine compared with baclofen. Acta Neurol Scand 1987:75:190.
620. Mathias CJ, Luckitt J, Desai P et al. Pharmacodynamics and pharmacokinetics of the oral antispastic agent tizanidine in patients with spinal cord injury. J Rehabil Res Dev 1989;26:9.
621. Azoury FJ. Double-blind comparison of Parafon forte and Flexeril in the treatment of acute musculoskeletal disorders. Curr Ther Res 1979;26:189.
622. Nibbelink DW, Strickland SC. Cyclobenzaprine (Flexeril™): Report of a postmarketing surveillance program. Curr Ther Res 1980;28:894.

623. Beeber AR, Manring JM. Psychosis following cyclobenzaprine use. J Clin Psychiatry 1983;44:151.
624. Cohen DA, Savino PJ, Stern MB, Hurtig Hl. Botulinum injection therapy for blepharospasm: a review of 75 patients Clin Neuropharmacol 1986;9:415.
625. Stell R, Coleman R, Thompson P, Marsden CD. Botulinum toxin treatment of spasmodic torticollis (Letter to Editor). Br Med J 1988;297:616.
626. Koay CE, Alun-Jones T. Pharyngeal paralysis due to botulinum toxin injection. J Laryngol Otol 1989;103:698.
627. Rudick RA, Breton D, Krall RL. The GABA-agonist progabide for spasticity in multiple sclerosis. Arch Neurol 1987;44:1033.
628. Powers BJ, Cattau EL, Zimmerman HJ. Chlorzoxazone hepatotoxic reactions: an analysis of 21 identified or presumed cases. Arch Intern Med 1986;146:1183.
629. Rosin MA. Chlorzoxazone-induced spasmodic torticollis (Letter to Editor). J Am Med Assoc 1981;246:2575.

Meyler's Side Effects of Drugs, 13th Edition
M.N.G. Dukes, editor

SECTION EDITOR: C.J. VAN BOXTEL

M.N.G. Dukes*

13 Drugs affecting autonomic functions or the extrapyramidal system

Editorial note *Certain sympathicomimetic drugs, used commonly as stimulants or anorectic agents, are dealt with primarily in Chapter 1. β-Adrenergic receptor blockers are reviewed in Chapter 18. The reader is also referred to other chapters for adrenergic receptor blockers used mainly as peripheral vasodilators (Chapter 19) or as antihypertensive agents (Chapter 20), or drugs which affect the autonomic system but are used in gastrointestinal disorders (Chapter 36) or ophthalmology (Chapter 47).*

GENERAL

Despite the large number of compounds which have become available for the stimulation or inhibition of autonomic functions, the pattern of their side effects is relatively simple. Most of these agents have been developed to promote, imitate or antagonize the effects of adrenaline or dopamine on the one hand, or those of acetylcholine on the other. Provided, therefore, one bears in mind the pharmacological properties of these three physiological substances, it is possible to anticipate what many of the effects, wanted or unwanted, of drugs influencing the autonomic system are likely to be.

It is true that within the last 20 years numerous compounds have been developed which are intended to act more selectively than their predecessors, affecting, for example, primarily the adrenergic receptors in the respiratory system. What has actually been achieved, however, is only a partial dissociation of effect; the degree of selectivity claimed for some of these compounds reflects in part wishful thinking, and the physician should be hesitant to assume that a particular effect truly has been eliminated until long experience in the field has been gained.

No classification of drugs affecting autonomic functions is entirely satisfactory. The presentation in Table 1 is intended to help the reader to find his way in the present chapter and to locate those drugs which, by reason of their special applications (e.g. in ophthalmology or in treating hypertension), are dealt with primarily in other parts of this book. It should always be borne in mind that agonists and antagonists tend to be close cousins and share to some extent each other's properties, in this as in other fields of pharmacology.

Anti-Parkinson drugs are included in this chapter because the key element in parkinsonism is a disorder of central nervous transmission of dopamine, which is one of the mediators of autonomic functions.

SYMPATHICOMIMETIC DRUGS

Sympathicomimetic drugs evoke physiological responses similar to those produced by stimulation of adrenergic nerves or physiological release of adrenaline (see Table 2). For many of these responses it is currently possible to conclude that only an α- or β-adrenergic receptor is involved, and in some cases one can distinguish a β_1 from a β_2 response. In some situations, however, the distinction is not clear: e.g. most sympathicomimetic drugs, however specific to a particular receptor type they are claimed to be, will on occasion stimulate the central nervous functions, resulting in nervousness, insomnia, tremors, dizziness or headache. In some organ systems both α- and β- adrenergic receptors are present; the nature of the response produced when a drug of this type is given will depend either on the concentrations achieved or on other factors; whether, for example, the uterus contracts or relaxes in response to an adrenergic drug depends in part on the hormonal balance in the system at that moment.

* The author would like to acknowledge the assistance of Mr Knud Enevoldsen, Denmark, in the compilation of this Chapter.

Table 1. *Prinicipal types of drugs affecting autonomic functions*

I: Sympathicomimetic agents
A. *Drugs stimulating both* α- and β-adrenergic receptors, e.g. adrenaline, ephedrine
B. Drugs predominantly stimulating α-adrenergic receptors, e.g. noradrenaline, metaraminol
C. Drugs predominantly stimulating β-adrenergic receptors (β_1 and β_2) e.g. isoprenaline, methoxyphenamine
D. Drugs predominantly stimulating β_1-adrenergic receptors
  i. Direct stimulants used in shock and hypertension, e.g. dopamine, dobutamine
  ii. Indirect stimulants used in parkinsonism, e.g. levodopa, amantadine
  iii. Drugs stimulating dopaminergic-receptors, e.g. bromocriptine
E. Drugs predominantly stimulating β_2-adrenergic receptors, e.g. salbutamol, terbutaline
F. Drugs predominantly stimulating receptors in the central nervous system, e.g. amphetamines and anorectics (see Chapter 1)
G. Drugs stimulating atypical β-receptors
H. Drugs stimulatinmg 5-hydroxytryptamine receptors

II: Sympathicolytic agents
A. Drugs blocking α-adrenergic receptors
  i. The haloalkylamines, e.g. phenoxybenzamine, dibenamine
  ii. The ergot alkaloids and related agents, e.g. ergotamine, methylsergide
  iii. The 2-substituted imidazoline vasodilators, e.g. tolazoline, phentolamine (see Chapter 19)
  iv. The adrenergic neuron blockers used in hypertension, e.g. guanethidine (see Chapter 20)
B. Drugs blocking β-adrenergic receptors, e.g. propranolol (see Chapter 17)
C. Drugs blocking dopa formation (α-methyl-*p*-tyrosine)

III: Agents with cholinergic effects
A. Drugs stimulating acetylcholine receptors (choline alfoscerate)
B. Acetylcholine and related substances, e.g. choline, carbachol
C. Alkaloids used in ophthalmology, e.g. pilocarpine (see Chapter 47)
D. Acetylcholinesterase inhibitors, e.g. neostigmine, edrophonium

IV: Agents with anticholinergic effects
A. Atropine-like drugs, e.g. hyoscine, ipratropium
B. Synthetic quaternary ammonium compounds, e.g. xanthine, propantheline

Sympathicomimetic drugs, however diverse, also tend to have interactions in common, particularly those with other drugs which produce central stimulant effects and with monoamine-oxidase (MAO) inhibitors.

DRUGS STIMULATING BOTH α- AND β-ADRENERGIC RECEPTORS

Adrenaline (epinephrine)

At the present day, the use of adrenaline itself is largely limited to subcutaneous administration for the immediate relief of severe conditions, particularly anaphylactic shock. Doses of 0.1 ml of a 1:1000 solution are often given repeatedly, up to a maximum of some 2 ml in 5 minutes. Although the sensitivity of individuals to adrenaline varies considerably, the adverse reactions to such doses are generally limited to mild cardiovascular effects; where the limits of tolerance are approached, there may be *palpitations*, *extrasystoles* and a *rise in blood pressure*. In sensitive individuals or with high doses, *ventricular fibrillation*, *pulmonary edema*, *subarachnoid hemorrhage* and even *hemiplegia* have been known to occur. It is possible that in at least some of these cases the drug has been inadvertently injected intravenously. Intravenous administration of adrenaline for treatment of systemic anaphylactic shock should be undertaken with extreme caution, even in patients without a history of cardiovascular disease. At all times the patient must be monitored and emergency treatment should be available. Even the infiltration of low doses of adrenaline for local hemostasis can be attended by these risks; one patient developed ventricular tachycardia and severe hypertension after receiving 3.75 μg locally for this purpose (SEDA-17, 160), the value of the treatment today being regarded as dubious (SEDA-17, 161).

Adrenaline was still until recently a component of some old asthma sprays, and *dilated cardiomyopathy* has been described after many years of use (1[C]).

If in healthy subjects one compares the effects of giving adrenaline by subcutaneous injection or by high-dose inhalation, one finds surprisingly that while absorption from an injection is variable (and sometimes very slow) the inhaled dose is absorbed rapidly and reliably. The main side effect of the inhaled form, e.g. in a dose of 3—4.5 mg, is *gastrointestinal discomfort*, with nausea and sometimes vomiting; this seems to be a local effect since it does not occur with injections. Both forms however produce *mild tremor* and *palpitations* in some individuals.

Since adrenaline is so short acting, the metabolic and other adrenergic effects which it can produce are unlikely to be elicited unless a depot preparation is used; in the latter event, *hyperglycemia* may occur. *Lactic acidosis* has been observed, persisting for some hours after deliberate intravenous misuse of 20 mg adrenaline by an addict (SED-12, 308). Facial swelling due

Table 2. *Adrenergic and cholinergic receptors and effects**

Organ or system	Adrenergic impulses		Cholinergic impulses
	Receptor	Response	Response
Cardiovascular			
Heart			
Sinoatrial node	β_1	Increased heart rate	Decreased heart rate; vagal arrest**
Atria	β_1	Increased contractility and conduction velocity	Decreased contractility; usually increased conduction velocity
Atrioventricular node and conduction system	β_1	Increased conduction velocity and automaticity	Decreased in conduction velocity; atrioventricular block
Ventricles	β_1	Increased contractility, conduction velocity, automaticity, rate of idiopathic pacemakers	Slight decrease in contractility(?)
Blood vessels			
Coronary	α,β_2	Constriction	Dilatation
Skin, mucosa	α	Constriction	Slight dilatation
Skeletal muscle	α	Constriction *or*	Dilatation
	β_2	Dilatation	
Cerebral	α	Slight constriction	Dilatation
Pulmonary	α	Constriction *or*	Slight dilatation
	β_2	Dilatation	
Abdominal viscera	α	Constriction *or*	—
	β_2	Dilatation	
Salivary glands	α	Constriction	Dilatation
Respiratory			
Bronchial muscle	β_2	Relaxation	Contraction
Bronchial glands	α_1, β_2	Decreased *or* increased secretion	Stimulation
Nervous system			
Cerebral function		Stimulation	
Liver			
Glycogenolysis and gluconeogenesis	α_1, β_2	Stimulation	—
Gallbladder, ducts	β_2	Relaxation	Contraction
Gastrointestinal			
Salivary glands	α_1	Potassium and water secretion	Potassium and water secretion
	β	Amylase secretion	(marked)
Motility and tone	α_1, β_1, β_2	Decrease (usually)	Increase
Sphincters	α	Contraction (usually)	Relaxation (usually)
Secretion		Inhibition?	Stimulation
Urinary system			
Ureter; tone, motility		Increase (usually)	Increase (?)
Bladder; detrusor	β	Relaxation (usually)	Contraction
Trigone, sphincter	α	Contraction	Relaxation
Renal vessels	α_1, β_1, β_2	Primary constriction	—
Skin			
Pilomotor muscles	α	Contraction	—
Sweat glands	α	Slight local secretion	Generalized secretion
Special senses; eye			
Radial muscle, iris	α	Contraction (mydriasis)	—
Sphincter muscle, iris		—	Contraction (meiosis)
Ciliary muscle	β	Relaxation for far vision (slight)	Contraction for near vision

Table 2. *(continued)*

Organ or system	Adrenergic impulses		Cholinergic impulses
	Receptor	Response	Response
Other systems			
Uterus	α,β_2	Variable effect**	Variable effect**
Male sex function		Ejaculation	Ejaculation
Spleen capsule	α	Contraction	—
Muscle glycogenolysis	β	Stimulation	—

* Adapted and condensed from; Goodman LS, Gilman A. The Pharmacological Basis of Therapeutics, 7th edn. New York—Toronto—London: MacMillan, 1985.
** Response depends inter alia on hormonal status.

to a drug-induced *sialadenosis* was repeatedly observed in one patient controlling her asthma symptoms with an adrenaline inhaler (SEDA-14, 119).

Adrenaline has been largely abandoned as an adjuvant to local anesthetics, though in 1:80 000 concentration it is still sometimes used in dental and in epidural anesthesia; in a sensitive subject, a life-threatening *torsade de pointes* was observed when an epidural anesthetic was giving using 20 ml bupivacaine containing only 1:200 000 adrenaline (2^R).

Risk situations In subjects with *angina pectoris*, an attack may be induced, and it is evident that in any form of cardiac disease caution is indicated; at one time an attempt was made to use high doses of adrenaline for the early treatment of *ventricular fibrillation*, but the pharmacological effects of the drug swing the balance against its use, the immediate survival rate actually decreasing. *Thyrotoxic patients* are unduly sensitive to the drug's effects. (SEDA-14, 179).

Interactions *Halothane* and some other anesthetics sensitize the patient to the risk of adrenaline-induced ventricular arrhythmias and acute pulmonary edema, especially if hypoxia is present (see Chapter 10). *Tricyclic antidepressants* inhibit the uptake of catecholamines such as adrenaline into the sympathetic neurons and can enhance the cardiovascular effects so that even the small amounts of adrenaline present as additives in some local anesthetics exert a marked effect on the cardiovascular system.

Similarly these small quantities present in local anesthetics can be dangerously potentiated by β-adrenoceptor blockers; propranolol should be discontinued at least 3 days in advance of administering such products for local anesthesia. A combined infusion of adrenaline and propranolol has indeed been used for diagnosing insulin resistance, but it may evoke cardiac arrhythmias even in patients without signs of coronary disease. (3^c).

The control of diabetes by *antidiabetic drugs* may be briefly deranged because of adrenaline's hyperglycemic effects. *MAO inhibitors* can dangerously potentiate the hypertensive effects of the drug (see Chapter 2). Adrenaline is physically incompatible with *sodium warfarin*, *hyaluronidase* and *sodium novobiocin*.

Ephedrine

Ephedrine is longer-acting than adrenaline and can exert any type of adrenergic effect (see Table 2), including metabolic changes and dysuria. It has somewhat less effect on the cardiovascular system than does adrenaline but relatively more on the central nervous system; even low doses may, in sensitive patients, cause *tremor*, *insomnia* and *anxiety*, and such problems are clearly much more marked if ephedrine is given together with caffeine, as it sometimes is for appetite control (SEDA-17, 161). In children, ephedrine sometimes paradoxically induces *sedation*. *Psychosis* has resulted from excessive self-medication (4^C).

Oral doses of 25—30 mg ephedrine are often prescribed, e.g. for orthostatic hypotension. Lower oral doses, present in some 'cold remedies' in tablet form, are unlikely to be useful although they are risky where the drug is contraindicated, e.g. in cardiac patients. Ephedrine used in nasal sprays and drops can have systemic effects in the doses normally used.

Risk situations See under Adrenaline, above. It should be noted that in patients on prescribed *antihypertensive therapy* the patient's use of ephedrine-containing self-medication remedies can result in an increase in blood pressure.

Interactions These are as for adrenaline, including the risk of combination with *MAO inhibitors*. In intravenous solutions, ephedrine is physically incompatible with *hydrocortisone* and several *barbiturates*.

Isometheptene

One report (5[C]) describes an autonomic *dysreflexic syndrome* following the use of an isometheptene combination to treat migraine.

Oxyfedrine

Impairment of the sense of taste is a complication of oxyfedrine therapy, and 21 such cases were reviewed as early as 1985 (6[R]); they continue to be reported to national monitoring centres. The side effect usually occurs within 4 weeks after the start of therapy; it is slowly reversible after the drug is withdrawn.

Pseudoephedrine (D-isoephedrine)

Although the dosage and properties resemble those of ephedrine, this compound appears to be slightly less active. Both *fixed eruptions* and generalized *rash* have been reported. It can elevate *blood pressure*, especially in children. In one patient with Graves' disease who used the drug a *thyroid storm* developed, suggesting that hyperthyroidism constitutes a special risk situation (7[cr]); in another, a form of *toxic shock syndrome* appeared on more than one occasion (SEDA-18, 158).

Pseudoephedrine is a component of some non-prescription basal decongestants given by mouth; even quite ordinary doses of such products (e.g. 120 mg) can cause a hypertensive reaction in sensitive subjects, namely those with a pheochromocytoma and those with at least a family history of hypertension (SEDA-17, 162).

DRUGS PREDOMINANTLY STIMULATING α-ADRENERGIC RECEPTORS

Noradrenaline (norepinephrine)

Noradrenaline is still occasionally used to maintain blood pressure in acute situations. Extraordinary care is needed to avoid *local damage* at the site of the intravenous infusion, which can readily result in skin necrosis as a consequence of ischemia. The infusion should always be ended very gradually, since otherwise a catastrophic *fall in blood pressure* may occur. Like adrenaline, the drug is also sometimes added to local anesthetics (e.g. in 1:250 000 concentration) to prolong their effect; it should not be injected into extremities (finger, penis) for this purpose since dangerous *ischemia* can result.

The systemic adverse reactions are typically adrenergic, involving primarily the central nervous system and the vessels (see Table 2); there is very little effect on the β-adrenergic receptors of the heart, but there tends to be some *bradycardia* as a reflex consequence of the drug-induced rise in blood pressure. *Retrosternal pain* may be caused, as with the amphetamines. A paradoxical but transient *engorgement of the thyroid* has occurred.

Risk situations See under Adrenaline, above. As with adrenaline, *individual sensitivity* to the effects of noradrenaline varies markedly, hence problems can occur unexpectedly. If used late in *pregnancy*, the drug can induce contractions of the uterus.

Other drugs mainly used systemically

Metaraminol Metaraminol (2—10 mg i.m.) is used in treating seriously hypotensive states. When so used, there is no noticeable central nervous effect and the β-adrenergic receptors of the heart usually do not react. The maximum effect of a dose is not at once apparent and one should wait for some 10 minutes before deciding to give a further dose. Intravenous infusion, used in two published cases to treat paroxysmal supraventricular tachycardia resulted in *acute hypertension* and *pulmonary edema* (8[C]). Subcutaneous administration is risky; it can result in dangerous *sloughing*.

Interactions If *guanethidine* or related drugs are being given, the adrenergic receptors will be rendered highly sensitive to metaraminol.

Methoxamine Methoxamine (10—20 mg i.m., 5—10 mg i.v.) is another compound still primarily used in the emergency treatment of hypotension; when so used it has little other effect. It has also been given locally as a nasal decongestant. Active doses given by any route can result in adrenergic type effects including *coldness of the extremities*, *pilomotor stimulation*, and a *desire to micturate*. *Tachyphylaxis* has been seen in experimental animals.

Phenylephrine Phenylephrine (up to 10 mg i.m.) has similar properties and uses to the above congeners. When employed as a nasal decongestant, it can cause *local nasal irritation*. Like most other drugs in this class, it has occasionally been *abused* by those dependent on stimulants. Use in eyedrops has in a long series of cases led to *blepharoconjunctivitis* (SEDA-17, 162).

Phenylpropanolamine (norephedrine) This drug is mainly used in mixtures given orally to produce nasal decongestion, e.g. in doses of 25 mg; in some countries it is still used as a free-sale anorectic agent (see Chapter

1). Although it has been thought to have relatively little stimulant effect on the central nervous system, doses such as these can produce *restlessness*, *anxiety*, *insomnia* and *tremor*; its central stimulant effects are in practice often masked by the manufacturers' practice of combining it with an antihistamine, but marked *psychic depression* has on occasion been observed. Phenylpropanolamine can also give rise to severe *allergic reactions* with dyspnea, urticaria and facial swelling (9[C]).

Much of the concern expressed with respect to the free sale of this drug relates to its cardiovascular effects. Work in healthy volunteers (10[CR]) shows that although the commonly recommended 75-mg dose has no significant effect on *blood pressure* in such individuals, ingestion of double this dose (150 mg) causes a significant though transient hypertension lasting several hours; *hypertensive crises* have been reported (e.g. after a 600-mg overdose—see SEDA-18, 158). Field experience suggests that, because of individual variations in sensitivity, the risks to some patients are greater than these findings would suggest, doses of 50 mg phenylpropanolamine sometimes having caused significant hypertension. In addition it can on occasion cause *cardiac dysrhythmias* in mild overdosage; a transient *cardiomyopathy* without hypertension occurred in a girl of 14 who had taken only a slight overdose (11[c]) and another in an adult woman (SEDA-17, 163).

Occasional reports of the more severe type of reaction continue to cause concern, though the drug has found its champions (see SEDA-18, 158). Because of these problems, the occurrence of misuse, the fact that the effect of prescribed antihypertensive medication can be disrupted and the possibility of potentiation by caffeine-containing drinks, tighter restrictions on the use of phenylpropanolamine in free-sale products have often been advocated.

Interactions *Indomethacin* even in a single dose has been found to potentiate the hypertensive effect of phenylpropanolamine, and the volunteer study cited above confirmed that *caffeine* has something of the same effect; a normal 75-mg dose of phenylpropanolamine induces marked hypertension if taken along with several cups of strong coffee or a corresponding dose of caffeine. The drug can also counter the effects of *simultaneous antihypertensive therapy*.

Other drugs mainly used topically

Propylhexedrine In the form of the volatile base, propylhexedrine is used in nasal inhalers; it is also a component of some liquid decongestant mixtures. When inhaled, and especially if over-used, it can cause *nasal irritation*, *rebound congestion* and *chronic rhinitis*. There are several reports of *abuse* by addicts who extract the contents of the cotton wad (250 mg propylhexedrine with added aromatics) and take them either orally or intravenously. In a few reported cases, fatalities have occurred in abusers because of myocardial infarct or pulmonary hypertension, and psychoses of the amphetamine type have been induced (SED-9, 216, 217).

Naphazoline (Privine) Privine is used as a 0.05% intranasal solution. *Local irritation*, *headache* and *rebound effects* can all occur, and *rhinorrhea* can follow prolonged use. It has been suggested that such effects are more common with naphazoline than with other decongestants. In one case reported in 1992, nasal drops containing naphazoline had been given to an infant of 12 weeks; he experienced what was apparently severe depression of the CNS with pallor followed by apnea, then tachycardia with hypertension; the condition responded to treatment. Though the reaction is unusual, all nasal decongestants should be regarded as contraindicated in young infants.

Oxymetazoline and xylometazoline These drugs seem to be better tolerated, although *nasal irritation* with *dryness of the mouth and throat* can occur; a *rebound effect* on the nasal mucosa was found in some 5% of cases studied (12[C]).

Overdosage An unusual response to an overdose of oxymetazoline (0.05% nasal spray) occurred in an elderly patient who used the product several times daily; the patient, who had pre-existing cerebellar degeneration and peripheral neuropathy, developed severe *bradycardia* and *systolic pressure oscillations* between 236 and 60 mmHg. Withdrawal of the spray resulted in complete recovery (13[Cr]).

The development of an acute *retinal artery obstruction* in a young, otherwise healthy man was associated with his excessive use of an oxymetazoline nasal spray. Platelet coagulation studies indicated a platelet aggregation hypersensitivity to adenosine diphosphate and adrenaline. Predisposition to sympathomimetic drug-induced platelet fibrin embolus formation may have played a role in this case (14[C]).

Overdose and withdrawal symptoms The interruption of a high dose nasal spray therapy precipitated a prolonged *panic disorder* in a healthy man (SEDA-13, 109).

Use during pregnancy Repeated use of an oxymetazoline nasal spray has been associated with changes in fetal heart rate demonstrated as a non-reactive, non-stress test and late decelerations in a patient at 41 weeks of gestation. Six hours after the last dose these changes gradually disappeared (15[C]).

DRUGS PREDOMINANTLY STIMULATING β-ADRENERGIC RECEPTORS

The drugs developed some 35 years ago as general β-adrenergic receptor stimulants have to some extent fallen into the background with the development of more selective β_1 stimulants (for use in respiratory disease) and β_2 stimulants (for use in threatened premature labor).

The possibility of a causal relation between the administration of β-adrenergic drugs and *decreasing serum immunoglobulin levels* has been raised in various papers. In one study, adult asthmatic patients receiving steroid treatment were compared with patients receiving β-adrenergic agents. It was found that the patients receiving β-adrenergic agents had significantly lower serum IgG levels. This effect was seen irrespective of any history of steroid use, but in patients receiving both treatments this depressive effect was indeed even more pronounced; its mechanism is unclear (16[C]).

Isoprenaline (isoproterenol)

As a non-selective β-adrenergic receptor stimulant, isoprenaline produces a wide range of adrenergic effects (as defined in Table 2), those involving the heart presenting the most marked problems in practice. Doses of up to 10 μg/minute are used to improve peripheral circulation in shock. In respiratory disease, sublingual tablets (up to 10 mg) and oral inhalers continue to be used to some extent despite the advent of selective stimulants; the inhalers sometimes provide more than the 20 μg which are needed for a maximum effect on the bronchi, resulting in unnecessary adverse effects.

Cardiovascular *Tachycardia*, *arrhythmias*, *palpitations*, *flushing* and induction of *anginal pain* are disadvantages of the drug when used in respiratory disease. Users tend to raise the dose (hence increasing the degree of cardiac toxicity), possibly because a metabolite (3-α-methylisoprenaline), which may act as a weak β-blocker, accumulates and renders the original doses ineffective. The drug has been clearly shown to produce *ECG changes compatible with myocardial infarction* or to lead to *ventricular fibrillation* or even *cardiac muscle necrosis* if infusions are not given with the utmost caution (SED-12, 312; 17[C], 18[C]). Exceptionally, the tachycardia produced by an infusion of the drug may be overshadowed by a reflex *bradycardia*, even while the drug is being given (SEDA-17, 163).

Respiratory In relaxing bronchial smooth muscle, isoprenaline may impair the ventilation perfusion ratio and aggravate *hypoxemia* even as it diminishes airway resistance; the patient may feel better but be worse off. In addition, paradoxical *bronchospasm* can occur, a response of this type having been found in 30% of patients in one series.

Nervous system *Headache*, *tremor*, *apprehension*, *dizziness* and *faintness* are common problems with isoprenaline treatment.

Gastrointestinal Quite apart from the fact that systemic adverse reactions appear to be more common when the drug is given in the form of sublingual tablets, these commonly induce *mouth ulcers*. Their long-term use has also been reported on one occasion to result in tooth destruction (SED-8, 305), but this was probably coincidental.

Risk situations Isoprenaline can better be avoided wherever stimulation of the heart or the central nervous system is undesirable, e.g. in *angina* or *thyroid disease*. There is no reliable information on the risks in liver or renal disease.

Second-generation effects The drug has often been given in pregnancy, and animal studies do not suggest that it is specifically teratogenic.

Interactions The toxicity of isoprenaline will be increased if it is given alongside other drugs stimulating the heart or central nervous system (*e.g. sympathicomimetics*, *theophylline*, *thyroid*).

Orciprenaline (metaproterenol) Orciprenaline is somewhat β_2-selective compared with isoprenaline, but is by no means free of cardiac effects. Individual susceptibility to these varies, but it would seem that about one individual in 10 will experience *tachycardia* after normal therapeutic doses. At normal doses (e.g. 20 mg q.i.d.) '*jitteriness*' and *nervousness* are not uncommon, and one repeatedly finds that about one patient in 12 suffers from *cramps* or *numbness* in the extremities. *Lactic acidosis* has been described in one published case as a result of concomitant use of orciprenaline, theophylline and glucocorticoids. Other risk situations and interactions are as listed for isoprenaline. The drug has recently been approved in some countries for use in acute asthma in children, and it will be necessary to monitor its safety again in this new target group

Methoxyphenamine hydrochloride This agent is claimed to be relatively free of cardiostimulant and psychomotor effects, but there is little published evidence suggesting a marked β_2-selectivity, and the normal oral dose of 50—100 mg can in a minority of cases produce *tightness of the chest* and *palpitations*. *Drowsi-*

ness, *mouth dryness*, *nausea* and *faintness* have been anecdotally reported.

Isoxsuprine Isoxsuprine has been variously presented as a strong β-sympathicomimetic agent, a specific vasorelaxant, a uterine relaxant and an agent reducing blood viscosity. Since its efficacy has been doubted with respect to both its vascular and its obstetric use, one must suspect that underdosage of the drug is the best explanation for the low incidence of adverse reactions reported; the latter are generally of the type regarded as anecdotal (nausea, vomiting, palpitations, dizziness, weakness). The sympathicomimetic effect is sufficient to cause *fetal tachycardia* when the drug is given intravenously in late pregnancy, although one large survey suggests that it may be better tolerated by the mother (as regards cardiac and stimulant effects) than salbutamol (SED-12, 313), The fact that maternal *blood pressure can fall* may indeed reflect a direct relaxant effect on the blood vessels.

Isoethamine Isoethamine is given in 10—20-mg oral doses as a slow-release tablet. It is slightly more β_2-selective than isoprenaline but has a β-blocking metabolite. *Tremor*, *palpitations*, *tiredness* or *cramps* are not unexpected effects; in long-term use, *tachyphylaxis* can occur.

DRUGS PREDOMINANTLY STIMULATING β_1-ADRENERGIC RECEPTORS

Dopamine

This natural catecholamine and central nervous transmitter is capable of raising cardiac output, decreasing peripheral resistance and specifically increasing the renal blood flow. Infusions (generally up to 10 μg/kg per hour) have proven valuable in shock and congestive heart failure.

Common adverse reactions during this (life-saving) procedure include *ectopic beats*, *tachycardia* and *palpitations*. *Anginal pain*, *bradycardia*, *derangement of cardiac conduction*, *nausea* and *vomiting*, *headache and dyspnea* can occur; *pilo-erection* and *azotemia* have been reported and *blood pressure* may either rise or fall.

The major risk during dopamine treatment is that of severe peripheral *ischemia*, particularly in patients in whom the peripheral circulation is already impaired, since dopamine is converted in the body to noradrenaline; gangrene has repeatedly resulted. In some of the reported cases the error lay in extravasation of dopamine from a peripheral venous infusion site; in others the dosage had been high and prolonged, or ergometrine had also been given. In cases of pre-existing vascular damage from arteriosclerosis, diabetes, Raynaud's disease or frostbite, particular care must be taken. If discoloration appears, the infusion should be stopped and 5—10 mg phentolamine given intravenously. Nitroprusside may fail to prevent the onset of gangrene.

When used for the treatment of low-output congestive heart failure, dopamine has been shown to *inhibit platelet aggregation* in vivo and in vitro. This is in contrast to the platelet-aggregating properties of many catecholamines (19[C]).

In one reported case, dopamine was considered to have produced *myoclonic encephalopathy* (20[C]).

Risk situations For obvious reasons, use of dopamine may be dangerous in cases of *coronary or peripheral vascular disorders*. Dopamine used for hypotension during *percutaneous transluminal angioplasty* (PTCA) may be associated with the development of diffuse coronary spasms, and it should therefore be employed with caution, particularly if high doses are required. In cases where dopamine aggravates pulmonary hypertension and right ventricular failure, isoproterenol must be considered as an alternative inotropic drug.

Interactions Dopamine appears to be unstable in the presence of *alkali*. One might expect its hypertensive effect to be counteracted by *phentolamine* and strongly prolonged by *MAO inhibitors*. Potentiation could occur with cyclopropane or halogenated hydrocarbon anesthetics.

Dobutamine

Dobutamine is a relatively selective β_1-adrenergic receptor antagonist with only slight β_2- and α-adrenergic activity. It has been developed as a positive inotropic agent with less vasoconstrictive effects than high doses of dopamine.

Dobutamine appears to augment cardiac output after acute myocardial infarction without exacerbating myocardial infarction or ventricular arrhythmias. However, a mild increase in heart rate occurs routinely, and occasionally a more marked *tachycardia* is induced.

Cardiac *arrhythmias* of various types (including occasional ventricular dysrhythmias when the drug is used as a stress-inducing agent during echocardiography—see SEDA-18, 158) have been described; *angina* and *coronary artery spasm* (21[c]) have also occurred under these and other conditions. Some 10% of patients may require treatment for angina occurring during the test, but up to a quarter may show ischemic changes on the ECG (SEDA-17, 163), while others experience *headache*, *palpitations*, *anxiety*, *nausea*, *tingling* and *flushing*.

One study showed that of patients undergoing dobutamine stress echocardiography, 37.5% actually developed *hypotension*. Increases in blood pressure are more in line with what one would expect; although dobutamine does not as a rule cause a marked increase in systolic blood pressure in normotensive patients, hypertensive patients can develop marked *systolic hypertension* during an infusion of the drug. When stress echocardiography with dobutamine is performed in subjects who prove to be entirely healthy, an audible *Still's-like vibratory systolic ejection murmur* is nevertheless produced.

Whilst the drug has indeed proved valuable, it became evident early in its use that severe *peripheral ischemia* (even leading to dermal necrosis) could occur, as with dopamine (22[C]).

A non-cardiovascular side effect attributed to dopamine is *urinary urgency* during infusion of a relatively high dose (15 μg/kg per minute).

Ibopamine

Ibopamine is an orally active dopamine derivative which has been studied in patients with congestive heart failure (23[R]). In theory most, if not all, of the reported side effects can be considered to result from the drug's known pharmacological actions. The *gastrointestinal reactions* could be interpreted as dopaminergic in nature, the occasional *dizziness*, *flushing* and *tremor* as β_2-adrenergic agonist effects, the *tachycardia* as an effect of β_1-adrenergic stimulation or a reflex response to β_2-adrenergic agonism. A reversible *leukopenia* has been described but the relationship to the drug is uncertain (24[c]).

Prenalterol

This agent of the dobutamine type has been used in severe heart failure. It can produce *cardiac arrhythmia* (SEDA-6, 135).

Xamoterol

This partial agonist has been used in milder cases of cardiac failure, but in more severe cases it may actually increase *mortality*; for this reason it has been withdrawn from general sale in many countries (SEDA-18, 2).

Levodopa

Dopamine is known to be depleted in cases of Parkinson's disease, but it cannot be used in treating the disease since, because of its low lipid solubility, it is poorly absorbed from the gastrointestinal tract and hardly penetrates the central nervous system. Levodopa, a precursor which is decarboxylated to dopamine but is much more lipid soluble, was developed to overcome this problem. The drug was originally given alone, but because of the extent to which it was decarboxylated outside the central nervous system, large doses had to be given and gastrointestinal intolerance was a problem. By combining levodopa with a decarboxylase inhibitor (carbidopa or benserazide) tolerance is improved and the dose can be lowered. In the following monograph, both the use of levodopa alone and with enzyme inhibitors will be covered.

ADVERSE REACTION PATTERN

General and toxic reactions When levodopa is given alone, severe gastrointestinal upsets are very common during the first year of treatment; they are much less common when enzyme inhibitors are also given. Postural hypertension is not uncommon. Dyskinesias occur in some patients only after starting therapy. Some mental changes are seen in a high proportion of cases. Psychological dependence occurs in a small subset of patients (25[C]). Effects on the liver, renal function and hematological parameters are normally slight. Individual prescribers and clinics tend to develop their own approaches to obtaining the best balance between effects and adverse reactions; a 'drug holiday' (e.g. 2 days per week) has long been recommended by some workers to reduce the incidence of adverse effects (26[C]), but others have described a neuroleptic malignant syndrome when the administration of the drug was temporarily discontinued (SEDA-17, 147; 27[CR]).

Hypersensitivity reactions Allergic type reactions do not seem to occur, but carbidopa has been reported to produce a fixed drug eruption.

Tumor-inducing effects Cases of malignant melanoma (on one occasion within a congenital nevus) have been described in patients taking levodopa; the causal link has not been established, but patients should be monitored for skin changes (28[C]).

ORGANS AND SYSTEMS

Cardiovascular *Postural hypotension* has been estimated to occur in some 15% of cases on plain levodopa during the first year of treatment, and in 10% of patients treated with the levodopa/carbidopa mixture; it would seem doubtful whether the difference is significant. Some patients on the other hand become *hypertensive*; they may be individuals who absorb or metabolize the drug at an abnormal rate. Levodopa can cause *ventricular arrhythmias* in patients with existing cardiac disorders. Transient *flushing* of the skin is common; *palpitations* are unusual.

Respiratory An isolated case of *respiratory dysrhythmia* has been reported (29[C]); it was dose-related and impeded adequate treatment but was ultimately suppressed with tiapride.

Nervous system Dyskinesias occurring during long-term use of levodopa have been classified in various ways. One system presents them as falling broadly into three groups:

'On' dyskinesias These coincide with periods of clinical response to the drug; they include chorea, myoclonus and dystonic movements. They are enhanced by dopamine agonists and reduced by dopamine antagonists

'Off' dyskinesias These coincide with periods of poor response and comprise mainly dystonic postures, affecting in particular the feet; they are inhibited both by dopamine agonists and antagonists.

'Dysphasic dyskinesias' These occur at the beginning and end of 'on' period. They involve repetitive stereotyped movements of the lower limbs, and they too react well to both dopamine agonists and antagonists.

Currently work is being undertaken to find an explanation for the emergence of dyskinesias during prolonged levodopa treatment; there is reason to believe that they result from an interaction between the levodopa and the underlying condition rather than from one or the other. In many cases of severe parkinsonism one can speak of a 'peak dose dyskinesia' which is only problematical when the patient is treated at a relatively high dose, which tends to be most marked on the most severely diseased side, and which responds to dose reduction (30[CR]).

There is some evidence that the atypical neuroleptic clozapine may help to alleviate levodopa-induced dyskinesia while itself providing additional relief of parkinsonism (SEDA-18, 159); clozapine may also relieve levodopa-induced psychosis (SEDA-17, 166).

'Start hesitation' (*akinesia paradoxical*) is the name given to sudden episodes during which the patient may experience a sensation of extreme heaviness of the feet and find himself unable to start walking; the legs tremble and the patient may fall forward; the condition can improve if the levodopa dose is reduced.

Asterixis, a jerky relaxation of tonically contracted postural muscles, was observed in some patients with structural lesions of the brain or metabolic encephalopathy who were taking levodopa, but not in Parkinson patients (31[C]).

The *'on-off effect'*, seen after prolonged therapy in some patients, has been referred to above; it is characterized by sudden swings between severe parkinsonian symptoms (with freedom from side effects) and normal mobility (but with marked adverse drug effects). It would seem likely that unexplained variations in dopamine levels in the central nervous system are responsible; the condition has been seen less often since the combination with a decarboxylase inhibitor came into general use.

Toxic psychoses and toxic *delirium* can occur, particularly in individuals with a history of postencephalitic parkinsonism or psychiatric disease. Much more common are such symptoms as *confusion* (13% of cases), *depression* (9% of cases, often requiring antidepressant drugs), and *sleep disturbances* (20% of cases). Vivid *hallucinations* are common. *Psychotic symptoms* appear to be more common when enzyme inhibitors are used or anticholinergic drugs given. *Panic attacks* seem to occur in some 20% of cases during the 'off' phases of 'off/on' fluctuation (32[CR]).

Libido has been found to increase, at least for some time, in a proportion of patients; whilst perhaps in part reflecting the improved mobility and sense of well-being, a causative relation with prolactin inhibition by levodopa has been suggested.

Headache and *peripheral neuropathy* are rare complications.

Endocrine, metabolic Occasional increases in *protein-bound iodine* have occurred. Elevated *uric acid* levels can occur and in some cases frank gout appears, occasionally within a few days of starting treatment. Levodopa slightly raises plasma *growth hormone* levels. *Carbohydrate tolerance* is slightly impaired.

Disruption of the diurnal *cortisol* rhythm has been detected; it could explain some of the sleep disturbances and psychic side effects noted above (SEDA-8, 143).

Mineral and fluid balance There is a tendency to *potassium loss* with hypokalemia, less frequent since the combination with enzyme inhibitors came into use. *Hyponatremia* has been reported in one published case, but the patient had earlier experienced the same reaction with amantadine (SEDA-18, 159).

Hematological Very occasional falls in *white blood cell count*, *hemoglobin* and *hematocrit* occur. The *Coombs test* can be positive and there is an isolated report of *hemolytic anemia*, and another of *thrombocytopenia* with a positive antinuclear antibody test (SED-12, 315). An otherwise unexplainable acute severe *non-hemolytic anemia* in an elderly man taking levodopa with benserazide has also been observed (SEDA-12, 124).

Liver Liver function tests are as a rule unchanged, but isolated changes in *SGOT*, *SGPT*, *bilirubin* and *LDH* have been recorded.

Gastrointestinal Despite the fact that gastrointestinal tolerance can be improved by cautious dosage, very gradual dose increases and the use of antiemetics, *anorexia*, *nausea* and *vomiting* were estimated to occur in between 36 and 83% of patients taking levodopa alone, and some 10% of patients never succeeded in tolerating the dose which was optimally effective for them. Gastrointestinal tolerance is substantially better with the combined products in use today; provided the combination is taken during meals, digestive disturbances are usually mild and transitory, only a few patients requiring antiemetics.

Urinary system *Blood urea nitrogen* levels occasionally increase. One report suggested darkening of the urine; this seems to have been coincidental, but it is striking that darkening of the sweat and of cartilage has also been described (see below). *Urinary retention* has been described in a case of hypertonic bladder; again the association may have been fortuitous.

There are several reports of a *diuretic effect* of levodopa; although seldom recognized, the effect is probably fairly consistent and not limited, as was at one time suggested, to obese subjects (33[r]).

Skin One case of *pemphigus erythematosus* after 18 months of treatment with levodopa/carbidopa has been reported (34[C]). Darkening of the *sweat fluid* has been described. Darkening of the white *hair* of a patient who was treated with levodopa in combination with bromocriptine for parkinsonism has also been reported (SEDA-15, 1). Strikingly, there is also a little scattered evidence suggesting a link between levodopa and the development of *melanoma* (SEDA-17, 167), but a prior history of melanoma should not be regarded as a contra-indication to levodopa treatment.

Skeletal system There seems to be no doubt that patients treated in this way are more prone to sustain *fractures* (35[R]). The most likely explanation is simply that they are more mobile and thus more likely to fall than before treatment was instituted, but it should be borne in mind that benserazide did cause skeletal changes in rats used for the original toxicity investigations.

'*Black cartilage*' (intense black pigmentation confined to the costal cartilage) has been found at necropsy in a man after 13 years of levodopa/carbidopa treatment (SED-12, 316).

Risk situations Because of the cardiovascular effects, patients with *cardiac disorders* are at risk. This treatment should not be used in patients with a history of *mental illness*, *hemolytic anemia*, or any serious *organic disease*.

Withdrawal effects A serious relapse of parkinsonism can occur after withdrawal. At least two reports also describe an incident reminiscent of the *neuroleptic malignant syndrome* with hyperthermia, semistupor, rigidity and tremor (36[C]; see also above).

Second-generation effects These have not been described.

Interactions *Monoamine-oxidase inhibitors* given with levodopa will lead to hypertension. *Pyridoxine* interferes with the desired CNS effect of levodopa, since it is itself a co-decarboxylase which facilitates the transformation of levodopa to dopa outside the central nervous system. *Papaverine* can reduce the effects of levodopa treatment. *Orphenadrine* may potentiate the effects, while *propranolol* improves the effect on tremor. *Neuroleptics* can aggravate parkinsonism, and if antiemetics are required non-phenothiazines should therefore be chosen.

Interference with diagnostic routines Treatment with levodopa results in false-positive tests for urinary glucose and ketone bodies.

Long-term safety In view of the fundamental nature of the therapy involving, on the one hand, interference with central nervous transmitters and, on the other, the chronic inhibition of an enzyme system widely distributed in the body, the very long-term safety of this approach must remain a matter of study. To date there seems to be good reason for optimism.

OTHER DRUGS INCREASING DOPAMINE ACTIVITY

Amantadine

Originally developed as an antiviral agent, amantadine appears to promote the release of dopamine from nerve endings, but it may delay their re-uptake into synaptic vesicles. Doses of 100—200 mg daily are often used and are usually well tolerated. The best-documented adverse reactions to amantadine are *nausea*, *psychotic episodes* (mania, hallucinations, agitation, confusion), *restless legs* and *convulsions*. In one case, an elderly man developed the 'Othello syndrome'—a severe delusion of marital infidelity; it receded with drug withdrawal (SEDA-17, 170). The risk of mental complications seems to increase substantially if doses of 200 mg or more are given. In bipolar patients, in whom it can trigger mania, amantadine is contraindicated. Resistant *edema* of the ankles in the absence of cardiac disease has repeatedly been described and well documented by rechallenge (37[CR]). *Livedo reticularis* has been stated to occur in as many as 90% of patients; certainly it is very common in female patients. Although neither edema nor livedo reticularis has been shown to be a sign of a serious systemic disorder, suspicion has been raised that the drug could be mildly *cardiotoxic*, and a case of reversible congestive failure during amantadine treatment is on record (38[R]). Minor adverse reactions often resemble those caused by anticholinergic agents, e.g. *blurred vision*, *dryness of the mouth*, *insomnia*, *lethargy* and *rash*. In rare cases, *photosensitization* has been described. Rarely, amantadine causes *visual impairment* due to corneal abrasions, local edema and superficial keratitis (39[c]). In a case of end-stage renal failure, the drug caused *coma*, though drug plasma levels were not grossly increased (SEDA-18, 160).

Apomorphine *(SEDA-17, 167)*

This old drug has been reassessed with some success for use in Parkinsonism. It is a very potent non-selective dopamine agonist, acting on both D_1 and D_2 receptors. Because of the first-pass effect it has to be used subcutaneously, sublingually or intranasally. Its adverse effects resemble those of levodopa.

Yawning, *somnolence*, *nausea* and *vomiting* can all result from use of apomorphine; they respond to naloxone.

A paradoxical *akinetic response* has been reported in a middle-aged man, probably with nigrostriatal degeneration, who became both immobile and mute 15 minutes after taking 4 mg of the drug; the effect was seen again on rechallenge with doses as low as 2 mg. The mechanism is not clear.

Local reactions to administration in the nose and throat can include swelling of the nose and lips, stomatitis and buccal mucosal ulceration.

Memantine

Memantine is an amantadine derivative which has been studied in patients with parkinsonism. Side effects have included *agitation*, *restlessness*, *insomnia*, *pronounced delirious states* and *muscular hypotonia*. All were reversible after reduction of dosage or discontinuation of therapy. A *toxic psychosis* has been reported in two patients (40[c]).

Rimantadine

Rimantadine, an amantadine analog (α-methyl-1-adamantanemethylamine hydrochloride), has been found to be more active than amantadine against influenza A viruses in vitro and in laboratory animals. Clinically, side effects have been considered to be less common with rimantadine (SEDA-8, 143).

Precursor amino acids

Tyrosine, 5-hydroxytryptamine and carbidopa have in the past been given experimentally in an attempt to provide oral replacement therapy for the cerebral neurotransmitters serotonin, dopamine and noradrenaline. The treatment produced *frequent stools* or frank diarrhea in all patients, *nausea* and *drowsiness* in the majority, *agitation* and *restlessness* in 50% and *hyperventilation*, *confusion* and *hallucination* in some cases. There was little evidence of improvement (SEDA-3, 125).

Selegiline

The therapeutic merits of this selective inhibitor of monoamine oxidase type B are currently disputed following further clinical study. Rarely, selegiline has reactivated pre-existing *peptic ulcer* disease. Through its metabolism to amphetamine and methamphetamine it may cause *insomnia* (SEDA-17, 167).

Interactions can be of importance: selegiline seems to exacerbate adverse reactions induced by concurrent levodopa therapy and is known to inhibit dopamine metabolism; when given alongside fluoxetine it has produced a sudden increase in blood pressure.

DRUGS STIMULATING DOPAMINERGIC RECEPTORS

Bromocriptine

Bromocriptine is an ergot derivative. High doses (e.g. 30—75 mg daily p.o.) are used in parkinsonism; low doses (2.5—5.0 mg daily) are used in prostatic tumors and to suppress lactation. The adverse reactions are dose-dependent and, so far as is known, reversible, but they are frequent, being experienced in up to 50% of cases.

ADVERSE REACTION PATTERN

General and toxic reactions With any dose, nausea, vomiting and postural hypotension are problematical in some patients, especially those given high doses from the start; the gastrointestinal symptoms tend to become less as treatment is continued, but other symptoms, e.g. peripheral circulatory disturbances, can set in later. Psychic and psychiatric changes can be troublesome in a proportion of patients on high doses. Constipation tends to be a frequent and persistent complication.

Hypersensitivity reactions These have not been reported.

Tumor-inducing effects In rats (but not in mice) high doses induced malignant uterine tumors within 2 years (SEDA-3, 122). Tumor induction has not been seen in man, but enlargement of a non-invasive pituitary tumour has been observed on more than one occasion.

ORGANS AND SYSTEMS

Cardiovascular Occasional patients on low doses experience *postural hypotension* leading to dizziness or syncope. A *Raynaud-type syndrome* with blanching of the extremities in response to cold is a rare occurrence. With high doses some 30% may suffer a peripheral cold reaction of this type, which may not become manifest for a time, while *leg cramps* appear in some 10% of cases. Rather less than 10% of patients suffer *flushing* or *erythromelalgia*, and *hypotension* appears in some 5%. Occasional cases of *bradycardia* or acute *left ventricular failure* have been described. Cases of *angina pectoris* can experience aggravation of the condition (SED-12, 317). Even acute *myocardial infarction* following coronary spasm has been reported (SEDA-12, 123, 317). *Edema* can occur with this and other dopamine agonists, the association easily being overlooked (SEDA-18, 159). The fibrotic complications noted below can extend to the heart, resulting in *constrictive pericarditis*.

Respiratory Pulmonary reactions are rare. *Pleural thickening and effusions* and *pleuropulmonary fibrosis* have been observed in a number of cases (SEDA-11, 130); other forms of fibrosis are noted above and below. *Nasal catarrh* is not uncommon even with low doses.

Nervous system High doses given in parkinsonism are perhaps slightly less well tolerated than equi-effective doses of levodopa, and up to 10% of cases may have to be withdrawn from treatment because of *psychiatric symptoms*. Bromocriptine-induced *psychosis* is well known and it seems that particular caution is warranted in patients having a family history of mental disorders (41[C]). Even very low doses of bromocriptine can induce psychotic reactions (SEDA-9, 126; SEDA-10, 117), and well-recognized problems include confusion, hallucinations, delusions and paranoia.

Syncope, *headache* and *migraine* can all occur in a minority of cases on low doses, and even where there is no hypotensive reaction some 30% of cases will experience *dizziness*. *Dyskinesias* have been described as complicating the treatment of parkinsonism in a high proportion of cases, but more especially if the drug is used alongside levodopa. Occasionally, *paresthesia* and *bad dreams* have been described. When the manufacturer examined reports from physicians on adverse effects occurring with the use of bromocriptine for the inhibition of lactation, 38 cases of *seizures* were prominent in the analysis.

An interesting but highly unusual sequel of bromocriptine administration may be *CSF rhinorrhea* (SEDA-8, 143). The reverse effect—air aspiration through a sellar-pharyngeal leak—has also been encountered (SEDA-9, 126).

Gastrointestinal *Nausea* and *vomiting* are common.

Liver In one series six of 18 patients on high doses for parkinsonism developed isolated and asymptomatic increases in *serum transaminases* (SED-12, 317). Other patients have also shown this reaction, which is reversible (SEDA-17, 168).

Hematological One case of *leukocytopenia* and *thrombocytopenia* has been described (42[Cr]).

Endocrine, metabolic A 1993 case report describes *inappropriate secretion of ADH* in a single patient (43[c]).

Skin and appendages *Alopecia*, reversible after drug withdrawal, has been reported as a rare effect of the drug (SEDA-18, 159).

Local effects Intravaginal administration, sometimes used to reduce gastric adverse effects, has in a few patients caused intravaginal 'burning'.

Special senses In one series three of 18 patients developed *blurred vision* during high-dose treatment of parkinsonism (SEDA-3, 124). *Diplopia* has been incidentally reported. In three patients with chronic hepatic encephalopathy, reversible *ototoxicity* developed following the administration of bromocriptine (44[C]).

Musculoskeletal system *Dysarthria* has been occasionally described. Three cases of *contractures* of the extremities were possibly caused by bromocriptine (SEDA-14, 119).

Fibrotic reactions *Retroperitoneal fibrosis* (SEDA-12, 123; 45[c]) and *pulmonary fibrosis* (SEDA-11, 130) during treatment with high doses of bromocriptine have been observed. The drug's structural relationship to methysergide clearly has to be borne in mind.

Sexual function Increased *sexual drive* in patients with Parkinson's disease is common, but *impotence* can also be induced by bromocriptine therapy. Dose reduction may be helpful in this situation (SEDA-13, 111).

Risk situations If bromocriptine is to be used to treat infertility, the presence of a *pituitary adenoma* must be excluded, since this may otherwise undergo suprasellar extension during pregnancy. Because of its adverse reaction profile, bromocriptine can better be avoided in patients with *cardiac disease* or *peripheral vascular impairment*. *Acromegalics with a history of gastrointestinal ulceration or bleeding* should not be treated; generally, however, bromocriptine seems to be rather better tolerated by acromegalics, postmenopausal women and patients with a raised serum prolactin than by other individuals.

In *hypertension of pregnancy*, the impression is that bromocriptine may have an aggravating effect (SEDA-15, 2); this has led to hesitation as regards the continued use of bromocriptine for suppression of lactation, especially in patients with a history of pregnancy-induced hypertension.

A new risk group for bromocriptine could be *cocaine abusers*, who it is suspected might develop *cerebrovascular and cardiovascular disorders*.

Second-generation effects Because of its use in the treatment of female infertility, which inevitably involves early exposure of some embryos, the safety of bromocriptine in early pregnancy was systematically evaluated in a large multicenter study with prolonged follow-up (SEDA-13, 112). No evidence was found that this use of bromocriptine was associated with an increased risk of spontaneous abortion, multiple pregnancy or the occurrence of congenital malformation; nor did exposure to this drug in utero seem to produce any adverse effect on postnatal development. Cervical incompetence may be a problem at the time of delivery, but this may well be due to a long history of infertility rather than to the drug. In other work, no chromosomal changes were found in 19 children born after bromocriptine-induced ovulation (46[C]).

Use in lactation Bromocriptine suppresses lactation and the infant should not be breast-fed from the moment the treatment is instituted. If the drug is deliberately (and successfully) used to suppress lactation, *breast tenderness* and *milk leakage* can ensue. It has been suggested that use of bromocriptine for this purpose raises the risk of post-puerperal seizures, but the evidence is equivocal (SEDA-17, 146).

Effects on fertility Sudden induction of fertility in sterile women may occasionally be an embarrassing adverse reaction if the drug is being use for other purposes, e.g. parkinsonism.

Interactions Bromocriptine can cause intolerance to *alcohol* resulting in alcohol-induced migraine. The response to bromocriptine, at least in acromegaly, can be blocked by *griseofulvin*. *Tamoxifen* can resolve some of the drug's side effects, offering perhaps a possibility of bromocriptine treatment to patients who cannot otherwise tolerate it (SEDA-8, 144). Dangerous hypertensive reactions can result from interaction with *sympathicomimetic drugs* isometheptene and phenylpropanolamine (SEDA-17, 168).

Carbergoline

This later ergoline derivative has been tried in hyperprolactinemic patients (SEDA-15, 2). Side effects observed were *nausea*, *hypotension*, *headache*, *gastric pain*, *dizziness* and *weakness* which as a rule resolved over time.

Cases have been described in which patients who developed retroperitoneal or pleural *fibrosis* on bromocriptine experienced a further aggravation of the condition after switching to carbergoline; the latter drug may well prove to share this risk with bromocriptine, though it has to date apparently not been reported in patients in whom carbegoline therapy was not preceded by use of bromocriptine (SEDA-17, 169).

Ergoline

8-α-Ergoline (CU 32-085) was compared in an open study with bromocriptine. It appeared to be more effective and to have fewer side effects.

Lisuride (Lysuride)

Lisuride is used as an alternative drug in the treatment of parkinsonism. The pattern of side effects is similar to that seen with most of the ergot alkaloids (SEDA-10, 118). In one instance to date, *pleuropulmonary disease* has been observed. Effusions were present but apparently there was no significant fibrosis, and the condition was almost completely reversible.

Mesulergine (8-α-aminoergoline)

Mesulergine is an ergoline derivative acting as a dopamine agonist. The most frequent side effect is *dyskinesia*, mostly in patients who have had similar reactions with levodopa. *Orthostatic light-headedness* and *visual hallucinations* were also frequently observed. Other side effects included *anorexia*, *nausea*, *drowsiness*, *ankle swelling*, *insomnia*, *confusion*, *irritability*, *visual disturbance*, *chest pain*, *rash* and augmented *body odor*. One study of 17 patients with mild Parkinson's disease who were given either mesulergine or pergolide concluded that mesulergine impaired the quality of life; frequent side effects were *vomiting*, *lassitude*, *abdominal discomfort*, *depression*, *right bundle-branch block*, *fuzzy-headedness*, and *increasing insulin requirement in a diabetic patient* (SEDA-13, 313).

It was recommended in 1985 that clinical research with mesulergine be discontinued, following the finding that an increased prevalence of interstitial testicular tumors occurred in male rats treated lifelong with the drug. This seems to be a sex-related toxicity specific for the male rat; there is no evidence of carcinogenic potential in mice or female rats (SED-12, 319).

Pergolide

The adverse reactions to pergolide resemble those of bromocriptine (SEDA-10, 118; SEDA-13, 113). Long-term assessment (SEDA-15, 3) pointed to *confusion* and *hallucinations* as the side effects most likely to require discontinuation of the drug. Symptoms suggestive of dose-related *angina pectoris* were observed in a number of patients, either early or late in treatment, but they were easily controlled by dose reduction of pergolide, without sequelae.

Dose-related *leukopenia* developed in one patient.

Pergolide can cause severe *hypotension* in patients already receiving antihypertensive agents (47^C).

Piribedil

Hallucinations and *confusion* as well as *nausea*, *vomiting* and *hypotension* may occur during treatment with piribedil. *Sleepiness* has also been described (SEDA-10, 119).

Ropinrole

This selective dopamine D_2 agonist appears so far to have effects similar to its congeners.

Terguride

This compound has produced epigastric distress, transient orthostatic hypotension, headache and nausea.

CV 205-502

This is an interesting innovation in that it is a potent non-ergot benzoquinoline dopamine D_2 receptor agonist. To date, the adverse effects reported are limited to gastrointestinal upsets and weight loss.

DRUGS PREDOMINANTLY STIMULATING β_2-ADRENERGIC RECEPTORS

Drugs predominantly stimulating β_2-adrenergic receptors are employed primarily for the treatment of asthma on the one hand and the arrest of premature labor on the other; not all of them have been developed for both purposes.

Salbutamol

Salbutamol (albuterol) is employed in asthma orally, in nebulized form and by injection; for obstetric use it is usually given by injection. The question as to whether resistance to the bronchodilator effect develops with repeated use is disputed. The nebulized form is generally found to have the fewest side effects, apparently because the dosage can be more finely adjusted and not because of any preferential local effect on the airways; adverse reactions may be even less when the drug is given by intermediate positive pressure breathing, for similar reasons.

ADVERSE REACTION PATTERN

General and toxic reactions Since the drug is not entirely selective in its β_2-stimulating action, it retains some stimulant effects on cardiac sensitivity and activity, on the central nervous system, and on carbohydrate and fat metabolism; these only become troublesome with relative overdosage or in particularly susceptible subjects. Surprisingly, one large survey suggests that when used in pregnancy salbutamol may be less well tolerated by the mother (stimulation, cardiovascular effects) than the much less selective isoxsuprine (SED-12, 321).

Hypersensitivity reactions These are rare, but one well-documented case of allergy against salbutamol has been described (SEDA-13, 109).

Tumor-inducing effects These have not been reported in man. Chronic administration to rats produces mesovarian leiomyomas, a form of tumor not known in human subjects. The findings might reflect a species-specific consequence of prolonged

β_2-adrenergic stimulation of the rat estrous cycle; no tumors developed in mice similarly treated (SEDA-3, 118).

ORGANS AND SYSTEMS

Cardiovascular In many subjects, slight *palpitations* and some peripheral *vasodilatation* occur; more marked cardiovascular effects usually appear only with high doses or rapid administration, or in the presence of predisposing factors. Inhalation of 400 μg was found not to affect the heart rate, whereas inhalation of 5 mg raised it by 15/minute (48[C]) and an infusion of 25 μg/minute, studied by others, had a similar effect. This slight *tachycardia* can result in a mild rise in blood pressure. With more extreme dosage, the vasodilatation predominates and the *blood pressure may fall*, e.g. infusion of 125 μg/minute reduced blood pressure by 30 mmHg. In those patients in whom there is a marked rise in free fatty acids, a fall in serum potassium or severe hypoxemia, the chance of *ectopic beats* and cardiac *dysrhythmias* is increased (SEDA-2, 121). Salbutamol is known to cause an increase in the activity of the MB isoenzyme of creatine kinase, suggesting that it might be cardiotoxic (49[C]).

Respiratory Although the drug generally improves respiratory activity in the asthmatic, arterial *hypoxemia* can be aggravated if salbutamol is used to excess, or if parenchymal lung infection is present (50[C]). In patients with bronchiectasis, salbutamol may aggravate hemoptysis (SEDA-9, 125). A feeling of *'thick neck'*, *chest heaviness*, *erythema and edema of the face* experienced in one reported case after the third dose could be reproduced by re-administration of the drug (SEDA-10, 116). *Pulmonary edema* may occur, even hours after discontinuation of β_2-adrenergic receptor stimulants (SEDA-13, 110).

Nervous system A fine *muscular tremor* is common and a few patients experience *headache*. With overdosage there can be *agitation* and even *psychotic manifestations*. In susceptible persons, *hallucinations* can develop, particularly in children but also in adults (51[C]).

Endocrine, metabolic Salbutamol causes a *rise in blood glucose* which is usually of no consequence except in the pregnant diabetic. There are also changes in *blood lipids* (see Table 3). *Perspiration* may reflect a general increase in sympathetic tonus.

Mineral and fluid balance Serum *potassium* can fall (see Table 3) and a mild *acidosis* can be induced. The former effect is potentiated by the concurrent use of theophylline (SEDA-17, 164); it does not normally have serious consequences.

Gastrointestinal High doses can produce mild *nausea*.

Special senses Salbutamol has been given in the eye for glaucoma, but has very often produced *local irritation*.

Risk situations Because of its cardiac and metabolic effect, salbutamol should be given only very cautiously and under strict control in *cardiovascular disease*, *diabetes* and *hyperthyroidism*. Since 50% of the drug is excreted renally, adjustment of the dose will be needed if *renal function* is markedly impaired.

Some risk situations for β_2-adrenergic stimulants as such are mentioned when discussing other members of the group (below).

Second-generation effects Should an abortion occur in pregnant asthmatic patients taking this drug, the relaxant effect on the uterine wall is likely to result in marked *bleeding*. When salbutamol is used to arrest premature labor, effective doses are likely to produce mild *fetal tachycardia* (e.g. an increase of 20/minute).

Overdosage A dose of 200 mg p.o. has resulted in *agitation*, *tachycardia* and *peripheral vasodilatation*, amenable to treatment with β-blockers and benzodiazepines.

Interactions The risk of hyperglycemia or hypokalemia will be increased if *corticosteroids* are given simultaneously (e.g. for asthma). Salbutamol has additive effects with *other sympathicomimetics* and *theophylline*. Its effects are naturally antagonized by the β-blockers. Treatment with *bendrofluazide* and presumably other *diuretics* augments the hypokalemic and ECG effects of high-dose inhaled albuterol; the arrhythmogenic potential of this interaction may be important in patients with acute exacerbations of chronic airflow obstruction, who have concomitant hypoxemia and ischemic heart disease (SEDA-15, 3).

Table 3. *Metabolic effects of intravenous salbutamol in healthy pregnant women and pregnant diabetics (for sources, see SEDA-3, 119)*

	Healthy women (n = 5)			Diabetics (n = 7)
	Lunell et al.*	Thomas et al.**	Fredholm et al.***	Fredholm et al.***
Glucose (mmol/l)	+1.8	−4.0	+1.7	+4.0
Insulin (mU/I)	+30	−26	+47	
Free fatty acids (mmol/l)	+0.5		+0.4	+0.9
Glycerol (mmol/l)	+0.11		+0.10	+0.22
Hydroxybutyrate (mmol/l)	+0.6		+0.45	+1.05
Potassium (mmol/l)		−0.6		

Values are maximal mean changes in plasma levels. * Salbutamol, 15 μg/min for 45 min. ** Salbutamol, 16—36 μg/min for 2 h. *** Salbutamol in progressive doses up to 22.5 μg/min for 80 min.

OTHER DRUGS PREDOMINANTLY STIMULATING β_2-ADRENERGIC RECEPTORS

Bitolterol
Broxaterol
Carbuterol
Clenbuterol
Dopexamine
Fenoterol
Formoterol
Hexoprenaline
Isoetharine
Pirbuterol
Procaterol
Reproterol
Rimiterol
Ritodrine
Salmefamol
Terbutaline
Tulobuterol

It is impossible to find sufficient evidence to assess the relative merits of the β_2-sympathicomimetic drugs as regards the specificity of their action, although for each enthusiastic claims are made in this regard. Some of them have only been compared directly with drugs having no β_1/β_2 dissociation, such as isoprenaline, rather than with other β_2-mimetic agents. Often the doses used in comparisons are not truly comparable. Apart from a few minor points (e.g., hexoprenaline may be marginally better tolerated than fenoterol, but the latter may tend to be used in more severe cases), these drugs all appear to have a similar safety/efficacy ratio. It is probable that in the interests of safety all these agents (or at least the longer-acting compounds) should be used intermittently rather than continuously (52[R]), since with continuous use their efficacy may decline and the chance of paradoxical bronchial hyperreactivity increase.

Clenbuterol Clenbuterol may have a somewhat higher incidence of adverse reactions than some other members of the series and its long half-life could perhaps explain this. *Dyskinetic movements* have been reported as an adverse effect in one elderly patient (SEDA-17, 164).

Dopexamine Dopexamine, though related structurally to dopamine, is a potent β_2-receptor antagonist. Adverse effects reported to date include cases of *atrial fibrillation* and single instances of *supraventricular tachycardia* and *hypotension*.

Isoetharine Isoetharine is primarily a β-adrenergic bronchodilator given orally. In several patients, described by Hooper et al. (53[C]), administration of isoetharine resulted in a *pink coloration of the sputum*, due to the presence of a reddish metabolite; in such cases, hemoptysis may wrongly be suspected.

Ritodrine Ritodrine has been used mainly in obstetrics; the side effects are discussed below. Ritodrine can produce *bradycardia* instead of the expected tachycardia (SEDA-3, 145); an unexpected *hypertensive crisis* has also been reported (SEDA-8, 145). *ST-segment depression* is a consistent finding in patients during ritodrine infusion, and should therefore not always be interpreted as an indication of myocardial ischemia. The ECG changes are unrelated to the more generally accepted changes in heart rate, glucose and potassium levels and are probably an intrinsic effect of the drug. A curious finding is that brief infusions of ritodrine (150 μg/minute for 4 hours) rapidly raise *plasma melatonin* levels in healthy women (54[C]). *Palmar erythema* was observed in 12 of 209 patients who were treated with ritodrine for more than 7 days (SEDA-12, 123). There are two well-documented independent reports of *severe ketoacidosis* in non-diabetic pregnant subjects; both the

β-agonist therapy and inadequate dietary intake could have played a role (55[Cr]).

Agranulocytosis and a petechial rash due to *vasculitis* have both been documented in individual pregnant women (SEDA-17, 165).

As regards the offspring: *neonatal jaundice* is considered to be more frequent in the babies of mothers receiving ritodrine during the second or third trimesters of pregnancy (56[R]).

Rimiterol Rimiterol is metabolized to a 3-*O*-methyl derivative with weak β-blocking and anticholinesterase activity, and the drug also has α-adrenergic effects. This may explain the paradoxical increase in airway resistance that can occur following initial bronchodilatation.

Salmeterol Salmeterol has an adverse reaction pattern closely similar to that of its congenors. A single case of a *pruritic burning maculopapular rash* has been documented and confirmed by patch testing with the active component (SEDA-17, 165).

Terbutaline With terbutaline, *somnolence* has been reported in some studies, and it may be characteristic for this drug, apparently occurring in some 25% of patients. In pregnant patients with a history of *migraine or vascular headache* the use of terbutaline (and its congeners) should be avoided because of the risk of cerebral ischemia (SEDA-8, 145). One pregnant asthmatic patient suffered a *hypotensive* episode after treatment with subcutaneous terbutaline (SEDA-12, 123); a severe and life-threatening hypotensive reaction in patients with quadriplegia after terbutaline medication warrants a warning against indiscriminate use of β-adrenergic agents in the absence of autonomic spinal functions (SEDA-8, 145). The possibility of paradoxical *bronchospasm* due to terbutaline must be taken into consideration (SEDA-8, 145).

Use of β_2-sympathicomimetic agents in premature labor

None of the β_2-sympathicomimetic agents used to delay delivery can be given in effective doses either orally or by injection without affecting the *maternal heart rate* (and to a lesser extent the *fetal heart rate*) in a high proportion of cases. It is not possible to say whether this effect is more prone to occur with certain drugs of this type than with others (particularly because the obstetric situation itself affects the fetal heart rate (see SEDA-17, 145), but in effective doses a maternal heart rate increase of some 30 beats/minute or more is common, with a fetal heart rate increase of up to 20 beats/minute. A substantial proportion of mothers (with intravenous use up to 30%) experience such symptoms as *headache*, *tremulousness*, *tightness of the chest*, *palpitations* and flushing; *pulmonary edema* may occur in one of 20 cases (57[C]), There is clear and direct evidence that tocolytics also exert toxic effects on the myocardial tissue of the infant, especially if given for long periods (58[C], 59[C]), The calcium antagonist, verapamil, does not protect either the maternal heart or the fetal heart against the toxic effects of tocolysis (SEDA-9, 126). A rare, but potentially life-threatening complication of the β_2-stimulants is the development of pulmonary edema (SEDA-10, 115).

All these drugs can exercise the metabolic effects described in the salbutamol monograph above. The effects on glucose metabolism may be absent or harmless in the non-diabetic, but dangerous in the diabetic woman; the hyperglycemic effect can be aggravated if glucocorticoids are given (as they may be to prevent hyaline membrane disease in prematurity).

It has been found that when ritodrine is used to alleviate fetal distress, atropine premedication prior to cesarean section must be avoided; the vagolytic action of atropine is synergistic with the action of ritodrine, resulting in severe maternal tachycardia and systolic hypertension (60[C]); it would seem very likely that the same problem exists with other sympathicomimetic drugs.

Pressurized aerosols

The rapid increase in mortality among asthmatic patients—particularly children and young adults—which occurred in England and Wales and to a lesser extent elsewhere during the period 1959—1966 is now historical (SED-8, 306). Pressurized aerosol vasodilators had been used in 84% of the cases, and sometimes there was evidence of overuse followed by sudden death. Warnings and restrictions on the supply of these aerosols put an end to the epidemic. In 1980—1981, however, a new series of fatalities in The Netherlands and the United Kingdom gave rise to renewed concern, all involving overdosage. Elements involved probably included:

(a) the use of higher concentration products;

(b) a delayed effect due to tolerance developing during long-term treatment, tempting the patient to take an additional dose during the waiting period;

(c) an exaggerated reaction because of derangement of vagal sympathetic equilibrium as a result of long-term use;

(d) addiction and potentiation resulting from simultaneous use of stimulants including ephedrine.

The role of the freons used as propellants is disputed; it is apparently not impossible to attain dangerous cardiac concentrations of a freon if such an aerosol is intensively overused; apart from the fact that this could further sensitize the heart to the sympathicomimetic agent, freons are capable of producing sudden death when abused on their own.

There are however many other theories (SEDA-17, 164) including the possible role of paradoxical broncho-spasm, the involvement of sulfites or other excipients, changes in genetic susceptibility, mucus plugging, hypo-kalemia and hypomagnesemia; some workers have sought an explanation in the fact that the established sympathicomimetics are racemic mixtures; the levorotatory enantiomer is reponsible for the desired effect, but the dextrorotatory component does have its own specific activity, as demonstrated in animal studies.

To these possible causative factors, that of overt abuse must be added. It certainly occurs and is not always possible to trace. When inhalers are used, careful monitoring and advice are needed, especially in young people, although the elderly are certainly not immune to abuse. It might be advisable to prescribe salbutamol in a rotacap inhaler, as fluorocarbon use is thereby avoided and the dosage is better controlled (61[Cr]).

When salbutamol is used in a nebulizer, a marked increase in dosage often occurs. The dose from a pressurized aerosol dispenser amounts to 200—400 μg, while a nebulizer yields much more, up to 10 mg. Such a dose produces tachycardia and palpitations. As tachycardia shortens diastole, the time for coronary perfusion is shortened, and in cases of existing coronary disease this may result in an anginal attack or even a myocardial infarct. Three such cases have been recently published, but it is suspected that many other cases go unrecognized. Caution is therefore recommended when salbutamol is used in nebulized form in older patients or in individuals with known coronary disease. The dose must be kept low, initially not more than 1 mg, increasing it only until adequate bronchodilatation is achieved (62[c]).

The entire debate as to the (historic) problem with asthma aerosols must now be viewed against a more general background, namely the continuing increase in asthma mortality in general, despite ever better treatment. The discussion of that topic goes beyond the scope of the present volume, but it is clear that type of therapy currently in use could paradoxically be contributing to the rising mortality.

DRUGS STIMULATING ATYPICAL β-RECEPTORS

Stimulation of β-adrenoceptors on the cell surface of adipocytes promotes lipolysis and energy expenditure. These receptors, neither β_1- nor β_2-, have been termed atypical or β_3-receptors. Some atypical agonists (BRL 26830A, BRL 35135, CL 316243 and D 7114) have now been developed and assessed for their ability to stimulate these receptors and hence induce weight loss. The BRL compounds appear to *exaggerate physiological tremor*, presumably through an effect on the β_2-receptors; the two other compounds are said to be more selective.

SYMPATHICOLYTIC AGENTS

DRUGS BLOCKING α-ADRENERGIC RECEPTORS

The haloalkylamines and related agents

Alfusozin This selective α-adrenoceptor antagonist is used to relieve the symptoms of prostatic hypertrophy. *Dizziness*, *headache*, *postural hypertension* and other symptoms familiar from the older α-blockers (see phenoxybenzamine below) occur primarily during the first 2 weeks of treatment.

Phenoxybenzamine This agent is given orally in total daily doses up to 60 mg in pheochromocytoma, and lower doses have been used to relieve bladder obstruction before surgery; the maximum effect may be delayed because of irregular absorption, and even after intravenous use it may not be attained for an hour; some of the most severe effects, i.e. *hypotension* and *syncope* with tachycardia, may thus occur unexpectedly. In patients with myocardial infarction, where the drug has been used to improve circulation, it has been found to induce or aggravate *pulmonary edema*; this could be explained by an observation of severe hyponatremia during treatment with phenoxybenzamine (SEDA-13, 113).

Troublesome but frequent adverse reactions are *inhibition of ejaculation* and *nasal stuffiness*; the drug can also cause *miosis*, *lassitude* and *gastrointestinal upsets*. *Panic attacks* have been described in one case, a week after withdrawal of the drug; the causal association is not certain (SEDA-17, 163). When the drug is injected intradermally or when it is extravasated during intravenous administration, it can cause both extremely severe *necrotic reactions* and an *allergic response*.

In view of the nature of its effects the drug should be used sparingly in cardiovascular disease; because a large proportion is renally excreted, renal disease is a reason for reducing dosage. Long-term use seems to destroy the α-adrenergic receptors.

Dibenamine This agent is structurally closely related to phenoxybenzamine and has very similar effects.

Phentolamine, papaverine, and indoramin These agents are used as bronchodilators and vasodilators. Intracavernous administration of papaverine with phentolamine is currently used in the diagnosis and treatment of erectile dysfunction. The major local side effect is *prolonged erection* which usually occurs early during diagnostic testing and is reduced after dose adjustment; furthermore, local *hematomas* have been reported in a number of patients. It may be that cases most prone to priapism can be identified in advance by testing their erectile abilities in response to erotic stimulation (63[C]). Long-term therapy can also cause *intracavernous fibrosis* but it may also lead to development of tolerance to the desired effect. Systemic side effects reported are *hypotension* and *dizziness* and, in rare cases, abnormal results of *liver function tests* (SEDA-15, 3).

Thymoxamine (moxysylate) In separate publications from France in 1991, three instances of *hepatitis* have been reported with this drug (SEDA-17, 163).

Tolazoline This agent has a pulmonary vasodilator action and is therefore used to improve arterial oxygenation in infants. However, it also has a histamine-like action, increasing gastric juice secretion. This property apparently led to *duodenal perforation* in a 31-hour-old infant treated with tolazoline for 6 hours because of meconium aspiration; the defect required surgical correction (64[c]).

THE ERGOT ALKALOIDS AND RELATED AGENTS

Ergotamine

Total daily doses of up to 6 mg ergotamine tartrate are given orally in migraine, generally together with caffeine; injections and suppositories are also in use. If the drug is chronically used (which is in any case undesirable because of the vascular effects), a *vicious circle* can arise, withdrawal headaches leading to the use of ever-increasing doses (SEDA-13, 113). In this situation tolerance can develop to the point at which the doses being used exceed what are normally regarded as safe limits. The only possible treatment for the condition is to withdraw the drug; the withdrawal symptoms tend to be poorly responsive to alternative medication, but they usually recede within 72 hours, after which the patient can be treated with other anti-migraine drugs. The best means of preventing ergotamine 'dependence' is to limit the use of ergotamine tartrate to no more than 2 days per week and to ensure that the drug is not used unnecessarily for plain headaches which have all too readily been labelled as 'migrainous'.

Cardiovascular The *vasoconstrictive effects* present a greater risk. The extremities become pale and cold, and arterial spasm in the upper and lower limbs has been demonstrated; even the face can be affected by the ischemic state. The condition can develop acutely even after brief use of the drug, and there is real risk of *gangrene*; if given early, intra-arterial infusion of prostaglandin E_1 can reverse the spasms. Protracted *coronary spasm* due to the use of ergotamine has also been reported in some cases (SEDA-14, 122), as has severe cardiac valvular disease of the fibrotic type. *Renal arterial spasm* has been found after a dose of 10 mg in the form of suppositories given over a 60-hour period (SED-8, 308) and bilateral *papillitis* with ischemia of the periaxial fibers has resulted from 2 weeks of maximum-dose treatment. High doses have also led on occasion to *mesenteric vascular constriction*, *ischemic bowel disease* and partial *necrosis of the tongue*. Arterial stenosis can even result in *aneurysm* formation (65[C]). The absence of symptoms does not mean that there is no adverse effect; in a group of 30 patients who had taken 1–5 mg daily for a year all were found to exhibit lowered systolic blood pressures in the foot. Treatment of migraine can lead to subclinical ergotism for a prolonged period, and thence to occlusive peripheral vascular disease; peripheral systolic pressure (and liver function tests) should be monitored in patients taking ergotamine regularly (SEDA-15, 135). The degree of tolerance of patients to these vasoconstrictive effects, however, varies widely; such symptoms as *cyanosis* of the limbs, *syncope*, *hypotension* and *paresthesia* have been seen in sensitive subjects after doses of up to 8 mg taken over as little as 10 days. The Swedish drug authorities have recommended that treatment should not be continued for more than 7 days (SEDA-13, 113).

Gastrointestinal *Nausea* and *vomiting* are common problems with effective doses. *Rectal stenosis* demanding treatment has several times been described after prolonged use or overuse (66[CR]). This pattern of use can also cause reversible *gastrointestinal ischemia*, presenting as lower abdominal pain (SEDA-17, 146).

Risk situations The risk of severe vascular reactions is increased in the presence of *peripheral vascular disease* or when *sympathicomimetic agents* are given at the same time. In *angina-prone subjects*, ECG changes and angina pectoris have been induced. Some *combined therapies* may cause risks; painful superficial phlebitis (in some cases with positive rechallenge) was observed in seven patients after treatment with ergotamine tartrate, isobutyl allylbarbital and caffeine; however, most of these patients had a *history of varicosis* as a predisposing factor (SEDA-12, 124).

There are special risks in giving ergotamine in *liver disease* (since a large part of the drug is probably metabolized by the liver), *renal* or *cardiovascular disorders* or *sepsis* (which seems to increase the risk of gangrene).

Second-generation effects A report on a child born with microcephaly whose mother had used ergotamine and caffeine (during the first trimester) and propranolol (during the second) for the relief of migraine suggest the possibility of congenital defects (SEDA-13, 114). Ergotamine should clearly not be used in *pregnancy* in view of its oxytocic effects (SEDA-8, 147) which can lead to fetal stress requiring cesarean section (67[cr]); teratogenicity data in animals are not consistent. If used during *lactation*, the infant may suffer gastrointestinal upsets, cardiovascular instability and even convulsions.

Miscellaneous *Retroperitoneal fibrosis*, as produced classically by methysergide, has been reported following the administration of ergotamine (SEDA-8, 147). A case of *portal hypertension* (SEDA-11, 131) and one of *diverticulum formation in the internal carotid artery* following 4 years of treatment with ergot might be due to a similar mechanism (SEDA-10, 119). Anocutaneous ergotism (characterized by *anal ulceration*) has been observed (in one case) after excessive application of ergot suppositories (SEDA-10, 119).

Overdosage Ergot poisoning can be caused by ergotamine, as well as by other ergot alkaloids. Signs of poisoning initially include *dizziness*, *frontal headache*, *depression*, and *leg and low back pain*; more severe poisoning results in *formication*, *severe cyanosis* of the extremities, *muscular twitching*, *tonic spasms*, *convulsions*, *delirium* and ultimately *death* (68[R]). A symptom resembling reversible *dementia* has been described in chronic ergotamine intoxication (SEDA-3, 121). Long-term abuse of the drug has in a small number of published cases induced *fibrosis of the cardiac valves* (SEDA-18, 160).

Dihydroergotamine

Dihydroergotamine is used for preventing migraine attacks, but also in the treatment of hypotension (either orthostatic or caused by spinal or epidural anesthesia), because of its strong constrictor effect on capacitance vessels. When dihydroergotamine was given intravenously after coronary bypass surgery, it was found that despite increased filling pressure there was no rise in cardiac output, and that in spite of increased cardiac work the bypass flow significantly decreased. The significant decrease in regional myocardial vascular resistance found after the administration of dihydroergotamine may explain the absence of the expected increase in cardiac output and coronary bypass flow.

The combination of heparin with dihydroergotamine is frequently used for the prevention of thromboembolic complications. It is claimed that these two components act synergistically, allowing a lower dosage of heparin to be used. However, the lower risk of hemorrhagic complications is certainly not counterbalanced by a lowered risk of *ergotism*, despite the claims of manufacturers (SEDA-8, 147). *Vasospastic reactions* after giving heparin with dihydroergotamine seem to occur particularly in traumatized patients or when a limb is injured, and in these patients another antithrombotic drug should be the first choice. Since the risk of vasospasms increases with treatment time, the Swedish Adverse Reactions Committee recommends that the duration of treatment with dihydroergotamine with heparin should not exceed 7 days (SEDA-15, 135). It is also known that patients taking oral contraceptives and pregnant women are more susceptible to vasospasm, as are patients in shock, with sepsis and with Raynaud's or Burger's disease. Dihydroergotamine should also be avoided after vascular surgery or angioplasia.

In one instance, dihydroergotaine has been incriminated in the causation of *retroperitoneal fibrosis* (SEDA-17, 170).

During intranasal administration for migraine, inconveniences can include *nasal congestion or irritation* and *sneezing*. In daily use, with administration by injections, there is an ill-defined frequency of *nausea*, *vomiting*, *abdominal pain* and *diarrhea*, but also a high incidence of *muscle cramps* and some occurrence of *lethargy* and *peripheral edema* (SEDA-17, 171).

'Codergocrine mesylate' and components

This curious mixture of dihydrogenated ergot alkaloids is claimed to have some effect in brain ageing, but it has also been used experimentally in various other age groups. In the elderly, the drug has a low incidence of *diarrhea*, *nausea*, *gastric pain*, *orthostatic hypotension* and *headache*. When the side effects of codergocrine were studied in a group of 40 children, *nasal stuffiness* and *anorexia* were most frequently encountered.

Dihydroergocristine mesylate and dihydroergocryptine mesylate are components of 'co-dergocrine mesylate' and have similar actions. When the latter was studied in normal subjects, and in hyperprolactinemic and acromegalic patients, it caused a marked fall in blood pressure in one (hyperprolactinemic) woman in the total group of 22 patients.

Ergometrine (ergonovine)

Ergometrine is used in obstetrics (e.g. in injections of up to 1 mg) since its oxytocic effects are relatively more marked than its vascular effects. *Nausea* and *vomiting* can occur if the drug is given orally. Slight *bradycardia* is common, but *tachycardia* occurs in some patients, and some changes in intracardiac conduction and pacemaker function may be traced on the electrocardiogram. Very rarely, *hypertensive reactions* and *cardiac arrest* have been described and there are two reports of myocardial infarction in women who were healthy, but who were known smokers (SEDA-18, 160). A newborn infant inadvertently injected with ergometrine and oxytocin was found to develop *depression of respiration* and *convulsions* (69[C]).

If there are predisposing factors, adverse reactions of the type described in connection with ergotamine can occur; a patient with Raynaud's disease has been found to develop impalpable arterial pulses, and the peripheral vasoconstrictor effect can be potentiated by general anesthesia.

The 'ergonovine provocation test' for the diagnosis of angina pectoris (by producing vasospasm during angiography) should be used with extreme caution and only in expert hands; *myocardial* infarctions and even *fatalities* have resulted from its use (SED-12, 324; 70[C]).

Methylergometrine

Transient *cortical blindness*, with severe *headache* and *hallucinations*, has been associated with the intravenous injection of 0.2 mg methylergometrine in a postpartum patient; in another similar situation, acute *hypertensive encephalopathy* has been seen (SED-3, 121).

Methysergide

Although this semisynthetic ergot derivative is structurally very similar to ergometrine, its spectrum of activity differs substantially. Its strong anti-serotonin activity is used prophylactically in migraine patients, with oral daily doses up to 6 mg. Its vasoconstrictor and oxytocic effects are generally slight, but it can better be avoided in pregnancy.

Although a third of patients experience some side effects, only about 10–15% have to stop treatment acutely for this reason. Mild *gastrointestinal upsets*, *abdominal cramping* and a tendency to *dizziness*, *lightheadedness* and *nervousness* are the most frequent complaints. Less frequent but more serious symptoms, including those attributable to fibrosis, are listed below.

Cardiovascular Symptoms include *tachycardia*, *postural hypotension* and *angina pectoris*. Reversible murmurs may be heard; in at least as many cases, however, the murmurs reflect organic changes affecting the valves. *Aortic and mitral valvular fibrosis* can lead to *congestive cardiac failure*; fibrosis may rarely affect the endocardium more extensively (extending into the myocardium) or the pericardium (resulting in *constrictive pericarditis*). *Vasospastic effects* may in occasional susceptible subjects be as severe as with ergotamine; especially dangerous are combinations with ergotamine tartrate, as are combinations of ergot alkaloids with β-blockers (SEDA-9, 128).

Nervous system In addition to the milder changes mentioned above, one may observe *restlessness*, *insomnia*, *drowsiness* or mild *psychic changes*. An *LSD-like reaction* has been observed with as little as 2 mg. There is a risk of dependence and the drug can better be avoided in patients with a history of mental disorder.

Hematological *Hemolytic anemia*, *neutropenia* and *eosinophilia* have all been described. A case of postpartum *hemolytic-uremic syndrome* has been observed (SEDA-12, 124).

Skin Various dermatological disorders have been described and in a single case the drug has been held responsible for hair loss.

Fibrotic symptoms Serious *fibrotic changes* seem to occur in about 1% of patients given methysergide continuously for a year or more, and provide the main reason for reducing doses and withdrawing the drug at intervals. Most commonly the fibrosis is *retroperitoneal* and starts in the pelvis or the lumbar region, where it can constrict the ureters, arteries, veins and lymph vessels; both infarction and obstruction of the bowel have occasionally been described. Fibrotic syndromes elsewhere can involve the heart (see above) *pleura*, *chest wall* and *pulmonary tissue*.

Risk situations In view of its properties, methysergide should not be used in patients with any serious organic disease, and regular checking for complications is essential. Most or all patients taking methysergide can equally well be treated with an alternative and safer drug.

DRUGS STIMULATING 5-HYDROXY-TRYPTAMINE RECEPTORS

Sumatriptan

Sumatriptan is a 5-hydroxytryptamine (5-HT) agonist effective in the treatment of all features of the headache phase of an acute attack of migraine (71[CR]); the way in which it exerts this effect is not clear; it penetrates the blood—brain barrier poorly. A detailed review will be found in SEDA-18 (see pp. 171—173).

Cardiovascular Particularly when injected the drug can cause a transient *increase in both systolic and diastolic blood pressure*; the (usually higher) oral dose, e.g. 200 mg, has this effect to a lesser extent; it would be unwise to use the drug in cases with uncontrolled severe hypertension. Some of the minor discomfort often experienced (*tingling*, *flushing*, *sensations of heat or cold*) may also reflect cardiovascular effects. There is a fairly high incidence of *discomfort in the chest* ('tightness', 'need to breathe') and this may or may not correlate with the fact that i.v. sumatriptan induces some *coronary constriction* during diagnostic angiography. At least during clinical studies it was prudent to exclude patients with a history of cardiovascular disease, and this view was then extended into the field (72[R]). *Myocardial infarction* has been described in a patient who had received 6 mg sumatriptan s.c., but the causal association was not clear.

Nervous system At least a third of users experience *recurrent headache* but without the migraine aura, occurring within the first 24 hours of treatment; it can be severe but usually responds to a further dose.

Gastrointestinal *Nausea*, *vomiting and taste disturbances* clearly occur more often in sumatriptan users than in a placebo group.

Risk situations As noted above, it is unwise at present to use sumatriptan in patients with *cardiovascular disorders*. Because of limited experience it is also best avoided in *children* or the *elderly*, in *pregnancy* or during *lactation*.

On theoretical grounds, it should not be used alongside *ergotamine*, *monoamine oxidase inhibitors*, *5-HT re-uptake inhibitors* or *lithium*.

DRUGS BLOCKING DOPA FORMATION

α-Methyl-*p*-tyrosine

This agent is sometimes used to prepare pheochromocytoma patients for surgery. It appears to induce *sedation*, *drowsiness*, *insomnia* and *tremor*. It can cause crystalluria unless there is a high fluid intake.

When tested in 21 healthy subjects, the drug produced *panic attacks* on several occasions in three of them.

AGENTS WITH CHOLINERGIC EFFECTS

DRUGS STIMULATING ACETYLCHOLINE RECEPTORS

α-Glycerylphosphorylcholine (choline alfoscerate)

This drug increases cerebral acetylcholine synthesis and release. In the light of animal studies it is under investigation as a possible treatment for vascular dementia. To date, adverse effects have been few, notably *headache* and *flushing*.

ACETYLCHOLINE AND SUBSTANCES WITH RELATED EFFECTS

Acetylcholine
Carbachol

Neither acetylcholine itself nor carbachol is generally used outside the field of ophthalmology (see Chapter 47), but it has been used systematically (subcutaneously, e.g. in doses of 2 mg daily) for urinary retention. Severe *cholinergic effects* can result. In one instance they primarily involved the gastrointestinal tract and the patient died of *esophageal rupture* (73[c]). In other instances patients have experienced extreme *bradycardia with hypotension*, demanding treatment with intravenous atropine. It should be noted that, as carbachol is not destroyed by cholinesterase, a cumulative effect is possible in patients receiving regular doses at shorter intervals; in one case, hypotension only developed on the third treatment day (74[C]).

Choline

Choline has been given in the past as an acetylcholine precursor to raise acetylcholine levels in the brain in dyskinesias; occasionally, doses rising to 9 grams daily have been found to produce severe *depression*, no doubt as a result of derangement of the adrenaline/acetylcholine balance.

Bethanecol

An acute *dystonic reaction* to bethanecol has been reported in a 10-month-old boy (SEDA-12, 124). This reaction was unexpected since it is a quaternary ammonium compound which does not normally penetrate the blood—brain barrier; the authors assumed that the barrier may not be impenetrable to the drug in young infants.

During a controlled clinical trial of intraventricular bethanecol in patients with Alzheimer's disease, reversible drug-induced *parkinsonism* was observed in one patient (SEDA-15, 5). The frequent coexistence of Alzheimer's disease and Parkinson's disease presents potential problems for therapy and side effects when the cholinergic system is manipulated.

ACETYLCHOLINESTERASE INHIBITORS

Ambenonium
Distigmine
Edrophonium
Neostigmine
Physostigmine
Pyridostigmine
Tacrine

These and related cholinesterase inhibitors with a reversible effect are, apart from their ophthalmic uses (see Chapter 47), mainly employed in myasthenia gravis and in the treatment of atony of the intestine or bladder.

General pattern of adverse effects These drugs have the nicotinic and muscarinic effects which one would expect to result from their promoting cholinergic activity (see Table 2), and those cholinergic effects which in the circumstances of the case are unwanted comprise their side effects, e.g. *bradycardia*, *miosis*, *colic*, *hypersalivation*. Adverse reactions have been stated to be relatively more common with neostigmine than with some other drugs such as pyridostigmine or ambenonium, but it is doubtful whether the therapeutic index indeed differs, since neostigmine also tends to be more effective in certain patients. Ambenonium seems relatively prone to cause *headache*. When either neostigmine or pyridostigmine is used in the form of their bromide, *bromide rashes* can appear.

Some particularly serious problems which can occur with these drugs are defined in the paragraphs below.

Cardiovascular With any of these drugs, the bradycardia can, with excessive dosage, proceed to *dysrhythmias* (SEDA-13, 114) and even *asystole*. With physostigmine, *hypertension* has been both demonstrated in animal experiments and observed in a series in patients after intravenous use in relatively high doses; it has also occurred during use of low doses of orally administered physostigmine in an elderly patient with Alzheimer's disease (SEDA-12, 125). During another experimental trial of oral physostigmine *myoclonus* was observed in two patients with probable Alzheimer's disease (SEDA-12, 125).

Muscular function Any of these drugs can produce *muscular fasciculation* followed by *voluntary muscle paralysis*, and these muscular effects can serve as a valuable sign of approaching overdosage. Two patients, one with dystrophia myotonica and the other with progressive muscular dystrophy, presented with *respiratory difficulties*, necessitating prolonged mechanical ventilation; as these difficulties are as good as impossible to predict, short-acting neuromuscular blockers should preferably be used, thus avoiding the need for pharmacological reversal (75[Cr]).

Liver The authors of a study evaluating the side effects of tacrine (tetrahydroaminoacridine) in Alzheimer's disease recommend regular monitoring for *hepatotoxicity* (SEDA-15, 136; see also below).

Second-generation effects Cholinesterase inhibitors can probably be safely used in pregnancy when needed, provided dosage is carefully regulated; a case of reversible myasthenia in a newborn infant has been attributed to relative overdosage of the mother with pyridostigmine bromide (76[C]).

Risk situations Special caution is recommended when cholinesterase inhibitors are given in patients with *inflammatory*, *infiltrative or degenerative disease of the conduction system*, patients being treated with *digitalis*, *calcium channel antagonists* or β-blockers, patients with *myocardial ischemia* and *elderly* patients. Appropriate resuscitative equipment should be readily available. Neostigmine or other anticholinesterase preparations are regularly used in anesthesiology to reverse neuromuscular block; however, in patients suffering from *neuromuscular disorders* this reversal may present unforeseen difficulties. All these drugs must be *cautiously dosed* if severe adverse reactions are to be avoided. When given orally, administration should be suspended during periods of *severe constipation*, in the light of one reported case in the past where neostigmine accumulated in the gastrointestinal tract of a child during a constipative phase and was thereafter rapidly absorbed with fatal results (SED-12, 326). Anticholinesterase drugs are contraindicated in *bronchial asthma*.

The *elderly* may need to be treated with caution because of their greater susceptibility to cardiovascular effect; this is relevant in connection with the experimental use of centrally acting cholinergic agonists such as physostigmine in Alzheimer's disease.

Interactions Although *diazepam* does not have anticholinergic properties, it is possible to reverse diazepam-induced delirium by the use of cholinesterase inhibitors such as physostigmine; the latter treatment can, however, on occasion induce severe arterial hypertension, especially if the dose exceeds 2 mg i.v. In healthy volunteers sedated with diazepam an increase in awareness was established with the use of physostigmine, but there was also a decrease in ventilatory drive (SEDA-10, 119).

The effect of cholinesterase inhibitors may be modified if a patient is taking a drug with strong anticholinergic effects, notably an *antihistamine* or a *neuroleptic*.

Tacrine
7-Methoxytacrine

These drugs are currently being investigated for use in cases of Alzheimer's disease and in AIDS. In 12–30% of Alzheimer patients, tacrine caused an increase in hepatic transaminase activity, but this was not seen in a (younger) group of AIDS patients given twice the dose (SEDA-17, 174). The peripheral cholinomimetic effects of tacrine occur in a very high proportion of patients, probably the majority. The hepatic effects seem to be such that the use of these experimental drugs would not be justified in any less serious disease states than the two at present under study, but they appear to reversible if the drug is withdrawn. With methoxytacrine, current reports point primarily to the classic cholinomimetic effects.

AGENTS WITH ANTICHOLINERGIC EFFECTS

There are vast numbers of anticholinergic drugs on sale; although many of them are claimed to be superior as regards their efficacy, specificity or tolerance, few have ever been critically compared with others. As so often happens, the so-called freedom from side effects claimed for many of these compounds can often be traced to uncritical clinical work, the use of ineffective dose levels, or mere lack of activity of the compound.

Table 4. *General classification of anticholinergic drugs*

Atropine and closely related agents	
Atropine	(Natural alkaloid)
Hyoscine	(Natural alkaloid)
Ipratropium	(Semisynthetic)
Synthetic quaternary ammonium compounds	
Clidinium	
Emepronium bromide	
Isopropamide	
Methantheline	
Mepenzolate	
Oxyphenonium	
Poldine	
Propantheline	
Tertiary amines used in visceral disorders	
Adiphenine	
Dicyclomine	
Oxyphencyclimine	
Piperidolate	
Drugs with primarily anticholinergic effects used mainly in Parkinson's disease	
Tertiary amines related to diphenhydramine	
Chlorphenoxamine	
Orphenadrine	
Trihexyphenidyl-related compounds	
Biperiden	
Procyclidine	
Trihexyphenidyl (benzhexol)	
Compounds related both to atropine and to diphenhydramine	
Benzatropine	
Ethybenztropine	

General pattern of adverse effects An indication of what may be expected in the way of adverse reactions can be obtained by fitting a drug into its structural class (see Table 4), since the pattern of effects of drugs in each class is generally very similar. The drugs closely related to atropine have the full range of antinicotinic and antimuscarinic activity of atropine itself. Of the synthetic compounds used in visceral disorders, the quaternary compounds are fully ionized in the pH range found in body fluids and are therefore less lipid-soluble than the corresponding tertiary amines. This means that they penetrate physiological barriers less readily; less drug is absorbed in the intestine, less enters the cerebrospinal fluid and aqueous humor, and less enters the cells. Consequently, these drugs tend to be relatively less active by mouth and to have less effect on the brain and the eye than the tertiary amines. Of the latter, some have little antimuscarinic activity and indeed probably very little useful activity at all; they may have some specific relaxant effect on smooth muscle, but it seems to be of little clinical significance.

Of the drugs in this class used largely in parkinsonism, the tertiary amines related to diphenhydramine seem to have some antihistamine activity, as one would expect; some of these drugs are also related to atropine. The derivatives of trihexyphenidyl are also pharmacologically closely similar: e.g. they have some excitatory effects if given in sufficient dosage.

To complement Table 4, a number of specific problems with these drugs are outlined below.

Dyskinesias *Orofacial dyskinesia*, though familiar with dopaminergic drugs, can apparently also occur with some anticholinergic agents; it has been described with trihexyphenidyl in a patient who did not experience this reaction with levodopa (SEDA-18, 160).

Effects on memory From recent work it now seems clear that anticholinergic drugs can impair *short-term memory* (which was long suspected), but that the effects in non-demented patients are reversible, receding within a few weeks of discontinuing treatment (77[C])

Anticholinergic intoxication The clinical manifestations of overdosage with atropine-like drugs, as recorded in a series of 119 such patients, are presented in Table 5. Death, when it occurs, is due primarily to the effects on the central nervous system; a stage of excitement is followed by drowsiness, stupor and coma, with generalized central depression.

Risk situations Anticholinergic drugs clearly may cause problems in patients with *closed-angle glaucoma* (or a narrow angle between the iris and cornea), *paralytic ileus*, *pyloric stenosis* or *urinary retention*. Because of their effects on temperature control they may be undesirable in cases with *pyrexia* (especially children) and during *very hot weather*. In fact, not all these situations necessarily result in contraindications; everything will depend on the drug to be used and the circumstances of the case; these situations call for caution rather than for the complete avoidance of anticholinergic therapy if there is a serious indication for the latter.

Psychotic reactions and misuse The ability of anticholinergic drugs to cause vivid and sometimes exotic *hallucinations* is well-known and has led to their misuse; plants containing atropine and related substances were used in witches' brews in the Middle Ages to conjure up the devil, but even synthetic tertiary amines given in eyedrops and depot plasters containing atropine (SEDA-13, 114) have caused hallucinations (see Chapter 49). *Postoperative confusion* in elderly patients has been clearly correlated with drugs having anticholinergic properties (SEDA-13, 114). Patients on long-term anticholinergic treatment can develop drug *dependence* (SEDA-15, 136).

Table 5. *Clinical manifestations of anticholinergic intoxication in 71 adults and 48 children (77[R])*

	Adults (%)	Children (%)
Pupils widely dilated and poorly reactive	79	88
Flushed facies; dry mucous membranes	55	90
Tachycardia (greater than 100/minute)	44	65
Incoherence, confusion or disorientation	66	56
Restlessness, hyperactivity or agitation	39	58
Auditory or visual hallucinations	52	27
Ataxia or motor incoordination	35	48
Picking, plucking, grasping or gathering movements	37	44
Hyperreflexia, twitching or increased muscle tone	25	35
Apprehension, fear or paranoid ideation	23	14
Somnolence or coma	34	16
'Toxic delirium'	14	40
Giddiness; labile or inappropriate affect	18	13
Dysarthria or slurred speech	14	14
Fever greater than 100°F	18	25
Complaint of thirst or dry mouth	18	14
Complaint of blindness or blurred vision	20	13
Return to normal sensorium in 24 hours	35	40
Retrograde amnesia	18	13

Infrequent manifestations (less than 10% of cases): seizures, convulsions, vomiting, rash, urinary retention, abdominal distress, paralytic ileus, constipation.

Risk of unrecognized exposure Drugs with anticholinergic activity may be promoted and employed variously as antidepressants, antipsychotic agents, antihistamines, antispasmodics or anti-Parkinson agents; consequently, unless the prescriber stops to consider the total anticholinergic barrage to which a patient is being exposed, he may inadvertently produce anticholinergic overdosage.

ATROPINE-LIKE SUBSTANCES

Atropine

Atropine itself is mainly used today in premedication, e.g. in doses of 0.3—0.6 mg, but is also employed in the acute phase of myocardial infarction and (as methylnitrate) in bronchodilator aerosols.

Cardiovascular One classic study, a generation ago, of patients given atropine sulfate intravenously as premedication in a total dose of 1 mg showed that *arrhythmias* occurred in over one-third of the subjects, and in over half of those younger than 20. In adults, atrioventricular dissociation was common and in children atrial rhythm disturbances (78[Cr]). In volunteers it has been found that atropine in doses of 1.6 mg/70 kg tends to cause episodes of nodal rhythm with absent P-waves on the electrocardiogram (79[C]); the episodes occurred before the heart rate had increased under the influence of the drug. In healthy males being anesthetized for dental surgery it was found that a dose of only 0.4 mg atropine i.v. 5 minutes before induction caused a *depression of mean arterial pressure, stroke volume and total peripheral resistance* (80[C]).

The above-mentioned use of atropine in myocardial infarction is intended to increase the heart rate; as a rule, this succeeds, but in some patients with second-degree heart block the ventricular rate is slowed by atropine resulting in *bradycardia*. Other patients may experience *tachycardia* and even *ventricular fibrillation* has been seen, occasionally even in doses as low as 0.5 mg (81[C]).

Respiratory Atropine increases the *rate and depth* of respiration, probably as a reaction to the increase in the dead space resulting from bronchodilatation.

Nervous system Some recent work points to *memory impairment*, although this only became apparent if special studies of mental function were performed. This is true also for benzatropine (SEDA-13, 115).

Hypothermia Atropine was considered to have produced hypothermia in a boy aged 14 who was being treated with paracetamol and cooling blankets for hyperthermia (82[C]). As atropine can produce hypothermia in animals, a causal relationship cannot be excluded, even if a concomitant action with acetaminophen is assumed.

Special senses *Transient central blindness* has been seen to follow an intravenous injection of 0.8 mg atropine in the course of spinal anesthesia; blink reflex and pupillary response to light and accommodation were lost; vision returned slowly after some hours following the instillation of pilocarpine (83[C]).

Allergy Hypersensitivity to atropine can occur, it is most usually seen in the form of *contact dermatitis* and *conjunctivitis* (see Chapter 47). One case of *anaphylactic shock* after intravenous injection of atropine has been reported (SEDA-14, 122).

Risk situations In *Down's syndrome*, atropine produces an abnormally large degree of pupillary dilatation, probably because of a genetically abnormal response; there is also a much greater acceleration of the heart rate than that produced by atropine in normal subjects. In *congenital albinism*, by contrast, the duration of dilatation of the pupil is much shorter than usual; the response to homatropine, scopolamine and pilocarpine appears to be normal.

Interactions Atropine can, by slowing intestinal passage, increase the degree of absorption of drugs which undergo prolonged dissolution in the gastrointestinal tract, e.g. *digoxin*, but the absorption of *paracetamol* can be retarded. It also has additive effects with other *sedatives* and other drugs with anticholinergic properties. The addition of atropine to antidiarrheal agents to prevent abuse would appear pointless and dangerous.

Salts and congeners of atropine and hyoscine

Atropine methylbromide This is a quaternary ammonium derivative, and it seems to cross the placenta less readily than atropine; when given close to term, it has much less effect on the fetal heart rate than on the maternal heart rate.

Benztropine

A paradoxical *sinus bradycardia* in a psychotic patient was attributed to beztropine since it receded when this drug (but not others) were withdrawn (SEDA-17, 174). A similar effect has been described with trihexyphenidyl.

Hyoscine butylbromide

When given parenterally this is effective but very short-acting; given by mouth it is virtually inactive, even in doses up to 1 gram. An isolated case of *angioneurotic edema* has been described during the use of this salt (SEDA-8, 148).

Hyoscine hydrobromide

Hyoscine hydrobromide is used primarily in motion sickness; doses of 0.6 mg appear to be effective, particularly in combination with drugs having a mild central stimulant effect such as ephedrine. The doses used unfortunately produce *somnolence* and *dryness of the mouth* in a high proportion of patients, and where ephedrine is not given the somnolence is likely to be present in the majority; some individuals also experience *headache*, *giddiness* and *blurred vision*. One study showed that hyoscine premedication had detrimental effects on *memory* and on *motor tasks* compared with placebo, while atropine did not (84[C]), though the difference is unlikely to be absolute. In view of certain of these effects, hyoscine hydrobromide is not a suitable antiemetic for those likely to drive vehicles before the effect has worn off, e.g. air passengers.

Ipratropium bromide

Ipratropium is the semisynthetic isopropyl derivative of atropine and it is used in the form of a spray for inhalation in chronic bronchitis, the metered dose being some 20 μg. The risk of using most traditional atropine-like drugs in asthmatics and chronic bronchitis lies in the possibility of a 'drying effect', as a result of which the airways may become blocked with viscous secretions; with local use of ipratropium this does not appear to constitute a problem (SEDA-17, 147), the bronchodilator effect being the dominant one. Only if substantial overdosage occurs (e.g. 1 mg by inhalation) do traces of generalized atropine-like effects begin to appear. In some patients with atopic asthma, *bronchoconstriction* can follow the use of ipratropium (SEDA-9, 127).

One case of *paralytic ileus* has been reported (SEDA-15, 137).

Pupillary dilatation has several times been reported, possibly because the spray enters the eye; it is risky in cases of glaucoma (85[C]).

In elderly males, who may have prostatic hypertrophy, ipratropium bromide should be used with caution since it can produce *urinary retention* (SEDA-14, 122).

Pilocarpine

While mainly used in the eye (see Chapter 47) pilocarpine is still occasionally employed for other purposes, e.g. for treating salivary gland hypofunction and xerostomia. When used in this way, cardiovascular tolerance was good but there was a high incidence of sweating, flushing, frequency of micturition, increased nasal secretion and lacrimation (SEDA-18, 174),

Terodiline

This drug, used for urinary incontinence, was withdrawn in most countries in 1991 because of multiple reports of drug-related *cardiac dysrhythmias* (SEDA-17, 174).

Transdermal scopolamine

In recent years, scopolamine has been marketed as a transferral delivery system, using an adhesive patch for postauricular application; the drug is released at a uniform rate for 72 hours. The main indication is prevention of motion sickness and vomiting.

The side effects of this application form are qualitatively typical of those reported for the oral and parenteral formulations of scopolamine and its congeners, although comparative studies suggest the incidence is reduced with transdermal administration. *Dry mouth* occurs in about 67% of subjects and *drowsiness* in approximately 16%. Transient effects on ocular *accommodation*, including blurred vision and mydriasis, have also been observed, in some cases possibly due to finger-to-eye contamination. Adverse effects on the central nervous system including *toxic psychosis* (in three elderly patients), *hallucinations* (in a child) have been reported only occasionally, as have other adverse reactions, such as *dry*, *itchy eyes*, *difficulty in urinating*, *rashes* and *erythema* (86[R]).

Propiverine

Propiverine is a spasmolytic drug for the bladder. Its effect on the eye has been investigated in normal and glaucomatous eyes. A considerable *reduction in accommodation* has been found in younger individuals in both groups. The drug should therefore be given to younger patients only on very strict indications (87[Cr]).

Asthma cigarettes

This traditional remedy is discussed in Chapter 16.

SYNTHETIC QUATERNARY AMMONIUM COMPOUNDS

The effects of the synthetic quaternary ammonium compounds are those of anticholinergic drugs in general, subject to the reservation raised in the introduction: i.e., they tend to be less readily absorbed and hence to have less central effect than other substances in this pharmacological group.

Bornaprine

The side effects of bornaprine, sometimes used as an anticholinergic in parkinsonism, are those characteristic of this class of drugs.

Cimetropium bromide

Cimetropium bromide is a relatively new anticholinergic drug belonging to a series of scopolamine quaternary salts with strong antimuscarinic effects.

Clinidium bromide

Clidinium is best known as a component of Librax (chlordiazepoxide 5 mg, clidinium bromide 2.5 mg); the dose used is sufficient to produce typical anticholinergic side effects. Since here it is combined with a benzodiazepine, it would seem most unwise to allow patients taking Librax to drive motor vehicles or to ingest alcohol.

Emepromium bromide

Doses of 200 mg given 3 times daily (sometimes with double dosage in the evenings) are useful in relieving urinary frequency.

Quite apart from the milder anticholinergic adverse reactions, which are as one would anticipate, emepromium has repeatedly been proven to cause *ulceration of the mouth and esophagus* and widespread *esophagitis* (88[Cr]); the buccal irritation is particularly marked if the tablets are retained in the mouth instead of being swallowed, and the problem as a whole is greater if the drug is not taken with sufficient fluid.

Central effects are only serious in gross overdosage; in one case of attempted suicide with 100 tablets, there was severe confusion and derangement of breathing (due to neuromuscular paralysis) demanding mechanical ventilation (SED-12, 330).

Isopropamide iodide

A 5—10-mg oral dose produces typical anticholinergic effects, but with this compound one should also bear in mind the possibility of interfering with thyroid function tests or inducing reactions in patients sensitive to iodine. The presence of this anticholinergic agent in some over-the-counter 'cold remedies', e.g. alongside antihistamines, should be borne in mind as a hidden cause of urinary retention.

Mepenzolate

The 25-mg dose of mepenzolate bromide often given several times a day for gastrointestinal disorders is sufficient to induce anticholinergic side effects, but the compound may itself be a cause of *gastric pain*, and one must hence realize the risk of creating a vicious circle.

Methantheline

Oral doses of 25—100 mg methantheline have typical anticholinergic side effects; the compound is considered to be more toxic than propantheline, mainly because its ganglion-blocking activity is relatively more marked than its antimuscarinic effect. Perhaps for this reason, *impotence* has appeared to be a greater problem with this drug; central nervous adverse reactions, even including psychosis, have been reported in the past.

Oxybutynin

Oxybutynin is an anticholinergic and spasmolytic agent, first described in the mid-sixties, but apparently little used. It has typical anticholinergic side effects when given in effective doses (89[cr]).

Oxyphenonium

Like methantheline, this drug has relatively marked ganglion-blocking effects, but it seems to have little effect on the central nervous system; an oral dose of 5—10 mg given several times a day produces typical anticholinergic effects.

Pinaverium bromide

Like emepromium, this drug can cause *inflammation and ulceration in the mouth and esophagus* (SEDA-6, 143).

Poldine methylsulfate

A total oral daily dose of some 10—30 mg is sufficient to produce typical anticholinergic side effects.

Propantheline

Oral doses range from 7.5 to 30 mg, the latter being used at bedtime; injections of 15 mg have been used in radiology. The persisting doubt as to the incidence of adverse reactions probably reflects the poor and variable bioavailability of the oral form, which also seems to account for conflicting reports on efficacy. All typical anticholinergic effects can occur if effective doses are given, but the pharmacokinetic factors referred to earlier mean that central nervous and ocular effects are relatively slight. The drug, like others of this type, is not contraindicated in glaucoma or prostatic hyperplasia, but it may influence the response of these conditions to other treatment and hence should be used with some caution.

The *interactions* are similar to those of atropine, e.g. the absorption of nitrofurantoin and digoxin can be enhanced, that of paracetamol reduced and retarded, and the anticholinergic effects of other drugs can be supplemented.

TERTIARY AMINES USED IN VISCERAL DISORDERS

Adiphenine
Dicyclomine hydrochloride (dicycloverine)

Adiphenine and dicyclomine are again drugs which, in the doses generally used (up to 60 mg of the former and as much as 450 mg of the latter), are of disputed value. Both may have a non-specific relaxant action on the gastrointestinal muscle, while adiphenine has some local anesthetic effect on the buccal mucosa. The evidence on the effects of these two drugs is meager and it would again seem that one is dealing with anticholinergic agents which have been promoted in doses which are often too low to result in either a useful therapeutic effect or in side effects.

Dicyclomine was formerly combined with doxylamine succinate and sometimes with pyridoxine in Debendox (Bendectin) tablets which were used in certain countries for the treatment of nausea and vomiting in pregnancy. There has been a widely discussed suggestion that Debendox might cause a range of fetal malformations, but a number of large studies failed to confirm this; however, the sporadic reports of such problems sometimes involved women who took the product in high doses for long periods in early pregnancy and there is some doubt as to the dosage schedule used in the larger studies. Particularly since the pattern of supposed malformations was highly variable, and they were of types which tend to occur spontaneously, the point cannot be considered settled. Any teratogenic effect must have been very slight.

Oxyphencyclamine

Here again, the wide range of oral doses used (10—50 mg daily) indicate doubt as to the potency of the compound, which is claimed to act for some 12 hours.

Piperidolate

Doses of 50 mg of piperidolate are usual for treating pyloric spasm; the effects and side effects at this dose level are both weak.

DRUGS WITH PRIMARILY ANTICHOLINERGIC EFFECTS USED MAINLY IN PARKINSON'S DISEASE

Studies in normal volunteers comparing dopaminergic drugs with anticholinergic drugs have shown that while taking anticholinergic drugs there was significant impairment of memory function, more confusion and dysphoria (SEDA-13, 115). The authors recommend that every effort be made to treat parkinsonism with dopaminergic agents and to avoid anticholinergic drugs, a trend in therapy which has in any case been developing strongly in recent years.

Tertiary amines related to diphenhydramine

Orphenadrine and chlorphenoxamine These agents are both related to an antihistamine (diphenhydramine), and appear to have been developed in the hope of producing a greater effect in parkinsonism by combining both anticholinergic and antihistaminic effects in a single molecule.

In the doses usually used, any of the well-recognized *anticholinergic effects* can occur. Some patients experience drowsiness, whilst others are stimulated; with increasing dosage, some patients may go into coma; others exhibit agitation, convulsions and marked euphoria, perhaps with hallucinations and disorientation.

In *overdosage*, orphenadrine has been stated to be a relatively toxic substance (SEDA-3, 124). Although some patients have survived doses grossly in excess of the usual maximum of 400 mg daily, the therapeutic margin may vary; on occasion doses of as little as 2—3 grams have produced a fatal outcome within 6—12 hours. The clinical picture of intoxication tends to be characterized by coma together with seizures, apnea, disturbances of cardiac rhythm, and shock; physostigmine should only be used cautiously and preferably after the most severe toxic phase has been overcome (90[R]). Orphenadrine *abuse* has been described (SEDA-14, 122).

Chlorphenoxamine is very similar to orphenadrine, as one would expect. Its adverse reactions are described as mild, but it is not at all clear whether this indeed reflects a more favorable therapeutic index than is found with orphenadrine or merely a lesser potency in all respects.

Trihexyphenidyl-related compounds

Trihexyphenidyl (benzhexol) This agent is given in oral doses rising from 2 to 20 mg daily. A wide range of anticholinergic adverse reactions can be produced, but the drug is apparently particularly prone to cause *excitement*. As little as 8 mg daily combined with levodopa has been found to produce an acute toxic confusional state in some patients. High doses could potentially impair learning in children, but a careful study of this question suggests that there is in practice little interference (91[c]). Impairment of *memory* was observed in a group of healthy volunteers (SEDA-13, 115). In the elderly, it may occasionally cause *irreversible brain failure* (SEDA-2, 126).

Glaucoma is prone to be precipitated in patients predisposed to this condition and blindness has resulted (92[C]). One case of paradoxical *bradycardia* has been reported; the reaction was specific to trihexyphenidyl and was not observed while the patient was given other anticholinergic drugs (SEDA-12, 125).

The drug has been *misused* by drug addicts to produce elation or relieve depression.

In one reported case where a dose of 300 mg was taken with suicidal intent the patient survived the resultant toxic psychosis (93[C]).

Biperiden This drug is given orally in doses rising from 2–6 mg daily, more being given in individual cases. Of the anticholinergic effects which biperiden can induce, *drowsiness* seems to be one of the most prominent, and the drug should not be given to patients who have to drive motor vehicles. A dose of 12 mg has been reported to precipitate *involuntary movements* in some cases of parkinsonism (SEDA-1, 120).

Procyclidine The usual oral dose, which lies between 20 and 30 mg daily, is likely to produce only mild anticholinergic side effects at this dose level, but *involuntary movements* with chewing and sucking have been described in some patients at this dose level (SEDA-1, 120); even small doses have produced *toxic confusional states* when combined with phenothiazines for schizophrenia. Procyclidine is more likely to produce *sedation* than stimulation.

Compounds related to both atropine and diphenhydramine

Benzatropine and ethylbenzatropine These drugs represent further attempts to combine atropine-like and antihistaminic effects in single molecules. The dose is determined individually and varies from 0.5 to 6 mg daily for the former drug and 6 to 30 mg daily for the latter. Though the adverse reactions are essentially those of the anticholinergic drugs as such, *sedation* seems very prone to occur and the drugs should not be used in patients who need to drive motor vehicles. Benzatropine has also been reported to cause *rash*, *peripheral numbness* and *muscular weakness*. These drugs, because of their double-barrelled effect, are particularly prone to *interact* additively with other drugs having both anticholinergic and antihistaminic activity, such as the neuroleptic agents; complications such as *hyperpyrexia*, *coma* and *toxic psychosis* have several times been reported when such combinations were used. A series of cases have also been reported in which *heat stroke* occurred during hot weather, probably due to impaired heat adaptation (94[cR]); this can occur with other anticholinergic and neuroleptic drugs as well (see Chapter 6). Considerable *memory impairment* was observed in normal volunteers after short-term administration of benzatropine (SEDA-13, 115; SEDA-15, 137).

As to possible *second-generation effects*, two cases of 'small left colon' have been described in infants whose mothers had taken various psychotropic drugs, including benzatropine, late in pregnancy. The causal link is not at all clear (SEDA-6, 142).

REFERENCES

1. Stewart MJ, Fraser DM, Boon N. Dilated cardiomyopathy associated with chronic oveuse of an adrenaline inhaler. Br Heart J 1992;68:221–222.
2. Jackman WM, Friday KJ, Anderson JL et al. The long QT syndromes; a critical review, new clinical observations and a unifying hypothesis. Prog Cardiovasc Dis 1988; 31:115–172.
3. Lampman M, Santinga T, Basset DR, Savage PF. Cardiac arrhythmias during epinephrine–propranolol infusions for measurements of in vivo insulin resistance. Diabetes 1981;30:618.
4. Herridge CF, Brook MF. Ephedrine psychosis. Br Med J 1968;2:160.
5. Wineinger MA, Basford JR. Autonomic dysreflexia due to medication: misadventure in the use of an isometheptene combination to treat migraine. Arch Phys Med Rehabil 1985;60:645.
6. von Rüdiger F, Lantzsch W. Schmeckstörungen als Nebenwirkung des Myofedrin. HNO Praxis 1985;10:201.
7. Blackard WG. Edema—an infrequently recognized complication of bromocriptine and other ergot dopaminergic drugs. Am J Med 1993;94:445.
8. Lamado S, Kronzon I, Mehta SS. Pulmonary edema: a complication of metaraminol treatment of paroxysmal supraventricular tachycardia. Isr J Med Sci 1974;10:504.
9. Speer F, Carrasco LC, Kimura CC. Allergy to phenylpropanolamine. Ann Allergy 1978;40:32.
10. Lake CR, Zalaga G, Clymer R et al. A double dose of phenylpropanolamine causes transient hypertension. Am J Med 1988;85:339.
11. Chin C, Choy M. Cardiomyopathy induced by phenylpropanolamine. J Pediatr 1993;123:825–827.
12. Feinberg AR, Feinberg SM. The 'nose drop nose' due to oxymetazoline (Afrin) and other topical vasoconstrictors. Ill Med J 1971;140:50.
13. Glazener F, Blake K, Gradman M. Bradycardia, hypotension, and near-syncope associated with Afrin (oxymetazoline) nasal spray. N Engl J Med 1983;309:731.

14. Magargal LE, Sanborn GE, Donoso LA, Gonder JR. Branch retinal artery occlusion after excessive use of nasal spray. Ann Ophthalmol 1985;17:500.
15. Baxi LV, Gindoff PR, Pregenzer GJ, Parras MK. Fetal heart rate changes following maternal administration of a nasal decongestant. Am J Obstet Gynecol 1985;153:799.
16. Mansfield LE, Nelson HS. Effect of beta-adrenergic agents on immunoglobin G levels in asthmatic subjects. Int Arch Allergy Appl Immunol 1982;68:13.
17. Pentele L. Unsere Erfahrungen mit der Verwendung von Isoproterenol in der Behandlung des Schocks. Bruns Beitr Klin Chir 1969;271:355.
18. Jacobs RL, Koppes GM. Myocardial necrosis associated with isoproterenol abuse: a ten-year follow-up. Tex Med 1982;78:58.
19. Smith RE, Briggs B, Unverferth DV, Leier CV. Dobutamine-induced inhibition of platelet function. Intensive Care Med 1982;8:155.
20. Boudouresques G, Tafani B, Benichou M, Sarlon B. Encéphalopathie myoclotuque à la dopamine. Sem Hop Paris 1982;58:2729.
21. Friart A, Hermans L, De Valeriola Y. Unusual side-effect of a dobutamine stress echocardiography. Am J Noninvasive Cardiol 1993;7:63–64.
22. Hoff JV, Peatty PA, Wade JL. Dermal necrosis from dobutamine. N Engl J Med 1979;May:31.
23. Nausiede PA. Sinemet 'Abusers'. Clin Neuropharmacol 1985;8:318.
24. Said SAM, Bucx JJJ, Dankbaar H et al. Ibopamine-induced reversible leukopenia during treatment during treatment for congestive heart failure. Eur Heart J 1993;14:999–1001.
25. Barbeau A, Roy M. Six-year results of treatment with levodopa plus benserazide in Parkinson's disease. Neurology 1976;26:399.
26. Goetz G, Tanner M, Nausieda A. Weekly drug holiday in Parkinson's disease. Neurology 1981;31:1460.
27. Vlay SC. Isoprotorenol-induced brady-arrhytmias. Am Heart J 1991;122:1169.
28. Rosin MA, Braun M. Malignant melanoma and levodopa. Cutis 1984;33:572.
29. DeKeyser J, Vincken W. L-Dopa-induced respiratory disturbance in Parkinson's disease suppressed by tiapride. Neurology 1985;35:235.
30. Horstink MWIM, Zijlmans JCM, Pasman JW et al. Severity of Parkinson's disease is a risk factor for peak-dose dyskinesia. J Neurol Neurosurg 1990;53:224–226.
31. Glantz R, Weiner WJ, Goetz CG et al. Drug-induced asterixis in Parkinson disease. Neurology 1982;32:553.
32. Vazques A, Jimenez-Jimenez FJ, Garcia-Ruiz P et al. 'Panic attacks' in Parkinson's disease. A long-term complication of levodopa therapy. Acta Neurol Scand 1993;87:14–19.
33. Goldberg LI. L-Dopa effects on renal function. N Engl J Med 1977;297:112.
34. Lisi P. Pemfigo eritemosa indotto dall'associazione levodopa-carbidopa. Ann Ital Dermatol Clin Sper 1983;37.
35. Barbeau A, Roy M. Six-year results of treatment with levodopa plus benserazide in Parkinson's disease. Neurology 1976;26:399.
36. Toru M, Matsuda O, Maklguchi K et al. Neuroleptic malignant syndrome-like state following a withdrawal of anti-Parkinsonian drugs. J Nerv Ment Dis 1981;169:324.
37. New Approvals/Indications. Pediatric indication for metaproterenol. Drug Ther 1992;Feb 22 and 38.
38. Vale JA, Maclean KS. Amantadine-induced heart failure. Lancet 1977;i:548.
39. Nogaki H, Morimatsu M. Superficial punctate keratitis and corneal abrasion due to amantadine hydrochloride. J Neurol 1993;240:388–389.
40. Riederer P, Lange KW, Kornhuber J et al. Pharmacotoxic psychosis after memantine in Parkinson's disease. Lancet 1991;338:1022–1023.
41. Le Feuvre CM, Isaacs AJ, Frank OS. Bromocriptine-induced psychosis in acromegaly. Br Med J 1982;285:1315.
42. Giampietro O, Ferdeghini M, Petrini M. Severe leukopenia and mild thrombocytopenia after chronic bromocriptine (CB-154) administration. Am J Med Sci 1981;281:169.
43. Damase-Michel C, Sarrail E, Laens J et al. Hyponatraemia in a patient treated with bromocriptine, Drug Invest 1993;5:285–287.
44. Lanthier PL, Morgan MY, Ballantyne J. Bromocriptine-associated ototoxicity. J Laryngol Otol 1984;98:399.
45. Hardy JC, Chevalier C, Kains JP. Fibrose rétropéritonéale. A propos de troi cas dont deux induits par la bromocriptine. Acta Urol Belg 1991;59:95–103.
46. Schellekens LA, Snuiverink H, Van den Berghe H. Chromosomal patterns of children born after induction of ovulation with bromocriptine. Arzneim-Forsch 1977;27:2151.
47. Kando JC et al. Pergolide and hypertension. Drug Intell Clin Pharm 1990;24:543.
48. Scherrer M, Bachofen H. Vergleich der Wirkung einer 4.5 Minuten dauernden Aerosolinhalation von Salbutamol und von Trimetoquinol mit derjenigen einer 10–15 Minuten dauernden Tacholiquin–Orciprenalin-Inhalation bei Bronchialasthma. Schweiz Med Wochenschr 1972;102:909.
49. Chazan R, Tadeusiak W, Jaworski A et al. Creatine kinase (CK) and ceeatine kinase isoenzyme (CK-MB) activity in serum before and after intravenous salbutamol administration of patients with bronchial asthma. Int J Clin Pharmacol Ther Toxicol 1992;30:371–373.
50. Connett G, Lenney W. Prolonged hypoxaemia after nebulized salbutamol. Thorax 1993;48:574–575.
51. Khanna PB, Davies R. Hallucinations associated with administration of salbutamol via a nebulizer. Br Med J 1986;292:1430.
52. Skorodin MS. Beta-adrenergic agonists: a problem. Chest 1993;103:1587–1590.
53. Hooper PL, Harrelson LK, Johnson GE. Pseudohemoptysis from isoetharine. N Engl J Med 1983;1:1602.
54. Desir D, Kirkpatrick C, Fevre-Montange M et al. Ritodrine increases plasma melatonin in women. Lancet 1983; i:184.
55. Land JM, A'Court CHD, Gillmer MDG et al. Severe non-diabetic ketoacidosis causing intrauterine death. Br J Obstet Gynaecol 1992;99:77–79.
56. Rugolo S, Russo S, Di Stefano F et al. Influenza di alcuni farmaci sull'ittero fisiologico del neonato. Min Ginecol 1991;43:569–572.
57. Wagner JM, Morton MJ, Johnson KA et al. Terbutaline and maternal cardiac function. J Am Med Assoc 1981; 246:2698.
58. Böhm N, Adler CP. Focal necrosis, fatty degeneration and subendocardial nuclear polyploidization of the myocardium in newborns after beta-sympathicomimetic suppression of premature labour. Eur J Pediatr 1981;136:149.
59. Fletcher SE, Fyfe DA, Case CL et al. Myocardial necrosis in a newborn after long-term maternal subcutaneous terbutaline infusion for suppression of pre-term labor. Am J Obstet Gynecol 1991;165:1401–1404.

60. Sheybany S, Evans D, Nwcombe RG, Pearson JF. Ritodrine in the management of fetal distress. Br J Obstet Gynaecol 1982;89:723.
61. Pratt HF. Abuse of salbutamol inhalers in young people. Clin Allergy 1982;12:203.
62. Neville E, Corris PA, Vivian J et al. Nebulized salbutamol and angina. Br Med J 1982;285:796.
63. Fouda A, Hassounda M, Beddoe E. Priapism: an avoidable complication of pharmacologically induced erection. J Urol 1989;142:995–997.
64. Matsuo M, Yamada T, Takemine N et al. Duodenal perforation with tolazoline therapy. J Pediatr 1982;100:1005.
65. Pajewski M, Modai D, Wisgarten J. Iatrogenic arterial aneurysm associated with ergotamine therapy. Lancet 1981;ii:934.
66. Gordon RD, Ballantine DM, Bachmann AW. Effects of repeated doses of pseudoephedrine on blood pressure and plasma catecholamines in normal subjects and in subjects with phaeochromocytoma. Clin Exp Pharmacol Physiol 1992;19:287–290.
67. De Groot ANJA, van Dongen PWJ, Van Roosmalen J et al. Ergotamine-induced fetal stress: review of side-effects of ergot alkaloids during pregnancy. Eur J Obstet Gynecol Reprod Biol 1993;51:73–77.
68. Loew DM, Van Deusen EB, Meier-Ruge W. Effect on the central nervous system. In: Berde B, Schild HO, eds. Handbook of Experimental Pharmacology, Vol 49: Ergot Alkaloids and Related Compounds, Ch. 6. Berlin–Heidelberg–New York: Springer-Verlag, 1978;421.
69. Kenna AP. Accidental administration of syntometrine to a newborn infant. J Obstet Gynaecol Br Commonw 1972;79:764.
70. Hays JT, Hamill RD, DeFelice CA et al. Coronary artery spasm culminating in thrombosis following ergonovine stimulation. Catheter Cardiovasc Diagn 1993;28:221–224.
71. Morley J. Beta agonist and asthma mortality: déja vu. Clin Exp Allergy 1992;22:724–725.
72. Committee on Safety of Medicines. Sumatriptan (Imigran) and chest pain. Curr Probl 1992;34:2.
73. Cochrane P. Spontaneous oesophageal rupture after carbachol therapy. Br Med J 1973;1:463.
74. Van der Meer FJM, Van der Vijver JCM. Bradycardie en cardiogene shock veroorzaakt door carbachol. Ned Tijdschr Geneeskd 1982;126:1010.
75. Buzello W, Krieg N, Schlickewei A. Hazards of neostigmine in patients with neuromuscular disorders. Br J Anaesth 1982;54:529.
76. Blackhall MI, Buckley GA, Roberts DV et al. Drug-induced neonatal myasthenia. J Obstet Gynaecol Br Commonw 1969;76:157.
77. Van Herwaarden G, Berger HJC, Horstink MWIM. Short-term memory in Parkinson's disease after withdrawal of long-term anticholinergic therapy. Clin Neuropharmacol 1993;16:438–443.
78. Dauchot P, Gravenstein JS. Effects of atropine on the electrocardiogram in different age groups. Clin Pharmacol Ther 1971;12:274.
79. Gravenstein JS, Ariet M, Thornby JI. Atropine or the electrocardiogram. Clin Pharmacol Ther 1969;10:660.
80. Allen G, Everett GB, Kennedy WF Jr. Cardiorespiratory effects of general anaesthesia in outpatients: the influence of atropine. J Oral Surg 1972;30:576.
81. Lunde P. Ventricular fibrillation after intravenous atropine for treatment of sinus bradycardia. Acta Med Scand 1976;199:369.
82. Lacouture PG, Lovejoy FN Jr, Mitchell AA. Acute hypothermia associated with atropine. Am J Dis Child 1983; 137:291.
83. Gooding JM. Holcomb MC. Transient blindness following intravenous administration of atropine. Anesth Analg 1977;56:872.
84. Anderson S, McGuire R, McKeown D. Comparison of the cognitive effects of premedication with hyoscine and atropine. Br J Anaesth 1985;57:169.
85. Mulpeter KM, Walsh JB, O'Connor M et al. Ocular hazards of nebulized bronchodilators. Postgrad Med J 1992;68:132–133.
86. Clissold SP, Heel RC. Transdermal hyoscine (scopolamine): a preliminary review of its pharmacodynamic properties and therapeutic efficacy. Drugs 1985;29:189.
87. Priz U. Die Nebenwirkungen des Urologikums Mictonorm aud das Auge. Folia Opthalmol 1985;10:105.
88. Puhakka NJ. Drug-induced corrosive injury of the oesophagus. J Laryngol Otol 1978;42:927.
91. General Practitioner Research Group. Mepenzolat bromide in mucomembranous colitis. Practitioner 1974;212:890.
89. Parma A, Visentini E, Bondavalli C. Impiego de cloruro di ossibutinina nella sindrome post-TUR nell'uretrocistalgia femminile. Urologia 1983;48:1001.
90. Sangster B, van Heijst ANP, Zimmerman ANE. Treatment of orphenadrine overdose. N Engl J Med 1977;296:1006.
91. Marsden CD, Marion MH, Quinn N. The treatment of severe dystonia in children and adults. J Neurol Neurosurg Psychiatry 1984;47:1166.
92. Friedman Z. Neumann E. Benzhexol-induced blindness in Parkinson's disease. Br Med J 1972;1:605.
93. Ananth JV, Lehmann HE, Ban TA. Toxic psychosis induced by benzhexol hydrochloride. Can Med Assoc J 1970;103:771.
94. Adama BE, Manoguerra AS, Lilja GP et al. Heat stroke associated with medications having anticholinergic effects. Min Med 1977;60:103.

Meyler's Side Effects of Drugs, 13th Edition
M.N.G. Dukes, editor

SECTION EDITOR: P.I. FOLB

Anton C. de Groot

14 Dermatological drugs, topical agents and cosmetics

This chapter presents a selection of adverse reactions to dermatological drugs, topical agents and cosmetics. For more information the reader is referred to Reference 4, which provides an encyclopedic survey of side effects of cosmetics and drugs used in dermatology.

Photochemotherapy (PUVA)

Photochemotherapy, which consists of the oral (and sometimes topical) administration of psoralens (usually 8-methoxypsoralen) plus long-wave ultraviolet radiation, known as PUVA, is a well-established effective treatment for psoriasis; it may also be used for vitiligo, mycosis fungoides, alopecia areata, dyshidrotic eczema, atopic dermatitis, and certain other dermatoses. Guidelines for treatment have been recommended (171[R]).

ADVERSE REACTION PATTERN (141[R])

General and toxic reactions Short-term reactions are well known and not infrequent, including erythema, burns, nausea, pruritus, headache and dizziness.

Hypersensitivity reactions Hypersensitivity reactions, occurring infrequently, have included drug fever (54[C]), skin rashes and bronchial asthma.

Tumor-inducing effects Long-term treatment increases the risk of non-melanoma skin cancers.

ORGANS AND SYSTEMS

Cardiovascular A rise in ambient temperature may exert a definite cardiovascular stress. Under high-risk conditions, cardiovascular monitoring during treatment has been advised (SEDA-6, 148), although patients with cardiovascular disease and hypertension are also reported to tolerate PUVA therapy without evidence of cardiovascular stress (155[C]). Edema of the legs has been noted occasionally. Temporal arteritis has been reported (SEDA-6, 147).

Respiratory Bronchial asthma and coughing attacks have been attributed to methoxsalen allergy (55[C]).

Nervous system Dizziness, headache and itching are well-known immediate side effects (SEDA-3, 132). Persistent *skin pain* may pose a serious problem (22[Cr]).

Hematological Preleukemia (SEDA-4, 105, dubious report), acute leukemia (SEDA-10, 125) and neutropenia (SEDA-5, 151) have been reported to occur during PUVA. Transformation of stable chronic myelomonocytic leukemia to acute myeloid leukemia has been attributed to PUVA (SEDA-14, 124). These events may all have been purely coincidental and not causally related to PUVA.

Liver *(SEDA-5, 150; SEDA-6, 147)* Slight and transient elevations of liver enzymes during PUVA treatment have been reported, but they were usually attributable to pre-existing liver disease or intake of alcohol or other drugs. However, two reports of liver damage clearly attributable to PUVA have been presented (198[C], 199[C]).

Gastrointestinal Nausea and diarrhea sometimes occur.

Urinary system In 12 of 106 patients treated with PUVA an increase in serum creatinine to abnormal values was noted. A renal biopsy showed uncharacteristic glomerulonephritis in one patient (SEDA-5, 151). Nephrotic syndrome in a patient treated with PUVA for polymorphic light eruption has been reported (SEDA-9, 132).

Skin and appendages Well-known immediate side-effects are erythema, burns, localized edema, and blistering. Other side-effects (possibly) related to PUVA are listed in Table 1.

Cutaneous carcinogenicity A review of the English language literature on the risk of non-melanoma skin cancer from photochemotherapy in the treatment of psoriasis resulted in the following conclusions and recommendations (63[R]).

Table 1. *Dermatological side effects related to PUVA therapy*

Acne (SEDA-3, 132)
PUVA keratoses (156[CR])
Actinic lichenoid dermatitis (SEDA-12, 130)
Allergic contact dermatitis to methoxsalen (8-methoxypsoralen) (162[C])
'Allergic' cutaneous vasculitis (SEDA-6, 146)
Bacterial infections such as folliculitis and erysipelas
Bowen's disease and Bowenoid lesions (160[C])
Bullous eruptions (SEDA-8, 152; SEDA-10, 126; 17[illegible][C])
Disseminated epidermolytic acanthoma (SEDA-12, 130)
Disseminated superficial actinic porokeratosis (SEDA-6, 147; SEDA-11, 136)
Exacerbation of polymorphic light eruption
Granuloma annulare (SEDA-4, 105)
Herpes simplex, Kaposi's varicelliform eruption (165[C])
Herpes zoster (164[c])
Keratoacanthoma (SEDA-9, 131; 160[C], 163[R])
Lichen planus (SEDA-6, 147)
Lupus erythematosus (SEDA-15, 140; SEDA-17, 183)
Lymphomatoid papulosis (SEDA-16, 151)
Neurofibroma (SEDA-15, 142)
Papular phototoxic reaction (163[R])
Pemphigus vulgaris (19[Cr])
Photoallergic dermatitis (SEDA-15, 141)
Pigment alterations, notably PUVA lentigines (SEDA-9, 130). Absence of PUVA lentigines may be an indicator of a lower risk of PUVA malignancy (145[Cr])
Pustular psoriasis
Rosacea
Scleroderma-like alterations (157[C])
Seborrhoeic dermatitis of the face
Suppression of induction and expression of delayed cutaneous hypersensitivity (161[C])
Toxic pustuloderma (SEDA-16, 151)
Urticaria (25[Cr])
Appendages
Hirsutism (SEDA-6, 146)
Hypertrichosis (62[CR])
Nail pigmentation (SEDA-8, 152)
Photo-onycholysis (SEDA-3, 132; SEDA-4, 105)
Psoriasis of the nails
Subungual bleeding
Miscellaneous
Epidermal dystrophy
Senile elastoidosis

(1) PUVA is an independent carcinogen in a dose-related fashion in humans and is capable of initiating and promoting the formation of squamous cell carcinoma (SCC, 145[Cr]). The relation of basal cell carcinoma to PUVA alone is not well established.
(2) The carcinogenic risk of PUVA is not simply dose-related and skin type and geographic location in addition to other well-established cocarcinogenic risk factors must be taken into account.
(3) Three factors are important cocarcinogens with PUVA. They include history of arsenic exposure, ionizing radiation therapy, and skin cancer. Other factors believed to be related to increased risk include skin types I and II.
(4) Factors that appear to be associated with little or no risk of increased PUVA-related carcinogenesis include methotrexate (although a study from Sweden (90[Cr]) suggests otherwise), topical tar, and ultraviolet B (UVB). Exceptions to this include simultaneous use of methotrexate and PUVA, as well as high exposure to UVB/tar to genital skin. Retinoids may prove to be negatively correlated with skin cancer.
(5) The dose-related increased risk of cutaneous SCC from PUVA is independent of skin type (I—IV), although the absolute risk is much higher in skin types I and II.
(6) Men treated with PUVA without genital protection are at high risk of developing invasive SCC of the penis and the scrotum in a dose-related fashion (SEDA-15, 141).
(7) PUVA-induced SCC does not appear to be biologically aggressive. Nevertheless, metastases have been observed in four patients, which emphasizes the need for continued monitoring.
(8) There is no definitive level of cumulative PUVA exposure above which carcinogenicity can be predicted. However, trends from recent studies indicate that patients with skin types II, III and IV and no risk factors are at relatively low risk of SCC below 1000 J/cm^2 cumulative exposure. Of patients treated with over 2000 J/cm^2 even those without risk factors, at least 20% will develop squamous cell carcinomas and 50% atypical squamous keratoses (145[Cr]). Patients with skin type I should be monitored more rigorously.

The following recommendations were given:

(1) Whenever possible, exclude patients with a history of ionizing radiation therapy, skin cancer, or arsenic exposure.
(2) Shield the male genital skin at all times during PUVA treatment.
(3) Use the European dosage protocol (lower doses and less frequent irradiations than the US protocol) whenever possible.
(4) Reduce PUVA dosage by combining or cycling with other treatments. Avoid maintenance if possible.
(5) Use PUVA in younger patients only when necessary.
(6) Monitor patients with skin type I closely.
(7) Monitor patients prospectively and at least annually for keratoses and cutaneous carcinoma, particularly after cumulative exposure of more than 1000 J/cm^2.

Special senses *Eyes* Although several cases of cataracts presumably or probably induced by PUVA therapy have been reported (10[CR], 84[C]), the risk appears to be small when recommendations to prevent ocular complications (201[C]) are strictly adhered to (158[Cr], 169[Cr]).

Other ocular symptoms after PUVA treatment include photophobia, conjunctivitis, keratitis and dry eyes (SEDA-7, 166; 166[C]). Visual field defects have been described in three patients (202[Cr]).

Antinuclear antibodies induced by PUVA Concerns about the ability of PUVA therapy to induce systemic lupus erythematosus (SLE) and other connective tissue diseases (CTD) have been raised by several case reports describing the development of CTDs in close temporal relation to PUVA therapy for psoriasis (SED-12, 336; SEDA-15, 139; SEDA-17, 183).

As a consequence, several studies have evaluated the incidence of antinuclear antibodies (ANAs) in the serum of PUVA-treated patients, with both positive and negative results.

Current evidence suggests that a frequent evaluation of ANAs during treatment of patients with uncomplicated psoriasis with a test initially negative for ANA and with no symptoms of connective tissue diseases is unnecessary (42[Cr]).

Risk situations Relative contraindications to PUVA therapy include a history of arsenic intake, previous ionizing radiation, long-term use of cytostatic drugs, skin cancer, cataracts, and severe cardiovascular disease.

In patients known to suffer from photosensitive dermatoses and in patients using systemic photosensitizing drugs, PUVA therapy should be administered with caution. The possible long-term side effects should be taken into consideration, especially when young patients are candidates for photochemotherapy.

Second-generation effects Although PUVA therapy should not be instituted in pregnancy or during lactation, the theoretical mutagenic and teratogenic effect of PUVA treatment does not carry any significant risk for abnormal delivery outcome (21[R], 100[r]).

Interactions Phenytoin may cause low serum levels of methoxsalen, possibly by induction of the hepatic enzyme system leading to increased metabolism of methoxsalen (159[C]).

Oral retinoids

Vitamin A (retinol) is a known key regulator of epithelial cell proliferation and differentiation. Aberrations in these processes are a feature of many skin diseases; dermatologists have therefore long taken an interest in vitamin A as a therapeutic agent. However, marginal efficacy and unacceptable side effects (Table 2) have minimized the usefulness of vitamin A per se.

Table 2. *Clinical findings in chronic hypervitaminosis A, in order of decreasing frequency (178[R], 190[R])*

Scaling of skin, erythema, pruritus, disturbed hair growth
Dry mucuous membranes, cheilitis, angular stomatitis, gingivitis, glossitis
Pain and tenderness of the bones, restricted movement
Occipital headache
Hyperirritability, sleep disturbance
Papillary edema, diplopia
Anorexia, loss of weight
Hepatomegaly, sometimes with splenomegaly
Edema, swelling
Fatigue, lassitude, occasionally somnolence
Hemorrhages, epistaxis, increased menstrual bleeding

Tretinoin (all-*trans*-retinoic acid), a natural metabolite of vitamin A, was used orally at first with some dermatological success, but its general therapeutic ratio did not differ markedly from that of vitamin A itself (186[C]). More recently, two new synthetic retinoids, etretinate (the ethyl ester of trimethoxymethylphenyl retinoic acid; Tigason; Tegison) and isotretinoin (13-*cis*-retinoic acid; Acutane, Roaccutane), have been successfully administered for a variety of dermatological disorders, all of which display disordered epidermal or epithelial cell growth and differentiation as a prominent pathogenic feature, e.g. psoriasis, ichthyosis, Darier's disease, lichen planus and pityriasis rubra pilaris.

Isotretinoin has been of great value for the treatment of cystic acne and acne conglobata, with no serious long-term side effects (20[Cr]).

In 1990, etretinate (Tigason) was replaced by acitretin (Neo-Tigason), the main and active metabolite of etretinate. Its main advantage is its short elimination half-life of 50 hours (versus more than 80 days for etretinate) (239[CR]).

ADVERSE REACTION PATTERN

General and toxic reactions Although the various retinoids show similar toxicity spectra, they differ in the extent to which they affect various body systems. Cutaneous and mucous membrane symptoms (up to 70%) are by far the most prominent side effects, patients receiving isotretinoin having a 50% incidence of conjunctivitis and irritation of the eyes.

Hypersensitivity reactions Hypersensitivity reactions are rare.

Tumor-inducing effects Retinoids may prevent or even cure certain malignancies (189).

ORGANS AND SYSTEMS *(64[R], 68[R], 203[R])*

Respiratory Exercise-induced bronchoconstriction has been reported (197[C]). Eosinophilic pleural effusion has been attributed to isotretinoin (179[Cr]).

Nervous system (167[CR]) Nervous system disturbances reported include fatigue, lassitude, vertigo, sweating, hypesthesia, paresthesia, dizziness, fever, amnesia, delirium, flu-like symptoms, somnolence, pseudotumor cerebri, hyperirritability, sleep disturbance, lethargy, depression (168[Cr]) and psychological changes. The relationship between isotretinoin and seizures is still unclear (SEDA-18, 169). Rare cases of peripheral neuropathy have been observed (SEDA-17, 183).

Cardiovascular One case of myocardial infarction may have been related to etretinate.

Respiratory The manufacturers have on record in the USA several pulmonary adverse effects during isotretinoin therapy, including worsening of asthma, recurrent pneumothorax, pleural effusion, interstitial fibrosis, pulmonary granuloma and deterioration in lung function test. Exercise-induced bronchoconstriction was probably caused by isotretinoin in one patient. Pneumonia has also been reported as a possible side effect (69[Cr]).

Endocrine, metabolic (174[R]) Frequently, alterations in lipid metabolism are noted: increase in triglycerides (174[R]), increases in cholesterol levels, sometimes persisting after discontinuation of the therapy, and a decrease in high-density lipoprotein and HDL-cholesterol.

The consequences of hypertriglyceridemia are not well understood, but it may increase the cardiovascular risk status and induce pancreatitis (SEDA-13, 123). Patients with an increased tendency to develop hypertriglyceridemia include those with diabetes mellitus, obesity, increased alcohol intake, and a positive family history.

With a short course (16 weeks) of isotretinoin it is sufficient to ensure there is no hyperlipidemia prior to the onset of therapy, and to determine the triglyceride response to therapy on one occasion after 4 weeks' treatment (57[Cr]).

An increase in calcium, small decreases in indices of thyroid function (182[C]) and decreased albumin concentrations (182[C]) have been observed.

Breast discharge has been reported (200[C]). Menstrual disturbances occur, and may be under-reported (SEDA-13, 121, 123). Thyrotoxicosis may have been triggered by isotretinoin in one patient (SEDA-12, 136).

Side effects of isotretinoin affecting the male reproductive system reported to the manufacturer include gynecomastia, local inflammation/discomfort, potency disorders, reduced fertility, ejaculatory failure (SEDA-18, 168; 47[C])

Hematological Increased menstrual bleeding, disturbed blood clotting due to hypoprothrombinemia, elevated erythrocyte sedimentation rate (190[R]), decreased red cell parameters (190[R]), decreased white cell count (190[R]), thrombocytopenia (SEDA-12, 136) and eosinophilia (SEDA-13, 122) have all been observed incidentally (SEDA-17, 184).

Mineral and fluid balance Generalized edema has been caused by etretinate.

Liver (175[R]) Hepatomegaly is a known side effect of retinol and tretinoin. Transient slight elevation of liver enzymes, notably ASAT, ALAT and alkaline phosphatase, are frequent (184[C], 188[C]), but some cases of hepatotoxicity due to etretinate and acitretin (SEDA-17, 185) have also been reported (187[CR]). Cholestatic jaundice due to etretinate has been reported (213[CR]). Liver failure leading to death has been reported (187[C]) in which etretinate may have played a role.

Gastrointestinal (167[CR]) Gastrointestinal side effects of retinoids include anorexia, nausea, vomiting, loss of weight, stomach pain, thirst and splenomegaly. Proctosigmoiditis has been reported (SEDA-13, 123).

Urinary system Impaired renal function and hypercalcemia have (not very convincingly) been ascribed to etretinate (236[C]). Abnormalities in urinary protein, inflammation of the urethral meatus and nephrolithiasis have rarely occurred.

Skin and appendages Adverse effects on the skin are frequent (up to 70%). Symptoms and signs are listed in Table 3.

Bones (*SEDA*-17, 183; 70[Cr], 215[R]) Skeletal abnormalities associated with retinoid therapy have included: achilles tendonitis (SEDA-17, 185); acute arthritis (SEDA-18, 168; 56[Cr]); bridging of vertebral bodies; diffuse idiopathic skeletal hyperostosis (DISH); disc narrowing; nasal bone osteophytosis; osteoma cutis; ossification of tendons and ligamentous insertions; ossification of the posterior longitudinal ligament; periosteal thickening, premature epiphyseal closure; reduced bone density/osteoporosis; skeletal aches and pains; slender long bones; Tietze's syndrome.

Special senses *Eyes* (183[R], 214[R]) Ocular findings are among the more frequent side effects in patients taking isotretinoin, the most common being blepharoconjunctivitis.

Table 3. *Symptoms and signs of adverse effects of oral retinoids on the skin*

Abnormal skin odor
Acne fulminans (SEDA-11, 137)
Angular stomatitis
Balanitis (rare)
Bullous pemphigoid (SEDA-17, 184)
Cheilitis
Cystic and comedonal acne (SEDA-15, 142)
Delayed wound healing
Dissemination of herpes simplex
Disturbed hair growth
Dry mucous membranes
Epistaxis
Eruptive xanthomas (1 report, 173[C])
Erythema multiforme (SEDA-14, 124)
Erythema nodosum
Erythroderma (237[C])
Excess granulation tissue (SEDA-9, 134)
Generalized edema (1 report, 180[c])
Gingivitis, bleeding of the gums
Glossitis
Hirsutism
Hyperhidrosis (rare)
Hypo/hyperpigmentation
Mucosal erosions
Mycosis fungoides-like dermatitis (SEDA-10, 125)
Nasal carriage of *Staphyloccucus aureus* (SEDA-12, 131)
Nummular eczema (SEDA-12, 136)
Papulopustular palmoplantar eruption (218[Cr])
Paronychia
Petechiae
Phototoxicity/allergy (SEDA-17, 184)
Pityriasis rosea-like dermatitis
Porokeratosis (exacerbation of) (SEDA-16, 152)
Prurigo nodularis (SEDA-12, 131)
Pruritus
Pseudoporphyria (SEDA-17, 184)
Psoriasis as a Koebner phenomenon (1 case, SEDA-13, 123)
Rosacea-like eruption (1 report, 172[C])
Ruptured striae atrophicae (238[C])
Scaling of the skin
Skin erosions (217[Cr])
Sticky skin (185[R])
Thinning of the hair
Toxic epidermal necrolysis
'Unruly' hair (216[C], SEDA-11, 136)
Various nail deformities(181R):
Chronic paronchyia
Nail dystrophies
—Softening
—Fragility
—Beau's lines
—Onychomadesis
—Onychoschizia
—Transverse leukonychia
—Onycholysis
—Curly fingernails
Pyogenic granuloma
Nail growth disturbance (decreased growth)
Vasculitis (176[CR], 177[C])
Vulvitis
Worsening of pre-existing osteoma cutis (219[C])

Table 4. *Possible adverse ocular effects associated with isotretinoin exposure in 236 patients (220[R])*

Adverse effects	No. of patients
Eyelids	
Blepharoconjunctivitis or meibomianitis (193[C])	88
Photodermatitis	6
Cornea	
Corneal opacities	12
Dry eyes	47
Contact lens intolerance	19
Optic nerve	
Papilledema or pseudotumor cerebri	18
Optic neuritis	3
Congenital abnormalities	
Microphthalmos	5
Orbital hypertelorism	2
Optic nerve hypoplasia	4
Cortical blindness	1
Others	
Blurred vision	39
Myopia	5
Decreased night vision and dark adaptation (SEDA-10, 25)	3
Ocular inflammation (uveitis, scleritis, retinitis, ophthalmitis, iritis)	7

In one article (220[R]) 236 cases of adverse ocular reactions possibly associated with isotretinoin were evaluated (Table 4).

Ocular side effects secondary to isotretinoin are generally benign in nature and reversible on reduction or cessation of drug therapy. However, papilledema necessitates discontinuation of the drug. Corneal opacities should be monitored closely. Although they do not usually interfere with vision, prudence dictates discontinuation of isotretinoin or reduction of the dosage when corneal opacities develop (220[R]). Etretinate has caused photophobia and decreased night vision (SEDA-17, 183), possibly ectropion (SEDA-16, 152).

Ears Unilateral earache has been reported in two patients (SEDA-9, 134). Excessive cerumen production and otitis externa have also been reported.

Taste and smell may be altered by isotretinoin (SEDA-16, 153).

Muscles Muscle aches occur in 15% of patients. Elevation of creatine phosphokinase may be observed, especially in individuals engaging in strenuous physical activity (SEDA-10, 124). Clinical and subclinical muscle damage has been reported (SEDA-12, 131, 136; SEDA-14, 124).

Second-generation effects Retinoids are teratogenic

(5[Cr]). Prior to institution of therapy, pregnancy should be ruled out. An effective form of contraception must be used for at least 1 month prior to initiation of therapy, during therapy, and for at least 1 month (isotretinoin)/2 years (acitretin) after therapy is stopped. For a review of retinoid teratogenicity see Ref. 144[R].

Overdosage The possible symptoms and signs of overdosage, the effect of which is the same as in hypervitaminosis A (see Table 2).

Drug interactions Combination with tetracyclines increases the risk of pseudotumor cerebri. The concomitant medication of phenytoin or barbiturates should be avoided, since altered serum concentration of either medication may occur.

CONTACT ALLERGY

Contact allergy is the most frequently described adverse reaction of topical drugs and cosmetics; the diagnosis of a contact allergic reaction may be established by patch testing. Patch testing techniques have been discussed in classic textbooks (1[R]—4[R]) and review articles (17[R]).

In allergic contact dermatitis due to topical medicaments (18[R]), it should be appreciated that *any* constituent of the preparation may be responsible for the adverse event, e.g. the vehicle, preservative, emulsifier, perfume and, of course, the active drug. Hence, patch tests should be carried out with all active and 'inactive' ingredients of the incriminated topical drug.

Where cosmetic allergy is suspected (SEDA-11, 142; SEDA-13, 117; 273[R]), it is also advisable to test all ingredients of the cosmetic product separately; patch-testing with cosmetics 'as such' will often give unsatisfactory results since both false-negative and false-positive patch test reactions frequently occur. Ingredient labelling which will be mandatory in the European Union from January 1, 1997, will greatly facilitate investigating patients with suspected cosmetic dermatitis (26).

Table 5 lists alphabetically a large number of ingredients of cosmetics and topical drugs which may act as (possible) sensitizers; some drugs are accidental contactants, e.g. in the pharmaceutical industry or in health personnel. For each compound the concentration and vehicle for patch testing, known or generally held to be adequate, are mentioned; unless otherwise indicated, the data in the column 'Reference' are obtained from De Groot (3[R]).

Substances not listed in any standard table should be patch tested with great caution; control tests are mandatory when positive reactions are obtained, so as to exclude false-positive irritant patch test reactions.

We have attempted to estimate the sensitizing potential of each particular drug using the following scale: (1) sensitization is common; (2) sensitization may occur; (3) sensitization is unusual; (4) sensitization is rare/nonexistent. These estimates are based on literature data and our personal experience (4[R]).

CONTACT URTICARIA (IMMEDIATE CONTACT REACTIONS) *(SEDA-7, 159; 4[R], 38[R]–40[R])*

Contact urticaria refers to a wheal-and-flare response to the application of chemicals to intact skin. A variety of cutaneous and extracutaneous symptoms and signs has been described, justifying the term 'contact urticaria syndrome'. The broad spectrum of clinical manifestations is classified in Table 6. The symptoms usually develop within 20—30 minutes after contact with the offending chemical, but 'delayed' reactions after several hours have also been recorded.

Most cases of contact urticaria are of non-immunological origin, presumably due to the direct release of histamine, slow-reacting substance of anaphylaxis (SRS-A), bradykinin or other vasoactive compounds. Topical drugs and ingredients of cosmetics that have caused 'non-immunological' contact urticaria are listed in Table 7.

Contact urticaria of immunological origin is apparently less frequent, although many topical drugs have caused this condition in previously sensitized individuals. In a number of reports, positive passive-transfer tests were noted; specific antibodies have occasionally been demonstrated, indicating an immunological phenomenon. Topical drugs and ingredients of cosmetics that have caused 'immunological' contact urticaria are listed in Table 8; in most of these cases, the contact urticaria was of probable immunological origin.

Some cases of contact urticarial reactions cannot be ascribed with certainty either to 'immunological' or to 'non-immunological' mechanisms; the classical example of this category of contact urticaria of uncertain mechanism is that caused by the bleaching agent, ammonium persulfate. Also belonging to this category are a number of topical substances which have caused contact urticaria upon patch testing, the clinical significance of which is uncertain, e.g. nickel sulfate, butylated hydroxyanisole (BHA), butylated hydroxytoluene (BHT), ethyl vanillin, potassium bichromate, parabens and ethylenediamine (274[C]).

The diagnosis of contact urticaria can usually be confirmed by an open test; however, these tests should be performed with great caution since anaphylactoid

Table 5. *Patch test concentrations and vehicles for dermatological testing of ingredients of topical drugs and cosmetics*

Chemical	Patch-test concentration and vehicle*	Frequency of sensitization*	References	Comment
Acetylsalicylic acid	2% pet.	4	SEDA-18, 164; 146[R]	
Acyclovir	5% pet.	4	SEDA-14, 125	
Aescin	2% aqua	4	SEDA-17, 188	
Alcohol, ethyl [‡]	10% aqua, pure	4	SEDA-12, 133; 316[R]	b,d
Alkylammonium amidobenzoate	0.1% pet.	3	SEDA-17, 188	
Alprenolol	0.25–1% aqua	4	SEDA-4, 107	c
Ambroxol hydrochloride	0.5% aqua	4	SEDA-14, 125	
Amcinonide[†]	1% epi	3	SEDA-15, 140	
Amerchol CAB	pure	2	SEDA-17, 188	
p-Aminobenzoic acid[§]	2–5 % pet.	2	SEDA-18, 171	a
ϵ-Aminocaproic acid[§]	1% aqua	4	SEDA-17, 189	
3-(Aminomethyl)-pyridyl salicylate	1% aqua	3	SEDA-14, 125	
Aminophylline	2% pet.	3		c
Amlexanox	0.01–1% aqua/pet.	3	SEDA-16, 155	
Ammoniated mercury	1% pet.	2	SEDA-13, 127	d
Ammonium persulfate	2.5% pet.	4		e,b
Ampicillin	5% pet.	4	SEDA-9, 136	b
α-Amylcinnamic alcohol	2% pet.	2	SEDA-8, 158	
α-Amylcinnamic aldehyde	2% pet.	2	SEDA-8, 158; 12[CR]	
Apomorphine	0.05% ?	4	SEDA-17, 188	
Arnica, tincture of	20% pet.	3		
Atropine sulfate[§]	1% pet.	4		
Avocado oil	pure	4	SEDA-12, 134	
Azidamfenicol	5% pet.	3	SEDA-12, 132	
Azulene	1% pet.	4	SEDA-11, 140	
Bacitracin[§]	20% pet.	2	SEDA-18, 171	b
Basic blue 99	0.5% pet.	4	267[C]	
Beclomethasone dipropionate[†]	5% pet.	4	SEDA-15, 140	
Beeswax	30% pet.	2		
Befunolol[§]	1% aqua	3	SEDA-17, 188	
Benzalkonium chloride[‡§]	0.05% aqua	3	SEDA-7, 161	
Benzarone	2% pet. and pure	4	SEDA-10, 127	
Benzidine	1% pet. or MEK	2	SEDA-7, 163	
Benzocaine[§]	5% pet.	1		a,b
Benzoic acid[‡]	5% pet.	2		b
Benzoin tincture	10% alc./glyc.	3	SEDA-10, 127	b
Benzoxonium chloride[‡]	0.05% aqua	3	SEDA-13, 127	
Benzoyl peroxide	1% pet.	2	SEDA-9, 152	b,e
Benzydamine hydrochloride	5% pet.	3	SEDA-17, 188; 146[R]	a
Benzyl alcohol[‡]	5% pet.	3	SEDA-8, 154	b
Benzyl benzoate	5% pet.	3	SEDA-8, 154	
Benzyl salicylate	1% pet.		3	
Betamethasone 17-valerate[†]	5% pet.	3	SEDA-15, 140	
Betamethasone sodium phosphate[†]	5% pet.	4	SEDA-15, 140	
Betaxolol hydrochloride	1–5% aqua	4	SEDA-17, 188	
Bismuth tribromophenol	pure	4	SEDA-9, 136	
Bornelone	5% pet.	4	SEDA-9, 140	
2-Bromo-2-nitropropane-1,3-diol[‡]	0.25–0.5% pet.	3	SEDA-9, 136	
Budesonide	1% pet.	2	SEDA-17, 185	
Bufexamac	5% pet.	3	SEDA-18, 164; 146[R]	
Buphenine hydrochloride	1% alc.	4	SEDA-10, 127	
Bupivacaine			see SEDA-18 172 under Lidocaine	
Butoxyethyl nicotinate	2.5% pet.	4	SEDA-15, 146	
t-Butyl alcohol	70% aqua	4	SEDA-8, 159; 16[R]	b
Butylated hydroxyanisole (BHA)[‡]	2–5% pet.	3		b
Butylated hydroxytoluene (BT)[‡]	2–5% pet.	3		b
Butyl aminobenzoate	2% pet.	2	SEDA-16, 155	

* For key to abbreviations, see page 389. *(continued)*

Table 5. *(continued)*

Chemical	Patch-test concentration and vehicle*	Frequency of sensitization*	References	Comment
Butyl methoxydibenzoylmethane	2% pet.	3	SEDA-18, 171	a
Calcipotriol	2–10 μg/ml isopropanol	4	SEDA-18, 172	d,e
Carbarsone	1–5% pet.	4	SEDA-7, 161	
Carprofen	10% pet.	4	SEDA-18, 164; 146[R]	a
Carvone	1% pet.	4	SEDA-11, 140	
Castor oil	pure	4	SEDA-10, 130	
Centelase®	1% powder in pet.	3	SEDA-12, 132	
Cetrimonium bromide‡	0.05% aqua	3	SEDA-8, 126	
Cetyl alcohol	30% pet.	2		b
Cetylpyridinium chloride‡	0.05% aqua	3	SEDA-9, 136	
Cetylstearyl alcohol (Lanette®)	30% pet.	2	SEDA-9, 136; 14[Cr]	
Chamomile, oil of	25% o.c.	3		
Chloral hydrate	1–5% MEK	4	SEDA-12, 132	
Chloramine	2% aqua	3		b
Chloramphenicol§	1% alc./5–10% pet.	2	SEDA-10, 127	b
Chlordantoin	0.1–1% pet.	4		
Chlorhexidine‡§	1% aqua	3	SEDA-13, 125	a,b
Chloroacetamide‡	0.2% pet./aqua	2	SEDA-12, 134	
4-Chloro-*m*-cresol‡	1–2% pet.	3		b
Chloro-2-phenylphenol‡	1% aqua	3		a
Chloroquine diphosphate	5% aqua	4		c
Chloroquine sulfate	1% pet.	4	SEDA-10, 127	
p-Chloro-*m*-xylenol‡	0.5–1% pet.	3	SEDA-15, 148	
Chlorphenesin	1% pet.	4	SEDA-12, 134	
Chlorpheniramine maleate§		4	SEDA-17, 191	f
Chlorquinaldol	5% pet.	2	SEDA-9, 136	
Chromium hydroxide	potassium bichr. 0.5% pet.	?	SEDA-7, 164	
Cinnamic alcohol	1% pet.	2	SEDA-2, 140; 12[Cr]	
Cinnamic aldehyde	1% pet.	2	SEDA-12, 134;12[Cr]	a,b
Cinoxicam	2% pet.	4	SEDA-18, 164; 146[R]	
Clindamycin phosphate	1% aqua	3	SEDA-15, 146	d
Clobetasol-17-propionate†	0.05–10% pet.	3	SEDA-15, 140	b
Clobetasone butyrate†	0.5% pet.	3	SEDA-9, 137	
Clonidine	1% pet.	1	SEDA-15, 144; 270[R], 271[R]	
Clotrimazole	1% MEK/pet.	4	SEDA-12, 132	
Cocamide DEA	0.5% pet.	4	SEDA-12, 134	
Cocamidopropyl betaine§	1% pet.	2	SEDA-16, 155	
Cocobetaine	2% aqua	4	SEDA-8, 158	
Codeine	0.001–0.033% aqua	4	SEDA-11, 139	
Corticosteroids†	1% alc. 94%	2	48[R], 49[R], 50[R]	d
Crotamiton	10% aqua	4	SEDA-15, 146	
Crystal violet	2% aqua	3		
Cyclomethycaine	1% pet.	3		
Cyclopyroxolamine	10% pet.	4	SEDA-12, 132	
D&C Red No. 17	2% pet	4	SEDA-7, 164	
D&C Red No. 36	2% pet	3	SEDA-11, 140	
D&C Yellow No. 11	0.1% pet.	3	SEDA-14, 129	
Decyl oleate	1% pet	4	SEDA-17, 188	
Desoximetasone†	1% epi	4	SEDA-15, 140	a
Dexchlorpheniramine maleate	1% aqua	4	SEDA-15, 146	
Dexpanthenol	5% pet	3	SEDA-14, 125	
Diazolidinyl urea‡	2% aqua or pet.	3	SEDA-15, 148	
1,2-Dibromo-2,4-dicyanobutane‡	0.3% pet.	2	SEDA-16, 150	
Dibromopropamidine	5% pet	4	SEDA-13, 125	
Dibutyl phthalate	5% pet	4	SEDA-17, 188	
Dichlorodifluoromethane	pure	4	SEDA-13, 127	
Dichlorophene‡	1% pet.	4		a

Table 5. *(continued)*

Chemical	Patch-test concentration and vehicle*	Frequency of sensitization*	References	Comment
Diclofenac sodium	10% pet.	3	SEDA-18, 164; 146[R]	
Diethyl sebacate	1% pet./10% alc	3		
Diethylstilbestrol	1% pet.	4		b,d
Diflucortolone 21-valerate†	1% pet.	4	SEDA-10, 127	
Dihydrostreptomycin	1% pet.	2		
Dihydroxyacetone	10% aqua	4	SEDA-16, 155	
Diisopropanolamine	1% pet.	3	SEDA-15, 146	
Diisopropyl sebacate	3%—10% alc.	4	SEDA-16, 155	
Dimethindene maleate	comm. prep.	4	SEDA-18, 172	
Dimethyl sulfoxide	90% aqua	4		b,d,e
Dioxybenzone	2% pet.	3	SEDA-2, 137	
Diphenhydramine	1% pet.	3		a
Dipicolinic acid	0.1% pet.	3	SEDA-14, 125	
Dipivalyl epinephrine hydrochloride	0.5% aqua	4	SEDA-17, 188	
Dipropylene glycol	0.5% pet. and aqua	4	SEDA-18, 172	
Dithranol (cignolin, anthralin)	0.03% acet.	4	SEDA-7, 161	e
Dodecyl (= lauryl) gallate	0.25% pet.	3	SEDA-12, 132	
Dodecyl maleamic acid	1% pet.	4	SEDA-8, 154	
Drometrizole	5% pet.	4	SEDA-9, 140	
Dyclonine hydrochloride	1% pet.	4	SEDA-10, 128	
Econazole nitrate	2% alc	3	SEDA-14, 126	
Enilconazole	2% pet.	4	SEDA-8, 154	
Enoxolone	10% pet.	4	SEDA-17, 188	
Epinephrine (adrenalin)§	0.1—1% aqua	4		
Erythromycin	5% pet.	3	SEDA-8, 154	a
Esculin	1% pet.	4	SEDA-5, 155	
Essential oils	2% pet.317-β-Estradiol?	4	SEDA-17, 189	
Estradiol benzoate	0.05% MEK	4	SEDA-14, 126	b,d
Ethambutol	1% pet. or aqua	4	SEDA-12, 133	f
2-Ethoxyethyl-*p*-methoxycinnamate	2% pet.	3	SEDA-18, 171	a
Ethoxyquin	0.5% alc. or pet.	1	SEDA-9, 137	
Ethyl chloride	pure	4	SEDA-15, 146	
Ethylenediamine tetraacetate (EDTA)‡§	1% pet.	4	SEDA-12, 132	
Ethyl lactate	1% pet.	4	SEDA-13, 125	
Ethylmercuric chloride‡	0.05% pet.	2	SEDA-18, 174; 52[CR]	
Ethyl sebacate	1% pet.	4	SEDA-15, 146	
Etofenamate	2% pet.	4	SEDA-18, 164; 146[R]	b
Eucerin	pure	3		
Eugenol	5% pet.	1	12[CR]	b
Eusolex 8021®	2% pet.	2	SEDA-7, 164	
Fepradinol	5% DMSO 2% alc	3	SEDA-18, 172	
Feprazone	5% pet.	4	SEDA-18, 164; 146[R]	
Flufenamic acid	2—5 % pet.	4	SEDA-18, 164; 146[R]	
Fluocinolone acetonide†	1% pet.	4	SEDA-9, 137	
Fluocortin butyl†	1% alc.	3	SEDA-15, 140	
Fluorouracil	5% pet.	4	SEDA-10, 128	a,e
Flurandrenolide	1% pet.	3	SEDA-10, 128	
Gallate esters	0.1—1% pet.	3		
Gelatin	pure	4	SEDA-8, 155	
Gentamicin§	20% pet.	2	SEDA-14, 126	b,d
Gentian violet	1% aqua	4	SEDA-8, 155	b,d (under tri-phenyl-methane dyes)
Geraniol	2% pet.	4	SEDA-7, 164; 12[CR]	

(continued)

Table 5. *(continued)*

Chemical	Patch-test concentration and vehicle*	Frequency of sensitization*	References	Comment
Glutaraldehyde[‡]	1% aqua	3	SEDA-8, 155	
Glycerol	1–10% aqua	4		
Glyceryl *p*-aminobenzoate	5% pet.	3	SEDA-2, 137	a
Glyceryl diisostearate	2% pet.	4	SEDA-18, 172	
Glyceryl stearate	30% pet.	4	SEDA-14, 128	
Glyceryl thioglycolate	1% pet.	3	SEDA-10, 128	
Guaiazulene	1% pet.	4	SEDA-10, 130	
Heparin	comm. prep.	4	SEDA-14, 126	
Hexachlorophene[‡]	1% pet.	4		a,d,e
Hexamidine[‡]	0.15% aqua	3	SEDA-10, 128	
cis-3-Hexenyl salicylate	3% pet.	4	SEDA-8, 158	
Hexetidine	0.1% pet.	4	SEDA-7, 161	
Hexyl laurate	30% pet.	4	SEDA-15, 146	
Hinokitiol	0.1% alc.	4	SEDA-8, 158	
Homomenthyl salicylate	2% pet.	4	SEDA-3, 131	
4-Homosulfanilamide (mafenide)	5% pet.	2	SEDA-17, 189	d
Hydrocortisone acetate[†]	25% pet.	3		a
Hydrocortisone-17-butyrate[†]	1% alc.	2	SEDA-17, 185	
Hydroquinone	1% pet.	3	SEDA-9, 137	
Hydroxycitronellal	5% pet.	1	SEDA-2, 140; 12[CR]	
17-α-Hydroxyprogesterone	1% alc.	3	SEDA-18, 170	
Hydroxypropylcellulose	5% aqua	4	SEDA-13, 125	
Ibuprofen	5% pet.	3	SEDA-18, 164; 146[R]	f
Ibuprofen piconol	1–5% pet.	3	SEDA-13, 125	
Ibuproxam	2.5% pet.	3	SEDA-18, 164; 146[R]	
Ichthyol (ichthammol)	5% pet.	3	SEDA-9, 136	
Idoxuridine[§]	1% pet.	3	SEDA-7, 162	
Indomethacin	5% pet.	4	SEDA-18, 164; 146[R]	
Interferon-β-hydrochloride	eyedrops pure and diluted 1:32	4	SEDA-16, 155	
Iodine, tincture of	0.5% aqua (open test)	3		b,d,e
Isoconazole	2% alc.	4	SEDA-14, 126	
Isoeugenol	5% pet.	1	12[CR]	
Isopropyl alcohol[‡]	20% aqua	3	SEDA-7, 162; 16[R]	b
4-Isopropyl dibenzoylmethane	2% pet.	2	SEDA-18, 171	a
Isopropyl myristate	20% pet.	4		
Isopropyl palmitate	2% pet.	4	SEDA-8, 155	
Isostearyl alcohol	5% alc.-pure	4	SEDA-12, 135	
Isothipendyl hydrochloride	1% pet.	4	SEDA-9, 137	
Jasmin synthetic	10% pet.	2		
Jojoba oil	20% o.o.	3	SEDA-7, 164	
Kanamycin[§]	20% pet.	3		
Kathon® CG	100 ppm aqua	1	SEDA-11, 134; 212	
Ketoconazole	1% pet.	4	SEDA-15, 146	
Ketoprofen	5% pet.	3	SEDA-18, 164; 146[R]	a,f
Lactic acid	3% aqua	4	SEDA-18, 172	
Lanette N®	20% pet.	3	14[Cr]	
Lanette wax	30% paraff.liq.	3	SEDA-2, 139	
Lanolin	pure	3		
Laurylpyridinium chloride[‡]	0.1% aqua		SEDA-13, 127	
Lawsone (2-hydroxy-1,4-naththoquinone)	5% pet.	4	SEDA-12, 135	
Lead acetate	0.5% pet. or aqua		SEDA-8, 158	
Levobunolol hydrochloride[§]	1% aqua	3	SEDA-17, 189	
Lidocaine	2% aqua	3	SEDA-18, 172	b,d
Lilial	1% pet.	4	SEDA-8, 159	
Linalozol	30% pet.	3	SEDA-9, 140	
Lincomycin hydrochloride	1% aqua	4	SEDA-10, 128	

Table 5. *(continued)*

Chemical	Patch-test concentration and vehicle*	Frequency of sensitization*	References	Comment
Malathion	0.5% pet.	4	SEDA-2, 136	d
Mandelic acid	5% pet.	4	SEDA-18, 172	
Masoprocol (nordihydroguaiaretic acid)	1% "cream"	2	SEDA-18, 171	e
Mechlorethamine hydrochloride (nitrogen mustard)	0.02% aqua (open test)	1	SEDA-6, 149b	
Mephenesin	5% pet.	3	SEDA-9, 137	
Mepivacaine	1% aqua	4	SEDA-16, 155	
Mercuric chloride	0.05% pet.	3	SEDA-17, 186	
Mesulfen	5% pet.	4	SEDA-8, 155	e
Metaoxedrine (phenylephrine hydrochloride)	5% aqua	4		
8-Methoxypsoralen	0.1% alc.	4	SEDA-11, 139	a
3-(4-Methylbenylidene)-camphor	2% pet.	3	SEDA-18, 171	a
Methyl(chloro)isothiazolinone	100 ppm aqua	1	SEDA-4, 134; 212	a
6-Methylcoumarin	1% pet.	3		
Methyl glucose sesquistearate	5% pet.	4	SEDA-10, 130	
Methylionone	10% pet.	4	SEDA-14, 128	
Methyl octine carbonate	1% MEK	4	SEDA-13, 125	
Methyl salicylate	2% pet.	4		b
Metipranolol§	2% aqua	4	SEDA-13, 125	
Metoprolol§	3% aqua	4		
Mexenone (benzophenone-10)	2% pet.	3	SEDA-18, 171	a
Miconazole nitrate	2% pet. or alc.	3	SEDA-14, 126	
Microcrystalline wax	pure	3	SEDA-10, 130	
Minoxidil	1% alc.	3	SEDA-11, 139	a,d
Monobenzylether of hydroquinone	1% pet.	3		
Monotertiary butyl hydroquinone	1% pet.	4	SEDA-9, 140	
Musk ambrette	5% pet.	3	SEDA-7, 164	a
Mycanodin	2% pet.	4		a
Naftifine	1% pet.	3	SEDA-15, 147	
Neomycin§	20% pet.	2		
Nicotine	10% aqua	2	SEDA-18, 170	b
Nifuratel	1% acet.	3	SEDA-15, 147	
Nitrofurazone	1% pet.	2		
Nitroglycerin	2% pet.	3	SEDA-15, 144, 270[R], 271[R]	
Nonoxynols	2% aqua	3	268[R]	
Nystatin	100 000 U/g in PEG-400	3	266[R]	
Oak moss	2% pet.	1	12[CR]	
Octyl dimethyl PABA	2% pet.	3	SEDA-18, 171	a
Oleamidopropyl dimethylamine	0.1% aqua	2	SEDA-14, 128	
Olive oil	pure	3	SEDA-15, 147	
Omeprazole	0.25–1% pet.	4	SEDA-12, 133	
Oxiconazole	1% alc. or MEK	4	SEDA-12, 133	
Oxybenzone	2% pet.	3	SEDA-18, 171	a
Oxyphenbutazone	1% pet.	3	SEDA-18, 164; 146[R]	b,f
Palmitoyl hydrolyzed milk protein	10% pet.	4	SEDA-13, 126	
Patchouli oil	10% pet.	4	SEDA-17, 189	
d-Panthenyl ethyl ether	30% pet.	4	SEDA-9, 141	
Pecilocin	10% pet.	4		
Penicillin	pure (comm. prep.)	1		b
Petrolatum	pure	4	SEDA-9, 138	
Phenobarbital	0.1% aqua 20% prop glyc.	4	SEDA-12, 133	
Phenothiazine derivatives	2% pet.	1		a
Phenoxybenzamine	1% aqua	4	SEDA-1, 136	c
Phenoxyethanol‡	1% pet.	4	SEDA-10, 128	
Phenylbutazone	5% pet.	3	SEDA-18, 164; 146[R]	

(continued)

Table 5. *(continued)*

Chemical	Patch-test concentration and vehicle*	Frequency of sensitization*	References	Comment
Phenyl dimethicone	2% pet.	4	SEDA-10, 130	
Phenylephrine	0.5% pet.	4	SEDA-9, 138	
Phenylmercuric acetate‡	0.01% aqua	2		b,d
Phenylmercuric borate‡	0.01% aqua	2		b,d
2-Phenyl-5-methylbenzoxazol	2% pet.		SEDA-14, 128	a
Phenyl salicylate (salol)	1% pet.	4	SEDA-7, 165	
Picric acid	1% aqua	4	SEDA-16, 155	
Pigment red 57:1	1% pet.	4	SEDA-18, 172	
Pilocarpine§	1% ?	4	SEDA-18, 172	
Piperazine	1% pet.	3	SEDA-8, 156	c
Piroxicam	0.5% pet.	2	SEDA-18, 164; 146[R]	a
Pivampicillin	5–10% ?	1	SEDA-17, 189	c
Polidocanol	5% pet.	3	269[CR]	
Polyethylene glycol	pure	3	SEDA-15, 144	b
Polymyxin B§	3% pet	4		
Polysorbate 40 (Tween 40®)	5% pet.	3	SEDA-2, 139	
Polysorbate 80 (Tween 80®)	10% pet.	3	SEDA-2, 139; 14[Cr]	
Potassium coco-hydrolyzed animal protein	5 and 30% aqua	4	SEDA-14, 129	
Povidone-iodine	10% aqua/pet.	3	SEDA-18, 172	d
Pramocaine	2% aqua	4	SEDA-9, 138	
Prednisolone (pivalate)†	1% epi	4	SEDA-13, 126	
Prilocaine	2% aqua	3	SEDA-18, 172	
Procaine§	1% pet.	1		
Proflavine dihydrochloride	1% pet.	1	SEDA-13, 126	
Promethazine hydrochloride	1% pet.	1		a,b,d
Propantheline bromide	5% pet.	3	SEDA-9, 141	
Propolis	10% pet.	2	SEDA-17, 181	
Propylene glycol	2% pet.	4	SEDA-7, 162; 15[R]	e
Propyl gallate	1% pet.	3	SEDA-14, 126, 129	a
Pyrazinobutazone	?	4	SEDA-17, 191	f
Pyridoxine 3,4-dioctanoate	1% pet.	4	SEDA-8, 159	
Pyridoxine hydrochloride	10% pet.	4	SEDA-10, 128	
Pyrocatechol	2% pet.	4	SEDA-14, 129	
Pyrrolnitrin	1% pet.	3	SEDA-9, 138	
Quinidine sulfate	1% aqua	3	SEDA-7, 163	a,c
Quinine	1% aqua	4	SEDA-18, 173	a,c
Ranitidine (base)	2–5 % w/w pet.	4	SEDA-10, 128	
Resorcinol	2% pet.	3	SEDA-18, 173	b,d,e
Rhus aculeatus	0.8–1.6% alc.	4	SEDA-2, 138	e
Rifamycin	0.5% pet.	4	SEDA-11, 139	b
Salbutamol sulfate	5% pet./aqua	4	SEDA-18, 173	
Salicylates	2% pet.	3	SEDA-7, 165	
Salicylic acid	2% pet.	4	SEDA-2, 137	b,d,e
Scopolamine§	1% pet.	3	SEDA-15, 144; 270[R], 271[R]	
Sesame oil	pure	3	SEDA-13, 127	
Shellac	20% alc and pure	4	SEDA-12, 135	
Silicic acid	5% pet. and pure	4	SEDA-14, 133	
Silver nitrate	?	4	SEDA-17, 189	
Silver sulfadiazine cream	pure	3	SEDA-10, 129	
Sodium benzoate‡	1–2% aqua/pet.	3	SEDA-17, 189	
Sodium cromoglycate§	2% aqua	4	SEDA-14, 127	
Sodium fusidate	2% pet.	3	SEDA-8, 156	
Sodium ricinoleic monoethanol-amidosulfosuccinate derivative	5% pet.	4	SEDA-15, 148	
Sodium sulfite	2–5% pet.	4	SEDA-17, 190	
Solvent Red 3	1% pet	4	SEDA-16, 156	

Table 5. *(continued)*

Chemical	Patch-test concentration and vehicle*	Frequency of sensitization*	References	Comment
Sorbic acid[‡§]	2% pet.	3	SEDA-17, 190	b
Sorbitan laurate	5% aqua	4	SEDA-9, 139	b
Sorbitan oleate	5% pet.	4	SEDA-8, 156; 14[Cr]	
Sorbitan sesquioleate	2% pet.	3	SEDA-18, 173; 14[Cr]	
Sorbitan stearate	5% pet.	3	14[Cr]	
Spiramycin	10% aqua/pet.	3		c
Spironolactone	1% alc. or pure	4	SEDA-9, 138	
Squaric acid dibutyl ester	0.05% acet.	1	SEDA-9, 138	b
Stearic acid	5% pet.	4	SEDA-14, 129	
Stearyl alcohol	30% pet.	3		b
Storax (styrax)	2% pet.	2		
Streptomycin	1% pet.	2		b
Sulfonamides	5% pet.	1		a
Suprofen	0.1% pet.	3	SEDA-18, 164; 46[R]	a
Tannin	1–10% pet./aqua	4	SEDA-17, 156	
TEA-PEG-3 cocamide sulfate	1% aqua	4	SEDA-10, 130	
Tea tree oil	1% pet. and pure	3	SEDA-18, 170; 51[CR]	f
Tetracaine	1% pet.	2	SEDA-9, 138	
Tetracyclines	3% pet.	4		b
Thiabendazole	2% pet.	4	SEDA-17, 190	a?
Thimerosal[‡§]	0.1% pet.	2	SEDA-18, 171; 13[R], 52[CR]	b,d
Thioxolone	0.5% alc.	4	SEDA-13, 126	
Thuja essential oil	pure	4	SEDA-18, 173	
Tiaprofenic acid	1% pet.	3	SEDA-18, 164; 146[R]	a,f
Timolol maleate[§]	0.5% pet.	4	SEDA-16, 156	
Tioconazole	1% pet.	4	SEDA-15, 147	
Tixocortol pivalate[†]	1% pet.	1	SEDA-17, 185	
Tobramycin	20% aqua/pet.	3	SEDA-15, 147	
Tocopherols	10% pet.	3	272[CR]	b
Tolazoline[§]	<10% aqua	4	SEDA-11, 139	
Tolnaftate	1% pet.	4	SEDA-11, 139	
Toluene sulfonamide/formaldehyde resin	10% pet.	2	SEDA-17, 186	
Transdermal therapeutic systems		1–4	270[R], 271[R]	
Tretinoin	0.005% alc.	4	SEDA-2, 138	e
Triamcinolone acetonide[†]	1% alc.	3		
Triclosan	2% pet.	3		
Triethanolamine	2.5% pet.	2	SEDA-15, 143	
Triethanolamine polypeptide oleate condensate	1% pet.	4		
Triethanolamine stearate	5% pet.	4	SEDA-8, 159	
Trifluorothymidine[§]	1% pet.	4	SEDA-6, 149	
Trilaureth-4-phosphate	0.5 and 1% pet.	4	SEDA-10, 130	
Triphenylmethane dyes	2% aqua	3		d
Tromantadine hydrochloride	1% pet.	2	SEDA-9, 138	
Tropicamide	5% aqua	4	SEDA-18, 173	
Tylosin	5% pet.	3	SEDA-9, 138	
Tyrothricin	20% pet.	3		
Undecylenamide diethanolamide	0.1 and 1% aqua	4	SEDA-17, 190	
Undecylenic acid	2% pet.	4		
Virginiamycin	5% pet.	3		b
Vitamin A (retinol palmitate)	0.1% pet.	4	SEDA-10, 129	
Vitamin B_1	10% pet.	4		c
Vitamin E	10% pet.	3	SEDA-10, 129	c
Vitamin K_4	0.1% pet.	4		c

(continued)

Table 5. *(continued)*

Chemical	Patch-test concentration and vehicle*	Frequency of sensitization*	References	Comment
Xanthocillin	1–10% pet.	3		
Zinc pyrithione	1% pet.	3	SEDA-10, 130	a
Zinc ricinoleate	comm. prep.	3	SEDA-12, 135	

**Key to abbreviations:* acet. = acetone; alc. = alcohol; comm. ointm. base = commercial ointment base; epi = 45% alcohol, 10% propylene glycol, 45% isopropyl alcohol; glyc. = glycerol; MEK = methyl ethyl ketone; m.o. = mineral oil; o.o. = olive oil; paraff. liq. = paraffinum liquidum; pet. = petroleum.

In the column 'Comment' the following symbols are used: a = photosensitivity reported; b = immediate contact reactions reported; c = accidental contactant; d = see section on systemic side effects; e = has also caused irritant dermatitis; f = systemic contact dermatitis reported; prop. glyc. = propylene glycol.

In the column 'Frequency of sensitization' the following scale for the occurrence of sensitization is used: 1 = common; 2 = may occur; 3 = unusual; 4 = rare/non-existent.

†For corticosteroid allergy, see Refs. 48[R]–50[R].
‡For allergy to preservatives, see Refs. 6[R] and 7[R].
§For allergy to ophthalmic drugs, see Ref. 8[R].

Table 6. *Staging and symptomatology of the contact urticaria syndrome (39[R]–40[R])*

Cutaneous reactions only		Extracutaneous reactions	
Stage 1	Localized urticaria Dermatitis/dermatosis Non-specific symptoms (itching, tingling, burning, etc.)	Stage 3	Bronchial asthma Rhinoconjunctivitis Otolaryngeal symptoms Gastrointestinal symptoms
Stage 2	Generalized urticaria	Stage 4	Anaphylactoid reactions

Table 7. *Agents that have caused non-immunological contact urticaria (4[R], 40[R])*

Alcohols
Balsam of Peru
Benzaldehyde
Benzocaine
Benzoic acid
Camphor
Cantharides
Capsaicin
Chlorocresol
Cinnamic acid
Cinnamic aldehyde (SED-9, 249)
Cinnamon oil
Diethyl fumarate (SEDA-16, 153)
Dimethyl sulfoxide (SED-9, 249)
Eugenol
Formaldehyde
Iodine
Methyl green
Methyl salicylate
Monoethyl fumarate (SEDA-16, 153)
Nicotinic acid esters (SEDA-17, 187)
Parabens
Phenol
Resorcinol
Sodium benzoate
Sorbic acid
Sulfur
Tincture of benzoin

reactions due to the testing procedure have been described several times (39[R], 40[R]).

PHOTOCONTACT DERMATITIS *(2[R], 4[R], 99[R], 102[R])*

Photocontact dermatitis may be toxic or allergic in nature.

Phototoxicity can occur in anybody if enough light energy and photosensitizer are present in the skin.

Photoallergy is due to a cell-mediated hypersensitivity response, and therefore occurs in sensitized individuals only. Compared to contact allergy, photocontact allergy is uncommon, though a large number of chemicals has been responsible for photoallergic reactions.

Topical photosensitizers are listed in Table 9.

CORTICOSTEROIDS: LOCAL SIDE EFFECTS *(4[R], 191[R])*

In this section, the *local* side effects of topical corticosteroids are discussed; systemic adverse reactions are discussed elsewhere in this Chapter. Local side effects are listed in Table 10.

Table 8. *Agents known or believed to have caused immunological contact urticaria (4[R], 39[R], 49[R], 257[R])*

Acetylsalicylic acid
Acrylic acid (SEDA-18, 175)
Albendazole
p-Aminophenylamine (SEDA-5, 152)
Aminophenazone
Aminopyrine
Ampicillin
Amyl alcohol

Bacitracin
Balsam of Peru
Benzocaine
Benzoic acid
Benzophenone (SED-9, 249)
Benzoyl peroxide
Benzyl alcohol
Buserelin acetate
Butyl alcohol
Butylated hydroxyanisole
Butylated hydroxytoluene

Caraway seed oil
Cefotiam hydrochloride
Cephalosporins
Cetyl alcohol
Chamomile
Chloramine (SEDA-9, 139)
Chloramphenicol
Chlorhexidine (SEDA-13, 125; SEDA-15, 145)
Chlorocresol (SEDA-12, 137)
Chlorproethazine* (SEDA-17, 187)
Chlorpromazine* (259[c])
Clobetasol 17-propionate (SEDA-8, 153)
Clioquinol (SEDA-5, 152)
Colophony
Corn starch

Denatonium benzoate
Diethyl fumarate
Diethyl toluamide (SEDA-8, 153)
1,3-Diiodo-2-hydroxypropane
Dinitrochlorobenzene
Diphenylcyclopropenone (SEDA-14, 132)
Dipyrone
Disodium cromoglycate (SEDA-12, 137)

Emulgade F
Estrogen cream
Ethyl alcohol
Ethylenediamine dihydrochloride
Etofenemate
Formaldehyde (SEDA-8, 153)

Gelatine
Gentamicin (SEDA-12, 139)
Gentian violet

Hamamelis
Henna
Hexantriol
p-Hydroxybenzoinc acid

Iodochlorhydroxyquin
Isopropyl alcohol
4-Isopropyl dibenzoylmethane*

Labetalol
Lanolin alcohol (SEDA-5, 152)
Latex
Lidocaine (SEDA-15, 149)
Lindane

Mechlorethamine hydrochloride (SEDA-6, 149)
Menthol
Merbromin
Methamizole
Methotrimeprazine
Methyl ethyl ketone
Mexiletine hydrochloride (SEDA-18, 175)
Mezlocillin (SEDA-15, 149)
Monoamylamine
Myrrh

Neomycin
Nickel sulfate
Nicotine
Nicotinyl alcohol
Nifurozime
Nitroglycerin

Oxyphenbutazone

Parabens
Penicillin
Pentamidine isethionate
p-Phenylene diamine (derivatives)
Phenylmercuric salts
o-Phenylphenate
Polyethylene glycol (SED-9, 250)
Polypropylene
Polysorbate 60 (SED-9, 250)
Pristinamycin
Procaine hydrochloride
Promethazine hydrochloride
Propipocaine hydrochloride (SEDA-15, 149)
Propyl alcohol
Propylene glycol
Protein hydrolysate (SEDA-15, 149)
Pyrazolone derivatives (SEDA-9, 139)
Pyrethrin (SEDA-15, 149)

Rifamycin (SEDA-17, 191)

Salicyclic acid
Sisomycin (SEDA-12, 139)
Sodium hypochlorite
Sodium sulfite
Sorbitan laurate (SEDA-9, 139)
Squaric acid dibutyl ester
Stearyl alcohol
Streptomycin
Sulfur

Tetracycline (SEDA-9, 139)
Thimerosal
Thuja
α-Tocopherol
Tropicamide

Vanillin
Virginiamycin

*Photocontact urticaria

Table 9. *Topical photosensitizers* (2^{R}, 4^{R}, 99^{R}, 102^{R}, 275^{R}, 276^{Cr})

6-Acetoxy-2,4-dimethyl-*m*-dioxane (SEDA-10, 131)	(a)
p-Aminobenzoic acid (derivatives) (SEDA-17, 187)	(a)
Amyl dimethyl PABA (SEDA-10, 131)	(b)
Balsam of Peru (SEDA-8, 160)	(b)
Benoxaprofen*	(b)
Benzocaine	(a)
Benzydamine (SEDA-18, 164)*	(a)
Brilliant lake red R	(a)
Bithionol	(a)
5-Bromo-4′-chlorsalicylanilide	(a)
Buclosamide (Jadit®)	(a,b)
Butyl methoxydibenzoylmethane	(a)
Cadmium sulfide	(b)
Carbimazole (SEDA-10,131)	(a)
β-Carotene (SEDA-5, 153)	(a)
Chlorhexidine	(a)
Chlormercaptodicarboximide	(a)
Chloro-2-phenylphenol	(a)
Cinnamates	(a)
Cinnamic aldehyde (SEDA-8, 153)	(a)
Cinoxate	(a)
Coal tar (derivates) (SEDA-8, 160)	(a,b)
Coumarin (derivatives) (SEDA-4, 106)	(a)
Desoximetasone (SEDA-14, 130)	(b)
Dibenzthione (sulbentine)	(b)
Dibromsalan	(a)
Dibucaine hydrochloride (SEDA-5, 155)	
Dichlorophene	(a)
Digalloyl trioleate	(a)
Dimethoxane (SEDA-8, 153)	(a)
Dimethoxydibenzoylmethane	(a)
Dyes, e.g. methylene blue, fluorescein (SEDA-15, 150) rose bengal, acridine orange, acriflavin, neutral red	(a)
Diphenhydramine	(b)
Erythromycin	(a)
Essential oils: Bergamot oil, cedar oil, citron oil, lavender oil, lime oil, neroli oil, petitgrain oil, sandalwood oil	(b)
2-Ethyoxyethyl-*p*-methoxycinnamate (cinoxate) (SEDA-10, 131; SEDA-12, 134)	(a,b)
Fenofibrate (SEDA-17, 187)	(a)
Fenticlor (SEDA-14, 130)	(a,b)
Fluorouracil	(b?)
Formaldehyde (SEDA-7, 161)Formaldehyde (SEDA-7, 161)	(b)
Furocoumarins	(b)
Glyceryl PABA (SEDA-10, 131)	(a)
Hexachlorophene	(a)
Homosalate	(a)
Hydrocortisone	(a)
2-Hydroxy-4-methoxybenzophenone (SEDA-8, 158)	(a)
Isoamyl-*p*-*N*,*N*-dimethylaminobenzoate	(b)
Isoamyl-*p*-methoxycinnamate	(a)
Isobutyl PABA	(a)
4-Isopropyl dibenzoylmethane (SEDA-15, 150)	(a,b)
Ketoprofen (SEDA-10, 131)*	(a,b)
Lithiol red-CA (D&C Red No. 11)	(a)
8-Methoxypsoralen (SEDA-15, 150; SEDA-17, 187)	(a,b)
4-Methylbenzylidene camphor	(a,b)
6-Methylcoumarin (SEDA-17, 187)	(a)
Mexenone	(a)
Minoxidil (SEDA-11, 139)	(a)
Musk ambrette (SEDA-15, 150)	(a,b)
Musk moskene	(a)
Musk xylene	(a)
Mycanodin	(a)
Octyl dimethyl PABA (SEDA-10, 131)	(a)
Octyl methoxycinnamate	(a)
Oxybenzone (SEDA-15, 150)	(a,b)
Permanent orange (D&C Orange No. 17)	(a)
Phenothiazines	(a,b)
2-Phenylbenzimidazole-5-sulfonic acid (SEDA-10, 131)	(a)
p-Phenylene diamine	(a)
2-Phenyl-5-methylbenzoxazol (witisol)	(a)
Piroxicam (SEDA-15, 150)*	
Procaine hydrochloride	(a)
Sulfanilamide	(a,b)
Sulfisoxasole (260^{Cr})	(b)
Sulizobenzone (benzophenone-4)	(a)
Suprofen*	(a)
Tetrachlorosalicylanilide	(a,b)
Tiaprofenic acid (SEDA-15, 150)*	(a,b)
Thiocolchicoside	(a)
Toluidine red (D&C Red No. 35)	(a)
Tribromsalan	(a,b)
Triclocarban	(a,b)
Triclosan	(a,b)
Selenium disulfide (?) (SEDA-16, 157)	(?)
Zinc pyrithione	(a?)

(a) = photoallergic; (b) = phototoxic.
*See SEDA-18, 164; 146^{R}

Local side effects of *intralesional* corticosteroid therapy include (192^{R}, 261^{R}): transient local erythema, calcinosis cutis, cramps (due to injection of crystals into a vessel), amaurosis (dubious report), depigmentation, cutaneous atrophy and cutaneous necrosis.

DISCOLORATION, NECROSIS, MISCELLANEOUS SIDE EFFECTS

Drugs causing discoloration of the skin and appendages are listed in Table 11, necrosis of the skin and mucous membranes in Table 12. Other side effects of topical drugs and cosmetics are listed in Table 13.

Table 10. *Local side effects of topical corticosteroids*

Effects on the pilosebaceous unit
Perioral dermatitis (SEDA-5, 151)
Steroid rosacea or rosacea-like dermatitis, cannot be differentiated from perioral dermatitis and may be identical
Steroid acne
Exacerbation of pre-existing rosacea
Hypertrichosis of the face

Atrophy
Cigarette-paper wrinkling of the skin
Telangiectasia (SEDA-6, 153)
Petechiae, ecchymoses
Striae rubrae distensae, mainly occurring in the inguinal and axillary region (occlusion effect)
Susceptibility of the skin to minor trauma
Fragile skin in surgery
Delayed wound-healing
Worsening of existing ulceration

Effects on skin color
Hypopigmentation
Hyperpigmentation

Effects on the immunological system (SEDA-7, 167)
Masking of pre-existing disease
Aggravation of pre-existing disease
Inhibition of immunological mechanisms

Clinical examples of the effects on the immunological system:
Aggravation of pre-existing folliculities
Development of extensive, but unrecognized dermatophytic infections, so-call 'tinea incognito'
Perpetuation of masked infections with *Candida albicans*
Conversion of scabies into the 'Norwegian' type
Extensive mollusca contagiosa eruption
'Galloping' impetigo
(Possibly) exacerbation or dissemination of viral skin infections
Development of generalized pustural psoriasis
Spreading of malignant skin lesions
Suppression of pruritus

Ocular and nasal effects
Ocular hypertension
Open-angle glaucoma (SEDA-9, 143)
Uveitis
Posterior subcapsular cataracts
Nasal septal perforation (steroid aerosol)

Allergic effects
Allergic contact dermatitis (SEDA-15, 139)
Cross-allergy between various corticosteroids appears to be infrequent (196[c]); the literature has been reviewed (48[R]–50[R])
Generalized urticaria

Miscellaneous side effects
Tachyphylaxis: acute tolerance to the vasoconstrictor effect of topically applied corticosteroids
Milia (147[C])
Granuloma gluteale infantum
Pseudo-cicatrices stellaires spontanées
Avascular necrosis of the bones (223[Cr]) (clobetasol propionate)
Eczema craquelatum after discontinuation of corticosteroids (256[C])
Elastoidosis cutanée nodulaire à cystes et à comédones Favré-Racouchot
Erythrosis interfollicularis colli
Cutis linearis punctate colli or 'stippled skin'
Photosensitivity: Long-term topical corticosteroid treatment leads to atrophy of the epidermis which in turn increases its sensitivity to light

SYSTEMIC SIDE EFFECTS OF TOPICAL DRUGS

In this section, the *systemic* side effects of topical drugs are discussed.

Whether a topically applied drug will cause systemic effects depends largely on the ability of the drug to pass the skin barrier. Factors influencing percutaneous absorption have been extensively discussed by De Groot (4[R]) and by Wester and Maibach (194[R]). Systemic anaphylactoid reactions to topical drugs as part of the 'contact urticaria syndrome' are discussed on page 389.

Boric acid *(111[CR], 112[CR], 113[Cr]) (see also Chapter 24)*

Boric acid scarcely penetrates the intact skin, but is readily absorbed through inflamed or otherwise damaged skin or through mucous membranes.

The skin, which is unlikely to react unfavorably to topical application of boric acid, can react strongly if the substance is absorbed systemically; the redness may mimic scarlet fever, and psoriasiform lesions, bullae and alopecia can occur. Other effects of systemic absorption involve particularly the central nervous system and the gastrointestinal tract; they are dealt with in Chapter 24.

Benzocaine

Several cases of methaemoglobinaemia from topical application of benzocaine to mucous membranes or skin have been reported, especially in children (41[Cr]).

Calcipotriol *(SEDA-17, 191; SEDA-18, 176)*

Topical calcipotriol (a vitamin D analogue) is now established as an effective and safe treatment for mild to moderate psoriasis vulgaris. During initial investigation, there was concern that percutaneous absorption might result in vitamin D intoxication and hypercal-

Table 11. *Discoloration of the skin and appendages*

Drug	Side effect	References
Ammoniated mercury	Grey-brown discoloration of skin and fingernails; depigmentation	
Benzoyl peroxide	Discoloration of hair and post-inflammatory pigmentation; hypopigmentation	
Butylated hydroxyanisole (BHA)	Depigmentation	
Butylated hydroxytoluene (BHT)	Depigmentation (?)	
Carmustine (BCNU)	Pigmentation	
Chlorhexidine	Discoloration of the teeth and tongue	SED-9, 249
Chrysarobin	Brown-purplish discoloration of the skin, nails and hair	
Cinnamic aldehyde	Depigmentation	SEDA-6, 153
Clioquinol	Red discoloration of white hair	SEDA-9, 143
Cloflucarban	Contact allergy has caused pigmentation of the skin	
Coal tar dyes	'Pigmented cosmetic dermatitis'	
Corticosteroids	Hyper- and hypopigmentation	
Dihydroxyacetone	Brown discoloration	
Dinitrochlorobenzene (DNCB)	Yellow discoloration of grey hair	SEDA-4, 107
Diphencyprone	Triggering of vitiligo	SEDA-14, 132
Dithranol	Brown-purplish discoloration of skin, nails and hair	
Fluorouracil	Hyperpigmentation	SEDA-5, 155
	Melanonychia	241[cr]
Glutaraldehyde	Brown discoloration	SED-9, 249
Hydroquinone	Pigmentation and depigmentation; nail staining	9[Cr], 23[Cr]
Hydroxyquinoline sulfate	Leukoderma	
Iron salts	Brown discoloration (sometimes permanent)	
4-Isopropylcatechol	Reticular hyperpigmentation and depigmentation	
Mechlorethamine hydrochloride	Pigmentation	
Monobenzylether of hydroquinone	Depigmentation and pigmentation	
Monomethylether of hydroquinone	Depigmentation	SEDA-8, 161
Perfume ingredients	Contact allergy has caused pigmentation of the face	
Benzyl alcohol		
Benzyl salicylate		
Cananga oil		
Cinnamic alcohol		
Geraniol		
Hydroxycitronellal		
Jasmin absolute		
Lavender oil		
Methoxycitronellal		
Musk moskene (295[Cr])		
Red zig		
Sandalwood oil		
Petrolatum	Hyperpigmentation	
Phenolic compounds	Depigmentation and hyperpigmentation	SEDA-7, 166
Resorcinol (and -monoacetate)	Darkens fair hair; orange-brown discoloration of lacquered nails	
Silver nitrate	Grey-brown discoloration of conjunctiva	
Stilbestrol	Brown discoloration of nipples and linea alba; systemic effects, caused by percutaneous absorption	SED-9, 250
Thiotepa	Periorbital leukoderma	SEDA-5, 155
Tretinoin	Hypopigmentation	
Triclocarban	Contact allergy has caused pigmentation of the face	
Vitamin K_3	Dark-brown staining in factory workers	

cemia, but throughout extensive clinical trials no alteration in serum calcium levels was detected. The maximum weekly dose of calcipotriol in these studies was 100 grams, but most subjects used only 30–40 grams per week. There are few available data concerning the safety of doses greater than the recommended maximum of 100 grams/week, and the manufacturers strongly advise against exceeding this dose. Indeed, there have been several reports of hypercalcemia in patients who had used higher doses of calcipotriol (29[C]–31[C]). However, hypercalcemia has also been reported in a few patients using no more than the recommended doses (33[Cr], 34[Cr]). Patients with extensive psoriasis, who may require a dose rate approaching 100 grams/week should be screened for hypercalciuria before starting treatment, and urine calcium should be

Table 12. *Drugs that have caused necrosis of the skin and mucous membranes*

Drug	References
Adrenalin	SEDA-10, 131
Arsenious oxide	SED-9, 249
Cetrimonium bromide	SED-9, 249
Chlorhexidine	
Corticosteroids	SEDA-7, 166
Crystal violet	
Dequalinium	
Fluorouracil	SEDA-5, 155
Fuchsin-silver nitrate	
Gentian violet	SEDA-12, 138
Phenol	SED-9, 250
Povidone-iodine	SEDA-5, 152
Triclocarban	

monitored if their dose rate is continued for more than a few weeks, as a statistically significant rise in calcium urinary excretion has been observed (37[CR]). These changes could be of potential concern to patients with pre-existing hypercalciuria or a history of stone formation. Local side effects of calcipotriol are mostly perilesional irritation at the site of application. Contamination of the facial skin may result in frank irritant contact dermatitis. Allergic contact dermatitis has been observed in some patients (58[Cr]).

Camphor

The symptomatology of *systemic* camphor poisoning has been reviewed (35[R]).

Skoglund et al. (36[C]) reported systemic adverse reactions after *cutaneous* contact with camphor. A 15-month-old child had crawled through spirits-of-camphor containing 10% camphor. Over the ensuing 48 hours the child became progressively ataxic and had several brief generalized motor seizures. The seizures persisted for 2 days despite appropriate therapy. Over a 15-day period he slowly improved; recovery in motor and mental function was eventually complete. The child had no further seizures until 1 year later when a camphorated vaporizer preparation containing 4.81% camphor was administered by the mother. Concurrent with this inhalation there was a brief major motor seizure. Breathing difficulties, convulsions and coma have been reported after repeated topical application of camphor-containing agents for external application (254[R]).

Carmustine (BCNU)

Of 91 patients treated topically with the nitrosourea cytostatic, carmustine (BCNU), three developed reversible bone marrow depression (252[CR]). Local side effects included tender erythema, superficial denudation or bullae, contact allergy, pigment alterations, and patchy telangiectasia.

Clindamycin *(SEDA-6, 152)*

Dermal application of this drug is considered efficacious in acne vulgaris and without significant side effects (43[R]). However, percutaneous absorption does occur (SEDA-8, 160) and several cases of associated diarrhea have been reported (44[c]) including two cases of *pseudomembranous colitis* (45[C], 221[CR]).

Local adverse effects, e.g. contact allergic reactions, are infrequent (46[C]).

Clonidine transdermal therapeutic system (clonidine TTS)

Clonidine TTS has been used with some success for the treatment of mild hypertension. Systemic side effects are similar to those seen after oral administration of clonidine, but less frequent and milder. They include (246[C], 247[C], 248[c]) dry mouth, drowsiness, headache, sexual disturbance, cold extremities, obstipation and fatigue. These adverse effects rarely necessitate discontinuation of clonidine TTS. However, a high percentage of patients treated with the drug (up to 38%) (270[R]) may develop contact allergic reactions, usually due to the active ingredient, clonidine.

Corticosteroids *(80[Cr]–83[Cr])*

Systemic side effects of topical corticosteroids include: (1) growth retardation (SEDA-6, 151); (2) suppression of the hypophyseal-pituitary-adrenal axis; (3) glycosuria and hyperglycemia; (4) benign intracranial hypertension after withdrawal of topical steroids; (5) Cushing's syndrome: benign intracranial hypertension, glaucoma (24[C]), subcapsular cataract (24[C]), pancreatitis, avascular necrosis of the bones (24[C]), obesity, facial rounding, psychiatric symptoms, edema, delayed wound healing, hypertension (SEDA-7, 167), acne, disorders of sexual function, hirsutism, virilism, striae, ecchymoses and plethora.

Diachylon ointment

A 64-year-old woman had treated extensive ulcers of both legs with daily dressings of diachylon ointment, containing 15% lead oxide, for more than a year. She then developed general weakness, loss of weight, anemia, hypotension, and neuropathy. Lead levels in blood were increased 3-fold and urinary lead levels 10-fold, and a diagnosis of percutaneous lead intoxication was

Table 13. *Miscellaneous side effects of topical drugs (for additional references, see SED-9, 249—250)*

Drug	Common uses	Side effects	References
Benzoyl peroxide	Acne treatment	Co-carcinogenic (?)	SEDA-7, 168
Benzyl benzoate	Antiscabietic drug	Pemphigoid (?)	
Cetrimonium bromide	Antiseptic	'Matting' of hair	
Clonidine (in TTS)	Antihypertensive drug	Activation of herpes simplex; hyperpigmentation	SEDA-13, 128
Coal tar	Psoriasis; eczema	Carcinogenic?	10[Cr], 11[r]
Dinitrochlorobenzene (DNCB)	Treatment of alopecia areata	Yellow discoloration of grey hair; enhancement of allergy to non-related allergens; mutagenic(?), carcinogenic(?)	SEDA-4, 107; SEDA-6, 149; 61[C]; SEDA-10, 131; 195
5-Fluorouracil	Topical antimitotic drug	Telangiectasia; bilateral cicatrical ectropion; exacerbation of herpes labialis; pain, edema, livedo reticularis; erosion	SEDA-7, 166; SEDA-7, 166; SEDA-5, 155
Fusidic acid	Antibacterial agent	Acanthosis nigricans	SEDA-17, 192
Idoxuridine	Antiviral drug	Carcinogenic(?), mutagenic(?), teratogenic(?)	
Lindane	Antiscabietic drug	Morphea	SEDA-16, 159
Mechlorethamine hydrochloride (nitrogen mustard)	Topical antimitotic drug	Carcinogenic; suppression of immunological defence	SEDA-6, 153
Nicotinic acid	Treatment of alopecia	Acanthosis nigricans	SEDA-11, 142
Petrolatum	Vehicle constituent	Comedogenic; lipogranuloma	235[C]; SEDA-6, 154
Phenol	Face-peeling; Antipruritic	Milia; persistent erythema; skin pore prominence; telangiectasia; scarring; pigment alterations	SEDA-7, 166
Podophyllin	Treatment of condylomata acuminata	Carcinogenic(?)	240[C]
Polyethylene glycol	Vehicle constituent	Carcinogenic(?)	SEDA-6, 153
Salicylic acid	Keratolytic drug	Thinning of the skin, telangiectasia and (de)pigmentation after prolonged use	SEDA-15, 151
Selenium sulfide	Antiseborrheic drug	Reversible hair loss; structural defects of the hair(?); oiliness of the scalp	263[C]
Tretinoin	Acne treatment	Ectropion; Eruptive pyogenic granuloma	SEDA-17, 185; SEDA-15, 151

made. Treatment with dimercaptopropane sulfonic acid resulted in considerable reduction of the lead deposits, and the symptoms of poisoning subsided (227[CR]).

Diethyltoluamide (DEET)

Toxic encephalopathy has been reported in children sprayed repeatedly with DEET 10—15%, an insect repellant (60[Cr]). Acute manic psychosis has also been attributed to percutaneous absorption of DEET (SEDA-12, 138).

Dinitrochlorobenzene

Generalized urticaria, pruritus and dyspepsia developed in a previously healthy individual treated with dinitrochlorobenzene (DNCB) for alopecia totalis; after the therapy was stopped, all symptoms disappeared within 10 days. The symptomatology returned after reinstitution of the DNCB applications (255[c]).

Diphenhydramine

Acute anticholinergic toxicity with fever, hallucination and tachycardia has been described in a 2.5-year-old boy from applications of calamine-diphenhydramine lotion (140[Cr]).

Ethyl alcohol

Twenty-eight children from Argentina were intoxicated by ethyl alcohol applied in alcohol-soaked cloths to the abdomen, as a home-remedy for disturbance of the gastrointestinal tract (86[C]). Symptoms and signs included CNS depression (100%), abdominal erythema (89%), alcoholic breath (86%), miosis (86%), hypoglycemia (54%), convulsions (18%), respiratory depression (18%), mydriasis (14%), acidosis (11%) and death (7%).

Fumaric acid monethyl ester (ethyl fumarate)

The effect of systemically and/or topically administered ethyl fumarate on psoriasis was studied in six patients. Two patients who had been treated with locally applied ointments, consisting of 3 or 5% ethyl fumarate in petrolatum, developed symptoms of renal toxicity (85[C]).

Gentamicin

Topical application of gentamicin to large burns has caused ototoxic effects, ranging from mild to severe loss of hearing, with decrease of vestibular function (87[C]). Positional vertigo has been recorded in one patient (262[C]).

A female patient experienced tinnitus each time she treated her paronychia with gentamicin cream (88[C]).

Glycopyrrolate

Twenty-two patients suffering from the Frey syndrome (localized facial gustatory sweating and flushing) were treated with topical glycopyrrolate, a quaternary ammonium compound, 0.5–2% in a solution, cream or roll-on lotion. A total of 1012 applications was recorded, and seven episodes of side effects were noted: blurred vision (one), minor eye infections (two), itchy or dry eyes (one) and dry mouth (three). It should be noted that in the control group blurred vision and dry mouth were also recorded as side effects (SEDA-8, 160).

Henna and *p*-phenylenediamine *(SEDA-9, 142)*

The combination of henna and *p*-phenylenediamine for coloring nails, skin and hair appears to be very toxic, and 20 cases of toxicity, some fatal, have been noted in Khartoum (Sudan) over a 2-year period. Initial symptoms are those of angioneurotic edema with massive edema of the face, lips, glottis, pharynx, neck and bronchi. These occur within hours of the application of the dye-mix to the skin. The symptoms may then progress on the second day to anuria and acute renal failure with death occurring on the third day. Dialysis has helped some patients, but others have died from renal tubular necrosis.

Deliberate ingestion of *p*-phenylenediamine with suicidal attempt leads to similar toxic symptoms, death being mainly due to respiratory distress.

Table 14. *Distribution of symptoms and signs in 224 hexachlorophene poisoning episodes among 204 children (94[CR])*

Symptons and signs	No. (%)
Systemic and skin features	
Erythema of buttocks	209 (93)
Other cutaneous signs	38 (17)
Fever	99 (44)
Vomiting	77 (34)
Refusal of food	75 (33)
Diarrhea	65 (29)
Neurological features	
Drowsiness	83 (37)
Irritability	75 (33)
Coma	55 (25)
Seizures	39 (17)
Babinski sign	24 (11)
Decerebration	22 (10)
Weakness or paralysis	17 (8)
Opisthotonus	9 (4)

Hexachlorophene *(94[CR], 98[R], 205[C]) (see also Chapter 24)*

This antiseptic readily penetrates excoriated or otherwise damaged skin, but absorption through intact skin has also been described. The most dramatic complication reported was that due to accidental use in talcum powder in the newborn, with neurological and other features and many fatalities (Table 14) (94[CR]); particularly since then there has been reticence in using hexachlorophene in young infants at all, and certainly the customary 3% emulsion is too strong (97[C]). Optic atrophy has been described after oral or topical use (206[C]) and teratogenicity has been described in a report (95[C]) which was however not confirmed by an expert review (96[R]). The antiseptic is dealt with more fully in Chapter 24.

4-Homosulfanilamide (mafenide)

4-Homosulfanilamide is a topical sulfonamide which has been used for the treatment of burns; nowadays the drug has been largely replaced by sulfadiazine silver. Side effects reported include hyperchloremic metabolic acidosis and (possibly) methemoglobinemia (89[C]). Pulmonary insufficiency has been ascribed to mafenide acetate cream (SEDA-8, 160).

Iodine

Skin disinfection with iodine has caused goiter and hypothyroidism in five of 30 newborns under intensive care (91[C]). See also under 'Povidone-iodine'.

Iodochlorohydroxyquinoline (clioquinol, Vioform)

A study (242[C]) has demonstrated that up to 40% of topically applied iodochlorohydroxyquinoline may be absorbed percutaneously in man. In an animal study (243) significant toxicity (loss of weight, lethargy, paralysis, hepatoxicity) was noted in dogs treated with 5 grams of a topical iodochlorohydroxyquinoline 3% preparation twice daily over a 28-day period, which resulted in a dose of approximately 17 mg/kg per day.

Preparations containing the drug are frequently used to treat diaper rash; when a child of 10 kg is treated with 1 gram of iodochlorohydroxyquinoline 3% preparation 3 times daily, the amount of the drug applied would be 9 mg/kg per day. It has been found that 35% of patients who received between 12.5 and 25 mg/kg per day of oral iodochlorohydroxyquinoline developed symptoms of subacute myelo-optic neuropathy (SMON) (244[R]). The absorption of the oral dose is approximately 46% compared with the 40% found in the adult human study (242[C]). However, it is quite possible that in infants with diaper rashes the actual absorption of the drug would exceed this figure, since absorption through inflamed skin occurs more readily than through intact skin, and infant skin is more permeable than adult skin (245[Cr]).

Thrombocytopenia has (unconvincingly) been ascribed to topical iodochlorohydroxyquinoline (65[C]).

Lead

See Diachylon ointment.

Lidocaine (lignocaine) *(66[CR], 251[Cr])*

Lidocaine has been used as a local anaesthetic agent since 1948. Lidocaine is also prescribed as a local anesthetic preparation for application to the mucous membranes and the skin. Cutaneous absorption of lidocaine is negligible through normal skin after short-term application. However, when applied to erosive lesions over large body areas, significant absorption may occur. When the drug is applied to mucous membranes, blood levels simulate those resulting from intravenous injection. The major toxic effects of lidocaine involve the central nervous system. Toxic manifestations first appear at a serum lidocaine concentration of 5 mg/l and worsen progressively at higher levels (66[CR]). Early symptoms (at serum lidocaine concentrations of 5—10 mg/l) are dizziness, drowsiness, tinnitus and perioral paresthesia. More severe symptoms are disorientation, delirium, convulsions, coma (at concentrations of 10—20 mg/l) and cardiorespiratory arrest (>20 mg/l). Lidocaine intoxication has been reported with various routes of administration; severe and even lethal intoxications have been described after local application to mucous membranes or after ingestion.

Topical administration of lidocaine to the nasal mucosa occasionally causes severe methemoglobinemia in patients who have the heterozygous form of NADH-methemoglobin reductase deficiency (79[Cr]). See also under Prilocaine.

Lindane (γ-benzene hexachloride) *(SEDA-5, 154; 103[R], 104[R], 105[CR], 106[Cr])*

Lindane is the γ-isomer of 1,2,3,4,5,6-hexachlorocyclohexane; this pesticide is widely used in the treatment of scabies and pediculosis, usually in a 1% lotion. Lindane is a potentially toxic agent and the hazards of excessive industrial exposure and accidental ingestion have been well documented (105[R]).

In 1976, the US Food and Drug Administration (FDA) published a 'Gamma Benzene Hexachloride (Kwell) Alert' based in part on 'several poorly documented cases of convulsions following topical treatment with the drug' (107[r]). Indeed, several authors have reported lindane-induced convulsions (108[c], 109[C], 110[c]); however, it should be appreciated that in most cases lindane had been inappropriately used (106[Cr], 108[c]), while another case (109[C]) took place in an unusual therapeutic situation (prematurity, marasmus, pneumonia, congestive heart failure, ventricular septal defect).

The child with convulsions following lindane application reported by Matsuoka (110[c]) was suffering from tuberous sclerosis and may therefore have had a decreased threshold for convulsions.

Rasmussen (103[R]) and Kramer et al. (208[R]) feel that 1% lindane is safe *when used properly*, but agree with some recommendations made by Solomon et al. (105[R]):

(1) A hot soapy bath prior to the treatment is not necessary.

(2) The regimen of application for 24 hours may be too long, 6 hours having a cure rate of 96%.

(3) A concentration weaker than 1% may be adequate.

(4) Lindane treatment should not be repeated within 8 days, and then only if active parasites can still be demonstrated.

(5) Lindane 1% should be used with extreme caution, if at all, in pregnant women, very small infants, and people with massively excoriated skin (Rasmussen (103[R]) apparently does not agree with this item).

There has been concern from animal experiments that lindane may be carcinogenic, mutagenic and teratogenic; in therapeutic situations, however, such hazards seem to be highly unlikely (103[R], 104[R]).

Anemia and Henoch-Schönlein purpura possibly caused by topical lindane have been described (209[C], 210[c]). Retention of urine has been ascribed to lindane (SEDA-10, 131).

Malathion

Malathion is used for the treatment of lice, a single application of 0.5% in a solution being customary. Used in this way, it is generally safe, although the same compound has caused fatal poisoning when used as a pesticide in the environment.

Ramu et al. (92[C]) reported on four children with intoxication following hair-washing with a solution containing malathion (50% in xylene) for the purpose of louse control. One case is described in detail. The patient was in coma and did not respond to pain stimuli. Other symptoms included: severe dyspnea; extensive, moist rales over both lung fields; voluminous frothy saliva and mucus filling the nose, mouth and pharynx; pinpoint pupils not responding to light; excess lacrimation and fasciculation in the upper eye lids; flaccid limbs and absence of tendon reflexes. Hyperglycemia and glycosuria were found in all cases.

Mercury and mercurials

With a few exceptions, the use of mercury in medicine is considered to be outdated. Symptoms of chronic mercurial poisoning include (151[R], 152[R], 153[CR]):

Cardiovascular Hypertension, hypotension, arteritis of the legs.

Nervous system Emotional deviations, irritability, hypochondria, psychosis, impaired memory, insomnia, tremors, dysarthria, involuntary movements, vertigo, hypacusis, polyneuropathy, paresthesiae of the extremities, headache.

Endocrine Dysmenorrhea, hyperthyroidism.

Hematological Hypochromic anemia, erythrocytosis, lymphocytosis, neutropenia, aplastic anemia.

Gastrointestinal Anorexia, nausea, vomiting, epigastric pain, diarrhea, constipation, discoloration of the gums and mucosa of the mouth, stomatitis, ulcerations of the mouth, fetor ex ore.

Urinary system Nephrotic syndrome.

Skin Tylotic eczema, dryness of the skin, skin ulcerations, erythroderma.

Eye Corneal opacities and ulcerations, conjunctivitis.

Miscellaneous Acrodynia (153[CR]), loose teeth.

In a series of 70 psoriatic patients treated with an ointment containing ammoniated mercury, symptoms and signs of mercurial poisoning were detected in 33 (154[Cr]): albuminuria, headache, gingivitis, erythroderma, nausea, dizziness, precordial pain, contact dermatitis, conjunctivitis, epistaxis, keratitis, tremor, neuritis, hematological changes, metallic taste in mouth, and purpura.

The use of mercury in dermatological therapy should be abandoned. Even nowadays cases of mercury intoxication from use of topical mercurials still occur (150[Cr]).

Minoxidil *(225[R])*

Minoxidil (2,4-diamino-6-piperidinopyrimidine 3-oxide) is a potent vasodilator effective in severe hypertension irrespective of the cause. Hypertrichosis occurs in approximately 70% of patients taking *oral* minoxidil, usually within 2 months of the start of therapy. Isolated case reports have been published of hair growth in areas of male pattern baldness in patients treated with oral minoxidil. Because of this side effect, *topical* minoxidil has been used for the treatment of alopecia areata and alopecia androgenica with some success.

Local side effects of therapy with topical minoxidil (usually in an alcohol-propylene glycol base) have included dryness, irritation, pruritus, contact allergy (SEDA-11, 139), photocontact allergy (SEDA-11, 139). Minoxidil is poorly absorbed through the skin (<4%) (231[Cr]); blood levels of minoxidil are far less than 10% of the mean minoxidil blood level present 2 hours after oral ingestion of a 5.0 mg pill, the lowest dose for the treatment of hypertension (226[Cr]). Nevertheless, in seven out of 30 non-hypertensive patients treated with 3% minoxidil solution twice daily, a 'significant' decrease in blood pressure was noted (232[c]).

Also, a hypertensive crisis occurred in one patient following withdrawal of topical minoxidil (SEDA-16, 158).

Also, some patients treated with minoxidil solution showed increased hair growth outside the area of drug application (SEDA-18, 175), which suggests a systemic effect (224[CR]). The sudden death of a patient on topical minoxidil (233[c]) was probably not drug-related but due to cardiovascular disease and hypertension. Nevertheless, in patients who are known to be hypertensive and who are also receiving other antihypertensive medication extra caution is warranted when topical minoxidil is used (234[Cr]). Smoking intolerance possibly related to topical minoxidil has been observed rarely (53[Cr]). A 'polymyalgia syndrome'' characterized by fatigue, anorexia, weight loss, and severe pain in the shoulders and the pelvic girdle was attributed to minoxidil in four male patients (228[CR]).

Monosulfiram

Monosulfiram (sulfiram, tetraethyl thiurammonosulfide) is used for the topical treatment of scabies. After repeated treatment the ingestion of alcohol may rarely lead to an antabuse effect with generalized flushing, malaise and rhinorrhea (148[C]).

2-Naphthol

2-Naphthol (β-naphthol) is sometimes used for the treatment of acne. It has been estimated that 5–10% of the drug is absorbed after topical application (114[C]).

A brownish-red discoloration of the urine may be noted and fatal poisoning from external administration has been reported (115[C]).

Neomycin

Not only is ototoxicity a well-known hazard of *parenteral* neomycin administration, but loss of hearing has also been reported after *topical* treatment with this drug, e.g. for burns (116[Cr]), wounds (117[C]), decubitus ulcers (118[C]) and otitis (119[C]).

Prolonged application of 1% neomycin ointment (also containing 11% dimethyl sulfoxide) to intact skin in a girl with dermatomyositis (approx. 30% of the body surface) led to vertigo, nystagmus and complete loss of hearing (120[C]).

Nitroglycerin

Nitroglycerin transdermal therapeutic system is used for the treatment (prophylaxis) of angina pectoris. Side effects include: headache, pressure feeling in the head, nausea, vomiting, dizziness, tiredness, blackouts and, possibly, penile erection and ageusia (248[Cr], 249[Cr]).

Phenol (carbolic acid) *(SEDA-6, 152; SEDA-7, 166)*

Serious adverse reactions due to percutaneous absorption may occur and death has been described several times.

Signs and symptoms of phenol toxicity include (73[C]–75[C], 76[c], 77[R], 78[C]):

Cardiovascular Cyanosis, cardiac arrhythmias, ECG abnormalities, circulatory failure, collapse.

Respiratory Respiratory failure leading to death.

Nervous system Death, dizziness, coma.

Hematological Methemoglobinemia.

Gastrointestinal Abdominal pain.

Urinary system Hemoglobinuria.

Skin Darkening of the face and hands.

Special senses Darkening of the cornea.

Currently, complications of topical phenol (including acute death) are caused by phenol face peels, notably cardiac arrhythmias (28[r]).

Podophyllum resin *(SEDA-4, 108; SEDA-6, 152; SEDA-7, 167; 72[R], 32[R])*

Podophyllum resin is a powerful skin irritant and antimitotic agent, widely used for the treatment of condylomata acuminata.

Signs and symptoms of systemic toxicity include:

Cardiovascular Cyanosis, tachycardia, abnormal ECG readings.

Respiratory Stertorous respiration.

Nervous system Polyneuritis, ataxia, coma, agitation, delirium, confusion, lethargy, death, muscular weakness, paresthesias.

Hematological Leukopenia, leukocytosis, thrombopenia, anemia.

Liver Elevation of liver enzymes.

Gastrointestinal Nausea, vomiting, abdominal pain, paralytic ileus.

Urinary system Oliguria, anuria, hematuria.

Miscellaneous Fever, urticaria.

Second-generation effects Intrauterine death and teratogenicity have not been demonstrated convincingly.

Povidone-iodine *(see also Chapter 24)*

Povidone-iodine is a water-soluble iodine complex which is said to be free of the undesirable effects of iodine tincture. However, iodine may be absorbed from it through burned areas (121[C]), vaginal mucosa (122[C]), oral mucosa (123[C]) and in children even with normal skin (124[C]). Adverse reactions include goiter and hypothyroidism (124[C], 207[C]), hyperthyroidism (SEDA-18, 176), neutropenia (125[C]), metabolic acidosis (126[C]) and generalized iododerma (121[C]). Treatment of vaginitis in pregnant women may lead to goiter and hypothyroidism in the infant (122[C]). The antiseptic is further discussed in Chapter 24.

Prilocaine

A mixture of prilocaine and lidocaine (25 g/l in an oily base) is used for reducing pain and other minor skin procedures in children. Several cases of methemoglobinemia have been reported (71[CR]).

Promethazine

Promethazine intoxication from topical application has been observed in children (204[C]) and adults (230[C]). Symptoms include disorientation, hallucinations, hyperactivity, convulsions and coma.

Resorcinol

Formerly also applied to leg ulcers, resorcinol is nowadays mainly used for the treatment of acne vulgaris as a peeling agent.

In the older literature (but even nowadays, (27[C])), several cases of systemic toxicity from percutaneous absorption were reported and some fatalities occurred (129[CR]).

Signs and symptoms of resorcinol intoxication include (127[C], 128[C], 129[CR], 130[C]):

Cardiovascular Pallor, dizziness, cold sweat, collapse, cyanosis.

Nervous system Tremors, death.

Endocrine Hypothyroidism.

Hematological Methemoglobinemia, hemolytic anemia.

Urinary system Hemoglobinuria, violet-black urine.

Skin Maculopapular eruption, ochronosis, myxedema.

The use of resorcinol in the treatment of acne is considered safe (SEDA-9, 142).

Salicylic acid

Salicylic acid is widely used in dermatology because of its keratolytic properties.

Numerous reports have described 'salicylism'—intoxication due to percutaneous absorption. The first symptoms of salicylism (131[Cr]) are pallor, fatigue and drowsiness, and a modification of the respiration, which becomes more frequent and at the same time deeper, and which can be heard from a distance. Other early signs of intoxication with salicylic acid are nausea, vomiting, changes in the ability to hear, and mental confusion (132[CR]). Several deaths have been recorded, mainly in children.

Other signs and symptoms of salicylism have included (132[CR], 133[CR], 134[C], 135[C]):

Respiratory Frequent deep respiration, Cheyne-Stokes respiration, dyspnea, hyperpnea.

Nervous system Drowsiness, mental confusion, stupor, hallucinations, headache, dizziness, tinnitus, slurred speech, agitation, disorientation, lethargy, delusions, aggression, retrograde amnesia, depression, coma, somnolence.

Gastrointestinal Nausea, vomiting, thirst, anorexia, diarrhea.

Miscellaneous Fatigue, changes in hearing ability, nuchal rigidity, fever, profuse sweating, pallor, metabolic acidosis (211[C]), hypoglycemia (SEDA-16, 158).

Scopolamine (Hyoscine) *(222[Cr], 93[Cr])*

The use of scopolamine for prevention of motion-sickness is well established. In tablet or injectable form scopolamine frequently causes (in addition to the intended antiemetic effect) adverse effects due to its anticholinergic action: dry mouth, hypotension, drowsiness, cycloplegia, bradycardia (low doses), and tachycardia (high doses). These frequently occurring adverse reactions stimulated the development of a transdermal delivery system, which is also used to prevent postoperative emesis. Transdermal scopolamine is reported to have a lower incidence of adverse effects than the oral form. Nevertheless, side effects involving the central nervous system (CNS), vision, bladder, and skin have been described, as have withdrawal symptoms that occur after the patch is removed.

The most common side effects are dry mouth (65%), drowsiness, mydriasis and impaired ocular accommodation. Toxic psychosis has been reported several times. Several factors predispose to CNS side effects, including advanced age, pre-existing psychiatric disease, and concurrent treatment with medications that possess anticholinergic activity. Children may also be more susceptible to unwanted effects.

Sex hormones

Topical application of estrogen-containing preparations and testosterone (SEDA-16, 158) may lead to absorption of these hormones and systemic effects.

Transdermal absorption of estrogen may lead to pseudoprecocious puberty in young girls and gynecomastia in young boys and adult men. Other symptoms in men may include loss of libido, impotence and galactorrhea (199[Cr], 138[Cr]).

Table 15. *Side effects of transdermal scopolamine (59[CR])*

CNS effects	Urinary retention
Confusion	
Disorientation	Dry mouth
Dizziness	
Drowsiness	Constipation
Excitability	
Hallucinations	Cutaneous effects
Memory disturbances	Irritant dermatitis
Restlessness	Allergic contact dermatitis
Ocular effects	Withdrawal symptoms
Cycloplegia	Disturbances of equilibrium
Mydriasis	Dizziness
Acute narrow-angle glaucoma	Headaches
Impaired ocular accommodation	Nausea
	Vomiting

Transdermal absorption of testosterone (usually from treatment of vulvar lichen sclerosus et atrophicus) may lead to increased libido, clitoral hypertrophy, pubic hirsutism, thinning of the scalp hair, facial acne, voice change, hirsutism and even virilization (139[CR]).

Silver nitrate

Silver nitrate has been a popular topical therapy for burns, but its use has been largely replaced by sulfadiazine silver.

Several reports have described methemoglobinemia due to topical silver nitrate, in one case apparently leading to death (142[C]).

Another complication of silver nitrate is electrolyte disturbances, especially in children, due to the hypotonicity of the silver nitrate dressings (143[Cr]). Local and systemic argyria and renal damage have also been observed.

Sulfadiazine silver *(SEDA-4, 108; SEDA-5, 152; SEDA-7, 167)*

Sufadiazine silver cream is widely used for the topical treatment of burns. Silver intoxication in such patients from pharmaceuticals containing silver is well known. Silver from silver sulfadiazine cream is rapidly absorbed and deposited in large amounts throughout the body (59[Cr]). Deposition in the skin leads to argyria (157[C]).

Nephrotic syndrome following topical therapy with this drug has been reported by Owens et al. (67[C]), but this observation has not been confirmed since. Several authors have however reported *leukopenia* during treatment with sulfadiazine silver (265). This side effect appears to run a typical course: sulfadiazine-induced leukopenia reaches a nadir within 2–4 days of starting therapy, with a characteristic drop in the neutrophil count and a relative increase in the number of band forms. The erythrocyte count is not affected. Two to 3 days after the onset of leukopenia, the leukocyte count returns to normal levels. Recovery is not affected by the continuation of therapy.

Peripheral neuropathy from long-term treatment of venous leg ulcers with silver sulfadiazine cream has been observed in one patient (157[C]).

Miscellaneous side effects attributed to silver sulfadiazine include respiratory tract infections and pneumonia, toxicity against human protozoa and acute hemolytic anemia (257[Cr]).

Transdermal therapeutic systems

See under Clonidine, Glycopyrrolate, Nitroglycerin and Scopolamine.

Tretinoin

Tretinoin cream is used extensively for the treatment of acne and photodamaged skin. Local irritant dermatitis occurs frequently. With normal use, absorption is minimal and systemic side effects are therefore not expected. The risk of teratogenicity of topical tretinoin, if any, appears to be minimal (SEDA-18, 164; 229[Cr]) even though it is a well-known potent teratogen. However, vaginal bleeding in a 64-year-old woman was convincingly ascribed to the use of tretinoin cream 0.05% daily to her face, suggesting a systemic effect (SEDA-16, 159).

REFERENCES

1. Rycroft RJG, Frosch PJ, Menné T, ed. Textbook of Contact Dermatitis, 2nd edition. Berlin: Springer-Verlag, 1995.
2. Fisher AA. Contact Dermatitis, 3rd edn. Philadephia: Lea and Febiger, 1986.
3. De Groot AC. Patch Testing. Test concentrations and vehicles for 3700 allergens. Amsterdam: Elsevier, 1994.
4. De Groot AC, Weyland JW, Nater JP. Unwanted Effects of Cosmetics and Drugs used in Dermatology, 3rd edn. Amsterdam: Elsevier, 1994.
5. Dai WS, Labraico JM, Stern RS. Epidemiology of isotretinoin exposure during pregnancy. J Am Acad Dermatol 1992;26:599—606.
6. Fransway AF, Schmitz NA. The problem of preservation in the 1990s. II. Formaldehyde and formaldehyde-releasing biocides: Incidence of cross-reactivity and the significance of the positive response to formaldehyde. Am J Contact Dermatol 1991;2:78—88.
7. Fransway AF. The problem of preservation in the 1990s. III. Agents with preservation function independent of formaldehyde release. Am J Contact Dermatol 1991;2:145—174.
8. Herbst RA, Maibach HI. Contact dermatitis caused by allergy to ophthalmic drugs and contact lens solution. Contact Dermatitis 1991;25:305—312.
9. Coulson IH. 'Fade Out' photochromonychia. Clin Exp Dermatol 1993;18:87—88.
10. Jemec, GBE, Østerlind, A. Cancer in patients treated with coal tar: a long-term follow up study. J Eur Acad Dermatol Venereol 1994;3:153—156.
11. Goldman WJ. Carcinogenicity of coal-tar shampoo. Lancet 1995;345:326 .
12. Johansen JD, Menné T. The fragrance mix and its constituents: a 14-year material. Contact Dermatitis 1995;32: 18—23.
13. Möller H. All these positive tests to thimerosal. Contact Dermatitis 1994;31:209—213.
14. Pasche-Koo F, Piletta PA, Hunziker N, Hauser, C. High sensitization rate to emulsifiers in patients with chronic leg ulcers. Contact Dermatitis 1994;31:226—228.
15. Funk JO, Maibach HI. Propylene glycol dermatitis: reevaluation of an old problem. Contact Dermatitis 1994; 31:236—241.
16. Ophaswongse S, Maibach HI. Alcohol dermatitis: allergic contact dermatitis and contact urticaria syndrome. Contact Dermatitis 1994;30:1—6.
17. Fischer T. Design considerations for patch testing. Am J Contact Dermatitis 1994;5:70—75.
18. Angelini G, Vena GA, Grandolfo, M, Mastrolonardo, M. Iatrogenic contact dermatitis and eczematous reactions. Clin Dermatol 1993;11:467—477.
19. Fryer EJ, Lebwohl M. Pemphigus vulgaris after initiation of psoralen and UVA therapy for psoriasis. J Am Acad Dermatol 1994;30:651—653.
20. Goulden V, Layton AM, Cunliffe WJ. Long-term safety of isotretinoin as a treatment for acne vulgaris. Br J Dermatol 1994;131:360—363.
21. Gunnarskog JG, Kallén AJB, Lindelof BG, Sigurgeirsson B. Psoralen photochemotherapy (PUVA) and pregnancy. Arch Dermatol 1993;129:320—323.
22. Burrows NP, Norris PG. Treatment of PUVA-induced skin pain with capsaicin. Br J Dermatol 1994;131:584—585.
23. Camarasa JG, Serra-Baldrich E. Exogenous ochronosis with allergic contact dermatitis from hydroquinone. Contact Dermatitis 1994;31:57—58.
24. McLean CJ, Lobo RFJ, Brazier DJ. Cataracts, glaucoma and femoral avascular necrosis caused by topical corticosteroid ointment. Lancet 1995;345:330.
25. Bech-Thomsen N, Wulf HC. 8-Methoxypsoralen urticaria. J Am Acad Dermatol 1994;31:1063—1064.
26. Elsner P. What is the state of cosmetic labelling in Europe? Am J Contact Dermatitis 1993;4:198—200.
27. Bontemps H, Mallaret M, Besson G, Bochaton H, Carpentier F. Confusion after topical use of resorcinol. Arch Dermatol 1995;131:112.
28. Botta SA, Straith RE, Goodwin HH. Cardiac arrhythmias in phenol face peeling: a suggested protocol for prevention. Aesth Plast Surg 1988;12:115—117.
29. Cunliffe WJ, Berth-Jones J, Claudy A et al. Comparative study of calcipotriol (MC903) ointment and betamethasone 17-valerate ointment in patients with psoriasis vulgaris. J Am Acad Dermatol 1992;26:736—743.
30. Dwyer C, Chapman RS. Calcipotriol and hypercalcaemia. Lancet 1991;338:764—765.
31. Bourke JF, Berth-Jones J, Hutchinson PE. Hypercalcaemia associated with calcipotriol (Dovonex) treatment. Br Med J 1993;306:1344—1345.
32. Miller RA. Podophyllin. Int J Dermatol 1985;24:491—498.
33. Hardman KA, Heath DA, Nelson HM. Hypercalcaemia associated with calcipotriol (Dovonex) treatment. Br Med J 1993;306:896.
34. Russell, S, Young MJ. Hypercalcaemia during treatment of psoriasis with calcipotriol. Br J Dermatol 1994;130:795—796.
35. Committee on Drugs. Camphor—Who needs it? Pediatrics 1978;62:404.
36. Skoglund RR, Ware LL Jr, Schanberger JE. Prolonged seizures due to contact and inhalation exposure to camphor Clin Pediatr 1977;16:901.
37. Berth-Jones J, Bourke JF, Iqbal SJ, Hutchinson PE. Urine calcium excretion during treatment of psoriasis with topical calcipotriol. Br J Dermatol 1993;129:411—414.
38. Von Krogh G, Maibach HI. The contact urticaria syndrome—an updated review. J Am Acad Dermatol 1982; 5:328.
39. Katchen BR, Maibach HI. Immediate-type contact reaction: immunologic contact urticaria. In: Menné T, Maibach HI, eds. Exogenous Dermatoses: Environmental Dermatitis, Chapter 4. Boston: CRC Press, 1991;51.
40. Lahti A, Maibach HI. Immediate contact reactions. In: Menné T, Maibach HI, eds. Exogenous Dermatoses: Environmental Dermatitis, Chapter 2. Boston: CRC Press, 1991;21.
41. Olson ML, McEvoy GK. Methemoglobinemia induced by local anesthetics. Am J Hosp Pharm 1981;38:89.
42. Calzavara-Pinton P, Fransceschini F, Rastrelli P et al. Antinuclear antibodies are not induced by PUVA treatment in patients with uncomplicated psoriasis. J Am Acad Dermatol 1994;30:955—958.

43. Stoughton RB. Topical antibiotics for acne vulgaris: current usage. Arch Dermatol 1979;115:486.
44. Becker LE, Bergstresser PR, Whiting DA et al Topical clindamycin therapy for acne vulgaris. Arch Dermatol 1981;117:482.
45. Milstone EB, McDonald AJ, Scholhamer CF Jr. Pseudomembranous colitis after topical application of clindamycin. Arch Dermatol 1981;117:154.
46. De Groot AC. Contact allergy to clindamycin. Contact Dermatitis 1982;8:428.
47. Coleman, R, MacDonald D. Effects of isotretinoin on male reproductive system. Lancet 1994;344:198.
48. Dooms-Goossens A. Corticosteroid contact allergy, a challenge to patch testing. Am J Contact Dermatitis 1993;4:120—122.
49. Lauerma AI, Reitamo S. Contact allergy to corticosteroids. J Am Acad Dermatol 1993;28:618—622.
50. Wilkinson SM. Hypersensitivity to topical corticosteroids. Clin Exp Dermatol 1994;19:1—11.
51. Knight TE, Hausen BM. Melaleuca oil (tea tree oil) dermatitis. J Am Acad Dermatol 1994;30:423—427.
52. Pirker C, Moslinger T, Wantke F, Gotz, M, Jarisch R. Ethylmercuric chloride, the responsible agent in thimerosal hypersensitivity. Contact Dermatitis 1993;29:152—154.
53. Trattner A, Ingber A. Topical treatment with minoxidil 2% and smoking intolerance. Ann Pharmacother 1992; 26:198—199.
54. Toth Kasa J, Dobozy A. Drug fever caused by PUVA treatment. Acta Derm-Venereol 1985;65:557.
55. Ramsay B, Marks JM. Bronchoconstriction due to 8-methoxypsoralen. Br J Dermatol 1988;119:83—86.
56. Hughes RA. Arthritis precipitated by isotretinoin treatment for acne vulgaris. J Rheumatol 1993;20:1241—1242.
57. Barth JH, MacDonald-Hull SP, Mark J, Jones RG, Cunliffe WJ. Isotretinoin therapy for acne vulgaris: a re-evaluation of the need for measurements of plasma lipids and liver function tests. Br J Dermatol 1993;129:704—707.
58. De Groot AC. Contact allergy to calcipotriol Contact Dermatitis 1994;30:242—243.
59. Coombs CJ, Wan AT, Masterson JP, Conyers RAJ, Pedersen J, Chia YT. Do burn patients have a silver lining? Burns 1992;18:179—184.
60. Edwards D, Johnson CE. Insect-repellent-induced toxic encephalopathy in a child. Clin Pharm 1987;6:496—498.
61. De Groot AC, Nater JP, Bleumink E, De Jong MCJM. Does DNCB therapy potentiate epicutaneous sensitization to non-related contact allergens? Clin Exp Dermatol 1981;6:139.
62. Rampen FHJ. Hypertrichosis in PUVA-treated patients. Br J Dermatol 1983;109:657.
63. Studniberg HM, Weller P. PUVA, UVB, psoriasis and nonmelanoma skin cancer. J Am Acad Dermatol 1993; 29:1013—1022.
64. Landon RK. Etretinate: a clinician's view. Dermatol Clin 1988;6:553.
65. Khaleeli AA. Quinaband-induced thrombocytopenic purpura in a patient with myxoedema. Br Med J 1976;2:562.
66. Lie RL, Vermeer BJ, Edelbrock PM. Severe lidocaine intoxication by cutaneous absorption. J Am Acad Dermatol 1990;23:1026—1028.
67. Owens CJ, Yarbrough DR, Brackett NR. Nephrotic syndrome following topically applied sulfadiazine therapy. Arch Intern Med 1974;134:332.
68. Lowe NJ, David M. New retinoids for dermatologic diseases: uses and toxicity. Dermatol Clin 1988;6:539.
69. Bunker CB, Tomlinson MC, Johnson NM, Dowd PM. Isotretinoin and the lung. Br J Dermatol 1991;125(Suppl 38):29.
70. Tangrea JA, Kilcoyne RF, Taylor PR et al. Skeletal hyperostosis in patients receiving chronic, very-low-dose isotretinoin. Arch Dermatol 1992;128:921—925.
71. Frayling IM, Addison GM, Chatterjee K et al. Methaemoglobinaemia in children treated with prilocaine-lignocaine cream. Br Med J 1990;301:153.
72. Cassidy DE, Drewry J, Fanning JP. Podophyllum toxicity: a report of a fatal case and a review of the literature. J Toxicol Clin Toxicol 1982;19:35.
73. Truppman ES, Ellerby JD. Major electrocardiographic changes during chemical face peeling. Plast Reconstr Surg 1979;63:44.
74. Delpizzo A, Tanski E. Chemical face peeling: malignant therapy for benign disease (Editorial)? Plast Reconstr Surg 1980;66:121.
75. Ruedemann R, Deichmann WB. Blood phenol level after topical application of phenol-containing preparations. J Am Med Assoc 1953;152:506.
76. Woolley PB. Exogenous ochronosis. Br Med J 1952; 4:760.
77. Deichmann WB. Local and systemic effects following skin contact with phenol—a review of the literature. J Ind 1949;31:146.
78. von Hinkel GK, Kintzel HW. Phenolvergiftungen bei Neugeborenen durch kutane Resorption. Dtsch Gesundheidswes 1968;23:240.
79. Kotler RL, Hansen-Flaschen J, Casey MP. Severe methaemoglobinaemia after flexible fiberoptic bronchoscopy. Thorax 1989;44:234—235.
80. Walsh P, Aeling JL, Huff L, Weston WL. Hypothalamus-pituitary-adrenal axis suppression by superpotent topical steroids. J Am Acad Dermatol 1993;29:501—503.
81. Dhein S. Cushing-Syndrom nach externer Glukokortikoid-Applikation bei psoriasis. Z Hautkr 1986;61:161—166.
82. Lawlor F, Ramabala K. Iatrogenic Cushing's Syndrome—A cautionary tale. Clin Exp Dermatol 1984;9:286—289.
83. Olsen EA, Cornell RC. Topical clobetasol-17-propionate: Review of its clinical efficacy and safety. J Am Acad Dermatol 1986;15:246—255.
84. Lerman S, Megaw J, Gardner K. Psoralen-long-wave ultraviolet therapy and human cataractogenesis. Invest Opthalmol Vis Sci 1982;23:801.
85. Dubiel W, Happle R. Behandlungsversuch mit Fumarsäure monoäthylester bei Psoriasis vulgaris. Z Haut-Geschlechtskr 1972;47:545.
86. Giménez ER, Vallejo NE, Roy E et al. Percutaneous alcohol intoxication. Clin Toxicol 1968;1:39.
87. Dayal VS, Smith EL, McCain WG. Cochlear and vestibular gentamicin toxicity: a clinical study of systemic and topical usage. Arch Otolaryngol 1974;100:338.
88. Drake TE. Reaction to gentamicin sulfate cream. Arch Dermatol 1974;110:638.
89. Ohlgisser M, Adler M, Ben-Dov B et al. Methaemoglobinaemia induced by mafenide acetate in children. Br J Anaesth 1978;50:299.
90. Lindelof B, Sigurgeirsson B. PUVA and cancer: a case control study. Br J Dermatol 1993;129:39—41.

91. Chabrolle JP, Rossier A. Goitre and hypothyroidism in the newborn after cutaneous absorption of iodine. Arch Dis Child 1978;53:495.
92. Ramu A, Slonim AE, Eyal F. Hyperglycemia in acute malathion poisoning. Isr J Med Sci 1973;9:631.
93. Parrot AC. Transdermal scopolamine: effects of single and repeated patches upon psychological task performance. Neuropsychobiology 1987;17:53—59.
94. Martin-Bouyer G, Lebreton R, Toga M et al. Outbreak of accidental hexachlorophene poisoning in France. Lancet 1982;i:91.
95. Halling H. Suspected link between exposure to hexachlorophene and malformed infants. Ann NY Acad Sci 1979;320:426.
96. Källen B et al. Delivery outcome in women employed in medical occupations in Sweden. J Occup Med 1979;21:542.
97. García-Buñuel L. Toxicity of hexachlorophene (Letter to Editor). Lancet 1982;i:1190.
98. Editorial. Hexachlorophene today. Lancet 1982;i:87.
99. Maibach HI, Marzulli FN. Phototoxicity (photoirritation) of topical and systemic agents. In: Marzulli FN, Maibach HI, eds. Dermatotoxicology, 2nd edn. Washington: Hemisphere Publishing Corporation, 1983;375.
100. Garbis H, Elefant E, Bertolotti E et al. Pregnancy outcome after periconceptional and first-trimester exposure to methoxsalen photochemotherapy. Arch Dermatol 1995; 131:492—493.
101. Woo T, Wong RC, Wong JM, Anderson TF, Lerman S. Lenticular psoralen photoproducts and cataracts of a PUVA-treated psoriatic patient. Arch Dermatol 1985;1985:1307—1308.
102. Frain-Bell W. What is that thing called light? Clin Exp Dermatol 1979;4:1.
103. Rasmussen JE. The problem of lindane. J Am Acad Dermatol 1981;5:507.
104. Shachter B. Treatment of scabies and pediculosis with lindane preparation: an evaluation. J Am Acad Dermatol 1981;5:517.
105. Solomon LM, Fahrner L, West DP. Gamma benzene hexachloride toxicity: a review. Arch Dermatol 1977;113: 353.
106. Telch J, Jarvis D. Acute intoxication with lindane (gamma benzene hexachloride). J Can Med Assoc 1982;126:662.
107. Food and Drug Administration. Gamma benzene hexachloride (Kwell) alert. FDA Drug Bull 1976;6:28.
108. Lee B, Groth P. Transcutaneous poisoning during lindane treatment. Pediatrics 1977;59:643.
109. Pramanik AK, Hansen RC. Transcutaneous gamma benzene hexachloride absorption and toxicity in infants and children. Arch Dermatol 1979;115:1224.
110. Matsuoka LY. Convulsions following application of gamma benzene hexachloride (Letter to Editor). J Am Acad Dermatol 1981;5:98.
111. Valdes-Dapena MA, Arey JB. Boric acid poisoning: three fatal cases with pancreatic inclusions and a review of the literature. J Pediatr 1962;61:531.
112. Schillinger BM, Bernstein M, Goldberg LA, Shalita AR. Boric acid poisoning. J Am Acad Dermatol 1982;7:667.
113. Siegel E, Wason S. Boric acid toxicity. Ped Clin N Am 1986;33:363—367.
114. Hemels HGWM. Percutaneous absorption and distribution of 2-naphthol in man. Br J Dermatol 1972;87:614.
115. Merck Index, 9th edn. Rahway NJ: Merck and Co Inc, 1976.
116. Bamford MFM, Jones LF. Deafness and biochemical imbalance after burns treatment with topical antibiotics in young children. Arch Dis Child 1978;53:326.
117. Martin J, Heidemüller B, Berger K, Dietel K. Hörschäden nach Lokalbehandlung von thermischen Schäden der Haut am Beispiel ototoxischer Erscheinungen durch Neomycin. Kinderärztl. Praxis 1985;53:597—601.
118. Kelly DR, Nilo ER, Berggren RB. Deafness after topical neomycin wound irrigation. N Engl J Med 1969;280:1338.
119. Kellerhals B. Hörschäden durch ototoxische Ohrtropfen: Ergebnisse einer Umfrage. HNO 1978;26:49.
120. Herd JK, Cramer A, Hoak FC, Norcross BN. Ototoxicity of topical neomycin augmented by dimethysulfoxide. Pediatrics 1967;40:905.
121. Bishop ME, Garcia RL. Iododerma from wound irrigation with povidone-iodine. J Am Med Assoc 1978;240:249.
122. Vorherr H, Vorherr UF, Mehta P et al. Vaginal absorption of povidone-iodine. J Am Med Assoc 1980;244:2628.
123. Ferguson MM, Geddes DAM, Wray D. The effect of a povidone-iodine mouthwash upon thyroid function and plaque accumulation. Br Dent J 1978;144:14.
124. Block SH. Thyroid function abnormalities from the use of topical betadine solution on intact skin of children. Cutis 1980;26:88.
125. Alvarez E. Neutropenia in a burned patient being treated topically with povidone-iodine foam. Plast Reconstr Surg 1979;63:839.
126. Pietsch J, Meakins JL. Complications of povidone-iodine absorption in topically treated burn patients. Lancet 1976;ii:280.
127. Berthezène F, Fournier M, Bernier, E, Mornex, R. L'Hypothyroidie induite par la résorcine. Lyon Méd 1973;230:319.
128. Thomas AE, Gisburn MA. Exogenous ochronosis and myxoedema from resorcinol. Br J Dermatol 1961;73:378.
129. Cunningham AA. Resorcin poisoning. Arch Dis Child 1956;31:173.
130. Wuthrich B, Zabrodsky S, Storck H. Percutaneous poisoning by resorcinol, salicylic acid, and ammoniated mercury. Pharm Acta Helv 1972;45:453.
131. Gorter E. On salicylate poisoning in children. Acta Paediatr (Uppsala) 1949;37:170.
132. Von Weiss JF, Lever WF. Percutaneous salicylic acid intoxication in psoriasis. Arch Dermatol 1964;90:614.
133. Young CJ. Salicylate intoxication from cutaneous absorption of salicylic acid. South Med J 1952;45:1075.
134. Lindsey CP. Two cases of fatal salicylate poisoning after topical application of an antifungal solution. Med J Aust 1968;1:353.
135. Treguer G, Le Bihan G, Coloignier M et al. Intoxication salicylée par application locale de vaseline salicylée à 20% chez un psoriasique. Nouv Presse Méd 1980;9:192.
136. Scharpf LG, Hill ID, Maibach HI. Percutaneous penetration and disposition of triclocarbon in man. Arch Environ Health 1975;30:7.
137. Rozzini R, Inzol M, Trabucchi M. Delirium from transdermal scopolamine in an elderly woman. J Am Med Assoc 1988;260:478.
138. Gottswinto JM, Korth-Schütz S, Tümmers B, Ziegler R. Gynäkomastie durch östrogen-haltiges Haarwasser. Med Klin 1984;79:181—183.
139. Parker LU, Bergfeld WF. Virilization secondary to topical testosterone. Clev Clin J Med 1991;58:43—46.
140. Reilly JF, Weisse ME. Topically induced diphenhydramine toxicity. J Emerg Med 1990;8:59.

141. Gupta AK, Anderson TF. Psoralen photochemotherapy. J Am Acad Dermatol 1987;17:703.
142. Ternberg JL, Luce, E. Methemoglobinemia: a complication of the silver nitrate treatment of burns. Surgery 1968;63:328.
143. Connelly DM. Silver nitrate—ideal wound therapy? NY State J Med 1970;70:1642.
144. Teelman, K. Retinoids: toxicology and teratogenicity to date. Pharmacol Ther 1989;40:29.
145. Lever LR, Farr PM. Skin cancers or premalignant lesions occur in half of high-dose PUVA patients. Br J Dermatol 1994;131:215–219.
146. Ophaswongse S, Maibach HI. Topical nonsteroidal anti inflammatory drugs: allergic and photoallergic contact dermatitis and phototoxicity. Contact Dermatitis 1993;29:57–64.
147. Iacobelli D, Hashimoto K, Kato I et al. Clobetasol-induced milia. J Am Acad Dermatol 1989;21:215.
148. Blanc D, Deprez PH. Unusual adverse reaction to an acaricide. Lancet 1990;i:1291–1292.
149. Langer J. Gynäkomastie durch Pharmaka. Dermatosen 1989;37:121–147.
150. Kern F, Roberts N, Ostlere L, Langtry J, Staughton RCD. Ammoniated mercury ointment as a cause of peripheral neuropathy. Dermatologica 1991;183:280–282.
151. LeClercq A, Melennec J, Proteau J. Intoxication mercurielle. Concours Méd 1973;95:6055.
152. Ciaccio EI. Mercury: therapeutic and toxic aspects. Semin Drug Treatm 1971;1:177.
153. Ward OC, Hingerty D. Pink disease from cutaneous absorption of mercury. J Ir Med Assoc 1967;60:94.
154. Young E. Ammoniated mercury poisoning. Br J Dermatol 1960;72:449.
155. Chappe SG, Roenigk HH Jr, Miller AJ et al. The effect of photochemotherapy on the cardiovascular system. J Am Acad Dermatol 1981;4:561.
156. van Praag MCG, Bouwes Bavinck JN, Bergman W et al. PUVA keratosis. J Am Acad Dermatol 1993;28:412–417.
157. Rowland Payne CMI, Bladin C, Colcester ACF, Bland J, Lapworth R, Lane D. Argyria from excessive use of topical silver sulphadiazine. Lancet 1992;340:126.
158. Boukes RJ, Bruynzeel BP. Ocular findings in 340 long-term treated PUVA patients. Photodermatology 1985; 2:178–180.
159. Staberg B, Hueg B. Interaction between 8-methoxypsoralen and phenytoin: consequence for PUVA therapy. Acta Derm-Venereol 1985;65:553.
160. Hofmann C, Plewig G, Braun-Falco O. Bowenoid lesions, Bowen's disease and keratoacanthomas in long-term PUVA-treated patients. Br J Dermatol 1979;101:685.
161. White SI, Friedmann PS, Moss C et al. Recovery of cutaneous immune responsiveness after PUVA therapy. Br J Dermatol 1988;118:403.
162. Weismann I, Wagner G, Plewig G. Contact allergy to 8-methoxypsoralen. Br J Dermatol 1980;102:113.
163. Stüttgen G. The risk of photochemotherapy. Int J Dermatol 1982;21:198.
164. Roenigk HH, Martin JS. Photochemotherapy for psoriasis. Arch Dermatol 1977;113:1667.
165. Segal RJ, Watson W. Kaposi's varicelliform eruption in mycosis fungoides. Arch Dermatol 1978;114:1067.
166. Backman HA. The effects of PUVA on the eye. Am J Optom Physiol Opt 1982;59:86.
167. Strauss JS, Rapini RP, Shalita AR et al. Isotretinoin therapy for acne: results of a multicenter dose-response study. J Am Acad Dermatol 1984;10:490.
168. Hazen PG. Depression—a side effect of 13-*cis*-retinoic acid therapy. J Am Acad Dermatol 1983;9:278.
169. Stern RS, Parrish JA, Fitzpatrick TB. Ocular findings in patients treated with PUVA. J Invest Dermatol 1985;85:269–273.
170. Heidbreder G. Lokalisierte Blasen bei Fotochemotherapie. Eine akrobullöse Fotodermatose. Z Hautkr 1980;55:84.
171. Drake LA, Ceilley RI, Dormer W et al. Guidelines of care for phototherapy and photochemotherapy. J Am Acad Dermatol 1991;31:643–648.
172. Crivellato E. A rosacea-like eruption induced by Tigason (Ro 10-9359) treatment. Acta Derm-Venereol 1982; 62:450.
173. Dicken CH, Connolly SM. Eruptive xanthomas associated with isotretinoin (13-*cis*-retinoic acid). Arch Dermatol 1980;116:951.
174. Marsden JR. Lipid metabolism and retinoid therapy. Pharmacol Ther 1989;1:55.
175. Roenigk HH Jr. Liver toxicity of retinoid therapy. Pharmacol Ther 1989;1:145.
176. Dwyer JM, Kenicer K, Taylor Thompson B et al. Vasculitis and retinoids. Lancet 1989;ii:494.
177. Reynolds P, Fawcett H, Waldram R et al. Delayed onset of vasculitis following isotretinoin. Lancet 1989;ii:1216.
178. Silverman AK, Ellis CN, Voorhees JJ. Hypervitaminosis A syndrome: a paradigm of retinoid side effects. J Am Acad Dermatol 1987;16:1027–1039.
179. Bunker CB, Sheron N, Maurice PDL et al. Isotretinoin and eosinophilic pleural effusion. Lancet 1989;i:435.
180. Lauharanta J. Oedema, a rare adverse reaction to etretinate (Tigason). Br J Dermatol 1982;106:251.
181. Baran R. Retinoids and the nails. J Derm Treatm 1990;1:151–154.
182. Lyons F, Laker MF, Marsden JR et al. Effect of oral 13-*cis*-retinoic acid on serum lipids. Br J Dermatol 1982; 107:591.
183. Lebowitz MA, Berson DS. Ocular effects of oral retinoids. J Am Acad Dermatol 1988;19:209.
184. Orfanos CE, Mahrle G, Goerz G et al. Laboratory investigations in patients with generalized psoriasis under oral retinoid treatment. Dermatologica 1979;159:62.
185. Pochi PE. Oral retinoids in dermatology. Arch Dermatol 1982;118:57.
186. Stüttgen G. Oral vitamin A acid therapy. Acta Derm-Venereol 1975;55(Suppl 74):174.
187. Sanchez MR, Ross B, Rotterdam H et al. Retinoid hepatitis. J Am Acad Dermatol 1993;28:853–858.
188. Van der Rhee HJ, Tijssen JGP, Herrmann WA et al. Combined treatment of psoriasis with a new aromatic retinoid (Tigason) in low dosage orally and triamcinolone acetonide cream topically: a double blind trial. Br J Dermatol 1980;102:203.
189. Peck GL. Therapy and prevention of skin cancer. In: Saurat JH, ed. Retinoids. Basel: S. Karger. 1985;345.
190. Windhorst DB, Nigra Th. General clinical toxicology of oral retinoids. J Am Acad Dermatol 1982;6:675.
191. Miller JA, Munro DD. Topical corticosteroids: clinical pharmacology and therapeutic uses. Drugs 1980;19:119.
192. Rimbaud P, Meynadier J, Guilhou JJ, Meynadier, J. Complications dermatologiques locales secondaires aux injections cortisonées. Nouv Presse Méd 1974;3:665.

193. Blackman HJ, Peck GL, Olsen TG, Bergsma DR. Blepharoconjunctivitis: a side effect of oral 13-*cis*-retinoic acid therapy for dermatologic diseases. Ophthalmology 1979; 86:753.
194. Wester RC, Maibach HI. In vivo percutaneous absorption. In: Marzulli FN, Maibach HI, eds. Dermatotoxicology, 2nd edn, Ch. 5. Washington: Hemisphere Publishing Corporation. 1983:131.
195. Summer KH, Gogglemann W. 1-Chloro-2,4-dinitrobenzene depletes glutathione in rat skin and is mutagenic in *Salmonella typhimurium*. Mutat Res 1980;77:91.
196. Van Ketel WG, Swain AF. Allergy to clobetasol-17-propionate (Dermovate®). Contact Dermatitis 1981;7:278.
197. Fisher DA. Exercise-induced bronchoconstriction related to isotretinoin therapy (Letter to Editor). J. Am Acad Dermatol 1985;13:524 .
198. Bjellerup M, Bruze M. Liver injury following administration of 8-methoxypsoralen during PUVA therapy. Acta Derm-Venereol 1979;59:371.
199. Pariser DM, Wyles RJ. Toxic hepatitis from oral methoxsalen photochemotherapy (PUVA). J Am Acad Dermatol 1980;3:248.
200. Larsen KE. Iatrogenic breast discharge with isotretinoin (Letter to Editor). Arch Dermatol 1985;121:450.
201. Lerman S, Megaw J, Willis I. Potential ocular complications from PUVA therapy and their prevention. J Invest Dermatol 1980;74:197.
202. Fenton DA, Wilkinson DJ. Dose-related visual-field defects in patients receiving PUVA therapy. Lancet 1983; i:1106.
203. David M, Hodak E, Lowe NJ. Adverse effects of retinoids. Med Toxicol 1988;3:273.
204. Shawn DH, McGuigan MA. Poisoning from dermal absorption of promethazine. Can Med Assoc J 1984;130:1460–1461.
205. Anderson JM, Cockburn F, Forfar JO et al. Neonatal spongiform myelinopathy after restricted application of hexachlorophene skin disinfectant. J Clin Pathol 1981;34:25.
206. Slamovits TL, Burde RM, Klingele TG. Bilateral optic atrophy caused by oral ingestion and topical application of hexachlorophene. Am J Ophthalmol 1980;89:676.
207. Safran M, Braverman LF. Effect of chronic douching with polyvinyl-pyrrolidone-iodine on iodine absorption and thyroid function. Obstet Gynecol 1982;60:35.
208. Kramer MS, Hutchinson TA, Rudnick SA et al. Operational criteria for adverse drug reactions in evaluating suspected toxicity of a popular scabicide. Clin Pharmacol Ther 1980;27:149.
209. Morgan DP, Roberts RJ, Walter AW et al. Anemia associated with exposure to lindane. Arch Environ Health 1980;35:307.
210. Fagan JE. Henoch-Schönlein purpura and gamma-benzene-hexachloride (Letter to Editor). Pediatrics 1981;67:310.
211. Smith WO, Lyons D. Metabolic acidosis associated with percutaneous absorption of salicylic acid. J Oklahoma State Med Assoc 1980;73:7.
212. De Groot AC, Bos JD. Preservatives in the European standard series for epicutaneous testing. Br J Dermatol 1987;116:289.
213. Gavish D, Katz M, Gottehrer N et al. Cholestatic jaundice, an unusual side effect of etretinate. J Am Acad Dermatol 1985;13:669.
214. Gold JA, Shupack JL, Nemec MA. Ocular side effects of the retinoids. Int J Dermatol 1989;28:218.
215. White SI, Mackie RM. Bone changes associated with oral retinoid therapy. Pharmacol Ther 1989;1:137.
216. Mortimer PS. Unruly hair. Br J Dermatol 1985;113:467.
217. Ramsay B, Bloxham C, Eldred A et al. Blistering, erosions and scarring in a patient on etretinate. Br J Dermatol 1989;121:397.
218. David M, Ginzburg A, Hodak E et al. Palmoplantar eruption associated with etretinate therapy. Acta Derm-Venereol 1986;66:87.
219. Brodkin RH, Abbey AA. Osteoma cutis: a case of probable exacerbation following treatment of severe acne with isotretinoin. Dermatologica 1985;170:210.
220. Fraunfelder FT, LaBraico JM, Meyer SM. Adverse ocular reactions possibly associated with isotretinoin. Am J Ophthalmol 1985;100:534.
221. Parry MF, Rha, C-K. Pseudomembranous colitis caused by topical clindamycin phosphate. Arch Dermatol 1986; 122:583.
222. Ziskind AA. Transdermal scopolamine-induced psychosis. Postgrad Med 1988;84:73.
223. Hogan DJ, Sibley JT, Lane PR. Avascular necrosis of the hips following long-term use of clobetasol propionate (Letter to Editor). J Am Acad Dermatol 1986;14:515.
224. Gonzalez M, Landa N, Gardeazabal J et al. Generalized hypertrichosis after treatment with topical minoxidil. Clin Exp Dermatol 1994;19:157–158.
225. Savin RC, Atton AV. Minoxidil. Update on its clinical role. Dermatol Clin 1993;11:55–64.
226. Vanderveen EE, Ellis CN, Kang S et al. Topical minoxidil for hair regrowth. J Am Acad Dermatol 1984;11:416.
227. Bialonczyk C, Partsch H, Donner A. Bleivergiftung durch langzeitanwendung von Diachylonsalbe. Z Hautkr 1989;64:118–120.
228. Colamarino R, Dubost D, Brun P et al. Etats polyalgiques induits par le minoxidil topique. Ann Med Int 1990;141:425–428.
229. Jick SS, Terris BZ, Jick H. First trimester topical tretinoin and congenital disorders. Lancet 1993;341:1181–1182.
230. Gonzalez Quintela A, Anuncibay PG. Topical promethazine intoxication. DICP Ann Pharmacother 1989;23:89.
231. Franz TJ. Percutaneous absorption of minoxidil in man. Arch Dermatol 1985;121:203.
232. Ranchoff RE, Bergfeld WF. Topical minoxidil reduces blood pressure (Letter to Editor). J Am Acad Dermatol 1985;12:586.
233. Baral J. Minoxidil and sudden death (Letter to Editor). J Am Acad Dermatol 1985;13:297.
234. Vanderveen EE. Minoxidil and sudden death: reply (Letter to Editor). J Am Acad Dermatol 1985;13:298.
235. Frankel EB. Acne secondary to white petrolatum use (Letter to Editor). Arch Dermatol 1985;121:589.
236. Horber FF, Zimmermann A, Frey FJ. Impaired renal function and hypercalcaemia associated with etretinate (Letter to Editor). Lancet 1984;ii:1093.
237. Levin J, Almeyda J. Erythroderma due to etretinate (Letter to Editor). Br J Dermatol 1985;112:373.
238. Bordier C, Flechet M-L, Thomine E et al. Rupture de vergetures au cours d'un psoriasis pustuleux traité par étrétinate (Tigason). Ann Dermatol Vénéréol 1984;11:929.
239. Pilkington T, Brogden RN. Acitretin. A review of its pharmacology and therapeutic use. Drugs 1992;43:597–627.
240. Svindland HB. Malignant transformation of condyloma acuminata after treatment with podophyllin. Eur J Sex Transm Dis 1984;1:165.

241. Baran R, Laugier P. Melanonychia induced by topical-5-fluorouracil. Br J Dermatol 1985;112:621.
242. Stohs SJ, Ezzedeen FW et al. Percutaneous absorption of iodochlorhydroxyquin in humans. J Invest Dermatol 1984;82:195.
243. Ezzedeen FW, Stohs SJ. Percutaneous absorption and disposition of iodochlorhydroxyquin in dogs. J Pharm Sci 1984;73:1369.
244. Oakley GP. The neurotoxicity of the halogenated hydroxyquinolines. J Am Med Assoc 1973;225:395.
245. Public Citizen, Health Research Group. Clioquinol (Letter to FDA). Public Citizen 1985;July 24.
246. Weber MA, Drayer JIM, Brewer DD et al. Transdermal continuous antihypertensive therapy. Lancet 1984;i:9.
247. Groth H, Vetter H, Knüsel J et al. Clonidin-TTS bei essentieller Hypertonie: Wirkung und Verträglichkeit. Schweiz Med Wochenschr 1983;113:1841.
248. Olivari MT, Cohn JN. Cutaneous administration of nitroglycerin: a review. Pharmacotherapy 1983;3:149.
249. Ewing RC, Janda SM, Henann NE. Ageusia associated with transdermal nitroglycerin. Clin Pharm 1989;8:146—147.
250. [Deleted]
251. Mofenson HC, Caraccio TR, Miller H et al. Lidocaine toxicity from topical mucosal application. Clin Pediatr 1983;22:190.
252. Zackheim HS, Epstein EH Jr, McNutt NS et al Topical carmustine (BCNU) for mycosis fungoides and related disorders: a 10-year experience. J Am Acad Dermatol 1983;9:363.
253. [Deleted]
254. Gossweiler B. Kampfervergiftungen heute. Schweiz Rundsch Med (Praxis) 1982;71:1 .
255. McDaniel DH, Blatchley DM, Welton WA. Adverse systemic reaction to dinitrochlorobenzene (Letter to Editor). Arch Dermatol 1982;118:371.
256. Björnberg A. Erythema craquelé provoked by corticosteroids on normal skin. Acta Derm-Venereol 1982;62:147.
257. Eldad A, Neuman A, Weinberg A et al. Silver sulphadiazine induced haemolytic anaemia in a glucose-6-phosphatase dehydrogenase deficient burn patient. Burns 1991; 17:430—432.
258. Edwards EK Jr. Allergic reactions to benzyl alcohol in a sunscreen. Cutis 1981;28:332.
259. Lovell CR, Cronin E, Rhodes EL. Photocontact urticaria from chlorpromazine. Contact Dermatitis, 1985;14:290.
260. Flach AJ, Peterson JS, Mathias CG. Photosensitivity to topically applied sulfisoxazole ointment: evidence for a phototoxic reaction. Arch Ophthalmol 1982;100:1286.
261. Davy A, Guillerdt E, Boyer C. An iatrogenic complication subsequent to an injection of corticoids into the instep. Phlébologie 1986,39:527.
262. LeLiever WC. Topical gentamicin-induced positional vertigo. Otolaryngol. Head Neck Surg 1985;93:553.
263. Chetty GN, Kamalan A, Thambiah AS. Acquired structural defects of the hair. Int J Dermatol 1981;20:119.
264. Lockhart SP, Rushworth A, Azmy AAF, Raine AM. Topical silver sulphadiazine: side effects and urinary excretion. Burns 1984;10:9.
265. Hollis Caffee H, Bingham HG. Leukopenia and silver sulfadiazine. J Trauma 1982;22:586.
266. De Groot AC, Conemans JMH. Nystatin allergy. Petrolatum is not the optimal vehicle for patch testing. Dermatol Clin 1990;8:153.
267. De Groot AC, Weyland JW. Cosmetic allergy from the aminoketone colour Basic Blue 99 (CI 56059). Contact Dermatitis 1990;23:56.
268. Dooms-Goossens A, Deveylder H, Gidi de Aslam A et al. Contact sensitivity to nonoxynols as a cause of intolerance to antiseptic preparations. J Am Acad Dermatol 1989; 21:723.
269. Frosch PJ, Schulze-Dirks A. Kontaktallergie durch Polidocanol (Thesis). Hautarzt 1989;40:146.
270. Holdiness MR. A review of contact dermatitis associated with transdermal therapeutic systems. Contact Dermatitis 1989;200:3.
271. Hogan DJ, Maibach HI. Adverse dermatologic reactions to transdermal drug delivery systems. J Am Acad Dermatol 1990;22:811
272. De Groot AC, Berretty PJM, van Ginkel CJW et al. Allergic contact dermatitis from tocopheryl acetate in cosmetic creams. Contact Dermatitis 1991:25:302—304.
273. De Groot AC. Adverse Reactions to Cosmetics. Thesis, University of Groningen, 1988.
274. Warin RP, Smith RJ. Chronic urticaria; investigations with patch and challenge tests. Contact Dermatitits 1982; 8:117.
275. Dromgoole SH, Maibach HI. Sunscreening agent intolerance, contact and photocontact sensitization and contact urticaria. J Am Acad Dermatol 1990;22:1068.
276. Thune P, Jansen C, Wennersten G et al. The Scandinavian multicenter photopatch study: final report. Photodermatology 1988;2:561.

Meyler's Side Effects of Drugs, 13th Edition
M.N.G. Dukes, editor

SECTION EDITOR: M.N.G. DUKES

Carsten Bindslev-Jensen

15 Antihistamines (H_1-receptor antagonists)

GENERAL CONSIDERATIONS

The antihistamines discussed in this chapter are the H_1-receptor blocking agents, which are among the most commonly used drugs. H_1-receptor antagonists bear some structural resemblance to histamine and, like histamine, contain an ethylamine group. The traditional classification of H_1-receptor antagonists according to chemical structure: ethanolamine, ethylene diamine, alkylamine, piperazine and phenothiazine, is becoming anachronistic, since some of the second-generation H_1-receptor antagonists such as terfenadine or astemizole do not readily fit into the old classification system (1[r]).

H_1-receptor antagonists act by competitively inhibiting the interaction between the H_1-receptor and histamine, thus especially exerting effects on H_1-mediated reactions such as vasodilatation, sneezing and itching. The new second-generation H_1-receptor antagonists are more selective H_1-receptor antagonists, and many of them have additional anti-allergic properties in vivo, e.g. decrease release of inflammatory mediators or inhibit recruitment of inflammatory cells (2[C]–6[C]).

The classic antihistamines Besides the interaction with the H_1-receptor, the classic antihistamines also have affinity to the serotonin, the α-adrenergic and the muscarinic receptors. In addition, they decrease cyclic GMP, increase atrial-ventricular node conduction and may inhibit activation of airway vagal afferent nerves. The incidence of side effects—especially sedation and antimuscarinic effects—to the classic antihistamines is very high, perhaps up to 50%. Although these side effects are rarely serious, and often disappear with continued therapy, they are often so troublesome that medication must be discontinued.

The second-generation antihistamines This group contains astemizole, terfenadine, loratadine, cetirizine, acrivastine, ebastine and azelastine together with Levocabastine, used for local application in the nose and eye (1[r], 7[R]) (SEDA-12, 142–143; SEDA-13, 131; SEDA-14, 135–137; SEDA-17, 199–200). These agents are relatively free from anticholinergic, anti-serotoninergic and α-adrenergic activity. They cause markedly less sedation, perhaps due to their relative lipophobicity, penetrating less extensively into the central nervous system than the classic antihistamines (8[r]–10[r]).

Antihistamines

ADVERSE REACTION PATTERN

General and toxic reactions Sedation is common but varies in severity from compound to compound and from individual to individual. Also, in the second-generation group of antihistamines, sedation is sometimes seen. Central nervous system stimulation may however, also occur, particularly in children. Especially with the classic antihistamines, concomitant ingestion of alcohol and other CNS depressants increases the risk of more serious reactions. Neuroleptic and anticholinergic side effects are also prominent with the classic antihistamines. Gastrointestinal side effects occur, but may be reduced by taking the drug with meals. Blood dyscrasies are rare but may be fatal (SEDA-16, 162). Teratogenicity is poorly documented, but there are no clear guidelines for safe use of antihistamines in pregnant women.

In the second-generation antihistamines cases of cardiac arrythmias have been reported, especially in children taking terfenadine or astemizole and in particular when taken in overdose (11[C]–13[C]; SEDA-17, 196–197).

Hypersensitivity reactions Antihistamines may *per se* act as allergens, and any of the usual manifestations of drug allergy may develop when antihistamines are given orally.

Direct application to the skin carries a risk of sensitization. Haemolytic anaemia may be of immunological origin.

Tumor-inducing effects Such effects have been reported in animal studies on methapyriline; the significance of this finding is not clear (see SEDA-4, 171).

ORGANS AND SYSTEMS

Cardiovascular *Tachycardia* and *hypertension* have been incidentally reported with various classic antihistamines. Overdoses of astemizole have been reported to induce ventricular arrhythmias (*torsade de pointes*) or prolonged Q—T interval, accompanied by syncope and cardiac arrest especially in children (SEDA-12, 142; SEDA-14, 135; SEDA-17, 196—197; 11[C], 12[C]). Overdoses of terfenadine may cause similar episodes (SEDA-14, 137; SEDA-17, 196—197) and a case of *torsade de pointes* was described in a patient taking the prescribed dose of terfenadine together with cefachlor, ketoconazole and medroxyprogesterone (14[C]). These effects of astemizole and terfenadine are probably due to saturation or interaction with the P_{450} system, leading to increased and cardiotoxic plasma concentrations of the unmetabolized parent compound.

Respiratory Phenothiazines are known to be capable of aggravating asthma. The use of the classic antihistamines in asthma was hampered by induction of coughing when inhaled and by the sedative properties when given orally. Furthermore, the dessicating and thickening effect on the airway mucus is undesirable. The effect of the second-generation antihistamines for the treatment of asthma is under current investigation, and so far results clearly demonstrate a moderate, bronchodilating effect as well as an effect on exercise-induced asthma, hyperventilation and cold-air breathing, and to a varying degree some protection against the early and late responses to allergen (1[r]; SEDA-14, 135). Ketotifen is discussed in Chapter 16. Second-generation H_1-receptor antagonists are not first-choice drugs in asthma; however previous concerns about their potential adverse effects in asthma has been exaggerated. The American Academy of Allergy and Immunology (15[R]) has stated that antihistamines are not contraindicated in patients with asthma, unless previous adverse reactions to this treatment have been demonstrated (SEDA-14, 135).

Nervous system Central nervous depression causing sedation is the most common side effect of the classic antihistamines. This drowsiness has been attributed to inhibition of histamine *N*-methyltransferase and to blockage of central histaminergic receptors together with action on other receptors, in particular the receptor for serotonin (1[r], 8[R]—10[R]). Daytime drowsiness may be a problem above all when driving or operating machinery. This side effect forms the basis of the use of these preparations as preoperative medication. As with many other CNS depressants, this effect may decrease or disappear after several days of use, but unintentional combination with other agents or a short discontinuation of therapy may reactivate the sedative effect.

The relative lack of sedative properties in the second-generation antihistamines has been ascribed to the relative lipophobicity of the agents, but no data concerning the actual concentrations of the agents and, even more important, their active metabolites have been published.

A grouping of the antihistamines into those with marked, moderate and very low sedative effect is possible. The dividing lines are not sharp and classification often depends on how many studies are taken into account. Pharmacokinetic studies, penetration into CNS and rate of elimination are important, but, particularly with the older preparations, not always well known. Dosage per administration and total daily dosage do play a role as does the age of the patient, since the sedative effect is often more pronounced in the elderly patient. In a recent study on children, even the classical and sedating drug chlorpheniramine failed to induce significant sedation in a group of children (16[C]) In adults, the sedative effect is marked and common, the incidence being 25—60% or even higher, with substances like bromipheniramine, chlorpheniramine, cyproheptadine, diphenhydramine, hydroxyzine and pitozifen.

Acrivastine is a derivative of triprolidine. When compared with diphenhydramine it has a small but significant additive effect with alcohol at a dose of 8 mg (17[C]). The usual clinical dose is 8 mg three times daily: this dose is effective in treating seasonal allergic rhinitis and is without clinical sedative effect (18[c]). In another study, five of 35 patients receiving acrivastine reported drowsiness as opposed to none in the placebo group (SEDA-14, 135). In patients with urticaria, Acrivastine produced a lower rate of sedation (four of 18) than did Cyproheptadine (12 of 18) (SEDA-17, 197). In recent years, very little new data on sedation induced by acrivastine has been published. Further studies are needed before Acrivastine can be fully evaluated.

The incidence of sedation with astemizole has been reported to be similar to placebo in most studies (7[R], 19[R]). Sedation does, however, occur in some patients (SEDA-12, 142) sometimes after several weeks of treatment. In terms of its psychomotor effects a study of the effect of astemizole compared with terfenadine on visuo-motor coordination, arithmetic ability and digit signal substitution and on mood was carried out by Nicholson (20[C]): triprolidine 10 mg in the sustained release form was used as a positive control. Triprolidine caused a decrement in performance and motor coordination, but neither 60 mg terfenadine nor 10 and 20 mg astemizole had any effect on these performance tests.

In most studies azatadine has been shown only rarely to cause sedation (21[cr]; SEDA-14, 1136), whereas some studies report sedation in 30% of the patients (see SED-11, 317; SEDA-9, 149; SEDA-10, 135).

In a recent study, 10 mg cetirizine was shown to elicit acute sedating effects impairing driving performance (22[C]), whereas loratadine in the same study was devoid of sedating potential. Furthermore an additive effect of alcohol and cetirizine but not loratadine was found. In another study using a driving simulator, however, 10 mg cetirizine did not affect driving abilities (23[C]). In a number of studies, a dose of 20 mg has been demonstrated to cause significant sedation and, in one study, a dose-dependent sedation of 10 and 20 mg but not 5 mg was found (24[C]). Pooling available data (SEDA-16, 163) reveals cetirizine to be little more sedating than loratadine and terfenadine.

Bradley and Nicholson (25[C]) studied the effects of 10, 20 and 40 mg loratadine on tests of visuo-motor coordination, dynamic visual acuity, short-term memory, digit signal substitution and subjective assessments of mood: trioprolidine was used as an active control and impaired performance on all the tasks presented. The 40 mg dose of loratadine caused a significant impairment of the Digit Symbol Substitution Test and the Dynamic Visual Acuity Test, but the 10 and 20 mg doses were without effect. Loratadine did not affect objective sleepiness as measured by Multiple Sleep Latency Test (26[R]). Other investigations studying loratadine in the normal 10 mg dose have also failed to demonstrate a sedation rate different to placebo (SEDA-12, 143; SEDA-14, 136).

Terfenadine has been investigated in several thousands of patients with a sedation rate comparable to placebo (27[R]). It has not been demonstrated to impair driving performance (28[R]).

Clemastine fumarate was reported to have a percentage of sedation between 9 and 50 (29[r]), whereas 10 mg mequitazine, but not 5 mg, seems to have central effects (21[CR]), and oxatomide has been reported to cause drowsiness in 37—56% of treated patients (21[CR], 30[c]). Loss of memory, confusion and disorientation has been ascribed to meclozine in an 85-year-old female (SEDA-13, 132).

Thus, the second-generation antihistamines generally seem to be free of sedative effects when administered in the recommended dosage (1[r], 7[R]). It should be borne in mind, however, that sedative effects in an individual can never be entirely excluded in advance.

CNS stimulation is less frequent but, when it occurs, is present in the form of insomnia, irritability and tremor; nightmares and hallucinations have occasionally been reported with the classic antihistamines. In overt intoxication, they may well be related to the anticholinergic effect. Intoxication leading to CNS stimulation in children is not frequent. An analysis of 113 200 admissions to a pediatric hospital revealed only two patients with excitation, insomnia, visual hallucinations and seizures, followed by coma (31[CR]).

Prolonged use of antihistamine-containing decongestants may produce *facial dyskinesia* including blepharospasm, swallowing difficulties and dysarthria. As these patients have frequently been taking combined products containing antihistamines, proper evaluation of interactions is needed before final assessment is possible. As the dyskinesia may be unilateral, a neurological disorder should be diagnosed prior to thinking about a side effect (SEDA-1, 144). Marked dyskinesia in an 18-month-old girl followed an overdose of a combination of dexbrompheniramine and pseudoephedrine (32[C]). Cyproheptadine has been described as causing reversible toxic *psychosis* in a patient with renal impairment and low body weight after an incidental overdose of 24 mg within 24 hours (SEDA-2, 150).

Methapyrilene is a relatively strong sedative and therefore a constituent in many sedative and sleep-inducing OTC preparations. Due to easy access and abuse, intoxications with fatal outcome have been reported (33[C]).

Autonomic effects are connected with the marked anticholinergic properties of the classical antihistamines, resulting in dessication of the oral and respiratory mucosa. Other antimuscarinic effects are less common, but nasal stuffiness, blurring of vision, urinary retention and constipation may all occur, relative to the dosage.

Appetite stimulation and resulting *weight gain* is a well-known feature of cyproheptadine, but astemizole also causes weight gain in approximately 3% of patients within weeks of treatment (7[R], 19[R]). Cetirizine also has been reported to induce weight gain (approx. 2.8%) when used for a prolonged time (SEDA-17, 200)

Cinnarizine and flunarizine are piperazine derivatives with antihistaminic properties and calcium channel blocking activity. Several reports have described *extrapyramidal reactions* and *depression* associated with their use (SEDA-14, 136) and *worsening of motility* in Parkinson patients (SEDA-13, 391).

Endocrine, metabolic Occasional reports of antihistamine-induced *hypoglycemia* may well reflect mere coincidence. *Hyperpyrexia* is an occasional complication of treatment.

Hematological Blood *dyscrasias* are infrequent, but agranulocytosis, hemolytic anemias and thrombocytopenia have been described; the latter may be more common with antazoline, whereas chlorpheniramine was ascribed to produce agranulocytosis in a patient (SEDA-16, 1162). Aplastic anemia has been described (34[C]). Mebhydrolin has been reported to produce granulocytopenia (35[C]). Blood viscosity may be reduced by some of these compounds when given in high doses (see Chapter 19).

Liver Repeated reports of changes in liver function may reflect sheer coincidence, in view of the widespread use of these drugs. Occasionally, however, hepatitis (56[c]) or cholestatic jaundice seems to have occurred.

Gastrointestinal Gastrointestinal effects are not very common, but may manifest themselves as *nausea*, *vomiting*, *gastric pain*, *diarrhoea* or *constipation*. *Appetite* may be increased (see earlier), but anorexia may also occur.

Skin and appendages Although H_1-antagonists are often used in the treatment of allergic conditions, their topical use frequently produces skin *sensitization* and subsequent contact dermatitis. This effect occurs more frequently with the use of ethylenediamines and phenothiazines, the latter also producing photoallergic cutaneous reactions. Cross-reactions between phenothiazine tranquillizers and classic H_1-antagonists are possible, as well as reactions between H_1-antagonists and the ethylenediamine present in some creams and ointments. As local sensitization is quite common, topical use of H_1-antagonists is not recommenced. Despite these disadvantages they are still available in many countries as OTC products. It should also be noted, that topical administration of antihistamines in sufficient doses can result in adverse systemic reactions.

Terfenadine has been reported to cause skin reactions, notably urticaria and rashes in a number of cases (SEDA-11, 148; SEDA-13, 132). A photoallergic reaction to terfenadine has also been reported (SEDA-12, 143), and so have severe exacerbations of psoriasis possibly due to terfenadine (SEDA-14, 137). A lichen planus pemphigoides-like eruption following the use of cinnarizine has been reported in a Japanese woman (SEDA-11, 146). PLEVA (pityriasis lichenoides et varioliformis) has been convincingly (by reappearance after rechallenge) ascribed to intake of astemizole in a patient (SEDA-18, 4)

Special senses Dimenhydrinate has been studied in healthy volunteers. The drug was found to affect colour discrimination, night vision, reaction time and stereopsis (36[c]). Other (classic) antihistamines are likely to have similar effects, due in whole or in part to their anticholinergic or sedative effects (see also 'Risk situations' below). Azelastine has been reported to alter taste perception for several hours after ingestion (37[c]).

Incidental and unverified reports Headache, extrasystoles and anaphylactoid reactions have all been reported.

Risk situations In view of the anticholinergic effects, H_1-antagonists should be avoided in cases of *glaucoma* and *prostatism*. It has been reported that antihistamines can provoke release of catecholamines from a *pheochromocytoma*. The possibility of circulatory effects means that antihistamines should be used with caution in patients with *cardiac diseases* or *hypertension*. H_1-antagonists may be dangerous to *drivers* and people *operating machinery*, primarily because of the sedative effects but also due to blurring of vision.

Withdrawal effects Since dyskinesia may occur after withdrawal of phenothiazine neuroleptic drugs (see Chapter 6), it is not unlikely that the same problem may follow termination of prolonged antihistamine therapy. A case of cyproheptadine *dependence* has been reported (SEDA-12, 142).

Second generation effects *Teratogenic* effects are not proven in man, although some piperazine derivatives display teratogenic properties in laboratory animals. Cleft palate is seen more frequently in infants whose mothers have used H_1-antagonists for the treatment of hyperemesis gravidarum (4.44 per 1000 births) than in infants of mothers without hyperemesis gravidarum and not treated with antihistamines (0.78 per 1000). However, children of mothers suffering from hyperemesis gravidarum but not treated also showed a high incidence of cleft palate (3.14 per 1000). It would seem that cleft palate could be a consequence of the maternal condition rather than of drug teratogenicity. However, until more evidence is available, the possibility of palate malformation with at least some of these drugs must be borne in mind (38[C]–40[C]).

Teratogenic activity has been attributed to doxylamine, a constituent of many combinations with vitamin B_6 and antispasmodic agents, and used in the treatment of hyperemesis gravidarum. Extensive studies and reviews seem to indicate, however, that the incidence of malformations is not higher in children whose mothers have taken preparations containing doxylamine (41[R], see also Chapter 36).

Hydroxyzine used in a fairly high dose (600 mg/day) in pregnancy has been reported to produce a *neonatal withdrawal syndrome* after delivery; this was characterized primarily by hyperactivity and irritability (SEDA-2, 151).

There have been no specific reports of harm resulting from the use of antihistamines during *lactation*, but in view of the special sensitivity of children to the central nervous effects of these drugs, caution is clearly advisable. Cyproheptadine is stated by the manufacturer to inhibit lactation.

Overdosage and abuse Overdosage problems arise particularly in children (CNS effects and cardiac effects) and in drug abusers. It is notable in this connection that abuse of antihistamines in Scandinavia is often found in school children, and particularly involves diphenhydramine (alone or in combination with caffeine). As a consequence such preparations were changed from OTC preparations to POM (42, 43). A total of 136 diphenhydramine poisonings (with suicidal intent) has been evaluated. The most common symptom seen was impaired consciousness followed by psychotic behaviour resembling catatonic stupor. Other symptoms included hallucinations, mydriasis, tachycardia and, less frequently, diplopia, respiratory insufficiency and seizures (SEDA-13, 132). A 5-year-old patient treated with a topical lotion containing 1% diphenhydramine for pruritic vesicular exanthema developed disorientation, agitation, dilated pupils accompanied by ataxis (SEDA-13, 132).

Some antihistamines, e.g. tripellenamine (often used in combination with pentazocine) have a particular abuse potential and are used by drug addicts. Psychiatric disturbances, dysphoria, depression, confusion and hallucinations can occur while under the influence of a H_1-antagonist or during drug withdrawal. Chronic parenteral abuse may cause skin lesions, muscular fibrosis and vasculitis.

Interactions Drugs with a CNS-depressive effect (hypnotics, sedatives, narcotic analgesics, neuroleptics, alcohol, etc.) will have an increase in effect vaused by interaction with especially the classic antihistamines. The second-generation antihistamines have not yet been proven to interact with CNS-depressants such as alcohol or diazepam (44[C]–47[C]).

Drugs with anticholinergic effects (anticholinergics, phenothiazines, tricyclic antidepressants) will have their effects increased by antihistamines.

Antihistamines will antagonize the effect of betahistine. It has been claimed that antihistamines should not be given less than 2 days after withdrawal of monoamine oxidase inhibitors because of a marked potentiation of the sedative effects.

When diphenhydramine was mixed with *meglumine iodopamide* to prevent an allergic reaction to the latter, a precipitate was formed. These two drugs should be regarded as incompatible for in vitro mixing.

To counteract the sedative effects of the classic antihistamines, combinations with stimulants have been tried. The efficacy of such combinations has not been proved, but additional side effects such as irritability has been observed (48[C]).

Combinations with decongestants such as *pseudoephedrine* have been advocated for upper respiratory conditions, but the latter drug may cause additional side effects such as nervousness and elevated blood pressure (49[c]–50[c]).

When used for the treatment of common cold and allergic upper airways disorders, antihistamines (alone or in combination with decongestants) may produce a decrease in mucociliary motility in the middle ear, thus contributing to the development of otitis media (51[cr]).

Metabolism of drugs with an extensive liver metabolism (e.g. terfenadine and astemizole) will be influenced by other extensively metabolized drugs, e.g. ketoconazole, leading to increased concentration of the unmetabolized drug in plasma.

Interference with diagnostic routines Since H_1-antagonists inhibit the cutaneous response to *histamine* and *allergens*, they should be withdrawn (usually for a week, astemizole for up to 8 weeks) before skin testing for allergy is undertaken.

INDIVIDUAL H_1-ANTAGONISTS

A comparison of the clinical efficacy of the newer antihistamines can be found in SEDA-17, 197–199 and SEDA-18, 1–3.

Variations in the spectrum of wanted and unwanted effects of H_1-antagonists, other than listed above, are poorly documented.

Acrivastine *(SEDA-14, 135; SEDA-15, 155; SEDA-17, 199)*

In the recent years, very little new data on sedation induced by acrivastine has been published. Further studies are needed before acrivastine can be truly classified as being non-sedating.

Antazoline (Antistin) *(SED-9, 783; SEDA-7, 172)*

Antazoline has sometimes produced thrombocytopenic purpura when used in normal doses. Antibodies to antazoline were present, obviously as a result of previous, yet uneventful, use.

Astemizole *(SEDA-12, 142; SEDA-14, 135)*

Weight gain after prolonged use occurs. In overdose, cardiac arrythmias occur particularly in children (1[r], 12[C], 19[R]).

Azelastine *(SEDA-12, 375; SEDA-15, 155; SEDA-17, 199; SEDA-18, 2, 4) (see also Chapter 16)*

In controlled studies, azelastine nasal spray produces a high incidence of itching and burning of the nasal mucosa together with taste perversion and sometimes unpleasant smell. Sedation does not seem to be frequent.

Cinnarizine and flunarizine *(SEDA-13, 131; SEDA-14, 136) (see also Chapter 17)*

Seventy reports of development of tremor and Parkinsonism in patients treated with cinnarizine and eleven reports of development of tremor and parkinsonism in patients treated with flunarizine have been reported in a Spanish study (52[C]).

Clemastine fumarate *(SEDA-7, 172)*

Clemastine belongs to the benzhydryl ether group and was developed in the hope of lessening sedative effects. No significant difference as compared with other antihistamines was noted.

Cyproheptadine

Cyproheptadine and other H_1-antagonists with antiserotoninergic effects are frequently used because of their appetite-stimulating capacity. This effect is present during regular use, but disappears after withdrawal. Drowsiness and other side effects common to the classic antihistamines are frequently seen. A case of dependence has been reported (SEDA-12, 142).

Dexchlorpheniramine maleate

Dexchlorpheniramine maleate produced hemolytic anaemia in a 47-year-old woman ingesting 4 mg/day for 3 days. The direct antiglobulin test was found to be positive, and circulating antibodies were detected in serum, which reacted in vitro with other antihistamines as well (53[C]).

Levocabastine *(SEDA-17, 201; SEDA-18, 4)*

Since the drug is applied locally in the eye or nose, local reactions are seen most often. Most frequent is ocular irritation followed by nasal irritation. Sedation does not seem to be frequent.

Mequitazine

In a comparative study with placebo, no significant difference was seen in the incidence of drowsiness, while dry mouth was reported in nine of 23 mequitazine patients versus six of 25 placebo patients. Accomodation disturbance was seen in three patients treated with mequitazine (53[c]).

Oxatomide *(SED 12, 371; SEDA-18, 5)*

In some cases of asthma an exacerbation of the bronchospasm has occurred (54[c], 55[R]).

Acute cytolytic hepatitis (56[c]) and drug eruptions has been described.

Pitozifen *(see also Chapter 2)*

Pitozifen is chemically and pharmacologically similar to cyproheptadine and shares its side effects. When used for migraine an increase in weight occurs; conversely, when used to improve appetite, sleepiness and dizziness frequently occur.

Phenindamine

Phenindamine is reputed to cause stimulation rather than sedation in some patients, but good documentation is lacking.

Terfenadine *(SEDA-12, 143; SEDA-13, 132; SEDA-14, 137; SEDA-16, 165; SEDA-17, 196—197; SEDA-18, 6)*

Sedation rate is low with terfenadine (1[r], 26[R]). An important interaction seems to exist between the unmetabolized terfenadine and other drugs, which are metabolized by the cytochrome P_{450} system (CYP2A4). Inhibition of metabolization of terfenadine leads to cardiotoxic concentrations of the parent compound; this is probably the reason for the cardiac arrhythmias seen at overdoses (25[R]). A single case of cardiac arrhythmia in a woman receiving normal doses of terfenadine together with cefachlor, ketoconazole and medroxyprogesterone has been reported—the authors demonstrated excessive plasma levels of parent terfenadine (14[C]).

Two cases of excacerbation of psoriasis have been reported (57[Cr]).

Thiazinanium

Thiazinanium can cause attacks of sternal and epigastric pain, perhaps due to spasm of the oesophagus or cardia.

REFERENCES

1. Simmonds FER, Simons K. Second-generation antihistamines. Ann Allergy 1991;66:5.
2. Temple DM, McCluskey M. Loratadine, an antihistamine, blocks antigen- and inophore-induced leukotriene release from human lung in vitro. Prostaglandins 1988;35:549.
3. Little MM, Wood DR, Casale TB. Azelastine inhibits stimulated histamine release from human lung tissue in vitro but does not alter cyclic nucleotide content. Agents Actions 1988;28:16.
4. Charlesworth EN, Kagey-Sobotka A, Norman PS, Lichtenstein LM. Effect of cetirizine on mast cell mediator release and cellular traffic during the cutaneous late phase reaction. J Allergy Clin Immunol 1989;83:905.
5. Michel L, De Vos C, Rihoux J-P et al. Inhibitory effect of oral cetirizine on in vivo antigen-induced histamine and PAF-acether release and eosinophil recruitment in human skin. J Allergy Clin Immunol 1988;82:101.
6. Leprevost C, Capron M, De Vos C, Tomassini M, Capron A. Inhibition of eosinophil chemotaxis by a new antiallergic compound (cetirizine). Int Arch Allergy Appl Immunol 1988;87:9.
7. Kunkel G, ed. Antihistamines reassessed. Clin Exp Allergy 1990;20:1.
8. Simons FER. H_1-receptor antagonists: clinical pharmacology and therapeutics. J Allergy Clin Immunol 1989; 84:845.
9. Trzeciakowski JP, Mendelsohn N, Levi R. Antihistamines. In: Middleton E, Reed CE, Ellis EF, Adkinson NF, Yunginger JW, eds. Allergy Principles and Practice, 3rd ed. St Louis: C.V. Mosby Company, 1988;715.
10. Druce H. Impairment of function by antihistamines. Ann Allergy 1990;64:403.
11. Craft TM. Torsade de pointes after astemizole overdose. Br Med J 1986;292:660.
12. Simons FER, Kesselman MS, Giddins NG, Pelech AN, Simons KJ. Astemizole-induced torsade de pointes. Lancet 1988;ii:624.
13. Davies AJ, Harindra V, McEwan A, Ghose RR. Cardiotoxic effect with convulsions in terfenadine overdose. Br Med J 1989;298:325.
14. Monahan BP, Ferguson CL, Killeavy ES et al. Torsade de pointes occurring in association with terfenadine use. J Am Med Assoc 1990;264(21):2788.
15. Sly RM, Kemp JP. The use of antihistamines in patients with asthma. J Allergy Clin Immunol 1988;82:101.
16. Feldman W, Shanon A, Leiken L et al. Central nervous system side-effects of antihistamines in schoolchildren. Rhinology 1992;13:13.
17. Cohen A, Hamilton M, Peck A. The effects of acrivastine (BW825C), diphenhydramine and terfenadine in combination with alcohol on human C.N.S. performance. Eur J Pharmacol 1987;32:279.
18. Gibbs T, Irander K, Salo O. Acrivastine in seasonal allergic rhinitis: two randomised crossover studies to evaluate efficacy and safety. J Int Med Res 1988;16:431.
19. Richards D et al. Astemizole. Drugs 1984;28:38.
20. Nicholson AN, Stone BM. Performance studies with the H_1-histamine receptor antagonists, astemizole and terfenadine. Br J Clin Pharmacol 1982;13:199.
21. Barlow JLR, Beitman RE, Tsai TH. Terfenadine, safety and tolerance in controlled clinical trials. Arzneim-Forsch/-Drug Res 1982;32:1215.
22. Ramaekers JG, Uiterwijk M, O'Hanlon JF. Effects of larattadine and cetirizine on actual driving and psychometric test performance, and EEG durung driving. Eur J Clin Pharmacol 1992;42:363.
23. Gengo FM, Gabos C, Mechtler L. Quantitative effects of cetirizine and diphenhydramine on mental performance measured using an automobile driving simulator. Ann Allergy 1990;64:520.
24. Seidel WF, Cohen S, Bliwise NG, Dement WC. Cetirizine effects on objective measures of daytime sleepiness and performance. Ann Allergy 1987;59:58.
25. Bradley CM, Nicholson AN. Studies on the central effects of the H_1-antagonist, loratadine. Eur J Clin Pharmacol 1987;32:419
26. Roth T, Roehis T, Kusthurek G, Sicklesteel J, Zurick M. Sedative effects of antihistamines. J Allergy Clin Immunol 1987;80:94.
27. Mctavish D, Goa KL, Ferrill M. Terfenadine, an updated review of its pharmacological properties and therapeutic efficacy. Drugs 1990;39:552.
28. Nicholson A. Antihistaminic activity in central effects of terfenadine. A review of European studies. Arzneim-Forsch/Drug Res 1982;32(ii):1191.
29. Kriz RJ. Patient evaluation of clemastine fumarate and comparison with other antihistamines. Wisc Med J 1981;80:31.
30. Brompton Hospital Medical Research Council Collaborative Trial. A controlled trial of oxatomide in the treatment of asthma with or without perennial rhinitis. Clin Allergy 1981;2:483.
31. Reyes-Jacang A, Wenzl JE. Antihistamine toxicity in children. Clin Pediatr (Philadelphia) 1969;8:297.
32. Barone DA, Raiolo J. Facial dyskinesia from overdose of an antihistamine. N Engl J Med 1980;303:107.
33. Winek CL, Fochtman FW, Frogus WJ et al. Methapyriline toxicity. Clin Toxicol 1977;11:287.
34. Kanoh T, Jingami H, Uchino H. Aplastic anaemia after prolonged treatment with chlorpheniramine. Lancet 1977;i:546.
35. Current Problems Committee on Safety of Medicine. Mebhydrolin (Fabahistin) and white cell depression. Committee on Safety of Medicine 1981;7 December.

36. Luria SM, Kinney JAS, McKay CL et al. Effects of aspirin and dimenhydrinate (Dramamine) on visual processes. Br J Clin Pharmacol 1979;7:585.
37. Meltzer EO, Storms WW, Pierson WE et al. Efficacy of azelastine in perennial allergic rhinitis: clinical and rhinomanometric evaluation. J Allergy Clin Immunol 1988;82:447.
38. Saxen I. Cleft palate and maternal diphenhydramine intake. Lancet 1974;i:407.
39. McBride WG. An aetiological study of drug ingestion by women who gave birth to babies with cleft palate. Aust NZ J Obstet Gynaecol 1969;9:103.
40. Sadusk JF Jr, Palmisano PA. Teratogenic effect of meclizine, cyclizine and chlorcyclizine. J Am Med Assoc 1965; 194:987.
41. Henderson IWD. Congenital deformities associated with Bendectin. Can Med Assoc J 1977;117:721.
42. Bjoeldager AL, Jensen K, Nielsen K et al. Forgiftningstilfaelde med antihistaminer. Ugeskr Laeg 1980;142:2140.
43. Gullmann NC, Petersen E, Nielsen V. En epidemi af antihistaminmisbrug på en psykiatrisk afdeling. Ugeskr Laeg 1980;142:2542.
44. Bhatti JA, Hindmarch I. The effects of terfenadine with and without alcohol on an aspect of car driving performance. Clin Exp Allergy 1989;19:609.
45. Moser L, Hüther KJ, Koch-Weser J, Lundt PV. Effects of terfenadine and diphenhydramine alone or in combination with diazepam or alcohol on psychomotor performance and subjective feelings. Eur J Clin Pharmacol 1978;14:417.
46. Rombaut N, Heykants, J, Vanden Bussche G. Potential of interaction between the H_1-antagonist astemizole and other drugs. Ann Allergy 1986;57:321.
47. Doms M, Vanhulle G, Baelde Y et al. Lack of potentiation by cetirizine of alcohol-induced psychomotor disturbances. Eur J Clin Pharmacol 1988;34:619.
48. Newlands WJ. The effect of pemoline on antihistamine-induced drowsiness. Practitioner 1980;224:1199.
49. Falliers CJ, Redding MA. Controlled comparison of a new antihistamine-decongestant combination to its individual components. Ann Allergy 1980;45:75.
50. Tarasiso JC. Azatadine maleate/pseudoephedrine sulfate repetabs versus placebo in the treatment of severe seasonal allergic rhinitis. J Int Med Res 1980;8:391.
51. Peerless SA, Noiman AH. Etiology of otitis media with effusion: antihistamine-decongestants. Laryngoscope 1980; 90:1852.
52. Capella D, Laporte JR, Castel JM et al. Parkinsonism, tremor and depression induced by cinnarizine and flunarizine. Br Med J 1988;297:722.
52. Duran-Suarez JR, Martin-Vega C, Argelagues E et al. The I antigen as an immune complex receptor in the case of haemolytic anaemia induced by an antihistaminic agent. Br J Haematol 1981;49:153.
53. Dry J, Pradalier A, Di Palma H, Lanoue R. Essai clinique en double aveugle contre placebo de la méquitazine chez des patients non hospitalisés. Thérapie (Paris) 1980; 35:189.
54. Banham SW, Moran F. A clinical trial of oxatomide in asthma. Br J Clin Pract 1980;34:323.
55. Castaner J. Oxatomide. Drugs Future 1978;3:465.
56. De Parades V, Roulot D, Neyrolles N et al. Hepatite cytolotique au cours de l'administration d'oxatomide. Gastroenterol Clin Biol 1994;18:294.
57. McKenna KE, McMillan JC. Excacerbation of psoriasis, liver dysfunction and thrombocytopenia associated with mebhydrolin. Clin Exp Dermatol 1993;18:131.

Meyler's Side Effects of Drugs, 13th Edition
M.N.G. Dukes, editor

SECTION EDITOR: M.N.G. DUKES

J.W. Paterson and K.M. Lulich

16 Antiallergic drugs and antitussives

GENERAL PROBLEMS

In asthma, it may be necessary to treat a patient with two or more drugs at the same time. Thus, bronchodilator therapy using combinations of β-adrenoceptor agonists with theophylline or antimuscarinics has been shown to be beneficial. Bronchodilators may be combined with cromolyn sodium and/or corticosteroids (1[R]). However, the use of fixed-dose combinations (e.g. ephedrine, barbiturate and theophylline) has no place in modern asthma therapy and is not without risk.

Cough is a symptom of a variety of different underlying problems ranging from the common cold to bronchial carcinoma and may be productive or non-productive. *Treatment of cough is often inappropriate*, e.g. suppression of a productive cough, *or illogical*, where agents to promote expectoration are given with others designed to suppress it; this is a particular problem with fixed-combination cough or expectorant mixtures.

Another problem in children is that *cough may be a major symptom of asthma*, even in the absence of appreciable wheeze (2[C]). This is best treated by the administration of bronchodilators or other antiasthmatic therapy and there is a specific danger of respiratory depression if asthmatics are given cough mixtures containing opioids.

Several surveys have shown that, in asthma, patients who are symptomatically and spirometrically severely incapacitated may be *inadequately treated* (3[C], 4[C]). Another problem is that many drugs used in the treatment of obstructive lung disease are given by inhalation and patients will not benefit if they do not use the inhaler correctly. It has been shown that even doctors and nurses may make mistakes in the use of an inhaler (5[C]). Only a minority of hospitalized patients were found to be using a completely correct technique despite reading the package insert, whereas those who received instructions at the start of treatment were more likely to use the inhaler correctly (6[C]). The increases in death rates among asthmatic patients in several countries led to concern about the safety of β-adrenoceptor agonist aerosols. However, it is probable that death is due to suboptimal treatment or patients reaching hospital too late to be responsive to intensive treatment (SEDA-15, 1). Investigation of patients requiring admission for severe, life-threatening asthma has shown that they have deteriorated over a number of days without adequate treatment being given (1[R], 7[C]). This highlights the dangers of inadequate or inappropriate therapy rather than drug toxicity in asthma. The powerful bronchodilator action of β_2-adrenoceptor agonists may mask the onset and/or exacerbation of airway inflammation in asthmatics, resulting in the under-utilization of effective anti-inflammatory drugs. Thus β_2-adrenoceptor agonists need to be combined with adequate doses of anti-inflammatory drugs (1[R]). The new generation long acting β_2-adrenoceptor agonists such as salmeterol or formeterol can provide symptomatic relief for up to 12 hours without exerting a clinically significant anti-inflammatory effect (8[R]). This may result in a greater tendency to underestimate the need for anti-inflammatory treatment than occurs with the shorter acting agents such as salbutamol and terbutaline.

As inflammation is now recognised as the central lesion in asthma, there should be a greater emphasis on trying to control or reverse inflammation at an early stage of the disease. Inhaled corticosteroids are very effective in treating the underlying airway inflammation (9[R]).

Patients with bronchial asthma have been shown to be *more hypersensitive to drugs* than other people. Up to 26% of asthmatic patients were shown to be hypersensitive to one or more drugs, whereas in healthy controls, 4.5% were hypersensitive (SEDA-5, 169). Asthmatics may also be sensitive to acetylsalicylic acid, which may be given alone or as a constituent of a combination medicine. The association between aspirin sensitivity, nasal polyps and rhinitis in asthma is well known. Asthma induced by aspirin may be very severe and resistant to treatment. Estimates of the prevalence of so-called aspirin asthma vary from 3.3 to as high as 44% in different series (SEDA-5, 169). Aspirin-sensitive subjects may have attacks induced by other non-steroidal anti-inflammatory drugs (10[C]). It is thought that the basis of this reaction is inhibition of prostaglandin synthetase by aspirin or other non-steroidal anti-inflammatory drugs. Tartrazine, which is commonly included as coloring matter in foodstuffs and drugs, may also induce hypersensitivity that can lead to asthma, angio-edema and uticaria (SEDA-1, 149). Cross-sensitivity between tartrazine and aspirin exists. The problem is compounded because colorants are still not listed as constituents on drug packaging in many countries. An additional problem with asthmatics is sensitivity to sulfur dioxide and metabisulfite. Patients may be exposed to this agent in various foodstuffs and drinks, where the agent is used as a preservative. Asthma has been reported to be induced by injections of drugs containing metabisulfite as a preservative (11^C).

ANTIALLERGIC DRUGS

Cromolyn sodium (sodium cromoglycate)

Cromolyn sodium is administered as a powder for inhalation using a 'spinhaler'. Recently it has been dispensed in a multidose pressurized aerosol. Cromolyn is a prophylactic drug and is not effective in the acute attack. If it is ceased abruptly, asthma may recur quite rapidly. A liquid form is available for use in rhinitis and ocular conditions. Some gastrointestinal uses are dealt with in Chapter 36. The solution is also effective in the treatment of atopic dermatitis (SEDA-17, 205).

Cromolyn sodium inhibits mast-cell degranulation and the histamine release induced by phospholipase A_2; it does not interfere with the interaction of antigen and reaginic antibodies. Evidence is accumulating that cromolyn sodium has an important stabilising action on leukocytes apart from mast cells such as neutrophils, eosinophils and monocytes, and that it also affects nerve reflexes in the lung (12^R).

ADVERSE REACTION PATTERN

General and toxic reactions These seem to be very rare. Cromolyn is a safe drug; most of the observed side effects are mild, often transient and usually do not require cessation of therapy. With over 20 years of widespread use the safety of cromolyn sodium is established. Adverse effects such as laryngeal edema, swollen parotid gland, bronchospasm, joint swelling, nausea, cough, headache, nasal congestion, rash and urticaria are reported in only one in 10 000 patients (SEDA-12, 142). The excellent safety record has led to cromolyn being preferred to corticosteroids in the cases of asthma which respond to it. The American Academy of Allergy and Immunology reported two 10-year safety reports involving 424 and 85 patients, respectively. These emphasised the safety of long term use. The only serious side effects were three cases of pulmonary infiltration and eosinophilia (SEDA-6, 171). In another series of 375 patients, only eight experienced adverse reactions. These included dermatitis with pruritus, myositis and gastroenteritis (SEDA-4, 120). A double-blind study compared a cromolyn sodium preparation with lactose and one without lactose. It was found that after 3 months of treatment there was no significant clinical difference in their effects or tolerance, but after 6 months there was a slight subjective preference for the lactose-free formulation of cromolyn sodium (SEDA-15, 2).

Hypersensitivity reactions (or pseudo-allergic reactions) These are rare but can occur, both in immediate form with bronchospasm, aggravation of existing asthma and a progressive fall in FEV_1, resulting in dyspnea and also in delayed forms with, for example, fever and dyspnea (13^C). A survey of the world literature up to 1982 (14^R) detected 13 cases of facial rash, urticaria and/or generalised dermatitis, one of nasal congestion, 19 of severe bronchospasm and/or pulmonary edema, eventually culminating in shock, four of eosinophilic or granulomatous pulmonary infiltration, one of liver disease and vasculitis, one of pericarditis and three of polymyositis. The overall incidence was about 2% when using inhalation therapy. At present there is no proof that the adverse reactions to cromolyn which mimic allergic processes of the immediate or delayed type are in fact mediated by IgE and/or specifically reactive lymphocytes; consequently these reactions fulfil the criteria which characterize pseudoallergic reactions (14^R, 15^R). There is a much higher incidence of such adverse reactions when cromolyn is used orally (50—100 mg q.i.d.) to prevent food allergic reactions, perhaps as high as 29% of cases treated (14^R, 15^R).

Tumor inducing effects These have not been reported.

ORGANS AND SYSTEMS

Cardiovascular A single case report of a woman developing peripheral eosinophilia and pericarditis with cardiac tamponade has been noted. Cellular and humoral sensitivity to cromolyn were demonstrated and the patient recovered following pericardiocentesis (SEDA-4, 120).

Respiratory Initial *bronchospasm* which is seen in some patients is thought to be due to the irritative effect of the powder. This type of bronchospasm can be prevented by prior inhalation of a β-adrenoceptor agonist aerosol. In one case-report a severe asthmatic reaction occurred and was thought to be reflexogenic in origin (SEDA-4, 120). A 1% nebulizer solution (20 mg cromolyn sodium dissolved in 2.5 ml distilled water and nebulized over a 15-minute period) has the same effect as the substance given by the use of the 'spinhaler' (16[c]). A randomized double-blind placebo-controlled cross-over study in children with chronic asthma showed that nebulized cromolyn sodium caused a reduction in forced mid-expiratory flow rate (between the 25th and 75th percentiles). The effect was equivalent to that seen with distilled water. It was concluded that inhalation of the *current hypotonic* solution may be hazardous (SEDA-17, 205). Bronchospasm and *breathlessness* as a result of hypersensitivity are rare, but do occur. A case of a 7-year-old asthmatic child sensitive to timothy grass in whom a single inhalation (following 1 week's treatment) caused cyanosis, hypotension and cardiopulmonary arrest has been reported. IgE involvement was demonstrated by passive transfer of the patient's serum to the mother producing positive results (17[c]). As indicated above, pulmonary infiltration and eosinophilia are other possible manifestations of hypersensitivity.

Intranasal use of cromoglycate can cause *sneezing* and *nasal congestion*. In a double-blind trial in hay fever patients, comparing flunisolide and cromolyn, both groups reported a large number of minor side effects. Of the 29 patients using cromolyn, 10 had nasal irritation, five swollen sore eyes and six sore throat. The authors indicate that the sensitive nasal mucosa may be very susceptible to irritation by any nasal spray (18[c]).

Nervous system *Headaches* have been referred to by most investigators. Dizziness has been reported, but may be connected with hyperventilation during the inhalation of the powder.

Liver Minor abnormalities of liver function have been described when the drug is used orally for ulcerative colitis (19[C]). A single case has been reported of a 45-year-old woman who developed liver disease, vasculitis and peripheral eosinophilia. Liver biopsy showed inflammatory changes with infiltration of eosinophils. Discontinuation of the medication markedly improved the symptoms (SEDA-4, 120).

Gastrointestinal *Nausea* can occur. A case of esophagitis following inhalation of cromolyn has been reported. This was much improved by prophylactic antacids before each inhalation (SEDA-5, 169). In a patient with lactose intolerance cromolyn sodium capsules with lactose produced nausea, bloating and flatulence while lactose free preparations produced no such symptoms (SEDA-13, 135).

Urinary system There is no evidence of renal toxicity. Premarketing evidence of renal arteriopathy in monkeys used in toxicity studies appears to have had no relevance to man.

Skin Skin reactions including *dermatitis* with pruritic symptoms have been reported. In addition, *urticaria* or *maculopapular rashes* may occur, but rarely.

Special senses The irritant effect of cromoglycate can induce *lacrimation* and some *inflammatory change in the eye*.

Musculoskeletal *Joint swelling and pain* have been reported and the USA Food and Drug Administration have issued a report (SEDA-7, 1) on a suspected case of cromolyn-induced systemic lupus erythematosus (SLE) syndrome. Six months therapy induced arthritis, positive LE cells and a positive antinuclear factor. After withdrawal of cromolyn, signs and symptoms regressed. Although this does not prove cause and effect, the report indicates similarity between SLE and some of the adverse reactions listed earlier in the USA data sheet (SEDA-3, 48).

Withdrawal effects True withdrawal reactions have not been described, but withdrawal of the drug can be dangerous, particularly where its introduction has made it possible to reduce the requirement for steroids. If suitable precautions are not taken, a very severe attack may follow withdrawal of cromolyn in this situation.

Second-generation effects The drug probably does not reach the fetus following inhalation as systemic blood levels are extremely low (20[c]). Animal testing gives no reason to anticipate that adverse effects involving the fetus would occur.

Interactions No interactions have been reported.

Nedocromil (Tilade)

Nedocromil sodium is classified as an antiallergic drug (12[R]). It is inhaled as a metered dose aerosol and is used prophylactically in asthma. In the laboratory, nedocromil has a greater potency than cromolyn for inhibiting lung mast-cell secretions, stabilizing neutrophils, eosinophils and platelets and it appears to affect nerve reflexes in the lung in a similar manner to cromolyn (12[R]). A number of clinical studies comparing inhaled nedocromil with cromolyn have failed to show any difference between the two drugs (21[R]). A more recent multicentre study was carried out in 132 patients requiring β_2-adrenoceptor agonists and inhaled steroids for treatment of asthma. Cromolyn was compared with nedocromil after a 50% reduction in steroid dosage. Both drugs caused significant symptomatic improvement compared to placebo, with nedocromil appearing more effective (22[C]). Nedocromil 2% ophthalmic solution was found to be as effective as cromolyn in allergic conjunctivitis and more effective in peak periods of pollen challenge (23[C]). 1552 patients were treated with 2% nedocromil eye drops and 5% noticed a distinct taste while, minor irritation was noted frequently just after application of the drops (24[R]).

Though less extensively used so far than cromolyn, nedocromil apparently has a similarly high degree of safety; nausea (3.8% of patients) and headaches (4.8%) are the most commonly observed side effects. These adverse effects are mild and tend to diminish during chronic therapy (SEDA-13, 135). Fourteen percent of patients report that nedocromil has a distinctive bitter taste (25[R]). Throat irritation is another frequent complaint with nedocromil therapy and less common side effects include tremor, chest tightness, yellow mucus and dizziness (SEDA-15, 2).

Nedocromil, 4 mg, four times daily, was examined in an open study of 55 patients over 12 months. No serious adverse effects were ascribed to the treatment. Eleven patients reported throat irritation which was usually mild and of short duration. Two patients were withdrawn because of this symptom (SEDA-12, 142).

Azelastine (E-0659) *(SEDA-13, 135)*

Azelastine is a phthalazinone compound with antiallergic and bronchodilator properties. It is available as a nasal spray and in oral form for the prophylactic treatment of allergic rhinitis and asthma as well as dermatoses. This drug can inhibit histamine release from mast cells and inhibit histamine- and leukotriene-mediated bronchospasm (26[C]). The kinetics of single doses of azelastine hydrochloride tablets were studied in normal volunteers. Dose linearity for C_{max} and $AUC_{0-\infty}$ was seen for doses of 2.2—17.6 mg, whereas t_{max} and terminal half life were not dose related and averaged 4.6 and 25.5 h, respectively. Overall tolerance was good and the therapeutic range was wide enough to recommend 4.4 mg b.i.d. or single doses of 8.8 mg azelastine hydrochloride per day in adults (27[C]). In 14 volunteers over 65 years in age, $t_{1/2}$ was significantly greater than in young volunteers, single dose 38.5 ± 15.3 vs 25.0 ± 5.2 h; multiple dose: 55.4 ± 24.9 vs 35.5 ± 16.3 h resulting in approximately twice as much accumulation in the elderly subjects. The N-demethylated metabolite is pharmacologically active and has an even longer half life which is relevant in chronic dosing (28[C]).

Azelastine has been shown to be effective against exercise-induced asthma and allergen challenge in patients with extrinsic asthma. Patients report there is a bitter taste, but overall there is a low incidence of side effects. In most studies, the frequency of fatigue and drowsiness was not significantly different from placebo. In an open trial in which 119 patients with various types of pruritic dermatosis were treated orally with azelastine, 27 patients reported mild side effects such as drowsiness (15 cases) and bitter aftertaste (six cases) and in four patients the treatment was discontinued because of side effects (SEDA-15, 2). The nasal spray was compared with budesonide in 193 patients with perennial allergic rhinitis. Efficacy was equivalent and both drugs were well tolerated. The most frequent complaint reported with azelastine was an 'unpleasant' taste or smell (29[C]).

Ketotifen (Zaditen) *(SEDA-7, 189)*

Ketotifen is an orally active antihistamine which blocks H_1-receptors, has mast cell stabilising properties, inhibits eosinophil accumulation in lungs of animals exposed to platelet-activating factor and reverses β-adrenoceptor tachyphylaxis (12[R]). It is classified, like cromolyn, as an antiallergic and is used long term in a prophylactic role. Its adverse effects are more typical of other antihistamines. There is some discussion about its efficacy, but a number of trials have suggested that it has a similar efficacy to that of cromolyn sodium (30[C]) and also has a small steroid sparing effect (31[C]). It is also more effective than placebo in the treatment of atopic dermatitis (32[C]). The normal therapeutic dose is 1—2 mg/day.

The most common side effects noted in long-term clinical trials have been sedation and weight gain (SEDA-7, 1). There is considerable controversy about the frequency of sedation and about its severity. In a study involving 1791 patients, with allergic paroxysmal asthma, somnolence occurred in 13%. This effect started early in treatment and wore off in more than one third of the patients (33[C]). In a smaller series, Clarke and May found that 10 of 35 patients complained of drowsiness while on ketotifen, although this was not severe enough to stop treatment; the same symptom was reported in five of the 10 patients when they were on cromolyn (30[C]).

Although sedation is initially common (e.g. 23% in one study), its incidence falls during the first 2 months to about 6%; only 2—3% of patients seem likely to discontinue therapy for this reason (34[C]). A rare side effect reported in one patient was drug-induced cystitis. The patient had never taken tranilast, and symptoms resolved on stopping the drug and recurred when the drug was restarted. Aseptic pyuria was found and cystoscopy revealed remarkable reddening over the urinary bladder (35[c]).

In 74 young children (average age 16 months) ketotifen was given in the form of a syrup at a dosage of 0.02—0.03 mg/kg body weight twice daily over a period of 12 weeks, the most frequently reported adverse effect (in 21 patients) was dry mouth. In six patients the mothers reported that their children had increased appetite (36[C]). In a series of 257 older children (average age 6 years and 8 months) increased weight was reported in 17, sedation in 13 and nausea in three (37[C]). However, an interim evaluation of post-marketing surveillance of ketotifen in the United Kingdom showed the percentage of adverse effects reported in children to be lower than in adults, sedation occurring in only 6% at the beginning of treatment; the corresponding figure in adults was 14.2% (38[R]).

In the United Kingdom, eight cases of overdose have been reported in which the patients took doses ranging from 10 to 120 mg. The plasma level after a therapeutic dose is 1—4 mg/l and the levels measured in four of the eight patients ranged from 5 to 122 mg/l. The symptoms of overdose were drowsiness, confusion, coma, dyspnea, bradycardia and tachycardia, hyperexcitability, convulsions and nystagmus. Six patients received gastric lavage and following supportive treatment all eight patients made a full recovery within 12 hours of admission (39[C]). Ketotifen produced seizures in a 5-year-old epileptic boy with allergic rhinitis. This was not specific to ketotifen but the result of H_1 receptor blockade and administration of *d*-chlorpheniramine increased the number of epileptic discharges seen on electroencephalography. It is recommended that centrally-acting H_1 antagonists should be avoided in epileptic patients, especially children (40[c]).

Respirinast

The anti-allergic drug respirinast was given to 56 asthmatic patients for 6 months. It was effective in 47% and moderately effective in 81%. Two patients complained of sleepiness but the drug was continued with or without reduction of dose (SEDA-17, 205).

Tranilast (Rizaben)

Tranilast is an orally active antiallergic agent. The mechanism of action may be analogous to that of cromolyn sodium, but reliable documentation is sparse.

Some patients taking tranilast have developed severe bladder symptoms which could not be relieved by antibiotic treatment (42[C]). The symptoms disappeared after discontinuation of the drug. In two patients, cystitis symptoms occurred as early as 11 and 18 days after the beginning of tranilast therapy (SEDA-12, 145). Bladder biopsy on six of eight patients with cystitis believed to be caused by tranilast showed an eosinophilic cystitis in three cases (SEDA-14, 139). A further three cases of eosinophilic cystitis have been reported. Biopsy in one case revealed eosinophilic cystitis. Symptoms ceased within 2 to 3 days after stopping the drug. Drug-induced lymphocytic stimulation showed that both tranilast and its major metabolite are causative agents (SEDA-17, 205).

A number of adverse reactions that may occur have been incidentally mentioned; they include liver function abnormalities, anorexia, nausea, vomiting, abdominal pain, decrease in the red blood cell count and hemoglobin, headache, drowsiness, insomnia, dizziness and general malaise.

Fenspiride (Pneumorel 80)

An overview of findings from 800 general practitioners in several thousand patients treated with this bronchodilator/anti-inflammatory drug in doses claimed to be effective noted mild adverse effects in 10%; they were not very specific (gastrointestinal, neurovegetative) (43[R]). The drug is poorly documented in the accessible literature.

DESENSITIZATION *(SEDA-7, 190)*

Controversy still exists about the efficacy and side effects of allergenic extracts used in desensitizing patients, particularly with bronchial asthma and rhinitis. Problems in assessing efficacy are due to the differences in the extracts used, variation in desensitization schedules, differing duration of therapy, and criteria for final assessment of therapeutic response. A meta analysis of 20 randomized placebo controlled double-blind trials of allergen immunotherapy for asthma has been reported. The mean effect for any allergen immunotherapy on all continuous outcomes was 0.71 (0.43—1) which would correspond to a mean rise in predicted FEV_1 of 7.1%. It was concluded that immunotherapy was a treatment option in highly selected patients with extrinsic allergic asthma where a clinically relevant and unavoidable allergen can be identified (44[C]).

The most obvious side effect is immediate anaphylactic sensitivity following administration of an extract. Adequate facilities for resuscitation including adrenaline injection should be available when an extract is given. The US Food and Drug Administration appointed a panel of experts to review this area of therapy in 1974. The panel concluded that extracts used in accordance with generally accepted principles are associated with a minimal and acceptable risk of immediate reaction. There is at present no evidence of any undesirable long-term adverse effect resulting from repeated courses of allergenic extracts, although non-allergic individuals may have hypersensitivity induced, particularly when they receive aluminum-containing extracts. It has been suggested that tyrosine-absorbed preparations with relatively short half-lives may be more dangerous in terms of immediate anaphylaxis. The alumpyridine preparation, Allpyral, has a long half-life and in the United Kingdom over 4 million injections have been given with no deaths reported. A report of 23 patients receiving specific freeze-dried insect venoms for *Hymenoptera* sensitivity is available. Systemic reactions occurred in three patients (13%). These reactions were all milder than the systemic reactions that the patients experienced when stung. A study of reactions to insect venoms during desensitization in 3236 individuals showed that most systemic reactions occurred during maintenance treatment at doses between 1 and 50 μg, and that wasp and honey bee venoms were most likely to cause reactions (SEDA-17, 206). In the meta analysis of allergen treatment of asthma, systemic reactions occurred in a mean of 32% (20—44%) of patients but anaphylaxis was only reported on four occasions (44[C]).

The Committee on Safety of Medicines reviewed the UK experience with desensitization in 1986, weighing efficacy against risk. They considered the evidence for efficacy and found it convincing for ragweed pollen, bee and wasp venoms and some antibiotics but thought the evidence for grass pollen and housedust mite less convincing. The Committee warned of the dangers of anaphylaxis and bronchospasm and noted that 26 patients had died since 1957, five in the preceding 18 months. With different products the risk of death varied from one in 8000 to one in 321 750 with no deaths recorded for some preparations. Anaphylaxis and bronchospasm occurred with all preparations, the incidence varying from one in 300 to one in 14 998. The Committee recommended that physicians carefully weigh the potential benefits against the known risks. Allergenic products should only be given where facilities for full cardiopulmonary resuscitation are immediately available and patients should be kept under medical observation for at least 2 hours after receiving an injection (45[R]). The Committee on Allergen Standardization of the American Academy of Allergy and Immunology investigated 46 fatalities that occurred during immunotherapy or skin testing since 1945 and remarked that the nature and severity of the initial symptoms did not appear to predict the fatal outcome or indicate the cause of death (SEDA-13, 136). In the 5 years from 1985 to 1989, 17 deaths due to allergen immunotherapy were reported. None occurred with skin testing. Sixteen deaths were in asthmatic patients. Unstable asthma or accidental overdose were major contributory factors. The annual fatality rate in the United States from administration of allergenic extracts remains low at one fatality per 2 million doses (46[R]). In 419 patients treated with aluminum hydroxide adsorbed extracts of grass pollen or house dust mite, local reactions occurred in 10.5% and systemic reactions in 4.8% (47[C]). A survey of 27 806 injection visits noted 143 (0.51%) systemic reactions. Of these 83% were mild and 17% (i.e. five reactions) needed adrenaline treatment (48[C]).

The Canadian Society of Allergy and Clinical Immunology have published guidelines for the use of allergen immunotherapy and these are similar to others being developed by the American Academy of Allergy, Asthma and Immunology. They recommend therapy with specific, standardized allergenic materials, administered in high dose schedules, to patients with allergy to insect stings or allergic rhinoconjunctivitis, and in some patients with asthma. The latter should be correctly diagnosed by a meticulous history, confirmed by positive skin tests and be insufficiently controlled by allergen avoidance and appropriate drug treatment (49[R]).

INHALANTS AND AEROSOLS FOR ASTHMA

OLDER ATROPINE-LIKE AGENTS

Stramonium

Asthma cigarettes, asthma pipe mixture or powder burnt like incense represent the oldest type of inhalation used in the treatment of bronchial asthma. A typical preparation contains stramonium 50%, potassium nitrate 25% (to facilitate the burning) and *Grindelia* or tobacco to make up the desired bulk. Stramonium, like belladonna, contains the alkaloids, scopolamine and atropine. Side effects seen following administration of this type of medication are irritation and drying of the mouth and trachea.

When taken orally, stramonium powder can produce hallucinations which may also occur after excessive smoking of asthma cigarettes. Abuse leads to hallucination and disorientation in a high percentage of cases. Other symptoms occur which would be anticipated from the components, viz. amnesia, anxiety, paranoia, hyperactivity and aggression, ataxia, dryness of skin and mucous membranes, flush, fever and tachycardia. The dilated pupils which are often present can be helpful in the diagnosis. There is no longer any real need for stramonium preparations in the treatment of asthma, as atropine and ipratropium provide adequate antimuscarinic therapy when this approach to asthma is needed.

ATROPINE-LIKE INHALATIONS *(see also Chapter 13)*

Three muscarinic receptor subtypes have been demonstrated in airways: M_1 receptors (which are excitatory on airway ganglia); M_2 receptors (which inhibit acetylcholine release at cholinergic nerve terminals); and M_3 receptors (which mediate contraction of airway smooth muscle) (50[R]). Antimuscarinics such as atropine and ipratropium have equal affinity for the different muscarinic receptor subtypes and thus may increase the amounts of acetylcholine released from cholinergic nerve terminals resulting in postjunctional muscarinic blockade being overcome to some extent. It may be advantageous to introduce antimuscarinic drugs clinically that are selective for M_3 receptors (50[R]).

Atropine

Atropine administered by aerosol will exert some selective effect on the airways because of the low systemic absorption. Side effects seen will be those of atropine and atropine-like drugs but systemic effects are unlikely after topical administration. In a child suffering regular akinetic seizures atropine sulfate eye drops increased the frequency of fits (51[c]). Two patients have been reported who developed the signs and symptoms of angle closure glaucoma after receiving aerosolized atropine. Patients with shallow anterior chambers or possible prior angle closure glaucoma are probably at greater risk (52[c]). Atropine methyl nitrate, a quaternary ammonium derivative, may be somewhat more selective than atropine sulfate because it is less readily absorbed.

Ipratropium hydrobromide (Atrovent; *N*-isopropylnortropine tropic ester methylbromide)

Ipratropium hydrobromide is a quaternary amine, which has low lipid solubility and is poorly absorbed. This limited bioavailability would account for relative bronchial selectivity when given in low doses by the aerosol route. In normal volunteers, 0.12–0.28 mg i.v. decreased salivary secretion and increased heart rate, but inhaled doses up to a total of 1.2 mg had no significant effects on heart rate, although some patients reported dryness of the mouth (53[R]). The drug appears to have established a place in the therapy of asthma as an alternative to β-adrenoceptor agonist aerosols in patients who fail to respond adequately to these agents. It is usually not possible to predict which patients will respond well and therefore use of the drug has been suggested in patients not responding adequately to β-adrenoceptor agonists. Ipratropium may be somewhat more effective than β-adrenoceptor agonists in patients with non-atopic asthma and chronic bronchitis. The drug has been reported to augment the effects of β_2-adrenoceptor-agonists when given by nebulized inhalation in acute asthma (54[R]). A nasal spray (isotonic aqueous iptatropium pump) has been used in allergic and non-allergic rhinitis as well as the common cold. In perennial non-allergic rhinitis 233 patients experienced a 30% reduction in rhinorrhea as compared to a saline placebo. Both treatments caused a modest reduction in post nasal drip, sneezing and congestion attributable to the saline solution. There was a reduction in interference with daily activities and mood. There was no nasal rebound after treatment stopped, no systemic side effects and minor infrequent episodes of nasal dryness and epistaxis which did not limit treatment (55[C]). Sixty-three patients with perennial allergic rhinitis were treated for 1 year with the nasal spray with similar results (56[C]). In patients with the common cold the spray significantly reduced rhinorrhea, 82 μg per nostril dose was better than 42 μg and almost as good as 168 μg per nostril but with fewer adverse effects none of which were serious (57[C]).

The drug has been well tolerated in most studies. Usual inhaled doses appear to be free of important systemic side effects, no doubt as a result of the very low blood concentration achieved by this mode of administration. Transient dryness of the mouth and scratching in the trachea have been reported by some patients and can occur in up to 25% of patients receiving wet nebulizer treatment with the drug. A bad taste in the mouth has also been reported by 20–30% of patients. Systemic anticholinergic effects do not usually occur with the normal inhaled dose (53[R]). The normal contraindications for atropine-like drugs should be observed. A case report of angle-closure glaucoma precipitated by the drug has been made. This patient was given the drug in a wet nebulizer solution over a 3-day period and angle-closure glaucoma was precipitated. The authors pointed out that the complication may occur when the drug is given as a nebulizer since droplets of the solution could enter the eye, particularly with an ill-fitting mask (58[c]). This effect has now been reported in one patient after ipratropium given by metered-dose inhaler (59[c]). Thirty children were systematically studied to evaluate the risk of this side effect. Before and 30 minutes after nebulized drug intraocular pressures, pupillary size and pupillary responses were measured and no changes occurred. It was concluded that in asthmatic children with no pre-existing ocular abnormalities the risk of an ocular adverse effect from nebulized ipratropium is extremely small (60[C]). A case report of urinary retention caused by nebulized drug which resolved after stopping the drug was reported in a 69-year-old man. This is a rare complication and as all the cases described in the literature have been elderly men with prostatic hypertrophy, the drug should be used cautiously in this group (61[cr]). Concern has been expressed that ipratropium and other antimuscarinics may cause drying and inspissation of sputum. In vitro studies show no effect on ciliary activity. In normal subjects and in patients with chronic bronchitis, inhaled ipratropium did not affect the rate of tracheobronchial clearance of a previously inhaled radioactive carrier; in studies using therapeutic doses for 2—14 days sputum volume and viscosity remained unaltered (53[R]).

SYMPATHOMIMETICS AND PROPELLANTS *(see also Chapter 13)*

Sympathomimetics are extensively used in the form of aerosols: originally these were hand-pumped, but in recent years pressurized aerosols using Freon (chloro-fluorocarbons) propellants have become widely used. In addition, the drugs may be given by various types of wet nebulizer.

Adverse reactions to sympathomimetic drugs are referred to in Chapter 13. The risk of the propellant Freon gases is the subject of some controversy. In animal studies, plasma levels of Freon 11 and Freon 12 of 20—35 mg/l were shown to sensitize the heart to adrenaline and exercise. In a clinical study where severely-ill asthmatic subjects (mean oxygen tension, 55 mmHg, range 50—80) were studied following therapeutic doses of aerosol, plasma levels of Freon 11 up to 4.53 mg/l and of Freon 12 up to 4.73 mg/l were measured after two inhalations. The authors concluded that a toxic level could only be reached if the aerosol was taken on every breath for over 12 consecutive breaths (62[C]).

Other constituents are present in these aerosols in addition to the propellant gases. The effects of some of these were investigated in 11 850 asthmatic patients. Three aerosols were compared. Two different placebo metered-dose inhalers contained the same freons but different dispersant chemicals, one oleic acid (MDI-OA) and the other lecithin NF (MDI-L), the third contained salmeterol xinafoate (25 μg) and lecithin NF (MDI-S). Peak expiratory flow was measured before and 5 min after inhalation, a 20% fall in PEF was defined as clinically significant bronchoconstriction. Overall, 180 (1.5%) patients developed bronchoconstriction, 43 in the MDI-S group, 67 in the MDI-L group and 70 in the MDI-OA group. Thus bronchoconstriction was significantly less with the salmeterol aerosol. It was suggested that one of the inert constituents currently present in metered-dose aerosols is the likely irritant causing occasional acute bronchoconstriction, the risk of which increased with age and decreasing pretreatment PEF (63[C]).

Because of the proposed international ban on freons (chloro-fluorocarbons), due to their effect on the ozone layer, non-chlorinated propellants are being trialled in asthma metered-dose aerosols. Salmeterol has been reformulated with such a propellant, HFA134a. This aerosol was compared with a placebo containing only HFA134a in 12 healthy volunteers. The new inhaler showed no differences from the current salmeterol inhaler for pulse rate, blood pressure, tremor, QTc interval and plasma glucose levels and had significantly less effect on plasma potassium levels. It was concluded that in healthy volunteers the new salmeterol inhaler is at least as safe and well tolerated as the current one and has similar pharmacodynamic activity (64[C]).

In a further study salbutamol in a conventional chloro-fluorocarbon propellant system (Ventolin, CFC-11/12) was compared with salbutamol in a novel CFC free (HFA-134a) system (Airomir in the 3M CFC-Free System). The two aerosols were compared in 26 patients with chronic stable asthma. The bronchodilator effects of the two preparations were significant and equivalent and there were no clinically meaningful differences in the safety parameters measured (65[C]).

An increase in sudden deaths among asthmatic patients using aerosol therapy was noted in the United Kingdom in the 1960s. A number of reasons were advanced to explain this, including toxicity of β-adrenoceptor agonists or even the propellant gases. A number of authors, however, feel that the major reason for the rise in deaths was too great a reliance on β-adrenoceptor agonist aerosols leading to neglect of other measures which are required to prevent deterioration in a severely-ill asthmatic patient (66[R]).

A further 'epidemic' was reported in New Zealand in the early 1980s. This was attributed to the use of the inhaled β_2-adrenoceptor agonist fenoterol (67[CR]). A Canadian study showed an increased risk of death or near death from asthma associated with β-adrenoceptor agonist use. The risk was greater for fenoterol than albuterol but when the doses were corrected to allow for the higher dose per puff in the fenoterol aerosol there was no difference between the two drugs. The authors concluded that regular use of any inhaled β-adrenoceptor agonist was associated with an increased risk of death or near death. It was not possible to decide if the association was due to direct adverse effects of the drugs or whether increased drug use indicated more severe asthma. However it was concluded that heavy use of these drugs should alert clinicians to the need for urgent re-evaluation of the patient (68[CR]). There is general agreement that the increased use of β_2-adrenoceptor agonists should result in urgent action and it remains possible that very high doses could cause adverse effects in severe asthma (67[CR]).

In hospitals, it is common to give bronchodilators and other therapeutic agents from wet nebulization inhalation devices. Inhalation of distilled water will cause bronchoconstriction in 60% of infants with a history of wheeze (SEDA-17, 212).

In addition, if nebulizer solutions are hypotonic, hypertonic or contain preservative (such as benzalkonium chloride, edetic acid, sulfites and metabisulfite) they may cause paradoxical bronchoconstriction. A *Lancet* editorial concluded that all nebulizer solutions should be isotonic and preservative free (SEDA-13, 132).

Nebulizer therapy also carries the risk of contamination of the airways with hospital bacterial flora. The heavier the environmental contamination, the greater the risk. Flora carried by the aerosol will closely resemble those of the room where the appliance has been handled (SEDA-2, 154).

CORTICOSTEROIDS

Adverse reactions to corticosteroids are reviewed in Chapter 39. The orally active corticosteroids (hydrocortisone, prednisolone, dexamethasone) have all been given in the form of aerosols in the hope of attaining a local effect on the airways with minimal systemic absorption of the drug and hence fewer systemic side effects.

The dose of steroid needed to produce a therapeutic effect in the patient when an aerosol is used is similar to that needed when the same drug is given by other routes. As the majority of an aerosol is swallowed, oral therapy is being given. This situation has changed with the development of topically active steroid aerosols. These have high local activity and low bioavailability when swallowed. All of them are steroid esters, i.e. a combination of a steroid alcohol with an acid, e.g. beclomethasone combined with propionic acid to form beclomethasone dipropionate. Due to the high local activity and reduced bioavailability of the swallowed fraction, a selective effect is obtained. There are local side effects due to deposition of relatively high concentrations in the oro-pharynx and upper airways.

If sufficient is taken, enough is absorbed after swallowing to produce the systemic side effects associated with oral steroids. Inhaled steroids work best after several days and their major therapeutic effect is to suppress airway inflammation. Because of the delay in onset of effect patients may not persist with them and if they stop the loss of effect is also gradual and so patient education is essential if patients are to achieve the maximum benefit from this very effective therapy.

When a patient is switched from oral or parenteral therapy to inhalation therapy, this should be considered as systemic dose reduction and appropriate precautions taken. In particular, if the asthma deteriorates suddenly, the aerosol may no longer be effective, as there will be very poor penetration in a severe attack. Thus, one of the greatest risks of this therapy may be death from asthma in an exacerbation if systemic steroids are not immediately restarted. If any degree of adrenal suppression exists following cessation of oral steroids, it will not be counteracted by an aerosol steroid.

Administration of potent corticosteroids in high local dose may increase the risk of local fungus infection and perhaps atrophy of the mucosa. The latter is a theoretical risk which has not been demonstrated in practice, but an increased presence of oropharyngeal *Candida albicans* has been reported by several groups. The incidence varied greatly depending on the patients studied and the method of detection, ranging from 13% to as much as 71% with the use of a daily dose up to 800 μg. The condition rarely requires treatment or cessation of the drug. Local measures such as gargling immediately following inhalation of the aerosol may be effective in reducing the incidence of this complication.

Candidiasis may result in dysphonia, but one report suggests a local myopathy caused by inhaled steroids can also cause dysphonia. Nine of 14 asthmatic patients with persistent dysphonia while taking inhaled corticosteroids had a bilateral adductor vocal cord deformity causing the dysphonia. The effect was related to the dose and potency of the inhaled steroid and was reversed when the steroid was stopped, although recovery could take weeks to occur. Candidiasis may have contributed in two out of nine patients. In nine patients started on a steroid aerosol and examined at monthly intervals, three developed a vocal cord deformity but only one had persistent dysphonia (69[C]).

Beclomethasone dipropionate

There are now three preparations available; 50 μg per puff, 100 μg per puff and 250 μg per puff. It is important that the dose is titrated to the patient's needs as it is easy to overdose with the stronger preparations and induce systemic side effects. Guidelines, such as those issued by the British Thoracic Society, recommend that stepwise increments in inhaled steroid are titrated against parameters of disease activity and that the dose is then gradually lowered to achieve an individualized maintenance dose (SEDA-17, 4). In our experience practitioners are not aware of the doses available and tend to start patients on the 250 μg aerosol thus exceeding a daily dose of 1 mg (1000 μg) after four puffs. Doses above 1 mg per day have an increased likelihood of systemic side effects. Of particular concern recently has been the possibility of impaired growth in children. This is difficult to investigate as poorly controlled asthma can also lead to impaired growth. In 94 children aged 7—9 years, beclomethasone dipropionate (BDP) 400 μg per day was given for 7 months in a double-blind placebo-controlled trial. The BDP-treated children grew significantly less than the children on placebo, mean 2.66 vs 3.66 cm. During a wash-out period of 4 months there was no significant catch up growth (70[C]). In adults significant adrenal suppression can occur at a daily dose of 1.5 mg or six puffs per day of high strength BDP (71[C]). In another series, 100 adults were treated for 3 months with BDP 1.5—2.0 mg (1500—2000 μg) per day. There was mild suppression of the hypothalamo-pituitary-adrenal axis and 8% of patients complained of dysphonia. Twenty-five percent suffered from oropharyngeal candidiasis (72[C]). Two hundred and two respiratory patients using inhaled steroids were compared with 204 patients not on inhaled steroids. The patients on steroids reported easy bruising. The patients with bruising tended to be older (61 vs 52 years), on higher daily doses (1388 vs 1067 μg) and had been on treatment longer (55 vs 43 months) (73[C]). The efficacy of inhaled steroids can be increased by the use of a spacer device, or other devices such as the 'Diskhaler', 'Nebuhaler' or 'Turbohaler' which will reduce oropharyngeal deposition, increase the lung dose and lower the total body dose hence increasing the efficacy and reducing the risk of systemic side effects. Although individual patients vary in their dose requirements, if a spacer is used to optimize lung dose, higher doses give little additional therapeutic effect. In 143 severe steroid-dependent asthmatics high dose, 1500 μg/day of BDP, was compared with low dose, 300 μg/day. There was no difference in efficacy between the two regimes as assessed by reduction in systemic steroids, PEF readings, asthma symptoms and use of on-demand β-adrenoceptor agonist aerosols (74[C]).

Budesonide

Budesonide, like BDP, is a corticosteroid with high topical potency (75[R]). It is available in three strengths 50, 200 and 400 μg per puff. It is used in the treatment of asthma and allergic rhinitis. Side effects are similar to those reported with beclomethasone dipropionate. In 38 steroid dependent patients, a dose-dependent effect was seen between 200 and 1600 μg per day. Four patients were eventually able to decrease the inhaled dose of budesonide when asthma control was optimal. Ten patients reported hoarseness and sore throat (76[C]). In a double-blind study of two parallel groups of 15 allergic asthmatics, the patients were treated with either 200 or 800 μg of inhaled budesonide per day and it was demonstrated that bronchial hyperreactivity was reduced in a dose-dependent manner and bronchial hyperreactivity improved with longer duration of treatment (77[R]). Two cases of psychic disturbances have been reported with inhaled budesonide (SEDA-13, 356).

Fluticasone propionate

This is another topically active steroid which it was hoped would have greater potency in the lung, compared to its predecessors, resulting in a more favourable therapeutic ratio. It is available as a pressurized aerosol, 250 μg per puff, and powder for inhalation as 'Diskhaler' containing 500 μg per puff. In a study 585 patients with moderate asthma and receiving 400—1000 μg inhaled steroid daily were treated for 6 weeks in a double-blind study comparing fluticasone propionate 500 μg daily by either pressurized aerosol or Diskhaler, and beclomethasone dipropionate 1000 μg daily by pressurized aerosol. It was concluded that fluticasonate propionate 500 μg (by pressurized aerosol or Diskhaler) was equivalent to 1000 μg of beclomethasone dipropionate in the treatment of moderate asthma. Adverse events were equivalent with either drug (59 and 63% with fluticasone and beclomethasone dipropionate, respectively) leading to 11% of patients withdrawing in each group (SEDA-17, 4). In perennial rhinitis 251 patients were studied for 1 year and were treated with either 200 μg fluticasone propionate aqueous spray daily or beclomethasone dipropionate 250 μg aqueous spray twice daily. There was no clinically significant difference between the two treatments and they were equally well tolerated (SEDA-17, 4).

We believe inhaled steroids are a highly effective

treatment in asthma. Local side effects due to deposition of high local concentrations can be reduced by various devices such as the spacer which increase lung dose and reduce deposition in the oro-pharynx. These should also help to reduce the chances of systemic side effects although there are no long-term trials which show this. There is considerable discussion about the dose above which systemic side effects will occur and there are variables such as efficiency of inhalation and use of spacer devices. For beclomethasone dipropionate and budesonide, systemic side effects probably start in the dose range 800—1600 μg per day, and in children 400-800 μg per day, while the equivalent doses for fluticasone propionate would be approximately 50% of these. Large multicentre studies are needed to evaluate the long-term use of varying doses of inhaled steroids. The major danger of sudden cessation is more likely to be a serious flare-up of asthma than adrenal insufficiency.

EXPECTORANT AND MUCOLYTIC DRUGS

IODINES AND IODIDES (*see also Chapter* 41)

Iodine, mainly in the form of potassium iodide, has been widely used in asthma and chronic bronchitis as an expectorant. There is considerable controversy about its efficacy. It should not be used in adolescent patients because of its potential to aggravate and induce acne and its effect on the thyroid gland; indeed, in view of its doubtful effectiveness and definite toxicity, our recommendation is that physicians should cease prescribing it as an expectorant.

Allergic reactions Allergy to iodide may occur with fever, general malaise, diffuse myalgia, rash and lymphadenopathy. In addition, arthritis has been reported as has angio-edema. Occasionally, after a high dose of iodine, sudden swelling of the partoid and submandibular glands can be seen. This is thought to be a hypersensitivity reaction due to formation of a complex between iodides and plasma proteins.

Cardiovascular system Arrhythmias have been seen after accidental ingestion of a large amount of potassium iodide solution. A case has been described in which administration of iodide was associated with pulmonary edema and ioderma of the skin (SEDA-7, 190).

Endocrine system Estimations of protein-bound iodine and tracer studies for the estimation of thyroid function are interfered with by the use of iodine-containing compounds.

In a number of patients, iodine-induced hypothyroidism has been described as the result of prolonged intake. It may be that patients with an underlying disorder of the thyroid gland are predisposed to this complication.

Urinary system A very rare side effect is hypersensitivity causing acute nephropathy.

Skin Induction and aggravation of acne is a typical reaction to iodide. The more serious skin condition, ioderma, starts with an acneiform lesion, localised in the area of the sebaceous glands which spreads to form verrucous granulomatous lesions. After discontinuation of iodide, the skin clears over a few weeks. It is thought that ioderma is an allergic hypersensitivity. In addition to this typical picture of iodide sensitivity, iodide can cause different types of skin reactions: urticaria, erythema and even hemorrhagic rashes have been described. In order to be sure of the etiology of the skin conditions in certain cases, sensitivity testing may be required, but this is not without risk.

Teratogenic effects The regular use of iodide during pregnancy may cause development of a goiter in the fetus. The size of the goiter in the child can be large enough to cause difficulties during delivery.

MUCOLYTIC AGENTS

Mucolytic agents have often been marketed after only cursory clinical work has been done, throwing little real light either on their supposed efficacy or on their safety. Like antitussive agents (see below) some are probably quite without effect in the clinical situation, whatever their properties in vitro.

N-Acetylcysteine

This compound acts as a mucolytic by splitting disulfide bonds in mucoproteins to lower mucus viscosity. As with other mucolytic agents, a larger volume of sputum may be produced following its administration. It is normally administered by inhalation as a nebulized solution or aerosol, although it can also be prescribed in an oral form. Oral administration introduces the possibility of interaction, e.g. interference with absorption of drugs, including antibiotics.

As a 5% solution for inhalation, it almost completely inactivates penicillin and cephalosporins in vitro and the activity of tetracycline is somewhat reduced. Aerosol therapy with *N*-acetylcysteine is often stated to be free from side effects, but a degree of bronchoconstriction has been reported following administration of the aerosol. In a series of 31 ambulant asthmatics using 10% *N*-acetylcysteine solution, there was a mean reduction of 55% in the FEV_1 in 19 of the subjects. The addition of 0.05% isoprenaline lowered the number of patients from 19 to five (SEDA-5, 170). In two placebo-controlled studies with over 700 patients, there was no difference in side effects between oral acetylcysteine and a placebo (SEDA-6, 171) (78[C]), but there was no improvement in FEV_1 in these studies.

The compound is used intravenously as an antidote for severe paracetamol poisoning. Hypersensitivity reactions have been reported in this situation, a generalized erythematous rash may develop, and complaints of itching, nausea, vomiting, dizziness and severe breathlessness with bronchospasm and tachycardia have been reported (SEDA-5, 170). Other features reported included angio-edema, hypotension and bronchospasm (79[C]). Wheal responses to high concentrations of *N*-acetylcysteine (20 mg/ml) were significantly greater in reactors. In two patients with a positive reaction the effects could be inhibited by prior therapy with an antihistamine. As hypersensitivity reactions have been reported in up to 3% of patients receiving intravenous *N*-acetylcysteine for paracetamol overdose, it has been emphasized that physicians need to prepare for these reactions and consider the use of antihistamines for their treatment (80[cr]). A pseudo-allergic reaction on the basis of histamine liberation rather than an immunological etiology is suggested as the mechanism (81[C], 82[c], 83[c]).

Bromhexine hydrochloride (Bisolvon)

This compound can be administered orally and absorbed from the gastrointestinal tract. There has been some controversy about the clinical significance of its effects on sputum viscosity measured in vitro. It has been reported to increase the concentration of amoxycillin in sputum (SEDA-17, 208) and promote the diffusion of antibiotics into lung tissue (84[R]). Because it may cause gastrointestinal tolerance and possibly impair the mucous barrier in the stomach, it has been suggested it should not be given to patients with gastric ulceration. Reactivation of intestinal ulcers certainly can occur, but has only been described in a few patients. No hematemesis, melena or other complications appear to have been described (85[R]). Following oral administration of the drug, nausea and transient increases in serum transaminases have been occasionally reported.

Administration of the drug by inhalation aerosol or nasal spray produces a local expectorant-mucolytic action (84[R]). A study of 21 patients indicated that inhaled bromhexine (Paxirasol) reduced the amount of sputum, but did not reduce symptoms noticeably (SEDA-17, 208). There was no evidence for hemopoietic or liver damage.

Carbocysteine

Carbocysteine is administered orally or from a metered dose inhaler as a mucolytic. Side effects include headache, nausea, vomiting, gastric discomfort and bleeding, diarrhea and skin rash. It has been shown to be an effective mucolytic which is generally well tolerated with few side effects (SEDA-17, 208).

Letosteine (Viscotiol) *(SEDA-5, 170: SEDA-7, 191)*

Letosteine is taken orally to loosen bronchial secretions and facilitate expectoration. In 37 patients, two experienced gastralgia and vomiting, severe enough to stop therapy (SEDA-7, 191). In a further series of 40 patients, five patients also experienced gastralgia and nausea requiring cessation of therapy in three.

Mesna (Mistabron, sodium mercaptoethanesulfonate)

Mesna is used mainly to prevent or ameliorate hemorrhagic cystitis produced by the anticancer drugs cyclophosphamide and ifosfamide, but it can be administered as a mucolytic. Like other mucolytics, this drug is used to liquefy sputum and facilitate expectoration. In a few cases, a so-called bronchorrhea has been described which may be the result of mucolysis, but could also be caused by stimulation of bronchial secretions. Application by aerosol or nebulizer is occasionally followed by bronchospasm, but the compound is usually well tolerated by asthmatic subjects. The other side effect which has been documented is a skin rash which occurs very rarely.

Sfericase

Sfericase is a crystallised alkaline protease showing ability to breakdown various protein bases; it is given in enterolytic tablets containing 10 000 units of sfericase. One is bound to wonder whether such a protease can be absorbed from the intestine. When sfericase was prescribed at a dosage of two tablets 3 times daily to 73 patients with chronic respiratory diseases, no significant side effects were observed (86[c]).

Other expectorants

A number of compounds such as creosote, ammonium chloride, squill and ipecacuanha are traditional ingredients with an expectorant property in cough mixtures. The dosage used in cough mixtures is unlikely to cause problems and in the event of overdosage will lead to vomiting prior to toxicity occurring.

ANTITUSSIVE AGENTS

Many patients with varying types of respiratory disorders cough. Treatment is aimed at suppressing the cough reflex itself or countering factors which trigger it, or may be given to relieve the subjective discomfort. The agents used commonly have been designed and developed to suppress the mechanism of coughing and this can have undesirable consequences. It may indeed be fortunate that many so-called antitussives are not effective, at least in the doses usually employed.

Cough is essentially a protective reflex, its purpose being to expel, from the upper airways, material which may obstruct breathing. If the primary treatment of the disorder does not result in the disappearance or liquefaction of this material, it is necessary for the patient to continue to cough. He should be advised to do so at intervals to clear his airways. Thus, to a certain extent, cough has a physiological function. Even in subjects with no pathological disorder, cough occurs at intervals, since coughing and the activity of the ciliary escalator complement one another in disposing of approximately 100 ml of secretion which is estimated to be produced daily by the mucosa of the trachea and bronchi. An antitussive agent which also suppresses ciliary action therefore induces a double risk.

Nevertheless, the physician is faced with patients who cough persistently and unproductively and demand relief. This may involve the use of centrally acting antitussives. These agents should be used in effective doses only if there is little or no sputum, otherwise there is a definite risk of sputum retention and resulting pneumonia. Suppression of cough is particularly dangerous in patients with chronic bronchitis and impaired carbon dioxide sensitivity.

An ideal antitussive would reduce the frequency of cough and render it less distressing but leave the cough reflex unimpaired. **Codeine** in lower doses appears to help patients, whilst not greatly affecting the central control of ventilation.

Dextromethorphan is a non-narcotic agent which seems to suppress cough but not greatly impair ciliary activity. This property is also found in **noscapine**.

Many so-called antitussive agents have never been shown to suppress the cough reflex. Some may be mere placebos (which would explain their absence of adverse effects), whereas others, like small doses of opiates, may alleviate the distress of cough in an ill-defined manner which is appreciated by the patient subjectively but where objective measurements show that cough has not been diminished.

Although generally safe dextromethorphan can cause CNS side effects including hyperexcitability, increased muscle tone and ataxia. Respiratory depression can occur with excessive doses. Intentional dextromethorphan overdose has been reported to cause two deaths (SEDA-17, 210).

Particular caution is necessary in treating patients in whom the central depressant effects of an effective antitussive agent may be markedly potentiated by other agents being given. Caution is also necessary in the debilitated and in patients confined to the supine position. Another problem in the elderly and debilitated is the constipating effects of drugs like codeine, which may result in the administration of laxatives to an already debilitated patient.

In addition, great care should be taken in using centrally active agents in children. A specific cause for cough can usually be found in a child, and if it needs to be treated, a bland sugar-based cough syrup is safe and soothing and has a useful placebo effect where acute cough may be only due to a cold.

Various ingredients not mentioned above may be found in over-the-counter and prescribed cough remedies:

Alcohol This can induce central depression or even addiction to the product, as up to 40% alcohol can be present in some cough mixtures. Pregnant or nursing mothers and patients on disulfiram should be advised to avoid cough mixtures containing alcohol.

Ammonium chloride This can cause acidosis and hypokalemia in large doses.

Antihistamines and anticholinergic agents These can, in larger doses, inhibit secretion of the bronchial glands and also will cause central depression.

Azipranone (RU-20201) This is a cough suppressant claimed to have effects comparable to those of codeine. Some very limited evidence suggests that its side effects are similar to those of placebo (SEDA-9, 157).

Benzocaine This can cause allergic reactions or sensitize a patient. It should not be given to patients with a known hypersensitivity to para-aminobenzoic acid.

Clofedanol This is a centrally acting cough suppressant with mild local anesthetic properties. In an open clinical study 30 patients were treated with the agent for a period of 14 days in the recommended dose. Two patients were withdrawn from the study because of tiredness and vomiting. These side effects disappeared immediately after interruption of the therapy (87[c]).

Eprazinone, eprozinol, zipeprol A retrospective study of the cases of eprazinone, eprozinol and zipeprol intoxication collected at the Poison Control Center in Paris from 1975 to 1982 noted 199 cases of accidental or intentional acute poisoning. In seven cases, seizures were observed. They resolved rapidly and without recurrence under symptomatic treatment. The seizures were observed at 8 times the therapeutic dose (88[C]). Abuse to zipeprol can become a problem (SEDA-17, 211).

Glaucine This is a non-narcotic antitussive agent. The D-isomer of glaucine is an alkaloid from *Glaucium flavum* Crantz, a species of Papaveraceae. Glaucine was compared with codeine in a double-blind trial in 90 patients. In doses claimed to be equieffective with codeine, it is claimed to be better tolerated, but in an open trial with glaucine (30 mg capsules 3 times daily for 28 days) mild constipation was reported by five patients (89[c]).

Iodide This is toxic for certain patients and can cause allergic reactions in others.

Licorice A number of preparations contain enough licorice to cause water and salt retention in susceptible people because of the mineralocorticoid-like property. Headache is another side effect of this agent.

Noscapine (narcotine) This is an alkaloid from the poppy which does not possess much analgesic or sedative effect. It is thought to be capable of modifying cough, although, as with other antitussives, it is difficult to say whether cough is genuinely suppressed or merely better tolerated. Headache and drowsiness can occur in a minority of patients and skin rash has been reported rarely.

In vitro work indicates that noscapine can produce spindle inhibition and polyploidy suggesting it may be genotoxic or carcinogenic (SEDA-17, 210). Its danger to humans when used as a cough mixture remains to be established. Nevertheless, as there are alternative drugs we recommend that noscapine should be avoided in women of child-bearing potential.

Opiates These can cause central depression and addiction.

Oxolamine (Bredon) This is a structurally unusual substance which has been in use in some European countries for rather more than two decades for the treatment of cough. Quite early in its use there were ill-defined reports that a substance related to oxolamine (perhaps the mild analgesic benzydamine) was being misused, together with alcohol, as a hallucinogen. Gradually, enough evidence has accumulated from several countries to make it quite clear that oxolamine can cause hallucinations in young children, including those without fever (90[C], 91[R]). Some cases have been confirmed by rechallenge. Hallucinations due to oxolamine tended to be reported in children under 10 years of age rather than older children or adults (91[R]).

Sugar It is often forgotten that the amount of sugar in a cough mixture may be responsible for complications in a diabetic patient. The use of sugar-containing mixtures, particularly at bedtime, over a long period may promote dental caries, particularly in children. This effect is enhanced if drugs which depress salivation such as antihistamines are also present. It is most important that the teeth are brushed immediately after taking such mixtures.

Sympathomimetics These can cause a number of side effects (see Chapter 13)

MISCELLANEOUS PRODUCTS

Camphor, menthol and eucalyptus These are often found as constituents of cold remedies in the form of ointments designed to be rubbed onto the chest or applied around and even into the nostrils (Vicks Vaporub, Obat Macjan, etc.). Locally, they serve as rubefacients and counterirritants, but substantial concentrations of volatile oil can be inhaled from them. In young children, menthol can induce reflex apnea or laryngospasm and application of the compound to the nostrils can result in instant collapse. Hypersensitivity reactions to menthol are well recognized and comprise urticaria and flushing. Twelve cases of contact sensitivity to the flavoring agents menthol and peppermint oil were reported in patients presenting with intra-oral symptoms in association with burning mouth syndrome, recurrent oral ulceration or a lichenoid reaction (92[C]). In the five patients with burning mouth syndrome, one was sensitive to both agents, three were sensitive to menthol only and one was sensitive to peppermint only. The four cases with recurrent intra-oral ulceration were sensitive to both menthol and peppermint. The three patients with an oral lichenoid reaction were positive to menthol with two also sensitive to peppermint. Of the nine patients who could be contacted afterwards, six described clearance or improvement of their symptoms as a result of avoidance of menthol/peppermint. Overdose of menthol, particularly over long periods, e.g. overuse of mentholated cigarettes, can result in gastrointestinal distress, ataxia, stupor and convulsions—even blood dyscrasias have been reported.

Camphor is readily absorbed from mucous membranes. A large spoonful of 3—10% camphor—an amount present in many over-the-counter products—may cause intoxication in a child. A considerable number of cases of accidental ingestion of camphor-containing products, usually involving children under 4 years of age have been reported (93[R], 94[cr]). In some instances the products have been mistaken for cough syrups (94[cr]). It is not only following ingestion that toxic symptoms (convulsions) have resulted: cutaneous and nasal application may be dangerous as well. Blood and especially urine levels can give information on the degree of exposure.

Symptoms of camphor toxicity can occur within 5 to 15 minutes of ingestion (93[R]). Mild poisoning generally causes gastrointestinal symptoms, which include burning of the mouth, nausea, vomiting and epigastric distress. In severe poisoning, CNS signs of restlessness, excitement, confusion, vertigo, delirium and seizures, which result in apnea and asystole, are observed. The ingestion of 2 g of camphor generally causes dangerous toxicity, but an adult can ingest as much as 42 g and recover. In children, ingestions of only 0.7—1.0 g of camphor have been shown to cause death, usually from seizures and apnea (93[R]). *Four teaspoons* (*20 ml*) of 5% camphor if ingested by a child is a potentially lethal dose.

All camphor ingestions estimated to be 2 mg/kg or greater reported between 1980 and 1983 have been reviewed to determine guidelines for treatment of camphor toxicity (95[R]). Seventy-three patients (90%) remained asymptomatic, three (4%) developed minor symptoms and five (6%), who ingested over 59 mg/kg, developed major symptoms. There were no deaths observed. A literature review of six deaths indicated the mean fatal dose was 199 mg/kg (range 64—570, median 113). The results obtained indicated it was appropriate to manage asymptomatic patients who ingested less than 10 mg/kg of camphor by observation only. If 10—30 mg/kg were ingested, treatment with 1 g/kg activated charcoal or emesis was given. For doses over 30 mg/kg, gastric decontamination and referral were recommended

As small children are particularly sensitive, camphor-containing preparations should not be used for them; the danger outweighs the slight subjective relief that may be provided (96[R]). It has been argued that, as camphorated oil provides doubtful benefits and poses a danger to the public, it should be avoided (93[R]) or even be removed from the market (94[cr]).

Almitrine bimesilate This is a respiratory stimulant that improves hypoxemia in about 80% of patients with severe chronic obstructive pulmonary disease (COPD) (SEDA-17, 212). A 1-year investigation showed oral almitrine bimesilate (100 mg/day) increased Pa_{O_2} in patients with severe COPD without altering mean pulmonary artery pressure (97[C]). Side effects to almitrine were rarely observed and it was concluded that long-term treatment was safe. In other studies, respiratory, digestive and neurological symptoms have been noted but were often pre-existent. Mild gastrointestinal symptoms sometimes occurred (nausea, accelerated intestinal transit) but regressed spontaneously or after brief symptomatic therapy (98[c], 99[c]).

REFERENCES

1. Paterson JW, Tarala RA. Asthma: Common pitfalls in management. Curr Ther Aug 1981;33—43.
2. Cloutier MM, Loughlin GM. Chronic cough in children: a manifestation of airway hyperreactivity. Paediatrics 1981;67:6—12.
3. Speight ANP, Lee DA, Hey EN. Underdiagnosis and undertreatment of asthma in childhood. Br Med J 1983; 286:1253—1256.
4. Stellman JL, Spicer JE, Cayton RM. Morbidity from chronic asthma. Thorax 1982;37:218—221.
5. Fryd V, Keiding LM, Tonnesen P. Årsager til forkert anvendelse af asthma-spray (dosis-aerosol). Ugeskr Læg 1986;148:1395—1397.
6. Tonnesen P, Odum L. Hospitalspersonalets kendskab til brugen af asthma-spray (dosis-aerosol). Ugeskr Læg 1986;148:1397—1399.
7. Davis B, Gett PM, Sherwood-Jones E. A service for the adult asthmatic. Thorax 1980;35:111—113.
8. Goldie RG, Lulich KM, Paterson JW. Bronchodilators: β-agonists. Med J Aust 1995;162:100—102.
9. Paterson JW, Lulich KM, Goldie RG. Pharmacology of asthma treatment: an overview. Med J Aust 1995;162:42—43.
10. Martelli NA. Bronchial and intravenous provocation tests with indomethacin in aspirin-sensitive asthmatics. Am Rev Respir Dis 1979;120:1073—1079.
11. Baker GJ, Collett P, Allen DH. Bronchospasm induced

by metabisulphite-containing foods and drugs. Med J Aust 1981;2:614—617.
12. Garland LG. Pharmacology of prophylactic anti-asthma drugs. In: Page CP, Barnes PJ, eds. Pharmacology of Asthma. Berlin: Springer-Verlag, 1991;261—290.
13. Repo UP, Neiminen P. Pulmonary infiltrates with eosinophilia and urinary symptoms during disodium cromoglycate treatment. A case report. Scand J Respir Dis 1976;57:1—4.
14. Kallós P, Kallós L. Pseudo-allergic reactions due to disodium cromoglycate. In: Dukor P, Kallós P, Schlumberger HD, West GB, eds. Pseudo-Allergic Reactions. Involvement of Drugs and Chemicals. Basel: Karger, 1982;122—132.
15. Scheffer AL, Rocklin RE, Goetzl EJ. Immunologic components of hypersensitivity reactions to cromolyn sodium. N Eng J Med 1975;293:1220—1224.
16. Marks MB. Nebulized cromolyn sodium: efficacy and safety. Immunol Allergy Pract 1984;6:130—134.
17. Brown LA, Kaplan RA, Benjamin PA, Hofman LS, Shearer WT. Immunoglobulin E-mediated anaphylaxis with inhaled cromolyn sodium. J Allergy Clin Immunol 1981;68:416—420.
18. Brown HM, Engler C, English JR. A comparative trial of flunisolide and sodium cromoglycate nasal sprays in the treatment of seasonal allergic rhinitis. Clin Allergy 1981;11:169—173.
19. Mani V, Lloyd G, Green FH, Fox H, Turnberg LA. Treatment of ulcerative colitis with oral sodium cromoglycate. A double-blind controlled trial. Lancet 1976;i:439—441.
20. Walker SR, Evans ME, Richards AJ, Paterson JW. The fate of [^{14}C]disodium cromoglycate in man. J Pharm Pharmacol 1972;24:525—531.
21. Geddes DM, Turner-Warwick M, Brewis RAL, Davies RJ. Nedocromil sodium workshop. Respir Med 1989; 83:265—267.
22. Lal S, Dorow PD, Venho KK, Chatterjee SS. Nedocromil sodium is more effective than cromolyn sodium for the treatment of chronic reversible obstructive airway disease. Chest 1993;104:438—447.
23. Alexander M. Comparative therapeutic studies with Tilavist. Allergy 1995;50:23—29.
24. Kjellman NI, Stevens MT. Clinical experience with Tilavist: an overview of efficacy and safety. Allergy 1995;50:14—22.
25. Thomson NC. Nedocromil sodium: an overview. Respir Med 1989;83:269—276.
26. Kemp JP, Meltzer EO, Orgel AH et al. A dose-response study of the bronchodilator action of azelastine in asthma. J Allergy Clin Immunol 1987;79:893—899.
27. Riethmuller-Winzen H, Peter G, Buker KM, Romeis P, Borbe HO. Tolerability, pharmacokinetics and dose linearity of azelastine hydrochloride in healthy subjects. Arzneimittel-Forschung 1994;44:1136—1140.
28. Peter G, Romeis P, Borbe HO, Buker KM, Riethmuller-Winzen H. Tolerability and pharmacokinetics of single and multiple doses of azelastine hydrochloride in elderly volunteers. Arzneimittel-Forschung 1995;45:576—581.
29. Gastpar H, Aurich R, Petzold U et al. Intranasal treatment of perennial allergic rhinitis. Comparison of azelastine nasal spray and budesonide nasal aerosol. Arzneimittel-Forschung 1993;43:475—479.
30. Clarke CW, May CS. A comparison of the efficacy of ketotifen (HC20—511) with sodium cromoglycate (SCG) in skin test positive asthma. Br J Clin Pharmacol 1980;10:473—476.
31. Lane DJ. A steroid sparing effect of ketotifen in steroid-dependent asthmatics. Clin Allergy 1980;10:519—525.
32. Falk ES. Ketotifen in the treatment of atopic dermatitis. Results of a double blind study. Riv Eur Sci Med Farmacol 1993;15:63—66.
33. Lebeau B, Gence B, Bourdain M, Loria Y. Preventive treatment of asthma with ketotifen: an analysis of 1791 cases treated in general practice. Poumon Coeur 1982;38:125—129.
34. Tinkelman DG, Moss BA, Bukantz SC et al. A multicenter trial of the prophylactic effect of ketotifen, theophylline and placebo in atopic asthma.. J Allergy Clin Immunol 1985;76:487—497.
35. Hara H, Kurita M, Morioka H et al. [Drug induced cystitis due to ketotifen fumarate—a case report]. [Japanese]. Nippon Hinyokika Gakkai Zasshi (Jpn J Urol) 1992;83:1906—1909.
36. El-Hefny A. Treatment of wheezy infants and children with ketotifen. Pharmatherapeutica 1983;3:388—392.
37. Saintmont C, Duprat P, Bourdain M, et al. Etude clinique du kétotifène solution buvable chez l'enfant. Résultats préliminaires sur 257 observations. Ann Pédiatr 1984;31:81—84.
38. Craps L. Prophylaxis of asthma with ketotifen in children and adolescents a review. Pharmatherapeutica 1983;3:314—326.
39. Jeffreys DV, Volans GN. Ketotifen overdosage: surveillance of the toxicity of a new drug. Br Med J 1981;282:1755—1756.
40. Yokoyama H, Iinuma K, Yanai K, Watanabe T, Sakurai E, Onodera K. Proconvulsant effect of ketotifen, a histamine H1 antagonist, confirmed by the use of *d*-chlorpheniramine with monitoring electroencephalography. Methods Findings Exp Clin Pharmacol 1993;15:183—188.
41. Reference deleted.
42. Nishida T, Kusakai Y, Ogoshi R. Four cases of cystitis induced by the anti-allergic drug tranilast. Acta Urol Jpn 1985;31:1813—1817.
43. Brems H, Pauly N, Thomas J. Fenspiride (Pneumorel 80) dans le traitement des affections aiguës des voies respiratoires. Ars Med 1984;39:55—58.
44. Abramson MJ, Puy RM, Weiner JM. Is allergen immunotherapy effective in asthma. A meta-analysis of randomized controlled trials. Am J Respir Crit Care Med 1995;74:969—974.
45. CSM Update. Desensitising vaccines. Br Med J 1986;293:948
46. Reid MJ, Lockey RF, Turkeltaub PC, Platts-Mills AE. Survey of fatalities from skin testing and immunotherapy 1985—1989. J Allergy Clin Immunol 1993;92:6—15.
47. Tabar AI, Garcia BE, Rodriguez A, Olaguibel JM, Muro MD, Quirce S. A prospective safety-monitoring study of immunotherapy with biologically standardized extracts. Allergy 1993;48:450—453.
48. Matloff SM, Bailit IW, Parks P, Madden N, Greineder DK. Systemic reactions to immunotherapy. Allergy Proc 1993;14:347—350.
49. Anonymous. Guidelines for the use of allergen immunotherapy. Canadian Society of Allergy and Clinical Immunology (Review). Can Med Assoc J 1995;152:1413—1419.
50. Barnes PJ. Neural mechanisms in asthma. In: Page CP,

Barnes PJ, eds. Pharmacology of Asthma. Berlin: Springer-Verlag, 1991;143–166.
51. Wright BD. Exacerbation of akinetic seizures by atropine eye drops. Br J Ophthalmol 1992;76:179–180.
52. Berdy GJ, Berdy SS, Odin LS, Hirst LW. Angle closure glaucoma precipitated by aerosolized atropine. Arch Int Med 1991;151:1658–1660.
53. Pakes GE, Brogden RN, Heel RC, Speight TM, Avery GS. Ipratropium bromide: A review of its pharmacological properties and therapeutic efficacy in asthma and chronic bronchitis. Drugs 1980;20:237–266.
54. Delacourt C, de Blic J, Lebourgeois M, Scheinmann P. [Value of ipratropium bromide in asthma crisis in children—in French]. Arch Pediatr 1994;1:87–92.
55. Bronsky EA, Druce H, Findlay SR et al. A clinical trial of ipratropium bromide nasal spray in patients with perennial nonallergic rhinitis. J Allergy Clin Immunol 1995;95:17–22.
56. Kaiser HB, Findlay SR, Georgitis JW et al. Long-term treatment of perennial allergic rhinitis with ipratropium bromide nasal spray 0.06%. J Allergy Clin Immunol 1995;95:28–32.
57. Diamond L, Dockhorn RJ, Grossman J et al. A dose-response study of the efficacy and safety of ipratropium bromide nasal spray in the treatment of the common cold. J Allergy Clin Immunol 1995;95:39–46.
58. Malani JT, Robinson GM, Seneviratine EL. Ipratropium bromide induced angle-closure glaucoma. NZ Med J 1982;95:749
59. Hall SK. Acute angle-closure glaucoma as a complication of combined beta-agonist and ipratropium bromide therapy in the emergency department. Ann Emerg Med 1994; 23:884–887.
60. Watson WT, Shuckett EP, Becker AB, Simons FE. Effect of nebulized ipratropium bromide on intraocular pressures in children. Chest 1994;105:1439–1441.
61. Pras E, Stienlauf S, Pinkhas J, Sidi Y. Urinary retention associated with ipratropium bromide. DICP 1991;25:939–940.
62. Dollery CT, Williams FM, Draffan GH et al. Arterial blood levels of fluorocarbons in asthmatic patients following use of pressurized aerosols. Clin Pharmacol Ther 1974; 15:59–66.
63. Shaheen MZ, Ayres JG, Benincasa C. Incidence of acute decreases in peak expiratory flow following the use of metered-dose inhalers in asthmatic patients. Eur Respir J 1994;7:2160–2164.
64. Kirby SM, Smith J, Ventresca GP. Salmeterol inhaler using a non-chlorinated propellant, HFA134a: Systemic pharmacodynamic activity in healthy volunteers. Thorax 1995;50:679–681.
65. Dockhorn R, Vanden Burgt JA, Ekholm BP, Donnell D, Cullen MT. Clinical equivalence of a novel non-chlorofluorocarbon-containing salbutamol sulfate metered-dose inhaler and a conventional chlorofluorocarbon inhaler in patients with asthma. J Allergy Clin Immunol 1995;96:50–56.
66. Paterson JW, Woolcock AJ, Shenfield GM. State of the art: bronchodilator drugs. Am Rev Respir Dis 1979; 120:1149–1188.
67. Beasley R, Burgess C, Pearce N, Woodman K, Crane J. Confounding by severity does not explain the association between fenoterol and asthma death. Clin Exp Allergy 1994;24:660–668.
68. Spitzer WO, Suissa S, Ernst P et al. The use of beta-agonists and the risk of death and near death from asthma. New Engl J Med 1992;326:501–506.
69. Williams AJ, Baghat MS, Stableforth DE, Cayton RM, Shenoi PM, Skinner C. Dysphonia caused by inhaled steroids: recognition of a characteristic laryngeal abnormality. Thorax 1983;38:813–821.
70. Doull IJ, Freezer NJ, Holgate ST. Growth of prepubertal children with mild asthma treated with inhaled beclomethasone dipropionate. Am J Respir Crit Care Med 1995;151:1715–1719.
71. Brown PH, Greening AP, Crompton GK. Hypothalamo-pituitary-adrenal axis suppression in asthmatic adults taking high dose beclomethasone dipropionate. Br J Clin Pract 1992;46:102–104.
72. Dong JC, Shen ZY, Wang WJ. [The investigation on 100 bronchial asthma and asthmatic bronchitis cases treated with high dose beclomethasone dipropionate aerosol—Chinese]. Chung Hua Chieh Ho Ho Hu Hsi Tsa Chih 1993;16:33–35.
73. Mak VH, Melchor R, Spiro SG. Easy bruising as a side-effect of inhaled corticosteroids. Eur Respir J 1992;5:1068–1074.
74. Hummel S, Lehtonen L. Comparison of oral-steroid sparing by high-dose and low-dose inhaled steroid in maintenance treatment of severe asthma. Lancet 1992;340:1483–1487.
75. Andersson PT, Persson CGA. Developments in anti-asthma glucocorticoids. Agents Actions 1988;23:239–260.
76. Adelroth E, Rosenthall L, Glennow C. High dose inhaled budesonide in the treatment of severe steroid-dependent asthmatics. Allergy 1985;40:58–64.
77. Kraan J, Koeter GH, van der Mark THW et al. Dosage and time effects of inhaled budesonide on bronchial hyperreactivity. Am Rev Respir Dis 1988;137:44–48.
78. British Thoracic Society Research Committee. Oral *N*-acetylcysteine and exacerbation rates in patients with chronic bronchitis and severe airways obstruction. Thorax 1985; 40:832–835.
79. Mant TGK, Tempowski JH, Volans GN, Talbot JC. Adverse reactions to acetylcysteine and effects of overdose. Br Med J 1984;289:217–219.
80. Bonfiglio MF, Traeger SM, Hulisz DT, Martin BR. Anaphylactoid reaction to intravenous acetylcysteine associated with electrocardiographic abnormalities. Ann Pharmacother 1992;26:22–25.
81. Aylward M, Davies DE, Dewland PM. Clinical evaluation of carbocisteine (Mucolex) in the treatment of patients with chronic bronchitis: a double blind trial with placebo control. Clin Trials J 1984;22:36
82. Bateman DN, Woodehouse KW, Rawlins MD. Adverse reactions to *N*-acetylcysteine. Lancet 1984;ii:228.
83. Tenenbein M. Hypersensitivity-like reactions to *N*-acetylcysteine. Vet Hum Toxicol 1984;26:3–5.
84. Nagy G. The use of Paxirasol in clinical practice (Review). Ther Hung 1993;41:100–106.
85. Jørgensen PH. Bromhexin. En genvurdering ud fra litteraturen. Ugeskr Læg 1982;144:1327–1329.
86. Itoh K, Kounou O, Morise M et al. Clinical effects of proteinase, sfericase (AL-794), on chronic bronchitis and similar diseases. Int J Clin Pharmacol Ther Toxicol 1984;22:32–38.
87. Cosmi F, Mollaioli M, Aimi M et al. Attivatà antitussigena del clofedanolo. Eur Rev Med Pharmacol Sci 1983; 5:239–242.
88. Merigot PH, Garnier R, Efthymiou ML. Les convulsions avec trois antitussifs dérivés substitués de la pipérazine (zipeprol, eprazinone,eprozinol). Ann Pédiatr 1985;32:504–506.

89. Gastpar H, Criscuolo D, Dieterich HA. Efficacy and tolerability of glaucine as an antitussive agent. Curr Med Res Opin 1984;9:21—27.
90. Anonymous. Hallucinaties door oxolamine (Bredon). Bull Bijwerk Geneesmd 1986;2:10—11.
91. McEwen J, Meyboom RH, Thijs I. Hallucinations in children caused by oxolamine citrate. Med J Aust 1989;150:449—452.
92. Morton CA, Garioch J, Todd P, Lamey PJ, Forsyth A. Contact sensitivity to menthol and peppermint in patients with intra-oral symptoms. Contact Dermatitis 1995;32:281—284.
93. Anonymous. Camphor revisited: focus on toxicity. Committee on Drugs. American Academy of Pediatrics. Pediatrics 1994;94:127—128.
94. Theis JG, Koren G. Camphorated oil: still endangering the lives of Canadian children. Can Med Assoc J 1995;152:1821—1824.
95. Geller RJ, Spyker DA, Garrettson LK, Rogol AD. Camphor toxicity: development of a triage strategy. Vet Hum Toxicol 1984;26:8—10.
96. Bavoux F, Bodiou C, Castot A et al. Le camphre en pédiatrie. Son intérêt thérapeutique et ses risques. Thérapie 1985;40:25—30.
97. Weitzenblum E, Schrijen F, Apprill M, Prefaut C, Yernault JC. One year treatment with almitrine improves hypoxaemia but does not increase pulmonary artery pressure in COPD patients. Eur Respir J 1991;4:1215—1222.
98. Ansquer JC, Bertrand A, Blaive B et al. Intérêt thérapeutique et acceptabilitié du Vectarion 50mg comprimés enrobés (bismésilate d'almitrine) à la dose de 100mg/jour. Etude des resultats gazometriques, cliniques et biologiques en traitement prolonge pendant 1 an. Rev Mal Respir 1985;2:S61—S67.
99. Grassi V, Bottino G, Blasi A, Grassi C. Première expérience clinique italienne du bismésilate d'almitrine. Rev Mal Respir 1985;2:S53—S60.

Meyler's Side Effects of Drugs, 13th Edition
M.N.G. Dukes, editor

SECTION EDITOR: J.K. ARONSON

J.K. Aronson

17 Positive inotropic drugs and drugs used in dysrhythmias

Cardiac glycosides

Many aspects of the pharmacology and clinical pharmacology of cardiac glycosides have been reviewed in the proceedings of various symposia (1^{CR}–4^{CR}). There have also been specific reviews of digitalis intoxication and its treatment (5^{R}–9^{R}).

Mechanisms of digitalis toxicity There is a large amount of circumstantial evidence that the mechanisms of action of cardiac glycosides are mediated directly or indirectly by inhibition of the sodium/potassium pump enzyme, Na/K-ATPase (10^{R}). Their toxic effects on the myocardium may be due to excessive inhibition of cardiac Na/K-ATPase, although there is also evidence that effects on the nervous input to the heart may be involved (11^{R}), and it is not clear to what extent such an effect is mediated by inhibition of Na/K-ATPase. There is also evidence that color vision disturbances due to cardiac glycosides are due to inhibition of Na/K-ATPase (12^{C}).

Epidemiology of digitalis toxicity Digitalis toxicity is common, since all cardiac glycosides have a low therapeutic index. Estimates vary widely from study to study, but in large prospective studies of hospital in-patients the frequency of digitalis toxicity has been as high as 29% (13^{C}). In out-patients the figure may be as high as 16% (7^{R}). The lower frequency in out-patients may be due partly to poor compliance and partly to the fact that digitalis toxicity may be a reason for admission to hospital, thus increasing the numbers of toxic in-patients. The risk of toxicity may be lower with digitoxin than with digoxin (4^{R}), but when toxicity occurs it lasts longer, because of the very long half-life of digitoxin.

The overall mortality from digitalis toxicity also varies widely, having been reported as low as 4% and as high as 36% (7^{R}). However, it varies with dysrhythmias, and for paroxysmal supraventricular tachycardia with block may be as high as 50% (7^{R}).

ADVERSE REACTION PATTERN

General and toxic reactions Adverse reactions to cardiac glycosides may be cardiac or non-cardiac, and are dose-related. Frequent non-cardiac reactions include gastrointestinal effects (anorexia, nausea, vomiting, and diarrhea), central nervous system effects (drowsiness, dizziness, confusion, delirium), and less commonly visual effects (color vision abnormalities, photophobia, and blurred vision). Frequent cardiac adverse effects include heart block and ectopic dysrhythmias (ventricular extra beats, other ventricular tachydysrhythmias, and paroxysmal supraventricular tachycardia). The combination of heart block with an ectopic dysrhythmia, e.g. paroxysmal supraventricular tachycardia with block, is particularly suggestive of toxicity due to cardiac glycosides. Any other dysrhythmia can occasionally be caused by cardiac glycosides.

Hypersensitivity reactions Hypersensitivity reactions are rare and include thrombocytopenia and skin rashes.

Tumor-inducing effects Tumor-inducing effects have not been reported.

ORGANS AND SYSTEMS

Cardiovascular *Dysrhythmias and heart block* Percentage incidence figures for digitalis-induced dysrhythmias were given by Chung in his review of 726 patients (5^{R}). The commonest dysrhythmias are ventricular extra beats (54% of all dysrhythmias), coupled ventricular extra beats (25%), and *supraventricular tachycardia* (33%). Sinus tachycardia was not common (3.4%). *Atrial fibrillation* (1.7%) or *atrial flutter* (1.8%) can cause difficulty in diagnosis, since digitalis is often used to treat those dysrhythmias. *Atrioventricular block* was common (42%: first-degree, 14%; second-degree,

17%; and complete, 11%). However, first-degree heart block (i.e. prolongation of the PR interval) without higher degrees of atrioventricular nodal block may occur in the absence of digitalis intoxication.

The dysrhythmias that digitalis can cause can be classified according to their sites of origin as follows.

Sinoatrial node Digitalis can cause *sinus bradycardia* as a toxic effect, although patients with sinus bradycardia who are at rest often have no other evidence of digitalis toxicity, and this effect may simply represent increased vagal tone (14[C]). Digitalis inhibits conduction through the sinoatrial node and has been reported to cause a syndrome mimicking that of the sick sinus syndrome (15[C]—17[C]), although it is not clear whether or not it can impair sinus node function in patients who have previously normal sinoatrial nodes (18[C], 19[C]). In other cases digitalis can worsen sinus node function that has been otherwise impaired, e.g. by hyperthyroidism (20[c]) or endotracheal suction (21[c]).

Atria and atrioventricular node Digitalis can cause *supraventricular extra beats* or tachycardia. The combination of such dysrhythmias with atrioventricular block is particularly suggestive of digitalis toxicity and carries a high mortality rate (22[C], 23[C]). Rarely atrial fibrillation (24[C]) and atrial flutter (25[CR]) may be attributed to digitalis toxicity. The risks of atrioventricular nodal block are mentioned above.

Ventricles *Ventricular extra beats*, including coupled beats (i.e. ventricular bigeminy), are the most common effects of digitalis toxicity, although they are not specific. In more severe cases *ventricular tachycardia*, *bidirectional tachycardia*, and *ventricular fibrillation* may occur. There have also been reports of *accelerated idioventricular rhythm* (26[c], 27[c]).

Effects of digitalis on the electrocardiogram Digitalis can prolong the PR interval in the absence of toxicity. It also causes shortening of the QT interval, depression of the ST segment, and asymmetrical T wave inversion. These effects are non-specific and can occur in the absence of toxicity. However, there is evidence that the effects on the ST segment and T wave may be more common in patients with co-existing ischemic heart disease (28[C]). Digitalis can also rarely cause both left (29[C]) and right (30[cr]) bundle branch block.

Heart failure In toxic doses digitalis may impair myocardial contractility and cause or worsen heart failure. In one series of 148 patients with digitalis intoxication, worsening heart failure was diagnosed in 7.5% (31[C]). In some cases worsening heart failure may be attributable to a cardiac dysrhythmia (32).

Vasoconstrictor and hypertensive effects Giving a cardiac glycoside rapidly intravenously causes a transient increase in blood pressure, which has been attributed to an increase in peripheral resistance (33[C]). However, digitalis does not seem to increase the blood pressure during long-term treatment.

Myocardial ischemia Subacute digitalis intoxication in dogs causes myocardial damage (34), and after intravenous administration there is increased CPK activity in the plasma in man (35[C]), suggesting ischemic damage. There is no direct evidence of this, but during long-term administration of digitalis in patients who have had an acute myocardial infarction there may be an increased rate of mortality (discussed in the next section), which might be attributable to myocardial ischemia. An alternative explanation would be cardiac dysrhythmias.

Long-term use and cardiovascular adverse effects of cardiac glycosides There have been many studies of the long-term efficacy of digitalis in patients in heart failure in sinus rhythm and also in patients with atrial fibrillation. These have been reviewed in the Side Effects of Drugs Annuals (SEDA-4, 123; SEDA-14, 145; SEDA-18, 196). The following is a brief resumé.

Atrial fibrillation is not necessarily an indication for long-term therapy with digitalis. In patients with controlled atrial fibrillation whose plasma digitalis concentration is below the lower end of the therapeutic range (0.8 ng/ml for digoxin and 10 ng/ml for digitoxin) withdrawal rarely if ever results in deterioration. However, in those who have plasma digitalis concentrations within the therapeutic range withdrawal should not be attempted, since the risk of worsening of atrial fibrillation outweighs the risk of toxicity, if careful monitoring of the plasma concentration is possible.

In patients with heart failure in sinus rhythm there is no way of predicting which patients will benefit from long-term therapy, but the following recommendations may be made:

- If the plasma digitalis concentration is below the therapeutic range (see above) withdrawal is very likely not to produce deterioration.
- If a patient's condition is stable, with the plasma digitalis concentration in the therapeutic range, and little risk of toxicity, withdrawal is probably not worth while because of the risk of deterioration.
- However, if there is an increased risk of toxicity (e.g. because of renal impairment or if potassium balance is difficult to maintain) careful withdrawal of digitalis may be worth attempting.
- In patients who have evidence of poor left ventricular function it may be better to continue therapy, even if there is an increased risk of toxicity, since these patients are very likely to deteriorate following withdrawal. In these cases careful monitoring of therapy will help to reduce the risk of toxicity.

The long-term adverse cardiovascular effects of digitalis have been discussed in several editions of the Side

Effects of Drugs Annuals (SEDA-10, 142; SEDA-11, 153; SEDA-15, 165). Briefly, in a number of retrospective studies, although mortality in the digitalis-treated patients was generally higher than in those not treated with digitalis, the difference was reduced when allowance was made for other confounding factors, such as the degree of heart failure, a history of dysrhythmias, and the use of other drugs. This is currently the subject of a prospective clinical study, due to be published in 1996. There may also be a higher mortality rate in patients who take long-term digitalis therapy after coronary artery bypass graft surgery (36[C]) and in patients who have had a cardiac arrest (37[C]). In both of these studies the risk was increased further among those who were taking digitalis with diuretics, and it may be that these effects are due to digitalis toxicity secondary to potassium depletion, although it may simply indicate a greater prevalence of hypertension or heart failure among those treated with digitalis and diuretics.

Until the results of prospective studies are available, digitalis is best reserved in long-term treatment for patients with chronic heart failure due to mitral valvular, ischemic, or hypertensive heart disease, particularly in those in whom there is evidence of left ventricular dysfunction. A trial of withdrawal of digitalis therapy can be considered in some cases (see above).

Of course, there are alternatives to the use of digitalis in the long-term treatment of heart failure in sinus rhythm. However, it is not clear that any of these offers any particular advantage over digitalis in terms of therapeutic efficacy, although there may be fewer problems with toxicity. The comparative studies have been reviewed in SEDA-14 (p. 141), and the conclusions can be briefly summarized as follows.

(1) *Sinus rhythm* Other positive inotropic drugs carry no extra benefit, and there is no evidence that the combination of two drugs with positive inotropic actions is beneficial in chronic congestive heart failure. Vasodilators are as efficacious as digitalis, but there is a rationale for combining digitalis and a vasodilator, since by doing so it is possible to affect simultaneously the three important factors determining cardiac output, namely contractility, pre-load, and after-load. Furthermore, a vasodilator will oppose the small effect that digitalis has in increasing peripheral resistance, and which may reduce the beneficial effect of digitalis on cardiac output.

(2) *Atrial fibrillation* In uncomplicated atrial fibrillation a cardiac glycoside such as digoxin remains the drug of first choice. However, in those in whom digitalis is not completely effective or in whom symptoms (e.g. bouts of palpitation) persist despite adequate digitalization, a calcium antagonist, such as verapamil or diltiazem, may be added, or amiodarone used as an alternative. In patients with atrial fibrillation due to hyperthyroidism, a β-adrenoceptor antagonist should be used in preference to digitalis, but digitalis may be added if there is an incomplete effect. In patients with atrial fibrillation secondary to an anomalous conduction pathway (e.g. Wolff-Parkinson-White syndrome) in most of whom digitalis is contraindicated, a calcium antagonist would be the treatment of choice. Paroxysmal atrial fibrillation generally does not respond to digitalis, and digitalis may in fact prolong the duration of a paroxysmal attack when it occurs. The treatment of paroxysmal atrial fibrillation is problematic, but my current preference is for amiodarone or sotalol. Propafenone and flecainide are useful alternatives, but there are current doubts about the long-term safety of flecainide, particularly in those who have had an acute myocardial infarction (see below).

Cardioversion and digitalis The presence of digitalis increases the risk of serious dysrhythmias following electrical cardioversion, even in the absence of frank toxicity (38[CR]). In order to minimize the risk of dysrhythmias in these circumstances digitalis should be withdrawn if possible a day or two before cardioversion and potassium depletion should be corrected. If cardioversion is required acutely then it has been recommended that one should start with low energies (e.g. 10 J) (39[C]).

Nervous system Toxic effects of digitalis on the nervous system occur relatively frequently. Although in severe toxicity the incidence may be as high as 65% (40[C]), in most series it has been below 25% (41[r]).

Anorexia, *nausea*, and *vomiting* (discussed below) are gastrointestinal effects mediated by the central nervous system. Other common nervous system effects of digitalis include *confusion*, *dizziness*, *drowsiness*, *bad dreams*, *restlessness*, *nervousness*, *agitation*, and *amnesia*. *Acute psychosis* and *delirium* may occur, particularly in elderly people (42[C], 43[CR], 44[cr]), and may be accompanied by visual or auditory hallucinations (45[c], 46[c]). *Epilepsy* occurs rarely and may be accompanied by EEG changes (47[C], 48[c], 49[cr]). Other reported effects include *chorea* (50[C]), *transient global amnesia* (51[C]), *trigeminal neuralgia* (52[C], 53[C]), *nightmares* (54[c]), *organic brain syndrome* (including impairment of long- and short-term memory) (55[c]), and *impairment of learning and memory* (56[C]).

Endocrine, metabolic *Digitalis has effects on sexual function*. It causes increased serum concentrations of FSH and estrogen and reduced concentrations of LH and testosterone (57[C]–60[C]). These effects are probably not related to any direct estrogen-like structure of digitalis (despite structural similarities), but rather to some effect involving the synthesis or release of sex hormones. The clinical results of these effects are:

- *Gynecomastia in men and breast enlargement in women* These may be associated with demonstrable histological changes (61[C], 62[C]).
- *Stratification of the vaginal squamous epithelium in postmenopausal women* This may cause difficulty in the pathological interpretation of vaginal smears for cancer diagnosis (63[C]).
- *A possible modifying effect on breast cancer* (64[C]).

Digitalis may reduce the heterogeneity of breast cancer cell populations and reduce the rate of distant metastases. There is also evidence that the 5-year recurrence rate after mastectomy is lower in women who have been treated with digitalis (65[c]). However, more evidence is required to support these suggestions, which have been by no means proven.

Mineral and fluid balance The normal increase in plasma potassium concentration during exercise may be exacerbated by digoxin (66[C]). Although this might increase the risk of dysrhythmias, only one case of an exercise-associated dysrhythmia attributed to digitalis has been reported (67[c]).

Hematological *Thrombocytopenia* has been reported in patients taking digitoxin, acetyldigoxin, and digoxin (68[c], 69[c], 70[cr], 71[c]).

There have been rare reports of *eosinophilia* in patients taking cardiac glycosides (72[c]).

Gastrointestinal Gastrointestinal symptoms are common in digitalis toxicity. They include *anorexia*, *nausea*, and *vomiting* (73[R]), and these probably result from stimulation of the chemoreceptor trigger zone in the brain. *Diarrhea* can occur occasionally (74[C]). Other gastrointestinal effects are rare, and include *dysphagia* (75[C]), *intestinal ischemia* (76[R], 77[c]), and *hemorrhagic intestinal necrosis* (78[c]). Intestinal ischemia has been reported to respond to treatment with verapamil and to antidigoxin antibody (78[c]).

Skin and appendages Digitalis rarely affects the skin, but has been reported to cause pruritus, *erythematous rashes*, *papules*, *vesicles*, *bullae*, and *angio-edema* (79[R]). In some cases positive skin reactions to the implicated glycoside have been demonstrated and there may also be cross-sensitization to other glycosides (79[R]). Some cases have been associated with circulating antibodies (80[C]). Cutaneous *vasculitis* has also been reported (81[C], 82[cr]). Other rare effects of digitalis on the skin include a *psoriasiform eruption* (83[c]), *excessive sweating* (84[c]), and a *pemphigus foliaceus-like eruption* (85[c]).

Special senses Cardiac glycosides have several effects on the eyes, including photophobia, *blurred vision*, *scotomata*, *flickering sensations*, and *flashes of light before the eyes* (86[R]). *Color vision disturbances* are also well known effects of digitalis toxicity. They most commonly take the form of yellow vision (xanthopsia) and other forms occur more rarely (86[R]). However, even in patients *without* any visual symptoms digitalis intoxication frequently causes impairment of color vision discrimination, which is measurable using sensitive techniques, although it may not be apparent to the patient (87[Cr]). *Pain during eye movement* has been reported with digoxin (88[c]).

Muscle Intramuscular injection of digitalis can be painful and may cause local muscle necrosis, sometimes with pyrexia (89[CR]). In addition, the systemic availability of digitalis after intramuscular injection is poor (90[R]), and this route of administration should be avoided if possible.

Risk factors Several factors increase the risk of digitalis intoxication. They can be considered in three groups (91[R]):

(1) *Factors that alter the amount of drug that accumulates in the body or the plasma concentration at a fixed dose.*

Alterations in tissue distribution The apparent volume of distribution of digoxin is reduced in hypothyroidism (92[R]) and in renal failure (93[R]). This leads to increased plasma concentrations after a loading dose and hence an increased risk of toxicity, but does not affect the plasma concentration at steady-state. The opposite occurs in hyperthyroidism.

Alterations in renal elimination The effects of renal failure on the pharmacokinetics of cardiac glycosides have been reviewed (93[R]). The most important effect of renal failure is a reduced rate of elimination of digoxin, leading to increased accumulation during steady-state treatment. The same applies to some other glycosides, including β-methyldigoxin, β-acetyldigoxin, ouabain, and κ-strophanthin, but not to glycosides that are mostly metabolized, such as digitoxin, the proscillaridins, and peruvoside (4[R]). Drug interactions can also lead to reduced digoxin renal elimination (see below).

Alterations in non-renal elimination See 'Interactions' below.

(2) *Factors that alter the clinical response to digoxin at a fixed amount of digoxin in the body and a fixed plasma concentration.*

Electrolyte disturbances Of these, hypokalemia is the most important. It has been estimated that a fall in plasma potassium concentration from 3.5 to 3.0 mmol/l is associated with a 50% increase in sensitivity to digoxin (see Ref. 91[R]). Total body potassium depletion, even in the absence of hypokalemia, has a similar effect (94[C]).

There is evidence that hypomagnesemia has the same effect as hypokalemia (95[C]).

Hypercalcemia has the same effects as hypokalemia; hypocalcemia has the opposite effect, i.e. it causes resistance to the effects of digitalis.

There is evidence that hypoxia and acidosis increase the risk of digitalis intoxication.

Age Old people are more sensitive to the effects of digitalis for reasons that are not entirely clear. Of course, renal function tends to be impaired in elderly people, and hypokalemia is more likely, but there also seems to be a true increase in the sensitivity of their tissues to digitalis, perhaps because of reduced Na/K-ATPase activity.

Matters are also more complicated in young people. Firstly, the pharmacokinetics of cardiac glycosides are different (96[R]): the apparent volume of distribution of digoxin is higher in neonates, infants, and older children than in adults, and renal digoxin clearance is lower in children under 4–6 months. However, there may also be increased resistance to the effects of digoxin in infants because of changes in digitalis tissue receptors (97[C]). Seriously ill low birth weight children may be particularly at risk, even when low dosages of digitalis are used (98[C]).

The risk of digitalis toxicity during the therapeutic use of cardiac glycosides is similar in children to that in adults, ranging in 12 separate published series from 12 to 50% (median 21%) (99[R]). The most common non-cardiac effects are vomiting and feeding problems, and the most common cardiac effects are conduction defects, particularly atrioventricular block and ectopic rhythms, although (as in adults) any dysrhythmia can occur.

Thyroid disease Apart from the pharmacokinetic differences in thyroid disease (mentioned above), there may also be changes in tissue responsiveness, with decreased sensitivity in hyperthyroidism and the reverse in hypothyroidism (92[R]). The reasons for these changes are not known, but may be related to differences in tissue Na/K-ATPase activity.

Cardiac disease Cardiac glycosides are better avoided in patients with acute myocardial infarction, since they increase oxygen demand in ischemic tissue, increase peripheral vascular resistance, and carry an increased risk of dysrhythmias, especially in the presence of tissue hypoxia and acidosis. Furthermore, there is evidence that digitalis is of little value in patients with acute myocardial infarction and either left ventricular failure or cardiogenic shock (100[R]). The evidence that mortality in patients who take digitalis after an acute myocardial infarction is increased is discussed above.

Cardiac glycosides are contraindicated in conditions in which there is obstruction to ventricular outflow, e.g. hypertrophic obstructive cardiomyopathy, constrictive pericarditis, and cardiac tamponade. Acute myocarditis may also increase the risk of toxicity.

Direct current cardioversion increases the risk of digitalis-induced dysrhythmias, but digitalis treatment is not a contraindication to cardioversion (see above and Ref. 101[C]).

Renal failure In addition to its effect in reducing the elimination of digoxin, renal failure may be associated with an increased sensitivity to the actions of digitalis (102[C]).

Second-generation effects Digoxin crosses the placenta and enters the neonatal circulation (103[R]). It has therefore been used, for example, to improve fetal cardiac function (104[R]). However, in normal circumstances there seem to be no adverse effects on the neonate, and neonatal plasma concentrations are below those generally considered to be therapeutic. There has been one report of fatal toxicity in the fetus of a woman who took an overdose of digitoxin (105[c]).

Overdosage The most important complication of overdosage in all age groups is disturbance of cardiac conduction, but in addition any dysrhythmia may occur. Death may occur from asystole or ventricular fibrillation. Hyperkalemia is common and the higher the plasma potassium concentration the poorer the prognosis (106[C]).

Other common effects of overdosage are nausea, vomiting, and central nervous system and visual disturbances (40[C]).

The pharmacokinetics of digoxin are altered after overdosage, the half-life being rapid, but there is too little information to define the kinetics precisely (106[R]).

Treatment of toxicity and overdosage These topics have been reviewed in SEDA-5 (p. 172) and SEDA-12 (p. 149). In summary, the following measures should be taken:

(1) *Remove digitalis from the stomach* If the patient is seen within 1–2 hours of overdosage one would try to remove whatever drug still remains in the stomach by either gastric lavage or ipecacuanha-induced emesis. Gastric lavage is likely to produce a better result, but some recommend emesis as the preferred method, since lavage may carry a higher risk of inducing cardiac dysrhythmias.

(2) *Prevention of further absorption* Activated charcoal should be given orally or by nasogastric tube. It binds digitalis and therefore reduces both primary absorption and reabsorption after excretion via the bile (digitoxin) or the intestinal mucosa (digoxin) (107[C]). To be fully

Table 1. *Methods for calculating the required dose of anti-digoxin antibody fragments in cases of digoxin or digitoxin intoxication*

Digoxin

(1) When the ingested dose is known:

(a)	Tablets	— dose in mg × 40
(b)	Elixir	— dose in mg × 48
(c)	Capsules	— dose in mg × 55
(d)	Intravenous	— dose in mg × 60

(2) When the plasma or serum concentration is known:
ng/ml × lean body weight × 0.34
or
nmol/l × lean body weight × 0.26

Example Plasma (or serum) digoxin concentration = 24 ng/ml in a patient with an estimated lean body weight of 75 kg.
Dose of antibody fragments = 24 × 75 × 0.34 = 612 mg.
Give 640 mg (e.g. 16 ampoules of Digibind).

Digitoxin

(1) When the ingested dose is known (all formulations):
Dose in mg × 60

(2) When the plasma or serum concentration is known:
ng/ml × lean body weight × 0.034
or
nmol/l × lean body weight × 0.026

Example Plasma (or serum) digitoxin concentration = 280 ng/ml in a patient with an estimated lean body weight of 70 kg.
Dose of antibody fragments = 280 × 70 × 0.034 = 666 mg.
Give 680 mg (e.g. 17 ampoules of Digibind).

effective charcoal should be given at regular intervals (e.g. 50 grams hourly).

(3) *Correct potassium disturbances* Hypokalemia should be treated with potassium chloride. Hyperkalemia carries a poor prognosis and is usually an indication for antidigoxin antibody (see next section).

(4) *Give antidigoxin antibody* Antidigoxin antibody (Fab fragments) is the treatment of choice in patients with severe digitalis toxicity due to any cardiac glycoside. It is effective after self-poisoning with digitoxin, lanatoside C, and acylated forms of digoxin, as well as digoxin itself. It should be used when there are life-threatening dysrhythmias or heart block, and when the plasma potassium concentration is above 5.0 mmol/l or is rising, since hyperkalemia is evidence of serious toxicity and carries a poor prognosis. The role of antidigoxin antibody fragments in treating milder forms of digitalis toxicity has not been fully assessed. The dose of antidigoxin antibody should be based on the dose of digitalis taken and, where possible, the plasma digitalis concentration. The recommended doses for cases of poisoning with digoxin and digitoxin are given in Table 1. Although the clearance of the fragments is reduced in patients who also have severe renal impairment (108[c], 109[c]), there is no need to reduce the dose of antibody in such patients (for more details see Refs. 110[R]–111[R]).

(5) *Treat dysrhythmias* Cardiac dysrhythmias in digitalis overdose should only be treated if they are life-threatening. Phenytoin is probably the treatment of choice for ventricular tachydysrhythmias, but lidocaine or a β-adrenoceptor antagonist, such as practolol or propranolol, are good alternatives. Sinus bradycardia and heart block may respond to atropine, but a temporary pacemaker may be required.

Heart block is the most serious consequence of digitalis poisoning and should be anticipated by the insertion of a temporary pacemaker. If this is delayed until heart block or dysrhythmias occur, there may be difficulty in inserting the pacemaker (because of ventricular excitability), and delay in treatment may be deleterious.

(6) *Other measures* Hemoperfusion has been used to treat digitalis overdose (see SEDA-5, 174). There may be a case for its use very soon after digitalis overdose, but once a cardiac glycoside has been distributed to the body tissues the value of hemoperfusion is limited. For digitoxin, which has a lower apparent volume of distribution than digoxin, charcoal hemoperfusion may be more valuable. Hemofiltration has also been used (see SEDA-12, 149), but there is no convincing evidence of its efficacy.

Monitoring digitalis therapy *Plasma concentrations* The use of plasma digitalis concentrations in monitoring therapy has been reviewed elsewhere (91[R], 114[R]). The underlying principles are as follows:

- The plasma digitalis concentration must be considered in conjunction with other pieces of information about the patient, i.e. symptoms, the signs of possible intoxication, the stability of the underlying condition, age, renal function, the dosage, and biochemical measurements such as the plasma potassium concentration.
- At plasma digitalis concentrations above 3.0 ng/ml (digoxin) or 30 ng/ml (digitoxin) toxicity is highly likely. At concentrations below 1.5 or 15 ng/ml, respectively, toxicity is unlikely. However, toxicity can occur even with low concentrations and should particularly be suspected if there is hypokalemia.
- Certain factors increase the risk of digitalis toxicity at a given plasma concentration (see above under 'Risk factors'). These factors will alter the interpretation of the plasma digitalis concentration and lower one's threshold for suspicion.
- When in doubt it is far better to withhold digitalis and monitor progress than to continue treatment, thereby running the risk of perpetuating toxicity.

The following are the main uses of plasma digitalis concentration measurements:

Individualizing therapy In the absence of factors that alter the response to digitalis it is worth measuring the plasma concentration during the initial stages of therapy to ensure that a reasonable concentration has been achieved (1.0–1.5 ng/ml for digoxin, 10–15 ng/ml for digitoxin). In cases where there is still a poor response to treatment it is justifiable to increase digitalis dosages cautiously, but the risk of toxicity starts to rise markedly at plasma concentrations above 2.0 and 20 ng/ml, respectively. If there are subsequent changes in the patient's condition, e.g. renal impairment, then plasma concentration measurement may help in readjusting dosages.

Diagnosis of toxicity The principles of using plasma concentrations of digitalis to diagnose toxicity are discussed above.

Monitoring compliance The presence of a cardiac glycoside in a blood sample confirms that the drug has at least been taken recently.

The treatment of overdosage The use of the plasma digitalis concentration in the calculation of the appropriate dose of antidigoxin antibody is discussed above.

Deciding therapy after long-term treatment In patients whose condition is satisfactory and stable and whose plasma digoxin concentration is low (below 0.8 ng/ml), withdrawal of digoxin is recommended and is highly unlikely to affect the patient's condition (discussed above). Probably the same applies for digitoxin at concentrations below 8.0 ng/ml, although that has not been demonstrated.

Salivary digitalis concentration This has not been well studied and cannot be recommended as an alternative to plasma digitalis concentration measurement.

Salivary electrolyte concentrations The results of salivary electrolyte (potassium and calcium) concentration measurements in diagnosing digitalis toxicity, although initially encouraging, have not lived up to expectations (see SEDA-7, 193).

Erythrocyte electrolyte concentrations Although attractive in principle and based on the observation that digitalis inhibits the transport of sodium and potassium across cell membranes, the measurement of intra-erythrocytic sodium concentrations has not been widely enough studied to be recommended as a routine test either in the diagnosis of digitalis toxicity or in routine monitoring (see SEDA-5, 176).

Color vision measurement Because color vision is impaired in digitalis toxicity (12[C]) its measurement might be helpful in diagnosis. However, this has proved disappointing in practice (115[Cr]).

Interactions Interactions with cardiac glycosides can be subdivided into six types, according to mechanism: (1) absorption; (2) protein binding (digitoxin); (3) metabolism; (4) renal excretion (digoxin); (5) uptake by the end-organ; (6) response of the end-organ.

Interactions with digoxin have been reviewed elsewhere (SEDA-6, 173; 116[R]–118[R]).

Absorption Absorption interactions are probably not of great clinical importance, since (a) the dosages of drugs that reduce the absorption of digitalis are usually larger than those used clinically, and (b) the major effect on absorption probably occurs only if the two drugs are taken together.

The effect of activated charcoal in reducing digitalis absorption has been mentioned above under the treatment of poisoning, and binding resins, such as cholestyramine and colestipol have similar actions (119[c], 120[cR]). Since digitoxin and digoxin are excreted via the bile and the intestinal mucosa, respectively, concurrent administration of digitalis with charcoal or the binding resins is not necessary for the interaction to occur.

Certain combinations of cytotoxic drugs (cyclophosphamide, vincristine, and prednisone, with and without procarbazine) reduced plasma digoxin concentrations by about 50% during treatment with β-acetyldigoxin, perhaps through impaired absorption of β-acetyldigoxin (121[C]); digitoxin was not affected (122[C]).

Absorption interactions involving altered gastrointestinal motility have been described. These include interactions of digoxin with propantheline (123[C]), metoclopramide (123[C]), and cisapride (124[C]). However, the clinical relevance of these interactions is unclear and they are probably unimportant.

Some antacids, such as magnesium trisilicate, may reduce the absorption of digoxin slightly, but these interactions are probably of no clinical importance (125[R]).

Protein-binding displacement Interactions of this kind are of no importance for digoxin, which is only about 20% bound and has a high apparent volume of distribution. An interaction of heparin with digitoxin has been described and ascribed to altered protein binding, secondary to changes in fatty acid concentrations, but the clinical relevance, e.g. in patients undergoing hemodialysis, is unclear (116[R]).

Renal clearance Digoxin is cleared by the kidneys by glomerular filtration and active secretion, and retained by passive reabsorption, the last two roughly balancing each other, so that clearance is usually proportional to creatinine clearance.

Some drugs inhibit the active secretion of digoxin; these include quinidine, verapamil, and spironolactone; they probably do this by inhibiting the P glycoprotein, which is responsible for the active renal tubular secretion of digoxin. Vasodilators may increase the active secretion of digoxin.

Quinidine The quinidine—digoxin interaction was reviewed in SEDA-6 (p. 173) and further information was added in later Annuals (SEDA-7, 195; SEDA-9, 159; SEDA-10, 145; SEDA-15, 166; SEDA-18, 198). Although the major mechanism of the interaction is probably inhibition of the active secretion of digoxin by quinidine, other mechanisms are involved, including reduced non-renal clearance and displacement of digoxin from the tissues. The reduction in non-renal clearance is at least partly due to a reduction in biliary clearance. This interaction affects most patients and on average causes a two-fold increase in steady-state plasma digoxin concentrations. Because both clearance and apparent volume of distribution are reduced, the half-life of digoxin is either unaffected or perhaps slightly prolonged.

In addition to the pharmacokinetic interaction there may be a pharmacodynamic interaction, since there is some evidence that quinidine may reduce the positive inotropic effect of digoxin on the heart, in addition to having a negative inotropic effect of its own. Thus, the outcome of the interaction is a 24-fold increased risk of digoxin toxicity and a reduction in its beneficial effect on the heart, at least in sinus rhythm. If the two drugs are used together, the digoxin dosage should be reduced by a half at first and adjusted subsequently on the basis of the patient's clinical condition and the plasma digoxin concentration.

Lanatoside C and *β*-methyldigoxin are theoretically likely to be similarly affected by quinidine, and there is anecdotal evidence of this.

The pharmacokinetic interaction of quinidine with digoxin also occurs with *quinine* and *hydroxychloroquine*. However, the effects of these drugs are smaller than those with quinidine, and quinine does not reduce the biliary excretion of digoxin.

Either quinidine does not interact pharmacokinetically with *digitoxin* or the interaction is of little importance.

Amiodarone Amiodarone reduces both the renal and non-renal clearances of digoxin and prolongs its half-life, without changing its apparent volume of distribution. It has also been suggested that amiodarone increases the absorption of digoxin (see SEDA-10, 144 and SEDA-12, 150). Digoxin dosages should be halved as soon as amiodarone is introduced. This interaction may also occur with acetyldigitoxin (126[c]).

Calcium antagonists *Verapamil* increases plasma digoxin concentrations at steady state by inhibiting the active tubular secretion and non-renal clearance of digoxin (127[C], 128[C]). There is anecdotal evidence that this may result in digitalis toxicity (129[R], 130[c]). Diltiazem may do the same (131[c]). Other calcium antagonists have varying effects on the disposition of digoxin, but any effects they have are probably small enough to ignore in practice. The calcium antagonists for which varying amounts of information are available include cinnarizine, felodipine, fendiline, gallopamil, isradipine, lidoflazine, nicardipine, nifedipine, nitrendipine, and tiapamil (132[C]).

Verapamil and tiapamil have both been reported to reverse digoxin-induced splanchnic vasoconstriction in healthy men (133[C]), but this has no direct effect on systemic hemodynamics.

Spironolactone Spironolactone inhibits the active secretion of digoxin by about 25% and in some cases digoxin dosages may have to be reduced (134[C]).

Vasodilators Nitroprusside and hydralazine increase the renal clearance of digoxin, perhaps by increasing renal blood flow and therefore renal tubular secretion (135[C]). This causes a small fall in plasma digoxin concentration the clinical significance of which is unclear.

Indomethacin Indomethacin increased plasma digoxin concentrations in premature neonates with a patent ductus arteriosus (136[C]), but a formal study in healthy adults showed no interaction (137[C]). It may be that pre-existing impairment of renal function is required for this interaction, but this remains to be elucidated.

Itraconazole Itraconazole increases plasma concentrations of digoxin, perhaps by reducing its renal clearance (138[c], 139[c]).

Metabolism The metabolism of digitoxin can be increased, with resulting increasing dosage requirements, by rifampicin (140[C]) and other enzyme-inducing drugs (119[R]). For example, phenobarbital 100 mg daily reduces steady-state serum digitoxin concentrations by 50%.

Although digoxin is not extensively metabolized in the majority of patients, it may be metabolized before its absorption from the gut by two mechanisms, hydrolysis by gastric acid and hydrogenation by intestinal bacteria. In patients who have hypochlorhydria this presystemic metabolism is reduced and increasing concentrations of digoxin achieved systemically. This means that drugs that reduce gastric acid secretion, such as cimetidine, ranitidine, other H_2 receptor antagonists, and omeprazole would be expected to increase the systemic availability of digoxin, and there is some evidence of that (141[C], 142[C]), albeit not conclusive (SEDA-17, 216).

The antibiotics *erythromycin* and *tetracycline* may also increase the systemic availability of digoxin, by inhibiting its breakdown by intestinal bacteria, mainly

Eubacterium glenum (143[C]). There is anecdotal evidence that this interaction may be clinically important.

Uptake by the end-organ The interaction of *quinidine* with digoxin, in which there may be displacement of digoxin from tissues, is discussed above. *Hyperkalemia*, due to potassium chloride, potassium-retaining diuretics, or ACE inhibitors, may reduce the apparent affinity of digitalis for Na/K-ATPase and thereby reduce its tissue binding.

Response of the end-organ Interactions involving changes in the response of the end-organ to digitalis are the most common of all interactions with cardiac glycosides.

Potassium depletion, e.g. due to *diuretics* or *corticosteroids*, potentiates the effects of cardiac glycosides on the myocardium and may also have a small effect in reducing the renal tubular secretion of digoxin (144[C], 145[C]).

Magnesium depletion, e.g. due to diuretics, may have a similar effect (146[C]), but the data are not as clear-cut as for potassium.

Anecdotal reports suggest that intravenous infusion of *calcium salts* in patients taking digitalis may result in dangerous cardiac dysrhythmias. This may also be the basis of the report that *edrophonium* and *suxamethonium* may enhance the actions of digitalis, since both of these drugs might cause altered disposition of calcium. Conversely, there is good anecdotal evidence that hypocalcemia causes reduced plasma responsiveness to digoxin (147[c]).

Miscellaneous interactions *Propafenone* causes a small increase in plasma digoxin concentrations by an unknown mechanism (148[C], 149[C]). Although this effect is perhaps not clinically significant, in patients with dysrhythmias it was accompanied by an increase in the PR interval (149[C]).

Non-interactions Digoxin has been reported not to interact with a variety of antidysrhythmic drugs, including ajmaline, aprindine, lidocaine, lidoflazine (150[C]), and moricizine (151[C]). Other drugs that may have minor and clinically unimportant interactions include captopril, carvedilol, disopyramide, and flosequinan.

INDIVIDUAL CARDIAC GLYCOSIDES

There are major pharmacokinetic differences among the different cardiac glycosides, the principal difference being between those that are mainly excreted via the kidneys (e.g. digoxin, β-methyldigoxin, β-acetyldigoxin, ouabain, and κ-strophanthin) and those that are mainly excreted via hepatic metabolism (including digitoxin, gitoxin, pengitoxin (16-acetyldigoxin), and gitoformate).

It has also been suggested that there may be some pharmacodynamic differences among different cardiac glycosides (152[R]), but these may at least partly be determined by differences in tissue distribution.

It is debatable whether any of these differences makes any particular cardiac glycoside preferable to another. The most strongly argued case is that digitoxin is preferable to digoxin in patients with renal failure, since digitoxin is metabolized and digoxin is excreted by the kidneys. However, digitoxin has a much longer duration of action, and if toxicity occurs it will take longer to resolve. Furthermore, determining the effective dose of digitoxin is much more difficult, since there is great variability in the extent to which digitoxin is metabolized from patient to patient, and hepatic function in regard to this metabolism cannot be measured. Although digoxin excretion also varies from patient to patient, it can at least be gauged by measurement of creatinine clearance. The arguments for and against these preferences have been outlined (4[R], 153[R]) and it may be that it would be best to choose particular patients depending on their individual requirements.

Adverse effects of antidigoxin antibody fragments Antidigoxin antibody fragments cause adverse events in about 7% of cases, including allergic responses, possible *recurrence of digitalis toxicity* after treatment, and some effects attributable to the withdrawal of digitalis, such as *worsening of heart failure*. In one series (154[R]) allergic reactions occurred in only six of 717 patients reviewed, and consisted of pruritic rash and flushing or facial swelling. The risk of an allergic reaction was increased in patients who had a history of previous allergy or asthma. Recurrence of digitalis toxicity after treatment was usually due to inadequate treatment with the antibody.

OTHER POSITIVE INOTROPIC DRUGS

The pharmacology, clinical pharmacology, uses, and adverse effects of positive inotropic drugs other than digitalis have been reviewed (155[R]–157[R]). The therapeutic value of positive inotropic drugs other than digitalis has been reviewed (158[R], 159[R]), as has the suggestion that their long-term use may be deleterious (159[R]).

DRUGS ACTING AS β-ADRENOCEPTOR AGONISTS

These positive inotropic drugs include dobutamine, dopamine, ibopamine, pirbuterol, prenalterol, and xamoterol. The β-adrenoceptor agonists and dopamine receptor agonists are dealt with in Chapter 13.

SELECTIVE PHOSPHODIESTERASE INHIBITORS

There is a range of bipyridines that are inhibitors of a specific isoenzyme of phosphodiesterase, F-III. These include amrinone, enoximone (fenoximone), milrinone, sulmazole, and vesnarinone. Their clinical pharmacology has been reviewed (160[R]).

Although the phosphodiesterase inhibitors are effective in the treatment of acute cardiac failure in various settings, overall mortality during long-term treatment of heart failure is increased, and they should not be used for that purpose (161[R]).

Amrinone

The adverse effects of amrinone (162[C]—166[C]) include thrombocytopenia (10%), *hypotension*, *tachydysrhythmias* (sometimes resulting in syncope and death) (9%), worsening *cardiac ischemia* (7%), worsening *heart failure* (15%), *gastrointestinal disturbances* (39%), *neurological complications* (17%), *liver damage* (7%), *fever* (6%), *nephrogenic diabetes insipidus*, *hyperuricemia*, *flaking of the skin*, *brown discoloration of the nails*, and *reduced tear secretions*. (The figures in parentheses are taken from a study of the use of amrinone in 173 patients with chronic ischemic heart disease or idiopathic cardiomyopathies (164[C]).)

Other reported adverse effects include acute *pleuropericardial effusions*, *perforated duodenal ulcer*, *acute myositis and pulmonary infiltrates*, *vasculitis* with pulmonary infiltrates and jaundice, *influenza-like illnesses*, *chest pain*, *headache*, *dizziness*, *anxiety*, *maculopapular rash*, and *night sweats* (167[C]). There has also been one report of a *paroxysmal supraventricular tachycardia* in one of 16 patients with cardiogenic shock (168[C]).

The effect of amrinone on liver function has also been reported to have reduced the metabolism of *aminopyrine* (169[C]). However, the relevance of this observation to drug interactions with amrinone is not clear.

Enoximone

The most common adverse effects of enoximone are gastrointestinal and cardiac.

The gastrointestinal effects include *anorexia*, *nausea*, *vomiting*, and *diarrhea* (170[C]—171[C]).

The cardiac effects include *hypotension*, transient *atrial fibrillation*, and *bradycardia* (174[C]). *Ventricular tachydysrhythmias* have been reported in about 4% of patients (171[C]) and *myocardial ischemia* may also occur (175[C], 176[C]). In a study of 102 patients taking digoxin and diuretics the addition of enoximone did not confer any therapeutic advantage and there was a significantly higher drop-out rate and a significantly higher mortality rate in those taking enoximone (177[C]).

Other rarely reported adverse effects include *thrombocytopenia*, *leukocytosis*, *increased appetite*, *increased serum AlT activity*, *hyperglycemia*, *headache*, *lethargy*, *anxiety*, *dyspnea*, and *skin rash* (171[C]—175[C]).

Milrinone

Milrinone may occasionally cause *ventricular dysrhythmias* (178[C]—180[C]) and *sudden death* has occurred (178[C]). In one series *fluid retention* was very common (178[C]). Falls in platelet counts have been seen (181[C]), but there have been no reports of frank thrombocytopenia.

Sulmazole

Sulmazole commonly causes adverse gastrointestinal effects. Dose-related *anorexia*, *nausea*, and *vomiting* have been reported in about 50% of patients given an intravenous infusion (182[C], 183[C]) and also after single oral doses (184[C]). Cardiac *dysrhythmias*, mostly ventricular, have been reported occasionally with sulmazole. Other reported adverse effects in small numbers of patients include *headache* (182[C]), temporary *visual disturbances* (183[C], 186[C]), *discoloration of the urine* (attributed to a metabolite) (181[C], 183[C]), and a small *reduction in platelet count* (182[C]).

Vesnarinone

Although it is safe in low dosages, in high dosages vesnarinone increases mortality (187[C], 188[C]). It causes reversible *neutropenia* in 2.5% of patients (189[C]).

Table 2. *Classification of antidysrhythmic drugs*

Class I	*Ia*	*Ib*	*Ic*
	Quinidine	Lidocaine	Lorcainide
	Procainamide	(lignocaine)	Flecainide
	Disopyramide	Phenytoin	Encainide
		Mexiletine	Propafenone
		Aprindine	(also has Class
		Tocainide	II activity)
Class II	Beta-adrenoceptor antagonists		
	Bretylium		
Class III	Amiodarone		
	Sotalol (also has Class II activity)		
Class IV	Verapamil		

Table 3. *Sites of action of antidysrhythmic drugs*

Sinus node	*Anomalous pathways*
Class Ic	Class Ia
Flecainide	Quinidine
Propafenone	Procainamide
Class II	Disopyramide
β-adrenoceptor antagonists	Class Ic
Class IV	Propafenone
Verapamil	Class III
	Amiodarone
Atrria	
Class Ia	
Quinidine	
Procainamide	*Ventricles*
Disopyramide	Class Ia
Class Ic	Quinidine
Lorcainide	Procainamide
Encainide	Disopyramide
Flecainide	Class Ib
Propafenone	Lidocaine
Class III	Phenytoin
Amiodarone	Mexiletine
Tocainide	Class Ic
	Lorcainide
Atrioventricular node	Encainide
Class Ic	Propafenone
Lorcainide	Class III
Flecainide	Amiodarone
Propafenone	
Class II	
β-adrenoceptor antagonists	
Class IV	
Verapamil	

DRUGS USED IN DYSRHYTHMIAS

Drugs used in dysrhythmias may be classified in different ways, the usual classification being according to their effects on the cardiac action potential (190^R), as shown in Table 2.

The Class I antidysrhythmic drugs reduce the rate of the fast inward sodium current during Phase I of the action potential and increase the duration of the effective refractory period expressed as a proportion of the total action potential duration. The action potential duration is itself affected in different ways by subgroups of the Class I drugs. Class Ia drugs, of which quinidine is the prototype, prolong the action potential; Class Ib drugs, of which lidocaine is exemplary, shorten the action potential; Class Ic drugs do not alter action potential duration.

The β-adrenoceptor antagonists (Class II) and bretylium inhibit the effect of catecholamines on the action potential. The β-adrenoceptor antagonists are dealt with in Chapter 18.

Class III antidysrhythmic drugs prolong the total action potential duration. They probably act by effects on potassium channels, altering the rate of repolarization.

Class IV antidysrhythmic drugs prolong total action potential duration by prolonging the plateau phase (Phase III) of the action potential via calcium channel blockade.

Other classifications of antidysrhythmic drugs have been proposed, but the most useful clinical classification relates to the sites of action of the antidysrhythmic drugs on the various cardiac tissues, as shown in Table 3. The patterns of adverse effects of the antidysrhythmic drugs depend on three features.

• All antidysrhythmic drugs have effects on the cardiac conducting tissues and can all therefore cause cardiac dysrhythmias.

• All antidysrhythmic drugs have a negative inotropic effect on the heart, which can result in heart failure. However, the degree of negative inotropy varies from drug to drug; for example, it is less marked with drugs such as lidocaine and phenytoin and very marked with the β-adrenoceptor antagonists.

• Each antidysrhythmic drug has its own non-cardiac effects, which may result in adverse effects. These are summarized in Table 4.

Cardiovascular adverse effects of antidysrhythmic drugs *Cardiac dysrhythmias* The risk of antidysrhythmic-induced cardiac dysrhythmias (prodysrhythmic effects) has been estimated at about 11–13% in non-invasive studies (191^C, 192^C) and up to 20% in invasive electrophysiological studies. The prodysrhythmic effects of antidysrhythmic drugs have been extensively reviewed (193^R–208^R).

There are four major mechanisms whereby antidysrhythmic drugs may cause dysrhythmias (193^R):

• Worsening of a pre-existing dysrhythmia. For example, ventricular extra beats may be converted to ventricular tachycardia or the ventricular rate in atrial flutter may be accelerated when slowing of the atrial

Table 4. *Non-cardiac effects of some antidysrhythmic drugs*

Drug	Common non-cardiac adverse effect(s)
Acecainide	Gastrointestinal and CNS effects
Ajmaline derivatives	Liver damage, agranulocytosis, neurological symptoms
Amiodarone	Corneal microdeposits, effects on skin, thyroid, lungs, liver, nerves, muscles
Aprindine	Agranulocytosis, CNS effects, liver damage.
Cibenzoline	Gastrointestinal and CNS effects, hypoglycaemia
Disopyramide	Anticholinergic effects
Encainide	CNS effects
Flecainide	CNS effects
Lidocaine	CNS effects
Lorcainide	CNS effects
Mexiletine	CNS effects
Phenytoin	see Chapter 7
Procainamide	Lupus-like syndrome, neutropenia
Propafenone	Gastrointestinal and CNS effects, asthma
Quinidine	Anticholinergic effects, hypersensitivity reactions
Tocainide	CNS effects

rate results in the conduction of an increased number of atrial impulses through the AV node.

• The induction of heart block or suppression of an escape mechanism. For example, slowing of conduction through the AV node may impair a mechanism that allows the conducting system to escape a re-entry mechanism.

• The uncovering of a hidden mechanism of dysrhythmia. For example, antidysrhythmic drugs may cause early or delayed afterdepolarizations, which may result in dysrhythmias.

• The induction of a new mechanism of dysrhythmia. For example, a patient in whom myocardial ischemia has predisposed to dysrhythmias may be more at risk when an antidysrhythmic drug alters conduction.

Combinations of these different mechanisms are also possible.

Dysrhythmias secondary to antidysrhythmic drugs are arbitrarily defined as either early (within 30 days of starting treatment) or late (194[R], 195[R]). A lack of early dysrhythmias in response to antidysrhythmic drugs does not predict the risk of late dysrhythmias (196[C]).

Ventricular dysrhythmias due to drugs may be either monomorphic or polymorphic. The class Ia drugs are particularly likely to cause polymorphic dysrhythmias, as is amiodarone (although to a lesser extent). In contrast, the class Ic drugs are more likely to cause monomorphic dysrhythmias (197[cR]).

There are no good predictors of the occurrence of dysrhythmias, but there are known to be several risk factors (198[R], 199[R]), including a history of sustained tachydysrhythmias, poor left ventricular function, and myocardial ischemia. Potassium depletion and prolongation of the QT interval are particularly important, and these may particularly predispose to polymorphous ventricular dysrhythmias (e.g. *torsade de pointes*). Altered metabolism of antidysrhythmic drugs (e.g. liver disease, polymorphic acetylation or hydroxylation, and drug interactions) can also contribute.

The methods for minimizing the risks of prodysrhythmic effects of antidysrhythmic drugs (193[R]) are as follows:

• Care in choosing those who are likely to benefit from antidysrhythmic drug therapy.

• Identification and correction, if possible, of impaired pump function and ischemic damage.

• Correction of electrolyte abnormalities.

• Exercise testing before and during the early stages of drug therapy: widening of the QRS complex during exercise predicts a high risk of ventricular tachycardia as does an increase in the QT_c interval.

• Instruction of patients about the signs and symptoms that may occur with dysrhythmias.

• Monitoring of renal or hepatic function in order to predict reduced drug elimination.

• Avoiding drug interactions or changing the dosage of the antidysrhythmic drug in anticipation of a change in its disposition secondary to an interaction.

Measurement of the concentrations of antidysrhythmic drugs and their metabolites in the plasma may be useful in recognizing the need for changing dosage requirements when cardiac, hepatic, or renal dysfunction occurs and to maintain serum drug or metabolite concentrations within optimal ranges, and for predicting dosage changes required when interacting drugs are added (200[R]).

Another strategy for reducing the risk of prodysrhythmias is to use combinations of different classes of antidysrhythmic drugs in lower dosages than one would use with monotherapy.

Torsade de pointes can be prevented by withholding antidysrhythmic drug therapy from patients who have pre-existing prolongation of the QT interval, and by correction of low serum potassium and magnesium concentrations before therapy. During therapy patients at risk should have frequent monitoring of the ECG and serum electrolytes. Established *torsade de pointes* should be treated with intravenous magnesium sulfate (209[R]). The dose is 2 grams intravenously given over 2–3 minutes followed by continuous intravenous infusion at a rate of 2–4 mg/minute); if the dysrhythmia recurs, another bolus of 2 grams should be given and the infusion rate increased to 6–8 mg/min; rarely, a third bolus of 2 grams may be required. If magnesium is ineffective, cardiac pacing should be tried.

Adverse hemodynamic effects of antidysrhythmic drugs Many antidysrhythmic drugs have negative inotropic effects (210[R]–212[R]). This means that they should be avoided in patients with a history of heart failure, a low left ventricular ejection fraction, or a cardiomyopathy; the general risk of induction or a worsening of heart failure is up to about 5%, but those who have these risk factors have a risk of up to 10%. The negative inotropic effects are most marked with drugs of Classes Ia, Ic, II, and IV. For Class I drugs there is a strong relation between their negative inotropic effect and the extent to which they block the inward sodium current (212[R]). Thus, the drugs of Class Ib that are associated with a short recovery time of sodium channels have a smaller negative inotropic effect than drugs of Class Ia, which in turn have less of an effect than drugs of Class Ic. However, the overall hemodynamic effects of antidysrhythmic drugs depend not only on their negative inotropic effects on the heart, but also on their effects on the peripheral circulation (213[R]). Thus, although all Class I drugs have similar negative inotropic effects on the heart, disopyramide has large hemodynamic effects (because it increases peripheral resistance) and its hemodynamic effect is therefore greater than that of mexiletine, for example. Similarly the adverse hemodynamic effects of encainide and tocainide are greater than those of procainamide (214[C]).

General adverse effects of antidysrhythmic drugs There have been several reviews of the pharmacology, clinical pharmacology, pharmacokinetics, and adverse effects of antidysrhythmic drugs (215[R]–223[R]).

The safety of antidysrhythmic drugs in children has not been thoroughly studied. However, the risk of prolongation of the QT interval seems to be considerably less than in adults (224[R]), although it has been reported with quinidine, disopyramide, amiodarone, sotalol, and diphemanil.

Drug interactions with antidysrhythmic drugs Some important drug/drug interactions with antidysrhythmic drugs are summarized in Table 5.

Acecainide (*N*-acetylprocainamide; NAPA)

Acecainide is the main metabolite of procainamide, and it has antidysrhythmic activity (225[R]). However, in contrast to procainamide, which has Class Ib activity, the main action of acecainide is of Class III.

Cardiovascular Acecainide prolongs the QT interval and may therefore cause *ventricular dysrhythmias* (226[C]). The risk of this is increased in renal failure, since acecainide is mainly eliminated unchanged via the kidneys.

Lupus-like syndrome The main advantage of acecainide over procainamide is the reduced incidence of the *lupus-like syndrome*. Many fewer patients develop antinuclear antibodies during long-term treatment with acecainide than during long-term treatment with procainamide (227[C]).

There are also reports of remission of lupus-like syndrome without recurrence in patients in whom acecainide has been used as a replacement for procainamide (228[C]–230[C]). Furthermore, patients in whom procainamide has previously caused a lupus-like syndrome have been reported not to suffer from the syndrome on subsequent long-term treatment with acecainide (228[C]). However, in one case a patient suffered mild arthralgia while taking acecainide, having had a more severe arthropathy while taking procainamide (228[C]).

Other adverse effects The other adverse effects of acecainide are as common as those of procainamide. The commonest are those affecting the gastrointestinal tract and the central nervous system. *Anorexia*, *nausea*, *vomiting*, *diarrhea*, and *abdominal pain* are common, as are *insomnia*, *dizziness*, *light-headedness*, *tingling sensations*, and *blurred vision*. Other reported unwanted effects include *skin rashes*, *constipation*, and *reduced sexual function* (231[C]–234[C]).

Risk situations Because acecainide is eliminated mostly unchanged by renal excretion, with a half-life of about 7 hours, its clearance is reduced in patients with renal impairment, and they are at increased risk of adverse effects. This means that elderly people, who generally also have a degree of renal impairment, are also at increased risk.

Interactions Because acecainide may prolong the QT interval it should not be used in combination with other antidysrhythmic drugs that do likewise.

Drugs that inhibit the renal tubular secretion of other drugs may inhibit the renal clearance of acecainide, and this happens with *cimetidine* (235[C]) and *trimethoprim* (236[C]). However the effects of these drugs are rather small and probably have little clinical significance.

Monitoring therapy The therapeutic plasma concentration range of acecainide is 15–25 μg/ml. Adverse effects are dose-related and increase in frequency at concentrations above 30 μg/ml (237[R]).

Adenosine and adenosine triphosphate

Several reviews of the clinical pharmacology, actions, therapeutic uses, and adverse reactions and interactions

Table 5. *Some important drug/drug interactions with antidysrhythmic drugs*

Object drug(s)	Precipitant drug(s)	Result of interaction
Adenosine	Dipyridamole	Increased effect
Adenosine	Theophylline	Reduced effect
Anticholinergic drugs	Disopyramide, quinidine	Potentiation
Antihypertensive drugs	Bretylium	Severe hypotension
Beta-adrenoceptor antagonists	Propafenone	Potentiation
Class I drugs	β-adrenoceptor antagonists	Negative inotropy
Class I drugs	Class I drugs	Potentiation
Class I drugs	Drugs causing potassium depletion	Prodysrhythmic effects
Digoxin	Amiodarone, quinidine, verapamil	Digoxin toxicity
Disopyramide	Enzyme-inducing drugs	Increased metabolism
Neuromuscular blockers	Quinidine	Potentiation
Phenytoin	Various	See Chapter 7
Procainamide	Cimetidine, trimethoprim	Reduced metabolism
Quinidine	Enzyme-inducing drugs	Increased metabolism
Theophylline	Mexiletine	Cardiac dysrhythmias
Verapamil	β-adrenoceptor antagonists	Negative inotropy/bradycardia/asystole
Warfarin	Amiodarone, quinidine	Warfarin toxicity

of adenosine and adenosine triphosphate (ATP) have appeared (238[R]—241[R]). The adverse effects of adenosine triphosphate are similar to those of adenosine.

Although the adverse effects of adenosine and ATP are very common they are generally mild, and because adenosine is rapidly eliminated from the blood (with a half-life of less than 10 seconds) they are generally transient. Adverse effects have been reported in 81% of patients given adenosine and 94% of patients given ATP (242[C]).

Cardiovascular The most common cardiac effects are *atrioventricular block*, *sinus bradycardia*, and *ventricular extra beats*. Occasionally serious dysrhythmias occur (SEDA-17, 219). ATP has been reported to cause transient *atrial fibrillation*. *Chest pain* occurs in 30—50% of patients and *dyspnea* and *chest discomfort* in 35—55%. Chest pain can occur in patients with and without coronary artery disease, and the symptoms are not always typical of cardiac pain.

Respiratory Adenosine may cause *bronchoconstriction* with asthma (243[C]) and a history of bronchoconstriction should be considered as a possible contraindication to intravenous adenosine.

Nervous system Adenosine has been reported to cause *increased intracranial pressure* (244[c]).

Gastrointestinal Adenosine can cause transient *epigastric pain* mimicking that of peptic ulceration (245[c]).

Miscellaneous Other reported adverse effects include *flushing* (23%), *headache* (32%), *nausea* (14%), *abdominal discomfort* (5%), and *light-headedness*. The figures in parentheses are from a study of 55 patients (246[C]). Rarer effects include *anxiety*, *dizziness*, and *seizure*.

Interactions Antagonists at adenosine receptors should inhibit the action of adenosine, and *theophylline* increases the dose of adenosine needed for conversion of supraventricular tachycardia (247[C]). *Dipyridamole* inhibits the uptake of adenosine by cells and thus increases its effects; this causes a large reduction in the effective dose of adenosine (248[C]). Adenosine does not interact with digoxin, disopyramide, flecainide, and quinidine.

Ajmaline and its derivatives

Ajmaline and its derivatives, prajmalium (*N*-propylajmaline), chloroacetylajmaline, and diethylaminohydroxypropylajmaline, are *Rauwolfia* alkaloids. Their use is restricted by serious adverse effects, which have been reviewed (222[R]).

Cardiovascular Ajmaline has prodysrhythmic effects. Of 1995 patients who were given ajmaline (1 mg/kg intravenously) during an electrophysiological study, 63 developed a *supraventricular tachydysrhythmia* (atrial flutter, fibrillation, or tachycardia), and seven an *atrioventricular re-entrant tachycardia* (249[C]). Those most at risk were the older patients, those with underlying cardiac disease, and those with a history of dysrhythmias or sinus node dysfunction. Ajmaline may also occasionally cause *hypotension* after intravenous administration.

Nervous system Neurological effects have been reported occasionally and include *confusion* and *cranial nerve palsies* (250[C], 251[c]).

Hematological *Neutropenia* is a relatively common and important adverse effect of ajmaline (252[R]). Of the three main mechanisms that can cause neutropenia (immune, toxic, and autoimmune) two have been associated with aprindine: immune and autoimmune neutropenia.

Liver Ajmaline may cause a *hepatitis* or *cholestasis*. Cholestasis has been reported with neutropenia (253[cr]) and with fever and eosinophilia (254[cr]). Although acute liver damage due to ajmaline is usually reversible there has been a report of persistent jaundice due to long-lasting cholestasis (255[c]).

Hypersensitivity reactions Hypersensitivity to ajmaline is rare, but there has been a report of an immune *interstitial nephritis* in association with fever (256[C]).

Other adverse effects include *dizziness*, *headache*, and a *sensation of warmth* after intravenous injection.

Overdosage In overdosage ajmaline may cause heart block and dysrhythmias, hypotension, malaise, vertigo, respiratory depression, and coma (257[R]). In one series of 38 cases there were nine deaths (24%) (258[C]). Treatment of overdosage includes gastric lavage, the intravenous administration of molar sodium lactate for dysrhythmias, conduction disturbances, and circulatory failure, and the insertion of a pacemaker if required.

Amiodarone

Amiodarone is highly effective in treating both ventricular and supraventricular dysrhythmias (259[CR]). Its pharmacology, therapeutic uses, and adverse effects and interactions have been extensively reviewed (260[R]–268[R]).

ADVERSE REACTION PATTERN

General and toxic reactions Amiodarone prolongs the QT interval and may therefore cause dysrhythmias; there have also been reports of conduction disturbances. Abnormalities of thyroid function tests can occur without thyroid dysfunction, typically increases in serum T_4 and reverse T_3 and a decrease in serum T_3. However, in up to 6% of patients frank thyroid dysfunction can occur (either hypothyroidism or hyperthyroidism). Several of the adverse effects of amiodarone are attributable to deposition of phospholipids in the tissues. These include its effects on the eyes, nerves, liver, skin, and lungs. Almost all patients develop reversible corneal microdeposits, which may occasionally interfere with vision. There are reports of peripheral neuropathy and other neurological effects. Changes in serum activities of aspartate aminotransferase and lactate dehydrogenase may occur without other evidence of liver disease, but liver damage may occur in the absence of biochemical evidence. Skin sensitivity to light occurs commonly, possibly due to phototoxicity. There may also be a bluish pigmentation of the skin. Interstitial pneumonitis and alveolitis have been reported and may be fatal.

Hypersensitivity reactions Lung damage due to amiodarone may be partly due to hypersensitivity.

Tumor-inducing effects Tumor-inducing effects have not been reported.

ORGANS AND SYSTEMS

Cardiovascular The incidence of *dysrhythmias* with amiodarone is under 3% (269[C]), lower than with many other antidysrhythmic drugs. It can prolong the QT interval and this can be associated with *torsade de pointes*, although this is uncommon. This effect is potentiated by hypokalemia (270[R]).

Other cardiac effects that have been reported include *sinus bradycardia*, *atrioventricular block*, *infra-His block*, *asystole*, and *refractoriness to DC cardioversion* (SEDA-10, 147).

There is a risk of *hypotension* and *atrioventricular block* when amiodarone is given intravenously (see below).

Respiratory There are many anecdotal reports that amiodarone may cause *interstitial pneumonitis* or *alveolitis*, and there have been reviews of the lung complications of amiodarone toxicity (271[R], 272[R]) and of its mechanisms (273[R]).

The risk of lung toxicity is about 5–6% (274[C]) and the risk is greatest during the first 12 months and among patients over 40 years of age. The effect may be dose-related. The mortality rate is about 9% (about 0.5% of the total).

The commonest form of lung damage is an interstitial alveolitis, although pneumonitis and bronchiolitis obliterans have also been reported, as have solitary localized fibrotic lesions, non-cardiac pulmonary edema, acute respiratory failure, acute pleuritic chest pain, and adult respiratory distress syndrome (SEDA-17, 220; SEDA-18, 201).

Amiodarone causes lung damage either by direct deposition of phospholipids in the lung tissue or by some immunologically mediated reaction. Other mechanisms have also been proposed, including oxidant-mediated damage, a direct detergent effect, and a direct toxic effect of iodide (SEDA-15, 168).

Diagnosis can be difficult. The clinical symptoms and signs, the changes on chest radiography, and abnormalities of lung function tests are all non-specific. The presence of lymphocytes and foamy macrophages in bronchial lavage fluids and of phospholipidosis in lung biopsies are all suggestive. Measurement of the diffusing capacity of carbon monoxide and lung scanning with gallium-67 have been used, but are unreliable. Computed tomography may show a typical pattern of basal peripheral high-density pleuroparenchymal linear opacities, although these may be absent (275[C]).

Although early reports suggested that corticosteroids might be beneficial in management, this has not been subsequently confirmed (276[C]).

Amiodarone has also been reported to cause impairment of lung function, even in patients who do not develop pneumonitis (277[c]), and pre-existing impairment of lung function may constitute a contraindication to amiodarone.

Nervous system The most common forms of neurological damage attributed to amiodarone are tremor, peripheral neuropathy, and ataxia (278[Cr]). Other effects that have been reported include delirium (279[c]), a Parkinsonian tremor (280[cr]), and pseudotumor cerebri (281[c]).

The peripheral neuropathy is probably due to intracellular lipidosis (282[C]).

Endocrine, metabolic There have been several reviews of the effects of amiodarone on thyroid function (283[R]–286[R]). Amiodarone causes *altered thyroid function tests*, with rises in serum concentrations of T_4 and reverse T_3 and a fall in serum T_3 concentration. This is due to inhibition of the peripheral conversion of T_4 to T_3, causing a preferential conversion to reverse T_3. These changes may occur in the absence of symptomatic abnormalities of thyroid function.

However, the use of amiodarone is also associated with both functional *hyperthyroidism* or *hypothyroidism*, in up to 6% of patients. These effects may be partly due to the excess intake of iodine present in the molecule of amiodarone or because amiodarone affects autoimmunity, either through its iodine content or through some other aspect of its structure. Patients with a history or a family history of thyroid abnormality are more susceptible to these effects.

Iodine intake may be important in determining the type of amiodarone-induced thyroid disease, since in one study amiodarone-induced hyperthyroidism was more common in an area of low iodine intake and hypothyroidism more common in an area of high iodine intake (287[C]). The risk of hypothyroidism may also be greater in patients who have pre-existing thyroid autoimmune disease (288[C]).

The diagnosis of amiodarone-induced thyroid disorders can be difficult, because amiodarone often alters thyroid function tests without disturbing clinical thyroid function. Although radio-iodine uptake by the thyroid gland is not helpful in making a diagnosis, the discharge of iodine from the thyroid gland in response to perchlorate is reduced in patients with hypothyroidism (289[C]). The test is not abnormal in patients with hyperthyroidism and it is not clear how helpful it is in hypothyroidism.

Since the measurement of serum T_3 and T_4 concentrations may not be helpful, an alternative would be to measure metabolic status. Measurement of the serum concentration of co-enzyme Q_{10} may distinguish patients with clinical thyroid dysfunction from those who simply have abnormalities of thyroid function tests (290[C]), but this remains to be better established.

The treatment of amiodarone-induced hyperthyroidism is difficult. It often does not respond to conventional therapy with carbimazole, methimazole, or radioiodine. However, corticosteroids and the combination of methimazole with potassium perchlorate have been reported to be effective (291[C]), even if the amiodarone is continued (292[c]). Other regimens that may be helpful include combinations of corticosteroids with carbimazole and benzylthiouracil, or with propylthiouracil (SEDA-15, 170). Other forms of treatment that have been successful have been plasma exchange and in very severe cases subtotal or total thyroidectomy (SEDA-17, 221).

There have also been reports of painful thyroiditis associated with amiodarone (SEDA-15, 170).

Amiodarone may cause *altered serum lipid concentrations* (293[C]). Serum cholesterol rises, as may the blood glucose and serum triglyceride concentrations. The mechanisms of these effects are not known; nor is it known to what extent they are due to changes in thyroid function.

Amiodarone may cause *endocrine testicular dysfunction*, judged by increases in serum concentrations of FSH and LH and hyper-responsiveness to GnRH (294[C]).

Hematological Although phospholipid inclusion bodies commonly occur in the neutrophils of patients taking amiodarone (295[C]), adverse hematological effects have rarely been attributed to amiodarone. However, there have been reports of *thrombocytopenia* (296[c]) and of impaired platelet aggregation, associated with gingival bleeding and ecchymoses of the legs (297[c]). Coombs'-positive *hemolytic anemia* has also been reported (298[c]).

Liver Amiodarone often causes rises in the serum activities of aspartate aminotransferase and lactate dehydrogenase to about twice normal, without changes in alkaline phosphatase or bilirubin, and without clinical evidence of liver dysfunction (299[C]). Changes of this kind were originally reported to be transient and dose-related, returning to normal when the dose was reduced

(300[R]). However, amiodarone may also cause *liver damage*, which usually takes the form of a hepatitis associated with phospholipid deposition, and there may be changes similar to those of alcoholic hepatitis (301[R]—303[R]). In some cases there may be progression of cirrhosis (304[c]). Other forms of liver damage that have been reported include cholestasis (305[c], 306[c]), and a syndrome resembling that of Reye's syndrome (307[c]). Acute hepatitis with liver failure can occur after intravenous administration and may be due to the solvent, polysorbate (308[c]).

The risk of hepatic impairment in patients taking amiodarone is not known, but it is clear that relatively severe liver damage can occur even in the absence of symptoms and with only minor associated changes in liver function tests.

Pancreas There has been one case report of *pancreatitis* in a patient who died of progressive liver failure (309[c]). Whether this was a direct effect of amiodarone or not is not clear.

Urinary system Increases in serum creatinine concentrations, correlated with serum amiodarone concentrations, have been reported (310[C]).

Skin and appendages Amiodarone commonly causes *photosensitivity* reactions in the skin (311[R], 312[C]). The risk of photosensitivity increases with the duration of the exposure. Window glass and sun screens do not give protection, although zinc or titanium oxide formulations may help (313[c], 314[C]). For most patients this adverse effect will be no more than a nuisance, and the benefit of therapy may be worth while. In a few cases, however, treatment may have to be withdrawn. There has also been a single report of a severe case of photosensitivity in conjunction with a syndrome resembling porphyria cutanea tarda, resulting in bullous lesions (315[c]).

Amiodarone may also cause a cosmetically annoying *bluish pigmentation* of the skin (316[c]). Other skin reactions which have been reported include *iododerma* (317[C]), *erythema nodosum*, *psoriasis* (see Ref. 318[c]), and *exfoliative dermatitis* (319[c]).

Amiodarone may increase the risk of mucosal and cutaneous toxicity due to radiotherapy and may rarely cause *hair loss* (SEDA-17, 221), and vasculitis (320[c]).

Histological examination of skin biopsies shows intracytoplasmic inclusions of phospholipids (321[c]).

Special senses In almost all patients (322[C], 323[C]) *corneal microdeposits* of lipofuscin occur secondary to the deposition of amiodarone. These are generally of no clinical significance, but occasionally patients may complain of haloes, photophobia, blurring of vision, or lid irritation. In some cases chronic *blepharitis* and *conjunctivitis* have been reported (324[C]), but the relation of these to amiodarone is not clear. Amiodarone has been reported to cause impaired color vision associated with *keratopathy* (325[C]).

A more serious effect of amiodarone on the eye is an *optic neuropathy* (326[c]). Although this resolves on withdrawal there may be residual field defects (327[c], 328[c]).

Rare effects include *raised intracranial pressure* with papilledema (329[c]) and *retinal maculopathy* (330[c]).

Sexual function *Epididymitis* has been reported in patients taking high dosages of amiodarone, resolving with dosage reduction or withdrawal (SEDA-18, 203).

Musculoskeletal A proximal *myopathy* has occasionally been reported in patients taking amiodarone (277[Cr]) and there has been a report of an acute necrotizing myopathy (331[c]).

Intravenous administration In contrast to its effects during oral administration, the therapeutic and short-term unwanted effects of amiodarone during intravenous administration come on within minutes or hours (260[R]). The reason for this is not clear; plasma concentrations after single oral and intravenous doses of 400 mg are very similar (260[R]), but that does not rule out a pharmacokinetic explanation for the paradox. The possible role of the solvent used in the intravenous formulation, polysorbate (Tween) 80, has not been fully elucidated.

After rapid intravenous administration *hypotension*, *shock*, and *atrioventricular block* may occur and may be fatal (260[R]). The rate of infusion should not exceed 5 mg/min. Other adverse effects reported during intravenous infusion include *sinus bradycardia* (332[C]), *facial flushing*, and *thrombophlebitis* (332[C], 333[C], 334[c], 335[c]). The risk of this last complication can be reduced by infusing the drug into as large a vein as possible and preferably via a central venous catheter, or perhaps by using a very dilute solution of the drug (336[c]).

Risk situations There is some evidence that the risk of hypothyroidism due to amiodarone is increased in elderly patients (337[C]), but the data are not conclusive.

In children under 10 years of age the risk of adverse effects seems to be *less* than in adults (338[C], 339[C]). It is not clear whether older children are at greater or lesser risks of adverse effects than adults.

There appears to be an increased risk of some of the adverse effects of amiodarone (including dysfunction of the liver and lungs) in patients who have had or who are having surgery (340[C]). In addition the perioperative mortality in these patients is higher than in controls (341[C]).

The factors that increase the risks of amiodarone-associated adverse cardiovascular effects during surgery

(342[R]) include pre-existing ventricular dysfunction, too rapid a rate of intravenous infusion, hypocalcemia, and an interaction between amiodarone and both the general anesthetics used and other drugs with negative inotropic or chronotropic effects. It has therefore been recommended (342[R]) that serum concentrations of calcium, amiodarone, and digoxin should be within the reference or therapeutic ranges before operation, and that other drugs with negative inotropic or chronotropic effects should be withdrawn before surgery.

Second-generation effects There are no major teratogenic effects of amiodarone (343[cR]). However, there have been individual reports of neonatal *hyperthyroxinemia* (344[c]), *goiter* (345[C]), and *hypothyroidism* (346[c]). In the case with goiter there was associated hypotonia, bradycardia, large fontanelles, and macroglossia (345[C]). There have also been reports of *sinus bradycardia* (345[C], 347[c]) and *prolongation of the QT interval* (343[cR]).

Overdosage There has been a report of acute self-poisoning with 8 grams of amiodarone orally (348[c]). On admission, the only abnormal physical sign was profuse sweating; the electrocardiogram showed sinus rhythm with a normal QT_c interval and the blood pressure was normal. No active measures were taken. The QT_c interval was subsequently prolonged on the third and fourth days after overdosage, and there was sinus bradycardia between the second and fifth days. Over 3 months of follow-up there were no effects on thyroid or liver function and no evidence of lung, skin, or corneal involvement.

Interactions Drug interactions with amiodarone have been reviewed (349[R]).

The interaction of amiodarone with digoxin is discussed in the section on cardiac glycosides above; dosages of digoxin should be reduced during amiodarone therapy.

Amiodarone potentiates the effects of the anticoagulants *warfarin* and *acenocoumarol*, probably by inhibiting their metabolism.

Amiodarone increases the plasma concentrations of *phenytoin*, probably by inhibiting its metabolism, while phenytoin increases the metabolism of amiodarone and perhaps also of its metabolite desethylamiodarone.

The clearance of *phenazone* (antipyrine) is reduced by amiodarone.

Because it prolongs the QT_c interval, amiodarone may potentiate the dysrhythmogenic actions of some *Class I antidysrhythmic drugs*.

The risks of cardiovascular adverse effects in patients undergoing surgery, mentioned above, may be partly related to an interaction of amiodarone with *anesthetics*, either directly or via some interaction with the catecholamines that are released during anesthesia. The risk of hypotension during cardiopulmonary bypass in patients taking amiodarone may be increased by the concurrent administration of an *ACE inhibitor*. There is a high incidence of lung complications when patients treated with amiodarone are ventilated with 100% *oxygen*, including acute adult respiratory distress syndrome.

The combination of amiodarone with β-adrenoceptor antagonists may be beneficial in the treatment of refractory ventricular tachycardia, especially when low doses of the β-blockers are used. However, there have also been reports of *adverse* interactions in these circumstances.

Sinus arrest and hypotension has been reported in a patient with a congestive cardiomyopathy when *diltiazem* was added to amiodarone therapy.

Amiodarone may increase the blood concentrations of *ciclosporin* and thus impair renal function.

Interference with diagnostic routines The effects of amiodarone on thyroid function tests have been mentioned above. Amiodarone has also been reported to cause a small and reversible increase in serum creatinine and blood urea nitrogen concentrations (350[c]). It is not clear whether this effect is due to true renal impairment, or to some effect on either the kinetics of creatinine or urea or their measurement in the blood.

Monitoring therapy It follows from the differences in the rates of onset of effects of amiodarone after oral and intravenous administration in the face of similar plasma concentrations (see above) that there can be no simple relation between the plasma concentrations of amiodarone and its therapeutic effects. Matters are further complicated by the fact that amiodarone is metabolized to desethylamiodarone, which has pharmacological activity. Thus, there is no value of the plasma amiodarone concentration above which it can be clearly stated that a therapeutic effect can be expected in the individual (260[R]), although current evidence (260[R], 351[C]) suggests that a plasma amiodarone concentration of around 1.0–2.5 μg/ml is associated with a high likelihood of therapeutic efficacy in patients with dysrhythmias. However, adverse effects may still occur when the plasma concentration is within this range, and there is no clear limit to the concentration above which toxicity starts to become important. Similarly, it is not clear what the therapeutic range of concentrations for desethylamiodarone is, although the therapeutic range seems to be around 0.5–1.0 μg/ml (SEDA-10, 146).

In one careful study EC_{50} values for certain effects of amiodarone were calculated on the basis of concentration–effect relations (352[C]). The concentrations of amiodarone and desethylamiodarone, respectively, that were associated with certain effects were as follows: reduction in heart rate 1.2 and 0.5 μg/ml; QT_c prolongation 2.6 and 1.4 μg/ml; corneal microdeposits 2.2 and 1.1 μg/ml.

Because amiodarone prolongs the QT_c interval, it has been suggested that that might be a useful measure of its efficacy. The percentage prolongation of the QT_c interval has been found to correlate well with both daily dose and the plasma and myocardial concentrations of amiodarone (353[C]), although this is not a universal finding during long-term administration (333[C], 354[C]), and the QT_c interval is not prolonged after short-term intravenous use (260[R]).

Since amiodarone inhibits the peripheral conversion of thyroxine (T_4) to tri-iodothyronine (T_3) there is an increase in serum concentrations of reverse tri-iodothyronine (rT_3). However, there have been conflicting results in studies of the relation between serum concentrations of rT_3 and the therapeutic and adverse effects of amiodarone (SEDA-15, 172).

Aprindine

The clinical pharmacology, clinical uses, efficacy, and adverse effects of aprindine have been extensively reviewed (220[R], 222[R], 355[R], 356[R]).

The adverse effects of aprindine are usually dose-related and most commonly affect the central nervous system. However, other less common but serious and potentially fatal adverse effects (neutropenia and liver damage) occur, and these limit its usefulness.

Nervous system Central nervous system adverse effects are common, particularly if a loading dose is given. These include *tremor* of the hands and fingers, *dizziness*, *ataxia*, *diplopia*, *nervousness*, *memory impairment*, *hallucinations and acute psychosis*, *convulsions*, *headache*, *nausea*, and *vomiting* (220[R]). There effects tend to wear off with continued treatment.

Hematological *Neutropenia* has often been reported, and is probably due to a direct toxic effect. Although its incidence is not known it may be as high as 1.3%; the incidence of leukopenia may be as high as 2.9% (356[R], 357[R]). Pancytopenia has also been reported (358[C]).

Liver *Liver damage* has been reported in association with aprindine, but the exact incidence is not known. In a report of five cases, three patients had a moderate hepatitis and two had cholestatic jaundice. The effects were confirmed by rechallenge in the three patients with hepatitis (359[C]). Granulomatous hepatitis has also been reported (360[c]).

Bepridil

Bepridil has been the subject of a brief general review (361[R]) and its pharmacokinetics have been specifically reviewed (362[R]).

Cardiovascular Bepridil may cause *hypotension* after rapid intravenous injection (363[C], 364[C]), but not during long-term oral therapy (365[C], 366[C]).

Bepridil prolongs the QT interval (367[C]–370[C]), an effect that is dose-related (368[C]). It may therefore cause *dysrhythmias*, including polymorphous ventricular tachycardia, the risk of which is greater in patients with potassium depletion, those with a pre-existing prolongation of the QT interval, those with a history of serious ventricular dysrhythmias, and those who are also taking other drugs that prolong the QT interval (371[R]).

Other After intravenous infusion bepridil may cause *local reactions* (370[C]) and *phlebothrombosis* (372[C]). Other minor adverse effects that have been reported include *urticaria* (373[C]), gastrointestinal disturbances (especially *diarrhea*) (363[C], 369[C]), and *dizziness* (363[C], 367[C], 369[C]).

Interactions Because it prolongs the QT interval, bepridil may potentiate the effects of other drugs which do the same (e.g. other *Class I antidysrhythmic drugs* and *amiodarone*).

Bepridil increases the rate of *antipyrine* clearance and might therefore be expected to enhance the rate of clearance of other drugs that are metabolized (374[c]).

Bepridil does not interact with digoxin (375[C]) or propranolol (367[C]). Although it is highly protein-bound, it seems not to take part in protein-binding displacement interactions (362[R]).

Bretylium

Bretylium, originally introduced as a hypotensive agent, but no longer used as such, has not been extensively used as an antidysrhythmic drug. Its clinical pharmacology, uses, efficacy, and adverse effects have been reviewed (222[R], 376[R]–378[R]). Adverse effects have reportedly caused the need for withdrawal in about 7% of patients (377[R]).

Bretylium is poorly absorbed and is therefore given parenterally. After intravenous administration it may cause *nausea*, *vomiting*, and *diarrhea*. *Postural hypotension* is common, and a significant fall in arterial pressure may occur even in patients who are supine (379[C]). Bretylium should be infused over 30–60 minutes to minimize these effects.

Occasionally there may be a transient *rise in blood pressure* after intravenous administration, due to the release of noradrenaline from sympathetic nerve-endings.

Ventricular tachydysrhythmias have been reported occasionally (380[Cr]).

Intravenous bretylium can cause severe *hyperthermia* (381[c], 382[c]).

Long-term treatment with bretylium can cause *parotid pain and swelling* and *pain in the tongue* (383[C]).

Cibenzoline

The electrophysiological effects, therapeutic effects and indications, pharmacokinetics, and adverse effects of cibenzoline have been reviewed (384[R]).

Cardiovascular Cibenzoline prolongs the PR interval, the QRS interval, and the QT_c interval (385[C]–388[C]). It also prolongs the AH and HV intervals (386[c], 389[C]) and shortens the sinus cycle length (386[c], 389[C]). Because of these effects it can cause *dysrhythmias*, as has been reported in several studies (385[C], 387[C], 388[C], 390[C]). *Right bundle branch block* has also been reported (387[C]).

Cibenzoline has a negative inotropic effect and may therefore cause *hypotension* (387[C], 388[C], 391[C], 392[C]) and *worsening heart failure* (385[C]).

Nervous system Various nervous system complaints have been reported in occasional patients, including *headache* (393[C]), *disturbances of visual accommodation* (393[C]), and *tremulousness* (394[C]). *Dizziness* and *light-headedness* have more commonly been reported, sometimes in association with *hypertension* (388[C], 395[C]).

There have been frequent reports of anticholinergic adverse effects, including *dry mouth* (388[C], 390[C], 391[C]), *blurred vision* (385[C], 390[C]), and *difficulty in micturition* (396[C]).

Endocrine, metabolic Several cases of *hypoglycemia* attributed to cibenzoline have been reported (397[C]–399[C]).

Liver There has been one report of slight rises in the activities of serum aminotransferases (394[C]), and one of ischemic *hepatitis* (400[c]).

Gastrointestinal Various gastrointestinal adverse effects have been reported not infrequently, including *nausea* (393[C]), sometimes in association with *abdominal pain* (388[C], 390[C], 391[C]), *vomiting*, and *diarrhea* (388[C], 389[C], 392[C], 394[C]).

Risk situations Cibenzoline is mainly cleared by the kidneys (392[C], 401[C], 402[C]). Its renal clearance falls with age (401[C]), which is attributable to renal impairment.

Monitoring therapy In most studies plasma cibenzoline concentrations have been around 200–400 μg/ml on average (385[C], 387[C], 389[C], 395[C]). Plasma concentrations correlate well with the electrophysiological effects of cibenzoline on the ECG (387[C]), its hemodynamic effects on the heart (403[C]), and the reduction in ventricular extra beats that it causes during therapy (404[C]).

It has been suggested that plasma concentrations of 100–200 μg/ml are associated with efficacy and that at concentrations over 400 μg/ml there is an increased risk of adverse reactions (388[C]). In one study, the patients who suffered adverse effects had a mean concentration of 913 μg/ml compared with 312 μg/ml in those who did not (389[C]).

Disopyramide

The use, clinical pharmacology, and adverse effects of disopyramide have been reviewed thoroughly (405[R], 406[R]).

ADVERSE REACTION PATTERN

General and toxic reactions The adverse effects of disopyramide are dose-related and are mostly mediated by its effects on the cardiovascular system and by its anticholinergic effects. Disopyramide has a strong negative inotropic effect on the myocardium and can cause heart failure and hypotension. It prolongs the QT_c interval and can cause serious ventricular tachydysrhythmias. Its anticholinergic effects can cause dry mouth, blurred vision, urinary retention, glaucoma, and erectile impotence. Hypoglycemia may also occur. Disopyramide may cause uterine contractions and should not be used during pregnancy.

Hypersensitivity reactions Angio-edema has been reported rarely.

Tumor-inducing effects Tumor-inducing effects have not been reported.

ORGANS AND SYSTEMS

Cardiovascular Disopyramide has three effects that can lead to cardiovascular complications (407[CR]).

(1) *Anticholinergic* The anticholinergic effects of disopyramide on the vagus have been reported to cause tachycardia with bundle branch block or conversion to

1:1 conduction of a supraventricular tachycardia with block.

(2) *QT_c interval prolongation* There have been several reports of ventricular dysrhythmias (e.g. polymorphous ventricular tachycardia, ventricular fibrillation, ventricular tachycardia) in association with a prolonged QT_c interval (SEDA-5, 180).

(3) *Negative inotropic effect* Disopyramide may cause worsening of cardiac failure and occasionally hypotension.

Current evidence suggests that the risk of adverse cardiac effects of disopyramide during intravenous administration relates to the *speed* of its administration rather than to the total dose given (SEDA-10, 149).

Nervous system Through its anticholinergic effects disopyramide causes *dry mouth* and *blurred vision* and occasionally may cause serious adverse effects, including *glaucoma* and *acute urinary retention* (405[R]). *Erectile impotence* (408[C]) and *acute psychosis* (409[C], 410[C]) have also been reported.

Endocrine, metabolic Disopyramide can cause *hypoglycemia* (411[C]) and it may also potentiate the effects of conventional hypoglycemic drugs (412[c]). This effect may be due to its chief metabolite mono-*N*-dealkyldisopyramide, since most of the reported cases of hypoglycemia have been in patients with renal impairment, in which the metabolite accumulates.

Hematological Disopyramide has been reported to cause *neutropenia* (413[c]) and a *coagulopathy* (414[c]).

Liver *Liver damage* was reported in 22 (0.35%) of 6294 patients given disopyramide, with jaundice in six (0.09%) (415[Cr]). Liver damage due to disopyramide may be associated with direct hepatocellular damage (416[c]) and intrahepatic cholestasis (417[c], 418[c]). However, it may also occur indirectly because of heart failure and hepatic congestion (419[c]). Thus, the incidence of direct liver damage quoted above may be an overestimate.

Sexual function Disopyramide may cause *uterine contractions* and should be avoided during pregnancy (420[C]). Transient *erectile impotence* has also been reported (421[c]).

Hypersensitivity *Angio-edema* has been attributed to disopyramide (422[c]).

Risk situations The risk of myocardial depression with consequent hypotension is greatest when disopyramide is infused rapidly intravenously. Loading doses of disopyramide should therefore be infused slowly (over 30–60 minutes).

Because of its anticholinergic effects, care should be taken both in patients with symptoms of prostatic hyperplasia (because of the risk of urinary retention) and in patients with glaucoma.

In renal failure there are complex changes in the pharmacokinetics of disopyramide, but the overall effect is accumulation due to reduced renal clearance (405[R]).

Disopyramide is highly bound to plasma proteins and this binding is saturable within the therapeutic range. Thus, at high dosages there may be an increase in the unbound fraction of drug in the plasma with proportionately greater effects.

Second-generation effects Although disopyramide and its *N*-monodesalkyl metabolite are both excreted in breast milk the amounts are probably too small to be of importance (423[c]).

Overdosage Overdosage of disopyramide is associated with apnea, loss of consciousness, loss of spontaneous respiration, hypotension, and cardiac dysrhythmias (424[C], 425[CR]). Suggested treatment (426[R]) includes arterial blood pressure monitoring, correction of acidosis and hypokalemia, and the intravenous infusion of a pressor agent for severe hypotension. Cardiac depressant drugs (e.g. Class I antidysrhythmics) should not be used to treat dysrhythmias, and the use of pyridostigmine to reverse the anticholinergic effects of disopyramide (427[C]) is not recommended (SEDA-10, 149).

Interactions There is an increased risk of dysrhythmias if disopyramide is used in conjunction with other drugs that prolong the QT interval, e.g. *Class I antidysrhythmic drugs* (428[CR]).

Disopyramide may potentiate the effects of *warfarin* (429[c]), although it is not known whether or not this is of any importance (430[c]).

The combination of disopyramide and *practolol* has been reported to cause profound sinus bradycardia and asystole (431[c], 432[c]).

Hyperkalemia has been reported to increase the risk of dysrhythmias in patients taking disopyramide (433[c]), and disopyramide should therefore be used with caution in patients who are taking drugs that can increase body potassium, such as *potassium-sparing diuretics* and *ACE inhibitors*.

Encainide

In the wake of the preliminary and final reports of the results of the Cardiac Arrhythmia Suppression Trial (CAST) (434[C], 435[C]) that there was an increased risk of death among patients being treated with encainide and flecainide after myocardial infarction, there have been numerous publications in which the implications of these findings have been thoroughly discussed (436[R]–439[R], 440[C]).

The relative risk of death or cardiac arrest due to dysrhythmia in the treated patients was 2.6 and the relative risk due to all causes was 2.38. The risk of non-fatal cardiac adverse effects was no different in the treated patients to those taking placebo and there was no difference in the use of other drugs across the groups.

Although there is a consensus that encainide and flecainide were associated with an increase in the rate of mortality in CAST, there are still some open questions. First, the patients recruited to CAST all had asymptomatic ventricular dysrhythmias after myocardial infarction, and it is not clear whether the results can be extrapolated to other patients. Second, the reasons for the increased mortality in the treated patients are not clear: ventricular dysrhythmias and worsening of left ventricular function are both possible. Third, it is not clear whether the results of CAST in patients with asymptomatic ventricular dysrhythmias after myocardial infarction can also be applied to other Class I antidysrhythmic drugs.

Other reviews of the clinical pharmacology, clinical use, efficacy, and adverse effects of encainide have appeared elsewhere (223[R], 441[R]–444[R], 445[CR]).

Cardiovascular The increased risk of cardiovascular death when encainide is used in patients who have had a myocardial infarction has been mentioned above. Separate studies have confirmed the *prodysrhythmic* actions of encainide (446[CR], 447[C]–449[C]). The incidence of prodysrhythmias is much higher in patients being treated for ventricular dysrhythmias than in those being treated for supraventricular dysrhythmias (450[C]).

Encainide has also been reported to cause *sinus node arrest* in association with prolonged sinus node recovery time (451[c]). It may also raise the pacing threshold in patients with chronic implanted pacemakers (452[C]), although this has not been reported to increase the failure rate of pacemakers.

Encainide has a negative inotropic effect on the heart and may cause *hypotension* (191[C]) or *worsening heart failure*.

Nervous system The most common non-cardiac effects of encainide affect the central nervous system, and include *abnormal or blurred vision* (10.6%), *dizziness* (7.3%), *headaches* (6.0%), *nausea* (4.3%), *vertigo* (2.3%), *insomnia*, and *fatigue*. The figures in parentheses are taken from a review of 349 patients with supraventricular dysrhythmias treated with encainide (446[CR]). These effects are common during long-term therapy but may also occur transiently during intravenous administration and appear to be dose-related (453[C], 454[C]).

A case of *encephalopathy* has also been attributed to encainide (455[c]).

Endocrine, metabolic Encainide can cause *hyperglycemia* (456[c]), perhaps due to insulin resistance.

Gastrointestinal *Nausea* may occur during long-term therapy, probably due to a central nervous effect (see above).

Skin and appendages *Skin rashes* have been reported occasionally during long-term therapy (457[C]).

Other There have been reports of *leg cramps* and of a *metallic taste* in the mouth after intravenous treatment (454[C]).

Risk situations Encainide is metabolized, at least partly, by hydroxylation, and it is possible that poor hydroxylators may be at greater risk from adverse effects than extensive hydroxylators. However, this has not been formally proven.

Children under the age of 6 months may be more liable to the prodysrhythmic effects of encainide than older children (458[C]).

Flecainide

The clinical pharmacology, clinical use, and adverse effects of flecainide have been reviewed (459[R]–461[R]).

In a review of 60 original articles detailing 1835 courses of intravenous and/or oral flecainide in both placebo-controlled and comparative studies as well as a large number of uncontrolled studies, unwanted cardiac events occurred in 8% of patients (462[R]). The cardiac events were *hypotension* (1.3%), *heart failure* (0.4%), *sinus node dysfunction* (1.6%), *bundle branch block* (1.0%), *atrial dysrhythmias* (1.6%), and *ventricular dysrhythmias* (1.3%). However, in a series of 8505 patients, 5507 of whom took flecainide for more than 4 weeks and most of whom took dosages of 100–300 mg/day, cardiac adverse effects occurred in only about 2% and non-cardiac effects in about 10% (463[C]). The most common cardiac adverse effects were *angina pectoris*, *dysrhythmias*, *worsening of heart failure*, and *hemodynamic changes*. Of the long-term non-cardiac adverse effects the most common were nausea and vomiting, dizziness, bowel disturbances, headache, and visual disturbances.

The increased mortality rate in patients taking flecainide after an acute myocardial infarction in the CAST study has been mentioned above under encainide.

Cardiovascular The *prodysrhythmic effects* of flecainide, by prolongation of the QT_c interval, have been widely discussed (SEDA-15, 175; 464[C], 465[R], 466[Cr], 467[R], 468[c]).

Flécainide has also been reported to cause acute *hypotension* after intravenous administration (469[C]).

Nervous system The most common non-cardiac adverse effects of flecainide are on the central nervous system and include *dizziness*, *drowsiness*, *visual disturbances*, *headache*, *nausea*, *paresthesia*, *nervousness*, and *tremor*. The incidence of these adverse effects has varied widely from report to report (470[CR], 471[CR]). Other reported effects of flecainide include *dysarthria* and *visual hallucinations* (472[C]), *abnormal taste sensations*, *flushing*, a glove-and-stocking type of *peripheral neuropathy*, and *dystonia* (SEDA-17, 223).

Hematological Flecainide can cause *neutropenia* (473[C]).

Liver Flecainide can cause increases in the serum concentrations of aminotransferases (474[c]), in one case with *cholestasis* and jaundice (475[c]).

Urinary system Flecainide can cause acute *urinary retention*, perhaps due to a local anesthetic effect on the bladder mucosa (476[c]).

Skin and appendages Flecainide can cause a *psoriasiform eruption* (477[c]).

Genital system Flecainide inhibits sperm motility in vitro (478[c]), but this has not been reported to be of clinical relevance. It can cause *erectile impotence* (479[C]).

Risk situations Reports of the use of flecainide in children suggest that the risk of adverse effects is low, although these studies have been very small (480[C]—482[C]).

Flecainide is cleared partly by dose-dependent metabolism and partly unchanged via the kidneys. As one would therefore expect, severe renal impairment and hepatic impairment both cause a reduction in its rate of clearance (483[C], 484[C]). Dosages should therefore be reduced in these circumstances.

Flecainide is metabolized by hydroxylation in the liver. Its half-life is therefore prolonged in poor hydroxylators (485[c]) and poor metabolizers may be at an increased risk of adverse effects.

Overdosage There have been a few reports of the effects of overdosage of flecainide (486[cr], 487[c], 488[C], 489[C], 490[c], 491[c]). Various treatments have been used in these circumstances, but nothing specific can be recommended.

Interactions Despite an early report that flecainide might alter the pharmacokinetics of *digoxin*, there is evidence that whatever action it has is minimal and probably of no clinical significance (492[C]). However, the combination does cause a significant increase in the PR interval; although the clinical significance of this is unclear, it may be important for patients with impaired sinus node function (493[c]).

The combination of flecainide with *propranolol* results in additive hypotensive and negative inotropic effects.

The combination of flecainide with *amiodarone* may result in reduced conduction, predisposing to bundle branch block and dysrhythmias (494[C], 495[c]).

Although *verapamil* reduces the clearance of flecainide, this is probably not clinically important (496[C]). However, there is also a pharmacodynamic interaction, since both drugs increase the PR interval and have additive effects on myocardial contractility and atrioventricular conduction (497[c]).

Flecainide is metabolized by CYP2D6, and is subject to polymorphic metabolism. In extensive metabolizers its clearance is reduced by *quinine* (498[C]). *Quinidine* reduces the clearance of R-flecainide but not that of S-flecainide (499[C]).

Lidocaine (lignocaine)

The use of lidocaine as a local anesthetic is covered in Chapter 11.

The incidence of adverse effects to lidocaine in antidysrhythmic dosages is low. In one series of 750 patients given lidocaine intravenously for cardiac dysrhythmias, adverse reactions occurred in only 47 (6.3%) and were thought to have been life-threatening in 12 (1.6%) (500[CR]). However, the risk of adverse effects is dose-related and increases at intravenous infusion rates of around 3 mg/minute (501[C]). Most of the adverse effects are on the cardiovascular and central nervous systems.

ADVERSE REACTION PATTERN

General and toxic reactions The adverse effects of lidocaine are dose-related and occur more commonly at higher rates of infusion (around 3 mg/minute or more). Most commonly they affect the central nervous system and include headache, dizziness, tremor, confusion, tinnitus, dysarthria, paresthesia, alterations in the level of consciousness from drowsiness to coma, respiratory depression, and convulsions. Cardiac adverse effects are less common, although lidocaine may occasionally cause dysrhythmias and very rarely worsening of cardiac function. Its active metabolites are also toxic and infusion should not continue for more than 24—48 hours.

Hypersensitivity reactions Hypersensitivity reactions have not been reported.

Tumor-inducing effects Tumor-inducing effects have not been reported.

ORGANS AND SYSTEMS

Cardiovascular Lidocaine can cause *dysrhythmias* and *hypotension*. The dysrhythmias that have been reported include sinus bradycardia, supraventricular tachycardia (500[CR]), and rarely *torsade de pointes* (502[CR]). There have also been rare reports of *cardiac arrest* (500[CR]) and *worsening heart failure* (503[c]). Lidocaine may also cause an increased risk of *asystole* after repeated attempts at defibrillation (504[C]). After acute myocardial infarction lidocaine may increase mortality, and it should be used only in patients with specific so-called warning dysrhythmias (i.e. frequent or multifocal ventricular extra beats, or salvos) (505[R]).

Nervous system Nervous system toxicity is most often seen with rapid intravenous infusion (501[C], 506[CR], 507[C]). The effects include *headache*, *dizziness*, *tremor*, *confusion*, *tinnitus*, *dysarthria*, *paresthesia*, *respiratory depression*, *altered level of consciousness* (from drowsiness to coma), and *convulsions*.

Risk situations The adverse effects of lidocaine are dose-related, and are more common in elderly people, in people of light weight, and in patients with acute myocardial infarction or congestive cardiac failure. There is also an increased risk of central nervous system effects during cardiopulmonary bypass (508[C]).

Because lidocaine is metabolized to two toxic metabolites with longer half-lives than lidocaine, it should not be infused for more than 24—48 hours at a time.

In cardiac failure, shock, and postoperatively, there are reductions in both the metabolism and the apparent volume of distribution of lidocaine. Dosages should be altered accordingly (509[R]).

Interactions *Propranolol* reduces the clearance of lidocaine (510[C], 511[C]), and one would therefore expect this combination to increase the chance of adverse effects of lidocaine.

The combination of lidocaine with β-adrenoceptor antagonists is associated with an increased risk of some minor non-cardiac adverse events (dizziness, numbness, somnolence, confusion, slurred speech, and nausea and vomiting), although the difference is very small (512[C]). The combination is not associated with an increased risk of dysrhythmias.

The histamine (H_2) receptor antagonists *cimetidine* and *ranitidine* inhibit the clearance of lidocaine, but it is not clear if this is clinically important (513[R]).

Propafenone reduces the clearance of lidocaine, a small and probably clinically unimportant effect; however, there may also be a pharmacodynamic interaction, with increased central nervous system adverse effects (514[C]).

Lorcainide

The clinical pharmacology, clinical use, efficacy, and adverse effects of lorcainide have been reviewed (515[R]—517[R]).

Cardiovascular Cardiovascular effects of lorcainide are reportedly uncommon (under 1% of cases) and have mostly been associated with intravenous administration. They include *hypotension* (515[R]) and *heart block*. Pre-existing sinoatrial disease and heart block are contraindications to the use of lorcainide (518[R]).

Nervous system Nervous system effects account for most adverse reactions to lorcainide after both intravenous and oral administration. During intravenous treatment patients may complain of *vertigo*, *feeling hot*, and *numbness of the feet* (519[C]), *dizziness*, *blurred vision*, and *muscle tremor* (520[C]), and *tingling sensations in the fingers or tongue* (521[C]). All of these effects are transient.

During long-term oral therapy the most frequent adverse effect is of *sleep disturbances* of one kind or another, the frequency being anything up to 45% (520[C], 522[C]—527[C]). The main types of disturbance are difficulty in falling asleep, nightmares, and lively dreams. In about half of the patients affected there is also *excessive sweating* (524[C], 525[C]). These effects become less severe after a week or two of therapy, and during that time benzodiazepines may give symptomatic relief (528[R]). In contrast, these patients do not suffer drowsiness or other central nervous system effects during the day.

Seizures and *hallucinations* have been rarely reported (528[R]).

Endocrine, metabolic Lorcainide has been reported to cause *hyponatremia*, attributed to inappropriate secretion of ADH (529[C]).

Gastrointestinal *Nausea* occurs in about 5% of patients during long-term oral therapy. It is probably of central nervous origin (528[R]).

Skin and appendages There have been a few reports of mild *allergic skin reactions* (528[R]).

Risk situations The adverse effects of lorcainide are dose-related and may be partly caused by its active metabolite, norlorcainide, which accumulates during treatment.

Magnesium sulfate

Magnesium sulfate in bolus doses of 2—4 grams over up to 5 minutes causes feelings of *warmth*, *flushing*, and sometimes *sweating* (530[C]—533[C]). Transient *nausea* has also been reported (531[C], 533[C]). Some patients develop mild transient *hypotension* (531[C], 533[C]).

Adverse effects are uncommon during prolonged intravenous infusions in doses of 0.5—8 mmol/hour (60—1000 mg/hour).

Mexiletine

Mexiletine is similar in action to lidocaine, but it can be given orally. Its adverse effects are dose-related. They may occur in up to 50% of patients (534[C]) and require to be withdrawn in a higher proportion (535[C]). Its most common adverse effects are on the cardiovascular and central nervous systems. Its pharmacokinetics, clinical use, and adverse effects and interactions have been widely reviewed (222[R], 536[R]—539[R], 540[cR]).

Cardiovascular *Prodysrhythmic* effects of mexiletine have been reported in up to 29% of cases, although it has been suggested that on average the incidence is lower than has been reported with other antidysrhythmic drugs (541[R]).

Circulatory depression with *bradycardia* and *hypotension* have also been reported (542[C]—544[C]), and it may have major hemodynamic effects in patients with preexisting impairment of left ventricular dysfunction (545[C]). Other cardiovascular effects include *widening of the QRS complex*, *atrioventricular dissociation*, *heart block*, *sinus arrest*, and *cardiac arrest* (544[C], 546[C]). *Angina-like pain* has also been reported.

Respiratory Mexiletine has been associated with *pulmonary fibrosis* and eventual respiratory failure (547[c]).

Nervous system The commonest adverse effects of mexiletine are on the nervous system and include *gastrointestinal distress* (38%), *light-headedness* (20%), *tremor* (12%), and *co-ordination difficulties* (11%). The figures in parentheses are quoted from a study in which mexiletine was compared with quinidine (548[C]). Other reported adverse effects include *changes in sleep habit*, *weakness*, *headache*, *visual problems*, and *nervousness*. *Slurred speech*, *dysarthria*, *diplopia*, and *ataxia* have also been reported (549[R]).

Hematological Mexiletine can cause a spuriously low platelet count as a result of clumping of platelets due to antibodies (550[c]); however, it can also cause a true *thrombocytopenia* (551[c], 552[c]).

Liver Changes in liver function tests, resolving on withdrawal, have been reported (553[C]). In one case there was histological evidence of *cholestasis*.

Gastrointestinal *Nausea* and *vomiting* are common and probably central in origin, since they occur with intravenous as well as oral therapy (542[c]).

Mexiletine also affects the esophagus, and may cause *heartburn* (534[C]) and *esophageal spasm and ulceration* (534[C], 554[c]).

Skin and appendages Mexiletine can occasionally cause generalized *rashes* (SEDA-17, 224; 548[C]), *pseudolymphomatous change with erythroderma* (555[cr]), and *contact urticaria* (556[c]).

Risk situations Mexiletine is mainly cleared polymorphically by CYP2D6 in the liver, and poor metabolizers and the slower among the extensive metabolizers have a higher incidence of mild adverse effects (nausea and light-headedness) (557[C]). However, it has also been reported that renal failure may be associated with an increase in plasma mexiletine concentrations (558[c]).

Overdosage Overdosage with mexiletine in two cases resulted in death due to cardiovascular effects (559[C], 560[c]).

Interactions Interactions of mexiletine with other cardioactive drugs have been reviewed (561[R]). The most important are the beneficial interactions with β-adrenoceptor antagonists, *quinidine*, and *amiodarone* in the suppression of ventricular tachydysrhythmias. During these interactions the adverse effects of mexiletine may also be reduced in frequency, although that has not always been found (562[C]).

Mexiletine reduces the clearance of *theophylline*, and this combination has been reported to cause ventricular tachycardia (563[c]). The interaction of mexiletine with *caffeine* is similar (564[c]).

Other interactions have been reported (for example, with antacids, rifampicin, and phenytoin), but they are unlikely to be clinically important (561[R]).

Interference with diagnostic routines Mexiletine caused an increased incidence of positive antinuclear antibody (ANA) titers in some studies (540[cR], 565[C]) but not in others (566[C], 567[C]). The clinical significance of this effect is not clear. For example, there have been no reports of a lupus-like syndrome attributable to mexiletine.

Mexiletine causes increases in the serum activities of AsT, AlT, and alkaline phosphatase in a few patients (540[cR]).

Moricizine (moracizine, ethmozine)

Moricizine has class I antidysrhythmic actions that cannot be easily further subclassified. Its pharmacology, clinical pharmacology, clinical uses, and adverse effects and interactions have been the subject of several reviews (568[R]–570[R]).

Cardiovascular The overall risk of *dysrhythmias* with moricizine seems to be similar to that of other antidysrhythmic drugs, at around 10% (571[R]), although lower rates have been reported. Moricizine increases mortality in patients with asymptomatic ventricular dysrhythmias after myocardial infarction, as shown by CAST-II (572[C]).

There have also been anecdotal reports of *conduction defects* (SEDA-17, 225).

Moricizine has little or no effect on hemodynamics, but it sometimes has adverse hemodynamic effects and may *exacerbate heart failure* (SEDA-17, 225).

Hematological Moricizine has an antiaggregatory effect on platelets, and *thrombocytopenia* has been reported (573[C]).

Liver Moricizine can cause increased serum bilirubin concentrations and serum aminotransferase activities (573[C]).

Risk situations Moricizine is cleared by the liver, and dosages should be reduced in liver disease (574[C]).

Interactions Moricizine is an enzyme-inducer and it increases the rates of clearance of *antipyrine* (575[C]) and *theophylline* (576[C]).

Cimetidine inhibits the metabolism of moricizine, but the effect is probably clinically unimportant (577[C]).

Procainamide

In a prospective study of 488 in-patients there were adverse reactions in 45 cases (9.2%), thought to have been life-threatening in seven (1.4%), none of whom died (578[C]). The seven patients all had cardiovascular effects. Common adverse effects included gastrointestinal upsets (19 cases) and fever (eight cases). Reactions were more common at daily dosages of 3 grams and more.

ADVERSE REACTION PATTERN

General and toxic reactions Dose-related adverse effects of procainamide predominantly affect the heart, causing reduced myocardial contractility and hypotension, prolongation of the QT_c interval with consequent dysrhythmias, and conduction defects. Also dose-related is the lupus-like syndrome, which most commonly causes polyarthralgia, myalgia, fever, and pleurisy. Neutropenia has been relatively commonly reported in patients taking modified-release formulations. Other adverse effects are uncommon; they include muscle weakness, ataxia, mental confusion, cholestasis, and skin rashes.

Hypersensitivity reactions Hypersensitivity reactions include fever and hematological reactions including neutropenia, pancytopenia, and pure red cell aplasia.

Tumor-inducing effects Tumor-inducing effects have not been reported.

ORGANS AND SYSTEMS

Cardiovascular Procainamide has a negative inotropic effect and can cause *hypotension* after both intravenous and oral administration (579[C], 580[C]). For this reason it should be infused slowly when given intravenously, at no more than 20 mg/minute. In patients with poor cardiac function procainamide may *worsen heart failure*, and it may reduce survival after myocardial infarction (581[C]).

Procainamide prolongs the QT interval (582[C]) and can cause *dysrhythmias*. It can also impair cardiac conduction and can cause *bradycardia* and *heart block* (578[C]). In the sick sinus syndrome it may alter sinus node recovery time (583[C]), although the clinical significance of this is not clear.

Pericarditis and *tamponade* have been reported as rare complications of procainamide-induced lupus-like syndrome (584[c]).

Respiratory Procainamide can cause *lung damage* in the context of a lupus-like syndrome (SEDA-17, 226).

Nervous system Procainamide rarely causes nervous system effects. *Acute confusion* (585[C]), *cerebellar ataxia* (586[c]), *tremor* (587[c]), and *muscle weakness* (588[c]–591[c]) have all been reported occasionally. In high dosages procainamide has *anticholinergic effects* (592[c]).

Hematological Hematological abnormalities can occur in the absence of a lupus-like syndrome (see below). *Hemolytic anemia* (593[C]), *thrombocytopenia* (594[C], 595[C]), and *pancytopenia* (596[C]) have all been reported occasionally. Thrombocytopenia may be more common in patients taking modified-release formulations (595[C]). *Pure red cell aplasia* has also been reported (597[c], 598[c]), but it was not clear whether or not there was an associated lupus-like syndrome.

However, the most common adverse hematological effect of procainamide is *neutropenia*, which has been frequently reported in recent years, particularly in patients taking modified-release formulations. In one case-control study 4.4% of 114 patients taking modified-release formulations had neutropenia, compared with none in a control group of 509 patients (599[C]). However, a larger subsequent case-control study failed to confirm this association (600[C]). Nonetheless, reports of neutropenia attributed to procainamide continue to appear (601[c]).

There was a positive direct antiglobulin (Coombs') test in about 20% of elderly patients taking procainamide (602[C]). Although a positive Coombs' test may occur in association with a lupus-like syndrome, there was no relation in these cases between positive tests and the presence of antinuclear antibodies. Three of the patients had an autoimmune hemolytic anemia.

Gastrointestinal *Pseudo-obstruction* has been attributed to the use of a modified-release formulation of procainamide, perhaps due to its anticholinergic effects (603[c]).

Liver Procainamide may cause intrahepatic *cholestasis*, perhaps as part of a hypersensitivity reaction (604[cr]).

Gastrointestinal *Nausea*, *vomiting*, and *diarrhea* in response to procainamide are dose-related and are common with dosages of 4 grams a day or more (605[C]).

Skin and appendages *Lichen planus* has been attributed to procainamide as part of a lupus-like syndrome (606[c]).

Angio-edema has been reported in a patient who had no history of hereditary angio-edema (607[c]).

Procainamide has also been reported to cause *urticarial vasculitis*, although it was not clear whether or not this was part of a lupus-like syndrome (608[c]).

Special senses *Scleritis* has been reported as part of a procainamide-induced lupus-like syndrome (609[c]).

Musculoskeletal Procainamide can cause an *arthropathy* as part of a lupus-like syndrome, and the histological findings are indistinguishable from those in idiopathic SLE (610[cr]).

Procainamide has occasionally been reported to cause *muscle weakness* (SEDA-14, 152; SEDA-16, 183), and it may also cause or *exacerbate myasthenia gravis* (611[c]). Necrotizing *myopathy of the diaphragm* has also been reported, perhaps as part of a lupus-like syndrome (612[c]).

Lupus-like syndrome Procainamide is one of the common causes of drug-induced lupus-like syndrome (613[R]), which is contrasted with idiopathic lupus erythematosus in Table 6. About 29—35% of patients taking procainamide for at least a year will be affected and the effect is dose-related. The average age of onset is 59—68 years and 35—58% of the subjects are women. The syndrome can come on within a few weeks, but has been reported as late as 9 years after starting treatment.

Antinuclear antibody is usually present (in 83% of cases), but antibodies to native DNA are not found, although there may be antibodies to single-stranded DNA. Patients taking procainamide may have antinuclear antibodies without developing a lupus-like syndrome.

Because this adverse effect is dose-related, it is more likely to occur in slow acetylators than in fast acetylators (614[R]), and the rate of development of antinuclear antibody depends on acetylator status (615[C]). Acecainide (see above) probably does not cause the syndrome, which is therefore attributable to either procainamide itself or a metabolite other than acecainide, such as a hydroxylated derivative (616[R]). The syndrome usually regresses rapidly after withdrawal of procainamide, but in a few patients recovery may be delayed; if there are serious effects oral corticosteroid therapy may be required.

The most common feature is arthralgia, in about 77% of cases, with *pleural or lung involvement* in about 75%. Other common features include *myalgia*, *fever*, *hepatomegaly*, *pericarditis*, *arthritis*, and *splenomegaly*. *Skin rashes*, *adenopathy*, and *Raynaud's phenomenon* occur in 5—10% of cases, and neuropsychiatric and renal involvement are rare. *Thrombotic problems* may occur because of the properties of anti-DNA and antiphospholipid antibodies (see below). The so-called lupus anticoagulant may be detected in people taking procainamide even without clinical evidence of lupus (617[c]).

The mechanisms whereby procainamide causes this lupus-like syndrome are not clear. It is, of course, associated with the production of many antibodies, including antihistone, antiguanosine, anti-DNA, and antiphospholipid antibodies (618[R]). The production of autoantibodies may be due to one of two major mechanisms: first, procainamide may act as a hapten, binding to DNA, nuclear protein, or some membrane constituent, the hapten—protein complex stimulating the production of antibodies; second, it may alter suppressor cell function (619[C]). There is also evidence that procainamide can combine with ribonucleoprotein from damaged myocardium after myocardial infarction, thus precipitating the production of antibodies to ribonucleoprotein (620[C]).

The antinuclear antibody is positive in virtually all cases and the ESR is often raised. Antihistone antibodies are also present in most cases. The prevalence of serum autoantibodies to high-mobility group (HMG) proteins in the serum of patients with drug-induced lupus-like syndrome varies from protein to protein: 67% for HMG-14 and/or HMG-17, compared with 21% for HMG-1 and/or HMG-2. Procainamide-induced lupus is also associated with antibodies to the H2A-H2B dimer (621[C]).

In procainamide-induced lupus there is an increase in the number of B cells in both blood and pleural fluid

Table 6. *Contrast between drug-induced lupus-like syndrome and idiopathic lupus erythematosus*

Feature	Idiopathic lupus erythematosus	Drug-induced lupus-like syndrome
Age and sex	Typically young women	Any (depends on use)
Acetylator status	Any	More likely in slow acetylators
Organs	Any	Kidneys usually spared
Antinuclear antibody	Usually present	Usually present
Complement	May be reduced	Usually normal
Anti-DNA antibodies	Usually present (native DNA)	Only to single-stranded DNA

to about 80% (normal 10—25%). Concentrations of IL-6 and soluble IL-2R are also increased (622[c]).

Risk situations Care must be taken in patients with pre-existing conduction tissue disease or heart failure. Loading dosages should be reduced in cardiac failure, because of a lowered apparent volume of distribution (509[R]). Maintenance dosages should also be reduced in the presence of renal or hepatic impairment, including hepatic congestion due to cardiac failure (509[R]).

Interactions The effects of procainamide on the QT interval may be potentiated by other drugs with this action, i.e. other *Class I antidysrhythmic drugs* and *amiodarone* (623[C]). It has also been reported that the pharmacokinetics of procainamide are altered by *amiodarone*, with a reduction in clearance of about 25% due to changes in both renal and non-renal clearances (619[C]).

The renal clearance of procainamide is inhibited by *cimetidine* (235[C], 624[C]), and by *trimethoprim* (236[C]).

Monitoring therapy The use of serum procainamide concentration measurements in monitoring therapy has been reviewed (509[R], 625[R]). Serum concentrations of 4—10 μg/ml are associated with therapeutic benefit in over 90% of ventricular tachydysrhythmias, and toxicity becomes highly likely over 12 μg/ml. However, the main metabolite of procainamide, acecainide (see above), has antidysrhythmic activity of its own; thus, because metabolism varies widely between individuals and because acecainide is eliminated by the kidneys, serum concentration measurement of procainamide alone has limited usefulness, particularly in renal failure. There is currently little information on the interpretation of combined measurement of the two compounds.

Propafenone

The pharmacological effects, clinical pharmacology, therapeutic uses, adverse effects, and interactions of propafenone have been reviewed (626[R]—629[R]).

The main adverse effects of propafenone are cardiovascular (27%), central nervous (21%), and gastrointestinal (20%) (figures taken from Ref. 630[CR]). Other adverse effects occur in under 6% of cases. The overall risk of non-cardiac effects is around 14%. These adverse effects are dose-related: the incidence is 11% at 300 mg/day, 22% at 450 mg/day, 33% at 600 mg/day; and 48% at 900 mg/day (630[CR]).

Cardiovascular Cardiovascular adverse effects have been reported in 13—27% of patients and ventricular dysrhythmias in 8—19% in small studies. However, in large studies the risk has been reported to be about 5%.

Conduction disturbances are common and can result in sinus bradycardia, sinoatrial block, sinus arrest, any degree of atrioventricular block, and right or left bundle-branch block (SEDA-10, 151; SEDA-15, 179). *Dysrhythmias* may occur, including ventricular tachycardia, ventricular flutter, and atrial fibrillation (631[C]—633[C]). *Hypotension* and *worsening of heart failure* have occasionally been reported (SEDA, 151).

Respiratory Since propafenone is a β-adrenoceptor antagonist as well as a Class I antidysrhythmic drug, it may cause shortness of breath or worsening of asthma (634[c]).

Nervous system Adverse effects on the nervous system are common and include *somnolence*, *weakness and disorientation*, *dizziness and vertigo*, *tremor*, *visual disturbances*, and *convulsions* (SEDA-10, 151).

Mineral and fluid balance Propafenone can cause *hyponatremia* due to inappropriate secretion of ADH (635[C]).

Hematological Propafenone can occasionally cause *neutropenia*, with a calculated incidence of about one in 10 000 prescriptions per year (636[c]).

Liver Propafenone can increase the serum activities of aminotransferases and other enzymes associated with liver function (637[C]). There have also been reports of *cholestatic jaundice* (638[r]).

Gastrointestinal Unwanted gastrointestinal effects are the most common, occurring in up to 30% of cases. These include *anorexia*, *nausea and vomiting*, *dry mouth*, a *metallic or bitter taste* in the mouth, *abdominal discomfort*, and *constipation* (SEDA-10, 151).

Skin and appendages *Skin rashes* have been reported occasionally (635[C]), including an acneiform rash and urticaria.

Genital system *Impotence* has occasionally been reported, in one case with a reduced sperm count (639[c], 640[C]).

Lupus-like syndrome Propafenone may cause a rise in antinuclear antibody titers (640[C]) and has once been reported to have caused a *lupus-like syndrome* (641[c]).

Risk situations The incidence of adverse effects of propafenone in children have varied from study to study, but have sometimes been as high as 25% and requiring withdrawal in 6% of cases (642[C]). Elderly people are at increased risk of adverse effects.

Propafenone has been given to a pregnant woman from the fifth month to term in a dosage of 300 mg t.d.s. (643[c]). Her dysrhythmias responded satisfactorily and the neonate was healthy.

Interactions Propafenone reduces the apparent oral clearance of metoprolol, but it is not clear whether it does this by reducing its true clearance or by increasing its systemic availability (644[C]). In addition the β-blocking action of *metoprolol* is increased by propafenone, and this could be due either to reduced clearance of metoprolol or to a true pharmacodynamic interaction between the two drugs, since propafenone has β-blocking activity.

Monitoring therapy Therapeutic benefit is most likely when the plasma propafenone concentration is in the range 0.5–2.0 μg/ml, although the correlation is poor (645[R]), and there is a large overlap between therapeutic and toxic concentrations (635[C]). The therapeutic effect of propafenone correlates better with the prolongation of the PR and QRS intervals that it causes (646[CR]).

Quinidine

In a group of 652 consecutive in-patients (647[CR]) 91 adverse reactions to quinidine occurred in as many patients (14%); of these, 51 were gastrointestinal, 16 dysrhythmic, 11 febrile, six dermatological, and one hematological, and there were six cases of cinchonism. Although there were four cases of potentially fatal dysrhythmias, there were no deaths.

In another study of 245 patients, the most common adverse effects were diarrhea (35%), upper gastrointestinal distress (22%), and light-headedness (15%). Other common adverse effects included fatigue (7%), palpitation (7%), headache (7%), angina-like pain (6%), weakness (5%), and rash (5%) (548[C]).

The actions, clinical use, interactions, and adverse effects of quinidine have been reviewed elsewhere (648[R]).

ADVERSE REACTIONS PATTERN

General and general toxic reactions Gastrointestinal symptoms, including anorexia, nausea, and vomiting, are common. Quinidine has a negative inotropic effect on the heart and may cause heart failure and hypotension. It prolongs the QRS complex and QT_c interval and may cause cardiac dysrhythmias, which may result in syncope (so-called 'quinidine syncope'). 'Cinchonism' is the term used to describe a cluster of adverse effects that occur at high dosages, including nausea, vomiting, diarrhea, tinnitus, dizziness, and blurred vision; in severe cases there may be deafness and toxic amblyopia in addition to cardiac abnormalities. Other adverse effects that have been described include dementia, psychosis, esophagitis, sometimes resulting in stricture, and exacerbation of myasthenia.

Hypersensitivity reactions Various hypersensitivity reactions have been attributed to quinidine, including fever, skin rashes, various types of hematological abnormalities (particularly thrombocytopenia), hepatitis, asthma, and anaphylactic shock. Quinidine has rarely been reported to cause a lupus-like syndrome.

Tumor-inducing effects Tumor-inducing effects have not been reported.

ORGANS AND SYSTEMS

Cardiovascular Quinidine prolongs the QRS complex and QT_c interval, the effect being related to plasma quinidine concentrations (649[C]). As a result, *torsade de pointes* or other *ventricular tachydysrhythmias* may occur and may lead to syncope ('quinidine syncope'). The minimum risk of *torsade de pointes* has been estimated at 1.5% per year (650[C]). Quinidine has also been incriminated in cases of *sinoatrial block* and *sinus arrest*, but it was not clearly established that quinidine was responsible (651[C], 652[C]). The anticholinergic effects of quinidine may increase the risk of dysrhythmias (653[C]).

Treatment of tachydysrhythmias secondary to quinidine is problematic. Other Class I antidysrhythmic drugs are theoretically contraindicated. Some success has been reported with bretylium and with a combination of a β-adrenoceptor antagonist and phenytoin (654[C], 655[CR]). Overdrive pacing has also been reported to be of value (656[C]).

Quinidine has a negative inotropic effect on the heart

and causes peripheral vasodilatation. *Hypotension* may occur secondary to these effects (657).

Nervous system Quinidine rarely causes effects on the nervous system when used in therapeutic dosages, although there have been occasional reports of *dementia* (658[C], 659[c], 660[c]). In toxicity, however, it can cause *vertigo* and *tinnitus* (661[C]).

Hematological Hypersensitivity reactions to quinidine include *thrombocytopenia*, *hemolytic anemia*, and *neutropenia*.

The overall annual incidence of acute thrombocytopenia has been estimated at 18 cases per million (662[C]), and two possible mechanisms have been invoked: first, that the drug combines with platelets, causing the production of antibodies, which then cause platelet lysis; second, that drug-antibody complexes are first formed and then deposited on the platelet (the so-called 'innocent bystander' mechanism). There is evidence in favor of both of these mechanisms (663[R]).

Other hematological effects are much less common, and include *hemolytic anemia* (663[R], 664[C]), *neutropenia* (665[C], 666[C]), and *eosinophilia* (667[c]).

Withdrawal of quinidine and the administration of corticosteroids is the usual treatment for thrombocytopenia (668[c]), although intravenous immune globulin has also been used (669[c]).

Liver Hypersensitivity reactions to quinidine include granulomatous hepatitis, reports of which keep appearing. In one retrospective series of 487 patients, 32 had evidence of hypersensitivity, 10 of whom had hepatotoxicity (670[CR]). In another series of 1500 patients, quinidine-induced hepatitis was identified in 33 (2.2%) (671[C]); these represented a third of all cases of drug-induced hepatitis in those patients. In all cases the liver damage resolved on withdrawal.

Gastrointestinal *Anorexia*, *nausea*, *vomiting*, and *diarrhea* are common adverse effects of quinidine and may occur in up to 30% of patients (647[C], 672[C]). These effects may be minimized by the use of modified-release formulations (673). In one series diarrhea was reported commonly (674[C]), and it may occur late in treatment (675[c]).

Quinidine may sometimes cause *esophagitis* (676[R], 677[c]), especially when there is some abnormality of the esophagus or cardiomegaly. This may sometimes result in esophageal stricture (678[C]).

A *blue-black pigmentation of the oral mucosa* has been reported (679[C]).

Urinary system *Glomerulonephritis* has been reported in association with *Henoch-Schönlein purpura* (680[c]) and *nephrotic syndrome*, possibly as part of a lupus-like syndrome (see below) (681[c]).

Skin and appendages *Skin rashes* are uncommon (682[R]), but may occur as part of a hypersensitivity reaction. Several different kinds of rash have been reported occasionally, including *photosensitivity* (683[cr]), which can result in a variety of types of rash, *contact dermatitis* (684[cr]), *pigmentation* (685[c]), *urticaria* (686[c]), *exfoliative dermatitis* (687[c], 688[c]), *granuloma annulare* (689[c]), and exacerbation of *psoriasis*.

Special senses Quinidine may rarely affect vision, and can cause *scotomata*, *impaired color vision*, and *toxic amblyopia* (690[C]), *altered vision* (691[c]), *sicca syndrome* (692[c]), *keratopathy* (693[c]), and *granulomatous uveitis* (694[c]).

Musculoskeletal Quinidine is a neuromuscular blocking drug and it may exacerbate *myasthenia gravis* (695[c]). It may also cause an increase in the serum activity of the muscle-specific isozyme of creatine phosphokinase (696[c], 697[c]).

Quinidine may cause *polyarthropathy* (698[c]), both in association with and independently of a lupus-like syndrome.

Lupus-like syndrome A *lupus-like syndrome* has occasionally been reported (699[cr]). It usually presents with a polyarthralgia, a raised erythrocyte sedimentation rate, and a raised antinuclear antibody titer. It may occasionally be associated with antihistone antibodies and a circulating coagulant. In two cases (700[c]) the syndrome was associated with quinidine and not with procainamide.

Risk situations Care must be taken in patients with pre-existing conduction tissue disease or heart failure. Loading doses should be reduced in cardiac failure, because of a lowered apparent volume of distribution (509[R]). Maintenance dosages should be reduced if hepatic metabolism is reduced, for example in congestive cardiac failure and hepatic disease and in elderly people (509[R]).

Overdosage In acute overdosage the chief effect of quinidine is profound hypotension, due to the combination of peripheral vasodilatation and a negative inotropic effect on the heart (701[c], 702[c]). Charcoal hemoperfusion has been successfully used in the treatment of quinidine overdose (703[C]).

Interactions Quinidine potentiates the effects of *warfarin* (704[c]) and of *neuromuscular blocking drugs* (705[R]).

The metabolism of quinidine is enhanced by drugs that induce hepatic microsomal drug-metabolizing enzymes (509[R]), such as *rifampicin* (706[C]) and *phenytoin* and *phenobarbitone* (707[C]). This leads to an increase in the first-pass metabolism of quinidine, and thus increased requirements of oral quinidine but little change in intravenous dosages.

Quinidine itself inhibits drug hydroxylation and can thus convert extensive hydroxylators to poor hydroxylators, as in the case of *metoprolol* (708[C]). Inhibition of hydroxylation does not occur in poor hydroxylators.

Quinidine prolongs the QT interval and will therefore potentiate the effects of other antidysrhythmic drugs that do likewise (e.g. *Class I antidysrhythmic drugs* and *amiodarone*). Specific interactions of this kind have been reported with *tocainide* (709[C]) and *mexiletine* (710[C]); in these cases the interactions were reported to be beneficial in terms of antidysrhythmic effects.

The combination of quinidine with *timolol* causes an increased risk of bradycardia (711[c]).

Quinidine has a pharmacodynamic interaction with *amiloride*, further prolonging the duration of the QRS complex, but not the QT interval (712[C]).

The interactions of quinidine with *antacids* have been reviewed (713[R]). Although the data are inconclusive, it has been suggested that at least 2 hours should elapse between quinidine and antacid doses.

The quinidine—*digoxin* interaction is discussed above under 'Cardiac glycosides'.

Tocainide

The clinical pharmacology, uses, efficacy, and adverse effects of tocainide have been extensively reviewed (222[R], 714[R]—721[R]).

The adverse effects of tocainide are dose-related, and occur with increasing frequency above plasma concentrations of 10 μg/ml. They are mostly related to the nervous system. In two large series withdrawal of tocainide was required in 11—16% of patients because of adverse effects (722[C], 723[C]). The high incidence of blood dyscrasias (see below) now severely limits the use of tocainide.

Cardiovascular Adverse cardiovascular effects have been reported in 6—55% of cases. After a single dose of tocainide the most common effect has been *hypotension* with *bradycardia* (501[C]). *Angina pectoris* has also been reported (724[C]).

During repeated administration cardiovascular adverse effects have been relatively uncommon. *Increasing heart failure* (725[C], 726[C]), *worsening dysrhythmias* (726[C], 727[c]), *pericarditis* (726[C], 728—729[C]), and *sinus arrest with sinoatrial block* (730[c]) have all been reported. Tocainide may also worsen *ventricular tachycardia* (731[c]).

Respiratory There have been several reports of *interstitial pneumonitis* attributable to tocainide (732[Cr], 733[c]), and it may also cause severe *pulmonary fibrosis* (734[c], 735[c]).

Nervous system A wide variety of central nervous system symptoms has been reported in almost every study, varying in incidence from 10 to 100%. Common reactions include *dizziness*, *tremor and tremulousness*, *dysesthesia and paresthesia*, *light-headedness*, and *blurred vision*. Various mental changes have been described, including *paranoid psychosis* (736[c]—738[c]). *Nausea* is common and probably central in origin, since it occurs after intravenous as well as oral administration. These adverse effects can be reduced in frequency during oral administration by taking the tablets with food.

Hematological Tocainide may cause blood dyscrasias (*neutropenia*, *thrombocytopenia*, *pancytopenia*, and *aplastic anemia*) in one in 300 patients (739[r], 740[r], 741[c], 742[c]). Isolated cases of *eosinophilia* with an allergic rash, and *anemia* with pericarditis have also been reported (728[C], 743[C]).

Liver Tocainide may increase the activities of serum aminotransferases (744[cr]), and may cause fatty change (744[cr]) and granulomatous *hepatitis* (745[c]).

Gastrointestinal *Nausea* is very common, as noted above, particularly during the initial stages of treatment, after which it may tend to disappear (725[C]). There have been occasional reports of *constipation* (728[C]) and of *anorexia and vomiting* (725[C]).

Urinary system A case of non-membranous *glomerulonephritis* has been reported (746[C]).

Skin There have been a few reports of skin rashes attributed to tocainide (728[C], 747[C]). *Night sweats* have been reported in three patients (728[C]). Cross-reactivity with lidocaine has been reported (748[c]).

Special senses There have been not infrequent reports of *odd taste sensations* (peppermint and menthol) and of coolness of the throat, hands, and feet.

Lupus-like syndrome *Arthralgia* has been reported in two cases with positive antinuclear antibody titers, suggesting the possibility of a *lupus-like syndrome* (749[C]). In another case tocainide treatment was associated with both a lupus-like syndrome and neutropenia (750[C]).

Overdosage Convulsions, complete heart block, and asystole developed in a case of fatal self-poisoning with 400 mg of tocainide (751[c]).

Interaction Tocainide reduces the clearance of theophylline and increases its half-life, but to an extent that is probably clinically insignificant (752[C]).

REFERENCES

1. Various authors. Digoxin symposium. Br Heart J 1985;54:227.
2. Fisch C, ed. William Withering: An account of the foxglove and some of its medical uses 1785–1985. J Am Coll Cardiol 1985;5:(Suppl A).
3. Erdmann E, Greeff K, Skou JC, eds. Cardiac Glycosides 1785–1984. Biochemistry, Pharmacology, Clinical Relevance. Darmstadt: Steinkopff Verlag, 1985.
4. Rietbrock N, Woodcock BG. Handbook of Renal-Independent Cardiac Glycosides: Pharmacology and Clinical Pharmacology. Chichester: Ellis Horwood, 1989.
5. Chung EK. Digitalis Intoxication. Amsterdam: Excerpta Medica, 1969.
6. Smith TW, Antman EM, Friedman PL, Blatt CM, Marsh JD. Digitalis glycosides: mechanisms and manifestations of toxicity. Prog Cardiovasc Dis 1984;26:413–458(Part II) and 27:21–56(Part III).
7. Aronson JK. Digitalis intoxication. Clin Sci 1983; 64:253–258.
8. Buchanan JF, Olson KR. Current management of digitalis toxicity. Part I: Clinical manifestations. Prac Cardiol 1988;14:75–79.
9. Buchanan JF, Olson KR. Current management of digitalis toxicity. Part II: Treatment of digitalis intoxication. Pract Cardiol 1988;14:92–95.
10. Schwartz A, Lindenmayer GE, Allen JC. The sodium-potassium adenosine triphosphatase: pharmacological, physiological and biochemical aspects. Pharmacol Rev 1975;27:3–134.
11. Levitt B, Cagin N, Kleid J, Somberg J, Gillis R. Role of the nervous system in the genesis of cardiac rhythm disorders. Am J Cardiol 1976;37:1111–1113.
12. Aronson JK, Ford AR. The use of colour vision measurement in the diagnosis of digoxin toxicity. Q J Med 1980;NS49:273–282.
13. Beller GA, Smith TW, Abelmann WH, Haber E, Hood WB Jr. Digitalis intoxication: a prospective clinical study with serum level correlations. New Engl J Med 1971; 284:989–997.
14. Williams P, Aronson JK, Sleight P. Is a slow pulse rate a reliable sign of digoxin toxicity? Lancet 1978;ii:1340–1342.
15. Hamer, SS, Lemberg L. Digitalis excess mimicking the sick sinus syndrome. Heart Lung 1976;5:652–656.
16. Di Giacomo V, Carmenini G, Sciacca A. Su un caso di malattia del nodo del seno insorto in corso di trattamento digilatico. Progr Med 1977;33:775.
17. Margolis JR, Strauss HC, Miller HC, Gilbert J, Wallace AG. Digitalis and the sick sinus syndrome: clinical and electrophysiologic documentation of a severe toxic effect on sinus node function. Circulation 1975;52:162–169.
18. Engel TR, Schaal SF. Digitalis in the sick sinus syndrome: the effects on sinoatrial automaticity and atrioventricular conduction. Circulation 1973;48:1201–1207.
19. Vera Z, Miller RR, McMillin D, Mason DT. Effects of digitalis on sinus nodal function in patients with sick sinus syndrome. Am J Cardiol 1978;41:318–323.
20. Talley JD, Wathen MS, Hurst JW. Hyperthyroid-induced atrial flutter-fibrillation with profound sinoatrial nodal pauses due to small doses of digoxin, verapamil, and propranolol. Clin Cardiol 1989;12:45–47.
21. McCauley CS, Boller LR. Bradycardiac responses to endotracheal suctioning. Crit Care Med 1988;16:1165–1166.
22. Lown B, Wyatt NF, Levine HD. Paroxysmal atrial tachycardia with block. Circulation 1960;21:129–143.
23. Agarwal BL. Agarwal BV. Digitalis induced paroxysmal atrial tachycardia with AV block. Br Heart J 1972;34:330–335.
24. Tawakkol AA, Nutter DO, Masumi RA. A prospective study of digitalis toxicity in a large city hospital. Med Ann DC 1967;36:402–409.
25. Agarwal BL, Agarwal BV, Agarwal RK, Kansal SC. Atrial flutter. A rare manifestation of digitalis intoxication. Br Heart J 1972;34:392–395.
26. Pellegrino L. Ritmo idioventriculare accelerato da intoxicazione digitalica. Studio clinico ed elettrocardiografico su due casi. G Ital Cardiol 1976;6:527–531.
27. Castellanos A, Shin E-K, Luceri RM, Myerburg RJ. Parasystolic accelerated idioventricular rhythms producing bidirectional tachycardia patterns. J Electrophysiol 1988; 2:296.
28. Lehmann H-U, Witt E, Hochrein H. Zunahme von Angina pectoris und ST-Strecken-Senkung im EKG durch Digitalis. Z Kardiol 1978;67:57–66.
29. Singh RB, Agarwal BV, Somani PN. Left bundle branch block: a rare manifestation of digitalis intoxication. Acta Cardiol (Brussels) 1976;31:175–179.
30. Gould L, Patel C, Betzu R, Judge D, Lee J. Right bundle branch block: a rare manifestation of digitalis toxicity-case report. Angiology 1986;37:543–546.
31. Von Capeller D, Copeland GD, Stern TN. Digitalis intoxication: a clinical report of 148 cases. Ann Intern Med 1959;50:869–878.
32. Somlyo AP. The toxicology of digitalis. Am J Cardiol 1960;5:523–533.
33. Braunwald E, Bloodwell RD, Goldberg LI, Morrow AG. Studies on digitalis. IV. Observations in man on the effects of digitalis preparations on the contractility of the non-failing heart and on total vascular resistance. J Clin Invest 1961;40:52–59.
34. Teske RH, Bishop SP, Righter HF, Detweiler DK. Subacute digoxin toxicosis in the beagle dog. Toxicol Appl Pharmacol 1976;35:283–301.
35. Varonkov Y, Shell WE, Smirnov V, Gukovsky D, Chazov EI. Augmentation of serum CPK activity by digitalis in patients with acute myocardial infarction. Circulation 1977;55:719–727.
36. Eaker ED, Kronmal R, Kennedy JW, Davis K. Comparison of the long-term, postsurgical survival of women and men in the Coronary Artery Surgery Study (CASS). Am Heart J 1989;117:71–81.
37. Ross DL, Davis KB, Pettinger MB, Alderman EL, Killip T, Mason JW. Features of cardiac arrest episodes with and without acute myocardial infarction in the Coronary Artery Surgery Study (CASS). Am J Cardiol 1987;60:1219–1224.
38. Deglin S, Deglin J, Chung EK. Direct current shock and digitalis therapy. Drug Intell Clin Pharm 1977;11:76.
39. Ali N, Dais K, Banks T, Sheikh M. Fit rated electrical cardioversion in patients on digoxin. Clin Cardiol 1982;5:417.
40. Lely AH, Van Enter CHJ. Large-scale digitoxin intoxication. Br Med J 1970;3:737–740.
41. Lely AH, Van Enter CHJ. Non-cardiac symptoms of digitalis intoxication. Am Heart J 1972;83:149–152.
42. Singh RB, Singh VP, Somani PN. Psychosis: a rare mani-

festation of digoxin intoxication. J Indian Med Assoc 1977;69:62–63.
43. Shear MK, Sacks MH. (a) Digitalis delirium: reports of two cases. Am J Psychiatry 1978;135:109–110; (b) Digitalis delirium: psychiatric considerations. Int J Psychiatry Med 1978;8:371–381.
44. Portnoi VA. Digitalis delirium in elderly patients. J Clin Pharmacol 1979;19:747–750.
45. Gorelick DA, Kussin SZ, Kahn I. Paranoid delusions and auditory hallucinations associated with digoxin intoxication. J Nerv Ment Dis 1978;166:817–819.
46. Volpe BT, Soave R. Formed visual hallucinations as digitalis toxicity. Ann Intern Med 1979;91:865–866.
47. Miller S, Forker AD. Digitalis toxicity: neurologic manifestations. J Kans Med Soc 1974;75:263–264.
48. Kerr DJ, Elliott HL, Hillis WS. Epileptiform seizures and electroencephalographic abnormalities as manifestations of digoxin toxicity. Br Med J 1982;284:162–163.
49. Douglas EF, White PT, Nelson JW. Three per second spike-wave in digitalis toxicity. Report of a case. Arch Neurol 1971;25:373–375.
50. Mulder LJMM, Van der Mast RC, Meerwaldt JD. Generalized chorea due to digoxin toxicity. Br Med J 1988;296:1262 (erratum in 297:562).
51. Greenlee, JE, Crampton RS, Miller JQ. Transient global amnesia associated with cardiac arrhythmia and digitalis intoxication. Stroke (New York) 1975;6:513–516.
52. Bernat JL, Sullivan JK. Trigeminal neuralgia from digitalis intoxication. J Am Med Assoc 1979;241:164.
53. Batterman RC, Guter LB. Hitherto undescribed neurological manifestations of digitalis toxicity. Am Heart J 1984;36:582–586.
54. Brezis M, Midhaeli J, Hamburger R. Nightmares from digoxin. Ann Intern Med 1980;93:639–640.
55. Eisendrath SJ, Gersgengorn KN, Unger R. Digoxin-induced organic brain syndrome. Am Heart J 1983;106:419–420.
56. Tucker AR, Ng KT. Digoxin-related impairment of learning and memory in cardiac patients. Psychopharmacology 1983;81:86–88.
57. Donat J, Jirkalova V, Havel V, Milulecka D. Kotazce estrogenniho ucinku digitalisu u zen po menopauze. Cesk Gynekol 1980;45:19–23.
58. Burckhardt D, Vera CA, LaDue JS. Effect of digitalis on urinary pituitary gonadotrophine excretion. A study in postmenopausal women. Ann Intern Med 1968;68:1069–1071.
59. Stoffer SS, Hynes KM, Jiang NS, Ryan RJ. Digoxin and abnormal serum hormone levels. J Am Med Assoc 1973;225:1643–1644.
60. Neri A, Aygen M, Zuckerman Z, Bahary C. Subjective assessment of sexual dysfunction of patients on long-term administration of digoxin. Arch Sex Behav 1980;9:343–347.
61. Le Winn EB. Gynecomastia during digitalis therapy: report of 8 additional cases with liver function and studies. New Engl J Med 1953;248:316–320.
62. Calov WL, Whyte HM. Oedema and mammary hypertrophy: toxic effect of digitalis leaf. Med J Aust 1964;1:556–557.
63. Navab A, Koss LG, La Due, JS. Estrogen-like activity of digitalis: its effect on the squamous epithelium of the female genital tract. J Am Med Assoc 1965;194:30–32.
64. Stenkvist B, Bengtsson E, Eklund G, Eriksson O, Holmquist J, Nordin B, Westman-Naeser S. Evidence of a modifying influence of heart glucosides on the development of breast cancer. Anal Quant Cytol 1980;2:49–54.
65. Stenkvist B, Bengtsson E, Dahlqvist B, Eriksson O, Jarkrans T, Nordin B. Cardiac glycosides and breast cancer, revisited. New Engl J Med 1982;306:484.
66. Nørgaard A, Bøtker HE, Klitgaard NA, Toft P. Digitalis enhances exercise-induced hyperkalaemia. Eur J Clin Pharmacol 1991;41:609–611.
67. Gosselink ATM, Crijns HJGM, Wiesfeld ACP, Lie KI. Exercise-induced ventricular tachycardia: a rare manifestation of digitalis toxicity. Clin Cardiol 1993;16:270–272.
68. Karpatkin S. Drug-induced thrombocytopenia. Am J Med Sci 1971;262:68–78.
69. Schneider A-W, Gilfrich H-J, Fechler L. Thrombozytopenie bei Digitoxin-Intoxikation. Dtsch Med Wochenschr 1992;117:337–340.
70. Forzy P, Joram F. Thrombopénie severe en rapport avec une intoxication a l'acetyl digitoxine. Sem Hôp Paris 1989;65:235–236.
71. Pirovino M, Ohnhaus EE, Von Felten A. Digoxin-associated thrombocytopenia. Eur J Clin Pharmacol 1981; 19:205–207.
72. Almeyda J, Levantine A. Cutaneous reactions to cardiovascular drugs. Br J Dermatol 1973;88:313–319.
73. Holt DW, Volans GN. Gastrointestinal symptoms of digoxin toxicity. Br Med J 1977;2:704.
74. Willems J, De Geest H. Digitalis intoxicatie. Ned Tijdschr Geneeskd 1968;24:617.
75. Kelton JG, Scullin DC. Digitalis toxicity manifested by dysphagia. J Am Med Assoc 1978;239:613–614.
76. Cordeiro MF, Arnold KG. Digoxin toxicity presenting as dysphagia and dysphonia. Br Med J 1991;302:1025.
77. Adar R, Salzman EW. Intestinal ischemia and digitalis. J Am Med Assoc 1974;229:1577.
78. Bourhis F, Riard P, Danel V, Hostein J, Fournet J. Intoxication digitalique avec ischémie colique grave: évolution favorable après traitement par anticorps spécifiques. Gastoenterol Clin Biol 1990;14:95.
79. Brobmann GF, Milosch H, Mayer M. Glykosidbedingte Durchblutungsstörungen des Darms und Möglichkeiten therapeutischer Beeinflüssung. Med Klin 1976;71:2066–2071.
80. Wolanski A, Kardaszewixz S, Jazanek E. Algeria po naparstnicy. Pol Tyg Lek 1971;26:441–443.
81. Brauner GJ, Geene MH. Digitalis allergy: digoxin induced vasculitis. Cutis (New York) 1972;10:441–443.
82. Wagner G, Lubach D. Über die Vasculitis allergica als unerwartete Nebenwirkung einer Digitalis-Therapie. Aktuel Dermatol 1986;12:125–127.
83. David M, Livni E, Stern E, Feurerman EJ, Grinblatt J. Psoriasiform eruption induced by digoxin: confirmed by re-exposure. J Am Acad Dermatol 1981;5:702–703.
84. Lofgren RP. Diaphoresis with digoxin. New Engl J Med 1979;302:919.
85. Inadomi T, Aoki M, Ishizaka S, Kurihara H, Suzuki H. Pemphigus foliaceus-like eruption due to digoxin. Eur J Dermatol 1993;3:33–35.
86. Robertson DM, Hollenhorst RW, Callahan JA. Ocular manifestations of digitalis toxicity. Discussion and report of three cases of central scotomas. Arch Ophthalmol 1966;76:640–645.
87. Haustein K-O, Schmidt C. Differences in color vision discrimination between three cardioactive glycosides. Int J Clin Pharmacol Ther Toxicol 1988;26:517–520.
88. Mermoud A, Safran AB, de Stoutz N. Pain upon eye

movement following digoxin absorption. J Clin Neuro-ophthalmol 1992;12:41–42.
89. Andersen KE, Damsgaard T. The effect on serum enzymes of intramuscular injections of digoxin, bumetanide, pentazocine and isotonic sodium chloride. Acta Med Scand 1976;199:317–319.
90. Lewis WS, Doherty JE. Another disadvantage of intramuscular digoxin. New Engl J Med 1973;288:1077.
91. Aronson JK. Digoxin: clinical aspects. In: Richens A. Marks V, eds. Therapeutic Drug Monitoring, Ch 17A. London, Edinburgh: Churchill-Livingstone, 1981;404.
92. Shenfield GM. Influence of thyroid dysfunction on drug pharmacokinetics. Clin Pharmacokin 1981;6:275–297.
93. Aronson JK. Clinical pharmacokinetics of cardiac glycosides in patients with renal dysfunction. Clin Pharmacokin 1983;8:155–178.
94. Brater DC, Morrelli HF. Digoxin toxicity in patients with normokalemic potassium depletion. Clin Pharmacol Ther 1977;22:21–33.
95. Young IS, Goh EML, McKillop UH, Stanford CF, Nicholls DP, Trimble ER. Magnesium status and digoxin toxicity. Br J Clin Pharmacol 1991;32:717–721.
96. Steinberg C, Notterman DA. Pharmacokinetics of cardiovascular drugs in children. Inotropes and vasopressors. Clin Pharmacokin 1994;27:345–367.
97. Kearin M, Kelly JG, O'Malley K. Digoxin receptors in neonates: an explanation of less sensitivity to digoxin in adults. Clin Pharmacol Ther 1980;28:346–349.
98. Johnson GL, Desai NS, Pauly TH, Cunningham MD. Complications associated with digoxin therapy in low-birthweight infants. Pediatrics 1982;69:463.
99. Hastreiter AR, Van der Horst RL, Chow-Tung E. Digitalis toxicity in infants and children. Pediatr Cardiol 1984;5:131–148.
100. Hamer J. The paradox of the lack of the efficacy of digitalis in congestive heart failure with sinus rhythm. Br J Clin Pharmacol 1979;8:109–113.
101. Hagemeijer F, Van Houwe E. Titrated energy carddioversion of patients on digitalis. Br Heart J 1975;37:1303.
102. Piergies AA, Worwag EM, Atkinson AJ Jr. A concurrent audit of high digoxin plasma levels. Clin Pharmacol Ther 1994;55:353–358.
103. Aronson JK. Clinical pharmacokineticxs of digoxin. Clin Pharmacokin 1980;5:137–149.
104. Rotmensch HH, Rotmensch S, Elkayam U. Management of cardiac arrhythmias during pregnancy. Drugs 1987;33:623–633.
105. Nishimura H, Tanimura T. Clinical Aspects of the Teratogenicity of Drugs. Amsterdam: Excerpta Medica, 1976.
106. Bismuth C, Gaultier M, Conso F, Efthymicu ML. Hyperkalemia in acute digitalis poisoning: prognostic significance and therapeutic implications. Clin Toxicol 1973;6:153–162.
107. Lalonde RL, Deshpande R, Hamilton PP, McLean WM, Greenway DC. Acceleration of digoxin clearance by activated charcoal. Clin Pharmacol Ther 1985;37:367–371.
108. Erdmann E, Mair W, Knedel M, Schaumann W. Digitalis intoxication and treatment with digoxin antibody fragments in renal failure. Klin Wochenschr 1989;67:16–19.
109. Clifton GD, McIntyre WJ, Zannikos PN, Harrison MR, Chandler MH. Free and total serum digoxin concentrations in a renal failure patient after treatment with digoxin immune Fab. Clin Pharm 1989;8:441–445.
110. Proudfoot AT. A star treatment for digoxin overdose? Br Med J 1986;293:642–643.
111. Butler VP, Smith TW. Immunologic treatment of digitalis toxicity: a tale of two prophecies. Ann Intern Med 1986;105:613–614.
112. Robinson CP. Digoxin immune Fab (ovine). Drugs Future 1986;11:922–926.
113. Aronson J. Digitalis intoxication and its treatment. Top Circ 1987;2:9–12.
114. Aronson JK. Digoxin. In: Widdop B, ed. Contemporary Issues in Biochemistry, 3: Therapeutic Drug Monitoring, Ch 10. Edinburgh: Churchill Livingstone, 1985.
115. Le Sage J. Color vision testing to assist in diagnosis of digitalis toxicity. Nurs Res (New York) 1984;33:346–351.
116. Binnion PF Drug interactions with digitalis glycosides. Drugs 1987;15:369–380.
117. Brown DD, Spector R, Juhl RP. Drug interactions with digoxin. Drugs 1980;20:198–206.
118. Lampe D, Lampe H, Banaschak H. Arzneimittelwechsel-Wirkungen mit Herzglykosiden. Dtsch Gesundheitsw 1980;35:1081–1087.
119. Bazzano G, Bazzano GS. Digitalis intoxication. Treatment with a new steroid-binding resin. J Am Med Assoc 1972;220:828–830.
120. Fresard F, Balant L, Noble J, Garcia B, Muller AF. Cholestyramine et intoxication a la digoxine: éfficacité therapeutique? Schweiz Med Wschr 1979;109:431–436.
121. Kuhlmann J, Zilly W, Wilke J. Effects of cytostatic drugs on plasma level and renal excretion of beta-acetyldigoxin. Clin Pharmacol Ther 1981;30:518–527.
122. Kuhlmann K, Wilke J, Rietbrock N. Cytostatic drugs are without significant effect on digitoxin plasma level and renal excretion. Clin Pharmacol Ther 1982;32:646.
123. Manninen V, Apajalahti A, Melin J, Karesoja M. Altered absorption of digoxin in patients given propantheline and metoclopramide. Lancet 1973;i:398–400.
124. Kirch W, Janisch HD, Santos SR, Duhrsen U, Dylewicz P, Ohnhaus EE. Effect of cisapride and metoclopramide on ditgoxin bioavailability. Eur J Drug Metab Pharmacokin 1986;11:249–250.
125. D'Arcy PF, McElnay JC. Drug-antacid interactions: assessment of clinical importance. Drug Intell Clin Pharm 1987;21:607–617.
126. Lelarge P, Bauer P, Royer-Morrot MJ, Meregnani JL, Larcan A, Lambert H. Intoxication digitalique aprés administration conjointe d'acétyl digitoxine et d'amiodarone. Ann Méd Nancy Est 1993;32:307.
127. Pedersen KE, Dorph-Pedersen A Hvidt S, Klitgaard NA, Nielsen-Kudsk F. Digoxin-verapamil interaction. Clin Pharmacol Ther 1981;30:311–316.
128. Klein HO, Lang R, Weiss E, Didegni E, Libhaber C, Guerrero J. The influence of verapamil on serum digoxin concentration. Circulation 1982;665:998–1003.
129. Klein HO, Lang R, Weiss E, Di Segni E, Libhaber C, Guerrero J, Kaplinsky E. The influence of verapamil on serum digoxin concentration. Circulation 1982;65:998–1003.
130. Zatuchni J. Verapamil-digoxin interaction. Am Heart J 1984;108:412–413.
131. King T, Mallet L. Diltiazem-digoxin interaction in an elderly woman: a case report. J Geriatr Drug Ther 1991;5:79–83.
132. Pliakos ChC, Papadopoulos K, Parcharidis G, Styliadis J, Tourkantonis A. Effects of calcium channel blockers on serum concentrations of digoxin. Epitheorese Klin Farmakol Farmakokinetikes 1991;9:118–125.
133. Gasic S, Eichler HG, Korn A. Effect of calcium anta-

gonists on basal and digitalis-dependent changes in splanchnic and systemic hemodynamics. Clin Pharmacol Ther 1987;41:460–466.

134. Waldorff S, Anderson JD, Heeboll-Nielsen N, Nielson OG, Molthe E, Sorensen U, Steiness E. Spironolactone-induced changes in digoxin kinetics. Clin Pharmacol Ther 1978;24:162–167.

135. Cogan JJ, Humphreys MH, Carlson CJ, Benowitz NL, Rapaport E. Acute vasodilator therapy increases renal clearance of digoxin in patients with congestive heart failure. Circulation 1981;64:973–976.

136. Schimmel MS, Inwood RJ, Eidelman AI, Eylath U. Toxic digitalis levels associated with indomethacin therapy in a neonate. Clin Pediatr 1980;19:768–769.

137. Finch MB, Kelly JG, Johnston GD, McDevitt DG. Evidence against a digoxin-indomethacin interaction. Br J Clin Pharmacol 1983;16:212P–213P.

138. Alderman CP, Jersmann HPA. Digoxin-itraconazole interaction. Med J Aust 1993;159:838–839.

139. Sachs MK, Blanchard LM, Green PJ. Interaction of itraconazole and digoxin. Clin Infect Dis 1993;16:400–403.

140. Boman G, Eliasson K, Odar-Cederlof I. Acute cardiac failure during treatment with digitoxin-an interaction with rifampicin. Br J Clin Pharmacol 1980;10:89–90.

141. Fraley DS, Britton HL, Schwinghammer TL, Kalla R. Effect of cimetidine on steady-state serum digoxin concentrations. Clin Pharmacol 1983;2:163–165.

142. Osterhuis B, Jonkman JHG, Andersson T, Zuiderwijk PBM, Jedema JN. Minor effect of multiple dose omeprazole on the pharmacokinetics of digoxin after a single oral dose. Br J Clin Pharmacol 1991;32:569–572.

143. Lindenbaum J, Rund DG, Butler VP, Tse-Eng D, Saha JR. Inactivation of digoxin by the gut flora: reversal by antibiotic therapy. New Engl J Med 1981;305:789–794.

144. Shapiro W. Correlative studies of serum digitalis level and the arrhythmias of digitalis intoxication. Am J Cardiol 1978;41:852–859.

145. Steiness E. Suppression of renal excretion of digoxin in hypokalemic patients. Clin Pharmacol Ther 1978;23:511–514.

146. Storstein O, Hansteen V, Hatle L, Hillestad L, Storstein L. Studies on digitalis. XIII. A prospective study of 649 patients on maintenance treatment with digoxin. Am Heart J 1977;93:434–443.

147. Chopra D, Janson P, Sawin CT. Insensitivity to digoxin associated with hypocalcemia. New Engl J Med 1977; 296:917–918.

148. Cardaioli P, Compostella L, De Domenico R, Papalia D, Zeppellini R, Libardoni M, Pulido E, Cucchini F. Influenza del propafenone sulla farmacocinetica della digossina somministrata per via orale: studio su volontari sani. G Ital Cardiol 1986;16:237–240.

149. Palumbo E, Svetoni N, Casini M, Spargi T, Biagi G, Martelli F, Lancetta T. Interazione digoxina-propafenone: valori e limiti del dosaggio plasmatico dei due farmaci. Efficacia antiaritmica del propafenone. G Ital Cardiol 1986; 16:855–862.

150. Doering W. Quinidine-digoxin interaction. Pharmacokinetics, underlying mechanism and clinical implications. New Engl J Med 1979;301:400–404.

151. Antman EM, Arnold MO, Friedman PL, White H, Bosak M, Smith TW. Drug interactions with cardiac glycosides: evaluation of a possible digoxin-ethmozine pharmacokinetic interaction. J Cardiovasc Pharmacol 1987;9:622–627.

152. Joubert PH. Are all cardiac glycosides pharmacodynamically similar? Eur J Clin Pharmacol 1990;39:317–320.

153. Aronson JK. Book review. Lancet 1990;ii:1130–1131.

154. Kelly RA, Smith TW. Recognition and management of digitalis toxicity. Am J Cardiol 1992;69:108G–119G.

155. Colucci WS, Wright RF, Braunwald E. New positive inotropic agents in the treatment of congestive heart failure: mechanisms of action and recent clinical developments. New Engl J Med 1986;314:290–299(Part I); 1986;314:349–358(Part 2).

156. Webster MWI, Sharpe DN. Adverse effects associated with the newer inotropic agents. Med Toxicol 1986;1:335–342.

157. Rocci ML, Wilson H. The pharmacokinetics and pharmacodynamics of newer inotropic agents. Clin Pharmacokin 1987;13:91–109.

158. Leier CV. Current status of non-digitalis positive inotropic drugs. Am J Cardiol 1992;69:120G–129G.

159. Sasayama S. What do the newer inotropic drugs have to offer? Cardiovasc Drugs Ther 1992;6:15–18.

160. Frielingsdorf J, Kiowski W. Pharmacology and clinical use of newer inotropic agents. Anaesth Pharmacol Rev 1994;2:332–341.

161. Nony P, Boissel J-P, Lievre M, Leizorovicz A, Haugh MC, Fareh S, de Breyne B. Evaluation of the effect of phosphodiesterase inhibitors on mortality in chronic heart failure patients. A meta analysis. Eur J Clin Pharmacol 1994;46:191–196.

162. Wilmshurst PT, Webb-Peploe MM. Side effects of amrinone therapy. Br Heart J 1983;49:447–451.

163. Di Bianco R, Shabetai R, Silverman BD, Leier CV, Benotti JR, with the Amrinone Multicenter Study Investigators. Oral amrinone for the treatment of chronic congestive heart failure: results of a multicenter randomized double-blind and placebo-controlled withdrawal study. J Am Coll Cardiol 1984;4:855–866.

164. Johnstone DL, Humen DP, Kostuk WJ. Amrinone therapy in patients with heart failure: lack of improvement in functional capacity and left ventricular function at rest and during exercise. Chest 1984;86:394–400.

165. Packer M, Medina N, Yushak M. Hemodynamic and clinical limitations of long-term inotropic therapy with amrinone in patients with severe chronic heart failure. Circulation 1984;70:1038–1047.

166. Klepzig M, Kleinhans E, Bull U, Strauer BE. Amrinone in Akut- und Langzeittherapie. Z Kardiol 1985;74:85–90.

167. Leier CV, Dalpiaz K, Huss P, Hermiller JB, Magorien DB, Bashore TM, Unterverth DV. Amrinone therapy for congestive heart failure in outpatients with idiopathic dilated cardiomyopathy. Am J Cardiol 1983;52:304–308.

168. Bichel T, Steinbach G, Olry L, Lambert H. Utilisation de l'amrinone intraveineux dans le traitement du choc cardiogenique. Agressologie 1988;29:187–192.

169. Manzione NC, Goldfarb JP, LeJemtel TH, Maskin CS, Sternlieb I. The effects of two new inotropic agents on microsomal liver function in patients with congestive heart failure. Am J Med Sci 1986;291:88–92.

170. Shah PK, Amin DK, Hulse S, Shellock F, Swan HJ. Inotropic therapy for refractory congestive heart failure with oral fenoximone (MDL-17, 043): poor long-term results despite early hemodynamic and clinical improvement. Circulation 1985;71:326–331.

171. Kereiakes D, Chatterjee K, Parmley WW, Atherton B, Curran D, Kereiakes A. Intravenous and oral MDL 17043 (a

new inotrope-vasodilator agent) in congestive heart failure: hemodynamic and clinical evaluation in 38 patients. J Am Coll Cardiol 1984;4:884—889.
172. Rubin SA, Tabak L. MDL 17,043: short- and long-term cardiopulmonary and clinical effects in patients with heart failure. J Am Coll Cardiol 1985;5:1422—1427.
173. Uretsky BF, Generalovich T, Verbalis JG, Valdes AM, Reddy PAS. MDL 17,043 therapy in severe congestive heart failure: characterization of the early and late hemodynamic, pharmacokinetic, hormonal and clinical response. J Am Coll Cardiol 1985;5:1414—1421.
174. Leeman M, Lejeune P, Melot C, Naeije R. Reduction in pulmonary hypertension and in airway resistances by enoximone (MDL 17,043) in decompensated COPD. Chest 1987;91:662—666.
175. Martin JL, Likoff, MJ, Janicki JS, Lasskey WK, Hirshfeld JWJR. Myocardial energetics and clinical response to the cardiotonic agent MDL 17043 in advanced heart failure. J Am Coll Cardiol 1984;4:875—883.
176. Amin DK, Shah PK, Hulse S, Shellick FG, Swan HJ. Myocardial metabolic and hemodynamic effects of intravenous MDL-17,043, a new cardiotonic drug, in patients with chronic severe heart failure. Am Heart J 1984;108:1285—1292.
177. Uretsky BF, Jessup M, Konstam MA, Dec GW, Leier CV, Benotti J, Murali S, Herrmann HC, Sandberg JA. Multicenter trial of oral enoximone in patients with moderate to moderately severe congestive heart failure: lack of benefit compared with placebo. Circulation 1990;82:774—780.
178. Simonton CA, Chatterjee K, Cody RJ, Kubo SH, Leonard D, Daly P, Rutman H. Milrinone in congestive heart failure: acute and chronic hemodynamic and clinical evaluation. J Am Coll Cardiol 1985;6:453—459.
179. Jaski BE, Fifer MA, Wright RF, Braunwald E, Colucci WS. Positive inotropic and vasodilator actions of milrinone in patients with severe congestive heart failure: dose-response relationships and comparison to nitroprusside. J Clin Invest 1985;75:643—649.
180. Anderson JL, Askins JC, Gilbert EM, Menlove RL, Lutz JR. Occurrence of ventricular arrhythmias in patients receiving acute and chronic infusions of milrinone. Am Heart J 1986;111:466—474.
181. Timmis AD, Smyth P, Jewitt DE. Milrinone in heart failure: effects on exercise haemodynamics during short term treatment. Br Heart J 1985;54:42—47.
182. Renard M, Jacobs P, Dechamps P, Dresse A, Bernard R. Hemodynamic and clinical response to three day infusion of sulmazol (AR-L 115 BS) in severe congestive heart failure. Chest 1983;84:408—413.
183. Renard M, Jacobs P, Melot C, Dresse A, Bernard R. Le sulmazol: un nouvel agent inotrope positif. Ann Cardiol Angéiol 1984;33:219—222.
184. Berkenboom GM, Sobolski JC, Depelchin PE, Contu E, Dieudonne PM, Degre SB. Clinical and hemodynamic observations on orally administered sulmazol (ARL 115BS) in refractory heart failure. Cardiology 1984;71:323—330.
185. Haemeijer F, Segers A, Schelling A. Cardiovascular effects of sulmazol administered intravenously to patients with severe heart failure. Eur Heart J 1984;5:158—167.
186. Thormann J, Schlepper M, Kraamer W, Gottwik M, Kindler. Effects of AR-L115 BS (sulmazol), a new cardiotonic agent, in coronary artery disease: improved ventricular wall motion, increased pump function and abolition of pacing-induced ischemia. J Am Coll Cardiol 1983;2:332—337.
187. Feldman AM, Baughman KL, Lee WK, Gottlieb SH, Weiss JL, Becker LC, Strobeck JE. Usefulness of OPC-8212, a quinolinone derivative, for congestive heart failure in patients with ischemic heart disease or idiopathic dilated cardiomyopathy. Am J Cardiol 1991;68:1203—1210.
188. Feldman AM, Bristow MR, Parmley WW, Carson PE, Pepine CJ, Gilbert EM, Strobeck JE, Hendrix GH, Powers ER, Bain RP et al. Effects of vesnarinone on morbidity and mortality in patients with heart failure. Vesnarinone Study Group. New Engl J Med 1993;329:149—155.
189. Feldman AM, Bristow MR, Parmley WW, Carson PE, Pepine CJ, Gilbert EM, Strobeck JE, Hendrix GH, Powers ER, Bain RP, White BG. Effects of vesnarinone on morbidity and mortality in patients with heart failure. New Engl J Med 1993;329:149—155.
190. Vaughan Williams EM. A classification of antiarrhythmic actions reassessed after a decade of new drugs. J Clin Pharmacol 1984;24:129—147.
191. Rinkenberger RL, Prystowsky EN, Jackman WM, Naccarelli GV, Heger JJ, Zipes DP. Drug conversion of nonsustained ventricular tachycardia to sustained ventricular tachycardia during serial electrophysiological studies: identification of drugs that exacerbate tachycardia and potential mechanisms. Am Heart J 1982;103:177—184.
192. Velebit V, Podrid P, Lown B, Cohen BH, Graboys TB. Aggravation and provocation of ventricular arrhythmias by antiarrhythmic drugs. Circulation 1982;65:886—894.
193. Wellens HJJ, Smeets JL, Vos M, Gorgels AP. Antiarrhythmic drug treatment: need for continuous vigilance. Br Heart J 1992;67:25—33.
194. Morganroth J. Early and late proarrhythmia from antiarrhythmic drug therapy. Cardiovasc Drugs Ther 1992; 6:11—14.
195. Morganroth J. Proarrhythmic effects of antiarrhythmic drugs: evolving concepts. Am Heart J 1992;123:1137—1139.
196. Hilleman DE, Mohiuddin SM, Gannon JM. Adverse reactions during acute and chronic class I antiarrhythmic therapy. Curr Ther Res 1992;51:730—738.
197. Hilleman DE, Larsen KE. Proarrhythmic effects of antiarrhythmic drugs. PT 1991;June:520—524.
198. Libersa C, Caron J, Guedon-Moreau L, Adamantidis M, Nisse C. Adverse cardiovascular effects of antiarrhythmic drugs. Part 1: proarrhythmic effects. Thérapie 1992;47:193—198.
199. Podrid PJ, Fogel RI. Aggravation of arrhythmia by antiarrhythmic drugs, and the important role of underlying ischemia. Am J Cardiol 1992;70:100—102.
200. Follath F. Clinical pharmacology of antiarrhythmic drugs: variability of metabolism and dose requirements. J Cardiovasc Pharmacol 1991;17(Suppl 6):S74—S76.
201. Cowan JC, Coulshed DS, Zaman AG. Antiarrhythmic therapy and survival following myocardial infarction. J Cardiovasc Pharmacol 1991;18(Suppl 2):S92—S98.
202. Friedman L, Schron E, Yusuf S. Risk-benefit assessment of antiarrhythmic drugs. An epidemiological perspective. Drug Safety 1991;6:323—331.
203. Furberg CD, Yusuf S. Antiarrhythmics and VPD suppression. Circulation 1991;84:928—930.
204. Lüderitz B. Möglichkeiten und Grenzen der Arrhythmiebehandlung. Z Ges Inn Med 1991;46:425—430.
205. Podrid PJ. Safety and toxicity of antiarrhythmic drug therapy: benefit versus risk. J Cardiovasc Pharmacol 1991;17(Suppl 6):S65—S73.
206. Zimmermann M. Antiarrhythmic therapy for ventricu-

lar arrhythmias. J Cardiovasc Pharmacol 1991;17(Suppl 6):S59–S64.
207. Fauchier JP, Babuty D, Fauchier L, Rouesnel P, Cosnay P. Les effets proarythmiques des antiarythmiques. Arch Mal Coeur 1992;85:891–897.
208. Leenhardt A, Coumel P, Slama R. Torsade de pointes. J Cardiovasc Electrophysiol 1992;3:281–292.
209. Banai S, Tzivoni D. Drug therapy for torsades de pointes. J Cardiovasc Electrophysiol 1993;4:206–210.
210. Scholz H. Antiarrhythmischer Substanzen. Z Kardiol 1988;77(Suppl 5):113–119.
211. Luderitz B, Manz M. Hämodynamic bei ventrilularen Rhythmusstörungen und bei ihrer Behandlung. Z Kardiol 1988;77(Suppl 5):143–149.
212. Schleper M. Cardiodepressive effects of antiarrhythmic drugs. Eur Heart J 1989;10(Suppl E):73–80.
213. Seipel L, Hoffmeister HM. Hemodynamic effects of antiarrhythmic drugs: negative inotropy versus influence on peripheral circulation. Am J Cardiol 1989;64:37J–40J.
214. Hammermeister KE. Adverse hemodynamic effects of antiarrhythmic drugs in congestive heart failure. Circulation 1990;81:1151–1153.
215. Mason DT, DeMaria AN, Amsterdam EA, Zelis R, Massumi RA. Antiarrhythmic agents. I. Mechanisms of action and clinical pharmacology. II. Therapeutic considerations. Drugs 1973;5:261–291 and 292–317.
216. Winkle RA, Glantz SA, Harrison DC. Pharmacologic therapy of ventricular arrhythmias. Am J Cardiol 1975; 36:629–650.
217. Singh BN. Side effects of antiarrhythmic drugs. Pharmacol Ther 1977;2:151.
218. Harrison DC, Meffin PJ, Winkle RA. Clinical pharmacokinetics of antiarrhythmic drugs. Prog Cardiovasc Dis 1977;20:217–242.
219. Anderson Jl, Harrison DC, Meffin PJ, Winkle RA. Antiarrhythmic drugs: clinical pharmacology and therapeutic uses. Drugs 1978;15:271–309.
220. Zipes DP, Troup PJ. New anti-arrhythmic agents: amiodarone, aprindine, disopyramide, ethmozin, mexitetine, tocainide, verapamil. Am J Cardiol 1978;41:1005–1024.
221. Nattel S, Zipes DP. Clinical pharmacology of old and new antiarrhythmic drugs. Cardiovasc Clin 1980;11:221–248.
222. Schwartz JB, Keefe D, Harrison DC. Adverse effects of antiarrhythmic drugs. Drugs 1981;21:23–45.
223. Keefe DLD, Kates RE, Harrison DC. New antiarrhythmic drugs: their place in therapy. Drugs 1981;22:363–400.
224. Villain E. Les syndromes de QT long chez l'enfant. Arch Fr Pédiatr 1993;50:41–47.
225. Atkinson AJ, Ih Ruo T, Piergies AA. Comparison of the pharmacokinetic and pharmacodynamic properties of procainamide and *N*-acetylprocainamide. Angiology 1988;39:655–667.
226. Piergies AA, Ih Ruo T, Jansyn EM, Belknap SM, Atkinson AJ. Effect kinetics of *N*-acetylprocainamide-induced interval prolongation. Clin Pharmacol Ther 1987;42:107–112.
227. Lahita R, Kluger J, Drayer DE, Koffler D, Reidenberg MM. Antibodies to nuclear antigens in patients treated with procainamide or acetyl-procainamide. New Engl J Med 1979;301:1382–1385.
228. Kluger J, Leech S, Reidenberg MM, Lloyd V, Drayer DE. Long-term antiarrhythmic therapy with acetylprocainamide. Am J Cardiol 1981;48:1124–1132.
229. Kluger J, Drayer DE, Reidenberg MM, Lahita R. Acetylprocainamide therapy in patients with previous procainamide-induced lupus syndrome. Ann Intern Med 1981; 95:18–23.
230. Stec GP, Lertora JJL, Atkinson AJ Jr, Nevin MJ, Kushner W, Jones C, Schmid FR, Askenazi J. Remission of procainamide-induced lupus erythematosus with *N*-acetylprocainamide therapy. Ann Intern Med 1979;90:799–801.
231. Roden DM, Reele SB, Higgins SB, Wilkinson GR, Smith RF, Oates JA, Woosley RL. Antiarrhythmic efficacy, pharmacokinetics and safety of *N*-acetyl-procainamide in human subjects: comparison with procainamide. Am J Cardiol 1980;46:463–468.
232. Winkle RA, Jaillon P, Kates RE, Peters R. Clinical pharmacology and antiarrhythmic efficacy of *N*-acetylprocainamide. Am J Cardiol 1981;47:123–130.
233. Atkinson AJ, Lertora JJL, Kushner W, Chao GC, Nevin MJ. Efficacy and safety of *N*-acetylprocainamide in long-term treatment of ventricular arrhythmias. Clin Pharmacol Ther 1983;33:565–576.
234. Domoto DT, Brown WW, Bruggensmith P. Removal of toxic levels of *N*-acetylprocainamide with continuous arteriovenous hemofiltration or continuous arteriovenous hemodiafiltration. Ann Intern Med 1987;106:550–552.
235. Somogyi A, McLean A, Heinzow B. Cimetidine-procainamide pharmacokinetic interaction in man: evidence of competition for tubular secretion of basic drugs. Eur J Clin Pharmacol 1983;25:339–345.
236. Kosoglou T, Rocci ML, Vlasses PH. Trimethoprim alters the disposition of procainamide and *N*-acetylprocainamide. Clin Pharmacol Ther 1988;44:467–477.
237. Connolly SJ, Kates RE. Clinical pharmacokinetics of *N*-acetylprocainamide. Clin Pharmacokin 1982;7:206–220.
238. Camm AJ, Garratt CJ. Adenosine and supraventricular tachycardia. New Engl J Med 1991;325:1621–1629.
239. Harper KJ. Adenosine in the acute treatment of PSVT. Drug Ther 1992;March:53–72.
240. Rankin AC, Brooks R, Ruskin JN, McGovern BA. Adenosine and the treatment of supraventricular tachycardia. Am J Med 1992;92:655–664.
241. Hori M, Kitakaze M. Adenosine, the heart, and coronary circulation. Hypertension 1991;18:565–574.
242. Rankin AC, Oldroyd KG, Chong E, Dow JW, Rae AP, Cobbe SM. Adenosine or adenosine triphosphate for supraventricular tachycardias? Comparative double-blind randomized study in patients with spontaneous or inducible arrhythmias. Am Heart J 1990;119:316–323.
243. Ng WH, Polosa R, Church MK. Adenosine bronchoconstriction in asthma: investigations into its possible mechanism of action. Br J Clin Pharmacol 1990;30:89S–98S.
244. Clarke KW, Brear SG, Hanley SP. Rise in intracranial pressure with intravenous adenosine. Lancet 1992;339:188–189.
245. Watt AH, Lewis DJM, Horne JJ, Smith PM. Reproduction of epigastric pain of duodenal ulceration by adenosine. Br Med J 1987;294:10–12.
246. Abe S, Takeishi Y, Chiba J, Ikeda K, Tomoike H. Comparison of adenosine and treadmill exercise thallium-201 stress tests for the detection of coronary artery disease. Jpn Circ J 1993;57:1111–1119.
247. DiMarco AH, Sellers TD, Lerman BB, Greenberg ML, Berne RM, Belardinelli L. Diagnostic and therapeutic use of adenosine in patients with supraventricular tachyarrhythmias. J Am Coll Cardiol 1985;6:417–425.

248. Watt AH, Bernard MS, Webster J, Passani SL, Stephens MR, Routledge PA. Intravenous adenosine in the treatment of supraventricular tachycardia: a dose-ranging study and interaction with dipyridamole. Br J Clin Pharmacol 1986;21:227—230.
249. Brembilla-Perrot B, Terrier de la Chaise A. Provocation of supraventricular tachycardias by an intravenous class I antiarrhythmic drug. Int J Cardiol 1992;34:189—198.
250. Aquaro G, Marra S, Paolillo V, Pavia M. Complicanze neurologiche in corso di terapia con 17-MDCAA. G Ital Cardiol 1977;7:304—308.
251. Lessing JB, Copperman IJ. Severe cerebral confusion produced by prajmalium bitartrate. Br Med J 1977;2:675.
252. Brna TG. Agranulocytosis from antiarrhythmic agents. Postgrad Med 1991;89:181—188.
253. Offenstadt G, Boisante L, Onimus A, Amstutz P. Agranulocytose et hepatite cholestatique au cours d'un traitement par l'ajmaline. Ann Méd Interne 1976;127:625—627.
254. Buscher HP, Talke H, Rademacher HP, Gesner U, Oehlert W, Gerok W. Intrahepatische Cholestase durch *N*-Propyl-Ajmalin. Dtsch Med Wschr 1976;101:699—703.
255. Chammartin F, Levillain P, Silvain C, Chauvin C, Beauchaut M. Hepatite prolongée a l'ajmaline-description d'un cas et revue de la litterature. Schweiz Rundsch Med (Prax) 1989;78:582—584.
256. Dupond JL, Herve P, Saint-Hillier Y, Guyon B, Colas JM, Perol C, Leconte des Floris R. Anurie recidivant a 3 reprises; complication exceptionelle d'un traitement antiarythmique. J Med Besançon 1975;11:231.
257. Tempe JD, Jaeger A, Beissel J et al. Intoxications aiguës par trois drogues cardiotropes: l'ajmaline, la chloroquine, la digitaline. J Med Strasbourg (Eur Med) 1976;7:569.
258. Conso F, Bismuth C, Riboulet G, Efthymiou ML. Intoxication aiguë par l'ajmaline. Thérapie 1979;34:529—530.
259. Rosenbaum MB, Chiale PA, Halpern MS, Nau GJ, Przybylski J, Levi RJ, Lazzari JO, Elizari MV. Clinical efficacy of amiodarone as an antiarrhythmic agent. Am J Cardiol 1976;38:934—944.
260. McGovern B, Garan H, Ruskin JN. Serious adverse effects of amiodarone. Clin Cardiol 1984;7:131—137.
261. Latini R, Tognoni G, Kates RE. Clinical pharmacokinetics of amiodarone. Clin Pharmacokin 1984;9:136—156.
262. Heger JJ, Prystowsky EN, Miles WM, Zipes DP. Clinical use and pharmacology of amiodarone. Med Clin North Am 1984;68:1339—1366.
263. Cetnarowski AB, Rihn TL. A review of adverse reactions to amiodarone. Cardiovasc Rev Rep 1985;5:1206—1222.
264. Kadish A, Morady F. The use of intravenous amiodarone in the acute therapy of life-threatening tachyarrhythmias. Prog Cardiovasc Dis 1989;31:281—294.
265. Kopelman HA, Horowitz LN. Efficacy and toxicity of amiodarone for the treatment of supraventricular tachyarrhythmias. Prog Cardiovasc Dis 1989;31:355—366.
266. Heger JJ. Monitoring and treating side effects of amiodarone therapy. Cardiovasc Rev Rep 1988;9:47.
267. Kerin NZ, Aragon E, Faitel K, Frumin H, Rubenfire M. Long-term efficacy and toxicity of high- and low-dose amiodarone regimens. J Clin Pharmacol 1989;29:418—423.
268. Somani P. Basic and clinical pharmacology of amiodarone: relationship of antiarrhythmic effects, dose and drug concentrations to intracellular inclusion bodies. J Clin Pharmacol 1989;29:405—412.
269. Kerin NZ, Blevins RD, Kerner N, Faitel K, Frumin H, Maciejko JJ, Rubenfire M. A low incidence of proarrhythmia using low-dose amiodarone. J Electrophysiol 1988;2:289—295.
270. Krikler DM, McKenna WJ, Chamberlain DA, eds. Amiodarone and Arrhythmias. Oxford: Pergamon Press, 1983.
271. Dunn M, Glassroth J. Pulmonary complications of amiodarone toxicity. Prog Cardiovasc Dis 1989;31:447—453.
272. Kennedy JI. Clinical aspects of amiodarone pulmonary toxicity. Clin Chest Med 1990;11:119—129.
273. Martin WJ. Mechanisms of amiodarone pulmonary toxicity. Clin Chest Med 1990;11:131—138.
274. Dusman RE, Stanton MS, Miles WM, Kleijn LS, Zipes DP, Fineberg NS, Heger JJ. Clinical features of amiodarone-induced pulmonary toxicity. Circulation 1990;82:51—59.
275. Nicholson AA, Hayward C. The value of computed tomography in the diagnosis of amiodarone-induced pulmonary toxicity. Clin Radiol 1989;40:564—567.
276. Biour M, Hugues FC, Hamel JD, Cheymol G. Les effets indesirables pulmonaires de l'amiodarone: analyse de 162 observations. Thérapie 1985;40:343—348.
277. Kudenchuk PJ, Pierson DJ, Greene HL, Graham EL, Sears GK, Trobaugh GB. Prospective evaluation of amiodarone pulmonary toxicity. Chest 1984;86:541—548.
278. Palakurthy PR, Iyer V, Meckler RJ. Unusual neurotoxicity associated with amiodarone therapy. Arch Intern Med 1987;147:881—884.
279. Trohman RG, Castellanos D, Castellanos A, Kessler KM. Amiodarone-induced delirium. Ann Intern Med 1988;108:68—69.
280. Werner EG, Olanow CW. Parkinsonism and amiodarone therapy. Ann Neurol 1989;25:630—632.
281. Borruat F-X, Regli F. Pseudotumor cerebri as a complication of amiodarone therapy. Am J Ophthalmol 1993; 116:776—777.
282. Jacobs JM, Costa-Jussa FR. The pathology of amiodarone neurotoxicity. II. Peripheral neuropathy in man. Brain 1985;108:753—769.
283. Wiersinga WM, Trip MD. Amiodarone and thyroid hormone metabolism. Postgrad Med J 1986;62:909—914.
284. Mason JW. Amiodarone. New Engl J Med 1987; 316:455—466.
285. Tajiri J, Higashi K, Morita M, Umeda T, Sato T. Studies of hypothyroidism in patients with high iodine intake. J Clin Endocrinol Metab 1986;63:412—417.
286. Nademanee K, Piwonka RW, Singh BN, Hershman JM. Amiodarone and thyroid function. Prog Cardiovasc Dis 1989;31:427—437.
287. Martino E, Safran M, Aghini-Lombardi F, Rajatanavin R, Lenziardi M, Fay M, Pacchiarotti A, Aronin N, Macchia E, Haffajee C, et al. Environmental iodine intake and thyroid dysfunction during chronic amiodarone therapy. Ann Intern Med 1984;101:28—34.
288. Martino E, Aghini-Lombardi F, Bartalena L, Grasso L, Loviselli A, Velluzzi F, Pinchera A, Braverman LE. Enhanced susceptibility to amiodarone-induced hypothyroidism in patients with thyroid autoimmune disease. Arch Intern Med 1994;154:2722—2726.
289. Martino E, Bartalena L, Mariotti S, Aghini-Lombardi F, Ceccarelli C, Lippi F, Piga M, Loriselli A, Braverman L, Safran M. Radioactive iodine thyroid uptake in patients with amiodarone-iodine-induced thyroid dysfunction. Acta Endocrinol (Copenhagen) 1988;119:167—173
290. Mancini A, De Mainis L, Calabro F, Sciuto R, Oradei

A, Lippa S, Sandric S, Littaru GP, Barbarino A. Evaluation of metabolic status in amiodarone-induced thyroid disorders: plasma coenzyme Q_{10} determination. J Endocrinol Invest 1989;12:511–516.
291. Martino E, Aghini-Lombardi F, Mariotti S, Lenziardi M, Baschiere L, Braverman LE, Pinchera A. Treatment of amiodarone associated thyrotoxicosis by simultaneous administration of potassium perchlorate and methimazole. J Endocrinol Invest 1986;9:201–207.
292. Reichert LJM, de Rooy HAM. Treatment of amiodarone induced hyperthyroidism with potassium perchlorate and methimazole during amiodarone treatment. Br Med J 1989;298:1547–1548.
293. Pollak PT, Sharma AD, Carruthers G. Elevation of serum total cholesterol and triglyceride levels during amiodarone therapy. Am J Cardiol 1988;62:562–565.
294. Dobs AS, Sarma PS, Guarnieri T, Griffith L. Testicular dysfunction with amiodarone use. J Am Coll Cardiol 1991;18:1328–1332.
295. Adams PC, Sloan P, Morley AR, Holt DW. Peripheral neutrophil inclusions in amiodarone treated patients. Br J Clin Pharmacol 1986;22:736–738.
296. Weinberger I, Rotenberg Z, Fuchs J, Ben-Sasson E, Agmon J. Amiodarone-induced thrombocytopenia. Arch Intern Med 1987;147:735–736.
297. Berrebi A, Shtalrid M, Vorst EJ. Amiodarone-induced thrombocytopathy. Acta Haematol 1983;70:68–69.
298. Arpin MP, Alt M, Kheiralla JC, Chabrier G, Welsch M, Imbs JL, Imler M. Hyperthyroïdie et anémie hémolytique immune après traitement par amiodarone. Rev Méd Interne 1991;12:309–311.
299. Heger JJ, Prystowsky EN, Jackman WM, Naccarelli GV, Warfel KA, Rinkenberger RL, Zipes DP. Amiodarone. New Engl J Med 1982;305:539–545.
300. Bexton RS, Camm AJ. Drugs with a Class III antiarrhythmic action. Pharmacol Ther 1982;17:315–355.
301. Freneaux E, Larrey D, Pessayre D. Phospholipidose et lesions pseudoalcooliques hepatiques medicamenteuses. Rev Fr Gastro-enterol 1988;24:879–884.
302. Adams PC, Bennett MK, Holt DW. Hepatic effects of amiodarone. Br J Clin Pract 1986;40(Suppl 44):81–92.
303. Geneve J, Zafrani ES, Dhumeaux D. Amiodarone-induced liver disease. J Hepatol 1989;9:130–133.
304. Harrison RF, Elias E. Amiodarone-associated cirrhosis with hepatic and lymph node granulomas. Histopathology 1993;22:80–82.
305. Tilz GP, Liebig E, Pristautz H. Cholestase bei Amiodaron-eine seltene Komplikation der antiarrhythmischen Therapie. Med Welt 1989;40:985.
306. Salti Z, Cloche P, Weber P, Houssemand G, Vollmer F. A propos d'un cas d'hepatite cholestatique a l'amiodarone. Ann Cardiol Angéiol 1989;36:13–16.
307. Jones DB, Mullick FG, Hoofnagle JH, Baranski B. Reye's syndrome-like illness in a patient receiving amiodarone. Am J Gastroenterol 1988;83:967–969.
308. Rhodes A, Eastwood JB, Smith SA. Early acute hepatitis with parenteral amiodarone: a toxic effect of the vehicle? Gut 1993;34:565–566.
309. Sastri SV, Diaz-Arias AA, Marshall JB. Can pancreatitis be associated with amiodarone hepatotoxicity? J Clin Gastroenterol 1990;12:70–73.
310. Pollak PT, Sharma AD, Carruthers SG. Creatinine elevation in patients receiving amiodarone correlates with serum amiodarone concentration. Br J Clin Pharmacol 1993;36:125–127.
311. Anonymous. Amiodarone—a new type of antiarrhythmic drug. Drug Ther Bull 1981;19:86–88.
312. Chalmers RJG, Muston HL, Srinivas V, Bennett DH. High incidence of amiodarone-induced photosensitivity in North-West England. Br Med J 1982;285:341.
313. Ferguson J, De Vane PJ, Wirth M. Prevention of amiodarone-induced photosensitivity. Lancet 1984;ii:414.
314. Ferguson J, Addo HA, Jones S, Johnson BE, Frain-Bell W. A study of cutaneous photosensitivity induced by amiodarone. Br J Dermatol 1985;113:537–549.
315. Parodi A, Guarrera M, Rebora A. Amiodarone-induced pseudoporphyria. Photodermatology 1988;5:146–147.
316. Beukema WP, Graboys TB. Spontaneous disappearance of blue-gray facial pigmentation during amiodarone therapy (out of the blue). Am J Cardiol 1988;62:1146–1147.
317. Zantkuyl CF, Weemers M. Iododerma caused by amiodarone (Cordarone). Dermatologia (Basel) 1975;151:311.
318. Muir AD, Wilson M. Amiodarone and psoriasis. NZ Med J 1982;95:711.
319. Moots RJ, Banerjee A. Exfoliative dermatitis after amiodarone treatment. Br Med J 1988;296:1332–1333.
320. Dootson G, Byatt C. Amiodarone-induced vasculitis and a review of the cutaneous side-effects of amiodarone. Clin Exp Dermatol 1994;19:422–424.
321. Waitzer S, Butany J, From L, Hanna W, Ramsay C, Downar E. Cutaneous ultrastructural changes and photosensitivity associated with amiodarone therapy. J Am Acad Dermatol 1987;16:779–787.
322. Ingram DV, Jaggarao NSV, Chamberlain DA. Ocular changes resulting from therapy with amiodarone. Br J Ophthalmol 1982;66:676–679.
323. Ingram DV. Ocular effects in long-term amiodarone therapy. Am Heart J 1983;106:902–905.
324. Duff GR, Fraser AG. Impairment of colour vision associated with amiodarone keratopathy. Acta Ophthalmol 1987;65:48–52.
325. Feiner LA, Younge BR, Kazmier FJ, Stricker BH, Fraunfelder FT. Optic neuropathy and amiodarone therapy. Mayo Clin Proc 1987;62:702–717.
326. Mansour AM, Puklin JW, O'Grady R. Optic nerve ultrastructure following amiodarone therapy. J Clin Neuro-ophthalmol 1988;8:231–237.
327. Dewachter A, Lievens H. Amiodarone and optic neuropathy. Bull Soc Belge Ophtalmol 1988;227:47–50.
328. Garret SN, Kearney JJ, Schiffman JS. Amiodarone optic neuropathy. J Clin Neuro-ophthalmol 1988;8:105.
329. Fikkers BG, Bogousslavsky J, Regli F, Glasson S. Pseudotumor cerebri with amiodarone. J Neurol Neurosurg Psychiatry 1986;49:606.
330. Thystrup JD, Fledelius HC. Retinal maculopathy possibly associated with amiodarone medication. Acta Ophthalmol 1994;72:639–641.
331. Clouston PD, Donnelly PE. Acute necrotising myopathy associated with amiodarone therapy. Aust NZ J Med 1989;19:483–485.
332. Morady F, Scheinman M, Shen E, Shapiro W, Sung RJ, DiCarlo L. Intravenous amiodarone in the acute treatment of recurrent symptomatic ventricular tachycardia. Am J Cardiol 1983;51:156–159.
333. Holt P, Curry PVL, Way B, Storey G, Holt DW. Intravenous amiodarone in the management of tachyarrhythmias. In: Breithardt H, Loogen F, eds. New Aspects in the Medical Treatment of Tachyarrhythmas. Munich; Urban and Schwartzenberg, 1983; 136–141.

334. Faniel R, Schoenfeld P. Efficacy of i.v. amiodarone in converting rapid atrial fibrillation and flutter to sinus rhythm in intensive care patients. Eur Heart J 1983;4:1880—1885.
335. Antonelli D, Barzilay J. Acute thrombophlebitis following IV amiodarone administration. Chest 1983;84:120.
336. Kerin NZ, Blevins R, Rubenfire M, Faital K, Householder S. Acute thrombophlebitis following IV amiodarone administration. Chest 1983;84:120.
337. Hyatt RH, Sinha B, Vallon A, Bailey RJ, Martin A. Noncardiac side-effects of long-term oral amiodarone in the elderly. Age Ageing 1988;17:116—122.
338. Garson A, Gillette PC, McVey P, Hesslein PS, Porter CJ, Angell LK, Kaldis LC, Hittner HM. Amiodarone treatment of critical arrhythmias in children and young adults. J Am Coll Cardiol 1984;4:749—755.
339. Guccione P, Paul T, Garson A. Long-term follow-up of amiodarone therapy in the young: continued efficacy, unimpaired growth, moderate side effects. J Am Coll Cardiol 1990;15:1118—1124.
340. Kupferschmid JP, Rosengart TK, McIntosh CL, Leon MB, Clark RE. Amiodarone-induced complications after cardiac operation for obstructive hypertrophic cardiomyopathy. Ann Thorac Surg 1989;48:359—364.
341. Andersen HR, Bjorn-Hansen LS, Kimose H-H et al. Amiodaronebehandling og arytmikirurgi. Ugeskr Laeg 1989;151:2264.
342. Perkins MW, Dasta JF, Reilley TE, Halpern P Intraoperative complications in patients receiving amiodarone: characteristics and risk factors. DICP Ann Pharmacother 1989;23:757—763.
343. Foster CJ, Love HG. Amiodarone in pregnancy: case report and review of the literature. Int J Cardiol 1988;20:307—316.
344. Tubman R, Jenkins J, Lim J. Neonatal hyperthyroxinaemia associated with maternal amiodarone therapy: case report. Ir J Med Sci 1988;157:243.
345. De Wolf D, De Schepper J, Verhaaren H, De Meyer M, Smitz J, Sacre-Smits L. Congenital hypothyroid goiter and amiodarone. Acta Paediatr Scand 1988;77:616—618.
346. De Catte L, De Wolf D, Smitz J, Bougatef A, De Schepper J, Foulon W. Fetal hypothyroidism as a complication of amiodarone treatment for persistent fetal supraventricular tachycardia. Prenat Diag 1994;14:762—765.
347. Hamer A, Peter T, Mandel WJ Scheinman MM, Weiss D. The potentiation of warfarin anticoagulation by amiodarone. Circulation 1982;65:1025.
348. Bonati M, D'Aranno V, Galletti F, Fortunati MT, Tognoni G. Acute overdosage of amiodarone in a suicide attempt. J Toxicol Clin Toxicol 1983;20:181—186.
349. Marcus FI. Drug combinations and interactions with class III agents. J Cardiovasc Pharmacol 1992;20(Suppl 2):S70—S74.
350. Jacobs MB. Serum creatinine increase associated with amiodarone therapy. NY State J Med 1987;87:358—359.
351. Rotmensch HH, Belhassen B, Swanson BN, Shoshani D, Spielman SR, Greenspon AJ, Greenspan AM, Vlasses PH, Horowitz LN. Steady-state serum amiodarone concentrations: relationships with antiarrhythmic efficacy and toxicity. Ann Intern Med 1984;101:462—469.
352. Pollak PT, Sharma AD, Carruthers SG. Correlation of amiodarone dosage, heart rate, QT interval and corneal microdeposits with serum amiodarone and desethylamiodarone concentrations. Am J Cardiol 1989;64:1138—1143.
353. Debbas NMG, Du Cailar C, Bexton RS, Demailler JG, Camm AJ, Puech P. The QT interval: a predictor of the plasma and myocardial concentrations of amiodarone. Br Heart J 1984;51:316—320.
354. Primeau R, Agha A, Giorgi C, Shenasa M, Nadeau R. Long term efficacy and toxicity of amiodarone in the treatment of refractory cardiac arrhythmias. Can J Cardiol 1989;5:98—104.
355. Danilo P Jr Aprindine. Am Heart J 1979;97:119—124.
356. Zipes DP, Elharrar V, Gilmour RF, Heger JJ, Prystowsky EN. Studies with aprindine. Am Heart J 1980;100:1055—1062.
357. Opie LH. Aprindine and agranulocytosis. Lancet 1980;ii:689—690.
358. Casteels-Van Daele M, Beirinckx J, De Cock P, Peetes M, Corbeel L. Pancytopenia under treatment with aprindine, a new anti-arrhythmic drug. Acta Paediatr Belg 1977; 30:247—248.
359. Elewaut A, Van Durme JP, Goethals L, Kauffman JM, Mussche M, Elinck W, Roels H, Bogaer M, Barbier F. Aprindine-induced liver damage. Acta Gastroenterol Belg 1977;40:236—243.
360. Elisaf M, Stefanaki-Nikou S, Voulgarelis M, Masalas C, Tsianos EV. Aprindine-induced hepatic granulomata. J Hepatol 1992;14:276—279.
361. Anonymous. Bepridil. Lancet 1988;i:278.
362. Benet LZ. Pharmacokinetics and metabolism of bepridil. Am J Cardiol 1985;55:8C—13C.
363. Faauchier JP, Cosnay P, Neel C, Rouesnel P, Bonnet P, Quilliet L. Traitement des tachycardies supraventriculaires et ventriculaires paroxystiques par le bépridil. Arch Mal Coeur 1985;78:612—619.
364. Flammang D, Waynberger M, Jansen FH, Paillet R, Courne P. Electrophysiological profile of bepridil, a new anti-anginal drug with calcium blocking properties. Eur Heart J 1983;4:647—654.
365. Canicave JC, Deu J, Jacq J, Paillet R. Un nouvel antiangoreux, le bépridil: appreciation de son efficacité par l'epreuve d'effort au cours d'un essai a double insu contre placébo. Thérapie 1980;35:607—612.
366. Upward JW, Daly K, Campbell S, Bergman G, Jewitt DE. Electrophysiologic, hemodynamic and metabolic effects of intravenous bepridil hydrochloride. Am J Cardiol 1985;55:1589—1595.
367. Frishman WH, Charlap S, Farnham DJ, Sawin HS, Michelson EL, Crawford MH. Combination propranolol and bepridil therapy in stable angina pectoris. Am J Cardiol 1985;55:43C—49C.
368. Perelman MS, McKenna WJ, Rowland E, Krikler DM. A comparison of bepridil with amiodarone in the treatment of established atrial fibrillation. Br Heart J 1987;58:339—344.
369. Roy D, Montigny M, Klein GJ, Sharma AD, Cassidy D. Electrophysiologic effects and long-term efficacy of bepridil for recurrent supraventricular tachycardias. Am J Cardiol 1987;59:89—92.
370. Ponsonnaille J, Citron B, Thriel F, Heiligenstein D, Gras H. Etude des effets electrophysiologiques du bepridil utilisé par voie veineuse. Arch Mal Coeur 1982;75:1415—1423.
371. Singh BN. Bepridil therapy: guidelines for patient selection and monitoring of therapy. Am J Cardiol 1992;69:79D—85D.
372. Rowland E, McKenna WJ, Krikler DM. Electrophysiologic and antiarrhythmic actions of bepridil: comparison with

verapamil and ajmaline for atrioventricular reentrant tachycardia. Am J Cardiol 1985;55:1513–1519.
373. Brembilla-Perrot B, Aliot E, Clementy J, Cosnay P, Djiane P, Fauchier JP, Kacet S, Lellouche D, Mabo P, Richard M, Victor J. Evaluation of bepridil efficacy by electrophysiologic testing in patients with recurrent ventricular tachycardia: comparison of two regimens. Cardiovasc Drugs Ther 1992;6:187–193.
374. Funck-Brentano C, Chaffin PL, Wilkinson GR, McAllister B, Woosley RL. Effect of oral administration of a new calcium channel blocking agent, bepridil on antipyrine clearance in man. Br J Clin Pharmacol 1987;24:559–560.
375. Stern H, Aust P, Belz GG, Schneider HT. Interaction entre bepridil et digoxine. Rev Med 1983;24:1279.
376. Cooper JA, Frieden J. Bretylium tosylate. Am Heart J 1971;82:703–706.
377. Koch-Weser J. Bretylium. New Engl J Med 1979; 300:473–477.
378. Rapeport WG. Clinical pharmacokinetics of bretylium. Clin Pharmacokin 1985;10:248–256.
379. Taylor SH, Saxton C, Davies PS, Stoker JB. Bretylium tosylate in prevention of cardiac arrhythmias after myocardial infarction. Br Heart J 1970;32:326–329.
380. Anderson JL, Popat KD, Pitt B. Paradoxical ventricular tachycardia and fibrillation after intravenous bretylium therapy. Report of two cases. Arch Intern Med 1981;141:801–802.
381. Thibault J. Hyperthermia associated with bretylium tosylate injection. Clin Pharm 1989;8:145–146.
382. Perlman PE, Adams WG, Ridgeway NA. Extreme pyrexia during bretylium administration. Postgrad Med 1989;85:111–114.
383. Heinrich KW, Effert S. Bretylium-Tosylat zur Behandlung maligner Arrhythmien: erste Resultate. Med Welt 1973;24:1000–1002.
384. Miura DS, Dangman KH, Berchin B, Somberg J. New antiarrhythmic agents. VII. The pharmacology and clinical use of cibenzoline. Pract Cardiol 1985;11:103–117.
385. Miura DS, Keren G, Torres V, Butler B, Aogaicki K, Somberg JC. Antiarrhythmic effects of cibenzoline. Am Heart J 1985;109:827–833.
386. Thizy JF, Jandot V, Andre-Fouet X, Viallet M, Pout M. Etude electrophysiologique de l'UP 339–01 chez l'homme. Lyon Med 1981;245:119–122.
387. Hoffmann E, Mattke S, Haberl R, Steinbeck G. Randomized crossover comparison of the electrophysiologic and antiarrhythmic efficacy of oral cibenzoline and sotalol for sustained ventricular tachycardia. J Cardiovasc Pharmacol 1993;21:95–100.
388. Kostis JB, Davis D, Kluger J, Aogaicki K, Smith M. Cifenline in the short-term treatment of patients with ventricular premature complexes: a double-blind placebo-controlled trial. J Cardiovasc Pharmacol 1989;14:88–95.
389. Kushner M, Magiros E, Peters R, Carliner N, Plotnik G, Fisher M. The electrophysiologic effects of oral cibenzoline. J Electrocardiol 1984;17:15–23.
390. Browne KF, Prystowsky EN, Zipes DP, Chilson DA, Heger JJ. Clinical efficacy and electrophysiologic effects of cibenzoline therapy in patients with ventricular arrhythmias. J Am Coll Cardiol 1984;3:857–864.
391. Humen DP, Lesoway R, Kostuk WJ. Acute, single intravenous doses of cibenzoline: an evaluation of safety, tolerance, and hemodynamic effects. Clin Pharmacol Ther 1987;41:537–545.
392. Katoh T, Ishihara S, Tanaka T, Kobagasi Y, Takada K, Shimai S, Seino Y, Tanaka K, Takano T, Hayakawa H. Hemodynamic effects of intravenous cibenzoline, a new antiarrhythmic agent. Jpn J Clin Pharmacol Ther 1988; 19:707–716.
393. Cocco G, Strozzi C, Pansini R, Rochat N, Bulgarelli R, Padula A, Sfrisi C. Antiarrhythmic use of cibenzoline, a new class 1 antiarrhythmic agent with class 3 and 4 properties, in patients with recurrent ventricular tachycardia. Eur Heart J 1984;5:108–114.
394. Klein RC, House M, Rushforth N. Efficacy and safety of oral cibenzoline in treatment of ventricular ectopy. Clin Res 1984;32:9A.
395. Lee MA, Fenster PE, Garcia ZM, Kipps JE, Huang SK. Cibenzoline for symptomatic ventricular arrhythmias: a prospective, randomized, double-blind, placebo controlled trial and a long term open label study. Can J Cardiol 1989;5:295–298.
396. Miura D, Torres V, Butler B, Gottlieb S, Aogaicki K, Somberg J. Effects of cibenzoline in patients with ventricular tachycardia. J Clin Pharmacol 1984;24:413.
397. Lefort G, Haissaguerre M, Floro J, Beauffigeau P, Warin JF, Latapie JL. Hypoglycémies au cours de surdosages par un nouvel anti-arythmique: la cibenzoline; trois observations. Presse Méd 1988;17:687–691.
398. Jeandel C, Preiss MA, Pierson H, Penin F, Cuny G, Annwarth B, Netter P. Hypoglycaemia induced by cibenzoline. Lancet 1988;ii:1232–1233.
399. Gachot BA, Bezier M, Cherrier J-F, Daubeze J. Cibenzoline and hypoglycaemia. Lancet 1988;2:280.
400. Gutknecht J, Larrey D, Ychou M, Fedkovic Y, Janbon C. Ischémie hépatique grave après prise de cibenzoline. Ann. Gastroentérol. Hépatol 1990;27:269–270.
401. Canal M, Flouvat B, Tremblay D, Dufour A. Pharmacokinetics in man of a new antiarrhythmic drug, cibenzoline. Eur J Clin Pharmacol 1983;24:509–515.
402. Brazzell RK, Rees MMC, Khoo K-C, Szuna AJ, Sandor D, Hannigan J. Age and cibenzoline disposition. Clin Pharmacol Ther 1984;36:613–619.
403. van den Brand M, Serruys P, de Roon Y, Aymard MF, Dufour A. Haemodynamic effects of intravenous cibenzoline in patients with coronary heart disease. Eur J Clin Pharmacol 1984;26:297–302.
404. Khoo K-C, Szuna AJ, Colburn WA, Aogaicki K, Morganroth J, Brazzell RK. Single-dose pharmacokinetics and dose proportionality of oral cibenzoline. J Clin Pharmacol 1984;24:283–288.
405. Heel RC, Brogden RN, Speight RM, Avery GS. Disopyramide: a review of its pharmacological properties and therapeutic use in treating cardiac arrhythmias. Drugs 1978;15:331–368.
406. Koch-Weser J. Disopyramide. New Engl J Med 1979; 300:957–962.
407. Warrington SJ, Hamer J. Some cardiovascular problems with disopyramide. Postgrad Med J 1980;56:229–233.
408. McHaffie DJ, Guz A, Johnston A. Impotence in patient on disopyramide. Lancet 1977;i:859.
409. Falk RH, Nisbet PA, Gray TJ. Mental distress in patient on disopyramide. Lancet 1977;i:858–859.
410. Padfield PL, Smith DA, Fitzsimons EJ, McCruden DC. Disopyramide and acute psychosis. Lancet 1977;i:1152.
411. Otsu T, Ito T, Inagaki Y, Amano I, Masamoto S, Niwa M. Accumulation of a disopyramide metabolite in renal failure. Jpn J Nephrol 1993;35:1065–1071 and Asaio J 1993;39:M609–613 (Japanese and English, respectively).

412. Series C. Hypoglycémie induite ou favorisée par le disopyramide. Rev Med Interne 1988;9:528–529.
413. Conrad ME, Cumbie WG, Thrasher DR, Carpenter JT. Agranulocytosis associated with disopyrmide therapy. J Am Med Assoc 1978;240:1857–1858.
414. Handa SP. Disopyramide-induced toxic cutaneous blisters and coagulopathy. Dialysis Transplant 1982;11:706–707.
415. Anonymous. Hepatic damage due to disopyramide. Jpn Med Gaz 1981;June 20:11.
416. Doody PT. Disopyramide hepatotoxicity and disseminated intravascular coagulation. South Med J 1982;75:496–498.
417. Meinertz T, Langer KH, Kasper W, Just H. Disopyramide-induced intrahepatic cholestasis. Lancet 1977;ii:828–829.
418. Riccioni N, Bozzi L, Susini N, Roni P. Disopyramide-induced intrahepatic cholestasis. Lancet 1977;ii:1362–1363.
419. Scheinman SJ, Poll DS, Wolfson S. Acute cardiac failure and hepatic ischemia induced by disopyramide phosphate. Yale J Biol Med 1980;53:361–366.
420. Tadmor OP, Keren A, Rosenak D, Gal M, Shaia M, Hornstein E, Yaffe H, Graff E, Stern S, Diamant YZ. The effect of disopyramide on uterine contractions during pregnancy. Am J Obstet Gynecol 1990;162:482–486.
421. Hasegawa J, Mashiba H. Transient sexual dysfunction observed during antiarrhythmic therapy by long-acting disopyramide in a male Wolff-Parkinson-White patient. Cardiovasc Drugs Ther 1994;8:277.
422. Porterfield JG, Antman EM, Lown B. Respiratory difficulty after use of disopyramide. New Engl J Med 1980;303:584.
423. Barnett DB, Hudson SA, McBurney A. Disopyramide and its *N*-monodesalkyl metabolite in breast milk. Br J Clin Pharmacol 1982;14:310–312.
424. Hayter AM, Holt DW, Volans GN. Fatal overdosage with disopyramide. Lancet 1978;i:968–969.
425. Larcan A, Lambert H, Laprevote-Heully MC, Delorme N, Royer MJ, Guillet J. Les intoxications aiguës volontaires au disopyramide: à propos de 20 observations. Ann Med Nancy 1981;20:901–917.
426. Hayler AM, Medd RK, Holt DW, O'Keefe BD. Treatment of disopyramide overdosage. Vet Hum Toxicol 1979;12(Suppl):93–95.
427. Teichman SL, Fisher JD, Matos JA, Kim SG. Disopyramide-pyridostigmine: report of a beneficial drug interaction. J Cardiovasc Pharmacol 1985;7:108–113.
428. Ellrodt G, Singh BN. Adverse effects of disopyramide (Norpace): toxic interactions with other antiarrhythmic agents. Heart Lung 1980;9:469–474.
429. Haworth E, Burroughs AK. Disopyramide and warfarin interaction. Br Med J 1977;2:866–867.
430. Sylven C, Anderson P. Evidence that disopyramide does not interact with warfarin. Br Med J Clin Res Ed 1983;286:1181.
431. Cumming AD, Robertson C. Interaction between disopyramide and practolol. Br Med J 1979;2:1264.
432. Gelipter D, Hazell M. Interaction between disopyramide and practolol. Br Med J 1980;280:52.
433. Maddux BD, Whiting RB. Toxic synergism of disopyramide and hyperkalaemia. Chest 1980;78:654–656.
434. The Cardiac Arrhythmia Suppression Trial (CAST) Investigators. Preliminary report: effect of encainide and flecainide on mortality in a randomized trial of arrhythmia suppression after myocardial infarction. New Engl J Med 1989;321:406–412.
435. Echt DS, Liebson PR, Mitchell LB, Peter RW, Obias-Manno D, Barker AH, Arensberg D, Baker A, Friedman L, Greene HL, Huther ML, Richardson DW, The CAST Investigators. Mortality and morbidity in patients receiving encainide, flecainide, or placebo. The Cardiac Arrhythmia Suppression Trial. New Engl J Med 1991;324:781–788.
436. Gottlieb SS. The use of antiarrhythmic agents in heart failure: implications of CAST. Am Heart J 1989;118:1074–1077.
437. Podrid PJ, Marcus FI. Lessons to be learned from the Cardiac Arrhythmia Suppression Trial. Am J Cardiol 1989;64:1189–1191.
438. Bigger JT. The events surrounding the removal of encainide and flecainide from the Cardiac Arrhythmia Suppression Trial (CAST) and why CAST is continuing with moricizine. J Am Coll Cardiol 1990;15:243–245.
439. Tast Force of the Working Group on Arrhythmias of the European Society of Cardiology. CAST and beyond. Implications of the cardiac arrhythmia suppression trial. Circulation 1990;81:1123–1127.
441. Harrison DC, Winkel R, Sami M, Mason J. Encainide: a new and potent antiarrhythmic agent. Am Heart J 1980;100:1046–1054.
442. Lynch JJ, Lucchesi BR. New antiarrhythmic agents. II. The pharmacology and clinical use of encainide. Pract Cardiol 1984;10:109–132.
443. Roden DM, Woosley RL. Clinical pharmacology of the new antiarrhythmic encainide. Clin Prog Pacing Electrophysiol 1984;2:112–119.
444. Rinkenberger RL, Naccarelli GV, Dougherty AH. New antiarrhythmic agents. X. Safety and efficacy of encainide in the treatment of ventricular arrhythmias. Pract Cardiol 1987;13:110–132.
445. Naccarelli GV, Wellens HJJ. eds. A symposium: the use of encainide in supraventricular tachycardias. Am J Cardiol 1988;62:1L.
446. Soyka LF. Safety considerations and dosing guidelines for encainide in supraventricular arrhythmias. Am J Cardiol 1988;62:63L–68L.
447. Miles WM, Zipes DP, Rinkenberger RL, Markel ML, Prystowsky EN, Dougherty AH, Heger JJ, Naccarelli GV. Encainide for treatment of atrioventricular reciprocating tachycardia in the Wolff-Parkinson-White syndrome. Am J Cardiol 1988;62:20L–25L.
448. Rinkenberger RL, Naccarelli GV, Miles WM, Markel ML, Dougherty AH. Encainide for atrial fibrillation associated with Wolff-Parkinson-White syndrome. Am J Cardiol 1988;62:26L–30L.
449. Naccarelli GV, Jackman WM, Akhtar M, Rinkenberger RL, Friday KJ, Dougherty AH, Tchou P, Yeung-Lai-Wah JA. Efficacy and electrophysiologic effects of encainide for atrioventricular nodal reentrant tachycardia. Am J Cardiol 1988;62:31L–36L.
450. The Encainide-Ventricular Tachycardia Study Group. Treatment of life-threatening ventricular tachycardia with encainide hydrochloride in patients with left ventricular dysfunction. Am J Cardiol 1988;62:571–575.
451. Lemery R, Talajic M, Nattel S, Theroux P, Roy D. Sinus node dysfunction and sudden cardiac death following treatment with encainide. Pace 1989;12:1607–1612.
452. Salel AF, Seargren C, Pool PE. Effects of encainide on the function of implanted pacemakers. Pace 1989;12:1439–1444.

453. Kesteloot H, Stroobandt R. Clinical experience of encainide (MJ 9067): a new antiarrhythmic drug. Eur J Clin Pharmacol 1979;16:323–326.
454. Sami M, Mason JW, Peters, F, Harrison DC. Clinical electrophysiologic effects of encainide, a newly developed antiarrhythmic agent. Am J Cardiol 1979;44:526–532.
455. Tartini A, Kesselbrenner M. Encainide-induced encephalopathy in a patient with chronic renal failure. Am J Kidney Dis 1990;15:178–179.
456. Winter WE, Funahashi M, Koons J. Encainide-induced diabetes: analysis of islet cell function. Res Commun Chem Pathol Pharmacol 1992;76:259–268.
457. Sami M, Harrison DC, Kraemer H, Houston N, Shimasaki C, De Busk RF. Antiarrhythmic efficacy of encainide and quinidine: validation of a model for drug assessment. Am J Cardiol 1981;48:147–156.
458. Strasburger JF, Smith RT Jr, Moak JP. Encainide for resistant supraventricular tachycardia in children: follow-up report. Am J Cardiol 1988;62:50L–54L.
459. Anderson JL, Pritchett ELC, eds. International symposium on supraventricular arrhythmias: focus on flecainide. Am J Cardiol 1988;62:1D.
460. Schneeweiss A. New antiarrhythmic drugs. II. Flecainide. Pediatr Cardiol 1990;11:143–146.
461. Falk RH, Fogel RI. Flecainide. J Cardiovasc Electrophysiol 1994;5:964–981.
462. Hohnloser SH, Zabel M. Short- and long-term efficacy and safety of flecainide acetate for supraventricular arrhythmias. Am J Cardiol 1992;70:3A–10A.
463. Schulze JJ, Inhester B. Arrhythmiebehandlung unter Praxisbedingungen. Therapiewoche 1985;35:5898.
464. Anderson JL, Jolivette DM, Fredell PA. Summary of efficacy and safety of flecainide for supraventricular arrhythmias. Am J Cardiol 1988;62:62D–66D.
465. Morganroth J, Horowitz LN. Flecainide: its proarrhythmic effect and expected changes on the surface electrocardiogram. Am Heart J 1984;53:89B–94B.
466. Nathan AW, Hellerstrand KJ, Bexton RS, Spurrell RA, Camm AJ. The proarrhythmic effects of flecainide. Drugs 1985;29(Suppl 4):45–53.
467. Podrid PJ, Morganroth J. Aggravation of arrhythmia during drug therapy: experience with flecainide acetate. Pract Cardiol 1985;11:55–70.
468. Wehr M, Noll B, Krappe J. Flecainide-induced aggravation of ventricular arrhythmias. Am J Cardiol 1985;55:1643–1644.
469. Saishu T, Iwatsuki N, Tajima T, Hashimoto Y. Flecainide is effective against premature supraventricular and ventricular contractions during general anesthesia. J Anesth 1994;8:284–287.
470. Gentzkow GD, Sullivan JY. Extracardiac adverse effects of flecainide. Am J Cardiol 1984;53:101B–105B.
471. Epstein M, Jardine RM, Obel IWP. Flecainide acetate in the treatment of resistant supraventricular arrhythmias. S Afr Med J 1988;74:559.
472. Ramhamadany E, Mackenzie S, Ramsdale DR. Dysarthria and visual hallucinations due to flecainide toxicity. Postgrad Med J 1986;62:61–62.
473. Samlowski WE Frame RN, Logue GL. Flecainide-induced immune neutropenia: documentation of a hapten-mediated mechanism of cell destruction. Arch Intern Med 1987;147:383–384.
474. Kuhlkamp V, Haasis R, Seipel L. Flecainidinduzierte Hepatitis. Z Kardiol 1988;77:678–680.
475. Mikloweit P, Bienmuller H. Medikamentös induzierte intrahepatische Cholestase durch Flecainidacetät und Enalapril. Internist Berlin 1987;28:193–195.
476. Ziegelbaum M, Lever H. Acute urinary retention associated with flecainide. Cleveland Clin J Med 1990;57:86–87.
477. Mancuso G, Tampieri E, Berdondini RM. Eruzione psoriasiforme da flecainide. G Ital Dermatol Venereol 1988;123:171–172.
478. Penhall RK, Hong CY, Muhiddin KA. The effect of flecainide on human sperm motility. Br J Clin Pharmacol 1982;14:147P.
479. Zehender M, Treese N, Kasper W, Pop T, Meinertz T. Effectiveness and tolerance in long-term treatment with flecainide. Circulation 1982;66(Suppl II):144.
480. Musto B, D'Onfrio A, Cavallaro C, Musto A, Greco R. Electrophysiologic effects and clinical efficacy of flecainide in children with recurrent paroxysmal supraventricular tachycardia. Am J Cardiol 1988;62:229–233.
481. Priestly KA, Ladusans EJ, Rosenthal E, Holt DW, Tynan MJ, Jones OD, Curry PV. Experience with flecainide for the treatment of cardiac arrhythmias in children. Eur Heart J 1988;9:1284–1290.
482. Perry JC, McQuinn RL, Smith RT, Gothing C, Fredell P, Garson A. Flecainide acetate for resistant arrhythmias in the young: efficacy and pharamacokinetics. J Am Coll Cardiol 1989;14:185–191.
483. Williams AJ, McQuinn RL, Walls J. Pharmacokinetics of flecainide acetate in patients with severe renal impairment. Clin Pharmacol Ther 1988;43:449–455.
484. McQuinn RL, Pentikainen PJ, Chang SF, Conard GJ. Pharmacokinetics of flecainide in patients with cirrhosis of the liver. Clin Pharmacol Ther 1988;44:566–572.
485. Beckmann J, Hertrampf R, Gundert-Remy U, Mikus G, Gross AS, Eichelbaum M. Is there a genetic factor in flecainide toxicity? Br Med J 1988;297:1316.
486. Rodin SM, Johnson BF, Wilson J, Ritchie P, Johnson J. Comparative effects of verapamil and isradipine upon steady-state digoxin kinetics. Clin Pharmacol Ther 1988;43:668–672.
487. Kirch W, Logemann C, Heiemann H, Santos SR, Ohnhaus EE. Nitrendipine/digoxin interaction. J Cardiovasc Pharmacol 1987;10(Suppl 10):S74–S75.
488. Dunselman PHJM, Scaf AHJ, Kuntze CEE, Lie KI, Wesseling H. Digoxin-felodipine interaction in patients with congestive heart failure. Eur J Clin Pharmacol 1988;35:461–465.
489. Bruserud O, Skadberg BT, Ohm OJ. Combined intoxication with digitoxin and verapamil: the possible inhibition of sensitisation to digitalis-specific antiserum by toxic drug concentrations. J Lab Clin Immunol 1988;25:167–171.
490. Ferrari E, Fournier JP, Gibelin P, Drici MD, Morand P. Le traitement par le lactate molaire de l'intoxication par le flecainide est-il sans danger? Presse Méd 1989;18:1395.
491. Xing-sheng Y, Jing-ping S, Guang Z. Acute flecainide toxicity. Chin Med J 1990;103:606–607.
492. Lewis GP, Holtzman JL. Interaction of flecainide with digoxin and propranolol. Am J Cardiol 1984;53:52B–57B.
493. Hellestrand KJ, Nathan AW, Bexton RS, Camm AJ. Response of an abnormal sinus node to intravenous flecainide acetate. Pace 1984;7:436–439.
494. Chouty F, Coumel P. Oral flecainide for prophylaxis of paroxysmal atrial fibrillation. Am J Cardiol 1988;62:35D–37D.

495. Saoudi N, Galtier M, Hidden F, Gerber L, Letac B. Bundle-branch reentrant ventricular tachycardia: a possible mechanism of flecainide proarrhythmic effect. J Electrophysiol 1988;2:365–371.
496. Holtzman JL, Finley D, Mottonen L, Berry DA, Ekholm BP, Kram DC, McQuinn RL, Miller AM. The pharmacodynamic and pharmacokinetic interaction between single doses of flecainide acetate and verapamil: effects on cardiac function and drug clearance. Clin Pharmacol Ther 1989;46:26–32.
497. Buss J, Lasserre JJ, Heene DL. Asystole and cardiogenic shock due to combined treatment with verapamil and flecainide. Lancet 1992;340:546.
498. Munafo A, Reymond-Michel G, Biollaz J. Altered flecainide disposition in healthy volunteers taking quinine. Eur J Clin Pharmacol 1990;38:269–273.
499. Birgersdotter UM, Wong W, Turgeon J, Roden DM. Stereoselective genetically-determined interaction between chronic flecainide and quinidine in patients with arrhythmias. Br J Clin Pharmacol 1992;33:275–280.
500. Pfeifer HJ, Greenblatt DJ, Koch-Weser J. Clinical use and toxicity of intravenous lidocaine. A report from the Boston Collaborative Drug Surveillance Program. Am Heart J 1976;92:168–173.
501. Greenspon AJ, Mohiuddin S, Saksena S, Lengerich R, Snapinn S, Holmes G, Irvin J, Sappington E, et al. Comparison of intravenous tocainide with intravenous lidocaine for treating ventricular arrhythmias. Cardiovasc Rev Rep 1989;10:55–59.
502. Krikler DM, Curry PVL. Torsade de pointes, an atypical ventricular tachycardia. Br Heart J 1976;38:117–120.
503. Gottlieb SS, Packer M. Deleterious hemodynamic effects of lidocaine in severe congestive heart failure. Am Heart J 1989;118:611–612.
504. Weaver WD, Fahrenbruch CE, Johnson DD, Hallstrom AP, Cobb LA, Copass MK. Effect of epinephrine and lidocaine therapy on outcome after cardiac arrest due to ventricular fibrillation. Circulation 1990;82:2027–2034.
505. Tisdale JE. Lidocaine prophylaxis in acute myocardial infarction. Henry Ford Hosp Med J 1991;39:217–225.
506. Stargel WW, Shand DG, Routledge PA, Barchowsky A, Wagner GS. Clinical comparison of rapid infusion and multiple injection methods for lidocaine loading. Am Heart J 1981;102:872–876.
507. von Olthoff D, Vetter B, Deutrich C, Burkhardt U. Pharmakokinetische Untersuchungen zu den Ursachen der erhoten Neurotoxizität des Lidokains wahrend kardiochirurgischer Operationen. Anästhesiol Reanim 1989;14:207–214.
508. Bauer LA, Brown T, Gibaldi M, Hudson L, Nelson S, Raisys V, Shea JP. Influence of long-term infusion of lidocaine kinetics. Clin Pharmacol Ther 1982;31:433–437.
509. Kumana CR. Therapeutic drug monitoring-antidysrhythmic drugs. In: Richens A, Marks V, eds. Therapeutic Drug Monitoring. Ch 16A. London, Edinburgh: Churchill-Livingstone. 1981;370.
510. Ochs HR, Carstens G, Greenblatt DJ. Reduction in lidocaine clearance during continuous infusion and by coadministration of propranolol. New Engl J Med 1980; 303:373–377.
511. Bax NDS, Tucker GT, Lennard MS, Woods HF. The impairment of lignocaine clearance by propranolol—major contribution from enzyme inhibition. Br J Clin Pharmacol 1984;19:597–603.
512. Wyse DG, Kellen J, Tam Y, Rademaker AW. Increased efficacy and toxicity of lidocaine in patients on beta-blockers. Int J Cardiol 1988;21:59–70.
513. Kowalsky SF. Lidocaine interaction with cimetidine and ranitidine: a critical analysis of the literature. Adv Ther 1988;5:229–244.
514. Ujhelyi MR, O'Rangers EA, Fan C, Kluger J, Pharand C, Chow MSS. The pharmacokinetic and pharmacodynamic interaction between propafenone and lidocaine. Clin Pharmacol Ther 1993;53:38–48.
515. Amery WK, Heykants JJP, Xhonneux R, Iowse G, Oettel P, Gough DA, Janssen PA. Lorcainide (R15889), a first review. Acta Cardiol 1981;36:207–234.
516. Anonymous. Lorcainide hydrochloride. Medicam Actual/Drugs Today 1982:18:12–16 (Spanish) and 1982;18:17–22 (English).
517. Eiriksson CE, Brogden RN. Lorcainide. A preliminary review of its pharmacodynamic properties and therapeutic efficacy. Drugs 1984;27:279–300.
518. Kasper W, Meinertz T, Kersting F, Loppgen H, Lang K, Just H. Electrophysiological actions of lorcainide in patients with cardiac disease. J Cardiovasc Pharmacol 1979;1:343–352.
519. Shita A, Bernard R, Mostinckx R, De Backer M. Haemodynamic reactions after intravenous injection of lorcainide hydrochloride in acute myocardial infarction. Eur J Cardiol 1981;12:237–242.
520. Kesteloot H, Stroobandt R. Clinical experience with lorcainide (R15889), a new anti-arrhythmic drug. Arch Int Pharmacodyn Ther 1977;230:225–234.
521. Somani P. Pharmacokinetics of lorcainide, a new antiarrhythmic drug, in patients with cardiac rhythm disorders. Am J Cardiol 1981;48:157–163.
522. Klotz U, Muller-Seydlitz P, Heimburg P. Disposition and antiarrhythmic effect of lorcainide. Int J Clin Pharmacol Biopharm 1979;17:152–158.
523. Cocco G, Strozzi C. Initial clinical experience of lorcainide (Ro 13–1042), a new antiarrhythmic agent. Eur J Clin Pharmacol 1978;14:105–109.
524. Klotz U, Muller-Seydlitz PM, Heimburg P. Lorcainide infusion in the treatment of ventricular premature beats (VPB). Eur J Clin Pharmacol 1979;16:1–6.
525. Meinertz T, Kasper W, Kersting F, Bechtold H, Just H, Jahnchen E. Antiarrhythmic effect of lorcainide during chronic treatment. Arzneim-Forsch Drug Res 1980; 30:1593–1595.
526. Myburgh DP, Goldman AP, Schamroth JM. Lorcainide—an anti-arrhythmic agent for ventricular arrhythmias. S Afr Med J 1980;57:236–239.
527. Keefe DL, Peters F, Winkle RA. Randomized double-blind placebo controlled crossover trial documenting oral lorcainide efficacy in suppression of symptomatic ventricular tachyarrhythmias. Am Heart J 1982;103:511–518.
528. Somani P, Temesy-Armos PN, Leighton RF, Goodenday LS, Fraker TD Jr. Hyponatremia in patients treated with lorcainide, a new antiarrhythmic drug. Am Heart J 1984;108:1443–1448.
529. Meinertz T, Kasper W, Kersting F, Just H, Bechtold H, Jahnchen E. Lorcainide II. Plasma-concentration effect relationship. Clin Pharmacol Ther 1979;26:196–204.
530. Étienne Y, Blanc JJ, Boschat J, Le Potier J, Jobic Y, Le Grand O, Penther P. Effets antiarythmiques du sulfate de magnésium intraveineux dans les tachycardies supraventriculaires paroxystiques. Ann Cardiol Angéiol 1988; 37:535–538.

531. Wesley RC, Haines DE, Lerman BB, DiMarco JP, Crampton RS. Effect of intravenous magnesium sulfate on supraventricular tachycardia. Am J Cardiol 1989;63:1129–1131.
532. Gullestad L, Birkeland K, Mølstad P, Høyer MM, Vanberg P, Kjekshus J. The effect of magnesium versus verapamil on supraventricular arrhythmias. Clin Cardiol 1993; 16:429–434.
533. Gurfinkel E, Alvarez Pazos A, Mautner B. Abnormal QT intervals associated with negative T waves induced by antiarrhythmic drugs are rapidly reduced using magnesium sulfate as an antidote. Clin Cardiol 1993;16:35–38.
534. Kerin NZ, Aragon E, Marinescu G, Faitel K, Framin H, Rubenfire M. Mexiletine. Long-term efficacy and side effects in patients with chronic drug-resistant potentially lethal ventricular arrhythmias. Arch Intern Med 1990; 150:381–384.
535. Murray KT, Barbey JT, Kopelman HA, Siddoway LA, Echt DJ, Woosley RL, Roden DM. Mexiletine and tocainide: a comparison of antiarrhythmic efficacy, adverse effects, and predictive value of lidocaine testing. Clin Pharmacol Ther 1989;45:553–561.
536. Grech-Belanger O. Clinical pharmacokinetics of mexiletine. Clin Prog Electrophysiol Pacing 1986;4:553.
537. Roden DM. Use of mexiletine in combination with other antiarrhythmic drugs. Clin Prog Electrophysiol Pacing 1986;4:561–567.
538. Halinen MO. Mexiletine for the management of ventricular arrhythmias in ischemic heart disease. Clin Prog Electrophysiol Pacing 1986;4:580–581.
539. Sami MH. Mexiletine: its role in the management of chronic ventricular arrhythmias. Clin Prog Electrophysiol Pacing 1986;4:582–588.
540. Flaker GC, Beach CL, Chapman D. Adverse side effects associated with mexiletine. Clin Prog Electrophysiol Pacing 1986;4:602–607.
541. Manolis AS, Deering TF, Cameron J, Estes NAM. Mexiletine: pharmacology and therapeutic use. Clin Cardiol 1990;13:349–359.
542. Poole JE, Werner JA, Bardy GH, Graham EL, Pulaski WP, Fahrenbruch CE, Greene HL. Intolerance and ineffectiveness of mexiletine in patients with serious ventricular arrhythmias. Am Heart J 1986;112:322–326.
543. Talbot RG, Nimmo J, Julian DG, Clark RA, Neilson JMM, Prescott LF. Treatment of ventricular arrhythmias with mexiletine (Ko 1173). Lancet 1973;ii:399–404.
544. Campbell NPS, Kelly JG, Shanks RG, Chaturvedi NC, Strong JE, Pantridge JF. Mexiletine (Ko 1173) in the management of ventricular dysrhythmias. Lancet 1973;ii:404–407.
545. Gottlieb SS, Weinberg M. Cardiodepressant effects of mexiletine in patients with severe left ventricular dysfunction. Eur Heart J 1992;13:22–27.
546. Campbell NPS, Kelly JG, Chaturvedi NC, Strong JE, Shanks RG, Adgey AAJ. The development of mexiletine in the management of ventricular dysrhythmias. Postgrad Med J 1977;53(Suppl 1):114–119.
547. Bero CJ, Rihn TL. Possible association of pulmonary fibrosis with mexilitine. DICP Ann Pharmacother 1991; 25:1329–1331.
548. Roos JC, Paalman DCA, Dunning AJ. Electrophysiological effects of mexiletine in man. Postgrad Med J 1977;53(Suppl 1):92–96.
549. Morganroth J for the Mexiletine-Quinidine Research Group. Comparative efficacy and safety of oral mexiletine and quinidine in benign or potentially lethal ventricular arrhythmias. Am J Cardiol 1987;60:1276–1281.
550. Girmann G, Pees H, Scheurlen PGH. Pseudothrombocytopenia and mexiletine. Ann Intern Med 1984;100:767.
551. Campbell NPS, Pantridge JF, Adgey AAJ. Long-term oral antiarrhythmic therapy with mexiletine. Br Heart J 1978;40:796–801.
552. Fasola GP, d'Osualdo F, De Pangher V, Barducci E. Thrombocytopenia and mexiletine. Ann Intern Med 1984;100:162.
553. Pernot C, Marcon F, Weber JL, Nether P, Trechot P. Effects indésirables hépatiques de la mexiletine. Thérapie 1983;38:695–700.
554. Rudolph R. Seggewiss H, Seckfort H. Ösophagus-Ulcus durch Mexiletin. Dtsch Med Wochenschr 1983;108:1018–1020.
555. Sigal M, Pulik M. Pseudo-lymphomes médicamenteux à expression cutanée prédominante. Ann Dermatol Venéreol 1993;120:175–180.
556. Yamazaki S, Katayama I, Kurumaji Y, Yokozeki H, Nishioka K. Contact urticaria induced by mexiletine hydrochloride in a patient receiving iontophoresis. Br J Dermatol 1994;130:538–540.
557. Lledó P, Abrams SML, Johnston A, Patel M, Pearson RM, Turner P. Influence of debrisoquine hydroxylation phenotype on the pharmacokinetics of mexiletine. Eur J Clin Pharmacol 1993;44:63–67.
558. Nora MO, Chandrasekaran K, Hammill SC, Reeder GS. Prolongation of ventricular depolarization. ECG manifestation of mexiletine toxicity. Chest 1989;95:925–928.
559. Jequier P, Jones R, Mackintosh A. Fatal mexiletine overdose. Lancet 1976;i:429.
560. Mackintosh AF, Jequier P. Fatal mexiletine overdose. Postgrad Med J 1977;53(Suppl 1):134.
561. Bigger JT. The interaction of mexiletine with other. cardiovascular drugs. Am Heart J 1984;107:1079–1085.
562. Poole JE, Werner JA, Bardy GH, Graham EL, Pulaski WP, Fahrenbruch CE. Intolerance and ineffectiveness of mexiletine in patients with serious ventricular arrhythmias. Am Heart J 1986;112:322–326.
563. Kessler KM, Interian A Jr, Cox M, Topaz O, de Marchena EJ, Myerburg RJ. Proarrhythmia related to a kinetic and dynamic interaction of mexiletine and theophylline. Am Heart J 1989;117:964–966.
564. Joeres R, Richter E. Mexiletine and caffeine elimination. New Engl J Med 1987;317:117.
565. Stein J, Podrid PJ, Lampert S, Hirsowitz G, Lown B. Long-term mexiletine for ventricular arrhythmia. Am Heart J 1984;107:1091–1098.
566. Johansson BW, Stavenow L. Long-term clinical effects and side effects of mexiletine in patients with ventricular arrhythmias. Clin Prog Electrophysiol Pacing 1986;4:589–594.
567. Johansson BW, Stavenow L, Hanson A. Long-term clinical experience with mexiletine. Am Heart J 1984; 107:1099–1102.
568. Carnes CA, Coyle JD. Moricizine: a novel antiarrhythmic agent. DICP Ann Pharmacother 1990;24:745–753.
569. Podrid PJ. Moricizine (ethmozine HCl)—a new antiarrhythmic drug: is it unique? Am J Cardiol 1991;68:1521–1525.
570. Clyne CA, Estes NAM, Wang PJ. Moricizine. New Engl J Med 1992;327:255–260.

571. Podrid PJ, Lampert S, Graboys TB, Blatt CM, Lown B. Aggravation of arrhythmia by antiarrhythmic drugs—incidence and predictors. Am J Cardiol 1987;59:38E—44E.
572. The Cardiac Arrhythmia Suppression Trial II Investigators. Effect of the antiarrhythmic agent moricizine on survival after myocardial infarction. New Engl J Med 1992;327:227—233.
573. Kennedy HL. Noncardiac adverse effects and organ toxicity of moricizine during short- and long-term studies. Am J Cardiol 1990;65:47D—50D.
574. Kurapov AP, Nekrasova OV, Gneushev ET, Ryzhenkova AP, Kukes VG. Farmokokinetika etmozina pri nedostatochnosti funkstii pecheni. Sov Med 1990;5:34—36.
575. Benedek IH, Davidson AF, Pieniaszek HJ Jr. Enzyme induction by moricizine: time course and extent in healthy subjects. J Clin Pharmacol 1994;34:167—175.
576. Pieniaszek HJ, Davidson AF, Benedek IH. Effect of moricizine on the pharmacokinetics of single-dose theophylline in healthy subjects. Ther Drug Monit 1993;15:199—203.
577. Biollaz J, Shaheen O, Wood AJJ. Cimetidine inhibition of ethmozine metabolism. Clin Pharmacol Ther 1985; 37:665—668.
578. Lawson DH, Jick H. Adverse reactions to procainamide. Br J Clin Pharmacol 1977;4:507—511.
579. Koch-Weser J, Klein S W, Foo-Canto LL, Kastor JA, De Sanctis RW. Antiarrhythmic prophylaxis with procainamide in acute myocardial infarction. New Engl J Med 1969;281:1253—1260.
580. Kosowsky BD, Taylor J, Lown B, Ritchie RF. Long-term use of procainamide following acute myocardial infarction. Circulation 1973;47:1204—1210.
581. Hallstorm AP, Cobb LA, Yu BH, Weaver WD, Fahrenbruch CE. An antiarrhythmic drug experience in 941 patients resuscitated from an initial cardiac arrest between 1970 and 1985. Am J Cardiol 1991;68:1025—1031.
582. Miller RR, Hilliard G, Lies JE, Massumi RA, Zelis R, Mason DT, Amsterdam EA. Hemodynamic effects of procainamide in patients with acute myocardial infarction and comparison with lidocaine. Am J Med 1973;55:161—168.
583. Goldberg D, Reiffel JA, Davis JC. Electrophysiologic effects of procainamide on sinus node function in patients with and without sinus node disease. Am Heart J 1982;103:75—79.
584. Mohindra SK, Udeani GO, Abrahamson D. Cardiac tamponade associated with drug-induced systemic lupus erythematosus. Crit Care Med 1989;17:961—962.
585. McCrum ID, Guidry JR. Procainamide-induced psychosis. J Am Med Assoc 1978;240:1265—1266.
586. Schwartz AB, Klausner SC, Yee S, Turchyn M. Cerebellar ataxia due to procainamide toxicity. Arch Intern Med 1984;144:2260—2261.
587. Rubinstein A, Cabili S. Tremor induced by procainamide. Am J Cardiol 1986;57:340—341.
588. Miller B, Skupin A, Rubenfire M, Bigman O. Respiratory failure produced by severe procainamide intoxication in a patient with preexisting peripheral neuropathy caused by amiodarone. Chest 1988;94:663—665.
589. Godley PJ, Morton TA, Karboski JA, Tami JA. Procainamide-induced myasthenic crisis. Ther Drug Monit 1990;12:411—414.
590. Putnam JB, Bolling SF, Kirsh MM. Procainamide-induced respiratory insufficiency after cardiopulmonary bypass. Ann Thorac Surg 1991;51:482—483.
591. Sayler DJ, DeJong DJ. Possible procainamide-induced myopathy. DICP Ann Pharmacother 1991;25:436.
592. Prendergast MD, Nasca TJ. Anticholinergic syndrome with procainamide toxicity. J Am Med Assoc 1984; 251:2926—2927
593. Prince RA, Brown BT, Jacknowitz AI. Agranulocytosis associated with procainamide therapy report of a case. Am J Hosp Pharm 1977;34:1362—1365.
594. Galanakis DK, Newman J, Summers D. Circulating thrombin time anticoagulant in a procainamide-induced syndrome. J Am Med Assoc 1978;239:1873—1874.
595. Meisner DJ, Carlson RJ, Gottlieb AJ. Thrombocytopenia following sustained-release procainamide. Arch Intern Med 1985;145:700—702.
596. Bluming AZ, Plotkin D, Rosen P, Thiessen AR. Severe transient pancytopenia associated with procainamide ingestion. J Am Med Assoc 1976;236:2520—2521.
597. Giannone L, Kugler JW, Krantz SB. Pure red cell aplasia associated with administration of sustained-release procainamide. Arch Intern Med 1987;147:1179—1180.
598. Agudelo CA, Wise CM, Lyles MF. Pure red cell aplasia in procainamide induced systemic lupus erythematosus. Report and review of the literature. J Rheumatol 1988; 15:1431—1432.
599. Ellrodt AG, Murata GH, Riedinger MS, Stewart ME, Mochinzuki C, Gray R,. Severe neutropenia associated with sustained-release procainamide. Ann Intern Med 1984;100:197—201.
600. Meyers DG, Gonzalez ER, Peters LL, David RB, Feagler JR, Egan JD, Nair CK. Severe neutropenia associated with procainamide: comparison of sustained release and conventional preparations. Am Heart J 1985;109:1393—1395.
601. Hoffman HS. Severe neutropenia with procainamide therapy. Conn Med 1990;54:59—61.
602. Kleinman S, Nelson R, Smith L, Goldfinger D. Positive direct antiglobulin tests and immune hemolytic anemia in patients receiving procainamide. New Engl J Med 1984; 311:809—812.
603. Peterson AM, Conrad SD, Bell JM. Procainamide-induced pseudo-obstruction in a diabetic patient. DICP Ann Pharmacother 1991;25:1334—1335.
604. Chuang LC, Tunier AP, Akhtar N, Levine SM. Possible case of procainamide-induced intrahepatic cholestatic jaundice. Ann Pharmacother 1993;27:434—437.
605. Bigger JT, Heissenbuttel RH. The use of procaineamide and lidocaine in the treatment of cardiac arrhythmias. Prog Cardiovasc Dis 1969;11:515—534.
606. Sherentz EF. Lichen planus following procainamide-induced lupus erythematosus. Cutis 1988;42:51—53.
607. Ponte CD, Horner P. Suspected procainamide-induced angioedema. Drug Intell Clin Pharm 1985;19:139—140.
608. Knox JP, Welykyi SE, Gradini R, Massa MC. Procainamide-induced urticarial vasculitis. Cutis 1988;42:469—472.
609. Turgeon FW, Slamovits TL. Scleritis as the presenting manifestation of procainamide-induced lupus. Ophthalmology 1989;96:68—71.
610. Vivino FB, Schumacher HR. Synovial fluid charcteristics and the lupus erythematosus cell phenomenon in drug-induced lupus. Findings in three patients and review of pertinent literature. Arthr Rheum 1989;32:560—568.
611. Miller CD, Oleshansky MA, Gibson KF, Cantilena LR. Procainamide-induced myasthenia-like weakness and dysphagia. Ther Drug Monit 1993;15:251—254.

612. Venkayya RV, Poole RM, Pentz WH. Respiratory failure from procainamide-induced myopathy. Ann Intern Med 1993;119:345—346.
613. Yung RL, Richardson BC. Drug-induced lupus. Rheum Dis Clin North Am 1994;20:61—86.
614. Uetrecht JP, Woosley RL. Acetylator phenotype and lupus erythematosus. Clin Pharmacokin 1981;6:118—134.
615. Woosley RL, Drauer DE, Reidenberg MM, Nies AS, Carr K, Oates JA. Effect of acetylator phenotype on the rate at which procainamide induces antinuclear antibodies and the lupus syndrome. New Engl J Med 1978;298:1157—1159.
616. Sim E. Drug-induced immune-complex disease. Complem Inflamm 1989;6:119—126.
617. Heyman MR, Flores RH, Edelman BB, Carliner NH. Procainamide-induced lupus anticoagulant. South Med J 1988;81:934—936.
618. Smiley JD, Moore SE. Molecular mechanisms of autoimmunity. Am J Med Sci 1988;295:478—496.
619. Green BJ, Wyse DG, Duff HJ, Mitchell LB, Matheson DS. Procainamide in vivo modulates suppressor T lymphocyte activity. Clin Invest Med 1988;11:425—429.
620. Burlingame RW, Rubin RL. Drug-induced anti-histone autoantibodies display two patterns of reactivity with substructures of chromatin. J Clin Invest 1991;88:680—690.
621. Klimas NG, Patarca R, Perez G, Garcia-Morales R, Schultz D, Schabel J, Fletcher MA. Case report: distinctive immune abnormalities in a patient with procainamide-induced lupus and serositis. Am J Med Sci 1992;303:99—104.
622. Winfield JB, Koffler D, Kunkel HG. Development of antibodies to ribonucleoprotein following short-term therapy with procainamide. Arthr Rheum 1975;18:531—534.
623. Windle J, Prystowsky EN, Miles WM, Heger JJ. Pharmacokinetic and electrophysiologic interactions of amiodarone and procainamide. Clin Pharmacol Ther 1987;41:603—610.
624. Bauer LA, Black D, Gensler A. Procainamide-cimetidine drug interaction in elderly male patients. J Am Geriatr Soc 1990;38:467—469.
625. Koch-Weser J. Serum procainamide levels as therapeutic guides. Clin Pharmacokin 1977;2:389—402.
626. Birgersdotter-Green U. Propafenone for cardiac arrhythmias. Am J Med Sci 1992;303:123—128.
627. Bryson HM, Palmer KJ, Langtry HD, Fitton A. Propafenone. A reappraisal of its pharmacology, pharmacokinetics and therapeutic use in cardiac arrhythmias. Drugs 1993;45:85—130.
628. Cobbe SM. Drug therapy of supraventricular tachyarrhythmias-based on efficacy or futility? Eur Heart J 1994; 15(Suppl A):22—26.
629. Paul T, Janousek J. New antiarrhythmic drugs in pediatric use: propafenone. Pediatr Cardiol 1994;15:190—197.
630. Ravid S, Podrid PJ, Novrit B. Safety of long-term propafenone therapy for cardiac arrhythmia-experience with 774 patients. J Electrophysiol 1987;1:580—590.
631. Antman EM, Beamer AD, Cantillon C, McGowan N, Friedman PL. Therapy of refractory symptomatic atrial fibrillation and atrial flutter: a staged care approach with new antiarrhythmic drugs. J Am Coll Cardiol 1990;15:698—707.
632. Escande M, Diadema B, Maarek-Charbit M. Etude a long terme de la propafenone dans l'extrasystolie ventriculaire grave du sujet age. Ann Cardiol Angéiol 1989;38:555—560.
633. Colas A, Maarek-Charbit M. Propafenone per os dans les troubles du rhythme ventriculaire. Cah Anesthésiol. 1989;37:241—244.
634. Veale D, McComb JM, Gibson GJ. Propafenone. Lancet 1990;335:979.
635. Hammill SC, Sorenson PB, Wood DL, Sugrue DD, Osborn MJ, Gersh BJ, Holmes DR Jr. Propafenone for the treatment of refractory complex ventricular ectopic activity. Mayo Clin Proc 1986;61:98—103.
636. Miwa LJ, Jolson HM. Propafenone-associated agranulocytosis. PACE 1992;15:387—390.
637. Connolly SJ, Kates RE, Lebsack CS, Harrison DC, Winkle RA. Clinical pharmacology of propafenone. Circulation 1983;68:589—596.
638. Mondardini A, Pasquino P, Bernardi P, Aluffi E, Tartaglino B, Mazzucco G, Bonino F, Verme G, Negro F. Propafenone-induced liver injury: report of a case and review of the literature. Gastroenterology 1993;104:1524—1526.
639. Korst HA, Brandes J-W, Litmann K-P. Potenz- und Spermiogenesestorungen durch Propafenon. Dtsch Med Wochenschr 1980;105:1187—1189.
640. Gaita F, Richiardi E, Bocchiardo M, Asteggiano R, Pinnavaia A, Di Leo M, Rosettani E, Brusca A. Short- and long-term effects of propafenone in ventricular arrhythmias. Int J Cardiol 1986;13:163—170.
641. Guindo J, Rodriguez de la Serna AR, Borja J, Oter R, Jane F, Bayes de Luna A. Propafenone and a syndrome of the lupus erythematosus type. Ann Intern Med 1986;104:589.
642. Vignati G, Mauri L, Figini A. The use of propafenone in the treatment of tachyarrhythmias in children. Eur Heart J 1993;14:546—550.
643. Brunozzi LT, Meniconi L, Chiocchi P, Liberati R, Zuanetti G, Latini R. Propafenone in the treatment of chronic ventricular arrhythmias in a pregnant patient. Br J Clin Pharmacol 1988;26:489—490.
644. Wagner F, Kalusche D, Trenk D, Jahnchen E, Roskamm H. Drug interaction between propafenone and metoprolol. Br J Clin Pharmacol 1987;24:213—220.
645. Dinh H, Murphy ML, Baker BJ, De Soyza N. Propafenone: a new antiarrhythmic for treatment of chronic ventricular arrhythmias. Clin Prog Electrophysiol Pacing 1986;4:535—545.
646. De Soyza N, Murphy M, Sakhaii M, Treat L. The safety and efficacy of propafenone in suppressing ventricular ectopy. In: Shlepper M. Olsen B, eds. Cardiac Arrhythmias. Berlin: Springer Verlag: 1983;221.
647. Cohen S, Jick H, Cohen SI. Adverse reactions to quinidine in hospitalized patients: findings based on data from the Boston Collaborative Drug Surveillance Program. Prog Cardiovasc Dis 1977;20:151—167.
648. Malcolm AD, David GK. Quinidine in cardiology. Acta Leiden 1987;55:87—98.
649. White NJ, Looareesuwan S, Warrell DA, Chongsuphajaisiddhi T, Bunnag D, Harinasuta T. Quinidine in falciparum malaria. Lancet 1981;ii:1069—1071.
650. Roden DM, Woosely RL, Primm RK. Incidence and clinical feature of the quinidine-associated long QT syndrome: implications for patient care. Am Heart J 1986;111:1088—1093.
651. Grayzel J, Angeles J. Sino-atrial block in man provoked by quinidine. J Electrocardiol 1972;5:289—294.
652. Jeresaty RM, Kahn AH, Landry AB. Sinoatrial arrest due to lidocaine in a patient receiving quinidine. Chest 1972;61:683—685.
653. Cappato R, Alboni P, Codecà L, Guardigli G, Toselli

T, Antonioli GE. Direct and autonomically mediated effects of oral quinidine on RR/QT relation after an abrupt increase in heart rate. J Am Coll Cardiol 1993;22:99–105.

654. Van der Ark CR, Reynolds EW, Kahn DR. Quinidine syncope. A report of successful treatment with bretylium tosylate. J Thorac Cardiovasc Surg 1976;72:464.

655. Koster RW, Wellens HJJ. Quinidine-induced ventricular flutter and fibrillation without digitalis therapy. Am J Cardiol 1976;38:519–523.

656. Di Segni E, Klein Ho, David D, Libhaber C, Kaplinsky E. Overdrive pacing in quinidine syncope and other long QT-interval syndromes. Arch Intern Med 1980;140:1036–1040.

657. Luchi RJ, Helwig J, Conn HL. Quinidine toxicity and its treatment. An experimental study. Am Heart J 1963; 65:340–348.

658. Gilbert GJ. Quinidine dementia. J Am Med Assoc 1977;237:2093–2094.

659. Billig N, Buongiorno P. Quinidine-induced organic mental disorders. J Am Geriatr Soc 1985;33:504–506.

660. Deleu D, Schmedding E. Acute psychosis as idiosyncratic reaction to quinidine: report of two cases. Br Med J 1987;294:1001–1002.

661. Abrams J. Quinidine toxicity: a review. Rocky Mount Med J 1973;70:31–34.

662. Kaufman DW, Kelly JP, Johannes CB, Sandler A, Harmon D, Stolley PD, Shapiro S. Acute thrombocytopenic purpura in relation to the use of drugs. Blood 1993;82:2714–2718.

663. Garratty G. Review: immune hemolytic anemia and/or positive direct antiglobulin tests caused by drugs. Immunohematology 1994;10:41–50.

664. Barzel US. Quinidine sulfate induced hypoplastic anemia and agranulocytosis. J Am Med Assoc 1967;201:325–327.

665. Castro O, Nash I. Quinidine leukopenia and thrombocytopenia with a drug-dependent leukoagglutinin. New Engl J Med 1977;296:572.

666. Eisner EV, Carr RM, MacKinney AR. Quinidine induced agranulocytosis. J Am Med Assoc 1977;238:884–886.

667. Religa H, Rozniecki J, Szmidt M. Eozynofilia w przezbiegu leczenia lanatozydem C i siarczanem chinidyny jako jedyny przejaw nadwrazliwoski polekowej. Pol Tyg Lek 1972;27:1727–1729.

668. Saleh MN, Dhodaphar N, Allen K, LoBuglio AF. Quinidine-induced immune thrombocytopenia. Henry Ford Hosp Med J 1989;37:28–32.

669. Redell MA, Moore BR, Fass L. Use of i.v. immune globulin for presumed quinidine-induced thrombocytopenia. Clin Pharm 1989;8:89.

670. Geltner D, Chajek T, Rubinger D, Levij IS. Quinidine hypersensitivity and liver involvement: a survey of 32 patients. Gastroenterology 1976;70:650–652.

671. Knobler H, Levij IS, Gavish D, Chajek-Shaul T. Quinidine-induced hepatitis: a common and reversible hypersensitivity reaction. Arch Intern Med 1986;146:526–528.

672. Rokseth R, Storstein O. Quinidine therapy of chronic auricular fibrillation. The occurrence and mechanism of syncope. Arch Intern Med 1963;111:184–189.

673. Mahon WA, Mayersohn M, Inaba T. Disposition kinetics of two oral forms of quinidine. Clin Pharmacol Ther 1972;19:566–575.

674. Kennedy HL, DeMaria AN, Sprague MK, Wiens RD, Redd RM, Janosik DL, Buckingham TA. Comparative efficacy of moricizine and quinidine for benign and potentially lethal ventricular arrhythmias. Am J Noninvas Cardiol 1988;2:98–105.

675. Zahger D, Gilon D, Gotsman MS. Delayed quinidine-induced diarrhea after five years of treatment. Chest 1992;101:296.

676. Bott SJ, McCallum RW. Medication-induced oesophageal injury: survey of the literature. Med Toxicol 1986;1:449–457.

677. Wong RKH, Kikendall JW, Dachman AH. Quinaglute-induced esophagitis mimicking an esophageal mass. Ann Intern Med 1986;105:62–63.

678. Bonavina L, DeMeester TR, McChesney L, Schwizer W, Albertucci M, Bailey RT. Drug-induced esophageal strictures. Ann Surg 1987;206:173–183.

679. Birek C, Main JH. Two cases of oral pigmentation associated with quinidine therapy. Oral Surg Oral Med Oral Pathol 1988;66:59–61.

680. Aviram A. Henoch-Schönlein syndrome associated with quinidine. J Am Med Assoc 1980;243:432–433.

681. Chisholm JC Jr. Quinidine-induced nephrotic syndrome. J Natl Med Assoc 1985;77:920–922.

682. Pariser DM, Taylor JR. Quinidine-induced photosensitivity. Arch Dermatol 1975;111:1440–1443.

683. Lang PG. Quinidine-induced photodermatitis confirmed by photopatch testing. J Am Acad Dermatol 1983;9:124–128.

684. Fowler JF. Allergic contact dermatitis to quinidine. Contact Dermatitis 1985;13:280–281.

685. Mahler R, Sisson W, Watters K. Pigmentation induced by quinidine therapy. Arch Dermatol 1986;122:1062–1064.

686. Shaftel N, Halpern A. The quinidine problem. Angiology 1958;9:34–46.

687. Taylor DR, Potashnick R. Quinidine-induced exfoliative dermatitis with a brief review of quinidine idiosyncrasies. J Am Med Assoc 1951;145:641–642.

688. Gouffault J, Pawlotsky Y, Morel H, Bourel M. Erythrodermie d'origine quinidinique. Sem Hôp Paris 1965; 41:1350–1353.

689. Ross V, Cobb M. Generalized granuloma annulare associated with quinidine therapy. J Assoc Military Dermatol 1991;17:16–17.

690. Bolton FG. Thrombocytopenic purpura due to quinidine, serologic mechanisms. Blood 1956;2:547–564.

691. Fisher CM. Visual disturbances associated with quinidine and quinine. Neurology 1981:31:1569–1571.

692. Naschitz JE, Yeshurun D. Quinidine induced sicca syndrome. J Toxicol Clin Toxicol 1983;20:367–371.

693. Zaidman GW. Quinidine keratopathy. Am J Ophthalmol 1984;97:247–249.

694. Hustead JD. Granulomatous uveitis and quinidine hypersensitivity. Am J Ophthalmol 1991;112:461–462.

695. Stoffer SS, Chandler JH. Quinidine-induced exacerbation of myasthenia gravis in a patient with Graves disease. Arch Intern Med 1980;140:283–284.

696. Weiss M, Hassin D, Eisenstein Z, Bank H. Elevated skeletal-muscle enzymes during quinidine therapy. New Engl J Med 1979;300:1218.

697. Ramsey R, Higbee M, Wood JS. Quinidine-induced creatine phosphokinase elevations: case report and prospective case survey in the elderly. J Geriatr Drug Ther 1989;3:97.

698. Yagiela JA, Benoit PW. Skeletal-muscle damage from quinidine. New Engl J Med 1979;301:437.

699. Tebas P, Lozano I, de la Fuente J, Ortigosa J, Pérez Maestu R, Masa C, de Leonta JML. Lupus inducido por quinidina. Rev Clin Esp 1991;189:123–124.
700. Amadio P, Cummings DM, Dashow L. Procainamide, quinidine, and lupus erythematosus. Ann Intern Med 1985;145:446–448.
701. Kerr F, Kenoyer G, Bilitch M. Quinidine overdose. Neurological and cardiovascular toxicity in a normal person. Br Heart J 1971;33:629–631.
702 Woie L, Oyri A. Quinidine intoxication treated with hemodialysis. Acta Med Scand 1974;195:237–239.
703. Haapanen EJ, Pellinen TJ. Hemoperfusion in quinidine intoxication. Acta Med Scand 1982;210:515–516.
704. Koch-Weser J. Quinidine-induced hypoprothrombinemic hemorrhage in patients on chronic warfarin therapy. Ann Intern Med 1968;68:511–517.
705. Hartshorn EA. Interactions of cardiac drugs. Drug Intell Clin Pharm 1970;4:272.
706. Twum-Barima Y, Carruthers SG. Quinidine-rifampin interaction. New Engl J Med 1981;304:1466–1499.
707. Data JL, Wilkinson GR, Nies AS. Interaction of quinidine with anticonvulsant drugs. New Engl J Med 1976; 294:699–702.
708. Leemann T, Dayer P, Meyer UA. Single-dose quinidine treatment inhibits metoprolol oxidation in extensive metabolizers. Eur J Clin Pharmacol 1986;29:739–774.
709. Barbey JT, Thompson KA, Echt DS. Tocainide plus quinidine for treatment of ventricular arryhthmias. Am J Cardiol 1988;61:570–573.
710. Giardina E-GV, Wechsler ME. Low dose quinidine-mexiletine combination therapy versus quinidine monotherapy for treatment of ventricular arrhythmias. J Am Coll Cardiol 1990;15:1138–1145.
711. Dinai Y, Sharir M, Naveh N, Halkin H. Bradycardia induced by interaction between quinidine and ophthalmic timolol. Ann Intern Med 1985;103:890–891.
712. Wang L, Sheldon RS, Mitchell LB, Wyse DG, Gillis AM, Chiamvimonvat N, Duff HJ. Amiloride-quinidine interaction: adverse outcomes. Clin Pharmacol Ther 1994; 56:659–667.
713. Sadowski DC. Drug interactions with antacids. Mechanisms and clinical significance. Drug Safety 1994;11:395–407.
714. Danilo P Jr. Tocainide. Am Heart J 1979;97:259–262.
715. Holmes B, Brodgen RN, Heel RC, Speight TM, Avery GS. Tocainide: a review of its pharmacological properties and therapeutic efficacy. Drugs 1983;26:93–123.
716. ADIS Editors and Consultants. Tocainide (Tonocard): a review of its pharmacological properties and therapeutic efficacy. Curr Ther 1984;July:17–25.
717. Schweyen DH. Tocainide: a new antiarrhythmic. Hosp Pharm 1984;19:558–565.
718. Keefe DL, Somberg JC. New therapy focus: tocainide. Cardiovasc Rev Rep 1984;5:1023–1030.
719. Lynch JJ, Lucchesi BR. New antiarrhythmic agents. IV. The pharmacology and clinical use of tocainide. Pract Cardiol 1985;II:108–137.
720. Hasegawa GR. Tocainide: a new oral antiarrhythmic. Drug Intell Clin Pharm 1985;19:514–517.
721. Kutalek SP, Morganroth J, Horowitz LN. Tocainide: a new oral antiarrhythmic agent. Ann Intern Med 1985;103:387–391.
722. Horn HR, Hadidian Z, Johnson JL, Vassallo HG, Williams JH, Young MD. Safety evaluation of tocainide in the American Emergency Use Program. Am Heart J 1980;100:1037–1040.
723. Young MD, Hadidian Z, Horn HR, Johnson JL, Vassallo HG. Treatment of ventricular arrhythmias with oral tocainide. Am Heart J 1980;100:1041–1045.
724. Winkle RA, Anderson JL, Peters F, Meffin PJ, Fowles RE, Harrison DC. The hemodynamic effcts of intravenous tocainide in patients with heart disease. Circulation 1978;57:787–792.
725. Maloney JD, Nissen RG, McColgan JM. Open clinical studies at a referral centre: chronic maintenance tocainide therapy in patients with recurrent sustained ventricular tachycardia refractory to conventional antiarrhythmic agents. Am Heart J 1980;100:1023–1030.
726. Cheesman M, Ward DE. Exacerbation of ventricular tachycardia by tocainide. Clin Cardiol 1985;8:47–50.
727. Winkle RA, Meffin PJ, Harrison DC. Long-term tocainide therapy for ventricular arrhythmias. Circulation 1978;57:1008–1016.
728. Roden DM, Reele SB, Higgins SB, Carr RK, Oates JA, Woosley RL. Tocainide therapy for refractory ventricular arrhythmias. Am Heart J 1980;100:15–22.
729. Gould LA, Betzu R, Vacek, Muller R, Pradeep V, Downs L. Sinoatrial block due to tocainide. Am Heart J 1989;118:851–853.
730. van Natta B, Lazarus M, Li C. Irreversible interstitial pneumonitis associated with tocainide therapy. West J Med 1988;149:91–92.
731. Perlow GM, Jain BP, Pauker SG, Zarren HS, Wistran DC, Epstein RL. Tocainide-associated interstitial pneumonitis. Ann Intern Med 1981;94:489–490.
732. Braude AC, Downar E, Chamberlain DW, Rebuck AS. Tocainide-associated interstitial pneumonitis. Thorax 1982; 37:309–310.
733. Anonymous. Tocainide hydrochloride pulmonary fibrosis. Swed Adv Drug React Advis Comm Bull 1988;54.
734. Feinberg L, Travis WD, Ferrans V, Sato N, Bernton HF. Pulmonary fibrosis associated with tocainide: report of a case with literature review. Am Rev Respir Dis 1990;141:505–508.
735. Currie P, Ramsdale DR. Paranoid psychsosis induced by tocainide. Br Med J 1984;288:606–607.
736. Harrison DJ, Wathen CG. Paranoid psychosis induced by tocainide. Br Med J 1984;288:1010–1011.
737. Clarke CWF, El-Mahdi EO. Confusion and paranoia associated with oral tocainide. Postgrad Med J 1985;61:79–81.
738. Woosley RL, McDevitt DG, Nies AS, Smith RF, Wilkinson GR, Oates JA. Suppression of ventricular ectopic depolarizations by tocainide. Circulation 1977;56:980–984.
739. Anonymous. Tocainide and blood disorders. Aust Adv Drug React Bull 1986;April.
740. Drost RA. Voorzorgen bij gebruik van Tonocard® (tocainide). Meded Coll Geoord Geneesmidd 1986;121:167.
741. Soff GA, Kadin ME. Tocainide-induced reversible agranulocytosis and anemia. Arch Intern Med 1987;147:598–599.
742. Morrill GB, Gibson SM. Tocainide-induced aplastic anemia. DICP Ann Pharmacother 1989;23:90–91.
743. Engler R, Ryan W, Le Winter M, Bluestein H, Karliner JS. Assessment of long-term antiarrhythmic therapy: studies on the long-term efficacy and toxicity of tocainide. Am J Cardiol 1979;43:612–618.
744. Farquhar DL, Davidson NMcD. Possible hepatotoxicity of tocainide. Scott Med J 1984;29:238.
745. Tucker LE. Tocainide-induced granulomatous hepatitis. J Am Med Assoc 1986;255:3362.

746. Winkle RA, Mason JW, Harrison DC. Tocainide for drug-resistant ventricular arrhythmias: efficacy, side effects, and lidocaine responsiveness for predicting tocainide success. Am Heart J 1980;100:1031–1036.
747. Nyquist O, Forssell, G, Nordlander R, Schenck-Gustafsson K. Hemodynamic and antiarrhythmic effects of tocainide in patients with acute myocardial infarction. Am Heart J 1980;100:1000–1005.
748. Duff HJ, Roden DM, Marney S, Colley DG, Maffucci R, Primm RK, Oates JA, Woosler RL. Molecular basis for the antigenicity of lidocaine analogs: tocainide and mexiletine. Am Heart J 1984;107:585–589.
749. Mohiuddin SM, Esterbrooks D, Mooss AN, Dahl JM, Hilleman DE. Efficacy and tolerance of tocainide during long-term treatment of malignant ventricular arrhythmias. Clin Cardiol 1987;10:457–462.
750. Oliphant LD, Goddard M. Tocainide-associated neutropenia and lupus-like syndrome. Chest 1988;94:427–428.
751. Barnfield C, Kemmenoe AV. A sudden death due to tocainide overdose. Hum Toxicol 1986;5:337–340.
752. Loi C-M, Wei X, Parker BM, Korrapati MR, Vestal RE. The effect of tocainide on theophylline metabolism. Br J Clin Pharmacol 1993;35:437–440.

Meyler's Side Effects of Drugs, 13th Edition
M.N.G. Dukes, editor

SECTION EDITOR: J.K. ARONSON

Pitt O. Lim and Thomas M. MacDonald

18 Antianginal and β-adrenoceptor blocking drugs

SAFETY FACTORS GOVERNING THE CHOICE OF ANTIANGINAL THERAPY

In recent years we have gained further insights into the epidemiology, physiology, cell and molecular biology, and treatment of ischemic heart disease. The three major modifiable risk factors, hypertension, hypercholesterolemia, and smoking, remain the mainstay of our preventive strategies, but evidence that intervention is beneficial has been considerably strengthened.

Hypertension Studies in the high-risk elderly population have shown that treatment of hypertension does indeed prevent coronary events (1[C], 2[C]).

Hypercholesterolemia A landmark study of cholesterol-lowering therapy has convincingly shown the effectiveness of treating patients with high serum cholesterol concentrations and ischemic heart disease (3[C]) and has scotched much of the heated debate on this topic (4[R]).

Smoking The risks of smoking have been highlighted (5[R]), evidence has emerged that changing from high-tar to low-tar cigarettes is ineffective in reducing myocardial infarction (6[C]), and the anti-smoking lobby has become more vocal (7[r], 8[r]).

The role of cigarette smoking as a major factor in myocardial infarction has been further emphasized by a study of the survivors of the ISIS studies (9[Cr]). Smoking increased the risk of a non-fatal myocardial infarction 5-, 3- and 2-fold in the age ranges 30–49, 50–59 and 70–79, respectively. In addition, the results of this study suggested that enforcement of a European Union upper limit of cigarette tar at 12 mg will result in only modest reduction in myocardial infarction. Preventing adolescents from smoking seems to be the only strategy, as few adults start smoking after the age of 18 (10[Cr]). The US ruling in July 1995 that nicotine is an addictive substance (11) was a monumental advance in fighting smoking, since cigarettes are considered to be nicotine delivery systems. If the FDA gains legal jurisdiction in regulating tobacco, active steps will be taken to reduce smoking among children.

The roles of these modifiable risks have thus become more important, and others, such as dietary antioxidants (12[r]) and physical activity (13[Cr]), have also been highlighted.

In recent years potassium channel activators have been added to our armamentarium for treating angina. In addition, the line between anti-anginal drugs and drugs used to prevent angina has become somewhat blurred. Aspirin has now become a mainstay drug in the treatment of ischemic heart disease (14[R]), as have lipid-lowering drugs (3[C]). In the United Kingdom, the angiotensin-converting-enzyme inhibitor enalapril has gained a licence for the prevention of coronary ischemic events in patients with left ventricular dysfunction following the Studies of Left Ventricular Dysfunction Trials (15[C]), and heparin is now a potent weapon in the treatment of unstable angina (16[C]). We are thus in a position to achieve much more with medical therapy than previously, and treatment can be tailored to meet the needs of individual patients.

Our view of drug therapy has subtly changed with this. Before the advent of invasive techniques the physician's role was to use drugs to relieve the symptoms of angina. Nowadays, drugs must not only relieve symptoms but also, where possible, improve life expectancy. We are also more concerned with the quality of symptomatic relief. The notion of 'well-being' is now more important and has been assessed in 'quality-of-life' comparisons of different agents (17[R]). Subtle effects that individually might not be detected have been highlighted in such studies and can modify our view of a drug's adverse effects profile. As the subtle adverse effects of drugs become more important, serious drug toxicity becomes even more unacceptable.

A further consideration, the economic evaluation of drugs, has also crept up on us, although not without criticism (18[R]). In its most rigorous form the cost of drug therapy is measured against the aggregate number of years of improved health that such therapy might be expected to bring (19[R]). These so-called 'quality-adjusted life years' (QUALYs) are reduced if a drug has an adverse effect, so that the net benefit of a drug that prolongs life but makes that life miserable may well be a negative number of QUALYs. Such studies have put a price-tag on mild adverse events as well as on beneficial effects. In time we may pay increasing attention to the price of adverse effects when choosing a drug.

To list a drug's adverse effects profile in isolation is now less appropriate, as its potential benefits may well be far in excess of other drugs of its class. In practice, the drug treatment of angina is time-consuming, empirical, and often relatively unrewarding. Drug treatment simply palliates the underlying disease, and no symptomatic treatment has been shown to improve survival or to prevent myocardial infarction. This is in contrast to surgical intervention, which, in good hands, prolongs survival (20[C]) and improves its quality. The three main comparisons of coronary surgery with medical therapy (21[C]—23[C]) are now out of date, since both medical therapy and surgical techniques have improved considerably since they were completed. However, long-term medical therapy is now more often being reserved for patients who for one reason or another are unsuitable for surgery or percutaneous coronary angioplasty, which, at least for single-vessel disease, is superior to medical treatment (24[C]). The three main choices of drugs for symptomatic control are the nitrates, the β-adrenoceptor antagonists, and the calcium antagonists, with a fourth more recently introduced class, the potassium-channel activators. New agents such as L-carnitine and trimtazidine are being developed (25[R]).

β-Adrenoceptor antagonists Despite the fact that β-blockers have been available for many years, new members of this class with interesting pharmacological profiles continue to be developed. These new drugs are claimed to have either greater cardioselectivity or vasodilating and β_2-agonist properties. The claimed advantages of these new drugs serve to highlight the supposed disadvantages of the older members of the class (their adverse constricting effects on the airways and peripheral blood vessels). Strong commercial emphasis is being placed on these new properties, and papers extolling these effects often appear in non-peer-reviewed supplements or even in reputable journals (26[r]). Whether these new β-blockers will in practice be any better than the older drugs remains to be seen.

Although the toxicity of the β-adrenoceptor antagonists has been fairly well documented, there has been a subtle change in perceptions of their potential benefits and drawbacks. The cardioprotective effect of β-blockers after myocardial infarction and their efficacy in reducing 'silent' myocardial ischemia have persuaded some clinicians to use them preferentially. On the other hand, they may significantly impair the quality of life (27[R]) and are contraindicated in some patients. A few patients cannot tolerate β-blockade per se. These include patients with bronchial asthma, patients with established or incipient cardiac failure, patients with second- or third-degree heart block, and those with seriously compromised limb perfusion causing claudication, ischemic rest pain, and pre-gangrene. β-Blockers are also relatively contraindicated in patients with diabetes, in whom they may mask the metabolic and autonomic responses to hypoglycemia.

β-Blockers that have some degree of intrinsic sympathomimetic activity (i.e. are partial agonists at β-adrenoceptors) may be of some use in patients in whom symptomatic bradycardia occurs and may also reduce coldness of the extremities. In contrast to other β-blockers, these agents are not cardioprotective after myocardial infarction (28[R]). Drugs that are water-soluble are less likely to enter the brain than those that are lipid-soluble and may cause less disturbance of sleep (but see below). Some β-blockers are relatively cardioselective, with less of an effect on β_2 (bronchial) receptors than on β_1 receptors. Whilst these drugs may have relatively less effect on the airways they are in no way *cardiospecific* and they should be used with great care in patients with evidence of reversible obstructive airways disease.

Nitrates Traditionally, nitrates have been first-line therapy in angina. They can be given to treat acute attacks, can be taken prophylactically before exertion or other stimuli known to provoke an attack, or can be used as continuous prophylaxis over 24 hours. Since angina is an episodic symptom, the first two methods of use have merit, as continuous prophylaxis requires treatment over long periods when there are no symptoms. Tempering this argument is the realization that there may be silent myocardial ischemia, especially overnight, and morning angina on waking can be troublesome. In practice, a combination of continuous prophylaxis and 'as required' therapy is often used.

The nitrates are now believed to work by releasing nitric oxide, which relaxes vascular smooth muscle. The discovery that endothelium-derived relaxing factor (EDRF) is nitric oxide (29[R]) has stimulated new interest in these drugs, as nitric oxide not only controls local vessel wall tension in response to shear stress but also plays a role in regulating the interaction of platelets with blood vessel walls. The release of nitric oxide from the walls of atheromatous arteries is reduced, because of malfunctioning or absent endothelium. Atheromatous arteries behave differently from healthy arteries, in that they vasoconstrict rather than vasodilate when stimulated by acetylcholine. This impairment of the acetylcholine vasomotor response appears to be related to serum cholesterol (30[C]). Functional abnormalities of the endothelium are thus assuming a more important role in the possible etiology of angina, and the organic nitrates, which reverse these abnormalities by substituting for nitric oxide, are being examined with renewed interest.

The renewed enthusiasm for nitrates must be viewed along with the realization that nitrate tolerance is a significant drawback, although it occurs not only to the beneficial but also to the adverse effects. At first it was thought that tolerance was due to the depletion of the intracellular endothelial cell sulfhydryl groups (31[R]) that are necessary for the biotransformation of organic nitrates to nitric oxide. However, the precise mechanisms of tolerance are still uncertain (32[R]). What has been convincingly shown is that a nitrate-free period reduces nitrate tolerance (33[CR]). The modern strategy is to have a nitrate-free period when the patient is asleep. However, one problem with this is the increasing worry of reduced protection from ischemia in the early morning, the time when most episodes of silent ischemia and myocardial infarction occur (32[R]). This makes interval monotherapy less attractive.

Nitrates are the drugs of choice in patients with left ventricular impairment, in whom the Veterans Administration Co-operative Study showed nitrate vasodilators to be of benefit (34[C]), and they should be used in preference to the calcium antagonists, which cause deterioration in myocardial function by an as yet unknown mechanism (35[R]).

Calcium antagonists The number of calcium antagonists reaching the market continues to increase. They fall into three groups, the dihydropyridines (e.g. nifedipine), the phenylalkylamines (e.g. verapamil), and the benzothiazepines (e.g. diltiazem). The properties of these drugs vary widely (36[R]). Nifedipine is said to have little negative inotropic effect and no effect on the atrioventricular node; verapamil is a potent cardiac depressant, with a marked effect on the atrioventricular node; and diltiazem has less cardiac depressant effect but inhibits atrioventricular nodal activity.

That calcium antagonists are effective in relieving the symptoms of angina pectoris is beyond doubt, but recently attention has focused on 'silent' ischemia. The Angina and Silent Ischemia Study (37[C]), in which nifedipine, diltiazem, and propranolol were compared with placebo in a crossover study, produced conflicting results. Only diltiazem improved treadmill exercise time and only propranolol convincingly reduced the number of silent ischemic episodes during ambulatory monitoring. These surprising findings are difficult to explain (38[R]). Their clinical importance is that β-blockers may be cardioprotective and therefore a better choice than calcium antagonists (39[CR]). This may also go some way to explaining the clinically significant deterioration seen in patients with impaired left ventricular function taking calcium antagonists (34[C]). This is important, as many patients with angina have previously had a myocardial infarction or have poor left ventricular function. Like β-adrenoceptor antagonists, calcium antagonists can no longer be assumed to be safe second-line drugs for angina in patients with poor cardiac reserve, although newer agents may prove to be safer (40[C]).

Calcium antagonists are very effective in controlling variant angina, and are often used during coronary angioplasty and after coronary artery surgery. They are also useful in patients who are intolerant of β-blockers (41[R]), or who have a poor response to nitrates, or who have concurrent hypertension. They relax the lower esophageal sphincter and may worsen symptoms of reflux esophagitis in those prone to it. Minor unwanted effects, such as headache, flushing, tachycardia, and ankle edema (resistant to diuretics), are relatively common, and some patients find them intolerable.

Potassium channel activators The potassium channel activators are relatively new drugs in Europe, although they have been in use in Japan for over 8 years. They cause both arterial and venous dilatation. Their place in therapy is not yet clear and their use should perhaps be restricted to those patients who are intolerant of or gain inadequate symptomatic relief from the other three classes of drugs.

Unstable angina The term 'unstable angina' has many synonyms, but it describes the syndrome in which angina becomes increasingly severe. This may mean that there is a rapid reduction in exercise tolerance or that pain occurs at rest. Its pathophysiology is different from that of chronic stable angina, in that there is nearly always atheromatous coronary narrowing, with fissuring of one or more of the atheromatous plaques or ulceration with overlying thrombus (42[R]). The vessel lumen is markedly reduced in cross-sectional area by the thrombus and this critically reduces flow, causing ischemia. Distal embolization of platelet aggregates may lead to patchy necrosis downstream, and if the remaining walls of the partially-occluded lumen contain vascular muscle, this may go into spasm, further reducing coronary flow. Treatment of unstable angina should therefore not only reduce myocardial oxygen consumption and (where possible) dilate coronary arteries, but also prevent spasm and reverse coagulation and platelet activation. Antiplatelet drugs, such as aspirin, are of proven benefit in both low dosages (43[C]) and high dosages (44[C]). Intravenous anticoagulation with heparin may also be of use. Intravenous nitrates and oral β-blockers are the medical treatments of choice; calcium antagonists given alone should probably be avoided, as they are of little or no value (45[R]). Repeated episodes of ischemia should be avoided, as they are thought to have a cumulative adverse effect (46[C]).

In summary, it is clear that the selection of prophylactic drug therapy for angina pectoris requires careful appraisal of both the patient and the therapeutic options, particularly with respect to adverse drug reactions. The initial choice lies among long-acting organic nitrates, β-adrenoceptor antagonists, and calcium antagonists. The nitrates are safe and effective. The β-blockers have a good record of efficacy and safety. The role of the calcium antagonists in specific patients is now clearly defined: these include patients with variant angina or those in whom intolerance of β-blockers can be easily predicted. However, there is concern over the safety profile of short-acting calcium antagonists in these patients. Despite some methodological inconsistencies, a recent meta-analysis has suggested that nifedipine may increase mortality dose-dependently (47[R]). This conclusion cannot be generalized to other groups of calcium antagonists or modified-release formulations, and the results of other studies, such as INSIGHT (European, long-acting nifedipine versus a thiazide diuretic) and ALLHAT in the US, are awaited. In the meantime, the US National Heart, Lung, and Blood Institute has issued an official statement urging physicians to use "short-acting nifedipine with caution, especially at higher doses in the treatment of hypertension, angina and myocardial infarction" (48[r]).

For many patients for whom angioplasty or surgery is not appropriate a combination of drugs has traditionally been recommended. However, combinations of β-blockers and calcium channel antagonists probably do not produce additive effects but do increase adverse effects (49[R]), and the efficacy of 'triple therapy' with nitrate, β-blocker, and calcium antagonist may not be superior to optimum β-blockade as monotherapy (50[C]).

β-ADRENOCEPTOR ANTAGONISTS

There are now many β-adrenoceptor antagonists on the market and their adverse effects were comprehensively reviewed in 1988 (51[R]). The spectrum of adverse effects is broadly similar for them all, although differences in their pharmacological properties have been described, notably cardioselectivity, partial agonist activity, membrane-stabilizing activity, and lipid solubility (see Table 1). The influence of these is mentioned in the general discussion when appropriate and is summarized at the end of the section. Individual drug differences in toxicity are largely unimportant but will be mentioned briefly.

ADVERSE REACTION PATTERN

Toxic reactions These are usually mild, with occurrence rates between 10 and 20% for the most common in the majority of studies. Most are predictable from the pharmacological and physicochemical properties of these drugs. Examples include fatigue, cold peripheries, bradycardia, heart failure, sleep disturbances, bronchospasm, and altered glucose tolerance. Gastrointestinal upsets are also relatively common. Serious adverse cardiac effects and even sudden death may follow the abrupt withdrawal of therapy in patients with ischemic heart disease. The majority of severe adverse reactions can be avoided by careful selection of patients and consideration of individual β-blockers.

Hypersensitivity reactions These have been relatively rare since the withdrawal of practolol over 10 years ago.

Tumor-inducing effects These have not been established in man.

ORGANS AND SYSTEMS

Cardiovascular *Heart failure* β-Adrenoceptor antagonists reduce cardiac output through their negative inotropic and negative chronotropic effects. They may therefore cause worsening systolic heart failure or the development of heart failure in patients who depend on high sympathetic drive to maintain cardiac output. Plasma noradrenaline is increased in patients with heart failure, and the extent of this increase is directly related to the degree of ventricular impairment (52[C]). Since the greatest effect on sympathetic activity occurs with the first (and usually the lowest) doses, heart failure associated with β-blockade is independent of dosage. Heart failure is one of the most serious adverse effects of the β-adrenoceptor antagonists (53[R]), but it is usually predictable and can be attenuated by pre-treatment with diuretics and angiotensin-converting enzyme inhibitors in patients who are considered to be at risk. Against this, there are some patients with systolic heart failure who may benefit, at least symptomatically, from a β-blocker (54[R]), although the evidence is strongest

Table 1. *Properties of β-adrenoceptor agonists*

Drug	Lipid solubility[a]	Cardioselectivity	Partial agonist activity	Membrane-stabilizing activity
Acebutolol	0.7	±	+	+
Alprenolol	31	−	+	+
Amosulalol		−		
Atenolol	< 0.02	+	−t−	
Betaxolol		+	−	±
Bevantolol	low	+	−	+
Bisoprolol		++	−	−
Bufuralol	+	−	+	
Bunitrolol	+	−	++	±
l-Bunolol		−		
Carteolol	−	+		
Carvedilol	++	−	−	
Celiprolol		±	+[b]	−
Epanolol	minimal	+	+	−
Esmolol	−	+	−	
Flestolol	−	−	−	
Labetalol	+	−	−	
Metoprolol	0.2	+	−	±
Nadolol	0.03	−	−	−
Nevibolol		+	−	−
Oxprenolol	0.7	−	+	+
Penbutolol	−	−	+	+
Pindolol	0.2	−	++	±
Practolol	< 0.02	+	+	−
Propranolol	4.3	−	−	++
Sotalol	0.02	−	−	−
Talinolol		+		
Timolol	0.03	−	±	±
Xamoterol		+	++	

[a] Octanol:water partition coefficient.
[b] Partial β_2-agonist.

for idiopathic dilated cardiomyopathy rather than ischemic heart disease (55[C]). These drugs cannot currently be recommended for routine use, and their prescription in heart failure should probably be confined to hospital physicians with a special interest in heart failure.

It has been suggested that drugs with partial agonist activity (see Table 1), which have a minimal depressant effect on normal resting sympathetic tone, might cause lesser reductions in cardiac output (56[R]) and thus protect against the development of cardiac decompensation (57[R]). However, this has not been satisfactorily demonstrated for drugs with high partial agonist activity, e.g. acebutolol, oxprenolol, and pindolol (58[C]), and these drugs should therefore be given with the same caution as others in compromised patients. Xamoterol, a β-adrenoceptor antagonist with substantial β_1 partial agonist activity, is thought to be of benefit in mild congestive heart failure (59[R]), but its widespread use by non-specialists in more severe degrees of heart failure has resulted in many reports of worsening heart failure (60[R]). Heart failure has also been produced by labetalol (61[C]) and after the use of timolol eye-drops in the treatment of glaucoma (62[C]).

With the advent of echocardiography, it has become possible to assess systolic and diastolic function of the heart non-invasively in patients presenting with symptoms and signs of heart failure. It is now realized that the above comments are particularly relevant for patients with systolic dysfunction, but probably not for those with diastolic dysfunction, which may lead to congestive heart failure even when systolic function is normal (63[Cr], 64[Cr]). Diastole is the phase of myocardial relaxation allowing ventricular filling. Failure of intraventricular pressure to fall appropriately during this part of heart cycle leads to increased atrial pressure, which eventually leads to increased pulmonary and systemic venous pressure, causing a syndrome of congestive heart failure indistinguishable clinically from that caused by systolic pump failure (65[R]). Diastolic dysfunction occurs in systemic arterial hypertension, hypertrophic obstructive cardiomyopathy, and infiltrative heart diseases, which reduce ventricular compliance or increase ventricular 'stiffness' (66[R]). As energy is required for active diastolic myocardial relaxation, a relative shortage of adenosine triphosphate in ischemic heart disease also often leads to co-existing diastolic and systolic dysfunction (67[C]). β-Blockers improve diastolic function in general, and this may be beneficial in this subset of patients with congestive heart failure but with normal systolic function (66[R]); however, more research is needed to clarify this situation. The risks of β-blockade in acute myocardial infarction are considered below (see 'Risk situations').

Hypotension β-Adrenoceptor antagonists lower blood pressure by about 15–25 mmHg on average, probably by a variety of mechanisms, including reduced cardiac output. More severe reductions of blood pressure can occur and may be associated with syncope (53[R]). It has been suggested that this is more likely to occur in old people, but comprehensive studies in this age group have stressed their safety (68[C]). Profound hypotension resulting in renal failure after the administration of atenolol 100 mg orally has been reported in a single patient (69[C]); however, large doses of furosemide and diazoxide were also given, and this appears more likely to have been a consequence of a drug interaction.

Cardiac dysrhythmias β-Blockade may result in sinus bradycardia, because blockade of sympathetic tone allows unopposed parasympathetic activity. Drugs with partial agonist activity may prevent bradycardia (70[C]). However, heart rates under 60 beats/min often worry the physician more than the patient. Confirmation for this comes from a retrospective study of nearly 7000 patients taking β-adrenoceptor antagonists: apart from dizziness in patients with heart rates under 40 beats/min (0.4% of the total group), slow heart rates were well tolerated (71[C]).

All β-adrenoceptor antagonists cause an increase in atrioventricular conduction time, which in clinical practice means advancing atrioventricular block; this is most pronounced with drugs that have potent membrane-depressant properties and no partial agonist activity (Table 1). Sotalol differs from other β-adrenoceptor antagonists, in that it increases the duration of the action potential in the cardiac Purkinje fibers and ventricular muscle at therapeutic doses. This is a Class III antidysrhythmic effect, and because of this sotalol has been used to treat ventricular (72[C], 73[C], 74[R]) and supraventricular dysrhythmias (75[C]) with varying success. The main serious adverse effect of sotalol is that it is prodysrhythmic in certain circumstances, and can cause the polymorphous ventricular tachycardia known as *torsade de pointes* (76[C], 77[C]). In a recent survey of 1288 patients taking sotalol, dysrhythmias occurred in 56, 24 of which were *torsade de pointes* (78[R]). There was no relation between these dysrhythmias and previously associated factors, such as bradycardia, a long QT interval, and hypokalemia. The β-adrenoceptor antagonist properties of *d,l*-sotalol reside in the *l*-isomer, the *d*-isomer having Class III antidysrhythmic activity but no clinically significant β-blocking action (79[C]). In clinical trials *d*-sotalol has a low incidence of adverse events, but *torsade de pointes* occurred in 1.2% of those exposed (data on file, Bristol-Myers Squibb, Princeton, New Jersey). A trial to test the efficacy of *d*-sotalol in reducing mortality in patients with left ventricular dysfunction was recently mounted (80[R]), but was discontinued early when an interim analysis of 2762 patients showed an overall mortality of 3.9% in the *d*-sotalol group, compared with 2% in the placebo group (81[r]).

An unusual dysrhythmia has been attributed to propranolol therapy for angina pectoris: *alternating sinus rhythm with intermittent sinoatrial block*. The authors suggested that this was accounted for by the existence of sinoatrial conduction via two pathways, the first with 2:1 block and the second with a slightly longer conduction time and intermittent 2:1 block (82[c]).

Acute chest pain Worsening of angina pectoris has been attributed to β-blocker therapy. The reports include 35 cases in a series of 296 elderly patients admitted to hospital with suspected myocardial infarction; in these 35 the pain disappeared within 7 hours of discontinuing β-blocker therapy (83[C]). Worsening of angina has been reported at very low heart rates (84[c]). Propranolol resulted in vasotonic angina in six patients during a double-blind trial, with prolongation of the duration of pain and electrocardiographically assessed ischemia. It has been suggested that this reflects a reduction in coronary perfusion as a result of reduced cardiac output, and also that non-selective agents may provoke coronary arterial spasm by inhibiting β_2-mediated vasodilatation (85[C]). The latter explanation is controversial, and the use of β-blockers in patients with arteriographic evidence of coronary artery spasm has not consistently caused worsening of the disorder (86[r]). In addition, unstable angina has also followed the initiation of treatment for hypertension with cardioselective drugs such as betaxolol (87[C]). Finally, β-adrenoceptor antagonists may cause non-anginal chest pain because of esophagitis (88[C]), due to adherence of the tablet mass resulting in esophageal spasm, inflammatory change, and even perforation. The occurrence of chest pain by this mechanism may be more common than has been recognized in the past.

Fatigue and reduced work capacity This is one of the most commonly reported adverse effects of β-adrenoceptor antagonists, with reported occurrence rates of up to 20% or more, particularly in those who exert themselves. It has to be viewed alongside the ability to produce fatigue and lethargy by a possible effect on the nervous system (see below). The precise cause of physical fatigue, whether due to hemodynamic upset, metabolic effects in muscle, or both, is unknown and it is not clear if drugs with β_1-selectivity or partial agonist activity are to be preferred in this respect. A variety of mechanisms have been proposed to explain reduced left ventricular work capacity and exercise tolerance: reduced cardiac output, impaired muscle blood supply, effects on intermediary metabolism, and a direct effect on muscle contractility (89[R]).

Theoretically, β_1-selective drugs are less likely to alter these variables, and they might therefore have an advantage over non-selective drugs. However, this has not always been demonstrated in single-dose studies in volunteers (90[C], 91[C]), although in two such studies atenolol was considered to have produced less exercise intolerance than propranolol, in comparable dosages (92[C], 93[C]). For an unexplained reason, cardioselectivity appeared to impair performance relatively less in subjects with a high proportion of slow-twitch muscle fibers than it did in those whose muscle biopsy specimens showed a high percentage of fast-twitch fibers (94[R]). The muscle fibers of long-distance runners (joggers) are predominantly of the slow-twitch type, and this probably explains the superiority of atenolol over propranolol when exercise performance was assessed in such subjects (92[C]). Other studies have shown that the release of lactic acid from skeletal muscle cells is impaired to a greater extent by non-selective β-blockers than by cardioselective drugs, and furthermore that cardioselectivity was associated with a less marked fall in blood glucose during and after maximal and submaximal exercise (95[C], 96[C]). Partial agonist activity might have been the reason for the superiority of oxprenolol over propranolol in terms of exercise duration (97[C]).

Peripheral vascular effects Cold extremities or exacerbation of Raynaud's phenomenon are amongst the commonest adverse effects reported with β-adrenoceptor antagonists (5.8% of nearly 800 patients taking propranolol) (53[R]); Raynaud's phenomenon occurs in 0.5–6% of patients (98[C]). The mechanism may be potentiation of the effects of a cold environment on an already abnormal circulation, but whether symptoms can be produced de novo is more difficult to determine. However, a retrospective questionnaire study of 758 patients taking hypotensive drugs showed that 40% of patients taking β-blockers noted cold extremities compared with 18% of those taking diuretics; there were no significant differences among propranolol, alprenolol, pindolol, atenolol, and metoprolol (99[C]). Similarly, a large randomized study showed that the incidence of Raynaud's phenomenon was the same for atenolol and pindolol (100[C]). In another study vasospastic symptoms improved when labetalol was substituted for a variety of β-blockers (101[C]). On the other hand, a small, double-blind, placebo-controlled study in patients with established Raynaud's phenomenon showed that the prevalence of symptoms with both propranolol and labetalol was no greater than with placebo (102[C]).

Intermittent claudication has also been reported to be worsened by the use of β-adrenoceptor antagonists, but has been difficult to document because of study design in patients with advanced atherosclerosis. As early as 1975 it was reported from one small placebo-controlled study that propranolol did not exacerbate symptoms in patients with intermittent claudication (103[C]). This has subsequently been supported by the results of several large placebo-controlled trials of β-blockers in mild hypertension and by the fact that reports of trials of the secondary prevention of myocardial infarction did not mention intermittent claudication as an adverse effect, even though it was not a specific contraindication to inclusion (104[R]). In addition, a comprehensive study of the effects of β-adrenoceptor antagonists in patients with intermittent claudication did not show β-blockade to be an independent risk factor for the disease (105[C]). A study of atenolol (50 mg bd) in men with chronic stable intermittent claudication showed no effect on walking distance or foot temperature (106[C]). These findings have been confirmed in a recent meta-analysis of 11 randomized controlled trials to determine whether β-blockers exacerbate intermittent claudication (SEDA-17, 234). However, it should not be forgotten that patchy skin necrosis has been described in hypertensive patients with small-vessel disease in the legs who were taking β-adrenoceptor antagonists. Characteristically, pedal pulses remained palpable and the lesions occurred during cold weather and healed on withdrawal of the drugs (107[C]–109[C]). Similarly, three cases have been reported in which long-lasting incipient gangrene of the leg was immediately overcome when treatment with a β-adrenoceptor antagonist was stopped (110[C], 111[C]), showing how easily the use of these drugs is overlooked in such circumstances. In several cases of β-adrenoceptor antagonist-induced gangrene, recovery has not followed withdrawal of therapy and amputation has been necessary (112[CR], 113[CR]). Thus, where possible, alternative forms of therapy should be used in patients at risk.

There is also a suggestion that β-blockade may compromise the splanchnic vasculature. Intravenous propranolol has been shown experimentally to reduce splanchnic blood flow by 29% whilst reducing cardiac output by only 6% (114[CR]), and five patients have been described who developed *mesenteric ischemia*, four with ischemic colitis, and one with abdominal angina, while taking β-adrenoceptor antagonists (115[CR]). Although causation is not proven, a possible relation must be allowed.

Respiratory *Increased airways resistance* Since the introduction of propranolol into clinical practice, it has been recognized that patients with bronchial asthma treated with β-adrenoceptor antagonists can develop severe airways obstruction (116[C]), which may be fatal (117[C]) or near fatal (118[C], 119[C]), and which has even followed the use of eye-drops containing timolol (120[C]) (see also Chapter 47). β-Blockers may upset the balance of bronchial smooth muscle tone, presumably by blocking the bronchial β_2-adrenoceptors responsible for bronchodilatation. They may also promote degranulation of mast cells and depress central responsiveness to carbon dioxide (121[C], 122[C]). Although β_1-selective drugs are theoretically safer, there are occasions when they have caused serious reductions in ventilatory function (123[C], 124[C]), even when used as eye-drops (125[C]). However, it has recently been concluded that if β-blockade is necessary in the treatment of glaucoma, cardioselective β-blocking drugs should be used in preference (126[Cr]). Cardioselectivity has been considered to be dose-dependent (127[C]), and higher dosages might therefore be expected to produce adverse effects. However, it has recently been shown that the cardioselective drugs metoprolol and bevantolol, even in dosages that are lower than those usually required for a therapeutic effect, may be poorly tolerated by patients with asthma (128[C]). Whether drugs with partial agonist activity confer any advantage is still uncertain. Some of the evidence that asthmatic patients may tolerate β-blockers is probably misleading, relating to patients with chronic obstructive airways disease who have irreversible changes and who fail to respond either to bronchoconstricting or bronchodilating drugs (129[C]). In contrast, a few patients who have never had asthma or chronic bronchitis may develop severe bronchospasm when given a β-adrenoceptor antagonist. Some, but not all, of these cases (130[C]) may represent an allergic reaction to the dyes (e.g. tartrazine) that are used to color some formulations. Other patients, who may not have a history of chest disease, will only develop increased airways resistance with β-adrenoceptor antagonists during respiratory infections. It is against this potentially hazardous background that claims that some asthmatic subjects will tolerate certain β-blockers (131[C]) must be viewed. Some asthmatic patients may indeed tolerate either cardioselective β-blockers (such as atenolol and metoprolol) or labetalol (132[C], 133[C]), and in patients taking atenolol β_2-adrenoceptor agonists may continue to produce bronchodilatation (134[C]), but in most instances there are therapeutic alternatives and they should be preferred (135[R]). Celiprolol is a β_1-adrenoceptor antagonist that has partial β_2-agonist activity, and small studies have suggested that it may be useful in asthmatic patients (136[C]). However, worsening airways obstruction has been reported with celiprolol (137[C]), and it has been concluded that it has no advantage over existing β-blockers in the treatment of hypertension (138[R]). Attention has also been drawn recently to the increased risks of the adverse effects of β-blockers on respiratory function in old people (139[R]).

Central ventilatory suppression Reduced sensitivity of the respiratory center to carbon dioxide has been reported (140[C], 141[C]). The clinical significance of this phenomenon is unknown, but a lethal synergism between morphine and propranolol in suppressing ventilation in animals has been described (142[C]).

Pneumonitis, pulmonary fibrosis, and pleurisy Pulmonary fibrosis (143[C]) and pleural fibrosis (144[C]) have both been described as infrequent complications associated with practolol. Pulmonary fibrosis has also occurred during treatment with pindolol (145[C]) and acebutolol (146[C], 147[C]). Pleuritic and pneumonitic reactions to acebutolol have been reported (147[C], 148[C]).

Nervous system *Minor psychiatric symptoms* Some minor neuropsychiatric adverse effects, such as lightheadedness, visual and auditory hallucinations, illusions, sleep disturbances, vivid dreams, and changes in mood and affect, have been causally related to long-term treatment with β-adrenoceptor antagonists (149[C], 150[R]). In addition, tiredness, fatigue, and lethargy, probably the commonest troublesome adverse effects of β-blockers and often the reason for their withdrawal (151[r]), may have a contributory CNS component, although they are primarily due to reduced cardiac output and altered muscle metabolism (98[R]) (see also 'Fatigue and reduced work capacity' above). In general, a definite neurological association has been difficult to prove, and studies of patients taking β-adrenoceptor antagonists for hypertension, which incorporated control groups of patients taking either other antihypertensive drugs or a placebo, appear to have shown that the incidence of symptoms that can be specifically attributed to β-adrenoceptor antagonists is lower than anticipated (151[r], 152[C]).

The more lipophilic drugs, such as propranolol and oxprenolol, would be expected to pass the blood-brain barrier more readily than hydrophilic drugs, such as atenolol and nadolol, and there is some evidence that they do so (153[C]). In theory, therefore, hydrophilic drugs might be expected to produce fewer neuropsychiatric adverse effects. A double-blind, placebo-controlled evaluation of the effects of four β-blockers (atenolol, metoprolol, propranolol, and pindolol) on central nervous function (154[C]) showed that disruption of sleep was similar with the three lipid-soluble drugs, averaging six to seven wakenings per night, compared with an average of three wakenings per night for atenolol and placebo. Only pindolol significantly altered rapid eye movement sleep and latency, and it is known to have a higher CSF/plasma concentration ratio than metoprolol and propranolol (155[CR]). Pindolol and propranolol also had high depression scores. In another placebo-controlled sleep laboratory study of atenolol, propranolol, metoprolol, and pindolol, the three lipophilic drugs reduced dreaming (equated with rapid eye movement sleep) but increased the recollection of dreaming and the amount of wakening; in contrast, although atenolol also reduced sleep it had no effect on subjective measures of sleep (156[C]).

All the published data on the CNS effects of β-blockers have been extensively reviewed (157[R]). The overall incidence of CNS effects was low, but it was lowest with the hydrophilic drugs. However, a meta-analysis of 55 studies of the cognitive effects of β-blockade did not show any firm evidence that lipophilic drugs caused more adverse effects than hydrophilic ones (158[R]). Recent data confirming a correlation between lipophilicity and serum concentrations on the one hand and CNS effects on the other (159[R]) have fuelled this controversy.

Disturbances of psychomotor function β-Adrenoceptor antagonists impair performance in psychomotor tests after single doses. These include effects of atenolol, oxprenolol, and propranolol on pursuit rotor and reaction times (160[C]—161[C]). However, other studies with the same drugs have failed to show significant effects (162[C]—166[C]), and the issue has remained controversial. A report that sotalol improved psychomotor performance in 12 healthy individuals in a dose of 320 mg daily but impaired it at 960 mg daily (167[C]) has been interpreted to indicate that the water-soluble β-adrenoceptor antagonists would be less likely to produce CNS effects than the fat-soluble drugs. However, recently both atenolol and propranolol have been shown to modify the electroencephalogram, atenolol affecting body sway and alertness and propranolol impairing short-term memory and the ability to concentrate (168[C], 169[C]). These results suggest that both lipophilic and hydrophilic β-adrenoceptor antagonists affect the central nervous system, although their effects may be subtle and difficult to demonstrate.

Car-driving and other specialized skills In view of the large numbers of people who currently take β-blockers regularly for hypertension or ischemic heart disease, the question arises whether they may impair performance in tasks requiring psychomotor co-ordination. The occupations under scrutiny include car-driving, the operation of industrial machinery, and the piloting of aeroplanes. Again, the current evidence is conflicting and controversial. One report suggested that propranolol and pindolol given for 5 days impaired ability for slalom driving in a manner comparable with the co-ordination defects caused by alcohol (170[C]). In contrast, other studies have shown that driving skills were not impaired during long-term β-adrenoceptor antagonist therapy and might even be enhanced (171[C]—173[C]). There is also a suggestion that tolerance to the central effects of these drugs may develop within 3 weeks of starting therapy, provided the dosage does not change (174[C]). Until more information is available from well-controlled studies, it is probably prudent to inform patients who are starting treatment with β-adrenoceptor antagonists that they should exercise special care in the performance of skills requiring psychomotor co-ordination for the first 1 or 2 weeks.

Psychosis, depression, and other CNS effects The development of a severe organic brain syndrome has been reported in several patients taking β-adrenoceptor antagonists regularly without a previous history of psychiatric illness (175[C]—177[C]). A similar phenomenon was seen in a young healthy woman who took propranolol 160 mg daily in a drug trial (178[C]). The psychosis may follow initial therapy or dosage increases during long-term therapy (179[C]). The symptoms, which include agitation, confusion, disorientation, anxiety, and hallucinations, may not respond to treatment with neuroleptic drugs (179[C]) but subside rapidly when the β-adrenoceptor antagonists are discontinued. They have also been shown to respond to changing from propranolol to atenolol (180[r]). A schizophrenia-like illness has also been seen in close relation to the initiation of propranolol therapy (181[C]). Anxiety and depression have been reported after the use of nadolol, which is hydrophilic (182[C]). In a recent study of the co-prescribing of antidepressants in 3218 new β-blocker takers (183[C]), 6.4% had prescriptions for antidepressant drugs within 34 days compared with 2.8% in a control population. Propranolol had the highest rate of co-prescribing (9.5%). It was followed by other lipophilic β-blockers (3.9%) and then hydrophilic β-blockers (2.5%). In propranolol users the risk of antidepressant use was 4.8-times (95% CI 4.1—5.5) greater than the control group, and appeared to be highest in those aged 20—39 (relative risk 17.2, 95% CI 13.7—21.5).

Other occasional CNS effects of β-blockers have been reported, including *hearing impairment* (184[C]), *episodic diplopia* (185[C]), and *myotonia* (186[c]).

Although some migraine sufferers use β-adrenoceptor antagonists prophylactically, there are also reports of the development of migraine on exposure to propranolol or rebound aggravation when the drug is withdrawn (187[C]). Stroke, a rare complication of migraine, has been reported in three patients using propranolol for prophylaxis (188[C]—190[C]). Seizures have been reported with the short-acting β-blocker, esmolol, usually with excessively high doses (191[C]). *Myasthenia gravis* has been associated with labetalol (192[C]), oxprenolol, and propranolol (193[C]), and *carpal tunnel syndrome* has been reported with long-term β-blockade, the symptoms gradually disappearing on withdrawal of therapy (194[C]). Pindolol, which has substantial partial agonist activity, may cause tremor (195[C]).

Endocrine, metabolic *Hypoglycemia*, producing loss of consciousness in some cases, may occur in non-diabetic individuals who are taking β-adrenoceptor antagonists, particularly those who undergo prolonged fasting (196[C]) or severe exercise (197[C], 198[C]). Patients on maintenance dialysis also seem to be at risk of this adverse effect (199[C]). It has been suggested that non-selective drugs are most likely to produce hypoglycemia and that cardioselective drugs are to be preferred in at-risk patients (200[C]), but the same effect has been reported with atenolol under similar circumstances (198[C]).

Type II diabetics taking β-adrenoceptor antagonists do not seem to have an increased risk of developing hypoglycemia: indeed, in 20 such patients treated with diet or diet plus oral hypoglycemic agents, both propranolol and metoprolol produced small but significant *increases* in blood glucose concentrations after 4 weeks of treatment (201[C]). The rise was considered clinically important in only a few patients.

Contrary to popular belief, β-adrenoceptor antagonists have not been shown to increase the risk of hypoglycemic episodes in insulin-treated diabetics, in whom their use was concluded to be generally safe (202[C]). However, in the insulin-treated diabetic who becomes hypoglycemic, non-selective β-adrenoceptor antagonists may mask the adrenaline-mediated symptoms, such as palpitation, tachycardia, and tremor; they may result in a rise in mean and diastolic blood pressures, due to unopposed α-stimulation from the adrenaline, because the β_2-adrenoceptor-mediated vasodilator response is blocked (203[C]); they may also impair the rate of rise of blood glucose towards normal (203[C], 204[C]). In contrast, cardioselective drugs appear to mask hypoglycemic symptoms less (205[C]); because of vascular sparing, their use is less likely to result in a diastolic pressor response in the presence of adrenaline (205[C]), although this has been reported with metoprolol (206[C]); and delay in recovery from hypoglycemia is either less marked or undetectable with cardioselective drugs, such as atenolol or metoprolol (203[C], 204[C]). Thus, if insulin-requiring diabetics need to be treated with a β-adrenoceptor antagonist, a cardioselective agent should always be chosen for reasons of safety, while allowing that this type of β-blocker is associated with *insulin resistance* and may impair insulin sensitivity by 15—30% (SEDA-17, 235), which might increase insulin requirements.

A recent observational study following up 686 hypertensive men for 15 years found that β-blockers were associated with a higher incidence of diabetes than thiazide diuretics (207[Cr]). This was an uncontrolled study, but the observation deserves further study.

Thyroid disease Propranolol inhibits the conversion of thyroxine (T_4) to triiodothyronine (T_3) by peripheral tissues (208[C]), resulting in increased formation of inactive reverse T_3. This seems unlikely to play a significant role in the use of β-adrenoceptor antagonists in hyperthyroidism. Since *d*-propranolol has similar effects on thyroxine metabolism to those seen with the conventionally-used racemic mixture, membrane-stabilizing activity may be involved (209[C]). In one case β-adrenoceptor blockade, given for an entirely different purpose, masked an unexpected thyroid crisis, resulting in severe cerebral dysfunction before the diagnosis was made (210[C]). There have now been several reports of hyperthyroxinemia in clinically euthyroid patients taking propranolol for non-thyroid reasons in high dosages (320—480 mg/day) (211[C], 212[C]). The incidence was considered to be higher than could be accounted for by the development of spontaneous hyperthyroidism, but the mechanism is unknown.

Prolactin A case of reversible *hyperprolactinemia* with *galactorrhea* has been described in a 38-year-old woman taking atenolol for hypertension (213[c]).

Blood lipids There is increasing evidence to suggest that β-adrenoceptor antagonists increase total triglyceride concentrations in blood and reduce high-density lipoprotein (HDL) cholesterol. Comparison of non-selective and cardioselective drugs shows that although the lipid derangements are less marked with β_1-selective agents, they are nevertheless still present (214[R]). The importance of these effects for the long-term management of patients with hypertension or ischemic heart disease is unknown, but it is recognized that a high serum total cholesterol and a low HDL cholesterol are associated with an increased risk of ischemic heart disease. However, it has recently been concluded that a significant reduction in HDL cholesterol after treatment for 1 year with timolol was of no prognostic significance and did not attenuate the protective effect of the drug (215[R]). In a 4-year randomized, placebo-controlled, follow-up study of six antihypertensive monotherapies, acebutolol produced a only small and probably clinically irrelevant (0.17 mmol/l) reduction in total cholesterol (216[C]), which was not statistically different from four of the other antihypertensive drugs.

Current information suggests that β_1-selective drugs may be preferable in patients with hypertriglyceridemia (217[C]).

Obesity It has been suggested that β-blockers may predispose to obesity by reducing basal metabolic rate via β-adrenoceptor blockade (218[C]). Thermogenesis in response to cold and heat exposure, meals, stress, and anxiety is also reduced by β-adrenoceptor blockade, promoting weight gain (SEDA-16, 193). The β_3-adrenoceptor has been implicated in this mechanism (219[C], 220[Cr]). Since propranolol blocks the β_3-receptor in vivo (221[c]), it would be wise on theoretical grounds to avoid propranolol in obese patients, nadolol being an alternative non-selective β-blocker which does not antagonize β_3-receptors.

Mineral and fluid balance *Hypokalemia* Adrenaline by infusion produces a transient increase in plasma potassium, followed by a prolonged fall; pretreatment with β-adrenoceptor antagonists results in a rise in plasma potassium (222[C]). These effects may be mediated via β_2-adrenoceptors (223[C]), and cardioselective drugs should have less of an effect (222[C]). In the Treatment of Mild Hypertension Study (TOMHS), acebutolol did not change serum potassium after 4 years (216[C]).

It has been argued that drug combinations that contain a β-adrenoceptor antagonist in combination with a thiazide diuretic may minimize the hypokalemic effect of the latter; however, a case of marked hypokalemia in the absence of primary hyperaldosteronism has been reported in a patient taking Sotazide (a combination of hydrochlorothiazide and the non-selective drug sotalol) (224[C]). The use of a combination formulation of chlorthalidone and atenolol has also produced hypokalemia (225[c]), in one case complicated by ventricular fibrillation after myocardial infarction (226[c]).

In addition to a rise in serum potassium, timolol has also been shown to increase plasma *uric acid* concentrations (227[C]). A fall in serum *calcium* has been reported (228[C]) with atenolol, but whether this is causal has been disputed (229[C]). In the TOMHS study, acebutolol increased serum urate by 7 μmol/l (216[C]).

Hematological *Thrombocytopenia* has been reported in patients taking oxprenolol (230[C], 231[C]) and alprenolol (232[C], 233[C]); it may recur with rechallenge. This effect is presumed to have an immunological basis. In the International Agranulocytosis and Aplastic Anemia Study the relation between cardiovascular drugs and agranulocytosis was examined: there was a relative risk of 2.5 (95% CI 1.1–6.1) for propranolol (234[C]). Other β-blockers had no increased risk and propranolol had no association with aplastic anemia. There are also anecdotal reports of this association (235[C]).

Liver *Biliary cirrhosis* was reported as part of the practolol syndrome, but there have been no comparable reports with other β-adrenoceptor antagonists. Many β-adrenoceptor antagonists undergo substantial first-pass hepatic metabolism, e.g. alprenolol, metoprolol, oxprenolol, and propranolol. Hepatic cirrhosis, with consequent portosystemic shunting, may therefore result in increased systemic availability and higher plasma concentrations, perhaps resulting in adverse effects. β-Adrenoceptor antagonists may also reduce liver blood flow and cause interactions with drugs whose hepatic clearance is flow-dependent (see 'Interactions' below). The oxidative clearance of the lipophilic drugs metoprolol, timolol, and bufuralol is influenced by the debrisoquine hydroxylation gene locus, resulting in polymorphic metabolism (236[R]). This might result in an increase in the adverse effects of these β-blockers in poor metabolizers, but to date there is no objective evidence of such an association (237[C]).

The role of β-adrenoceptor antagonists in the prevention of bleeding from esophageal varices in patients with hepatic cirrhosis is under evaluation, but their use has been considered to be the cause of *hepatic encephalopathy* in several patients (238[C], 239[r], 240[R], 241[C], 242[C]). Thus, extreme caution is required, particularly because resuscitation may be difficult when β-blockers are given to patients with bleeding or encephalopathy (243[R]).

Gastrointestinal Mild gastrointestinal adverse effects, such as *nausea*, *dyspepsia*, *constipation* or *diarrhea*, have been reported in 5–10% of patients taking β-adrenoceptor antagonists (53[R]). A reduction in dosage or a change to another member of the group will usually produce amelioration. Severe reactions of this type are very infrequent, but severe diarrhea, dehydration, hypokalemia, and weight loss, recurring after rechallenge, occurred with propranolol in a single case (244[C]).

Sclerosing peritonitis and retroperitoneal fibrosis Sclerosing peritonitis was described as part of the practolol syndrome (245[C]–247[C]) and it may also occur with other β-adrenoceptor antagonists (248[C], 249[C]).

Retroperitoneal fibrosis has been reported in patients taking oxprenolol (250[C]), atenolol (251[C]), propranolol (252[C]), metoprolol (253[C]), sotalol, and timolol (including eye-drops) (254[C]–256[C]). However, this disorder often occurs spontaneously and has been reported very infrequently in patients taking β-adrenoceptor antagonists (257[C]). Thus, in the absence of any causal relation it seems most likely to reflect the spontaneous incidence in patients taking a commonly prescribed therapy. This conclusion has been supported by an analysis of 100 cases of retroperitoneal fibrosis (258[R]).

Urinary system *Renal function* Propranolol reduces renal blood flow and glomerular filtration rate after acute administration, associated with, and probably partly due to, falls in cardiac output and blood pressure (259[C], 260[C]). There has been some argument about whether these effects persist during chronic therapy or not (260[C], 261[C]). Despite early suggestions that renal function might be worsened by such therapy, particularly in patients with chronic renal failure (262[C]), the clinical significance of these changes is now considered debatable (263[R]). Claims that nadolol actually increases renal blood flow (264[C]) and that cardioselective drugs such as atenolol reduce renal blood flow less than non-selective agents in old people (265[C]) are thus probably relatively unimportant. The vasodilating β-blocker carvedilol maintains renal blood flow whilst reducing glomerular filtration rate, suggesting that renal vasodilatation occurs (266[C]).

Skin and appendages *Exanthemata* are part of the practolol syndrome. They appear to be an established but infrequent adverse effect of the other β-adrenoceptor antagonists. The eruptions may be urticarial, morbilliform, eczematous, vesicular, bullous, psoriasiform, or lichenoid (267[C]—272[C]). Some patients show positive patch tests and/or a positive response to oral rechallenge. There may also be cross-sensitivity to other β-adrenoceptor antagonists in a compromised patient. The mechanisms appear to include both immunological and pharmacological responses; in the latter case the suggestion is that the drug may modify growth regulation in the epidermis (273[R]). In a recent review of 588 patients with established psoriasis it was concluded that about two-thirds of these patients are likely to experience a flare-up with a β-adrenoceptor antagonist regardless of the agent used (274[R]).

Alopecia There have been single case reports of alopecia in association with propranolol (275[C]) and metoprolol (276[C]).

Special senses *Eyes* Keratopathy in association with the practolol syndrome is the major serious ocular effect ascribed to β-adrenoceptor antagonists. Conjunctivitis and visual disturbances have also been reported, and recently a case of ocular pemphigoid has been described in a patient taking timolol eye-drops for glaucoma (277[C]). Anterior uveitis has been reported in patients taking betaxolol (278[c]) and metipranolol (279[c], 280[c]).

A case of recurrent retinal arteriolar spasm with associated visual loss has been described in a 68-year-old man with hypertension treated with atenolol (SEDA-17, 236).

Nasal polyps, rhinitis and *sinusitis* resistant to long courses of antibiotics and surgical intervention have been described in five patients taking non-selective β-adrenoceptor blockers (propranolol and timolol). The symptoms resolved when the drugs were discontinued and did not recur when β_1-selective adrenoceptor blockers (metoprolol or atenolol) were given instead (281[C]).

Musculoskeletal It was suggested in 1983 that *arthralgia* is a not uncommon adverse effect of β-adrenoceptor antagonists, particularly metoprolol (282[R]), although the association was not confirmed by rechallenge in any patient. However, a later case-control study of 127 patients attending a hypertension clinic who had arthropathy showed no significant relation between the arthropathy and the use of β-blockers (283[CR]). On the other hand, five cases of metoprolol-associated arthralgia, most with negative serological tests for collagenases, have been reported to the FDA (284[C]).

Muscle cramps have been reported in patients taking β-blockers with partial agonist activity (285[C]); it has been suggested (286[C]) that this might be a β_2-partial agonist effect, although this has not subsequently been supported (287[C]).

Sexual function Uncontrolled studies of the effect of β-adrenoceptor antagonists on sexual function have often shown a high incidence of absence of erections, reduced potency, and reduced libido (288[C]). Several large controlled trials in hypertension and ischemic heart disease have provided more exact information. A single-blind comparison of placebo and propranolol in the treatment of mild hypertension in over 3000 men showed that although impotence was not reported as an adverse effect more often in the active treatment group at either 12 weeks or 2 years of therapy, impotence was a cause of withdrawal of therapy, significantly more often in the propranolol than the placebo group (147[C]). Similarly, in another large-scale prospective placebo-controlled study, reduced sexual activity was an adverse effect of sufficient severity to lead to the withdrawal of some patients in the propranolol-treated group (289[C]). In the TOMHS study the incidence of difficulty in obtaining and maintaining an erection over 48 months was 16.5% in placebo-treated patients and 17.3% in acebutolol-treated patients, a difference that was not statistically significant (216[C]). In the TIAM study (290[C]), a randomized placebo-controlled study lasting 6 months, atenolol did not cause a significant increase in erectile problems in men (11%; 95% CI 2—

20%) compared with placebo (3%; 0–9%). Loss of libido and difficulty in sustaining an erection can even be reproduced in young healthy volunteers (291[C]); although these effects may be more common with lipophilic drugs, such as propranolol (292[C]) and pindolol (293[C]), they have also been reported with atenolol (294[C]).

Peyronie's disease This fibrotic condition of the penis has been associated with β-blockers, such as propranolol (295[C]) or metoprolol (296[C]), as well as with labetalol (297[C]). However, 100 consecutive cases of Peyronie's disease included only five men who had taken a β-blocker before the onset of the condition (298[R]); the authors concluded that the syndrome was likely to be associated with chronic degenerative arterial disease and not with β-adrenoceptor antagonists.

Immunological and hypersensitivity reactions *Antinuclear antibodies* in high titers were detected in a number of patients with the practolol oculomucocutaneous syndrome. Tests in patients taking acebutolol (299[C], 300[C]) and celiprolol (301[c]) have also shown a high frequency of antinuclear antibodies. Positive lupus erythematosus cell preparations have been observed in patients taking acebutolol (300[C]).

The *lupus-like syndrome* was part of the practolol syndrome and has also been attributed to pindolol (302[C]), acebutolol (303[R], 304[R]), propranolol (305[C]), atenolol (SEDA-16, 194), and labetalol (306[C]). However, apart from practolol, it seems to be very rare during treatment with β-adrenoceptor antagonists.

Anaphylactic reactions have been attributed to β-adrenoceptor antagonists only very infrequently (307[C]). However, it appears that anaphylactic reactions precipitated by other agents may be particularly severe in patients taking β-blockers, especially non-selective drugs, and may require higher-than-usual doses of adrenaline for treatment (308[CR], 309[CR], 310[C], 311[r]). The view that allergy skin testing or immunotherapy is inadvisable in such patients (312[CR]) has been disputed, bearing in mind the low incidence of this adverse effect (313[r]).

Risk situations Untreated *congestive heart failure secondary to systolic pump failure* is an absolute contraindication to the use of β-adrenoceptor antagonists. Patients in frank or incipient heart failure have reduced sympathetic drive to the heart and therefore acute life-threatening adverse effects may follow β-adrenoceptor blockade. This is one of the recognized potentially serious complications of using these drugs in the management of thyrotoxic crisis (314[R]). Hence, patients with congestive heart failure should have their systolic function assessed objectively before a decision is made to use β-adrenoceptor antagonists.

Second-degree or third-degree heart block is a contraindication to β-adrenoceptor blockade. If it is considered necessary for the control of dysrhythmias, a β-blocker may be given after the institution of pacing.

Acute myocardial infarction After many trials including thousands of patients it is becoming increasingly accepted that treatment of acute myocardial infarction with β-adrenoceptor antagonists may have beneficial effects. Given intravenously within 4–6 hours of the onset of the infarction they may prevent ventricular dysrhythmias and cardiac rupture (315[CR], 316[C]). When given orally during the first year after infarction, they reduce mortality by about 25% (317[R]). Since heart failure, hypotension, and bradycardia are complications both of myocardial infarction and of β-adrenoceptor blockade, it might be assumed that these effects would be seen more commonly when the two are combined. However, reviews of the relevant studies (318[C], 319[R], 320[C]–327[C]) do not suggest that β-adrenoceptor antagonists, given after acute myocardial infarction either acutely intravenously or for secondary prophylaxis, increase the incidence of adverse effects or the risk of any particular adverse effect. Nevertheless, it must be recognized that patients were rigorously selected for inclusion in these trials; less careful decisions to treat may carry increased risks.

Bronchial asthma β-Adrenoceptor antagonists should not, as pointed out above, be given to patients with bronchial asthma or obstructive airways disease unless there are no other treatment alternatives, because of the risk of precipitating bronchospasm resistant to bronchodilators. If used, cardioselective drugs should be chosen in the lowest possible dosages and in conjunction with a β_2-adrenoceptor agonist, such as salbutamol or terbutaline, to minimize bronchoconstriction.

Stress It is now recognized that some common activities, such as mental effort (328[C]), cigarette smoking, and coffee drinking (329[C], 330[C]), may produce stress associated with increased adrenaline secretion. In the presence of a non-selective β-adrenoceptor antagonist a marked diastolic pressor response may result from mechanisms identical to those described above in the hypoglycemic diabetic patient. This effect may be attenuated with a cardioselective drug (329[C]). Theoretically, frequent rises in diastolic blood pressure associated with smoking whilst taking a non-selective β-adrenoceptor antagonist could be harmful; in a patient with ischemic heart disease or hypertension a cardioselective drug might offer advantages. There is no evidence of differences in morbidity or mortality in patients taking non-selective and cardioselective agents, but it has recently been pointed out that both the MRC and IPPPSH trials of mild hypertension showed increases in the incidence of coronary events in patients taking β-adrenoceptor antagonists who were also cigarette smokers (331[R]). This may be explained by an inhibitory effect of cigarette smoking on the metabolism of β-adrenoceptor blockers, which are metabolized by the liver, reducing their effectiveness (332[C]).

Insulin-treated diabetes β-Adrenoceptor antagonists may mask the symptoms of hypoglycemia, result in an adrenaline-mediated rise in diastolic blood pressure, and delay the return of blood glucose concentrations to normal. These effects are minimized or abolished by using a β_1-selective drug and this type of drug should always be used in preference to a non-selective drug in insulin-treated diabetes.

Renal impairment The hydrophilic drugs atenolol and sotalol are eliminated largely unchanged in the urine; with deteriorating renal function their half-lives can be prolonged as much as ten-fold (333[C], 334[C]). Other β-adrenoceptor antagonists, e.g. acebutolol and metoprolol, have active metabolites that may accumulate (335[R]). Massive retention of the metabolite propranolol gluconate has also been reported in patients with renal failure taking long-term oral propranolol (336[C]); this metabolite is deconjugated, and unchanged propranolol concentrations may be significantly increased in these patients. Thus, in a patient with a low creatinine clearance, either dosage adjustment or a change of β-adrenoceptor antagonist may be necessary.

Anaphylaxis β-Blockers may make anaphylactic reactions more difficult to diagnose and treat (311[r]). Even patients with spontaneous attacks of angioedema or urticaria may be at risk when given β-blockers (337[R]).

Withdrawal effects Interest in the possible effects of the sudden withdrawal of β-adrenoceptor antagonists followed a 1975 report of two deaths and four life-threatening complications of coronary artery disease within 2 weeks of withdrawal of propranolol (338[C]). Subsequent analyses did not always confirm these findings (339[C], 340[C]), and it has not been easy to distinguish between natural progression and deterioration caused by drug discontinuation under such circumstances. However, a recent case-control study in hypertensive patients showed a relative risk of 4.5 (95% CI 1.1—18.5) associated with recent withdrawal of β-blockers and the development of myocardial infarction or angina (341[C]).

The symptoms attributed to the sudden withdrawal of β-adrenoceptor antagonists (severe exacerbation of angina pectoris, acute myocardial infarction, sudden death, malignant tachycardia, sweating, palpitation, and tremor) could be consistent with transient adrenergic hypersensitivity. Unequivocal signs of rebound hypersensitivity have been observed after drug withdrawal in patients with ischemic heart disease (342[C]), but not in hypertensive patients (343[C]—345[C]). The density of β-adrenoceptors on human lymphocyte membranes increased by 40% during treatment with propranolol for 8 days (346[C]) and hypersensitivity to isoprenaline can be shown in hypertensive patients after the discontinuation of different β-adrenoceptor antagonists, including propranolol (347[C]), metoprolol (348[C]), and atenolol (349[C]). This hypersensitivity occurs within 2 days of drug withdrawal, may persist for up to 14 days, and is presumed to reflect the upregulation of β-adrenoceptors that occurs with prolonged treatment. This phenomenon is said to be diminished by gradual withdrawal of therapy and by the use of drugs with partial agonist activity, such as pindolol (350[C]). Whether this is directly relevant to the effects of the sudden withdrawal of β-adrenoceptor antagonists in patients with ischemic heart disease is still speculative.

Current information suggests that discontinuation of β-adrenoceptor antagonists, particularly in patients with ischemic heart disease, should be accomplished by gradual dosage reduction over 10—14 days, but there is some evidence that abrupt withdrawal of long-acting β-blockers may protect against the development of the β-blocker withdrawal syndrome (351[C]). However, even gradual withdrawal may not always prevent rebound (352[C]).

Second-generation effects *Pregnancy* Great concern at one time accompanied the increasing use of β-adrenoceptor antagonists in pregnancy, particularly in the management of hypertension. On theoretical grounds β-adrenoceptor antagonists might be expected to increase uterine contractions, impair placental blood flow, cause intrauterine growth retardation, accentuate fetal and neonatal distress, and increase the risk of neonatal hypoglycemia and perinatal mortality. The literature is replete with anecdotal reports describing such complications and attributing them to treatment with β-adrenoceptor antagonists, often propranolol. However, many of the adverse effects listed above are also potential complications of hypertension in pregnancy, and in the absence of a properly controlled trial of therapy, definite conclusions of cause and effect have been impossible on the basis of these anecdotes alone.

Many of the fears expressed were set aside when a double-blind, randomized, placebo-controlled trial of atenolol in pregnancy-associated hypertension in 120 women (352[C]) showed that: babies in the placebo group had a higher morbidity; atenolol reduced the occurrence of respiratory distress syndrome; intrauterine growth retardation and neonatal hypoglycemia and hyperbilirubinemia were equally common in the treated and placebo groups. Although bradycardia was more common with atenolol, it appeared to have no deleterious consequences.

It is currently reasonable to consider that β-adrenoceptor antagonists may be used in pregnancy without serious risks, provided patients are kept under careful clinical observation. Since all β-adrenoceptor antagonists cross the placenta freely, major differences in effects or toxicity among the various drugs are unlikely, and in a review of β-blockers in pregnancy it was concluded that no single β-blocker is superior (353[CR]).

Lactation The list of β-adrenoceptor antagonists that have been detected in breast milk includes atenolol (354[C]), acebutolol and its active *N*-acetyl metabolite (355[C]), metoprolol (356[C]), nadolol (357[C]), oxprenolol and timolol (358[C]), propranolol (359[C]), and sotalol (360[C]). Most authors have concluded that the estimated daily infant dose derived from breast feeding is likely to be too low to produce untoward effects in the suckling infant, and indeed such effects were not noted in the above cases. However, in the case of acebutolol it was considered that clinically important amounts of drug could be transferred after increasing plasma concentrations were noted in two breast-fed infants.

Overdosage The increasing use of β-adrenoceptor antagonists appears to have resulted in more frequent reports of severe high-dose intoxication (361[R], 362[R]), in which β-adrenoceptor antagonists are often taken in combination with sedatives or alcohol. There may be a very short latency from intake of the drug until fulminant symptoms occur (363[C]). The clinical features seem well established. Cardiovascular suppression results in bradycardia, heart block, and congestive heart failure, and intraventricular conduction abnormalities are common (364[C]). Ventricular tachycardias with sotalol intoxication may reflect its Class III antidysrhythmic properties, leading to prolongation of the QT_c interval (365[C]). Bronchospasm and occasionally hypoglycemia can also occur. Coma and epileptiform seizures are frequently seen (364[C], 366[C]) and may not be secondary to circulatory changes. The outcome is seldom fatal, but it can be, and 16 fatal cases of intoxication with talinolol (which is β_1-selective) have been described. Deaths have also occurred with metoprolol and acebutolol. Acebutolol has membrane-stabilizing activity, and it has been suggested that drugs with this property carry greater risk when taken in overdose (367[R]). Lipid solubility influences the rate of CNS penetration of a drug, and overdosage with highly lipophilic drugs, such as oxprenolol and propranolol, has been associated with rapid loss of consciousness and coma (368[C], 369[R], 370[C]).

Treatment should include isoprenaline (although massive doses may be required), glucagon, and atropine. If a β_1-selective antagonist has been taken, isoprenaline may reduce diastolic blood pressure by its unopposed vasodilator effect on β_2-adrenoceptors (371[C]). The β_1-selective agonist dobutamine may be preferable in such patients (372[C]). A temporary transvenous pacemaker should be inserted if significant heart block or bradycardia occur. Seizures in overdose with a β-adrenoceptor antagonist respond poorly to diazepam and barbiturates; they may require muscle relaxants and artificial ventilation. In general, the lipid-soluble drugs are highly protein bound with a large apparent volume of distribution; forced diuresis or hemodialysis are therefore unlikely to be of use.

Interactions Drug interactions with β-adrenoceptor antagonists can be pharmacokinetic or pharmacodynamic (366[C], 373[R], 374[C], 375[R]).

Pharmacokinetic interactions These include interactions in which the absorption of a β-adrenoceptor antagonist is altered by *aluminium hydroxide*, *ampicillin* and *food*; these interactions are of doubtful clinical relevance.

β-Adrenoceptor antagonists that are cleared predominantly by the liver (e.g. propranolol, oxprenolol, metoprolol, and timolol) are more likely to participate in drug interactions involving changes in liver blood flow, hepatic drug metabolism, or both. Thus, *enzyme--inducing drugs*, such as *phenobarbital* and *rifampicin*, increase the clearance of drugs such as propranolol and metoprolol and reduce their systemic availability (376[C], 377[C]). Similarly, the H_2-receptor antagonist *cimetidine* increases the systemic availability of propranolol, labetalol, and metoprolol by inhibiting hepatic mono-oxygenase systems (378[C], 379[C], 380[CR], 381[R]). *Chlorpromazine* also inhibits the metabolism of propranolol (382[C], 383[C]). The disposition of drugs with high extraction ratios, such as propranolol and metoprolol, is also affected by changes in liver blood flow, and this may be the mechanism by which hydralazine reduces the first-pass clearance of oral propranolol and metoprolol (384[C]).

Lipophilic β-adrenoceptor antagonists are metabolized to varying degrees by oxidation by liver microsomal cytochrome P-450 (e.g. propranolol by CYP1A2 and CYP2D6 and metoprolol by CYP2D6). They may therefore reduce the clearance and increase the steady-state plasma concentrations of other drugs undergoing similar metabolism, potentiating their effects. Drugs that may interact in this way include: *theophylline* (385[C]), *thioridazine* (386[C]), *chlorpromazine* (387[C]), *warfarin* (388[C]), *diazepam* (389[C]), *isoniazid* (390[C]), and *flecainide* (391[C]). These interactions are most likely to be of clinical significance when the affected drug has a variable therapeutic ratio, e.g. theophylline or warfarin.

β-Blockers can also affect the clearance from the plasma of other drugs by altering hepatic blood flow. This occurs when propranolol is co-administered with *lidocaine* (392[C]), but it appears that this interaction is due more to inhibition of enzyme activity than to a reduction in hepatic blood flow (393[C]). Atenolol inhibits the clearance of *disopyramide*, but the mechanism is unknown (394[C]). Conversely, *quinidine* doubles propranolol plasma concentrations in extensive but not poor metabolizers (395[C]) and *oral contraceptives* increase metoprolol plasma concentrations (396[C]).

Pharmacodynamic interactions These can be predicted from the pharmacology of β-adrenoceptor antagonists. Thus, the antihypertensive effect of β-blockers may be impaired by the concurrent administration of some *non-steroidal anti-inflammatory drugs* (NSAIDs), possibly because of inhibition of the synthesis of renal vasodilator prostaglandins. This interaction is probably common to all β-blockers, but may not occur with all NSAIDs; for example, *sulindac* appears to affect blood pressure less than indomethacin (397[C], 398[R], 399[CR]).

The bradycardia produced by *digoxin* may be enhanced by β-adrenoceptor antagonists. *Neostigmine* enhances vagal activity and may also aggravate bradycardia (400[C]).

The negative inotropic effect of Class I antidysrhythmic agents, such as *quinidine*, *procainamide*, *tocainide*, and *disopyramide*, may be accentuated; this is most pronounced in patients with pre-existing myocardial disease and can result in left ventricular failure or even asystole (401[C]). The apparent interaction between sotalol and *thiazide*-induced hypokalemia resulting in *torsade de pointes* has already been mentioned.

The hypertensive crisis that may follow the withdrawal of *clonidine* may be accentuated in the presence of β-blockers. It has also been reported that when β-blockers are used in conjunction with *drugs that cause arterial vasoconstriction* they may have a synergistic effect on peripheral perfusion which may be hazardous. Thus, combining β-blockers with *ergot alkaloids*, as has been recommended for the treatment of migraine, may cause severe peripheral ischemia and even tissue necrosis (402[C]).

Anesthesia The hypotensive effects of *halothane* and *barbiturates* may be exaggerated by β-adrenoceptor antagonists. However, they are not contraindicated in anesthesia, provided the anesthetist is aware of what the patient is taking.

The interaction with *calcium antagonists* is discussed below.

DIFFERENCES AMONG β-ADRENOCEPTOR ANTAGONISTS

Although there are now many different β-adrenoceptor antagonists, and the number is still increasing, there are only a few important characteristics that distinguish them in terms of their physicochemical and pharmacological properties: lipid solubility, cardioselectivity, partial agonist activity, and membrane-stabilizing activity. The characteristics of the currently available compounds are shown in Table 1.

Lipid solubility (403[R]) Lipid solubility determines the extent to which a drug partitions between an organic solvent and water. Propranolol, oxprenolol, metoprolol, and timolol are the most lipid-soluble β-adrenoceptor antagonists, and atenolol, nadolol, and sotalol are the most water-soluble; acebutolol and pindolol occupy intermediary positions (404[C]). The more lipophilic drugs are extensively metabolized in the gut-wall and liver (first-pass metabolism). This first-pass clearance is variable and may result in 20-fold differences in plasma drug concentrations between patients taking a fixed dose. It also produces susceptibility to drug interactions with agents that alter hepatic drug metabolism, e.g. cimetidine, and may result in altered kinetics and hence drug response in patients with hepatic disease, particularly cirrhosis. Lipid-soluble drugs pass the blood—brain barrier more readily (153[C]) and may be more likely to cause adverse CNS effects, but the evidence for this is not very convincing (see above).

In contrast, water-soluble drugs are cleared more slowly from the body by the kidneys. They will therefore tend to accumulate in patients with renal disease and adverse effects may result. They do not interact with drugs that affect hepatic metabolism and gain access to the brain less readily.

Cardioselectivity (405[R]) Cardioselectivity, or more properly β_1-receptor selectivity, is the term used to indicate that there are at least two types of β-adrenoceptors, and that whilst some drugs are non-selective (i.e. they are competitive antagonists at both β_1- and β_2-adrenoceptors), others appear to be more selective antagonists at β_1-adrenoceptors, which are predominantly found in the heart. Bronchial tissue, peripheral blood vessels, the uterus, and pancreatic β-cells contain principally β_2-adrenoceptors. Thus, cardioselective β-adrenoceptor antagonists, such as atenolol and metoprolol, might offer theoretical benefits to patients with bronchial asthma, peripheral vascular disease, and diabetes mellitus. As already indicated, cardioselective drugs are less likely to produce adverse effects in patients with obstructive airways disease and Type I diabetes than non-selective drugs. However, benefits in patients with Raynaud's phenomenon or intermittent claudication have been difficult to prove. Because of vascular sparing, cardioselective agents may also be preferable in stress when adrenaline is released. At present, however, hypoglycemia in Type I diabetics is the only clinical problem in which cardioselectivity is considered important. Any potential advantages of cardioselective drugs in minimizing adverse effects apply only at low dosages, since cardioselectivity is known to be dose-dependent.

Partial agonist activity (406[R], 407[C]) Partial agonist activity is the property whereby a molecule occupying the β-adrenoceptor exercises agonist effects of its own at the same time as it competitively inhibits the effects of other extrinsic agonists. Thus, drugs with this property, such as oxprenolol, acebutolol, practolol and pindolol, may produce less resting bradycardia. It has also been claimed that they cause less of an increase in airways resistance in asthmatics, less reduction in cardiac output and consequently congestive heart failure, and fewer adverse effects in patients with cold hands, Raynaud's phenomenon, or intermittent claudication: however, none of these advantages has been convincingly demonstrated in clinical practice, and patients with bronchial asthma or incipient heart failure must be considered at risk with this type of compound. Drugs with partial agonist activity may produce tremor. Drugs that combine β_1-antagonism or partial agonism with β_2-agonism (celiprolol, dilevalol, labetalol, pindolol) or α-antagonism (labetalol, carvedilol) have been developed (408[R]). Both of these classes have significant peripheral vasodilating effects. Drugs with significant agonist activity at β_1-receptors have poor antihypertensive properties (409[CR]).

Membrane-stabilizing activity Drugs with membrane-stabilizing activity reduce the rate of rise of the cardiac action potential and have other electrophysiological effects. Membrane-stabilizing activity has only been shown in human cardiac muscle in vitro in concentrations of 100 times greater than those produced by therapeutic doses (410[C]). Thus, it is likely to be of clinical relevance only if large overdoses are taken.

INDIVIDUAL β-ADRENOCEPTOR ANTAGONISTS

Certain characteristics of individual β-adrenoceptor antagonists have been delineated during the general discussion; the notes which follow are only supplementary.

Acebutolol

Acebutolol is sometimes cited as being cardioselective, but it has considerable effects on bronchioles and peripheral blood vessels. Patients taking acebutolol commonly develop antinuclear antibodies (299[C], 300[C]). A case of bronchiolitis obliterans has been reported (411[C]) as well as six cases of reversible hepatitis (412[C]).

Atenolol

Although atenolol is generally regarded as one of the safest β-blockers, severe adverse effects are occasionally reported. These include profound hypotension after a single oral dose (413[C]), organic brain syndrome (414[C]), cholestasis (415[C]), and cutaneous vasculitis (416[C]).

Bevantolol

This cardioselective β-blocker may have a higher incidence of fatigue, headache, and dizziness than atenolol or propranolol (417[C], 418[C]).

Bisoprolol

This is a highly selective β_1-antagonist. It may increase serum triglycerides and reduce HDL cholesterol (419[R]). Its adverse effect profile is similar to that of atenolol (420[C]), and despite theoretical advantages there is no convincing clinical evidence that this drug has any benefit over atenolol (421[C]).

Carvedilol

Carvedilol is a non-selective β-adrenoceptor blocker with α_1-blocking action, promoting peripheral vasodilatation. In addition, it also has free radical scavenging and antimitogenic effects. As with other α_1-blockers, postural hypotension is quite common, especially in elderly people (422[R]). In a comparison of carvedilol with pindolol in elderly patients, postural hypotension occurred even with small doses (12.5 mg) of carvedilol (423[C]). The authors concluded that lower starting doses should be used in elderly people, in patients taking diuretics, and in patients with heart failure.

Celiprolol

Celiprolol is a β_1-selective antagonist with partial β_2-agonist activity. In healthy volunteers it was reported to cause 'particularly unpleasant' subjective adverse effects, including headache, sleepiness, and feeling cold and generally unwell (424[C]). However, it has beneficial effects on lipids, reducing total cholesterol by 6% and low density lipoproteins by 10% (SEDA-17, 235). Whether this will translate into clinical benefit is not known, but at present no convincing advantages over other β-blockers have been demonstrated (138[R]).

There has been a report of hypersensitivity pneumonitis secondary to celiprolol (425[c]).

Dilevalol

Dilevalol is one of the four enantiomers of labetalol. It was withdrawn from the market by its manufacturers in early 1991 because of an unacceptably high incidence of liver damage (426[r]).

Esmolol

Esmolol is a β_1-selective agent with an extremely short half-life (about 10 min) because of extensive metabolism by esterases in blood, liver, and other tissues. It causes hypotension, sometimes symptomatic, in up to 44% of patients (427[R], 428[C]—430[C]). It has been reported to increase digoxin concentrations by 10—20% in healthy volunteers, and co-administration with morphine resulted in increased steady-state concentrations of esmolol (431[Cr]).

Irritation at the infusion site occurs in up to 9% of patients and relates to the duration of the infusion (432[R]).

Labetalol

Labetalol is an α- and β_1-adrenoceptor antagonist. It appears to be less likely to increase airways resistance in patients with bronchial asthma or to reduce peripheral blood flow. However, it may produce dose-dependent postural hypotension, and paresthesia of the scalp and perioral numbness have been described. Antinuclear and antimitochondrial antibodies develop not uncommonly during long-term administration (433[r]). In addition, 11 cases of hepatotoxicity have been reported in patients taking labetalol (434[C]). Two children developed a proximal myopathy and rhabdomyolysis, which resolved on stopping the drug (435[C]). Three cases of severe hyperkalemia have been reported in renal transplant recipients taking labetalol for acute hypertension (436[C]).

Labetalol has a high transplacental transfer rate. A single 30 mg intravenous dose administered to a woman with severe pregnancy-related hypertension 20 minutes before Cesarean section was associated with significant neonatal β-adrenoceptor blockade (hypoglycemia, bradycardia, and hypotension), and high labetalol concentrations were found in the umbilical cord blood (150—180 ng/ml) (437[C]). In a similar case, an infant was born dead to a woman given 50 mg of intravenous labetalol, which lowered her blood pressure from 170/110 to 115/85 mmHg before surgery (438[C]). In another case, neonatal cardiac arrest was precipitated (439[c]). Oral labetalol is well tolerated in pre-eclampsia, but if intravenous treatment is necessary a small dose (5—10 mg) should be used initially and titrated up as necessary.

Metoprolol

Metoprolol administration was associated with hepatitis, which reappeared on rechallenge, in a patient who was a poor metabolizer (440[C]). A metoprolol-induced polymyalgia-like syndrome (441[C]) has also been described. A modified-release formulation of metoprolol has been associated with more skin reactions, probably due to the succinate component instead of the tartrate component used in the old fast-acting formulation (SEDA-16, 195).

Pindolol

Because of its partial agonist activity, and β_2-receptor stimulating action (442[C]), pindolol may produce resting tremor in some patients.

Practolol

Although practolol has long been withdrawn from general oral use (because of the oculomucocutaneous syndrome and sclerosing peritonitis), it is still available for intravenous administration in some countries. The practolol syndrome included a psoriasiform rash, xerophthalmia due to lachrymal gland fibrosis, secretory otitis media, fibrinous peritonitis, and a lupus-like syndrome. The pathogenesis of this adverse effect remains unknown, but it appears to have been unique to practolol.

Propranolol

Propranolol has been implicated in hypersensitivity pneumonitis (443[Cr], 444[C]), although other β-blockers have also been associated with this.

Sotalol

As discussed above, sotalol has Class III antidysrhythmic action and may predispose to *torsade de pointes* (78[R]), sustained ventricular tachycardia, and cardiac arrest, especially in those taking 160 mg of sotalol a day or more (SEDA-16, 191). In a recent review it was concluded that *torsade de pointes* is also more likely in patients with depressed left ventricular function and a history of sustained ventricular tachydysrhythmias (445[R]). In the US, the manufacturer's recommendations include initiating therapy in a setting in which the patient can be monitored.

Timolol *(see also Chapter 47)*

The development of liver tumors in mice and an increased incidence of mammary fibroadenomata in female rats at one time caused concern in the US, although animal studies elsewhere and clinical studies have shown no evidence of tumor-forming potential.

Organic nitrates

Drugs of this group have been in use for over 100 years and their adverse effects are therefore well documented. Nitrates have been produced in many chemical forms, but the current choice lies between the rapid-onset, short-acting glyceryl trinitrate (nitroglycerin) and the longer-acting isosorbide mononitrate and isosorbide dinitrate. Nitrates can be administered by various routes. For example, glyceryl trinitrate is used not only as traditional sublingual tablets but also in the form of modified-release tablets, buccal tablets, aerosolized oral spray, intravenous injection, and topical ointment or skin patches intended for percutaneous absorption (446[R]). These different formulations have been developed largely as a means of controlling the onset and duration of action of glyceryl trinitrate, since in conventional oral form its duration of action is severely limited by marked hepatic first-pass metabolism. The toxicity of the nitrates is unaffected by the chemical form or by the route of administration and so they can all be considered as a single group.

ADVERSE REACTION PATTERN

Toxic reactions Generalized vasodilatation predictably produces mild adverse effects commonly. These include headache, flushing, and palpitation, which are most often experienced during the early treatment period and to which a degree of tolerance invariably occurs. More severe adverse effects, including syncope, transient cerebral ischemic attacks, and peripheral edema, are less common. Sublingual glyceryl trinitrate tablets produce a characteristic local burning or tingling sensation. Adverse cardiac effects may follow abrupt withdrawal of treatment after long-term exposure or high-dose therapy.

Hypersensitivity reactions Contact irritation and allergic contact dermatitis may follow the use of cutaneous glyceryl trinitrate in ointment or skin patches, and may be attributed to the drug itself or an inactive excipient such as an adhesive agent.

Tumor-inducing effects No excess risk of cancer has been demonstrated in a historical cohort study involving 2023 male fertilizer workers exposed to industrial nitrates at work in Norway during 1945–79 (447[C]).

ORGANS AND SYSTEMS

Cardiovascular *Hypotension* is a frequent adverse effect of nitrate therapy (448[C]), resulting from dilatation of arteries and veins. It may be associated with *reflex tachycardia* and *palpitation*, and even *syncope* on assuming an upright posture. It occurs particularly in old people, especially those with recurrent falls (SEDA-16, 196), and more commonly with the oral glyceryl trinitrate spray than with sublingual tablets, because of its faster onset of action (449[r]). It tends to occur more commonly in those who take nitrates infrequently. Alternatively *bradycardia* may accompany hypotension or syncope (450[C], 451[C], 452[Cr]), presumably due to a vagal effect (it is responsive to atropine); complete heart block has also been reported (453[C]). Occasionally, similar events can occur in patients without ischemic heart disease (454[CR]), suggesting a mechanism similar to vasovagal syncope or coronary artery spasm (455[C], 456[C]) rather than a coronary steal. Nitrates can precipitate myocardial infarction in susceptible patients (457[C]), and occasionally they can worsen myocardial infarction, producing asystole (458[C]) or ventricular fibrillation (459[C], 460[C]), possibly due to coronary steal or reperfusion of ischemic myocardium.

In one case a small explosion occurred when a patient

was defibrillated with the paddle placed over a glyceryl trinitrate patch (461[C]). The authors felt that this was probably due to arcing of the electrical current from the aluminium backing of the patch, but they advised that patches and gel should be removed before defibrillation.

Throbbing headache as a result of dilatation of cerebral vessels (462[R], 463[R]) is common, although it often recedes as tolerance develops. The once-a-day modified-release formulations of oral isosorbide mononitrate are particularly likely to cause headache on first exposure and have accounted for premature withdrawal in about 1% of cases in some trials (464[C], 465[C]).

Peripheral edema occurred in patients treated for left ventricular failure with isosorbide dinitrate (466[C]). This disappeared on withdrawal of treatment. The mechanism is unclear, in common with fluid retention reported with other vasodilators.

Organic nitrates should be used with caution in patients with hypertrophic obstructive cardiomyopathy, as they reduce afterload and venous return, which may exacerbate intraventricular obstruction and reduce left ventricular filling (SEDA-16, 196).

Respiratory Transient hypoxemia may complicate the use of glyceryl trinitrate and has been described after sublingual (467[C]) and intravenous administration (468[r]). In patients with ischemic heart disease this may result in a paradoxical response, with further angina pectoris and ST segment depression on the ECG (467[C]). A possible explanation is vasodilatation of pulmonary arteries, leading to relative hypoventilation in some areas of the lungs, and it may be especially common and troublesome when glyceryl trinitrate is being tried for pulmonary hypertensive disease (468[R], 470[R]).

Nervous system *Transient cerebral ischemic attacks*, unrelated to blood pressure changes, have been described with isosorbide dinitrate and glyceryl trinitrate ointment in a patient with previous cerebrovascular disease; they disappeared on discontinuation of therapy (471[C]). Such changes may be more frequent than is realized and, added to the risk of hypotension, suggest that nitrates should be used with great caution in patients with cerebrovascular disease.

Isosorbide mononitrate precipitated pituitary apoplexy in a patient with an unsuspected pituitary macroadenoma (472[C]). In an elderly woman isosorbide dinitrate caused visual hallucinations and subsequent suicidal ideation, thought to be due to hypotension and cerebral ischemia (473[C]). Intracranial hypertension associated with glyceryl trinitrate has also been reported and attributed to cerebral vasodilatation (474[C]). However, it may occasionally be a consequence of hyperosmolality, hemolysis, and lactic acidosis caused by the excipient ethylene glycol used with intravenous isosorbide dinitrate. The risk of this may be greatest in patients with renal impairment (475[C]).

Hematological *Methemoglobinemia* has been reported after overdosage of sublingual glyceryl trinitrate (476[C]). However, it does not occur with normal doses, and prolonged intravenous infusion (up to 128 μg/min) was not associated with pathological concentrations of methemoglobin (477[C]). Even higher mean infusion rates (290 μg/min) (478[C]), or occasionally lower rates in a patient with reduced drug clearance (479[C]), may result in higher methemoglobin concentrations and could conceivably cause a clinical problem, although recovery is rapid after injection of methylene blue (480[R]).

Organic nitrates inhibit platelet aggregation in response to a wide variety of stimuli and prolong bleeding time.

Skin and appendages In a multicenter comparison of two transdermal nitrate delivery systems there were skin problems at the application site in 20—39% of cases (481[C]).

Allergic *contact dermatitis* has been reported with the use of an ointment containing glyceryl trinitrate (482[C]), and its development should be suspected if persistent erythema, vesicles, papules, hyperpigmentation, or edema follow the use of such formulations. Allergy may be due to the drug itself or to an excipient in the ointment base. However, erythema and pruritus produced by glyceryl trinitrate ointment may also result from the pharmacological action of the drug. The use of transdermal nitrate patches has also resulted in allergic contact dermatitis which, after testing, has been attributed both to the active drug (483[C]) and to an inactive component of the delivery system or adhesive (484[Cr]).

A causal relation between *rosacea* and the facial flushing seen with vasodilators such as glyceryl trinitrate seems probable (485[C]).

An unusual *skin burn* resulted from the application of a glyceryl trinitrate transdermal patch in a patient who was subsequently exposed to radiation that leaked from a damaged microwave oven. The patient sustained a second-degree burn of the size and shape of his skin patch, probably due to a reaction with a metallic element in the adhesive strip (486[C]).

Increased frequency of *dental caries* with the use of buccal glyceryl trinitrate formulations have been reported in Sweden (SEDA-17, 237).

Special senses *Taste* Glyceryl trinitrate in sublingual tablets cause a burning sensation under the tongue, an indication of the activity of the formulation. Altered and later absent taste sensation developed in a patient taking long-term transdermal glyceryl trinitrate patches. This improved on withdrawal, only to recur on rechallenge (487[C]).

Eyes On the basis of animal experiments it has been suggested that nitrates could increase intraocular pressure and should therefore not be used in the presence of glaucoma (488[C]). However, both intravenous glyceryl trinitrate and oral isosorbide dinitrate actually lower the intraocular pressure both in healthy individuals and in patients with open-angle and closed-angle glaucoma (489[C]).

Risk situations The problems that can complicate the use of nitrates in patients with *acute myocardial infarction*, severe *coronary atherosclerosis*, and *prior cerebrovascular disease* have already been stressed. *Hypotension*, *reflex tachycardia*, or *bradycardia* may all prove hazardous in individual patients.

Myocardial infarction Although meta-analysis of studies in acute myocardial infarction had suggested that nitrates protected from death and reinfarction (490[R]), the recent ISIS-4 study found no such protection at 1 month after infarction (491[C]). However, this study did demonstrate the safety and adverse effects of nitrates in suspected myocardial infarction, even though 14.2% of patients who received nitrates had heart failure. Compared with placebo-treated patients there was an excess of hypotension considered severe enough to withdraw the drug in 15 per 1000 patients; in about half the cases it occurred soon after the start of treatment; the excess risk for headache was 18.7 per 1000 and of dizziness 1.6 per 1000, 0.8 per 1000 being associated with profound hypotension. The authors concluded that nitrate therapy started early in acute myocardial infarction was safe and well tolerated but that there was no clear survival advantage.

Congestive heart failure Large studies of isosorbide dinitrate with hydralazine have shown that the combination is safe in systolic heart failure. Only headache and palpitation necessitated drug withdrawal and were more common compared with treatment with enalapril (492[C]).

A paradoxical increase in pulmonary vascular resistance has been reported after intravenous infusion of glyceryl trinitrate, and one needs to be careful when giving potent vasodilators to patients with *idiopathic pulmonary hypertension* (493[C]).

The presence of high concentrations of ethanol and glycerol in intravenous glyceryl trinitrate formulations has led to alcohol intoxication after high-dose therapy (494[Cr], 495[C], 496[C]). In one case, a 74-year-old man developed Wernicke's encephalopathy, which required treatment with intravenous thiamine after discontinuation of the glyceryl trinitrate infusion. Thus, high-dose intravenous therapy should be given with caution to patients with prior *vitamin deficiency* or a history of *alcohol abuse* (497[C]). Ethanol has also been implicated as the cause of *acute gout* in four patients with unstable angina who received intravenous infusions of glyceryl trinitrate (498[C]).

A dramatic rise in plasma glyceryl trinitrate concentrations occurred after exercise in healthy subjects following transdermal administration (499[C]). This altered systemic availability could cause adverse effects.

Withdrawal effects and tolerance Exposure to organic nitrates, e.g. in workers in the explosives industry, may result in profound vascular changes after departure from the environment (500[C]). Non-exertional ischemic cardiac pain may occur, occasionally resulting in myocardial infarction, as may peripheral ischemia, with Raynaud's phenomenon and gangrene of the extremities (501[C]). The development of tolerance to the vasodilatory effects of glyceryl trinitrate, with arterial spasm when exposure ceases, has been postulated as the mechanism (502[CR]). Tolerance may also be seen in patients who are given long-term continuous treatment with nitrates in high dosages for angina pectoris (see Introduction). Harmful withdrawal symptoms can be avoided by gradual dosage reduction, but high dosages should be avoided where possible (503[R]). Likewise, abrupt withdrawal of intravenous glyceryl trinitrate in treating patients with unstable angina precipitates further angina (SEDA-16, 196).

In a review of a transdermal nitrate system the disappointing duration of action of the formulation was ascribed to the development of tolerance (504[R]). In an assessment of how nitrate tolerance might be avoided, the efficacy of thrice-daily buccal glyceryl trinitrate and that of 4 times a day oral isosorbide dinitrate were compared (505[c]); over 2 weeks, prolonged antianginal efficacy was maintained only with thrice-daily buccal administration. None-the-less, in another study transdermal glyceryl trinitrate seemed to offer a sufficiently prolonged effect to wean patients with unstable angina from intravenous nitrate therapy (506[c]).

One possible mechanism of tolerance has been elucidated (507[CR]). Organic nitrates are converted to *S*-nitrosothiols when combined with sulfhydryl moieties in smooth muscles. These compounds activate guanylate cyclase, leading to an increase in the intracellular concentration of cyclic GMP, with resultant vascular relaxation and vasodilatation. As the supply of sulfhydryl within the smooth muscles is limited, prolonged exposure to organic nitrates results in its depletion and hence tolerance (508[R]). However other mechanisms of nitrate tolerance have been proposed, including neurohumoral adaptation and a plasma volume-dependent mechanism (509[R]). It seems likely that tolerance occurs through several mechanisms.

Interactions Severe postural hypotension has been observed in patients given both isosorbide dinitrate and *hydralazine* for chronic heart failure (451[C]), although this has not been borne out in large studies (492[C]). The combination of isosorbide dinitrate with *clonidine* also predisposes to postural hypotension (510[C]). In addition, undue dizziness or faintness has been claimed to follow the use of sublingual nitrate in patients taking the β-adrenoceptor antagonist *metoprolol* (511[Cr]).

A case of laryngeal edema has been reported with the use of isosorbide dinitrate spray followed shortly by sublingual *nifedipine* in an attempt to reduced high blood pressure (230/130 mmHg) in a 65-year-old woman who presented with coma secondary to a large intracerebral hemorrhage. The patient needed tracheal intubation. The same complication recurred when the patient was rechallenged with the same sequence of drugs (512[C]).

Complete atrioventricular block has been reported after the use of sublingual nitrates in patients receiving *lidocaine* by infusion (513[R], 514[C]) and can result in asystole. *Disopyramide*, by producing xerostomia, may prevent the dissolution of sublingual isosorbide tablets (515[R]). *Alcohol* potentiates the hypotensive effects of sublingual glyceryl trinitrate (516[C]). Finally, there have been case reports of heparin resistance associated with glyceryl trinitrate (517[C]), (SEDA-16, 196), but subsequent review of this interaction showed no clinical relevance provided heparin anticoagulation is monitored closely (518[C], 519[C]).

INDIVIDUAL ORGANIC NITRATES

The spectrum and frequency of adverse effects for the individual drugs, such as glyceryl trinitrate, isosorbide dinitrate, and isosorbide-5-mononitrate, appear to be similar. Misuse of amyl nitrite is referred to in Chapters 4 and 48.

Calcium antagonists

Several drugs are currently classified as calcium antagonists and various others are under development, such has been the impact that drugs of this group have made during the past 10 years. The main calcium antagonists currently in use are verapamil, diltiazem, and the dihydropyridines, including nifedipine, felodipine, nicardipine, nimodipine, nitrendipine, and amlodipine. Other agents, e.g. prenylamine and lidoflazine, are now rarely used, and perhexiline, having failed to reach the market at all in some countries, was withdrawn in the UK after continuing concern about its safety (520[R]). The currently used calcium antagonists are generally well tolerated.

Although chemically a heterogeneous group, many adverse effects are common to all calcium antagonists and these may be predicted from their main pharmacological actions. Calcium plays a role in the functions of contraction and conduction in the heart and in the smooth muscle of arteries; drugs that interfere with its availability (of which there are many, the calcium antagonists being the most specific) will therefore be expected to act in all these tissues. A few idiosyncratic and hypersensitivity reactions have also been reported with individual calcium antagonists.

ADVERSE REACTION PATTERN

Toxic reactions Mild reactions are relatively common. Dizziness, facial flushing, leg edema, postural hypotension, and constipation have been reported in up to one-third of patients. These are rarely severe and often diminish on continued therapy. More serious adverse effects, mainly those affecting cardiac conduction, are much less common, and only rarely is it necessary to discontinue treatment. In general the calcium antagonists are relatively safe drugs.

Hypersensitivity reactions Verapamil, nifedipine, and diltiazem have all been associated with allergic reactions, including skin eruptions and effects on liver and kidney function. Nifedipine has also been reported to cause a febrile reaction (521[CR]) and diltiazem was associated with fever, lymphadenopathy, hepatosplenomegaly, an erythematous maculopapular rash, and eosinophilia in a 50-year-old man (522[C]).

Tumor-inducing effects These have not been described.

ORGANS AND SYSTEMS

Cardiovascular *Myocardial failure* Although acute hemodynamic studies suggested that calcium antagonists might be beneficial in cardiac failure (523[C]), long-term treatment has been associated with clinical deterioration. Calcium antagonists should therefore be prescribed with caution for patients with impaired cardiac function, who should be regularly reassessed; treatment should be withdrawn if the signs or symptoms of cardiac failure appear. In some cases heart failure may be predictable, as in the case of a patient with aortic stenosis who developed left ventricular failure after treatment with nifedipine (524[C]). Increased sympathetic activity may also compensate for the myocardial suppressant effects of calcium antagonists, and the combination of these drugs (particularly verapamil) with β-adrenoceptor antagonists has therefore given cause for concern in the past (see 'Interactions'), although this combination is now considered relatively safe for the majority of patients with normal cardiac function (525[C]–527[C]).

Myocardial infarction There have been many studies of the efficacy of calcium antagonists in early and late intervention (528[C]) in myocardial infarction. These studies have failed to show convincing benefits. Indeed, in the nifedipine intervention studies there was a consistent trend towards higher mortality in the treated patients than in those taking placebo. A more recent study, in which patients were randomized to placebo or nifedipine within 48 hours of admission, was terminated after 1358 patients had been recruited, because mortality at 6 months was 15.4% on nifedipine and 13.3% on placebo (529[C]).

It has been argued that dihydropyridine calcium antagonists that increase the heart rate may all increase the risk of death and reinfarction (530[R], 531[R]). Early beneficial results with diltiazem in patients with non-Q-wave infarction (532[C]) were not confirmed in the Multicenter Diltiazem Postinfarction Trial (533[C]). In patients with pulmonary congestion, diltiazem was associated with an increase in cardiac events, and a similar result was seen in patients with low ejection fractions. Verapamil, however, does appear to reduce reinfarction (534[C]), a benefit that is more marked in those without heart failure (535[C]). Nifedipine may also have a detrimental effect in unstable angina: it certainly appears to offer no benefit (536[C]) (see under unstable angina).

A recent retrospective case-control study (537[Cr]) has sparked controversy concerning the use of short-acting calcium antagonists in treating hypertension. The study involved 623 cases of fatal and non-fatal myocardial infarction over a period of 8 years, and 2032 age- and sex-matched controls. The risk of myocardial infarction in patients taking calcium antagonists was 16 per 1000 compared with 10 per 1000 in patients taking β-blockers or thiazides. However, this result may have been an example of confounding by indication, since patients exposed to calcium antagonists will have been more likely to have had peripheral vascular disease, lung disease (a low forced expiratory volume being a risk factor for cardiovascular disease), higher serum cholesterol concentrations, and diabetes mellitus. Careful statistical analysis was carried out in an attempt to control for some of the confounding, but such confounding can only be properly controlled for in a randomized study. The current guideline of the Joint National Committee on the Detection, Evaluation and Treatment of High Blood Pressure, recommending diuretics and β-blockers as first-line agents, should continue to be followed. Pending the results of current studies, long-acting calcium antagonists may still be used if required, as the adverse effects of uncontrolled hypertension exceed the increased risk of myocardial infarction suggested by this study.

Disturbances of cardiac rhythm Calcium antagonists differ in their effects on the myocardial conduction system. Thus, both verapamil and diltiazem have significant inhibitory effects on both sinoatrial and atrioventricular nodal function, whereas nifedipine has little or no effect. Nevertheless, nifedipine can on occasion cause troublesome bradydysrhythmias (538[c], 539[C]).

Relatively harmless and asymptomatic disturbances of heart rhythm are common during treatment with verapamil. For example, Wenckebach phenomenon (Mobitz Type I second-degree atrioventricular block), sinus bradycardia and junctional escape, and accelerated junctional rhythm have been seen during the treatment of angina pectoris (540[C]). In the DAVIT II study (530[C]), 23 of 878 patients who received verapamil and seven of 897 who received placebo in a post-myocardial infarction survival study developed second- or third-degree AV block. It has been suggested that the extent of PR prolongation may be proportional to the pharmacological effect of verapamil in patients with sinus rhythm (541[C]). Patients with diseased conduction systems may develop atrioventricular block, sinoatrial block, sinus arrest, or sinus bradycardia with verapamil (542[R]).

Therapy with diltiazem can be associated with similar adverse reactions (543[CR], 544[C]). In a randomized trial of diltiazem in patients with non-Q-wave myocardial infarction, 38 of 287 patients who received diltiazem developed some degree of AV block at some time. Of these 32 were first degree, eight second degree, and only two third degree. In the placebo-treated group there were 10 events in 289 patients; eight were first degree, two second degree, and none third degree. Problems may also occur in patients with aberrant conduction pathways; for example, verapamil caused an increased ventricular response in patients with the Wolff-Parkinson-White syndrome associated with atrial fibrillation (545[C]–547[C]). The danger lies in provocation of ventricular fibrillation from advanced anterograde conduction in accessory pathways (548[C]). Severe conduction disturbances may also occur if calcium antagonists are used in hypertrophic cardiomyopathy (549[C]), but these drugs have become increasingly used in this condition (550[C]). Ventricular tachycardia associated with QT prolongation (*torsade de pointes*) has been described with prenylamine (551[C], 552[C]), but a causal relation between *torsade de pointes* and nifedipine (553[C]) has been questioned (554[C]).

There are many case reports of symptomatic *hypotension*, usually in hypertensive patients treated with large dosages of calcium antagonists (555[C], 556[C]) or in patients with myocardial infarction (557[C]). These may represent injudicious prescribing rather than true adverse drug effects. In the DAVIT II study, 1.9% of the verapamil-treated group versus 1.6% of the placebo-treated group developed hypotension or dizziness (535[C]); the figures for hypotension in a randomized study of diltiazem after infarction were 0.6% in the drug-treated group and 0.2% in the placebo-treated group (532[C]).

Ischemic chest pain This is an infrequent but well-documented adverse effect of initiating therapy with nifedipine (558[R]). Its mechanism is unclear, but it may arise from reduced overall coronary blood flow or a coronary steal phenomenon (559[Cr]). Ischemic ECG changes without pain have also been reported (560[C]).

There has been a report of *cardiovascular collapse* following uncomplicated coronary artery bypass surgery in patients taking nifedipine preoperatively (561[Cr]); the condition responded to intravenous calcium chloride in three patients and adrenaline in four.

Respiratory Adverse respiratory effects appear to be uncommon with calcium antagonists. However, three cases of acute bronchospasm accompanied by urticaria and pruritus have been reported in patients taking verapamil (562[R]), and a patient with Duchenne-type muscular dystrophy developed respiratory failure during intravenous verapamil therapy for supraventricular tachycardia (563[C]).

In *pulmonary hypertension* both verapamil and nifedipine increase mean right atrial pressure in association with hypotension, chest pain, dyspnea, and hypoxemia; the severe hemodynamic upset resulted in cardiac arrest in two patients after verapamil and death in another after nifedipine (564[CR]). A patient with pulmonary hypertension also developed pulmonary edema whilst taking nifedipine (565[C]) and another seems to have developed this as an allergic reaction (566[C]).

Nervous system *Transient cerebral ischemia* with aphasia and hemiparesis in one patient and *cerebellar dysfunction* and *loss of consciousness* in another have been observed with nifedipine (567[C]). In addition, rapidly progressive hemiparesis, aphasia, and confusion, accompanied by a substantial fall in blood pressure, occurred in a patient whose hypertension (230/136 mmHg) was treated with sublingual nifedipine (568[CR]). *Transient retinal ischemia*, which may be recurrent, has also been attributed to nifedipine (569[C], 570[Cr]). Hypotension or a steal phenomenon seem the likely mechanisms of these ischemic events involving the nervous system.

Cerebral vasodilatation might have contributed to a subarachnoid hemorrhage in a 32-year-old woman with a berry aneurysm (571[C]).

Hyperactivity has been attributed to diltiazem therapy. In one case this appeared as akathisia (572[C]), another patient showed signs and symptoms of mania (573[C]), and another developed mania with psychotic features (574[C]). There have also been reports that nifedipine can cause agitation, tremor, belligerence, and depression (575[Cr]), and that verapamil can cause toxic delirium (576[c]). Nightmares and visual hallucinations have also been associated with nifedipine (577[c]). *Depression* has also been reported as a possible adverse effect of nifedipine (578[C]).

Fasciculation occurred when a patient with background peripheral neuropathy was given verapamil (SEDA-16, 197). *Paresthesia* of hands and feet have been reported with diltiazem and nifedipine (SEDA-17, 237).

Myoclonic dystonia has been described in a 70-year-old man treated with verapamil for supraventricular tachycardia for 10 months; the abnormal movements disappeared within 3 weeks of substituting diltiazem, but rechallenge was not attempted (579[C]).

Calcium antagonists may cause *Parkinsonism*. Of 32 patients with this complication, only three patients had made a full recovery 18 months after drug withdrawal; patients under 73 years of age tended to have a better prognosis (580[CR]). It is not known if these patients would have developed Parkinsonism anyway, and whether these drugs only act as precipitants.

A patient with Lambert-Eaton syndrome and a small-cell carcinoma of the lung developed respiratory failure within hours of starting treatment with verapamil for atrial flutter, and required assisted ventilation (581[Cr]). Only after verapamil had been withdrawn did her breathing improve. Verapamil influences calcium channels in nerve membranes in animal studies, but the experimental concentrations used exceed those found in clinical practice (581[Cr]). Thus, the evidence for a drug-related effect is circumstantial. In another case, diltiazem triggered Lambert-Eaton syndrome, which improved with drug withdrawal (582[cr]). Myasthenia gravis may deteriorate with oral verapamil (583[cr]).

Endocrine, metabolic *Carbohydrate metabolism*

Calcium transport is essential for insulin secretion, which is therefore inhibited by calcium antagonists (584[CR]). Despite this, calcium antagonists generally have minimal effects on glucose tolerance in both healthy and diabetic subjects. Oral glucose tolerance is not affected by verapamil, and basal blood glucose concentrations were not altered during long-term verapamil administration (585[C]). Similarly, neither nifedipine nor nicardipine produced significant hyperglycemic effects in either diabetic or non-diabetic patients (586[C], 587[c], 588[CR]). In 117 hypertensive patients nifedipine caused a significant rise in mean random blood glucose of only 0.3 mmol/l (589[C]), an effect which was clearly of no clinical relevance. In the Treatment of Mild Hypertension Study, 4 years of monotherapy with amlodipine maleate caused no change compared with placebo in the serum glucose of 114 hypertensive patients (216[C]). In a recent review (590[R]) it was concluded that in usual dosages calcium antagonists do not alter glucose handling. However, in a few patients diabetes has been found to appear de novo or to worsen considerably on starting nifedipine (589[C], 591[C]), so that there may be a small potential risk in some individuals.

Other possible unusual adverse effects of calcium antagonists include *menorrhagia* (592[C]) and *gynecomastia* (593[c]).

Calcium antagonists have a minor inhibitory effect on aldosterone secretion (see 'Miscellaneous').

Mineral and fluid balance *Hypokalemia* associated with muscle weakness was described in a 56-year-old man after 2 weeks of nifedipine treatment for angina; the potassium concentration rose on withdrawal of therapy but fell rapidly again on rechallenge (594[CR]). Nifedipine may enhance urinary *potassium loss* in patients treated with a thiazide diuretic (595[C]), but it has no effect on adrenaline-induced hypokalemia (596[C]). In the Treatment of Mild Hypertension Study, 4 years of monotherapy with amlodipine maleate caused no change compared with placebo in the serum potassium, uric acid, aspartate aminotransferase, or creatinine of 114 hypertensive patients (216[C]).

There was a significant rise in *serum alkaline phosphatase* of skeletal origin in a group of patients treated with verapamil for hypertension. It was associated with a slight increase in parathyroid hormone, indicating involvement of bone metabolism, although there was no change in the urinary excretion of calcium, phosphate, or potassium. It has yet to be demonstrated whether verapamil causes osteopenia in man as it does in animals (SEDA-16, 197).

Hematological Hematological effects are rare. Nifedipine has been reported to cause *agranulocytosis* (597[C]) and a case of *leucopenia* was attributed to diltiazem; the latter patient had scleroderma, active rheumatoid disease, and pulmonary fibrosis, but the white cell count fell after 3 weeks of diltiazem therapy, recovered on drug withdrawal, and fell on rechallenge (598[cr]). Diltiazem has also been reported to cause *immune thrombocytopenia* in a 68-year-old man with angina (599[C]).

Liver *Mild hepatic reactions* have been observed in association with the use of verapamil, nifedipine (600[C]–603[C]), and diltiazem (604[r], 605[r]). In some instances fever, chills, and sweating have been associated with right upper quadrant pain, hepatomegaly, and mild increases in serum bilirubin and aminotransferase activity; in others, patients have remained asymptomatic. One patient had granulomatous hepatitis with diltiazem (606[C]); another had a periportal infiltrate rich in eosinophils while taking verapamil (607[C]). The increase in liver enzyme activities is generally transient, although mild persistent abnormalities have been seen. Occasionally, extreme increases in hepatic enzyme activities have been reported (598[r], 605[C]). Their frequency appears to be low, and since the symptoms and signs are mild they could easily be overlooked.

Gastrointestinal Because of their effects on smooth muscle, the calcium antagonists can cause *constipation*, particularly verapamil (608[r]) but also diltiazem. Gastroesophageal reflux is known to occur and the calcium antagonists should be avoided in patients with symptoms suggesting this (609[R]).

Urinary system Several reports have linked *renal dysfunction* with nifedipine. In a study of hypertensive diabetics with renal insufficiency it increased proteinuria and made renal function worse (SEDA-16, 196). Others have reported mild reversible renal impairment in patients with chronic renal insufficiency taking nifedipine for angina or hypertension; a biopsy in one of the patients, who had heavy proteinuria, showed focal and segmental glomerulosclerosis (610[C]). Immune-complex nephritis was reported in a patient taking nifedipine, but the proteinuria persisted (and indeed worsened) on changing to verapamil (611[C]). Diltiazem was also associated with the development of acute renal failure in a patient being treated for severe retrosternal chest pain who had neither primary kidney disease nor urinary tract obstruction (612[C]).

Nifedipine was associated with an apparent *diuresis* within a short time of the first dose in 14 of 24 patients (613[C]) and with *nocturia* which ceased or improved markedly on withdrawal of therapy in nine patients (614[C]). The latter was considered to reflect an effect of calcium channel blockade on detrusor function.

Skin and appendages Feelings of '*painful coldness*

and numbness' in the legs, in the absence of neurological deficit, have been reported with verapamil (615[C]); the symptoms disappeared with drug withdrawal and recurred with rechallenge. An *erythematous rash with painful edema* has been described with nifedipine (616[Cr]) and also with diltiazem, but without the edematous element (617[C]). Photosensitivity (618[C]) and a generalized bullous eruption (619[C]) have also been attributed to nifedipine. Mild *erythema multiforme* and the *Stevens-Johnson syndrome* have been reported as probable reactions to diltiazem (598[r]). However, apart from minor *flushing* and *leg erythema* associated with edema, skin reactions with calcium antagonists seem to be infrequent and have been estimated at 1.3% for diltiazem (620[C]). Acute generalized *exanthematous pustular dermatitis* has been reported after diltiazem (621[C]), and nifedipine, verapamil, and diltiazem have all been implicated as possible causes of *toxic epidermal necrolysis* (Lyell's syndrome) and/or *exfoliative dermatitis* from FDA data. *Psoriasiform eruptions* have been reported in patients taking verapamil and nicardipine (SEDA-16, 199).

Telangiectasia and *spider nevi* have been associated with treatment with nifedipine, and *increased hair growth* with modified-release verapamil (SEDA-17, 238).

Special senses *Dysosmia and dysgeusia* Transient disturbances of taste and smell, without other signs of neurological deficit, have been reported after nifedipine and diltiazem. The time to the onset of symptoms after nifedipine varied from days to months, and symptoms regressed within 24 hours of discontinuation (622[Cr]). With diltiazem the effect gradually diminished over 10 weeks, despite continuation of therapy (623[Cr]).

Painful eyes occurred in 14% of patients taking nifedipine compared with 9% in captopril-treated patients in a post-marketing surveillance study (624[C]). The mechanism is unknown but is not via ocular vasodilatation (625[Cr]).

Musculoskeletal Severe *muscle cramps* in the legs and hands may occur during nifedipine treatment (626[C]).

Miscellaneous *Peripheral edema* Edema of the legs is a well-recognized reaction to nifedipine therapy and it may also occur with verapamil and diltiazem (627[Cr], 628[C]). The mechanism is unclear.

Gingival hyperplasia, similar to that seen with phenytoin and ciclosporin, is a rare but well-recognized adverse effect of nifedipine (629[C]). It has also been reported in patients taking felodipine (630[C]), nitrendipine (SEDA-16, 200), and verapamil (631[C]). Only one case of gingival hyperplasia related to calcium antagonists had been reported to the Norwegian Adverse Drug Reaction Committee up to 1991, despite their widespread use (632[Cr]). However, subclinical gingival hyperplasia on tissue histology was found in 83 and 74% of patients taking nifedipine and diltiazem, respectively (633[Cr]). The reaction generally occurs within a few months of starting treatment, and drug withdrawal produces marked regression of clinical hyperplasia in some cases. The mechanism of this adverse effect is unclear, but has been proposed to involve a hormonal imbalance in the hypothalamus-pituitary-adrenal axis (634[R]). The calcium-dependent pathway of aldosterone synthesis in the zona glomerulosa is blocked by calcium antagonists, producing a negative feedback increase in pituitary secretion of ACTH, which in turn causes hyperplasia of the zona glomerulosa. This leads to increased production of androgenic steroid intermediate products and subsequently testosterone, which acts on gingival cells and matrix, giving rise to gingival hyperplasia. In a study of six hypertensive patients given nitrendipine 20 mg a day for 30 days, there was inhibition of aldosterone response but no significant change in ACTH secretion in response to corticotrophin-releasing hormone (635[C]).

Minor complaints Throbbing headache, facial warmth, and dizziness are minor complaints associated with the use of calcium antagonists. These effects are dose-related and are believed to be caused by inhibitory actions on smooth muscle (636[C]).

Risk situations Patients with *impaired function of the sinus node* or *impaired atrioventricular conduction* may develop sinus bradycardia, sinus arrest, heart block, hypotension and shock, and even asystole, with verapamil (637[C]) or diltiazem. These drugs should not be given to patients with aberrant conduction pathways associated with broad-complex tachydysrhythmias, and severe conduction disturbances may occur with their use in hypertrophic cardiomyopathy.

Similarly, verapamil should be used with caution in patients with *heart failure*, and both diltiazem and nifedipine can cause problems in patients with poor cardiac reserve. Calcium antagonists should be avoided where possible in the *peri-infarction period*.

Rapid lowering of the blood pressure with nifedipine, particularly sublingually, may precipitate cerebral ischemia with confusion, loss of consciousness, and stroke. Cases of cortical blindness with macular sparing secondary to occipital lobe infarction have been reported (SEDA-17, 238).

The use of calcium antagonists in patients with *pulmonary hypertension* (see 'Respiratory' above) has been associated with cardiac arrest and sudden death.

Caution should be exercised in using verapamil in

patients with liver cirrhosis, as its metabolism is reduced, leading to high plasma concentrations and potential toxicity (SEDA-16, 198). This also applies to patients with chronic renal insufficiency, especially those taking the modified-release formulation of verapamil (SEDA-17, 238).

Withdrawal effects The possibility of a calcium antagonist withdrawal syndrome has been raised (638[C], 639[C], 640[CR], 641[C]—647[C]), and it has been reported that withdrawal of verapamil, nifedipine, and diltiazem can worsen angina or even cause myocardial infarction. However, in a randomized double-blind study of withdrawal of nifedipine in 81 patients before coronary artery bypass surgery, angina at rest occurred only in patients who had experienced similar symptoms previously, and there were no early untoward effects of drug withdrawal (640[C]). If a withdrawal syndrome does exist, it could be due to rebound coronary vasospasm, but the present weight of evidence suggests that withdrawal results in no more than the loss of a useful therapeutic effect or the unmasking of progressive disease (647[C]).

Second-generation effects These drugs have so far had very limited use in pregnancy. The absence of reports of fetal deaths, malformations, or other maternal or neonatal adverse effects cannot therefore be construed as indicating their safety in this area. However, a comparison of nifedipine and hydralazine in 54 patients with severe pre-eclampsia showed that nifedipine is more effective, allowing delivery of more mature infants (648[CR]). Both verapamil (649[R]) and diltiazem (650[R]) are excreted in breast milk, but the risk to the suckling infant is unclear.

Overdosage The treatment of overdosage with calcium antagonists has recently been reviewed (651[R]). The features appear to be arterial hypotension, bradycardia due to sinus node depression and atrioventricular block, and congestive cardiac failure and angina (652[c]—654[c], 655[R]). Although the therapeutic effects are different according to the drug, in overdosage the effects are similar (656[cr]). Severe metabolic acidosis (usually lactic acidosis) and generalized convulsions may also occur (657[C]) and hypoglycemia has been reported (658[CR]). Non-cardiogenic pulmonary edema has been reported with diltiazem (659[Cr]). Several fatalities have now occurred with verapamil. Treatment consists of gastric lavage, activated charcoal, and cathartics. Contrary to popular belief, significant overdosage of immediate-release verapamil may be associated with delayed absorption, as suggested by a recent case report, the authors of which suggested the use of repeated doses of activated charcoal (660[Cr]). In severe cases total gut lavage should be considered. Intravenous calcium gluconate (661[cR]), glucagon (662[Cr]), pressor amines (isoprenaline, adrenaline, and dobutamine have all been tried), artificial ventilation, and cardiac pacing may all be required. Hemoperfusion does not appear to influence the clinical course, but 4-aminopyridine reversed the features of a modest accidental overdose of verapamil in a patient on maintenance hemodialysis (663[C]). The rationale for the use of aminopyridine, an antagonist of non-depolarizing neuromuscular blocking agents, supported by prior animal experiments, was the enhancement of transmembrane calcium flux and the facilitation of synaptic transmission. This is of potential interest, in view of the apparent unresponsiveness of some patients to supportive measures. An overdose of 280 mg of nifedipine produced marked vasodilatation in a young patient with advanced renal insufficiency; it was successfully treated with intravenous calcium (664[C]). Other reports have reviewed poisoning with verapamil (660[Cr], 665[C], 666[cR]) and other calcium antagonists (656[R], 667[R]).

Interactions The greatest potential for serious mishap arises from interactions between calcium antagonists (especially verapamil and related compounds) and β-adrenoceptor antagonists (668[R]). This combination may cause severe hypotension and cardiac failure, particularly in patients with poor myocardial function (669[c]—671[c]). The major risk appears to be associated with the intravenous administration of verapamil to patients who are already taking a β-blocker (672[R]), but a drug like tiapamil, which closely resembles verapamil in its pharmacological profile, might be expected to carry a similar risk (673[CR]). Conversely, intravenous diltiazem does not produce deleterious hemodynamic effects in patients treated with long-term propranolol (674[CR]).

The concurrent use of oral calcium antagonists and β-adrenoceptor antagonists in the management of angina pectoris or hypertension is less likely to result in heart block or other serious adverse effects (675[c]), and these two drug groups are now commonly used together. However, caution is still advised, and nifedipine or other dihydropyridine derivatives would be preferred in this type of combination (676[R]—678[R]). Nevertheless, the combination of nifedipine and atenolol in patients with stable intermittent claudication resulted in a reduction in walking distance and skin temperature, whereas either drug alone produced benefits (106[C]). It should also be remembered that oral verapamil may interact with topical β-blockers (679[C]).

Calcium antagonists also interact with *cardiac glycosides* (see also Chapter 17). Verapamil suppresses renal digoxin elimination acutely, but this suppression disappears over a few weeks (680[C]). However, the inhibition of the extrarenal clearance of digoxin persists, and the result of this complex interaction is an increase in plasma digoxin concentrations. As a result, patients taking both drugs should be carefully monitored. However, the effects of digoxin are apparently reduced by verapamil (681[C]), so that dosage adjustment may be unnecessary.

The interaction of digoxin with nifedipine increases plasma digoxin concentrations by only about 15% (682[C], 683[c]) and is less important. The interaction of digoxin with diltiazem increases digoxin concentrations by 20–50% (684[CR], 685[C]). Interactions of digoxin with nitrendipine (686[C]) and bepridil (687[C]) have also been described. Verapamil and diltiazem, but not nifedipine, also increase steady-state plasma *digitoxin* concentrations (688[R]).

In a review of the interactions of calcium antagonists with digoxin, in which their clinical relevance was assessed, it was concluded that serious consequences can be prevented by careful monitoring, especially in patients whose serum digoxin concentration is already near the upper end of the therapeutic range (689[R]).

Cardiovascular collapse and/or asystole has followed the use of intravenous verapamil in patients taking oral *digoxin* alone (690[C]) or in combination with *quinidine*, *propranolol*, or *disopyramide* (673[R]). Nifedipine may enhance the elimination of *quinidine* (691[C]) and result in hypotension and a loss of antidysrhythmic effect (692[c]).

An interaction of *prazosin* with nifedipine or verapamil resulted in acute hypotension (693[C], 694[c]). The mechanism appears to be partly kinetic (the systemic availability of prazosin increasing by 60%) and partly dynamic.

Theophylline toxicity has been reported in several patients, apparently stabilized on theophylline, after the introduction of verapamil (695[C]) or nifedipine (696[C]).

The H_2-receptor antagonist *cimetidine* increases plasma concentrations of nifedipine and delays its elimination by inhibition of hepatic mono-oxygenases. Maximum plasma nifedipine concentrations and AUC may be increased by as much as 80% and this results in a significant enhancement of the antihypertensive and antianginal effects of nifedipine and also toxicity (697[C], 698[C]). Cimetidine also increases plasma concentrations of nitrendipine and nisoldipine (699[C], 700[C]). Ranitidine, which inhibits the microsomal mono-oxygenase system only slightly, does not alter plasma dihydropyridine concentrations to the same extent (701[R]).

A pharmacokinetic interaction has been described between the anticonvulsant drug *carbamazepine* and the calcium antagonists verapamil (555[C]) and diltiazem (702[C]). With both drugs, inhibition of the hepatic metabolism of carbamazepine resulted in increased serum carbamazepine concentrations and neurotoxicity, with dizziness, nausea, ataxia, and diplopia. Adding nifedipine to carbamazepine was not associated with alterations in steady-state carbamazepine concentrations (703[C]). However, increased serum *phenytoin* concentrations have been reported after the introduction of nifedipine (704[C], 705[C]).

A substantial increase in the systemic availability of nifedipine occurs when either alcohol (706[C]) or citrus fruit juice is taken at the same time (707[C]).

Nine kidney transplant recipients experienced an increase in trough whole blood *ciclosporin* concentrations of 24–341% after the introduction of nicardipine (708[C]). A similar interaction has been reported with diltiazem (709[C]) but not with nifedipine.

Treatment of osteoporosis with *calcium adipinate* and *calciferol* counteracts the antidysrhythmic effect of verapamil (710[C]). The enzyme-inducing antibiotic rifampicin reduces the systemic availability of verapamil (711[C]).

Dantrolene interacts with both verapamil and diltiazem, causing myocardial depression and cardiogenic shock (SEDA-16, 199).

INDIVIDUAL CALCIUM ANTAGONISTS

Amlodipine

This long-acting calcium antagonist has an adverse effects profile similar to those of other dihydropyridines, but at a lower rate (712[R]).

Bepridil

Bepridil (see also Chapter 17) has an effect on the resting electrocardiogram, producing dose-related reduction of the sinus rate and prolongation of the QT and QT_c intervals (713[C], 714[c]). Bepridil also appears to be associated with *torsade de pointes*, commonly in association with hypokalemia (715[C]). Minor complaints, including headache, dizziness, tremor, and dyspepsia, are not uncommon, and hepatic enzymes may be increased (714[c], 716[c]).

Diltiazem

Cardiovascular Following the publication of a report of serious dysrhythmias (717[C]), further cases (junctional bradycardia, sinoatrial block) have been reported (718[C]).

Skin and appendages Two cases of cutaneous vasculitis (719[C]) and two cases of angioedema (720[C]) have been reported with diltiazem. In 1988, the Federal German Health Authorities imposed a warning of dermal hypersensitivity reactions (including erythema multiforme) with diltiazem.

Felodipine

Felodipine is a dihydropyridine derivative with diuretic properties (721[R]). Its vasodilator-related adverse effects include flushing, headache, and tachycardia (722[r], 723[c]). Reduced arterial oxygen saturation has been seen in patients given intravenous felodipine for pulmonary hypertension (724[C]). Its metabolism is inhibited by erythromycin (SEDA-17, 239).

Nifedipine

Cardiovascular Nifedipine may facilitate cardiac arrest during induction of anesthesia by sensitizing the carotid sinus (725[C]).

Gastrointestinal Acute abdominal pain due to mesenteric ischemia has been described with nifedipine (726[C]).

Liver Hepatic steatosis with Mallory inclusion bodies has been reported with nifedipine (727[C]).

Interactions *Lithium* clearance is reduced about 30% by co-administration of nifedipine (728[C]). *Ciclosporin* significantly inhibits the metabolism of nifedipine, leading to increased effects (729[C]).

Lidoflazine

The use of lidoflazine in patients with microvascular angina has been associated with malignant ventricular dysrhythmias (SEDA-16, 199).

OTHER CALCIUM ANTAGONISTS

Nicardipine, nisoldipine, nitrendipine, isradipine, and lacidipine are dihydropyridine derivatives with typical minor adverse effects: headache, facial flushing, palpitation, muscle cramps, and pedal edema (730[C]—736[C]).

Potassium channel activators

The potassium channel activators include cromakalim and its levorotatory isomer lemakalim, bimakalim, nicorandil, and pinacidil (737[R]). Older drugs with this property include minoxidil and diazoxide. Nicorandil, a nicotinamide derivative is the only drug in the group to be specifically designed as one of this new fourth class of agents in the management of angina pectoris after organic nitrates, β-blockers, and calcium antagonists.

Nicorandil

Apart from being an arterial/coronary vasodilator through its modulation of ATP-sensitive potassium channels, nicorandil also contains a nitrate moiety, giving it properties similar to organic nitrates but lacking the disadvantages of drug tolerance (see below). In addition, it also has a vasospasmolytic action (738[R]), and in animal studies it is cardioprotective in induced myocardial ischemia (739[C]). Theoretically, it is a promising agent for treating anginal syndromes. In clinical practice it is effective in controlling 69—80% of cases of chronic stable angina when used as a monotherapy (740[R]).

Clinical experience with nicorandil is still limited, although it has been in general use in Japan for over 8 years. An overview of toxicity data has been published (741[R]).

ADVERSE REACTION PATTERN

Toxic reactions The arterial and venous vasodilatory properties of nicorandil precipitate postural hypotension, leading to dizziness, syncope, palpitation, and headache through a mechanism similar to that of organic nitrates. Other minor gastrointestinal symptoms, such as nausea, vomiting, abdominal pain, and diarrhea, and flushing due to cutaneous vasodilatation have been reported.

Hypersensitivity reactions There have been no reported cases of hypersensitivity reactions in humans.

Tumor-inducing effects None have been reported in animal or human studies.

ORGANS AND SYSTEMS

Cardiovascular Nicorandil causes venodilatation, reducing preload, and systemic arterial vasodilatation, reducing systemic vascular resistance and afterload, by its nitrate-like and potassium channel opening effects, respectively. In the heart it has a selective effect on coronary vasculature over myocardial muscle (742[R]), and it does not appear to affect the sinus node or atrioventricular conduction in animal studies (743[Cr]). However, its systemic hemodynamic actions are occasionally associated with a transient increase in heart rate of up to 18% (744[C], 745[C]). Larger doses are associated with cardiac depression, a dose-dependent fall in the sinus rate and atrioventricular conduction velocity (746[R]), and a shortening of the cardiac action potential duration (747[c]), but no prodysrhythmic effects have been observed in man (748[CR], 749[C]). Single oral doses over 40 mg have been associated with severe postural hypotension, dizziness, and syncope (745[C], 750[C]).

Nicorandil is not associated with an excess of sudden deaths complicating acute myocardial infarction in a Japanese series of 1000 sudden deaths between 1983 and 1987 (751[c]).

Respiratory Experimental asthma caused by IgE antibodies in animals is inhibited by nicorandil (752[C]). The relevance of this in humans is not known.

Nervous system Headache occurs in up to one-third of cases in dosages of 10—20 mg twice daily (753[C], 754[C]), but it is usually mild to moderate, necessitating withdrawal in about 5% of cases. It is more common at the start of therapy and is dose-dependent; it gets better with continued therapy or progressive dose titration (755[CR], 756[R]).

Endocrine, metabolic Nicorandil suppresses the release of insulin from isolated animal pancreatic cells. However, this effect is 4-times weaker than that of diazoxide and its effect in man is not known (757[C]).

Hematological Nicorandil has an inhibitory effect on platelet aggregation by increasing intracellular platelet cyclic GMP concentrations (758[C]). Whether this effect will potentiate bleeding or protect against myocardial infarction in patients with coronary heart disease is not known.

Liver Nicorandil is denitrated in the liver. Its half-life was slightly prolonged in eight patients with cirrhotic liver impairment given a single intravenous bolus of nicorandil (0.1 mg/kg for 5 min, half-life 1 7 hours versus 1.1 hours in controls) (759[c]). This is unlikely to have any significance in adjusting dosages in patients with stable liver disease.

Gastrointestinal Nausea, vomiting, gastralgia, diarrhea, and abdominal pains have been reported in some studies (740[R], 745[C]).

Skin and appendages Nicorandil, like minoxidil, appears to enhance the incorporation of cysteine into hair shafts (760[R]). However, hypertrichosis has not been reported.

A case of anal eczema, which resolved after the withdrawal of nicorandil, has been reported (755[CR]).

Sexual function Nicorandil's potassium channel opening action and its ability to release nitric oxide promotes tumescence in isolated human penile corpus cavernosum (761[C]). This effect is currently being exploited to provide treatment for erectile dysfunction by local injection. Whether oral nicorandil is associated with enhanced erectile function has not been assessed.

Risk situations The use of nicorandil in *elderly patients* with *chronic renal failure* and (as discussed above) in patients with stable *cirrhotic liver disease* is not associated with any significant alteration in its pharmacokinetics. In addition, its metabolism is not affected by drugs that interfere with drug-metabolizing liver enzymes (762[R]).

There is a theoretical contraindication to nicorandil in patients with *cardiogenic shock*, *acute left ventricular failure with low filling pressure*, and *hypotension*. A sublingual dose of 20 mg in patients with coronary artery disease and normal left ventricular function was associated with a 12% fall in left ventricular end-systolic pressure, a 3% fall in left ventricular end-diastolic pressure, accentuated diastolic filling, a 13% reduction in mean aortic pressure, and a reduced cardiac output at rest (744[C], 763[C]). However, cardiac output may be augmented by up to 60% in patients with congestive cardiac failure or with a previous history of myocardial infarction, principally by reduced preload, reduced afterload, and improved myocardial oxygen supply (764[CR], 765[C], 766[c]).

Withdrawal effects and tolerance Adverse effects have not been observed with the withdrawal of nicorandil after long-term therapy.

Unlike organic nitrates, there is no drug tolerance with prolonged use of nicorandil (767[Cr]), and there does not appear to be any cross-tolerance (768[R]). The effects of organic nitrates depend solely on the activation of cyclic GMP in smooth muscles, but this is not the case with nicorandil. In a comparison of intravenous nicorandil and glyceryl trinitrate it took twice as long for blood concentrations of cyclic GMP to return to baseline after the latter, but the hemodynamic effects of the former continued for longer (769[c]). This may be because of the additional non-nitrate potassium channel opening effect of nicorandil when further formation of cyclic GMP ceases.

Interactions *Food* reduces the rate but not the extent

of absorption of nicorandil following an oral dose (770[C]). Its systemic availability is good and is generally greater than 75% in healthy volunteers, suggesting limited first-pass hepatic metabolism, unlike the organic nitrates (771[C]). *Cigarette* exposure in animals suppresses and delays the absorption of nicorandil from the gastrointestinal tract (772[C]), but this has yet to be investigated in man.

The combination of nicorandil and β-blockers (atenolol/propranolol) potentiates hypotension, with attenuation of reflex tachycardia (740[R]).

The coronary vasodilator response of nicorandil is potentiated by *dipyridamole* (773[R]).

REFERENCES

1. Dahlof B, Lindholm LH, Hansson L, Schersten B, Ekbom T, Wester P-O. Morbidity and mortality in the Swedish Trial in Old Patients with Hypertension (STOP-hypertension). Lancet 1991;338:1281.
2. The Systolic Hypertension in the Elderly Program (SHEP) Cooperative Research Group. Prevention of stroke by antihypertensive drug treatment in older persons with isolated systolic hypertension: final results of SHEP. J. Am Med Assoc 1991;265:3255.
3. Scandinavian Simvastatin Survival Study Group. Randomized trial of cholesterol lowering in 4444 patients with coronary heart disease: the Scandinavian Simvastatin Survival Study (4S). Lancet 1994;344:1383.
4. Davey-Smith G, Pekkanen J. Should there be a moratorium on the use of cholesterol lowering drugs? Br Med J 1992;304:431.
5. Bartecchi CE, MacKenzie TD, Schrier RW. The human cost of tobacco use: (first of two parts). New Engl J Med 1994;330:907.
6. Negri E, Franzosi MG, Vecchia CL, Santoro L, Nobili A, Tognoni G, on behalf of the GISSI-EFRIM investigators. Tar yield of cigarettes and risk of acute myocardial infarction. Br Med J 1993;306:1567.
7. Vickers A. Why cigarette advertising should be banned. Br Med J 1992;304:1195.
8. Anonymous. Enlightenment on the road to death. Lancet, 1994;343:1109.
9. Parish S, Collins R, Youngman L, Barton J, Jayne K et al. Cigarette smoking, tar yields, and non-fatal myocardial infarction: 14 000 cases and 32 000 controls in the United Kingdom. Br Med J 1995;311:471.
10. McNeill AD, Jarvis MJ, Stapleton JA, Russell MAH, Eiser JR et al. Prospective study of factors predicting uptake of smoking in adolescents. J Edipemiol Community Health 1988;43:72.
11. Anonymous. Nicotine is addictive, rules FDA. Br Med J 1995;311:211.
12. Steinberg D. Antioxidant vitamins and coronary heart disease. New Engl J Med 1993;328:1487.
13. Lakka TA, Venalainen JM, Rauramaa R, Salonen R, Tuomilehto J, Salonen JT. Relation of leisure-time physical activity and cardiorespiratory fitness to the risk of acute myocardial infarction in men. New Engl J Med 1994; 330:1549.
14. Willard JE, Lange RA, Hillis LD. The use of aspirin in ischemic heart disease. New Engl J Med 1992;327:175.
15. Yusuf S, Pepine CJ, Garces C et al. Effect of enalapril on myocardial infarction and unstable angina in patients with low ejection fractions. Lancet 1992;340:1173.
16. Gensini GF, Branzi A, Melandri G et al. Randomised comparison of subcutaneous heparin, intravenous heparin, and aspirin in unstable angina. Lancet 1995;345:1201.
17. Fitzpatrick R, Fletcher A, Gore S, Jones D, Spiegelhalter D, Cox D. Quality of life measures in health care. I: Applications and issues in assessment. Br Med J 1992;305:1074
18. Meynard J. Oil and water? Economic advantage and biomedical progress do not mix well in a government guidelines committee. Am J Hypertens 1994;7:877.
19. Fletcher A. Pressure to treat and pressure to cost a review of cost-effectiveness analysis J Hypertens 1991;9:193.
20. Myers WO, Davis K, Foster ED, Maynard C, Kaiser GC. Surgical survival in the coronary artery surgery study (CASS) registry. Ann Thorac Surg 1985;40:245.
21. Detre K, Murphy ML, Hultgren H. Effect of coronary bypass surgery on longevity in high and low risk patients. Report from the VA Cooperative Coronary Surgery Study. Lancet 1977;ii:1243.
22. European Coronary Surgery Study Group. Long-term results of prospective randomised study of coronary artery bypass surgery in stable angina pectoris. Lancet 1982;ii:1173.
23. CASS Principal Investigators and their Associates. Coronary artery surgery study (CASS): a randomised trial of coronary artery bypass surgery. Survival data. Circulation 1983;68:939.
24. Parisi AF, Folland ED, Hartigan PA. A comparison of angioplasty with medical therapy in the treatment of single-vessel coronary artery disease. New Engl J Med 1992;326:10.
25. Chierchia SL, Fragasso G. Metabolic management of ischaemic heart disease. Eur Heart J 1993;14(Suppl G):2.
26. Brennan TA. Buying editorials. New Engl J Med 1994;331:673.
27. Croog SH, Levine S, Testa MA, Brown B, Bulpitt CJ, Jenkins CD, Klerman GL, Williams GH. The effects of antihypertensive therapy on the quality of life. New Engl J Med 1986;314:1657.
28. Pearce DL. Pharmacologic management of ischemic heart disease with β-blockers and calcium channel blockers. Am Heart J 1990;120:739.
29. Palmer RMJ, Ferrige AG, Moncada S. Nitric oxide release accounts for the biological activity of endothelium derived relaxing factor. Nature 1987;327:524.
30. Leung W-H, Lau C-P, Wong C-K. Beneficial effect of cholesterol-lowering therapy on coronary endothelium-dependent relaxation in hypercholesterolaemic patients. Lancet 1993;341:1496.
31. Cowan JC. Nitrate tolerance. Int J Cardiol 1986;12:1.
32. Cowan JC. Antianginal drug therapy. Curr Opin Cardiol 1990;5:453.

33. Abrams J. Management of myocardial ischemia: role of intermittent nitrate therapy. Am Heart J 1990;120:762.
34. Cohn JN, Archibald DG, Ziesche S et al. Effect of vasodilator therapy on mortality in chronic congestive heart failure: results of a Veterans Administration Cooperative Study. New Engl J Med 1986;314:1547.
35. Anonymous. Calcium antagonist caution. Lancet 1991; 337:885.
36. Wood AJJ. Calcium antagonists. Pharmacologic differences and similarities. Circulation 1989;80(Suppl IV):184.
37. Stone PH, Gibson RS, Glasser SP et al. Comparison of propranolol, diltiazem and nifedipine in the treatment of ambulatory ischemia in patients with stable angina. Differential effects on ambulatory ischemia, exercise performance, and anginal symptoms. The ASIS Study Group. Circulation 1990;82:1962.
38. Maseri A. Medical therapy of chronic stable angina pectoris. Circulation 1990;82:2258.
39. Psaty BM, Koepsell TD, LoGerfo JP, Wagner EH, Inui TS. β-blockers and primary prevention of coronary heart disease in patients with high blood pressure. J Am Med Assoc 1989;261:3087.
40. Packer M, Nicod P, Khanderia BR et al. Randomised multicenter double-blind placebo controlled evaluation of amlodipine in patients with mild to moderate heart failure. J. Am Coll Cardiol 1991;17(Suppl 1):274A.
41. Vetrovec GW, Parker VE. Alternative medical treatment for patients with angina pectoris and adverse reactions to β-blockers. Am J Med 1986;81(Suppl 4A):20.
42. Chesebro JH, Fuster V. Thrombosis in unstable angina. New Engl J Med 1992;327:192.
43. ISIS-2 Collaborative Group. Randomised trial of intravenous streptokinase, oral aspirin, both or neither among 17,187 cases of suspected acute myocardial infarction: ISIS 2. Lancet 1988;ii:349.
44. Theroux P, Ouimet H, McCans J et al. Aspirin, heparin or both to treat acute unstable angina. New Engl J Med 1988;319:1105.
45. Held PH, Yusuf S, Furberg CD. Calcium channel blockers in acute myocardial infarction and unstable angina: an overview. Br Med J 1989;299:1187.
46. Geft IL, Fishbein MC, Ninomiya K et al. Intermittent brief periods of ischemia have a cumulative effect and may cause myocardial necrosis. Circulation 1982;66:1150.
47. Furberg CD, Psaty BM, Meyer JV. Nifedipine. Dose-related increase in mortality in patients with coronary artery disease. Circulation 1995;92:1326.
48. McCarthy M. NIH issues warning on nifedipine. Lancet 1995;346:689.
49. Packer M. Combined β-adrenergic and calcium-entry blockers in angina pectoris. New Engl J Med 1989;320:709.
50. Akhras F, Jackson G. Efficacy of nifedipine and isosorbide mononitrate in combination with atenolol in stable angina. Lancet 1991;338:1036.
51. Cruickshank JM, Prichard BNC. β-Blockers in Clinical Practice. Edinburgh: Churchill Livingstone, 1988.
52. Thomas JA, Marks BH. Plasma norepinephrine in congestive heart failure. Am J Cardiol 1978;41:233.
53. Greenblatt DJ, Koch-Weser J. Clinical toxicity of propranolol and practolol: a report from the Boston Collaborative Drug Surveillance Program. In: Avery GS, ed. Cardiovascular Drugs, Vol 2. β-Adrenoceptor Blocking Drugs, Ch. VIII. Sydney: Adis Press, 1977;179.
54. Barnett DB. Beta blockers in heart failure: a therapeutic paradox. Lancet 1994:343:557.
55. Wagstein F, Bristow MR, Swedberg K et al. Beneficial effects of metoprolol in idiopathic dilated cardiomyopathy. Lancet 1993;342:1441.
56. Aelig WH. Pindolol—a β-adrenoceptor blocking drug with partial agonist activity: clinical pharmacological considerations. Br J Clin Pharmacol 1982;13:187S.
57. Imhof P. The significance of β-blockers with particular reference to antihypertensive treatment. Adv Clin Pharmacol 1976;11:26.
58. Davies B, Bannister R, Mathias C et al. Pindolol in postural hypotension: the case for caution. Lancet 1981; ii:982.
59. Anonymous. Xamoterol: stabilising the cardiac β-receptor? Lancet 1988;ii:1401.
60. Anonymous. New evidence on xamoterol. Lancet 1990;336:24.
61. Frais MA, Bayley TJ. Left ventricular failure with labetalol. Postgrad Med J 1979;55:567.
62. Britman NA. Cardiac effects of topical timolol. New Engl J Med 1979;300:800.
63. Dougherty AH, Naccareli GV, Gray EL et al. Congestive heart failure with normal systolic function. Am J Cardiol 1984;4:778.
64. Wheeldon NM, MacDonald TM, Flucker CJ et al. Echocardiography in chronic heart failure in the community. Q J Med 1993;86:17.
65. Clarkson PBM, Wheeldon NM, MacDonald TM. Left ventricular diastolic dysfunction. Q J Med 1994;87:143.
66. Wheeldon NM, Clarkson P, MacDonald TM. Diastolic heart failure. Eur Heart J 1994;15:1689.
67. Pouler H. Diastolic dysfunction and myocardial energetics. Eur Heart J 1990;11(Suppl C):30—34.
68. Wikstrand J, Berglund J. Antihypertensive treatment with β-blockers in patients aged over 65. Br Med J 1982;285:850.
69. Montolin J, Botey A, Durnell A et al. Hipotension prolongada tras la primera dosis de atenolol. Med Clin (Barcelona) 1981;76:365.
70. McNeill JJ, Louis WJ. A double-blind crossover comparison of pindolol, metoprolol, atenolol and labetalol in mild to moderate hypertension. Br J Clin Pharmacol 1979;8:163S.
71. Cruickshank JM. β-Blockers, bradycardia and adverse effects. Acta Ther 1981;7:309.
72. Anastasiou-Nana MI, Anderson JL, Askins JC et al. Long-term experience with sotalol in the treatment of complex ventricular arrhythmias. Am Heart J 1987;114:288.
73. Obel IW, Jardine R, Haitus B, Millar RN. Efficacy of sotalol in re-entrant ventricular tachycardia. Cardiovasc Ther 1990;4(Suppl 13:613.
74. Griffith MJ, Linker NJ, Garratt CJ et al. Relative efficacy and safety of intravenous drugs for termination of sustained ventricular tachycardia. Lancet 1990;336:670.
75. Juul-Moller S, Eduardsson N, Relinquist-Ahlberg N. Sotalol versus quinidine for the maintenance of sinus rhythm after direct current conversion of atrial fibrillation. Circulation 1990;82:1932.
76. Desoutter P, Medioni J, Lerasle S et al. Bloc auriculoventriculaire et torsade de pointes après surdosage par le sotalol. Nouv Presse Med 1982;11:3855.
77. Belton P, Sheridan J, Mulcahy R. A case of sotalol poisoning. Ir J Med Sci 1982;151:126.

78. Soyka LF, Wirtz C, Spargenberg RB. Clinical safety profile of sotalol in patients with arrhythmias. Am J Cardiol 1990;65:74A.
79 Yasuda SU, Barbey JT, Frunck-Brentano C, Wellstein A, Woosley RL. *d*-Sotalol reduces heart rate in vivo through a β-adrenergic receptor-independent mechanism. Clin Pharmacol Ther 1993;53:436.
80 Waldo AL, Camm J, deRuyter H, Friedman PL, MacNeil DJ, Pitt B, Pratt CM, Rodda BE, Schwartz PJ. Survival with oral *d*-sotalol in patients with left ventricular dysfunction after myocardial infarction: rationale, design and methods (the SWORD trial). Am J Cardiol 1995;75:1023.
81 Choo V. SWORD slashed. Lancet 1994;344:1358.
82. Ozturk M, Demiroglu C. Alternating sinus rhythm and intermittent sinoatrial block induced by propranolol. Eur Heart J 1984;5:890.
83. Pathy MS. Acute central chest pain in the elderly: a view of 296 consecutive hospital admissions during 1979 with particular reference to the possible role of β-adrenergic blocking agents in inducing substernal pain. Am Heart J 1979;98:168.
84. Warren V, Golberg E. Combined therapy with propranolol and permanent pervenous pacemaker. J Am Med Assoc 1976;235:841.
85. Robertson RM, Wood AJJ, Vaughan WK et al. Exacerbation of vasotonic angina pectoris by propranolol. Circulation 1982;65:281.
86. McMahon MTV, McPherson MA, Talbot RL et al. Diagnosis and treatment of Prinzmetal's variant angina. Clin Pharmacol 1982;1:34.
87. Aubran M, Trigano JA, Allard-Laour G et al. Angor accelere sous βbloquants. Ann Cardiol Angéiol 1985;35:99.
88. Carlborg B, Kumlien A, Olsson H. Medikamentella esofagusstrikturen. Lakartidningen 1978;75:4609.
89. Anonymous. Fatigue as an unwanted effect of drugs. Lancet 1980;i:1285.
90. Pearson SB, Banks DC, Patrick JM. The effect of β-adrenoreceptor blockade on factors affecting exercise tolerance in normal man. Br J Clin Pharmacol 1979;8:143.
91. Anderson SD, Bye PTP, Perry CP et al. Limitation of work performance in normal adult males in the presence of β-adrenergic blockade. Aust NZ J Med 1979;9:515.
92. Kaiser P. Running performance as a function of the dose-response relationship to β-adrenoreceptor blockade. Int J Sports Med 1982;3:29.
93. Kaijser L, Kaiser P, Karlsson J et al. β-Blockers and running. Am Heart J 1980;98:542.
94. Bowman WC. Effect of adrenergic activators and inhibitors on the skeletal muscles. In: Szekeres L, ed. Adrenergic Activators and Inhibitors. Berlin Springer Verlag, 1980.
95. Frisk-Holmberg M, Jorfeldt L, Juhlin-Dannfelt A. Metabolic effects in muscle during antihypertensive therapy with β1- and $\beta 1/\beta 2$-adrenoceptor blockers. Clin Pharmacol Ther 1981;30:611.
96. Koch G, Franz IW, Lohmann FW. Effects of short-term and long-term treatment with cardioselective and non-selective β-receptor blockade on carbohydrate and lipid metabolism and on plasma catecholamines at rest and during exercise. Clin Sci 1981;65(Suppl 7):433S.
97. Franciosa JA, Johnson SM, Tobian LJ. Exercise performance in mildly hypertensive patients. Chest 1980;78:291.
98. Hall PE, Kendall MJ, Smith SR. β-Blockers and fatigue. J Clin Hosp Pharm 1984;9:283.
99. Feleke E, Lyngstrum O, Rastam L et al. Complaints of cold extremities among patients on antihypertensive treatment. Acta Med Scand 1983;213:381.
100. Greminger P, Vetter H, Boerlin JH et al. A comparative study between 100 mg atenolol and 20 mg pindolol slow release in essential hypertension. Drugs 1983;25(Suppl 2):38.
101. Eliasson K, Danielson M, Hylander B et al. Raynaud's phenomenon caused by β-receptor blocking drugs. Acta Med Scand 1984;215:333.
102. Steiner JA, Cooper R, Gear JS et al. Vascular symptoms in patients with primary Raynaud's phenomenon are not exacerbated by propranolol or labetalol. Br J Clin Pharmacol 1979;7:401.
103. Reichert N, Shibolet A, Adar R et al. Controlled trial of propranolol in intermittent claudication. Clin Pharmacol Ther 1975;17:612.
104. Breckenridge A. Which β blocker? Br Med J 1983; 286:1085.
105. Lepantalo M. β-Blockade and intermittent claudication. Acta Med Scand 1985;217(Suppl 700):3–48.
106. Solomon S, Ramsay LE, Yeo WW et al. β-Blockade and intermittent claudication: placebo controlled trial of atenolol and nifedipine and their combination. Br Med J 1991;303:1100.
107. Gokal R, Dornan TL, Ledingham JGG. Peripheral skin necrosis complicating β-blockade. Br Med J 1979;1:721.
108. Hoffbrand BI. Peripheral skin necrosis complicating β blockade. Br Med J 1979;2:1082.
109. Rees PJ. Peripheral skin necrosis complicating β-blockade. Br Med J 1979;2:955.
110. O'Rourke DA, Donahue MF, Hayes JA. β-Blockers and peripheral gangrene. Med J Aust 1979;2:88.
111. Fogoros RN. Exacerbation of intermittent claudication by propranolol. New Engl J Med 1980;302:1089.
112. Stringer MD, Bentley PG. Peripheral gangrene associated with β-blockade. Br J Surg 1986;73:1008.
113. Dompmartin A, Le Maitre M, Letessier D et al. Necrose digitales sous béta-bloquants. Ann Dermatol Vénéréol 1988;115:593.
114. Price HL, Cooperman HL, Warden JC. Control of the splanchnic circulation in man: role of β-adrenergic receptors Circ Res 1967;21:333.
115. Schneider R. Do β-blockers cause mesenteric ischaemia? J Clin Gastroenterol 1986;8:109.
116. McNeill RS. Effect of a β-adrenergic blocking agent, propranolol, on asthmatics. Lancet 1964;ii:1101.
117. Harries AD. β-Blockade in asthma. Br Med J 1981; 2:1321.
118. Australian Adverse Drug Reactions Advisory Committee. β-Blockers. Med J Aust 1980;2:130.
119. Raine JM, Palazzo MG, Kerr JH et al. Near fatal bronchospasm after oral nadolol in a young asthmatic and response to ventilation with halothane. Br Med J 1981;1:548.
120. McMahon CD, Shaffer RN, Hoskins HD et al. Adverse effects experienced by patients taking timolol. Am J Ophthalmol 1979;88:736.
121. Mustchin CP, Gribbin HR, Tattersfield AE, George CF. Reduced respiratory response to carbon dioxide after propranolol: a central action? Br Med J 1976;2:1229.
122. Trembath PW, Taylor EA, Varley J, Turner P. Effect of propranolol on the ventilatory response to hypercapnia in man. Clin Sci 1979;57:465.
123. Chang LCT. Use of practolol in asthmatics: a plea for caution. Lancet 1971;ii:321.
124. Waal-Manning HJ, Simpson FO. Practolol treatment in asthmatics. Lancet 1971;ii:1264.

125. Harris LS, Greenstein SH, Bloom EF. Respiratory difficulties with betaxolol. Am J Ophthalmol 1986;102:274.
126. Diggory P, Cassels-Brown A, Vail A, Abbey LM, Hillman JS. Avoiding unsuspected respiratory side effects of topical timolol with cardioselective or sympathomimetic agents. Lancet 1995;345:1604.
127. Formgrein H. The effect of metoprolol and practolol on lung function and blood pressure in hypertensive asthmatics. Br J Clin Pharmacol 1976;3:1007.
128. Wilcox PG, Ahmad D, Darke AC et al. Respiratory and cardiac effects of metoprolol and bevantolol in patients with asthma. Clin Pharmacol Ther 1986;39:29.
129. Nordstrom LA, MacDonald F, Gobel FL. Effect of propranolol on respiratory function and exercise tolerance in patients with chronic obstructive lung disease. Chest 1975;67:287.
130. Fraley DS, Brutis FJ, Segel DP et al. Propranolol-related bronchospasm in patients without history of asthma. South Med J 1980;73:238.
131. Mue S, Sasaki T, Shibahara S et al. Influence of metoprolol on hemodynamics and respiratory function in asthmatic patients. Int J Clin Pharmacol 1979;17:346.
132. Assaykeen TA, Michell G. Metoprolol in hypertension—an open evaluation. Med J Aust 1982;1:73.
133. Jackson SHD, Beevers DG. Comparison of the effects of single doses of atenolol and labetalol on airways obstruction in patients with hypertension and asthma. Br J Clin Pharmacol 1983;15:553.
134. Ellis ME, Sahay JN, Chatterjee SS et al. Cardioselectivity of atenolol in asthmatic patients. Eur J Clin Pharmacol 1981;21:173.
135. Committee on Safety on Medicines. Fatal bronchospasm associated with β-blockers. Curr Probl 1987 20:2.
136. Van Zyl AI, Jennings AA, Bateman ED, Opie LH. Comparison of the respiratory effects oftwo cardioselective β-blockers, celiprolol and atenolol, in asthmatics with mild to moderate hypertension. Chest 1989;95:209.
137. Waal-Manning HJ, Simpson FO. Safety of celiprolol in hypertensives with chronic obstructive respiratory disease. NZ Med J 1990;103:222.
138. Anonymous. Celiprolol—a better β-blocker? Drug Ther Bull 1992;30:35.
139. Tattersfield AD. Respiratory function in the elderly and the effects of β-blockade. Cardiovasc Drugs Ther 1991; 4(Suppl 6):1229.
140. Mustchin CP, Gribbin HR, Tattersfield AE et al. Reduced respiratory responses to carbon dioxide after propranolol: a central action? Br Med J 1976;2:1229.
141. Campbell SC, Lauver GL, Cobb RB. Central ventilatory depression by oral propranolol. Clin Pharmacol Ther 1981;30:758.
142. Davis WM, Hatoum NS. Lethal synergism between morphine or other narcotic analgesics and propranolol. Toxicology 1979;14:141.
143. Erwteman TM, Braat MCP, Van Aken WG. Interstitial pulmonary fibrosis: a new side effect of practolol. Br Med J 1977;2:297.
144. Marshall AJ, Barritt DW, Griffiths DA et al. Respiratory disease associated with practolol therapy. Lancet 1977; ii:1254.
145. Musk AW, Pollard JA. Pindolol and pulmonary fibrosis. Br Med J 1979;2:581.
146. Wood GM, Bolton RP, Muers MF et al. Pleurisy and pulmonary granulomata after treatment with acebutolol. Br Med J 1982;285:936.
147. Akoun GM, Herman DP, Mayaud CM. Acebutolol-induced hypersensitivity pneumonitis. Br Med J 1983; 286:266.
148. Akoun GM Touboul JL, Mayaud CM et al. Pneumopathie d'hypersensibilité à l'acébutolol: données en faveur d'un mécanisme immunologique et médiation cellulaire. Rev Fr Allergol 1985;75:85.
149. Fleminger R. Visual hallucinations and illusions with propranolol. Br Med J 1978;1:1182.
150. Greenblatt DJ, Shader RI. On the psychopharmacology of β-adrenergic blockade. Curr Ther Res 1972;14:615.
151. Medical Research Council Working Party on Mild to Moderate Hypertension. Adverse reactions to bendrofluazide and propranolol for the treatment of mild hypertension. Lancet 1981;ii:539.
152. Bengtsson C, Lenartsson J, Lindquist O et al. Sleep disturbances, nightmares and other possible central nervous disturbances in a population sample of women with special reference to those on antihypertensive drugs. Eur J Clin Pharmacol 1980;17:173.
153. Neil-Dwyer G, Bartlett J, McAinsh J et al. β-adrenoceptor blockers and the blood-brain barrier. Br J Clin Pharmacol 1981;11:549.
154. Kostis JB, Roseu RC. Central nervous system effects of β-adrenergic blocking drugs: the role of ancillary properties. Circulation 1987;75:204.
155. Patel L, Turner P. Central actions of β-adrenoceptor blocking drugs in man. Med Res Rev 1981;1:387.
156. Betts TA, Alford C. β-Blocking drugs and sleep: a controlled trial. Drugs 1983;25(Suppl 2):268.
157. McAinsh J, Cruickshank JM. β-Blockers and central nervous system side-effects. Pharmacol Ther 1990;46:163.
158. Dimsdale JE, Newton RP, Joist T. Neuropsychological side-effects of β-blockers. Arch Intern Med 1989;149:514.
159. Dohlof C, Dimenas E. Side-effects of β-blocker treatments as related to the central nervous system. Am J Med Sci 1990;229:236.
160. Bryan PC, Efiong DO, Stewart-Jones J et al. Propranolol on tests of visual function and central nervous activity. Br J Clin Pharmacol 1974;1:82.
161. Glaister DH, Harrison MH, Allnutt MF. Environmental influences on cardiac activity. In: Burley DM, Frier JH, Rondel RK, Taylor SH, eds. New Perspectives in β-Blockade. Horsham, UK: Ciba Laboratories, 1973;241.
162. Landauer AA, Pocock DA, Prott FW. Effects of atenolol and propranolol on human performance and subjective feelings. Psychopharmacology 1979;60:211.
163. Salem SA, McDevitt DG. Central effects of β-adrenoceptor antagonists. Clin Pharmacol Ther 1983;33:52.
164. Ogle CW, Turner P, Markomihelakis H. The effects of high doses of oxprenolol and of propranolol on pursuit rotor performance, reaction time and critical flicker frequency. Psychopharmacologia 1976;46:295.
165. Turner P, Hedges A. An investigation of the central effects of oxprenolol. In: Burley DM, Frier JH, Rondel RK, Taylor SH, eds. New Perspectives in β-Blockade. Horsham, UK: Ciba Laboratories, 1973;269.
166. Tyrer PJ, Lader MH. Response to propranolol and diazepam in somatic and psychic anxiety. Br Med J 1974;2:14.
167. Greil W. Central nervous system effects. Curr Ther Res 1980;28:106.
168. Currie D, Lewis RV, McDevitt DG et al. Central effects of β-adrenoceptor antagonists. I. Performance and subjective assessments of mood. Br J Clin Pharmacol 1988;26:121.

169. Nicholson AN, Wright NA, Zetlein MB et al. Central effects of β-adrenoceptor antagonists. II. Electroencephalogram and body sway. Br J Clin Pharmacol 1988;26:129.
170. Braun P, Reker K, Friedel B et al. Driving tests with β-receptor blockers. Blutalkohol 1979;16:495.
171. Moser L, Schmidt U, Lundt PV. Die Auswirkungen eines β-Rezeptorenblockers auf die Kraftfahreignung. Med Klin 1979;74:1134.
172. Betts TA. Effects of β-blockade on driving. Aviat Space Environ Med 1981;58:40.
173. Panniza D, Lecasble M. Effect of atenolol on car drivers in a prolonged stress situation. Eur J Clin Pharmacol 1985;28(Suppl):97.
174. Broadhurst AD. The effect of propranolol on human psychomotor performance. Aviat Space Environ Med 1980;57:176.
175. Topliss D, Bond R. Acute brain syndrome after propranolol treatment. Lancet 1977;ii:1133.
176. Helson L, Duquc L. Acute brain syndrome after propranolol. Lancet 1978;i:98.
177. Kurland ML. Organic brain syndrome with propranolol. New Engl J Med 1979;300:366.
178. Gershon ES, Goldstein RE, Moss AJ et al. Psychosis with ordinary doses of propranolol. Ann Intern Med 1979;90:938.
179. Kuhr BM. Prolonged delirium with propranolol. J Clin Psychiatry 1979;40:198.
180. McGahan DJ, Wojslaw A, Prasad V et al. Propranolol-induced psychosis. Drug Intell Clin Pharm 1984;18:601.
181. Steinhert J, Pugh CR. Schizophrenia-like psychosis after treatment with β-blockers. Br Med J 1979;1:790.
182. Russel JW, Schickt MA. Anxiety and depression in a patient on nadolol. Lancet 1982;ii:1286.
183. Thiessen BQ, Wallace SM, Blackburn JL et al. Increased prescribing of antidepressants subsequent to β-blocker therapy. Arch Intern Med 1990;150:2286.
184. Faldt R, Liedholm H, Aursnes J. β-Blockers and loss of hearing. Br Med J 1984;289:1490.
185. Weber JCP. β-Adrenoceptor antagonists and diplopia. Lancet 1982;ii:826.
186. Turkenitz LJ, Sahgal V, Spiro A. Propranolol induced myotonia. Mt Sinai J Med 1980;51:207.
187. Robson RH. Recurrent migraine after propranolol. Br Heart J 1977;39:1157.
188. Prendes JL. Considerations in the use of propranolol in complicated migraine. Headache 1980;20:93.
189. Gilbert GJ. An occurrence of complicated migraine during propranolol therapy. Headache 1982;22:81.
190. Bardwell A, Trott JA. Stroke in migraine as a consequence of propranolol. Headache 1987;27:381.
191. Das G, Ferris JC. Generalised convulsions in a patient receiving ultra-short acting β-blocker infusion. DICP Ann Pharmacother 1988;22:484.
192. Leys D, Pasquier F, Kermerch P et al. Possible revelation of latent myasthenia gravis by labetalol chlorohydrate. Acta Clin Belg 1987;42:475.
193. Komar J, Szalay M, Szel I. Myasthenische Episode nach Einnahme grosser Mengen β-blocker. Fortschr Neurol Psychiatr 1987;55:201.
194. Emara MK, Saadah AM. The carpal tunnel syndrome in hypertensive patients treated with β-blockers. Postgrad Med J 1988;64:91.
195. Hod H, Kaplinsky N, Har-Zahav J et al. Pindolol-induced tremor. Postgrad Med J 1980;56:346.
196. Gold LA, Merimee TJ, Misbin RI. Propranolol and hypoglycemia: the effects of β-adrenergic blockade on glucose and alanine levels during fasting. J Clin Pharmacol 1980;20:50.
197. Uusitupa M, Aro A, Pietikainen M. Severe hypoglycaemia caused by physical strain and pindolol therapy: a case report. Ann Clin Res 1980;12:25.
198. Holm G, Herlitz J, Smith U. Severe hypoglycaemia during physical exercise and treatment with β-blockers. Br Med J 1981;282:1360.
199. Zarate A, Gelfand M, Novello A et al. Propranolol-associated hypoglycemia in patients on maintenance hemodialysis. Int. J. Artif Organs 1981;4:130.
200. Belton P, Carmody M, Donohoe J et al. Propranolol-associated hypoglycaemia in non-diabetics. J Ir Med Assoc 1980;73:173.
201. Wright AD, Barber SG, Kendall MJ et al. β-Adrenoceptor blocking drugs and blood sugar control in diabetes mellitus. Br Med J 1979;1:159.
202. Barnett AH, Leslie D, Watkins PJ. Can insulin-treated diabetics be given β-adrenergic blocking drugs? Br Med J 1980;280:976.
203. Davidson NMCD, Corrall RJM, Shaw TRD et al. Observations in man of hypoglycaemia during selective and non-selective β-blockade. Scot Med J 1976;22:69.
204. Deacon SP, Barnet D. Comparison of atenolol and propranolol during insulin-induced hypoglycaemia. Br Med J 1976;2:272.
205. Blohme G, Lager I, Lonnroth P, Smith U. Hypoglycaemic symptoms in insulin-dependent diabetics: a prospective study of the influence of β-blockade. Diabetes Metab 1981;7:235.
206. Shepherd AMM, Keeton TK. Hypoglycemia-induced hypertension in a diabetic patient on metoprolol. Ann Intern Med 1981;94:358.
207. Samuelsson O, Hedner T, Berglund G, Persson B, Andersson OK, Wilhelmsen L. Diabetes mellitus in treated hypertension: incidence, predictive factors and the impact of non-selective β-blockers and thiazide diuretics during 15 years treatment of middle-aged hypertensive men in the Primary Prevention Trial Goteborg, Sweden. J Hum Hypertens 1994;8:257.
208. Harrower ADB, Fyffe JA, Hom DR et al. Thyroxine and triiodothyronine levels in hyperthyroid patients during treatment with propranolol. Clin Endocrinol 1977;7:41.
209. Heyma P, Larkins RG, Higginbotham L et al. *d*-Propranolol and *dl*-propranolol both decrease conversion of L-thyroxine to L-triiodothyronine. Br Med J 1980;281:24.
210. Jones DK, Solomon S. Thyrotoxic crisis masked by treatment with β-blockers. Br Med J 1981;283:659.
211. Cooper DS, Daniels GH, Ladenson PW et al. Hyperthyroxinemia in patients treated with high dose propranolol. Am J Med 1982;73:G867.
212. Mooradian A, Morley JE, Simon G et al. Propranolol-induced hyperthyroxinemia. Arch Intern Med 1983; 143:2193.
213. Lee ST. Hyperprolactinemia, galactorrhea, and atenolol. Ann Intern Med 1992;116:522.
214. Van Brammelen P. Lipid changes induced by β-blockers. Curr Opin Cardiol 1988;3:513.
215. Northcote RJ. β-Blockers, lipid and coronary atherosclerosis: fact or fiction? Br Med J 1988;296:731.
216. Neaton JD, Grimm RH, Prineas RJ, Stamler J et al. Treatment of mild hypertension study. J Am Med Assoc 1993;270:713.

217. Bielmann P, Leduc G, Jequier JC et al. Changes in the lipoprotein composition after chronic administration of metoprolol and propranolol in hypertriglyceridemic-hypertensive subjects. Curr Ther Res 1981;30:956.
218. Astrup A. Obesity and diabetes as side-effects of β-blockers. Ugeskr Laeg 1990;152:2905.
219. Connacher AA, Jung RT, Mitchell PEG. Weight loss in obese subjects on a restricted diet given BRL26830A, a new atypical β-adrenoceptor agonist. Br Med J 1988; 296:1217.
220. Wheeldon NM, McDevitt DG, McFarlane LC, Lipworth BJ. Do β-3 adrenoceptors mediate the metabolic responses to isoprenaline? Q J Med 1993;86:595.
221. Emorine LJ, Marullo S, Briend-Sutren MM et al. Molecular charecterisation of the human β3-receptor. Science 1989;245:1118.
222. Saunders J, Prestwich SA, Avery AJ et al. The effect of non-selective and selective β-1 blockade on the plasma potassium response to hypoglycaemia. Diabetes Metab 1981;7:239.
223. Arnold JMO, Shanks RG, McDevitt DG. β-Adrenoceptor antagonism of isoprenaline induced metabolic changes in man. Br J Clin Pharmacol 1983;16:621P.
224. Skehan JD, Barnes JN, Drew PJ et al. Hypokalaemia induced by a combination of a β-blocker and a thiazide. Br Med J 1982;284:83.
225. Walters EG, Horsweill CE, Shelton JR et al. Hazards of β-blocker/diuretic therapy. Lancet 1985;ii:220.
226. Odugbesan O, Chesner IM, Bailey G et al. Hazards of combined β-blocker/diuretic tablets. Lancet 1985;i:1221.
227. Pedersen LO, Mikkelsen E. Serum potassium and uric acid changes during treatment with timolol alone and in combination with diuretics. Clin Pharmacol Ther 1979; 26:339.
228. Bushe CJ. Does atenolol have an effect on calcium metabolism? Br Med J 1987;294:1324.
229. Freestone S, MacDonald TM. Does atenolol have an effect on calcium metabolism? Br Med J 1987;295:53.
230. Dodds WN, Davidson RJL. Thrombocytopenia due to slow-release oxprenolol. Lancet 1978;ii:683.
231. Hare DL, Hicks BH. Thrombocytopenia due to oxprenolol. Med J Aust 1979;2:259.
232. Caviet NL, Klaasen CHL. Thrombocytopenia brought about by alprenolol. Ned Tijdschr Geneeskd 1979;123:18.
233. Magnusson B, Rodjer S. Alprenolol-induced thrombocytopenia. Acta Med Scand 1980;207:231.
234. Kelly JP, Kaufman DW, Shapiro S. Risk of agranulocytosis and aplastic anemia in relation to the use of cardiovascular drugs: The International Agranulocytosis and Aplastic Anemia Study. Clin Pharmacol Ther 1991;49:330.
235. Nawabi IU, Ritz ND. Agranulocytosis due to propranolol. J Am Med Assoc 1973;223:1376.
236. Mahgoub A, Idle JR, Dring LG et al. Polymorphic hydroxylation of debrisoquine in man. Lancet 1977;ii:584.
237. Smith RL. Polymorphic metabolism of the β-adrenoceptor blocking drugs and its clinical relevance. Eur. J Clin Pharmacol 1985;28(Suppl):72.
238. Sherlock S. In: Diseases of the Liver and Biliary System, 6th edn. Oxford: Blackwell Scientific Publications, 1981;163.
239. Conn HO. Propranolol in the treatment of portal hypertension: a caution. Hepatology 1982;2:641.
240. Hayes PC, Shepherd AN, Bouchier IAD. Medical treatment of portal hypertension and oesophageal varices. Br Med J 1983;287:733.
241. Tarver D, Walt RP, Dunk AA et al. Precipitation of hepatic encephalopathy by propranolol in cirrhosis. Br Med J 1983;287:585.
242. Watson P, Hayes JR. Cirrhosis, hepatic encephalopathy and propranolol. Br Med J 1983;287:1067.
243. Anonymous. β-Adrenergic blockers in cirrhosis. Lancet 1985;i:1372.
244. Robinson JD, Burtner DE. Severe diarrhea secondary to propranolol. Drug Intell Clin Pharm 1981;15:49.
245. Windsor WO, Kurrein F, Dyer NH. Fibrous peritonitis: a complication of practolol therapy. Br Med J 1975;2:68.
246. Eltringham WK, Espiner HJ, Windsor CWO et al. Sclerosing peritonitis due to practolol: a report of 9 cases and their surgical management. Br J Surg 1977;64:229.
247. Marshall AJ, Baddeley H, Barrit DW et al. Practolol peritonitis: a study of 16 cases and a survey of small bowel function in patients taking β-adrenergic blockers. Q J Med 1977;46:135.
248. Ahmad S. Sclerosing peritonitis and propranolol. Chest 1981;79:361.
249. Nillson BV, Pederson KG. Sclerosing peritonitis associated with atenolol. Br Med J 1985;290:518.
250. McCluskey DR, Donaldson RA, McGeown MG. Oxprenolol and retroperitoneal fibrosis. Br Med J 1980;2:1459.
251. Johnson JN, McFarland J. Retroperitoneal fibrosis associated with atenolol. Br Med J 1980;1:864.
252. Pierce JR, Trostle DC, Warner JJ. Propranolol and retroperitoneal fibrosis. Ann Intern Med 1981;95:244.
253. Thompson J, Julian DG. Retroperitoneal fibrosis associated with metoprolol. Br Med J 1982;284:83.
254. Laakso M, Arvala I, Tervonen S et al. Retroperitoneal fibrosis associated with sotalol. Br Med J 1982;285:1085.
255. Rimmer E, Richens A, Forster ME et al. Retroperitoneal fibrosis associated with timolol. Lancet 1983;i:300.
256. Benitah E, Chatelain C, Cohen F et al. Fibrose retroperitoneale: effet systemique d'un collyre béta-bloquant? Presse Méd 1987;16:400.
257. Bullimore DW. Retroperitoneal fibrosis associated with atenolol. Br Med J 1980;2:564.
258. Pryor JP, Castle WM, Dukes DC et al. Do β-adrenoceptor blocking drugs cause retroperitoneal fibrosis. Br Med J 1983;284:347.
259. Falch DK, Odegaard AE, Norman N. Decreased renal plasma flow during propranolol treatment in essential hypertension. Acta Med Scand 1979;205:91.
260. Baver JH, Brooks CS. The long-term effect of propranolol therapy on renal function. Am J Med 1979;66:405.
261. Kincaid-Smith P, Fang P, Laver MC. A new look at the treatment of severe hypertension. Clin Sci Mol Med 1973;45(Suppl 1):75S.
262. Warren DJ, Swainson CP Wright N. Deterioration in renal function after β-blockade in patients with chronic renal failure and hypertension. Br Med J 1974;2:193.
263. Wilkinson R. β-Blockers and renal function. Drugs 1982;23:195.
264. Britton KE, Gruenwald SM, Nimmon CC. Nadolol and renal haemodynamics. In: International Experience With Nadolol, No. 37, International Congress and Symposium Series. London: Royal Society of Medicine, 1981;77.
265. O'Malley K, O'Callaghan WG, Laher MS et al. Adrenoceptor blocking drugs and renal blood flow with special reference to the elderly. Drugs 1983;25(Suppl 2)103.
266. Dupont AG. Effects of carvedilol on renal function. Eur J Clin Pharmacol 1990;38(Suppl 2):596.

267. Hawk JLM. Lichenoid drug eruption induced by propranolol. Clin Exp Dermatol 1980;5:93.
268. Guillet G, Chouvet V, Perrot H. Un accident des bétabloquants: lichen induit par le pindolol avec anticorps pemphigus-like. Bordeaux Med 1981;14:95.
269. Faure M, Hermier CI, Perrot H. Accidents cutanés provoqués par le propranolol. Ann Dermatol Vénéréol 1979;106:161.
270. Newman BR, Schultz LK. Epinephrine-resistant anaphylaxis in a patient taking propranolol hydrochloride. Ann Allergy 1981;47:35.
271. Kauppinen K, Idanpaan-Heikkila J. Cutaneous reactions to β-blocking agents. In: Proceedings, XV International Congress of Dermatology, Mexico, 1977. 1979;702.
272. Halevy S, Fuererman EJ. Psoriasiform eruption induced by propranolol. Cutis 1979;24:95.
273. Neumann HAM, Van Joost TH. Dermatitis as a side-effect of long-term treatment with β-adrenoceptor blocking agents. Br J Dermatol 1980;103:566.
274. Gold MH, Holy AK, Roenigk HH Jr. β-Blocking drugs and psoriasis. A review of cutaneous side-effects and a retrospective analysis of their effects on psoriasis. J Am Acad Dermatol 1988;19:837.
275. Hilder RJ. Propranolol and alopecia. Cutis 1979;24:63.
276. Graeber CW, Lapkin RA. Metoprolol and alopecia. Cutis 1981;28:633.
277. Fiore PM, Jacobs IH, Goldberg DB. Drug-induced pemphigoid: a spectrum of diseases. Arch Ophthalmol 1989;105:1660.
278. Jain S. Betaxolol-associated anterior uveitis. Eye 1994;8:708–709.
279. Schultz JS, Hoenig JA, Charles H. Possible bilateral anterior uveitis secondary to metipranolol (optipranolol) therapy. Arch Ophthalmol 1993;111:1606.
280. O'Connor GR. Granulomatous uveitis and metipranolol. Br J Ophthalmol 1993;77:536.
281. Bergsmark J, Gadeholt G. Nesepolypper og kronisk sinusitt som mulig bivirkning av uselektive betablokkere. Tidsskr Nor Laegeforen 1994;114:2116.
282. Savola J. Arthropathy induced by β-blockade. Br Med J 1983;287:1256.
283. Walker PC, Ramsay LE. Do β-blockers cause arthropathy? A case controlled study. Br Med J 1985;291:1684.
284. Sills JM, Bosco L. Arthralgia associated with β-adrenergic blockade. J. Am Med Assoc 1986;255:198.
285. Zimlichmann R, Krauss S, Paran E. Muscle cramps induced by β-blockers with intrinsic sympathomimetic activity properties: a hint of a possible mechanism. Arch Intern Med 1991;151:1021.
286. Tomlinson B, Cruickshank JM, Hayes Y et al. Selective β-adrenoceptor partial agonist effects of pindolol and xamoterol on skeletal muscle assessed by plasma creatinine kinase changes in healthy subjects. Br J Clin Pharmacol 1990;30:665.
287. Wheeldon NM, Newnham DM, Fraser GC et al. The effect of pindolol on creatine kinase is not due to β_2-adrenoceptor partial agonist activity. Br J Clin Pharmacol 1991;31:723.
288. Burnett WC, Chahine RA. Sexual dysfunction as a complication of propranolol therapy in man. Cardiovasc Med 1979;4:811.
289. β-Blocker Heart Attack Trial Research Group. A randomised trial of propranolol in patients with acute myocardial infarction. 1. Mortality results. J Am Med Assoc 1982;247:1707.
290. Wassertheil-Smoller S, Blaufox MD, Oberman A, Davis BR et al. Effect of antihypertensives on sexual function and quality of life: the TAIM study. Ann Intern Med 1991;114:613.
291. Kostis JB, Rosen RC. Central nervous system effects of β-adrenergic blocking drugs: the role of ancillary properties. Circulation 1987;75:204.
292. Croog SH, Levine S, Sudilowsky A et al. Sexual symptoms in hypertensive patients. A clinical trial of antihypertensive medication. Arch Intern Med 1988;148:788.
293. Kostis JB, Rosen RC, Holzer BC et al. CNS side effects of centrally-active antihypertensive agents: a prospective, placebo controlled study of sleep, mood state and cognitive and sexual function in hypertensive males. Psychopharmacology 1990;102:163.
294. Sayuki H, Taminaga T, Kamagai H, Soruta T. Effects of first-line antihypertensive agents on sexual function and sex hormones. J Hypertens 1988;6(Suppl 4):S649.
295. Osborne DR. Propranolol and Peyronie's disease. Lancet 1977;i:311.
296. Yudkin JS. Labetalol-induced Peyronie's disease. Lancet 1977;ii:1335.
297. Kristensen BO. Labetalol-induced Peyronie's disease. Acta Med Scand 1979;206:511.
298. Pryor JP, Castle WM. Peyronie's disease associated with chronic degenerative arterial disease and not with β-adrenoceptor agents. Lancet 1982;i:917.
299. Booth RF, Bullock JY, Wilson JD. Antinuclear antibodies in patients on acebutolol. Br J Clin Pharmacol 1980;9:515.
300. Cody RJ, Calabrese L, Clough JD et al. Development of antinuclear antibodies during acebutolol therapy. Clin Pharmacol Ther 1979;25:800.
301. Huggins MM, Menzies CW, Quail D, Rumfitt IW. An open multicenter study of the effect of celiprolol on serum lipids and antinuclear antibodies in patient with mild to moderate hypertension. J Drug Dev 1991;4:125–133.
302. Clerens A, Guilmot-Bruneau MM, Defresne C et al. β-blocking agents: side effects. Biomedicine 1979;31:219.
303. Trenque T, Bigot M-C, Moulin M et al. Syndrome lupique induits par les béta-bloquants. Ouest Méd 1984;37:711.
304. Hourdebaigt-Larrusse P, Grivaux M. Une nouvelle obscuration de lupus induit par un béta-bloquant. Sem Hôp 1984;60:1515.
305. Harrison T, Sisca TS, Wood WH. Propranolol-induced lupus erythematosus syndrome? Postgrad Med 1976;59:24.
306. Griffiths ID, Richardson J. Lupus-like illness associated with labetalol. Br Med J 1979;2:496.
307. Holzbach E. Ein β-blocker als Zusatztherapie beim Delirium tremens. Münch Med Wochenschr 1980;122:847.
308. Jacobs RL, Rake GW, Fournier DC et al. Potential anaphylaxis in patients with drug-induced β-adrenergic blockade. J Allergy Clin Immunol 1981;68:125.
309. Hannaway PJ, Hopper GDK. Severe anaphylaxis and drug induced β-blockade. New Engl J Med 1983;308:1536.
310. Cornaille G, Leynadier F, Modanio F et al. Gravité du choc anaphylactic chez les malades traités par béta-bloqueurs. Presse Méd 1985;14:790.
311. Raebel MA. Potentiated anaphylaxis during chronic β-blocker therapy. DICP Ann Pharmacother 1988;22:720.
312. Toogood JH. β-Blocker therapy and the risk of anaphylaxis. Can Med Assoc J 1989;136:929.
313. Arkinstall WW, Toogood JH. β-Blocker therapy and the risk of anaphylaxis. Can Med Assoc J 1989;137:370.

314. McDevitt DG. β-Adrenoceptor blockade in hyperthyroidism. In: Shanks RG, ed. Advanced Medicine: Topics in Therapeutics 3. London: Pitman Medical, 1977;100.
315. Rossi PRF, Yusuf S, Ramsdate D et al. Reduction of ventricular arrhythmias by early intravenous atenolol in suspected acute myocardial infarction. Br Med J 1983 286:506.
316. Ryden L, Ariniego R, Arnman K et al. A double-blind trial of metoprolol in acute myocardial infarction. Effects on ventricular tachyarrhythmias. New Engl J Med 1983 308:614.
317. Anonymous. Long-term and short-term β-blockade after myocardial infarction. Lancet 1982;i:1159.
318. Rossi PRF, Yusuf S, Rawsdak D et al. Reduction of ventricular arrhythmias by early intravenous atenolol in suspected acute myocardial infarction. Br Med J 1983 286:506.
319. Baber NS, Wainwright Evans D, Howitt G et al. Multicentre post-infarction trial of propranolol in 49 hospitals in the United Kingdom, Italy and Yugoslavia. Br Heart J 1980;44:96.
320. β-Blocker Heart Attack Study Group. The β-blocker heart attack trial. J Am Med Assoc 1981;246:2073.
321. Wilhelmsson C, Vedin JA, Wilhelmsen L et al. Reduction of sudden deaths after myocardial infarction by treatment with alprenolol. Lancet 1974;ii:7890.
322. Anderson MD, Bechsgaard P, Fredriksen J et al. Effect of alprenolol on mortality among patients with definite or suspected myocardial infarction. Lancet 1979;ii:865.
323. Ahlmark G, Saetre H, Korsgren M. Reduction of sudden deaths after myocardial infarction. Lancet 1974; ii:1563.
324. Hjalmarson A, Elmfeldt D, Herlitz J et al. Effect on mortality of metoprolol in acute myocardial infarction. Lancet 1981;ii:823.
325. Norwegian Multicentre Study Group. Timolol-induced reduction in mortality and reinfarction in patients surviving acute myocardial infarction. New Engl J Med 1981;304:801.
326. Julian DG, Prescott RJ, Jackson FS et al. Controlled trial of sotalol for one year after myocardial infarction. Lancet 1982;i:1142.
327. Hansteen V, Moinicken E, Lorensten E et al. One year's treatment with propranolol after myocardial infarction: preliminary report on Norwegian multicentre trial. Br Med J 1982;284:155.
328. Heidbreder E, Pagel G, Rockel A et al. β-Adrenergic blockade in stress protection: limited effect of metoprolol in psychological stress reaction. Eur J Clin Pharmacol 1978; 14:391.
329. Trap-Jensen J, Carlsen JE, Svendsen TL et al. Cardiovascular and adrenergic effect of cigarette smoking during immediate non-selective and selective β-adrenoceptor blockade in humans. Eur J Clin Invest 1979;9:181.
330. Freestone S, Ramsay LE. Effect of coffee and cigarette smoking in untreated and diuretic-treated hypertensive patients. Br J Clin Pharmacol 1981;11:428.
331. Ramsay LE. Antihypertensive drugs. Curr Opin Cardiol 1987;1:524.
332. Deanfield J, Wright C, Krikler S. Cigarette smoking to the treatment of angina with propranolol, atenolol and nifedipine. New Engl J Med 1984;310:951.
333. McAinsh J, Holmes BF, Smith S et al. Atenolol kinetics in renal failure. Clin Pharmacol Ther 1980;28:302.
334. Berglund G, Descamps R, Thomis JA. Pharmacokinetics of sotalol after chronic administration to patients with renal insufficiency. Eur J Clin Pharmacol 1980;18:321.
335. Verbeeck RK, Branch RA, Wilkinson GR. Drug metabolites in renal failure: pharmacokinetic and clinical implications. Clin Pharmacokin 1981;6:329.
336. Stone WJ, Walle T. Massive retention of propranolol metabolites in maintenance hemodialysis patients. Clin Pharmacol Ther 1980;27:288.
337. Howard PJ, Lee MR. Beware β-adrenergic blockers in patients with severe urticaria. Scot Med J 1988;33:344.
338. Miller RR, Olson HG, Amsterdam FA et al. Propranolol-withdrawal rebound phenomenon. New Engl J Med 1975;293:416.
339. Myers MG, Wisenberg G. Sudden withdrawal of propranolol in patients with angina pectoris. Chest 1977;71:24.
340. Shiroff RA, Mathis J, Zelis R et al. Propranolol rebound: a retrospective study. Am J Cardiol 1978;41:778.
341. Psaty BM, Koepsell TD, Wagner EH et al. The relative risk of incident coronary heart disease associated with recently stopping the use of β-blockers. J Am Med Assoc 1990;263:1653.
342. Olsson G, Hjemdahl P, Rehnquist M. Rebound phenomena following gradual withdrawal of chronic metoprolol treatment in patients with ischemic heart disease. Am Heart J 1984;108:454.
343. Maling TJB, Dollery CT. Changes in blood pressure, heart rate and plasma noradrenaline concentration after sudden withdrawal of propranolol. Br Med J 1979;2:366.
344. Lederballe Pedersen O, Mikkelsen E, Nielsen J et al. Abrupt withdrawal of β-blocking agents in patients with arterial hypertension: effects on blood pressure, heart rate and plasma catecholamines and prolactin. Eur J Clin Pharmacol 1979;15:215.
345. Webster J, Hawksworth GM, Barber HE et al. Withdrawal of long-term therapy with atenolol in hypertensive patients. Br J Clin Pharmacol 1981;12:211.
346. Aarons RD, Nies AS, Gal J et al. Elevation of β-adrenergic receptor density in human lymphocytes after propranolol administration. J Clin Invest 1980;65:949.
347. Nattel S. Rangno RE, Vanloon G. Mechanism of propranolol withdrawal phenomena. Circulation 1979;59:1158.
348. Rangno RE, Langlois S, Lutterodt A. Metroprolol withdrawal phenomena: mechanism and prevention. Clin Pharmacol Ther 1982;31:8.
349. Walden RJ, Bhattacharjee P, Tomlinson B et al. The effect of intrinsic sympathomimetic activity on β-adrenoceptor blockade withdrawal. Br J Clin Pharmacol 1982;13:359S.
350. Rango RE, Langlois S. Comparison of withdrawal phenomena after propranolol, metoprolol and pindolol. Br. J Clin Pharmacol 1982;13:345S.
351. Krukemyer JJ, Boudoulas H, Binkley PF, Lema JJ. Comparison of hypersensitivity to adrenergic stimulation after abrupt withdrawal of propranolol and nadolol: influence of half-life differences. Am Heart J 1990;120:572.
352. Rubin PC, Butters L, Clark DM et al. Placebo-controlled trial of atenolol in treatment of pregnancy-associated hypertension. Lancet 1983;i:431.
353. Lowe SA, Rubin PC. The pharmacological management of hypertension in pregnancy. J Hypertens 1992;10:201.
354. White WB, Andreoli JW, Wong SH et al. Atenolol in human plasma and breast milk. Obstet Gynecol 1984; 62(Suppl 3):42S.
355. Bianchetti G, Dubruc C, Vert P et al. Placental transfer and pharmacokinetics of acebutolol in newborn infants. Am Soc Clin Pharmacol Ther 1981;29:223.
356. Sanderstrom B. Metoprolol excretion into breast milk. Br J Clin Pharmacol 1980;9:518.

357. Devlin RG, Duchin KL, Fleiss PM. Nadolol in human serum and breast milk. Br J Clin Pharmacol 1981;12:393.
358. Fidler J, Smith V, De Swiet M. Excretion of oxprenolol and timolol in breast milk. Br J Obstet Gynaecol 1983; 90:961.
359. Smith MT, Livingstone L, Hooper WD et al. Propranolol, propranolol glucuronide, and naphthoxylactic acid in breast milk and plasma. Ther Drug Monit 1983;5:87.
360. O'Hare MF, Murnaghan GA, Russell CJ et al. Sotalol as a hypertensive agent in pregnancy. Br J Obstet Gynaecol 1980;87:814.
361. Anonymous. Self-poisoning with β-blockers. Br Med J 1978;1:1010.
362. Anonymous. β-Blocker poisoning. Lancet 1980;i:803.
363. Tynan RF, Fisher MMcD, Ibles LS. Self-poisoning with propranolol. Med J Aust 1981;1:82.
364. Buiumsohn A, Eisenberg ES, Jacob H et al. Seizures and intraventricular conduction defect in propranolol poisoning. Ann Intern Med 1979;91:860.
365. Neuvonen PJ, Elonen E, Vuorenmaa T et al. Prolonged Q-T interval and severe tachyarrhythmias: common features of sotalol intoxication. Eur J Clin Pharmacol 1981;20:85.
366. Lagerfelt J, Matell G. Attempted suicide with 5.1 g of propranolol. Acta Med Scand 1976;199:157.
367. Henry JA, Cassidy SL. Membrane stabilising activity: a major cause of fatal poisoning. Lancet 1986;i:1414.
368. Aura ED, Wexler LF, Wirtzburg RA. Massive propranolol overdose: successful treatment with high dose isoproterenol and glucagon. Am J Med 1986;80:755.
369. Weinstein RS. Recognition and management of poisoning with β-adrenergic blocking agents. Ann Emerg Med 1984;13:1123.
370. Nicholas F, Villers D, Rozo L et al. Severe self-poisoning with acebutolol in association with alcohol. Crit Care Med 1987;15:173.
371. Richards DA, Prichard BWC. Self-poisoning with β-blockers. Br Med J 1978;1:1623.
372. Freestone S, Thomas HM, Bhamra RK, Dyson EH. Severe atenolol poisoning: treatment with prenalterol. Hum Toxicol 1986;5:343.
373. McDevitt DG. Clinically important adverse drug interactions. In: Petrie JC, ed. Cardiovascular and Respiratory Disease Therapy, Vol. 1. Amsterdam: Elsevier/North Holland, Biomedical Press, 1980;21.
374. Lewis RV, McDevitt DG. Adverse reactions and interactions with β-adrenoceptor blocking drugs. Med Toxicol 1986;1:343.
375. Kendall MJ, Beeley L. β-Adrenoceptor blocking drugs: adverse reactions and drug interactions. Pharmacol Ther 1983;21:351.
376. Alvan G, Piafsky K, Lind M et al. Effect of pentobarbital on the disposition of alprenolol. Clin Pharmacol Ther 1977;22:316.
377. Bennett PN, John VA, Mutmarsh VB. Effects of rifampicin on metoprolol and antipyrine kinetics. Br J Clin Pharmacol 1982;13:387.
378. Feely J, Wilkinson GR, Wood AJJ. Reductions of liver blood flow and propranolol metabolism by cimetidine. New Engl J Med 1981;304:692.
379. Daneshmend TK, Roberts CJC. Cimetidine and bioavailability of laβlol. Lancet 1981;i:565.
380. Kirch W, Kohler H, Spahn H, Mutschler E. Interaction of cimetidine with metoprolol, propranolol or atenolol. Lancet 1981;ii:531.
381. Sax MJ. Analysis of possible drug interactions between cimetidine (and ranitidine) and β-blockers. Adv Ther 1988;5:210.
382. Vestal RE, Kornhauser DM, Hollifield JW et al. Interaction between chlorpromazine and propranolol in man. Clin Res 1978;26:277A.
383. Peet M, Middlemiss DN, Yates RA. Pharmacokinetic interaction between propranolol and chlorpromazine in schizophrenic patients. Lancet 1980;ii:978.
384. McLean AJ, Skews H, Bobik A, Dudley FJ. Interaction between oral propranolol and hydralazine. Clin Pharmacol Ther 1980;27:726.
385. Conrad KA, Nyman DW. Effects of metoprolol and propranolol on theophylline elimination. Clin Pharmacol Ther 1980;28:463.
386. Greendyke RM, Kanter DR. Plasma propranolol levels and their effect on plasma thioridazine and haloperidol concentrations. J Clin Psychopharmacol 1987;7:178.
387. Peet M, Middlemiss DN, Yates RA. Pharmacokinetic interaction between propranolol and chlorpromazine in schizophrenic patients. Lancet 1980;ii:978.
388. Bax NDS, Lennard MS, Tucker GT et al. The effect of β-adrenoceptor antagonists on the pharmacokinetics and pharmacodynamics of warfarin after a single dose. Br J Clin Pharmacol 1984;17:553.
389. Ochs H, Greenblatt D, Verbing-Ochs B. Propranolol, interactions with diazepam, lorazepam and alprazolam. Clin Pharmacol Ther 1984;36:451.
390. Sautoso B. Isoniazid clearance by propranolol. Int J Clin Pharmacol 1985;23:134.
391. Lewis GP, Holtzman JC. Interaction of flecainide with digoxin and propranolol. Am J Cardiol 1984;53:52B.
392. Ochs HR, Carstens G, Greenblatt DJ. Reduction in lidocaine clearance during continuous infusion and by coadministration of propranolol. New Engl J Med 1980;303:373.
393. Bax NDS, Tucker GT, Lennard MS et al. The impairment of lignocaine clearance by propranolol: major contribution from enzyme inhibition. Br J Clin Pharmacol 1984; 19:597.
394. Bonde J, Botker S, Angelo HR et al. Atenolol inhibits the elimination of disopyramide. Eur J Clin Pharmacol 1985;28:41.
395. Leeman T, Dayer P, Meyer UA. Single dose quinidine treatment inhibits metoprolol oxidation in extensive metabolisers. Eur J Clin Pharmacol 1986;29:739.
396. Kendall MJ, Jack DB, Quarterman CP et al. β-adrenoceptor blocker pharmacokinetics and the oral contraceptive pill. Br J Clin Pharmacol 1984;17(Suppl 1):875.
397. Watkins J, Abbott EC, Hensby C et al. Attenuation of hypotensive effect of propranolol and thiazide diuretics by indomethacin. Br Med J 1980;281:702.
398. Wong DG, Spence JD, Lamki L et al. Effect of nonsteroidal anti-inflammatory drugs on control of hypertension by β-blockers and diuretics. Lancet 1986;i:997.
399. Lewis RV, Tower JM, Jackson PR et al. Effects of sulindac and indomethacin on the blood pressure of hypertensive patients. Br Med J 1986;292:934.
400. Eldor J, Hoffman B, Davidson JT. Prolonged bradycardia and hypotension after neostigmine administration in a patient receiving atenolol. Anaesthesia 1987;42:1294.
401. Ikram H. Hemodynamic and electrophysiologic interactions between antiarrhythmic drugs and β blockers with special reference to tocainide. Am Heart J 1980;100:1076.

402. Venter CP, Joubert PH, Buys AC. Severe peripheral ischaemia during concomitant use of β-blockers and ergot alkaloids. Br Med J 1984;289:788.
403. McDevitt DG. Differential features of β-adrenoceptor blocking drugs for therapy. In: Laragh J, Buhler F, eds. Frontiers in Hypertension Research. New York: Springer Verlag, 1981;473.
404. Woods PB, Robinson ML. An investigation of the comparative liposolubilities of β-adrenoceptor blocking agents. J Pharm Pharmacol 1981;33:172.
405. McDevitt DG. Clinical significance of cardioselectivity: state of the art. Drugs 1983;25(Suppl 2):219.
406. McDevitt DG. β-Adrenoceptor blocking drugs and partial agonist activity: is it a clinical reality? Drugs 1983;25:331.
407. Cruickshank JM. Measurement and cardiovascular relevance of partial agonist activity (PAA) involving β_1 and β_2-adrenoceptors. Pharmacol Ther 1990;46:199.
408. Pritchard BNC. β-Blocking agents with vasodilating actions. J Cardiovasc Pharmacol 1992;19(Suppl D):S1.
409. Pritchard BNC, Owens CWI. Mode of action of β-adrenergic blocking drugs in hypertension. Clin Physiol Biochem 1990;8(Suppl 2):1.
410. Coltart DJ, Meldrum SJ. The effect of propranolol on human and canine transmembrane action potential. Br J Pharmacol 1970;40:148P.
411. Camus P, Lombard JN, Perrichan M et al. Bronchiolitis obliterans organising pneumonia in patients taking acebutolol or amiodarone. Thorax 1989;44:711.
412. Tanner LA, Bosco LA, Zimmerman HJ. Hepatic toxicity after acebutalol therapy. Ann Intern Med 1989;111:533.
413. Kholeif M, Isles C. Profound hypotension after atenolol in severe hypertension. Br Med J 1989;298:161.
414. Arber N. Delirium induced by atenolol. Br Med J 1988;297:1048.
415. Schwartz MS, Frank MS, Yanoff A, Morecki E. Atenolol-induced cholestasis. Am J Gastroenterol 1989;84:1084.
416. Wolf R, Ophir J, Elman M, Krakowski L. Atenolol-induced cutaneous vasculitis. Cutis 1989;43:231.
417. Maclean D. Bevantolol vs propranolol: a double-blind controlled trial in essential hypertension. Angiology 1988; 39:387.
418. Rodrigues EA, Lawrence JD, Dasgupta P et al. Comparison of bevantolol and atenolol in chronic stable angina. Am J Cardiol 1988;61:1204.
419. Lancaster SG, Sorkin EM. Bisoprolol: a preliminary review of its pharmacodynamic and pharmacokinetic properties, and therapeutic efficacy in hypertension and angina pectoris. Drugs 1988;36:256.
420. Neutel JM, Smith DHG, Venkata C et al. Application of ambulatory blood pressure monitoring in differentiating between antihypertensive agents. Am J Med 1993;94:181.
421. Wheeldon NM, MacDonald TM, Prasad N, Maclean D, Peebles L, McDevitt DG. A double-blind comparison of bisoprolol and atenolol in patients with essential hypertension. Q J Med 1995;88:565.
422. Louis WJ, Krum H, Conway EL. A risk-benefit assessment of carvedilol in the treatment of cardiovascular disorders. Drug Safety 1994;11:86.
423. Krum H, Conway EL, Broadbear JH, Howes LG, Louis WJ. Postural hypotension in elderly patients given carvedilol. Br Med J 1994;309:775.
424. Busst CM, Bush A. Comparison of the cardiovascular and pulmonary effects of oral celiprolol, propranolol and placebo in normal volunteers. Br J Clin Pharmacol 1989; 27:405.
425. Lombard JN, Bonnotte B, Maynadie M et al. Celiprolol pneumonitis. Eur Respir J 1993;6:588.
426. Harvengt C. Labetalol hepatoxicity. Ann Intern Med 1990;114:341.
427. Benfield P, Sorkin EM. Esmolol: a preliminary review of its pharmacodynamic and pharmacokinetic properties and therapeutic efficacy. Drugs 1987;33:392.
428. Gray RJ, Bateman TM, Czer LSC et al. Esmolol: a new ultrashort-acting β-adrenergic blocking agent for rapid control of heart rate in post-operative supraventricular tachycardia. J Am Coll Cardiol 1985;5:1451.
429. Morganroth J, Horowitz LM, Anderson J et al. Comparative efficacy and tolerance of esmolol to propranolol for control of supraventricular tachyarrhythmia. Am J Cardiol 1985;56:33F.
430. The Esmolol vs Placebo Multicentre Study Group. Comparison of the efficacy and safety of esmolol, a short-acting β-blocker with placebo in the treatment of supraventricular tachyarrhythmias. Am Heart J 1986;111:42.
431. Lowenthal DT, Porter S, Saris SD et al. Clinical pharmacology, pharmacodynamics and interactions with esmolol. Am J Cardiol 1985;56:14F.
432. Angaran DM, Schultz NJ, Tschida VH. Esmolol hydrochloride: an ultrashort-acting β-adrenergic blocking agent. Clin Pharmacol 1988;5:288.
433. Kanto JH. Current status of labetalol, the first α- and β-blocking agent. Clin Pharmacol Ther Toxicol 1985;23:617.
434. Clark JA, Zimmerman HJ, Tanner LA. Labetalol hepatotoxicity. Ann Intern Med 1990;113:210.
435. Willis JK, Tilton AH, Harkin JC, Boineau FG. Reversible myopathy due to labetalol. Pediatr Neurol 1990;6:275.
436. Arthur S, Greenberg A. Hyperkalemia associated with intravenous labetalol therapy for acute hypertension in renal transplant recipients. Clin Nephrol 1990;33:269.
437. Klarr JM, Bhatt-Mehta, Donn SM. Neonatal adrenergic blockade following single dose maternal labetalol administration. Am J Perinatol 1994;11:91.
438. Olsen KS, Beier-Holgersen R. Fetal death following labetalol administration in pre-eclampsia. Acta Obstet Gynecol Scand 1992;71:145.
439. Sala X, Monsalve C, Comas C et al. Paro cardiaco en neonato de madre tratada con labetalol. Rev Esp Anestesiol Reanim 1993;40:146.
440. Larrey D, Henrion J, Heller F et al. Metoprolol-induced hepatitis: rechallenge and drug oxidation phenotyping. Ann Intern Med 1988;108:67.
441. Snyder S. Metoprolol-induced polymyalgia-like syndrome. Ann Intern Med 1991;114:96.
442. Aellig WH, Clark BJ. Is the ISA of pindolol β_2-selective? Br J Clin Pharmacol 1987;24:21S.
443. Akoun GM, Milleorom BJ, Maythus CM et al. Provocation test coupled with bronchoalveolar lavage in the diagnosis of propranolol induced hypersensitivity pneumonitis. Ann Rev Respir Dis 1989;139:247.
444. Gauthier-Rahman S, Akoun GM, Milleron BJ, Mayaud CM. Leukocyte migration inhibition in propranolol-induced pneumonitis. Evidence of an immunologic cell-mediated mechanism. Chest 1990;97:238.
445. Hohnloser SH, Woosley RL. Sotalol. New Engl J Med 1994;331:31.
446. Abrams J. Nitrate delivery systems in perspective. Am J Med 1984;76:38.

447. Amlie E. Incidence of cancer among workers in a Norwegian nitrate fertiliser plant. Br J Ind Med 1993; 50:647–652.
448. Sporl-Radun S, Betzien G, Kaufmann B et al. Effects and pharmacokinetics of isosorbide dinitrate in normal man. Eur J Clin Pharmacol 1980;18:237.
449. Anonymous. Buccal nitroglycerin spray. Adverse Reactions Newsletter, Nos 3 and 4. Uppsala: WHO Collaborating Centre for International Drug Monitoring, 1988.
450. Nemerovski M, Shah PK. Syndrome of severe bradycardia and hypotension following sublingual nitroglycerin administration. Cardiology 1981;67:180.
451. Massie B, Kramer B, Haughom F. Postural hypotension and tachycardia during hydralazine-isosorbide dinitrate therapy for chronic heart failure. Circulation 1981;63:658.
452. Lamaud M, Duranton B, Verneyre H. Une syncope nitrée. Lyon Méd 1985;253:39.
453. Viskin S, Heller K, Porat R, Belhassen B. Complete atrioventricular block due to sublingual isosorbide dinitrate. South Med J 1991;84:369.
454. Brandes W, Santiago T, Limacher M. Nitroglycerin-induced hypotension, bradycardia, and asystole: report of a case and review of the literature. Clin Cardiol 1990;13:741.
455. Feldman RL, Pepine CJ, Conti CR. Neuronal vasomotor coronary arterial responses after nitroglycerin. Am J Cardiol 1978;42:517.
456. Curry RC. Coronary vasoconstriction following nitroglycerin. Catheter Cardiovasc Diagn 1980;6:211.
457. Scardi S, Zigone B, Pandullow C. Myocardial infarction following sublingual administration of isosorbide dinitrate. Int J Cardiol 1990;26:378.
458. Ong EA, Canlas C, Smith W et al. Nitroglycerin induced asystole. Arch Intern Med 1985;145:954.
459. Quigley PJ, Maurer BJ. Ventricular fibrillation during coronary angiography: association with potassium-containing glyceryl trinitrate. Am J Cardiol 1985;56:101.
460. Berisso MZ, Cavallini A, lannetti M. Sudden death during continuous Holter monitoring out of hospital after nitroglycerin consumption. Am J Cardiol 1984;54:677.
461. Wrenn K. The hazards of defibrillation through nitroglycerin patches. Ann Emerg Med 1990;19:1327.
462. Iversen HK, Olesen J, Tfelt-Hansen P. Intravenous nitroglycerin as an experimental model of vascular headache. Basic characteristics. Pain 1989;38:17.
463. Asmark H, Lundberg PO, Olsson S. Drug-related headache. Headache 1989;29:441.
464. Herrmann H, Kuhl A, Maier-Lenz H. Der Einfluss des Dosierungszeitpunktes von Isosorbidmononitrat auf objektive und subjektive Parameter der Angina pectoris. Arzneim Forsch 1988;38:694.
465. Ankier S, Fay L, Warrington SJ, Woodings DF. A multicentre open comparison of isosorbide-5-mononitrate and nifedipine given prophylactically to general practice patients with chronic stable angina pectoris. J Int Med Res 1989;17:172.
466. Rodger JC. Peripheral oedema in patients with isosorbide dinitrate. Br Med J 1981;283:1365.
467. Kopiman ES. Hypoxemia after sublingual nitroglycerin. Prim Cardiol 1981;7:105.
468. Jaffe AS, Roberts R. The use of intravenous nitroglycerin in cardiovascular disease. Pharmacotherapy 1982; 2:273.
469. Pepke-Zaba J, Higgenbottam JW, Dinh-Xuan AT et al. Inhaled nitric oxide as a cause of selective pulmonary vasodilatation in pulmonary hypertension. Lancet 1991; 338:1173.
470. Packer M, Halpeim JL, Brooks KM et al. Nitroglycerin therapy in the management of pulmonary hypertensive disease. Am J Med 1984;76:67.
471. Purvin VA, Dunn DW. Nitrate-induced transient ischemic attacks. South Med J 1981;74:1130.
472. Bevan JS, Oza AM, Burke CW, Adams CBT. Pituitary apoplexy following isosorbide administration. J Neurol Neurosurg Psychiatry 1987;50:636.
473. Rosenthal R. Visual hallucinations and suicidal ideation attributed to isosorbide dinitrate. Psychosomatics 1987; 28:555.
474. Ahmad S. Nitroglycerin and intracranial hypertension. Am Heart J 1991;121:1850.
475. Demey HE, Daelemans RA, Verpoorten GA et al. Propylene glycol-induced side-effects during intravenous nitroglycerin therapy. Intens Care Med 1988;14:221.
476. Marshall B, Ecklund E. Methemoglobinemia from overdose of nitroglycerin. J Am Med Assoc 1980;244:330.
477. Kaplan JA, Finlayson DC, Woodward S. Vasodilator therapy after cardiac surgery: a review of the efficacy and toxicity of nitroglycerin and nitroprusside. Can Anaesth Soc J 1980;27:254.
478. Kaplan KJ, Taber M, Teguarden JR et al. Association of methemoglobinemia and intravenous nitroglycerin administration. Am J Cardiol 1985;55:181.
479. Zurick AM, Wagner RH, Starr NJ et al. Intravenous nitroglycerin, methemoglobinemia and respiratory distress in a post-operative cardiac anginal patient. Anesthesiology 1984;61:464.
480. Buenger JW, Mauro VF. Organic nitrate-induced methemoglobinemia. DICP Ann Pharmacother 1989;23:283.
481. Chinoy DA, Camp J, Elchahal S et al. A multicenter comparison of adhesion, preference, tolerability, and safety characteristics of two transdermal nitroglycerin delivery systems: Transderm-Nitro and Deponit. Clin Ther 1989;11:678.
482. Hendricks AAH, Dee GW Jr. Contact dermatitis due to nitroglycerin ointment. Arch Dermatol 1979;115:853.
483. Rosenfeld AS, White WB. Allergic contact dermatitis secondary to transdermal nitroglycerin. Am Heart J 1984;108:1061.
484. Letendre PW, Barr C, Wilkens K. Adverse dermatologic reaction to transdermal nitroglycerin. DICP Ann Pharmacother 1984;18:69.
485. Wilkin JK. Vasodilator rosacea. Arch Dermatol 1980; 116:598.
486. Murray KB. Hazard of microwave ovens to transdermal delivery systems. New Engl J Med 1984;310:721.
487. Erwith RC, Janda SM, Henann NE. Ageusia associated with transdermal nitroglycerin. Clin Pharmacol 1989;8:146.
488. Needleman P, Johnson EM Jr. Vasodilators in the treatment of angina. In: Gilman AG, Goodman LS, Gilman A, eds. The Pharmacological Basis of Therapeutics, 6th edn, Ch. 33. New York: MacMillan, 1980;819.
489. Wizemann AJS, Wizemann V. Organic nitrate therapy in glaucoma. Am J Ophthalmol 1980;90:106.
490. De Caterina R. Nitrate als Thrombocytenfunktionskemmer. Z Kardiol 1994;83:463–473.
491. ISIS-4 (Fourth International Study of Infarct Survival) Collaborative Group. ISIS-4: a randomised factorial trial assessing early oral captopril, oral mononitrate, and intravenous magnesium sulphate in 58,050 patients with suspected acute myocardial infarction. Lancet 1995;345:669.

492. Cohn JN, Johnson G, Ziesche SZ et al. A comparison of enalapril with hydralazine-isosorbide dinitrate in the treatment of chronic congestive heart failure. New Engl J Med 1991;325:303.
493. Hoit B, Gregoratos G, Shabete IR. Paradoxical pulmonary vasoconstriction induced by nitroglycerin in idiopathic pulmonary hypertension. J. Am Coll Cardiol 1985;6:490.
494. Korn SH, Comer JB. Intravenous nitroglycerin and ethanol intoxication. Ann Intern Med 1985;102:274.
495. Shook TL, Kirshenbaum JM, Hundley RF et al. Ethanol intoxication complicating intravenous nitroglycerin therapy. Ann Intern Med 1984;101:498.
496. Anderson P, Lemberg L. An unusual complication of intravenous nitroglycerin. Heart Lung 1986;15:534
497. Shorey J, Bhardwal N, Loscalzo J. Acute Wernicke's encephalopathy after intravenous infusion of high-dose nitroglycerin. Ann Intern Med 1984;101:500.
498. Shergy WJ, Gilkeson GS, German DC. Acute gouty arthritis and intravenous nitroglycerin. Arch Intern Med 1988;148:2505.
499. Lefebvre RA, Bogaert MG, Teirlynck O et al. Influence of exercise on nitroglycerin plasma concentrations after transdermal application. Br J Clin Pharmacol 1990;30:292.
500. Hogstedt C, Axelson O. Nitroglycerine nitroglycol exposure and the mortality in cardio-cerebrovascular diseases among dynamite workers. J Occup Med 1977;19:675.
501. Lange RL, Reid MS, Tresch DD et al. Non-atheromatous ischemic heart disease following withdrawal from chronic industrial nitroglycerin exposure. Circulation 1972; 46:666.
502. Danahy DT, Aronow WS. Hemodynamics and antianginal effects of high dose oral isosorbide dinitrate after chronic use. Circulation 1977;56:205.
503. Aronow WS. Nitrates as antianginal agents. Prim Cardiol 1980;6:46.
504. Anonymous. Transdermal glyceryl trinitrate patches (Transiderm-Nitro). Drug Ther Bull 1986;24:5.
505. Parker JO, Vankoughnett KA, Farrel IB. Comparison of buccal nitroglycerin and oral isosorbide dinitrate for nitrate tolerance in stable angina pectoris. Am J Cardiol 1985;56:724.
506. Lin S-G, Flaherty JT. Crossover from intravenous to transdermal nitroglycerin therapy in unstable angina pectoris. Am J Cardiol 1985;56:742.
507. Needleman P, Johnson EM Jr. Mechanism of tolerance development to organic nitrates. J Pharmacol Exp Ther 1971;184:709.
508. Elkayam U. Tolerance to organic nitrates: evidence, mechanisms, clinical relevance, and strategies for prevention. Ann Intern Med 1991;114:667.
509. Cowan JC. Avoiding nitrate tolerance. Br J Clin Pharmacol 1992;34:96.
510. Tongia SK. Exaggerated tendency to postural hypotension with isosorbide dinitrate on clonidine's background activity. J Assoc Phys India 1994;42:580.
511. Hyldstrup L, Morgensen NB, Nillsen PE. Orthostatic response before and after nitroglycerin in metoprolol and verapamil-treated angina pectoris. Acta Med Scand 1983;214:131.
512. Silfast T, Kinnunen A, Varpula T. Laryngeal oedema after isosorbide dinitrate spray and sublingual nifedipine. Br Med J 1995;311:232.
513. Lancaster L, Forster PE. Complete heart block after sublingual nitroglycerin. Chest 1983;84:111.
514. Antonelli D, Barzilay J. Complete atrioventricular block after sublingual isosorbide dinitrate. Int J Cardiol 1986;10:71.
515. Barletta MA, Eisen H. Isosorbide dinitrate-disopyramide phosphate interaction. DICP Ann Pharmacother 1985; 19:764.
516. Abrams J, Schroeder K, Raizada V. Potentially adverse effects of sublingual nitroglycerin during consumption of alcohol. J Am Coll Cardiol 1990;15:226A.
517. Habbab MA, Haft JI. Intravenous nitroglycerin and heparin resistance. Ann Intern Med 1986;105:305.
518. Pye M, Oldroyd KG, Conkie JA. A clinical and in vitro study on the possible interaction of intravenous nitrates with heparin anticoagulation. Clin Cardiol 1994;17:658.
519. Bechtold H, Kleist P, Landgraf K. Effect of low-dosage intravenous nitrate therapy on the anticoagulant effect of heparin. Med Klin 1994;89:360–366.
520. Committee on Safety of Medicines. Perhexiline maleate (Pexid): adverse reactions. Curr Probl 1983;11.
521. Carraway RD. Febrile reaction following nifedipine therapy. Am Heart J 1984;108:611.
522. Scolnick B, Brinberg D. Diltiazem and generalised lymphadenopathy. Ann Intern Med 1985;102:558.
523. Matsumoto S, Ito T, Sada T et al. Hemodynamic effects of nifedipine in congestive heart failure. Am J Cardiol 1980;46:476.
524. Gillmer DJ, Kark P. Pulmonary oedema precipitated by nifedipine. Br Med J 1980;280:1420.
525. Balasubramanian V, Bowles MJ, Davies AB et al. Combined therapy with verapamil and propranolol in chronic stable angina. Am J Cardiol 1982;49:125.
526. Bassan M, Weiler-Ravell D, Shalev O. Additive antianginal effect of verapamil in patients receiving propranolol. Br Med J 1982;284:1067.
527. Terry RW. Nifedipine therapy in angina pectoris: evaluation of safety and side effects. Am Heart J 1982;104:681.
528. Yusuf S, Wittes J, Friedman L. Overview of results of randomized clinical trials in heart disease. I. Treatments following myocardial infarction. J. Am Med Assoc 1988;260:2088.
529. Goldbourt U, Behar S, Reicher-Reiss H, Zion M, Mandelzeig L, Kaplinsky E, for the SPRINT study group. Early administration of nifedipine in acute myocardial infarction. Arch Intern Med 1993;152:345.
530. Held PH, Yusuf S, Fruberg CD. Calcium channel blockers in acute myocardial infarction and unstable angina: an overview. Br Med J 1989;299:1187.
531. Held PH, Yusuf S. Effects of β-blockers and calcium channel blockers in acute myocardial infarction. Eur Heart J 1993;14(Suppl F):18.
532. Gibson RS, Boden WE, Theroux P et al. Diltiazem and reinfarction in patients with non-Q wave myocardial infarction. New Engl J Med 1986;315:423.
533. The Multicentre Diltiazem Postinfarction Trial Research Group. The effect of diltiazem on mortality and reinfarction after myocardial infarction. New Engl J Med 1988;319:385.
534. The Danish Study Group on Verapamil in Myocardial Infarction. Verapamil in acute myocardial infarction. Eur Heart J 1984;5:516.
535. The Danish Study Group on Verapamil in Myocardial Infarction. Effect of verapamil on mortality and major events after acute myocardial infarction (The Danish Verapamil Infarction Trial II-DAVIT II). Am J Cardiol 1990;66:779.

536. Lubsen J, Tijssen JGP, Kerkkamp HJJ. Early treatment of unstable angina in the coronary care units: a randomised, double-blind, placebo controlled comparison of recurrent ischaemia in patients treated with nifedipine, metoprolol or both. Br Heart J 1986;56:400.
537. Psaty BM, Heckbert SR, Koepsell TD, Siscovick DS, Raghunathan TE et al. The risk of myocardial infarction associated with antihypertensive drug therapies. J Am Med Assoc 1995;274:620.
538. Zangerie KF, Wolford R. Syncope and conduction disturbances following sublingual nifedipine for hypertension. Ann Emerg Med 1985;14:1005.
539. Villani GQ, del Giudice S, Arruzzoli S, Dieci G. Blocco seno-atriale dopo somministrazione orale di nifedipina. Descrizione di un caso. Minerva Cardioangiol 1985;33:557.
540. Pine MB, Citron PD, Bailly DI et al. Verapamil versus placebo in relieving stable angina pectoris. Circulation 1982;65:12.
541. Dominic JA, Bourne DWA, Tan TG et al. The pharmacology of verapamil. III. Pharmacokinetics in normal subjects after intravenous drug administration. J Cardiovasc Pharmacol 1981;3:25.
542. Opie LH. Drugs and the heart. III. Calcium antagonists. Lancet 1980;i:806.
543. Hossack KF. Conduction abnormalities due to diltiazem. New Engl J Med 1982;307:953.
544. Schroeder JS, Feldman RL, Giles TD et al. Multiclinic controlled trial of diltiazem for Prinzmetal's angina. Am J Med 1982;72:227.
545. Harper R, Whitford E, Middlebrook K et al. Verapamil in patients with Wolff-Parkinson-White syndrome-a potential hazard? NZ J Med 1981;11:456.
546. Strasberg B, Sagie A, Rechvia E et al. Deleterious effects of intravenous verapamil in Wolff-Parkinson-White patients and atrial fibrillation. Cardiovasc Drugs Ther 1989;2:801.
547. Garratt C, Ward D, Antoniou A, Camm AJ. Misuse of verapamil in pre-excited atrial fibrillation. Lancet 1989;i:367.
548. Jacob AS, Neilsen DH, Gianelly RE. Fatal ventricular fibrillation following verapamil in Wolff-Parkinson-White syndrome with atrial fibrillation. Ann Emerg Med 1985; 14:159.
549. Epstein SE, Rosing DR. Verapamil: its potential for causing serious complications in patients with hypertrophic cardiomyopathy. Circulation 1981;64:437.
550. Hopf R, Rodrian S, Kaltenbach M. Behandlung der hypertrophen Kardiomyopathie mit Kalziumantagonisten. Therapiewoche 1986;36:1433.
551. Riccioni N, Bartolomei C, Soldani S. Prenylamine-induced ventricular arrhythmias and syncopal attacks with Q-T prolongation. Cardiology 1980;66:199.
552. Burri CH, Ajdacic K, Michot F. Syndrom der verlangerten QT-Zeit und Kammer-Tachykardie 'en torsade de pointe' nach Behandlung mit Prenylamin (Segontin). Schweiz Rundsch Med 1981;70:717.
553. Grayson HA, Kennedy JD. Torsade de pointes and nifedipine. Ann Intern Med 1982;97:144.
554. Krikler DM, Rowland E. Torsade de pointes and nifedipine. Ann Intern Med 1982;97:618.
555. Wachter RM. Symptomatic hypotension induced by nifedipine in the acute treatment of severe hypertension. Arch Intern Med 1987;147:556.
556. Schwartz M, Naschitz JE, Yesharun D, Sharf B. Oral nifedipine in the treatment of hypertensive urgency: cerebrovascular accident following a single dose. Arch Intern Med 1990;150:686.
557. Shettiger UR, Laungani R. Adverse effects of sublingual nifedipine in acute myocardial infarction. Crit Care Med 1989;17:196.
558. Committee on Safety of Medicines. Nifedipine (Adalat) and myocardial ischaemia. Curr Probl 1979;4:1.
559. Deanfield J, Wright C, Fox K. Treatment of angina pectoris with nifedipine: importance of dose titration. Br Med J 1983;286:1467.
560. Yagil Y, Kobrin I, Leibel B et al. Ischemic ECC changes with initial nifedipine therapy of severe hypertension. Am Heart J 1982;103:310.
561. Goiti JJ. Calcium channel blocking agents and the heart. Br Med J 1985;291:1505.
562. Graham CF. Intravenous verapamil-isotopin (Calan): acute bronchospasm. ADR Highlights 1982;868:82.
563. Zalman F, Perloff JK, Durant NN et al. Acute respiratory failure following intravenous verapamil in Duchenne's muscular dystrophy. Am Heart J 1983;105:510.
564. Packer M, Medina N, Yushak M. Adverse hemodynamic and clinical effects of calcium channel blockade in pulmonary hypertension secondary to obliterative pulmonary vascular disease. J Am Coll Cardiol 1984;4:890.
565. Baltra AK, Segall PH, Ahmed T. Pulmonary oedema with nifedipine in primary pulmonary hypertension. Respiration 1985;47:161.
566. Hasebe N, Fijikana T, Wantanabe M et al. A case of respiratory failure precipitated by injecting nifedipine. Kokya To Junkan 1988;36:1255.
567. Mobile-Orazio E, Sterzi R. Cerebral ischemia after nifedipine treatment. Br Med J 1981;283:948.
568. Ellrodt AG, Ault MJ, Riedinger MS et al. Efficacy and safety of sublingual nifedipine in hypertensive emergencies. Am J Med 1985;79(Suppl 4A):19.
569. Pitlick S, Manor RS, Lipshitz I et al. Transient retinal ischaemia induced by nifedipine. Br Med J 1983;287:1845.
570. Bertel O, Conen LD. Treatment of hypertensive emergencies with the calcium channel blocker nifedipine. Am J Med 1985;79(Suppl 4A):31.
571. Gill JS, Zezulka AU, Horrocks PM. Rupture of cerebral aneurysm associated with nifedipine treatment. Postgrad Med J 1986;62:1029.
572. Jacobs MB. Diltiazem and akathisia. Ann Intern Med 1983;99:794.
573. Brink DD. Diltiazem and hyperactivity. Ann Intern Med 1984;100:459.
574. Ahmad S. Nifedipine associated acute psychosis. J Am Geriatr Soc 1984;32:408.
575. Palat GK, Hooker EA, Movahed A. Secondary mania associated with diltiazem. Clin Cardiol 1984;7:611.
576. Jacobsen FM, Sack DA, James SP. Delirium induced by verapamil. Am J Psychiatry 1987;144:248.
577. Pitlick S, Manor RS, Lipshitz I et al. Transient retinal ischaemia induced by nifedipine. Br Med J 1983;287:1845.
578. Eccleston D, Cole AJ. Calcium channel blockade and depressive illness. Br J Psychiatry 1990;156:889.
579. Hicks CB, Abraham K. Verapamil and myoclonic dystonia. Ann Intern Med 1985;103:154.
580. Garcia-Ruiz PJ, Garcia de Yebenes J, Jimenez-Jimenez FJ. Parkinsonism associated with calcium channel blockers: a prospective follow-up study. Clin Neuropharmacol 1992; 15:19.
581. Krendel DA, Hopkins LC. Adverse effect of verapamil

in a patient with the Lambert-Eaton syndrome. Muscle Nerv 1986;9:519.
582. Ueno S, Hara Y. Lambert-Eaton myasthenic syndrome without anti-calcium channel antibody: adverse effect of calcium antagonist diltiazem. J Neurol Neurosurg Psychiatry 1992;55:409.
583. Swash M, Ingram DA. Adverse effect of verapamil in myasthenia gravis. Muscle Nerv 1992;15:396.
584. Malaisse WJ, Sener A. Calcium antagonists and islet function. XII. Comparison between nifedipine and chemically related drugs. Biochem Pharmacol 1981;30:1039.
585. Giugliano D, Gentile S, Verza M et al. Modulation by verapamil of insulin and glucagon secretion in man. Acta Diabetol 1981;18:163.
586. Donnelly T, Harrower ADB. Effect of nifedipine on glucose tolerance and insulin secretion in diabetic and non-diabetic patients. Curr Med Res Opin 1980;6:690.
587. Abadie E, Passa PH. Diabetogenic effect of nifedipine. Br Med J 1984;289:438.
588. Collings WCJ, Cullen MJ, Feely J. The effect of therapy with dihydropyridine calcium channel blockers on glucose tolerance in non-insulin dependent diabetes. Br J Clin Pharmacol 1986;21:568P.
589. Zezulka AV, Gill JS, Beevers DG. Diabetogenic effects of nifedipine. Br Med J 1984;289:437.
590. Trost BN. Glucose metabolism and calcium antagonists. Horm Metab Res 1990;22(Suppl):48.
591. Bhatnagar SK, Amin MMA, Al-Yusuf AR. Diabetogenic effects of nifedipine. Br Med J 1984;289:19
592. Rodger VC, Torrance TC. Can nifedipine provoke menorrhagia? Lancet 1983;ii:460.
593. Clyne CAC. Unilateral gynaecomastia and nifedipine. Br Med J 1986;292:380.
594. Tishler M, Armon S. Nifedipine-induced hypokalemia. DICP Ann Pharmacother 1986;20:370.
595. Murphy MB, Scriven AJI, Brown MJ et al. The effects of nifedipine and hydralazine induced hypotension on sympathetic activity. Eur J Clin Pharmacol 1982;23:479.
596. Struthers AD, Reid JL. Nifedipine does not influence adrenaline induced hypokalaemia in man. Br J Clin Pharmacol 1983;16:342.
597. Voth AJ, Turner RH. Nifedipine and agranulocytosis. Ann Intern Med 1983;99:882.
598. Quigley MA, White KL, McGraw BF. Interpretation and application of world-wide safety data on diltiazem. Acta Pharmacol Toxicol 1985;57(Suppl 2):61.
599. Baggot LA. Diltiazem-associated immune thrombocytopenia. Mt Sinai J Med 1987;54:500.
600. Rotmensch HH, Roth A, Livon M et al. Lymphocyte sensitisation in nifedipine-induced hepatitis. Br Med J 1980;2:976.
601. Davidson AR. Lymphocyte sensitisation in nifedipine-induced hepatitis. Br Med J 1980;2:1354.
602. Centrum Voor Geneesmiddelenbewaking. Nifedipine en hepatitis. Folia Pharmacother 1981;8:7.
603. Stern EH, Pitchon R, King BD et al. Possible hepatitis from verapamil. New Engl J Med 1982;306:612.
604. Tartaglione TA, Pepine CJ, Pieper JA. Diltiazem: a review of its clinical efficacy and use. Drug Intell Clin Pharm 1982;16:371.
605. McGraw BF, Walker SD, Hemberger JA. Clinical experience with diltiazem in Japan. Pharmacotherapy 1982; 2:156.
606. Sarachek NS, London RL, Matulewicz TJ. Diltiazem and granulomatous hepatitis. Gastroenterology 1985; 88:1260.
607. Guarascio P, D'Amato C, Sette P et al. Liver damage from verapamil. Br Med J 1984;288:362.
608. Hedback B, Hermann LS. Antihypertensive effect of verapamil in patients with newly discovered mild to moderate essential hypertension. Acta Med Scand 1984;215(Suppl 681):129.
609. Ganginella TS, Maxfield DL. Calcium channel blocking agents and chest pain. DICP Ann Pharmacother 1988; 22:623.
610. Diamond JR, Cheung JY, Fang LST. Nifedipine-induced renal dysfunction in man. Am J Med 1984;77:905.
611. Hall-Craggs M, Light PD, Peters RW. Development of immune complex nephritis during treatment with the calcium channel-blocking agent nifedipine. Hum Pathol 1984;15:691.
612. Ter Wee PM, Rosman JB, Van der Geest J. Acute renal failure due to diltiazem. Lancet 1984;ii:1337.
613. Groth H, Foerster EC, Neyses L et al. Nifedipine beim hypertensiven Notfall und bei schwerer Hypertonie. Schweiz Rundsch Med Prax 1984;73:45.
614. Williams G, Donaldson RM. Nifedipine and nocturia. Lancet 1986;i:738.
615. Kumana CR, Mahon WA. Bizarre perceptual disorder of extremities in patients taking verapamil. Lancet 1981; i:1324.
616. Grunwalk Z. Painful edema, erythematous rash, and burning sensation due to nifedipine. DICP Ann Pharmacother 1982;16:492.
617. Wirebaugh SR, Geraets DR. Reports of erythematous macular skin eruptions associated with diltiazem therapy. DICP Ann Pharmacother 1990;24:1046.
618. Wood TML. Photosensitivity reaction associated with nifedipine. Br Med J 1986;292:992.
619. Alcalay J, David M. Generalised fixed drug eruption associated with nifedipine. Br Med J 1986;292:450.
620. Wirebaugh SR, Ceraets DR. Reports of erythmatous macular skin eruptions associated with diltiazem. Drug Intell Clin Pharm 1990;24:1046.
621. Lambert DG, Dalac S, Beer F et al. Acute generalised exanthematous pustular dermatitis induced by diltiazem. Br J Dermatol 1988;116:308.
622. Levenson JC, Kennedy K. Dysosmia, dysgeusia and nifedipine. Ann Intern Med 1985;102:135.
623. Berman JL. Dysosmia, dysgeusia and diltiazem. Ann Intern Med 1985;103:154.
624. Coulter DM. Eye pain with nifedipine and disturbance of taste with captopril: a mutually controlled study showing a method of post-marketing surveillance. Br Med J 1988;296:1086.
625. Kelly SP, Walley TJ. Eye pain with nifedipine. Br Med J 1988;296:1401.
626. Keidar S, Binenboim C, Palant A. Muscle cramps during treatment with nifedipine. Br Med J 1982;285:1241.
627. Lindenberg BS, Weiner DA, McCabe CH et al. Efficacy and safety of incremental doses of diltiazem for the treatment of stable angina pectoris. J Am Coll Cardiol 1983;2:1129.
628. Petru MA, Crawford MH, Sorensen SG et al. Short and long-term efficacy of oral diltiazem for angina due to coronary artery disease: a placebo-controlled, randomiseddouble-blind cross-over study. Circulation 1983;68:139.
629. Ramon Y, Behar S, Kishon Y et al. Gingival hyperplasia caused by nifedipine-a preliminary report. Int J Cardiol 1984;5:195.

630. Lombardi T, Fiore-Donno G, Belser U et al. Felodipine-induced gingival hyperplasia: a clinical and histological study. J Oral Pathol Med 1991;20:89–92.
631. Cucchi G, Giustiniani S, Robustelli F. Gengivite ipertrofica da verapamil. G Ital Cardiol 1985;15:556.
632. Lokken P, Skomedal T. Kalsiumkanalblokkerindusert gingival hyperplasi. Sjelden, eller tusener av tilfeller i Norge? Tidsskr Nor Laegeforen 1992;112:1978.
633. Fattore L, Stablein M, Bredfeldt G et al. Gingival hyperplasia: a side effect of nifedipine and diltiazem. Spec Care Dentist 1991;11:107.
634. Nyska A, Shemesh M, Tal H. Gingival hyperplasia induced by calcium channel blockers: mode of action. Med Hypotheses 1994;43:115.
635. Rocco S, Mantero F, Boscaro M. Effects of a calcium antagonist on the pituitary-adrenal axis. Horm Metab Res 1993;25:114.
636. Andersson K-E. Effects of calcium and calcium antagonists on the excitation-contraction coupling in striated and smooth muscle. Acta Pharmacol Toxicol 1978;43(Suppl 1):5.
637. Hagemeijer F. Verapamil in the management of supraventricular tachyarrhythmias occurring after a recent myocardial infarction. Circulation 1978;57:751.
638. Offerhaus L, Dunning AJ. Angina pectoris: variaties op het thema nifedipine. Ned T Geneeskd 1980;124:2097.
639. Lederballe Pedersen O, Mikkelsen I, Andersson KE. Paradoks angina pectoris efter nifedipin. Ugeskr Laeg 1980;142:1883.
640. Gottlieb SO, Gerstenblith G. Safety of acute calcium antagonist withdrawal from nifedipine. Am J Cardiol 1985; 55(Suppl):27E.
641. Gottlieb SO, Ouyang P, Achuff SC et al. Acute nifedipine withdrawal: consequences of preoperative and late cessation of therapy in patients with prior unstable angina. J Am Coll Cardiol 1984;4:382.
642. Kay R, Blake J, Rubin D et al. Possible coronary spasm rebound to abrupt nifedipine withdrawal. Am Heart J 1982;103:308.
643. Engelman RM, Hadji-Rousou I, Breyer Rli et al. Rebound vasospasm after coronary revascularization in association with calcium antagonist withdrawal. Ann Thorac Surg 1984;37:469.
644. Lette J, Gagnon RM, Lemire JG et al. Rebound of vasospastic angina after cessation of long-term treatment with nifedipine. Can Med Assoc J 1984;130:1169.
645. Mysliwiec M, Rydzewski A, Bulhak W. Calcium antagonist withdrawhal syndrome. Br Med J 1983;286:1898.
646. Schick EC, Liang C-S, Heupler FA et al. Randomized withdrawal from nifedipine: placebo-controlled study in patients with coronary artery spasm. Am Heart J 1982;104:690.
647. Balasubramanian V, Bowles MJ, Khurmi NS et al. Calcium antagonist withdrawal syndrome: objective demonstration with frequency-modulated ambulatory ST-segment monitoring. Br Med J 1983;286:520.
648. Fenakel K, Fenakel G, Appelman Z et al. Nifedipine in the treatment of severe preeclampsia. Obstet Gynecol 1991;77:331.
649. lnove H. Excretion of verapamil in human milk. Br Med J 1984;288:645.
650. Okada M, Inove H, Nakamura Y et al. Excretion of diltiazem in human milk. New Engl J Med 1985;312:992.
651. Kenny J. Treating overdose with calcium channel blockers: It's their cardiovascular effects that kill. Br Med J 1994;308:992.
652. Perkins CM. Serious verapamil poisoning: treatment with intravenous calcium gluconate. Br Med J 1978;2:1127.
653. DaSilva DA, De Melo RA, Filho JPJ. Verapamil acute self-poisoning. Clin Toxicol 1979;14:361.
654. Candell J, Valle V, Soler M et al. Acute intoxication with verapamil. Chest 1979;75:200.
655. Kenney J. Calcium channel blocking agents and the heart. Br Med J 1985;291:1150.
656. Ramoska EA, Spiller HA, Myers A. Calcium channel blocker toxicity. Ann Emerg Med 1990;19:649.
657. Borkje B, Omvik P, Storstein L. Fatal verapamilforgiftning. Tidsskr Nor Laegeforen 1986;106:401.
658. Zogubi W, Schwartz JB. Verapamil overdose: report of a case and review of the literature. Cardiovasc Rev Rep 1984;5:356.
659. Humbert VH, Munn NJ, Hawkins RF. Non-cardiogenic pulmonary oedema complicating massive diltiazem overdose. Chest 1991;99:258.
660. Buckley CD, Aronson JK. Prologned half life of verapamil in a case of overdose: implications for therapy. Br J Clin Pharmacol 1995;39:680.
661. Pearingen PD, Benowitz NJ. Poisoning due to calcium antagonists. Drug Safety 1991;6:408.
662. Walter FG, Frye G, Mullen JT, Ekins BR, Khasigian PA. Amelioration of nifedipine poisoning associated with glucagon therapy. Ann Emerg Med 1993;22:1234.
663. Ter Wee PM, Kremer Hovings TIC, Uges DRA et al. 4-Aminopyridine and haemodialysis in the treatment of verapamil intoxication. Hum Toxicol 1985;4:327.
664. Schiffl H, Siupa J, Schollmeyer P. Clinical features and management of nifedipine overdosage in a patient with renal insufficiency. Clin Toxicol 1984;22:387.
665. Sauder P, Kopferschmitt J, Dohlet M et al. Acute verapamil poisoning: 6 cases. Review of literature. J Toxicol Clin Exp 1990;10:261.
666. McMillan R. Management of severe verapamil intoxication. J Emerg Med 1988;6:193.
667. Howarth DM, Dawson AH, Smith AJ. Calcium channel blocking drug overdose: an Australian series. Hum Exp Toxicol 1994;13:161.
668. Klieman RL, Stephenson SH. Calcium antagonists-drug interactions. Rev Drug Metab Drug Interact 1985;5:193.
669. Opie LH, White DA. Adverse interaction between nifedipine and β-blockade. Br Med J 1980;2:1462.
670. Staffurth JS, Emery P. Adverse interaction between nifedipine and β-blockade. Br Med J 1981;1:225.
671. Anastassiades CJ. Nifedipine and β-blocker drugs. Br Med J 1980;2:1251.
672. Young GP. Calcium channel blockers in emergency medicine. Ann Emerg Med 1984;13:172.
673. Saini RK, Fulmor IE, Antonaccio MJ. Effect of tiapamil and nifedipine during critical coronary stenosis and in the presence of adrenergic β-receptor blockade in anaesthetized dogs. J Cardiovasc Pharmacol 1982;4:770.
674. Rocha P, Baron B, Delestrain A. Hemodynamic effects of intravenous diltiazem in patients treated chronically with propranolol. Am Heart J 1986;111:62.
675. Leon MB, Rosing DR, Bonow RO. Clinical efficacy of verapamil alone and combined with propranolol in treating patients with chronic stable angina pectoris. Am J Cardiol 1981;48:131.
676. Sorkin EM, Clissold SP, Broaden RN. Nifedipine: a review of its pharmacodynamic and pharmacokinetic properties, and therapeutic efficacy, in ischaemic heart disease,

hypertension and related cardiovascular disorders. Drugs 1985;30:12.
677. Goa KL, Sorkin EM. Nitrendipine: a review of its pharmacodynamic and pharmacokinetic properties, and therapeutic efficacy in the treatment of hypertension. Drugs 1987;33:123.
678. Sorkin EM, Clissold SP. Nicardipine: a review of its pharmacodynamic and pharmacokinetic properties, and therapeutic efficacy, in the treatment of angina pectoris, hypertension and related cardiovascular disorders. Drugs 1987;33:206.
679. Pringle SD, MacEwen CJ. Severe bradycardia due to interaction of timolol eye drops and verapamil. Br Med J 1987;294:155.
680. Pedersen K, Dorph-Pedersen A, Hvidt S et al. The long term effect of verapamil on plasma digoxin concentration and renal digoxin clearance in healthy subjects. Eur J Clin Pharmacol 1982;22:123.
681. Schwartz JB, Keefe D, Kates RE et al. Acute and chronic pharmacodynamic interaction of verapamil and digoxin in atrial fibrillation. Circulation 1982;65:1163.
682. Kleinbloesem CH, Van Brummelen P, Hillers J et al. Interaction between digoxin and nifedipine at steady state in patients with atrial fibrillation. Ther Drug Monit 1985;7:372.
683. Kirch W, Hutt HJ, Dylewizc D. Dose dependence of the nifedipine-digoxin interaction. Clin Pharmacol Ther 1986;39:35.
684. Dyama Y, Fujii S, Kanda K et al. Digoxin-diltiazem interactions. Am J Cardiol 1984;53:1480.
685. D'Arcy PF. Diltiazem-digoxin interactions. Pharm Int 1985;6:148.
686. Kirch W, Hutt HJ, Heidemann H et al. Drug interactions with nitrendipine. J Cardiovasc Pharmacol 1984; 6(Suppl):S982.
687. Belz GG, Wistuba S, Matthews JH. Digoxin and bepridil: pharmacokinetic and pharmacodynamic interactions. Clin Pharmacol Ther 1986;39:65.
688. Kuhlmann J. Effects of verapamil, diltiazem and nifedipine on plasma levels and renal excretion of digitoxin. Clin Pharmacol Ther 1985;38:667.
689. De Vito JM, Frieman B. Evaluation of the pharmacodynamic and pharmacokinetic interaction between calcium antagonists and digoxin. Pharmacotherapy 1986;6:73.
690. Kounis NG. Asystole after verapamil and digoxin. Br J Clin Pract 1980;34:57.
691. Green JA, Clementi WA, Porter C et al. Nifedipine-quinidine interaction. Clin Pharmacol 1983;2:461.
692. Farringer JA, Green JA, O'Rourke RA et al. Nifedipine-induced alterations in serum quinidine concentrations. Am Heart J 1984;198:1570.
693. Jee LD, Opie LH. Acute hypotensive response to nifedipine added to prazosin in treatment of hypertension. Br Med J 1983;287:1514.
694. Pasanisi F, Meredith PA, Elliott HL et al. Verapamil and prazosin: pharmacodynamic and pharmacokinetic interactions in normal man. Br. J Clin Pharmacol 1984 18:290P.
695. Burnakis TG, Seldon M, Czaplicki AD. Increased serum theophylline concentrations secondary to oral verapamil. Clin Pharmacol 1983;2:458.
696. Parillo SJ, Venditto M. Elevated serum theophylline levels from institution of nifedipine therapy. Ann Emerg Med 1984;13:216.
697. Kirch W, Janisch HD, Heidemann H et al. Einfluss von Cimetidin und Ranitidin auf Pharmakokinetik und antihypertensiven Effect von Nifedipin. Dtsch Med Wochenschr 1983;108:1757.
698. Dylewicz P, Kirch W, Benesch L, Ohnhaus EE. Influence of nifedipine with and without cimetidine on exercise tolerance in patients after myocardial infarction. In: Proceedings 6th International Adalat Symposium, Geneva, 1985. ICS 71. Amsterdam: Excerpta Medica, 1986.
699. Van Harten J, Van Brummelen P, Michiel M et al. Pharmacokinetics and hemodynamic effects of nisoldipine and its interaction with cimetidine. Clin Pharmacol Ther 1988;43:332.
700. Kirch W, Hutt JH, Heidemann H et al. Drug interactions with nitrendipine. J Cardiovasc Pharmacol 1984;6:S982.
701. Kirch W, Kleinblocsein CH, Belz GG. Drug interactions with calcium antagonists. Pharmacol Ther 1990;45:109.
702. MacPhee GJA, Mclnnes GT, Thompson GG et al. Verapamil potentiates carbamazepine neurotoxicity: a clinically important inhibitor interaction. Lancet 1986;i:700.
703. Brodie MJ, MacPhee GJA. Carbamazepine neurotoxicity precipitated by diltiazem. Br Med J 1986;292:1170.
704. Ahmad S. Nifedipine-phenytoin interaction. J Am Coll Cardiol 1984;3:1582.
705. Bahls FH, Ozuna J, Ritchie DE. Interactions between calcium channel blockers and the anticonvulsants carbamazepine and phenytoin. Neurology 1991;41:740.
706. Qureshi S, Langaniere S, McGilveray IJ et al. Nifedipine-alcohol interaction. J Am Med Assoc 1990;264:1660.
707. Bailey DG, Spence JD, Muroz C, Arnold JMO. Interaction of citrus juices with felodipine and nifedipine. Lancet 1991;337:268.
708. Boubigot E, Guiseri J, Airan J. Nicardipine increases cyclosporin blood levels. Lancet 1986;i:1447.
709. Pochet JM, Pirson Y. Cyclosporin-diltiazem interaction. Lancet 1986;i:979.
710. David D, Yoel G. Calcium and calciferol antagonise effect of verapamil in atrial fibrillation. Br Med J 1981; 282:1585.
711. Barborash RA, Bauman JL, Fischer JH et al. Near-total reduction in verapamil bioavailability by rifampicin: electrocardiographic correlates. Chest 1989;94:954.
712. Osterloch I. The safety of amlodipine. Am Heart J 1989;118:1114.
713. Hill JA, Pepine CJ. Effects of bepridil on the resting electrocardiogram. Int J Cardiol 1984;6:319.
714. DiBanco R, Alpert J, Katz RJ et al. Bepridil for chronic stable angina pectoris: results of a prospective multicenter, placebo-controlled dose-ranging study in 77 patients. Am J Cardiol 1984;53:35.
715. Leclerq JF, Kural S, Valere PE. Bepridil and torsade de pointes. Arch Mal Coeur Vaiss 1983;76:341.
716. Hill JA, O'Brien JT, Alpert JS et al. Effect of bepridil in patients with chronic stable angina: results of a multicenter trial. Circulation 1985;71:98.
717. Waller PC, Inman WHW. Diltiazem and heart block. Lancet 1989;i:617.
718. Nagle RE, Low-Beer T, Horton R. Diltiazem and heart block. Lancet 1989;i:907.
719. Sheehan-Dare RA, Goodfield MJD. Widespread cutaneous vasculitis associated with diltiazem. Postgrad Med J 1988;64:467.
720. Sadick NS, Katz AS, Schreiber TH. Angioedema from calcium channel blockers. J Am Acad Dermatol 1989;21:132.
721. Edgar B, Bengtsson B, Elmfeldy D et al. Acute diuretic/natriuretic properties of felodipine in man. Drugs 1985; 29(Suppl 2):176.

722. Sluiter HE, Huysmans FTM, Timen TA et al. Haemodynamic effects of intravenous felodipine in normotensive and hypertensive subjects. Drugs 1985;29(Suppl 2):144.
723. Agner E, Rehling M, Trap-Jensen J. Haemodynamic effects of single dose felodipine in normal man. Drugs 1985;29(Suppl 2):36.
724. Bratel T, Hodenstierna G, Nyquist O et al. The effect of a new calcium antagonist on pulmonary hypertension and gas exchange in chronic obstructive lung disease. Eur J Respir Dis 1985;67:244.
725. Plotkin CN, Eckenbrecht PD, Waldo DA. Consecutive cardiac arrests on induction of anesthesia associated with nifedipine-induced carotid sinus hypersensitivity. Anesth Analg 1989;68:402.
726. Goglin WK, Elliot BM, Deppe SA. Nifedipine-induced hypotension and mesenteric ischemia. South Med J 1989; 82:274.
727. Babany G, Uzzan F, Larrey D et al. Alcoholic-like liver lesions induced by nifedipine. J Hepatol 1989;9:252.
728. Bruun NE, Ibsen H, Skott P et al. Lithium clearance and renal tubular sodium handling during acute and long-term nifedipine treatment in essential hypertension. Clin Sci 1988;75:609.
729. McFadden JP, Pantin JE, Parkes AV et al. Cyclosporin decreases nifedipine metabolism. Br Med J 1989;299:1224.
730. Jones RI, Hornung RS, Sonecha T et al. The effect of a new calcium blocker, nicardipine, on 24-hour ambulatory blood pressure and the pressor response to isometric and dynamic exercise. J Hypertens 1983;1:85.
731. Bellinetto A, Lessem J. Excretion of verapamil in human milk. Br Med J 1984;288:645.
732. Stoefel K, Deck K, Corsing C. Safety aspects of long-term nitrendipine therapy. J Cardiovasc Pharmacol 1984; 6(Suppl 7):1063.
733. Dubois C, Blanchard D, Loria Y, Moreau M. Clinical trial of new antihypertensive drug nicardipine: efficacy and tolerance in 29,104 patients. Curr Ther Res 1987;42:727.
734. De Wood MA, Wolbach RA. Randomised double-blind comparison of side-effects of nicardipine and nifedipine in angina pectoris. Am Heart J 1990;19:468.
735. Sorkin EM, Chissold SP. Nicardipine. A review of its pharmacodynamic and pharmacokinetic properties and therapeutic efficacy in the treatment of angina pectoris hypertension and related cardiovascular disorders. Drugs 1987;33:296.
736. Sundstedt C, Ruegg P, Keller A, Waite R. A multicenter evaluation of the safety tolerability and efficacy of isradipine in the treatment of essential hypertension. Am J Med 1989;86(Suppl 4A):98.
737. Hamilton TC, Weston AH. Cromakalim, Nicorandil, and Pinacidil: Novel drugs which open potassium channels in smooth muscle. Gen Pharmacol 1989;20:1.
738. Feldman RL. A review of medical therapy for coronary artery spasm. Circulation 1987;75(Suppl V):V96.
739. Pieper GM, Gross GJ. Salutary action of nicorandil, a new antianginal drug, on myocardial metabolism during ischemia and post ischemic function in a canine preparation of brief, repetitive coronary artery occlusions: comparison with isosorbide dinitrate. Circulation 1987;76:916.
740. Krumenacker M, Roland E. Clinical profile of nicorandil: An overview of its hemodynamic properties and therapeutic efficacy. J Cardiovasc Pharmacol 1992;20:S93.
741. Roland E. Safety profile of an anti-anginal agent with potassium channel opening activity: an overview. Eur Heart J 1993;14(Suppl B):48.
742. Sakai K. Nicorandil: animal pharmacology. Am J Cardiol 1989;63:2J.
743. Taira N, Satoh K, Yanagisawa T et al. Pharmacological profile of a new coronary vasodilator drug, 2-nicotinamidoethyl nitrate (SG-75). Clin Exp Pharmacol Physiol 1979;6:301.
744. Coltart DJ, Signy M. Acute hemodynamic effects of single-dose nicorandil in coronary artery disease. Am J Cardiol 1989;63:34J.
745. Camm AJ, Maltz MB. A controlled single-dose study of the efficacy, dose response and duration of action of nicorandil in angina pectoris. Am J Cardiol 1989;63:61J.
746. Taira N. Nicorandil as a hybrid between nitrates and potassium channel activators. Am J Cardiol 1989;63:18J.
747. Fenici RR, Melillo G. Effects of nicorandil on human cardiac electrophysiological parameters. Cardiovasc Drugs Ther 1991;5(Suppl 3:367.
748. Gross GJ, Auchampach JA. Role of ATP dependent potassium channels in myocardial ischaemia. Cardiovasc Res 1992;26:1011.
749. Mitrovic V, Neuss H, Kindler M. Elektrophysiologische Auswirkungen einer Vasodilatation durch Nicorandil. Herz/Kreislauf 1986;18:403.
750. Galie N, Varani E, Maiello L et al. Usefulness of nicorandil in congestive heart failure. Am J Cardiol 1990;65:343.
751. Kambara H, Kinoshita M, Nakagawa M. Sudden death among 1, 000 patients with myocardial infarction: incidence and contributory factors. KYSMI Study Group (Japanese). J Cardiol 1995;25:55.
752. Nagai H, Kitagaki K, Goto S. Effect of three novel K^+ channel openers, cromakalim, pinacidil and nicorandil on allergic reaction and experimental asthma. Jpn J Pharmacol 1991;56:13.
753. Doring G. Antianginal and anti-ischemic efficacy of nicorandil in comparison with isosrbide-5-mononitrate and isosorbide dinitrate: results from two multicenter, double-blind, randomized studies with stable coronary heart disease patients. J Cardiovasc Pharmacol 1992;20(Suppl 3):S74.
754. Ulvenstam G, Diderholm E, Frithz G et al. Antianginal and anti-ischemic efficacy of nicorandil compared to nifedipine in patients with angina pectoris and coronary heart disease: a double-blind randomized multi-center study. J Cardiovasc Pharmacol 1992;20(Suppl 3):S67.
755. Wagner G. Selected issues from an overview on nicorandil: tolerance, duration of action and long-term efficacy. J Cardiovasc Pharmacol 1992;20(Suppl 3):S86.
756. Roland E. Safety profile of an anti-anginal agent with potassium channel opening activity: an overview. Eur Heart J 1993;14(Suppl B):48.
757. Garrino MG, Plant TD, Henquin JC. Effects of putative activators of K^+ channels in mouse pancreatic β-cells. Br J Pharmacol 1989;98:957.
758. Jaraki O, Strauss WE, Francis S. Antiplatelet effects of a novel antianginal agent, nicorandil. J Cardiovasc Pharmacol 1994;23:24.
759. Jungbluth GL, Della-Coletta AA, Blum RA et al. Comparative pharmacokinetics (PK) and bioavailability of nicorandil (NI^C) in subjects with stabilized cirrhosis and matched healthy volunteers. Clin Pharmacol Ther 1991;49:181.
760. Buhl AE, Waldon DJ, Conrad SJ. Potassium channel conductance: a mechanism affecting hair growth both in vitro and in vivo. J Invest Dermatol 1992;98:315.
761. Hedlund P, Holmquist F, Hedlund H, Andersson KE. Effects of nicorandil on human isolated corpus cavernosum and cavernous artery. J Urol 1994;151:1107-13.

762. Frydman A. Pharmacokinetic profile of nicorandil in humans: an overview. J Cardiovasc Pharmacol 1992; 20(Suppl 3):S34.
763. Suryapranata H, MacLeod D. Nicorandil and cardiovascular performance in patients with coronary artery disease. J Cardiovasc Pharmacol 1992;20(Suppl 3):S45.
764. Solal AC, Jaeger P, Bouthier J. Hemodynamic action of nicorandil in congestive heart failure. Am J Cardiol 1989;63:44J.
765. Tice FD, Binkley PF, Cody RJ et al. Hemodynamic effects of oral nicorandil in congestive heart failure. Am J Cardiol 1990;65:1361.
766. Murakami M, Takeyama Y, Matsubara H et al. Effects of intravenous injection of nicorandil on systemic and coronary hemodynamics in patients with old myocardial infarction. A comparison with nifedipine and ISDN. Eur Heart J 1989;10:426.
767. Guermonprez JL, Blin P, Peterlongo F. A double-blind comparison of the long-term efficacy of a potassium channel opener and a calcium antagonist in stable angina pectoris. Eur Heart J 1993;14(Suppl B):30.
768. Frampton J, Buckley MM, Fitton A. Nicorandil, a review of its pharmacology and therapeutic efficacy in angina pectoris. Drugs 1992;44:625.
769. Tsutamoto T, Miyauchi N, Kanamori T et al. Mechanism of nicorandil intolerance in patients with heart failure. Circulation 1991;84(Suppl 11):58.
770. Horii D, Ishibashi A, Iwamoto. Bioavailability study of nicorandil before and after meals. Rinsho Yakuri 1984; 15:489.
771. Frydman AM, Chapelle P, Diekmann H et al. Pharmacokinetics of nicorandil. Am J Cardiol 1989;63:25J.
772. Gomita Y, Eto K, Furuno K et al. Influences of cigarette smoke on concentration of nicorandil in plasma of rats. J Pharm Sci 1992;81:228.
773. Sakai K, Shiraki Y, Nabata H. Cardiovascular effect of a new coronary vasodilator *N*-(2-hydroxyethyl)nicotinamide nitrate (SG-75): comparison with nitroglycerin and diltiazem. J Cardiovasc Pharmacol 1981;3:139.

Meyler's Side Effects of Drugs, 13th Edition
M.N.G. Dukes, editor

SECTION EDITOR: J.K. ARONSON

R. Verhaeghe

19 Drugs acting on the cerebral and peripheral circulations and drugs used in the treatment of migraine

Many drugs are still being prescribed for treating patients with chronic obstructive arterial disease of the legs, with Raynaud's arteriospastic phenomenon, and with reduced cerebral function ascribed to impaired cerebral blood flow. Each new compound is claimed to be superior to drugs that have already been marketed. However, the stringent rules of clinical pharmacology have drastically reduced the introduction of new compounds in recent years, and new literature is becoming relatively sparse.

Atherosclerotic disease of the arteries of the legs has a relatively benign local course, with stabilization and even improvement of functional capacity in most patients, despite progression of the underlying disease with time. On the other hand, because of a high prevalence of concomitant coronary and cerebrovascular disease, the general outlook for patients with arterial disease in the legs is rather poor. Ideally, management of patients with arterial disease in the legs should take into account the general prognosis as well as the local progression of the disease. Reducing the known risk factors for the development of atherosclerosis is still the mainstay of therapy. Vascular surgery and percutaneous revascularization procedures, such as balloon angioplasty, relieve the symptoms of ischemia, and their use therefore depends in the first place on the severity of these symptoms.

Two classes of pharmacological agents are being used: first, antithrombotic drugs, which are increasingly being prescribed in the hope of improving the general prognosis and of retarding the local progression of atherosclerosis in the legs (1[r]); second, drugs that are used in an attempt to alleviate the pain of claudication and other symptoms of leg ischemia. These are commonly referred to as vasodilators, but since the old concept of vasodilatation as a unique remedy for all the symptoms of arterial obstruction has been abandoned, characteristics other than vasodilatation are now being emphasized and the term 'anticlaudication agent' may be preferable (2[R]).

Raynaud's phenomenon still cannot be classified clinically in such a way as to make the choice of treatment straightforward (3[r]). Conventionally, a distinction is made between primary Raynaud's disease and secondary Raynaud's phenomenon. Primary Raynaud's disease is a benign disorder, and most patients learn to cope with their problems by keeping warm. Symptomatic relief with drugs is reserved for those with severe complaints, and many of them have secondary Raynaud's phenomenon. Apart from the drugs that come under the broad heading of vasodilators, a few other types of treatment can be considered in resistant cases. However, the benefit of systemic vasodilatation may be tempered by systemic adverse effects, such as dizziness and faints secondary to hypotension, tachycardia, palpitation, flushing, headache, nausea, and vomiting (4[r]).

Critical reviews of the therapeutic role of drugs in the treatment of cerebrovascular disorders have correctly stressed that most such drugs hardly rate a mention in textbooks (4[r], 5[r]). However, mental impairment is a steadily increasing problem in the ageing population, so that pressure to use these drugs in old people is increasing. However, the current working premise is that the pathology of the ageing brain is more often related to *non-vascular* metabolic disturbances of brain-cell function than to *cerebrovascular* insufficiency. Approximately 75% of people with dementia have senile dementia of the Alzheimer type, and only 15% have a vascular type of dementia or multi-infarct dementia secondary to atherosclerotic changes in the extracranial or intracranial arteries. If drugs that are thought to affect the cerebral circulation have any beneficial effect in patients with mental impairment, it probably has little to do with their effects on the cerebral circulation. Indeed, experts in the field remain sceptical about the contribution that vascular drugs can make to the care of demented patients.

Thus, a critical attitude towards the use of drugs acting on the cerebral and peripheral circulations remains justified. Furthermore, even minor adverse reactions to this class of drugs may overshadow their limited benefits and make the benefit/risk ratio unacceptable.

Any pharmacological classification of vasoactive agents will be inadequate, since each drug has several properties, the relative importance of which is still uncertain with regard to the clinical aim. For this reason the various drugs have been listed here in alphabetic order.

DRUGS USED IN THE TREATMENT OF ARTERIAL DISORDERS OF THE BRAIN AND LIMBS

Adenosine *(see also Chapter 17)*

Exercise myocardial perfusion scintigraphy using thallium-201 is a major non-invasive diagnostic method for assessing coronary artery disease. In patients who cannot perform an exercise test, dipyridamole can be used to induce coronary vasodilatation. As an alternative, adenosine has recently been introduced to provoke maximal controlled vasodilatation in the coronary circulation (6^r).

Adenosine is a ubiquitous substance that is of physiological importance in many tissues. It has an extremely short half-life in the blood. Exogenous adenosine is therefore administered as a continuous infusion in order to maintain maximal coronary blood flow for a few minutes during thallium-201 scintigraphy. Adverse effects are very common and can be attributed to the potent vasodilator action of adenosine: *chest pain* (often typical of angina pectoris), *hypotension*, cutaneous *flushing*, and *headache*. In addition, *dyspnea* may occur as a result of hyperventilation induced by the interaction of adenosine with carotid chemoreceptors. Although they are frequent, the adverse effects are rarely serious and disappear within a few minutes of discontinuing the infusion (SEDA-17, 243).

Bencyclane

The main properties of bencyclane are its papaverine-like spasmolytic action, antagonism of the effects of 5-hydroxytryptamine (serotonin), and weak inhibition of platelet aggregation. Although it is still available in a few European countries, evidence of its clinical usefulness in patients with claudication or rest pain is meagre. Its main adverse effects are *gastrointestinal* or *neurological* (dizziness, hand tremor, memory problems) and occur in a quarter of the patients taking 400 mg/day (SEDA-3, 175).

Buflomedil

Buflomedil appears to be safe and has generally been well tolerated by the majority of patients in clinical trials (7^r). The most frequently reported adverse effects include *flushing*, *headache*, *vertigo*, *gastrointestinal discomfort*, and *dizziness*. They rarely require discontinuation of treatment. In controlled trials, they occur in 20% of patients assigned to buflomedil and 18% of those assigned to placebo; only gastrointestinal discomfort occurred more frequently in buflomedil-treated patients (3.4 vs 2%) (8^r). *Extrapyramidal symptoms* and *depression* have been reported in a few frail elderly women (SEDA-13, 169). A few cases of *myoclonic encephalopathy* have been observed at therapeutic dosages; old people, patients of low body weight, and patients with renal failure due to dehydration appear to be especially vulnerable (SEDA-9, 189; SEDA-10, 172; SEDA-11, 179). Overdosage of buflomedil causes convulsions, and a few cases of myoclonic encephalopathy have been observed in elderly people and in patients with renal failure.

Cetiedil

This β_2-adrenoceptor agonist also has papaverine-like properties, possibly through one of its metabolites. Some anticholinergic activity has also been noted. Originally used as a vasodilator in Raynaud's phenomenon and intermittent claudication, it has been used to treat the vaso-occlusive crises of sickle-cell disease.

After oral administration of cetiedil minor *abdominal symptoms* may occur. *Disorientation* in time and place may be more disturbing, particularly at a dosage of over 400 mg/day.

The intravenous infusion of cetiedil may elicit the atropine-like adverse effects of *dryness of the mouth* and *altered visual accommodation*. With repeated infusions the incidence and duration of the adverse effects fall, suggesting the development of tolerance (SEDA-2, 184; SEDA-3, 176). Cetiedil should not be given to patients with urinary retention or glaucoma.

Cinnarizine and flunarizine

Cinnarizine is a well-established histamine (H_1) receptor antagonist, as is its difluoro-derivative, flunarizine; both are considered to act by selective blockade of calcium influx into depolarized smooth muscle cells in arterial walls.

A few controlled clinical trials of flunarizine in patients with intermittent claudication have suggested significant improvements in subjective signs and some objective measurements. Its clinical effectiveness in patients with cerebrovascular insufficiency has not been clearly demonstrated, but its use in the prevention of migraine and other forms of common headache has been studied extensively in recent years. Several controlled, double-blind studies have suggested that flunarizine in a daily dose not exceeding 10 mg reduces the frequency of headaches (SEDA-11, 179).

With a daily maintenance dose of 10 mg, the main adverse effects of flunarizine are *somnolence*, *sedation*, *fatigue*, and *drowsiness* during the first few days in up to 10% of patients. During prolonged treatment some patients note difficulty in sleeping, lethargy, and decreased motivation. A daily dose of 20 mg or more may induce drowsiness, increasing sweating, peripheral edema, and fatigue (SEDA-7, 229).

Flunarizine has a piperazine radical, in common with some neuroleptics and antihistamines. *Parkinsonism*, *tardive dyskinesia*, and *depression* have been described in a number of mostly elderly patients taking flunarizine (SEDA-12, 170; SEDA-13, 169; SEDA-14, 167; SEDA-15, 198). These symptoms appear to be resistant to anticholinergic drugs, L-dopa, and bromocriptine, but regress within a few weeks to months after withdrawal of flunarizine; however, mild rigidity and bradykinesia may persist in some patients. The daily recommended dose of 10 mg should never be exceeded, and in elderly patients doses higher than 5 mg may lead to an increased risk of extrapyramidal symptoms. Patients who take flunarizine to prevent migraine are usually some 25—30 years younger than those with cerebrovascular and peripheral vascular disease and appear to be at less risk of developing extrapyramidal symptoms with flunarizine (9[C]).

Co-dergocrine (Hydergine®)

Ergoloid mesylates are marketed under the trade name of Hydergine®, a mixture of the methane sulfonates of the dihydrogenated derivatives of the three alkaloids of ergotoxin (dihydroergocornine, dihydroergocristine, and dihydroergocryptine). Dihydrogenation eliminates the vasoconstrictor effects of ergotoxine and enhances the α-adrenoceptor antagonist and 5-HT receptor antagonist properties. Co-dergocrine has in addition other pharmacological effects, including inhibition of brain-specific phosphodiesterases, several of which are still poorly described. In recent years it has also been promoted as a 'metabolic enhancer', mainly because it protects against metabolic alterations induced by hypothermia and ischemia in animal experiments (10[r]).

Over 20 double-blind, controlled clinical trials have been conducted with co-dergocrine in senile dementia, and almost all have reported improvement in scores on at least one psychomotor test scale. Despite this evidence of short-term efficacy, many sceptical clinicians still consider it to be no better than placebo, and find support in a double-blind, placebo-controlled trial in which a group treated with the recommended dosage of 1 mg t.i.d. for 24 weeks did not perform better after treatment than the placebo-treated group (11[c]). However, none of the alternative drug treatments for senile dementia is very effective either.

The clinical value of co-dergocrine in patients with claudication and rest pain is poorly documented. Although the recommended dosage has been tripled in the last few years (from 0.5 to 1.5 mg t.i.d.) significant unwanted effects are rare. *Vomiting*, *blurred vision*, *skin rashes*, *nasal stuffiness*, *bad taste*, *postural hypotension*, *and vasospastic reactions* are all uncommon (SED-12, 472). Diffuse fibrotic processes (e.g. retroperitoneal fibrosis), as repeatedly reported with other ergot derivatives, such as methysergide and dihydroergotamine, have not to our knowledge been observed with co-dergocrine.

Cyclandelate

The spasmolytic action of this ester of mandelic acid was described as early as 1959, but only in later years have its properties been more fully investigated. It appears to act as a calcium antagonist in smooth muscle and platelets, this effect being partly due to inhibition of phosphodiesterase(s). It also produces increased deformability of red blood cells; the mechanism responsible is so far unknown, although phosphodiesterase inhibition may again be responsible. Cyclandelate also reduces the activity of the rate-limiting enzyme for the biosynthesis of cholesterol (HMG-CoA), and its 'antidiabetic' properties may be due to inhibition of aldose reductase.

Major adverse effects have not been reported at daily doses of 1.6 g; *gastrointestinal upset*, *flushing*, and *tingling* are rare and minor complaints. Even elderly patients apparently tolerate 3.2 g/day without problems (SEDA-9, 189).

Ginkgo biloba

Extracts from the leaves of *Ginkgo biloba*, the maiden-hair tree, are marketed in some countries for the treatment of cerebral dysfunction and of intermittent claudication. In a recent review it was concluded that seven out of eight controlled trials of good quality showed positive effects of *Ginkgo biloba* compared with placebo on the following symptoms: memory difficulties, dizziness, tinnitus, headache, and emotional instability with anxiety (12[r]). For intermittent claudication, the evidence for efficacy was judged unconvincing. No serious adverse effects have been noted in any trial.

Iloprost

Iloprost is an analog of prostacyclin whose pharmacodynamic properties it mimics, namely inhibition of platelet aggregation, vasodilatation, and cytoprotection (as yet ill-defined). Iloprost has greater chemical stability than prostacyclin, which facilitates its clinical use (13[r]).

Most clinical experience with iloprost has been gained in patients with critical leg ischemia. An intermittent intravenous infusion of up to 2 ng/kg/min for 2–4 weeks reduced rest pain and improved ulcer healing in roughly half of the patients with critical leg ischemia, including diabetics. Compared with placebo, the improvement obtained with iloprost was significant in most but not all individual clinical trials. In addition, a meta-analysis showed a 15% reduction in major amputation rate in comparison with placebo (14[r]).

The adverse effects of iloprost are clearly dose-related and predictable from its pharmacological effects. Minor vascular reactions during infusion (characterized by *facial flushing and headache*) are so common as to make double-blind trials impossible. Gastrointestinal effects become more prevalent at higher dosages and include *nausea*, *vomiting*, *abdominal cramps*, *and diarrhea*. Less common adverse effects include *restlessness*, *sweating*, *local erythema* along the infusion line, *wheals*, *fatigue*, and *muscle pain*. Clinically significant *hypotension* is rare with the doses tested. The untoward effects resolve rapidly after the infusion is discontinued.

Therapy with iloprost is usually started at a dosage of 0.5 ng/kg/min and increased in increments until either minor vascular reactions occur or a dosage of 2 ng/kg/min has been reached. The optimal total dose remains to be established.

Isoxsuprine

Isoxsuprine is a β_2-adrenoceptor agonist which also has antagonist action at α-adrenoceptors. In high dosages it also lowers blood viscosity and inhibits platelet aggregation. There is slim evidence that isoxsuprine may improve cognitive function and mental performance in a limited number of patients, but the practical benefit is minor. There is no convincing proof of its efficacy in patients with claudication.

The main adverse reactions of isoxsuprine are *tachycardia* and *orthostatic hypotension*, but only at high dosages. Minor *facial flushing* and *tremor* are quite common. As patients tend gradually to increase their dosage, *diarrhea*, *vomiting*, *headache*, *vertigo*, and *rash* may occur (SEDA-3, 177; SEDA-7, 228).

Ketanserin

Ketanserin is a selective 5-HT_2 receptor antagonist with antihypertensive action. Because it antagonizes vasoconstriction and platelet aggregation induced by 5-HT and increases erythrocyte deformability, its potential usefulness in peripheral vascular disease has been extensively investigated but never convincingly demonstrated. Most of the adverse effects attributable to ketanserin seem, not surprisingly, to affect the central nervous system. They include *drowsiness*, *fatigue*, *headache*, *sleep disturbances*, and *dry mouth*. Other complaints include *dizziness*, *light-headedness*, *lack of concentration*, and *dyspepsia*. A gradual increase in dosage is therefore recommended. These adverse effects occur in about 10% of patients and lead to withdrawal of the drug in 3–4% (SEDA-17, 243).

A dose-related prolongation of the QT_c interval on the ECG occurs in roughly one-third of patients taking ketanserin (15[r]). Several cases of ventricular dysrhythmias with QT_c prolongation, leading to loss of consciousness, have been reported (SED-11, 392; SED-12, 473), but the exact incidence of significant ventricular dysrhythmias on the basis of QT_c prolongation during ketanserin therapy remains unknown. In an international study on the prevention of atherosclerotic complications with ketanserin (PACK) almost 4000 patients with claudication were randomized to take ketanserin or placebo for at least 1 year (16[C]). There was an excess of deaths (mainly sudden) in the patients treated with ketanserin and diuretics, and more than 300 patients were therefore withdrawn from the trial. A secondary analysis indicated that this effect was associated with the combined use of potassium-wasting, but not potassium-sparing, diuretics. Prolongation of the QT_c interval induced by ketanserin was more pronounced when potassium-wasting diuretics were also prescribed. Ketanserin must therefore not be combined with potassium-wasting diuretics.

Naftidrofuryl oxalate

Naftidrofuryl is a complex acid ester of diethylaminoethanol, with direct vasodilating properties and antagonistic effects on 5-HT (via 5-HT_2 receptors) and bradykinin. It also causes an intracellular increase in ATP concentrations, improves cellular oxidative metabolism (by activating succinate dehydrogenase), and reduces blood and plasma viscosity and fibrinogen concentrations.

Naftidrofuryl has been marketed in Europe for over 20 years for the treatment of peripheral and cerebrovascular diseases and for senile dementia. A few placebo-controlled studies have reported increases in walking distance in patients with claudication, but no substantial hemodynamic improvement. Subjective improvement with naftidrofuryl was also noted in patients with Raynaud's phenomenon, but it had variable effects on digital blood flow and pressure during cold provocation. In patients with an acute ischemic stroke, there was better neurological progress leading to a shorter hospital stay in three studies but not in a fourth (17[C]). Several double-blind clinical trials have reported improvements in the deficits associated with mild senile organic brain syndrome.

Oral naftidrofuryl (300—600 mg/day) was generally well tolerated in the controlled trials: gastrointestinal complaints were as frequent with placebo as with the drug. *Esophageal ulceration* has been ascribed to naftidrofuryl in a few patients. Rare cases of reversible *liver dysfunction* have been reported. Several adverse effects have been noted with parenteral administration, including *intracardiac conduction defects*, *epileptic seizures*, severe *anaphylactic reactions*, and *acute renal failure* secondary to deposition of oxalate crystals in the tubules (SED-12, 473; SEDA-17, 244). Bolus injections either intravenously or intra-arterially may be particularly dangerous. A recent reappraisal of the benefit:risk ratio of parenterally administered naftidrofuryl led to withdrawal of all parenteral forms of the drug from the market.

Nicotinic acid derivatives

Nicotinic acid (niacin) is a potent vasodilator, probably by a direct effect on vascular smooth muscle mainly of the skin vessels of the face and trunk. It also interferes with the metabolism of carbohydrates, lipids, and fibrinogen. Nicotinic acid acts as a source of the physiologically active amide nicotinamide before incorporation into essential nucleotide co-enzymes; however, it has no vasodilating properties. Nicotinic acid also briefly stimulates fibrinolysis and reduces blood viscosity, surface tension, and density. Niacin is an effective hypolipidemic agent.

However, nicotinic acid has to be given in large doses, at which adverse effects are a frequent nuisance. It has therefore been combined in lower dosages with another agent (e.g. pentoxifylline), its molecular structure modified (e.g. as xanthinol nicotinate), or chemically changed in order to obtain a modified release of nicotinic acid (e.g. inositol hexanicotinate, tetranicotinoylfructose, and β-pyridylcarbinol).

The clinical value of nicotinic acid derivatives in patients with organic vascular disease of the brain or limbs is doubtful. They may be effective in the treatment of cutaneous vasospasm, but they do not produce consistent increases in muscle blood flow.

Nicotinic acid is well absorbed from the gastrointestinal tract, but produces *facial flushing*, *pounding in the head*, *a sensation of heat*, *gastric irritation*, and *diarrhea*. Less common adverse effects include *pruritus*, *skin lesions*, *blurring of vision*, *abdominal pain* and *activation of peptic ulcer*, *jaundice* and *impairment of liver function*, *reduced glucose tolerance*, and *hyperuricemia*.

Cholestatic and hepatocellular reactions have been described clinically, with biopsy findings of parenchymal necrosis and centrilobular cholestasis in most cases. The mechanism by which hepatic injury occurs is unknown, but a dose-related direct toxic effect is more likely than an idiosyncratic reaction. Most cases occur with daily doses over 3—4 g, but occasionally liver toxicity has been observed at lower dosages (SEDA-14, 168; 18[c]). The liver injury is usually mild and reversible, although fulminant hepatic failure has been reported. Modified-release niacin appears to be more hepatotoxic than crystalline niacin (19[c]).

Inositol hexanicotinate Inositol hexanicotinate is a long-acting derivative of nicotinic acid, incorporating six nicotinic acid moieties in its molecule. It causes fewer and milder adverse effects than nicotinic acid, and they are mainly limited to *a feeling of warmth*, *pruritus*, *dyspepsia*, *moderate sweating*, *headache*, and *cough*. With 1.2 g of inositol hexanicotinate adverse effects have been noted in 8% of patients, *gastrointestinal symptoms* predominating (SEDA-3, 177; SEDA-5, 207).

Tetranicotinoylfructofuranose (Nicofuranose®) Tetranicotinoylfructofuranose is a fructose ester of nicotinic acid which releases nicotinic acid mainly in the small intestine. The gradual release of the active substance avoids gastric irritation and reduces flushing. A feeling of warmth may be experienced, especially if the tablets are taken before patients enter a warm room, or on a warm day, or together with alcohol (SEDA-3, 179).

Nicotinyl alcohol tartrate (β-pyridylcarbinol) Nicotinyl alcohol tartrate is an alcohol of nicotinic acid, to which it is metabolized. Adverse effects with this compound are mainly limited to transient *facial flushing*. Nicotinyl alcohol or its tartrate can cause a *rise in fasting blood sugar*. When the maximum recommended oral dosage of 1200 mg/day is exceeded impairment of liver function may occur (SEDA-3, 175).

Xanthinol nicotinate Xanthinol nicotinate consists of a xanthine base chemically combined with nicotinic acid. Adverse effects are frequent, more particularly when the drug is taken on an empty stomach, and include *flushing of the skin*, *abdominal pain*, and *hypotension*. Xanthinol nicotinate has been reported to *reduce placental blood flow pooling* during the third trimester of pregnancy and may thus create a risk to the fetus.

Nylidrin (buphenine) There is a striking structural similarity between nylidrin and isoxsuprine, and they have similar pharmacological effects.

Available for many years, nylidrin was described provisionally by the FDA as "possibly effective for peripheral vascular disease and circulatory disturbances of the inner ear".

The positive inotropic effect of nylidrin may produce *palpitation* and *dizziness*. It may cause *tremulousness* and *nervousness* as well as *nausea* and *vomiting*; an increase in intraocular pressure and gastric secretion have also been described. Blood glucose concentrations may be increased in pregnant woman and diabetics. Nylidrin should not be used in patients with myocardial infarction, hypothyroidism, peptic ulcer, paroxysmal dysrhythmias, or severe angina pectoris (SEDA-3, 175).

Pentoxifylline

Pentoxifylline is a methylxanthine which antagonizes the vasoconstrictor effects of catecholamines and increases cyclic AMP concentrations, causing smooth muscle to relax. It has also been claimed to correct impaired microcirculation by improving various factors that disturb blood rheology: it reduces whole blood viscosity, lowers the plasma fibrinogen concentration, and increases the filterability of blood cells, particularly of lymphocytes with a high viscosity (20[R], 21[r]). Recently, pentoxifylline has been shown to reduce the generation of toxic free radicals from leucocytes during ischemic leg exercise in patients with intermittent claudication (22[c]).

The efficacy of pentoxifylline in treating claudication has been evaluated in double-blind controlled trials in Europe and in the US. Several of these trials have shown that 400 mg t.i.d. increases the walking distance in patients with claudication significantly more than in similar patients on placebo. However, critics remain sceptical about the real value of pentoxifylline, because of a negative correlation between the trial sample sizes and its effects, reflecting an overestimate of drug effect in highly selected trial populations (23[R]). In a trial in almost 300 patients with acute ischemic stroke, the neurological deficit improved more rapidly with pentoxifylline in the initial phase, but the difference was not significant at the end of 1 week (24[C]).

Unwanted effects of pentoxifylline recognized in the double-blind studies are *gastrointestinal symptoms* (chiefly *nausea*, *vomiting*, and *bloating*) and *dizziness*. Although common, they required discontinuation of the drug in only about 3% of patients. The incidence of adverse effects was reportedly higher with the capsule formulation than with commercially available modified-release tablets. A single case of bleeding duodenal ulcer following a single dose of pentoxifylline was reported as possibly secondary to disturbed platelet function induced by the drug (25[c]). However, the effects of pentoxifylline on platelet function have not been very consistent and the role of pentoxifylline in causing the bleeding may have been purely incidental. Rare cases of hallucinations in elderly people have been ascribed to a stimulant effect on the central nervous system (SEDA-18, 219).

In recent years, a continuous intravenous infusion of pentoxifylline has been tested in patients undergoing allogeneic bone-marrow transplantation, in an effort to reduce transplant-related morbidity and mortality. The results have not been impressive, and the amount of pentoxifylline infused has been limited by *nausea and vomiting*, *increased serum creatinine concentrations*, or central nervous system toxicity manifesting as *acute obtundation* and *myoclonic jerks* (26[c]—28[c]).

Piridoxilate

Piridoxilate, an equimolar mixture of glyoxylic acid and pyridoxine, is marketed in a few countries (e.g. France) for peripheral arterial occlusive disease and functional venous disorders.

A few reports have dealt with the occurrence of calcium oxalate *renal calculi* associated with prolonged long-term piridoxilate, and one case of *acute renal failure* due to hyperoxaluria and intratubular deposits of oxalate crystals has been reported in a 23-year-old man who attempted suicide with an overdose of piridoxilate (SEDA-11, 180). There has been one report of an old woman with end-stage chronic renal failure and histological evidence of renal oxalosis ascribed to 10 years of piridoxilate treatment. Her renal function did not improve after withdrawal of the drug, and chronic hemodialysis was required (29[c]).

Pyridinol carbamate

Pyridinol carbamate, a bradykinin antagonist, is in clinical use mainly in Japan. Studies conducted in the West in patients with intermittent claudication have shown little success and no dose-related drug effects.

With a daily dose of 1.5 g minor *gastrointestinal* adverse effects occur in about 1% of patients, mainly in the early treatment period, and tend to subside during further medication. At a daily dose of 2 g the incidence of adverse effects increases, and may include *gastric upset*, *nausea*, *anorexia*, *fatigue*, *weakness*, *hyperhidrosis*, and mild *sleep disturbances*. There have been rare reports of *liver dysfunction* in Japan and a few cases of drug-induced hepatitis have been reported in other countries as well (SEDA-10, 172).

Tolazoline

Tolazoline blocks autonomic ganglia and peripheral α-adrenoceptors and has also a histamine-like effect. It increases skin blood flow in healthy subjects, in patients without rest pain, and occasionally in patients with Raynaud's phenomenon. However, convincing evidence of its therapeutic value in patients with claudication is not available and is at least conflicting with regard to the treatment of patients with cerebrovascular problems. Tolazoline seems to be a useful adjunct in the management of neonates with persistent fetal circulation.

The most common adverse effects are *palpitation*, *tachycardia*, *flushing*, *sweating*, *headache*, and *paresthesia* of the skin with pilo-erection. Unwanted *gastrointestinal effects* are nausea, vomiting, and diarrhea. Postural hypotension and failure to ejaculate have also been reported. Tolazoline can also produce disulfiram-like effects in the presence of alcohol. It may antagonize the effects of clonidine and prevent the brief hypertensive reaction often observed after the intravenous administration of this drug (SEDA-2, 192; SEDA-3, 180).

Vincamine

Vincamine is an alkaloid extracted from the plant *Vinca minor*. Ethyl apovincaminate is a related synthetic ethyl ester of vincaminic acid. These drugs have spasmolytic effects similar to those of reserpine, but also have metabolic effects, including, in high doses, inhibition of phosphodiesterase.

Although increased cerebral blood flow has been reported after the intravenous administration of vincamine, there have been no reliable studies of blood flow after oral medication. Improvement in scores on some psychometric tests have been obtained in some patients with cerebrovascular disease, but no clear-cut practical benefit has been demonstrated.

Commercial formulations obtained from the alkaloids in *Vinca minor* may not be free from adverse effects. *Ventricular dysrhythmias* have been observed, but only after intramuscular or intravenous administration, and they seem to reflect a direct effect on myocardial cells. Hypokalemia and a prolonged QT interval seem to be predisposing factors. Vincamine should therefore be avoided in patients with a prolonged QT interval. Vincamine has a very minor sedative effect (SEDA-2, 183; SEDA-5, 206, 207; SEDA-7, 228).

Vitamin E nicotinate (di-α-tocopheryl nicotinate)

The suggestion that vitamin E could be useful in patients with peripheral arterial disease was made many years ago, but the available evidence is meagre and incomplete. However, vitamin E is in widespread use in high dosages among the general public. This would be a minor problem were it not that the drug is not completely innocuous. A daily dose of 3 g can cause *abdominal discomfort*, *thrombophlebitis*, and *skin disorders*, and can raise the *serum cholesterol* concentration (SEDA-3, 180).

DRUGS USED IN THE TREATMENT OF VENOUS DISORDERS

The aim of using drugs in patients with venous disorders is to prevent, retard, or reverse varicose degenerative changes in the vessel wall. These changes primarily involve the connective tissues, with fibrous tissue largely replacing muscle tissue. The clinical usefulness of these agents is limited and in most cases poorly demonstrated. The following review is not exhaustive.

Benzbromarone (Benzarone)

Benzarone is a benzofuran derivative chemically related to amiodarone, a drug with well-known hepatotoxicity (see Chapter 9.2). Benzarone has for a long time been considered to be innocuous, but several cases of acute *hepatitis* have been reported in recent years (SEDA-16, 205). Consequently the drug was withdrawn from the market in several European countries (SEDA-17, 244).

β-Aescin

β-Aescin is a natural mixture of saponins from the horse chestnut. It often causes abdominal discomfort and can precipitate *renal failure* when combined with aminoglycoside antibiotics (SEDA-3, 180; SEDA-9, 189).

Calcium dobesilate

Calcium dobesilate is a synthetic compound which has been claimed to preserve endothelial integrity and to reduce capillary permeability. It has been recommended in diabetic retinopathy and venous disorders. After oral intake *gastrointestinal disturbances* and occasionally *nervousness* and *fever* have been described but are rare effects. Intramuscular calcium dobesilate may be painful (SEDA-3, 181; SEDA-16, 204).

Cyclo-3 fort

Cyclo-3 fort is a flavonoid derivative marketed in France. It is usually well tolerated. Hesperidine, an extract of *Ruscus aculeatus*, and ascorbic acid are the active ingredients. Increasingly, patients who develop chronic *diarrhea* with this drug are being discovered; disturbance of gastrointestinal motility appears the most likely mechanism (SEDA-16, 205; SEDA-17, 244).

Dimethylaminoethanol

Several esters and salts of dimethylaminoethanol have been used in patients with venous disorders without much success. It can cause serious *cardiac dysrhythmias* and is therefore not to be recommended.

Diosmine

This extract of *Rutacea* is well tolerated. *Nausea* and *epigastric discomfort* are rare (SEDA-3, 181).

Troxerutin

This flavonoid derivative, which is claimed to reduce capillary fragility, is generally well tolerated. The active ingredient is a yellow substance (SEDA-13, 170), and a few cases of *yellow discoloration of the skin*, but not of the sclerae, have been observed. The discoloration, which may be mistaken for jaundice, vanishes when the drug is stopped.

DRUGS USED IN THE TREATMENT OF MIGRAINE

Ergotamine *(see also Chapter 13)*

Ergot poisoning from food has almost disappeared, but the therapeutic use of ergot alkaloids remains responsible for occasional reports of severe *vasospasm*. In one study of 1500 consecutive patients with acute leg ischemia admitted to a vascular unit, four were due to ergotamine intoxication (30[c]). Arterial spasm can be due to ergotamine overdose, but some patients develop an exaggerated response to a normal therapeutic dose. Pregnant women and patients with hyperthyroidism, acute infections, and shock appear to be particularly vulnerable.

In recent years, dihydroergotamine has been used to improve the effect of heparin in preventing deep vein thrombosis. However, the use of this combination occasionally results in leg ischemia due to arterial spasm, especially in patients with pre-existing obstructive arterial disease. The risk of vasospasm may also outweigh the potential benefit of the combination over heparin alone in trauma patients (SEDA-14, 167). The advent of low-molecular-weight heparin formulations has largely obviated the need for the combination of heparin with dihydroergotamine. In consequence, the combination has been removed from the market in some countries.

Ergotamine taken for migraine can also cause spasm in other vascular beds. In the coronary arteries this can lead to acute myocardial infarction. In a review of 168 patients under the age of 40 years with cerebral ischemia, 18 developed their symptoms in connection with attacks of migraine and five had taken ergotamine before the ischemic symptoms. In addition, similar symptoms occurred in two other patients who took ergotamine for alleged hypotension (31[r]). Vasospasm in the carotid territory has been documented, and occasionally venous problems may arise as well (SEDA-16, 204; SEDA-17, 243).

A less well known complication of the rectal use of ergotamine is the occurrence of *anorectal ulcers*, eventually leading to necrosis and stenosis of the rectum. Reduced blood flow to the rectal wall secondary to vasospasm locally induced by ergotamine suppositories is thought to be the cause.

Sumatriptan

Sumatriptan is a 5-HT receptor agonist, highly selective for a 5-HT_1 receptors, which mediate constriction of some (dilated) cranial blood vessels in animal studies.

According to extensive clinical trials, sumatriptan is highly effective in the treatment of acute attacks of migraine.

The drug is available as film-coated tablets of 200 mg and as prefilled syringes of 6 mg for self-administered subcutaneous injection. An intranasal formulation has also been tested in clinical trials. The systemic availability of sumatriptan is high (96%) after subcutaneous injection, but rather low (14%) after oral administration because of first-pass metabolism. The elimination half-life is short (2 h) and 80% of the drug is removed by metabolism. The principal metabolite is an inactive indole acetic acid analog. Propranolol, flunarizine, and pizotifen, all drugs commonly used in migraine prophylaxis, do not affect the pharmacokinetics of sumatriptan (32^R, 33^R).

A high proportion of patients respond to a single standard dose of therapy with minor or mild adverse effects. Because of the short half-life, recurrence of headache within 24 h is common (50%) but can be effectively treated by a second dose of the drug. At the same time, any adverse effect is likely to be brief as well. The most commonly experienced adverse effects are a *feeling of pressure/stiffness* in the neck and throat or of pressure/tightness or pain in the chest. *Tingling sensations* in head and arms, *dizziness*, and *tiredness* are also commonly reported. *Dyspnea* appears to be associated with obstructive lung disease. *Local reactions* at the injection site are usually mild. The reported frequencies of these adverse effects vary widely between clinical trials and post-marketing surveys. This may be due to selection of patients in trials and to differences in the questionnaires used to evaluate unwanted effects (34^R, 35^R).

Sumatriptan-induced coronary artery spasm is often suspected as the cause of the feeling of chest pressure or chest pain. Evidence in favor of this concept is derived from in vitro studies on coronary artery rings, from a few small human studies with a reduction of coronary artery diameter after sumatriptan injection, and from a few case reports with cardiac disturbances attributed to the administration of sumatriptan. As a consequence, the use of sumatriptan is contra-indicated in patients with coronary artery disease. However, an alternative hypothesis has been advanced to explain the chest syndromes: abnormal esophageal motility and contraction (36^R).

REFERENCES

1. Verhaeghe R. Prophylactic antiplatelet therapy in peripheral arterial disease. Drugs 1991;42(Suppl 5):51.
2. Verstraete M. Peripheral vasodilator drugs: a misnomer. Drugs 1980;19:81.
3. Roath S. Management of Raynaud's phenomenon. Focus on newer treatments. Drugs 1989;37:700.
4. Lowe GDO. Drugs in cerebral and peripheral arterial disease. Br Med J 1990;300:524.
5. Spagnoli A, Tognoni G. 'Cerebroactive' drugs. Clinical pharmacology and therapeutic role in cerebrovascular disorders. Drugs 1983;26:44.
6. Verani MS, Mahmarian JJ. Myocardial perfusion scintigraphy during maximal coronary artery vasodilation with adenosine. Am J Cardiol 1991;67:12D.
7. Clissold SP, Lynch S, Sorkin EM. Buflomedil. A review of its pharmacodynamic and pharmacokinetic properties, and therapeutic efficacy in peripheral and cerebral vascular diseases. Drugs 1987;33:430.
8. Bachand RT, Dubourg AY. A review of long-term safety data with buflomedil. J Int Med Res 1990;18:245-252.
9. Bono G, Martucci N, Merlo P et al. Safety profile of flunarizine. A retrospective study in migraine and cerebrovascular disorders. Ann NY Acad Sci 1988;522:712.
10. Hollister LE, Yesavage J. Ergoloid mesylates for senile dementias: unanswered questions. Ann Intern Med 1984; 100:894.
11. Thompson TL, Filley CM, Mitchell WD et al. Lack of efficacy of hydergine in patients with Alzheimer's disease. New Engl J Med 1990;323:445 (erratum 691).
12. Kleijnen J, Knipschild P. *Ginkgo biloba*. Lancet 1992;340:1136.
13. Grant SM, Goa KL. Iloprost. A review of its pharmacodynamic and pharmacokinetic properties, and therapeutic potential in peripheral vascular disease, myocardial ischemia and extracorporeal circulation procedures. Drugs 1992; 43:889.
14. Dormandy JA. Limb salvage with iloprost. Crit Ischaemia 1992;3(Suppl 1):45.
15. Zehender M, Meinertz T, Hohnloser S et al. Incidence and clinical relevance of QT prolongation caused by the new selective serotonin antagonist ketanserin. Am J Cardiol 1989;63:826.
16. Prevention of Atherosclerotic Complications with Ketanserin Trial Group. Prevention of atherosclerotic complications: controlled trial of ketanserin. Br Med J 1989;298:424 (erratum 644).
17. Gray CS, French JM, Venables GS et al. A randomized double-blind controlled trial of naftidrofuryl in acute stroke. Age Ageing 1990;19:356.
18. Hodis HN. Acute hepatic failure associated with the use of low-dose sustained-release niacin. J Am Med Assoc 1990;264:181.
19. Henkin Y, Johnson KC, Segrest JP. Rechallenge with crystalline niacin after drug-induced hepatitis from sustained-release niacin. J Am Med Assoc 1990;264:241.
20. Ward A, Clissold SP. Pentoxifylline. A review of its pharmacodynamic and pharmacokinetic properties, and its therapeutic efficacy. Drugs 1987;39:50.
21. Verhaeghe R, Verstraete M. Pentoxifylline in arterial disease of the legs. Eur J Clin Pharmacol 1991;41:507.
22. Ciuffetti G, Mercuri M, Ott C et al. Use of pentoxifylline

as an inhibitor of free radical generation in peripheral vascular disease. Results of a double-blind placebo-controlled study. Eur J Clin Pharmacol 1991;41:511.
23. Cameron HA, Waller PC, Ramsay LE. Drug treatment of intermittent claudication: a critical analysis of the methods and findings of published clinical trials, 1965–1985. Br J Clin Pharmacol 1988;26:569.
24. Hsu CY, Norris JW, Hogan EL et al. Pentoxifylline in acute nonhemorrhagic stroke. A randomized, placebo-controlled double-blind trial. Stroke 1988;19:716.
25. Oren R, Yishar U, Lysy J, Livshitz T, Ligumsky M. Pentoxifylline-induced gastrointestinal bleeding. Drug Intell Clin Pharm Ann Pharmacother 1991;23:315.
26. Sempere AP, Garcia FM, Duarte J et al. Impotence associated with cinnarizine. Ann Pharmacother 1993;27:370.
27. Pitner J, Simpson W, Gutierrez S, Mintzer J. Pentoxifylline (Trental)-induced visual hallucinations. J Am Geriatr Soc 1993;42:782.
28. Gilbert GJ. Pentoxifylline induced musical hallucinations. Neurology 1993;43:1621.
29. Stockshläder M, Kalhs P, Peters S et al. Intravenous pentoxifylline failed to prevent transplant-related toxicities in allogeneic bone marrow transplant recipients. Bone Marrow Transplant 1993;12:357.
30. Beelen DW, Sayer HG, Franke M et al. Constant intravenous pentoxifylline infusions in allogeneic marrow transplant recipients: results of a dose escalation study. Bone Marrow Transplant 1993;12:363.
31. Berlit P, Endemann B, Better P. Zerebrale Ischämien bei jungen Erwachsenen. Fortschr Neurol Psychiatr 1991;59:322.
32. Rose FC. Sumatriptan: an overwiew. Headache Q 1993;4(Suppl 2):37.
33. Scott AK. Sumatriptan clinical pharmacokinetics. Clin Pharmacokin 1994;27:337.
34. Dahlöf C, Ekbom K, Persson L. Clinical experiences from Sweden on the use of subcutaneously administered sumatriptan in migraine and cluster headache. Arch Neurol 1994;51:1256.
35. Ottervanger JP, van Witsen TB, Valkenburg HA et al. Adverse reactions attributed to sumatriptan. A postmarketing study in general practice. Eur J Clin Pharmacol 1994;47:305.
36. Houghton LA, Foster JM, Whorwell PJ et al. Is chest pain after sumatriptan oesophageal in origin? Lancet 1994;344:985.

Meyler's Side Effects of Drugs, 13th Edition
M.N.G. Dukes, editor

SECTION EDITOR: J.K. ARONSON

H.L. Elliott

20 Antihypertensive drugs

INTRODUCTION

The selection of a first-line antihypertensive agent is increasingly being shared among the traditional drugs, thiazide diuretics and β-adrenoceptor antagonists (see Chapters 21 and 18, respectively), and the relatively newer drugs, the angiotensin-converting enzyme (ACE) inhibitors and calcium antagonists (see Chapter 18), which are progressively achieving increased importance as first-line agents. Within these established classes the only significant recent change has been a clear preference for long-acting, once-daily calcium antagonist drugs and formulations. However, a new class of drug has emerged as a possible alternative to ACE inhibitors, the selective angiotensin II receptor antagonists, losartan being the prototype.

The emergence of ACE inhibitors and calcium antagonists as alternative first-line agents possibly reflects continuing concerns about adverse effects that interfere with patients' quality of life, and also the possible adverse metabolic consequences of long-term treatment with thiazide diuretics and β-blockers. Whilst this includes overt drug-induced changes in glucose and lipid metabolism, there is accumulating evidence to suggest that there may be a more fundamental metabolic abnormality in hypertensive patients (i.e. insulin resistance), which is exacerbated by both thiazides and β-blockers (but not by ACE inhibitors or calcium antagonists), and which in the long term may lead to several adverse cardiovascular effects. The effects of antihypertensive treatments on insulin responsiveness and insulin resistance have been the subject of several recent reviews (1^R–3^R).

As a result of the increased use of the newer agents there have been significant further reductions in the use of conventional vasodilators (such as hydralazine, minoxidil, and diazoxide) and of the centrally-acting agents (such as α-methyldopa and clonidine). There have therefore been few recent new reports of adverse effects attributable to these drugs.

ANGIOTENSIN-CONVERTING ENZYME (ACE) INHIBITORS

In recent years there have been several reviews of ACE inhibitors in their major therapeutic areas of hypertension and heart failure (4^R, 5^R). In general these articles have highlighted the increasing use of ACE inhibitors and an expanding knowledge of the renin–angiotensin system, particularly the importance of 'tissue' renin–angiotensin systems.

ADVERSE REACTION PATTERN

General and toxic reactions The commonest unwanted effects of ACE inhibitors are related to their pharmacological actions (i.e. inhibition of the angiotensin-converting enzyme and kininase II): renal failure, potassium retention, pronounced first-dose hypotension, cough, and angioedema. Skin rashes and taste disturbances are uncommon, but they may be more likely with sulfhydryl-containing drugs, particularly captopril. However, the exacerbation of pre-existing skin conditions is being increasingly reported with all types of ACE inhibitors. Again, this is suggestive of a class effect mediated via a pharmacological mechanism.

Hypersensitivity reactions It has proved difficult to classify skin rashes clearly as toxic or hypersensitivity reactions, and occasional instances of bone-marrow suppression have been similarly difficult to classify. Cases of hepatitis and alveolitis, presumably hypersensitivity reactions, have rarely been described.

Tumor-inducing effects No tumor-inducing effects have been reported.

Second-generation effects A syndrome of fetal growth retardation, renal impairment, and hypocalvaria is now recognized (6^R).

ACE INHIBITOR CLASS EFFECTS

Cardiovascular *First dose hypotension* The initiation of ACE inhibitor treatment is occasionally associated with marked reductions in blood pressure, without any significant change in heart rate. Such reductions, which are not orthostatic, are sometimes symptomatic but rarely fatal. The volume of evidence is greatest with the longer established agents, but continues to suggest that the problems of first-dose hypotension are most likely to occur in 'complex' patients. From a multivariate analysis of 269 unselected hypertensive patients the largest falls in blood pressure after 25 mg of captopril occurred in patients with a past history of renovascular hypertension or with previous vasodilator treatment, which was assumed by the authors to be an indication of the presence of severe hypertension (7[Cr]). Similar hypotensive problems associated with initiating captopril for the treatment of severe heart failure have also been the subject of two recent case reports (8[c]). This potential problem of first-dose hypotension has been confirmed with enalapril in heart failure (8[C]—10[C]) and with lisinopril (11[C]). Similar problems have occurred in the treatment of hypertensive neonates and infants (12[C]), but again were particularly likely in the setting of high plasma renin activity associated with either renovascular disease or concurrent diuretic treatment.

The use of very low doses to avoid first-dose hypotension is common, although the rationale remains unclear (13[r]). It is even less clear whether or not there are differences between different ACE inhibitors, i.e. whether first-dose hypotension is agent-specific or a class effect (14[Cr], 15[c]). For example, in a well-designed study in patients with heart failure first-dose hypotension occurred with both captopril and enalapril but not with perindopril (14[Cr]). Similarly, first-dose hypotension after enalapril (10 mg) has been reported in a 52-year-old male hypertensive who had previously taken captopril 75 mg daily with no satisfactory blood pressure response (15[c]).

Respiratory *Cough* A non-productive irritant cough is associated with ACE inhibitor treatment (16[r], 17[R]). However, there is still controversy about the absolute incidence (which ranges from 0.7 to 48%), the discontinuation rate (which ranges from 1 to 10%), and the relative incidences with different ACE inhibitors (17[R], 18[r]). Cough appears to be more common in non-smokers (19[r]) and in women (19[r], 20[R]).

The pharmacology of this response has been explored in several reviews (21[R]—23[R]). In general, bronchial hyper-reactivity has been causally implicated and may also be associated with exaggerated dermal responses to histamine (23[R]). However, in one report airways hyper-responsiveness was not a consistent finding (24[r]).

It has recently been suggested that ACE inhibitors are also associated with an increased incidence of symptomatic obstructive airways disease, leading to bronchospasm and asthma (25[cR]). However, a prescription event monitoring study of more than 29 000 patients taking ACE inhibitors, compared with 278 000 patients taking other drugs, failed to confirm this association (26[cR]).

Endocrine, metabolic Gynecomastia has been reported in a patient taking captopril 75 mg daily; it resolved when the captopril was withdrawn but recurred when the patient was given enalapril (27[c]). This suggests that gynecomastia may not be simply attributable to the sulfhydryl group of captopril.

Hematological Some further reports of a bone-marrow suppressive effect of captopril have been published, including a case of aplastic anemia. The patient was a 78-year-old woman who had been taking captopril for 2 years, but since other causes of aplastic anemia (including other drug therapy) were not excluded, clear interpretation is difficult (28[c]). Further cases of neutropenia (29[c]) and agranulocytosis (30[c], 31[c]) have also been reported, although in some of these there were similar complicating issues, making a clear association difficult to establish. Nevertheless, in one of the cases of agranulocytosis the white cell count returned to normal when captopril was withdrawn (30[c]). Agranulocytosis has also been reported with enalapril (32[c]).

Autoimmune thrombocytopenia, gradually reversible on withdrawal of captopril, has been reported in three patients taking captopril (33[c]). Thrombocytopenia has also been reported with enalapril in a report of two elderly sisters (34[c]). Ten days after starting enalapril a 76-year-old woman became thrombocytopenic and recovered when enalapril was stopped; her 75-year-old sister had a similar response to captopril. Both sisters had the same HLA phenotype (B8DR3), which the authors postulated may reflect a genetic predisposition to this reaction

Liver and pancreas Hepatic injury has become a well-recognised albeit rare adverse effect of the ACE inhibitors (35[c], 36[R]). Although this was originally attributed to a hypersensitivity reaction, it now appears that the mechanism is idiosyncratic, that both acute and chronic hepatitis may be precipitated (37[r], 38[r]), and that cross-reactivity may also occur, as identified in a case report involving enalapril and captopril (39[c]).

There is also a growing list of reports of acute pancreatitis with both enalapril and lisinopril (40[r]).

Urinary system *Impairment of renal function* The dangers of ACE inhibition, particularly in the context of renovascular disease, are well established (41[R]). In a review of the factors that predispose to renal insufficiency it has been suggested that hyponatremia, high dosages of diuretics, severe heart failure, and diabetes mellitus are the most important contributory factors (42[R]). However, there is increasing evidence that ACE inhibition itself provokes hyponatremia (43[c]). A 63-year-old white woman presented with a serum sodium concentration of 109 mmol/l after the introduction 6 weeks before of lisinopril, 10 mg/day. Initially the hyponatremia was considered to reflect a pneumonia-induced syndrome of inappropriate ADH secretion and, because blood pressure control was deteriorating, lisinopril was reintroduced. Subsequently, the serum sodium concentration fell from 134 to 126 mmol/l. After the withdrawal of lisinopril there was no further hyponatremia, despite further episodes of chest infection. An interaction of ACE inhibitors with lithium has also been identified, leading to both lithium toxicity (44[c]) and renal dysfunction, including hyponatremia (45[c]).

Skin and appendages *Angioedema* This potentially fatal complication has now been associated with several different ACE inhibitors, with a reported incidence of 0.1–0.5% (46[c]–48[c]). The problem may manifest as recurrent episodes of facial swelling, which resolves with withdrawal (47[c]), or as acute oropharyngeal edema and airways obstruction, which requires emergency treatment with an antihistamine and corticosteroids, and which is occasionally fatal (49[c], 50[r]). A variant form is angioedema of the intestine, which may present clinically as an 'acute abdomen', which has tended to occur within the first 24–48 h of treatment (51[c]–53[c]).

Rashes There has now been a sufficient number of case reports of different skin rashes developing in association with ACE inhibitor drugs to indicate that this is a significant adverse effect. The most common skin reaction is a pruritic, maculopapular eruption, which is reportedly more common with captopril (2–7%) than with enalapril (about 1.5%). The incidence appears to be dose-related and is higher in patients with renal insufficiency (54[r]). Lichenoid reactions, bullous/pemphigoid lesions, exfoliative dermatitis, flushing and erythroderma, vasculitis/purpura, subcutaneous lupus erythematosus, and reversible alopecia have all been reported (55[r]–57[r]). It now appears that the ACE inhibitors are pharmacologically implicated, particularly with respect to psoriasis, by a mechanism mediated by inhibition of the activity of leukotrienes, which are implicated in the pathogenesis of psoriasis (58[c]).

Taste disturbance Dysgeusia (taste disturbance and taste loss) appears to be particularly associated with captopril. However, a recent report from the Australian Drug Evaluation Committee has confirmed that this complication is more likely to complicate treatment with captopril than with other ACE inhibitors. In this report, captopril was the drug most commonly associated with taste disturbance and it accounted for more than half the cases of taste loss (59[R]). Taste loss was dose-related, insofar as more than 90% of reports detailed a daily dose of 50 mg or more. Most cases recovered on withdrawal, although the sense of taste had not returned 7 months after discontinuation in one case, and in two of the reports there was associated anosmia. Although there was no significant difference between captopril and lisinopril (60[c]), it appears that captopril, presumably via its sulfhydryl group, has an increased likelihood of provoking dysgeusia.

Immunological and hypersensitivity reactions Two cases of alveolitis have been reported with captopril, one associated with eosinophilia (61[c]) and the other with a lymphocytic pulmonary infiltrate (62[c]). There has also been a report of a captopril-associated lupus-like syndrome (63[c]).

Second-generation effects It is now established in humans that enalapril, captopril, and lisinopril (and presumably other ACE inhibitors) cross the placenta in pharmacologically significant amounts (6[R], 64[c]). Inevitably, pregnancies will occur in women taking ACE inhibitors, but although there is clear evidence of a teratogenic syndrome it has been suggested that this is not necessarily an indication for termination of pregnancy. However, since continuation of treatment beyond the first trimester carries an excess risk of low fetal birth weight and other more severe complications, it is important to withdraw the ACE inhibitor at this time. Intrauterine growth retardation, oligohydramnios, and neonatal renal impairment, frequently with a serious outcome, are characteristic (65[c]); failure of ossification of the skull or hypocalvaria also appear to be part of the pattern (6[R]). There is also evidence that persistence of a patent ductus arteriosus is also more likely to occur.

Risk situations Enalapril has been specifically studied in patients resistant to other drugs and intolerant of captopril (66[C]) and in patients with collagen vascular disease and renal disease known to be at high risk of adverse effects (67[C]). In the first study (66[C]) the major reasons for discontinuing captopril were a low white blood cell count, proteinuria, taste disturbance, and skin rash. In the vast majority of the 281 patients these adverse effects did not recur during enalapril treatment; instead, the main adverse events that warranted discontinuation of enalapril were impairment of renal function (5%), hypotension (2%), and skin rashes (2%). The authors noted that patients with angioedema should not be given alternative ACE inhibitors.

In the second study (67[C]), of 738 high-risk patients the main reasons for the discontinuation of enalapril were increases in serum creatinine (4%), hypotension (1%), and nausea (1%).

INDIVIDUAL ACE INHIBITORS

Benazepril

Headache, upper respiratory tract infections, fatigue, and dizziness were identified in a review of 1595 hypertensive patients treated with benazepril (68[R]). Orthostatic hypotension, ventricular tachycardia, and urinary tract infection were considered the most frequent adverse events in a study of 26 patients with moderate/severe cardiac failure (69[c]).

Cilazapril

A case of subacute cutaneous lupus erythematosus has been associated with cilazapril treatment in a previously healthy 64-year-old white woman. The authors speculated that genetically predisposed individuals would be at risk from such skin reactions, irrespective of the choice of ACE inhibitor (70[r]).

Perindopril

In two reviews of the safety and efficacy of perindopril the main adverse effects that forced drug withdrawal were cough and gastrointestinal disturbances (71[c], 72[c]). In another study of hypertensive subjects the most frequently reported adverse effects were dizziness, headache, mood/sleep disturbance, asthenia, and muscle cramps (73[c]).

Quinapril

A 68-year-old woman treated with quinapril reportedly developed a cough that later resolved when her treatment was changed to fosinopril (74[r]).

Ramipril

Dizziness, weakness, upper abdominal pain, and headache were reported from a trial of 331 hypertensive subjects (75[C]), and hypotension, diarrhea, and dizziness were reported in a study of 27 patients with heart failure (76[c]).

ANGIOTENSIN II RECEPTOR ANTAGONISTS

The action of angiotensin II (AII) at the AII subtype 1 receptor is of critical importance in cardiovascular regulation, and blockade of this receptor interferes with processes that include vasoconstriction, salt and water retention, sympathetic nervous system activity, and cellular growth. Losartan potassium is the prototype of a new class of antihypertensive drug, the selective and competitive angiotensin II antagonists. However, the pharmacological activity of losartan mainly depends on its active metabolite (E3174), which is a non-competitive and longer-lasting angiotensin II antagonist. The preliminary data obtained in patients with a range of cardiovascular disorders, including hypertension, cardiac failure, and left ventricular hypertrophy, suggest that losartan has efficacy comparable to that of ACE inhibitors and other antihypertensive drugs. It remains to be established whether or not the overall therapeutic profile is superior to other agents that are widely used in clinical practice. These preliminary studies, however, have suggested that losartan has an acceptable profile of adverse effects and, of particular interest, is not associated with the non-productive cough that is a well-recognized feature of ACE inhibitor treatment.

The data presented in a recent overview have been derived from clinical trials involving about 3000 patients with mild, moderate, or severe hypertension who took losartan with or without a thiazide diuretic (77[R]).

ADVERSE REACTION PATTERN

General and toxic reactions To date, losartan is reported to have a relatively low incidence of adverse effects, comparable with most commonly used antihypertensive drugs. There are no obvious toxic reactions and the overall profile of adverse effects is non-specific, headache, dizziness, and asthenia/fatigue being the most common.

Hypersensitivity reactions As yet there have been no reports indicative of an obvious hypersensitivity pattern, but there have been reports of raised liver enzymes, which necessitated drug withdrawal in one patient (78[c]).

Tumor-inducing effects No tumor-inducing effects have been reported.

Second-generation effects No second-generation effects have been reported.

ANGIOTENSIN II ANTAGONISM: PREDICTABLE CLASS EFFECTS

Cardiovascular The action of losartan to interfere with the activity of the renin—angiotensin system is sufficiently similar to the action of the ACE inhibitor drugs that episodes of first-dose hypotension, renal impairment, and hyperkalemia would be anticipated. There have been only a few such reports to date, although this may reflect the careful screening of patients for clinical trials, from which, by inference, obviously high-risk patients may have been excluded.

Respiratory *Cough* Cough has been specifically studied, because the mechanism of action of losartan differs from the ACE inhibitor group, in that there is no accumulation of kinins, which have been implicated in the non-productive cough associated with ACE inhibitors (79[R], 80[R]). The most convincing proof comes from a study of 135 patients known to suffer from ACE inhibitor-induced cough who were then rechallenged with lisinopril, losartan, or hydrochlorothiazide. Of the patients rechallenged with lisinopril, 72% developed a cough compared with only 29 and 34% in the losartan and hydrochlorothiazide groups, respectively (81[c]).

Immunological and hypersensitivity reactions To date there have been two reports of angioedema during losartan treatment. A patient known to be hypersensitive to penicillin and aspirin developed facial rash and swelling, which was considered by the investigator to be angioedema (78[c]). Facial swelling and flushing, without dyspnea, occurred within 30 min of ingesting 50 mg losartan in another patient with glomerulosclerosis and no history of angioedema when previously treated with captopril (78[c]).

DRUGS ACTING ON THE SYMPATHETIC NERVOUS SYSTEM

CENTRALLY-ACTING AGENTS

These agents, particularly α-methyldopa and clonidine, have been widely used for many years. Their mechanisms of action depend on reducing sympathetic nervous outflow from the CNS by interference with regulatory neurotransmitter systems in the brain stem. These effects were originally attributed to agonist actions at central α_2-adrenoceptors, and because none of the drugs was selective or specific for circulatory control systems the hypotensive effects were invariably accompanied by other CNS effects. However, the identification of imidazoline receptors has suggested that it may be possible to develop drugs, such as moxonidine, which have greater selectivity for circulatory control mechanisms and a reduced likelihood of unwanted CNS depressant effects.

ADVERSE REACTION PATTERN

General and toxic reactions In general, treatment with centrally-acting agents is characterized by a relatively high incidence (up to 60% in some studies) of CNS depressant effects (dizziness, drowsiness, tiredness, dry mouth, headache, depression), particularly during the initial period of treatment or following dosage increments.

A withdrawal syndrome with marked rebound hypertension (attributed to increased sympathetic nervous activity as a result of drug-modified receptor responses) is an occasional but well-recognized complication of the abrupt cessation of treatment, particularly with clonidine.

Hypersensitivity reactions Hypersensitivity reactions are particularly well-recognised with α-methyldopa: Coombs positivity (asymptomatic) in about 20% of patients, hepatitis in about 6%, fever, eosinophilia, and skin rash in about 3%. Rarely (0.02%) a Coombs-positive hemolytic anemia develops.

Tumor-inducing effects Tumor-inducing effects have not been reported.

Second-generation effects There have been no consistent reports of second generation effects.

α-Methyldopa

Cardiovascular Although postural hypotension is often quoted as a complication of treatment with methyldopa there is no convincing evidence that this unwanted effect is more likely with methyldopa than with other commonly used antihypertensive drugs. Complete heart block, which resolved following the withdrawal of methyldopa but reappeared on rechallenge, has been reported in two elderly patients and attributed to the central sympatholytic effect of methyldopa (82[c]).

Nervous system Sedation, drowsiness, forgetfulness, depression, and tiredness are common. These are dose-related. Some tolerance develops during long-term treatment, but the insidious presence of these depressant effects may not be fully apparent until the patient is given alternative treatment.

Methyldopa should probably be avoided in patients with Parkinsonism, because in theory the production of α-methyldopamine may worsen the disease, and there have indeed been reports of exacerbation (83[c]).

Endocrine, metabolic Acutely methyldopa promotes the release of growth hormone and prolactin, but the long-term significance of this is unclear. However, there have been case reports of hyperprolactinemia, leading to amenorrhea and galactorrhea (84[c]).

Hematological Coombs positivity and Coombs-positive hemolytic anemia are well recognized. For example, a syndrome of hemolytic anemia, arthritis, photosensitivity, and high titers of antinuclear antibody (1:256) and of IgG antibodies to class I histones were found in a 55-year-old man who took methyldopa 250 mg b.d. for 13 months. All of these changes resolved spontaneously when methyldopa was withdrawn (85[c]). Anemia, reticulocytosis, and a positive Coombs test were seen in a 64-year-old woman taking methyldopa 1000 mg b.d.; these problems resolved after withdrawal (86[c]).

Liver Hepatotoxicity due to methyldopa is most often an acute hepatitis, which resolves when the drug is withdrawn. It may start at any time after the start of therapy, but usually within the first few weeks, and it ranges in severity from a minor disturbance of liver function tests to acute hepatic necrosis. There has been a report of a fatal toxic hepatitis in a 22-year-old woman treated with methyldopa in late pregnancy (87[c]). Sometimes, a more chronic picture develops after treatment for 2 or 3 years, with features of chronic active hepatitis (88[r]).

Gastrointestinal Dry mouth occurred twice as often with methyldopa (41%) as with atenolol (21%) in a crossover comparison in 69 hypertensive patients (89[C]). The well-recognized association between methyldopa and diarrhea was further confirmed by the case of an 84-year-old black woman who over a period of 7 years was free of diarrhea during periods when methyldopa was stopped but suffered diarrhea as soon as methyldopa was re-introduced (90[c]). Similar recurrences on repeated exposure were identified in a 71-year-old man who took methyldopa 250 mg b.d. (91[c]).

Withdrawal effects A withdrawal syndrome with rebound hypertension has been reported with methyldopa. Although it is similar to that associated with clonidine, it is less well-defined, less severe, and less frequent.

Withdrawal of methyldopa has also been associated with the development of an acute manic syndrome in a 62-year-old man who had had methyldopa withdrawn 4 weeks before. There had been no previous history of psychiatric disorder (92[c]).

Clonidine

The advantages and disadvantages of clonidine and other α_2-adrenoceptor agonists have recently been reviewed (93[R]), as has their effect on respiratory function in asthmatics (94[R]). Inhaled α_2-adrenoceptor agonists may reduce the bronchial response to allergens, and if ingested they may aggravate the bronchial response to histamine.

Cardiovascular Clonidine causes sinus bradycardia and atrioventricular block, as illustrated by two cases, one a 10-year-old boy (95[c]) and the other a 71-year-old woman (96[c]) who developed Wenckebach's phenomenon. Clonidine was also studied in seven patients subjected to electrophysiological studies after 5 weeks of therapy (97[C]). Clonidine slowed the sinus rate and increased the atrial pacing rate, producing AV nodal Wenckebach in these patients, indicating depressed function of the sinus and AV nodes.

Nervous system Sedation, lethargy, and tiredness are common, particularly at the start of treatment.

Endocrine, metabolic Clonidine stimulates growth hormone release (and has been used as a provocation test of growth hormone reserve) and reduces plasma renin activity and aldosterone and catecholamine concentrations.

Gastrointestinal Dry mouth is common with clonidine. Constipation is frequent and one case of pseudo-obstruction of the bowel has been reported (98[c]).

Skin and appendages Rashes occur in about 5% of patients taking clonidine.

Transdermal clonidine formulated in adhesive skin patches has been used for long-term treatment with once weekly application. Systemic adverse effects are the same as those with oral administration, and in addition contact dermatitis has been reported (99[c]).

Immunological and hypersensitivity reactions A 46-year-old woman took clonidine 25 mg b.d. for menopausal flushing She developed depigmentation and swelling of her forearms. She also had the symptoms and signs of a median nerve palsy. A skin biopsy showed a pattern consistent with immune complex disease, with IgG, IgM, Clq, C2c, and C4 complement between muscle fibers and at the dermo-epidermal junctions. All of these abnormalities disappeared after withdrawal of clonidine (100[c]).

Withdrawal effects In its most florid form, the clonidine withdrawal syndrome is characterized by a pronounced increase in blood pressure, tachycardia, tremulousness, and sweating. There is an associated marked increase in catecholamine output and the features are reminiscent of pheochromocytoma or accelerated hypertension. Milder cases may pass unnoticed, unless the patient is being carefully monitored. The syndrome begins within 48 hours of clonidine withdrawal, and although the exact incidence is unknown it is more likely if the patient has been taking a high dosage. There has even been a case report of rebound hypertension in association with transdermal clonidine (101[c]). Treatment is by combined α- and β-blockade, and it is important to avoid monotherapy with a β-blocker, since this may exacerbate the syndrome by promoting unopposed α-adrenergic effects.

There have also been two case reports of serious complications arising from the acute withdrawal of clonidine. Neuropsychiatric disturbance with self-injury occurred in a child (102[c]) and myocardial infarction developed in a patient with no history of ischemic heart disease (103[c]).

OTHER CENTRALLY-ACTING AGENTS

Guanabenz, guanfacine, and tiamenidine appear to be qualitatively similar to clonidine. Clear evidence of quantitative differences remains to be confirmed.

Rilmenidine

In a number of trials in hypertension the adverse effects profile of rilmenidine was qualitatively similar to that of clonidine, although the overall incidence of adverse events appeared to be lower. The main complaints were of dry mouth, drowsiness, and constipation (104[C]–106[C]). In one of these reviews, in which the impact on vigilance was particularly examined, it was concluded that although there were dose-related effects there was no statistically significant difference between rilmenidine and placebo in relation to sedation and drowsiness. However, these results consistently showed a rank order among placebo, rilmenidine, and clonidine, progressively leading to greater degrees of sedation (107[r]).

Reserpine (and Rauwolfia alkaloids)

These agents are now little used. They act by depleting neurotransmitter storage systems and reducing sympathetic nervous activity, but their effects are non-specific and CNS adverse effects (depression, drowsiness, tiredness, confusion) are prominent. There is also a troublesome incidence of diarrhea, hyperprolactinemia, and gynecomastia. There is also a possible withdrawal syndrome. For example, a 66-year-old woman was admitted to hospital suffering from an agitated depressive psychosis. This settled with standard antipsychotic therapy. It was subsequently found that she had been taking reserpine in an over-the-counter formulation and had stopped this a week before her admission (108[c]). Her doctor felt that the syndrome had occurred as a result of CNS hypersensitivity after reserpine withdrawal.

POSTSYNAPTIC α_1-ADRENOCEPTOR ANTAGONISTS

These drugs block α_1-adrenoceptor-mediated vasoconstriction of peripheral blood vessels (both arterial and venous) and are effectively peripheral 'vasodilators'.

α-blockers have recently been reviewed (109[R], 110[R]). Qualitatively and quantitatively their common adverse effects are generally similar, although indoramin has additional effects on other neurotransmitter systems and therefore tends to be considered separately.

ADVERSE REACTION PATTERN

General and toxic reactions The 'first-dose response' (profound postural hypotension and reflex tachycardia) is a well-recognized complication of the initiation of treatment with prazosin and related agents. This phenomenon is dose-related and can usually be avoided by appropriate titration of the initial dosages, which are preferably taken at bedtime.

During long-term treatment orthostatic hypotension and dizziness is reported by about 10% of patients.

Hypersensitivity reactions There have been no consistent reports of hypersensitivity reactions.

Tumor-inducing effects No tumor-inducing effects have been reported.

Prazosin

Cardiovascular Postural hypotension and reflex tachycardia, particularly on standing, are features of the first-dose response to prazosin, but adaptive receptor responses lead to 're-setting' of the reflex mechanisms within the first few days of treatment, and there are therefore generally no significant changes in heart rate during long-term treatment. An orthostatic component to the hypotensive response persists during long-term treatment, and this may be significant and symptomatic if high dosages are used.

Endocrine, metabolic Prazosin and other quinazolines are associated with small but significant changes in plasma lipid profiles. Generally these are potentially beneficial changes, with reductions in LDL/total cholesterol and triglycerides and increases in HDL cholesterol.

Urinary system Blockade of the α_1-adrenoceptors

in the urinary tract leads to smooth muscle relaxation and improvement in urinary flow, and this pharmacological action has been harnessed to ameliorate the urinary symptoms of benign prostatic hyperplasia. Conversely, prazosin may occasionally lead to urinary incontinence, particularly stress incontinence in women (111[C]).

Sexual function There is some evidence that male sexual dysfunction occurs less often with α-blockers than with other types of antihypertensive drug (112[C]). For example, in a comparison of the effects of prazosin and hydrochlorothiazide on sexual function in 12 hypertensive men, plethysmographic measurements and subjective assessments indicated less dysfunction with prazosin than with hydrochlorothiazide (113[C]). There is no evidence that this effect can be used therapeutically, but cases of priapism have been reported: for example, a 55-year-old man presented with priapism having taken prazosin 7.5 mg t.d.s. for 4 months. After a further 3 months, prazosin was discontinued and his erections became normal (114[c]).

OTHER α_1-ANTAGONISTS

Doxazosin and terazosin are quinazoline derivatives whose adverse effects profiles are similar to that of prazosin.

The safety and tolerability of doxazosin has been the subject of several reviews (115[R]) and the long-term efficacy and safety of terazosin have been reviewed, in both monotherapy and combination therapy in whites and blacks (116[Cr], 117[Cr]).

Indoramin is a post-synaptic α_1-adrenoceptor antagonist (and chemically distinct from the quinazolines), which penetrates the CNS to a significant extent. It is reported to have a relatively high incidence of adverse effects, including sedation, dizziness, depression, headache, palpitation, dry mouth, and constipation (118[R]).

DIRECT VASODILATORS

Direct vasodilators act on vascular smooth muscle to produce systemic vasodilatation. As a result there is baroreceptor-mediated activation of the sympathetic nervous system and the renin—angiotensin system. These drugs are therefore generally reserved for second- or third-line antihypertensive use, particularly in combination with β-adrenoceptor antagonists and thiazide diuretics.

ADVERSE REACTION PATTERN

General and toxic reactions Vasodilator drugs (as monotherapy) are associated acutely with flushing, headache, dizziness, and reflex tachycardia and palpitation. Chronic treatment may be complicated by fluid retention.

Hypersensitivity reactions The drug-induced lupus-like syndrome, with fever, arthralgia, and anemia, is well recognized (particularly in slow acetylators) but uncommon. Seropositivity for antinuclear antibody is relatively common (about 20%) but its significance is debatable.

Tumor-indu[...] effects Although tumors have been reporte[...] have been no reports in hum[...]

Hydralazin[...]

Cardiova[...] [...]nably as a result [...]ported (119[c]).

Nervous system Periph[...]een described in association with pyridoxine [...] B$_6$) deficiency in slow acetylators (120[Cr]).

Endocrine, metabolic Salt and water retention mediated by secondary hyperaldosteronism may complicate hydralazine treatment, leading to weight gain and peripheral edema, loss of blood pressure control, and rarely cardiac failure.

Liver There have been several reports of acute hepatitis (usually with negative antinuclear antibodies) (121[c]–125[c]).

Gastrointestinal Anorexia, nausea, and vomiting may complicate hydralazine treatment, particularly initially.

Immunological and hypersensitivity reactions The lupus-like syndrome (see SED-9, 318) with hydralazine occurs particularly in slow acetylators (and only rarely in fast acetylators) and in patients with the HLA-DR4 antigen. Blood dyscrasias and necrotizing vasculitis are rare additional features.

Second-generation effects Thrombocytopenia has been reported in infants whose mothers were taking hydralazine with no evidence of the lupus-like syndrome (126[c]). The administration of hydralazine 25 mg b.d. at 34 weeks to a hypertensive pregnant woman was associated, within 1 week, with atrial extra beats in the fetus. These subsided when hydralazine was stopped, and the rest of the pregnancy and delivery were uneventful (127[c]).

A 29-year-old woman, 26 weeks pregnant, was treated with hydralazine for toxemia of pregnancy. She developed arthralgia and dyspnea and was subsequently found to be antinuclear antibody-positive. Following an induced labor, a low-birth-weight infant was born but died aged 36 hours. At autopsy the neonate was found to have a pericardial effusion and tamponade (128[c]). Although hydralazine was implicated as the cause of a maternal and neonatal lupus-like syndrome, the toxemia and low-birth weight of the child make interpretation of the case difficult.

OTHER DIRECT VASODILATORS

Minoxidil

The pattern of adverse vasodilator effects with minoxidil is similar to, but more severe than that of hydralazine, and fluid retention may be troublesome. A particular feature of minoxidil is excessive hair growth. For example, severe hypertrichosis, including excessive hair on the face, ears, and forehead, developed in a 57-year-old man who took minoxidil 5 mg t.d.s. for refractory hypertension. He developed hypertrichosis of the external auditory meatus, which led to chronic otitis externa, chronic otitis media, and mastoiditis, and eventually led to permanent severe deafness (129[c]). Severe hypertrichosis, unacceptable even to men, has complicated the otherwise successful antihypertensive treatment of six patients after renal transplantation, for which ciclosporin was also used. Since hypertrichosis has also been described with ciclosporin, there may be an additive pharmacodynamic interaction (130[C]).

Diazoxide

The peripheral vasodilator effect of diazoxide produces a pattern of adverse effects similar to that of minoxidil. An additional feature is hyperglycemia and diabetes mellitus. Diazoxide is used to treat hyperinsulinism in infancy, but its use may be hazardous (131[c], 132[c]).

REFERENCES

1. Ferrannini E, Buzzigoli G, Bonadonwa R. Insulin resistance in essential hypertension. New Engl J Med 1987; 317:350–357.
2. Berne C, Pollare T, Lithell H. Effects of antihypertensive treatment on insulin sensitivity with special reference to ACE inhibitors. Diabetes Care 1991;14(Suppl 4):39–47.
3. Moller DE, Flier JS. Insulin resistance—mechanisms, syndromes and implications. New Engl J Med 1991;325: 938–948.
4. Kostis JB. Angiotensin converting enzyme inhibitors. II. Clinical use. Am Heart J 1988;116:1591.
5. Dzau VJ, Creager MA. Progress in angiotensin-converting enzyme inhibition in heart failure: rationale, mechanisms and clinical responses Cardiol Clin 1989;7:119.
6. Barr M Jr. Teratogen update: angiotensin-converting enzyme inhibitors. Teratology 1994;50:399–409.
7. Scott RA, Barnett DB. Lower than conventional doses of captopril in the initiation of converting enzyme inhibition in patients with severe congestive heart failure. Clin Cardiol 1989;12:225.
8. Kjekshus J, Swedberg K. Enalapril for congestive heart failure. Am J Cardiol 89;63:26D.
9. Warner JN, Rush JE, Keegan ME. Tolerability of enalapril in congestive heart failure. Am J Cardiol 1989;63:33D.
10. Francis GS, Rucinska EJ. Long-term effects of a once-a-day versus twice-a-day regimen of enalapril for congestive heart failure. Am J Cardiol 1989;63:17D.
11. Lewis GR. Comparison of lisinopril versus placebo for congestive heart failure. Am J Cardiol 1989;63:12D.
12. Perlman JM, Volpe JJ. Neurologic complications of captopril treatment of neonatal hypertension. Pediatrics 1989; 83:47.
13. Reznik V, Griswold W, Mendoza S. Dangers of captopril therapy in newborns. Pediatrics 1989;83:1076.
14. MacFadyen RJ, Lees KR, Reid JL. Differences in first dose response to angiotensin converting enzyme inhibition in congestive cardiac heart failure: a placebo controlled study. Br Heart J 1991;66:206–211.
15. Mullen PJ. Unexpected first dose hypotensive reaction to enalapril. Postgrad Med J 1990;66:1087.
16. Strocchi E, Valtancoli G, Ambrosioni E. The incidence of cough during treatment with angiotensin converting enzyme inhibitors. J Hypertens 1989;7(Suppl 6):S308-S309.
17. Yeo WW, Ramsay LE. Persistent dry cough with enalapril: incidence depends on method used. J Hum Hypertens 1990;4:517–520.
18. Sharif MN, Evans BL, Pylypchuk GB. Cough induced by quinapril with resolution after changing to fosinopril. Ann Pharmacother 1994;28:720–721.
19. Os I, Bratland B, Dahlof B, Gisholt K, Syvertsen J, Tretli S. Female sex as an important determinant of lisinopril induced cough. Lancet 1992;339:372.
20. Israili ZH, Hall WD. Cough and angioneurotic edema associated with angiotensin-converting enzyme inhibitor therapy: a review of the literature and pathophysiology. Ann Intern Med 1992;117:234–42.
21. Lindgren BR, Andersson RGG. Angiotensin-converting enzyme inhibitors and their influence on inflammation, bronchial reactivity and cough. A research review. Med Toxicol Adv Drug Exp 1989;4:369.

22. Kaufman J, Casanova JE, Rienal P, Schlueter DP. Bronchial hyperreactivity and cough due to angiotensin-converting enzyme inhibitors. Chest 1989;95:544.
23. Lindgren BR, Rosenqvist U, Ekström T et al. Increased bronchial reactivity and potentiated skin responses in hypertensive subjects suffering from coughs during ACE inhibitor therapy. Chest 1989;95:1225—1230.
24. Boulet L-P, Milot J, Lampron N, Lacourciere Y. Pulmonary function and airway responsiveness during long-term therapy with captopril. J Am Med Assoc 1989;261:413—416.
25. Lunde H, Hedner T, Samuelsson O, Lotvall J, Andren L, Lundholm L et al. Dyspnoea, asthma, and bronchospasm in relation to treatment with angiotensin converting enzyme inhibitors. Br Med J 1994;308:18—21.
26. Inman WH, Pearce G, Wilton L, Mann RD. Angiotensin converting enzyme inhibitors and asthma. Drug Safety Research Unit, Southampton, 1994.
27. Nakamura Y, Yoshimoto K, Saima S. Gynaecomastia induced by angiotensin converting enzyme inhibitor Br Med J 1990;300:541.
28. Kim CR, Maley MB, Mohler ER. Captopril and aplastic anemia. Ann Intern Med 1989;111:187.
29. Husain IS, Akhtar MJ. Neutropenia related to captopril. Saudi Med J 1989;10:111.
30. Gomez-Martino Arroyo JR, Jorquesa Plaza F, Ordonez Gonzalez R, Granda Rodriguez M. Agranulocitosis inducida por el uso de captopril. An Med Interna 1989;6:387.
31. Pillans PI, Koopowitz A. Captopril-associated agranulocytosis. A report of 3 cases. S Afr Med J 1991;79:390—400.
32. Elis A, Lishner M, Lang R, Ravid M. Agranulocytosis associated with enalapril. Drug Intell Clin Pharm 1991; 25:461—462.
33. Pujol M, Duran-Suarez JR, Vega CM et al. Autoimmune thrombocytopenia in three patients treated with captopril. Vox Sang 1989;57:218.
34. Grosbois B, Milton D, Beneton C, Jacomy D. Thrombocytopenia induced by angiotensin converting enzyme inhibitors. Br Med J 1989;298:189.
35. Hagley MT, Hulisz DT, Burns CM. Hepatotoxicity associated with angiotensin-converting enzyme inhibitors. Ann Pharmacother 1993;27:228—231.
36. Stricker BHCh, Biour M, Wilson JHP. ACE inhibitors. In: Stricker BHCh, ed.; Dukes MNG, series ed. Drug-Induced Hepatic Injury, 2nd edn. Amsterdam: Elsevier, 1992;323—327.
37. Valle R, Carrascosa M, Cillero L, Perez-Castrillon JL. Enalapril-induced hepatotoxicity. Ann Pharmacother 1993; 27:1405.
38. Droste HT, de Vries RA. Chronic hepatitis caused by lisinopril. Neth J Med 1995;46:95—98.
39. Hagley MT, Benak RL, Hulisz DT. Suspected cross-reactivity of enalapril and captopril-induced hepatotoxicity. Ann Pharmacother 1992;26:780—781.
40. Standridge JB. Fulminant pancreatitis associated with lisinopril therapy. South Med J 1994;87:179—181.
41. Burnier M, Waeber B, Nussberger J, Brunner HR. Effect of angiotensin converting enzyme inhibition in renovascular hypertension. J Hypertens 1989;7(Suppl 7):S27.
42. Packer M. Identification of risk factors predisposing to the development of functional renal insufficiency during treatment with converting enzyme inhibitors in chronic heart failure. Cardiology 1989;76(Suppl 2):50.
43. Hume AL, Jack BW, Levinson P. Pharmacotherapy case reports: severe hyponatremia: an association with lisinopril? Ann Pharmacother 1990;24:1169—1171.
44. Baldwin CM, Safferman AZ. A case of lisinopril-induced lithium toxicity. Ann Pharmacother 1990;24:946—947.
45. Lehmann K, Ritz E. Occasional hypothesis: angiotensin-converting enzyme inhibitors may cause renal dysfunction in patients on long-term lithium treatment. Am J Kidney Dis 1995;25:82—87.
46. Israeli Z, Hall W. Cough and angioneurotic edema associated with angiotensin converting enzyme inhibitor therapy. Ann Intern Med 1992;117:234—242.
47. Frontera Y, Piecuch JF. Multiple episodes of angioedema associated with lisinopril, an ACE inhibitor. J Am Med Assoc 1995;126:217—220.
48. Hedner T, Samuelson O, Lunde H, Lindholm L, Andren L, Weholm BE. Angioedema in relation to treatment with angiotensin-converting enzyme inhibitors. Br Med J 1992; 304:941—5.
49. Ulmer JL, Garvey MJ. Fatal angioedema associated with lisinopril. Ann Pharmacother 1992;26:245—246.
50. Giannocaro PJ, Wallace GJ, Higginson LAJ, Williams WL. Fatal angioedema associated with enalapril. Can J Cardiol 1989;5:335.
51. Fernandez-Diaz ML, Herranz P, Suarez-Marrero MC, Borbujo J, Manzano R, Casado M. Subacute cutaneous lupus erythematosus associated with cilazapril. Lancet 1995;345:398.
52. Jacobs RL, Hoberman LJ, Goldstein HM. Angioedema of the small bowel caused by an angiotensin-converting enzyme inhibitor. Am J Gastroenterol 1994;39:127—128.
53. Dupasquier E. Une forme clinique rare d'oedéme angioneurotique sous énalapril: l'abdomen aigu. Arch Mal Coeur 1994;87:1371—1374.
54. Roten SV, Mainetti C, Donath R, Saurat J-H. Enalapril-induced lichen planus-like eruption. J Am Acad Dermatol 1995;32:293—295.
55. Kuechle M, Hutton KP, Muller SA. Angiotensin-converting enzyme inhibitor-induced pemphigus: three case reports and literature review. Mayo Clin Proc 1994;69:1166—1171.
56. Gilleaudeau P, Vallat VP, Carter DM, Gottlieb AB. Angiotensin-converting enzyme inhibitors as possible exacerbating drugs in psoriasis. J Am Acad Dermatol 1993; 28:490—493.
57. Butt A, Burge SM. Pemphigus vulgaris induced by captopril. Dermatology 1993;186:315—315
58. Ikai K. Exacerbation and induction of psoriasis by angiotensin-converting enzyme inhbitors. J Am Acad Dermatol 1995;???:819.
59. Boyd I. Captopril-induced taste disturbance. Lancet 1995;342:304.
60. Neil-Dwyer G, Marus A. ACE inhibitors in hypertension: assessment of taste and smell function in clinical trials. J Hum Hypertens 1989;3:169—176.
61. Schatz PL, Mesologites D, Hyun J et al. Captopril-induced hypersensitivity lung disease. An immune-complex mediated phenomenon. Chest 1989;95:685.
62. Kidney JC, O'Halloran DJ, Fitzgerald MX. Captopril and lymphocytic alveolitis. Br Med J 1989;299:981.
63. Sieber C, Grimm E, Follath F. Captopril and systemic lupus erythematosus syndrome. Br Med J 1990;301:669.
64. Pryde PG, Sedman AB, Nugent CE, Barr M. Angioten-

sin-converting enzyme inhibitor fetopathy. J Am Soc Nephrol 1993;3:1575–1582.
65. Martin T, Taupignon A, Graf E, Perrin D. Pancréatite et hépatite chez une femme traitée par maléate d'énalapril. Un cas. Thérapie 1989;44:449.
66. Rucinska EJ, Small R, Mulcahy WS et al. Tolerability of long term therapy with enalapril maleate in patients resistant to other therapies and intolerant to captopril. Med Toxicol Adv Drug Exp 1989;4:144.
67. Rucinska EJ, Small R, Irvin J. High-risk patients treated with enalapril maleate: safety considerations. Int J Cardiol 1989;22:249.
68. Whalen JJ. Definition of the effective dose of the converting enzyme inhibitor benazepril. Am Heart J 1989; 117:728.
69. Insel J, Mirvis DM, Boland MJ et al. A multicenter study of the safety and efficacy of benazepril hydrochloride, a long acting angiotensin-converting enzyme inhibitor in patients with chronic congestive heart failure. Clin Pharmacol Ther 1989;45:312.
70. Fernandez Diaz ML, Herranz P, Suarez Marrero MC, Borbujo J, Manzano R, Casado M. Subacute cutaneous lupus erythematosus associated with cilazapril. Lancet 1995;345:398
71. Sharif MN, Evans BL, Pylypchuk GB. Cough induced by quinapril with resolution after changing to fosinopril. Ann Pharmacother 1994;28:720–722.
72. Brichard S, Lambert AE. Perindopril safety and tolerance in at-risk patients. Drugs 1990;39(Suppl 1):64.
73. Santoni JPh, Richard Ch, Pouyollon F et al. Tolérance et sécurité d'emploi du périndopril. Arch Mal Coeur 1989;82:87.
74. Lees KR, Reid JL, Scott MGB et al. Captopril versus perindopril: a double blind study in essential hypertension. J Hum Hypertens 1989;3:17.
75. Bauer B, Lorenz H, Zahltern R. An open multicenter study to assess the long-term efficacy, tolerance, and safety of the oral angiotensin converting enzyme inhibitor ramipril in patients with mild to moderate essential hypertension. Clin Pharmacol Ther 1989;13(Suppl 3):S70.
76. Gerckens V, Grube E, Mengden T et al. Pharmacokinetic and pharmacodynamic properties of ramipril in patients with congestive heart failure. (NYHA III–IV). J Cardiovasc Pharmacol 1989;13(Suppl 3):S49.
77. Goldberg AI, Dunlay MC, Sweet CS. Safety and tolerability of losartan potassium, an angiotensin II receptor antagonist, compared with hydrochlorothiazide, atenolol, felodipine ER and angiotensin-converting enzyme inhibitors for the treatment of systemic hypertension. Am J Cardiol 1995;75:793–795.
78. Merck & Co Inc. Losartan potassium prescribing information. West Point, PA 19486, USA, April 1995.
79. Karlberg BE. Cough and inhibition of the renin angiotensin system. J Hypertens Suppl 1993;S49–S52.
80. Lacourciere Y, Lefebvre J. Modulation of the renin angiotensin aldosterone system and cough. Can J Cardiol 1995;11(Suppl F):33F–39F.
81. Lacourciere Y, Brunner H, Irwin R, Karlberg BE, Ramsay LE, Snavely DB, Dobbins TW, Faison EP, Nelson EB. Effects of modulators of the renin angiotensin aldosterone system on cough. Losartan Cough Study Group. J Hypertens 1994;12:1387–1393.
82. Rosen B, Ovsyshcher IA, Zimlichman R. Complete atrioventricular block induced by methyldopa. Pace 1988; 11:1555.
83. Rosenblum AM, Montgomery EB. Exacerbation of Parkinsonism by methyldopa. J Am Med Assoc 1980;244:2727.
84. Arze RS, Ramos JM, Rashid HV, Kerr DNS. Amenorrhoea, galactorrhoea and hyperprolactinaemia induced by methyldopa. Br Med J 1981;283:194.
85. Nordstrom DM, West SG, Rubin RL. Methyldopa-induced systemic lupus erythematosus. Arthr Rheum 1989; 32:205.
86. Egbert D. Congestive heart failure and respiratory arrest secondary to methyldopa-induced hemolytic anemia. Ann Emerg Med 1988;17:525.
87. Picaud A, Walter P, de Preville G, Nicolas Ph. Hépatite toxique mortelle au cours de la grossesse. J Gynecol Obstet Biol Reprod 1990;19:192.
88. Arranto AJ, Sotaniemi EA. Morphologic alterations in patients with alpha-methyldopa-induced liver damage after short- and long-term exposure. Scand J Gastroenterol 1981;16:853.
89. Glazer N, Goldstein RJ, Lief PD. A double blind, randomized, crossover study of adverse experiences among hypertensive patients treated with atenolol and methyldopa. Curr Ther Res 1989;45:782.
90. Gloth FM, Busby MJ. Methyldopa-induced diarrhea: a case of iatrogenic diarrhea leading to request for nursing home placement. Am J Med 1989;87:480.
91. Troster M, Sullivan SN. Acute colitis due to methyldopa. Can J Gastroenterol 1989;3:182.
92. Labbate LA, Holzgang AJ. Manic syndrome after discontinuation of methyldopa. Am J Psychiatry 1989;146:1075.
93. Dollery CT. Advantages and disadvantages of alpha$_2$-adrenoceptor agonists for systemic hypertension. Am J Cardiol 1988;61:1D.
94. Xuan ATD, Lockhart A. Bronchial effects of alpha$_2$-adrenoceptor agonists and of other antihypertensive agents in asthma. Am J Med 1989;87(Suppl 3C):34S.
95. Dawson PM, Zanden JAV, Werkman SL et al. Cardiac dysrhythmia with the use of clonidine in explosive disorder. Ann Pharmacother 1989;23:465.
96. Marini M, Cavani E, Abbatangelo R, Mascelloni R. Periodismo di Luciani Wenckeback e clonidina. Presentazione di un caso. Clin Ther 1989;126:273.
97. Roden DM, Nadeau JHJ, Primm RK. Electrophysiologic and hemodynamic effects of chronic oral therapy with the alpha$_2$-agonists clonidine and tiamenidine in hypertensive volunteers. Clin Pharmacol Ther 1988;43:648.
98. Kellaway GSM. Adverse drug reactions during treatment of hypertension. Drugs 1976;11(Suppl 1):91.
99. Boekhorst JC. Allergic contact dermatitis with transdermal clonidine. Lancet 1983;ii:1031.
100. Petersen HH, Hansen M, Albrectsen JM. Clonidine-induced immune complex disease. Acta Dermatol-Venereol (Stockholm) 1989;69:519.
101. Schmidt GR, Schuna AA. Rebound hypertension after discontinuation of transdermal clonidine. Clin Pharm 1988; 7:772–774.
102. Dillon JE. Self-injurious behavior associated with clonidine withdrawal in a child with Tourette's disorder. J Child Neurol 1990;5:308–310.
103. Berge KH, Lanier WL. Myocardial infarction accompanying acute clonidine withdrawal in a patient without a history of ischemic coronary artery disease. Anesth Analg 1991;72:259–261.
104. Ostermann G, Brisgand B, Schmit J, Fillastre J-P. Ef-

ficacy and acceptability of rilmenidine for mild to moderate systemic hypertension. Am J Cardiol 1988;61:76D.
105. Beau B, Mahieux F, Paraire M et al. Efficacy and safety of rilmenidine for arterial hypertension. Am J Cardiol 1988;61:95D.
106. Fillastre J-P, Letac B, Galinier F et al. A multicenter double-blind comparative study of rilmenidine and clonidine in 333 hypertensive patients. Am J Cardiol 1988,61:81D.
107. Mahieux F. Rilmenidine and vigilance Am J Med 1989;87(Suppl 3C):67S.
108. Samuels AH, Taylor AJ. Reserpine withdrawal psychosis. Aust NZ J Psychiatry 1989;23:129.
109. Grimm RH. Alpha$_2$-antagonists in the treatment of hypertension. Hypertension 1989;13(Suppl 1):1–131.
110. Luther RR. New perspectives on selective alpha$_1$ blockade. Am J Hypertens 1989;2:729.
111. Wall LL, Addison WA. Prazosin-induced stress incontinence. Obstet Gynecol 1990;75:558.
112. Neaton JD, Grimm RH Jr, Prineas RJ, Stamler J, Grandits GA, Elmer PJ, Cutler JA, Flack JM, Schoenberger JA, McDonald R, Lewis CE, Liebson PR. Treatment of mild hypertension study. J Am Med Assoc 1993;270:713–724.
113. Scharf MB, Mayleben DW. Comparative effects of prazosin and hydrochlorothiazide on sexual function in hypertensive men. Am J Med 1989;86(Suppl 1B):110.
114. Bullock N. Prazosin-induced priapism. Br J Urol 1988;62:487.
115. Brown MJ. Efficacy and tolerance of doxazosin: a review J Hum Hypertens 1990;4(Suppl 3):34–38.
116. Saunders E. The safety and efficacy of terazosin in the treatment of essential hypertension in blacks. Am Heart J 1991;122:936–942.
117. Cohen JD. Long-term efficacy and safety of terazosin alone and in combination with other antihypertensive agents. Am Heart J 1991;122:919–925.
118. Marshall AJ, Kettle MA, Barritt DW. Evaluation of indoramin added to oxprenolol and bendrofluazide as a third agent in severe hypertension. Br J Clin Pharmacol 1980; 10:217.
119. Kuchel OG, Mahon WA, McKenzie JK, Ogilvie RI. Approach to drug therapy for hypertension. Can Med Assoc J 1979;120:565.
120. Raskin N, Fishman R. Pyridoxine-deficiency neuropathy due to hydralazine. New Engl J Med 1965;273:1182.
121. Bartoli E, Massarelli G, Solinas A et al. Acute hepatitis with bridging necrosis due to hydralazine intake. Arch Intern Med 1979;139:698.
122. Forster HS Hepatitis from hydralazine. New Engl J Med 1980;302:1362.
123. Itoh S, Ichinoe A, Tsukada Y, Itoh Y. Hydralazine-induced hepatitis. Hepato-Gastroenterology 1981;28:13.
124. Itoh S, Yamaba Y, Ichinoe A, Tsukada Y. Hydralazine-induced liver injury. Dig Dis Sci 1980;25:884.
125. Barnett DB, Hudson SA, Golightly PW. Hydralazine-induced hepatitis? Br Med J 1980;281:1165.
126. Widerlöv E, Karlman I, Storsater J. Hydralazine-induced neonatal thrombocytopenia. New Engl J Med 1980; 303:1235.
127. Lodeiro JG, Feinstein SJ, Lodeiro SB. Fetal premature atrial contractions associated with hydralazine. Am J Obstet Gynecol 1989;160:105.
128. Yemini M, Shoham Z, Dgani R et al. Lupus-like syndrome in a mother and newborn following administration of hydralazine: a case report. Eur J Obstet Gynecol Reprod Biol 1989;30:193.
129. Torumi DM, Konior RJ, Berktold RE. Severe hypertrichosis of the external ear canal during minoxidil therapy. Arch Otolaryngol Head Neck Surg 1989;114:918.
130. Sever MS, Sonmez YE, Kocak N. Limited use of minoxidil in renal transplant recipients because of the additive side effects of cyclosporine on hypertrichosis. Transplantation 1990;50:536.
131. Low LCK, Yu ECL, Chow OKW et al. Hyperinsulinism in infancy. Aust Paediatr J 1989;25:174.
132. Abu-Osba YK, Manasra KB, Mathew PM. Complications of diazoxide treatment in persistent neonatal hyperinsulinism. Arch Dis Child 1989;64:1496.

Meyler's Side Effects of Drugs, 13th Edition
M.N.G. Dukes, editor

SECTION EDITOR: J.K. ARONSON

Gordon T. McInnes

21 Diuretics

GENERAL CONSIDERATIONS

Diuretics remain among the most widely used of drugs, particularly for the treatment of hypertension and of various conditions associated with sodium retention. Considering their widespread use over a long period—the earliest thiazides have been in use for more than 30 years—their safety record is remarkable, and reports of side effects of any significance with the best known drugs of this type are uncommon.

Where problems do arise they usually reflect either interactions, which with caution could have been avoided, or relative overdosage. In the course of time the recommended doses of diuretics have been reduced, and some adverse effects which were noted in the early years are now of less significance; they include hypotension, dehydration, reduction of the glomerular filtration rate and severe hypokalemia. Continued use of thiazides in excessive doses may reflect ignorance of their very flat dose—response curve (1[C]). One other prescribing fault is a discernible shift in some countries from the thiazides and related compounds to the more potent loop diuretics which for most patients offer little advantage but can disrupt daily life by increasing urinary frequency.

RISK VERSUS BENEFIT

Despite their safety record, speculation persists that the metabolic effects of long-term diuretic treatment may predispose to myocardial infarction or sudden death and that diuretic treatment may therefore be hazardous. It is worth noting that much of this speculation is found outside the columns of the legitimate medical press (SEDA-10, 185). The supposed risks of diuretics are broadcast in countless symposium proceedings, monographs and such like, which are sponsored by pharmaceutical companies with a vested interest in diverting prescriptions from diuretics to other drugs. Needless to say, these publications do not present a balanced view. Studies of dubious quality are published repeatedly without ever appearing in a refereed journal, and eventually come to be cited in independent reviews and articles. There can be no doubt that these publications have a large impact on prescribing practice.

It is relatively easy to foster these concerns, particularly since antihypertensive therapy would be expected to prevent myocardial infarction and sudden death, but in selected studies does not appear to do so. To explain this, it is suggested that the beneficial effects of lowering blood pressure are offset in part by adverse effects related to thiazide-induced biochemical disturbances. Hypokalemia and hypomagnesemia might, for example, be dysrhythmogenic and cause sudden death, or hyperlipidemia and impaired glucose tolerance might be atherogenic and promote myocardial infarction. A vocal rump continues to support these views (2[cR], 3[R], 4[r]). These authors suggest that thiazides should certainly be avoided in left ventricular hypertrophy and coronary heart disease because of an increased risk of ventricular ectopy (3[R], 4[r], 5[r]), and that diuretics are not appropriate options in those who already have hyperglycemia, hyperuricemia, or hyperlipidemia (5[r]). Poulter et al. (6[r]) take the argument ad absurdum by declaring that the use of diuretics as first-line treatment of hypertension is illogical. Others have argued effectively that we should not be impressed by such speculations and that treatment should be based on long-term experience (7[R]—9[R]), a conclusion similar to that reached in SEDA-9 to 19. It had been evident for some time that this impasse would be resolved satisfactorily only by the outcome of large, long-term, controlled trials in hypertension, trials which particularly would examine the incidence of coronary events in relation to thiazide and other antihypertensive agents.

In the United Kingdom Medical Research Council (MRC) trial (10[C]) trial, the outcome of antihypertensive treatment based on diuretics was compared with placebo treatment in a very large number of hypertensive subjects. Treatment based on a thiazide did not increase the incidence of coronary events or sudden death; indeed, thiazide-based treatment reduced the incidence of strokes by 67% and of all cardiovascular complications by 20%. It should be noted that the dose of bendrofluazide used in the MRC trial (10 mg/day) is now known to be unnecessarily high and that it was used without prophylaxis against hypokalemia. Even so, a subgroup analysis of data from the MRC Trial provided no evidence that the association between major ECG abnormalities and increased likelihood of a clinical event was strengthened by bendrofluazide treatment (11[C]). A series of trials in elderly hypertensive subjects has shown a very pronounced reduction in cardiac events as a result of treatment based on thiazide diuretics (12[C]—15[C]). In the European Working Party on Hypertension in the Elderly (EWPHE) trial (12[C]), total cardiovascular deaths were reduced by 38%, all cardiac deaths by 43% and deaths due to myocardial infarction by 60%. Benefits in the Systolic Hypertension in the Elderly Program (SHEP) included a reduction in fatal and non-fatal myocardial infarction of 25% and major cardiovascular events of 32% (13[C]) and were seen in those with and without ECG abnormalities at entry. The Swedish Trial of Old Patients with Hypertension (STOP-Hypertension) reported a significant reduction in myocardial infarction and all cause mortality (14[C]). In the MRC Trial in elderly adults (15[C]), diuretic treatment reduced coronary events by 44% and fatal cardiovascular events by 35%.

In the MRC trials (10[C], 15[C]), the IPPSH trial (16[C]) and the HAPPHY trial (17[C]), antihypertensive treatment based on a thiazide diuretic were compared with treatment based on a β-blocker. The results with diuretic treatment were no less favourable as regards cardiac events than those when using a 'cardioprotective' β-blocker. In the IPPPSH trial, the group using no β-blockers (but having a higher incidence of diuretic use and of hypokalemia) showed no excess of cardiac events, even in patients who had an abnormal electrocardiogram when they entered the study. The MRC trial in elderly adults (15[C]) indicated a significantly lower risk of cardiovascular events with the diuretic compared with the β-blocker, raising the possibility that diuretics confer benefit through a mechanism other than the reduction of blood pressure.

In the MAPHY study (18[C]), total mortality was significantly lower for metoprolol than for thiazide, because of fewer deaths from coronary heart disease and stroke. However, the MAPHY study population comprised a subgroup of about half of the patients from the HAPPHY trial followed up for an extended period. The difference in mortality between metoprolol and diuretics did not emerge during this extended follow-up but was present during the first period of observation (i.e. during the HAPPHY trial) when there was no overall difference between β-blockers and thiazides. Therefore, patients treated with atenolol in the HAPPHY trial must have fared worse than those treated with thiazides and much worse than those treated with metoprolol. Since there was no prior hypothesis for a difference between atenolol and metoprolol (and no plausible explanation for it), it seems reasonable to conclude that the apparent advantage of metoprolol was a chance finding produced by post hoc subgroup analysis. The MAPHY study should be interpreted with extreme caution.

Two retrospective case-control studies have reported an increased risk of cardiac arrest in hypertensive patients treated with thiazide-type diuretics (19[CR], 20[C]). The risk was less among those treated with low dose thiazides (equivalent to hydrochlorothiazide 25 mg daily) or with thiazides plus potassium-sparing agents. The case-control design lacks one of the major advantages of randomized clinical trials, the tendency to equalize unknown, but important, differences between the comparison groups. Underadjustment is usual in case-control studies; for example, patients with more severe hypertension were more likely to have been treated with higher doses and less likely to have received potassium-sparers because of renal dysfunction. Failure to randomize treatment tends to exaggerate differences between groups.

A detailed examination of all the evidence (21[R]) concluded that controlled clinical trials have shown beyond all reasonable doubt the benefit of treating hypertension with diuretics. Regardless of metabolic disturbances, which are in any case of uncertain clinical significance, there is no valid evidence that diuretics contribute to myocardial infarction, sudden death, or to a failure to antihypertensive treatment or other risk factor interventions to prevent coronary deaths. An association between diuretics and sudden death has been suggested only in selected subset analyses which allow no valid conclusions. Even in subjects with ECG abnormalities before treatment, there is no sound or consistent evidence to support the suggestion that diuretics predispose to sudden death. The case for a cardiotoxic risk of thiazides has been constantly overstated. It simply does not withstand scrutiny.

A review of the large trials indicates that the reduction in the incidence of events with usually thiazide-based treatment is 16% (with 95% confidence interval 8,23%) against the prediction from epidemiological studies of 20—25% (22[R]). Thus, the shortfall in benefit could easily be due to chance. Critics of diuretic use in hypertension are '. . . concerned that a non-existing phenomenon (long-term raising of cholesterol concentrations by thiazides) causes a problem that may not exist (a shortfall in coronary prevention) and that if it did exist could not be explained by the non-existent phenomenon' (23[R]).

One must conclude that the hypothesis that thiazide diuretics cause or predispose to myocardial infarction and sudden death has been put to the test and has been disproved. A strong case can be made for considering thiazide diuretics to be the drugs of first choice for hypertension when there is no contraindication to their use.

The Fifth Joint Committee Report on Detection, Evaluation and Treatment of High Blood Pressure (24[r]) has concluded that since diuretics are one of the only two classes of drugs (the other being β-blockers) that have been shown in long-term treatment trials to reduce cardiovascular mortality, a diuretic (or a β-blocker) should be the first-step drug of choice unless there are specific indications for other drugs. This recommendation has been echoed by other authoritative articles (25[r], 26[r], 27[Cr]). Although other drugs may have an impact on coronary heart disease greater than that with diuretics, none of the new agents has been subjected to the rigorous tests that are required for the confirmation of cardiovascular disease prevention. Therefore, a general switch from diuretics to new antihypertensive drugs would represent a triumph of hope over experience.

DIURETICS IN PREGNANCY

For theoretical reasons discussed in earlier volumes, there has been some reluctance to use diuretics in pregnancy. Essentially it was feared that if they were used in pre-eclampsia, a further reduction in the already reduced cardiac output would result, leading to inadequate perfusion of the uterus and placenta. There was also concern that biochemical derangement might harm either the mother or the foetus. The results of large-scale trails must weigh more heavily than these theoretical forebodings.

Collins et al. (28[CR]) have analyzed all the randomized controlled studies of the use of diuretics in pre-eclampsia. The nine studies which they reviewed involved almost 7000 subjects in whom thiazides had been compared either with placebo or with no treatment. In the pooled analysis, diuretic treatment was found to be associated with a nonsignificant reduction in perinatal mortality (about 10%) and stillbirths (about 33%). There was no excess of serious adverse reactions either in the mothers or the neonates. These findings thus give no support to the belief that diuretics are harmful in pregnancy. It should not be concluded that diuretics ought to be used in pre-eclampsia in preference to other well-established agents, but they certainly can be employed with confidence when they are really needed, e.g. in patients with severe hypertension which predates pregnancy and in heart failure.

DIURETICS IN THE ELDERLY

There has been much discussion about the safety or risks of diuretics in the elderly. Although diuretic use has been implicated as a cause of urinary incontinence, no evidence has been presented to confirm this. An epidemiological survey of 1956 respondents aged at least 60 years showed no significant difference between diuretic-users and non-users in the prevalence of incontinence (29[C]).

Orthostatic hypotension, though often loosely referred to in older literature (SED-10, 370), is in fact only likely to become a problem in very old subjects indeed, aged 90 or more, even if a potent loop diuretic is used; this was the clear conclusion of a good prospective study published in 1978 (30[C]). In 843 independent living men and women aged between 60 and 87 years, postural fall in systolic blood pressure was not related to treatment with diuretics, after correction for initial blood pressure (31[C]). At currently recommended doses, older subjects do not generally experience particular problems from hypokalemia and do not appear to be at special risk of cardiac dysrhythmias in the face of diuretic-induced hypokalemia (SEDA-15, 218).

Recent reviews of the age-related effects of diuretics in hypertensive subjects (32[r], 33[R]) have concluded that symptomatic adverse reactions are not more frequent in older patients and that some trials suggest a lower frequency than in younger subjects. Although the elderly may be susceptible to some metabolic effects of diuretics, the evidence for cardiotoxic potential is not definitive.

The best overall evidence of the safety of diuretics in old people comes from the large scale outcome trials in hypertensive patients (12[C]–15[C]). These studies in over 10 000 subjects aged over 60 years of age demonstrated clearly that thiazide-based treatment reduces the risk of stroke, coronary heart disease events, and cardiovascular events in older hypertensive patients. The beneficial effects noted in these trials should dispel any doubts as to the safety and efficacy of diuretics in old people.

The only specific problems which are more likely to be encountered in the elderly than in other groups are those reflecting the general pathology of this age group. For example, since a degree of diabetes is more common, the effects on glucose metabolism may be problematical, and since cardiac glycosides are often being taken, the possibility of interaction must be kept in mind. Both these matters are dealt with in the appropriate sections below.

It is important to recognise the major role that diuretics play in the treatment of elderly patients by relieving symptoms, reducing disability, preventing morbidity, and prolonging life. Compared with those who enjoy these benefits, only a minority develop significant biochemical abnormalities, and an even smaller group suffer significant side effects.

ABUSE OF DIURETICS

Where diuretics are abused it is mostly in the course of a misguided attempt to lose weight; in the past, various 'slimming remedies' offered for sale outside normal trading channels have been found to contain diuretics, sometimes with such components as thyroid extract. The unnecessary use of diuretics by a healthy individual, perhaps in excessive doses, can clearly lead to dehydration, hypokalemia and hypotension; when furosemide is abused, even tetany can occur because of hypocalcemia (34[R]). The weight loss achieved by using diuretics as 'slimming agents' is purely due to dehydration and will soon be annulled by extra fluid intake. One complication can, however, be edema, and it has been suggested that surreptitious use of diuretics can explain some otherwise paradoxical cases of 'idiopathic' edema; presumably the diuretic induces a persistent increase in plasma renin activity and secondary hyperaldosteronism, and attempts to stop the diuretic intake may at first actually aggravate the condition (35C). Three studies have furnished strong evidence that diuretic abuse is not an important cause of idiopathic edema (36[C]—38[C]).

In some patients the secret use of diuretics leads to a complete replica of Bartter's syndrome, characterized by hypokalemia and hyper-reninemia without hypertension (39[C], 40[C]). In a patient who denies having taken diuretics, the true diagnosis may only be made by finding the drug or its metabolites in the urine, although challenge with diuretic may provoke the syndrome while withdrawal leads to body weight gain and disappearance of metabolic alkalosis.

EFFECT OF DIURETICS ON THE KIDNEY

Since diuretics act primarily on the kidney, it is hardly surprising that renal damage can ensue. As indicated in the monographs which follow, toxic damage is very rare in relation to the number of patients treated. However, diuretics are a prominent cause of drug-induced interstitial nephritis (41[C]—42[C]). The problem is more likely to arise in patients with pre-existing glomerular disease. It tends to present 4—10 weeks after starting treatment with non-oliguric acute renal failure and, in some cases, pyrexia and eosinophilia. This complication probably always recovers spontaneously and completely although some consider it prudent to give high doses of steroids.

DIURETICS IN FIXED COMBINATIONS

As a matter of principle, it is generally better for a prescriber to use a single-component drug than a combination. There are however some exceptions to the rule, particularly where two drugs are likely to be used by large numbers of patients in the same dosage ratio, and where a single dosage form is likely to improve compliance.

Diuretics have been combined variously with potassium, with potassium-sparing diuretics, and with β-blockers. From the point of view of drug safety, each of these types of combination can be viewed differently.

Fixed combinations of thiazides and loop diuretics with potassium serve no useful purpose and in fact do harm. As pointed out elsewhere in this Chapter, oral potassium does not provide a satisfactory means of countering hypokalemia, and its use introduces the risk of esophageal ulceration, which has repeatedly been documented when such combinations have been used.

Combinations of thiazides and loop diuretics with potassium-sparing diuretics serve the needs of the small minority of patients who develop clinically significant hypokalemia when given diuretics alone, or in whom hypokalemia is particularly risky. In fact, these combinations are much too widely used, and since individual needs vary so much there is a spectrum of risk, ranging from hypokalemia to hyperkalemia (SEDA-10, 370, 371).

The fixed combinations of thiazides with β-blockers similarly represent a solution which is tailored to the needs of a minority. Bearing in mind that many hypertensive patients will respond adequately to a thiazide or a β-blocker alone, there can be no justification for giving both from the outset of treatment, yet this is often the case. Interactions between the components include a greater risk of hyperglycemia than if either component were given separately.

BIOCHEMICAL CHANGES

All diuretics cause an array of effects on body chemistry. To what extent these represent important adverse events or merely biochemical changes of little clinical significance is variable and in some cases controversial.

Mineral and fluid balance Diuretics are used with the intention of removing water and salt from the body; problems arise when they do this to excess or when they exert unwanted effects on other minerals. The effects of thiazides and loop diuretics on mineral balance differ somewhat in character and degree.

Hyponatremia Hyponatremia was a not uncommon problem with the old mercurial diuretics and during the first few years of use of the thiazides, when they were often used in excessive doses. It has become much less of a problem with the dosages now used.

Two major surveys have reviewed the features of diuretic-induced hyponatremia (43[R], 44[cR]). Thiazide-like diuretics alone or in combination with potassium-sparing diuretics are responsible for more than 90% of cases. It occurs mainly in elderly females, although the relation with age probably merely reflects the widespread use of diuretics in older subjects. In the vast majority of cases, the interval between starting thiazide and clinical presentation is less than 2 weeks; serum sodium may fall by 5 mmol/l or more in 24 hours or less in those patients who develop severe hyponatremia. In contrast, where loop diuretics cause hyponatremia, the lag period is usually several months. Hypertension is the indication for diuretics in over 80% of cases. The patient is clinically euvolumic, but in the majority excess antidiuretic hormone (ADH) activity, hypokalemia, excess water intake and increased free water clearance singly or together appear to contribute to the development of hyponatremia. The urine is inappropriately concentrated and contains moderately large amounts of sodium. It may be clinically indistinguishable from the syndrome of inappropriate ADH. Severe neurological complications are seen in about 60%; seizures (30%), stupor or coma (30%) and death (5–10%). The extent of irreversible loss of intellectual function is unknown. Serum sodium concentration is usually in the range 105–120 mmol/l. If diuretics are discontinued, serum sodium concentration returns to normal, but hyponatremia is reproducible on rechallenge.

Comprehensive accounts of the pathophysiology, etiology and management of hyponatremia have stressed the care required in correction of symptomatic hyponatremia (44[cR], 45[r]). Neurological signs are an indication for active sodium replacement using hypertonic saline. Correction should be planned over 24–48 hours to increase serum sodium by 1 mmol/l each hour with a target increase of 20–25 mmol/l, a serum sodium concentration of 130 mmol/l or abolition of symptoms. If onset is within 24 hours of starting diuretics, correction should be rapid but within a total elevation of 20 mmol/l in the first 24 hours. If onset is over several days or longer, correction should be slower aiming for 12–15 mmol/l in 24 hours. There is concern that rapid correction of hyponatremia and a relatively high total correction (more than 20 mmol/l in the first 24 h) may be associated with higher morbidity or a demyelinating syndrome (44[cR]), but the rate of correction does not appear to be important in outcome if the absolute increase is limited to 25 mmol/l over 48 hours (45[r]). An extensive review of the literature suggests that rate of correction is not a factor in the genesis of hyponatremic brain syndrome (45[r]).

Use of fixed combination of a thiazide and a potassium-sparing drug, often Moduretic (hydrochlorothiazide 50 mg with amiloride 5 mg), has been implicated consistently in diuretic-induced hyponatremia. Treatment with chlorpropamide (200–800 mg/day) along with Moduretic has precipitated hyponatraemia in a number of cases (46[C]). Simultaneous use of Moduretic with trimethoprim has also been reported to increase the risk (47[Cr]). The mechanism appears to be impairment of the clearance of free water, resulting in dilutional hyponatremia. Whether data such as these point to a special risk of Moduretic as a product or merely reflect its extraordinarily widespread use in old people is not clear. In a survey of electrolyte disturbances in 1000 geriatric admissions, Byatt et al. (48[C]) found that the incidence of hyponatremia with the combination of hydrochlorothiazide and amiloride was twice that with other diuretics, although the difference failed to reach statistical significance.

Hypokalemia The loss of potassium caused by diuretics is their most intensively debated adverse effect, and the extent and significance of the problem has long been disputed.

Changes in potassium metabolism are claimed to cause electrical instability in the heart, certain cardiac arrhythmias and increased mortality; replacement of potassium is said to eliminate the risk of dysrhythmias (49[R], 50[r], 54[R]). The arguments are based on theoretical considerations supported by selective and uncritical reviews of the literature; the clinical evidence is far from compelling (SEDA-12, 182; SEDA-13, 184; SEDA-15, 179). Two large studies employing 24-hour ECG monitoring have failed to demonstrate a relation between diuretic-induced hypokalemia and ventricular arrhythmias (27[Cr], 52[Cr]). The effect of diuretics on potassium balance and their clinical consequences have recently been extensively reviewed (21[R], 53[r], 54[r], 55[R]–57[R], 58[r]). A fall in plasma potassium is common, but sound studies are consistent in showing that diuretics do not deplete body potassium or cause potassium deficiency in hypertensive patients (21[R]). Potassium depletion may occur in cardiac failure when neurohumoral systems are stimulated by diuretics and may be especially profound when skeletal muscle wasting is advanced (58[r]). However, since heart failure itself, independent of diuretic treatment, is associated with loss of total body potassium, it is difficult to assess the independent contribution of diuretic treatment to this potassium deficit. The risks of diuretic-induced hypokalemia have been greatly exaggerated (21[R], 55[R], 56[R]). The evidence linking thiazide-induced hypokalemia with dysrhythmias and sudden death is indirect and tenuous at best (21[R], 53[r]). Diuretics are not responsible for the relation between hypokalemia and ventricular fibrillation in acute myocardial infarction (21[R]). Neither is chronic preoperative hypokalemia due to diuretics a risk factor for intraoperative dysrhythmias (57[R]). In most patients, routine monitoring of serum potassium and routine administration of potassium-sparing diuretics is unnecessary (55[R], 56[R]), although patients at special risk require particular attention. Diuretic-induced hypokalemia may be hazardous in the presence of digitalis (53[r]). In heart failure, depletion of potassium can provoke fatigue and lethargy, and may cause ventricular dysrhythmias in the failing heart (53[R]). Routine administration of potassium-sparing diuretics may have some justification in such patients. The following postulates seem to summarize the present position:

(1) The thiazides do increase potassium excretion, but rarely to such an extent that total body potassium stores are appreciably affected. In most patients there is no reason to think that long-term diuretic treatment will deplete body potassium at all.
(2) The risk of a clinically important degree of hypokalemia is increased in patients with liver cirrhosis and those with severe cardiac failure complicated by secondary hyperaldosteronism.
(3) Relatively mild degrees of hypokalemia can be dangerous in patients taking cardiac glycosides because their effects on the myocardium are potentiated in the absence of potassium. It is less well recognised that diuretic-induced hypokalemia should also be carefully avoided in patients taking drugs known to prolong QT interval, e.g. some antiarrhythmics (quinidine, procainamide, disopyramide, encainide, sotalol, amiodarone), some psychotropics (thioridazine, imipramine, phenothiazines), the lipid lowering drug probucol, the antibiotic erythromycin and the 5-HT_2 receptor antagonist, ketanserin.
(4) Similarly, mild hypokalemia might be expected to cause dysrhythmias in patients with serious organic heart disease (cardiomegaly, abnormal ECG, frequent ventricular extra beats before treatment). However, the available evidence suggests that hypokalemia after myocardial infarction is not the cause of arrhythmias but that both are the result of excess catecholamines. Furthermore, although hypertensive patients with left ventricular hypertrophy have an increased frequency of ventricular arrhythmias, ectopy does not increase during diuretic treatment even in the face of profound hypokalemia (59[CR]).
(5) When severe hypokalemia is found, one should not immediately attribute it to diuretic treatment. It may well be due to primary hyperaldosteronism, occult chronic liver disease, or abuse of licorice or laxatives.

Critical reviews thus conclude that in most patients (i.e. in the absence of the occasional risk factors listed above) diuretics can be prescribed alone, and that there is no need to take precautions against hypokalemia (60[R], 61[R]). Precautions, including the monitoring of serum potassium, will have to be taken when there are risk factors or when symptoms (e.g. muscular pain) occur, or in those patients who require aggressive treatment with both a thiazide and a loop diuretic; such a combination is indeed likely to provoke considerable falls in serum potassium, e.g. even to concentrations below 2.5 mmol/l (62[c]).

Recent studies (63[C], 64[C]), have underlined the dissociation of the dose-response curves for lowering blood pressure and lowering plasma potassium during diuretic treatment. There is little if any loss of antihypertensive effect with low doses of diuretics, whereas hypokalemia is much less prominent. It is now clear that low doses of diuretics are to be preferred in uncomplicated hypertension. However, very low doses of thiazides may lack antihypertensive effects equivalent to those of higher doses (65[Cr]).

The current widespread use of fixed combinations of thiazides with potassium-sparing diuretics is indefensible; they are useful products for a minority only. In those patients in whom hypokalemia needs to be prevented or corrected, the potassium-sparing diuretics should be used. Potassium supplements do not provide an answer and they are relatively ineffective even in high doses (SEDA-14, 180; SEDA-15, 214). Potassium, given separately or in combination with a diuretic, also introduces the added risk of esophageal injury (see Chapter 49); attempts to provide potassium in slow-release formulations seem only to have transposed the site of injury from the esophagus to the small bowel (SEDA-10, 187). Finally, there is little point in trying to compensate for potassium losses by changes in the diet; Kopyt and co-workers have calculated that to provide 60—80 mmol of extra potassium daily in this way one would have to eat 100 cm of bananas daily (66[C]).

Angiotensin-converting enzyme inhibitors are widely believed to attenuate diuretic-induced falls in plasma potassium. However, captopril 25 mg twice daily had no effect on plasma potassium in hypertensive patients treated with bendrofluazide 5 mg daily (67[c]).

Hyperkalemia All potassium-sparing diuretics can

cause hyperkalemia (68[c], 69[C], 70[R]). This complication is particularly likely in diabetics, in patients with renal dysfunction, in elderly patients, and in those receiving additional potassium supplements. Commonly forgotten is the patient for whom these diuretics are prescribed as a precautionary measure and who for many years has been flavouring a low-salt diet with 'salt substitutes' which are often based on potassium chloride (70[R]). Life-threatening hyperkalemia has been observed in patients receiving potassium-sparing diuretics (71[C]). The most distressing finding in this study was that these agents were far more often prescribed in patients with abnormal kidney function than were other diuretics. Combining potassium-sparing diuretics with potassium supplements borders on malpractice; regular monitoring of serum potassium is mandatory in all patients treated with potassium-sparing diuretics, particularly if they are elderly or have abnormal renal or hepatic function.

Hypomagnesemia There has been much interest in diuretic-induced magnesium loss, and this phenomenon has been heavily stressed both by some independent investigators and by those seeking for commercial reasons to discredit the diuretics; there are, unhappily, far more reviews on the subject than sound original studies. Reyes and Leary (72[R]) have declared that diuretic-induced magnesium deficiency 'positively contributes' to myocardial infarction, delayed infarct healing, coronary and cerebral arterial spasm, hyperlipidemia, and cardiac dysrhythmias; they have added a horrific catalog of clinical manifestations including ataxia, delirium, convulsions, coma and ventricular fibrillation. Ramsay has remarked that this review, and others like it, belong to the category of science fiction rather than that of serious medical writing (SEDA-10, 187).

Most reviews of the effects of diuretics on magnesium metabolism are uncritical and extrapolate wildly from the little sound evidence that is available (21[R]). Several uncontrolled studies and very few controlled studies have suggested that long-term thiazide treatment causes a small fall in serum magnesium within the reference range. There is absolutely no evidence that diuretic treatment reduces intracellular magnesium, and the few competent investigations have suggested that it does not. Diuretic-induced disturbances of magnesium balance do not cause depletion of intracellular potassium. The clinical significance of the small diuretic-induced alterations in magnesium balance, if any, is obscure. There is no satisfactory evidence that diuretic-induced magnesium disturbances cause or predispose to cardiac dysrhythmias, either in general or specifically after myocardial infarction (73[r]).

The most balanced account so far published (74[R]) concluded that the controlled trials, of which there are few, do not substantiate a role of diuretics in causing magnesium deficiency. Consequently, the vast majority of patients taking conventional doses of thiazides do not need magnesium supplements. On balance, potassium-sparing diuretics tend to increase serum and intracellular magnesium content, but this should not be taken as evidence of prior magnesium deficiency. It remains theoretically possible that large doses of loop diuretics given more than once daily for long periods could induce negative magnesium balance and magnesium deficiency. However, it is difficult to conduct appropriately controlled trials in heart failure where such treatment is needed and, until more reliable information becomes available, no absolute recommendation can be made. The complex relation between intracellular free and total magnesium content remains to be clarified. In any case, magnesium depletion should be regarded as no more than a possible, as yet unproven, risk factor for cardiovascular morbidity and mortality (75[r]). Future work involving the effect of diuretics on magnesium balance should make every attempt to avoid the errors of trial design and multiple publication that litter the current and past literature.

In ordinary practice, serum magnesium need not be monitored in patients taking diuretics, and potassium-sparing drugs should not be used to prevent magnesium problems which do not exist (SEDA-10, 190).

Calcium metabolism Thiazides and related diuretics reduce the renal clearance of calcium by inhibiting tubular secretion of calcium ions. This property has been used successfully in preventing stone formation in idiopathic hypercalciuria (SED-9, 345, 366). Hypercalcemia is generally present in mild degree although severe symptomatic hypercalcemia has been reported in elderly patients taking thiazides together with vitamin D preparations (76[C]).

It has been suggested that the tendency to increased serum calcium might help to counter osteoporosis. Several large studies have reported that thiazide use is associated with a reduction in the risk of hip and other fractures (77[CR], 78[Cr], 79[CR]–81[CR]). In contrast, a case–control study of 462 elderly hospitalized patients and an equal number of age- and sex-matched population-based controls revealed a significant 60% increased risk of hip fracture, after adjustment for potentially confounding variables, in current thiazide and furosemide users (82[C]). The authors speculated that these drugs may predispose to falls but they provided no evidence. Browner et al. (83[c]) found a strong association between diminished bone density and death from stroke in 970 ambulatory women aged at least 65 years. This relation was not confounded by treatment with thiazide diuretics, casting doubt on reports that these drugs are associated with increased bone density.

The author of a thoughtful review of the controversy surrounding the potential role of thiazides in protecting against osteoporosis in elderly people (84[R]) considered it premature to prescribe thiazides for this indication and called for a randomized controlled clinical trial. If benefit were confirmed, this would be an important factor in the choice of antihypertensive drugs for elderly people, and low doses might avoid unacceptable adverse effects in normotensives. However, the discrepancies between the results of the available studies of thiazides may be attributable to differences in the effects of high and low doses (79[CR]); beneficial effects on calcium metabolism may accrue only for those taking high doses, with concomitant metabolic risks, popular lower dose regimens may have little effect on bone mass. Broken bones and especially hip fractures are major causes of morbidity and mortality in elderly people. Given the limited number of candidate therapies for osteoporosis in this group, the high cost of hip fractures, and the growth of the population at risk, clinical trials are urgently needed (84[R]).

Unlike the thiazides, furosemide (which does not promote reabsorption of calcium in the distal tubule) causes transient hypercalciuria, an effect which has been exploited on occasion in the treatment of hypercalcemia (SED-9, 346). In premature infants, the drug seems to cause secondary hyperparathyroidism, which leads to skeletal calcium loss with calcium excretion rates 10—20 times those in normal children and a real risk of renal calcification (SEDA-8, 219; SEDA-9, 208; SEDA-14, 182). The latter can be detected by ultrasound examination. If stones are present, the drug should be withdrawn, the secondary sepsis which is often present treated, and a thiazide given; the stone will often later be passed or will disintegrate. Continued treatment with furosemide in children of low birth weights is associated with persistent glomerular and tubular dysfunctions as well as with nephrocalcinosis. The high risk of renal morbidity necessitates long-term follow-up (SEDA-18, 263). The above findings are the more disturbing in view of the evidence that prophylactic use of furosemide in newborn infants with severe respiratory distress syndrome is of no benefit on any measure of pulmonary function and may be harmful (85[C]). Therefore, furosemide appears to expose the infant to the risk of nephrocalcinosis without benefit. It appears that a large intake of sodium can override the normal tendency of thiazides to promote calcium reabsorption in the distal tubules (86[CR]). Therefore, thiazides too may increase the risk of nephrocalcinosis in premature infants.

Renal calcification has also been described in children who were not low birth weight infants but who were treated with furosemide for congestive heart failure (87[C]). Residual renal morbidity included reduced creatinine clearance, microscopic hematuria and hypercalciuria. The phenomenon of renal calcification with furosemide treatment is more frequent than previously recognized and can arise with initiation of treatment well after the neonatal period.

Endocrine, metabolic *Glucose metabolism* There is little doubt that diuretics carry an appreciable risk of impairing diabetic control in patients with established diabetes mellitus. However, their role in causing de novo glucose intolerance is not clear (60[R]). Long-acting diuretics are more likely to alter glucose metabolism. Impaired glucose tolerance is a relatively rare complication with loop diuretics, although isolated cases of non-ketotic hyperglycemia in diabetics have been described (SED-9, 350).

The effects of thiazide-type diuretics on carbohydrate tolerance cannot be ignored (21[R]). There is a definite relation between diuretic treatment, impaired glucose tolerance, and biochemical diabetes, and a possible relation with insulin resistance (88[R]). It is well established that the effect of thiazides on blood sugar is dose-related, probably in a linear fashion, while the antihypertensive effect has little relation to dose (56[R], 63[C], 89[Cr]). There is relatively little information on the time course; numerous short-term studies have shown that the blood sugar concentration increases in 4—8 weeks (90[R]). The evidence that current low dosages impair glucose tolerance in the long-term is not entirely consistent, perhaps because of differences between studies in dosages, diuretics used, durations of treatment, and types of patient (89[R], 91[R]). The apparent differences between diuretics may be due to comparisons of dosages which are not equivalent (85[R]). Important differences between individual diuretics will be established only when their complete dose-responses for metabolic variables and blood pressure have been defined (90[R]).

In contrast to the wealth of evidence on impaired glucose tolerance with diabetic treatment, sound clinical trials of the effect on insulin resistance are difficult to find, considering the amount of comment and speculation on the topic (SEDA-15, 216). It is not known whether insulin resistance is completely or even partly responsible for the changes in glucose tolerance which occur during long-term thiazide treatment; impaired insulin secretion may also have a role (92[R]). Hypokalemia or potassium depletion may contribute to impaired glucose tolerance by inhibiting insulin secretion rather than by causing insulin resistance, but is not the only or even the main cause of impaired glucose tolerance during long-term diuretic treatment (90[R], 91[R]). The routine use of potassium-sparing diuretics with relatively low dosages of thiazides does not prevent impaired glucose tolerance.

Diuretic treatment worsens metabolic control in established diabetes, but it is not known whether this adversely affects prognosis (90[R]). Disturbances of carbohydrate homeostasis have been detected by detailed biochemical testing but their clinical importance is uncertain (88[R]). The major clinical trials have not shown a major risk of diabetes mellitus. The incidence of diabetes mellitus in diuretic-treated subjects is only about 1%, even when large dosages are used (93[R]). Prospective studies have yet to show that glucose intolerance short of diabetes mellitus and increased insulin concentrations are independent risk factors for coronary heart disease (21[R]). It is now established that biochemical diabetes, glucose intolerance, and insulin resistance probably do not increase the risk of coronary heart disease in treated hypertensive patients (88[R]).

While thiazides may be best avoided in patients with diabetes mellitus there is as yet no good evidence that effects on carbohydrate metabolism should limit their use in non-diabetics. Since changes in glucose balance after diuretics tend to be reversible on discontinuation, measures of carbohydrate homeostasis should be assessed after several months of thiazide treatment to detect those few patients who experience significant glucose intolerance (94[R]). With this approach, the small risk of diabetes mellitus secondary to diuretic therapy can be minimized.

Hyperuricemia Most diuretics cause hyperuricemia. Increased reabsorption of uric acid (along with other solutes) in the proximal tubule as a consequence of volume depletion is one reason for the hyperuricemia; however, diuretics also compete with uric acid for excretory transport mechanisms. In the large outcome trials, about 3–5% of subjects treated with diuretics for hypertension developed clinical gout (95[R]).

In those with acute gout during diuretic treatment, attacks were more strongly related to loop diuretics than to thiazides (96[CR]). Gout was significantly associated with obesity and a high alcohol intake in the subgroup taking only a thiazide diuretic. About 40% of cases of acute gout may have been prevented by avoiding thiazides in those 20% of men who weighed over 90 kg and/or who consumed more than 56 units of alcohol per week.

Potassium-sparing diuretics have little effect on uric acid metabolism. After spironolactone, uric acid concentrations are slightly, but significantly, lowered. However, Myers (97[c]) noted that the increase in serum uric acid was greater with hydrochlorothiazide plus amiloride than with hydrochlorothiazide alone providing evidence that amiloride agent also impairs uric acid handling.

Recent well-conducted studies have demonstrated that diuretic-induced changes in serum uric acid are dose-related (63[C], 64[C]). In low dose regimens, as currently recommended, alterations are minor and other than the risk of gout, the long-term consequences of an increased serum uric acid are unknown.

Hyperuricemia is not an independent risk factor for coronary heart disease (21[R]). Obsessive monitoring and aggressive therapy of diuretic-induced hyperuricemia are unnecessary. Apart from a small increased risk of acute gout in susceptible subjects (93[R]), this metabolic disturbance is of little clinical consequence (12[R]).

Lipid metabolism Reviews of the influence of diuretics on serum lipids (98[R]–102[R]) are in broad agreement as regards the short-term effects. Thiazide and loop diuretics increase low-density lipoprotein cholesterol (LDL-C), very-low-density lipoprotein cholesterol (VLDL-C), total cholesterol (TC) and triglycerides. The effect on high-density lipoprotein cholesterol (HDL-C) has been variable. The LDL-C/HDL-C or TC/HDL-C ratio is generally increased, but not in all studies. Spironolactone at a dose of 50 mg b.i.d. causes modest falls of high-density lipoprotein cholesterol and triglyceride (103[c]). The effect of other potassium-sparing drugs on lipid metabolism has not been well documented. Weidmann et al. (102[R]) have discussed the possible mechanisms of these various short-term effects.

It is now quite clear that diuretic-induced effects on lipid metabolism are dose-dependent (48[C], 63[Cr], 89[Cr]): at low doses of thiazides, changes are very slight while antihypertensive efficacy is well maintained. Diuretic-induced lipid changes have not been prominent in studies lasting one year or longer (10[C], 17[C], 98[R], 102[R], 104[Cr]). An association between thiazide use or antihypertensive treatment and changes in serum lipids has been shown in some population surveys (105[C], 106[C]) but not in others (107[C]).

Most studies of the effects of diuretics on serum lipids have lacked a placebo control group to allow identification of time-dependent or environmental changes, or have been confounded intentionally or unknowingly by life-style interventions, including weight loss, diet, and exercise (91[R]). The argument that the effects of diuretics on lipids may limit the beneficial effect of blood pressure reduction is difficult to sustain (21[R]). The effect of thiazides is largely transient and in the long-term, total cholesterol and LDL-cholesterol are raised only slightly and HDL-cholesterol is unchanged. It is not known whether diuretic-induced changes in cholesterol carry the same prognostic significance as naturally occurring hyperlipidemia (21^{R}, 108^{R}). Attempts to calculate a potential impact of diuretic-induced increases in total cholesterol and LDL-cholesterol on coronary prognosis are premature. Observations have so far been limited largely to serum concentrations. However, binding of lipids to vascular cells rather than in the blood stream is decisive for atherogenesis, and the effect at the cellular level remains to be investigated. Johnston (92^{r}) has accurately summed up current knowledge: 'There is little or no evidence that thiazide diuretics have long-term adverse effects on plasma lipids and no evidence whatsoever that these supposed changes have any detrimental effect on cardiovascular mortality'.

There is little or no evidence that thiazides should be avoided in patients with hyperlipidemia (94^{R}), although some physicians continue to make this recommendation. Serum lipids should be checked within 3–6 months of starting thiazides to detect the very few patients who experience an increase in total cholesterol or LDL-cholesterol. This should not add to the cost of care since serum chemistry need only be obtained once or twice per year and is no reason to avoid the use of these agents as initial monotherapy.

Impotence Anecdotal reports have for a long time suggested a link between diuretics (generally thiazides, if only because of their widespread use) and impotence. However, analysis of the question has been hampered by the fact that impotence is common in men beyond middle age and the likelihood that it is even more common in hypertension, treated or otherwise. The United Kingdom MRC trial (10^{C}) was the first to provide quantified evidence of a link with diuretics; in men on 10 mg bendroflumethiazide daily, the withdrawal rate for impotence was 19.6 cases per 1000 treatment years, compared with 0.9 cases on placebo. These figures may however exaggerate the effect since the trial was single-blind. A questionnaire pointed to a less striking difference; after 3 months impotence was noted in 16% of diuretic-treated patients and 9% of those on placebo, and the roughly 2:1 ratio was again noted after 2 years of treatment.

More recent studies (104^{cr}, 109^{C}, 110^{C}, 111^{CR}) have pointed to a similar effect. Weight reduction appears to ameliorate diuretic-induced sexual dysfunction (111^{CR}). Smith and Talbert (112^{R}) have reviewed the epidemiology and pathophysiology of sexual dysfunction related to antihypertensive drugs, including diuretics. They point to major differences between surveys, with the prevalence of impotence during diuretic therapy ranging from 4 to 32%. It remains unclear whether younger men and women are similarly affected; whether lower dosages cause less sexual dysfunction; whether patients find these adverse effects, which may be mild, more troublesome than those caused by other antihypertensive drugs; and whether normotensive men have fewer such problems. No convincing mechanism has been proposed. Most investigations of the effects of diuretics on sexual function have been characterized by poor study design (113^{r}); the majority had no placebo control group and relied on comparisons against baseline. The best studies have suggested an increase in erectile dysfunction in thiazides users compared with placebo. Bearing in mind all the confounding factors, it can be concluded that diuretics will sometimes cause impotence, but that in the population as a whole the effect is slight compared with other causes (SEDA-11, 197, 198).

MODERATELY POTENT DIURETICS

The thiazide diuretics

Although one thiazide may be 100 times more potent than another weight-for-weight, all these products have essentially the same properties. Their mechanism of action (inhibition of sodium and chloride reabsorption in the distal convoluted tubule of the kidney) is identical and they can therefore be dealt with as a group.

ADVERSE REACTION PATTERN

General and toxic reaction Like all diuretics, the thiazides can cause altered electrolyte balance (with hypokalemia as the best-known) and dehydration. These complications are rare when treating uncomplicated hypertension, but they are more common when treating heart failure or decompensated hepatic cirrhosis with secondary hyperaldosteronism. Until a patient is accustomed to the effect of a diuretic he may experience some dizziness. Serum lipid concentrations are slightly raised acutely and hyperglycemia can arise on long-term therapy. Rare effects are thrombocytopenia, rashes, drug fever, cholestatic jaundice, pancreatitis, and precipitation of hepatic encephalopathy in patients with hepatic cirrhosis.

Hypersensitivity reactions Skin rashes are common but they are usually mild. Generalized allergic vasculitis has been described occasionally; other reactions are even more rare.

Tumor-inducing effects There is no evidence that the thiazides induce tumors.

Second generation effects These have not been reported.

ORGANS AND SYSTEMS

Cardiovascular Although dizziness is a fairly frequent complaint at the beginning of diuretic treatment (114[C]), postural hypotension is rarely reported. Ischemic complaints (mesenteric infarction and transient cerebral ischemic attacks) have been observed in elderly patients, but it is not clear whether this resulted from diminished organ perfusion or from an effect of the drug itself. The former would appear more likely since similar problems have arisen with any form of antihypertensive treatment in old people who have to some degree become dependent on their hypertension to ensure a blood supply through sclerotic vessels.

Criticism directed against the diuretics in recent years has among other things sought to demonstrate that they increase the risk of coronary events, including acute myocardial infarction. As pointed out in the introductory section of this Chapter, there is no real basis for such criticism; properly used in hypertension the diuretics produce a beneficial effect out of all proportion to any incidental adverse cardiac events which they may provoke.

Respiratory In the older literature there were various reports of acute allergic interstitial pneumonitis caused by the thiazides, sometimes confirmed by rechallenge. Recent work has confirmed this as a rare complication. Typically, it presents with chest pain, breathlessness or both within an hour of taking the drug; the chest X-ray is characteristic (115[C], 116[C]). Recovery is rapid, but assisted ventilation may be needed. Most cases in the recent literature relate to hydrochlorothiazide, but that may simply reflect the wide use of that particular thiazide. The first reported incident precipitated by chlorothiazide (117[C]) suggests that this syndrome may arise with any drug of the thiazide group although it sometimes occurs after the first dose of hydrochlorothiazide when other thiazides have been well tolerated. The incidence of this reaction is unknown and no risk factors have been identified. It may occur on initial exposure, or on subsequent rechallenge. The mechanism remains obscure but an immunological basis has been suggested.

The reason for concern about this adverse reaction is that it may easily be mistaken for myocardial infarction or acute left ventricular failure, conditions which are not uncommon in patients requiring diuretics.

One case of diffuse interstitial pulmonary fibrosis has been reported after treatment with cyclopenthiazide and triamterene (118[C]).

Nervous system Impotence is discussed in the introductory section.

Endocrine, metabolic The effects of thiazide diuretics on endocrine and metabolic function are reviewed in the general introduction to this Chapter.

Mineral and fluid balance The effects of thiazide on sodium, potassium, magnesium and calcium metabolism are covered in the introduction to this Chapter.

Zinc metabolism Thiazide diuretics apparently promote zinc loss in the urine and may reduce the zinc content of hair in the long run (119[C]). It has sometimes been suggested that changes in zinc equilibrium could be responsible for the (supposed) effects on sexual potency, noted above. Geissler et al. (120[C]) investigated the hypothesis that diuretics deplete body zinc which in turn interferes with testosterone production and causes impotence; this, eventually, did not prove to be the case.

Hematological Thrombocytopenia has been regularly reported, but its incidence seems to be quite low (SED-8, 484). Even rarer complications are autoimmune hemolytic anemia, granulocytopenia and agranulocytosis (SED-9, 354).

Acute intravascular hemolysis has been described in a single case, and in this instance antibodies to hydrochlorothiazide were demonstrable; the suggestion was made that methyldopa, which had been given concurrently, might have facilitated antibody formation (121[C]).

Liver The use of thiazide diuretics in hepatic cirrhosis is associated with a high incidence of severe hypokalemia, asterixis and precipitation of encephalopathy. No new cases of jaundice due to 'second generation' thiazide diuretics have been reported since 1964.

Gastrointestinal Nausea and vomiting have been rather frequently reported, but if the incidence is compared to that in a suitable control group on placebo (114[C]), it seems to be negligible, even in a hospital population (122[R]), and such complaints rarely necessitate a change of therapy. The high incidence reported in the past (SED-9, 354) was probably related to the sheer size of chlorothiazide tablets, and it has almost disappeared since the general changeover to more potent thiazides and related drugs. Pancreatitis has been reported occasionally (SED-9, 354; SEDA-5, 228; SEDA-17, 263).

Studies of the relation between diuretic use and cholecystitis have yielded conflicting results. Van der Linden et al. report a significant association of thiazide use with acute cholecystitis in a case—control study (123[Cr]). However, Kakar et al. (124[C]) have examined further the association between thiazide use and cholecystectomy; and have failed to show a relation between thiazide use and gallstone disease, except possibly in women who are not overweight.

Urinary system (see also general section) Toxic damage to the kidney has occasionally been reported, but it seems to be quite rare, and it is not clear whether such effects were caused by severe hypokalemia or by the drug itself. Uric acid precipitation is not normally a problem, although it was with the uricosuric drug, tienilic acid (see below). Renal vasculitis due to thiazides is rare but cannot be ignored (SEDA-18, 234).

Skin and appendages Skin rashes are common but only very occasionally are they severe and disabling (SEDA-11, 198). A state of chronic photosensitivity may persist for many years after drug withdrawal and is difficult to treat (121[C]); the condition may mimic contact dermatitis, and there may be cross-reaction with sulfonamides and phenothiazines. Patients who develop photosensitivity to thiazides should never take them again. Several cases of a reaction resembling systemic lupus erythematosus have been described (126[cF], 127[C]). It remains uncertain whether thiazides cause a lupus-like syndrome or activate latent disease in predisposed individuals. Two of nine patients with drug-induced toxic epidermal necrolysis (128[CR]) were taking hydrochlorothiazide, one with triamterene and allopurinol, the other with reserpine and hydralazine. Both died. In a patient who developed an allergic vasculitis affecting the skin during long-term treatment with hydrochlorothiazide (129[c]) the findings suggested that immediate (Type I) hypersensitivity may be involved in the induction of vasculitis. Baker et al. (130[c]) reported the first case of pseudoporphyria caused by chlorthalidone.

Special senses Visual disturbances caused by dehydration of lens tissue or by retinal edema have been reported, particularly in the first few weeks of treatment. On the whole these effects are innocuous and transient (SED-9, 354). Presenile cataract has been attributed to long-standing use of hydrochlorothiazide (131[c]).

Risk situations Thiazides should be used with caution in patients with a history of gout or diabetes They should be avoided altogether in advanced hepatic insufficiency. In patients taking digitalis, or drugs which prolong QT interval, hypokalemia should be avoided.

Withdrawal effects Risks from withdrawal of diuretics are discussed under the 'Furosemide' monograph below.

Second-generation effects In the past, thiazide diuretics have been considered as being contraindicated in pregnancy because of risk to the mother and fetus. However, more recent evidence suggests that their use need not be contraindicated.

Overdosage This topic is dealt with in the introductory section.

Interactions Thiazide drugs may oppose the blood sugar-lowering effects of oral hypoglycemics and insulin (although these effects are rarely serious) and have additive potassium-lowering effects with other drugs which decrease serum potassium such as corticosteroids and carbenoxolone. Profound hypokalemia due to the latter combination has been reported to cause massive rhabdomyolysis and acute tubular necrosis (132[c]).

A 47-year-old man developed the milk-alkali syndrome while being treated with chlorothiazide 500 mg daily for hypertension and calcium carbonate 7.5—10 g daily for heartburn (133[C]).

The thiazide diuretics inhibit the tubular excretion of lithium ions and may thus cause frank lithium intoxication. This is a potentially serious and well-documented interaction.

In addition, even low doses of angiotensin-converting enzyme (ACE) inhibitors such as enalapril can cause profound first-dose hypotension in hypertensive patients treated with a thiazide (134[C]). ACE inhibitors can cause renal failure in patients with bilateral renal artery stenosis, or stenosis of the artery supplying a single functioning kidney. Concomitant diuretic treatment may play an important role in this adverse reaction (135[c]).

Several non-steroidal anti-inflammatory drugs (NSAIDs) have been reported to interfere with the natriuretic and antihypertensive effects of thiazides (SED-11, 423). The salt-retaining properties of the NSAIDs probably play the central role in this interaction.

Pharmacokinetic interactions between thiazides and diflunisal, propantheline, amantidine, colestipol and colestyramine (SED-11, 424) are of uncertain clinical significance.

Patients taking diuretics and cyclosporin may be at higher risk of hyperuricemia and gouty complications, perhaps because of the tissue breakdown caused by cyclosporin (136[C]).

Since thiazides are often used along with β-blockers, the possibility that the two may act together to produce hyperglycemia must be borne in mind (SEDA-10, 191, 192).

Adverse reactions to allopurinol, particularly toxic epidermal necrolysis and a hypersensitivity syndrome, are reputed to be more common in patients taking thiazides, but evidence to support this is hard to find (SEDA-11, 198; SEDA-13, 188).

Interference with diagnostic routines Apart from the well-known metabolic changes there are no recent reports on in vitro interference of thiazides and their metabolites with diagnostic routines.

OTHER MODERATELY POTENT DIURETICS

Although these drugs are chemically unrelated to the thiazide drugs proper, they share many of their actions and adverse effects.

Bemetizide

In 1988 the Federal German Health Authorities imposed a 'warning' on fixed combinations of the thiazide bemetizide and triamterene that they could cause allergic vasculitis (137[r]). It is well documented that thiazides can occasionally cause allergic vasculitis (see p. 569) and it is not clear on what basis the combination might be more prone to cause the same problem.

Chlorthalidone

Chlorthalidone is so closely similar to the thiazide diuretics in most respects that data have generally been regarded as interchangeable and some have indeed already been cited in the thiazide monograph. In the past (see, e.g. SED-8, 488) chlorthalidone was though to carry a greater risk of hypokalemia and hyponatremia, but this probably reflected relative overdosage with accumulation because of its long half-life. With the much lower doses now in use one can discern no clear difference from the thiazides.

Indapamide

Although it was introduced as a specific antihypertensive without appreciable diuretic action, the hypotensive effects of indapamide are no different from those of bendrofluazide (138[C]). Cases of severe indapamide-induced hypokalemia have also been reported (SED-11, 424; SEDA-15, 213) and other metabolic effects appear to be as common with indapamide as with thiazides (SEDA-14, 185; SEDA-15, 216). Hypersensitivity to indapamide may provoke serious adverse skin reactions (SEDA-17, 260; SEDA-18, 234) and interstitial nephritis leading to acute renal failure has been reported (139[c]).

Metolazone

Metolazone seems to occupy an intermediate position between the thiazide diuretics and the more potent loop diuretics. It is more effective than the thiazides in moderate to advanced renal failure (SED-8, 488; SED-9, 355). In patients with normal renal function its antihypertensive effect compares favourably with bendrofluazide—albeit causing a greater degree of potassium depletion and more adverse effects (SED-11, 424). Where severe heart failure is refractory to conventional triple therapy (high-dose loop diuretic, digoxin, and angiotensin-converting enzyme inhibitor) metolazone can restore diuresis, with weight loss and clinical improvement. However, hypokalemia, hyponatremia and renal impairment are frequent complications. To avoid serious electrolyte disturbances, additional metolazone (preferably in low doses) should be given in hospital and, at the same time, the dose of loop diuretics should be reduced under careful biochemical monitoring (SEDA-16, 225). Neutropenia appears to be a real but rare complication (140[c]).

Quinethazone

Quinethazone is chemically related to the thiazides; early work suggested that it was in all essential respects identical with them (SED-8, 488), and there is no newer evidence that it has any special characteristics.

Tienilic acid (ticrynafen)

Although it is no longer marketed, tienilic acid deserves mention, both because it was a promising uricosuric drug and because it had to be withdrawn so soon after release (in 1980) after causing several hundred cases of severe liver damage, many of them fatal (SEDA-5, 229). Other adverse effects, including acute renal failure, the formation of urate stones, and a stereoselective interaction with oral anticoagulants and with other drugs (e.g. phenytoin) helped ticrynafen to its early demise. For a time it was considered that the hepatic complication might be geographically limited (e.g. because of differences in manufacturing in different countries), but there is now no doubt that the drug itself was responsible. The hepatic complication has been thoroughly studied in retrospect (SED-11, 424). In France, where tienilic acid was still sold until recently, almost 500 reports of liver injury were received. Tienilic acid had no advantage over other diuretics; it certainly had the worst risk:benefit ratio (SEDA-17, 269).

Xipamide

Xipamide is a non-thiazide diuretic acting mainly on the distal tubule. It maximal diuretic effect is as great as that of furosemide, but its duration of action is longer and similar to that of the thiazides; like metolazone it thus seems to occupy an intermediate position between the two main groups of diuretics and again, like metolazone, it can be used in renal failure. However, xipamide does appear to present some risks, and it is not clear that these are outweighed by any advantages. At equivalent therapeutic doses, metabolic effects are greater than those seen with thiazides or furosemide (SED-11, 425). A photo-allergic skin reaction has been described (SEDA-16, 222).

CARBONIC ANHYDRASE INHIBITORS

Acetazolamide

The carbonic anhydrase inhibitors, of which acetazolamide is the prototype, are not suitable for normal diuretic use, because tolerance to their effect soon develops. They are, however, well suited to intermittent employment, particularly in the relief of glaucoma; acetazolamide is for that reason discussed primarily in Chapter 47.

Various adverse effects common to diuretics can occur. Acetazolamide has occasionally caused hepatic failure, formation of renal calculi, nephrocalcinosis and blood disorders; mild effects such as paresthesias, drowsiness, rash and fever are repeatedly encountered. Hypokalemia is not a problem during longer-term administration because of compensatory potassium retention secondary to acidosis (141[C]). Metabolic acidosis may be present in 50% of elderly patients (SEDA-11, 199); occasionally (particularly if salicylates are being given or renal function is poor) the acidosis can become severe. Two elderly patients developed lethargy, confusion and incontinence attributed to interaction between acetazolamide and salicylate (142[c]).

Two unusual adverse effects were reported in SEDA-15, 219. Thyrotoxic periodic paralysis occurs only occasionally in Caucasians but, for unknown reasons, it may be worsened by administration of acetazolamide. The mechanism for altered taste perception for carbonated drinks is unknown, but carbonic drinks may be a source of high concentrations of carbonic acid, which otherwise exist at much lower concentrations due to carbonic anhydrase activity.

Eleven cases of acetazolamide-associated aplastic anemia were reported in Sweden during a 17-year period (143[CR]). The median dose was 500 mg daily and the median duration of therapy was 3 months (2—71 months). Ten of the 11 patients died within 8 weeks of diagnosis. The relative risk of aplastic anemia with acetazolamide was 13.3 (95% confidence interval 6.8, 25.3) and the estimated frequency was one in 18 000. These findings suggest that acetazolamide is associated with a substantial increased risk of aplastic anemia.

POTENT DIURETICS

Furosemide (frusemide)

Furosemide is the classic member of the group of 'high ceiling' or 'loop' diuretics which can achieve a much greater peak diuresis than the thiazides. It is widely and frequently used both orally and parenterally over a rather wider dosage range than the thiazide diuretics, because its dose—effect curve is steeper and because it is effective in patients with moderate renal insufficiency (creatinine clearance 5—25 ml/min), in whom the thiazide diuretics and most related compounds fail. The drug is quickly and almost completely excreted by kidney in the unmetabolized form. Because of this much wider range of application it is not surprising that adverse effects are rather frequently reported, although serious adverse effects seem to be uncommon. The usual oral dose is 20—120 mg, but much larger doses (e.g. 1000 mg) have been used in renal failure. It is very effective after intravenous injection, and doses of 500 mg and more may be used in emergencies (renal failure, pulmonary edema). The majority of adverse effects occur with the use of high doses, 95% of the reactions being dose dependent (144[C]).

ADVERSE REACTION PATTERN

General and toxic reactions Disturbances of fluid and electrolyte balance such as hyponatremia, hypokalemia, and dehydration with circulatory disturbances (such as dizziness, postural hypotension and syncope) have been reported. Rarely gastrointestinal symptoms are problems with high dosages and in the elderly. Pancreatitis and jaundice seem to occur more frequently than with the thiazide diuretics, but deterioration of glucose tolerance seems to be less common. At serum concentrations over 50 μg/ml, tinnitus, vertigo and deafness, sometimes permanent, have been reported. Hematological disorders, particularly thrombocytopenia, and serious skin disorders occur occasionally.

Hypersensitivity reactions These are discussed

below under 'Urinary system' and 'Skin and appendages'.

Tumor-inducing effects These have not been documented.

Second-generation effects These have not been reported.

ORGANS AND SYSTEMS

Cardiovascular Because furosemide, apart from its diuretic effect, has transient but pronounced vasodilator properties (changes in both venous capacitance and peripheral arteriolar resistance have been described in anephric patients), it may cause postural hypotension and syncope, particularly if given together with other hypotensive drugs (SED-8, 458; SED-9, 349, 350). Ischemic complications have been reported in elderly patients. Reactions due to extracellular volume depletion accounted for 9.0% of all adverse effects observed in 535 patients treated with furosemide in a clinical setting (144[C]).

When administered in cardiac failure, furosemide acts in two ways: besides it diuretic effect it also produces an immediate fall in left ventricular filling pressure which is independent of diuresis and precedes it. If furosemide is given intravenously in stable chronic heart failure (which it normally is not), this may be an unwanted effect, causing deterioration (SEDA-11, 199).

Nervous system Visual disturbances and drowsiness have been described, but it is not clear whether these were caused by decreased cerebral perfusion or by an effect of the drug itself.

Endocrine, metabolic The influence of loop diuretics on lipid, carbohydrate and uric acid metabolism is discussed under general considerations.

Other effects Furosemide may rarely cause inappropriate antidiuretic hormone secretion syndrome (IADHS) (although it has been found useful to treat IADHS of other origin). In furosemide-induced cases (SEDA-7, 246), serum ADH concentrations were elevated, total body sodium was normal, total body potassium grossly decreased and intracellular water increased at the expense of extracellular fluid volume. However, such cases seem to be decidedly rare, and no new cases have been published since this complication was reported in SEDA-7.

Mineral and fluid balance The effect of furosemide and other loop diuretics on sodium, potassium, magnesium and calcium metabolism is described in the introductory section of this Chapter.

Hematological Agranulocytosis, thrombocytopenia and hemolytic anemia have occasionally been reported (SED-8, 484; SED-9, 350; SEDA-1, 180). The commonest complication is thrombocytopenia (145[c]), although it is often mild and asymptomatic (146[R]).

Liver Though furosemide is extremely hepatotoxic in experimental animals only a few cases of jaundice have been reported (SED-8, 484, 485), and no fully documented cases have so far been published. However, in patients with hepatic cirrhosis the drug may readily precipitate hepatic encephalopathy (SED-8, 485), even when low doses are used (144[c]).

Gastrointestinal With normal doses, nausea, vomiting and diarrhea are extremely uncommon, accounting for less than 1% of all adverse reactions (SED-9, 350). The incidence rises with higher doses and in the presence of uremia. Increases in serum isoamylase (SEDA-6, 213) and pancreatitis have been reported. Biliary colic has also been described (SED-11, 427).

Urinary system Excessive diuresis and dehydration often cause a transient decrease in glomerular filtration rate and elevation of serum BUN (approx. 8% of all adverse reactions) (SED-8, 350). Particularly in elderly patients the sudden diuresis may cause loin pain, and, in elderly men with prostatic hypertrophy, acute urinary retention and overflow incontinence. Interstitial nephritis, discussed in the general section above, can be caused by any diuretic, including furosemide (SED-11, 427).

Skin and appendages Rashes seem to be just as common (SED-8, 484) as with other oral diuretics, but severe skin reactions (exfoliative dermatitis, erythema multiforme, acquired epidermolysis bullosa), which are quite rare with other diuretics, have been reported occasionally with the use of high doses in renal failure (SED-12, 503; SEDA-18, 234). Cases of furosemide-induced lupus-like syndrome (147[Cr]), bullous pemphigoid (148[c], 149[C]) and lichenoid drug eruption (150C) have been reported. Cobb (151[cR]) reviewed furosemide-induced cutaneous reactions and described a unique case of an 88-year-old man who developed an eruption that clinically and histologically simulated Sweet's syndrome (acute febrile neutrophilic vasculitis) after 6 weeks' treatment. Atypical features and the rapid resolution suggested a drug eruption rather than true Sweet's syndrome. However, a similar mechanism may be implicated—a hypersensitivity reaction involving immune complexes.

Special senses At high doses, and especially if serum concentrations are over 50 μg/ml, furosemide may cause ototoxic reactions such as tinnitus, vertigo and even deafness, sometimes permanent (SED-9, 351). Subclinical, audiometrically determined, high-tone deafness has been reported to occur in 6.4% of furosemide-treated patients (152[r]). It is generally considered advisable to use another diuretic in patients whose hearing is already impaired, and to avoid using furosemide along with other ototoxic drugs such as the aminoglycosides.

Risk situations Although high-dose furosemide therapy can be very useful in incipient acute renal failure, the drug should be used with extreme caution in patients with severe hepatic insufficiency (SEDA-14, 183) and not at all in hepatic coma. High doses in uremia are potentially ototoxic. The risks of hypercalciuria and stone formation in premature infants are discussed in connection with mineral effects above. A second well-documented risk in premature infants is persistence of a patent ductus arteriosus (SEDA-9, 208). It seems clear that the use of the drug at all in this age group needs at least careful re-evaluation (SEDA-14, 182; SEDA-15, 217).

Withdrawal effects The more intensive diuretic treatment is, the greater the risk from sudden withdrawal. In one reported series of 38 patients, treatment had been with 20—40 mg furosemide or equivalent, generally for heart failure. When all had been free of heart failure or hypertension for at least 3 months, withdrawal was attempted; it was followed by clinical or radiological relapse in 29% and one of the patients died (153[C]). In another series of five patients, withdrawal in three cases led to severe symptoms necessitating admission to hospital (SEDA-10, 192, 193). The best advice is to withdraw intensive diuretic treatment only with the utmost caution and not to attempt withdrawal at all if there is any radiological evidence of heart failure. In patients with congestive heart failure, independent predictors of the need for continued diuretic were furosemide dose greater than 40 mg daily, left ventricular ejection fraction less than 0.27 and hypertension (154[C]).

Second-generation effects Although furosemide has embryotoxic properties in some animal species, it has been widely used in pregnant women without any adverse effects. Nevertheless, it should be used with great caution since hypovolemia may lead to decreased uterine and placental blood flow. Careful monitoring of fetal heart action is necessary. Furosemide passes the placenta and increases fetal urine production. It may also increase acid concentrations in maternal serum, fetal serum and amniotic fluid, thus masking a useful index for the development of pre-eclampsia (155[R]). Its use in pregnant patients should therefore be restricted to the treatment of cardiac failure (see section 'Diuretics in pregnancy' above). The drug passes into breast milk at a concentration of 80% of the serum value at pH 7.0, but the total amount of drug ingested is probably too low to affect the neonate (156[R]).

Overdosage Overdosage of diuretics is discussed in the introductory section of this Chapter and in connection with diuretic abuse.

Interactions The use of thiazide and loop diuretics in combination to treat resistant hypertension often causes a severe deterioration in renal function (157[C], 158[C]). It is not clear whether this is the result of excess diuresis or excessive blood pressure reduction.

Furosemide increases the ototoxic risks of aminoglycoside antibiotics (159[c], 160[c]) by decreasing their clearance by approximately 35% (161[c]); permanent deafness has resulted from the use of this combination.

The nephrotoxic effects of cefaloridine are potentiated by concurrent administration of furosemide (162[c]—164[c]), perhaps by a direct interaction and probably also because furosemide lowers the clearance of the antibiotic (165[c]). Such combinations are better avoided.

The combination of furosemide and mannitol may rapidly lead to acute renal failure (166[c]) and may potentiate the effect of curare (167[c]).

Furosemide may induce lithium toxicity by inhibiting tubular excretion of lithium ions (168[c]).

Acute renal failure with severe hyponatremia has been attributed to vigorous diuretic treatment (metolazone, furosemide + spironolactone) and an ACE inhibitor (169[C]).

In congestive heart failure, single conventional doses of captopril (25—75 mg) attenuated the natriuretic response to furosemide while low dose captopril (1 mg) significantly enhanced furosemide-induced natriuresis (SEDA-17, 268; SEDA-18, 236). The mechanism of this interaction is uncertain but captopril did not affect delivery of furosemide to its site of action (170[C]). In the long-term intensive treatment with captopril enhanced the natriuretic response to furosemide (SEDA-17, 268).

The diuretic response to furosemide is reduced by approximately 50% during concurrent administration of phenytoin (171[c]), probably through reduction of furosemide absorption (172[c]).

Furosemide inhibits the absorption of indomethacin (173[c]), while the diuretic and hypotensive effects of most diuretics are blunted by indomethacin and probably also other non-steroidal anti-inflammatory drugs (174[c]). Similar observations have been made with aspirin (175[c]). This interaction is further discussed at the end of this Chapter.

Mousson et al. (176[c]) report a patient with both interstitial nephritis and granulomatous hepatitis which they attribute to a furosemide—allopurinol interaction. As in previous reports (SEDA-11, 198) the evidence for this interaction is not convincing. The role of allopurinol in causing the illness is credible, but the role of furosemide is doubtful.

Intravenous frusemide may increase steady-state theophylline concentrations (SED-11, 428).

Although furosemide does not alter the pharmacokinetics of digoxin, it is advisable to closely monitor serum potassium values if furosemide is combined with any cardiac glycoside.

Potentiation of the potassium-lowering effects of other drugs (corticosteroids, licorice, carbenoxolone) should be kept in mind.

Bumetanide

Bumetanide is a furosemide analog which has been extensively studied and used. It is very similar in most respects to furosemide, although it is, mol for mol, much more potent—an oral dose of 1—4 mg often sufficing for ordinary use.

One advantage which it appears to have is a lesser degree of ototoxicity (152[r], 177[R], 178[R]). It is sensible to prefer bumetanide to furosemide in patients with hearing problems or concurrently needing ototoxic drugs, such as the aminoglycoside antibiotics.

All the other evidence points to furosemide-like adverse effects and interactions. Occasional drug rashes including pseudoporphyria (SEDA-16, 222) and a case of Stevens-Johnson syndrome have been reported (SED-10, 376). A patient in whom pancreatitis was induced by both furosemide and bumetanide has been documented (SEDA-14, 184). Very high doses used for renal failure have sometimes produced colic (SED-10, 376). It has been suggested that the drug has less effect on blood glucose than does furosemide, but this is not at all clear. Bumetamide has been implicated in the development of pulmonary fibrosis (SEDA-16, 223) but causality could not be determined with certainty.

Etacrynic acid

The absence of new reports on the adverse effects of etacrynic acid probably reflects the declining popularity of the drug, which is more toxic than either furosemide or the newer derivatives, and offers no clear advantages. Its adverse effects are very similar to those of furosemide (precipitation of hepatic coma, pancreatitis, ototoxicity, hematological disturbances, skin reactions), but it causes more gastrointestinal problems (nausea, vomiting, diarrhea, gastrointestinal hemorrhage and jaundice) (SED-9, 351, 352).

Mefruside

Mefruside is an intermediate-acting diuretic closely related to furosemide, and earlier literature showed that it was clinically also very similar (SED-8, 488). More recent work, relating, for example, to its effects on serum lipids (SEDA-11, 196) or serum magnesium (SEDA-10, 188), has confirmed this.

Muzolimine

Muzolimine has an action of long duration and it seems to be slightly more effective than furosemide. In 29 patients with chronic renal insufficiency treated with high doses of muzolimine, five subjects developed a neurological syndrome very similar to multiple sclerosis (179[c]). Further reports of severe neurotoxicity with muzolamine followed (SEDA-16, 225). The drug was withdrawn from use in Germany in 1989, two years after its introduction.

Piretanide

Piretanide is a close relative of furosemide; its diuretic and kinetic properties are very similar to those of furosemide and bumetanide, and its potency lies somewhere between the two.

As in the case of some other diuretics, attempts have been made to demonstrate and claim specific advantages for piretanide (e.g. that it is a 'potassium-stable diuretic') but there is no good evidence that it has such advantages (SEDA-10, 188; SEDA-15, 213).

Torasemide

Torasemide is a new long-acting loop diuretic which has no structural similarities with other diuretics. It is promoted for use in hypertension and, like piretanide, is claimed to be potassium neutral. The assertion is premature. Current evidence indicates no metabolic advantages over thiazides (SEDA-16, 226; SEDA-17, 264; SEDA-18, 237).

POTASSIUM-SPARING AGENTS

Spironolactone

Spironolactone is a competitive antagonist of aldosterone and it has therefore been used as a potassium-sparing diuretic in cardiac failure and in the management of ascites and edema associated with hepatic cirrhosis with secondary hyperaldosteronism. It is also used to treat hyperaldosteronism due to adrenal tumours or hyperplasia. It has a weak positive isotropic effect and a modest antihypertensive effect in keeping with its natriuretic action.

ADVERSE REACTION PATTERN

General and toxic reactions The major limitation to the use of spironolactone is its liability to cause (sometimes lethal) hyperkalemia, particularly in the elderly, in patients with decreased renal function, and in patients who are simultaneously given potassium supplements or ACE inhibitors. As with other diuretics, hyponatremia and dehydration can occur. Other less frequent adverse effects are gastrointestinal intolerance, neurological symptoms and skin rashes.

Hypersensitivity reactions These are described below under 'Skin and appendages'.

Tumor-inducing effects Spironolactone possesses antiandrogenic properties and it frequently causes gynecomastia in men. In women, it causes breast enlargement and soreness; five cases of mammary carcinoma have been reported. It increases the peripheral metabolism of testosterone to estradiol (180[C]). Potential human metabolic products of spironolactone have proven to be carcinogenic in rodents and the United Kingdom Committee on Safety of Medicines in 1988 restricted the approved indications for the drug, removing the indications of essential hypertension and idiopathic edema (181[r]).

Second-generation effects These have not been reported.

ORGANS AND SYSTEMS

Nervous system Central nervous system effects such as weakness, drowsiness and confusion have been reported. Because most patients experiencing such adverse effects were treated with spironolactone for edema and ascites in hepatic cirrhosis, it is not yet clear whether they were caused by the drug itself or by hepatic encephalopathy. The incidence of these complaints in such patients is quite high (9.8%) (SED-9, 357).

Endocrine, metabolic *Antiandrogenic effects* Because of its antiandrogenic action, spironolactone causes gynecomastia, decreased libido and erectile failure in 4—30% of men. Such effects on sexual function seem to be both dose- and time-dependent. It causes breast tenderness and enlargement, mastodynia, infertility, chloasma, altered vaginal lubrication and decreased libido in women, probably because of estrogenic effects on target tissue. Menstrual irregularities were experienced by almost all women treated with spironolactone 400 mg daily and most developed amenorrhea at doses of 100—200 mg daily. Normal menstruation was resumed within 2 months of discontinuation. Very high doses of spironolactone (over 450 mg daily) can cause infertility, but such doses are rarely employed. As with other diuretics, studies with spironolactone were not placebo controlled, small and often anecdotal (SEDA-18, 235).

Other effects Spironolactone effects on carbohydrate, uric acid and lipid metabolism are discussed in the introduction to this Chapter.

Mineral and fluid balance The effect of spironolactone on potassium and magnesium metabolism are described under general considerations.

Hematological One case of agranulocytosis has been reported (SED-11, 430).

Gastrointestinal Nausea and vomiting are more common than with other diuretics (SED-9, 358) and were reported in 11% of patients in the Boston Collaborative Drug Surveillance Program (182[R]).

Liver One case of spironolactone-induced parenchymal hepatitis with a positive rechallenge has been reported (183[c]). The patient recovered uneventfully.

Urinary system There is no firm evidence that spironolactone has any nephrotoxic properties.

Skin and appendages Rashes (sometimes with eosinophilia) lichen planus (SED-9, 358), and a lupus-like syndrome with a positive rechallenge (SEDA-5, 230) have been reported, but on the whole skin reactions seem to be rare. Cutaneous vasculitis has been attributed to spironolactone (SED-11, 430). It is unclear whether a patient presenting with erythema annulare centrifugum while taking spironolactone (184[C]) suffered a similar reaction. Other adverse reactions reported include urticaria, alopecia and chloasma (SEDA-14, 185).

Risk situations Renal failure, co-medication with potassium salts or other potassium-sparing agents, dosages over 200 mg/day, hepatic failure and use in elderly patients carry unwarranted risk unless serum potassium is regularly monitored.

Second-generation effects There are no reliable data on the use and safety of spironolactone in pregnant women. It is not known whether the drug passes into breast milk.

Interactions Several interactions of spironolactone with other drugs have been reported, not all of them being clinically significant.

Spironolactone has a weak enzyme-inducing effect, and it enhances the metabolic breakdown of antipyrine and digitoxin (SED-9, 358).

Spironolactone raises steady-state digoxin concentrations by approximately 30% and it may also be involved in a pharmacodynamic interaction with digoxin. The clinical importance of these observations is uncertain (SEDA-9, 209).

The secretion of the main metabolite, canrenone, in the renal tubules is blocked by aspirin (185[r]), abolishing the diuretic response, although the antihypertensive effect is apparently not affected (186[c]).

Some non-steroidal anti-inflammatory drugs, notably indomethacin and mefenamic acid, have been shown to inhibit the excretion of canrenone (187[c]). The interaction with NSAIDs is further discussed at the end of the Chapter.

Spironolactone abolishes the ulcer-healing properties of carbenoxolone (188[c]). It has been suggested that spironolactone may reduce the anticoagulant effect of warfarin (SED-11, 430).

Interference with diagnostic routines Spironolactone has been reported to interfere with the radioimmunological assay of digoxin when poorly specific antidigoxin antibodies are used.

Potassium canronate

The main metabolite of spironolactone (canrenone) has been in use for a number of years as a potassium-sparing diuretic for intravenous use. More recently, the potassium salt has been used orally in the hope of avoiding the hormonal adverse effects exerted by spironolactone. In patients with hepatic cirrhosis, gynecomastia was twice as common during treatment with spironolactone than with potassium canrenoate (42 vs 20%) at equiactive doses (189[cr]).

The difference in propensity to gynecomastia may be related to structural characteristics unique to metabolites of spironolactone, viz. a thiol group at the 7-α position (SEDA-11, 200).

OTHER POTASSIUM-SPARING AGENTS

Neither triamterene nor amiloride is an aldosterone antagonist, but both have similar effects on the distal tubules. They carry the risk of causing hyperkalemia and should not be used in renal insufficiency or combined with potassium supplements or other potassium-sparing agents (SED-9, 358).

Amiloride

Amiloride does not influence renal function (190[c]), but does block the tubular secretion of creatinine, leading to falsely elevated measurements of creatinine clearance; inulin clearance is not affected similarly (191[R]). It is otherwise a relatively safe drug with few reported adverse effects. Skin rashes, diarrhea and eosinophilia have been reported (191[R]). Amiloride has a specific effect on sodium flux in the renal tubules; severe hyponatremia has been reported with the use of the combination of a thiazide diuretic and amiloride. The involvement of amiloride in the genesis of diuretic-induced hyponatremia is discussed under general considerations.

It has been argued that potassium-sparing diuretics present a real risk of renal failure when they are used in elderly people (192[R]). In large-scale studies involving elderly hypertensive patients there is indeed some slight increase in the incidence of renal failure when combinations including potassium-sparing diuretics are used. Although the overall incidence of nephrotoxicity is quite low, elderly patients and those with prior renal dysfunction are at particular risk. Special care is necessary in these circumstances.

Sweden's National Adverse Reaction Monitoring System has called the attention of physicians to a case in which a woman of 73 developed anaphylactic shock after taking only a single tablet of Moduretic (193[c]). The National System had three other reports on anaphylactic reactions to this combination and, by 1988, the World Health Organisation System had eight others from other countries. Except for mild skin reactions hypersensitivity reactions to hydrochlorothiazide alone are highly unusual and not of this type (see 'Thiazide' monograph).

An isolated report (194[c]) suggests that amiloride may have prodysrhythmic potential in a small proportion of patients with inducible sustained ventricular tachycardia.

Like spironolactone, but unlike triamterene, amiloride inhibits the ulcer-healing properties of carbenoxolone (195[c]). Amiloride appears to be free of the troublesome interaction with lithium which complicates the use of thiazides and loop diuretics.

Triamterene

Of the milder adverse effects of triamterene, nausea, vomiting and diarrhea are fairly common; rashes including photodermatitis (196[C]) sometimes occur; drug fever has been reported (197[c]). Pseudoporphyria has been attributed to Dyazide (hydrochlorothiazide + triamterene) in a patient with vitiligo (198[c]). It is uncertain which constituent was responsible.

Triamterene blocks dihydrofolate reductase and may cause folate deficiency with megaloblastic anemia and pancytopenia, particularly in patients with hepatic cirrhosis, who show reduced clearance of the drug (SED-11, 431). Where this has been reported, all patients were taking doses of 150—600 mg daily for treatment of ascites and all had hepatic cirrhosis, often due to alcohol abuse (SEDA-17, 269). It would seem advisable to use spironolactone rather than triamterene in cirrhotic patients. Because of this potential risk of folate deficiency it would also seem sensible to avoid triamterene in pregnancy.

Like other diuretics, triamterene occasionally causes interstitial nephritis (199[C]), but it has also been responsible for other renal problems, notably reversible non-oliguric renal failure when it is given along with indomethacin (or presumably any other inhibitor of prostaglandin synthesis) (200[c]). More questionable is whether triamterene indeed causes crystals, casts and frank stones in the urinary tract, as has long been believed. The phenomenon has often been reported anecdotally in SEDAs and it has been shown that microcrystals of the parahydroxy metabolite form a particularly suitable nucleus for crystalline calcium oxalate deposition (201[c]); however, this does not prove that the stones would not have formed in the absence of triamterene treatment. The cause-and-effect relationship has been questioned on epidemiological grounds and in the light of a controlled study which found no link (202[C]), and the drug could still prove to be an 'innocent bystander' in stone formation (SEDA-11, 200). Other aspects of possible renal complications are discussed under 'Amiloride' above.

INTERACTIONS WITH POTASSIUM-SPARING DIURETICS *(see also 'Thiazide' monograph)*

Two reviews (192[R], 203[R]) have considered the interaction between non-steroidal anti-inflammatory drugs (NSAIDs) and potassium-sparing diuretics. Both types of drugs can cause nephrotoxicity and, in combination, the effects appear to be additive. This is a particular problem in the elderly where serum creatinine may be in the normal range even in the face of marked renal impairment. The availability of over-the-counter NSAIDs has increased the importance of this interaction. Plasma potassium and renal function should be monitored closely. Potassium-sparing diuretics and NSAIDs should be prescribed together only when both are essential, and only with very careful monitoring of renal function and serum potassium. Elderly patients and those with even very mild renal impairment may be at very high risk (SED-11, 431).

Coadministration of angiotensin-converting enzyme inhibitors and potassium-sparing diuretics can cause severe hyperkalemia, which resulted in complete heart block in two patients (204[C], 205[C]).

REFERENCES

1. Cranston WI, Juel-Jensen BE, Semmence AM et al. Effects of oral diuretics on raised arterial pressure. Lancet 1963;ii:966.
2. Hollifield JW. Thiazide treatment of systemic hypertension: effects on serum magnesium and ventricular ectopic activity. Am J Cardiol, 1989;63:22G.
3. Kaplan NM. How bad are diuretic-induced hypokalaemia and hypercholesterolaemia? Arch Intern Med 1989;149; 2649.
4. Weinberger MH. Selection of drugs for initial treatment of hypertension. Pract Cardiol 1989;15;81.
5. Lipsitz LA. Hypertension in the elderly. Hosp Pract 1989;April 15:119.
6. Poulter N, Sever P, Thom S. Antihypertensive and adverse biochemical effects of bendrofluazide. Br Med J 1990;300;1465.
7. Moser M. In defence of traditional antihypertensive therapy. Hypertension 1988;12;324.
8. Gifford RW, Borazanian RA. Traditional first-line therapy. Overview of medical benefits and side effects. Hypertension 1989;13(Suppl 1):I—119.
9. Thompson WG. Review: an assault on old friends: thiazide diuretics under siege. Am J Med Sci 1990;300;152—158.
10. Medical Research Council Working Party. MRC trial of treatment of mild hypertension: principal results. Br Med J 1985;291;97.
11. Medical Research Council Working Party on Mild Hypertension. Coronary heart disease in the Medical Research Council trial of treatment of mild hypertension. Br Heart J 1988;59;364.
12. Amery A, Birkenhäger W, Brixko P et al. Mortality and morbidity results from the European Working Party on High Blood Pressure in the Elderly trial. Lancet 1985;i:1349.
13. SHEP Cooperative Research Group. Prevention of stroke by antihypertensive drug treatment in older persons with isolated systolic hypertension. Final results of the Systolic Hypertension in the Elderly Program (SHEP). J Am Med Assoc 1991;265;3255—3264.
14. Dahlöf B, Lindholm LH, Hansson L, Schersten B, Ekbom T, Wester P-O. Morbidity and mortality in the Swedish Trial in Old Patients with Hypertension (STOP-Hypertension). Lancet 1991;338;1281—1285.

15. MRC Working Party. Medical Research council trial of treatment of hypertension in older adults: principal results. Br Med J 1992;304;405–412.
16. The IPPPSH Collaborative Group. Cardiovascular risk and risk factors in a randomized trial of treatment based on the beta-blocker oxprenolol: the International Prospective Primary Prevention Study in Hypertension (IPPPSH). J Hypertens 1985;3;379.
17. Wilhelmsen L, Berglund G, Elmfeldt D et al. Beta-blockers versus diuretics in hypertensive men: main results from the HAPPHY trial. J Hypertens 1987;5;561.
18. Wikstrand J, Warnold I, Olsson G et al. Primary prevention with metoprolol in patients with hypertension. Mortality results from the MAPHY study. J Am Med Assoc 1988;259;1976.
19. Hoes AW, Grobbee DE, Lubsen J, Man in't Veld AJ, Van der Does E, Hofman A. Diuretics, β-blockers, and the risk for sudden cardiac death in hypertensive patients. Ann Intern Med 1995;123:481–487.
20. Siskovick DS, Raghunathan TE, Psaty BM, Koepsell TD, Wicklund KG, Lin X, Cobb L, Rautaharju PM, Copass MK, Wagner EH. Diuretic therapy for hypertension and the risk of primary cardiac arrest. New Engl J Med 1994;330;1852–1857.
21. McInnes GT, Yeo WW, Ramsay LE, Moser M. Cardiotoxicity and diuretics: much speculation—little substance. J Hypertens 1992;10;317–335.
22. Collins R, MacMahon S. Blood pressure, antihypertensive drug treatment and the risks of stroke and of coronary heart disease. Br Med Bull 1994;50;272–298
23. Ramsay LE, Yeo WW. Antihypertensive and adverse biochemical effects of bendrofluazide. Br Med J 1990; 301;240.
24. Joint National Committee on Detection, Evaluation, and Treatment of High Blood Pressure. The fifth report of the Joint National Committee on Detection, Evaluation and Treatment of High Blood Pressure. Arch Intern Med 1993;153;154–183.
25. Swales JD. Pharmacological treatment of hypertension. Lancet 1994;344;380–385.
26. The Systolic Hypertension in the Elderly Program Cooperative Research Group. Implications of the Systolic Hypertension in the Elderly Program. Hypertension 1993; 21;335–343.
27. Neaton JD, Grimm RH, Prineas RJ, Stamler J, Grandits GA, Elmer PJ, Cutler JA, Flack JM, Schoenberger JA, McDonald R, Lewis CE, Liebson PR. Treatment of Mild Hypertension Study. Final results. J Am Med Assoc 1993;270;713–714.
28. Collins R, Yusuf S, Peto R. Overview of randomised trials of diuretics in pregnancy. Br Med J 1985;290;17.
29. Diokno AC, Brown MB, Herzog AR. Relationship between use of diuretics and continence status in the elderly. Urology 1991;38;39–42.
30. Myers MG, Kearns PM, Kennedy DS et al. Postural hypotension and diuretic therapy in the elderly. Can Med Assoc J 1978;119;581.
31. Burke V, Beilin LJ, Gerrman R, Grosskopf S, Ritchie J, Puddey IB, Rogers P. Postural fall in blood pressure in the elderly in relation to drug treatment and other factors. Q J Med 1992;84;583–591.
32. Applegate WB. Hypertension in elderly patients. Ann Intern Med 1989;110;901.
33. Nicholls MG. Age-related effects of diuretics in hypertensive subjects. J Cardiovasc Pharmacol 1988;12(Suppl 8):S51.
34. Kaufmann H, Elijovitch F, Yahr MD. An unusual cause of tetany: surreptitious use of furosemide. Mt Sinai J Med 1984;51;625.
35. De Wardener HE. Idiopathic oedema: role of diuretic abuse. Kidney Int 1981;19;881.
36. Dunnigan MG, Denning DW, Henry JA et al. Idiopathic oedema and diuretics. Postgrad Med J 1987;63;25.
37. Pelosi AJ, Sykes RA, Lough JRM et al. A psychiatric study of idiopathic oedema. Lancet 1986;ii:999.
38. Young JB, Browjohn AM, Lee MR. Diuretics and idiopathic oedema. Nephron 1986;43;311.
39. Marty H. Pseudo-Bartter Syndrom bei Diuretika-Abusus. Schweiz Med Wochenschr 1985;115;250.
40. Jiminez ML, Barbado FJ, Mateos F et al. Sindrome de Bartter factitio inducido por la ingestion subrepticia de diureticos. Med Clin (Barcelona) 1985;84:23.
41. Jennings M, Shortland JR, Maddocks JL. Interstitial nephritis associated with frusemide. J R Soc Med 1986; 79;239.
42. Magil AB. Drug induced acute interstitial nephritis with granulomas. Hum Pathol 1983;14;36.
43. Fernandez P, Choi M. Thiazide-induced hyponatraemia. In: Puschett JB, Greenberg A, eds. Diuretics IV: Chemistry, Pharmacology and Clinical Applications. Amsterdam: Elsevier, 1993;199–209.
44. Sonnenblick M, Friedlander Y, Rosin AJ. Diuretic-induced severe hyponatraemia. Review and analysis of 129 reported cases. Chest 1993;103;601–606,
45. Arieff AI. Management of hyponatraemia. Br Med J 1993;307;305–308.
46. Zalin AM, Hutchinson CE, Jong M et al. Hyponatraemia during treatment with chlorpropamide and Moduretic (amiloride plus hydrochlorothiazide). Br Med J 1984;289;659.
47. Hart TJ, Johnston LJ, Edmonds MW, Brownscombe L. Hyponatraemia secondary to thiazide-trimethoprim interaction. Can J Hosp Pharm 1989;42;243–246.
48. Byatt CM, Millard PH, Levin GE. Diuretics and electrolyte disturbances in 1000 consecutive geriatric admissions. J R Soc Med 1990;83;704.
49. Andersson OK, Gudbrandsson T, Jamerson K. Metabolic adverse effects of thiazide diuretics: the importance of normokalemia. J Intern Med 1991;229(Suppl 2):89–96.
50. Dyckner T. Relation of cardiovascular disease to potassium and magnesium deficiency. Am J Cardiol 1990;65:44K–46K.
51. Schulman M, Narins RG. Hypokalemia and cardiovascular disease. Am J Cardiol 1990;65:4E–9E.
52. Kostis JB, Lacy CR, Hall WD, Wilson AC, Borhani NO, Krieger SD, Cosgrove NM. The effect of chlorthalidone on ventricular ectopic activity in patients with isolated systolic hypertension. Am J Cardiol 1994;74;464–467.
53. Papademetriou V. Diuretics in hypertension; clinical experiences. Eur Heart J 1992;13(Suppl G):92–95.
54. Frohlich ED. Current issues in hypertension. Old questions with new answers and new questions. Med Clin North Am 1992;76;1045–1056.
55. McInnes GT. Potassium and diuretics—when does it matter? Med Resource 1992;6;21–24.
56. Saunders A, Wilson SM. Do diuretics differ in degree of hypokalaemia, and does it matter? Aust J Hosp Pharm 1991;21;120–121.
57. Restrick IJ, Huddy N, Hofbrand BI. Diuretic-induced

hypokalaemia and surgery: much ado about nothing? Postgrad Med J 1992;68;318–320.
58. Nicholls MG. Interaction of diuretics and electrolytes in congestive heart failure. Am J Cardiol 1990;65:17E–21E.
59. Papademetriou V, Burris JF, Notargiacomo A et al. Thiazide therapy is not a cause of arrhythmia in patients with systemic hypertension. Arch Intern Med 1988;148:1272.
60. Anonymous. Potassium-sparing diuretics: when are they really needed? Drugs Ther Bull 1985;23;17.
61. Kassirer JP. Does the benefit of aggressive potassium replacement in diuretic-induced patients outweigh the risk? J Cardiovasc Pharmacol 1984;6:S488.
62. Shintani S, Shiigai T, Tsukagoshi H. Marked hypokalaemic rhabdomyolysis with myoglobinuria due to diuretic treatment. Eur Neurol 1991;31;396–398.
63. Carlsen JE, Kober L, Torp-Pederson C, Johansen P. Relation between dose of bendrofluazide, antihypertensive effect, and adverse metabolic effects. Br Med J 1990;300;975.
64. McVeigh G, Galloway D, Johnston D. The case for low dose diuretics in hypertension: comparison of low and conventional doses of cyclopenthiazide. Br Med J 1988;297;95.
65. Harper R, Ennis CN, Sheridan B, Atkinson AB, Johnston GD, Bell PM. Effects of low dose versus conventional dose thiazide diuretic on insulin action in essential hypertension. Br Med J 1994;309;226–230.
66. Kopyt N, Dalal F, Narins RG. Renal retention of potassium in fruit. N Engl J Med 1985;313;582.
67. Murdoch DL, Gillen GJ, Morton JJ, Leckie E, Murray GD, Davies DL, McInnes GT. Twice-daily low-dose captopril in diuretic-treated hypertensives. J Hum Hypertens 1989;3;29–33.
68. Hollenberg NK, Michiewicz CW. Postmarketing surveillance in 70,898 patients treated with a triamterene/hydrochlorothiazide combination (Maxzide). Am J Cardiol 1989; 63:37B.
69. Hollenberg NK, Michiewicz C. Hyperkalaemia in diabetes mellitus. Effect of a triamterene-hydrochlorothiazide combination. Arch Intern Med 1989;149;1327.
70. McCaughan D. Hazards of non-prescription potassium supplements. Lancet 1984;i:513.
71. Lawson DH, O'Connor PC, Jick H. Drug attributed alterations in potassium handling in congestive heart failure. Eur J Clin Pharmacol 1982;23;21.
72. Reyes AJ, Leary WP. Cardiovascular toxicity of diuretics related to magnesium depletion. Hum Toxicol 1984;3;351.
73. Gettes LS. Electrolyte abnormalities underlying lethal and ventricular arrhythmias. Circulation 1992;85(Suppl I):I-70–I-76.
74. Davies DL, Fraser R. Do diuretics cause magnesium deficiency? Br J Clin Pharmacol 1993;36;1–10.
75. Leary WP. Diuretics and increase in urinary magnesium excretion: possible clinical relevance. In: Puschett JB, Greenberg A, eds. Diuretics IV: Chemistry, Pharmacology and Clinical Applications. Amsterdam: Elsevier, 1993;261–265.
76. Boulard JC, Hanslik T, Alterescu R, Baglin A. Symptomatic hypercalcaemia after thiazide diuretics and vitamin D: 2 cases in elderly women. Presse Med 1994, 23, 95.
77. La Croix AZ, Wienpahl J, White LR et al. Thiazide diuretic agents and the incidence of hip fracture. New Engl J Med 1990;322;286.
78. Ray WA, Griffin MR, Downey W, Melton LJ. Long-term use of thiazide diuretics and risk of hip fracture. Lancet 1989;i:687.
79. Felson DT, Sloutskis D, Anderson JJ, Anthony JM, Kiel DP. Thiazide diuretics and the risk of hip fractures. Results from the Framingham Study. J Am Med Assoc 1991; 265;370–373.
80. Wasnick R, Davis J, Ross P, Vogel J. Effect of thiazides on rates of bone mineral loss: a longitudinal study. Br Med J 1990;301;1303–1305.
81. Cauley JA, Cummings SR, Seeley DG, Black D, Browner W, Kuller LW, Nevitt MC. Effects of thiazide diuretic therapy on bone mass, fractures and falls. Ann Intern Med 1993;188;656–673.
82. Heidrich FE, Stergachis A, Gross KM. Diuretic drug use and the risk of hip fracture. Ann Intern Med 1991;115;1–6.
83. Browner WS, Seeley DG, Vogt TM, Cummings SR. Non-trauma mortality in elderly women with low bone mineral density. Lancet 1991;338;355–358.
84. Ray WA. Thiazide diuretics and osteoporosis: time for a clinical trial? Ann Intern Med 1991;115;64–65.
85. Green TP, Johnson DE, Bass JL et al. Prophylactic furosemide in severe respiratory distress syndrome: Blinded prospective study. J Paediatr 1988;12;605.
86. Atkinson SA, Shah JK, McGee C Steele BT. Mineral excretion in premature infants receiving various diuretic therapies. J Paediatr 1988;113;540.
87. Alon US, Scagliotti D, Garola RE. Nephrocalcinosis and nephrolithiasis in infants with congestive heart failure treated with furosemide. J Paediatr 1994, 125, 149–151.
88. Ramsay LE, Yeo WW, Jackson PR. Diuretics, impaired glucose tolerance and insulin resistance with diuretics. Eur Heart J 1992;13(Suppl G):68–71.
89. McVeigh GE, Dulie EB, Ravenscroft A et al. Low and conventional dose cyclopenthiazide on glucose and lipid metabolism in mild hypertension. Br J Clin Pharmacol 1989; 27;523.
90. Ramsay LE, Yeo WW, Jackson PR. Influence of diuretics, calcium antagonists, and α-blockers on insulin sensitivity and glucose tolerance in hypertensive patients. J Cardiovasc Pharmacol 1992;20(Suppl 11):S49–S54.
91. Weinberger MH. Mechanisms of diuretic effects on carbohydrate tolerance, insulin sensitivity and lipid levels. Eur Heart J 1992;13(Suppl G):5–9.
92. Johnston GD. Treatment of hypertension in older adults. Br Med J 1992;304;639.
93. Moser M. Diuretics and cardiovascular risk factors. Eur Heart J 1992;13(Suppl G):72–80.
94. Moser M. Diuretics should continue to be recommended as initial therapy in the treatment of hypertension. In: Puschett JB, Greenberg A, eds. Diuretics IV: Chemistry, Pharmacology and Clinical Applications. Amsterdam: Elsevier, 1993;465–476.
95. Moser M. Do different haemodynamic effects of antihypertensive drugs translate into different safety profiles? Eur J Clin Pharmacol 1990;38:S134–S138.
96. Waller PC, Ramsay LE. Predicting acute gout in diuretic-treated hypertensive patients. J Hum Hypertens 1989;3;457.
97. Myers MG. Hydrochlorothiazide with or without amiloride for hypertension in the elderly. A dose-titration study. Arch Intern Med 1987;147;1026.
98. Freis ED, Papademetriou V. How dangerous are diuretics? Drugs 1985;30;469.
99. Miller NE Plasma lipoproteins, antihypertensive drugs and coronary heart disease. J Cardiovasc Pharmacol 1985; 7:S105.

100. Spence JD. Effects of antihypertensive drugs on atherogenic factors: possible importance of drug selection in prevention of atherosclerosis. J Cardiovasc Pharmacol 1985; 7:S121.
101. Weinberger MH. Antihypertensive therapy and lipids: evidence, mechanisms and implications. Arch Intern Med 1985;145;1102.
102. Weidmann P, Ferrier C, Saxenhofer M et al. Serum lipoproteins during treatment with antihypertensive drugs. Drugs 1988;35(Suppl 6):118.
103. Falch DK, Schreiner A. The effect of spironolactone on lipid, glucose and uric acid levels in blood during long-term administration to hypertensives. Acta Med Scand 1983; 213;27.
104. The Treatment of Mild Hypertension Research Group. The Treatment of Mild Hypertension Study. A randomized, placebo-controlled trial of a nutritional-hygienic regimen alone with various drug monotherapies. Arch Intern Med 1991;151;1413–1423.
105. MacMahon SW, Macdonald GJ, Blacket RB. Plasma lipoprotein levels in treated and untreated hypertensive men and women. Arteriosclerosis 1985;5;391.
106. Wallace RB, Hunninghake DB, Chambless LE et al. A screening survey of dyslipoproteinaemias associated with prescription drug use. Circulation 1986;73(Suppl 1):I–70.
107. Tuomilehto J, Salonen JT, Nissenen A. Factors associated with changes in serum cholesterol during a community-based hypertension programme. Acta Med Scand 1985; 217;243.
108. Weidmann P, de Cousten M, Ferrari P. Effect of diuretics on the plasma lipid profile. Eur Heart J 1992;13(Suppl G):61–67.
109. Grimm RH, Cohen JD, McFate Smith W et al. Hypertension management in the Multiple Risk Factor Intervention Trial (MRFIT). Arch Intern Med 1985;145;1191.
110. Helgeland A, Strommen R, Hagelund CH et al. Enalapril, atenolol, and hydrochlorothiazide in mild to moderate hypertension. Lancet 1986;i:872.
111. Wassertheil-Smoller S, Blaufox MD, Oberman A, Davis BR, Swencionis C, Knerr MO'C, Hawkins CM, Langford HG. Effect of antihypertensives on sexual function and quality of life: the TAIM Study. Ann Intern Med 1991; 114;613–620.
112. Smith PJ, Talbert RL. Sexual dysfunction with antihypertensive and antipsychotic agents. Clin Pharm 1986;5;373.
113. Prisant LM, Carr AA, Bottini PS, Solursh DS, Solursh LP. Sexual dysfunction with antihypertensive drugs. Arch Intern Med 1994;154;730–736.
114. Medical Research Council Working Party on Mild to Moderate Hypertension. Adverse reactions to bendrofluazide and propranolol for the treatment of mild hypertension. Lancet 1981;ii:539.
115. Wagner AC. Interstitial pulmonary oedema due to hydrochlorothiazide: case report. Virginia Med 1983;110;715.
116. Parfrey NA, Herlong HF. Pulmonary oedema after hydrochlorothiazide. Br Med J 1984;288;1880.
117. Bowden FJ. Non-cardiogenic pulmonary oedema after ingestion of chlorothiazide. Br Med J 1989;298;605.
118. Kheir A, Chabot F, Lesur O, Gerard H, Delorme N, Polu JM. Cyclothiazide-induced fibrosing pneumonitis. Rev Mal Respir 1992;9;208–212.
119. Mountokalakis T, Dourakis S, Karatzas N et al. Zinc deficiency in mild hypertensive patients treated with diuretics. J Hypertens 1984;2(Suppl 3):571.
120. Geissler AH, Turnlund JR, Cohen RD. Effect of chlorthalidone on zinc levels, testosterone, and sexual function in man. Drug-Nutrient Interact 1986;4;275.
121. Beck ML, Clive JF, Hardman JT et al. Fatal intravascular immune haemolysis induced by hydrochlorothiazide. Am J Clin Pathol 1984;81;791.
122. Greenblatt DJ. Diuretics. In: Miller RR, Greenblatt DJ, eds. Drug Effects in Hospitalized Patients, Ch 10. New York: John Wiley and Sons, 1976;80.
123. Van der Linden W, Ritter B, Edlund G. Acute cholecystitis and thiazide. Br Med J 1984;289;654.
124. Kakar F, Weiss NS, Strite SA. Thiazide use and the risk of cholecystectomy in women. Am J Epidemiol 1986; 124;428.
125. Robinson HN, Morison WL, Hood AF. Thiazide diuretic therapy and chronic photosensitivity. Arch Dermatol 1985;121;522.
126. Parodi A, Romagnoli M, Rebora A. Subacute cutaneous lupus erythmatosus-like eruption caused by hydrochlorothiazide. Photodermatology 1989;6;100.
127. Reed BR, Huff JC, Jones SK et al. Subacute cutaneous lupus erythematosus associated with hydrochlorothiazide therapy. Ann Intern Med 1985;103;49.
128. Westly ED, Wechsler HL. Toxic epidermal necrolysis: granulocytic leukopenia as a prognostic indicator. Arch Dermatol 1984;120;721.
129. Grunwald MH, Halevy S, Livni E. Allergic vasculitis induced by hydrochlorothiazide: confirmation by mast cell degranulation test. Isr J Med Sci 1989;25;572.
130. Baker EJ, Reed KD, Dixon SL. Chlorthalidone-induced pseudoporphyria: clinical and microscopic findings of a case. J Am Acad Dermatol 1989;5;1026.
131. Kang JS, Kim TH, Park KB. Hydrochlorothiazide-induced phototoxic reaction. Korean J Dermatol 1992; 30;529–534.
132. Descamps C. Rhabdomyolysis and acute tubular necrosis associated with carbenoxolone and diuretic treatment. Br Med J 1977;1;272.
133. Gora ML, Seth SK, Bay WH, Visconti JA. Milk-alkali syndrome associated with the use of chlorothiazide and calcium carbonate. Clin Pharm 1989;8;227.
134. Webster J, Robb OJ, Witte K, Petrie JC. Single doses of enalapril and atenolol in hypertensive patients treated with bendrofluazide. J Hypertens 1987;5;457.
135. Watson ML, Bell GM, Muir AL. Captopril-diuretic combinations in severe renovascular disease: a cautionary note. Lancet 1983;ii:404.
136. Tiller DJ, Hall BM, Horvarth JS et al. Gout and hyperuricaemia in patients on cyclosporin and diuretics. Lancet 1985;i:453.
137. Anonymous. Bemetizide/triamterene: warning of allergic vasculitis. WHO Drug Inform 1988;2;148.
138. Bing RF, Russell GI, Swales JD et al. Indapamide and bendrofluazide: a comparison in the management of essential hypertension. Br J Clin Pharmacol 1981;12;883.
139. Newstead CG, Moore RH, Barnes AJ. Interstitial nephritis associated with indapamide. Br Med J 1990;300;1344.
140. Donovan KL. Neutropenia and metolazone. Br Med J 1989;299;981.
141. Critchlow AS, Freeborn SF, Roddie RA. Potassium supplements during treatment of glaucoma with acetazolamide. Br Med J 1984;289;21.
142. Sweeney KR, Chapron DJ, Brandt JL et al. Toxic interaction between acetazolamide and salicylate: case reports

and a pharmacokinetic explanation. Clin Pharmacol Ther 1986;40;518.
143. Keisu M, Wilholm B-E, Öst A, Mortimer Ö. Acetozalamide-associated aplastic anaemia. J Intern Med 1990; 228;627–632.
144. Naranjo CA, Busto U, Cassis L. Furosemide-induced adverse reactions during hospitalization. Am J Hosp Pharm 1978;35;794.
145. Böttiger LE, Westerholm B. Thrombocytopenia. II. Drug-induced thrombocytopoenia. Acta Med Scand 1972; 191;541.
146. De Gruchy GC. Thrombocytopenia. In: Drug-induced Blood-Disorders. Ch 6. Oxford: Blackwell, 1975:118.
147. Lin RY. Unusual autoimmune manifestations in furosemide-associated hypersensitivity angiitis. NY State J Med 1988;88;439.
148. Ihu H, Shimozuma H. Bullous pemphigoid induced by furosemide. Nishinihon J Dermatol 1993;55;890–893.
149. Guerrera V, Carbone RL. Bullous pemphigoid induced by furosemide. G Ital Dermatol Venereol 1994, 129, 239–241.
150. Eom SC, Chae YS, Suh KS, Kim ST. The clinical features of lichenoid drug eruption and the histopathological differentiation between lichenoid drug eruption and lichen planus. Korean J Dermatol 1994, 32, 1019–1025.
151. Cobb MW. Furosemide-induced eruption simulating Sweet's syndrome. J Am Acad Dermatol 1989;21;339.
152. Tuzel IH. A comparison of adverse reaction to bumetanide and furosemide. J Clin Pharmacol 1981;21;615.
153. Taggart AJ, McDevitt DG. Diuretic withdrawal—a need for caution. Curr Med Res Opin 1983;8;501.
154. Grinstead WC, Francis MJ, Marks GF, Tawa CB, Zoghbi WI, Young JB. Discontinuation of chronic diuretic therapy in stable congestive heart failure secondary to coronary artery disease or to idiopathic dilated cardiomyopathy. Am J Cardiol 1994, 73, 881–886.
155. Berkowitz RL, Coustan DR, Mochizuki TK. Furosemide (Lasix). In: Handbook for Prescribing Medications during Pregnancy. Boston, MA: Little, Brown and Co, 1981;95.
156. Dailey JW. Anticoagulant and cardiovascular drugs. In: Wilson JT, ed. Drugs in Breast Milk, Ch 10. Lancaster: MTP Press, 1981;61.
157. Freestone S, Ramsay LE. Frusemide and spironolactone in resistant hypertension: a controlled trial. J Hypertens 1983;1(Suppl 2):326.
158. Wollam GL, Tarazi RC, Bravo EL. Diuretic potency of combined hydrochlorothiazide and furosemide therapy in patients with azotemia. Am J Med 1982;72;929.
159. Brown CB, Ogg CS, Cameron JS et al. High dose frusesmide in acute reversible intrinsic renal failure. Scott Med J 1974;19;35.
160. Thomsen J, Bech P, Szpirt W. Otological problems in chronic renal failure: the possible role of aminoglycoside-furosemide interaction. Arch Oto-Rhino-Laryngol 1976; 214;71.
161. Lawson DH, Tilstone WJ, Gray JMB et al. Effect of furosemide on the pharmacokinetics of gentamicin in patients. J Clin Pharmaocl 1982;22;254.
162. Dodds MG, Foord RD. Enhancement by potent diuretics of renal tubular necrosis induced by cephaloridine. Br J Pharmacol 1970;40;227.
163. Kleinknecht D, Jungers P, Fillastre J-P. Nephrotoxicity of cephaloridine. Ann Intern Med 1974;80;421.
164. Simpson IJ. Nephrotoxicity and acute renal failure associated with cephalotin and cephaloridine. NZ Med J 1971;74;312.
165. Norrby R, Stenqvist K, Elgefors B. Interaction between cephaloridine and furosemide in man. Scand J Infect Dis 1976;8;209.
166. Plouvier B, Baclet P, De Coninck P. Une association néphrotoxique: mannitol et furosémide. Nouv Presse Méd 1981;10;1744.
167. Miller RD, Sohn YJ, Matteo RS. Enhancement of *d*-tubocurarine neuromuscular blockade by diuretics in man. Anaesthesiology 1976;45;422.
168. Hurtig HI, Dyson WL. Lithium toxicity enhanced by diuresis. N Engl J Med 1974;290;748.
169. Hogg KJ, Hillis WS. Captopril/metolazone induced renal failure. Lancet 1986;i:501.
170. Reed S, Greene P, Ryan T, Cerimele B, Schwertschlag U, Weinberger M, Voelker J. The renin angiotensin aldosterone system and frusemide response in congestive heart failure. Br J Clin Pharmacol 1995;39;51–57.
171. Ahmad S. Renal insensitivity to frusemide caused by chronic anticonvulsant therapy. Br Med J 1974;3;657.
172. Fine A, Henderson IS, Morgan DR et al. Malabsorption of frusemide caused by phenytoin. Br Med J 1977;4;1061.
173. Brooks PM, Bell P, Lee P et al. The effect of frusemide on indomethacin plasma levels. Br J Clin Pharmacol 1974;1;485.
174. Benet LZ. Pharmacokinetics pharmacodynamics of furosemide in man: a review. J Pharmacokinet Biopharm 1979;7;1.
175. Bartoli E, Arras S, Faedda R et al. Blunting of furosemide diuresis by aspirin in man. J Clin. Pharmacol 1980;20;452.
176. Mousson C, Justrabo E, Tanter Y et al. Néphrite interstitielle et hépatite aigués granulomateuses d'origine médicamenteuse: rôle possible de l'association allopurinol-furosémide. Néphrologie 1986;5;199.
177. Halstenson CE, Matzke GR. Bumetanide: a new loop diuretic. Drug Intell Clin Pharm 1983;17;786.
178. Ward A, Heel RC. Bumetanide: a review of its pharmacodynamic and pharmacokinetic properties and therapeutic use. Drugs 1984;28;426.
179. Gilli M, Papurello D, Cutin IC et al. Azione neurotossica della muzolimina ad alte dosi in pazienti uremica. Osservazione su un gruppo di 29 soggetti. Minerva Urol Nefrol 1989;41;215.
180. Rose LI, Underwood RH, Newmark SR et al. Pathophysiology of spironolactone-induced gynecomastia. Ann Intern Med 1977;87:398.
181. Committee on Safety of Medicines. Spironolactone. Curr Probl 1988;21.
182. Ochs HR, Greenblatt DJ, Bodem G et al. Spironolactone. Am Heart J 1978;96;389.
183. Shuck J, Shen S, Owensby L et al. Spironolactone hepatitis in primary hyperaldosteronism. Ann Intern Med 1981;95;708.
184. Carsuzaa F, Pierre C, Dubegny M. Erythème annulaire centrifugé à l'aldactone. Ann Dermatol Venereol 1977; 114:375.
185. McInnes GT, Shelton JR, Ramsay LE. Evaluation of aldosterone antagonists in healthy man. Methods Find Exp Clin Pharmacol 1982;4;49.
186. Hollifield JW. Failure of aspirin to antagonize the antihypertensive effect of spironolactone in low-renin hypertension. South Med J 1976;69;1034.
187. Tweeddale MG. Antagonism between antipyretic anal-

gesic drugs and spironolactone in man. Clin Res 1974;22:727A.
188. Doll R, Langman MJS, Shawdon HH. Treatment of gastric ulcer with carbenoxolone: antagonistic effects of spironolactone. Gut 1968;9;42.
189. Emili M, Cuppone R, Ricci GL. Comparative clinical study of spironolactone and potassium canrenoate. A randomised evaluation with double cross-over. Arzneim Forsch 1988;38;1492.
190. Maronde RF, Milgrom M, Vlachakis ND. Response of thiazide-induced hypokalaemia to amiloride. J Am Med Assoc 1983;249;237.
191. Vidt DG. Mechanisms of action, pharmacokinetics, adverse effects, and therapeutic uses of amiloride hydrochloride, a new potassium-sparing diuretic. Pharmacotherapy 1981;1;179.
192. Bailey RR. Adverse renal reactions to non-steroidal anti-inflammatory drugs and potassium-sparing diuretics. Adverse Drug Reaction Bull 1988;131;492.
193. Anonymous. Moduretic—anaphylactic shock. Adverse Reactions Newsletter, Nos. 3—4. Uppsala: WHO Collaborating Centre for Adverse Drug Reaction Monitoring, 1988.
194. Duff HJ, Mitchell LB, Kavanagh KM et al. Amiloride. Antiarrhythmic and electrophysiologic actions in patients with inducible sustained ventricular tachycardia. Circulation, 1989;79;1257.
195. Reed PI, Lewis SI, Vincent-Brown A et al. The influence of amiloride on the therapeutic and metabolic effects of carbonoxolone in patients with gastric ulcer. Scand J Gastroenterol 1980;15(Suppl 65):51.
196. Fernandez de Corres, Berneola G, Fernandez E et al. Photodermatitis from triamterene. Contact Dermatitis 1978;17;114.
197. Safdi AM. Fever secondary to triamterene. N Engl J Med 1980;303;701.
198. Motley RJ. Pseudoporphyria due to Dyazide in a patient with vitiligo. Br Med J 1990;300;1468.
199. Bailey RR, Lynn KL, Drennan CJ et al. Triamterene-induced acute interstitial nephritis, Lancet 1982;i:226.
200. Favre L, Glasson P, Valloton MB. Reversible acute renal failure from combined triamterene and indomethacin. Ann Intern Med 1982;96;317.
201. White DJ, Nancollas GH. Triamterene and renal stone formation. J Urol 1982;127;593.
202. Jick H, Dinan BJ, Hunter JR. Triamterene and renal stones. J Urol 1982;127;224.
203. Sica DA, Gehr TWB. Triamterene and the kidney. Nephron 1989;51;454.
204. Lo TCN, Cryer RJ. Complete heart block induced by hyperkalaemia associated with treatment with a combination of captopril and spironolactone. Br Med J 1986;292;1672.
205. Lakhani M. Complete heart block induced by hyperkalaemia associated with treatment with a combination of captopril and spironolactone. Br Med J 1986;293;271.

Meyler's Side Effects of Drugs, 13th Edition
M.N.G. Dukes, editor

SECTION EDITOR: P. FOLB

M.N.G. Dukes

22 Metals

GENERAL INTRODUCTION

Metals and their derivatives have always played a role in medicine but the uses to which are (or have been) put and the risks which their use entails are extremely diverse. Some—and particularly the inorganic compounds—have had their day, generally because the dangers which they introduced were disproportionate to any medical benefit which they may have offered. Others, in one form or another, still have their place. The fact must not be overlooked that metal compounds are often encountered in a number of non-prescription and 'alternative' remedies, often without justification. It should also be noted that in spite of the diversity there are some parallels between the adverse effects produced by metals which can be useful in assessing reports; the encephalopathies produced by aluminium, bismuth and lead are a case in point.

This Chapter will not deal with the substitution of trace metal deficiencies, with the adverse effects of excessive sodium or potassium levels, or with adverse effects due to non-medical exposure to metal compounds, e.g. as a result of environmental contamination. It has to be borne in mind, however, that the effects of combined medical and non-medical exposure may have to be considered (1^R).

Aluminium *(see also Chapter 36)*

Aluminium is widely used in medicine, pharmacy, food technology and cosmetics. While the aluminium load from environmental sources is still small, increasing concern has developed about the risk—benefit relationship of aluminium preparations used for therapeutic purposes.

External use Water-soluble aluminium compounds such as aluminium acetate, aluminium chlorate, basic aluminium chloride, potassium aluminium sulfate (alum) and others have long been used as mild external antiseptic, astringent, antihydrotic or styptic agents, administered to the skin or mucous membranes. Some remain in popular use. Aluminium chloride is also a constituent of many deodorant and antiperspirant sprays. These compounds may occasionally cause skin irritation in sensitive individuals. Wound dressings and sheets impregnated with metallic aluminium are considered useful in the management of burns and oozing wounds.

Significant adverse effects are rare unless the circumstances lead to a high degree of absorption. Acute aluminium toxicity in one reported case, for example, followed introduction of aluminium sulphate (alum) into the urinary tract to treat hemorrhagic cystitis; here there was apparently both increased absorption, due to the mucosal lesion of the bladder wall, and an increased susceptibility due to pre-existing renal failure (SED-12; 2^C).

Internal use Aluminium is employed for its adsorptive capacities in antidiarrheal drugs and vaccines, while its use in antacids exploits its pH-modifying properties. Furthermore, aluminium compounds are prescribed on a large scale to patients with chronic renal insufficiency. Aluminium forms poorly soluble phosphates in the gastrointestinal tract and thereby decreases the serum phosphate level, which is frequently elevated in chronically uremic patients. Aluminium preparations for internal use primarily comprise aluminium hydroxide, basic aluminium carbonate and aluminium phosphate, although the use of the latter in hyperphosphatemia seems irrational.

Aluminium hydroxide

When used as a prescribed antacid, administration of the hydroxide is usually limited in time, but the total daily dose may attained 10 grams or more; in self-medication it may be used for years at a time. When it is prescribed for hyperphosphatemia in chronic renal failure, chronic administration is usually necessary; the average total daily dose required here is 6—8 grams (SED-12, 513).

The amount of aluminium in the body is normally very low because the gastrointestinal tract, skin and lungs are excellent barriers to its entry, and the small amounts which pass these barriers are efficiently eliminated by the kidneys. However, problems can arise if the natural protective barriers are bypassed and/or there is impaired renal function (see 'Risk situations' below).

Nervous system In 1976, aluminium was first incriminated as a cause of *dialysis encephalopathy*. This syndrome can occur in chronically dialyzed patients and has often proved fatal within a few months of the appearance of the initial symptoms. Difficulties in speech, disturbances of consciousness, and ataxia were followed by psychotic episodes, personality changes, myoclonic jerks, EEG abnormalities, convulsions and dementia. Accumulation of aluminium could be demonstrated in the grey matter of the brain and in other tissues.

The fact that aluminium is involved is demonstrated by the diminution of symptoms which usually occurs after reduction of the oral aluminium in hemodialysis solutions (and use of deferoxamine therapy). and supported by the occurrence of a progressive encephalopathy in aluminium plant workers and miners exposed to aluminium dust, as well as by animal experiments. However, not every instance of dialysis encephalopathy can be considered due to aluminium. The condition appears to fall into three categories: (a) a sporadic endemic type of unknown origin and having no known association with aluminium; (b) an epidemic type often related to levels of aluminium in the dialysis fluid; (c) a childhood type possibly due to uremia and having no known link to aluminium.

In recent years the theory has been advanced that aluminium may be linked to the etiology of *Alzheimer's disease* (2[R]), the suggestion being that the mechanism could be inhibition of tetrahydrobiopterin synthesis in the temporal cortex. Others have rejected an association between the metal and the disease, but the debate continues (3[R]).

Metabolic *Hypophosphatemia, hypophosphaturia and hypercalciuria* are consequences of chronic ingestion of aluminium hydroxide. Symptoms of phosphorus depletion include *bone pain*, *debility*, *muscle weakness*, *anorexia and malaise*. Even relatively small doses of commonly used aluminium-containing fluid antacids (90—120 ml/day) can lead to adverse effects on calcium and phosphorus metabolism. During long-term therapy, a considerable loss of calcium may occur, resulting in *skeletal demineralization* (4[R]). Aluminium overload may in addition have a toxic effect on the bones: collagen synthesis and matrix mineralization are affected, resulting in a vitamin D-resistant osteomalacia (5[R]). These effects of aluminium overload on the bones respond to reduction in aluminium exposure; in chronic hemodialysis, it is clear that aluminium-related bone disease can be prevented by diminishing aluminium exposure (6[C]).

Hematological Aluminium overload in uremic patients may lead to a *microcytic hypochromic anemia* (7[C]). The mechanism is unknown, but it appears to involve inhibition of heme synthesis, either by inhibition of enzyme activity or by interference with the incorporation or utilization of iron. The anemia can be reversed by lowering the aluminium intake or by chelation therapy with deferoxamine.

Gastrointestinal Aluminium hydroxide may cause *constipation*. Large doses may be associated with fecal impaction and the development of intestinal obstruction in uremic patients. Animal experiments suggest that aluminium may play a role in the pathogenesis of parenteral nutrition-induced *hepatobiliary dysfunction* (8).

Urinary system Irrigation of the urinary bladder with alum successfully controls vesical hematuria but it can cause *bladder spasm* (9[c]), and in patients with renal disease it can undesirably increase the aluminium load to the point where an encephalopathy is induced (SEDA-17, 273).

Effect on the immune response Aluminium has a non-specific immunosuppressive action which results in a lower incidence of transplant rejection in patients with high aluminium concentrations in the tissues; in the first instance one might consider this a reason for seeking to maintain a particularly high aluminum level in transplant patients. However, there are good reasons not to do so. Firstly, should infection occur, this immunosuppressive effect can lead to increased risk and even greater mortality. Secondly, after transplantations there already is a high aluminium level because of mobilization of aluminium from the storage pool. Aluminium loading before transplant should therefore be avoided and excessive levels countered (10[r]). Other work, in dialysis patients, has confirmed the fact that an increased aluminium load raises the risk of infections (11[C])

Risk situations As noted above, the principle risk situations are those in which an *unusual amount* of aluminium enters the system or the body cannot handle its aluminium load because of *impaired renal function*. A high level of medical intake is sometimes overlooked; toxic effects of aluminium have for instance been identified in patients treated with total parenteral nutrition contaminated with aluminium (12[R]); high levels of aluminium have been detected in some intravenously administered solutions, such as human serum albumin (13[c]); finally, the possibility of unnoticed self-medication with antacids needs to be considered.

In many patients with severe renal disease there is a double risk: they are exposed to aluminium as a part of their treatment (in agents given for the control of serum phosphate levels, in aluminium-containing dialysis fluids and, in a recent case, in the form of bladder irrigation with alum (14[c]), and at the same time they have little ability to eliminate it. Aluminium-containing phosphate binders are especially risky if used in combination with an alkalinizing citrate solution (Sohl's solution) (15[c], 16[r]); due to the formation of an aluminium citrate complex in the gastrointestinal tract aluminium is absorbed more readily. In addition, aluminium citrate complex has a synergistic inhibition action on bone growth and thus exacerbates aluminium-associated osteomalacia in chronic renal failure. Unsuspected intake of citrate from other sources has also apparently promoted appearance of aluminium encephalopathy in a case of renal failure (17[c]).

Children with impaired renal function may be particularly susceptible to aluminium intoxication solely from oral aluminium loading (18[R]). As noted above, these situations are avoidable and the harm thus preventible. In all patients with chronic renal failure, strict supervision of the total aluminium intake is vital. The administration of aluminium should be stopped as soon as the serum level exceeds 150 μg/ml or at the appearance of the first symptoms of encephalopathy (19[R]). According to current recommendations, dialyzate solutions should contain less than 10 μg of aluminium per liter (20[c]). There is some controversy as to the belief that aluminium-containing medications used to control serum phosphate levels in uremic subjects should be replaced by calcium-containing phosphate binders (21[R]). Another approach used to reduce the toxic risks of aluminium hydroxide may be the adaptation of the prescribed doses to the phosphate concentration in serum, i.e. individualizing aluminium gel therapy (SED-12, 515). Deferoxamine has been proved to be an effective treatment for aluminium overload in uremic patients (SEDA-11, 204), but several reports have shown that deferoxamine can induce an exacerbation of aluminium encephalopathy (22[C]); see also Chapter 23), possibly due to increased aluminium levels in the cerebrospinal fluid (23, 24[C]). In addition, treatment with deferoxamine has been associated with other risks which justify its cautious use (see Chapter 23). During treatment, plasma aluminium levels should be monitored, as levels exceeding 800—1000 μg/l might exacerbate the encephalopathy.

Interactions The laboratory finding that aluminium hydroxide will bind a variety of drugs, thus forming poorly absorbable salts or complexes, has led to a general rule of thumb that the patient should wait 1—2 hours after taking aluminium compounds before other drugs are taken. The reduced absorption of tetracyclines under these conditions is of proven significance, but in most other instances the theoretical interactions seem to be clinically irrelevant and result in delayed rather than reduced drug absorption. It is still prudent to take the traditional precaution where one is taking any drug with a steep dose-response curve and narrow therapeutic margin, such as *digitalis*. Interactions with *diflunisal* and with *prednisone* may be of clinical importance in cases of chronic liver disease (SEDA-6, 315). The interaction with *citrate* is discussed under 'Risk situations' above.

Arsenic

Arsenic and arsenicals must be considered obsolete in medicine because of their limited therapeutic value, their multi-system toxicity, and their apparent carcinogenic properties. The interested reader is referred to reviews in much earlier editions of this volume (SED-8, 502; SED-9, 368). Cases are still experienced of patients with late effects of obsolete preparations such as Fowler's solution or Neosalvarsan (SEDA-16, 231).

Chronic arsenic poisoning is marked by edema of the eyelids and face, mucosal inflammation, pruritus, anorexia, vomiting and diarrhea. Long-term use of small doses may produce keratinization and dryness of the skin, sometimes with frank dermatitis and pigmentation; alopecia can follow, and basal cell epithelioma is a late effect (25[Cr]). In the long run there is serious damage to the internal organs.

Bismuth

Despite the declining role of bismuth, the remarkable data on *bismuth encephalopathy* which emerged some 25 years ago need to be recalled briefly here, if only because a recurrence might be anticipated if bismuth in some form were to enjoy a revival.

Bismuth enjoyed great popularity down to the early 20th century; thereafter it continued to be used in the form of insoluble bismuth compounds, employed for their supposed effects on the gastric wall as antacids, protective 'coatings' or inhibitors of proteolytic activity. The use of bismuth remained particularly heavy in Australia, where bismuth subgallate was commonly used in post-colectomy or post-ileostomy patients, and in France where bismuth subnitrate and other salts were widely self-administered for both gastric and intestinal conditions. Though organic injury, skin disorders and blue-line coloration of the gums were attributed to parenteral bismuth, these oral preparations were regarded as safe.

In 1973 and later however, both countries experienced numerous cases of an encephalopathy among bismuth users. By 1979, 945 cases had been recorded in France alone, 72 of them fatal; the worldwide total exceeded 1000 cases.

Three phases of this toxic brain syndrome may be distinguished (SEDA-4 167; 26[R]):

(*a*) *Prodromal phase* This is characterized by such vague complaints as asthenia, mental slowness, short memory, decreased working capacity, insomnia, headache and anxiety; they may easily be dismissed as non-specific, and may persist for more than 2 years before further signs develop. In general, however, the course is gradually progressive towards the symptoms of the next phase.

(*b*) *Acute phase* Sudden deterioration to an acute encephalopathy occurs over a period ranging from several hours to 1–2 days. Patients develop dysarthria, severe locomotor disturbances such as ataxia, difficulty in walking, intention tremor, myoclonic jerks (especially of the upper limbs, face and trunk), incontinence due to loss of sphincter control, hyperreflexia and sometimes generalized convulsions. The patient may be confused, disoriented and agitated. Excitation, hallucinations, delirium and fluctuations of mental alertness ranging from dizziness to loss of consciousness and coma may occur. In about 7–9% of cases the outcome is fatal due to bronchopulmonary, cardiovascular, thromboembolic or infectious complications.

(*c*) *Recovery phase* After the withdrawal of bismuth the toxic symptoms usually recede rapidly, though physical and psychic asthenia, depressive mood alterations, memory impairment, intellectual deterioration, sleep disturbances, headache and other symptoms may occasionally persist for several months, and in isolated cases for more than a year. Exceptionally, psychic and intellectual capacity may remain permanently impaired.

The reason for the suddenness of the outbreak of bismuth encephalopathy after the drug had been used for so many years remains uncertain. A major French epidemiological study undertaken at the time by INSERM (SEDA-6, 217) failed to detect any clear link to particular dosage habits, topographical factors or drug interactions. Unknown environmental factors may have affected either the effects of bismuth itself or the sensitivity of the brain. More recently it has been suggested that a change in intestinal flora converted bismuth salts into more soluble neurotoxic compounds (27[C]), though it is not clear why this should have happened during the 1970s. Since measures were taken to counter the traditional use of bismuth, only very occasional new cases of encephalopathy have been reported. It is unresolved at present whether the lower doses of bismuth in gastric powders, antacids, astringents, demulcents, purgatives or antidiarrheal preparations which are still in use are in the long run innocuous; if an unknown environmental factor indeed led to toxic manifestations with the older products, it might similarly modify the effects of others; watchfulness is therefore essential. Following the literature, indeed, one suspects something of a renaissance of bismuth encephalopathy in the 1990s; in 1993 cases were reported from several countries, associated inter alia with abuse of bismuth subsalicylate ('Pepto-Bismol') (28[c]) and use of bismuth subgallate (29[C]).

Gastrointestinal *Constipation* is an occasional side effect of bismuth therapy. The *feces are grey- or black-colored* which may be mistaken for melena.

Musculoskeletal *Osteoarthropathy* was associated with bismuth encephalopathy (see above) in some 3% of reported cases of the latter. However, at least one case is on record in which a bismuth osteoarthropathy developed without any manifestation of encephalopathy. The symptoms mainly involve one or both shoulders, of which a painful restriction of movement is usually the first sign in the post-acute phase of bismuth encephalopathy. This may persist for several months after the intake of bismuth has been stopped. X-ray examination reveals an osteolytic, deforming glenohumeral osteoarthropathy with necrosis of the humeral head. Unilateral or bilateral fractures may occur. The lesions described can regress without sequelae over a period of several months, or osteonecrosis may also proceed to complete lysis of the humeral head.

The fact that much bismuth is ordinarily stored in the skeleton may be relevant in the etiology of bismuth osteoarthropathy. It may be noted that in two reported cases a differing type of osteopathy has occurred, associated with a different localization of the pathological lesions and with unusually high bismuth concentrations in the bone: both patients had received bismuth injections for syphilis many months or even years before (SEDA-4, 169).

Risk situations Bismuth is predominantly excreted via the kidney and it would be expected to accumulate in patients with *renal insufficiency*. It is not impossible that combined exposure to bismuth and *other metals* could render the patient more susceptible to bismuth toxicity; the parallels between the complications seen here and with other light metals (zinc, aluminium) are striking.

Second-generation effects Very little is known about the use of bismuth in pregnancy, but in documented cases mothers affected with bismuth encephalopathy during pregnancy gave birth to healthy infants.

Topical preparations Severe systemic intoxications have in the past been observed following incautious use of bismuth salts on extensive wound areas.

Newer bismuth preparations and anti-ulcer

drugs Approximately at the time when the epidemic of bismuth encephalopathy occurred, some new types of bismuth preparation appeared, and the question naturally arose—and is still not entirely solved—whether these might in some situations produce the same complication. *Tripotassium dicitratobismuthate* (*DeNol®*) and *bicitropeptide* are both intended for treating gastric disorders. Due to the formation of an insoluble bismuth chloride complex in the gastric juice, the diffusion of the bismuth ion into the circulation is delayed. During treatment with DeNol plasma concentrations of bismuth rise to 10—20 μg/l which is not regarded as toxic. From field experience over somewhat more than 20 years it would seem that the inherent risks of bismuth intoxication are relatively small if these compounds are used within the recommended ranges of dosage and length of treatment. Since they belong to the small group of anti-ulcer products which have been shown to act against *Campylobacter pylori* medical opinion has generally favoured their retention. However they too can be abused, resulting in renal tubular damage (SEDA-18, 241) and attention has been drawn to the possible risks resulting from the ready absorption of citrate (30[R]).

Cobalt

Cobalt has been used in the treatment of anemia because of its erythropoietic action. It is toxic to many organs, and its medicinal benefits have repeatedly been questioned. In most countries the use of cobalt in anemia has been abandoned, though it is possible that in very rare cases there may be a need for it. If it is still to be used at all, the administration of cobalt ought to be entrusted to the experienced clinical hematologist. References to possible adverse reactions may be found in older editions of this volume. One tragic case in 1989 concerned a 13-month-old baby treated with a commercial iron-cobalt preparation which was still on sale, resulting in *hypothyroidism*, *cardiomyopathy*, *polycythemia* and *hypertrichosis* (SEDA-16, 231).

Metallic cobalt is referred to under 'Metal implants and prostheses' (see below).

Copper

Copper in intrauterine devices (IUDs) Mechanical problems associated with the use of IUDs are the field of the gynecologist and will only marginally be referred to this section (see also Chapter 48).

There is a steady loss of copper with increasing duration of IUD use, though the rate of loss shows a marked individual variation. Copper may act rather aggressively on tissue. Its ability to induce the generation of free radicals and malonaldehyde may contribute to its contraceptive effect and likewise to the low-level inflammatory reaction which is likely to be encountered shortly after the insertion of the device and which is presumbly also of contraceptive significance. A positive correlation has been shown between high copper loss and development of *menorrhagia* or pathological lesions such as *cervical dysplasia and endometrial cytopathology* (31[Cr]). Evidence of endometrial carcinoma was not found in endometrial aspirates from 189 women who had used Copper-T-200 devices for 1—10 years, but five cases of *endometrial hyperplasia* (2.67%) were encountered in women in the series, all of whom had worn copper IUDs for 6 years or more. Inflammatory changes in the endometrial cells were found in 12 cases (6.2%), 11 of 12 being wearers for over 3 years. It is conceivable that the constant exposure to copper may be responsible for persistence of chronic inflammatory changes in the endometrial cells, which could be the precursors of hyperplastic changes. It is not clear whether the dissolved copper is also responsible for the temporarily increased predisposition to *bacterial contamination* and the somewhat increased risk of *pelvic inflammatory disease*, seen especially in young nulliparous women using this contraceptive method.

If copper-containing fragments of IUDs perforate the uterine wall and enter the peritoneal cavity, acute inflammatory reactions and *peritoneal adhesions* may occur. Laparoscopic removal is then not only as a rule impossible but may also be dangerous because of the marked peritoneal reaction surrounding the copper part of the IUDs. Laparotomy has therefore been suggested as the primary measure in such cases. Whether copper IUDs result more commonly in perforation than non-copper devices is not entirely clear, nor is the question answered whether copper increases the risk of extra-uterine pregnancies, though older evidence suggested this as a risk (SED-9, 371).

Skin rash, *generalized urticaria* and *eczematoid eruptions* have occurred as a result of allergy to the copper released from IUDs, although they are extremely rare (SEDA-11, 204; SEDA-12, 186).

Second-generation effects The estimated frequency of pregnancy in women using copper IUDs is 2—3 per 100 woman-years; a significant number of early pregnancies are thus likely to be exposed to the influence of copper in the uterus. In a case where pregnancy occurred in the presence of such a device the neonate showed significantly increased copper and ceruloplasmin levels, whereas maternal levels were within the normal range. Whether such exposure to copper can cause harm is not clear; because of the pharmacological effects mentioned above, it has been suspected of having mutagenic and carcinogenic potential. Until now, there is no clear evidence that harm is actually done. Five published cases scattered throughout the literature in which incomplete closure of the neural tube was found (32[Cr]) could have been coincidental, bearing in mind the large number of pregnancies in which exposure to copper must occur in this way. In various species of animals which have been studied (rat, rabbit, hamster, sheep) no teratogenicity of intrauterine copper was detected (SED-11, 442).

Edetic acid *(see also Chapter 23)*

Ethylene diaminetetra-acetic acid (EDTA) is an anticoagulant used in the vials in which specimens for blood cell counting are collected. In vitro appearances suggesting pseudothrombocytopenia caused by EDTA-induced platelet clumping was first described in 1973. The phenomenon seems to be more frequent with blood from hospitalized and ill patients (1.9%) than in outpatients (0.09%) (33[R]). When pseudothrombocytopenia is suspected and a stained smear of blood containing EDTA shows platelet clumping, testing should be repeated with blood collected in a tube containing 3.8% sodium citrate solution as anticoagulant.

Gallium

Gallium has been used both in the form of a radiopharmaceutical (^{67}Ga as the citrate) and experimentally as a therapeutic agent in certain malignancies since gallium nitrate has been shown to be concentrated in various neoplasms in both animals and man. This compound has proved effective in animal tumor screening and was found to possess preclinical anti-tumor activity in man. A Phase I clinical evaluation in 58 patients, however, indicated dose-related *nephrotoxicity*; as a consequence, doses of 700 mg/m^2 should not be exceeded. Hematological toxicity was minimal, but *ototoxicity* was observed in one patient. Nephrotoxicity was again the major adverse effect in a Phase II evaluation with 700 mg/m^2 administered at intervals of 2—3 weeks. One death was considered to have been due to kidney damage by gallium nitrate. Other adverse effects observed were *nausea and/or vomiting* (33%), *maculopapular skin rash* (5%), a metallic taste (4%) and diarrhea (3.4%) (34[Cr]).

In a Phase II study in advanced breast cancer (35[Cr]) toxic reactions were mild; five of 26 women developed mild nausea, while minimal renal dysfunction was found in six patients. In this study an adequate diuresis was ensured with 5% dextrose/saline, and this may reduce the risk of nephrotoxicity. In a study of the use of gallium nitrate in malignant lymphoma (a constant infusion in doses ranging from 200 to 400 mg/m^2 daily for 7 days) reversible mild increases in serum creatinine concentration occurred in 20% of the patients. Other toxic effects included *diarrhea*, *hypocalcemia* and *hypomagnesemia*. Concomitant treatment with aminoglycoside antibiotics in two cases resulted in acute *renal failure* (36[C]).

The pharmacokinetics of gallium have been reported to be altered in patients with acute renal dysfunction, and in patients who have received multiple doses of gallium or other metal-based chemotherapy. This clearly suggests situations in which the treatment should be used reluctantly or not at all (SED-12, 519).

Germanium

In several countries, organic or inorganic germanium has acquired a remarkable reputation in self-medication as a widely useful prophylactic and therapeutic, with little scientific evidence to support it. Some germanium compounds, particularly spirogermanium, do have certain immunoregulatory activities, but germanium itself does not seem to play a role in this. Some severe *nephrotoxic reactions* have been described, and it has become clear that these can occur both with inorganic and organic germanium compounds. One middle-aged woman who had taken germanium lactate-citrate for at least a year (with an estimated cumulative dose of 32.1 grams germanium) developed renal insufficiency with a creatinine clearance of 10 ml/min, elevated creatine kinase and moderately *elevated liver enzymes*. Biopsy showed highly vacuolated cytoplasm of the epithelial cells of the distal renal tubules and micro- and macrovesicular steatosis of centrilobular hepatocytes. After discontinuation of the germanium the laboratory values normalized but moderately severe renal impairment persisted (SEDA-16, 231—232).

Gold

Metallic gold is used in dentistry, whilst gold compounds still form a mainstay of treatment for rheumatoid arthritis. In Japan, chrysotherapy has a reputation for efficacy in bronchial asthma and some recent work elsewhere suggests that this may be justified (SEDA-26, 235).

In the treatment of rheumatism, the most commonly administered gold preparations are sodium aurothiomalate and aurothioglucose. Both are water-soluble and administered intramuscularly; sodium aurothiomalate is usually employed as an aqueous solution, but aurothioglucose is also available as an oily suspension. There is some reason to believe that adverse effects are less frequent with the suspensions (of aurothioglucose or aurothiosulfate) than with the more rapidly absorbed solution (of sodium gold thiomalate) (SEDA-16, 233; 37[Cr]). For oral use, a triethylphosphine gold compound (auranofin) is available; it is discussed separately below.

Whereas gold was previously regarded as one of the most toxic drugs in the pharmacopoeia, many authors now share the view that the incidence of severe toxic events or fatalities due to gold has fallen in comparison with older reports. This seems to reflect a greater awareness by clinicians of the need to monitor for potential dangers and the development of more flexible and individually adapted therapeutic regimens (SEDA-10, 203; 38[r]). The experience of the physician in the correct use of gold compounds, and regular examination of the skin, buccal mucosa, urine and blood including cell and platelet counts, are the prerequisites in order to minimize the risks associated with chrysotherapy.

In the patient population as a whole, the prevalence of adverse gold reactions seems to be similar in patients given 25 or 50 mg of gold weekly (SED-12, 520; 39[cr]), and it is impossible to predict which patients will develop complications due to gold or when this will happen. Some studies suggest that the frequency of mucocutaneous and renal adverse reactions may be higher in the initial months of treatment, while hematological complications may occur at any stage in the course of chrysotherapy, but there are sufficient exceptions to maintain careful monitoring throughout treatment. In one series of 200 patients receiving gold sodium thiomalate, a plateau in the cumulative incidence of withdrawals due to rash was reached only after 40 months (45% of all patients), while withdrawals due to proteinuria reached a plateau after 18 months (15%) (40[Cr]).

It is widely considered that the patients most prone to develop adverse effects are those who react most favourably to the treatment. In the past, many rheumatologists indeed intensified treatment with high doses of gold salts until a skin eruption occurred, only then seeking to reduce dosage to a maintenance level.

After discontinuation due to adverse reactions, treatment with gold compounds may be cautiously reintroduced without the previous side effects necessarily reappearing; clearly one will not take this course for life-threatening (e.g. hematological) reactions.

It should always be borne in mind that many adverse reactions allegedly due to chrysotherapy may have other possible causes, particularly in the case of skin reactions. Most patients have been or are using other drugs at the same time. The concomitant use of penicillamine can be particularly confusing since its pattern of side effects closely resembles that produced by gold.

ADVERSE REACTION PATTERN

General and toxic reactions Side effects of gold appear in approximately one-third of systemically treated patients, the incidence varying from 25 to 40%. The drop-out rate due to adverse reactions has been assessed as 22–26% (41[R]). Children are considered to show the same pattern of adverse reactions as adults.

Cutaneous lesions are the most frequent side effects of gold, followed by involvement of the mucous membranes and kidneys. Pruritus and a wide range of skin reactions may occur; the gastrointestinal system may exhibit inflammation at all levels from the buccal cavity to the colon. Glossitis, cheilitis and stomatitis are less common than dermatitis. Enterocolitis is a rare though very serious complication. Mild proteinuria is frequently seen in patients receiving chrysotherapy, while severe nephrotic syndrome is much less common. Blood dyscrasias of any type can occur either during therapy or after its withdrawal. Leukopenia and thrombocytopenia are the most common hematological complications, although both are clearly less common than the mucocutaneous and renal side effects. Unusual reactions include pulmonary infiltration, intrahepatic cholestasis and peripheral neuropathy. By and large, undesirable effects are transient and mild, but occasional fatalities continue to be reported, usually because of hematological complications.

Apart from the 'nitritoid' cardiovascular reaction, which is unique to sodium aurothiomalate, and possible differences between slowly and rapidly absorbed gold preparations in the relative frequency of side effects, the general pattern of adverse reactions is similar for all parenteral gold compounds. In contrast, auranofin, the first oral gold preparation, exhibits a different pattern of side effects from the parenterally administered agents, with gastrointestinal reactions predominating.

Hypersensitivity reactions Though most side effects have traditionally been characterized as 'toxic', various factors suggest that the complications due to chrysotherapy are, at least in part, manifestations of hypersensitivity reactions to gold. Eosinophilia, raised IgE levels, immune complexes and a positive reaction to gold in the lymphocyte transformation test have been observed in association with many adverse reactions to chrysotherapy and point to immunological mechanisms (42[R]). It may be that gold facilitates the development of autoimmunity in patients with rheumatoid arthritis. Gold-induced membranous glomerulonephritis is believed to be an immune complex (Type III) reaction, although the role of gold in the development of proteinuria has not yet been clarified.

Metallic gold used in dentistry may cause allergic reactions, including contact stomatitis as well as skin eruptions at sites not usually associated with dentistry; contact dermatitis to metallic gold, e.g. in jewellery, has also been observed (SED-8, 510). A gold surgical clip has also caused an apparently allergic reaction, characterized by sterile abscess formation (43[c]). However, such reactions are rare and may in part be due to other metals contained in the alloy.

Tumor-inducing effects These have not been observed.

ORGANS AND SYSTEMS

Cardiovascular *Acute vasodilatory* (*nitritoid*) *reactions* may occur in a minority of patients on parenteral gold, especially sodium aurothiomalate. A few minutes after injection, the patient experiences weakness, flushing, hypotension, tachycardia, palpitations, sweating and sometimes syncope. Very rarely indeed, *myocardial infarction* and *stroke* follow (44[R]). The mechanism is unknown, but it has been suggested that the vehicle might be responsible, and that aurothioglucose might therefore be preferable to sodium aurothiomalate in elderly patients or in those with a history of cardiovascular disease.

Respiratory About 60 cases of '*gold lung*' have been reported. Beginning as a rule some weeks or months after starting treatment, the patient develops dyspnea on exertion, weakness, dry cough and malaise. Chest X-rays show bilateral pulmonary infiltrates of varying. If chrysotherapy is continued, pulmonary insufficiency can ensue. In fact two types of process need to be distinguished; fibrosing alveolitis and obliterative bronchiolitis occur and may exist together (45[R]); some patients develop proliferative and immunoallergic changes, perhaps even mimicking malignant processes. Bronchoalveolar lavage in 'gold lung' tends to show an increase in the total cell count and predominance of the percentage of lymphocytes with an inverse helper/suppressor ratio (46). The prognosis is generally good; if gold is immediately withdrawn, the pulmonary lesions as a rule subside, though incomplete regression or even persistence of dyspnea and impaired lung function despite glucocorticoid therapy have been described (SEDA-10, 204).

Nervous system Gold can damage nervous tissue. *Peripheral neuropathy* due to gold is possibly not as rare as was previously assumed and can co-exist with a neuroencephalopathy (see below). Damage can also take other forms; *peripheral pain*, *general malaise*, *psychic disorders* and *insomnia* may be the first uncharacteristic symptoms and can easily be overlooked as adverse effects. Acute polyneuropathy of the *Guillain-Barré* type (SED-12, 521; 47[CR]), *myokymia* (Morvan-type fibrillating chorea) (SEDA-6, 216; 48[R]) and *gold encephalopathy* (49[cr]) are rare neurological complications of chrysotherapy which have however all been well-documented from different sources (50[R]).

Hematological The hematological effects of gold are such that full blood counts should be monitored regularly at least during the first 2 years of gold treatment (51[CR]). *Eosinophilia* in the peripheral blood has been considered to be the most frequent hematological change, affecting up to 40% of patients. It is no longer believed that it is a reliable advance marker of more serious reactions of any type (52[CR]). Among the latter are severe *blood dyscrasias*, sometimes appearing unexpectedly despite regular blood counts.

Thrombocytopenia occurs in 1–3% of cases, presenting with petechiae, hematuria, oral mucosal bleeding and other hemorrhagic phenomena; some cases represent immune reactions, others a direct toxic effect of gold on the megakaryocytes. It is important to distinguish the two types. For an immunologically mediated thrombocytopenia, one may choose high-dose steroid therapy, if necessary followed or accompanied by immunosuppressive drugs, infusions of fresh-frozen plasma or high-dose immunoglobulin, and even splenectomy. Toxic thrombocytopenia probably demands gold chelator therapy. There is no correlation between the appearance of thrombocytopenia and effect on the skin or kidney (53[R]).

Leukopenia is rare, sometimes very mild, and not always related to the gold treatment which is being given (SED-12, 522).

Granulocytopenia may evolve slowly or suddenly, and its course may be transient or prolonged. Some workers have found gold-associated granulocytopenias to be brief and self-limiting; indeed, if other marrow elements are unimpaired, full recovery even from severe agranulocytosis can occur. Fully-fledged aplastic anemia and pancytopenia are the most serious and feared conditions, and although they are today uncommon, fatalities continue to occur (SEDA- 13, 192), particularly because of superimposed infections or hemorrhages. Pure *red cell aplasia* (in a patient also suffering from cholestatic jaundice) is on record (SEDA-17, 275). It has been postulated that early treatment with very high doses of intravenous *N*-acetylcysteine and the use of immunomodulatory drugs, such as antithymocyte globulin and ciclosporin, might improve the recovery of hematological parameters, even in the case of pancytopenia (54[cR]). One case of gold-induced aplastic anemia, unresponsive to various treatments, recovered after therapy with antithymocyte globulin (ATG) (SED-12, 522).

Liver Liver injury is an extremely rare complication (SEDA-14, 189; 55[Cr]); the underlying mechanisms are probably complex and certainly variable. Overdosage (see below) may cause *centrilobular necrosis* and *bile stasis*. With normal doses one is more likely to encounter intrahepatic *cholestasis* with an absence of necrosis, though there can be both bile duct damage and canicular damage (56[cr]); an immunological etiology of this disorder has been suggested. Several cases of a severe form of *idiosyncratic hepatonecrosis* soon after starting chrysotherapy have been described (57[c], 58[c]). Most hepatic lesions however as a rule resolve rapidly after cessation of chrysotherapy, and mild or moderate liver injury of any type is not necessarily a contraindication for gold treatment.

Gastrointestinal A *metallic taste* can precede the onset of *stomatitis*, which is a frequent complication of gold; it may take the form of superficial erosions producing mild symptoms but tending to run a protracted course (59[CR]).

Fulminant enterocolitis or *panenteritis* are fortunately rare manifestations of gold intolerance; more than 30 cases have been published since 1945 (60[R]), and one third of them prove fatal. One should alert for such presenting symptoms as *diarrhea*, *rectal bleeding* and *vomiting*. Bowel dilatation may develop. The course of the disease is occasionally complicated by overwhelming infection. The X-ray picture sometimes simulates regional or ischemic enteritis. Pathological findings include intense mucosal edema, ulceration, hemorrhage, and lymphocytic and plasma cell infiltration. No treatment is known. There is however a milder *eosinophilic type of enterocolitis* due to gold, which, it has been suggested, responds to treatment with cromolyn sodium.

Urinary system Mild *proteinuria* develops in 2—3% of patients on chrysotherapy; it is usually benign and reversible within a few weeks after discontinuation of chrysotherapy (61[R]). No deterioration in creatinine clearance has been found at periodic follow-up. It is not always necessary to stop gold treatment if a patient develops a proteinuria; provided there is no marked loss of renal function loss, and proteinuria is not in the nephrotic range, gold therapy can be continued under close monitoring for at least 10 months without causing permanent renal damage (62[R]).

Microhematuria has long been considered a manifestation of nephrotoxicity from chrysotherapy, but one multicenter study found no higher an incidence than in patients receiving placebo (SED-12, 522).

Serious nephrotoxicity is uncommon, but *nephrotic syndrome* can develop in about 0.3% of patients treated, generally among some of the patients who have experienced mild proteinuria earlier in treatment. Very exceptionally, *acute renal failure* may occur; peritoneal dialysis has been reported to promote recovery. The histological findings in cases of gold nephropathy may range from essentially normal glomeruli to a focal increase in mesangium, glomerular basement membrane thickening or splitting, membranous glomerulonephritis, periglomerular fibrosis with proliferation of Bowman's capsule or even hyalinization of glomeruli. Chronic interstitial nephritis has also been added to the pattern of gold nephropathy (63[CR]).

Gold nephropathy is often considered to be an immunological disorder, and IgG and C3 are usually present in fine granular immune complex deposits along the capillary walls of the glomeruli. Oddly however, X-ray microanalysis fails to detect gold as a component of the deposited immune complexes, throwing doubt on the concept of gold itself acting as an antigen or a hapten. Gold might however alter the proximal tubular cells in such a way that tubular autoantigens are released, resulting in the development of antigen—antibody complexes; these would then become attached to the glomerular basement membrane, hence inducing membranous glomerulopathy and proteinuria. That gold does damage the tubular cells is well known, although there appears to be no correlation with the dosage and duration of therapy. Gold-containing, electron-dense filamentous cytoplasmic inclusions have been found in proximal tubular cells. The urinary excretion of β-glucosaminidase, leucine aminopeptidase, β2-microglobulin and other tubular proteins has frequently been found to be increased in patients treated with gold compounds (SEDA-15, 229). Tubular dysfunction may persist for up to 2 years after the cessation of chrysotherapy.

Skin and appendages *Toxic/immune skin reactions* are the most frequent of all clinical side effects of gold; they develop in about 25% of patients, sometimes in association with other forms of gold intolerance. These skin reactions seem to involve both a toxic and an immune mechanism. No increase in gold concentration in the skin has been found in patients, nor is there any correlation with blood levels of gold. Skin biopsies indicate that both macrophages and Langerhans cells are actively involved in the pathogenesis of gold dermatitis (64). *Pruritus* is the commonest and earliest manifestation of such reactions, and may precede an eruption by some weeks. *Subsequent lesions are of every conceivable type*; they range from transient, non-specific, localized or generalized dermatitis (eczema) and erythematous, maculopapular rash to lichen planus-like eruptions, discoid eczema, pityriasis rosacea, erythema multiforme, erythema nodosum, scaling eruptions, urticaria, photosensitivity, hyperkeratosis, seborrheic dermatitis and toxic epidermal necrolysis (Lyell syndrome), granuloma annulare and exacerbation of pre-existing psoriasis. Patients on aurothioglucose treatment have sometimes presented a dermatitis with a close resemblance to contact dermatitis (SED-12, 523). More than one of these effects may occur in the same patient. Not every gold-induced skin disorder is necessarily wholly disfiguring; in one curious case, the patient was found to 'glitter' with tiny specks of a gold-coloured (and gold-containing) material covering the skin of the neck, upper arms and back (65[c]).

If toxic/immune skin reactions are not serious, the withdrawal of gold is not essential, and as noted above some physicians have deliberately intensified dosage to the point where some skin reaction does appear as a means of securing the best possible therapeutic effect. Once troublesome reactions have appeared they can often be relieved simply by reducing the dosage or the frequency of administration. More troublesome reactions will demand withdrawal of gold, and in that case most skin lesions will begin to subside within a few days or a week, and disappear within several weeks more. On the other hand, some gold-induced skin lesions can run a protracted course, necessitating in certain cases topical or systemic glucocorticoid treatment. A patchy, brown discoloration may persist after the disorders have resolved. When gold has been discontinued it may often be restarted later without inducing recurrence of the lesion.

Chrysiasis, a grey, blue or purple pigmentation of the light-exposed skin areas, is a rare but dose-dependent complication which tends to be permanent.

In patients with a history of localized hypersensitivity to metallic gold, *allergic skin reactions* may develop in the sensitized region following gold injections (SEDA-13, 193).

Alopecia is a most uncommon side effect of gold, but it clearly does occur. The same applies to *onycholysis* followed by *irreversible nail dystrophy* (SED-9, 373).

As noted above, a case of pre-existing *psoriasis* seems to have been exacerbated by gold therapy (66[cR]).

Special senses *Chryseosis corneae*, i.e. deposition of gold crystals in the cornea, is dose-dependent. Such deposits are rarely found in patients treated with a cumulative dose of 500 mg gold or less, but they occur in nearly all patients who have received 1500 mg or more. Deposition of gold as such has no clinical consequences. Gold may occasionally cause a *keratitis* or *keratoconjunctivitis*, but these are usually associated with skin involvement and are not a consequence of gold deposits in the cornea.

Miscellaneous *Polyarteritis* and *systemic lupus erythematosus* have been reported following the administration of gold compounds. *Pyrexia* and a transient *exacerbation of rheumatoid symptoms* can develop before a therapeutic response to gold occurs.

An increased incidence of *herpes zoster* was found in a series of patients receiving sodium aurothiomalate; the mechanism is unknown, but herpes also occurs in association with some other heavy metals, e.g. in environmental poisoning.

One published case describes the appearance of *axillary lymphadenopathy* in association with gold therapy for rheumatoid arthritis; biopsy of the nodes detected crystalline material containing gold (SEDA-16, 234).

Several patients with selective *IgA deficiency* and even a *panhypogammaglobulinemia* during intramuscular gold treatment have been described (SEDA-14, 190; SEDA-15, 230). A *lymphadenopathy* related to intramuscular gold treatment and disappearing after withdrawal has been reported (SEDA-12, 188).

Risk situations (67[R]) Gold is considered to be contraindicated in *active hepatic disease*, *impaired renal function*, *colitis*, *cases with a history of hematological disorders*, and in patients who have recently had *radiotherapy* (because of the depressant action of the latter on hematopoietic tissue). *Elderly patients* were formerly stated to be more prone than younger individuals to develop severe reactions (68[R]) but more recent work seems to show that this is not the case. There is firm evidence that *rheumatoid arthritis patients carrying the DR3 antigen* run a greater risk of proteinuria (69[Cr]), mucocutaneous reactions (70[C]) and hematotoxic actions (71[C]) to parenteral gold compounds as well as to penicillamine, though such patients also tend to react rather better than others to aurothioglucose (72[C]). The same applies to the B8, DR3 haplotype (73[C]). The prevalence of the HLA antigens DR2 and DR7 is lower among rheumatoid arthritis patients with toxic reactions than among patients without toxic reactions or among controls (74[c]). Due to conflicting results on the one hand

and the low relative risk on the other, HLA typing is so far not of much practical help as a guide to therapy risk forecasting.

It has been shown that rheumatoid arthritis patients with a *poor sulfoxidation state* are six times more susceptible than others to appearance of toxic effects of sodium aurothiomalate (75[c]); this parallels an earlier finding to the same effect regarding treatment with penicillamine which has the same sulfhydryl group in its structure.

Second-generation effects In 1980 alarm was caused by a report on a seriously malformed child born to a mother treated with sodium gold thiomalate during pregnancy (76[C]), particularly since a partially congruent pattern of neural abnormalities had earlier been described in rats and rabbits, and the fact that gold crosses the placenta. On the other hand, a Danish team in 1983 studied eight children born after exposure to gold in utero from weeks 2–9 or longer; no abnormalities were found, and the children appeared to develop normally during a follow-up period averaging 8.6 years (77[C]). In view of the lack of further incriminating evidence some physicians today adopt the view that chrysotherapy may be continued in selected pregnant women whose rheumatoid arthritis is of such severity as to warrant the treatment.

Breast feeding is not recommended since gold salts are excreted in the milk (SEDA-12, 188; SEDA-13, 193).

Overdosage (78[cr]) In a reported case, severe overdosage of sodium aurothiopropanol sulfonate (1.1 gram daily for 13 days) led to jaundice and skin eruptions. Liver biopsies revealed modest centrilobular necrosis and significant bile stasis. Hepatic enzyme levels in serum were increased. The patient was treated with dimercaprol and recovered after 2 months, although alkaline phosphatase and γ-glutamyltransferase levels remained high for 6 months. Other literature is scarce but in line with this history. It seems advisable in cases of acute gold intoxication to adopt a conservative strategy; should severe complications set in, supportive therapy can be given if necessary in combination with such treatments as chelation, corticosteroids or gammaglobulin.

Interactions Although there is no direct evidence of potentiation of hematological toxicity, the concomitant use of *drugs with a recognized potential to cause blood dyscrasias* is unwise. Simultaneous use of *corticosteroids* in small doses is not thought to detract from the beneficial effects of gold and may delay the onset of adverse reactions (79[CR]).

Oral gold (auranofin)

Much of what has been said about gold applies to any of its medicinal compounds, but auranofin—the only available gold product for oral use—has certain striking differences from the remainder. Some 25% of an oral dose is absorbed through the intestinal wall; the blood levels attained are some 15–25% those reached with parenteral therapy. Auranofin is bound to cellular elements of the blood, is excreted mainly in the feces, and exhibits less tissue retention and total body gold accumulation than the parenteral products. It is more effective in acute inflammatory models and is a potent inhibitor of lysosomal enzyme release, antibody-dependent cellular toxicity and superoxide production; auranofin also affects humoral and cellular immune reactions. However, some work has found auranofin to be rather less effective than parenteral gold. The drug is today used in doses of 2–9 mg daily (generally 6 mg), which is less than the dose level originally recommended.

In view of all this it is not surprising that auranofin has a distinct profile, both as regards its therapeutic and adverse effects, the differences being so great that one actually suspects differences in the mechanism of action between the oral and parenteral products. Like the latter, however, auranofin shows no clear correlation between whole blood gold concentrations and either toxic reactions or clinical efficacy.

ADVERSE REACTION PATTERN

General and toxic reactions Auranofin has been well tolerated by most patients; the adverse effects resemble those of the parenteral compounds, but are generally less severe. Where serious side effects have been attributed to the drug, cause and effect has usually remained in doubt. Side effects affecting the lower gastrointestinal tract are the most common; the original studies showed a change in bowel habit in some 40% of cases, but it does not often amount to frank diarrhea (80). The same study noted proteinuria (4%) and hematotoxic reactions (2%). Mucocutaneous reactions (pruritus, conjunctivitis, stomatitis) often occur but are rarely severe and are less problematical than with sodium aurothiomalate. Most side effects have occurred during the first few months; age, sex and duration of disease did not influence the risk of developing an adverse effect. The side effect-related withdrawal rates for injectable gold, auranofin and placebo were found to be 40, 14 and 6%, respectively.

Hypersensitivity reactions Rash has been found to occur in some 20% of cases but is rarely a reason for withdrawal.

Tumor-inducing effects These have not been observed.

ORGANS AND SYSTEMS

Hematological *Anemia* has been reported to occur occasionally (0.1%) either as a direct effect or secondary to auranofin-associated hematuria. Auranofin has also been associated with *leukopenia* (0.1%), *lymphopenia*, *neutropenia* and *eosinophilia* (range of incidence in various reports 0.1—13%). Early eosinophilia is not a reliable indicator of potential toxicity. *Thrombocytopenia* is known but rare (0.5%); after withdrawal, platelet counts returned to the normal range within 1—2 weeks.

Respiratory A case of *interstitial pneumonia* has been described in an adult who had taken auranofin for only 6 days; corticosteroids were required (SEDA-17, 276).

Liver Mild and transient abnormalities in *serum transaminase and alkaline phosphatase* levels have been reported. during therapy with auranofin (0.4%). This is noteworthy since almost all patients were receiving acetylsalicylic acid or other non-steroidal anti-inflammatory drugs, which also can elicit transaminase increases. Early in 1985 there was a brief report on two cases of *toxic hepatosis* (81[Cr]) but it seems to have remained unique.

Gastrointestinal About half of all users have *loose stools* at some time during treatment; the effect can be transient, can occur at any time, and is rarely severe. In cases which have been studied, no infective cause or signs of malabsorption could be found, nor was gold absorption adversely affected. In a long-term study using auranofin 6 mg daily, diarrhea was mainly observed in the first 6 months of therapy; in 8% of the cases this was a reason for withdrawal (82[Cr]). There is animal experiment evidence for a direct effect of auranofin on ion and water absorption from the intestine with a concentration-dependent inhibition of enterocyte Na^+/K^+-ATPase activity (SED-12, 525).

Stomatitis is experienced in about 10% of cases, generally early in treatment, demanding withdrawal only rarely (0.3%).

Two patients have been described who developed a *fulminant colitis* with *toxic megacolon* during treatment with auranofin (83[c], 84[c]). Both recovered completely within 4—6 weeks with supportive treatment including high doses of prednisone.

Urinary system *Proteinuria* has been observed in many clinical trials, but in contrast to cases associated with parenteral gold it has only rarely progressed to nephrotic syndrome. Of 1283 auranofin-treated patients surveyed, 38 had a raised protein level, but only in nine was it heavy, and in most patients who continued treatment the proteinuria did not persist beyond the first 12 months of treatment; seven of eight who were rechallenged after the drug had been withdrawn and the protein had cleared were able to continue treatment without relapse. Biopsy showed membranous glomerulonephritis, indicating an underlying immunopathological mechanism (85[cR]).

Hematuria associated with auranofin has been reported in a few patients, generally following at least 2—3 months of treatment. Other abnormalities in renal function, such as elevation in *blood urea nitrogen*, *serum creatinine* or *uric acid*, have been reported and led to withdrawal in 0.1%.

Endocrine, metabolic In one recently documented case, *diabetes was destabilized* after 3 weeks of auranofin treatment (86[c]).

Skin and appendages Some 18—24% of patients on auranofin develop *rash* or *pruritus*, meriting discontinuation in some 4% of cases. Worldwide experience with auranofin points to a 2% incidence of *alopecia*, but this included older experience; at current dose levels, alopecia is rather less common.

Special senses *Conjunctivitis* has occurred in some 10% of patients, either early or late in treatment, and has led to withdrawal in about 1%.

Miscellaneous The incidence of *herpes zoster* in auranofin-treated patients was slightly higher (0.9%) than in patients with rheumatoid arthritis not receiving gold therapy (0.4%), but less frequent than in patients given parenteral gold compounds (3.1%).

Use in children Several studies show that in juvenile chronic arthritis auranofin gives rise to even fewer adverse reactions than in adults, but the therapeutic effect is dubious and variable (SEDA-17, 277). In one documented case there was an acute reaction to aurothioglucose but when this was withdrawn the patient not only recovered but exhibited improvement in the joint condition (SEDA-17, 276).

Risk situations The general contraindications as for gold therapy (see monograph above).

Interactions A 1992 placebo-controlled study has concluded that auranofin is capable of reducing the doses of *corticosteroids* needed in asthma (87[C]). This is perhaps a parallel effect rather than an interaction since, as noted above, gold itself may have an effect in asthma.

Iron

The body has no physiological route for the excretion of excess iron, and a constant risk of therapy is that of iron overload. Long-term use of iron by any route in large amounts can lead to *hemosiderosis*, clinically simulating hemochromatosis; the danger is greatest when the mucosal barrier is bypassed by parenteral injection. Even the safety of iron-fortified food is uncertain (SEDA-4, 171). These things are important since iron is often given unnecessarily, in excessive amounts, and without respect for contraindications such as the iron-loading anemias (thalassemia and sideroblastic anemia). In the elderly, iron deficiency is usually a sign of bleeding, and it is wiser to track down and correct the hemorrhage (e.g. gastric malignancy) than lightly to prescribe iron which may merely mask the problem and delay diagnosis.

In cases of *erythropoietic protoporphyria*, iron is capable of inducing a relapse of clinical symptoms (88[C]); an involvement of iron overload in the pathogenesis of some cases of *porphyria cutanea tarda* has been suggested (89[CR]).

Oral iron

Iron and the gastrointestinal system Though iron clearly does have the ability to irritate the mucous membranes, its widespread reputation for poor gastric tolerance is undeserved, generally reflecting its having been given to excess. Of patients taking up to 200 mg of elemental iron daily, only a few highly susceptible individuals will develop gastrointestinal side effects, and *constipation* is then the most usual feature. Higher doses may indeed give rise to *gastric discomfort*, *nausea*, *ructus* or *vomiting*, or in the lower gastrointestinal tract to either *constipation* or *diarrhea*. Oral iron can also *color the feces black*, which may be mistaken for melena. Fewer gastrointestinal side effects occur if the iron dose is gradually increased to the desired level or if iron is taken with food, but since insoluble iron complexes may be formed with food it has been recommended that iron salts be taken between meals. Despite many claims for the better tolerance of expensive iron preparations it is still not entirely proven that these are any better tolerated than plain ferrous sulfate if the latter is properly dosed, though research by enthusiastic manufacturers continues. A 1990 paper concluded that iron supplementation via a gastric delivery system did not produce any gastrointestinal adverse reactions while the efficacy was similar to that of a ferrous sulfate elixir (90). Carbonyl iron has also been studied, though mainly as a means of reducing acute toxicity if such a product is accidentally taken by children (SEDA-16, 235).

True gastrointestinal risks arise if a solid dosage form becomes lodged in the pharynx, esophagus or intestinal diverticula; severe *erosion* may ensue (SEDA-6, 224); *necrosis* is also possible. An accumulation of ferrosulfate tablets with a non-soluble matrix has been the source of *ileus* in a case of Crohn's disease (SEDA-16, 236). This sort of risk is greatest with slow-release formulations (see below) and absent with liquid iron preparations; the latter should therefore be preferred in cases of delayed gastric emptying, pyloric stenosis or known diverticula of the alimentary tract.

Effect on rheumatoid arthritis Although total dose infusions of iron (see below) can cause rheumatoid arthritis to flare up, this has not been demonstrated with oral iron.

However, a patient who has reacted in this way to an infusion can subsequently relapse if given oral iron.

Sustained-release oral preparations Although slow-release preparations seem to be better tolerated this is almost certainly a reflection of their less complete absorption. Iron is best absorbed in the duodenum, and most of the iron in sustained-release tablets is released only when the tablets reach the lower parts of the gastrointestinal tract (91[r]). Risks of such preparations becoming lodged in the gastrointestinal tract are noted above.

Risks of aspiration Aspiration of iron tablets can produce an acute reaction in the airways since they are highly irritative; immediate removal bronchoscopy is necessary to avoid permanent damage (SEDA-16, 236).

Liquid preparations for oral use Most liquid ferrous products *stain dental enamel*, but this is usually reversible.

Overdosage (*SEDA*-11, 208; 92[R], 124[R]) *Acute poisoning* due to sudden accidental ingestion of iron-containing preparations has repeatedly been reported in childhood; this acute toxicity is associated with free radical formation. Emetics, gastric lavage and even surgery may be called for to remove the excess. Much more common is *chronic poisoning* due to excessive intake over a long period, with deposition of iron within the cells. Iron exerts a toxic effect in almost all organs, especially the liver, heart and the endocrine glands. Histological evidence of iron-mediated tissue damage can be obtained before the clinical picture becomes evident. Combined management with ascorbic acid and deferoxamine may yield high rates of deferoxamine-induced urinary iron excretion without obvious adverse effects on the heart (93[R]).

Interactions Concomitant administration of oral *tetracyclines* and oral iron will grossly disturb absorption because complexes are formed; there should be an interval of 2—3 hours between the use of the two. Iron absorption may also be impaired by *antacids* (e.g. magnesium trisilicate and carbonates), *tea* and *cholestyramine*. Concomitant ingestion of iron has been found to reduce the cupruretic effect of *penicillamine* (SED-12, 527) and penicillamine also seems to reduce iron absorption as one would expect.

Parenteral iron

General considerations Like oral iron, parenteral iron is probably used too widely. Intractable gastrointestinal intolerance to the oral product, hyperemesis in pregnancy, very severe blood loss and possibly ulcerative colitis are some of the few valid indications for parenteral iron. A low iron-binding capacity (e.g. due to prior saturating iron therapy or malnutrition), folic acid deficiency and an allergic constitution predispose the patient to adverse reactions to parenteral iron. Iron injections have been reported to provoke *hemolytic anemia* in cases of paroxysmal nocturnal hemoglobinuria.

Effect on immunological defense mechanisms Single dose infusions of iron dextran appear to have increased the occurrence of *malaria* in regions where this disease is endemic. A raised mortality was found after oral or parenteral iron therapy in children with severe malnutrition (*kwashiorkor*), perhaps due to overwhelming infections (94[C]). Reactivation of quiescent infections of various other types has been observed in African nomads following ferrous sulfate therapy (SEDA-4, 171). Iron dextran has similarly been associated with a flaring up of latent *tuberculosis* in children.

It may be noted that persistent *hypogammaglobulinemia* has been described in a patient receiving gold; a year after drug withdrawal the gamma-globulin levels were still unchanged (95[c]). An *insulin autoimmune syndrome*, marked by presence of insulin antibodies and of small granulomas in the skin, has also been documented in Japanese cases, many of whom had also received pencillamine (96[c], 97[cr]).

Interference with diagnostic routines *Urine* may be dark in color in the first 24 hours after parenteral iron injection. The reddish-brown colour, which has been observed after the intramuscular injection of iron sorbitol-citric acid complex (SED-8, 515), is due to urinary excretion of part of the iron compound. It has to be distinguished from the black discoloration which may develop if urine of iron—sorbitex-treated patients is allowed to stand and which is assumed to be due to production of iron sulfide by bacterial growth. Phenomena of this kind are unlikely to appear after use of iron dextran which does not pass a healthy glomerular filter. If *blood grouping* is to be performed, samples should be taken prior to the intravenous iron dextran injection, since the latter interferes with the reading. Single-dose infusion of iron dextran may cause *plasma discoloration* which may be misinterpreted as a sign of severe hemolysis.

Effects in folic acid deficiency Latent folic acid deficiency can become manifest during iron therapy due to additional demand for the vitamin secondary to increased erythropoietic activity (98[Cr]).

Intramuscular iron Iron compounds for intramuscular use are iron sorbitol—citric acid complex (iron sorbitex), iron dextran, iron glycerin—citric acid complex and iron polyisomaltose. The work on these preparations is largely old and has been reviewed in much earlier volumes in this series.

Intramuscular iron injections are often *painful*, can produce topical *discoloration of the skin* and some *local inflammation* with lymphadenopathy. Rarely, more severe local reactions follow (SEDA-6, 224) such as transient *lipomyodystrophy*. An unpleasant *metallic taste* in the mouth is common and can persist for some hours or days. Repeatedly one encounters patients who develop general symptoms such as *headache*, *flushing*, *sweating*, *nausea*, *vomiting*, *dizziness*, *generalized aches and pains*, *malaise*, *arthralgia*, *palpitation*, and *pericardial or abdominal pain*. Although very rare, a severe *anaphylactic reaction* to intramuscular iron dextran can occur.

The major hazard of the i.m. use of iron sorbitex is presented by *severe systemic reactions with cardiac involvement*, which may be fatal; they occur in up to 1% of cases, the onset occurring 10—30 minutes after injection and a patient who has received an injection must be monitored for an hour. The patient may develop *nausea*, *chest pain*, *profuse sweating*, *cardiac dysrhythmias* and *loss of consciousness*. Cardiac complications may include *complete atrioventricular block*, *ventricular tachycardia* and *ventricular fibrillation*.

After i.m. iron dextran, a symmetrical *allergic purpura* of the lower limbs due to hypersensitivity vasculitis has been observed in a child (99[C]).

The possible *sarcoma-inducing* potential of intramuscular iron was fully discussed 15 years ago (SED-9, 375—376; 100[R]) and no new information on the topic has come to light to resolve the issue.

Intravenous iron Iron dextran is now the most commonly employed iron compound for intravenous use, and most reported adverse reactions to i.v. iron relate to this preparation.

Local reactions to intravenous iron dextran include transient *pain* (in some 4% of cases) and *phlebitis*. The risk of the latter may be reduced by using saline instead of 5% dextrose as diluent. Nevertheless, *deep vein thrombosis* has been observed in a few patients infused with a dilution of iron dextran in normal saline (SED-8, 514).

Systemic reactions to iron dextran given intravenously are more common than those to intramuscular iron; they include non-immunological and immunological, immediate and delayed reactions. *Flushing*, a *sensation of warmth* and a *metallic taste* are frequently associated with excessively rapid injection, but usually subside within less than a minute after slowing or stopping the injection. In about 1% of cases, including patients with no known prior exposure to dextran, life-threatening *anaphylactoid reactions* present at once with *hypotension*, *cardiovascular shock*, *syncope*, *cyanosis*, *bronchospasm*, *respiratory arrest*, *urticaria* and *angioneurotic edema*; fatalities have ensued.

Milder allergic reactions comprise *mild and transient hypotension*, *malaise*, *itching* and *urticaria*. Desensitization under an umbrella of corticosteroids, antihistamines and ephedrine has been carried out successfully (101^{C}).

Delayed systemic reactions to i.v. iron dextran appear to be more common, the reported incidence ranging from 5 to 15%; they start within 4—48 hours of injection and may last for 3—7 days. Characteristic symptoms are *fever*, *arthralgia*, *myalgia*, *headache* and *lymphadenopathy*, singly or in combination, and a classic *serum sickness* has been seen (SEDA-16, 26). *Chills* may also occur and individual patients may experience *dizziness*, *tinnitus*, *paresthesias*, a feeling of *stiffness in the arms and neck*, *pruritus*, *urticarial* or other *cutaneous eruptions*, *pallor*, *nausea*, *vomiting* and *nasal irritation*. *Hepatosplenomegaly* may be found on examination. These delayed reactions appear to be more frequent in children and, for some reason, in patients of Chinese origin. They tend to be more severe in patients with low body weight given higher doses, and in patients with rheumatoid arthritis or other types of inflammatory disease.

Other iron compounds for intravenous use Saccharated iron oxide is strongly alkaline and hypertonic; if injected outside the vein, it may give rise to marked *local reactions*. Significant serum *hypophosphatemia* has on occasion been observed during treatment, accompanied by decreased renal tubular reabsorption of phosphate. The mechanism of these changes, which were reversible after stopping the iron injections, has not been clarified (102^{C}).

Total dose-infusion of iron With this technique, the amount of iron which is required is delivered in a single infusion rather than by intermittent therapy. Although iron levels may rise to very high values, e.g. 100 000 μg/ml (103^{CR}), there are unlikely to be signs of iron intoxication (SED-8, 513). Toxic reactions to intravenously administered iron do occur when ionized iron exceeds plasma binding capacity. With iron dextran, the iron moiety seems to be so firmly bound to dextran that ionized iron does not exceed plasma iron-binding capacity even when total plasma iron levels are extremely high. All the same there are adverse effects which were at first underestimated, and today it would be fair to say that whenever possible other routes or methods of iron dextran administration should be preferred (104^{Cr}).

Immediate reactions occurred in nine of one series of 40 adults, variously in the form of *anaphylaxis*, *chills*, *malaise*, *hypertension*, *gastrointestinal reactions*, *epistaxis* or *chest pain*. Monitoring for these early reactions is always necessary, but elderly patients require particular attention since they are more prone to react in this way.

Symmetric allergic purpura following the intravenous infusion of iron dextran has exceptionally been noted. In children, *transient hepatosplenomegaly* has been described as a common finding.

An *adverse effect on rheumatic disorders* is well documented (SEDA-12, 190), the injections exacerbating the joint symptoms, perhaps by promoting lipid peroxidation (105^{C}). Of 11 rheumatoid arthritis patients who received a total dose infusion of iron for anemia, nine experienced an exacerbation of the synovitis, and the two other patients had an anaphylactic reaction. The exacerbations occurred 24—48 hours after completion of the iron dextran infusion and settled in all patients within 11 days. One of these patients had synovial flares when challenged with oral ferrous sulfate. In a single reported case, total dose iron infusion was followed by prolonged polyarthritis, mainly of the large joints, in a patient with no previous evidence of rheumatoid arthritis or ankylosing spondylitis (106^{C}). Despite prolonged corticosteroid therapy, clinical resolution of the problem took 5 months. It may also be relevant that when an iron infusion was given to 20 dialysis patients several of them developed muscular aches, an influenza-like condition or joint pain (SEDA-17, 278).

Organ calcification has very rarely been described after use of iron dextran in uremic patients (SED-8, 515).

Risk situations in use of intravenous iron *Age* as a

possible risk factor regarding adverse reactions to total-dose infusions of iron dextran has been referred to above. In addition, patients with a history of *allergy* may be at risk of developing undesired immunological reactions, e.g. asthma attacks, following parenteral iron dextran administration; however, the incidence of such reactions seems to be low, and the risk probably also exists with other iron compounds as well. A small test infusion may or may not detect susceptibility to immediate reactions and can itself elicit a violent reaction.

There was at one time impressive but limited case evidence that systemic reactions to iron dextran might be more frequent in *patients with rheumatic or other inflammatory diseases*; no further evidence has been published. There might be confusion with the ability of i.v. iron to induce a flare-up of an existing rheumatic condition (see above).

The case once made against use of iron dextran in *pregnancy* because of a supposed risk of possible uterine cramps (SED-9, 377) or a greater risk of systemic reactions (SED-8, 513) has not been substantiated.

As noted above, iron toxicity may be expected if the amount of free iron which is released into the plasma exceeds plasma iron-binding capacity. This is more likely to occur when using iron sorbitol—citric acid complex (iron sorbitex), since the iron is here less firmly bound than with iron dextran. Several conditions associated with low iron-binding capacity such as *malnutrition* (kwashiorkor, malnutrition syndrome) and *previous or simultaneous oral iron therapy* appear to predispose to the development of these toxic reactions. In addition, *folic acid deficiency* has been reported to be a predisposing factor (SED-9, 516); the likely mechanism here is a disturbance of iron utilization secondary to folic acid deficiency, which results in an increased saturation of iron-binding capacity.

Iron overload due to transfusions Symptoms and signs of iron overload in transfusion-dependent anemias occur after a total transfusion burden of approximately 100—150 units of blood.

Topical iron

Iron chloride is sometimes used topically as a hemostyptic after minor surgery. It can result in persistent *brown staining* at the site of application. Use of Monsel's solution (ferric subsulfate), another hemostyptic agent, may after an interval of up to 3—5 weeks lead to *fibrovascular proliferation* accompanied by strongly pigmented macrophages; the condition may be mistaken for malignant melanoma.

Lead

Lead has no place in internal medical treatment, though lead acetate has retained a very small place as an astringent. Its toxic effects are known primarily from environmental and occupational exposure and occasionally from the use of 'alternative' remedies or cosmetics; lead sulphide in eyedrops originating in India has for example led to lead poisoning, and lead has been found in some 'aphrodisiacs' from India. Children with circulating lead levels in excess of 600 ng/ml have been found to show impaired intellectual performance and changes in the electrocardiogram, and at any age excessive intake can cause encephalopathy, neuropathies, anemia, anorexia, colic and renal damage.

Magnesium

Since magnesium salts are used for gastric disorders they are considered primarily in the relevant chapter. Magnesium is however also in use in infusions and cardiac disorders, and intoxication can be a consequence of overdosage or of intestinal or renal disease. The main symptoms are neuromuscular (paralysis) and cardiac (ECG changes, hypotension, bradycardia, heart block). In more severe cases there will be CNS or respiratory depression, hypomotility of the bowel, muscle paralysis and hyporeflexia.

Mercury

The use of mercury in medicine is generally considered to be outdated; the few exceptions include its use in certain preservatives and in dental amalgam. The move away from mercury has been catalyzed by knowledge of its environmental toxicity.

Inorganic mercury

Although calomel (mercurous chloride) is obsolete as a laxative in official medicine, non-prescription laxatives containing it are still sold in some countries. Similarly, there is some residual use of mercurial ointments as antiseptics or ectoparasiticides, and mercury is present in some contraceptive jellies, hemorrhoidal remedies and cosmetics (bleaching creams). The presence of mercury may not be divulged on the labelling.

Cases have been described of chronic mercurialism with *CNS involvement*, *renal failure* and *progressive colitis* following the long-term use of such remedies.

They may also explain the persistence of other unexplained disorders such as *pink disease* (see below). Inorganic mercury salts may cause *allergic dermatitis*. Frank *poisoning* from these sources, although uncommon today, is still possible, and occasional case reports appear (SEDA-13, 195). Inhalation of mercury vapor from broken thermometers by persons allergic to mercury allergy may give rise to *allergic contact dermatitis*.

Dental amalgam *(SEDA-10, 210; SEDA-15, 233; 107ʳ)*

Dental amalgam is still used for about 75—80% of single-tooth restorations. The modern amalgam consists of a metallic alloy (silver, tin and copper, sometimes with small amounts of zinc, indium and/or palladium) mixed with mercury in a percentage of 40— 54% mercury by weight. The resultant plastic mass sets and hardens over a period of 8—24 hours.

Contrary to previous belief, measurable amounts of mercury escape from dental amalgam fillings in the form of vapor, ions and abraded particles, and individuals who are accustomed to chew their food thoroughly are exposed to particularly high levels of mercury. This finding has led to a widespread belief in some countries, supported by certain scientific workers (108ʳ), that mercury released from amalgam may be the cause of some hitherto unexplained diseases, and a demand has arisen for the removal of amalgam fillings. A number of case histories have been published of individuals in whom chronic (primarily neurological) disorders appear to have responded to removal of amalgam.

Although it is acknowledged that occasional individuals are allergic to mercury, the view that it presents any other risk has generally been contested by the dental profession, citing evidence that the mercury released from amalgam will not accumulate in the body as long as there is adequate renal function. The debate however continues at the time of writing.

Organic mercury

Aryl mercury Aryl mercurials used in medicine include phenylmercuric acetate, phenylmercuric nitrate, nitromersol, thiomersal, merbromin (mercurochrome) and mercurobutol. They compounds are variously used as preservatives in drugs, for skin disinfestation, the treatment of infections of the skin and mucosa, and in contraceptive jellies and hemorrhoidal remedies. The aryl mercurials are better absorbed across the mucous membranes than most inorganic mercury salts. There is controversy as to whether the elevated mercury levels which may be found in blood and urine after the external application of such compounds as mercurochrome are as ominous as comparable levels of inorganic mercurials. Notwithstanding some arguments that the toxicity of absorbed merbromin might be lower than previously assumed, an undeniable risk remains associated with its application, e.g. in burn patients, which is not offset by the weak bacteriostatic effect of this compound (SEDA-8, 232). Young children run a particular risk of *renal damage* from absorption of organic mercury compounds used as antiseptics; in one reported case, frequent application of merbromin to an omphalocele apparently resulted in anuria, respiratory arrest and death (SED-8, 520).

Long-term use of eyedrops containing phenylmercuric nitrate as a preservative may cause *pigmentation of the anterior lens capsule*. However, the pigmentation does not seem to be associated with visual impairment.

Allergic reactions The presence of aryl mercurials as preservatives in many drugs, in which they may easily be overlooked, is important in view of their sensitizing properties. Some reagents for intracutaneous testing (tuberculin, etc.) may contain thiomersal, which may cause sensitization and thus elicit *false-positive delayed-type skin reactions*. *Asthmatic attacks* have been attributed to aryl mercurials. Organomercurials are a common cause of *allergic contact dermatitis*. The thiomersal content of eyedrops may be the unsuspected cause of chronic *conjunctivitis* or *blepharoconjunctivitis*.

Acrodynia ('pink disease') is thought to be a particular form of mercury hypersensitivity which can be caused by organic or inorganic mercury; it formerly occurred in young children exposed to 'teething preparations' containing mercury compounds. Typical signs include pink scaling palms and soles, flushed cheeks, pruritus, photophobia, profuse irritability and insomnia. A modern case of acrodynia involved a patient with congenital agammaglobulinemia who had received merthiolate-containing gammaglobulin injections for 15 years (SEDA-6, 225).

Nickel

Various medical and surgical routines expose the body to metallic nickel. The influence of the drug in prostheses is dealt with at the end of this Chapter. Nickel-plated artificial kidney devices have also been in use and proved to give rise to nickel poisoning in 23 patients in a hemodialysis unit. They developed *nausea*, *vomiting*, *weakness*, *headache* and *palpitation*, all of which remitted 3—13 hours after cessation of dialysis (SEDA-6, 225). *Contact dermatitis* to nickel is well-known but usually reflects non-medical exposure (109[CR]); nickel released from injection needles and from Dermojets may however also give rise to cutaneous hypersensitivity reactions. Occupational exposure explains most cases of nickel-associated *asthma* (110[C]) and *rhinitis* (111[C]). Exposure to nickel is not always readily traced, e.g. nickel may be present in contaminated cosmetics (SEDA-12, 531).

The commonly recommended patch test procedure is not fully reliable for diagnosing nickel allergy. The lymphocyte transformation test has been suggested as a useful additional tool (112[R]); an increased incidence of HLA-B21 was found in patients with cutaneous nickel hypersensitivity (113[CR]).

Platinum

Organic platinum compounds used as cytostatic agents are discussed in Chapter 45.

Selenium *(SEDA-12, 190)*

Selenium has gained undeserved popularity as a constituent of health-food preparations and alternative tonics, perhaps because selenium deficiency has been implicated in the pathogenesis of some forms of malnutrition in children. However even in these children the therapeutic benefit and safety margin of selenium dosage have not yet been established—indeed in protein deficiency it seems to be particularly toxic. Nor is there any serious basis for the reputation of selenium as a remedy for cystic fibrosis, a prophylactic against ageing or a sexual stimulant. Perhaps somewhat arbitrarily, the US Food and Nutrition Board's Committee on Dietary Allowances has proposed a recommended daily intake of selenium of 50—200 μg/day.

As is evident from veterinary practice and animal studies, selenium has both acute and chronic toxic effects on many organs. Endemic selenium poisoning of populations in an area of China produced a picture resembling arsenic poisoning (114[C]). It is not possible to say what effects have gone unrecorded, or perhaps what irregular use in alternative medicines might have at various ages in human subjects.

An FDA overview describes 12 cases of selenium intoxication in the US due to ingestion of 'superpotent' selenium tablets, the estimated total ingested doses ranging from 27 to 2310 mg. (115[C]). *Nausea*, *vomiting*, *nail changes*, *fatigue* and *irritability* were the most common symptoms; some subjects had *watery diarrhea*, *abdominal cramps*, *dryness of the hair*, *paresthesias and a garlic-like breath odor*. Many of these resemble the pattern of endemic poisoning seen in China and noted above. A case of fatal suicidal selenium *poisoning* has been described (116[C]), though that patient had ingested not only selenious acid 90 mg/kg but also cupric sulfate 60 mg/kg. At autopsy, pulmonary edema, congestion of the kidneys, and hemorrhagic and erosive gastric mucosa were found. Finally, daily selenium doses of 400 and 25 μg daily for 2 weeks or 2 months, respectively, have been suggested as the cause of *kidney damage* in a 17-year-old boy and an 11-month-old girl (117[C]).

In countries where selenium is in vogue, physicians should be aware of the potential risks of this element and should enquire as to the possible use of selenium products in the home, either in adults or children.

Silver

Silver compounds are still used to a limited extent, notably in dermatologicals, certain nasal drops and eye-drops. If sufficient is absorbed, e.g. from long use or application to extensive burns, there can be accumulation in many tissues. As with other metals, there is also some unwitting exposure to silver, e.g. in certain obscure or outdated free-sale remedies or some anti-smoking preparations designed to alter taste sensations.

Argyrosis—a characteristic smoke-grey discoloration of the skin—is one permanent consequence. In the same subjects the visible mucosal membranes exhibit a bluish discoloration reminiscent of cyanosis (118[CR]). The deposited pigment may be partly silver sulfide and partly metallic silver, formed by photoactivated reduction.

Accumulation in the deeper tissues occurs at the same time, but probably has no clinical consequences. One disputed report dating from 1984 (119[Cr]) concerned two patients with what was regarded as systemic argyrosis following the uncontrolled use for several years of nasal drops containing silver salts; they suffered dyspnea, palpitations, asthenia, a slightly reduced CO_2 diffusion capacity and in one case 'functional adrenal hypofunction'.

Intrapelvic instillation of silver nitrate is sometimes still used in the treatment of essential hematuria. A patient has been described who developed ureteral stenosis as a consequence (120[c]).

Ophthalmic use of silver nitrate solution for prophylaxis of *gonorrhea ophthalmia* in the newborn should be considered as obsolete; it is highly irritant and there are better alternatives. The same applies to the use of silver nitrate as an astringent on skin burns, as opposed to the (well-documented) use of silver sulfadiazine for this purpose; the latter has the adverse effects of the sulfonamides, not those of silver.

Zinc *(SEDA-11, 208)*

In recent years, oral zinc sulphate has been overused in many fields of therapy, particularly in dermatology, despite the fact that some of the indications once claimed for it have been discredited and only a few disorders have been clearly shown to result from zinc deficiency. Dosage has often been high, e.g. the equivalent of 45 mg of metallic zinc three times daily. Once more, one must draw attention to the largely unrecorded use of this metal in some free-sale 'alternative' remedies.

If zinc sulfate is given on an empty stomach, gastric acid can convert it to zinc chloride, which is a powerful caustic agent; it is therefore not surprising that *gastric irritation, nausea, vomiting, hemorrhagic erosive gastritis* and *diarrhea* are common adverse reactions. In the above dosage, zinc sulfate may also produce *copper deficiency* by inducing the production of metallothionein in intestinal cells and thus lowering copper absorption; the copper deficiency may lead in turn to *sideroblastic anemia* (121[c]), *neutropenia* and *osteopenia* (122[C]). Interestingly, this interaction is used constructively to reduce body copper levels in Wilson's disease. It is not clear whether zinc itself also causes anemia directly, or whether the effect is exerted solely through this interaction with copper, but with the increasingly popular sale of zinc supplements for obscure reasons this side effect merits attention as a possible cause of unexplained blood disorders (123[r]).

The dosage of zinc cited above considerably exceeds the recommended daily allowance of 15 mg zinc for healthy adults. In view of the adverse effects, it would seem advisable to limit dosage to two or three times this level. To reduce the unwanted gastrointestinal effects it may prove helpful to use zinc acetate rather than zinc sulphate (124[C]).

Use of topical zinc is considered elsewhere in this volume.

METAL IMPLANTS AND PROSTHESES

Metals used in orthopedic surgery are generally stainless steel (10—14% nickel, 17—20% chromium) or one of the cobalt chrome alloys (27—30% chromium, 57—68% cobalt, and up to 2.5% nickel). All these metals can produce sensitization or elicit toxic reactions when they are solubilized and come into contact with tissue; it can be difficult or impossible to differentiate between hypersensitivity and toxic reactions. Nickel plays a major role in sensitization of patients, even the small amount present in cobalt chrome alloys often sufficing to elicit allergic reactions; reactions to cobalt are more generally toxic in nature (125[C]). An increased rate of allergy to cobalt and nickel has been found in those patients bearing metallic implants who have developed bone infection in the surroundings of osteosynthesis material.

Metals from prostheses can continue to be released into the system for many years. The development of hypersensitivity takes time, and allergic reactions are usual delayed for weeks, months or 1—2 years. The symptoms may assume a variety of forms. Local reactions may cause loosening of the device or local pain. Dermatological reactions include eczema, bullous pemphigoid, urticaria and 'muscle tumors'.

Attempts continue to predict metal sensitivity in the individual patient so that the choice of material can be made accordingly. In vitro tests for metal allergies have been developed on the basis of lymphokinine (MIF) release from sensitized T-lymphocytes exposed to metal—protein complexes (126[CR]). About 6% of patients without a previous metal implant showed positive reactions to nickel, chromium or cobalt. For the present, however, it is still not clear whether such a positive reaction is a reliable predictor of clinical problems. In practice few patients exhibit either local or systemic reactions; where symptoms indeed occur and other causes are ruled out, the implant should be removed. Some workers recommend removal of an implant wherever there is both a positive MIF test and a positive skin test, even in the current absence of a serious reaction. Allergic dermatitis will clear up as soon as the metal has begun to be cleared from the tissue. The type of metal and the amount released into the tissue will affect the time taken for the disappearance of toxic dermatological phenomena.

REFERENCES

1. Veeman GE. De gecombineerde effccten van enkele zware metalen. Pharm Weekbl 1980;115:293.
2. Martyn C, Osmond C, Edwardson JA et al. Geographical relation between Alzheimer's disease and aluminium in drinking water. Lancet 1989;i:5.
3. Kawachi I, Pearce N. Aluminium in the drinking water—is it safe? Austr J Public Health 1991;154:84—87.
4. Spencer H, Kramer L. Antacid-induced calcium loss. Arch Intern Med 1983;143:657.
5. Goodman WG. Bone disease and aluminium: pathogenetic considerations. Am J Kidney Dis 1985;VI:336.
6. Moriniére P, Cohen-Solal M, Belbrik Set al. Disappearance of aluminic bone disease in a long term asymptomatic dialysis population restricting $Al(OH)_3$ intake: emergence of an idiopathic adynamic bone disease not related to aluminium. Nephron 1989;53:93.
7. Shah N, Oberkircher O, Lobel J. Aluminium-induced mcirocytosis in a child with moderate renal insufficiency. Am J Pediat Hematol 1990;12:77—79.
8. Klein GL, Heyman MB, Lee TC et al. Aluminium-associated hepatobiliary dysfunction in rats: relationships to dosage and duration of exposure. Pediatr Res 1988;23:275.
9. Praveen BV, Sankaranarayanan A, Vadiyanathan S. A comparative study of intravesical instillation of 15(s) 15 Me alpha and alum in the management of persistent hematuria of vesical origin. Int J Clin Pharmacol Ther Toxicol 1992;30:7—12.
10. Winterberg B, Korte R, Lison AE. Clinical impact of aluminium load in kidney transplant recipients. Trace Elem Med 1991;8(Suppl 1):46—48.
11. Solkova S, Valek A. Aluminium elimination in patients receiving regular dialysis treatment for chronic renal failure. Trace Elem Med 1991;8(Suppl 1):26—30.
12. Klein GL. Aluminium in parenteral products: medical perspective on large and small volume parenterals. J Parenter Sci Technol 1989;43:120.
13. Milliner DS, Shinaberger JH, Shuman P et al. In advertent aluminium administration during plasma exchange due to aluminium contamination of albumin-replacement solutions. N Engl J Med 1985;312:165.
14. Murphy CP, Cox RL, Harden EA et al. Encephalopthy and seizures induced by intravesical alum irrigation. Bone Marrow Transplannt 1992;10:383—385.
15. Bakir AA, Hryhorczuk DO, Ahmed S et al. Hyperalbuminemia in renal failure: tbe influence of age and citrate intake. Clin Nephrol 1989;31:40.
16. Hewitt CD, Poole CL, Westervelt FB et al. Risks of simultaneous therapy with oral aluminium and citrate compounds. Lancet 1988;ii:849.
17. Sherrard DJ. Aluminium—much ado about something. New Engl J Med 1991;324:558—559.
18. Freunlich M. Tbe spectrum of aluminium toxicity in pediatrics. Int J Pediatr 1988;3:41.
19. Rottembourg J, Jaudon MC, Lagrain M et al. Les gels d'alumine chez les insuffisants rénaux chroniques. Ann. Méd. Interne 1980;131:71.
20. Sideman P, Manor D. Tbe dialysis dementia syndrome and aluminium intoxication. Nephron 1982;31:1.
21. Arief AI. Aluminium and the pathogenesis of dialysis encephalopathy. Am J Kidney Dis 1985;VI:317.
22. Campistol JM, Cases A, Botey A et al. Acute aluminium encephalopathy in an uremic patient. Nephron 1989;51:103.
23. Ellenberg R, King A, Sica D et al. Cerebrospinal fluid aluminium levels following deferoxamine. Am J Kidney Dis 1991;XVI:157.
24. Warady BA, Ford DM, Gaston CE et al. Aluminium intoxication in a child: treatment with intraperitoneal desferrioxamine. Pediatrics 1986;78:651.
25. Feinsilber D, Cha D, Lemos A et al. Arsenicismo cronico medicamentoso. Rev Argent Dermatol 1990;71:178—184.
26. Martin-Boyer G. Intoxications par les sels de bismuth administrés par voie orale. Gastroenterol Clin Biol 1978;2:349
27 Menge H, Gregor M, Brosius B et al. Pharmacology of bismuth. Eur J Gastroenterol Hepatol 1992;4(Suppl 2):41—47.
28. Jungreis AC, Schaumberg HH. Encephalopathy from abuse of bismuth subsalicylate (Pepto-bismol). Neurol 1993;43:1265.
29. Friedland RP, Lerner AJ, Hedra P et al. Encephalopathy associated with bismuth subgallate therapy. Clin Neuropharmacol 1993;16:173—176.
30. Slikkerveer A, De Wolff FA. Bismuth: Biokinetics and neurotoxicity. In: Vinken PJ, Bruyn GW, eds. Handbook of Clinical Neurology, Vol. 64: Intoxication of the Nervous System Part I. Amsterdam: Elsevier, 1994;331—351.
31. Engineer AD. Misra JS. Tandon P. Copper loss and cytopathological changes associated with copper IUD use. Indian J Med Res 1983;78:42.
32. Graham D, Enkin M. DeSa D. Neural tube defects in association with copper intrauterine devices. Int J Gynaecol Obstet 1980;18:404.
33. Payne BA, Pierre RV. Pseudothrombocytopenia: a laboratory artefact with potentially serious consequences. Mayo Clin Proc 1984;59:123.
34. Samson MK. Fraile RJ. Baker LH. O'Bryan R. Phase I-II clinical trial of gallium nitrate (NSC-15200). Cancer Clin Trials 1980;3:131.
35. Fabian CJ. Baker LH, Vaughan CB, Hynes HE. Phase II evaluation of gallium nitrate in breast cancer: a Southwest Oncology Group study. Cancer Treat Rep 1982;66:1591.
36. Warrell RP. Coonley CJ. Straus DJ et al. Clinical evaluation of gallium nitrate (NSC-15200) by 7-day continuous infusion in advanced malignant lymphoma. Proc Am Assoc Cancer Res 1982;1:160.
37. Rothermich NO, Philips VK, Bergen W et al. Chrysotherapy. A prospective study. Arthr Rheum 1976;19:1321—1327.
38. McMahon JM. Gold therapy for rheumatoid arthritis Ann Intern Med 1992;117:169—170.
39. Griffin AJ, Gibson T, Huston G. A comparison of conventional and low dose sodium aurothiomalate treatment in rheumatoid arthritis. Br J Rheumatol 1983;22:82.
40. Sambrook PN, Brouwne CD, Champion GD et al. Terminations of treatment with gold sodium thiomalate in rheumatoid arthritis. J Rheumatol 1982;9:932.
41. Arrigoni-Martelli E. Antirheumatic drugs. Med Actual 1982;18:461.
42. Rau R. Hepatotoxicity of gold compounds. In: Schattenkirchner M, Müller W, eds. Modern Aspects of Gold Ther-

apy. Rheumatology, An Annual Review, 8. Basel—New York: Karger, 1983;188.
43. Trathen WT, Stanley RJ. Allergic reaction to Hulka clips. Obstet Gynecol 1985;66:743.
44. Gottlieb NL, Gray RG. Diagnosis and management of adverse reactions from gold compounds. J Anal Toxicol 1978;2:173.
45. Evans RB, Ettensohn DB. Fawaw-Estrup F et al. Gold lung: recent developments in pathogenesis, diagnosis, and therapy. Arthr Rheum 1987;16:196.
46. Shannon RL, Strayer DS. Arsenic-induced skin toxicity. Hum Toxicol 1989;8:99.
49. Dick DJ, Raman D. The Guillain-Barré syndrome following gold therapy. Scand J Rheumntol 1982;11:119.
50. Fam AC, Gordon DA, Sarkozi J et al. Neurologic complications associated with gold therapy for rheumatoid arthritis. J Rheumatol 1984;11:700.
51. Cervi PL, Wright P, Casey EB. Audit of full blood count monitoring in patients on long term gold therapy for rheumatoid arthritis. Ir J Med Sci 1992;161:73—74.
52. Edelman J, Davis P, Owen ET. Prevalence of eosinophilia during gold therapy for rheumatoid arthritis. J Rheumatol 1983;10:121.
53. Davis P. Undesirable effects of gold salts. J Rheumatol Suppl 1979;5:18.
54. Yan A, Davis P. Gold induced marrow suppression: a review of 10 cases. J Rheumatol 1990;17:47.
55. Harats N, Shalit M, Ehrenfeld M et al. Gold-induced granulomatous hepatitis. Isr J Med Sci 1985;21:753.
56. Murphy M, Hunt S, McDonald GSA et al. Intrahepatic cholestasis secondary to gold therapy. Eur J Gastroenterol Hepatol 1991;3:855—859.
57. Watkins PB, Schade R, Mills AS et al. Fatal hepatic necrosis associated with parenteral gold therapy. Dig Dis Sci 1988;33:1025.
58. Van Linthoudt D, Buss W, Beyner F. et al. Nécrose hépatique fatale au cours d'un traitement aux sels d'or d'une polyarthrite rheumatoide. Schweiz Med Wochenschr 1991;121:1099—1102.
59. Glenert U. Drug stomatitis due to gold therapy. Oral Surg Oral Med Oral Pathol 1984;58:52.
60. Jackson CW, Haboubi NY, Whorwell PJ et al. Gold induced enterocolitis. Gut 1986;27:452.
61. Hall CL, Fothergill NJ, Blackwell MM et al. The natural course of gold nephropathy: long term study of 21 patients. Br Med J 1987;295:745.
62. Hall CL, Tighe R. The effect of continuing penicillamine and gold treatment on the course of penicillamine and gold nephropathy. Br J Rheumatol 1989;28:53.
63. Cramer CR, Hagler HK, Silva FG et al. Chronic interstitial nephritis associated with gold therapy. Arch Pathol Lab Med 1983;107:258.
64. Ranki A, Niemi KM, Kanerva L. Clinical, immunohistochemical and electron-microscopic findings in gold dermatitis. Am J Dermatopathol 1989;11:22.
65. Michalski JP, Isphording W, Parker S. All that glitters may be gold. Arthr Rheum 1991;43:514—516.
66. Smith DL, Wernick R. Exacerbation of psoriasis by chrysotherapy. Arch Dermatol 1991;127:268—269.
67. Wijnands MJH, Van Riel PLCM, Gribnau FWJ et al. Risk factors of second-line antirheumatic drugs in rheumatoid arthritis. A review of the literature. Semin Arthr Rheum 1990;19:337.
68. Prupas HM. Stroke-like syndrome after gold sodium thiomalate induced vasomotor reaction. J Rheumatol 1984:11:235.
69. Hakala M, Van Assendelt AHW, Ilonen J et al. Association of different HLA antigens with various toxic effects of gold salts in rheumatoid arthritis. Ann Rheum Dis 1986:45:177.
70. Speerstra F, Van Riel PLCM, Reekers P et al. The influence of HLA phenotypes on the response to parenteral gold in rheumatoid arthritis. Tissue Antigens 1986;28:1.
71. Speerstra F, Reekers P, Van de Putte LBA et al. HLA associations in aurothioglucose and D-penicillamine induced haematotoxic reactions in rheumatoid arthritis. Tissue Antigens 1985;26:35.
72. Van Riel PLCM, Reekers P, Van de Putte LBA. Association of HLA antigens, toxic reactions and therapeutic response to auranofin and aurothioglucose in patients with rheumatoid arthritis. Tissue Antigens 1983;22:194.
73. Singal DP, Green D, Reid B et al. HLA-D region genes and rheumatoid arthritis (RA): importance of DR and DQ genes in conferring susceptibility to RA. Ann Rheum Dis 1992;51:23—28.
74. Rodriguez Perez M, Gonzalez Dominquez J, Mataran Perez L et al. HLA DR7 como factor de proteccion frente a la toxicidad por sales de oro en la artritis reumatoide. An Med Interna 1993;10:484—486.
75. Madhok R, Capell HA, Waring R. Does sulphoxidation state predict gold toxicity in rheumatoid arthritis? Br Med J 1987;294:483.
76. Rogers JG, Anderson RMcD, Chow CW et al. Possible teratogenic effects of gold. Aust Pediatr J 1980;16:194.
77. Tarp U, Graudal H, Møller-Madsen B, Danscher G. A follow-up study of children exposed to gold salts in utero. In: Abstracts, X European Congress of Rheumatology, Moscow, 1983, Abstract No. 646. Moscow, 1983.
78. Jaeger A, Leroy M, Sander Ph et al. Hepatitis after gold oerdose. Treatment with chelating agents. Toxicol Lett 1980;6:65.
79. Corkill MM, Kirkham BW, Chikanza IC et al. Intramuscular depot methylprednisolone induction of chrysotherapy in rheumatoid arthritis: a 24-week randomized controlled trial. Br J Rheumatol 1990;29:274.
80. Heuer MA, Pietrusko RG, Morris RW. An analysis of worldwide safety experience with auranofin. J Rheumatol 1985;15:695.
81. Goebel KM, Storck U, Kohl FV et al. Klinischer Effekt und unerwünschte Arzneimittelwirkungen von Auranofin bei rheumatoider Arthritis. Inn Med 1985;12:39.
82. Wallin BA, McCafferty JP, Fox MJ et al. Incidence and management of diarrhea during longterm auranofin therapy. J Rheumatol 1988;15:1755.
83. Horing E. Goldinduzierte kolitis. Med Welt 1989;40:876.
84. Jarner D, Nielsen AM. Auranofin (SK+F39162) induced enterocolitis in rheumatoid arthritis. Scand J Rheumatol 1983;12:254.
85. Katz WA, Blodgett RC, Pietrusko RG. Proteinuria in gold-treated rheumatoid arthritis. Ann Intern Med 1984;101:176.
86. Auranofin—Diabetes situation impaired/hypoglycemia. Bull SADRAC, June/October (English version), 3.
87. Nierop G, Gijzel WP, Bel EH et al. Auranofin in the treatment of steroid dependent asthma: a double blind study. Thorax 1992;47:349—354.

88. Millagan A, Graham-Brown RAC, Sarkany I et al. Erythropoietic protoporphyria exacerbated by oral iron therapy. Br J Dermatol 1988;119:63.
89. Ivanov E, Adjarov D, Kerimova M et al. Rare cases of porphyria cutanea tarda associated with additional iron overload. Dermatologia 1982;164:127.
90. Cook JD, Carriaga M, Kahn SG et al. Gastric delivery system for iron supplementation. Lancet 1990;i:1136.
91. Begemann H. Praktische Hämatologie, 8th edn. Stuttgart—New York: Thieme, 1982;355.
92. Marcus RE, Huehns ER. Transfusional iron overload. Clin Lab Haematol 1985;7:195.
93. Van der Weyden MB. Vitamin C, desferrioxamine and iron loading anemias. Aust NZ J Med 1984;14:593.
94. McFarlane H, Reddy S, Adcock KJ et al. Immunity, transferrin, and survival in kwashiorkor. Br Med J 1970;4:268.
95. Weber MH, Ammon A, Oppermann M et al. Panhypogammaglobulinämie: eine seltene Komplikation der parenteralen Gold-Therapie. Z Rheumatol 1991;50:207—210.
96. Yao K, Uchigata Y, Kyono H et al. Human insulin-specific immunoglobulin G antibody and hypoglycemic attacks after the injection of gold thioglucose. J Endocrin Invest 1992;15:43—47.
97. Hirata Y. Autoimmune insulin syndriome 'up to date'. In: Andreani D, Marks V, Lefebvre PH, eds. Hypoglycemia. New York: Raven Press, 1987;105.
98. Scott JM. Iron-sorbitol-citrate in pregnancy anaemia. Br Med J 1963;2:354.
99. Amitai I, Acker M. Adverse effects of intramuscular iron injections. Acta Haematol 1982;68:341.
100. IARC Monographs on the Evaluation of Carcinogenic Risk of Chemicals to Man. Iron-Carbohydrate Complexes, International Agency for Research on Cancer, Lyon. 1973;161.
101. Altman LC, Petersen PE. Successful prevention of an anaphylactoid reaction to iron dextran. Ann Intern Med 1988;109:346.
102. Okada M, Imamura K, Lida M et al. Hypophosphatemia induced by intravenous administration of saccharated iron oxide. Klin Wochenschr 1983;61:99.
103. Marchasin S, Wallerstein RO. The treatment of iron deficiency anaemia with intravenous iron dextran. Blood 1964;23:354.
104. Shimada A. Adverse reactions to total-dose infusion of iron dextran. Clin Pharm 1952;1:248.
105. Blake DR, Lunec J, Ahern M et al. Effect of intravenous iron dextran on rheumatoid synovitis. Ann Rheum Dis 1985;44:183.
106. Brighton SW, De la Harpe AL. Development of an inlammatory synovitis following total-dose infusion of iron dextran. S Afr Med J 1982;62:141.
107. Lorscheider F, Vimy M. Mercury exposure from 'silver' fillings. Lancet 1991;337:1103.
108. Kupsinel R. Mercury amalgam toxicity: a major common denominator of degenerative disease. J Orthomol Psychiatr 1984;13:240.
109. Wahlberg JE. Nickel allergy in hairdressers. Contact Dermatitis 1981;7:358.
110. Block 6T, Yeung M. Asthma induced by nickel. J Am Med Assoc 1982;247:1600.
111. Niordson AM. Nickel sensitivity as a cause of rhinitis. Contact Dermatitis 1981;7:273.
112. Al-Tawil PIG, Marcusson JA, Miiller E. Lymphocyte transformation test in patients with nickel sensitivity: an aid to diagnosis. Acta Dermatol-Venereol 1981;61:511.
113. Kapoor-Pillarisetti A, Mowbray JF et al. HLA dependence of sensitivity to nickel and chromium. Tissue Antigens 1982;17:261.
114. Yang G, Wang S, Zhou R et al. Endemic selenium intoxication of humans in China. Am J Clin Nutr 1984;37:872—881.
115. Anonymous. Toxicity with superpotent selenium. FDA Drug Bull 1984;14:19.
116. Matoba R, Kimura H, Uchima E et al. An autopsy case of acute selenium (selenious acid) poisoning and selenium levels in human tissues. Forensic Sci Int 1986;31:87.
117. Snodgrass W, Rumack BH, Sullivan JB. Selenium: childhood poisoning and cystic fibrosis. Clin Toxicol 1981;18:211.
118. Tanner L, Gross D. Generalized argyria. Cutis 1990;45:237—239.
119. Dupont T, Gomez J, Cuvillier P et al. Argyrie généralisée médicamenteuse: intérêt des dosages sériques et urinaires i propos de 2 cas. LARC Méd 1984;4:103.
120. Vijan SR, Keating MA, Althausen AF. Ureteral stenosis after silver nitrate instillation in the treatment of essential hematuria J Urol 1988;139:1015.
121. Fiske DN, McCoy HE III, Kitchens CS. Zinc-induced sideroblastic anemia. Am J Hematol 1994;46:147—150.
122. Patterson WP, Winkelmann M, Perry MC. Zinc-induced copper deficiency: megamineral sideroblastic anemia. Ann Intern Med 1985;103:385.
123. Frambach D, Bendel R. Zinc supplementation and anemia. J Am Med Assoc 1991;265:869.
124. Mahajan SK, Abbasi AA, Prasad AS et al. Effect of oral zinc therapy on gonadal function in hemodialysis patients. Ann Intern Med 1982;97:357.
125. Waterman AH, Schrik JJ. Allergy in hip arthroplasty. Contact Dermatitis 1985;13:294.
126. Hierholzer S, Hierholzer G. Untersuchungen zur Metallallergie nach Osteosynthesen. Unfallchirurgie 1982;8:347.

Meyler's Side Effects of Drugs, 13th Edition
M.N.G. Dukes, editor

SECTION EDITOR: P. FOLB

R.H.B. Meyboom and C.C.E. Brodie-Meijer

23 Metal antagonists

Metal antagonists are usually chelate-producing drugs such as deferoxamine, penicillamine and salts of edetic acid. These drugs have a strong affinity for metals necessary for the function of many important enzymes, and have been shown experimentally to have strong influences on biological systems and pathophysiological processes. In addition to metal poisoning, the use of chelators has been extended to diseases not related to metal toxicity, e.g. rheumatoid arthritis.

Penicillamine *(SED-11, 461; SEDA-14, 194; SEDA-13, 198)*

Penicillamine is dimethylcysteine or 2-amino-3-mercapto-3-methylbutyric acid. It has three functional groups: an α-amine, a carboxyl and a sulfhydryl, which largely determine the pharmacological effects of the drug. L-Penicillamine is a pyridoxine antagonist and a toxic drug. The racemic mixture has, therefore, been replaced in medicine by purified D-pencillamine. In this volume the word 'penicillamine' refers to the D-isomer unless otherwise specified. As the name indicates, penicillamine is a degradation product of penicillin. Several reviews of the chemistry, kinetics and pharmacology of penicillamine have been provided (SED-12, 537; 1[R]). After oral administration approximately two-thirds (50—70%) of a penicillamine dose are absorbed. As much as 33% may be degraded in the gut before absorption can take place. With a half-life of less than 1 hour, penicillamine is after oral administration rapidly cleared, largely by the formation of disulfides with plasma albumin and with low molecular weight thiols such as cysteine and glutathione. The low molecular disulfides constitute the major urinary metabolites. The penicillamine-albumin disulfide, on the other hand, has a long half-life. The consequence of this is slow accumulation: in healthy volunteers pseudo-steady-state plasma concentrations of penicillamine-albumin disulfide are not reached until the second week of daily administration. Peak plasma concentrations of penicillamine occur at 1.5—4 hours after ingestion and range from 5.0 μM after 150 mg to 27.5 μM after 800 mg (when conventional release oral preparations are used). About 80% of penicillamine is protein-bound; approximately 7% occurs as L-cysteine-D-penicillamine disulfide, 5% as penicillamine disulfide and 6% as free penicillamine. A large proportion is rapidly excreted in the urine, mainly as the disulfide or as the disulfide metabolite conjugated with cysteine; the latter may lead to cysteine depletion. Another part is converted to *S*-methyl-penicillamine and is either excreted by the kidney or metabolized in the liver. Although *S*-methylation is a quantitatively minor elimination pathway, the *S*-methyl-penicillamine produced is a potential substrate for sulfoxide formation and it has been found that patients with rheumatoid arthritis who form the sulfoxide at a reduced rate are at greater risk of side effects (2[CR]). The concentrations of penicillamine and metabolites within cells and at the cell surface are largely unknown, but may (in the case of a cellular site of action) be relevant to variability in response. In clinical trials about 50% of patients experienced one or more side effects and discontinuation was necessary in about one-third (3—6, 7[C]). Long-term follow-up studies have shown that, indeed, many patients—up to 80%—stop taking penicillamine, either because of side effects or lack of efficacy (8[C], 9[R], 10[C]). The frequency, diversity and severity of side effects of penicillamine are impressive. Side effects are less frequent when small doses are used, when increments are made only slowly, when patients are closely monitored and when penicillamine has been tolerated for some years. In a meta-analysis of a large series of clinical trials, on the other hand, there was no evidence found for a dose-related toxicity in patients taking penicillamine (dose range 500—1250 mg/day) (7[C]). Anyone responsible for a patient taking penicillamine must bear in mind that serious adverse reactions may occur even with very small doses (as low as 125 mg daily), suddenly, and at any time during treatment, even after many years. Penicillamine may be the unexpected cause of serious adverse reactions as an additive to 'Chinese herbs' (11[c]).

With regard to the safe use of penicillamine the words of Huskisson are still very true (12): 'Perhaps the most important aspect of the surveillance of patients receiving penicillamine is the need for physician and patient to be able to contact each other. The physician must find the patient if his blood count changes. The patient must find the physician if he becomes ill. Disasters have occurred when patients consulted physicians who were unaware of the problems of penicillamine and instituted unwise therapy for them. Penicillamine can only be used by those who know how to use it and skilful management of the side effects is a most important aspect, perhaps *the* most important aspect of the treatment.'

ADVERSE REACTION PATTERN

General and toxic effects Untoward effects are frequent, occurring in about half the patients and leading to discontinuation in one-third. In long-term follow-up studies an even greater proportion of the patients stopped penicillamine, either because of side effects or lack of efficacy. Early effects are gastrointestinal upset and, more characteristically, loss of taste. Although a decline in the number of thrombocytes is common, serious thrombocytopenia is less frequent. After long-term use of high doses, skin collagen and elastin are impaired, resulting in increased friability and sometimes in disorders such as perforating elastoma or cutis laxa; the latter has also been observed in neonates.

Hypersensitivity reactions These are frequent early in a course of penicillamine, with urticarial or maculopapular rashes, fever and lymphadenopathy. Cross-allergy to penicillin may occur. In addition, the use of penicillamine may be complicated by a unique variety of often serious hypersensitivity reactions, involving the skin, kidneys, liver, lungs, muscular system or other organs, which are frequently accompanied by autoimmune phenomena. Proteinuria is found in more than 10% of patients and sometimes develops into a nephrotic syndrome. Pemphigus, myasthenia gravis, polymyositis or systemic lupus erythematosus occur in a small percentage of users. Rare reactions such as aplastic anemia, Goodpasture's syndrome or thrombotic thrombocytopenic purpura (Moschcowitz's syndrome) have a high fatality rate.

Tumor-inducing effects Although lymphatic malignancies have been described in a few patients using penicillamine, a causal relationship is considered unlikely.

ORGANS AND SYSTEMS

Cardiovascular *(SED-12, 539)* Penicillamine has no effect on cardiovascular function. Although *hypersensitivity reactions* are frequent, systemic *anaphylaxis* has only been reported rarely (13[C]). The effect of penicillamine on collagen and elastin fibers, causing characteristic skin lesions, was found also to include the vascular wall (see 'Skin and appendages'). Clinical manifestations of vascular insufficiency have, however, not been reported. Penicillamine-associated *polymyositis* may also involve the heart muscle and cause *arrhythmia*, *Adams-Stokes attacks*, and death (see 'Musculoskeletal').

Respiratory *(SED-12, 539; SEDA-18, 246)* Although penicillamine has no direct effects on the lungs (14[c]), its use is nevertheless associated with a spectrum of pulmonary injury: *interstitial and alveolar reactions*, *pulmonary fibrosis*, *bronchiolitis obliterans and pulmonary/renal syndromes* (15[R]–18[R]). The differentiation between drug reactions and pulmonary disorders secondary to rheumatic or other underlying diseases, however, is often difficult. In addition, several autoimmune reactions to penicillamine can secondarily affect pulmonary function. Penicillamine-induced *polymyositis* (19[C]) or *myasthenia gravis* can cause *respiratory failure*, even requiring ventilatory support (20[C]) (see below). Although the causal role of penicillamine has never been proven, *obliterating bronchiolitis* is usually included in the list of its possible adverse reactions (SED-12, 539; 18, 21[CR], 22[cR]). The principal lesion is a stenosis of the small bronchioles throughout the lung, causing severe respiratory failure. Obliterating bronchiolitis can be severely debilitating and often has a fatal course.

Alveolar hemorrhage may occur in connection with penicillamine as part of a life-threatening pulmonary-renal syndrome, resembling Goodpasture's syndrome (23[CR]) (see 'Urinary system').

Rhinitis, *bronchospasm and asthma* may occur as a manifestation of hypersensitivity to penicillamine (SEDA-5, 248; 24[C], 25[C], 26[c]) and rarely of the *Churg-Strauss syndrome* (see 'Multisystem reactions') (27[CR]). Rhinitis may also be a symptom of penicillamine-induced pemphigus (28[C]) (see 'Skin and appendages'). In one patient a large *pulmonary cyst* developed concomitantly with skin lesions characteristic of the use of large doses of penicillamine (29[C]) (see 'Skin and appendages'). Microscopic derangement of the elastic fibers predominated. Although the frequency is uncertain, penicillamine may be associated with recurrent respiratory tract infections, i.e. secondary to IgA deficiency (30[CR], 31[CR]) or as part of the 'yellow nail syndrome' (SEDA-9, 223) (see 'Skin and appendages').

Nervous system *(SED-12, 539; SEDA-16, 242; SEDA-17, 281; SEDA-18, 246)* L-Penicillamine and the racemic mixture strongly inhibit pyridoxal-dependent enzymes, cause pyridoxine deficiency in animal experiments, and are neurotoxic. Although this effect is much weaker with D-penicillamine, a few case-reports have shown that D-penicillamine may also occasionally cause *polyneuropathy*, either as a toxic or allergic reaction (32[C]–34[C], 35[c]). Rarely *optic neuropathy* (36[C]) or *polyradiculoneuritis* (37[C], 38[C]) have been reported. When penicillamine therapy is started in patients with Wilson's disease, pre-existing neurological involvement may be acutely aggravated; convulsions, muscle spasms and coma can occur and death may follow (39[C]–42[C], 43[R], 44[C]). Worsening of the neurological syndrome on starting therapy with penicillamine may occur in up to 50% of neurologically affected patients with Wilson's disease (42[C], 43[R]) and penicillamine may precipitate serious neurological injury in a previously asymptomatic patient (45[C]). It is uncertain if this results from alterations of copper distribution at submolecular, subcellular, transcellular or transorganic levels, or whether it results from some other property of penicillamine (e.g. its capacity to donate sulfhydryl groups). Since the initial damage may be caused by copper decompartmentalization it has been suggested that pretreatment with lipid-soluble antioxidants such as vitamin E may be useful (40), whereas at least some of these effects may reflect secondary pyridoxine deficiency. Supplementary oral pyridoxine may be advisable (43[R]).

Penicillamine can induce a *myasthenia gravis*-like reaction which is clinically indistinguishable from idiopathic myasthenia gravis (11[CR], 20[C], 45[CR]–54[CR], 55[C]–58[C], 59[c]). It develops in up to 4% of patients using penicillamine. The reaction often starts with involvement of ocular muscles, but all striated muscles may become involved. The antigenic properties of circulating acetylcholine receptor antibodies in penicillamine-induced and idiopathic myasthenia are similar to those in recent-onset cases of spontaneous mysasthenia gravis (51[C], 58[C], 60[CR]). Antistriational and antinuclear antibodies (61[C]) may be present, and a sensitive immunoassay for striational autoantibodies may be used to monitor patients on penicillamine for developing myasthenia (53[c]). In one study, the measurement of AChR antibodies was considered to be of little or no use in routine monitoring of patients using penicillamine, because in 20% of patients AChR antibodies were detected at least on one occasion, although none of the patients had signs or symptoms of myasthenia and the antibody tests returned to normal despite continuation of the drug (62[CR]). Others have advised annual monitoring of every patient taking penicillamine, to detect subclinical changes in neuromuscular transmission and by AChR antibody testing (63[C], 64[CR]). In spite of the clinical similarities, there are some differences between spontaneous and penicillamine-induced myasthenia in respect to genetics. Myasthenic reactions to penicillamine appear to occur in a special genetic subgroup of patients; the prevalence of the HLA antigens DRI and Bw35 is higher in these patients, whereas that of antigens DR3 (which is associated with idiopathic myasthenia) and DR4 (which is increased in rheumatoid arthritis) is lower (65[CR], 66[CR]). Myasthenia usually improves rapidly after stopping penicillamine, but it may have a protracted course; fatal cases have occurred. Unrecognized myasthenia may present with prolonged paralysis after general anesthesia. For this reason, for all patients on penicillamine undergoing anesthesia the same precautions are necessary as for patients with known myasthenia gravis (67[C]). Penicillamine may be the unexpected cause of myasthenia gravis as an additive to 'Chinese herbs' (11[c]).

Isolated cases have been described of *myasthenic pseudo-internuclear ophthalmoplegia* (68[C]), *neuromyotonia* (69[C]) and *diffuse fasciculations* (70[C]), attributed to the use of penicillamine.

Endocrine, metabolic; mineral and fluid balance *(SED-11, 463; SEDA-13, 199) Metals* Penicillamine is a potent chelator of metals. The stability of complexes of metals and penicillamine decreases in the following order: Hg, Pb, Ni, Cu, Zn, Cd, Co, Fe, Mn (71[C]–73[C]). Most human data refer to copper, lead and mercury. Because of the strong affinity of penicillamine for copper and other metals, the drug is used in the treatment of Wilson's disease and lead poisoning. In other patients, however, this effect may sometimes induce deficiencies (SED-8, 531), especially of *copper*. The prevalence and consequences of copper deficiency in patients receiving penicillamine need further study (SEDA-10, 223). Copper deficiency has been thought to play a role in the occasionally reported alopecia and in the loss of taste which is often experienced by patients with rheumatoid arthritis receiving penicillamine (but rarely in Wilson's disease; see 'Gastrointestinal'), but this could not be confirmed (74[C]). Penicillamine-induced deficiency of both copper and *iron* has been held responsible for the development of anemia (75[C]), but serum iron levels do not usually change in patients using penicillamine (SED-8, 535). The influence on metals such as copper and *zinc* may be difficult to assess, since penicillamine not only increases the excretion but also the absorption of these metals (76[C]). Although this patient had a greatly increased excretion of copper, penicillamine did not influence that of calcium, magnesium or iron. A zinc deficiency syndrome, with skin lesions, alopecia, granulocytopenia and eye damage, has nevertheless been described in association with penicillamine (77[CR]).

Vitamins L-Penicillamine strongly inhibits pyridoxal-dependent enzymes and causes manifest *pyridoxine* deficiency in animal experiments. Although D-penicillamine is much less active in this respect, some decline in the pyridoxine effect is measurable, and in a report describing penicillamine-associated polyneuropathy, pyridoxine supplements for patients receiving D-penicillamine were advised (32[C]); see 'Nervous system').

Proteins and enzymes In in vitro studies penicillamine was found to have an inhibiting effect on angiotensin-converting enzyme (ACE) and carboxypeptidase (78[c]). Penicillamine interferes with the functions of the copper-containing enzyme ceruloplasmin and some of the penicillamine- and copper-containing complexes formed in vivo have superoxide dismutase effects (1[r]). The effects of penicillamine on collagen and elastin are reviewed below (see 'Skin and appendages').

Autoimmune hypoglycemia One of the remarkable autoimmune phenomena that penicillamine may elicit is the induction of anti-insulin antibodies with resultant clinical hypoglycemia (autoimmune hypoglycemia). In these patients, high concentrations of immunoreactive insulin are found, despite undetectable free insulin. Four such patients have so far been described (79[CR], 80[CR]). When penicillamine is discontinued the antibody titers fall sharply. (The occurrence of hypo- rather than hyperglycemia is not fully understood but well known with spontaneous 'autoimmune hypoglycemia' (81[r]). In addition, hypoglycemia developed in two previously well-controlled diabetic patients while taking penicillamine; however no reference was made to anti-insulin antibodies in these patients (82[c]). In a study using a competitive radiobinding assay, as many as 43% of rheumatoid patients using penicillamine had autoantibodies against insulin (83[C]). These antibodies did not appear to be deleterious to pancreatic β-cells, as the response to intravenous glucose was normal and no episodes of hypoglycemia were observed. Other sulfhydryl compounds occasionally reported in association with autoimmune hypoglycemia are tiopronin, pyritinol and methimazol (84[CR]).

Thyroiditis Two patients are on record with suspected penicillamine-induced thyroiditis, one case being associated with a myasthenic reaction (85[C], 86[C]).

Enlargement of the breasts and gynecomastia These are discussed below (see 'Genital system').

Hematological *(SED-12, 541; SEDA-16, 242; SEDA-17, 282; SEDA-18, 246)* Eosinophilia may be encountered in about 25% of patients using penicillamine, but is of little value in predicting serious hypersensitivity reactions (87[C]). The use of penicillamine is often associated with changes in platelet or white cell counts. In the ARAMIS PMS Program, hematological events regarded as side effects of penicillamine, calculated per 1000 person-years, were as follows: pancytopenia 10, low white blood cells 8, low platelets 18 and polycythemia 2 (88[c]). Serious blood dyscrasias, although rare, belong to the most important adverse reactions to penicillamine (SED-12, 541; 89[C], 90[c]). The assessment of the frequency of penicillamine-related hematological reactions may be hindered by the use of other potentially hematotoxic drugs, such as analgesics or gold compounds. The pathogenesis of hematological reactions to penicillamine is uncertain, but the available evidence suggests that pharmacological as well as immunological processes may be involved (91[CR]–94[CR]).

Thrombocytopenia occurs in about 10–16% of patients treated, needing withdrawal in up to 10% (3, 4, 95[c]), but these percentages vary considerably, presumably reflecting the use of different doses of penicillamine and different definitions of thrombocytopenia. The decrease in platelets is usually transient, but occasionally it is a warning for impending profound and dangerous thrombocytopenia or serious hematological disorders such as aplastic anemia or thrombotic thrombocytopenic purpura. Thrombocytopenia mainly develops during the first 6 months of penicillamine administration and appears to be associated with certain HLA antigens (i.e. DRA4, A1, C4BQO). Platelet counts fall to some extent in about 75% of patients receiving penicillamine and it may be difficult to decide when to stop drug therapy. Platelet counts are recommended initially at 2-weekly intervals and subsequently each month, in addition to clear instructions to the patient. When the counts fall to between 100 and 70 × 10^9/l, weekly checks are needed and daily checks when below 70. If platelet counts show an obvious progressive decline or fall below 70 × 10^9/l, penicillamine should be immediately discontinued (96). Several cases are on record of *thrombotic thrombocytopenic purpura* or *Moschcowitz's syndrome*, characterized by intravascular coagulation, thrombocytopenia and hemolysis, as a rare but life-threatening complication of penicillamine (SEDA-9, 224; SEDA-14, 195; 97[CR], 98[cR]).

Penicillamine is a well-known and relatively frequent cause of other serious hematological reactions such as *agranulocytosis* and *aplastic anemia*, but the number of well-documented observations concerning such patients described in the literature is small (89, 94, 99–103, 104[c], 105[c]). *Pure red cell aplasia* developed in a 40-

year-old woman as a rare idiosyncratic hematological reaction to penicillamine (61[C]). Discontinuation of the drug, which had been taken in a daily dose of 500 mg for rheumatoid arthritis, and a short treatment with corticosteroids was followed by permanent recovery. *Evans' syndrome*, i.e. thrombocytopenic purpura in combination with autoimmune hemolytic anemia, developed in a patient receiving treatment with penicillamine (300 mg daily for 11 months) for rheumatoid arthritis (106[C]). Anti-platelet antibodies as well as antibodies against erythrocytes were detected. The condition persisted despite discontinuation of penicillamine, but finally recovered in the course of 1 year and following treatment with danazole and hydrocortisone. Because of its effect on the enzyme ceruloplasmin and, in turn, the utilization of stored iron, penicillamine is considered to be able to cause *iron deficiency anemia* (75[C], 107[R], 108[R]). Penicillamine may also elicit *hemolytic anemia* (SEDA-8, 535; 109[c]), although good clinical support for this is lacking. A positive Coomb's test may occur as part of a lupus syndrome (110[C]). *Polycythemia* (88[c]), *leukocytosis* and *thrombocytosis* have been mentioned in association with penicillamine, but data are lacking.

For *lymphatic malignancies* see Tumor-inducing effects (page 606).

Liver *(SED-11, 464; SEDA-13, 199)* Several case reports have demonstrated that penicillamine can cause liver injury (SEDA-13, 199; 111[R]), mainly *cholestatic hepatitis*, often associated with other signs of hypersensitivity such as fever, rash (112[CR]) and pulmonary (100[CR], 113[CR]) or hematological reactions (103[C]). In two children with Wilson's disease, penicillamine was thought to have caused persistence of a pre-existing increase in aminotransferase activity (114[c]).

Gastrointestinal *(SED-12, 541; SEDA-16, 243; SEDA-17, 282)* Gastrointestinal complaints, including *nausea*, *vomiting*, *heartburn*, *abdominal distress or diarrhea*, occur in up to one-third of patients starting penicillamine and may account for up to half of the withdrawals in the first 3 months of treatment (SED-12, 541; 3, 4). For *taste disturbances*, see 'Special senses'. Withdrawal of penicillamine was required because of nausea and vomiting in five of 98 patients (115[c]). Penicillamine is not known to be ulcerogenic, however (SED-8, 535; SEDA-2, 217; 116), and the nature of this reaction is not clear. Sulfhydryl compounds can damage the gut mucosa, but examination of the mucosa of cysteinuric patients who reported gastrointestinal upset while on penicillamine, revealed no evidence of structural damage (117[c]). Gastrointestinal symptoms are less frequent with initially low doses which are slowly increased. Taking penicillamine with food improves tolerance but decreases absorption (see introductory section). *Ulcers of the oral mucosa* are not uncommon in patients on penicillamine, occurring in about 10% of patients. Oral ulcers occurred in two of 25 patients with systemic sclerosis and necessitated withdrawal in one (118[C]), whereas in a series of 98 rheumatoid arthritis patients withdrawal of penicillamine because of mouth ulcers was required in three (115[c]). On the other hand, aphthous stomatitis occurs frequently in users of non-steroidal anti-inflammatory drugs (119[r]). In seven cases in 56 consecutive patients on penicillamine, *oral lichen planus* was a frequent phenomenon (120[Cr]) (see also 'Skin and appendages'). Most patients have erosive oral lichen planus but also bullous, plaque-like or 'classic' lichen planus may occur. *Cheilosis* has been reported (121[c]). Oral lesions may constitute a pemphigus, in the absence of lesions outside the oral cavity. Penicillamine-induced cicatricial pemphigoid may be associated with *oral ulcers or lesions of the esophagus*, and stenosis may occur (see 'Skin and appendages'). An unusual case attributed to the use of penicillamine concerned a woman with dysphagia, heartburn and weight loss in whom numerous large *aphthoid ulcerations* were found in the esophagus (122[C]). When high doses are used, stomatitis may reflect impaired collagen synthesis. In one such patient mucosal ulcerations were associated with *leiomyomatosis* in the peripheral serosa which in turn caused *intestinal obstruction* (123[CR]). In another patient treated with penicillamine for Wilson's disease the removal of an impacted maxillary third molar was followed by the development of an oroantral fistula, presumably as a result of impaired collagen synthesis and *disturbed wound healing* (124[C]). Oral ulcers may be an important warning sign for penicillamine-induced agranulocytosis.

Although less well-documented than with gold, penicillamine may also occasionally cause life-threatening colitis (125[CR]). Three poorly documented cases have been reported of *pancreatitis* attributed to the use of penicillamine (SED-8, 385; SEDA-2, 217). For *Sjögren syndrome*, see Immune system and autoimmune reactions.

Kidney and urinary system *(SED-12, 542; SEDA-13, 199; SEDA-14, 196; SEDA-16, 243; SEDA-17, 282; SEDA-18, 247)* The administration of penicillamine is frequently associated with renal injury. Some *proteinuria* is encountered in about 10—25% of patients receiving penicillamine (SED-11, 464; 3[c], 4[c], 88[C], 95[c], 118[C], 126[C], 127[C], 128[Cr]) and occurs in 50% of patients with cysteinuria (SEDA-8, 236). In about 5% of patients, proteinuria is the reason for withdrawing penicillamine. To avoid renal damage, response-dependent prescribing is recommended in rheumatoid arthritis, starting with only a small dose and making increments at intervals of at least 1—2 months. Frequent urine testing is necessary, particularly during the first 18 months. Mild proteinuria (<1 g/24 hours) occurs most frequently, is often transient, and may be coincidental. Moderate proteinuria may be penicillamine-induced but may not be progressive and not clinically harmful; close monitoring is indicated in such an event, and a temporary decrease of the dose is advisable, although withdrawal of penicillamine may not be needed. When proteinuria increases, the development of a nephrotic syndrome and serious renal injury may occur, necessitating discontinuation of the drug (129[C]). In cysteinuria it is advisable to stop penicillamine when proteinuria exceeds 5 g/24 hours (130), but in rheumatoid arthritis a lower limit of 2 g/24 hours has been proposed (131).

Nephropathy mainly develops during the second 6 months of treatment with penicillamine (131). It is more frequent in patients with a low sulfoxidation capacity (132[CR], 133[R]) and with the HLA antigens DR3 and B8 (SEDA-11, 212; 134[C]). Although nephropathy is thought to be rare in Japanese people (SEDA-8, 235; 6[C]), it has been encountered in Japan (135[C]). The principal lesion is *membranous glomerulopathy* or *minimal-change glomerulitis* (127[C], 131[R], 136[C], 137[C]), characterized by little (some thickening of the basal membrane) or no changes on light-microscopic examination, but striking disturbances of the glomerular structures on electron microscopy (fusion of epithelial cell foot processes, subepithelial electron-dense deposits and mesangial cell hyperactivity). Immunofluorescence microscopy shows granular deposits containing IgG and C3 (138[C]). These immunoglobulin deposits are not the result of precipitation of circulating immune complexes, as was previously thought. The available evidence indicates that the nephritogenic antigen, although still not identified, is expressed in the glomerulus and the immune complexes are formed in situ (136[C], 139[R]). Although nephrosis may be profound, serum creatinine is usually unaltered and penicillamine glomerulopathy has a good prognosis. Proteinuria may nevertheless continue for longer than 12 months after stopping and microscopic lesions may persist for longer. Although penicillamine nephropathy is more frequent when high doses are taken, it can also occur with small doses (e.g. 125 mg daily). On rechallenge, nephropathy does not necessarily relapse (SEDA-10, 218), and a history of previous gold nephropathy is not thought to be a risk factor (134[C]). In one study, titers of anti-galactosyl antibodies were correlated with the prior development of penicillamine (or gold) nephropathy (140[C]).

Occasionally penicillamine-associated renal injury may be proliferative and progressive, extending beyond the basement membrane, with crescent formation in the glomeruli, and encompassing other renal structures, e.g. in the case of *renal vasculitis*, *IgM nephropathy* (141[C]) or as part of a more general reaction; persistent renal failure may develop and death may follow (127[cR], 142[CR], 143[CR], 144[c], 145[C]—147[C]). Penicillamine-induced systemic lupus erythematosus may be associated with *proliferating glomerulonephritis* with mesangial involvement and interstitial infiltrates (148[CR], 149[CR]). In such cases anti-native DNA antibodies may be found. A rare but life-threatening complication of penicillamine is the development of a *Goodpasture's syndrome-like reaction*, characterized by alveolar hemorrhage, glomerulonephritis and fever (23, 150[C], 151[CR], 152[CR], 153[C]). Plasmapheresis and immunosuppressive therapy may be needed. In contrast with genuine Goodpasture's syndrome, circulating antiglomerular basement membrane antibodies are not detected (151), perhaps because the antigen concerned is not present in the test extracts used (152). Since it is transient or coincidental in the majority of patients receiving penicillamine (SEDA-7, 260), microscopic *hematuria* has limited predictive value. It may nevertheless be an important sign heralding serious renal complications requiring the immediate discontinuation of the drug.

The diagnosis of penicillamine-induced renal injury is often difficult because of the frequent association of rheumatoid arthritis with renal disorders (135[CR], 154[R], 155[CR]—157[CR]), including spontaneous membranous glomerulopathy (158), or with injury caused by concomitant analgesics (159[C]). Ultimately the course in time-relation to penicillamine exposure may be indicative of the role of penicillamine (159).

In a recent study of 84 children with low-level lead poisoning, *urinary incontinence* was mentioned as a suspected side effect of penicillamine (160[c]). For three of these children the parents spontaneously reported the onset or worsening of urinary incontinence during treatment with penicillamine, which improved or resolved once treatment was terminated. In contrast, there were no unsolicited reports of enuresis in the control group. Unfortunately, no more details were given and the issue remains unclear.

Skin and appendages *(SED-12, 543; SEDA-16, 244; SEDA-17, 283; SEDA-18, 247)* There is probably no other medicine that causes skin reactions at such a high frequency and of such striking diversity as penicillamine (see Table 1). During the first few weeks of treatment, allergic reactions occur in about one patient in five (SED-11, 465; 6[c]).

Maculopapular or urticarial rashes are frequent and may be associated with *pruritus*, *edema*, *lymphadeno-*

Table 1. *Penicillamine-associated skin disorders, reported in the literature*

Maculopapular or urticarial rashes
Hemorrhagic bullous lesions, miliary papules, increased friability
Elastosis perforans serpiginosa
Pseudoxanthoma elasticum
Cutis laxa (hyperelastica)
Pemphigus vulgaris
Pemphigus erythematosus
Pemphigus foliaceus
Bullous pemphigoid
Cicatricial pemphigoid
Systemic lupus erythematosus
Discoid lupus; subacute cutaneous lupus
Circumscribed scleroderma (morphea)
Dermatomyositis
Erythema annulare
Lichen planus-like eruptions
Graft-versus-host-like reactions
Erythema multiforme
Toxic epidermal necrolysis
Photosensitivity
Seborrheic dermatitis
Cutaneous pseudolymphoma
Alopecia
Nail dystrophy; yellow nail syndrome

pathy, *arthralgia*, *fever* and *eosinophilia*. Patients with previous hypersensitivity to penicillin are particularly likely to experience a rash when taking penicillamine; cross-allergy may occur (161). Skin reactions may be more common in the presence of the HLA antigen DRw6 (162[cr]) and rashes and febrile reactions were more frequent in patients with anti-Ro(SSA) antibodies (163[Cr]). Early allergic reactions do not usually necessitate permanent withdrawal of penicillamine, and can frequently be overcome by lowering the dose or by timely stopping of the drug and the use of a corticosteroid. A non-specific eruption may, on the other hand, be the first sign of a serious penicillamine-induced skin disorder, e.g. pemphigus. A rash or *photosensitivity* may also occur as part of the penicillamine-induced *SLE syndrome* (164[CR], 165[C], 166[C]) (see 'Immune system'). In one case report, a hypersensitivity reaction to penicillamine with a skin rash and fever was associated with low back pain (167[C]; see 'Musculoskeletal system'). There is a report of a man with a history of penicillin allergy who developed a hypersensitivity reaction of the penis when his wife was taking penicillamine (168[C]).

When penicillamine is administered for a long time and in high doses (for Wilson's disease) it may cause a characteristic *delayed skin eruption*, with increased friability, hemorrhagic bullous lesions and miliary papules (169–174[C], 175[R]). The lesions develop predominantly in those parts of the skin that are frequently exposed to trauma. This disorder is a manifestation of the effects of penicillamine on collagen and elastin. Occasionally, these eruptions imitate other rare dermatological diseases and take the shape of *elastosis perforans serpiginosa*, *pseudoxanthoma elasticum* (176[CR]–178[CR]) or *cutis hyperelastica* (*cutis laxa*) (179[c]); the histological and ultrastructural characteristics of the penicillamine variants differ, however, from those of the spontaneous disorders. Elastosis perforans serpiginosa starts as red umbilicated papules that coalesce to form annular (serpiginous or arcuate) lesions with clear centres. Pseudoxanthoma elasticum is characterized by coalescent yellow waxy papules with a 'plucked chicken' appearance (because of the prominence of follicular orifices in the papules) and a marked laxity and wrinkling of the skin, resulting in redundant skin folds. In delayed penicillamine skin disorders gross abnormalities of elastic and collagen fibers are seen electron-microscopically. Elastic fibers have 'moth-eaten', 'saw-toothed' or 'bramble bush thorns' appearances. Collagen fibers show large differences in thickness. Elastic tissue stains show an increase in the number of elastic fibers and irregular serrated fibers. Elastin content of lesional skin is three times greater than normal, whereas the number of elastin cross-links is only 15% of normal. In electron photomicrographs, dermal elastic fibers are studded with multiple perpendicular buds of different sizes and shapes, described as 'lumpy-bumpy' and show varying degrees of fragmentation. Aggregations of granular elastinophilic material surround the central core of normal mature elastic tissue. In contrast to spontaneous pseudoxanthoma elasticum there is no calcium deposition in elastic fibers. In elastosis perforans serpiginosa-like lesions, there are microscopically thickened coarse elastic fibers, extruding through narrow epidermal channels. In delayed penicillamine skin disorders abnormal elastic tissue also exists in non-lesional skin, and has occasionally been documented in other organs (lungs, blood vessels, ileum, visceral adventitia, joint tissue), but the clinical implications of these findings are uncertain. In one study, multiple lymphangiectases and blood vessel-lymphatic anastomoses were observed (171[C]). Clinically manifest impairment of collagen and elastin has been reported in association with much lower penicillamine doses than had previously been recognized (180[C]–182[C]). In five of eight patients receiving penicillamine for rheumatoid arthritis, elastic fiber damage existed in joint capsules (but in only one also in a skin biopsy), suggesting that penicillamine-associated collagen injury may be common (182[C]). The fact that the lesions in delayed penicillamine skin disorders concentrate in flexural areas (neck, axillae, antecubital fossae and buttocks) may reflect the accelerated turnover rate of elastin in these areas, secondary to shearing stresses and stretching.

The development of a *pemphigus-like eruption* (183—193) in 1—2% of the users of penicillamine (SEDA-11, 213) is probably a cutaneous manifestation of the autoimmunogenic properties of the drug. The available evidence suggests that the penicillamine-induced variant of pemphigus is essentially the same as idiopathic pemphigus. The disease usually recedes when penicillamine is stopped, but may persist for many years (192[C], 194[CR]), and recur on rechallenge (195[C]); fatal cases have occurred (196[C], 197[R]). The entire clinical and pathological spectrum of pemphigus has been reported in association with penicillamine, i.e. *p. erythematosus*, *p. foliaceus*, *p. vulgaris*, and *bullous pemphigoid* (193[C]). In this order of sequence the level of blister formation descends from the superficial layers to deeper layers of the epidermis towards the basal membrane and subepidermal tissue. Penicillamine-induced pemphigus is often of the foliaceus type, whereas spontaneous pemphigus is usually of the vulgaris type. Another feature of penicillamine reactions is that characteristics of pemphigus, bullous or cicatricial pemphigoid (see below), lupus erythematosus, discoid lupus or seborrheic dermatitis may occur concomitantly in the same patient (SEDA-11, 213; SEDA-15, 239; 195[CR]). This suggests differences in the pathogenic process rather than several different reactions. As in spontaneous pemphigus, by indirect immunofluorescence antibodies against intercellular substance may be detected, although these may not be found in early stages. Different antibodies suggest that different antigens are involved in the development of p. foliaceus and p. vulgaris (198[CR], 199[CR]).

Penicillamine has epidermotropic properties and accumulates in the skin. There are several possible mechanisms involved in penicillamine-induced pemphigus (SED-12, 544): (1) penicillamine may cause acantholysis by direct destruction of epidermal intercellular attachment (without pemphigus antibodies) (200[C], 201[C], 202[Cr]); (2) the drug may induce autoantigens through modification of epidermal differentiation or interaction with epidermal tissues; and (3) penicillamine may change immunological tolerance and influence T-suppressor cells and elicit autoimmune responses (203[R], 204[R]). There is still uncertainty with regard to the precise underlying processes. Apart from an association with a reduced frequency of the rheumatoid-associated antigen B15, penicillamine-induced pemphigus does not appear to be strongly associated with a characteristic HLA antigen pattern (205[CR], 206[CR]). Penicillamine-induced pemphigus may pose diagnostic difficulties, e.g. because it may present as a *non-specific rash*, *seborrheic dermatitis*, *erythema annulare* (207[C]), *isolated stomatitis* or even *rhinitis* (28[C]). Because of the friability of the superficial blisters, the bullous nature of p. erythematosus and p. foliaceus may be overlooked.

Although many different drugs have been described as a cause of pemphigus, there is a remarkably strong predominance of penicillamine (and other sulfhydryl compounds) (203[CR], 204[CR], 208[R], 209[CR]). Since also β-lactam antibiotics appear to be associated with pemphigus reactions, especially ampicillin and amoxicillin, the earlier hypothesis (SEDA-5, 244) that this (and perhaps other reactions) to β-lactam antibiotics may in fact be induced by the hydrolytic metabolite penicillamine, has received renewed attention (203[r], 209).

A rare but potentially serious skin reaction to penicillamine is *cicatricial-pemphigoid* (210[CR], 211[CR]). These patients may suffer from symblepharon and entropion of the eyes, ulcers in the mouth and blistering lesions on trunk, extremities and perineum (212[C]). Involvement of the esophageal or vaginal epithelium may result in the development of a stenosis.

Lichen planus-like reactions are known to occur in association with penicillamine. With seven cases in 56 consecutive patients on penicillamine in one study, oral lichen planus may be a fairly frequent phenomenon (120[Cr]). Most patients have erosive oral lichen planus but bullous, plaque-like or 'classic' lichen planus may occur. Another major category of cutaneous reactions to penicillamine (and other sulfhydryl compounds) are *graft-versus-host-like eruptions*, often presenting as a lichen-like reaction or mimicking other eruptions (213[CR]).

Paradoxically, penicillamine is occasionally involved in the development of rare diseases for which it is also sometimes used, such as *circumscribed scleroderma* (*or morphea*) (214[C], 215[R]). Penicillamine-induced *dermatomyositis*, with its characteristic facial rash, is reviewed below (see 'Musculoskeletal system'). *Erythema multiforme and toxic epidermal necrolysis* are considered to occur as adverse reactions to penicillamine (SEDA-12, 465), but recent case-reports of such patients do not appear to have been published. In a female patient *acne and hirsutism* developed in association with breast enlargement, probably induced by penicillamine (see 'Genital system').

The peculiar *yellow nail syndrome* (SEDA-9, 223), characterized by dystrophy of the nails, lymphedema, pleural effusion and bronchial involvement, has occasionally been reported in association with penicillamine and also with bucillamine (216[C], 217[CR], 218[CR]). It has been suggested that penicillamine and bucillamine, because of their structural similarity to cysteine, might disturb nail growth by interfering with keratin synthesis. Although the nail changes and injury to other organs probably develop by different mechanisms, in patients with nail changes a careful search for possible systemic disorders is needed. Monosymptomatic *nail changes*, with longitudinal ridging, transverse or longitudinal defects of the nailplate, absence of lunulae and a tendency towards onychoschizia, can occur as side effects of penicillamine (219[CR]).

Alopecia has occasionally been reported in association with penicillamine (88[c]), but is ill-understood; hair loss may occur in association with polymyositis (220[CR]; see 'Musculoskeletal').

Special senses *(SED-12, 544; SEDA-16, 243)* Alterations or loss of taste is a characteristic and dose-dependent side effect of penicillamine. In a study of rheumatoid arthritis it occurred in 10% of patients and none withdrew (4). Depending on the doses used, taste impairment (dysgeusia) occurs in 10—25% of patients and when daily doses in excess of 900 mg are used this increased to over 50% (SED-11, 466; 4, 95[c]). It usually develops in about the 6th week of treatment. Patients complain of requiring increasing amounts of sugar and spices. Food does not taste normal, but salty or metallic, or tastes like cotton wool or blotting paper; identification of certain foods becomes difficult. Absolute taste loss may ensue, but the sense of smell remains unaltered. Spontaneous recovery usually follows within 6—8 weeks, despite continuation of the drug. Dysgeusia may occur at any time and may be persistent (4). In patients with Wilson's disease, penicillamine is rapidly attached to copper and, although higher doses are used, taste disturbances develop in a lower frequency of about 4% (SED-8, 536). It has been suggested that dysgeusia is related to deficiency of copper or zinc, but a strong connection between taste impairment and urinary copper excretion has not been demonstrated (221). Serum copper levels remained within normal limits and copper supplements were not successful in prevention (222). In another study, an association was found with decreased serum zinc levels and taste recovered after zinc supplements (it should be remembered that spontaneous recovery occurs in most patients) (223[C]). Taste alterations have been reported with other sulfhydryl compounds, including pyritinol, captopril and propylthiouracil (224[R]), suggesting that the thiol moiety may be involved. Dysgeusia has not been observed in many studies on the use of penicillamine in children (SEDA-7, 258; 225[c]).

Optic neuropathy has only rarely been reported in association with penicillamine (36[C], see 'Nervous system'). In a case-report, blurred vision occurred as a result of development of bilateral choroidal hemorrhage complicating penicillamine-induced thrombocytopenia (226[C]). The patient recovered after discontinuation of penicillamine.

Genital system *(SED-12, 545; SEDA-17, 284; SEDA-18, 248)* *Gigantism of the breasts* is an example of the bizarre and little understood complications that occur with penicillamine (SEDA-8, 238; 227[CR]—229[CR], 230[cr], 231[CR]). About 16 cases have been described. The condition usually develops in women and very rarely, as *gynecomastia*, in men (231[R], 232[C]). There is resemblance to the pubertal form of massive breast enlargement. It may be painful and has been encountered in pre- and postmenopausal women, with normal and increased prolactin levels. Histological examination mainly shows increased connective tissue, and no changes of the glandular tissue. In one patient, the breasts were tender and grew progressively larger during each menstrual period. In another patient, a 25-year-old woman with Wilson's disease, treatment with penicillamine (1.5 grams daily) was first followed by the development of hirsutism, mainly of the face (229[C]). After starting the use of an oral contraceptive, her breasts enlarged rapidly and she experienced cyclic mastodynia; in addition, gingival hyperplasia developed. All symptoms improved on discontinuation of penicillamine, but additional mammoplasty was needed. The sequence of events in that patient suggested that the use of the oral contraceptive contributed to the development of macromastia. Danazole often causes regression of breast size, but surgical intervention may be necessary.

Ulcerative lesions of the vagina may occur in patients taking penicillamine, as a manifestation of pemphigus or cicatricial pemphigoid or following impaired collagen synthesis (SED-8, 533; see 'Skin and appendages). There is the unusual report of a man with a history of penicillin allergy who developed *a hypersensitivity reaction of the penis* when his wife was taking penicillamine (168[C]).

Musculoskeletal system *(SED-12, 545; SEDA-16, 244; SEDA-17, 284; SEDA-18, 248)* In addition to *myasthenia gravis*, which has been reviewed above (see 'Nervous system'), penicillamine can cause other serious autoimmune reactions involving the muscles: *dermatomyositis*, with its characteristic facial rash (233[C]), and *polymyositis* (19[C], 55[C], 220[CR], 234—243, 244[CR], 245[CR], 246[C]). Effects vary from only biochemical deviations, through moderate muscular weakness to severe polymyositis with myolysis and sometimes myocarditis; arrhythmia, heart block and *Adams-Stokes attacks* may develop (241[C], 247[C]), and fatal cases have occurred (55[C]). Muscular weakness may cause secondary respiratory failure (19[C], 220[CR]). The clinical, pathological and electromyographic features are similar to those of idiopathic polymyositis. Antinuclear antibodies are found in about 90% of cases of penicillamine-induced polymyositis, a finding which may be helpful in distinguishing this condition from true polymyositis (236). In one patient anti-Jo-1 antibodies were found, which was thought to be an epiphenomenon and not pathogenic (41). Myositis may occur in approximately 1% of patients receiving penicillamine and appears to be relatively frequent in Japanese and Indian patients (SEDA-15, 240; 4[c], 234[CR], 243[cR]). HLA investigations showed that the antigens DR2 and DQwl are increased in patients with penicillamine-induced myositis, suggesting that myositis occurs in a specific genetic subgroup (243). Of interest is the case-report on a patient with penicillamine-associated polymyositis who had a relapse after administration of ampicillin (237; see also page 615). In penicillamine-induced polymyositis *weakness* may be the presenting symptom and it may at first be mistaken for myasthenia reaction (19[C]).

Joint symptoms in patients taking penicillamine vary from 'creaking' and subjective discomfort and worsening of joint pain to severe *arthralgia* (248[c], 249[c]). An important observation concerned the paradoxical acute and severe *exacerbation of rheumatoid arthritis* in three patients, probably induced by penicillamine (250[C]). *Arthritis* may also be a manifestation of penicillamine-induced systemic lupus erythematosus (see below). Isolated cases have been described *of myasthenic pseudo-internuclear ophthalmoplegia* (68[C]), *neuromyotonia* (69[C]) and diffuse *fasciculations* (70[C]) attributed to the use of penicillamine (see 'Nervous system'). An unusual case report showed that *low back pain* can be a manifestation of drug hypersensitivity (167[C]). *Demineralization osteopathy* has been reported in a study on the use of D-penicillamine in Wilson's disease (SED-8, 536).

Immune system and autoimmune reactions *(SED-12, 545; SEDA-16, 245; SEDA-17, 285; SEDA-18, 248)* Several experimental studies in humoral and cell-mediated immune systems have demonstrated numerous effects of penicillamine on the immune system, which are in keeping with a reduction of helper T-lymphocyte overactivity which is found in rheumatoid arthritis (1[R], 251[C]). There is a decline in numbers of immunoglobulin-secreting cells and cultured mononuclear cells produce less IgA, IgG and IgM. There is suppression of the autologous mixed lymphocyte reaction (252) and a decreased hydroxyl radical generation from polymorphonuclear leukocytes (253). Penicillamine decreases the clearance of immune complexes and inhibits the complement cascade (254, 255).

Penicillamine has a unique power to induce *autoimmune reactions* (see Table 2). Clinically and biochemically, these variants of autoimmune disorders are closely similar to the true diseases. The patients usually recover when the drug is stopped. This is the principal difference between penicillamine-induced and spontaneous diseases. Different HLA configurations suggest that penicillamine-induced and spontaneous autoimmune disorders occur in different populations. Serological features of *systemic lupus erythematosus* develop in about 7% of patients taking penicillamine (110[C], 157[C], 165[c], 166[C], 256[CR]–257[CR]). A clinical SLE syndrome is less frequent (about 2%) and is as equally frequent in rheumatoid arthritis as in Wilson's disease. Characteristic phenomena are (increased) polyarthritis, a rash, pleurisy, fever, leukopenia, thrombocytopenia, antinuclear antibodies and LE cells. Rarely, the syndrome may be associated with anti-native DNA antibodies, renal injury (see 'Urinary system') or neurological symptoms. The disorder usually recovers in the first few weeks or months after stopping penicillamine, but serological tests may remain abnormal for a longer period. Another interesting penicillamine-induced immune disorder, although rarely described, is *IgA deficiency*, accompanied with recurrent upper respiratory tract infections (258[CR], 259[CR], 260[C]). IgA deficiency is likely to develop when there is an improvement of rheumatic disease activity, together with other side effects (e.g. rash, thrombocytopenia, proteinuria). Two cases has been reported of *Sjögren's syndrome* (keratoconjunctivitis sicca, xerostomia, swelling of the parotids) in suspected association with penicillamine (261[C], 262[C]). In one study reference is made to a patient with a *Henoch-Schönlein-like syndrome* as a suspected adverse reaction to penicillamine, but no details were given (263[c]).

An autoimmune phenomenon which has recently been described with penicillamine is the development of *anti-centromere antibodies* (264[CR], 265[c]). Although

Table 2. *Autoimmune-like reactions reported in suspected association with penicillamine*

Pemphigus (erythematosus, foliaceus, vulgaris)
Bullous pemphigoid, cicatricial pemphigoid
Graft-versus-host-like skin eruptions
Myasthenia gravis
Dermatomyositis/polymyositis
Glomerulonephritis
Systemic lupus erythematosus
Goodpasture's syndrome
Autoimmune hypoglycemia
Thyroiditis
Sjögren's syndrome
Aplastic anemia
Thrombocytopenia
Agranulocytosis
Thrombotic thrombocytopenic purpura (Moschcowitz's syndrome)

Table 3. *Examples of simultaneous multiple reactions reported with penicillamine*

Pulmonary alveolitis, pancytopenia, cholestatic hepatitis, stomatitis, proctitis, skin rash, proteinuria, renal failure (269[C])
Cholestatic hepatitis with allergic pneumonitis (113[C])
Pemphigus and nephrosis (minimal change nephropathy) (270[C])
Pemphigus and myasthenia gravis (268[CR])
Thyroiditis and myasthenia gravis (85[C])
Polyradiculopathy and nephrosis (33[C])
Aplastic anemia and cholestatic hepatitis (103[C])
Gingival hyperplasia, acne, hirsutism, breast gigantism (229[C])

these are usually a marker of serious autoimmune diseases, in association with penicillamine the phenomenon was not accompanied by clinical symptoms and disappeared after stopping the drug. In the serum of three patients with acute hypersensitivity reactions to penicillamine, complement-binding antibodies against penicillamine were detected (266[c]). The striking variability of penicillamine-induced pathology, including autoimmune reactions, is also seen in patients with Wilson's disease, but the proportion of these patients in whom discontinuation is necessary is much smaller, about 2–8% (35[CR], 42[CR], 43[R], 267[R]). Patients with Wilson's disease are not known to have an abnormal immune status, and it is noteworthy that autoimmune reactions (e.g. lupus-like syndrome) are also encountered in these patients.

Multisystem reactions *(SEDA-8, 239; SEDA-13, 200; SEDA-14, 198; SED-12, 547; SEDA-16, 246; SEDA-18, 248)* Penicillamine has a remarkable potency to elicit *multiple adverse reactions in the same patient*. Examples are listed in Table 3. In a long-term prospective study in a series of 69 patients receiving penicillamine (750 mg/day) for progressive systemic sclerosis, 27 (39%) patients experienced adverse effects requiring either temporary reduction or complete cessation of therapy. Five of these patients had two or even three (in one case) different reactions (95[c]). Another study described a 47-year-old female patient with concurrent pemphigus and myasthenia gravis (with ptosis and diplopia), apparently induced by penicillamine (500 mg daily for rheumatoid arthritis) (268[CR]). The capacity of penicillamine to elicit more than one autoimmune reaction simultaneously illustrates the immunomodulatory action of the drug. Penicillamine-induced IgA deficiency is likely to develop together with other side effects (e.g. rash, thrombocytopenia, proteinuria) and when there is improvement in rheumatic disease activity (see 'Immune system and autoimmune reactions'). The Churg-Strauss syndrome is a rare disease, with eosinophilia, vasculitis and granulomas, involving many organ systems (skin, lungs, kidneys, gastrointestinal tract, joints, heart and central nervous system); rhinitis and asthma are often an early manifestation. In one of two patients with the syndrome, penicillamine might have triggered its development (27[CR]); however, stopping the drug had no effect on the course of the disease and the relationship therefore remained uncertain.

Use in children *(SED-12, 547)* Although published experience is limited, penicillamine has the same pattern of side effects when used in children. An interesting difference is, however, that taste dysfunction has so far not been reported in children (SED-10, 221; SEDA-14, 198). In two children with Wilson's disease, penicillamine was thought to have caused persistence of a pre-existing increase in aminotransferase activity (114[c]).

Tumor-inducing effects *(SED-11, 464; SED-12, 547)* There are a few case reports describing lymphatic malignancies in patients using penicillamine, but epidemiological data in support of the association are lacking (SEDA-7, 259; 271[C]–273[C], 274[R]). In one experimental study it has been suggested that penicillamine may be mutagenic (275).

Miscellaneous *(SED-12, 547)* In a study in scleroderma patients, penicillamine was found to have a normalizing effect on the collagen metabolism, via a decrease in β-galactosidase activity (276[C]). Penicillamine was found to cause an artificially abnormal α-antitrypsin protein pattern, which may be the cause of diagnostic errors (277[C]).

Risk situations, genetic factors, rechallenge *(SED-12, 547; SEDA-13, 201; SEDA-14, 198; SEDA-16, 246; SEDA-17, 285)* An important measure to decrease the frequency of adverse reactions of penicillamine is to start with a small daily dose (e.g. 125 mg in rheumatoid arthritis), to increase the dose only slowly, and to maintain treatment with the lowest effective dose. Nevertheless, serious complications such as nephrosis, pemphigus, alveolitis and polymyositis have occurred while only 250 mg penicillamine or less was used (SEDA-8, 235; 17[C], 117[c], 234).

The absorption of penicillamine can be significantly altered by *alimentary factors*. Changing habits, e.g. taking penicillamine between meals instead of with food, or stopping iron supplements, may precipitate adverse reactions by increased absorption (see 'Interactions'). Certain side effects occur predominantly during the first few months of treatment, e.g. taste alterations or non-specific hypersensitivity reactions, whereas others are more frequent during the second half-year of treatment (thrombocytopenia, proteinuria) or become apparent even later (e.g. collagen insufficiency). However, almost the entire spectrum of possible adverse reactions can occur at any time and without warning throughout a course of treatment with penicillamine. Although different schemes may be used, the monitoring of penicillamine treatment usually includes regular testing of platelet and white cell counts, a blood smear, proteinuria and hematuria.

A basic consideration in drug prescription is the history of *previous drug exposure*, but with penicillamine this information may be difficult to interpret. 'Early' hypersensitivity reactions are usually transient and, although there is undoubtedly an increased risk, several experiences have shown that in patients with a history of previous adverse reactions to penicillamine (or gold), re-exposure may not be followed by a relapse (SEDA-10, 218). In the case of serious complications, such as *agranulocytosis, profound thrombocytopenia, polymyositis or Goodpasture's syndrome*, the repeated use of penicillamine carries unacceptable risks for the patient. Commencing penicillamine in patients with *Wilson's disease* may aggravate or even precipitate neurological involvement (see 'Nervous system'). Several studies have shown an increased frequency of penicillamine adverse effects in patients with low sulfoxidation activity, especially with regard to proteinuria and probably thrombocytopenia and myasthenia gravis (SED-12, 547; 2[CR], 278[r], 279[CR], 280[CR]). The sulfoxidation capacity is expressed as the sulfoxidation index (SI), calculated as the percentage of administered *S*-carboxymethyl-L-cysteine (750 mg), excreted as sulfoxides in the urine in 8 hours. An SI above 6% is taken as indicative of a relative impairment of sulfoxidation capacity.

Antibodies to the Ro(SSA) cellular antigen (163[C], 281[CR]) and *circulating cryoglobulins* (163[C]) seem to be other risk factors for adverse reactions to penicillamine. AntiRo(SSA) antibodies seem to characterize a distinct group of RA patients who are almost exclusively female, express more activated B-cell function, have a high prevalence of Sjögren's features, and commonly develop adverse reactions to penicillamine. Rashes and febrile reactions were especially associated with anti-Ro(SSA) antibodies, and renal pathology was more frequent in *male patients* (163[c]).

Many studies have shown that certain adverse reactions to penicillamine are associated with increased or decreased frequencies of HLA antigens (SEDA-8, 235; SEDA-11, 212; 3[cr], 282, 283–289). Most consistently reported are the associations between proteinuria and the antigens B8 and DR3 and between thrombocytopenia and DR4. These associations are not strong enough to include HLA typing into the routine of treatment with penicillamine. The relative risk of toxicity for patients possessing either HLA-DR3 or *poor sulfoxidation* appeared to be 25 as compared with those possessing neither; if these tests could be simplified, a valuable opportunity would become available for identifying patients at risk (278[r], 279[CR]). *Racial factors* may be involved: proteinuria is less frequent in Japanese people (see 'Urinary system'), whereas polymyositis occurs at an increased frequency in India and Japan (250, 278).

In the past, penicillamine, because of its effects on collagen synthesis, has been suspected of interfering with normal wound healing. Experience in 217 operations in 150 patients did not show such effects and, consequently, there does not seem to be a need for stopping penicillamine before surgery (290[CR]). A small number of case-reports, on the other hand, suggest that penicillamine may, at least in some patients, have deleterious effects on wound healing (291[C], 292[C]). Removal of an impacted maxillary third molar in a patient with Wilson's disease (which was treated with penicillamine) was followed by the development of an oroantral fistula, presumably as a result of impaired collagen synthesis (292[C]).

Second-generation effects Whereas the benefits of penicillamine outweigh the risk in patients with Wilson's disease and probably cysteinuria, a small number of case-reports concerning congenital injury attributed to the use of penicillamine—notably *congenital cutis hyperelastica* with a fatal course in three infants—are a reason for stopping the drug during pregnancy in patients with rheumatoid arthritis (293[R], 294[R]).

Interactions and combinations *(SED-11, 469; SEDA-13, 201)* Only a few adverse drug–drug interactions with penicillamine have been documented. When taken concomitantly with *iron compounds*, the bioavailability of penicillamine is reduced to about 35% and copper excretion to about 28%, probably as a result of catalyzation of the oxidation of penicillamine to its disulfide (1[r], 295[C], 296). Even the iron present in certain multivitamin preparations may be sufficient to cause interference, and when a patient who has regularly taken iron stops taking it, increased absorption of penicillamine and side effects can ensue (297[cr], 298[cr]). Also, *aluminum- and magnesium-containing antacids* may lower absorption by up to 45% presumably because increased gastric pH favors oxidation to the poorly absorbed disulfide (117, 296, 299). When *probenecid* is administered to a patient taking penicillamine for cysteinuria, the efficacy of the latter is significantly reduced (300[C]). Chloroquine or hydroxychloroquine in combination with penicillamine in the management of rheumatoid arthritis probably offers no therapeutic advantages, produces more side effects and may even be less effective (SEDA-10, 223; 301[R], 302[C], 303[C], 304). A combination of penicillamine and sulfasalazine seems to be more effective, although the extent of the advantage is uncertain, and side effects are more frequent (301[R]). In one study penicillamine and intramuscular gold together produced a much earlier improvement, but efficacy and side effects did not differ significantly compared with either drug given alone. In an open and uncontrolled study the combination of penicillamine and intramuscular gold yielded the highest proportion of remissions in a group of patients with refractory rheumatoid arthritis (301[R]). The possible consequences of previous intolerance to *gold compounds* in association with adverse reactions to penicillamine administration have been reviewed in SEDA-8 (p. 236); at present no firm conclusions can be made. Penicillamine does not chelate gold stores in the body.

RELATED COMPOUNDS

The side-effect patterns of other sulfhydryl compounds used in rheumatoid arthritis—i.e. bucillamine, pyritinol and tiopronin—show remarkable similarities to those of penicillamine (SED-12, 548; 305[R]). These drugs have probably similar mechanisms of action on the rheumatoid process. Most information regarding side effects is extracted from efficacy studies, however, and well-documented case observations, which are necessary for a proper study of the various adverse reactions, are rare.

Acetylpenicillamine *(SED-10, 416; SEDA-16, 246)*

Acetylpenicillamine is a weaker chelating agent than penicillamine, has no influence on collagen cross-links and is not effective in rheumatoid arthritis. It was used in three children for mercury poisoning without side effects (306[c]).

Bucillamine *(SEDA-16, 246; SEDA-17, 285)*

Bucillamine (mercapto-methylpropanoyl-cysteine) is chemically related to penicillamine and is used in rheumatoid arthritis; their patterns of adverse reactions are roughly similar. Most of the information on bucillamine comes from Japan, its country of origin. In a study of 55 patients, 32 episodes of suspected side effects occurred in 25 patients: *rashes and/or itching* in 12 (22%), *proteinuria* in four (7%), *liver dysfunction* in three (5%), and *eosinophilia* in three (5%); *hemorrhagic gastritis, stomatitis, alopecia, loss of appetite, nausea, soft stools, epigastric pain, increased serum creatinine concentration, reduced serum γ-globulin*, and *increased serum potassium* were seen in single cases, but no details were given (307[c]).

Respiratory In 10 patients with bucillamine-associated *interstitial pneumonitis* the HLA antigen DR4 was present in all and a positive lymphocyte stimulation test was found in three of six (308[CR]).

Nervous system There has been a report of what may be the first case of bucillamine-induced *myasthenia gravis* in a 36-year-old woman (309[C]). Since the disease persisted despite withdrawal, the role of the drug was uncertain.

Urinary system Proteinuria was reported in four (7%) of 55 patients using bucillamine (307[c]). The case has been reported of a 34-year-old Japanese woman, receiving bucillamine and amfenac for rheumatoid arthritis. Five months later *proteinuria* developed and a *membranous nephropathy* was diagnosed (310[C]). Both drugs were discontinued and the patient recovered. Because of the drug's similarity to penicillamine, bucillamine was suspected to have caused the reaction, but a role of amfenac could not be excluded. In a study of 11 patients with membranous nephropathy, bucillamine was included as one of the suspected causes (135[c]; see 'Penicillamine, Urinary system'). In two additional studies, 11 further cases of a *nephrotic syndrome* were suspected to be induced by bucillamine (311[C], 312[C]). Light microscopy, electron microscopy, and immunofluorescence investigations showed stage I—III membranous glomerulonephritis (Ehrenreich and Churg's classification), with diffuse fine granular precipitations of IgG and C3 around the capillary walls, electron-dense deposits at the subepithelial side of the basement membrane, and effacement of foot processes.

Skin and appendages *Rashes and/or itching* occurred in 12 (22%) and *eosinophilia* in three (5%) of 55 patients receiving bucillamine (307[c]). Two reports are on record of bucillamine-associated *pemphigus*. In a 57-year-old woman a generalized itchy rash developed 9 months after she started to take bucillamine (313[c]). A skin biopsy showed spongiosis, lymphocytic infiltration in the epidermis, and intercellular deposition of IgG, and a diagnosis of pemphigus was made. Another patient had a pemphigus foliaceus-like eruption on three different occasions, in association with penicillamine, auranofin, and bucillamine, respectively (314[c]). In a study of 13 patients with the peculiar *yellow nail syndrome* bucillamine was the suspected cause in seven (218[CR]) (see Penicillamine, Skin and appendages for further details).

Pyritinol (pyrithioxine) *(SED-12, 549; SEDA-11, 214; SEDA-14, 199; SEDA-16, 246; SEDA-17, 285)* (See also Chapter 10)

Especially in France, the sulfhydryl compound pyritinol (the dimer of 5-thiopyridoxine), is used as an alternative to penicillamine. In the usual doses, 600–800 mg daily, this drug has a profile of side effects reminiscent of that of penicillamine (305[R], 315[R]). Some 40% of users experience adverse effects, leading to withdrawal in about 23% (of the total). Most frequent are nonspecific *rashes* and *stomatitis*; in addition, *pemphigus*, *lichen planus* and *photosensitivity* have occurred. Other complications of interest are *hematological reactions* (*thrombocytopenia*, *agranulocytosis*), *myasthenia*, *nephrosis* and *polymyositis*. Also *disturbances of taste* may occur, but are less frequent than those seen with penicillamine. Valuable information on the occurrence of adverse reactions with this drug has been provided by a collaborative study of the French Pharmacovigilance Centers. Twenty-three collected reports of suspected reactions to pyritinol included four cases of pemphigus, three of agranulocytosis (but other drugs taken were oxyphenbutazone or clomipramine), two of *nephrosis*, and two of a *lupus syndrome* (316[c]). In another study, the development of a high titer of *antinuclear antibodies* and *anti-double-stranded native DNA antibodies* during treatment with pyritinol, 400 mg daily, was described in a woman with rheumatoid arthritis (246[C]). A clear temporal relationship and a decrease in antinuclear antibody titers and disappearance of anti-DNA antibodies after stopping the drug strongly suggested a causal relationship.

The first report has been published of *autoimmune hypoglycemia*, with demonstrated anti-insulin antibodies, probably induced by pyritinol (317[C]). This syndrome has previously been described in connection with other thiol compounds, i.e. penicillamine, methimazol and tiopronin (see Penicillamine, Immunological reactions). Finally, a patient has been described with pyritinol-induced acute hepatitis (318[C]).

Tiopronin (mercaptopropionylglycine) *(SED-12, 549; SEDA-15, 242; SEDA-16, 246; SEDA-17, 286; SEDA-18, 249)*

Tiopronin appears to be used extensively in France and Japan. The drug has a roughly similar pattern of side effects as penicillamine (319–323[CR]). Side effects occur in about 45% of patients and lead to withdrawal in approximately one fifth. Tiopronin may cause *fever*, with or without a *rash* (324[C])

Endocrine *(SED-12, 549)* Autoimmune hypoglycemia with anti-insulin antibodies, a recently discovered complication of penicillamine (see above), has also been reported with tiopronin (325[C]). One case has been described of a patient (a 49-year-old woman, with regular menstrual periods) with marked *enlargement of the breasts*, probably induced by tiopronine (326[C]; see also Penicillamine, Genital system). The breasts were red and painful; histological examination showed extensive lymphocytic inflammation and edema in the connective tissue. She recovered after stopping tiopronin and administering danazol.

Hematological *(SED-12, 549; SEDA-17, 286)* Hematological reactions, e.g. *thrombocytopenia* and *leukopenia*, occur in about 6–9% of patients using tiopronin (319[cr], 320[cr]). *Aplastic anemia* with fever and *pancytopenia* developed in a 29-year-old woman, probably as a reaction to tiopronin, 500 mg daily for 71 days for seronegative rheumatoid arthritis (327[C]). A bone-marrow examination confirmed acute marrow aplasia. She recovered within 5 weeks after withdrawal. Another detailed case report described profound *granulocytopenia*, probably induced by tiopronin (328[CR]).

Liver *(SEDA-16, 247)* In a review of 140 patients using tiopronin three had cholestasis (320[cr]). A case has been described of *liver injury*, with *steatosis*, *intrahepatic cholestasis* and *centrilobular inflammation*, in association with tiopronin (329[C]). In one patient *cholestatic hepatitis* as well as *toxic epidermal necrolysis* developed in suspected association with tiopronin (330[C]).

Gastrointestinal Gastrointestinal side effects of tiopronin include *impaired taste and ageusia*, *nausea*, *vomiting*, *oral ulcers and stomatitis* (319–323[cr]).

Urinary system *(SED-12, 549; SEDA-16, 246; SEDA-17, 286)* Some degree of *renal injury* occurs in about 10% of patients on tiopronin (319–323[cr]). As with penicillamine, *proteinuria* may progress to a *nephrotic syndrome* (331[CR], 332[CR]). A biopsy may reveal minimal change membranous glomerulonephritis and granular depositions of IgG and C3 (331[C], 333[C]).

Skin *(SED-12, 549; SEDA-16, 246; SEDA-17, 286; SEDA-18, 249)* Cutaneous or mucous reactions occur in about 15–30% of patients using tiopronin. *Alopecia*, *erythema*, *eczema*, *cutaneous vasculitis*, *lichenoid eruptions*, *skin wrinkling and perforating elastoma* may develop (319–323[cr]). Several cases have been described of tiopronin-induced *pemphigus*, characterized by intra-epidermal bullae with acantholysis and epidermal intercellular deposition of IgG and C3 (334[c], 335[C]). The eruption may present as multiple red crusted macules. One patient first had *pemphigus* in association with penicillamine and later had a relapse when tiopronine was taken (336[c]). In skin explant cultures tiopronin can cause acantholysis with intra-epidermal splits and bullae formation (200). In a patient with a tiopronin-associated *lichenoid skin eruption* the rash was associated with *alopecia* (337[C]). In another report of a lichenoid eruption a positive rechallenge confirmed the role of tiopronin (338[C]). In four patients with pluriform skin eruptions in association with tiopronin, the pathological findings were characteristic of a *graft-versus-host reaction* (213[CR]).

In one patient *cholestatic hepatitis* as well as *toxic epidermal necrolysis* developed in suspected association with tiopronin (330[C]).

Musculoskeletal system *(SEDA-17, 286; SED-12, 549)* A few cases have been reported of *myasthenia gravis* in association with tiopronin (339[C], 340[C]). Also *polymyositis* may be induced by tiopronin (1 g/day) (SED-12, 549; 341[CR]).

Tiobutarit *(SED-12, 549)*

Tiobutarit or *N*-(2-mercapto-2-methylpropionyl)-L-cysteine is a new penicillamine analog, used experimentally in Japan in the treatment of rheumatoid arthritis; it is considered to cause *skin reactions* in about 5% of patients (342[r]). A recent case report described *bullous pemphigoid* probably induced by tiobutarit (200 mg daily) (342[CR]). In addition to the skin of chest, abdomen and axilla, the mouth, pharynx, larynx and conjunctiva were also involved. Indirect immunofluorescence revealed circulating antibodies against the basement membrane zone. This observation may suggest that tiobutarit could have a profile of adverse reactions similar to that of penicillamine.

IRON CHELATORS

Deferoxamine (Desferrioxamine) *(SED-12, 550; SEDA-16, 247; SEDA-17, 286; SEDA-18, 249; 343[CR]–345[CR])*

Deferoxamine is a polyhydroxamine acid and a naturally occurring siderophore produced by *Streptomyces pilosus*. Deferoxamine is usually administered subcutaneously or intravenously. After subcutaneous infusions of deferoxamine many patients experience some local irritation and swelling (see Skin and appendages). Rapid intravenous injection may be followed by flushing, wheals, tachycardia and hypotension; shock or convulsions may also occur. Headache, blurred vision, dysuria, diarrhea, and leg or hand cramps have been reported in the past. Intramuscular injection can be painful. Hypersensitivity reactions occasionally occur, with rash, fever and edema; anaphylactic shock has been encountered (SEDA-7, 262; 346[C], 347[C]).

An important concern relates to the safety of high-dose deferoxamine regimens. The administration of 25–50 mg/kg by daily 10- to 12-hour subcutaneous infusion to patients with substantial iron overload is associated with little serious toxicity. However, a wide range of previously undescribed toxicities has in recent years been associated with deferoxamine doses in excess of 50 mg/kg per 12 hours, and with lower 'standard' doses administered to patients with minimal iron burdens (SED-12, 550). A further major problem associated with deferoxamine therapy, especially in countries with limited medical and financial resources, is its expense and complexity of administration. The problem of the safe use of deferoxamine in patients with minimal iron loads is important. The fear of toxicity may delay initiation of chelation therapy in young patients and restrict deferoxamine doses in older children with low iron loads. Since even a little excess of iron can produce serious toxicity, such as delayed puberty, limiting chelation therapy may have far-reaching consequences for these patients.

ADVERSE REACTION PATTERN

General and toxic reactions Deferoxamine is only used parenterally. When effective amounts are administered, side effects are frequent. Deferoxamine is more toxic when used in patients without metal overload (e.g. rheumatoid arthritis). Of special importance are visual and auditory neurotoxicity. When given early in childhood, osteopathy and growth impairment may occur. Hypotension, acute adult respiratory distress and renal failure may develop. Local reactions are frequent after subcutaneous infusion.

The use of deferoxamine is associated with an increased risk of life threatening opportunistic infections, notably yersiniosis and mucormycosis; such infections may affect various organ systems and pose diagnostic problems. Deferoxamine is teratogenic in animals.

Hypersensitivity reactions These can occur but have infrequently been reported. Rare cases of anaphylactic shock, thrombocytopenia and bone marrow failure have been described.

Tumor-inducing effects These have not been reported.

ORGANS AND SYSTEMS

Cardiovascular Although rarely described, *hypotension* seems to be a significant problem in patients receiving deferoxamine, especially when an intravenous injection is administered too rapidly (343[r]), and is possibly due to histamine release (348[cr]). Dose reduction alleviated the hypotension, but there was no strong link between deferoxamine doses and the occurrence of hypotension. *Anaphylactic shock* has only rarely been reported (SEDA-7, 262). In a single case-report, *soft tissue swelling* around the elbow and localized mild pitting edema were thought to have been induced by desferoxamine (349[cr]). Although the clinical features suggested a deep-vein thrombosis, this was ruled out by a phlebogram. In iron storage disease *ascorbic acid* should be given only after adequate serum levels of deferoxamine have been attained, in order to prevent serious cardiac arrhythmia (130[cR]). Opportunistic fungal infections associated with deferoxamine may also involve the heart muscle and have usually a fatal outcome (350[C]—352[C]) (see 'Opportunistic infections'). In a series of nine cancer patients receiving deferoxamine (50 mg/kg given daily as an i.v. infusion over 72 h) and iron sorbitol citrate in an attempt to enhance doxorubicin activity, severe *phlebitis* occurred in five (353[C]). Dilution of the drug in large volumes of saline did not prevent this side effect.

Respiratory Deferoxamine in continuous infusion may induce life threatening *acute adult respiratory distress syndrome*, with respiratory failure, hypoxia, pulmonary edema, low pulmonary compliance, and pulmonary capillary wedge pressures below 18 mmHg as observed in four (355[C]—357[C]). Respiratory distress may start 32—72 hours after the infusion and lung biopsy shows diffuse abnormalities with alveolar damage, interstitial fibrosis and inflammatory infiltrates with lymphocytes, eosinophils, mast cells and some erythrocytes. It is therefore recommended that deferoxamine should not be given as a continuous infusion for longer than 24 hours (357[C]). Although the mechanism is unknown, it has been suggested that deferoxamine may cause damage in the lungs by increasing paradoxically the production of free radicals, as a result of extended exposure of the lungs to ferrioxamine (357). However, others have emphasized that pulmonary endothelial cells are sensitive to macrophage-generated oxidants, and have proposed that in chelating intracellular iron deferoxamine may acutely reduce the synthesis of catalase and heme, and that readily available extracellular heme subsequently enters cells, is broken down, and releases iron in the presence of low concentrations of catalase, which catalyses oxidant damage (358[R]).

Similar effects of deferoxamine (respiratory distress and interstitial infiltrates) have been reported in children receiving deferoxamine for iron poisoning or refractory cancer (359[C], 360[C]).

In another patient, pulmonary symptoms occurred after 7 days of continuous deferoxamine infusion (dyspnea, tachypnea, tachycardia, pleuritic chest pain, and fever) and were diagnosed as *pulmonary microembolism* (361[C]).

Pneumonia occurring during treatment with high doses of deferoxamine (2—2.5 grams by continuous infusion) in a patient with thalassemia major, was found to be induced by *Pneumocystis carinii* (362[CR]). The lungs may also be involved in deferoxamine-associated *systemic mucormycosis*, which usually runs a fatal course (363[C], 364[C]) (see also 'Opportunistic infections').

Nervous system and special senses *(SED-12, 551; SEDA-16, 250; SEDA-17, 287; SEDA 18, 249)* In many studies, *sensorineural toxicity* of deferoxamine, leading to *deafness* or *visual impairment*, has been documented, although the reported frequencies differ considerably. Some degree of visual and auditory toxicity may occur in about one third of patients, and impairment of vision and hearing may occur simultaneously. In many studies much lower frequencies were found. Acute visual injury in aluminium-overloaded dialysis patients may occur following the administration of only a first or second intravenous test dose of 40 mg/kg deferoxamine (365[Cr], 366[CR], 367[CR]). Careful estimation of the necessary doses of deferoxamine (see above) and monitoring of the patients may often prevent serious injury. Ocular and auditory disturbances are not infrequent in patients with thalassemia, iron storage (368, 369) or uremia (370[CR]), and they may be coincidental (371[CR]). The sensorineural toxicity of deferoxamine is much more pronounced in patients without iron storage (e.g. rheumatoid arthritis). In aluminium-overloaded dialysis patients acute visual injury may occur already following the administration of the first or second intravenous test dose of 40 mg/kg deferoxamine (365[r], 366[CR], 367[CR]). Visual symptoms are of retinal origin and include impairment of color vision, night blindness and decreased visual acuity; serious and persistent visual loss may occur (365[C], 370[C], 372[CR], 373[C], 374[C]). Color blindness is of the tritan type, involving the blue-yellow axis (375). A light- and electron-microscopic study revealed loss of microvilli from the apical surface, patchy depigmentation, vacuolation of the cytoplasm, swelling and calcification of mitochondria, and thickening of Bruch's membrane (376[CR]). Optic neuritis and pigmentary retinal degeneration may develop (377[CR]—379[CR]). Visual evoked potentials may be used to monitor patients receiving high doses of deferoxamine (380[CR]). Perhaps the retinal abnormalities found may be related to the concomitant depletion of metals such as zinc, copper and/or iron (381[CR]). Ocular toxicity of deferoxamine in patients without iron storage was also apparent in cancer patients receiving deferoxamine and iron sorbitol citrate in an attempt to enhance doxorubicin activity (353[CR]). Ototoxicity ranges from a subclinically abnormal audiogram, mid- to high-frequency neurosensorial hearing loss of the cochlear type, to acute deafness (SED-12, 552; 372[CR]). There are two apparent risk factors: a high total cumulative dose and a low serum ferritin level. For the prevention of deferoxamine ototoxicity a therapeutic index (TI) has been proposed, defined as the daily dose of deferoxamine (in mg/kg/day) divided by the serum ferritin level (ng/ml) (SED-12, 552; 382[CR]). A TI of 0.027 is considered to be associated with a low risk of hearing impairment.

The use of deferoxamine in aluminum overload in hemodialysis may precipitate *dialysis dementia* and exacerbation of pre-existing aluminum encephalopathy (383[CR]—386[CR]). Aluminium may be more neurotoxic than was previously thought (28). Confusion, disorientation, agitation, aggression, abnormal behavior, speech arrest and myoclonus may develop and deterioration of neurological symptoms with seizures and hallucinations may occur. Some patients may be very sensitive to this effect and it has been advised to give a test dose of deferoxamine to ascertain whether aluminum is excessively mobilized when deferoxamine is used experimentally for immunosuppression in aluminum-burdened renal transplant patients (387). Deferoxamine can modify the electroencephalogram (progressive EEG slowing and bilateral paroxysms) (388[C]).

Nausea and vomiting developed frequently in rheumatoid arthritis patients after 4—12 days of treatment with deferoxamine, presumably as a result of chelation of iron from the central nervous system (389[cr]). Two patients who received the phenothiazine derivative, prochlorperazine, during deferoxamine therapy lost consciousness for 48—72 hours, possibly because this combination of drugs removes essential iron from the nervous system. Deferoxamine and phenothiazine derivatives should not be used concomitantly (390[C]).

Headache, loss of vision, disturbed consciousness and various other neurological symptoms may be alarming signs of deferoxamine-associated *systemic mucormycosis with cerebral involvement*, a condition which is usually fatal (391[C]—393[C]) (see 'Opportunistic infections').

Cataract has been observed in animals, but in man only rarely and after prolonged use of deferoxamine (394[c], 395[r]).

Endocrine, metabolic The administration of deferoxamine to dialysis patients in order to chelate aluminum is often associated with asymptomatic *hypocalcemia*, which may in turn aggravate hyperparathyroidism (348[CR]). Deferoxamine-induced hypocalcemia could be corrected with supplements of vitamin D and calcium carbonate. In an 8-month-old child the administration of deferoxamine caused sustained hypocalcemia without concomitant hypercalciuria (396[C]). In this patient deferoxamine was used for chelation of aluminum, which had accumulated as a result of total parenteral nutrition. Presumably the decreased calcium levels reflected bone regeneration following the disappearance of aluminum from the bone.

When used in patients without iron overload, deferoxamine may cause *iron deficiency* (348). In one study a marked decline in ferritin levels in six out of 20 patients required the interruption of deferoxamine and parenteral administration of iron dextran (348[c]). In patients receiving deferoxamine for aluminium overload the monitoring of ferritin levels is therefore recommended.

Hematological Rare cases have been reported of *thrombocytopenia* and fatal *pancytopenia*, attributed to the use of deferoxamine (397[C], 398[CR]). For iron depletion induced by deferoxamine see 'Endocrine, metabolic'. Deferoxamine may perhaps accumulate in the case of renal failure if repeated doses are given, and it has been advised that platelet counts in such patients be monitored (397). Deferoxamine has a strongly depressing effect on proliferation of *bone marrow* cultures in vitro (399). On the other hand, deferoxamine may improve hematopoiesis in anemia or hemolysis (400[C]—403[C]). The mechanism is unknown, but may perhaps refer to a decreased toxic effect of iron overload on the red-cell membrane (401) or to the chelation of aluminium (402) or other toxic substances (403).

Gastrointestinal *(SED-12, 553; SEDA-18, 250) Gastrointestinal upset* occurred in seven in a series of 28 patients after intravenous administration of deferoxamine and seems to be a frequent problem (404[CR]). In addition to *nausea, vomiting and abdominal cramps*, passage of *black stools* may occur, the latter perhaps representing an increase in stool iron content induced by deferoxamine. Nausea and vomiting developed frequently in rheumatoid arthritis patients after 4—12 days of treatment with deferoxamine, presumably as a result of chelation of iron from the central nervous system (385[CR]). One pathway in deferoxamine metabolism, involving the enzyme monoamine oxidase, is oxidative deamination and the production of an intermediate aldehyde which is further metabolized to MFO1 (a carboxylic acid end product) and excreted as such in the urine (405[C]). The aldehyde formation is thought to be responsible for the side effects such as nausea and vomiting. Another metabolite, MFO2, which probably does not cause side effects, is generated through acetylation of the amino terminal of deferoxamine. Kruck et al. proposed an MFO1/TOT index as a predictor for the occurrence of gastrointestinal side effects—anorexia, stomach upset and weight loss—of deferoxamine (250 mg daily by i.m. injection), in patients with Alzheimer's disease (405[C]). The MFO1/TOT index is the ratio of the urinary excretion of MFO1 and the total excretion of MFO1 plus MFO2.

Urinary system *(SED-12, 553; SEDA-17, 287)* The iron—deferoxamine complex gives the urine a reddish-brown color. In a series of 27 patients with thalassemia subcutaneous deferoxamine was found to cause a clinically significant reduction in renal glomerular filtration rate in 40% of the patients and a mild reduction in another 40% (406[CR]). In all cases of severe reductions the glomerular filtration rate tended to return to baseline on discontinuation of deferoxamine. There was also a significant increase in urine volume during deferoxamine therapy. Deferoxamine has occasionally been reported to cause *renal failure* (407[C], 408[Cr]) and adequate hydration and repeated measurements of renal function are recommended in patients on intravenous deferoxamine therapy. Perhaps the inability to reabsorb sodium and to concentrate urine during administration of deferoxamine may be caused by a diuretic effect of ferrioxamine (409[c]).

Skin and appendages Subcutaneous administration of deferoxamine often causes *local irritation* of the skin at infusion sites (343[r], 410[c]). The addition of 1—2 mg hydrocortisone to the deferoxamine solution and/or dilution with additional sterile water may alleviate this problem. If not, the patient may develop disfiguring *lumps* that can serve as foci for *bacterial infections*. Proper needle placement in deep subcutaneous sites and rotation of sites among the lower abdomen, thighs, buttocks and arms usually allows sufficient time for one area to heal before it is used again. Another concern is that rapid intravenous infusion of deferoxamine (greater than 25 mg/kg per 30 min) may cause *vertigo, hypotension, diffuse erythema and generalized pruritus* (343[r]). Such reactions reverse with cessation of the infusion, although occasionally a fluid bolus and/or diphenhydramine may be needed to reverse symptoms more rapidly. This reaction is considered to be due to histamine release and not to be immunological in nature; patients may be safely treated at a lower dose rate of deferoxamine later on. An edematous, erythematous and itching *rash* of the legs developed in a 62-year-old woman within 48 hours after the infusion of deferoxamine (411[c]). A recent and interesting observation concerned three patients in a series of 28, with *porphyria cutanea tarda-like skin lesions* developing on the dorsum of the hands and forearms and worsening with sun exposure (404[cR]). The skin eruption resolved in all three patients after completion of deferoxamine therapy. By contrast, in another study, deferoxamine was used successfully as a treatment for hemodialysis-related porphyria cutanea tarda (412[c]).

Skin lesions imitating *vasculitis or cutaneous infarction* may be the first manifestation of life-threatening *mucormycosis* (413[CR], 414[CR]) (see 'Opportunistic infections').

Genital system A repetitive association of *monilial vaginitis* with deferoxamine administration was reported in patients receiving the drug for dialysis-related aluminum overload (348[cr]) (see also 'Opportunistic infections').

Musculoskeletal system *(415[C], 416[CR]—420[CR])* In children deferoxamine has been found to cause *bone dysplasia*, especially when the use is started at a young age. Injury to the metaphyseal growth plate cartilage affects the development of tubular bones and vertebra. The lesions are reminiscent of scurvy but the mechanism involved is uncertain. Perhaps a combination of mechanisms is involved, of which the most relevant seem to be the defective function of iron-dependent enzymes and the chelation of other minerals, such as zinc, copper, and aluminium. Deferoxamine-induced bone dysplasia may cause *decreased body height and spinal deformities*. Metaphyseal changes may be detected at an early stage with serial radiographs. When they are found the nightly dose of deferoxamine should be reduced to the lowest level that results in a negative iron balance and growth rate should be carefully observed. Instead of the previous sequelae of marrow hyperplasia secondary to hemolysis, skeletal deformities in thalassemia patients may now be dominated by the spinal and metaphyseal changes associated with deferoxamine-induced growth failure.

Opportunistic infections *(SED-12, 553; SEDA-16, 252; SEDA-17, 288; SEDA-18, 250)* Iron is an essential metabolic agent and the extremely low free iron content of the blood is an important antimicrobial factor. Many micro-organisms do not produce siderophores and are entirely dependent on the iron content in their direct environment; usually their inability to produce siderophores is associated with low virulence. In the case of increased availability of iron, e.g. in iron storage diseases, the patient may have increased susceptibility to infectious diseases (421—423). Furthermore, iron has been found to impair granulocyte function (424, 425) and monocytic function (414[r]). An abundance of publications has revealed that the use of deferoxamine—in iron storage disease, dialysis patients or acute iron poisoning (426[R])—may promote the development of infections, notably with micro-organisms that are iron dependent and known to be otherwise only slightly virulent (SED-12, 553; 427[CR]—431[CR]). Besides the provision of iron by acting as a siderophore to these micro-organisms, deferoxamine may deplete the pool of iron available to the macrophage cytotoxic system (432), and adversely influence the immune system (387[R], 362[C]). *Yersinia enterocolitica* or *Y. pseudotuberculosis*, *Pneumocystis carinii* (362[C]), *Staphylococcus aureus* (433[C]), *Cunninghamella bertholletiae* (432[C]), *Rhizopus oryzae* and *microsporus* (mucormycosis) have been involved. (In other species, e.g. *Plasmodium falciparum*, on the other hand, deferoxamine has an opposite effect.) The diagnosis of these spontaneously rare diseases may be even more difficult because the deferoxamine-associated form may have an unusual and atypical course. Infections with *Y. enterocolitica*, a gram-negative aerobic and facultatively anaerobic, non-spore-forming bacterium, are known to occur in immune compromised patients, and enteritis and lymphadenopathy are characteristic. In deferoxamine-treated patients, however, septicemia predominates, and also peritonitis and intestinal perforation (428[C]) have been reported; the fatality rate is high (424[C], 426[C], 434[C]—441[C]). In all patients receiving deferoxamine, children and adults, the appearance of fever and other non-specific signs of infection should be a reason to think of yersiniosis. Another risk situation is when deferoxamine is used in children with acute iron poisoning. In view of the severity of a possible *Yersinia* sepsis, the prophylactic use of antibiotics has been advised whenever deferoxamine is administered to children from areas with a high incidence of yersiniosis (426[R]). Many reports of fatal cases of mucormycosis also underline the danger of acquiring disseminated fungal infection in patients receiving deferoxamine (350[C]—352[C], 413[C], 414[C], 442[C]—449[C]). Boelaert and co-workers of the International Registry of Mucormycosis in Dialysis Patients (Algemeen Ziekenhuis Sint Jan, B-8000 Brugge, Belgium) have been able to collect data on a total of 62 cases of mucormycosis, of which 59 were studied in detail (450[CR]). Seventy-eight percent of these patients were on treatment with deferoxamine. The infection presented as disseminated mucormycosis in 44%, rhinocerebral in 31% and other forms in 25%, and ran a fatal course in 52 (86%) of the patients. The fungus (cultured in only 36%) was always *Rhizopus* (in spite of the fact that human mucormycosis can be caused by various other fungal genera (e.g. *Mucor*, *Absida* and *Cunninghamella*). The finding that the species was *R. microsporus* in all identified cases is at variance with the usual predominance of *R. oryzae* in diabetes mellitus patients.

Patients using deferoxamine who present with fever, sinusitis or neurological symptoms should undergo evaluation for mucormycosis. Occasionally such conditions may start with skin lesions imitating vasculitis (413[CR]) or cutaneous infarction (414[CR]), or present with cavernous sinus or carotid arterial thrombosis (445[CR]).

Use in children The administration of high subcutaneous doses to young children with thalassemia before iron overload has been established is associated with a significant decrease in mean body length (451[CR], 452[cr]). Impairment of growth is associated with a rickets-like syndrome and joint stiffness. Metabolic studies have revealed a reduction of hair and leucocyte zinc levels and leucocyte alkaline phosphatase activity. Retardation of growth may be related to chelation of trace elements (e.g. zinc), to a direct toxic effect of unchelated deferoxamine by inhibiting critical iron-dependent enzymes, or to both. It is advised that in thalassemia major, treatment with deferoxamine be initiated only after iron accumulation is established, i.e. around 3 years of age, after 20—30 blood transfusions, when ferritin levels are in the range of 800—1000 ng/ml. Deferoxamine doses should be established on the basis of iron-balance studies and dose-response curves, and longitudinal growth monitoring is warranted.

The vulnerability of children to opportunistic infections (see above) is illustrated in a small series in The Netherlands of 10 children receiving intravenous deferoxamine (25 mg/kg); unexpected infections were observed in four; three patients had episodes of fever and *Staphylococcus aureus* in blood cultures and one patient had *Yersinia enterocolitica* sepsis (433[c]). In France another two children with *Y. enterocolitica* infections were reported—mesenteric adenitis in one and septicemia in the other. A review was also given of 28 literature cases, mostly children, of deferoxamine-associated *Yersinia* septicemia (439[CR]). The authors concluded that, because of the possibility of septicemic dissemination secondary to digestive *Y. enterocolitica* infections, the occurrence of febrile diarrhea in a child with thalassemia necessitates the immediate discontinuation of deferoxamine and the administration of antimicrobial therapy (co-trimoxazole).

Second-generation effects *(SED-12, 554)* Deferoxamine is teratogenic in animals. McElhatton et al. evaluated the outcome of pregnancy in women with iron poisoning, many of whom had been treated with deferoxamine (453[C]). Of 49 pregnancies, 43 resulted in live babies, two had spontaneous abortions and there were four elective terminations. Of the live babies, three were premature and three other babies had malformations. A total of 25 patients had been treated with deferoxamine; two of the babies with malformations occurred in this group, but it was concluded that the drug had probably not been the cause. In another seven cases of prenatal exposure to deferoxamine no morphological malformations were found (454[cR]).

Interactions There is a complex interaction between *ascorbic acid*, *iron* and deferoxamine (455[R]). Ascorbic acid appears to be essential for the mobilization of stored iron into a labile pool, available for chelation therapy. As a result, the administration of deferoxamine to patients with ascorbic acid deficiency will have a limited effect. On the other hand, ascorbic acid increases the toxic effects of iron, especially on the heart. In order to prevent serious cardiac arrhythmia, ascorbic acid should only be given after deferoxamine infusion has been started and adequate serum levels of deferoxamine have been attained (SEDA-8, 239; 456[cR]). Ascorbic acid reduces ferric to ferrous iron, and it is the reduced iron which is responsible for the generation of highly reactive free radicals, causing tissue injury (455[R]). Ascorbic acid up to 2 g/day stimulates deferoxamine-mediated urinary iron excretion, probably without adverse cardiac results (457[r]). A case report describing the precipitation of cardiomyopathy with a dose of 1 g/day of ascorbic acid in a patient with hemochromatosis not receiving deferoxamine, on the other hand, provides reason for caution in this respect (458[C]). Interestingly, this patient later showed a rapid beneficial effect of deferoxamine on the heart, even before significant iron chelation could have been established. Presumably deferoxamine detoxifies iron by the inhibition of Fe^{2+}-induced hydroxyl radical generation and lipid peroxidation.

The combination of *prochlorperazine*, and deferoxamine may cause loss of consciousness (390[C], see Nervous system).

Interference with diagnostic and laboratory tests *(SEDA-16, 252)* Experience in a patient with a cerebral hemorrhage showed that chelation of gallium by deferoxamine may interfere with the diagnostic value of a ^{67}Ga scan (459[C]). Bentur et al. have discussed the possible misinterpretation of the measurement of the iron-binding capacity in the presence of deferoxamine (430).

Deferiprone (L1, DMPH or dimethylhydroxypyridone) *(SEDA-17, 288)*

So far, most experience in humans with iron chelating agents for oral administration concerns deferiprone. The fact that toxic manifestations and iron excretion with deferiprone occur in the same dose range suggests that the drug interferes with cell proliferation by removing iron needed in this process. The avidity of deferiprone for iron is lower than that of deferoxamine and since circulating deferiprone—iron complexes can easily dissociate, deferiprone may redistribute iron in the body (460[R]). It is suggested that iron redistribution might play a role in certain suspected adverse reactions, such as arthralgia and perhaps the precipitation or aggravation of heart failure (460[R]).

Hematological *(SEDA-18, 251)* Since their previous report (461[C]), Al-Refaie et al. observed a third patient with deferiprone-associated agranulocytosis and an additional three patients with milder decreases in granulocytes in whom the causal role of deferiprone was demonstrated in a positive rechallenge (SEDA-17, 288; 462[CR]). Granulocytopenia occurred in patients with different indications for deferiprone (Blackfan-Diamond anemia, thalassamia major and myelodysplasia). There are presumably two patterns of deferiprone myelotoxicity. The first is agranulocytosis, usually occurring about 6 weeks from the commencement of deferiprone administration. The second may be less severe neutropenia (neutrophils $<1.5 \times 10^9$/l), occurring at any time. Reintroduction of deferiprone appears to cause neutropenia to recur, but at the same pace as for the original development of neutropenia. This pattern is more in favour of a toxic than immune mechanism. In the three patients with agranulocytosis there was no in vitro or in vivo evidence for an immune mechanism (462[CR]). Culture of bone marrow myeloid progenitor cells did not provide evidence for an increased sensitivity to deferiprone, however, and the mechanism involved remains obscure. The frequency of neutropenia in deferiprone users is estimated to be 2.4% and of agranulocytosis 2% (462[CR]).

Musculoskeletal Arthralgia in association with deferiprone has been reported in 16.5—38% of patients (463[CR], 464[c], 465[C], 466[r]—468[r]). Berkovitch et al. have reported more in detail on the three patients with deferiprone-induced arthropathy, already referred to in SEDA 18 (p. 251), occurring in a series of 16 patients with thalassemia (466[C]). Deferiprone dose was 75 mg/kg/day. Three to 8 months after the start of therapy, these patients, aged 17, 20 and 27 years, complained of severe bilateral knee pain at rest, worsening with exertion, morning stiffness, joint warmth and swelling.

One patient also had similar symptoms in the fingers and wrists of both hands. Rheumatoid factor, anti-DNA and anti-histone antibodies were negative and arthralgia was not part of an SLE reaction. Knee radiographs in one patient showed thalassemic changes, joint effusions and minor degenerative changes in the patellofemoral joint. Magnetic resonance imaging confirmed effusions, with no evidence of synovial hypertrophy or cartilage abnormalities. Aspiration of synovial fluid revealed a sterile transudate without inflammatory cells and low concentrations of deferiprone uncomplexed to iron. Arthroscopy showed mild synovial hypertrophy and hyperplasia, with iron staining. Synovial biopsy revealed mild synovial lining cell proliferation and extensive iron deposition, without evidence of an inflammatory or allergic reaction. High concentrations of iron relative to deferiprone were detected in synovial fluid, suggesting that iron is shifted by deferiprone from body stores to the joints and that incomplete complexation may result in the formation of catalytic iron. This, in turn, accelerates the formation of hydroxyl radicals that peroxidase synovial membranes. Alternatively, deferiprone might merely worsen underlying thalassemic osteoarthropathy.

Immunological reactions In two patients the use of deferiprone was associated with a lupus-like reaction (469[C]). One patient had nausea, abdominal pain, muscle and joint pains, and a low-grade fever. A test for anti-ds-DNA antibodies was negative, but there were antinuclear antibodies and antibodies to histones. The patient died of a cardiac arrest, perhaps as a complication of the lupus-like reaction. In the other patient antinuclear and antihistones antibodies developed, without clinical symptoms. The possible association between deferiprone and ANA and antihistone antibodies (AHA) and the possible occurrence of a serious lupus syndrome, however, is still a matter of controversy). Mehta et al. have reported on their observations in 90 thalassemia patients (470[CR]). ANA were found in seven (25.9%) of 27 patients using deferiprone and four of these seven also had AHA. In two of these patients deferiprone was stopped and the antibodies disappeared. In 63 patients not receiving deferiprone, only two (3.2%) had antinuclear antibodies and none had antihistone antibodies. Since there is a low background ANA positivity in thalassemia patients and AHA are characteristic of drug-induced lupus, the authors concluded that deferiprone seems to cause systemic autoimmunity in a substantial proportion of users. In the series of Olivieri et al., on the other hand, a weakly positive test for ANA developed in two out of 13 patients during deferiprone treatment (465[C]). Al-Refaie et al. emphasized that the question of whether deferiprone can cause an SLE syndrome is unproven (471).

Second-generation and tumor-inducing effects Deferiprone inhibits intracellular ribonucleotide reductase, a rate-limiting enzyme in DNA synthesis, and in animal experiments deferiprone is toxic to proliferating tissues, especially the bone marrow. It has a pattern of toxicities similar to that of cytotoxic drugs and is embryotoxic and teratogenic in animals (460[R], 472[r]).

Desferrithiocin

An in vitro study shows that the new oral iron chelator desferrithiocin is, like deferoxamine, a potent and reversible inhibitor of T-cell proliferation and subsequent T-cell function (473). This effect may have clinical potential, e.g. to inhibit graft rejection.

OTHER METAL ANTAGONISTS

Dimercaprol (BAL) *(SED-12, 555)*

Dimercaprol or BAL (British Anti-Lewisite) was originally developed to counteract arsenic-containing war gases. Dimercaprol is used for the treatment of poisoning with heavy metals such as arsenic, gold, lead or mercury, and is administered by intramuscular injection. Side effects include nausea, vomiting, a burning sensation in the mouth, throat, eyes and sometimes limbs, muscle pain and spasms, lacrimation, rhinorrhea and hypersalivation. Of importance are elevation of the blood pressure and tachycardia. Pain in head, teeth or abdomen can occur. The symptoms develop soon after injection and subside within about 2 hours. Injections may be painful and give rise to sterile abscesses. Fever can occur. Dimercaprol is contraindicated in patients with glucose-6-phosphate dehydrogenase deficiency, because of the risk of hemolysis (474[C], 475[r]).

Dimercaptopropanesulfonate

Dimercaptopropanesulfonate (2,3-dimercapto-1-propanesulfonate) is used in heavy metal poisoning. The drug, a water-soluble and possibly less toxic derivative of dimercaprol, appears to be little used in Western countries. Reported side effects are nausea, vertigo, weakness, skin itching and allergic reactions (476[r]).

Edetic acid *(SED-12, 555)*

Edetic acid is ethylenediamine tetraacetic acid. The effect of an intravenous dose of 1 gram of calcium disodium edetate on the urinary excretion on the elements Al, B, Ba, Cu, Fe, Mn, Pb, Si, Sr, Zn, Na, K, Ca, Mg, S, and P was measured in healthy volunteers. The ratio of the increase of urinary elimination was about 2 for Fe, 5 for Al, Pb and Mn, and 15 for Zn (477). In spite of the established dangers and lack of efficacy, salts of edetic acid are still used in intravenous 'chelation therapy' as an alternative treatment of atherosclerotic disease in several countries (SEDA-10, 225; 478[R], 479[C], 480[R], 481[CR], 482[R], 483[C]). Much of the data on side effects are derived from older studies.

Adverse effects of disodium edetate include *hypocalcemia*, *tetany*, *convulsions*, *cardiac arrhythmia*, *respiratory arrest* and *renal failure*. Other possible symptoms are *nausea*, *vomiting*, *diarrhea*, *fever*, *headache* and *urinary urgency*. *Pain* and *phlebitis* at the site of injection can occur. The sodium load of 'chelation therapy' may precipitate *heart failure*. *Renal tubular necrosis* may occur (478). Sodium calcium edetate can cause the same adverse effects as the disodium salt, with the exception of hypocalcemia. Administration by mouth may cause *vomiting*, *diarrhea* and *abdominal cramps*. *Bone marrow depression* and a *histamine-releasing reaction* (*sneezing*, *lacrimation*) have been reported (484[r]). Salts of edetic acid have been reported in association with symptomatic *zinc deficiency*, abnormalities of the skin (crusted lesions of mouth and eyelids, leukokeratosis of the tongue, stomatitis, a papular, pustular and erosive rash of the face and perianally), alopecia, and white bands on the nails (485, 486[cr]).

In three of six children receiving disodium ethylenediaminetetraacetate by intravenous infusion, an *influenza-like syndrome* developed, characterized by *lacrimation, rhinorrhea, sneezing and cough* (487[CR]). Additional symptoms were *malaise*, *fatigue*, *nausea* and *vomiting*; one patient had a *fever* of 39.2°C. The symptoms disappeared within 24 h and did not recur when sodium citrate was given instead of EDTA.

Hematological When edetate is used as an in vitro anticoagulant, artifactual *pseudothrombocytopenia* may occur in about 0.1% of blood samples (488[R]–491[C], 492[CR]–494[CR], 495[C]). The phenomenon is more frequently encountered in severely ill patients and during hospitalization, suggesting that the antibody involved is an acquired one. Unlike true thrombocytopenia, edetate-induced pseudothrombocytopenia is associated with a normal mean platelet volume. Plasma or serum from these patients agglutinates homologous and autologous platelets, and the presence of other anticoagulants does not inhibit the coagulation induced by EDTA. The serum factor responsible for agglutination is an immunoglobulin which acts as a drug-dependent antibody. It is usually an IgG antibody, but IgM or IgA may also be found (489[R], 494[CR]). Presumably the strong calcium chelator EDTA modifies the calcium content of the platelet membrane, changing its physical properties and exposing a hidden antigenic determinant of platelet membrane glycoproteins IIb/IIIa. The immunoglobulin reacts (as has been shown in vitro) with this antigen, causing agglutination. The diagnosis of pseudothrombocytopenia should be suspected in patients lacking signs of an increased tendency to bleed. The diagnosis includes: (a) the demonstration of platelet clumps in the sample by examination of the histogram display or the peroxidase display, or by microscopic examination of a peripheral blood sample; (b) a normal platelet count using alternative anticoagulants; (c) the demonstration of EDTA-dependent platelet antibodies (although this is usually not necessary because the diagnosis is already obvious).

When automated cell counters interpret platelet clumps as leukocytes, *pseudoleukocytosis* (489, 495[C]) may also occur in association with edetic acid. By contrast, in blood samples edetate may also induce *agglutination of neutrophil granulocytes* and cause *pseudoleukocytopenia*, presumably also as an immunological phenomenon involving IgM antibodies (496[CR], 497[CR]).

The importance of a correct and early diagnosis of edetate-induced pseudothrombocytopenia follows from the fact that it may avoid expensive and disturbing investigations (e.g. bone-marrow puncture), delay of surgery, unnecessary transfusions, unnecessary stopping of wrongly suspected drugs, and potentially harmful treatment (e.g. steroids, splenectomy). It should be added that similar antibodies may occur that are *not* edetate dependent (598[C]). There has been some discussion that edetate, as a reagent red cell diluent, may, on rare occasions, cause inhibition of anti-Al (of the ABO system) antibodies, but the case has not yet been settled (499[C], 500[R]).

Urinary system Intravenous administration of disodium edetate may cause *renal failure* and *acute tubular necrosis* (478). In a study of children with subclinical lead-poisoning the administration of sodium calcium edetate and dimercaprol together was associated with mild and transient biochemical evidence of renal damage in 13% of patients, whereas another 3% had acute renal failure (501[CR]).

Immunological reactions Edetic acid is allergenic and can elicit *allergic reactions*, *with rashes*, *fever*, *edema* and *arthralgia*. There can be cross-allergy to ethylenediamine which is a constituent of various drugs (e.g. aminophylline, some ointments) (SED-8, 538). In addition, edetic disodium is found in small amounts in certain drugs, i.e. as a result of the removal of trace quantities of heavy metals.

In a 4-year-old child with a known allergy to ethylenediamine hydrochloride, patch testing showed a strong reaction to ethylenediamine hydrochloride, but ethylenediamine tetra-acetate petrolatum (1%) gave negative results (502[C]). The patient was subsequently treated with ethylenediamine tetra-acetate for lead poisoning without ill effects. Ethylenediamine tetra-acetate is presumably not a sensitizer and does not cross-react with ethylenediamine hydrochloride, and the tetra-acetate can be safely given to patients who are allergic to the hydrochloride.

Interactions The activity of *phenylmercuric preservatives* may be reduced by interaction with disodium edetate (503[r]).

Second generation effects Salts of edetic acid are *teratogenic* in animals, probably by causing zinc deficiency (504, 505).

Methyl *tert*-butyl ether

Methyl *tert*-butyl ether (MTBE) with or without ethylenediamine tetra-acetate (EDTA) is used, via transhepatic catheterization of the gallbladder, for direct chemical dissolution of cholesterol and pigment gallstones. Janowitz et al. reported on a series of 42 patients, 19 received MTBE alone and 23 MTBE and bile acid-EDTA (506[CR]). Mild complications occurred in 40 of the 42 patients: vomiting in 12, pain on commencement of treatment in 32, elevation of liver enzymes in six and fever and leukocytosis in five. In the MTBE group, there were two serious complications (gallbladder wall necrosis with perforation in one and catheter dislocation in the other). In the MTBE BA-EDTA group there were five serious complications: pericystic extravasation in two and catheter dislocation, sterile perihepatic abscess and perihepatic biloma each in one. Post-treatment CT examination after intravenous application of contrast medium was performed in 27 patients and revealed gallbladder mural hyperemia and edematous swelling of the pericystic tissue layer in 26 cases.

Succimer

Succimer, is the meso isomer of 2,3-dimethylmercaptosuccinic acid (DMSA). It is used as a lead chelator for oral administration. *Nausea*, *vomiting*, *diarrhea*, and *anorexia* are common. *Rashes*, sometimes necessitating withdrawal, have been reported in up to 10% of adults and 5% of children, and mild transient elevations of serum aminotransferase activity in 6—10% (mostly adults) (507[R], 508[r]). Life-threatening hyperthermia occurred on two occasions in one subject, but no details were given. Mild to moderate neutropenia has been reported (509[c]), and thrombocytopenia has occurred in some animals (510).

Iron can be safely and effectively given to patients receiving succimer, which (unlike dimercaprol) does not appear to deplete iron stores or to form a toxic chelate that would preclude the parenteral administration of iron (508[r]).

Urea-edetate

Urea-edetate (with methylhexyl ether) was used without side effects for the dissolution of calcified gallbladder stones in two patients (511).

Triene (trientine, triethylene tetramine dihydrochloride) *(SED-12, 556)*

Triene seems to be a safer drug in Wilson's disease than penicillamine, but experience with it is still limited (512[CR], 513[R]—515[R]). The modes of action of these drugs are complex, somewhat different, and in some respects unclear. Transient *aggravation of neurological symptoms* occurred in two of four Japanese patients with Wilson's disease receiving triene because of intolerance to penicillamine (516[c]). Triene, like penicillamine, should be started in small doses and be gradually increased.

Excessive excretion of metals (zinc, iron) may occur and is a potential cause of deficiency symptoms (517[CR]). A 44-year-old woman developed *antinuclear and anti-ds-DNA antibodies* (without clinical signs) while using penicillamine; the antibodies disappeared after withdrawal, but recurred when the patient was subsequently given triene (110[C]).

Sideroblastic anemia results from defective iron utilization in erythropoietic cells, secondary to a failure of heme synthesis or abnormal mitochondrial iron metabolism. It is characterized by an excess of ringed sideroblasts in the bone marrow. Condamine et al. described the development of *microcytic sideroblastic anemia* in a girl of about 15 years of age, 3 months after starting the use of triene, 2250 mg/day, for Wilson's disease (518[CR]). Perls staining showed 85% sideroblasts, with 30% ringed sideroblasts. There was increased bone marrow iron incorporation, with increased intramedullary abortion and slow red cell incorporation. No cause of the anemia was found; neither iron nor pyridoxine corrected the microcytosis and medullary sideroblastosis. The patient recovered when the dose of triene was decreased to 1000 mg/day. Walshe and Yealland in their review on a series of 137 patients with Wilson's disease also referred to the occurrence of sideroblastic anemia during treatment with triene (600 mg t.i.d.) together with zinc (354[cR]). These three patients were also females in their mid-teens and they had a marked increase in neurological symptoms together with the anemia.

Teratogenic effects of triene have not been observed (517[r]).

Tetrathiomolybdate

Tetrathiomolybdate may be used as a chelator of copper in Wilson's disease. It is reported to have caused reversible bone marrow depression in two patients, but details were not given (354[c]). This drug should not be used in children, because of its toxic effect on the epiphyses in growing bone (354[r]).

Dimercaptosuccinic acid

2,3-Dimercaptosuccinic acid (DMSA) is an orally active chelating agent, used in the treatment of lead poisoning (475[R]). The manufacturer has accumulated data on approximately 200 children treated with DMSA (475[r]). Approximately 10% of these children experienced an adverse event. Gastrointestinal symptoms and elevated serum transaminases were most frequently observed. Several episodes of neutropenia, possibly related to DMSA administration, have been reported.

REFERENCES

1. Joyce DA. D-Penicillamine pharmacokinetics and pharmacodynamics in man. Pharmacol Ther 1989;42:405–428.
2. Madhok R, Zoma A, Torley Hl et al. The relationship of sulfoxidation status to efficacy and toxicity of penicillamine in the treatment of rheumatoid arthritis. Arthr Rheum 1990;33:574–577.
3. Bernelot Moens HJ, Ament BJW, Feltkamp BW, Van der Korst JK. Longterm followup of treatment with D-penicillamine for rheumatoid arthritis: effectivity and toxicity in relation to HLA antigens. J Rheumatol 1987;14:1115–1119.
4. Cooperative Systematic Studies of Rheumatoid Disease Group. Toxicity of longterm low dose D-penicillamine therapy in rheumatoid arthritis. J Rheumatol 1987;14:67–73.
5. Kutsuna T, Maeda K, Okamoto T. Long term results of D-penicillame treatment in rheumatoid arthritis. Ryumachi 1986;26:270.
6. Kashiwazaki S. Current status of D-peniciliamine therapy in Japan. Z Rheumatol 1988;47(Suppl 1):38–40.
7. Felson DT, Anderson JJ, Meenan RF. The comparative efficacy and toxicity of second-line drugs in rheumatoid arthritis. Arthr Rheum 1990;33:1449–1459.
8. Wolfe F, Hawley DJ, Cathey MA. Termination of slow acting antirheumatic therapy in rheumatoid arthritis: a 14-year prospective evaluation of 1017 consecutive starts. J Rheumatol 1990;17:994–1002.
9. Taylor HG, Samanta A. Penicillamine in rheumatoid arthritis; a problem of toxicity. Drug Safety 1992;7:46–53.
10. Pincus T, Marcum SB, Callahan LF. Longterm drug therapy for rheumatoid arthritis in seven rheumatology private practices: II. Second line drugs and prednisone. J Rheumatol 1992;19:1885–1894.
11. Raynauld JP, Lee YSL, Kornfeld P, Fries JF. Unilateral ptosis as an initial manifestation of D-penicillamine induced myasthenia gravis. J Rheumatol 1993;20:1592–1593.
12. Huskisson EC. Side effects of penicillamine therapy in RA. J Rheumatol 1981;8(Suppl 7):181.
13. Tanphaichitr K. D-penicillamine-induced bronchial spasm. S Med J 1980;73:788.
14. Haerden J, Coolen L, Dequeker J. The effect of D-penicillamine on lung function parameters (diffusion capacity) in rheumatoid arthritis. Clin Exp Rheumatol 1993; 11:509–513.
15. Turner-Warwick M. Adverse reactions affecting the lung: possible association with penicillamine J Rheumatol 1981;8(Suppl 7):166.
16. Camus P. Manifestations respiratoires associées aux traitements par la D-penicillamine. Rev Fr Mal Respir 1982;10:7.
17. Shettar SP, Chattaopadhyay C, Wolstenholme RJ, Swinson DR. Diffuse alveolitis on a small dose of penicillamine. Br J Rheumatol 1984;23:220.
18. Canon GW. Antirheumatic drug reactions in the lung. Ballières Clin. Rheumatol 1993;7:147–171.
19. Jenkins EA, Hull RG, Thomas AL. D-Penicillamine and polymyositis: the significance of the anti-Jo-1 antibody. Br J Rheumatol 1993;32:1109–1110.
20. Drosos AA, Christou L, Galanopoulou V, Tzioufas AG, Tsiakou EK. D-Penicillamine induced myasthenia gravis: Clinical, serologic and genetic findings. Clin Exp Rheumatol 1993;11:387–391.
21. Padley SPG, Adler BD, Hansell DM, Müller NL. Bronchiolitis obliterans: high resolution CT findings and correlation with pulmonary function tests. Clin Radiol 1993; 47:236–240.
22. Honda T, Hachiya T, Hayasaka M, Morita M, Nakagawa S, Kusama Y, Kubo K, Sekiguchi M, Kobayashi O. A case of rheumatoid arthritis with obstructive bronchiolitis appearing after D-penicillamine therapy. Jpn. J Thorac Dis 1993; 31:1195–1200.
23. Lauque D, Courtin JP, Fournie B et al. Syndrome pneumo-rénal induit par la D-penicillamine: syndrome de Goodpasture ou polyartérite microscopique? Rev Méd Int 1990;11:168–171.
24. Storch W. Seltene immunologisch bedingte Asthmaformen. Atemw-Lungenkrkh 1990;16:271- 272.

25. Lagier F, Cartier A, Dolovich J, Malo J-L. Occupational asthma in a pharmaceutical worker exposed to penicillamine. Thorax 1989;44:157—158.
26. Grobbelaar J, Meyers OL. Penicillamine therapy in rheumatoid arthritis. South Afr Med J 1984;65:175.
27. Stockmann G. Die Stellung des Churg-Strauss-Syndrome zwischen anderen hypereosinophilen, granulomatösen und vaskulitischen Erkrankungen. Z Rheumatol 1988;47:388—396.
28. Presley AP. Penicillamine induced rhinitis. Br Med J 1988;296:1332—1333.
29. Bardach H, Gebhart W, Niebauer G. 'Lumpybumby' elastic fibers in the skin and lungs of a patient with penicillamine-induced elastosis perforans serpiginosa. J Cutan Pathol 1979;6:243.
30. Stanworth DR. D-Penicillamine-induced immunodeficiency. In: Dawkins RL, Christiansen FT, Zilko PJ, eds. Immunogenetics in Rheumatology: Musculoskeletal Disease and D-Penicillamine, p. 358. Amsterdam: Excerpta Medica, 1982;358.
31. Negishi M, Kobayashi K, Ide H et al. A case report of selective IgA deficiency in rheumatoid arthritis treated with D-penicillamine. J Showa Med Assoc 1990;50:205—209.
32. Pool KD, Feit H, Kirkpatrick J. Penicillamine-induced neuropathy in rheumatoid arthritis. Ann Intern Med 1981;95:457.
33. Pedersen PB, Hogenhaven H. Penicillamine-induced neuropathy in rheumatoid arthritis. Acta Neurol Scand 1983;81:188—190.
34. Mayer N, Graninger W, Wessicy P. Polyneuropathie bei chronischer Polyarthritis unter D-Penicillamin: medikamentös induziert? Wien Klin Wochenschr 1983;95:86.
35. Stremmel W, Meyerrose KW, Niederau C, Hefter H, Kreuzpaintner G, Strohmeyer G. Wilson's disease: clinical presentation, treatment and survival. Ann Intern Med 1991;115:720—726.
36. Klingele TG, Burde RM. Optic neuropathy associated with penicillamine therapy in a patient with rheumatoid arthritis. J Clin Neuro-Ophthalmol 1984;4:75.
37. Knezevic W, Mastaglio FL, Quinter J, Zilko PJ Guillain-Barré syndrome and pemphigus foliaceus associated with D-penicillamine therapy. Aust NZ J Med 1984;14:50.
38. Matsubara K, Noda T, Nakano I, Shikano Y, Maeda M, Mori S. A case of progressive systemic sclerosis with acute polyradiculoneuropathy during D-penicillamine therapy. Nishinihon J Dermatol 1990;52:1120—1126.
39. Hilz MJ, Druschky K-F, Bauer J et al. Morbus Wilson—kritische Verschlechterung unter hochdosierter parenteraler Penicillamin-Therapie. Dtsch Med Wochenschr 1990;115: 93—97.
40. Pall HS, Williams AC, Blake DR. Deterioration of Wilson's disease following the start of penicillamine therapy. Arch Neurol 1989;46:359.
41. Veen C, Van den Hamer CJ, De Leeuw PW. Zinc sulphate therapy for Wilson's disease after acute deterioration during treatment with low-dose D-penicillamine. J Intern Med 1991;229:549—552.
42. Barbosa ER, Scaff M, Canelas HM. Degeneraçao hepatolenticular. Arq Neuro-Psiquiatr 1991;49:399—404.
43. Tankanow RM. Pathophysiology and treatment of Wilson's disease. Clin Pharm 1991;10:839—849.
44. Kehr A, Bharucha BA, Kumta NB. Wilson's disease: initial worsening of neurologic syndrome with penicillamine therapy. Indian Pediatr 1992;29:927—929.
45. Glass JD, Reich ST, Mahlon R, De Long MP. Wilson's disease—development of neurological disease after beginning penicillamine therapy. Arch Neurol 1990;47:595—596.
46. Liu GT, Beinfang DC. Penicillamine-induced ocular myasthenia gravis in rheumatoid arthritis. J. Clin. NeuroOphthalmol 1990;10:2—15.
47. Katz LJ, Lesser RL, Merikangas JR, Silverman JP. Ocular myasthenia gravis after D-penicillamine administration. Br J Ophthalmol 1989;73:1015—1018.
48. Ferbert A. D-Penicillamin-induzierte okuläre Myasthenie bei Psoriasisarthritis. Nervenartzt 1989;60:576—579.
49. Chapat-Jolivet F, Wendling D, Moulin T et al. Myasthénie induite par la D-pénicillamine au cours du traitement de la polyarthrite rhumatoïde. Rhumatologic 1989;41:181—188.
50. Zakarian H, Viallet F, Acquaviva PC, Khalil R. Syndrome myasthénique induit par la D-pénicillamine au cours de la polyarthrite rhumatoïde. Sem. Hôp. Paris 1989; 65:2052—2056.
51. Tzartos SJ, Morel E, Efthimiadis A et al. Fine antigenic specificities of antibodies in sera from patients with D-penicillamine-induced myasthenia gravis. Clin Exp Immunol 1988;74:80—86.
52. Paladini G, Mazzanti G, Mysco G et al. La sindrome miastenica indotta da D-penicillamina nell'artrite reumatoide: carateri clinici e genetici. Reumatismo 1988;40:139—144.
53. Cikes N, Momoi MY, Williams CL et al. Striational autoantibodies: quantitative detection by enzyme immunoassay in myasthenia gravis, thymoma and recipients of D-penicillamine or allogeneic bone marrow. Mayo Clin Proc 1988;63:474—481.
54. Derman H, Theron HP. A propos de trois observations de syndrome myasthénique induit par la D-pénicillamine. Bull Soc Ophthalmol Fr 1987;11:1235—1243.
55. Dubost JJ, Soubrier M, Bouchet F, Kemeny JL, Lhopitaux R, Bussiere JL, Sauvezie B. Complications neuromusculaires de la D-pénicillamine dans la polyarthrite rhumatoide. Rev Neurol Paris 1992;148:207—211.
56. Norscini N, Lancman M, Doctorovich D, Poeraniec C, Bauso Toselli L, Granillo R. Miastenia gravis inducida por D-penicilamina. Presentacion de un caso y revision de la literatura. Rev Neurol Argent 1990;15:59—62.
57. Kuriyama S, Hosoya T, Sakai O. D-Penicillamine induced myasthenia gravis in a patient with rheumatoid arthritis. Ryumachi 1991;31:298—302.
58. Voltz R, Hohlfeld R, Fateh-Moghadam, Witt ThN, Wick, M, Reimers C, Siegele B, Wekerle H. Myasthenia gravis: measurement of anti-AChR autoantibodies using cell line TE 671. Neurology 1991;41:1836—1838.
59. Hanabusa K, Ohtsuki H, Watanabe S, Okano M, Hasebe S, Tadokoro Y. D-Penicillamine-induced ocular myasthenia gravis in rheumatoid arthritis. Folia Ophthalmol Jpn 1993;44:1306—1310.
60. Kawano M, Nomura H, Iwainaka Y, Nakashima A, Koni I, Tofuku Y, Takeda R. Bucillamine-associated membranous nephropathy in a patient with rheumatoid arthritis. Jpn J Nephrol 1990;32:817—821.
61. Morel E, Feuillet-Fieux MN, Vernet-der Garabedian B, Raimond F, D'Anglejan J, Bataille R, Sany H, Bach JF. Autoantibodies in D-penicillamine-induced myasthenia

gravis: a comparison with idiopathic myastenia and rheumatoid arthritis. Clin Immunol Immunopathol 1991;583:18–30.
62. Kolarz G, El-Shohoumi M, Maida EM, Scherak O. Azetylcholin rezeptor-Antikorper unter D-Penicillamin-Therapie. Ther Oesterr 1991;6:735–742.
63. Dominkus M, Chlud K, Maida EM, Grisold W. Monitoring of patients with rheumatoid arthritis in long term administration of D-penicillamine. J Rheumatol 1992;19:1648–1650.
64. Dominkus M, Grisold W, Albrecht G. Stimulation single fiber EMG study in patients receiving a long-term D-penicillamine treatment for rheumatoid arthritis. Muscle Nerv 1992;15:1300–1301.
65. Garlepp MJ, Dawkins RL, Christiansen FT. HLA antigens and acetylcholine receptor antibodies in penicillamine-induced myasthenia gravis. Br Med J 1983;286:338–340.
66. Andonopoulos AP, Terzis E, Tsibri E, Papasteriades CA, Papapetropoulos T. D-Penicillamine induced myasthenia gravis in rheumatoid arthritis: an unpredictable common occurrence? Clin Rheumatol 1994;13:586–588
67. Fried MJ, Protheroe DT. D-Penicillamine-induced myasthenia gravis: its relevance for the anaesthesist. Br J Anaesth 1986;58:191.
68. George J, Spokes EGS. Myasthenic pseudointernuclear ophthalmoplegia due to penicillamine. J Neurol Neurosurg Psychiatry 1984;47:1044.
69. Reeback J, Benton S, Swash M, Schwartz MS. Penicillamine-induced neuromyotonia. Br Med J 1979;1:1465.
70. Pinals RS. Diffuse fasciculations induced by D-penicillamine. J Rheumatol 1983;10:809.
71. Doornbos DA, Faber JS. Studies on the metal complexes of drugs D-penicillamine and *N*-acetyl-D-penicillamine. Pharm Weekbl 1964;99:289.
72. Doornbos DA. Stability constants of metal complexes of L-cysteine, D-penicillamine, *N*-acetyl-D-penicillamine and some biguanides. Pharm Weekbl 1968;103:213.
73. Kuchinskas EJ, Rosen Y. Metal chelates of DL-penicillamine. Arch Biochem Biophys 1962;97:370.
74. Knudsen L, Weisman K. Taste dysfunction and changes in zinc and copper metabolism during penicillamine therapy for generalized scleroderma. Acta Med Scand 1987;204:75.
75. Cutolos M, Accardo S, Cimmino MA et al. Hypocupremia-related hypochromic anemia during D-penicillamine treatment. Arthr Rheum 1982;25:119.
76. Datsych M, Jezek P, Richtrova M. Der Einfluss einer Penicillamintherapie auf die Konzentration von Zink, Kupfer, Eisen, Kalzium und Magnesium in Serum und auf deren Ausscheidung in Urin. Z Gastroenterol 1986;24:157.
77. Klingberg WG, Prasad AS, Oberleas D. Zinc deficiency following penicillamine therapy. In: Prasad AS, ed. Trace Elements in Human Health and Disease. New York: Academic Press, 1979.
78. Sheikh IA, Kaplan AP. Assessment of kininases in rheumatic diseases and the effect of therapeutic agents. Arthr Rheum 1987;30:138.
79. Benson EA, Healy LA, Barron EJ. Insulin antibodies in patients receiving penicillamine. Am J Med 1985;78:857.
80. Herranz L, Rovira A, Grande C, Suarez A, Martinez-Ara J, Pallardo LF, Gomez-Pan A. Autoimmune insulin syndrome in a patient with progressive systemic sclerosis receiving penicillamine. Horm Res 1992;37:78–80.
81. Becker RC, Martin R. Penicillamine-induced insulin antibodies. Ann Intern Med 1986;104:128.
82. Elling P, Elling H. Penicillamine, captopril and hypoglycemia. Ann Intern Med 1985;103:644.
83. Vardi P, Brik R, Barzilai D, Lorber M, Scharf Y. Frequent induction of insulin autoantibodies by D-penicillamine in patients with rheumatoid arthritis. J Rheumatol 1992; 19:1527–1530.
84. Faguer de Moustier B, Burgard M, Boitard C, Desplanque N, Fanjoux J, Tchobroutsky G. Syndrome hypoglycémique auto-immun induit par le pyritinol. Diabète Metab Paris 1988;14:423–429.
85. Deldrieu F, Menkes CJ, Sainte-Croix A et al. Myasthénie et thyroidite auto-immune au course du traitements de la polyarthrite rhumatoïde par la D-pénicillamine. Ann Méd Interne 1976;127:739.
86. Bertrand JL, Rousset H, Quenceau P et al. Thyroïdite auto-immune, une complication rare du traitement à la D-pénicillamine. Thérapie 1981;36:337.
87. Edelman J, Maguire KF, Owen ET. Eosinophilia of rheumatoid patients treated with penicillamine. J Rheumatol 1984;11:624.
88. Singh G, Fries JF, Willams CA, Zatarain E, Spitz P, Bloch DA. Toxicity profiles of disease modifying antirheumatic drugs in rheumatoid arthritis. J Rheumatol 1991; 1:188–194.
89. Kay AGL. Myelotoxicity Of D-penicillamine. Ann Rheum Dis 1979;38:232.
90. Netter P, Trechot P, Bannwarth B et al. Effets secondaires de la D-pénicillamine et du pyritinol. Thérapie 1985;40:475.
91. Hammond WP, Miller JE, Starkebaum G, Zweerink HJ, Rosenthal AS, Dale DC. Suppression of in vitro granulocytopoiesis by captopril and penicillamine. Exp Hermatol 1988;16:674–680.
92. Hamilton JA, Williams N. In vitro inhibition of myelopoiesis by gold salts and D-peniciliamine. J Rheumatol 1985;12:892.
93. Thomas D, Gallus AS, Brooks PM et al. Thrombokinetics in patients with rheumatoid arthritis treated with D-penicillamine. Ann Rheum Dis 1984;43:402.
94. Thomas D, Gallus AS, Brooks PM et al. Thrombokinetics in patients with rheumatoid arthritis treated with D-penicillamine. Ann Rheum Dis 1984;43:402.
95. Jimenez SA, Sigal SH. A 15 year prospective study of treatment of rapidly progressive systemic sclerosis with D-penicillamine. J Rheumatol 1991;18:1496–1503.
96. Hill HFH. Treatment of rheumatoid arthritis with penicillamine. Semin Arthr Rheum 1977;6:361.
97. Trice JM, Pinals RS, Plitman GI. Thrombotic thrombocytopenic purpura during penicillamine therapy in rheumatoid arthritis. Arch Intern Med 1983;143:1487.
98. Holdrinet RSG, Namdar Z, Haanen C. Thrombotic thrombocytopenic purpura: clinical course and response to therapy in twelve patients. Neth J Med 1988;33:113–132.
99. Henzgen M, Hein G. Agranulozytose und andere Nebenwirkungen. Erfahrungen mit der D-penicillamintherapie bei der Rheumatoidarthritis. Z Klin Med 1985;40:521.
100. Umeki S, Konishi Y, Yashuda T et al. D-Penicillamine and neutrophilic agranulocytosis. Arch Intern Med 1985; 145:2271.
101. Ramselaar ACP, Dekker AW, Huber-Bruning 0, Bijlsma JWJ. Acquired sideroblastic anemia caused by D-penicillamine therapy for rheumatoid arthritis. Ann Rheum Dis 1987;46:156.
102. Ehrlich JC, Van Paasen HC. Een dodelijke bijwerking van penicillamine. Ned Tijdschr Geneeskd 1984;128:1790.

103 Fishe IB, Tishler M, Caspi D, Yaron M. Fatal aplastic anaemia and liver toxicity caused by D-penicillamine treatment of rheumatoid arthritis. Ann Rheum Dis 1989;48:609–610.
104. Petrides PE, Gerhartz HH. D-Penicillamine-induced agranulocytosis: hematological remission upon treatment with recombinant GM-CSF. Z Rheumatol 1991;50:328–329.
105. Lowenthal RM, Cohen ML, Atkinson K, Biggs JC. Apparent cure of rheumatoid arthritis by bone marrow transplantation. J Rheumatol 1993;20:137–140.
106. Masson C, Brégeon C, Ifrah N, Berton V, Housseau F, Rénier JC. Syndrome d'Evans sous D-pénicillamine au cours d'une polyarthrite rhumatoïde. Inter–t de l'association corticoïdes-danazol. Rev Rhum 1991;58:519–522.
107. Williams DM. Copper deficiency in humans. Semin Hematol 1983;20:118.
108. Frieden E. The copper connection. Semin Hematol 1983;20:114.
109. Larusso NF, Wiesner RH, Ludwig J et al. Prospective trial of penicillamine in primary selerosing cholangitis. Gastroenterology 1988;95:1036–1042.
110. Demelia L, Vallebona E, Perpignano G, Pitzus F. Positivizzazione di sierologia lupica in corso di morbo di Wilson in trattamento con penicillamina. Reumatismo 1991;43: 119–124.
111. Roux H, Bonnefoy-Cudraz M, Antipoff GM. Les complications hépatiques de la D-penicillamine. Rhumatologie 1984;36:233.
112. Gefel D, Harats N, Lijovetsky G, Eliakim M. Cholestatic jaundice associated with D-penicillamine therapy. Scand J Rheumatol 1985;14:303.
113. Kumar A, Bhat A, Gupta DK et al. D-Penicillamine-induced acute hypersensitivity pneumonitis and cholestatic hepatis in a patient with rheumatoid arthritis. Clin Exp Rheumatol 1985;3:337.
114. Menara M, Sturniolo GC. Penicillamine hepatotoxicity in the treatment of Wilson's disease. J Pediatr Gasterentorol Nutr 1992;14:353–354.
115. Capell HA, Marabani M, Madhok R, Torley H, Hunter JA. Degree and extent of response to sulphasalazine or penicillamine therapy for rheumatoid arthritis: results from a routine clinical environment over a two-year period. Q J Med 1990;75:335–344.
116. Lyle WH. Peptic ulceration and D-penicillamine. Lancet 1974;ii:285.
117. Perret D. The metabolism and pharmacology of D-penicillamine in man. J Rheumatol 1981;8(Suppl 7):41.
118. Rook AH, Freundlich B, Jegasothy BV, Perez MI, Barr WG, Jimenez SA, Rietschel RL, Wintroub B, Kahaleh B, Varga J, Heald PW, Steen V, Massa MC, Murphy GF, Perniciaro C, Istfan M, Ballas SK, Edelson RL. Treatment of systemic sclerosis with extracorporeal photochemotherapy (Japan) (Switzerland). Arch Dermatol 1992;128:337–346.
119. Fenton DA, Young ER, Wilkinson JD. Recurrent aphthous ulceration. Br Med J 1983;286:1062.
120. Blasberg B, Dorey JL, Stein HB et al. Lichenoid lesions of the oral mucosa in rheumatoid arthritis patients treated with penicillamine. J Rheumatol 1984;11:348.
121. Rajendran N, Koteeswaran A, Kala M. Penicillamine-induced cheilosis. Indian J Dermatol Venereol Leprol 1985;51:50.
122. Ramboer C, Verhamme M. D-Penicillamine-induced oesophageal ulcers. Acta Clin Belg 1989;44:189–191.
123. Wassef M, Galian A, Pepin B et al. Unusual digestive lesions in a patient with Wilson's disease treated with long-term penicillamine. N Engl J Med 1985;313:49.
124. Greene MW, King RC, Alley RS. Management of an oroantral fistula in a patient with Wilson's disease: case report and review of the literature. Oral Surg Oral Med Oral Pathol 1988;66:293–296.
125. Houghton AD, Nadel S, Stringer MD. Penicillamine-associated total colitis. Hepato-Gastroenterology 1989;36: 198.
126. Stein HB, Schroeder ML, Dillon AM. Penicillamine-induced proteinuria: risk factors. Semin Arthr Rheum 1986;15:282.
127. Hall CL, Jawas D, Harrison PR et al. Natural course of penicillamine nephropathy: a long term study of 33 patients. Br Med J 1988;296:1083.
128. Combe C, Deforges-Lasseur C, Chehab Z, De Précigout, Aparicio M. La lithiase cystinique et son traitement par la D-pénicillamine. Sem Hop 1992:68:746–750.
129. DeSilva RN, Eastmond CJ. Management of proteinuria secondary to penicillamine therapy in rheumatoid arthritis. Clin Rheumatol 1992;11:216–219.
130. Stephens AD. Cystinuria and its treatment: 25 years experience at St Bartholomew's Hospital. J Inherit Metab Dis 1989;12:197–209.
131. Hill GS. Drug-associated glomerulopathies. Toxicol Pathol 1986;14:37.
132. Madhok R, Zoma A, Torley HI et al. The relationship of sulfoxidation status to efficacy and toxicity of penicillamine in the treatment of rheumatoid arthritis. Arthr Rheum 1990;33:574–577.
133. Emery P, Panayi G. Penicillamine nephropathy. Br Med J 1988;296:1538.
134. Speerstra F, Van de Putte LBA, Rasker JJ et al. The relationship between aurothioglucose- and D-penicillamine-induced proteinuria. J Rheumatol 1984;13:363.
135. Yoshida A, Morozumi K, Suganuma T, Aoki J, Sugito K, Koyama K, Oikawa T, Fujinimi T, Matsumoto Y. Clinicopathological study of nephropathy in patients with rheumatoid arthritis. Ryumachi 1991;31:14–21.
136. Verroust PJ. Kinetics of immune deposits in membranous nephropathy. Kidney Int 1989;35:1418–1428.
137. Isenring P, René de Cotret P, Delage C, Kingma I, Lebel M. D-Penicillamine induced reversible minimal change nephropathy in rheumatoid arthritis. J Nephrol 1991;4:245–248.
138. Dische FE. Immunopathology of penicillamine-induced glomerular disease. J Rheumatol 1984;11:584.
139. Druet P, Kleinknecht D. Les néphropathics glomérulaires d'origine toxique. Presse Méd 1989;18:1840–1845.
140. Malaise MG, Davin JC, Mathieu PR, Franchimont P. Elevated antigalactosyl antibody titers reflect renal injury after gold or D-penicillamine in rheumatoid arthritis. Clin. Immunol. Immunopathol 1986;40:356.
141. Rehan A, Johnson K. IgM nephropathy associated with penicillamine. Am J Nephrol 1986;6:71.
142. Ntoso KA, Tomaszewski JL, Jimenez SA, Neilson EG. Penicillamine-induced rapidly progressive glomerulonephritis in patients with progressive systemic sclerosis: successful treatment of two patients and a review of the literature. Am J Kidney Dis 1986;8:159.
143. Williams AJ, Fordham JN, Barnes CH, Goodwin FJ. Progressive proliferative glomerulonephritis in a patient with rheumatoid arthritis treated with D-penicillamine. Ann Rheum Dis 1986;45:82.

144. Suda M, Yoshikawa Y, Suzuki T, Dohi Y, Shibata T. A case report of rheumatoid arthritis which showed acute renal failure, nephrotic syndrome and drug-related lupus-like syndrome caused by D-penicillamine. Nippon Jinzo Gakkai Shi 1990;32:1235–1241.
145. Donnelly S, Levison DA, Doyle DV. Systemic lupus erythematosus-like syndrome with focal proliferative glomerulonephitis during D-penicillamine therapy. Br J Rheumatol 1993;32:251–253.
146. Rejchrt S, Hrncir Z, Pinterova E. Transformation of rheumatoid arthritis into systemic lupus erythematosus during long-term penicillamine and sulfasalazine. Vnitrni Lékarstvi 1991;37:597–603.
147. Almirall J, Alcorta I, Botey A, Revert L. Penicillamine-induced rapidly progressive glomerulonephritis in a patient with rheumatoid arthritis. Am J Nephrol 1993;13:286–288.
148. Gaertner H-V. Drug-associated nephropathy. In: Grundman E ed. Drug-induced Pathology. Current Topics in Pathology, Vol. 69. Berlin: Springer-Verlag, 1980.
149. Ntoso KA, Tomaszewski JE, Jimenez SA, Neilson EG. Penicillamine-induced rapidly progressive glomerulonephritis in patients with progressive systemic sclerosis: successful treatment of two patients and a review of the literature. Am. J. Kidney Dis 1986;8:159–163.
150. Sadjadi SA, Seelig MS, Berger AR, Milstoc M. Rapidly progressive glomerulonephritis in a patient with rheumatoid arthritis during treatment with high dosage D-penicillamine. Ann Rheum Dis 1985;45:82.
151. Devogelaer JP, Pirson Y, Vandenbroucke JM et al. D-Penicillamine induced crescentic glomerulonephritis: report and review of the literature. J Rheumatol 1987;14:1036–1041.
152. Leatherman JW, Davies SF, Hoidal JR. Alveolar hemorrhage syndromes. Medicine 1984;63:343.
153. Macarron P, Garcia Diaz JE, Azofra JA, Martin de Francisco J, Gonzalez E, Fernandez G, Sampedro J. D-Penicillamine therapy associated with rapidly progressive glomerulonephritis. Nephrol Dial Transplant 1992;7:161–164.
154. Scherberig JE, Sniehotta KP, Miehlke K, Schoeppe W. Nierenbeteiligung bei rheumatoider Arthritis. Nieren Hochdrukkr 1987;16:69.
155. Boers M, Croonen AM, Dijkmans BAC et al. Renal findings in rheumatoid arthritis; clinical aspects of 132 autopsies. Ann Rheum Dis 1987;46:658–663.
156. Cantagrel A, Fournie B, Pourrat J, Conte JJ, Fournie A. Hématurie microscopique d'origine rénale au cours de la polyarthrite rhumatoïde. Rev Méd Intern 1991;12:31–36.
157. Boers M, Croonen AM, Dijkmans BAC et al. Renal findings in rheumatoid arthritis: clinical aspects of 132 autopsies. Ann Rheum Dis 1987;46:568.
158. Honkanen E. Toernroth T, Petterson E, Skrifvars B. Membraneous glomerulonephritis in rheumatoid arthritis not related to gold or D-penicillamine therapy: a report of four cases and review of the literature. Clin Nephrol 1987;27:87.
159. Feehally J, Wheeler DC, Mackay EH et al. Recurrent acute renal failure with interstitial nephritis due to D-penicillamine. Renal Failure 1987;10:55.
160. Shannon M, Graef J, Lovejoy FH. Efficacy and toxicity of D-penicillamine in low-level lead poisoning. J Pediatr 1988;112:799–804.
161. Oliver L, Liberman UA, De Vries A. Lupus-like syndrome induced by penicillamine in cystinuria. J Am Med Assoc 1972;220:588.
162. Pachoula-Papasteriades C, Boki K, Varla-Leftherioti M et al. HLA-A, -B and -DR antigens in relation to gold and D-penicillamine toxicity in Greek patients with RA. Dis Markers 1986;4:35–41.
163. Vlachoyiannopoulos PG, Zerva LV, Skopouli FN, Drosos AA, Moutsopoulos HM. D-Penicillamine toxicity in Greek patients with rheumatoid arthritis: anti-Ro(SSA) antibodies and circulating cryoglobulins are predictive factors. J Rheumatol 1991;18:44–49.
164. Enzenauer RJ, West SG, Rubin RL. D-Penicillamine-induced lupus erythematosus. Arthr Rheum 1990;33:1582–1585.
165. Chin GL, Kong NCT, Lee BC, Rose IM. Penicillamine induced lupus-like syndrome in a patient with classical rheumatoid arthritis. J Rheumatol 1991;18:947–948.
166. Tsankov NK, Lazarova AZ, Vasileva SG, Obreshkova EV. Lupus erythematosus-like eruption due to penicillamine in progressive systemic sclerosis. Int J Dermatol 1990; 29:571–574.
167. Bannwarth B, Schaeverbeke T, Dehais J. Low back pain associated with penicillamine. Br Med J 1991;303:525.
168. Newbold PCH. Contact reaction to penicillamine in vaginal secretions. Lancet 1979;i:1344.
169. Dootson G, Sarkany I. D-Penicillamine induced dermopathy in Wilson's disease. Clin Exp Dermatol 1987;12:66–68.
170. Galassi G. Dermal alterations in patients with Wilson's disease treated with D-penicillamine. J Submicrosc Cytol Pathol 1989;1:131–139.
171. Goldstein JB, Scott McNutt N, Hambrick GW, Hsu A. Penicillamine dermatopathy with lymphangiectases. Arch Dermatol 1989;125:92–97.
172. Bardach H, Gebhart W, Niebauer G. 'Lumpybumpy' elastic fibers in the skin and lungs of a patient with penicillamine-induced elastosis perforans serpiginosa. J Cutan Pathol 1979;6:243.
173. Light N, Meyrick Thomas RH, Stephens A et al. Collagen and elastin changes in D-penicillamine-induced pseudoxanthoma elasticum-like skin. Br J Dermatol 1986;114:381.
174. Camus JP, Kroeger AC. D-Pénicillamine et collagène. Ann Biol Clin 1986;44:296.
175. Nimni ME. Penicillamine and collagen metabolism. Scand J Rheumatol Suppl 1979;28:71.
176. Narron GH, Zec N, Neves RI, Manders EK, Sexton FM. Penicillamine-induced pseudoxanthoma elasticum-like skin changes requiring rhytidectomy. Ann Plast Surg 1992; 29:367–370.
177. Bolognia JL, Braverman I. Pseudoxanthoma-elasticum-like skin changes induced by penicillamine. Dermatology 1992;184:12–18.
178. Layton AM, Cunliffe WJ. Electrocautery as a successful treatment for penicillamine-induced elastosis perforans serpiginosa. J Dermatol Treat 1991;2:111–112.
179. Buckley C, Sankey EA, Harris D, Wright S. Case update—progressive skin laxity secondary to penicillamine treatment. Clin Exp Dermatol 1991;16:310–312.
180. Dalziel KL, Burge SM, Frith PA et al. Elastic fibre damage induced by low-dose D-penicillamine. Br J Dermatol 1990;123:305–312.
181. Sahn E, Maize JC, Garen PD, Mullins SC, Silver RM. D-Penicillamine-induced elastosis perforans serpiginosa in a child with juvenile rheumatoid arthritis. J Am Acad Dermatol 1989;20:979–988.
182. Price RG, Prentice RSA. Penicillamine-induced elas-

tosis perforans serpiginosa—tip of the iceberg? Am J Dermatopathol 1986;8:314—330.
183. Verret JL, Avene IM, Smulevici A, Esparbès M. Les pemphigus induits par la peniciliamine á propos de trois cas. J Agrégrés 1983;16:209.
184. Hashimoto K, Shafran KM, Webber PS et al. Anticell surface pemphigus autoantibody stimulates plasminogen activator activity of human epidermal cells; a mechanism for the loss of epidermal cohesion and blister formation. J Exp Med 1983;157:259.
185. Hashimoto K, Singer K, Lazarus GS. Penicillamine induced pemphigus. Arch Dermatol 1984;120:762.
186. Bahmer FA, Bambauer R, Stenger D. Penicillamine-induced pemphigus foliaceus-like dermatosis. Arch Dermatol 1985;121:665.
187. Tholen S. Arzneimittelbedingter Pemphigus. Z Hautkr 1987;61:719.
188. Walton S, Keczkes K, Robinson AE. A case of penicillamine-induced pemphigus, successfully treated by plasma exchange. Clin Exp Dermatol 1987;12:275—276.
189. Kind P, Goerz G, Gleichmann E, Piewig G. Penicillamin induzierter Pemphigus. Hautartz 1987;21:548—552.
190. Buckley C, Barry C, Woods R, Dervan P, O'Loughlin S. Penicillamine induced pemphigus—a report of 2 cases. Indian J Med Sci 1988;August:267—268.
191. Civatte J. Durch Medikamente induzierte Pemphigus-Erkrankungen. Dermatol Mon Schr 1989;175:1—7.
192. Willemsen MJ, De Coninck AL, De Raeve LE, Roseeuw DI. Penicillamine-induced pemphigus erythematosus. Int J Dermatol 1990;29:193—197.
193. Rasmussen HB, Jepsen LV, Brandrup F. Penicillamine-induced bullous pemphigoid with pemphigus like antibodies. J Cutan Pathol 1989;16:154—157.
194. Willemsen M, De Coninck AL, De Raeve LE, Roseeuw DI. Penicillamine-induced pemphigus erythematosus. Int J Dermatol 1990;29:193—197.
195. Verma KK, Pasricha JS. Pemphigus foliaceous induced by penicillamine. Indian J Dermatol Venereol Leprol 1990; 56:234—235.
196. Piette-Brion B, De Bast C, Chamoun E et al. Pemphigus superficial apparu lors du traitement d'une polyarthrite rhumatoïde par D-pénicillamine et piroxicam. Dermatologica 1985;170:297.
197. Kohn SR. Fatal penicillamine-induced pemphigus foliaceus-like dermatosis. Arch Dermatol 1986;122:17.
198. Korman NJ, Eyre RW, Zone J, Stanley JR. Drug-induced pemphigus: autoantibodies directed against the pemphigus antigen complexes are present in penicillamine and captopril-induced pemphigus. J Invest Dermatol 1991; 96:273—276.
199. Bedane C, Bernard P, Dang PM, Amici JM, Catanzano G, Bonnetblanc JM. Étude ultrastructurale des antigènes-cibles du pemphigus foliacé et du pemphigus vulgare. Ann Dermatol Venereol 1991;118:888—890.
200. Ruocco V, De Angelis E, Lombardi ML, Pisani M. In vitro acantholysis by captopril and thiopronine. Dermatologica 1988;176:115—123.
201. Yokel BK, Hood AF, Anhalt GJ. Induction of acantholysis in organ explant culture by penicillamine and captopril. Arch Dermatol 1989;125:1367—1370.
202. Lombardi LM, De Angelis E, Rossano F, Ruocco V. Imbalance between plasminogen activator and its inhibitors in thiol-induced acantholysis. Dermatology 1993;186:118—122.
203. Mutasim DF, Pelc NJ, Anhalt GJ. Drug-induced pemphigus. Dermatol Clin 1993;11:463—471.
204. Brenner S, Livni E, Sandbank M, Halevy S. Macrophage migration inhibition test in patients with drug-induced pemphigus. Isr J Med Sci 1993;29:44—46.
205. Bauer-Vinassac D, Menkes CJ, Muller JY, Escande JP. HLA system and penicillamine induced pemphigus in nine cases of rheumatoid arthritis. Scand J Rheumatol 1992; 21:17—19.
206. Wilkinson SM, Smith AG, Davis MJ, Hollowood K, Dawes PT. Rheumatoid arthritis: an association with pemphigus foliaceous. Acta Dermato-Venereol 1992;72:289—291.
207. Aydemir EH,Isçimen A, Aksoy F. D-Penisilamin'e bagli eritem anuler benzeri pemfigus. Deri Hast Frengi Ars 1988;22:247—250.
208. Wolf R, Brenner S. Arzneimittelbedingter Pemphigus—Uebersicht. Z Hautkrankh 1991;66:289—293.
209. Zillikens D, Zentner A, Burger M, Hartmann A, Burg G. Pemphigus foliaceus durch Penicillamin. Hautarzt 1993;44:167—171.
210. Shuttleworth D, Graham-Brown RA, Hutchinson PE, Joliffe DS. Cicatricial pemphigoid in D-penicillamine treated patients with rheumatoid arthritis: a report of three cases. Clin Exp Dermatol 1985;10:392.
211. Peyri J, Servitje O, Ribera M et al. Cicatricial pemphigoid in a patient with rheumatoid arthritis treated with D-penicillamine. J Am Acad Dermatol 1986;14:681.
212. Marti-Huguet T, Quintana M, Cabiro I. Cicatricial pemphigoid associated with D-penicillamine treatment. Arch Ophthalmol 1989;107:1115.
213. Kitamura K, Aihara M, Osawa J et al. Sulfhydryl drug-induced eruption: a clinical and histological study. J Dermatol 1990;17:44—51.
214. Liddle BJ. Development of morphea in rheumatoid arthritis treated with penicillamine. Ann Rheum Dis 1989; 48:963—964.
215. Schachter RK. Localized seleroderma. Curr Opin Rheumatol 1990;2:947—955.
216. Ilchyshyn A, Vickers CFH. Yellow nail syndrome associated with penicillamine therapy. Acta Derm Venereol 1983;63:554.
217. Dubost JJ, Fraysse P, Ristori JM, Rampon S. Syndrome des ongles jaunes avec dilatation des bronches après traitement d'une polyarthrite rhumatoïde par la D-pénicillamine. Semin Hôp Paris 1988;64:1548—1551.
218. Ichikawa Y, Shimizu H, Arimori S. 'Yellow nail syndrome' and rheumatoid arthritis. Tokai J. Exp Clin Med 1991;16:203—209.
219. Bjelierup M. Nail changes induced by penicillamine. Acta Dermatol Venereol 1989;69:339—341.
220. Jimenez-Balderas FJ, Rangel J, Mintz G. Penicillamine-induced myositis: correlation between urinary zinc excretion and serum creatine. J Rheumatol 1991;18:945—947.
221. Knudsen L, Weismann K. Taste dysfunction and changes in zinc and copper metabolism during penicillamine therapy for generalized scleroderma. Acta Med Scand 1978;204:75.
222. Tausch G, Bröll H, Eberl R. D-Penicillamin (Artamin) als Basistherapie bei chronischer Polyarthritis. Wein Klin Wschr 1973;85:59.
223. Fuentes JAG, Gallega MCV, Remis JEF. Ageusia como manifestacti—n secundaria del tratiamento con D-penicillamina. Rev Clin Esp 1984;172:149.

224. Schiffman SS. Taste and smell in disease. N Engl J Med 1983;308:1275.
225. Prieur AM, Piussan C, Manigne P et al. Arthrite chronique juvénile. Arch Fr Pédiatr 1985;42:91.
226. Klepach GL, Wray SH. Bilateral serous retinal detachment with thrombocytopenia during penicillamine therapy. Ann Ophthalmol 1981;February:201.
227. Kahl LE, Medsger TA, Klein I. Massive breast enlargement in a patient receiving D-penicillamine for systemic sclerosis. J Rheumatol 1985;12:990.
228. Craig HR. Penicillamine induced mammary hyperplasia: report of a case and review of the literature. J Rheumatol 1988;15:1294–1297.
229. Rose BI, LeMaire WJ, Jeffers LJ. Macromastia in a woman treated with penicillamine and oral contraceptives. J Reprod Med 1990;35:43–45.
230. Spaeth M, Berkl M, Miehle W. Mammahyperplasie und D-penicillamin. Aktuel Rheumatol 1991;16:214–216.
231. Caballeria J, Caballeria L, Cabre J, Bruguera M, Rodes J. Mammary hyperplasia secondary to treatment with D-penicillamine in a patient with Wilson's disease. Gastroenterol Hepatol 1993;16:607–609.
232. Sallière D, Clerc C, Bisson M, Massias P. Gynécomastie transitoire an course d'un traitement par la D-penicillamine. Presse Méd 1984;13:2265.
233. Kolsi R, Bahloul Z, Hachicha J, Gouiaa R, Jarraya A. Dermatopolymyosite induite par la D-pénicillamine au cours de la polyarthrite rhumatoide. Rev Rhum Mal Osteo-Articulaires 1992;59:341–344.
234. Takahashi D, Ogita T, Okudaira H et al. D-Penicillamine-induced polymyositis in patients with rheumatoid arthritis. Arthr Rheum 1986;29:560.
235. Matsumura T, Yuhara T, Yamane K et al. D-Penicillamine-induced polymyositis occurring in patients with rheumatoid arthritis: a report of two cases and demonstration of a positive lymphocyte stimulation test to D-penicillamine. Henry Ford Hosp Med J 1986;34:123.
236. Masson CJ, Ménard HA, Audran M et al. Polymyosite induite par la D-pénicillamine lors d'arthrite rhumatoïde: A propos de deux cas avec des anticorps antinucléaire. Un Méd Can 1986;115:855.
237. Ostensen M, Husby G, Aarli J. Polymyositis with acute myolysis in a patient with rheumatoid arthritis treated with penicillamine and ampicillin. Arthr Rheum 1980;23:375.
238. Car J, Lorette G, Jacob C. Dermatomyosite induite par la D-pénicillamine. Sem Hôp 1987;63:399.
239. Leden I, Libelius R. Penicillamine-induced polymyositis. Scand J Rheumatol 1985;14:90.
240. Carroll GJ, Will RK, Peter JB et al. Penicillamine induced polymyositis and dermatomyositis. J Rheumatol 1987;14:995–1001.
241. Christensen PD, Sorensen KE. Penicillamine induced polymyositis with complete heart block. Eur Heart J 1989;10:1041–1044.
242. Derman H, Theron HP. A propos de trois observations de syndrome myasthénique induit par la D-pénicillamine. Bull Soc Ophthalmol Fr 1987;11:1235–1243.
243. Taneja V, Mehra N, Singh YN et al. HLA-D region genes and susceptibility to D-penicillamine-induced myositis. Arthr Rheum 1990;33:1445–1446.
244. Santos JC, Velasco JA. Polymyositis due to D-penicillamine in a patient with systemic sclerosis. Clin Exp Dermatol 1991;16:76.
245. Fukuda S, Murata Y, Takahashi T, Hatada Y, Tsushima Y, Takemori H, Yoshida Y, Okushima T. D-Penicillamine-induced polymyositis in a patient with rheumatoid arthritis. Saishin-Igaku 1990;45:1854–1859.
246. Larbre JP, Perret P, Collet P, Llorca G. Antinuclear antibodies during pyrithioxine treatment. Br J Rheumatol 1990;29:496–497.
247. Christensen PD, Sorensen KE. Penicillamine-induced polymyositis with complete heart block. Eur Heart J 1989;19:1041–1044.
248. Sturrock RD, Brooks PM. Penicillamine and creaking joints. Br Med J 1974;3:575.
249. Stein HB, Patterson CA, Offer RC, Atkins CJ, Teufel A, Robinson HS. Adverse effects of *d*-penicillamine in rheumatoid arthritis. Ann Intern Med 1980;92:24.
250. Butler D, Tiliakos NA. Penicillamine-induced exacerbation of rheumatoid arthritis. South Med J 1986;79:778.
251. Rosada M, Fiocco U, De Silverstro G, Doria A, Cozzi L, Favaretto M, Todesco S. Effect of D-penicillamine on the T cell phenotype in scleroderma. Comparison between treated and untreated patients. Clin Exp Rheumatol 1993;11:143–148.
252. Panayi GS, McKenzie Mills M. Second-line drug treatment in rheumatoid arthritis associated with depressed autologous mixed lymphocyte reaction. Rheumatol Int 1986;6:25.
253. Miyachi Y, Yoshioka A, Imamura S, Niwa Y. Decreased hydroxyl radical generation from polymorphonuclear leucocytes in the presence of D-penicillamine and thiopronine. J Clin Lab Immunol 1987;22:81.
254. Sim E, Dodds AW, Goldin A. Inhibition of the covalent binding reaction of complement component C4 by penicillamine, an anti-rheumatic agent. Biochem J 1989;259:415–419.
255. Sim E. Drug-induced immune-complex disease. Complement Inflammation 1989;6:119–126.
256. Enzenauer RJ, West SG, Rubin RL. D-Penicillamine-induced lupus erythematosus. Arthr Rheum 1990;33:1582–1585.
257. Chalmers A, Thompson D, Stein HE et al. Systemic lupus erythematosus during penicillamine therapy for rheumatoid arthritis. Ann Intern Med 1982;97:659–663.
258. Stanworth DR. D-Penicillamine induced immunodeficiency. In: Dawkins RL, Christiansen FT, Zilko PJ, eds. Immunogenetics in Rheumatology: Musculoskeletal Disease and Penicillamine. Amsterdam: Excerpta Medica, 1982;358.
259. Negishi M, Kobayashi K, Ide H et al. A case report of selective IgA deficiency in rheumatoid arthritis treated with D-penicillamine. J Showa Med Assoc 1990;50:205–209.
260. Ibel H, Feist D, Enderes W, Belohradsky BH. D-Penicillamin-induzierter IgA-Mangel bei der Therapie der Wilsonschen Erkrankung. Klin Pädiatr 1990;202:427–429.
261. May V, Aristoff H, Lecoq G. Syndrome of Gougerot-Sjögren induced by D-penicillamine. Rev Rhum 1977;44:497.
262. Pruzanski W, ed. Proceedings, International Symposium on Penicillamine, Miami, 1980. J Rheumatol 1981; 8(Suppl 7):181.
263. Dubois RS, Rodgerson DO, Hambridge KM. Treatment of Wilson's disease with triethylene tetramine hydrochloride (trientine). J Pediatr Gastroenterol Nutr 1990; 10:77–81.
264. Haberhauer G, Bröll H. Drug-induced anticentromere antibody? Z Rheumatol 1989;48:99–100.
265. Haberhauer G. D-Penicillamine (DPA)-induced anticentromere antibody (ACA). Int J Rheum Connective Tissue Dis 1989;7:332–334.

266. Storch W. Antikörper gegen D-Penicillamin bei primär biliärer Zirrhose. Immun Infekt 1990;18:22–23.
267. Yarze JC, Martin P, Munos SJ. Wilson's disease: current status. Am J Med 1992;292:643–654.
268. Jones E, Sobkowski WW, Murray SJ, Walsh NMG. Concurrent pemphigus and myasthenia gravis as manifestations of penicillamine toxicity. J Am Acad Dermatol 1993;28:655–656.
269. Bauer P, Bollaert PE, Dopff C et al. Syndrome de détresse respiratoire aiguë d'évolution fatale au cours d'un traitement par D-pénicillamine. Presse Méd 1988;17:961–962.
270. Savill JS, Chia Y, Pusey CD. Minimal change nephropathy and pemphigus vulgaris associated with penicillamine treatment or rheumatoid arthritis. Clin Nephrol 1988; 29:267–270.
271. Gilman PA, Holtzman NA. Acute lymphoblastic leukemia in a patient receiving penicillamine for Wilson's disease. J Am Med Assoc 1982;248:467.
272. Clausen JE, Arndal JCK, Gram L, Kudahl SB, Fog P. Chronic lymphocytic leukemia after treatment with penicillamine. Lancet 1978;ii:152.
273. Sheldon P, Wood JK. Remission of arthritis and radiological improvement after combination therapy for non-Hodgkin's lymphoma in a patient with rheumatoid arthritis undergoing treatment with *d*-penicillamine. Ann Rheum Dis 1985;44:556.
274. McDuffie FC, ed. Neoplasm in rheumatoid arthritis: update on clinical and epidemiologic data. Am J Med 1985;78(Suppl 1A):1.
275. Speit G, Haupter S. Cytogenetic effects of penicillamine. Mutat Res 1987;190:197.
276. Schulze E, Herrmann K, Haustein U-F et al. Einfluss von Penicillin und D-Penicillamin auf die Betagalactosidaseaktivität bei Patienten met progressiver Sklerodermie. Dermatol Monatsschr 1988;174:661–666.
277. Whithouse DB, Lovegrove JU, Hopkinson DA. Variation in alpha-1-antitrypsin phenotypes associated with penicillamine therapy. Clin Chim Acta 1989;179:109–116.
278. Emery P, Panayi G. Penicillamine nephropathy. Br Med J 1988;296:1538.
279. Emery P, Panayi GS, Huston G et al. D-Penicillamine induced toxicity in rheumatoid arthritis: the role of sulfoxidation status and HLA-DR3. J Rheumatol 1984;11:626–632.
280. Seideman P, Ayesh R. Reduced sulphoxidation capacity in D-penicillamine induced myasthenia gravis. Clin Rheumatol 1994;13;435–437.
281. Skopouli FN, Andonopoulos AP, Moursopoulos HM. Clinical implications of the presence of anti-Ro (SSA) antibodies in patients with rheumatoid arthritis. J Autoimmun 1988;3:381–388.
282. Dawkins RL, Christiansen FT, Zilko PJ, eds. Immunogenetics in Rheumatology: Musculoskeletal Disease and D-Peniciliamine. Amsterdam: Excerpta Medica, 1982 358.
283. Speerstra F, Reekers T, Van de Putte LBA, Vandenbroucke JP. HLA associations in aurothioglucose- and D-penicillamine-induced haematotoxic reactions in rheumatoid arthritis. Tissue Antigens 1985;26:35.
284. Welsh KI, Black CM. The major histocompatibility system and its relevance to rheumatological disorders. In: Carson DW, Moll JMH, eds. Recent Advances in Rheumatology. Edinburgh: Churchill Livingstone, 1983;147.
285. Scherak O, Smolen JS, Mayer WR et al. HLA antigens and toxicity to gold and penicillamine in rheumatoid arthritis. J Rheumatol 1984;11:610.
286. Dequeker J, Van Wanghe P, Verdickt W. A systematic survey of HLA-A, B, C, and D antigens and drug toxicity in rheumatoid arthritis. J Rheumatol 1984;11:282.
287. Ford PM. HLA antigens and drug toxicity in rheumatoid arthritis. J Rheumatol 1984;11:259.
288. Bardin T, Dryll A, Ryckewaert A. Système HLA et accidents du traitement de la polyarthrite rhumatoïde par la D-peniciliamine Rev Rhum 1986;53:27.
289. Perrier P, Raffoux C, Thomas P et al. HLA antigens and toxic reactions to sodium aurothiopropanolsulphonate and D-penicillamine in patients with rheumatoid arthritis. Ann Rheum Dis 1985;44:621.
290. Zacher J, Spath S, Wessinghage D, Waertel G. Basistherapie der chronisch-entzündlichem Gelenkerkrankungen met D-Penicillamin und Wundheilungsstörungen bei rheumaorthopädischen Eingriffen. Z Rheumatol 1988;47(Suppl 1):41–43.
291. Burry HC. Penicillamine and wound healing—a potential hazard? Postgrad Med J 1974;50(Suppl):75.
292. Greene MW, King RC, Alley RS. Management of an oroantral fistula in a patient with Wilson's disease: case report and review of the literature. Oral Surg Oral Med Oral Pathol 1988;66:293–296.
293. Miehic W. Aktuelles zu D-Peniciliamin and Schwangerschaft. Z Rheumatol 1988;47(Suppl 1):20–23.
294. Rosa FW. Teratogen update: penicillamine. Teratology 1986;33:127.
295. Lyle WH, Pearcey DF, Hui M. Inhibition of penicillamine-induced cupruresis by oral iron. Proc R Soc Med 1977;70(Suppl 3):48–49.
296. Osman MA, Patel RB, Schuna A et al. Reduction in oral penicillamine absorption by food, antacids and ferrous sulphate. Clin Pharm Ther 1983;33:465–470.
297. Harkness JA, Blaki DR. Penicillamine nephropathy and iron. Lancet 1982l;ii:1368–1369.
298. Muijsers AO, Van de Stadt FJ, Henrichs AMA et al. D-Penicillamine in patients with rheumatoid arthritis. Serum levels, pharmacokinetic aspects and correlation with clinical course and side effects. Arthr Rheum 1984;27:1362–1369.
299. Ifan A, Welling PG. Pharmacokinetics of oral 500 mg penicillamine: effect of antacids on absorption. Biopharm Drug Disposit 1986;7:401.
300. Yu T-F, Roboz HJ, Johnson S, Kaung C. Studies on the metabolism of D-penicillamine and its interaction with probenecid in cystinuria and rheumatoid arthritis. J Rheumatol 1984;11:467.
301. Jaffe IA. Combination therapy of rheumatoid arthritis —rationale and overview. J Rheumatol 1990;17(Suppl 25):24–27.
302. Bunch TW, O'Duffy JD, Tompkins RB, O'Fallon WM. Controlled trial of hydroxychloroquine and D-penicillamine singly and in combination in the treatment of rheumatoid arthritis. Arthr Rheum 27, 267–276.
303. Gibson T, Emery P, Armstrong RD et al. Combined D-penicillamine and chloroquine treatment of rheumatoid arthritis—a comparative study. Br J Rheumatol 1987; 26:279–284.
304. Dijkmans BA, De Vries E, De Vreede TM. Synergistic and additive effects of disease modifying anti-rheumatic drugs combined with chloroquine on the mitogen-driven stimulation of mononuclear cells. Clin Exp Rheumatol 1990;8:455–459

305. Jaffe IA. Adverse effects profile of sulfhydrylcompounds in man. Am J Med 1986;80:471.
306. Florentine MJ, Sanfilippo DJ. Elemental mercury poisoning. Clin Pharm 1991;10:213—221.
307. Takahashi C, Murasawi A, Nakazono K, Yoshida K, Sekiguchi H, Kikuchi M. An open clinical study of bucillamine in uncontrollable rheumatoid arthritis. Int J Immunother 1991;7:95—98.
308. Negishi M, Kaga S, Kasama T, Hashimoto M, Fukushima T, Yamagata N, Tabata M, Kobayashi K, Ide H, Takahashi T. Lung injury associated with bucillamine therapy. Ryumachi 1992;32:135—139.
309. Fujiyama J, Tokimura Y, Ijichi S, Arimura K. Bucillamine may induce myasthenia gravis. Jpn J Med 1991;30:101.
310. Kawano M, Nomura H, Iwainaka Y, Nakashima A, Koni I, Tofuku Y, Takeda R. Bucillamine-associated membranous nephropathy in a patient with rheumatoid arthritis. Jpn J Nephrol 1990;817—821.
311. Yoshida A, Morozumi K, Suganuma T, Sugito K, Ikeda M, Oikawa T, Fujinami T, Takeda A, Koyama K. Clinicopathological findings of bucillamine-induced nephrotic syndrome in patients with rheumatoid arthritis. Am J Nephrol 1991;11:284—288.
312. Baba N, Nomura T, Sakemi T, Uchida M, Watanabe T. Membranous glomerulonephritis probably related to bucillamine therapy in two patients wtih rheumatoid arthritis. Nippon Jinzo Gakkai Shi 1991;33:629—634.
313. Amasaki Y, Sagawa A, Atsumi T, Jodo S, Nakabayashi T, Watanabe I, Mukai M, Fujisaku A, Nakagawa S, Kobayashi H. A case of rheumatoid arthritis developing pemphigus-like skin lesion during treatment with bucillamine. Ryumachi 1991;31:528—534.
314. Takashima T, Tani M. Antirheumatics-induced pemphigus foliaceus-like lesions. Hihu 1990;32:205—208.
315. Crouzet J, Beraneck L. Pyrithioxine et polyarthrite rhumatoide. Rev Rhum 1986;53:45.
316. Netter P, Trechot P, Bannwarth B et al. Effects secondaires de la D-pénicillamine et du pyritinol. Thérapie 1985;40:475.
317. Faguer de Moustier B, Burgard M, Boitard C et al. Syndrome hypoglycémique auto-immune induit par le pyritinol. Diabète Métabol 1988;14:423—429.
318. Macedo G, Sarmento JA, Allegro S. Acute hepatitis due to pyritinol. Gastroenterol Clin Biol 1992;16:186—187.
319. Ehrhart A, Chicault P, Fauquert P, Le Goff P. Effets secondaires dus au traitement par la tiopronine de 74 polyarthrites rhumatoïdes. Rev Rhum 1991;58:193—197.
320. Sany J, Combe B, Verdie-Petibon D et al. Etude de la tolérance á long terme de la thiopronine dans le traitement de la polyarthrite rhumatoïde. Rev Rhum 1990;57:105—111.
321. Sigaud M, Maugars Y, Maisonneuve H, Prost A. Tiopronine dans 69 cas de polyarthrite rhumatoïde traités antérieurement par la D-pénicillamine. Rev Rhum 1988;55:467—471.
322. Amor B, Mery C, De Gery A. L'acadione, un nouveau traitement de fond de la polyarthrite rhumatoïde. Rev Rhum 1988;55:462—466.
323. Pak CYC, Fuller C, Sakhace K et al. Management of cystine nephrolithiasis with alpha-mercaptopropionylglycine J Urol 1986;136:1003—1008.
324. Komura A, Tamaki. Clinical analysis of drug allergy due to tiopronin. Skin Res 1988;30(Suppl 4):197—199.
325. Faguer de Moustier B, Burgard M, Boitard C et al. Syndrome hypoglycémique auto-immune induit par le pyritinol. Diabète Métabol 1988;14:423—429.
326. Gregoir C, Hilliquin P, Acar F, Lessana-Leibowitch M, Renoux M, Menkès CJ. Mastite aiguë au cours d'une polyarthrite rhumatoïde avec syndrome de Gougerot-Sjögren traitée par tiopronine (acadione). Rev. Rhum 1991;58:203—206.
327. Taillan B, Nectoux F, Vinti H, Fuzibet JG, Verdier JM, Dujardin P, Chichmanian RM, Viteta A. Aplasie médullaire au cours d'une polyarthrite rhumatoïde traitée par tiopronine. Rev Rhum 1990;57:443—444.
328. Corda C, Tavernier C, Oriol P et al. Thiopronin-induced agranulocytosis. Thérapie 1990;45:161—166.
329. Mori T, Ohta M, Nakagawa Y, Hayashi K, Sobajima J, Okuda M, Mochi T, Shimamoto K, Kagawa K, Okanoue T, Kashima K. A case report of non-alcoholic steatohepatitis associated with tiopronin-induced liver injury. Acta Hepatol Jpn 1990;31:449—453.
330. Matsueda K, Matsuoka Y, Mizuno M et al. A case of drug-induced toxic epidermal necrolysis complicated with severe liver injury. Acta Hepatol Jpn 1988;29:949—955.
331. Lindell Å, Denneberg T, Eneström S, Fich C, Skogh T. Membranous glomerulonephritis induced by 2-mercaptopropionylglycine (2MPG). Clin Nephrol 1990;34:108—115.
332. Shibasaki T, Murai S, Kodama K, Nakano H, Ishimoto F, Sakai O. A case of nephrotic syndrome due to alpha-mercaptopropionyl glycine in a patient with familial cystinuria. Jpn J Nephrol 1990;32:933—937.
333. Azar R, Mercier D, Codaccioni MX. Néphropathie a lésions glomérulaires minimes secondaire a un traitement par la triopronine. Semin Hôp 1992;68:209—210.
334. Ohno S, Fujita M, Miyachi Y. Tiopronine-induced pemphigus-like lesions. 532—537.
335. Meunier L, Combes B, Marck V, Barneon G, Sany J, Meynadier J. Pemphigus induit par l'alpha-mercaptopropionylglycine (Acadione). Ann Dermatol Vénéréol 1990; 117:959—961.
336. Meunier J, Krause E, Guillot B et al. Pemphigus induit par l'alpha-mercaptopropionylglycine. Presse Méd 1988; 17:647.
337. Kawabe Y, Mizuno N, Yoshikawa K, Matsumoto Y. Lichenoid eruption due to mercaptopropionylglycine. J Dermatol 1988;15:434—439.
338. Kurumaji Y, Miyazaki K. Tiopronin-induced lichenoid eruption in a patient with liver disease and positive patch test reaction to drugs with sulfhydryl group. J Dermatol 1990;17:176—181.
339. Menkes CJ, Job-Deslander C, Bauer-Vinassac D et al. Myasthénie induite par la tiopronine au course du traitement de la polyarthrite rhumatoïde. Presse Méd 1988;17:1156—1157.
340. Arfi S, Caplanne D, Jean-Baptiste G, Habault Ch, Panelatti G, Vernant JC. Myasthénie induite par la tiopronine au cours du traitement d'une polyarthrite rhumatoïde. Bull SMNFI 1991;12:489.
341. Koeger AC, Rozenberg S, Chaibi P, Camus JP, Bourgeois P. Polymyosite induite par la tiopronine, confirmée par l'histologie. Rev Rhum Mal Osteo-Articulaires 1992;59:78—79.
342. Ymaguchi R, Oryu F, Hidano A. A case of bullous pemphigoid induced by tiobutarit (D-penicillamine analogue). J. Dermatol 1989;16:308—311.
343. Fosburg MT, Nathan DG. Treatment of Cooley's anemia. Blood 1990;76:435—444.
344. Giardina PJ, Grady RW, Ehlers KH, Burstein S, Graziano JH, Markenson AL, Hilgartner MW. Current therapy of Cooley's anemia. Ann NY Acad Sci 1990;612:275—285.

345. Gabutti V. Current therapy for thalassemia in Italy. Ann NY Acad Sci 1990;612:268—274.
346. Athanasion A, Shepp MA, Necheles TF. Anaphylactic reaction to deferoxamine. Lancet 1977;ii:616.
347. Miller KB, Rosenwasser LJ, Besette JM, et al. Rapid desensitisation for desferrioxamine anaphylactic reaction. Lancet 1981;i:1059.
348. McCarthy JT, Milliner DS, Johnson WJ. Clinical experience with desferrioxamine in dialysis patients with aluminium toxicity. Q J Med New Ser 1990;74:257—276.
349. Jacobs P, Wood L, Bird AR, Ultmann JE. Pseudo deep-vein thrombosis following desferrioxamine infusion: a previously unreported adverse reaction? Lancet 1990;336:815.
350. Harndy NAT, Andrew SM, Shortland JR et al. Fatal cardiac zygomycosis in a renal transplant patient treated with desferrioxamine. Nephrol Dial Transplant 1989;4:911—913.
351. Daly AL, Velasquez LA, Bradley SF, Kaufmann CA. Mucormycosis: association with deferoxamine therapy. Am J Med 1989;87:468—471.
352. Arizono K, Fukui H, Miura H, Hayano K, Otsuka Y, Tajiri M. A case report of rhinocerebral mucormycosis in hemodialysis patient receiving deferoxamine. Jpn J Nephrol 1989;31:99—103.
353. Voest EE, Neijt JP, Keunen JEF, Dekker AW, Van Asbeck BS, Nortier JWR, Ros FE, Marx JJM. Phase I study using desferrioxamine and iron sorbitol citrate in an attempt to modulate the iron status of tumor cells to enhance doxorubicin activitiy. Cancer Chemother Pharmacol 1993;31:357—362.
354. Walshe JM, Yealland M. Chelation treatment of neurological Wilson's disease. Q J Med 1993;86:197—204.
355. Freedman MH, Grisaru D, Olivieri N, MacLusky I, Thorner PS. Pulmonary syndrome in patients with thalassemia major receiving intravenous deferoxamine infusions. Am J Dis Child 1990;144:565—569.
356. Castriota Scanderberg A, Izzi GC, Butturini A, Benaglia G. Pulmonary syndrome and intravenous high-dose desferrioxamine. Lancet 1990;336:1511.
357. Tenenbein M, Kowalski S, Sienko A, Bowden DH, Adamson IYR. Pulmonary toxic effects of continuous desferrioxamine administration in acute iron poisoning. Lancet 1992;339:699—701.
358. Weitman SD, Buchanan GR, Kamen BA. Pulmonary toxicity of deferoxamine in children with advanced cancer. J Natl Cancer Inst 1991;83:1834—1835.
359. Helson L, Helson C, Braverman S, Deb G, Donfrancesco A. Desferrioxamine in acute iron poisoning. Lancet 1992;339:1602—1603.
360. Anderson KJ, Rivers RPA. Desferrioxamine in acute iron poisoning. Lancet 1992;339:1602.
361. Cianciulli P. Pulmonary embolism and intravenous high-dose desferrioxamine. Haematologica 1992;77:368—369.
362. Kouides PA, Slapak CA, Rosenwasser LJ, Miller KB. *Pneumocystis carinii* pneumonia as a complication of desferrioxamine therapy. Br J Haematol 1988;70:383—384.
363. Arizono K, Fukui H, Miura H et al. A case report of rhinocerebral mucormycosis in hemodialysis patient receiving deferoxamine. Jpn J Nephrol 1989;31:99—103.
364. Arden GB, Wonke B, Kennedy C, Huehns ER. Ocular changes in patients undergoing long term desferrioxamine treatment. Br J Ophthalmol 1984;68:873.
365. Yaqoob M, Ahmad R, Roberts N, Helliwell T. Low-dose desferrioxamine test for the diagnosis of aluminium-related bone disease in patients on regular haemodialysis. Nephrol Dial Transpl 1991;6:484—486.
366. Rivera CF, Fontan MP, Cabanas M, Moncalian J, Arrojo F, Valdes F. Toxicidad ocular irreversible tras administratión de una dosis aislada de desferroxiamina en hemodiálisis. Nefrologia 1990;10:431—434.
367. Ravelli M, Scaroni P, Mombelloni S, Movilli E, Feller P, Apostoli P, De Maria G, Valotti C, Sciuto G, Maiorca R. Acute visual disorders in patients on regular dialysis given desferrioxamine as a test. Nephrol Dial Transplant 1990; 5:945—949.
368 Barratt PS, Toogood RG. Hearing loss attributed to desferrioxamine in patients with beta-thalassaemia major. Med J Austr 1987;147:177—179.
369. Gelmi C, Borgna-Pignatti C, Franchin S et al. Electroretinographic and visual-evoked potential abnormalities in patients with beta-thalassemia major. Ophthalmologica 1988;196:29—34.
370. Hamed LM, Winward KE, Glaser JS, Schatz NJ. Optic neuropathy in uremia. Am J Ophthalmol 1989;108:30—35.
371. Rinaldi M, Della Corte M, Ruocco V, D'Onofrio C, Zanotta G, Romano A. Ocular involvement correlated with age in patients affected by major and intermedia β-thalassemia treated or not with desferrioxamine. Metab Pediatr Syst Ophthalmol 1993;16:23—25.
372. Cases A, Kelly J, Sabater F, Torras A, Grino MC, Lopez-Pedret J, Revert L. Ocular and auditory toxicity in hemodialyzed patients receiving desferrioxamine. Nephron 1990;56:19—23.
373. Bournerais F, Monnier N, Dufier JL, Réveillaud FJ. Toxicité oculaire sévère de la desferrioxamine chez l'hémodialysé. Néphrologie 1987;8:27.
374. Bene C, Manzler A, Bene D, Kranias G. Irreversible ocular toxicity from single 'challenge' dose of deferoxamine. Clin Nephrol 1989;31:45—48.
375. Cases A, Kelly J, Sabater J et al. Acute visual and auditory neurotoxicity in patients with end-stage renal disease receiving desferrioxamine. Clin Nephrol 1988;29:176—178.
376. Rahi AH, Hungerford JL, Ahmed AI. Ocular toxicity of desferrioxamine: light microscopic, histochemical and ultrastructural findings. Br J Ophthalmol 1986;70:373.
377. Lakhanpal V, Schocket SS, Jiji R. Deferoxamine (Desferal)-induced toxic retinal pigmentary degeneration and presumed optic neuropathy. Ophthalmology 1984; 91:443.
378. Schindléry C, Macarol V. Serial studies of auditory neurotoxicity in patients receiving deferoxamine therapy. Am J Med 1989;86:365.
379. Borgna-Pignatti C, De Stefano P, Broglia AM. Visual loss in a patient on high dose subcutaneous desferroxamine. Lancet 1984;i:681.
380. Marciani MG, Ciaciulli P, Stefani N, Stefanini F, Peroni L, Sabbadini M, Maschio M, Trua G, Paga G. Toxic effects of high-dose deferoxamine treatment in patients with iron overload: an electrophysiological study of cerebral and visual function. Haematologica 1991;76:131—134.
381. De Vergillis S, Congia M, Turco MP et al. Depletion of trace elements and acute ocular toxicity induced by desferrioxamine in patients with thalassaemia. Arch Dis Child 1988;63:250—255.
382. Sacco M, Meleleo D, Tricario N, Greco Miani A, Serra E, Parlatore L. Valutazione dell' ototossicita della desferrioxamina in pazienti talasemici. Minerva Pediatr 1994; 46:225—230
383. Ogborn MR, Dorcas VC, Crocker JF. Deferoxamine

and aluminum clearance in pediatric hemodialysis patients. Pediatr Nephrol 1991;5:62–64.
384. Sherrard DJ, Walker JV, Boykin JL. Precipitation of dialysis dementia by deferoxamine treatment of aluminum-related bone disease. Am J Kidney Dis 1988;12:126–130.
385. McCauley J, Sorkin MI. Exacerbation of aluminium encephalopathy after treatment with desferrioxamine. Nephrol Dial Transplant 1989;4:110–114.
386. Lillevang ST, Bangsgaard Pedersen F. Exacerbation of aluminium encephalopathy after treatment with desferrioxamine. Nephrol Dial Transplant 1989;4:676.
387. Weinberg K. Novel uses of deferoxamine. Am J Pediatr Hematol Oncol 1990;12:9–13.
388. Brancaccio D, Avanzini G, Padovese P, Gallieni M, Franceschetti S, Panzica F, Anelli A, Colantonio G, Martinelli D, Bugiani O. Desferrioxamine infusion can modify EEG tracing in haemodialysed patients. Nephrol Dial Transpl 1991;16:264–268.
389. Polson RJ, Jawed A, Bomford A et al. Treatment of rheumatoid arthritis with desferrioxamine: relation between stores of iron before treatment and side effects. Br Med J 1985;291:448.
390. Blake DR, Winyard P, Lunec J et al. Cerebral and ocular toxicity induced by desferrioxamine. Q J Med New Ser 1985;86:345.
391. Daly AL, Velasquez LA, Bradley SF, Kaufmann CA. Mucormycosis: association with deferoxamine therapy. Am J Med 1989;87:468–471.
392. Arizono K, Fukui H, Nflura H et al. A case report of rhinocerebral mucormycosis in hemodialysis patient receiving deferoxamine. Jpn J Nephrol 1989;31:99–103.
393. Hamdy NAT, Andrew SM, Shortland JR et al. Fatal cardiac zygomycosis in a renal transplant patient treated with desferrioxamine. Nephrol Dial Transplant 1978;4:911–913.
394. Caballero LG. Toxicidad auditiva, visual y neurologica de la desferroxamina. Rev Med Chil 1989;117:557–561.
395. Bloomfield SE, Markenson AL, Miller DR, Peterson CM. Lens opacities in thalassemia. J Pediatr Ophthalmol Strabismus 1978;15:154.
396. Klein GL, Snodgrass WR, Griffin MP et al. Hypocalcemia complicating deferoxamine therapy in an infant with parenteral nutrition-associated aluminum overload: evidence for a role of alumimum in the bone disease of infants. J Pediatr Gastroenterol 1985;9:400–403.
397. Walker JA, Sherman RA. Thrombocytopenia associated with intravenous desferrioxamine. Am J Kidney Dis 1985;6:254–256.
398. Sofroniadou K, Drossou M, Foundoulaki L et al. Acute bone marrow aplasia associated with intravenous administration of deferoxamine (desferrioxamine). Drug Safety 1990;5:152–154.
399. Nocka KH, Pelus LM. Cell cycle specific effects of deferoxamine on human and murine hematopoietic progenitor cells. Cancer Res 1988;48:3571.
400. Praga M, Andrés A, De la Serna J et al. Improvement of anaemia with desferrioxamine in haemodialysis patients. Nephrol Dial Transplant 1987;2:243–247.
401. Swartz R, Dombrouski J, Burnatowska-Hledin M, Mayor G. Microcytic anemia in dialysis patients: reversible marker of aluminum toxicity. Am J Kidney Dis 1987;9:217–223.
402. Felipe C, Rivera M, Orofino L et al. Effect of desferrioxamine on anaemia of haemodialysis patients. Nephrol Dial Transplant 1988;3:105–106.
403. Cuvelier R, Deceuninck P. Desferrioxamine improves anaemia in haemodialysis patients without aluminium or iron overload. Nephrol Dial Transplant 1988;3:104.
404. McCarthy JT, Milliner DS, Johnson WJ. Clinical experience with desferrioxamine in dialysis patients with aluminium toxicity. Q J Med New Ser 1990;74:257–276.
405. Kruck TPA, Fisher EA, McLachlan DRC. A predictor for side effects in patients with Alzheimer's disease treated with deferoxamine mesylate. Clin Pharm Ther 1993;53:30–37.
406. Koren G, Kochavi-Atiya Y, Bentur Y, Olivieri NF. The effects of subcutaneous deferoxamine administration on renal function in thalassemia major. Int J Hematol 1991;54:371–375.
407. Batey R, Scott J, Jain S, Sherlock S. Acute renal insufficiency occurring during intravenous desferrioxamine therapy. Scand Haematol 1979;22:277–279.
408. Koren G, Bentur Y, Strong D et al. Acute changes in renal function associated with deferoxamine therapy. Am J Dis Child 1989;143:1077–1080.
409. Koren G, Bentur Y, Li Volti S et al. Comments. Am J Dis Child 1990;144:1096–1070.
410. Brittenham GM, Griffith PM, Nienhuis AW, McLaren CE, Young NS, Tucker EE, Allen CJ, Farrell DE, Harris JW. Efficay of deferoxamine in preventing complications of iron overload in patients with thalassemia major. N Engl J Med 1994;331:567–573.
411. Venencie P-Y, Rain B, Blanc A, Tertian G. Toxidermie á la déferoxamine (Desféral). Ann Dermatol Vénéréol 1988;115:1174.
412. Praga M, Enriques de Salamanca R, Andres A et al. Treatment of hemodialysis-related porphyria cutanea tarda with deferoxamine. N Engl J Med 1987;316:547.
413. Sombolos K, Kalekou H, Barboutis K, Tzarou V. Fatal phycomycosis in a hemodialyzed patient receiving deferoxamine. Nephron 1988;49:169–170.
414. Sane A, Manzi S, Perfect J et al. Deferoxamine treatment as a risk factor for zygomycete infection. J Infect Dis 1989;159:151–152.
415. Brill PW, Winchester P, Giardina PJ, Cunningham-Rundles S. Deferoxamine-induced bone dysplasia in patients with thalassemia major. Am J Radiol 1991;156:561–565.
416. Orzincolo C, Castaldi G, De Sanctis V, Scutellari PN, Ciaccio C, Vullo C. Lesioni scheletriche simil-rachitiche e/o scorbutiche nella β-talassemia major. Radiol Med 1990;80:823–829.
417. Orzincolo C, Scutellari PN, Castaldi G. Growth plate injury of the long bones in treated β-thalassemia. Skeletal Radiol 1992;21:39–44.
418. Olivieri NF, Koren G, Harris J, Khattak S, Freedman MH, Templeton DM, Bailey JD, Reilly BJ. Growth failure and bony changes induced by deferoxamine. Am J Pediatr Hematol Oncol 1992;14:48–56.
419. Hartkamp MJ, Babyn PS, Olivieri F. Spinal deformities in deferoxamine-treated homozygous beta-thalassemia major patients. Pediatr Radiol 1993;23:525–528.
420. Miller TT, Caldwell G, Kaye JJ, Arkin S, Burke S, Bril PW. MR imaging of deferoxamine-induced bone dysplasia in an 8-year-old female with thalassemia major. Pediatr Radiol 1993;23:523–524.
421. Seifert A, Von Herrath D and Schaefer K. Iron overload, but not treatment with desferrioxamine favours the development of septicemia in patients on maintenance hemodialysis. Q J Med New Ser 1987;65:1015–1024.

422. Chiu HY, Flynn DM, Hoffbrand AV, Politis D. Infections with *Yersinia enterocolitica* in patients with iron overload. Br Med J 1986;292:97.
423. Mofenson HC, Caraccio TR, Sharieff N. Iron sepsis: Yersinia enterocolitica septicemia possibly caused by an overdose of iron. N. Engl J Med 1987;316:1092.
424. Waterlot Y, Caninieaux B, Hariga-Muller C. Impaired phagocytic activity of neutrophils in patients receiving haemodialysis: the critical role of iron overload. Br Med J 1985;291:501.
425. Emami A, Fagundus DM. Granulocyte dysfunction in patients with iron overload. Br J Haematol 1990;74:546.
426. Hadjiminas JM. Yersiniosis in acutely iron-loaded children treated with desferrioxamine. J Antimicrob Chemother 1988;21:680—681.
427. Abcarian PW, Demas BE. Systemic *Yersinia enterocolitica* infection associated with iron overload and deferoxamine therapy. Am J Roentgenol 1991;157:773—775.
428. Mazzoleni G, Desa D, Gately J, Riddell RH *Yersinia enterocolitica* infection with ileal perforation associated with iron overload and deferoxamine therapy. Dig Dis Sci 1991;36:1154—1160.
429. Nouel O, Voisin PM, Vaucel J, Dartois-Hoguin M, Le Bris M. Association d'une septicémie á *Yersinia enterocolitica*, d'une hémochromatose idiopathique et d'un traitement par deferoxamine. Un cas. Presse Méd 1991;20:1494—1496.
430. Pierron H, Gillet R, Perrimond H, Broudeur JC, Soudry G. Yersiniose et dyshémoglobinose. Á propos de 4 observations. Pédiatrie 1990;45:379—382.
431. Kaneko T, Abe F, Ito Makoto, Hotchi M, Yamada K, Okada Y. Intestinal mucormycosis in a hemodialysis patient treated with desferrioxamine. Acta Pathol Jpn 1991;41:561—566.
432. Rex JH, Ginsberg AM, Fries LF, Pass HI, Kwon-Chung KJ. *Cunninghamella bertholletiae* infection associated with deferoxamine therapy. Rev Infect Dis 1988;10:1187—1194.
433. Eijgenraam FJ, Donckerwolcke RA. Treatment of iron overload in children and adolescents on chronic haemodialysis. Eur J Pediatr 1990;149:359—362.
434. Boyce N, Wood C, Holdsworth S et al. Life-threatening sepsis complicating heavy metal chelation therapy with desferrioxamine. Aust NZ J Med 1985;15:654.
435. Melby K, Slordahl S, Gutteberg TJ, Nordbo SA. Septicaemia due to *Yersinia enterocolitica* after oral overdoses of iron. Br Med J 1982;285:467.
436. Robins-Browne RM, Prpic JK. Desferrioxamine and systemic yersiniosis. Lancet 1983;ii:1372.
437. Waterlot Y, Vanherweghem J-L. Desferrioxamine en hémodialyse á l'origine d'une septicémie á Yersinia enterocolitica. Presse Méd 1985;14:699.
438. Gallant TSVI, Freedman MH, Vellend H et al. *Yersinia* sepsis in patients with iron overload treated with deferoxamine. N Engl J Med 1986;314:1643.
439. Chirio R, Collignon A, Sabbah L et al. Infections á *Yersinia enterocolitica* et thalassémie majeure chez l'enfant. Ann Pédiatr 1989;36:308—314.
440. Masters AP, Hopkinson RB. *Yersinia enterocolitica* septicaemia. Intensive Care Med 1988;14:585—587.
441. Hoen B, Renoult E, Jonon B, Kessler M. Septicemia due to Yersinia enterocolitica in a long-term hemodialysis patient after a single desferrioxamine administration. Nephron 1988;50:378—379.
442. Goodill JJ, Abuelo JG. Mucormycosis—a new risk of deferoxamine therapy in dialysis patients with aluminum or iron overload? N Engl J Med 1987;317:54—55.
443. Daly AL, Velasquez LA, Bradley SF, Kaufmann CA. Mucormycosis: association with deferoxamine therapy. Am J Med 1989;87:468—471.
444. Boelaert JR, Van Roost GF, Vergauwe PL et al. The role of desferrioxamine in dialysis-associated mucor mycosis: report of three cases and review of the literature. Clin Nephrol 1988;29:261—266.
445. Johnson EV, Kline LB, Julian BA, Garcia JH. Bilateral cavernous sinus thrombosis due to mucormycosis. Arch Ophthalmol 1987;106:1089—1092.
446. Veis JH, Contiguglia R, Klein M et al. Mucormycosis in deferoxamine-treated patients on dialysis. Ann Intern Med 1987;107:258.
447. Anonymous. Mucormycosis induced by deferoxamine mesylate. Information on Adverse Reactions to Drugs, No. 89, February 1988, Pharmaceutical Affairs Bureau, Ministry of Health and Welfare, Japan.
448. Boelaert JR, Fenves AZ, Coburn JW. Mucormycosis among patients on dialysis. N Engl J Med 1989;321:190—191.
449. Nakamura M, Weil WB, Kaufman DB. Fatal fungal peritonitis in an adolescent on continuous ambulatory peritoneal dialysis: association with deferoxamine. Pediatr Nephrol 1989;3:80—82.
450. Slade MP, McNab AA. Fatal mucormycosis associated with deferoxamine therapy. Am J Ophthalmol 1991;112: 594—595.
451. De Virgillis S, Congia M, Frau F et al. Deferoxamine-induced growth retardation in patients with thalassemia major. J Pediatr 1988;113:661—669.
452. Piga A, Luzzatto L, Capalbo P et al. High dose desferrioxamine as a cause of growth failure in thalassemic patients. Eur J Haematol 1988;40:380.
453. McElhatton PR, Roberts JC, Sullivan FM. The consequences of iron overdose and its treatment with desferrioxamine in pregnancy. Hum Exp Toxicol 1991;10:251—259.
454. Briggs GG, Freeman RK, Yaffe SJ. Drugs in Pregnancy and Lactation, 2nd edn. Baltimore: Williams and Wilkins, 1986;121.
455. Roeser HP. The role of ascorbic acid in the turnover of storage iron. Semin Hematol 1983;20:91.
456. Nienhuis AW. Vitamin C and iron. N Engl J Med 1981;304:170.
457. Van der Weyden MB. Vitamin C, desferrioxamine and iron loading anemias. Aust NZ J Med 1984;14:593.
458. Rowbotham B, Roeser HP. Iron overload associated with congenital pyruvate kinase deficiency and high dose ascorbic acid ingestion. Aust NZ J Med 1984;14:667.
459. Baker DL, Manno CS. Rapid excretion of gallium-67 isotope in an iron-overloaded patient receiving high-dose intravenous deferoxamine. Am J Hematol 1988;29:230—232.
460. Berdoukas V, Bentley P, Frost H, Schnebli HP. Toxicity of oral iron chelator L1. Lancet 1993;341:1088.
461. Al-Refaie FN, Veys PA, Wilkes S, Wonke B, Hoffbrand AV. Agranulocytosis in a patient with thalassaemia major during treatment with the oral iron chelator, 1,2-dimethyl-3-hydroxypyrid-4-one. Acta Haematol 1993;89: 86—90.
462. Al-Refaie FN, Wonke B, Hoffbrand AV. Deferiprone-associated myelotoxicity. Eur J Haematol 1994;53:298—301.
463. Bartlett AN, Hoffbrand AV, Kontoghiorghes GJ. Long-term trial with the oral iron chelator 1,2-dimethyl-3-hydroxypyrid-4-one (L1). Br J Haematol 1990;76:301—304.
464. Agarwal MB, Viswanathan C, Ramanathan J, Massil

DE, Shah S, Gupte SS, Vasandani D, Puniyani RR. Oral iron chelation with L1. Lancet 1990;335:601.

465. Olivieri NF, Matsui D, Liu PP, Blendis L, Cameron R, McClelland RA, Templeton DM, Koren G. Oral iron chelation with 1,2 dimethyl-3-hydroxypyridin-4-one (L1) in iron loaded thalassemia patients. Bone Marrow Transplant 1993;12(Suppl 1):9–11.

466. Berkovitch M, Laxer RM, Inman R, Koren G, Pritzker KPH, Oliviery NF. Arthropathy in thalassaemia patients receiving deferprone. Lancet 1994;343:1471–1472.

467. Al-Refaie FN, Wonke B, Hoffbrand AV. Arthropathy in thalassaemia patients receiving deferiprone. Lancet 1994;344:262–263.

468. Olivieri NF. Arthropathy in thalassaemia patients receiving deferiprone. Lancet 1994;344:263

469. Mehta J, Singhal S, Revankar R, Walvalkar A, Chablani A, Mehta BC. Fatal systemic lupus erythematosus in patients taking oral iron chelator L1. Lancet 1991;337:298.

470. Mehta J, Singhal S, Mehta BC. Oral iron chelator L1 and autoimmunity. Blood 1993;81:1970–1971.

471. Al-Refaie FN, Hoffbrand AV, Nortey P, Wonke B, Wickens DG. Oral iron chelator L1 and autoimmunity. Blood 1993;81:1971–1972.

472. Hershko C. Development of oral iron chelator L1. Lancet 1993;341:1088–1089.

473. Bierer BE, Nathan DG. The effect of desferrithiocin, an oral iron chelator, on T-cell function. Blood 1990;76:2052–2059.

474. Janakiraman N, Seeler RA, Royal JE, Chen MF. Hemolysis during BAL chelation therapy for high blood lead levels in two G6PD deficient children. Clin Pediatr 1978;17:485.

475. Glotzer D. The current role of 2,3 dimercaptosuccinic acid (DMSA) in the management of childhood lead poisoning. Drug Safety 1993;9:85–92.

476. Hruby K, Donner A. 2,3-Dimercapto-1-propanesulphonate in heavy metal poisoning. Med Toxicol 1987;2:317–323.

477. Allain P, Mauras V, Premel-Cabic A, Islam S, Herve JP, Cledes J. Effects of an EDTA infusion on the urinary elimination of several elements in healthy subjects. Br J Clin Pharmacol 1991;31:347–349.

478. Magee R. Chelation treatment of artherosclerosis. Med J Aust 1985;142:514.

479. McGillem MJ, Mancini GBJ. Inefficacy of EDTA chelation therapy for coronary artherosclerosis. N Engl J Med 1988;318:1618–1619.

480. Scott J. Chelation therapy—evolution or devolution of a nostrum? NZ Med J 1988;9:109–110.

481. Sloth-Nielsen J, Guldager B, Mouritzen C, Lund EB, Egeblad M, Norregaard O, Jorgensen SJ, Jelnes R. Arteriographic findings in EDTA chelation therapy on peripheral arteriosclerosis. Am J Surg 1991;162:122–125.

482. Anonymous. EDTA-chelatie behandeling. Ned Tijdschr Geneeskd 1991;135:2296.

483. Guldager B, Jelnes R, Jorgensen SJ, Nielsen JS, Klaerke A, Mogensen K, Larsen KE, Reimer E, Holm J, Ottesen S. EDTA treatment of intermittent claudication a double-blind, placebo controlled study. J Intern Med 1992; 231:261–267.

484. Reynolds JEF, ed. Martindale. The Extra Pharmacopoeia, 28th edn. 1993;681–682 and 693–694.

485. Ridley CM. Zinc deficiency developing in treatment for thalassaemia. J R Soc Med 1982;75:38.

486. Vicari A, Banfi G, Bonini PA. EDTA-dependent pseudothrombocytopaenia: a 12-month epidemiological study. Scand J Clin Lab Invest 1988;48:537–542.

487. Ramirez JA, Goodman WG, Menezes C, Segre GV, Salusky IB. Disodium ethylenediaminetetraacetate: adverse effects in children. Pediatr Nephrol 1993;7:182–184.

488. Lippi U, Schinelia M, Nicoli M et al. EDTA-induced platelet aggregation can be avoided by a new anticoagulant also suitable for automated complete blood count. Haematologica 1990;75:38–41.

489. Lavender RC, Salmon JS, Golden WE. Pseudothrombocytopenia in an elderly preoperative patient. Anesth Analg 1989;69:396–397.

490. Lombarts AJPF, De Kieviet W. Recognition and prevention of pseudothrombocytopenia and concomitant pseudoleukocytosis. Am J Clin Pathol 1988;89:634–639.

491. Perrier JF, Nace L, Mariot J et al. Pseudothrombopénie en présense d'ETDA évoquant une thrombopénie á l'héparine. Réanim Soins Intens Méd Urg 1988;4:313–315.

492. Berkman N, Michaeli V, Or R, Eldor A. EDTA-dependent pseudothrombocytopenia: a clinical study of 18 patients and a review of the literature. Am J Hematol 1991;36:195–201.

493. Foresti V, Parisio E, Tronci M, Casati O, Zubani R, Pedretti D. Pseudothrombocitopenia da EDTA. Rec Prog Med 1990;81:661–662.

494. Pestana D, Marcote C, De Castro MF. EDTA-dependent pseudothrombocytopenia in a preoperative patient. Acta Anaesthesiol Scand 1992;36:328–330.

495. Angelo G, Calvano D, Mattaini R, Cosini I, Giardini C. Platelet aggregation in presence of anticoagulant dependent pseudothrombocytopenia. Minerva Med 1993;84:399–402.

496. Hillyer CD, Knopf AN, Berkman EM. EDTA-dependent leukoagglutination. Am J Clin Pathol 1990;94:458–461.

497. Kobayashi S, Seki K, Yamguchi M, Maruta A, Kodama F. Studies on EDTA-dependent pseudoleukocytopenia. Rinsho Ketsueki 1991;32:205–211.

498. Hoyt RH, Durie BGM. Pseudothrombocytopenia induced by a monoclonal IgM Kappa platelet agglutinin. Am J Hematol 1989;31:50–52.

499. Tedrow HE, Zeigler ZR. Evidence of anti-A1 inhibited by EDTA. Transfusion 1988;28:177–178.

500. Judd WJ, Barnes BA. EDTA-saline and ABO system antibodies. Transfusion 1989;29:84.

501. Moel DI, Kumar K. Reversible nephrotoxic reactions to a combined 2,3-dimercapto-1-propanol and calcium disodium ethylenediamine tetra-acetate regimen in asymptomatic children with elevated blood lead levels. Pediatrics 1982; 70:259.

502. Fisher AA. Safety of ethylenediamine tetraacetate in the treatment of lead poisoning in persons sensitive to ethylenediamine hydrochloride. Cutis 1991;48:105–106.

503. Reynolds JEF, ed. Martindale. The Extra Pharmacopoeia, 28th edn. 1993;1138.

504. March L, Fraser FC. Chelating agents and teratogenesis. Lancet 1973;ii:846.

505. Swenerton H, Harley LS. Teratogenic effects of a chelating agent and their prevention by zinc. Science 1971;173:62.

506. Janowitz P, Schumacher KA, Swobodnik W, Kratzer W, Tudyka J, Wechsler G. Transhepatic topical dissolution of gallbladder stones with MTBE and EDTA. Dig Dis Sci 1993;38:2121–2129.

507. Mann KV, Travers JD. Succimer, an oral lead chelator. Clin Pharm 1991;10:914–922.
508. Anonymous. Drug reviews from the Formulary. Succimer Hosp Pharm 1991;26:974–976.
509. Mann KV, Travers JD. Succimer, an oral lead chelator Clin Pharm 1992;11:388.
510. Marcus SM, Ruck B. Use of succimer. Clin Pharm 1992;11:387–388.
511. Swobodnik W, Baumgaertel H, Janowitz P et al. Dissolution of calcified gallbladder stones by treatment with methyl-hexyl ether and urea-EDTA. Lancet 1988; i:216
512. Dubois RS, Rodgerson DP, Hambidge KM. Treatment of Wilson's disease with triethyiene tetramine hydrochloride. J Pediatr Gastroenterol Nutr 1990;10:77–81.
513. Siegemund R, Loessner J, Guenther K, Kuehn HJ, Bachmann H. Mode of action of triethylenetetramine dihydrochloride on copper metabolism in Wilson's disease. Acta Neurol Scand 1991;83:364–366.
514. Kiechl SG, Willeit J, Aichner F, Felber S. Treatment of Wilson's disease: penicillamine or triene (Letter to the Editor). Acta Neurol. Scand 1991;84:154–155.
515. Siegemund R. Reply. Acta Neurol Scand 1991;84:155–157.
516. Saito H, Watanabe K, Sahara M, Mochizuki R, Edo K, Ohyama Y. Triethylene-tetramine (trien) therapy for Wilson's disease. Tohoku J Exp Med 1991;164:29–35.
517. Walshe JM. Treatment of Wilson's disease with trientine (triethylene tetramine) dihydrochloride. Lancet 1982; i:643.
518. Condamine L, Hermine O, Alvin P, Levine M, Rey C, Courtecuisse V. Acquired sideroblastic anaemia during treatment of Wilson's disease with triethylene tetramine dihydrochloride. Br J Haematol 1993;83:166–168.

Meyler's Side Effects of Drugs, 13th Edition
M.N.G. Dukes, editor

SECTION EDITOR: C.B.M. TESTER-DALDERUP

F. Hackenberger

24 Antiseptic drugs and disinfectants

Antiseptics are substances that kill or inhibit the growth of micro-organisms, especially in preparations applied to living tissue. In contrast, disinfectants are substances that prevent infection by the destruction of pathogenic micro-organisms, but are used especially in preparations applied to inanimate objects. Because disinfectants may also cause side effects directly or indirectly, due to residues originating from objects that have been sterilized, the commonly used disinfectants are also discussed in this Chapter.

Contamination with micro-organisms It is too often not realized that an antiseptic or disinfectant solution that is left standing can provide culture ground for bacteria, and these can be pathogenic. In this manner the antiseptic or disinfectant solution may become the source of an infection.

ACIDS

BORIC ACID *(SED-11, 478; SEDA-8, 243; SEDA-10, 229)*

In the past, boric acid was falsely considered a relatively non-toxic substance, and had an unwarranted reputation as a germicide. It is only bacteriostatic, even in a saturated aqueous solution. Boric acid has often proved poisonous, either by ingestion or following local use. Goldbloom and Goldbloom and Valdes-Dapena and Arey have given detailed reviews of cases from the world literature. The latter covers 172 cases of boric acid intoxication, including 83 deaths. In this series there were 37 deaths after external use of boric acid, including 23 children with diaper rashes. From 1974 to March 1984, 134 cases of intoxication by boric acid or borates were recorded by the Poison Center in Paris, 88 of which were accidental, and 31 due to iatrogenic measures.

Boric acid penetrates even intact skin, but it is readily absorbed through inflamed or otherwise damaged skin and through mucous membranes. Schuppli et al. applied wet compresses of boric acid to the intact and eczematous skin of 21 patients over several days and generally did not find elevated blood levels of boric acid. One patient, however, did show a significant rise in blood level of boric acid which the authors ascribed to pre-existing kidney insufficiency.

Acute intoxication In acute intoxication a progressive development of symptoms occurs.

After ingestion the typical clinical picture begins with persistent vomiting and diarrhea (mucous and blood, with a bluish-green color).

Shortly after the onset of the gastrointestinal symptoms, in some intoxications even earlier, a rash appears (with macules and/or papules), beginning on the abdomen, genitals and head, and rapidly spreading, followed by excoriation and intensive desquamation after 1—2 days. Mucous membranes are often involved, especially in young infants, in whom the mouth, pharynx and conjunctivae are often inflamed.

Later one sees central nervous system symptoms with headache and mental confusion followed by convulsions. In children there is meningism, and twitching of the facial muscles and extremities, followed by convulsions.

Acute tubular necrosis may occur with oliguria or anuria, hypernatremia, hyperchloremia and hyperkalemia, proteinuria, erythrocyturia and cylindruria.

Finally hyperthermia, a fall in blood pressure, tachycardia and shock ensue.

Pinto has described 14 cases of acute boric acid ingestion reported to the New York City Poison Control Center over $2\frac{1}{2}$ years. In these patients the urinary riboflavin (vitamin B_2) excretion was determined, and in approximately two-thirds of the cases it was significantly elevated. This is not surprising, since riboflavin and boric acid are known to form a water-soluble complex. The range of lethal doses is held to be 1—3 grams for babies, 5 grams for infants and 15—20 grams for adults. Skipworth et al. reported severe acute boric acid poisoning in a 3-year-old boy after application of a boric acid-containing talcum powder. Baliah et al. reported a similar case in a 27-day-old baby girl. Hilman et al. reported generalized erythema and skin desquamation, fever convulsions, and diarrhea following repeated boric acid applications to a denuded umbilical stump.

Fatal intoxication has followed prostatectomy and subsequent bladder irrigation with 3% boric acid.

Chronic intoxication Prolonged absorption of boric acid causes anorexia, weight loss, Vomiting, mild diarrhea, skin rash, diffuse alopecia, convulsions and anemia.

On account of the high toxicity and limited therapeutic value of boric acid, borates appear in many countries to have been abandoned as obsolete.

ALCOHOLS

Ethanol, isopropanol(2-propanol), *N*-propanol(1-propanol)

The lower aliphatic alcohols are widely used, specially for skin antisepsis. In appropriate concentrations these alcohols are bactericidal to most of the common pathogenic bacteria, but some rare species survive and can grow, especially since these alcohols are inactive against dried spores. Seven cases of gaseous edema were observed in the former GDR following intramuscular injections after rubbing of the skin with *N*-propanol (SED-11, 474); this has led to a national recommendation that alcohols should not be used for rubbing of the skin prior to intramuscular injections, injections of vasoconstrictive agents, injections in patients with disturbed peripheral circulation, or before lumbar, paraneural and intra-articular injection and puncture (SED-11, 474).

Skin reactions Skin reactions are extremely rare, although allergic contact dermatitis due to lower aliphatic alcohols has been described in the literature (SED-11, 474). However, in premature infants of very low birth weight, second- and third-degree chemical skin burns were reported after the use of isopropanol either for conduction in electrocardiography, for the preparation of the umbilical stump for arterial catheterization, or for cleansing before herniotomy (SED-11, 474). Possible causes are hypoperfusion of the skin by local pressure and general hypoperfusion derived from hypoxia, hypothermia and acidosis. Immediate drying of the skin of small premature infants after antisepsis with alcoholic preparations and carefully avoiding that the alcohol is absorbed by the diapers is recommended.

Use of ethanol in local treatment of omphaloceles When it is not possible to perform surgical treatment for omphalocele, ethanol application is probably the safest method. Dosage and frequency of application, however, should be as limited as possible since absorption with clinical intoxication may be observed (SED-11, 474; 1[C]).

Intoxications Intoxications can only occur after ingestion or inhalation of large amounts of ethanol. The fatal dose by ingestion for an average adult is 300—400 ml and for a small child approximately 14 ml/kg of pure ethanol.

The Drug Monitoring Centers of the Parisian hospitals have reported a case of acute ethanol intoxication (blood alcohol level 2948 mg/l) in a pre-term infant of 180 grams, due to local application of ethanol-imbued compresses on the legs as a treatment for puncture hematomas. The US National Poison Center Network collected reports of 422 cases of mouthwash ingestion in a total of 128 370 poisonings in children under 6 years of age. Mouthwashes may contain up to 27% ethanol and are dangerous in the sense that people are unaware of their toxicity, and that they are both highly accessible and attractive to children (SED-11, 475).

N-Propanol and isopropanol are about twice as toxic as ethanol. The fatal dose by ingestion for adults is approximately 250 ml (2[R]). About 15% of an ingested dose of isopropanol is metabolized to acetone; ingestion produces ketosis without acidosis and with hypoglycemia. Because the toxicity of *N*-propanol and isopropanol is greater than ethanol, the enzymatic (alcohol dehydrogenase) method for ethanol determination may give erroneous results (SED-11, 475).

Benzyl alcohol *(SEDA-7, 265; SEDA-12, 201; SEDA-14, 205)*

Benzyl alcohol is commonly used as preservative in multidose injectable pharmaceutical preparations. For this purpose, concentrations in the range of 0.5—2% are used and the whole amount of benzyl alcohol injected is generally very well tolerated. Concentrations of 0.9% are used in Bacteriostatic Sodium Chlorine (USP), which is frequently used in the management of critically ill patients to flush intravascular catheters after the addition of medications or the withdrawal of blood and in Sterile Bacteriostatic Water for injection (USP), used to dilute or reconstitute medications for intravenous use. The content of benzyl alcohol in a lot of injectable pharmaceutical preparations is to be considered carefully. Unfortunately the view still taken in many countries that the identity of the additives and excipients in medicines are a trade secret must be deplored. The duty to declare them is only realized in some countries.

Toxicity of benzyl alcohol caused by use of preserved solutions *Use in newborn infants* In 1981 a gasping syndrome in small premature infants who had been exposed to intravenous preparations containing benzyl alcohol 0.9% as preservative was described. The affected infants presented with metabolic acidosis, seizures, neurological deterioration, hepatic and renal dysfunction and cardiovascular collapse. Death was reported in 16 cases, who received a minimum of 99 mg/kg body weight per day of benzyl alcohol (SED-11, 475).

Toxic effects of benzyl alcohol including respiratory vasodilation, hypotension, convulsions and paralysis have been known for years. However, little is known about the toxic effects or levels of benzyl alcohol and the metabolic acidosis caused by accumulation of the metabolite benzoic acid in neonates, especially in sick premature infants (see SED-10, 421; SED-11, 475). It is mainly related to an excessive body burden relative to body weight, so that the load of this metabolite may exceed the capacity of the immature liver and kidney for detoxication.

Based on reports, the FDA has recommended that neither intramuscular flushing solutions containing benzyl alcohol nor dilutions with this preservative should be used in newborn infants (SED-11, 475).

Jardine and Rogers (3^{C}) reviewed the hospital and autopsy records of infants admitted to a nursery during the previous 18 months. The 218 patients had been administered fluids still containing benzyl alcohol as flush solutions and were compared with 218 neonates admitted during the following 18 months. Withdrawal of benzyl alcohol as preservative had no demonstrable effect on mortality, but the development of kernicterus was significantly associated in 15 out of 49 patients exposed to benzyl alcohol, and no cases occurred after withdrawal of this preservative (3^{CR}).

However, this apparent association has not been confirmed in a 5-year study of the use of benzyl alcohol as a preservative in intravenous medications in a neonatal intensive care unit (4^{C}). In this study, including 129 neonates who died between the ages of 2 and 28 days, there was no difference in the rate of kernicterus and the exposure to benzyl alcohol between neonates who developed kernicterus and the control group of unaffected infants who were born during the same period and who were of the same birth weight and gestational age. In this study only estimates of the extent of exposure to benzyl alcohol were given rather than exact doses and serum concentrations.

Use in intrathecal agents When reporting a case of flaccid paraplegia following intrathecal administration of cytosine arabinoside diluted in bacteriostatic water containing 1.5% benzyl alcohol (SEDA-8, 243), Hahn et al. (5^{CR}) reviewed clinical data in other reported cases of neurological disorders after intrathecal chemotherapy with methotrexate or cytosine arabinoside that could be attributed to benzyl alcohol or to other preservatives (SEDA-9, 225). Most commonly, flaccid paraparesis with absence of reflexes developed rapidly, often with pain and anesthesia. Very often there was full recovery, the prognosis depending mainly on the concentration of the preservative and on the time of exposure. In some cases, the paralysis ascended to cause respiratory distress, cardiac arrest, and death. Only preservative-free sterile CSF-substitute or saline, or preferably the patient's own CSF, should be used to dilute chemotherapeutic agents (SED-11, 475).

Hypersensitivity Grant et al. 6^{C}) described the occurrence of hypersensitivity in a 55-year-old man who developed fatigue, nausea and diffuse angio-edema shortly after an intramuscular injection of vitamin-B_{12}-containing benzyl alcohol. Wilson et al. (7^{C}) reported on a hypersensitivity reaction with fever and maculopapular rash on the chest and arms after an injection of cytarabine, vincristine and heparin using a dilution solution containing benzyl alcohol.

Skin reactions Shmunes (8^{Cr}) observed a case of an allergic contact dermatitis traceable to benzyl alcohol; it was characterized by erythema, palpable edema, and raised borders. In this case, the benzyl alcohol was present as a preservative in an injectable solution of sodium tetradecyl sulfate, a sclerosing agent used for the treatment of varicose veins. The author provided a list of 151 injectable preparations, 48 of which were for subcutaneous administration, that contained benzyl alcohol as a preservative in the range 0.5–2%. The list included hormones and steroids, antihypertensives (reserpine), vitamin preparations (vitamins B_{12} and B_6), acid-base chemicals (ammonium sulfate), antihistamines, antibiotics, heparin (17 brands), tranquilizers and sclerosing agents (sodium morrhuate and sodium tetradecyl sulfate).

ALDEHYDES

Formaldehyde and glutaraldehyde are used as solutions and vapours for disinfection and sterilization. The solid paraformaldehyde is used as a source of formaldehyde vapor for the disinfection of rooms. Noxythiolin, polynoxylin, hexamidine and taurolidine act by slow release of formaldehyde.

Formaldehyde

Formaldehyde solution contains 34–38% of formaldehyde methanol as a stabilizing agent to delay polymerization of the formaldehyde. Formaldehyde solutions have to be diluted before use to a 2–8% solution to disinfect inanimate objects and to a 1—2% solution for disinfection by scrubbing. For fumigation of air a concentration of 1—2% is used.

Because of its aggressive properties, formaldehyde cannot be applied safely to the skin or the mucous membranes in the concentration necessary to rapidly kill microbes.

The intensive current discussion about the toxicity, mutagenicity and potential carcinogenicity of formaldehyde is more a problem of occupational and environmental exposure, caused by its release from urea formaldehyde resins used for wood products and from foams for cavity-wall insulation, than a problem of its use for disinfection (SED-11, 476; SED-12, 569).

However, Ponsold et al. (9^{C}) found that the air concentrations for formaldehyde can be several hundred percent higher than the maximum safe workplace concentration, even when disinfection by scrubbing is carried out properly. Very high concentrations have also been established in the workrooms of pathologists. De Zotti et al. (10^{C}) measured formaldehyde pollution in the pathology departments in two Italian hospitals. The highest values of 2.6 and 6.0 ppm were measured in the dissection laboratories. In the histology and cytology laboratories, levels were less than 1 ppm, except when technicians handled formaldehyde solutions.

Acute toxicity and primary irritant effects of formaldehyde The minimum amount of formaldehyde that can be detected by odor varies considerably between individuals and ranges from 1.12 to 1.2 mg/m^3 (0.1—1.0 ppm), close to the level at which minimal irritant effects are felt in the eyes and in the pulmonary airways (10^{R}). Thus the fundamental toxicity of the compound lies in producing primary irritation to the eyes, nose and throat when the subject is exposed to concentrations in the range of 1—5 ppm. Concentrations above 2—5 ppm cause irritation of the pharynx, lungs and eyes and some erythema of vaporized areas of the skin such as the face and neck. Acute exposure to concentrations of formaldehyde in the order of 3 times the maximum threshold of detection of the odor will most likely produce severe acute pulmonary edema after only a few minutes.

Acute toxicity after local administration of formaldehyde-containing solutions *Instillation of dilute solutions of formalin into the bladder* as a treatment for inoperable, profusely bleeding tumors or intractable hemorrhagic cystitis has been described. Dilutions of 1—10% of formalin (an aqueous solution of 37% formaldehyde) were used in this procedure. Anuria was a severe complication. This was due either to edematous obstruction of the ureter or to tubular or papillar necrosis, probably caused by resorptive intoxication. Bladder perforation with intraperitoneal spillage, peritonitis and finally death was described in an elderly patient with a cervix carcinoma (SED-11, 476).

In 1983, Godec and Gleich reviewed all available published results of treatment of intractable hematuria with formalin (37% formaldehyde). Dilutions of 1—10% formalin (containing 0.37—3.7% formaldehyde) were used, most often the dilution to 10% was used. The authors conclude that formalin was probably the most effective tool for controlling massive hematuria, but also probably the most dangerous. The review covers 23 articles and 118 patients; in 104 cases the treatment was successful. But in only 10 reports had the treatment been used without serious side effects; four deaths and numerous serious local and systemic complications were listed in the remaining 13 articles. The complication rate increased when the formalin concentration was higher but the contact time and the volume instilled did not influence the occurrence of side effects. The most frequent local complications were reflux and hydronephrosis. Fibrosis of the bladder with reduced capacity was the usual clinical sequel. A systemic effect was tubular necrosis with anuria; two fatal cases were reported. Another complication was ureteric obstruction, which was not related to ureteric fibrosis or to bladder wall fibrosis obstructing the intramural ureter; in two cases the obstruction appeared to be due to retroperitoneal fibrosis (SED-11, 476).

In 1989, Donahue and Frank (SED-11, 476; SED-12, 569; SEDA-14, 205; 12^{R}) published an analysis of the literature; 235 cases of intravesical hemorrhagic cystitis were treated with intravesical instillations of diluted formalin in concentrations of 1, 5 or 10% formalin. Complete response rates are given at 71, 78 and 83%, and these rates were practically independent of the concentration of formalin used. The average duration of a complete response was 3—4 months; the recurrence rate was decreased gradually with the use of higher concentrations.

Complications were divided into two groups: '*minor complications*' included all mild or transient problems not requiring surgical intervention (fever, tachycardia, transient or minor elevations of blood urea nitrogen or creatinine, mild hydronephrosis, grades I and II urico-urethral reflux, frequency, urgency, incontinence, supra pubic pain or a decrease in bladder capacity not requiring urinary diversion); '*major complications*' comprised those requiring surgical intervention, resulting in the loss of renal function or inducing damage to the supravesical urinary tracts (stricture formation), including anuria, acute tubular necrosis, papillary necrosis, ureteral or retroperitoneal fibrosis, uterovesical or uteropelvic junction obstruction, severe hydronephrosis, grades III or IV vesicoureteral reflux, any vesical fistula or a decrease in bladder capacity requiring urinary diversion.

Major complications occurred in all treatment groups, including the group treated with 1% formalin. The higher rate observed with 10% formalin was not significantly different from the rate after the use of 5 or 1% formalin.

The mortality rates were 2.2% for all the formalin groups, but the rates are not significantly different. A 10% formalin solution resulted in a higher and favorable response rate, a lower recurrence rate, equal 'major complications' and mortality rate and a 3-fold higher minor complications rate than 5% formalin in patients with hemorrhagic cystitis due to radiotherapy for bladder tumor. In contrast, 5% formalin was more effective than the 10% solution in treating patients with intractable hematuria due to unresectable bladder tumors or cyclophosphamide cystitis.

The use of 2 or 4% formaldehyde solutions as a *scolecidal agent for injection in hydatid cysts* and for *peritoneal lavage* was followed by shock in seven cases and resulted in death in three. All three patients who died had undergone a peritoneal lavage with 2—8 liters of a 2 or 4% formaldehyde solution (SED-11, 476).

Borries et al. reported three cases of secondary sclerosing cholangitis which developed during the early postoperative phase of surgical treatment of hydatid liver cysts; one patient died within 3 months and the remaining two underwent liver transplantation following biliary sclerosis. Belghiti et al. also reported three cases with sclerosing cholangitis and both groups of authors conclude that because of the risk of complication and the unproven efficacy of intracystic injection of a scolecidal solution in preventing the dissemination of the parasite, this technique should be abandoned in the surgical treatment of hydatid disease of the liver. Bourgeon has, however, noted that he observed no sclerosing cholangitis in a series of 560 patients when the concentration was not more than 2% and the solution was injected only into cysts which contained clear fluid content (SED-14, 476).

Immunogenically mediated responses to formaldehyde Formaldehyde is one of the most frequent contact allergens. It is released by numerous agents, such as paraformaldehyde, dichlorophen, Dowicil 75 and Dowicil 200 (*cis*-1-(3-chloroalkyl)-3,5,7-triaza-L-azonia-adamantane chloride), bronopol, Biocide DS 52-49 (1,2-benzoisothiazoline-3-one plus a formaldehyde releaser) and Bakzid (cyclic aminoacetal). Free formaldehyde is used in cosmetics, especially in hair shampoos, and in many disinfectants and antiseptics.

If the responses in some individuals to acute exposure to formaldehyde are immunogenically mediated, they are of serious clinical significance. These individuals should not be exposed to any concentration of the agent. However, the intensity and nature of the immunogenic response may so resemble a primary irritant effect that a different diagnosis is not possible.

Allergic dermatitis Allergic dermatitis has been demonstrated from direct skin contact and from exposure to gaseous formaldehyde in the air. Varied forms of reaction occur, from simple erythema to maculopapular lesions, hyperesthesia and angioneurotic edema. Five patients have been reported who developed an allergic contact dermatitis to plaster casts, caused by free formaldehyde released by a melamine-formaldehyde resin incorporated in the plaster. Urticaria with acute Quincke edema was reported following the use of a formaldehyde-containing dental paste (SED-11, 477).

Photosensitivity The first published case of photosensitivity to formaldehyde was reported by Shelley (13^c). A 48-year-old man experienced pruritus, burning and redness of the skin within minutes of exposure to sunlight. Photopatch tests revealed a specific photosensitivity to formaldehyde.

Formaldehyde-induced bronchial asthma Sakrila reported formaldehyde-induced asthma in a laboratory technician and in a neurologist preparing brain specimens for a student demonstration. Hendrik and Lane found that in a renal dialysis unit, five of 28 members of the staff had respiratory symptoms associated with formaldehyde, and that in two cases attacks of wheezing could be provoked by exposure to formaldehyde. One nurse was particularly affected, the asthmatic wheeze persisting for 8 days after exposure. Nordman et al. examined 230 persons who had been exposed to formaldehyde and suffered from asthma-like respiratory symptoms with a bronchial provocation test; 12 cases were considered to be caused by specific sensitization to formaldehyde, 11 were triggered by 2.5 mg/m^3 and one by 1.2 mg/m^3. They conclude that formaldehyde asthma, although apparently a rare disease, is under-reported (SED-11, 477).

Formation of an anti-N-like antibody in hemodialysis patients Fassbinder et al. have detected in the sera of 68 (20.9%) of 325 hemodialysis patients a specific cold agglutinin, cross-reacting with anti-N. Each patient showing this anti-N-like antibody used a formaldehyde-sterilized dialyzer. Results of transfusion experiments indicated an in vivo hemolytic activity of this antibody. It has been postulated that such in vivo exposure might affect the MN-receptor of the erythrocytes, rendering it immunogenic, and thus inducing the formation of this hemodialysis-associated anti-N-like antibody.

Maurice et al. reported on an immediate-type allergy

to formaldehyde mediated by IgE during the use of a formaldehyde reconditioned dialyzer in a 20-year-old woman without a personal or familiar history of atopy. Friedman and Lundin pointed to the problem that the commonly used Clinitest-reaction for residual formaldehyde in re-used dialyzers fails to detect concentrations below 50 ppm. Zasuwa and Lewin recommended the use of Schiff reagent in ratios of 1:1 to 3:1, which may detect formaldehyde at a concentration of 3.6–5 p.p.m. It may also be used in combination with a glucose-containing dialysate (SED-12; 571).

Mutagenicity Formaldehyde has long been known to be mutagenic. Positive findings have been reported in numerous laboratory test systems, e.g. fruit flies (*Drosophila*), grasshoppers, flowering plants, fungi, bacteria, and cultured human bronchial fibroblasts.

Grafstrom et al. found that formaldehyde may cause genotoxicity by a dual mechanism of directly damaging DNA and inhibiting repair of mutagenic and carcinogenic DNA lesions by other chemical and physical carcinogens.

Goh investigated chromosomal patterns in bone marrow from 40 patients who were undergoing maintenance hemodialysis. During the period of these cytogenetic studies the dialyzers were re-used after sterilization with formaldehyde, and each patient may have received residual amounts as much as 127 ± 51 mg of formaldehyde during each dialysis. Marked chromosomal abnormalities and chromosomal breaks were found in metaphases from direct bone marrow preparations (SED-11, 477; 14[R]).

Carcinogenicity Evidence of possible carcinogenicity of formaldehyde was produced by two inhalation studies on rats and mice (SED-10, 423; SED-11, 477; SED-12, 571; 14[R]).

In man a number of epidemiological studies using different designs have been conducted to date (14[R]) on the health risks of non-medical exposure to formaldehyde and also to health-professionals (15[C]–20[C]) with contradictory results. Cancers in excess in more than one study were: Hodgkin's disease (21[C], 22[C]), leukemia (15[C], 16[C], 19[C], 20[C], 23[C]), cancers of the buccal cavity and pharynx (particular nasopharynx) (15[C], 16[C], 22[C], 24[C], 25[C]), lung (15[C], 21[C], 24[C], 26[C]–28[C]), nose (29[C]–31[C]) prostate (16[C], 21[C], 23[C]), bladder (16[C]), 20[C], 23[C]), brain (17[C]), colon (15[C]–17[C], 22[C], 24[C]), skin (15[C], 22[C]) and kidney (24[C]).

No association between formaldehyde exposure and lung cancer was observed in a case-referral study among Danish physicians working in pathology, forensic medicine and anatomy departments (18[C]).

Mortality from *prostatic cancer* has been found to be elevated among embalmers (16[C]) and industrial workers (21[C], 23[C]), but the excess was statistically significant only among embalmers (16[C]). A slight excess of mortality from *bladder cancer* (16[C], 19[C], 23[C]), a significant excess of *colon cancer* (15[C], 16[C], 24[C]) and a significant excess mortality from *skin cancer* (15[C], 22[C]) were noted among British pathologists (19[C]), embalmers (15[C], 16[C]) and among industrial workers (22[C]–24[C]).

The excess mortalities from *leukemia* and from *cancer of the brain* were generally not seen among industrial workers, which suggests that the excess for these cancers among professionals (anatomists (17[C]), pathologists (19[C]), embalmers (15[C], 16[C]), undertakers (20[C])) is due to factors other than just formaldehyde.

It is of course possible that the studies providing positive evidence of a link between formaldehyde and cancer related to more intensive (e.g. industrial) exposure than did those resulting in negative findings.

A critical review of the available reports on the risk connected with chronic exposure to low concentrations of formaldehyde leads us to the conclusion that formaldehyde cannot be a potent carcinogen; if it were, the high incidence of exposure in the human environment would result in much clearer evidence of risk. However, and although human subjects and animals may differ in their susceptibility to formaldehyde, any compound that produces cancer in experimental animals or mutagenicity in several test systems should be considered as a potential cancer risk to human subjects; even the contradictory evidence from human studies should therefore be taken seriously and efforts made to reduce exposure.

Lewis and Chestner (20[R]) pointed to the necessity to re-evaluate the rationale underlying the use of formaldehyde, formocresol and paraformaldehyde in dentistry, since the clinical use and delivery of these products are considered to be arbitrary and unscientific.

Glutaraldehyde (glutaral)

The safety and biocidal efficacy of glutaraldehyde has led to its endorsement by CDC and WHO (35, 36) as a substitute to formaldehyde in high-level disinfection and cold sterilization. Glutaraldehyde is used in a 2% aqueous solution buffered to a pH of about 8 for sterilization of endoscopic and dental equipment, and for other equipment that cannot be sterilized by heat. Mwaniki et al. (37[r]) pointed out that occupational safety considerations for glutaraldehyde largely relate to its volatility and stringent precautions in handling are needed in warm tropical climates. The lack of precautionary details for glutaraldehyde fumes, especially in warm climates is inadequate. Manufacturers should provide details of possible side effects that could arise from glutaraldehyde vapor, and of the precautions that should be taken to keep the air concentration below the recommended limit. There is an urgent need to develop affordable and effective methods of containing glutaraldehyde fumes.

Contact dermatitis Glutaraldehyde can cause contact dermatitis (SED-11, 478; SED-12, 572). The threshold concentration for glutaraldehyde aqueous solution to induce dermal sensitization is in the range of 0.1 to 1.0%.

Local irritation (*SED*-12, 572) Calder et al. reported on an inquiry which included 169 nurses working in 17 hospitals, especially in endoscopy units. From the nurses who participated, 68% had symptoms, 38% two or more. The major complaints were eye irritation in 49%, skin discoloration or irritation in 41%, and cough or shortness of breath in 34%. Complaints were not related to habits, atopic status or duration of exposure. In two hospitals the time-weighted average concentrations were estimated. The 10-minute time-weighted average was below the UK occupational exposure standard of 0.2 ppm. Waldron reported on a similar survey of 150 staff of two Middlesex hospitals who were exposed to glutaraldehyde. The rate of complaints reported was in the same range.

Corrado et al. have described nurses working in endoscopy units who complained of respiratory symptoms on exposure to glutaraldehyde. The provocation test was positive in two of these patients. Small reported a case of an anaphylactic reaction in a woman after the fourth intramuscular injection of a glutaraldehyde-containing pollen preparation (SED-11, 478).

Jonas et al. observed a unique form of colitis during endoscopy of the lower gastrointestinal tract in 21 patients. They were found to have discrete or confluent white plaques adherent to the colonic mucosa, mild to severe erythema of surrounding mucosa, and variable amounts of foam liquid upon withdrawal of the endoscope. Some patients developed rectal bleeding, tenesmus, and increased frequency of stools, lasting 12 days. Durande et al. reported the occurrence of bloody diarrhea after sigmoidoscopy, associated with residuals of a 2% glutaraldehyde-containing endoscope cleaning solution in the endoscopes. The toxic effects were confirmed in animal experiments subsequently performed.

Acute eye injury was reported, caused by a leakage of retained glutaraldehyde in an anesthesia mask.

Wright and Newman recorded nine instances of periprosthetic incompetence (all in mitral valves) in a series of 184 implantations of glutaraldehyde-preserved valve bioprostheses. Since this incidence of dehiscence substantially exceeded that previously noted with synthetic valves, it has been suggested that incomplete removal of glutaraldehyde from the prosthesis might have contributed to the failure of healing. Collagen-ultrastructure investigations of glutaraldehyde-treated porcine aortic valve tissue demonstrated that the long-term mechanical durability of treated aortic valves can be substantially increased if careful consideration is given to the pressure at which initial fixation of glutaraldehyde is carried out.

DYES

ACRIDINE DERIVATIVES

These include acriflavine, aminacridine, ethacridine, euflavine and proflavine.

Acrisorcin

Acrisorcin (aminoacridine 4-hexylresorcinolate), has been used for induction of abortion in mid-trimester pregnancies. Abortion was produced when a 0.1% solution of acrisorcin was introduced into the extra-amniotic space in 23 women. All patients aborted after a mean induction-delivery interval of 59 hours (SED-11, 474).

Ethacridine

Ethacridine (6,9-diamino-2-ethoxyacridine) is widely used in the local treatment of inflammatory or ulcerative conditions of the skin, particularly crural eczema due to venous stasis. Many publications point to the high frequency of exacerbation involving local allergic reactions and also generalized eczematous reactions (SED-11, 474).

Ethacridine was also applied by slow extra-amniotic instillation of 150 ml of a 0.1% solution to induce abortion or delivery in patients with missed abortion or fetal death, and during the second and third trimester without or in combination with drip infusion of oxytocin or dinoprost (prostaglandin $F_2\alpha$) (SED-11, 474). No side effects were reported.

Triphenylmethane dyes

These include brilliant green, crystal violet (SED-9, 249) gentian violet (SED-9, 249), Castellani's solution ('Margenta pain') (SED-11, 302), and the main side effects are contact allergies and irritations of the skin.

Brilliant green and gentian violet are potent inhibitors of wound healing, and cause necrosis of the skin at higher concentrations. Necrotic skin or mucous membrane reactions have been reported: a severe hemorrhagic cystitis followed the accidental injection of gentian violet solution through the urethra; keratoconjunctivitis was induced by the accidental or voluntary instillation of gentian violet solution in the eyes, and a tattoo effect was observed after application of this dye to a deep burn on the face (39[R]).

Gentian violet is a mixture of crystal violet (hexamethyl-*p*-rosaniline; at least 96%) and methyl-violet (tetramethyl- and pentamethyl-*p*-rosaniline). It is a mitotic poison, and a clastogen. Carcinogenic effects of gentian violet in rodents have been reported. These findings are not surprising, a number of triphenylmethane-classed dyes, of which gentian violet is a member, have been recognized as animal and human carcinogens (39[R], 40[R]). The Department of Health in Great Britain recommends that it should not be used on mucous membranes or open wounds, but be restricted to topical application on unbroken skin (41[r]). Even for this purpose there are more effective antiseptics.

Oral administration as an anthelminthic can cause gastrointestinal irritation, and intravenous injection can cause depression in the white blood cell count. More recently gentian violet has been used as a blood additive to prevent transmission of Chagas' disease. Surprisingly, no acute toxic effects were reported after administration of large amounts of gentian violet-treated blood to date, but no studies have been done on long-term effects of gentian violet-treated blood either in humans or in laboratory animals.

ETHYLENE OXIDE

Ethylene oxide is a gas utilized in the sterilization of equipment too large for other techniques, as well as for sterilization of rubber, plastic goods and other materials which are damaged by heat and not adequately disinfected by other cold methods.

Ethylene oxide is highly toxic and, if not eliminated after sterilization, may produce severe irritation and burns. In addition, it forms ethylene glycol with moisture and ethylene chlorhydrine with free chlorine atoms. Both products, also irritants, are absorbed by the sterilized object from which they elute very slowly. The rate of elimination of ethylene oxide and its irritant reaction products depends on a variety of factors, such as the nature and thickness of the material, the duration and temperature of aeration, and the material used for wrapping the sterilized item.

Human exposure to ethylene oxide should be kept as low as feasible given present-day technology. Health personnel working in close proximity to ethylene oxide should be given information to the dangers of this compound, and be informed of the known and uncertain risks of being exposed to it. The function of sterilizing equipment should be regularly assessed, proper ventilation established, and alarm systems installed. These procedures must guarantee that the content of ethylene oxide is lower than 1 ppm, and that the content of halogenated ethylene hydrines is lower than 150 ppm on material sterilized by ethylene oxide at the time of use. The manufacturer of each device or instrument which should be sterilized by ethylene oxide must declare the conditions necessary for sterilization and decontamination (SED-11, 479).

Occupational exposure of the sterilizing staff with ethylene oxide in hospitals, tissue banks and research facilities may result during any of the following operations and conditions: changing pressurized ethylene oxide gas cylinders; leaking valves, firrings and piping; leaking sterilizer door gaskets; opening of sterilizer doors at the end of a cycle; improper ventilation at the sterilizer door; improperly or unventilated air gap between the discharge line and the sewer drain; removal of items from the sterilizer and transfer of the sterilized load to aerator; improper ventilation of aerators and aeration areas; incomplete aeration items; inadequate general room ventilation; passing near sterilizers and aerators during operation (42[CR]). In most studies, exposure appears to result mostly from peak emissions during such operations as opening the door of sterilizer, and unloading and transferring sterilized material. Although much smaller amounts are used in sterilizing medicinal instruments and supplies in hospitals and industrially, it is during these uses that the highest occupational exposure levels have been measured. On the other hand, proper engineering controls and work practices are reported to result in full-shift exposure levels of less than 0.1 ppm (0.18 mg/m^3) and short-term exposure levels of less than 2 ppm (3.6 mg/m^3) (42[CR]). A regular medical follow-up is advisable for the sterilizing staff.

Uptake and elimination Ethylene oxide is readily taken up by the lung. At steady state, 20–25% of inhaled ethylene oxide reaching the alveolar space is exhaled as unchanged compound and 75–80% is taken up by the body and metabolized. Aqueous ethylene oxide solutions can penetrate human skin. The compound is rapidly and uniformly distributed throughout the body. It is eliminated metabolically by hydrolysis and by conjugation with glutathione and glycol. The elimination half-life has been estimated as between 14 minutes and 3.3 hours in the human (43[C]–47[C]). It is excreted mainly in the urine as thioethers; at higher doses, the proportion of thioethers is reduced, while the proportion of ethylene glycol increases. Ethylene oxide alkylates nucleophilic groups in biological macromolecules. Hemoglobin adducts have been used to monitor tissue doses of ethylene oxide (48^R).

Irritating effects caused by residue in ethylene oxide-sterilized materials Some communications report irritating effects caused by liberation of residue of ethylene oxide and its reaction products in industrial materials, e.g. tracheal stenosis by tracheotomy cannulae, severe bronchospasms and asthmatic attacks after endotracheal anesthesia by endotracheal tubes, anaphylaxis in a hemodialysis patient from plastic and rubber connecting tubes in an arteriovenous shunt, postoperative inflammatory reactions to intraocular lenses, allergic contact dermatitis and hemolysis of blood following exposure to plastic tubing sterilized with ethylene oxide (SED-11, 479).

Dialyzer hypersensitivity syndrome *(SED-11, 219, 479)* This syndrome presents as an acute anaphylactoid reaction, the symptoms of which may range from mild to life threatening in severity. The cause of the syndrome is unknown, but affected patients appear to have a high incidence of positive radioabsorbent tests to a conjugate of human serum albumin and ethylene oxide used to sterilize artificial kidneys. This conjugate may be the allergen responsible. Leitman et al. observed the syndrome in six of 600 donors who underwent automated platelet pheresis procedures. In skin-prick testing, four of the six donors (but none of the 40 controls) had positive tests when an ethylene oxide-human serum albumin reagent was used. Radioallergosorbent testing revealed that serum from four of the six donors, but only one of 145 controls, contained IgE antibodies to ethylene oxide-albumin.

Acute toxicity Jay et al. examined 12 men who were exposed to ethylene oxide after a sterilizer developed a leak. Although the levels of ethylene oxide were not monitored, all four operators intermittently smelled the ethylene oxide gas, roughly indicating a level of more than 700 ppm. All four operators developed neurological disorders. One operator who had been working for only 3 weeks, developed headaches, nausea, vomiting and lethargy followed by major motoric seizures. The other three had all been working for more than 2 years and experienced headache, limb numbness and weakness, increased fatigue, trouble with memory and slurred speech. Three of them developed cataracts, and one required bilateral cataract extractions. Four men, two of whom had not worked directly with the leaking sterilizer, had increased central corneal thickness with normal endothelial cell counts (SED-11, 479).

Carcinogenicity Ethylene oxide is carcinogenic, assigned to Group 1 of the International Agency for Research of Cancer (IARC) (48^R). However, while there is limited evidence in humans for carcinogenicity, there is sufficient evidence in experimental animals.

The overall evaluation of the Working group of the IARC, updated in 1995, is based on following supporting evidence. Ethylene oxide is a directly acting alkylating agent that:
(a) induces a sensitive, persistent dose-related increase in the frequency of chromosomal abberations and sister chromatid exchange in peripheral lymphocytes and micronuclei in bone marrow cells of exposed workers;
(b) has been associated with malignancies of the lymphatic and hemopoietic system in both humans and experimental animals;
(c) induces a dose-related increase in the frequency of hemoglobin adducts in exposed humans and a dose-related increase in the numbers of adducts in both DNA and hemoglobin in exposed rodents;
(d) induces gene mutations and heritable translocations in germ cells of exposed rodents;
(e) is a powerful mutagen and clastogen at all phylogenetic levels.

In 1979, Hogsted et al. (56^C) reported three cases of hematopoietic cancer that had occurred between 1972 and 1977 in workers at a Swedish factory where 50% ethylene oxide and 50% methyl formate had been used since 1968 to sterilize hospital equipment. In epidemiological studies of exposure to ethylene oxide, the most frequently reported association has been with lymphatic and hematopoietic cancer. Two populations were studied, people using ethylene oxide as a sterilant and chemical workers manufacturing or using the compound. Of the *studies of sterilization personnel*, the largest and most informative is that conducted in the USA (57^C, 58^C). Overall, mortality from lymphatic and hematopoietic cancer was only marginally elevated, but a significant trend was found, especially for lymphatic leukemia and non-Hodgkin's lymphoma, in relation to estimated cumulative exposure. For exposure at a level of 1 ppm (1.8 mg/m^3) over a working lifetime of 45 years, a ratio of 1.2 was estimated for lymphatic and hematopoietic cancer. The other studies of workers involved in sterilization in Sweden (59^C–61^C) and in the United Kingdom (62^C) each showed nonsignificant excess of lymphatic and hematopoietic cancer.

Because of the possibility of confounding occupational exposures in the studies of chemical workers exposed to ethylene oxide (59^C, 60^C, 62^C–72^C) less weight can be given to the positive findings. Nevertheless, they are compatible with the small but consistent excess of lymphatic and hematopoietic cancer found in the studies of sterilization personnel. Some of the epidemiological studies show an additional risk for cancer of the stomach, which was significant only in one study from Sweden (59[C], 60[C], 63[C]).

Mutagenicity There is overwhelming evidence that ethylene oxide produces genetic damage in a wide range of organisms including somatic cells of exposed humans. A detailed review is given by Dellarco et al. (48[R], 73[R]):

> Ethylene oxide is a germ-cell mutagen in rodents In male mice it is an inducer of chromosome breaks leading to dominant-lethal mutations and heritable translocations, sensitive stages appear to be restricted to late spermatides and early spermatozoa. In females, ethylene oxide also induces presumed dominant-lethal mutations.
>
> When females are exposed shortly after mating or during the early pronuclear stage of the zygote, high frequencies of fetal anomalies are induced.
>
> Ethylene oxide was found ineffective in inducing morphological-specific locus mutations in spermatogonial-stem cells; however, it produced dominant visible and electrophoretic-specific locus mutants in male mice, which are assumed be derived from post-stem cells.
>
> The effectiveness of ethylene oxide in inducing chromosome breaks in germ cells of male mice is strongly influenced by varying levels or rates of exposure. Since a dose-rate effect for ethylene oxide-induced dominant lethal mutations was observed at high concentrations and long exposure periods, considering the short burst exposure and low TWA exposure in humans, the question of whether significant dose-rate effects also exist at low-exposure levels remain unanswered.

Cytogenetic studies in peripheral lymphocyte of humans exposed to ethylene oxide (*SED*-12, 574) Several studies were performed involving workers in hospital ethylene oxide sterilization units or plants. In general, the studies indicate that these workers display elevated frequencies of chromosomal aberrations, including micronuclei and sister chromatid exchanges in peripheral lymphocytes.

The IARC-Working Group reviewed the published studies of workers exposed to ethylene oxide in hospital and factory sterilization units and in ethylene manufacturing and processing plants (49[R]). The studies consistently showed chromosomal damage in peripheral blood lymphocytes, including chromosomal aberrations in 11 of 14 studies, sister chromatid exchange in 20 of 23 studies, micronuclei in three of eight studies, and gene mutation in one study. In general the degree of damage is correlated with level and duration of exposure. The induction of sister chromatid exchange appears to be more sensitive to exposure to ethylene oxide than is that of either chromosomal aberrations or micronuclei. In one study, chromosomal aberrations were observed in the peripheral emphocytes of workers 2 years after cessation of exposure to ethylene oxide, and sister chromatid exchanges 6 months after cessation of exposure. But, in one study (72[C]), Tates et al. show that an incidental exposure to high concentrations of ethylene oxide did not cause any measurable permanent mutational/cytogenetic damage in lymphocytes of exposed persons.

Teratogenicity In animal experiments ethylene oxide exerts toxic effects at the reproduction process and is teratogenic, but the consequences of the animal and epidemiological studies in relation to occupational exposure levels of humans in the environment of sterilization units are unclear at times (SED-12, 576; 74[R]).

CHLORHEXIDINE (HIBITANE) *(SEDA-5, 254)*

Chlorhexidine (1,1′-hexamethylene-bis[5-(*p*-chlorophenyl)biguanice]) is a widely used antibacterial agent with activity against gram-positive and gram-negative bacteria (less against *Pseudomonas* species) as well as yeasts. It was introduced as an antiseptic in the early 1950s. Primarily it has been used for topical antisepsis, e.g. preoperative skin disinfection, and for disinfection of materials, mainly in combination with cetrimide. Long-term experience has demonstrated a low incidence of sensitization and a low irritant potential (SED-111, 480).

Unwanted effects have resulted from undue reliance on the disinfecting properties of chlorhexidine. Hospital-acquired infections have been caused by infected chlorhexidine used for bladder irrigation and for storage or disinfection of catheter spigots and needles (SED-11, 480). A microbiological analysis of chlorhexidine-cream tubes, repeatedly used by patients with indwelling urethral catheters, demonstrated high contamination with potential pathogens in 32% of cream samples and in 35% of swabs taken from the outside of the tubes beneath the screw cap (SED-11, 480).

Use of chlorhexidine in dentistry In recent years, chlorhexidine has been used as an adjuvant for plaque control and in the treatment of gingival inflammation. Generally, chlorhexidine is considered to be effective in the control of plaque, and may be helpful in the treatment of gingivitis. The agent can be applied in the form of a solution, used as a mouthrinse or with a toothbrush, in dentifrice or as a gel. The concentrations used are between 0.05 and 2% chlorhexidine (SED-11, 480). It is very difficult to summarize the effect of chlorhexidine on oral hygiene, since studies differ markedly as regards the population studied, the occurrence of gingival lesions, the application of other oral hygiene regimens, previous scaling, and polishing of the teeth, etc. The most frequently reported side effects of oral use are discoloration of the teeth, tongue and buccal mucosa, taste disorders and desquamation of the oral mucosa. A mild increase in gingival bleeding was reported after use of chlorhexidine mouthwash as compared with mechanical cleaning methods (SEDA-8, 244).

Staining of teeth, tongue and oral mucosal surfaces Staining of the teeth was the first and principal side effect observed. Fløtra et al. demonstrated, by a 4-month study of soldiers who applied chlorhexidine mouthwashes in concentrations of 0.1 and 0.2% chlorhexidine, that 15% of the interproximal surface and 62% of the fillings, especially the old and porous ones, were discolored. The stain intensity seems to be directly correlated to the concentration of the applied chlorhexidine preparation and to the frequency and duration of usage. The type of administration—0.2% mouthwash or 0.2% spray or 1% gel—does not seem to influence the amount of tooth staining. The initial discoloration is yellow-brown, but prolonged use and stronger concentrations result in a dark-brown color. Extensive investigations have been performed to evaluate factors that influence tooth-staining and the possibilities of their avoidance. The etiology of extrinsic tooth discoloration is not fully understood. However, the available evidence indicates that browning and formation of pigmented metal sulfides are the most likely causes of staining, while dietary factors (such as beverages or red wine) and smoking may play an aggravating role only (see SED-10, 427).

A discoloration of the dorsum of the tongue occurs in up to one-third of subjects using chlorhexidine mouthrinses. It does not occur during the use of chlorhexidine-containing dentifrices or gels (SED-11, 481).

Taste impairment and/or a disturbance of taste sensations These are especially seen with the chlorhexidine mouthwashes (SED-11, 481; SED-12, 577). It occurs in approximately one-third of the subjects and is perhaps the main complaint. Symptoms comprise a burning sensation, feeling of soreness, dryness in the mouth, and a bitter aftertaste lasting from a few minutes up to several hours. It is worth mentioning that symptoms also occur, but to a lesser extent, in placebo or control groups.

Desquamation and ulceration of the oral mucosa This has been observed after the use of chlorhexidine mouthwashes. The frequency of this side effect must be very low. Histological and histochemical examination of mucosal biopsies taken after 18 months of daily exposure to chlorhexidine did not reveal any adverse effect on the oral mucosa. Heideman et al. found *increased keratinization of human gingiva cells* in vitro in cell cultures, if the chlorhexidine concentration exceeded 25 μg/ml, and he found the same acceleration of keratinization of human gingiva cells in gingival swabs after rinsing with 0.025, 0.05, and 0.1% chlorhexidine solutions. Furthermore, he reported on one case with excessive disturbances in the wound-healing process after daily rinses with a 0.1% chlorhexidine solution following oral surgery (SED-11, 481).

Finally, reversible swelling of the *parotid glands* has been reported occasionally after use of chlorhexidine mouthwashes; this is probably due to mechanical obstruction of the parotid duct by over-rigorous rinsing (SED-11, 481).

Atrophic gastritis This was reported in a 72-year-old man with Parkinson's disease. He had used a 4% chlorhexidine solution for a daily mouthwash and swallowed it. Gastroscopy showed multiple erosions in the lower part of his stomach and the first part of the duodenum (75^C).

In summary, it must be pointed out that with excessive long-term use of chlorhexidine as a mouthwash, gel or dentifrice no deleterious side effects have been reported, and from the point of view of human safety chlorhexidine seems to be suitable for long-term oral use. However, the development of tooth-staining imposes a practical cosmetic limitation to such use.

Neurotoxicity after topical exposure in the middle ear Bicknell observed 14 patients who suffered from a severe sensorineural deafness among 97 patients who underwent a myringoplasty operation. The only common factor in all these patients was the preoperative skin disinfection of the ear with 0.5% chlorhexidine in a 70% alcoholic solution.

Parker and James and Aurnes performed extensive investigations of the ototoxicity caused by chlorhexidine after introducing it into the middle ear of guinea-pigs. The extent of severe vestibular and cochlear damage was related to the concentration of chlorhexidine, to the duration of exposure and to the time-lapse after exposure.

The middle ear should be carefully protected against chlorhexidine solutions in preoperative skin disinfection in otolaryngology (SED-11, 481).

Effects on olfactory senses after topical use Yamagishi et al. reported a reversible hyposmia after Hardy's operation for pituitary adenomas following preoperative disinfection of the nasal cavity with chlorhexidine. The olfactory disturbance improved after 3–7 weeks. Degeneration of the olfactory epithelium was also seen in guinea-pigs when the nasal cavities were irrigated 3 times with 5 ml 0.5% chlorhexidine solution; regeneration of the epithelium started after 14 days and the surfaces appeared normal after 1 month (SED-11, 481).

Use of chlorhexidine in neonatal skin care The withdrawal of hexachlorophene-containing products for routine neonatal skin care stimulated investigations into the possible use of chlorhexidine in this field. Its activity range includes effectiveness of high dilutions against gram-positive and gram-negative bacteria, yeast and molds. In studies of nursery populations chlorhexidine appears to be as effective as hexachlorophene in preventing staphylococcal colonization and infection. Until now, there is no evidence suggesting that chlorhexidine promotes gram-negative colonization in neonates bathed in water containing chlorhexidine (SED-11, 482).

Data presented in three studies provide substantial evidence in support of very low percutaneous absorption in fullterm infants and also in excessively exposed newborn rhesus monkeys. However, traces of chlorhexidine were found in adipose tissue (two of five monkeys), kidneys (five of five), and liver (one of five), indicating some absorption percutaneously or by oral ingestion, following the rigorous bathing procedure in the above study. The grooming habits of the monkeys could have played a role (SED-12, 578).

Use of chlorhexidine in routine neonatal cord care About 0.2 ml of undiluted 4% chlorhexidine solution with a detergent was included in the daily routine of rubbing the dry cord stump and the surrounding skin, which were then rinsed and dried. No chlorhexidine was detectable in the blood samples of the neonates, taken on the fifth day (76[C]).

Use of chlorhexidine in spermicides This has been promoted as a strategy for protection against sexually transmitted diseases including HIV. But both the claim of protection and the cytotoxicity of chlorhexidine, with a risk of damage to the epithelia of the vagina, cervix and glans penis due to chronic exposure, have to be further validated (77[C]).

Contact sensitivity and allergic reactions Allergic reactions to chlorhexidine such as contact dermatitis, contact urticaria and photosensitive dermatitis are relatively rare.

In a collaborative Danish study, 2061 patients were patch-tested which chlorhexidine gluconate 1% in water. A positive reaction was found in 2.3% of the patients. This was more common in patients with leg eczema (6.8%) or leg ulcer (10.6%) than in those with eczema of the hands (1.9%) or at other sites (1.6%). Of the 14 patients who were retested with chlorhexidine only one was positive to the 1% solution and none to a 0.01% solution. This apparent loss of sensitivity may be due to irritable skin at the initial testing, the so-called excited skin syndrome. This study suggests that the sensitizing potential of chlorhexidine is very low, but that it should be used with caution in dressings for leg ulcers.

Andersen and Brandrup tested 1063 consecutive eczema patients with the ICDRG standard series, supplemented with chlorhexidine gluconate 1% in water and 1% in petrolatum. The frequency of positive reactions was similar to that in the collaborative study.

Osmundsen observed 14 patients with a strong and obviously relevant reaction among 551 who patients who were patch-tested with chlorhexidine. Severe dermatitis had developed in 10 patients with venous or traumatic ulcers of the leg, and in four patients with skin infections on the face and/or scalp.

Bergqvist-Karlsson et al. (78[CR]) described a case with both contact urticaria and delayed-type contact allergy to chlorhexidine.

Rare but *life-threatening anaphylactic reactions* with generalized urticaria, dyspnea, and shock were reported by Okano et al. (79[Cr]) in six patients after use of 0.05, 0.5 or 1% chlorhexidine, and in one patient reported by Ohtoshi et al. (80[C]) following topical use of an alcoholic 0.5% chlorhexidine digluconate solution. A severe systemic allergic response was observed in a patient in whom the large donor area of skin graft was dressed with Bactigras which contains 0.5% chlorhexidine acetate (83[C]).

Evans (69[c]) reported an acute anaphylactic reaction in a 19-year-old man after cleaning of burns on the left arm. In this case the scratch test with chlorhexidine acetate 0.05% was positive.

An earlier report to the Japanese Ministry of Welfare about reactions observed between 1967 and 1984 included 22 cases with a fall of blood pressure, 13 with dyspnea, nine with anaphylactic shock, four with cyanosis, 19 cases showed erythema, 11 urticaria, nine pruritus, and seven facial wheals. Following this report, in 1984, the Japanese Ministry of Welfare recommended that the use of chlorhexidine on mucous membranes be prohibited because of the evidence that this application could provoke anaphylactic shock. Application of chlorhexidine on wound surfaces appears to be safe, but it should be used at the lowest bactericidal concentration of 0.05% (79[Cr]).

Occupational asthma Waclawski et al. (82[c]) described three well-documented case reports of occupational asthma in nurses, caused by chlorhexidine-alcohol disinfectant spray.

Sclerosing peritoneal disease This occurred in peritoneal dialysis patients in whom the tubing connection had been disinfected with chlorhexidine (84[C]–86[C]). Cases (214) were reported from 112 centers in European countries up to 1984 (SEDA-15, 250).

Toxic effects A newborn showed cyanotic spells associated with sinus bradycardia but not with apnea on the third day of life. The mother had used a chlorhexidine spray on her breasts from the third feed onwards. Bradycardia became less frequent and less severe from day 4 after the spray was stopped, and had abated completely by day 6. The serum chlorhexidine concentration was estimated at 11 pg/l on day 5 (87[C]).

In 1988 five normal newborn breast-fed babies were accidentally fed a dilute antiseptic solution containing chlorhexidine 0.05% with cetrimide 1% instead of sterile water They developed caustic burns of the lips, mouth and tongue within minutes. One baby became severely ill due to acute pulmonary edema, but all survived without sequelae (88[c]).

Risk of an accidental contamination of the eye by preoperative face disinfection Tabor et al. (89[c]) described four patients in whom accidental cornea exposure to Hibiclens, containing 4% chlorhexidine formulated with a detergent, resulted in keratitis, with severe and permanent corneal opacification.

Epithelial and stromal edema of the cornea and a diffuse bullous keratopathy developed in a 39-year-old woman 2 weeks after a preoperative disinfection of the face with an alcoholic chlorhexidine solution. This led to penetrating keratoplasty 10 months later (90[C]). Varley et al. (91[C]) described the histopathological findings of the cornea in such cases. They include epithelial edema with bullous changes marked loss of keratocytes, a thickened Descemet's membrane, and an attenuated, disrupted cell layer.

Care should be taken during preoperative skin preparation to keep chlorhexidine out of the eye and to flush copiously with sterile saline solution or sterile water if contact accidentally occurs.

HEXETIDINE

Hexetidine (5-amino-1,3-bis(2-ethylhexyl)hexahydro-5-methylpyrimidine) has in recent years been more widely advertized as an oral-cavity antiseptic. At the concentration normally employed (1 mg/ml), it is effective against gram-positive bacteria and *Candida albicans* in vitro, but insufficiently active against most gram-negative bacteria, but the duration of the germ count reduction is not longer than 1 hour. When applied to the mucosa it also appears to have mild local anesthetic properties. Very little critical clinical work on the substance has been published (SED-11, 482). A review of five studies of the prophylactic intravaginal use of chlorhexidine vaginal suppositories before delivery and in obstetrics was published in 1991 by Weidinger et al. (92[R]). No severe adverse reactions are reported. Plath and Otten, who used the preparation as a buccal and pharyngeal antiseptic in 61 patients, noted that a minority of individuals, generally those who had just undergone tonsillectomy, complained of a burning sensation and a salty taste.

It is not clear whether the use of the product as a spray, of which some elements will certainly be inhaled, affects its clinical tolerance or not. Mann and Wagner did not record side effects when reporting on 81 patients treated in this way, but their report is not sufficiently detailed for a full assessment. Merk et al. refer to a case of allergic contact dermatitis (SED-11, 482).

HALOGENS

Chlorine compounds

Chlorine compounds are used for disinfection of relatively clean impervious surfaces, water in small swimming pools and drinking water. Solutions containing 10 000 ppm 'available chlorine' are effective against hepatitis B and HIV-virus and are used to disinfect surfaces contaminated with body fluids.

Hypochloride

Alkaline hypochloride solutions with 0.25% 'available chlorine' were used to clean and disinfect wounds, but it was shown that their toxicity to wound cells could delay healing.

Use as an irrigating solution during endodontic treatment Linn et al. (93[c]) reported one patient who developed ulceration and paresthesia of the lip with facial swelling following the accidental injection of Milton solution (sodium hypochloride 1%, sodium chloride 16,5%) into the upper lip when a sharp needle was used for irrigation. The ulceration healed within 6 weeks, the paresthesia within 3 months. A similar case was reported by Becker et al. (94[C]) with an accidental injection of a solution (25 mg NaClO) into periapical tissue, and also by Herrmann et al. (95[c]) after an injection (90 mg) into the mandibular branch of the facial nerve.

Accidental intraperitoneal infusion Accidental intraperitoneal infusion of hypochloride solution on two occasions (the first time with about 10 ml of a 5% solution the second time more diluted) was reported by Dedhia et al. (96[C]). Following infusion the patient felt severe abdominal pain accompanied by nausea but not by vomiting. Elevated peritoneal solute transport rates and reduced ultrafiltration gradually subsided, but they did not return to pre-infusion values.

Accidental intravenous infusions These were reported from Marroni et al. (97[cr]), Froner et al. (98[c]) and Hoy et al. (99[c]).

A 68-year-old man with a *Listeria monocytogenes* infection received accidental infusion of a 1% sodium hypochlorite solution. After 1 hour and an infusion volume of 150 ml, the infusion (1500 mg NaClO) was stopped. The patient had a slow heart rate, mild hypotension, and an increased respiratory rate. The blood cell count, hemoglobin, serum electrolytes, creatine, urea, and aminotransferase activity were normal were and hemolysis did not occur. Treatment with NaCl 0.9% and dextrose solutions at an infusion rate of 300 ml/hour was started immediately with the goal of maintaining adequate diuresis. Furosemide and dopamine hydrochloride also were administered. Blood pressure and respiratory rate promptly returned to normal, but the bradycardia persisted for 3 days despite atropine sulfate administration. The patient was discharged from the hospital after 58 days with a diagnosis of *L. monocytogenes* meningoencephalomyelitis and had persistent lower limb paralysis on physical examination at follow-up 2 months later (97[cr]).

One patient received an accidental infusion of a large dose during hemodialysis (30 ml of a 5.25% solution, 1500 mg NaClO). This led to more significant toxicity characterized by cardiorespiratory arrest and massive hemolysis with hyperkalemia, although the patient eventually recovered (99[c]).

The intravenous infusion of 60 ml of an oral and 0.3 ml of a parenteral 5.25% solution in a suicide attempt did not result in any serious effects (98[c]).

Chloramine T

Chloramine T (tosylchloramide) has been used as a wound disinfectant, a general surgical antiseptic and for the disinfection of water. It seldom causes side effects. Urticaria and rhinitis, dyspnea and edema in the face were reported in a female nurse following contact. Specific IgE antibodies to chloramine T were demonstrated (SED-11, 492).

IODOPHORS *(SED-11, 487)*

Iodophors are labile complexes of elemental iodine with macromolecular carriers that not only serve to increase the solubility of iodine but rather to provide a sustained release of iodine.

Povidone-iodine (PVP-I)

Povidone-iodine is the most widely used iodophor, with the carrier molecule PVP-I (poly-I(I-vinyl-2-pyrrolidinone)). PVP-I is used as a 10% applicator solution, a 2% cleansing solution and in many preparations administered topically, e.g. aerosol sprays, aerosol foams, vaginal gels, ointments and mouthwashes. Because of the very low amount of free iodine—less than 1 ppm in a 10% solution—antibacterial effectiveness is only moderate compared with that of an iodine solution.

Absorption (*SED*-11, 487; *SEDA*-10, 230; *SEDA*-11, 220) Repeated surgical skin antisepsis and hand washing did not elevate serum iodine concentrations, but produced a low increase in iodine content in the 24-hour urine (100[CR]).

The extent of systemic absorption of PVP-I depends on the localization and the conditions of its use (area, skin surface, mucous membranes, wounds, body cavities).

The use of PVP-I for the treatment of burns, for peritoneal lavage in the treatment of purulent peritonitis, or as a rinsing solution for body cavities, may increase serum iodine concentrations associated with elevation of urinary excretion of iodine. In burn victims the extent of iodine resorption depends on the size of the burned body surface. More than 1000 μg/ml iodine are not uncommon. If renal function is intact, the iodine elimination with the urine may exceed this level and is proportional to the serum levels. The serum iodine level is normalized about 1 week after the last application of PVP. When PVP is used as a rinsing solution in body cavities, the absorption of the whole macromolecular PVP-I complex is also possible. The complex-compound PVP-I has a molecular weight of about 60 000 and cannot be eliminated by the kidneys or metabolically. It is filtered by the reticuloendothelial system (100[CR], 101[C], 102[C]).

Colcleuth (103[C]) tested the penetration of PVP in vivo on rabbits. The penetration from third-degree burns on the back was measured autoradiographically in tissue as well in blood, in urine and in bandages. The results indicate that approximately 20% of iodine is absorbed through a fresh necrosis, whereas only 5% is absorbed through a clean wound or a 24-hour old necrosis. The passage through a burn necrosis was faster than through vital tissue.

In repeated topical use on burns the extent of absorption seems to decrease with the treatment time.

Effects on the thyroidal system The extensive iodine absorption connected with the use of PVP-I in burns and body cavities may cause the well-known side effects on thyroidal regulation, namely a passing hypothyroidism or, in cases with latent hypothyroidism, the danger of destabilization and thyrotoxic crises.

Especially at risk are patients with an autonomous adenoma, a localized diffuse autonomy of the thyroid gland, a nodular goiter, a latent hyperthyroidism of autoimmune origin, or with an endemic iodine deficit (100[R]).

Hematological side effects Alvarez reported a case of severe neutropenia in a patient in whom serious burns (deep, second-degree burns, involving about 50% of the body surface) were being treated with Betadine Helafoam twice a day.

Neurological side effects Seizures were described in a 62-year-old man treated with continuous mediastinal irrigation with a 1:10 solution of PVP (104[c]) on the fifth day of drainage. After the seizure, his serum iodine levels were found to be elevated (120 μg/ml). Renal failure developed at the same time. The EEG showed no evidence of epileptic activity or other abnormalities. The PVP-I irrigation was replaced by continuous irrigation with a solution of neomycin and polymyxin B. Renal function improved, with the creatinine concentration returning to normal 3 days after the seizure.

Effect of PVP-I on wound healing PVP-I causes a concentration-dependent damage to cells and clusters. The effect is most pronounced for isolated cells, but it is also detectable in the more complex tissues. Clinical experiences with burn victims cannot rule out the probability that the healing process might be slightly retarded. However, this deficiency might be balanced by an appropriate microbicidal effect on the healing edge (105[R]).

Allergic reactions In principle, all forms of the well-known iodine-induced allergic reactions such as iododerma tuberosum, dermatitis, petechiae and sialadenitis are possible, but the incidence seems to be very low (SED-11, 488; SED-12, 586). A severe anaphylactoid reaction was reported immediately after the instillation of a 10% PVP-I solution into a hydatid cyst cavity during surgery. A severe bronchospasm developed immediately and was followed by a coagulopathy and subsequent liver and renal failure (106[c]).

Interference with laboratory tests Van Steirtegham et al. investigated the influence of PVP-I used for skin disinfection before skin puncture blood was taken. The levels of potassium, phosphate and uric acid were changed after the use of PVP-I, but a wide range of other tests were unaffected. PVP-I gives a positive reaction with an orthotoluidine reagent, e.g. Hematest reagent tablets or dipsticks (SED-11, 488).

Intravaginal and obstetric use Routine vaginal douching with PVP-I during pregnancy induces maternal iodine overload and markedly increases the iodine content in amniotic fluid and of the fetal thyroid, as soon as the trapping mechanism of iodine by the thyroid has started to develop. The vaginal application of PVP-I is therefore not recommended during pregnancy (107[CR], 108[CR]).

The fetal thyroid starts with the storage of iodine between the 10th and 13th weeks of gestation, and with thyroid hormone secretion between the 18th and 24th weeks. Especially after intravaginal administration during pregnancy, PVP-I may induce an iatrogenic congenital goiter and hypothyroidism in newborn infants. However, hyperthyroidism can also be induced.

Jacobsen et al. (109[C]) published the first case on iodine absorption after intravaginal PVP-I administration.

Vorherr et al. (110[C]) reported a distinct increase in iodine, protein-bound iodine and inorganic iodine, but not in serum thyroxine, after a 2-minute vaginal administration of PVP-I in non-pregnant women.

Grüters et al. (111[C]) reported that 99 of 9320 newborns exhibited TSH concentrations above the normal value (20 μU/ml) on the fifth day of life, but during a control examination between the 10th and 21st day all these infants displayed normal TSH levels and normal thyroid function. In 76 of the newborns with hyperthyrotropinemia, urinary iodine excretion was significantly elevated (above 16 μg/ml). Most of them were born in obstetric departments where iodophores were routinely used for disinfection during labor. The same authors (112[c]) therefore performed a controlled study in 66 mothers and their infants who were exposed to PVP-I during labor and delivery.

Following the technique of Saling, a plastic catheter was inserted into the portio with a ring pessary or attached to the scalp electrode for fetal heart rate monitoring, and a 1 or 2% solution of PVP-I was pumped through until delivery; the duration of treatment varied from 5 to 30 hours. Urinary iodide concentrations on the first and the fifth day and the serum iodine levels at birth were significantly elevated in the mothers as well as in their neotates. At birth, TSH concentrations of mothers and infants were no different from those of the control group, but on the third and fifth days they were significantly higher. Thyroxine (T4) levels were significantly lower in exposed mothers and infants (at birth, on the third and on the fifth days). One-fifth of the infants had high TSH concentrations ($>$20 μU/ml) and low T4 values ($<$7 μg/ml), which is suggestive of hypothyroidism, but none of the infants developed clinical symptoms, and on the 14th day the values were normal again. In the iodine-exposed mothers and infants liothyronine (T3) concentrations were significantly decreased at birth, but not thereafter. The reverse T3 concentrations did not differ from the controls at birth, but were significantly lower on the following days. This decrease in reverse T3 values in the iodine-exposed infants is probably a result of reduced T4 levels, causing a lack of substrate for monodeiodination to reverse T3.

It must be concluded that perinatal iodine exposure causes a transient hypothyroidism in a significant number of newborn infants. In these neonates, careful monitoring and follow-up of thyroid gland function are needed. For convenience and for safety, iodine-containing antiseptics should not be used in pregnancy or neonatology, especially if this follow-up cannot be guaranteed.

Use in newborn infants A number of cases of hypothyroidism in the newborn have been related to the use of small doses of iodine as an antiseptic. The high vulnerability of the newborn thyroid is a reason to avoid the use of PVP-I for the care of the umbilical stump or omphaloceles (SED-11, 488; SED-12, 585).

Arena et al. studied blood TSH and T4 concentrations 5–7 days after birth in 365 healthy newborns whose umbilical stump had been treated with 10% PVP-I. The prevalence of high TSH levels was higher in this group than in the general population (3.09 vs 0.417%, $P<0.001$), as was the rate of transient hypothyroidism (2.73 vs 0.25%, $P<0.001$). All children were found to be normal at retesting 1 week later. Tummers et al. reported a transient hypothyroidism due to skin contamination with PVP-I in a newborn infant with an omphalocele.

Castaing et al. studied the postnatal iodine overload after cutaneous application of PVP-I (0.96% I_2; Betadine) in 11 neonates. The mean iodine was 1297 μg/24 hours in the PVP-I group and 1253 μg/24 hours in the second group; in the control group 64% of the newborns showed an ioduria of less than 100 μg/24 hours, and of the 10 other patients (mean ioduria 1212 μg/24 hours) three were born by cesarean section: in these cases the mothers received an iodine-containing curariform agent. There were 12 cases of hypothyroidism among the newborns exposed to iodine-containing antiseptics, but none in the control group (SED-11, 488).

Smerdely et al. compared 29 very low-birth-weight infants admitted to a neonatal intensive care unit who had been administered chlorhexidine-containing antiseptics with a group of 54 infants in a comparable unit who had been administered routinely iodinated antiseptic agents. The latter showed an up to 50-fold higher increase in the urinary iodine excretion than the controls. The median of the serum TSH concentrations was significantly higher in the iodine-exposed (4.6 mIU/ml) than in the control infants (2.4 IU/ml). At day 14, TSH levels in nine of the 36 iodine-exposed infants were above 20 mIU/ml, their mean thyroxine level was significantly lower (44.1 nmol/l) than that in exposed infants with normal TSH levels (83.1 nmol/l) and in the control group (83.0 nmol/ml).

Use in mouthwash Ferguson et al. measured the influence of a PVP-I mouthwash on thyroid function in 16 medically healthy volunteers. After using the mouthwash 4 times daily for a period of 14 days all thyroid tests revealed significant changes, but the study did not show any suppression of thyroid function. This was not to be expected, considering the short test period.

Use in preoperative wound disinfection PVP-I may inhibit the leukocyte migration and fibroblast aggregation in wounds. Viljanto studied the influence of PVP-I on the wound healing process in 294 pediatric surgical patients, 283 of whom had undergone appendectomy.

In a first series using 5% PVP-I aerosol for preoperative disinfection the postoperative wound infection rate was 19% in the test group and only 8% in the controls. When a 1% PVP-I solution was applied, only 2.6% of the patients were infected (control group 8.5%). Using a drain with a cellulose viscose sponge, Viljanto found that the 5% PVP-I aerosol inhibited leukocyte migration, but no cell aggregates or fibroblasts were detected. The 5% PVP-I solution allowed better cellular movement and attachment on the framework, polymorphonuclear leukocytes predominating. The excipients of the aerosol formula must be more toxic to the cell than those of the solution. If a 1% PVP-I solution was absorbed by the sponge, the aggregation phenomenon was only slightly averted and cell morphology was similar to that of the saline control.

A decrease in the number of wound infections was noted only in those patients with appendicitis in whom neither peritonitis nor a peri-appendicular abscess had yet developed (SED-11, 489).

Peritoneal dialysis Although PVP-I is no longer used in dialyzates, a PVP-I-containing cap is used to seal the Tenckhoff catheter during the day. Vulsma et al. (113[c]) reported an iodine-induced hypothyroidism in a 3-year-old boy and an 18-month-old girl. In both cases the iodine source was shown to be the sealing cap. The PVP-I inside the cap diffused into the catheter and flushed into the peritoneal cavity at the next dialysis session.

Bacterial contamination of PVP-I preparations *Pseudomonas cepacia* was discovered in the blood cultures of 52 patients in four hospitals in New York over 7 months, and of 16 patients in a Boston hospital over a 10-week period in 1980 (114[C], 115[C]). A contaminated PVP-I solution produced by one manufacturer was implicated as the source of the pseudobacteria. The question remains why this solution was contaminated, whereas other currently marketed PVP-I solutions showing equivalent levels of available or free iodine remain sterile.

Guidelines for the use of PVP-I complexes In 1985 a working group of the Federal German Medical Association issued a number of recommendations for the safe use of PVP-I complexes (116). They can be summarized as follows:

(a) The application of PVP-I formulations cannot be recommended for *surgical hand disinfection* since active iodine-free preparations are available.

(b) The activity of PVP-I in case of *preoperative skin disinfection* in adults is well proven.

(c) PVP-I is appropriate for *skin disinfection* before an incision, a puncture, with use of intravenous or arterial

catheters, and for the prophylaxis of iatrogenic clostridial infections.
(d) In the case of *superficial wounds*, PVP-I can be applied occasionally or also repeatedly in spite of increased iodine absorption through the broken skin surfaces.
(e) *Lavage of wound and body cavities* with PVP-I or its instillation is not indicated due to increased iodine absorption.
(f) *Routine body washing* of patients in intensive care units should be avoided for cost-benefit considerations.
(g) PVP-I for *vaginal application* in infection or on hygienic grounds is not recommended.
(h) Due to the special risks for *premature and newborn infants and babies* the application of PVP-I is contraindicated in this age group. This also applies to prophylactic disinfection of the umbilical stump.
(i) The clinical usefulness of PVP-I in the treatment of *burns* is well proven.
(j) Local *mouth* antiseptics serve no therapeutic purpose. This is also true for PVP-I preparations.

MERCURY COMPOUNDS

INORGANIC MERCURY COMPOUNDS *(SEDA-8, 246; SEDA-9, 227; SEDA-10, 231)*

Repeated cutaneous application of inorganic mercury results in absorption and if applied on large body surfaces in *mercury poisoning*.

Yellow mercuric oxide

A 4-month-old boy was hospitalized with a weeping eczema covering more than the half of the body surface and complicated by skin hemorrhage and infection by *Klebsiella pneumoniae* and *Proteus mirabilis*. Apart from the general therapy, the following ointment was applied twice daily on the skin: zinc oxide 10 grams, salicylic acid 0.5 grams, yellow mercuric oxide 2 grams, zinc sulfate 0.5 grams, resorcine 1 gram, lanolin 40 grams. After 12 days, cardiovascular collapse, acute pulmonary edema and coma Stage II with right hemiparesis, generalized hypertonia and muscular tremor developed rapidly. Mercury levels in blood, urine and CSF were 12 μg/100 ml (normal <1 μg/100 ml), creatinine 260 μg/g (normal <5 μg/g) and 4.8 μg/l (normal <0.1 μg/l), respectively. Despite BAL therapy and vigorous supportive measures, the child's condition deteriorated, he developed a *Klebsiella aerogenes* septicemia and died 6 weeks later (117[Cr]).

Mercuric chloride *(SEDA-8, 246; SEDA-10, 231)*

Despite several warnings over many years, the use of mercuric chloride solutions during operations in an attempt to kill cancer cells implanted on healthy tissue persists in some countries. Especially intraperitoneal application, where seeding of a visceral cancer is feared, carries the risk of mercury absorption and nephrotoxicity. Laundy et al. (118[CR]) described the tenth reported case and the fifth known death of intoxication after peritoneal lavage with a mercuric chloride solution. *The characteristic clinical picture of acute mercury poisoning* includes sudden, profound circulatory collapse with tachycardia, hypotension and peripheral vasoconstriction, vomiting, and bloody diarrhea due to hemorrhagic colitis. Renal failure usually develops within 24 hours and is associated with albuminuria, epithelial cell casts and red cells in the urine, glycosuria, aminoaciduria. Oliguria may proceed to complete anuric failure. There is further, a neutrophil leukocytosis due to tissue necrosis (SED-11, 483).

ORGANIC MERCURY COMPOUNDS

Merbromin *(SEDA-8, 246)*

Merbromin (mercurochrome, disodium salt of 2,7-dibromo-4-hydroxymercurifluorescein) is the oldest organic mercurial antiseptic in use but it is active only as a bacteriostatic agent. In contrast to earlier assumptions, it is absorbed through burned or otherwise absorptive surfaces, and may cause severe and lethal intoxications. High mercury concentrations in blood, urine and organs have been demonstrated (SED-11, 483).

Use in local treatment of omphaloceles Neither merbromin nor thiomersal can today be considered the remedy of choice for the conservative management of large omphaloceles.

Use in local treatment of burns Weber reported on a 37-year-old patient with burns involving 50% of the body surface, who was treated by Grob's 3-phase method (2% merbromin, 5% tannic acid and 10% silver nitrate solutions). By the sixth day of treatment the patient had pink-colored urine and he progressively developed motoric unrest, confusion, and coma with hypothermia on the eight day. He died on the tenth day with respiratory arrest. The mercury concentration of the urine had been 2170 μg/l on the sixth day and 1250 μg/l on the ninth day. The authors pointed out that merbromin should no longer be used in the treatment of burns. However, Hiemer et al. reported good results in a retrospective study on the treatment of second-degree burns in 129 children using the same method (solutions with 7% silver nitrate and 2% merbromin). The authors pointed out that the indication is given only in second-degree burns, with burned surfaces of maximally 10—20% of the body surface, preferably in burn injuries of the trunk and non-mobile areas of the extremities. The most important factor seems to be careful attention to the serum sodium concentration and sufficient substitution with infusion therapy (SED-11, 483).

Hematological side effects Slee et al. described a patient suffering from mercury intoxication caused by the local application of merbromin to an operation wound; the patient developed aplastic anemia most probably connected with the antiseptic (SED-11, 483).

Risk situations Camarasa reported an anaphylactic reaction after local use of merbromin in one patient, and very virulent local reactions in patch-tests of several mercury-sensitive patients (SED-11, 483).

Thiomersal (SED-*10, 231)*

The danger of toxic effects and the efficacy of thiomersal (*O*-(ethylmercurithio)benzoic acid) are similar to those of merbromin. The problem of absorption of toxic amounts during omphalocele treatment has been discussed above. A case of fatal mercury (and borate) intoxication has been reported following ear irrigations with 0.1% thiomersal and 0.14% sodium borate for a purulent otitis media which was refractory to antibiotic therapy over 4 weeks (SED-11, 483).

Chemical burns by preoperative skin preparation Hodgkinson et al. have reviewed the histories of 25 patients with chemical burns caused by preoperative skin preparation. Thiomersal was the most common agent implicated. The burns did not occur in the main area of the preparation, but more peripherally where the solution was in close contact with the skin in the drapes or was more closely applied to the skin by pressure, either due to the patient's own weight or to tourniquet dressings. No burning occurred under a sterile wound drape (although solutions stagnate at this site and do not evaporate), perhaps because there is no pressure. There are particular risks in patients placed in the lithotomy position to undergo gynecological operations (the burns being on the buttocks), and in those undergoing orthopedic operations (the burns then being on the extremities and under a tourniquet) (SED-11, 483).

Use as a preservative in medical products Thiomersal is one of the most frequent sensitizers throughout the world (118[R]). It is used as an effective preservative in vaccines, test solutions as well as in topically administered applications, e.g. creams and solutions used on eczematous skin, ophthalmics, rhinologics and cleanser solutions for ocular contact lenses. Thiomersal concentration varies between 0.0005 and 0.01% in these preparations.

Sensitization is most likely provoked by immunization with thiomersal-containing vaccines. Even in sensitized patients, thiomersal-induced side effects due to vaccination has not been shown to be a severe risk and patch-test positively to thiomersal does not represent a contraindication to immunization with thiomersal-containing vaccines. Many of the reactions seen in patch-tests with 0.1% thiomersal are probably caused by the irritant nature of thiomersal. Lisi et al. (120[C]) pointed out that only half of a series of subjects tested with a solution of 0.1% thiomersal had a positive reaction in patch tests with concentrations of 0.05 and 0.01%.

Thiomersal included in patch-test series has given varying frequencies of positive reactions. Cross-reactions occur to a few organic mercurials, but not to inorganic or metallic mercury. The allergic determinant seems to be the ethylmercury radical of thiomersal.

Frequencies of positive reactions have been reported in the following countries: 13.4% in 1967 (121[c]) and 8% in 1972 (122[c]) in the US; 5.6 (123[c]) and 16.3% positive tests (130[c]) in Japan; 2.0% (124[c]) in Finland; 1.3% (125[c]) in Denmark; 6.9% (126[c]) in the GDR; 5.3% in a group of infant inpatients in Czechoslovakia (127[c]); 2.3% in a multicenter study on 200 adult patients submitted to routine patch-testing in France and Belgium (128[c]); and 5.3% in Italy (129[c]).

Möller (131[C]) found a very high peak frequency of positive patch tests in the 20—30 years age group in Sweden: 16% of male recruits and 10% of other healthy subjects in nursing schools and among medical students. A common reason for sensitization to thiomersal in the younger generation in Sweden arises from intracutaneous testing with tuberculin, containing thiomersal as a preservative. It was shown experimentally that tuberculin could act as adjuvant during sensitization to thiomersal. The iatrogenic occurrence of thiomersal allergy in the Swedish population does not result in eczematous reactions, but merely in false-positive cutaneous tests.

Thiomersal takes second place, after nickel, as a contact allergen in Austria. As in Sweden this high incidence is probably due also to frequent vaccination with vaccines containing thiomersal (132[C]).

Mackenzie and Vlahevic reported a *generalized allergic reaction* in a 50-year-old nurse with a documented allergy to thiomersal, who received 10 ml of human γ-globulin with thiomersal as a preservative. Maibach described a 38-year-old man who treated a mild sore throat himself with a thiomersal spray. Approximately 30 hours after the second application a severe laryngeal obstruction developed, and emergency tracheotomy was necessary. A subsequent patch-test produced a severe disseminated allergic reaction to thiomersal (SED-

11, 484). Serious allergic reactions are reported in 18 patients after Japanese encephalitis vaccine (133[C]). Reactions in 15 patients were thought to be related to the vaccine, 13 of these patients had urticaria affecting the whole body, one had erythema multiforme, and one had rash. Fourteen reactions arose after the second vaccination. Seven of the 13 urticaria reactions began within 24 hours of vaccination, the remaining six within 72 hours. In five patients encephalitis vaccine was the only vaccination given. It was noted that thiomersal concentration was increased from 0.0005% in previous vaccine batches, to 0.0067% in the batch used. The concentration of thiomersal was, however, that used in most vaccines.

In topical preparations thiomersal may lead to an *allergic contact dermatitis*. Möller (131[C]) found a high incidence of thiomersal allergy in patients with pompholyx, i.e. vesicular eruptions on the palms and soles.

A large number of cases of *allergic conjunctivitis* which have been reported were caused by thiomersal as a constituent of a solution for preserving soft contact lenses (SED-11, 484).

PARABENS *(SEDA-8, 246; SEDA-11, 221)*

Parabens (alkyl esters—methyl, ethyl, propyl and butyl—of *p*-hydroxybenzoic acid) are employed as preservatives in concentrations between 0.1 and 0.3% in pharmaceutical preparations, and in concentrations between 0.01 and 0.1% in cosmetics and foods. In such concentrations the parabens are devoid of systemic toxic effects, but allergic reactions have been reported. Parabens may cause allergic contact dermatitis which may run an insidious course, especially when the parabens are an ingredient of a steroid ointment. In such cases, treatment leads to a protracted dermatitis without acute exacerbation, so that neither the patient nor the physician suspects parabens as a possible cause. Schott obtained a sensitization index of 0.8% in 273 chronic dermatitis patients.

In 1973, a 10-center study of 1200 individuals carried out by the North American Contact Dermatitis Group found a 3% incidence of delayed hypersensitivity to parabens. General allergic reactions have also been reported following injections of parabens-containing preparations of lidocaine, hydrocortisone and after oral use of barium sulfate contrast suspension, haloperidol syrup and an antitussive syrup, all of which contained parabens (SED-11, 484).

PEROXIDES *(SEDA-12, 203; SEDA-14, 208; SEDA-16, 260; SEDA-17, 295)*

Hydrogen peroxide solution containing 5—7% H_2O_2 is used for cleansing wounds and ulcers. The disinfectant and deodorant action occurs by oxidation of cell materials during the rapid release of oxygen during contact of hydrogen peroxide with tissue. The solution does not penetrate well but the effervescence provides a mechanical means for detachment of necrotic tissue from inaccessible parts of wounds. It should not be used in closed body cavities. The germicidal action of hydrogen peroxide is relatively weak and of short duration.

A case of pneumomediastinum caused by subcutaneous emphysema has been reported in a 30-year-old man after the application of hydrogen peroxide solution to a root canal. The patient had acute pulpitis of the lower right third molar, treated by extirpation followed by irrigation with 3% hydrogen peroxide solution. Soon after irrigation, subcutaneous emphysema developed (134[c]).

Residues on insufficiently rinsed equipment disinfected by hydrogen peroxide may provoke local irritation, burns and general reactions. Non-specific *inflammation* has been reported with instantaneous blanching and effervescence on the surfaces of the intestinal mucosa during endoscopy (135[c]). *Hemolysis* was reported after hemodialysis therapy with a dialysis fluid inadvertently contaminated with hydrogen peroxide (136[C]).

PHENOL AND DERIVATIVES

The permeability of the human epidermis to many phenolic compounds is correlated with their lipophilic pattern. However, phenolic compounds appear to produce denaturation in the skin, and an additional increase in permeability is attributed to the resulting damage to the epidermis. Severe intoxications after skin administration of phenol or derivatives are possible.

Neonatal jaundice has been associated with the use of phenolic disinfectants in nurseries, not only when used in excessive concentrations (SEDA-4, 182), but also when applied in the recommended dilution (SEDA-5, 258; SEDA-8, 246; SED-11, 484).

Phenol

Phenol can be fatal in the newborn as shown by case histories. A 1-day-old child died 11 hours after 2%

phenol had been applied to the umbilicus. The post-mortem blood level of phenol was 12.5 mg/100 ml. A 6-day-old child developed cerebral symptoms, circulatory failure and methemoglobinemia after application of a phenol camphor solution (30% phenol, 60% camphor) to a skin ulcer. The child recovered after exchange transfusion (SED-11, 485).

Paratertiary butyl- and amylphenol

Depigmentation has been observed to be caused by germicides (O-Syl and Ves-Phene), containing a mixture of phenol derivatives, in five hospital workers and in seven other patients who had used these preparations as household disinfectants. Patch-tests with the phenolic components of the disinfectants on the patients and controls showed that virtually any moderately irritating phenolic compound can apparently depigment the skin, but of those tested, paratertiary butyl- and amylphenol most often depigmented the skin without producing a toxic inflammation. Initial signs of depigmentation appeared 6 months after using the phenolic mixtures. Within 1 year, two of five patients noted a spontaneous return of pigment; in another the use of the product was continued and there was no evidence of repigmentation (SED-11, 485).

Pentachlorophenol

This phenolic disinfectant is used in commercial laundries.

Intoxications after skin contact in newborn infants In 1967 a hospital laundry accidentally employed a product containing sodium pentachlorophenolate for a final rinse in the laundering of diapers and infants' bed linen. Twenty newborn infants developed sweating, tachycardia, tachypnea, hepatomegaly and metabolic acidosis. Six severe cases were subjected to exchange blood transfusion and in each instance there was a dramatic improvement. Two babies died before the exchange blood transfusion could be carried out; post-mortem examination showed fatty metamorphosis of the liver and hydropic and fatty degeneration of the renal tubules and myocardium. Toxic levels of pentachlorophenol were found in the serum of one patient and in autopsy tissue of another. Brandt reported chronic liver disease caused by long-term household poisoning with pentachlorophenol.

Immunosuppressive effects caused by chemical properties of pentachlorophenol Evidence of immunosuppressive effects and other clinicopathological symptoms has been discussed, suggested by interference by dibenzo-*p*-dioxin and/or dibenzofuran with the chemical properties of pentachlorophenol (SED-11, 485).

Chloroxylenol (PCMX) *(SED-11, 485)*

Since the withdrawal of hexachlorophene from the non-prescription drug market in the United States, PCMX (4-chloro-3,5-dimethylphenol) has been a substitute in a large number of products. PCMX apparently far exceeds hexachlorophene in its antigenic potential. Allergic contact dermatitis caused by PCMX is well known in Europe. In 1975, for example, Stors described seven individuals who developed allergic contact dermatitis following sensitization to PCMX, contained either in medicated vaseline or in electrocardiographic paste.

Myatt and Beck published the results of a retrospective analysis of patch tests in 951 patients; 1.8% had positive reactions to PCMX. Most of the patients had been sensitized by popular proprietary preparations containing PCMX (SEDA-11, 221).

Intoxications Intoxications were reported to be caused by oral ingestion and after skin administration.

Kumar et al. reported a 10-day-old baby who was given a bath in a 25% Dettol solution containing 1.2% PCMX. The child became hydrated and toxemic; it developed a diffuse erythema and vesicles, and afterwards an exfoliative dermatitis. The patient responded well to therapy with systemic steroids and supportive measures.

Chan et al. (137^C-139^C) published experiences from a relatively large number of oral Dettol liquid intoxications, a widespread household disinfectant, containing 4.8% chloroxylenol, pine oil and isopropyl alcohol and involved in 10% of self poisoning-related hospital admissions in Hong Kong. In a retrospective study of 67 cases, serious complications were relatively common (8%) and these included aspiration of Dettol with gastric contents resulting in pneumonia, cardiopulmonary arrest, bronchospasm, adult distress syndrome, and sever laryngeal edema with upper airway obstruction. In a group of 89 patients, five (5.6%) developed minor hematemesis, in the form of coffee-coloured or blood-stained vomitus (139^C). One patient had a gastroscopy performed on the day after admission, the examination demonstrated signs of chemical burns in the esophagus and stomach. Gastroscopy in one other patient on day 11, done to rule out esophageal stricture; showed no abnormality. All patients with hematemesis completely recovered. The authors suggest that upper gastrointestinal hemorrhage following Dettol ingestion tends to be mild and self-limiting. Gastroscopy, which may increase the risk of aspiration in patients with impaired consciousness, is not required unless other causes of gastrointestinal bleeding are suspected. Further, Dettol poisoning may be associated with an increased risk of aspiration, possibly caused by the use of gastric lavage in 88% of the patients and the occurrence of vomiting in 62% (140^C). Of 121 patients who ingested Dettol, three (2.5%) developed a renal impairment as evidenced by raised plasma urea and creatinine following ingestion of about 200–500 ml Dettol (140^C. Two of these patients also had serious complications, including aspiration leading to pneumonia and adult respiratory distress syndrome, one died. The renal impairment only appears to be observed when relatively large amounts of Dettol are ingested (140[C]).

Hexachlorophene (HCP) *(SED-11, 485)*

Hexachlorophene (2,2′-methylene-bis(3,4,6-trichlorophenol) has been extensively used as an ingredient of innumerable kinds of consumer goods and medical preparations. Since 1961, when it was reported that daily bathing of newborn infants with a 3% HCP suspension prevented colonization of the skin by coagulase-positive staphylococci, HCP has been widely used in hospital nurseries. As a result of investigations on the toxicity of HCP in animals and reports of accidental intoxications in France, the FDA in 1972 banned all non-prescription use of this drug, restricting HCP to prescription use only, as a surgical scrub and handwash product for health-care personnel. HCP was excluded from cosmetics, except as a preservative in levels not exceeding 0.1%. Other countries followed. An extensive critical review of HCP is given by Delcour-Firquet.

Neurotoxicity HCP treatment can induce cerebral edema, affecting exclusively the white matter of the brain and spinal cord and producing a spongiform encephalopathy which transforms the white matter into an almost unbelievable network of cystic spaces lined by fragments of myelin. Electron-microscopic studies demonstrated an intramyelinic location of the edema with splitting and separation of the myelin lamellae. Nerve damage appears to be reversible, although it takes many weeks for all the holes in the white matter to disappear. However, extensive edema occurring within a rigid structure such as the spinal canal can result in infarction of nervous tissue. The clinical symptoms resemble those of the intracranial hypertension.

Animal studies In animal experiments, there seems to be a clear relationship between dosage, blood levels, duration of treatment and morphological and functional disturbances of the nervous system. In the lower dose range, unequivocal histological evidence of neurotoxicity is produced, but without clinical symptoms of neurotoxicity (SED-9, 397; SED-11, 486).

Human studies and clinical experience The absorption of HCP by the intact skin has been demonstrated extensively. However, clinical symptoms of neurotoxicity have been observed only after dermal application of HCP to large areas of burned or otherwise excoriated skin, and on intact skin after accidental use of extremely high concentrations or after ingestion. It should be taken into consideration that, if HCP is applied in high concentrations or at frequent intervals to the intact skin, excoriation will result.

Neurotoxicity and use of HCP in newborn skin care The HCP concentrations in the blood, determined during newborn skin care with HCP bathing, cover a range which varies between studies but is similar to a level associated with neurotoxicity in rats, mice and monkeys (SED-9, 397, cf. Tables 2 and 3). In interpreting the HCP plasma levels we have to consider that the majority of HCP is probably distributed very rapidly in the lipophilic tissue compartments and low plasma concentrations may correspond to high tissue levels.

In 1969, Herter reported topical toxicity in a newborn infant treated with a 3% HCP lotion which had not been rinsed off. Four days later, the infant's skin was excoriated and there was muscular twitching which progressed to convulsions. Four days after discontinuation of HCP application the convulsions disappeared; recovery was complete.

The potential hazard connected with the use of HCP in nurseries is furthermore indicated by the results of several extensive studies.

A critical review of the available data on the risk of HCP bathing or other kinds of HCP use in newborn skin care suggests that there is ample evidence for the toxic potential of this disinfectant. Absolutely contraindicated is the use in infants with a low birth weight (under 2000 grams), excoriated areas of the skin and raised serum bilirubin. The use of a dusting powder with maximal 0.3–0.5% HCP seems to be connected with a lower toxicity risk, but there is a need for further information, especially about the pharmacokinetic patterns of HCP in newborns. A marked absorption of HCP after application of 0.33% HCP dusting powder was also shown unequivocally. The view that a small degree of edematous change in the central nervous system caused by HCP use in newborn infants should be reversible and with high probability is without influence on the further development of the child, cannot be accepted because these changes are certainly the first signs of central nervous system toxicity. A detailed discussion of the problem can be found in the literature.

In assessing the use of HCP in the nursery one also has to consider the fact that infections with virulent strains of *Staphylococcus* producing serious life-threatening diseases do not appear to be prevented or aborted by HCP bathing, and the problem that, as the staphylococcal colonization of the infant is diminished by HCP, gram-negative bacteria may cause an increased number of clinical infections.

Neurotoxicity of HCP after application on burned or otherwise excoriated skin In 1968, Larson reported on eight burned children, including four with a history of convulsive seizures following HCP use. Serum levels of HCP in six of these patients ranged from 4 to 74 ng/ml (approximately equivalent to blood levels of 2—37 ng/ml). In 1972, Lockart reported six deaths registered by the FDA and related to the use of HCP preparations in burn patients. Mullick reported four children; two of these were being treated with 3% HCP baths for burns and two for severe congenital ichthyosis. The interval between exposure and symptoms ranged from 6 hours to 10 days. All children showed severe vacuolation of the white matter in different areas of the cerebrum and cerebellum.

In 1977, Chilcote et al. reported a 10-year-old boy who had sustained 25% first- and second-degree burns, and was treated with frequent daily applications of a 3% HCP emulsion (diluted and undiluted); he developed a fatal encephalopathy.

Due to the high resorption rate of HCP and the high danger of fatal absorptive intoxications the use of HCP in the treatment of burns or on otherwise excoriated skin is strongly contraindicated.

Use in clinical vaginal lubricants HCP present in vaginal lubricants is variably absorbed from the vaginal mucosa, and HCP can be identified in maternal and cord serum in an appreciable number of women in whom vaginal examinations during labor were carried out with an HCP-containing antiseptic lubricant. Because of the potential for neonatal HCP toxicity, the use of alternative lubricants for pelvic examinations is recommended.

Overdosage *Accidental HCP poisoning after dermal application* In France in 1972, 6% HCP was accidentally included in the preparation of certain batches of a baby talcum powder. French law prohibited publication of the detailed report on the consequences of this contamination, until litigation was concluded. In 1977 Goutières and Aicardi published a detailed report on 18 children involved in this accidental poisoning. In 1982, Boyer et al. published a scientific report, which included 204 children (SED-10, 433).

Follow-up investigations have likewise been published only by Goutières and Aicardi of 14 surviving children. No obvious cerebral sequelae were noted, but follow-up was not long enough to exclude the possibility of more subtle damage, which may be manifest by learning difficulties or behavior disorders.

Toxicity after oral use In 1963, Chung reported on the treatment of five Chinese patients, aged 14—39 years, for *Clonorchiasis sinensis* infection with 20 mg/kg HCP given for 5—6 days orally. They developed nausea, vomiting, diarrhea, abdominal pain, general muscle weakness and soreness in the eyeballs and lower limbs. All patients recovered. Liu et al. treated eight children in a similar way. One became comatose on the fourth day, with temporary loss of light reflex, alternating dilatation and contraction of the pupils, and positive cerebrospinal tract signs. The fundus showed papillary edema. Recovery followed symptomatic treatment.

Toxicity after ingestion of high doses In 1962, Wear et al. summarized four cases of accidental ingestion of HCP in human subjects with anorexia, nausea, vomiting, abdominal cramps and diarrhea. No neurological symptoms were reported.

Bilateral atrophy of the optic nerve was reported in a 31-year-old who had ingested 10—15 ml of a 3% HCP emulsion orally each day for 10—11 months. She had also applied large amounts of HCP solution to her face every day as a self-treatment for pimples. She was depressed during this period, noted no headache, diplopia or dizziness, but may have had intermittent numbness of the left foot. Another case of acute bilateral optic nerve necrosis was reported in a 7-year-old boy, who accidentally received 3% HCP emulsion during a 52-hour period, an approximate amount of 12 grams HCP. After the last dose the child complained of intermittent blindness. Peritoneal dialysis was ineffective, and the child died 98 hours after the last dose. Other cases have been reported since.

Teratogenicity In 1977, Halling published a study on Swedish medical personnel, suggesting that repeated handwashing with HCP-containing detergents during the first trimester of pregnancy could be associated with a greatly increased incidence of both major and minor birth defects in the offspring. This publication has been the subject of extensive discussion, but in view of several serious methodological deficiencies the suggested teratogenicity of HCP has not been proven. There has been neither confirmation nor denial concerning this issue in the past 15 years.

HCP crosses the placenta and accumulates in fetal neural tissue in mice and rats, and the administration of toxic doses was associated with birth defects including cleft palate, hydrocephalus, anophthalmia and microphthalmia in rats.

Topical exposure of male neonate rats to a commercial HCP preparation produced a significantly reduced fertility, resulting in inability to ejaculate. It was possibly caused by dioxin, an 'androgenic' contaminant of HCP, responsible for permanent disruption of the integrated ejaculatory reflex. However, in subneurotoxic levels HCP did not seem to induce significant impairment of spermatogenesis in rats or dogs. HCP is also secreted by rats in milk.

Allergy A case of occupational asthma was reported in a pediatric nurse who had been working in contact with HCP for 15 years. The initial symptom was rhinitis but at the time of diagnosis she was also suffering from asthmatic attacks.

QUATERNARY AMMONIUM COMPOUNDS *(SED-11, 480)*

Quaternary ammonium compounds are surface-active agents. Some of these compounds have the ability to precipitate or denature protein and to destroy microorganisms. The most important disinfectants in this group are cationic surface-active agents such as benzalkonium chloride, benzethonium chloride, cetylpyridinium chloride and methylbenzethonium chloride; the problems they cause are similar. An advantage of this group is the low local and systemic toxicity. Depending on the concentration of the solution, local irritant effects can occur. Solutions should not be used in the eye.

Benzalkonium

Benzalkonium chloride is composed of a mixture of alkyldimethylbenzylammonium chlorides. The hydrophobic alkyl residues are paraffinic chains with 8–18 carbon atoms.

Limited antibacterial effectiveness of benzalkonium chloride The bactericidal activity of benzalkonium chloride is limited to the gram-positive and some of the gram-negative bacteria, but especially *Pseudomonas* species are resistant and have caused many severe infections in the past. Too often it is not realized that the disinfectant can be contaminated with active multiplying resistant organisms.

Pseudomonas bacteremia has been reported to be caused by the use of material in open-heart surgery that was stored in accidentally contaminated benzalkonium solutions, and following cardiac catheterization caused by inadequate disinfection of the catheters with benzalkonium solutions. In 1961, about 15 patients were reported with *Pseudomonas* infections caused by cotton pledgets kept in a contaminated aqueous solution used for skin antisepsis before intravenous and intramuscular injection; 1976 witnessed outbreaks of *Pseudomonas cepacia* infections in two American general hospitals. In 1976, Kaslow reported a pseudobacteremia (*Pseudomonas cepacia* or *Enterobacter*), caused by contamination of blood cultures in 79 patients in whom contaminated aqueous benzalkonium solutions were used for skin and antisepsis before venipuncture and due to contamination of the samples (SED-11, 490).

Benzalkonium chloride in eyedrops (*See also Chapter 48*) Benzalkonium chloride is used in eyedrops in concentrations of 0.033 or 0.025%. At a dilution of 1:1000 (or 0.1% concentration), a drop applied to the human cornea causes mild discomfort which persists for 2 or 3 hours. Slit-lamp examination within 90 seconds shows fine gray clots (epithelial keratitis) in the corneal epithelium. Within 10 minutes a gray haze may be seen in the corneal surface; superficial desquamation of the conjunctival epithelium may follow. The superficial irritation and disturbances disappear in a day or less. It must be realized that patients with glaucoma, dry eyes, infections, iritis, etc., use solutions containing benzalkonium chloride frequently and long enough to cause damage. In these patients, a higher incidence of endothelial damage, epithelial edema, and bullous keratopathy is seen, and because of the severity of the disease, additional damage from the medication might be overlooked. This is especially true in patients with defective epithelia or corneal ulcers in whom medication might penetrate best and who may well be most vulnerable. Analogous results have been given by investigations of benzethonium chloride, cetrimonium bromide, cetylpyridinium chloride, decyldodecylbromide, hexadecyl- and tetradecyltrimethylammonium bromide (SED-11, 490).

Allergic reactions in topical use Allergic reactions may occur, but are fairly rare. Allergic contact dermatitis has been reported in some cases. Allergic rhinitis on contact has also been reported.

In a study on the efficacy and acceptability of benzalkonium chloride-containing contraceptives (vaginal sponge, pessary and cream) an allergic reaction with vulva edema occurred in one woman out of 56 studied. Non-allergic local irritation, itching and a burning sensation were reported in nine women and nine husbands (141[c]).

Benzalkonium chloride as preservative in nebulizer solutions This induces a secondary paradoxical bronchoconstriction due to the administration of bronchodilators by inhalation in patients with bronchial asthma. Although the nebulizers with sympathomimetic agents may contain the same preservative, reports are more common with the anticholinergic agents. This is probably caused by a rapid onset and higher intensity of the sympathomimetic-induced bronchodilatation response than after anticholinergics (141[R]).

Benzethonium chloride and methylbenzethonium chloride

An extensive report by the Expert Panel of the American College of Toxicology (142[R]) has concluded that both these compounds can be regarded as safe when applied to the skin at a concentration of 0.5% or when used around the eye in cosmetics at a maximum concentration of 0.02%. In clinical studies, benzethonium chloride produced mild skin irritation at 5%, but not at a lower concentration. Neither ingredient is considered to be a sensitizer.

Intoxication The Paris Poison Centre has received reports on 45 cases of acute accidental poisoning, with 18 deaths. All the victims were mentally disturbed patients who had ingested Airsane HP 800, a powder packed in a water-soluble sachet; it contains a mixture of quaternary ammonium compounds and was left in the patient's rooms by hospital workers. Symptoms were corrosive burns of the mouth, pharynx, esophagus and sometimes of the respiratory tract (145[Cr])

Cetrimonium bromide (cetrimide)

Baraka et al. described a case of severe methemoglobinemia after excision of hydatid cysts and a liberal irrigation of the cysts in the liver with a 0.1% cetrimide solution. Frayha et al. reported the experience in three hospitals of 378 surgically treated patients with hydatid cysts including irrigation with cetrimide solutions in concentrations between 0.05 and 1%. No side effects were observed. Momblano et al. described a case of severe metabolic acidosis without signs of peritonitis; more than 1 liter of 1% cetrimide was instilled into the cysts (SED-11, 490).

SALICYLANILIDES *(SED-11, 490)*

Photocontact dermatitis still occurs following the use of halogenated salicylanilides in soaps. Cases have been described due to tribromosalicylanilide, but also to bithionol in first-aid creams. Many halogenated salicylanilides have been used in disinfectants. They have varying abilities to produce photocontact dermatitis.

Tetrachlorosalicylanilide produced many cases in 1961 and has now been withdrawn from use. Photosensitivity has also been reported to other analogs which are in widespread use, such as the tribromo and dibromo derivatives. The photoallergy is localized, but transient generalized reactions may occur.

Smith and Epstein observed a reduction in the number of patients with positive photopatch-tests to salicylanilides occurring after 1970. They concluded that these results were most likely due to removal from the market of the more potent photosensitizing chemicals and increased physician familiarity with the disease process.

SILVER NITRATE *(SED-11, 490)*

Silver nitrate is used as a caustic, antiseptic and astringent agent. The silver ion is precipitated by the chloride in tissue fluids, so that it does not readily penetrate.

Use in the eye (*See Chapter 47*) Silver nitrate is effective in vitro against *Neisseria gonorrhoeae* and *Staphylococcus aureus* at a concentration of 0.1% and against *E. coli* at about 0.01%.

The use of 1% silver nitrate eyedrops in Crede's prophylaxis of ophthalmia neonatorum has been periodically reviewed and compared with other prophylactic measures. The critical review by Barsam and several other reviews and extensive clinical studies support the conclusion that there seems to be no case in which permanent damage to the eye was actually proven to have been caused by a single application of a correctly used 1% silver nitrate solution.

In a blind study, Graf et al. (164[C]) examined the reaction of the ophthalmic front-region in the first 5 days after delivery in 40 neonates with and without Crede's-prophylaxis with silver nitrate solution. They found no significant differences in the frequency of pathological changes in the palpebrae, conjunctiva bulbi et tarsi and cornea between the two groups. There was the same frequency of palpebral edema and conjunctival hyperemia in both groups.

Nishida and Risemberg investigated the clinical significance and incidence of chemical conjunctivitis in 1000 newborn infants. Rinsing after instillation does not reduce the conjunctival irritation. Although 90% of the infants had conjunctivitis in the first 6 hours of life, in the majority it cleared within 24 hours. Chemical conjunctivitis did not increase the incidence of secondary infections. In 1980 the American Academy of Pediatrics pointed out the need for continued prophylaxis for all newborn infants; a 1% silver nitrate solution in single dose ampules or single-use tubes of an ophthalmic ointment 1% tetracycline or 0.5% erythromycin are proposed. However, in infants of mothers with clinically apparent gonorrhea aqueous crystalline penicillin G should be injected.

Hick et al. published a double-blind controlled study of a possible causal relationship between the use of 1% silver nitrate solution or 1% tetracycline solution in Crede's prophylaxis and the subsequent development of nasolacrimal duct obstructions. No statistically significant difference was found in the incidence between the two groups at either 2 weeks or 2 months of age.

Concentrations of silver nitrate of 5—50% applied accidentally in the eye have caused severe injuries with permanent corneal opacification and cataract in some cases. Repeated application of silver nitrate solutions in low concentrations may induce discoloration of the conjunctiva due to argyrosis.

Use on mucous membranes Raghavaiah and Soloway reported a case of anuria following silver nitrate irrigation for intractable bladder hemorrhage caused by cyclophosphamide chemotherapy. The level of obstruction was the ureterovesical junction, on the one hand, and the collecting ducts of the renal papillae, on the other. Therapy consisted of rigorous endoscopic evacuation of deposited coagulate from the bladder, after which the urinary output rapidly returned to normal.

Frost described a case with severe ulceration of the anterior ventral surface of the tongue, caused by ill-advised cauterization of a small ulcer with a silver nitrate stick. Only silver nitrate solutions of 5—10% should be used to cauterize mucous membranes or when a strong germicidal action is desired.

Use on burned skin Silver nitrate (147^R) is effective against most strains of *Staphylococcus aureus* and epidermidis, has also activity against *Pseudomonas aeruginosa*, but is less active against other gram-negative species such as *Enterobacter* and *Klebsiella*. It does not penetrate the burns eschar to any significant degree. The non-histotoxic concentrations of 0.5% used in burns are bacteriostatic. Thick cotton dressings saturated with the solution are applied to thoroughly debrided areas. The dressings must be rewetted every 2—3 hours with fresh solution to prevent development of histotoxic concentrations over 2% at the wound surface.

Electrolyte imbalances, secondary to the hypotonicity of the silver nitrate solution, are the major adverse effect of its use in burns. They result from the hypotonicity of the distilled water vehicle used to carry the silver nitrate, and from the insolubility of the silver salts which are formed in the tissues, primarily silver chloride and sulfide. The hypotonicity produces absorption of large amounts of water into the body with its dilutional effect and the leaking of significant quantities of body minerals, including sodium, potassium, magnesium, calcium and chloride. Deficiency of chloride is caused by the formation of silver chloride on the treated surface. Up to 350 mmol/day of sodium may be lost per square meter of treated body surface area. Problems occur particularly in patients with burns exceeding 20% of the body surface and in infants, unless a regular replacement schedule is established. Maximum deficiency can occur within a matter of 6—8 hours after initiation of therapy. A continuous oral or intravenous electrolyte supplementation and a careful monitoring of electrolyte balance is necessary.

Methemoglobinemia occurs via bacterial reduction of nitrate to nitrite, which is subsequently absorbed. The diagnosis should be suspected if the skin or blood appear cyanotic or gray in the presence of normal arterial Po_2. The diagnosis should always be confirmed with measurement of blood methemoglobin level. The silver nitrate should be discontinued if this complication occurs. A treatment of the methemoglobinemia with reducing agents is rarely required.

Ternberg and Luce observed fatal methemoglobinemia in a 3-year-old caucasian girl, who had suffered extensive burns involving 82% of the body surface and had been treated by painting the burns with silver nitrate solution. By the fourth day, low-grade fever was evident and *Aerobacter cloacae*, which was resistant to silver nitrate in 0.5% concentration, was cultured from the scar tissue. From the 14th to the 24th days of treatment onwards the child became cyanotic and she died on the 27th hospital day. Methemoglobin was found to constitute 70% of the hemoglobin; there was no other evident cause of death. The *Aerobacter cloacae* cultured from the skin was tested and found to reduce nitrate to nitrite. In the treatment of burns with silver nitrate solutions, the possible occurrence of methemoglobinemia must be considered, especially when organisms are cultured from the wounds.

Silver sulfadiazine

Silver sulfadiazine (147^R) is a white highly insoluble compound synthesized from silver nitrate and the sulfonamide sodium sulfadiazine. It is used in burns as a 1% preparation in a water-soluble cream base. It has in vitro activity against a wide range of burn wound microbial pathogens including *Staphylococcus aureus*, *Escherichia coli*, *Klebsiella* species, *Pseudomonas aeruginosa*, *Proteus* species, other Enterobacteriaceae and *Candida albicans*. Its penetration in the eschar is considered to be better than that of silver nitrate.

Transient leukopenia with a disproportionate decrease of neutrophil leukocytes appears typically 2—3 days after initiation of the therapy. The leukocyte count tends to recover whether or not the agent is withdrawn and may also be an intrinsic response to burn injury and unrelated to the use of silver sulfadiazine.

Cutaneous sensitivity reactions, typically a maculopapular rash, occur in less than 5% of patients and rarely require discontinuation of the use of silver sulfadiazine.

A modification of silver diazine by the incorporation of cerium nitrate is believed to enhance the clinical effectivity. Methemoglobinemia from reduction of nitrate to nitrite has been observed, as seen with silver nitrate.

TRICLOCARBAN (TCC) *(SED-11, 491; SEDA-4, 182)*

Triclocarban (3,4,4′-trichlorocarbanilide) is mainly used as an antibacterial agent in soaps and antiperspirants. Two types of toxic reaction caused by TCC have been reported.

Ponte et. al. observed a methemoglobinemia in seven newborn infants in connection with the use of TCC. There was no history of familial methemoglobinemia, but in one case the mother had been taking phenacetin before labor and this was most probably the cause. In five of the six other cases the lesion was considered to be due to the use of disinfecting solutions or ointments containing TCC which had been used as a vaginal disinfectant in four cases and as a powder for the umbilicus in one case. The authors advise against the use of this compound in maternity units and by those dealing with newborn infants. Cutaneous lesions have also been reported. Barrière described several patients presenting with relatively minor dermatological problems which were treated with TCC. Three cases developed very extensive erosive cutaneo-mucosal lesions following the use of TCC for periods ranging from 20 days to 3 months.

In recent years, several observations of allergic contact dermatitis after use of TCC and propylene glycol-containing antiperspirants have been published.

SULFITES

Sulfites and bisulfites are used extensively in the food industry but also as preservatives in drugs and bronchodilator inhalant solutions. The major symptoms of an adverse reaction are flushing, acute bronchospasm and hypotension. The incidence of sulfite sensitivity in an asthmatic population is estimated at about 10%; it is mainly reported in patients with a history of asthma. It is a cause that needs to be considered in cases of paradoxical reaction to a bronchodilator spray and in cases with a history of reported adverse reaction to foods (SED-11, 492; SEDA-8, 246; SEDA-10, 232; SEDA-11, 221; 148[R]).

REFERENCES

Editorial note *For reasons of space this list includes only more recent references. For a more complete list the reader is referred to SED-11 and SED-12.*

1. Schröder CH, Severijnen RSVM, Monnens LAH. Vergiftiging door desinfectans bij conservatieve behandeling van twee patiënten met omfalokele. Tijdschr Kindergeneeskd 1985;53:76.
2. Dreisbech RH. Handbook of Poisoning: Diagnosis and Treatment, 9th edn. Los Altos, CA: Lenge Medical Publications, 1977;159.
3. Jardine DS, Rogers K. Relationship of benzylalcohol to kernicterus, intraventricular hemorrhage, and mortality in preterm infants. Pediatrics 1989;83:153.
4. Cronin CM, Brown DR, Ahdab-Barmada M. Risk factors associated with kernicterus in newborn infant: importance of benzyl alcohol exposure. Am J Perinatol 1991; 8:80–85.
5. Hahn AF, Feasby TE, Gilbert JJ. Paraparesis following intrathecal chemotherapy. Neurology 1983;33:1032
6. Grant JA, Bilodeau PA, Buernsey BG et al. Unsuspected benzyl alcohol hypersensitivity. N Engl J Med 1982;306:108.
7. Wilson JP, Solimando DA, Edwards MS. Parenteral benzyl alcohol-induced hypersensitivity reaction. Drug Intell Clin Pharm 1986;20:689.
8. Shmunes E. Allergic dermatitis to benzyl alcohol in an injectable solution. Arch Dermatol 1984;120:1200.
9. Ponsold B, Schulze B, Kirsch H. Hygenic problems in the use of formaldehyde containing disinfectants. Zentralbl Gesamte Hyg 1977;23:408.
10. De Zotei R, Petronio L, Negro C et al. Inquinamento da formaldeide in anatomia patologica: esperienze in due ospedali regionali. Med Lav 1986;77:523.
11. Leonardos G, Kendak D, Barnard N. Odor threshold determinations of 53 odorant chemicals. J Air Pollut Control Assoc 1969;19:51.
12. Donahue LA, Frank IN. Ineravesical formalin for hemorrhagic cystitis: analysis of therapy. J Urol 1989; 141:809.
13. Shelly WB. Immediate sunburn like reaction in a patient with formaldehyde photosensitivity. Arch Dermatol 1982;118:117.
14. IARC Monographs updating of Vol. 1 to 42, Supplement 7. 1987;211–216.
15. Walrath J, Fraumeni JF Jr. Mortality patterns among embalmers. Int J Cancer 1983;31:407–411.
16. Walrath J Fraumeni JF Jr. Cancer and other causes of death among embalmers. Cancer Res 1984;44:4638–4641.
17. Stroup NE, Blair A, Erikson GE. Brain cancer and other causes of death in anatomists. J Natl Cancer Inst 1986; 77:121–1224.
18. Jensen 0M, Andersen SK. Lung cancer risk from formaldehyde. Lancet 1982;i:913.
19. Harrington JM, Oakes D. Morality study of British pathologists 1974–80. Br J Indust Med 1984;41:188–191.
20. Levine RJ, Andjelkovich DA, Shaw LK. The mortality of Ontario undertakers and a review of formaldehyde-related mortality studies. J Occup Med 1984;26:740–746.
21. Blair A, Stewart P, O'Berg M et al. Mortality among industrial workers exposed to formaldehyde. J Natl Cancer Inst 1986;76:1071–1084.

22. Stayner L, Smith AB, Reeve G et al. Proportionate mortality study of workers in the garment industry exposed to formaldehyde. Am J Indust Med 1985;7:229—240.
23. Fayerweather WE, Pell S, Bender JB. Case-control study of cancer deaths in DuPont workers with potential exposure to formaldehyde. In: Clary JJ, Gibson JE, Waritz RS, eds. Formaldehyde: Toxicology, Epidemiology, mechanisms. New York: Marcel Dekker, 1983;47—125.
24. Liebling T, Rosemann KD, Pastides H et al. Cancer mortality among workers exposed to formaldehyde. Am J Indust Med 1984;5:423—428.
25. Vaughan TL, Strader C, Davis S et al. Formaldehyde and cancers of the pharynx, sinus and nasal cacity. I. Occupational exposures. Int J Cancer 1986;38:677—683.
26. Partanen T, Kauppinen T, Nurminen M et al. Formaldehyde exposure and respiratory and related cancers: a case-referent study among Finnish woodworkers. Scand J Work Environ Health 1985;11:409—415.
27. Coggon D, Pannett B, Acheson ED. Use of job-exposure matrix in an occupational analysis of lung and bladder cancers on the basis of death certificates. J Natl Cancer Inst 1984;72:61—65.
28. Bertazzi PA, Pesatori AC, Radice L et al. Exposure to formaldehyde and cancer mortality in a cohort of workers producing resins. Scand J Work Environ Health 1986; 12:461—468.
29. Heayes RB, Raatgever JW, De Bryn A et al. Cancer of the nasal cavity and paranasal sinuses, and formaldehyde exposure. Int J Cancer l986;37:487—492.
30. Olsen JH, Jensen SP, Hine M et al. Occupational formaldehyde exposure and increased nasal risk in man. Int J Cancer 1984;34:639—644.
31. Olsen JH, Asnaes S. Formaldehyde and the risk of squamous cell carcinoma of the sinonasal cavities. Br J Indust Med 1986;43:769—774
32. Acheson ED, Gardner MJ, Panett B et al. Formaldehyde in the British chemical industry. Lancet 1984;i:611—616.
33. Vaughan TL, Strader C, Davis S et al. Formaldehyde and cancers of the pharynx, sinus and nasal cavity. II. Residential exposures. Int J Cancer 1986;38:685—688.
34. Lewis BB, Chestner SB. Formaldehyde in dentistry: a review of mutagenic and carcinogenic potential. J Am Dent Assoc 1981;103:429.
35. Guidelines on sterilization and disinfection effective against human immunodeficiency virus (HIV). WHO AIDS series 2. Geneva: WHO, 1989.
36. Editorial. Recommendations for preventing transmission of infection with human T-lymphotropic virus Type III/Lymphadenopathy-associated virus in the workplace. MMWR 1985;34:684.
37. Mwaniki DL, Guthua SW. Occupational exposure to glutaraldehyde in tropical climates. Lancet 1992; 340(8833):1476—1477.
38. Ballanty B, Berman B. Dermal sensitization potential of glutaraldehyde: A review and recent observations. J Toxicol Cut Ocul Toxicol 1984;3:251—262.
39. Drinkwater P. Gentian violet—Is it safe? Austr NZ Obstet Gynecol 1990;30:65—66.
40. Docampo R, Moreno SNJ. The metabolism and mode of action of gentian violet. Drug Metab Rev 1990;22:161—178.
41. Niedner R, Pfister-Wartha A. Farbstoffe in der Dermatologie. Akt Dermatol 1990;16:255—261.
42. Mortimer VD Jr, Kercher SL. Control Technology for Ethylene Oxide Sterilization in Hospitals. NIOSH Publ No 89-120, Cincinnati, 0H, National Institute for Occupational Safety and Health. 1989.
43. Brugnone F, Perbellini L, Faccini G et al. Concentration of ethylene oxide in the alveolar air of occuoationally exposed workers. Am J Indust Med 1985;8:67—72.
44. Brugnone F, Perbellini L, Faccini G et al. Ethylene oxide exposure. Biological monitoring by analysis of alveolar air and blood. Int Arch Occup Environ Health 1986;58:105—112.
45. Ostermann-Golkar S, Bergmark E. Occupational exposure to ethylene oxide. Relation between in vivo dose and exposure dose. Scand J Work Environ Health 1988;14:372—377.
46. Osterman-Golkar S. Dosimetry of ethylene oxide. In: Bartsch H, Hemminki K, O'Neill IK, eds. Methods for Detecting DNA Damaging Agents in Humans: Applications in Cancer Epidemiology and Prevention (IARC Scientific Publications No. 89). Lyon: IARC 1988;249—257.
47. Filser JG, Denk B, Tonqvist M et al. Pharmacokinetics of ethylene oxide and hydroxyethylation of hemoglobin due to endogeneous and environmental ethylene. Arch Toxicol 1992;66:157—163.
48. WHO International Agency for Research of Cancer. Ethylene oxide. IARC Monographs on the Evaluation of Carcinogenic Risks to Humans 1994;60:73—159.
49. Schroder JM, Hohneck M, Weis M et al. Ethylene oxide polyneuropathy: clinical follow-up study with morphometric and electron microscopic findings in a sural nerve biopsy. J Neurol 1985;232:83—90.
50. Fukushima T, Abe K, Nakagawa A et al. Chronic ethylene oxide poisoning in a factory manufacturing medicinal applicances. J Soc Occup Med 1986;36:118—123.
51. Estrin WJ, Cavalieri SA, Wald P et al. Evidence of neurologic dysfunction related to long-term ethylene oxide exposure. Arch Neurol 1987;44:1283—1286.
52. Estrin WJ, Bowler RMI, Lash A et al. Neurotoxicological evaluation of hospital sterilizer workers exposed to ethylene oxide. Clin Toxicol 1990;28:1—20
53. Crystal A, Schaumberg HH, Grober E et al. Cognitive impairment and sensory loss associated with chronic low-level ethylene oxide exposure. Neurology 1988;38:567—569.
54. Klees JE, Lash A, Bowler RM et al. Neuropsychologic 'impairment' in a cohort of hospital workers chronically exposed to ethylene oxide. Clin Toxicol 1990;28:21—28.
55. Grober E, Crystal H, Lipton RB et al. EtO is associated with cognitive dysfunction. J Occup Med 1992;34:1114—1116.
56. Hogsted C, Malmqvist N, Wadman B. Leukemia in workers exposed to ethylene oxide. J Am Med Assoc 1979; 241:1132—1123.
57. Stayner L, Steenland K, Greife A et al. Exposure-response analysis of cancer mortality in a cohort of workers exposed to ethylene oxide. Am J Epidemiol 1993;138:787—798.
58. Steenland K, Stayner L, Greife A et al. Mortality among workers exposed to ethylene oxide. New Engl J Med 1991;324:1402—1407.
59. Hogstedt C, Aringer L, Gustavsson A. Epidemiologic support for ethylene oxide as a cancer-causing agent. J Am Med Assoc 1986;255:1575—1578.
60. Hogstedt C. Epidemiological studies on ethylene oxide and cancer: an updating. In: Bartsch H, Hemminki K, O'Neill, eds. Methods for Detecting DNA damaging Agents in

Humans: Applications in Cancer Epidemiology and Prevention (IARC Scientific Publications No. 89). Lyon: IARC 1988;265–270.
61. Hagmar L, Welinder H, Linden K et al. An epidemiological study of cancer risk among workers exposed to ethylene oxide using haemoglobin adducts to validate environmental exposure assessments. Int Arch Occup Environ Health 1991;63:271–277.
62. Gardner MJ, Coggon D, Pannett B et al. Workers exposed to ethylene oxide: a follow up study. Br J Indust Med 1989;46:860–865.
63. Hogstedt C, Rohlen O, Berndtsson BS et al. A cohort study of mortality and cancer incidence in ethylene oxide production workers. Br J Indust Med 1979;36:276–280.
64. Morgan RW, Claxon KW, Divine BJ et al. Mortality among ethylene oxide workers. J Occup Med 1981;23:767–770.
65. Shore RE, Gardner MJ, Pannet B. Ethylene oxide: an assessment of epidemiologic evidence on carcinogenicity. Br J Indust Med 1993;50:971–997.
66. Kiesselbach N, Ulm K, Lange H et al. A multicentre mortality study of workers exposed to ethylene oxide. Br J Indust Med 1990;47:182–188.
67. Benson LO, Teta MJ. Mortality due to pancreatic and lymphopoietic cancers in chlorohydrin production workers. Br J Indust Med 1993;50:710–716.
68. Teta MJ, Benson LO, Vitale JN. Mortality study of ethylene oxide workers in chemical manufacturing: a 10 year update. Br J Indust Med 1993;50:704–709.
69. Bisanti L, Maggini M, Raschetti R et al. Cancer mortality in ethylene oxide workers. Br J Indust Med 1993;50:317–324.
70. Thiess AM, Frentzel-Beyme R, Link R et al. Mortality study of workers exposed to alkylene oxides (ethylene oxide/propylene oxide) and derivatives. J Occup Med 1981; 23:343–347.
71. Greenberg HL, Ott MG, Shore RE. Men assigned to ethylene oxide production or other ethylene oxide related chemical manufacturing: a mortality study. Br J Indust Med 1990;47:221–230.
72. Tates AD, Boogaard PJ, Darroudi F et al. Biological effect monitoring in industrial workers following incidental exposure to high concentrations of ethylene oxide. Mutation Res 1995;329:63–77.
73. Dellarco VL, Generoseo WM, Sega GA et al. Review of mutagenicity of ethylene oxide. Environ Mol Mutagen 1990;16:85–103.
74. Florack EIM, Zielhuis GA. Occupational ethylene oxide exposure and reproduction. Int Arch Occup Environ Health 1990;62:273–277.
75. Roche S, Chinn R, Webb S. Chlorhexidine-induced gastritis. Postorad Med J 1991;67:210–211.
76. Johnsson J, Kjelner I, Seeberg S. Blood concentrations of chlorhexidine in neonates undergoing routine cord care with chlorhexidine gluconate solution. Acta Paediatr Scand 1987;76:675.
77. Salole EG. Sheperd AJ. Spermicides: anti-HIV activity and cytotoxicity in vitro. AIDS 1993;7:293–295.
78. Bergqvist-Karlsson A. Delayed and immediate-type hypersensitivity of chlorhexidine. Contact Dermatitis 1988; 18:84.
79. Okano M, Nomura M, Hata S et al. Anaphylactic symptoms due to chlorhexidine gluconate. Arch Dermatol 1989;125:50.
80. Ohtoshi T, Yamauchi N, Tadokoro K et al. IgE antibody-mediated shock reaction caused by topical application of chlorhexidine. Clin Allergy 1986;16:155.
81. Evans RJ. Acute anaphylaxis due to topical chorhexidine acetate. Br Med J 1992;304:68.
82. Waclawski ER, McAlpine LG, Thomson NC. Occupational asthma in nurses caused by chlorhexidine and alcohol aerosols. Br Med J 1989;298:929–930.
83. Cheung J, O'Leary JJ. Allergic reaction to chlorhexidine in an anaesthetised patient. Anaesth Intens Care 1985; 13:429.
84. Junor BJR, Briggs JD, Forwell MA et al. Sclerosing peritonitis—the contribution of chlorhexidine in alcohol. Periton Dial Bull 1985;5:101.
85. Oules R, Challah S, Brunner FP. Case control study to determine cause of sclerosing peritoneal disease. Nephrol Dial Transplant 1988:3:66.
86. Lo W-K, Chan K-T, Leung ACT et al. Sclerosing peritonitis complicating prolonged use of chlorhexidine in alcohol in the connection procedure for peritoneal dialysis. Periton Dial Int 1991;11:166–176.
87. Quinn MW, Bini RM. Bradycardia associated with chlorhexidine spray. Arch Dis Child 1989;64:892.
88. Macklow ES. Accidental feeding of dilute antiseptic solution (chlorhexidine 0.05% with cetrimide 1%) to five babies. Hum Taxicol 1988;7:567–569.
89. Tabor E, Bostwick DC, Evans CC. Corneal damage due to eye contact with chlorhexidine gluconate. J Am Med Assoc 1989;261 557–558.
90. Phinney RB, Mondino BJ. Hofbauer JD. Corneal edema related to accidental Hibiclens exposure. Am J Ophthalmol 1988;106:210–215.
91. Varley GA, Meisler DM, Benes SC et al. Hibiclens keratopathy Cornea 1990;9:341–346.
92. Weidinger H, Passloer HJ, Kovacs L et al. Nutzen der prophylaktischen vaginalantiseptik mit Hexetidin in Geburtshilfe und Gynäkologie. Geburtsh Frauenheilkd 1991; 51:929–935.
93. Linn JL, Messer HH. Hypochlorite injury to the lip following injection via labial perforation. Case report. Aust Dent J 1993;38:280–282.
94. Becker G, Cohen S, Borer R. The sequelae of accidentally injection sodium hypochlorite beyond the root apex. Oral Surg Oral Med Oral Pathol 1974;38:633–638.
95. Herrmann JW, Heicht RC. Complications in therapeutic use of sodium hypochlorite (Letter to Editor). J Endodontol 1979;5:160.
96. Dedhia NM, Schmidt LM, Twardowski ZJ et al. Long-term increase in peritoneal membrane transport rates following incidental intraperitoneal sodium hypochlorite infusion. Int J Artif Organs 1989;12:711–714.
97. Marroni M, Menichetti F. Accidental intravenous infusion of sodium hypochlorite DICP. Ther Ann Pharmacother 1991;25:1008.
98. Froner GA, Rutherford GW, Rokeach M. Injection of sodium hypochloride of intravenous drug users (Letter to Editor). J Am Med Assoc 1987;258:325.
99. Hoy RH. Accidental systemic exposure to sodium hypochlorite. Am J Hosp Pharm 1981;38:1512–1514.
100. Gortz G, Haring R. Wirkung und Nebenwirkung von Polyvinylpyrrolidon-Jod (PVP-Jod). Therapiewoche 1981; 31:4364.
101. Glick PL, Guglielmo BJ, Tranbaugh RF et al. Iodine toxicity in a patient treated by continuous povidine-iodine mediastinal irrigation. Ann Thorac Surg 1985;39:478–480.

102. Campistol JM, Abad C, Nogue S et al. Acute renal failure in a patient treated by continuous povidine-iodine mediastinal irrigation. J Cardiovasc Surg 1988;29:410—412.
103. Colcleuth RG. Distribution protein binding of betadine ointment in burn wounds. In: Altemeier WA, ed. II World Congress/Antisepsis Proceedings. New York: HP Publishing Co, 1980;122—123.
104. Zec N, Ward Donovan J, Autiero TX. Seizures in a patient treated with continuous povidone-iodine mediastinal irrigation. New Engl J Med 1992;326:1784.
105. Kobayashi H. Review of the use of povidone-iodine (PVP-I) in the treatment of burns. Postgrad Med J 1993;69:584—592.
106. Okten F, Oral M, Canakici N et al. An anaphylactoid induced with polyvinylpyrrolidone iodine. A case report. Turk Anesteziyol Reanim 1993;21:118—122.
107. Melvin GR, Aceto T, Barlow J et al. Iatrogenic congenital goiter and gypothyroidism with respiratory distress in a newborn. SD J Med 1978;31 15.
108. Mahillon J, Peers W, Bourdoux P et al. Effect of vaginal douching with povidone-iodine during early pregnancy on the iodine supply to mother and fetus. Biol Neonate 1989;56:210.
109. Jacobsen JM, Hankins GV, Murray JM et al. Self-limited hyperthyroidism following intravaginal iodine administration. Am J Obstet Gynecol 1981;140:472.
110. Vorherr H, Vorherr UF, Menta P et al. Vaginal absorption of povidone-iodine. J Am Med Assoc 1980;244:2628.
111. Grüters A, l'Allemand D, Heidemann PH et al. Incidence of iodine contamination in neonatal transient hyperthyrotropinemia. Eur J Pediatr 1983;140:299.
112. l'Allemand D, Grüters A, Heidemann PH et al. Iodine induced alterations of thyroidfunction in newborn infants after prenatal and perinatal exposure to povidone iodine. J Pediat 1983;102:935.
113. Vulsma Th, Menzel D, Abbad FCB et al. Iodine-induced hypothyroidism in infants treated with continuous cyclic peritoneal dialysis. Lancet 1990;336:812.
114. Berkelman RL, Lewin S, Allen JR et al. Pseudobacteremia caused by povidone-iodine solution contamination with *Pseudomonas cepacia*. N Engl J Med 1981;305:621.
115. Craven DE, Moody B, Connolly MG et al. Pseudobacteremia caused by povidone-iodine solution contamination with *Pseudomonas cepacia*. N Engl J Med 1981;305:621.
116. Wissenschaftlicher Berat der Bundesärztakammer. Für Anwendung von Polyvinylpyrolidon-Jod Komplexen. Dtsch Ärztebl 1985;82:1434.
117. De Bont B, Lauwers R, Govaerts H et al. Yellow mercuric oxide ointment and mercury intoxication. Eur J Pediatr 1986;145:217.
118. Laundy T, Adam AE, Kershaw JB et al. Deaths after peritoneal lavage with mercuric chloride solutions: case report and review of the literature. Br Med J 1984;289:96.
119. Gille J, Goerz G. Thiomersal: Ein häufiges Kontaktallergen. Z Hautkr 1992;67:1049—1054.
120. Lisi P, Perno P, Ottaviani M et al. Minimum eliciting patch test concentration of thiomersal. Contact Dermatitis 1991;24:22—16.
121. Epstein S. Sensitivity to merthiolat: a cause of false delayed intradermal reactions: clinical and histological investigations. J Allergy Clin Immunol 1963;34:225.
122. Rudner EJ, Clendenning WE, Epstein E. Epidemiology of contact dermatitis in North America. Arch Dermatol 1973;108:537.
123. Massuda T, Honda S, Nakauchi Y et al. Patch test: the data at the Allergy Clinic of Department of Dermatology of Tokyo University Hospital for the past three years. Jpn J Dermatol Ser B 1970;80:133.
124. Hannuksela M, Kousa R, Pirila V. Allergy to ingredients of vehicles. Contact Dermatitis 1976;2:205.
125. Hjorth N. Sensitivity to organic mercury compounds. Contact Dermatitits Newsletter 1976;1:15.
126. Loechel J, Zschunke E. Zur Aktualisät der Quecksilberallergie. Dermatol Monatssschr 1971;157:570.
127. Novak M, Kvicalova E, Friedlanderova B. Reactions to merthiolate in infants. Contact Dermatitis 1986;15:304—310.
128. LaChapelle J-M, Chabeau G, Ducombs G et al. Enquète multicentrique relative à la fréquence des tests épicutanés positifs au mercure et au thiomersal. Ann Dermatol Vénéréol 1988;155:793—796.
129. Lisi P, Perno P, Ottaviani M et al. Minimum eliciting patch test concentration of thiomersal. Contact Dermatitis 1991;24:22—26.
130. Osawa J, Kitamura K, Ikezawa Z et al. A probable role for vaccines containing thiomersal in thimersal hypersensitivity. Contact Dermatitis 1991;24:178—182.
131. Möller H. Merthiolate allergy: a nationwide iatrogenic sensitization. Acta Dermatol-Venereol 1977;57, 509.
132. Aberer W. Vaccination despite thiomersal sensitivity. Contact Dermatitis 1991;23:381—382.
133. Andersen MM, Ronne T. Side-effects with Japanese encephalitis vaccine. Lancet 1991;337:l044.
134. Nahliedi O, Neader A. Iatrogenic pneumomediastinum after endodontic therapy. Oral Surg Oral Med Oral Pathol l991;71:618—619.
135. Bilotta JJ, Waye JD. Hydrogen peroxide enteritis: the 'snow white' sign. Gastrointest Endosc 1989;35:428—430.
136. Gordon SM, Bland LA, Alexander SR et al. Hemolysis associated with hydrogen peroxide at a pediatric dialysis center. Am J Nephrol 1990;10:123—127.
137. Chan TY, Lau MS, Critchley JA. Serious complications associated with Dettol poisoning. Quart J Med 1993;86:735—l38.
138. Chan TY, Critchley JA. Is chloroxylenol nephrotoxic like phenol? A study of patients with Dettol poisoning. Veter Human Toxicol 1994;36:250—251.
139. Chan TY, Critchley JA, Lau JT. The risk of aspiration in Dettol poisoning: a retrospective cohort study. Human Exp Toxicol 1995;14:190—191.
140. Chan TY, Suno JJ, Critchley JA. Chemical gastro-oesophgitis, upper gastrointestinal haemorrhage and gastroscopic findings following Dettol poisoning. Human Exp Toxicol l995;14:18—19.
141. Meyer U, Gerhard I, Runnebaum B. Benzalkonium-Chlorid zur vaginalen Kontrazeption—der Scheidenschwamm. Geburtsh Frauenheilk 1990;50:542—547.
142. Worthington I. Bronchoconstriction due to benzalkonium chloride in nebulizer solutions. Can J Hosp Pharm 1989;42:165.
143. Anonymous. Final report on the safety assessment of benzethonium chloride and methylbenzethonium chloride. J Am Coll Toxicol 1985;4:65.
144. Monafio WW, West M. Current treatment recommendations for topical burn therapy. Drugs 1990;40:364—373.
145. Chataigner D, Garnier R, Sans S et al. Intoxication aigue accidentelly par un desinfectant hospitalier. Presse Med 1991;20:741—743.
146. Graf H, Retzke U, Schilling C et al. Die Reaktion

des vorderen Augenabschnittes auf die Crede-Prophylaxe. Zentralbl Gynekol 1994;116:639–642.

147. Monafio WW, West M. Current treatment recommendations for topical burn therapy. Drugs 1990;40:364–373.

148. Gunnison AF, Jacobsen DW. Sulfite hypersensivity: a critical review. CRC Crit Rev Toxicol 1987;17:185.

Meyler's Side Effects of Drugs, 13th Edition
M.N.G. Dukes, editor

SECTION EDITOR: R. HOIGNÉ

P. Cottagnoud, A. Cerny and K.A. Neftel

25.1 β-Lactam antibiotics

GENERAL CONSIDERATIONS

The β-lactam antibiotics still comprise roughly half of the antibiotic market worldwide. Despite their growing chemical diversity, their side effect profiles continue to share various common aspects which will be discussed collectively in Chapters 25.1 and 25.2.

The common structure defining the whole family of β-lactam antibiotics is the four-membered, highly reactive β-lactam ring, which is essential for anti-microbial activity (1[R]). For discussing side effects the following simplifying classification is practical: (1) penicillin-structured compounds; (2) cephalosporin-structured compounds; (3) monobactams (containing no second ring system besides the β-lactam ring); (4) carbapenems; (5) β-lactamase inhibitors (representing a chemically heterogeneous group). The crucial event initiating the antimicrobial effects of β-lactam antibiotics is binding to and inhibition of bacterial enzymes located in the cell membrane, the so called penicillin-binding proteins (PbPs) (2[R]). This happens by covalent binding through opening of the β-lactam ring. Enzyme activities of PbPs are involved in the last steps of bacterial cell wall (peptidoclycan-) synthesis and their inhibition leads to halt of cell growth, and consequent cell death and lysis (3[R]). Functioning of β-lactamase inhibitors exhibits some analogies in that β-lactamases are genetically and structurally closely related to PbPs, and clinically useful β-lactamase inhibitors are so far β-lactam compounds with particularly high affinity to β-lactamases (4[R]). Obviously, β-lactamase inhibitors having no clinically relevant antimicrobial activity, are only given to patients in combination with another β-lactam compound.

IMMUNOGENICITY, ALLERGENICITY, TOXICITY

β-Lactam antibiotics, and penicillin in particular, seemed initially to fulfil almost perfectly the ideal conception of what a clinically useful antibiotic should do, i.e. specifically inhibit vital functions of the pathogenic micro-organisms without affecting whatsoever functions of the infected host. Not so surprisingly, the relevant iatrogenicity of early penicillin use consisted almost exclusively of clearly immune-mediated anaphylaxis, albeit with a disturbingly high mortality. This, in turn, stimulated extensive research on the immune responses associated with penicillin use and made penicillin the most prominent model for immune reactions to drugs.

The pathogenesis of many presumably immunologically mediated reactions to β-lactam antibiotics is still unknown. Reliable and standardized tests to predict hypersensitivity only exist for a minority of allergic reactions, i.e. IgE-mediated reactivity against penicillins. The matter is further complicated by the fact that β-lactams can readily induce immune responses which by themselves do not necessarily result in disease. This is the case in many instances where anti-erythrocyte antibodies directed against β-lactam bound to the red cell surface are detected. This biological property (immunogenicity) has to be distinguished from allergenicity, i.e. immune responses causing disease. A detailed description of the spectrum of β-lactam-associated hypersensitivity reactions is presented in Chapter 26.

Cross-reactivities, i.e. hypersensitivity reactions initially induced by one compound but triggered by another are an important and not yet resolved problem. The study of the issue is complicated by the fact that β-lactams undergo structural modifications within the organism and that different parts of the molecule such as the nucleus or the side chains can be involved. Data from cross-exposed patients (skin tests or drug challenge) presented in detail in the subsequent chapters suggest a high degree of cross-reactivity between compounds belonging to the same class and between the penicillins and carbapenems but a low cross-reactivity between penicillins and cephalosporins and between monobactams and the remaining β-lactams.

Mechanisms of hypersensitivity Drug allergy or hypersensitivity represents an acquired capacity of the organism to mount an immunologically mediated reaction to a given compound. This ultimately involves covalent or exceptionally non-covalent binding to and modification of host molecules (presumably proteins) by β-lactams to which the host becomes sensitized (induction phase). Re-exposure to the sensitizing drug may trigger a series of immunological effector mechanisms (effector phase). The latter can be defined as pathways of inflammation or tissue injury but they also represent mechanisms of immune protection from infectious agents.

The classification scheme defined by Coombs and Gell (5[R]) distinguishes between four different types of reactions. Briefly, Type I are IgE-mediated immediate hypersensitivity reactions, Type II are reactions mediated by cytotoxic IgM and/or IgG, Type III consist of immune complex-mediated reactions and Type IV are cell-mediated hypersensitivity responses. The classification may be useful to describe hypersensitivity reactions in a first approximation but fails to account for the complex and sequential involvement of several cell types and mediators in the immune response as recognized today (6[R]).

IgE mediated adverse reactions IgE antibody-mediated hypersensitivity can serve as a paradigm to demonstrate some important features of β-lactam hypersensitivity. β-Lactams are small molecules that have to combine with a host macromolecule to be recognized by the immune system. In the case of penicillin this reaction involves coupling of reactive degradation products to a protein-containing carrier (7[R]). Several degradation pathways have been described resulting in the formation of reactive compounds most importantly penicilloyl (8[C]). The penicilloyl determinant is also called the *major determinant*. Other less abundant degradation products include penilloate, benzylpenicilloate and benzylpenilloate forming so called *minor determinants*.

The complex contains often multiple haptens coupled to a protein-containing carrier molecule and is capable of inducing a T-cell-dependent B-cell activation leading to the formation of anti-hapten antibodies. The mechanisms governing the selection of the different immunoglobulin isotypes are reviewed elsewhere (6[R]).

The time required for sensitization is called latency and is variable depending on a number of parameters such as route of exposure, hapten dose and chemical reactivity of the drug as well as genetic and acquired host factors. The period between the last exposure to the drug and the first appearance of symptoms has been termed reaction time. It is part of the clinical description of an adverse event and may help to attribute it to a specific drug (SED-12, 594; see Chapter 25.3).

Once sensitivity has been established, i.e. hapten-specific IgE-producing B-cells have been formed, exposure to even small amounts of hapten may induce a cascade of events leading to immediate reactions such as anaphylaxis (9[R]). Briefly, preformed IgE antibodies to drug determinants recognize the hapten carrier complex and fix to the surface of mast cells or basophils triggering the release of a series of mediators such as histamine, neutral proteases, biologically active arachidonic acid products and cytokines. This ultimately leads to a clinical spectrum ranging from a mild local reaction to anaphylactic shock.

Non-IgE-mediated immunological adverse reactions Modification of erythrocyte surface components due to binding of β-lactams or their metabolic products is thought to be the cause of the formation of anti-red cell antibodies and the development of a positive Coombs test implicated in the development of immune hemolytic anemia (10[C]). Approximately 3% of patients receiving large doses of intravenous penicillin (10—20 million units per day) will develop a positive direct Coombs test (11[C]). Only a small fraction of Coombs positive patients will develop frank hemolytic anemia (12[C]). Elimination of antibody-coated erythrocytes most likely occurs via elimination by the reticulo-endothelial system (extravascular hemolysis) (13[C]) or less frequently by complement-mediated intravascular erythrocyte destruction (14[C]). Another mechanism implicates circulating (anti-β-lactam antibody—β-lactam) immune complexes resulting in erythrocyte elimination by an 'innocent bystander' mechanism (15[C]). Similar mechanisms have been implicated in β-lactam associated thrombocytopenia (16[C], 17[C]).

Contact dermatitis was frequently observed when penicillin was used in topical formulations and still continues to be described in cases of occupational exposure to β-lactams (18[C], 19[Cr]). The underlying mechanism is thought to involve chemical modification of antigen presenting cells in the epidermis leading to the sensitization of drug specific T-cells (20[C], 21[R]).

The underlying mechanism of a series of clinical entities associated with β-lactam usage such as maculopapular rash, drug fever, eosinophilia, serum sickness-like disease, vesicular and bullous skin reactions, erythema nodosum and acute interstitial nephritis is suspected to be immunological but is still largely unknown.

Side chain-specific reactions Apart from epitopes generated by the β-lactam nucleus, side chains attached to it may serve as additional epitopes recognized by the host immune response. Side-chain specific antibodies can be detected in β-lactam-allergic patients even in the absence of reactivity against the mother compound. The clinical importance of this is currently subject to debate. The occurrence of serious anaphylactic reactions to amoxicillin in three patients tolerating challenge with benzylpenicillin has been reported (22[C]). The phenomenon is mostly relevant for patients treated with semisynthetic penicillins, cephalosporins, carbapenems and monobactams: compounds derived from each of these classes of drugs share certain side chains that may be cross-recognized by preformed antibody. Diagnosis of side chain-specific allergy requires a panel of diagnostic tools available only at selected research centers.

Features of hypersensitivity reactions and their distinction from dose-dependent reactions The requirement for sensitization explains why a drug may be administered for a variable length of time without adverse effects. Once the organism is sensitized, manifestation of hypersensitivity will depend on the route and dose of the allergen as well as the type of effector mechanism involved in hypersensitivity, preformed IgE being the most rapid, others evolving more slowly typically over days. Generally far lower amounts of drug are required to trigger a hypersensitivity reaction in a sensitized subject than for induction. Cases of anaphylactic reactions have been described occurring after ingestion of meat from penicillin-fed animals or after intercourse in a penicillin-sensitive patient (23[C], 24[C]).

The time of sensitization is often difficult to establish in a patient developing symptoms during continuous therapy. A classification scheme distinguishing between immediate, accelerated and late reactions is of limited clinical use since it will only allow distinction between IgE, i.e. rapidly developing and non-IgE-mediated, i.e. more slowly evolving reactions in the setting of re-exposure of a sensitized subject (25[C]).

Hypersensitivity reactions have to be distinguished from dose-dependent drug toxicity-related adverse reactions. In contrast to hypersensitivity, the most important features of dose-dependent adverse reactions are: (a) lack of requirement for sensitization; (b) re-induction of toxicity typically requires similar doses of drug.

A special case is a syndrome (Hoigné's syndrome) resembling an immediate allergic reaction combined with hallucinations, aggressive behaviour, anxiety and auditory as well as visual disturbances that has been described after intramuscularly administered procaine or benzathine penicillin. It is most likely due to accidental intravascular injection and results from microemboli of the penicillin depot preparation (26[C]–29[C], 30[R]).

Non-immune-mediated reactions While the presumptive immunological basis of various reactions remains unproven or doubtful, in parallel to the growth of the β-lactam family, many reactions were observed being clearly not immune mediated. These include among others bleeding disorders, neurotoxicity, and most cases of diarrhea. In addition, many reactions, the pathogenesis of which are still being discussed, are clearly dependent upon the daily and the cumulative dose of β-lactam antibiotics given and hence the duration of treatment. Although the rare but well-understood immune hemolysis following penicillin is seen mostly with high-dose and long-term treatment, dose and time dependency as a general phenomenon point to direct toxicity rather than to immunological mechanisms. Indeed, direct toxic effects of β-lactam antibiotics on eukaryotic cells and specific interactions with receptor- and enzyme-proteins have been shown (31[R]) and might underlie particular reactions (see Chapter 25.2).

Incidence and cause-effect relationship Although β-lactam antibiotics are the most widely used and in some respects the best investigated antibiotics, some particularities still make it difficult to clearly establish the incidence and cause-effect relationship of many reactions and hence identifying patients at risk.

(1) The range of recommended daily dose may vary by more than one order of magnitude, according to clinical necessity. Hence, the incidence of some dose dependent reactions may vary greatly among different populations.

(2) Combinations of β-lactam antibiotics with antimicrobials from other molecular classes are frequently used especially in severe infection.

(3) The spectrum of potential β-lactam antibiotic-induced reactions is especially broad, and in a majority no test procedure is available to distinguish β-lactam antibiotics from other causes of a given reaction, in particular from consequences of the treated infection.

MICROBIOLOGICAL RESISTANCES ASSOCIATED WITH β-LACTAM USE

The introduction of penicillin G into clinical use more than 50 years ago is still one of the milestones in the treatment of infectious diseases, leading to a drastic decrease of mortality of severe infections (32[R], 33[c], 34[C]). Two years later the emergence of the first penicillin-resistant *Staphylococcus aureus* rapidly cooled the enthusiasm of clinicians. During the following years micro-organisms developed various mechanisms in order to survive the antibiotic pressure. Basically, micro-organisms have developed several strategies.

(1) They are able to modify the targets of β-lactam antibiotics, i.e. the PbP (35[R], 36[R]), resulting in a reduced affinity of the antibiotic to its target.

(2) In certain cases the micro-organisms have acquired a completely new PbP with a very low affinity to the antibiotic providing a high level of resistance.

(3) By producing and secreting β-lactamases in the periplasmic space, i.e. enzymes sharing structural analogies with the PbPs without fulfilling any function in

the cell wall synthesis but hydrolyzing and inactivating the β-lactam ring. The genes encoding for these β-lactamases are usually located on a plasmid but also might be anchored in the bacterial genome (37[R], 38[R]).

(4) Another way to increase resistance is to prevent the antibiotics reaching their targets (the PbPs) by decreasing their penetration through channels of the outer membrane by structural modification of the porines (porines are proteins forming channels in the outer membrane of gram-negative bacteria) (39[R], 40[R]).

All these mechanisms are mainly based on interbacterial exchange of DNA or on point mutations (41[R]), the predominant mechanisms for genetic exchange being *transformation*, *transduction* and *conjugation* (42[R]). Transformation is the simplest way to transfer DNA to another bacterium, provided that this is ready to accept foreign DNA (= competent bacteria). This mechanism of genetic transfer is mostly used by several human pathogens i.e. *Streptococcus pneumoniae*, *Haemophilus influenzae*, *Neisseria meningitidis*, *Neisseria gonorrhoeae*, and *Bacillus subtilis*. The transduction needs a bacteriophage (= virus) as a vector to inject DNA into a bacteria. This elaborate system is limited by the restricted specificity of the vectors for few micro-organisms. The most sophisticated system is conjugation. This mechanism was first observed in *E. coli* 1952 by Hayes who described the first transfer of genetic material (F-Factor: fertility factor) by conjugation (43[r]). Micro-organisms used conjugation to transfer several types of genetic material, either extra-chromosomal, i.e. plasmids or intra-chromosomal, i.e. transposons. In summary, micro-organisms are able to exchange and acquire genetic material in order to adapt to a changing environment, i.e. the antibiotic pressure. Furthermore, DNA exchange between procaryotes and eukaryotic cells (yeasts) and some plants have been observed (44[R]). A recent review has addressed in detail the problem of emergence and spread of resistance among clinical isolates (45[R]). Here, development of resistance by two major pathogens, i.e. *S. pneumoniae* and *S. aureus* will only briefly be discussed as examples.

One of the most striking features in microbiology is the rapid emergence and worldwide spread of penicillin-resistant pneumococci, mainly due to the uncontrolled use of penicillin in certain countries (46[R]). The first cases of penicillin-resistant pneumococci were reported in the 1960s in New Guinea and Australia. Penicillin-resistant pneumococci have now been registered in all continents. The highest rate has been reported in 1989 in Hungary, amounting to 57% of all clinical isolates (47[C]). Until now pneumococci have not acquired the genes encoding for β-lactamases. Accordingly, the underlying mechanism of penicillin-resistance is the structural modification of PbPs, leading to a decreased affinity to the penicillin molecule (see above). These PbP-modifications usually require several genetical steps. Moreover, horizontal transfer of pieces of PbP genes has been described between *Streptococcus mitis* and pneumococci (48[R]). Such modifications of PbPs lead to a decreased affinity of these enzymes for their natural substrates, (disaccharide-pentapeptides) (49[R]) and eventually to the synthesis of a structurally different cell wall harboring more branched peptides. This is the biological price that pneumococci pay to survive the antibiotic pressure (50[r]). Usually, in an epidemic area, a few clones of penicillin-resistant pneumococci are responsible for the majority of the registered cases (51[R]). Furthermore it has been shown by DNA-polymorphism analysis that isolates have been imported from one continent to another, causing new epidemics (52[r], 53[c], 54[c], 55[r]).

Staphylococcus aureus, another major pathogen has developed two different mechanisms of resistance: (1) synthesis of β-lactamase (nowadays more than 80% of *S. aureus* secrete β-lactamase); (2) furthermore so-called methicillin-resistant *S. aureus* (MRSA) are able to grow even in the presence of high concentrations of methicillin (up to 800 μg/ml). This unique feature is based on the acquisition of a low-affinity PbP for β-lactam antibiotic molecules (the PbP 2A) which allows the bacteria to carry on the synthesis of the cell wall, whereas the other PbPs are already inactivated by the high concentration of methicillin or other β-lactamase-resistant β-lactam antibiotics. The origin of the PbP 2A remains a matter of debate. Until now the only antibiotic class inhibiting MRSA is that of the glycopeptides, e.g. vancomycine. A nightmare scenario would be the transfer of vancomycine-resistance from enterococci to MRSA, causing a major epidemiological and therapeutical problem in the treatment of staphylococcal infections. Few cases of vancomycin-resistant coagulase-negative *S. aureus* have been registered (56[C], 57[c]) but until now vancomycin-resistant MRSA have not been reported in the literature, although the transfer of the vancomycin-resistance to staphylococci has experimentally succeeded (58[r]).

The continuous spread of resistance among clinical isolates, especially of multiresistant micro-organisms (i.e. pneumococci) represents a unique challenge in the treatment of infectious diseases. The detection of asymptomatic carriers of pneumococci—especially young children in day care centers—makes early detection even more difficult (59[C]). Uncontrolled utilization of antibiotics in the agriculture selects for a multiresistant fecal flora in animals and consumable meat can be contaminated by imperfect processing.

The problem of increasing resistance of micro-organisms is a worldwide major issue which necessitates the close collaboration of clinicians, epidemiologists and basic research laboratories. Newer and fast diagnostic tools (i.e. polymerase chain reaction), routinely introduced in clinical laboratories, and better understanding at the molecular level of mechanisms of resistance of micro-organisms are key-prerequisites in order to prevent further spread of resistant microorganisms. Additional measures, e.g. broad use of vaccines; restrictions on antibiotic use imposed by health authorities might require global cooperation and will have to be addressed by international organizations (e.g. WHO).

REFERENCES

1. Morin RB, Gorman M, eds. The Chemistry and Biology of the Beta-lactam Antibiotics. Vol 1–3. New York: Academic Press, 1982.
2. Waxman DJ, Strominger JL. Penicillin-binding proteins and mechanism of action of beta-lactam antibiotics. Annu Rev Biochem 1983;52:825.
3. Frère J-M, Joris B. Penicillin-sensitive enzymes in peptidoglycan biosynthesis. CRC Crit Rev Microbiol 1985;11:299.
4. Rolinson GN. Evolution of beta-lactamase inhibitors. Rev Inf Dis 1991;13:727.
5. Gell PGH, Coombs RRA. Classification of allergic reactions responsible for clinical hypersensitivity and disease. In: Gell PGH, Coombs RRA, Lachmann PJ, eds. Clinical Aspects of Immunology. Oxford: Blackwell Scientific Publications, 1975;761.
6. Plaut M, Zimmerman EM. Allergy and mechanisms of hypersensitivity. In: Paul WE, ed. Fundamental Immunology, 3rd edn. New York: Raven Press, 1993;1399.
7. de Weck AL. Pharmacologic and immunochemical mechanisms of drug hypersensitivity. Immunol Allergy Clin N Am 1991;11:461.
8. Lafaye P, Lapresle C. Fixation of penicilloyl groups to albumin and appearance of anti-penicilloyl antibodies in penicillin-treated patients. J Clin Invest 1988;82:7.
9. Bochner BS, Lichtenstein LM. Anaphylaxis. N Engl J Med 1991;324:1785.
10. Levine B, Redmond A. Immunochemical mechanisms of penicillin-induced Coombs positivity and hemolytic anemia in man. Int Arch Allergy 1967;21:594.
11. Abraham GN, Petz LD, Fudenberg HH. Immunohaematologic cross-allergenicity between penicillin and cephalothin in humans. Clin Exp Immunol 1968;3:343.
12. Garratty G, Petz LD. Drug-induced immune hemolytic anemia. Am J Med 1975;58:398.
13. Worledge SM. Immune drug-induced hemolytic anemias. Semin Hematol 1973;10:327.
14. Kerr RO, Cardamone J, Dalmassa AP et al. Two mechanisms of erythrocyte destruction in penicillin-induced hemolytic anemia. N Engl J Med 1972;287:1322.
15. Funicella T, Weinger RS, Moake JL et al. Penicillin-induced immunohemolytic anemia associated with circulating immune complexes. Am J Hematol 1977;3:319.
16. Christie DJ, Lennon SS, Drew RL. Cefotetan-induced immunologic thrombocytopenia. Br J Haematol 1988;70:423.
17. Gharpure V, O'Connell B, Schiffer CA. Mezlocillin-induced thrombocytopenia. Ann Intern Med 1993;119:862.
18. Moller NE, von Wurden K, Nielsen B. Contact dermatitis to semisynthetic penicillins in factory workers. Contact Dermatitis 1986;14:307.
19. Tadokoro K, Niimi N, Ohtoshi T et al. Cefotiam-induced IgE-mediated occupational contact anaphylaxis of nurses; case reports, RAST analysis, and a review of the literature. Clin Exp Allergy 1994;24:127.
20. Hertl M, Boecker C, Merk HF. Selective generation of CD8+ T-cell clones from the peripheral blood of patients with cutaneous reactions to beta-lactam antibiotics. Br J Dermatol 1993;128:619.
21. Scheper RJ, von Blomberg BM. Immunoregulation of T-cell mediated skin hypersensitivity. Arch Toxicol 1994;16:63.
22. Blanca M, Perez E, Garcia J et al. Anaphylaxis to amoxicillin but good tolerance for benzyl penicillin. Allergy 1988;43:508.
23. Kanny G, Puygrenier J, Beaudoin E et al. Choc anaphylactique alimentaire: implication des résidues de penicilline. Allerg Immunol 1994;26:181.
24. Green RL, Green MA. Postcoital urticaria in a penicillin-sensitive patient. J Am Med Assoc 1985;254:531.
25. Levine BB, Redmond AP, Fellner M et al. Penicillin allergy and the heterogeneous immune responses of man to benzylpenicillin. J Clin Invest 1966;45:1895.
26. Hoigné R. Akute Nebenreaktionen auf Penicillinpräparate. Acta Med Scand 1962;171:201.
27. Silber TJ, D'Angelo L. Psychosis and seizures following the injection of penicillin G procaine: Hoigné's syndrome. Am J Dis Child 1985;139:335.
28. Kraus SJ, Green RL. Pseudoanaphylactic reactions with procaine penicillin. Cutis 1976;17:765.
29. Kryst L, Wanyura H. Hoigné's syndrome—its course and symptomatology. J Maxillofac Surg 1979;7:320.
30. Tompsett R. Pseudoanaphylactic reactions to procaine penicillin G. Arch Intern Med 1967;120:565.
31. Neftel KA, Hafkemeyer P, Cottagnoud P et al. Did evolutionary forerunners of betalactam antibiotics bind to nucleid acid replication enzymes? In: 50 Years of Penicillin Application. Berlin-Prague: Technische Universität Berlin, Public Ltd, 1993;394.
32. Fleming A. On the bactericidal action of cultures of a Penicillium with a special reference to their use in the isolation of B. Influenzae. Br J Exp Pathol 1929;10:226.
33. Abraham E.P. Further observation on penicillin. Lancet 1941;16:177.
34. Florey HW. Penicillins in war wounds. A report from the Mediterranean. Lancet 1943;ii:742.
35. Tomasz A. Penicillin-binding proteins and the antibacterial effectiveness of beta-lactam antibiotics. Rev Infect Dis 1986;3:260.
36. Georgopapadakou NH. Penicillin-binding proteins and

bacterial resistance to beta-lactams. Antimicrob Agents Chemother 1993;10:2045.
37. Ghuysen JM. Serine Beta-lactamases and penicillin binding proteins. Ann Rev Microbiol 1991;45:37.
38. Philippon A, Labia R, Jacoby G. Extended-spectrum β-lactamases. Antimicrob Agents Chemother 1989;33:1131.
39. Nikaido H. Prevention of drug access to bacterial targets: permeabilitiy barriers and active flux. Science 1994;264:382.
40. Livermore DM. Interplay of impermeability and chromosomal Beta-lactamase activity in imipenem-resistant *Pseudomonas aeruginosa*. Antimicrob Agents Chemother 1992; 36:2046.
41. Moreillon P. La résistance bactérienne aux antibiotiques. Schweiz Med Wochenschr 1995;125:1151.
42. Watson JD, Hopkins NH, Roberts JW et al. The genetic systems provided by *E. coli* and its viruses. In: Gillen JR, ed. Molecular Biology of the Gene. Menlo Park: Benjamin/Cummings, 1987;176.
43. Hayes W. Recombination in Bact. coli K-12: Unidirectional transfer of genetic material. Nature 1952;169:118.
44. Amabilie-Cuevas CF. Bacterial plasmids and gene flux. Cell 1992;70:189.
45. Neu H. The crisis in antibiotic resistance. Science 1992; 257:1064.
46. Friedland IR, McCracken GH. Management of infections caused by antibiotic-resistant *Streptococcus pneumoniae*. N Engl J Med 1994;331:377.
47. Marton A. Extremely high incidence of antibiotic resistance in clinical isolates of *Streptococcus pneumoniae* in Hungary. J Infect Dis 1991;161:542.
48. Coffey TJ. Genetics and molecular biology of Beta-lactam resistant pneumococci. Microb Drug Resist 1995;1:29.
49. Tomasz A. Multiple antibiotic-resistant pathogenic bacteria—a report on the Rockefeller University Workshop. N Engl J Med 1994;330:1247.
50. Garcia-Bustos J. A biological price of antibiotic resistance. Major changes in peptidoglycan structure of penicillin-resistant pneumococci. Proc Natl Acad Sci USA 1990; 87:5415.
51. Appelbaum PC. Antimicrobial resistance in *Streptococcus pneumoniae*: an overwiew. Clin Infect Dis 1992;15:77.
52. Barnes DM. Transmission of multridrug-resistant serotype 23 F *Streptococcus pneumoniae* in group day care: evidence suggesting capsular transformation in resistant strain in vivo. J Infect Dis 1995;171:890.
53. Munoz R. Intercontinental spread of a multiresistant clone of serotype 23 F *Streptococcus pneumoniae*. J Infect Dis 1991;164:302.
54. Soares S. Evidence for the introduction of a multiresistant clone of serotype 6B *Streptococcus pneumoniae* from Spain to Iceland in the late 1980. J Infect Dis 1993;168:158.
55. Tomasz A. The pneumococcus at the gates. N Engl J Med 1995;333:514.
56. Cherubin CE. Susceptibility of gram-positive cocci to various antibiotics, including cefotaxime, moxalactam, *N*-formimidoyl thienamycin. Antimicrob Agents Chemother 1981;20:553.
57. Schwalbe R. Emergence of vancomycin resistance in coagulase-negative staphylococci. N Engl J Med 1987;316:927.
58. Noble WC. Co-transfer of vancomycin and other resistance genes from *Enterococcus faecalis* NCTC 12201 to *Staphylococcus aureus*. FEMS Microbiol Lett 1992;93:195.
59. Reichler MR. The spread of multiply resistant *Streptococcus pneumoniae* at a day care center in Ohio. J Infect Dis 1992;166:1346.

Meyler's Side Effects of Drugs, 13th Edition
M.N.G. Dukes, editor

SECTION EDITOR: R. HOIGNÉ

K.A. Neftel, M. Zoppi, A. Cerny and P. Cottagnoud

25.2 Reactions typically shared by more than one class of β-lactam antibiotics

There are various reasons why β-lactam antibiotics belonging to different classes can induce comparable reactions. Besides the β-lactam ring, other structural similarities (e.g. the side chains) or the antimicrobial activity itself may be relevant. However, the incidence and, in particular instances also, the severity of a given reaction may vary among β-lactam classes.

The reactions dealt with in this chapter include (following the order in 'Organs and systems'): anaphylactic reactions, serum sickness-like syndromes, neurotoxicity, effects on mineral and fluid balance, immune hemolysis, agranulocytosis and leukopenia, bleeding disorders, hepatitis, diarrhea and colitis, acute interstitial nephritis, maculopapular rash and some other skin manifestations, carnitine loss with pivaloyl containing compounds, and the Jarisch-Herxheimer-reaction.

This list is not intended to be complete and some more rare reactions and additional aspects as well as adverse reaction summaries are dealt with in Chapters 25.1—25.5.

DOSE-DEPENDENT REACTIONS TO β-LACTAM ANTIBIOTICS

There are three lines of evidence that β-lactam antibiotics induce a variety of different reactions by dose-dependent, and hence probably toxic, mechanisms: (1) certain reactions are overwhelmingly reported to occur in a dose- and time-dependent manner; (2) particular compounds have been shown to induce side effects with unexpectably high frequency in certain clinical situations, e.g. cystic fibrosis, bacterial endocarditis and osteomyelitis, requiring particularly high-dose, prolonged treatment; (3) β-lactam antibiotics have been found to affect a variety of cultured eukaryotic cells.

Particular dose-dependent reactions For some reactions a strictly dose-dependent mechanism is accepted largely based on stringent in vivo and in vitro models. These include, among others, neurotoxic reactions (1^{C}), inhibition of platelet aggregation (2^{R}) and, to some extent, interaction with vitamin K-dependent synthesis of coagulation factors (3^{R}). The occurrence of such reactions and effects appears to depend directly on high serum levels maintained for a sufficiently long time. Renal failure may thus be a risk factor for dose-dependent reactions (4^{R}, 5^{C}).

For other reactions the underlying mechanisms are less clear. The body of individual reports and some published series suggest that their incidence increases disproportionally with prolonged, high-dose treatment, i.e. with high cumulative doses. This is particularly the case in the following reactions: (a) severe neutropenia up to total agranulocytosis as observed with virtually all β-lactam antibiotics; (b) acute interstitial nephritis previously seen with meticillin but more rarely also with other β-lactams, e.g. penicillin G; (c) hepatitis induced by isoxazolyl-penicillins; and (d) varying combinations of symptoms positively referred to or not as 'serum sickness-like syndromes'.

Neutropenia While in large series studying several thousand patients each, neutropenia has generally been reported as a side effect in less than 0.1—1.0% (SEDA-13, 212). An overview in 1985 estimated that neutropenia (neutrophil count $<1000/\mu l$) occurs in up to >15% of all patients treated with high-dose intravenous β-lactam antibiotics for more than 10 days (6^{C}). Indeed, in subsequent series of patients treated for several weeks with various β-lactam antibiotics, up to >25% developed neutropenia (7^{C}—11^{C}).

In one series, 22 out of 128 patients receiving cloxacillin for staphylococcal infections became neutropenic (7^{C}). Neutropenia appeared on average 23.2 days after starting therapy. The same authors, in a somewhat enlarged population, found neutropenias in 1.1% receiving cumulative doses of less than 150 grams of oxacillin, but in 43.1% (22 out of 51) with more than 150 grams (8^{C}). Similarly in 132 patients, cefapirin did not induce neutropenia after less than 90 grams cumulative dose, but did in 26.3% (five out of 19) of those receiving higher total doses (9^{C}).

In addition, for a given compound higher daily doses may increase the risk of developing neutropenia. In one study seven out of 14 patients became neutropenic with a mean of 16.7 grams penicillin G daily after 9–23 days (10[C]). While in another only 12 out of 193 patients developed neutropenia with a mean of 11.2 grams a day for an average duration of 20 days (11[C]).

No clear documentation exists so far showing different risks for different compounds. The data best fit the assumption that the risk for developing neutropenia correlates with the cumulative dose of a given compound, or probably more precisely with the area under the serum level curve (AUC). Hence, renal insufficiency is a potential risk factor. In addition, β-lactam antibiotic-induced leukopenia has been found associated with hepatic dysfunction (12[c]). Recovery in most cases is rapid and uneventful. In cases that have been re-exposed later to the same or other β-lactam antibiotics, a similar dependence of neutropenia upon duration and cumulative dose of treatment has again been observed (6[C]). Whether application of GMCSF is useful remains unclear. There are case reports of positive clinical effects (13[c], 14[c]). However, the recovery time in these reports did not differ from those observed in a large population of untreated cases (6[C]). Theoretically, early application of GMCSF could even be contra-productive since the toxicity of β-lactam antibiotics for bone marrow cells appears to be related to the S-phase of the cell cycle (15[R]).

Nephritis Methicillin-induced acute interstitial nephritis follows a similar pattern of dose and time dependency to that of neutropenia (16[R], 17[C]). In a pediatric series this reaction occurred in 16% of all patients treated with high-dose methicillin (18[C]). Nephritis manifested after a mean of 17 days and a mean cumulative dose of 120 grams. With other β-lactams, mainly penicillin G, acute interstitial nephritis is only rarely seen, but again follows the same pattern (19[R]).

Hepatitis One type of hepatitis, mainly associated with oxacillin (20[C], 21[c]), also parallels the dose-dependent pattern described above. Eight out of 54 patients developed this reaction after a mean cumulative dose of 157 grams oxacillin (22[C]). Accordingly, prolonged duration of treatment—besides increasing age—was found to be a risk factor for the development of flucloxacillin-induced jaundice (23[C]).

Besides this rapidly reversible variant, another type of prolonged, but not apparently dose-dependent, cholestatic liver injury has been described most frequently with flucloxacillin (24[C], 25[C]) and other isoxazolylpenicillins (26[C]). Whether cholestatic hepatitis following the amoxicillin + clavulanic acid combination belongs to one of these categories is so far unclear (see Chapters 25.3 and 25.5).

In addition to their comparable dose dependency each of the three reactions is accompanied by fever, eosinophilia and/or rash in more than 80% of cases. This hints (a) to the possibility of overlapping pathogenetic steps and (b) sheds some doubt on the reliability of these accompanying symptoms as indicators of immune-mediated reactions, e.g. 'serum sickness-like syndromes'.

High frequency of side effects with high cumulative doses An increasing number of reports document an astonishingly high overall frequency of side effects to very high cumulative doses of β-lactam antibiotics in patients with, e.g. chronic osteomyelitis, pulmonary exacerbations in cystic fibrosis, bacterial endocarditis and in healthy volunteers (8[C], 10[C], 27[C], 28[C]).

In one series 22.8% of patients treated with an average cumulative dose of 924.6 grams carbenicillin and 67.7% of those treated with 328.9 grams of ureidopenicillins developed side effects including rash, fever, leukopenia, eosinophilia, thrombocytopenia and hepatic damage, requiring change of therapy in 51.6% of cases in the latter group (29[C]). In another series, 15 out of 29 consecutive patients with high-dose penicillin G or other β-lactam antibiotics, treatment had to be discontinued due to side effects, such as neutropenia (eight cases), fever and rash (seven cases) (10[C]). Fourteen out of 44 patients receiving up to 900 mg/kg per day of piperacillin for acute pulmonary exacerbations in cystic fibrosis developed a syndrome 'which resembled a serum sickness reaction'; mainly the symptoms fever, malaise, anorexia, eosinophilia and cutaneous manifestations (27[C]). The reaction occurred after a minimum of 9 days of therapy and the frequency of observed symptoms appeared to be dose-dependent. All patients who developed the reaction were re-admitted to the same hospital between 4 and 28 months after the initial episode and in every case the re-exposure to piperacillin did not evoke the reaction again.

The dose dependency of reactions to piperacillin in patients with cystic fibrosis has, indeed, created a debate about its usefulness in this condition (30[c], 31[c], 32[r], 33[c], 34[C]). However, comparable dose-dependent patterns and frequencies of side effects were found in other series treated with piperacillin (34[C]) and with other β-lactam antibiotics (35[C]), as well as in patients with both cystic fibrosis and other conditions (10[C], 29[C], 35[C]). A recent study found piperacillin along with imipenem/cilastatin to more frequently induce fever and/or rash per treatment course in patients with cystic fibrosis as compared to carbenicillin, mezlocillin, ticarcillin, cefazolin, ceftazidime and nafcillin (36[C]). Of particular interest is a study from 1974 where volunteers developed comparable syndromes in those treated for up to

4 weeks with high doses of cephalotin or cephapirin reaching eventually an overall incidence of side effects of 100%!! (28[C]). Despite these astonishingly high frequencies, these reactions were predominantly regarded as 'allergic', albeit their pathogenesis is mostly unclear.

Thus a disproportionally high frequency of various, apparently unrelated, side effects occurs in a relatively small group of patients; those needing high-dose prolonged treatment, hence those who are at particular risk.

Effects on eukaryotic cells The selectivity of β-lactam antibiotics for bacterial target proteins is not absolute. A specific interaction of modified cephalosporins with mammalian serine proteases has been demonstrated (37[r]) and the affinity of various penicillins for the benzodiazepine receptor may be part of the chain of events leading to neurotoxicity (38[C]). Most intriguing, however, are the observations made in proliferating cultured cells. Biological activities associated with proliferation were dose-dependently inhibited by a large array of β-lactam antibiotics in a variety of cells from both human and animal sources (15[R], 39[R]). Resting cells, on the other hand, were unsusceptible even to very high concentrations.

Degradation products as spontaneously formed in aqueous solutions, e.g. culture media, may be responsible for the observed effects rather than the parent molecules themselves (15[R]). Antiproliferative activities were generally more pronounced with cephalosporins than with penicillins, while monobactams appear to be practically free from such effects. Carbapenems have not been thoroughly studied in this respect and some recent data on clavulanic acid and two other β-lactamase inhibitors do not clearly reflect the same kind of toxicity as observed with penicillins and cephalosporins (40[C]).

The impact of the inhibitory effects of β-lactam antibiotics on proliferating eukaryotic cells for the clinical situation is so far unknown and formal proof of a toxicity correlation in patients is lacking. There are reasons, however, to consider this type of toxicity as the cause of neutropenia and thrombocytopenia (SEDA-13, 230). In dogs, high-dose treatment with cefonicid and cefazedone for up to several months induced bone marrow damage, which can explain peripheral cytopenias and resembles the bone marrow findings in clinical cases of neutropenia (41[C]–43[C]). In addition, mild thrombocytopenia and reticulocytopenia which have each been concomitantly found in 30 and 17% of neutropenia cases each (6[C]) are also paralleled by results in the dog experiments. On the other hand, in the same dog model, erythrocyte-, neutrophil- and platelet-associated IgG were found following high-dose treatment with cefazedone (44[C]). Anti-granulocyte IgG antibodies in β-lactam-induced neutropenia have also been described in man (45[C]–47[C]). The relevance of these findings, however, remains unclear since high cumulative β-lactam doses frequently induce β-lactam-specific IgG antibodies regardless of whether side effects are present or not (48[C]). Hence, there remains to date a controversy about whether β-lactam-antibiotics can induce neutropenias by both toxic and immunological mechanisms and how both mechanisms may act in concert with each other.

In summary, the direct toxic effects of penicillins and cephalosporins and possibly other β-lactams—or rather of some of their degradation products—must be considered to be involved in the pathogenesis of various side effects.

HYPERSENSITIVITY REACTIONS

Incidence of hypersensitivity reactions The true incidence of immunologically mediated reactions to β-lactam antibiotics is difficult to evaluate. This is mainly due to problems associated with the case definition of hypersensitivity reactions. The pathogenetic mechanism for a significant number of reactions presumed to be immunological in nature has not yet been conclusively determined. Studies addressing incidences of adverse reactions are furthermore facing the problem of dealing with heterogeneous patient populations treated with different types of β-lactams administered by diverse routes in various dosages. The issue may be illustrated by reviewing data derived from four pharmaco-epidemiological studies:

- The International Rheumatic Fever Study A prospective multicenter study recording allergic reactions defined as hypotension, dyspnea, pruritus, urticaria, angioedema, arthralgia and maculopapular rash in a cohort of 1790 patients treated with monthly intramuscular benzathine penicillin for prophylaxis of rheumatic fever (32 430 injections during 2736 patient years) reported a 3.2% case incidence of allergic reactions and a 0.2% case incidence of anaphylaxis (1.2/10 000 injections) including one fatality (0.05% equivalent to 0.31/10 000 injections) (49[C]).
- A large national study of venereal disease clinics in the United States included four cooperative surveys conducted at 5-year intervals (1954, 1959, 1964 and 1969). The study included data on a total of 94 655 patients unselected with regard to a history of penicillin allergy. The total frequency of occurrence of anaphylaxis was 0.055% including one death (50[C]).
- Pleasants and colleagues conducted a retrospective analysis of allergic reactions, i.e. drug-induced fever

and rash observed in 90 adult patients with cystic fibrosis. Twenty-six of the 90 patients (28.8%) developed probable allergic reactions to parenteral β-lactams. Drug-induced fever was seen in 54 and dermatological reactions in 28 of 897 treatment courses (6 and 3.1%, respectively). One case of non-fatal anaphylaxis was observed. The number of allergic reactions per number of patients receiving specific antibiotics were carbenicillin (4/56), mezlocillin (7/42), piperacillin (11/31), ticarcillin (1/20), cefazolin (0/24), ceftazidime (1/35), imipenem-cilastatin (4/16) and nafcillin (3/36) (36[C]) (see also above 'Dose-dependent reactions to β-lactam antibiotics').

• The Boston Collaborative Drug Surveillance Program: This classic study was conducted in in-patients over the period of 1966 to 1982 and was published in two consecutive reports. β-Lactams head the list of drugs causing presumably allergic skin reactions. The overall reaction rate (number of drug-related skin reactions per 1000 treated patients) was 51 for amoxicillin, 42 for ampicillin, 29 for semisynthetic penicillins, 16 for penicillin G and 13 for cephalosporins (51[C], 52[C]).

These four sets of data illustrate a spectrum of diverse settings of β-lactam use ranging from single course parenteral (venereal disease clinics study), intermittent parenteral (rheumatic fever study) to continuous high-dose parenteral application (cystic fibrosis study). Factors other than route of application and dosing such as drug history, underlying disease, co-administered drugs, risk profile of a particular compound, etc., will be important to assess the risk of administrating a β-lactam to a given patient as discussed in more detail below.

Table 1 contains a list of presumably immunologically mediated manifestations of β-lactam hypersensitivity according to their estimated frequency of occurrence. It has to be noted that the mechanism of most reactions is not completely understood, which also implies that some of the clinical entities listed may be due to a non-immunological underlying mechanism. The frequency of occurrence of the various side-effects varies among different β-lactams and depends on a number of additional factors discussed below. A compilation of reported frequencies of occurrence related to different compounds has been published and was used and extended to prepare Table 1 (53[R]).

Factors affecting hypersensitivity reactions Several factors influencing hypersensitivity have been recognized and reviewed (92[R]).

Patient-related factors include increased incidences of allergic reactions to β-lactams in patients with systemic lupus erythematosus (93[C]) but not with atopic diseases (94[C]). Genetic factors influencing drug metabolism and excretion as well as the underlying disease of the patient and host immune reactivity are likely to modulate the risk and severity of hypersensitivity reactions.

A history of prior penicillin reaction increases the risk of a subsequent exposure. A classic study by Rodolph and Price reported a frequency of occurrence of

Table 1. *Presumably immunologically mediated adverse reactions to β-lactams: clinical entity*

(1) Frequency of occurrence	References
Expected in one or more of 100 treatment courses	
Maculopapular rash[a]	51[C]–53[C], 54[R]
Expected once in 100–1000 treatment courses	
Urticaria, angioedema	53[C]–56[C]
Drug fever[b]	36[C], 57[C]
Eosinophilia[c]	58[C], 59[R], 60[C]
Expected once in 1000–10 000 treatment courses	
Anaphylactic shock	61[C]–63[C]
Bronchospasm and acute severe dyspnoea	64[C], 65[C]
Thrombocytopenia	66[C], 67[R]
Serum sickness-like disease[d]	68[C]–71[C]
Vasculitis	68[C]
Expected less than once in 10 000 treatment courses	
Hemolytic anemia	72[R], 73[C], 74[C], 75[c]–77[c]
Vesicular and bullous skin reactions (including Stevens-Johnson syndrome and toxic epidermal necrolysis)	78[C]–81[C], 82[c], 83[c], 84[C]
Erythema multiforme[e]	78[C], 85[R]
Erythema nodosum	78[C], 85[R]
Interstitial nephritis[f]	86[R]
(2) Observed after occupational exposure	
Contact sensitivity	87[C], 88[C]
Anaphylaxis	63[C]
Asthma, pneumonitis	89[C]–91[C]

[a] Occurs with all β-lactams, more frequently with aminopenicillins, penicillinase-resistant penicillins and antipseudomonas penicillins.
[b] Occurs with all β-lactams, probably more frequently with piperacillin/tazobactam and aztreonam.
[c] Occurs with all β-lactams, probably more frequently with meticillin, nafcillin, oxacillin, second- and third-generation cephalosporins, aztreonam and imipenem.
[d] Occurs with all β-lactams, probably more frequently with penicillin G and V, antipseudomonas penicillins, cefaclor, cefadroxil, cephalexin, loracarbef, aztreonam and imipenem.
[e] Occurs probably with all β-lactams, more frequently with penicillin G and V, cefuroxime, cefoperazone, cefaclor and imipenem.
[f] Occurs probably with all β-lactams, well documented for meticillin.

allergic reactions to penicillin of 0.62% (155 out of 24 906 treatment courses) in patients without history of penicillin allergy compared to 12.8% (10 out of 78 treatment courses) in patients with a history of penicillin allergy (50[C]). Reaction rates are higher in patients with histories suggesting IgE-mediated reactions (95[C]).

Patients with concurrent EBV- or HIV-infection or chronic lymphatic leukemia have increased frequency of occurrence of ampicillin- and amoxicillin-associated rashes (96[C]).

Drug dose, mode of application and duration of treatment probably influence the frequency of occurrence of allergic reactions. Topical administration of drug has been associated with a high incidence of sensitization in contrast to a low incidence with the oral route. For IgE-mediated reactions a frequent and intermittent course of treatment is more likely to induce allergy than a prolonged course without drug-free interval (97[R]). High doses of parenteral β-lactam are usually required for the induction of penicillin-induced hemolytic anemia (98[C]). Similarly, it is likely that the high doses of β-lactams used in patients with cystic fibrosis result in the high incidence of drug fever in that patient population (36[C]).

Co-administration of β-blocker drugs has been associated with an increased risk of severe allergic drug reactions and reduces the effect of epinephrine as immediate treatment for anaphylactic shock. The mechanism involves changes in the regulation of anaphylactic mediators (99[C]).

Evidence for a role of allopurinol in potentiating skin reactions to ampicillin remains controversial (100[C], 101[C]).

The Jarisch-Herxheimer reaction This is a systemic reaction occurring hours after initial treatment of spirochetal diseases such as syphilis, leptospirosis, Lyme disease, relapsing fever and presents with fevers, rigors, hypotension and flushing (102[Cr]). In the case of syphilis the reaction is more frequent in secondary syphilis and may cause additional manifestations such as flare-up of cutaneous lesions, sudden aneurysmal dilatation of the aortic arch (103[c]) or angina pectoris or acute coronary occlusion (SED-8, 559). It is mentioned here since it may easily be mistaken for a drug-induced hypersensitivity reaction. The underlying mechanism is initiated by the antibiotic-induced release of spirochete-derived pyrogens. Transient elevations of TNF, IL-6 and IL-8 have been detected in patients with the Jarisch-Herxheimer reaction (104[Cr]). The reaction lasts 12 to 24 hours and can be alleviated by the use of aspirin. Alternatively prednisone can be used and is recommended as adjunctive treatment of symptomatic cardiovascular syphilis or neurosyphilis.

ANTIBIOTIC-RELATED DIARRHEA AND COLITIS

Almost all antibacterial chemotherapeutic agents have been observed to induce diarrhea in a very variable proportion of patients (105[R], 106[R]). This proportion varies not only depending on the antibiotic, but also on the clinical setting (in/out-patient, age, race) and the definition of diarrhea. In a variable proportion of cases, severe colonic inflammation will develop and, in some of them, pseudomembranes. Patients treated with lincomycin or clindamycin, cephalosporins, penicillinase-resistant penicillins or multiple antibiotic regimens seem to be at especially high risk (107[C], 108[C], 109[R]). A low risk usually is associated with sulfonamides, cotrimoxazole, chloramphenicol and tetracyclines (111[R]). Although little data have yet been published on this subject for the quinolines, this relatively new class of antimicrobial agents seldom seems to cause diarrhea and pseudomebranous colitis (PMC) (110[C]). PMC represents the most severe form of antibiotic colitis (for extensive reviews see: 111[R]—114[R]). PMC was known before the introduction of antimicrobial agents and still may occur without previous antibiotic use, e.g. after antineoplastic chemotherapy (115[R]) or even 'spontaneously'. However, the number of cases has increased dramatically since antibiotics began to be used (116[R]).

In PMC the stools are generally watery with occult, but seldom gross, blood loss. Common findings include abdominal pain, cramps, fever and leukocytosis. Especially severe forms may run such a rapid course that diarrhea does not occur, they present with symptoms of severe toxicity and shock (117[c]). As a rare complication, marked dilatation of the colon and paralytic ileus may develop, i.e. toxic megacolon.

Pseudomembranes are described as initially punctuate creamy to yellow plaques, 0.2—2.0 cm in size, which may be confluent, with 'skip areas' of edematous mucosa. Histologically, they are composed of fibrin, mucous, necrotic epithelial cells, and leukocytes.

Until the late 1970s, PMC was thought to be caused by mucosal ischemia, viral infection or *Staphylococcus aureus*. Since 1977 much evidence has accumulated indicating that the etiological agent of PMC is an anerobic gram-positive, toxin-producing bacterium, *Clostridium difficile* (118[C], 119[R], 120[r]).

The appearance of PMC in clusters of patients (121[C], 122[C], 123[C]) may explain the wide variation in occurrence and suggests that the disease may result from cross-contamination among patients rendered susceptible by antibiotic treatment. An additional possible explanation for the large differences in reported frequency may be the use of different methods for detection and differences in the definition of the disease. In fact, the rate of diarrhea associated to clindamycin varies from zero to 20% (124[C]) and also varies considerably with the other antibiotics (125[C]). If proctosigmoidoscopy was routinely performed in all patients with diarrhea under clindamycin, PMC could be found in as many as 10% of the patients (126[R]). Among predisposing factors to the development of PMC, age of the patient, severity of the underlying disease, colonic stasis, cytostatic therapy, surgical interventions and gastrointestinal manipulations are mentioned in the literature (127[C]—131[C]).

After adjustment for age and severity of disease, multivariate analysis showed acute (1—7 days) exposure to cephalosporins, exposure to penicillins (8—14 days), use of gastrointestinal stimulants and use of enemas to be single risk factors associated with *Clostridium difficile*-related diarrhea. A possible explanation for these risk factors is that all these conditions can alter the normal gastrointestinal flora, which is normally able to protect the host from colonisation with *Clostridium difficile* (122[C]).

There have been several reports of frequent diarrhea in patients treated with combinations of ampicillin or amoxicillin with β-lactamase-inhibitors such as sulbactam or clavulanic acid (132[C], 133[r], 134[C], 135[R], 136[R]). A double-blind cross-over study on healthy volunteers showed disturbances of small-bowel motility in healthy volunteers after oral administration of the combination amoxicillin/clavulanic acid (137[C]).

Although the first antibiotics correlated to PMC were lincomycin and clindamycin, the disease has later been described with all other antimicrobial agents, even topical applications (138[c]). Ironically, intravenous vancomycin (139[c]) and metronidazole (140[c]), which may be used as specific therapy of the condition, have also been implicated.

Clostridium difficile has been isolated in 11—33% of patients with antibiotic-associated diarrhea, 60—75% of the patients with antibiotic-associated colitis, and 96—100% of cases with PMC (112[R], 141[R], 142[C]). There is, however, a certain number of asymptomatic carriers judged to be about 2% of the adult population (107[C]). Infants up to 2 years seem to be refractory to PMC, although a high percentage may be carriers of the toxigenic *Clostridium difficile* (142[C], 143[C]). The reasons for this are unknown. It has been speculated that infants may lack the receptors for the toxin.

Clostridium difficile produces two well-characterized toxins (120[R], 144[R]). Toxin A, an enterotoxin, and toxin B, an extremely potent cytotoxin are thought to be ultimately responsible for the disease. The toxigenicity between different *Clostridium difficile* strains for toxins A and B may vary, and seems to correlate with symptomatic disease (145[C]). Pseudomembranes were found in a higher percentage of patients with stools positive for cytotoxin than in patients whose stools were positive for *Clostridium difficile*, but toxin-negative (128[C]).

Although there is also a high association with *Clostridium difficile* toxin (about 20% are toxin positive) in antibiotic-associated diarrhea without pseudomembranes, it is possible that this micro-organism plays no pathogenic role in this disease. Rather, it may be due to an impaired metabolism of carbohydrates, altered fatty acid profiles, and/or the composition and deconjugation of bile acids by quantitatively and qualitatively altered fecal flora (105[R], 106[R], 142[C]).

Diagnosis

The diagnosis of antibiotic-related colitis should be considered in any patient with severe diarrhea during or within 4—6 weeks after antibiotic therapy. The single most diagnostic procedure is sigmoidoscopy, although in a number of cases the typical pseudomembranous lesions may be seen only above the rectosigmoid area (146[c]). Radiographic investigations (barium enema and air contrast) may show typical findings, but are dangerous procedures in advanced cases and should therefore be avoided. Computerized tomography has been described to show typical, although not pathognomonic patterns in two patients (147[c]).

An acute colitis, different from PMC, was described by Toffler et al. (148[C]). It was observed in five patients under treatment with penicillin and penicillin derivatives. Considerable rectal bleeding occurred. The radiographical findings were those of ischemic colitis (spasm, transverse ridging, 'thumbprinting' and punctuate ulcerations). On sigmoidoscopy and biopsy, the mucosa was normal except for the inflammatory cell infiltration seen in one case. Conservative treatment resulted in rapid clinical remission of the hemorrhagic diarrhea and radiological changes.

Clostridium difficile may be cultured from stool, and toxin B may assessed by different techniques (111[R]). The most accurate method is still a cytotoxin tissue culture assay. This test detects the cytopathic effect of cytotoxin B, which can be neutralized by *Clostridium sordellii*-antitoxin, but requires 24-48 hours to show a result. Alternative tests that produce faster results have been developed. A latex agglutination test may have a similar sensitivity, but is less specific than the cytotoxin tissue culture assay. The same seems true for the enzyme immunoassay. Dot immunobinding assay has not yet been extensively studied (149[C]).

Treatment

Therapy consists in discontinuing—whenever possible—the antibiotic when diarrhea occurs, and replacement of fluid and electrolyte loss. In the less severe cases of antibiotic-associated diarrhea no further treatment may be needed. A more intensive approach is usually needed in all patients with PMC. When a toxic syndrome develops, the fluid losses within the bowel may be very large. In these cases, a central venous line is usually helpful offering the opportunity to measure central venous pressure. Usually there is also a loss of serum proteins, and in some cases, of blood, which need appropriate replacement. In the rare cases with fulminant colitis and development of a toxic megacolon, a surgical intervention may be necessary (150[R], 151[c]).

In the case of PMC (typical endoscopic findings, positive test for *Clostridium difficile* or its toxin) the most effective treatment is oral administration of vancomycin for 7—14 days. A regimen of 125 mg q.i.d. has been shown to be as effective as the formerly employed high-dose regimen of 500 mg qid (152[C]). Oral metronidazole (250 mg t.i.d. or q.i.d.) has proved to be as effective as vancomycin and shows comparable relapse rates (153[C]). It may be preferred in all less severe forms because of the very high cost of vancomycin. Oral bacitracin 25 000 U q.i.d. (154[R]) and oral teicoplanin (155[r]) have been shown to be acceptable alternatives.

The role of anion-exchange resins (i.e. cholestyramine and colestipol), which may bind *Clostridium difficile* toxin, is still controversial (156[r]). If ion exchange resins are given at all, they should not be given together with vancomycin, because of their ability to bind this antibiotic (157[C]). Attempts to restore the intestinal flora with *Lactobacillus* GG (158[C]), or with fecal enemas (159[C]) from healthy volunteers have shown some favorable results in less severe cases. Esthetic and infectious concerns may be an obstacle to the latter. It also has been suggested that treatment with *Saccharomyces boulardii* may help prevent the development of antibiotic-associated diarrhea (160[r]). Its value in the prevention and treatment of relapses has still to be demonstrated. Antimotility agents have been associated with an increased incidence of antibiotic-related diarrhea and may worsen symptoms when the disease is already established (161[C]). They should therefore be avoided.

Relapses are similarly frequent after treatment with metronidazole and vancomycin (111[R]). In a survey of 189 adult patients a first relapse occurred in up to 24%, a second relapse in 46% of this subpopulation (154[R]), and may be due to sporulation of *Clostridium difficile*. They usually respond to further courses of the initial treatment. Some further alternative treatments have been proposed for repeatedly relapsing cases, including the combination of vancomycin and rifampicin (162[C]).

There is little evidence that re-exposure to the same antibiotic which caused PMC comprises a further risk for relapse. Still, it would seem wise to avoid antibiotics most often related to PMC in a patient who experienced this complication.

ORGANS AND SYSTEMS (*for single classes of β-lactam antibiotics and particular compounds see Chapters* 25.3—25.5)

Cardiovascular Anaphylactic shock and other anaphylactic reactions see 'Hypersensitivity reactions' above and Chapter 25.1—25.5.

Respiratory Anaphylactic reactions see 'Hypersensitivity reactions' above and Chapter 25.1—25.5.

Allergic bronchospasm can principally be a consequence of IgE-antibody-mediated allergy to all β-lactam antibiotics.

Nervous system Since the first observation of convulsions following intraventricular administration of penicillin more than 50 years ago (163[c]), neurotoxicity has been attributed to the majority of β-lactam antibiotics. Its manifestations are considered to be the consequence of GABAergic inhibition (164[r], 165[r]) and include clear epileptic manifestations as well as more atypical reactions such as asterixis, drowsiness, hallucinations and others. Epileptogenic activity of β-lactam antibiotics is also documented in animals and, e.g. in brain slices in vitro (for review see 166[R]). The integrity of the β-lactam ring is a prerequisite and, accordingly, epileptogenic activity is extinguished by β-lactamase (167[R], 168[R]). Clinical manifestations are clearly dose dependent and brain tissue fluid concentrations appear to be more relevant than CSF- or blood-levels (166[R]). Accordingly the major risk factor is impaired renal function, particularly when not recognized. Further risk situations are in the very young or very old, ongoing meningitis, intraventricular therapy and a history of epilepsy (169[cR]). The neurotoxic potential differs considerably among the various β-lactam antibiotics, and experimental models have been developed for investigating this aspect (170[cr], 171[cR]). Currently, imipenem/cilastatin appears to cause the highest frequencies of neurotoxicity observed (172[C], 173[C]) and the above-mentioned risk factors have been confirmed particularly with use of this compound (174[C]) (SEDA-18, 261). Quinolone-antibiotics, which by themselves have a proconvulsant activity, can potentiate excitation of the central nervous system by β-lactam antibiotics at least in animals (175[c], 176[c]).

Endocrine, metabolic Pivaloyl-containing compounds such as pivmecillinam, pivampicillin and cefetamet-pivoxil can induce significant increase of urinary carnitine excretion (177[C], 178[C]). There are esterified prodrugs which become only effective after release of pivalic acid which in turn is esterified with carnitine. Carnitine loss was initially described in children and may produce symptoms similar to other types of carnitine deficiency, e.g. secondary to organic acidurias (177[C]). A recent report, however, describes slow replenishment of carnitine deficiency after cessation of long-term treatment with pivaloyl-containing antibiotics. Structural alteration as shown by muscle biopsy and functional carnitine deficiency of the liver with reduced ketogenesis in one patient were reversible upon carnitine replenishment (179[C]). Another 51-year-old female developed a skeletal muscle myopathy after 3 months of pivampicillin therapy which only improved after oral carnitine replacement (180[c]). As long as the risk potential of pivaloyl-induced urinary loss of carnitine as well as particularly risk situations are not better defined, it is prudent to use pivaloyl-containing prodrugs only for short-term treatment.

Mineral and fluid balance Since β-lactam antibiotics contain sodium or potassium, they can cause or at least aggravate electrolyte disturbances when given in sufficiently high doses. The most frequently seen manifestations are hypernatremia and hypokalemia (see also Chapter 25.3). The sodium content of injectable β-lactam antibiotics per gram active compound may vary by up to a factor of three (181[r]).

Hematological Immune hemolytic anemia has originally been described with penicillin G but later on with other penicillins and also cephalosporins. It is usually seen during treatment with very high doses following the so-called 'drug absorption' mechanism. The β-lactam antibiotic binds covalently to the erythrocyte surface forming thereby complete antigens which in turn can bind drug-specific circulating IgG antibody. Typically direct and indirect Coombs tests are positive but complement is not activated (55[C], 72[R], 74[C]). Rarely, other immunological mechanisms have been observed, e.g. the so-called 'innocent bystander type' of hemolysis (74[C]). Here, complement can be detected on the erythrocyte surface (see also Chapters 25.3 and 25.4). Some cephalosporins, clavulanic acid and imipenem/cilastatin can cause positive direct antiglobulin tests (183[C]). The phenomenon is due to unspecific serum protein absorption on to the erythrocyte membrane and is not related to immune hemolytic processes. Detection of non-immunologically bound serum proteins is improved if the reagents used include additional anti-albumin activity (184[R]). The phenomenon is a known source of difficulties in evaluating suspected immune hemolysis or routine cross-matching of blood products (185[C]). The true frequency of the phenomenon remains unclear, since it has not been positively sought.

Agranulocytoses and leukopenia have been observed with virtually all β-lactam antibiotics. For further discussions see 'dose-dependent reactions' above.

Thrombocytopenia (see Chapters 25.3 and 25.4).

Thrombocytosis is frequently mentioned as a side effect. It has been suggested, however, that this rather reflects healing from infection than toxicity (186[R]).

Virtually all cephalosporins can cause eosinophilia, isolated or in the context of very different reactions (see also above 'Dose-dependent reaction' and 'Hypersensitivity reactions').

Bleeding disorders Treatment with β-lactam antibiotics may result in impaired haemostasis and bleeding. The true incidence of bleeding is however difficult to assess in a clinical setting, since many non-antibiotic factors may be involved, such as malnutrition with vitamin K depletion (187[C]), renal failure (188[C]), serious infection (189[C]), cancer, and use of cytotoxic drugs, or surgery, and have made conclusive interpretation difficult (190[C]). Between the different β-lactam antibiotics, the reported incidence of clinical bleeding varies widely and was highest (22.2% of the patients) with moxalactam, now withdrawn from the market (cf. SED-12). For the other cephalosporins, clinical bleeding was observed with frequencies ranging from 2.7 (cefazolin/cephalothin) to 8.2% (cefoxitim) (191[C]). Two basic mechanisms have been proposed:

Alteration of coagulation Both direct inhibition of hepatic production of vitamin K-dependent clotting factors as well as alterations in the intestinal flora with subsequent reduction of microbial supply of vitamin K have been implicated (192[C], 193[c]). The relative role of either mechanism is difficult to assess, but experimental support for the flora theory is weak (194[R], 195[R]).

Several of the cephalosporins containing either a non-substituted *N*-methylthiotetrazole side chain (NMTT) such as cefamandole, cefamazole, cefmenoxime, cefoperazone, cefotetam, and moxalactam as well as a substituted NMTT side chain (i.e. ceforanide, ceforicid or cefotiam), or the structurally similar *N*-methylthiotriazine ring in ceftriaxone as well as the 2-methyl-1,2,4-thiadiazole-5-thiol (MTD) ring of cefazolin have been shown to interfere with vitamin K-dependent clotting factor synthesis. The molecular mechanism involves a dose-dependent inhibition of microsomal carboxylase function as shown in vitro in animal studies (196[C]) as well as inhibition of the epoxide reductase system in both animal models and humans or in both (197[C]–200[C]). Interestingly, cefoxitin, a non-NMTT compound, was implicated significantly more often than the NMTT-containing cefamandole or cefoperazone (201[C]).

NMTT must leave the parent antibiotic to inhibit the γ-carboxylation reaction (202[C]). The NMTT molecule may leave the parent cephalosporin either during spontaneous hydrolysis in the blood or during nucleophilic cleavage of the β-lactam ring by intestinal bacteria, followed by resorption from the gut into the portal circulation (203[C]). Studies in normal volunteers indicate compound-related differences in the ability of NMTT antibiotics to generate free NMTT, reflecting drug-specific differences in the susceptibility to in vitro hydrolysis or differences in gut NMTT production which may be a function of biliary excretion of the drug (204[C]).

Alteration of platelet number and platelet function Platelet dysfunction occurs primarily with carbenicillin, ticarcillin and infrequently other broad-spectrum penicillins in a dose-dependent fashion (205[C]), but the NMTT cephalosporin, moxalactam, has also been associated with altered platelet function in both normal subjects and patients treated with standard therapeutic regimens (206[C]–210[C]). In contrast, clinical studies including cefotaxime, ceftizoxime, cefoperazone and ceftracone did not reveal platelet dysfunction attributable to these compounds (209[C]–211[C]). There is evidence that β-lactam antibiotic-induced platelet dysfunction is at least partially irreversible (212[C]).

From a practical point of view it can be concluded that: (a) Use of NMTT side chain-containing cephalosporins is associated with the risk of a dose-dependent inhibition of vitamin K-dependent clotting factor synthesis. (b) Platelet dysfunction occurs primarily with the broad-spectrum penicillins, but the NMTT cephalosporins, notably moxalactam, have also been associated with altered platelet function. Monitoring of bleeding times should be considered in patients at risk (bleeding history, clinical bleeding, concomitant thrombocytopenia or use of other drugs known to interfere with platelet function. (c) The presence of non-antibiotic factors such as therapy with vitamin K antagonists, renal failure, hepatic dysfunction, impaired gastrointestinal function, and malnutrition may increase the risk of bleeding in cephalosporin-treated patients. Close monitoring of homeostasis (prothrombin time, template bleeding time), as well as prophylactic supplementation with vitamin K or, if necessary, therapeutic administration of fresh-frozen plasma and/or platelets is warranted according to the clinical context.

Liver Increases in serum transaminases and alkaline phosphatase, largely without additional symptoms, have been reported with the majority of β-lactam antibiotics. With different compounds the estimated frequencies vary by up to a factor of 10 (186[R]). The frequencies observed, however, may also depend on patient-related factors; in one particular study it was shown that only a minority of transaminase increases could not be explained by factors other than antibiotic treatment (213[C]).

More severe liver disease presenting as hepatitis and/or intrahepatic cholestasis has been seen with β-lactam antibiotics belonging to various classes, the isoxazolyl-penicillins being most frequently involved. More recently amoxicillin-clavulanate has repeatedly been found associated with cholestatic hepatitis (see 'Dose-dependent reactions' above and Chapters 25.3–25.5).

Gastrointestinal Gastrointestinal upset, nausea and vomiting have been observed under treatment with virtually all β-lactam antibiotics, both oral and parenteral. Even when comparing analogous applications and doses, no particular risk can be clearly ascribed to a given compound.

Urinary system Acute renal failure, with or without skin rash and eosinophilia has been reported with various β-lactam antibiotics, most frequently with meticillin. Hence, the designation 'methicillin-nephritis' is still sometimes used (see 'Dose-dependent reactions' above). The pathogenesis is largely unknown and is different from the nephrotoxicity of older cephalosporins namely cephaloridine and cephalotin. (see also Chapters 25.3–25.5).

Skin and appendages The majority of distinct mucocutaneous reactions which can be induced by drugs has been associated with the use of individual β-lactam antibiotics. These reactions include urticaria, angioedema, maculopapular exanthema, fixed drug eruption, erythema multiforme, Stevens-Johnson syndrome and TEN (toxic epidermal necrolysis), pruritus, eczematous lesions, and stomatitis (recently reviewed in 214[R]). However, the maculopapular rash is more frequent than all other skin manifestations taken together (51[C]–54[C]). In addition, an indistinguishable rash accompanies frequently various reactions manifesting on other organs (see 'Hypersensitivity reactions' and 'Dose-dependent reactions' above).

Musculoskeletal system Urinary carnitine loss with pivaloyl-containing compounds, see 'Endocrine, metabolic' above.

Serum sickness-like syndrome See 'Dose-dependent reactions' and 'Hypersensitivity reactions' above as well as Chapters 25.3 and 25.4.

Host defense mechanisms β-Lactam antibiotics like

many other antimicrobials have been studied with regard to immunomodulating properties and other influences on the host-parasite interaction. Although there is a large body of information from studying effects of β-lactam antibiotics on living cells or in animal models (e.g. 215[R], 216[R], 217[r], 218[r], 219[R]) it is not yet possible to clearly define 'side effect syndromes' paralleling these findings in patients.

RISK SITUATIONS (*see 'Dose-dependent reactions and Hypersensitivity reactions' and Chapters* 25.3 *and* 25.4)

Interactions and interference with diagnostic routines

Nearly 100 possible drug—drug interactions of 50 clinically used β-lactam preparations have recently been compiled (220[R]) (see also Chapters 25.3—25.5).

REFERENCES

1. Schliamser SE, Bolander H, Kourtopoulos H et al. Neurotoxicity of benzylpenicillin: correlation to concentrations in serum, cerebrospinal fluid and brain tissue fluid in rabbits. J Antimicrob Chemother 1988;21:365.
2. Bang NU, Kammer RB. Hematologic complications associated with betalactam antibiotics. Rev Infect Dis 1983; 5(Suppl):380.
3. Sattler FR, Weitekamp MR, Ballard JO. Potential for bleeding with new betalactam antibiotics. Ann Intern Med 1986;105:924.
4. Fossieck B Jr, Parker RH. Neurotoxicity during intravenous infusion of penicillin: a review. J Clin Pharmacol 1974; 14:504.
5. Andrassy K, Weischedel E, Ritz E et al. Bleeding in uremic patients after carbenicillin. Thromb Haemost 1976; 36:115.
6. Neftel KA, Hauser SP, Müller MR. Inhibition of granulopoiesis in vivo and in vitro by betalactam antibiotics. J Infect Dis 1985;52:90.
7. Gatell JM, Rello J, Miro JM et al. Cloxacillin-induced neutropenia. J Infect Dis 1986;154:372.
8. Rello J, Gatell JM, Miro JM et al. Effectos secundarios associados a la cloxacillina. Med Clin (Barcelona) 1987; 89:631.
9. Vidal Pan C, Gonzalez Quintela A, Roman Garcia J et al. Cephapirin-induced neutropenia. Chemotherapy 1989; 35:449.
10. Olaison L, Alestig K. A prospective study of neutropenia induced by high doses of betalactam antibiotics. J Antimicrob Chemother 1990;25:449.
11. Neftel KA, Wälti M, Schulthess HK et al. Adverse reactions following intravenous penicillin-G related to degradation of the drug in vitro. Klin Wochenschr 1984;62:25.
12. Oldfield EC. Leukopenia associated with the use of betalactam antibiotics in patients with hepatic dysfunction. Am J Gastroenterol 1994;89:1263.
13. Ramos-Fernandez de Soria R, Martin Nunez G, Sanchez Gil F. Agranulocitosis inducida por drogas. Rapida recuperacion con el uso precoz de G-CSF. Sangre 1994;39:145.
14. Bradford CR, Ong EL, Hendrick DJ, Saunders DWG. Use of colony stimulating factors for the treatment of drug-induced agranulocytosis. Br J Haematol 1993;84:182.
15. Neftel KA, Hafkemeyer P, Cottagnoud P, et al. Did evolutionary forerunners of betalactam antibiotics bind to nucleid acid replication enzymes? In: 50 Years of Penicillin Application. Technische Universität Berlin, Public Ltd Prag, 1993;394.
16. Ditlove J, Weidmann P, Bernstein M et al. Methicillin nephritis. Medicine 1977;56:483.
17. Galpin JE, Shinaberger JH, Stanley TM et al. Acute interstitial nephritis due to methicillin. Am J Med 1978; 65:756.
18. Sanjad SA, Haddad GC, Nassar VH. Nephropathy, an underestimated complication of methicillin therapy. J Pediatr 1974;84:873.
19. Neftel KA. Verträglichkeit der hochdosierten Therapie mit Betalactam-Antibiotika—Pathogenese der Nebenwirkungen insbesondere der Neutropenie. Fortschr Antimikr Antineoplast Chemother 1984;3-1:71.
20. Olans RN, Weiner LB. Reversible oxacillin hepatotoxicity. J Pediatr 1976;89:835.
21. Michelson PA. Reversible high dose oxacillin-associated liver injury. Can J Hosp Pharm 1981;34:83.
22. Onorato IM, Axelrod AL. Hepatitis from intravenous high-dose oxacillin therapy. Ann Intern Med 1978;89:497.
23. Fairley CK, McNeil JJ, Desmond P et al. Risk factors for development of flucloxacillin associated jaundice. Br Med J 1993;306:233.
24. Turner IB, Eckstein RP, Riley JW et al. Prolonged hepatic cholestasis after flucloxacillin therapy. Med J Aust 1989;151:701.
25. Devereaux BM, Crawford DHG, Purcell P et al. Flucloxacillin associated cholestatic hepatitis: an Australian and Swedish epidemic? Eur J Clin Pharmacol 1995;49:81.
26. Kleinmann MS, Presberg JE. Cholestatic hepatitis after dicloxacillin-sodium therapy. J Clin Gastroenterol 1986;8:77.
27. Reed MD, Stern RC, Myers CM et al. Therapeutic evaluation of piperacillin for acute pulmonary exacerbation in cystic fibrosis. Pediatr Pulmonol 1987;3:101.
28. Sanders WW, Johnson JE, Taggart JG. Adverse reactions to cephalotin and cephapirin. N Engl J Med 1974; 290:424.
29. Lang R, Lishner M, Ravid M. Adverse reactions to prolonged treatment with high doses of carbenicillin and ureidopenicillins. Rev Infect Dis 1991;13:68.
30. Stead RJ, Kennedy HG, Hodson ME et al. Adverse reactions to piperacillin in cystic fibrosis (Letter to Editor). Lancet 1984;i:857.
31. Strandvik B. Adverse reactions to piperacillin in patients with cystic fibrosis (Letter to Editor). Lancet 1984;i:1362.
32. Brock PG, Roach M. Adverse reactions to piperacillin in cystic fibrosis (Letter to Editor). Lancet 1984;i:1070.
33. McDonnell TJ, Fitzgerald MX. Cystic fibrosis and penicillin hypersensitivity (Letter to Editor). Lancet 1984;i:1301.

34. Stead RJ, Kennedy HG, Hodson ME et al. Adverse reactions to piperacillin in adults with cystic fibrosis. Thorax 1985;40:184.
35. Koch C, Hjelt K, Pedersen SS et al. Retrospective clinical study of hypersensitivity reactions to aztreonam and six other beta-lactam antibiotics in cystic fibrosis patients receiving multiple treatment courses. Rev Infect Dis 1981;13(Suppl 7):608.
36. Pleasants RA, Walker TR, Samuelson WM. Allergic reactions to parenteral beta-lactams in patients with cystic fibrosis. Chest 1994;106:1124.
37. Doherty JB, Ashe BM, Argenbright LW et al. Cephalosporin antibiotics can be modified to inhibit human leukocyte elastase. Nature 1986;322:192.
38. Antoniadis A, Müller WE, Wollert V. Benzodiazepine receptor interactions may be involved in the neurotoxicity of various penicillin derivatives. Ann Neurol 1980;8:71.
39. Neftel KA, Hübscher U. Effects of betalactam antibiotics on proliferation of eukaryotic cells. Antimicrob Agents Chemother 1987;31:1657.
40. Yamabe S, Adachi K, Watanabe M et al. The effects of three betalactamase inhibitors: YTR 830 H, sulbactam and clavulanic acid on the growth of human cells in culture. Chemotherapia 1987;6:337.
41. Bloom JC, Lewis HB, Sellers TS et al. The hematologic effects of cefonicid and cefazedone in the dog: a potential model of cephalosporin hematotoxicity in man. Toxicol Appl Pharmacol 1987;90:135.
42. Bloom JC, Lewis HB, Sellers TS et al. The hematopathology of cefonicid- and cefazedone-induced blood dyscrasias in the dog. Toxicol Appl Pharmacol 1987;90:143.
43. Deldar A, Lewis H, Bloom J et al. Cephalosporin-induced changes in the ultrastructure of canine bone marrow. Vet Pathol 1988;25:211.
44. Bloom JC, Thiem PA, Seller TS et al. Cephalosporin-induced immune cytopenia in the dog: demonstration of erythrocyte-, neutrophil-, and platelet-associated IgG following treatment with cefazedone. Am J Hematol 1988;28:71.
45. Rouveix B, Lassoued K, Regnier B et al. Neutropénies induites par les betalactamines: mécanisme toxique ou immun? Thérapie 1988;43:489.
46. Murphy MF, Riordan T, Minchinton RM et al. Demonstration of an immune-mediated mechanism of penicillin-induced neutropenia and thrombocytopenia. Br J Haematol 1983;55:155.
47. Murphy MF, Metcalfe P, Grint PCA et al. Cephalosporin-induced immune neutropenia. Br J Haematol 1985;59:9.
48. Lee D, Dewdney JM, Edwards RG et al. Measurement of specific IgG antibody levels in serum of patients on regimens comprising high total dose betalactam therapy. Int Arch Allergy Appl Immunol 1986;79:344.
49. International rheumatic fever study group. Allergic reactions to long-term benzathine penicillin prophylaxis for rheumatic fever. Lancet 1991;337:1308.
50. Rudolph AH, Price EV. Penicillin reactions among patients in veneral disease clinics. J Am Med Assoc 1973; 223:499.
51. Arndt KA, Jick H. Rates of cutaneous reactions to drugs. A report from the Boston Collaborative Drug Surveilllance Program. J Am Med Assoc 1976;235:918.
52. Bigby M, Jick S, Hershel J, Arndt K. Drug-induced cutaneous reactions. A report from the Boston Collaborative Drug Surveilllance Program on 15438 consecutive in patients, 1975 to 1982. J Am Med Assoc 1986;256:3358.
53. Hunziker T, Hoigné RV, Küenzi UP et al. Comprehensive hospital drug monitoring (CHDM), the adverse skin reactions, a 20-years survey, Abstract. Pharmacoepidemiology 1995;4(Suppl 1):S13.
54. Shepherd GM. Allergy to β-lactam antibiotics. Immunol Allergy Clin North Am 1991;11:611.
55. Levine BB, Redmond AP, Fellner M et al. Penicillin allergy and the heterogeneous immune responses of man to benzylpenicillin. J Clin Invest 1966;45:1895.
56. Hantson P, de Coninck B, Horn JL et al. Immediate hypersensitivity to aztreonam and imipenem. Br Med J 1991;302:294.
57. Mackowiak PA, LeMaistre CF. Drug fever: a critical appraisal of conventional concepts. Ann Int Med 1987;106:728.
58. Calandra GB, Wang C, Aziz M, Brown KR. The safety profile of imipenem/cliastin: worldwide clinical experience based on 3470 patients. J Antimicrobial Chemother 1986; 18(Suppl E):193.
59. Sanders CV, Greenberg MD, Marier RL. Cefamandole and cefoxitin. Ann Intern Med 1985;103:70.
60. Swabb EA. Review of the clinical pharmacology of the monobactam aztreonam. Am J Med 1985;78(Suppl 2A):11.
61. Delage C, Irey NS. Anaphylactic deaths: a clinico-pathologic study of 43 cases. J Forensic Sci 1972;17:525.
62. Weiss ME, Adkinson NF. Immediate hypersensitivity reactions to penicillin and related antibiotics. Clin Allergy 1988;18:515.
63. Bochner BS, Lichtenstein LM. Anaphylaxis. N Engl J Med 1991;324:1785.
64. Hoigné RV, Braunschweig S, Zehnder D et al. Abstract, Pharmaco-epidemiology 1994;4(Suppl 1):S90.
65. Hoigné R, D'Andrea Jaeger M, Hess T et al. Akute schwere Dyspnoe als Medikamentennebenwirkung. Schweiz Med Wochenschr 1990;120:1211.
66. Adkinson NF Jr. Immunogenicity and cross-allergenicity of aztreonam. Am J Med 1990;88:12S–38S.
67. Hicks MJ, Flaitz CM. The role of antibiotics in platelet dysfunction and coagulopathy. Int J Antimicrob Agents 1993;2:129.
68. Platt R, Dreis MW, Kennedy DL et al. Serum sickness-like reactions to amoxicillin, cefaclor, cephalexin and trimethoprim-sulfamethoxazole. J Infect Dis 1988;158:474.
69. Levine LR. Quantitative comparison of adverse reactions to cefaclor vs amoxicillin in a surveillance study. Pediatr Infect Dis 1985;4:358.
70. Moskovitz BL. Clinical adverse effects during ceftriaxone therapy. Am J Med 1984;77:84.
71. Stricker BH, Tijssen JG. Serum sickness-like reactions to cefaclor. J Clin Epidemiol 1992;45:1177.
72. Petz LD, Fudenberg HH. Coombs-positive hemolytic anemia caused by penicillin administration. N Engl J Med 1966;274:171.
73. White JM, Brown DL, Hepner GW et al. Penicillin-induced haemolytic anaemia. Br Med J 1968;3:26.
74. Funicella T, Weinger RS, Moake JL et al. Penicillin-induced immunohemolytic anemia associated with circulating immune complexes. Am J Hematol 1977;3:219.
75. Tuffs L. Flucloxacillin-induced haemolytic anaemia. Med J Aust 1986;144:559.
76. Garratty G, Postoway N, Schwellenbach J, McMahill PC. A fatal case of ceftriaxone (Rocephin)-induced hemolytic anemia associated with intravascular immune hemolysis. Transfusion 1991;31:176.

77. Chambers LA, Donovan LM, Kruskall MS. Ceftazidime-induced hemolysis in a patient with drug-dependent antibodies reactive by immune complex and drug adsorption mechanisms. Am J Clin Pathol 1991;95:393.
78. Fellner MJ. Adverse reactions to penicillin and related drugs. Clin Dermatol 1986;4:133.
79. Schöpf E, Stühmer A, Rzany B et al. Toxic epidermal necrolysis (TEN) and Stevens-Johnson syndrome (SJS): an epidemiological study from West Germany. Arch Dermatol 1991;127:839.
80. Kauppinen K, Stubb S. Drug eruptions: causative agents and clinical types. Acta Derm-Venereol 1984;64:320.
81. Fellner MJ, Mark AS. Penicillin- and ampicillin-induced pemphigus vulgaris. Int J Dermatol 1980;7:392.
82. Manders SM, Heymann WR. Acute generalized exanthemic pustulosis. Cutis 1994;54:194.
83. McDonald BJ, Singer JW, Bianco JA. Toxic epidermal necrolysis possibly linked to aztreonam in bone marrow transplant patients. Ann Pharmacother 1992;26:34.
84. Brenner S, Wolf R, Ruocco V. Drug-induced pemphigus. I. A survey. Clin Dermatol 1993;11:501.
85. Blacker KL, Stern RS, Wintroub BU. Cutaneous reactions to drugs. In: Fitzpatrick TB, ed. Dermatology in General Medicine, 4th Edition. New York: McGraw-Hill, Inc, 1993;1783.
86. Murray KM, Keane WR. Review of drug-induced acute interstitial nephritis. Pharmacotherapy 1992;12:462.
87. Tadokoro K, Niimi N, Ohtoshi T et al. Cefotiam-induced IgE-mediated occupational contact anaphylaxis of nurses; case reports, RAST analysis, and a review of the literature. Clin Exp Allergy 1994;24:127.
88. Schulz KH, Schöpf E, Wex O. Allergische Berufsekzeme durch Ampicillin. Berufsdermatosen 1970;18:132.
89. Davies RJ, Hendrick DJ, Pepys J. Asthma due to inhaled chemical agents: ampicillin, benzylpenicillin, 6-aminopenicillanic acid, and related substances. Clin Allergy 1974;4:227.
90. Wengrover D, Tzfoni EE, Drenger B, Leitersdorf E. Erythroderma and pneumonitis induced by penicillin. Respiration 1986;50:301.
91. De Hoyos A, Holness DL, Tarlo SM. Hypersensitivity pneumonitis and airway hyperreactivity induced by occupational exposure to penicillin. Chest 1993;103:303.
92. Van Arsdel PP Jr. Classification of risk factors for drug allergy. Immunol Allergy Clin North Am 1991;11:475.
93. Petri M, Albritton J. Antibiotic allergy in systemic lupus erythematosus: a case control study. J Rheumatol 1992; 20:399.
94. Capaul R, Maibach R, Kuenzi UP et al. Atopy, bronchial asthma and previous adverse drug reactions (ADRs): risk factors for ADRs? Post Marketing Surveillance 1993;7:331.
95. Green GR, Rosenblum RH, Sweet LC. Evaluation of penicillin hypersensitivity: value of the clinical history and skin testing with penicilloyl-polylysine and penicillin G: a cooperative prospective study of the penicillin study group of the American Academy of Allergy. J Allergy Clin Immunol 1977;60:339.
96. Battegay M, Opravil M, Wüthrich B, Lüthy R. Rash with amoxicillin-clavulanate therapy in HIV-infected patients. Lancet 1989;ii:1100.
97. de Weck AL. Pharmacologic and immunochemical mechanisms of drug hypersensitivity. Immunol Allergy Clin North Am 1991;11:461.
98. Abraham GN, Petz LD, Fudenberg HH. Immunohaematologic crossallergenicity between penicillin and cephalothin in humans. Clin Exp Immunol 1968;3:343.
99. Toogood JH. Risk of anaphylaxis in patients receiving beta-blocker drugs. J Allergy Clin Immunol 1988;81:1.
100. Jick H, Porter J. Potentiation of ampicillin skin reactions by allopurinol or hyperuricemia. J Clin Pharmacol 1981;21:456.
101. Hoigné R, Sonntag MR, Zoppi M et al. Occurrence of exanthems in relation to aminopenicillin preparations and allopurinol. N Engl J Med 1987;316:1217.
102. Friedland JS, Warrell DA. The Jarisch-Herxheimer reaction in leptospirosis: possible pathogenesis and review. Rev Infect Dis 1991;13:207.
103. Young EJ, Weingarten NM, Boughn RE et al. Studies on the pathogenesis of the Jarish Herxheimer reaction. J Infect Dis 1982;146:606.
104. Detection of plasma tumor necrosis factor, interleukins 6, and 8 during the Jarish-Herxheimer reaction in relapsing fever. J Exp Med 1992;175:1207.
105. Ewe K. Diarrhoea and constipation. Ballière's Clin. Gastroenterol 1988;2:353.
106. Hooker KD, Di Piro JT. Effect of antimicrobial therapy on bowel flora. Clin Pharm 1988;7:878.
107. Aronsson B, Möllby R, Nord CE. Antimicrobial agents and *Clostridium difficile* in acute enteric disease: epidemiological data from Sweden, 1980—1982. J Infect Dis 1985; 151:476.
108. Aronsson B, Möllby R, Nord CE. *Clostridium difficile* and antibiotic associated diarrhoea in Sweden. Scand J Infect Dis 1982;35(Suppl)35:53.
109. Fekety MB, Akshay BS. Diagnosis and treatment of *Clostridium difficile* colitis. J Am Med Assoc 1993;269:71.
110. Zehnder D, Künzi UP, Maibach R et al. Die Häufigkeit der Antibiotika-assoziierten Kolitis bei hospitalisierten Patienten der Jahre 1974—1991 im 'Comprehensive Hospital Drug Monitoring' Bern/St. Gallen. Schweiz Med Wschr 1995;125:676.
111. Bartlett JG. Antibiotic-Associated diarrhea. Clin Infect Dis 1992;15:573.
112. Kelly CP, Pothoulakis C, LaMont JT. *Clostridium difficile* colitis. N Engl J Med 1994;330:257.
113. George WL. Antimicrobial agent-associated colitis and diarrhea: historical background and clinical aspects. Rev Infect Dis 1984;6(Suppl 1):S208.
114. Talbot RW, Walker RC, Beart jr RW. Changing epidemiology, diagnosis, and treatment of *Clostridium difficile* toxin-associated colitis. Br J Surg 1986;73:17.
115. Anand A, Glatt Aaron E. *Clostridium difficile* infection associated with antineoplastic chemotherapy: A review. Clin Infect Dis 1993;17:109.
116. Bartlett JG. Antibiotic-associated pseudomembranous colitis. Rev Infect Dis 1979;1:530.
117. Burke GW, Wilson ME, Mehrez IO. Absence of diarrhea in toxic megacolon complicating *Clostridium difficile* pseudomembranous colitis. Am J Gastroenterol 1988;83:304.
118. Larson HE, Price AB. Pseudomembranous colitis: presence of clostridial toxin. Lancet 1977;ii:1312.
119. Borrelio SP. Pathogenesis of *Clostridium difficile* infection of the gut. J Med Microbiol 1990;33:207.
120. Bartlett JG. *Clostridium difficile*: History of its role as an enteric pathogen and the current state of knowledge about the organism. Clin Infect Dis 1994;18(Suppl 4):S265.
121. Cerquetti M, Pantosti A, Gentile G et al. Epidemie ospedaliere di diarrea da *Clostridium difficile*: dimostrazione di infezione crociata mediante tecniche di tipizzazione. Ann Ist Super Sanità 1989;25:327.

122. McFarland LV, Suravwicz CM, Stamm WE. Risk Factors for *Clostridium difficile* carriage and *C. difficile*-associated diarrhea in a cohort of hospitalized patients. J Infect Dis 1990;162:678.
123. Nolan NPM, Kelly CP, Humphreys JFH et al. An epidemic of pseudomembranous colitis: importance of person to person spread. Gut 1987;28:1467.
124. Friedman GD, Gérard MJ, Ury HK. Clindamycin and diarrhea. J Am Med Assoc 1976;236:2498.
125. Stergachis A, Perera DR, Schnell MM, Jick H. Antibiotic-associated colitis. West J Med 1984;140:217.
126. Tedesco FJ. Clindamycin and colitis: A Review. J Infect Dis 1977;135(Suppl):S95.
127. Brown E, Talbot GH, Axelrod P et al. Risk factors for *Clostridium difficile* toxin-associated diarrhea. Infect Control Hosp Epidemiol 1990;11:283.
128. Gerding DN, Olson MM, Peterson LR et al. *Clostridium difficile*-associated diarrhea and colitis in adults. Arch Intern Med 1986;146:95.
129. Church JM, Fazio VW. A role for colonic stasis in the pathogenesis of disease related to *Clostridium difficile*. Dis Colon Rectum 1986;29:804.
130. Pierce PF Jr, Wilson R, Silva J Jr et al. Antibiotic-associated pseudomembranous colitis: an epidemiologic investigation of a cluster of cases. J Infect Dis 1982;145:269.
131. DeLalla F, Privitera G, Ortisi G et al. Third generation cephalosporins as a risk factor for *Clostridium difficile*-associated disease; a four-year survey in a general hospital. J Antimicrob Chemother 1989;23:623.
132. Bäumler C, Doller P, Decker K, Hirsch HA. Comparative study of ciprofloxacin and ampicillin with clavulanic acid for treatment of salpingitis and infections after gynaecological surgery. Personal communication, 1988.
133. Pitts NE, Gilber GS, Knirsch AK, Noguchi Y. Worldwide clinical experience with sultamicillin. APMIS 1989; 5(Suppl):23.
134. McLinn SE, Moskal M, Goldfarb J et al. Comparison of cefuroxime axetil and amoxicillin-clavulanate suspensions in treatment of acute otitis media with effusion in children. Antimicrob Agents Chemother 1994;38:315.
135. Todd PA, Benfield P. Amoxicillin/clavulanic acid. An update of its antibacterial activity, pharmacokinetic properties and therapeutic use. Drugs 1990;39:264.
136. Friedel HA, Campoli-Richards DM, Goa KL. Sultamicillin. A review of its antibacterial activity, pharmacokinetic properties and therapeutic use. Drugs 1989;37:491.
137. Caron F, Ducrotte P, Lerebours E et al. Effects of amoxicillin-clavulanate combination on the motility of the small intestine in human beings. Antimicrob Agents Chemother 1991;35:1085.
138. Milstone EB, McDonald AJ, Scholhamer CF Jr. Pseudomembranous colitis after topical application of clindamycin. Arch Dermatol 1981;117:154.
139. Hecht JR, Olinger EJ. *Clostridium difficile* colitis secondary to intravenous vancomycin. Digest Dis Sci 1989; 34:148.
140. Saginur R, Hawley CR, Bartlett JG. Colitis-associated with metronidazole therapy. J Infect Dis 1980;141:772.
141. Finegold SM. Clinical considerations in the diagnosis of antimicrobial agent-associated gastroenteritis. Diagn Microbiol Infect Dis 1986;4:87S.
142. Viscidi R, Willey S, Bartlett JG. Isolation rates and toxigenic potential of *Clostridium difficile* isolates from various populations. Gastroenterology 1981;81:5.
143. Mårdh PA, Helin I, Colleen I et al. *Clostridium difficile* toxin in faecal specimens of healthy children and children with diarrhoea. Acta Paediatr Scand 1982;71:275.
144. Lyerly DM, Krivan HC, Wilkins TD. *Clostridium difficile*: Its disease and toxins. Clin Microbiol Rev 1988;1:1.
145. Wren B, Heard SR, Tabaqchali S. Association between production of toxins A and B and types of *Clostridium difficile*. J Clin Pathol 1987;40:1397
146. Seppälä K, Hjelt L, Sipponen P. Colonoscopy in the diagnosis of antibiotic-associated colitis. Scand J Gastroent 1981;16:465.
147. Mukay JK, Janower ML. Diagnosis of pseudomembranous colitis by computed tomography: A report of two patients. J Can Assoc Radiol 1987;38:62.
148. Toffler RB, Pingoud EG, Burrell MI. Acute colitis related to penicillin and penicillin derivatives. Lancet 1978; ii:707.
149. Woods GL, Iwen PC. Comparison of a dot immunobinding assay, latex agglutination and cytotoxin assay for laboratory diagnosis of *Clostridium difficile*-associated diarrhea. J Clin Microbiol 1990;28:855.
150. Morris JB, Zollinger RM, Stellato TA. Role of surgery in antibiotic-induced pseudomembranous enterocolitis. Am J Surgery 1990;160:535.
151. VanNess MM, Cattau EL Jr. Fulminant colitis complicating antibiotic-associated pseudomembranous colitis: Case report and review of the clinical manifestations and treatment. Am J Gastroenterol 1987;82:374.
152. Fakety R, Silva J, Kauffman C et al. Treatment of antibiotic-associated *Clostridium difficile* colitis with oral vancomycin: comparison of two dosage regimens. Am J Med 1989;86:15.
153. Teasley DG, Gerdin DN, Olson MM et al. Prospective randomised trial of metronidazole versus vancomycin for *Clostridium difficile*-associated diarrhea and colitis. Lancet 1983;ii:1043.
154. Bartlett JG. Treatment of antibiotic-associated pseudomembranous colitis. Rev Infect Dis 1984;6(Suppl 1):S235.
155. DeLalla F, Santoro D, Rinaldi E et al. Teicoplanin in the treatment of infections by staphylococci, *Clostridium difficile* and other gram-positive bacteria. J Antimicrob Chemother 1989;23:131.
156. Ariano RE, Zhanel GG, Harding GKM. The role of anion-exchange resins in the treatment of antibiotic-associated pseudomembranous colitis. Editorial. Can Med Assoc J 1990;142:1049.
157. Taylor NS, Bartlett JG. Binding of *Clostridium difficile* cytotoxin and vancomycin by anion-exchange resins. J Infect Dis 1980;141:92.
158. Gorbach SL, Chang TW, Goldin B. Successful treatment of relapsing *Clostridium difficile* colitis with *Lactobacillus* GG. Lancet 1987;ii:1519.
159. Bowden TA Jr, Mansberger AR Jr, Lykins LE. Pseudomembraneous enterocolitis: mechanism of restoring floral homeostasis. Am Surgeon 1981;47:178.
160. McFarland LV, Surawicz CM, Greenberg RN et al. Prevention of beta-lactam-associated diarrhea by *Saccharomyces boulardii* compared with placebo. Am J Gastroenterol 1995;90:439.
161. Novak E, Lee JG, Seckmann CE, Phillips JP, DiSanto AR. Unfavorable effects of atropine-diphenoxylate (Lomotil) therapy in lincomycin-caused diarrhea. J Am Med Assoc 1976;235:1451.
162. Buggy BP, Fekety R, Silva J. Therapy of relapsing *Clostridium difficile*-associated diarrhea and colitis with the com-

bination of vancomycin and rifampin. J Clin Gastroenterol 1987;9:155.
163. Johnson HC, Walker A. Convulsive factor in commercial penicillin. Arch Surg 1945;50:69.
164. Macdonald RL, Barker JL. Pentylenetetrazol and penicillin are selective antagonists of GABA-mediated post-synaptic inhibition in cultured mammalian neurons. Nature, 1977;267:720.
165. Chow P, Mathers D. Convulsant doses of penicillin shorten the lifetime of GABA-induced channels in cultured central neurons. Br J Pharmacol 1986;88:541.
166. Schliamser SE, Cars O, Norrby SR. Neurotoxicity of betalactam antibiotics: predisposing factors and pathogenesis. J Antimicrob Chemother 1991;27:405.
167. Gutnick MJ, Prince DA. Penicillinase and the convulsant action of penicillin. Neurology, 1971;21:759.
168. Sobotka P, Safanda J. The epileptogenic action of penicillins: structure-activity relationship. J Mol Med 1976;1:151.
169. Barrons RW, Murray KM, Richey RM. Populations at risk for penicillin-induced seizures. Ann Pharmacother 1992;26:26.
170. Grondahl TO, Langmoen IA. Epileptogenic effect of antibiotic drugs. J Neurosurg 1993;78:938.
171. De Sarro A, Ammendola D, Zappala M et al. Relationship between structure and convulsant properties of some β-lactam antibiotics following intracerebroventricular microinjection in rats. Antimicrob. Agents Chemother 1995; 39:232.
172. Winston DJ, Ho WG, Brukner DA, Champlin RE. Beta-lactam antibiotic therapy cefoperazone plus piperacillin, ceftazidime plus piperacillin, and imipenem alone. Ann Intern Med 1991;115:849.
173. Rolston KVI, Berkey P, Bodey GP et al. A comparison of imipenem to ceftazidime with or without amikacin as empiric therapy in febrile neutropenic patients. Arch Intern Med 1992;152:283.
174. Pestotnik SL, Classen DC, Evans RS et al. Prospective surveillance of imipenem/cilastatin use and associated seizures using a hospital information system. Ann Pharmacother 1993;27:497.
175. De Sarro A, Zappala M, Chimirri A et al. Quinolones potentiate cefazolin-induced seizures in DBA/2 mice. Antimicrob Agents Chemother 1993;37:1497.
176. De Sarro A, Ammendola D, De Sarro G. Effects of some quinolones on imipenem-induced seizures in DBA/2 mice. Gen Pharmacol 1994;25:369.
177. Holme E, Greter J, Jacobsen CE et al. Carnitine deficiency induced by pivampicillin and pivmecillinam therapy. Lancet 1989;ii:469.
178. Melegh B, Kerner J, Bieber L. Pivampicillin-promoted excretion of pivaloyl carnitine in humans. Biochem Pharmacol 1987;63:3405.
179. Diep QN, Bohmer T, Holme JI et al. Slow replenishment of carnitine deficiency after cessation of long-term treatment with pivaloyl-containing antibiotics. Pharm World Sci 1993;15:225.
180. Rose SJ, Stokes TC, Patel S et al. Carnitine deficiency associated with long-term pivampicillin treatment: the effect of a replacement therapy regime. Postgrad Med J 1992; 68:932.
181. Baron DN, Hamilton-Miller JMT, Brumfitt W. Sodium content of injectable betalactam antibiotics. Lancet 1984; i:1113.
182. White JM, Brown DL, Hepner GW et al. Penicillin-induced haemolytic anaemia. Br Med J 1968;3:26.
183. Garratty G. Review: Immune hemolytic anemia and/or positive direct antiglobulin tests caused by drugs. Immunohematology 1994;10/2:41.
184. Petz LD, Garratty G. Acquired Immune Hemolytic Anemias. New York: Churchill Livingstone, 1980.
185. Williams ME, Thomas D, Harman CP et al. Positive direct antiglobulin tests due to clavulanic acid. Antimicrob Agents Chemother 1985;27:125.
186. Norrby SR. Side effects of cephalosporins. Drugs 1987;34(Suppl 2):105.
187. Barza M, Furie B, Brown AE, et al. Defects in vitamin K-dependent carboxylation associated with moxalactam treatment. J Infect Dis 1986;153:1166.
188. Andrassy K, Koderisch J. An open study on hemostasis in 20 patients with normal and impaired renal function treated with cefotetan alone or combined with tobramycin (Abstract). In: Proceedings, 15th International Congress of Chemotherapy, Istanbul, 1987.
189. Conly JM, Ramotar K, Chubb H et al. Hypoprothrombinemia in febrile, neutropenic patients with cancer: association with antimicrobial suppression of intestinal microflora. J Infect Dis 1984;150:202.
190. Holt J. Hypoprothrombinemia and bleeding diathesis associated with cefotetan therapy in surgical patients. Arch Surg 1988;123:523.
191. Hicks MJ, Flaitz CM. The role of antibiotics in platelet dysfunction and coagulopathy. Int J Antimicrob Agents 1993;2:129.
192. Shirakawa H, Komai M, Kimura S. Antibiotic-induced vitamin K deficiency and the role of the presence of intestinal flora. Int J Vit Nutr Res 1990;60:245.
193. Williams KJ, Bax RP, Brown H, Machin SJ. Antibiotic treatment and associated prolonged prothrombin time. J Clin Pathol 1991;44:738.
194. Lipsky JJ. Antibiotic associated hypoprothrombinaemia. J Antimicrob Chemother 1988;21:281.
195. Sattler FR, Weitekamp MR, Sayegh A et al. Impaired hemostasis caused by betalactam antibiotics. Am J Surg 1988;155(SA):30.
196. Lipsky JJ. Mechanism of the inhibition of the gamma carboxylation of glutamic acid: possible mechanism for antibiotic associated hypoprothrombinaemia. Proc Natl Acad Sci USA 1984;81:2893.
197. Suttie JW, Engelke JA, McTigue J. Effect of *N*-methylthiatetrazole on rat liver microsomal Vit K-dependent carboxylation. Biochem Pharmacol 1986;35:2429.
198. Uchida K, Yoshida T, Komeno T. Mechanism for hypoprothrombinemia caused by *N*-methyltetrazolethiol (NNTT)-containing antibiotics. Abstracts, 15th International Congress of Chemotherapy, Istanbul, 1987;Abstr 1153.
199. Shearer MJ, Bechtold H, Andrassy K et al. Mechanism of cephalosporin-induced hypoprothrombinemia: relation to cephalosporin side chain, vitamin K metabolism and vitamin K status. J Clin Pharmacol 1988;28:88.
200. Jones P, Bodey GP, Rolston K et al. Cefoperazone plus mezlocillin for empiric therapy of febrile cancer patients. Am J Med 1988;85(Suppl 1A):3.
201. Brown RB, Klar J, Lemeshow S et al. Enhanced bleeding with cefoxitin or moxalactam: statistical analysis within a defined population of 1493 patients. Arch Intern Med 1986;146:2159.
202. Boyd DB, Lunn WH. Electronic structures of cephalosporins and penicillins. 9. Departure of a leaving group in cephalosporins. J Med Chem 1979;22:778.

203. Mizojirik K, Norikura R, Takashima A et al. Disposition of moxalactam and N-methyltetrazolethiole in rats and monkeys. Antimicrob Agents Chemother 1987;31:1169.
204. Schentag JJ, Welage LS, Williams JS et al. The kinetics and actions of *N*-methylthiotetrazole (NMTT) in volunteers and patients and population-based clinical comparisons of NMTT-containing antibiotics with those lacking this moiety. Am J Surg 1988;15(Suppl).
205. Fletcher C, Pearson C, Choi SC et al. In vitro comparison of antiplatelet effects of β-lactam penicillins. J Lab Clin Med 1986;108:217.
206. Bang NU, Tessler SS, Heidenreich RO et al. Effects of moxalactam on blood coagulation and platelet function. Rev Infect Dis 1982;4(Suppl):5546.
207. Weitekamp MR, Aber RC. Prolonged bleeding times and bleeding diathesis associated with moxalactam administration. J Am Med Assoc 1983;249:69.
208. Weitekamp MR, Caputo GM, Al-Mondhiry HAB et al. The effect of latamoxef, cefotaxime and cefoperazone on platelet function and coagulation in normal volunteers. J Antimicrob Chemother 1985;16:95.
209. Weitekamp MR, Holmes P, Walker ME. A double blind study on the effects of cefoperazone (CPZ), ceftizoxime (CTZ), moxalactam (MOX) on platelet function and prothrombin time in normal volunteers. In: Abstracts, 25th Interscience Conference on Antimicrobial Agents and Chemotherapy, Minneapolis, Minnesota, 1985;Abstr 959.
210. Fass RJ, Copelan EA, Brandt JT et al. Platelet-mediated bleeding caused by broad-spectrum penicillins. J. Inf. Dis. 1987;155(6):1242.
211. Norrby SR, Foord RD, Price JD et al. Pharmacokinetics and clinical studies on cefuroxime. Proc R Soc Med 1977;70(Suppl 9):25.
212. Burroughs SF, Johnson GJ. β-Lactam antibiotic-induced platelet dysfunction: evidence for irreversible inhibition of platelet activation in vitro and in vivo after prolonged exposure to penicillin. Blood 1990;7:1473.
213. Norrby SR. Side effects of cephalosporins. Drugs 1987;34(Suppl 2):105.
214. Zürcher K, Krebs A. Cutaneous Drug Reactions. Basel: Karger-Verlag, 1991.
215. Korzeniowski OM. Effects of antibiotics on the mammalian immune system. Infect Dis Clin North Am 1989; 3:469.
216. Van den Brock PJ. Antimicrobial drugs, microorganisms, and phagocytes. Rev Infect Dis 1989;11:213.
217. Labro MT, el Benna J, Charlier N et al. Cefdinir (CI-983), a new oral amino-2-thiazolyl cephalosporin, inhibits human neutrophil myeloperoxidase in the extracellular medium but not the phagolysosome. J Immunol 1994;152:2447.
218. Villa ML, Armelloni S, Ferrario E et al. Interference of cephalosporins with immune response: effects of cefonicid on human T-helper-cells. Int J Immunopharmacol 1991; 13:1099.
219. Furuhama K, Benson RW, Knowles BJ, Roberts DW. Immunotoxicity of cephalosporins in mice. Chemotherapy 1993;39:278
220. Strehl E, Ibrom W. Arzneimittelwechselwirkungen bei der Antibiotikatherapie. Chemother J 1995;2:73.

Meyler's Side Effects of Drugs, 13th Edition
M.N.G. Dukes, editor

SECTION EDITOR: R. HOIGNÉ

R. Hoigné, A. Cerny and R. Sonntag

25.3 Penicillins

The penicillin preparations are among the few antibiotics with bactericidal effect that, as a rule, are hardly toxic in man even when given in high doses. They show an excellent distribution in the various body tissues. Today, their costs are reasonable or even low compared to other antibiotics. Penicillins may also be used in pregnant women and in children. The development of newer semisynthetic penicillins has rendered the production of penicillinase-resistant preparations (isoxazolyl penicillins, meticillin and nafcillin) and broad-spectrum penicillins possible. The former have proven themselves effective in most cases against penicillinase-producing staphylococci. The later (amino- and amidopenicillins) are effective against gram-negative bacteria including *Pseudomonas aeruginosa*, *Proteus* (carbenicillin, ticarcillin, ureidopenicillins, thienamycins, including the more recently developed β-lactam antibiotics (see Chapter 25.1)) and *Bacteroides*. β-Lactamase-susceptible penicillins such as aminopenicillins, ticarcillin, and possibly other preparations, can be combined with β-lactamase inhibitors such as clavulanic acid or sulbactam.

On the other hand, all the penicillin preparations available today have produced so-called penicillin *allergies* which cross-react mainly within the family of penicillins.

ADVERSE REACTION PATTERN

General and toxic reactions These reactions to penicillin G appear mainly with high doses or are related to renal insufficiency. They consist of convulsions or electrolyte disturbances with hyperkalemia, hypokalemia or sodium retention. The penicillinase-resistant and broad-spectrum penicillins may show specific adverse reactions. Embolic-toxic reactions due to accidental intravascular administration are encountered with penicillin depot preparations, mainly procaine penicillin. Under certain circumstances, intra-arterial injections with tissue necrosis may occur. Based on recent research, agranulocytosis, leukopenia, thrombocytopenia, hepatopathy and nephropathy are considered to be due to toxic rather than to allergic mechanisms (see Chapters 25.1 and 25.2). Diarrhea is a common complication, whereas antibiotic-associated colitis is rare.

Hypersensitivity reactions Hypersensitivity reactions occur in about 1—10% of patients treated. In view of their great importance, they are dealt with in a special section (see Chapters 25.1 and 25.2). They range from mostly harmless skin reactions to life threatening immediate reactions including anaphylactic shock, acute bronchial obstruction and other rare severe skin reactions. Type 1-reactions (classification by Coombs et al.) in particular may also be initiated by a pseudoallergic pathomechanism, if all kinds of drugs are taken into account (2^R, 3^R) (Chapter 25.2).

It is important to distinguish hypersensitivity reactions from the Jarisch-Herxheimer reaction, which often presents with the same symptoms, mainly exanthema, fever and cardiovascular reactions (SED 12, 607).

Tumor-inducing effects These have not been described.

CLINICAL SYNDROMES OF PREDOMINANTLY DOSE-DEPENDENT PENICILLIN REACTIONS

These reactions occur in patients treated with high doses of penicillins, e.g. bacterial endocarditis, osteomyelitis and septicemia with gram-positive and gram-negative bacteria. They are presented in detail in the section 'Organs and symptoms' and concern the nervous system, blood, liver and kidney (urinary tract) (see Chapter 25.1).

HYPERSENSITIVITY REACTIONS

In penicillin allergies an entire series of penicillins and penicillin metabolites may play the role of a hapten. The complete antigen results from 'binding' of the hapten with a protein or cellular component, as discussed in Chapter 25.2. Therefore, allergy to any one of the penicillin preparations indicates to the clinician that an allergy to most other penicillin preparations, and in rare patients also to the related cephalosporins and carbapenems, must be assumed. Hypersensitivity reactions are often classified according to the four pathomechanisms proposed by Coombs and Gell (1[R]). In practice, however, the proof that any of these mechanisms is responsible for individual observations may often be impossible. Only for reactions of the immediate type, hemolytic anemia and allergic contact eczema, can the allergic mechanism usually be demonstrated. Mixed-type immunological reactions also occur frequently.

Reaction time and exposure time in allergic drug reactions Frequently there is a definite relationship between the *reaction time* (the time between the last drug exposure and appearance of the first symptoms) and the *type of clinical symptom*. This relationship was described by von Pirquet and Schick (4[C]) as early as 1905 with respect to anaphylactic shock and serum sickness due to foreign sera. The chronological sequence is still a part of the clinical description of a drug 'allergy' (see Chapter 25.1) (5[C]–7[C]).

The reaction times in allergies to small molecular drugs, however, have generally been found to be shorter than those in allergies to complete antigenic substances. This has prompted us, on the basis of clinical experience with drug treatment and re-exposure, to differentiate the following three types of reactions: (a) immediate within 1 hour (acute allergic reactions); (b) between 1 and 24 hours (subacute allergic reactions); (c) more than 24 hours to weeks (latent-type allergic reactions) (5[C], 6[C], 7). This classification is virtually independent of the type of drug involved.

The reaction time for anaphylactic shock ranges generally from a few minutes to 30–60 minutes. The frequent maculo-papular exanthemas, allergic pneumopathies and the hematological syndromes usually occur after 1–24 hours. The lag time for reactions primarily affecting other specific organs and for pancytopenia is often longer than 1 day. Upon critical evaluation, the reaction times for urticaria, angioedema and an attack of bronchial asthma are found to be spread among all three groups (6[C], 7[C]). The serum-sickness syndrome has a reaction time of hours to weeks.

The classification of reaction times in drug allergy is of practical significance, especially in patients exposed to several drugs. It helps to determine the most probable causative agent. Test methods often either do not exist or are available only in highly specialized institutions. Furthermore, reaction times are often different from the time of peak pharmacological activity.

The *exposure time* (time from the first to the last application of the drug) is usually at least several days in patients developing reactions after exposure to drugs given for the first time. This is the time necessary for development of sensitization. Sensitization to penicillin is, in the vast majority of patients, initiated through the therapeutic use of this antibiotic rather than through exposure in other ways, e.g. residues in milk.

PENICILLIN 'ANTIGEN' AND ANTIBODY *(see Chapter 25.1)*

DIAGNOSTIC EVALUATION OF IgE-MEDIATED PENICILLIN HYPERSENSITIVITY

The two most important elements in the evaluation of an individual for the presence or absence of β-lactam hypersensitivity are the drug history and skin tests. Other diagnostic tools such as measurement of drug-specific antibodies, lymphocyte transformation tests, etc. remain investigational. It should be noted that standardized and widely applied protocols for skin testing only exist for the penicillins and only allow assessment of IgE-mediated hypersensitivity.

The most commonly used reagents are penicilloyl-polylysine (PPL, containing multiple penicilloyl molecules coupled to a polylysine carrier) and fresh penicillin followed by minor determinant mixtures (MDM), containing penilloate, benzylpenicilloate and benzylpenilloate. A recent survey conducted among members of the American Academy of Allergy and Immunology reports the use of PPL and fresh penicillin by 86% and MDM by 40% of those responding to the questionnaire (8[C]). Skin tests are first applied as a prick test for safety. In the absence of a local or systemic reaction an intradermal test is performed and interpreted as described elsewhere (9[C], 10[C]). The experience with skin testing in penicillin allergy has been reviewed recently by Lin (11[R]). Properly performed sequential testing is considered a safe procedure and only an estimated 1% or less of penicillin allergic patients will experience systemic symptoms while undergoing skin tests. However, at least three fatalities have been reported with both epicutaneous and intradermal testing (12[C]).

In a recent collaborative study by the National Institute of Allergy and Infectious Diseases (N/A/D), hospitalized patients were tested with major and minor skin test reagents in order to assess the predictive value of skin testing. Among 600 history-negative patients, 568 were also skin test-negative and none (0%) had a reaction to penicillin administration. Among 726 history-positive patients, 566 had a negative skin test and received penicillin, seven of whom (1.2%) experienced a possibly IgE-mediated reaction. Nine of the 167 skin test-positive patients were exposed to penicillin two of which (22%) had reactions compatible with IgE-mediated reactions. The data suggests that, overall, 99% of patients with negative skin tests to PPL and MDM can safely receive penicillin. A history of a previous reaction increases the risk of an adverse reaction slightly to 1.2%. Most positive skin tests were detected with PPL with or without MDM, and an additional 16% reacted to MDM alone (13[C]).

Another recent study conducted in an outpatient STD clinic setting tested a total of 5063 consecutive patients with PPL with and without MDM skin tests (14[C]). The role of the history of a previous penicillin reaction is emphasized in this study: 1.7% of history-negative subjects had a positive skin test, in contrast 7.1% of history-positive patients had a positive skin test, and a previous history of anaphylaxis or urticaria was associated with positive skin tests in 17.3 and 12.4%, respectively. Similar to the NIAID study, penicillin administration was safe in more than 99% of history- and skin test-negative patients. Reaction on exposure was higher (2.9%) in history-positive, skin test-negative subjects. The reactions observed were mild and self limited. Two patients with a history of severe IgE-mediated reaction experienced a mild anaphylactic reaction.

Based on this, patients with a history of penicillin allergy should undergo skin testing with both PPL and MDM. Skin test-positive patients should be treated with another immunologically unrelated compound or undergo desensitization. The management of skin test-negative patients with a history of a severe IgE-mediated reaction has to be individualized, options include the use of an alternative compound, desensitization or the controlled administration of a test dose.

Relatively 'safe' doses for skin testing, provided that one begins with a prick test, are 25 nmol/ml of PPL and purified benzyl-penicillin. Positive skin tests of the immediate type with PPL are usually obtained 2 weeks to 3 months after the clinical reaction (15[C]).

The safety of such an approach has been challenged by a recent report by Blanca et al. These investigators describe three patients negative by skin tests for PPL and MDM tolerating therapeutic doses of benzylpenicillin, but reacting upon exposure to amoxicillin (16[C]). In an extension of that study, 177 β-lactam-allergic patients were identified using clinical history, a skin test panel including PPL and MDM as well as ampicillin and amoxicillin and drug-specific radio-allergosorbent tests. Fifty-four patients (30.5%) tolerated penicillin G but reacted to amoxicillin with anaphylaxis, urticaria or angioedema. Skin tests with PPL and MDM failed to detect those patients but tests using amoxicillin were positive in 63% (17[C]). Data obtained by Silviu-Dan and colleagues confirm these findings in part. In this Canadian study, skin tests using both benzylpenicillin derivatives as well as semisynthetic penicillins were applied to 112 patients with a history of an allergic reaction to penicillins. They identified 21 patients (18.8%), out of whom 10 reacted against the semisynthetic penicillin reagents only (47%). The report contains no challenge data however (18[C]). Further studies are required to define the importance of such side chain-specific hypersensitivity reactions.

PROPHYLACTIC MEASURES

Taking a careful medical history before every new course of penicillin treatment is of great importance for the prevention of allergic penicillin reactions. If there is any evidence at all for the presence of allergy, the patient is for all practical purposes to be considered as allergic to penicillin. The same is valid for the appearance of any suspiciously allergic reaction in a patient undergoing penicillin therapy in combination with other drugs (19[C]–25[C]).

There is no question that the use of penicillin in the form of ointments for skin application or solutions as inhalation aerosol for treating bronchitis should have been discontinued long ago. This is also true for other antibiotics which are used systemically. Sensitization which develops through such topical use may lead to severe allergic reactions if the drug is later given systemically.

For high-dose intravenous therapy with penicillin G, the solutions should be made from single-dose vials, freshly prepared every time and not by a continuous infusion (26[C]).

The type of penicillin used plays some role in the initial evaluation, as the allergy may involve various penicillins, partly without cross-reactions and one or more penicillin metabolites. The consequences of penicillin re-exposure are hardly predictable. An apparently harmless initial exanthema, a local edema, a transient erythema, an Arthus phenomenon or even an episode of drug fever may be followed by life-threatening anaphylactic shock if penicillin is re-administered (27[C], 28[C]). Special caution seems to be vital in dealing with asthmatics (2[R], 27[C]–31[C]). According to several studies, atopic persons as a group do not appear to be more susceptible to drug sensitization than non-atopics (7[C], 29[C], 30[C], 32[r]) (see also Chapter 25.2). It has been stated with some justification that the appearance of maculo-papular rash during ampicillin treatment is rarely followed by severe reactions to subsequent penicillin exposure. Nevertheless, reactions with anaphylactic shock have also been initiated by ampicillin (11[C], 16[C], 33[c], 34[c]). If penicillin allergy is suspected or proven, the indications for the use of penicillin preparations and even cephalosporins must be carefully weighed (see Chapter 25.2). Even cross-reactions with the monobactam aztreonam have occasionally been observed (35a[C], 35b[C]).

For most infectious diseases other unrelated antibiotics or chemotherapeutic agents are available. If the institution of penicillin therapy is considered to be of vital importance and the history of penicillin allergy not convincing, skin testing should be carried out as described above.

DESENSITIZATION IN THE PRESENCE OF PENICILLIN ALLERGY

In a clinical situation requiring the administration of a β-lactam to a patient at high risk of experiencing an IgE-mediated reaction, desensitization may be attempted. β-Lactam desensitization requires an intensive care setting and any concomitant risk factors for anaphylaxis such as use of β-blocker drugs should be corrected. Protocols based on incremental application of the drug using the oral or parenteral route have been described (36[R]). The oral route is preferable and is associated with a lower incidence of adverse events but mild transient reactions are frequent (37[C], 38[C]). Also, pregnant women with limited antibiotic choices have been treated with immunotherapy (39[C]). Continuous administration of the drug will maintain a state of anergy which is often lost after discontinuation (40[C]). At the conclusion of therapy, the patient must be informed that after discontinuing penicillin, he may once again become allergic to penicillin with a new reaction to the first subsequent application (40[C]).

Desensitization has not been shown to be effective in non-IgE-mediated reactions and should therefore not be attempted, e.g. in cases of serum sickness or Stevens-Johnson syndrome.

It is advantageous to carry out desensitization rapidly under protective antihistamine therapy.

ORGANS AND SYSTEMS

Cardiovascular *Anaphylactic shock* may occur even after oral administration of penicillin and skin testing. The occurrence of anaphylactic shock seems to be lower after oral than after parenteral administration of the allergenic substance (37[C]). A lethal course is rare, but has also been observed after oral application (SEDA-4, 185) and exceptionally after skin test (12[C]).

In nearly half of the cases, the course of anaphylactic shock in man, especially that induced by penicillin and other small molecular substances, is that of a cardiovascular reaction without any additional clinical symptoms suggestive of an allergic mechanism (16[C], 24[C], 41[C]).

There is an extensive list of articles on anaphylactic shock to penicillins (11[C], 16[C], 24[C], 29[C], 30[C], 42[C], 43[c], 44[C]).

It has to be kept in mind that arterial hypotension in relation to penicillin can be secondary to other organ manifestations, such as a severe attack of bronchial asthma, fluid albumin and electrolyte loss in severe general skin reactions, diarrhea and vomiting, etc., with important therapeutic implications (45[C], 46[C]).

General anesthesia does not inhibit the development of anaphylactic shock in penicillin allergy (47[C]). Immediate treatment with adrenaline, followed by intravenous H_1 or H_2 blockers, corticosteroids, fluids and electrolytes is essential. In view of the frequency of cardiac arrhythmias and conduction disturbances in patients with anaphylactic shock, they should immediately be monitored (48[C], 49[C]). The incidence of anaphylactic shock is 0.04% of all patients treated with penicillin in a Swiss population (43[C]). It is also low in patients receiving long-term benzathine penicillin therapy (1.2 million units administered every 4 weeks). Four episodes of anaphylaxis occurred in 0.012% of injections (1.2 reactions to 10 000 injections) (50[C]). Anaphylactic shock resulting in death has been observed in 0.002% of all patients treated with penicillin (43[C]) and in 0.003% of the cohort treated with benzathine penicillin (50[C]).

Embolic toxic reactions with shock See 'Special problems of penicillin depot preparations' (p. 700). Combinations of embolic toxic and allergic reactions may also occur (51[C], 52[C], Case 3).

Respiratory *An attack of allergic bronchospasm* may be a consequence of penicillin allergy (29[C], 30[C], 42[C], 43[C], 53a[C], 53b[C]). The patient is not always a known asthmatic with extrinsic (reaginic or atopic) or intrinsic (idiopathic or cryptogenic) asthma. Acute severe dyspnea with cyanosis has also been observed without clinical symptoms of bronchial obstruction or pulmonary edema (6[C], 54[C]). Specific mechanisms for such cases have yet to be identified (54[C]).

Hypersensitivity *Allergic pneumonitis* or *transient eosinophilic pulmonary infiltrate* (*Loeffler's syndrome*) is rare. These syndromes have also been observed with penicillin hypersensitivity (55[C], 56[c], 57[c]). A possibly related interstitial pneumonitis has been described as cheese washer's disease in relation to exposure to the mould *Penicillium casei* (58). An alveolar allergic reaction, probably to ampicillin, showed features of an adult respiratory distress syndrome (59[c]).

Nervous system Administration of higher doses of penicillin, in the order of several 10 million units daily, may produce *myoclonic jerks*, *hyperreflexia*, *seizures* or *coma*. Also, *drowsiness* and *hallucinations* may occur occasionally (60[C]—62[C]). Such reactions due to a toxic effect, are apparently favored by high concentrations as seen with intravenous administration (63[C], 64[C]) as well as with cardiopulmonary bypass in open heart surgery (65[C], 66[C]).

Intrathecal instillation of more than 10 000 units of penicillin as well as local application of higher penicillin concentrations to the nervous system, especially the brain, during surgery have also produced comparable reactions (67[C]). Nearly all penicillin preparations may produce this kind of reaction, even ampicillin (SEDA-10, 235) (see Chapter 25.1).

Benign intracranial hypertension is an extremely rare, probably allergic reaction, if caused by penicillins (68[c]) (see Chapter 26, Tetracyclines, and Chapter 29.1, Sulfonamides).

Endocrine, metabolic The possibility of *vitamin deficiencies resulting from destruction of vitamin-producing intestinal bacteria* has been discussed for a long time. It is true that vitamin K and the vitamin B complex are produced by intestinal bacteria. Newer studies, however, have shown that in comparison to the amount of these vitamins present in food, the quantity produced by intestinal bacteria is indeed very small and hardly of practical significance, except for patients receiving oral anticoagulants. The concomitant antibiotic therapy may substantially reduce the amount of vitamin K levels and make it difficult to control the degree of anticoagulation. The massive administration of additional vitamins in patients undergoing antibiotic therapy would, therefore, not seem to be indicated as long as normal nutrition is maintained. (For further details and literature references, see 'Hematological' below.)

Mineral and fluid balance Potassium penicillin G and sodium penicillin G are capable of significantly altering the electrolyte balance when administered in very high doses: 20 million units of potassium penicillin G contains approximately 30 mmol of potassium. In patients with renal failure, this amount may decisively aggravate a potentially lethal *hyperkalemia*. In a similar fashion, large doses of sodium penicillin G, carbenicillin or tricarcillin may lead to *hypernatremia* with all its consequences (69[R], 70[C]). Penicillin and particularly carbenicillin, ticarcillin and nafcillin, induce urinary *potassium loss*, presumably by acting as a non-adsorbable anion in the distal tubule (70[C], 71[c], 72[C]). Also mezlocillin and pipercillin preparations may induce *hypokalemia*, mainly in severely sick patients (73a[C], 73b[C]).

Hematological An immunologically induced *hemolytic anemia* is rare. It usually occurs during treatment with high doses (over 10 million units daily) of penicillin (74[C]—76[C], 77[c]). It can also occur with other penicillins such as ampicillin, oxacillin, flucloxacillin, meticillin and ticarcillin (78[c]). As a rule, other allergic symptoms are not present. Microangiopathic hemolysis and thrombocytopenia related to penicillin drugs have also been described (79[C], 80[c], 81[c]).

During penicillin treatment the erythrocytes are normally coated with penicillin. Penicillenic acid seems to form a penicilloyl bond on the erythrocyte surface (82[C]). In patients with a penicillin-induced hemolytic anemia the pertinent specific IgG antibody is found in the blood. It is directed against the complete antigen penicillin-erythrocyte complex and may be demonstrated in the direct and indirect Coombs test. A second, less frequent immunological mechanism may also be involved. This is a so-called 'innocent bystander reaction' (77[C], 82[C], 83[C]). Penicillin-antibody complexes which are only loosely bound to the erythrocytes activate complement (82[C]). Complement may be detected on the erythrocyte surface with the complement antiglobulin test ('complement' or 'non-γ' type). This latter mechanism plays the decisive role in immune-hemolytic anemias due to drugs other than penicillin. In the first mentioned situation, the hemolytic reaction may continue for weeks, after discontinuation of the penicillin therapy or as long as sufficient penicillin-coated erythrocytes and specific antibodies remain in circulation.

Penicillin can probably also cause, exceptionally, a *hemolytic uremic syndrome* (84[c]). According to the newer literature, bacterial cytotoxins, mainly of Coli 0157-H_7, are considered to be the usual cause of the hemolytic-uremic syndrome (85[R]).

Agranulocytosis and leukopenia related to isoxazolylpenicillins have been observed (SEDA-4, 185; 86[C]—90[C]). Benzylpenicillin (91[C]—96[C]) and other penicillins, such as ampicillin, azlocillin, mezlocillin, carbenicillin, ticarcillin, meticillin, nafcillin and piperacillin, have also been implicated (90[C], 97[c], 98[C]—100[C]).

In other studies, a dose-dependent inhibition of in

vivo and in vitro granulocytopoiesis by β-lactam antibiotics has been demonstrated by Neftel et al., thus indicating a toxic effect (91[C], 101[C]). This fact does not affect the high rate of concomitant 'allergic' symptoms, such as that of exanthema and blood eosinophilia, which may have an immunological pathomechanisms (see also Chapters 25.1 and 25.2).

The development of a positive LE-cell phenomenon has been observed in patients with penicillin hypersensitivity (102[c], 103[c]).

Thrombocytopenia related to penicillins seems to occur very rarely (79[C], 80[c], 81[C], 104[c]—106[c]).

Bleeding disorders see Chapter 25.2, p. 685.

Liver *Hepatitis* and *intrahepatic cholestasis* have been observed with various penicillin preparations. Even if this reaction is only rarely encountered, oxacillin has more frequently been implicated as the cause than other penicillins (see also 'Dose-dependent reactions', Chapter 25.2; 107[C]—110[C]). Comparable reactions were also observed under flucloxacillin (109[c], 111[c], 112[c]), carbenicillin (113[C]) and ticarcillin with clavulanic acid (114[C]). The combination of amoxicillin with clavulanate potassium has rarely been associated with cholestatic reactions (see Chapter 25.5; 115[C]).

Critical evaluation of such reactions is problematic in that liver damage can also result from bacterial infections, especially staphylococcal septicemia. Hepatitis and active chronic (lupoid) hepatitis, probably as a hypersensitivity reaction, is only very rarely seen.

Gastrointestinal A whole series of penicillins, usually oral preparations, has produced *diarrhea* in certain patients. This is often associated with mild nausea and less frequently with vomiting (116[C], 117[C]). If the gastrointestinal symptoms occur immediately upon drug ingestion, then they are usually due to a direct toxic side effect. Even in such cases, a bacterial enterocolitis should be promptly ruled out or proven. Special forms of reactions are *pseudomembranous colitis* and *acute hermorrhagic colitis* (118[C]) (see Chapter 25.2).

Urinary system *Nephropathy* or *interstitial nephritis* has been described in a number of reports in relation to methicillin (119[C]—121[C], 122[R], 123[C], 124[c]). However, nafcillin (125[c], 126[C]), penicillin G, ampicillin, amoxicillin (127[C]—129[C], 130[c]), oxacillin (122[R]), dicloxacillin (131[C]) and piperacillin (132[C], 133[C]) may also be the cause.

Fever and hematuria (macroscopic or microscopic) are the dominating symptoms. Exanthema, eosinophilia in the blood, possibly eosinophiluria and signs of non-oliguric renal failure may be found but are not always present (122[R]). Acute anuric/oliguric renal failure is rare.

The frequency and degree of *renal failure* may be increased with the combination of methicillin and gentamicin (134[C]). In patients where aminoglycoside treatment is undesirable because of pre-existing renal damage, ureidopenicillins may be used (69[R], 135[R]). Acute interstitial nephritis has the confusing potential of being cured and caused by the same agent (136a[R]). Patients with recurrent symptoms upon re-exposure to methicillin or another penicillin preparation provide clinical proof of the drug association (136b[C], 137a[c], 137b[C]). The presence of tubular basement membrane antibodies in a few cases (121[C], 122[R]) could be an epiphenomenon resulting from the renal damage (119[C], 120[C], 129[C], 138a[c]). Prudence would dictate to stop all penicillin and cephalosporin treatment in a situation with otherwise unexplained progressive renal failure or hematuria.

Hemorrhagic cystitis has been observed in connection with meticillin (138b[C]) and with carbenicillin (139[c]).

Skin and appendages Penicillin allergy may present an entire spectrum of symptoms and syndromes. Especially in penicillin allergy, symptoms as described in cases of sensitization to foreign complete antigenic substances dominate (4[C]). Skin manifestations, primarily *urticaria* and most frequently *maculopapular exanthemas* (usual rash) are observed (21[C], 23[C], 24[C], 140[C]). In some cases, urticaria is combined with angioedema. But the last can also be observed without urticarial lesions. Less frequently, *allergic vasculitis* (44[C], 141[C]), *erythema multiforme* (142[C]—145[C]), *fixed drug eruption* (23[C], 24[C], 145[C]), *'erythema nodosum-like' lesions*, *purpuric reactions* (23[C], 24[C], 141[C]), *exfoliative dermatitis*, *Stevens-Johnson syndrome* and *toxic epidermal necrolysis* are encountered (142[C]—144[C], 146[C], 147[c], 148[c], 149[R]). In extremely rare cases, *pemphigus vulgaris* (150[c]) and *acquired cutis laxa* (151[c]) have been described.

In a group of patients with chronic urticaria, penicillin allergy was demonstrated by epicutaneous and intracutaneous tests. A diet free from dairy products seemed to have a curative effect in 30 of 70 patients with positive skin tests to penicillins (152[C]). Penicillin-contaminated milk or meat may induce itching or generalized skin reactions (153[C]) and even anaphylaxis (154[c], 155[c]). Allergic contact dermatitis has been observed with a number of different penicillins (146[C], 156[C], 157[C]).

Preventive measures in usual exanthemas: see 'Risk situations', p. 699. The treatment of toxic epidermal necrolysis has improved, but a persisting mortality of up to 20—30% mandates early and close multidisciplinary management (burn unit) (45[C]). As a preventive measure, the suspected drug should be stopped at the beginning of any maculopapular exanthema or generalized erythema (24[C]).

Local reactions to parenteral penicillin applica-

tions Intramuscular injection of high doses of depot preparations may lead to *painful swelling* especially when over 600 000—1 000 000 units are given at a single site (158[R], 159[c]). Such reactions appeared in two of 878 patients (0.2%) with intramuscular procaine penicillin (160a[C]). Arthus phenomenon seems to be rare (28[C], 146[C]). Allergic contact dermatitis usually is induced by topically applied drugs, but is also seen in connection with ingested, injected or inhaled substances (146[C], 156[C], 157[C]).

Serum sickness-like syndrome The diagnosis of serum sickness-like syndrome should be limited to patients with at least three of the classical symptoms of real serum sickness: fever, exanthema, arthritis, lymphadenitis and leukopenia (SED-8, 553; 4[C], 7[C], 45[C]). In more severe cases, the syndrome is associated with histological findings of allergic vasculitis (45[C]). It may be accompanied by specific IgE antibodies (160b[C]).

Similar symptoms are encountered in Henoch-Schönlein purpura defined to be associated with involvement of more than one other organ. In all 16 observations of palpable purpura related to penicillin or sulfonamide compounds, the criteria of Henoch-Schönlein purpura were not fulfilled (CHDM Bern/St. Gallen, 1974—1991; 141[C]).

In some infectious diseases, e.g. meningococcal septicema, complications such as arthritis, cutaneous vasculitis and episcleritis may develop as a reaction to the microorganism.

Drug fever may develop also without a generalized exanthema (5[C], 27[C]).

Secondary reactions *Jarisch-Herxheimer reaction* This should be distinguished from allergic drug reactions. The reaction usually starts 2—12 hours after administration of the first dose of penicillin (or of any other drug) in the treatment of syphilis. Some patients develop fever with shaking chills. This is often accompanied by an aggravation of the syphilitic symptoms (161[C]). Also cardiovascular, psychic and neurological reactions may occur. The fever rarely lasts longer than 28 hours (see Chapter 25.2).

Prevention To prevent this type of reaction, penicillin, when used in syphilis, is started at low doses. If the first dose is limited to 20 units/kg body weight, such reactions are rare. Despite this, they may still appear later when the dose is increased, for example, to 10 000 units/kg body weight (162[C]). Corticosteroids may be given simultaneously with penicillin to further reduce the incidence of the Jarisch-Herxheimer reaction (SEDA-8, 559; 162[C]).

Antibiotic-associated colitis This reaction form may also represent a secondary reaction (118[C]) (see Chapter 25.2).

Risk situations Despite their rarity, several situations must be considered.

Anaphylactic shock may begin immediately or mostly within minutes to an hour, mainly after re-instituting penicillin treatment in a *previously sensitized patient.* The situation is life-threatening. Allergic cross-reactions may occur with cephalosporins in penicillin-allergic patients (69[R], 163[C]) (Chapter 25.4) and occasionally also with the monobactam aztreonam (35a[C], 35b[C]).

Based on a number of studies, there is no evidence that atopy favors sensitization with anaphylactic shock or an attack of bronchial asthma (2[R], 29[C], 30[C], 32[r]). However, the most severe and the lethal reactions seem to occur mainly in patients with a history of atopy (2[R], 31[C]).

The risk of developing a rash is high in HIV-infected patients treated with amoxycillin clavulate (164[C]) (Chapter 25.2) and cotrimoxazole (Chapter 29.1). This is especially true in patients with low CD_4 counts (164[C]). Also, the most severe reactions, including anaphylactic shock, seem to be prevalent in this situation.

Patients with *cystic fibrosis* show a relatively high rate of IgE-mediated and other, less well understood, adverse drug reactions (see Chapters 25.1 and 25.2).

Anaphylactic shock is reported to be potentiated by drug-induced β-adrenergic blockade (165[c]). This is now a generally accepted fact, substantiated by the diminished effectiveness of epinephrine in this situation.

Prevention of the most severe skin reactions In patients with any kind of Type 1-reaction, even uncomplicated urticaria, the culprit drug is usually stopped. This is not yet routinely so in cases of maculopapular rash or erythema. The fact that no skin reactions such as erythema multiforme major, Stevens-Johnson syndrome or toxic epidermal necrolysis were registered in 48 005 hospitalized patients, despite wide use of drugs known to potentially cause such reactions, may warrant the more recent concept of discontinuing the suspected drug in all kinds of common exanthema (24[C]). Further studies on this subject are needed to prove this hypothesis.

The *transfer of penicillin preparations* (ampicillin, pivampicillin, phenoxymethyl-penicillin) through the milk of nursing mothers with puerperal mastitis *to the breast-fed infant* seems to be minimal (166[C]). Therefore, the risk of adverse drug reactions due to penicillins seems to be negligible unless the infant is hypersensitive to penicillin.

Toxic reactions may occur either in patients with *renal failure* if the dosage is not adapted or in patients with special predispositions such as *cerebral damage*, *cardiopulmonary bypass*, etc. *Embolic toxic* reactions may have severe consequences in patients with pre-existing *cardiac or possibly pulmonary disease*.

Myasthenia gravis seem to be aggravated by ampicillin (167[c]), a reaction well known for aminoglycosides and some other antibiotics.

Second-generation effects In earlier studies it was thought, mainly on the basis of animal studies, that malformations could be induced by penicillins. This could not be confirmed by later, more extensive evaluations (168[R]). Penicillin G, ampicillin and probably most other penicillin preparations can be used in pregnant women and children. Experience with the newer semisynthetic penicillins might not be large enough to allow for definite conclusions regarding their safety for mother and fetus during pregnancy.

Overdosage See 'Risk situations' above as well as Chapter 25.2.

Interactions Renal excretion is lowered when *probenecid* (Benemid) is used in combination with penicillins. This results in higher plasma levels. The resorption of oral penicillin preparations may be hampered if certain other drugs are given simultaneously.

If penicillins are given in higher doses by the intravenous route (penicillin G, carbenicillin, ticarcillin, azlocillin, mezlocillin and piperacillin), *aminoglycosides* may be inactivated (169[R], 170[C]–172[C]). Especially in patients with reduced renal function receiving adapted smaller aminoglycoside doses, this interaction is probably of clinical significance (170[C], 173[c]). Combinations of two β-lactams offer an antimicrobial spectrum similar to that of an aminoglycoside and β-lactam combination, but without the renal or 8th nerve toxicity (135[R], 174[R]). However, they may be less active against *Pseudomonas* (174[R]).

Some reports suspect a possible interaction of penicillin-preparations with methotrexate therapy (175[c]). In lung transplant recipients, cyclosporin nephrotoxicity is potentiated by nafcillin (126[C]).

In our experience, rashes are not more frequently induced by ampicillins in patients also treated with allopurinol (19[C], 20[C]). This had been suspected in earlier reports (176[C]). In more recent data of the CHDM Bern, exposure time to the aminopenicillins has been taken into consideration and was equal for both groups of patients, with and without allopurinol (20[C]).

The opinion that ampicillin may reduce the effect of contraceptives appears to be rather unlikely (177[C]) (see Chapter 40.1).

Interference with diagnostic methods *Positive direct anti-globulin test* Under β-lactam antibiotics this test is often falsely positive, especially under cephalosporins as well as clavulanic acid (see Chapters 25.4 and 25.5). *Pseudo-proteinuria* has been described in patients treated with penicillin G or ureido penicillin derivatives at doses in excess of 5 g/day. Proteinuria should be excluded using either a bromphenol-blue test (Albustix) or other methods after urine dialysis (SEDA-3, 219).

Urine samples containing β-lactams should be tested for *glucose* by the glucose-oxidase method. Falsely elevated values are generally observed with the copper reduction method (SEDA-10, 236; 178[R]).

Aminoglycoside inactivation by antipseudomonal penicillins and cephalosporins may occur in serum if it is stored for 24 hours or longer before testing (173[C], 174[R], 179[C]–181[C]). In *chronic hemodialysis patients* the same effect was observed for tobramycin, but not for netilmicin (173[C], 181[C]).

In the light of early studies it must be accepted that high-dosage penicillin therapy procludes abnormally *elevated 17-ketogenic steroid levels* in the blood and high 17-keto-steroid values in the urine (182[C]).

Penicillins may interfere with typing of *HLA antigens* (SEDA-8, 248).

SPECIAL PROBLEMS OF PENICILLIN DEPOT PREPARATIONS

Embolic-toxic reactions to penicillin depot preparations The symptoms are quite characteristic and different from those of inadvertent intra-arterial injections. The term 'embolic-toxic reaction' is proposed by the authors to realize a unified terminology. Up to now, the syndrome has been called 'pseudo-anaphylactic reaction' or 'acute non-allergic reaction' (41[C], 183[C]–185[C], 186[c], 187[C], 188[C], 189a[C], 189b[C]), 'panic attack syndrome' and 'acute psychotic reaction' (190[C], 195[C]). The pathomechanism is probably embolic-toxic (50[C], 186[C], 189a[C], 196[c], 197[C]). In several countries, the term 'Hoigné syndrome' is used. The first observations were in syphilitic patients and published by Batchelor et al. (197[C]).

The symptoms comprise fear of death, confusion, acoustic and visual hallucinations, and possibly palpitations, tachycardia and cyanosis (SEDA-8, 559; 41[C], 183[C]–185[C], 197[C], 198[C]). Generalized seizures or twitching of the extremities have been observed in children and adults (185[C], 190[C], 193[C], 199[C]–201[C]). As a rule the symptoms diminish and disappear within several minutes to an hour. They rarely persist up to 24 hours. A few patients continue to complain of milder symptoms for weeks and months. These are usually intermittent. Ilechukwu described seven patients with complete or partial recurrence of the experience containing elements of the original reaction following the injection of another drug or any injection at all (195[C]).

If a cardiovascular reaction with a drop in blood pressure occurs simultaneously with typical symptoms of an embolic-toxic reaction, a combination with anaphylactic shock must be considered (51[C], 52[C], Case 3).

The reports show the rate with procaine penicillin preparations to be about one to three reactions per 1000 intramuscular injections, the usual dose being about 0.6—1.2 million units (41[C], 192[C], 194[C], 196[c], 201[C]). Eight of 920 patients with venereal disease were reported to have a definite toxic-like reaction with a dose of 4.8 million units of procaine-penicillin G, corresponding to approximately one in 120 patients (202[C]). In a series of 7700 intramuscular injections with only 400 000 units of procaine-penicillin, not a single episode of embolic-toxic reaction was observed (188[C]).

Reports, mainly from the United States, consider the procaine component in this situation to be especially important (189[C], 201[C]). Procaine esterase activity was low in the plasma of patients with systemic toxic reactions (201[C]).

There is no preference of the reaction for race or sex (203[C]).

The same symptoms occurred in three patients after erroneous administration of procaine-penicillin G by intravenous infusion (189a[C]), but also in two after procaine-free antihistamine penicillin was injected intramuscularly (50[C], 196[c]). The theory that procaine was the only factor responsible could be largely discarded after convincing observations of similar symptoms occurring with a procaine-free antihistamine penicillin preparation (41[C], 51[C], 187[c], 188[C], 196[c]) and benzathine penicillin (SED-8, 560) were documented. The embolic pathogenesis of such reactions was proven in a patient at autopsy. Emboli of benzathine penicillin crystals were demonstrated in the lungs (186[c]).

It is noteworthy that reactions which should be considered of embolic-toxic origin have followed the use of procaine-free benzathine penicillin in several patients with severe cardiac disease (204[C], 205[C], 206[c]). Visual and acoustic hallucinations, however, have been described in this situation by only a few observers. Dyspnea, pulmonary edema and collapse seem to be predominant (204[C]—207[C], Cases 2, 3 and 4). A number of these patients were subsequently treated with oral penicillin without side effects (206[C]). For practical purposes, this virtually excludes the possibility of anaphylactic sensitization. Among the reactions encountered with depot penicillins containing a local anesthetic, allergic phenomena or cardiac arrhythmias due to the anesthetic must still be borne in mind as additional possibilities (5[C], 197[C], 208[C]).

Prophylaxis of embolic-toxic reactions, especially in patients with cardiac disease, relies mainly on using oral and intravenous penicillins instead of depot penicillins (204[C], 206[C], 207[C]).

Based on the type of symptoms involved and the rapidity of their appearance as well as by a few situations of erroneously intravenous administration, the hypothesis that an inadvertent intravascular injection is responsible was obviously attractive to most observers.

Arterial vascular damage and emboli (Nicolau syndrome and 'embolia medicamentosa cutis') Occlusion and thrombosis following penicillin injection into arteries is rare. The consequences of such complications, however, may be severe. As a rule, injection of depot penicillin preparations into the gluteal area is involved, the superior gluteal artery having been entered. The complication is also encountered with injections into the thigh.

Possibly the rules for intragluteal injection as given by von Hochstetter (209[C]) were not always followed in such cases. Only the ventral portions of the small gluteal muscles should be used for injection or, for injection into the thigh, the middle of the vastus lateralis muscle (210[C]). This will probably prevent contracture of the most important portions of the quadriceps femoris muscle as well as damage to the sciatic nerve. On the other hand, the development of local gangrene in children has been described, despite careful injection at the proper anatomical site (211[c], 212[C]). In other publications the quadriceps femoris (213[C], 214[c]) or the forearm muscles (215[c]) were used for injection. Surprisingly, ischemic reactions followed by gangrene have been described, not only after the injection of oily procaine penicillin, aluminium stearate penicillin, depot penicillin combined with streptomycin preparations and benzathine penicillin, but also after injection of water-soluble penicillin solutions (213[C], 216[c]). It may be difficult to differentiate this from a local Arthus phenomenon (28[C], 146[C]). A highly vascular *granulomatous inflammation* may develop at the site of injection. Fibrous scar tissue is found at surgery and histologically (159[C]).

Repeated intramuscular injections into the thighs of newborns and infants may cause severe and widespread *muscular contractures* of the quadriceps femoris (SEDA-8, 560). In a number of cases injections of penicillin preparations were the cause.

This clinical picture following intra-arterial injection of depot preparations has been called 'Nicolau syndrome' (217[C]). In 1925 this author reported an arterial bismuth embolus followed by gangrene in the gluteal area. A probably milder reaction, also due to a bismuth preparation, was described as early as 1924 by Freudenthal (218[C]). In the following discussion we shall limit ourselves strictly to arterial vascular damage caused by penicillin preparations.

The first symptom to appear is a local mottling of the skin over the injected region. The high pressure necessary for injection of viscous fluids may produce a retrograde flow of the drug into the larger arteries as high as the common iliac, abdominal aorta, renal and spinal cord vessels. Complications may therefore include everything from an ischemic syndrome with local necrosis of the skin, sub-cutaneous tissue and muscle, often combined with vascular and nervous system involvement of greater extent such as intestinal and renal hemorrhage, necrosis of the entire lower extremity and even paraplegia from spinal cord damage (211[c], 212[C], 213[C], 219[c], 220[C], 221[C], 222[c]). Necrosis of the forearm has been described in two patients following inadvertent intra-arterial administration of dicloxacillin (223[C]).

Local hemorrhagic-necrotic reactions limited to the skin (224[c], 225[c]), called 'embolia medicamentosa cutis' (226[C]) have also been described (see 'Skin reactions').

At autopsy, benzathine penicillin crystals were found in the artery of a child who died of shock following arterial emboli (227[C]).

SPECIAL PROBLEMS WITH SPECIFIC GROUPS OF PENICILLINS

Penicillin G (benzylpenicillin) and penicillin V (phenoxymethylpenicillin)

Benzylpenicillin-Na or -K salts As these preparations may be administered in doses of 10–50 million units daily to adult patients, the cations sodium and potassium take on a significant role. This is especially true for patients with cardiac or renal disease and may favour the occurrence of hyperkalemia or hypernatremia (see also p. 693 and Chapter 25.2).

Long-acting benzylpenicillin preparations Procaine penicillin, antihistamine penicillin, benzathine penicillin and possibly other depot penicillins may lead to embolic-toxic reactions following accidental intravascular injection (see above).

Penicillin V (phenoxymethylpenicillin) These preparations can be used orally. Other drugs, even sodium bicarbonate, seem to markedly influence the absorption of oral penicillin preparations (SED-8, 562; 228[C]).

β-Lactamase-resistant penicillin preparations

Isoxazolyl penicillins (oxacillin, cloxacillin, dicloxacillin, flucloxacillin) Side effects on the gastrointestinal tract are seen in a small percentage of treated patients. Generalized skin reactions are observed with about the same frequency as with penicillin-G. In several papers, oxacillin-, cloxacillin-, dicloxacillin- or flucloxacillin-treated patients were shown to develop agranulocytosis or neutropenia (86[C], 88[C]–90[C], 93[R]). If neutropenia was found later than the critical phase of staphylococcal infection, the drug relationship had to be seriously considered (88[C]).

In all these observations, neutropenia and in the majority also leukopenia, evolved slowly after 6–30 days of isoxazolyl penicillin treatment. Immune hemolytic anemia occurred under oxacillin and flucloxacillin (166[c]).

Rarely, hepatitis and intrahepatic cholestasis may occur during treatment with various penicillin preparations, mainly oxacillin (107[C]–110[C]) and flucloxacillin (111[c], 112[c]).

Interstitial nephritis has also been described in relation to oxacillin and dicloxacillin therapy (122[c], 131[C]).

Methicillin Whereas penicillin G seems to produce nephropathy only in rare and exceptional cases, there can be no doubt as to the existence of meticillin-induced nephritis (119[R], 120[C], 121[C], 122[R], 123[C], 124[C], 137b[c]). In the study by Baldwin et al. (121[C]) histological examinations in four patients showed a characteristic interstitial nephritis without glomerulonephritis or arteritis. Two of these patients were undergoing treatment with penicillin G and two others with methicillin. Similar findings were reported by other authors (SED-8, 562; 119[R], 120[C], 122[R], 138a[c]). Severe acute oliguric or non-oliguric renal failure may occur. The differential diagnosis of renal failure must include the infectious process for which the penicillin was given (122[R], 136a[R], 229[C]).

Agranulocytosis or leukopenia, in some cases combined with anemia, have been observed during methicillin treatment (SEDA-11, 225; 99[C]) (see 'Agranulocytosis', p. 697. Also, methicillin-induced thrombocytopenia has been observed (80[c]).

Used intramuscularly, methicillin is more painful than most of the other penicillins. Local thrombosis is not infrequent following intravenous administration.

Sodium nafcillin Granulocytopenia has been observed (90[C], 93[C], 98[C]). Platelet dysfunction and bleeding may also be encountered (see Chapter 25.2). Nausea and diarrhea occur occasionally following oral intake. The increased sulfobromphthalein (BSP)-retention and SGOT levels in some patients may be due to hepatic toxicity. To our knowledge, interstitial nephritis is rare as compared with methicillin (122[R], 137a[c]). Staphylococcal infections may of themselves cause nephritis (136a[R]).

In lung transplant patients, nafcillin seems to potentiate cyclosporin nephrotoxicity during the week following transplantation (126[C]).

The local toxic side effects of intravenous nafcillin seem to be more pronounced than those of methicillin (230[C]).

Aminopenicillins

Ampicillin, amoxycillin, and their congeners A high percentage of patients (approximately 3—10%) treated with ampicillin or amoxycillin develop a rash (SEDA-8, 563; 7[C], 19[C]—22[C]). If several other drugs were also given to the patient during the same period, a relative frequency for the most commonly used drugs can be calculated by the method of weighted attributions (21[C]) or on the basis of the Euler-Venn diagram (7[C]). Anaphylactic shock see 'Cardiovascular reactions', p. 696. The occurrence rate of the reaction depends largely on time of exposure (20[C]). This observation is compatible with an allergic pathomechanism. Positive results with the lymphocyte transformation test may support this interpretation (231[C]).

For over 20 years the use of ampicillin in the presence of mononucleosis can no longer be defended since (SED-8, 563). The incidence of maculopapular, frequently purpuric rashes in such cases was between 42 and 100%. The frequency of exanthemas in infectious mononucleosis without antibiotic treatment is only 3—15%. An increase in the occurrence rate of rashes if ampicillin is combined with allopurinol (176[C]) could not be confirmed by our group which took the exposure time for both treatment groups into account (19[C], 20[C]).

New combinations of amoxicillin with the β-lactamase inhibitor, potassium clavulanate, or ampicillin with sulbactam, a penicillanic acid sulfone, seem to have a spectrum of adverse reactions similar to that of the aminopenicillins (232[R]) (see Chapter 25.5). Clavulanate might increase the frequency of the gastrointestinal adverse effects of amoxicillin alone, especially diarrhea and nausea (116[C], 117[C], 233[R]). In a recent paper, a difference in frequency between the single and the combined preparation (amoxicillin and clavulanate) could not be confirmed for diarrhea (118[C]) (see Chapters 25.1 and 25.5).

Aminopenicillin with added clavulanic acid proved capable of inducing cholestatic hepatitis which did not reappear after a second exposure to amoxicillin alone, but did recur with amoxicillin and clavulanic acid (234[C]). Aminopenicillin preparations can also induce interstitial nephritis (122[R], 128[c], 129[C], 137b[c]). A positive direct Coombs test and hepatitis in relation to the combination of amoxicillin and clavulanate has been demonstrated (see Chapter 25.5).

Bacampicillin, *pivampicillin* and *talampicillin* also belong to the *individual ampicillin analogs* and show properties similar to ampicillin. These are called 'prodrugs' (SEDA-9, 232).

Amdinocillin (formerly *mecillinam*) and *pivmecillinam* are newer penicillanic acid derivatives. They have effects and probably adverse reactions comparable to ampicillin.

Antipseudomonal penicillins

Carboxypenicillins and ureidopenicillins *Carbenicillin* It is employed parenterally in high doses for generalized infections. Excretion is markedly retarded in the presence of renal insufficiency, whereas hepatic disease has little effect on its halflife (SED-8, 564). It is often combined with gentamicin. As a result of the high doses of carbenicillin which are necessary, the sodium content may lead to acute pulmonary edema in patients with cardiac failure. Hypokalemia, such as has been described in isolated cases with sodium penicillin G treatment, has also been observed (235[C], 236[C]).

In a few isolated instances, a rise in the serum glutamic oxalacetic transaminase (SGOT) has been documented. Episodes of mild, reversible anicteric hepatitis have been described (113[C]).

An apparently specific side effect of carbenicillin is a bleeding disorder seen primarily in patients with renal insufficiency. The clinical manifestations comprise purpura, mucous membrane bleeding, epistaxis, and bleeding from injection sites or minor surgical procedures (SED-8, 564).

Interference with platelet aggregation and anticoagulant action through interference with conversion of fibrinogen to fibrin have been considered as possible mechanisms (see Chapter 25.2). An analogous coagulation disorder has been described in connection with ticarcillin and high doses of penicillin G.

Granulocytopenia also can be associated with carbenicillin and ticarcillin (93[C], 100[C]).

Disodium carbenicillin given intramuscularly may

cause particularly severe pain at the injection site (237[C]).

Carbenicillin indanyl-Na (carindacillin) This was introduced for the treatment of persistent or recurrent urinary tract infections due to *Pseudomonas* and indole-positive *Proteus*, but is no longer used in many countries. Peak concentrations in the serum achieved with oral indanyl carbenicillin are low. In patients with marked renal insufficiency, urine concentrations of the drug are probably inadequate (238[C]). The most commonly reported side effects are a bad or bitter taste, nausea, diarrhea, flatulence, abdominal cramps and, rarely, vomiting. Occasional elevations of the SGOT levels have also been noted.

Ticarcillin Ticarcillin is α-carboxy-3-thienyl-methyl-penicillin used parenterally. Hypokalemia (169[R], 239[C]), prolongation of bleeding time and anticoagulant actions (see Chapter 25.1) have been noted, as with carbenicillin.

Ticarcillin also exists in a combination with clavulanate (240[C]).

Ureidopenicillins: azlocillin, mezlocillin, piperacillin

These preparations show a wide antibacterial spectrum comparable to carbenicillin and ticarcillin. So far the side effects appear to be similar to those of other penicillin preparations (241[C], 242[C]). A case of allergic thrombocytopenia related to mezlocillin has been described (106[c]). Ureidopenicillins are often used in combination with either a second β-lactam antibiotic or with an aminoglycoside (135[C], 173[C], 174[R]), e.g. in patients with neutropenia or malignant tumors and gram-negative bacteria, possibly *Pseudomonas*. In this situation, the combination with an aminoglycoside seems to be more effective than a double β-lactam combination.

Other types of adverse drug reactions with both combinations may include bleeding or hypokalemia. Both are often associated with a reduced general condition and possibly undernourishment (73a[C], 73b[C], 243[C], 244[C]). The bleeding may be induced by a coagulation or by a platelet disorder (73a[C], 243[C], 244[C]). These complications seem less pronounced than with carbenicillin or ticarcillin (see Chapter 25.2).

Clavulanic acid

The principles are discussed in Chapter 25.5.

REFERENCES

1. Coombs RRA, Gell PGH. Classification of allergic reactions responsible for clinical hypersensitivity and disease. In: Gell PGH, Coombs RRA, eds. Clinical Aspects of Immunology, 2nd edn. Oxford, Edinburgh: Blackwell Scientific Publications, 1968;575.
2. Hoigné R, Schlumberger HP, Vervloet D et al. Epidemiology of allergic drug reactions. In: Burr M, ed. Epidemiology of Allergic Disease. Monogr. Allergy, 31. Basle: S. Karger AG, 1993;147.
3. Dewdney JM. Pseudo-allergic reactions to antibiotics. In: Dukor P, Kallos P, Schlumberger HD, eds. PAR. Pseudo-Allergic Reactions. Involvement of Drugs and Chemicals, Vol. 1. Basel: S. Karger, 1980;273.
4. Von Pirquet C, Schick B. Die Serumkrankheit. Leipzig/Vienna: Franz Deuticke, 1905.
5. Hoigné R. Arzneimittelallergien. Bern/Stuttgart: Hans Huber Verlag, 1965.
6. Hoigné R, D'Andrea Jaeger M, Wymann R et al. Time pattern of allergic reactions to drugs. In: Weber E, Lawson DH, Hoigné R, eds. Risk Factors for Adverse Drug Reactions, Agents Actions, Vol 29 (Suppl). Basel/Boston/Berlin: Birkhäuser-Verlag, 1990.
7. Hoigné R, Stocker F, Middleton P. Epidemiology of drug allergy: drug monitoring. In: de Weck AL, Bundgaard H, eds. The Handbook of Experimental Pharmacology, Vol. 63. Allergic Reactions to Drugs. Berlin/Heidelberg: Springer-Verlag, 1983;187.
8. Wickern GM, Nish WA, Bitner AS et al. Allergy to β-lactams: a survey of current practices. J Allergy Clin. Immunol 1994;94:725.
9. Levine BB, Redmond AP, Fellner M et al. Penicillin allergy and the heterogeneous immune responses of man to benzylpenicillin. J Clin Invest 1966;45:1895.
10. Van Arsdel PP Jr, Larson EB. Diagnostic tests for patients with suspected allergic diseases. Ann Intern Med 1989;110:304.
11. Lin RY. A perspective on penicillin allergy. Arch Intern Med 1992;152:930.
12. Ressler C, Mendelson L. Skin tests for diagnosis of penicillin allergy—current status. Ann Allergy 1987;59:167.
13. Sogn DD, Evans R III, Shepherd GM et al. Results of the National Institute of Allergy and Infectious Diseases collaborative clinical trial to test the predictive value of skin testing with major and minor penicillin derivatives in hospitalized adults. Arch Intern Med 1992;152:1025.
14. Gadde J, Spence M, Wheeler B et al. Clinical experience

with penicillin skin testing in a large inner-city STD clinic. J Am Med Assoc 1993;270:2456.
15. Erffmeyer JE. Adverse reactions to penicillin. Ann Allergy 1981;47:288.
16. Blanca M, Perez E, Garcia J et al. Anaphylaxis to amoxicillin but good tolerance for benzyl penicillin. Allergy 1988;43:508.
17. Vega JM, Blanca M, Garcia JJ et al. Immediate allergic reactions to amoxicillin. Allergy 1994;49:317.
18. Silviu-Dan F, McPhillips S, Warrington RJ. The frequency of skin test reactions to side-chain penicillin determinants. J Allergy Clin Immunol 1993;91:694.
19. Sonntag MR, Zoppi M, Fritschy D et al. Exantheme unterhäufig angewandten Antibiotika und antibakteriellen Chemotherapeutika (Penicilline, speziell Aminopenicilline, Cephalosporine und Cotrimoxazol sowie Allopurinol). Schweiz Med Wochenschr 1986;116:142.
20. Hoigné R, Sonntag MR, Zoppi M et al. Occurrence of exanthems in relation to aminopenicillin preparations and allo purinol. N Engl J Med 1987;316:1217.
21. Arndt KA, Jick H. Rates of cutaneous reactions to drugs. A report from the Boston Collaborative Drug Surveillance Program. J Am Med Assoc 1976;235:918.
22. Bigby M, Jick S, Jick H et al. Drug-induced cutaneous reactions. A report from the Boston Collaborative Drug Surveillance Program on 15 438 consecutive patients, 1975 to 1982. J Am Med Assoc 1986;256:3358.
23. Green GR, Rosenblum A. Report of the penicillin study group American Academy of Allergy. J Allergy Clin Immunol 1971;48:331.
24. Hunziker Th, Hoigné R, Künzi UP et al. Comprehensive Hospital Drug Monitoring (CHDM), the adverse skin reactions, a 20-year study. Abstract 033. Pharmacol Drug Safety 1995;4:S13.
25. Hoigné R, Hunziker T, Künzi UP. Risikofaktoren und epidemiologische Aspekte unerwünschter Arzneimittelwirkungen unter besonderer Berücksichtigung der allergischen und pseudo-allergischen Reaktionen. Allergologie 1995; 18:320.
26. Neftel KA, Wälti M, Spengler H et al. Effect of storage of penicillin-G solutions on sensitisation to penicillin-G after intravenous administration. Lancet 1982;i:986.
27. Mackowiak PA, Le Maistre CF. Drug fever: A critical appraisal of conventional concepts. Ann Int Med 1987; 106:728.
28. Girard JP, Zawodnik S. Diagnostic procedures in drug allergy. In: de Weck AL, Bundgard H., eds. Handbook of Experimental Pharmacology, Vol 63. Berlin: Springer-Verlag, 1983;207.
29. Capaul R, Maibach R, Künzi UP et al. Atopy, bronchial asthma and previous adverse drug reactions (ADRs): risk factors for ADRs? Post Marketing Surveillance 1993;7:331.
30. Bertelsen K, Dalgaard JB. Penicillin-dodsfad. Nord Med 1965;73:173.
31. Delage C, Irey NS. Anaphylactic deaths: a clinicopathologic study of 43 cases. J Forensic Sci 1972;17:525.
32. Horowitz L. Atopy as a factor in penicillin reactions. N. Engl J Med 1975;292:1243.
33. Bajoghli M. Anaphylactoid reaction immediately after opening of ampicillin bottle. N Engl J Med 1975;293:1153.
34. Pietzcker F, Kuner V. Anaphylaxie nach epicutanem Ampicillin-Test. Z Hautkr 1975;50:437.
35a. Moss RB. Sensitization to aztreonam and cross-reactivity with other beta-lactam antibiotics in high-risk patients with cystic fibrosis. J Allergy Clin Immunol 1991;87:78.
35b. Adkinson NF. Immunogenicity and cross-allergenicity of Aztreonam. Am J Med 1990;88:3C.
36. Sullivan TJ. Management of patients allergic to antimicrobial drugs Allergy Proc 1991;12:361.
37. Bochner BS, Lichtenstein LM. Anaphylaxis. N. Engl J Med 1991;324:1785.
38. Sullivan TJ, Yecies LD, Shatz GS et al. Desensitization of patients allergic to penicillin using orally administered beta-lactam antibiotics. J Allergy Clin Immunol 1982;69:500.
39. Wendel DG Jr, Stark BJ, Jamison RB et al. Penicillin allergy and desensitization in serious infections during pregnancy. N Engl J Med 1985;312:1229.
40. Naclerio R, Mizrahi EA, Adkinson NF. Immunologic observations during desensitization and maintenance of clinical tolerance to penicillin. N Engl J Med 1983;71:294.
41. Hoigné R. Akute Nebenreaktionen auf Penicillin-präparate. Acta Med Scand 1962;171:201.
42. Hoffman DR, Hudson P, Carlyle SJ et al. Three cases of fatal anaphylaxis to antibiotics in patients with prior histories of allergy to the drug. Ann Allergy 1989;62:91.
43. Idsoe O, Guthe T, Willcox RR et al. Art und Ausmass der Penizillinnebenwirkungen unter besonderer Berücksichtigung von 151 Todesfällen nach anaphylaktischem Schock. Schweiz Med Wochenschr 1969;99:1190.
44. Spark RP. Fatal anaphylaxis due to oral penicillin. Am J Clin Pathol 1971;56:407.
45. Hoigné R. Drug therapy of allergic states with special reference to anaphylactic shock, serum sickness and organ manifestations. Allergol Immunopathol 1976;4(Suppl 3):125.
46. Revuz J, Roujeau J-C, Guillaume J-C. Treatment of toxic epidermal necrolysis. Arch Dermatol 1987;123:1156.
47. Cullen DJ. Severe anaphylactic reaction to penicillin during halothane anaesthesia: a case report. Br J Anaesth 1971;43:410.
48. Booth BH, Patterson R. Electrocardiographic changes during human anaphylaxis. J Am Med Assoc 1970;211:627.
49. Petsas AA, Kotler MN. Electrocardiographic changes associated with penicillin anaphylaxis. Chest 1973;64:66.
50. Markowitz M, Kaplan E, Cuttica R et al. Allergic reactions to long-term benzathine penicillin prophylaxis for rheumatic fever. Lancet 1991;337:1308.
51. Hoigné R, Krebs A. Kombinierte anaphylaktische und embolisch-toxische Reaktion durch akzidentelle intravaskuläre Injektion von Procain-Penicillin. Schweiz Med Wochenschr 1964;94:610.
52. Kryst L, Wanyura H. Hoigné's syndrome—its course and symptomatology. J Maxillofac Surg 1979;7:320.
53a. Davies RJ, Hendrik DJ, Pepys J. Asthma due to inhaled chemical agents: ampicillin, benzyl penicillin, 6-aminopenicillanic acid and related substances. Clin Allergy 1974;4:227.
53b. Hoigné R, Braunschweig S, Zehnder D et al. Drug-induced bronchial asthma attack: epidemiological aspects (communication of CHDM Berne/St. Gallen, Switzerland). Pharmacoepidemiol Drug Safety 1994;3:S90(abstract).
54. Hoigné R, D'Andrea Jaeger M, Hess T. et al. Akute schwere Dyspnoe als Medikamentennebenwirkung. Schweiz Med Wochenschr 1990;120:1211.
55. Reichlin S, Loveless MH, Kane EG. Loeffler's syndrome following penicillin therapy. Ann Intern Med 1953;38:113.
56. Wengrower D, Tzfoni EE, Drenger B et al. Erythro-

derma and pneumonitis induced by penicillin. Respiration 1986;50:301.
57. de Hoyos A, Holness L, Tarlo SM. Hypersensitivity pneumonitis and airways hyperreactivity induced by occupational exposure to penicillin. Chest 1993;103:303.
58. Minnig H, de Weck AL. Die 'Käsewascherkrankheit': immunologische und epidemiologische Studien. Schweiz Med Wochenschr 1972;102:1205.
59. Poe RH, Condemi JJ, Weinstein SS et al. Adult respiratory distress syndrome related to ampicillin sensitivity. Chest 1980;77:449.
60. New PS, Wells CE. Cerebral toxicity associated with massive intravenous penicillin therapy. Neurology 1965;15:1053.
61. Nicholls PJ. Neurotoxicity of penicillin. J Antimicrob Chemother 1980;6:161.
62. Schliamser SE, Bolander H, Kourtopoulos H et al. Neurotoxicity of benzylpenicillin: correlation to concentrations in serum, cerebrospinal fluid and brain tissue fluid in rabbits. J Antimicrob Chemother 1988;21:365.
63. Boston Collaborative Drug Surveillance program. Drug-induced convulsions. Lancet 1972;ii:677.
64. Smith H, Lerner PI, Weinstein L. Neurotoxicity and 'massive' intravenous therapy with penicillin. Arch Intern Med 1967;120:47.
65. Currie TT, Hayward NJ, Westlake G et al. Epilepsy in cardiopulmonary bypass patients receiving large intravenous doses of penicillin. J. Thorac Cardiovasc Surg 1971;62:1.
66. Seamans KB. Gloor P, Dobell ARC et al. Penicillin-induced seizures during cardiopulmonary bypass: a clinical and electroencephalographic study. N Engl J Med 1968;278:861.
67. Reuling JR, Cramer C. Intrathecal penicillin. J Am Med Assoc 1947;134:16.
68. Schmitt BD, Krivit W. Benign intracranial hypertension associated with a delayed penicillin reaction. Pediatrics 1969;43:50.
69. Wright AJ, Wilkowske CJ. The penicillins. Mayo Clin Proc 1987;62:806.
70. Brunner FP, Frick PG. Hypokalaemia, metabolic alkalosis, and hypernatraemia due to 'massive' sodium penicillin therapy. Br Med J 1968;4:550.
71. Mohr JA, Clark RM, Waack TC et al. Nafcillin-associated hypokalaemia. J Am Med Assoc 1979;242:544.
72. Wade JC, Schimpff SC, Newman KA. Piperacillin or ticarcillin plus amikacin. Am J Med 1981;71:983.
73a. Rotstein C, Cimino M, Winkey K et al. Cefoperazone plus piperacillin versus mezlocillin plus tobramycin as empiric therapy for febrile episodes in neutropenic patients. Am J Med 1988;85(Suppl 1A):36.
73b. Kibbler CC, Prentice HG, Sage RJ et al. A comparison of double beta-lactam combinations with netilmicin/ureidopenicillin regimens in the empirical therapy of febrile neutropenic patients. J Antimicrob Chemother 1989;23:759.
74. Petz LD, Fudenberg HH. Coombs-positive hemolytic anemia caused by penicillin administration. N. Engl J Med 1966;274:171.
75. Spath P, Garratty G, Petz LD. Immunhämatologische Reaktionen bei Penizillinbehandlung. Schweiz Med Wochenschr 1973;103:383.
76. White JM, Brown DL, Hepner GW et al. Penicillin-induced haemolytic anaemia. Br Med J 1968;3:26.
77. Funicella T, Weinger RS, Moake JL et al. Penicillin-induced immunohemolytic anemia associated with circulating immune complexes. Am J Hematol 1977;3:219.
78. Tuffs L. Flucloxacillin-induced haemolytic anemia. Med J Aust 1986;144:559.
79. Parker JC, Barrett DA II. Microangiopathic hemolysis and thrombocytopenia related to penicillin drugs. Arch Intern Med 1971;127:474.
80. Schiffer CA, Weinstein HD, Wiernik PH. Methicillin-associated thrombocytopenia. Ann Intern Med 1976;85:338.
81. Lee M, Sharifi R. Severe thrombocytopenia due to apalcillin. Urol Int 1987;42:313.
82. Kerr RO, Cardamone J, Dalmasso AP et al. Two mechanisms of erythrocyte destruction in penicillin-induced hemolytic anemia. N Engl J Med 1972;287:1322.
83. Harris JW. Studies on the mechanism of a drug-induced hemolytic anemia. J Lab Clin Med 1956;47:760.
84. Brandslund I, Petersen PH, Strunge P et al. Haemolytic uraemic syndrome and accumulation of haemoglobin—haptoglobin complexes in plasma in serum sickness caused by penicillin drugs. Haemostasis 1980;9:193.
85. Boyce TG, Swerdlow DL, Griffin PM. Escherichia coli 0157:H7 and the hemolytic-uremic syndrome. N. Engl J Med 1995;333:364.
86. Gatell JM, Rello J, Miro JM et al. Cloxacillin-induced neutropenia. J Infect Dis 1986;154:372.
87. Rello J, Gatell JM, Miro JM et al. Effectos secundarios associados a la cloxacilina. Med Clin (Barcelona) 1987; 89:631.
88. Ahern MJ, Hicks JE, Andriole VT. Neutropenia during high dose intravenous oxacillin therapy. Yale J Biol Med 1976;49:351.
89. Teyssier G, Frappaz D, Blanc JP et al. Neutropénies sous oxacilline: 3 observations pédiatriques. Pédiatrie 1984; 39:451.
90. Schmid L, Heit W, Flury R. Agranulocytosis associated with semisynthetic penicillins and cephalosporins. Blut 1984;48:11.
91. Neftel KA, Hauser SP, Müller MR. Inhibition of granulopoiesis in vivo and in vitro by betalactam antibiotics. J Infect Dis 1985;52:90.
92. Olaison L, Alestig K. A prospective study of neutropenia induced by high doses of betalactam antibiotics. J Antimicrob Chemother 1990;25:449.
93. Rouveix B, Lassoued K, Regnier B et al. Neutropénies induites par les betalactamines: mécanisme toxique ou immun? Thérapie 1988;43:489.
94. Murphy MF, Riordan T, Minchinton RM et al. Demonstration of an immune-mediated mechanism of penicillin-induced neutropenia and thrombocytopenia. Br J Haematol 1983;55:155.
95. Colvin B, Rogers M, Layton C. Benzylpenicillin-induced leucopenia, complication of treatment of bacterial endocarditis. Br Heart J 1974;36:216.
96. Al-Hadramy MS, Aman H, Omer A et al. Benzylpenicillin-induced neutropenia. J Antimicrob Chemother 1986; 17:251.
97. Wilson C, Greenhood G, Remmington JS et al. Neutropenia after consecutive treatment courses with nafcillin and piperacillin. Lancet 1979;i:1150.
98. Zakhireh B, Root RK. Unusually high occurrence of drug reactions with nafcillin. Yale J Biol Med 1978;51:449.
99. Mallouh AA. Methicillin-induced neutropenia. Pediatr Infect Dis J 1985;4:262.
100. Reyes MP, Palutke M, Lerner AM. Granulocytopenia associated with carbenicillin. Five episodes in two patients. Am J Med 1973;54:413.

101. Neftel KA, Mueller MR, Widmer U et al. Beta-lactam antibiotics inhibit human in vitro granulopoiesis and proliferation of some other cell types. Cell Biol Toxicol 1986; 2:513.
102. Miescher P, Delacretaz J. Démonstration d'un phénomène 'L.E.' positif dans deux cas d'hypersensibilité médicamenteuse. Schweiz Med Wochenschr 1954;83:536.
103. Walsh JR, Zimmerman HJ. The demonstration of the 'L.E.' phenomenon in patients with penicillin hypersensitivity. Blood 1953;8:65.
104. Brocks AP. Thrombocytopenia during treatment with ampicillin. Lancet 1974;ii:273.
105. Hsi YJ, Kuo HY, Ouyang A. Thrombocytopenia following administration of penicillin. Clin Med J 1966;85:249.
106. Gharpure V, O'Connell B, Schiffer CA. Mezlocillin-induced thrombocytopenia. Ann Int Med 1993;119:862.
107. Olans RN, Weiner LB. Reversible oxacillin hepatotoxicity. J Pediatr 1976;89:835.
108. Onorato IM, Axelrod AL. Hepatitis from intravenous high-dose oxacillin therapy. Ann Intern Med 1978;89:497.
109. Lobatto S, Dijkmans BAC, Mattie H et al. Flucloxacillin-associated liver damage. Neth J Med 1982;25:4.
110. Pollock AA, Berger SA, Simberkoff MS et al. Hepatitis associated with high-dose oxacillin therapy. Arch Intern Med 1978;138:195.
111. Turner IB, Eckstein RP, Riley JW et al. Prolonged hepatic cholestasis after flucloxacillin therapy. Med J Aust 1989;151:701.
112. Miros M, Walker N, Kerlin P et al. Flucloxacillin-induced delayed cholestatic hepatitis. Aust NZ J Med 1990;20:251.
113. Wilson FM, Belamaric J, Lauter CB et al. Anicteric carbenicillin hepatitis. J Am Med Assoc 1975;232:813.
114. Auwera P, van der Legand JC. Ticarcillin-clavulanic acid therapy in severe infections. Drugs Exp Clin Res 1985;11:805.
115. Reddy KR, Brillant P, Schiff ER. Amoxicillin-clavulanate potassium-associated cholestasis. Gastroenterology 1989; 96:1135.
116. Leigh DA, Freeth M, Bradnock K et al. Augmentin (amoxycillin and clavulanic acid) therapy in complicated urinary tract infections due to beta-lactamase-producing bacteria. In: Rolinson GN, Watson A, eds. Augmentin Clavulanate-Potentiated Amoxycillin. Proceedings, First Symposium. Amsterdam: Excerpta Medica, 1980;145.
117. Stein GE, Gurwith MJ. Amoxicillinpotassium clavulanate, a beta-lactamase-resistant antibiotic combination. Clin Pharm 1984;3:591.
118. Zehnder D, Künzi UP, Maibach R et al. Die Häufigkeit der Antibiotika-assoziierten Kolitis bei hospitalisierten Patienten der Jahre 1974—1991 im 'Comprehensive Hospital Drug Monitoring' Bern/St. Gallen. Schweiz Med Wochenschr 1995;125:676.
119. Ditlove J, Weidmann P, Bernstein M et al. Methicillin nephritis. Medicine 1977;56:483.
120. Galpin JE, Shinaberger JH, Stanley TM et al. Acute interstitial nephritis due to methicillin. Am J Med 1978; 65:756.
121. Baldwin DS, Levine BB, McCluskey RT et al. Renal failure and interstitial nephritis due to penicillin and methicillin. N Engl J Med 1968;279:1245.
122. Appel GB. A decade of penicillin related acute interstitial nephritis: more questions than answers. Clin Nephrol 1980;13:151.
123. Woodroffe AJ, Thomson NM, Meadows R et al. Nephropathy associated with methicillin administration. Aust NZ J Med 1974;4:256.
124. Sommer Hansen E, Tauris P. Methicillin-induced nephropathy. Acta Pathol Microbiol Scand 1976;84:440.
125. Parry MF, Ball WD, Conte JE Jr et al. Nafcillin nephritis. J Am Med Assoc 1973;225:178.
126. Jahansouz F, Kriett JM, Smith CM et al. Potentiation of cyclosporine nephrotoxicity by nafcillin in lung transplant recipients. Transplantation 1993;55:1045-1048.
127. Ruley EJ, Lisi M. Interstitial nephritis and renal failure due to ampicillin. J Pediatr 1974;84:878.
128. Tannenberg AM, Wicher KJ, Rose NR. Ampicillin nephropathy. J Am Med Assoc 1971;218:449.
129. Kleinknecht D, Vanhille P, Morel-Maroger L et al. Acute interstitial nephritis due to drug hypersensitivity. An up-to-date review with a report of 19 cases. In: Advances in Nephrology. Chicago: Year Book Medical Publisher, 1983; 277.
130. Gilbert DN, Gourley R, D'Agostino A et al. Interstitial nephritis due to methicillin, penicillin and ampicillin. Ann Allergy 1970;28:378.
131. Hedsttöm SA, Hybbinette CH. Nephrotoxicity in isoxazolylpenicillin prophylaxis in hip surgery. Acta Orthop Scand 1988;59:144.
132. Dörner O, Piper C, Dienes HP et al. Akute interstitielle Nephritis nach Piperacillin. Klin Wochenschr 1988;67:682.
133. Soto J, Bosch JM, Alsar Ortiz MJ et al. Piperacillin-induced acute insterstitial nephritis. Nephron 1993;65:154.
134. Iver L, Berg-Giraudion B, Pourrat O et al. La néphrotoxicité de l'association méthicilline-gentamycine. Sem Hôp Paris 1976;52:1903.
135. Barriere SL. Therapeutic considerations in using combinations of newer beta-lactam antibiotics Clin Pharm 1986; 5:24.
136a. Fried T. Acute interstitial nephritis. Postgrad Med 1993;93:105.
136b. Lamy P, Anthoine D, Rebeix G et al. Néphropathies par intolérance à la méthicilline. Ann Méd Nancy 1963;2:1489.
137a. Parry MF, Ball WD, Conte JE Jr et al. Nafcillin nephritis, J Am Med Assoc 1973;225:178.
137b. Gilbert DN, Gourley R, D'Agostino A et al. Interstitial nephritis due to methicillin, penicillin and ampicillin. Ann Allergy 1970;28:378.
138a. Border WA, Lehman DH, Egan JD et al. Antitubular basement-membrane antibodies in methicillin-associated interstitial nephritis. N Engl J Med 1974;291:381.
138b. Bracis R, Sander CV, Gilbert DN. Methicillin hemorrhagic cystitis. Antimicrob Agents Chemother 1977; 12:438.
139. Moller NE. Carbenicillin-induced haemorrhagic cystitis. Lancet 1978;ii:946.
140. Stubb S, Heikkilä H, Kauppinen K. Cutaneous reactions to drugs: a series of in-patients during a five-year period. Acta Dermatol Venereol (Stockholm) 1994;74:289.
141. Hoigné R, Hunziker T. Editorial 'Palpable Purpura'. Schweiz Med Wochenschr 1992;122:1271.
142. Schöpf E, Stühmer A, Rzany B et al. Toxic epidermal necrolysis (TEN) and Stevens-Johnson syndrome (SJS): an epidemiological study from West Germany. Arch Dermatol 1991;127:839.
143. Roujeau J-C, Chosidow O, Saiag P, Guillaume J-C. Continuing medical education. J Am Acad Dermatol 1990;23:1039.
144. Bastuji-Garin S, Rzany B, Stern RS et al. Clinical classi-

fication of cases of toxic epidermal necrolysis, Stevens-Johnson syndrome, and erythema multiforme. Arch Dermatol 1993;129:92.
145. Kauppinen K, Stubb S. Drug eruptions: causative agents and clinical types. Acta Dermatol-Venerol 1984; 64:320.
146. Fellner MJ. Adverse reactions to penicillin and related drugs. Clin Dermatol 1986;4:133.
147. Tagami H, Tatsuta K, Iwatski K et al. Delayed hypersensitivity in ampicillin-induced toxic epidermal necrolysis. Arch Dermatol 1983;119:910.
148. Amon RB, Dimond RL. Toxic epidermal necrolysis. Rapid differentiation between staphylococcal- and drug-induced disease. Arch Dermatol 1975;111:1433.
149. Zürcher K, Krebs A. Antiinfectious drugs. In: Zürcher K, Krebs A, eds. Cutaneous Drug Reactions. Basel/Munich: Karger, 1993;54.
150. Fellner MJ, Mark AS. Penicillin- and ampicillin-induced pemphigus vulgaris. Int J Dermatol 1980;7:392.
151. Kerl H, Burg G, Hashimoto K. Fatal, penicillin-induced, generalized, postinflammatory elastolysis (cutis laxa). Am J Dermatopathol 1983;5:267.
152. Boonk WJ, Van Ketel WG. Chronische urticaria, penicilline-allergie en melkprodukten in de voeding. Ned Tijdschr Geneeskd 1980;124:1771.
153. Lindemayr H, Knobler R, Kraft D et al. Challenge of penicillin-allergic volunteers with penicillin-contaminated meat. Allergy 1981;36:471.
154. Schwartz HJ, Sher TH. Anaphylaxis to penicillin in a frozen dinner. Ann Allergy 1984;52:342.
155. Tscheuschner I. Anaphylaktische Reaktion auf Penicillin nach Genuss von Schweinefleisch. Z Haut Geschlechtskr 1972;47:591.
156. Schulz KH, Schöpf E, Wex O. Allergische Berufsekzeme durch Ampicillin. Berufsdermatosen 1970;18:132.
157. Calkin JM, Maibach HI. Delayed hypersensitivity drug reactions diagnosed by patch testing. Contact Dermatitis 1993;29:223.
158. Fishman LS, Hewitt WL. The natural penicillins. Med Clin North Am 1970;54:1081.
159. Lloyd-Roberts GC, Thomas TG. The etiology of quadriceps contracture in children. J Bone Joint Surg 1964; 46B:498.
160a. Greenblatt DJ, Allen MD. Intramuscular injection-site complications. J Am Med Assoc 1978;240:542.
160b. Kraft D, Werner HP, Stemberger H et al. Immunglobulin-E-Nachweis mittels Immunfluoreszenztechnik bei Penicillinallergie vom Typ der Serumkrankheit. Wien Klin Wochenschr 1971;83:758.
161. Wolters EC. Treatment of neurosyphilis. Clin Neuropharmacol 1987;10:143.
162. Gudjonsson H, Skog E. The effect of prednisolone on the Jarisch-Herxheimer reaction. Acta Dermatol-Venereol 1968;48:15.
163. Audicana M., Bernaola G, Urrutia I et al. Allergic reactions to betalactams: Studies in a group of patients allergic to penicillin and evaluation of cross reactivity with cephalosporin. Allergy 1994;49:108.
164. Battegay M, Opravil M, Wüthrich B et al. Rash with Amoxycillin-Clavulanate therapy in HIV-infected patients. Lancet 1989;2:1100.
165. Jacobs RL, Rake GW, Fournier DC et al. Potentiated anaphylaxis in patients with drug-induced beta-adrenergic blockade. J Allergy Clin Immunol 1981;68:125.
166. Matheson I, Samseth M, Sande HA. Ampicillin in breast milk during puerperal infections. Eur J Clin Pharmacol 1988;34:657.
167. Argov Z, Brenner T, Abramsky O. Ampicillin may aggravate clinical and experimental myastenia gravis. Arch Neurol 1986;43:255.
168. Heinonen OP, Slone D, Shapiro S. Antimicrobial and antiparasitic agents. In: Birth Defects and Drugs in Pregnancy, 4th ed. Boston: John Wright PSG, 1982;296.
169. Brogden RN, Heel RC, Speight TM et al. Ticarcillin: a review of its pharmacological properties and therapeutic efficacy. Drugs 1980;20:325.
170. Henderson JL, Polk RE, Kline BJ. In vitro inactivation of gentamicin, tobramycin, and netilmicin by carbenicillin, azlocillin, or mezlocillin. Am J Hosp Pharm 1981;38:1167.
171. Noone P, Pattison JR. Therapeutic implications of interactions of gentamicin and penicillins. Lancet 1971;ii:575.
172. Thompson MIB, Russo ME, Saxon BJ et al. Gentamicin inactivation by piperacillin or carbenicillin in patients with end-stage renal disease. Antimicrob Agents Chemother 1982;21:268.
173. Halstenson CE, Hirata CA, Heim-Duthoy KL et al. Effect of concomitant administration of piperacillin on the disposition of netilmicin and tobramycin in patients with end-stage renal disease. Antimicrob Agents Chemother 1990; 34:128.
174. Giamarellou H. Aminoglycosides plus beta-lactams against gram-negative organisms: evaluation of in vitro synergy and chemical interactions. Am J Med 1986;80:126.
175. Dean R, Nachman J, Lorenzana AN et al. Possible methotrexate-mezlocillin interaction. Am J Pediatr Hematol Oncol 1992;14:88.
176. Jick H, Porter J. Potentiation of ampicillin skin reactions by allopurinol or hyperuricemia. J Clin Pharmacol 1981;21:456.
177. Friedman CI, Huneke AL, Kim MH et al. The effect of ampicillin on oral contraceptive effectiveness. Obstet Gynecol 1980;55:33.
178. Le Bel M, Paone RP, Lewis GP. Effect of ten new betalactam antibiotics on urine glucose test methods. Drug Intell Clin Pharm 1984;18:617.
179. Tindula RJ, Ambrose PJ, Harralson AF. Aminoglycoside inactivation by penicillins and cephalosporins and its impact on drug-level monitoring. Drug Intell Clin Pharm 1983;17:906.
180. Pickering LK, Rutherford I. Effect of concentrations and time upon inactivation of tobramycin, gentamicin, netilmicin and amikacin by azlocillin, carbenicillin, mecillinam, mezlocillin and piperacillin. J Pharmacol Exp Ther 1981; 217:345.
181. Blair DC, Duggan DO, Schroeder ET. Inactivation of amikacin and gentamicin by carbenicillin in patients with end-stage renal failure. Antimicrob Agents Chemother 1982; 22:376.
182. Bower BF, McComb R, Ruderman M. Effect of penicillin on urinary 17-ketogenic and 17-ketosteroid excretion. N Engl J Med 1967;277:530.
183. Hoigné R, Schoch K. Anaphylaktischer Schock und akute nichtallergische Reaktionen nach Procain-Penicillin. Schweiz Med Wochenschr 1959;89:1350.
184. Dry J, Leynadier F, Damecour C et al. Réaction pseudo-anaphylactique à la procaine-pénicilline G. Nouv Presse Méd 1976;22:1401.
185. Schmied C, Schmied E, Vogel J et al. Syndrome de

Hoigné ou réaction pseudo-anaphylactique à la procaine pénicilline G: un classique d'actualité. Schweiz Med Wochenschr 1990;120:1045.
186. Ernst G, Reuter E. Nicht-allergische tödliche Zwischenfälle nach Depot-Penicillin. Beitrag zur Pathogenese und Prophylaxe. Dtsch Med Wochenschr 1970;95:618.
187. Bornemann K, Schulz E, Heinecker R. Akute, nicht-allergische Reaktionen nach i.m. Gabe von Clemizol-Penicillin G und Streptomycin. Münch Med Wochenschr 1966; 108:834.
188. Bredt J. Akute nicht-allergische Reaktionen bei Anwendung von Depot-Penicillin. Dtsch Med Wochenschr 1965;90:1559.
189a. Galpin JE, Chow AW, Yoshikawa TT et al. 'Pseudo-anaphylactic' reactions from inadvertent infusion of procaine penicillin G. Ann Intern Med 1974;81:358.
189b. Kraus SJ, Green RL. Pseudoanaphylactic reactions with procaine penicillin. Cutis 1976;17:765.
190. Silber TJ, D'Angelo L. Psychosis and seizures following the injection of penicillin G procaine: Hoigné's syndrome. Am J Dis Child 1985;139:335.
191. Björnberg A, Selstam J. Acute psychotic reaction after injection of procaine penicillin. Acta Dermatol-Venereol 1957;37:50.
192. Utley PM, Lucas JB, Billings TE. Acute psychotic reactions to aqueous procaine penicillin. South Med J 1966; 59:1271.
193. Silber TJ, D'Angelo LJ. Panic attack following injection of aqueous procaine penicillin G (Hoigné syndrome). J Pediatr 1985;107:314.
194. Randazzo SD, Di Prima G. Psicosi allucinatoria acuta da penicillina-procaina in sospensione acquosa. Minerva Dermatol 1959;34:422.
195. Ilechukwu STC. Acute psychotic reactions and stress response syndromes following intramuscular aqueous procaine penicillin. Br J Psychiatry 1990;156:554.
196. Clauberg G. Wiederbelebung bei embolisch-toxischer Komplikation. Anaesthesist 1966;15:284.
197. Batchelor RCL, Horne GO, Rogerson HL. An unusual reaction to procaine penicillin in aqueous suspension. Lancet 1951;ii:195.
198. Lewis GW. Acute immediate reactions to penicillin. Br Med J 1957;1:1153.
199. Berger H, Juchinka H, Tomczyk D et al. Pseudo-anaphylactic syndrome after procaine penicillin in children. In: Abstracts, 10th Jubilee Congress. Bialystok: Polish Neurology Society, 1977;82.
200. Menke HE, Pepplinkhuizen L. Acute non-allergic reaction to aqueous procaine penicillin. Lancet 1974;ii:723.
201. Downham TF II, Cawley RA, Sailey SO et al. Systemic toxic reactions to procaine penicillin G. Sex Transm Dis 1978;5:4.
202. Green RL, Lewis JE, Kraus SJ et al. Elevated plasma procaine concentrations after administration of procaine penicillin G. N Engl J Med 1974;291:223.
203. Menke HE, Pepplinkhuizen L. Reaction to aqueous procaine penicillin G. Arch Dermatol 1973;108:856.
204. Albert M, Tiehle E. Erfahrungen mit Karditisrezidivprophylaxe im Erwachsenenalter. Wiss Z Friedrich-Schiller Univ Jena Math Naturwiss Reihe 1976;16:119.
205. Steigmann F, Suker JR. Fatal reactions to benzathine penicillin G. Report of three cases and discussion of contributory factors. J Am Med Assoc 1962;179:288.
206. Mozziconacci P, Nouaille J. Allergie à la pénicilline au cours de la prophylaxie continue du rhumatisme. Rev Fr Allergie 1965;5:302.
207. Gautier M, Fidelle J, Dagonet Y. La prophylaxie antistreptococcique dans la maladie de Bouillaud. Sem Hôp 1966;42:1513.
208. Dübi B, Wortman F, Wüthrich B et al. Unerwünschte Reaktionen auf die örtliche Anwendung von Lokalanästhetika, Antibiotika und Vasokonstriktoren im Bereich der Mundhöhle. Schweiz Monatschr Zahnheilkd 1973;83:543.
209. Von Hochstetter A. Ueber Probleme und Technik der intraglutäalen Injektion. I. Der Einfluss des Medikamentes und der Individualität des Patienten auf die Entstehung von Spritzenschäden. Schweiz Med Wochenschr 1955;85:1138.
210. Von Hochstetter A. Eine sichere Technik in der intramuskulären Injektion in den Oberschenkel: 'Laterale Vastus-Injektion'. Schweiz Med Wochenschr 1969;99:266.
211. Schanzer H, Gribetz I, Jaccobson JH. Accidental intra-arterial injection of penicillin G: a preventable catastrophe. J Am Med Assoc 1979;242:1289.
212. Vivell O, Hennewig J. Infarktähnliche Nekrosen nach intramuskulärer Injektion von Antibiotika. Pädiatr Prax 1963;2:415.
213. Friederiszick FK. Embolien während intramuskulärer Penicillinbehandlung. Klin Wochenschr 1949;27:173.
214. Talbert JL, Haslam RHA, Haller JA. Gangrene of the foot following intramuscular injection in the lateral thigh: a case report with recommendations for prevention. J Pediatr 1967;70:110.
215. Sengupta S. Gangrene following intra-arterial injection of procaine penicillin. Aust NZ J Med 1976;6:71.
216. Darby CP, Bradham G, Waller CE. Ischemia following an intragluteal injection of benzathine-procaine penicillin G mixture in a one-year-old boy. Clin Pediatr 1973;12:485.
217. Nicolau S. Dermite livédoide et gangréneuse de la fesse, consécutive aux injections intra-musculaires, dans la syphilis: à propos d'un cas d'embolie artérielle bismuthique. Ann Mal Vénér 1925;20:321.
218. Freudenthal W. Lokales embolisches Bismogenol-Exanthem. Arch Dermatol Syph (Berlin) 1924;147:155.
219. Deutsch J. Schwere lokale Reaktion nach Benzathin-Penizillin. Dtsch Gesundheitswes 1966;21:2433.
220. Gerbeaux J, Couvreur J, Lajouanine P et al. Sur deux cas d'ischémie étendue transitoire après injection intramusculaire de benzathine-pénicilline chez l'enfant. Presse Méd 1966;74:299.
221. Müller-Vahl H. Adverse reactions after intramuscular injection. Lancet 1983;i:1050.
222. Shaw EB. Transverse myelitis from injection of penicillin. Am J Dis Child 1966;111:548.
223. Ehringer H, Fischer M, Holzner JH et al. Gangrän nach versehentlicher intraaerterieller Injektion von Dicloxacillin. Dtsch Med Wochenschr 1971;96:1127.
224. Rubens E. Local hemorrhagic-necrotic skin reaction following penicillin. J Pediatr 1951;38:630.
225. Marie J, Lévêque B, Debauchez C et al. Accident hémorragique et nécrotique loco-régional à la suite d'une injection de benzathine-pénicilline. Sem Hôp. Paris 1964; 40:2517.
226. Kienitz Th, Braun-Falco O. Umschriebene Hautnekrosen nach intramuskulärer Injektion. Münch Med Wschr 1976;118:1515.
227. Stiehl P, Weissbach G, Schröter K. Das Nicolau-Syndrom: zur Pathogenese und Klinik arteriell-embolischer Penizillin-Zwischenfälle. Schweiz Med Wochenschr 1971; 101:377.

228. Blanc MH, Berthoud S, Rudhardt M et al. Pénicilline V et interactions médicamenteuse. Praxis 1973;62:861.
229. Nolan CM, Abernathy RS. Nephropathy associated with methicillin therapy. Arch Intern Med 1977;137:997.
230. Tilden SJ, Craft JC, Cano R et al. Cutaneous necrosis associated with intravenous nafcillin therapy. Am J Dis Child 1980;134:1046.
231. Koponen M, Pichler WJ, De Weck AL. T cell reactivity to penicillin: phenotypic analysis of in vitro activated cell subsets. J Allergy Clin Immunol 1986;78:645.
232. Baltzer B, Binderup E, Von Daehne W et al. Mutual pro-drugs of beta-lactam antibiotics and beta-lactamase inhibitors. J Antibiot 1980;33:1183.
233. Brodgen RN, Carmine A, Heel RC et al. Amoxycillin/clavulanic acid: a review of its antibacterial activity, pharmacokinetics and therapeutic use. Drugs 1981;22:337.
234. Stricker BHC, van den Broek JWG, Keuning J et al. Cholestatic hepatitis due to antibacterial combination of amoxicillin and clavulanic acid (Augmentin). Dig Dis Sci 1989;34:1576.
235. Hoffbrand BI, Stewart JDM. Carbenicillin and hypokalaemia. Br Med J 1970;4:746.
236. Stapleton FB, Nelson B, Vats TS et al. Hypokaelemia associated with antibiotic treatment. Am J Dis Child 1976;130:1104.
237. Cahn MM, Levy EJ. A study of the local reaction to intramuscular disodium carbenicillin (Geopen). Curr Ther Res 1972;14:573.
238. Cox CE. Pharmacology of carbenicillin indanyl sodium in renal insufficiency. J Infect Dis 1973;127(Suppl):S157.
239. Titanji R, Trofa A. Hypokalemia associated with ticarcillin-clavulanic acid. Md Med J 1993;42:1013.
240. Roselle GA, Bode R, Hamilton B et al. Clinical trial of the efficacy and safety of ticarcillin and clavulanic acid. Antimicrob Agents Chemother 1985;27:291.
241. Parry MF. The tolerance and safety of azlocillin. J Antimicrob Chemother 1983;11(Suppl B):223.
242. Winston DJ, Murphy W, Lowell SY et al. Piperacillin therapy for serious bacterial infections. Am J Med 1980; 69:255.
243. Gentry LO, Jemsek JG, Natelson EA. Effects of sodium piperacillin on platelet function in normal volunteers. Antimicrob Agents Chemother 1981;19:532.
244. Fass RJ, Copelan EA, Brandt JT et al. Platelet-mediated bleeding caused by broad-spectrum penicillins. J Infect Dis 1987;155:1242.

Meyler's Side Effects of Drugs, 13th Edition
M.N.G. Dukes, editor

SECTION EDITOR: R. HOIGNÉ

K.A. Neftel, A. Cerny and P. Cottagnoud

25.4 Cephalosporins

The cephalosporins represent a still-growing family of β-lactam antibiotics originally derived from the naturally occurring cephalosporin C. Isolation of the cephalosporin C nucleus, i.e. 7-aminocephalosporanic acid, made it possible to introduce new groups into this molecule to obtain ultimately the current variety of cephalosporin-structured compounds (1[R]). Actual cephalosporins vary widely in their antibacterial properties, β-lactamase stability and pharmacokinetic behavior, but there is no unequivocal classification so far (2[R]). For reasons more practical than biological, cephalosporins are often classified into first-, second-, third- and fourth-generation compounds (following their sequence of development), a fifth generation now being added.

Large multicenter reviews, which include several thousand patients each, have been published on all cephalosporins. They are generally congruent in many respects and will be mentioned here only exceptionally in reference to certain aspects. In view of the ever-growing literature we prefer to summarize selected information under more comprehensive headings, thus avoiding dealing with individual compounds in detail.

Various aspects of toxicity and hypersensitivity are common to both penicillins and cephalosporins. In so far as they are dealt with in Chapters 25.1—25.5, they will not be discussed further here.

ADVERSE REACTION PATTERN

Anaphylactic shock and other IgE-antibody-mediated reactions are rare but analogous to those experienced with the penicillins. Sufficiently reliable tests to predict or prove these reactions are still lacking for cephalosporins.

Other reactions paralleling those observed with penicillins include local reactions to parenteral application, epileptogenicity, effects on sodium and potassium balance, immune hemolytic anemia, neutropenia, thrombocytopenia and altered platelet function, acute interstitial nephritis, the majority of drug-inducible mucocutaneous manifestations and various combinations of symptoms often referred to as 'serum sickness-like reactions'.

More specifically associated with cephalosporins are: false-positive Coombs-tests (also seen with clavulanic acid and imipenem/cilastatin), impaired vitamin K-dependent clotting factor synthesis with cephalosporins containing the *N*-methylthiotetrazole side chain, biliary sludge formation with ceftriaxone, tubular nephrotoxicity of the older compounds, cefaloridine, cefaloglycine and cefalotin, and disulfiram-like interaction with alcohol.

ORGANS AND SYSTEMS

Cardiovascular Anaphylactic shock (see 'Hypersensitivity reactions' below and Chapters 25.1 and 25.2).

Thrombophlebitis is a common reaction to administration of cephalosporins into peripheral veins. Use of buffered solutions mitigated the reaction with cefalotin (3[C]). Published trials have mainly compared older cephalosporins, but the overall results are still contradictory (4[C], 5[R]). Pain and inflammatory reactions following intramuscular injection are also common. Ceftriaxone is probably given more often intramuscularly now than any other cephalosporin. Its local tolerability does not differ from that of other compounds (6[R]).

Respiratory Anaphylactic reactions (see 'Hypersensitivity reactions' below and Chapters 25.2 and 25.3).

Diffuse pulmonary inflammation as documented by gallium scanning in one case was possibly caused by ceftriaxone (7[c]). Recently cefotiam and in another case cefotiam followed by ceftazidime were suspected to be the cause of pulmonary hypersensitivity (8[c], 9[c]).

Nervous system In a rat model using intraventricular administration, marked differences in epileptogenic potential were found among 15 cephalosporins (10[CR]), and were recently confirmed with a total of 15 compounds (11[CR]). Compounds having two heterocyclic rings both at position 3 and position 7 of the cephalosporin molecule, e.g. ceftriaxone, cefoperazone, and ceftazidime, were even more epileptogenic than benzylpenicillin, while others having only one heterocyclic ring at position 7, e.g. cefotaxime and cefonicid, were less potent. Cefazolin, as a tetrazol derivative exhibiting similarity to the convulsant phenyltetrazol, was most potent.

Recent cases of neurotoxicity have been reported with cefazolin (after both intraventricular (12[c]) and systemic (13[c]—19[c]) application), cefotaxime (16[c]—18[c]) and ceftazidime (15[c]—20[c]). The latter also caused truncal asterixis (21[c]) as well as absence status and toxic hallucinations (22[c]). The least epileptogenic of 15 cephalosporins (11[CR]), namely cefonicid, was also reported to induce seizure (23[c]); the case however was disputed (24[c]). As expected, cases with systemic treatment were predominant in uremic patients and neurotoxicity has been associated with intraperitoneal ceftazidime therapy in a CAPD patient (25[c]). Of practical interest is a patient treated with intravenous cefmetazole in whom the CSF-level was found to be twice as high as the corresponding blood level (236 μg/ml versus 103 μg/ml) (26[c]). Uremia may have contributed to this unusual distribution pattern.

Hematological Immune hemolytic anemia has rarely been reported with the older cephalosporins, cefalotin (27[c]—29[c]), cefazolin (29[c]), cefalexin (30[c]), and cefaloridine (31[c]). The main laboratory findings correspond to the 'drug adsorption' mechanism classically found in benzylpenicillin-induced immune hemolysis. Antibodies cross-reacting with cefalotin and benzylpenicillin were found in both benzylpenicillin- and cefalotin-induced hemolysis (29[c], 32[c]). More recently new cases were reported with cefamandole (33[c]), cefalexin (34[c]), ceftriaxone (35[c]), cefotaxime (36[c], 37[c]), cefotetan (38[c], 39[c]) and ceftazidime (40[c]).

In addition to the so-called 'drug-adsorption' mechanism, findings were in some instances consistent with formation of concomitant auto-antibodies (38[c]) or the so called 'innocent bystander' mechanism, leading to acute intravascular hemolysis, one with ceftriaxone being fatal (35[c]).

Cefalotin and other cephalosporins can cause positive direct antiglobulin tests (DAT) (41[C], 42[R]). This phenomenon is due to unspecific serum protein adsorption on to the erythrocyte membrane and is not related to immune hemolytic processes. Detection of non-immunologically bound serum proteins is improved if DAT reagents include additional anti-albumin activity (43[R]). The phenomenon is a known source of difficulties in evaluating suspected immune hemolysis or routine cross-matching of blood products (44[C]). The true frequency with many individual cephalosporins remains unclear, since it has not been positively sought.

Virtually all cephalosporins can induce neutropenia up to agranulocytosis (45[C]). Additional cases have been reported in the last few years associated with ceftriaxone (46[c]—48[c]), cefmenoxime (49[c]), moxalactam (50[c]), cefapirin (51[C]), and cefmetazole (52[c]) among others. All of these cases were seen after high cumulative doses given in one treatment course. In one series cefapirin-induced neutropenia occurred in five out of 19 patients receiving a total of 90 grams or more but not in 113 patients receiving smaller cumulative cefapirin doses (51[C]). It remains unsettled whether toxic or immunological mechanisms are involved and how both principal ways could perhaps act in concert (see also Chapter 25.2 'Dose-dependent reactions').

Only three cases of thrombocytopenia have previously been reported, all associated with cefalotin (53[c]—55[c]). In one of them drug-dependent antibodies were detected. In two recent cases the role of drug-dependent antibodies was further evaluated. In one case the antibodies only reacted with platelets in the presence of exogenous cefotetan, but not with cefotetan-coated platelets (56[c]). In another cefamandole-induced case, antibodies cross-reacted with two cephalosporins which also had a thiomethyltetrazole group at position 3 but not with others (57[c]). In about one-third of cases with cephalosporin-induced neutropenia, slight concomitant thrombocytopenia has been found (45[C]).

Bleeding disorders As with other β-lactam antibiotics, treatment with cephalosporins can result in impaired hemostasis and clinical bleeding by alterations of (1) coagulation and (2) platelet function. For details see Chapter 25.2.

Liver As with all β-lactam antibiotics, slight increases in serum transaminases and alkaline phosphatase have been reported with cephalosporins. In contrast to the isoxazolylpenicillins and the amoxicillin/clavulanate combination, only very sporadic cases with more severe liver disease have occurred (58[R], 59[c], 60[c]).

Ceftriaxone-associated biliary complications Ceftriaxone has been associated with mostly asymptomatic and reversible biliary sludge. The condition is defined by the presence of low amplitude echoes with absent post-acoustic shadows in the gallbladder in ultrasonographic examination and has also been called 'biliary pseudolithiasis' (61[C]). Findings consistent with the presence of cholelithiasis (high amplitude echoes with acoustic shadowing) have also been reported (62[C]).

The frequency of occurrence of biliary sludge in children was 40% in a series of 37 children treated for serious infections and seems to be lower in adults (about 20%) (61[C], 63[C], 64[C]). The condition usually runs a benign course and ultrasounds become normal after discontinuation of ceftriaxone administration in a mean of 15 days (61[C]). Clinical signs of cholecystitis have however been reported (65[C]). The occurrence of at least partly reversible gallstones containing mostly ceftriaxone have been described (66[C]). In a recent case-control study of patients treated with ceftriaxone for Lyme disease, more serious biliary complications (cholecystitis, cholelithiasis and cholecystectomy) were observed in 2%. An age of >18 years as well as female sex were risk factors for the development of biliary complications (67[C]).

Ceftriaxone treatment does not seem to predispose to subsequent gallbladder stone formation as assessed 6 and 12 months later (68[C]). The pathogenesis of the phenomenon relates to the drug's high rate of biliary excretion and subsequent formation of calcium-containing precipitates (69[C]). Thus, apart from the risk factors mentioned, the risk of biliary sludge may increase with the use of high doses, rapid bolus injection, gall bladder stasis, as well as renal failure associated with enhanced biliary excretion. Routine ultrasound scans are not required in patients treated with ceftriaxone. In the presence of clinical symptoms possibly related to ceftriaxone-associated sludge or cholelithiasis, confirmed by ultrasonography, the drug should be stopped. Surgery is mostly unnecessary.

Gastrointestinal (*see also Chapter* 25.2) Cefotetan-induced singultus recurred after each cefotetan infusion and disappeared immediately after discontinuation. Singultus recurred after re-administration of cefotetan but not of another antibiotic (70[c]).

Urinary system Two of the older cephalosporins, namely cefaloridine and cefalotin are nephrotoxic and have induced renal dysfunction in a substantial number of cases (71[R], 72[R]). Nephrotoxicity of cefaloridine is related to its unusual renal transport resulting in higher intracellular concentrations in the proximal tubular cells than with other cephalosporins (5[R]). With less toxic cephalosporins available, the clinical use of cefaloridine is no longer justified. Cefalotin can induce two types of renal disease in man (72[R]): the first is acute tubular necrosis, apparently similar to that seen with cefaloridine, although less frequently observed. The second is acute interstitial nephritis and is often accompanied by a rash, fever or eosinophilia resembling the same disorder induced by meticillin (see Chapters 25.2 and 25.3). A somewhat different tubular toxicity has been described with cefaloglycin (5[R]). In animals, cefazolin has been reported to be the second most nephrotoxic cephalosporin and to induce similar lesions as cefaloridine (5[R], 73[C]). A clear correlate to this, however, is unknown in man.

It has been proposed that, although in much higher doses or concentrations, basically all cephalosporins may cause nephrotoxicity corresponding either to the cefaloridine type or the cefaloglycin type (5[R]). Broad clinical use, however, of second- and third-generation cephalosporins has not produced clear evidence for a significant nephrotoxic potential. In two groups of 10 and 17 patients treated with 3 and 4 grams each of ceftazidime a day, decreases in glomerular filtration rate of about 10 ml/min were seen after treatment courses of 4—9 days or 7—31 days, respectively (74[C], 75[C]). For many other cephalosporins comparable data are lacking. Furthermore, an increase of aminoglycoside nephrotoxicity can only be documented for cefalotin and cefaloridine when used in combination (71[R], 76[R]). Nevertheless, adjustment of cephalosporin dosages in cases with renal insufficiency is justified and acute tubular necrosis may indeed occur with very high doses of cephalosporins other than cefaloridine and cefalotin (77[c]). Recently isolated cases of acute interstitial nephritis have been related to cefaclor (78[c]), cefoxitin (79[c]), cefamandole (80[c]), cefotetan (81[c]), cefuroxim (82[c]) and ceftriaxone (83[c]). Ceftriaxone, on the other hand, has proved to protect against tobramycin nephrotoxicity in rats (84[c]). In addition to biliary sludge and stone formation with ceftriaxone occasional patients developing urinary stones have been described (85[C], 86[C]).

Skin and appendages (*see also Chapter* 25.2) More recently generalized pustular eruptions—very rarely seen with other drugs so far (87[C])—have repeatedly been reported with cefazolin (88[c], 89[c]), cefradine (90a[c]), cefalexin (90b[c]) and cefaclor (91[c]). Skin biopsies showed subcorneal pustules with neutrophiles and leukocytoclastic vasculitis.

Cefaclor treatment was the common denominator in three pediatric cases presenting at one institution (92[C]). All had intraoral ulcers covered with a thick pseudomembrane together with various skin lesions, suggesting viral diseases at first sight.

Isolated cases of the following syndromes have been reported more recently in connection with cephalosporins: pemphigus vulgaris with cefadroxil (93[c]) and cefalexin (94[c]); erythema multiforme with cefotaxime (95[c]); adult linear IgA disease associated with an erythema multiforme-like reaction with cefamandole (96[c]); Stevens-Johnson-syndrome with cefalexin (97[c]); toxic epidermal necrolysis ('Lyell's syndrome') with cefsulodin (98[c]) and cefazolin (99[c]); a photo-recall-like phenomenon, with cefazolin (100[c]); photosensitivity due to ambulatory intravenous ceftazedim in a cystic fibrosis patient (101[c]) and a fixed drug eruption presenting as an acute paranychea with cefalexin (102[c]).

Serum sickness-like syndromes Skin manifestations and arthralgia/arthritis along with fever, eosinophilia or some other symptoms are frequently referred to as 'serum sickness-like syndromes' (see also Chapter 25.2). True serum sickness is classically the consequence of an interaction of specific antibodies with foreign proteins. The majority of cephalosporins has sporadically been reported to induce reactions closely resembling classical serum sickness, but there is no clear evidence, so far, for drug-specific antibodies generating those reactions and the outcome has always been benign. Earlier suspicions that cefaclor carries an excess risk of 'serum sickness-like syndromes' (103[C]) have subsequently been confirmed (104[C]–109[C]). It still remains open whether cefaclor-associated 'serum sickness-like reactions' correspond to true hypersensitivity. It has indeed been suggested that they may result from inherited defects in the metabolism of reactive intermediates and may be a unique adverse reaction that requires biotransformation of the parent drug (110[C]). However, comparable syndromes were seen with other cephalosporins (111[c], 112[c]) and especially in the majority of a series of volunteers treated for up to 4 weeks with high doses of cefalotin and cefapirin (113[C]).

Hypersensitivity reactions Immediate hypersensitivity reactions, mediated through IgE antibodies to cephalosporin determinants are a major factor limiting their use. Early cases of anaphylaxis to cephalosporins were probably due to a contamination with trace amounts of penicillin (114[R]). These studies may thus over-report cross-sensitivity.

A retrospective study reported a frequency of systemic anaphylaxis to cephaloridine, cefalotin and cephalexin of two out of 9388 patients (0.02%) without a history of penicillin allergy (115[R]). Both patients received cefalotin (2/1983). The incidence of systemic anaphylaxis (to cephaloridine, cefalotin and cephalexin) was two out of 450 patients (0.4%) with a history of penicillin allergy.

Solley et al. prospectively evaluated 178 patients (116[C]). Of these, 151 patients had a history of penicillin allergy but were negative on penicillin skin testing. Two had reactions upon treatment with a cephalosporin. Twenty-seven had a positive penicillin skin test but did not react after cephalosporin administration. Similar results were found by others (117[C]).

A history of penicillin allergy, however, is often vague and numerous studies have suggested that it is an unreliable indicator as confirmed recently (118[C]). Saxon et al. treated 62 penicillin skin test-positive patients with cephalosporins and observed only one reaction of 'mild urticaria and bronchospasm' (119[C]).

An accurate molecular definition of cephalosporin allergy is not available at this time. Relevant determinants for cephalosporin-induced anaphylaxis may not reside in the bicyclic core but rather in the side chain structure (120[C], 121[R]). Neither currently available in vitro tests nor skin tests can reliably predict cephalosporin allergy (122[R]). The true frequency of clinical allergic reactions in penicillin-allergic patients exposed to cephalosporins has been estimated to be 1 or 2% (123[C]). Nevertheless, in the presence of a history of penicillin anaphylaxis or other severe IgE-mediated reaction it seems wise to avoid the use of a cephalosporin.

Primary cephalosporin allergy in patients not allergic to penicillin has been reported, but the exact frequency is not clear (124[R], 125[R]). The true incidence of allergic reactions may differ within the group of cephalosporins. Several reports implicating particular compounds have been published (126[C]–130[C]).

Loracarbef is a newly introduced β-lactam belonging to the carbacephem group. Its structure resembles cefaclor, a first generation cephalosporin, except for the presence of a methylene group instead of the sulfur atom in the dihydrothiazine ring forming the tetrahydropyridine compound. Until more clinical data is available it seems prudent to avoid using this compound in β-lactam-allergic subjects.

Risk situations Penicillin hypersensitivity see 'Hypersensitivity reactions' above.

Renal insufficiency, in particular deterioration of renal function during ongoing treatment (see Chapter 25.2 'Dose-dependent reactions' and 'Nervous system').

Second-generation effects Sporadic reports on findings in cell culture (131[C]) or animals (132[C]) have pointed to potential second-generation effects of cephalosporin; however, no such effects are known in man.

Interactions Alcohol intolerance manifesting with reactions as produced by disulfiram is well known under treatment with cephalosporins containing the methyltetrazole side chain on position 3 of the cephalosporin nucleus, i.e. cefamandol, cefoperazone, cefmethazole, cefmenoxime and moxalactam (133[R]). Cefotiam, ceforanide and cefonizid, having a substituted methylthiotetrazole side chain, can also cause the reaction (134[C]). Ceftriaxone, with a different side chain at position 3, has nevertheless been reported to induce a disulfiram-like reaction, possibly by structural analogy (6[R]). The structural requirements for a cephalosporin to induce the reaction have been reviewed (135[R]). Alcohol intolerance requires some time to build up after starting cephalosporin treatment and alcohol ingestion before the first cephalosporin administration has not been reported to cause a reaction (136[C]).

In parallel to penicillins, probenecid interferes with the renal excretion of many cephalosporins (137[R]).

An unexpectedly high frequency of side effects has

been observed in a pediatric intensive care unit with the combination of high-dose phenobarbital and β-lactam antibiotics (138[C]). Most reactions included exanthematic skin manifestations, and cephalosporin treatment in most cases was with cefotaxime. The impact of these observations, encompassing 24 out of a total of 49 children, is unclear and has not been confirmed so far.

In contrast to, e.g. nafcillin, ceftriaxone may increase ciclosporin blood levels (139[c]). Ceftazidime was found to form microprecipitations when mixed together with vancomycin, e.g. for intravitreal injection (140[c]). Verapamil toxicity was possibly precipitated by intravenous administration of ceftriaxone together with clindamycin, the high affinity to serum proteins of these drugs being a presumable explanation (141[c]).

Interference with diagnostic routines Cephalosporins may interfere with the Jaffé-technic for analysis of creatinine resulting in falsely elevated values (142[C]). False positive tests for glucosuria may result with reduction technics, but not with enzymatic tests (143[C]).

REFERENCES

1. Abraham EP. Cephalosporins 1945—1986. Drugs 1987;34(Suppl 2):1.
2. Williams JD. Classification of cephalosporins. Drugs 1987;34(Suppl 2):15.
3. Berger S, Ernst EC, Barza M. Comparative incidence of phlebitis due to buffered cephalotin, cephapirin, and cefamandole. Antimicrob Agents Chemother 1976;9:575.
4. Cole DR. Double-blind comparison of phlebitis associated with cefazolin and cephalothin. Int J Clin Pharmacol 1976;14:75.
5. Browning MC, Tune BM. Toxicology of betalactam antibiotics. In: Demain AL, Solomon NA, eds. Antibiotics, Containing the Betalactam Structure, Part II. Berlin: Springer-Verlag, 1983;371.
6. Moskovitz BL. Clinical adverse effects during ceftriaxone therapy. Am J Med 1984;7:84.
7. Krasnow AZ, McNamara M, Akhtar R et al. Cephalosporin-induced diffuse pulmonary inflammation depicted by Ga-67 scintigraphy. Clin Nucl Med 1989;14:379.
8. Irie M, Teshima H, Matsuura T et al. Pulmonary infiltration with eosinophilia possibly induced by cefotiam in a case of steroid-dependent asthma. Nippon Kyobu Shikkan Gakkai Zasshi 1990;28:1353.
9. Suzuki K, Inagaki T, Adachi S et al. A case of ceftazidime-induced pneumonitis. Nippon Kyobu Shikkan Gakkai Zasshi 1993;31:512.
10. De Sarro A, De Sarro GB, Ascioti C et al. Epileptogenic activity of some betalactam derivatives: structure—activity relationship. Neuropharmacology 1989;28:359.
11. De Sarro A, Ammendola D, Zappala M et al. Relationship between structure and convulsant properties of some β-lactam antibiotics following intracerebroventricular microinjection in rats. Antimicrob Agents Chemother 1995;1:232.
12. Manzella JP, Ronald LP, Butler IL. CNS toxicity associated with intraventricular injection of cefazolin. J Neurosurg 1988;68:970.
13. Herd AM, Ross CA, Bhattacharya SK. Acute confusional state with postoperative intravenous cefazolin. Br Med J 1989;299:393.
14. Josse S, Godin M, Fillastre JP. Cefazolin-induced encephalopathy in a uraemic patient. Nephron 1987;45:72.
15. Geyer J, Höffler D, Demers HG et al. Cephalosporin-induced encephalopathy in uremic patients. Nephron 1988; 48:237.
16. Vincent JP, Dervanian P, Bodak A. Encéphalopathie sous céfotaxime Une observation chez un sujet âgé insuffisant rénal. Ann Méd Intern 1989;332.
17. Pascual J, Liaño F, Ortuño J. Cefotaxime-induced encephalopathy in an uremic patient. Nephron 1990;54:92.
18. Wroe SJ, Ellershaw JE, Whittaker JA et al. Focal motor status epilepticus following treatment with azlocillin and cefotaxime. Med Toxicol 1987;2:233.
19. Douglas MA, Quandt CM, Stanley DA et al. Ceftazidime-induced encephalopathy in a patient with renal impairment. Arch Neurol 1988;45:936.
20. Höffler D, Demers HG, Niemeyer R. Neurotoxizität moderner Cefalosporine. Dtsch Med Wochenschr 1986; 5:197.
21. Hillsley RE, Massey EW. Truncal asterixis associated with ceftazidime, a third-generation cephalosporin. Neurology 1991;41:2008.
22. Jackson G, Berkovic SF. Ceftazidime encephalopathy: absence status and toxic hallucinations (letter). J Neurol Neurosurg Psychiatry 1992;56:333.
23. Tse CST, Madura AJ, Vera FH. Suspected cefonicid-induced seizure. Clin Pharm 1986;5:629.
24. Higbee M, Ramsey RA. Cefonicid-induced seizure. Clin Pharm 1987;6:271.
25. Lye WC, Leong SO. Neurotoxicity associated with intraperitoneal ceftazidime therapy in a CAPD patient (4). Perit Dial Int 1994;14:408.
26. Uchihara T, Tsukagoshi H. Myoclonic activity associated with cefmetazole, with a review of neurotoxicity of cephalosporins. Clin Neurol Neurosurg 1988;90:369.
27. Gralnick HR, MacGinniss M, Elton W et al. Hemolytic anemia associated with cephalorin. J Am Med Assoc 1971;217:1193.
28. Jeannet M, Block A, Dayer JM et al. Cephalotin-induced immune hemolytic anemia. Acta Haematol 1976;55:109.
29. Moake JL, Butler CF, Hewell GM et al. Hemolysis induced by cefazolin and cephalotin in a patient with penicillin sensitivity. Transfusion 1977;18:369.
30. Forbes CD, Craig JA, Mitchell R et al. Acute intravascular hemolysis, associated with cephalexin therapy. Postgrad Med J 1972;48:186.
31. Kaplan K, Reisberg B, Weinstein L. Cephaloridine studies of therapeutic activity and untoward effects. Arch Intern Med 1968;121:17.

32. Nesmith LW, Davis JW. Hemolytic anemia caused by penicillin. Report of a case in which antipenicillin antibodies cross-reacted with cephalotin sodium. J Am Med Assoc 1968;203:27.
33. Branch DR, Berkowitz LK, Becker RL et al. Extravascular hemolysis following the administration of cefamandole. Am J Hematol 1985;18:213.
34. Manoharan A, Kot T. Cephalexin-induced haemolytic anaemia. Med J Aust 1987;147:202.
35. Garratty G, Postoway N, Schwellenbach J, McMahill PC. A fatal case of ceftriaxone (Rocephin)-induced hemolytic anemia associated with intravascular immune hemolysis. Transfusion 1991;31:176.
36. Shulman IA, Arndt PA, McGehee W et al. Cefotaxime-induced immune hemolytic anemia due to antibodies reacting in vitro by more than one mechanism. Transfusion 1990; 30:263.
37. Salama A, Göttsche B, Schleiffer T et al. 'Immune complex' mediated intravascular hemolysis due to IgM cephalosporin-dependent antibody. Transfusion 1987;27:460.
38. Chenoweth CE, Judd WJ, Steiner EA, Kauffman CA. Cefotetan-induced immune hemolytic anemia. Clin Infect Dis 1992;15:863.
39. Eckrich RJ, Fox S, Mallory D. Cefotetan-induced immune hemolytic anemia due to the drug-adsorption mechanism. Immunohematology 1994;10/2:51.
40. Chambers LA, Donovan LM, Kruskall MS. Ceftazidime-induced hemolysis in a patient with drug-dependent antibodies reactive by immune complex and drug adsorption mechanisms. Am J Clin Pathol 1991;95:393.
41. Molthan L, Reidenberg MM, Eichmann MF. Positive direct Coombs tests due to cephalotin. N Engl J Med 1967;277:123.
42. Garratty G. Review: Immune hemolytic anemia and/or positive direct antiglobulin tests caused by drugs. Immunohematology 1994;10/2:41.
43. Petz LD, Garratty G. Acquired Immune Hemolytic Anemias. New York: Churchill Livingstone, 1980.
44. Williams ME, Thomas D, Harman CP et al. Positive direct antiglobulin tests due to clavulanic acid. Antimicrob Agents Chemother 1985;27:125.
45. Neftel K, Hauser S, Müller M. Inhibition of granulopoiesis in vivo and vitro by betalactam antibiotics. J Infect Dis 1985;152:90.
46. Rey D, Martin T, Albert A et al. Ceftriaxone-induced granulopenia related to a peculiar mechanism of granulopoiesis inhibition. Am J Med 1989;87:591.
47. Baciewicz AM, Skiest DJ, Weinshel EL. Ceftriaxone-associated neutropenia. Drug Intell Clin Pharm 1988;22:826.
48. Beq-Giraudon B, Cazenave F, Breux J-Ph. Agranulocytose aiguë réversible au cours d'un traitement par la ceftriaxone. Pathol Biol 1986;34:534.
49. Lucht F, Guy C, Perrot JL et al. Agranulocytose à la cefménoxime. Thérapie 1988;43:506.
50. Miyano T, Kawauchi K, Suto Y et al. Latamoxef-induced agranulocytosis—direct inhibition of CFU-C by in vitro colony assay. Jpn. J Clin Hematol 1988;29:174.
51. Pan CV, Quintela AG, Garcia JR et al. Cephapirin-induced neutropenia. Chemotherapy 1989;35:449.
52. Sugimoto M, Saito K, Hashimoto et al. Antibiotic-induced agranulocytosis. Patient's IgG inhibits a GM colony formation. Jpn J Clin Hematol 1989;30:768.
53. Gralnick HR, McGinnis M, Hatterman R. Thrombocytopenia with sodium cephalothin therapy. Ann Intern Med 1972;77:401.
54. Sheiman L, Spielvogel AR, Horowitz HI. Thrombocytopenia caused by cephalothin sodium. J Am Med Assoc 1968;203:159.
55. Naraqi S, Raiser M. Nonrecurrence of cephalothin-associated granulocytopenia and thrombocytopenia. J Infect Dis 1982;145:281.
56. Christie DJ, Lennon SS, Drew RL et al. Cefotetan-induced immunologic thrombocytopenia. Br J Haematol 1988;70:423.
57. Lown J, Barr A. Immune thrombocytopenia induced by cephalosporins specific for thiomethyltetrazole side chain. J Clin Pathol 1987;40:700.
58. Horsmans Y, Larrey D, Pessayre D et al. Hépatotoxicité des médicaments anti-infectieux. Gastroentérol Clin Biol 1990;14:911.
59. Ammann R, Neftel K, Hardmeier T et al. Cephalosporin-induced cholestatic jaundice. Lancet 1982;ii:336.
60. Kojima N, Kumamoto I, Masumoto T, Onji M. A case report of drug-induced allergic hepatitis probably due to the *N*-methyltetrazolethiol group cephalosporin. Arerugi 1994; 43:511.
61. Schaad UB, Wedgwood-Krucko J, Tschaeppeler H. Reversible ceftriaxone-associated biliary pseudolithiasis in children. Lancet 1988;ii:1411.
62. Sahni PS, Patel PJ, Kolawole TM et al. Ultrasound of ceftriaxone-associated reversible cholelithiasis. Eur J Radiol 1994;18:142.
63. Heim-Duthoy KL, Caperton EM, Pollok R et al. Apparent biliary pseudolithiasis during ceftriaxone therapy. Antimicrob Agents Chemother 1990;34:1146.
64. Pigrau C, Pahissa A, Gropper S et al. Ceftriaxone-associated pseudolithiasis in adults. Lancet 1989;ii:165.
65. Jacobs RF. Ceftriaxone-associated cholecystitis. Pediatr Infect Dis J 1988;7:434.
66. Lopez AJ, O'Keefe P, Morrissey M, Pickleman J. Cefriaxone-induced cholelithiasis. Ann Intern Med 1991;115:712.
67. Genese C, Finelli L, Parkin W, Spitalny KC. Ceftriaxone-associated biliary complications of treatment of suspected disseminated lyme disease. J Am Med Assoc 1993;269:979.
68. Cometta A, Gallot-Lavallée-Villars S, Iten A et al. Incidence of gallbladder lithiasis after ceftriaxone treatment. J Antimicrob Chemother 1990;25:689.
69. Shiffman ML, Keith FB, Moore EW. Pathogenesis of ceftriaxone-associated biliary sludge. Gastroenterology 1990; 99:1772.
70. Morris JT, McAllister CK. Cefotetan-induced singultus. Ann Intern Med 1992;116:522.
71. Zhanel GG. Cephalosporin-induced nephrotoxicity: does it exist? Drug Intell Clin Pharm 1990;24:262.
72. Foord RD. Cephaloridine, cephalothin and the kidney. J Antimicrob Chemother 1975;1(Suppl):119.
73. Silverblatt F, Harrison WO, Turck M. Nephrotoxicity of cephalosporin antibiotics in experimental animals. J Infect Dis 1973;182(Suppl):367.
74. Norrby SR, Burman LA, Linderholm H et al. Ceftazidime: pharmacokinetics in patients and effects on the renal function. J Antimicrob Chemother 1982;10:199.
75. Alestig K, Trollfors B, Anderson R et al. Ceftazidime and renal function. J Antimicrob Chemother 1984;13:177.
76. Rankin GO, Sutherland CH. Nephrotoxicity of aminoglycosides and cephalosporins in combination. Adverse Drug React Acute Poison Rev 1989;8:73.
77. Lentnek AL, Rosenworcel E, Kidd L. Acute tubular

necrosis following high-dose cefamandole therapy for Haemophilus parainfluenzae endocarditis. Am J Med Sci 1981;281:164.
78. Pommer W, Krause PH, Berg PA et al. Acute interstitial nephritis and non-oliguric renal failure after cefaclor treatment. Klin Wochenschr 1986;64:290.
79. Toll LL, Lee M, Sharifi R. Cefoxitin-induced interstitial nephritis. South Med J 1987;80:274.
80. Csanyi P, Rado JP, Hormay M. Acute renal failure due to cephamandole. Br Med J 1988;296:433.
81. Nguyen VD, Nagelberg H, Agarwal BN. Acute interstitial nephritis associated with cefotetan therapy. Am J Kidney Dis 1990;16:259.
82. Goddard JK, Janning SW, Gass JS, Wilson RF. Cefuroxime-induced acute renal failure. Pharmacotherapy 1994; 14:488.
83. Mancini S, Iacovoni R, Fierimonte V et al. Drug induced interstitial nephritis. A case report. Minerva Pediatr 1994; 46:557.
84. Beauchamp D, Thériault G, Grenier L et al. Ceftriaxone protects against tobramycin nephrotoxicity. Antimicrob Agents Chemother 1994;38:750.
85. Schaad UB, Suter S, Gianella-Borradori A, P et al. A comparison of ceftriaxone and cefuroxime for the treatment of bacterial meningitis in children. N Engl J Med 1990; 322:141.
86. Cochat P, Cochat N, Jouvenet M et al. Ceftriaxone-associated nephrolithiasis. Nephrol Dial Transplant 1990; 5:974.
87. MacMillan AL. Generalized pustular drug rash. Dermatologica 1973;146:285.
88. Stough D, Guin JD, Baker GF et al. Pustular eruptions following administration of cefazolin: a possible interaction with methyldopa. J Am Acad Dermatol 1987;16:1051.
89. Fayol J, Bonnetblanc JM. Pustular eruption following administration of cefazolin: a second case report. J Am Acad Dermatol 1988;19:571.
90a. Kalb RE, Grossman ME. Pustular eruption following administration of cephradine. Cutis 1986;38:58.
90b. Jackson H, Vion B, Levy PM. Generalized eruptive pustular drug rash due to cephalexin. Dermatologica 1988; 177:292.
91. Ogoshi M, Yamada Y, Tani M. Acute generalized exanthematic pustulosis induced by cefaclor and acetazolamide. Case report. Dermatology 1992;184:142.
92. Blignaut E. Cefaclor associated with intra-oral ulceration. South Afr Med J 1990;77:426.
93. Wilson JP, Koren JF, Daniel RC et al. Cefadroxil induced ampicillin-exacerbated pemphigus vulgaris: case report and review of the literature. Drug Intell Clin Pharm 1986;20:219.
94. Wolf R, Dechner E, Ophir J et al. Cephalexin: a nonthiol drug that may induce pemphigus vulgaris. Int J Dermatol 1991;30:213.
95. Green ST, Natarajan S, Campbell JC. Erythema multiforme following cefotaxime therapy. Postgrad Med J 1986; 62:415.
96. Argenyi ZB, Bergfeld WF, Valenzuela R et al. Adult linear IgA disease associated with an erythema multiforme-like drug reaction. Cleveland Clin J Med 1987;54:445.
97. Murray KM, Camp MS. Cephalexin-induced Stevens-Johnson syndrome. Ann Pharmacother 1992;26:1230.
98. Okano M, Kitano Y, Ohzono K. Toxic epidermal necrolysis due to cephem. Int J Dermatol 1988;27:183.
99. Julsrud ME. Toxic epidermal necrolysis. J Foot-Ankle Surg 1994;33:255.
100. Flax SH, Uhle P. Photo recall-like phenomenon following the use of cefazolin and gentamicin sulfate. Cutis 1990;46:59.
101. Vinks SATMM, Heijerman HGM, de Jonge P, Bakker W. Photosensitivity due to ambulatory intravenous ceftazidime in cystic fibrosis patient. Lancet 1993;341:1221.
102. Baran R, Perrin C. Fixed-drug eruption presenting as an acute paronychia. Br J Dermatol 1991;125:592.
103. Murray DL, Singer DA, Singer AB et al. Cefaclor a cluster of adverse reactions (Letter to Editor). N Engl J Med 1980;303:1003.
104. Platt R, Dreis MW, Kennedy DL et al. Serum sickness-like reactions to amoxicillin, cefaclor, cephalexin, and trimethoprim-sulfamethoxazole. J Infect Dis 1988;158:474.
105. Heckbert SR, Stryker WS, Coltin KL et al. Serum sickness in children after antibiotic exposure: estimates of occurrence and morbidity in a health maintenance organization population. Am J Epidemiol 1990;132:336.
106. Stricker BH, Tijssen JG. Serum sickness-like reactions to cefaclor. J Clin Epidemiol 1992;45:1177.
107. Vial T, Pont J, Pham E et al. Cefaclor-associated serum sickness-like disease: eight cases and review of the literature. Ann Pharmacother 1992;26:910.
108. Hebert AA, Sigman ES, Levy ML. Serum sickness-like reactions from cefaclor in children. J Am Acad Dermatol 1991;25:805.
109. Parra FM, Igea JM, Martin JA et al. Serum sickness-like syndrome associated with cefaclor therapy. Allergy 1992;47:439.
110. Kearns GL, Wheeler JG, Childress SH et al. Serum sickness-like reactions to cefaclor: role of hepatic metabolism and individual susceptibility. J Pediatr 1994;125:805.
111. Lowery N, Kearns GL, Young RA, Wheeler JG. Serum sickness-like reactions associated with cefprozil therapy. J Pediatr 1994;125:325.
112. Plantin P, Milochau P, Dubois D. Drug induced serum sickness after ingestion of cefatrizine. First reported case (letter). Presse Med 1992;21:1915.
113. Sanders WW, Johnson JE, Taggart JG. Adverse reactions to cephalotin and cephapirin. N Engl J Med 1974; 290:424.
114. Pedersen-Ejergaard J. Cephalotin in the treatment of penicillin-sensitive patients. Acta Allergol 1967;22:299.
115. Petz LD. Immunologic reactions of humans to cephalosporins. Postgrad Med J 1971;47(Suppl):64.
116. Solley GO, Gleich GJ, Van Dellen RG. Penicillin allergy: clinical experience with a battery of skin-test reagents. J Allergy Clin Immunol 1982;69:238.
117. Van Arsdel PP Jr, Miller S. Antimicrobial treatment of patients with a penicillin allergy history. J Allergy Clin Immunol 1990;85:188.
118. Surtees SJ, Stockton MG, Gietzen TW. Allergy to penicillin: fable or fact? Br Med J 1991;302:1051.
119. Saxon A, Beall GN, Rohr AS et al. Immediate hypersensitivity reactions to beta-lactam antibiotics (clinical conference). Ann Intern Med 1987;107:204.
120. Blanca M, Fernandez J, Miranda A et al. Crossreactivity between penicillin and cephalosporins: clinical and immunologic studies. J Allergy Clin Immunol 1989;83:381.
121. Anderson JA. Cross-sensitivity to cephalosporins in patients allergic to penicillin. Pediatr Infect Dis 1986;5:557.
122. Saxon A, Beall GN, Rohr AS et al. Immediate hyper-

sensitivity reactions to beta-lactam antibiotics. Urology 1988;31(Suppl):14.
123. Saxon A. Antibiotic choices for the penicillin-allergic patient. Postgrad Med J 1988;83:135.
124. Abraham GN, Petz LD, Fudenberg HH. Cephalothin hypersensitivity associated with anti-cephalothin antibodies. Int Arch Allergy 1968;34:65.
125. Ong R, Sullivan T. Detection and characterization of human IgE to cephalosporin determinants (Abstract). J Allergy Clin Immunol 1988;81:222.
126. Nishioka K, Katayama I, Kobayashi Y et al. Anaphylaxis due to cefaclor hypersensitivity. J Dermatol 1986; 13:226.
127. Hama R, Mori K. High incidence of anaphylactic reactions to cefaclor (Letter to Editor). Lancet 1988;i:1331.
128. Levine LR. Quantitative comparison of adverse reactions to cefaclor vs amoxycillin in a surveillance study. Pediatr Infect Dis 1985;4:358.
129. Bloomberg RJ. Cefotetan-induced anaphylaxis. Am J Obstet Gynecol 1988;159:125.
130. Hashimoto Y, Soeda Y, Takarada M et al. Anaphylaxis to moxalactam: report of a case. J Oral Maxillofac Surg 1990;48:1004.
131. Jaju M, Ahuja YR. Effect of cephaloridine on human chromosomes in vitro in lymphocyte cultures. Mutat Res 1982;101:57.
132. Hoover DM, Buening MK, Tamura RN et al. Effects of cefamandole on spermatogenic development of young CD rats. Fundam Appl Toxicol 1989;13:737.
133. Norrby SR. Side effects of cephalosporins. Drugs 1987; 34(Suppl 2:105.
134. Fromtling RA, Gadebusch HH. Ethanol-cephalosporin antibiotic interactions: an animal model for the detection of disulfiram (Antabuse)-like effects. Methods Find Exp Clin Pharmacol 1983;5:595.
135. Kitson TM. The effect of cephalosporin antibiotics on alcohol metabolism: a review. Alcohol 1987;4:143.
136. Buening MK, Wold JS. Ethanol moxalactam interactions in vivo. Rev Infect Dis 1982;4(Suppl):555.
137. Young DS. Effects of Drugs on Clinical Laboratory Tests. 3rd edn. Washington: AACC Press, 1990.
138. Harder S, Schneider W, Bae ZU et al. Unerwünschte Arzneimittel-reaktionen bei gleichzeitiger Gabe von hochdosiertem Phenobarbital und Betalaktam-Antibiotika. Klin Pädiatr 1990;202:404.
139. Soto Alvarez J, Sacristán Del Castillo JA, Alsar Ortiz MJ. Interaction between ciclosporin and ceftriaxone. Nephron 1991;59:681.
140. Fiscella RG. Physical incompatibility of vancomycin and ceftazidime for intravitreal injection. Arch Ophthalmol 1993;111:730.
141. Kishore K, Raina A, Misra V, Jonas E. Acute verapamil toxicity in a patient with chronic toxicity: possible interaction with ceftriaxone and clindamycin (see comments). Ann Pharmacother 1993;27:877.
142. Kroll MH, Elin RJ. Mechanism of cefoxitin and cephalothin interference with the Jaffé method for creatinine. Clin Chem 1983;29:2044.
143. Kowalsky SF, Wishnoff FG. Evaluation of potential interaction of new cephalosporins with Clinitest. Am J Hosp Pharm 1982;39:1499.

Meyler's Side Effects of Drugs, 13th Edition
M.N.G. Dukes, editor

SECTION EDITOR: R. HOIGNÉ

K.A. Neftel, P. Cottagnoud and A. Cerny

25.5 β-Lactam antibiotics other than penicillins and cephalosporins

In more recent years compounds other than penicillins and cephalosporins, but still containing the β-lactam ring, have been developed for antimicrobial chemotherapy, some of them now being in routine clinical use. These include (a) monocyclic β-lactams, (b) carbapenems and other penems, and (c) compounds acting as β-lactamase inhibitors.

MONOBACTAMS

In the monobactams there is no second ring fused to the β-lactam ring. However, the highly active compounds of this group do, as a rule, contain the aminothiazole side chain, known to be associated with good antimicrobial activity and β-lactamase stability in cephalosporins (1^R). Aztreonam was the first monobactam marketed in 1984. Further compounds such as carumonam, pirazmonam and tigemonam have been developed (2^R), but so far only aztreonam is more widely used. Monobactams are almost exclusively active against gram-negative bacteria and their clinical usefulness lies particularly in their antipseudomonas activity.

Like 6-aminopenicillanic acid for the penicillins and 7-amino-cephalosporanic acid for the cephalosporins, 3-aminomonobactamic acid is the basic compound for the monobactam family.

In clinical trials the safety profile of aztreonam has been found to be similar to or better than that of other, more conventional β-lactam antibiotics, in adult patients with both normal (3^R, 4^R) and impaired renal function (5^R). More recently, these findings have been confirmed in pediatric patients (6^R).

ORGANS AND SYSTEMS

Hematological In a child with typhoid fever, severe leukopenia and neutropenia necessitated discontinuation of aztreonam treatment (150 mg/kg/day) on the tenth day, followed by recovery (7^C). However, acute reversible neutropenia has been otherwise reported in fewer than 0.1% of aztreonam-treated patients (6^R). Three out of 28 patients receiving high-dose aztreonam (300 mg/kg/day) for cystic fibrosis developed mild and transient thrombocytopenia (8^C).

Liver The frequency of liver function test abnormalities does not differ from other β-lactam antibiotics (3^R, 6^R, 8^C).

Urinary system Acute renal failure, skin rash and eosinophilia associated with aztreonam has been reported in a 70-year-old man after 9 days of treatment (9^C). No significant nephrotoxicity, however, has been documented in larger patient series.

Skin and appendages Aztreonam has been the suspected cause of toxic epidermal necrolysis in two patients undergoing bone marrow transplantations (10^C). Graft-versus-host disease seemed a less likely diagnosis of the cutaneous manifestations.

Hypersensitivity reactions The prototype substance aztreonam has a minor immunogenicity in animal studies and was associated with a 2% incidence of all presumably immunologically mediated drug reactions in early phase I and II trials (11^R).

Negligible cross-reactivity has been reported in both animal and human studies involving hapten inhibition, skin tests, as well as treatment of penicillin-allergic patients with therapeutic doses of aztreonam (11^R—14^R, 15^C, 16^c, 17^C).

Aztreonam thus seems to be a safe alternative for the penicillin-allergic patient. However, the numbers of safely treated patients reported are still small and immediate type hypersensitivity to aztreonam has been reported to occur in penicillin-allergic patients (18^c, 19^c, 20^C, 21^c).

Several cephalosporins, e.g. ceftazidime, share the same amino-thiazole side chain as aztreonam. Sensitization with either drug involving side chain-specific antibodies may thus predispose to allergy to the other. Clinical data on this problem are at present not available.

Carbapenems

Carbapenems differ from penicillins and cephalosporins by a methylene substitution for sulfur in the five-membered α-ring structure. Imipenem and the more recently introduced meropenem belong to this class of compounds. In the last 15 years various natural carbapenems have been discovered (22[R]). Their clinical potential, however, is limited by chemical instability. Imipenem (*N*-formimidoylthienamycin), the first carbapenem in clinical use, is therefore a stabilized synthetic compound. To overcome a second difficulty, namely inactivation by a kidney dehydropeptidase, imipenem has to be combined with cilastatin, a competitive inhibitor of that enzyme. Meropenem is a new compound in clinical evaluation having improved stability in the presence of renal dehydropeptidase I (23[R]). Carbapenems exhibit the broadest antibacterial spectrum of all clinically used β-lactam antibiotics, including gram-positive as well as gram-negative aerobic and anaerobic pathogens, and have good stability against many β-lactamases.

ADVERSE REACTIONS PATTERN

The safety profile of imipenem + cilastatin is comparable to that of other β-lactam antibiotics, in particular with regard to laboratory abnormalities, the most common ones being those related to liver function (24[R]–26[R]). Seizures appear to be more common than with other β-lactam antibiotics.

ORGANS AND SYSTEMS

Nervous system Seizures associated to imipenem + cilastatin treatment have repeatedly been reported (27[C]–29[C], 30[c]). As with other β-lactam antibiotics, it is difficult to assess clearly the etiology of a seizure in patients exhibiting a cluster of other predisposing factors for neurotoxicity (31[R]) and hence to reach clear estimates of frequency. In a review of 1754 patients a similar incidence of seizures was found with imipenem + cilastatin as with other antibiotic regimens usually containing another β-lactam (32[R]). In rabbits imipenem + cilastatin and another penem were more neurotoxic than benzylpenicillin (33[C]). In one mouse model, ataxia and seizures were seen with much lower blood levels of imipenem than cefotaxime or benzylpenicillin (1900 μg/ml versus 3400 μg/ml and 5800 μg/ml) (28[C]). In another mouse model imipenem lowered the convulsive threshold of pentylenetetrazole more than cefazolin or two other penems (34[C]). Cilastatin alone was not proconvulsive, but increased the effects of imipenem when co-administered.

All recent reports confirm a relatively high imipenem-related seizure activity as compared to other β-lactam antibiotics, particularly when high doses are given (35[C], 36[C], 37[c]). In one study seven of 21 children developed seizure activity while treated with imipenem-cilastatin for bacterial meningitis, a recognized risk factor (35[C]). However, computer-assisted monitoring of imipenem-cilastatin dosages in relation to renal function resulted in a reduced incidence of seizures (38[C]).

In animal models meropenem (39[C]) and also other carbapenems (40[C], 41[C]) were less epileptogenic than imipenem. In a series of 403 children no meropenem-associated neurotoxicity was observed (42[C]) and meropenem was well tolerated in a pediatric series with bacterial meningitis (43[C]).

Special senses Taste alterations were seen in some earlier cases (47[C]); these observations have not subsequently been confirmed.

Hematological As with some cephalosporins and clavulanic acid, the Coombs test was positive in a number of instances, without the presence of hemolysis (25[R]).

Urinary system In animals, the tubular toxicity of imipenem was completely abrogated by co-administering cilastatin. Accordingly, definite nephrotoxicity of this combination has not been documented in patients (25[R]) or in volunteers (44[C]). The cilastatin component may even reduce the nephrotoxic effects ciclosporin after kidney transplantation (45[C]).

Skin A pustular rash as repeatedly observed with cephalosporins has been described in one case (46[c]). The frequency of rash, urticaria and pruritus was similar to that seen with other β-lactam antibiotics (25[R]).

Hypersensitivity reactions Saxon et al. reported a high degree of cross-reactivity between imipenem determinants analogous to the penicillin determinants in penicillin-allergic patients. They found that nine out of 20 penicillin skin test-positive patients had positive skin reactions to analogous imipenem determinants (48[C]). Immediate hypersensitivity related to imipenem has been reported in a patient allergic to penicillin and aztreonam (21[c]). In view of this appreciable cross-reactivity, imipenem should be withheld from the penicillin-allergic patient.

Interactions Possible imipenem-cilastatin-associated neurotoxicity was observed in five recipients of various allografts who were on ciclosporin. Interestingly, toxicity occurred immediately after the first dosage in one patient and only one day after the onset of imipenem-cilastatin treatment in three others (49[C]).

Interference with diagnostic routines Imipenem has been reported to induce positive dipstick-tests for leukocytes in agranulocytotic patients with normal urinary sediments. The phenomenon could be reproduced in standardized artificial urine with imipenem and meropenem as well as with clavulanic acid. However, sulbactam and tazobactam, three penicillins and three cephalosporins as well as the basic structures, 6-aminopenicillanic acid, 7-aminocephalosporanic acid and 3-amino-monobactamic acid, tested negative (50[C]).

β-Lactamase inhibitors

Structural variation is the main way to overcome inactivation of β-lactam antibiotics by bacterial β-lactamases. Another is co-administration of effective β-lactamase inhibitors. Among various compounds having inhibitory activity, only those containing a β-lactam ring themselves have proved to have a potential clinical value so far (1[R]). Clavulanic acid, produced naturally by *Streptomyces clavuligerus*, was the first compound in clinical use in combination with amoxicillin or ticarcillin. Sulbactam, another inhibitor, has been combined with ampicillin or cefoperazone, and more recently tazobactam with piperacillin (sulbactam and tazobactam are halogenated derivatives of penicillanic acid). In order to improve insufficient enteral absorption, sulbactam has been bound to ampicillin in the single molecule sultamicillin, which is again hydrolyzed to the active components after absorption. Other β-lactamase inhibitors are under evaluation.

An inherent obstacle in evaluating side effects to β-lactamase inhibitors is that such compounds are only co-administered with other antimicrobially active β-lactams, the absolute dose of which is usually several times higher.

ADVERSE REACTION PATTERN

Combinations basically produced the side effects of the β-lactam antibiotic combined with the β-lactamase inhibitor. In addition clavulanic acid can cause a positive direct antiglobulin test and when combined with amoxicillin or ticarcillin, cholestatic hepatitis.

ORGANS AND SYSTEMS

Hematological Parallel to a well-known phenomenon seen with cephalosporins, clavulanic acid can be associated with a positive direct antiglobulin test (DAT). In three patient series antibiotic courses including intravenous ticarcillin + clavulanic acid were associated in up to more than 50% of cases with positive DATs (51[C]–53[C]). In vitro studies showed that clavulanic acid causes non-immunological absorption of plasma proteins onto the erythrocyte surface (51[C]). There seems to be no clinical impact of the phenomenon, but it may interfere with cross-matching of blood products or with work up of true hemolysis.

Liver The causal relationship of the amoxicillin/clavulanic acid combination to a particular type of cholestatic hepatitis is now firmly established. Although the first case-report only appeared in 1988 (54[c]), several hundreds of cases possibly associated to amoxicillin/clavulanate have been reported, e.g. to health authorities (55[C]), and subsequently over 100 cases have been described in detail in the literature (e.g. 56[C]–62[C], 63[c], 64[C]–66[C]). Considering, however, the high number of patients treated with this very widely used combination, the risk of developing hepatitis was still estimated to be very low, probably below 1/100 000 (64[C]). Hepatitis usually manifests acutely, although a time interval up to 4 weeks between end of treatment and clinical manifestation of hepatitis is frequent and may obscure a rapid diagnosis. Liver biopsy shows predominantly centrilobular or panlobular cholestasis. Occasionally granulomatous hepatitis was present (67[c]). Although clinical manifestations may be impressive, the condition is usually reversible within 4–6 weeks. One fatal outcome was described in a patient under concurrent administration of ethinylestradiol for prostatic cancer, a potentially cholestatic agent by itself (68[c]).

The mechanism of the syndrome and its possible relationship to liver injury seen with other β-lactam antibiotics, particularly isoxazolylpenicillins, are unclear. Slight eosinophilia has been seen in many cases (63[c], 67[c], 69[c]) and some of the sporadic rechallenges were positive (56[C]). But there is no further evidence indicating an immuno-allergic basis. Clavulanic acid is instrumental, either alone or together with amoxicillin, since a similar reaction is practically unknown with amoxicillin alone. Gastroenteral passage of the drug may play some role, however hepatic accumulation or biliary secretion of clavulanic acid or its metabolites have not been demonstrated (70[R]). Increasing age (over 55 years) and male sex were recognized as risk factors for the development of amoxicillin-clavulanate-associated jaundice (64[C], 71[C]), while drug dose, route and duration of therapy, other medications, previous drug allergies, or prior use of amoxicillin/clavulanate were not significantly associated with the reaction. The syndrome is practically unknown in children and one pediatric case reported so far in a 4-year-old boy with spherocytosis (56[C]) has been disputed (57[c]).

Ticarcillin/clavulanate which is only used intravenously, besides having aggravated pre-existing hepatitis (72[C]), has recently also been reported to induce a similar syndrome (73[c], 74[c]). One cholestatic reaction has been reported with the intravenously administered sulbactam/ampicillin combination (75[C]).

In isolated cases, the Stevens-Johnson syndrome together with cholestasis and bone marrow aplasia have been associated with either amoxicillin alone (76[c]) or with the amoxicillin/clavulanic acid combination (77[c]).

Gastrointestinal Two cases of hemorrhagic colitis, apparently not related to *Clostridium difficile*, following amoxicillin + clavulanate have been reported (78[c], 79[c]). The same type of colitis, however, has repeatedly been observed with aminopenicillins alone (79[c]).

The amoxicillin + clavulanate combination is often reported to induce diarrhea and other gastrointestinal problems (see Chapter 25.2). Interestingly, oral administration was found to be associated with the occurrence of small-intestinal motor disturbances (80[C]).

Miscellaneous Behavioral changes occurred in four children aged 1.5—10.5 years while taking amoxicillin + clavulanate (81[C]). A woman immediately developed hyperpyrexia up to 40—C after the first dose of intravenous ampicillin + sulbactam, having previously tolerated ampicillin alone for 10 days. Hyperpyrexia was repeatedly observed after six more sulbactam-containing doses (82[c]).

Hypersensitivity reactions Clavulanic acid has been shown to have a very low immunogenic and allergenic potential in animal models. The possible impact of its co-administration with other β-lactam antibiotics is unknown (83[C]). Recently Fernandez-Rivas et al. described two patients presenting with IgE-mediated hypersensitivity to oral amoxicillin/clavulanic acid and positive skin tests for clavulanic acid but not for penicillins. Both patients tolerated oral challenge with amoxicillin. One patient was also challenged with clavulanic acid and developed urticaria, conjunctivitis and broncho-obstruction (84[C]). Given the fact that the drug has been widely used since its introduction in 1981, the frequency of occurrence of hypersensitivity reactions seems low. The clinical data available on sulbactam and tazobactam are still limited and do not allow an assessment of the frequency and pattern of associated hypersensitivity reactions (85[R]).

Interference with diagnostic routines False positive outcomes of urine dipstick-tests for leukocytes could be induced by adding clavulanic acid to standardized artificial urine (50[C]). Sulbactam and tazobactam on the other hand tested negative (see above 'Carbapenems').

REFERENCES

1. Hoover JRE. Betalactam antibiotics: structure-activity relationships. In: Demain AL, Solomon NA, eds. Antibiotics, Containing the Betalactam-Structure, Part II. Berlin. Springer-Verlag: 1983;119.
2. Kirrstetter R, Dürckheimer W. Development of new betalactam antibiotics derived from natural and synthetic sources. Pharmazie 1989;3:177.
3. Newman TJ, Dreslinski GR. Safety profile of aztreonam in clinical trials. Rev Infect Dis 1985;7(Suppl 4)S648.
4. Scully BE, Neu HC. Use of aztreonam in the treatment of serious infections due to multiresistant gram-negative organisms, including *Pseudomonas aeruginosa*. Am J Med 1985;78:251.
5. Sattler FR, Schramm M, Swab EA. Safety of aztreonam and SQ 26,992 in elderly patients with renal insufficiency. Rev Infect Dis 1985;7(Suppl 4):S622.
6. Chartrand SA. Safety and toxicity profile of aztreonam. Pediatr Infect Dis J 1989;8:S120.
7. Tanaka-Kido J, Ortega L, Santos JL. Comparative efficacies of aztreonam and chloramphenicol in children with typhoid fever. Pediatr Infect Dis J 1990;9:44.
8. Schaad UB, Wedgwood-Krucko J, Guenin K et al. Antipseudomonal therapy in cystic fibrosis. Aztreonam and amikacin versus ceftazidime and amikacin administered intravenously followed by oral ciprofloxacin. Eur J Clin Microbiol Infect Dis 1989;8:858.
9. Pazmiño P. Acute renal failure, skin rash and eosinophilia associated with aztreonam. Am J Nephrol 1988;8:68.
10. McDonald BJ, Singer JW, Bianco JA. Toxic epidermal necrolysis possibly linked to aztreonam in bone marrow transplant patients. Ann Pharmacother 1992;26:34.
11. Adkinson NF Jr. Immunogenicity and crossallergenicity of aztreonam. Am J Med 1990;88(125):38S.
12. Adkinson NF Jr, Swabb EA, Sugerman AA. Immunology of the monobactam aztreonam. Antimicrob Agents Chemother 1984;25:933.
13. Saxon A, Beall GN, Rohr AS et al. Immediate hypersensitivity reactions to beta-lactam antibiotics. Urology 1988; 31(Suppl):14.
14. Saxon A, Beall GN, Rohr AS et al. Immediate hypersensitivity reactions to beta-lactam antibiotics (clinical conference). Ann Intern Med 1987;107:204.
15. Adkinson NF Jr, Wheeler B, Swabb EA. Clinical tolerance of the monobactam aztreonam in penicillin-allergic subjects. In: Proceedings, 14th International Congress of Chemotherapy, Kyoto, Japan, 1985, Abstract. WS-26-4, 1985.
16. Loria RC, Finnerty N, Wedner HJ. Successful use of

aztreonam in a patient who failed oral penicillin desensitization. J Allergy Clin Immunol 1989;83:735.
17. Jensen T, Koch C, Pedersen SS et al. Aztreonam for cystic fibrosis patients who are hypersensitive to other betalactams (Letter to Editor). Lancet 1987;i:1319.
18. Iglesias-Cadarso A, Saez-Jimenez SA, Vidal-Pan C et al. Aztreonam-induced anaphylaxis (Letter to Editor). Lancet 1990;336:746.
19. Soto-Alvarez J, Sacristan del Castillo JA, Sampedro-Garcia I et al. Immediate hypersensitivity to aztreonam. Lancet 1990;335:1094.
20. Moss RB, McClelland E, Williams RR et al. Evaluation of the immunologic cross-reactivity of aztreonam in patients with cystic fibrosis who are allergic to penicillin and/or cephalosporin antibiotics. Rev Infect Dis 1991;13(Suppl 7): S598.
21. Hantson P, de Coninck B, Horn JL et al. Immediate hypersensitivity to aztreonam and imipenem. Br Med J 1991;302:294.
22. Birnbaum J, Kahan FM, Kropp H. Carbapenems, a new class of betalactam antibiotics; discovery and development of imipenem/cilastatin. Am J Med 1985;78(Suppl 6A):3.
23. Fukusawa M, Sumita Y, Harabe ET et al. Stability of meropenem and effect of 1β-methyl substitution on its stability in the presence of renal dehydropeptidase I. Antimicrob Agents Chemother 1992;36:1577.
24. Calandra GB, Brown KR, Grad IC et al. Review of adverse experiences and tolerability in the first 2516 patients treated with imipenem/cilastatin. Am J Med 1985;78:73.
25. Calandra GB, Wang C, Aziz M et al. The safety profile of imipenem/cilastatin: worldwide clinical experience based on 3470 patients. J Antimicrob Chemother 1986;18(Suppl E):193.
26. Ahonkhai VI, Cyhan GM, Wilson SE et al. Imipenem-cilastatin in pediatric patients; an overview of safety and efficacy in studies conducted in the United States. Pediatr Infect Dis J 1989;8:740.
27. Brotherton TJ, Kelber RL. Seizure-like activity associated with imipenem. Clin Pharmacol 1984;3:536.
28. Eng RHK, Munsif AN, Yangco BG et al. Seizure propensity with imipenem. Arch Intern Med 1989;149:1881.
29. Job ML, Dretler RH. Seizure activity with imipenem therapy: incidence and risk factors. Drug Intell Clin Pharm 1990;24:567.
30. Tse CS, Hernandez-Vera F, Desai DV. Seizure-like activity associated with imipenem-cilastin. Drug Intell Clin Pharm 1987;21:659.
31. Schliamser SE, Cars O, Norrby SR. Neurotoxicity of betalactam antibiotics: predisposing factors and pathogenesis. J Antimicrob Chemother 1991;27:405.
32. Calandra G, Lydick E, Carrigan J et al. Factors predisposing to seizures in seriously infected patients receiving antibiotics: experience with imipenem/cilastatin. Am J Med 1988;84:911.
33. Schliamser SE, Broholm KA, Liljedahl AL et al. Comparative neurotoxicity of benzylpenicillin, imipenem/cilastatin und FCE 22101, a new injectable penem. J Antimicrob Chemother 1988;22:687.
34. Williams PD, Bennett DB, Comereski CR. Animal model for evaluating the convulsive liability of betalactam antibiotics. Antimicrob Agents Chemother 1988;5:758.
35. Wong VK, Wright HT Jr, Ross LA et al. Imipenem/cilastatin treatment of bacterial meningitis in children. Pediatr Infect Dis J 1991;10:122.
36. Winston DJ, Ho WG, Bruckner DA, Champlin RE. Beta-lactam antibiotic therapy in febrile granulocytopenic patients. A randomized trial comparing cefoperazone plus piperacillin, ceftazidime plus piperacillin, and imipenem alone. Ann Intern Med 1991;115:849.
37. Leo RJ, Ballow CH. Seizure activity associated with imipenem use: clinical case reports and review of the literature. DICP Ann Pharmacother 1991;25:351.
38. Pestotnik SL, Classen DC, Evans RS et al. Prospective surveillance of imipenem/cilastatin use and associated seizures using a hospital information system. Ann Pharmacother 1993;27:497.
39. Patel JB, Giles RE. Meropenem evidence of lack of proconvulsive tendency in mice. J Antimicrob Chemother 1989;24:(Suppl A):307.
40. Kurihara A, Hisaoka M, Mikuni N, Kamoshida K. Neurotoxicity of panipenem/betamipron, a new carbapenem, in rabbits: correlation to concentration in central nervous system. J Pharmacobiodyn 1992;15:325.
41. Sunagawa M, Matsumura H, Fukasawa M. Structure-activity relationships of carbapenem and penem compounds for the convulsive property. J Antibiot 1992;45:1983.
42. Fujii R, Pediatric Study Group of Meropenem. Pharmacokinetic and clinical studies with meropenem in the pediatric field. Jpn J Antibiot 1992;45:697.
43. Klugman KP, Dagan R. Meropenem meningitis study group. Randomized comparison of meropenem with cefotaxime for treatment of bacterial meningitis. Antimicrob Agents Chemother 1995;39:1140.
44. Drusano GL, Standiford HC, Bustamante C et al. Safety and tolerability of multiple doses of imipenem/cilastatin. Clin Pharmacol Ther 1985;37:539.
45. Hammer C, Thies JC, Mraz W et al. Reduction of cyclosporin (CSA) nephrotoxicity by imipenem/cilastatin after kidney transplantation in rats. Transplant Proc 1989;21:931.
46. Escallier F, Dalac S, Foucher JL et al. Pustulose exanthématique aiguë généralisée: imputabilité à l'imipénème (Tienam). Ann Dermatol Vénéréol 1989;116:407.
47. Ribner BS, Donabedian H, Raeder R et al. Empirical use of imipenem as the sole antibiotic in the treatment of serious infections. J Antimicrob Chemother 1985;16:499.
48. Saxon A, Adelman DC, Patel A et al. Imipenem cross-reactivity with penicillin in humans. J Allergy Clin Immunol 1988;82:213.
49. Bösmüller C, Steurer W, Königsrainer A et al. Increased risk of central nervous system toxicity in patients treated with ciclosporin and imipenem/cilastatin (Letter to the Editor). Nephron 1991;58:362.
50. Beer JH, Vogt A, Neftel K, Cottagnoud P. False positivity for leucocytes of the urine stix test induced by commonly used antibotics. Br Med J 1996;313:25.
51. Williams ME, Thomas D, Harman CP et al. Positive direct antiglobulin tests due to clavulanic acid. Antimicrob Agents Chemother 1985;27:125.
52. Finegold SM, Johnson CC. Lower respiratory tract infection. Am J Med 1985;79(Suppl 5B):73.
53. Blanchard M, Oppliger R, Bucher U. Positiver direkter Coombs-Test bei akuten Leukämien und anderen Hämoblastosen: Zusammenhang mit clavulansäurehaltigen Antibiotika? Schweiz Med Wschr 1989;119:39.
54. Van den Broek JWG, Buennemeyer BLM, Stricker

BHCh. Cholestatische hepatitis door de combinatic amoxicilline en clavulaanzuur (Augmentin). Ned Tijdschr Geneeskd 1988;132:1495.

55. Thomson JA, Fairley CK, McNeil JJ, Purcell P. Augmentin-associated jaundice. Med J Aust 1994;160:733.

56. Stricker BHCh, Van den Broek JWG, Keuning J et al. Cholestatic hepatitis due to antibacterial combination of amoxicillin and clavulanic acid (Augmentin). Dig Dis Sci 1989;34:1576.

57. Reddy KR, Brillant P, Schiff ER. Amoxicillin-clavulanate potassium-associated cholestasis. Gastroenterology 1989; 96:1135.

58. Reddy KR, Schiff ER. Hepatitis and Augmentin (Letter to the Editor). Dig Dis Sci 1990;35:1045.

59. Verhamme M, Ramboer C, Van de Bruane P et al. Cholestatic hepatitis due to an amoxycillin/clavulanic preparation. J Hepatol 1989;9:260.

60. Dowsett JF, Gillow T, Heagerty A et al. Amoxycillin/clavulanic acid (Augmentin)-induced intrahepatic cholestasis. Dig Dis Sci 1989;34:1290.

61. Schneider JE, Kleinmann MS, Kupiec JW. Cholestatic hepatitis after therapy with amoxicillin/clavulanate potrassium. NY State J Med 1989;89:355.

62. Pelletier G, Ink O, Fabre M et al. Hépatite cholestatique probablement due à l'association d'amoxilline et d'acide clavulanique. Gastroentéral Clin Biol 1990;14:601.

63. Alexander P, Roskams T, Van Steenbergen W et al. Intrahepatic cholestasis induced by amoxicillin/clavulanic acid (Augmentin): a report on two cases. Acta Clin Belg 1991;46:327.

64. Larrey D, Vial T, Micaleff A et al. Hepatitis associated with amoxycillin-clavulanic acid combination report of 15 cases. Gut 1992;33:368.

65. Hanssens M, Mast A, Van Maele, Pauwels W. Cholestatische icterus door amoxicilline-clavulaanzuur bij 4 patiënten. Ned Tijdschr Geneeskd 1994;138:1481.

66. Wong FS, Ryan J, Dabkowski P et al. Augmentin-induced jaundice. Med J Aust 1991;154:698.

67. Silvain C, Fort E, Levillain P et al. Granulomatous hepatitis due to combination of amoxicillin and clavulanic acid. Dig Dis Sci 1992;37:150.

68. Hebbard GS, Smith KGC, Gibson PR, Bhathal PS. Augmentin-induced jaundice with a fatal outcome. Med J Aust 1992;156:285.

69. Belknap MK, McClelland KJ. Cholestatic hepatitis associated with amoxicillin-clavulanate. Wis Med J 1993; 92:241.

70. Reading C, Slocombe B. Augmentin: clavulanate-potentiated amoxicillin. In: Queener SF, Webber JA, Queener SW, eds. Betalactam Antibiotics for Clinical Use. New York: Marcel Dekker, 1986;527.

71. Thomson JA, Fairley CK, Ugoni AM et al. Risk factors for the development of amoxycillin-clavulanic acid associated jaundice. Med J Aust 1995;162:638.

72. Van der Auwera P, Legrand JC. Ticarcillin-clavulanic acid therapy in severe infections. Drugs Exp Clin Res 1985;11:805.

73. Ryan J, Dudley FJ. Cholestasis with ticarcillin-potassium clavulanate (Timentin). Med J Aust 1992;156:291.

74. Sweet JM, Jones MP. Intrahepatic cholestasis due to ticarcillin-clavulanate (Letter to the Editor). AJG 1995; 90:675.

75. Lode H, Springsklee M et al. Klinische Ergebnisse mit Sulbactam/Ampicillin in einer multizentrischen Studie an 425 Patienten. Med Klin 1989;84:235.

76. Cavanzo FJ, Garcia CF, Botero RC. Chronic cholestasis, paucity of bile ducts, red cell aplasia, and the Stevens-Johnson syndrome. Gastroenterology 1990;99:854.

77. Escallier F, Dalac S, Caillot D et al. Erythàme polymorphe, aplasie, hépatite cholestatique au cours d'un traitement par Augmentin (amoxicilline + acide clavulanique). Rev Méd Intern 1990;11:73.

78. Klotz F, Barthet M, Perreard M. A propos d'un cas de colite aiguë hémorragique après la prise orale d'Augmentin. Ann Méd Intern 1990;141:276.

79. Heer M, Sulser H, Hany A. Segmentale, hämorrhagische Kolitis nach Amoxicillin-Therapie. Schweiz Med Wschr 1989;119:733.

80. Caron F, Ducrotte PH, Lerebours E et al. Effects of amoxicillin-clavulanate combination on the motility of the small intestine in human beings. Antimicrob Agents Chemother 1991;35:1085.

81. Macknin ML. Behavioral changes after amoxicillin-clavulanate. Pediatr Infect Dis J 1987;6:873.

82. Olivencia-Yurvati AH, Sanders SP. Sulbactam-induced hyperpyrexia. Arch Intern Med 1990;150:1961.

83. Edwards RG, Dewdney JM, Dobrzanski RJ et al. Immunogenicity and allergenicity studies on two beta-lactam structures, a clavam, clavulanic acid, and a carbapenem: structure-activity relationships. Int Arch Allergy Appl Immunol 1988;85:184.

84. Fernandez-Rivas M, Carral CP, Cuevas M et al. Selective allergic reactions to clavulanic acid. J Allergy Clin Immunol 1995;95:748.

85. Wilson SE, Nord CE. Clinical trials of extended spectrum penicillin/beta-lactamase inhibitors in the treatment of intra-abdominal infections. European and North American experience. Am J Surg 1995;169(Suppl 5A):21S.

Meyler's Side Effects of Drugs, 13th Edition
M.N.G. Dukes, editor

SECTION EDITOR: M.N.G. DUKES

C. Ruef, J. Blaser, P. Maurer, H. Keller and F. Follath

26 Miscellaneous antibiotics

Tetracyclines

The tetracyclines are a closely related group of antibiotics with comparable pharmacological, however somehow different kinetic properties. They possess both the advantages and disadvantages of broad-spectrum antibiotics. Tetracyclines are effective not only against bacteria and spirochetes, but also against some *Mycoplasma*, *Chlamydia* and *Rickettsia*, as well as protozoa. By the inhibition of ribosomal protein synthesis they affect merely multiplying microorganisms. Their main effect is therefore bacteriostatic rather than bactericidal, depending on the kind of microorganism.

Most of the side effects are of toxic nature and dependent on the concentration of the antibiotic in the organ affected. The newer, more lipophilic preparations are more potent with regard to their bacteriostatic efficacy and hence usually require daily doses below 1 gram. Side effects affecting hemopoiesis are hardly ever seen with the tetracyclines.

The syndrome of benign intracranial hypertension, which is also encountered in adults, is extremely rare.

A common and nearly unique feature of all the tetracyclines is the formation of drug—melanin complexes, resulting in pigment deposition at various sites. Except from enamel defects and presumable disturbances of osteogenesis these deposits do not give rise to organ function abnormalities.

ADVERSE REACTION PATTERN

General and toxic reactions These may occur if the dosage is not adapted in patients with renal insufficiency. The syndrome of fatty liver degeneration is rarely encountered today because risk situations such as pregnancy are respected and preparations with lower dosage are available. Slight gastrointestinal intolerance is not infrequently seen. In view of tooth discoloration and enamel hypoplasia with a tendency to caries formation, children under 8 years of age and women after the third month of pregnancy should be given tetracyclines only when there is no alternative. The risk of photosensitivity reactions depends largely on the dose of the drug and the degree of exposure to sunlight. It may be elevated in long-term treatments purely by an increased drug—radiation dose product. Skin, nail and other organ pigmentation is encountered frequently, even with low-dose long-term treatment.

Hypersensitivity reactions Allergic reactions to tetracycline preparations are less than half as common as allergic reactions to penicillin. For this reason, tetracyclines may offer an alternative for the treatment of patients with allergic reactions to one or more of other antibiotic groups. Exceptional observations of anaphylactic shock have been reported (1[C], 2[C]). In a few cases tetracycline preparations were assumed to be the cause of hypersensitivity myocarditis (3[C]). Pneumonitis with eosinophilia has been described in recent years (4[c]). In a newly published observation a serum sickness-like syndrome was probably associated with minocycline therapy in a 19-year-old youth treated for acne (5[c]). Allergic as well as toxic reactions may in some special cases have been caused by degraded preparations or additives (6a[C]).

Tumor-inducing effects These have not been reported.

ORGANS AND SYSTEMS

Cardiovascular reactions These were often associated with other symptoms of hypersensitivity, such as urticaria, allergic angioedema, attack of bronchial obstruction and arterial hypotension (1[C], 6b[c]). They occurred in patients who had tolerated tetracyclines previously and therefore were considered as anaphylactic or anaphylactoid reactions.

Respiratory A few cases with an acute reaction of bronchial obstruction following the administration of a tetracycline preparation have been published (7a[c]). Pneumonitis with eosinophilia has also been described recently (4[c], 7b[C]).

Where pleural tetracycline instillation is used for pleurodesis in spontaneous pneumothorax, no severe short- or long-term side effects, besides the therapeutically expected local inflammation, could be observed (8[C]).

Nervous system Tetracyclines can induce the syndrome described as *benign intracranial hypertension*, which represents a seldom, but nearly unique complication of tetracycline therapy.

The appearance of this clinical syndrome in association with tetracycline therapy has primarily involved children (9[c], 10[c]). Predominantly in later years, benign intracranial hypertension has also been observed in adults (11[R], 12[c], 13[C]—16[C], 17[c]—19[c]). Re-exposure resulting in recurrence of the syndrome was also reported (8[c]). As a rule, the symptoms develop between days and as long as months after initiation of therapy. In one case they appeared only after 18 months of tetracycline therapy for acne (18[c]). The syndrome includes headache, nausea and vomiting, dizziness, tinnitus, papilledema and visual disturbances caused by scotoma or optic nerve damage. Intracranial pressure may be elevated up to three times normal. Distinct intracerebral lesions, are however, lacking in the CT scan or angiography and enlargement of the ventricular spaces is absent (11[R]). With the exception of intracranial pressure, all findings including cell count and protein content in cerebrospinal fluid examination are normal. After the drug is discontinued, symptoms resolve over a period of hours to days or occasionally weeks. Broadly applied long-term therapy with tetracyclines for acne may contribute to a higher prevalence of this syndrome (20[C]).

Reactions in myasthenia gravis and neuromuscular block In early studies it was shown that curare block was increased with tetracyclines (21[C]—23[C]). This effect can be antagonized by calcium ions (24[C]). A short time increase in muscular weakness in patients with myasthenia gravis following intravenous administration of tetracycline preparations was observed. The clinical finding might be due to a calcium-antagonizing effect of magnesium ions present in the tetracycline solvent, as the symptoms could be provoked by similar amounts of magnesium alone. The formation of calcium complexes with non-protein-bound tetracycline, thus lowering serum concentration of free calcium, may also be involved, as suggested by experimental investigations (25[R]).

Endocrine, metabolic Tetracyclines may increase blood urea nitrogen or urea in the serum without a corresponding increase of serum creatinine. The reason for this constellation is an excess nitrogen load of metabolic origin accompanied by a negative nitrogen balance. This effect is termed 'anti-anabolic'; it is in fact the result of the therapeutically desired inhibition of protein synthesis, which affects not only microorganisms but to some degree also mammalian cells.

Hormone production in patients with 'black thyroid' (see 'Pigmentation' in 'Skin and appendages') treated for a long time with a tetracycline preparation, was normal (26[C], 27[C]).

Mineral and fluid balance A few observations of a nephrogenic *diabetes insipidus-like syndrome* with demeclocycline (demethylchlortetracycline hydrochloride) and resistance to exogenous vasopressin suggest an impairment of renal concentrating function by tubular damage (28[C]). The use of this preparation has therefore been proposed to treat inappropriate antidiuretic hormone secretion (29[C]—33[C]).

Interstitial nephritis seems to be extremely rare (34[c], 35[c], 36[R]).

An *azotemic effect*, which may be at least partly due to a decrease in renal function, has been observed in patients with liver cirrhosis (37[C], 38[C], 39[R]), with cardiac failure and interstitial nephritis (40[c]). (For acquired *Lignac-De Toni-Fanconi syndrome* see 'Urinary system'.)

Hematological Hematological changes with tetracycline preparations are extremely rare. However, in individual cases, *hemolytic anemia* (41[C]), *neutropenia* or slight *leukopenia*, *thrombocytopenia* (42[C]) and even *aplastic anemia* have all been described. In view of the fact that such blood changes may be found in patients without any evidence of their etiology, the relationship to the drug often remains doubtful, especially if reactions are listed in tabular form and lacking information of specific details or concomitant drug therapy.

Bleeding with *thrombocytopenia* and signs of intravascular clotting in patients treated for louse-borne relapsing fever may be due to a Jarisch-Herxheimer reaction via the release of endotoxins from dying spirochetes (43[C]).

Liver and pancreas A clinical syndrome with often fatal outcome has become recognized as a complication of high tetracycline doses. It is characterized by nausea, vomiting, spiking fever, frequently also jaundice, acidosis, uremia, possibly hematemesis and melena and terminal hypotensive shock. The histopathological findings are those of diffuse *fatty liver degeneration* (44[C]—46[C]). Though the syndrome was primarily described in pregnant women, it is not restricted to this patient group. Diminished renal function and thus impaired renal elimination of tetracyclines as well as serious infections may increase the risk of this complication (44[C], 46[C]). Since the introduction of tetracycline preparations effective in a dosage below 1 gram per day, the syndrome of fatty liver with severe hepatic insufficiency due to tetracyclines has become rare (45[C]). But liver enzymes and renal function should be controlled, especially in risk situations.

Pancreatitis is a common feature of the clinical syndrome, though it has also been observed without overt liver disease in a patient following two separate exposures (47[C]).

Gastrointestinal The syndrome of *stomatitis*, other signs of *irritation of the oropharynx* as well as *a rash* in and around the orifices have been described. They may partly be considered as mucous membrane manifestation of allergic or toxic origin. The overgrowth of pathogenic organisms as fungal strains, mainly *Candida albicans*, viral or bacterial infections has always to be considered (48[C]).

Nausea, *vomiting* and *epigastric burning* represent the most common side effects seen with tetracycline therapy. This is also true for the lower-dosed preparations. The symptoms are usually mild and seldom necessitate discontinuation of treatment. Nausea occurs in 8—15% of treated patients according to these reports.

Esophageal ulcers have been described in association with oral doxycycline or tetracycline therapy in several patients by a number of gastroenterologists. The symptoms were acute substernal burning pain and dysphagia within hours of taking the last capsule (49[C], 50[R], 51[C]—53[C]). Often, remaining parts of the ingested capsule have been identified by esophagoscopy.

Hence, patients should not lie down immediately after taking a tetracycline capsule and the preparation should be swallowed with generous quantities of water (50[C], 54[C]).

Enterocolitis See 'Diarrhea and antibiotic-associated colitis' in Chapter 25.2.

Urinary system *Renal insufficiency and anti-anabolic effect* Patients with renal insufficiency are particularly prone with most tetracycline preparations to develop an elevation of blood urea nitrogen, serum phosphate and sulfate. These changes may be associated with acidosis and even symptoms of uremia. By measurement of diuresis alone, renal dysfunction may be missed, since cases of non-oliguric renal failure have been reported (55[C]). Interstitial nephritis is an extremely rare complication (34[c], 35[c], 36[R]).

It is characteristic for many cases of uremia that the serum creatinine remains unchanged during tetracycline therapy whereas blood urea values rise temporarily. All tetracycline preparations have an anti-anabolic effect. They inhibit the synthesis of protein from amino acids in the patient, just as they do in bacteria. Several studies report increased urea production resulting in a negative nitrogen balance during tetracycline therapy and the phenomenon was hence termed 'anti-anabolic effect' (56[C], 57[C]). Azotemia may be increased additionally by water and sodium depletion due to the diuretic effect of some tetracyclines (57[C]).

Most observations indicate that a determining factor for the risk of renal insufficiency is a relative overdose of the drug in patients with pre-existing renal damage (38[C], 39[C]) (see also 'Mineral and fluid balance'). The half-life values of tetracyclines eliminated by the kidney are thereby increased to several times normal (58[C]). With normal renal function, 20—70% of an intravenously applied tetracycline dose is eliminated through the kidney by glomerular filtration. Maintenance therapy must be adjusted to the degree of renal impairment. Tetracyclines are removed by hemodialysis, however to a significantly lesser degree than creatinine or urea (44[C], 58[C]). Only doxycycline and minocycline are almost completely eliminated through the liver and the biliary tract.

For intravenous application, doxycycline is rendered soluble with polyvinylpyrrolidone. The clearance of this substance is less than that of doxycycline. In patients with a creatinine serum level of more than 250 μmol/l (3 mg/100 ml) it is therefore advisable to limit the duration of treatment to a few days.

Acquired *Lignac-De Toni-Fanconi syndrome* with polyuria, polydipsia, glucosuria, aminoaciduria, hyperphosphaturia and hypercalciuria was described in a number of patients treated with outdated tetracycline preparations. The degeneration products responsible for the toxic action probably are epitetracycline, anhydro-4-epitetracycline and anhydrotetracycline (59[C]) as similar renal damage could be produced in rats with anhydro-4-epitetracycline (60[C]).

Skin and appendages Pronounced *photosensitivity of the skin* and also, if exposed to sunlight, of the *nails* is a complication of systemic therapy with tetracyclines. It has been described with various tetracyclines and presumably may occur with any preparation. The skin changes resemble those of minor to severe sunburn with erythema, edema or even papules and blisters as well as urticaria (61[C], 62[C]). In some circumstances they may resemble cutaneous porphyria and therefore were described as 'porphyria-like cutaneous changes' (63[C]). *Onycholysis* is associated with nail discolouration. Dystrophy is usually preceded by photosensitivity reactions of the skin (64[C]). According to the degree and area of light exposure, onycholysis may affect also the toe nails (61[C]) and, in contrast to idiopathic onycholysis, it affects not only women, but men as well (65[R]).

As a rule, the *pathogenesis* of skin reactions promoted by sunlight exposure are probably phototoxic. This is supported by the high occurrence rate (up to nine out of 10 patients), depending on sun exposure and drug dosage. From experimental studies a wavelength close to 320 nm within the ultraviolet spectrum was identified as the most potential to induce phototoxic reactions (66[C]).

Pigmentation due to tetracyclines is frequently encountered in patients treated with tetracyclines, however the real risk remains unknown. In contrast to phototoxic reactions, pigmentations may appear even without light exposure and present no signs of inflammation. Pigment deposits were observed in the light-exposed and non exposed skin, the conjunctiva, in the oral mucosa, on the tongue, as well as in inner organs such as the thyroid and heart valve endothelium (26[C], 27[c], 67[C]—74[C]). The pigment is presumed to be a drug—melanin—calcium complex and depends on the chelating properties of the tetracycline molecule. Tetracycline-induced pigmentation has been observed with the newer and lower-dose preparations as well as with the former preparations and presumably occurs with all tetracyclines. Though pigmentation usually tends to persist after termination of tetracycline therapy, it does not provoke any symptoms or organ dysfunction, except for cosmetic problems. A number of recent observations published, often concerning patients treated for acne, may possibly be due to a higher incidence of long-term treatments (75[C]), though there is no evidence that the true risk has really changed.

Tooth discoloration is due to deposition of tetracyclines in the form of calcium complexes in the mineralizing zones of the teeth and hence seems pathogenically related to the pigmentation of other organs. It occurs when tetracyclines are present during the formation of the teeth. Tetracyclines pass through the placenta and can be found in considerable amounts in the mother's milk (76[C]). As mineralization of the deciduous teeth takes place from the fourth month of intrauterine life until 1 year after birth and continues for the permanent teeth up to the age of 7—8 years (77[C]), pregnant women after the third month of pregnancy, nursing women and children under the age of 8 years should not be treated with tetracyclines. Discoloration of the teeth following intrauterine exposure to tetracyclines was observed in up to 50% of children at risk and was especially high when tetracyclines were administered during the last trimester (77[C]). Besides its merely cosmetic aspect, tooth discoloration in children is associated with enamel defects and hypoplasia in severe cases (78[C]). Adult-onset tooth discoloration coincident with minocycline administration has been observed in four of 72 patients (79[C]).

Allergic skin and mucous membrane reactions are observed with a very low incidence in the range of 0.3%, which lies about 10-fold below the incidence of such reactions in patients treated with other antibiotics (80[C]). A generalized rash may appear during tetracycline treatment. Various forms have been described including generalized urticaria, maculopapular rash, erythema exsudativum multiforme-like eruptions and rare cases of Stevens-Johnson syndrome (64[C], 81[C], 82[C], 83a[R]). Even acute generalized exanthematous pustulosis has been described (83b[c]). Fixed drug eruptions due to the systemically applied drug are rare (84[C]—86[C]) as is serum sickness-like syndrome (5[c], 87[C]).

Allergic *contact dermatitis* induced by local application of a tetracycline preparation with positive patch tests is an exception compared to other antibiotics (64[C], 88[C]—90[C]).

Genital system *Monilial infections of the vulva and vagina* seem to appear more frequently, even without other predisposing factors such as diabetes, pregnancy, immunodeficiency, oral contraceptives and corticosteroids. They are also found in patients treated with other antibiotics (91[C]). *Candida albicans* is not always the cause of vaginitis. The same holds true for balanitis observed in men (92[C]). If symptoms persist or change in patients treated for urethritis or adnexitis, this may be due to a treatment failure, because the putative microorganism is resistant to tetracyclines, rather than an adverse effect (93[R]).

Eyes Acute transitory myopia was described as an effect of tetracycline therapy, probably due to changes in refractive power (94[C]). Tetracyclines, especially demeclocycline, are among the most effective ocular hypotensive agents according to studies in rabbits and cats, whatever the biochemical mechanism of the action is. The prolonged effect and apparent lack of adverse ocular side effects suggest their possible usefulness for antiglaucoma therapy in man (SEDA-15, 260).

Bone The *deposition* of tetracycline in bone tissue has been demonstrated by early animal studies (95[C]) and was shown to occur in men as well (96[C]).

Whereas the bone of adult patients treated with tetracycline has shown depositions of the drug only in areas of repair or remodelling, the bones of children contain extensive areas. Tetracycline deposition in bone has been reported to have an effect on longitudinal bone growth (97[C]). In experimental studies on tissue cultures it was shown that osteogenesis is impaired by tetracyclines in concentrations similar to that considered to be a normal therapeutic serum level (i.e. 1 μg/ml) (98[C]). The deposition of tetracyclines in human bone begins in utero as early as in the first trimester of pregnancy (96[C]). With regular tissue turn-over the depositions disappear.

Jarisch-Herxheimer reaction It is common in patients treated for louse-borne relapsing fever (43[C]).

Two forms of reaction are described at the beginning of tetracycline therapy: (a) fever, rigor, increase of respiratory and pulse rates, perhaps with delirium and coma (99[R]); (b) fever and disseminated intravascular clotting (100[R]). A Jarisch-Herxheimer type of reaction seems likely, since at about the time the temperature reaches its peak, spirochetes disappear from the peripheral blood (99[R]). Meptazinol, a partial opioid antagonist, diminishes the Jarisch-Herxheimer reaction of relapsing fever (101[C]).

Risk situations The risk situations include inadequate dosage adaptation in patients with renal insufficiency and the appearance of liver damage and nephropathy in pregnant women. Tetracycline metabolism and excretion do not seem altered per se in pregnancy. The severe effects occur almost exclusively with doses over 1.0 g/day (45[C]) or in the treatment of pyelonephritis with concomitantly impaired renal function. In addition, during pregnancy the liver may be more sensitive to disturbances in protein synthesis.

Intensive irradiation with sunlight may produce a photo-sensitivity reaction of the skin, especially under demeclocycline. A pigmentation of the skin is also favoured by the interaction of sunlight and relatively high doses or long-term treatment with tetracyclines.

Second-generation effects Discoloration of the milk teeth is particularly likely if tetracycline therapy is given to the mother after the third month of pregnancy (102[C]). In any case, the tetracyclines pass through the placental barrier and reach therapeutic concentrations in the fetal circulation (77[C], 103[C]). Embryotoxic effects were demonstrated as evidenced by higher intrauterine death rate and rate of congenital anomalies in general (104[C]) and congenital cataracts (105[C]) in fetuses exposed to tetracyclines. The distinction between the drug and an underlying, unidentified virus infection as culprit is often impossible.

In view of their effects on the teeth and similarly on the bones, as well as in view of an increased risk of potentially fatal fatty liver degeneration in pregnant women, tetracycline preparations should not be prescribed during pregnancy with the exception of a vital indication. They should equally be avoided in children younger than 8 years.

Interactions Combining the tetracyclines with *antacids* or other drugs containing bi- or trivalent cations such as calcium, magnesium or iron is contraindicated. Tetracycline preparations combine with such bi- and trivalent cations to form complexes which are very poorly or not at all absorbed (25[C]). The same holds true for simultaneously administered oral iron preparations (106[C]). Both, tetracyclines as well as iron, are scarcely absorbed in this condition (107[C]). *Antidiarrheal drugs* such as kaolin-pectin and bismuth products (108[C], 109[C]) impair the absorption of tetracyclines in the same way. Besides chelation of drug metal complexes, a direct inhibition of active mucous membrane transports may be effected by the complexes. To avoid the interaction a time interval of 2–3 hours between the ingestion of the tetracycline and iron preparation is recommended (107[C]). Similarly decreased bioavailability results from simultaneous intake of abundant quantities of milk or milk products.

The combination of tetracyclines with *diuretics* is especially detrimental to renal function (110[C]). Though not described so far, the same may be true for angio-converting enzyme inhibitors or other drugs which often impair renal function.

In patients treated with oral or parenteral tetracyclines and *methoxyflurane anesthesia* renal failure and oxalate crystal formation in renal tissue was described as an interacting effect of the combination (111[c], 112[C], 113[C]). Therefore tetracycline administration in preoperative patients is not recommended.

Black galactorrhea under minocycline and a *phenothiazine* combined in a lactating mother was described (114[c]).

In patients under anticoagulant therapy with *vitamin K antagonists*, the use of tetracyclines does not interfere with anticoagulation as vitamin K production by intestinal bacteria is of little importance compared with that obtained through food intake (115[C]).

INDIVIDUAL TETRACYCLINES

The spectrum of bacterial effectiveness is fairly similar for the various tetracyclines. Metabolism and excretion may, however, vary. In general, preference is currently given to those preparations requiring relatively low dosage (not over 1.0 g daily).

Tetracycline (chlortetracycline) and oxytetracycline These are incompletely absorbed from the gastrointestinal tract. Plasma concentration declines with a half-life of 6–12 hours. Both are predominantly excreted by the kidney, extrarenal elimination amounting at most to 10–20% of the ingested drug. For chemical reasons the two preparations have lower affinity for fat and membranes, so that in fact higher doses are required for effectiveness. This, however, may contribute to an increased risk of systemic toxic effects and, as absorption from oral administration is incomplete, also to an increased risk of gastrointestinal adverse reactions.

Demeclocycline (demethylchlortetracycline) produces a significantly higher rate of phototoxic skin reactions than do other preparations, presumably due to its long half-life of about 16 hours with effective plasma concentrations to 24 to 48 hours and an even longer lasting accumulation of the drug in membranes and fatty tissue. Demeclocycline is eliminated to about 20 to 40% by glomerular filtration. In patients with liver cirrhosis, with cardiac failure or decreased renal function, it should be used cautiously because of its pronounced effect on electrolyte and fluid balance (28[C]).

Doxycycline and minocycline These are more lipophilic.They are absorbed well after oral administration. Serum concentration is halved only after 16 to 18 hours. The higher affinity to fatty tissue of both preparations improves their effectiveness and also their risk benefit profile with regard to side effects. Especially local gastrointestinal irritation and biological disturbance of the intestinal bacterial flora are less frequent compared to the more hydrophilic preparations which have to be administered in higher oral doses for sufficient absorption. Nevertheless, the toxic effects similar to any tetracycline preparation, which arise from accumulation of the drugs in fatty tissue and go in parallel with effective concentrations at the site of wanted action are not at all eliminated. Accumulation of the drug in a third space and its hereby resulting long half-life time in long-term treatment may contribute to increased incidence of various toxic side effects, even if lower daily doses are administered. This seems to be true at least for pigmentation disorders and possibly for neurological disturbances (18[C]).

Minocycline and doxycycline are eliminated predominantly (70—90%) by the liver and biliary tract so that no dose adaption in impaired renal function is needed. However, it has to be considered that hepatic elimination of doxycyline or minocycline may be accelerated when agents that induce liver enzymes are administered simultaneously.

Methacycline Methacycline is eliminated to about equal parts by the hepatic and renal pathway. Special problems of therapy with this rarely used tetracycline derivate have not been reported (116[R]).

Resistance Resistance to tetracyclines shows marked inter-regional variations and changes rapidly in the course of time. With regard to tetracyclines the selection of resistant bacterial strains may be favoured by widespread, often prophylactic, use in veterinary medicine and by long-term therapy for acne, periodontal disease or symptomatic *Borrelia* infections. Much of the proven resistances have lesser practical significance, since the tetracyclines are merely one of a number of different therapeutic alternatives. The problem may be pronounced in situations where they represent the chemotherapeutic of the first choice, i.e. in chronic *Borrelia* infections, especially Lyme arthritis and pulmonary or bubonic plague due to *Yersinia pestis* (117[R]). Even in the case of mere suspicion of plague and its possible epidemiological impact, immediate initiation of tetracycline treatment is recommended, although the microbiological proof of *Yersinia pestis* infection takes several days (117[R]). For chlamydial or mycoplasma infections, effective alternative antibiotics are nowadays available, and increasing frequency of resistant strains of genital mycoplasma may be the reason for treatment failures (93[C], 118[C]). A rather high amount 25 to 50% of resistant *Haemophilus* species is reported (119[C]), which has to be taken into consideration if tetracyclines are administered in chronic pulmonary diseases or for treatment of acute respiratory infections. For *Neisseria gonorrhoea* infections, tetracyclines are not indicated, due to the higher prevalence of resistance, especially among penicillinase-producing strains (120[C]). For these patients, better alternatives of antibiotics are usually available.

CHLORAMPHENICOL AND THIAMPHENICOL

Chloramphenicol

Chloramphenicol is one of the older broad-spectrum antibiotics which, after its introduction in 1948, grew in popularity because of its high antimicrobial activity against a wide range of gram-negative and gram-positive bacteria, rickettsial organisms, *Chlamydia* and *Mycoplasma*. It is particularly useful in infections due to *Salmonella typhi* and *Haemophilus influenzae*. The effect of chloramphenicol is mainly bacteriostatic. It readily crosses tissue barriers and diffuses rapidly through nearly all tissues and body fluids. The main route of elimination is metabolic transformation by glucuronidation. The microbiologically inactive metabolites are excreted rapidly and there is only a small proportion of unchanged drug excreted in the urine. The usual daily dose is 1—2 grams for adults and 50 mg/kg for children over 2 months. The total dose should not exceed 3.0—3.5 g/70 kg body weight. The recommendation that neither the dose nor the interval of chloramphenicol administration needs to be adjusted in patients with significant renal dysfunction (121[R]), probably has to be modified in view of recent findings (122[C]).

By 1950, it became evident that the drug could cause serious and fatal blood dyscrasias. Its use has therefore steadily declined during the past 25—30 years. Since the risk of serious chloramphenicol toxicity, however, is so small (1:18 000 or probably less) the drug is of more than historical interest. There are still many areas where its benefits outweigh its risks. These include: (a) typhoid and paratyphoid fever; (b) other septic forms of *Salmonella* infections; (c) meningitis due to *H. influenzae*, *Streptococcus pneumoniae* and *Neisseria meningitidis* when the patient is allergic to β-lactam antibiotics or when the strains (*H. influenzae*, Enterobacteriaceae) are resistant to amino-penicillins and cephalosporins; (d) brain abscess; and (e) serious infections caused by *Bacteroides fragilis* (as an alternative to clindamycin or metronidazole). Since chloramphenicol is still one of the cheapest antibiotics ever made, in developing countries, where chloramphenicol may be more readily available than the expensive newer antibiotics, this list of indications is rightly longer. In conditions, however, which can be readily, safely and effectively treated with alternative antimicrobial agents, these should be preferred.

Chloramphenicol and its metabolites act primarily on the 50S ribosomal subunit with suppression of the activity of the enzyme, peptidyltransferase. The drug has been found to inhibit mitochondrial membrane protein synthesis, leading to suppression of mitochondrial respiration and ultimately to cessation of cell proliferation (123[C]). Analogous mechanisms may be operative in production of the reversible type of bone marrow depression, which is the most prominent toxic effect in patients being treated with chloramphenicol. Its potency to induce toxic effects on mitochondria in maturing or rapidly proliferating eukaryotic cells is very close to that for inhibiting prokaryotic cells (bacteria and blue-green algae). Little progress, however, has been made in elucidation of the pathogenesis of irreversible marrow aplasia (123[C]—125[C]) (see below).

ADVERSE REACTION PATTERN

General and toxic reactions Chloramphenicol has been associated with two serious but rare toxic effects, each with a high mortality. One is the 'gray syndrome', a vasomotor collapse in newborn infants caused by excessive parenteral doses. The second is bone marrow aplasia which is not dose dependent (see also under 'Hypersensitivity reactions'). Prolonged use can result in neuropathies. Mild gastrointestinal disturbances are common. Jarisch-Herxheimer reactions can occur.

Hypersensitivity reactions These are commonly mild and more frequent with topical use (allergic contact dermatitis, rashes, glossitis). The late, severe type of bone marrow reaction may be of allergic origin.

Tumor-inducing effects These have not been described; a statement that chloramphenicol might induce cancer in the fetus appears to be purely speculative.

ORGANS AND SYMPTOMS

Cardiovascular, respiratory Systemic reactions with collapse, bronchial spasm, angioedema and urticaria occur only rarely (126[R], 127[C]).

Nervous system and special senses Local application of chloramphenicol preparations may cause *hearing defects*. After treatment of chronic bilateral otitis media with chloramphenicol powder, asymmetrical hearing loss with lowered perception of high tones has been documented (128[R]). For chloramphenicol eardrops, propylene glycol is often used as a vehicle. Ototoxicity may then be due to chloramphenicol and/or to propylene glycol which itself is strongly ototoxic. A recent report shows that ototoxic effects can also occur after systemic drug application (129[c]).

Neurological and ocular effects Optical and peripheral neuropathy have been seen after prolonged courses of treatment with chloramphenicol. Alterations in color perception and optical neuropathy, in some cases resulting in optic atrophy and blindness, have been observed, especially in children with cystic fibrosis receiving relatively high doses for many months (130[C], 131[C]). Most of these complications were reversible and have been attributed to a deficiency of B-vitamins.

Hematological Chloramphenicol may produce two types of bone marrow damage: (a) a frequent early and dose-dependent reversible suppression of the formation of erythrocytes, thrombocytes and granulocytes ('early toxicity') and (b) a rare, late type of bone marrow aplasia, which is unrelated to dosage, is generally irreversible and has a high mortality rate ('aplastic anemia').

Early toxicity The early, dose-dependent type of chloramphenicol toxicity is usually seen after the second week of treatment and is characterized by inhibited proliferation of erythroid cells and decreased incorporation of iron into heme. The clinical correlates in the peripheral blood are anemia, reticulocytopenia, normoblastosis and a shift to early erythrocyte forms. The plasma iron concentration is increased. Early erythroid forms and granulocyte precursors show cytoplasmic vacuolation. After cessation of therapy, complete recovery is the rule. Leukopenia and thrombocytopenia are less frequent.

Although there is no evidence that these abnormalities may progress to frank bone-marrow aplasia, continuation of chloramphenicol therapy after the appearance of early toxicity is thought to be hazardous. Preexisting liver damage due to infectious hepatitis or alcoholism and impaired kidney function may lead to decreased elimination of chloramphenicol and its metabolites, thereby aggravating marrow toxicity. As a rule, this is not the irreversible type.

Aplastic anemia Although bone marrow aplasia has not been related with certainty either to the daily or total dose of chloramphenicol or to the sex or age of the patients, it has occurred almost exclusively in individuals who were undergoing prolonged therapy, particularly if they had been exposed to the drug on more than one occasion (132[R]). The condition has been quite rare, occurring about once in every 18 000–50 000 subjects in various countries. These variations may depend on ethnic factors (133[C], 134[C]). There have been very few blacks among the victims (135[C]). Bone marrow aplasia due to chloramphenicol has usually resulted in aplastic anemia with pancytopenia; other forms such as red cell hypoplasia, selective leukopenia or thrombocytopenia are less common.

When bone marrow aplasia was complete, the fatality rate approached 100%. As a rule, it has been found that the longer the interval between the last dose of chloramphenicol and the appearance of the first sign of a blood dyscrasia, the more severe the resulting aplasia. Nearly all patients in whom the interval was longer than 2 months have died as a result of this complication. Fatal aplastic anemia may, however, also occur shortly after the administration of normal doses of chloramphenicol (136[C]).

The pathogenesis of bone marrow aplasia following chloramphenicol treatment is still uncertain. Compared with normal cells, bone marrow aspirates from patients with the clinical manifestation of marrow aplasia have been found to be relatively resistant to the toxic effects of chloramphenicol in vitro. This observation has been explained by the suggestion that during treatment with chloramphenicol, the sensitive cells had been eliminated, leaving behind only a chloramphenicol-insensitive population of blood cell precursors with poor proliferative capacity (137[C]).

Since thiamphenicol, which causes very few cases of aplastic anemia, differs from chloramphenicol by substitution of the *p*-nitro group by a methylsulfonyl group, interest has focused on the *p*-nitro group and metabolites of that part of the molecule: nitrosochloramphenicol and chloramphenicol hydroxylamine.

In human bone marrow, nitrosochloramphenicol inhibited DNA synthesis at 10% of the concentration of chloramphenicol required for the same effect. Proliferation of myeloid progenitors was irreversibly inhibited by that metabolite. The covalent binding of nitrosochloramphenicol to marrow cells was 15 times greater than that of chloramphenicol (138[R]). This fact has lent support to the hypothesis that abnormal metabolism may contribute to the susceptibility to bone marrow aplasia. The production of reductive derivatives by intestinal microbes may contribute to the toxicity, but the oral administration of chloramphenicol is not essential for the development of aplastic anemia (139[C]). Slight evidence has been advanced that a genetic predisposition may play a role (140[C], 141[R]). The wide geographical variations in incidence of aplastic anemia may also reflect environmental factors.

For many years, it had been stated that there were no cases of aplastic anemia following parenteral administration of chloramphenicol. However, a few cases of aplastic anemia due to parenteral chloramphenicol have been reported (142[C]). There have also been two reports of bone marrow hypoplasia following the use of chloramphenicol eyedrops (143[C], 144[c]).

Development of leukemia In a small fraction of those patients who survive the chronic type of bone marrow damage, a myeloblastic leukemia may develop (145[R], 146[C]). In most instances, this complication appeared within a few months of the diagnosis of aplasia and was considered to be a sequel to chloramphenicol treatment; the delay has sometimes been shorter. The majority were either children or adults aged between 50 and 70 years.

Gastrointestinal Mild, dose-dependent gastrointestinal disturbances are common.

Skin and appendages Hypersensitivity seems to develop about four times more frequently after topical than after oral use. In fact, there has been a continuous increase in chloramphenicol hypersensitivity due to the application of dermatological preparations (147[R]). The symptoms of allergic contact dermatitis and macular or vesicular skin rashes are usually limited to skin areas previously exposed to the drug. Contact conjunctivitis has also been reported.

Gray syndrome This syndrome is characterized by an ashen gray, cyanotic color of the skin, a fall in body temperature, vomiting, a protuberant abdomen, refusal to suck, irregular and rapid respiration, and lethargy. It is mainly seen in newborn infants, particularly when premature. It usually begins 2–9 days after the start of treatment.

Inadequate glucuronyl transferase activity combined with decreased glomerular filtration in the neonatal period is responsible for a longer half-life and accumulation of the drug. In addition, the potency of chloramphenicol to inhibit protein synthesis is higher for proliferating cells and tissues. The most important abnormality seems to be a respiratory deficiency of mitochondria, due, for example, to suppressed synthesis of cytochrome oxidase. In the light of the data now available, the dose should be adjusted according to the age of the neonate and blood levels should be monitored. In most cases of gray syndrome, the daily dose of chloramphenicol has been higher than 25 mg/kg (148[R], 149[R]).

Occasionally, treatment of older children and teenagers with large doses of chloramphenicol (approx. 100 mg/kg) has resulted in a similar form of vasomotor collapse (150[c]) (see 'Second-generation effects').

Jarisch-Herxheimer reaction Patients with typhoid fever receiving full doses of chloramphenicol at the start of treatment may run the risk of a Herxheimer reaction. The shock-like symptoms may be due to the release of bacterial endotoxins.

Adverse microbiological effects The number and types of microorganisms that constitute the normal microflora of the alimentary, respiratory and genital tracts are changed during therapy with chloramphenicol. Superinfections may then develop with *Staphylococcus aureus*, *Pseudomonas*, *Proteus*, and fungi. The changes in intestinal flora may be partly responsible for a decrease in synthesis of vitamin K-dependent clotting factors, especially in patients with severe illness and malnutrition or during administration of oral anticoagulants.

Bacterial resistance Reports of chloramphenicol-resistant *H. influenzae* are available from various countries, but cases are very few in number (151[c]). Outbreaks of chloramphenicol-resistant *Salmonella typhi* have been observed in several countries (152[C], 153[C]).

Risk situations Chloramphenicol should be avoided in *premature infants* and the *newborn* as well as in the *late phase of pregnancy* (see below) (154[R]). Pre-existing *blood dyscrasia* is generally considered to be an absolute contraindication. *Liver damage* with a reduced clearance of chloramphenicol, and *impaired kidney function* may also be risk factors.

In pediatric patients, a high cumulative dose seems to be an important factor of risk. As leukopenia can start early in treatment, a complete blood count every third day is recommended (SEDA-15, 267).

Second-generation effects Chloramphenicol penetrates into the fetal circulation and has been found in relatively large amounts in maternal milk. It should, therefore, be avoided during the last phase of pregnancy and during breast-feeding (155[C]). The gray syndrome has been observed in babies born to mothers who had received chloramphenicol in the final stage of pregnancy (see 'Gray syndrome').

The drug is not regarded as embryotoxic in man, clinical experience outweighing some animal evidence to the contrary.

Interactions Chloramphenicol may interfere with the elimination of those drugs which are inactivated by hepatic metabolism probably through a mechanism involving inhibition of microsomal enzymes. The ability of chloramphenicol to retard the biotransformation of *tolbutamide*, *phenytoin*, *oral anti-coagulants* and *cyclophosphamide* is well established and clinically relevant (156[C], 157[R]). The mechanism has been claimed to be an inactivation of microsomal enzymes via an intermediate reactive metabolite which covalently binds to the protein moiety of cytochrome P-450 (157[R]). If this is so, chloramphenicol should interact with the metabolism of other drugs dealt with by the P-450 system. On the other hand, *paracetamol* leads to a prolongation of the half-life of chloramphenicol. The interaction is of importance in developing countries where chloramphenicol, as the usual treatment of typhoid fever, is often combined with an antipyretic. Conversely, *phenytoin*, *phenobarbital* and *rifampicin* (158[c], 159[C]) may increase the rate of chloramphenicol metabolism and thus lead to abnormally low serum chloramphenicol levels.

Thiamphenicol

Thiamphenicol is a semisynthetic derivative of chloramphenicol. It differs in that the NO_2 group in the *para*-position is replaced by a methylsulfonyl group. Investigational data so far available seem to show that the substitution of the *para*-position of the molecule has not influenced its effect on either protein or DNA synthesis in any recognizable way. The antibacterial spectrum is almost identical to that of chloramphenicol. The two drugs are employed in similar dosages, although there are great differences between thiamphenicol and chloramphenicol with regard to their mode of elimination. Glucuronidation is unimportant for thiamphenicol. Over 90% of a therapeutic dose is excreted by the kidneys in unchanged form, whereas the corresponding figure for chloramphenicol is only about 10%. Thus, in contrast to chloramphenicol, the half-life of thiamphenicol is prolonged in patients with reduced renal function in whom cumulation can occur.

Although the mechanism by which chloramphenicol induces aplastic anemia is not exactly known, all the available evidence suggests that the biochemical consequences of thiamphenicol administration and the risk of serious complications differ from those of chloramphenicol (160[R]).

It does not seem unreasonable, therefore, to use thiamphenicol with wider indications than chloramphenicol, provided the creatinine level is used for dosage adjustments. At the same time, thiamphenicol does have adverse effects on bone marrow, calling for a degree of caution in its use; the general rule that thiamphenicol treatment should not exceed 10—14 days has been accepted by many authors.

The most important adverse effects are an immediate dose-dependent and reversible disturbance of erythropoiesis (161[R], 162[R]) and peripheral neuropathy. In contrast to chloramphenicol, aplastic anemia and the gray syndrome do not seem to occur after thiamphenicol.

Nervous system Several observations of peripheral neuropathy following the administration of thiamphenicol for periods of 3—5 months have been reported and were thought to be due to a vitamin deficiency. In most cases, the sensory function of the nerves of the lower extremities was primarily affected. When discovered early, the damage was reversible, but in other cases it tended to persist (163[R]).

Hematological Concerning the early dose-dependent, and therefore predictable, type of hematotoxicity, evidence is accumulating that thiamphenicol is more potent than chloramphenicol. Many studies clearly show that thiamphenicol in therapeutic doses of 1.5 grams and to a much lesser extent at a dose of 0.75 g/day, causes an immediate disturbance of erythropoiesis in almost every instance (164[C]). Alteration of the bone marrow becomes most evident in patients with renal disease and in elderly subjects, probably because of the physiological decrease in renal function. Leukocytes and thrombocytes are affected only to a slight degree (165[c]).

Most reviewers have been impressed by the fact that the cases of peripheral cytopenia reported in the literature were never accompanied by an aplastic bone marrow (124[C]). In the literature, there are some doubtful case reports of marrow aplasia in which factors such as advanced age (predisposing to antibiotic accumulation), neoplasia, concurrent treatment (myelotoxic drugs, anticoagulants) and major surgical interventions have to be mentioned. Even if these cases are to be ascribed to thiamphenicol, they fall within the normal spontaneous incidence of aplastic anemia (132[R], 166[r], 167[c], 168[C]).

The most severe hematological changes reported following treatment of typhoid fever and sepsis with relatively high doses of thiamphenicol have always been reversible upon withdrawal of the drug. The serum iron concentration returned to normal within a few days and was rapidly followed by reticulocytosis. Experimental results strongly suggest that the toxic effect of thiamphenicol is temporary and that the bone marrow recovery following the drug-induced suppression is complete with no subsequent risk of myelodysplasia or leukemic transformation (169[C]).

Depression of antibody formation Thiamphenicol has been demonstrated to possess immunosuppressive properties which are less well documented for chloramphenicol. These are ascribed to an effect on immunocompetent cells rather than on immunoglobulin synthesis. In animals, thiamphenicol prolonged the survival of skin homografts.

Gray syndrome No cases of gray syndrome have ever been observed with thiamphenicol, although there is no reason why it should not occur if pregnant women or infants receive sufficiently excessive doses.

Gastrointestinal Diarrhea, nausea or constipation occur in less than 10% of cases and are usually mild.

Skin and appendages Alopecia has been reported in patients with renal insufficiency. It may lead to complete baldness (164[c]). After withdrawal of the antibiotic, normal hair growth will recover. Reactions of the skin seem to be rare.

Risk situations Pre-existing bone marrow dysfunction, impaired renal function and prolonged treatment are considered to be the main risk factors.

Second-generation effects Although thiamphenicol penetrates into the fetal circulation and is distributed evenly in the tissues of the fetal compartment, no fetal abnormalities could be related to thiamphenicol administration during pregnancy. Since mitochondrial protein synthesis in the fetal liver has been shown to be inhibited at the drug levels normally attained, repeated administration of thiamphenicol to pregnant women is not recommended.

Interactions Biotransformation of other drugs may be retarded although this has not been so well documented as with chloramphenicol.

MACROLIDES

The group of macrolide antibiotics has established itself anew and firmly as an important pillar in the treatment of community-acquired infections. In addition, certain macrolides have found new indications in the treatment of opportunistic infections in HIV-infected patients (170[R]). Lastly, new macrolides have become popular due to their remarkable pharmacokinetic and safety features (171[R]). It comes therefore as no surprise that the leading product of past decades, erythromycin, has met fierce competition and has, at least in some health care systems, lost its place as the most important macrolide.

Parallel with this shift of attention to newer macrolides, attention has to shift to the discussion of adverse events and drug interactions experienced with the use of these compounds. In many instances, this discussion will sound familiar to physicians with knowledge of the profile of adverse events of erythromycin. Some new kinds of adverse events and drug interactions have been reported recently, while others may only become known in the future with our growing experience in the clinical use of these drugs.

The focus of this section will be on macrolides which are widely used in clinical practice. These include erythromycin, clarithromycin, roxithromycin and azithromycin. Other less frequently used macrolides, i.e. spiramycin, dirithromycin, flurithromycin, miocamycin, and rokitamycin, will be discussed to the extent that valid and clinically relevant information is available

The antibacterial spectrum of macrolides covers a broad range of pathogens. Most macrolides are active against gram-positive cocci, some gram-negative bacteria, including *Campylobacter*, *Haemophilus*, but not most Enterobacteriaceae. They are however very active against *Mycoplasma*, *Ureaplasma*, *Chlamydia*, *Legionella* and *Coxiella*. The activity against *Mycobacterium avium* complex, *Cryptosporidia* and *Toxoplasma* is quite variable between the newer macrolides (170[R]). Clinical experience regarding treatment of *Mycobacterium avium* complex (MAC) infections is largest with clarithromycin. The antibacterial activity of macrolides is based on the interference with protein synthesis by combining with a subunit of bacterial ribosomes. This generally results in a bacteriostatic effect.

ADVERSE REACTION PATTERN

The following paragraphs summarize the most important adverse reactions associated with the use of macrolides. While some of these reactions are common to several or all of the currently available macrolides, other reactions have only been reported with one particular drug. In addition to differences in the pattern of adverse reactions, there are differences in the rate of occurrence of these untoward events. Table 1 summarizes the frequency and rate of adverse reactions and premature discontinuation of the most widely used macrolides.

Table 1. *Frequency of adverse reactions to macrolides*

Drug (No. of patients)	Adverse reaction (%)	Premature discontinuation (%)	References
Erythromycin (112)	33	18.7	Anderson (180[C])
Clarithromycin (4291)	19.6	3.5[a]	Peters (304[R])
Roxithromycin (2917)	4.1	0.9	Young (298[R])
Azithromycin (3995)	12	0.7	Peters (307[R])
Dirithromycin (2825)	33.1	3.1	Brogden (181[R])

[a]Frequency dose related: At high doses (2000 mg/day) discontinuation rate 22%.

General and toxic reactions Macrolides are in general well tolerated and are clinically used over a fairly wide dose range, as is exemplified by the total daily dose range of clarithromycin (500–2000 mg). The rate of adverse reactions is dose-dependent as exemplified by the rate of adverse events to clarithromycin, which was higher with 2000 or 4000 mg in two doses per day than with 500 or 1000 mg per day (170[R]). A single oral dose of 3000 mg clarithromycin resulted in severe abdominal pain within 1 hour of administration in two patients (172[r]). Severe toxicity is very rarely observed with macrolides. Most adverse reactions are rated as either mild or moderate, regardless of the macrolide used.

Among 245 patients who were hospitalized because of toxic epidermal necrolysis or Stevens-Johnson syndrome, six patients had had exposure to macrolides within the week preceding the onset of illness (173[R]). The following antibiotics were used: erythromycin, roxithromycin (171[R]) and spiramycin (171[R]). Based on the results of a case-control study, the conclusion emerges that macrolides do not pose an excess risk for the development of this toxic complication (173[R]).

Hypersensitivity reaction Allergic anaphylactic reactions to macrolides are exceedingly uncommon, but anaphylaxis and acute respiratory distress have been reported (174[R], 175[R]). Skin tests with erythromycin were found positive for the immediate and or delayed type of hypersensitivity (176[r]). Also, a fixed drug eruption due to erythromycin has been observed (177[c]). A peculiar hypersensitivity reaction was reported in an employee of a pharmaceutical company. He developed attacks of

Table 2. *Frequency of organ system specific adverse events*[a]

Drug (No. of patients)	Gastrointestinal (%)	Nervous system (%)	Skin (%)
Erythromycin (112)	27	4	1
Clarithromycin (96)	6	2	0
Roxithromycin (2917)	3.9	0.4	0.7
Azithromycin (3995)	9.6	1.3	0.6
Dirithromycin (4263)	5.6	4.5	0.4

[a]For References see Table 1.

sneezing, coughing and breathlessness while working with spiramycin. The patient showed immediate positive skin prick tests to spiramycin and developed blood eosinophilia during asthma attacks (178[c]).

Tumor-inducing effects These have not been reported.

ORGANS AND SYSTEMS

Cardiovascular Cardiovascular reactions are rare, if macrolides are used in the absence of other drugs. Intravenous administration of erythromycin into peripheral veins results relatively frequently in thrombophlebitis, although the lactobionate form of erythromycin may be less irritating to veins than are other parenteral forms of erythromycin (179[R]). Clinically relevant cardiac adverse events may occur as a consequence of interactions between macrolides and other drugs (see 'Drug interactions' below).

Respiratory Adverse events involving the respiratory system were reported in 2% of patients receiving treatment with erythromycin stearate (180[C]). Similar rates of dyspnea, increased cough or asthma were reported for dirithromycin (181[R]). Recently, a beneficial effect on sputum rheology by low doses of clarithromycin was reported in patients with chronic pulmonary diseases such as chronic bronchitis (182[C]). Similar beneficial effects on sputum volume were observed with erythromycin in a patient with severe airway obstruction due to bronchorrhea (183[c]).

Nervous system and special senses Erythromycin has been associated with complications such as confusion, paranoia, visual hallucinations, fear, lack of control and nightmares. These suspected psychiatric side effects were seen within 12—48 hours of starting therapy with conventional doses. Such complications may even be under-reported (184[c], 185[C], 186[c], 187[c]). Table 2 lists the rates of adverse events affecting the nervous system attributed to erythromycin and newer macrolides.

Endocrine, metabolic Serum TSH levels are moderately but significantly decreased by troleandomycin compared with josamycin or placebo administered over a 10-day period. At the same time serum estradiol concentration was also significantly increased (188[C]).

Mineral and fluid balance There is no evidence for adverse effects of macrolides on these systems.

Hematological Hematological changes with macrolides are extremely rare. Isolated instances of neutropenia are occasionally reported.

Liver Cholestatic hepatitis, which is associated primarily with the use of erythromycin estolate, may be caused by other forms of erythromycin as well (189[C]). Symptoms usually begin after 10—20 days of treatment. The clinical presentation with nausea, vomiting and abdominal cramps may mimic acute cholecystitis or cholangitis. Fever, jaundice, leukocytosis, elevated serum transaminase levels and eosinophilia may be observed as well. In spite of histological changes compatible with cholestasis, such as periportal inflammatory infiltrates and occasionally hepatic necrosis, cessation of therapy is usually rapidly followed by the disappearance of symptoms. While it was speculated that a hypersensitivity reaction to the estolate ester rather than to the erythromycin itself was responsible for this adverse reaction (179[R], 190[C]), a more recent review lists erythromycin among the drugs that inhibit bile flow, without proposing a mechanism for this interference (191[r]). Although cholestatic hepatitis has been typically described in association with erythromycin use, newer macrolides are not totally free of this risk. A recent case report describes a gradual increase of bilirubin and transaminase levels during treatment of a *Mycobacterium chelonae* infection with clarithromycin. These alterations were quickly reversible after interruption of treatment but re-appeared with re-exposure of the patient to 1 gram of clarithromycin (192[C]).

Similar involvement of the liver has been seen with the ester of triacetyl oleandomycin, but not with the unesterified antibiotic. Macrolides such as josamycin, midecamycin and spiramycin, which do not form stable complexes with cytochrome P-450, rarely, if ever, produce cholestatic hepatitis.

Gastrointestinal The gastrointestinal adverse events are the most common untoward effects of this otherwise well-tolerated class of drugs (Table 2). Nausea and vomiting associated with abdominal pain and occasionally diarrhea may be minor and transitory or, in a small percentage of patients, become severe enough to result in premature discontinuation of the drug. The rate of these adverse events varies among the different antibiotics. In general, newer macrolides such as roxithromycin, clarithromycin or azithromycin are better tolerated and cause fewer adverse events than erythromycin.

Several studies have demonstrated that erythromycin

acts as a motilin receptor agonist (193[c], 194[c], 195[c]). This mechanism may be at least partially responsible for the gastrointestinal adverse events observed with macrolides. Clarithromycin and azithromycin may act on gastrointestinal motility in a similar way to erythromycin. In dogs, clarithromycin caused contractions and discomfort, as did erythromycin (196[c]). In healthy volunteers, oral clarithromycin (250 mg twice a day) resulted in a statistically significant increase in the number of postprandial antral contractions and antral motility (197[c]). Azithromycin also results in a significant increase in postprandial antral motility (198[c]).

Based on observations made in dogs and rabbits, clarithromycin is significantly less potent than azithromycin and erythromycin as an agonist for stimulation of smooth muscle contraction (199[c]). Therefore, a lower rate of gastrointestinal adverse events would be expected with clarithromycin than with azithromycin. As is shown in Table 2, this is the case. Since most of these data reflect data compiled from several studies, and since most have not been obtained by direct comparison of the various macrolides in single studies, the rates should be interpreted with caution. They most likely provide only an approximate indication of the rate of adverse events. Small differences in rates between individual macrolides will in most cases not be clinically useful indicators of the true risk for the occurrence of adverse events.

In contrast to the macrolides mentioned above, macrolides with a 16-membered lactone ring (josamycin, spiramycin, acetylspiramycin, leucomycin, tylocin, midecamycin, miocamycin, rokitamycin) have little, if any, motor-stimulating effects (196[c], 200[r]).

Urinary system There is no evidence for adverse effects of macrolides on this system.

Skin and appendages Skin rashes and fixed drug eruptions may occur during treatment with various macrolides but are considered to be rare (<1%).

Genital system There is no evidence for adverse effects of macrolides on this system.

Bone There is no evidence for adverse effects of macrolides on bone.

Eyes There is no evidence for adverse effects of macrolides on the visual system.

Pharmacokinetic drug interactions of macrolides

Although macrolides are in general well tolerated, the potential for adverse drug interactions should be kept in mind and the prescribing physician should be familiar with the drugs incriminated in such interactions. The following paragraphs will describe the mechanisms of drug interaction and provide a general overview of relevant drug interactions known so far.

The frequency and pattern of drug interactions is influenced by the chemical structure of the macrolide. The most important mechanism determining many drug interactions is the effect of macrolides on the hepatic cytochrome P-450 system. This system oxidizes macrolides following binding of the drug to oxidized (Fe^{3+}) cytochrome P-450 (201[R]). Binding of the macrolide to group IIIA cytochrome P-450 may have one of several consequences: oxidation may result in formation of a stable iron—metabolite complex, induction of cytochrome P-450 and metabolism of the antibiotic, or inactivation of cytochrome P-450 (201[R]).

Structural properties of the macrolides determine whether the drug metabolizing enzyme is induced or inactivated. Macrolides with a 14-membered lactone ring have a bigger potential of inhibition of cytochrome P-450 than bulkier macrolides with 15- or 16-membered lactone rings. Therefore it is useful to group the macrolides according to their molecular structure and their potential for drug interactions via the P-450 system (Table 3).

The differences regarding interaction with cytochrome P-450 are quite marked and may even be substantial between drugs categorized in the same group. Troleandomycin is a more potent inhibitor of microsomal drug metabolism than erythromycin, while josamycin, midecamycin and spiramycin have not been incriminated so far in causing drug interactions (202[c], 203[R]).

The clinical occurrence of interactions in a particular patient is difficult to predict. The effect of erythromycin on the cytochrome P-450 system plays an important role in determining various drug interactions (Table 4). Hepatic levels of cytochrome P-450 IIIA4 vary at least 10-fold among patients (204[c], 205[c]). The activity of this enzyme can be estimated by a erythromycin breath test (202[c]). In addition to the liver, mucosal cells of the small intestine commonly express cytochrome P-450 IIIA4, where it is responsible for significant first-pass metabolism of orally administered substrates (205[c]).

The following discussion will focus on interactions with drugs which are frequently prescribed in clinical practice. It is beyond the scope of this chapter to review all studies of drug interactions in detail. Instead, pertinent conclusions will be summarized here, while aspects particular to individual macrolides will be described below.

Ergotamine Clinically severe interactions between troleandomycin and ergotamine (206[C]—209[C]) resulting in ischemia of extremities are probably the consequence of raised serum levels of dihydroergotamine (210[c], 211[c]).

Table 3. *Molecular structure of macrolides and degree of interaction with cytochrome P-450*

Degree of interaction	Macrolide ring: 14-membered	15-membered	16-membered
High degree (Group 1)	Troleandomycin Erythromycin		
Low degree (Group 2)	Flurithromycin Clarithromycin Roxithromycin		Josamycin Midecamycin Miocamycin
Not incriminated (Group 3)	Dirithromycin	Azithromycin	Rokitamycin Spiramycin

Adapted from Periti et al. (201)

Table 4. *Drug interactions between macrolides and other drugs*

Interacting Drug	Erythromycin	Roxithromycin	Clarithromycin	Azithromycin	References
Theophylline	++	(+)	+	–	(201[R], 303[c], 301[C])
Methylprednisolone	+	ND	ND	–	(213[c])
Oral contraceptives	ND	–	–	ND	
Carbamazepine	++	–	++	–	(301[C], 225[C])
Triazolam, Midazolam	++	(+)	ND	–	(230[C])
Alfentanil	++	ND	ND	ND	(293[C])
Warfarin	++	–	–	–	(233[c], 306[C])
Cyclosporin	++	(+)	ND	+	(239[c], 309[c])
Digoxin	++	ND	++	ND	(242[C], 244[C])
Disopyramide	++	(+)	ND	ND	(246[C], 247[C])
Terfenadine Astenizole	++	ND	++	ND	(251[C])
Rifampicin Rifabutin	ND	ND	++	+?	(253[C]–257[C])
Zidovudine	ND	ND	+	–	(310[C])

++, clinically relevant; –, documented lack of interaction; +, potentially clinically relevant, ND, no published data; (+), probably insignificant interaction; ?, insufficient information to definitely judge relevance.

Although interactions between other macrolides and ergotamine have not been reported, current recommendations are to avoid the concomitant use of any macrolide and drugs containing ergotamines.

Theophylline and other xanthines The most frequently observed effects of macrolides on theophylline pharmacokinetics are increases of serum half-life ($t_{1/2}$), serum theophylline levels and reduction of serum clearance (201[R]). The interaction with theophylline is mainly seen with higher doses of macrolides and may result in theophylline toxicity (212[c]).

Methylprednisolone Some macrolides exert a dosage- and time-related effect on methylprednisolone elimination resulting in an increase in the $t_{1/2}$ and a decrease in clearance (213[c]). These changes were considered advantageous ('steroid sparing') in patients with asthma because of the possibility of using lower doses (214[C], 215[c]).

Oral contraceptives Most reports associating the occurrence of cholestatic jaundice with the concomitant use of oral contraceptives and macrolides mention troleandomycin as the causative agent (216[c]–219[c]). The exact mechanism of this interaction has not been established. Troleandomycin possibly inhibits the metabolism of estrogens and progestational agents (201[R]). In most patients jaundice persisted for more than a month after the antibiotic was discontinued.

Carbamazepine Significant increases in serum concentrations of carbamazepine due to decreased clearance (220[C]) and prolonged $t_{1/2}$ (221[c]–223[c]) resulting in toxicity manifested by confusion, somnolence, ataxia, vertigo, nausea and vomiting, have been observed in patients during treatment with macrolides (224[c], 225[C], 226[C]). Toxicity may become manifest rapidly after addition of the macrolide and abates quickly following discontinuation of the antibiotic (201[R]).

Triazolam, midazolam Interactions of macrolides with

these benzodiazepines are clinically relevant. Increases in serum concentration, area under the plasma concentration-time curve (AUC), serum $t_{1/2}$ and a decrease in clearance have been documented (227[C] 228[C], 229[c]). These changes may result in clinical signs such as prolonged psychomotor impairment, amnesia or loss of consciousness (230[C]).

Alfentanil The metabolism of alfentanil, a short-acting potent narcotic is inhibited by macrolide antibiotics, resulting in significant changes in $t_{1/2}$ and clearance (231[C]).

Warfarin Despite only modest effects of macrolides on warfarin serum concentrations and increases in prothrombin time (232[C]), morbidity caused by hemorrhage may be significant as illustrated by several case reports (233[c], 234[C]—237[C]). It is likely that this interaction may be potentiated by additional factors such as old age or dietary restrictions (232[C]).

Ciclosporin The pharmacokinetics of ciclosporin may also be altered by the co-administration of macrolides. Commonly observed changes include increases in ciclosporin AUC, peak plasma concentration and reductions in time to C_{max} and clearance (238[R], 239[c]—241[c]). Ciclosporin concentrations should therefore be monitored to minimize the risk of toxicity in patients receiving certain macrolides.

Digoxin Unlike the interactions mentioned above, the interaction between macrolide and digoxin is not a consequence of alterations of the cytochrome P-450 system. Increased digoxin plasma concentrations with subsequent severe nausea, vomiting and arrhythmia were associated with macrolide therapy (242[C]—244[C]). Digoxin is metabolized in the gastrointestinal tract by *Eubacterium lentum* (245[C]). The direct antibacterial effect of macrolides on *Eubacterium lentum* may decrease digoxin metabolism and increase digoxin bioavailability (203[R]).

Disopyramide The interaction between erythromycin and disopyramide was potentially fatal in two cases (246[C]). Disopyramide was shown to alter protein binding of both disopyramide and roxithromycin and this resulted in increased plasma concentrations of both drugs in vitro (247[C]). However, this effect has not been observed with roxithromycin in vivo.

Terfenadine, astemizole Toxic effects of both drugs have been reported in patients receiving concomitant treatment with macrolides, especially with clarithromycin (248[r], 249[r], 250[C], 251[C]). These toxicities were typically manifested by cardiac arrhythmias (torsades de pointes) and prolongation of the QT interval (252[c]).

Rifampin, rifabutin A new drug interaction involving mainly clarithromycin and possibly also azithromycin in interaction with rifabutin, and less commonly rifampin, was observed in patients receiving treatment for *Mycobacterium avium* complex (MAC) infections (253[C]). The interaction resulted in uveitis, probably as a result of increased rifabutin levels (254[C]—257[C]). On the other hand, drug interactions between rifabutin or rifampin and clarithromycin were proposed as explanation for reduced clarithromycin serum levels, if both drugs were used concomitantly (258[C]).

Miscellaneous drugs Based on case reports or small studies the potential for drug interactions between macrolides and the following drugs should be considered when using any one of these drugs together with a macrolide: bromocriptine (259[C]), lovastatin (260[c]), zidovudine and possibly other antiretroviral agents.

INDIVIDUAL MACROLIDES

Erythromycin

ADVERSE REACTION PATTERN

General and toxic reactions Erythromycin has been relatively well tolerated with the exception of gastrointestinal side effects (see below). Cholestasis resulting from the use of all forms of erythromycin is virtually the only serious illness induced by the drug. Local irritation (affecting the gastrointestinal system, the muscles or the veins, depending on the route of administration), is however common. Erythromycin may increase serum theophylline concentrations and occasionally cause symptoms of theophylline toxicity. Simultaneous use of triacetyloleandomycin and ergotamine in low doses may cause ergotism.

Hypersensitivity reactions These are rare, unless the above-mentioned liver reaction is to be regarded as allergic. They probably become clinically manifest in less than 0.5% of treated patients, and consist mainly of maculopapular rashes, pruritus, urticaria, and angioedema, but anaphylaxis and acute respiratory distress have also been reported. Skin tests with erythromycin were found positive for the immediate and/or delayed type of hypersensitivity (176[r]). Also, fixed drug eruption due to erythromycin has been observed (177[c]).

ORGANS AND SYSTEMS

Nervous system In addition to the symptoms of confusion, paranoia, visual hallucinations, etc., described earlier, ototoxicity resulting in hearing loss has been reported in patients treated with 4 grams or more per day of erythromycin lactobionate or the oral administration of large doses of erythromycin estolate (261[C]). This adverse event may be more likely in the presence of diminished renal function, but is usually reversible after therapy is discontinued.

Liver During treatment with erythromycin two different reactions are thought to occur (189[C], 262[R]). Administration of erythromycin as base or salt may be followed in 0—10% of cases by apparently benign increases in the transaminases ALT or AST, which may or may not recur upon rechallenge. In children, elevated transaminases were noted when daily doses of 40 mg/kg were given but not after 20 mg/kg. It is now recognized that reversible cholestatic jaundice may occur with all forms of erythromycin, including the base, propionate, stearate, ethylsuccinate and estolate (263[C]).

Most probably the differences in hepatotoxicity between the various erythromycin derivatives are of a quantitative rather than a qualitative nature (264[C], 265[C]). The potentially severe but rare cholestatic liver injury occurs perhaps in up to 2—4% of treated patients. This reaction generally starts 10—14 days after the beginning of therapy, but earlier after re-exposure, sometimes within 12—24 hours (266[R]).

The clinical presentation of erythromycin-induced cholestasis may be quite variable. It is rare in children under the age of 12 years, but it has also occurred in infants at 6 weeks of age. In infants, this syndrome of biliary obstruction may mimic acute cholecystitis, biliary atresia or neonatal hepatitis (267[c]). The syndrome at all ages often begins with abdominal pain, nausea, vomiting, pyrexia, pruritus and jaundice. It may, however, also be ushered in with severe acute upper abdominal pain or right subcostal tenderness simulating an acute abdomen, or it may resemble the clinical picture of obstructive jaundice. It may be associated with a skin rash and blood eosinophilia. Serum bilirubin, alkaline phosphatase and the transaminases are elevated. Histological examination typically shows intrahepatic cholestasis and periportal inflammatory infiltration with lymphocytes, neutrophils and disproportionate numbers of eosinophils (268[C]). These histological findings could be interpreted as reflecting a hypersensitivity reaction, but a recent review (191[r]) does not support this hypothesis. If erythromycin is promptly stopped, clinical signs often improve rapidly, although prolonged jaundice has been reported.

Cholestasis seems to be more frequent with the estolate of erythromycin than with erythromycin given as the base or its salts. This difference has been explained by better intestinal absorption of the ester.

Gastrointestinal The incidence of gastrointestinal symptoms including nausea, vomiting, abdominal discomfort, cramps, diarrhea and rectal irritation is higher than with tetracyclines and may range from 5 to 30% of patients, depending on the dosage. They seem to occur more frequently with 500 than with 250 mg doses. Usually they disappear within 24—48 hours after cessation of the antibiotic.

Erythromycin given intravenously should be restricted to as few patients as possible. It may cause severe abdominal cramps, probably by direct action on smooth muscle (269[c]—271[c]). Pylorospasm or even pyloric stenosis has been observed in neonates, manifesting after 1—2 days of treatment with erythromycin (272[C]).

Pseudomembranous colitis This complication is relatively rarely seen with macrolide use. Nevertheless, it has been reported in patients being treated with clarithromycin (see also SED-12, 597; 273[C]; 274[C]).

Special senses *Ototoxicity* High parenteral doses of erythromycin have resulted in transient perceptive deafness (275[R], 276[C], 277[r], 278[C]). Since renal and hepatic disease was a prominent feature of these patients, ototoxicity was thought to result from high blood levels (279[c]). The phenomenon differs from the permanent type of ototoxicity caused by aminoglycosides. Ototoxic reactions have also been observed after the use of esters of erythromycin such as stearate, ethylsuccinate and propionate (280[c]). Recovery occurred within a few days after cessation of drug administration. Especially in the elderly, erythromycin should not be given together with other potentially ototoxic drugs and hearing acuity should be monitored during erythromycin therapy. A recent report describes acute psychotic reactions related to ototoxicity and high-dose erythromycin therapy (186[c]).

Bacterial resistance Development of resistance to erythromycin may occur rapidly and is usually associated with bacterial cross-resistance to the other macrolide antibiotics, and also to the chemically unrelated lincomycins. Resistance has been detected in strains of staphylococci, Group A hemolytic streptococci, viridans streptococci, *Streptococcus pyogenes*, *Neisseria gonorrhoeae*, *Bacteroides fragilis* and *Clostridium difficile* (179[R]). It has tended to occur in hospitals, where either erythromycin or the lincomycins were used extensively, but may also result from multiple drug resistance where other antibiotics were used. Subinhibitory concentrations of erythromycin may induce resistance in staphylococci.

Miscellaneous A myasthenia-like clinical picture has been documented by electromyography in adult patients treated with 1.5 grams of erythromycin. The phenomenon disappeared after withdrawal of the antibiotic. Aggravation of myasthenia has also been reported (281[C]).

Acute renal insufficiency has been observed in a patient with Henoch-Schönlein syndrome. Another case presented as interstitial nephritis with acute renal failure (282[C]).

Intravenous infusions of 1-gram doses of erythromycin tend to produce thrombophlebitis. Intramuscular injection of more than 100 mg may produce severe local pain for some hours.

Drug interactions Erythromycin being bacteriostatic, may inhibit the bactericidal action of simultaneously administered penicillins or cephalosporins. Antagonism in vitro has also been described with the lincomycins. Competition between macrolides and lincomycins for similar binding sites at bacterial ribosomes probably underlies this phenomenon.

Erythromycin may increase the serum levels of theophylline. Asthmatics, therefore, could experience problems if this antibiotic is added to an already established treatment with theophylline. However, patients with an average serum concentration of theophylline under 15 μg/ml will probably only experience a small increase in their serum theophylline concentration during erythromycin therapy, whereas patients with steady-state concentrations above 15 μg/ml deserve careful monitoring and close observation for symptoms of theophylline toxicity during treatment with erythromycin (283[C], 284[C]).

In corticosteroid-dependent asthmatic patients, macrolides seem to have a steroid-sparing effect due to undefined mechanisms (213[c]), but possibly related to the rate of metabolism of corticosteroids in the liver.

The simultaneous use of troleandomycin and ergotamine in low doses may cause ergotism. Ischemia involving all four limbs has been described (285[c]). This observation led to the recommendation that ergotamine should be avoided in all patients receiving any kind of macrolide including erythromycin.

In patients treated with carbamazepine because of epilepsy, erythromycin may result in acute carbamazepine intoxication, probably due to inhibited metabolism of carbamazepine in the liver (286[C]). In a controlled study of the effects of erythromycin on carbamazepine pharmacokinetics in healthy volunteers (220[C]), clearance of a single dose of carbamazepine was reduced by 19% during erythromycin treatment. In contrast, the single-dose pharmacokinetics of phenytoin were not affected by erythromycin (287[c], 288[c]). After withdrawal of the macrolide, carbamazepine levels quickly return to normal (289[C]).

Erythromycin may also interact with warfarin (290[C]). The interaction with digoxin (245[C], 291[C]) is probably due to interference with the intestinal flora. A marked reduction in the excretion of reduced metabolites of digoxin in the urine and feces results in increased plasma concentration of digoxin and toxicity.

Interactions with quinidine, disopyramide, alfentanil, nifedipine, ciclosporin, triazolam and midazolam have also been reported (227[C], 230[C], 246[C], 292[c], 293[C], 294[c]).

In erythromycin-treated patients interactions with ciclosporin resulted in renal insufficiency. Other symptoms such as abdominal pain and periorbital edema have also been reported. In addition to interference with hepatic metabolism, improved oral absorption of ciclosporin has been documented (239[c], 295[C], 296[C]). Ventricular tachycardia has been associated with intravenous erythromycin (297[C]).

Roxithromycin

Adverse events Adverse events were examined in 2917 adults and observed in 4.1% at a dosage of 150 mg twice a day (298[R]). Nausea (1.3%), abdominal pain (1.2%) and diarrhea (0.8%) were the most frequently reported events, whereas rash, vomiting, headache, dizziness, pruritus, urticaria and constipation were reported only rarely. Treatment had to be discontinued in 0.9% of the patients because of adverse events.

In infants and children under 14 adverse events occurred in 6.9% of 304 patients (299[C]). Treatment was discontinued in 10 children (two vomiting, two diarrhea, six rash). In 480 elderly patients (>65 years old), adverse events were observed in 3.1% and treatment was discontinued in 1.9%. The gastrointestinal tract was most frequently affected, whereas laboratory changes (increases in bilirubin, ALT, AST, alkaline phosphatase) were seen in less than 0.7% of the patients. In one study lymphopenia or eosinophilia were observed in two of 37 patients (300[c]). However, this finding could not be confirmed in other studies.

Drug interactions Roxithromycin did result in alterations of the pharmacokinetic profile of theophylline, mainly raising the maximum concentration from 9.6 to 11.07, prolonging the half-life from 6.14 to 6.66 hours, enlarging the area under the curve from 63.9 to 74, and increasing renal clearance from 0.185 to 0.292 (301[C]). While these changes are statistically significant, they are considered clinically irrelevant. There was no effect of roxithromycin on trough concentrations of theophylline.

Roxithromycin did not alter the pharmacokinetic profile of carbamazepine (301[C]) or interact with warfarin, ranitidine and antacids containing hydroxides of aluminium and magnesium (298[R]).

Clarithromycin

Adverse events Variable rates of adverse events are reported with clarithromycin, ranging between 4 and 30%. In a direct comparison of clarithromycin with erythromycin stearate, the rate of adverse events was 19% in 96 patients receiving clarithromycin and 35% in 112 patients receiving erythromycin (180[C]). The majority of adverse events associated with clarithromycin affect the gastrointestinal tract (7%). In some patients adverse events located in the nervous system were observed (3%). A case report describes the development of progressive loss of strength, difficulties with swallowing and eye opening after the first dose of clarithromycin (2 g/day) in a patient with cerebral toxoplasmosis and AIDS (302[C]). This myasthenic syndrome resolved within 6 hours following withdrawal of clarithromycin and administration of pyridostigmine. The authors postulate that this adverse event may be the consequence of a neuromuscular blockade through inhibition of the presynaptic release of acetylcholine. In patients without neuromuscular disease erythromycin induced subclinical loss of motor unit contractions, which improved with intravenous administration of edrophonium or neostigmine (303[c]). Elevations of liver function tests, bilirubin as well as hepatomegaly have been described (304[R]). In an analysis of 4291 treated patients, the frequency of increased alanine aminotransferase levels was 5% (304[R]).

Drug interaction Clarithromycin results in a decrease of P-450 activity. This affects the metabolism of theophylline and carbamazepine. The results of several studies of the effect of clarithromycin on theophylline levels are conflicting. While the total body clearance of theophylline decreased (305[c]) and plasma theophylline level increased by 18% (306[C]), mean theophylline concentrations remained within the therapeutic range (306[C]). Based on these data it appears prudent to monitor serum theophylline concentrations in patients receiving high doses of theophylline or in patients with theophylline concentrations in the upper therapeutic range (304[R]). Furthermore, clarithromycin decreases C_{max} and AUC of zidovudine (172[r]). A different mechanism is responsible for clarithromycin-induced digoxin toxicity. This may be clinically relevant in patients receiving clarithromycin while being treated with digoxin. Normally, a proportion of digoxin is metabolized by gut flora. Antibiotics result in alteration of these bacteria. As a consequence more digoxin becomes biologically available. This may result in a significant increase in the serum concentration of digoxin and potential toxic adverse events (244[C]).

Another important interaction is observed with terfenadine, resulting in increased terfenadine levels, if used together with clarithromycin. This kind of interaction is also observed with erythromycin, but not with azithromycin. Since elevated terfenadine levels may cause or contribute to cardiac arrhythmia, especially torsades de pointes, this antihistamine should not be used in combination with clarithromycin (249[r]). Clarithromycin was also associated with cholestatic hepatitis (192[C]).

In recent years clarithromycin has become one of the core drugs to treat *Mycobacterium avium* complex (MAC) infections in both HIV-infected and non-infected patients. For this indication, doses of up to 2000 mg clarithromycin daily are used, typically in combination with other drugs. Clinically relevant drug interactions have been reported between clarithromycin and rifampicin and rifabutin respectively (253[C], 258[C]). Following addition of rifampin peak serum levels of clarithromycin are markedly reduced from a mean of 5.8 to 2.5 μg/ml (258[C]). At the same time the ratio of the serum concentrations of clarithromycin and its 14-OH metabolite was reversed from 3.3:1 to 1:2.7. Similar, although less marked changes were observed following the addition of rifabutin 600 mg daily to a regimen containing clarithromycin at 1000 mg daily.

The reason for this change in pharmacokinetics is a complex interaction of these drugs on the cytochrome P-450 system in the liver. Clarithromycin inhibits P-450 IIIA4 (CYP3A4), while both rifampin and rifabutin induce P-450 cytochromes, including CYP3A4, which results in enhanced metabolism of drugs by this mechanism. The observed changes in serum concentrations of clarithromycin and its metabolite, in the presence of the enzyme inducers rifampin and rifabutin, suggest that the metabolism of clarithromycin by the P-450 system is increased. Whether or not these changes in serum concentrations are clinically relevant regarding antimicrobial activity is unknown, since prediction of clinical efficacy based on serum concentrations of clarithromycin is probably not justified, given the fact that this class of drugs accumulates to a large degree in tissue and macrophages.

The interactions between rifabutin and clarithromycin are manifold. In addition to the effect of rifabutin on clarithromycin serum concentration, clarithromycin interacts with rifabutin to cause uveitis (254[C]—256[C]), especially if rifabutin at doses of 600 mg daily or higher is used. In addition, it was recently reported that if both clarithromycin or azithromycin were administered concomitantly with rifabutin, rifabutin-related adverse events occurred in 77% of patients (253[C]). The principal adverse events were hematological (neutropenia), gastrointestinal (nausea, vomiting, diarrhea) and abnormal liver enzyme levels. In addition, a diffuse polyarthralgia syndrome (19%) and anterior uveitis (8%) were also observed in this population of HIV-negative patients with *Mycobacterium avium* complex lung disease. Since inhibition of the cytochrome P-450 system by clarithromycin may interfere with rifabutin metabolism, as possibly illustrated by a report documenting a 77% increase of the area under the curve for rifabutin during treatment with clarithromycin (253[C]), the recommendation of the authors, to use rifabutin at a dose of 300 mg/day in multidrug regimens including a macrolide, seems prudent. This recommendation seems to be especially pertinent in light of the report of a 40% rate of uveitis in patients treated with the combination of clarithromycin and rifabutin (600 mg/day) for disseminated MAC disease (255[C]).

Azithromycin

Adverse events Studies on the tolerability of azithromycin encompass 3995 patients who were treated with 1.5 grams in divided doses over 5 days, or who received 1 gram as a single dose for treatment of urethritis/cervicitis (307[R]). Adverse effects were observed in 12% of the patients. In patients older than 65 years this rate was 9.3%, and in children under 14 years of age the corresponding rate was 5.4%.

The most common adverse events were gastrointestinal (9.6%), whereas central nervous system and peripheral nervous system adverse events were reported in 1.3% of the patients. Overall, only 6% of the adverse events were considered severe, involving mainly the gastrointestinal tract, and in 0.7% of treated patients adverse events resulted in discontinuation of the drug. This rate was lower than the rate reported with other macrolides. Fifty-nine percent of adverse events were considered mild and 34% moderate. Treatment-related elevations of liver function tests (ALT, AST) were rare (<2%) as was leukopenia (1.1—1.5%).

Drug interactions Azithromycin is contraindicated in patients receiving ergot alkaloids. This 15-membered macrolide does not induce or inhibit the cytochrome P-450 enzymes in rats. A retrospective analysis of 3995 patients treated with azithromycin did not reveal any pharmacokinetic interactions in patients who were also receiving theophylline, warfarin, cimetidine, carbamazepine or methylprednisolone (307[R], 308[C]). In two double-blind, placebo-controlled randomized studies no inhibition of the metabolism of theophylline was observed (309[c], 310[C]).

When azithromycin is used concomitantly with ciclosporin or digoxin, serum levels of these drugs need to be monitored (311[C]). While data on the effects of azithromycin on the intestinal metabolism of digoxin have not been reported so far, it appears likely that *Eubacterium lentum* is also affected by azithromycin. This would likely ensue similar consequences regarding serum digoxin levels as seen with erythromycin or clarithromycin.

Due to interference of food or antacids, it is necessary to give azithromycin at least 1 hour before or 2 hours after food or antacids. Antacids containing aluminium and magnesium result in decreased peak serum levels, but the total extent of the absorption of azithromycin is not altered (308[C]).

Since azithromycin is used in HIV-infected patients with various infections, the potential for drug interactions with antiretroviral drugs needs to be considered. Studies show that zidovudine does not affect azithromycin levels and azithromycin does not influence serum levels of zidovudine (312[c]). No data are available on potential interactions between azithromycin and didanosine, zalcitabine, stavudine, 3TC, delavirdine, indinavir and other protease inhibitors.

Dirithromycin

Adverse events Adverse events were studied in 4263 patients (181[R]). Abdominal pain was noted in 5.6%, diarrhea in 5.0% and nausea in 4.9%. Headache was relatively commonly reported (4.5%). In 63.2% of the instances the adverse events were considered mild, in 30.5% moderate and in 6.3% severe. The adverse event resulted in discontinuation of the drug in 3.1%, mainly because of gastrointestinal symptoms such as nausea and abdominal pain.

Drug interactions Drug interactions were rarely reported, since dirithromycin does not interact with the cytochrome P-450-system. Nevertheless, a 10-day treatment with 500 mg daily resulted in a significant decrease by 18% of the average steady-state plasma theophylline concentration and a 26% decrease of C_{max}, while at the same time a 14—15% increase of its clearance was observed in 13 healthy volunteers (313[C]). In contrast, steady-state pharmacokinetic characteristics of theophylline did not change in 14 patients with COPD receiving a 10-day course of dirithromycin (314[C]). Ciclosporin levels remain unaffected as well. Oral dirithromycin resulted in a small decrease in the mean ethinylestradiol 24-hour area under the curve and an increase in oral clearance in women using an oral contraceptive. However, since there was no effect on the inhibition of ovulation, the clinical importance of this interaction may be negligible (315[c]). No data on interactions with other drugs, i.e. carbamazepine are available (181[R]).

Miocamycin

Adverse events The reported rates of adverse events among 1565 patients treated with 900—1800 mg miocamycin daily are similar to the rate observed with other macrolide antibiotics (316[R]). The profile of adverse events is also similar, but precise data are not available. In 12 053 pediatric patients under age 15 in Japan the rate of adverse events was 0.54% (317[c]). Very young children (<1 year) experienced adverse events in 0.97%. These adverse events affected mainly the skin and the gastrointestinal tract. However, this very low rate of adverse events must be interpreted with caution, since lower dosage (21—40 mg/kg/day) were used than typically prescribed (50 mg/kg/day) (316[R]).

Drug interactions Some drug interactions may be caused by weak induction of P-450 by miocamycin (201[R]). The pharmacokinetics of theophylline are not significantly affected (318[C]). No significant change in this respect was observed with the anticoagulant nicoumalone in six volunteers (316[R]). However miocamycin at 1600 mg daily increased the steady-state level of ciclosporin 2-fold (241[c]). The elimination half-life of carbamazepine given as a single daily dose (13% increase) and the area under the curve were significantly affected (222[c]), whereas the trough levels and mean AUC-levels of nine patients treated with 400, 600 or 1200 mg carbamazepine increased only minimally (319[C]).

Spiramycin Spiramycin is a macrolide antibiotic with activity primarily against *Staphylococcus aureus*, β-hemolytic streptococci and viridans streptococci. Since spiramycin is retained in bone and in the salivary glands and reaches prolonged high levels in the saliva, it is used mainly by dentists and otorhinolaryngologists. Because of high concentration in the tonsillar lymphoid tissue it has been proposed that spiramycin be used in the prevention of meningococcal infections. It does not reach the cerebrospinal fluid. Its toxicity is very low. Adverse effects may comprise nausea, vomiting, diarrhea and skin reactions (320[c]).

AMINOGLYCOSIDE GROUP

Aminoglycosides

Ten aminoglycosides have been, or are still, important in medical practice: gentamicin, tobramycin, sisomicin, netilmicin, kanamycin, amikacin, streptomycin, dihydrostreptomycin, neomycin and paromomycin. In accordance with their chemical similarity, they have many features in common, in particular the mechanism of antibacterial action, a broad antibacterial spectrum, partial or complete cross-resistance, bactericidal action in a slightly alkaline environment, poor absorption from the gastrointestinal tract, elimination by glomerular filtration, nephrotoxicity, ototoxicity, a potential ability to cause neuromuscular blockade, and partial or complete cross-allergy (321[R]).

The aminoglycosides have probably more than one mechanism of action on bacterial cells. They cause misreading of the RNA code and/or inhibition of the polymerization of amino acids.

For the clinician, it is important to know that all aminoglycosides exhibit a similar pattern of adverse reactions, although there are important differences with regard to their frequency and severity (Table 5).

Strategies for minimizing aminoglycoside toxicity include early bedside detection of cochlear and vestibular dysfunction, which should lead to prompt cessation of the aminoglycoside, use of short periods of treatment, dosing intervals of at least 12 hours, monitoring of serum levels, and awareness of relative contraindications such as renal or hepatic dysfunction, old age, hearing impairment and previous, recent aminoglycoside exposure (322[R]).

ONCE VERSUS MULTIPLE DAILY DOSING

Twice or thrice daily administration has been the standard dosing regimen during aminoglycoside therapy of systemic bacterial infections in patients with normal renal function. However, in vitro, in vivo and clinical studies suggest that once-daily dosing of the same total daily dose might be more beneficial with respect to both efficacy and toxicity (323[R]—325[R]).

Less frequent administration of higher doses results in higher peak concentrations. Due to the pronounced

Table 5. *Main adverse reactions of aminoglycosides*

Antibiotic	Usual parenteral dose (mg/kg per day)*	Localization of adverse reaction**			
		Vestibulum	Cochlea	Kidney	Neuromuscular transmission
Low-dose aminoglycosides					
Gentamicin	3–6	++	++	++	+
Tobramycin	3–6	++	++	++	+
Sisomicin	2–4	++	++	++	+
Netilmicin	3–6	+	+	++	+
High-dose aminoglycosides					
Kanamycin	10–15	+	+++	++	+
Amikacin	10–20	+	++	++	+
Antituberculous aminoglycosides					
Streptomycin	10–20	+++	+	+	++
Dihydrostreptomycin	10–20	+	+++	+	+
Oral aminoglycosides					
Neomycin Paromomycin	Only accidental absorption after topical or gastrointestinal use	+	+++	+++	++

* In general older patients require lower doses. Low doses are required during therapy of enterococcal endocarditis with an aminoglycoside given in combination with a penicillin. Monitoring of serum levels should be considered, particularly when using multiple-daily dosing regimens and administering high doses for several days.
** The number of + signs indicates the relative clinical importance of each reaction.

concentration dependence of bacterial killing higher peaks may potentiate the efficacy of aminoglycosides. The importance of a high ratio of peak concentration to the minimal inhibitory concentration (MIC) has been shown in vitro for both bactericidal activity and prevention of emergence of resistance (326[C]). Clinically the predictive value of the peak to MIC ratio could be documented for aminoglycoside therapy of gram-negative bacteremia (327[C]). Once-daily dosing may result in prolonged periods of subinhibitory concentrations. However, bacterial regrowth does not occur immediately after the aminoglycoside concentration drops below the MIC. The term 'post-antibiotic effect' has been suggested to describe the persistent suppression of bacterial regrowth after cessation of exposure of bacteria to an active antibiotic. This phenomenon has been observed both in vitro and in vivo (328[C]).

Various in vivo models have been used to study the effect of the dosing regimen on aminoglycoside nephro- and ototoxicity. Renal uptake of aminoglycosides is not proportional to serum concentrations due to saturation at high concentrations achieved during once-daily regimens. The degree of renal injury increased the more frequently the aminoglycoside was administered to humans, dogs, rabbits, guinea-pigs and rats as long as the total daily dose was kept constant (329[C], 330[C]). Development of early auditory alterations also occurred more frequently, or to a greater extent, the more frequently the aminoglycoside was administered.

Once-daily versus multiple-daily dosing regimens have been compared for amikacin, netilmicin, and gentamicin in 24 randomized, clinical trials including a total of 3181 patients (325[R]). An analysis of these studies revealed superior results for once-daily regimens with respect to clinical efficacy (89.5 vs. 84.7%, $p<0.001$) as well as bacteriological efficacy (88.6 vs. 83.4%, $p<0.01$). No statistically significant differences were noted for toxicity. Nevertheless, both nephrotoxicity and ototoxicity occurred less frequently during once-daily dosing (4.5 vs. 5.5% and 4.2 vs. 5.8%, respectively). Finally, once-daily dosing is more economical, since less nursing time and infusion material are required and the efforts for drug monitoring can be reduced. In conclusion, amikacin, netilmicin, and gentamicin can be administered once a day.

IMPORTANCE OF PLASMA LEVEL DETERMINATIONS

Serum concentrations have been frequently monitored during multiple-daily dosing of aminoglycosides, particularly when high doses are administered and also during prolonged therapy. The main goals of individual dosing and monitoring are to reach high, bactericidal drug concentrations and to avoid drug accumulation in serum to minimize the risk of toxicity. Since both goals are much more likely to be met with once-daily dosing it may be feasible to reduce the monitoring efforts during such dosing regimens. However, more clinical experience needs to be accumulated to establish solid guidelines for monitoring once-daily dosing regimens. Although an increasing number of clinicians is nowadays switching to once-daily dosing of aminoglycosides there is still a coexistence in the administration of once- and multiple-daily dosing regimens. Therefore two separate concepts of aminoglycoside monitoring have to be considered, depending on the dosing schedule.

Monitoring multiple-daily dosing regimens Peak serum concentrations of gentamicin and tobramycin >5—7 g/ml and of amikacin >20—28 g/ml have been shown to be associated with improved survival in patients with septicemia and pneumonia caused by gram-negative bacteria (331[C], 332[C]). On the other hand, excessive peak (>10—12 g/ml) and trough (>2 g/ml) concentrations of gentamicin and tobramycin increase the risk of oto- and nephrotoxicity (333[R]). Dose requirements to obtain aminoglycoside concentrations in the desired therapeutic range may differ considerably, even in patients with normal renal function (334[R]). Due to the great individual variability in pharmacokinetics, dosage adjustment with the commonly used nomograms often results in suboptimal or potentially toxic aminoglycoside concentrations (335[R]). An individualized treatment based on serum concentration monitoring is therefore necessary to achieve maximum bactericidal efficacy without a concomitant high risk of adverse reactions. Measurements of peak and trough serum levels should be carried out during the initial 24—48 hours in all patients and repeated after 3—5 days to detect any tendency to abnormal drug accumulation. However, one must realize that close monitoring alone cannot completely eliminate the danger of oto- and nephrotoxicity since aminoglycoside drug concentrations progressively increase in renal tissue and in the inner ear with repeated administration, even if optimum serum concentrations are maintained. The relationship between serum concentration of aminoglycosides and the two clinically important side effects, ototoxicity and nephrotoxicity, has been debated for many years. Whereas some authors have found a definite relationship between the frequency of side effects and serum concentrations, others have not (333[R]). This controversy can be partly explained by the pharmacokinetic behavior common to all aminoglycosides, which leads to drug accumulation in deep compartments, particularly in the renal cortex. Assuming that the extent of accumulation is a factor which relates to the frequency of side effects, it is not surprising to find a correlation between serum concentrations and toxicity in one group of patients but not in another. The amount accumulated depends not only on the dosing schedule and the serum concentration achieved during treatment, but also on the duration of drug administration. The same concentration in the same patient can be associated with a significantly different amount of drug in the body, depending on whether it was sampled during the second or the tenth day after the beginning of treatment.

Monitoring once-daily dosing regimens In general, both peak and trough concentrations are determined during monitoring of multiple-daily dosing regimens and doses are subsequently adjusted to achieve the recommended levels. However, peak and trough levels do not necessarily offer the most valuable information for dose adjustments during once-daily dosing. The indication and frequency of monitoring and the timing of serum levels within the interval, along with their target ranges, have yet to be established. At present, different targets have been proposed and used clinically (336[C]—338[C]). In one prospective study 8-hour levels have been considered for monitoring as an alternative to the measurement of peaks and troughs (339[C]). Fifty-one adult patients received an average dose of 400 mg given once a day. Doses were adjusted during therapy if 8-hour levels were not within the target range of 1.5—6.0 mg/l. Concentrations above or below this target range correlated significantly with nephrotoxicity, 24-hour trough levels and AUC values, respectively. Determination of 8-hour levels was therefore useful for identifying patients with either low AUCs or increased risk of nephrotoxicity. In other studies, aminoglycoside serum levels have been determined in the second half of the dosing interval (336[C], 338[C], 340[C]—342[C]). Trough levels, however, do not allow for extrapolations of levels achieved in the period after infusion. Thus, patients with very low peak concentrations due to unusually high volumes of distribution cannot be identified to possibly increase the dose. Similarly, patients with very rapid elimination, as frequently observed in burn-injured patients or in children, may not be noticed.

Depending on the goals of drug monitoring, peak 8-, 12- or 24-hour levels might be more important (325[R]). The correlation of efficacy with high peak levels, high ratios of peak to MIC and high AUC values suggests that drug concentrations should be determined within the first part of the dosing interval. In order to minimize toxicity, drug accumulation should be avoided. Therefore early detection of increased trough levels is of importance. It has been strongly suggested to lower the threshold values for troughs during once-daily compared to multiple-daily dosing (340[C], 343[C]). To reduce the cost of aminoglycoside therapy, indication and frequency of monitoring serum levels should be minimal. Instead, serum creatinine concentrations might be used to monitor renal function. The strategy selected for monitoring an aminoglycoside therapy must consider a number of factors, including the type and severity of infection, the duration of therapy or the presence of parameters associated with increased risk of toxicity. In addition, local factors should be considered for the timing of blood samples, including the sensitivity of the drug assay available (344[C]) and the time required for processing the specimens in order to modify the subsequent dose, if necessary.

Table 6. *Risk factors for aminoglycoside toxicity*

Patient factors	Drug-related factors
Prior renal insufficiency/abnormal audiogram	Dose (blood level exceeding the therapeutic range)
Age (mainly older patients)	Duration of therapy (2–3 weeks) and total dose
Septicemia	Prior aminoglycoside exposure
Dehydration	
High temperature	

* Adapted from Moore et al. (348[C], 367[C])

ADVERSE REACTION PATTERN *(see also Table 5)*

General and toxic reactions The main adverse reactions of aminoglycosides consist of kidney damage (often presenting as non-oliguric renal insufficiency) and ototoxicity, including vestibular and/or cochlear dysfunction. Neuromuscular transmission may also be inhibited.

Hypersensitivity reactions These are most frequent after topical use, which should be avoided (see 'Skin and appendages'): anaphylactic reactions can occur.

Tumor-inducing effects These have not been reported.

ORGANS AND SYSTEMS

Cardiovascular Anecdotal reports refer to tachycardia, ECG changes, hypotension and even cardiac arrest. In practice, effects on the cardiovascular system are unlikely to be of any significance. Rare observations of anaphylactic shock have been reported.

Respiratory Severe respiratory depression due to neuromuscular blockade (see below) has been observed (335a[C]). Bronchospasm can occur as part of a hypersensitivity reaction.

Nervous system and special senses Ototoxicity is a clinically important, major side effect of aminoglycoside antibiotics. The incidence of this complication varies in different studies, depending on the type of patients treated, the methods used to monitor cochlear and vestibular function, and the aminoglycoside prescribed (345[R]). Clinically recognizable hearing loss and vestibular damage occur in about 2–4% of patients, but pure-tone audiometry, particularly at high frequencies, and electronystagmography may show hearing loss and/or vestibular damage in up to 26 and 10%, respectively, despite careful dosage adjustment (346[C]). In patients with *Pseudomonas* endocarditis receiving prolonged high-dose treatment with gentamicin, auditory toxicity was found in 44% (347[R], 352[R]).

There is a discrepancy between clinical observations, in which very few patients receiving aminoglycosides actually complain of developing a hearing loss, and the reported incidences of ototoxicity in studies considering audiometry thresholds. A major reason for this discrepancy relates to the fact that aminoglycosides cause high-frequency hearing loss well before they affect the speech frequency range in which they can be detected by the patient (346[C]).

Clinically, ototoxicity is more frequent and easier to detect than vestibular toxicity; combined defects are relatively rare. Symptoms of cochlear damage include tinnitus, hearing loss, pressure and sometimes pain in the ear. The manifestations of vestibular toxicity are dizziness, vertigo, ataxia and nystagmus. These are often overlooked in severely ill, bed-ridden patients.

Symptoms of ototoxicity may occur within 3–5 days of starting treatment, but most patients with severe damage have received prolonged courses of aminoglycosides. In some cases, hearing loss may progress after the administration of the causative drug has been interrupted. The ototoxicity is reversible only in about 50% of patients. Permanent deafness is often seen in patients with delayed onset of symptoms, progressive deterioration after discontinuation of treatment and hearing loss of >25 db (346[C]).

There are a number of factors which predispose the patient to ototoxic effects (Table 6). Drug-related toxicity is influenced by the quality of prescribing. Overdosage in patients with impaired renal function, unnecessary prolongation of treatment and the concomitant administration of other potentially ototoxic agents should be avoided. The exact mechanism of increased toxicity in patients with septicemia and high temperature is not clear; the possible relevance of additive damage by bacterial endotoxins has been discussed (348[C]). Dehydration with hypovolemia is probably the main reason for the increased toxicity experienced when aminoglycosides are given together with loop diuretics, but furosemide treatment itself does not seem to be an independent risk factor of the diuretic effect (349[C], 350[C]).

The mechanism of ototoxicity by aminoglycosides is still not fully clarified. Most of the experimental data have been gained in the guinea-pig model which seems to resemble the human situation. Traditionally, toxic damage is considered to be the consequence of drug accumulation in the inner ear fluids (351[R], 353[R]). After a period of reversible functional impairment, a destruction of outer hair cells in the basilar turn of the cochlear duct occurs and proceeds to the apex. Similar changes are found in the hair cells of the vestibular system.

Ototoxicity does not necessarily correlate with plasma perilymph or whole-tissue levels of aminoglycosides (353[C]).

There is evidence that the site of ototoxic action is the mitochondrial ribosome (354[R]). A point mutation in the mitochondrial 12S ribosomal RNA gene has been shown to be common in all pedigrees with maternally inherited ototoxic deafness (354[C]). The recent findings might create a molecular baseline for preventive screening of patients when aminoglycosides are going to be used (SEDA-18, 1; 354[R]).

There are interesting differences in the toxicity patterns of aminoglycosides in animal models. Gentamicin and tobramycin affect the cochlear and vestibular systems to a similar extent, while amikacin, kanamycin and neomycin preferentially damage the cochlear and streptomycin the vestibular system. Netilmicin appears to be the least toxic (355[R]–357[R]).

In man, differences in the ototoxic risks of the currently used aminoglycosides are difficult to evaluate (345[R]). No prospective studies comparing more than two drugs using the same criteria in similar patient populations have been performed. However, several controlled trials with two aminoglycosides are available and provide some information. A survey of 24 such trials by Cone (358[R]) showed the following mean frequencies of ototoxicity: gentamicin 7.7%, tobramycin 9.7%, amikacin 13.8% and netilmicin 2.3%. A lower incidence of netilmicin-induced inner ear damage as compared to tobramycin has also been demonstrated in two studies (359[C], 360[C]).

To recognize auditory damage at an early stage and avoid severe irreversible toxicity, repeated tests of cochlear and vestibular function should be carried out in all patients needing prolonged aminoglycoside treatment. Pure-tone audiometry at 250–8000 Hz and electronystagmography with caloric testing are the standard methods. The first detectable audiometric changes usually occur in the high-tone range (>4000 Hz) and then progress to lower frequencies. Hearing loss of >15 db is usually considered as evidence of toxicity. Brainstem auditory-evoked potentials have been recommended as a means of monitoring ototoxicity in non-cooperative, comatose patients (361[C], 362[C]). This technique is time consuming and requires some expertise, but may become a useful tool for detecting damage at an early stage. It also provides information on preexisting changes which is otherwise rarely available in intensive care patients (362[C]).

Neuromuscular blockade The aminoglycosides have a curare-like action which can be antagonized by calcium ions and prostigmine. In cases requiring general anesthesia, the effect of muscle relaxants of the nondepolarizing type such as *d*-tubocurarine and succinylcholine may be potentiated by aminoglycosides.

Aminoglycoside-induced neuromuscular blockade may be clinically relevant in patients with respiratory acidosis, in myasthenia gravis and in other neuromuscular diseases. Severe illness, the simultaneous use of anesthetics, e.g. in the immediate postoperative phase, and application of the antibiotic to serosal surfaces are predisposing factors to be considered (363[R]).

With regard to this reaction, neomycin is the most potent member of the group. Several deaths and cases of severe respiratory depression due to neomycin have been reported. Severe clinical manifestations are rare in patients treated with those aminoglycosides which are administered in low dose, such as gentamicin, tobramycin and netilmicin. In some of the cases reported the paralysis was successfully reversed by prostigmine.

Endocrine, metabolic Neomycin and presumably other aminoglycosides reduce the absorption of cholesterol from the intestine by disruption of the intestinal micelles which normally play a role in its absorption. The point is further referred to in the section on neomycin.

Hypomagnesemia Hypomagnesemia is a well-recognized side effect of treatment with various drugs, including aminoglycosides (SEDA-16, 279). Gentamicin-induced magnesium depletion is most likely to occur when the drug is given to older patients in large doses over extended periods of time (346[C]). Under these circumstances, serum concentrations and urinary wasting of electrolytes should be monitored.

Hematological Occasional hematological complications can occur with individual drugs in this series (see individual drug sections).

Liver Certain drugs in this group can affect liver function tests. Increases in alkaline phosphatase after gentamicin and tobramycin have been described.

Urinary system The impairment of kidney function is a major side effect of aminoglycoside antibiotics. The incidence of this complication in different studies is highly variable. It depends on the study population and definition of toxicity and may range from a few percent to more than 30% in severely ill patients (365[C], 366[C]). As in the case of ototoxicity, certain risk factors could be identified for nephrotoxicity (367[C], 368[C]). The 1-hour post-dose and trough aminoglycoside serum levels, duration of treatment, total dose, age, abnormal initial creatinine clearance and co-existent liver disease were found to be predictors for subsequent kidney damage. However, the clinical significance and utility of such predictive risk nomograms have been challenged by some authors (369[C]).

Nephrotoxicity may present clinically as an acute tubular necrosis or, more commonly, as a gradually evolving non-oliguric renal failure. The time course of toxicity is variable, but it usually develops only after several days of treatment. Early diagnosis is difficult since a decrease in glomerular filtration may be present before a significant rise in serum creatinine concentration is found (370[C]). An increased number of casts in the urinary sediment can also precede the increase in serum creatinine (371[C]). Measurement of phospholipids and urinary enzymes, such as β_2-microglobulin or alanine-aminopeptidase, has been proposed as a means of detecting early toxicity (372[C], 373[C], 374[R]). Data on these enzymes are however not very useful clinically, since they can be increased for various other reasons and elevated levels do not reliably predict pending renal toxicity. Fortunately, recovery of renal function nearly always follows the discontinuation of aminoglycoside therapy, although serum creatinine concentrations may continue to rise for several days after the last dose of the aminoglycoside has been given.

The mechanism of nephrotoxicity has been studied in animal models, in in vitro systems, and in man. The data indicate that accumulation of aminoglycosides in the renal cortex is an important reason for functional damage. In addition, aminoglycoside-induced alterations of glomerular ultrastructure have been described (375[C]). Tissue uptake is predominantly mediated by proximal tubular reabsorption of the filtered drug. The degree of renal injury caused by an aminoglycoside correlates with the amount of drug accumulated in the renal cortex. However, the intrinsic toxicity may differ between the aminoglycosides. Endotoxin may increase intracortical accumulation (376[C]). After binding to a amino acid receptor site pinocytotic entry into the tubular cells takes place. Once the drug is within the cell, it persists there for a long time and is liberated only slowly with an elimination half-life of several days (377[r], 378[r]). Direct toxicity to tubular cells is mainly explained by an inhibition of lysosomal activity with accumulation of lamellar myeloid bodies consisting of phospholipids. The inhibition of lysosomal phospholipids can also be demonstrated in purified liposomes in vitro (379[R]). In renal biopsy specimens, vacuolization of the proximal tubular epithelium, clumped nuclear chromatin and swollen mitochondria are seen. Patchy tubular cell necrosis, desquamation and luminal obstruction are found at later stages.

A comparison of the nephrotoxic potential of the various aminoglycosides has been carried out in many animal experiments. The following order of relative nephrotoxicity was found: neomycin > gentamicin > tobramycin > amikacin > netilmicin (380[C], 381[C]).

In man, conclusive data regarding the relative toxicity of the various aminoglycosides are still lacking. The analysis by Cone (358[R]) of 24 controlled trials showed the following average rates for nephrotoxicity: gentamicin, 11%; tobramycin, 11.5%; amikacin, 8.5%; and netilmicin, 2.8%. In contrast to this survey, direct comparison in similar patient groups showed no significant differences between the various agents in most trials (382[C]—388[C]). In fact, the relative advantage of lower nephrotoxicity rates observed with netilmicin in some studies may be limited to administration of low doses. Noone and co-workers demonstrated in a prospective study significantly lower nephrotoxicity with daily doses of 15 mg/kg of amikacin (4% toxicity) as compared with 7 mg/kg of netilmicin (12%) (389[C]). One prospective trial (390[C]) indicated a significant advantage of tobramycin over gentamicin. Subsequently these findings could not be confirmed (391[C]). Nephrotoxicity remains a serious risk with all the currently available aminoglycoside antibiotics and no drug in this series can be regarded as safe.

Skin and appendages *Topical application* It is generally accepted that antibiotics which are important for systemic use should not be administered topically. This rule applies particularly to the aminoglycoside antibiotics. Even though neomycin and streptomycin are no longer frequently used systemically, the frequency of sensitization after topical administration of these drugs is particularly high.

The risk of sensitization by topically administered gentamicin seems to be smaller. Nevertheless, also in order to avoid resistance, its topical use should be restricted to life-endangering thermal burns and to severe dermatological infections in which pseudomonal strains resistant to other antibiotics are involved.

Bacterial resistance Differences between resistance of the chromosomal type and the type mediated by R-factors are mentioned in Chapter 25.2.

Streptomycin and dihydrostreptomycin differ from the other members of the group by not having the 2-deoxystreptamine moiety in their molecule. Accordingly, the mechanism by which bacterial resistance arises is different. Whereas resistance to the streptomycins is often of the chromosomal type (one-step resistance by mutation), resistance to the other aminoglycosides is usually mediated by R-factors. The latter type of resistance, occurring mainly in gram-negative bacteria, is associated with the production of several bacterial enzymes which inactivate aminoglycosides by acetylation, phosphorylation and adenylation.

During treatment of either gram-negative or gram-positive bacteria, resistant subpopulations emerge unless the peak to MIC ratio is high enough to reduce drastically the bacterial inoculum within a few hours (392[C]). Similarly, rapid emergence of resistant subpopulations has been reported during aminoglycoside treatment in neutropenic animals. The virulence and clinical relevance of the relatively slow-growing resistant subpopulations (small colony variants) have been documented in both animal and clinical studies (393[C], 394[C]). The presence of resistant subpopulations can be detected only by direct plating of specimens on aminoglycoside-containing agar plates, since resistance may be lost within one subculture. Combination therapy of an aminoglycoside plus a β-lactam antibiotic has been successfully used to prevent selection of resistant subpopulations (395[C]).

Risk situations The main risk situations are summarized under 'Organs and systems' and in Table 6. The most important factors are prior or concomitant renal insufficiency, high serum drug levels and long duration of treatment.

Second-generation effects During pregnancy the aminoglycosides cross the placenta and they might theoretically be expected to cause otological and perhaps nephrological damage to the fetus. No proven cases of intrauterine damage by gentamicin and tobramycin have been recorded. In 135 mother/child pairs exposed to streptomycin during the first 4 months of pregnancy, no increase in the risk of any malformation was found (396[R]). Streptomycin and dihydrostreptomycin have given rise to severe otological damage.

Overdosage Although aminoglycoside antibiotics are dialyzable, peritoneal dialysis may not remove sufficient amounts of gentamicin or of other aminoglycosides from the blood after overdosage. Hemodialysis has been reported to be an efficient method of treatment.

Interactions There are many reports describing cases of acute renal failure resulting from combined treatment with gentamicin (or another aminoglycoside) and one of the cephalosporins (397[C]—399[C]). The potential nephrotoxic effect of the combinations seems to be related mainly to the nephrotoxic effect of the aminoglycosides. In contrast, there is some experimental (400[C]) and clinical evidence (401[C]) that ticarcillin might attenuate the renal toxicity of the aminoglycosides.

Among the agents promoting the nephrotoxicity of the aminoglycosides, strong diuretics such as furosemide and ethacrynic acid are often mentioned. However, the existence of this interaction is by no means clearly established (355[R]). Some of these agents, e.g. furosemide, are not truly nephrotoxic in themselves. The so-called interaction may only be a consequence of sodium and volume depletion. Other types of diuretics such as mannitol hydrochlorothiazide and acetazolamide do not produce this 'interaction' (355[R]).

Similarly, combined use of vancomycin and an aminoglycoside may increase the risk of toxicity (402[C]—404[C]). Also, the nephro- and ototoxic side-effects of cisplatin and carboplatin may be potentiated by concurrent administration of aminoglycosides, as shown in animal studies (405[C], 406[C]).

It is established that an in vitro interaction exists between aminoglycoside antibiotics and carbenicillin or ticarcillin, leading to a significant loss of aminoglycoside antibacterial activity (407[c]) if these antibiotics are mixed in the same infusion bottle. The extent of inactivation is dependent upon penicillin concentration, contact time and temperature. Azlocillin and mezlocillin inactivate aminoglycosides in a similar manner to that described for carbenicillin (408[c], 409[c]). Aminoglycosides should not be mixed with penicillins or cephalosporins in the same infusion bottle.

The clinical significance of the presence of both groups of antibiotics in the organism of the patient is debatable. Several authors have shown that in patients receiving a combination of gentamicin and carbenicillin the measured serum gentamicin levels were lower than the pharmacokinetically predicted values. Especially in patients with severe renal impairment where long in vivo incubation of these drug combinations takes place before supplemental doses of the aminoglycoside drugs are given, this interaction may be important (410[c]).

INDIVIDUAL DRUGS OF THE AMINOGLYCOSIDE GROUP

Gentamicin

Gentamicin is a well-established antibiotic for the treatment of several bacterial infections, especially those caused by gram-negative bacteria, including

Pseudomonas aeruginosa, *Klebsiella* and *Serratia marcescens*. In adults, gentamicin is usually given in daily amounts of 240—360 mg.

Nervous system and special senses In many studies of serious neonatal infections treated with gentamicin there have been very few cases providing unequivocal evidence of gentamicin-induced ototoxicity. Gentamicin can be an excellent drug in neonatal sepsis, and its potential toxicity should not preclude its use where it is needed. There are indications that its tolerance in children is better than in adults. Whether or not ototoxicity in elderly patients is particularly frequent is still a matter of discussion. Recent authors contest the view that age above 60 is per se a factor predisposing to the ototoxic effects of aminoglycosides.

Audiometric monitoring has been recommended in patients receiving aminoglycosides for more than 7—10 days. Since gentamicin-induced ototoxicity in the majority of cases only involves vestibular function, the symptoms are easily overlooked in severely ill patients who are unable to sit. If diagnosed early, the vestibular damage is usually reversible. In some cases, severe long-term disability has been described (411[c]).

Even if the tympanic membrane is intact, one should hesitate to use the drug in ear-drops or in other topical forms for the treatment of otitis media.

There are several case reports of acute toxic psychosis due to gentamicin (412[c]). Intrathecal gentamicin may cause neurotoxic lesions (413[c]).

Urinary system Two clinical types of gentamicin-induced nephrotoxicity have become recognized which may also be relevant to other aminoglycosides:

(1) A gradual decrease in creatinine clearance, occurring after about 2 weeks, in about 5—10% of patients receiving the drug in full doses, the decrease being rapidly reversible in most cases as soon as gentamicin is withdrawn.

(2) An acute renal failure due to tubular necrosis usually associated with oliguria lasting 10—12 days, followed by a diuretic phase. This type of nephrotoxicity occurs far less frequently than the first type.

In a few cases, gentamicin nephrotoxicity was associated with a Fanconi syndrome with elevated levels of serum enzymes in the urine. Among these, muramidase seemed to be especially useful in checking for proximal tubular dysfunction (414[c]).

Adequate antibiotic therapy is in most cases attainable with multiple daily dosing regimens producing maximum serum concentrations of 6—10 g/ml and trough levels <2 g/ml.

Gentamicin is of considerable value for the management of sepsis in the immunosuppressed renal-transplant recipient. Although it has been suggested that gentamicin should be avoided in such patients because of potential renal toxicity in the allograft, experienced physicians have felt that gentamicin may be given, provided the dosage schedule is adapted to the level of allograft function and that blood levels are monitored.

Problems with special applications *Oral administration* of gentamicin in low dosage to reduce the intestinal flora is rarely practised although it is probably as effective as neomycin. In these cases it should be noted that in the presence of an intestinal mucosal inflammation more than 10% of the dose may be absorbed.

Endotracheal administration may be used for tracheotomized patients in intensive care units. This route of administration does not produce effective antibiotic plasma concentrations. However, in cases with renal failure the absorption of a certain amount via the respiratory tract should be taken into account.

Tobramycin

Tobramycin closely resembles gentamicin in its microbiological and toxicological properties. The drugs have similar half-lives, peak serum levels, lack of protein binding, volumes of distribution and predominantly renal excretion by glomerular filtration. Its main advantage may be its greater intrinsic activity against *Pseudomonas aeruginosa*. Not all bacterial strains resistant to gentamicin are invariably also resistant to tobramycin. Because of its inherent potential for ototoxicity and nephrotoxicity, renal and 8th-nerve functions should be closely monitored (415[R], 416[R]).

As with gentamicin, peak plasma concentrations over 10—12 g/ml should be avoided and trough levels should not exceed 2 g/ml during administration of multiple daily dosing regimens.

Nervous system and special senses Clinical studies comparing tobramycin and gentamicin show a similar frequency of auditory damage (7—8%). Vestibular disturbances may be somewhat less frequent with tobramycin, but several cases of reversible vestibular dysfunction have been described after tobramycin.

Toxic psychosis As with gentamicin, toxic psychosis may also occur with tobramycin (417[c]).

Neuromuscular blockade As with other aminoglycosides, circumstances such as high doses, anesthesia, intrapleural and intraperitoneal application probably increase the risk of neuromuscular blockade. Nevertheless, the phenomenon is rare in patients treated with tobramycin. In one reported case the paralysis was successfully reversed by prostigmine (SEDA-3, 231).

Urinary system In some retrospective and prospective studies assuring reasonably comparable conditions, nephrotoxicity induced by tobramycin was reported to be slightly less frequent than that following the use of gentamicin, but these observations could not be generally confirmed (390[C], 391[C]).

Sisomicin

Sisomicin is a dehydrogenated gentamicin derivative with similar pharmacokinetic, toxicological and microbiological properties. Cross-resistance to sisomicin, gentamicin and tobramycin may occur, but is incomplete. The only major difference in spectrum is that sisomicin is approximately twice as active against *Pseudomonas aeruginosa* as gentamicin.

Local tolerance of intramuscular injection is remarkably good.

At present, it is not possible to evaluate adequately the frequency of side effects in comparison with gentamicin and the other aminoglycosides (418[c], 419[R]).

In experimental animals, the neuromuscular blocking activity was slightly higher than with gentamicin. Because of the slightly lower therapeutic doses this difference probably has no clinical relevance (420[R]). The compound is removed by hemodialysis.

Netilmicin

Netilmicin is resistant to two of the enzymes that inactivate gentamicin. It seems to be as efficacious as amikacin with susceptible pathogens, possibly with the exception of *Pseudomonas aeruginosa* (389[C]). The multidose pharmacokinetics of netilmicin and gentamicin are similar and the data also confirm the presence of a deep tissue compartment. In experimental animals its ototoxicity and nephrotoxicity was significantly lower than that of gentamicin. The relatively low incidence of high-frequency changes in audiograms suggests that it might be preferred to other aminoglycosides in patients with impaired hearing or at risk for hearing loss (358[R], 359[C], 360[C]).

Kanamycin

In most hospitals kanamycin has largely been replaced by gentamicin, tobramycin or netilmicin. Amikacin, a semisynthetic derivative of kanamycin, is a further alternative. Kanamycin may be used for short-term treatment of severe infections caused by susceptible strains (e.g. *Escherichia coli*, *Proteus* species, *Enterobacter aerogenes*, *Klebsiella pneumoniae*, *Serratia marcescens* and *Mima-Herellea*) resistant to other less ototoxic aminoglycosides. The drug is not indicated for long-term therapy, e.g. in tuberculosis. The dosage level and the adverse reaction pattern are indicated in Table 5.

Nervous system and special senses Like dihydrostreptomycin and neomycin, kanamycin causes mainly auditory damage. After prolonged administration (e.g. 1 gram for periods of 30–180 days) the frequency of this adverse reaction is higher than 40%. Vestibular toxicity occurs in less than 10% of cases treated with usual doses and is generally reversible soon after the cessation of therapy.

Neuromuscular blockade Like the other aminoglycosides, kanamycin has neuromuscular blocking properties, particularly if administered directly into the peritoneum. Clinically, however, this drug seems to be less dangerous in this respect than neomycin or streptomycin. Paresthesia may occur on rare occasions.

Gastrointestinal tract Presurgical bowel preparation by oral doses of kanamycin is seldom practised; it may be followed by an intestinal malabsorption syndrome. Only negligible amounts of kanamycin are absorbed through an intact intestinal mucosa, but increased systemic availability and potential toxicity may result from the presence of ulcerated or denuded areas.

Urinary system Nephrotoxicity has been relatively low after short courses of treatment with daily doses of less than 15 mg/kg. If total doses of 30 grams or more are given, the incidence of renal damage may be 50% or higher.

Allergic reactions Sensitization after parenteral administration (skin rash, drug fever) is less frequent than with streptomycin. Anaphylaxis has only rarely been described. Cross-allergy with the other aminoglycosides is frequent.

Amikacin

Amikacin is a semisynthetic derivative of kanamycin with similar pharmacokinetic properties and dosage. It is resistant to many of the bacterial R-factor-mediated enzymes that inactivate kanamycin and gentamicin. Noteworthy is its effect against *Pseudomonas aeruginosa* and against most gram-negative aerobes that are resistant to gentamicin and tobramycin. Strains of *Staphylococcus aureus* have been found which were able to inactivate amikacin by phosphorylation and adenylation. Ticarcillin or azlocillin plus amikacin is considered as one of the most efficacious empiric antibiotic combinations in febrile granulocytopenic cancer patients. On a weight basis it is less active than gentamicin; the usual dose, therefore, is 10–20 mg/kg daily (Table 5). Wherever possible, peak levels of 40 g/ml and troughs of 10 g/ml should not be exceeded during twice-daily dosing regimens.

Nervous system and special senses The ototoxicity, is primary cochlear. In comparative studies with equipotent dosages, ototoxicity due to amikacin was of the same order as that caused by gentamicin (383[C], 388[C], 421[R]).

Neuromuscular blockade

The blocking potency of amikacin in rabbit experiments has been found to be less than one-tenth that of kanamycin.

Urinary system

After administration of the recommended doses of amikacin for 10 days renal damage probably occurs in less than 10% of cases. In several prospective randomized studies the liability of amikacin to cause nephrotoxicity was no greater than that of gentamicin or tobramycin (365[C], 382[C], 383[C]). As with other aminoglycosides, the renal toxicity is reversible in most cases (422[R]).

Miscellaneous Amikacin may be inactivated by penicillins. This inactivation occurs not only with a mixture of the agents in solution but also in vivo, particularly in patients with renal failure. Amikacin offers, at least in vitro, the advantage of being much less inactivated than tobramycin or gentamicin (423[R]).

Streptomycin; dihydrostreptomycin

Since the advent of less toxic and orally active antituberculous drugs such as isoniazid, rifampicin and ethambutol, the use of the streptomycins has declined considerably. For good reasons, there are countries, however, in which streptomycin is still an important standard drug in programs for the treatment of tuberculosis.

A usual dose has been 1 gram daily. In bacterial endocarditis, especially that caused by an enterococcus, streptomycin is often administered concomitantly with penicillin (in a dose of 1 gram twice daily for 2 weeks, followed by 0.5 gram twice daily for 4 weeks). Ototoxicity may require withdrawal of streptomycin prior to completion of the 6-week course of treatment.

As with other aminoglycosides, the most important adverse effects are ototoxicity, neuromuscular blockade, hypersensitivity reactions and rarely nephrotoxicity.

Nervous system and special senses It is generally accepted that in patients with normal kidney function the main factors involved in the ototoxicity of the streptomycins are the daily dose and the total amount received during a certain period. Clinically, the toxicity of dihydrostreptomycin has been much more significant since this drug may easily cause partial or complete loss of hearing, whereas the toxicity of streptomycin tends to be limited to the vestibular apparatus, thereby being less incapacitating. For this reason, dihydrostreptomycin is now obsolete.

In the absence of renal failure, amounts of streptomycin up to 30 grams have been reported as relatively safe in the older literature. Nonetheless, vestibular damage has been observed after administration of no more than 5–30 grams in daily doses of 1 gram. A familial incidence of damage to the inner ear after even smaller doses of streptomycin is due presumably to hereditary susceptibility in some patients. Toxicity resulting from 'small' doses of streptomycin has also occurred in patients with otitis media or with a history of otitis media.

After daily doses of 1 gram of streptomycin for 4 months vestibular damage could be documented in about 30% of cases, whereas impaired hearing in the high-frequency range occurred in 5–15%, although this can easily be overlooked. Without adequate explanation, ototoxicity was found in many studies to be more frequent in children than in adults (424[c]).

Complete or partial anosmia (disappearance of olfactory function) has been reported to occur after treatment with streptomycin over prolonged periods of time and in particular after administration of dihydrostreptomycin. Shortly after injection some patients develop circumoral anesthesia; others rarely show a temporary loss of mental concentration (425[c]).

Intratympanic administration of streptomycin has exceptionally been used in the treatment of Ménière's disease. In 95% of the treated cases the attacks of dizziness disappeared while the auditory functions were maintained. This might have been the spontaneous course of the syndrome.

Neuromuscular blockade Neuromuscular blockade with respiratory depression may occur, especially after intrapleural or intraperitoneal use. Peripheral neuritis is rare during streptomycin therapy, but in some series a disturbance of vision has been observed in more than 50% of cases. In a few instances, intrathecal application was followed by the occurrence of radiculitis, myelitis and other neurological complications.

Allergic reactions Exanthematous cutaneous reactions seem to occur in about 5% of patients 7–9 days after the first injection. A case of Stevens-Johnson syndrome caused by streptomycin has been described (426[c]). Development of streptomycin-specific antibodies of the IgG class causing hemolytic anemia and renal failure has been reported, but this appears to be a very rare effect.

Persons regularly handling streptomycin (nurses, employees in pharmaceutical firms) quite often develop hypersensitivity to streptomycin due to skin contact or inhalation of the drug. In such subjects, skin tests may be dangerous and may precipitate an anaphylactic or anaphylactoid reaction. Specific hyposensitization with slowly increasing doses of streptomycin has been effective. Due to the high incidence of streptomycin allergy, local administration in dermatological preparations or inhalation is to be condemned.

Second-generation effects Severe hearing loss and deficient vestibular function has been reported in children after the use of streptomycin in pregnancy (427[C]). The fact that streptomycin crosses the placenta has been used to explain the severe damage to the inner ear which has been observed in children exposed in utero. Possible hearing loss has been associated with the use of streptomycin during administration in the first trimester of pregnancy (SEDA-17, 305; 428[C]).

Neomycin; paromomycin

The parenteral use of neomycin and paromomycin is associated with such a high risk of toxicity that these antibiotics are now applied only locally or orally to decontaminate the gastrointestinal tract. More than 45 years ago neomycin was used for a short period of time as a tuberculostatic drug and as a result of this practice the full spectrum of toxicity is well known. Even though systemic use has now been abandoned, reports of nephrotoxic and ototoxic reactions continue to appear.

For special indications, neomycin continues to be a frequently prescribed drug. When neomycin is used as an irrigating solution in surgery, e.g. after total hip replacement, it may easily lead to toxic serum levels.

Inadequate attention is often paid to the drug's potential for ototoxicity and nephrotoxicity despite the fact that about 0.5—3% of an orally or rectally administered dose of neomycin is absorbed, potentially leading to peak serum levels of up to 6 g/ml. Furthermore, in patients with pre-existing renal disease, toxic concentrations may develop. Once renal damage is induced, further accumulation of the drug will lead to a vicious circle.

Adverse effects of paromomycin given by mouth are mainly limited to diarrhea.

Nervous system and special senses Clinical records of deafness due to neomycin are now becoming scarce, probably as a result of the growing awareness of the high ototoxicity of the systemically distributed drug. Frequently oto- and nephrotoxicity are noted simultaneously. The inner ear damage appears initially as high-tone hearing loss, then rapidly progresses to complete deafness.

Vestibular dysfunction has only been noted in the presence of concurrent auditory involvement. Damage to the inner ear is usually permanent.

There are reports related to ototoxicity following use of neomycin-containing ear-drops for conditions such as otitis externa and chronic otitis media with or without a perforated tympanic membrane. Inner ear damage was reported in about one case per 1000—3000 treatments (429[r], 430[r]).

Neomycin-induced deafness has been reported after virtually any form of topical use, e.g. in skin infections and burns and as a result of instillation into cavities or irrigation of large wounds, etc. In patients with cystic fibrosis and complicated bronchiectases, treatment for several months with aerosols containing neomycin has resulted in hearing loss.

Neuromuscular blockade Of the aminoglycosides, neomycin is the most potent with regard to the blocking effect on neuromuscular transmission. Many cases of severe respiratory depression, including fatalities, have been reported.

Allergic reactions Hypersensitivity to neomycin, usually of the delayed type, is one of the most common findings in dermatological departments. About 50% of patients sensitive to neomycin show cross-allergy with other aminoglycoside antibiotics. Many pharmaceutical preparations of neomycin also contain a corticosteroid component which may mask the manifestations of hypersensitivity. Neomycin is among the first 10 drugs or chemicals listed as being responsible for contact allergy. Hypersensitivity of the eyelids and the cheeks has been observed after administration of eye-drops containing neomycin. Cross-sensitization to framycetin, kanamycin, gentamicin and other related antibiotics does occur (431[r]).

Problems arising with special applications *Gastrointestinal tract* Neomycin is a valuable antibiotic for the prevention and treatment of portal systemic encephalopathy. When given orally in doses of 4—12 grams per day, neomycin may induce a malabsorption syndrome with steatorrhea (432[R]). This condition has also been evaluated experimentally in healthy volunteers.

Special indication As a lipid-lowering drug in hyperlipoproteinemia, neomycin is not to be recommended since it favors the emergence of multiresistant coliform bacteria (SEDA-2, 234).

POLYMYXINS

Polymyxin B and colistin (formerly known as 'polymyxin E') are effective against gram-negative bacteria with the exception of *Proteus* and *Neisseria* (*Branhamella*). They have in the past been used particularly to treat infection due to *Pseudomonas*. Both antibiotics combine with phospholipids in the bacterial cell wall, thereby changing the latter's permeability. This mode of action may explain the fact that the polymyxins can be bactericidal even for resting bacteria. Alteration of the cell wall is also thought to explain the damage to renal epithelia and to the nervous system which these drugs may induce.

When comparing doses, it should be noted that 1 mg of polymyxin B corresponds to 10 000 units and 1 mg of colistin to 20 000–30 000 units.

Even in patients with normal renal function, adverse reactions have occurred in up to 25%, contributing to death in 5% (433[C]). At therapeutically equivalent doses, allegations of differences in nephrotoxicity or neurotoxicity between polymyxin B and colistin are not convincing. In view of their adverse reaction potential the polymyxins have now been largely replaced by aminoglycosides, carboxypenicillins, ureidopenicillins and cephalosporins.

Bacterial resistance Acquired bacterial resistance is not a problem since extrachromosomal resistance (R-factor) has not yet been found.

Allergy Compared with the toxic effects of these drugs, allergic reactions to the polymyxins are relatively unimportant. Nevertheless, drug fever, maculopapular eruptions and other skin lesions have been observed in approximately 4% of treated patients (438[C]). Polymyxin is a bronchial irritant probably due to its well-known pharmacological histamine release. The reaction may be very rapid and resistant to bronchodilator treatment.

Nervous system During treatment with any one of the polymyxins, neurotoxicity may occur in up to 7% of patients with normal renal function.

Circumoral paresthesias, vasomotor instability, ataxia, dizziness, convulsions of varying severity and apnea have been reported.

Meningeal irritation rarely occurs in daily doses of 50 000 units (5 mg) given intrathecally, but higher doses may cause a stiff neck with liquor pleocytosis.

Neuromuscular blockade In animal models the polymyxins can produce a neuromuscular blockade similar to that observed with aminoglycosides which is aggravated by curare, ether and suxamethonium and antagonized by calcium. In patients the reaction may be noted first as fatiguability 1–26 hours after dosing, and may progress to severe muscular weakness including respiratory paralysis (434[c]). This complication has been reported in neurologically normal subjects exposed to high plasma concentrations of the antibiotic, but also in some individuals with concentrations that were considered to be in the therapeutic range. Particularly at risk are patients with myasthenia gravis, who may require increased doses of neostigmine. In patients with chronic pulmonary disease, a polymyxin-induced neuromuscular block may result in fatal apnea. Finally, after anesthesia involving muscle relaxants the polymyxins may induce a relapse in muscular weakness and inadequate ventilation (435[c]).

Effective treatment of polymyxin-induced neuromuscular blockade requires awareness of the complication with appropriate supervision and, if required, immediate ventilatory support. Calcium gluconate and neostigmine are not of proven efficacy against the blockade and should not be relied upon (434[c]).

Urinary system Adverse reactions involving the kidneys have occurred in about 20% of patients (433[C]). In man, the potential for kidney damage seems to be related to the age group. Whereas in the newborn and young infants 20 mg/kg of colistin methanesulfonate may be well tolerated, children over 2 years should not receive more than 10 mg/kg per day and adults even less.

Hyponatremia, hypokalemia and hypocalcemia with the corresponding clinical manifestations have occurred in patients treated for 3 weeks with polymyxin B, whenever the total dose exceeded 2 g/m^2 body surface. These electrolyte abnormalities were interpreted as consequences of polymyxin-induced nephrotoxicity. Hyperchloremia and a negative anion gap seem to result from the polycationic properties of polymyxin B.

Overdosage If patients have high plasma concentrations of the antibiotic, neither hemodialysis nor peritoneal dialysis is effective in eliminating the drug. Exchange transfusion has been proposed for treatment.

Second-generation effects Colistin and probably also polymyxin B may cross the placenta. Although the teratogenicity of these antibiotics has not been documented, treatment of pregnant patients exposes the fetus to these rather toxic drugs.

Problems with special applications Intramuscular injection of the sulfates of polymyxin B or of colistin often causes pain at the site of injection. With sodium colistin methanesulfonate this adverse reaction is largely absent.

Intratympanic administration of polymyxin B or of colistin to guinea-pigs has caused cochlear damage. On the basis of weight, both antibiotics are even more toxic than neomycin. They should not be used in ear-drops if the tympanon is not intact.

Lincomycins

Two members of this group—lincomycin and the semisynthetic derivative, clindamycin—have become established drugs. Both have a narrow antibacterial spectrum involving mostly gram-positive species and some obligate anaerobes such as *Bacteroides*. Like chloramphenicol and erythromycin, they combine with a subunit of bacterial ribosomes, thereby interfering with protein synthesis. Whereas oral lincomycin has a systemic availability of about 40%, which may be further compromised by food, clindamycin is absorbed from the gastrointestinal tract to the extent of 90—100%. Both are eliminated mainly by hepatic metabolism and biliary excretion.

ADVERSE REACTION PATTERN

General and toxic reactions The direct toxicity of the lincomycins is relatively low (SED-7, 389; 436[R]). Clindamycin has not been given in similar high amounts as lincomycin. The most common adverse reaction is diarrhea which occurs in as many as 10—20% of patients. The most serious gastrointestinal complication is *Clostridium difficile*-induced colitis which arises with about equal frequency after oral and parenteral treatment (437[R]; 438[C]) (see Chapter 25.2).

Hypersensitivity reactions Skin rashes, urticaria and angioedema have been reported with lincomycin, but are apparently rare. In contrast, maculopapular and pruritic eruptions seem to occur after 1—2 weeks of treatment in up to 10% of patients receiving clindamycin. This drug has also been incriminated in one case of Stevens-Johnson syndrome and in one of anaphylaxis. In the latter patient, hemagglutinating antibodies were found against clindamycin and lincomycin (439[R]). Leukoclastic angiitis associated with clindamycin seems to be a rather rare event. If a similar angiitis can also occur in the colon, the question arises whether some cases of antibiotic-associated colitis might be caused by the drug itself rather than by bacterial toxins.

Tumor-inducing effects These have not been reported.

ORGANS AND SYSTEMS

Cardiovascular Rapid intravenous infusion of large doses of lincomycin (600 mg given in 5—10 min) may cause flushing and a sensation of warmth for about 10 min. A patient receiving 200 mg/kg experienced nausea, vomiting, hypotension, dyspnea and ECG changes for 20 min (SED-7, 389). Rapid intravenous infusions of 1—2 grams of lincomycin may cause phlebitis. A case of cardiac arrest associated with rapid intravenous administration of clindamycin has been reported (440[C]; SEDA-8, 258).

Hematological Granulocytopenia and thrombocytopenia have been described in a few patients. The cause-and-effect relationship, however, has not been unequivocally established.

Liver and kidney Abnormal liver tests during treatment with lincomycin have been noted rarely only in cases who had received large doses (>4 g/day) for more than 3 weeks (436[R]). In another series, intravenous administration of lincomycin in doses of 4—18 g/day was not associated with renal or hepatic toxicity (SED-7, 388). High doses of clindamycin may be hepatotoxic. Since the lincomycins are eliminated from the organism by biliary excretions, toxicity may be expected particularly in patients with liver disease.

Gastrointestinal The most prominent adverse reaction of the lincomycins is diarrhea, which may vary from mildly loose bowel movements to life-threatening pseudomembranous colitis (see Chapter 25.2). Almost all antimicrobial drugs have been associated with severe diarrhea and colitis; lincomycin and clindamycin, however, have been particularly incriminated. The incidence of clindamycin-induced diarrhea has been reported to be 23% in hospitals. Diarrhea resolves promptly after drug withdrawal in most cases. It seems to be dose-related and may result from a direct action on the intestinal mucosa. Severe *Clostridium difficile*-induced colitis is not dose-related and arises in 0.01—10% of recipients. Clustering of cases in time and place suggests the possibility of cross-infection (see Chapter 25.2).

Even low doses of clindamycin—in one reported case topical administration (441[C])—may cause marked alterations in several intestinal flora-related functions (442[R]). Most antibiotics have been associated with the development of antibiotic-associated colitis.

As with other antibiotics, esophageal ulcers have been observed due to delayed passage of clindamycin capsules through the esophagus. The drug should be taken with a meal or followed by a glass of water (443[R]).

Skin and appendages Typical sunlight sensitivity

with a maculopapular eruption has been observed with lincomycin in two patients treated by the intramuscular route (436[R]). Lincomycin reaction may also present as rosacea (444[C]).

Bacterial resistance and superinfections In vitro *Staphylococcus aureus*, *pneumococci*, *Group A streptococci* and *viridans streptococci* acquire resistance to the lincomycins regularly, easily and quickly (SED-8, 638). In endometrial cultures taken following clindamycin therapy the occurrence of clindamycin-resistant anaerobic bacteria was significantly higher than before therapy (445[C]). Their similar mechanism of action has been used to explain cross-resistance between the macrolide antibiotics and the lincomycins. Among erythromycin-resistant *staphylococci* 50% of the isolated strains were also resistant to lincomycin (SED-6, 304). In patients who need long-term suppressive therapy, but who are allergic to penicillin, the development of such combined resistance of the oropharyngeal flora may present a serious clinical problem.

Superinfection with resistant strains of *Pseudomonas*, *Proteus* or *staphylococci* has been observed. Suppression of *Bacteroides* in the intestinal flora may be related to the proliferation of *Clostridium difficile* which is important for the production of pseudomembranous colitis. Excessive growth of *Candida* on the skin has occurred when lincomycin was applied topically (436[R]).

Second-generation effects Although lincomycin penetrates into the fetal circulation, no fetal abnormalities could be related to lincomycin administration in a series of 302 women who had completed a course of lincomycin therapy (500 mg every 6 h) for 1 week. All three trimesters of pregnancy were included (446[R]).

Interactions Sodium or calcium cyclamate may retard (but do not prevent) lincomycin absorption.

Antagonism between the lincomycins and the macrolide antibiotics has been observed in vitro and was explained also by their binding to the same subunit of bacterial ribosomes. This mechanism of bacteriostatic action also suggests that the lincomycins might prevent the bactericidal action of the penicillins and the cephalosporins.

Clindamycin may potentiate the effects of some ganglion blocking agents.

Clindamycin and lincomycin have been found to potentiate the action of non-depolarizing myorelaxants, such as pancuronium and *d*-tubocurarine. The lincosamide-induced block cannot be reliably reversed by pharmacological means (447[R]). Treatment with clindamycin may increase the plasma concentration of digoxin.

GLYCOPEPTIDES

Vancomycin

Vancomycin is a narrow-spectrum glycopeptide antibiotic with potent antistaphylococcal activity. It was developed in the early 1950s. Early preparations of the compound contained substantial impurities. These impurities were presumably responsible for some of the adverse reactions reported (449[R]). When rapid infusion rates are avoided, vancomycin is rarely associated with serious toxicity. Recent reviews suggest that the potential for vancomycin to cause significant oto- or nephrotoxicity has been exaggerated (450[R], 451[R]).

Vancomycin inhibits bacterial cell-wall synthesis and is bactericidal during cell division at therapeutic concentrations. Bacterial resistance to vancomycin has been no issue during the first decades of clinical use. More recently, vancomycin-resistant enterococci have been recovered with increasing frequency from hospitalized patients. In some institutions multidrug-resistant and vancomycin-resistant enterococci have become important nosocomial pathogens that are difficult to treat. For example, vancomycin-resistant enterococcal bacteremia is associated with a poor prognosis. Judicious use of vancomycin and broad-spectrum antibiotics is recommended, and strict infection control measures must be implemented to prevent nosocomial transmission of these organisms (452[R]). Vancomycin is particularly useful in infections caused by meticillin-resistant or penicillinase-producing staphylococci and diphtheroids, as well as in the prophylaxis of bacterial endocarditis and in the treatment of antibiotic-associated colitis. Sufficient fecal concentrations can be achieved with oral therapy. Poorly absorbed from the gastrointestinal tract, it is painful when injected intramuscularly.

ORGANS AND SYSTEMS

Cardiovascular Severe anaphylactic reactions are rare.

Nervous system It is still controversial whether vancomycin can indeed cause ototoxicity when administered alone. However, vancomycin can augment the ototoxicity of aminoglycosides (453[R]). Tinnitus and dizziness has been noted, resolving on withdrawal of vancomycin (454[C]). Hearing loss may be transient or permanent. If vancomycin is combined with aminoglycosides, toxicity may be additive (455[C]).

Hematological Neutropenia has also been observed (456[R], 457[C]). It occurs after prolonged treatment with high doses in patients with normal renal function (e.g.

more than 20 days of more than 15 or 20 mg/kg) or in the prolonged presence of high serum levels in patients with severe renal insufficiency (458[C]). After withdrawal of vancomycin, neutropenia disappeared promptly. The bone marrow seemed to be unaffected. A direct toxic effect of vancomycin and/or an immune reaction have been discussed as causative mechanisms. Cases of agranulocytosis related to vancomycin therapy have been reported (459[C]–461[C]).

Urinary system Vancomycin is eliminated almost exclusively by renal excretion. In oliguria a 1-gram dose may produce therapeutic plasma concentrations for 10–14 days. Hemodialysis fails to remove vancomycin from the body to any significant degree. If the renal function is compromised, even oral therapy with vancomycin may lead to high and potentially toxic serum and CSF drug levels (462[C]). Nephrotoxicity of vancomycin, once thought to be a major problem, is often mild and reversible after cessation of therapy. It occurs in 6–17% of therapies (463[R]). Higher frequencies of nephrotoxicity have been reported when vancomycin was used in combination with an aminoglycoside, which is consistent with toxicological data obtained in rats (464[C]). Nevertheless the evidence of synergistic toxicity between vancomycin and aminoglycosides is controversial (450[R], 454[C], 463[C]). Endotoxins seem to potentiate the nephrotoxic effect of vancomycin, at least in rats (465[R]).

Skin and appendages A unique and peculiar adverse reaction related to the rapid infusion of large doses is the so-called red neck or red man syndrome. It is the most common adverse reaction to vancomycin, characterized by fever, chills, paresthesia, and erythema at the base of the neck and the upper back, and may be followed by a hypotensive episode (466[C]). It is not a true allergic reaction. It seems to be due to vancomycin-induced release of histamine and possibly other vasoactive substances without the involvement of preformed antibodies (467[C], 468[C]). Antihistamine H1 blocking agents are effective in preventing the anaphylactoid reactions to vancomycin (469[R]). A 0.25–0.5% solution given over 60 minutes is recommended and patients have to be monitored closely. A possible red man syndrome has also been associated with systemic absorption of oral vancomycin in a patient with normal renal function (470[C]). Allergic reactions such as skin rashes, chill, fever and eosinophilia may occur in up to 5% of patients. Vancomycin can lead to the development of Stevens-Johnson syndrome (471[C]). Some authors stress the fact that vancomycin may interact with anesthetic drugs, particularly muscle relaxants. In the reported cases anaphylactoid reactions were seen with intense erythema and marked permeability changes (472[C]). Even when given slowly by the intravenous route, it may cause phlebitis.

Therapeutic drug monitoring Monitoring of serum levels has been advocated to reduce potential nephro- and ototoxicity due to interpatient variability in vancomycin pharmacokinetics. However, routine monitoring might be unnecessary in the majority of patients (451[R], 473[R]). Clinical settings in which therapeutic monitoring of vancomycin may be prudent include combination therapies with an aminoglycoside and treatments of patients with poor or unstable renal function (450[R]). There is evidence that the risk of toxicity increases with higher serum concentrations, but there are no firm data for defining a therapeutic range.

Teicoplanin

The glycopeptide teicoplanin has been used as an alternative drug to vancomycin for the treatment of gram-positive infections. Its pharmacological properties permit once-a-day dosing. The safety profile of this compound has been thoroughly investigated. It is generally well tolerated, but physicians should be familiar with potential adverse drug reactions.

ADVERSE REACTION PATTERN

General and toxic reactions The well described 'red man syndrome' associated with rapid infusion of vancomycin resulting in histamine release is very rarely seen with teicoplanin. In a double-blind, randomized, two-way crossover study comparing the effects of vancomycin (15 mg/kg over 60 minutes) and teicoplanin (15 mg/kg over 30 minutes), erythema and pruritus were observed in 11 of 12 subjects receiving vancomycin, but not in patients given teicoplanin. While plasma histamine levels increased significantly following vancomycin infusion, histamine levels remained essentially unchanged after teicoplanin (475[C]). Although the reported very high rate of red man syndrome in these healthy volunteers appears to be unusual and does not correlate with clinical experience of vancomycin, the study nevertheless shows that this particular histamine-mediated toxic reaction is less likely with teicoplanin use than with vancomycin.

Local reactions at the injection site including pain, redness or discomfort following intramuscular injection, or phlebitis following intravenous injection may be observed in approximately 3% of patients (476[R]). The overall rate of adverse reactions in comparative trials was 18.9%, which is comparable with the rate observed with β-lactams, but lower than the corresponding rate (38.9%) associated with vancomycin use (476[R]).

Hypersensitivity reaction Allergic reactions have been reported following administration of teicoplanin. Erythroderma during infusion of teicoplanin with fever and hypotension was described in a single patient. Re-exposure to the drug again elicited the same reaction (477[C]). Allergic cross-reactivity between teicoplanin and vancomycin has been reported (478[C], 479[C]). This cross-reactivity was documented by in vitro studies showing IgE release by basophils in response to stimulation by both vancomycin and teicoplanin in a further patient who experienced a clinically relevant allergic reaction to vancomycin (480[c]). In other studies the second drug did not elicit allergic reactions in patients known to be allergic to one of the two compounds (481[C]—483[C]). Based on these small studies and individual case reports one can conclude that allergic hypersensitivity reactions to teicoplanin may occur in patients with known allergic reactions to vancomycin, but the frequency of occurrence of this type of cross-reaction appears to be low. Therefore, known hypersensitivity to vancomycin is not a contraindication for teicoplanin use.

Tumor-inducing effects None reported.

ORGANS AND SYSTEMS

Cardiovascular As mentioned above, hypotension has been observed as part of the manifestations of a hypersensitivity reaction (477[C]).

Respiratory Bronchospasm as a result of teicoplanin administration required discontinuation of the drug in two out of 310 patients (484[C]).

Nervous system and special senses Ototoxicity has been reported during treatment with teicoplanin (485[C]). A decrease in high-frequency auditory threshold has been observed in one patient treated with teicoplanin for a serious gram-positive infection (486[C]). However, the causal relationship between teicoplanin use and alterations of auditory function has not been established in controlled clinical studies (487[R]). Guinea-pigs treated for 28 days with a maximum dose of 75 mg/kg/day remained without any evidence of functional, morphological, or histological changes indicative of ototoxicity (488[R]). Davey reported 11 cases of ototoxicity among 3377 patients treated with teicoplanin (487[R]). Details of the treatment regimens used in these patients are not provided. Therefore it can be concluded that teicoplanin-associated ototoxicity is rare.

Endocrine, metabolic No adverse events are reported.

Mineral and fluid balance No adverse events are reported.

Hematological Neutropenia developed in a patient after 20 days of treatment with teicoplanin (489[C]). However, this appears to be a rare occurrence. In patients undergoing bone marrow transplantation receiving teicoplanin for the treatment of severe sepsis, the duration of neutropenia was not prolonged by teicoplanin in a small open trial (490[C]). Thrombocytopenia was associated on two consecutive occasions with teicoplanin therapy in a patient with acute myeloid leukemia (491[C]). The exact mechanism for this adverse event is unknown. Teicoplanin does not alter platelet function or blood coagulation (492[C]). Teicoplanin may also rarely cause eosinophilia (493[C]). Overall, the rate of hematological alterations was 2.2% in 1431 patients participating in a large multicentre non-comparative study (494[c]).

Liver Transient elevations of liver enzymes were observed in 2.3% of patients in one study (484[C]). Other authors also reported abnormal liver enzymes in some patients treated with teicoplanin (486[C], 495[c], 496[C], 497[c]).

Gastrointestinal Adverse events involving the gastrointestinal system appear to be rather rare. Diarrhea has been listed among the nonspecific events observed in 5.1% of the patients (494[c]).

Urinary system Nephrotoxicity may result from teicoplanin therapy, but this occurs less frequently with teicoplanin than with vancomycin (476[R]). However, the concomitant aminoglycoside therapy in some patients makes the contribution of the glycopeptide antibiotic difficult to assess. Renal toxicity was observed more frequently in patients receiving the combination of netilmicin/vancomycin than in patients treated with netilmicin and teicoplanin (498[C]). Similar differences in nephrotoxicity between vancomycin and teicoplanin were observed in febrile neutropenic patients receiving concomitant tobramycin and piperacillin (499[C]). Kureishi described a significant deterioration of renal function when vancomycin and ciclosporin A, but not teicoplanin and ciclosporin A, were used together. The mechanism responsible for this drug interaction is unknown (499[C]).

Skin and appendages Observed skin reactions included pruritus, urticaria and rash in 2.4% of patients (494[c]).

Genital system No adverse events are reported.

Bone No adverse events are reported. Teicoplanin has been successfully used to treat bone and joint infections without any adverse reactions affecting bones or joints (500[c]).

Eyes No adverse events are reported.

Interactions Nephrotoxicity may occur during treatment with teicoplanin as noted above. The risk of nephrotoxicity may increase with the concomitant use of other nephrotoxic drugs, especially aminoglycosides. In addition, a possible drug interaction with enalapril was reported (501[C]). A diabetic patient receiving teicoplanin therapy for osteomyelitis developed renal insufficiency requiring dialysis following the addition of enalapril to his regimen (501[C]). Since cholestyramine binds teicoplanin in vitro and reduces its activity against *Clostridium difficile* almost completely, there is a potential for a clinically relevant interaction between these drugs (502[c]). Teicoplanin should be administered separately from ciprofloxacin since precipitation has been provoked by concomitant parenteral administration (503[r]).

Monitoring of serum teicoplanin levels In severe infections monitoring of serum teicoplanin levels is indicated to assure adequate trough concentrations (>10 mg/l) (504[R]). For the treatment of *S. aureus* endocarditis trough levels should exceed 20 mg/l (504[R]). Inadequately low serum levels of teicoplanin may have been responsible for the high failure rate observed in intravenous drug users treated with teicoplanin for right-sided endocarditis (505[C]). The fact that teicoplanin pharmacokinetics are quite variable and relatively unpredictable in intravenous drug users adds further weight to the importance of monitoring serum drug levels in this population during treatment of severe infections such as endocarditis (506[C]). Since the elimination half-life of teicoplanin also varies greatly in patients with various degrees of renal insufficiency, monitoring of serum levels may also be helpful in guiding therapy in some patients with markedly reduced creatinine clearance (507[C]).

OTHER ANTIMICROBIAL DRUGS

Bacitracin

Bacitracin has mostly dermatological applications. It may cause allergic reactions of the delayed type. A shock-like picture after local application has occurred in a hypersensitive individual (508[C]). Since bacitracin is nephrotoxic, it should also not be administered intraperitoneally to patients with renal impairment.

Fosfomycin

Fosfomycin has relatively low toxicity. Its penetration into tissues, including bones and joints, and into the cerebrospinal fluid is good. When given orally (2—3 grams/day), it can produce gastrointestinal distress; when injected intramuscularly, it may cause local pain. Fosfomycin is now recommended in daily doses of 4—16 grams i.v. for the treatment of severe infections resistant to other commonly used antibiotics. During systemic administration, elevation of serum GOT, GPT, LDH, skin reactions, eosinophilia and derangement of vision have been noted (509[R]).

Fusidic acid

Fusidic acid is the best-known representative of a group of antibiotics having a steroid structure and which are eliminated primarily by biliary excretion as microbiologically inactive metabolites. The antibacterial action of fusidic acid is bacteriostatic and limited to gram-positive cocci, particularly staphylococci. The drug is adequately absorbed from the gastrointestinal tract, but has also been used topically. It has the important property of good tissue penetration, including entry into the bones and joints, but does not reach the cerebrospinal fluid. Fusidic acid may also have a role as a clinically useful suppressor of immunoinflammatory processes (510[R]).

Fusidic acid has detergent properties and may cause hemolysis when injected intravenously or may induce tissue damage when given intramuscularly. The systemic toxicity is relatively low, but development of bacterial resistance has been a obstacle to its widespread use.

Hematological Rare cases of granulocytopenia have been reported (511[R]).

Liver Raised transaminases occurred in some patients on 1.5—3 grams of fusidic acid per day and normalized rapidly upon cessation of therapy. Since hepatic metabolism and biliary excretion are the main routes of elimination, toxicity may be expected in patients with liver or biliary tact disease leading to accumulation of the drug. In some reports relating to both the oral and the intravenous form, several cases of jaundice have been described (512[c]—514[c]). In one report, jaundice developed in 34% of patients with staphylococcal bacteremia treated intravenously with fusidic acid. Although experimental evidence suggests that the intravenous preparation may cause hemolysis, this was not considered a likely explanation for the liver damage in these observations. An alternative explanation may lie in the steroid structure of fusidic acid (515[r], 516[r]). It is recommended that patients receiving intravenous fusidic acid should be changed to oral therapy as soon as their condition has improved.

Gastrointestinal Epigastric pain, nausea and possibly vomiting may be regarded as signs of gastrointestinal irritation. These symptoms are markedly reduced if the drug is taken with meals. Mild constipation or diarrhea have been observed.

Skin and appendages Allergic exanthematous skin reactions and contact dermatitis are rare. Also, development of a widespread macular rash has been described; it seemed to be a genuine reaction to intravenous fusidic acid (517^C, 518^R, 519^C).

Bacterial resistance and interactions Bacterial resistance may be an important problem with this antibiotic. It develops in a single step in vitro and has also been observed in patients, particularly during prolonged administration (520^R). Combined administration with some other antibiotics, however, requires caution. Being bacteriostatic, fusidic acid may prevent the bactericidal action of penicillin, and increased survival of staphylococci may occur. Hydrocortisone, which is chemically similar to fusidic acid, inhibits its antibacterial activity in vitro.

Spectinomycin

Spectinomycin is an aminocyclitol antibiotic, thereby differing from the aminoglycosides. It has been mainly used in single-dose (2 grams i.m.) treatment of gonorrhea, also in those forms complicated by multiple antibiotic resistance. Apart from indurations at the site of injection, tolerance in otherwise healthy individuals has been good even with doses of 8 g/day for 21 days. Allergic reactions have been observed, but are rare. Spectinomycin-resistant gonococci have already been found (521^R, 522^R).

REFERENCES

1. Sastre Dominguez J, Sastre Castillo A, Marin Nunez F. Anafilaxia sistémica a tetraciclinas. Rev Clin Esp 1984; 174:135.
2. Golbert TM, Patterson R, Pruzansky JJ. Systemic allergic reactions to ingested antigens. J Allergy 1969;44:96.
3. Fenoglio JJ, McAlister HA, Mullick FG. Hypersensitivity mocarditis. Hum Pathol 1981;12:900.
4. Guillon J-M, Joly P, Autran B et al. Minocycline-induced cell-mediated hypersensitivity pneumonitis. Ann Int Med 1992;117:476.
5. Puyana J, Ureña V, Quirce S et al. Serum sickness-like syndrome associated with minocycline therapy. Allergy 1990;45:313.

6a. Sulkowsky SR, Haserick JR. Simulated systemic lupus erythematosus from degraded tetracycline. J Am Med Assoc 1964;189:179.

6b. Pollen RH. Anaphylactoid reaction to orally administered demethylchlortetracycline. N Engl J Med 1964; 271:673.

7a. Menon MPS, Das AK. Tetracycline asthma—a case report. Clin Allergy 1977;7:285.

7b. Sitbon O, Bidel N, Dussopt C et al. Minocycline pneumonitis and eosinophilia. A report on eight patients. Arch Intern Med 1994;154:1633.

8. Almind M, Lange P, Viskum K. Spontaneous pneumothorax: comparision of simple drainage, talc pleurodesis, and tetracycline pleurodesis. Thorax 1989;44:627.
9. Fields JP. Bulging fontanelle: a complication of tetracycline therapy in infants. J Pédiatr 1961;58:74.
10. Maroon JC, Mealy J. Benign intracanial hypertension. Sequel to tetracycline therapy in a child. J Am Med Assoc 1971;216:1479.
11. Rush MA. Pseudotumor cerebri: clinical profile and visual coutcom in 63 patients. Mayo Clin Proc 1980;55:541.
12. Koch-Weser J, Gilmor EB. Benign intracranial hypertension in an adult after tetracycline therapy. J Am Med Assoc 1967;200:345.
13. Bowmick BK. Benign intracranial hypertension after antibiotic therapy. Br Med J 1972;3:30.
14. Meacock DJ, Hewer RL. Tetracycline and benign intracranial hypertension. Br Med J 1981;282:1240.
15. Walters BNJ, Gubbay SS. Tetracycline and benign intracranial hypertension: report of five cases. Br Med J 1981;1282:19.
16. Pearson MG, Littlewood SM, Bowden AN. Tetracycline and benign intracranial hypertension. Br Med J 1981;282:4.
17. Lubetzki C, Sanson M, Cohen D et al. Hypertension intracrÂnienne bénigne et minocycline. Rev Neurol (Paris) 1988;144:218.
18. Lander CM Minocycline-induced benign intracranial hypertension. Clin Exp Neurol 1989;26:161.
19. Haenggeli ChA, Laufer D. Pseudotumeur cérébrale chez un jeune homme traité aux tétracyclines pour une acne. Schweiz Med Wochenschr 1990;120(Suppl 34):25.
20. Askmark H, Lundberg PO, Olsson S. Drug-related headache. Headache 1989;29:441.
21. Bezzi G, Gesa GL. Rapporti tra antibiotici e curarismo (III). Tetraciciline e curarismo. Boll Soc Ital Biol Sper 1960;36:374.
22. Baïsset A, Lareng L, Puig G. Incidence d'une thérapeutique antibiotique sur la curarisation. In: Comptes-Rendus, XII Congrès Francais d'Anesthésiologie, Monpellier, 1962;813.
23. Snavely SR, Hodges GR. The neurotoxicity of antibacterial agents. Ann Intern Med 1984;101:92.
24. Kubiowski P, Szreniawski Z. The mechanism of the neuromuscular blockade by antibiotics. Arch Int Pharmacodyn 1963;146:549.
25. Lambs L, Venturini M, Decock-Le Révérend et al. Metal ion—tetracycline interactions in biological fluids. Part

8. Pontentiometric and spectroscopic studies on the formation of Ca(II) and Mg(II) complexes with 4-dedi-methylamino-tetracycline and 6-desoxy-6-demethyl-tetracycline. J Inorg Biochem 1988;33:193.
26. Billano RA, Ward WQ, Little WP. Minocycline and black thyroid. J Am Med Assoc 1983;249:1887.
27. Reid JD. The black thyroid associated with minocycline therapy. Am J Clin Pathol 1983;79:738.
28. Maxon HR, Rutsky EA. Vasopressin-resistant diabetes insipidus associated with short-term demethyl-chlortetracycline (Declomycin) therapy. Milit Med 1973;138:500.
29. Cherril DA, Stote RM, Birge JR, Singer I. Demeclocycline treatment in the syndrome of inappropriate antidiuretic hormone secretion. Ann Intern Med 1975;83:654.
30. Forrest JN, Cox M, Hong C et al. Superiority of demeclocycline over lithium in the treatment of chronic syndrome of inappropiate secretion of antidiuretic hormone. N Engl J Med 1978;298:173.
31. Singer I, Rotenberg D. Demeclocycline-induced nephrogenic diabetes insipidus. Ann Intern Med 1973; 79:679.
32. De Troyer A, Pilloy W, Broeckaert I, Demanet JC. Correction of antidiuresis by demeclocycline. N Engl J Med 1976;239:915.
33. De Troyer A, Pilloy W, Broeckaert I, Demanet JC. Demeclocycline treatment of water retention in cirrhosis. Ann Intern Med 1976;85:336.
34. Walker RG, Thomson NM, Dowling JP, Ogg CS. Minocycline-induced acute interstitial nephritis. Br Med J 1979;1:524.
35. Wilkinson SP, Stewart WK, Spiers EM. Protracted systemic illness and interstitial nephritis due to minocycline. Postgrad Med J 1989;65:53.
36. Murray KM, Keane WR. Review of drug-induced acute interstitial nephritis. Pharmacotherapy 1992;12:462.
37. Carrilho F, Bosch J, Arroyo V et al. Renal failure associated with demeclocycline in cirrhosis. Ann Intern Med 1977;87:195.
38. Miller PD, Linas SL, Schrier RW. Plasma demeclocycline levels and nephrotoxicity: correlation in hyponatremic cirrhotic patients. J Am Med Assoc 1980;243:2513.
39. Geheb M, Cox M. Renal effects of demeclocycline. J Am Med Assoc 1980;243:2519.
40. Zegers de Beyl D, Naeije R, De Troyer A. Demeclocycline treatment of water retention in congestive heart failure. Br Med J 1978;1:760.
41. Simpson MB, Pryzbylik J, Innis B et al. Hemolytic anemia after tetracycline therapy. N Engl J Med 1985;312:840.
42. Kounis NS. Oxytetracycline-induced thrombocytopenic purpura. J Am Med Assoc 1975;231:734.
43. Zein ZA. Louse borne relapsing fever (LBRF): Mortality and frequency of Jarisch-Herxheimer reaction. J R Soc Health 1987;107:146.
44. Dowling JF, Lepper MH. Hepatic reactions to tetracycline. J Am Med Assoc 1964;188:307.
45. Peters RL, Edmondson HG, Mikkelsen WP, Tatter D. Tetracycline-induced fatty liver in nonpregnant patients: a report of six cases. Am J Surg 1967;113:622.
46. Burette A, Finet C, Prigogine T et al. Acute hepatic injury associated with minocycline. Arch Intern Med 1984;144:1491.
47. Elmore MF, Rogge JD. Tetracycline-induced pancreatitis. Gastroenterology 1981;81:1134.
48. Topoll HH, Lange DE, Müller FR. Multiple periodontal abscesses after systemic antibiotic therapy. J Clin Periodontol 1990;17:268.
49. Bonavina L, DeMeester TR, McChesney L et al. Drug-induced esophageal strictures. Ann Surg 1987;206:173.
50. Baeriswyl G, Bengoa J, De Peyer R et al. Importance des ulcérations médcamenteuses dans les lésions endoscopiques de l'oesophage. Schweiz Med Wochenschr 1985; 114(Suppl 19):6.
51. Zijnen-Suyker MP, Hazenberg BP. Oesophagusbeschadiging door doxycycline. Ned Tijdschr Geneeskd 1981;125:1407.
52. Schneider R. Doxycycline esophageal ulcers. Digest Dis 1977;22:805.
53. Crowsen TD, Head LH, Ferrante WA. Esophageal ulcers associated with tetracycline therapy. J Am Med Assoc 1976;235:2747.
54. Kobler E, Nüesch HJ, Bühler H et al. Medikamentös bedingte Oesophagusulzera. Schweiz Med Wochenschr 1979;109:1180.
55. Gant NF, Whalley PJ, Baxter CR. Nonoliguric renal failure: report of a case. Obstet Gynecol 1969;34:675.
56. Korkeila J. Antianabolic effect of tetracaclines. Lancet 1971;i:974.
57. Morgan T, Ribush N. The effect of oxytetracycline and doxycycline on protein metabolism. Med J Austr 1972;1:55.
58. Kunin CM, Rees SB, Merrill JP et al. Persistence of antibiotics in blood of patients with acute renal failure. I. Tetracycline and chlortetracycline. J Clin Invest 1959; 38:1487.
59. Carey BW. Abnormal urinary findings and achromycin V. Pediatrics 1963;31:697.
60. Lowe MB, Tapp E. Renal damage caused by anhydro-4-epitetracycline. Arch Pathol 1966;81:362.
61. Frank SB, Cohen HJ, Minkin W. Photo-onycholysis due to tetracycline hydrochloride and doxycycline. Arch Dermatol 1971;103:520.
62. Frost P, Weinstein GD, Gomez EC. Phototoxic potential of minocycline and doxycycline. Arch Dermatol 1972; 105:681.
63. Epstein JH, Tuffanelli DL, Seibert JS et al. Porphyria-like cutaneous changes induced by tetracycline hydrochloride photosensitization. Arch Dermatol 1976;112:661.
64. Shelley WB, Heaton CL. Minocycline sensitivity. J Am Med Assoc 1973;224:125.
65. Samman PD. The nails; onchylosysis. In: Rook A, Welkinson DS, Ebling FJG, eds. Textbook of Dermatology. Oxford: Blackwell Scientific Publications, 1972;1647.
66. Jones HE, Lewis CW, Reisner JE. Photosensitive lichenoid eruption associated with demeclocycline. Arch Dermatol 1972;106:58.
67. Fenske NA, Millns JL, Greer KE. Minocycline-induced pigmentation at sites of cutaneous inflammation. J Am Med Assoc 1980;244:1103.
68. Möller H, Rausing A. Methacycline hyperpigmentation: a five-year follow-up. Acta Dermatol-Venereol 1980;60:495.
69. Messmer E, Font RL, Sheldon G et al. Pigmented conjunctival cysts following tetracycline/minocycline therapy. Ophthalmology 1983;90:1463.
70. Beehner ME, Houston GD, Young JD. Oral pigmentation secondary to minocycline therapy. J Oral Maxillofac Surg 1986;44:582.
71. Basler RSW. Minocycline related hyperpigmentation. Arch Dermatol 1985;121:606.
72. Hanzlick R, Wilson R. Monocycline-related black thyroid. Am J Forensic Med Pathol 1988;9:201.

73. Mooney E, Bennett RG. Periungual hyperpigmentation mimicking Hutchinson's sign associated with minocycline administration. J Dermatol Surg Oncol 1988;14:1001.
74. Butler JM, Marks R, Sutherland R. Cutaneous and cardiac valvular pigmentation with minocycline. Clin Exp Dermatol 1985;10:432.
75. Shum DT, Smout MS, Pace WE et al. Unusual skin pigmentation from long-term methacycline and minocycline therapy. Arch Dermatol 1986;122:17.
76. Charles D, Obst D. Placental transmission of antibiotics. J Obstet Gynaecol Br Emp 1954;61:750.
77. Seeliger HPR, Ronde G. Die Wirkung von Tetracyclingaben auf das kindliche Gebiss bei Listeriosebehandlung von Schwangeren. Geburtshilfe Frauenheilk 1968;28:209.
78. Witkop CT, Wolf RO. Hypoplasia and intrinsic staining of enamel following tetracycline therapy. J Am Med Assoc 1963;185:1008.
79. Poliak SC, Di Giovanni JJ, Gross EG et al. Minocycline-associated tooth discoloration in young adults. J Am Med Assoc 1985;254:2930.
80. Arndt KA, Jick H. Rates of cuteaneous reactions to drugs. J Am Med Assoc 1976;235:918.
81. Fawcett IW, Pepys J. Allergy to a tetracycline preparation: a case report. Clin Allergy 1976;6:301.
82. Shoji A, Someda Y, Hamada T. Stevens-Johnsons syndrome due to minocycline therapy. Arch Dermatol 1986;123:18.
83a. Curley RK, Verbov JL. Stevens-Johnson syndrome due to tetracyclines—a case report (doxycycline) and of the literature. Clin Exp Dermatol 1987;12:124.
83b. Trüeb RM, Burg G. Acute generalized exanthematous pustulosis due to doxycycline. Dermatology 1993;136:75.
84. Fiumara NJ, Yaqub M. Pigmented penile lesions (fixed drug eruptions) associated with tetracycline therapy for sexually transmitted disease. Sex Transm Dis 1981;8:23.
85. Pasricha JS. Drugs causing fixed eruptions. Br J Dermatol 1979;100:183.
86. Kanwar AJ, Bharija SC, Singh M et al. Ninety-eight fixed drug eruptions with provocation test. Dermatologica 1988;177:274.
87. Domz CA, McNamara DH, Holzapfel HF. Tetracycline provocation on lupus erythematosus. Ann Intern Med 1959;50:1217.
88. Bojs G, Möller H. Eczematous contact allergy to oxytetracycline with cross-sensitivity to other tetracyclines. Berufs-Dermatosen 1974;22:202.
89. Mahaur BS, Sharma VK, Kumar B et al. Prevalence of contact hypersensitivity to common antiseptics, antibacterials and antifungals in normal persons. Indian. J Dermatol Venerol. Leprol. 1987;53:269.
90. Burton J. A placebo-controlled study to evaluate the efficacy of topical tetracycline and oral tetracycline in the treatment of mild to moderate acne. J Int Med Res 1990;18:93.
91. Gilgor RS. Complications of tetracycline therapy of acne. NC Med J 1972;33:331.
92. Csonka GW, Rosedale N, Walkden L. Balanitis due to fixed drug eruption associated with tetracycline therapy. Br J Vener Dis 1971;47:42.
93. Elsner P, Hartmann AA, Burg G. Experiences with oxytetracycline treatment of non-gonorrhea urethritis caused by *Ureaplasma urealyticum*. Hautarzt 1990;41:94.
94. Edwards TS. Transient myopia due to tetracycline. J Am Med Assoc 1963;186:69.
95. Rall DP, Loo Ti Li, Lane M et al. Appearance and persistence of fluorescent material in tumor tissue after tetracycline administration. J Natl Cancer Inst 1975;19:79.
96. Tötterman LE, Saxén L. Incorporation of tetracycline into human foetal bones after maternal drug administration. Acta Obstet Gynecol Scand 1969;48:542.
97. Cohlan SQ. Bevelander G, Tiamsic T. Growth inhibition of prematures receiving tetracycline. Am J Dis Child 1963;105:453.
98. Kaitila I, Wartiovaara J, Laitinen O et al. The inhibitory effect of tetracycline on osteogenesis in organ culture. J Embryol Exp Morphol 1970;23:185.
99. Bryceson ADM, Parry EHO, Perine PL et al. Louse-borne relapsing fever. A clinical and labaoratory study of 62 cases in Ethiopia and a reconsideration of the literature. Q J Med 1970;39:129.
100. Perine PL, Kidan TG, Warrel DA et al. Bleeding in louse-borne relapsing fever. II. Fibrinolysis following treatment. Trans R Soc Trop Med Hyg 1971;65:782.
101. Teklu B, Habte-Michael A, Warrel DA et al. Meptazinol diminishes the Jarisch-Herxheimer reaction of relapsing fever. Lancet 1983;i:835.
102. Anthony JR. Effect on deciduous and permanent teeth of tetracycline deposition in utero. Postgrad Med 1970; 48:165.
103. Briggs GG, Freeman RK, Yaffe SJ. Drugs in Pregnancy and Lactation, 2nd edn. Baltimore, MD: Williams and Wilkins, 1986.
104. Skosyreva AM. Comparative evaluation of the embryotoxic effect of various antibiotics. Antibiot Khimioter 1989;34:779.
105. Krejci L, Brettschneider I. Congenital cataract due to tetracycline. Ophthalmic Paediatr Genet 1983;3:59.
106. Neuvonen PJ, Gothoni G, Hackman R, Af Björksten K. Interference of iron with the absorption of tetracyclines in man. Br Med J 1970;4:532.
107. Gothoni G, Neuvonen PJ, Mattila M et al. Iron-tetracycline interaction: effect of time interval between the drugs. Acta Med Scand 1972;191:409.
108. Albert KS, Welch RD, De Sante KA et al. Decreased tetracycline bioavailabilitiy caused by bismuth subsalicylate antidiarrheal mixture. J Pharm Sci 1970;68:586.
109. Ericsson CD, Feldman S, Pickering LK et al. Influence of subsalicylate bismuth on absorption of doxycycline. J Am Med Assoc 1982;247:2266.
110. Boston Collaborative Drug Surveillance Program. Tetracycline and drug-attributed rises in blood urea nitrogen. J Am Med Assoc 1972;220:377.
111. Albers DD, Leveret L, Sandin JH. Renal failure following prostatovesiculectomy related to methoxyflurane anesthesia and tetracycline complicated by candida infection. J Urol 1971;106:348.
112. Kzucu EY. Methoxyflurane, tetracycline, and renal failure. J Am Med Assoc 1970;211:1162.
113. Proctor EA, Barton FL. Polyuric acute renal failure after methoxyflurane and tetracycline. Br Med J 1971;4:661.
114. Basler RSW, Lynch PJ. Black galactorrhea as a consequence of minocycline and phenothiazine therapy. Dermatology 1985;121:417.
115. Koch-Weser J, Sellers EM. Drug interactions with coumarin anticoagulants. Part I. N Engl J Med 1971;285:487.
116. Sande MA, Mandel GL. Tetracyclines. In: Goodman and Gilman's The Pharmacological Basis of Therapeutics, 8th edn. 1990;1117.

117. Crook LD, Tempest B. Plague: A review of 27 cases. Arch Intern Med 1992;152:1253.
118. Jones RB, Van der Pol B, Martin DH et al. Partial characterization of *Chlamydia trachomatis* isolates resistant to multiple antibiotics. J Infect Dis 1990;162:1309.
119. Ling JM, Khin Thi Oo H, Hui YW et al. Antimicrobial susceptibilities of Haemophilus species in Hong Kong. J Infect 1989;19:135.
120. Schläpfer G, Eichmann A. Penicillinase-producing strains of *N. gonorrhoeae* (PPNG) in the Zürich area, 1981—1988: incidence, antibiotic sensitivity and plasmid profile (3). Schweiz Med Wochenschr 1990;120:92.
121. Bennett Wm, Aronoff GR, Morrison G et al. Drug prescribing in renal failure: dosing guidelines for adults. Am J Kidney Dis 1983;3:155.
122. Phelps SJ, Tsiu W, Barrett FF et al. Chloramphenicol-induced cardiovascular collapse in an anephric patient. Pediatr Infect Dis J 1987;6:285.
123. Yunis AA. Effects of chloramphenicol on erythropoiesis. In: Dimitrov NV, Nodine JH, eds. Drugs and Hematological Reactions. London, New York: Grune and Stratton, 1974;133.
124. Keiser G. Co-operative study of patients treated with thiamphenicol: comparative study of patients treated with chloramphenicol and thiamphenicol. Postgrad Med J 1974;50(Suppl 5):143.
125. Polin HB, Plaut ME. Chloramphenicol. NY State J Med 1977;77:378.
126. Palchick BA, Funk EA, McEntire JE et al. Anaphylaxis due to chloramphenicol. Am J Med Sci 1984;288:43.
127. Liphshitz I, Loewenstein A. Anaphylactic reaction following application of chloramphenicol eye ointment. Br J Ophthalmol 1991;75:64.
128. Editorial. Ear drops and iatrogenic deafness. Med J Aust 1975;2:626.
129. Iqbal S, Strivatsav CBP. Chloramphenicol toxicity: a case report. J Laryngol Otol 1984;98:523.
130. Beyer CR. Chloramphenicol-induced acute bilateral optic neuritis in cystic fibrosis. J Pediatr Ophthalmol Strabismus 1978;15:291.
131. Murayama E, Miyakawa T, Sumiyoshi S et al. Retrobulbar optic neuritis and polyneuritis due to prolonged chloramphenicol therapy. Clin Neurol 1973;13:213.
132. Najean Y, Guérin MN, Chomienne C. Etiology of acquired aplastic anemia. In: Najean Y, Tognoni G, Yunis AA, eds. Safety Problems Related to Chloramphenicol and Thiamphenicol Therapy. New York: Raven Press, 1981;61.
133. Wallerstein RO, Condit PK, Brown JW, Morrison FR. Statewide study of chloramphenicol-therapy and fatal aplastic anemia. J Am Med Assoc 1969;208:2045.
134. Mary JY, Baumelou E, Guinet M et al. Epidemiology of aplastic anemia in France: a prospective multicentric study. Blood 1990;75:1646.
135. Froese EA. Chloramphenicol-associated aplastic anemia: its occurrence in Africans and with parenteral administration. Cent Afr J Med 1978;24:58.
136. Daum RS, Cohen DL, Smith L. Fatal aplastic anemia following apparent 'dose-related' chloramphenicol toxicity. J Pediatr 1979;94:403.
137. Yunis AA, Mayan DR, Arimura GK. Comparative metabolic effects of chloramphenicol and thiamphenicol in mammalian cells. J Pediatr 1974;94:403.
138. Murray TR, Downey KM, Yunis AA. Chloramphenicol-mediated DNA damage and its possible role in the inhibitory effects of chloramphenicol on DNA synthesis. J Lab Clin Med 1983;102:926.
139. Chaplin S. Bone marrow depression due to mianserin, phenylbutazone, oxyphenbutazone, and chloramphenicol. II. Adv Drug React Acute Poison Rev 1986;3:181.
140. Nagao T, Mauer AM. Concordance for drug-induced aplastic anaemia in identical twins. N Engl J Med 1969;281:7.
141. Yunis AA. Differential in-vitro toxicity of chloramphenicol, nitroso-chloramphenicol and thiamphenicol. Sex Transm Dis 1985;11:340.
142. Fink TJ, Gumps DW. Chloramphenicol: an inpatient study of use and abuse. J Infect Dis 1978;138:690.
143. West BC, De Vault GA, Clement JC et al. Aplastic anemia associated with parenteral chloramphenicol: review of 10 cases, including the second case of possible increased risk with cimetidine. Rev Infect Dis 1988;10:1048.
144. Brodsky E, Biger Y, Zeidan Z et al. Topical application of chloramphenicol eye ointment followed by fatal bone marrow aplaxia. Isr J Med Sci 1989;25:54.
145. Baumelou E, Najean Y. Why still prescribe chloramphenicol in 1983? Blut 1983;47:317.
146. Shu XO, Gao YT, Linet MS et al. Chloramphenicol use and childhood leukemia in Shanghai. Lancet 1987;ii:934.
147. Van Joost T, Dikland W, Stolz E, Prens E. Sensitization to chloramphenicol: a persistent problem. Contact Dermatitis 1986;14:176.
148. Lietman PS. Chloramphenicol and the neonate—1979 view. Clin Pharmacol 1979;6:151.
149. Nahata MC. Lack of predictability of chloramphenicol toxicity in pediatric patients. J Clin Pharmacol Ther 1989;14:297.
150. Brown RT. Chloramphenicol toxicity in an adolescent. J Adolesc Health Care 1982;3:53.
151. Kinmonth M-L, Storrs CN, Mitchell RG. Meningitis due to chloramphenicol-resistant *Haemophilus influenzae* type b. Br Med J 1978;1:694.
152. Butler T, Link NN, Arnold K, Pollack M. Chloramphenicol resistant typhoid fever in Vietnam associated with R-factor. Lancet 1973;ii:983.
153. Cherubin CE, Neu HC, Rahal JJ, Sabath LD. Emergence of resistance to chloramphenicol in Salmonella. J Infect Dis 1977;135:807.
154. Kunz J, Schreiner WE. Breitspektrumantibiotika. In: Kunz J, Schreiner WE, eds. Pharmakotherapie während Schwangerschaft und Stillperiode. Stuttgart, New York: Thieme Verlag, 1982;28.
155. Havelka J, Frankova A. A study of side effects of chloramphenicol therapy in newborns. Cs Pediatr 1972;27:31.
156. Rose JA, Choi HK, Schentag JJ et al. Intoxication caused by interaction of chloramphenicol and phenytoin. J Am Med Assoc 1977;237:2630.
157. Halpern J, Naslund B, Betner I. Suicide inactivation of rat liver cytochrome P-450 by chloramphenicol in vivo and in vitro. Mol Pharmacol 1983;23:445.
158. Prober CG. Effect of rifampicin on chloramphenicol levels. N Engl J Med 1985;312:788.
159. Kelly HW, Couch RC, Davis RL et al. Interaction of chloramphenicol and rifampicin. J Pediatr 1988;112:817.
160. Yunis AA. Chloramphenicol: relation of structure to activity and toxicity. Ann Rev Pharmacol Toxicol 1988;28:83.
161. International Symposium on Chloramphenicol, Thiamphenicol, Known and Unknown Aspects of Drug—Host Interactions, January 10—12, 1973, Sils-Maria, Switzerland.

162. Ferrary V. Salient features of thiamphenicol: review of clinical pharmacokinetics and toxicology. Sex Transm Dis 1984;11(Suppl 4):336.
163. Japanese Ministry of Health and Welfare. Information on adverse reactions to drugs (27). Peripheral nerve damage due to thiamphenicol. Jap Med Gaz Dec 1977;20:12.
164. Sotto J-J, Simon P, Subtil E, Rozenbaum A. Toxicité hématologique du thiophénicol. Nuov Presse Méd 1976; 5:2163.
165. Moeschlin S, Novotny Z, Koller F, Rüefli P. Zytostatische Nebenwirkungen des Thiamphenicols: Alopezie, reversible Zytopenien. Schweiz Med Wochenschr 1974;104:384.
166. De Renzo A, Fromisano S, Rotoli B. Bone marrow aplasia and thiamphenicol. Haematologica 1981;66:98.
167. Keiser G. Toxizität von Choramphenicol und Thiamphenicol (CAP und TAP). In: Löhr GW, Arnold H et al, eds. Probleme der Erythrozytopoese, Granulozytopoese und des malignen Melanoms. Berlin, Heidelberg: Spring Verlag, 1978;179.
168. Martinez Dalman A, Fernandez MH, Barbolla L. Haematological toxicity of thiamphenicol: analysis of a case with total irreversible bone marrow aplasia and general review of the problem. Sangre 1972;17:59.
169. Yunis AA, Miller AM, Salem Z et al. Chloramphenicol toxicity: pathogenetic mechanisms and the role of the p-NO_2 in aplastic anemia Clin Toxicol 1980;17:359.
170. Barradell L, Plosker G, McTavish D. Clarithromycin. A review of its pharmacological properties and therapeutic use in *Mycobacterium avium-intracellulare* Complex infection in patients with acquired immune deficiency syndrome. Drugs 1993;46:289.
171. Schlossberg D. Azithromycin and clarithromycin. Med Clin North Am 1995;79:803.
172. Polis M, Haneiwich S, Kovacs J et al. Dose escalation study to determine the safety, maximally tolerated dose and pharmacokinetics of clarithromycin with zidovudine in HIV-infected patients. In: Interscience Conference on Antimicrobial Agents and Chemotherapy, American Society for Microbiology, 1991.
173. Roujeau J-C, Kelly J, Naldi L et al. Medication use and the risk of Stevens-Johnson syndrome or toxic epidermal necrolysis. N Engl J Med 1995;333:1600.
174. Periti P, Mazzei T, Mini E, Novelli A. Adverse effects of macrolide antibacterials Drug Safety 1993;9:346.
175. Slater J. Hypersensitivity to macrolide antibiotics. Ann Allergy 1991;66:193.
176. Van Ketel W. Immediate and delayed-type allergy to erythromycin. Contact Dermatitis 1976;2:363.
177. Pigatto P, Riboldi A, Riva F, Altmare G. Fixed drug eruption to erythromycin. Acta Dermatol-Venereol 1984; 64:272.
178. Davies R, Pepys J. Asthma due to inhaled chemical agents—the macrolide antibiotic spiramycin. Clin Allergy 1975;5:99.
179. Washington J, Wilson W. Erythromycin: a microbial and clinical perspective after 30 years of clinical use (two parts). Mayo Clin Proc 1985;60:189.
180. Anderson G, Esmonde T, Coles S et al. A comparative safety and efficacy study of clarithromycin and erythromycin stearate in community-acquired pneumonia. J Antimicrob Chemother 1991;27(Suppl A):117.
181. Brogden R, Peters D. Dirithromycin. A review of its antimicrobial activity, pharmacokinetic properties and therapeutic efficacy. Drugs 1994;48:599.
182. Tamaoki J, Takeyama K, Tagaya E, Konno K. Effect of clarithromycin on sputum production and its rheological properties in chronic respiratory tract infections. Antimicrob Agents Chemother 1995;39:1688.
183. Marom Z, Goswami S. Respiratory mucus hypersecretion (bronchorrhea): a case discussion—possible mechanisms and treatment. J Allergy Clin Immunol 1991;87:1050.
184. Black R, Dawson T. Erythromycin and nightmares. Br Med J 1988;296:1070.
185. Murdoch J. Psychiatric complications of erythromycin and clindamycin. Can J Hosp Pharm 1988;41:277.
186. Umstead G, Neumann K. Erythromycin ototoxicity and acute psychotic reaction in cancer patients with hepatic dysfunction. Arch Intern Med 1986;146:897.
187. Williams N. Erythromycin: a case of nightmares. Br Med J 1988;296:214.
188. Uzzan B, Nicolas P, Perret G et al. Effects of troleandomycin and josamycin on thyroid hormone and steroid serum levels, liver function tests and microsomal monooxygenases in healthy volunteers: a double blind placebo-controlled study. Fundam Clin Pharmacol 1991;5:513.
189. Braun P. Hepatotoxicity of erythromycin. J Infect Dis 1969;119:300.
190. Tolman K, Sannella J, Freston J. Chemical structure of erythromycin and hepatotoxicity. Ann Intern Med 1974; 81:58.
191. Lee W. Drug-induced hepatotoxicity. N Engl J Med 1995;333:1118.
192. Yew W, Chau C, Lee J, Leung C. Cholestatic hepatitis in a patient who received clarithromycin therapy for a *Mycobacterium chelonae* lung infection. Clin Infect Dis 1994;18:1025.
193. Lin H, Sanders S, Gu Y, Doty J. Erythromycin accelerates solid emptying at the expense of gastric sieving. Dig Dis Sci 1994;39:124
194. Hasler W, Heldsinger A, Owyang C. Erythromycin contracts rabbit colon myocytes via occupation of motilin receptors. Am J Physiol Gastrointest Liver Physiol 1992;262:G50.
195. Kaufman H, Ahrendt S, Pitt H, Lillemoe K. The effect of erythromycin on motility of the duodenum, sphincter of Oddi, and gallbladder in the prairie dog. Surgery 1993;114:543.
196. Nakayoshi T, Izumi M, Tatsuta K. Effects of macrolide antibiotics on gastrointestinal motility in fasting and digestive states. Drugs. Exp Clin Res 1992;18:337.
197. Sifrim D, Janssens J, Vantrappen G. Comparison of the effects of midecamycin acetate and clarithromycin on gastrointestinal motility in man. Drugs Clin Res 1992;18:337.
198. Sifrim D, Matsuo H, Janssens J, Vantrappen G. Comparison of the effects of midecamycin acetate and azithromycin on gastrointestinal motility in man. Drugs Exp Clin Res 1994;20:121.
199. Nellans H, Petersen A. Stimulation of gastrointestinal motility: clarithromycin significantly less potent than azithromycin. In: Seventh International Congress of Chemotherapy, Berlin, 1991.
200. Peeters T. Erythromycin and other macrolides as prokinetic agents. Gastroenterology 1993;105:1886.
201. Periti P, Mazzei T, Mini E, Novelli A. Pharmacokinetic drug interactions of macrolides. Clin Pharmacokinet 1992;23:106.
202. Watkins P, Murray S, Winkelmann L. Erythromycin breath test as an assay of glucocorticoid-inducible liver cytochromes P-450. J Clin Invest 1989;83:688.

203. Ludden T. Pharmacokinetic interactions of the macrolide antibiotics. Clin Pharmacokinet 1985;10:63.
204. Lown K, Kolars J, Turgeon K et al. The erythromycin breath test selectively measures P450IIIA in patients with severe liver disease. Clin Pharmacol Ther 1992;51:229.
205. Lown K, Kolars J, Thummel K et al. Interpatient heterogeneity in expression of CYP3A4 and CYP3A5 in small bowel. Lack of prediction by the erythromycin breath test. Drug Metab Dispos 1994;22:947.
206. Bacourt F, Couffinhal J. Ischémie des membres par association dihydroergotamine-triacetyloléandomycin. Nouv Presse Méd 1978;7:1956.
207. Franco A, Boulard P, Massot C et al. Ergotamine par association dihydroergotamine-triacetyloléandomycin. Nouv Presse Méd 1978;7:205.
208. Hayton A. Precipitation of acute ergotism by triacetyloleandomycin. NZ Med J 1969;69:42.
209. Matthews N, Havill J. Ergotism with therapeutic doses of ergotamine tartrate. NZ Med J 1979;89:476.
210. Azria M, Kiechel J, Lavenne D. Contribution à l'étude de l'interaction de la triacetyloléandomycine avec l'ergotamine ou la dihydroergotamine. J Pharmacol 1979;10:431.
211. Martinet M, Kiechel J. Interaction of dihydroergotamine and triacetyloleandomycin in the minipig. Eur J Drug Metab Pharmacokinet 1983;8:261.
212. Parrish R, Haulman N, Burns R. Interaction of theophylline with erythromycin base in a patient with seizure activity. Pediatrics 1983;72:828.
213. La Force C, Szefler S, Miller M et al. Inhibition of methylprednisolone elimination in the presence of erythromycin therapy. J Allergy Clin Immunol 1983;72:34.
214. Spector S, Katz F, Farr R. Troleandomycin: effectiveness in steroid-dependent asthma and bronchitis. J Allergy Clin Immunol 1974;54:367.
215. Ziger R, Schatz M, Sperling W et al. Efficacy of troleandomycin in outpatients with severe, corticosteroid-dependent asthma. J Allergy Clin Immunol 1980;66:438.
216. Claudel S, Euvrard P, Borx R et al. Cholestase intrahépatique après aasociation triacetyloléandomycine-estroprogestatif. Nouv Presse Med 1979;8:1182.
217. Fevery J, Van Steenbergen W, Desmet V et al. Severe intrahepatic cholestasis due to the combined intake of oral contraceptives and triacetyloleandomycin. Acta Clin Belg 1983;38:242.
218. Haber I, Hubens H. Cholestatic jaundice after triacetyloleandomycin and oral contraceptives: the diagnostic value of gammaglutamyl transpeptidase. Acta Gastroenterol Belg 1980;43:475.
219. Miguet J, Vuitton D, Pessayre D et al. Jaundice from troleandomycin and oral contraceptives. Ann Intern Med 1980;92:434.
220. Wong Y, Ludden T, Bell R. Effect of erythromycin on carbamazepine kinetics. Clin Pharmacol Ther 1983;33:460.
221. Albin H, Vincon G, Pehourcq F, Dangoumau J. Influence de la josamycine sur la pharmacokinétique de la carbamazepine. Thérapie 1982;37:151.
222. Couet W, Istin B, Ingrand L et al. Effects of ponsinomycin on single-dose kinetics and metabolism of carbamazepine. Ther Drug Monitoring 1990;12:144.
223. Barzaghi N, Gatti G, Crema F et al. Effect of flurithromycin, a new macrolide antibiotic, on carbamazepine disposition in normal subjects. Int J Clin Pharmacol Res 1988;8:101.
224. Mesdjian E, Dravet C, Cenraud B, Roger J. Carbamazepine intoxication due to triacetyloleandomycin administration in epileptic patients. Epilepsia 1980;21:489.
225. Berrettini W. A case of erythromycin-induced carbamazepine toxicity. J Clin Psychiatry 1986;47:147.
226. Carranco E, Kareus J, Co S et al. Carbamazepine toxicity induced by concurrent erythromycin therapy. Arch Neurol 1985;42:187.
227. Warot D, Bergougnan L, Lamiable D. Troleandomycin-triazolam interaction in healthy volunteers: pharmacokinetic and psychometric evaluation. Eur J Clin Pharmacol 1987;32:389.
228. Phillips J, Antal E, Smith R. A pharmacokinetic drug interaction between erythromycin and triazolam. J Clin Psychopharmacol 1986;6:297.
229. Gascon M, Dayer P, Waldvogel F. Les interactions médicamenteuses du midazolam. Schweiz Med Wochenschr 1989;119:1834.
230. Hiller A, Olkkola K, Isohanni P, Saarnivaara L. Unconsciousness associated with midazolam and erythromycin. Br J Anaesth 1990;65:826.
231. Bartkowski R, Goldberg M, Larijani G, Boerner T. Inhibition of alfentanyl metabolism by erythromycin. Clin Pharmacol Ther 1989;46:99.
232. Weibert R, McQuade L, Townsend R et al. Effect of erythromycin in patients receiving long-term warfarin therapy. Clin Pharm 1989;8:210.
233. Bartle W. Possible warfarin-erythromycin interaction. Arch Intern Med 1980;140:985.
234. Grau E, Fontcuberta J, Felez J. Erythromycin-oral anticoagulants interaction. Arch Intern Med 1986;146:1639.
235. Husserl F. Erythromycin-warfarin interaction. Arch Intern Med 1983;143:1831.
236. Sato R, Gray D, Brown S. Warfarin interaction with erythromycin. Arch Intern Med 1984;144:2413.
237. Schwartz J, Bachmann K. Erythromycin-warfarin interaction. Arch Intern Med 1984;144:2094.
238. Yee G, McGuire T. Pharmacokinetic drug interactions with cyclosporin (Part I and Part II). Clin Pharmacokinet 1990;19:319.
239. Wadhwa N, Schroeder T, O'Flaherty E et al. Interaction between erythromycin and cyclosporin in a kidney and pancreas allograft recipient. Ther Drug Monit 1987;9:123.
240. Azanza J, Catalan M, Alvarez P et al. Possilbe interaction between cyclosporine and josamycin. J Heart Transplant 1990;9:265.
241. Couet W, Istin B, Seniuta P et al. Effect of ponsinomycin on cyclosporin pharmacokinetics. Eur J Clin Pharmacol 1990;39:165.
242. Friedman H, Bonventre M. Erythromycin induced digoxin toxicity. Chest 1982;82:202.
243. Maxwell D, Gilmour-White S, Hall M. Digoxin toxicity due to interaction of digoxin with erythromycin. Br Med J 1989;298:572.
244. Ford A, Crocker Smith L, Baltch A, Smith R. Clarithromycin-induced digoxin toxicity in a patient with AIDS. Clin Infect Dis 1995;21:1051.
245. Lindenbaum J, Rund D, Butler V. Inactivation of digoxin by the gut flora: reversal by antibiotic therapy. N Engl J Med 1981;305:789.
246. Ragosta M, Weihl A, Rosenfeld L. Potentially fatal interaction between erythromycin and disopyramide. Am J Med 1989;86:465.
247. Zini R, Fournet M, Barre J et al. In vitro study of roxithromycin binding to serum proteins and erythrocytes in man. Br J Clin Pract 1987;42(Suppl 5):54.

248. Tran H. Torsades de pointes induced by nonantiarrhythmic drugs. Conn Med 1994;58:291.
249. Zechnich A, Hedges J, Eiselt-Proteau D, Haxby D. Possible interactions with terfenadine or astemizole. West J Med 1994;160:321.
250. Jurima-Romet M, Crawford K, Cyr T, Inaba T. Terfenadine metabolism in human liver. In vitro inhibition by macrolide antibiotics and azole antifungals. Drug Metab Dispos 1994;22:849.
251. Honig P, Wortham D, Zamani K, Cantilena L. Comparison of the effect of the macrolide antibiotics erythromycin, clarithromycin and azithromycin on terfenadine steady-state pharmacokinetics and electrocardiographic parameters. Drug Invest 1994;7:148.
252. Botstein P. Is QT interval prolongation harmful? A regulatory perspective. Am J Cardiol 1993;72:50.
253. Griffith D, Brown B, Girard W, Wallace R Jr. Adverse events associated with high-dose rifabutin in macrolide-containing regimens for the treatment of *Mycobacterium avium* Complex lung disease. Clin Infect Dis 1995;21:594.
254. Fuller J, Stanfield L, Craven D. Rifabutin prophylaxis and uveitis. N Engl J Med 1994;330:1315.
255. Shafran S, Deschênes J, Miller M et al. Uveitis and pseudojaundice during a regimen of clarithromycin, rifabutin, and ethambutol. N Engl J Med 1994;330:438.
256. Frank M, Graham M, Wispelway B. Rifabutin and uveitis. N Engl J Med 1994;330:868.
257. Havlir D, Torriani F, Dubé M. Uveitis associated with rifabutin prophylaxis. Ann Intern Med 1994;121:510.
258. Wallace R Jr, Brown B, Griffith D et al. Reduced serum levels of clarithromycin in patients treated with multidrug regimens including rifampin or rifabutin for *Mycobacterium avium-M. intracellulare* infection. J Infect Dis 1995;171:747.
259. Nelson M, Berchou R, Kareti D, Lewitt P. Pharmacokinetic evaluation of erythromycin and caffeine administered with bromocriptine. Clin Pharmacol Therapeut 1990;47:694.
260. Ayanian J, Fuchs C, Stone R. Lovastatin and rhabdomyolysis. Ann Intern Med 1988;109:682.
261. Eckman M, Johnson T, Riess R. Partial deafness after erythromycin. N Engl J Med 1975;292:649.
262. Ginsburg C, Eichenwald H. Erythromycin: a review of its uses in pediatric practice. J Pediatr 1976;89:872.
263. Ginsburg C, and the Multicenter Pneumonia Study Group. A prospective study on the incidence of liver function abnormalities in children receiving erythromycin estolate, erythromycin ethylsuccinate or penicillin V for treatment of pneumonia. Pediatr Infect Dis 1986;5:151.
264. Funck-Brentano C, Pessayre D, Benhamou J. Hépatites dues à divers dérivés de l'érythromycine. Gastroentérol Clin Biol 1983;7:362.
265. Inman W, Rawson I. Erythromycin estolate and jaundice. Br Med J 1983;286:1954.
266. Eichenwald H. Adverse reactions to erythromycin. Pediatr Infect Dis 1986;5:147.
267. Krowshuk D, Seashore J. Complete biliary obstruction due to erythromycin estolate administration in an infant. Pediatrics 1979;64:956.
268. Lunzer M, Huang S, Ward K, Sherlock S. Jaundice due to erythromycin estolate. Gastroenterology 1975;68:1284.
269. Tomomasa T, Kuroume T, Arai H. Erythromycin induces migrating motor complex in human gastrointestinal tract. Dig Dis Sci 1986;31:157.
270. Omura S, Tsuzuki K, Sunazuka T. Macrolides with gastrointestinal motor stimulating activity. J Med Chem 1987;30:1941.
271. Lehtola J, Jauhonen P, Kesäniemi A. Effect of erythromycin on the oro-caecal transit time in man. Eur J Clin Pharmacol 1990;39:555.
272. San Filippo J. Infantile hypertrophic pyloric stenosis related to ingestion of erythromycin estolate: a report of five cases. J Pediatr Surg 1976;11:177.
273. Teare J, Booth J, Brown J et al. Pseudomembranous colitis following clarithromycin therapy. Eur J Gastroenterol Hepatol 1995;7:275.
274. Gantz N, Zawacki J, Dickerson J. Pseudomembranous colitis associated with erythromycin. Ann Intern Med 1978;91:866.
275. Brummett R, Fox K. Minireviews. Vancomycin- and erythromycin-induced hearing loss in humans. Antimicrob Agents Chemother 1989;33:791.
276. Haydon R, Thelin J, Davis W. Erythromycin ototoxicity: analysis and conclusions based on 22 case reports. Otolaryngol Head Neck Surg 1984;92:678.
277. Hyang M, Schacht J. Drug induced ototoxicity. Med Toxicol Adverse Exp 1989;4:452.
278. Agusti C, Ferran F, Gea J, Picado C. Ototoxic reaction to erythromycin. Arch Intern Med 1991;151:380.
279. Quinnan G, McCabe W. Ototoxicity of erythromycin. Lancet 1978;i:1160.
280. Schweitzer V, Olson N. Ototoxic effect of erythromycin therapy. Arch Otolaryngol 1984;100:298.
281. May E. Aggravation of myasthenia gravis by erythromycin. Ann Neurol 1990;28:577.
282. Rosenfeld J, Gura V, Boner G. Interstitial nephritis with acute renal failure after erythromycin. Br Med J 1983;286:938.
283. Zarowitz B, Szefler S, Lasezkay G. Effect of erythromycin base on theophylline kinetics. Clin Pharmacol Ther 1981;29:601.
284. Paulsen O, Höglund P, Nilsson L-G. The interaction of erythromycin with theophylline. Eur J Clin Pharmacol 1987;32:493.
285. Bigorie B, Aimez P, Soria R. L'association triacétyloléandomycine-tartrate d'ergotamine, est-elle dangereuse? Nouv Presse Méd 1975;4:2723.
286. Hedrick R, Williams F, Morin R. Carbamazepine-erythromycin interaction leading to carbamazepine toxicity in four epileptic children. Ther Drug Monit 1983;5:405.
287. Bachmann K, Schwartz J, Forney R Jr, Jauregui L. Single dose phenytoin clearance during erythromycin treatment. Res Commun Chem Pathol Pharmacol 1984;4:207.
288. Milne R, Coulthard K, Nation R et al. Lack of effect of erythromycin on the pharmacokinetics of single oral doses of phenytoin. Br J Clin Pharmacol 1988;26:330.
289. Wroblenski B, Singer W, Whyte J. Carbamazepine-erythromycin interaction. J Am Med Assoc 1986;255:1165.
290. Bachmann K, Schwarz J, Forney R. The effect of erythromycin on the disposition kinetics of warfarin. Pharmacology 1984;28:171.
291. Morton M, Cooper J. Erythromycin-induced digoxin toxicity. Ann Pharmacother 1989;23:668.
292. Guengerich F, Muller-Enoch D, Blair I. Oxidation of quinidine by human liver cytochrome P-450. Mol Pharmacol 1986;30:287.
293. Bartkowski R, McDonnel T. Prolonged alfentanil effect following erythromycin administration. Anesthesiology 1990;73:566.
294. Kronbach T, Fischer V, Meyer R. Cyclosporin metabolism in human liver: Identification of a cytochrome P-450 III

gene family as the major cyclosporin-metabolizing enzyme explains interactions of cyclosporin with other drugs. Clin Pharmacol Ther 1988;43:630.
295. D'Arcy P. Cyclosporin-erythromycin interaction. Pharm Int 1986;7:164.
296. Jensen C, Flechner S, Van Buren C. Exacerbation of cyclosporin toxicity by concomitant administration of erythromycin. Transplantation 1987;43:263.
297. Schoenenberger R, Haefeli W, Weiss P, Ritz R. Association of intravenous erythromycin and potentially fatal ventricular tachycardia with Q-T prolongation (torsades de pointes). Br Med J 1990;300:1375.
298. Young R, Gonzalez J, Sorkin E. Roxithromycin. A review of its antibacterial activity, pharmacokinetic properties and clinical efficacy. Drugs 1989;37:8.
299. Kafetzis D, Blanc F. Efficacy and safety of roxithromycin in treating paediatric patients: a European multicentre study. J Antimicrob Chemother 1987;20(Suppl B):171.
300. Agache P, Amblard P, Moulin G et al. Roxithromycin in skin and soft tissue infections. J Antimicrob Chemother 1987;20(Suppl B):153.
301. Saint-Salvi B, Tremblay D, Surjus A, Lefebure M. A study of the interaction of roxithromycin with theophylline and carbamazepine. J Antimicrob Chemother 1987;20(Suppl B):121.
302. Pijpers E, van Rijswijk R, Takx-Köhlen B, Schrey G. A clarithromycin-induced myasthenic syndrome. Clin Infect Dis 1996;22:175.
303. Herishanu Y, Taustein I. The electromyographic changes induced by antibiotics: a preliminary study. Confin Neurol 1971;33:41.
304. Peters D, Clissold S. Clarithromycin. A review of its antimicrobial activity, pharmacokinetic properties and therapeutic potential. Drugs 1992;44:117.
305. Niki Y, Nakajima M, Tsukiyama K et al. Effect of TE-031(A-56268), a new oral macrolide antibiotic on serum theophylline concentration. Chemotherapy 1988;36:515.
306. Ruf F, Chu S, Sonders R, Sennello L. Effect of multiple doses of clarithromycin on the pharmacokinetics of theophylline. In: International Conference on Antimicrobial Agents and Chemotherapy. Atlanta, Georgia/USA: American Society for Microbiology, 1990.
307. Peters D, Friedel H, McTavish D. Azithromycin. A review of its antimicrobial activity, pharmacokinetic properties and clinical efficacy. Drugs 1992;44:750.
308. Hopkins S. Clinical toleration and safety of azithromycin. Am J Med 1991;91(Suppl 3A):40.
309. Gardner M, Coates P, Hilligoss D, Henry E. Lack of effect of azithromycin on the pharmacokinetics of theophylline in man. In: Proceedings of the Mediterranean Congress of Chemotherapy, Athens, 1992.
310. Clauzel A, Visier S, Michel F. Efficacy and safety of azithromycin in lower respiratory tract infections. Eur Resp J 1990;3(Suppl 10):89.
311. Ljutic D, Rumboldt Z. Possible interaction between azithromycin and cyclosporin: a case report. Nephron 1995;70:130.
312. Chave J-P, Munafo A, Chatton J-Y et al. Once-a-week azithromycin in AIDS patients: tolerability, kinetics, and effects on zidovudine disposition. Antimicrob Agents Chemother 1992;36:1013.
313. Bachmann K, Nunlee M, Martin M. Changes in the steady-state pharmacokinetics of theophylline during treatment with dirithromycin. J Clin Pharmacol 1990;30:1001.
314. Bachmann K, Jauregui L, Sides G. Steady-state pharmacokinetics of theophylline in COPD patients treated with dirithromycin. J Clin Pharmacol 1993;33:861.
315. Wermeling D, Chandler M, Sides G et al. Dirithromycin increases ethinyl estradiol clearance without allowing ovulation. Obstet Gynecol 1995;86:78.
316. Holliday S, Faulds D. Miocamycin. A review of its antimicrobial activity, pharmacokinetic properties and therapeutic potential. Drugs 1993;46:720.
317. Mayama T, Maruyama K, Nakazawa T, Iida M. A survey of the side effects of midecamycin acetate (Miocamycin) dry syrup after marketing. Int J Clin Pharmacol Ther Toxicol 1990;28:245.
318. Couet W, Ingrand I, Reigner B et al. Lack of effect of ponsinomycin on the plasma pharmacokinetics of theophylline. Eur J Clin Pharmacol 1989;37:101.
319. Zagnoni P, De Luca M, Casini A. Carbamazepine-miocamycin interaction. Epilepsia 1991;32(Suppl 1):28.
320. Johnson R, Rozanis J, Shofield I. The effect of spiramycin on plaque accumulation and gingivitis. J Can Dent Assoc 1979;44:456.
321. Brewer NS. The aminoglycosides. Mayo Clin Proc 1977;52:675.
322. John JF Jr. What price success? The continuing saga of toxic: therapeutic ratio in the use of aminoglycoside antibiotics. J Infect Dis 1988;158:1.
323. Mattie H, Craig WA, Pechere JC. Determinants of efficacy and toxicity of aminoglycosides. J Antimicrob Chemother 1989;24:293.
324. Gilbert DN. Once-daily aminoglycoside therapy. Antimicrob Agents Chemother 1991;35:3.
325. Blaser J, König C. Once-dailey dosing of aminoglycosides. Eur J Clin Microbiol Infect Dis 1995;14:1029.
326. Blaser J, Stone BB, Groner MC, Zinner SH. Effect of the ratio of antibiotic peak concentration to MIC on bactericidal activity and emergence of resistance: a comparative study with enoxacin and netilmicin in a pharmacodynamic model. Antimicrob Agents Chemother 1987;31:1054.
327. Moore RD, Lietman PS, Smith CR. Clinical response to aminoglycoside therapy: importance of the ratio of peak concentration to minimal inhibitory concentration. J Infect Dis 1987;I55:93.
328. Vogelman B, Gudmundsson S, Turnidge J et al. In vivo postantibiotic effect in a thigh infection in neutropenic mice. J Infect Dis 1988;157:287.
329. Powell SH, Thompson WL, Luthe MA et al. Once-daily vs. continuous aminoglycoside dosing: efficacy and toxicity in animal and clinical studies of gentamicin, netilmicin, and tobramicin. J Infect Dis 1983;147:918.
330. De Broe ME, Verbist L, Verpooten G. Influence of dosage schedule on renal cortical accumulation of amikacin and tobramycin in man. J Antimicrob Chemother 1991; 27(Suppl C):41.
331. Moore RD, Smith CR, Lietman PS. The association of aminoglycoside plasma levels with mortality in patients with gram-negative bacteremia. J Infect Dis 1984;149:443.
332. Moore RD, Smith CR, Lietman PS. Association of aminoglycoside plasma levels with therapeutic outcome in gram-negative pneumonia. Am J Med 1984;77:657.
333. Wenk M, Vozeh S, Follath F. Serum level monitoring of antibacterial drugs. Clin Pharmacol Ther 1984;9:475.
334. Zaske DE, Cipolle RJ, Rotschafer JC et al. Gentamicin pharmacokinetics in 1640 patients: method for control of serum concentrations. Antimicrob Agents Chemother 1982;21:407.

335. Lesar TS, Rotschafer JC, Strand LM et al. Gentamicin dosing errors with four commonly used nomograms. J Am Med Assoc 1982;248:1190.
335a. Emery ERS. Neuromuscular blocking properties of antibiotics as a cause of post-operative apnoea. Anesthesia 1963;18:57.
336. Konrad F, Wagner R, Neumeister B et al. Studies on drug monitoring in thrice and once daily treatment with aminoglycosides. Intens Care Med 1993;19:215.
337. Janknegt R: Aminoglykoside monitoring in the once- or twice-daily era. The Dutch situation considered. Pharm World Sci 1993;15:151.
338. Parker SE, Davey PG. Practicalities of once-daily aminoglycoside dosing. J Antimicrob Chemother 1993;31:4.
339. Blaser J, König C, Simmen H.P et al. Monitoring serum concentrations for once-daily dosing regims of netilmicin. J Antimicrob Chemother 1994;33:349.
340. MacGowan AP, Reeves DS. Serum monitoring and practicalities of once-daily aminoglycoside dosing. J Antimicrob Chemother 1993;33:349.
341. Giamarellou H, Yiallouros K, Petrkkos G, et al. Comparative kinetics and efficacy of amikacin administered once or twice daily in the treatment of systemic Gram-negative infections. J Antimicrob Chemother 1991;27(Suppl C):73.
342. Maller R, Ahrne H, Holmen C et al. and the Scandinavian Amikacin Once Daily Study Group. Once- versus twice-daily amikacin regimen: efficacy and safety in systematic Gram-negative infections. J Antimicrob Chemother 1993;31:939.
343. Reeves DS, MacGowan AP. Commentary on once-daily aminoglycoside dosing. Lancet 1993;341:896.
344. Blaser J, König C, Fatio R et al. and members of the IATCG-EORTC. Multicenter quality control study of amikacin assay for monitoring once-daily dosing regimens. Ther Drug Monitoring 1995;17:133.
345. Brummet RE, Fox KE. Aminoglykoside-induced hearing loss in humans. Antimicrob Agents Chemother 1989; 33:6.
346. Fee WE. Aminoglycoside ototoxicity in the human. Laryngoscope, 1980;90(Suppl 24):1.
347. Tablan OC, Reyes MP, Rintelmann WF et al. Renal and auditory toxicity of high-dose, prolonged therapy with gentamicin and tobramycin in *Pseudomonas* endocarditis. J Infect Dis 1984;149:257.
348. Moore RD, Smith CR, Lietman PS. Risk factors for the development of auditory toxicity in patients receiving aminoglycosides. J Infect Dis 1984;149:23.
349. Smith CR, Lietman PS. Effect of furosemide on aminoglycoside-induced nephrotoxicity and auditory toxicity in humans. Antimicrob Agents Chemother 1983;23:133.
350. Schonenberger U, Streit C, Hoigné R. Nephro- und Ototoxizitat von Aminoglykosid-Antibiotica unter besonderer Berücksichtigung von Gentamicin. Schweiz Rundsch Med Praxis 1981;70:169.
351. Federspil P. Zur Ototoxizitat der Aminoglykosid-Antibiotika. Infection 1976;4:239.
352. Federspil P, Schatzle W, Tiesler E. Pharmakokinetische, histologische und histochemische Untersuchungen zur Ototoxizitat des Gentamicins, Tobramycins und Amikacins. Arch Oto-Rhino-Laryngol 1977;217:147.
353. Hently III CM, Schacht J. Pharmacokinetics of aminoglycoside antibiotics in blood, inner ear fluids and tissues and their relationship to ototoxicity. Audiology 1988;27:137.
354. Fischel-Ghodsian N, Prezant TR, Bu X et al. Mitochondrial ribosomal RNA gene mutation in a patient with sporadic aminoglycoside ototoxicity. Am J Otolaryngol 1993;14:399.
355. Brummett RE, Fox KE. Studies of aminoglycoside ototoxicity in animal models. In: Whelton A, Neu HC, eds. The Aminoglycosides. New York, Basel: Marcel Dekker, Inc., 1982;419.
356. Brummett RE, Fox KE, Bendrick TW, Himes DL. Ototoxicity of tobramycin, gentamicin, amikacin and sisomicin in the guinea pig. J Antimicrob Chemother 1978;4(Suppl A):73.
357. Brummett RE, Fox KE, Brown RT et al. Comparative ototoxic liability of netilmicin and gentamicin. Arch Otolaryngol 1978;104:579.
358. Cone LA. A survey of prospective, controlled clinical trials of gentamicin, tobramycin, amikacin, and netilmicin. Clin Ther 1982;5:155.
359. Lerner AM, Cone LA, Jansen W et al. Randomized, controlled trial of the comparative efficacy, auditory toxicity, and nephrotoxicity of tobramycin and netilmicin. Lancet 1983;i:1123.
360. Gatell JM, SanMiguel JG, Araujo V et al. Prospective randomized double-blind comparison of nephrotoxicity and auditory toxicity of tobramycin and netilmicin. Antimicrob Agents Chemother 1984;26:766.
361. Guerit JM, Mathieu P, Houben-Giurgea S et al. The influence of ototoxic drugs on brainstem auditory evoked potentials in man. Arch Otolaryngol 1981;233:189.
362. Hotz MA, Allum JH, Kaufmann G et al. Shifts in auditory brainstem response latencies following plasma-level-controlled aminoglycoside therapy. Eur Arch Otorhinolaryngol 1990;247:202.
363. Holtzman JL. Gentamicin and neuromuscular blockade. Ann Intern Med 1976;84:55.
364. Kes P, Reiner Z. Symptomatic hypomagnesia associated with gentamicin therapy. Magnesium Trace Elem 1990;9:54.
365. Plaut ME, Schentag JJ, Jusko WJ. Aminoglycoside nephrotoxicity: comparative assessment in critically ill patients. J Med 1979;10:257.
366. Schentag JJ, Plaut ME, Cerra FB. Comparative nephrotoxicity of gentamicin and tobramycin: pharmacokinetic and clinical studies in 201 patients. Antimicrob Agents Chemother 1981;19:859.
367. Moore RD, Smith CR, Lipsky JJ et al. Risk factors for nephrotoxicity in patients treated with aminoglycosides. Ann Intern Med 1984;100:352.
368. Sawyers CL, Moore RD, Lerner SA et al. A model for predicting nephrotoxicity in patients treated with aminoglycosides. J Infect Dis 1986;153:1062.
369. Lam YWF, Arana CJ, Shikuma LR et al. The clinical utility of a published nomogram to predict aminoglycoside nephrotoxicity. J Am Med Assoc 1986;255:639.
370. Keys TF, Kurtz SB, Jones JD et al. Renal toxicity during therapy with gentamicin or tobramycin. Mayo Clin Proc 1981;56:556.
371. Schentag JJ, Gengo FM, Piaut ME et al. Urinary casts as an indication of renal tubular damage in patients receiving aminoglycosides. Antimicrob Agents Chemother 1979; 16:468.
372. Schentag JJ, Sutfin TA, Plaut ME et al. Early detection of aminoglycoside nephrotoxicity with urinary beta-2-microglobulin. J Med 1978;9:201.
373. Tulkens PM. Pharmacokinetic and toxicologiacal evaluation of a once-daily regimen versus conventional schedules

of netilmicin and amikacin. J Antimicrob Chemother 1991;27(Suppl C):29.
374. Mondorf AW. Urinary enzymatic markers of renal damage. In: Whelton A, Neu HC, eds. The Aminoglycosides. New York, Basel: Marcel Dekker, Inc., 1982;283.
375. Luft FC, Evan AP. Comparative effects of tobramycin and gentamicin on glomerular ultrastructure. J Infect Dis 1980;142:6.
376. Tardif D, Beauchamp D, Bergeron MG. Influence of endotoxin on the intracortical accumulation kinetics of gentamicin in rats. Antimicrob Agents Chemother 1990;34:4.
377. Appel GB. Aminoglycoside nephrotoxicity: physiologic studies of the sites of nephron damage. In: Whelton A, Neu HC, eds. The Aminoglycosides. New York, Basel: Marcel Dekker, Inc., 1982;269.
378. Whelton A. Renal tubular transport and intrarenal aminoglycoside distribution. In: Whelton A, Neu HC, eds. The Aminoglycosides. New York, Basel: Marcel Dekker, Inc., 1982;191.
379. Carlier MB, Laurent G, Claes PJ et al. Inhibition of lysosomal phospholipases by aminoglycoside antibiotics: in vitro comparative studies. Antimicrob Agents Chemother 1983;23:440.
380. Luft FC, Yum MN, Kleit SA. Comparative nephrotoxicities of netilmicin and gentamicin in rats. Antimicrob Agents Chemother 1976;10:845.
381. Hottendorf GH, Gordon LL. Comparative low-dose nephrotoxicities of gentamicin, tobramycin and amikacin. Antimicrob Agents Chemother 1980;18:176.
382. Smith CR, Baughman KL, Edwards CQ et al. Controlled comparison of amikacin and gentamicin. N Engl J Med 1977;296:349.
383. Feld R, Valdivieso M, Bodey GP et al. Comparison of amikacin and tobramycin in the treatment of infection in patients with cancer. J Infect Dis 1977;135:61.
384. Love LJ, Schimpff SC, Hahn DM et al. Randomized trial of empiric antibiotic therapy with ticarcillin in combination with gentamicin, amikacin or netilmicin in febrile patients with granulocytopenia and cancer. Am J Med 1979;66:603.
385. Lau WK, Young LS, Black LE et al. Comparative efficacy and toxicity of amikacin/carbenicillin vs. gentamicin/carbenicillin in leukopenic patients. Am J Med 1979;62:959.
386. Fong IW, Fenton RS, Bird R. Comparative toxicity of gentamicin vs. tobramycin: a randomized prospective study. J Antimicrob Chemother 1981;7:81.
387. Bock BV, Edelstein PH, Meyer RD. Prospective comparative study of efficacy and toxicity of netilmicin and amikacin. Antimicrob Agents Chemother 1980;17:217.
388. Barza M, Lauermann MW, Tally FP, Gorbach SL. Prospective, randomized trial of netilmicin and amikacin, with emphasis on eight-nerve toxicity. Antimicrob Agents Chemother 1980;17:707.
389. Noone M, Pomeroy L, Sage R et al. Prospective study of amikacin versus netilmicin in the treatment of severe infection in hospitalized patients. Am J Med 1989;86:809.
390. Smith CR, Lipsky JJ, Laskin OL et al. Double-blind comparison of the nephrotoxicity and auditory toxicity of gentamicin and tobramycin. N Engl J Med 1980;302:1106.
391. Matzke GR, Lucarotti RL, Shapiro HS. Controlled comparison of gentamicin and tobramycin nephrotoxicity. Am J Nephrol 1983;3:11.
392. Blaser J, Stone BB, Zinner SH. Efficacy of intermittent versus continuous administration of netilmicin in a two compartment in vitro model. Antimicrob Agents Chemother 1985;27:343.
393. Gerber AU, Craig WA. Aminoglycoside selected subpopulations of *P. aeruginosa*: characterisation and virulence in normal and leukopenic mice. J Lab Clin Med 1982;100:671.
394. Olson B, Weinstein RA, Nathan C et al. Occult aminoglycoside resistance in *Pseudomonas aeruginosa*: epidemiology and implications for therapy and control. J Infect Dis 1985;152:769.
395. Hilf MS, Yu VL, Sharp JA et al. Antibiotic therapy for *Pseudomonas aeruginosa* bacteremia: Outcome correlations in a prospective study of 200 patients. Am J Med 1989;87:540.
396. Heinonen OP, Slone D, Shapiro S. Birth defects and drugs in pregnancy. In: Kaufmann DW, ed. Antimicrobial and Parasite Agents. Littleton, MA: John Wright, 1982;296, 435.
397. Bailey RR. Renal failure in combined gentamicin and cephalothin therapy. Br Med J 1973;2:776.
398. Cabamilas F, Burgos C, Rodriguez C, Baldizon C. Nephrotoxicity of combined cephalothin-gentamicin regimen. Arch Intern Med 1975;135:850.
399. Tobias JS, Whitehouse JM, Wrigley PFM. Severe renal dysfunction after tobramycin/cephalothin therapy. Lancet 1976;i:425.
400. English J, Gilbert DN, Kohlhepp PW et al. Attenuation of experimental tobramycin nephrotoxicity by ticarcillin. Antimicrob Agents Chemother 1985;27:897.
401. Wade JC, Schimpff SC, Wiernik PH. Antibiotic combination-associated nephrotoxicity in granulocytopenic patients with cancer. Arch Intern Med 1981;141:1789.
402. Ryback MJ, Albrecht LM, Boike SC, Chandrasekar PH. Nephrotoxicity of vancomycin, alone and with an aminoglycoside. J Antimicrob Chemother 1990;25:679.
403. de Lemos E, Pariat C, Piriou A et al. Variations circadiennes de la nephrotoxicite de 1'association vancomycine-gentamicine chez le rat. Pathol Biol 1991;39:12.
404. Pauly DJ, Musa DM, Lestico MR et al. Risk of nephrotoxocity with combination vancomycin-aminoglycoside antibiotic therapy. Pharmacotherapy 1990;10:6.
405. Bregman CL, Williams. Comparative nephrotoxicity of carboplatin and cisplatin in combination with tobramycin. Cancer Chemother Pharmacol 1986;18:117.
406. Caston J, Doinel L. Comparative vestibular toxicity of dibekacin, habekacin and cisplatin. Acta Otolaryngol 1987;104:315.
407. Holt HA, Broughale JM, McCarthy M, Reeves DS. Interactions between aminoglycoside antibiotics and carbenicillin or ticarcillin. Infection 1976;4:107.
408. Adam D, Haneder J. Studies on the inactivation of aminoglycoside antibiotics by acylureidopenicillins and piperacillin. Infection 1981;9:182.
409. Henderson JL, Polk RE, Kline BJ. In vitro inactivation of gentamicin, tobramycin and netilmicin by carbenicillin, azlocillin or mezlocillin. Am J Hosp Pharmacol 1981; 38:1167.
410. Thompson MIB, Russo ME, Saxon BJ et al. Gentamicin inactivation by piperacillin or carbenicillin in patients with end-stage renal disease. Antimicrob Agents Chemother 1982;21:268.
411. Dayal VS, Chait GE, Fenton SSA. Gentamicin vestibulotoxicity: long term disability. Ann Otol Rhinol Laryngol 1979;88:36.
412. Kane FG, Byrd G. Acute toxic psychosis associated with gentamicin therapy. South Med J 1975;68:1283.

413. Watanabe I, Hodges GR, Dworzack DL et al. Neurotoxicity of intrathecal gentamicin: a case report and experimental study. Ann Neurol 1978;4:564.

414. Russo JC, Adelman RD. Gentamicin-induced Fanconi syndrome. J Pediatr 1980;96:151.

415. Bendush CL, Weber R. Tobramycin sulfate: a summary of world wide experience. J Infect Dis 1976;123(Suppl).

416. Neu HC. Tobramycin: an overview. J Infect Dis 1976;134(Suppl):3.

417. McCartney CF, Hatley LH, Kessler JM. Possible tobramycin delirium. J Am Med Assoc 1982;247:1319

418. Feld R, Valdivieso M, Bodey GP, Rodriguez V. A comparative trial of sisomicin therapy by intermittent versus continuous infusion. Am. J Med Sci 1977;274:179.

419. Lode H, Kemmerich B, Koeppe P, Langmack H. Vergleichende Pharmakokinetik und klinische Erfahrungen mit einem neuen Aminoglykosid-Derivat, Sisomicin. Dtsch Med Wochenschr 1975;100:2144.

420. Gruenwaldt G, Arcieri G, Gionti A. Klinische Erfahrungen mit Sisomicin: Zusammenfassung der Ergebnisse. Infection 1976;4(Suppl 4):505.

421. Matz GJ, Lerner SA. Prospective studies of aminoglycoside ototoxicity in adults. In: Lerner SA, Matz GJ, Hawkins JE, eds. Aminoglycoside Ototoxicity. Boston: Little, Brown and Co., 1981;327.

422. Lane AZ, Wright GE, Blair DC. Ototoxicity and nephrotoxicity of amikacin. Am J Med 1977;62:911.

423. Meyer RD. Amikacin. Ann Intern Med 1981;95:328.

424. Prazic M, Salaj B. Ototoxicity with children caused by streptomycin. Audiology 1975;14:173.

425. Kushimoto H, Aoki T. Toxic erythema with generalized follicular pustules caused by streptomycin. Arch Dermatol 1981;17:444.

426. Sarker SK, Purohit SD, Sharma TN et al. Stevens-Johnson-syndrome caused by streptomycin. Tubercle 1982; 63:137.

427. Robinson G, Cambon KG. Hearing loss in infants of tuberculosis mothers treated with streptomycin during pregnancy. N Engl J Med 1964;271:949.

428. Donald PR, Doherty E, Van Zyl FJ. Hearing loss in the child following streptomycin administration during pregnancy. Cent Afr J Med 1991;37:268.

429. Kellerhals B. Hörschaden durch ototoxische Ohrtropfen. HNO 1978;26:49.

430. Smith BM, Myers MG. The penetration of gentamicin and neomycin into perilymph across the round window membrane. Otolaryngol Head Neck Surg 1979;87:888.

431. Forstrom L, Pirila V. Cross-sensitivity within the neomycin group of antibiotics. Contact Dermatitis 1978;4:312.

432. Weinstein L. Neomycin. In: Goodman LS, Gilman A, eds. The Pharmacological Basis of Therapeutics, 5th ed. New York: Macmillan Publishing Co., Inc., 1975;1173.

433. Koch-Weser J, Sidel VW, Federman EB et al. Adverse effects of colistimethate: manifestations and specific reaction rates during 317 courses of therapy. Ann Intern Med 1970;72:857.

434. Lindesmith LA, Baines RD, Bigelow DB, Petty TL. Reversible respiratory paralysis associated with polymyxin therapy. Ann Intern Med 1968;68:318.

435. Sobek V. Arrest of respiration induced by polypeptide antibiotics. Arzneim-Forsch 1982;32:235.

436. Herrell WE. Considerations of toxicity of lincomycin. In: Herrell WE, ed. Lincomycin. Chicago: Modern Scientific Publications Inc., 1969;147.

437. Klainer AS. Clindamycin. Med Clin North Am 1987;1:1169.

438. Zehnder D, Künzi UP, Maibach R et al. Die Häufigkeit der Antibiotika-assoziierten Kolitis bei hospitalisierten Patienten der Jahre 1974–1991 im 'Comprehensive Hospital Drug Monitoring' Bern/St. Gallen. Schweiz Med Wochenschr 1995;125:676.

439. Lochmann O, Kohout P, Vymola F. Anaphylactic shock following the administration of clindamycin. J Hyg Epidemiol Microbiol 1977;21:441.

440. Aucoin PA, Beckner R, Nelson MG. Clindamycin-induced cardiac arrest. South Med J 1982;75:768.

441. Parry MF, Rha C-K. Pseudomembranous colitis caused by topical clindamycin phosphate. Arch Dermatol 1986; 122:583.

442. Midtvedt T, Carlstedt-Duke B, Höverstad T et al. Influence of peroral antibiotics upon the biotransformatory microflora in healthy subjects. Eur J Clin Invest 1986;16:11.

443. Bott SJ, McCallum RW. Medication-induced oesophageal injury. Survey of the literature. Med Toxicol 1986;1:499.

444. De Kort WJA, De Groot AC. Clindamycin allergy presenting as rosacea. Contact Dermatitis 1989;20:72.

445. Ohm-Smith M, Sweet RL, Hadley WK. Occurrence of clindamycin-resistant anaerobic bacteria isolated from cultures taken following clindamycin therapy. Antimicrob Agents Chemother 1986;30:11.

446. Mickal A, Dildy GA, Miller HJ. Lincomycin in the treatment of cervicitis and vaginitis in pregnancy. South Med J 1966;59:567.

447. Marshall IG, Henderson F. Drug interactions at the neuromuscular junction. Clin Anaesthesiol 1985;3:261.

448. Johnson RH, Rozanis J, Shofield IDF. The effect of spiramycin on plaque accumulation and gingivitis. J Can Dent Assoc 1979;44:456.

449. Griffith RS. Introduction to vancomycin. Rev Infect Dis 1981;3:S200.

450. Moellering RC. Monitoring serum vancomycin levels: climbing the mountain because it is there? Clin Infect Dis 1994;18:544.

451. Cantu TG, Yamanaka-Yuen NA, Lietman PS. Serum vancomycin concentrations: reappraisal of their clinical value. Clin Infect Dis 1993;18:533.

452. Hospital Infection Control Practices Advisory Committee. Recommendations for preventing the spread of vancomycin resistance. Am J Infect Control 1995;23:87.

453. Brummett RE. Ototoxicity of vancomycin and analogues. Otolaryngol Clin North Am 1993;26:821.

454. Mellor JA, Kingdom J, Cafferkey M, Keane CT. Vancomycin toxicity: a prospective study. J Antimicrob Chemother 1985;15:773.

455. Cook FV, Farsar WE. Vancomycin revisited. Ann Intern Med 1978;88:813.

456. Weitzman SA, Stossel TP. Drug-induced immunological neutropenia. Lancet 1978;i:1068.

457. Keith H, Steinberg I, Crossley KB. Vancomycin-induced neutropenia during treatment of osteomyelitis in an outpatient. Drug Intell Clin Pharm 1986;20:783.

458. Eich G, Neftel KA. Hämatologische Nebenwirkungen der antiinfektiösen Therapie. Infection 1991;19;S1–S35.

459. Adrouny A, Meguerditchian S, Chae HK et al. Agranulocytosis related to vancomycin therapy. Am J Med 1986;81:1059.

460. West BC. Vancomycin-induced neutropenia. South Med J 1981;74:1255.

461. Koo KB, Bachand RL, Chow AW. Vancomycin-induced neutropenia. Drug Intell Clin Pharm 1986;20:780.
462. Thompson CM, Long SS, Gilligan PH et al. Absorption of oral vancomycin—possible associated toxicity. Int J Pediatr Nephrol 1983;4:1.
463. Downs NJ, Neihart RE, Dolezahl JM, Hodges GR. Mild nephrotoxicity associated with vancomycin use. Arch Intern Med 1989;149:1777.
464. Wold JS, Turnipseed SA. Toxicology of vancomycin in laboratory animals. Rev Infect Dis 1981;3:S224.
465. Ngeleka M, Auclair P, Tardif D et al. Intrarenal distribution of vancomycin in endotoxic rats. Antimicrob Agents Chermother 1989;33:1575.
466. Newfield P, Roizen MF. Hazards of rapid administration of vancomycin. Ann Intern Med 1979;91:981.
467. Davis RL, Smith AL, Koup JR. The 'red-man syndrome' and slow infusion of vancomycin. Ann Intern Med 1986;104:285.
468. Healy DP, Sahai JV, Fuller SH, Polk RE. Vancomycin-induced histamin release and 'red-man syndrome': comparison of 1- and 2-hour infusion. Antimicrob Agents Chemother 1990;34:550.
469. Polk RE. Anaphylactoid reactions to glycopeptide antibiotics. J Antimicrob Chemother 1991;27S.B:17.
470. Bergeron L, Boucher FD. Possible red man syndrome associated with systemic absorption of oral vancomycin in a child with normal renal function. Ann Pharmacother 1994;28:581.
471. Packer J, Olshan AR, Schwarts AB. Prolonged allergic reaction to vancomycin in endstage renal disease. Dialysis Transplant 1987;16:87.
472. Symons NLP, Hobbes AFT, Leaver H. Anaphylactoid reactions to vancomycin during anesthesia: two clinical reports. Can Anaesth Soc J 1985;32:178.
473. Freeman CD, Quintiliani R, Nightingale CH. Vancomycin therapeutic monitoring: is it necessary? Ann Pharmacother 1993;27:594.
474. Reference deleted.
475. Sahai J, Healy D, Shelton M et al. Comparison of vancomycin- and teicoplanin-induced histamine release and 'red man syndrome'. Antimicrob Agents Chemother 1990;34:765.
476. Campoli-Richards D, Brogden R, Faulds D. Teicoplanin. A review of its antibacterial activity, pharmacokinetic properties and therapeutic potential. Drugs 1990;40:449.
477. Paul C, Janier M, Carlet J et al. Erythroderma induced by teicoplanin. Ann Dermatol Venereol 1992;119:667.
478. McElrath M, Goldberg D, Neu H. Allergic cross-reactivity of teicoplanin and vancomycin. Lancet 1986;i:47.
479. Davenport A. Allergic cross-reactivity to teicoplanin and vancomycin. Nephron 1993;63:482.
480. Knudsen J, Pedersen M. IgE-mediated reaction to vancomycin and teicoplanin after treatment with vancomycin. Scand J Infect Dis 1992;24:395.
481. Smith S, Cheesbrough J, Makris M, Davies J. Teicoplanin administration in patients experiencing reactions to vancomycin. J Antimicrob Chemother 1989;23:810.
482. Wood G, Whitby M. Teicoplanin in patients who are allergic to vancomycin. Med J Aust 1989;150:668.
483. Schlemmer B, Falkman H, Boudjadja A et al. Teicoplanin for patients allergic to vancomycin. N Engl J Med 1988;318:1127.
484. Stille W, Sietzen W, Dieterich H, Fell J. Clinical efficacy and safety of teicoplanin. J Antimicrob Chemother 1988;21(Suppl A):69.
485. Maher E, Hollman A, Gruneberg R. Teicoplanin-induced ototoxicity in Down's syndrome. Lancet 1986;i:613.
486. Bibler M, Frame P, Hagler D et al. Clinical evaluation of efficacy, pharmacokinetics, and safety of teicoplanin for serious gram-positive infections. Antimicrob Agents Chemother 1987;31:207.
487. Davey P, Williams A. A review of the safety profile of teicoplanin. J Antimicrob Chemother 1991;27(Suppl B):69.
488. Brummett R, Fox K, Warchol M, Himes D. Absence of ototoxicity of teichomycin A2 in guinea pigs. Antimicrob Agents Chemother 1987;31:612.
489. Del Favero A, Patoia L, Bucaneve G et al. Leukopenia with neutropenia associated with teicoplanin therapy. DICP 1989;23:45.
490. Lang E, Schmid J, Fauser A. A clinical trial on efficacy and safety of teicoplanin in combination with beta-lactams and aminoglycosides in the treatment of severe sepsis of patients undergoing allogeneic/autologous bone marrow transplantation. Br J Haematol 1990;76(Suppl 2):14.
491. Terol M, Sierra J, Gatell J, Rozman C. Thrombocytopenia due to use of teicoplanin. Clin Infect Dis 1993;17:927.
492. Agnelli G, Longetti M, Guerciolini R. Effects of the new glycopeptide antibiotic teicoplanin on platelet function and blood coagulation. Antimicrob Agents Chemother 1987;31:1609.
493. Del Favero A, Menichetti F, Guerciolini R et al. Prospective randomized clinical trial of teicoplanin for empiric combined antibiotic therapy in febrile, granulocytopenic acute leukemia patients. Antimicrob Agents Chemother 1987;31:1126.
494. Lewis P, Garaud J-J, Parenti F. A multicentre open clinical trial of teicoplanin in infections caused by Gram-positive bacteria. J Antimicrob Chemother 1988;21(Suppl A):61.
495. Bochud-Gabellon I, Regamey C. Teicoplanin, a new antibiotic effective against gram-positive bacterial infections of the skin and soft tissues. Dermatologica 1988;176:29.
496. Verhagen D, De Pauw B. Teicoplanin for therapy of gram-positive infections in neutropenic patients. Int J Clin Pharm Res 1987;8:491.
497. Webster A, Russell S, Souhami R et al. Use of teicoplanin for Hickman catheter associated staphylococcal infection in immunocompromised patients. J Hosp Infect 1987;10:77.
498. Charbonneau P, Garaud J, Aubertin J et al. Efficiency and safety of teicoplanin plus netilmicin compared to vancomycin plus netilmicin in the treatment of severe gram-positive infections. In: 27th Interscience Conference on Antimicrobial Agents and Chemotherapy, American Society for Microbiology, 1987;110.
499. Kureishi A, Jewesson P, Rubinger M et al. Double-blind comparison of teicoplanin versus vancomycin in febrile neutropenic patients receiving concomitant tobramycin and piperacillin: effect on cyclosporin A-associated nephrotoxicity. Antimicrob Agents Chemother 1991;35:2246.
500. Weinberg W. Safety and efficacy of teicoplanin for bone and joint infections: results of a community-based trial. South Med J 1993;86:891.
501. Frye R, Job M, Dretler R. Teicoplanin nephrotoxicity: first case report. Pharmacotherapy 1990;10:234.
502. Pantosti A, Luzzi I, Cardines R, Gianfrilli P. Comparison of the in vitro activities of teicoplanin and vancomycin against *Clostridium difficile* and their interactions with cholestyramine. Antimicrob Agents Chemother 1985;28:847.

503. Jim L. Physical and chemical compatibility of intravenous ciprofloxacin with other drugs. Ann Pharmacother 1993;27:704.
504. Brogden R, Peters D. Teicoplanin. A reappraisal of its antimicrobial activity, pharmacokinetic properties and therapeutic efficacy. Drugs 1994;47:823.
505. Fortun J, Perez-Molina J, Anon M et al. Right-sided endocarditis caused by *Staphylococcus aureus* in drug abusers. Antimicrob Agents Chemother 1995;39:525.
506. Rybak M, Lerner S, Levine D et al. Teicoplanin pharmacokinetics in intravenous drug abusers being treated for bacterial endocarditis. Antimicrob Agents Chemother 1991;35:696.
507. Lam Y, Kapusnik-Uner J, Sachdeva M et al. The pharmacokinetics of teicoplanin in varying degrees of renal function. Clin Pharmacol Therapeut 1990;47:655.
508. Kanof HB. Bacitracin and tyrothricin. Med Clin N Am 1970;54:1291.
509. Reports of fosfomycin (76 laboratory and clinical studies in Japanese, with summaries in English). Chemotherapy (Tokyo) 1975;23:1649.
510. Bendtzen K, Diamant M, Faber V. Fusidic acid, an immunosuppressive drug with functions similar to cyclosporin A. Cytokine 1990;2:423.
511. Revell P, Nicholson F, Pearson TC. Granulocytopenia due to fusidic acid. Lancet 1988;ii:454.
512. McAreavey D, Redding PJ. Staphylococcal septicaemia complicated by probable cloxacillin neurotoxicity and by jaundine induced by fusidic acid. Scott Med J 1983;28:179.
513. Talbot J, Beely L. Fusidic acid and jaundice. Br Med J 1980;2:308.
514. Kutty KP, Nath IVS, Kothandaraman KR et al. Fusidic acid-induced hyperbilirubinemia. Dig Dis Sci 1987;32:32.
515. Humble MW, Eykyn SJ, Phillips I. Staphylococcal bacteriaemia, fusidic acid and jaundice. Br Med J 1980;1:1495.
516. Wynn V. Metabolic effects of the steroid antibiotic fusidic acid. Br Med J 1965;1:1400.
517. De Groot AC. Contact allergy to sodium fusidate. Contact Dermatitis 1982;8:429.
518. Goh CL. Contact sensitivity to topical antimicrobials. Contact Dermatitis 1989;21:46.
519. Stonelake PS. Rash with intravenous fusidic acid (Letter to Editor). Br Med J 1990;301:1281.
520. Shanson DC. Clinical relevance of resistance to fusidic acid in *Staphylococcus aureus*. J Antimicrob Chemother 1990;25(Suppl B):15.
521. Zenilman JM, Nims LJ, Menegus MA et al. Spectinomycin-resistant gonococcal infections in the United States 1985–1986. J Infect Dis 1987;156:1002.
522. Boslego JW, Tramont EC, Takafuji ET et al. Effect of spectinomycin use on the prevalence of spectinomycin-resistant and of penicillinase-producing *Neisseria gonorrhoeae*. N Engl J Med 1987;317:272.

Meyler's Side Effects of Drugs, 13th Edition
M.N.G. Dukes, editor

SECTION EDITOR: P.K.M. LUNDE

C.B.M. Tester-Dalderup

27 Antifungal drugs

While fungus infections have always been prevalent, there seems to be a current increase, especially in systemic infections and those involving a greater variety of fungi. Fungus infections are more readily diagnosed than in the past which makes comparisons difficult. Most of these infections are seen in patients with underlying illnesses and during the use of multiple medications. Organ transplant patients on immunosuppressive drugs, cancer treatment cases on high doses of chemotherapy, the immune deficient patient on experimental antiviral drugs and the low weight new-born infant with systemic candida infections: each such group brings its own challenge. In all cases, knowledge of the pharmacology and the interactions of the drugs used is essential. Facts about medication used by the patient during prior episodes of the same illness or for other conditions (drug, dosage used, total dosage, adverse effects) will help to prevent toxicity and especially nephrotoxicity. Newly developed antifungal drugs should be tested or otherwise followed at an early phase to detect drug interactions early in the course of development; this applies particularly to systemic antifungal drugs which are so often used concomitantly with other medications. Pharmacokinetic and pharmacodynamic interactions may and do occur.

Amphotericin B

ADVERSE REACTION PATTERN

General and toxic reactions Amphotericin B is an effective but also a toxic agent. Intravenous administration—the only possible method of systemic treatment—is in almost all cases followed by a generalized reaction with chills, fever, rigor, nausea, vomiting, abdominal pains, headache and muscle and joint pains. The incidence and severity of the reaction is highest with the initial doses. Starting treatment with a low dosage will mitigate the severity of the reaction. The use of liposomes as a drug carrier for the amphotericin may reduce the immediate reaction. Phlebitis at the site of injection occurs frequently. Nephrotoxicity is unavoidable at dosages in current use and often results in permanent renal damage. The renal damage may bring about hypokalemia and hypomagnesemia. The concomitant or even prior use of other nephrotoxic drugs enhances the risk of serious renal damage. Close attention to amphotericin serum levels and early signs of nephrotoxicity with appropriate adjustment of dosages does help in preventing permanent renal damage. The lipid formulations exhibit a lesser degree of nephrotoxicity. The pharmacokinetics in young children differ from those in the adult; higher serum levels and longer elimination times have been demonstrated and, for these reasons, lower doses should be used than those which would be anticipated if extrapolating from adult experience. Some reports indicate that prophylactic sodium supplementation may provide protection against the development of amphotericin nephrotoxicity.

Hypersensitivity reactions Possible hypersensitivity reactions have been described in case reports. Reports of rashes have been rare. The UK Committee on Safety of Medicine received 20 reports of the occurrence of rash over a 17-year period (SEDA-16, 289). With the increased use of the lipid formulations this could change.

Tumor-inducing effects No carcinogenic effects have been demonstrated either in animals or in man.

PHARMACOKINETICS

Amphotericin is highly protein bound, primarily to lipoproteins, erythrocytes and cholesterol in plasma (1^R) Concentrations in peritoneal, pleural and synovial fluids are usually less than half those in serum, while cerebrospinal fluid levels range from the undetectable to some 4% of the serum concentration; the findings are dependent upon the sensitivity of the analytical method used. The serum $T_{1/2}$ is 1—2 days. Levels in bile are detectable for up to 12 days, and in urine for 27—35 days. There is marked tissue storage. Amphotericin can be detected in liver and kidney tissue for as long as 12 months after therapy has been terminated. Up to 40% of the amphotericin is excreted unchanged in the urine. The metabolism of amphotericin is largely unknown; it could be that storage is a more important factor than metabolism. Each lipid formulation of amphotericin has distinct pharmacokinetic properties; in general these formulations distribute the amphotericin preferentially to organs rich in reticuloendothelial cells, leading to higher levels in the liver, spleen and lung and lower levels in the kidneys. With the lipid formulation, higher doses can be given without the restrictions imposed by renal toxicity. Some data suggest an enhanced and prolonged activity when using this form, but a number of reports suggest that there is an increased variability in the serum levels attained (1[R]). Studies of the pharmacokinetics of—AmBisone (the unilamellar liposomal formulation of amphotericin) showed that there was a large inter-patient variability, and that at a dose of 3 mg/kg serum concentrations were 8-fold greater than after conventional amphotericin 1 mg/kg (SEDA-18, 279). Accumulation in serum was seen in nearly half of the patients, and in this study the half-life was longer (SEDA-18, 279). The serum half-life is increased with AmBisome as well as with Amphocil (a colloidal dispersion, an equimolar mixture of amphotericin B and cholesteryl sulphate) Complexing amphotericin with lipids or entrapping it in liposomes may increase its efficacy by reducing toxicity and affecting distribution, it may also influence the nature of the side effects which occur. Depending on the lipids involved, interference with antifungal activity has been shown (SEDA-17, 319; SEDA-18, 3; 1[R], 2, 3[R]).

The primary mechanism of action of amphotericin B is due to binding to ergosterol, the principal sterol present in the cell membrane of sensitive fungi. it also binds to a lesser extent to other sterols such as cholesterol, which accounts for much of the toxicity associated with its use (1[R]).

Immunomodulating activity Amphotericin has immunostimulatory properties. Polymorphonuclear leukocytes are activated by amphotericin. Amphotericin induces production of tumor necrosis factor by macrophages, and the ability of (viable or heat-killed) *Candida albicans* to induce in vitro macrophage production of tumor necrosis factor(SEDA-18, 279). *Candida albicans* may resist intracellular killing by macrophages through the formation of germ tubes; in a study specifically set up to study the effects of different antifungal drugs on this process, amphotericin blocked germ tube formation completely, both in macrophages and extracellularly. In this set-up, amphotericin was fungicidal (3). This effect on host cells has also been mentioned in other publications (1[R], 5—7).

ORGANS AND SYSTEMS

General reactions The concentration of amphotericin in the infusion fluid and the rate of infusion have been considered important factors in determining the incidence of reactions, though reports are conflicting. Rapid infusion over 45 minutes to 2 hours has been advocated (SEDA 16, 286) A more recent double-blind randomized trial covering the first 5—7 days of treatment showed a statistically higher rating for 7-day mean chill scores, pethidine requirements and increases in pulse rate for the rapid (45 minutes) infusion as compared with slow (4 hours) infusion (SED-17, 320). These acute reactions can be tempered using by pethidine, codeine, paracetamol or corticosteroids. Diphenhydramine has been found useful as an anti-emetic in this situation (SED-16, 286; SED-17, 320; 1[R]). The use of liposomes as drug carriers may mitigate the immediate reaction.

Cardiovascular *Changes in blood pressure*, hypotensive as well as hypertensive, cardiac *arrhythmias* and even (rare) instances of *cardiac arrest* have been reported. These immediate reactions follow the intravenous administration and occur particularly with excessively rapid injection. The description of the occurrence of an arrhythmia in a neonate and of *torsade de pointes* in an adult during a controlled infusion suggest that arrhythmias may occur more frequently than is generally believed, and may be detected if the patient is monitored. Ventricular dysrhythmias have been reported after rapid infusion of large doses of amphotericin in patients with hyperkalemia and renal failure, but not in patients with normal serum creatinine and potassium levels, even if they have received the drug over a period of 1 hour (SEDA-18, 278). A case of fatal cardiac arrest due to ventricular fibrillation was seen during an infusion of liposomal amphotericin; serum creatinine and electrolytes were normal in this case (SEDA-18, 278). Dysrhythmia was reported earlier in one out of 71 patients treated with AmBisome (SEDA-17, 319). Acute hypertension during amphotericin infusion was observed in a 68-year-old woman, and in a 64-year-old female. In both cases a further dose of amphotericin after recovery again provoked a hypertensive reaction. No obvious mechanism causing this acute hypertension was evident, and it was therefore considered to be an idiosyncratic reaction (SED-12, 672; SEDA-16, 285). The frequency with which this adverse effect occurs is unknown.

Amphotericin B is increasingly being administered on an out-patient basis with less intensive monitoring during the actual infusion. This can introduce risks, since an acute hypertension can easily be fatal if it is not immediately and adequately treated.

Electrolyte disturbances (hypo- and hyperkalemia due to renal toxicity, but also hypomagnesemia and hypovolemia) can be additional factors precipitating cardiac reactions.

Thrombophlebitis at the site of injection is common and even more frequent in children than in adults.

Extravasation may cause severe local reactions including tissue necrosis. Good puncture techniques, use of special needles and buffered solutions, and the use of heparin sodium is essential in minimizing the risk of phlebitis.

Respiratory The possibility of occurrence of *pulmonary infiltrates* caused by amphotericin B when given in combination with granulocyte infusions was mentioned in SED-11 (p. 169).

Acute dyspnea, mild hemoptysis, new infiltrates on chest films and intra-alveolar hemorrhage diagnosed by lung biopsy were seen in a granulocytopenic patient with undifferentiated myeloid leukemia who was given amphotericin B and transfusions of blood and platelets. A second identical episode occurred 4 days later after the second dose of amphotericin B, this time in combination with a platelet infusion (SEDA-12, 227).

A retrospective study over the period 1973—1980 by the National Institutes of Health showed that 14 of the 22 patients who received granulocyte transfusion and amphotericin B showed *respiratory deterioration*, while only two of the 25 cases who received granulocyte infusion alone experienced such respiratory distress. The data on 20 profoundly neutropenic patients given amphotericin alone however showed no reports of adverse pulmonary reactions (SEDA-16, 288).

Amphotericin B can damage *pulmonary surfactant* (SED-12, 673). Reversible abnormalities in pulmonary gas exchange and cardiopulmonary hemodynamics were seen in a patient receiving high dose liposomal amphotericin B; the effects were transient but reproducible. Clinical symptoms were absent when lower doses were administered over longer periods of time (SEDA-16, 289).

The possibility of a liposome overload, as the explanation of this reaction should be considered. Inhalation treatment with amphotericin B has been tried in order to prevent pulmonary fungus infections in patients with prolonged neutropenia (SEDA-18, p. 3). Side effects seen in 29 patients on a dose of 30 mg in 3 ml of sterile water, daily for 7 days, thereafter every second or third day.

Table 1. *Adverse effects of inhaled amphotericin*

Adverse effect	% of patients
Cough	100
Aftertaste	100
Nausea/vomiting	69
Wheezing	17
Dysphagia	14
Epistaxis	3
Dyspnea/Rigors	0
Renal insufficiency	0

Nervous system *Headaches* are common during the immediate infusion reaction. *Neuropathy, convulsions, tremors and paresis* have been attributed to the use of amphotericin B. It is difficult to assess these findings because in systemic fungus infections with the possibility of central nervous system involvement the symptoms may be due to the underlying disease.

Amphotericin B given intravenously does not lead to adequate CSF levels, and the drug has to be given intrathecally in cases of cerebral infection. *Complications after intrathecal injection* are manifold and frequent; irritative symptoms, local pain, radiculitis, arachnoiditis and even meningitis can occur, while myelopathy and neuropathy have been described (SED-12, 673). Impairment of vision can complicate the intrathecal use of amphotericin B.

Endocrine, metabolic A reduction in ketogenic steroid excretion was recorded in the past (SED-11, 569). There has been no more recent confirmation of this finding.

Mineral and fluid balance See 'Kidney and urinary system'.

Hematological A normochromic, normocytic, and usually mild *anemia* is the rule rather than the exception. The anemia may be due to suppression of erythrocyte production and inhibition of erythropoietin production. *Hemolysis, leukopenia and thrombocytopenia* have been reported (SED-12, 673). Concentrations of amphotericin of more than 5 mg/l have been shown to have deleterious effects on normal *neutrophil function* in vitro (1^R). Amphotericin B in combination with flucytosine gives an increased risk of hematological complications.

Liver A rare case of *acute hepatic toxic degeneration* is to be found in the literature. Asymptomatic *elevation of hepatic serum enzyme levels* was seen in one case. *Cholestasis* has been reported in infants treated with amphotericin B for systemic candida infections (SEDA-14, 230). Most of the above reports are incidental and amphotericin B cannot in the overall view be regarded as a known cause of liver damage. This does not necessarily also apply to the liposomal amphotericin preparations; increases in serum bilirubin, alkaline phosphatase, transaminases and γ-GT levels have been seen during administration of liposomal amphotericin (SEDA-17, 319; SEDA-18, 278—279). Hay (2) sees a link between these changes and high doses of liposomal amphotericin. It is difficult to interpret their importance; they could reflect the greater uptake in the liver of the liposomal amphotericin but liver function changes are not uncommon in patients with invasive fungal disease (2). What is more these liposomal preparations are more likely used in those patients who are more seriously ill or have already run into treatment complications.

Gastrointestinal *Anorexia, nausea and vomiting* are common after effects of parenteral administration. *Gastrointestinal bleeding* has been reported on rare occasions as part of the generalized reaction. Gastrointestinal complaints are markedly less common with the use of liposomal amphotericin (SEDA-17, 319; 1[R], 2), the differences being more pronounced with AmBisone than with Amphocil (2, 3[R]).

Kidney and urinary system Nephrotoxicity is inherent to the use of amphotericin B. Both *glomerular and tubular damage* can be caused. The clinical and laboratory findings may include a decrease in glomerular filtration rate and renal plasma flow, proteinuria, cylindruria and hematuria; the latter three are frequent but usually discrete. The decrease in renal plasma flow and filtration fraction is seen early. Increased excretion of the renal enzymes *N*-acetyl-β-D-glucosaminidase and alanine aminopeptidase suggests damage to the proximal tubular cells (SEDA-14, 233). Changes in tubular function can cause an increased excretion of uric acid (an effect which can be used to monitor the tubular damage), an excessive loss of potassium resulting in hypokalemia and or an excessive loss of magnesium. With severe renal damage *hyperkalemia* may develop. The exact mechanisms involved in amphotericin-induced azotemia are not yet fully understood. Changes in tubular cell permeability for ions have been demonstrated both in vitro and in vivo (1[R], 8). The *azotemia* can be caused by a tubular-glomerular feedback, a mechanism whereby increased delivery and re-absorption of chloride ions in the distal tubule initiates a decrease in the glomerular filtration rate of the nephron. Tubular-glomerular feedback is amplified by sodium deprivation and suppressed by sodium loading. Other possible mechanisms are; renal arteriolar spasm, calcium deposition during periods of ischemia and direct cellular toxicity (1[R]). Yet other lines of research have looked at the roles of prostaglandins and tumor necrosis factor-α. *Hypomagnesemia*, as described in one case after only 8 days of amphotericin treatment, may also have been promoted by a prior treatment with gentamycin (SEDA-12, 226). Hypomagnesemia should be suspected in the patient not doing so well—with general tiredness and malaise and muscle weakness complaints—especially when the infection seems to have come under control.

It is well known that the concomitant use of aminoglycosides increases kidney damage but it is also necessary to watch for the cumulative impact of renal toxic drugs, even if no clinical evidence has been found of renal damage and serum levels have been within so-called safe limits during drug administration. For the aminoglycosides, a progressive increase in drug concentration in renal tissue and the inner ear has been demonstrated (SED-11, 547); it is to be expected that such drug accumulation in a 'deep compartment' occurs with other nephrotoxic agents too. With amphotericin itself, high kidney tissue levels have been found. Acknowledging the fact that patients treated with antifungal drugs are often also at risk for bacterial infections and the treatment thereof, especially if they are on immunosuppressive drugs or cancer chemotherapy as well, it becomes even more important to keep an accurate record of all the drugs used (actual amounts, recorded serum levels and toxic effects). A drug given last year may influence this year's toxic adverse effects.

The renal failure of amphotericin B is to some extent reversible and recovery can be rapid, indicating an important functional component (SED-12, 672). Vasoconstriction has been advanced as a possible cause of the renal damage during amphotericin B administration (SED-11, 569). Circulatory dynamics and hypovolemia may also play a role. It was observed that the combination treatment of amphotericin B and ticarcillin in leukemia patients seemed to have a lower incidence of nephrotoxicity. This may reflect the fact that ticarcillin treatment in higher doses creates a considerable salt load; the use of a direct salt load (500—1000 ml of normal saline or 150 mEq of 0.9% sodium chloride) has been found to have a protective effect (SED-12, 673). The use of infusions of mannitol, saralasin or theophylline is of no proven benefit (SEDA-14, 229). Clearly, administration of other nephrotoxic drugs should be avoided wherever possible. Pentoxifylline decreases the effect of amphotericin on the leukocytes and was found to decrease renal toxicity in animal experiments (SED-12, 674). HWA-138, a pentoxifylline analog, has been shown to prevent amphotericin B-induced acute renal failure in rats. HWA-138 was also shown to increase yeast urinary clearance and reduce yeast counts in rats infected with *Candida albicans*. Co-administration of amphotericin B and HWA-138 resulted in an increased survival time (SED-12, 674).

The induction of *nephrocalcinosis* during amphotericin treatment was reported during the early years of use of amphotericin. More recently, development of pelvic-calyceal fungal concretions with calcification was seen in two neonates with renal candidiasis during amphotericin treatment (SEDA-16, 288).

Liposomal amphotericin B is markedly less nephrotoxic than the plain drug. It makes possible the use of dosages that cannot be tolerated with the use of ordinary amphotericin. In some cases existing renal dysfunction improved following the switch to a liposomal preparation. Hypokalemia and hypomagnesemia may and do occur during the use of liposomal amphotericin (SEDA-17, 319).

Amphotericin B in infants and children The high incidence of fungal infections, especially systemic candida infections, in newborn infants at risk because of prematurity, low birth weight or immune deficiency syndrome, and in infants who have undergone surgery or transplant, can make it necessary to use amphotericin B treatment very early in infancy. Such use has shown the presence of differences in the kinetics and safety of amphotericin B in this age group. Elimination of the drug is slower, the $T_{1/2}$ being inversely correlated with the patient's age. Serum levels may go well above those required; merely monitoring nephrotoxicity is not adequate. With changes in renal function, significant differences in hemoglobin, platelets and serum potassium and liver enzyme levels were seen in these young patients (SEDA-14, 231). However not all reports indicate similar changes in kinetics (1^R). Information on the use of liposomal amphotericin in children is very limited, but general and renal toxicity seem to be less in this age group. In one of a series of 10 children, age range 4—16 years, an elevation of alkaline phosphatase was seen (SEDA-18, 279).

Skin Skin reactions are rare and in the cases described it is often questionable if the exanthema was indeed caused by the amphotericin or by other drugs given concomitantly. An immediate reaction to infusion named the '*grey syndrome*' is characterized by an ashen color, acral cyanosis and a general feeling of prostration. It is not a true skin reaction.

Special senses *Dysgeusia* and *hypogeusia* have been reported (76^r).

Risk situations Patients with renal impairment are obviously at risk, as are neonates and elderly patients with a limited renal reserve. It is probable that patients who suffered seemingly transient renal damage have a decreased tolerance as well. There is no information available indicating specific adverse effects with the use of amphotericin in the pregnant woman.

Second-generation effects Teratogenic effects have not been reported. It is not known if the fetal kidney could be damaged during treatment of the pregnant woman.

Interactions Concomitant use of other known nephrotoxic agents clearly does increase the risk and severity of amphotericin renal damage. Goren et al. (SED-12, 674) showed increases in the half-life of *aminoglycosides* (amikacin and gentamycin) and higher serum levels requiring dosage adjustments of the aminoglycosides when amphotericin B was added to the treatment regimen even prior to the appearance of significant increases in serum creatinine, thus demonstrating once again that monitoring serum creatinine alone is not an adequate guarantee of safety. Because *ciclosporin* causes a reduction in renal function there is increased nephrotoxicity if amphotericin B is given to a patient already receiving ciclosporin.

Tacrolimus (*FK* 506), a macrolide immunosuppressant, has adverse effects similar to those of ciclosporin including the nephrotoxicity. Increased nephrotoxicity can be expected when it is given alongside amphotericin (9^R). Amphotericin-induced hypomagnesemia may be more profound in patients who develop a divalent cation-losing nephropathy associated with the anti-neoplastic drug *cisplatin* (1^R). Induced hypokalemia may enhance the toxicity of *digitalis* and *neuromuscular blocking agents* (SED-12, 674; 1^R, 10^R). The hypokalemia may also further augment the potassium excretion produced by *corticosteroids*, *thiazides and loop diuretics*, and possibly *NSAIDs*. Amphotericin B may increase the curariform effect of *skeletal muscle relaxants* and may enhance the potential for adverse effects related to *antineoplastic agents* (10^R). The combination with *flucytosine* increases the effectivity against yeast infections, augmenting fungal membrane penetration but it enhances the toxicity of the flucytosine because renal dysfunction leads to higher flucytosine levels (SED-12, 674). The combination of amphotericin B with *ketoconazole* appears to lead to antagonism (SED-12, 674). A study of the effects of combinations of amphotericin B with *fluconazole*, *itraconazole or ketoconazole* against *Aspergillus fumigatus* strains in vitro showed antagonistic effects in some strains, but indifferent combination effects in other strains (11). An in vitro study of the effects of amphotericin in combination with miconazole, itraconazole or fluconazole on *Pseudallescheria boydii* did not demonstrate an antagonism (12). In one group of mice infected with *Candida* combinations of amphotericin with *fluconazole* were more effective than fluconazole alone. In the second group the combination showed no interaction, but was not better than either of the drugs given alone (13). It seems that the result of the combination of amphotericin with any of the azoles depends to a large extent on the type of fungus infection being treated.

Flucytosine (5-fluorocytosine, 5F-C)

Flucytosine is an antimetabolite of the fluoropyrimidine type. Flucytosine enters the fungal cell by means of the enzyme cytosine permease; it is de-aminated to 5-fluorouracil which is metabolized to 5-fluorouridine. Replacement of 5-fluorouracil in RNA results in the disruption of protein synthesis in the sensitive fungus. Flucytosine has a selective activity against such pathogenic yeasts as *Candida*, but only moderate activity against such as *Aspergillus* and chromoblastomycosis. There is synergism between flucytosine and amphotericin B and the combination has been shown to be effective against meningeal cryptococcosis and pheohyphomycosis of the central nervous system, specifically disease caused by *Xylohypha bantiana* (SED-12, 674; 1[R], 14[R], 15[R]). Flucytosine can be given orally as well as parenterally. It should not be given as a single agent because of the frequent development of secondary drug resistance.

ADVERSE REACTION PATTERN

General toxic reactions Nausea and vomiting, gastrointestinal discomfort and (infrequently) enterocolitis occur. Hepatic dysfunction, hepatitis and even hepatic necrosis and blood disorders including fatal bone marrow aplasia may occur. The severe reactions were seen mainly at the time when the importance of high serum levels (in excess of 100 μg/ml) of flucytosine in the occurrence of these side effects was not recognized. Myelosuppression and hepatotoxicity in most patients appear to be concentration dependent. Patients have been described who suffered such adverse effects as hepatotoxicity or eosinophilia that were idiosyncratic and not related to flucytosine levels. Hypersensitivity reactions may occur.

Teratogenic effects These have not been recorded.

Tumor-inducing effects These have not been described.

PHARMACOKINETICS

Flucytosine can be given orally; peak serum concentrations are seen within 1—2 hours in patients with normal renal function. Absorption of flucytosine can be delayed by food or antacids. Flucytosine is poorly bound to protein. It penetrates CSF, vitreous, peritoneal fluid, inflamed joints and other fluid compartments. Serum levels are clearly dose related. There are several methods for determining serum levels. Francis and Walsh (14[R]) describe in their 1992 paper various assays and, particularly, the creatinine iminohydrolase assay which makes use of the spurious creatinine elevation in sera as measured by the Kodak Ektachem analyzer, an apparatus widely available and providing a low cost method as compared with the HPLC technique. The compound accumulates in patients with impaired renal function, resulting in potentially toxic serum levels. Approximately 90% of the dose is excreted unchanged in the urine.

Flucytosine does penetrate into the central nervous system.

ORGANS AND SYSTEMS

Nervous system Mention has been made of *headaches, confusion, hallucinations, somnolence and vertigo*; there have also been a few reports of peripheral neuropathy; however, it is difficult to establish the role of flucytosine in these adverse reactions (SED-12, 674).

Hematological Bone marrow depression is recognized; *anemia, leukopenia and thrombocytopenia* occur in about 5% of cases. The hematological effects are related to prolonged high blood levels of flucytosine, the critical toxic level in serum being around 100 μg/ml. However such serum levels can also occur without any sign of hematotoxicity. Hematotoxicity is seen more often in the presence of renal impairment and hence during the use of flucytosine in combination with amphotericin B. If the bone marrow reserve has already been depleted by underlying disease or by medication, the risk of hematotoxicity increases. Monitoring of blood levels is advisable to allow adjustment of the dosage to maintain peak levels of 40—60 mg/l. Patients with AIDS treated for antifungal disease with flucytosine and amphotericin B may be particularly prone to develop bone marrow depression (SED-12, 675; 1[R], 14[R], 15[R]).

Liver *Abnormal liver function tests*, mainly comprising raised serum alkaline phosphatase and transaminases and, less frequently, elevated serum bilirubin levels have been reported. The hepatic involvement is rarely serious (SED-12, 675). Liver cell *necrosis*, detected by means of a liver biopsy has been described (SED-9, 477); such necrosis seems to be very rare and there are no recent reports. The reason for antifungal treatment and the concurrent use of other medication may contribute to hepatotoxicity (SED-12, 675; 14[R], 15[R]).

Gastrointestinal *Nausea, vomiting and diarrhea* are the most common side effects with flucytosine. *Nausea* occurs in almost all patients. *Enterocolitis*, usually sparing the rectosigmoid, has been described in some cases. Bennett (SED-12, 675) first suggested that this type of flucytosine toxicity may be associated with deamination of flucytosine to 5-fluorouracil in the gut by an enzyme derived from bacteria, such as *Escherichia coli*, present in the bowel. Subsequent work has confirmed this (1[R]). Two more recent studies using 19-F-magnetic resonance spectroscopy have confirmed the presence of several detectable metabolites of flucytosine in addition to fluorouracil in body fluids (16, 17). Potentially fatal *ulcerative colitis* has been suspected in a few patients; however in most cases there were no diagnostic data to back up the diagnosis. *Bowel lesions and perforations* have been described in a few cases.

Urinary system There is no evidence of renal toxicity with flucytosine given alone.

Skin Maculopapular and also urticarial rashes severe enough to require discontinuation of treatment have been reported. The incidence is low. Acquired photosensitivity was described in two cases (SED-12, 675).

Risk situations Caution is advised in treating patients with renal dysfunction and in patients with a reduced bone marrow reserve (see under 'Hematological' above).

Second-generation effects Flucytosine is teratogenic in the rat, and the close chemical relationship to antimetabolites, plus the simple fact that 5-fluorouracil is a metabolite of flucytosine, make it inadvisable to administer this drug during pregnancy or to fertile women taking no precautions to prevent pregnancy.

Development of resistance It is essential to maintain adequate serum levels, above 25 μg/ml, if one is to prevent the development of resistant yeasts. *Candida albicans* and *Cryptococcus neoformans* readily become resistant. Naturally resistant fungus strains are also found among normally flucytosine-sensitive species; 1—2% of strains of *Candida neoformans* are resistant. The addition of amphotericin B can prevent the emergence of resistant mutants (SED-12, 675).

Interactions The combination with *amphotericin B* enhances the efficacy but also the toxicity. Flucytosine has been successfully used in combination with *ketoconazole*, *fluconazole* and *itraconazole*. *Flucytosine* and *ketoconazole* were found to be synergistic in about 40% of yeast isolates resistant to flucytosine alone. The synergistic action of flucytosine with the triazoles against *Candida* spp. was seen both in vitro and in vivo (14[R], 15[R]). The combination of flucytosine with fluconazole is potentially promising as an alternative to the standard treatment for cryptococcal meningitis (14[R]). *Itraconazole* might be a good alternative to amphotericin in the therapy of chromocytosis and pheohyphomycosis when combined with flucytosine (15[R]). Flucytosine should not be used in combination with *cytosine arabinoside* since this may interfere with its metabolism; cytosine arabinoside may also interfere with the antifungal activity of flucytosine by competitive inhibition (SED-12, 675; 10[R]). The combination of *interferon-*α_{2b} with 5-fluorouracil has been shown to lead to significant change in the kinetics of 5-FU, the bioavailability being elevated to 80% and plasma levels increased; a similar interaction with flucytosine could well be possible in view of the metabolism of flucytosine (18). Fluorocytosine in serum interferes with the *enzymatic iminohydrolase methods for creatinine determination*; this may lead to a pseudo elevation of creatinine levels (SEDA-16, 296; 14[R]). On theoretical grounds it is suspected that drugs like the *aminoglycosides*, *NSAIDs* and *thiazide diuretics* may affect flucytosine excretion.

Griseofulvin

Griseofulvin is a metabolic product of *Penicillium griseofulvin*. Discovered in 1939, its activity in dermatophytosis was only found in 1958 when it was used orally in the treatment of ringworm. Griseofulvin is fairly well absorbed from the gastrointestinal tract and is distributed into body fluids and tissues. The penetration in the skin is slow. Griseofulvin could be detected in the base of the stratum corneum 48—72 hours after ingestion and at 12—19 days in the middle layer of the horny layer. The slow penetration rate may explain the difficulties and delays in eradication of infection in nails (SED-12, 676).

With the coming of the triazoles, a comparison of the ease of use, efficacy and adverse effects between griseofulvin and the newer azoles for recalcitrant skin and nail fungus infections is warranted. Itraconazole is effective in these conditions and seems to be better tolerated. It appears questionable whether griseofulvin can any longer be considered the 'gold standard' for the treatment of conditions such as nail tinea (SEDA-18, 283).

ADVERSE REACTION PATTERN

General and toxic reactions Headache and central nervous system disturbances and also gastrointestinal upset can be serious enough to enforce discontinuation of treatment.

Hypersensitivity reactions These, mainly in the form of skin rashes, are not uncommon but rarely severe. A serum sickness-like illness has been described and, in rare instances, angioedema.

Tumor-inducing effects Hepatomas have been produced in mice in experimental settings. Evidence of carcinogenicity in man is lacking.

ORGANS AND SYSTEMS

Nervous system *Headache* is the most common side-effect with griseofulvin; it occurs in about 50% of patients and can be severe. *Drowsiness*, *dizziness*, *fatigue*, *confusion* and *depression*, as well as *irritability* and *insomnia*, have been observed. The psychic symptoms can be very disturbing and are aggravated by the use of alcohol (SED-12, 676). *Impaired coordination and unsteadiness while walking* have been reported in some cases where there was confusion. *Visual disturbances* may occur. *Peripheral neuritis* has been attributed to griseofulvin, but with little proof of a causal relationship.

Endocrine, metabolic An *estrogen-type effect* has been reported in children, affecting the genitals and the breasts (SED-11, 567).

Hematological *Leukopenia*, *neutropenia* and *monocytosis* have been reported. There is no evidence that griseofulvin can cause serious blood disorders. The triggering of *systemic lupus erythematosus* by griseofulvin, by way of an allergic type reaction, has been described, but this is rare. A patient with pre-existing lupus erythematosus may be more prone to the development of skin manifestations from griseofulvin.

Liver While there have been anecdotal reports of *hepatitis*, *cholestasis* and *increased sulfobromphthalein retention*, a causal relationship has never been shown. Griseofulvin does however induce hepatic microsomal enzyme; it is this mechanism that probably explains the interaction with warfarin cited below (SEDA-12, 236). In mice an increased occurrence of hepatomas has been observed (SED-12, 676).

Endocrine, metabolic Griseofulvin interferes with *porphyrin metabolism*; in man, transient increases in erythrocyte proto-porphyrin levels have been demonstrated and the production and excretion of porphyrins is increased. Acute intermittent porphyria is an absolute contraindication for griseofulvin treatment. In patients with other forms of porphyria the drug should be avoided or, if essential, only administered under strict clinical supervision.

Gastrointestinal *Anorexia*, *a feeling of bloating* and mild *nausea* are common, as is mild *diarrhea*. *Vomiting*, *abdominal cramps* and severer forms of diarrhea are rare. *Black furry tongue*, *glossodynia*, *angular stomatitis* and *taste disturbances* have been described. *Dysgeusia* is also known to occur; both taste and smell disturbances may occur more frequently than realized (SED-12, 676; 76[r]).

Urinary system Non-specific urinary sediment abnormalities have been reported but there is no evidence of renal toxicity.

Skin Dermatological side effects are not uncommon and are of considerably variety, including *urticaria*, *photosensitivity eruptions*, *lichen planus*, *erythema multiforme*, *vesicular* and *morbilliform rashes*. *Serum sickness-like reactions* and *angioedema* have been observed. *Stevens-Johnson syndrome*, *cutaneous vasculitis* and *toxic epidermal necrolysis* have been described in case histories (SED-11, 568; SEDA-13, 236; SEDA-16, 296). The downgrading of clinically subpolar tuberculoid *leprosy* towards subpolar lepromatous leprosy was reported in 1982 in a 29-year-old male (SED-11, 568). With the present general increase in sun exposure levels due to climatological changes photosensitivity effects may be seen more often and in more severe form than in the past.

Risk situations Patients with *porphyria* are at risk; acute intermittent porphyria is an absolute contraindication for the use of griseofulvin. Exposure to intense natural or artificial *sunlight* should be avoided during treatment with griseofulvin.

Second-generation effects Embryotoxicity and mutagenicity have been demonstrated in animal experiments using high doses of griseofulvin. Though most handbooks and drug formularies for this reason warn against the use of griseofulvin during pregnancy, there are no reports of any adverse influence on the human fetus—this despite the fact that griseofulvin has been on the market since the early 1960s and has been used extensively and, no doubt, during many pregnancies during that time (SED-12, 676).

Interactions The effects of *alcohol* are potentiated and the use of alcohol increases the risk and severity of psychic disturbances. The concomitant use of *phenobarbital* reduces griseofulvin levels, an effect attributed to the induction of liver enzymes by the phenobarbital.

Griseofulvin is a potent inducer of cytochrome P450-dependent xenobiotic metabolism and has a significant effect on P450 expression in the hepatocyte, consequently griseofulvin influences the effect of *coumarin* (warfarin). It can enhance the metabolism of coumarin anticoagulants, but both increases and decreases in prothrombin time have been reported (SED-12, 676). Again, because of its ability to induce cytochrome P450, griseofulvin can be expected to reduce the concentration/effect of *ciclosporin* if this drug is given concomitantly. The combination of griseofulvin treatment and *oral contraceptives* may lead to oligomenorrhea, amenorrhea and breakthrough bleeding; unintended pregnancies have been reported. In a more recently described case of oligomenorrhea following treatment with griseofulvin, the use of a higher estrogen oral contraceptive restored regularity of the menstrual cycle (SEDA-12, 237). The fact that, as noted above, griseofulvin has an estrogen-like effect in children suggests that it may affect the rate of estrogen metabolism (SED-12, 676; 10[R]).

THE AZOLES

IMIDAZOLE DERIVATIVES FOR SYSTEMIC USE

Ketoconazole

While ketoconazole was not the first of the imidazole derivatives, it was the earliest member of this group to exhibit reasonably reliable absorption when given orally, and it has become the best known. Even after years of usage, new side effects (often related to high doses and/or newer indications) continue to be reported. Ketoconazole is water soluble at a pH of <3. Oral absorption is influenced by the acidity of the stomach content and, not surprisingly, the concomitant administration of H_2-antagonists or antacids and food affects the drug's absorption. A high carbohydrate meal ingested with ketoconazole may decrease total drug absorption, while a high lipid meal may increase it. Erratic resorption is particularly apparent in AIDS patients (SED-12, 676; 1[R]). Peak serum levels are seen 2–3 hours after ingestion; the half-life is about 8 hours. CSF penetration is less than 10%. According to findings in animal experiments, ketoconazole does penetrate into ocular fluids and tissues in cases of candida endophthalmitis (19).

Ketoconazole is extensively metabolized in the liver and excreted with the bile in an inactive form; less than 1% of the active drug is excreted in the urine. Clearance is not significantly altered by renal dialysis (SED-12, 676; 1[R]).

Ketoconazole interferes with the ergosterol biosynthesis by a selective interaction with cytochrome P450-dependent α-demethylase. In the fungus it inhibits the 14α-demethylation of lanosterol and the uptake of triglycerides and phospholipids through the cell membrane. In man, higher doses of ketoconazole have been shown to influence cortisol/cortisone and androgen/testosterone substrates. This finding has led to the use of ketoconazole in Cushing's disease and prostate cancer, but the phenomenon is also responsible for some of the side effects, especially those associated with higher doses and prolonged use (SED-12, 677). The possibility of these hormonal effects should be borne in mind when contemplating the prolonged use of ketoconazole in the prevention of fungus infections in the immune compromised patient. The hormonal effects are also dose related; the high doses required, for example, to treat meningitis due to *Coccidioides immitis*, make ketoconazole in these cases the least desirable of the available azoles (20[R]).

It seems possible that the azoles have an influence on the immune system. Pawelec et al. (21) found an inhibitory effect on the proliferative responses in human mixed lymphocyte cultures. The mechanism of inhibition did not involve blockade of T-cell growth factor production. The hierarchy of inhibitory activity was itraconazole > ketoconazole > miconazole > fluconazole. Interleukin 2-dependent T-cell clone proliferation was blocked by these agents in the same order of decreasing activity (21).

The potency of ketoconazole in inhibiting of P450 isozymes (like cytochrome 3A4), is a cause of interactions with several other drugs, discussed below.

ADVERSE REACTION PATTERN

General and toxic reactions Gastrointestinal complaints ranging from anorexia, nausea and gastralgia to constipation are the most frequently occurring side effects. Hepatotoxicity, varying in degree from mild disturbances of liver function tests to clinical hepatitis and the rare case of fulminating hepatic necrosis has been reported. Some cases have been reported in the first weeks of treatment; there is however a strong impression that duration of treatment is of importance, and in prolonged courses of treatment monitoring is advisable. With the use of high doses, especially for longer periods of time, the effects of interference of hormonal balance should be watched for. Adrenal insufficiency has been reported even on low-dose treatment. Pruritus and skin reactions have been reported but do not, in general, cause major problems.

Hypersensitivity reactions These are rare.

Tumor-inducing effects have not been reported.

ORGANS AND SYSTEMS

Nervous system *Headache*, *dizziness*, *nervousness* and *somnolence* have been reported (SED-11, 573). The incidence is low. In one patient on high dosage for prostate cancer, asthenia was associated with mental disturbances, notably *confabulation and disorientation* in time and space (SEDA-13, 233). *Encephalopathy* can be seen as a result of severe liver damage. *Dysgeusia* has been mentioned.

Endocrine, metabolic *Gynecomastia* was observed occasionally in male patients during the first years that ketoconazole was available. In more recent years it has been shown that ketoconazole has a marked and determinable *effect on steroid levels*, which include a change in the testosterone/estradiol ratio; this is most likely to underlie the base of the observed gynecomastia. A lowering of testosterone serum levels and a diminished response of testosterone levels to human gonadotrophin has been shown (SED-11, 573). This demonstrated effect of ketoconazole has led to the use of high doses in the treatment of prostatic cancer, and under these conditions a rapid fall in testosterone levels was observed during the first few days of treatment. After a month, a slow rise in testosterone levels was seen until a low normal was attained (SEDA-13, 234). Various studies have demonstrated a suppression of testosterone, androstenedione and dehydro-epiandrosterone with reciprocal elevation of gonadotrophins.

The influence on the hormonal balance is however not restricted to the testosterone/androgen hormones; there is also a marked effect on corticosteroids. *Decreases in serum and urinary cortisol levels* were found. Clinical signs of hypoadrenalism have been seen during high-dose treatment. It is not clear from the reports whether the *asthenia syndrome*, described in the past, (severe muscle weakness most pronounced in the legs, fatigue, apathy and anorexia) is connected with the hypoadrenalism or not. In some cases, hypoadrenalism has been described shortly after low-dose treatment had been initiated. Substitution therapy may be required, since simple discontinuation of ketoconazole treatment may not redress the hormonal balance quickly enough.

Various studies have shown that ketoconazole interferes with 17- and 20-hydroxylase and inhibits mitochondrial 11β-hydroxylase. In vitro studies showed ketoconazole to be a potent inhibitor of the 16α-, 17α- and 21-hydroxylases, and an inhibitor of cytochrome P450-dependent steroid hydroxylase enzymes (SED-12, 677; SEDA-12, 228; SEDA-14, 234).

Ketoconazole has been tried in the treatment of hypercalcemia of sarcoidosis on the basis of its influence upon the over-production of 1,25-dihydroxyvitamin D. Serum 1,25-dihydroxyvitamin D levels were reduced in two patients so treated, but serum calcium was not affected and in both patients renal function deteriorated (SEDA-16, 291).

Because of its effects on the pituitary/adrenal system, ketoconazole has been used in the treatment of Cushing's syndrome not responding to other treatment and it may be useful in patients needing pre-operative treatment (SED-12, 677; SEDA-12, 228; SEDA-17, 323). The drug may, however, cause such a rapid reduction in serum cortisol levels that a crisis is precipitated, and patients should be carefully monitored for adrenal function. While ketoconazole used in doses between 400 and 800 mg daily may indeed be a good alternative to other adrenal steroid inhibitors, patients should be observed for signs of hepatotoxicity.

Because of the drug's antiandrogenic properties ketoconazole is particularly suitable for women, in whom it has few effects on menstrual disturbances and does not cause hirsutism. In men, however, the long-term inhibition of androgen production may be disruptive, especially if it leads to gynecomastia and hypogonadism. Combination with aminoglutethimide and metyrapone has been advocated in order to avoid these effects (SEDA-17, 323).

Delayed puberty was reported in a young patient with chronic candidiasis treated with ketoconazole (SEDA-16, 291).

Hypoglycemia was reported in a case history; because of the use of multiple medications, it is difficult to attribute this, with any degree of certainty, to the ketoconazole (SEDA-13, 234).

Ketoconazole has been given in low doses (400 mg/day) for the treatment of hirsutism and acne in women.

Table 1 shows the side effects noted in a group of 20 such women over a period of 6 months (SEDA-16, 290).

In another study of this form of treatment, 17 women were treated for acne and 36 for hirsutism over a 6-month period. Acne improved in all cases, but an effect on hirsutism was only seen in 14 of the 36. Marked side effects were reported, arising during the first 60 days and affecting 23 patients. Loss of scalp hair occurred in six, and became progressively worse in

Table 1. *Side effects of ketaconazole treatment in 20 hirsute women*

Symptoms	No. of patients	%
Polymenorrhea (transient)	7	35
Gastrointestinal (mild)	4	20
Somnolence (transient)	3	18
Pruritus (transient)	2	10
Headache (mild)	1	5
Liver function abnormalities	1	5
Dropout rate	4	20

four subjects. Some patients complained of nausea, headache, dryness of the skin, desquamation, asthenia and itching. One subject had acute hepatitis after 30 days of treatment and another developed a toxic erythema on the legs. Mean triglycerides and cholesterol values decreased during treatment. Three subjects had AST and ALT levels above normal (SEDA-16, 291). Thirteen subjects experienced polymenorrheic anovulatory cycles.

In a third study, a dose of 600 mg/day was used. Ketoconazole effectively inhibited androgen synthesis in hirsute women but side effects were severe and frequent (22).

Hematological There is no evidence of undesirable effects on the hematopoietic and lymphatic systems.

Liver Mild and often transient *elevation of serum liver enzyme values* are not uncommon; the incidence is reported to be about 10–15% (SEDA-12, 229). This figure is higher than quoted in SED-11 (p. 573) and by Lewis et al. (1984), the newer figures probably representing a greater awareness of the risk rather than a true increase; it is however possible that use of higher doses does play a role (SED-12, 678). *Toxic hepatitis* has now been described in many cases. The incidence of symptomatic hepatic injury associated with the use of ketoconazole is estimated to be about one in 10 000 treated cases (SEDA-18, 284). Again there has been a steady trickle of reports over the years (SEDA-16, 290; SEDA-17, 323; SEDA-18, 284). Because the liver damage is now a recognized entity, cases occurring are less likely to be reported in the literature, so there is probably considerable under-reporting. The histological picture is usually one of hepatocellular damage with (in some cases) also evidence of cholestasis. *Cholestatic hepatitis* was reported after the withdrawal of ketoconazole in two cases, but both recovered spontaneously (SEDA-16, 290). *Acute hepatic necrosis* was reported on several occasions (SED-11, 573, SEDA-12, 229, SEDA-13, 234). Less usual was the case reported in 1990 with massive *fatty changes in the liver*, seen histologically (SEDA-16, 290).

While some cases of hepatic complications have been described in the early days of treatment, most cases have been observed after weeks or months of therapy. While the duration of treatment seems to be a factor, a relationship to high dosages has not been shown in the literature. Studies suggest a higher risk in the elderly and in females. Other factors mentioned were a history of idiosyncrasy, prior hepatic reactions and a history of alcoholism. Milder cases of hepatitis are usually reversible on discontinuation of treatment.

Gastrointestinal *Nausea*, mild *gastrointestinal symptoms* and *vomiting* may occur; *diarrhea* has been reported but the incidence is low (SED-12, 678). Incidence of gastrointestinal complaints is higher with the use of daily doses above 800 mg (1^R).

Skin *Pruritus* and occasional *rashes* may occur. Rare cases of a fixed drug eruption have been reported (SED-12, 678; SEDA-17, 323).

Special senses *Papilledema* was reported in one case. The condition cleared on withdrawal of ketoconazole and recurred on resumption of the medication 2 months later (SEDA-18, 284).

Musculoskeletal *Muscle weakness* and diffuse *myalgia* was reported in a 17-year-old male with multiple endocrine neoplasia syndrome type 1, while being treated with ketoconazole for oral candidiasis. The electromyogram showed a distinct myopathic pattern. Withdrawal of the ketoconazole was followed by a rapid improvement (SEDA-17, 323).

Toxicity studies in rats with high doses indicated that ketoconazole leads to increased *bone fragility* in females, which presumably could be related to the hormonal changes discussed above. There are no reports of this effect in humans.

Second-generation effects In the rat, feeding of high doses (80 mg/kg) induced syndactyly in one experiment (SED-11, 574). There are insufficient data to determine whether there might be a harmful effect in humans. Ketoconazole can be found in the milk of the lactating dog receiving ketoconazole; again there are insufficient data to decide whether harm might ensue to the breastfed child.

Risk situations Because of the ability of ketoconazole to interfere with steroid synthesis and vitamin D metabolism, long-term ketoconazole treatment *in children* should be undertaken with great caution.

The prolonged prophylactic use of ketoconazole to prevent fungus infections in *immune compromised patients* may bring about severe hormonal changes.

Liver complications may, as noted above, be more common in the *elderly*, in *women*, or in subjects in whom liver function is already compromised for other reasons.

Interactions As noted above, the azoles, including ketoconazole, have an inhibitory potential for microsomal liver enzymes, a capability which leads to a multitude of interactions with other drugs though of varying degree.

Concomitant administration of *antacids*, *bicarbonate or* $H_{2\text{-antagonists}}$, such as cimetidine and ranitidine, decreases the absorption. Because this effect is connected with the low pH required in the stomach contents for optimal ketoconazole resorption, it is to be expected that a similar effect will be seen with the concomitant use of *omeprazol* (SED-12, 678; 1[R]).

If ketoconazole is given concomitantly with *dideoxyinosine*, the absorption of ketoconazole will be deranged by the citrate phosphate buffer present in the preparation; administering the ketoconazole 2 hours before the dideoxyinosine will allow for normal resorption of the ketoconazole (23).

The influence of ketoconazole on steroid metabolism is reflected in other interactions; ketoconazole increases the total presence of *methylprednisone* and causes a decrease of its clearance with a resulting additional suppression of cortisol levels and an extension of the adrenal suppressive effects (SED-12, 678). The reported decrease in the effect of *oral contraceptives* when ketoconazole is taken (SEDA-12, 231) fits well with the drug's influence on steroid metabolism, as reported; the effect seems to be mild and may be mainly of importance during the use of those preparations with a low estrogen content (SED-12, 678). There have been reports of decreased *insulin* need in diabetic patients treated with ketoconazole. It is questionable if this is a drug interaction; it may be related rather to food intake and tighter control of the diabetes, but it could also be a consequence of the steroid effects, since estrogen tends to improve the effect of insulin (SED-12, 678).

As noted above, ketoconazole interferes with *vitamin D* metabolism; no clear clinical interaction has been described but conceivably the effect of vitamin D given during ketoconazole treatment could be less than expected. The practical importance of this interaction is likely to be nil, except possibly in the case of prolonged use of ketoconazole in a child with an organ transplant. However, ketoconazole does lower serum levels of 1,25-dihydroxyvitamin D in normal subjects and in patients with primary hyperparathyroidism (SEDA-16, 291).

Ketoconazole can reverse acquired resistance to *retinoid* therapy, potentially important when tretinoin (all-*trans*-retinoic acid) is used to induce remission in patients with acute promyelocytic leukemia). Ketoconazole probably attenuates the accelerated catabolism of retinoid during continuous treatment, this again probably being related to the oxidation of retinoid by cytochrome P450 (SEDA-18, 284).

Serum concentrations of ketoconazole are decreased by concomitant use of drugs that induce hepatic microsomal enzymes, such as *rifampicin*, *phenytoin* and *carbamazepine*. There may at the same time be a change in serum levels of these drugs (SED-12, 678, 1[R], 10[R] 24[c]).

Combined administration of ketoconazole with *isoniazid* may lead to increased levels of the latter, but there may possibly also alterations in ketoconazole levels (SED-12, 678; 10[R], 24[c]).

Ketoconazole reduces the clearance of *antipyrine* (SED-11, 574).

Combination of ketoconazole with *amphotericin B* reportedly leads to antagonism (25[R]). This could be on account of the type of sensitivity of the fungus. Maesaki et al. (11) tested the in vitro activity of amphotericin in combination with azoles and found antagonistic effects in five of 15 strains of *Aspergillus fumigatus*. The effect of combinations with the azoles were indifferent or even antagonistic; pre-treatment with amphotericin followed by the azole agent was more effective than simultaneous use of the combination (11).

Potentiation of the effects of *warfarin* was reported in one case, but absence of interference with anticoagulants was claimed in a review by Drouhet et al. (SED-12, 678; 25[R]).

A disulfiram-type reaction with *alcohol* has been reported (SEDA-12, 231).

The combination of ketoconazole with *theophylline* was reported to cause a decrease in the theophylline levels following the ketoconazole dose (SEDA-13, 234). This is surprising in view of the reported inhibition of theophylline metabolism by fluconazole.

Ketoconazole seems to have a synergistic antiviral effect when administered concurrently with *acyclovir* (10[R]).

The fact that ketoconazole is a cytochrome P450 inhibitor accounts for its interactions with various concomitantly given drugs. Ketoconazole given alongside *ciclosporin* will lead to a sharp increase in ciclosporin levels with, as a further consequence, the possibility of a marked influence upon renal function as demonstrated by a decrease in the creatinine clearance; this seems to be connected with the dose-dependent nephrotoxicity of ciclosporin (SED-12, 678; 1[R], 10[R]).

Ketoconazole, given with the combination with *astemizole* or *terfenadine* may lead to an increased level of these two substances due to inhibition of cytochrome 3A4. High levels of terfenadine may cause cardiac toxicity. Increased plasma levels of unmetabolized terfenadine prolong the QT interval carry the risk of torsade de pointes and fatal ventricular arrhythmias (10[R], 26[c]).

By the same mechanism ketoconazole also inhibits

the metabolism of *midazolam* and *triazolam*, causing a dramatic increase in the hypnotic effect of these normally very short-acting drugs.

If *erythromycin*, also a cytochrome 3A4 inhibitor, is being given in combination with ketoconazole this would have an even more dramatic effect on terfenadine, astemizole, midazolam and triazolam levels, and probably also on ciclosporin levels.

Clotrimazole

Clotrimazole was the first oral azole. While it was effective in deep mycosis, its only moderate absorption and the fact that there was induction of liver microsomal enzymes after a few days (leading to a need for increasing amounts of the drug) impeded clinical use. Clotrimazole also proved rather toxic. Clotrimazole should therefore not be used for systemic infections and the oral form can be considered obsolete at this time (SED-12, 678). With the number of other azoles now available for external use it is even doubtful whether the intravaginal and local application of this compound is advisable in view of the occurrence of contact dermatitis.

Nervous system *Tiredness*, *drowsiness*, *depression* and occasional *hallucinations* and *disorientation* occur. Stimulation of the adrenal cortex was recorded in animal studies.

Hematological Mild neutropenia, but no more serious hematological effect, has been reported.

Liver A rise in levels of liver enzymes was noted in most studies.

Gastrointestinal *Anorexia*, *nausea*, *vomiting*, *epigastric pains* and *diarrhea* are common.

Urinary system *Pollakisuria* and a *burning sensation on micturition* are mentioned in many reports. *Albuminuria* and *hematuria* have been reported, but without evidence of more serious renal damage.

Skin Macular and urticarial *rashes* occur. Allergic *contact dermatitis* has been reported. With vaginal use a *local burning sensation*, *edema of the vulva and perianal rash* were reported.

Risk situations No specific risk group is recognized. Oral use has generally been for short periods of time only.

Second-generation effects No information is available (SED-12, 679).

Miscellaneous A recent study, comparing fluconazole 200 mg daily with clotrimazole 10 mg taken 5 times daily in the prevention of fungus infections in patients with advanced AIDS, showed little difference in the occurrence of undesirable effects and abnormalities in laboratory measurements. In a subgroup of patients receiving aerosolized pentamidine, relatively more of the patients assigned to fluconazole required transfusions than among those in the clotrimazole group. Treatment compliance was markedly less in the clotrimazole group (27[C]).

Miconazole

Miconazole has been evaluated as a topical, oral and intravenous agent. Resorption is slightly better than with clotrimazole, with 25—30% of the administered doses being detectable. The main advantage of the drug is the possibility of intravenous and intrathecal administration. Like ketoconazole it is highly protein bound. Miconazole does not diffuse well into the CSF, but it does penetrate readily into synovial and vitreous fluids. The half-life of miconazole is rather short, necessitating at least three intravenous injections a day (25[R]).

Oral miconazole is better tolerated than clotrimazole but probably less well than ketoconazole. Parenteral administration carries a higher frequency of side effects, some probably being caused by the Cremophor El (the carrier). Adverse effects include fever, chills, pruritus, rash, nausea and vomiting, diarrhea and hyponatremia, cardiac toxicity, phlebitis, hyperlipidemia and central nervous system disturbances. Hypersensitivity reactions may occur. Tumor-inducing effects have not been demonstrated.

Cardiovascular Local phlebitis is not uncommon; the type of intravenous solution used is of importance. Collapse after rapid intravenous injection was described, as were some cases of tachycardia, ventricular tachycardia and even, in a few instances, cardiac/respiratory arrest; the latter were attributable to the histamine-releasing properties of Cremophor (SED-12, 679; 25[R]). In a low-weight infant a rather high dose of miconazole, 150 mg/kg/day, led within 2 days to bradycardia with an ectopic atrial rhythm and delayed intraventricular conduction in the presence of electrolyte disturbances (SED-12, 679).

Nervous system Arachnoiditis has been described after intrathecal injection. Hyperesthesia, euphoria, and light-headiness have been mentioned, as well as drowsiness. Acute toxic psychosis is a rare consequence of miconazole administration (SED-12, 679).

Hematological Erythrocyte aggregation in blood smears was seen after the i.v. use of miconazole; the clinical significance of this finding is not clear. Thrombocytosis was reported in isolated cases.

Hyperlipidemia has been described in many instances, this may be caused by the solvent used (SED-12, 679).

Liver Enzyme induction, demanding increased doses to maintain effectivity is seen, as with clotrimazole. Drouhet (25[R]) mentions hepatotoxicity without specifying the type of liver damage.

Gastrointestinal On oral administration, complaints are usually mild. Nausea, vomiting, discomfort and diarrhea occur more easily after parenteral administration.

Mineral and water balance Hyponatremia can occur and may possibly be explained by the gastrointestinal effects, in the absence of evidence of nephrotoxicity, but this explanation is not quite satisfactory.

Skin Pruritus and rashes have been reported but do not seem to be frequent.

Second-generation effects No information is available.

Interactions A pattern of interaction such as occurs with ketoconazole can be expected for miconazol as well, be it that absorption of oral miconazole is likely less affected by those substances changing the pH of the stomach content. Miconazole may potentiate the effects of coumarin-anticoagulants and warfarin (SED-12, 679). Enhancement of the effects of hypoglycemic sulfonamides was reported (SED-12, 679). An apparent interaction between intravenous miconazole and tobramycin, with a reduced effect of tobramycin, was reported in SEDA-12 (p. 235), but details are lacking. Miconazole in combination with phenytoin may lead to increased levels of the phenytoin (SED-12, 679).

THE TRIAZOLES

Itraconazole

Itraconazole is poorly soluble in water and highly lipophilic. The oral absorption of the solution in dimethyl-β-cyclodextrin is good with a T_{max} at 1.5—2 hours; when polyethylene glycol is used as a solvent the absorption is not as good. Bioavailability of the capsules is enhanced by taking the capsules with food when it approaches that seen with the solution. The absorption of capsules containing itraconazole-coated sugar spherules is also markedly influenced by the presence of food and this too attains the absorption levels seen with solution. Conversely, inadequate plasma concentrations are often found in patients receiving antineoplastic therapy which predisposes them to a poor food intake or to frequent vomiting. The absorption of oral itraconazole seems to be reduced in AIDS patients; a study by Smith et al. demonstrated a 50% reduction for steady state-serum levels; in fact levels after a 200-mg dose once daily schedule resulted in levels seen in healthy controls after a 100-mg daily dose (35[C], 36[c]).

The normal T_{max} of itraconazole is 1.5—4 hours and serum levels are dose related. Steady-state levels are reached after about 10—14 days and are high in comparison with those attained after single doses. Using single daily dose treatment the half-life is 20—30 hours.

Itraconazol is strongly bound in blood/serum. The tissue concentrations in lung, kidney, liver, bone, spleen and muscle are 2—3 times higher than the corresponding serum levels. Concentrations in omentum and adipose tissue are particularly high and higher levels were also found in various parts of the genital tract. Itraconazole is markedly keratinophilic; after discontinuation of treatment it will take 1—2 weeks before levels in the skin start to decline. Itraconazole levels in urine, saliva, eye fluids and cerebrospinal fluid are low. Penetration of itraconazole into ocular tissues is low compared with that of ketoconazole and fluconazole (19, 28[R], 29—34). Itraconazole incorporated into multilamellar liposomes may be useful; in murine models of cryptococcosis and pulmonary aspergillosis an enhancement of the concentration in infected tissues was seen, accompanied by improved in vivo efficacy (37).

The drug is degraded in the liver and excreted via the bile and to some extent in the urine. Metabolism of the drug is not altered by renal dysfunction (1[R], 28[R], 29—34).

In vitro studies of neutrophil and lymphoproliferative responses have shown that itraconazole, like ketoconazole, suppresses neutrophil chemotaxis, random movement, deoxyglucose uptake and hexose-monophosphate shunt activity (38).

ADVERSE REACTION PATTERN

General and toxic Itraconazole appears in general to be well tolerated. Most of the adverse reactions reported are transient. Gastrointestinal reactions, mild dyspepsia, pyrosis, nausea, vomiting, diarrhea and epigastric pain are not uncommon. In many of the published reports mention is made of increases in serum liver enzyme levels and hypertriglyceridemia. Symptomatic cases with evidence of liver toxicity have been reported, but serious hepatic injury has not been described, so far as is known. The incidence of liver toxicity cannot be determined from available data. Itraconazole does not induce drug-metabolizing enzymes and is a weaker inhibitor of microsomal enzymes than ketoconazole (1^R, 28^R). In the rat given doses of up to 160 mg/kg, no induction or inhibition of the metabolism of xenobiotics was seen (SEDA-16, 285). Hypokalemia was mentioned in several reports without an explanation as to the mechanism. The use of higher doses (400 or even 600 mg/day) gives rise to an increased incidence in side effects; among those documented at these dose levels are severe hypokalemia, reversible adrenal insufficiency and (in one published case) arrhythmias, the latter being connected with an interaction with terfenadine (SEDA-16, 295; SEDA-18, 198).

Hypersensitivity reactions Skin rashes and pruritus were reported.

ORGANS AND SYSTEMS

Cardiorespiratory *Pleural* and subsequent *pericardial effusion* developed in a patient treated with itraconazol 200 mg b.d. for a localized pulmonary *Aspergillus fumigatus* infection. After more then 9 weeks of treatment the patient developed a pericardial effusion which necessitated drainage. Itraconazole was discontinued at this time. Six weeks later, and 2 weeks after the resumption of itraconazole treatment, she developed signs of *pulmonary edema* and *cardiac enlargement*. These signs disappeared rapidly on discontinuation of itraconazole (SEDA-18, 282).

Nervous system The occurrence of *headaches* was mentioned in some reports; *dizziness* is an uncommon complaint and so are *mood disturbances*. *Nervousness* and *tinnitus* continue to be described. More specific disorders of the nervous system do not appear to have been described. *Visual hallucination* with *confusion* has however been reported in a patient as occurring on three separate occasions, each time appearing about 2 hours after the ingestion of a 200-mg dose of itraconazole in a 75-year-old woman. Symptoms abated spontaneously over about 8 hours (77^c).

Endocrine, metabolic *Sexual impotence* with normal steroid levels has been reported in one recent case and a *decrease in libido* in another (SEDA-17, 321), and some similar reports appeared earlier. There are, however, inconsistent reports as to the effects on steroids. Levels of testosterone, corticosterone and progesterone remained unchanged in a group of rats and in six dogs in which possible endocrine effects were studied (SED-12, 680). On the other hand, administration of itraconazole to seven male volunteers for 2 weeks did not produce detectable changes in plasma testosterone or cortisol levels. It should be remembered that the marked influence of ketoconazole on steroid levels described in some rather older papers was only reported after several years of usage and mainly in connection with higher doses and prolonged treatment. A slightly reduced cortisol response to ACTH stimulation 2 weeks after the start of high dose (600 mg/day) itraconazol therapy was seen in one of eight patients with severe mycosis.

After 6 weeks the patient experienced weakness, fatigue, orthostatic dizziness, heat intolerance and edema prominent in the face and lower extremities. The cortisol response was markedly blunted by this time. Dose reduction was associated with a resolution of symptoms of adrenal insufficiency. Measurements of urinary metabolites demonstrated normal levels of 17-ketosteroids, depressed levels of free cortisol, and reduced levels of 17-hydroxycorticosteroids (SED-12, 680). It was thought that the pattern of endocrine suppression was different from that seen with ketoconazole, the data being consistent with a greater sensitivity of the 11α-hydroxylase and a relative sparing of the C_{17-20} lyase enzyme activity (and androgen synthesis).

Another patient was noted to have hypokalemia, hypertension and mild edema with mildly depressed aldosterone concentrations after 8 months of treatment, again with a high doses (SED-12, 680; SEDA-16, 295).

Mineral and fluid balance *Hypokalemia*, occurring either in isolation or along with hypertension, has been seen in some cases. Marked ankle *edema* with weight gain was seen in a patient on 400 mg itraconazole daily, in whom there was no explanation other than the use of the drug; after withdrawal of the itraconazole these symptoms disappeared. Hypokalemia and edema have also been observed in a number of patients on high dose (600 mg/day) itraconazole therapy (SED-12, 680; SEDA-16, 295; SEDA-17, 321; 1^R, 39^C).

Liver In most of the available clinical reports there were some cases reported with *elevated liver enzyme* levels; the changes were transient or disappeared after discontinuation of the itraconazole. More serious instances of hepatic toxicity were not reported.

Gastrointestinal *Dyspepsia*, *pyrosis*, *nausea*, *vomiting*, *mild epigastric discomfort* and *diarrhea* may occur. These gastrointestinal complaints are generally mild but they seem to be the most frequent side effects noticed during treatment. The total incidence of side effects was 3—5% in patients treated for superficial mycosis and 8% in 99 patients treated for deep mycosis (SED-12, 680). An incidence closer to 15% was reported in a multicenter trial (SEDA-17, 321). In a group of 50 women treated for acute vaginal candidiasis, side effects were reported in 17 (35%), nausea in seven, headache in six, dizziness in three and bloating in three patients, while elevated SGOT levels were found in one (40[c]).

Urinary system In an older report, increased levels of urea nitrogen were seen after 2 weeks of treatment, the values remaining within normal limits. These increases occurred primarily in men older than 60 years of age (SED-12, 680). There has been no further mention of this side effect in the recent literature.

Skin The occurrence of different types of *rash*, including a case of an acneiform rash, has been mentioned in the literature. In one case the appearance of bloody *bullae* was reported (SED-12, 680).

Second-generation effects Since embryotoxicity and teratogenicity have been found in the rat, albeit after the administration of high doses, itraconazole should be avoided during pregnancy (SED-12, 681).

Interactions The activity of itraconazole against black fungi may be augmented by the combination with *flucytosine*; the combination has prevented the development of flucytosine resistance (15[R]). The in vitro effects of the combination of *amphotericin* and itraconazole was tested using 15 strains of *Aspergillus fumigatus*, and an antagonistic effect was found in four of the strains (11). The combination of itraconazole with *ciclosporin* treatment leads to a marked elevation of ciclosporin levels and this may result in a rise of serum creatinine, clearly pointing to renal damage as a result of the high ciclosporin concentrations (SED-12, 681; SEDA-17, 322; 10[R], 20, 41[C], 42[C]). Itraconazole may also inhibit the metabolism (or elimination?) of *digoxin*, leading to digitalis toxicity (10[R]; see also case reported in SEDA-18 (p. 198). Low and sometimes very low serum levels of itraconazole have been seen during concurrent therapy with *rifampicin*, *phenytoin* or *carbamazepine*. Barbiturates may also cause a lowering of itraconazole levels (SED-12, 681; 1[R], 28[R], 24, 39[C]). At the same time, levels of phenytoin and rifampicin themselves may be lowered when they are used alongside itraconazole.

The *citrate-phosphate buffer* used to facilitate the absorbtion of dideoxyinosine, used in the treatment of AIDS, may interfere with the absorption of itraconazole if these medications are taken at the same time (18). Itraconazole added to anti-coagulant treatment may influence *warfarin* levels; following the addition of itraconazole to a treatment regimen comprising warfarin, ranitidine and terfenadine, cardiac dysrhythmias developed in a 62-year-old man. The signs and symptoms included prolongation of the QT interval and ventricular fibrillation (see SEDA-18, 198 or 282?). This particular regimen apparently resulted in a second interaction since unexpectedly very high levels of *terfenadine* were found (SEDA-18, 283). The phenomenon has been described by others, referring to a marked rise in terfenadine serum levels and increased the toxicity of the drug during concurrent ingestion of itraconazole. The mechanism is not known, but it is likely to be related to inhibition of the cytochrome 3A4 liver enzymes (10[R]). It seems likely that the combination of itraconazole with *astemizole* and short-acting benzodiazepine derivatives such as *midazolam* and *triazolam* will lead to increased activity of the latter drugs, as is seen with terfenadine (10[R]).

Inhibition of the activity of *oral hypoglycaemic agents* can be expected.

Second-generation effects Itraconazole was embryotoxic and teratogenic when given in high doses to rats (SEDA-16, 295).

Fluconazole

Fluconazole, derived from the older imidazoles, is the product of extensive research and of fundamental molecular changes. Fluconazole has a lower molecular weight and is better soluble in water than ketoconazole; it can be administered orally and parenterally. After oral administration the bio-availability is about 90%; maximum plasma concentrations are seen in 1—2 hours, the half life time is about 30 hours and a steady state is reached within 5—7 days. Fluconazole has a low protein binding of about 12%, is hardly metabolized, and about 80% of it is excreted in the urine. Hemodialysis reduces plasma concentration by about half in 3 hours (43, 44[C]). Tissue and body fluid penetration is good (45, 46); the CSF levels ratio is 0.5—0.9, the resultant levels being adequate for the treatment of cryptococcal meningitis. Penetration in the eye, studied in rabbits was found to be good in acute treatment of *Candida* infection; ketoconazole was better in the longer established infection (19). In a patient in whom the levels of fluconazole in bile were studied, the concentrations attained after the first dose were about the same as in serum levels, but 10—12 hours after the fluconazole dose the bile levels were found to be higher than the serum levels (47[c]). Sputum levels are about equal to plasma levels (48). Levels in vaginal secretion are slightly lower than in plasma but persist over a longer period of time (49, 50). Like ketoconazole, fluconazole is a highly selective inhibitor of the fungal cytochrome P450, and it inhibits the demethylase enzyme involved in the synthesis of ergosterol (SED-12, 681; 1[R], 46[R]).

ADVERSE REACTION PATTERN

General and toxic reactions Fluconazole is generally well tolerated. The most common side effects are nausea and vomiting. Abnormal liver function tests and mild increases in hepatic enzymes have been reported, but there have been no reports about life-threatening liver toxicity connected with fluconazole treatment; it is still not known whether toxic hepatitis and liver cell necrosis may occur after high and/or prolonged dosage regimes. Early studies have shown no changes in testosterone levels or in the adrenal response to ACTH. Skin rashes and a few cases of exfoliative skin disorder have been reported (SED-12, 681). Alopecia has been reported in a few cases on high doses for prolonged periods of time (SEDA-18, 281).

Hypersensitivity reactions An anaphylactoid reaction was reported in a patient with AIDS (SED-12, 681) Rare instances of hypersensitivity reactions have occurred in other individuals (SEDA-16, 293; SEDA-17, 320). Skin rashes may occur and have been seen more frequently in AIDS patients.

Tumor-inducing effects No information is available.

ORGANS AND SYSTEMS

Nervous system *Dizziness*, *headaches* and the occurrence of *seizures* were seen in 2—5% of a group of 232 cases with severe systemic fungus infections. In the same group there were three cases each of *delirium* and *dysesthesias* (1.3%). A possible influence of the underlying illness has to be considered. In a small group of 14 patients treated with fluconazole for cryptococcal meningitis dizziness was reported in 14% of cases (SED-12, 691). The more recent literature points to *dizziness* and *headaches* but not of a severe nature.

Endocrine and metabolic Preliminary studies concerning a possible effect on testosterone levels and adrenal response to adrenocorticotropic hormone did not demonstrate such changes; determinations were however performed after only 14 days of fluconazole administration. Even with the use of high doses there has to date been no mention of an endocrine influence.

Mineral and fluid balance The occurrence of *hypokalemia* was observed in a few cases only, which contrasts with experience as regards itraconazole. *Hyperkalemia* was however reported in one paper (SED-12, 681).

Hematological *Cytopenia* does occur but it seems to be mild. The few more marked changes which have occasionally been described could have been connected with the disease treated as much as with the treatment (SED-12, 681; 51[C]).

Liver Elevation of *liver enzyme levels* is reported in most studies. In some articles this effect is described as transient during therapy, in others as disappearing after discontinuation of treatment. The incidence varies from a few percent of cases to 35—45%, but occasionally the effect has been recorded in all cases treated. The temporal relationship between these liver function changes and the fluconazole treatment has been shown in many cases. Severe liver toxicity has not been reported (SED-12, 681; 1[R], 52[R]). Lee et al. (53[C]) noted asymptomatic AST and ALT elevation in three out of 12 children in a group with neoplastic disease who were treated concomitantly with fluconazole.

Gastrointestinal The occurrence of *nausea* and *vomiting* is mentioned in most reports (SED-12, 682, 1[R]). The incidence is low, some 10—15%. *Anorexia*, *mild abdominal pains* and *diarrhea* have been reported, but none of these symptoms was severe.

Urinary system There is no indication of renal toxicity. In the presence of a creatinine clearance below 40 ml/min, however, fluconazole doses should be adjusted (SED-12, 682; 43, 44[C]).

Skin *Rashes* of several types occur and seem to be more frequent in immune compromised patients. *Pruritus* was reported as well. Sugar et al. noted in a paper published in March 1990 that up to that time three cases of *Stevens-Johnson disease* had been reported worldwide (SED-12, 682). A case of *toxic epidermal necrolysis* running a clinically mild course has been described (SEDA-18, 281).

Risk factors As noted above, in patients with *impaired renal function* it is prudent to reduce the dosage of fluconazole because of the primary role of the kidney in clearance of the drug. There is as yet little information about tolerance of this drug by *children*; in the group of children with fever, neutropenia and neoplastic disease referred to above, an increased renal clearance was found (53[C]). Pharmacokinetic findings in the adult should not be assumed to hold good for children.

Second-generation effects No relevant information appears to be available.

Interactions Since a drug like fluconazole will inevitably often be used in combination with other medications, it was evaluated for its interactions in the early stages of clinical trials. Fluconazole absorption after oral administration was not influenced by *cimetidine* or a *magnesium/aluminum hydroxide* formulation, this finding being in accordance with the solubility of fluconazole in water; nor is to be expected that other H_2 receptor antagonists or *omeprazole* will influence absorption (SED-12, 682; 54). Since then, however, a review by Bickers (10[R]) has stated that cimetidine may decrease the bioavailability of fluconazole; it is not clear how solid the evidence is for this belief.

The concurrent use of fluconazole with *flucytosine* may have a synergistic effect; (55) this combination could be useful in the treatment of cryptococcal meningitis (14[R], 15[R], 56).

Fluconazole did not significantly alter the pharmacokinetics of *ethinylestradiol* or *norgestrel*, and this finding was interpreted by the investigators concerned as suggesting that treatment with fluconazole in a user of oral contraceptives would not increase the risk of pregnancy (57); the study in question was however carried out using a 50-mg dose of fluconazole; clinical experience with therapeutic dosage show different results (SED-12, 682). Again according to the review by Bickers, fluconazole decreases the bioavailability of ethinylestradiol in an oral contraceptive, but this author provides no source of information as to the doses involved (10[R]).

There are conflicting reports about the influence upon *ciclosporin* levels from fluconazole administration. In some reports minimal changes or none at all in the ciclosporin level are recorded, but in other work ciclosporin levels were found to be elevated. Differences in the dosage and duration of fluconazole treatment could explain these apparent discrepancies (SED-12, 682; 1[R], 10[R], 41[C], 58[C]—61[C]). In a study of ciclosporin-treated patients who had undergone bone marrow transplantation, in which prophylactic use of a high dose of fluconazole (400 mg/day) was compared with placebo, no increase in ciclosporin toxicity was found in the patients receiving fluconazole (78[C]).

The concurrent administration of fluconazole with *tolbutamide* resulted in an increase of tolbutamide levels (SED-12, 682). A similar rise in drug levels, with a consequent risk of hypoglycemia, can be expected with *glipizide* and *glibenclamide*.

Administration of fluconazole and *phenytoin* together resulted in markedly higher phenytoin levels (SED-12, 682; 1[R], 10[R]).

Co-administration of fluconazole and *warfarin* led, in some cases, to an increase in prothrombin time (SED-12, 682; 1[R], 10[R]).

The combination of *rifampicin* with fluconazole has been found to result in lower levels of fluconazole than expected, but the alteration of fluconazole pharmacokinetics was considerably smaller than the effect of rifampicin on ketoconazole in similar circumstances (SED-12, 682; 1[R], 10[R], 24[C], 62[C]).

Antipyrine concentration levels and clearance were not altered by fluconazole (SED-12, 682).

The combination with the diuretic *hydrochlorothiazide* resulted in mild increases of fluconazole levels which were of little significance.

The prescribing information leaflet for fluconazole in Canada indicates that *zidovudine* and *pentamidine isothionate* used together with fluconazole do not result in an altered adverse reaction pattern. In a study by Bozzette et al. (SED-12, 682) concerning preventive maintenance therapy with fluconazole after cryptococcal meningitis in AIDS patients, a higher rate of hematological toxicity was seen in the fluconazole group than in the placebo group, but this probably reflected the greater proportional and absolute amounts of zidovudine used in the fluconazole group. There was no serious hematotoxicity (SED-12, 682).

Fluconazole, like other azoles can inhibit hepatic cytochrome P4503A4 and this can result in various drug interactions. Concurrent use of *terfenadine* may lead to dangerously high levels of the terfenadine with resulting cardiotoxicity. It is suspected that the same may happen with concurrent use of *astemizol* (10[R]). The further addition of *erythromycin* to the joint medication would further enhance the risks.

Cross-hypersensitivity and cross-resistance With the increasing number of azoles available in the market for systemic and for local use, the question should be raised whether there is cross-hypersensitivity for the different compounds and also whether there is cross-resistance. Cross-sensitivity between several of the imidazoles including sulconazole has been observed. Cross-sensitivity between miconazole, econazole and sulconazole and a lack of cross-sensitivity with clotrimazole are understandable if the chemical structure is considered: the cross-reactions are all between β-substituted 1-phenethyl imidazoles, whilst clotrimazole has an altogether different ring structure (SEDA-14, 234). If this explanation is correct one could expect cross-sensitivity between ketoconazole and itraconazole and terconazole but not with fluconazole. There are on the other hand some indications that cross-resistance does occur; a resistant strain of *Candida albicans* was isolated from a patient with mucocutaneous candidiasis who relapsed after receiving ketoconazole and failed to improve on itraconazole. The fluconazole concentration required to inhibit this *Candida* strain was 4—70 times higher than that needed for two other typical strains (SED-12, 682).

Saperconazole

Saperconazole is a water-insoluble, lipophilic fluorinated triazole. The structure resembles that of itraconazole. It has a broad antifungal spectrum including *Cryptococcus* spp. and *Aspergillus* spp. Saperconazole has a long clearance time. Side effects are not yet known, but one would expect them to resemble those of itraconazole (1^R).

SCH-39304

This is an N-substituted triazole with a wide antifungal spectrum. Absorption appeared rather slow with peak levels 2—4 hours after a single dose and mean peak levels markedly higher after 16 days of administration. The mean elimination $T_{1/2}$ thereafter is about 90—100 hours (63). It has high levels of tissue penetration, including the CNS, and a good broad spectrum antifungal activity. SCH-39304 has been shown to cause hepatocellular carcinoma in animals (1^R).

ICI-195739

This bis-triazole has a broad antifungal spectrum as well. It is an inhibitor of fungal C-14 sterol demethylation. The drug penetrates the fungal cell wall better than ketoconazole or fluconazole (1^R).

ZD0870

This is a further new triazole which has been shown in vitro to be active against a wide range of fungi ranging from *Candida* species, to *Torulopsisglabrata*, *Aspergillus*, *Trichosporon beigelii*, and *Coccidioides immitis*. In general, it was found to be more potent in vitro than fluconazole and also active against fluconazole-resistant candida strains (64, 65). In animal experiments, too, ZD0870 was found more active than established azoles (66—69). Early human pharmacokinetic studies showed good absorption, a dose-related increase in maximum blood levels, absence of urinary excretion and a possible enterohepatic circulation. The half-life was very variable with a mean of 79 hours (range 27—193 hours) (70). Initial clinical studies in the treatment of oral candidiasis showed good tolerance with minor adverse effects in a total of 39 patients with HIV infections (71^C, 72^C)

SDZ-89-485

This is another triazole with demonstrated activity against fungi and a sufficient selectivity for fungal (as compared with human) P450 enzymes to preclude toxicity at therapeutic doses. The pharmacokinetics and side effects in humans are not yet known (1^R).

Electrazole (3.4.4. Bay-R-3783)

This azole, which is transformed in vivo to three primary metabolites, has not been further developed. One of the two active metabolites with a very long half life had a structure which was considered potentially hepatotoxic (1^R).

OTHER ANTIFUNGAL DRUGS FOR SYSTEMIC USE

Echinocandins

Echinocandin B, which is produced by some species of *Aspergillus*, has a candidicidal activity but it is toxic, notably causing hemolysis.

LY-121019

This is a semi-synthetic lipopeptide derived from echinocandin B; it is active against *Candida* species and in high doses against *aspergillosis*. It acts on the cell wall of *candida albicans* by modulating the incorporation of glucon-associated proteins (73) LY-121019 is lipophilic and can only be administered intravenously. High doses were found to result in non-linear saturation plasma pharmacokinetics. The carrier used, polyethylene glycol, was shown to be the cause of a metabolic acidosis (1^R).

L-693989

This is a water soluble, semi-synthetic cyclic lipopeptide, the phosphorylated derivative of an echinocandin-like natural product. This too is active only against *Candida* species, but in vivo it is more active than ketoconazole or fluconazole. The drug is converted back to the natural pro-drug in plasma and is excreted via the biliary route. The clinical usefulness and adverse reactions are still largely undefined (1^R).

The allylamine antifungal drugs

The allylamine derivatives are derived from heterocyclic spironaphthalenes. *Terbinafine* can be used orally or topically. *Natifine* is for topical administration. *Terbinafine* is effective against a broad range of fungi. The clinical studies have been mainly in the treatment of dermatophytes. The allylamines do not inhibit cytochrome P450. In vitro studies (74) demonstrated that the allylamines enhance selected functions of the human polymorphonuclear leukocytes in contrast to the findings with the imidazoles which in varying degree inhibit these same functions. Terbinafine appears to be well tolerated. Gastrointestinal complaints, dyspepsia, nausea, diarrhea) were the commonest reasons for withdrawal of treatment. Abdominal pain and loss of taste were reported. Mild CNS symptoms, headaches and dizziness comprise most of the adverse effects reported. There were no changes seen in hematological variables. Changes in liver biochemical tests were generally not considered clinically relevant (SEDA-16, 297; SEDA-18, 7; 1[R]); mild liver dysfunction has however incidentally been reported. Kovacs et al. (75[C]) recorded two cases with hematological abnormalities associated with the use of terbinafine.

A 53-year-old woman was found to have developed a neutropenia after 5 months of treatment for tinea pedis and onychomycosis caused by *Trichophyton rubrum*. The bone marrow study showed an absolute and relative decrease in granulocytes. The terbinafine was discontinued and the patient was treated with granulocyte colony-stimulating factor for 5 days. Seven days after discontinuation of the drug the neutrophil count was normal.

The second (male) case with onychomycosis had been treated with tioconazol, and cicloprox olamine creams before he started on terbinafine 250 mg daily. After 63 days of treatment he had complaints of nausea, vomiting, diarrhea, abdominal pain, fever, chills and rigors, and appeared acutely ill and dehydrated. He was found to have a pancytopenia. Following discontinuation of the terbinafine and rehydration he recovered rapidly and after 4 days WCB and platelet count had normalized (75[C]).

Interactions The concomitant use of rifampicin may lead to lower terbenafine levels.

Pradimicins and benanomicin

Both these are sterol-like molecules with amino acids in their side chains, which can form calcium-linked complexes with mannose-containing components of the fungal cell membrane. Both are fungicidal against a wide variety of fungi. The toxicity seems to be low (1[R]). Pradimicin A inhibits influenza virus replication and could possibly have an anti-HIV effect at the stage of viral adsorption and cell-to-cell infection (1[R]).

Hamacin

This tetraene antibiotic, resembling amphotericin B, can be given orally but it is too toxic for parenteral use. It appears to be little used (SED-12, 683).

Nystatin

Nystatin, the earliest antifungal antibiotic, is used today primarily by the oral route to treat gastrointestinal mycosis and topically for mucocutaneous candidiasis (SED-11, 576; 1). Absorption in the gut is insufficient to produce systemic activity. Nausea, vomiting and diarrhea are reported after oral administration, possibly due to the drug but perhaps also ascribable to the underlying disease. These effects are more marked with use of doses exceeding 5 M units a day (SED-11, 576). Allergic reactions to topical use are rare (SED-11, 576). In a 14-month-old child who had experienced skin rash on two occasions after treatment with nystatin, a third course of treatment was followed by Stevens-Johnson syndrome (SEDA-16, 297).

Potassium iodide

The therapeutic effect of potassium iodide is mediated through the direct antifungal effect of the molecular iodide. It is actually only effective against sporotrichosis. Apart from its influence on the thyroid, various side effects have been recorded after oral use, including fever, lymphadenopathy, parotitis, increased lacrimation, acneiform rashes and the exacerbation of dermatitis herpetiformis (SED-11, 577).

Saramycitin

This polypeptide antibiotic, is only employed parenterally and can be used in the treatment of histoplasmosis and blastomycosis. Injection may cause a local inflammatory reaction. Febrile reactions and urticaria have been reported. Saramycitin may cause a liver function disturbance with rises in serum alkaline phosphatase, bilirubin and transaminases and a delay in sulfobromphthalein excretion. Saramycitin often causes marked eosinophilia (SED-11, 577).

Saramycitin, as well as hamycin and the oral antibiotic ambrucitin, (a cyclopropanyl-pyran acid) have all been further developed but no references throwing light on their safety have been found in the literature down to mid-1995.

Stilbamidine diisothionate and hydroxystilbamidine diisothionate

Both of these drugs are given intravenously. Rapid injection may cause hypotension and complaints such as dizziness, pruritus, tachycardia and circulatory collapse with a warm red skin. Anorexia, nausea and vomiting, diarrhea, general malaise, weakness, fever, myalgia, headache and paresthesia have been noted. Mild hepatic dysfunction, as demonstrated by mild rises in serum transaminase levels, is not uncommon; the potentially more dangerous hepatotoxicity is fortunately rare (SED-11, 577).

ANTIFUNGAL DRUGS FOR TOPICAL USE

IMIDAZOLES

All the topically used imidazoles may cause local irritation, burning, and if used intravaginally, burning, swelling and discomfort with micturition. There is cross-hypersensitivity between econazole, enilconazole, miconazole and probably all other β-substituted 1-phenethyl imidazoles.

Bifonazole

This is reported to be more effective in a 2% cream than miconazole. No specific side effects have been reported.

Econazole

Econazole is used topically on the skin but it is also used intravaginally. With intravaginal application, about 3–7% of the applied dosage is absorbed. General tolerance is good. Redness, burning and pruritus seems to occur more readily on inguinal application.

Enilconazole

This is used in 10% solution/cream. No specific adverse effects have been described.

Isoconazole

This is mainly used for vaginal infections with *Candida albicans*; it is generally well tolerated.

Latoconazole

Used in a 1% cream, this imidazole has been shown to be effective in vitro and also in vivo against *tinea*, and more active than clotrimazole or bifonazole. No specific side effects were reported in the only (early) study available.

Nimorazole

This agent is believed to be active against *Trichomonas vaginalis*. No specific adverse effects have been described.

Ornidazole

Complaints of mild nausea and headache during treatment were reported, suggesting relatively marked absorption of this intravaginally applied imidazole.

Terconazole

This is prepared in creams and ovules for intravaginal use. Besides local irritation this imidazole was found to cause more marked reactions; headaches were reported in over a quarter of patients. Other effects reported include hypotension, fever and chills. It is reasonable to conclude that terconazole is resorbed to a greater extent than the other locally used azoles (SED-12, 684).

Tioconazole

This compound too is mainly used for vaginal or inguinal *Candida* infections. It is reported to have less local side effects than some of the older preparations. There is evidence of significant resorption. The local irritation, burning, rash, erythema and pruritus usual with products of this type have been reported. In a few female patients, marked burning on micturition was described; these women all showed signs of vaginal epithelial atrophy (SED-12, 684).

OTHER ANTIFUNGAL DRUGS FOR TOPICAL USE

Like the topical imidazoles all these preparations may cause local irritation (with or without pruritus) and eczematous reactions; some however can cause photosensitivity.

5-Bromo-4′-chlorosalicylamide (Multifungin)

This is one of a group of local antiseptics and fungistatics that is capable of inducing photosensitization. There is cross-sensitization with bithionol, fenticlor and tribromosalicylanide.

Buclosamide (*N*-butyl-4-chlorosalicylamide)

Photocontact dermatitis has been described. There is a cross-reaction with a number of drugs, notably oral antidiabetics, diuretics and sulfonamides, and because of these reactions buclosamide is not recommended for topical treatment.

Captan (Orthocide-406)

This is one of the older fungicides in use for pityriasis versicolor, and included in some soaps and cosmetics to provide bactericidal and fungicidal effects. It has been shown to be allergenic. It also has been found to be carcinogenic in mice, and in several countries control agencies have taken steps to prohibit the use of captan in cosmetics and non-drug products (SEDA-13, 236).

Ciclopirox

Ciclopirox, a substituted pyridone unrelated to the imidazoles, has proven to be effective against a wide variety of dermophytes, yeasts, actinomycetes, moulds and other fungi. Ciclopirox olamine is generally well tolerated locally, with reactions occurring in only 1—4% of cases (SEDA-12, 684).

Clodantoin

Contact dermatitis has been reported, but it is rare.

Fluonilid (4-fluoro-3′,5′-thiocarbanilide)

Contact dermatitis has been reported.

Gentian violet

Gentian violet was at one time the treatment of choice for vaginal and oral candidiasis. The main problem is the staining and the messiness of the application since the fluid has to be brushed on the skin.

Hachimycin (Trichomycin)

Contact dermatitis has been reported.

KP-363

This benzylamine derivative is used in creams and solution in 0.1 and 0.6% concentrations. It is reported to cause less irritation than bifonazole and tolciclate (SEDA-14, 235).

Naftifine

Naftifine is one of a series of allylamine antifungal agents. Both naftifine and terbinafine (the latter also being effective orally) are normally sold in the form of a 1% cream for the topical treatment of dermatomycoses, dermatophytes and yeasts. The efficacy is claimed to be better than with the imidazoles. Local irritation and a burning sensation, if they occur, are only mild (SED-12, 684; SEDA-16, 297).

Natamycin (Pimaricin)

Contact dermatitis was described in industrial workers in frequent contact with this agent.

Nifuratel

Contact dermatitis with facial edema and a generalized erythema was described in the partner of a woman treated with nifuratel vaginal suppositories (SED-11, 578).

Niphimycin

This antimycotic and antibiotic derived from *Actinomyces hygroscopicus* is reportedly effective against both dermatomycosis and onychomycosis with a 16—26% success rate for the latter indication. Tolerance is reported to be good, but there is a notable lack of recent data (SEDA-12, 236).

Pecitocin (Variotin)

Skin irritation was reported to occur in 2—6.5% of patients. Contact dermatitis has been described in a few cases.

Pyrrolnitrin (Miutrin, 3-chloro-4-(3-chloro-2-nitrophenyl) pyrrole)

Contact dermatitis with cross-reaction with dinitrochlorobenzene was reported in one case.

Salicylic acid 3% with benzoic acid 6% (Whitfield's ointment)

Used for *Trichophyton rubrum*. This combination also has a keratolytic effect and local irritation can occur (SED-12, 685).

Selenium sulfide (Versel, Selsun)

This is effective in the treatment of tinea versicolor in the form of a shampoo. It can cause local irritation (SED-12, 685).

Sulbentine (dibenzthion)

Photoallergic contact dermatitis has been described, probably due to a breakdown product; benzyl-isothiocyanate.

Tolciclate

This thiocarbamate is active against most common dermatophytes. Local irritation occurs, as with all of these preparations.

Tolnaftate

Tolerance is good. Local erythema has been described, as have some cases of allergic dermatitis.

REFERENCES

1. Lyman CA, Walsh ThJ. Systemically adminstered antifungal agents. A review of their clinical phamarcology and therapeutic applications. Drugs 1992;44(1):9—35.
2. Hay RJ. Liposomal amphotericin B, Ambisome. J Infection 1994;28(Suppl 1):35—43.
3. Stevens DA. Overview of amphotericin B colloidal dispersion (Amphocil). J Infection 1994;28:(Suppl 1):45—49.
4. Van 't Wout JW, Meynaar I, Linde I, Poell R, Mattie H, Van Furth R. Effect of amphothericin B, fluconazole and itraconazole on intracellular *Candida albicans* and germ tube development in macrophages. J Antimicrobial Chemother 1990;25:803—811.
5. Wilson E, Tharson L, Speert D.P. Enhancement of macrophage superoxide ion production by amphotericin B. Antimicrobial Agents Chemother 1991;35:796—800.
6. Sokol-Anderson ML, Brajtburg J, Medoff G. Amphotericin B induced oxidative damage and killing of *Candida albicans*. J Infect Dis 1986;154:76—83.
7. Bratjtburg J, Powderly WG, Kobayashi GS, Medoff G. Amphotericin B. Current understanding of mechanisms of action. Antimicrobial Agents Chemother 1990;34:183—188.
8. Warda J, Barriere SL. Amphotericin B nephrotoxicity. Drug Intell Clini Pharm 1985;19:25—26.
9. Peters DH, Fitton A, Plasker GL, Faulds D. Tacrolimus. A review of its pharmacology and therapeutic potential in hepatic and renal transplants. Drugs 1993;46(4):746—794.
10. Bickers DR. Antifungal therapy: potential interactions with other classes of drugs. J Am Acad Dermatol 1994; 31(3)2;S87-S90.
11. Maesaki S, Kohno S, Kaku M, Koga H, Hara Ko. Effects Of antifungal agent combinations administered simultaneously and sequentially against *Aspergillus fumigatus*. Antimicrobial Agents Chemother 1994;38(12):2843—2845.
12. Walsh ThJ, Peter J, Mcgough DA, Fothergill AW, Rinaldi MG, Pizzo PA. Activities of amphotericin B and antifungal azoles alone and in combination against *Pseudallescheria boydii*. Antimicrobial Agents Chemother 1995;39:136.
13. Sugar AM, Hitchcock ChA, Troke PF, Picard M. Combination therapy of murine invasive candidiasis with fluconazole and amphotericin B. Antimicrobial Agents Chemother 1995;39:598—601.
14. Francis P, Walsh ThJ. Evolving role of flucytosine in immunocompromised patients: new insights into safety, pharmacokinetics and antifungal therapy. Clin Infect Dis 1992;15:1003—1018.
15. Viviani MA. Leading Article: Flucytosine—what is the future? J Antimicrobial Chemother 1995;35:241—244.
16. Malet-Martino MC, Martino R, De Forni M, Andremont A, Hartman O et al. Flucytosine conversion to fluoroucil in humans: does a correlation with gut flora exist? A report of two cases using fluorine-19 magnetic resonance spectroscopy. Infection 1991;19:178—180
17. Vialaneix JP, Malet-Martino MC, Hoffmann JS, Pris J, Martino R. Direct detection of new flucytosine metabolites in human biofluids by ^{19}F-nuclear magnetic resonance. Drug Metabolism Dispos 1987;15:718—724.
18. Czejka MJ, Jaeger W, Schuller J, Fogl U, Schernhaner G. Pharmakokinetische Aspecte Der Kombination Von Interferon-Alpha-2β Und Folinsaure und Fluorouracil. Arzneim Forsch/Drug Res 1991;41(11):860—862.
19. Savani DV, Perfect JR, Cobo LM, Durack DT. Penetration of new azole compounds into the eye and efficacy in experimental *Candida* endophyhalmitis. Antimicrobial Agents Chemother 1987;31:6—19.
20. Stevens DA. Coccidiodomycosis. New Engl J Med 1995;332(16):1077—1082.
21. Pawelec G, Ehninger G, Rehbein A, Schaudt K, Jaschonek K. Comparison of the immunosuppresive activities of the antimycotic agents intraconazole, fluconazole, ketoconazole and miconazole on human T-cells. Int J Immunopharmac 1991;13:299—304.
22. Akalin S. Effects of ketoconazole in hirsute women. Acta Endocrinol 1991;124:19.
23. Metroka CE, Mcmechan MF, Rada R, Laubenstein LJ, Jacobus DP. Failure of prophylaxis with dapsone in patients taking dideoxyinosine. New Engl J Med 1991;325:737.

24. Tucker RM, Denning DW, Hanson LH, Rinaldi MG, Graybill JR et al. Interaction of azoles with rifampin, phenytoin and carbamazepine; in vitro and clinical observations. Clin Infect Dis 1992;14:165–74.
25. Drouhet E, Dupont B. Evolution of antifungal agents: past, present and future. Rev Infect Dis 1987;9(Suppl 1):S4.
26. Honig PK, Wortham DC, Zamani K. Conner DP, Mullin JC et al. Terfenadine-ketoconazole interaction. J Am Med Assoc 1993;269:1513–1518.
27. Powderly WG, Finkelstein DM, Feinberg J, Frame P, He W et al. A randomized trial comparing fluconazole with clotrimazole troches for the prevention of fungal infections in patients with advanced human immunodeficiency virus infection. New Engl J Med 1995;332:700–705.
28. Heykants J, Van Peer A, Van De Velde V, Van Rooy P, Meuldermans W et al. The clinical pharmacokinetics of itraconazole: an overview. Mycoses 1989;32(Suppl):67–87.
29. Barone JA, Koh JG, Bierman RH, Colaizzi JL. Swanson KA et al. Food interaction and steady-state pharmacokinetics of itraconazole capsules in healthy male volunteers. Antimicrobial Agents Chemother 1993;37(4):778–784
30. Hardin TC, Graybill JR, Fetchick R, Woestenborghs R, Rinaldi MG, Kuhn JG. Pharmacokinetics of itraconazole following oral adminstration to normal volunteers. Antimicrobial Agents Chemother 1988;32:1310–1313.
31. Watkins DN, Badcock NR, Thompson PJ. Itraconazole concentrations in airway fluid and tissue. Br J Clin Pharmac 1992;33:206–207.
32. Larosa E, Cauwenbergh G, Cilli P, Woestenborghs R, Heykants J. Itraconazole pharmacokinetics in the female genital tract: plasma and tissue levels in patients undergoing hysterectomy after a single dose of 200 mg itraconazole. Eur J Obstet Gynecol Reprod Biol 1986;23:85–89.
33. Cauwenbergh G, Degreef H, Heykants J, Woestenborghs R, Van Rooy P et al. Pharmacokinetic profile of orally adminstered intraconazole in human skin. J Am Acad Dermatol 1988;18:263–268.
34. Schaefer-Korting M, Korting HC, Lukacs A, Heykants J, Behrendt H. Levels of intraconazole in skin blister fluid after a single oral dose and during repetitive administration. J Am Acad Dermatol 1990;22:211–215.
35. Smith D, Van De Velde V, Woestenborghs R, Gazzard BG. The pharmacokinetics of oral itraconazole in AIDS patients. J Pharm Pharmacol 1992;44:618–619.
36. Denning DW, Follansbee SE, Scolaro N et al. Pulmonary aspergillosis in the acquired immunodeficiency syndrome. New Engl J Med 1991;324:654.
37. Leconte P, Joly V, Siant-Julien L, Gikkardin JM, Carbon D et al. Tissue distribution and antifungal effect of liposomal itraconazole in experimental cryptococcis and pulmonary aspergillosis. Am Rev Resp Dis 1992;145:424–429.
38. Vuddhakul V, Mai GT, McCormack JC, Seow WK, Thong YH. Suppression of neutrophil and lymphoproliferative responses in vitro by itraconazole but not fluconazole. Int J Immunopharmac 1990;12:639–645.
39. Wheat J, Hafner R, Wulfsohn M, Spencer P, Squires K et al. Prevention of relapse of histoplasmosis with itraconazole in patients with the acquired immunodeficiency syndrome. Ann Intern Med 1993;118:610–616.
40. Stein GE, Mummaw N. Placebo-controlled trial of intraconazole for treatment of acute vaginal candidiasis. Antimicrobial Agents Chemother 1993;37:89–92.
41. Kosely M, Bren A, Kandus A, Kovac D. Drug interactions between cyclosporine and rifampicin, erythromycin and azoles in kidney recipients with opportunistic infections. Transplant Proc 1994;25(5):2823–2824.
42. Sorenson AL, Lovdahl M, Hewitt JM, Granger DK, Almond PS et al. Effects of ketaconazole on cyclosporine metabolisme in renal allograft recipients. Transplant Proc 1994;26(5):2822.
43. Toon S, Ross CF, Gokal R, Rowland M. An assesment of the effects of impaired renal function and haemodialysis on the pharmacokinetics of fluconazole. Br J Clin Pharmacol 1990;29:221–226.
44. Debruyne D, Ryckelynck JP, Moulin M, Hurault De Ligny B, Levaltier B, Bigot MC. Pharmacokinetics of fluconazole in patients undergoing continuous ambulatory peritoneal dialysis. Clin Pharmacokinet 1990;18:491–498.
45. Fishman AJ, Alpert NM, Livni E, Ray S et al. Pharmacokinetics of 18-F-labeled fluconazole in healthy human subjects by positron emission tomography. Antimicrobial Agents Chemother 1993;37:1270–1277.
46. Brammer KW, Farrow PR, Faulkner JK. Pharmacokinetics and tissue penetration of fluconazole in humans. Rev Infect Dis 1990;12(Suppl 3):S318-S326.
47. Bozzette SA, Gordon RL, Yen A, Rinaldi M. Ito MK, Fierer J. Biliary concentrations of fluconazole in a patient with candidal cholecystitis: case report. Clin Infect Dis 1992;15:701–703.
48. Ebden P, Neill L, Farrow PR. Sputum levels of fluconazole in humans. Antimicrobial Agents Chemother 1989; 33:963–964.
49. Dellenbach P. Penetration of fluconazole into vaginal tissues and secretions. Roy Soc Med Serv Int Congress Symp Ser 1989;160.
50. Houang ET, Chappatte O, Byme D, Macrae PV, Thorpe JE. Fluconazole levels in plasma and vaginal secretions of patients after a 150 mg single oral dose and rate of eradication of infection in vaginal candidiasis. Antimicrobial Agents Chemother 1990;34:909–910.
51. Ellis ME, Clink H, Ernst P, Halim MA, Padmos A et al. Controlled study of fluconazole in the prevention of fungal infections in neutropenic patients with hematological malignancies and bone marrow transplant recipients. Eur J Clin Microbiol Infect Dis 1994;January:3–11.
52. Magino JE, Moser SA, Waites KB. When to use fluconazole. New Engl J Med 1995;345:6–7.
53. Lee JW, Seibel NL, Amantea M, Whitcomb P, Pizzo PA et al. Safety, tolerance and pharmacokinetics of fluconazole in children with neoplastic diseases. J Pediatr 1992;120:987–993.
54. Thorpe JE, Baker N, Bromet-Petit M. Effect of oral antacid administration on the pharmacokinetics of oral fluconazole. Antimicrobial Agents Chemother 1990;34:2032–2033.
55. Allendoerfer R, Marquis AJ, Rinaldi MG, Graybill JR. Combined therapy with fluconazole and flucytosine in murine cryptococcal meningitis. Thirteenth Interscience Conference on Antimicrobial Agents and Chemotherapy. Atlanta, Abstract, 1990,1160.
56. Larsen RA, Bozzetta SA, Jones BE, Haghighat D, Leal MA et al. Fluconazole combined with flucytosine for treatment of cryptococcal meningitis in patients with AIDS. Clin Infect Dis 1994;19:741–745.
57. Devenport MH, Crook D, Wynn V, Lees LJ. Metabolic effects of low dose fluconazole in healthy female users and

non-users of oral contraceptives. Br J Clin Pharmacol 1989;26:851–859.

58. Graves NM, Matas AJ, Hilligoss DM, Canafax DM. Fluconazole/cyclosporine interaction. Clin Pharmacol Ther 1990;47(2):208.
59. Krueger HU, Schuler U, Zimmermann R, Ehninger G. Absence of significant interaction of fluconazole with cyclosporine. J Antimicrobial Chemother 1989;24:781–786.
60. Sugar AM, Saunders C, Idelson BA, Bernard DB. Interaction of fluconazole and cyclosporine. Ann Intern Med 1989;110:844.
61. Kramer MR, Marshall SE, Denning DW et al. Cyclosporine and itraconazole interaction in heart and lung transplant recipients. Ann Intern Med 1990;113:327–329.
62. Coker RJ, Tomlinson DR, Parkin J, Harris JRW, Pinching AJ. Interaction between fluconazole and rifampicin. Br Med J 1990;301:818.
63. Hardin TC, Sharkey PK, Lam YF, Wallace JE, Rinaldi MG et al. Pharmacokinetics of Sch-39304 in human immunodeficiency virus-infected patients following chronic oral dosing. J Antimicrobial Chemother 1992;36:2790–2793.
64. Wardle HM, Law D, Moore CB, Mason C, Denning DW. In vitro activity of D0870 compared with those other azoles against fluconazole resistant *Candida* spp. Antimicrobial Agents Chemother 1995;39:868–871.
65. Barchiesi F, Colombo AL, Mvcough DA, Fothergill AW, Rinaldi MG. In vitro activity of a new antifungal triazole, D0870, against *Candida albicans* isolates from oral cavities of patients infected with human immunodeficiency virus. Antimicrobial Agents Chemother 1994);38:2553–2556.
66. Graybill JR, Najvar LK, Holmberg JD, Luther MF. Fluconazole, D0870, and flucytosine treatment of disseminated *Candida tropicallis* in mice. Antimicrobial Agents Chemother 1995;39:924–929.
67. Clemens KV, Stevens DA. Efficacy of the triazole D0870 in a murine model of systemic histoplasmosis. Antimicrobial Agents Chemother 1995;39:778–780.
68. Karyotakis NC, Anaissie EJ, Hachem R, Dignani MC, Samonis G. Comparison of the efficacy of polyenes and triazoles against hematogenous *Candida kruse* infections in neutropenic mice. J Infect Dis 1993;168:1311–1313.
69. Atkinson BA, Bocanerga R, Colombo AL, Graybill JR. Treatment of Disseminated *Torulopsis glabrata* Infection with D0870 and amphotericin B. Antimicrobial Agents Chemother 1994;38:1604–1607.
70. Burggraaf J, Van-Rooy J, Yates RA, Cohen AF. A placebo controlled study to assess the safety, tolerance and pharmokinetics of ascending single oral doses of Zeneca D0870 in fasted healthy male volunteers. Abstr Br Pharmacol Soc Winter Meeting 1994;December;13–16.
71. Cartledge JD, Denning D, Dupont B, Clumeck N, Hawkins DA et al. Treatment Of fluconazale (Fcz) resistant (Res) oral candidosis (Oc) with D0870 In patients with AIDS (Pwa). Program and Abstracts of the Annual Interscience Conference on Antimicrobial Agents and Chemotherapy, ABS M89 34th ICAAC, Florida, 1994;248.
72. De-Wit S, Dupont B, Cartledge JD, Hawkins DA, Denning D et al. Pilot study of new triazole derivative (D0870) in H.I.V. patients with oral candidiasis. Program and Abstracts of the Annual Interscience Conference on Antimicrobial Agents and Chemotherapy, ABS 1225 34th ICAAC, Florida, 1994;213.
73. Angiolella L, Simmonetti N, Cassone A. The lipopeptide antimycotic, cilofungin modulates the incorporation of glucan-associated proteins into the cell wall of *Candida albicans*. J Antimicrob Chemother 1994;33:1137–1146.
74. Vargo T, Baldi G, Colombo D, Barbareschi M, Norbiato G et al. Effects of naftifine and terbinafine, two allylamine antifungal drugs on selected functions of human polymorphonuclear leukocytes. Antimicrobial Agents Chemother 1994;38:2605–2611.
75. Kovacs MJ, Alshammari S, Guenther L, Bourcier M. Neutropenia and pancytopenia associated with oral terbinafine. J Am Acad Dermatol 1994;November;806.
76. Henkin RI. Drug induced taste and smell disorders. Drug Safety 1994;11:318–377.
77. Cleveland KO, Cambell JW. Hallucinations associated with itraconazole therapy. Clin Infect Dis 1995;21:456.
78. Slavin MA, Osborne B, Adams R, Levenstein MJ, Schoch HG et al. Efficay and safety of fluconazole prophylaxis for fungal infections after marrow transplantation—a prospective, randomized, double-blind study. J Infect Dis 19??;171:1545–1552.

Meyler's Side Effects of Drugs, 13th Edition
M.N.G. Dukes, editor

SECTION EDITOR: P.K.M. LUNDE

C.B.M. Tester-Dalderup

28 Antiprotozoal drugs

ANTIMALARIAL DRUGS

Malaria has been a world-wide problem for centuries. The influence of certain products of natural origin on fever was recognized long before the disease entity of malaria caused by hematozoon parasites was discovered by Laveran in 1890. In Europe the Cinchona (Jesuit bark) which contained quinine was introduced in the Middle Ages but the properties of the Cinchona to act against the classic pattern of fever now known to be typical of malaria tropica had been known long before that time. The Chinese herb *Artemisia annua*, sweet worm wood, with its healing properties in typical malaria-induced pyrexia, has also has been known for centuries, be it in a different part of the world. With the introduction of the synthetic antimalarials, plasmoquine in 1926, and Mepacrine (atebrine) shortly thereafter, and the development of the 4-aminoquinolines in the 1950s, preventive and curative treatment became possible. In combination with the use of the newly developed pesticides malaria was confidently believed to have become an illness of the past in the course of just a few years. Quinine was considered outdated and dangerous. Artemisin remained in use in those parts of the world where it had always been popular. The optimism lasted little more than two decades, the development of drug resistance, especially in the case of *Plasmodium falciparum* has made quinine and artemisin valuable drugs once more. Artemisin in particular has been studied extensively in recent years, though unfortunately the development of an easily and cheaply produced synthetic, semi-synthetic or more accurately assayed form of this product has been slow and not well co-ordinated.

Chloroquine-resistant *falciparum* malaria (CRFP) was first reported in 1960. As of 1996 chloroquine resistance is widespread throughout the world and in many areas there is multi-drug resistance. Preventative administration of drugs such as chloroquine, primaquine and pyrimethamine as well as the use of various sulfonamide mixtures and the combinations of sulfonamides with trimethoprim have progressively lost their usefulness. At the present time, hardly half a century after the therapeutic breakthroughs occurred, quinine is once more one of the most valuable drugs in the treatment of malaria and there is a desperate need for other effective drugs (SED-12, 687).

The advice given to travellers to countries where malaria is endemic has to be adapted to the local circumstances, as well as taking into account the fact that the antimalarial drugs cause a wide range of dose-dependent, idiosyncratic and also cumulative adverse effects (SEDA-17, 325).

In those areas where *P. vivax*, *P. ovale* and *P. malaria* occur, and in the very limited areas where *P. falciparum* is still sensitive and prophylaxis is indeed required, chloroquine or proguanil, or the combination of these two drugs, can be used. This approach would apply to Central America, as well as to malarial areas in the Middle East and North Africa (1, 2). The need for prophylaxis for the infections caused by *P. vivax*, *ovale* and *malaria*, all generally mild illnesses, is questionable. In low risk areas the traveller will be more at risk from the drug than the disease (SED-12, 687; SEDA-16, 301; SEDA-17, 325). *P. vivax* resistance to chloroquine has been reported (SED-12; 688; 3[C]).

Prophylaxis is advisable in areas of intense transmission and for short visits. Residents in malaria endemic areas often cannot afford chemoprophylaxis and this would in any case entail their virtually life-long use of one or more drugs. The population of an area where malaria is endemic however builds up an immunity, which disappears after an absence from the area for a longer period. It is not clear how soon the immunity would return on renewed exposure to *P. falciparum*, whether chemoprophylaxis would be useful in the transition period in order to prevent clinical malaria before immunity returns, and (if prophylactic chemotherapy is advisable) for how long a period it should be given.

For most areas the prophylactic use of mefloquine is advised, at a dose of 250 mg every week. This applies to the Amazon region of South America, tropical Africa and many areas in South East Asia (1, 2).

Mefloquine resistance is well developed in Thailand, Cambodia, Irian Jaya, Laos, Myanmar (Burma) and Papua New Guinea (1). For these regions The Netherlands Advisory Body indicates that the traveller should take medication with him to treat a malaria attack if there are no adequate treatment centers. In Thailand and Vietnam there are good functioning malaria clinics (1, 2).

With emergent resistance to drugs, the use of non-drug measures to prevent malaria have become more important than ever. Proper protective clothing should be worn to cover the greater part of the skin, especially in the evening hours; mosquito repellents (such as diethyltoluamide) can be applied to exposed areas of skin. Nets impregnated with permetrin are valuable; they can provide about 70% protection in small children (SED-12, 687; SEDA-17, 1; 1, 4, 5). Equally important is that the public be taught to recognize the early symptoms of malaria, since early treatment remains crucial. Last but not least the traveller should be told that malaria can show up after he is back home in a temperate climate and it is up to him to tell the physician about his journeys if he is subsequently taken ill.

In many urban areas of the tropics, where there is likely to be a low attack rate by mosquitoes such measures will provide adequate protection, albeit not a 100% guarantee. The effectiveness of these old-time measure has been demonstrated again in recent studies (SED-12, 687; 1, 4, 5).

For travellers having no immunity going to areas with a high attack rate the provision of medication for therapeutic use in case of the development of a fever may be the best approach. The seriousness of an attack of malaria tropica should not be underestimated (SED-12, 687). The medication to be chosen for treatment has to be adapted to the resistance pattern of *Plasmodium falciparum*. In view of the common resistance to chloroquine, this drug should not be used to treat the patient taken ill with *falciparum* malaria following a stay in an area where resistance is common; quinine, given parenterally or orally, is the better choice; but quinidine can be used instead. In treatment centers in areas where malaria is virtually unknown, quinidine may be available because of its use in cardiovascular medicine, while quinine is not. Mefloquine is at present another good choice, though in some regions lack of availability may be one problem, and resistance another; mefloquine may induce seizures in those with a predisposition.

One of the greatest risks is still that in non-endemic areas of the world the malaria may not be recognized, and/or that too much is relied on the effectiveness of a prophylactic method which is no longer sufficiently effective (SED-12, 687).

Prophylaxis during pregnancy Malarial infection in pregnant women may be more severe than in the non-pregnant individual. Semi-immune patients lose much of their resistance to local strains of *P. falciparum* during pregnancy; this commonly results in massive sequestration of organisms in the placenta, leading to maternal anemia, low birth-weight babies, pre-term deliveries and abortions. The pregnant state decreases the ability of the mother to mount an adequate IgG response, resulting in an increased level of malarial infestation. Malaria in pregnant women is associated with a higher than usual incidence of cerebral malaria, anemia and pulmonary edema (SEDA-16, 301; SEDA-17, 325). Chemoprophylaxis is advocated, despite the (small) risks of teratogenicity (SEDA-17, 325).

Pregnant travellers should be dissuaded from visiting areas of high transmission rates, particularly during the first trimester. If travel cannot be avoided, protective measures must be taken. Chloroquine and proguanil have no record of an increased risk of fetal malformations. Mefloquine is not recommended by the manufacturer for use during pregnancy (SEDA-16, 301; SEDA-17, 329), but Nosten et al. (8^C) reported no increase in fetal malformations in their study of the drug.

Prophylaxis while breast feeding The minute amounts of antimalarial drugs secreted in breast milk of lactating women are not considered harmful to the nursing infant (SEDA-16, 302); they may possibly even confer some protection on the infant. No hard facts are however available, and it is of utmost importance to shelter the infant from mosquito bites.

Use of newer drugs for prophylaxis A number of new drugs have been developed in recent years. The indiscriminate prophylactic use of these drugs should be discouraged, in line with the view taken by the WHO and many centers for the treatment of tropical diseases. However, the use of mefloquine is advocated by some authorities for travellers in Zone C regions (regions of the world where *Plasmodium falciparum* is resistant to chloroquine), while others would restrict its use to East Africa where the risk is highest. Outdated advice concerning the choice of drugs for chemoprophylaxis is common, and knowledge of their adverse effects often insufficient. Mefloquine resistance has become widespread in large areas in a few years. As with other drugs, adequate dosages should be used; the use of mefloquine every 2 weeks has been shown to be insufficient and in February of 1991 the American Centers for Disease Control recommended weekly administration (SED-12, 688). Campbell (7^R) states that *Plasmodium falciparum* resistance to available antimalarial drugs other than chloroquine, will evolve to an extent roughly proportional to the extent of their use.

Artemisin and its derivatives have been developed over the last years; their use for treatment is promising in areas like Thailand and Cambodia mainly in combination with mefloquine, despite the emergence of mefloquine resistance. Here again, indiscriminate use is a danger. Doxycycline has been used for prophylaxis among UN peace-keeping forces in Cambodia; it offers protection against initial infection, and according a 1992 report resistance had not been seen up to that date. The drawback of this agent is its unwanted effect on the bacterial flora (5).

WR 243251, a dihydroacridinedione, is a schizonticidal agent which is currently being developed (8). Dispiro-1,2,4,5-tetraoxane and the tricyclic 1,2,4-trioxanes are other potential new drugs (9, 10). All these are being studied in research projects of the Walter Reed Army Institute. A series of bisbenzylisoquinolines is being tested in the UK (11).

Progress in being made in research to develop a vaccine but practical application cannot be foreseen in the near future. A Colombian team is currently working on a synthetic vaccine; a phase III randomized double-blind controlled trial in volunteers showed an overall protective efficacy against *falciparum* malaria of 39%, Further independent trials in Ecuador and Venezuela confirmed the protective efficacy. A trial in Tanzania, an intense transmission area for *P. falciparum*, showed some effect but the results here are tantalizing, since they point only to a marginal effect. Avoidance of infection is however not the only valid criterion for the usefulness of a vaccine; a decrease in morbidity and or mortality of some 30% could be very worthwhile. Further studies are under way (12[R], 13[C]—18[C]).

In the field, prophylaxis with chloroquine is possible in some areas in middle America and the middle East, in other areas chloroquine in combination with proguanil, maloprim, or possibly fansidar, can be used with due regard for the toxicity of the two combination preparations. In high risk areas with CRFP (East Africa) mefloquine may be indicated either alone or in an attempt to prevent development of resistance in combination with doxycycline or pyrimethamine-sulfadoxine (SED-12, 686; SEDA-16, 301; SEDA-17, 325).

'Partial prophylaxis' and the use of quinine While *Plasmodium falciparum* has become resistant to chloroquine in most of the areas where it is endemic, chloroquine is still extensively used for prophylaxis, even in those areas. Chloroquine is often used to reduce the density of parasitemia and resolve fever, which can be valuable even though a high proportion of such patients remain parasitemic. Campbell (7[R]) provides the interesting comment that, since in areas of intense transmission some degree of parasitemia is required to sustain immunity, and frequent re-infection is to be expected, complete elimination of infection may not be desirable. A study of the influence of chronic parasitemia on childhood morbidity will be needed to provide firm data on this point. Relevant is a paper by Carme et al. (19[C]) who reported on the extensive use of chloroquine and amodiaquine in certain areas of Congo; little change in resistance was seen in groups of semi-immune children. The actual influence of chloroquine in the control of symptomatic malaria in these regions is however open to question, since even in a CRFP area resistance is not absolute.

Another interesting phenomenon was observed in Thailand where, following a widespread reduction in chloroquine usage, strains of *Plasmodium falciparum* sensitive to chloroquine are rapidly re-emerging. If this observation is confirmed it might be worthwhile to use the various drugs on a rotation basis in a specific region or country.

Efficacy/safety ratio of antimalarial prophylaxis

A survey of travellers to tropical East Africa between 1985 and 1991 provided some informative data concerning efficacy and side effects, though it should be remembered that resistance patterns have changed since that time (20[R]) (see Tables 1 and 2).

Chloroquine and congeners (4-aminoquinoline)

Chloroquine is rapidly and almost completely absorbed from the intestinal tract, peak serum levels being reached in 1—6 hours, (with an average of 3 hours). Chloroquine is extensively distributed, and redistribution follows. It is slowly metabolized by side chain de-ethylation. It is not possible to determine a clear half-life, but the presence of chloroquine has been demonstrated from 7—10 days to as exceptionally as long as 56 days after administration. The beta-phase half life of chloroquine has been established as being 30—60 days. Elimination is mainly via the kidney. Malnutrition may slow down the rate of metabolism.

Alongside the well-known development of resistance by *Plasmodium falciparum* to chloroquine, the emergence of chloroquine-resistant *Plasmodium vivax* is now clear (SED-12, 688; 3[C]).

In France an increased frequency of cerebral malaria

Table 1. *Effectiveness of malaria chemoprophylaxis*

Regimen	Malaria infections (deaths)	Person-months exposure	Effectiveness (95% CI)
No chemoprophylaxis	39	3137	0
Chloroquine 300 mg/week	43 (4)	3827	10 (−43 to 43)
Chloroquine 600 mg/week	35	4897	42 (6 to 64)
Chloroquine + proguanil	41 (1)	11912	72 (56 to 82)
Mefloquine	35	31412	91 (85 to 94)
Pyrimethamine + sulfadioxine	36	16206	82 (71 to 89)

Malaria incidence of 1.2%/month of stay, taken as baseline with 0% effectiveness.

Table 2. *Side effects*

Side-effect	No chemoprophylaxis	Chloroquine		Mefloquine	Chloroquine + proguanil	Pyrimethamine + sulfadioxine
		300 mg/week	600 mg/week			
	n = 4026	*n* = 3354	*n* = 3646	*n* = 50 053	*n* = 20 150	*n* = 8673
Nausea	2.0	10.8	10.8	12.3	18.8	7.5
Headache	1.3	6.4	6.0	6.2	7.6	4.4
Dizziness	1.2	5.3	6.4	7.6	5.5	3.3
Visual	1.0	3.5	4.2	2.2	2.8	1.6
Depression	0.3	1.4	1.0	1.8	1.7	0.7
Insomnia	0.5	4.5	5.0	4.2	6.3	2.4
Mouth ulcers	0.2	0.8	0.8	1.2	7.9	0.7
Pruritus	0.4	2.3	3.4	2.7	3.7	2.8
Other skin	1.1	4.2	6.5	5.5	6.0	5.4
% patients with side-effects	5.3	18.5	17.2	18.7	30.1	11.6

Rates corrected by subtracting the rate for no therapy.

appears to coincide with the growing emergence of the chloroquine resistant strains in Francophone Africa. The hypoxemic effects of chloroquine, reflecting cardiac and respiratory toxicity, pose a particular problem in the newborn, in whom existing malarial infection may not become clinically manifest until some months after birth (SEDA-16, 302).

ADVERSE REACTION PATTERN

General and toxic reactions Relatively few adverse effects are encountered with the doses prescribed for malaria prophylaxis and standard doses of treatment. The use of higher doses than those recommended, e.g. because of problems with resistance, can however cause problems. The infant is very easily overdosed (SEDA-16, 302). If given intravenously, chloroquine should be diluted and infused slowly, since rapid injection causes toxic concentrations. Toxicity and even death have been reported after intramuscular administration of larger doses; this is probably connected with rapid absorption in such cases (SEDA-17, 327). In the treatment of rheumatoid arthritis and lupus erythematosus larger doses are used, often for long periods of time and with this use the incidence of side effects is high. Neuromyopathy, neuritis, myopathy and cardiac myopathy may cause serious problems. Retinopathy may lead to blindness. Chloroquine with its long half life is liable to accumulate in the tissues including the brain. Levels in the brain may have a bearing on mental status and psychotic syndromes. Chloroquine interferes with the action of several enzymes including alcohol dehydrogenase and is able to block the sulfhydryl—disulfide interchange reaction.

Hypersensitivity reactions These are generally limited to rashes and pruritus; the latter seems to be more common in strongly pigmented races.

Tumor-inducing effects These have not been reported.

ORGANS AND SYSTEMS

Cardiovascular *Electrocardiographic changes*, comprising altered T-waves and prolongation of the QT interval, are not uncommon during high dose treatment. The clinical significance of this finding is uncertain. With chronic intoxication, a varying degree of *atrio-ventricular block* may be seen; first degree right bundle branch block but also total atrio-ventricular block have been described. Clinical symptoms depend on the severity of the effects: *syncope*, *Adam Stokes attacks*, but also signs of *cardiac failure* can be encountered. Acute intoxication may cause cardio-vascular collapse and/or respiratory collapse. Cardiac complications may prove fatal in both chronic and acute intoxication.

Intravenous administration may lead to arrhythmias and again cardiac arrest; the speed of administration is relevant, but also the concentration attained; deaths have been recorded with blood levels of 1 μg/ml; it may be noted that levels after a 300-mg dose are usually between 50 and 100 μg/l (SED-12, 689).

More than one mechanism may underlie the cardiac side effects. The occurrence of severe hypokalemia after ingestion of a single large dose of chloroquine has been documented; some studies show a correlation between plasma potassium concentrations and the severity of the cardiac effects (91[R]). Light and electron microscopic abnormalities were found on endometrial biopsy in two cases with clinically manifest cardiac failure. The first case had taken 200 mg hydroxychloroquine daily for 10 years then 400 mg daily for a further 6 years; the second patient received 400 mg hydroxychloroquine for 2 years (SEDA-13, 239). A similar case was reported after the use of 250 mg daily for 25 years (SEDA-18, 286).

Respiratory Respiratory collapse may occur with acute over-dosage (see also above).

Nervous system Chloroquine, especially in higher doses, can cause marked neurotoxicity. A range of mental changes attributed to chloroquine have been described, notably *agitation*, *aggressiveness*, *confusion*, *personality changes*, *psychotic symptoms* and *depression*. Acute *mania* has also been recognized (SEDA-18, 287). *Neuritis*, *neuromyopathy* and a *pyramidal tract syndrome* have been described. The mental changes may develop slowly and insidiously. Subtle symptoms such as fluctuating impairment of thought, memory and perception can be early signs, but may also be the only signs. The symptoms may be connected with the long half-life of chloroquine and its accumulation leading to high tissue concentrations (SED-11, 583). More recently it has been shown that chloroquine inhibits glutamate dehydrogenase activity and can reduce concentrations of the inhibitory transmitter γ-aminobutyric acid.

In an number of cases with psychosis following the administration of normal recommended doses, symptoms developed after the patients had received a total of 1.0–10.5 grams of the drug, the time of onset of behavioral changes varying from 2 hours to 40 days after initiation of therapy. The majority of cases occurred during the first week and lasted from 2 days to 8 weeks (SED-11, 583).

A case of transient global *amnesia* was seen in a 62-year-old healthy male 3 hours after he took 300 mg chloroquine prior to his departure to Zaire. Recovery was spontaneous after some hours (SEDA-16, 302).

In one centre, *toxic psychosis* was reported in four children over a period of 18 months. The children presented with an acute delirium, marked restlessness, outbursts of increased motor activity, mental inaccessibility and insomnia. One child seemed to have visual hallucinations. In each case chloroquine had been administered intramuscularly because of fever. The dosage was not recorded. The children returned to normal within 2 weeks (SEDA-16, 302).

Chloroquine, especially in higher doses, can cause marked *neurotoxicity* and *neuromyopathy*. The condition is characterized by the insidious onset of slowly progressive weakness. In many cases this weakness first affects the proximal muscles of the lower limb. Reduction in nerve conduction time and electromyographic abnormalities typical of both neuropathic and myopathic changes can be found. Increased serum levels of SGOT and SGPT may be present. Histologically the picture of a vacuolar myopathy is found. Neuromyopathy is a rare side effect usually limited to those patients receiving doses of 250–750 mg per day over prolonged periods. The symptoms may be accompanied by other manifestations of overall chloroquine toxicity (SED-11, 583). A recent case was described in an 80-year-old woman following 6 months treatment with chloroquine 300 mg daily (SEDA-16, 302), once more demonstrating that a standard dosage regime can be much too high for the elderly.

A spastic *pyramidal tract syndrome* of the lower limbs has been reported in relation to the use of chloroquine. In young children the features of an extrapyramidal syndrome may comprise abnormal eye movements, trismus, torticollis and torsion dystonia.

Mild myopathy may be difficult to distinguish from the original disease in cases of systemic lupus or severe rheumatoid arthritis, or from the muscle weakness induced by corticosteroid therapy. The incidence of reversible myopathy has been reported as 0.1%, but the paper did not consider the relationship to serum and/or tissue levels of chloroquine (SED-11, 583).

A *myasthenia like syndrome* was seen in a young woman on chronic corticosteroid therapy for systemic lupus erythematosus 7 weeks after starting chloroquine therapy; discontinuation of the chloroquine was followed by a remission. Ocular symptoms reappeared following a second short course of chloroquine. Pathology tests revealed a vacuolar myopathy with membranous bodies in intramuscular nerves (SEDA-13, 238).

The occurrence of tonic-clonic *convulsions* was reported in four cases in whom chloroquine was part of a prophylactic regimen. Anti-epileptic treatment was required to control the seizures. None had further seizures after discontinuation of the antimalarials (SEDA-13, 239; SEDA-14, 239).

Overdosage with chloroquine can cause *vertigo* and *headache*.

The incidence of serious CNS events among patients receiving chloroquine for less than a year has been estimated as one in 13 600 patients (90^R).

Endocrine, metabolic *Hypoglycemia* was reported in a fatal chloroquine intoxication in a 32-year-old black Zambian male (SEDA-13, 240). Hypoglycemia has also been seen in patients, especially children, with cerebral malaria and the possibility of a connection with the anti-malaria treatment and chloroquine was mentioned (SEDA-13, 240). Further studies have shown that the hypoglycemia in these African children was usually present before the antimalarials were started, but a study in The Gambia showed occurrence of hypoglycemia after treatment with the drug was started, though not necessarily connected with the treatment (SEDA-13, 240). Convulsions were more common in hypoglycemic children. This often not recognized complication of hypoglycemia contributes to the morbidity and mortality of cerebral *falciparum* malaria. Hypoglycemia is amendable to treatment with intravenous dextrose or glucose which may help to prevent brain damage (SED-12, 689).

Effects on *potassium* are noted under 'Cardiovascular' above.

Hematological Chloroquine inhibits human myelopoiesis in vitro at normal therapeutic concentrations and higher. In a special test procedure a short-lasting anti-aggregating effect could be seen with chloroquine concentrations of 3.2—32 mg/ml (SEDA-16, 303). These effects have clinical consequences. Chloroquine and related aminoquinolines have reportedly caused blood dyscrasias at antimalarial doses. *Leukopenia* and even *agranulocytosis* and the occasional case of *thrombopenia* were reported (SED-12, 690). There is some evidence that the myelosuppression is dose dependent. This is in line with the hypothesis that 4-aminoquinoline therapy merely accentuates the cytopenia linked with other forms of bone marrow damage (SED-11, 584; SEDA-16, 302).

Some studies in the past have pointed to inhibitory effects of chloroquine on platelet aggregability. In a new investigation this aspect of chloroquine was studied in vitro in a medium containing ADO, collagen and ristocin. A highly significant effect was recorded at concentrations of 3.2—32 mg/ml chloroquine. However no significant differences were observed in platelet responses to ADP or collagen 2 or 6 hours after adding chloroquine, as compared to pre-drug values. The investigators believed that these data provided no cause for concern in using chloroquine for malaria prophylaxis in patients with impaired hemostasis (SEDA-16, 303).

Gastrointestinal Gastrointestinal *discomfort* is not unusual and *diarrhea* may occur. Changes in intestinal motility may be to blame; intramuscular injection of chloroquine was shown to cause a shortening of oral-cecal time in the five cases in which this was measured. Over-dosage may give rise to *vomiting*. *Pigmentation of the palate* can occur as a part of a more generalized pigmentation; *stomatitis* occasionally with *buccal ulceration* has been mentioned (SED-11, 584).

Skin Skin lesions and eruptions of different types have been attributed to the use of chloroquine, including the occasional case of *epidermal necrolysis*.

Pruritus is not uncommon in malaria patients treated with chloroquine, the onset occurring about 10 hours after the start of treatment with a maximum intensity at about 25 hours. These times correspond with maximum serum concentrations of chloroquine and its metabolites after oral ingestion. In many cases the itch is confined to the palms of the hands and the soles of the feet. In a study carried out in Nigeria, the incidence of pruritus was reported to be 60—75%; the itch was considered unbearable in 40%, with 30% of the respondents refusing the further use of chloroquine. A second study showed an even higher incidence of pruritus. In a further study elsewhere the incidence of pruritus was 27% (SEDA-16, 304). Not surprisingly, pruritus is a major cause of non-compliance with treatment and its occurrence may contribute largely to the emergence and spread of resistant *Plasmodium falciparum* (SEDA-16, 304). Pruritus is more frequently seen in black- than in white-skinned people in Africa, a difference ascribed to the binding of chloroquine to melanin and hence a racial predisposition. No such reports have come from America (SED-11, 584; SEDA-16, 303; SEDA-17, 327; SEDA-18, 288).

Antihistamine treatment can have a preventive effect on pruritus. Other treatments which have been mentioned are with prednisone and niacin, but the results were not impressive.

A few cases of *psoriasis* or severe exacerbation of psoriasis shortly after the start of treatment, have been reported (SED-12, 690; SEDA-16, 304; SEDA-17, 327).

Photosensitivity and photo-allergic dermatitis have

been seen particularly during prolonged therapy with high doses.

Blue-black *pigmentation* involving the palate and facial, pretibial and subungual areas occurs rarely but it has been associated with the presence of retinopathy (see below) (SED-11, 584). The nail bed can turn blue-brown and the nail itself may develop longitudinal stripes and show a blue-grey fluorescence (SED-11, 584). Chloroquine can however also cause *vitiligo* (SEDA-17, 327).

There is some support for the contention that hydroxychloroquine causes skin reactions more often than chloroquine.

Special senses *Eyes* In man chloroquine and its congeners can cause two typical effects involving the eye, namely a *keratopathy* and a specific *retinopathy*. Both these effects are associated with the administration of the drug over longer periods of time. The keratopathy is limited to the corneal epithelium, where high concentrations of the drug are readily demonstrable. Slit lamp examination shows a series of punctate opacities scattered diffusely over the cornea; these are sometimes seen as lines just below the center of the cornea, while thicker yellow lines may be seen in the stroma. The keratopathy is often asymptomatic, fewer than 50% of patients having complaints. The commonest symptoms are the appearance of halos around lights and photophobia. Keratopathy may appear after 1—2 months of treatment, but doses of less than 250 mg per day usually do not cause it. Dust exposure may lead to similar changes. The incidence of keratopathy is high, in 30—70% of patients treated with higher doses of chloroquine. The condition is usually reversible on discontinuation of therapy. The condition does not seem to involve a threat to vision (SED-12, 690). There are differences in incidence between chloroquine and hydroxychloroquine. In a survey of 1500 patients, 95% of the patients on chloroquine demonstrated corneal deposition of the drug with the pupils dilated, while less than 10% of patients on hydroxychloroquine showed any corneal changes (SEDA-16, 303)

The retinopathy encountered with the prolonged use of chloroquine or related drugs is a much more serious side effect and can lead to irreversible damage to the retina and loss of vision. It is however not possible to predict in which patients and in what proportion of patients an early retinopathy will progress to blindness.

The typical picture is that of the 'bull's eye' an intact foveal area surrounded by a depigmented ring, the whole lesion being enclosed in a scattered hyperpigmented area. At this stage the retinal vessels are contracted, there are changes in the peripheral retinal pigment epithelium, and the optic disk is atrophic. In the early stages there are changes in the macular retinal pigment epithelium. The picture is however not always clear and peripheral retinal changes may appear as first symptom. Another sign may be a unilateral paramacular retinal edema.

The functional defects are varied: difficulty in reading, scotomas, defective color vision, photophobia, light flashes and a decrease in visual acuity. Symptoms do not parallel the retinal changes. By the time that visual acuity has become impaired irreversible changes will have taken place.

Testing of visual acuity, central fields (with or without the use of red targets), contrast sensitivity, dark adaptation and color vision provides no early indication of chloroquine retinopathy. Careful ophthalmoscopic examination of the macula can be a sensitive index when visual acuity remains intact. More sophisticated tests like the measurement of the critical flicker fusion frequency and the Amsler grid test (detection of small peripheral scotoma) can be useful. It is important to trace, if at all possible, the results of a pre-treatment ophthalmological examination after dilatation of the pupils, thus reducing the possibility of confusing senile degenerative changes with chloroquine-induced abnormalities.

It should be noted that the macular changes and the 'bull's eye' are occasionally seen in patients who have never been treated with chloroquine or related drugs (SED-12, 690).

Despite the fact that the retinopathy has been known for many years, it is still not clear why certain patients develop these changes while others do not. There clearly is a relation with the daily dosage of the drug. The retinopathy is rarely seen with doses of less then 250 mg of chloroquine or 400 mg of hydrochloroquine daily; the level of the daily dose seems more important then the total dosage. Nevertheless, cases have been described with retinopathy following the use of small doses for relatively short periods of time while, on the other hand, prolonged treatment and total doses of a kilogram or more have been used in many other patients without any evidence of macular changes. In the published cases there is usually no information about other treatments given previously or concomitantly. More cases are seen in the older age group. Patients with lupus erythematosus are more susceptible than patients with rheumatoid arthritis. The presence of nephropathy increases the likelihood of the development of a retinopathy, as does the concomitant use of probenecid. Exposure to sunlight may be of importance, since light amplifies the risk of retinopathy.

The changes with the retinopathy are probably connected with the concentrative capacity of the melanin-containing epithelium. Chloroquine has been shown to inhibit the incorporation of amino acids into the retinal pigment epithelium.

Little is yet known about the development of the retinopathy after discontinuation of treatment. Retinal changes in the early stages are likely reversible if the drug is withdrawn, and progression of a severe maculopathy to blindness seems to be less frequent than feared. A study involving 1650 patients showed that patients with 6/6 vision and relative scotomas did not suffer any further decline in visual acuity after drug withdrawal, but that 63% of patients who presented with absolute scotomas lost further vision over a median period of 6 years. This suggests that withdrawal of chloroquine at an early stage of retinopathy halts progression of the disease (SEDA-17, 327).

The need for routine ophthalmological testing of all patients using chloroquine is under discussion, an obvious element being its cost/benefit ratio. The best current opinion seems to be that with doses not exceeding 6.5 mg/kg per day of hydroxychloroquine, given for not longer than 10 years and with periodic checking of renal and hepatic function, the likelihood of retinal damage is negligible and ophthalmological follow-up is not required (SEDA-16, 303; SEDA-17, 327). Patients on higher doses or on chloroquine however should be checked.

Occasionally other ocular side effects are mentioned: *rhegmatogenous retinal detachment* has been associated with chloroquine retinopathy, and bitemporal *hemianopsia* has similarly been seen, occurring in association with chloroquine retinopathy. Bilateral *edema of the optic nerve* was observed in a woman treated with 200 mg of chloroquine daily for 2.5 months. *Diplopia* and *impaired accommodation* (characterized by difficulty in changing focus quickly from near to far vision and vice versa) also affect a minority of patients (SED-12, 691).

Ears Ototoxicity has been mentioned occasionally over the years; *tinnitus* and *deafness* can occur in relation to high doses; symptoms described after injections of chloroquine phosphate include a case of *cochlear vestibular dysfunction* in a child. All the same there is insufficient evidence to attribute ototoxicity to chloroquine in human subjects except as a rare individualized phenomenon. In guinea-pigs given chloroquine 25 mg/kg/day i.p. one of the first signs of intoxication was ototoxicity (SED-11, 586).

Other senses Disturbances of *taste* and *smell* have also been described.

Other organs and systems *Hemoglobinuria* was described in children with glucose-6-phosphate dehydrogenase deficiency following a single chloroquine dose. Generalized *immunoblastic lymphadenopathy* was described in one case after 4 months of hydrochloroquine 400 mg daily.

Risk situations *Small children* have usually been considered as being relatively more sensitive to the toxic effect of overdosage, but it has been calculated that on a mg/kg body weight basis adults in fact exhibit a similar sensitivity. Young children do seem to be truly more susceptible to gastric irritation. Patients with a history of *mania* or *epilepsy* should be careful in taking chloroquine (90[R]). Some of the possible risk factors as regards the eyes have been considered above. As noted below, overdosage may have more severe consequences in *children*.

Second-generation effects Chloroquine inactivates DNA and it has been shown in animal studies that it can cross the placenta. Caution has generally been advised with respect to the use of chloroquine and related compounds during pregnancy, but except for one (coincidental?) case there have been no reports of complications to mother or child from treatment with chloroquine during pregnancy (SEDA-14, 239; SEDA-17, 326).

Overdosage Acute intoxication, either accidental or in attempted suicide may cause a rapid onset of headache, drowsiness, vision disturbance, vomiting and diarrhea and cardiovascular and or respiratory collapse. Deaths have been recorded at blood levels of 1 μg/ml (SED-11, 286). As compared with adults, mortality in children following acute chloroquine poisoning is extremely high. Although the clinical presentation is mostly similar to that in adults (apnea, seizures, cardiac arrhythmias), ingestion of a single 300-mg chloroquine tablet by a 12-month-old female infant was enough to cause death (SEDA-16, 302).

Interactions Studies of chloroquine used in combination with antibiotics showed an antagonistic effect for *penicillin* but a synergistic effect with *chlortetracycline*. Urinary tests after a single administration of 1 gram of ampicillin and 1 gram of chloroquine showed a significant reduction in the bio-availability of the ampicillin.

Chloroquine given in a dose used for malaria prophylaxis, 300 mg/week, adversely influenced the antibody response to human diploid-cell *rabies vaccine* administered concurrently with the chloroquine. The mean rabies-neutralizing antibody titer was significantly lower in the chloroquine group than in the control group on each day of testing (SED-12, 691; 21–23). In contrast, retrospective studies of the response to pneumococcal polysaccharide in patients with systemic lupus erythematosus taking chloroquine or hydroxychloroquine, and of the response to tetanus-measles-meningococcal vaccine in a region of Nigeria where malaria is endemic did not demonstrate an influence on antibody reaction. However it was pointed out that the altered immune status of patients with systemic lupus erythematosus makes it difficult to compare their response to that of young healthy adults receiving rabies vaccine. With respect to the Nigerian study it has also been noted that illness and nutritional state could have influenced the findings (SED-12, 691).

There may be an interaction with *insulin*. An oral glucose load given to normal subjects and to patients with non-insulin-dependent diabetes mellitus before and during a short course of chloroquine demonstrated a small but significant reduction in fasting blood glucose concentration in the control group while the patients showed improvement in their glucose tolerance. The response seems to reflect decreased degradation of insulin rather than increased pancreatic output (SEDA-12, 240).

The combination of chloroquine with *recombinant murine* γ-interferon proved superior in the treatment of *Plasmodium vinckei* infections in mice, not only with respect to the parasitemia but also to the development of strain-specific immunity (SED-12, 691).

In vitro studies have shown that a number of compounds without any antimalarial activity can influence the susceptibility of *Plasmodium falciparum* for chloroquine. Ndifor et al. (24[c]) demonstrated an enhancement of chloroquine susceptibility in 60% of isolates when adding *cimetidine*. *Verapamil* completely reversed pre-existing resistance to below the cutoff point of 70 nM. Practical clinical application of these findings will be needed to determine whether such interactions can be put to practical use (24[c]).

Amodiaquine

While amodiaquine is related to chloroquine and considered generally equivalent to it, more recent studies have shown that amodiaquine is superior to chloroquine in tackling resistant strains of *falciparum malaria*. Because of its adverse effects, amodiaquine is no longer in use in the countries of the European Union or the USA, but remains in use in other areas, including Africa and Oceania (SEDA-18, 287).

The principle reason against recommending amodiaquine for malaria prophylaxis is the reporting of *agranulocytosis*, occasionally associated with *hepatitis* (SEDA-12, 241; SED-12, 692). An attempt was made to characterize the mechanism and conditions under which amodiaquine may bring about agranulocytosis. Amodiaquine is rapidly metabolized in the body to desmethyl-amodiaquine, a subsequent metabolite being quinonimin; this acts as a hapten and can initiate an immune response. Since specific IgG antibodies which lead to hemopathy and leukopenia can be detected, all this suggests that the agranulocytosis or hepatotoxicity is immune mediated.

It seems that it takes substantial doses for a couple of weeks to cause the adverse hematological effects (SEDA-16, 692; SEDA-17, 327). If this is correct amodiaquine still could be of use for short intensive courses of treatment in the presence of chloroquine resistance. Use in children of a dose of 35 mg/kg given over 3 days was studied by Raccurt et al. (SEDA-16, 306); in only one of the 69 children was the parasitemia not cleared. The tolerance was good except that a fairly high percentage of *conjunctival hyperemia* was noticed (SEDA-16, 306).

Gastrointestinal complaints (*nausea*, *vomiting*, *diarrhea* or *constipation*) are not uncommon (SED-11, 587).

Corneal and conjunctival changes, which included intralysosomal membranous and amorphous inclusions in the epithelial cells, as well as *abnormal retinal test responses* were reported in a man who received amodiaquine over a period of a year. Follow-up over the years after discontinuation of treatment showed a decrease in the abnormalities. There are no data as to possible retinal changes similar to those seen with chloroquine. Abnormal *pigmentation* of the palate, but also pigmentation of the nail beds and even the skin of face and neck, have been reported. The duration of such pigmentation after discontinuation of the drug is unknown. The effects on the nails resemble those seen with chloroquine (SED-12, 692; SEDA-12, 241).

Amopyroquin (ApQ)

Amopyroquin is a relatively new 4-aminoquinoline which is structurally related to Amodiaquine. Amopyroquin is not a new compound but is now of renewed interest as a result of the extensive occurrence of resistance to chloroquine and the side effects experienced with prophylactic amodiaquin. In a first clinical study involving 152 patients with malaria, the efficacy of a 12-mg/kg total dose, given as two 6-mg/kg intramuscular injections with a 24-hour interval, was described as good. All patients became apyretic and clearance of parasites on day 7 was obtained in 143 cases; the nine who retained a low level of parasitemia were all children. In 50% of the cases the *P. falciparum* had been chloroquine resistant. The drug was well tolerated, no major side effects being seen. Time will show the place of this 4-aminoquinoline in the therapeutic arsenal (25^C).

Mefloquine (Lariam; WR-142,490)

Mefloquine, a derivative of 4-quinoline methanol, is the product of the US Army's antimalarial research program. Mefloquine is a highly active schizontocide but is not gametocidal. It has been found active against chloroquine-resistant *falciparum* malaria, while it also has been found to have an excellent schizonticidal effect in the blood in experimentally induced *Plasmodium vivax* infections in volunteers. Clinical experience has shown that *Plasmodium vivax* infections can persist after successful treatment of the *falciparum* infection with other drugs; the fact that mefloquine is effective against both organisms is thus of practical importance (SED-12, 692).

Mefloquine is readily absorbed after oral administration; absorption is influenced by the tablet formulation and is more rapid from an aqueous solution. Maximum serum levels are seen after 1—4 hours. Resorption is hampered in the presence of diarrhea. The elimination half-life varies considerably and has been reported to lie between 6.5 and 22.7 days by one investigator, between 14.7 and 30 days by an other, and between 8 and 18 days by a third (SED-12, 692; SEDA-16, 308). Plasma protein binding is high. Clinically ill patients displayed a prolongation of the time needed to reach peak concentration and had significantly higher plasma levels in the first 2 days after administration of either the 750- or the 1500-mg dose (SEDA-16, 308). A study in children under the age of 5 demonstrated lower mefloquine plasma levels in those children who were still parasitemic on day 7. There was a higher incidence of vomiting among the children in this series (10%) but it is not clear whether this influenced the therapeutic result (SEDA-16, 308). Mefloquine is concentrated in the erythrocyte. Only about 5% of mefloquine is found unaltered in the urine over a period of 4 weeks; the drug is excreted predominantly in the feces and the bile. Five metabolites have been isolated, the inactive carboxylic acid metabolite being present in fairly high concentrations in plasma (SED-12, 692).

Mefloquine has a high cure rate after a single dose of 750—1000 mg. The use of combinations of mefloquine with other anti-malarials has been advocated in order to reduce the development of resistance. Mefloquine is effective as a prophylactic using a weekly dosage schedule, a dose of 250 mg being appropriate in adults. Because early reports also suggested that the drug was without serious side effects, mefloquine became widely advocated by various advisory bodies for prophylactic use, starting a week before travel to an endemic area where chloroquine resistance is common, and continuing for 4 weeks after departure from the area (SEDA-16, 306). Regrettably, but as might have been expected, it has also come into use for prophylaxis in areas where its use is unnecessary (SED-12, 692). Instances of mefloquine resistance were reported in Tanzania in 1983, in Thailand in 1989, and in Africa (Malawi) in 1991. Resistance to the combinations of mefloquine with sulfadoxine and pyrimethamine was reported in 1985 (SED-12, 692). The possibility of cross-resistance between mefloquine and halofantrine was raised in 1990 (SED-12, 692). At the present time there are very large areas, including Thailand, Cambodia, New Guinea, Laos and Myanmar where *P. falciparum* is resistant to mefloquine. High-dose mefloquine treatment has been tried in areas with mefloquine-resistant *P. falciparum*; a 25-mg/kg mefloquine dose has been found effective even in a multi-drug-resistant area.

ADVERSE REACTION PROFILE

Though mefloquine is generally well tolerated, particularly when used prophylactically, the list of adverse effects has grown with the accumulated experience. With therapeutic doses, e.g. 750—1000 mg up to 1500 mg given within 24 hours for the adult (20 mg/kg body weight in children) side effects are usually mild but with occasional occurrence of severe neuropsychiatric derangement. The overall incidence of side effects is about the same as with chloroquine, about 40—50%. Events most commonly reported include nausea, diarrhea, abdominal pain, dizziness, strange dreams and insomnia. Side effects were dose related with an increase in dizziness and gastrointestinal complaints and fatigue at higher dose levels.

Extensive acute, subacute and chronic studies of mefloquine in animal testing demonstrated that it was not phototoxic like some of the quinolone-methanols studied, nor was it *mutagenic*, *teratogenic* or *carcinogenic* in these studies (SED-12, 692).

ORGANS AND SYSTEMS

Cardiovascular *Sinus bradycardia* was seen in 18% of cases by Kofi-Ekue et al. (SED-12, 307), occurring some 4—7 days after drug administration; the bradycardia was asymptomatic and lasted about 3—4 days. Transient *sinus arrhythmias* were reported as well, again without a need for treatment (SED-12, 693), asymptomatic arrhythmia was also recorded in a dosage comparison trial (SEDA-16, 308).

Nervous system Neuropsychiatric reactions occur even on occasion during prophylactic use. *Headaches*, *dizziness*, *vertigo* and *light-headedness* are common (SED-12, 693; SEDA-16, 307), the incidence reported varying between 20 and 90%. Dizziness is to some extent dose related (26[C], 27[C]). *Ringing in the ears* and *vertigo* are less frequent complaints.

Less frequent still but of a much greater impact are the neuropsychiatric and neuro-vegetative reactions seen after the administration of mefloquine. At first thought to occur only after therapeutic doses of mefloquine it is now evident that these reactions do occur after prophylactic use as well. The incidence is estimated at about one in 13 000 with prophylactic use, but as high as one in 215 with therapeutic use (SEDA-17, 329). The combination with CNS active drugs may result in unpredictable reactions. The symptoms may vary in type and severity; *non-cooperation*, *disorientation*, *mental confusion*, *hallucinations*, *agitation* and *decreased consciousness*. An *acute psychiatric syndrome* with suicide attempt was reported in one case. A single dose can be all that is needed to evoke a mental reaction. The occurrence of *convulsions* was reported, with or without psychiatric symptoms; it seems that mefloquine can aggravate and perhaps even provoke, latent epilepsy (SED-12, 693; SEDA-16, 307; SEDA-17, 329).

A severe *psychiatric and neurological syndrome* with agitation, progressive delirium and generalized rigors was seen in a 47-year-old male after the first day of treatment with mefloquine, 750 mg followed by 500 and 250 mg in 24 hours. Because of aspiration, intubation and mechanical ventilation was required. An anticholinergic syndrome was suspected because of the persistence of stupor, rigors together with mydriasis, and hyperpyrexia. A dose of 2 mg of physostigmine was given intravenously and brought about an immediate improvement. It is of note that this patient had been treated with 750 mg of quinine and 450 mg of clindamycin t.i.d. for 5 days prior to the administration of the mefloquine (29[c]).

All reports indicate that the neuropsychiatric reactions to mefloquine are transient. There is some reason to think that they can be precipitated by alcohol (28[C]).

Endocrine A 30-year-old woman took mefloquine, 250 mg per week, and developed abdominal pain, palpitations and tremor; *thyroid function tests* were discovered to be abnormal. One month after withdrawal of the mefloquine, function tests had returned to normal (SEDA-18, 289).

Hematological *Agranulocytosis* was recorded in a 31-year-old male with *P. vivax* parasitemia given an initial dose of mefloquine followed by 500 mg 8 hours later. Mefloquine was the only drug used (SEDA-16, 307). There were no other reports of hematological toxicity.

Gastrointestinal Gastrointestinal complaints like *nausea*, *vomiting*, *abdominal discomfort* and (usually mild) *diarrhea* are mentioned in most reports, the incidence being given as 10–25% (SED-12, 693; SEDA-16, 307). The frequency increases with the use of higher doses, e.g. 25 instead of 15 mg/kg (27, 27).

Skin *Maculo-papular rash*, *urticaria* and *itching* have been reported; itching may be more common with mefloquine than with chloroquine. There are however isolated case reports concerning more serious skin conditions:

A 42-year-old male developed an *exfoliative dermatitis* while taking mefloquine prophylaxis. Three weeks before the onset of the rash he had used Naproxen (30[c]).

A 44-year-old male developed an itchy rash after the third dose of prophylactic mefloquine, later diagnosed as *cutaneous vasculitis* (SEDA-17, page 3).

A 23-year-old woman developed a bilateral facial rash, comprising raised *red lesions and flat bullae* after the second weekly dose of mefloquine (SEDA-17, 329).

A Stevens-Johnson syndrome-like condition was described in a 66-year-old woman during prophylactic therapy (SEDA-16, 307).

Special senses There has been no mention of either keratitis or retinal abnormalities such as are seen with some other antimalarials.

Interactions Mefloquine has been given in combination with other antimalarials with the aim of delaying the development of drug resistance. Combinations have been made on an empirical basis with pyrimethamine and sulfa drugs. There is however no known drug which has been proven to be synergistic with mefloquine, and mefloquine with its very long half-life time is difficult to match. The chemotherapeutic response of *P. berghei* to various combinations of mefloquine with other drugs (sulfadoxine-pyrimethamine, primaquine, floxacrine) have shown the desired effects to be purely additive (SED-12, 693), so the side effects too are probably only those of the individual compounds. Adverse reactions observed in the treatment of 400 patients with Fancimef (mefloquine, pyrimethamine and sulfadoxine) occurred in 45.8% of the patients. Of note were: dizziness (28.8%), nausea (9.5%), vomiting (7.3%), weakness/lassitude (5.8%), abdominal discomfort or pain (5.5%), diarrhea (3.8%), pruritus (3.0%), insomnia (2.0%) and headache (2.0%) (SED-12, 693).

The combination with *artesunate* seems to give improved tolerance for mefloquine and there is the suggestion of an synergistic effect.

As noted above, one case history suggests that the

combined use of *alcohol* and mefloquine may precipitate a neuropsychiatric reaction.

Second-generation effects Mefloquine prophylaxis was studied in a group of 339 pregnant women on the Thai-Burmese border in a double-blind placebo-controlled trial. Mefloquine gave 86% or better protection against *P. falciparum* at that time. According the conclusion there were no significant adverse effects, though transient dizziness was seen in some, and on first analysis both reduced birth weight in multigravida and raised infant mortality proved to be linked to maternal anemia rather than drug treatment. Further review of the data did however show some grounds for concern, since infants in the mefloquine group had a lower mean birth weight and a higher percentage with low birth weight. There was also a higher rate of stillbirths and congenital anomalies in the mefloquine class, though these differences were not statistically significant (31^{C}, 32^{R}).

Special risk groups Airline pilots should not be put on routine prophylaxis with mefloquine because of the (small) risk of neuropsychiatric reactions.

Overdosage Accidental ingestion of 5.25 grams of mefloquine over 6 days by a 36-year-old woman induced vertigo, difficulty in visual accommodation, myalgia, hypotension and tachycardia. Most of the anomalies disappeared in 2 weeks (SEDA-16, 307).

Piperaquine

Piperaquine is a synthetic 4-aminoquinoline with a high blood schizontocidal activity similar to that of chloroquine. Field studies were carried out in China. There is some evidence that piperaquine is active against chloroquine-resistant *falciparum* malaria but laboratory studies do suggest a degree of cross-resistance. Piperaquine in a dose of two 300-mg tablets per month was well tolerated. Reported side-effects comprise *headache*, *dizziness*, *vomiting* and *diarrhea* (SED-12, 693).

Triperaquine and dabequine

These are both 4-aminoquinoline derivatives, the adverse reaction patterns of which are as yet unknown. Dabequine appeared however in early studies to have shown cross-resistance with chloroquine. The WHO Scientific Group's report concerning these drugs dates from 1984 and there seems to be little or no newer information on them.

Primaquine and congeners (8-aminoquinolines)

The 8-aminoquinolines were the first synthetic antimalarials to be introduced into medicine. Pamaquine (plasmochin) was the first to be marketed in 1926, but primaquine proved to have the highest chemotherapeutic index of the many compounds tested. Primaquine is rapidly absorbed, extensively distributed and predominantly cleared by non-renal elimination. The principal metabolite is carboxyprimaquine. While primaquine itself is rapidly eliminated from plasma, the drug is clinically effective when given once daily or even once weekly (SED-12, 693). The pharmacokinetics in children, pregnant women, or patients with renal or hepatic dysfunction are unknown.

Primaquine is mainly used to eradicate the exo-erythrocyte stages of *P. vivax* and *P. ovale* which if untreated cause late relapse (SEDA-18, 287).

Primaquine base used in a dose of 0.5 mg/kg daily in the prophylaxis of *falciparum* and *vivax* malaria for a year did not cause noteworthy side effects. General complaints in the study were less than seen in the placebo group but about the same as seen in man treated with chloroquine (92^{c}). None of the volunteers (smokers or non-smokers) had a methemoglobin level greater then 13% (92^{c}).

Experience as a whole shows that primaquine and its congeners are also, as a rule, well tolerated in therapeutic doses. The main reactions are gastrointestinal; mild to moderate *abdominal cramps* and occasional *gastric distress* are experienced.

Mild *anemia*, *methemoglobinemia* and *leukocytosis* have been mentioned occasionally, as well as a very occasional case of *agranulocytosis*; the latter is usually associated with overdosage.

Primaquine and its congeners may induce *hemolytic anemia* in persons with glucose-6-phosphate dehydrogenase (G6PD) deficiency. The effects are more pronounced in the B-type (the Mediterranean type) than in the A-type G6PD. In a case reported in 1989 involving a 28-year-old Thai soldier (SEDA-16, 308) G6PD deficiency was not mentioned, but four cases reported in Vanuta in 1992 (SEDA-17, 328) all had G6PD deficiency; all four developed acute intravascular hemolysis resulting in anemia, hemoglobinuria and systemic illness after a single dose of the drug.

Severe *mental depression* and *confusion* was reported in one case; all symptoms disappeared on discontinuation of the drug; the patient had been treated with chloroquine beforehand (SED-11, 588).

Interactions The combination of primaquine with *clindamycin* is currently used as an agent of second choice for the treatment or prevention of *Pneumocystis carinii* pneumonia. If the patient has been treated immediately beforehand with *dapsone*, methemoglobinemia may result.

Pentaquine

Another 8-aminoquinoline in common use has a pattern of adverse reactions very similar to that of primaquine.

WR-238605

WR-238605 is a further 8-aminoquinoline derivative developed by the Walter Reed Army Institute for Research. It was found to be more active than primaquine (SED-12, 694). Details of its adverse reaction pattern are still unknown, and one must assume that it has been little used.

Proguanil

Proguanil is currently one of the antimalarial drugs most widely used for prophylactic purposes. A biguanide, it is rapidly absorbed in standard doses and mainly excreted via the urinary system. The antimalarial effect is due to its metabolite cycloguanil. This metabolism of proguanil has however been shown to vary individually, and this may be reflected in a variable degree of efficacy (SED-17, 328).

No serious side effects have been reported in otherwise healthy patients (SED-12, 694; SEDA-17, 328). *Skin rashes* may occur. *Hair loss* has been reported. The development of *mouth ulcers* was mentioned as well as *abdominal discomfort* and *vomiting*. A recent study showed the incidence of mouth ulcers in a group of soldiers to be 24% in those receiving proguanil only and 37% in those receiving proguanil 200 mg plus either 300 or 150 mg chloroquine weekly (SED-12, 694). With the use of large doses *hematuria* has been seen.

The urinary excretion path may mean that caution is advisable when treating patients with renal disorders. Two patients with renal insufficiency indeed became severely ill on standard doses of proguanil. One developed *anorexia*, *dizziness*, *vomiting*, *diarrhea*, *mouth ulcers*, *a low white cell count* and a *low platelet count*. The other developed extensive *purpura*, *epistaxis* and *vomiting*. Bone marrow studies demonstrated hypoplasia and gross megaloblastic changes. The relationship of these findings to the proguanil therapy is nevertheless questionable, and if the drug was causative the mechanism is not understood. While it is tempting to seek an explanation in the fact that these biguanides interfere with (plasmodial) folate synthesis; the serum folate and vitamin B_{12} levels were normal in both patients (SED-12, 694).

Pyrimethamine

Pyrimethamine is the most active antimalarial in a series of 2-4-diaminopyrimidines, its effect being due to inhibition of the conversion of folic acid in its active form folinic acid. It is also effective in toxoplasmosis. The drug's antiprotozoal and antimalarial activity is enhanced by the addition of sulfonamides. Pyrimethamine is well absorbed in healthy subjects, with maximal plasma concentrations reaching a peak in 2–6 hours; the subsequent decline of serum levels is slow with a half-life of 80–95 hours (SED-12–694). The absorption after intramuscular injection is slower; this may be of importance in patients with reduced muscle blood flow (SEDA-17, 328). Pyrimethamine does penetrate into the cerebro-spinal fluid.

ADVERSE REACTION PATTERN

With the usual antimalarial prophylactic dosage of 25 mg per week reactions are generally slight or absent. With intensive treatment in high cumulative doses, as employed in the treatment of toxoplasmosis, gastrointestinal intolerance, neurological symptoms and depression of hematopoiesis may occur.

Hypersensitivity reactions These do not appear to occur.

Tumor-inducing effects have not been reported.

ORGANS AND SYSTEMS

Nervous system High doses of pyrimethamine may cause rapid development of neurological symptoms such as *ataxia*, *tremors* and *convulsions*. This is probably a direct toxic effect (SED-11, 588).

Respiratory A case of non-cardiogenic *pulmonary edema* was reported with the use of pyrimethamine alone (SED-12, 694).

Hematological *Leukopenia*, *agranulocytosis* and *thrombopenia* have been reported and, as might be expected in view of the drug's folate antagonism, *megaloblastic anemia*. The latter is, not surprisingly, more common when high doses are used or pyrimethamine is given in combination with a drug such as trimethoprim. The bone marrow depression can be reversed using folic acid (SEDA-18, 287). *Pancytopenia* has been reported following the use of pyrimethamine alone but is more often the result of its use in combination with dapsone or sulfonamides (SED-11, 589; SEDA-14, 241; SED-17, 328). In combination with the blood dyscrasias, *fever* and *lymphadenopathy* have been reported.

Although the hematological complications are generally a consequence of therapeutic use, long-term prophylactic treatment with pyrimethamine and dapsone in malaria could well involve an increased risk of megaloblastic anemia in patients whose nutritional state is not optimal (SED-12, 694).

Liver Minor increases in *transaminase levels* have been found when these were looked for.

Gastrointestinal Gastric tolerance is dose dependent. The high doses used in the treatment of toxoplasmosis were reported to lead to *abdominal pains*, *vomiting* and *dizziness*. *Gastrointestinal bleeding* related to thrombocytopenia was also reported (SED-11, 589).

Skin Skin *rashes* are uncommon. A *lichen planus* type skin reaction has been described. *Photosensitivity* has been attributed to pyrimethamine treatment.

Risk situations Pyrimethamine should not be given to patients with depleted folic acid reserves.

Second-generation effects Pyrimethamine is an inhibitor of dihydrofolate reductase and induces tetrahydrofolate deficiency. In animal experiments, pyrimethamine has been shown to be teratogenic. In rats it produces limb defects, cleft palate and brachygnathia, and in chick embryo's micromelia. Fetal death was seen in rats and hamsters. Treatment for toxoplasmosis with pyrimethamine, with or without sulfonamide, has however been given to pregnant women without evidence of subsequent abnormalities. Supplementation of such treatment with folic acid has been advocated to prevent or reduce adverse effects (SED-12, 695), but it is not known if this could impair efficacy.

Pyrimethamine + dapsone (12.5 mg + 100 mg = Maloprim; 25 mg + 100 mg=Deltaprim)

The combination of these drugs causes a higher incidence of *blood dyscrasias* than seen with pyrimethamine alone; in particular the occurrence of the agranulocytosis increases and a number of fatalities have been reported (SED-12, 695; SEDA-18, 287).

Dapsone (alone or in combination with pyrimethamine) may cause *methemoglobinemia* and *hemolytic anemia*. These complications tend to be dose dependent and are more frequently encountered in G6PD-deficient subjects (SEDA-18, 287).

When the pyrimethamine-dapsone combination was used in the prophylaxis of *P. carinii* pneumonia in AIDS patients (173) clinical anemia was seen in about 20% (35) of cases, and in all 117 cases where data were available serum haptoglobin levels had dropped (SEDA-18, 287).

A '*dapsone syndrome*' was reported in a 30-year-old female treated with Maloprim and chloroquine base 300 mg once weekly after 4 weeks. The symptoms comprised fever, joint and muscle pain, dry cough and diffuse red urticarial rash, followed by generalized lymphadenopathy and a painful exudative tonsillitis and a prominent atypical lymphocytosis.

Maloprim given for antimalarial prophylaxis was associated with *immunosuppression*. In a study of military personnel in Singapore the incidence of upper respiratory tract infections was 64% higher than in the non-treated group.

A *stillborn* male infant with a severe defect of the abdominal and thoracic wall and a missing left arm was delivered at 26 weeks to a woman who used Maloprim on days 10, 20 and 30 after conception (SED-11, 589). The case is anecdotal and the relationship to medication uncertain.

In Britain, the retrospective reported rate for serious reactions with Maloprim was 1 in 9100, the incidence of blood dyscrasias being 1 in 20 000. These figures are lower than those reported with Fansidar (SEDA-16, 309).

Pyrimethamine 25 mg + sulfadoxine 500 mg (Fansidar)

The combination of these two drugs, while effective in the prevention and treatment of *falciparum* malaria, carries a high frequency of side effects; hematological and, more especially, serious cutaneous adverse reactions occur, but there are also incidents of polyneuritis, vasculitis and hepatic toxicity. Most of the severe cutaneous adverse reactions and the cases of vasculitis developed within less then 1 month of instituting treatment (SED-12, 695). The use of Fansidar for malaria prophylaxis has been virtually abandoned on account of the side effects, including the frequency of severe cutaneous reactions. Fansidar is however increasingly used for the treatment of *falciparum* malaria in Africa. With the higher dosage used for that purpose an increase in side effects, particularly hematological, can be expected. In Britain the retrospective reported rate for all serious reactions to Fansidar was found to be 1 in 2100 prescriptions and for cutaneous reactions 1 in

4900 prescriptions, the fatality rate being 1 in 11 100 (SEDA-16, 309).

Respiratory *Dyspnea* and *pleurisy* have been described. Of 52 travellers with adverse reactions to Fansidar recorded in Sweden, six had *pulmonary infiltrates* accompanied by fever (SEDA-13 241). Such pulmonary infiltrates have also been described in the past, and in one case the diagnosis of *eosinophilic infiltration* was made (SED-11, 590). A case of *non-cardiogenic pulmonary edema* was reported in 1989 (SED-12, 695).

Hematological The hematological adverse effects are largely those known from pyrimethamine, i.e. *leukopenia*, *agranulocytosis*, *thrombocytopenia* and *pancytopenia*, but the literature gives the impression that when using the combination these effects are more marked, with lower cell counts. Severe *megaloblastic anemia* was described as well. A *hemolytic-uremic syndrome* was reported in a 24-year-old male with a G6PD deficiency (SEDA-18, 288).

Liver Liver function abnormalities occur, varying from elevation of *serum transaminase* levels to more marked disturbances with *jaundice* and proven *granulomatous hepatitis*. An occasional case of fatal *hepatic failure* has been reported; this was the case in a young American white female who had taken three doses of Fansidar with chloroquine before traveling to Ecuador (SEDA-12, 242). Hepatic symptoms may be part of a vasculitis syndrome or can be seen in association with cutaneous reactions (SEDA-13, 241).

Skin Severe cutaneous adverse reactions (SCAR) have been reported from various countries. These included *erythema exudativum multiforme*, *Stevens-Johnson syndrome*, *toxic epidermal necrolysis*, *cutaneous vasculitis* and further a variety of *rashes*, *lichen planus*, a single case of *ectodermosis pluriorificialis* and some cases of *photosensitivity*. The incidence of such reactions seems to vary regionally with a low incidence in Switzerland and a high incidence reported by the US Centers for Disease Control. The latter group reported cutaneous reactions in 1:5000—1:8000 cases with fatal cutaneous reaction in 1:10 000—1:25 000 users (SEDA-12, 242). In Britain the retrospective reporting rate for all serious reactions was found to be 1:2100 and for cutaneous reactions 1:4900 prescriptions, with a fatality rate of 1:11 100 (SEDA-16, 309).

Other adverse reactions General *vasculitis* was reported in two cases in Sweden, one developed fever, jaundice, orchitis and gastrointestinal bleeding after 2 weeks of treatment, the other cutaneous vasculitis and rapid progressive nephritis after 3 weeks (SEDA-13, 241). An illness resembling the *Sézary syndrome* was seen after combined treatment with chloroquine, 150 mg every third day (total seven tablets), and Fansidar, one tablet weekly (total six tablets); the symptoms comprises fever, diarrhea, erythrodermia, jaundice, general lymphadenopathy and hepato-splenomegaly (SED-12, 696). *Exudative erythema multiforme* with a chronic proliferation of the conjunctiva causing *blindness* was described in a 24-year-old male who had taken one tablet of Fansidar at 6-day intervals on three occasions (SEDA-16, 309).

Risk factors Sulfonamide and or pyrimethamine sensitivity, pregnancy and G6PD deficiency are accepted contraindications. Use in young infants is considered inadvisable; the case history of an 8-month-old infant with *P. falciparum* malaria who developed high fever, tachycardia, hypotension, chills, jaundice and splenomegaly 48 hours after a single parenteral dose of Fansidar (SEDA-16, 309) seems to confirm the wisdom of this advice. It has been advocated that Fansidar should not be used prophylactically if exposure to malaria will last less then 3 weeks, in view of the incidence of severe cutaneous effects during the first month.

Interactions The combined use of Fansidar with *chloroquine* seems to result in more severe adverse reactions.

The concomitant use of *folinic acid* might be expected to reduce the effectiveness of the drug.

Both pyrimethamine and sulfonamides are liver enzyme inhibitors which may lead to interactions with drugs normally metabolized in the liver.

Pyrimethamine 25 mg + sulfadioxine 500 mg + mefloquine 250 mg (Fansimef)

The side effects characteristic of all three components can be expected.

Pyrimethamine + trimethoprim

With this combination the risk of *megaloblastic anemia* seems to be higher than with the use of pyrimethamine alone, which on theoretical grounds might be expected. Concomitant administration of folic acid has been recommended (SED-11, 590), but the effect on efficacy of adding folic acid to the medication is not known.

Pyrimethamine + clindamycin

Pyrimethamine 50 mg/day has recently been used in combination with clindamycin for the treatment of toxoplasmic encephalitis in AIDS. Side effects were common (*rash*, *diarrhea*, *nausea*), but the incidence of hematological reactions was lower than that seen with the combination of sulfadiazine and pyrimethamine (SEDA-16, 309).

Pyrimethamine + clarithromycin

Clarithromycin, a macrolide, and other macrolide and lincosamine antibiotics (azithromycin, clindamycin, spiramycin and roxitramycin) have been used in combination with pyrimethamine in the treatment of *Toxoplasma gondii* infections, especially cases of toxoplasma encephalitis.

The combination with clarithromycin was studied in a small group of AIDS patients with encephalitis, using 2 grams clarithromycin and 75 mg of pyrimethamine per day for 6 weeks. The side effects were many and severe; severe *thrombopenia* but also *anemia* and *neutropenia*, *liver toxicity* of varying degree, *nausea*, *vomiting*, *skin rashes* and *hearing loss* were found in two out of three patients tested in a group of 13.

The dose of clarithromycin given in the above study was the maximum dosage used in an earlier investigation of the treatment of mycobacterial infections in HIV-infected patients (SED-12, 696).

There has been no mention of this combination in some more recent reviews.

Quinine

Quinine has once again become the drug of first choice for malaria originating in areas with multiresistant *Plasmodium falciparum*. To be effective, quinine plasma concentrations greater than the minimal inhibitory level must be achieved and maintained. Quinine given orally is well absorbed and shows a rapid distribution phase and an elimination $T_{1/2}$ of about 11 hours. Clearance is predominantly by hepatic metabolism, urinary clearance accounting for only 20% of the total. Information on pharmacokinetics observed in healthy volunteers may however be misleading since plasma quinine levels are higher in the presence of malaria infection than in healthy subjects given the same dose (SED-12, 696). The dosage regimen needs to be adapted to the severity of the illness and amended as improvement occurs. General and toxic reactions are connected with the dosage used and side effects are common with a plasma level above 10 μg/ml. Studies in patients indicated that the dose often recommended, 10 mg/kg intravenously over 10—20 minutes, may be to high in patients with cerebral malaria (SEDA-14, 240). In the USA, intravenous administration of quinine has been discontinued in favour of quinidine (SEDA-17, 329).

In some areas, a high rate of recrudescence is seen after short-term treatment with quinine. The addition of specific antibiotics may improve the cure rate.

ADVERSE REACTION PATTERN

General and toxic reactions Overdosage may cause marked complaints of gastrointestinal intolerance, central nervous system disturbances, especially vertigo, visual disorders (very occasionally involving sudden blindness) and cardiovascular problems connected with the interference with intracardiac conduction. A major risk with quinine is that of direct intravenous injection which is given too fast. The prolonged use of normal or low doses of quinine may lead to ‘cinchonism’ in sensitive persons; this in mild form consists of ringing in the ears, headaches, nausea and some visual disturbances (SED-12, 696).

Hypersensitivity reactions These are not uncommon. They are usually limited to fever and rashes but angioneurotic edema and asthma has been seen. Thrombocytopenic purpura and thrombopenia are, at least in some cases, caused by an allergic reaction and the amounts of quinine present in some ‘tonics’ are sufficient to trigger the thrombopenic reaction in such patients. Anaphylactic shock has been reported in rare instances (SED-12, 696).

Tumor-inducing effects have not been reported.

ORGANS AND SYSTEMS

Cardiovascular *Atrio-ventricular conduction disturbances* may occur. In sensitive patients such changes may occur with normal dosage given over a prolonged period of time; in most cases cardiac effects are however the consequence of overdosage. *Electrocardiographic changes* such as prolongation of the QT interval and widening of the QRS complex, as well as T-wave flattening, can be seen with plasma levels above 15 μg/ml (SED-11, 590; SEDA-14, 239). An 8-year-old child given an incorrect dose of quinine sustained *ventricular tachycardia* and *status epilepticus* 48 hours after start of treatment; on admission the plasma quinine level was found to be 19.8 mg/l (SEDA-18, 288), compared with an accepted therapeutic range of 1.9—4.9 mg/l.

Respiratory An allergic *asthmatic reaction* may occur. Quinine poisoning can lead to *respiratory depression*.

Nervous system *Tinnitus* and *vertigo* are not uncommon effects, especially at the higher dosages. *Headache* and *tinnitus* are seen with cinchonism. Intoxication may be followed by *convulsions* and *coma*. A more general *organic brain syndrome* was observed in a 24-year-old woman with tropical malaria after the third day of treatment with quinine sulfate 500 mg t.i.d.; the symptoms comprised headache, blurred vision, vertigo, tinnitus, impaired hearing and, with ongoing treatment, increasing apathy, disorientation, speech changes and incoherent thinking and disorientation with respect to time and place. Recovery followed the discontinuation of the quinine therapy (SEDA-16, 305). A quinidine-induced *myopathy* has been reported in the past.

Endocrine, metabolic Clinical signs and symptoms of *hypoglycemia* are reported once in a while; most cases are subclinical, but severe cases have been described (SED-12, 697). A study of the effect of quinidine on the homeostasis of glucose, carried out in Thai volunteers with malaria demonstrated a near doubling of plasma insulin concentrations with a corresponding fall in serum glucose levels. An additional factor may have been impaired nutritional status and the effects of parenteral quinine in a severely ill patient, who is not taking food (SED-12, 697; SEDA-12, 243; SEDA-14, 240; SEDA-18, 288).

Hematological *Thrombocytopenia* is a regularly reported side effect with quinine. It is probably an allergic rather than a toxic effect since even the ingestion of minimal amounts of quinine, such as are present in commercial tonic waters, can cause an episode of thrombocytopenic purpura. A drug—antibody complex has been demonstrated in the past (SED-11, 591).

Acute intravascular *hemolysis* with renal involvement and even renal failure is known with quinine usage; again the reaction may follow relatively small doses of quinine. Quinine-induced hemolysis has probably played a role in the clinical syndrome of *black water fever* in the past. In a number of cases with quinine-induced thrombocytopenia there was autoantibody binding to the glycoprotein (GP) 1b-IX, 11b and 111a complexes. In three published cases quinine-dependent autoantibodies to GP 1b-IX and 11b/111A were associated with both thrombocytopenia and a *hemolytic-uremic syndrome* (SEDA-16, 305; SEDA-17, 329). In two further cases, women were described with a recurrent febrile illness characterized by *hypotension*, *pancytopenia*, *coagulopathy* and *renal failure* and both had high titers of quinine-dependent antibodies which showed cross-sensitivity with quinidine. In one case there was a connection with the drinking of tonic water, while the other woman had used a quinine sulfate tablet prescribed for leg cramps before each episode (33^{Cr}). A list of nine earlier published cases with antibody findings was added to these two case histories.

The combination of *renal failure* with *cortical necrosis*, *thrombopenia*, *intravascular coagulation* and *deposition of fibrin* was seen in a 63-year-old woman after the drinking of tonic water. Her prior history showed two other episodes of acute renal failure also connected with the ingestion of quinine-containing drinks; this most certainly reflects a hypersensitivity reaction (SED-12, 697).

Liver A case of *granulomatous hepatitis* in a patient taking quinine sulfate for night cramps was reported. A *cholestatic liver disorder* was reported in another case. This patient too had been treated with quinine for night cramps (SED-12, 697). Except for the occasional anecdotal case history there is no evidence that true hepatotoxicity occurs with quinine.

Gastrointestinal *Nausea* and *abdominal pain* may occur. With high doses *diarrhea* has been seen.

Urinary system *Renal damage* is seen accompanying hemolysis (see above). Renal failure in cases of quinine poisoning is probably due to circulatory collapse. Hypersensitivity reactions underlie at least some cases of renal impairment. The picture can be complex with the renal failure coming in association with cortical necrosis, thrombopenia, intravascular coagulation and deposition of fibrin.

Skin *Rashes* are a common feature of allergic reactions. *Photosensitivity induced* by quinine has been reported. Some of the cases reported occurred in elderly persons taking quinine for night cramps. Another form of hypersensitivity to quinine is *cutaneous neutrophilic vasculitis* which is a form of photosensitivity (SEDA-16, 305). Local *pigmentation* following intramuscular injection has been described (SEDA-12, 243).

Special senses *Eyes* *Amaurosis* connected with damage to the retina is most common with high plasma levels and thus following high dosage and especially overdosage. The outdated, but still practised, use of quinine to induce abortion is probably the most common cause. Quinine initially affects the photoreceptor and ganglion cell layers; retina vascular changes are a secondary phenomenon. Clinically a first sign may be widely dilated pupils still responding to light; later, visual field contraction and loss of vision can occur. In milder cases vision may return but possibly with a residual disturbance of dark adaptation and/or restricted visual fields. Loss of vision can however be permanent. In those cases suffering permanent damage, the classic late appearance of the fundus after quinine intoxication, with marked pallor and vascular narrowing, appears after some months (SED-12, 697). Loss of vision occurs mainly at serum concentrations of over 10 mg/l. Such concentrations are not thought to be toxic in patients with malaria, who have high circulating concentrations of α1-acid glycoprotein, resulting in a lower fraction of unbound drug in the plasma (SEDA-17, 329).

Ears A *ringing sound in the ears* (tinnitus) is a fairly frequent complaint and is not only seen after overdosage. Permanent impairment of hearing has long been thought to be a possible consequence of long-term use of quinine, but this belief has recently been challenged and the original description of it is questionable (SED-12, 697); the complication is certainly rare (90[R]).

When serial audiometry was performed in 10 patients receiving quinine treatment for acute *P. falciparum* malaria, a *reduction was found in high tone auditory acuity* in all patients, resulting in flattening of the audiogram. The onset of the effect was rapid and it resolved completely after completion of the treatment; only seven of these patients reported tinnitus. Hearing impairment was investigated in six volunteers after single doses of 5, 10 and 15 mg/kg quinine. A clear effect on hearing was found, but with a large variability (SEDA-17, 306).

Alteration or even loss of *smell* and *taste* has been mentioned.

Risk situations Treatment of *cerebral malaria* and to a lesser extent of patients *severely ill* with malaria with quinine has always been considered more risky than treatment of the common case of malaria. The changes in pharmacokinetics of quinine caused by the malaria provide an explanation: the standard dose of 10 mg/kg body weight is usually well tolerated in the patient with uncomplicated malaria but causes markedly higher plasma serum levels in the patient with cerebral malaria. Total quinine clearance and total apparent volume of distribution are significantly lower in this latter type of cases. After recovery the pharmacokinetics return to normal. Probably the first loading dose should be maintained at the level generally advised, but with a reduction in subsequent doses until the general condition has improved. Monitoring of plasma or red cell levels of quinine would of course be ideal but this luxury is seldom available (SED-12, 697).

The patient who is *allergic* to quinine is obviously at risk.

Second-generation effects Quinine crosses the placenta and can be found in relatively high concentrations in cord blood, it is also excreted in the breast milk. Data about possible teratogenicity related to the therapeutic use of malaria are scanty (SEDA-14, 239). Hypoplasia of the optic nerve and deafness have been reliably described in children born after failure to induce abortion with the drug.

Overdosage and acute intoxication Early symptoms of intoxication are unremarkable except for mild vision and hearing complaints. The principal sign is the sudden onset of bilateral pupil dilatation. Other symptoms are tinnitus, mild deafness, vertigo, mild drowsiness, vague disturbances of consciousness, headache, nausea, vomiting and abdominal pain. The electrocardiogram may show prolongation of the QT interval and ST wave abnormalities. Deafness may occur within hours or days of acute symptoms. Vision disturbances do not necessarily appear early. Acute intoxication can be seen after ingestion of doses of 4—12 grams, but a dose of 8 grams can prove lethal. Death is commonly caused by respiratory arrest, but is sometimes due to renal failure. Early treatment (forced diuresis, hemodialysis, acidification of urine and plasmapheresis) may prevent permanent visual damage.

Interactions Administration of quinine can result in augmentation of the action of *anticoagulants*, possibly by inhibition of prothrombin synthesis.

The interaction with *digitalis* is similar to that of quinidine (see Chapter 17).

Chloroquine has been reported to antagonize the anti-parasitic action of quinine against *Plasmodium falciparum* in vivo. However, no such evidence of antagonism was found in a clinical study in which Malawian children with cerebral malaria were treated with quinine. There was no difference in survival and rate of recovery in patients who had been given chloroquine as compared with those who had not taken chloroquine (SED-12, 698).

On theoretical grounds quinine should not be combined with *halofantrine*, since both drugs influence atrio-ventricular conduction. The combination of quinine with *clindamycin* was found to improve the cure rate after a short course of quinine (34[C]). The combination enhances parasite and fever clearance and it is of value in combating bacteremia, which according to the report in question is a common event in African children in the region of this study. According to the authors the increased cost of the medication would be equalized by a possible reduced hospitalization (35[C]).

The antimalarial effect of *tetracycline* is well known. The combination of quinine, 12 mg/kg every 12 hours plus doxycycline 2 mg/kg per dose × 6 also improved the cure rate (34, 35). However, none of the patients in this study taking quinine in combination with either clindamycin or tetracycline were suffering from a high grade resistant *falciparum* infection. The drawback of combining quinine with tetracycline is the longer period required for adequate treatment which in most cases demands supervision. The combination can be used in multi-resistant and mefloquine-resistant *falciparum* malaria (27). Tetracycline should preferably not be given to young children. When quinine is combined with *doxycycline*, the effects of the antibiotic itself may be enhanced.

Enzyme inhibitors like *cimetidine*, as well as *amiodarone* and *ketoconazole*, will tend to increase the toxicity of quinine or quinidine, while enzyme inducers such as rifampicin, will tend to reduce the toxic effects.

Quinidine interferes with the analgesic effect of *codeine*.

Quinoform

An injectable form of quinine can be prepared by preparing it as a lactate. Little has been published on the compound; the side effects can be expected to be the same as those of quinine itself.

Quinidine *(see also Chapter 17)*

Quinidine is at least as potent as quinine as an antimalarial but it tends to be more readily available in a form suitable for parenteral use when the need for injections arises. Quinidine is moderately well absorbed after oral administration with a mean bioavailabilty of 70—90%. Absorption is delayed in the presence of congestive heart failure.

The renal clearance of quinidine is only 15—40% and hepatic metabolism is the predominant route of elimination. As with quinine the metabolism of quinidine is altered in the presence of malaria, especially in severe cases, with prolongation of the half-life elimination time, reduction in systemic clearance and decrease in the apparent volume of distribution, proportional to the severity of the malaria infection. Overdosage may occur if this change in pharmacokinetics is not considered when determining dosages.

Quinidine has a more marked effect on the myocardium and the conduction time. It prolongs the refractory period. Intravenous quinidine is more likely to cause hypotension and may cause syncope and myocardial failure (see also Chapter 17). It should be used with care in the patient with a pre-existing cardiac condition and/or taking cardiac medication (SED-11, 592; SEDA-12, 243; 14).

Quinidine, like quinine, may cause hypoglycemia.

Interactions The combination of quinidine and *halofantrine* should be considered dangerous because both drugs interfere with atrioventricular conduction. The combination is likely to cause arrhythmias. (Also see quinine.)

Mepacrine (Quinacrine)

Mepacrine inhibits phospholipase A_2 and subsequently leukotrienes which are calcium ionophores. Mepacrine also has an inhibitory effect on phospholipase C and subsequent inositol phosphate formation which mobilizes cytosolic calcium from intracellular stores. It has been suggested that this might influence myocardial contractile function (SEDA-13, 241). The known side effects of mepacrine do not point to cardiac toxicity but problems could arise in the presence of a 'sick' myocardium.

ADVERSE REACTION PATTERN

General and toxic effects Following the administration of mepacrine in normal doses, adverse effects are usually limited to gastrointestinal upsets with nausea and sometimes vomiting. Yellow discoloration of the skin and conjunctiva is common but is usually considered more of a cosmetic problem.

Hypersensitivity reactions The aplastic anemia seen with the use of mepacrine may be caused by a hypersensitivity reaction.

Tumor-inducing effects These have not been reported with any degree of certainty, although mention has been made of squamous cell carcinomas in Australian servicemen who were treated with mepacrine for prolonged periods of time during the Second World War.

ORGANS AND SYSTEMS

Cardiovascular system Despite the theoretical considerations noted above, there has been no mention of cardiotoxicity in connection with the preventive use of mepacrine; when mepacrine was extensively used it was mainly in a younger age group, and the drug is little employed today.

Nervous system *Headaches* and complaints of *dizziness* are not uncommon with ordinary doses. Acute *psychosis* and signs of central nervous system *excitation* including *convulsions* have been seen with the use of large doses given parenterally in the treatment of malignancies (SED-11, 592). An acute transient psychosis (screaming, kicking and hallucinations) was seen in an 11-year-old boy 5 days after commencing the use of quinacrine 100 mg three times daily for *Giardia lamblia* infestation. Recovery occurred after discontinuation of the drug (SEDA-16, 309).

Hematological Mepacrine used in the prophylaxis of malaria may cause *aplastic anemia*. The incidence amongst soldiers during World War II was 2.84 per 100 000 as compared with only 0.66 per 100 000 in control groups. A skin rash or lichenoid eruption was often seen to precede the blood dyscrasia (SED-11, 593). More recently a case was reported in a 28-year-old woman given quinacrine, 100 mg po qd increased to 200 mg po qd for several months for the treatment of lupus erythematosus (SEDA-16, 309).

Liver Rare cases of *hepatitis* and even hepatic *necrosis* have been reported (SED-11, 593).

Gastrointestinal Complaints, if they occur, are usually mild.

Skin (*see also Hematological above*) Mepacrine causes a marked yellow *discoloration* of the skin and often also the conjunctiva. This is often combined with a blue-black discoloration of the palate and a curious discoloration of the nails which may be brownish-black, yellowish-green or sometimes white fluorescent in appearance. The phenomenon is related to the cumulative dose level, though it is occasionally also seen with short-term use. The discoloration disappears after discontinuation of the drug. Mepacrine-induced discoloration shows up under Wood's lamp as a brilliant yellow-green fluorescence of the nails and palms of the hands and also of the urine. Chronic *dermatosis* has been described after long-term use.

Skin changes attributed to mepacrine use include *lichen planus nodules*, *wart like growths*, *erosions* and *ulcerations*. The possibility of a relation to the incidence of squamous cell carcinoma was suspected in Australian ex-servicemen, but causality is not at all clear (SED-12, 699; SED-11, 593; SEDA-14, 241). A high sun exposure could be a factor and this would explain the difference in findings around the world.

Special senses Yellow *discoloration of conjunctiva and sclera* occurs. The corneal deposits and a mild diffuse cornea edema which may cause blurring of vision are reversible. There have been occasional reports of retinopathy. The effects resemble those seen with chloroquine (SED-11, 593). As a rule mepacrine is non-toxic to the retina (SEDA-14, 241).

Miscellaneous The local placing in the cornual portion of the fallopian tube of a 250 mg quinacrine pellet was found to cause necrosis of the epithelial lining and an acute inflammatory reaction with subsequent progressive fibrosis and occlusion of the lumen of the tube; in that particular study it was a desired effect (SEDA-16, 309).

WR-243251

This dihydroacridinedione is active in vitro against chloroquine-, mefloquine- and pyrimethamine-resistant malaria strains and is being developed further. By analogy to quinacrine and floxacrin there is concern about possible dermatological, cardiac and neuropsychiatric toxicity and vascular side effects. WR 243251 is under further development (8).

The endoperoxides

Artemisinin

The herb Qinghaosa (*Artemisea annua* L) has been known to Chinese medicine for centuries and was used in the treatment of fevers, in particular malaria fever; it is not clear why it did not become more widely used elsewhere in the world. In 1979 the Qinghaosu Antimalarial Co-ordinating Research group reported their experience with four formulations of qinghaosa in both *P. vivax* and *P. falciparum* malaria. Despite this, it is only in recent years that more has become known about the different preparations in existence (SED-12, 699; SEDA-17, 326; 36[R]).

The sesquiterpene lactone peroxide, artemisinin, is unique to the plant *Artemesia annua* L (Qinghoa). The plant can be grown in locations other than China, and field studies in propagating and growing the plant are now being carried out in many parts of the world (37[R]).

Artemisinic acid (qinghao acid), the precursor of artemisin, is present in the plant in a concentration up to ten times that of artemisinin.

Several semi-synthetic preparations have been developed on the basis of dihydroartemisinin (DHA) (36[R], 38).

Artesunate This is a water-soluble hemisuccinate derivative, is available in parenteral and oral formulation. The parenteral drug is dispensed as powdered artesunic acid. Neutral aqueous solutions are unstable. Artesunate is effective by the intravenous, intramuscular and oral routes in a dose of 10 mg/kg given for 5–7 days. The combination with mefloquine is very effective even against highly multi-resistant strains of *P. falciparum*; the combination must be given for at least 3 days.

Artemether Artemether is a methyl ether derivative

of DHA; the β-anomer is the more active. Artemether is dispensed in ampoules for intramuscular injection suspended in ground nut oil and in capsules for oral use. Like Artesunate and Artemisinin it has been used for both severe and uncomplicated malaria. Artesunate is probably faster acting than the other two.

Arteether This is the ethyl ether derivative of DHA. Arteether was the choice of the WHO for development; it was considered less toxic because one would expect it to be metabolized to ethanol rather than methanol. It is also more lipophilic than artemether, a possible advantage for accumulation in brain tissues. The β-anomer was chosen since it is a crystalline solid and relatively easy to separate from the α-anomer which is liquid; it was necessary to choose a single anomer because of the more complex rules for the development of a drug with two anomers in the United States.

All the three substances listed above are quickly hydrolyzed to the biological active substance dihydroartemisinin. In terms of parasite clearance. the artemisin derivatives produce a more rapid clinical and parasitological response than do other antimalarial drugs. There are no reports of significant toxicity, and as late as 1994 there was no convincing evidence of specific resistance, but chloroquine-resistant *Plasmodium berghei* is resistant to artemisinin as well (36[R]). The recrudescence rate is fairly high (39[R]).

The mode of action is not fully known. There is strong evidence that the antimalarial activity of these drugs is dependent on the generation of free radical intermediates; free radical scavengers such as ascorbic acid and vitamin E therefore antagonize the antimalarial activity.

Drug activation by iron and heme may explain why endoperoxides are selectively toxic to malaria parasites. The malaria parasites live in a surrounding of heme-iron (the erythrocyte is 95% hemoglobin, or 20 mM heme) which the parasite converts into insoluble hemozoin. Chloroquine, which binds heme, antagonizes the antimalarial activity of artemisinin.

In animal studies, high doses of Arteether and Arthemether have been associated with hematopoietic, cardiac and nervous system toxicity. Brewer et al. (40) reported some subclinical neurotoxicity, with a discrete distribution in the brain stems of rats and dogs after multiple (high) doses. Dogs given high doses (15 mg/kg arthemeter for 28 days) displayed a progressive syndrome of clinical neurological defects with terminal cardiorespiratory collapse and death. Further in vitro testing on fetal rat cells suggested a specific neuronal target. This in vitro toxicity was dose and time dependent (40, 41). There has been no evidence of neurotoxicity in man, but the human dosage of these ethers is of course lower, e g. with arteether 3.2 mg/kg on day one followed by 1.6 mg for a further 4 days.

Some impression of possible adverse effects in human subjects can be gained from a primarily pharmacokinetic study; in this study, arteether solution in sesame oil was given intramuscularly. Initially the effects of a single dose (from 0.3 up to 3.6 mg/kg weight) were tested in 23 subjects); thereafter multiple doses were studied (a first dose of 3.2 mg/kg followed by either 0.8 or 1.6 mg/kg per day given to 27 healthy volunteers over a period of 5 days). After multiple doses accumulation in plasma was demonstrated. The elimination half-life was shown to be 25—72 hours, with a rather wide spread. Adverse effects in these 23 subjects after the single dose comprised *local pain* in two, *bitter taste* and *dryness of the mouth* in one, and a mild but slightly itching *papular rash* that persisted for 14 days in one other subject. There were no changes in the biochemical parameters or the ECG. Similar adverse effects after the 5-day administration occurred in 14 of the 27 subjects; there was local pain in three, metallic taste in two, 'flu'-like symptoms in three, and a macular papular rash in two subjects which receded within 24 hours. One subject did develop shivering, clammy hands and feet, dizziness, headache, nausea and a metallic taste in the mouth, all lasting for about an hour, but the same reaction occurred after an injection of sesame oil only. Apart from some increase in eosinophil count in all groups, there were no significant hematological changes in this multiple-dose series. A slight *increase in SGOT and SGPT* levels was seen in one subject on day 6 and a marginal increase in SGPT in another on day 19. Low glucose levels, without symptoms, were recorded in two subjects after arteether but also in two after sesame oil injection. Transient *albuminuria* occurred in two cases. There were again no changes in the ECG or on neurological examination. There is a mention of audiometric tests having been done in five persons; in one a slight hearing loss was found in the ultrahigh tones but no details are given as to the dosage involved or the pretreatment status (42[C]).

Artesunate has been combined with mefloquine in areas with high multi-resistant *P. falciparum* in Thailand and the Thai-Burmese border. In the study reported in 1992 with a total of 127 patients who were followed for 28 days, group A received artesunate 100 mg immediately and thereafter 50 mg every 12 hours for 5 days (total 600 mg), Group M Received mefloquine 750 mg and another 500 mg 6 hours later. Group AM received first artesunate and after that course the two doses of mefloquine. Fever and parasite clearance

Table 3.

	M	A	AM
Total no. patients (m/f)	39/4	38/4	39/3
No. patients with 28-day follow-up	37	40	39
No. cured at 28 days	30 (81%)	35 (88%)	39 (100%)
Fever clearance time (h, mean)	69.7	35.1	37.5
Parasite clearance time (h)	63.5	35.9	37.5
Headache	17 (39)	14 (33)	12(28)
Dizziness	8 (18)	6 (14)	5 (11)
Nausea	9 (20)	6 (14)	9 (21)
Vomiting	7 (16)	8 (19)	11 (26)
Abdominal pain	1 (2)	2 (4)	1 (2)
Diarrhea	1 (2)	3 (7)	1 (2)
Itching and rash	0	3 (7)	1 (2)

Table 4.

	Artesunate n=31	Quinine + tetracycline n=33
Parasite clearance time (h)	36.5 (24–52)	73.2 (36–135
Cure rate on day 28 (%)	96.7	10
Nausea	14 (45)	20 (60)
Dizziness	16 (52)	16 (48)
Vomiting	8 (26)	30 (91)
Tinnitus	0	29 (88)
Convulsions	1 (3)	0
Bradycardia	7 (23)	not done

Figures in parentheses are percentages.

time were significantly shorter in the two groups treated with artesunate. Table 3 gives results and side effects.

The combination of artesunate and mefloquine was reported to be more effective then either drug given alone. However, the trial design was such that the patients receiving both drugs were in fact treated twice, so the findings do not prove synergism between the two drugs (43[C]).

In a second Thai study a group of 652 adults and children were treated with the combination of artesunate and mefloquine. A single dose of artesunate 4 mg/kg plus mefloquine 25 mg of base/kg gave a rapid response but did not improve cure rate. Artesunate given for 3 days in a total dose of 10 mg/kg plus mefloquine was 98% effective. The incidence of vomiting was reduced significantly by giving the mefloquine on day 2 of the treatment. There were no side effects attributed to artesunate (44[C]).

A further comparative clinical study between oral aresunate (700 mg over 5 days) on the one hand, and quinine (600 mg quinine sulfate at 8-hour intervals) plus tetracycline (250 mg at 6-hour intervals) for 7 days on the other, showed artesunate to be more effective and better tolerated in uncomplicated malaria (see Table 4).

The fact that convulsions occurred in one case was considered striking. Convulsions are uncommon in uncomplicated cases of malaria (45[C]).

Risk factors The demonstrated neurotoxicity in animals suggest that the artemesinin compounds should not be used for prolonged periods.

Interactions There appears to be a synergism between artemisinin and *mefloquine*. There seems to be antagonism between *chloroquine* and artemisinin.

Halofantrine

Halofantrine is a phenanthrene-methanol derivative of an amino alcohol, active against multiple-drug-resistant *falciparum* malaria. Developed as WR-171669 it was found to be very active in mouse screening tests; it was not phototoxic and it was effective in a single dose in Aotus monkeys with *falciparum* malaria. Halofantrine was known in World War II but was little used at that time. Preliminary pharmacokinetics studies performed later showed that halofantrine was slowly and incompletely absorbed with peak levels 3.5–6 hours after dosing. Resorption seemed to be unpredictable in the formulation used (SED-12, 699). Dose-finding studies showed treatment failures with one single dose but cures with two doses—one of 1000 mg and one of 500 mg. A regime using 500 mg at 6-hourly intervals was also effective. Three 500-mg doses at 6-hourly intervals were also used in a French study and treatment resulted in cure in semi-immune subjects. The dosage seemed to be insufficient in non-immune Caucasian patients.

Halofantrine is now available in a micronized form; early information suggested that this improved absorption, but two more recently published studies provide conflicting evidence. Fadat et al. (46[C]) used one half of the standard dose, Bouchaud et al. (47) the usual dose of 500 mg given three times with 6-hour intervals. Both studies show a wide range of serum levels of halofantrine and its main metabolite *N*-desbutyl-halofantrine but generally similar to those obtained with the older form. Taking the drug with food is thought to increase absorption.

Side effects of the doses originally recommended have in general been mild, no more than *nausea, diarrhea, headache and pruritus* (SED-12, 699; 46[C]–48[C]). Pruritus occurred markedly less often with halofantrine than with chloroquine (SEDA-16, 306). A comparison between high -dose chloroquine (35 mg/kg total in three daily doses) and halofantrine in standard dose (total 25 mg/kg given at 6-hour intervals) in patients between 4 and 14 years old showed a fairly similar frequency of adverse effects. Itching was a common side effect in the chloroquine group (48^{C}).

With the increase in multi-resistance, higher doses of halofantrine are now being used and for longer periods of time, and several incidents of cardiac complications have been reported (SEDA-18, 287). In 1993 the sudden *cardiac death* of a 37-year-old woman was reported after the ninth dose of halofantrine. A subsequent prospective study demonstrated that halofantrine was associated with a dose-related lengthening of the QT interval by more than 25% (SEDA-17, 328). Mefloquine did not cause such changes but the combination of mefloquine with halofantrine had a more pronounced effect on the ECG. However, in the region where this investigation was carried out (on the Thai-Burmese border area) thiamine deficiency is common and patients in this area have longer baseline QT intervals than usually reported (SEDA-17, 328). Two patients, mother and son, both with a congenital prolonged QT interval suffered sustained episodes of *torsades de pointes* ventricular tachycardia after a total dose of 1000 mg of halofantrine. *Arrhythmias* can occur but respond to propranolol (49^{C}). With peak levels of halofantrine in serum appearing about 6 hours after dosing, this is likely the most critical time for cardiac effects. Toivonen et al. (49^{C}) point out that several drugs lengthen the repolarization phase; they include phenothiazines, some antihistamines, cholinergics and antimicrobial agents, and if these have been taken this could set the stage for this uncommon side effect of halofantrine.

Halofantrine is not indicated for prophylactic use. Baudon et al. (SED-12, 700) however reported on the use of two doses of 1500 mg each in army personnel on the third and the tenth day following return to a non-malaria area. Only one in the 480 men had a *Plasmodium falciparum* malaria in the next 5 months. There were no side effects except for one case of a morbilliform rash possibly due to the halofantrine.

Risk factors Pre-existing *cardiac conduction abnormalities*, including those induced by other drugs (see above), are a definite risk. Due consideration should be given not only to the serum half-life of such drugs, but also to the tissue levels and total clearance of the agents involved.

Interactions Early laboratory studies indicated a cross-resistance with *mefloquine*, but in a later rodent model the cross-resistance was not absolute (SED-12, 700). Increased risk of arrhythmias when combined with quinine/quinidine or chloroquinine!

Pefloxin

This is one of the fluoroquinolone antibiotics which inhibits *P. falciparum* in vitro. Pefloxin is effective against *P. yoelii* infections in mice. In human subjects it was tested in a dosage of 400 mg every 12 hours for 3 days against chloroquine-resistant *falciparum* infections in Madagascar and this treatment schedule proved successful in nine out of 22 cases; seven further cases responded at first but recrudescence followed. The use of pefloxin as a complementary drug rather than as a primary antimalarial drug was suggested by the investigators.

Side effects are those of the fluoroquinolones. A review of the entire group of the fluoroquinolones, dealt with primarily in the antibiotic section of this volume, shows that these drugs are generally well tolerated. *Gastrointestinal* complaints occur in some 3–6%, and have included (in declining order) nausea, abdominal discomfort, vomiting and diarrhea. *Colitis* with *Clostridium difficile* infection has been reported infrequently after quinolone therapy. Symptoms referable to the *nervous system* have been less common; mention has been made of headaches, dizziness, agitation, sleep disturbances and, more rarely, seizures, delirium and hallucinations. *Allergic* reactions have been infrequent. With perfloxacin *photosensitivity reactions* were reported. The quinolones may cause *cartilage erosions* in weight bearing joints in young growing animals, and the long-term use of perfloxacin in growing children, such as would be required for prophylaxis, should be avoided (SED-12, 700). In bacteria which have developed resistance to fluoroquinolones, a cross-resistance with chemically unrelated antibiotics such as tetracycline and chloramphenicol is possible; when using perfoxacin instead of tetracycline in malaria the physician should be on the look-out for this phenomenon.

Ciprofloxacin, another of the fluoroquinolones, does have an inhibitory effect on *P. falciparum*, but it proved to be ineffective in a small clinical study, the red cell concentration being below the levels required for a 50% growth inhibition. Other fluoroquinolones are being tested.

Pentoxifylline

This methylxanthine, more widely known for its disputed use in cerebrovascular disorders (see Chapters 1 and 19) can protect mice infected with *Plasmodium berghei* from developing cerebral malaria.

As yet there is little human experience in its use for this purpose. Since pentoxifylline belongs to the group of vasoactive drugs it may influence blood pressure, but the main side effect is nausea and further flushing. The case history of a 34-year-old negro with a 16% parasitemia with *Plasmodium falciparum* and clinically cerebral malaria, treated with pentoxifylline 10 mg/kg/day in addition to quinine suggests that pentoxifylline may be of therapeutic value in cerebral malaria in men (SED-12, 700). In an open randomized controlled trial in which 56 children with cerebral malaria participated, the effects of pentoxifylline were tested. The 26 children who received pentoxifylline 10 mg/kg/day by continuous infusion had significantly shorter comas than the controls. The pentoxifylline recipients showed a trend towards a lower mortality, with a borderline significant difference. Pentoxifylline exerted an inhibitory effect on the synthesis of tumor necrosis factor. The better outcome in the treated group was associated with a decline in TNF serum levels on the third day of treatment in a few subjects; this was not seen in the controls (50[C]).

Malaria vaccine

For centuries attempts have been made to find a vaccine against malaria, especially malaria tropica. Most of these attempts have been costly yet unsuccessful. In 1987 however Pattaroyo et al. in Colombia conducted successful preliminary tests with a synthetic *falciparum* vaccine (12[R]). The results of a number of field studies have now been reported. SPf66 vaccine is a synthetic polypeptide based on pre-erythrocyte and asexual blood stage proteins of *P. falciparum*. In the first studies, carried out in Colombia, the vaccine proved to bring about an immune response and side effects were minimal. The first randomized double blind controlled trial in Colombia, in which 1548 Colombian volunteers participated, showed an overall efficacy of 39%. In a small selected group of volunteer soldiers a protective effect of 60—80% was attained. In 96% of cases there were no side effects and the side effects noted in the remainder were mainly localized erythema, discomfort and sometimes induration (16, 17). A study in Ecuador demonstrated 66.8% mean prophylactic efficacy against *P. falciparum*, but the 95% confidence interval was 2.7—89.3%. The vaccine was administered in three doses, at zero time and after 30 and 180 days. Side effects (local pain, erythema and local induration) occurred after the first dose in 6.2%, after the second dose in 19.4%, and after the third dose in 13.9%. The placebo group showed similar side effects but in a lower proportion of subjects and with fewer cases of induration. There was no protection against *P. vivax* infections (15). In the Venezuelan study 1442 villagers were vaccinated and vaccination was completed with the three doses in 976 subjects, while there was a comparison group of 938 subjects from the same area. Again the production of antibodies against the vaccine could be shown. The side effects were as in earlier work, but some contralateral induration was also noted, mainly after the third dose of vaccine, which was given alternately into the left and right arms. Five women experienced a generalized *pruritus*. Bronchospasm has been observed in one case (18). A trial in Tanzania, in an area were malaria is not only endemic but the parasite load heavy, showed an estimated efficacy of 30% (95% confidence interval 0—52%; p=0.046). The vaccine was immunogenic. There was also a difference in mortality between the groups, with one death amongst the vaccinated children and five in the control group. Side effects were in general mild and similar to those in earlier work (13, 14).

DRUGS USED IN THE TREATMENT OF *PNEUMOCYSTIS CARINII* INFECTIONS

Pneumocystis carinii pneumonia (PCP) is a serious infection with a mortality approaching 100%, if untreated. PCP is seen commonly in patients with AIDS and may be the first indication that the condition exists. It can occur in any immune compromised patient and it is seen in patients with cancer, especially during cancer chemotherapy or use of immunosuppressive drugs. Masur (51[R]) points out that the incidence of PCP in a given clinic fluctuates considerably over time in a manner that suggests person to person transmission.

Several drugs and drug combinations have been and are being tried in treatment and prophylaxis of *P. carinii* infections. Table 5 gives the relative potency of 10 drugs with anti-*P. carinii* activity as found in an animal model (52).

When treating patients, it can be difficult to distinguish between the symptoms of the primary disorder and the adverse effects of these drugs. The toxicity of

Table 5.

Trimethoprim + sulfamethoxazole (most effective)
Azithromycin + sulfamethoxazole
Clarithromycin+ sulfamethoxazole
Erythromycin + sulfisoxazole
Dapsone + trimethoprim
Atovaquone
P.S. 15
Sulfadioxine + pyrimethamine
Clindamycin + primaquine
Pentamidine i.v (least effective)

the sulfamethoxazole combinations in the patient with AIDS is markedly higher than the toxicity seen with the use of these combinations for other indications, which has its effects on compliance and switching to other treatments. There may be an explanation for this in the fact that in AIDS patients glutathione levels in both serum and broncheoalveolar lavage fluid were found to be reduced. Glutathione is an important antioxidant and plays a major role in scavenging the toxic hydroxylamine metabolites of sulfamethoxazole (SED-12, 703; SEDA-18, 291). However the AIDS patient seems to be more prone to adverse effects with nearly all drugs. Due attention should be given to interactions with the other medications used concomitantly.

Prophylaxis is indicated in the adult HIV patient if the CD4 count drops under the 200 per μl, while for infants the threshold has to be adapted to the much higher norm for children depending on the age. Prophylaxis is also indicated after a clinical PCP.

Information to date shows the trimethoprim + sulfamethoxazole combination (TMP-SMZ) to be the most effective for treatment and prophylaxis, closely followed by the combination of trimethoprim with dapsone and also dapsone alone. However, the TMP-SMZ combination also has the highest percentage of side effects and because of that the highest rate of treatment dropouts, especially in prophylactic use. In a study by Schneider et al. (53[C]) a patient receiving TMP-SMZ developed adverse effects in 50% of cases and 17% dropped out, generally because of fever, exanthema, nausea and vomiting. In their pentamidine group two out of 71 patients stopped treatment because of cough and bronchospasm after 313 and 456 days (53[C]). Hardy et al. (54[C]) noted similar problems; complications with TMP-SMZ included pruritus, fever, colitis, myopathy and intractable vaginal candidiasis (each in one case only). Their pentamidine patients were less prone to drop out but incidental side effects included persistent cough, pneumothorax, pancreatitis, hyperglycemia and a pruritic rash (54).

In the pentamidine group 24% of cases were seen with bacterial infections against only 12% in the TMP-SMZ group.

When Bozette et al. (55[C]) compared TMP-SMZ 960 mg twice daily (276 patients) with dapsone 50 mg twice daily (288 patients) and with aerosolized pentamidine 300 mg every 4 weeks (278 patients), the three regimes seemed to have a similar degree of efficacy. However only 21% of the TMP-SMZ group and 25% of the dapsone group completed the study on the original drug against 88% in the pentamidine group. Dose reduction allowed some patients to continue with the same drug. Adverse effects and their incidence were generally similar to those in other studies. Pancreatitis occurred in eight cases each in the TMP-SMZ and the dapsone group and in six in the pentamidine group. Torres et al. (56[C]) compared the effects of dapsone 10 mg twice weekly or aerosolized pentamidine 100 mg every 2 weeks for the prophylaxis of PCP and toxoplasmic encephalitis; the drugs showed similar efficacy. All these studies, and others reviewed in more detail in the *Side Effects of Drugs Annuals*, illustrate the difficulty in evaluating efficacy alongside adverse effects, survival rates and quality of life, and suggest that more attention should be given to refining dosage schedules (SED-12, 701; SEDA-16, 311; SEDA-17, 330; SEDA-18, 289).

Pentamidine

Pentamidine, an aromatic diamine, has been known since the late 1930s as a treatment for trypanosomiasis and some forms of leishmaniasis. In recent times it has been extensively used in the treatment of *Pneumocystis carinii* pneumonia (PCP). The mechanism of action is probably related to the inhibition of dehydrofolate reductase and inhibition of oxidative phosphorylation and nucleic acid synthesis as well as an influence on aerobic glycolysis. As with many older drugs the pharmacokinetics are still incompletely known. Pentamidine is not absorbed after oral administration and needs to be given parenterally or by aerosol. After intramuscular injection peak levels are seen after about 1 hour, with the serum concentration staying about the same over a 24-hour period. A study of multiple dosing over a 2-week period showed progressive accumulation in the plasma during that period. After multiple i.v. doses the elimination half-life was found to be 12.5 ± 2.4 days as estimated from serum levels. After a course of treatment decreasing amounts of pentamidine can be found in the urine for as long as 8 weeks. It seems that pentamidine is stored or bound in the tissues and excreted slowly via the urine with the amount excreted changing only marginally with repeated doses. The highest tissue concentrations have been found in the kidney, followed by the liver and then other tissues, but pentamidine was not found in the brain. Serum levels after aerosol therapy are markedly lower than those observed after intravenous therapy. The uptake via the lungs seems to be very limited which explains the lack of serious systemic toxicity seen with aerosol treatment but also explains the reported occurrence of extra-pulmonary *Pneumocystis* infections.

These pharmacokinetic data merit attention since they may be helpful in preventing toxicity; the latter seems to be dictated by tissue accumulation rather than the serum levels, with major toxic reactions usually occurring only after the first week of parenteral treatment. These pharmacokinetics may also explain the varied response on treatment with aerosol pentamidine and the more satisfactory results of 'prophylaxis' with the aerosol after initial parenteral treatment (SED-12, 701; SEDA-16, 312).

ADVERSE REACTION PATTERN

Pentamidine in therapeutic doses has a high rate of adverse effects (over 50%). As seen with several other drugs, toxicity seems to occur more frequently in patients with AIDS.

General and toxic reactions Hypotension subsequent to injection or infusion, hypoglycemia and nephrotoxicity are the major side effects. Hepatotoxicity and neutropenia are not uncommon. Compared with the general population there is a high incidence of cases of pancreatitis in AIDS patients, particularly when receiving aerosol treatment. Hypoglycemia too has been seen after aerosol treatment. Intermittent prophylactic aerosol use causes few side effects apart from cough and bronchial irritation following inhalation. Reports indicate a higher incidence of 'spontaneous' pneumothorax with aerosol prophylaxis. There is also a higher incidence of extrapulmonary infections with *Pneumocystis carinii* in patients treated with aerosolized pentamidine. Another disturbing finding was the higher incidence of other opportunistic infections in the pentamidine aerosol group versus the placebo aerosol group, while the pentamidine aerosol group showed a marked lesser recurrence rate of the *Pneumocystis carinii* pneumonitis in a controlled pentamidine aerosol-placebo aerosol comparative study of prophylaxis after initial treatment (SED-12, 702).

Intramuscular administration of pentamidine brings its own side effects; localized pain, erythema and the formation of sterile abscesses are frequent and troublesome (SED-12, 702; 51[R], 57[R], 58[R]). The use of the Z-track technique for the injection seems to mitigate the local effects.

Hypersensitivity reactions Skin rashes, but also the rare case of toxic epidermolysis and Stevens-Johnson syndrome have been described, as well as a case of a likely Herxheimer reaction.

Tumor-inducing effects No information is available.

Environmental problems The administration of nebulized pentamidine has an environmental impact; handling the nebulizer, preparing for use and cleaning, and assisting the patient exposes the health care worker to pentamidine. Adverse reactions like ocular and pulmonary irritation and irritation of exposed skin have been reported. Health workers also run the risk of being exposed to airborne infections of the organism harbored by the patient, which may include tuberculosis (SEDA-16, 314; SEDA-17, 331).

ORGANS AND SYSTEMS

Cardiovascular Severe *hypotension* may develop after a single intramuscular injection or with rapid intravenous administration, but has been seen with slow infusion as well. The practice of infusing the drug over 60 minutes or more may reduce this risk. Facial flushing, breathlessness, dizziness, nausea and vomiting may occur at the same time. Cardiac *arrhythmias* including ventricular tachycardia have been reported during treatment (SED-12, 702; SEDA-16, 331; 51[R], 58). Prolongation of the QT interval, which usually precedes the development of ventricular dysrhythmias with pentamidine occurs in one third of patients, most times within 2 weeks of starting therapy. Torsades de pointes has been described. Any dysrhythmia may recur many days after the pentamidine has been discontinued, which is not so surprising in view of the tissue accumulation and long elimination time. Several cases have again been reported over the last years. Electrolyte abnormalities, including low serum magnesium levels have been noticed at times of arrhythmias (SEDA-16, 315; SEDA-17, 331; 51[R], 59[C]).

Local *thrombophlebitis* may occur but problems are more often seen with intramuscular injection at the injection site.

Respiratory The inhalation of pentamidine may cause intolerable *coughing*. *Bronchospasm* may occur, especially in cases of asthma; tolerance of inhaled pentamidine is increased in nearly all patients by pretreatment with inhaled β_2 receptor antagonists (SEDA-16, 313; SEDA-17, 330; SEDA-18, 290; 51[R]). In lung function tests, high dose aerosolized pentamidine (600 mg/month) was associated with an increased pulmonary residual volume, decreased flow rates and increased airway reactivity (SEDA-18, 291). There seems to be an increased incidence of spontaneous *pneumothorax*, which may be connected with the influence on airway resistance. A particularly high frequency of spontaneous pneumothorax was observed in a group of hemophiliacs; the report suggests that PC infection and treatment resistance played a role (SEDA-16, 313).

A case of acute *eosinophilic pneumonia* after one

dose of inhaled pentamidine of 300 mg was reported; the reaction subsided within 2 weeks but recurred on rechallenge (SEDA-18, 292).

Dissemination of lung infection is a potentially serious matter, especially when using the aerosol route. While high alveolar drug concentration can be reached in the most accessible parts of the lung, the systemic resorption is minimal and the organism might spread through the lung and beyond despite containment of the initial pulmonary infection; cases have been described; some with extensive spread of the *Pneumocystis* into major organs and the bone marrow (SEDA-16, 313; SEDA-17, 332). Patients who have been treated with parenteral pentamidine are less at risk for disseminated *Pneumocystis carinii* than those given aerosol prophylaxis only (SEDA-16, 313; SEDA-17, 322).

Nervous system Mild *dizziness* may occur but nervous system adverse effects are uncommon; an occasional case of *confusion* and of *hallucinations* has been reported. *Magnesium deficiency* may affect mental function; a flat affect, slow speech and mental withdrawal are some of the typical effects (SED-12, 702; 59[R]). The symptoms of hypomagnesemia can be ill defined; unexplained symptomatology despite improvement of the *Pneumocystis carinii* infection demands a check of serum magnesium levels.

Endocrine, metabolic *Hypoglycemia* can be a serious and life-threatening effect of the administration of pentamidine. Hypoglycemia is seen in 10—30% of cases and has been seen mainly with parenteral use but may occur as well with inhalation therapy. In one 21-day study it appeared to be equally common with either form of therapy. Higher doses and longer duration of treatment increase the likelihood of this effect as does prior treatment with pentamidine (SEDA-16, 314); the presence of azotemia also increases the risk. In one study nephrotoxicity was seen in 100% of cases with hypoglycemia. The hypoglycemia is the result of a direct toxic effect on the pancreatic β cells resulting in insulin release with transient hypoglycemia, which is followed by β cell destruction and insulin deficiency, which in turn eventually can lead to an irreversible state of *diabetes* (SED-12, 702; SEDA-16, 315; SEDA-17, 331; 51[R]).

Hypocalcemia has been reported but not explained.

Hypomagnesemia connected with an excess urinary excretion of magnesium and clinical signs of magnesium deficiency has been referred to above in view of its neurological consequences. In one case (59[C]) hypomagnesemia was still present 2 months after intravenous pentamidine treatment though it must be noted that aerosol pentamidine was being continued, and the latter is known to be itself capable of causing hypomagnesemia, Some patients may be particularly sensitive to this effect, and previous renal damage (e.g. by other drugs) can be one risk factor (SED-12, 702).

Pancreas Episodes of *acute pancreatitis* and of *hemorrhagic pancreatitis* have been reported. This may or may nor be combined with evidence of damage to the β cells (SED-12, 702; SEDA-16, 315; SEDA-17, 331; 51[R]). It must be noted however that pancreatitis has been seen in patients with AIDS who did not receive the drug. The risk for the development of pancreatitis seems to be greater in children with CD 4 counts less than 100 cells/mm^3.

Hematological *Anemia*, *leukopenia* or *thrombopenia* occur in less than 5% of cases (SED-12, 702). Thrombopenia is more likely seen in prolonged therapy than initially. *Megaloblastic bone marrow changes* can occur with prolonged therapy (SED-11, 598). Low blood cell counts have been reported even following aerosolized application of pentamidine.

In one AIDS patient with severe but reversible thrombopenia after i.v. pentamidine, the serum during the acute phase contained antiplatelet antibodies which reacted with the glycoprotein llb/llla, similar to the reactions observed with quinine-induced thrombopenia (SEDA-18, 292). This would suggest that even aerosol treatment or environmental exposure will need to be avoided in such a patient.

Gastrointestinal Gastrointestinal complaints are usually minor. *Nausea* and *vomiting* may occur. *Dysgeusia* was reported in a few cases on intravenous therapy, but one study of aerosol administration specifically noted its absence (SED-12, 702).

Urinary system *Nephrotoxicity* is common. In a pharmacokinetic study in patients with *Pneumocystis carinii* infection, serum creatinine levels increased during the 2—3 weeks treatment period in nine out of the ten cases. The clinical literature mentions an incidence of 20—35% (SED-12, 702), and in AIDS it seems to be higher still, e.g. 50—65% (SEDA-17, 331; 51[R]). The renal toxicity is more pronounced in patients with diarrhea (SED-12, 702) and probably may also be more severe with i.m. use, perhaps because of dehydration which is more readily corrected if the drug is given in an infusion. Stahl-Bayliss et al. (SED-12, 702) noted evidence of renal toxicity in all cases with pentamidine-induced hypoglycemia in contrast to an incidence of 38% in the group who remained euglycemic. This is one of the situations noted above where knowledge of the drug's kinetics is valuable; because of the marked accumulation of pentamidine it is conceivable that, after an initial period of daily administration, a modified treatment regimen, every other day or even twice a week, may prevent renal and pancreatic permanent damage (SED-12, 702).

A defect in renal conservation of magnesium (see above) can result from the effects on the kidney.

Liver Occasionally elevated liver transaminase levels have been seen.

Skin *Rashes* may occur but are not common. *Local pain* at the injection place, local *infiltration* and *sterile abscess* have been reported. There has been a case of an *Herxheimer reaction* and a case with skin lesions resembling a *toxic epidermal necrolysis*; both cases concerned children (SED-12, 702).

Interactions There are no reports of undue effects from the combination of pentamidine with those antiviral agents commonly used in the treatment of AIDS.

Hypocalcemia was reported during the use of pentamidine and *foscarnet* in patients with AIDS (SED-12, 702).

Trimethoprim-sulfamethoxazole (co-trimoxazole) *(see also Chapter 29.1)*

Co-trimoxazole has the advantage of low cost, and can be administered in oral or intravenous form. However, its toxicity when used for treatment or prophylaxis of *Pneumocystis carinii* infection in the patient with AIDS is markedly higher than that seen when it is used in other indications; there is no complete explanation for this (SED-12, 703; SEDA-18, 293; 51[R], 58[R]). One reason could lie in the fact that in patients with AIDS, as well as in symptom-free HIV-positive individuals, glutathione levels in both serum and bronchoalveolar lavage fluid have been found to be reduced. Glutathione is an antioxidant and plays an important role in the scavenging of the metabolites of sulfamethoxazole (the hydroxylamine derivative) which are toxic. If this explanation for the increased toxicity is correct it could be helpful to add *N*-acetylcysteine to the treatment, since this replenishes cysteine and sustains glutathione synthesis. An alternate approach would be to select a sulfonamide not easily hydroxylated for use in the combination with trimethoprim (SED-12, 703). It would be interesting to know whether use of *N*-acetylcysteine could change the susceptibility of *Pneumocystis carinii* infection.

Adverse reactions occur in HIV-infected patients in 50—100% of cases. Their nature is as reviewed in the main co-trimoxazole monograph elsewhere in this volume. Serious reactions are infrequent but anaphylaxis and hyperdynamic shock have been reported; rechallenge after this type of reaction may result in severe toxicity (SEDA-18, 293).

Dosages used in treatment of PCP are high, while for prophylaxis lower dosages suffice. The incidence of most adverse effects seems in any case to some extent dose dependent, hence they are not true hypersensitivity reactions; patients who have reacted adversely to a higher dose may subsequently tolerate a lower one (SEDA-18, 293). A side effect attributed specifically to trimethoprim is *hyperkalemia* (SEDA-17, 332); various other adverse reactions, like anemia, neutropenia and azotemia, may be less frequent if the trimethoprim serum levels remain below 5—8 μg/ml. Those side effects which are a direct result of folate depletion may respond to leucovorin; it has been recommended that folic acid be added to the treatment regime to counteract some of the effects of trimethoprim (53[C]), but this may interfere with the efficacy of the drug, as strongly suggested by work performed by Safrin et al. (60[C]).

Markers have been sought for the development of hypersensitivity in AIDS patients with PCP. Carr et al. (61[C]) found that hypersensitivity occurred in 27% of patients who had significantly higher than average total lymphocyte and CD4 and CD8 cell counts and CD4:CD8 ratios. Clinical variables listed suggest that in those who did not develop hypersensitivity PCP was more severe (with a greater mortality), that they more often were on assisted ventilation, and were more likely to be receiving corticosteroid therapy (61[C]).

Unusual reactions and syndromes can occur:

One HIV-positive man, who was seen for a productive cough, headache and low grade fever, reacted well to erythromycin. A month later the symptoms recurred, now with myalgias, night sweats and anorexia. This time he was treated with a cephalosporin antibiotic and, because of a lack of response, given TMP-SMZ in a high dose. Within 72 hours all symptoms had resolved. After treatment had been continued for a total of 14 days he had a fine, diffuse rash. About 10 days later he was started on zidovudine and prophylactic TMP-SMZ; within 2 hours of the first tablet he experienced headache and fever, a rash appeared with periorbital swelling and generalized weakness. Twelve hours after this single dose he was seen with fever, hypotension and conjunctivitis. The chest X-ray revealed diffuse patchy infiltrates and he was found to be hypoxic and liver-associated enzymes and serum creatinine levels doubled, blood cultures remained sterile. The patient recovered on general supportive measures (62[c]).

Dapsone *(see also Chapter 30)*

Dapsone, given alone or in combination with trimethoprim in the treatment of PCP, has been increasingly used since it was thought to be to more effective and better tolerated than TMP-SMZ. Bozette et al. (55[C]) confirmed the similar efficacy in a large open study as did Torres et al. (56[C]), and both studies pointed to a greater ability to prevent toxoplasmosis encephalitis. However, Salmon et al. (93[C]) found, in a comparison between dapsone 50 mg/daily and aerosolized pentamidine, 300 mg every month for secondary prophylaxis, an excess mortality in the dapsone group. A negative interaction was observed between dapsone and zidovudine and the mean CD4 cell count was found to be lower in the group treated with dapsone. Suggested explanations were the oxidative effect of dapsone or the possible addition of iron protoxalate to the dapsone in this study (93[C]). In treatment dapsone alone may be less effective than TMP-SMZ, while dapsone plus trimethoprim seems as effective as TMP-SMZ (SEDA-18, 292).

The side effects of dapsone are well known and are reviewed in Chapter 30. The hemolysis is quite common and is markedly dose related; with a dose of 100 mg per day or less there may be a reduced red cell survival but as a rule no clinical hemolysis. In the patient with a G6PD deficiency hemolysis is seen with lower dosages. A daily dose of 200 mg or more causes hemolysis in varying degree. The hemolysis can be so marked that manifestations of hypoxia become apparent. Dapsone elimination is reduced in the presence of renal impairment; hemolysis may then be seen at dosage levels normally considered safe.

Methemoglobinemia may occur and severe methemoglobinemia is a feature of dapsone intoxication and is often accompanied by more or less marked hemolysis; in severe cases it may lead to a toxic psychosis. With the increased use of dapsone in the treatment of AIDS patients, methemoglobinemia may be encountered more frequently. Methemoglobin levels of 15—20% are seen with the clinical signs of cyanosis, ashen colour and the typical chocolate brown appearance of the blood, and at higher levels a wide range of symptoms occur.

While the serum half life of dapsone is about 22 ± 6 hours, the sulfones tend to be retained in the tissues, skin, muscles and especially liver and kidney (63). Because of the slow elimination of dapsone, treatment with methylene blue may have to be continued for several days. In a case of attempted suicide with an estimated 100 tablets, the continuous administration of methylene blue was required for a week (64). The toxic dose of dapsone is above 1.5 grams.

The combination of clindamycin with primaquine is being used in the treatment of PCP. This brings the possibility of the concurrent use or presence in the body of dapsone and primaquine. Primaquine too may cause hemolysis and methemoglobinemia; it was this combination that was considered the reason for the marked methemoglobinemia in another case of overdosage (64). Three cases of methemoglobinemia were seen in one clinic after change-over from dapsone treatment to clindamycin/primaquine treatment on account of a recurrence of *Pneumocystis carinii* infection (64).

The 'sulfone' syndrome has been described as connected with a dapsone-induced exacerbation of lepromatous leprosy. Bozette et al. (55[C]) reported 'the sulfone syndrome' in one patient in a comparison trial of TMP-SMZ, dapsone and pentamidine in PCP prophylaxis.

In a study of patients with AIDS receiving dideoxyinosine, those given dapsone for PCP prophylaxis showed a high failure rate of the prophylaxis. The likely reason was thought to be connected with the citrate-phosphate buffer contained in the packet of dideoxyinosine, a buffer facilitating the absorption of the dideoxyinosine. An influence on the resorption of other drugs in which resorption depends on gastric acidity such as ketoconazole, pyrimethamine, trimethoprim and itraconazole can then be expected. Administering the drugs 2 hours before the dideoxyinosine will allow normal resorption. Regretfully serum levels of dapsone were not determined in this early study (SED-12, 703).

Dapsone plus trimethoprim *(see Chapter 29.1)*

Little is known about this combination, and the possible advantages have not been demonstrated. The adverse effects are likely to be those of its components.

Epiroprim (Ro 11-8958)/dapsone plus epiroprim

Epiroprim, a dihydrofolate reductase inhibitor, was when given alone or in combination with dapsone in animals found to be highly effective in protecting against *Toxoplasma gondii* (65).

WR-6026, WR-238605 and WR-242511

These three 8-aminoquinolines are being tested for activity against *P. carinii*. There is no information about side effects as yet; in animal studies WR-242511 seems to have a greater potential for producing methemoglobinemia than does primaquine (SED-12, 703).

Pyrimethamine-sulfadoxine (Fansidar)

This combination has been stated to be successful in the prophylaxis of PCP (51[R]).

Pyrimethamine-dapsone

This mixture has not been mentioned as effective, but it has been proposed and could be expected to have useful activity.

Primaquine plus clindamycin

Primaquine on its own has some effect against *Pneumocystis carinii*, but at dosages of 0.25 or 0.5 mg/kg primaquine alone proved to be ineffective in the rat model, confirming earlier clinical experience. Clindamycin alone was also ineffective. The combination was effective both in vitro and in the animal study for treatment and prophylaxis.

Intravenous clindamycin, 900 mg every 8 hours, with oral primaquine, 26.3 mg, was found to be effective in a number of patients with active disease. A maintenance dose of 150 mg clindamycin 4 times daily orally plus primaquine 26.3 mg daily was shown to be adequate. The drugs are thought to be synergistic. In a second study clindamycin 600 mg four times daily was used intravenously with a maintenance dose of 300–400 mg orally and primaquine 15 mg base orally once a day. Tolerance was reasonably good, the most frequent side effect, seen in half of the patients, was a generalized maculopapular rash on the 10–12th day. Rash was accompanied by fever in three cases. Other side effects comprised leukopenia (two), nausea (two) and diarrhea (one) (SED-12, 703). In a third study using higher doses of primaquine, methemoglobinemia was a major side effect. In a fourth study clindamycin was given 900 mg t.i.d. with primaquine 30 mg daily except in three of 28 episodes of PCP treated in a total in 26 patients, who received 15 mg primaquine daily (two) or 30 mg on alternate days (one). In 11 episodes the patients had experienced intolerance for standard therapy, in 13 episodes conventional therapy had failed and in four episodes there had been treatment failure and intolerance. Twenty-four of the 28 episodes were successfully treated with clindamycin/primaquine, the most common adverse effect being a rash (66[C]). With the use of the higher doses of clindamycin gastrointestinal effects, especially diarrhea and colitis, can be expected. The primaquine component may cause hemolytic anemia and methemoglobinemia. Patients should be screened for G6PD deficiency.

Dapsone treatment given immediately prior to instituting clindamycin/primaquine therapy may cause methemoglobinemia.

There is no information about interactions with antiviral agents for this combination.

Atovaquone (Meprone, 566C80) (2-[*trans*-4-(4-chlorophenyl)cyclohexyl]-3-hydroxy-1,4-naphthoquinone)

This new hydroxynaphthaquinone compound has been shown to be effective in the prevention and treatment of murine *Pneumocystis carinii* pneumonitis. It also has an effect against *Toxoplasma gondii* and *Plasmodium falciparum*. A phase I study showed that oral absorption was improved by taking the drug after a meal. Fats enhance the absorption significantly. The maximum concentration in serum is dose dependent but with a suggested decrease of absorption at doses above the 750 mg. Maximum concentration occurs after 4–6 hours with a second peak occurring 24–96 hours later pointing to an entero-hepatic cycling. The serum half-life is 77 ± 43 hours. In a 3-week study with test doses varying from 100 to 3000 mg daily the drug was well tolerated. Three patients reported an increased appetite; two of these had transient sinus arrhythmia. One of the 24 patients had a transient maculopapular rash that resolved without discontinuation of the drug. No abnormalities were seen in hematological parameters or renal function,

Two cases had slightly elevated serum bilirubin levels and one each an elevated AST and ALT. Two additional patients showed mildly increased AST and ALT levels, but both were known to have a chronic hepatitis B (SED-12, 703). Clinical experience is still limited, but atovaquone seems to be well tolerated. Mild rashes are fairly common, but more serious rashes like an erythema multiforme are rare. Gastrointestinal upset including abdominal pain, nausea and diarrhea is common. Other adverse effects include fever and elevation of serum aminotransferase levels. Mild CNS disturbances have been mentioned (SEDA-18, 286; 51[R]).

Hughes et al. (67[C]) compared atovaquone 250 mg t.i.d. with TMP-SMZ 320+1600 mg daily for 21 days in the treatment of PCP in a total of 408 patients. Analysis of results were possible for 322 cases. The groups were well matched. The therapeutic efficacy of the two treatments was closely similar, but atovaquone was much better tolerated, with a far lower incidence of rash, liver dysfunction, fever, nausea and pruritus and no occurrence of neutropenia, chills, headache, renal impairment or thrombocytopenia. However, preexisting diarrhea was associated with increased mortality in the atovaquone group.

Appropriate plasma concentrations are important, and an improved formulation is being tested (67[C], 68[C]). In the meantime it might be necessary to look at a higher dosage.

There is no information about interactions as yet. Atovaquone is highly bound to protein.

Whether it is safe to take the drug during pregnancy is unknown.

When atovaquane was tested against i.v. pentamidine for the treatment of mild and moderate PCP in an open trial, the success rate was considered by the investigators to be similar for the two treatments. However, discontinuation of the original treatment was much more frequent in the pentamidine group (36%) than in the atovaquone group (4%) (69[c]). The authors' conclusion that the two approaches have a similar success rate has also been challenged, and their series was indeed a small one.

Treatment-limited adverse effects occurred in only 7% with atovaquone as compared with 41% with pentamidine. In both series they included cases of rash and an increase in creatinine levels; atavaquone (unlike pentamidine) produced no vomiting, nausea, hypotension, leukopenia, acute renal failure, ECG abnormalities, but atovaquone did produce one case of dementia (69[c]).

Ornidyl (DFMO, α-difluoromethylornithine) *(see page 835)*

Ornidyl, a decarboxylase inhibitor, has been tried as a therapeutic agent in open trials in patients with AIDS having *Pneumocystis carinii* pneumonia. While some patients showed improvement, ornidyl is not currently advocated for this treatment. Leukopenia, thrombopenia and even pancytopenia have been reported with the drug when so used (SED-12, 704). Besides the toxicity, which can be seen in up to 60% of patients, DFMO is markedly less effective than TMP-SMZ. Of a group of patients with histologically proven PCP 58% failed to respond to DFMO, but the drug can be considered as a reserve tool in patients with severe PCP who have failed on conventional therapy (58[R]).

Trimetrexate and piritrexim

The lipid-soluble anti-folate methotrexate analogues seem to be another useful therapeutic tool provided the host is protected with concomitant leucovorin. The use of trimetrexate is associated with neutropenia and/or thrombopenia (SED-12, 704). Fever and elevation of liver transaminases, while uncommon, have been noticed with the use of trimetrexate. The efficacy is not as high as that of TMP-SMZ. Leucovorin is given with trimetrexate to minimize the hematological toxicity. The adverse effects of piritrexim are similar, but in addition there is mention of facial flushing, peri-orbital edema and pruritus. The occurrence of an anaphylactic reaction has been reported (SEDA-18, 289).

Trimetrexate has been studied more extensively than piritrexin. The efficacy is high but not as high as with TMP-SMZ, and the recurrence rate is markedly higher (51[R], 58[R]). Trimetrexate has to be given parenterally. Noting the findings of Safrin et al. (60[C]) regarding the addition of folinic acid to TMP-SMZ therapy (see earlier) it will be important to determine if the concurrent administration of leucovorin unfavourably influences the treatment outcome for these drugs.

L-693,989

The pneumocandins are a new class of anti-*Pneumocystis* agents. These compounds are thought to work by inhibiting the synthesis of β-1,3-glucan, a component of the *P. carinii* cyst wall (humans lack β-1,3-glucan). Chemical modification of the poorly water-soluble pneumocandins resulted in L-693,989 which can be administered by aerosol. Studies in rats showed this compound to be effective in the prevention of PCP using daily or weekly administration. There was no evidence of toxicity. Since there is no known counterpart for β-1,3-glucan synthesis in humans, there are no obvious reasons to suspect mechanism-based toxicity with this class of compounds in man. More effective compounds are being studied (72).

Albendazole *(see page 830)*

Albendazole, a benzimidazole derivative widely used for treating helminth infections, seems to be active against *Pneumocystis carinii*. It was found to be effective for prophylaxis and for treatment in inoculated, immunosuppressed mice (73).

Deferoxamine *(see also Chapter 23)*

The iron-chelating drug deferoxamine mesylate (DFO, Desferal) was found to be effective against PCP in bolus dosages in immunocompromised rats (74). The mechanism is not clear; various explanations have been advanced. Salmon et al. (93[C]) have speculated on a possible harmful effect of the presence of 100 mg iron protoxalate (=30 mg of iron per day) in the dapsone tablets used in their comparative study of dapsone with aerosolized pentamidine in the secondary prophylaxis of PCP; the study was prematurely discontinued after 18 months due to an excess mortality in the dapsone group. In the rat model of PCP, a 3-week infusion of deferoxamine eliminated the trophozoite cycle stage (94).

DRUGS USED IN THE TREATMENT OF OTHER PROTOZOAL INFECTIONS

EMETINE AND RELATED SUBSTANCES

Emetine and dihydroemetine *(SED-12, 704)*

Emetine, once the drug of choice for the treatment of amebiasis despite its marked cardiotoxicity has largely been replaced by metronidazole and related compounds for this indication.

ADVERSE REACTION PATTERN

General and toxic reactions Emetine, if used in the correct dosage and with proper safeguards, causes only mild and transient side effects. Individual sensitivity, however, varies. Large doses may produce damage to heart, liver, kidney, intestinal tract and skeletal muscle.

Hypersensitivity reactions These have not been documented.

Tumor-inducing effects These have not been described.

ORGANS AND SYSTEMS

Cardiovascular Cardiotoxicity is the most serious and also dangerous side effect of the treatment with emetine. The clinical signs are *tachycardia, arrhythmia and hypotension*. Fatalities have been described. *Electrocardiographic abnormalities* are common and are seen in 60–70% of cases; increased T-wave amplitude, prolongation of the P-R interval, S-T segment depression and T-wave changes are all common. It seems possible that emetine influences the cell permeability of natrium and calcium ions and this could be the basis of its effect on cardiac automaticity, on contractility and on the electrocardiogram (SED-11, 594). The symptoms of emetine toxicity suggest that an influence on magnesium cell concentrations could be another possible explanation, but there are no factual data to back this hypothesis (SED-11, 594).

Nervous and musculoskeletal systems Complaints of *weakness, tenderness, and stiffness of skeletal muscles*, especially in the neck and shoulder, are common. *Paralysis* has been described but is rare, as is *peripheral neuritis*. Following emetine aversion therapy for alcohol abuse, muscle weakness and pathological changes in muscle biopsy specimens were described (SED-11, 594).

Fatigue, mood changes, sleep disturbances and *irritability* have been observed and are in their milder forms probably more common than appears from the reports.

Gastrointestinal *Nausea* and *vomiting* occur frequently, perhaps in as many as a third of all cases treated. In about half the cases, *diarrhea* is induced or existing diarrhea aggravated. *Melena* may occur, but this seems unlikely to be drug-induced (SED-11, 594).

Urinary system Degenerative changes in the kidneys are a manifestation of emetine poisoning.

Skin *Dermatitis* has been reported. *Cellulitis* at the site of injection has been seen.

Interactions No clear interactions have been documented. Interaction with those *cardiac drugs* influencing calcium ion transport might on theoretical grounds be expected. Concurrent use with those drugs causing a prolongation of the QT interval would be imprudent.

Dihydrometine

Dihydroemetine seems to be a little less toxic but also less effective than emetine itself. Side effects are similar to those of emetine (SED-11, 594).

Diloxanide furoate (Furamide)

Furamide often causes flatulence and occasionally nausea, vomiting, diarrhea, urticaria and pruritus. Furamide is an excellent luminal amebicide and is indicated following treatment with the 5-nitroimidazole compounds which have relatively weak activity on the cyst stage. Experience over 14 years has been summarized by the Atlanta Center for Disease Control, confirming the minimal toxicity of this drug. Fewer adverse effects were reported in the age group 20 months to 10 years than for those patients aged over 10 years. There is no record of interactions between furamide and metronidazole or tinidazole (SED-12, 704; SEDA-17, 333).

Iodoquinol (Yodoxin)

Iodoquinol may cause nausea, diarrhea and abdominal cramps. Rashes, acne and anal pruritus have been mentioned as well. The possibility of slight enlargement of the thyroid gland has been raised. Prolonged use in high doses has been connected with loss of vision and optic atrophy (SED-12, 705).

Quinfamide

Quinfamide acts on the trophozoites of *Entamoeba histolytica*, making the trophozoite incapable of propagation. It is not active against amebic cysts. With doses of 100–1200 mg, side effects have been frequent but mild, mainly comprising headaches and nausea (SED-12, 704).

Metronidazole and related compounds

Metronidazole

Metronidazole has proven to be effective in the treatment of many protozoal diseases notably trichomoniasis, amebiasis, schistosomiasis, strongyloidiasis and lambliasis, and has been in use for over 20 years. In recent years the use of metronidazole against infections with anaerobic bacteria has come to the fore, and with this indication the use of metronidazole in combination with a multitude of other drugs used by patients with conditions likely to develop secondary anaerobic bacterial infections. With the increased use there is also a widespread and increasing incidence reported of resistance of various strains of bacteria. The use of metronidazole as an added medication merely 'to make assurance doubly sure' is to be discouraged. It is to be especially discouraged in immune compromised patients because of the risk of emergence of resistant bacterial strains. With the increased use there is also an increased number of reports of some more unusual adverse effects. Overall the drug can still be considered safe, if used in generally recommended doses. For amebiasis there is still discussion about the use of a single high dose versus repeated lower doses, both as regards efficacy and side effects.

Metronidazole has excellent bioavailability, and absorption after oral administration is not significantly influenced by food. Peak serum levels (±10 μg/ml after a 500-mg dose) are seen about 1 hour after ingestion. Multiple doses every 6–8 hours result in some drug accumulation, the elimination half-life averaging about 8 hours. There is a linear relationship between doses and serum concentrations. Rectal administration results in serum levels about half those seen after oral administration. Systemic absorption after local use in the vagina is slow, maximum serum levels being reached only after 8–24 hours; they are only about 20% of those attained after oral administration. Metronidazole is extensively metabolized, with about 20% of the dose excreted unchanged with the urine. Tissue levels are similar to serum levels and the drug penetrates readily into the central nervous system. As with many metabolized drugs the elimination half-life is markedly prolonged in the neonate; there is an inverse relationship between gestational age and the drug half-life. Prolonged elimination times are also seen in the presence of serious liver disease (SED-12, 705; SEDA-16, 310; SEDA-17, 332; SEDA-18, 294).

ADVERSE REACTION PATTERN

General and toxic reactions Metronidazole is generally well tolerated. With high doses and high-dose prolonged treatment, nausea and vomiting and central nervous system symptoms ranging from headache and dizziness to neuritis may occur. The commonest reactions are nausea, a metallic taste in the mouth, furry tongue and vulvo-vaginal irritation in patients given metronidazole for the treatment of bacterial vaginosis (SED-12, 704; SEDA-18, 295). The number of reports about pancreatitis, neuropathy and optic neuritis calls for some caution.

Hypersensitivity reactions These are unusual, but rashes have been described.

Tumor-inducing effects Prolonged high-dose exposure of mice to metronidazole leads to an increased incidence of lung tumors, and in one study an increase in lymphoreticular neoplasia in female animals was observed. These results, which caused much concern when first published, are probably non-specific and not relevant for human subjects; these and other neoplasms have also been induced in mice merely by varying the diets consumed. Several long-term follow-up studies in men have failed to demonstrate an excess cancer risk (SED-12, 705). There has been a single report of cancers occurring in three patients with Crohn's disease who had taken metronidazole for years (SED-11, 595), but they had also been treated with sulfasalazine and corticosteroids and this cannot be regarded as constituting reasonable evidence of a causal link.

ORGANS AND SYSTEMS

Cardiovascular *Thrombophlebitis* may occur following intravenous administration; an incidence of 6% has been cited (SED-11, 595).

Respiratory A case of *pneumonitis* probably due to metronidazole use (since there was recurrence of symptoms after rechallenge) was discussed in SEDA-14 (p. 242).

Nervous system Symptoms relating to the central nervous system may occur on standard doses but they are mainly seen with high doses and especially when such doses are given for a long time. Under the latter conditions, a 25% incidence of such symptoms as *headaches*, *dizziness*, *tremors*, *ataxia* and *confusion* were observed.

A 6% incidence of *neuropathy* has been quoted; polyneuritis, mainly sensory in nature, has been recorded during the treatment of Crohn's disease but again in connection with the prolonged use of high doses (SED-12, 705). The complication is not restricted to patients with this bowel disease—it is also seen when metronidazole is given for other purposes such as radiosensitization. Electrophysiological studies suggest a distal sensory axonal degeneration showing loss of sensory nerve potential over the distal segment and normal motor nerve conduction studies. In some cases the severity of clinical and electrophysiological abnormalities is closely related to the total amount of metronidazole administered (SEDA-14, 242). Alston (SED-12, 706) has noted that the structure of metronidazole bears a resemblance to that of thiamine and that thiamine-synthesizing gut flora may synthesize a neurotoxic analogue of thiamine from ingested metronidazole. This hypothesis is, as the author points out, rather weakened by the fact that nitroheterocyclic drugs other than metronidazole are also neurotoxic, despite a much weaker structural analogy to thiamine precursors (SED-12, 706).

The use of high doses in combination with cefamandole and clindamycin has been associated with a case of *encephalopathy* (SED-12, 705).

A case of *grand mal seizures* was published some years ago (SED-11, 259); although this possibility is mentioned in reviews it is doubtful whether there are authoritative sources for a cause—effect relationship.

Aseptic meningitis is another (rare, possibly allergic) adverse effect following the use of metronidazole; the one published case is well documented, with positive rechallenge (75[c]).

Hematological Metronidazole can produce *leukocytopenia* and *neutropenia*, usually only associated with prolonged therapy; cases reported have been reversible on discontinuation of therapy (SED-12, 706). In SED-11 (p. 595) mention was made of one case each of *agranulocytosis* and of *aplastic anemia*. A single paper cited described the development of a *hemolytic-uremic syndrome* in six children (SEDA-15, 298).

Liver Elevated serum lever enzyme levels were reported in a case a decade ago (SED-11, 595) but there has been no more recent confirmation.

Gastrointestinal *Anorexia*, *nausea*, *vomiting*, *abdominal pain* and *diarrhea* have all been reported; use of a large single dose most commonly leads to these complaints. *Metallic taste* also seems to be quite common as is the occurrence of a *black tongue* (SED-12, 706).

Pancreas *Pancreatitis* has been reported in various individual case histories (SEDA-15, 298) but there is reason to think that some of these at least were due to other factors such as alcohol use (SED-12, 706). Corey et al. (76[c]) described pancreatitis in a 63-year-old woman with Crohn's disease, coinciding with the administration of metronidazole and disappearing 1—2 days after discontinuation of the metronidazole treatment, but even here there is little support for a causal link (76[c], 77, 78).

Urinary system *Darkening of the urine* may occur; this is a harmless discoloration, mostly seen on prolonged treatment.

Genital system A genital mucosal erosion was observed in a 38-year-old woman who had taken metronidazole 400 mg three times a day for 10 days to counter a bacterial vaginitis (SEDA-16, 310).

Skin *Pruritus* and *rashes* have been reported including a fixed drug eruption and a pityriasis rosea-like eruption. *Urticaria* after a single dose has been reported but could have been coincidental (SEDA-17, 333).

Special senses Acute *myopia* after 11 days of treatment with metronidazole for *Trichomonas* infection has been described; the myopia resolved in 4 days after discontinuation but re-occurred on rechallenge. The combined figures of two major American reporting systems for adverse reactions listed seven cases of *retrobulbar or optic neuritis* associated with the oral use of metronidazole; two of these cases had a peripheral neuropathy at the same time. There is however insufficient information to evaluate these reports (SEDA-17, 333).

Taste and *smell disturbances* may occur.

Second-generation effects Mutagenicity of metronidazole has been demonstrated with some bacterial systems (SED-12, 706). Studies on DNA single-strand breaks in the lymphocytes of patients treated with metronidazole for *Trichomonas* vaginitis indicated that such breaks were repaired after therapy ceased. A mutagenic effect would theoretically be possible in patients with a DNA repair defect (SEDA-16, 310). Tests for embryotoxicity and teratogenicity in different animal species have shown negative results and there have been no reports of adverse effects on the fetus in pregnant women given the drug for trichomoniasis. Despite this, it still would seem wise to avoid administration of metronidazole during the first trimester of pregnancy.

Metronidazole is excreted in the breast milk. No adverse effects were seen in a group of nursing infants (SED-12, 706), but one should still be cautious in using metronidazole in the nursing mother (SEDA-18, 295).

Interactions Metronidazole has an antabus (disulfiram)-like effect on users of *alcohol*, sufficiently frequent to justify a warning (SED-12, 706).

The effect of *warfarin* is potentiated (SED-12, 706).

In a patient on *phenytoin* a disproportionate increase in the hydroxy-metabolite of metronidazole was found in the serum, suggesting that phenytoin may induce metronidazole-metabolizing enzymes (SED-12, 706).

In vitro the combination of metronidazole with *antibiotics* has an additive effect against anaerobic bacteria (SED-12, 706).

Metronidazole may increase the toxicity of *lithium* and *carbamazepine*.

Benznidazole (benzoylmetronidazole)

Benznidazole is used in the treatment of *Trypanosoma cruzi* infections and Chagas-Mazza disease, and is recommended for use in urogenital trichomoniasis, all forms of amebiasis, giardiasis and also anaerobic infections. The side effects are similar to those of metronidazole. Drowsiness, dizziness, headache and ataxia occasionally occur. With prolonged and/or high doses, transient peripheral neuropathy and epileptiform seizures may be seen. Other frequently mentioned side effects are: unpleasant taste, furred tongue, nausea, vomiting and gastrointestinal disturbances. Skin rash and pruritus may occur. One case each of erythema multiforme and of toxic epidermolysis were reported in the past.

Like metronidazole, benznidazole has a mutagenic effect. On testing for chromosomal aberrations and induction of micronuclei in cultures of peripheral lymphocytes of children with Chagas disease, an increase of micronucleated interphase lymphocytes and of chromosomal aberrations was seen after treatment with benznidazole (SED-12, 706).

Like metronidazole, benznidazole has an antabus-like effect if *alcohol* is taken, and it may interact with *warfarin* treatment.

Albendazole

Albendazole is used in the treatment of hydatidosis and neurocysticercosis and also seems to be effective against *Strongyloides*. Provided that an adequate concentration is attained within the cyst, it is scolicidal. Used in the treatment of neurocysticercosis, albendazole (like praziquantel) may cause a CSF syndrome characterized by fever, headaches, meningismus and exacerbation of some or many of the neurological signs of the disease; it is considered due to a local reaction to dying and dead larvae and can be attenuated by concomitant administration of prednisone (SED-12, 707; 79[C]).

Interactions In hydatidosis a combination of albendazole and praziquantel seems effective when either of these agents has failed when used alone (SED-12, 707).

Carnidazole

In early studies the side effects were found to be mild; nausea/vomiting, abdominal discomfort, dry mouth, dizziness, headache and tiredness were reported (SED-12, 707). Metronidazole-like side effects should be anticipated.

Flubendazole; fenbendazole

The antiprotozoal activity of these two benzimidazole derivatives is similar to that of mebendazole; the target seems to be the microtubule protein β-tubulin. Side effects seem comparable to those of mebendazole (89).

Hemazole

Reportedly less toxic then metronidazole in the treatment of amoebiases, this drug needs further study.

Mebendazole

Mebendazole, one of the benzimidazoles, is poorly absorbed from the gut and is most useful for treating intestinal infections; it is essentially an anthelminthic, but is effective against *Giardia lamblia* while in vitro *Trichomonas vaginalis* is susceptible. Mebendazole does not interfere with the normal intestinal flora. Side effects are few and mild (SED-12, 707). A study comparing the effects of mebendazole with the much better absorbed albendazole showed the substantially better effects of the latter, though with both drugs relapses were common. Side effects were mild and reversible, consisting mainly of abdominal pains and raised serum transaminases (79[C]). Mebendazole is effective against enteric *Strongyloides* but it is not absorbed and ineffective against tissue forms (80[r]).

Miconazole

Urticaria, tachycardia and facial edema were seen in a child during intravenous administration (SED-12, 707). Thrombocytosis with platelet counts exceeding 400 000/mm^3 was reported (SEDA-18, 295).

Misonidazole

Misonidazole is used as a radiosensitizing agent. In one study it induced a rash in 3.9% of 380 cases. A higher incidence of neuropathy was mentioned as well, presumably dose dependent (SED-11, 596).

Ornidazole

Used in single large doses for the treatment of *Trichomonas urogenitalis* or *Giardia* infections this drug may cause gastrointestinal symptoms (SED-11, 597).

Niridazole

Used in the treatment of schistosomiasis (standard dose 25 mg/kg/day for 7 days), side effects were seen in 80% of inpatients and 33% of outpatients. Gastrointestinal effects were the most common with vomiting occurring in a 50% of cases. Other side effects reported were; insomnia, somnolence, vertigo, nightmares, headache, weakness, jaundice (not further specified) and muscular pains (SEDA-12, 244).

Satranidazole

Satranidazole is a highly active amebicidal agent and has a slightly wider spectrum then metronidazole against micro-aerophilic and anaerobic bacteria; it is also effective against *Giardia* and *Trichomonas*. In comparison with metronidazole, nimorazole, secnidazole, and ornidazole, it is less toxic. Gastrointestinal tolerability was good in early studies. Therapeutic doses did not cause adverse interaction with alcohol in phase III, clinical studies (SED-12, 707).

Secnidazole

Secnidazole is reported to be more active and give more prolonged blood levels then metronidazole; it is effective in hepatic amebiasis. Gastrointestinal side effects seem be less common (SED-11, 597).

Thiabendazole

This non-carbamate benzimidazole is active against *Giardia lamblia*, but less effective then albendazole and mebendazole; it is also the drug of choice against *Strongyloides stercoralis* both the enteric and tissue forms. Normally given orally, it is rapidly absorbed with peak serum levels 1–2 hours after ingestion and also rapidly metabolized and excreted with 40% of the drug and its metabolites excreted during the first 4 hours and 80% during the first 24 hours. The main metabolite, 5-hydroxy-thiabendazole is inactive. Somnolence has been described when a high dose was used rectally or orally. Marked peripheral eosinophilia is also described after rectal thiabendazole therapy (80[c]).

Tinidazole

Side effects resemble those of metronidazole. Tinidazole can be given intravenously and seems to be well tolerated, though thrombophlebitis has been reported. In one healthy volunteer, fainting with low blood pressure and nausea and tiredness for several hours was reported (SED-11, 597). Skin reactions may occur. A fixed eruption with pruritus was observed in a 27-year-old man treated for *Entamoeba histolytica* with tinidazole 500 mg, four tablets in a single dose for 3 days. An erythematous patch with a sensation of burning appeared over the left buttock in a 32-year-old man while taking tinidazole for giardiasis. The allergic lesion could be provoked by a challenge dose. Both these patients reacted with the same skin reaction on challenge with metronidazole (SEDA-16, 310).

MISCELLANEOUS DRUGS

Arsenobenzol

Like the other compounds with an arsenic base, arsenobenzol may cause gastrointestinal complaints, but also polyneuritis and encephalopathy.

Administration of adrenaline was shown to be preventive against the development of encephalopathy and helpful in treating hemorrhagic encephalopathy (SED-11, 597).

Difetarsone

This pentavalent arsenical often causes minor side effects such as rashes, nausea, vomiting and abdominal discomfort. Transient increases in the liver enzyme serum levels, AST and ALT, may occur (SED-12, 708).

A case of generalized angioedema was described in a patient receiving difetarsone 500 mg t.i.d. for *Entamoeba histolytica* infection (SED-11, 597).

Melarsoprol (Arsobal)

Melarsoprol given intravenously in patients with trypanosomiasis may cause peripheral neuropathy within 2–5 weeks (SEDA-14, 243). This trivalent arsenical is also known to cause a reactive arsenical encephalopathy in 3—5% of patients with trypanosomiasis (SED-12, 708). Myalgias, distal paresthesias and rapidly progressive weakness in all limbs developed in a young woman treated for 38 days with melarsoprol; massive distal Wallerian degeneration was found in the peripheral nerve as well as abnormalities in the dorsal ganglia and spinal cord. Very high concentrations of arsenic were found in the spinal cord. All findings were typical for a toxic arsenic accumulation; in this case, renal dysfunction was probably at the base of the arsenic poisoning (SEDA-16, 316).

In a group of patients with *Trypanosoma brucei gambiense* sleeping sickness, the incidence of drug-induced encephalopathy was increased in patients with trypanosomes present in the CNS, in patients with high CSF lymphocyte counts, and among those in whom no trypanosomes were found in either the blood or lymph node aspirate. The authors of this report considered that aggressive therapeutic schemes may result in higher toxicity especially in the patient with an impaired blood-brain barrier (SEDA-16, 316). Without data on dosage, renal function and cerebral involvement prior to the start of therapy it is impossible to assess this conclusion.

Difluoromethylornithine (eflornithine hydrochloride; Ornidyl; DFM)

DFM is a specific irreversible inhibitor of ornithine decarboxylase, the enzyme involved in the first step of the polyamine pathway. Decarboxylation of ornithine is an obligatory and rate-limiting step in the biosynthesis of polyamines such as putrescine, spermidine and spermine. These low-molecular weight polyamines play an essential role in the growth, differentiation and replication of the cell by participating in nucleic acid and protein synthesis and are needed in the process of decoding genetic messages. In vitro studies of different types of cell lines (including human malignant cells) exposed to DFM demonstrated inhibition of growth. DFM added to human *Plasmodium falciparum*-infected red cells decreased parasite growth and intracellular polyamine content. Polyamines play an important role in the cellular metabolism of trypanosomatids (SED-12, 708). DFM can arrest viral replication.

The drug hydrochloride can be given intravenously and orally. Absorption after oral administration is adequate. After intravenous administration 80% of the drug is excreted unchanged in the urine within 14 hours. Eflornithine does penetrate into the CNS, cerebrospinal fluid levels are 10—45% of serum levels. Eflornithine has been used in chemotherapy for different types of tumors including glioblastoma and carcinoma in the presence of polyposis coli. It has been employed in the treatment of malaria tropica; in AIDS and in *Pneumocystis carinii* infections with varied success. It more recently has been authoritatively approved for use in *Trypanosoma gambiense* (SED-12, 708).

ADVERSE REACTION PATTERN

The most important side effect is a natural consequence of the manner of action, myelosuppression being frequent and sometimes treatment limiting. Gastrointestinal toxicity, too, is common; it is more marked with oral administration. Seizures, hearing loss, alterations in liver function tests and rash were described in the treatment of *Pneumocystis carinii* infections in patients with AIDS (SED-12, 708). In a group of 31 patients with AIDS and PCP-intolerant of and/or unresponsive to co-trimoxazole or pentamidine, about 50% reacted favourably to DFMO treatment. The adverse effects were no different from those seen in non-AIDS patients, but the frequency of adverse effects was higher. The most common effects in this group were myelosuppression, thrombocytopenia being the most serious, with hepatitis (3%) and hearing loss (9%) among the others (SEDA-17, 332).

Second-generation and tumour-inducing effects In vivo animal studies have shown arrest of the growth of malignant cells and decrease in tumor size (SED-12, 708), but as one might expect there was also an arrest of embryonic growth if DFM was given in the first days of pregnancy (SED-12, 708). On theoretical grounds influence on development of the fast growing embryo could be expected; if this could lead to defects and/or deformations is not known.

ORGANS AND SYSTEMS

Cardiovascular Intravenous use may cause *thrombophlebitis*.

Nervous system *Tinnitus* has been reported in some studies. The occurrence of convulsions was mentioned during cancer therapy (SED-12, 708). Further studies have estimated the frequency of occurrence of seizures at 8% in patients with trypanosomiasis (SEDA-16, 316).

Hematological *Myelosuppression* as evidenced by anemia, leukopenia and thrombopenia is common. The manufacturer of eflornithine quotes incidence rates of 55, 37 and 14%, respectively. Other reports however suggest that the thrombopenia is the most frequent problem; a report by Ajani et al. indicates that thrombopenia is dose dependent and occurred in 90% of patients with cancer on a dose of 6—8 grams/m^2 with DFM levels >400 mmol/ml (SED-12, 709). Again the impression is gained that patients with AIDS have an higher incidence of side effects. The myelosuppression is reversible on discontinuation of treatment (SED-12, 708; SEDA-16, 316).

Gastrointestinal *Nausea, vomiting, abdominal pains* and *diarrhea*, mild or severe, are seen with parenteral and oral administration, but more markedly after oral administration (SED-12, 708).

Skin *Alopecia* has been reported. However, many of the patients with malignant conditions had received chemotherapy as well.

Special senses *Hypoacusia* was mentioned during therapy in some cases, again a reversible effect (SED-12—708). It is not clear what the mechanism might be.

Interactions No information is available.

Suramin *(SEDA-17, 333; see also Chapter 31)*

Suramin is used for the treatment of African trypanosomiasis, and more recently has been found to have new potential as a cancer chemotherapeutic agent. It is toxic and causes many serious adverse effects. They include neurological toxicity (e.g. a polyradiculopathy), liver function disturbances, nephrotoxicity and electrolyte abnormalities including hypocalcemia. Adrenocortical suppression may occur.

Blood coagulation can be deranged, since suramin may cause an accumulation of glycosaminoglycans, which have heparin-like properties. There also seems to be a direct inhibitory effect on various clotting factors, in particular factor V, where the inhibition is irreversible (SED-17, 333). Occasional cases of hemolytic anemia and agranulocytosis have been reported (SED-12, 780).

Skin reactions are of variable severity but occurred in one study in some 60% of the patients. Epidermal necrolysis has been reported. A single dose of intravenous hydrocortisone, 200 mg, was protective against skin complications in another small group of patients.

Suramin may have varied effects on the eye. Photophobia, lacrimation and palpebral edema are recognized late effects and there is evidence of a late optic atrophy. Suramin was tried in the treatment of AIDS. With this indication and with use as a treatment for adrenal carcinoma a high incidence of keratopathy was seen (SED-12, 780).

Hycanthone

Hepatitis was found to be the major complication with hycanthone in the treatment of schistosomiasis. Hycanthone has also been evaluated as a potential antitumor agent, being used as a radiosensitizer; here too, hepatitis was a dose-limiting effect, occurring in some patients with doses of 100 mg/m^2 per day. The lowest dose able to induce hepatitis was reported to be 70 mg/m^2 per day. In several cases the hepatotoxicity proved fatal (SED-11, 597).

Menichlopholan (Niclofolan)

Sweating, generalized pains and transient rises of serum transaminase levels were reported with the use of menichlopholan in the treatment of pulmonary infections due to *Paragonimus uterobilaterali* (SED-11, 597).

Metrifonate

Metrifonate, used in the treatment of urinary schistosomiasis and given in a single monthly dose, causes few side effects; gastrointestinal intolerance, headache, vertigo and, in children, a depression of anti-cholinesterase activity are recognized (SED-11, 597). When metrifonate was used in daily doses, as in the treatment of *Onchocerca volvulus* infections, muscarine like effects of acetylcholine were present, and in one published case proximal weakness due to a nicotine-like effect was describe. The combination of polyarthritis, fever and an elevated sedimentation rate was described in 11 patients out of 34 treated.

The birth of a hydrocephalic infant with a large meningomyelocele to a mother who had been treated with metrifonate for a *Schistosoma haematobium* infection during the second month of pregnancy has been reported, but the report is not recent and the association was probably co-incidental (SED-11, 598).

Nifurtimox

There are still few drugs available for the treatment of late stage sleeping sickness due to *Trypanosoma brucei gambiense*. Melarsaprol and difluoromethylornithine are equally efficacious, but both are toxic and DFMO is also expensive. High-dose nifurtimox (30 mg/kg per day) has been used in Zaire for the treatment of arsenic-resistant trypanosomiasis; this dose was more effective and also more toxic. Of the 30 patients, one died after a period of confusion and coma and eight developed neurological effects, namely confusion, tremor, vertigo and convulsions. One developed a rash and 12 had marked weight loss (SEDA-17, 333).

Acute polymyositis and toxic erythema purpura were described in a young woman treated with nifurtimox for Chagas disease; the patient died due to respiratory and renal failure (SED-11, 598). Chromosomal aberrations were found to be significantly increased in cultures of peripheral lymphocytes from a small group of chagasic children treated with nifurtimox. G-binding analysis of chromosomal aberration sites revealed that treated patients presented coincidence in the chromosome regions affected (SEDA-15, 298).

Furazolidone

Used in the treatment of giardiasis, side effects are usually mild and transient: abdominal discomfort, nausea and vomiting. Urine may be dark coloured (SED-11, 597).

Oxamniquine (Vancil)

Oxamniquine, an aminomethyl tetrahydroquinoline, is mainly used in the treatment of schistosomiasis at a dose of 15—20 mg/kg a day. Treatment periods are usually short. The incidence of side effects is to a large extent dose dependent. With the higher doses somnolence was reported in 25% of cases. Somnolence is reportedly more common if the drug is given just prior to a meal. In a study comparing oxamniquine with praziquantel side effects were seen in 45% of cases treated with oxamniquine and in 71% of patients given praziquantel; somnolence however occurred less frequently (11% of cases) with praziquantel (SED-12, 709).

Gastrointestinal complaints are common, taking the form of epigastric or abdominal discomfort and anorexia. Headache and dizziness were reported also, but with a lesser incidence.

Fever occurs in about a quarter of the patients (SED-11, 598; 107) and in some 15% of these a Löffler-like syndrome with eosinophilia and pulmonary infiltrates was seen when it was specifically looked for in a study (SED-11, 598).

Hepatic enzyme changes, initially reported as rare, may in fact prove frequent if looked for. In the study by Kilpatrick et al. changes were seen in 79% of the patients, with elevations of alkaline phosphatase in 36% and a raised eosinophil count in 52% (SED-12, 710). ECG and EEG changes have been reported as rare side effects (SED-11, 598).

Praziquantel (Biltricide, Cysticide)

Praziquantel is effective against schistosomiasis (including cerebral forms), cysticercosis, pulmonary paragonimiasis and *Opisthorchis viverrini* infections. Doses vary from 40 to 70 mg/kg per day depending on the infecting species. Evaluation of the result of praziquantel treatment in a study revealed a lower laboratory rate of success than reported in the literature for clinical response (SEDA-16, 311). Fallon et al. reported a diminished susceptibility to praziquantel of *Schistosoma mansoni* in an area in Northern Senegal (81).

While side effects are common, it is rarely necessary to discontinue treatment (SED-12, 710). The main side effects are abdominal discomfort, diarrhea, nausea and vomiting and also dizziness and somnolence (SED-12, 710; SEDA-16, 310). In a group of children treated with 40 mg/kg per day the incidence was 63, 18 and 8% for the gastrointestinal complaints. Dizziness and somnolence are mentioned in most reports; among children somnolence was seen in 11%. Headaches, skin rashes and fever are less common (SED-12, 710).

A delayed reaction with central nervous system involvement has been described in patients with cerebral cysticercosis; papilledema, evidence of hemorrhages, focal seizures, motor weakness (SEDA-13, 242) and in one case a hemiplegia from a vasculitic infarct occurred (SEDA-14, 243). The possibility of this reaction being caused by a massive inflammatory response was discussed (SEDA-14, 243). If this hypothesis is correct, corticosteroid treatment could be contemplated. A recent review indicates that the use of corticosteroids, although still controversial, is generally accepted as a means of alleviation of inflammatory complications (SED-12, 710); however, simultaneous use of a corticosteroid seems to reduce significantly the plasma praziquantel concentration (SED-12, 710). According to one group of investigators, no delayed reaction was seen in patients with cerebral schistosomiasis (SED-12, 710).

A case of acute respiratory failure with exudative polyserositis has been reported.

In a group of patients with neurocysticercosis treated with praziquantel in increasing doses of 10—50 mg/kg per day during the first week and maintenance therapy the second week, 27 (60%) presented with side effects, three requiring the interruption of therapy. Decompensation of the increased intracranial pressure occurred in two cases (one of them fatal). Exacerbation of the CSF pleocytosis was recorded in 26 patients (57%) (SEDA-16, 311).

Paromomycin (Aminosidine)

Paromomycin is an orally administered, poorly absorbed aminoglycoside antibiotic. Recent reports suggest that it could be useful in the treatment of intestinal cryptosporidiosis such as occurs in AIDS patients. In a small group of seven patients, paromomycin 500 mg every 6 hours for an average of 11.7 days decreased the frequency of diarrhea in all, with improvement in body weight, although recurrence of the presence of *Cryptosporidium* was noted in three cases. Adverse effects were nausea and abdominal discomfort in two patients (82[c]). Another group of 41 AIDS patients was treated with 2000 mg daily for 4 weeks followed by 1000 mg daily for another 4 weeks. Eleven of the 41 patients had, alongside the symptoms of an intestinal cryptosporidiosis, other opportunistic infections. Efficacy of treatment could be evaluated in 35 patients; a complete response was seen in seven, an additional 15 had a marked improvement, 10 did not respond and three patients died. Treatment was well tolerated, six patients complained about transient constipation. No significant change was observed in the clinical laboratory parameters. There is no separate mention of renal function tests in this short report (83[C]).

Especially in patients with AIDS due care should be taken in checking renal function, despite the comment of Bissuel et al. that only two of 12 volunteer patients on long-term high-dose oral paromomycin had traces of paromomycin in the blood on testing (84[C]).

ANTIMONY COMPOUNDS

Antimony compounds, trivalent or pentavalent stibium, are still the most effective treatment of leishmaniasis. Sodium stibogluconate is the most commonly used. All have a rather high rate of acute and also cumulative toxicity. Frequent side effects include myalgia, joint stiffness, bone pain, fever and headache. Sudden death connected with myocardial or hepatic failure has been reported.

Meglumine antimoniate (Glucantime)/sodium stibogluconate (Pentostam)

These two pentavalent antimonials are chemically similar and are considered to have similar efficacy and toxicity. Meglutamine antimoniate solution contains 8.5% pentavalent Sb, stibogluconate 10%. Antimony is excreted in the urine. Peak levels of antimony are seen about 1—2 hours after an intramuscular injection. Serum levels fall to about 10% of peak levels after about 8 hours. There is some accumulation of Sb on continued treatment. On a weight for weight basis children require a higher dose and tolerate antimony better. Tolerance is adversely affected by impaired renal function, as would be expected for a drug mainly excreted in the urine.

ADVERSE REACTION PATTERN

General and toxic reactions Common side effects are anorexia, nausea, vomiting, malaise, myalgia, headache and lethargy. Muscle, bone and joint-pains have been described (SED-11, 599; SED-12, 710). Cardiac toxicity demonstrated with ECG changes is dose dependent.

The general condition of the patient with visceral leishmaniasis probably plays a crucial role in these and other side effects; malnutrition is common, the immune status often severely impaired and patients are susceptible to intercurrent infections (SED-12, 710).

Hypersensitivity reactions Skin rashes do occur, but serious cutaneous effects have not been reported. Palindromic arthropathy and arthralgias are quite common; these are more likely to represent a reaction to the tissue of the dead or dying parasite than a true allergy against the drug.

Tumor-inducing effects These have not been described.

ORGANS AND SYSTEMS

Cardiovascular *ECG changes* are common; in one group an incidence of 7% was observed. The most common changes are ST-wave changes, T-wave inversions and a prolonged QT interval. The role of conduction disturbances in cases of *cardiac failure* and *sudden death* is not well known. Cases of sudden death have been seen early in treatment after a second injection (SED-12, 710; SEDA-16, 311).

Nervous system *Headaches* are a common complaint during treatment. Generalized *neuralgia* was reported in one study with an incidence of 4% (SED-12, 710; SEDA-16, 311).

Hematological Hematological effects are rare. A case of *auto-immune hemolytic anemia* was described with *N*-methylglucamine antimonate. *Thrombopenia* was reported in a patients with a *Leishmania donovani infection* and AIDS after receiving stibogluconate therapy for 7 days (SED-12, 710). There have been two further reports, one involving a patient with cutaneous leishmaniases (occurring after 19 days of treatment), the second case a man with kala-azar (who became thombocytopenic 11 days after starting therapy); it should be noted that a kala-azar patient commonly has a low thrombocyte count as a result of the illness and that the count normally rises with treatment (SEDA-18, 294).

Liver Hepatotoxicity has been described but the disease itself may play an over-riding role. In a group of 16 patients treated for mucosal leishmaniasis with Pentostan 20 mg/kg i.v. for 28 days *liver enzyme elevations* in conjunction with ECG abnormalities and or musculoskeletal complaints occurred in three subjects (SEDA-16, 311).

Gastrointestinal *Anorexia*, *nausea* and *vomiting* are common complaints. Less common but probably under-reported is the complaint of a *metallic taste* (SEDA-16, 311).

Pancreas *Pancreatitis* has occasionally been reported with the use of the antimony compounds. In 1993, four cases were described in three reports; two of the patients were immunocompromised. One of the patients was asymptomatic, while the other three complained of abdominal pain. Rechallenge with the drug with half of the standard dose was carried out in one of the cases and this resulted in an renewed increase of serum amylase levels. The mechanism and frequency of this side effect are unknown. It has been suggested that immunocompromised patients may be at a higher risk (SEDA-18, 294) but pancreatitis is in any case seen more frequently in AIDS patients, irrespective of drug treatment.

Musculoskeletal system *Arthralgia* is a common complaint during treatment with pentavalent antimonial compounds and is usually dose dependent. *Muscle pain* and *bone pain* have been described as well. A palindromic arthropathy with effusion and pancreatitis occurred in association with stibogluconate treatment for kala-azar in a 30-year-old male on hemodialysis for chronic renal failure (SEDA-16, 311).

Risk factors *Impaired renal function* is an obvious risk factor.

Stibocaptate

The toxicity of this trivalent antimony compound, especially the acute type of adverse problem, is similar to that of the pentavalent compounds. Sudden death has been reported with Stibocaptate (SED-11, 599).

Combined drug treatments for leishmaniasis

In visceral and dermal leishmaniasis, treatment failure is common and this is one reason for the use of combined drug regimens. Combined treatment of meglumine antimonate with γ-interferon in refractory visceral leishmaniasis was reported (SED-12, 711). The clinical results were good with a rapid improvement in general condition, weight gain and decrease of the size of the spleen. Not all cases became parasite free. Side effects known to occur with interferon were seen; fever, fatigue, myalgia, headache. There was no evidence of any change in toxicity of the antimony treatment; whether there was any change in kinetics is not known.

A further success of combined treatment using γ-interferon and an antimony drug was reported by Sundar et al. Fifteen patients with treatment failure after antimony and at least one additional course of treatment with either antimony or pentamidine were treated with stiboglucanate 20 mg/kg per day plus γ-interferon for a period of 30 days. Treatment had to be discontinued in two patients because of anemia and congestive failure in the one and intractable vomiting in the other. Both these patients died subsequently. After 30 days of treatment, nine of the 13 were apparently cured and 6 months after treatment all nine were healthy, had parasite-free bone marrow smears and were considered cured. Over the follow-up of about 15 months there had been no relapses (85^C).

An improved reaction to pentamidine treatment when it was combined with γ-interferon was seen in a patients with *Leishmania infantum* infection and AIDS. This suggests that the improved reaction is connected with a direct effect of the interferon rather than a change in pharmacokinetics of the antimony drug. One may note that γ-interferon alone has been shown to be effective in the treatment of cutaneous leishmania lesions (SED-12, 711).

In a comparative trial in visceral leishmaniasis carried out in southern Sudan, the effectiveness of sodium stibogluconate alone at a doses of 20 mg/kg per day for 30 days was compared with the same regime plus aminosidine 15 mg/kg per day for a period of 17 days for the treatment of visceral leishmaniasis. Treatment results were comparable. In the stibogluconate-only group (99 patients) 7% died, in the two drug group (101 patients) 4% died. All 184 patients who completed the treatment were clinically cured. Where microscopy of aspirates was performed, it was found that 95% of the group receiving the combination were clear as against 81% of those receiving stibogluconate only. Of importance is of course the duration of treatment, and as the authors note the combined treatment for 17 days was less expensive than the stibogluconate medication for 30 days. The oto- or nephrotoxicity that can occur with aminosidine was looked for but not detected; there seemed to be a lesser incidence of pneumonia in the group on aminosidine, and there was a beneficial effect on the frequency and duration of diarrhea (86^C).

Allopurinol Allopurinol, an analogue of purine, has an antileishmanial effect in vitro and in animal models, its effect being strongly increased by the addition of antimonial compounds. Allopurinol and the combination with meglumine antimoniate have been used in clinical studies. In a small human study of leishmaniasis and HIV infection, clinical and parasitological cure was achieved in four of five cases treated for 4 weeks but in only one of the six treated for 3 weeks (87[C]).

Amphotericin B This might be useful in the treatment of leishmaniasis, as suggested by a comparative study (amphotericin in 14 doses of 0.5 mg/kg infused in 5% glucose on alternate days) against sodium stibogluconate (20 mg/kg in two divided doses daily for 40 days). All 40 patients on amphotericin were cured, whereas in the stibium gluconate group 28 of the 40 showed an initial cure but only 25 a definite cure (88). Other work seems to confirm this impression. Side effects observed are those well known with amphotericin B (see Chapter 27).

REFERENCES

1. Dolmans WM, Van Der Kaay HJ, Leentvaar-Kuypers A, Stuiver PC, Wetsteyn JCFM, Warris-Versteegen AA. Malariaprofylaxe: adviezen weer aangepast. Ned Tydschr Geneesk 1994;138(34):1723–1724.
2. Editorial. Staatstoezicht op de Volksgezondheid. Malariaprofylaxe. Ryswyk Geneesm Bull 1994;August.
3. Murphy GS, Purnomo HB, Andersen EM, Bangs MJ, Mount DL et al. Vivax malaria resistant to treatment and prophylaxis with chloroquine. Lancet 1993;341:96–100.
4. Greenwood BM, Pickering H. A malaria control trial using insecticide-treated bed nets and targeted chemoprophylaxis in a rural area of The Gambia, West Africa. Trans R Soc Trop Med Hyg 1993;87(Suppl 2);3–11.
5. Noticeboard. Resistant malaria in Cambodia. Lancet 1992;339:735.
6. Nosten F, Karbwang J, White N, Honeymoon K, Bangchang K et al. Mefloquine antimalarial prohylaxis in pregnancy: dose finding and pharmacokinetic studies. Br J Clin Pharmacol 1990;30:79–85.
7. Campbell CC. Challenges facing antimalarial therapy in Africa. J Infect Dis 1991;163:1207.
8. Berman J, Brown L, Miller R, Andersen SL, McGreevy P et al. Antimalarial activity of WR-243251, a dihydroacridinedione. Antimicrobial Agents Chemother 1994;38:1753–1756.
9. Vennerstrom L, Hong-Ning Fu, Ellis WY, Ager AL, Wood JK et al. Dispiro-1,2,4,5-tetraoxanes: a new class of antimalarial peroxides. J Med Chem 1992;35(16);3023–3027.
10. Posner GH, Chang HOH, Webster K, Ager AL, Rossan RN. New antimalarial tricyclic 1,2,4-trioxanes: evaluations in mice and monkeys. Am J Trop Med Hyg 1994;50:522–526.
11. Marshal SJ, Russell PF, Wright CW, Anderson MM, Philipson JD, et al. In vitro antiplasmodial antiamoebic, and cytotoxic activities of a series of bisbenzylisoquinoline alkaloids. Antimicrobial Agents Chemother 1994;38:96–103.
12. White NJ. Tough test for malaria vaccine. Lancet 1994;344:1172–1173.
13. Alonso PL, Smith T, Schellenberg JR, Masanja H, Mwankusye S et al. Randomised trial of efficacy of SPf66 vaccine against Plasmodium falciparum in children in Southern Tanzania. Lancet 1995;344:1175–1181.
14. Alonso PL, Tanner M, Smith T, Hayes RJ, Schellenberg JA et al. A trial of the synthetic malaria vaccine SPf66 in Tanzania: rationale and design. Vaccine 1994;12:181–186.
15. Sempertequi F, Estrella B, Moscoso J, Piedrahita L et al. Safety immunogenicity and protective effect of SPf66 malaria synthetic vaccine against Plasmodium falciparum infection in a randomized double-blind placebo-controlled field trial. Vaccine 1994;12:337–342.
16. Amador R, Moreno A, Murillo LA et al. Safety and immunogenicity of the synthetic malaria vaccine SPf66 in a large field trial. J Infect Dis 1992;166:139–144.
17. Valero MV, Amador LR, Galindo C et al. Vaccination with SPpf66, a chemically synthesised vaccine against Plasmodium falciparum in Colombia. Lancet 1993;341:706–710.
18. Noya O, Berti YG, Alarcon De Noya B, Borges R, Zerpa N et al. A population based clinical trial with the SPf66 synthetic Plasmodium falciparum vaccine in Venezuela. J Infect Dis 1994;170:396–402.
19. Carme B, Moudzeo H, Mbitsi A et al. Stabilisation of drug resistance (chloroquine and amodiaquine) of Plasmodium falciparum in semi immune populations in The Congo. J Infect Dis 1991;164:437–438.
20. Steffen R, Fuchs E, Schildknecht J, Nael U et al. Mefloquine compared with other malaria chemoprophylactic regimens in tourists visiting East Africa. Lancet 1993;341:1299–1302.
21. Committee To Advise On Tropical Medicine And Travel. Statement on travellers and rabies vaccine. Can Med Assoc J 1995;152:1241–1242.
22. Pappaioanou M, Fishbein DB, Dreesen DW et al. Antibody response to preexposure of human diploid cell to rabies vaccine given concurrently with chloroquine. New Engl J Med 1986;314:280–284.
23. Editorial. Human rabies Kenya. MMWR 1983;32:494–495.
24. Ndifor AM, Howells RE, Bray PG, Ngu JL et al. Enhancement of drug susceptibility in Plasmodium falciparum in vitro and Plasmodium berghei in vivo by mixed-function oxidase inhibitors. Antimicrobial Agents Chemother 1993; 37:1318–1823.
25. Gaudebout C, Pussard E, Clavier F, Gueret D et al. Efficacy of intramuscular amopryoquin for treatment of Plasmodium falciparum malaria in The Gabon Republic. Antimicrobial Agents Chemother 1993;37:970–974.

26. Smithuis FM, Van-Woensel JBM, Nordlander E, Wanta WS et al. Comparison of two mefloroquine regimens for treatment of Plasmodium falciparum malaria on the Northern Thai-Cambodian Border. Antimicrobial Agents Chemother 1993;37:1977–1981.
27. Ter Kuile FO, Ter Nosten F, Thieren M, Luxemburger C et al. High dose mefloquine in the treatment of multiresistant falciparum malaria. J Infect Dis 1992;165:1399–1400.
28. Wittes RC, Saginur R. Adverse reactions to mefloquine associated with ethanol ingestion. Can Med Assoc J 1995; 152(4):515–517.
29. Speich R, Haller A. Central anticholinergic syndrome with the antimalarial drug mefloquine. New Engl J Med 1994;331:57–58.
30. Martin G, Malone J, Ross V. Exfoliative dermatitis during malaria prophylaxis with mefloquine. Clin Infect Dis 1993;16:341–342.
31. Nosten F, Ter-Kuile F, Maelankiri L, Chongsuphajaisiddhi T, Nopdonrattakoon L et al. Mefloquin prophylaxis prevents malaria during pregnancy: a double blind placebo-controlled study. J Infect Dis 1994;169:595–603.
32. Clinton-White A, Runnels JH. Mefloquine prophylaxis in pregnancy. J Infect Dis 1995;171:235–254.
33. Maguire RB, Stroneck DF, Campbell AC. Recurrent pancytopenia coagulopathy and renal failure associated with multiple quinine-dependent antibodies. Ann Int Med 1993;119:215–217.
34. Metzger W, Mordmuller B, Graninger W, Bienzle U, Kremser PG. High efficacy of short-term quinine-antibiotic combinations for treating adult malaria patients in an area in which malaria is hyperendemic. Antimicrobial Agents Chemother 1995;39:245–246.
35. Kremsner PG, Radloff P, Metzger W, Wildling E, Mordmuller B et al. Quinine plus clindamycin improves chemotherapy of severe malaria in children. Antimicrobial Agents Chemother 1995;39:1603–1605.
36. White NJ. Artemisinin: current status. Trans R Soc Trop Med Hyg 1994;88(Suppl 1):3–4.
37. Laughlin JC. Agricultural production of artemisinin—a review. Trans R Soc Trop Med Hyg 1994;88(Suppl 1):21–22.
38. Shmuklarsky MJ, Klayman DL, Milhous WK, Kyle DE, Rossan RN et al. Comparison of β-artemether and β-arteether against malaria parasites in vitro and in vivo. Am J Trop Med Hyg 1993;48(3):377–384.
39. Meshnick SR. The mode of action of antimalarial endoperoxides. Trans R Soc Trop Med Hyg 1994;88(Suppl 1): 31–32.
40. Brewer TG, Peggins JO, Grate SJ, Petras JM, Levine BS et al. Neurotoxicity in animals due to arteether and artemether. Trans R Soc Trop Med Hyg 1994;88(Suppl 1):33–36.
41. Wesche DL, DeCoster MA, Totella FC, Brewer TG. Neurotoxicity Of artemisinin analogs in vitro. Antimicrobial Agents Chemother 1994;38:1813–1819.
42. Kager PA, Schultz MJM, Zijlstra EE, Van Den Berg B, Van Boxtel ChJ. Arteether administration in humans: preliminary studies of pharmacokinetics safety and tolerance. Trans R Soc Trop Med Hyg 1994;88(Suppl 1):53–54.
43. Looareesuwam S, Viravan C, Vanijanonta S, Wilairatana P, Suntharasami P et al. Randomised trial of artesunate and mefloquine alone and in sequence for acute uncomplicated falciparum malaria. Lancet 1992;339:821–24.
44. Nosten F, Luxemburger C, Ter Kuile FO, Woodrow C, White NJ. Treatment of multi resistant Plasmodium falciparum malaria with 3 day artesunate-mefloquine combination. J Infect Dis 1994;170:971–977.
45. Karbwang J, Na-Bangchang K, Thanavibul A, Bunnag D et al. Comparison of oral artesunate and quinine plus tetracycline in acute uncomplicated falciparum malaria. WHO Bull OMS 1994;72:233–238.
46. Fadat G, Louis FJ, Louis J-P, Le Bras J. Efficacy of micronized halofantrine in semi-immune patients with acute uncomplicated falciparum malaria in Cameroon. Antimicrobial Agents Chemother 1993;37:1955–1957.
47. Bouchaud O, Basco LK, Gillotin C, Gimenez F et al. Clinical efficay and pharmacokinetics of micronized halofantrine for the treatment of acute uncomplicated falciparum malaria in nonimmune patients. Am J Trop Med Hyg 1994;51(2):204–213.
48. Wilding E, Jenne L, Graninger W, Bienzle U, Kremsner PG. High dose chloroquine versus micronized halofantrine in chloroquine resistant Plasmodium falciparum malaria. J Antimicrobial Chemother 1994;33:871–875.
49. Toivonen L, Vitasalo M, Siikamaki H, Raatikka M et al. Provocation of ventricular tachycardia by antimalarial drug halofantrine in congenital long QT syndrome. Clin Cardiol 1994;17:403–404.
50. Di Perri G, Di Perri IG, Monteiro GB, Bonora S et al. Pentoxifylline as a supportive agent in the treatment of cerebral malaria in children. J Infect Dis 1995;171:1317–1322.
51. Masur H. Prevention and treatment of Pneumocystis pneumonia. New Engl J Med 1992;327:1853–1859.
52. Hughes WT, Killmar JT, Helich S. Relative potency of 10 drugs with anti-Pneumocystis carinii activity in an animal model. J Infect Dis 1994;170:906–911.
53. Schneider MM, Hoepelman AI, Eeftinck Schattenkerk JK, Nielsen TL, Van Der Graaf Y et al. A controlled trial of aerosolised pentamidine or trimethoprim-sulfamethoxazole as primary prophylaxis against Pneumocystis carinii pneumonia in patients with human immunodeficiency virus infection. New Engl J Med 1992;327:1836–1841.
54. Hardy WD, Feinberg J, Finkelstein DM, Power ME, He W et al. A controlled trial of trimethoprim-sulfamethoxazole or aerosolized pentamidine for secondary prophylaxis of Pneumocystis carinii pneumonia in patients with the acquired immunodeficiency syndrome. New Engl J Med 1992; 327:1842–1848.
55. Bozzette SA, Finkelstein D, Spector SA, Frame P, Powderly WG et al. A randomised trail of three anti-Pneumocystis agents in patients with advanced human immunodeficiency virus infection. New Engl J Med 1995;332:693–698.
56. Torres RA, Barr M, Thorn M, Gregory G, Keily S et al. Randomised trial of dapsone and aerosolised pentamidine for the prophylaxis of Pneumocystis carinii pneumonia and toxoplasmic encephalitis. Am J Med 1993;95:573–583.
57. Cheung TW, Matta R, Neibart E, Hammer G, Chusid E et al. Intramuscular pentamidine for the prevention of Pneumocystis carinii pneumonia in patients infected with H.I.V. Clin Infect Dis 1993;16:22–25.
58. Tietjen PA, Stover DE. Pneumocystis carinii pneumonia. Semin Resp Crit Care Med 1995;16:173–186.
59. Gradon JD, Fricchione L, Sepkowitz D. Severe hypo-

magnesemia associated with pentamidine therapy. Rev Infect Dis 1991;13:511–512.

60. Safrin S, Lee BL, Sande MA. Adjunctive folinic acid with trimethoprim-sulfamethoxazole for Pneumocystis carinii pneumonia in A.I.D.S. patients is associated with an increased risk of therapeutic failure and death. J Infect Dis 1994;170:912–917.

61. Carr A, Swanson C, Penny R, and Cooper D.A. Clinical Laboratory markers of hypersensitivity to trimethoprim-sulfamethoxazole in patients with Pneumocystis carinii pneumonia and A.I.D.S. J Infect Dis 1993;167:180–184.

62. Martin GJ, Scott F, Paparello SF, Decker CF. A severe systemic reaction to trimethoprim-sulfamethoxazole in a patient infected with the H.I.V. Clin Infect Dis 1993;16:175–176.

63. Goodman Gilman A, Rall ThW, Nies AS, Taylor P, eds. Goodman And Gilman's The Pharmacological Basis Of Therapeutics. Reference Book, 8th edn, 1990;1160.

64. Unpublished Personal Communication. 1995.

65. Chang HR, Arsenijevic D, Comte R, Polak A, Then RL, Pechere J-C. Activity of epiroprim (Ro 11-8958), a dihydrofolate reductase inhibitor alone and in combination with dapsone against Toxoplasma gondii. Antimicrobial Agents Chemother 1994;38:1803–1807.

66. Noskins GA, Murphy RL, Black JR, Phair JP. Salvage therapy with clindamycin/primaquine for Pneumocystis carinii pneumonia. Clin Infect Dis 1992;14:183–184.

67. Hughes W, Leoung G, Kramer F, Bozzette SA, Safrin S et al. Comparison of atovaquone (566C80) with trimethoprim-sulfamethoxazole to treat Pneumocystis carinii pneumonia in patients with A.I.D.S. New Engl J Med 1993; 328:1521–1526.

68. Hughes WT, Lafon SW, Scott JD, Masur H. Adverse events associated with trimethoprim-sulfamethoxazole and atovaquone during the treatment of A.I.D.S.-related Pneumocystis carinii pneumonia. J Infect Dis 1995;171:1295–1301.

69. Dohn MN, Weinberg WGG, Torres RA, Follansbee SE, Caldwell PT et al. Oral atovaquone compared with intravenous pentamidine for Pneumocystis carinii pneumonia in patients with AIDS. Ann Intern Med 1994;121:174–180.

70. Lederman MM, Van Der Horst Ch. Atovaquone for Pneumocystis carinii pneumonia (Letter To The Editor). Ann Intern Med 1995;122(4):314.

71. Stoeckle M, Tennenberg A. Atovaquone for Pneumocystis carinii pneumonia (Letter To The Editor). Ann Intern Med 1995;122(4):314.

72. Powles MA, McFadden DC, Liberator PA, Anderson JW, Vadas EB et al. Aerosolised L-693,989 for Pneumocystis carinii prophylaxis in rats. Antimicrobial Agents Chemother 1994;38:1397–1401.

73. Bartlett MS, Edlind TD, Lee CH, Dean R, Queener SF, et al. Albendazole inhibits Pneumocystis carinii proliferation in innoculated immunosuppressed mice. Antimicrobial Agents Chemother 1994;38:1834–1837.

74. Merali S, Chin K, Grady RW, Weissberger L, Clarkson AB. Response of rat model of Pneumocystis carinii pneumonia to continuous infusion of deferoxamine. Antimicrobial Agents Chemother 1995;39:1442–1444.

75. Corson AP, Chretien JH. Metronidazole-associated aseptic meningitis. Clin Infect Dis 1994;19:974.

76. Corey WA, Doebbeling BN, DeJong KJ, Britigan BE. Metronidazole-induced acute pancreatitis. Rev Infect Dis 1991;13:1213–1215.

77. Britigan BE, Doebeling BN. Metronidazole and pancreatitis (Reply). Clin Infect Dis 1992;15:751.

78. Romero Y, Lacoma YF, Manzano L. Metronidazole and pancreatitis. Clin Infect Dis 1992;15:750–751.

79. Teggi A, Lastilla MG, De-Rosa F. Therapy of human hydatid disease with mebendazole and albendazole. Antimicrobial Agents Chemother 1993;37:1679–1684.

80. Boken DJ, Leoni PA, Preheim LC. Treatment of Strongyloides stercoralis hyperinfection syndrome with thiabendazole administered per rectum. Clin Infect Dis 1993;16:123–126.

81. Fallon PG, Sturrock RF, Capron A, Niang M, Doenhoff MJ. Short report: dimensioned susceptibility to praziquantel in a Senegal isolate of Schistosoma mansoni. Am J Trop Hyg 1995;53(1):61–62.

82. Fichtenbaum CJ, Ritche DJ, Powderly WG. Use of paromomycin for treatment of cryptosporidiosis in patients with AIDS. Clin Infect Dis 1993;16:298–300.

83. Scaglia M, Atzori C, Marchetti G, Orso M et al Effectiveness of aminosidine (paromomycin) sulfate in chronic Cryptosporidium diarrhea in AIDS patients: an open, uncontrolled prospective clinical trial. J Infect Dis 1994; 170:1349–1350.

84. Bissuel F, Cotte L, Demontclos M, Rabodonirina M, Trepo Ch. Oral paromomycin long term high doses treatment for cryptosporidiosis in AIDS (Letter To The Editor). J Infect Dis 1994;170:749–750.

85. Sundar S, Rosenkaimer F, Murray HW. Successful treatment of refractory visceral leishmaniasis in India using antimony plus interferon-gamma. J Infect Dis 1994;170:659–662.

86. Seaman J, Pryce D, Sondorp HE, Moody SA, Bryceson ADM, Davidson RN. Epidemic visceral leishmaniasis in Sudan: a randomised trial of aminosidine plus sodium stibogluconate versus sodium stibogluconate alone. J Infect Dis 1993;168:715–720.

87. Laguna F, Lopez-Velez R, Soriano V, Montilla P et al. Assessment of allopurinol plus meglumine antimoniate in the treatment of visceral leishmaniasis in patients infected with HIV. J Infect Dis 1994;28:255–259.

88. Mishra M, Biswas UK, Jha AM, Khan AB. Amphotericin versus sodium stibogluconate in first-line treatment of Indian kala-azar. Lancet 1994;344:1599–1600.

89. Katiyar SK, Gordon VR, McLaughlin GL, Edlind TD. Antiprotozoal activities of benzimidazoles and correlations with β-tubulin sequence. Antimicrobial Agents Chemother 1994;38:2086–2090.

90. Editorial. CNS adverse event with antimalarial drugs—assess the risk:benefit ratio individually. Drugs 1995;6(8).

91. Clemessy J-L, Favier Ch, Borrin SW, Hantson PE, Vicaut E, Baud FJ. Hypokalaemia related to acute chloroquine ingestion. Lancet 1995;346:877–880.

92. Fryauf DJ, Baird JK, Basri H, Sumawinata I, Purnomo et al. Randomised placebo-controlled trial of primaquine for prophylaxis of falciparum and vivax malaria. Lancet 1995; 346:1190–1193.

93 Salmon-Ceron D, Fontbonne A, Saba J, May T, Raffi F et al. Lower survival in AIDS patients receiving dapsone compared with aerosolized pentamidine for secondary prophylaxis of Pneumocystis carinii pneumonia. J Infect Dis 1995;172:656–664.

94 Merali S, Chin K, Grady R, Clarkson AB. Trophosoite elimination in a rat model of *Pneumocystis carinii* pneumonia. By clinically achievable plasma deferoxame concentrations. Antimicrobial Agents Chemother 1996; 40(5):1298–1300.

Meyler's Side Effects of Drugs, 13th Edition
M.N.G. Dukes, editor

SECTION EDITOR: R. HOIGNÉ

R. Malinverni, R. Hoigné and R. Sonntag

29.1 Sulfonamides, other folic acid antagonists and miscellaneous antibacterial drugs

GENERAL TOPICS

RISKS OF ANTIBACTERIAL THERAPY

Clinical and epidemiological studies of adverse drug reactions focus on side effects. However, antimicrobial treatment may have much greater consequences due to excessive use, underdosage and inadequate duration of treatment.

At present, sulfonamides alone occupy a relatively small place in the therapeutic armamentarium of the physician (1[R]). The combination of sulfonamides with a folic acid antagonist such as trimethoprim has widened their spectrum and provided synergism against a number of bacterial micro-organisms. For some indications, such as uncomplicated urinary tract infection with susceptible organisms, trimethoprim alone has been proven to be clinically effective compared to co-trimoxazole or other combinations. The use of trimethoprim alone, however, is rapidly followed by an increase in bacterial resistance (SEDA-5, 287; 1[R], 2[R]). This fact as well as the favorable pharmacokinetics of co-trimoxazole has resulted in the widespread use of the combination. Established indications are pulmonary, bronchial and urinary tract infections, otitis media, shigellosis, typhoid fever, infections due to *Pneumocystis carinii* and *Toxoplasma*.

Nitrofurantoin, with its low serum and high urinary levels, may be used in uncomplicated urinary tract infections where kidney function is not reduced. It shows a relatively high incidence of severe adverse drug reactions.

Nalidixic acid has been replaced by newer, more effective quinolone preparations. Fluoroquinolones exhibit markedly enhanced antimicrobial activity and have comparable pharmacokinetic properties. Adverse drug reactions similar to those of nalidixic acid are reported.

New data point to a higher risk of adverse drug reactions in immunocompromised HIV-infected patients (SEDA-16, 322).

SULFONAMIDES

'Sulfonamide' is a generic name for derivatives of *p*-aminobenzenesulfonamide (sulfanilamide). Sulfonamides have a wide range of antimicrobial activity against both gram-positive and gram-negative organisms (1[R]). However, they exert only a bacteriostatic and not a bactericidal effect.
The combination of sulfonamides with trimethoprim or trimethoprim analogs results in a synergistic effect against some bacterial organisms and decreases the risk of bacterial resistance. Sulfonamides, therefore, are usually combined with trimethoprim.

Old and new sulfonamides

Based upon their pharmacological properties and adverse reactions, the sulfonamides can be divided into various generations:

The earliest preparations included azosulfonamides (Prontosil, Neoprontosil), sulfapyridine (Dagenan), sulfathiazole (Cibazol), sulfanilamide und sulfadiazine. These are *short-acting sulfonamides* of which sulfadiazine is readily excreted by the kidney. This group, with the exception of sulfadiazine, is currently no longer used.

Sulfadiazine and the more recent compounds including sulfisoxazole, sulfamethoxazole, sulfametrol, sulfacytine and sulfamethizole have been described as being rapidly absorbed and rapidly eliminated sulfonamides. Sulfamethoxazole is an intermediate acting sulfonamide and can be given twice daily (1[R]). Compared with the older generation, they are also more readily soluble, less toxic and probably less allergenic. Since the late 1960s, these sulfonamides have often been used in combination (e.g. trimethoprim with sulfamethoxazole = co-trimoxazole) (2[C]).

A second group is represented by *ultra-long-acting sulfonamides*, e.g. sulfadoxine (*N*-[5,6-dimethoxy-4-pyrimidinyl]sulfanilamide; Fanasil[R]). The combination of sulfadoxine + pyrimethamine (Fansidar[R]) is used for malaria prophylaxis. The advantage of infrequent administration has to be weighed against the possibility of adverse reactions which will then persist proportionately longer.

A third group comprises the *sulfonamides with special uses*. Salazosulfapyridine (sulfasalazine) is composed of sulfapyridine and 5-aminosalicylate linked through an azobond. It is used for mildly-to-moderately ill patients with ulcerative colitis or regional ileitis (Crohn's disease). Salazosulfapyridine is broken down in the gut to sulfapyridine, which is absorbed systemically, and 5-aminosalicylate, which is unabsorbed but reaches high levels in the feces (3[C]). Adverse reactions are mostly similar to those found with other sulfonamides. The combination has been replaced in clinical practice by newer preparations containing only 5-aminosalicylic acid (mesalazine) (3[C]).

Sulfacetamide and sulfadicramide are still used topically for ophthalmic infections. The topical use of sulfonamides, however, should be discouraged because of the high risk of sensitization.

Topical application of silver sulfadiazine is, however, used successfully in burn therapy (4[C]). Since sulfonamide is absorbed systemically through the skin lesions, its adverse reactions are comparable to those observed with systemic application.

ADVERSE REACTION PATTERN

General and toxic reactions The frequency and severity of adverse reactions to sulfonamides correspond to those seen with other antibacterial agents. Purely toxic effects, which tend to be more troublesome than serious, include gastrointestinal symptoms, hepatocellular dysfunction, headache, possibly drowsiness and mild psychic changes. Crystalluria may occur, but urinary obstruction is rare. Hemolytic anemia can be due to enzyme deficiencies and pathological hemoglobins rather than to immunological mechanisms which are extremely rare with sulfonamides. Hematological adverse reactions may also be due to a direct pharmacological effect, e.g. by folic acid antagonism.

Hypersensitivity This is suspected to be the mechanism for a wide range of effects such as anaphylactic shock, serum sickness-like syndrome, systemic allergic vasculitis, drug fever, lupus-like syndrome, allergic pneumonitis or PIE syndrome (pulmonary infiltrations with eosinophilia), or the subgroup of *transient* pulmonary infiltrates with eosinophilia (Loeffler syndrome), interstitial nephritis, hepatitis, severe skin reactions, allergic agranulocytosis and thrombocytopenia, and, extremely rarely, pancytopenia. Even aseptic meningitis has been observed.

In contrast to β-lactam antibiotics, the sulfonamides are rarely the cause of allergic reactions of type I (classification by Coombs and Gell), induced by IgE antibodies. The toxic or allergic nature of most of the above reactions is often unclear.

Tumor-inducing effects These have not been reported.

Second-generation effects Sulfonamides should not be given to pregnant women in the third trimester of pregnancy. The administration of sulfonamides to premature infants may lead to the displacement of bilirubin from plasma albumin and produce a so-called *kernicterus*.

GENERAL TOXIC EFFECTS

General toxic effects consist of gastrointestinal intolerance, nausea, vomiting, anorexia, headache and possibly drowsiness, lowered mental acuity and other psychic alterations (1[R]). Crystalluria with deposits of crystalline aggregates in the renal parenchyma, calyces, pelvis, ureter or bladder produce a pathological urinary sediment. Urinary obstruction with anuria/oliguria was seen primarily with the earlier, less soluble sulfonamides. It may also occur with salazosulfapyridine. This complication is extremely rare with the readily soluble sulfonamides, e.g. sulfadiazine and the new sulfonamides now in use, provided that fluid intake is adequate (about 1.2 liters per 24 hours for adults) (SEDA-11, 259). Prophylaxis can be achieved by urine alkalinization.

For the diagnosis of sulfonamide crystalluria, urine should be examined at 37—C; at room temperature crystals may even be found in urine from patients treated with the readily soluble sulfamethoxazole (5[C]).

Idiosyncratic reactions show clinical symptoms and syndromes resembling either toxic or even allergic adverse reactions. Individual differences in metabolism predispose patients to idiosyncratic reactions, e.g. sulfonamides are metabolized by N-acetylation (mediated by a genetically determined polymorphic enzyme) and oxidation to potentially toxic metabolites (6[C], 7[C]). In a child with dihydropteridine reductase deficiency, a variant of phenylketonuria, adverse drug reactions occurred to co-trimoxazole (8a[c]). Patients who experience immediate hypersensitivity reactions to sulfonamides express IgE that can bind to an N^4-sulfonamidoyl determinant (N4-SM) (8b[C]).

GENERALIZED HYPERSENSITIVITY (ALLERGIC) REACTIONS

Allergic reactions are observed in a few percent of patients treated systemically with the newer sulfonamides. With the older sulfonamides, very severe reactions were described more frequently. The most common form of skin reactions to the newer sulfonamides is a generalized rash, usually maculopapular, sometimes a generalized urticaria. Also, photosensitivity reactions may occur. They are either of the allergic or the toxic type. On rare occasions, generalized erythema (erythroderma), erythema multiforme, erythema nodosum, exfoliative dermatitis, Stevens-Johnson syndrome and toxic epidermal necrolysis ("Lyell syndrome') occur. Even anaphylactic shock may be observed.

If drug fever is accompanied by a skin reaction, the diagnosis is more highly likely than in situations with fever without other manifestations. The diagnosis of serum sickness-like syndrome should be limited to patients with at least three of the symptoms of classical serum sickness, i.e. fever, exanthema, allergic arthritis, lymphadenopathy and possibly leuko- or neutropenia (see also Penicillins, Chapter 25.3). Histologically, a severe serum sickness syndrome seems to correspond to an allergic vasculitis (9[C], 10[C]). Hypersensitivity vasculitis, as induced by drugs, involves the smallest branches of both the arterial and venous vasculature (11[C], 12[C]). This is different from classical polyarteritis which involves arteries of medium and small caliber (12[C]).

Allergic pneumonitis is also found in patients with ulcerative colitis or Crohn's disease, treated with sulfasalazopyrine (see under Respiratory).

Aseptic meningitis, probably with an allergic mechanism, may also be due to a sulfonamide, trimethoprim or both drugs. Transient myopia was described in patients with and without symptoms of a hypersensitivity reaction (see co-trimoxazole).

In some extremely severe systemic allergic reactions, the serum sickness-like syndrome may be complicated by a number of unusual organ manifestations including not only lymphadenopathy with plasmocytosis and lymphocytosis (13[C], 14[C]), but also interstitial myocarditis (15[C], 16[c]), allergic pneumonitis, nephropathy and hepatopathy as well as nervous system disorders (9[C], 10[C]).

The earlier, mainly histopathological descriptions of serum sickness-like syndrome were associated with older sulfonamides which are no longer used (SED-11, 605; 11[C]).

For *reactions probably related to sulfonamide idiosyncrasy* or *hypersensitivity*, there is still little basis for an explanation in terms of differences in metabolite formation, and little current prospect of in vitro tests to predict the reaction (6[C], 7[C], 8a[c], 17[C], 18[C]). Fever and rash, also with severe skin reactions, were observed significantly more often in the slow- as compared to the fast-acetylator phenotype (6[C], 7[C]). For immediate reactions to sulfonamides, IgE was shown to bind to N4-SM (8b[C]) (see also under General toxic effects).

A lymphocyte toxicity assay (LTA) showed a positive result in about 70% of the patients with a common exanthema, an urticarial reaction or erythema multiforme (19a[C]). This biochemical test determines the percent of cell-death due to the drug's toxic metabolites. The same 'in vitro' reaction using the hydroxylamine metabolite of sulfamethoxazole gave significantly different results in six patients with fever, skin rash with or without hepatitis than in control patients (17[C]). Systemic glutathione deficiency with a consequently reduced capacity to scavenge such toxic metabolites might contribute to these adverse reactions (18[C]).

IgE-induced in vitro reactions to sulfonamides have mainly been studied in the last 10 years (8b[C], 19b[C], 20[C]). They are not yet generally used. This may partly be due to the rarity of immediate type reactions.

Although *cross-reactions* between different sulfonamides do occur, this is not a universal phenomenon (1[R]). However, they may even be observed with PAS (*p*-aminosalicylic acid) and local anesthetics of the procain type. The real frequency of cross-sensitivity is almost impossible to assess. Many patients with rash or agranulocytosis have recovered in spite of continued treatment with the same drug (21a[C]). Later re-exposures to the causative agent are often without consequences (possibly in some 50% of cases), especially if rash was the only symptom. One possible explanation for such observations, which were made at a time when the sulfonamides were the only anti-infectious agents available, may be a specific desensitization or tolerance to the drug.

HIV-infected patients receiving relatively high doses of co-trimoxazole often experience rather severe skin and other hypersensitivity reactions (21b[C]).

Desensitization This has been tried with sulfonamides and especially sulfonamide + trimethoprim. The combined preparation seems to be essential, mainly in patients with AIDS, used against *Pneumocystis carinii* infection and cerebral toxoplasmosis (20[C], 22[C]). In spite of the acquired immune deficiency, desensitization could be realized in three of four patients (23[C], 24[C]). The procedure is, however, not completely safe and even anaphylactic shock may occur (20[C], 22[c], 23[c], 24[C], 25[C]).

ORGANS AND SYMPTOMS

Cardiovascular *Anaphylactic shock* is very rarely seen in relation to sulfonamide therapy (8b[c], 17[C], 20[c], 22[c], 26[c], 27[c]). Other cardiovascular reactions may be a consequence of sulfonamide myocarditis (16[C]), widespread and severe skin disease, etc. Sulfonamide myocarditis has been described in relation to earlier sulfonamides and was combined with generalized hypersensitivity reactions (15[C]).

Respiratory Pulmonary infiltrations with eosinophilia (PIE syndrome) have been divided into six categories (28[R], 29[R], 30[C]).

(1) Allergic pneumonitis or the subgroup of transient pulmonary infiltrations associated with blood eosinophilia (Loeffler syndrome) (31[C], 32[C], 33[c]).

(2) Prolonged pulmonary eosinophilia (chronic eosinophilic pneumonia) (8b[C], 28[R]) or migratory pneumonia with eosinophilia (34[c]).

(3) Pulmonary eosinophilia associated with asthma (33[c], 35[c]—37[c]).

(4) Tropical eosinophilia.

(5) Allergic angiitis (see Skin and appendages, Serum sickness-syndrome).

(6) Allergic granulomatosis and angiitis (Churg-Strauss syndrome) (30[C]).

Wegener's granulomatosis is not included because eosinophilia is rare in this condition. Drugs are probably not involved in the pathogenesis of Churg-Strauss syndrome (30[C]).

For categories 1, 2, 3 and 5, a hypersensitivity reaction to a sulfonamide may be responsible.

The link to the drug has been proven in most cases by recurrence following re-exposure to the same sulfonamide or sulfonamide and trimethoprim (see p. 843).

Pyrimethamine + sulfadoxine (Fansidar[R]), used for malaria prophylaxis or treatment, also rarely causes pulmonary reactions, if so, especially with aggressive combined drug therapy (38[c]).

In patients with ulcerative or Crohn's colitis, the pulmonary syndrome was preceeded by treatment with salazosulfapyridine in some cases. Re-exposure to the whole drug again elicited parts of the syndrome (35[c]—37[c], 39[c], 40[C], 41[c]). The sulfapyridine moiety of the drug alone may produce the same reaction on re-exposure (36[c], 37[c]).

Treatment of Crohn's colitis could be continued with 5-aminosalicylic acid alone (37[c]).

Transient pulmonary eosinophilia usually starts with fever, dyspnea, cough, crepitations in the lungs and one or more radiological pulmonary infiltrates. Shortness of breath is the predominant symptom in many patients. The reaction time (time from the last exposure to the drug to the first clinical symptoms) varies from hours to 1 or 2 days. Leukocytosis is not always present. Blood eosinophilia may attain 8—58% (33[C], 34[c], 35[c], 37[c], 39[c], 40[c]). The reaction disappears in most patients within a few days after discontinuation of the drug.

Histologically, the alveoli contain numerous histiocytes and eosinophils in a protein-rich edema fluid; there are transitory pulmonary infiltrations with blood eosinophilia (32[C], 34[C], 42[C]). The interstitial lung tissue may also be involved. Pulmonary function tests may show bronchial obstruction (33[c], 35[c]—37[c]). Arterial hypoxemia has also been described (35[c], 36[c]). Whereas bronchial obstruction is probably an immediate reaction (type I, according to the classification of Coombs and Gell), infiltration may correspond to a type III reaction as observed in extrinsic allergic alveolitis (36[c], 37[c], 43[C]).

Nervous system *Headache*, *drowsiness*, *lowered mental acuity* and other psychic alterations are only exceptionally encountered in connection with the newer sulfonamides. The causative role of the drug is usually not clearly established. Also, *polyneuritis* and *neuritis*, even an *optic neuritis* occur (44[c], 45[c]). Tremor has been described under co-trimoxazole (46[C]). Intravenous co-trimoxazole was considered to be the cause of ataxia (47[c]). *Aseptic meningitis* can be caused by a sulfonamide and/or trimethoprim. The occurrence of *meningitis* has been verified in most patients with reappearance of the same symptoms upon re-exposure (16[c], 48a[c], 48b[c], 49[c]—52[c], 53[C]—55[C]).

Special senses Transient *myopia* may be induced by sulfonamides applied topically and systematically (56[c]—58[c]). Corneal ring formation has been described as starting simultaneously with an erythematous skin rash in a patient known for his skin hypersensitivity (59[c]).

Endocrine, metabolic *Metabolic acidosis* Sulfonamides given in high doses may produce hyperchloremic metabolic acidosis. This has been observed in patients with extensive burns undergoing topical treatment with mafenide (60[C]). Mafenide (Sulfamylon) as well as *p*-sulfamoylbenzoic acid, an important metabolite, is a carbonic acid anhydrase inhibitor. Inhibition of renal carbonic acid anhydrase decreases re-absorption of bicarbonate. These preparations have been replaced by other compounds with fewer risks of adverse reactions such as silver sulfadiazine (4[C]).

The observation that antibacterial sulfonamides can

produce hypoglycemia was the basis for the development of the anti-diabetic sulfonylurea preparations. A more important cause of hypoglycemia is the interaction of antibacterial sulfonamides with sulfonylurea compounds and antiepileptic drugs (see Interactions, below).

Hematological *Hemolytic anemia* Sulfonamide-induced hemolysis, as well as the hemolytic effect of many other drugs, may be related to one or more of several mechanisms (61^R):

(1) Abnormally high blood levels due to large doses or a decreased excretion of the drug in patients with renal disease (62^C).

(2) Acquired hypersensitivity as reflected by the development of a positive Coombs test (63^R, 64^C).

(3) Genetically determined abnormalities of red blood cell metabolism, e.g. deficiency of glucose-6-phosphate dehydrogenase or of diaphorase (65^C, 66^R).

(4) The presence of an abnormal so-called 'unstable' hemoglobin in the red blood cell, e.g. hemoglobin Zürich (67^C, 68^C), hemoglobin Torino (69^C), hemoglobin Hasharon (70^C), hemoglobin H and M (66^R).

Today, simple and readily available in vitro methods for demonstrating pathogenic mechanisms include Coombs test, a Harris test (71^C), a quantitative assay or screening for glucose-6-phosphate dehydrogenase activity after the patient's recovery (72^R, 73^C), a test for Heinz bodies, and the buffered isopropanol technique (74^R) to detect 'unstable' hemoglobins and hemoglobin electrophoresis (61^R, 66^R).

The direct antiglobulin test may be negative in spite of a drug immune mechanism. If such a mechanism is suspected and the direct Coombs test is negative, the indirect Coombs test on patient serum with the addition of the suspected sensitizing agent can be of diagnostic value (75^C).

Heinz bodies in the erythrocytes may be important for early differentiation of a sulfonamide-induced reaction, which could further progress into hemolytic anemia (76^C). This result may also be of help to distinguish this development from other kinds of anemia.

Megaloblastic anemia Inflammatory bowel disease (Crohn's regional enteritis, ulcerative colitis) can interfere with folate absorption. Folate absorption is also influenced by salazosulfapyridine. There is agreement that sulfonamides, in contrast to trimethoprim, do not interfere with the micro-biological assay for folate (77^C).

Leukopenia, agranulocytosis and thrombocytopenia While adverse drug reactions of the red cell system are rare, the occurrence rate of leukopenia, neutropenia and thrombocytopenia is extremely variable if laboratory results without clinical symptoms are also considered. The incidence varies according to the definition of normal limits and the frequency of hematological controls. In the Comprehensive Hospital Drug Monitoring Program in Bern (CHDM), we found leuko- or neutropenia in 0.4%, or thrombocytopenia of mild-to-moderate degree in 0.1%, of 1809 treatments with co-trimoxazole (78^C, 79^R). This rate is close to that recorded in clinical trials (80^C, 81^C). Similar findings were also reported in children by the Group Health Cooperative of Puget Sound, Seattle, Washington, and published by the Boston Collaborative Drug Surveillance Program (BCDSP) (82^C).

Agranulocytosis was not infrequent during the early sulfonamide era. The first cases were observed in association with the administration of sulfanilamide (83^C, 84^C, Cases 1, 3 and 5), prontosil (83^C), sulfapyridine (84^C, Cases 7 and 8; 85^C), sulfathiazole (86^C), sulfadiazine (86^C) and salazosulfapyridine (87^C).

Severe neutropenia frequently occurs in HIV-infected patients under co-trimoxazole therapy (88^C). It seems to be due to either folic acid deficiency or immunological mechanisms. It cannot be excluded that, in some of the instances, HIV infection itself is the cause.

The topical form of silver sulfadiazine is an effective prophylaxis for patients with burns. As a consequence of systemic absorption, however, leukopenia and even agranulocytosis have been shown after topical treatment (89^C).

Special observations in patients with agranulocytosis favor an immunological/allergic rather than a toxic mechanism. Several points justify this view:

(1) The sulfonamide is well tolerated by most patients during the initial phase of treatment.

(2) Sulfonamide levels in the serum, when determined, are not particularly high when evaluated in cases with hematological complications.

(3) In a number of patients, skin rash, fever and arthritis start concomitantly with or even before the appearance of leukopenia or agranulocytosis.

(4) Re-exposure to a single dose can be followed by a second episode of severe agranulocytosis.

(5) An agglutinin for leukocytes has been identified in patients' serum shortly after discontinuation of the drug (85^C).

(6) Using in vitro techniques, positive reactions to the drug with the lymphocyte transformation test or inhibition of colony growth in bone marrow were found (90^C, 91^C).

Results of lymphocyte transformation tests must be interpreted with caution. Sometimes they are positive in patients exposed to the drug without any clinical symptoms of a hypersensitivity reaction.

Thrombocytopenia Acute thrombocytopenia is

rarely associated with the newer sulfonamides (92[C], 93[c], 94[C]). The antidiabetic sulfonylurea compounds and the thiazide diuretics may also induce acute, probably allergic, thrombocytopenia (95[C]). Positive in vitro tests were found with some methods. None of these has the simplicity necessary for a routine procedure (96[C], 97[C]). Furthermore, a negative test result with any given drug does not definitely exclude it as the responsible allergen.

Pancytopenia This may be an extremely rare form of an adverse reaction to sulfonamides (98[C], Table 7, Pt. B.H.) (see also Co-trimoxazole).

Liver and pancreas There are three forms of liver injury which may be related to sulfonamides (99[C]):
(1) *Hepatitis of the hepatocellular type* (100[C], 101[C], 102[c], 103[C], 104[c]).
(2) *Hepatitis of the 'mixed hepatocellular type'* accompanied by cholestatic features (105[C]).
(3) *Chronic active hepatitis*, possibly leading to cirrhosis (106[C]).

The number of observations of sulfonamide hepatitis published annually markedly diminished after 1947 with the introduction of the newer short-acting derivatives (SEDA-9, 261; 105[C]). Children may also be affected by drug-induced liver disease (107a[R]).

Until now, the connection to a sulfonamide has always been investigated by administering a test dose. Immunological in vitro methods which demonstrate sensitization to the drug, e.g. the lymphocyte transformation test, are of limited value (see Agranulocytosis, above).

In a number of patients the hepatic injury developed in connection with a general reaction such as serum sickness-like syndrome, generalized vasculitis or an exanthema often differing from the usual skin reactions of viral hepatitis (107b[C], 108[c]).

In patients with re-exposure to the drug, generalized malaise, nausea, back pain and chills may start as early as in one to several hours (103[c], 106[C]), or may be delayed for as long as several days (105[C]). The daily control of liver function upon re-exposure seems to be important, since subjective signs may be absent despite rising levels of serum transaminases and possibly of alkaline phosphatase (101[c]).

In most of the more recent reports, the histopathology of the liver injury has been documented. Even in the patients with chronic active hepatitis, the changes were indistinguishable from non-drug-induced disease. The degree of piecemeal necrosis usually varies from one area to another. Antinuclear factors (ANF) and lupus erythematosus factor were positive in some observations (106[C]). Early recognition of drug-induced liver disease is of great importance since liver injury may be completely reversible after stopping the drug.

Pancreatitis has been observed in some patients in relation to a sulfonamide. A causal connection with sulfamethiazole (48a[c]) and salazosulfapyridine has been shown by re-exposure (109[C]). Even the 5-aminosalicylic acid of this combined drug alone can be the cause (110[c], 111[c]).

Gastrointestinal *Nausea, vomiting and anorexia* are observed in a few percent of patients treated with sulfonamides (1[R]). They are usually of toxic origin. Their occurrence depends largely on the dosage in relation to renal function, the disposition of the individual patient and how the question concerning side effects is asked.

A patient with repeated *salivary gland enlargement* upon repeated exposure to sulfisoxazole (sulfafurazole) has been described (112[c]).

Urinary system Two types of complications may occur.
(1) *Concretions of crystals* in the collecting tubules, calyces and pelvis of the kidney and possibly in the ureters.

Since the newer and more soluble sulfonamide compounds were introduced, concretion and crystal formation are rare, as is acute renal failure due to various other mechanisms. During the last years, these complications were seen more often in AIDS patients due to large doses of sulfonamides against *Pneumocystis carinii* infection or *Toxoplasma* encephalitis. The sulfonamide is usually combined with trimethoprim. Reduced fluid intake and low urinary pH are other favoring factors (88[C], 113[c], 114[c], 115[C], 116[c], 117[C], 118[C]). Acute renal failure is often followed, at least in the published cases.
(2) *Disorders of renal tissues and vessels*, classified mainly according to histological findings: (a) acute tubular necrosis or tubulo-interstitial nephritis (116[c], Pts. 14-16, 119[C]); (b) interstitial nephritis (120[C]), in some cases combined with granulomatous lesions (121[c], 122[c]); (c) acute vasculitis (10[C]); (d) acute renal failure in connection with serum sickness-like syndrome, generalized vasculitis or exanthema, possibly with a hepatic reaction (107b[C]) (see also Generalized hypersensitivity reactions, above).

Acute anuria or oliguria is often the first symptom, not only in patients with tubular necrosis or tubulo-interstitial nephritis, but also in those with allergic vasculitis. Non-oliguric renal failure may also occur (see Co-trimoxazole, below). This presents initially only as an increase in serum creatinine, urea or BUN. It is not yet clear whether tubular necrosis in connection with sulfonamides is due to an immunological mechanism or to a toxic effect (1[R]).

Skin and appendages *Rashes* are common and are

usually considered to be of allergic origin. Maculopapular exanthema is more frequent than generalized urticaria (123[C]—125[C]). The rate of cutaneous reactions increases with the duration of therapy, especially for maculopapular reactions. These occur in approximately 1—3% of the patients treated (123[C]—127[C]). We include here also reactions to co-trimoxazole.

Erythema-multiforme and *fixed drug eruptions* (128[C]) are not uncommon. More severe forms such as *exfoliative dermatitis, vesicular and bullous exanthemas, Stevens-Johnson syndrome* and *toxic epidermal necrolysis* (Lyell's syndrome) are observed extremely rarely (125[C], 129[C]—131[C], 132[c], 133[C]—138[C]). The last two syndromes are of great importance. The lethality of drug-induced Lyell's syndrome was estimated to be about 20—30% (139a[C], 139b[C]), that of Stevens-Johnson syndrome 1—10% (SEDA-11, 259; 129[C]—131[C], 135[C], 138[C]).

Based on reports and our own experience, one gets the impression that a number of severe skin reactions started with a common maculopapular rash or a generalized erythema. The culprit drug is often either a long-acting preparation or a short-acting drug which has been continued over a long period. The non-occurrence of any severe skin reactions in the present author's own comprehensive hospital drug monitoring system, including 48 005 consecutively registered in-patients of general internal medicine, in the years 1974—1993, could probably be explained by the fact that these risk situations were avoided. Although still hypothetical, this has led Hunziker et al. to propose prophylactically stopping the culprit drug (125[C]).

Pathomechanism Cutaneous adverse drug reactions to sulfonamides and anticonvulsants are associated with an increased in vitro reactivity to metabolites of the culprit drug. Some authors suggest the presence of a still unidentified deficiency in cell defense mechanisms. In some cases glutathione deficiency was proposed as a major mechanism (17[C]). Also, an association with the phenotypes HLA-A29, B-12 and DR-7 was found in patients with bullous cutaneous reactions to sulfonamides (140[C]). Moreover, a predominance of slow acetylator phenotype was also observed among patients with sulfonamide hypersensitivity reactions (6[C], 7[C], 18[C]).

Drug-induced and staphylococcal scaled skin syndrome 'toxic' epidermal necrolysis can be distinguished histologically. In the former, the split is subepidermal at the level of the basal cells, whereas in the latter the split occurs in the upper epidermis near the granular layer, just beneath the stratum corneum (141a[C], 141b[C]).

Immediate discontinuation of all non-essential drugs as well as adequate supportive therapy with fluids, proteins and electrolytes is essential for preventing renal failure ('shock kidney'), pulmonary edema or bronchopneumonia (139a[C], 139b[C]). The use of antibiotics is also recommended, based on bacterial superinfection and blood culture results. In various reports, some cases of the drug-induced form were probably linked with sulfonamides or trimethoprim (130[C], 131[C], 132[c], 135[C], 140[C]).

The importance of drugs as an etiological factor in the Stevens-Johnson syndrome is extremely difficult to evaluate, except for patients with re-exposure or in situations where the drug was given prophylactically for meningitis (129[C]) or pneumonia (130[C]). In the first statistical epidemiological study by Bergoend et al. (129[C]) in 1968, 100 000 persons were given prophylactic treatment with sulfadoxine (Fanasil[R]) and 997 persons (0.9%) were reported to have experienced skin reactions. Of these, approximately 100 had severe reactions such as erythroderma with icterus, Stevens-Johnson syndrome or Lyell's syndrome. Eleven died from these complications, i.e. about one in 10 000 patients treated with the probably causative drug. It is not known how many persons would have had similar skin reactions unrelated to the drug. The benefit/risk ratio of meningitis prophylaxis was, however, clearly in favor of the sulfonamide-treated groups, compared to the control group (129[C]).

The second report by Taylor (130[C]) showed an incidence of three cases with Stevens-Johnson syndrome in 480 healthy, newly recruited Bantu mineworkers treated prophylactically with sulfadimethoxine.

A third epidemiological study in Mozambique was published by Hernborg and Beira in 1981: 149 000 inhabitants in one town were given a single dose of sulfadoxine as mass prophylaxis in an attempt to stem an outbreak of cholera (131[C]). Twenty-two patients with typical Stevens-Johnson syndrome were admitted to the Central Hospital over a period of 18 days. Three patients died.

Erythema nodosum, another skin manifestation with many different etiological factors, was also found in connection with sulfathiazole (142[C]): 706 children were studied; 231 had tuberculosis and the others had various other infectious diseases. Administration of sulfathiazole was followed by the appearance of erythema nodosum in 45% of those with tuberculosis and in 5% of those with other disorders. The frequency of 'spontaneously' occurring erythema nodosum in primary tuberculosis was increased by administration of the sulfonamide (142[C]). Other sulfonamides can also cause this type of reaction (143[R]).

Fixed drug eruptions may be due to various drugs, including sulfonamides (125[C], 144[C]—146[C]).

Among the special uses of sulfonamides, *topical ap-*

plication of silver sulfadiazine to the skin in severe burns seemed to represent real progress (4[C]). This drug, unlike its precursor mafenide (sulfamylon), requires less frequent application, is painless and hardly produces metabolic acidosis (60[C]). Local reactions with silver sulfadiazine consisting of rash, pruritus or a burning sensation are observed in 2.5% of patients.

In general, *allergic contact dermatitis* to sulfonamides seems to be rare.

Photosensitivity reactions may also occur with antibacterial sulfonamides (147[C]). *Generalized skin reactions involving light-exposed sites* after systemic drug application have been observed (148[R], 149[R]).

Systemic lupus erythematosus (SLE) and drug-induced lupus-like syndromes Drugs may induce three different clinical and biological situations similar or identical to SLE (150[C], 151[C]): (a) an exacerbation of pre-existing SLE can be provoked; (b) SLE may be triggered in a patient with SLE disposition; and (c) an allergic reaction of the serum sickness-like syndrome resembling SLE not only clinically, but also serologically. Positive LE-cell phenomenon and antinuclear factors may occur.

For situations (a) and (b), two pathogenetic mechanisms may be involved: (i) a reaction to the pharmacological properties of the drug (hydralazine, diphenylhydantoin, procainamide, isoniazid and possibly salazosulfapyridine and practolol) (150[C]—152[C], 153[R]); (ii) a hypersensitivity to the drug as in other allergic drug reactions (to sulfonamides, penicillins, tetracyclines and other drugs (151[C]).

In type (i) reactions, exposure time and especially re-exposure time are usually longer than 1—2 months. In type (ii) reactions, exposure is more variable, lasting from hours to days or up to 1—2 months (150[C], 151[C], 154[C]). For sulfonamides, type (i) (152[C], 154[C], 155[C]) as well as type (ii) reactions (156[C], Cases 1, 2 and 4, 157[c]) may occur.

Some patients with ulcerative colitis have developed arthropathy, possibly polyserositis, hematological abnormalities and even loss of consciousness with positive LE-cell and antinuclear antibody tests during treatment with salazosulfapyridine (154[C], 155[C]).

Serum sickness-like syndrome, and allergic arthritis See above under 'Generalized hypersensitivity reactions'. Both may also occur with co-trimoxazole (14[C], 158[C]).

Risk situations It is our opinion that patients with *severe blood*, *kidney* or *liver disease* should not be treated with sulfonamides. Relative contraindications are *systemic lupus erythematosus* and a known *predisposition to lupus-like reactions*. Before beginning any sulfonamide treatment, the patient should be asked about earlier applications and tolerance.

The *acetylator phenotype* of a patient (slow or rapid acetylator) may influence the frequency and severity of adverse reactions to drugs metabolized by acetylation (6[C], 7[C], 66[R]). Healthy subjects (159[C]) and patients with either ulcerative colitis or Crohn's disease (160[C]) in the slow-acetylator group have been found to experience more pronounced side effects to salazosulfapyridine. The adverse reactions to this drug are probably due to the sulfapyridine component rather than to the complete molecule or 5-acetylsalicylic acid.

In patients with *porphyria*, sulfonamides should not be used (161[R]).

There is increasing evidence that patients with *HIV-infection* are more prone to develop crystal concretions in the urinary tract, often causing acute renal failure and also generalized allergic skin reactions.

Second-generation effects *Teratogenicity* The sulfonamides appear to have little if any effect on early human development. This is indicated by the absence of case reports or epidemiological survey data during pregnancy. In one study of 50 282 mother—child pairs, 1455 were exposed to sulfonamides during lunar months 1—4. There was no increase in the relative risk of any malformation (162a[R], 162b[R]).

Male infertility with oligospermia during treatment with salazosulfapyridine was observed by several authors (163[c], 164[c]). Other investigators, however, came to the conclusion that the inflammatory bowel disease itself influenced the maturation of spermatozoa (165[C]).

Kernicterus is precipitated in infants by a number of drugs, e.g. sulfonamides and salicylates, capable of displacing unconjugated bilirubin from the plasma albumin to which it is normally firmly bound. In this way, bilirubin may enter the tissues and induce bilirubin encephalopathy (166[C]—169[C]). Successful treatment of neonatal hyperbilirubinemia with higher bilirubin levels has been established using exchange transfusion and phototherapy (170[C]). Drugs capable of displacing unconjugated bilirubin from plasma albumin should not be given in the third trimester of pregnancy or to lactating women. Breast-feeding by itself is one of the common causes of jaundice in normal newborns (169[C], 171[R]).

Interactions Sulfonamides show a decreased absorption in combination with *antacids*. *Urine alkalinizers* increase the urinary excretion of sulfonamides.

An important interaction is the hypoglycemia induced by *sulfonylureas* during simultaneous sulfonamide administration (172[C]—174[C], 175a[C]). This hypoglycemic effect results from inhibition of carboxylation, leading to a decreased sulfonylurea metabolism (175b[C]). Interference of the sulfonamide with the protein binding of the sulfonylurea derivative may contribute to this effect. Most reports regard concomitant treatment with tolbutamide and sulfaphenazole (172[C], 175a[C], 176[C]), sulfafurazole (173[C]) or sulfamethoxazole with trimethoprim (175a[c], 177[c]). Chlorpropamide produces the same interaction (178[C]). Hypoglycemia may start early, during the first hours of combining the two drugs.

Sulfafurazole enhances the anesthetic effect induced by short-acting intravenous *barbiturates* through competitive displacement from binding sites on plasma albumin (179[C]).

Co-trimoxazole (trimethoprim + sulfamethoxazole) and trimethoprim or trimethoprim analogs in combination with various sulfonamides

These combinations, mainly co-trimoxazole, have been frequently used. They are clearly more effective and provide a broader antibacterial spectrum than a sulfonamide alone and, in special situations, than trimethoprim or a trimethoprim analogue alone even in comparable dosage. With the widespread use of co-trimoxazole for about 30 years, only some increase in bacterial resistance can be demonstrated. Important adverse reactions are rare, provided patients in special risk situations are not treated with this combination. Sulfadiazine or sulfamoxole can replace sulfamethoxazole (180[C]).

In patients with advanced HIV infection with a CD_4 lymphocyte count of <200/mm^3, co-trimoxazole is the preferred agent for primary prophylaxis of *Pneumocystis carinii* infection. Moreover, this combination also protects against toxoplasmosis (181[C]). While the adverse reaction profile of co-trimoxazole is similar to that in other therapeutic indications, quite different reactions seem to be more frequent and severe in HIV-infected patients (SEDA-16, 322; 21b[C]).

ADVERSE REACTION PATTERN

General and toxic reactions Overall, the picture of co-trimoxazole's adverse reactions corresponds with that expected from a sulfonamide of relatively low toxicity, provided the contraindications are strictly respected (182[R]). This is also true of its use in children (107a[R]).

Trimethoprim interferes with the tubular secretion of creatinine, causing an increased serum creatinine level and a lowered creatinine clearance without affecting renal function or true glomerular filtration rate.

Hematological disturbances due to co-trimoxazole are seldom of clinical relevance. Serum folate is generally not significantly reduced in western industrialized countries. Mild leukopenia has been reported in less than 1% up to 10% of patients. Platelet counts decrease in a minority of patients, but clinically significant thrombocytopenia is only very rarely seen. Crystalluria hardly occurs, except in patients with HIV infection and is then often combined with renal damage.

Hypersensitivity reactions These are the same as described under sulfonamides (see above). Generalized skin reactions, probably with an allergic pathomechanism, seem to predominate. Trimethoprim may also be the cause. Leukopenia and thrombocytopenia often seem to be of immunological origin. Desensitization, see under 'Generalized hypersensitivity reactions', p. 845.

Tumor-inducing effects These have not been reported.

ORGANS AND SYMPTOMS

Cardiovascular reactions Anaphylactic shock seems to be extremely rare (20[C], 183[c]) (see also Sulfonamides).

Respiratory Allergic pneumonitis or PIE-syndrome (pulmonary infiltration with eosinophilia) and the subgroup of transient pulmonary infiltrations with eosinophilia (Loeffler syndrome) have been observed. Pulmonary infiltrates may occur in patients with AIDS under co-trimoxazole, mimicking sepsis or clinical progression of underlying opportunistic pulmonary infections (184[c]) (see under Sulfonamides, p. 843).

Nervous system *Tremor* was induced by trimethoprim-sulfamethoxazole in patients with AIDS (46[C]). *Ataxia* was described in two patients with AIDS after intravenous use of the combined preparation (47[c]). Extrapyramidal symptoms developed under co-trimoxazole in a girl with dihydropteridine reductase deficiency and rapidly disappeared after the drug withdrawal. This variant of phenylketonuria should be considered in all infants found to have elevated phenylalanine concentrations during the neonatal period (8a[c]).

Aseptic meningitis has been observed under co-trimoxazole treatment (48a[c], 48b[c], 49[c]–51[c], 52[C], 53[C]) as well as with trimethoprim alone (16[c], 54[C], 55[C]). A case with three episodes in relation to re-exposure with co-trimoxazole has been reported (50[c]). Polymorphonuclear or mononuclear cells may preponderate (51[C]).

Endocrine, metabolic High-dose co-trimoxazole for treatment of *Pneumocystis carinii* in HIV-infected patients led to an increase in the serum potassium concentration and may result in a life-threatening hyperkalemia (185[C]). This effect is due to a decreased renal potassium excretion induced by trimethoprim (186[C]). Whether sulfonamide and trimethoprim or trimethoprim alone have antithyroid activity is still unclear (187[C], 188[C]).

Hematological Since both components alone affect hematopoiesis, the adverse reactions to this compound may just as well be due to trimethoprim as to the sulfonamide. The Swedish adverse reaction reporting system had been compulsory for 20 years for the most serious as well as new and unexpected adverse reactions at the time of the announcement. The overall frequency of reported blood dyscrasias under co-trimoxazole was 5.3 per million defined daily doses (189[C]). This result still seems to underestimate the frequency estimated in comparison to comprehensive hospital drug monitoring systems which also include asymptomatic cases.

Red blood cell system Megaloblastic anemia, aplastic anemia (red cell aplasia) and pancytopenia have been described in an extremely small number of patients (79[R], 190[C]). All three types of reaction can be induced by the folic acid antagonism of trimethoprim alone or in combination with the sulfonamide. The megaloblastic phase may be missed. If folic acid deficiency continues, aplastic anemia and pancytopenia may result (191[C], 192[c]). Patients with megaloblastic anemia should not be treated with co-trimoxazole. The possible mechanisms underlying hemolytic reactions have been discussed in connection with the sulfonamides.

White blood cell system Agranulocytosis, possibly as one of the symptoms of pancytopenia, is very rare. If leukocytes are routinely controlled under treatment (more often than clinically indicated), mild leukopenia may be encountered in about 0.4% up to 10% of cases receiving either the combination (78[C], 79[R], 192[c], 193[C], 194[C]) or trimethoprim alone at a dosage of 2×200 or 250 mg/day (81[C]).

Thrombocyte system Severe thrombocytopenia is also very rare. This reaction is likely to be of immunological origin in most patients (96[C], 97[C]), either to the sulfonamide (97[C], 195[c]), to trimethoprim (196[C]) or to both. Mild thrombocytopenia, however, seems to be quite common, affecting 0.1% to several percent of patients treated with co-trimoxazole (78[C], 80[C], 81[C], 192[C], 193[C], 197[C]).

Blood dyscrasias See also 'Sulfonamides'.

A decreased serum folate level seems to be exceptional and occurs mainly in association with other predisposing factors (198[C]) or together with other drugs, e.g. those with antimetabolite properties (199[C]) or anticonvulsants (200[C]) (see Drug interactions, below).

In patients with pre-existing folic acid deficiency or with HIV infection, the administration of folinic acid has been advised in order to reduce the hematological side effects. However, preliminary data suggest that adjunctive folinic acid may be associated with an increased risk of therapeutic failure and death (201[R]). Serum folate levels should not be measured by the radioisotope method in patients being given trimethoprim preparations (77[C]).

Liver and pancreas The same types of liver disease occur with co-trimoxazole as with sulfonamides alone (202[c]–204[c]). A case of intrahepatic cholestasis associated with phospholipoidosis was published (205[c]). Acute pancreatitis with relapse on re-exposure also has been observed (206[c]).

Gastrointestinal *Nausea* and possibly *vomiting* are noted in a few percent to 20% of adult patients on normal dosage (80[C], 182[R], 193[C]).

Antibiotic-associated colitis (see Chapter 25.1, General considerations) is only very rarely seen with co-trimoxazole (207[C], 208[C]).

Urinary system The effect of short- and long-term co-trimoxazole therapy has been studied in patients with normal kidney function and in those with kidney disease.

Extremely rare instances of *crystalluria* followed by renal insufficiency due to obstruction, or other forms of renal disease, have been described (see Sulfonamides, p. 845).

Co-trimoxazole occasionally exerts a *direct nephrotoxic effect*, mainly in patients with pre-existing renal impairment, receiving large dosages (118[C], 209[C], 210[C]). Usually no deterioration of renal function was observed, provided the dose was adapted to the degree of initial renal insufficiency (118[C], 211[C], 212[C]). If creatinine clearance is reduced to 25–15 ml/min, the standard dose of the combined preparation (800 mg sulfamethoxazole and 160 mg trimethoprim per day) should be reduced by half after an initial 3 days of treatment with the normal dose. A small increase in serum creatinine levels at the beginning of treatment is not necessarily indicative of a decreased glomerular filtration rate in patients without renal insufficiency (213[C], 214[C]).

Co-trimoxazole used in high-dosage can reduce potassium excretion and induce even reversible hyperkalemia (see Endocrine, metabolic) (185[C], 186[C]).

Trimethoprim/sulfamethoxazole was shown to be the probable cause of growth failure and renal tubular acidosis in a pediatric patient (215[c]).

Skin and appendages The frequency of *skin rashes*, mostly maculopapular, is related to the duration of treatment (216[C]). They occur in between 1.3 and 5.9% of patients (80[C], 123[C]–126[C], 182[R]). Severe reactions such as toxic epidermal necrolysis (*Lyell syndrome*, *Stevens-Johnson syndrome* and *erythema multiforme major*, are rare.

The combination of pyrimethamine and sulfadoxine used for prophylaxis of chloroquine-resistant malaria (*P. falciparum*) caused severe skin reactions in one per 5000–8000 users with fatal reactions and in one per 11 000–25 000 users, depending on different data (217[C]). Even at the stage of common rash or generalized erythema, the drug should be stopped (125[C]).

Risk situations The combination should not be given in situations of malnutrition, pregnancy, alcoholism, severe liver damage, chronic inflammatory bowel disease or megaloblastic anemia (194[C], 199[C], 218[C]). It should also not be used in combination with other folic acid antagonists, anticonvulsants and comparable compounds used for malarial prophylaxis (see Interactions, below).

Risk situations due to folate deficiency can be treated by folic acid. If the principle indication is to circumvent the action of dihydrofolate reductase, as in the situation with trimethoprim, folinic acid may be indicated. In HIV-infected patients preliminary data suggest that folinic acid may cause also an increased risk (201[R]) (see Hematological, p. 847).

In children found to have elevated phenylalanine concentrations during the neonatal period (the variant with dihydropterine reductase deficiency), extrapyramidal symptoms might develop under co-trimoxazole (8a[c]).

In AIDS patients, the incidence of side effects is exceptionally high (SEDA-9, 260; SEDA-10, 260; 219[C]–221[C]). Of 37 patients with AIDS treated for *Pneumocystis carinii* pneumonia, only five were able to complete treatment. Drug toxicity occurred in 29. In 19 of these patients treatment was changed due to adverse drug reactions including rash, fever, neutropenia, thrombocytopenia and transaminase elevation (219[C]). A similarly high occurrence rate of side effects (65%) was seen in other studies (220[C], 221[C]). High dosage of co-trimoxazole may increase the serum potassium concentration by a decreased potassium excretion caused by trimethoprim (185[C], 186[C]). HIV infection risk factor for hematological side effects of co-trimoxazole, especially *agranulocytosis*, is increased significantly (88[C]).

Pentamidine is an alternative drug used for *Pneumocystis carinii* pneumonia. In a comparative study, it produced a lower rate of rashes but a higher rate of serum creatinine elevation (222[C]). It may also induce hyperkalemia due to the effect on renal ion transport (223[C]). Co-trimoxazole, if tolerated, is the preferred agent for treatment and prophylaxis of *Pneumocystis carinii* pneumonia.

Low-dose co-trimoxazole for prevention of *Pneumocystis carinii* pneumonia (160 mg trimethoprim and 800 mg sulfamethoxazole twice weekly) proved to be effective (224[C]) and reduced side effects (225[C]) from 28 to 9% of patients (226[C]).

Oral desensitization to co-trimoxazole was successfully achieved in AIDS patients suffering from fever, rash and wheezing due to the drug (20[C], 22[C], 23[c], 24[C]) (see Sulfonamides, p. 845). The method has also been used in children (25[C]). A previous rash under co-trimoxazole should not prevent later re-administration of this preparation, possibly after a rapid test dose in urgent clinical situations (227[C]).

Second-generation effects Experience with therapy in pregnant women and the newborn is limited. The product information distributed by the pharmacological companies still mentions this limitation. The FDA does not approve the use of this combination in such cases (228[R]). However, after reviewing newer case reports and placebo-controlled trials involving several hundred patients, Brigg et al. failed to demonstrate an increase in fetal abnormalities (229[R]).

Whether male fertility is impaired either by treatment with co-trimoxazole or by the underlying urogenital infection cannot be determined with the present data (230[C], 231[C]).

Chromosome studies performed in cultures of peripheral blood lymphocytes did not show significant differences before and after treatment (SED-10, 549). Cytogenetic studies on bone marrow cells from 12 patients with urinary tract infections treated with trimethoprim + sulfamethoxazole did not show structural chromosomal aberrations. An increased number of micronuclei, however, was present in the patients as compared to controls (232[C]).

Interactions Most interactions with other drugs are due to folic acid antagonism. This may be more pronounced in the combination of trimethoprim and sulfonamide than with the sulfonamide part alone. Such interactions have already been suspected with an *antimalarial drug* and with *anticonvulsants* such as barbiturates, diphenylhydantoin and primidone (200[R]). These anticonvulsants may themselves produce folic acid deficiency with megaloblastic anemia. Comparable effects can occur in combination of co-trimoxazole with any of the *cytostatic* and *immunosuppressive drugs* or in patients with HIV (201[C]). In renal transplant patients azathioprine treatment with co-trimoxazole was followed by neutropenia and thrombocytopenia (199[C]).

Children with acute lymphoblastic leukemia showed an interference of co-trimoxazole with 6-mercaptopurine metabolism (233[C]). In another study, co-trimoxazole treatment produced a 66% increase in systemic exposure to methotrexate (234[C]). Pronounced nephrotoxicity resulted from the interaction of co-trimoxazole and ciclosporin in patients with a renal transplant (235[C], 236[C]).

Co-trimoxazole can significantly augment the hypoprothrombinemic effect of warfarin (237[C]).

In women taking oral contraceptive steroids short courses of co-trimoxazole are unlikely to cause any adverse effects on contraceptive control (238[C]).

Trimethoprim

Even before the marketing of co-trimoxazole, many investigators emphasized that the clinical advantages of the combined use of trimethoprim with a sulfonamide, compared to the use of trimethoprim alone, are limited. Co-trimoxazole, however, widens the spectrum of treatable infections beyond that of trimethoprim as single drug (2[R]). These infections include gonorrhea, brucellosis, *Pneumocystis carinii* pneumonia and nocardiosis (239[R]—241[R]). In the treatment of uncomplicated urinary tract infections, trimethoprim has proved quite as effective as the combination in several trials (1[R], 242[C]). In complicated urinary tract infections most studies showed better results with co-trimoxazole than with trimethoprim alone (243[R]). If both drugs are used in combination, the emergence of resistance in most studies stays relatively low (SEDA-5, 287; 244[C] for Stockholm; 245[C] for Zürich). At present, it appears that concerns about trimethoprim resistance emerging from single agent use in urinary tract infections (240[C], 246[C]) have been rather exaggerated (1[R], 180[C], 241[R], 242[C]).

Severe adverse drug reactions with trimethoprim are extremely rare. Some investigators came to the conclusion that with trimethoprim alone in a dose of up to 400 mg/day, gastrointestinal tolerance was better and skin reactions were less frequent than with the combination (180[C]). Another study concluded that there is no definite proof that substituting trimethoprim alone by the combination would significantly reduce the frequency of adverse reactions (242[C]), probably due to higher dosage of trimethoprim as single preparation. Brodgen and colleagues summarized the data from five different centers and found that skin rash and gastrointestinal complaints seemed to be less frequent with trimethoprim than with the combination (243[R]).

Aseptic meningitis with encephalopathy occurs also with trimethoprim alone (16[c], 54[C], 55[C], as does meningoencephalopathy (247[c]).

Trimethoprim has been associated with megaloblastic anemia, thrombocytopenia, leukopenia, hypersegmentation of leukocytes, and bone marrow toxicity (81[C], 180[C], 248[C]). With trimethoprim at a daily dose of 400—500 mg slight hematological side effects, such as leukopenia or thrombocytopenia, did not occur less frequently than with the combination (81[C]). That cholestatic hepatitis may be induced by trimethoprim was shown in a patient with re-exposure (249[c]). Severe skin reactions such as toxic epidermal necrolysis ("Lyell syndrome") can also be caused by trimethoprim as a single drug (250[c]).

Trimethoprim should not be given to children under the age of 12 years, as long as other alternatives are available.

For risk situations, second-generation effects and interactions, see also under co-trimoxazole (trimethoprim + sulfamethoxazole).

NITROFURANTOIN AND RELATED DRUGS

Nitrofurantoin

After almost complete absorption from the gastrointestinal tract, nitrofurantoin produces high urinary concentrations, but only low blood and tissue levels. Nitrofurantoin has been used almost exclusively for the treatment and prophylaxis of urinary tract infections. Because of the severity and frequency of side effects it should be used only in exceptional cases. The frequency of certain adverse reactions varies in different geographical areas (SEDA-7, 301; SEDA-8, 282). Lung reactions seem to be more prevalent in Scandinavia and South Africa than in the United Kingdom, whereas polyneuropathies or gastrointestinal reactions are more frequent in the UK than in Sweden. These discrepancies remain unexplained.

ADVERSE REACTION PATTERN

General and toxic reactions Harmless gastrointestinal side effects are most frequent. Polyneuropathy occurs mainly in patients with renal failure where nitrofurantoin is contraindicated.

Hypersensitivity reactions Exanthemas, generalized urticaria and acute lung reactions are observed.

Tumor-inducing effects In vitro, nitrofurantoin acts as a mutagen by inhibiting DNA synthetase and damages DNA in human fibroblast cultures (251[R]). Some studies indicate a similar metabolism of nitrofurantoin and other (carcinogenic) nitrofurans. Formation of carcinogenic nitrofurantoin metabolites may thus be possible (252[R]). However, a carcinogenic effect has not been proven for nitrofurantoin (253[r]).

ORGANS AND SYSTEMS

Respiratory *Acute lung reactions* Nitrofurantoin induces acute lung reactions probably more frequently than all other drugs combined. Since the first well-documented case of an acute lung reaction in 1962 (254[C], 255[C]), several hundred further observations have been published (256[R], 257[R]). The frequency of acute severe pulmonary disease has been estimated to be one in every 5000 first administrations (258[C]). Women between 40 and 50 years of age are mainly affected. The acute lung reactions are dose-independent and sensitization occurs at the earliest 1—2 weeks after the onset of exposure during the first course of therapy. Symptoms develop 2—10 hours after drug intake and consist of severe dyspnea, tachypnea, non-productive cough, high fever (usually with chills), cyanosis, chest pain, occasionally arthralgia, backache or headache, vomiting, rash, collapse and anaphylactic shock. Lung findings include dense crackling crepitation or moist rales, predominantly at the posterior base of the lung. X-ray examination may be normal, but more often shows bilateral interstitial lower lobe infiltrates frequently with pleural effusions.

Initially the leukocyte count is normal or elevated, with neutrophilia and lymphopenia. Later, eosinophilia is common. When nitrofurantoin is stopped clinical symptoms subside rapidly, usually within 1—3 days (257[C]). However, minor X-ray changes may still be found 2 months later. Re-exposure to 50 mg of nitrofurantoin re-induces the syndrome. Single cases of death due to heart failure have been reported in debilitated patients. Acute lung reactions to nitrofurantoin are extremely rare in children (259[r]).

Chronic lung reactions These are 10—20 times less frequent than acute reactions and mainly involve older patients. Reactions serious enough to require hospitalization occur in one out of 750 long-term users (258[C]). Acute reactions do not seem to predispose to the later occurrence of chronic reactions. During long-term treatment, dyspnea and usually non-productive cough without fever develop (260[C]).

Subacute highly febrile episodes during continued nitrofurantoin treatment have also been reported.

Restrictive respiratory impairment is common. X-Ray examinations show interstitial infiltrations, often in the middle and basal lung regions. Fibrotic changes, alveolar exudates and pleural effusions are rare. After nitrofurantoin withdrawal, clinical symptoms regress rapidly. However, in most cases X-ray findings recede slowly and clearing remains ultimately incomplete in at least 50% of patients. Occasional deaths due to cardiopulmonary failure have also been reported. The therapeutic benefit of corticosteroid treatment is controversial, but the bulk of experience indicates its usefulness.

Two *atypical courses* have been rarely described. The first is the *mixed type of reaction*: following an initial short fever peak, the patient becomes either afebrile or subfebrile despite continuing nitrofurantoin and unabated activity of the lung process, or a typical chronic reaction converts to a typical acute reaction upon re-exposure to nitrofurantoin after its withdrawal. The second is an *acute reaction without clinical symptoms*, which can be recognized only on X-rays.

The typical acute lung reaction is often associated with a rash and rarely with a *granulomatous hepatitis* (261[C]) or with isolated elevation of serum transaminase levels. In the protracted acute and in chronic lung reactions, accompanying liver injury (such as chronic active hepatitis) is more frequent than in acute reactions. Such cases usually show a broad spectrum of serological autoimmune reactions (lupus-like syndrome) (262[C], 263[C]). *Lung tissue findings* in acute reactions showed minor vasculitis, granulomatous vasculitis (hypersensitivity angiitis), proliferation of endothelial cells and empty alveoli (264[C]). Recently, rapidly progressing bronchiolitis obliterans with organizing pneumonia (BOOP) has been reported (265[C]). Chronic reactions most frequently showed chronic interstitial pneumonitis with varying degrees of fibrosis and in some instances desquamative alveolitis (260[C], 266[C]—268[C]). These alterations suggest an immunological mechanism.

According to several authors, the pathomechanism of the acute lung reaction may be allergic (type III reaction) (268[C], 269[C]). However, there is also some evidence that a cytotoxic immune mechanism (type II reaction (270[C]), cell-mediated immunity (type IV reaction) (271[c]), or direct toxic injury of lung tissue through the production of oxygen radicals (272[r], 273[R]) may be involved in the acute pulmonary reaction.

In the chronic lung reaction, the etiological role of nitrofurantoin is less evident. It is supported by analogy and by the clinical course. Sometimes the skin test is positive even in chronic lung reactions (268[C]). Lymphocyte transformation tests give variable results. A polyclonal hypergammaglobulinemia is always present, with IgG predominating. Precipitating serum antibodies have not been found. Recent data support a toxic pathogenesis similar to that of the herbicide, paraquat (272[R], 274[R]).

Nervous system More than 140 cases of toxic *polyneuropathy* have been reported. The frequency depends upon dose, tissue levels and renal function. In fact, in up to 90% of cases, polyneuropathy occurred in patients with impaired renal function. Symptoms usually start 9—45 days (at the earliest 3 days) after beginning nitrofurantoin. The neuropathy predominantly affects the limbs, starts peripherally and remains more severe distally. Initially, there is sensory loss with paresthesia. Later, motor loss develops, often with severe muscle atrophy. As a rule, no further deterioration occurs after withdrawal of nitrofurantoin and total (34% of cases) or partial regression (45% of cases) occurs (275[R]). In some severe cases invalidity remains. The motor loss recedes more slowly and less completely than the sensory impairment. Single cases of *retrobulbar optic neuritis* and *lateral rectus muscle palsy* have been reported (SEDA-8, 282). Rarely, concomitant dysphoric, euphoric or even psychotic reactions are seen. Polyneuropathy occurs even in children.

The lesions comprise degeneration of the myelin sheath of the nerves and nerve roots with degeneration of the corresponding anterior horn cells and muscle fibers. The pathogenesis is unclear. Impairment of glutathione reductase has been considered. Even in healthy persons, a daily dose of 400 mg nitrofurantoin for 2 weeks induces a significant increase in motor nerve conduction time. If strict attention is paid to the contraindication of renal failure, the risk of polyneuropathy can be reduced. Careful controls for the initial symptoms of paresthesia may prevent the development of severe disablement.

Single cases of *benign intracranial hypertension* (pseudotumor cerebri) with and without ocular palsy have been reported (276[C]). Uncharacteristic general symptoms with *dizziness, cephalgia or drowsiness* are more frequent. *Psychic reactions* such as visual and auditory hallucinations together with extreme restlessness were reported from China in 1960. Apparently only women were affected and the problem does not appear to have been noted since. Whether typical *trigeminal neuralgia* (one case) or *cerebellar symptoms* can be related to nitrofurantoin is uncertain.

Mineral and fluid balance One case of hyperlactatemic *metabolic acidosis* together with hemolytic anemia due to glucose-6-phosphate dehydrogenase deficiency was reported (277[c]).

Hematological Some cases of *hemolytic anemia* associated with glucose–6-phosphate dehydrogenase deficiency have been described. Single cases of nitrofurantoin-induced (or enhanced) hemolytic anemia with other erythrocyte enzyme deficiencies (enolase or glutathione peroxidase) and isolated cases of methemoglobinemia were observed (278[C]). Nitrofurantoin produces oxidant stress and cellular damage by different mechanisms (279[C]). It can disturb folate metabolism, leading to a megaloblastic component in pre-existing (mostly hemolytic) anemia which responds to folic acid treatment. Single cases of *thrombocytopenia* (258[R]) and of *severe hemorrhagic diathesis* with deficiency of factors II and VII due to a nitrofurantoin-induced hepatic disorder (280[C]) were reported. Furthermore, nitrofurantoin experimentally inhibits ADP-induced platelet aggregation (281[R]).

Allergic *agranulocytosis* or *neutropenia* have been proven in only a few cases (SEDA-10, 260; 282[C]). *Pancytopenia* is also rarely seen (257[R]).

Liver Hepatic reactions are rare and different forms can be distinguished (283[r]). Data from The Netherlands suggest that acute reactions are more common than chronic (284[C]). *Acute hepatic reactions* may be hepatocellular or cholestatic. In the vast majority of subjects, symptoms appear within the first 6 weeks of nitrofurantoin treatment, in half of the patients within the first week of treatment. Jaundice is most common, followed by abdominal pain, malaise and nausea. Hepatomegaly has been reported in nearly 50% of the cases, fever in 30—65%, eosinophilia in 15—50% and a rash in 12—60%. An immunological pathogenesis is assumed. Experimental data, however, point to a toxic mechanism involving the formation of glutathione—protein mixed disulfides and/or protein alkylation (285[C]). The prognosis after withdrawal of the drug is good, but fatal courses have been reported when the drug is continued or, rarely, after it has been discontinued.

Recently, endstage liver disease requiring liver transplantation possibly associated with nitrofurantoin (400 mg daily during 4 weeks) was reported (286[C]).

Chronic active hepatitis, icteric or anicteric, has been described almost invariably in women with long-term nitrofurantoin treatment. Most patients suffer from symptoms after a period of approximately 6 months of nitrofurantoin use. Fever (0—24%), rash (0—3%) and eosinophilia (9—23%) occur rarely when compared to acute cases. Hepatomegaly is observed in 30—60% of the chronic cases (284[C]). Sometimes a broad spectrum of autoimmune reactions, a lupus-like syndrome or a mild cholestasis may be present (287[C], 288[C]). Some of these cases occurred in combination with lung reactions of the protracted acute or chronic type, or in patients with ascites and liver cirrhosis. The clinical symptoms usually improve after withdrawal of the drug, but a few cases with extensive hepatocellular necrosis ended fatally (289[C]). The histological changes may persist. Re-exposure to nitrofurantoin has reproduced the pathological liver tests.

Granulomatous hepatitis has been demonstrated in cases with lung reactions and possibly drug fever (261[C], 290[C]) One case of *focal nodular hyperplasia* of the liver during long-term treatment has been reported (SEDA-8, 282).

Gastrointestinal These are the most frequent side effects of nitrofurantoin. They are toxic, dose-dependent and usually harmless. Manifestations occur mostly after absorption of the drug and are mediated by the central nervous system. Measures to delay resorption, such as sugar coating or the use of a macrocrystalline form of the drug, reduce side effects (291[R]). Nausea and anorexia were most frequently reported. Abdominal pain and diarrhea are rare.

Two cases of nitrofurantoin-induced *acute pancreatitis*, confirmed by rechallenge, were reported (SEDA-9, 261; 292[C]).

Urinary system Nitrofurantoin crystalluria leading to obstruction of indwelling catheters has been described in a few patients (293[C]).

Skin and appendages *Allergic skin reactions* occur in 1–2% of treated cases and comprise about 21% of all adverse reactions to nitrofurantoin. They often occur together with other reactions such as drug fever, lung or liver reactions. The lesions may present as pruritus, as macular, maculopapular or vesicular exanthema, as urticaria or as angio-edema. The frequency of serious cutaneous reactions (erythema multiforme, Stevens-Johnson syndrome or toxic epidermal necrolysis) after nitrofurantoin use has been estimated to be seven cases per 100 000 exposed individuals (294[C]). The transitory *alopecia* reported in a few cases has a toxic pathogenesis (295[C]).

Some cases of parotitis, rarely proven by rechallenge with the drug, have been associated with nitrofurantoin (SEDA-8, 282; 296[R]).

Lupus-like syndrome Approximately 20 cases have been described, mostly in the Scandinavian literature. The clinical picture consisted of arthralgia or, rarely, exacerbation of a pre-existing rheumatoid arthritis and generalized lymphadenopathy, mostly associated with chronic lung and/or liver reactions such as chronic active hepatitis (263[C]). In patients with the lupus-like syndrome at least two immunological tests (antinuclear factor, rheumatoid factor, Coombs test, antibodies against smooth muscle fibers, thyreoglobulin, thyroid cell cytoplasm or glomeruli) were positive. The lupus erythematosus-cell phenomenon, however, was always negative. The lymphocyte transformation test was always positive when performed. In these cases, as in other allergic nitrofurantoin reactions, circulating albumin IgG complexes were found by immune electrophoresis, with tailing of the albumin line (297[C]). The syndrome regresses after withdrawal of the drug.

Special senses One case of crystalline retinopathy has been associated with long-term nitrofurantoin therapy (298[C]).

Risk situations The main risk factor for toxic reactions, especially polyneuropathy and gastrointestinal symptoms, is *impaired renal function* (275[R]). Long-term treatment puts patients at risk for chronic lung reactions and chronic active hepatitis. *Glucose-6-phosphate dehydrogenase deficiency* is decisive for the development of hemolytic anemia. Nitrofurantoin is *contraindicated in the newborn* because of the danger of hemolytic anemia resulting from immature enzyme systems.

Pyridoxine might accelerate the renal elimination of nitrofurantoin (299[C]).

Second-generation effects *Pregnancy and lactation* Clinically, teratogenic effects of nitrofurantoin are not known and only very small amounts of the drug cross the placenta (300[C]). However, in vitro investigations indicate a mutagenic potential. Nitrofurantoin is not found in breast milk.

Spermatogenesis High-dose oral nitrofurantoin intake (10 mg/kg per day) transiently reduces the sperm counts in 30% of patients (301[C]). This is due to arrest of maturation. Depression of sperm motility or ejaculate volume might also occur with lower doses (302[C]).

Interactions Antagonism in antibacterial efficacy between nitrofurantoin and *nalidixic acid* has been observed (303[C]). Nitrofurantoin can diminish the enterohepatic circulation of *estrogens*.

Interference with diagnostic routines Nitrofurantoin may produce spurious positive or elevated values of *urine or blood glucose* if reducing reagents are used. The determination of *creatine* and *creatinine* may also result in slightly elevated values (color interaction).

NALIDIXIC ACID AND FLUOROQUINOLONES

Nalidixic acid

Nalidixic acid is only rarely used in clinical practice. It is almost completely absorbed from the gastrointestinal tract and rapidly eliminated through the kidneys, resulting in urinary levels 4–6 times higher than plasma levels. There are better drugs to treat urinary tract infections. Knowledge of adverse effects, however, is important since similar reactions may be encountered with the very popular derivatives, the fluoroquinolones.

ADVERSE REACTION PATTERN

General and toxic reactions Adverse reactions tend to be toxic rather than allergic. CNS toxicity is predominant, including disturbances of sensory perception and benign intracranial hypertension, which is nearly exclusively found in babies and young children. Gastrointestinal toxicity and skin reactions also occur and are mostly harmless.

Hypersensitivity reactions These mainly affect the skin. Drug fever is rare. Hematological and hepatic reactions are very rare.

Tumor-inducing effects These have not been reported but require further study since nalidixic acid, as a DNA-gyrase inhibitor, damages DNA (304[R], 305[R]).

ORGANS AND SYSTEMS

Nervous system *Benign intracranial hypertension* (*pseudotumor cerebri*) mainly affects babies, especially during the first 3 months of life. Occasionally even older children or, very rarely, adults with renal failure may be affected. In infancy, a delay of nalidixic acid elimination (underdeveloped ability to couple glucuronic acid), overdosage or prolonged treatment may be responsible. Metabolic acidosis is usually important in adults (306[C]). The symptoms are described under tetracyclines. A total of about 30 cases have been described. In babies, the first symptoms appear during the first 3 days of initial treatment, in older children and adults symptoms may not appear before a second or even later exposure to the drug. After withdrawal of the drug, most symptoms usually subside quickly. Papillary edema and ocular palsy recede more slowly, the latter not always completely. In adults, peripheral paresis or severe pyramidal and extrapyramidal symptoms, occasionally followed by a transitory psychotic syndrome, have been seen (306[C]). Also, benign intracranial hypertension has been observed. Re-exposure to nalidixic acid has reproduced the syndrome in several cases (307[C]).

Functional short-lasting phenomena such as sensations of overbright lights, blurred vision, alteration of color perception or difficulty in focusing are dose-dependent and have been observed in about 7% of treated cases. They begin 30–60 minutes after drug intake and subside within 20 minutes to 3 hours. Disturbances of body perception, hallucinations, confusion, confabulation and depression may rarely persist for a longer time.

Convulsions without benign intracranial hypertension have been reported in at least 15 cases. Affected patients usually had pre-existing cerebral disease or had received extremely high doses. Normal doses in otherwise healthy persons can exceptionally provoke convulsions (SEDA-3, 246).

Uncharacteristic general symptoms such as headache, dizziness, drowsiness, insomnia or restlessness may also occur.

Polyneuropathy has mainly been reported from Australia.

Endocrine metabolic *Hyperglycemia* associated with convulsions has been observed following the use of high single doses (308[C]).

Mineral and fluid balance Nalidixic acid can induce *metabolic acidosis* in infants. This has also been seen in older children and adults with renal failure and may result from a disturbed lactate metabolism. Extreme overdosage (attempted suicide) can induce metabolic acidosis in subjects with normal renal function.

Hematological *Toxic effects* Rarely, hemolytic anemia associated with glucose-6-phosphate dehydrogenase deficiency has been reported. Rare cases of hemolytic anemia in the newborn have been related to nalidixic acid ingested through breast milk (309[C]). One case of fatal acute immune hemolytic anemia caused by nalidixic acid in a patient previously suffering from recurrent episodes of hemolysis has been described (SEDA-8, 283).

Allergic reactions Isolated cases of transient neutropenia, thrombocytopenia, Coombs-positive hemolytic anemia (310[C]) and of pancytopenia (311[R]) are known.

Liver *Cholestatic hepatitis* has been reported in single cases.

Gastrointestinal Nausea, vomiting and occasionally diarrhea or abdominal pain occur in about 8% of treated cases.

Skin and appendages Skin reactions are described in approximately 5% of treated cases.

Allergic reactions These include urticaria, erythematous or maculopapular rash, isolated pruritus, purpura, lesions resembling pityriasis rosea, erythema multiforme or exfoliative dermatitis. Except for the latter, they usually run a benign course.

Bullous photodermatosis After normal or excessive sun exposure blisters appear upon the exposed areas. Sometimes the lesions develop only several days after nalidixic acid withdrawal. The skin eruptions always persist long beyond the drug intake, sometimes for up to 4 months. Mainly women are affected and a toxic pathogenesis is assumed.

Special senses Occasional cases of *tinnitus* have been related to nalidixic acid treatment.

Musculoskeletal system Large doses of nalidixic acid produce degenerative inflammatory damage of the large weight-bearing joints in animal experiments. The clinical symptoms of juvenile canine arthropathy recede after withdrawal of the drug, but the histological alterations remain for a long time (312[R]). Occasionally *arthritis*, *arthralgia* or *myalgia* occur in humans (311[R]). However, three retrospective controlled studies found no evidence of nalidixic acid-associated arthropathy in children (313[C], 314[R]).

Lupus-like syndrome One case has been reported (315[C]).

Risk situations *Premature infants* and *young babies* are at highest risk of toxic reactions such as metabolic acidosis and benign intracranial hypertension, since excretion of the drug is still inadequate at this age. Sister-chromatid exchange, an indicator of DNA damage, increases significantly in nalidixic acid-treated children (316[R]). The drug should not be given to children before puberty. *Renal failure* favors toxicity by increasing serum levels of nalidixic acid and its metabolites. *Glucose-6-phosphate dehydrogenase deficiency* is the basis for the development of hemolytic anemia.

Second-generation effects Even if there is no evidence of teratogenicity in man, nalidixic acid should be avoided during pregnancy. Very small amounts of nalidixic acid pass into the breast milk.

Interactions Alkalinization of urine increases the excretion of free active drug. Nalidixic acid can displace *warfarin* from its plasma albumin-binding sites, thus inducing a hemorrhagic diathesis (317[C]).

Interference with diagnostic routines If reducing reagents are given with nalidixic acid, *glucosuric* and *hyperglycemia* may be mimicked by the presence of nalidixic and glucuronic acid compounds in the blood and urine. The urine levels of C17-*ketosteroids* (not of C17-hydroxysteroids) may be falsely elevated during nalidixic acid treatment.

Fluoroquinolones

Fluoroquinolones are derivatives of nalidixic acid. Several modifications of the molecule have produced characteristics which made them very popular drugs with favorable pharmacokinetic properties. The broadened and enhanced antimicrobial spectrum includes *P. aeruginosa*, staphylococci and intracellular organisms such as *Legionella* spp. and *Chlamydia*. These agents include norfloxacin, ciprofloxacin, ofloxacin, fleroxacin, pefloxacin, lomefloxacin and others. More recently some compounds with increased activity against streptococci (sparfloxacin) and against anaerobic bacteria have been developed. Increasing resistance to fluoroquinolones has been observed worldwide especially among *P. aeruginosa*, coagulase-positive and -negative staphylococci (oxacillin-susceptible and -resistant).

These nalidixic acid analogs act by the same mechanism as nalidixic acid. They inhibit DNA synthesis by blocking the ATP-dependent DNA supercoiling reaction catalyzed by DNA-gyrase, and are often as much as 100 times more active (318[R], 319[R]).

The fluoroquinolones are well absorbed after oral administration. They are excreted in the urine and bile in high concentrations of bioactive drug. Achievable blood concentrations are higher than with nalidixic acid, and their use is not limited to urinary tract infections.

Some of these drugs (ciprofloxacin, ofloxacin, fleroxacin, pefloxacin) are also available for intravenous administration. Their long elimination half lives of 4–15 hours make frequent dosing unnecessary (320[R]). Since the largest clinical experience with fluoroquinolones to date has been with norfloxacin, ciprofloxacin, ofloxacin, pefloxacin and fleroxacin, the most extensive safety data are available for these agents. The safety profile may be different with newer quinolones. Temafloxacin has been withdrawn from the market worldwide because of very severe and, in some cases, fatal side effects such as hemolytic anemia with renal failure, anaphylactoid reactions and hypoglycemia. Marketing of sparfloxacin in Europe has been delayed following reports of a possibly higher incidence of phototoxic reactions.

ADVERSE REACTION PATTERN

General and toxic reactions Adverse reactions are mainly toxic. Harmless gastrointestinal toxicities include nausea, vomiting and abdominal discomfort. They occur in about 5% of patients and are the most frequent adverse reactions to fluoroquinolones.The central nervous system is rarely affected, but headache, dizziness and, very rarely, convulsions may occur in susceptible patients.

Hypersensitivity reactions These have rarely been reported and mostly affect the skin.

Tumor-inducing effects These have not been described. As with other DNA-gyrase inhibitors (nalidixic acid), this issue needs further investigation.

ORGANS AND SYSTEMS

Cardiovascular No specific side effects have been reported so far. For anaphylactic or anaphylactoid reactions see skin and appendages.

Nervous system Fluoroquinolone toxicity of the central nervous system occurs in approximately 0.5–1% of patients, and has been most frequently observed (1.9%) with fleroxacin (321[R]–325[R], 326[C]).

Uncharacteristic general symptoms, mainly headache, dizziness, sleep disorders, depression, restlessness or tremors have been described. They are usually dose-dependent and subside quickly after withdrawal of the drug.

Individual cases of *convulsions* have been reported, but some of these patients had concomitant treatment with theophylline or non-steroidal anti-inflammatory agents (see Interactions, below).

The mechanisms by which fluoroquinolones affect the central nervous system are not fully elucidated. They apparently do not interfere with cerebral glucose or oxygen metabolism (327[C]). However, they have a weak, direct inhibitory effect on GABA-induced currents at the GABA-A receptor which is enhanced by the presence of certain non-steroidal anti-inflammatory drugs (328[R]). In two patients with myasthenia gravis, ciprofloxacin and norfloxacin, respectively, exacerbated the symptoms (SEDA-16, 325, 326; 329[C]). Bilateral acute visual loss, possibly due to toxic optic neuropathy, was observed after a 4-week treatment with 1.5 grams ciprofloxacin daily and improved after withdrawal of the drug (330[C]).

Two cases of generalized painful dysesthesia associated with ciprofloxacin have been reported (331[c]).

Hematological Anemia, thrombocytopenia and thrombocytosis have only rarely been reported (321[R], 322[R], 324[R], 332[R]). Leukopenia has been observed in 0.1–0.7% of patients given fluoroquinolones in Japan and eosinophilia was observed in 0.5–2.2% of these patients (325[R]). Leukopenia was generally mild and was reversible after the drug was reduced or withdrawn (333[C], 334[C]).

Liver Transient elevation of serum *aminotransferase* and serum *alkaline phosphatase* levels have been observed with all fluoroquinolones. They occurred in 0.9–4.3% of patients in Japan. Elevated serum *alkaline phosphatase* levels were very rare (up to 0.3%) (325[R]). In the vast majority of the cases this alteration was self-limited and reversible and did not require withdrawal of the drug.

One case of acute hepatitis following norfloxacin treatment was reported (335[c]).

Gastrointestinal Disturbances of the gastrointestinal tract are the most frequent side effects observed with fluoroquinolones and occur in about 5% of treated patients. These reactions include *nausea and/or vomiting*, *abdominal discomfort*, *dyspepsia* or *diarrhea*. Nausea has rarely necessitated interruption of therapy and has often been controlled by dosage reduction (336[C]).

Diarrhea has been infrequently reported (in 1%) and some cases of colitis due to *C. difficile* following norfloxacin and ciprofloxacin treatment have been observed.

Urinary system Animal studies suggest that ciprofloxacin is relatively insoluble at alkaline pH values. This could lead to crystalluria (drug precipitation) and renal tubular damage. The acid urine of humans, however, seems to protect against this effect. Rare cases of possibly drug-related crystalluria have been described (337[C], 338[C], 339[r]). Single cases of reversible, acute non-oliguric or oliguric renal failure probably due to tubulo-interstitial nephritis have been reported (340[C], 341[C]), as well as isolated cases of hematuria (342[R]). Two cases of acute renal failure due to necrotizing vasculitis associated with ciprofloxacin treatment were reported in elderly patients (343[C]).

Elevated serum creatinine or blood urea nitrogen has been observed in 0.1–0.7% of patients (325[R]).

Skin and appendages Skin reactions have been described in approximately 1–2% of treated cases (325[R]).

Allergic reactions include maculopapular or erythematous rash and pruritus. Anaphylactoid reactions including hypotension, shock, asthma, laryngeal edema, urticaria and angio-edema have been reported in about 20 patients. The incidence has been estimated to be around 0.5–1 per 100 000 prescriptions. Most reports regard ciprofloxacin. The majority of patients were without previous exposure to the drug and the reactions occurred 5–60 minutes after the first ingestion (344[C]–346[C]).

Photodermatitis has been observed in patients during or a few days after treatment with any of the fluoroquinolones, with the development of erythematous eruptions on exposed areas. Bullae and eczematization may evolve. In some cases the reactions were associated with fever. Overall, phototoxic reactions are rare, occurring in 0—0.04% of patients in Japan (325[R]). Whether some compounds such as sparfloxacin cause phototoxic reactions more often is still unclear. An animal model to study phototoxic effects of quinolones has been described (347[c]).

Local phlebitis was reported after intravenous bolus injection of 50—100 mg ciprofloxacin. No significant local irritation has been observed when the drug was administered as a short infusion over 20 minutes.

Special senses In animal studies long-term treatment with fluoroquinolones produced cataracts. This has not been observed in humans. A series of 600 American patients treated with ciprofloxacin underwent ophthalmological examination before and after therapy and no significant eye alterations were reported (348[R]).

Musculoskeletal system As with nalidixic acid, chronic high-dose administration of fluoroquinolones produces cartilaginous damage in the large weight-bearing joints of juvenile dogs. Preliminary data from several centers showed unchanged normal magnetic resonance images of the knee in children examined before and after treatment with quinolones (349[R]).

Single cases of *arthralgia and muscle pain* have been described with norfloxacin. Several cases of arthralgia in adolescents with cystic fibrosis treated with ciprofloxacin (350[C]) or pefloxacin (351[C]) have been reported. No erosion of joint cartilage has been noted, and signs and symptoms resolved or improved after stopping the drugs.

Tendonitis has been reported with various fluoroquinolones, apparently with pefloxacin predominating (352[R]). This side effect is rare, occurring in 0.3% of reported adverse reactions associated with fluoroquinolones. Tendonitis followed by *tendon rupture* has been observed among these patients. About 30 cases have been observed, mainly in France (352[R], 353[C], 354[C]). Many of these patients had received concomitant corticosteroid therapy. The Achilles tendon was affected most often, and half the patients had bilateral tendonitis. The ruptures occurred 2—42 (average 13) days after the start of treatment. It is unknown whether there is some relationship between tendonitis and the cartilage injury seen in juvenile dogs.

Risk situations Until cartilage toxicities have been proven not to occur in man, it would seem prudent *not to administer the fluoroquinolones to patients whose skeletal growth is incomplete*. In such cases, quinolone use should be limited to specific infections with complicating underlying conditions (cystic fibrosis, urological abnormalities).

Following the reports on tendonitis and tendon rupture it is recommended *to discontinue treatment with quinolones at the first sign of tendon pain or inflammation* and to refrain from exercise until the diagnosis of tendonitis can be confidently excluded.

Patients with a previous *history of convulsive disorders* are possibly at increased risk for fluoroquinolone CNS toxicity. A careful risk/benefit evaluation of fluoroquinolone treatment has to be performed in such cases.

Fluoroquinolones are, in part, excreted by the kidney and *renal failure prolongs elimination* of these compounds. This may produce increased toxicity, in particular to the central nervous system. Ofloxacin dosage should be reduced in patients with renal failure (creatinine clearance of less than 30 ml/minute).

Second-generation effects Even if there is no proof of teratogenicity of fluoroquinolones in man, these compounds, like nalidixic acid, should be avoided during pregnancy. Similarly, because of experimentally induced cartilaginous damage, fluoroquinolones should not be given during lactation.

Evidence of impaired spermatogenesis was found in long-term toxicity studies in rats and dogs treated with high doses of fluoroquinolones. No evidence of such toxicity has been observed in humans so far.

Interactions *Physical incompatibility of fluoroquinolones with other drugs* causing precipitation in intravenous lines has been observed with pefloxacin-aminophylline and ciprofloxacin or pefloxacin-flucloxacillin, amoxicillin and amoxicillin-clavulanate. Fluoroquinolones should not be mixed in the same container with aminophylline or any penicillin, nor should they be infused simultaneously through the same tubing.

Alterations of absorption of all fluoroquinolones have been reported to occur with the administration of *antacid products and sucralfate* containing di- and trivalent cations (aluminum, magnesium, calcium) (355[R]). The mechanism seems to involve the formation of insoluble complexes or the chelation of drug and polyvalent cation. *Histamine type 2 receptor antagonists do not interfere* with absorption. Use of all antacid preparations and of sucralfate should be avoided during fluoroquinolone therapy. Studies in healthy volunteers have shown that antacids given 6 hours before the antibiotic had no significant effect. However, data from studies with patients are still lacking. *Food*, especially with a high fat content, delays the t_{max} for fluoroquinolones but the extent of absorption was not significantly altered.

Nutritional supplements such as *ferrous sulfate* or *multivitamins containing zinc* significantly reduced the absorption of fluoroquinolones. This might cause treatment failures in critically ill patients given fluoroquinolone combined with enteral nutrition by nasogastric tube.

Fluoroquinolones *may alter the metabolism of other drugs*. They are *potent inhibitors of subsets of hepatic microsomal enzymes* (355[R]). *Methylxanthine metabolism* (*theophylline*, *caffeine*) may be affected and serious side effects possibly due to this interaction have been reported (356[C], 357[C]). The extent of metabolization of fluoroquinolones dictates the degree of this interaction. Pefloxacin, enoxacin and, to a lesser degree, ciprofloxacin decrease theophylline clearance thus raising its blood levels and prolonging its half life. Norfloxacin, ofloxacin and fleroxacin have a lower potential for affecting the metabolism of theophylline and caffeine. The dose of enoxacin and pefloxacin should be reduced by 50 and 30%, respectively, when administered concomitantly with theophylline. Ciprofloxacin treatment requires careful monitoring of theophylline levels, and patients with initial theophylline serum levels at the upper end of the therapeutic range should have the daily dose reduced by 30—50%. No adjustment should be necessary for norfloxacin, ofloxacin and fleroxacin.

Certain fluoroquinolones might interact with *warfarin* decreasing its clearance and increasing the patients' prothrombin time. Such interactions have been described with norfloxacin, ofloxacin and enoxacin. It seems prudent to closely monitor patients receiving warfarin concomitantly with any fluoroquinolone.

H_2 receptor antagonists such as *cimetidine and ranitidine may alter the clearance of certain fluoroquinolones*. Preliminary data indicate that the interaction depends on the specific agent involved, with drugs undergoing significant metabolism (pefloxacin, enoxacin) most likely to be affected. Preliminary data show that omeprazole does not alter the pharmacokinetics of ciprofloxacin or lomefloxacin in single-dose studies (358[C]).

A potential interaction of ciprofloxacin with *ciclosporin* with increased nephrotoxicity was suggested in a case report of a cardiac transplant recipient (359[C]). The suspected potentiation of nephrotoxicity by fluoroquinolones was, however, not supported in further investigations (355[R]).

The renal excretion of norfloxacin, fleroxacin and, in particular, ofloxacin is decreased by *probenecid*. The change is not clinically relevant for drugs with significant non-renal elimination (enoxacin, pefloxacin, ciprofloxacin).

Co-administration of fenbufen, a non-steroidal anti-inflammatory agent, with enoxacin has been associated with seizures in Japanese patients (360[R]). Results of numerous animal experiments have shown that virtually all fluoroquinolones antagonize the GABA-A receptor and all are potentiated by an active metabolite of fenbufen and, to a lesser extent, other NSAIDs (328[R], 355[R]). Fluoroquinolones in combination with NSAIDs should be used with caution.

OTHER DRUGS USED IN URINARY TRACT INFECTIONS

Phenazopyridine hydrochloride

This azo-dye has an analgesic action and alleviates symptoms of urinary tract infections. It is also marketed in combination with sulfonamides. Nausea, occasionally dizziness and headache, hepatocellular jaundice or drug fever may occur (361[C]). After a large overdose methemoglobinemia and hemolytic anemia with Heinz-body formation occur. Phenazopyridine hydrochloride concrements have seldom been observed in the lower urinary tract. Recently methemoglobinemia has been described in a patient with normal renal function given normal doses of phenazopyridine (362[C]).

In some cases of intoxication, acute renal failure was reported (363[C], 364[C]). The drug should not be given to patients with renal failure.

Simultaneous intake of phenazopyridine hydrochloride and sulfur preparations can induce sulf-hemoglobinemia. The color of the drug can produce false-positive tests for acetoacetic acid (Ketostix, ferric chloride), for bilirubin and for glucose (Tes-tape). 17-Hydroxycorticosteroids and 17-ketosteroids in the urine show falsely elevated values.

REFERENCES

1. Mandell GL, Sande MA. Antimicrobial agents Sulfonamides, trimethoprim—sulfamethoxazole, quinolones, and agents for urinary tract infections. In: Goodman Gilman A, Rall TW, Nies AS, Taylor P, eds. Goodman and Gilman's The Pharmacological Basis of Therapeutics, 8th edn. New York: Pergamon Press, 1990;1047.
2. Editorial. Trimethoprim resistance. Lancet 1986;ii:791.
3. Sutherland LR, May GR, Shaffer EA. Sulfasalazine revisited: a meta-analysis of 5-aminosalicylic acid in the treatment of ulcerative colitis. Ann Int Med 1993;118:540.
4. Lowbury EJL, Babb JR, Bridges K et al. Topical chemoprophylaxis with silver sulphadiazine and silver nitrate chlorhexidine creams: emergence of sulfonamide- resistant gram-negative bacilli. Br Med J 1976;1:493.
5. Alfthan O, Liewendahl K, Ervast HS. Importance of temperature for the diagnosis of sulfonamide crystalluria in man. Ann Clin Res 1969;1:177.
6. Shear NH, Spielberg SP, Grant DM et al. Differences in metabolism of sulfonamides predisposing to idiosyncratic toxicity. Ann Int Med 1986;105:179.
7. Rieder MJ, Shear NH, Kanee A et al. Prominence of slow acetylator phenotype among patients with sulfonamide hypersensitivity reactions. Clin Pharmacol Ther 1991;49:13.

8a. Woody RC, Brewster MA. Adverse effects of trimethoprim—sulfamethoxazole in a child with dihydropteridine reductase deficiency. Dev Med Child Neurol 1990;32:639.

8b. Carrington DM, Earl HS, Sullivan TJ. Studies of human IgE to a sulfonamide determinant. J Allergy Clin Immunol 1987;79:442.

9. Rich AR. Additional evidence of the role of hypersensitivity in the etiology of periarteritis nodosa. Bull Johns Hopkins Hosp 1942;71:375.
10. Van Rijssel TG, Meyler L. Necrotizing generalized arteritis due to the use of sulfonamide drugs. Acta Med Scand 1948;132:251.
11. Zeek PM, Smith CC, Weeter JC. Studies on periarteritis nodosa. III. Differentiation between vascular lesions of periarteritis nodosa and of hypersensitivity. Am J Pathol 1948;24:889.
12. Kussmaul A, Maier R. Ueber eine bisher nicht beschriebene eigentümliche Arterienerkrankung (Periarteriitis nodosa), die mit Morbus Brightii und rapid fortschreitender allgemeiner Muskellähmung einhergeht. Dtsch Arch Klin Med (1866) 1, 484.
13. Delage C, Lagacé R. Maladie sérique avec hyperplasie ganglionnaire pseudo-lymphomateuse secondaire à la prise de salicylazosulfapyridine. Union Méd Can 1975;104:579.
14. Han T, Chawla PL, Sokal JE. Sulfapyridine-induced serum-sickness-like syndrome associated with plasmocytosis, lymphocytosis and multiclonal gamma-globulinopathy. N Engl J Med 1969;280:547.
15. French AJ, Weller CV. Interstitial myocarditis following the clinical and experimental use of sulfonamide drugs. Am J Pathol 1942;18:109.
16. Wahlström B, Nyström-Rosander C, Aberg H et al. Recurrent meningitis and perimyocarditis after trimethoprim. Lakartitingen 1982;79:4854.
17. Shear NH, Rieder MJ, Spielberg SP et al. Hypersensitivity reactions to sulfonamide antibiotics are mediated by a hydroxylamine metabolite. Clin Res 1987;35:717
18. Shear NH, Spielberg SP. In vitro evaluation of a toxic metabolite of sulfadiazine. Can J Physiol Pharmacol 1985;63:1370.

19a. Ghajar BM, Naranjo CA, Shear NH et al. Improving the accuracy of the differential diagnosis of idiosyncratic adverse drug reactions (IADRs): skin eruptions and sulfonamides. Clin Pharmacol Ther 1990;47:127.

19b. Gruchalla RS, Sullivan TJ. Detection of human IgE to sulfamethoxazole by skin testing with sulfamethoxazoyl-polytyrosine. J Allergy Clin Immunol 1991;88:784.

20. Sher MR, Suchar C, Lockey RF. Anaphylactic shock induced by oral desensitization to Trimethoprim/Sulfmethoxazole. J Allergy Immunol 1986;77:133.

21a. Nixon N, Eckert JF, Holmesk B. The treatment of agranulocytosis with sulfadiazine. Am J Med Sci 1943;206:713.

21b. Coopman SA, Johnson RA, Platt R et al. Cutaneous disease and drug reactions in HIV infection. N Engl J Med 1993;328:1670.

22. Torgovnick J, Arsura E. Desensitization to sulfonamides in patients with HIV infection. Am J Med 1990;88:548.
23. Finegold I. Oral desensitization to trimethoprim—sulfamethoxazole in a patient with acquired immunodeficiency syndrome. J Allergy Clin Immunol 1986;78:905.
24. Papakonstantinou G, Füessl H, Hehlmann R. Trimethoprim—sulfamethoxazole desensitization in AIDS. Klin Wochenschr 1988;66:351.
25. Kreuz W. 'Treating through' hypersensitivity to cotrimoxazole in children with HIV infection. Lancet 1990; 336:508.
26. Binns PM. Anaphylaxis after oral sulphadiazine: two reactions in the same patient within eight days. Lancet 1958; i:194.
27. Reichmann J. Anaphylaktischer Schock durch intravenöse Sulfonamidapplikation mit letalem Ausgang Dtsch Gesundheitswes 1960;15:1139.
28. Crofton JW, Livingstone JL, Oswald NC et al. Pulmonary eosinophilia. Thorax 1952;7:1.
29. Reeder WH, Goodrich BE. Pulmonary infiltration with eosinophilia (PIE syndrome). Ann Intern Med 1952;36:1217.
30. Chumbley LC, Harrison EG, Deremee RH. Allergic granulomatosis and angiitis (Churg-Strauss syndrome): report and analysis of 30 cases. Mayo Clin Proc 1977;52:477.
31. Loeffler W. Ueber flüchtige Lungenilfiltrate (mit Eosinophilie). Beitr Klin Tuberk 1932;79:368.
32. Ellis RV, McKinlay CA. Allergic pneumonia. J Lab Clin Med 1941;26:1427.
33. Klinghoffer JF. Löffler's syndrome following use of a vaginal cream. Ann Intern Med 1954;40:343.
34. Fiegenberg DS, Weiss H, Kirshmann H. Migratory pneumonia with eosinophilia. Arch Intern Med 1967;120:85.
35. Jones GR, Malone NS. Sulphasalazine induced lung disease. Thorax 1972;27:713.
36. Thomas P, Seaton A, Edwards J. Respiratory disease due to sulphasalazine. Clin Allergy 1974;4:41.
37. Scherpenisse J, van der Valk PDL, van den Bosch JMM et al. Olsalazine as an alternative therapy in a patient with sulfasalazine-induced eosinophilic pneumonia. J Clin Gastroenterol 1988;10:218.
38. Swanbom M. Unusual pulmonary reaction during short term prophylaxis with pyrimethamine-sulfadoxine (Fansidar®). Br Med J 1984;288:1876.
39. Berliner S, Neeman A, Shoenfeld Y et al. Salazopyrin-induced eospinophilic pneumonia. Respiration 1980;39:119.

40. Tydd TF, Dyer NH. Sulphasalazine lung. Med J Aust 1976;1:570.
41. Wang KK, Bowyer BA, Fleming CR et al. Pulmonary infiltrates and eosinophilia associated with sulfasalazine. Mayo Clin Proc 1984;59:343.
42. Von Meyenburg H. Das eosinophile Lungenilfiltrat: pathologische Anatomie und Pathogenese. Schweiz Med Wochenschr 1942;72:809.
43. Pepys J. Hypersensivitiy diseases of the lungs due to fungi and organic dusts. In: Monographs in Allergy, Vol 4. Basel/New York: S. Karger, 1969.
44. Plügge H. Ueber zentrale und periphere nervöse Schäden nach Eubasinummedikation. Dtsch Z Nervenheilkd 1940; 151:205.
45. Bucy PC. Toxic optic neuritis resulting from sulfanilamide. J Am Med Assoc 1937;109:1007.
46. Borucki M. et al. Tremor Induced by trimethoprim—sulfamethoxazole in patients with the acquired immunodeficiency syndrome (AIDS). Ann Intern Med 1988;109:77.
47. Liu LX, Seward SJ, Crumpacker CS. Intravenous trimethoprim—sulfamethoxazole and ataxia. Ann Intern Med 1986;104:448.
48a. Barrett PVD, Thier SO. Meningitis and pancreatitis associated with sulfamethizole. N Engl J Med 1963;268:36.
48b. Haas EJ. Trimethoprim—sulfamethoxazole: another cause of recurrent meningitis. J Am Med Assoc 1984; 252:346.
49. Kremer I, Ritz R, Brunner F. Aseptic meningitis as an adverse effect of co-trimoxazole. N Engl J Med 1983; 308:1481.
50. Auxier GG. Aseptic meningitis with administration of trimethoprim and sulfamethoxazole. Am J Dis Child 1990; 144:144.
51. Biosca M, de la Figuera M, Garcia-Bragado F et al. Aseptic meningitis due to trimethoprim—sulfamethoxazole. J Neurol Neurosurg Psychiatry 1986;49:332.
52. Joffe AM, Farley JD, Linden D et al. Trimethoprim—sulfamethoxazole-associated aseptic meningitis: case reports and review of the literature. Am J Med 1990;87:332.
53. Gordon MF, Allon M, Coyle PK. Drug-induced meningitis. Neurology 1990;40:163.
54. Derbes SJ. Trimethoprim-induced aseptic meningitis. J Am Med Assoc 1984;252:2865.
55. Carlson J, Wiholm B. Trimethoprim associated aseptic meningitis. Scand J Infect Dis 1987;19:687.
56. Bovino JA, Marcus DF. The mechanism of transient myopia induced by sulfonamide therapy. Am J Ophthalmol 1982;94:99.
57. Hook SR, Holladay JT, Prager TC et al. Transient myopia induced by sulfonamides. Am J Ophthalmol 1986; 101:495.
58. Carlberg O. Zur Genese der Sulfonamidmyopie. Acta Ophthalmol 1942;20:275.
59. Gutt L, Feder JM, Feder RS. Corneal ring formation after exposure to Sulfamethoxazole. Arch Ophthalmol 1988;106:726.
60. White MG, Asch MJ. Acid-base effects of topical mafenide acetate in the burned patient. N Engl J Med 1971; 284:1281.
61. Zinkham WH. Unstable hemoglobins and the selective hemolytic action of sulfonamides. Arch Intern Med 1977; 137:1365.
62. De Leeuw NKN, Shapiro L, Lowenstein L. Drug-induced hemolytic anemia. Ann Intern Med 1963;58:592.
63. Worlledge SM. Immune drug-induced haemolytic anaemias. Semin Hematol 1969;6:181.
64. Fishman FL, Baron JM, Orlina A. Non-oxidative hemolysis due to salicylazosulfapyridine: evidence for an immune mechanism. Gastroenterology 1973;64:727.
65. Cohen SM, Rosenthal DS, Karp PJ. Ulcerative colitis and erythrocyte G6PD deficiency. J Am Med Assoc 1968;205:528.
66. Meyer UA. Drugs in special patient groups: Clinical importance of genetics in drug effects. In: Melmon KL, Morelli HF, Hoffman BB et al, eds. Clinical Pharmacology, Basic Principles in Therapeutics, 3rd edn. New York—St Louis—San Francisco, etc: McGraw-Hill Inc., 1992;875.
67. Frick PG, Hitzig WH, Stauffer U. Das Hämoglobin-Zürich-Syndrom. Schweiz Med Wochenschr 1961;40:1203.
68. Hitzig WH, Frick PG, Betke K et al. Hämoglobin Zürich: eine neue Hämoglobinanomalie mit sulfonamid- induzierter Innenkörperanämie. Helv Paediatr Acta 1960;15:499.
69. Beretta A, Prato V, Gallo E et al. Haemoglobin Torino X 43 (CDI) phenylalanine-vaniline. Nature 1968;217:1016.
70. Adams JG, Heller P, Abramson RK et al. Sulfonamide-induced hemolytic anemia and hemoglobin Hasharon. Arch Intern Med 1977;137:1449.
71. Harris JW. Studies on the mechanism of a drug-induced hemolytic anemia. J Lab Clin Med 1956;47:760.
72. Beutler E. Red cell metabolism. In: Beutler E, ed. Methods in Hematology Series, Vol 16. Edinburgh/London: Churchill-Livingston, 1986.
73. Gaetani GD, Mareni C, Ravazzolo R et al. Haemolytic effect of two sulfonamides evaluated by a new method. Br J Haematol 1976;32:183.
74. Huisman THJ. Hemoglobinopathies. In: Huisman THJ, ed. Methods in Hematology Series, Vol 15. Edinburgh/London: Churchill-Livingston, 1986.
75. Shinton NK, Wilson C. Autoimmune haemolytic anaemia due to phenacetin and *p*-aminosalicylic acid. Lancet 1960;i:226.
76. Lyonnais J. Production de corps de Heinz associée à la prise de salicylazosulfapyridine. Union Méd Can 1976; 105:203.
77. Streeter AM, Shum HY, O'Neill BJ. The effect of drugs on the microbiological assay of serum folic acid and vitamin B12 levels. Med J Aust 1970;1:900.
78. Baumgartner A, Hoigné R, Müller U et al. Medikamentöse Schäden des Blutbildes: Erfahrungen aus dem Komprehensiven Spital-Drug-Monitoring Bern, 1974—1979. Schweiz Med Wochenschr 1982;112:1530.
79. Müller U. Hämatologische Nebenwirkungen von Medikamenten. Ther Umsch 1987;44:942.
80. Havas L. Fernex M, Lenox-Smith I. The clinical efficacy and tolerance of co-trimoxazole (Bactrim; Septrim). Clin Trials J 1973;3:81.
81. Hoigné R, Klein U, Müller U. Results of four-week course of therapy of urinary tract infections: a comparative study using trimethoprim with sulfamethoxazole (Bactrim® Roche) and trimethoprim alone. In: Hejzlar M, Semonsky M, Masak S, eds. Advances in Antimocrobial and Antineoplastic Chemotherapy. München—Berlin—Wien: Urban and Schwarzenberg, 1972;1283.
82. Jick SS, Jick H, Habakangas JAS, Dianan BJ. Cotrimoxazole toxicity in children. Lancet 1984;ii:631.
83. Johnston FD. Granulocytopenia following the administration of sulphanilamide compounds. Lancet 1938;ii:1044.
84. Rinkoff SS, Spring M. Toxic depression of the myeloid

elements following therapy with the sulfonamides: report of 8 cases. Ann Intern Med 1941;15:89.
85. Moeschlin S. Immunolgical granulocytopenia and agranulocytosis. Sang 1955;26:32.
86. Rios Sanchez I, Duarte L, Sanchez Medal L. Agranulocitosis: analisis de 29 episodios en 19 pacientes. Rev Invest Clin 1971;23:29.
87. Ritz ND, Fisher MJ. Agranulocytosis due to administration of salicylazosulfapyridine (azulfidine). J Am Med Assoc 1960;172:237.
88. Malinverni R, Blatter M. Ambulante Therapie und Prophylaxe der häufigsten HIV-assoziierten opportunistischen Infektionen. Schweiz Med Wochenschr 1991;121:1194.
89. Jarrett F, Ellerbe S, Demling R. Acute leukopenia during topical burn therapy with silver sulfadiazine. Am J Surg 1978;135:818.
90. Maurer LH, Andrews P, Rueckert F et al. Lymphocyte transformation observed in sulfamylon agranulocytosis. Plast Reconstr Surg 1970;46:458.
91. Rhodes EG, Ball J, Franklin IM. Amodiaquine-induced agranulocytosis, inhibition of colony growth in bone marrow by antimalarial agents. Br Med J 1986;292:717.
92. Böttiger LE, Westerholm B. Thrombocytopenia. II. Drug-induced thrombocytopenia. Acta Med Scand 1972; 191:541.
93. Janovsky RC. Fatal thrombocytopenic purpura after administration of sulfamethoxypyridazine. J Am Med Assoc 1960;172:155.
94. Gremse DA, Bancroft J, Moyer S. Sulfasalazine hypersensitivity with hepatotoxicity, thrombocytopenia, and erythroid hypoplasia. J Pediatr Gastroenterol Nutr 1989;9:261.
95. Böttiger LE, Westerholm B. Thrombocytopenia. I. Incidence and aetiology. Acta Med Scand 1972;191:535.
96. Kelton JG, Meltzer D, Moore J et al. Drug-induced thrombocytopenia is associated with increased binding of IgG to platelets both in vivo and in vitro. Blood 1981;58:524.
97. Kiefel V, Santoso S, Schmidt S et al. Metabolite-specific (IgG) and drug-specific antibodies (IgG, IgM) in two cases of trimethoprim—sulfamethoxazole-induced immune thrombocytopenia. Transfusion 1987;27:262.
98. Scott JL, Cartwright GE, Wintrobe MM. Acquired aplastic anemia: an analysis of thirty-nine cases and review of the perinent literature. Medicine 1959;38:119.
99. Rammelkamp CH. Jaundice and sulfonamide drugs. Blood 1948;3:1411.
100. Fried J, Siraganian R. Sulfonamide hepatitis: report of a case due to sulfamethoxazole and sulfisoxazole. N Engl J Med 1966;274:95.
101. Kaufmann SF. A rare complication of sulfadimethoxine (Madribon) therapy. Calif Med 1967;107:344.
102. Konttinen A. Hepatotoxicity of sulphamethoxypyridazine. Br Med J 1972;2:168.
103. Konttinen A, Peräsalo JOS, Eisalo A. Sulfonamide hepatitis. Acta Med Scand 1972;191:389.
104. Sotolongo RP, Neefe L, Rudzki C et al. Hypersensitivity reaction of sulfasalazine with severe hepatotoxicity. Gastroenterology 1978;75:95.
105. Dujovne CA, Chan CH, Zimmermann HJ. Sulfonamide hepatic injury: review of the literature and report of a case due to sulfamethoxazole. N Engl J Med 1967;277:785.
106. Tönder M, Nordöy A, Elgjo K. Sulfonamide induced chronic liver disease. Scand J Gastroenterol 1974;9:93.
107a. Gutman LT. The use of trimethoprim—sulfamethoxazole in children: a review of adverse reactions and indications. Pediatr Infect Dis 1984;3:349.
107b. Chester AC, Diamond LH, Schreiner GE. Hypersensitivity to salicylazosulfapyridine: renal and hepatic toxic reactions. Arch Intern Med 1978;138:1138.
108. Shaw DJ, Jacobs RP. Simultaneous occurrence of toxic hepatitis and Stevens-Johnson syndrome following therapy with sulfisoxazole and sulfamethoxazole. Johns Hopkins Med J 1970;126:130.
109. Block MB, Genant HK, Kirsner JB. Pancreatitis as an adverse reaction to salicylazosulfapyridine. N Engl J Med 1970;282:380.
110. Surypranata H, De Vries H et al. Pancreatitis associated with sulphasalazine. Br Med J 1986;292:732.
111. Deprez P, Descamps Ch, Fiasse R. Pancreatitis induced by 5-aminosalicylic acid. Lancet 1989;ii:445.
112. Nidus BD, Field M, Rammelkamp CH. Salivary gland enlargement caused by sulfisoxazole. Ann Intern Med 1965;63:663.
113. Oster S, Hutchison F, McCabe R. Resolution of acute renal failure in toxoplasmic encephalitis despite continuance of sulfadiazine. Rev Infect Dis 1990;12:618.
114. Christin S, Baumelou A, Bahri S et al. Acute renal failure due to sulfadiazine in patients with AIDS. Nephron 1990;55:233.
115. Simon DI, Brosius FC, Rothstein DM. Sulfadiazine crystalluria revisited. The treatment of toxoplasma encephalitis in patients with acquired immunodeficiency syndrome. Arch Int Med 1990;150:2379.
116. Miller MA, Gallicano K, Dascal A et al. Sulfadiazine urolithiasis during antitoxoplasma therapy. Drug Invest 1993;5:334.
117. Furrer HJ, von Overbeck J, Jaeger Ph et al. Sulfadiazin-Nephrolithiasis und -Nephropathie. Schweiz Med Wochenschr 1994;124:2100.
118. Craig WA, Kunin CM. Trimethoprim—sulfamethoxazole: pharmacodynamic effects of urinary pH and impaired renal function. Ann Intern Med 1973;78:491.
119. Robson M, Levi J, Dolberg L et al. Acute tubulo-interstitial nephritis following sulfadiazine therapy. Isr J Med Sci 1970;6:561.
120. Baker SB, Williams RT. Acute interstitial nephritis due to drug sensitivity. Br Med J 1963;1:1655.
121. Pursey CD, Saltissi D, Bloodworth L et al. Drug associated acute interstitial nephritis: clinical and pathological features and the response to high dose steroid therapy. Q J Med 1983;52:194.
122. Cryst C, Hammar SP. Acute granulomatous interstitial nephritis due to co-trimoxazole. Am J Nephrol 1988;8:483.
123. Bigby M, Jick S, Jick H et al. Drug-induced cutaneous reactions: a report from the Boston Collaborative Drug Surveillance Program on 15,438 consecutive inpatients, 1975 to 1982. J Am Med Assoc 1986;256:3358.
124. Sonntag MR, Zoppi M, Fritschy D et al. Exantheme unter häufig angewandten Antibiotika und anti-bakteriellen Chemotherapeutika (Penicilline, speziell Aminopenicilline, Cephalosporine und Cotrimoxazol) sowie Allopurinol. Schweiz Med Wochenschr 1986;116:142.
125. Hunziker T, Hoigné R, Künzi UP et al. Comprehensive Hospital Drug Monitoring (CHDM), the adverse skin reactions, a 20-years survey. Abstract 033. Pharmacoepidemiol Drug Safety 1995;4:S13.
126. Arndt KA, Jick H. Rates of cutaneous reactions to drugs: a report from the Boston Collaborative Drug Surveillance Program. J Am Med Assoc 1976;235:918.
127. Hoigné R, Stocker F, Middleton P. Epidemiology of

drug allergy; drug monitoring. In: Born GVR, Farah AE, Herken H et al, series eds. The Handbook of Experimental Pharmacology, Vol 63, De Weck AL, Bundgaard H, eds. Allergic Reactions to Drugs. Berlin—Heidelberg: Springer-Verlag, 1983;187.

128. Gomez B, Sastre J, Azofra J, Sastre A. Fixed drug eruption. Allergol Immunopathol 1985;13:87.

129. Bergoend H, Löffler A, Amar R et al. Réactions cutanées survenues au cours de la prophylaxie de masse de la méningite cérébrospinale par un sulfamide long-retard (à propos de 997 cas). Ann Dermatol Syphiligr 1968;95:481.

130. Taylor CML. Stevens-Johnson syndrome following the use of an ultra-long-acting sulfonamide. S Afr Med J 1968;42:501.

131. Hernborg A. Stevens-Johnson syndrome after mass prophylaxis with sulfadoxine for cholera in Mozambique. Lancet 1985;ii:1072.

132. Gottschalk HR, Stone OJ. Stevens-Johnson syndrome from ophthalmic sulfonamide. Arch Dermatol 1976;112:513.

133. Lyell A. A review of toxic epidermal necrolysis in Britain. Br J Dermatol 1967;79:662.

134. Björnberg A. Fifteen cases of toxic epidermal necrolysis (Lyell). Acta Dermatol (Stockholm) 1973;53:149.

135. Schöpf E. Stühmer A, Rzany B et al. Toxic epidermal necrolysis (TEN) and Stevens-Johnson syndrome (SJS): an epidemiological study from West Germany. Arch Dermatol 1991;127:839.

136. Kauppinen K, Stubb S. Drug eruptions: causative agents and clinical types. Acta Dermatol-Venereol 1984; 64:320.

137. Cohlan SQ. Erythema multiforme exudativum associated with use of sulfamethoxypyridazine. J Am Med Assoc 1960;173:799.

138. Böttiger LE, Strandberg I, Westerholm B. Drug-induced febrile mucocutaneous syndrome. Acta Med Scand 1975;198:229.

139a. Hoigné R. Interne Manifestationen und Labor-befunde beim Lyell-Syndrom. In: Braun-Falco O, Bandmann HJ, eds. Das Lyell-Syndrom. Bern—Stuttgart—Wien: Verlag H. Huber, 1970;27.

139b. Revuz J, Roujeau JC, Guillaume JC et al. Treatment of toxic epidermal necrolysis. Arch. Dermatol. 1987;123:1156.

140. Roujeau JC, Bracq C, Huyn NT et al. HLA phenotypes and bullous cutaneous reactions to drugs. Tissue Antigens 1986;28:251.

141a. Amon RB, Dimond RL. Toxic epidermal necrolysis. Arch Dermatol 1975;11:1433.

141b. Elias PM, Fritsch P, Epstein EH. Staphylococcal scalded skin syndrome. Arch Dermatol 1977;113:207.

142. Rollof SL. Erythema nodosum in association with sulfathiazole in children: clinical investigation with special reference to primary tuberculosis. Acta Tuberc Scand Suppl 1950;24:1.

143. Wintroub BU, Stern RS, Arndt KA. Cutaneous reactions to drugs. In: Fitzpatrick TB, Eisen AZ, Wolff K et al., eds. Dermatology in General Medicine, 7th edn, Vol 1. New York: McGraw-Hill Book Co, 1987;1353.

144. Kauppinen K, Stubb S. Fixed eruptions: causative drugs and challenge tests. Br J Dermatol 1985;112:575.

145. Pasricha JS. Drugs causing fixed eruption. Br J Dermatol 1979;100:183.

146. Sehgal VN, Rege VL, Kharangate VN. Fixed drug eruptions caused by medications: a report from India. Int J Dermatol 1978;17:78.

147. Kuokkanen K. Drug eruptions. Acta Allergol 1972; 27:407.

148. Epstein JH. Photoallergy. Arch Dermatol 1972;106:741.

149. Harber LC, Bickers DR, Armstrong RB et al. Drug photosensitivity: phototoxic and photoallergic mechanisms. Semin Dermatol 1982;1:183.

150. Lee SL, Rivero I, Siegel M. Activitation of systemic lupus erythematosus by drugs. Arch Intern Med 1966; 117:620.

151. Hoigné R, Biedermann HP, Naegeli HR. INH-induzierter systemischer Lupus erythematodes: 2 Beobachtungen mit Reexposition. Schweiz Med Wochenschr 1975;105:1726.

152. Alarcon-Segovia D. Drug-induced lupus syndromes. Mayo Clin Proc 1969;44:664.

153. Hess E. Drug-related lupus. N Engl J Med 1988; 318:1460.

154. Clementz GL, Dolin BJ. Sulfasalazine-induced lupus erythematosus. Am J Med 1988;84:535.

155. Griffith ID, Kane SP. Sulphasalazine-induced lupus syndrome in ulcerative colitis. Br Med J 1977;2:1188.

156. Cohen P, Gardner FH. Sulfonamide reactions in systemic lupus erythematosus. J Am Med Assoc 1966;197:817.

157. Honey M. Systemic lupus erythematosus presenting with sulfonamide hypersensitivity reaction. Br Med J 1956;1:1272.

158. Heckbert SR, Stryker WS, Coltin KL et al. Serum sickness in children after antibiotic exposure: estimates of occurrence and morbidity in a Health Maintenance Organization population. Am J Epidemiol 1990;132:336.

159. Schröder H, Evans DAP. Acetylator phenotype and adverse effects of sulphasalazine in healthy subjects. Gut 1972;13:278.

160. Das KM, Eastwood MA, McManus JPA et al. Adverse reactions during salicylazosulfapyridine therapy and the relation with drug metabolism and acetylator phenotype. N Engl J Med 1973;289:491.

161. Peterkin GAG, Khan SA. Iatrogenic skin disease. Practitioner, 1969;202:117.

162a. Heinonen OP, Slone D, Shapiro S. Antimicrobial and antiparasitic agents. In: Heinonen OP, Slone D, Shapiro S, eds. Birth Defects and Drugs in Pregnancy, 4th edn. Boston—Bristol—London: John Wright PSG Inc, 1982;296.

162b. Karkinen-Jääskeläinen M, Saxén L. Maternal influenza, drug consumption, and congenital defects of the central nervous syndrome. Am J Obstet Gynecol 1974;118:815.

163. Levi AJ, Toovey S, Hudson E. Male infertility due to sulphasalazine. Gastroenterology 1981;80:1208.

164. Tobias R, Sapire KE, Coetzee T et al. Male infertility due to sulphasalazine. Postgrad Med J 1982;58:102.

165. Karbach U. Ewe K, Schramm P. Samenqualität bei Patienten mit Morbus Crohn. Z Gastroenterol 1982;20:314.

166. Brodersen R. Prevention of kernicterus, based on recent progress in bilirubin chemistry. Acta Paediatr Scand 1977;66:625.

167. Diamond I, Schmid R. Experimental bilirubin encephalopathy: the mode of entry of bilirubin-14C into the central nervous system. J Clin Invest 1966;45:678.

168. Silverman WA, Andersen DH, Blanc WA et al. A difference in mortality rate and incidence of kernicterus among premature infants allotted to two prophylactic antibacterial regimens. Pediatrics 1956;18:614.

169. Wadsworth SJ, Bjungse S. In vitro displacement of bilirubin by antibiotics and 2-hydroxybenzoylglycine in newborns. Antimicrobial Agents Chemother 1988;10:1571.

170. Amato M, Carasso A, De Muralt G. Photothérapie intensive avec une double lampe bleue dans le traîtement de l'hyperbilirubinémie néonatale. Helv Paediatr Acta 1983; 38:467.
171. Schneider AP II. Breast milk jaundice in the newborn. J Am Med Assoc 1986;255:3270.
172. Christensen LK, Hansen JM, Kristensen M Sulphaphenazole-induced hypoglycaemic attacks in tolbutamide-treated diabetics. Lancet 1963ii:1298.
173. Soeldner JS, Steinke J. Hypoglycemia in tolbutamide-treated diabetes. J Am Med Assoc 1965;193:148.
174. Dubach UC, Bückert A, Raaflaub J. Einfluss von Sulfonamiden auf die blutzuckersenkende Wirkung oraler Antidiabetica. Schweiz. Med. Wochenschr 1966;44:1483.
175a. Wing LMH, Miners JO. Cotrimoxazole as an inhibitor of oxidative drug metabolism: effects of trimethoprim and sulphamethoxazole separately and combined on tolbutamide disposition. Br J Clin Pharmac 1985;20:482.
175b. Pond S, Birkett DJ, Wade DN. Mechanisms of inhibition of tolbutamide metabolism: phenylbutazone, oxyphenbutazone, sulfaphenazole. Clin Pharmacol Ther 1977;22:573.
176. Hansen JM, Christensen LK. Drug interactions with oral sulphonylurea hypoglycaemic drugs. Drugs 1977;13:24.
177. Schattner A, Rimon E, Green L et al. Hypoglycaemia induced by co-trimoxazole in AIDS. Br Med J 1988;297:742.
178. Baciemicz AM, Swafford WB Jr. Hypoglycemia induced by the interaction of chlorpropamide and co-trimoxazole. Drug Intell Clin Pharm 1984;18:309.
179. Csögör SI, Kerek SF. Enhancement of thiopentone anaesthesia by sulphafurazole. Br J Anaesth 1970;42 988.
180. Garg SK, Ghosh SS, Mathur VS. Comparative pharmakokinetic study of four different sulfonamides in combination with trimethoprim in human volunteers. Int J Clin Pharmacol Ther Toxicol 1986;24:23.
181. Bozzette SA, Finkelstein DM, Spector SA. A randomized trial of three antipneumocystis agents in patients with advanced human immunodeficiency virus infection. N Engl J Med 1995;332:693.
182. Bernstein LS. Adverse reactions to trimethoprim—sulfamethoxazole with particular reference to longterm-therapy. Can Med Assoc J 1975;112:96.
183. Johnson MP, Goodwin SD, Shands JW. Trimethoprim— sulfamethoxazole anaphylactoid reactions in patients with AIDS: case reports and literature review. Pharmacotherapy 1990;10:413.
184. Silvestri RC, Jensen WA, Zibrak JD, et al. Pulmonary infiltrates and hypoxemia in patients with the acquired immunodeficiency syndrome re-exposed to trimethoprim—sulfamethoxazole. Am Rev Respir Dis 1987;136:1003.
185. Greenberg S, Reiser IW, Chou S-Y et al. Trimethoprim—sulfamethoxazole induces reversible hyperkalemia. Ann Intern Med 1993;119:291.
186. Velazquez H, Perazella MA, Wright FS et al. Renal mechanism of trimethoprim-induced hyperkalemia. Ann Intern Med 1993;119:296.
187. Cohen HN, Pearson DWM, Thompson JA et al. Trimethoprim and thyroid function. Lancet 1981;i:676.
188. Smellie JM, Bantock HM, Thompson BD. Cotrimoxazole and the thyroid. Lancet 1982;ii:96.
189. Keisu M, Wiholm BE, Palmblad J. Trimethoprim—sulphamethoxazole-associated blood dyscrasias. Ten years' experience of the Swedish spontaneous reporting system. J Intern Med 1990;228:353.
190. Blackwell EA, Hawson GAT, Leer J et al. Acute pancytopenia due to megaloblastic arrest in association with cotrimoxazole. Med J Aust 1978;2:38.
191. Tulloch AL. Pancytopenia in an infant associated with sulfamethoxazole-trimethoprim therapy. J Pediatr 1976; 88:499.
192. Asmar BI, Maqbool S, Dajani AS. Hematologic abnormalities after oral trimethoprim—sulfamethoxazole therapy in children. Am J Dis Child 1981;135:1100.
193. Jick H. Adverse reactions to trimethoprim—sulfamethoxazole in hospitalized patients. Rev Infect Dis 1982;4:426.
194. Van Hove W, Hamers J, Vermeulen A. Hematologische bijwerkingen van trimethoprim—sulfamethoxazole. Acta Clin. Belg 1973:28:176.
195. Barr AL, Whineray M. Immune thrombocytopenia induced by co-trimoxazole. Aust NZ J Med 1980;10:54.
196. Claas FHJ, Van der Meer JWM, Langerak J. Immunological effect of co-trimoxazole on platelets. Br Med J 1979;2:898.
197. Böse W, Karama A, Linzenmeier G et al. Controlled trial of co-trimoxazole in children with urinary-tract infection Lancet 1974;ii:614.
198. Poskitt EME, Parkin JM. Effect of trimethoprim— sulphamethoxazole combination on folate metabolism in malnourished children. Arch Dis Child 1972;47:626.
199. Bradley PP, Warden GD, Maxwell JG et al. Neutropenia and thrombocytopenia in renal allograft recipients treated with trimethoprim—sulphamethoxazole. Ann Intern Med 1980;93:560.
200. Reynolds EH. Anticonvulsants, folic acid, and epilepsy. Lancet 1973;i:1376.
201. Safrin S, Lee BL, Sande MA. Adjunctive folinic acid with trimethoprim—sulfamethoxazole for *Pneumocystis carinii* pneumonia in AIDS patients is associated with an increased risk of therapeutic failure and death. J Infect Dis 1994;170:912.
202. Horak J, Mertl L, Hrabal P. Severe liver injuries due to sulphamethoxazole—trimethoprim and sulfamethoxydiazine. Hepato-Gastroenterology 1984;31:199.
203. Ransohoff DF, Jacobs G. Terminal hepatic failure following a small dose of sulphamethoxazole—trimethoprim. Gastroenterology 1981;80:816.
204. Thies PW, Dull WL. Trimethoprim—sulfamethoxazole-induced cholestatic hepatitis. Arch Intern Med 1984;144: 1691.
205. Munoz SJ, Martinez-Hernandez A, Maddrey WC. Intrahepatic cholestasis and phospholipidosis associated with the use of trimethoprim—sulfamethoxazole. Hepatology 1990;12:342.
206. Antonow DR. Acute pancreatitis associated with trimethoprim—sulphamethoxazole. Ann Intern Med 1986;104: 363.
207. Cameron A, Thomas M. Pseudomembranous colitis and co-trimoxazole. Br Med J 1977;1:1321.
208. Zehnder D, Künzi UP, Maibach R et al. Die Häufigkeit der Antibiotika-assoziierten Kolitis bei hospitalisierten Patienten der Jahre 1974-1991 im 'Comprehensive Hospital Drug Monitoring' Bern/St. Gallen. Schweiz Med Wochenschr 1995;125:676.
209. Bailey RR Little PJ. Deterioration in renal function in association with co-trimoxazole therapy. Med J Aust 1976;1:914.
210. Kalowski S, Nanra RS, Mathew TH et al. Deterioration in renal function in association with cotrimoxazole therapy. Lancet 1973;i:394.

211. Horn B, Cottier P. Kreatininkonzentration im Serum vor und unter Behandlung mit Trimethoprim—Sulfamethoxazol (Bactrim®). Schweiz Med Wochenschr 1974;104:1809.
212. Lawson DH, Jick H. Adverse reactions to cotrimoxazole in hospitalised medical patients. Am. J Med Sci 1978;275:53.
213. Trollfors B, Wahl M, Alestig K. Co-trimoxazole, creatinine and renal function. J Infect 1980;2:221.
214. Kainer G, Rosenberg AR. Effect of co-trimoxazole on the glomerular filtration rate of healthy adults. Chemotherapy 1981;27:229.
215. Murphy JL, Griswold WR, Reznik VM et al. Trimethoprim/sulfamethoxazole-induced renal tubular acidosis. Child Nephrol Urol 1990;10:49.
216. Hoigné R, Sonntag MR, Zoppi M et al. Occurrence rate of exanthems in relation to aminopenicillin preparations and allopurinol (Letter to Editor). N Engl J Med 1987;316:1217.
217. Miller KD, Lobel HO, Satriale RF et al. Severe cutaneous reactions among American travellers using pyrimethamine—sulfadoxine (Fansidar) for malaria prophylaxis. Am J Trop Med Hyg 1986;35:451.
218. Chanarin I, England JM. Toxicity of trimethoprim—sulfamethoxazole in patients with megaloblastic haematopoiesis. Br Med J 1972;1:651.
219. Gordin FM, Simon GL, Wofsy CB et al. Adverse reactions to trimethoprim—sulfamethoxazole in patients with the acquired immunodeficiency syndrome. Ann Intern Med 1984;100:495.
220. Kovacs JA, Heimenz JW, Macher AM et al. *Pneumocystis carinii* pneumonia: a comparison between patients with the acquired immunodeficiencies. Ann Intern Med 1984; 100:663.
221. Mitsuyasu R, Groopman J, Volberding P. Cutaneous reaction to trimethoprim—sulfamethoxazole in patients with AIDS and Kaposi's sarcoma. N Engl J Med 1983;308:1535.
222. Wharton JM, Coleman DL, Wofsy CB et al. Trimethoprim—sulfamethoxazole or pentamidine for *Pneumocystis carinii* pneumonia in the acquired immunodeficiency syndrome. Ann Intern Med 1986;105:37.
223. Kleyman TR, Roberts C, Ling BN. A mechanism for pentamidine-induced hyperkalemia: inhibition of distal nephron sodium transport. Ann Int Med 1995;122:103.
224. Hughes WT, Rivera GK, Schell MJ et al. Successful intermittent chemoprophylaxis for *Pneumocystis carinii* pneumonitis. N Engl J Med 1987;316:1627.
225. Wormser GP, Horowitz HW, Duncanson FP et al. Low-dose intermittent trimethoprim—sulfamethoxazole for prevention of *Pneumocystis carinii* pneumonia in patients with human immunodeficiency virus infection. Arch Intern Med 1991;151:689.
226. Ruskin J, LaRivière M. Low-dose co-trimoxazole for prevention of *Pneumocystis carinii* pneumonia in human immunodeficiency virus disease. Lancet 1991;337:468.
227. Greenberger PA, Patterson R. Management of drug allergy in patients with acquired immunodeficiency syndrome. J Allergy Clin Immunol 1987;79:484.
228. Finland M. Combinations of antimicrobial drugs: trimethoprim—sulfamethoxazole. N Engl J Med 1974;291:624.
229. Brigg GG, Freedman RK, Jaffe SJ. A Reference Guide to Fetal and Neontal Risk: Drugs in Pregnancy and Lactation, 3rd edn. Baltimore—Hongkong—London—Sydney: Williams and Wilkins, 1990;621.
230. Guillebaud J. Sulpha-trimethoprim combinations and male infertility. Lancet 1978;ii:523.
231. Murdia A, Mathur V, Kothari LK et al. Sulpha-trimethoprim combinations and male fertility. Lancet 1978;ii:375.
232. Sørensen PJ, Jensen MK. Cytogenetic studies in patients treated with trimethoprim—sulfamethoxazole. Mutat Res 1981;89:91.
233. Rees CA, Lennard L, Lilleyman JS et al. Disturbance of 6-mercaptopurine metabolism by cotrimoxazole in childhood lymphoblastic leukaemia. Cancer Chemother Pharmacol 1984;12:87.
234. Ferrazzini G, Klein J, Sulh H. Interaction between trimethoprim—sulfamethoxazole and methotrexate in children with leukemia. J Pediatr 1990;117:823.
235. Ringdén O, Myrenfors P, Klintmalm G et al. Nephrotoxicity by co-trimoxazole and cyclosporin in transplanted patients. Lancet 1984;i:1016.
236. Thompson JF, Chalmers DHK, Hunnisett AGW et al. Nephrotoxicity of trimethoprim and co-trimoxazole in renal allograft recipients treated with cyclosporine. Transplantation 1983;36:204.
237. O'Reilly RA, Motley CH. Racemic warfarin and trimethoprim—sulfamethoxazole interaction in humans. Ann Intern Med 1979;91:34.
238. Grimmer SFM, Allen WL, Back DJ et al. The effect of cotrimoxazole on oral contraceptive steroids in women. Contraception 1983;28:53.
239. Brumfitt W, Hamilton-Miller JMT. Cotrimoxazole or trimethoprim alone? A viewpoint on their relative place in therapy. Drugs 1982;24:453.
240. Grüneberg RN. The microbiological reationale for the combination of sulfonamides with trimethoprim. J Antimicrob Chemother 1979;5(Suppl B):27.
241. Turnidge JD. A reappraisal of co-trimoxazole. Med J Aust 1988;148:296.
242. Martin AJ, Lacey RW. A blind comparison of the efficacy and incidence of unwanted effects of trimethoprim and co-trimoxazole in the treatment of acute infection of the urinary tract in general practice. Br J Clin Pract 1983;37:105.
243. Brogden RN, Carmine AA, Heel RC et al. Trimethoprim: a review of is antibacterial activity, pharmacokinetics and therapeutic use in urinary tract infections. Drugs 1982;23:405.
244. Dornbusch K, Toivanen P. Effect of trimethoprim or trimethoprim/sulfamethoxazole usage on the emergence of trimethoprim resistance in urinary tract pathogens. Scand J Infect Dis 1981;13:203.
245. Wuest J, Kayser FH. Susceptibility of bacteria to chemotherapeutic agents (Zürich, 1993). Schweiz Rundsch Med Prax 1995;84:98.
246. Huovinen P, Toivanan P. Trimethoprim resistance in Finland after five years' use of plain trimethoprim. Br Med J 1980;280:72.
247. Hedlund J, Aurelius E, Andersson J. Recurrent encephalitis due to trimethoprim intake. Scand J Infect Dis 1990;22:109.
248. Sheehan. Trimethoprim-associated marrow toxicity. Lancet 1981;ii:692.
249. Tanner AR. Hepatic cholestasis induced by trimethoprim. Br Med J 1986;293:1072.
250. Nwokolo C, Byrne L, Misch KJ. Toxic epidermal necrolysis occurring during treatment with trimethoprim alone. Br Med J 1988;296:970.
251. Hirsch-Kauffman M, Herrlich P, Schweiger M. Nitrofurantoin damages DNA of human cells. Klin Wochenschr 1978;56:405.

252. Boyd MR, Stiko AW, Sasame HA. Metabolic activation of nitrofurantoin—possible implications for carcinogenesis. Biochem Pharmacol 1979;28:601.
253. Hasegawa R, Murasaki G, St John MK et al. Evaluation of nitrofurantoin on the two stages or urinary bladder carcinogenesis in the rat. Toxicology 1990;62:333.
254. Israel HL, Diamond P. Recurrent pulmonary infiltration and pleural effusion due to nitrofurantoin sensitivity. N Engl J Med 1962;266:1024.
255. Lübbers P. Allergische Reaktion gegen Furandantin. Dtsch Med Wochenschr 1962;87:2209.
256. Chudnofsky CR, Otten EJ. Acute pulmonary toxicity to nitrofurantoin. J Emerg Med 1989;7:15.
257. Holmbeag L, Boman G, Böttiger LE et al. Adverse reactions to nitrofurantoin: analysis of 921 reports. Am J Med 1980;69:733.
258. Jick SS, Jick H, Walker AM et al. Hospitalizations for pulmonary reactions following nitrofurantoin use. Chest 1989;96:512.
259. Fauroux B, Tournier G. Toxicité pulmonaire des drogues chez l'enfant. Méd Infant 1990;97:289.
260. Rosenow EC III, DeRemee RA, Dines DE Chronic nitrofurantoin pulmonary reaction. N Engl J Med 1968; 279:1258.
261. Strohscheer H, Wegener HH. Nitrofurantoin-induzierte, granulomatöse Hepatitis. Münch Med Wochenschr 1977;119:1535.
262. Bäck O, Lundgren R, Wiman LG. Nitrofurantoin-induced pulmonary fibrosis and lupus syndrome. Lancet 1974;i:930.
263. Selroos O, Edgren J. Lupus-like syndrome associated with pulmonary reaction to nitrofurantoin: report of three cases. Acta Med Scand 1975;197:125.
264. Taskinen E, Tukiainen P, Sovijärvi ARA. Nitrofurantoin-induced alterations in pulmonary tissue: a report on five patients with acute and subacute reactions. Acta Pathol Microbiol Scand Sect A 1977;85:713.
265. Cohen AJ, King TE Jr, Downey GP. Rapidly progressive bronchiolitis obliterans with organizing pneumonia. Am J Respir Crit Care Med 1994;149:1670.
266. Smith GJW. The histopathology of pulmonary reactions to drugs. Clin Chest Med 1990;11:95.
267. Bone RC, Wolfe J, Sobonya R et al. Desquamative interstitial pneumonia following long-term nitrofurantoin therapy. Am J Med 1976;60:697.
268. Müller U, Abbühl K, Bisig J et al. Ueberempfindlichkeitsreaktionen der Lunge auf Nitrofurantoin. Schweiz Med Wochenschr 1970;100:2206.
269. Larsson S, Cronberg S, Denneberg T et al. Pulmonary reaction to nitrofurantoin. Scand J Respir Dis 1973;54:103.
270. Back O, Liden S, Ahlstedt S. Adverse reactions to nitrofurantoin in relation to cellular and humoral immune response. Clin Exp Immunol 1977;28:400.
271. Pearsall HR, Ewalt J, Tsoi MS et al. Nitrofurantoin lung sensitivity: report of a case with prolonged nitrofurantoin lymphocyte sensitivity and interaction of nitrofurantoin-stimulated lymphocytes with alveolar cells. J Lab Clin Med 1974;83:728.
272. Boyd MR, Catignani GL, Sasame HA et al. Acute pulmonary injury in rats by nitrofurantoin and modification by vitamin E, dietary fat, and oxygen. Am Rev Respir Dis 1979;120:93.
273. Martin WJ. Nitrofurantoin-potential direct and indirect mechanisms of lung disease. Chest 1983;5:515.
274. Sasame HA, Boyd MR. Superoxide and hydrogen peroxide production and NADPH oxidation stimulated by nitrofurantoin in lung microsomes: possible implications for toxicity. Life Sci 1979;24:1091.
275. Toole J, Parrish ML. Nitrofurantoin polyneuropathy. Neurology 1973;23:554.
276. Mushed GR. Pseudotumor and nitrofurantoin therapy. Arch Neurol 1972;34:257.
277. Lavelle KJ, Atkinson K, Kleit SA. Hyperlactatemia and hemolysis in G6PD deficiency after nitrofurantoin ingestion. Am J Med Sci 1976;272:201
278. Waller DJ, Gerok W. Hämiglobinbildung durch Furadantin. Dtsch Med Wochenschr 1956;81:1707
279. Novak RF, Kharash ED, Wendel NK. Nitrofurantoin-stimulated proteolysis in human erythrocytes: a novel index of toxic insult by nitroaromatics. J Pharmacol Exp Ther 1988;247:439.
280. Murphy KJ, Junis MD. Hepatic disorder and severe bleeding diathesis following nitrofurantoin ingestion. J Am Med Assoc 1968;204:396.
281. Rossi EC, Levin NW. Inhibition of primary ADP-induced platelet aggregation in normal subjects after administration of nitrofurantoin. J Clin Invest 1973;52:2457.
282. Palva JP, Lehmola U. Agranulocytosis caused by nitrofurantoin. Acta Med Scand 1973;194:575.
283. Zimmerman HJ. Update of hepatotoxicitiy due to classes of drugs in common clinical use: non steroidal antiinflammatory drugs, antibiotics, antihypertensives, and cardiac and psychotropic agents. Semin Liver Dis 1990;10:322.
284. Stricker BHC, Blok APR, Claas FHJ et al. Hepatic injury associated with the use of nitrofurans: a clinico-pathological study of 52 reported cases. Hepatology 1988;8:599.
285. Silva JM, Khan S, O'Brien PJ. Molecular mechanisms of nitrofurantoin-induced hepatotoxicity in aerobic versus hypoxic conditions. Arch Biochem Biophys 1993;305:362.
286. Hebert MF, Roberts JP. Endstage liver disease associated with nitrofurantoin requiring liver transplantation. Ann Pharmacother 1993;27:1193.
287. Black M, Rabin L, Schatz N. Nitrofurantoin-induced chronic active hepatitis. Ann Intern Med 1980;92:62.
288. Fagrell A, Strandberg J, Wengle B. A nitrofurantoin-induced disorder simulating chronic active hepatitis. Acta Med Scand 1976;199:237.
289. Sharp JR, Ishak KG, Zimmerman HJ. Chronic active hepatitis and severe hepatic necrosis associated with nitrofurantoin. Ann Intern Med 1980;92:14.
290. Sippel PJ, Agger WA. Nitrofurantoin-induced granulomatous hepatitis. Urology 1981;18:177.
291. Kalowski S, Radford N, Kincaid-Smith P. Crystalline and macrocrystalline nitrofurantoin in the treatment of urinary tract infection. N Engl J Med 1974;290:385.
291. Christophe JL. Pancreatitis induced by nitrofurantoin. Gut 1994;35:712.
292. Macdonald JB, Macdonald ET. Nitrofurantoin crystalluria. Br Med J 1976;2:1044.
293. Chan HL, Stern RS, Arndt KA et al. The incidence of erythema multiforme, Stevens-Johnson syndrome, and toxic epidermal necrolysis. A population-based study with particular reference to reactions caused by drugs among outpatients. Arch Dermatol 1990;126:43.
295. Johnson SH, Marshall M. Prophylactic treatment of chronic urinary tract infection with nitrofurantoin: one to five years following studies. J Urol 1959;82:162.
296. Thompson DF. Drug-induced parotitis. J Clin Pharm Ther 1993;18:255.

297. Teppo AM, Haltia K, Wager O. Immunoelectrophoretic 'tailing' of albumin line due to albumin-IgG antibody complexes: a side effect of nitrofurantion treatment. Scand J Immunol 1976;5:249.
298. Ibanez. Crystalline retinopathy associated with long-term nitrofurantion. Arch Ophtalmol 1994;112:304.
299. Matthews A, Heise H. Die Erhöhung der Nitrofurantoin (Nifuratin®) Ausscheidung durch Vitamin B_6. Dtsch Gesundheitswes 1973;28:716.
300. Olshan AF, Faustman EM. Nitrosatable drug exposure during pregnany and adverse pregnany outcome. Int J Epidemiol 1989;18:891.
301. Nelson WO, Bunge RG. The effect of therapeutic dosages of nitrofurantoin (furadantin) upon spermatogenesis in man. J Urol 1957;77:275.
302. Iunda IF, Kushniruk IUI. Functional state of the testis after the use of certain antibiotics and nitrofuran preparations. Antibiotiki 1975;9:843
303. Stille W, Ostner HH. Antagonismus Nitrofurantoin—Nalidixinsäure. Klin Wochenschr 1966;44:155.
304. McCoy E, Lynn AP, Rosenkranz HS. Non-mutagenic genotoxicants: novobiocin and nalidixic acid, 2 inhibitors of DNA gyrase. Mutat Res 1980;79:33.
305. Wright HT, Nurse KC, Goldstein DJ. Nalidixic acid, oxolinic acid, and novobiocin inhibit yeast glycyl- and lecyl transfer RNA synthetase. Science 1981;213:455.
306. Mobbs JP, Balant L, Revillard C et al. Effets secondaires de l'acide nalidixique chez une patiente atteinte d'insuffisance rénale sévère: étude clinique et proposition d'un modèle pharmacocinétique. Schweiz Med Wochenschr 1977;107:300.
307. Boréus LO, Sundström B. Intracranial hypertension in a child during treatment with nalidixic acid. Br Med J 1967;2:744.
308. Islam MA, Sreedharan T. Convulsions, hyperglycemia and glycosuria from overdose of nalidixic acid. J Am Med Assoc 1965;192:1100.
309. Belton EM, Jones RV. Hemolytic anemia due to nalidixic acid. Lancet 1965;ii:691.
310. Tafani O, Mazzoli M, Landini G et al. Fatal acute immune haemolytic anaemia caused by nalidixic acid. Br Med J 1982;2:936.
311. Gleckman R, Alvarez S, Joubert DW et al. Drug therapy reviews: nalidixic acid. Am J Hosp Pharm 1979;36:1071.
312. Gough A, Barsoum NJ, Mitchell L et al. Juvenile canine drug-induced arthropathy: clinico-pathological studies on articular lesions caused by oxolinic and pipemidic acids. Toxicol Appl Pharmacol 1979;51:177.
313. Schaad UB, Wedgwood-Krucko J. Nalidixic acid in children: retrospective matched controlled study for cartilage toxicity. Infection 1987;15:165.
314. Adam D. Use of quinolones in pediatric patients. Rev Infect Dis 1989;11(Suppl 5):1113.
315. Rubinstein A. LE-like disease caused by nalidixic acid. N Engl J Med 1979;301:1288.
316. Kowalczyk J. Sister-chromatid exchange in children treated with nalidixic acid. Mutat Res 1980;77:371.
317. Hoffbrand BJ. Interaction of nalidixic acid and warfarin. Br Med J 1974;2:666.
318. Chu DT, Fernandes PB. Structure-activity relationships of the fluoroquinolones. Antimicrob Agents Chemother 1989;33:131.
319. Wolfson JS, Hooper DC. Fluoroquinolone antimicrobial agents. Clin Microbiol Rev 1989;2:378.
320. Hooper DC, Wolfson JS. Fluoroquinolone antimicrobial agents. N Engl J Med 1991;324:384.
321. Wang C, Sabbai J, Corrado M et al. World-wide clinical experience with norfloxacin: efficacy and safety. Scand J Infect Dis 1986;48(Suppl):81.
322. Ball P. Ciprofloxacin: overview of adverse experiences. J Antimicrob Chemother 1986;18(Suppl D):187.
323. Shah PM, Mulert R. Safety profile of quinolones. Eur Urol 1990;17(Suppl I):46.
324. Sawada M, Nakamura S, Yamada A et al. Phase IV study and post-marketing surveillance of ofloxacin in Japan. Chemotherapy 1991;37:134.
325. Shimada J, Hori S. Adverse effects of fluoroquinolones. Prog Drug Res 1992;38:133.
326. Bowie WR, Willetts V, Jewesson PJ. Adverse reaction in a dose ranging study with a new long-acting fluoroquinolone fleroxacin. Antimicrob Agents Chemother 1989; 33:1778.
327. Bednarcyk EM, Green JA, Nelson AD et al. Comparison of the effect of temafloxacin, ciprofloxacin, or placebo on cerebral blood flow, glucose, and oxygen metabolism in healthy subjects by means of positron emission tomography. Clin Pharmacol Ther 1991;50:165.
328. Halliwell RF, Davey PG, Lambert JJ. Antagonsim of GABA A receptors by 4-quinolones. J Antimicrob Chemother 1993;31:457.
329. Moore B, Safani M, Keesey J. Possible exacerbation of myasthenia gravis by ciprofloxacin, Lancet 1988;i:882.
330. Vrabec TA, Sergott RC, Jaeger EA et al. Reversible visual loss in a patient receiving high-dose ciprofloxacin. Ophthalmology 1991;97:707.
331. Zehnder D, Hoigné R, Neftel K et al. Painful dysaesthesia with ciprofloxacin. Br Med J 1995;310:1204.
332. Simos J. Guyot A. Pefloxacin: safety in man. J Antimicrob Chemother 1990;26:215.
333. Eron LJ, Harvey L, Hixon DL et al. Ciprofloxacin therapy of infections caused by *Pseudomonas aeruginosa* and other resitant bacteria. Antimicrob Agents Chemother 1985;27:308.
334. Patoia L, Guerciolini R, Menichetti F et al. Norfloxacin and neutropenia. Ann Intern Med 1987;107:788.
335. Lopez-Navidad A, Domingo P, Cadalfach J et al. Norfloxacin induced hepatotoxicity. J Hepatol 1990;11:277.
336. Scully BE, Parry ME, Neu HC et al. Oral ciprofloxacin therapy of infections due to *Pseudomonas aeruginosa*. Lancet 1986;i:819.
337. Svanson BN, Boppana VK, Vlasses PH et al. Norfloxacin disposition after sequentially increasing oral doses. Antimicrob Agents Chemother 1983;23:284.
338. Schaeffer AJ. Multiclinic study of norfloxacin for treatment of complicated or uncomplicated urinary tract infections. Am J Med 1987;82(Suppl 6B):53.
339. Campoli-Richards DM, Monk JP, Price A et al. Ciprofloxacin. A review of its antibacterial activity, pharmacokinetic properties and therapeutic use. Drugs 1988;35:373.
340. Hootkins R, Fenves AZ, Stephens MK. Acute renal failure secondary to ciprofloxacin therapy: a presentation of 3 cases and a review of the literature. Clin Nephrol 1989;32:75.
341. Hatton J, Haagensen D. Renal dysfunction associated with ciprofloxacin. Pharmacotherapy 1990;10:337.
342. Rastogi S, Atkinson JLD, McCarthy JD. Allergic nephropathy associated with ciprofloxacin. Mayo Clin Proc 1990;65:987.
343. Shih DJ, Korbert SM, Rydel JJ et al. Renal vasculitis associated with ciprofloxacin. Am J Kidney Dis 1995;26:516.

344. Miller MS, Gaido F, Rourk MH et al. Anaphylactoid reactions to ciprofloxacin in cystic fibrosis patients. Pediatr Infect Dis 1991;10:164.
345. Davis H, McGoodvin E, Reed TG. Anaphylactoid reactions reported after treatment with ciprofloxacin. Ann Int Med 1989;111:1041.
346. Kennedy CA, Goetz MB, Mathisen GE. Ciprofloxacin-induced anaphylactoid reactions. Ann Int Med 1990;112:564.
347. Shimod K, Yoshido M, Wagai N et al. Phototoxic lesions induced by quinolone antibacterial agents in auricular skin and retina of albino mice. Toxicol Pathol 1993;21:554.
348. Arcieri G, August R, Becker N et al. Clinical experience with ciprofloxacin in the USA. Eur Clin Microbiol 1986; 5:220.
349. Schaad UB. Use of quinolones in pediatrics. Eur J Clin Microb Infect Dis 1991;10:335.
350. Black A, Redmond AOB, Steen HJ et al. Tolerance and safety of ciprofloxacin in pediatric patients. J Antimicrob Chemother 1990;26:25.
351. Pertuiset E, Lenor G, Jehanne M et al. Joint tolerance of pefloxacine and ofloxacine in children and teenagers with cystic fibrosis. Rev Rhum Mal Osteoart 1989;56:735.
352. Meyboom RHB, Olsson S, Knol A et al. Achilles tendinitis induced by pefloxacin and other fluoroquinolone derivatives. Pharmacoepidemiol Drug Safety 1994;3:185.
353. Szarfman A, Chen M, Blum M. Letter. N Engl J Med 1995;332:193.
354. Pierfitte C, Gillet P, Royer RJ. Letter. N Engl J Med 1995;332:193.
355. Radandt JM, Marchbanks CR, Dudley MN. Interactions of fluoroquinolones with other drugs: mechanisms, variability, clinical significance, and management. Clin Infect Dis 1992;14:272
356. Wijnands WJA, Van Heerwarden CLA, Vree TB. Enoxacin raises plasma theophylline concentrations. Lancet 1984;ii:108.
357. Maesen FPV, Teengs JP, Baur C. Quinolones and raised plasma concentrations of theophylline, Lancet 1984;ii:530.
358. Stuht H, Lode H, Koeppe P et al. Interaction study of lomefloxacin and ciprofloxacin with omeprazole and comparative pharmacokinetics. Antimicrob Agents Chemother 1995;39:1045.
359. Avent CK, Krinsky D, Kirklin JD et al. Synergistic nephrotoxicity due to ciprofloxacin and cyclosporine. Am J Med 1988;85:452.
360. Christ W, Lehnert T, Ulbrich B. Specific toxicologic aspects of the quinolones. Rev Infect Dis 1988;10(Suppl I):141.
361. Badley BWD. Phenazopyridine-induced hepatitis. Br Med J 1976;2:850.
362. Conroy JM, Baker JD, Martin WJ et al. Acquired methemoglobinemia from multiple oxidans. South Med J 1995;86:1156.
363. Alano FA, Webster GD. Acute renal failure and pigmentation due to phenazopyridine. Ann Intern Med 1970; 72:89.
364. Feinfeld DA, Ranieri R, Lippner H et al. Renal failure in phenazopyridine overdose. J Am Med Assoc 1978; 240:2661.

Meyler's Side Effects of Drugs, 13th Edition
M.N.G. Dukes, editor

SECTION EDITOR: R. HOIGNÉ

D. Germann and K. Schopfer

29.2 Antiviral drugs

During the last 30 years of research in virology it has become clear that viruses replicate by processes other than simple appropriation of the host-cell metabolic mechanisms, as has been assumed for several decades. The search for selectivity and the avoidance of host-cell cytotoxicity, however, still present a major challenge to those involved in the development of antiviral compounds. Selectivity for viral replication can be enhanced by targeting agents to virus-specific processes. Potential targets include inhibition of attachment, penetration, uncoating, assembly, substrate competition for virus-encoded enzymes or specific host-cell processes that are greatly enhanced during viral replication (replication of viral nucleic acid, elaboration and processing of viral messenger RNA of virus-specific proteins) (1^R).

COMPOUNDS DIRECTED AGAINST DNA VIRUSES

Aciclovir

Aciclovir (9-[-2-hydroxyethoxymethyl]guanine, acyclovir, ACV), is an acyclic purine nucleoside analog (SED-12, 742; SEDA-18, 299). Its antiviral activity depends upon its intracellular phosphorylation to the triphosphate derivative. As viral thymidine kinase (TK) has a much higher affinity for aciclovir than does cellular TK, it is phosphorylated at a much higher rate by the viral enzyme. The antiviral compound is thus formed almost exclusively in infected cells, fulfilling one of the selectivity principles. In addition, aciclovir triphosphate serves as a better substrate for viral than for host-cell DNA-polymerase and thereby causes preferential termination of viral DNA synthesis (2^R).

Aciclovir is active against herpes simplex virus type 1 (HSV-1), HSV-2, varicella zoster virus (VZV), herpes virus simiae and to a lesser degree Epstein-Barr virus (EBV). Resistant strains of HSV may arise due to the emergence of TK-deficient mutants. Other forms of resistance patterns are less common (3^C, 4^C).

Aciclovir is applied topically or systemically, either orally or intravenously. Its therapeutic potential is most impressive in active parenchymal or systemic HSV infections. The latency of these infections is not affected. Since the blood—brain barrier is well penetrated, aciclovir is the treatment of choice for HSV encephalitis.

Very few side effects, generally of minor importance, have been reported (5^R). Renal impairment has been associated with the use of intravenous aciclovir. Transient increase in serum creatinine and urea nitrogen have been observed in 14% of patients treated with bolus injections (6^C). These are related to crystal formation in the lower renal tubules when the solubility of aciclovir in urine is exceeded. Slow (1-hour) intravenous infusion and adequate hydration are therefore mandatory. Bolus doses are to be avoided. Dose modifications for patients with renal impairment are based on creatinine clearance (5^R). Renal toxicity has not been described in infants treated with intravenous aciclovir, 5—10 mg/kg every 8 hours for 5—10 days (7^C), in children receiving 500 mg/m² intravenously (8^C) or with oral aciclovir (5^R).

Local necrosis and inflammation may occur due to extravasation of the drug at the site of injection (9^R). In immunosuppressed patients abnormal liver function, encephalopathy and myelosuppression have been observed; however, it is unclear at present whether these side effects are related to the drug itself or to the underlying immunological disorder (10^C—12^C).

Neurotoxicity secondary to aciclovir is rare and is associated with high plasma concentrations of the drug (SEDA 18, 299). One report described reversible psychiatric side effects in three dialysis patients receiving intravenous aciclovir (8—10 mg/kg daily) (13^C).

Local application of 3% ophthalmic ointment may cause mild transient stinging. Diffuse, superficial, punctate and non-progressive keratopathy may develop. This quickly resolves as soon as the drug is omitted (14^R, 15^R).

Animal data suggest that aciclovir is probably safe for use during pregnancy. There are no reports of teratogenicity in humans, and a report of 312 pregnant women exposed to aciclovir showed no increase in the number of birth defects compared with the numbers expected in the general population (16^C). Data from larger numbers of human pregnancies, however, are not available to draw reliable conclusions about the safety of aciclovir in pregnancy.

Ganciclovir *(SEDA-18, 301)*

Ganciclovir (dihydroxy-propoxymethyl guanine, DHPG) is a nucleoside analog with antiviral activity in vitro against members of the herpes group viruses. Intracellular phosphorylation of ganciclovir to the triphosphate derivative, which acts as a competitive inhibitor of deoxyguanosine triphosphate, leads to the inhibition of viral DNA synthesis. It should be considered a first-line treatment of life- or sight-threatening cytomegalovirus (CMV) infections in immunocompromised patients. Ganciclovir has been evaluated in such patients with CMV infections, including retinitis, pneumonia, gastrointestinal, hepatic, CNS and disseminated infections. It is administered by infusion or by intravitreal injections (17^R). Successful oral ganciclovir as maintenance therapy for CMV retinitis in AIDS patients has recently been reported (18^C).

Ganciclovir is a toxic drug with the proportion of patients in whom therapy is subsequently interrupted or withdrawn because of adverse effects being estimated at 32% (17^R). Neutropenia is the most frequent adverse effect associated with ganciclovir therapy and seems to depend on the total dose administered, usually occurring before a total dose of 200 mg/kg has been given. Other hematological side effects include thrombocytopenia, anemia and lymphopenia. Pure red cell aplasia has been reported in one bone marrow transplant recipient (19^C) and hemolysis has been observed in two other patients (20^C). The adverse hematological effects of ganciclovir are generally rapidly reversible following treatment withdrawal (17^R). Other adverse effects involving the central nervous system (CNS) occurred in about 5% of patients and include confusion, seizures, abnormal thinking, psychosis, hallucinations, nightmares, anxiety, tremor, dysesthesia, ataxia, coma, headache and somnolence (17^R, 20^C, 21^C). Fever, rash and abnormal liver function values are each reported to occur in about 2% of ganciclovir recipients (17^R). Other infrequently reported side effects which may or may not be associated with ganciclovir therapy include chills, edema, malaise, vomiting, anorexia, diarrhea, dyspnea, decreased blood glucose, alopecia, decreased kidney function, and inflammation, pain or phlebitis at the infusion site (17^R). These effects may also be due to the underlying illness in such patients.

Adverse effects reported in patients receiving intravitreal ganciclovir therapy include foreign body sensation, conjunctival hemorrhage, mild conjunctival scarring, scleral induration, bacterial endophthalmitis and retinal detachment (17^R).

Animal data indicate that ganciclovir may inhibit spermatogenesis and fertility, but one clinical study did not find significant changes in serum gonadotropin hormone levels in 32 men during ganciclovir therapy (22^C).

It is not recommended that drugs which inhibit the replication of rapidly dividing cells be administered concomitantly with ganciclovir unless potential benefits outweigh the risks. Zidovudine and ganciclovir have overlapping toxicity profiles with respect to the adverse hematological effects. Severe life-threatening hematological toxicity has been reported in 82% of patients treated with a combination of zidovudine and ganciclovir (23^C). The combination of ganciclovir with didanosine was found to be much better tolerated (24^C).

Foscarnet *(SEDA-18, 300)*

Foscarnet (trisodium phosphonoformate hexahydrate, PFA) is a pyrophosphate analog and thus interacts at the site on a polymerase where pyrophosphate is split off from a nucleoside triphosphate. Foscarnet is a noncompetitive inhibitor of herpesvirus DNA polymerase, hepatitis B virus DNA polymerase and reverse transcriptases (25^R). Intravenous foscarnet has been used for the treatment of mucocutaneous disease due to aciclovir-resistant HSV (26^C) and for the treatment of severe CMV infection (27^C, 28^C). Foscarnet has been shown to be equally effective as ganciclovir for the treatment of CMV retinitis in AIDS patients (29^C). The two drugs differ, however, in their respective toxicity profile.

Treatment-limiting adverse effects are renal toxicity, hypocalcemia and mucosal ulcerations. Alterations in creatinine clearance or acute renal failure has been observed in 10—20% of AIDS patients receiving intravenous foscarnet (30^C). It appears to be due to acute tubular damage but the precise mechanism is net yet clear. To minimize the incidence of nephrotoxicity, the foscarnet dose should be frequently recalculated, based on the estimated creatinine clearance. The second most common adverse effect is symptomatic hypocalcemia which may be responsible for arrhythmias and seizures observed with acute overdose or excessively rapid infusion of foscarnet. Painful oral, penile and vulvar ulcerations may occur during foscarnet therapy. The ulceration is presumed to be caused by high local concentrations of the drug which is largely excreted unchanged in the urine (SEDA-17, 338). Penile ulcers have been reported to be the reason for discontinuation of foscarnet therapy in up to 10% of patients (31^C). In addition, foscarnet stimulates the release of parathyroid hormone which raised concerns about long-term administration (32^R). However, in a study of seven patients receiving a 14-day foscarnet induction regimen, no changes in calcium or phosphate metabolism have been observed (29[C]).

Idoxuridine

Idoxuridine (5-iodo-2′-deoxyuridine, IDU) is a halogenated pyrimidine analog. It is mainly active against HSV-1, HSV-2 and VZV. Its mode of action is based upon enzyme inhibition of the DNA pathway. Moreover, it competes with thymidine for incorporation into newly synthesized DNA of viral or cellular origin (33[R]).

As systemic use causes unacceptable toxicity without proven value, its application has been limited to the treatment of localized herpetic infections, where it may cause slight irritation (SED-10, 559). To circumvent its poor water solubility, idoxuridine 40% in dimethylsulfoxide (DMSO) has been used topically in the treatment of mucocutaneous herpetic lesions or VZV infections of the skin. DMSO, which greatly augments cutaneous penetration, may enhance unwanted side effects such as visual disturbances, headache, nausea, diarrhea, taste disturbances, allergic contact dermatitis and teratogenicity as observed in certain animal species (34[R]). Topical cutaneous application of this drug should therefore be avoided. More potent and less harmful antiherpetic compounds are now available.

Vidarabine

Vidarabine (9-β-D-arabinofuranosyladenine, adenine arabinoside, ara-A) is a purine analog. It is phosphorylated intracellularly to the corresponding nucleotide and acts mainly by inhibiting DNA-polymerase (35[R]). It is active against HSV-1, HSV-2, VZV, poxviruses and probably hepatitis B virus (HBV).

Vidarabine, administered intravenously, is inferior to aciclovir in its antiherpetic efficacy. Its major toxicity is the effect on the central nervous system ranging from tremor and hallucinations to coma (SEDA-17, 339). A number of less frequent side effects, including gastrointestinal disturbances, rashes, as well as bone marrow and liver dysfunction, have also been observed (SEDA-17, 339). Vidarabine, when applied topically to the eye, may have side effects similar to those of idoxuridine.

Its poor solubility in water, and hence the large volumes which have to be infused, further complicate the management of certain patients, as in those suffering from herpes encephalitis with cerebral edema.

The parent compound of vidarabine, vidarabine 5′-monophosphate, is water-soluble and well absorbed after intramuscular injections. The side effects are comparable to those of vidarabine (36[R]).

Trifluorothymidine (5-trifluoromethyl-2′-deoxyuridine, F3TdR)

F3TdR is a synthetic halogenated pyrimidine analog active against HSV-1, HSV-2 and VZV (37[C]). It may have adverse effects similar to idoxuridine when applied as a 1% aqueous solution for topical ophthalmic use. Due to the drug's myelosuppressive and teratogenic effects its systemic use is contraindicated.

COMPOUNDS DIRECTED AGAINST RNA VIRUSES

Amantadine *(SEDA-17, 340)*

Amantadine is a symmetrical C10 tricyclic amine with an unusual structure (1-adamantanamine hydrochloride). Its mode of action has not been precisely elucidated, but it seems to interfere in some way with virus uncoating (38[R]). Most consistent antiviral activity has been observed against influenza A virus, but it has little or no activity against influenza B virus (39[R]). Influenza A virus may, however, become rapidly resistant to amantadine in vitro (40[C]).

The drug is generally well tolerated. Oral or aerosol administration of amantadine may be accompanied by gastrointestinal or minor neurological symptoms such as insomnia, light headedness, concentration difficulties, nervousness, dizziness and headache in individuals receiving 200 mg amantadine daily (41[R]). These symptoms disappear upon withdrawal of the drug. More severe but rare complications include convulsions and coma (42[C], 43[C]). Local nasal side effects of the aerosolized form may mimic the symptoms of infection of the upper respiratory tract. If used in Parkinson's disease, mainly in doses of 200 mg or more, minor side effects resembling those caused by anticholinergic agents, e.g. blurred vision, dryness of mouth, also livedo reticularis, rash and photosensitization have been described (SED-12, 316).

Rimantadine *(SEDA-18, 301)*

Rimantadine hydrochloride (α-methyl-1-adamantane methylamine hydrochloride) is closely related to amantadine. It seems to be somewhat more active against influenza A virus. Like amantadine, rimantadine interferes with uncoating of viral nucleic acid at an early stage of infection. It is not active against influenza B virus. Emergence of resistance to rimantadine of influenza A virus in vivo has recently been reported (44[C]). Rimantadine has side effects similar to those of amantadine, but they appear to be less frequent and are less pronounced.

Tromantadine

Tromatadine is closely related to the above-mentioned drug. It may cause eczema, apparently due to contact sensitization (SEDA-10, 264).

Zidovudine

Zidovudine (3′-azido-3′-deoxythymidine, azidothymidine, AZT) is a thymidine-analog antiretroviral drug active against human immunodeficiency virus (HIV). It is converted intracellularly to its triphosphate form which is utilized by retroviral reverse transcriptase. Cellular DNA polymerase-α is 100 times less susceptible to inhibition by zidovudine triphosphate than is HIV-1 reverse transcriptase (45[R], 46[R]). Some clinical trials have shown its beneficial effect in the treatment of HIV-1 infection (47[C]—49[C]), while others have questioned its efficacy (50[C]). The drug has been shown to reduce maternal-infant transmission of HIV-1 (51[C], 52[R]). Zidovudine may be administered orally or intravenously.

An evaluation of the adverse effects of an anti-HIV drug is complicated by the complexity of the underlying disease. It is sometimes difficult to determine whether the apparent adverse effect is caused directly by the drug or by exacerbation of the HIV infection or whether conditions other than HIV infection may be the cause of such adverse effects. Reviews of the toxicity profile of zidovudine have been published previously (SEDA-15, 320; SEDA-17, 343).

The main dose-limiting adverse reaction of zidovudine therapy in HIV-infected adults and children are hematological complications (53[R]). Serious hematological changes have been reported in a majority of zidovudine-treated patients in a large double-blind, placebo-controlled trial (54[C]). These include neutropenia, leukopenia and anemia which are indicative of bone marrow suppression. Other zidovudine-induced hematological side effects include a progressive increase in mean corpuscular volume and increased platelet counts. Hematological side effects resulted in dose adjustment in nearly 50% of zidovudine-treated patients. In a different study of 4085 patients with AIDS treated with zidovudine, 19.7% required one or more transfusions and 11.4% exhibited severe anemia, with serious granulocytopenia occurring in 8.3% of the patients (55[C]). In a third study, four patients with AIDS and a history of *Pneumocystis carinii* pneumonia developed severe pancytopenia with bone marrow aplasia after 14—17 weeks of zidovudine therapy (56[C]). Hematological effects of zidovudine therapy in children are similar to those seen in adults (53[R], 57[C], 58[C]).

The drug was relatively well tolerated in pregnancy (100 mg orally five times daily) with anemia, neutropenia, or thrombocytopenia occurring in 10% and abnormalities of serum electrolytes and liver function in 5% of the women in the treatment group (51[C]).

Oral zidovudine at a dose of 200 mg every 4 hours for 42 days was used as a prophylactic treatment of health care workers after percutaneous exposure to blood or body fluids of HIV-infected patients. Clinical adverse reactions occurred in 73%, with the most frequent being nausea (47%), headache (35%), and fatigue (30%). Of selected hematological laboratory markers only platelet counts increased significantly over a period of 4 weeks. Although clinical adverse reactions were not very severe and none of the laboratory changes was considered clinically significant, treatment was poorly accepted and stopped prematurely by 30% (59[C]).

Other adverse effects include severe headache, insomnia, confusion, nausea, vomiting, abdominal discomfort, myalgia (myopathy) and nail pigmentation (60[R]). Various CNS side effects of zidovudine have been reported which may or may not be related directly to the drug. These include seizures, confusion and acute encephalopathy occurring after zidovudine dosage reduction (45[R]).

The use of zidovudine and ganciclovir in combination is not recommended because the two drugs have overlapping toxicity profiles (45[R]).

Paracetamol used in combination with zidovudine has been reported to increase the occurrence of bone marrow suppression. Both zidovudine and paracetamol are metabolized by glucuronidation, suggesting that paracetamol may competitively inhibit this process. Theoretically, other drugs metabolized by glucuronidation, when combined with zidovudine, may also result in an increased incidence of side effects (45[R], 47[C], 54[C]).

Fewer side effects have been reported in two studies using lower-dose regimens of zidovudine in AIDS patients (61[C], 62[C]).

Didanosine *(SEDA-18, 302)*

Didanosine (2′,3′-dideoxyinosine, ddI) is a purine analog which, after intracellular metabolic conversion, suppresses the replication of HIV. The drug has been approved by the US Food and Drug Administration for the treatment of patients with advanced HIV infection who have become intolerant to, or are deteriorating on zidovudine therapy. The administration of didanosine was associated with statistically significant increases in the number of $CD4^+$ cells and decreases in the serum level of p24 antigen (63[C], 64[C]).

The major clinical adverse effects were acute pancreatitis and a painful neuropathic syndrome (peripheral neuropathy) that appeared to be related to both the cumulative dose of didanosine and the dosage intensity (65[C]). These major toxicities have been extensively reviewed recently (SEDA-17, 340). A personality change was observed in five of 151 participants in a study of didanosine in zidovudine-intolerant HIV-1-infected patients (66[C]). Retinal depigmentation has been described in children (53[R]). No dose-related toxicity of didanosine was noted regarding hematological laboratory indices (63[C]). Minor adverse effects included insomnia, headaches, anxiety, irritability, rash, increased uric acid in plasma and increased hepatic transaminase combined with a rash (67[R]).

Zalcitabine *(SEDA-18, 302)*

Zalcitabine (dideoxycytidine, ddC) is the most potent of the dideoxynucleosides in vitro. Its approved indication is for use in combination with zidovudine in patients with advanced HIV infection.

Side effects of zalcitabine have been reviewed previously (SEDA-17, 342). Its most common toxic effect is peripheral neuropathy which seems to be dose-related. In a study of 52 HIV-1-infected patients, neuropathy developed more rapidly and was more severe in patients receiving 0.03—0.06 mg/kg zalcitabine than in those receiving lower dosages (0.005—0.01 mg/kg). Pain dominated the syndrome with high-dose treatment, while lower doses resulted in paresthetic neuropathy (68[C]).

Investigational compounds

Lamivudine (2′-deoxy-3′-thiacytidine, 3TC), an analog of ddC and stavudine (2′,3′-didehydro-2′,3′-dideoxythymidine, D4T) These are other members of the dideoxynucleoside reverse-transcriptase inhibitor group of antiretroviral agents. Their dose-limiting toxicity in phase I clinical trials is peripheral neuropathy (53[R]).

SUBSTANCES WITH BROAD ANTIVIRAL ACTIVITY

Ribavirin *(SED-12, 744; SEDA-18, 301)*

The synthetic triazole nucleoside, ribavirin (1-β-D-ribofuranosyl-1,2,4-triazole-3-carboxamide, virazole), has a broad spectrum of antiviral activity including DNA as well as RNA viruses (69[R]). Ribavirin closely resembles guanosine and is converted intracellularly to mono-, di- and triphosphate derivatives which inhibit the virally induced enzymes involved in viral nucleic acid synthesis by different mechanisms which are not yet fully understood (70[R]). Of the DNA viruses, HSV seems to be the most sensitive to ribavirin; among the RNA viruses, good activity has been observed against orthomyxo-, paramyxo-, arena- and bunyaviruses. No clinical or laboratory benefit was reported in ribavirin therapy for HIV infection (71[r]). So far, development of resistance has not been described.

Ribavirin is absorbed orally but may be most effective when given in aerosol form, particularly for the treatment of respiratory syncytial virus (RSV) infections in immunocompromised patients, those with cardiopulmonary abnormalities, or in infants receiving mechanical ventilation (72[C], 73[C]).

Oral ribavirin has been successfully used for the treatment of Lassa fever (74[C]) and Crimean Congo-hemorrhagic fever (75[C]).

The substance is generally well tolerated. Time- and dose-dependent mild hemolytic anemia is the only major toxicity associated with oral or intravenous ribavirin therapy. Daily doses of 1 gram may cause elevated levels of unconjugated bilirubin and increased reticulocyte counts. All these side effects, however are reversible upon withdrawal of the drug (76[R], 77[R], 78[C], 79[R]). Since ribavirin is teratogenic and embryotoxic in laboratory animals, concern has been expressed about the safety of persons in the same room with patients being treated with ribavirin by aerosol, particularly women of child-bearing age. However, no ribavirin was detected in urine, plasma or red blood cells of 19 nurses exposed to ribavirin therapy over a 3-day period applied via ventilator, oxygen tent, or oxygen hood (80[C]). Nevertheless, the drug should not be given to pregnant women.

Interferons *(SEDA-18, 304; SED-12, 791)*

Interferons are a group of host-cell proteins. Three major classes are recognized: α-interferons (IFN-α), derived from B-lymphocytes, null lymphocytes and macrophages/dendritic cells; β-interferons (IFN-β), produced by epithelial cells and fibroblasts; and γ-interferons (IFN-γ) derived from T-lymphocytes and macrophages after antigenic or mitogenic stimulation. Recombinant interferons have been produced on an industrial basis and these preparations are commercially available.

The antiviral activity of interferons involves their reversible binding to cell surface receptors. This leads to activation of cytoplasmic enzymes affecting messenger RNA translation and protein synthesis (81[R]). The antiviral state takes hours to develop but may persist for days. Besides their broad antiviral activity, interferons are of major importance in regulating immunological functions.

Recombinant IFN-α_{2b} has been approved for intralesional treatment of condyloma accuminatum (82[C]).

Subcutaneous IFN-α_{2b} has successfully been used for treatment of chronic hepatitis C and chronic hepatitis B with rates of treatment-associated remissions of 25% or more (83[C], 84[C]).

Side effects have been extensively reviewed in this series (SEDA-17, 345). Contrary to earlier beliefs, the natural products seem to be less toxic than the pure synthetic compounds. The most common side effects as observed in earlier clinical trials include a flu-like syndrome with fever, chills, fatigue, myalgia, nausea and general malaise, as well as hematological disorders. Side effects, however, may also include neurotoxicity (paresthesia, polyneuropathy), hepatic toxicity, renal toxicity or an increase in eyelash growth (84[C]–88[C]).

The most common side effects reported in two large multicenter studies were fever (60%), leukopenia (43%), increase in serum aspartate aminotransferase (30%), anorexia (30%), thrombocytopenia (25%), fatigue (21%), nausea, and emesis (17%) (89[C], 90[C]).

Intranasal administration in order to prevent viral infection may lead to local side effects such as discharge of bloody mucus and mucosal erosions (91[C], 92[C]).

Side effects were much more common and serious after high-dose intravenous interferon than after subcutaneous administration of a lower dose; efficacy, however, was similar (93[C], 94[C]).

REFERENCES

1. van der Sijs IH, Wiltink EH. Antiviral drugs: present status and future prospects. Int J Biochem 1994;26:621.
2. Wagstaff AJ, Faulds D, Goa KL. Aciclovir. A reappraisal of its antiviral activity, pharmacokinetic properties and therapeutic efficacy. Drugs 1994;47:153.
3. Erlich KS, Mills J, Chatis P et al. Acyclovir-resistant herpes simplex virus infections in patients with the acquired immunodeficiency syndrome. N Engl J Med 1989;320:293.
4. Sacks SL, Wanklin RJ, Reece DE. Progressive esophagitis from acyclovir-resistant herpes simplex: clinical roles for DNA polymerase mutants and viral heterogenicity. Ann Intern Med 1989;111:893.
5. Drucker JL, Tucker WE, Jr. Szczech M. Safety studies of acyclovir: preclinical and clinical. In: Baker DA, ed. Acyclovir Therapy for Herpesvirus Infections. New York: Marcel Dekker, 1990;15.
6. Brigden D, Rosling AE, Woods NC. Renal function after acyclovir intravenous injection. Am J Med 1982;73(Suppl 1A):182.
7. Yeager AS. Use of acyclovir in premature and term neonates. Am J Med 1982;73(Suppl 1A):182.
8. Prober CG, Kirk LE, Keeney RE. Acyclovir therapy of chickenpox in immunosuppressed children—a collaborative study. Am J Pediatr 1982;101:622.
9. Sylvester RK, Ogden WB, Draxler CA et al. Vesicular eruption—a local complication of concentrated acyclovir infusions. J Am Med Assoc 1986;255:385.
10. Wade JC, Meyers JD. Neurologic symptoms associated with parenteral acyclovir treatment after marrow transplantation. Ann Intern Med 1983;98:921.
11. Wade JC, Hintz M, McGuffin RW et al. Treatment of cytomegalovirus pneumonia with high-dose acyclovir. Am J Med 1982;73(Suppl 1A):249.
12. Straus SE, Smith HA, Brickman C et al. Acyclovir for chronic mucocutaneous herpes simplex infection in immunosuppressed patients. Ann Intern Med 1982;96:270.
13. Tomson CR, Goodship THJ, Rodgers RSC. Psychiatric side-effects of acyclovir in patients with chronic renal failure. Lancet 1985;2:385.
14. McGill J, Tormey P. Use of acyclovir in herpetic ocular infection. Am J Med 1982;73(Suppl 1A):286.
15. Richards DM, Carmine AA, Brogden RN et al. Acyclovir: a review. Drugs 1983;26:378.
16. Andrews EB, Yankaskas BC, Cordero JF et al. Acyclovir in pregnancy registry: six years' experience Obstet Gynecol 1992;79:7.
17. Faulds D, Heel RC. Ganciclovir: a review of its antiviral activity, pharmacokinetic properties and therapeutic efficacy in cytomegalovirus infections. Drugs 1990;39:597.
18. Drew WL, Ives D, Lalezari JP et al. Oral ganciclovir as maintenance treatment for cytomegalovirus retinitis in patients with AIDS. N. Engl J Med 1995;333:615.
19. Emanuel D, Cunningham I, Jules-Elysee K et al. Cytomegalovirus pneumonia after bone marrow transplantation successfully treated with the combination of ganciclovir and high-dose intravenous immune globulin. Ann Intern Med 1988;109:777.
20. Thomson MH, Jeffries DJ. Ganciclovir therapy in iatrogenically immunosuppressed patients with cytomegalovirus disease. J Antimicrob Ther 1989;23(Suppl E):61.
21. Collaborative DHPG treatment study group. Treatment of serious cytomegalovirus infections with 9-(1,3-dihydroxi-

2-propoxymethyl)guanine in patients with AIDS and other immunodeficiencies. N Engl J Med 1986;314:801.
22. Dietrich DT, Chachona A, Lafleur F et al. Ganciclovir treatment of gastrointestinal infections caused by cytomegalovirus in patients with AIDS. Rev Infect Dis 1988;10(Suppl 3):532.
23. Hochster H, Dieterich D, Bozzette S et al. Toxicity of combined ganciclovir and zidovudine for cytomegalovirus disease associated with AIDS: an AIDS clinical trials group study. Ann Intern Med 1990;113:111.
24. Jacobson MA, Owen W, Campbell J et al. Tolerability of combined ganciclovir and didanosine for the treatment of cytomegalovirus disease associated with AIDS. Clin Infect Dis 1993;16(Suppl 1):S69.
25. Öberg B. Molecular basis of foscarnet action in human herpesvirus infections. In: Lopez C, Roizman B, eds. Human Herpesvirus Infections. New York: Raven Press, 1986;141.
26. Chatis PA, Miller CH, Schrager LE et al. Successful treatment with foscarnet of an acyclovir-resistant mucocutaneous infection with herpes simplex virus in a patient with the acquired immunodeficiency syndrome. N Engl J Med 1989;320:297.
27. Klinthalm GL, Lönnquist B, Öberg B et al. Intravenous foscarnet for the treatment of severe cytomegalovirus infection in allograft recipients. Scand J Infect Dis 1985;17:157.
28. Jacobson MA, Drew WL, Feinberg J et al. Foscarnet therapy for ganciclovir-resistant cytomegalovirus retinitis in patients with AIDS. J Infect Dis 1991;163:1348.
29. Jacobson MA. Maintenance therapy for cytomegalovirus retinitis in patients with acquired immunodeficiency syndrome: foscarnet. Am J Med 1992;92(Suppl 2A):26S.
30. Katlama C, Dohin E, Caumes E et al. Foscarnet induction therapy for cytomegalovirus retinitis in AIDS: comparison of twice-daily and three-times-daily regimens. J AIDS 1992;5(Suppl 1):S18.
31. Moyle G, Barton S, Gazzard BC. Penile ulceration with foscarnet therapy. AIDS 1993;7:140.
32. Richman DD. HIV and other human retroviruses. In: Galasso GJ, Whitley RJ, Merigan TC, eds. Antiviral Agents and Viral Diseases of Man. New York: Raven Press, 1990;581.
33. Bauer JD. Antiviral agents. 1. The antiviral nucleosides. In: Bauer DJ, ed. The Specific Treatments of Virus Diseases. Lancaster: MTP Press, 1977;19.
34. Anonymous. Dimethylsulfoxide (DMSO). Med Lett Drugs Ther 1980;22:94.
35. Sacks SL, Scullard GH, Pollard RB et al. Antiviral treatment of chronic hepatitis B-infection: pharmacokinetics and side effects of interferon and arabinoside alone or in combination. Antimicrobial Agents Chemother 1982;21:93.
36. Whitley RJ, Tucker BC, Kinkel AW et al. Pharmacology, tolerance and antiviral activity of vidarabine monophosphate in humans. Antimicrobial Agents Chemother 1980;18:709.
37. De Clerq E, Descamps J, Verhelst G et al. Comparative efficacy of antiherpes drugs against different strains of herpes simplex virus. J Infect Dis 1980;141:563.
38. Bukrinskaya AG, Vorkunova NK, Narmanbetova RA. Rimantadine hydrochloride blocks the second step of influenza virus uncoating. Arch Virol 1980;66:275.
39. Oxford JS, Galbraight A. Antiviral activity of amantadine: a review of laboratory and clinical data. Pharmacol Ther 1980;11:181.
40. Skider A, Adamczyt B, Presber HW et al. Occurrence of amantadine and rimantadine resistant influenza A strains during the 1980 epidemic. Arch Virol 1981;25:395.
41. Van Norris LP, Newell PM. Antivirals for the chemoprophylaxis and treatment of influenza. Semin Respir Infect 1992;7:61.
42. Bryson YJ, Monahan C, Pollack M et al. A prospective double-blind study of side effects associated with the administration of amantadine for influenza A virus prophylaxis. J Infect Dis 1980;141:543.
43. Ing TS, Davgirolas JT, Soung LS et al. Toxic effects of amantadine in patients with renal failure. Can Med Assoc J 1979;120:695.
44. Hayden FG, Belshe RB, Clover RD et al. Emergence and apparent transmission of rimantadine-resistant influenza A virus in families. N Engl J Med 1989;321:1696.
45. Langtry HD, Campoli-Richards DM. Zidovudine: a review of its pharmacodynamic and pharmacokinetic properties, and therapeutic efficacy. Drugs 1989;37:408.
46. Yarchoan R, Mitsuya H, Myers CE et al. Clinical pharmacology of 3′-azido-2′,3′-dideoxythymidine (zidovudine) and related dideoxynucleosides. N Engl J Med 1989;321:726.
47. Fischl MA, Richman DD, Grieco MH et al. The efficacy of azidothymidine (AZT) in the treatment of patients with AIDS and AIDS-related complex. N Engl J Med 1987; 317:185.
48. Fischl MA, Richman DD, Hansen N et al. The safety and efficacy od zidovudine (AZT) in the treatment of subjects with mildly symptomatic human immunodeficiency virus type 1 (HIV) infection. Ann Intern Med 1990;112:727.
49. Kinloch-de Loës S, Hirschel B, Hoen B et al. A controlled trial of zidovudine in primary human immunodeficiency virus infection. N Engl J Med 1995;333:408.
50. Volberding PA, Lagakos SW, Grimes JM et al. A comparison of immediate with deferred zidovudine therapy for asymptomatic HIV-infected adults with CD4 cell counts of 500 or more per cubic millimeter. N Engl J Med 1995; 333:401.
51. Connor EM, Sperling RS, Gelber R et al. Reduction of maternal-infant transmission of human immunodeficiency virus type 1 with zidovudine treatment. N Engl J Med 1994;331:1173.
52. Peckham C, Gibb D. Current concepts: mother-to-child transmission of the human immunodeficiency virus. N Engl J Med 1995;333:298.
53. Pizzo PA, Wilfert C. Antiretroviral therapy for infection due to human immunodeficiency virus in children. Clin Infect Dis 1994;19:177.
54. Richman DD, Fischl MA, Grieco MH et al. The toxicity of azidothymidine (AZT) in the treatment of patients with AIDS and AIDS-related complex. A double-blind, placebo-controlled trial. N Engl J Med 1987;317:192.
55. Creagh-Kirk T, Doi P, Andrews E et al. Survival experience in patients with AIDS receiving zidovudine. J Infect Dis 1988;260:3009.
56. Gill PS, Rarick M, Brynes RK et al. Azidothymidine associated with bone marrow failure in the acquired immunodeficiency syndrome (AIDS). Ann Intern Med 1987;107:502.
57. Pediatric Zidovudine Study Group. Safety and tolerance of zidovudine (ZDV, Retrovir) during a phase 1 study in children of 14 years or less. Pediatr Res 1988;23:379A.
58. Pizzo AP, Eddy J, Falloon J et al. Effects of continuous intravenous infusion of zidovudine (AZT) in children with symptomatic HIV infection. N Engl J Med 1988;319:889.
59. Forseter G, Joline C, Wormser GP. Tolerability, safety, and acceptability of zidovudine prophylaxis in health care workers. Arch Intern Med 1994;154:2745.

60. Neuzil KM. Pharmacologic therapy for human immunodeficiency virus infection: a review. Am. J Med Sci 1994;307:368.
61. Fischl MA, Parker CB, Pettinelli C et al. A randomized controlled trial of a reduced daily dose of zidovudine in patients with the acquired immunodeficiency syndrome. N Engl J Med 1990;323:1009.
62. Collier AC, Bozzette S, Coombs RW et al. A pilot study of low-dose zidovudine in human immunodeficiency virus infection. N Engl J Med 1990;323:1015.
63. Lambert JS, Seidlin M, Reichmann RC et al. 2′3′-Dideoxy-inosine (ddI) in patients with the acquired immunodeficiency syndrome or AIDS-related complex. A phase I trial. N Engl J Med 1990;322:1333.
64. Cooley TP, Kunches LM, Saunders CA et al. Once-daily administration of 2′,3′-dodeoxyinosine (ddI) in patients with the acquired immunodeficiency syndrome or AIDS-related complex. N Engl J Med 1990;322:1340.
65. Yarchoan R, Mitsuya H, Pluda JM et al. The National Cancer Institute phase I study of 2′,3′-dideoxyinosine administration in adults with AIDS or AIDS-related complex: analysis of activity and toxicity profiles. Rev Infect Dis 1990;12(Suppl 5):522.
66. Moyle GJ, Nelson MR, Hawkins D et al. The use and toxicity of didanosine (ddI) in HIV antibody-positive individuals intolerant to zidovudine (AZT). Q J Med 1993;86:155.
67. Franssen RME, Meenhorst PL, Koks CHW et al. Didanosine, a new retroviral drug. Pharm Weekbl-Sci 1992;14:297.
68. Berger AR, Arezzo JC, Schaumburg HH et al. 2′,3′-Dideoxycytidine (ddC) toxic neuropathy: a study of 52 patients. Neurology 1993;43:358.
69. Stapleton T, ed. Studies with a Broad Spectrum Antiviral Agent. International Congress and Symposium Series. London/New York: Royal Society of Medicine Services, 1986.
70. Couch RB. Respiratory disease. In: Galasso GJ, Whitley RJ, Merigan TC, eds. Antiviral Agents and Viral Diseases of Man. New York: Raven Press, 1990;327.
71. Editorial. Ribavirin for HIV—continuing smoke, not much fire. Lancet 1991;338:22.
72. Hall CB, McBride JT, Walsh EE et al. Aerosolized ribavirin treatment of infants with respiratory syncytial virus infection: a randomized double-blind study. N Engl J Med 1983;308:1443.
73. Smith DW, Frankel LR, Mathers LH et al. A controlled trial of aerosolized ribavirin in infants receiving mechanical ventilation for severe respiratory syncytial virus infection. N Engl J Med 1991;325:24.
74. McCormick JB, King IJ, Wepp PA et al. Lassa fever. Effective therapy with ribavirin. N Engl J Med 1986;314:20.
75. Fisher-Hoch SP, Khan JA, Rehman S et al. Crimean Congo-haemorrhagic fever treated with oral ribavirin. Lancet 1995;346:472.
76. Smith CB, Charette RP. Double-blind evaluation of ribavirin in naturally occurring influenza. In: Smith RA, Kirkpatrick W, eds. Ribavirin: A Broad Spectrum Antiviral Agent. New York: Academic Press, 1980;147.
77. Fernandez H. Ribavirin: a summary of clinical trials—herpes genitalis and measles. In: Smith RA, Kirkpatrick W, eds. Ribavirin: A Broad Spectrum Antiviral Agent. New York: Academic Press, 1980;215.
78. Hall CB, Walsh EE, Hruska JF et al. Ribavirin treatment of experimental respiratory syncytial virus infection. J Am Med Assoc 1983;249:2666.
79. Hillyard IW. The preclinical toxicology and safety of ribavirin. In: Smith RA, Kirkpatrick W, eds. Ribavirin: A Broad Spectrum Antiviral Agent. New York: Academic Press, 1980;59.
80. Rodriguez WJ, Dang Bui RHD, Conner JD et al. Environmental exposure of primary care personnel to ribavirin aerosol when supervising treatment of infants with respiratory syncytial virus infections. Antimicrobial Agents Chemother 1987;31:1143.
81. Stiehm ER, Kronenberg CH, Rosenblatt HM et al. Interferon: immunobiology and clinical significance. Ann Intern Med 1982;96:80.
82. Reichmann RC, Oakes D, Bonnez W et al. Treatment of condyloma accuminatum with three different interferons administered intralesionally: a double-blind, placebo-controlled trial. Ann Intern Med 1988;108:675.
83. Di Bisceglie AM, Martin P, Kassianides C et al. Recombinant interferon alfa therapy for chronic hepatitis C: a randomized, double-blind, placebo-controlled trial. N Engl J Med 1989;321:1506.
84. Korenmann J, Baker B, Waggoner J et al. Long-term remission of chronic hepatitis B after alpha-interferon therapy. Ann Intern Med 1991;114:629.
85. Scott GM, Ward RJ, Wright DJ et al. Effects of cloned interferon alpha 2 in normal volunteers: febrile reactions and changes in circulating corticosteroids and trace metals. Antimicrobial Agents Chemother 1983;23:589.
86. Ingimarsson S, Cantell K, Strander H. Side-effects of long-term treatment with human leukocyte interferon. J Infect Dis 1979;140:560.
87. Cheeseman SH, Rubin RH, Stewart JA et al. Controlled clinical trial of prophylactic human leukocyte interferon in renal transplantation. N Engl J Med 1979;300:1345.
88. Smedley H, Katrak M, Sikova K et al. Neurological effects of recombinant human interferon. Br Med J 1983;286:262.
89. Taguchi T. Clinical studies of recombinant interferon alfa-2a (Roferon®-A) in cancer patients. Cancer 1986;67:1705.
90. Umeda T, Niijima T. Phase II study of alpha interferon on renal cell carcinoma: summary of three collaborative trials. Cancer 1986;58:1231.
91. Samo TC, Greenberg SB, Couch RB et al. Efficacy and tolerance of intranasally applied recombinant leucocyte A interferon in normal volunteers. J Infect Dis 1983;148:535
92. Dunnick JK, Galasso GJ. Clinical trials with exogenous interferon: summary of a meeting. J Infect Dis 1979;139:109.
93. Mirro J, Dow LW, Kalwinsky DK et al. Phase I-II study on continuous-infusion of high-dose human lymphoblastoid interferon and the in vitro sensitivity of leukemic progenitors in nonlymphocytic leukemia. Cancer Treat Rep 1986;70:363.
94. Muss HB, Constanzi JJ, Leavit R et al. Recombinant alfa interferon in renal cell carcinoma: a randomized trial of two routes of administration. J Clin Oncol 1987;5:286.

Meyler's Side Effects of Drugs, 13th Edition
M.N.G. Dukes, editor

SECTION EDITOR: R. HOIGNÉ

P. Leuenberger and R. Sonntag

30 Drugs used in tuberculosis and leprosy

DRUGS USED IN TUBERCULOSIS

INTRODUCTION

Treatment of tuberculosis and other mycobacterial diseases generally poses specific therapeutic problems (1[R]). These usually are chronic conditions, but they may also run a fulminant course. In addition, they significantly contribute to mortality. Mycobacteria are often intracellular, showing long periods of metabolic inactivity. They tend to develop resistance to antimycobacterial drugs if used as monotherapy. The recent increase in the prevalence of tuberculosis is associated with an increased frequency of multidrug-resistant strains with resistance to both isoniazid and rifampicin.

After over four decades of clinical experience with antituberculous treatment, various alternative drug regimens with acceptable efficacy and safety have been established. The choice will depend upon the individual case, the local epidemiology, and the financial constraints (2[R]). Developing countries have often favored strategies that reduce the number of daily doses and the duration of hospitalization. They have sometimes also preferred drugs having a low unit cost even when they are poorly tolerated. Thus, thiacetazone continued to be used much longer in developing countries than elsewhere. The aim of any antituberculous treatment, however, is tissue sterilization attained by a short, inexpensive treatment. This concept is valid for all sites of tuberculosis (3[R]). It is best achieved by an early intensive regimen of three to four drugs, followed by a period of maintenance therapy with the two most effective drugs used in the initial phase (4[C]). Early reduction in the bacterial population diminishes the risk of developing drug resistance. The maintenance therapy ensures destruction of slowly multiplying tubercle bacilli (5[R]). Treatment of mycobacterial diseases has become a challenging problem with the present acquired immunodeficiency syndrome (AIDS) pandemic. This has been associated with an increased frequency of tuberculosis and diseases caused by *M. avium* complex. These chronic conditions present special therapeutic difficulties, regarding compliance, hypersensitivity reactions and drug toxicity (6[R]).

Three to four bactericidal drugs are necessary to eliminate both the rapidly multiplying bacteria and the slowly growing strains known as 'persisters' (7[C]). First-line antituberculous drugs are isoniazid (INH), rifampicin (RMP), pyrazinamide (PZ), ethambutol (EMB) and streptomycin (SM) (3[R]). Occasionally, it may be necessary to use second-line drugs because of microbial resistance or drug side effects. These include thioacetazone, ethionamide, prothionamide, cycloserine, viomycin, capreomycin and some large spectrum antibiotics (such as *clarithromycin*, *ciprofloxacin*, *sparfloxacin* and *ofloxacin*) (8[C]). *Clofazimine*, a drug used in the treatment of leprosy, may also be useful (9[R]).

The numerous clinical trials on the treatment of tuberculosis have all concerned pulmonary tuberculosis. A 6-month regimen combining isoniazid, rifampicin, pyrazinamide for 2 months followed by INH and RMP for 4 months is the preferred therapy for the patients with susceptible strains. Unless the risk of monoresistance is considered to be low, EMB or SM should be added during the initial phase until drug sensitivity is determined. With the exception of tuberculous meningitis or osteitis which may require prolonged therapy for as long as 12 months or more. Extrapulmonary tuberculosis does not require a different therapeutic strategy.

A 9-month bitherapy with isoniazid and rifampicin is also acceptable. Ethambutol (or streptomycin) can be added until drug sensitivity is known. In case of resistance to isoniazid, a bitherapy with rifampicin and ethambutol can be prescribed, but not for less than 12 months.

The new combined triple formulations of INH, RMP and PZ (10[C]) offer significant advantages for short-course chemotherapy and improve compliance (11[R], 12[C]). Whenever possible, it is recommended to administer antimycobacterial treatment under direct supervision. Directly observed therapy (DOT) has been shown to be very effective in increasing drug compliance and success rate.

AIDS patients can be similarly treated. However, the Centers for Disease Control advise a 9-month regimen: 2 months with isoniazid, rifampicin and pyrazinamide, followed by at least 7 months with isoniazid and rifampicin or for at least 6 months after three negative cultures have been obtained. If isoniazid or rifampicin cannot be used, antituberculous therapy should be continued for at least 18 months or 12 months after cultures become negative (6[R]).

Patients with advanced human immunodeficiency virus infection are more prone to develop adverse drug reactions (ADRs). In a recent report (13[C]), 18% of the treated patients had alterations in their therapy because of ADR. Of the patients treated with RMP, 12% had ADRs requiring the discontinuation of the drug. Such reactions were attributed less frequently to the other drugs (PZA in 6%, INH in 4%, and EMB in 2% of patients). Sixty percent of the reactions occurred within the first month of treatment, and 95% by the end of the second month.

Certain patients also benefit from a four-drug regimen to ensure that the mycobacteria will be susceptible to at least two of the drugs. These are: (1) patients with known exposure to drug-resistant microorganisms; (2) Asians, Hispanics and refugees from developing countries; (3) patients with miliary tuberculosis; (4) patients with meningitis; (5) patients with extensive cavitary pulmonary tuberculosis.

Children should be given the same treatment as adults, with proper adjustment of doses according to age and weight.

When tuberculosis relapses it is advisable, if the clinical evolution permits, to wait for the results of drug sensitivity determination before starting therapy. In rapidly evolving or severe cases therapy should be started immediately. A five-drug regimen including INH, RMP, PZ, EMB and SM is most often chosen. A three-drug regimen is then selected based upon the antibiogram. After 2 months of active drug regimen a bitherapy is administered for up to 12 months or for at least 6 months after negative cultures.

Primary and secondary bacterial resistance to antituberculous drugs still represents a major problem. This may be demonstrated in resistance tests, if available. When testing is not done, primary or secondary resistance may only be suspected when drug treatment fails. The incidence of bacterial resistance varies enormously from country to country and from population to population. In Tanzania (14[C]), where the WHO and the International Union against Tuberculosis and Lung Diseases (IUATLD) has developed antituberculosis programs, primary resistance to INH and/or streptomycin is found in 10% of cases (15[C]). In a French study the resistance of 853 *Mycobacterium tuberculosis* strains from French and non-French patients was tested between 1977 and 1984 (16[R]). Drug resistance was also found in nearly 10%. In contrast, South-East Asian and African patients harbored resistant bacteria markedly more often (SED-10, 572). Resistance tests therefore remain mandatory for good epidemiological and therapeutic control (17[r], 18[r]).

Multidrug-resistant tuberculosis most often results from inadequate therapy or lack of compliance to drug regimen. A strain of mycobacteria is called resistant when it is insensitive to isoniazid or rifampicin. It is called multiresistant when it is insensitive to both. In this case other antituberculous drugs may also be inactive (19[R]). In practice, two second-line antituberculous drugs, selected on the bases of individual drug susceptibility, are given in combination with one quinolone (20[R]).

Drug malabsorption may contribute to the emergence of acquired drug resistance. It has been described in HIV-infected patients with advanced disease (21[r]). Thus, in addition to the use of directly observed therapy to ensure compliance, it is advisable to routinely control antimycobacterial drug levels in such patients. Practical proposals for the choice of tuberculostatic drugs in special situations, including cases of drug resistance, have been made by Des Prez and Heim (22[R]).

Indications for *prophylactic antituberculous* drug treatment (3[R]) include cases of tuberculin conversion, accidentally discovered and clinically inactive minor pulmonary lesions, clinically stabilized fibrotic disease with intermittent mycobacteria production and cases with a prior history of pulmonary tuberculosis who are undergoing long-term corticosteroid treatment. More recently, intravenous drug abusers and AIDS patients who are predisposed to develop meningitis or generalized tuberculosis have been added (23[C]). Preference is given to a single-drug regimen, i.e. isoniazid, except in immunocompromised patients (24[C]) who may harbor non-tuberculous mycobacteria (MOTT or NTM) resistant to first-line drugs (25[R], 26[c], 27[R]–29[R]).

Prophylactic administration of INH reduces the risk of further development of tuberculosis. In HIV-positive subjects the duration of prophylaxis should be 12 months. In HIV-negative subjects 6 months appears to be sufficient. The American Academy of Pediatrics recommends a 9-month prophylaxis in children (3[R]).

The best approach to prophylaxis in subjects exposed to multiresistant infection is not well established. A combination of *quinolone* and *pyrazinamide* for 4 months has been proposed, as well as a pyrazinamide/ethambutol regimen (30[R]).

Treatment of NTM infections poses a major problem (29[R], 31[R]) *M. avium* infections may be life-threatening in immunocompromised patients (25[R], 32[R]). With the increasing incidence of *M. kansasii* infections a four-drug regimen over 18–24 months has been suggested (33[R]).

Diseases due to NTM require multiple drug combinations and, in addition, surgery in individual cases. With the exception of diseases due to *M. avium-intracellulare* (MAC) in immunosuppressed patients, the course is usually less severe than with tuberculosis. Treatment of disseminated MAC infection is based on a three or more drug regimen selected in accordance with drug sensitivity determination (N9). Preliminary results suggest that new *macrolides* (such as *clarithromycin* and *azithromycin*) may contribute to a prolonged survival (34[r]).

Prophylaxis of MAC infection is advisable in HIV-positive patients with a CD4 lymphocyte count <200/m^3. *Rifabutine* has been shown to significantly decrease the rate of MAC bacteremia in these patients without causing severe adverse reactions (35[R]).

Some of the well-known antituberculous drugs such as streptomycin and rifampicin are also widely used in non-tuberculous diseases. These include leprosy, kidney transplant cases treated with ciclosporin (36[C]), meningococcal diseases (37[r]) and cystic fibrosis (Chapter 25).

Close supervision and monitoring of signs and symptoms during therapy, as well as the addition of pyridoxine to isoniazid, has decreased the number of side effects to drug treatment of tuberculosis. Awareness of potentially severe hepatotoxic reactions is vital because hepatic failure may be a devastating and often fatal condition without liver transplantation. Fulminant hepatic failure caused by RMP, INH or both have recently been described (38[c]).

Isoniazid

Isoniazid is the hydrazide of isonicotinic acid (INH). It is the first-line drug for antituberculous chemotherapy and chemoprophylaxis. It is bactericidal for rapidly dividing mycobacteria, but bacteriostatic for 'resting bacilli'. Among the NTM-group only a few strains such as *Mycobacterium kansasii* are susceptible to INH. As a rule, sensitivity should always be tested *in vitro* since the inhibitory concentration required may vary greatly. INH diffuses rapidly into body fluids and cells, including cerebrospinal fluid. It is as effective against bacteria growing within cells as it is against bacteria in culture media. There is no cross-resistance known between INH and other antituberculous drugs.

The daily dose of INH is 5 mg/kg, with a maximum of 400 mg/day in adults with normal liver and kidney function. In children 8–10 mg/kg may be an appropriate dose with a maximum daily dose of 300 mg, since the metabolism of INH in children is rapid. After ingestion of a common dose, INH reaches a peak plasma level of 3–5 μg/ml within 1–2 hours. Its concentration equilibrates into all body fluids and tissues, 75–95% of INH is excreted in the urine within 24 hours. The most important urinary metabolites are products of acetylation (acetylisoniazid) and hydrolysis (isonicotinic acid). Isonicotinyl glycine, isonicotinyl hydrazones and *N*-methylisoniazid appear in only small amounts.

Humans are divided genetically into rapid and slow acetylators of INH, depending upon the activity of their *N*-acetyltransferase. The rate of acetylation of INH is dependent upon race but is not influenced by sex or by age after childhood. Fast acetylation is found in Eskimos and Japanese. Slow acetylation is the predominant phenotype in most Scandinavians, Jews and North African Caucasians (39[R]).

Slow acetylators are homozygous for an autosomal recessive gene, while fast acetylators are homozygous or heterozygous for a dominant gene. The rate of acetylation significantly alters the drug concentrations achieved in plasma and its half-life. The mean half-life of the drug in rapid acetylators is approximately 70 minutes, while a value of 3 hours is found in slow acetylators. Despite this, there is probably no difference in the effectiveness of INH in the two phenotypes. The relationship between INH toxicity and acetylator status continues to be discussed in the literature (SEDA-9, 268; 40[C], 41[r], 42[C]).

ADVERSE REACTION PATTERN

Untoward effects of INH as a single antituberculous drug may be evaluated in preventive tuberculosis therapy, since curative treatments usually consist of multiple drugs. The addition of pyridoxine to usual doses of 5 mg/kg/day in adults and 8–10 mg/kg/day in children markedly reduces the neurotoxicity of INH (39[R]) (for dosage see above).

General and toxic reactions In a survey of more than 2000 patients treated with INH, the most frequent side effects were rash (2%), fever (1.2%), jaundice (0.6%) and peripheral neuritis (0.2%). Untoward neurological effects, i.e. peripheral neuritis or focal seizures occur in 2% of treated patients if pyridoxine is not given. They occur in 12–20% receiving higher doses of INH (10–15 mg/kg) (39[R]). INH decreases the half life of RMP and other drugs metabolized by the liver.

Hypersensitivity reactions Hypersensitivity can complicate both the treatment and chemoprophylaxis of TB. *Morbilliform, maculopapular, purpuric* and *urticarial rashes* with or without fever are considered to be of allergic origin. Hematological side effects consist of *agranulocytosis, thrombocytopenia*, INH-induced pure red cell aplasia and eosinophilia (SEDA-9, 268; 41[r]). Dyspnea with thoracic pain, cough, fever and eosinophilia as well as micronodular densities in the lung X-ray may also be due to an immunological process (43[r]). *Vasculitis* associated with antinuclear antibodies has been observed during treatment, as well as arthritic symptoms (44[c]). Liver injury (mainly hepatocellular) has been considered another form of hypersensitivity reaction, but usually occurs on combined antituberculous treatment with RMP in combination with anticonvulsants or halothane, or in association with alcoholism. Some authors are of the opinion that the main factor inducing liver damage is the fast acetylator phenotype (SEDA-9, 268; 40[C], 41[c]). Others did not find a correlation with the acetylator phenotype (42[c]).

Desensitization to INH has been attempted in some patients with drug fever or exanthema. A procedure of rush desensitization over a few days or a week may be used starting with 1 mg orally with increasing dosage every second day (SED-9, 528; 45[R]) or even every few hours.

Tumor-inducing effects No increase in cancer deaths was observed in a series of 338 women treated with INH for pulmonary tuberculosis (46[c]).

ORGANS AND SYSTEMS

Cardiovascular *Vasculitis, erythema nodosum* and *purpura* are described later in this monograph (47[C]).

Respiratory Symptoms suggesting *broncho-obstruction* occur only very rarely during INH treatment (43[r]).

Nervous system *Peripheral neuropathy* is a well-recognized side effect, resulting from an interference with *pyridoxine* metabolism. Numbness or tingling of the extremities in the 'stocking-glove' distribution has appeared early during treatment with INH when no additional pyridoxine was given. Neuropathy was noted by several authors in undernourished patients and in fast acetylators undergoing INH treatment at doses higher than 5–6 mg/kg with a frequency of up to 20%. Only 2% of patients receiving 5 mg/kg of the drug with pyridoxine developed neuropathy. Symptoms generally consist of hyperesthesia, diminution of vibratory and position sense, and exaggerated or reduced tendon reflexes, but ataxia, muscle weakness and even paralysis may develop (48[C]). Shoulder-arm syndrome has also been described.

Histological findings show disappearance of synaptic vesicles, mitochondrial swelling or condensation and fragmentation of axon endings. Alterations in the lumbar and sacral spinal ganglia and the spinal cord have also been reported (49[C]). Malnourished, diabetic, uremic and alcoholic patients are particularly at risk and should be given *pyridoxine supplements*.

Optic neuritis and *atrophy* have occurred, as well as toxic *encephalopathy*. Isoniazid is known to cause neuropsychiatric syndromes. They include euphoria, transient impairment of memory, separation of ideas and reality, loss of self-control, psychosis (39[R]), and obsessive compulsive neurosis (50[c]). Isoniazid should be used with caution in patients with pre-existing psychosis as it was shown to induce a relapse of *paranoid schizophrenia* (51[c]). Patients on chronic dialysis appear vulnerable to neurological adverse drug reactions because of abnormal metabolism of uremic toxins. It is thus recommended that a higher dose than the customary dose of 100 mg of *pyridoxine* be given to patients on dialysis taking *isoniazid* (52[cR], 53[c]).

Vitamin B deficiency or interference with the metabolism of biological amines may possibly be involved. Patients with seizure disorders (with or without phenytoin treatment) may develop signs of carbamazepine intoxication (54[c]). Serum levels of this drug were increased, probably due to the enzyme-inhibitory effect of INH.

Pellagra encephalopathy has been suspected as a side effect of INH administration in several tuberculosis patients. Niacin (nicotinic acid) deficiency is characterized by dermatitis, diarrhea and dementia. Other symptoms may arise, such as seizures, hallucinations, spasticity and glossitis. Pellagra induced by INH is promoted by malnutrition or a vegetarian diet with low intake of the nicotinamide precursors tryptophan and nicotinic acid. Specific supplementation is essential (55[c]).

Endocrine, metabolic *Cushing's syndrome, gynecomastia, amenorrhea* and *pubertas praecox* are regarded as reflecting the enzyme-inhibiting activity of INH and the resulting derangement of hepatic hormone metabolism (see below). In diabetics strict control of glucose metabolism is necessary since *hyperglycemia* may occur. In a trial of five volunteers with INH intake of 15 mg/kg daily over a period of 6 weeks levels of serum cholesterol were found to be decreased (SEDA-9, 268). INH exerts an anti-vitamin B_6 effect increasing pyridoxine requirements (see above and below).

Mineral and fluid balance As long as renal and hepatic functions remain normal, no untoward effects of INH are to be expected.

Hematological *Agranulocytosis*, *thrombocytopenia*, *hemolytic anemia*, *sideroblastic anemia* (56[c]), *pure red cell aplasia* (57[c]), *methemoglobinemia* and *eosinophilia* can occur exceptionally during INH treatment (SEDA-9, 268; 41[R], 58[R]). An acquired coagulation factor XIII inhibitor has developed in a patient on isoniazid resulting in a bleeding disorder (59[c]).

Liver *Abnormal liver function* is the most commonly described untoward reaction. The possible relationship to acetylator phenotype is mentioned under 'General and toxic reactions' above. Hepatotoxicity caused considerable alarm following an episode in Washington, DC, where 19 of 2231 government employees given INH preventive therapy developed clinical signs of liver disease within 6 months of starting the drug. Thirteen were severely jaundiced and two died (60[r]). In another series of 13 838 prophylactically treated cases 114 also developed overt hepatic disease probably related to INH (SED-9, 574; SEDA-6, 276). In those cases, the characteristic pathological damage was centrilobular necrosis. There were 13 fatalities; four of these showed massive necrosis and nine had lesser changes in the liver. The mechanism responsible for this toxicity remains undetermined. A metabolite of INH, acetylhydrazine, causes hepatic damage and may play a role. Alcoholic hepatitis is an aggravating factor, whereas chronic carriers of hepatitis B virus seem to tolerate isoniazid. In a clinical investigation with assay of the urinary metabolic profile of INH in patients who developed INH-related liver damage, it was impossible to predict which patients would prove susceptible. It was also impossible to demonstrate that rifampicin plays a significant role in inducing liver damage when added to INH (60[r], 61[C]). Nevertheless, it is conceivable that enzyme induction by rifampicin may influence the metabolism of INH. Further risk factors are alcoholism, malnutrition, diabetes, previous liver damage, renal insufficiency and drug abuse. Age is certainly another risk factor for hepatotoxicity. Hepatic damage seems to be rare in patients under the age of 20. The incidence of liver toxicity is 0.3% between the ages of 20 and 34, and increases with age to 1.2% between 34 and 49 and 2.3% over the age of 50 (39[R]). Even in chemoprophylaxis with INH monotherapy, side effects have been found to be more frequent in patients over 35 years old (SED-9, 574).

In practice it is advisable to control the *liver enzymes* ASAT and ALAT before treatment and monthly thereafter, for as long as INH administration lasts. INH should be discontinued if the ASAT elevation is greater than 5 times normal (39[R]). Hepatic damage usually appears 1—2 months after the start of therapy. In children, elevation of liver enzymes is common during the first few months of treatment, but interruption is seldom necessary. A careful watch should be kept for early symptoms of INH-induced hepatitis, such as malaise, fatigue, nausea and epigastric distress. The dangers of continuing isoniazid after the onset of symptoms of toxicity are highlighted in a recent review (62[R]). The earliest symptoms of INH toxicity should be clearly described to the patient, particularly to the hepatitis B carriers who appear in this study to be more susceptible to hepatotoxicity than a control group (63[c]).

Gastrointestinal No severe gastrointestinal side effects of INH have been observed; symptoms are limited to *epigastric distress*, *gastric burning and dryness of the mouth*. *Nausea* may occur, particularly if the drug is taken before breakfast or in combination with other antituberculous drugs.

Adverse reactions during INH treatment have been noted after ingestion of several kinds of *cheese* (SED-9, 575; 64[r], 65[c]). *Flushing*, *palpitations*, *tachycardia* and *increased blood pressure* have been observed 0.5—2 hours after cheese intake. The symptoms generally disappear within 2—4 hours. Interference by INH with monoamine oxidase and hence with tyramine metabolism has been incriminated. Somewhat similar symptoms are known to occur with INH after eating skipjack fish (class of Thunnidae, on both coasts of North America and elsewhere) (64[r], 66[c]). The symptoms, notably *headache*, *palpitations*, *erythema*, *redness of the eyes*, *itching*, *diarrhea and wheezing*, are thought to be elicited mainly by the high histamine content of this fish. *Acute pancreatitis* has recently been described in association with INH therapy (67[c], 68[c]).

Urinary system Pre-existing renal failure necessitates adequate control of urea and creatinine serum levels. Nephrotoxicity is rarely observed, but may be induced in combined therapy (rifampicin, streptomycin) or in patients developing hypersensitivity reactions. Urinary retention is a rare complication.

Skin and appendages Morbilliform, maculopapular or urticarial rashes have been observed in up to 2% of patients (39[R]). *Pellagra* (55[C]), *encephalopathy* combined with *skin lesions* (dermatitis) as a consequence of niacin deficiency in INH treatment is augmented in undernourished people (see under 'Nervous system'). *Acquired cutis laxa* has been mentioned in a single observation of a child, but it probably was coincidental (69[R]).

Other organs and systems *Arthritic symptoms* with back pain, bilateral proximal interphalangeal joint involvement, arthralgia of the knees, elbows and wrists and the so-called *'shoulder-arm-syndrome'* with *cervico-bracheal neuralgia* can occur under INH treatment (39[R]). *Lupus erythematosus-like syndrome or vasculitis* with arthritis, rheumatic pain, fever, pleurisy and leukopenia may be induced by INH (70[c], 71[c]). Tests for antinuclear antibodies are useful to distinguish systemic lupus erythematosus (SLE) and drug-induced lupus erythematosus-like syndromes. However, many patients taking INH have antinuclear antibodies, usually without clinical symptoms of SLE. INH also may enhance pre-existing SLE (47[C], 70[c], 71[c]). Long-term corticosteroid treatment might be necessary if symptoms persist after interruption of INH.

Risk situations *Pre-existing liver damage*, *renal failure*, *diabetes*, *AIDS*, *age*, *alcoholism*, *enzyme-inducing drugs* and perhaps *fast acetylator phenotype* may all promote adverse reactions. Some foods like *cheese* and special kinds of *fish* are able to provoke acute generalized reactions (see 'Gastrointestinal').

Second-generation effects INH diffuses into the blastocytes when ingested after conception, but no teratogenic effects have been reported (72[C]). INH remains the safest antituberculous drug for use during pregnancy and lactation (22[R], 72[C]). During pregnancy INH with ethambutol is considered to be the preferred combination (22[R]). As the drug passes into the milk, however, a lookout must be kept for side effects of INH in the infant when a nursing mother is undergoing INH therapy (73[R]). The drug has no influence on fertility and is not mutagenic (SEDA-6, 276), but patients receiving combined INH and rifampicin therapy for 3—10 months developed an increased rate of chromosomal aberrations as evaluated in peripheral blood lymphocytes (SEDA-9, 276). This effect, however, is not known to have clinical consequences. If antituberculous treatment is needed for suspected congenital tuberculosis, the dosage of INH or other drugs has to be adapted to the liver and kidney function at this age.

Overdosage Acute poisoning in children has been described (74[c]). Overdose was also observed in adults attempting suicide with the drug. They developed coma, seizures, metabolic acidosis and hyperglycemia (51[R], 63[c]). INH overdosage has been treated with pyridoxine at doses between 20 and 1500 mg per 1000 mg INH ingested (75[c]).

Interactions Absorption of INH may be inhibited by *aluminium-containing antacids* (76[R]).

INH is considered to be a potent hepatic enzyme inhibitor and therefore interferes with the metabolism of many drugs (SEDA-8, 287; SEDA-11, 271). Studies in healthy volunteers showed prolongation of the half-life of *triazolam* from 2.5 to 3.3 hours when it was given with INH, whereas INH did not affect the kinetics of *oxazepam*. It seems that INH impairs the hepatic microsomal oxidation of *triazolam*, whereas the conjugation of *oxazepam* is not influenced (SEDA-9, 267).

INH and *antipyrine* administration results in a significant decrease in the hepatic clearance of antipyrine by approximately 40% (SEDA-9, 267).

Barbiturates as well as *narcotics* are among the best known liver enzyme inducers. Their use is not advisable during INH, rifampicin or combined antituberculous treatment, since they may result in accelerated breakdown of these drugs (77[R]).

Disulfiram treatment in alcoholics interferes with INH metabolism in various ways. Simultaneous therapy with these two drugs should be avoided or well monitored. Disulfiram notably inhibits hepatic microsomal drug-metabolizing enzymes and thereby interferes with many drugs, the toxicity and other effects of which may be potentiated (see Chapter 49).

INH interacts with the antiepileptic drugs *ethosuximide* and *phenytoin*. In one patient simultaneous treatment with ethosuximide and INH induced deterioration of his general condition and mental status (SEDA-9, 267). INH is known to inhibit the parahydroxylation of *phenytoin*. Symptoms of phenytoin intoxication, such as dizziness, incoordination or excessive sedation, may occur particularly in patients who are slow acetylators (SEDA-11, 271). Dosage of phenytoin should be adjusted according to plasma levels (78[r]).

The undesirable effects which occur when *monoamine oxidase inhibitors* are taken together with INH resemble the symptoms seen after the simultaneous ingestion of *certain foods* (see above).

INH exerts its *anti-vitamin* B_6 effect (see above) primarily by inhibiting the formation of the coenzyme form of the vitamin. Neuropathy during INH treatment is nearly 100% preventable by *pyridoxine* supplementation in daily doses of 15—100 mg. Compliance is improved by prescribing combined tablets containing 20 mg of pyridoxine per 100 mg INH. In otherwise normal persons, prescription of pyridoxine is not mandatory. However it should be routinely administered in malnourished patients and those predisposed to neuropathy (e.g. pregnant women, elderly, diabetics, alcoholics and uremics) (79[R]).

Rifampicin

Rifampicin or rifampin (RMP) is a semisynthetic derivative of rifamycin B produced by *Streptomyces medi-*

terranei. By suppressing the initiation of chain formation in RNA synthesis, RMP inhibits the DNA-dependent RNA polymerase of mycobacteria and other microorganisms (39[R]).

RMP inhibits the growth of most gram-positive and many gram-negative bacteria: *Escherichia coli*, some *Pseudomonas strains*, *Proteus*, *Klebsiella*, *Staphylococcus aureus*, *Neisseria meningitidis*, *Haemophilus influenzae* and *Legionella* species. *Mycobacterium tuberculosis*, *M. kansasii*, *M. scrofulaceum* and *M. intracellulare* are suppressed with increasing concentrations between 0.005 and 4 μg/ml. The drug is bactericidal for *M. leprae* at a concentration of less than 1 μg/ml. *M. fortuitum* is not susceptible to the drug. Primary resistance is very rare, but secondary resistance among mycobacteria and meningococci (used in meningococcal carriers) develops very rapidly when RMP is employed as a single drug (39[R]).

RMP is distributed to nearly all organs and body fluids in sufficient antibacterial concentrations. It is responsible for orange-red coloration of the urine, feces, saliva, tears, sputum and sweat, leading to the so-called 'red man syndrome' (SED-10, 579). Peak concentrations of up to 7 μg/ml are reached within 2—4 hours after ingestion of a dose of 600 mg before a meal. Following gastrointestinal absorption, RMP is quickly eliminated in the bile, following an enterohepatic circulation. The drug is progressively deacetylated, but this metabolite retains full antibacterial activity. The half-life of RMP varies between 2.5 and 5 hours. It is decreased to various degrees by INH and hepatic disorders (39[R]). There is a progressive shortening of the half-life of RMP by about 40% during the first 14 days of treatment due to its own hepatic microsomal enzyme induction. RMP and other antibiotics are concentrated several-fold in alveolar macrophages when incubated with RMP (80[r]). This explains the efficacy of such antibiotics against intracellular bacteria. A similar process is observed in granulocytes in which the highly lipid-soluble RMP is also concentrated (81[c]).

ADVERSE REACTION PATTERN

General and toxic reaction RMP given in usual doses (e.g. 10 mg/kg/day) is well tolerated and causes side effects in only about 4% of patients. Adverse reactions are predominantly hepatic and immunoallergic. Gastrointestinal symptoms are generally transient in nature. Risk factors are age, alcoholism and hepatic disorders (39[R], 82[r]).

Hypersensitivity reactions These are rashes in 0.8%, fever, flu-like syndrome (*malaise*, *headache*) eosinophilia, and much less often hemolytic anemia, hemoglobinuria and kidney damage with acute renal failure. They occur especially during intermittent treatment (less than twice weekly) or after re-institution of RMP therapy. *Anaphylactoid reactions* to RMP have been described in HIV-infected patients (83[c]). Light-chain proteinuria and concomitant kidney damage are attributed to an immunological process (SEDA-10, 273). RMP antibodies have been found using an antiglobulin test (84[C]). Hemolysis as a side effect seems to be mainly of the immune-complex type, exceptionally of the IgG-antibody type (85[C]) (see also 'Hematological').

As a potent microsomal enzyme inducer, RMP decreases the half-life of a large series of compounds (39[R]). This effect appears about 7 days after RMP administration and persists for a few days after it has been stopped.

Tumor-inducing effects Tumor-inducing effects or chromosome aberrations have not been noted in RMP treatment.

ORGANS AND SYSTEMS

Cardiovascular With intermittent RMP therapy or doses higher than 1000 mg/day, or upon reintroduction of RMP treatment, *shock reactions* together with a *'flu-like' syndrome* (fever, chills and myalgias) have been observed most frequently in patients receiving intermittent RMP therapy, doses higher than 1000 mg/day, or upon restarting RMP treatment (39[R], 86[c]). Local *thrombophlebitis* may appear during prolonged intravenous administration.

Respiratory Respiratory symptoms are very rare. They may be part of a *'flu-like' syndrome* with *bronchial obstruction*.

Nervous system RMP-induced neurological symptoms include *drowsiness*, *headache*, *dizziness*, *ataxia*, *generalized numbness*, *pain in the extremities*, *muscular weakness*, *confusion*, *inability to concentrate*, *delusions*, *disorientation*, *hallucinations* and *agitation* (39[R], 87[c]). RMP is widely used in tuberculous and meningococcal meningitis, since it passes into the cerebrospinal fluid (88[C]).

Endocrine, metabolic In patients treated receiving corticosteroids for Addison's disease the beginning of treatment with a drug combination including RMP may necessitate an increase in the corticosteroid dosage. Thus, incipient adrenal insufficiency may be unmasked by RMP (SEDA-13, 261). The phenomenon is due to liver enzyme induction (89[c]).

Combination of rifampicin and isoniazid reduces serum vitamin 25(OH)D_3 concentrations. Rifampicin acts by induction of an enzyme which promotes conversion of 25(OH)D_3 to an inactive metabolite and isoniazid by inhibition of 25- and 1-hydroxylation (SEDA-14, 258). Children or pregnant tuberculous patients have an increased need of calcium supply independent of RMP administration (90[r]). In a series of 132 children of Afro-Asian origin a significant *increase in serum alkaline phosphatase* levels was found. This was more pronounced in patients receiving both isoniazid and RMP, than with isoniazid alone (91[c]). In our opinion the rise in alkaline phosphatase could reflect either a reaction of the liver or of the bone. The possibility of a link between this effect and osteomalacia remains unclear.

Hematological *Thrombocytopenia*, *agranulocytosis*, *leukopenia* and *hemolysis* have been reported (SED-10, 578; 81[c]). Isolated cases of massive hemolysis with or without renal failure, have been observed (92[c], 93[C], 94[C]). Whereas RMP given continuously and in the usual dose is quite safe, it may induce intravascular hemolysis when given intermittently. Antibodies to RMP have been found by several authors, with a positive Coombs' test in the presence of the drug (SEDA-5, 291) more often of the immunocomplex type (89[c], 90[r]) than with IgG or IgM antibodies (93[C], 94[C]). An increased frequency of thrombocytopenia has also been found under intermittent therapy (95[r]). The occurrence of severe hematological disturbances, such as thrombocytopenia and agranulocytosis is a contraindication to continuation of RMP administration. Hemorrhagic states have been induced by RMP in pregnant women and their offspring because of the drug-induced hepatic breakdown of vitamin K (see below). A single case of *disseminated intravascular coagulation* has been reported (95[r]).

Liver RMP is rarely used as monotherapy. The risk of hepatotoxicity appears to be very low in patients with normal liver function, especially if the drug is given continuously. When given with isoniazid, RMP administration may be followed by a fulminant liver reaction. This may be attributable to the *enhancement of isoniazid hepatotoxicity* as a result of enzyme induction by RMP. In some cases the onset of jaundice occurred within 6–10 days after beginning isoniazid + RMP therapy. High serum transaminase levels, disturbances of consciousness and centrilobular necrosis were found. All patients recovered (96[R]).

In a large series of 50 000 patients treated with RMP, 16 deaths associated with jaundice were reported (0.03%) (SED-10, 578; 39[R]). A *rise of transaminase* values in children is very common but rarely necessitates discontinuation of therapy (97[C]).

Total serum bile acid levels have been found to be *elevated* in 72% of 61 patients treated with RMP and isoniazid. In some patients, levels were as much as 40 times above normal. In only four of the 61 patients was the serum bilirubin elevated (98[C]).

Controls of transaminase levels and other liver tests should be performed weekly in cases with liver dysfunction and every 4 weeks in patients with no known liver disease.

Gastrointestinal Intake of RMP during or just after breakfast delays absorption of the drug. Serum levels are lower and the renal secretion of RMP within 24 hours is diminished (99[c]). The reasons for this probably are retarded gastric passage, diminished solubility of the galenic form and perhaps a physical binding of the drug on food. RMP should therefore be taken 1 hour before or 2 hours after meals. *Nausea*, *vomiting*, *epigastric pain*, *diarrhea*, *loss of appetite*, *abdominal cramps* and *meteorism* are frequently restricted to the beginning of RMP therapy. *Gastric burning* may however oblige some patients to take the drug after meals. Upper GI hemorrhage from gastric erosions is a rare complication of RMP treatment (100[c]).

Recently, several authors have reported fairly severe cases of histologically confirmed *pseudomembranous colitis*. Bacteriology revealed mainly *Clostridium difficile* resistant to RMP and several other antibiotics. Discontinuation of RMP and the institution of vancomycin therapy has been helpful (see Chapter 25.2, antibiotic colitis) (SEDA-6, 275; SEDA-7, 310; 101[c]).

Urinary system *Acute renal failure* is a rare complication during continuous treatment but may occur after restarting treatment or during intermittent RMP therapy. This effect is attributed to an immunological process (103[r]). It may or may not be preceded by hemolysis, hemoglobinuria and light-chain proteinuria (104[c]).

A direct antiglobulin test using a whole blood—drug mixture has been recommended as a simple screening test (SEDA-8, 288; SEDA-9, 269; SEDA-10, 273; 105[c], 106[c]) (see also 'Hematological'). Early symptoms of renal failure are *oliguria* and *anuria*, *hematuria* or *hemoglobinuria*. These are very often preceded by hemolysis, or 'flu-like' syndrome. Acute interstitial nephritis has also been described (SEDA-12, 258).

Skin and appendages *Pruritus*, *rashes* and *urticaria* have been reported. *Acne* occurs more frequently in patients receiving RMP and INH combinations than those without RMP (SEDA-9, 270). RMP-induced *porphyria cutanea tarda* has been described in one case, combined with alteration of liver function (107[c]). A patient with *pemphigus foliaceus* induced by RMP (108[c]) and another with exacerbation of *pemphigus vulgaris* during RMP therapy (109[c]) have been observed. Both improved after discontinuation of the drug. Severe bullous reactions have been associated with sub-epidermal detachment typical of *toxic epidermal necrolysis*

(110[c]). After intravenous RMP, a severe cutaneous hypersensibility reaction was described similar to the pattern known as the '*red neck syndrome*' seen after rapid infusion of vancomycin. The reaction responded to an H_1-antagonist (111[c]).

Influenza syndrome Occurrence of *fever*, *headache*, *malaise* and *bone pain* shortly after administration of RMP is well recognized. This reaction has recently been observed in a man on RMP 600 mg monthly for multibacillary leprosy (112). However, the reaction usually occurs with higher doses given weekly or twice weekly. The usual procedure is to reduce the dose or increase the frequency of treatment. Antipyretics may be used to provide symptomatic relief.

Special senses When RMP is combined with isoniazid or with other antituberculous drugs, untoward effects may occur because of the toxicity of these other compounds. When RMP is given alone, no effects on special senses seem to occur.

Immune system In man, there is no evidence that RMP causes clinically significant deleterious effects involving the immune system (113[R]), whereas it may cause immunosuppression in animal models (114[r]). RMP partially suppresses cutaneous hypersensitivity to tuberculin and T-cell function (39[R]).

Local effects Intravenous RMP has been used for several reasons. It may cause *thrombophlebitis*, *local swelling* and *pain* (115[r]).

Risk situations *Intermittent RMP therapy* introduces risks of hematological and renal adverse reactions probably due to immunological mechanisms (see above). Restarting RMP therapy after a drug-free interval has to be carefully guided using small initial doses of about 75 mg/day and increasing to a final dose of about 500–600 mg/day. Monitoring of blood counts, coagulation factors and kidney function is essential. *Chronic alcoholism*, *liver or kidney disease*, *age*, and *immunocompromised conditions* are also important risk factors. Preexisting liver damage or impaired renal function have to be taken into consideration when calculating the dosage of RMP. Close supervision is essential during the entire duration of treatment.

In patients with suspected *disorders of vitamin D and calcium metabolism* caution has to be taken in RMP therapy (SEDA-9, 269), see also 'Interactions' below.

Second-generation effects Drug companies having much experience with this drug advise against using RMP during the first 3 months of pregnancy, even though deleterious effects on the fetus have not been confirmed in man. Indeed, the drug is known to cross the placenta but the teratogenicity of RMP is uncertain. RMP may not be as innocuous during pregnancy as isoniazid or ethambutol (SEDA-6, 277; 52[C]). During lactation there are no contraindications for RMP. Only small amounts of the drug pass into the milk with no relevant effects for the newborn.

The induction of hepatic microsomal enzymes by RMP is believed to be the cause of *vitamin K deficiency* which has led to *hemorrhagic disturbances* in pregnant women and newborns. Therefore, prophylactic treatment with vitamin K should be given to all mothers and their offspring when the mother has received RMP during late pregnancy. Blood coagulation tests should be done on both (SEDA-8, 288). No deleterious influence on fertility has been documented.

Overdosage Severe overdosage has been observed in inadvertent administration of an excessive dose of RMP in children (116[C]) and also in suicidal attempts (117[c]–119[c]). It can also occur when there is impaired hepatic function or severe renal insufficiency (see above). Symptoms are *nausea*, *vomiting*, *headache*, *abdominal pain*, *diarrhea*, *pruritus*. A '*red man syndrome*', simply caused by the red color of the drug, has been described (SED-10, 579).

Interactions Antacids lower the bioavailability of RMP. Aluminium hydroxide gel, magnesium trisilicate and sodium bicarbonate reduce bioavailability to a significant degree (102[c]). RMP itself interferes with the metabolism of many drugs due to its intense microsomal enzyme-inducing activity.

Resumption of RMP after general anesthesia is a high risk condition since narcotics themselves are enzyme inducers. *Digoxin* and *digitoxin* plasma levels may be lowered by RMP treatment and the dosage of these drugs has to be adjusted to the serum concentration (SEDA-10, 272). Similar controls have to be performed when *quinidine* is used. Elimination of *nifedipine* is enhanced by RMP (SEDA-14, 259).

It is well known that RMP enhances the catabolism of many *corticosteroids*. The interaction is highly significant. RMP increases the plasma clearance of *prednisolone* by 45% and may reduce the amount of drug available to the tissues by as much as 66% (SEDA-8, 288). Corticosteroid therapy for concomitant diseases should therefore be adjusted in the light of plasma levels and clinical effects during RMP treatment (see also 'Endocrine, metabolic') (SEDA-10, 272). For example, rejection of a kidney transplant has been observed 7 weeks after initiation of RMP (120[c]).

Ethinylestradiol and similar steroids used as contraceptives show reduced serum levels during RMP therapy. It is therefore not surprising that unexpected pregnancies have occurred (121[C]). Oral hypoglycemic agents and oral anticoagulants of the coumarin type undergo accelerated metabolism in patients on RMP treatment (122[c], 123[c]). This is also true for the β-blocker *propranolol* (SEDA-9, 269).

The antifungal agent *ketoconazole* interacts with RMP and serum levels of both drugs are decreased (SEDA-9, 269). *Methadone* metabolism is also increased and the precipitation of withdrawal syndromes has been reported (39[R]).

Blood levels of *haloperidol* are decreased during RMP administration due to shortening of haloperidol half-life (SEDA-12, 258, 124[c]).

Low cyclosporin blood levels and acute graft rejection in a renal transplant recipient during prophylactic RMP therapy has been observed (125[C]). RMP significantly decreases the half-life of *antipyrine* (phenazone) (126[c]). RMP was found to increase metabolic clearance of *theophylline* by 45% in a series of volunteers, especially after intravenous application (127[c]). In one patient with paroxysmal supraventricular tachycardia receiving *verapamil* and RMP the lack of clinical effect of verapamil was probably due to a similar interaction (128[c]). A complete review of interactions between RMP and many other drugs such as *clofibrate*, *clonidine*, *diazepam*, *mexiletine*, *probenecid*, *trimethoprim* and *dapsone* has been published (129[C]).

Interference with diagnostic procedures *Excretion of contrast media through the bile* may be impaired during RMP therapy (39[R], 130[R]).

Ethambutol

Ethambutol (EMB) is tuberculostatic and acts against *M. tuberculosis* and *M. kansasii* as well as number of strains of *M. avium* complex. It has no effect on other bacteria. The sensitivities of NTM are variable. EMB suppresses the growth of most isoniazid- and streptomycin-resistant tubercle bacteria (131[R]). About 80% of an oral dose of EMB is absorbed from the gastrointestinal tract. Plasma peak levels are reached in 2–4 hours and half-life is 3–4 hours. Within 24 hours, about 60% is excreted unchanged in the urine by tubular secretion and glomerular filtration. In persons with renal insufficiency the dose has thus to be adapted (39[R]). There is no indication for EMB monotherapy.

ADVERSE REACTION PATTERN

General and toxic reactions Side effects of ethambutol are mainly observed in patients treated with very high doses, i.e. over 25 mg/kg/day; doses below 20 mg are therefore recommended. Of the side effects, visual disturbances are the most common and also the most important. These include diminished visual acuity, retrobulbar neuritis, retinal pigment displacement and (rarely) hemorrhages.

Gastrointestinal symptoms with abdominal pain or vomiting, as well as headache, dizziness, mental confusion and hallucinations are all rarely seen. Side effects are more frequent in elderly patients, alcoholics, diabetics and in patients with renal failure.

Hypersensitivity reactions Various exanthemas, Stevens-Johnson syndrome (132[c]), 'toxic' epidermal necrolysis (133[c]), purpura-like vasculitis, acute thrombogenic purpura, joint pain, drug fever, tachycardia and leukopenia have been attributed to hypersensitivity. As these reactions often arise during combined treatment with other tuberculostatics, it is difficult or impossible to determine which drug is responsible.

Tumor-inducing and teratogenic effects These have not been described.

ORGANS AND SYSTEMS

Nervous system *Peripheral neuropathy* may precede or accompany ocular damage. These symptoms may possibly serve as warning of impending eye damage (134[c]). Loss of sensitivity with numbness and tingling of the fingers are relatively rare side effects (135[c]). Electroneuromyography in ethambutol-induced neuropathy has confirmed that elderly patients are at increased risk (136[c]). Sensory changes are more severe than motor dysfunction (135[c]).

Endocrine, metabolic *Blood urate levels* can be increased due to diminished excretion of uric acid in 66% of patients treated with ethambutol (137[c]). This tendency is probably enhanced in combined treatment with isoniazid and pyridoxine. Special attention should be paid when antituberculous drug combinations include pyrazinamide. However, severe untoward clinical effects are rare, except in patients with gout or impaired kidney function (39[R], 138[R]).

Hematological Acute *thrombocytopenia*, probably due to an immunological mechanism, has been described in a single patient (139[c]).

Liver Jaundice and non-icteric liver disturbances are probably seen in less than 0.1% of treated patients as long as INH and RMP are not given simultaneously.

Urinary system In patients with impaired glomerular filtration or any other renal dysfunction, ethambutol doses have to be adapted to the serum creatinine level (140[C]).

Special senses *Ocular disturbances* are, to a certain degree, dose-dependent (141[C]). Doses not exceeding 25 mg/kg/day during the first 2 months of treatment and 15 mg/kg/day thereafter are generally accepted as adequate by most therapeutic centers (142[R]). At a dose of 15 mg/kg/day, which should be regarded as a maximum for maintenance therapy, ocular toxicity developed in only 1.6% (143[r]). The earliest onset of visual disturbance was observed in a 26-year-old man 3 days after beginning combined treatment containing 15 mg/kg/day ethambutol. This suggests an idiosyncratic reaction to the drug (144[c]). Advanced age (145[c]), renal insufficiency or diabetes may enhance ocular damage.

Biochemical research has revealed the importance of zinc metabolism in the retina (145[c]). This metal is found in high concentrations in the choroid, the retina and especially the ganglion cells. Retinol dehydrogenase, itself a zinc-containing enzyme, interferes with the transformation of retinol (vitamin A_1), which is essential for the color sense and conal vision. Furthermore, zinc is involved in the biosynthesis of the specific transport protein of retinol from the liver to the effector cells. EMB is a chelating agent and makes zinc unavailable for axoplasmatic transport, provoking optic or retrobulbar neuritis (146[C]). Patients with zinc blood levels lower than 0.70 mg/l (normal 0.9–1.0 mg/l) before the onset of EMB compose a high-risk group for ocular disturbances (147[C]).

The onset of visual loss may be sudden and dramatic with color vision defects in the red–green or blue–yellow ranges as well as variable field defects. In acute cases, disc edema is accompanied by splinter hemorrhages. Retrobulbar neuritis in ethambutol treatment may be predominantly axial, presenting with reduced visual acuity and central scotoma, or periaxial with peripheral field defects. In non-acute types the fundi and discs appear normal (130[C]). Visual defects may be unilateral or bilateral.

Visual-evoked potential tests such as flash electroretinography, flash and pattern visual-evoked responses, flicker fusion thresholds and visual fields are reported to be the most reliable methods for early detection of ocular abnormalities (143[r], 146[C], 148[r]). The routine use of visual-evoked potentials in the systematic follow-up of ethambutol-treated patients has been recommended (148[r]).

Color vision as well as visual acuity should be examined before the onset of ethambutol treatment and every 2–4 weeks during treatment using color tables and reading tests (SED-9, 525). Computerized perimetry of the central visual fields is recommended by a number of authors (SED-10, 581). Early childhood, when visual examination is difficult or impossible, is a major indication for the electroretinogram. As a rule, EMB is not recommended for children under 5 years of age because of the difficulty to reliably test their visual acuity.

Side effects are slowly reversible after discontinuation of the drug. If the drug is not stopped, optic atrophy or permanent blindness may occur. Patients therefore have to be instructed to interrupt treatment if any visual abnormality is experienced. Hydroxocobalamin may accelerate recovery (149[c]).

Risk situations In *diabetics with retinopathy* monthly controls of the visual acuity and fundi are mandatory.

Second-generation effects No evident fetal damage or toxic effects in the newborn related to ethambutol treatment of the mother during pregnancy or lactation have been published (72[C], 150[C]). EMB administered in combination with INH in pregnancy has been suspected of causing one case of gastrointestinal malformation but other factors may have been implicated (SEDA-12, 256).

Overdosage Doses higher than 25 mg/kg/day should only be administered for about 2 weeks at the beginning of therapy. Treatment may then be continued at 15 mg/kg/day. If initial problems arise and EMB is essential, the daily dose should not exceed 10 mg/kg/day.

Interactions Untoward effects may be enhanced when ethambutol is combined with *isoniazid* or *rifampicin*.

Pyrazinamide

Pyrazinamide is a pyrazine analog of nicotinamide and is one of the first-line antituberculous drugs. It is bactericidal for *Mycobacterium tuberculosis* in an acid environment and inside macrophages (39[R]). A pyrazinamide-containing regimen has produced significantly more rapid rates of sputum conversion than any other combination. Pyrazinamide is therefore especially appropriate for the initial phase of treatment. In the 6-month regimen of the American Thoracic Society, pyrazinamide is proposed together with isoniazid and rifampicin during the first 2 months. This has been widely applied (6[R]).

Pyrazinamide is distributed throughout the body. Peak plasma levels are reached 2 hours after oral administration. Excretion is primarily by glomerular filtration. Serum concentrations generally range from 30 to 50 μg/ml with daily doses of 20—25 mg/kg. The maximum daily dose should not exceed 3 grams, regardless of weight. At a pH of 5.5, the minimal inhibitory concentration of pyrazinamide for *M. tuberculosis* is 20 μg/ml (39[R]).

ADVERSE REACTION PATTERN

General and toxic reactions Most of the side effects seem to be toxic rather than allergic. Particularly, reactions involving the liver, hyperuricemia with and without gout, and symptoms of pellagra have been recognized. *Fever* and *urticaria* are described. Also, *sideroblastic anemia*, *thrombocytopenia*, *anorexia*, *nausea and vomiting*, *dysuria*, *malaise* and aggravation of *peptic ulcer* may occur (SEDA-13, 261).

Hypersensitivity reactions and tumor-inducing effects These have not been reported.

ORGANS AND SYSTEMS

Endocrine, metabolic Pyrazinamide interferes with renal excretion of urates, resulting in hyperuricemia. Acute episodes of gout or arthralgia have occurred (151[C]).

Pyrazinamide as well as isoniazid can induce *pellagra* symptoms. However, the prophylactic administration of nicotinamide is not generally recommended. In case of pellagra manifestations a dose of 300 mg daily should be given (152[c]).

Pyrazinamide may aggravate *porphyria* (153[c]).

Liver *Liver damage* is the most common side effect of pyrazinamide (154[c]). It varies from an asymptomatic alteration of hepatic cell function detectable only by laboratory tests, through a mild syndrome characterized by fever, anorexia, malaise, liver tenderness, hepatomegaly and splenomegaly, to more serious reactions with clinical jaundice, and finally the rare form with progressive acute yellow atrophy and death. As most patients receive a combined regimen of pyrazinamide with isoniazid and rifampicin, it is difficult to determine which of the three drugs causes the hepatotoxicity. It could be due to a combined effect (155[R]). As with INH and RMP treatment, hepatic function should initially be monitored every few weeks.

Skin and appendages Urticaria and maculo-papular exanthema may occur. Photosensitization has been described rarely (156[R]).

Risk situations Pyrazinamide should be avoided in patients with *liver disease* and *porphyria* (39[R], 153[c]). Liver tests are to be repeated at frequent intervals during the entire period of treatment. The drug has to be used with extreme caution in patients with a history of *gout*, especially in the elderly in whom urinary urate stones may induce renal failure (151[c]). In patients with *hemoptysis* the possibility that pyrazinamide may have an adverse effect on blood clotting time or vascular integrity should be borne in mind (151[c]).

Streptomycin

See 'Aminoglycosides', Chapter 26.

MISCELLANEOUS ANTITUBERCULOUS DRUGS

Drugs of second and third order have been largely eliminated during the past years and partly replaced by first-order drugs. They are now only administered in combination for patients exhibiting adverse reactions to the usual first-order drugs or with multiresistant mycobacteria (see Introduction to this Chapter). In some parts of the world, they remain important because of their relatively low cost.

Ethionamide

Ethionamide is a synthetic derivative of thioisonicotinamide. It is only administered orally.

The initial dosage for adults is 250 mg daily. It is then slowly increased up to 15—20 mg/kg/day (maximum 1 gram).

Untoward effects involve several organ systems. *Nausea*, *vomiting* and *anorexia* reflect gastric intolerance. The drug is best taken with meals. *Mental depression*, *asthenia*, *drowsiness* and *hypotension* are not rare. Other neurological reactions include *diplopia*, *olfactory disturbances*, *metallic taste*, *dizziness*, *paresthesia*, *headache* and *tremor*. *Severe allergic skin reactions*, *alopecia*, *acne* and *purpura* may occur. Acute rheumatic symptoms and difficulty in the management of diabetes have been reported. Since hepatitis is seen in about 5% of the cases treated with ethionamide, frequent controls of liver function are compulsory (39[R]). As a rare side effect, a case of goitrous *hypothyroidism* has been described (157[c]). Recovery occurred after discontinuation. In vitro studies have shown that ethionamide inhibits both the uptake of iodine and its incorporation into trichloroacetic acid-precipitable protein (154[c]). *Gynecomastia*, *impotence* and *menorrhagia* have also been observed. For teratogenic effect, see under 'Prothionamide'. Ethionamide is not available in all countries.

Ethionamide and prothionamide have often proved to be effective in NTM infections.

Prothionamide

Prothianimide, a pyridine derivative of ethionamide, has better gastric tolerance than ethionamide. Patients with a history of stomach ulcer, however, are still susceptible to gastric problems. Control of liver function tests is necessary during long-term treatment. Thionamides lower the blood sugar level and also have an appetite-suppressant action which influences carbohydrate intake. Menstrual disturbances, gynecomastia and amenorrhea may occur. Prothionamide may cause acneform eruptions, photodermatitis and hair loss. The nervous system can be influenced in the same way as by ethionamide. In view of their *teratogenic* effect neither ethionamide nor protionamide should be administered during the first trimester of pregnancy.

Thioacetazone

Thioacetazone (thiacetazone, thiosemicarbazone, TSC) was received enthusiastically in 1946 as one of the first synthetic agents against tuberculosis. Its use rapidly diminished with the observation of increasing untoward effects, and partly to its chemical structure and partly due to overdosage. At present it is rarely used and, if at all, mostly for economical reasons. Doses should never exceed 200 mg/day. Side effects include bone marrow depression with anemia, leukopenia, agranulocytosis and thrombocytopenia (158[c], 159[c], 156[R]). Hemolytic anemia has also been described. Adverse reactions of the skin are of various types, mainly *erythematous* and *maculopapular exanthema*, *angioedema*, *purpura* (160[C]), *toxic epidermal necrolysis*, *Stevens-Johnson syndrome* and *pigmentation* (161[c]). *Anorexia*, *nausea* and *vomiting* are not uncommon. Hepatotoxicity with jaundice is frequent. For all these reasons, continuous laboratory and clinical observations are required (39[R]). *Cutaneous hypersensitivity in HIV-positive patients* is very frequent; in the order of 20%. EMB should therefore be used instead of thiacetazone in these patients (162[c]).

A chromosome-damaging action of thioacetazone combined with isoniazid (and possibly of thioacetazone alone) on human lymphocyte cultures has been reported (163[C]).

Thioacetazone is also effective against leprosy.

Rifabutin

Rifabutin, a spiropiperidyl derivative of rifamycin, is more effective in vitro against *M. tuberculosis* than rifampicin. This substance has a longer half-life, a better tissue penetration and a lower enzymatic inductive action than rifampicin. Rifabutin is well absorbed in the gastrointestinal tract and reaches a peak serum level of about 0.5 μg/ml 4 hours after a single dose of 300 mg.

A 300-mg dose of rifabutin is usually well tolerated. Adverse effects include neutropenia, thrombocytopenia, rash, and gastrointestinal disturbances (nausea, flatulence). Myositis (164[R]) and uveitis (165[cr]) are rarely observed.

Cycloserine

Cycloserine is an amino-isoxazolidone which shows no cross-resistance with other tuberculostatic agents. The drug is usually given orally and may accumulate to attain toxic concentrations in patients with renal failure. Untoward effects involve the central nervous system and appear as *headache*, *somnolence*, *tremor*, *mood*, *cognitive deterioration*, *dysarthria*, *confusion* and even *psychotic crises*. The drug is contraindicated in individuals with a history of epilepsy. Because of its high toxicity, cycloserine should only be used when microorganisms are resistant to other drugs (relapse or primary resistance) (166[R]).

Amikacin

See 'Aminoglycosides'. Chapter 26.

Capreomycin
Kanamycin

These two drugs are of very little use in tuberculosis and should never be combined with streptomycin or other aminoglycosides because of their nephro- and ototoxicity. Presently, they are hardly available on the market. A *Bartter-like syndrome* has been reported in a 25-year-old man receiving prolonged treatment with capreomycin for drug-resistant pulmonary tuberculosis (167[r]). Marked renal loss of sodium, chloride, potassium and magnesium with progressive metabolic alkalosis and hyperreninemia were recorded. In rare cases, capreomycin may be administered in NTM infections when multiple drug resistance to the first-order antituberculous drugs is present (39[R]).

PROBLEMS WITH COMBINED THERAPY

As a rule, a regimen of two or three of the five first-line tuberculocidal drugs (isoniazid, rifampicin, pyrazinamide, ethambutol and streptomycin) is used in tuberculosis (3[R]). The 6-month short-course regimen consists of isoniazid, rifampicin and pyrazinamide for 2 months, followed by isoniazid and rifampicin for 4 months (6[R]). It may be advisable to include ethambutol in the initial phase when isoniazid resistance is suspected. A 9-month regimen consisting of isoniazid and rifampicin is also highly successful (3[R]). In principle, treatment should always include at least two drugs to which the mycobacteria are susceptible.

Treatment problems that may arise are mainly of two types:
(a) Development of *secondary resistance of Mycobacterium tuberculosis*, *M. bovis* or NTM to one or more of the tuberculocidal drugs. This situation probably only occurs when the patient has not taken the full combination of drugs all the time. A mixed combination preparation is thus particularly useful.
(b) Adverse reactions, either of *toxic or allergic* origin.

As regards the second problem, reactions in a given organ may often be due to at least two different drugs. Even hypersensitivity reactions may occur to more than one agent.

If *liver damage* occurs, isoniazid is probably an important factor and should be stopped before rifampicin or pyrazinamide. In the case of *renal insufficiency*, streptomycin or second-order tuberostatic drugs with renal toxicity should be immediately discontinued.

In *nervous system disorders*, ethambutol is the most likely drug to cause visual disturbances. Isoniazid is associated with polyneuritis and reactions of the central nervous system. Streptomycin may cause eighth nerve toxicity.

These simple rules reflect the principle that the most probable causative agent (or agents) must be stopped.

In *allergic reactions*, the drug most probably responsible may be even more difficult to identify, since the same kind of reaction can occur independently of the chemical nature of the drug. For evaluation of allergic drug reactions, the analysis of time relationships (duration of exposure, reaction time, drug-free interval before re-exposure) are extremely important (see also Chapter 25.1). Particularly in allergic reactions to rifampicin, intermittent treatment or re-exposure after a drug free-interval may favor sensitization and occurrence. Depending upon the severity of the side effects one, two or all drugs must be stopped until the adverse reaction has completely disappeared. The use of second-order tuberculostatic drugs may sometimes be necessary. In patients with drug fever or common exanthematous reactions, specific desensitization under clinical conditions may be attempted, at least with isoniazid (168[c]). In more severe reactions with anaphylactic shock, agranulocytosis, thrombocytopenia, Lyell's syndrome (toxic epidermal necrolysis) or Stevens-Johnson syndrome, specific desensitization should not be considered (see isoniazid monograph) and the drug has to be definitively discarded from the combination.

DRUGS USED IN LEPROSY

GENERAL REMARKS ON LEPROSY

Leprosy presents a broad spectrum of clinical lesions, depending on the individual's resistance to the disease. Several clinical types are recognized (SED-12, 761; SEDA-15, 331; SEDA-17, 352; 39[R], 169[R], 170[R]).

Paucibacillary leprosy (*PB*): indeterminate (I); tuberculoid (TT); borderline tuberculoid (BT); primary neuritic (PN).

Multibacillary leprosy (*MB*): mid-borderline (BB); borderline lepromatous (BL); lepromatous (LL).

In 1982, the WHO Study Group on Chemotherapy of Leprosy for control programmes recommended classification of patients into paucibacillary and multibacillary leprosy for the purpose of administering multidrug therapy (MDT).

The above-mentioned types of leprosy show distinct cutaneous manifestations, histological findings and immune reactions to lepromin. The course of disease and the density of *Mycobacterium leprae* vary from one type to another.

With progressive untreated disease the highly bacilliferous lepromatous type may evolve from the untreated indeterminate, tuberculoid and borderline type of leprosy. A lepromatous case may regress to borderline type with adequate treatment or, if inadequately treated, resistant *M. leprae* may develop (171[R]—173[R]).

AVOIDANCE OF MONOTHERAPY

The WHO instructions as well as the worldwide opinion of clinicians dealing with large-scale leprosy therapy programs agree on the need for long-term multidrug treatment in order to avoid development of drug resistance (169[R], 174[C], 175[C]). The major antileprosy drugs are: dapsone, clofazimine (Lamprene®), rifampicin

(RMP), ethionamide and prothionamide (176[R]). Use of RMP is essential in the therapy of all types of leprosy. According to many authors, RMP given as little as 600 mg once monthly is as effective as the same daily dose. Also for economic reasons, this monthly schedule is now recommended for all types of leprosy in combination with other drugs (177[C]). Strains of *M. leprae* resistant to dapsone, RMP or ethionamide have been isolated from patients taking these drugs as monotherapy.

RMP given monthly does not seem to induce the 'flu-like' syndrome or acute allergic thrombocytopenia (SEDA-5, 297) which has been noted especially with RMP administered two to three times weekly in tuberculosis. RMP given alone, or with incorrect irregular or inadequate low doses of dapsone, results in secondary resistance to the drug (178[C]). RMP is strongly bactericidal, ethionamide intermediate, dapsone and clofazimine weakly bactericidal against *M. leprae*.

Leprosy in children (age 0–14) is well controlled with 1–2 mg/kg/day of dapsone plus 10–20 mg/kg/month of RMP and 1–2 mg/kg/day of clofazimine (179[C], 180[c]). The regression of the disease under this multidrug treatment program proves its effectiveness. No special side effects are noted with this combination.

Thalidomide has been found to be the drug of choice for the erythema nodosum leprosum type of reaction in leprosy (181[c]). Patients treated with this drug showed a significant increase in T-helper cell lymphocytes. The grave teratogenic effects of this drug naturally mean that strict precautions must be taken to avoid its use in women of child bearing age.

In relapsing patients, corticosteroid therapy may be useful. In a study of 36 patients with lepromatous leprosy, those with active disease showed a decrease in hydrocortisone reserve after a loading dose of insulin. In patients in remission, however, a partial restoration of reserve cortisol production could be demonstrated (182[c]).

Lepromatous leprosy patients may be immunocompromised due to the extensive disease or because of corticosteroid treatment for repeated reactions. Such patients are likely to be at higher risk for developing opportunistic infections. A patient with lepromatous leprosy and repeated lepra reactions has been reported who was found to have pulmonary infection due to *M. fortuitum*. It would therefore seem wise to recommend mycobacterial culture and sensitivity testing in immunocompromised patients whose pathological specimens contain acid-fast bacilli (183[c]).

Chemoprophylaxis with dapsone is a controversial issue. It is not recommended by the WHO for large-scale control programs.

Drugs available for the treatment of leprosy can be divided into three groups: primary, secondary and investigational.

The primary drugs include dapsone, clofazimine and rifampicin.

Dapsone

Dapsone is 4,4-diaminodiphenylsulfone (DDS, avlosulfone, disulfone) (SEDA-17, 352). It is a bacteriostatic antileprosy agent with a chemical structure resembling sulfonamides. The dosage of dapsone should be 50–100 mg daily for adults, based on body weight (184[c]). For children aged 3–5 years, the dose should be reduced according to weight to, e.g., 25 mg daily (185[R]).

To what extent phenotype differences (fast versus slow acetylators) influence the metabolism of dapsone remains controversial. Since dapsone is acetylated in the liver, an effect might be anticipated (SEDA-4, 217; 186[C]), but has not been demonstrated.

Studies of patients with borderline leprosy suggested that dapsone had mild immunosuppressive effects (SEDA 18, 30). Thus, dapsone was given with some success to patients suffering from dermatitis herpetiformis, subcorneal pustular dermatosis, bullous dermatoses, relapsing polychondritis, thrombocytopenic purpura (187[c]), giant cell arteritis (188[c]), rheumatoid arthritis and systemic lupus erythematosus (189[c]).

ADVERSE REACTION PATTERN

General and toxic reactions The most common untoward effect is hemolysis of varying degree, usually mild except in patients with glucose-6-phosphate deshydrogenase (G6PD) deficiency. Methemoglobinemia and Heinz-body formation are also found.

Mild gastrointestinal complaints and neurological side effects induced by dapsone are not uncommon. Dapsone may induce peripheral neuropathy in patients taking very large doses. However, this reaction is especially seen when dapsone is used for diseases other than leprosy.

The sulfones may occasionally provoke an exacerbation of lepromatous leprosy, the so-called '*sulfone syndrome*' or '*dapsone syndrome*' (SEDA-16, 347). This syndrome resembles mononucleosis and may develop 3–6 weeks after initiation of treatment in malnourished patients. It includes *fever, malaise, pruritis exfoliative dermatitis, polyarthritis* (190[c]), jaundice even with hepatic necrosis, lymphadenopathy, methemoglobinemia and anemia. This syndrome is accompanied by the formation of atypical T-lymphocytes with markedly increased spontaneous tritiated thymidine uptake (SEDA-8, 289). The full syndrome is probably rare, but it is important to recognize its partial expression (191[r], 189[c], 192[c]). A clinical resemblance of the *dapsone syndrome* and acute infectious mononucleosis has been noted (193[c], SEDA-16, 347). It has been suggested that the *dapsone syndrome* has become more common since the introduction of multidrug therapy (194[C]), especially since rifampicin and dapsone have been routinely used together. The '*dapsone syndrome*' usually resolves rapidly after discontinuation of dapsone therapy and with corticosteroid treatment. However, it may also end in a fatal hypersensitivity reaction (SEDA-12, 259).

Hypoalbuminemia has been seen after prolonged dapsone therapy of dermatitis herpetiformis (195[c]).

Erythema nodosum leprosum may be due to an immune complex mechanism. The antigen is provided by the bacteria and their degeneration products, possibly as a kind of Jarisch-Herxheimer reaction (196[R]).

Hypersensitivity reactions Anaphylactic shock and tachycardia are rare. Rashes, serious cutaneous reactions and erythema nodosum might have an immunological basis.

Tumor-inducing effects These have not been reported.

ORGANS AND SYSTEMS

Cardiovascular *Anaphylactic shock* and *tachycardia* are among the most severe hypersensitivity reactions (194[C]). Signs of heart failure with edema, ascites and severe hypoalbuminemia have been described in the treatment of dermatitis herpetiformis (195[c]).

Nervous system Isolated cases of dapsone-induced *peripheral neuropathy* have been published (197[C], 198[C]). Severe motor and minor sensory neuropathy in a patient who received dapsone for 16 years for dermatitis herpetiformis has been reported. The clinical characteristics of this manifestation include a motor neuropathy affecting the extremities with onset within 5 years after the initiation of dapsone therapy at doses of ≥300 mg/day. Almost always complete recovery from the neuropathy occurs after the dose is reduced or the drug withdrawn. It should be mentioned that infection with *M. leprae* affects the peripheral nerves and the dermis, causing an accumulation of macrophages and other immune cells at the infected site (199[R]).

Dapsone-induced *psychosis* has rarely been reported (SEDA-15, 331; 200[c]).

Hematological The most common side effect of dapsone therapy remains *hemolysis* (SEDA-15, 331). In varying degrees it develops in nearly all patients receiving dapsone in doses of 200—300 mg/day. Even with the usual dose of 100 mg/day in normal persons and 50 mg/day in patients with a G6PD deficiency, some degree of hemolysis may already occur (39[R], 201[C]). Red cell survival may be reduced in dapsone therapy depending upon the doses of the sulfones and their oxidizing activity, but hemolytic anemia generally does not occur without a pre-existing disorder of the erythrocytes or bone marrow. The hemolysis may be so severe that manifestations of hypoxia become striking (39[R]). Mild hemolytic anemia was found in a breast-fed infant and his mother who had continuously been taking 100—150 mg dapsone daily. Dapsone and its metabolite, monoacetyl dapsone, were identified in the infant's serum (SEDA-8, 290). Agranulocytosis is a rare complication of dapsone treatment (202[R]).

Dapsone is an oxidant and can trigger *methemoglobinemia* and delayed *sulfhemoglobinemia* formation (SEDA-8, 289). Methemoglobinemia remains subclinical in most cases. However, its presence can be accurately inferred by a discrepancy between oxygen saturation measured by pulse oximetry and the concentration of oxygen in the arterial blood (203[c]). *Methemoglobinemia* at concentrations over 10% produces a visible lavender-colored cyanosis and concentrations over 35% result in weakness and shortness of breath. Methemoglobinemia can be minimized by the administration of an antioxidant such as *vitamins* C or E (204[c]). *Methemoglobinemia* disappears after withdrawal of dapsone (SEDA-10, 273).

Liver Jaundice and hepatitis have rarely been mentioned as untoward reactions to dapsone. Previous liver damage may predispose to serious hepatic or other side effects.

Urinary system If impaired renal function is present, the dosage of dapsone has to be reduced. Renal failure may be associated with severe hemolytic conditions.

Skin and appendages *Pruritus* and various forms of *rash* may occur. Serious cutaneous reactions such as *exfoliative dermatitis*, '*toxic*' *epidermal necrolysis and erythema multiforme bullosum* are extremely rare. *Erythema nodosum leprosum* has been described during dapsone therapy, mostly in the lepromatous type of leprosy (196[c]). If *erythema nodosum* develops prior to the beginning of therapy, drug administration should be withheld until this reaction has disappeared. Severe *erythema nodosum* can be controlled by short-term *corticosteroid* therapy. Desensitization to dapsone in patients with hypersensitivity reactions has been proposed (205[C]).

Special senses Ocular toxicity is a rare untoward reaction to *dapsone*. Decreased visual acuity was described after an overdose during an attempted suicide (206[c]).

Intramuscular administration Aqueous or oily suspensions for intramuscular injection may be used for better compliance and to prevent resistance due to irregular drug intake of the drug. Therapeutic efficacy of intramuscular preparations lasts for 3—4 weeks (207[C]).

Risk situations *Undernourishment*, *immunodeficiency*, *previous liver damage* or *impaired kidney function* predispose to side effects during dapsone therapy. G6PD deficiency is a risk factor for hemolytic anemia. The acetylator type does not markedly influence the side effects of dapsone.

Second-generation effects Dapsone passes into the milk of nursing mothers but usually no side effects are noted in the newborn (see 'Hematological'). The use of antileprosy drugs during pregnancy depends upon the severity of the disease and the relative need for treatment. Even though untoward effects on the fetus have not been reported, leprosy treatment during pregnancy probably predisposes to *erythema nodosum leprosum*. If this is present during pregnancy, clofazimine is considered the best drug available today (208[R]).

Interactions In a series of 28 patients with lepromatous leprosy the patients were given dapsone. *Clofazimine* was added and did not influence urinary excretion except in one case. When *rifampicin* was given, dapsone blood levels were lowered and urinary excretion was increased during the first 2 days of administration. Blood levels, however, remained within the therapeutic range (209[C]).

Acedapsone (diacetyl derivative of dapsone, DADDS)

With this repository sulfone, plasma levels are much lower than with standard oral dapsone and could enhance the emergence of resistant strains of *M. leprae*.

The effects and adverse reactions are similar to those of dapsone.

Clofazimine

Clofazimine is weakly bactericidal against *M. leprae*. It is active in chronic skin ulcers (Buruli ulcer) and partly against *M. avium intracellulare*. The usual adult dosage is 50—100 mg daily. At higher doses, its anti-inflammatory effect seems to prevent the development of acute reactions such as erythema nodosum leprosum.

Intraneural deposition of a ceroid-like pigment has been observed following treatment of lepromatous leprosy with clofazimine (210[c]). This pigment does not affect the healing process. Treatment may be continued, provided that the dose is not too high.

Clofazimine is a strongly lipophilic dye and accumulates, especially in fat, bile, macrophages, the reticuloendothelial system and skin. This is the basis of adverse reactions, including skin discoloration (211[c]). *Pigmentation* as well as purple skin discoloration are the most frequent side effects of clofazimine therapy. The drug is therefore unacceptable to most light-skinned patients (212[C]). Ichthyosis is very frequent after clofazimine therapy at doses above 100 mg/day (SEDA-8, 290).

Nail changes, such as brown discoloration of the nail plate and onycholysis, were described in patients on high doses (300 mg/day) of clofazimine (213[c]). Clofazimine crystals were demonstrated in the nail and the nail bed.

In a series of 76 patients on MDT including clofazimine for at least 6 months, 46% had *conjunctival deposition*, 53% had deposition in the cornea, and crystals were found in the tears of 32% (214[C]). Conjunctival pigmentation has been reported, as well as reversible linear brownish corneal streaks. Two cases of macular pigmentation have also been described (SEDA-5, 294).

Clofazimine crystals were observed in the alveolar macrophages of a patient with AIDS. This is considered harmless (215[c]).

Lymphedema (216[c]), *diminished sweating* and *reduced tearing* have been observed (202[R]).

Other side effects are *nausea*, *vomiting*, *diarrhea*, *abdominal pain* and *anorexia*. Clofazimine may accumulate and precipitate in tissues, such as the wall of the small bowel, after prolonged administration. Enteropathy may develop if crystals are stored in the lamina propria of the jejunal mucosa and the mesenteric lymph nodes. These findings are dependent on the dose and duration of therapy. In cases where this complication is suspected jejunal biopsy is indicated. At laparotomy, all organs may have an orange—yellow color (SEDA-9, 272; 211[c], 217[r]). Upon drug withdrawal the enteropathy progressively improves.

According to clinical observations, clofazimine is able

to inhibit the liver damage associated with lepromatous leprosy and the leprosy reaction. It has only a minimal or no deleterious effect on liver function (218[C]).

Rifampicin *(see also 'Drugs used in tuberculosis')*

Hepatotoxicity of combined therapy for leprosy has been reported in a series of 39 patients treated with dapsone, prothionamide and rifampicin (RMP). A group of 50 patients treated with *dapsone*, *clofazimine*, *RMP* and *prothionamide* showed similar findings. Fatalities probably related to the drugs occurred in both groups after 3–4 months of treatment (219[C]). The drug responsible for liver injury may have been *prothionamide*, although RMP administered simultaneously could also have contributed (219[C]).

In 33 leprosy patients treated with a RMP drug combination no *'flu-like' syndrome* or antibodies to rifampicin-conjugated proteins were observed (220[C]). The case of a patient with acute renal failure attributed to monthly administered RMP in a multidrug regimen has been reported. *Renal failure* recovered after cessation of treatment (221[c]).

Probenecid given before administration of RMP may increase the serum level of RMP. Serum levels of the drug were comparable after 300 mg RMP and 1 gram of probenecid or 450 mg without probenecid. This may reduce costs and *hepatotoxicity* in long-term antileprosy therapy (222[cr]).

OTHER DRUGS USED IN LEPROSY

Secondary drugs consist of *ethionamide*, the *long-acting sulfonamides*, *thiacetazone*, and certain *aminoglucosides*.

Ethionamide

The dosage of ethionamide and prothionamide should be 250–300 mg daily. Gastrointestinal complaints are common. Hepatotoxicity occurs in about 5% of cases. When used in combination with RMP, hepatotoxicity is more common and severe (202[R], 223[c]).

Sufloxone sodium

This sulfone may replace dapsone if gastrointestinal symptoms become severe. It is an enteric-coated preparation given in a dose of 330 mg daily. This long-acting drug liberates dapsone in the tissues but produces low blood levels of dapsone. The effects and adverse reactions are similar to those of dapsone.

Thiacetazone and streptomycin are rarely used in the treatment of leprosy. They may only be useful in combination regimens.

Investigational drugs

The most promising seem to be the fluorinated quinolone derivatives, pefloxacin and ofloxacin. Clinical trials with these drugs are under way (224[CR]). *Minocycline* and one of the newer macrolides, *clarithromycin*, are also currently undergoing comparative trials. *Augmentin*®, a combination of amoxicillin and the β-lactamase inhibitor, clavulanate potassium, is active against *M. leprae* to about the same degree as *dapsone*. This raises the possibility that other β-lactamase inhibitors might also be active.

It appears that certain *ansamycins* with half lives much longer than that of rifampicin might also prove to be useful antileprosy drugs.

Adverse reactions to some of these newer agents are dealt with in earlier Chapters as they are not exclusively employed in the treatment of mycobacterial diseases.

REFERENCES

1. Hyman CL. Tuberculosis: a survey and review of current literature. Curr Opin Pulm Med 1995;1:234.
2. Perez-Stable EJ, Hopewel PhC. Current tuberculosis treatment regimens. Choosing the right one for your patient. Clin Chest Med 1989;10:323.
3. Statement of the American Thoracic Society. Treatment of tuberculosis and tuberculosis infection in adults and children. Am J Respir Crit Care Med 1994;149:1359.
4. Combs DL, O'Brien RJ, Geiter LJ. US PHS Tuberculosis short-course chemotherapy trial 21: effectiveness, toxicity, and acceptability. The report of final results. Ann Intern Med 1990;112:397.
5. Mitchison DA. The action of antituberculosis drugs in short-course chemotherapy. Tubercle 1985;66:219.
6. American Thoracic Society. Treatment of tuberculosis and tuberculous infection in adults and children: A joint statement of the American Thoracic Society and the Centers for Disease Control and Prevention. Am J Respir Crit Care Med 1994;149:1359.
7. Karrer W, Röthlisberger K, Bezel R et al. Welches ist die beste Medikamentenkombination für Kurzzeittherapie der Tuberkulose? Schweiz Med Wochenschr 1985;115:1353.
8. Tsukamura M, Nakamura E, Yoshii S et al. Therapeutic effects of a new antibacterial substance of ofloxacin (DL

8280) on pulmonary tuberculosis. Am Rev Respir Dis 1985;131:352.
9. Jagannath C, Reddy MV, Kailasam S, O'Sullivan JF, Gangadharam RJ. Chemotherapeutic activity of clofazimine and its analogues against *Mycobacterium* tuberculosis. In vitro, intracellular, and in vivo studies. Am J Respir Crit Care Med 1995;151:1083.
10. Ellard GA, Ellard DR, Allen BW et al. The bioavailability of isoniazid, rifampin, and pyrazinamide in two commercially available combined formulations designed for use in the short-course treatment of tuberculosis. Am Rev Respir Dis 1986;133:1076.
11. Braude AL, Davis Ch E, Fierer J. Infectious Diseases and Medical Microbiology, 2nd edn. Philadelphia: WB Saunders, 1966;841.
12. Mitchison DA, Nunn AJ. Influence of initial drug resistance in the response to short-course chemotherapy of pulmonary tuberculosis. Am Rev Resp Dis 1986;133:423.
13. Small PM, Schecter GF, Goodman PC, Sande MA, Chaisson RE, Hopewell PC. Treatment of tuberculosis in patients with advanced human imunodeficiency virus infection. N Engl J Med 1991;324:289.
14. Tanzanian/British Medical Research Council Collaborative Study. Tuberculosis in Tanzania—a national survey of newly notified cases. Tubercle 1985;66:161.
15. Glassroth J, Robins AG, Snider DE. Tuberculosis in the 1980s. N Engl J Med 1980;302:1441.
16. Livengood JR, Sigler TG, Foster LR et al. Isoniazid-resistant tuberculosis: a community outbreak and report of a rifampin prophylaxis failure. J Am Med Assoc 1985;253:2847.
17. Grzybowski S. Isoniazid chemoprophylaxis. J Am Med Assoc 1986;255:1615.
18. Snider DE, Caras GJ, Koplan JP. Preventive therapy with isoniazid. J Am Med Assoc 1986;255:1579.
19. Yew WW, Chan CH. Drug-resistant tuberculosis in the 1990s. Eur Respir J 1995;8:1184.
20. Iseman MD. Treatment of multidrug-resistant tuberculosis. N Engl J Med 1993;329:784.
21. Peloquin CA, MacPhee AA, Berning SE. Malabsorption of antimycobacterial medications. N Engl J Med 1993; 329:1122.
22. Des Prez RM, Heim CR. Mycobacterium tuberculosis. In: Mandell GL, Douglas RG Jr, Bennett JE, eds. Principles and Practice of Infections Diseases, 3rd edn. New York: Churchill Livingstone, 1990;1877.
23. Bishburg E, Sunderam G, Reichman LB et al. Central nervous system tuberculosis with the acquired immunodeficiency syndrome and its related complex. Ann Intern Med 1986;105:210.
24. Hawkins CC, Gold JW, Whimbey E et al. *Mycobacterium avium* complex infections in patients with the acquired immunodeficiency syndrome. Ann Intern Med 1986;105:184.
25. Greene JB, Sidhu GS, Lewin S et al. *Mycobacterium avium-intracellulare*: a cause of disseminated life-threatening infection in homosexuals and drug abusers. Ann Intern Med 1982;97:539.
26. Vonmoos S, Leuenberger P, Beer R et al. Infection pleuropulmonaire à *Mycobacterium smegmatis*. Schweiz Med Wochenschr 1986;116:1852.
27. Issac-Renton JL, Allen EA, Chao CW et al. Isolation and geographic distribution of *Mycobacterium* other than *Mycobacterium tuberculosis* in British Columbia. Can Med Assoc J 1985;133:573.
28. Small PM, Schecter GF, Goodman PC, Sande MA, Chaisson RE, Hopewell PC. Treatment of tuberculosis in patients with advanced human immunodeficiency virus infection. N Engl J Med 1991;324:289.
29. Statement of the Amercian Thoracic Society. Diagnosis and treatment of diseases causes by nontuberculosis mycobacteria. Am Rev Respir Dis 1990;124:940.
30. Passannante MR, Gallagher CT, Reichman LB. Preventive therapy for contacts of multidrug-resistant tuberculosis. A Delphi survey. Chest 1994;106:431.
31. Horsburgh CR, Mason UG, Farhi DC et al. Disseminated infection with *Mycobacterium avium-intracellulare*. Medicine 1985;64:36.
32. Masur H. Recommandations on prophylaxis and therapy for disseminated *Mycobacterium avium* complex disease in patients infected with the human immunodeficiency virus. N Engl J Med 1993;329:898.
33. Ahn CH, Lowel JR, Ahn SS et al. Short-course chemotherapy for pulmonary disease caused by *Mycobacterium kansasii*. Am Rev Respir Dis 1983;128:1048.
34. Ives DV, Davis RB, Currier JS. Impact of clarithromycin and azithromycin on patterns of treatment and survival among AIDS patients with disseminated *Mycobacterium avium* complex. AIDS 1995;9:261.
35. Olliaro P, Dolfi L, Morelli P, Della Bruna C, Strolin-Benedetti M, Sassela D. Rifabutin for prevention and treatment of mycobacterial diseases: a review of microbiology, clinical pharmacology, efficacy and tolerability data. Eur Respir Rev 1995;25:77.
36. Farge D, Charpentier B, Simonneau G et al. Réaction de rejet et utilisation de la rifampicine dans le traitement de la tuberculose en transplantation rénale. Néphrologie 1985;6:53.
37. Sande MA. The use of rifampin in the treatment of nontuberculous infections. Rev infect Dis 1983;5(Suppl 3):S399.
38. Mitchell I, Wendon J, Fitt S, Williams R. Anti-tuberculous therapy and acute liver failure. Lancet 1995;345:555.
39. Mandell GL, Sande MA. Antimicrobial agents: Drugs used in the chemotherapy of tuberculosis and leprosy. In: Goodman Gilman A, Rall TW, Nies AS, Taylor P, eds. Goodman Gilman's The Pharmacological Basis of Therapeutics, 8th edn, Ch. 49. New York: Pergamon Press, 1990;1146.
40. Mitchell JR, Thorgeirsson UP, Black M et al. Increased incidence of isoniazid hepatitis in rapid acetylators: possible relation to hydrazine metabolites. Clin Pharmacol Ther 1975;18:70.
41. Weber WW, Hein DW, Litwin A, Lower GM. Relationship of acetylator status to isoniazid toxicity, lupus erythematosus, and bladder cancer. Fed Proc 1983;42:3086.
42. Gurumurthy P, Krishnamurthy MS, Nazareth O. Lack of relationship between hepatic toxicity and acetylator phenotype in three thousand South Indian patients during treatment with isoniazid for tuberculosis. Am Rev Respir Dis 1984;129:58.
43. Schelling JL. Dyspnées médicamenteuses. Ther Umschau 1981;38:163.
44 Ueda Y, Fujita K, Kohno K, Ichinose K, Fukushima H, Nakotomi M. A case of isoniazid-induced lupus. Kekkaku 1988;64:19.
45. De Weck AL. Approaches to prevention and treatment of drug allergy. In: Turk JL, Parker D, eds. Drugs and Immune Responsiveness, 13. Baltimore, MD: University Park Press, 1979;211.

46. Boice ID, Fraumeni JF. Late effects following isoniazid therapy. Am J Public Health 1980;70:987.
47. Rothfield NF, Bierer WF, Garfield JW. Isoniazid induction of antinuclear antibodies: a prospective study. Ann Intern Med 1978;88:650.
48. Snider DE Jr. Pyridoxine supplementation during isoniazid therapy. Tubercle 1980;61:191.
49. Schröder JM. Zur Pathogenese der Isoniazid-Neuropathie. II. Phasen-kontrast- und elektronenmikroskopische Untersuchungen am Rückenmark, an Spinalganglien und Muskelspindeln. Acta Neuropathol 1970;16:301.
50. Bhatia MS. Isoniazid-induced obsessive compulsive neurosis. J Clin Psychiatry 1990;51:387.
51. Bernando M, Gatell JM, Parellada E. Acute exacerbation of chronic schizophrenia in a patient treated with antituberculosis drugs. Am J Psychiatry 1991;148:1402.
52. Siskind MS, Thienemann D, Kirlin L. Isoniazid-induced neurotoxicity in chronic dialysis patients: report of three cases and a review of the literature. Nephron 1993 64:303.
53. Cheung WC, Lo CY, Ip M, Cheng IKP. Isoniazid induced encephalopathy in dialysis patients. Tubercle Lung Dis 1993;74:136.
54. Valsalan VC. Carbamazepine intoxication caused by interaction with isoniazid. Br Med J 1982;285:261.
55. Ishii N, Nishihara Y. Pellagra encephalopathy among tuberculous patients: its relation to isoniazid therapy. J Neurol Neurosurg Psychiatry 1985;48:628.
56. Sharp RA, Lowe JG, Johnston RN. Antituberculous drugs and sideroblastic anaemia. Br J Clin Pharmacol 1990;44:706.
57. Johnsson R, Lommi J. A case of isoniazid-induced red cell aplasia. Respir Med 1990;84:171.
58. Goldman AL, Braman SS. Isioniazid: a review with emphasis on adverse effects. Chest 1972;62:71.
59. Krumdieck R, Shaw DR, Huany ST, Poon MC Rustagi PK. Hemorrhagic disorder due to an isoniazid-associated acquired factor XIII inhibitor in a patient with Waldenstrom's macroglobulinemia. Am J Med 1991;90:639.
60. Gangadharam PRJ. Isoniazid, rifampin and hepatotoxicity. Am Rev Respir Dis 1986;133:963.
61. Timbrell JA, Wright JM. Urinary metabolic profile of isoniazid in patients who develop isoniazid-related liver damage. Hum Toxicol 1984;3:485.
62. Halpern M, Meyers B, Miller C, Bodenheimer H, Thung SN, Adler J, Toth D, Cohen D, Baccardo L, Difeddinando G, Birkhead A. Severe isoniazid-associated hepatitis—New York (1990—1993). J Am Med Assoc 1993;270:809.
63. Amarapurkar DN, Prabhudesai PD, Kalro RH, Desai HG. Antituberculosis drug-induced hepatitis and Hbs Ag carriers. Tubercle Lung Dis 1993;74:215.
64. Hauser MJ, Baier H. Interactions of isoniazid with foods. Drug Intell Clin Pharm 1982;16:617.
65. Lejonc JL, Schaeffer A, Brochard P et al. Hypertension artérielle paro-xystique provoquée sous isoniazide par l'ingestion de gruyère: deux cas. Ann Méd Interne 1980;131:346.
66. Uragoda CG. Histamine poisoning in tuberculous patients after ingestion of tuna fish. Am Rev Respir Dis 1980;212:157.
67. Chan KL, Chan HS, Lui SF, Lai KN. Recurrent acute pancreatitis induced by isoniazid. Tubercle Lung Dis 1994;75:383.
68. Rabassa AA, Trey G, Shukla U, Samo T, Anand BS. Isoniazid-induced acute pancreatitis. Ann Intern Med 1994;121:433.
69. Koch SE, Williams ML. Acquired cutis laxa: case report and review of disorders of elastosis. Pediatr Dermatol 1985;2:282.
70. Hoigné R, Biedermann HP, Naegeli HR. INH-induzierter systemischer Lupus Erythematodes: 2 Beobachtungen mit Reexposition. Schweiz Med Wochenschr 1975;105:1726.
71. Rothfielf NF, Bierer WF, Garfield JW. Isoniazid: induction of anti-nuclear antibodies. Ann Intern Med 1978;88:650.
72. Kunz J, Schreiner WE. Pharmakotherapie während Schwangerschaft und Stillperiode. Stuttgart—New York: G. Thieme, 1982.
73. Olive G. Interactions médicamenteuses chez le nouveau né. In: Comptes Rendus, 25e Congrès de l'Association des Pédiatres de Langue Française, Tunis, 1978. Paris: Expansion Scientifique Française, 1978;57.
74. Miller J, Robinson A, Percy AK. Acute isoniazid poisoning in childhood. Am J Dis Child 1980;134:290.
75. Gilhotra R, Malik SK, Singh S et al. Acute isoniazid toxicity—report of 2 cases and review of literature. Int J Clin Pharmacol Ther Toxicol 1987;25:259.
76. Hurwitz A, Schlozman DL. Effects of antacids on gastrointestinal absorption of isoniazid in rat and man. Am Rev Respir Dis 1974;109:41.
77. Duroux P. Surveillance et accidents de la chimiothérapie antituberculeuse. Rev Prat 1979;29:33.
78. Miller RR, Porter J, Greenblatt DJ. Clinical importance of the interaction of phenytoin and isoniazid. Chest 1979;75:356.
79. Snider DE Jr. Pyridoxine supplementation during isoniazid therapy. Tubercle 1980;61:191.
80. Hand WL, Boozer RM, King-Thompson NL. Antibiotic uptake by alveolar macrophages of smokers. Antimicrob Agents Chemother 1985;27:42.
81. Knecht K. Rifampicin und menschliche Granulocyten. In: Aufnahme mechanismus und Beeinflussung biologischer Funktionen. Thesis. University of Zürich, 1983.
82. Grosset J, Leventis S. Adverse effects of rifampin. Rev Infect Dis 1983;5(Suppl 3):S440.
83. Wurtz RM, Abrams D, Beckers S, Jacobson MA, Mass MM, Marks SH. Anaphylactoid drug reactions to ciprofloxacin and rifampicin in HIV-infected patients Lancet 1989;i:955.
84. Pujet JC, Homberg JC, Decroix G. Sensitivity to rifampicin: incidence, mechanism, and prevention. Br Med J 1974;1:415.
85. Stevens E, Bloemmen F, Mbuyi JM et al. Immunological aspects of rifampicin side-reactions. Bull Int Union Tuberc 1979;54:170.
86. Ramachandran A, Bhatia VN. Rifamicin induced shock—a case report. Indian J Lepr 1990;62:228.
87. Pratt TH. Rifampin-induced organic brain syndrome. J Am Med Assoc 1979;241:2421.
88. Artaza A, Gallofre M, Arboix M et al. Niveles de la rifampicina en liquido cefalorraquideo en cuadros de inflammación meningea. Arch Farmacol Toxicol 1983;9:121.
89. Kyriazopoulou V, Parparousi O, Vagenakis AG. Rifampicin-induced adrenal crisis in Addisonian patients receiving corticosteroid replacement therapy. J. Clin Endocrinol Metab 1984;59:1204.
90. Williams SE, Wardman AG, Taylor GA et al. Long term study of the effect of rifiampicin and isoniazid on vitamin D metabolism. Tubercle 1985:66:49.
91. Toppet M, Vainsel M, Cantraine F et al. Evolution de la phosphatase alcaline sérique sous traitement d'isoniazide et de rifampicine. Arch Fr Pédiatr 1985;42:79.

92. Van Assendelft AHW. Leucopenia in rifampicin chemotherapy. J Antimicrob Chemother 1985;16:497.
93. Diamond JR, Tahan SR. Ig-G mediated intravascular hemolysis and no-noliguric acute renal failure complicating discontinuous rifampicin administration. Nephron 1984; 38:62.
94. Tahan SR, Diamond JR, Blank JM et al. Acute hemolysis and renal failure with rifampicin-dependent antibodies after discontinuous administration. Transfusion 1985;25:124.
95. Ip M, Cheng KP, Cheung WC. Disseminated intravascular coagulopathy associated with rifampicin. Tubercle 1991;72:291.
96. Pessayre D. Present views on isoniazid and isoniazid-rifampicin hepatitis. Agressologie 1982;23:13.
97. Linna O, Uhari M. Hepatotoxicity of rifampicin and isoniazid in children treated for tuberculosis. Eur J Pediatr 1980;134:227.
98. Berg JD, Pandov HI, Sammons HG. Serum total bile acid levels in patients receiving rifampicin and isoniazid. Ann Clin Biochem 1984;21:218.
99. Kuhlmann J. Beeinflussung der Arzneimittelwirkung durch die Ernährung. Med Monatsschr Pharm 1980;3:133.
100. Ali Zargar S, Thapa BN, Sahni A, Mehta S. Rifampicin-induced upper gastrointestinal bleeding. Postgrad Med J 1990;66:310.
101. Moriarty HJ, Scobie BA. Pseudomembranous colitis in a patient on rifampicin and ethambuthol. NZ Med J 1980;91:294.
102. Khalil SAH, El-Khordagui LK, El-Gholmy ZA. Effect of antacids on oral absorption of rifampicin. Int J Pharm 1984;20:99.
103. Mauri JM, Fort J, Bartolome J et al. Anti-rifampicin antibodies in acute rifampicin-associated renal failure. Nephron 1982;31:177.
104. Warrington RJ, Hogg GR, Paraskevas F, Tse KS. Insidious rifampin-associated renal failure with high-chain proteinuria. Arch Intern Med 1977;137:927.
105. Winter RJD, Banks RA, Collins CMP et al. Rifampicin induced light chain proteinuria and renal failure. Thorax 1984;39:952.
106. Cohn JR, Fye DL, Sills JM et al. Rifampicin-induced renal failure. Tubercle 1985;66:289.
107. Millar JW. Rifampicin-induced porphyria cutanea tarda. Br J Dis Chest 1980;74:405.
108. Lee CW, Lim JH, Kang HJ. Pemphigus foliaceus induced by rifampicin. Br J Dermatol 1984;111:619.
109. Miyagawa S, Yamashina Y, Okuchi T et al. Exacerbation of pemphigus by rifampicin. Br J Dermatol 1986;114:729.
110. Prazuck T, Fisch A, Simonnet F, Noat G. Lyell's syndrome associated with rifampicin therapy of tuberculosis in an AIDS patient. Scand J Infect Dis 1990;22:629.
111. Nahata MC, Fan-Havard P, Barson WJ, Bartkowski AM, Kosnik EJ. Pharmacokinetics, cerebrospinal fluid concentration, and safety of intravenous rifampicin in paediatric patients undergoing shunt placements. Eur J Clin Pharmacol 1990;38:515.
112. Vaz M, Jacob AJW, Rajendran A. 'Flu' syndrome on once monthly rifampicin: a case report. Lepr Rev 1989; 60:300.
113. Farr BF, Mandell GL. Rifampin. Med Clin North Am 1982;66:157.
114. Bassi L, DiBerardino L, Arioli V, Silvestri LG, Cherie Ligniere EL. Conditions for immunosuppression by rifampicin. J Infect Dis 1973;128:736.
115. Kissling M, Xilinas M. Rimactan parenteral formulation in clinical use. J Int Med Res 1981;9:45.
116. Bolan G, Laurie RE, Broome CV. Red man syndrome: inadvertent administration of an excessive dose of rifampin to children in a day-care center. Pediatrics 1986;77:633.
117. Broadwell RO, Broadwell SD, Comer PB. Suicide by rifampicin overdose. J Am Med Assoc 1978;240:2283.
118. Newton RW, Forrest ARW. Rifampicin overdosage—'The red man syndrome'. Scot Med J 1975;20:55
119. Meisel S. Brower R. Rifampin: a suicidal dose. Ann Intern Med 1980;92:262.
120. Pallardo L, Moreno R, Garcia Martinez J et al. Rechado agudo tardio del injerto renal inducido por rifampicina. Nefrologia 1987;7:93.
121. Skolnick JL, Stoler BS, Katz DB et al. Rifampin, oral contraceptives and pregnancy. J Am Med Assoc 1976; 236:1382.
122. Held H. Interaktion von Rifampicin mit Phenprocoumon: Beobachtungen bei tuberkulosekranken Patienten. Dtsch Med Wochenschr 1979;104:1311.
123. Michot F, Bürgi M, Büttner J. Rimactan (Rifampicin) und Antikoagulan-tientherapie. Schweiz Med Wochenschr 1970;100:583.
124. Takeda M, Nishinuma K, Yamashita S et al. Serum haloperidol level of schizophrenics receiving treatment for tuberculosis. Clin Neuropharmacol 1986;9:386.
125. Offermann G, Keller F, Molzahn M. Low cyclosporin A blood levels and acute graft rejection in a renal transplant recipient during rifampin treatment. Am J Nephrol 1985;5:385.
126. Teunissen MWE, Bakker W, Meerbrug-Van der Torren JE et al. Influence of rifampicin treatment on antipyrine clearance and metabolite formation in patients with tuberculosis. Br J Clin Pharmacol 1984;18:701.
127. Powell-Jackon PR, Jamieson AP, Gray BJ et al. Effect of rifampicin administration on theophylline pharmacokinetics in human. Am Rev Respir Dis 1985;131:939.
128. Barbarash RA. Verapamil—Rifampin interaction. Drug Intell Clin Pharm 1985;19:559.
129. Baciewicz AM, Self TH. Rifampin drug interactions. Arch Intern Med 1984;144:1667.
130. Baciewicz AM, Self TH, BeKemeyer WB. Update on rifampin drug interactions. Arch Intern Med 1987;147:565.
131. Dickinson JM, Aber VR, Mitchison DA. Bactericidal activity of streptomycin, isoniazid, rifampin, ethambutol, and pyrazinamide alone and in combination against *Mycobacterium tuberculosis*. Am Rev Respir Dis 1977;116:627.
132. Surjapranata FJ, Rahaju NN. A case of Stevens-Johnson's syndrome caused by ethambutol. Paediatr Indones 1979;19:195.
133. Pegram PS, Mountz JD, O'Bar PR. Ethambutol-induced toxic epidermal necrolysis. Arch Intern Med 1981;141:1677.
134. Nair VS, Le Brun M, Kass I. Peripheral neuropathy associated with ethambutol. Chest 1980;77:98.
135. Takeuchi H, Takahasi M, Tarui S et al. Peripheral nerve conduction function in patients treated with antituberculotic agents, with special reference to ethambutol and isoniazid. Folia Pscyatr Neurol Jpn 1980;34:57.
136. Takeuchi H, Takahashi M, Kang J et al. Ethambutol neuropathy: clinical and electroneuromyographic studies. Folia Psychiatr Neurol Jpn 1980;34:45.
137. Khanna BK, Gupta VP. Ethambutol-induced hyperuricemia. Tubercle 1984;65:195.

138. Khanna BK. Acute gouty arthritis following ethambutol therapy. Br J Dis Chest 1980;74:409.
139. Rabinovitz M, Pitlik SD, Halevy J. et al. Ethambutol-induced thrombocytopenia. Chest 1982;81:765.
140. Strauss I, Erhardt F. Ethambutol absorption, excretion and dosage in patients with renal tuberculosis. Chemotherapy 1970;15:148.
141. Seigneuric C, Portier H. Complications oculaires du traitement antituberculeux: à propos de 3 observations. Lyon Méd 1981;246:127.
142. Otori T. Drug-induced ocular side effects. Asian Méd J 1981;24:141.
143. Garrett CR. Optic neuritis in a patient on ethambutol and isoniazid evaluated by visual evoked potentials: case report. Mil Med 1985;150:43.
144. Karnik AM, Al-Shamali MA, Fenech FF. A case of ocular toxicity to ethambutol—an idiosyncratic reaction? Postgrad Med J 1985;61:811.
145. Cole A, May PM, Williams DR. Metal binding by pharmaceuticals. I. Copper (II) and zinc (II) interactions following ethambutol administration. Agents Actions 198[illegible]; 11:296.
146. Yolton DP. Nutritional effects of zinc on ocular and systemic physiology. J Am Optom Assoc 1981;52:409.
147. Delacoux E, Moreau Y, Godefroy A et al. Prévention de la toxicité oculaire de l'éthambutol: intérêt de la zincémie et de l'analyse du sens chromatique. J Fr Ophtalmol 1978;1:191.
148. Williams DE. Visual electrophysiology and psychophysics in chronic alcoholics and in patients on tuberculostatic chemotherapy. Am J Optom Physiol Opt 1984;61:576.
149. Guerra R, Casu L. Hydroxycobalamin for ethambutol-induced optic neuropathy. Lancet 1981;ii:1176.
150. Lewit T, Nebel L, Terracina S et al. Ethambutol in pregnancy: observations on embryogenesis. Chest 1974; 66:25.
151. Jenner PJ, Ellard GA, Allan WGL et al. Serum uric acid concentrations and arthralgia among patients treated with pyrazinamide-containing regimens in Hong Kong and Singapore. Tubercle 1981;62:175.
152. Jorgensen J. Pellagra probably due to pyrazinamide: development during combined chemotherapy of tuberculosis. Int J Dermatol 1983;83:44.
153. Treece GL, Magnussen R, Patterson J et al. Exacerbation of porphyria during treatment of pulmonary tuberculosis. Am Rev Respir Dis 1976;113:233.
154. Danan G, Pessayre D, Larrey D et al. Pyrazinamide fulminant hepatitis: an old hepatotoxin strikes again. Lancet 1981;ii:1056.
155. Pretet S, Perdrizet S. La toxicité du pyrazinamide dans les traitements antituberculeux. Rev Fr Mal Respir 1980;8:307.
156. Chan SL. Chemotherapy of tuberculosis. In: Davies PDO, ed. Clinical Tuberculosis. London: Chapman and Hall, 1994;141.
157. Drucker D, Eggo MC, Salit IE et al. Ethionamide-induced goitrous hypothyroidism. Ann Intern Med 1984; 100:837.
158. Gupta SK, Bedi RS, Maini VK. Agranulocytosis due to thiacetazone. Indian J Tubercl 1983;30:146.
159. Jaliluddin Mohsini AA. Fatal aplastic anaemia due to thiacetazone toxicity. J Indian Med Assoc 1982:77:176.
160. Naraqui S, Temu P. Thiacetazone skin reaction in Papua New Guinea. Med J Aust 1980;1:480.
161. Short GM. Side-effect of thiacetazone. S Afr Med J 1980;58:5.
162. Nunn P, Kibuga D, Gathua S, Brindle R, Imalingat A, Wasunna K, Lucas S, Gilks C, Omwega M, Were J, McAdam K. Cutaneous hypersensitivity reactions due to thiacetazone in HIV-1 seropositive patients treated for tuberculosis. Lancet 1991;337:627.
163. Ahuja YR, Jaju M, Jaju M. Chromosome-damaging action of isoniazid and thiacetazhone on human lymphocyte cultures in vivo. Hum Genet 1981;57:321.
164. Masur H. Recommandations on prophylaxis and therapy for disseminated *Mycobacterium avium* complex disease in patients infected with the human immunodeficiency virus. N Engl J Med 1993;329:898.
165. Havlir D, Torriani F, Dubé M. Uveitis associated with rifatubin prophylaxis. Ann Intern Med 1994;121:510.
166. Goodman Gilman A, Rall ThW, Nies AS, Taylor P. The Pharmacological Basis of Therapeutics, 8th edn. Elmsfort, NY: Pergamon Press, 1990.
167. Steiner RW, Omachi AS. A Bartter's-like syndrome from capreomycin, and a similar gentamicin tubulopathy. Am J Kidney Dis 1986;7:245.
168. Hoigné R. Allergische Erkrankungen. In: Stucki P, Hess T, eds. Hadorn, Lehrbuch der Therapie, 7th edn. Berne—Stuttgart—Vienna: Verlag Hans Huber, 1983;155.
169. World Health Organization. A Guide to Leprosy Control, 2nd edn. Geneva: World Health Organization, 1988.
170. Noordeen SK. A look at world leprosy. Lepr Rev 1991;62:72.
171. Ji B, Grosset JH. Recent advances in the chemotherapy of leprosy. Lepr Rev 1990;61:313.
172. WHO Study Group. Chemotherapy of leprosy. Am Rev Respir Dis 1982;133:963.
173. Hastings RC, Franzblau SG. Chemotherapy of leprosy. Ann Rev Pharmacol Toxicol 1988;28:231.
174. Ramanan R, Maglani PR, Ghorpade A, Bhagoliwal SK. Follow-up study of paucibacillary leprosy on multidrug regimen. Indian J Leprosy 1987;59:50.
175. Waters MFR, Rees RJW, Laing ABG. The rate of relapse in lepromatous leprosy following completion of 20 years of supervised sulfone therapy. Lepr Rev 1986;57:101.
176. Rees RJW. Chemotherapy of leprosy for control programmes: scientific basis and practical application. Lepr Rev 1983;54:81.
177. Bullok WE. Rifampin in the treatment of leprosy. Rev Infect Dis 1983;5(Suppl 3):S606.
178. Floch HA. Sulfono-résistance de *Mycobacterium leprae* monothérapie par la diaminodiphylsulfone—intérêt des associations médicamenteuses triples. Int J Lepr Other Mycobact Dis 1986;54:122.
179. Guillet G, Tillard JP, Helenon R et al. La lèpre chez le jeune enfant: deux observations à l'âge de 3 ans. Ann Dermatol Vénéréol 1985;112:353.
180. Keeler R, Deen RD. Leprosy in children aged 0—14 years: report of an 11-year control programme. Lepr Rev 1985;56:239.
181. D'Arcy PF, Griffin GP. Thalidomide revisited. Adv Drug React Toxicol Rev 1994;13:65.
182. Balybin ES, Nazarov KI. Hydrocortisone production in lepromatous patients with insulin load. Int J Leprosy Other Mycobact Dis 1983;51:18.
183. Katoch K, Katoch VM, Dutta AK et al. Chest infection due to *M. fortuitum* in a case of lepromatous leprosy: a case report. Indian J Lepr 1985;57:399.
184. Garg SK, Kumar B, Bakaya V, Lal R, Shukla VK, Kaur S. Plasma dapsone and its metabolite monoacetyldap-

sone levels in leprotic patients. Int J Clin Pharmacol Ther Toxicol 1988;26:552.
185. Thangaraj RH, Yawalkar SJ. Leprosy for Medical Practitioners and Paramedical Workers, 2nd edn. Basle: Ciba-Geigy, 1987.
186. Peters JH, Gordon GR, Levy L et al. Metabolic disposition of dapsone in patients with dapsone resistant leprosy. Am J Trop Med Hyg 1974;23:222.
187. Godeau B, Oksenhendler E, Bierling P. Dapsone for autoimmune thrombocytopenic purpura. Am J Haematol 1993;44:70.
188. Liozon F, Vidal E, Barrier JH. Dapsone in giant cell arteritis treatment. Eur J Intern Med 1993;4:207.
189. Kraus A, Jakez J, Palacios A. Dapsone induced sulfone syndrome and systemic lupus erythematosus. J Reumatol 1992;19:178.
190. Pavithran K. Dapsone syndrome with polyarthritis: a case report. Indian J Lepr 1990;62:230.
191. Johnson DA, Cattau EL, Kuritsky JN et al. Liver involvement in the sulfone syndrome. Arch Intern Med 1986;146:875.
192. Mohle-Boetani J, Akula SK, Holodniy M, Katzenstein D, Garcia G. The sulfone syndrome in a patient receiving dapsone prophylaxis for *Pneumocystis carinii* pneumonia. West J Med 1992;156:303.
193. Chan HL, Lee KO. Tonsillar membrane in the DDS (dapsone) syndrome. Int J Dermatol 1991;30:216.
194. Richardus JH, Smith TC. Increased incidence in leprosy of hypersensitivity reactions to dapsone after introduction of multidrug therapy. Lepr Rev 1989;60:267.
195. Cowan RE, Wright JT. Dapsone and severe hypoalbuminaemia in dermatitis herpetiformis. Br J Dermatol 1981;104:201.
196. Somorin AO. Erythema nodosum leprosum in Nigeria. Int J Dermatol 1975;14:664.
197. Waldinger TP, Siegle RJ, Weber W et al. Dapsone-induced peripheral neuropathy. Arch Dermatol 1984; 120:356.
198. Ahrens EM, Meckler RJ, Callen JP. Dapsone-induced peripheral neuropathy. Int J Dermatol 1986;25:314.
199. Kaplan G, Cohn ZA. The immunobiology of leprosy. Int Rev Exp Pathol 1986;28:45.
200. Balkrishna Bhatia MS. Dapsone-induced psychosis. J Indian Med Assoc 1989;5:120.
201. Byrd SR, Gelber RH. Effect of dapsone on haemoglobin concentration in patients with leprosy. Lepr Rev 1991;62:171.
202. Braude AL, Davis Ch E, Fierer J. Infectious Diseases and Medical Microbiology, 2nd edn. Philadelphia: WB Saunders, 1966;1171.
203. Trillo RA, Ankburg S. Dapsone-induced methemoglobinemia and pulse oxymetry. Anesthesiology 1992;77:594.
204. Prussich R, Ali MAM, Rosenthal D, Guyatl G. The protective effect of vitamine E on the hemolysis associated with dapsone treatment. Arch Dermatol 1992;128:210.
205. Browne SG. Desensitization for dapsone dermatitis. Br Med J 1963;2:664.
206. Alexander TA, Raju R, Kuriakose T, Cherian AM. Presumed DDS ocular toxicity. Indian J Ophthalmol 1989;37:150.
207. Modderman ES, Huikeshoven H, Zuidema J et al. Intramuscular injection of dapsone in therapy for leprosy: a new approach. Int J Clin Pharmacol Ther Toxicol 1982; 20:51.
208. Duncan ME, Pearson JMH. The association of pregnancy and leprosy. III. Erythema nodosum leprosum in pregnancy and lactation. Lepr Rev 1984;55:129.
209. Balakrishnan S. Seshadri PS. Drug interactions—the influence of rifampicin and clofazimine on the urinary excretion of DDS. Lepr India 1983;53:17.
210. McDougall AC, Jones RL. Intra-neural ceroid-like pigment following the treatment of lepromatous leprosy with clofazimine (B663; Lamprene). J Neurol Neurosurg Psychiatry 1981;44:116.
211. Merrett MN, King RWF, Farrell KF, Zeimer H, Guli E. Orange/black discolouration of the bowel (at laparotomy) due to clofazimine. Aust NZ Surg 1990;60:638.
212. Burte NP, Chandorkar AG, Muley MP et al. Clofazimine on liver function tests in lepra reaction. Lepr India 1983;55:265.
213. Dixit VB, Chandhary SD, Jain UK. Clofazimine induced nail changes. Indian J Lepr 1989;61:476.
214. Kaur I, Ram J, Kumar B, Kaur S, Sharma VK. Effect of clofazimine on eye in multibacillary leprosy. Indian J Lepr 1990;62:87.
215. Sandler ED, Ng UL, Hadley WK. Clofazimine crystals in alveolar macrophages from a patient with acquired immuno-deficiency syndrome. Arch Pathol Lab Med 1992;116:541.
216. Oommen T. Clofazimine-induced lymphoedema. Lepr Rev 1990;61:289.
217. Jost JL, Venencie PY, Cortez A et al. Entéropathie à la clofamine. J Chir 1986;123:7.
218. Bulakh PM, Kowale CN, Ranade SM et al. The effect of clofazimine on liver function tests in lepra reaction. Lepr India 1984;55:714.
219. Baohong J, Jiakun C, Chenmin W et al. Hepatotoxicity of combined therapy with rifampicin and daily prothionamide for leprosy. Lepr Rev 1984;55:283.
220. Rook GAW. Absence from sera from normal individuals or from rifampin-treated leprosy patients (thelep trials) of antibody to rifamycin-protein or rifamycin-membrane conjugates. Int J Lepr 1985;53:22.
221. Kar HK, Roy RG. Reversible acute renal failure due to monthly administration of rifampicin in a leprosy patient. Indian J Lepr 1984;56:835.
222. Pankaj R, Lal S, Rao RS. Effect of probenecid on serum rifampicin levels. Indian J Lepr 1985;57:329.
223. Pattyn SR, Janssens L, Bourland J et al. Hepatotoxicity of the combination of rifampin—ethionamide in the treatment of multibacillary leprosy. Int J Lepr 1984;52:1.
224. WHO Expert Committee on Leprosy. 6th Report. Techn Rep Series 768. Geneva: World Health Organization, 1988.

Meyler's Side Effects of Drugs, 13th Edition
M.N.G. Dukes, editor

SECTION EDITOR: M.N.G. DUKES

A.M.M. Kaddu

31 Anthelminthic drugs

GENERAL

There is a continuous process of change in the treatment of helminth infections, largely a consequence of the replacement of toxic older agents by newer compounds, some of which are also more effective. As in some other fields, the economy of some developing countries unfortunately still necessitates the widespread employment of agents which from the medical point of view could better be replaced. The World Health Organization's overviews provide a compact and regularly updated view of the situation (1^R).

It must be realized that many of the unpleasant effects which can develop after effective anthelminthic treatment result from the death of the parasite and the consequent release into the body of toxins and allergens; the result is not likely to be specific to a particular drug or its dosage, but is likely to be more severe where the number of parasites killed is higher. One will therefore expect the reaction to be greater where the drug is more effective and/or where the initial infestation is more severe.

USE OF ANTHELMINTHIC DRUGS IN PREGNANCY

As pointed out in various of the sections which follow, one should be hesitant to use anthelminthic drugs during pregnancy. Some have been shown to be embryotoxic or teratogenic during animal studies; others may induce cramping or their action may result in the release of toxic products as the parasite disintegrates. These factors and the generally toxic nature of the anthelminthics outweigh any optimism which might be distilled from the fact that adverse effects in human pregnancy have generally not been reported in the literature.

Levamisole *(See also Chapter 37)*

Originally used only as an anthelminthic drug, levamisole acts by paralyzing the musculature of susceptible nematodes so that they are expelled by peristalsis. The drug is rapidly metabolized and excreted, with a plasma half-life of only some 4 hours. Treatment of ascariasis with a single oral dose of 2.5 mg/kg of levamisole is effective, with evidence of toxicity in less than 1% of patients. More recently, it has been used extensively and for extended periods of time in various rheumatic and other chronic diseases, in nephrotic syndrome and in malignancies because of its immunostimulant properties. Under these conditions, its side effects are more frequent and rather different. Most of the material in the following monograph is necessarily derived from this long-term treatment, and where possible a distinction will be drawn between adverse effects occurring under these conditions and those experienced when treating tropical disorders.

Levamisole continues to be used experimentally in leprosy, particularly in combination with dapsone. This combination was used in a documented series of Indian patients, some currently lepromatous and others in the course of reaction (2^{Cr}). In doses sufficient to provide as good an effect as that obtained with clofazimine/dapsone in a comparison group, side effects were limited to gastrointestinal intolerance (which was usually mild) affecting only five of the 30 patients; an incidental case developed pyrexia.

ADVERSE REACTION PATTERN

General and toxic reactions Single-dose anthelminthic use rarely causes complications, adverse effects being limited to mild gastrointestinal symptoms. In contrast, some 25% of individuals treated for long periods experience side effects, notably gastrointestinal disturbances, CNS abnormalities (occasionally with convulsions), fevers and influenza-like states, agranulocytosis and skin disorders. Hematological complications are unusual, but may prove fatal and may be allergic rather than toxic.

Hypersensitivity reactions Hypersensitivity reactions including pruritic skin eruptions, arthritic pain and swelling, muscular pain and swelling, may occur and have been reported, especially in patients already suffering from rheumatoid arthritis, Sjögren's syndrome (3^C) and psoriatic arthropathy. Skin reactions of various types can occur and Type III reactions have been noted. Influenza-like symptoms might be an unusual form of Type I allergy or a consequence of restoration of cellular immunity.

Tumor-inducing effects These have not been reported.

ORGANS AND SYSTEMS

Cardiovascular *Cutaneous vasculitis* can occur (see 'Skin' below) and a healed *varicose ulcer* has been observed to break down following treatment (4^C). *Hypotension* has been reported and may cause faintness.

Nervous system In one large literature survey, 6% of patients on long-term treatment, mostly for malignancies, were found to have experienced '*sensory stimulation*', e.g. in the form of 'hyperalert states' or insomnia (5^R). *Diplopia* and *tremor* have been observed, whilst a number of children treated for juvenile rheumatoid arthritis or nephrotic syndrome have developed *generalized convulsions* and *coma*, with EEG abnormalities suggestive of *encephalitis* (SED-12, 771; 6^c); the condition recovers spontaneously, but for a time anti-epileptic drugs may be needed. A fatal viral encephalitis due to enterovirus type 71 has indeed been reported during use of the drug and might explain the course of events in these children.

Hematological *Agranulocytosis* has been frequently reported during long-term treatment. The literature survey cited above, covering 3900 patients on whom data were available to the manufacturers, included 88 cases of agranulocytosis as well as 43 of *leukopenia*; such dyscrasias occurred in 4% of rheumatoid patients and 2% of oncological cases. In other published material the incidence has sometimes been higher; such differences do not appear to be related to dose or duration of therapy. Agranulocytosis is more prevalent in those rheumatoid patients with a HLA-B27 genotype (SEDA-7, 317). Children are also susceptible and fatal outcomes because of hematological disorders have been described in cases of juvenile rheumatoid arthritis treated intermittently with levamisole. Other fatalities have been observed in adult patients concurrently taking corticosteroids for several years.

The agranulocytosis may be asymptomatic and since it occurs unpredictably, regular monitoring of leukocyte counts is advisable, especially in patients concurrently receiving combination chemotherapy. Whilst the mechanism is not clear, granulocyte-agglutinating antibodies have been found, suggesting that levamisole acts as a hapten on the leukocyte membrane.

Thrombocytopenia has been reported in one instance in a woman with rheumatoid arthritis; it recurred following a provocation test.

Liver Neither animal nor most human studies point to hepatotoxicity, but in a series of 11 patients treated for pyoderma two showed an increase in aspartate aminotransferase.

Gastrointestinal *Nausea*, *vomiting* and *diarrhea* are not uncommon, sometimes accompanied by *abdominal pain*, though when these occur during treatment of a nematode infection it is not always clear that they are due to the drug rather than to its interaction with the disease process. Exacerbation of *peptic ulceration* has been described and *mouth ulcers* as well as abnormalities of *taste* sensation may be troublesome in patients on long-term therapy.

Urinary system There is one published case of *uremia* on record as well as one of a *reversible nephropathy* in a patient with rheumatoid arthritis.

Skin and appendages Immediate-type hypersensitivity reactions have occurred with *pruritic rashes* and *urticaria*. Cutaneous *necrotizing vasculitis* with histological changes resembling a Type III hypersensitivity reaction has been described. In another well-documented case, a widespread vasculitic rash, chiefly affecting the limbs, appeared in a woman with rheumatoid arthritis treated for 2 months. In these cases, serum complement was normal and there were no circulating immune complexes, although a histamine skin wheal test produced a vasculitis at a clinically non-affected site. Both cases were reversible.

A single instance of *erythema multiforme* has been observed as well as one of *erythema nodosum* (SEDA-7, 317). Two patients developed *lichenoid skin eruptions* which subsided when the drug was stopped, although one of these was left with severe scarring, alopecia of the scalp and widespread atrophic and hyper-pigmented skin lesions.

Musculoskeletal *Arthritis* has occurred in patients with Crohn's disease or Behcet's disease treated with levamisole, although it is well known that this may occur with either disease irrespective of drug treatment.

Risk situations There are no absolute contraindications. In view, however, of its distribution and excretion pattern, levamisole should not be used in severe *hepatic* or *renal disease*, nor should it be combined with *hepatotoxic* anthelminthics or other drugs presenting risks to the liver. Both *Sjögren's syndrome* and *psoriatic arthropathy* are probably conditions in which levamisole is better avoided because of the risk of hypersensitivity reactions. There is much agreement that the possible benefits of levamisole in rheumatoid arthritis are often outweighed by its side effects (SEDA-11, 277). It has been found that in the treatment of the hyperimmunoglobulin E recurrent-infection syndrome (*Job's syndrome*), infectious complications are more serious when levamisole is given, even where normal chemotactic responsiveness has been found. The risk of severe adverse reactions generally seems to be greater in cases treated for *lymphatic filariasis* and apparently also in cases with AIDS.

Second-generation effects Available animal studies do not point to a teratogenic effect, but there are insufficient human data available to assess the safety of levamisole in pregnancy and the WHO recommends delaying treatment until after pregnancy where possible.

Bephenium hydroxynaphthoate

Bephenium hydroxynaphthoate is used in the treatment of hookworm infection in a single dose of 5 grams of the salt. It is well tolerated and reactions are confined to mild *gastrointestinal disturbance* (*unpleasant taste in the mouth*, *nausea*, *abdominal pain*, sometimes also *vomiting* and *diarrhea*) as well as *headache* and *dizziness*. It is reputed to be safe in pregnancy but contraindicated in conditions in which purgation is undesirable such as during the last few months of pregnancy.

Bithionol

Bithionol has been used since 1982 for the treatment of *Fasciola hepatica* infection, which remains problematical. An Egyptian report in 1991 on the use of bithionol in doses of 30 mg/kg every other day for five doses noted that unpleasant symptoms were common, but some or most of them were certainly due to the underlying disease and actually declined with treatment (7[c]). The only symptom the incidence of which actually increased as a result of treatment was *diarrhea*, which appeared in 12 of 14 users; one patient also developed *urticaria* with *pruritus*. It is not clear whether liver function was monitored during treatment. More work is still needed before the safety profile of bithionol can be said to have been defined.

Bitosconate

Bitosconate is used in the treatment of hookworm infection in a dose of 100 mg, 12-hourly for two or three doses. Over half of treated patients develop mild reactions comprising *gastrointestinal symptoms* and *dizziness*.

Dichlorophen

Dichlorophen is used in the treatment of tapeworms, on which it has a direct lethal action. During the first few hours after a 6-gram oral dose of dichlorophen a third of patients experience *nausea*, *diarrhea* or *abdominal pain* and some experience *vomiting*. *Urticaria*, *contact allergic dermatitis* and *photosensitivity* can occur. In the past, with larger doses, *jaundice* and even *hepatic necrosis* occurred.

Diethylcarbamazine

Diethylcarbamazine is used in the treatment of filarial infections. In some infecting species it is effective in both the adult and microfilarial stages, whilst in others it is active only against the microfilarial stages and does not eradicate the infection. The drug is extensively metabolized, the plasma half-life being 6—12 hours; the remainder enters the urine within 48 hours. Dosage should be increased slowly over the initial period slowly to avoid or reduce *allergic responses* occurring as a result of destruction of parasites and liberation of antigen, and then maintained at 3 mg/kg 3 times daily for 34 weeks. Not all the adverse effects noted below are necessarily due to destruction of the parasite; weakness, lethargy, anorexia and nausea may be due to the drug itself.

Adverse reactions to treatment vary with the infecting filarial species and are most severe in onchocerciasis (see below). Minor reactions include *malaise*, *nausea* and *headache*, but the drug also appears to depress the central nervous system in some individuals, resulting in *dizziness* and *somnolence*; indeed, reversible *coma* has been reported in the past in patients in poor physical condition. Nicotine-like properties can produce *autonomic* effects. A degree of *eosinophilia* during treatment is usual. When one is treating *Wuchereria bancrofti* and *Brugia malayi* infections, reactions again include headache and fever, sometimes accompanied by *malaise*, *nausea* and *vomiting*. *Urticarial* skin rashes may occur, and subsequently *lymphangitis* and *lymphadenopathy* often appear (SEDA-17, 357). Abscess formation may occur in association with adult worms.

B. malayi is more susceptible to diethylcarbamazine than *W. bancrofti*; a study of the former condition, undertaken to explain the very severe effects often associated with diethylcarbamazine treatment of lymphatic filariasis, provided evidence of the involvement of the cytokinin interleukin-6 (IL-6), levels of which were found to be raised during treatment (8).

Loa loa infections are treated with the same dosage regimen and both adult and microfilariae are susceptible. Here *encephalitis* is a major risk among patients with heavy infestation (SEDA-17, 356; 9[C]) and ivermectin should be preferred. Severe *allergic reactions* can demand treatment with antihistamines and corticosteroids. The risk of encephalitis has led to the recommendation that prophylactic use of the drug against Loa loa should only be used where the chance of infection is considerable.

In *Onchocerca volvulus* infections, severe reactions may occur in the initial stages of therapy, particularly since diethylcarbamazine only kills the microfilariae of *O. volvulus* (resulting in the release of toxins) and does not eradicate the infection. The *Mazzotti reaction*, a Herxheimer-type response, may be severe and even fatal; it comprises a pruritic papular dermatitis, urticaria, fever, malaise and postural hypotension; asthma and respiratory distress may occur and the hypotension may be associated with irreversible collapse. There may be painful *lymphadenopathy*. Ocular complications are of particular importance: development of *iritis*, induced by dying microfilariae, requires topical or systemic corticosteroids. Changes may also occur in the posterior segment (10[C]) with *visual field defects*. These changes comprise transient retinal pigment epithelial lesions at the posterior pole, globular infiltrates at the limbus and optic disk leakage (11[C]). Similar ocular lesions may develop after topical diethylcarbamazine therapy (SEDA-7, 316). Visual field defects are not reversible and limit the clinical value of diethylcarbamazine in this disease. A study of the mechanisms involved was carried out on 20 males treated over a 6-month period (12[C]). Major systemic complications of therapy included *proteinuria*, severe *pruritus*, *visual field constriction*, *optic nerve pallor*, *chorioretinitis*, *anterior uveitis* and *punctate keratitis*. Circulating immune complexes were increased in 14 individuals. Those with a CIq binding greater than 3% were at significantly increased risk of developing visual field constriction and proteinuria. It may be noted that proteinuria has even been seen in some patients receiving the drug topically.

The dosage of diethylcarbamazine should be reduced in the case of *renal impairment*. Treatment is not advisable in patients ill with *other serious conditions* or in *pregnant women*.

Ivermectin *(13[R])*

Over a number of years, ivermectin has shown excellent results in the treatment of onchocerciasis, both in controlled studies and in the field, including use in the WHO-sponsored program of treatment, and these experiences have provided what is probably a complete picture of its adverse reactions. The effective dosage is of the order of 50—200 μg/kg; Following a single oral dose, skin microfilariae remain at low levels for up to 9 months. Ivermectin has also been found useful in *Brugia malayi* infestations and in loiasis.

Clinical experience has often shown relatively little toxicity, though mild side effects, presumably due to the killing of the microfilariae, involve at least a third of patients; some work has suggested that neutrophil activation may play a role in the development of side effects (14). Ivermectin has been adequately shown to be a safe drug, and across the board it is generally better tolerated than diethylcarbamazine. The only reservation to be made is that the drug has a long half-life and that some late effects might in principle occur in certain individuals; during the early phases of study it was recommended that in areas where the drug had been widely administered the health workers involved should remain for a period in case problems did arise, but no problems have so far arisen.

Among the clinical papers published on ivermectin there are some specifically seeking to define the pattern of adverse effects, e.g. a study published by Moulia-Pelat and others in 1993 (15[CR]); though these particular authors used their single 400-μg/kg dose of the drug in some patients in combination with diethylcarbamazide, the side effect pattern was similar to that when ivermectin was used alone (SEDA-18, 312). Addiss et al. (16[C]) similarly used the drug (in 200- or 400-μg doses) with or without diethylcarbamazide.

ADVERSE REACTION PATTERN

General and toxic effects Acute symptoms are related almost entirely to the release of toxic products and allergens from the killed filariae; in conditions in which this type of reaction does not occur one may suspect that the drug is ineffective. The Addiss study, in *W. bancrofti* infection, showed a higher than average incidence of reactions (and a higher incidence with ivermectin than with diethylcarbamazide) and perhaps reflected an unusually high success rate or the severity of the original infection. For similar reasons, repeated courses of treatment tend to show a declining incidence of adverse effects. Normally, such general symptoms as fever, asthenia, anorexia, malaise and chills occur in a substantial minority of patients on a first course, while at least a third suffer from muscle and/or joint pain. Vertigo, dyspnea, diarrhea and abdominal disturbances affect a few percent of patients.

Hypersensitivity Some of the above acute reactions to the release of parasite material are undoubtedly allergic rather than toxic. In addition, sensitivity to the drug itself can exist but is probably very rare.

Tumor-inducing effects These do not seem to have been reported.

ORGANS AND SYSTEMS

Cardiovascular Supine and postural *tachycardia* with (postural) *hypotension* can occur; in one large study, such effects were found in three of 40 patients (SEDA-14, 262), but in some others they have not been observed at all (SEDA-17, 356). A massive community study in Ghana noted hypotension in only 37 of nearly 15 000 patients treated (17[C]). Transient *ECG changes* are sometimes seen.

Neurological *Headache* and *vertigo* are common. It is notable that when treating *Loa loa* infections on a large scale with ivermectin the encephalitis which is a dreaded consequence of treating it with diethylcarbamazine does not seem to occur (18[c]).

Respiratory In the treatment of *W. bancrofti* filariasis with single doses up to 200 μg/kg, respiratory capacity was evaluated in 23 patients; a transient but significant *fall in vital capacity* was found some 24–30 hours after drug administration, apparently due to bronchodilatation (19[C]). Frank *dyspnea* occurred in 2% of cases in the Moulia-Petat study. In other studies, a few patients have developed a transient *cough* and in others *pneumonitic patches* have been seen in the lung X-ray (SEDA-18, 313).

Skin and appendages A degree of *pruritus* is common and *rash* or *skin edema* may appear, while pre-existing conditions of this type may be aggravated (SEDA-17, 355). The skin over hematomas (see below) may be *discolored*.

Hematological When 28 Sudanese patients were treated with a single dose for onchocerciasis they developed a prolonged prothrombin time which continued to lengthen significantly during the next 4 weeks; there were no changes in other clotting parameters. After a month, two of them developed *hematomatous swellings* which continued to enlarge for the next 3–4 days; both these patients had received a 150-μg/kg dose (20[C]). One of them patients was given a transfusion; the swellings in both cases resolved within a week. For a time it was considered that the prothrombin changes observed in some such cases taking ivermectin were a potential problem; more recent work suggests that, in the class of patients being treated, the prolongation of prothrombin ratios is in fact little more evident than in a placebo group, and that in fact ivermectin merely has a mild effect on vitamin K metabolism and little effect on coagulation (21[cR]). *Lymphadenitis* has however been noted in a few patients. In one Guatemalan study of biannual treatment of the population to eradicate *Onchocerca volvulus* infection, *upper-limb edema* was noted in nearly a fifth of cases receiving the treatment for the first time (22[Cr]).

Urinary system *Proteinuria* is unusual but it has been described; it was detected 14 days after single-dose treatment and disappeared during follow-up (SEDA-18, 313).

Musculoskeletal system *Joint or bone pain* is common but usually mild; the Moulia-Petat study noted myalgia in 33% of cases and arthralgia similarly in 33%.

Sexual organs *Orchitis with scrotal tenderness* is one possible manifestation of the acute reaction as the parasite succumbs (SEDA-17, 356).

Special senses Careful ophthalmological examination may show a striking increase in the number of *microfilariae* in the anterior chamber of the eye in a significant minority of patients, and in already damaged areas of the retina a new inflammatory *infiltrate* can appear during treatment (SEDA-15, 334). It is however notable that no permanent ocular sequelae have been documented. Most of the other ophthalmic symptoms experienced, including edema and local inflammations, are those of the primary infection.

Miscellaneous *Gland tenderness* may be experienced.

Second-generation effects No evidence of second-generation injury has been reported, but it is regarded as prudent to avoid the drug in pregnant and lactating women and in young children. Some 2% of the administered dose is excreted in the breast milk.

Risk situations The drug is contraindicated in any patient who has shown signs of *hypersensitivity* to it.

Niridazole

Niridazole is used in the treatment of schistosomiasis and of guinea-worm (*Drocunculus medinensis*) infections, in divided daily doses of 25 mg/kg for 5–10 days depending on the infecting species. The drug is well tolerated in *Schistosoma haematobium* infections. It is metabolized in the liver, and metabolites color the urine dark brown. It has been largely superseded by alternative drugs in the treatment of schistosomiasis.

ADVERSE REACTION PATTERN

General and toxic reactions Toxic reactions are seen more frequently in *S. mansoni* infections, especially in patients with poor liver function or porto-caval shunts, when neuropsychiatric complications can be expected. Some toxicity is directly related to parasite destruction and liberation of antigen rather than to the drug itself. Common reactions include gastrointestinal disturbances, headache and dizziness. Neurotoxic and psychiatric effects, convulsions and cardiac effects are less common, except in patients with liver disease.

Hypersensitivity reactions Hypersensitivity reactions related to parasite destruction include urticaria, allergic conjunctivitis and fever with peripheral eosinophilia.

Tumor-inducing effects Niridazole is a potent carcinogen in mice and tumorigenic effects have been demonstrated in mice and hamsters. It is not clear what risks may exist in man, but it is of course usually administered only over a brief period.

ORGANS AND SYSTEMS

Cardiovascular Minor ECG abnormalities, especially T-wave changes, are probably of no functional significance. *Dysrhythmias* with prolonged Q-T interval may occur in a small minority.

Respiratory *Cough*, *fever* and *dyspnea* with *pulmonary infiltration* have been reported in two published cases.

Nervous system *Headache*, *drowsiness* and *dizziness* are common. More severe neuropsychiatric symptoms are more frequent in patients with liver disease, especially with porto-systemic shunts since the drug bypasses the liver. Symptoms in these cases include *insomnia*, *anxiety*, *depression*, *confusion*, *hallucinations* and *convulsions*; the reactions may prove fatal. The *electroencephalogram* may show slowed α-rhythms, β-waves and θ-waves as well as sharp wave and spike forms. A single case of *acute cortical necrosis* is recorded in the older literature and could have been coincidental (SED-8, 691). *Agitation* can occur in patients with abnormal liver function.

Hematological An increased peripheral eosinophilia is usual. Hemolysis has been reported once in glucose-6-phosphate dehydrogenase deficiency (SED-8, 691). See also 'Liver' below.

Liver *Prolongation of prothrombin time* may occur. Niridazole is contraindicated in liver disease.

Gastrointestinal *Bad taste*, *anorexia*, *nausea*, *vomiting*, *diarrhea* and *abdominal pain* are common. *Hematemesis* has been seen.

Urinary system Metabolites color the urine dark brown.

Sexual function Transient *reduction in spermatogenesis*, apparently reversible, can occur.

Musculoskeletal system The *muscular pain*, *joint pain* and *bone pain* commonly reported may be related to parasite destruction rather than direct toxicity.

Risk situations Niridazole has largely been superseded in the treatment of schistosomiasis. Because of its toxic effects on several systems, it should not be used in the presence of *hepatic*, *neuropsychiatric*, *cardiac* or *renal* disease. Caution is required in individuals with *glucose-6-phosphate dehydrogenase deficiency*.

Second-generation effects It is considered that niridazole should not be used in pregnancy; mutagenic effects have been seen in bacteria.

Oxamniquine

Given in doses of 15 mg/kg or in a single oral dose up to 15 mg/kg b.i.d. for 2 days, depending on the sensitivity of *Schistosoma mansoni* in the area concerned, oxamniquine is effective with minimal toxicity. It has no effect in *S. haematobium* infections. The drug is no longer given intramuscularly because of severe pain at the injection site. Reactions occur in up to a third of patients and comprise *dizziness*, *drowsiness*, *headache*, *amnesia*, *occasional behavioural disturbances* (*hallucinations*, *excitement*) and even *seizures* (SEDA-14, 262); there is often some *nausea*, *vomiting* and *diarrhea* (23[CR]). Allergic manifestations including *fever* and *pruritic skin rashes* may occur. Minor *abnormalities of liver function* and *creatine phosphokinase* have been reported; *proteinuria* and *hematuria* have been reported during treatment.

Piperazine

Piperazine seems to block selectively the neuromuscular cholinergic receptors of the worm. It is readily absorbed, but has a highly variable plasma half-life. The adult oral dose of 4 grams of piperazine hydrate has been used extensively in the treatment of ascariasis. Though it is a very old drug, it is still considered sufficiently safe for use, though in most industrialized countries it has been abandoned primarily because of concerns as to possible carcinogenicity and to changes on the electroencephalogram (SEDA- 12, 267).

ADVERSE REACTION PATTERN

General and toxic reactions In most patients, piperazine is free of adverse reactions. Mild gastrointestinal disturbances may occur; neurotoxicity is rare.

Hypersensitivity reactions Eczematous skin reactions, lacrimation, rhinorrhea, joint pains, productive cough and bronchospasm can develop after sensitization, especially with occupational exposure. Urticaria has also been reported. When hypersensitivity reactions occur the drug should be withdrawn and not used again in the same patient.

Tumor-inducing effects Mononitrosation of piperazine can occur in the stomach releasing the potential carcinogen *N*-mono-nitrosopiperazine, but there is no direct proof of risk in human subjects.

ORGANS AND SYSTEMS

Cardiovascular Cardiac *conduction defects* have been described (24[cr]).

Respiratory Allergic *respiratory reactions* can occur, resulting in cough and bronchospasm.

Nervous system *Headache*, *dizziness* and *somnolence* occur in a small proportion of treated individuals. More serious neurological reactions occur rarely but tend to be reported in young children, in persons with neurological or renal disease, or after overdosage. Symptoms in such cases include *ataxia*, *paresthesias*, *undue clumsiness*, *myoclonus* and *nystagmus*. *Choreiform movements* and an electroencephalogram with prominent slow waves have been reported as well as an *exacerbation of petit mal* (25[c]) and absence seizures (26[c]). In a child, horizontal nystagmus and hypotonia has been reported after a normal dose.

Hematological One suspected case of *hemolysis* following piperazine treatment has been published (27[C]) but it related to a case of G6PD deficiency. A case of temporary *thrombocytopenia* has been described (28[c]), probably due to prior sensitization by ethylenediamide (a stabilizer in some creams) with which piperazine cross-reacts.

Liver A single incident resembling viral *hepatitis* following piperazine and recurring after further dosage has been reported.

Gastrointestinal *Nausea*, *vomiting*, *abdominal pain* and *diarrhea* may occur occasionally.

Skin *Erythema* and rarely *allergic reactions* can occur.

Special senses Several reports of difficulty in visual *focusing* have been documented; reports of cataract after piperazine have not been authenticated.

Risk situations Although piperazine is usually well tolerated, patients with hepatic or renal disease or neurological disease and epilepsy are better treated with alternative anthelminthics.

Second-generation effects There is no evidence that piperazine has any second-generation effects; it has been used extensively in pregnancy without untoward incidents, but as a precaution WHO advises against administration in the first trimester.

Interactions High doses of piperazine can enhance the adverse effects of *chlorpromazine* and other phenothiazines. Piperazine may antagonize the anthelminthic efficacy of *pyrantel* and vice-versa. There is cross-reactivity with *ethylenediamide* (see above).

Praziquantel (and levopraziquantel)

Praziquantel, initially introduced as a veterinary cesticidal drug, was found to have efficacy against all the human species of schistosomes as well as fasciolopsiasis, paragonomiasis (lung fluke) and *Clonorchis sinensis* (oriental liver fluke) infections. It is administered in a dose of 40 mg/kg as a single oral dose except in infestations with *Schistosoma japonicum*, *Clonorchis* and *Paragonimus* where more prolonged administration is required. Praziquantel was originally introduced as a racemic mixture; there is now evidence that the levo-isomer is relatively more effective, but it seems to have the same incidence of adverse reactions (29[C]). Reactions are in either case generally mild and occur several hours after administration, but any of the effects associated with the death of a parasite can in principle occur.

General Non-specific effects observed in a minority of cases include generalized *weakness*, *swelling* (of the legs, epigastric area, scrotum or more generally) and *fatigue* (SEDA-16, 354).

Nervous system Dose-dependent *dizziness* is a recognized effect, e.g. in some 14% of cases in the higher doses (SEDA-12, 267). A patient predisposed to epilepsy may develop *convulsions*, again probably as a reaction to the death of the parasite (30[c]). *Headache* and *drowsiness* are common in some studies and the manufacturers warn against driving or operating machinery while under the influence of praziquantel.

Most patients treated for neurocysticercosis with praziquantel develop an early '*cerebrospinal fluid reaction*', though a similar late reaction appearing some 2 weeks after treatment has been completed has also been described (31[Cr]). In both situations there can be clinical signs and symptoms, which can include papilledema, headache, nausea, vomiting, neck stiffness and even focal seizures. Steroids can usually prevent or relieve both the early and the late reaction, but it seems that they can also reduce the efficacy by lowering plasma levels of the drug by some 50% (32[CR]).

Gastrointestinal Dose-dependent *nausea*, *vomiting* and *abdominal pain* can occur: e.g. at doses of 30 mg/kg in schoolchildren there was stomach ache in some 16% of cases (SED-12, 775). *Bloody diarrhea* occurs in some patients but it can be difficult to distinguish this as a side effect from pre-treatment symptoms; an Ethiopian study of the drug's use in suspected schistosomiasis found that prior to treatment there was blood in the stool in 55% of cases, diarrhea in 61% and abdominal discomfort in 80%, and the figures recorded the next day after treatment were not very different (33[C]).

Liver In the Ethiopian study cited above, *hepatomegaly* was seen in 2% of cases and *splenomegaly* in 3%.

Allergic reactions Allergic reactions due to parasite death may occur subsequently and include *fever*, *urticaria*, *pruritic skin rashes* and *eosinophilia*. In one violent reaction reported by Azher and others the elements included marked eosinophilia, pleuritic chest pain, cardiac effusion, ascites, and all the evidence of an exudative polyserositis (34[C]).

Risk situations There is clearly a risk that if patients treated with the drug for disease other than neurocysticercosis do in fact also have this disease, serious neurological reactions (notable seizures) can occur as the parasite is killed and toxins are released (35[CR]). The risk of convulsions in patients predisposed thereto has been noted above. It is widely considered that the drug should not be used in ocular cystericercosis because of the risk of inoperable lesions resulting from destruction of the parasite within the eye.

Second-generation effects The drug is excreted in the breast milk, and mothers should not breast feed for 72 hours after intake.

Pyrantel

The usual single dose of pyrantel is 10 mg/kg and reactions are rarely an impediment to treatment. They include *gastrointestinal disturbance* (*nausea. anorexia*, *abdominal pain*, *diarrhea*) as well as *headache* and *vomiting*, which are usually mild but may occur in up to 20% of patients. The drug should not be given when hepatic function is impaired since it can *raise transaminase levels*.

Pyrvinium embonate (viprynium pamoate)

This deep-red insoluble dye is well tolerated in doses up to 5 mg/kg. *Nausea*, *vomiting*, *diarrhea* and *cramping abdominal pain* are more frequent at higher doses.

Feces and vomit are *stained red*. Isolated cases of *severe allergy* (36[C]), transient *photosensitivity* and *Stevens-Johnson syndrome* (37[C]) have been reported.

Tetrachloroethylene

This heavy liquid is given orally in a dose of 0.1 ml/kg up to a maximum of 5 ml as a single dose on an empty stomach for hookworm infection. Usually formulated as capsules or emulsion, it is unstable, especially if exposed to light. Concurrent *Ascaris* infection should be treated first to avoid migration of worms and the risk of *peritonitis*.

ADVERSE REACTION PATTERN

General and toxic reactions These are similar to those of carbon tetrachloride, but less severe. The drug is hepatotoxic and neurotoxic, but gastrointestinal disturbance is the only common side effect when it is used carefully. There is some risk of addiction to the inhaled vapour: inhalation may result in vascular reactions, loss of consciousness, pulmonary edema, and in fatal hepatic and renal damage. Alcohol and fatty foods increase absorption and hepatic toxicity. Exposure to the drug has been known to lead to vinyl chloride disease.

Hypersensitivity reactions These have not been recorded.

Tumor-inducing effects These have not been recorded and would not be anticipated in a single-dose treatment regime.

ORGANS AND SYSTEMS

Cardiovascular In cases of poisoning, *hypotension* can occur; sympathicomimetic drugs should not be used to treat it, since ventricular fibrillation can follow.

Respiratory Damage is only likely to occur if the liquid is inhaled in a concentration of more than 200 p.p.m.

Nervous system *Headache* and *vertigo* are common. Patients should remain at rest for 3 hours following administration and take only water. Inhalation of vapor by addicts (see above) may cause *stupor*. Reversible *neuropsychiatric symptoms*, readily resembling alcoholic intoxication, have occurred after a single 5-ml dose.

Liver *Hepatotoxicity* is similar to that induced by carbon tetrachloride and can occur after oral treatment or even inhalation of the vapour.

Gastrointestinal *Nausea*, *vomiting*, *colicky abdominal pain* and *diarrhea* are common reactions.

Urinary system *Renal damage* may occur, especially after inhalation.

Skin and appendages *Toxic epidermal necrolysis* has followed oral therapy. If the liquid comes into contact with the skin, either directly or following vomiting, *burn-like* reactions may occur.

Risk situations Treatment should be avoided in patients with hepatic or renal damage, gastrointestinal inflammation or ulceration, in debilitated individuals and in young children. As noted above, heavy *Ascaris* infections should be treated before giving tetrachloroethylene in order to avoid peritonitis and intestinal obstruction.

Second-generation effects It is considered unwise to use this drug in pregnancy in view of the potential hepatotoxicity, but no specific information on risks to the fetus is available.

Tiabendazole (thiabendazole)

Tiabendazole is the classic benzimidazole derivative; it inhibits cellular enzyme systems specific to some species of helminth. The drug is given in a dose of 25 mg/kg twice daily for 3 days. It has been used principally in the treatment of *Strongyloides stercoralis* infection and cutaneous *larva migrans*. It is absorbed and therefore acts on adult and larval stages. It is also effective in *Enterobius* infection, hookworm and *Trichuris trichiura* infections.

Individual tolerance to the drug is unfortunately variable and side effects are common, as a result of which the newer benzimidazoles are now often preferred.

ADVERSE REACTION PATTERN

General and toxic reactions Common toxic effects include nausea, vomiting and dizziness. Malaise and drowsiness are also common. Liver disorders can occur and are the most serious complications seen. Most systems can on occasion be affected.

Hypersensitivity reactions These are essentially due to parasite destruction rather than a direct effect of the drug itself. Chills, fever, lymphadenopathy, angioneurotic edema and pruritic rashes may all occur; treatment should in that case be stopped since otherwise more serious reactions (Stevens-Johnson syndrome) can follow.

Tumor-inducing effects These have not been reported.

ORGANS AND SYSTEMS

Cardiovascular *Bradycardia*, *hypotension* and *syncope* may occur, even to the point of collapse.

Nervous system *Drowsiness*, *headache*, *malaise* and *fatigue* are common. More severe symptoms of neurotoxicity are not unusual and include *disorientation*, *confusional states*, *feelings of detachment*, overt *psychosis* (38^{C}), and possibly epileptiform *convulsions* (39^{Cr}), though the latter have been reported only in a case of Down syndrome.

Endocrine, metabolic *Hypoglycemia* has been recorded.

Liver Parenchymal *liver damage* may occur and abnormal liver function tests have been documented. Various cases of persistent cholestasis are on record (40^{C}) as well as well-studied cases of bile-duct injury which can lead to micronodular cirrhosis (41^{C}).

Gastrointestinal *Nausea*, *anorexia*, *vomiting*, *abdominal pain* and *diarrhea* are common and occur in a high proportion of patients.

Musculoskeletal system Severe *muscle pain on exercise* can occur.

Urinary system *Crystalluria* has been noted, sometimes with *hematuria*, and the urine may have an '*asparagus-like*' smell.

Skin and appendages An unusual body *odor* is produced. *Pruritus* and *skin rashes* can occur and a *perianal rash* induced by the excreted drug has been observed. Much more rarely, *toxic epidermal necrolysis* has occurred after a total dose of 1800 mg. *Stevens-Johnson syndrome* and *erythema multiforme* have also been reported (42^{CR}). Very occasionally a topical form of tiabendazole is used, e.g. to treat rosacea, and in such a case *contact dermatitis* aggravated by sunlight occurred as a complication, with positive tests for tiabendazole sensitivity (43^{C}).

Special senses *Vision* may be deranged with objects having a yellow tinge; hypersensitivity can cause *conjunctivitis*. *Tinnitus* has occurred.

Musculoskeletal system Several papers refer to severe *muscular pain* during treatment.

Risk situations Tiabendazole should be used with caution in hepatic or renal impairment. It should be discontinued if hypersensitivity reactions occur. Patients should be warned not to drive or to carry out other potentially hazardous pursuits during the course of treatment.

Second-generation effects There is no firm information on adverse reactions during pregnancy, but animal evidence points to teratogenicity and there have been official warnings against use by pregnant women (44[R]).

Interactions There is some evidence that the therapeutic efficacy of the drug is impeded by *corticosteroids*. Tiabendazole can seriously increase serum levels of *theophylline* and related substances.

OTHER BENZIMIDAZOLES

The newer broad-spectrum benzimidazoles have a wide spectrum of anthelminthic activity, killing larval and adult cestodes as well as intestinal nematodes with generally low mammalian toxicity apart from a potential for teratogenicity and embryotoxicity. The principal members of the group are mebendazole, its fluorine analog flubendazole and the better-absorbed albendazole. Mebendazole and albendazole are active orally in a single dose for a wide range of intestinal nematodes and are being used increasingly in the treatment of hydatid disease, where experience is rapidly advancing. Flubendazole is very poorly absorbed and induces local tissue reactions at the site of injection when given parenterally. None of the benzimidazoles is known to be safe in pregnancy; animal studies and their spectrum of toxicity suggest that they should be avoided. Absence of positive reports of harm in human pregnancy does not mean that no harm can occur.

High-dose treatment with the benzimidazoles is discussed in a separate section following discussion of the individual drugs.

Albendazole

Albendazole is closely related to mebendazole (see below) and has been used in the treatment of both intestinal helminthiasis and hydatid disease, and it is being increasingly used in high doses for prolonged periods; it has proven particularly valuable in echinococcosis. Reports such as that by Steiger et al. (45[C]) who used 200 mg 3 times daily in cycles of 4 weeks (with 2-week drug-free intervals) have quantified the adverse effects of such intensive treatment and shown that side effects can sometimes occur late and unpredictably. As with other anthelminthics, general reactions can occur which reflect the destruction of the parasite; pyrexia is likely to be seen even in the absence of other problems.

Gastrointestinal With single-dose 400-mg oral therapy alone, there is little more in the way of adverse effects than mild gastrointestinal disturbances (notably *epigastric pain*, *dry mouth*), occurring only in about 6% of patients in large series studied; a few patients suffer abdominal pain. With higher doses, the irritation of the central nervous system can lead to *nausea and vomiting* (see below).

Liver Even in low single doses a transient *increase in transaminase levels* has been repeatedly reported, generally affecting up to 13–16% of patients (SEDA-18, 315). At the higher doses evidence of moderate hepatitis is found in almost all patients, and an occasional individual develops *jaundice* (46[C]).

Respiratory *Rhinitis* can be associated with contact allergy as seen in occupational reactions (see 'Skin' below).

Neurological In more intensive treatment, e.g. with 1.5 mg/kg continued for some time for neurocysticercosis, a majority of patients may initially develop intolerance in the form of *headache*, *vomiting* and *fever*, and occasionally *diplopia* and *meningeal irritation* have been seen (47[C]). When treating this condition even shorter and less intensive treatment has produced similar effects; all these symptoms are probably due to the death of the parasite and if therapy is continued they usually disappear within a few days. Data from large studies mention *somnolence* and even transient *hemiparesis* as incidental adverse effects. Corticosteroids can be needed to relieve those few cases of headache or other neurological symptoms where an increase in intracranial pressure is suspected (SEDA-18, 315). Very rarely indeed, the reaction to the death of the parasite is extremely violent, and in a case of neurocysticercosis cerebral edema has resulted in permanent neurological damage (48[c]).

Hematological There have been various reports of bone marrow depression. In the study by Steiger et al. (see above) two of 20 patients experienced a reversible *drop in leukocyte counts*.

Skin and appendages Generalized *rash* has sometimes been seen (SEDA-15, 334), and skin complications (including urticaria and contact dermatitis) are clearly a potential problem in employees in the pharmaceutical industry if they undergo heavy exposure to the drug (49[c]). There are various well-documented reports in the literature of *alopecia* (SEDA-17, 358) which in one study occurred in 2% of cases (SEDA-18, 315). When one woman was treated with 400 mg b.i.d. for 10 months for hydatid disease, she lost much of her hair; no other likely cause could be identified, and the hair growth recovered when the drug was stopped (50[C]). Transient but complete alopecia was found in one of the 20 patients in the Steiger study (see above), yet half of the other patients when specifically questioned remarked that their hair growth had actually improved during treatment.

Special senses An allergic *conjunctivitis* was seen in the cases of industrial occupational skin reactions noted above.

Musculoskeletal As in other situations where parasites are killed, *myalgia* and *arthralgia* are common features of the reaction.

Second-generation effects Administration in pregnancy is inadvisable in view of potential teratogenic and embryotoxic effects, suspected because of findings in animals.

Mebendazole

Mebendazole has a wide spectrum of anthelminthic activity, being effective against hookworm, ascariasis, enterobiasis, and trichuriasis. The usual dose is 100 mg b.i.d. for 3 days; absorption is minimal, the plasma halflife some 2–9 hours. It is almost without severe adverse reactions. However, doses up to 50–60 mg/kg have been used in cases of cystic echinococcosis unsuitable for surgery, and here side effects need to be watched.

With normal doses, very slight *headache*, *dizziness* and *nausea or diarrhea* are common; in principle *hypersensitivity* can occur. Mild and reversible rises in *transaminases* can occur and need to be followed but even in high-dose treatment are only in a small percentage of patients sufficient to justify stopping treatment (51[c]). These high doses can also cause *granulocytopenia*, *alopecia* and *cough*. The use of mebendazole has been associated with extra-intestinal migration of *Ascaris* in heavily infected patients. In one Indian case, a *fixed drug eruption* appeared to be related to the drug (52[c]) and other forms of rash have been seen.

Evidence of teratogenicity in rats has not been accompanied by reports that it causes harm in human pregnancy, but WHO recommends avoidance during the first trimester. Mebendazole can derange lactation.

Flubendazole

Flubendazole is a further analog of mebendazole used in intestinal helminthiasis and hydatid disease. In trials of two-dose oral treatment for intestinal helminthiasis, reactions were mild and uncommon. They consisted of *nausea*, *abdominal pain*, *dyspepsia* and *sleepiness* (SEDA-6, 281).

Triclabendazole

This drug is primarily used in veterinary medicine but has also been used experimentally in man. *Chills*, *fever*, *leukopenia* and upper abdominal *colic* have been described (SEDA-14, 263).

High-dosage treatment of hydatid disease

Until about 1980, surgery was the only treatment available for larval infections with *Echinococcus granulosus* or *E. multilocularis*. However, cysts are not always amenable to surgical removal and operation is associated with the risk of rupture, leading to anaphylactic shock and reinfection; a proportion of cases are in any case not fit enough for surgery. The benzimidazoles have been used in varying high dosage over extended periods, initially to treat inoperable hydatid cysts and prior to surgery in attempts to sterilize cysts.

Although poorly absorbed following oral administration, mebendazole has been assessed at a range of dose levels and durations of treatment. Doses in the range of 16–60 mg/kg per day have been given, but subsequently wide variations in blood mebendazole levels have been recorded although the drug is known to enter the cyst fluid dependably. Variable clinical efficacy, however, probably reflects the sometimes poor absorption, resulting in low plasma levels and poor cyst penetration.

Apart from the poor chemotherapeutic response obtained in some 25% of cases, drug toxicity (especially at high, prolonged dosage) has led to discontinuation of therapy in a small proportion of patients. Some 3–4% develop fever which may be persistent and accompanied by respiratory symptoms and eosinophilia. Neutropenia has been noted and may be severe and persistent. Other side effects reported include pain over the site of the cyst, allergic reactions and alopecia. Glomerulonephritis has been observed in five patients from Kenya (53[C]); the same paper documented two cases of exfoliative dermatitis in a total of 131 cases treated. Various authors have reported spontaneous rupture of hydatid cysts while on mebendazole therapy and this event is probably more frequent than in untreated individuals. Pleural and peritoneal cysts appear more likely to rupture.

Use of mebendazole may result in the evolution of a more rapidly developing multilobular cyst which is less amenable to surgery. Studies with ultrasound show that both albendazole and mebendazole induce a transformation from a cystic to an ectogenic appearance in these cases.

Side effects severe enough to lead to discontinuation of therapy have included worsening of a pre-existing hyperlipidemia (Type IV), a progressive azotemia and a marked rise in liver enzymes (54^{C}). One individual treated by Von Seitz et al. (55^{C}) developed an exanthema accompanied by a striking rise in serum transaminases, which recurred on subsequent re-exposure to mebendazole.

Experience with the treatment of *E. multilocularis* infection is similar. One case of fatal *agranulocytosis* receiving mebendazole also had severe, probably unrelated, liver disease (SEDA-8, 292).

Albendazole is substantially better and more consistently absorbed after oral administration than mebendazole. At dosage levels of 10 mg/kg, blood levels are a hundred-fold those obtained using mebendazole. Pharmacokinetic studies suggest that albendazole is well absorbed in the blood, tissues and cyst fluid, and that the drug and its active metabolites (albendazole sulfoxide and albendazole sulfone) act gradually, possibly preventing any massive release of antigen and thus allergic reactions. The drug was found to be well tolerated in 30-day courses of 10—14 mg/kg per day separated by 2-week intervals. Side effects reported so far are similar to those seen with mebendazole therapy and are possibly more common due to the improved and more reliable absorption. They include early pyrexia, neutropenia (in three cases) and rising transaminase levels. Cyst rupture may also occur as with mebendazole therapy. Careful monitoring of white cell count, platelet count, and liver function tests is indicated, and the possibility of teratogenicity and embryotoxicity suggests that the drug should be avoided in pregnancy.

OTHER ANTHELMINTHIC DRUGS

Hexachloroparaxylene

Previously used in the treatment of infection due to *Clonorchis sinensis* and *Schistosoma japonicum*, hexachloroparaxylene gives rise to *gastrointestinal reactions*, *cardiac arrhythmias* (perhaps in over 50% of cases) and *nephrotoxicity*. Early and late-type drug-induced *hemolysis* occurs; death may occur from the hemolytic uremic syndrome (SED-4, 219). Late-onset hemolysis occurring after treatment is associated with β-thalassemia, whilst early-onset hemolysis is associated with hemoglobin-H disease. So far as is known, the drug is no longer used.

Hycanthone mesylate

Hycanthone is a derivative of lucanthone but has less gastrointestinal or CNS toxicity. It has largely been superseded in the treatment of schistosomiasis by more recent, less toxic compounds. It is effective in both *Schistosoma haematobium* and *S. mansoni* infections. It is given as a single intramuscular injection in doses ranging from 1.0 to 2.5 mg/kg. The most common reaction, occurring in up to half of patients treated with higher-dose regimens, is *vomiting* often associated with *abdominal colic* and *diarrhea*. There may be *muscular pain*, and *T-wave changes* have been observed on the electrocardiogram.

Hepatotoxicity occurs, with frequent evidence of increased serum transaminase levels and less commonly overt jaundice. Fatal liver cell necrosis has been described, and may be associated with pancreatitis.

Experimentally, the drug has been reported to be carcinogenic, mutagenic and teratogenic, although no human data on these matters are available (52).

Metrifonate

Metrifonate, which is administered orally, is effective in *Schistosoma haematobium* infections in a dose of 7.5—10 mg/kg, for three doses separated by 14-day intervals. It depresses *blood cholinesterase* activity for up to 48 hours and reactions commonly occurring which probably result from this effect comprise *nausea*, *vomiting* and *abdominal pain*, *diarrhea*, *dizziness*, *weakness* and *headache*. Theoretically, *suxamethonium* will be potentiated following administration and, in view of its enzymatic suppression, metrifonate should be used with great caution in areas where *organophosphorus insecticides* are used.

Niclosamide

Niclosamide, widely used in the treatment of tapeworm infestation, is well tolerated in doses of 2 grams taken orally before breakfast (as two doses of 1 gram separated by 1 hour). The drug is not absorbed and reactions consist of mild *gastrointestinal disturbances*. Alcohol is usually restricted during treatment since the drug can interfere with its metabolism. When treating *Taenia solium* infections an antiemetic is usually given prior to administration of niclosamide, and patients are subsequently purged to reduce the theoretical risk of cysticercosis; the latter risks exists because the dose of niclosamide active against *T. solium* does not destroy ova contained within the tapeworm.

Suramin

Used for more than 60 years in the treatment of trypanosomiasis and onchocerciasis, suramin is unfortunately toxic and particularly prone to cause adverse effects in the undernourished. For such reasons it has largely been abandoned for these purposes, but it still seems uniquely capable of killing the adult onchocerciasis worm, and there was for a time some hope of using it in AIDS (SEDA-10, 277; SEDA-15, 335); more recently it has been studied in the treatment of prostatic and other cancers.

In the traditional areas of use, *vomiting*, *loss of blood from the gastrointestinal tract* and resultant *shock* can occur very rapidly, but appear only in one case in every 300 or less. *Colic* and *allergic skin reactions* are more usual. Late reactions include various skin *eruptions*, *hyperesthesia* and *paresthesia* (particularly affecting the palms and soles of the feet). Certain effects on the eye (*photophobia*, *lacrimation* and *palpebral edema*) are recognized; as with some other drugs, however, successful treatment of ocular onchocerciasis can be followed much later by *ocular damage* because of parasital remnants in the eye. Finally, *renal damage* can occur and in occasional cases *agranulocytosis* and *hemolytic anemia*. Suramin has generally been avoided in pregnancy cause its safety is uncertain; it is teratogenic in mice but not in rats.

The first study of suramin in AIDS (56^C) was undertaken because of the proven ability of suramin to impair the in vitro infectivity (and inhibit the cytopathic effect) of human T-cell lymphotropic virus Type III (HTLV-III) or lymphadenopathy-associated virus (LAV). The adverse effects in such studies were more severe and numerous than in the drug's traditional field of use—two-thirds of patients proved to suffer malaise, fever and transaminase elevation, and a quarter *adrenal insufficiency*. Erythematous drug eruptions (particularly on sun-exposed surfaces) were common; some patients had a burning sensation of the skin, particularly in the extremities. The most common laboratory abnormalities were proteinuria, microscopic pyuria, trace hemoglobinuria, and occasional granular casts. Rises in hepatic aminotransferase levels occurred in some patients, usually during the second and third weeks and others had eosinophilia (maximum 14%) during a drug eruption. There was a high incidence of *keratopathy* (SEDA-14, 263).

Tested in prostatic cancer, suramin in a loading dose of 100 mg/m^2 followed by individual determined dose levels, the drug was found to have a favorable effect; however, dosage had to be pressed to the point where the bulk of the patients no longer tolerated the adverse effects. Malaise, fatigue and lethargy proceeded to *neuropathy* and *renal toxicity* (SEDA-18, 316). The development of neuropathy has also been reported in detail by others, who recorded it in four of 38 patients infused with suramin for various malignancies (57). In one cancer patient, an immunological complement-mediated *destruction of circulating platelets* was induced by suramin, demanding urgent treatment (58^C)

The toxic effect on the adrenals has been exploited therapeutically in treating adrenal carcinoma (59^C), but with the evident problem of the severe side effects, again including keratopathy.

REFERENCES

1. World Health Organization. WHO Prescribing Information: Drugs used in Parasitic Diseases. Geneva: WHO, 1990, onwards.
2. Sharma A, Thalliath GH, Girgia HS. A comparative evaluation of levamisole in leprosy. Indian J Leprosy 1985;57:11.
3. Balint G. El-Ghobarey A. Capell H et al. Sjögren's syndrome: a contraindication to levamisole treatment. Br Med J 1977;2:1386.
4. Scheinberg MA, Bezerra IBC. Almeida FA et al. Cutaneous necrotising vasculitis induced by levamisole. Br Med J 1978;1:408.
5. Symoens J Veys E, Mielants M et al. Adverse reactions to levamisole. Cancer Treat Rep 1978;65:1721.
6. Palcoux JB, Niaudet P, Goumy P. Side effects of levamisole in children with nephrosis. Pediatr Nephrol 1994;8:263—264.
7. Bassiouny HK, Solian NK, El-Daly SM et al. Human fascioliasis in Egypt; effect of infection and efficacy of bithionol treatment. J Trop Med Hyg 1991;94:333—337.
8. Yazdanbakhsh M, Duym L, Aarden L. Serum Interleukin-6 levels and adverse reactions to diethylcarbamazide in lymphatic filariasis. J Infect Dis 1992;166:453—453.
9. Carme B, Boulesteix J, Boutes H et al. Five cases of encephalitis during treatment of loiasis with diethylcarbamazine. Am J Trop Med Hyg 1991;44:684—690.
10. Bird AC, El-Sheikh H, Anderson J et al. Changes in visual function and in the posterior segment of the eye during treatment of onchocerciasis with diethylcarbamazine citrate. Br J Ophthalmol 1980;64:191.
11. Bird AC, El-Sheikh H, Anderson J, Fuglsang H. Visual loss during oral diethylcarbamazine treatment for onchocerciasis. Lancet 1979;ii:46.
12. Greene BM et al. Ocular and systemic complications of

diethyl carbamazine therapy for onchocerciasis: association with circulating immune complexes. J Infect Dis 1983; 147:890.
13. Van Laethem Y. Ivermectin and other new drugs for the treatment of filariasis. Curr Opin Infect Dis 1992;5:849–854.
14. Njoo FL, Hack CE, Oosting J et al. Neutrophil activation in ivermectin-treated onchocerciasis patients. Clin Exp Immunol 1993;94:330–333.
15. Moulia-Pelat JP, Nguyen LN, Glaziou P et al. Safety trial of single-dose treatments with a combination of ivermectin and diethylcarbamazide in bancroftian filariasis. Trop Med Paristol 1993;44:79–82.
16. Addiss DG, Eberhard ML, Lammie PJ et al. Comparative efficacy of clearing-dose and single high dose ivermectin and diethylcarbamazide against *Wuchereria bancrofti* microfilaremia. Am J Trop Med Hyg 1993;48:178–185.
17. De Sole G, Awadzi K, Runne J et al. A community trial of Ivermectin in the onchocerciasis focus of Asubende, Ghana. II: Adverse reactions. Trop Med Parasitol 1989; 40:375–382.
18. Chippoux JP, Ernould JC, Garon J et al. Ivermectin treatment of loiasis. Trans R Soc Trop Med Hyg 1992;86:289.
19. Kumaraswami V, Ottesen EA, Vijayaserakam V et al. Ivermectin for the treatment of *Wuchereria bancrofti* filariasis. Efficacy and adverse reactions. J Am Med Assoc 1988;259:3150.
20. Homeida MMA, Bagi IA, Ghalib HW et al. Prolongation of prothrombin time with ivermectin. Lancet 1988;i:1325.
21. Whitworth JAD, Hay CRM, Nicholas AM et al. Coagulation abnormalities and ivermectin. Ann Trop Med Hyg 1992;86:301–305.
22. Collins RCV, Gonzales-Peralta C, Castro J et al. Ivermectin: reduction in prevalence and infection intensity of *Onchocerca volvulus* following biannual treatments in five Guatemalan communities. Am J Trop Med Hyg 1992; 47:156–159.
23. De Carvalho SA, Shikanai-Yasuda MA, Amato Neto V et al. Neurotoxicidade do oxamniquine no tratamento da infecção humana pelo *Schistosoma mansoni*. Rev. Inst. Med. Trop. São Paulo 1985;27:132.
24. Gouffault J, Driessche J van D, Pony JC et al. Les troubles de conduction induits par la pipérazine: Étude clinique et expérimentale. Arch Mal Coeur 1973;66:1289.
25. Vallat JN, Vallat JM, Pexier J et al. Les signes neurologiques d'intoxication par la pipérazine. Bordeaux Méd 1972;5:394.
26. Yohai D, Barnett SH. Absence and atonic seizures induced by piperazine. Pediatr Neurol 1989;5:393.
27. Buchanan N, Cassel R, Jenkins T. G6PD deficiency and piperazine. Br Med J 1971;2:110.
28. Cork J, Cooke NJ, Mellor E. Pruritus ani, piperazine and thrombocytopenia. Br Med J 1990;301:1398.
29. Yue-Han L, Xiao-Gen W, Min-Xin Q et al. A comparative trial of single dose treatment with praziquantel and levopraziquantel in human *Schistosomiasis japonica*. Jpn J Parasitol 1988;37:331.
30. Bada JL, Traviño B, Cabezos J. Convulsive seizures after treatment with praziquantel. Br Med J 1988;296:646.
31. Ciferri F. Delayed CSF reaction to praziquantel. Lancet 1988;i:642.
32. Del Brutto OH. Delayed CSF reaction to praziquantel. Lancet 1988;i:341.
33. Fletcher M, Teklehaimanot A. *Schistosoma mansoni* infection in a new settlement in Metekel district, North Western Ethiopia: morbidity and side effects of treatment with praziquantel in relation to intensity of infection. Trans R Soc Trop Med Hyg 1989;83:793–797.
34. Azher ME, El Kasimi FA, Wright SG et al. Exudative polyserositis and acute respiratory failure following praziquantel therapy. Chest 1990;98:241–243.
35. Torres JR. Use of praziquantel in populations at risk of neurocysticercosis. Rev Inst Med Trop São Paulo 1989; 31:290.
36. Desser KB, Baden M. Allergic reaction to pyrvinium pamoate. Am J Dis Child 1969;117:589.
37. Coursin DB. Stevens-Johnson syndrome: nonspecific parasensitivity reaction. J Am Med Assoc 1966;198:113.
38. Schantz PM, Van den Bossche H, Eckert J. Chemotherapy for larval echinococcosis in animals and man. In: Parasitenkunde. Berlin: Springer-Verlag, 1982;5.
39. Tchao P, Templeton T. Thiabendazole-associated grand mal seizures in a patient with Down syndrome. J Pediatr 1983;102:317.
40. Ishizaki I, Kamo E, Boehme K. Double blind studies of tolerance to praziquantel in Japanese patients with *Schistosoma japonicum* infections. Bull World Health Org 1979; 57:787.
41. Manival JC, Bloomer JR, Shover DC. Progressive bile duct injury after thiabendazole administration. Gastroenterology 1989;93:245.
42. Humphreys F, Cox NH. Thiabendazole-induced erythema multiforme with lesions around melanocytic naevi. J Dermatol 1988;118:855.
43. Izu R, Aguirre A, Goicoechea A et al. Photoaggravated allergic contact dermatitis due to topical thiabendazole. Contact Dermatitis 1993;28:243–255.
44. Anonymous. Communication from the Department of Health and Social Security, London, February 22nd, 1988.
45. Steiger U, Cotting J, Reichen J. Albendazole treatment of echinococcosis in humans: effects on microsomal metabolism and drug tolerance. Clin Pharmacol Ther 1990;47:347.
46. Chouduri G, Nath Prasad R. Jaundice due to albendazole. Ind J Gastroenterol 1988;7:245.
47. Escobedo F, Penagos P, Rodriguez J et al. Albendazole therapy for neurocysticercosis. Arch Intern Med 1987; 147:738.
48. Noboa C. Albendazole therapy for giant subarachnoid cysticerci. Arch Neurol 1993;50:347.
49. Macedo NA, Piñeyro MI, Carmona C. Contact urticaria and contact dermatitis from Albendazole. Contact Dermatitis 1991;25:73–75.
50. Al Karawi M, Kasawy MI, Mohamed AL. Hair loss as a complication of albendazole therapy. Saudi Med J 1988;9:530.
51. Bartolini C, Tricerri A, Guidi L et al. The efficacy of chemotherapy with mebendazole in human cystic echinococcosis; long-term follow up of 52 patients. Ann Trop Med Parasitol 1992;86:249–256.
52. Nair LV, Devi U. Mebendazole induced fixed drug eruption. Ind J Dermatol Venereol Leprol 1991;57:19.1.
53. Kunga A. Glomerulonephritis following chemotherapy of hydatid disease with mebendazole. East Afr Med J 1982;59:404.
54. Gil-Grande LA et al. Treatment of liver hydatid disease with mebendazole: a prospective study of thirteen cases. Am J Gastroenterol 1983;73:584.
55. Seitz R, Schwerk W, Arnold R. Hepatocelluläre Arznei-

mittelreaktion unter Mebendazoltherapie bei *Echinococcus cystis*. Gastroenterology 1983;21:324.
56. Broder S, Collins JM, Markham IM et al. Effects of suramin on HTLV-III/LAV infection presenting as Kaposi's sarcoma or AIDS-related complex: clinical pharmacology. and suppression of virus replication in vivo. Lancet 1985; i:627.
57. La Rocca RV, Meer J, Gilliatt RW et al. Suramin-induced polyneuropathy. Neurology 1990;40:954–960.
58. Seidman AD, Schwarz M, Reich L et al. Immune-mediated thrombocytopenia secondary to suramin. Cancer 1993;71:851–854.
59. Holland EJ. Stein CA, Palestine AC et al. Suramin keratopathy. Am J Ophthalmol 1988;106:216.

Meyler's Side Effects of Drugs, 13th Edition
M.N.G. Dukes, editor

SECTION EDITOR: C.J. VAN BOXTEL

S. Dittmann

32 Immunobiological preparations

GENERAL

Adverse events and side effects following immunization In the early days of vaccine development the majority of untoward effects following immunization was associated with faulty production. It is a fact that the control of biological products as they exist today has been developed largely as a result of major accidents, e.g. the Cutter incident in the United States in 1955, in which a batch of 'inactivated' poliomyelitis vaccine containing live poliovirus was inadvertently released with devastating consequences. The World Health Organization subsequently took over the responsibility for international biological standardization. Currently, more than 50 WHO requirements for the manufacture and control of biological substances have been adopted and updated. As a result of the incorporation of WHO requirements, and their strict observance by manufacturers and control authorities, accidents due to faulty production of vaccines have become rare (SEDA 13, 271).

However, during the last two decades rapid increases in immunization coverage levels have been reported worldwide, and the growth of WHO's Expanded Programme on Immunization has sometimes resulted in extension of immunization work into areas where logistic support and training programmes not have been adequate. In such situations, avoidable programmatic events have been incurred due to improper or inadequate sterilization, incorrect doses and routes of vaccine administration, or substitution of drugs for diluents or vaccines (SEDA-15, 340).

The detection of untoward effects following immunization is important to the success of an immunization programme since the occurrence of such events can be influential in community acceptance of immunization. Increasing interest in this problem can therefore be observed in many developed and developing countries, and international institutions and organizations, e.g. the World Health Organization (WHO) and the United Nations Children's Fund (UNICEF).

Terms and definitions used in surveillance programmes of adverse events and side effects following immunization These are fundamental for the establishment of any functioning surveillance system. There must be different definitions for monitoring and evaluation.

Monitoring This is the first step in surveillance, that of data collection. Terms and definitions developed for monitoring purposes should be useful for practitioners and health workers; monitoring definitions have to cover a broad range. For monitoring purposes, the term *adverse event* has been introduced, defined as an untoward event temporally associated with immunization, that might or might not be caused by the vaccine or the immunization process. The term *side effect* does not seem useful for monitoring purposes. The term inevitably relates to an untoward effect following immunization which is linked to the vaccine (antigen or vaccine component) or the immunization process. The term and its definition imply a distinct degree of causality.

The 'Adverse Vaccine Reactions Workshop' held in Ottawa, Canada, 30—31 October 1991, cosponsored by WHO and Health and Welfare Canada, was a starting point for the elaboration of internationally agreed terms and definitions (1^R). Definitions for monitoring of adverse events following immunization have been elaborated, e.g. for local adverse events (injection-site abscess, suppurative lymphadenitis, severe local reaction), central nervous system adverse events (acute paralysis, encephalopathy, encephalitis, meningitis, seizures), other adverse events (allergic reaction, acute hypersensitivity reaction, anaphylactic shock, arthralgia, disseminated BCG-itis, hypotensive-hyporesponsive episode, osteitis/osteomyelitis, persistent screaming, sepsis, toxic shock syndrome).

Evaluation Statistical analysis and expert evaluation of the collected data should be carried out at central level. Expert evaluation of reports should be based on precise evaluation definitions, taking into account the current scientific knowledge.

The events should be classified according to causality, e.g. into: certain, probable, possible, unlikely, unclassified (where no attempt to classify has been made), and unclassifiable events (e.g. due to the lack of data) (2^R);

or alternatively into: no evidence bearing on a causal relation, evidence insufficient to indicate a causal relation, evidence does not indicate a causal relation, evidence is consistent with a causal relation, and evidence indicates a causal relation (3[R]). An evaluated adverse event classified as either 'certain' or 'probable' or 'consistent with a causal relation' or 'indicating a causal relation' fulfils the criteria established to recognize a 'side effect following immunization'.

Following WHO's proposal to distinguish four types of adverse events following immunization, the evaluation should furthermore try to distinguish between: (a) vaccine-induced adverse events (e.g. BCG lymphadenitis, BCG osteitis, vaccine-associated poliomyelitis, allergic reactions); (b) vaccine-precipitated events (e.g. a simple febrile seizure following DPT immunization in a predisposed child); (c) programmatic errors (e.g. an abscess due to improper sterilization): (d) coincidental events (4[R]).

Most commonly, passive surveillance systems are used for the surveillance of adverse events following immunization. Spontaneous reports from health care providers on temporally related adverse events suspected of being caused by the vaccine or the immunization procedure are collected and evaluated. Examples of passive surveillance systems used in different countries have been provided in various Annuals in this series.

Surveillance systems in different countries Some countries have long experience in monitoring adverse events following immunization, starting with smallpox vaccination.

The Netherlands A special committee of the Health Council of the Netherlands has been created with the task of analyzing, classifying and interpreting the side effects (2[R]) which are reported to the National Institute of Health and Environmental Protection in Bilthoven (see SEDA-12, 271; SEDA-13, 278; SEDA-14, 269; SEDA-15, 341; SEDA-16, 365; SEDA-17, 363; SEDA-18, 325).

USA Since March 21, 1988, health care providers and vaccine manufacturers have been required by law to report certain events following specific immunizations (see Table 1, SED-12, 792) to the US Department of Health and Human Services. The 'Vaccine Adverse Event Reporting System' (VAERS) accepts all reports of suspected adverse events after the administration of any vaccine, including but not limited to those certain events required by law to be reported. In 1991, VAERS replaced the Centers for Disease Control's 'Monitoring System for Adverse Events Following Immunization' (MSAEFI) and the Food and Drug Administration's 'Adverse Reaction Reporting System' for publicly and

Table 1. *Estimated rates of adverse reactions following DTP immunization compared to complications of natural whooping cough*

Adverse reaction	Whooping cough complication rates per 100 000 cases	DTP vaccine adverse reaction rates per 100 000 immunizations
Permanent brain damage	600–2000 (0.6–2.0%)	0.2–0.6
Death	100–4000 (0.1–4.0%)	0.2
Encephalopathy/ encephalitis*	90–4000 (0.09–4.0%)	0.1–3.0
Convulsions	600–8000 (0.6–8.0%)	0.3–90
Shock	–	0.5–30

*Including seizures, focal neurological signs, coma, and Reye's syndrome.

privately purchased vaccines (4[R]). Results of the MSAEFI have been published in SEDA-13 (p. 273, 2nd report) and SEDA-16 (p. 320, 3rd report).

Canada Surveillance for adverse events temporally associated with the administration of immunizing agents at the federal level is the responsibility of the Bureau of Communicable Disease Epidemiology (BCDE), Laboratory Centre for Disease Control, Ottawa. The main source of information is passive reporting by health-care providers to provincial or territorial authorities of events thought to be due to immunization. These data, as well as information from manufacturers and other agencies is forwarded to BCDE (5[R]). Results of the Canadian surveillance system have been provided in SEDA-16 (p. 367) and SEDA-17 (p. 363).

Further national surveillance programmes on adverse events following immunization exist, e.g. in Denmark, Sweden, United Kingdom, Hungary; developing countries such as India (see SEDA-17, 363) and Brazil (see SEDA-16, 367) have also already started to collect data on severe adverse events.

National compensation programmes for vaccine-related injuries The need for some form of compensation when an individual is seriously injured by vaccination, particularly when the immunization has been compulsory or recommended by the health authority, has been accepted in many countries:

Canada All vaccines licensed in Canada would be included. Compensation would be provided for costs and losses beyond the scope of existing health care and education plans, including costs of special remedial devices, therapy and transportation, caretaker's allowance in recognition of the extra costs of attending or caring for an injured person, disability pensions or awards, proportional to loss of capacity, and death benefits.

Denmark Covers damage caused by specified vaccines. A disability pension is paid after the age of 15. Lump sum for disability of 5–50%, pension for greater disability.

France Covers damage by compulsory immunization. Compensation is determined by a central tribunal and covers economic and non-economic losses, including future support and help for parents.

Germany Covers damage caused by all officially recommended vaccines, provides coverage for medical and other costs. A disability pension based on federal scheme for workers. Probability of causal relation is sufficient to establish a claim.

Japan Covers damage caused by compulsory immunizations. Provisions include medical allowance, caretaker's allowance, disability pension and funeral grant. A national expert committee reviews applications.

Switzerland Covers damage caused by recommended vaccines, insofar as expenses are not covered by another plan.

United Kingdom Single award of 20 000 English pounds to people severely disabled (80% disability) as a result of immunization against specific diseases. Includes a central expert review panel that examines independent assessments of case histories and disabilities. Appeal mechanisms provided.

United States The system is designed on a no-fault basis; manufacturers are no longer required to prove their lack of negligence. Any part injured by one of the listed vaccines used in childhood immunization programmes would be required to make their initial claim through the federal system. The National Childhood Vaccine Injury Act (1986) limits compensation that could be awarded by the court system (SEDA-12, 271–272; SEDA-14, 271).

Although not focusing primarily on vaccine-induced injury, attention should be paid to an important and novel contribution to the field of liability for *drug-induced disease*: the monograph 'Responsibility for Drug-Induced Injury' by Dukes and Swartz (6[R]).

Benefits and risks of immunization Risks of side effects following immunization against diphtheria, pertussis, tetanus, poliomyelitis, measles and tuberculosis have been discussed in the framework of the WHO Expanded Programme on Immunization and compared with the complication rate following natural disease by Galazka et al. (7[R]). Table 1 presents a comparison of estimated risks of adverse reactions following DTP immunization with the complication rate of natural whooping cough, while Table 2 shows a similar comparison for measles immunization and natural measles. The authors concluded that no vaccine is without side effects, but the risks of serious complications from vaccines used in WHO's Expanded Programme on Immunization are much lower than the risks from the natural disease.

Actual overviews on side effects following immunization The reports of the Institute of Medicine, National Academy of Sciences, Washington, are cited at length (adverse events following pertussis and rubella immunization) in SED-12 (pp. 817 and 825) and (adverse events following immunization against tetanus, diphtheria, measles, mumps, poliomyelitis, *Haemophilus influenzae* type b, and hepatitis B) in SEDA-18 (p. 325) and provide useful overviews (8[R], 9[R]). A condensed overview on risks following the administration of current childhood and adult vaccines has been published by Dittmann (10[R]).

INDIVIDUAL PREPARATIONS

Anthrax vaccine

The inactivated vaccine is mainly used for protection against occupational anthrax exposure. A complete vaccine series consists of three 0.5-ml subcutaneous doses at 2-week intervals, followed by three additional doses 6, 12, and 18 months after the first dose. Mild local reactions occur in 30% of vaccinees, including local erythema and tenderness occurring within 24 hours and beginning to subside by 48 hours.

The reactions tend to increase in severity by the fifth injection. Systemic reactions are rare and usually characterized by malaise and lassitude, chills and fever (11[R]).

Bacille Calmette-Guérin (BCG) vaccine

BCG vaccine is a suspension of living tubercle bacilli of the Calmette-Guérin strain. It is used mainly prophylactically against tuberculosis but also as a means of stimulating the immune response in malignant disease. There are variations in the characteristics of BCG vaccines, depending on the strain of BCG derived from the original BCG strain and used for vaccine production. BCG is generally used intradermally, except the instillation in intravesical immunotherapy. The risk of side effects following BCG immunization is related to the BCG strain, the dose, the age of the vaccinee, the technique of immunization, and the skill of the vaccinator.

Table 2. *Estimated rates of serious adverse reactions following measles immunization compared to complications of natural measles infection and background rate of illness*

Adverse reaction	Measles complication rates per 100 000 cases	Measles vaccine adverse reaction rates per 100 000 vaccinees	Background illness rate per 100 000
Encephalopathy/encephalitis	50–400 (0.05–0.4%)	0.1	0.1–0.3
Subacute sclerosing panencephalitis	0.5–2.0	0.05–0.1	–
Pneumonia	3800–7300 (3.8–7.3%)	–	–
Convulsions	500–1000 (0.5–1.0%)	0.02–190	30
Death	10–10.000 (0.01–10%)	0.02–0.3	

ADVERSE REACTION PATTERN

General and toxic reactions BCG immunization is generally well tolerated. Locally a small papule appears which scales and ultimately leaves a scar; however, abnormal reactions can occur.

The most common adverse *local* reaction, suppurative lymphadenitis, has been reported in 0.1–10% of immunized children under 2 years of age. Faulty immunization technique is the most frequent cause of severe abnormal BCG primary reactions (7^R).

The most serious *generalized* complications of BCG immunization involve disseminated infection with the BCG bacillus and BCG osteitis.

Hypersensitivity reactions These are unusual, but severe anaphylactic reactions can occur, especially when the product is used as an immunostimulant.

Tumor-inducing or preventive effects These effects of prophylactic immunization with BCG have been studied extensively by Skegg (12^R), Lilienfeld et al. (13^R), Snider et al. (14^R), and Kendrick et al. (15^R). The conclusion is justified that among vaccinees no less and no more cancer is found, with the exception of the group with lymphoma–Hodgkin's disease–leukaemia (SEDA-7, 323; 16^R, 17^R).

PRINCIPAL RISKS

The incidence of side effects following BCG immunization has been extensively investigated by the Committee on Prophylaxis of the International Union against Tuberculosis and Lung Disease (IUATLD). Retrospective studies including 51 countries worldwide and collecting data from 1948–1974, according to organ and system category, have been published (SED-12, 795; 18^C, 19^C). The IUATLD has carried out a second prospective study (20^C). Six European countries (Denmark, the former Eastern Germany, Hungary, Romania, Croatia, some parts of the Federal Republic of Germany) participated in the study. Nearly 5.5 million children and adolescents or young adults were immunized from 1979 to 1981 and followed up till the end of 1983. The classification system already used in the retrospective study had been applied. There were important discrepancies among participating countries regarding population size, target groups, immunization schedules, and biological qualities of the vaccines as regards both strains/substrains and modalities of preparation. The mean risk of *local complications and suppurative lymphadenitis* has been found low: 0.387 per 1000 vaccinees or 0.093 per 1000 with positive bacteriological/histological findings, respectively. Due to discrepancies mentioned above, the differences between the countries were remarkable. Twenty-one *disseminated BCG infections and hypersensitivity manifestations* were recorded in four countries. The authors concluded that the study has reaped much more information than those of the retrospective study. The estimated risks of serious disseminated BCG infection were higher than calculated previously (except for bone and joint lesions), but very low when comparing benefit and risks of BCG immunization, especially in infants (20^C).

Disseminated BCG infection (<0.1/100 000 vaccinees) is usually associated with severe abnormalities of cellular immunity. Data collected of cases immunized between 1948 and 1974 (from the retrospective IUATLD study mentioned above) are shown in Table 3. Many authors (21^C) have provided detailed case reports on disseminated BCG infection following BCG immunization at birth in newborns with various underlying immunodeficiency syndromes (severe combined immunodeficiencies, cellular immunodeficiency syndromes, X-linked chronic granulomatous disease or autosomal recessive chronic granulomatous disease) (21^C–23^C) and include patients with *AIDS* (see 'HIV infection and immunization').

Table 3. *Retrospective study on BCG side effect numbers and rates per 1 million vaccinees, 1948–1974, worldwide*

	All countries	Countries where some cases were recorded in any category
Number of countries	187	51
Number of vaccinees (all ages) (1948–1974)	1 470 208 160	1 053 402 835

Number of complications recorded until December, 1977, among cohorts vaccinated 1948–1974

Side effect category	All patients				Cases proven (bacteriologically and/or histologically)	
	In 187 countries as above		In 51 countries as above			
	No.	Rate	No.	Rate	No.	Rate
1. Abnormal BCG primary complex*	6602	4.49	6602	6.27	1100	1.04
2. and 3. Disseminated BCG infection: generalized and/or localized lesions (non-fatal and fatal cases)*	1072	0.73	1072	1.02	561	0.53
4. Syndromes or diseases clinically associated with BCG vaccination**	1838	1.25	1838	1.74	7***	0.01
All categories	9512	6.47	9512	9.03	1668	1.58

* Such cases have often been proven bacteriologically and/or histologically.
** Until now, such cases have never been proven either bacteriologically or histologically.
*** For these 7 cases, TB lesions were seen at postmortem examination, but BCG etiology is doubtful.

Case reports Case reports on disseminated BCG infection in children with *chronic granulomatous disease* (*CGD*) have appeared (24^R–26^C). CGD can result in prolonged and relapsing local complications to BCG immunization (26^C). In a series of child autopsies, 26 of 36 cases which had been given BCG shortly after birth showed *tuberculoid granulomas* at various sites. None of the infants had histological evidence of an immune deficiency (SEDA-8, 301; 27^R).

Cases of fatal *histiocytosis* have been reported in babies with immune defects immunized shortly after birth (28^C). One boy who had been immunized shortly after birth developed ipsilateral axillary lymphoma at the age of 6 months. Microscopically the picture was typical of BCG histiocytosis. The child survived. The underlying immunological disturbance was considered to be a temporary derangement of T-lymphocyte function (SEDA-8, 300; 29^C). A report on a recovery from BCG sepsis of a 7-year-old girl with immunodeficiency has been provided (30^C).

A girl in her third year, who had been immunized against tuberculosis at birth, developed an abscess of the associated lymph nodes (extirpated) and some weeks later intestinal BCG dissemination which seemed to be cured by tuberculostatic treatment.

At the age of 22 years a left-sided hemiplegia due to aneurysmas and thrombosis of cerebral arteries was seen, and 4 years later a nervus oculomotorius paralysis was diagnosed. The women died in her 27th year due to recurrent intestinal BCG dissemination which developed at the end of a pregnancy (a healthy premature child was born). The autopsy confirmed the diagnoses and revealed acid-fast bacilli in the adventitia of the arteria basilaris; the paralysis of the nervus oculomotorius was caused by the brain lesion. A defective function of macrophages was suggested to be the cause of the underlying immunological abnormality (31^C).

Two infants with severe combined immunodeficiency who had developed *BCG dissemination* following neonatal BCG immunization, have been treated successfully by bone marrow transplantation and tuberculostatic therapy (32*C*).

Osteitis (<0.1–30/100 000 vaccinees) has been reported mainly among infants immunized in the neonatal period in the Scandinavian countries. A retrospective study showed that BCG osteitis was present in Sweden from 1949 onwards. The reported incidence was one per 40 000 in children born between 1960 and 1969 (33^C, 34^C). The increase in incidence of BCG osteitis in Sweden and Finland had coincided with the replacement (1971) of BCG vaccine produced by the Swedish BCG laboratory in favor of a Statens Seruminstitut, Copenhagen, vaccine. Both vaccines were based on the Gotenberg strain. In Sweden, the reported osteitis incidence rose to one per 3000 and one per 4000 for children vaccinated in the neonatal period during 1972–1975. Compulsory notification of BCG side effects to the Swedish Adverse Drug Reaction Committee was introduced at that time. Peltola et al. (35^C) have reported 10 cases of BCG osteitis in Finland. In Czechoslovakia, osteitis was not diagnosed before 1981. From March, 1980, another BCG vaccine (Moscow strain) was introduced. Beginning in 1981, 12 cases of BCG osteitis were diagnosed. The majority of cases developed between 7 and 24 months following immunization, but the interval has also been longer. The risk of osteitis

Table 4. *BCG osteitis*

Country	No. of vaccinees (all age groups)	BCG osteitis	
		No.	Rate per million vaccinees
Finland	2 790.4	128	45.9 (43.4)
Sweden	3 420.8	121	35.4 (32.5)
Denmark	2 279.9	4	1.75 (1.75)
Germany (West)	9 026.9	14	1.55 (1.11)
Norway	2 321.8	2	0.86 (0.86)
Germany (East)	8 677.3	5	0.58 (0.23)
Switzerland	2 166.4	1	0.46 (0.46)
France	16 216.9	6	0.37 (0.18)
Austria	2 864.0	1	0.35 (0.35)
Yugoslavia	17 426.5	2	0.11(0.11)
Europe (33 countries)	498 472.9	284	0.57 (0.52)
Israel	1 923.1	3	1.56 (1.04)
Algeria	8 047.6	2	0.25 (0.25)
Japan	166 464.7	2	0.01 (0.01)

In parentheses: bacteriologically or histologically confirmed.

rose to 35 per million in the period 1982–1985. The health authorities decided to halve the vaccine dose (36[C], 37[C]). Comparing the period from 1980 to June, 1985, when Russian BCG vaccine containing a higher amount of culturable particles was used, and the period from July, 1985 to 1989, when the dose of vaccine had been halved, Krepela et al. (38[C]) found 28 cases of BCG osteomyelitis during the first period and 11 cases after reduction of the dose of vaccine. During the last 2 years of the second period only one case in each immunized birth cohort has been found.

Haniman et al. (39[C]) have reported six cases of BCG osteitis in Switzerland occurring in 1980–1985. These authors remark that osteitis following BCG immunization is not well known and often misdiagnosed. Concurrently, however, case reports from New Zealand (40[C]) and India (41[C]) have emphasized the increasing knowledge of BCG osteitis. BCG osteitis has never been reported in the United Kingdom with use of the Glaxo vaccine.

Table 4 shows rates of BCG osteitis in different countries (18[C]). An infant developed BCG osteomyelitis of the upper spine, a very rare complication described only three times before (42[C]).

Suppurative lymphadenitis Clinical trials in different countries found a dose-effect relationship (Croatia: SED-12, 799; French Guyana: SEDA-16, 373; Germany: SED-12, 798; Hong Kong: SED-12, 799; Hungary: SED-12, 798; India: SEDA-18, 328) and strain-dependent relationship (Austria: SEDA-16, 374, SEDA-17, 366; Germany: SED-12, 798; India: SEDA-18, 328; Saudi Arabia: SED-12, 799; Togo: SED-12, 799; Turkey: SED-12, 799; Zaire: SED-12, 799) in BCG-vaccinated newborns.

Since 1984, WHO's Expanded Programme on Immunization has received many reports from various countries of an increased incidence of *suppurative lymphadenitis* following BCG immunization. Careful investigations of risk factors have been carried out, particularly in Zimbabwe and Mozambique (1987, 1988). The studies established a strong association between an increased risk of developing lymphadenitis within 6 months of immunization and—on the one hand—the use of the Pasteur BCG strain, and—on the other hand—programmatic errors such as poor injection technique, poor technique in reconstituting and mixing the freeze-dried vaccine with diluent, or an incorrectly administered dose of vaccine. Comparing the use of Pasteur vaccine strain administered in clinic settings with that of two other strains used under the same conditions, the incidence of lymphadenitis was found to be 9.9% with the suspect Pasteur strain versus 0% with the other two.

Experiences gained in other countries suggests that when Pasteur strain BCG vaccine is administered properly, the rate of lymphadenitis in newborns should not exceed 1%. The increased occurrence of lymphadenitis may require a reactogenic strain in the presence of poor technique (43[C]).

The WHO view Taking into account the results of the investigations mentioned above, WHO made the following recommendations:

(a) Pasteur BCG vaccine should be supplied only to countries using the product without problems. In no case should the vaccine be sent to a country which has been successfully using another product unless the country specifically requests this product.

(b) UNICEF supplies of BCG vaccine should specify the doses to be given to infants (0.05 cc), and, where possible, 0.05 cc syringes should be supplied with the vaccine to reduce the likelihood of too large a dose being given.

(c) WHO will supply to country programmes a short protocol to assess the incidence of BCG-associated lymphadenitis using a standard case definition. Evidence of a rate greater than 1% would be the basis for investigating the problem and for reviewing the vaccine strain being used. Additionally it is recommended that training in the technique of BCG immunization should be re-emphasized (43*C*).

A rare case of BCG lymphangitis occurring 11 years and again 18 years after immunization has been reported (44[C]).

Anaphylactic and anaphylactoid reactions A paper originating from Swaziland describes three cases of *anaphylactic reactions* to BCG in young children, one (in a 3-month-old girl) being fatal (45[C]). Following BCG immunization of a newborn girl, 30 minutes later an acute shock-like syndrome developed. *Anaphylactoid reactions* suspected to be caused by dextran as used in BCG vaccines have been described in the Annuals (SEDA-16, 375).

Meningitis There are two remarkable reports on *tuberculous meningitis* following BCG immunization in immunocompetent individuals: Tardieu et al. (46[C]) described meningitis in two French children aged 5 and 4.5 years, respectively; Morrison et al. (47[C]) reported on a 22-year-old woman from Cambridge.

Lupus vulgaris Since the initial report of lupus vulgaris following BCG immunization in 1946, about 60 cases have been published, mostly following (multiple) revaccination. The risk of developing lupus vulgaris following primary immunization is extremely low. Kanwar et al. (48[C]) have reported a case of lupus vulgaris occurring in a 7-year-old girl after only a single BCG immunization. The patient was treated with conventional antitubercular therapy with an excellent response.

Miscellaneous side effects Case reports on miscellaneous side effects following BCG vaccination have been provided: *acute febrile neutrophilic dermatosis* (*AFND*) (49[C]), may be the first report of AFND following BCG vaccine, whereas other reports on AFND have been published in connection with smallpox vaccine and tuberculin tests (for details see SEDA-12, 273); *polyneuritis* (50[C]); *sudden infant death syndrome* (*SDI*) (a 7-week-old infant died under circumstances reminiscent of SDI; the histopathological examination revealed disseminated BCG infection no abnormalities of the immune system were detected (51[C])); *endogenous endophthalmitis* (the first report in the literature documented following BCG immunization (SEDA-15, 344)); *bilateral optic neuritis* (52[c]); *granulomatous neonatal hepatitis* (53[C]); *eczema vaccinatum* (54[C]); and *mediastinal tumor* (X-ray and CT scan examinations suggested a teratoma in a 1-year-old girl who had received BCG vaccine at birth; however, histology and microbiology revealed the diagnosis of mediastinal BCG-itis (55[C])).

Treatment of BCG side effects Power et al. (56[C]) successfully introduced *therapy with erythromycin* for a period of 2—4 weeks in six patients with troublesome post BCG-lesions. The effect of erythromycin on the atypical mycobacteria was described by Wolinsky and colleagues as early as 1957, but its use for treatment of BCG lesions has not previously been reported. Singh and Singh (57[C]) have used erythromycin for the treatment of cold abscesses.

Isoniazid therapy of suppurative lymphadenitis Akenzua and Sykes (58[C]) treated newborns with suppurative lymphadenitis with isoniazid (10 mg/kg/day for 3—9 months). The treatment resulted in complete resolution of the adenitis. There was no significant difference between infants with ruptured nodes and those with intact nodes.

Comparison of different treatment of suppurative lymphadenitis No statistical difference was found between groups with different suppurative lymphadenitis treatment (36 patients received erythromycin, 21 isoniazid, and 21 isoniazid + rifampicin; there was also a 'no therapy' group). If lymphadenitis developed rapidly (within 2 months), the incidence of spontaneous drainage and suppuration was reported to be significantly higher than in patients with slowly developing processes. Total surgical excision is recommended in these rapidly evolving cases (59*C*).

Risk situations Disseminated BCG infection and death is usually associated with severe abnormalities of immunity. BCG for prevention of tuberculosis should therefore not be given to persons with impaired immune responses such as occur with congenital immunodeficiency, leukemia, lymphoma, or generalized malignancy, and when immunological responses have been suppressed with steroids, alkylating agents, antimetabolites, or radiation (60[R]). The risks are greater in the debilitated or the very young.

The WHO has recommended that individuals with clinical (symptomatic) AIDS or other clinical manifestations of HIV-infection should not receive BCG (61[R]).

Second-generation effects No harmful effects of BCG vaccine on the fetus have been seen. Nevertheless, it is prudent to avoid immunization of women during pregnancies, unless there is immediate excessive risk of unavoidable exposure to infective tuberculosis (60*R*).

Use of BCG immunostimulation (immunomodulation, immunotherapy) *BCG immunotherapy in bladder tumours* Whereas BCG has generally been ineffective for treatment of human cancers, the intravesical instillation of BCG is the treatment of choice for recurrent superficial transitional-cell carcinoma of the bladder, and BCG instillation is described as effective for carcinoma in situ of the urinary bladder. Many reports confirming the efficacy and resulting side effects have been provided (SED-11, 674; SEDA-12, 273; SEDA-13, 278; SEDA-15, 344; SEDA-16, 375; SEDA-17, 366; SEDA-18, 328; 62[C]—82[C]). In general, BCG immunotherapy of the bladder cancer is considered to be relatively safe. Although the treatment is not free of side effects (fever, arthritis/arthralgia, bladder irritability, bladder contracture, cytopenia, cystitis, disseminated intravascular coagulation and respiratory failure, epididymitis, hepatitis, miliary tuberculosis, pneumonitis, polyarthritis, prostatitis, pyelonephritis, pseudotumoral granulomatous renal mass, rhabdomyolysis, renal granulomas, renal insufficiency, skin abscess, tuberculous aneurysm of the femoral artery, ureteral obstruction, vertebral osteomyelitis and psoas abscess), major side effects are thought to be very rare and often self-limiting. A few reports on life-threatenining side effects following BCG instillation have been provided by Steg et al. (83[C]) (five cases of *disseminated BCG infection*); Deresiewicz et al. (84[C]), Rawls et al. (85[C]), and Sakamoto et al. (86[C]) (three cases of *disseminated BCG infection* (two of them being fatal)). The tragic cases illustrate many points of critical importance to all urologists using BCG. BCG should never been given at the time of tumor resection or at the time of transurethral resection of the prostate. The dose of BCG given intravesically is a potentially lethal intravenous dose. Intravasation as a result of catheterization, tumor resection or biopsy, or cystitis has occurred in two-thirds of the reported cases of systemic BCG infection. The exact mechanism of antitumor activity is unknown, but live BCG provokes an inflammatory response that includes activation of macrophages, a delayed hypersensitivity reaction, and stimulation of T- and B-lymphocytes and natural killer cells.

In 1990, the US Food and Drug Administration approved marketing of BCG Live (intravesical) for use in the treatment of primary or relapsed carcinoma in situ of the urinary bladder, with or without associated papillary tumors. BCG is not recommended for treatment of papillary tumors occurring alone. The drug is marketed by Connaught Laboratories under the trade name 'TheraCys' and marketed by Organon under the trade name 'TiceBCG'. The manufacturers recommend a 6-week induction course of weekly intravesical BCG usually starting 1—2 weeks after biopsy or after transurethral resection of papillary tumors. Follow-up treatments (3, 6, 12, 24 months or monthly for 6—12 months after initial treatment) are recommended.

Different doses of BCG vaccine Ortiz et al. (87[C]) compared the prevention of tumor relapse in patients with superficial bladder cancer using different doses of BCG vaccine (100—120 and 20—50 mg, and a small dose of 1 mg). Adverse reactions were seen to be dose-dependent. The authors considered that endovesical instillation using 1 mg BCG vaccine would be the optimal dosage for prevention of relapse. Rivera et al. (88[C]) have reported similar experience treating 108 patients with bladder cancer. Tumor relapse has been prevented by the use of 1 mg BCG vaccine. One case of inguinal lymphadenitis and few cases of dysuria occurred.

Comparison of BCG strains Comparing 56 patients receiving BCG instillations using Berna strain BCG and 32 patients receiving Pasteur strain BCG for treatment of superficial bladder cancer, Lo Cigno et al. (89[C]) have found that the patients receiving Pasteur strain BCG had the highest tumor-free rate and a significantly higher toxicity. The answer to another difficult question connected with the use of intravesical BCG, i.e. whether the treatment increases the incidence of second primary malignancies was sought by Guinan et al. (90[C]) and by Khanna (91[C]). Khanna has drawn attention to the fact that BCG immunotherapy may *accelerate the growth and cause metastatic spread of a growing second primary malignancy* that has remained undetected at the start of BCG therapy. In his opinion, the time relationship between the starting point of second primary tumour development and the starting point of BCG treatment may be crucial in determining whether BCG will eradicate the tumor or accelerate its growth. Khanna's report has influenced Guinan et al. (90[C]) to review their own experience in 153 patients. They found no evidence suggesting that intravesical BCG does increase the incidence of second primary malignancies.

BCG is still used to some extent in the stimulation of the immune system to attack cancer and to prevent it, generally as an adjunct to other modalities of treatment (92[R]—98[C]).

Cholera vaccine (including combined vaccines which include the cholera component)

Parenteral immunization against cholera has yielded only modest and short-term protection. Oral vaccines give the most promising approach. An oral cholera vaccine consisting of the immunogenic but completely nontoxic B subunit of cholera toxin in combination with heat- and formalin-killed cholera vibrios has been developed and extensively tested in clinical trials including a large field trial in Bangladesh over the last several years. The results represent an improvement as compared to those achieved previously using parenteral vaccines (99[R]). Data collected indicate that the frequency of side effects (pain at the injection site, nausea, diarrhea) was low (100[C]).

A randomized, double-blind, placebo-controlled trial using a live oral cholera vaccine (strain CVD 103, derived from the *Vibrio cholerae* 01 classical Inaba strain 569 B by deletion of the genes encoding the A subunit of cholera toxin) was conducted in 50 healthy Swiss adults. Seventy-six percent of volunteers responded with a significant rise in serum antitoxin levels. Two vaccinees reported watery stools following immunization (101[R]).

However, cholera vaccine for parenteral injection is still used around the world. The vaccine consists of a heat-killed, phenol-preserved mixed suspension of the Inaba and Ogawa subtypes of *Vibrio cholerae*, Serovar 01. The vaccine is given subcutaneously or intramuscularly; for booster doses, the vaccine may be administered intradermally. About 1% of vaccinees develop mild local skin lesions comprising transitory soreness at the injection site within 5—7 days after injection, characterized by erythema, swelling, pain, induration, and rarely resulting in ulceration. More general reactions are allergic: as a rule, these amount at most to slight pyrexia, headache and malaise.

Severe complications connected with cholera (or combined) immunization are extremely rare and the causal relationship is always doubtful, but when they do occur they constitute a contraindication for further doses. There are occasional reports of *neurological and psychiatric reactions* (SED-8, 706; SEDA-1, 246), *Guillain-Barré syndrome* (SEDA-1, 246), *myocarditis* (102[C], 103[C]), *myocardial infarction* (SEDA-3, 261), a syndrome similar to *immune complex disease* (104[C]), *acute renal failure* accompanied by *hepatitis* (105[C]), and *pancreatitis* (106[C]).

Diphtheria vaccine (including diphtheria—tetanus vaccine)

Single antigen products are only available for situations where combined antigens should not be used. The preparations of choice used in routine immunization practice are DTP diphtheria and tetanus toxoids combined with pertussis vaccine), DT (diphtheria and tetanus toxoids) for pediatric use, and Td (tetanus and diphtheria toxoids with a limited amount of diphtheria antigen) for use in older children and adults. Some relevant side effect reports will be found in the sections dealing with pertussis and tetanus vaccines. Diphtheria vaccine contains diphtheria toxoid carried on aluminium hydroxide or phosphate. The usual types of *local intolerance* may be seen, e.g. some 5% of schoolchildren have developed redness and swelling, whilst some older children have developed enlargement of the regional lymph nodes. Such reactions are much less common in young children, and much more common in children given combined vaccines. *General reactions* (seen in some older children and adults) are usually limited to brief fever.

After the administration of DT vaccine, *local reactions*, generally erythema and induration with or without tenderness, can occur. Fever and other *systemic reactions* are uncommon, unless the person has been hyperimmunized. In such cases, *Arthus-type hypersensitivity reactions* may occur. These characteristically severe, local reactions generally start 2—8 hours after an injection. Persons having such reactions usually have very high serum antitoxin levels and one should be careful not to administer a booster more than once every 10 years.

Comparisons of immunogenicity and reactogenicity of different diphtheria vaccines (single or combined administration of diphtheria and/or tetanus toxoids) have been carried out (see SEDA-13, 279; SEDA-15, 345).

Van Ramshorst et al. collected several case reports on neurological side effects of diphtheria immunization, but a causal connection was unclear (107[C]). Ehrengut (108[C]) has analyzed five cases of neurological complications following diphtheria or diphtheria—tetanus immunizations. Two cases were classified as vaccine-induced *poliomyelitis*. The three other cases could be traced back to a hyperergic reaction to diphtheria toxoids in the cerebral vessels; such a reaction is typically seen in individuals immunized against diphtheria.

Case reports of severe complications following diphtheria (or DT/Td) immunization have been rarely published, the causal relationship of these cases seems to be doubtful: *Guillain-Barré syndrome* (109[C]), polyradiculoneuritis (110[C], 111[C]). A national *GBS* surveillance study in the United States revealed that 31 out of 998 cases of GBS developed the illness within 8 weeks following immunization. Of these 31 cases, five had been immunized with DT or DPT vaccine (112[C]). *Erythema multiforme* has been reported in a 9-month-old infant, developing 8 hours following DT immunization (113[C]). There have already been reports of erythema multiforme after the receipt of hepatitis B vaccine, MMR vaccine and DPT vaccine.

The bioelectric activity of the brain after DT immunization was studied in healthy children. EEGs showed significant changes in 13 out of 17 children, which disappeared within 3 weeks (114[C]).

Between 1980 and 1982 in the Campana region of Italy, several cases of encephalopathy in children who had been given DT immunization a week previously were reported to the health authorities. Summarizing the results of a case-control study, Greco (115[C]) pointed out that the statistical association which he found between the incidence of encephalopathy and DT administration did not imply a causal association. Data on adverse events following the receipt of diphtheria—tetanus vaccine in the United States 1982—1984 have been provided in detail in SEDA-13 (pp. 273—277).

Risk situations The only contraindication to administering single diphtheria toxoid or combined diphtheria and tetanus toxoids is a history of a severe hypersensitivity or neurological reaction after a previous dose.

Diphtheria—pertussis—tetanus vaccine

See 'Pertussis vaccine'.

Haemophilus influenzae vaccine (including combined vaccine against *H. influenzae* type b, diphtheria, tetanus, and pertussis, and simultaneous administration of *H. influenzae* vaccine together with other vaccines)

Haemophilus influenzae causes several infectious diseases of man, the most serious being meningitis. Most cases of *H. influenzae infection* are due to type b of *H. influenzae* (*Hib*).

Two types of Hib vaccines have been developed: *Hib capsular polysaccharide* (*PRP*) *vaccines* (Hib vaccines of the first generation) and *Hib conjugate vaccines* (Hib vaccines of the second generation). Hib capsular polysaccharide vaccines are unable to protect infants and children less than 18 months, whereas Hib conjugate vaccines have shown greater immunogenicity and induced a high rate of protection in infants under the age of 18 months.

Four different types of conjugated vaccines are commercially available:

(a) PRP-D Hib vaccine (a mutant polypeptide of diphtheria toxin covalently linked to PRP), e.g. ProHIBit (produced by Connaught Laboratories);

(b) HbOC vaccine (Hib oligosaccharides linked to the nontoxic diphtheria toxin variant CRM197), e.g. HibTITER (produced by Lederle-Praxis);

(c) PRP-OMC (PRP conjugated to outer membrane protein of *Neisseria meningitidis* group B), e.g. PedvaxHIB (produced by Merck Sharp & Dohme Research Laboratories);

(d) PRP-T Hib vaccine (tetanus toxoid linked to PRP), e.g. PRP-T (produced by Pasteur Merieux Connaught).

Conjugated *H. influenzae* type b vaccines (second-generation Hib vaccines) have replaced completely the Hib polysaccharide vaccine of the first generation. The four different types of conjugated Hib vaccines currently available, and their safety and efficacy, have been described in detail (SED-12, 803; SEDA-16, 377; SEDA-17, 367; SEDA-18, 330). Meanwhile, more than 25 million doses of conjugated vaccines were administered worldwide. There were no reports of death, anaphylaxis, and residual neurological damage causally connected with the use of vaccine.

Weinberg and Granoff (116[R]) summarized, among other adverse reactions, the *neurological complications* that have been reported. There was a single *convulsion* occurring 12 hours after immunization in a 3-month-old child and a hyporesponsive episode in another 3-month-old child. *Guillain-Barré syndrome* (*GBS*) has been reported following immunization with several different vaccines. D'Cruz et al. (117[C]) reported the first three cases suspected to be GBS following the receipt of Hib conjugate vaccine within 1 week. One patient had also received DTP and oral poliomyelitis vaccine. An additional report on GBS after Hib conjugate vaccine has been given (118[C]), making four in all.

Immunization of risk groups Jakacki et al. (119[C]) have reported on immunization with Hib conjugate vaccine in 23 patients with Hodgkin's disease and splenectomy. Most of the vaccinees responded although the antibody response was significantly lower than in healthy persons. Side effects have been registered in three vaccinees: in one case nausea, vertigo and weakness occurring 2—4 days after receipt of the vaccine; myalgias occurred in another case; and fever and myalgias after primary immunization, with milder symptoms following the booster, in a third case.

Combined vaccine and simultaneous administration of Hib vaccines and other vaccines

Since immunization against diphtheria, tetanus, and pertussis is recommended at the same age as immunization against *Haemophilus influenzae*, children must usually receive two intramuscular injections at separate sites during the same visit. Combined vaccines, e.g. DTP/Hib vaccines, requiring one injection could be preferable and are commercially available. Results of clinical trials comparing the safety and efficacy of combined and simultaneously administrated vaccines (Hib, DTP, MMR, IPV) have been described (SEDA-17,

369; SEDA-18, 330). In general, rates of local and systemic reactions and antibody responses did not differ significantly between the groups.

Summarizing the results of efficacy and safety trials using Hib conjugate vaccines of the second generation, the new types of vaccine could be considered to be highly immunogenic and safe.

Hepatitis A vaccine

The propagation of hepatitis A virus in cell culture has made development of hepatitis A vaccines a realistic possibility. Various candidate hepatitis A vaccines have been tested in clinical trials. In December 1991, the first hepatitis A vaccine has been licensed in Western European countries. Currently, two different hepatitis vaccines are commercially available and further products are under development. Results of safety and immunogenicity testing of hepatitis A vaccines developed by SmithKline-Beecham and by Merck Research Laboratories have been provided in the Annuals (SEDA-16, 384; SEDA-17, 373; SEDA-18, 333). The vaccines were highly immunogenic. There were mild transient reactions at the injection site, systemic reactions were minor and uncommon. Hughes et al. (120[c]) have reported a case of probable post-hepatitis A immunization encephalopathy.

Hepatitis B vaccine

Two types of hepatitis B vaccine are commercially available: *plasma-derived hepatitis B vaccine* and *yeast recombinant hepatitis B virus vaccine*. In general, both vaccines have been considered to be equally immunogenic, protective and safe. However, in the majority of developed countries the recombinant vaccine is the vaccine of choice.

Plasma-derived hepatitis B virus vaccine The vaccine is prepared from the plasma of chronic HBsAg carriers, and consists of purified, inactivated 20-nm HBsAg particles adsorbed to an aluminium adjuvant. The use of a vaccine produced with plasma-derived from infected individuals represented a major departure from conventional approaches, and safety testing has therefore been designed to cover the possibility of all risks and to ensure freedom from transmission of residual HBV and other blood-borne agents. Various clinical trials (SEDA-10, 289; SEDA-11, 289) have confirmed the safety of plasma-derived hepatitis B virus vaccines produced by different manufacturers. Fears that plasma-derived vaccine may transmit AIDS can be considered unfounded.

Subsequent to the identification of HIV and the growing knowledge of its relatively easy inactivation with procedures such as heat or triple-step chemical inactivation, the complete safety and suitability of those plasma-derived vaccines which meet WHO requirements has now been generally accepted. Francis et al. (121[C]) have demonstrated the safety in a special study (for details see SEDA-12, 279). The vaccine is generally well tolerated. The most common side effect has been local soreness at the injection site. Less common local reactions include erythema, swelling and induration all usually subside within 48 hours. Transient low-grade fever has occurred occasionally; malaise, fatigue, vomiting, dizziness, myalgias and arthralgias have been infrequent. Individual reports of more severe suspected side effects (erythema multiforme, hepatitis-like changes in liver function, hypersensitivity, lichen planus, menstrual abnormality, myasthenia gravis, neurological disorders including transverse myelitis and Guillain-Barré syndrome, reactive arthritis, Takayasu's arteritis, urticaria, uveitis) are very rare and are no more than could be expected by chance (SEDA-9, 283; SEDA-10, 289; SEDA-11, 288; SED-12, 804; SEDA-16, 384; SEDA-17, 373; SEDA-18, 334). In one reported case with neurological symptoms, a preceding viral illness was likely and in the patient with hepatitis-like symptoms mentioned above, the possibility of other causes was not excluded. In a case with urticaria, patch tests revealed a hypersensitivity to thiomersal, the preservative in the vaccine.

Quast and Freiburg (122[C]) have summarized the side effects reported following the distribution of over 1.8 million doses of plasma-derived hepatitis B vaccine (Table 5).

In 1982, the Centers for Disease Control, the Food and Drug Administration, and the manufacturer, Merck Sharp & Dohme, had created a special surveillance system to monitor spontaneous reports of plasma-derived hepatitis vaccine. During the first 3 years, approximately 850 000 persons have been immunized. A total of 41 reports were received for one of the following neurological adverse events: convulsion (five cases), Bell's palsy (10 cases), Guillain-Barré syndrome (nine cases), lumbar radiculopathy (five cases), brachial plexus neuropathy (three cases), optic neuritis (five cases), and transverse myelitis (four cases). Half of these events occurred after the first vaccine dose. However, no conclusive causal association could be made between any neurological adverse event and the vaccine (123[C]).

Intradermal administration of hepatitis B vaccines Aiming at cost reduction of hepatitis B immunization programmes, the administration of low doses (2 μg) of vaccine given intradermally has been evaluated

Table 5. *Side effects following immunization with recombinant and plasma-derived hepatitis B vaccine*

Side effect	Recombinant vaccine, over 200 000 doses distributed (August 1986—April 1987)		Plasma-derived vaccine, over 1.8 million doses distributed (July 1982-December 1987)	
	No. of reported side effects	Rate per doses distributed	No. of reported side effects	Rate per doses distributed
Pruritis	2	1:103 000	38	1: 48 000
Urticaria	2	1:103 000	23	1: 79 000
Exanthema	6	1: 34 000	58	1: 30 000
Angio-edema	—	—	8	1: 228 000
Edema facialis	1	1:205 000	10	1: 182 000
Eczema	—	—	2	1: 912 000
Nodule formation	—	—	3	1: 608 000
Erythema nodosum	1	1:205 000	1	1:1.823 000
Total	12	1: 17 000	99	1: 18 000

in clinical trials in health care workers (124[C]) and children (125[C]). Resulting seroconversion rates were 96 and over 90%, respectively. A minimum of local side effects occurred. Wahl and Hermodsson (126[C]) have compared antibody responses and side effects following intradermal or subcutaneous administration of 2 μg of a plasma-derived hepatitis B vaccine to intramuscular administration of 20 μg. The intradermal and intramuscular routes gave the highest seroconversion rates (100 and 96%, respectively) and the highest mean titers of anti-HBs. The aluminium adjuvant in the vaccine has been assumed to cause a substantial number of local reactions (37% discoloration, 17% itching and 13% nodule formation) following intradermal administration; other routes of administration showed side effects only rarely. Correct intradermal deposition of the vaccine is crucial.

Reactogenicity following revaccination Jilg et al. (127[C]) have revaccinated non-responders to primary hepatitis immunization (only 50—70% of immunocompromised persons, especially dialysis patients, develop antibodies, and the anti-HBs levels are low) with either a dose of 20 μg plasma-derived vaccine or a 10-μg dose of recombinant vaccine depending on the vaccine used for previous doses. The revaccinations were well tolerated. Only 6.6% of the vaccinees reported slight irritation at the injection site, tenderness, minimal pain, or swelling lasting for a few hours up to 2 days. Regarding efficacy of revaccination, this and other studies showed that a single revaccination cannot solve the problem of all non-responders to hepatitis B immunization.

Yeast recombinant hepatitis B vaccine The yeast-derived recombinant vaccines first licensed in 1986 represent the first vaccine of any kind manufactured by recombinant technology. The vaccines are prepared using antigen produced by recombinant technology in yeast (*Saccharomyces cerevisiae*). Hilleman (128[C]) found the recombinant vaccine produced by Merck, Sharp & Dohme to be as immunogenic and protective against hepatitis B as plasma-derived vaccine. Clinical reactions in his series were mild and transient. About 17% of all recipients experienced pain, soreness, and tenderness at the injection site. A smaller proportion reported headache, weakness, nausea or malaise. Between February 1984 and August 1986, 33 investigators in 19 countries carried out clinical trials with the yeast-derived recombinant hepatitis B vaccine produced by Smith Kline Biologicals. Among other risk groups neonates, patients with thalassemia and sickle cell anemia and hemodialysis patients have been vaccinated. All the results point to the safety and acceptability of a yeast-derived vaccine. The incidence of reported reactions varied widely in different studies depending on the scrupulousness with which minor signs were reported. No serious, severe, or anaphylactic reactions occurred. The incidence of local and systemic reactions reported in each study tended to decrease after successive doses, suggesting that immunization did not induce hypersensitivity (SEDA-12, 280—281).

Reports on further studies investigating efficacy and safety of recombinant hepatitis vaccines have been published (SED-12, 805; SEDA-14, 282; SEDA-15, 351; SEDA-16, 385; SEDA-17, 373; SEDA-18, 334; 129[C]). Table 5 shows the side effects reported following the distribution of 205 000 doses of recombinant vaccine.

Central nervous system demyelination Herroelen et al. (130[C]) have described two patients with neurological symptoms and signs of *central nervous system demyelination* 6 weeks after administration of recombinant hepatitis B vaccine. One had known multiple sclerosis but the other had no history of neurological diseases. Both had HLA haplotype DR2 and B7, which are associated with multiple sclerosis. A causal link between immunization and demyelination cannot be established from these two case reports, but the time interval would fit a proposed immunological mechanism. In addition, the Centers for Diseases Control (CDC), Atlanta, Georgia, received reports on four cases of 'chronic demyelinizing disease'. This initiated, in 1992, a CDC study on reported serious neurological events following all kinds of immunization including hepatitis B immunization (131). Mahassin et al. (132[C]) have reported a case of *acute myelitis* in a 56-year-old man occurring 3 weeks after hepatitis B immunization. Trevisani et al. (133[C]) provided a case of *transverse myelitis* developing 3 weeks after the first dose of hepatitis B vaccine in an 11-year-old girl. Three days after recombinant hepatitis B booster immunization, a 31-year-old man developed *acute posterior multifocal placoid pigment epitheliopathy* (visual loss) and eosinophilia (134[C]).

Tuohy (135[C]) has observed a case of Guillain-Barré syndrome (GBS) in a 7-year-old girl following the administration of recombinant hepatitis vaccine. The author mentioned that few such incidents have been reported after the use of recombinant vaccines (two reports of optic neuritis and one of Guillain-Barré syndrome).

Case reports on *acute glomerulonephritis* (136[C]), *febrile convulsion* (137[C]), *lichen planus* (138[C]), *neuralgic amyotrophy* (139[R]), *reactive arthritis* (140[C]), *systemic lupus erythematosus* (141[C]), and *urticaria* (142[C]) have been provided. A case of *erythema nodosum* and *polyarthritis* occurring the next day after Engerix-B vaccine administration have been reported by Rogerson and Nye (143[R]). The authors referred to reports of three other cases of polyarthritis in the literature.

Levy and Koren (144[C]) have reported on pregnancy outcome in ten women having received hepatitis B vaccine during the first trimester of pregnancy. No congenital abnormalities were observed and at 2–12 months the infants were physically and developmentally normal for their ages.

Analyzing 31 cases of suspected chronic fatigue syndrome (CFS) occurring associated with hepatitis B immunization, a workshop involving CFS experts did not identify a causal relationship (145[R]).

Simultaneous administration of hepatitis B vaccine together with other vaccines Giammanco et al. (146[C]) have administered recombinant hepatitis B vaccine simultaneously with diphtheria–tetanus vaccine and oral poliomyelitis vaccine. Comparing the results with the administration of hepatitis B vaccine alone, they found no evidence of an increased reactogenicity after simultaneous application.

Forty children born to HBsAg-positive mothers received the second and third dose of hepatitis B vaccine simultaneously with DTP vaccine and inactivated poliomyelitis vaccine. Immunogenicity and reactogenicity were comparable with non-simultaneous administration of the different vaccines (147[C]).

Hypersensitivity to thimerosal and aluminium Thimerosal has been used as a preservative in vaccines for many years and cases of *hypersensitivity to thimerosal* in vaccines are well known. Four cases with reactions to thimerosal in hepatitis B vaccines (both plasma-derived and recombinant) have been reported by Rietschel and Adams (148[C]) and Jungkunz et al. (149[C]). Although thimerosal is present in the vaccines at a concentration of only 1:20 000, it can induce severe cutaneous reactions of the delayed hypersensitivity type, sometimes the reactions can be very long lasting. To interpret strictly the package insert for hepatitis B vaccines would preclude its administration to persons with a history of ocular sensitivity to thimerosal. Kirkland (150[C]) has immunized nine persons with such a history, without untoward reactions, but this small series should not be overestimated. Cosnes et al. (151[C]) and Hütteroth and Quast (152[C]) have provided reports on three cases of inflammatory nodular reactions after hepatitis B immunization. *Aluminium hypersensitivity* was confirmed.

Human immunodeficiency virus (HIV) vaccine (AIDS vaccine)

The difficult problems connected with clinical trials in man which were not approved by independent authorities have been highlighted when Zagury carried out the first immunizations in humans using vaccinia vaccine expressing glycoprotein gp-160 (153, 154) (see subchapter smallpox vaccine).

The first HIV vaccine approved for clinical trial status (1989) by the US Food and Drug Administration (FDA) was a recombinant gp-160 vaccine produced in a baculovirus-insect cell expression system by MicroGeneSys (155[c]). Since then, various clinical trials using different HIV vaccines have been carried out. *All HIV vaccines are still in the experimental stage.*

Immunization of HIV-infected persons

This section does not deal with safety and immunogenicity of HIV vaccines but with the use of various vaccines in HIV-infected persons. It is well known that immune deficiency can play a distinct role in the development of side effects following immunization, particularly in connection with the administration of live-virus vaccines. The first such experience was with smallpox vaccine; persons with immunodefects were known to have a markedly increased complication risk, e.g. generalized vaccinia. Disseminated BCG infection is usually associated with severe abnormalities of cellular immunity. The risk of vaccine-associated poliomyelitis is increased in immunodeficient children. Several reports have been submitted on adverse events or death following measles immunization in immunodeficient children. Based on these experiences, there is a general consensus that *live vaccines should not be administered to persons with immune deficiency diseases or to persons whose immune response may be suppressed because of leukemia, lymphoma, generalized malignancy, or therapy with corticosteroids, alkylating agents, antimetabolic agents or radiation* (for details see SEDA-12, 268–269).

The immunological abnormalities associated with symptomatic HIV infection have raised concerns about the immunization of infected persons. Replication of live attenuated vaccine viruses may be enhanced in persons with immunodeficiency diseases and may produce complications following immunization of symptomatic HIV-infected patients.

HIV infection and BCG immunization Reports on such complications following BCG immunization in HIV-infected individuals and AIDS patients have been already provided: *disseminated BCG-itis* (156[C]–158[C]), disseminated BCG-itis involving the spleen and mediastinal and mesenteric lymph nodes in one case and the liver and the lung in another case (159[C]), and *pneumonitis* (160[C]). Reynes et al. (161[C]) have reported a case of BCG *lymphadenitis* occurring 30 years after BCG immunization in a 36-year-old patient with AIDS. Surgical excision and biopsy revealed a puriform abscess. Pathological examination established the diagnosis of Kaposi's sarcoma; no granulomatous changes were found. BCG was grown. The authors believe that the BCG lymphadenitis was due to a late reactivation of the bacillus.

BCG reactions in HIV-positive and HIV-negative children have been compared in African children. The rates of local adenitis were equal, no observation having been observed to date (162[C], 163[C]).

HIV infection and smallpox vaccination *Vaccinia generalisata* developed following smallpox vaccination (simultaneously administrated with other vaccines) of an army recruit with asymptomatic HIV infection. After 2–3 weeks he developed *cryptococcal meningitis* and a diagnosis of AIDS was made. While being treated for the meningitis he developed *generalized vaccinia*. He was treated with vaccinia immune globulin and recovered from his vaccinia generalisata (164[C]).

Side effects following administration of other vaccines in HIV infected individuals Various studies in both symptomatic and asymptomatic HIV-infected individuals have failed to demonstrate side effects following other immunizations, e.g. children receiving live oral or inactivated polio vaccine, DPT or DT vaccine or measles vaccine (165[C]–168[C]).

Conclusions and recommendations regarding HIV infection and immunization Recommendations of the (US) Immunization Practices Advisory Committee (ACIP), of WHO's Global Programme on Immunization, and of the European Advisory Group on Expanded Programme on Immunization have been published in detail (SEDA-12, 270; SEDA-13, 273). Based on the recommendations elaborated by WHO or ACIP, similar recommendations have been prepared in other countries. WHO recommends that nonimmunized individuals with symptomatic HIV infection should not receive BCG, but should receive the other vaccines (166, 167); whereas the ACIP (164) recommends that children with symptomatic HIV infection should not receive live-virus and live-bacterial vaccines. Taking into account the hazard of measles in children with AIDS and HIV-infection, the ACIP additionally recommends measles vaccine for all (both symptomatic and asymptomatic) HIV-infected children.

Immunization techniques and HIV transmission Nonsterile injection equipment can transmit HIV (but also other infectious agents including hepatitis viruses). There is also a possibility of needle stick transmission from an HIV-infected person to a vaccinator. Data from the United States show that the risk of transmission of HIV through needle stick is very low, perhaps 20 times lower than in the case of hepatitis B, in the order of one per 100 accidents. Furthermore, the types of injections given during immunization sessions do not as a rule cause bleeding. The risk of transmission is thus extremely low. No instances of immunization-related spread of HIV to other infants have been reported and if proper sterilization of needles and syringes is performed and vaccines are administered correctly the risk of HIV transmission is zero (164[R]).

Aiming at prevention of HIV transmission (as well as transmission of other infectious agents) through immunizations and other injections, WHO and UNICEF have published guidelines, which may be set out briefly as follows:

(a) A single sterile needle and a single sterile syringe should be used with each injection.

(b) Reusable needles and syringes are recommended for use in developing countries. They should be steam-sterilized between uses. Boiling is an acceptable alternative procedure until steam sterilization is available.

(c) Disposable needles and syringes should only be used if it can assured that they will actually be destroyed after a single use.

(d) Disease transmission by use of jet injectors is theoretically possible and has been demonstrated in human beings in a single situation (SEDA-11, 296). Until further studies clarify the risks of disease transmission with different types of injectors, their use should be restricted to special circumstances where large numbers of persons need to be immunized within a short period of time (169[R], 170[R]).

Influenza vaccine

Worldwide, inactivated flu vaccine is the vaccine of choice in immunization practice. Influenza vaccine viruses are propagated in embryonated chicken eggs. The virus-containing extra-embryonic fluid is harvested, purified, and inactivated with formalin. Inactivated flu vaccine is produced either as whole virus vaccine or ether-disrupted split or subunit preparations.

A clear picture of side effects following flu immunization is difficult to obtain because of the many types of vaccine (e.g. whole virus or split vaccine; different subtypes and variants of type A; adsorbed or fluid vaccine). Comparisons of reactogenicity (and immunogenicity) of different vaccine types have been provided (SED-12, 808; SEDA-8, 299; SEDA-10, 290; SEDA-11, 290; SEDA-12, 282; SEDA-13, 286; SEDA-14, 284; SEDA-15, 351; SEDA-16, 386; SEDA-17, 375; SEDA-18, 335). In general, local side reactions following flu immunization are few and infrequent. Slight to moderate tenderness, erythema, and induration at the injection site lasting 1—2 days may occur in 15—30% of the recipients. Fever, malaise, myalgia, and other symptoms of toxicity are rare (about 2%) and, most often, affect persons with no exposure to the flu antigens in the vaccine, e.g. young children. These reactions usually begin 6—12 hours post immunization and may last 1 or 2 days. They have been attributed to the vaccine, although the virus is inactivated. On the other hand, cases of respiratory diseases occurring among vaccinees are coincidental. Although current flu vaccines are highly purified, they can induce hypersensitivity reactions such as hives or angioedema, perhaps due to residual egg protein (171[C], 172[R]). Notwithstanding the fact that the egg protein content is small, in persons sensitive to the material one may see asthma or full anaphylactic reactions with vascular purpura and encephalopathy (173[C], 174[C]).

In another overview (175[R]) it was reported that general reactions were more frequent in children immunized with whole-virus vaccine, and sometimes were accompanied by febrile convulsions.

Results of various trials comparing the *reactogenicity* of different whole virus, split and subunit vaccines, either as adsorbed or fluid preparations, have been presented (SEDA-8, 299; SEDA-10, 290; SEDA-11, 290; SEDA-13, 286; SEDA 14, 284; SEDA-15, 351; SEDA-17, 375). In the majority of these trials the investigators found little difference in reactogenicity between the various vaccines.

The findings of a nationwide surveillance system for illness after flu immunization (United States, 1976—1977) are worth summarizing. For over 48 million persons immunized in 1976 with A/New Jersey/76 influenza vaccine (swine flu vaccine), a total of 4733 reports of illness were received including reports of 223 deaths. Since most of the reported deaths occurred within 48 hours after immunization, the rates for deaths per 100 000 vaccinees (by diagnosis) have been compared with the expected death rate (by the same diagnosis) per 100 000 population for a 2-day period. In general, the crude expected death rate was found to be much higher than the death rate of vaccinees. Other than *Guillain Barré syndrome* (see below) and rare cases of *anaphylaxis*, no serious illnesses seem to be causally associated with flu immunization. Widespread underreporting of illness and death in the passive phase of this surveillance system, however, have impaired the validity of the study. *Allergic skin reactions* were reported at a rate of 0.3 per 100 000 vaccinees, *severe anaphylaxis* at a rate of 0.024 per 100 000. A cluster of four *encephalitis* cases within 1 week of vaccine administration was noted in one state. Three deaths from *cardiovascular disease* were noted in chronically ill persons over 70 years of age immunized in one clinic. It was not possible to establish a causative link between immunization and death. Persons immunized in the clinic died at rate of five per 100 000 per day in contrast to the expected rate of 17 per 100 000 per day for persons 65 years and older in the respective state (176).

Neurological reactions These range from *polyneuropathy* to *meningoencephalitis* and *Guillain-Barré syndrome* (*GBS*). The latter syndrome was observed during the 1976/1977 mass immunization campaign in the United States. The vaccine then used was A/New Jersey/76 (H1N1) flu vaccine (swine influenza). The overall incidence of GBS cases attributed to the use of vaccine at that time was 4.9—5.9 per million vaccinees (177[C]). Various authors tried to settle the question of a cause and effect relationship. Detailed reports have been published (SEDA-10, 289; SEDA-11, 290) and the resulting litigation has been reviewed by Dukes and Swartz (6[R]).

Analyzing computerized summaries of 1300 cases, Langmuir et al. (177[R]) found that immunized cases with extensive paresis or paralysis occurred in a characteristic epidemiological pattern, suggesting a causal relationship between immunization and GBS. Cases with limited motor involvement showed no such pattern. Unlike the 1976 swine flu vaccine, vaccines used subsequently have not been associated with an increased frequency of GBS. It has been calculated that the risk of polyneuritis following immunization is one in 200 000 as compared with a population incidence of spontaneous GBS of one in 1 000 000 (178[R]). To exclude other causes than immunization each case of polyneuritis or GBS thus has to be investigated carefully. The original Centers for Disease Control study of the relation between A/New Jersey/876 (swine flu) vaccine and Guillain Barré syndrome (GBS) demonstrated a statistically significant association and suggested a causal relation between the two events. To reassess this association, Safranek et al. (179[C]) have evaluated the medical records of all previously reported adult patients with GBS in Michigan and Minnesota from October 1, 1976 through January 31, 1977. The authors have found that the relative risk of developing GBS during the 6 weeks following flu immunization in adults of these two states was 7.10 (excess cases of GBS attributed to the vaccine: 8.6 per million vaccinees in Michigan and 9.7 per million vaccinees in Minnesota), comparable to the relative risk of 7.60 found in the original study. No increase in relative risk for GBS was noted beyond 6 weeks after immunization.

A retrospective study (1980—1988) conducted to determine if the US Army's mass influenza immunization programme was associated with an increased incidence of GBS has found no temporally related increase in GBS during the study years (180[C]).

The number of new cases of *multiple sclerosis* among the 45 million swine flu vaccine recipients indicated no excess over the expected frequencies. Inactivated swine flu vaccine did not influence the onset or exacerbation of the disease (181[R]).

Case reports on complications suspected to be caused by flu vaccine have been provided: *acute disseminated encephalitis* (182[C]), *acute thrombocytopenic purpura* (183[C]), *aseptic meningitis* (184[C]), *encephalopathy* (185[C]), *optic neuritis* with reversible blindness (SEDA-4, 226), *optical atrophy* (SEDA-6, 287), *pericarditis* (SEDA-7, 324), *polymyalgia rheumatica* (186[c]), *systemic vasculitis* (187[c]), *trigeminal-neuralgia-like symptoms* (188[C]), and *vascular purpura* with histological features of cutaneous necrotizing vasculitis (189[c]).

Lung disease A special risk group might be patients with intestinal disorders leading to less selective absorption from the intestinal lumen; this possibility is suggested by a case report on a man with adult celiac disease in whom influenza immunization was followed by the development of diffuse interstitial lung disease; he may have absorbed chicken embryo antigen formed during previous immunizations (SEDA-3, 261).

Influenza immunization in cardiac transplant patients Influenza infection has been a significant problem in cardiac transplant patients. Thus, the use of influenza immunization in cardiac transplant patients could be beneficial. However, its use has been limited by concern that stimulation of the immune system could potentially cause increased cardiac rejection. In the renal transplant experience, influenza infection itself may trigger an immunological response to cause graft rejection as well as dispose to other infections. Another concern is whether an immunosuppressed cardiac transplant patient could seroconvert sufficiently. Therefore, Kobashigawa et al. (190[C]) undertook a case-control study in 18 cardiac transplant patients (and 18 control patients) 6 months or beyond transplant surgery to assess the safety and immunogenicity of influenza vaccine. No differences in the incidence of cardiac rejection and in immune responses have been found.

Drug interactions After influenza immunization one group of researchers found a decrease of blood theophylline levels in patients and volunteers treated with this substance. The authors concluded that flu vaccine may influence the pharmacokinetics of several drugs (191[C]). A second group could not confirm these results. Effects of flu vaccine on hepatic drug metabolism were investigated by Meredith et al. (192[C]). Lorazepam and chlordiazepoxide metabolism was not altered by immunization. Theophylline oxidation was significantly decreased at 1 day, but not at 7 days, after immunization. An 81-year-old patient who had been well controlled by anticoagulants for 12 years had an episode of gastrointestinal bleeding associated with an influenza immunization. A prospective study evaluating the effect of flu immunization on the prothrombin time of eight patients on long-term anticoagulant treatment showed that there was prolongation of prothrombin time by 40%. In healthy subjects no significant effect on warfarin metabolism was observed after immunization (SEDA-10, 289). Gomolin's investigations (193[C]) failed to support reports on flu inhibition of theophylline metabolism or vaccine-enhanced anticoagulation. Additionally, Grabowski et al. (194[C]) have found no evidence that split virus influenza vaccine affects theophylline pharmacokinetics. The lack of a clinical interaction with warfarin or theophylline has now also been confirmed by a report of the US Immunization Practices Advisory Committee (172).

Jann et al. (195[C]) compared serum concentrations of the anticonvulsants, phenytoin, phenobarbital, and carbamazepine, before and after mentally retarded patients received flu vaccine. The authors concluded that serum concentrations of these drugs may increase as a result of flu immunization, and dosage adjustments may be necessary.

Changes in lymphocyte population Gerth (196[C]) paid special attention to *changes in the lymphocyte* *population* similar to those observed during virus infections and occurring within the first 2 weeks after immunization. There were no reports describing more severe courses of infectious diseases during this period.

Risk situations Persons with known anaphylactic hypersensitivity to eggs should not be given influenza vaccine.

Immunoglobulins and other antibody preparations

Animal-specific immunoglobulins Animal-specific immunoglobulins and other globulins of animal origin still currently in use in some countries include antirabies immunoglobulin, diphtheria antitoxin, botulinal antitoxin, antivenins, antilymphocyte globulin, antithymocyte globulin. The administration of equine or other immunoglobulins is associated with a considerable risk of adverse side effects and can produce virtually any type of early or late hypersensitivity reaction ranging from asthma and urticaria to serum sickness and fatal anaphylaxis (197—200[C]). It should not be forgotten that encephalitis (201[C]), myocarditis (202[C]), nephritis (203[C]), and uveitis (204[C]) can all be manifestations of such reactions.

Administering different lots of the same product of equine rabies immunoglobulin, significant differences in adverse reactions reflecting differences in production or purification processes and protein content have been observed (205[C]). It has been concluded in the past that the incidence of reactions to antirabies immunoglobulin is particularly high, but any of these immunoglobulins may cause severe reactions. The WHO has recommended that animal immunoglobulins should be used only after tests to rule out hypersensitivity.

The risk of reactions to *antilymphocyte globulin* (*ALG*) is increased in patients with autoimmune disease (206[C]). Fever and chills, sometimes with extreme hyperpyrexia, nausea, vomiting and urticaria, decrease of platelet and granulocyte count were symptoms reported after the administration of horse antithymocyte globulin (ATG). Rabbit ATG side effects cited were pain and erythema at the injection site and in one instance polyarthritis with urticaria (207[C]). Four cases in which malignant lymphoma developed in renal transplant recipients treated with ATG of animal origin have been reported (208[C]).

An overview on the discovery of antitoxins, the development of antibody preparations and possible side-effects has been provided by Gronski et al. (209[R]).

Intravenous immunogobulin Pirofsky et al. (210[R]) reviewed the use of intravenous immunoglobulins in selected immunodeficiency and autoimmune diseases. In general, reactions to present preparations are minimal and restricted to mild discomfort. Although more common during the first two infusions, such reactions appear to be primarily related to the speed of infusion. When reactions are given over a 1—3-hour period, the incidence of reactions is less than 5% and occur during the transfusion; when infusions are given rapidly the reactions may appear soon after completing the infusion. Common reactions are pallor, sweating, nausea, vomiting, chills, low-grade fever, muscle aches or pains, back discomfort, tachycardia, elevation or reduction of blood pressure and tightness on the chest.

Allerglobuline is a human gammaglobulin preparation which has been reported to have a protective effect against Type I allergic diseases and chronic infection of the upper respiratory tract both in adults and children. Bunnag et al. (211[C]) have treated 64 patients with allerglobuline. Pain and inflammation at the injection site were the most common side-effects. Fever, drowsiness, headache, nausea, back pain and conjunctivitis occurred in only few patients. One patient experienced rash and myalgia after the third injection; when the rash occurred again after the fourth injection the patient was withdrawn.

Japanese encephalitis vaccine

In the last half century, Japanese encephalitis (JE) has been recognized as an important arboviral disease in man in Japan, China, Korea, Thailand, India, Nepal, Sri Lanka and Vietnam. In 1954, JE vaccine of the mouse brain type for human use was licensed in Japan. However, strong criticism on mouse brain vaccine was raised and has continued for many years. Therefore, in 1965 the Nippon Institute of Biological Products and the Biken Foundation implemented more advanced purification procedures, such as alcohol precipitation and ultracentrifugation. In 1965, a special surveillance team was formed by the Japanese Ministry of Health and Welfare to investigate adverse events following the administration of JE vaccine. No severe adverse event was reported among 21 396 vaccinees including 18 401 adolescents and children under 18 years of age. Some mild reactions (fever, malaise, abdominal symptoms) were noted in 1.2% of the vaccinees. Using a countrywide hospital network, the surveillance team studied any severe neurological disease occurring within 1 month after receipt of the vaccine. During 1957—1966, 26 cases (nine cases of meningitis, 10 cases of convulsions, five cases of polyneuritis, and two cases of demyelinization) could be analyzed. No evidence was provided showing an etiological relationship between these clinical syndromes and JE immunization. The incidence of neurological disease was considered minor

Table 6. *Hypersensitivity reactions (generalized urticaria or angioedema) following JE immunization*

Country	Vaccine lot number	Cases	Estimated number of vaccinees	Estimated rate per 100 000 vaccinees
Denmark	16	13	17 500	7
	32	2	7 500	3
	33	2	10 000	2
	12	4	6 500	6
Sweden	30	1	15 000	0.7
United Kingdom	13	1	1 950	5
Australia				
Nationwide	9, 17, 42	4	3 400	12
Fairfield Hosp.	17, 42	3	601	50
Canada				
Nationwide	32, 54	3		
Univ. of Calgary	32	1	96	104
United States				
Travelers		2	1 328	15
Army	29, 30, 31	1	526	19
Army and dependents (Okinawa)	49, 55	220	35 253	62

compared with the millions of doses distributed annually in Japan (212). An additional detailed report on two cases of *acute disseminated encephalomyelitis* following JE immunization have been provided from Japan. A 6-year-old girl and a 5-year-old boy showed drowsiness, paresthesias, and gait disturbance 14 and 17 days, respectively, after immunization. Treatment with prednisolone improved the clinical findings (213[C]).

Hypersensitivity reactions Hypersensitivity reactions following the use of Japanese encephalitis vaccine have been reported from some countries (see Table 6). The vaccine constituent(s) responsible for these events has (have) not been identified (214[R]).

Risk situations The Advisory Committee on Immunization Practices (ACIP) recommended that vaccinees should be observed for 30 minutes after immunization, medications to treat anaphylaxis should be available. A personal history of allergic disorders should be considered when weighing the risks and benefits of the vaccine for an individual. JE vaccine should not be given to persons who had a previous adverse reaction after receiving JE vaccine or a previous hypersensitivity reaction to other vaccines of neural origin. Hypersensitivity to thiomersal is a contraindication to immunization (214).

Malaria vaccine

The first field studies to assess the safety, immunogenicity and protectivity of the synthetic malaria vaccine SPf66 directed against the asexual blood stages of *Plasmodium falciparum* have been carried out in Colombia (215[C], 216[C]). The vaccine was considered to be safe and effective.

Measles vaccine

Live measles virus vaccine is available in monovalent (measles only) form and in combinations: measles—rubella (MR) and measles—mumps—rubella (MMR) vaccines. Measles vaccines based on further attenuated strains (beyond the level of the original strain, e.g. the Edmonston B strain) produces a mild or inapparent, non-communicable infection. About 5—15% of vaccinees may develop a temperature of >39.4°C (beginning about the 6th day after immunization and lasting up to 5 days). Transient rashes have been reported in approximately 5% of vaccinees. Hypersensitivity reactions very rarely follow the immunization. Most of these reactions are considered minor and consist of wheal and flare or urticaria at the injection site. Very few cases of immediate allergic reactions in children who had histories of anaphylactoid reactions to egg ingestion have been reported, but these reactions could potentially have been life-threatening (217[R]). This risk of egg allergy is excluded in modern vaccines where the virus is propagated in chicken or human fibroblast cell cultures (see below under 'MMR vaccines'). In Japan, there are three further attenuated live measles vaccines licensed for general use: AIK-C vaccine, Biken-CAM vaccine and Schwarz-FFB vaccine. No significant differences have been reported between the three vaccines as regards either immunogenicity or adverse reactions (218[R]).

Data on side effects following measles immunization reported in the framework of the (US) *Monitoring System on Adverse Events Following Immunization* to the Centers for Disease Control, Atlanta, have been published (SEDA-13, 274—277, Tables 1—4).

Central nervous system The long debate on the degree of risk to the CNS, especially *encephalitis* and *encephalopathy* (Landrigan and Witte, 219[C]; CDC analysis, 217[R], 220[C], 221[R]; Ministry of Health and Welfare, Japan, 218[R]; National Childhood Encephalopathy Study in the United Kingdom, SEDA-11, 285; Northwest Thames region of England, 222[C]) is not completely solved. However, most investigators having critically analyzed the studies carried out considered that the incidence of suspected encephalitis/encephalopathy cases following immunization still remains much lower than that of natural infection, suggesting that some or most of the reported neurological disorders may be only temporally and not causally related to measles immunization.

As with the administration of other agents that may produce fever, some children develop *febrile seizures* after receipt of measles vaccine. Most of these convulsions are simple febrile seizures and do not, in themselves, increase the probability of subsequent epilepsy or other neurological disorders. Recent data suggest that there is an increased risk of convulsions among children with a prior history of convulsions or those with a history of convulsions in siblings or parents. After analyzing data on the increased risk of such children, both the (US) Immunization Practices Advisory Committee (ACIP) and the Committee on Infectious Diseases of the American Academy of Pediatrics have recommended that children with a history of convulsions should be vaccinated because the benefits of immunization outweigh the risks. Children at risk could receive antipyretics before the expected onset of fever and continued for 5—7 days. However, the Committee on Infectious Diseases was reluctant about prevention with antipyretics because after onset of fever these are likely to be effective (221[R], 223[R]).

Subacute sclerosing panencephalitis (*SSPE*) may occur after immunization with live attenuated measles vaccine, but the possible role of measles virus vaccine in the pathogenesis of SSPE has been neither proved or disproved. However, the frequency seems to be lower than after natural measles. Hinman et al. (224[R]) reported a decline in the reported incidence of SSPE in the United States accompanying the decline in the reported incidence of measles and following it by approximately 7 years. Similar experience has been reported from Israel (225[R]), Japan (226[R]—227[R]), and the Eastern part of Germany (228). The results underline the opinion that SSPE may occur after measles immunization but that the frequency is apparently much lower than after natural measles. There is no evidence of an enhanced risk of SSPE on revaccination. A different note is sounded from Roumania where epidemiological investigation of SSPE indicated a yearly incidence of five to six cases per million inhabitants without any change due to the measles immunization programme implemented approximately 10 years earlier (229[R]).

Toxic shock syndrome Within 3 hours of measles immunization, four children developed *toxic shock syndrome* (TSS), three of them died. TSS was initially seen in women who were using tampons in the presence of vaginal colonization and/or infection with toxin-producing strains of *Staphylococcus aureus*. The hallmarks of TSS are high fever, diarrhea, vomiting, tachycardia, hypertension, mucocutaneous ulceration, rash, conjunctival injection, red palms and soles and bleeding diathesis. There was some evidence that a used vial of measles vaccine was kept in cold water in a pot and became contaminated (230[C]). Similar events from various developing countries have been reported to the World Health Organization. Careful investigations revealed secondary bacterial contamination as the cause of disease and death (231).

Hypersensitivity (*See under 'MMR vaccine'*)

Hematological changes following measles immunization have been found by Olivares et al. (232[R]). The vaccine induced a significant decrease in hemoglobin that may persist for 14—30 days and may be difficult to distinguish from iron deficiency.

Case reports on side effects Case reports on suspected *encephalitis* (including two cases with hearing loss) and *convulsions* have been reviewed (SEDA-8, 299; SEDA-9, 284; SEDA-11, 291; SEDA-12, 283; SEDA-16, 388); very rare individual case reports on *cerebellar ataxia*, *diffuse retinopathy*, *optic neuritis*, *regional lymphadenitis*, *thrombocytopenic purpura* (70% of *thrombocytopenic purpura* occur following viral diseases; *purpura* has been reported also following the receipt of measles vaccine), *paroxysmal cold hemoglobinuria*, *parkinsonism*, *pityriasis lichenoides et varioliformis acuta*, *nephrosis*, *and depression of the tuberculin skin test reaction* were cited (SED-11, 679; SED-12, 811; SEDA-12, 283; SEDA-16, 389; SEDA-17, 376).

High-titre Edmonston-Zagreb measles vaccine has been found to be more immunogenic in young infants than measles vaccine based on other strains. It was hoped that the use of such vaccines could help to reduce the incidence of measles in infancy in developing countries. But little was known about the long-term effects of high-titer measles vaccine given early in life. Recently, experience gained in Senegal, Guinea-Bissau and other developing countries seems to show that child mortality after immunization was significantly higher in the groups receiving high-titer Edmonston-Zagreb vaccine than in the group given standard vaccine. The higher risk of death remained significant in multivariate analyses (233[C], 234[C]). There is a reason for concern about the long-term safety of high-titer measles vaccine. The World Health Organization has suspended the use of high-titer measles vaccine.

Risk situations Live measles vaccine should not be given to pregnant women. This precaution is based on (the purely theoretical) risk of fetal infection. Persons who have experienced anaphylactoid reactions to measles vaccine or neomycin (measles vaccine contains a small amount of neomycin) should not be immunized. Replication of the measles vaccine virus may be potentiated in patients with immune deficiencies and by the suppressed immune responses that occur with leukemia, lymphoma or generalized malignancy, or during therapy with corticosteroids, alkylating drugs, antimetabolites or radiation. Such patients should not be immunized (218[R]).

Contraindications to measles immunization in AIDS patients and HIV-infected individuals have been reviewed in 'Immunization of HIV-infected persons'.

Hülsse et al. (235[C]) immunized 176 high-risk children to protect them against measles during an outbreak. All were children with pre-existing damage to the central nervous system. Only four children developed side effects following immunization (convulsions, transient EEG changes). Comparing the risks of immunization and of natural disease, the authors recommended measles immunization of neurologically high-risk children where an epidemic occurs.

Inactivated measles vaccine This was not distributed after 1967 (due to inefficacy). Reports on the *atypical measles syndrome* following immunization with this vaccine type have been reportedly previously (SED-11, 679; SEDA-8, 299; SEDA-11, 291).

Measles—mumps—rubella (MMR) vaccine (including measles—mumps and measles—rubella vaccine)

In most developed countries MMR vaccine has replaced the former use of single antigen vaccines against measles, mumps and rubella. Comparisons of efficacy and safety of different MMR vaccines and monovalent versus bi-/trivalent vaccines have been made in various clinical trials (SEDA-14, 285). Minor symptoms (fever, rash, malaise) occurred usually after 5—14 days and lasting for 2—3 days. Occasionally, febrile convulsions have been recorded within 3 weeks of immunization, and mild parotitis occurred rarely in the third week after immunization. On average, the seroconversion rates were between 95 and 99% for measles and rubella, and less against mumps.

In a cross-over study among 581 twin pairs aged between 14 months and 6 years only 0.5—4% experienced side effects to MMR vaccine. The difference between the reaction rate reported in the immunized members of the twin pairs and those reported in the placebo-injected twin sisters or brothers showed that the majority of the reactions are temporally and not causally related to immunization. Respiratory symptoms as well as nausea and vomiting were observed more frequently in the placebo-injected group than in the MMR-immunized group (236[C]).

Data on adverse reactions following MMR immunization reported in the framework of the MSAEFI to the Centers for Disease Control, Atlanta, Georgia, have been provided in detail (SEDA-13, Tables 1 and 3, pp. 274 and 276, respectively).

Hypersensitivity and allergic reactions There is a controversy in the literature about the safety of MMR vaccine in children with adverse reactions to egg. Investigating the vaccine produced by Merck Sharpe & Dohme (virus grown in chicken fibroblasts), O'Brien et al. (237) did not detect egg proteins. More recently, Fasano et al. (238) revealed 37 pg of ovalbumin/0.5 ml of the MMR vaccine produced by MSD using a competitive ELISA. This extremely low amount of ovalbumin appears to be unlikely to provoke allergic reactions. The results of a study carried out in 15 children with egg-positive skin results confirmed the concept that the MMR vaccine does not contain enough egg protein to cause reactions (239[C]).

Considering allergy to egg proteins as a contraindication against immunization using vaccines produced in chicken fibroblast cultures, Giampetro et al. (240[C]) administered Moraten vaccine, Berna (virus grown in human fibroblast cultures and therefore certainly ovalbumin-free) to a 2-year-old male suffering from atopic dermatitis since the age of 3 months. The skin tests were positive to cow's milk and egg. Within a few minutes after the receipt of the vaccine, the child developed severe dyspnea, rhinoconjunctivitis and lip cyanosis. The child was successfully treated for an acute anaphylactic reaction. The case seems to demonstrate that the very rare allergic reactions following the administration of measles and MMR vaccines could be due to other causes than egg protein. Kelso et al. (241[C]) have reported the case of a 17-year-old female who had an anaphylactic reaction to MMR vaccine. The investigations revealed that the vaccinee is allergic to *gelatin*. After eating gelatin she developed ear and throat pruritus and tongue swelling. Prick skin tests were positive for MMR vaccine and gelatin. Immunoblotting confirmed the presence of IgE antibodies to multiple gelatin components from a variety of animal sources. MMR vaccine contains gelatin as a stabilizer. The authors concluded that the anaphylaxis was caused by the gelatin component of the vaccine. Reporting a case of suspected *neomycin* allergy in a child receiving MMR vaccine, Kwittken et al. (242[C]) recommended that patients should be questioned regarding antibiotic allergy as well as tolerance of gelatin prior to immunization.

A series of 135 children with suspected or documented systemic allergy (atopic eczema, asthma, cow milk's allergy, severe systemic reactions following previous doses of different vaccines) has been prick-tested with undiluted MMR vaccine before immunization; 122 out of 126 prick-test-negative children received the MMR vaccine. No untoward reactions developed, except mild generalized urticaria or fever in two vaccinees. The author concluded that allergic diseases should not be considered as contraindications to MMR immunization (243[C]).

Case reports on adverse events following MMR immunization have been provided (SED-12, 810; SEDA-16, 389; SEDA-17, 376; SEDA-18, 336). Acute *pancreatitis* may result from viral infections, including mumps, coxsackie B, Epstein-Barr, and varicella. Although anecdotal reports of pancreatitis to viral vaccines exist, only few cases have been reported in the literature. Adler et al. (244[C]) have submitted a case report on a 19-year-old women who received MMR vaccine; 11 days later, pancreatitis was diagnosed. Other etiologies of pancreatitis could not be implicated in the case report.

Meningococcal vaccine

Two meningococcal polysaccharide vaccines, bivalent serotypes A and C vaccine and tetravalent A, C, Y, and W135 vaccine are commercially available; group B vaccines are under development. Adverse reactions are infrequent and mild, consisting of local soreness or localized erythema at the injection site, and systemic reactions (transient fever, headache, fatigue), lasting 1–2 days (245[R], 246[C]).

During an immunization campaign in Auckland, New Zealand, involving 130 000 children, there were 92 reports of apparent peripheral nerve involvement, including 80 reports of unexplained weakness and 57 reports of paresthesia or dysesthesia (247[C]). This was the first report indicating that short-term neurological symptoms could occur after meningococcal immunization.

During the efficacy trial using the Norwegian meningococcal group B vaccine carried out in Norwegian secondary schools from 1988 to 1991 seven of the reported events in vaccinees have been classified as serious, among them one case of acute transverse myelitis considered to be most likely a vaccine reaction. The remaining cases could have been triggered by the vaccine without being directly caused by the vaccine (248[C]).

Further reports on clinical trials in children, adults, and asplenic persons have been provided (249[C]) and surveyed (SEDA-9, 282; SEDA-10, 288; SEDA-11, 288; SEDA-16, 379; SEDA-17, 370; SED-12, 813).

Mumps vaccine

Live mumps virus vaccine is available in monovalent (mumps only) form and in combination with measles (MM vaccine) and with measles and rubella (MMR vaccine). Currently, there are vaccines based on the following mumps vaccine strains in use:

(a) The *Jeryl Lynn strain* is used mainly in vaccines prepared in the United States. The virus was isolated from a female patient in 1963. Vaccines based on Jeryl Lynn strain are mostly used worldwide.

(b) The Urabe Am 9 strain was attenuated in Japan and has been used for the preparation of MMR and other mumps-component-containing vaccines in Japan and Europe.

(c) The Rubini strain has been isolated in Switzerland and was attenuated by passage in human diploid cells for use in vaccine production.

(d) The L-3 (Leningrad) strain was derived by combining five isolates of mumps virus from sick children. The attenuated strain is used for vaccine production, especially in Russia.

(e) The L-3 strain has been further attenuated in Zagreb, Croatia, by adaptation and passage in SPF chick embryo fibroblast cell cultures (mumps vaccine strain L-Zagreb); L-Zagreb mumps vaccine has been prepared.

Various authors investigated the immunogenicity and reactogenicity of different mumps vaccine strains (see Annuals). Mainly episodes of *parotitis* and low-grade *fever* have been reported. Rash, pruritus, purpura and other *allergic reactions* are uncommon, usually mild and of brief duration (250[R]). Data on side effects following immunization with mumps-containing vaccines collected in the framework of MSAEFI have been provided (SEDA-13, 274–277, Tables 1–4).

Mumps vaccine-associated meningitis is a well-known side-effect of mumps (or MMR) immunization, but until 1991 the reported frequency rates were low. In 1991, Japanese researchers published the result of a nationwide survey started in 1989: incidence rates of vaccine-associated mumps meningitis varied from less than one per 7000 to one per 405 from prefecture to prefecture. Meningitis was generally mild and there were no sequelae from the illness. The vaccine used contained the Urabe Am9 strain (251[C], 252[C]).

MMR vaccine was introduced in the UK in October, 1988. Vaccines based on the Urabe Am9 strain (85% of vaccine doses distributed) and the Jeryl Lynn strain (15% of vaccine doses distributed) have been used. To assess the risk of mumps vaccine-associated meningitis, pediatricians were asked to report to the British Pediatric Surveillance Unit (BPSU) all confirmed and suspected cases during 1990—1991. The risk based on confirmed cases was estimated to be one per 250 000 doses distributed (253[C]). However, data from one district, based on two confirmed cases and one suspected case identified by the Nottingham Public Health Laboratory, suggested a much higher risk, about one in 4000 doses (254[C]). To investigate whether the risk observed in Nottingham was atypical or indicative of substantial under-reporting elsewhere, additional studies were initiated. A laboratory study including four independent laboratories identified 13 cases of vaccine-associated meningitis following immunization with Urabe strain vaccines; in one-third, mumps virus characterized as vaccine-like virus has been isolated. The risk estimate of one per 11 000 doses distributed is lower than in the Nottingham study but much higher than in the BPSU surveillance. Furthermore, children with a discharge diagnosis of viral meningitis were identified in the Oxford region and their immunization status ascertained. The estimated risk per 100 000 doses was 4.7. Because there have been no cases of proven vaccine-associated mumps meningitis with isolation of the Jeryl Lynn vaccine virus in the UK, a decision to change to Jeryl Lynn-containing vaccines has been made (253[C]).

Eight cases of mumps vaccine-associated meningitis have occurred in Canada. Mumps viruses have been isolated and characterized by nucleotide sequencing as Urabe Am9-like strains. Urabe mumps vaccine virus-containing vaccines are no longer licensed for sale in Canada (255[C]).

Forsey et al. (256[C]) have examined over 80 mumps viruses from around the world, including 20 isolates found in the cerebrospinal fluid of children with vaccine-associated meningitis in the UK and Ireland and isolates from parotitis and meningitis following mumps immunization from Australia, Belgium, Canada, France, Germany, and Japan. With the polymerase chain reaction and nucleotide sequencing (recent advances in using polymerase chain reaction and dideoxynucleotide sequencing for the differentiation of wild and attenuated mumps viruses have created the possibility of differentiating meningitis cases into wild and vaccine-associated cases) the isolates have been characterized as Urabe Am9-like vaccine strains. Forsey and his colleagues identified the Jeryl Lynn mumps vaccine strain in one vaccinee from Germany, but have received no virus of this type from a patient with meningitis (256[C]). Although one cannot conclude from this that Jeryl Lynn would be free of such side-effects, all the considerable evidence points toward a considerable difference between the mumps vaccine strains. The virological heterogeneity provides a clue for further investigation (257[R]). Commercial mumps vaccine of the Jeryl Lynn strain contains at least two distinct mumps viruses. Afzal (257a) suspects that this factor contributes significantly to the safeguard and efficacy of this vaccine.

On September, 1992, health authorities world-wide were informed by SmithKline Beecham Biologicals that the company had decided to suspend the distribution of its vaccines containing the Urabe Am9 strain, provided that alternative vaccines were available to maintain the immunization programmes established in the various countries (258). In April 1993, the Ministry of Health and Welfare in Japan also decided to interrupt the use of MMR vaccine containing mumps vaccine viruses because of a higher rate of vaccine-associated meningitis (259[r]).

Tesovic et al. (260[C]) reviewed recently cases of aseptic meningitis occurring 14—26 days after MMR immunization. All patients were immunized with the L-Zagreb mumps strain, Edmonston-Zagreb measles strain, and RA 27/3 rubella strain. The incidence of vaccine-associated meningitis in the study was nine per 10 000 doses. This finding is similar to the one reported for the same mumps vaccine strain by Cizman (261): 10 per 10 000 (SEDA-12, 815), but higher than that found by Kraigher (cited in 260[C]).

Sawada et al. (259[C]) have reported the transmission of Urabe mumps vaccine strain between siblings. A younger sister developed parotitis following immunization with Urabe mumps strain. Nineteen days later the older sister developed mumps. The strain isolated showed molecular biological characteristics typical for the Urabe strain.

Induction of type I diabetes mellitus A total of 20 cases of type I diabetes mellitus suspected to be induced by mumps (MMR) immunization have been reported to Behringwerke, Marburg, Germany. The earliest case occurred 3 days after receiving the vaccine and the latest 7 months after immunization. Twelve cases were diagnosed within 30 days of immunization. The investigators considered the cases of diabetes mellitus to have a temporal relationship to mumps immunization. For every 5 million children immunized against mumps 50 spontaneous cases of diabetes mellitus are to be expected by random coincidence within a period of 30 days after immunization. In fact, only 12 cases were reported within 30 days after immunization (262[C]). Mainly based on this analysis the 'Deutsche Vereinigung zur Bekämpfung der Viruskrankheiten' (DVV) could not confirm the relationship between mumps immunization and diabetes mellitus (263).

Case reports on *febrile convulsions*, *meningitis*, *orchitis*, *parotitis*, *swollen lymphnodes* and *thrombocytopenia* have been provided (SED-12, 813; SEDA-16, 389: SEDA-17, 377).

Risk situations See 'Measles vaccine'.

Pertussis (whole cell and acellular) vaccine (including diphtheria—tetanus—pertussis vaccine)

Two types of pertussis vaccines (and combined vaccines including the different types of pertussis components) are now commercially available: pertussis whole cell vaccine and acellular pertussis vaccine.

Pertussis whole cell vaccine is an adsorbed suspension of inactivated pertussis bacteria. The vaccine is available in monovalent form or in combination with diphtheria and tetanus toxoids (DTP). DTP vaccine is the preparation of choice in routine immunization practice.

Local reactions following DTP immunization are common (40—70% of the vaccinees) but are usually self-limiting. A nodule may be palpable at the injection site of adsorbed products for several weeks. Abscess at the injection site has been reported (6—10 per million vaccinees). Mild to moderate fever (38.0—40.4°C) occurs frequently (about 50% of vaccinated infants), generally within several hours of administration, persisting for 1—2 days. Fever and other systemic symptoms are much less common following immunization with preparations not containing the pertussis component. *Arthus-type hypersensitivity reactions* occur, particularly after booster doses. Rarely, severe systemic reactions (urticaria, anaphylaxis) have been reported.

Different vaccines and reactogenicity Investigating the rates of local and systemic reactions following 9920 DTP immunizations, Baraff et al. (264[C]) have found significant differences relating to different manufacturers and different vaccine lots.

Age and reactogenicity Reports from Alberta and British Columbia provinces, Canada, have suggested that the incidence rates of severe local adverse reactions may increase with each dose (3rd, 4th, 5th) in preschool children (265[C]).

Comparison of reactogenicity of DTP vaccine and DT vaccine An older study in the United States had compared the rates of both minor and more serious reactions in 15 752 children 0—6 years of age to DTP vaccine and in 784 children to DT vaccine. The ratio of minor reactions associated with DTP and DT, respectively, was: local redness 37.4%/7.6%; local swelling 40.7%/7.6%; pain 50.9%/9.9%; fever 46.5%/9.3%; drowsiness 31.5%/14.9%; fitfulness 53.4%/22.6%; vomiting 8.2%/2.6%; anorexia 20.9%/7.0%; persistent crying 3.1%/0.7%; high-pitched unusual cry 0.1%/0%. The reactions after DT were not only less frequent, but also less severe. Convulsions and hypotonic-hyporesponsive episodes each occurred in one per 1750 immunizations (266[C]).

Data from the Monitoring System for Adverse Events Following Immunization (MSAEFI) (SEDA-13, 274—277, Tables 1—4) show that the side effect rate for DTP was twice as high as that for DT vaccine. The most reported side effect was fever (59% of all reports) followed by local reactions (36%) (267[c]). Similar results have been published by Dittmann (13.5 severe side effects per million vaccinees following DTP immunization and 4.8 reactions per million vaccinees following DT immunization) (268[c]) and Pollock et al. (269[c]).

Sterile abscess Vulginity (270[R]) believes it is an idiosyncratic reaction of some individuals, perhaps genetically determined, which causes a granulomatous response to antigens, irrespective of the location of the vaccine. Others maintain that it is caused by a contaminated needle track or to vaccine material coating the outside of the needle) resulting from the lack of a proper injection technique. Salomon et al. (271[C]) have evaluated the 'two-needle strategy', the hypothesis that changing the needle on the syringe after drawing up the DTP vaccine and before injecting reduces local reactions by eliminating deposition of aluminium adjuvant in the subcutaneous track of the needle. Upon immunizing 223 children by this 'two-needle strategy' and 200 by the 'one-needle strategy', no significant difference was found in the occurrence of local or systemic reaction.

The long-lasting debate on CNS complications and persistent brain damage following pertussis (whole-cell vaccine) immunization During the 1980s, the question of side effects caused by pertussis whole-cell vaccine, and especially the severity and frequency of CNS complications, was debated by physicians as well as by the general public, in several countries. Following reports, publications and national evaluations regarding CNS complications, few countries changed their national pertussis immunization policy. In the autumn of 1981, Japan replaced the whole-cell vaccine by acellular pertussis vaccine developed by Sato in Japan. Sweden finished its pertussis (whole-cell vaccine) immunization programme in 1979. As a result of the prominence accorded to the risks involved, the pertussis vaccine coverage rates in the United Kingdom declined sharply in the beginning of the 1980s, but were increasing again when big pertussis epidemics started as a result of diminished population immunity. In the 1980s, in the Federal Republic of Germany, pertussis immunization was only recommended for children at special risk (changed in 1991: DTP recommended in united Germany).

In the last edition of Meyler's Side Effect of Drugs (1992) the discussion on severe neurological side effects of (whole cell vaccine) pertussis immunization has been provided in detail including reports on pertussis vaccine (High Court) trials. Now it seems that the debate is over. Reviewing information sources available worldwide, the report of the Institute of Medicine, National Academy of Sciences, Washington (8[C]) cited at length in SED-12 made the following conclusions:

A causal relation between DTP vaccine and *anaphylaxis*, *febrile seizures* and (a) *inconsolable crying* is indicated; (b) *acute encephalopathy* and *hypotonic-hyporesponsive episodes* is weaker but still indicated; and (c) *infantile spasms*, *afebrile seizures*, *hypsarrhythmia*, *Reye's syndrome*, and *sudden infant death syndrome* is not indicated. There is insufficient evidence to indicate either the presence or absence of a causal relation between DTP vaccine and *chronic neurological damage*, *epilepsy*, *aseptic meningitis*, *erythema multiforme or other rash*, *Guillain-Barré syndrome*, *hemolytic anemia*, *juvenile diabetes*, *learning disabilities and attention-deficit disorder*, *peripheral mononeuropathy*, or *thrombocytopenia*.

In 1993, Miller et al. (272[C]) and Madge et al. (273[R]) presented the results of a 10-year follow-up study of the National Childhood Encephalopathy Study (NCES) carried out in 1976—1979. The conclusions of the follow-up study were as follows: The NCES suggested a small excess risk of severe acute neurological events within 7 days of pertussis immunization, but the risk of permanent damage due to the vaccine, if any, was slight. Follow up of cases and controls from this study for some years has shown that significantly more children with such illnesses die or suffer subsequent educational, behavioural, or neurological deficits than expected by comparison with controls, but the number of cases associated with pertussis vaccine was small and statistically vulnerable.

In light of these new data from the NCES, the committee responsible for the report of the Institute of Medicine concluded in 1994 that the recent findings from the NCES necessitated a review of the conclusion that the evidence is insufficient to indicate a causal relation between DTP and permanent neurological damage.

After having reviewed the new NCES data the committee stated as follows: The balance of evidence is consistent with a causal relation between DTP vaccine and the forms of chronic nervous system dysfunction described in the NCES in those children who experience a serious acute neurological illness within 7 days after receiving DTP vaccine. This serious acute neurological response to DTP is a rare event. The estimated excess risk ranged from 0 to 10.5 per million immunizations. The evidence remains insufficient to indicate the presence or absence of a causal relation between DTP vaccine and chronic nervous system dysfunction under any other circumstances (274[R]).

Reports on non-neurological side effects of pertussis (whole-cell) immunization These have been provided (SED-12, 815; SEDA-16, 379; SEDA-17, 370; SEDA-18, 330).

Recommendations on the use of pertussis (whole-cell) vaccine Considering international experience, the WHO as well as many national immunization advisory committees (see SEDA-16, 379) reaffirmed the appropriateness of continued routine pertussis immunization using the currently available whole-cell pertussis vaccines.

Risk situations The (US) Immunization Practices Advisory Committee (ACIP) has recommended that a *personal history of a prior convulsion* should be evaluated before initiating or continuing immunization with vaccines containing a pertussis component. The presence of an *evolving neurological disorder* contraindicates pertussis immunization. Other contraindications to the receipt of pertussis vaccine are *hypersensitivity* to vaccine components or a *history of a severe reaction* following an earlier dose (275[R]). Reviewing the data on the relationship between the *family history of convulsions* and immunization with pertussis-containing vaccines, both the ACIP as well as the US Committee on Infectious Diseases considered a family history of convulsions in parents and siblings not as a contraindication to pertussis immunization. The ACIP (and other authors, e.g. Lewis (276[C])) believes that antipyretic use (e.g. acetaminophen given at a dose of 15 mg/kg at the time of DTP immunization and again 4 hours later) in conjunction with DTP vaccine may be reasonable in children with personal or family histories of convulsions since it will reduce the incidence of postimmunization fever (277[R]).

Details regarding the age-related efficacy of the use of acetaminophen and the inefficacy of prophylactic acetaminophen given in a single dose have been provided (SEDA-14, 277).

Pertussis (acellular) vaccine

The first generation of the new acellular vaccines was developed in Japan in the late 1970s (Sato). Since late 1981, acellular vaccines replaced the whole-cell pertussis vaccines for use in the Japanese immunization programme. Two types of acellular pertussis vaccine were then produced by six Japanese manufacturers (278[R], 279[R], for details see SEDA-12, 276; SEDA-13, 283; SEDA-14, 279). The rate of reported serious reactions decreased in Japan. During the period 1975—1981 when whole-cell vaccines were given, the rate was 0.4 per million doses, compared with a rate of 0.25 per million doses during the period 1982—1984 (279[R]). In 1988, Kumura and Kuno-Sakai (280[R]) have summarized the experience gained in Japan since the introduction in 1981 of new DTP vaccines containing acellular pertussis components. Acellular vaccines seem to be effective in Japan. In accordance with the increase of coverage, reported cases of pertussis and pertussis deaths have declined. Reactogenicity (fever, local reactions) was very low (for details see SEDA-14, 279, Table 6); additionally Kimura and Kuno-Sakei cited reports on Quincke's edema-like swelling of the whole arm following the third injection (0.17% of vaccinees) and the booster injection (2.61%), respectively. Data on more severe adverse events have been collected from 1970 to 1986 in the framework of the National Adverse Reaction Compensation System (SED-12, 818, 819). Kimura and Kuno-Sakei considered the vaccines to be safe and effective enough to eliminate pertussis in Japan in the future (281[C]).

Large-scale clinical trials in Germany, Italy, and Sweden The epidemiological circumstances in Sweden and in parts of Germany and Italy, where the immunization programmes against pertussis has been discontinued or carried out on low level (because of public concern about rare severe adverse events), offered good opportunities to assess clinical efficacy and safety of acellular pertussis vaccines by controlled field trials and a household contact study (Germany). Different mono- and multi-component acellular vaccines produced by European and US manufacturers have been evaluated, sometimes compared with whole-cell pertussis vaccines. In general, acellular vaccines have been found to be immunogenic, epidemiologically effective and less reactogenic than the currently used whole-cell pertussis-component vaccines as assessed in terms of fever, pain, fretfulness, and local reactions at the injection site. Based on the results, acellular pertussis vaccines have been already licensed for booster immunization in the US, Canada, and some Western European countries. In Germany and Switzerland, acellular pertussis vaccines are also licensed for primary immunization. Details regarding the results and conclusions of the large-scale field trials finished in 1994 and 1995 in Germany, Italy and Sweden will be published in SEDA-19. Reports on other clinical trials using acellular pertussis vaccines have been provided (SED-12, 818; SEDA-12, 277; SEDA-13, 283; SEDA-14, 279; SEDA-15, 350; SEDA-16, 382; SEDA-17, 370; SEDA-18, 332).

Risk situations The available data allow the evaluation of local and systemic side effects but not the evaluation of possible severe complications which could occur when millions of children have been immunized. Therefore, the risk situation described under the section on whole-cell pertussis vaccine will be used similarly for acellular pertussis vaccine.

Plague vaccine

Plague vaccine is a suspension of the formaldehyde-killed encapsulated form of *Yersinia pestis*. A primary series of immunization consists of three doses given intramuscularly. General malaise, headache, fever, mild lymphadenopathy, or erythema and induration at the injection site have been reported following the administration of plague vaccine (10% of vaccinees) and occurring more commonly with repeated injections. Sterile abscesses and hypersensitivity reactions (urticaria, asthma) occur rarely (282[R]).

Risk situations Known hypersensitivity to any of the plague vaccine constituents (beef protein, soy, casein, phenol) contraindicates immunization. Severe local or systemic reactions following previous doses contraindicates revaccination (282[R]).

Pneumococcal vaccine (including combined pneumococcal—influenza vaccine)

Pneumococcal vaccine is composed of a saline solution containing the purified capsular polysaccharides of 23 types of *Streptococcus pneumoniae*. Replacing a 14-valent vaccine since the beginning of the 1980s, the improved 23-valent vaccine contains antigens to pneumococcal types that are responsible for approximately 85% of bacteremic pneumococcal pneumonia.

Pneumococcal vaccines produced by different manufacturers are currently available, e.g. 'Pneumovax 23' produced by Merck Sharp & Dohme, and 'Pnu-Imune 23' produced by Lederle Laboratories. Each vaccine dose (0.5 ml) contains 25 μg of each polysaccharide antigen. Immunization is recommended for persons who are at increased risk of developing pneumococcal disease because of underlying chronic health conditions and for older persons. Approximately 50% of vaccinees develop mild side effects following the receipt of the vaccine, such as erythema and pain at the injection site. Fever, myalgia, and severe local reactions have been reported in <1% of vaccinees. Severe systemic reactions, such as anaphylaxis have been rarely reported.

Case reports These have been published on *small vessel vasculitis* after combined pneumococcal–influenza immunization (283[C]), *severe febrile reaction with leucocytosis* (284[C]), *Sweet's syndrome* (285[C]), *thrombocytopenia* (286[C], 287[C]), and *keratoacanthoma* at the injection site (288[C]).

Patients with AIDS have been shown to have an impaired antibody response to pneumococcal vaccine. Side effects in symptomatic and asymptomatic HIV-infected vaccinees were not different from HIV-negative persons (289[R]).

Revaccination Arthus reactions and systemic reactions have been reported commonly following booster doses and are thought to be the result of antigen–antibody reactions involving antibodies induced by the previous immunization (290[R]). Data on revaccination of children are not yet sufficient to provide a basis for recommendation.

Immunization of persons who are at increased risk for developing pneumococcal disease The immunogenicity and safety of pneumococcal vaccine were studied in *renal allograft recipients*, *dialysis patients* (291[C]), children and adolescents with *sickle-cell anemia* (SED-11, 682; SEDA-12, 277), *diabetics* (SED-11, 682), and children with nephrotic syndrome (292[C]). When comparing the results with healthy persons there were no significant differences.

Poliomyelitis vaccine

Two types of poliomyelitis vaccines are available. One is prepared from polioviruses which as a rule have been inactivated by formaldehyde. Inactivated poliomyelitis vaccine (IPV) is administered parenterally. The second group of poliovaccines comprises attenuated strains of live polioviruses (oral poliomyelitis vaccine: OPV) which are given orally; these live vaccines are the most widely used.

IPV Inactivated poliomyelitis vaccine produced by the improvements in manufacturing technology in recent years (potency-enhanced IPV–eIPV–was licensed in 1987) is used for routine immunization in several countries (e.g. in Finland, France, Iceland, Norway, Sweden) and is recommended in other countries for certain specific purposes, e.g. for persons with underlying immunological disorders or unimmunized adults exposed to high risk. There are few countries using a mixed schedule starting primary immunization by IPV followed by OPV, e.g. Denmark, Hungary, and Israel. Currently, some developed countries using OPV in their routine immunization programmes which had no wild poliomyelitis cases for many years but some vaccine-associated poliomyelitis are reassessing their immunization strategy. They are considering new concepts of shifting from OPV to IPV or from OPV to mixed schedules. This change could help to prevent vaccine-associated poliomyelitis mostly occurring after the first dose of OPV immunization. In the US, the shift from OPV to a mixed schedule has already been recommended officially (293).

Serious side effects following IPV immunization have not been documented (294[R]). Because IPV contains streptomycin and neomycin, there is a possibility of hypersensitivity reactions in persons sensitive to these antibiotics. There is inadequate evidence to accept or reject a causal relation between IPV immunization and the occurrence of Guillain-Barré syndrome (9).

Data on adverse events following IPV immunization collected in the framework of the US Monitoring System for Adverse Events Following Immunization (MSAEFI) have been published (SEDA-13, 274–277, Tables 1–4).

OPV The vaccine very rarely produces side effects: even mild allergic reactions and diarrhea, although they can occur, are exceptional.

Neurological complications Coincident with the nationwide OPV mass campaign which interrupted the transmission of wild poliovirus in Finland in 1985 (4.5 million doses of OPV administered), an unexpected rise in the occurrence of *Guillain-Barré syndrome* (*GBS*) has been reported. Kinnunen et al. (295[C]) carefully examined 10 cases of GBS with onset of symptoms within 10 weeks following OPV immunization. No specific agents were found in these cases. The authors concluded that the investigations suggested the ability of live attenuated polioviruses, like other viral infections, to trigger GBS. The report of the Institute of Medicine, cited at length in SEDA-18 (p. 325) (9) concluded that evidence favors a causal relationship between OPV and *GBS*, whereas the authors of the report considered the evidence inadequate to accept or to reject a causal relation between OPV and *transverse myelitis*.

Vaccine-associated poliomyelitis There is no doubt that OPV can cause *poliomyelitis* in a minority of recipients and their contacts. The risk is very low but can have severe individual consequences in patients developing *vaccine-associated poliomyelitis*. Various case reports and national surveys of vaccine-associated poliomyelitis as well as studies quantifying the risk of OPV have been published (SED-12, 820; SEDA-16, 390; SEDA-18, 336). The main conclusions from the *WHO* 15-*year field study in* 13 *countries starting in* 1973 are as follows:

(a) type 1 strain is almost never implicated in vaccine-associated poliomyelitis cases;

(b) type 2 strain is an occasional cause of paralysis, commoner in contacts of the vaccine than in recipients;

(c) most of the very small number of cases which do occur are due to type 3, both in vaccine recipients and in contacts.

In general, the risk of vaccine-associated poliomyelitis is less than one per million children immunized. Type 1 strain has been confirmed to be as safe and effective as any biological substance can be. Type 2 strain is safe for recipients of the vaccine but on rare occasions can cause paralysis in contacts, so that any contact whose immunization status is doubtful should be immunized at the same time as the original vaccinee. Type 3 strain is much less stable genetically than the two other strains and requires constant monitoring in the laboratory and in the field (296[R]).

US studies, 1961—1989 The risk of VAPP has remained exceedingly low but stable since the mid-1960s. A total of 260 cases of VAPP were reported in the United States between 1961 and 1989. Cases of VAPP appeared to occur randomly in time and space. One potential cluster of VAPP consisting of six cases occurring over an 18-month period in Indiana was investigated during the period 1980—1989. These cases were not shown to be epidemiologically related.

Using the total number of 80 VAPP cases in the United States from 1980 to 1989 as a numerator, the overall risk of VAPP was one case per 2.5 million doses of trivalent OPV distributed (Table 7). The overall risk of VAPP was 9.7 times greater following the first dose of OPV as compared to the risk following all subsequent doses. The overall risk of recipient VAPP was one case per 6.8 million doses. The risk among OPV recipients was 29.0 times higher following the first dose as compared to the risk following subsequent doses. Comparing the first dose of OPV to subsequent doses, the lowest relative risk was found in immunologically abnormal persons. The average annual rate of VAPP for the period 1980—1989 was 0.34 cases per million population (Table 8). The annual incidence of VAPP among immunologically competent infants, who were used as the reference group, was 7.6 cases per 10 million population. Children below 1 year of age with a primary immunodeficiency were at highest risk of VAPP (annual rate of 16 216 cases per 10 million population, or 0.16%), which is more than 2000 times higher than the rate in the reference group. Among household contacts of children below 6 years of age, the annual rate of contact VAPP was 0.45 cases per 10 million population. For the remaining United States population, the annual rate of VAPP was 0.14 cases per 10 million population. Summarizing their experience, the authors of the 1980—1989 study distinguish three *groups at risk of VAPP*: (1) recipients of OPV, especially infants receiving their first dose of OPV; (2) persons in contact with OPV recipients, mostly unimmunized or inadequately immunized adults; and (3) immunologically abnormal individuals (297[C]).

Etiology of vaccine-associated poliomyelitis Evans et al. (298[R]) have summarized molecular-biological findings connected with the occurrence of VAPP. Recent studies have provided convincing evidence that the Sabin 2 and 3 viruses themselves may revert to a neurovirulent phenotype on passage in man. The authors report that a point mutation in the 5′-non-coding region of the genome of the poliovirus type 3 vaccine consistently reverts to the wild type in viruses isolated from cases of VAPP.

Risk of injections in provoking paralytic poliomyelitis Sutter et al. (299[C]) have evaluated the *risk of DTP injection in provoking paralytic poliomyelitis* during a large poliomyelitis outbreak in Oman. Health center immunization records were reviewed for 70 children aged 5—24 months with confirmed poliomyelitis and from 692 control children. A significantly higher proportion of case-patients received a DTP injection within 30 days prior to onset of paralysis when compared with controls (42.9 vs 28.3%, respectively). All cases for whom this information was available had paralysis of the injected limb. The study—the first quantitative estimate in this respect—confirmed that injections are an important cause of provocative poliomyelitis and stressed the recommendation to avoid unnecessary injections during poliomyelitis outbreaks. Additionally, investigations carried out in 1994/1995 in Romania revealed evidence that multiple (unnecessary) injections can possibly even increase the risk of vaccine-associated poliomyelitis. The results of this study will be published in SEDA-19.

OPV immunization and pregnancy To interrupt poliovirus transmission during an outbreak of wild poliomyelitis in Israel in 1988, about 90% of the population, including pregnant women, were immunized with trivalent OPV. Ornoy et al. (300[C]) compared the abortions that occurred within 4 months of immunization

Table 7. *Ratio* of cases of vaccine-associated paralytic poliomyelitis to doses of trivalent OPV distributed, United States, 1980–1989*

Epidemiological classification	Overall		First dose		Subsequent doses		Relative risk**
	No.	Ratio	No.	Ratio	No.	Ratio	
Sporadic	66	1:3.1	46	1:0.8	16	1:10.4	12.8
Recipient	30	1:6.8	26	1:1.4	4	1:41.5	29.0
Contact	32	1:6.4	20	1:1.9	12	1:13.8	7.4
Community-acquired	4	1:50.9	—		—		—
Imm. abnormal	14	1:14.5	6	1:6.2	8	1:20.8	3.4
Total	80	1:2.5	52	1:0.7	24	1:6.9	9.7

* Ratio of cases: 10^6 doses.
** Relative risk = first dose ratio/subsequent doses ratio.

Table 8. *Annual rate of vaccine-associated paralytic poliomyelitis per 10 million population, United States, 1980–1989*

Category	Average no. of cases per year	Population at risk (1984)	Rate per 10 million per year	Rate ratio*
Primary immunodeficiency < 1 year of age	0.6	370	16216	2.142
Infant recipients	2.8	3.7×10^6	7.57	1.0
Household contacts	1.9	42.2×10^6	0.45	0.06
All other	2.7	190.3×10^6	0.14	0.02
Total	8.0	236.2×10^6	0.34	—

* Rate ratio = individual category rate/infant recipient rate.

with that in a similar period in the previous year to establish whether there were any abnormalities that might have been associated with polio immunization. The results showed that the number of spontaneous abortions did not differ between women immunized during the first trimester of pregnancy and the controls. The authors concluded that OPV administered during early pregnancy has no adverse effect on the embryo or placenta that would cause increased fetal deaths and spontaneous abortions, nor does it seem to cause a higher rate of congenital anomalies Analyzing the OPV mass campaign in Finland, Harjulehto et al. (301[C]) considered that OPV during early pregnancy had no harmful effects on fetal development. No significant deviations from the baseline prevalence for all malformations were observed. Burton et al. (302[C]) described a case of irreparable damage to the anterior horn cells of the cervical and thoracic cord in a 20-week-old fetus whose mother was immune to poliomyelitis before conceiving but who was inadvertently given OPV at 18 weeks gestation.

Poliovaccines as a possible cause of AIDS There is a hypothesis that the HIV virus might have jumped the species barrier from monkey to people via a contaminated poliovaccine because the vaccine was manufactured in primary monkey kidney tissue known to be sometimes contaminated with monkey viruses. The existing evidence, including tests of poliovirus seed stocks, more than 20 vaccine lots, and serum samples from vaccine recipients makes this hypothesis highly improbable (303, 304).

Risk situations There are no known contraindications to the use of *IPV*. *OPV* should not be given to persons who are immunocompromised due to immunodeficiency diseases, leukemia, lymphoma or generalized malignancy or immunosuppressed due to therapy with corticosteroids, alkylating drugs, antimetabolites, or radiation. If poliomyelitis immunization is indicated in such persons, IPV should be used. OPV should also not be used for immunization of household contacts of immunocompromised patients.

In the *WHO view*, live vaccines should in general not be given to immunocompromised individuals, but the point is made that in developing countries, the risk of poliomyelitis in non-immunized infants is high and the risk from these vaccines, even in the presence of symptomatic HIV infection, appears to be lower (305[R]).

The Immunization Advisory Committees of many developed countries recommend that OPV should not be given to children and young adults who are immunocompromised due to AIDS or other clinical manifestations of HIV infection. OPV can be given to asymptomatic infected persons. However, because family members may be immunocompromised due to AIDS or HIV infection, it may be prudent to use IPV (306[R]), for details see also 'Immunization of HIV-infected persons'. *Pregnancy* is not a contraindication for the use of IPV. Although there is no convincing evidence documenting adverse effects of OPV on the developing fetus, it is prudent to avoid immunizing pregnant women, especially during the first 4 months of pregnancy. However, if immediate protection against poliomyelitis is needed, poliomyelitis immunization is recommended (307[R], 308[R]).

Pseudomonas aeruginosa **vaccine**

Stanislavsky et al. (309[C]) have tested an experimental *Pseudomonas aeruginosa* vaccine on the basis of cell-wall protein protective antigens in 119 volunteers aged 19—40 years receiving three doses of vaccine subcutaneously at intervals of 7 days. There were only mild local and systemic reactions. The majority of vaccinees (96.7%) responded immunologically well to the vaccine.

Rabies vaccine

Rabies vaccine was for a long time prepared from infected brain tissue, and neurological complications were likely to occur in as many as one in 300 cases. A second-generation vaccine prepared from duck embryo tissue has been found to be better tolerated in this respect, and third-generation vaccines prepared in non-neural tissue cultures or in human diploid cells (HDC vaccines) with a progressive improvement in safety have now become the vaccines of choice.

Any rabies vaccine can apparently cause mild local discomfort and swelling, and either of the animal preparations can result in hypersensitivity reactions, e.g. pyrexia, serum sickness or urticaria; sensitization can occur.

Brain tissue rabies vaccine There are still many countries worldwide lacking financial resources which use first-generation brain tissue rabies vaccine and where neurological complications following immunization still do occur. The neurological picture produced by this type of vaccine is very variable; sometimes *peripheral neuritis* occurs, other vaccinees develop *encephalomyelitis, dorsolumbar myelitis, ascending myelitis, hemiplegia or general subjective neurological symptoms* such as stiffness of the neck or physical weakness.

Duck embryo rabies vaccine (DEV) CNS complications following the administration of DEV occurred, but in much lower rates than following brain tissue rabies vaccines. Cases of transverse myelitis and other neurological complications have been published (SEDA-8, 300). There were some efforts to develop purified DEV but the improvements of third-generation vaccines made them the vaccines of choice for rabies prevention and treatment (310[R]).

Human diploid cell (HDC) rabies vaccine The major advantage of third-generation rabies vaccines prepared in non-neural tissue cultures or in human diploid cells is the greatly reduced risk of neurological complications. Millions of doses of these vaccines have been administered worldwide since 1974, and only a few neurological complications have been reported. In recipients given primary courses of immunization, only mild local and systemic reactions were reported by about 20%. Systemic allergic reactions occurred in 11 per 10 000 vaccinees (311[R]).

Mild local and systemic reactions to third generation rabies vaccines are common. Two to 21 days after administration of HDCV, about 5% of patients receiving booster injections for pre-exposure prophylaxis and a few receiving post-exposure primary immunization have developed an immune complex (serum sickness)-like reaction including urticaria, fever, malaise, arthralgias, arthritis, nausea and vomiting. This syndrome may prove to be less common with RVA, but direct comparisons are lacking. Anaphylaxis has been reported rarely after HDCV prophylaxis (312[c]).

Neurological complications Neurological complications following the administration of third-generation rabies vaccines cultured in non-neural tissues have been very rarely reported. Case reports on *Guillain-Barré syndrome* following the receipt of HDC have been provided (SED-11, 684; SEDA-15, 356; 312[C]). A case of *polyneuropathy and oculomotor nerve impairment* following the receipt of Russian cell-culture vaccine has been published (SEDA-12, 284). Two weeks after the second injection of HDCV a 45-year-old farmer developed *meningoradiculitis*. The symptoms regressed spontaneously (313[C]). Tornatore and Richert (314[C]) reported on a 25-year-old veterinarian developing an *inflammatory demyelinating process* affecting the central nervous system 8 days after the second HDCV immunization. The overall risk of neurological complications connected with HDC rabies vaccines is estimated to be less than one per 150 000 (SEDA-15, 356).

Further improvements of third-generation rabies vaccines These include a purified vero-cell rabies vaccine (PVRV) and HDC vaccine purified by zonal centrifugation. In clinical trials (see SEDA-12, 284; SEDA-15, 357) the improved vaccines have been well tolerated.

In 1988, Rabies Vaccine Adsorbed (RVA), a new cell culture-derived rabies vaccine (Kissling strain of rabies virus adapted to a diploid cell line of the fetal rhesus lung cells in medium-free of human albumin and adsorbed on aluminium phosphate) for human use was licensed in the United States. Reactions after primary immunization are similar to those observed with HDC. Systemic allergic reactions have been reported at a rate <1% (HDC: 6%) (315[R]).

Rubella vaccine

Rubella vaccine is a live attenuated virus vaccine. The majority of the vaccines currently manufactured outside Japan are produced in human diploid cells and are based either on the RA 27/3 strain (most widely used) or the Cendehill strain. In Japan, five different vaccine strains (e.g. TO 336 and MEQ 11) are produced in two different non-human substrates. In China, another vaccine strain (BRD-2) has been developed and produced in human diploid cells. Its antigenicity and reactogenicity have been shown to be comparable to those of RA 27/3 strain (316[R]).

In most developed countries, measles—mumps—rubella (MMR) vaccine has replaced the former use of single antigen vaccines against measles, mumps and rubella in childhood immunization programmes. Single antigen rubella vaccines are still used in post-childhood rubella prevention.

Reactogenicity Subcutaneous injection is commonly followed by local soreness and induration. Children sometimes develop low grade fever, rash and lymphadenopathy following immunization.

Acute arthritis/arthralgia occurs more frequently and tends to be more severe in susceptible women than in children, usually involving the small peripheral joints. Joint symptoms generally begin 3—25 days (8—14) after immunization, persist for 1—11 days (2—4) and rarely recur. Incidence rates are estimated to average 13—25% (317[R], 318) among adult women following RA 27/3 immunization with much lower levels noted among children, adolescents, and adult males. The incidence of acute joint symptoms increases with increasing age.

Persistent/recurrent/chronic arthritis Small studies of adult female vaccinees in Canada have shown that the incidence of *persistent or recurrent arthritis* is as high as 5—11%. Peters and Horowitz (317[C]) have provided a case report on radiological bone changes after rubella immunization. The committee responsible for the report of the Institute of Medicine, National Academy of Sciences, Washington, DC (1991) entitled 'Adverse Effects of Pertussis and Rubella Vaccines' (8[R]) found: (a) that the evidence *indicates a causal relation between RA 27/3 rubella vaccine and acute arthritis*; and (b) that the available evidence was weaker but still *consistent with a causal relation between RA 27/3 rubella vaccine and chronic arthritis*.

Bayer et al. (319[R]) have reviewed critically the sectionon rubella immunization and chronic arthritis included in the report. In the opinion of Bayer and his colleagues it is not justified to conclude on the basis of very limited experience that 'the evidence is consistent with a causal relation between the currently used rubella vaccine strain (RA 27/3) and chronic arthritis in adult women.'

The Centers of Disease Control, Atlanta, Georgia, is currently attempting to determine whether the frequency of persistent or recurrent joint symptoms reported by Canadian investigators can be confirmed in other studies. A prospective study of persistent or recurrent arthropathy and other potential adverse events following rubella immunization of adult women has therefore been started (318). However, natural rubella infection in adults is associated with a higher incidence, increased severity, and more prolonged duration of joint manifestations than is seen after immunization.

Individual reports on temporally connected events These have been provided: *myelitis*, *myeloradiculitis* (SEDA-2, 268), *meningomyelitis* (SEDA-10, 291), *encephalitis* (SEDA-5, 308), *bilateral optic neuritis* (320[C]), *peripheral neuropathy* (SEDA-12, 284), *facial paresthesias* (SEDA-11, 295), neurological manifestations, consisting of *carpal tunnel syndrome* or *multiple paresthesiae* (SEDA-12, 284), and *thrombocytopenic purpura* (321[c]). The causal relationship seems to be always doubtful. The authors of the report of the Institute of Medicine, National Academy of Sciences, Washington, DC (1991) entitled 'Adverse Effects of Pertussis and Rubella Vaccines' (8[R]) considered insufficient evidence to indicate either the presence or absence of a causal relation between RA 27/3 rubella vaccine and radiculoneuritis and other neuropathies or thrombocytopenic purpura.

Allen (322[R]) has discussed the hypothesis that RA 27/3 rubella strain could play a role in the etiology of *chronic fatigue syndrome*. Patients with chronic fatigue syndrome have elevated IgG serum antibodies to multiple common viruses. Only IgG rubella antibodies are positively correlated with the intensity of symptoms and reach levels that are significantly higher than in healthy controls.

Use of rubella vaccines in pregnancy Based on CDC's careful analyses since 1979 and the evaluation of reports from Germany and the United Kingdom showing that infants born to susceptible mothers did not develop signs of congenital rubella syndrome (CRS) the Immunization Practices Advisory Committee has concluded that: (a) pregnancy remains as a contraindication to rubella immunization because of the theoretical, albeit small, risk of CRS; (b) reasonable precautions should be taken to preclude immunization of pregnant women; (c) rubella immunization of pregnant women should not ordinarily be a reason to consider interruption of pregnancy (323[R]).

Continued surveillance in the US (data collected through the Vaccine in Pregnancy Registry) has not shown evidence that RA 27/3 rubella vaccine, administered during pregnancy, can cause CRS (324[R]).

Risk situations Immunization of women known to be pregnant should be avoided (see above). The other contraindication to the use of rubella vaccine is an immunocompromised state (see the sections above dealing with other live virus vaccines, e.g. measles or mumps or oral poliomyelitis vaccine). It is recommended that rubella (or MMR) vaccine should not be given to persons who are immunosuppressed in association with AIDS or other clinical manifestations of HIV infection. The vaccine can be given to asymptomatic infected persons (325[R]).

Smallpox (vaccinia) vaccine

Since the eradication of smallpox (the last case occurred in 1977 and the eradication of smallpox was declared by the World Health Assembly in 1980) routine smallpox vaccination has been ceased in all countries since it is no longer required and serious adverse reactions sometimes occur following both primary vaccination and revaccination. For a full account of side effects following smallpox vaccination the reader is referred especially to a previous edition (SED-8, 709—710) and for additional reports to other previous volumes (SED-11, 685; SEDA-1, 247; SEDA-3, 262; SEDA-4, 227; SEDA-6, 289; SEDA-13, 289; SEDA-15, 357). Smallpox vaccination in HIV-infected individuals is also reviewed above under 'Immunization of HIV-infected persons'.

Recombinant DNA technology using vaccinia virus An approach using recombinant DNA technology in the production of vaccines is the use of vaccinia virus as a live vaccine vector. Vaccinia DNA can tolerate large insertions into non-essential regions of the genome; this opens the door to the making of polyvalent live vaccinia recombinations. A major obstacle to their use as vaccines is that severe complications can occur after immunization, especially in immunodeficient individuals. Furthermore, little is known of the ways in which orthopoxviruses are maintained in nature. The possibility that vaccinia strains used as vaccines may become established in nature, as vaccinia may have in Indian buffaloes, and/or undergo genetic hybridization with existing orthopoxviruses, should be considered (326[R]). Enthusiasm for these new prospects should not be allowed to compromise the requirement for obtaining additional scientific information essential to ensure safety, efficacy and the exercise of all reasonable caution in mounting field investigations (327[R]).

There were already accusations that two AIDS patients treated with an experimental vaccine (vaccinia virus which had been inactivated(?) and genetically engineered to express HIV proteins) may have died from *vaccinia gangrenosa* (328[C], 329[C]). On the other hand, there is evidence that recombinant vaccinia viruses have reduced pathogenicity (for details see e.g. SEDA-13, 289); another attempt is the use of low neurovirulent strains of vaccinia virus (for details see e.g. SEDA-15, 357).

Protection of laboratory workers occupationally exposed to orthopoxviruses In 1980, the US Public Health Service first recommended the use of vaccinia (smallpox) vaccine to protect laboratory workers occupationally exposed to orthopoxviruses. In 1991, the Centers for Disease Control, Atlanta, Georgia, published recommendations on vaccinia (smallpox) vaccine. From 1983 through 1991, 4649 doses of smallpox vaccine were administered, of which 57% were given in 1989—1991. The proportion of primary vaccinations increased from 4% in 1983—88 to 14% in 1989—91. Ninety-three percent of vaccinees reported no signs or symptoms following vaccination. Reported adverse reactions were mild: lymphadenopathy, fever or chills, and tenderness at the site of vaccination. No severe adverse effects were reported. However, one vaccinee reported a spontaneous abortion 5 months after primary vaccination (330[C]).

A somewhat different note has been sounded from the Committee on Occupational Medical Practice, American College of Occupational and Environmental Medicine. The committee considered that, presumably, the infrequent risks for the laboratory worker exists equally for intentional vaccination or accidental laboratory exposure. The risk of infection after immunization is absolute, whereas most laboratory workers will not become infected unless immunized. On the other hand, immunization does permit control over the time and initial site of entry of the virus. In the committee's opinion, it is important for scientists and technicians to understand the US Public Health Service recommendations (mentioned above) and to have the opportunity to receive vaccinia immunization. They should also understand the reservations and have the opportunity to refuse vaccination (331[R]). These different recommendations in the US are also reflected in different national recommendations of other countries.

Tetanus vaccine

Tetanus toxoid is prepared from *Clostridium tetani* and may be given either in a fluid (plain) or adsorbed form. The slight local reactions which tend to occur (induration, erythema, tenderness) are more common with the adsorbed type. Intramuscular injection of tetanus toxoid is generally the administration of choice, and the vaccine can best be injected into a large muscle.

Reactogenicity of plain and adsorbed tetanus toxoids In children aged 15—16 years receiving routine reinforcement tetanus immunization, adsorbed vaccine caused stronger and more frequent local reactions than did plain tetanus toxoid, and a higher incidence of pyrexia. The incidence of swelling and erythema at the inoculation site increased with serum antitoxin titre at the time of administration, whereas pain and tenderness were related to the presence of the aluminium hydroxide adjuvant (332[C]). Based on similar experiences it is widely recommended that plain and not adsorbed tetanus toxoid should be used when reinforcement of immunity to tetanus alone is desired.

Overall risk rates Data on adverse events following tetanus immunization have been collected by Behringwerke, Germany (SED-12, 826) and in the framework of the (US) Monitoring System for Adverse Events Following Immunization (MSAEFI) (SEDA-13, 274).

Hypersensitivity Hypersensitivity to reinforcing doses of tetanus toxoid has been described by different investigators (see also SEDA-8, 300; SEDA-11, 288). The association between high titers of antitoxin produced by active immunization and reactions is well established (333[C], 334[C]). Booster doses of tetanus toxoid are being given with unnecessary and indeed excessive frequency. Continuing to do this will produce a more highly toxoid-sensitive population without adding significantly to the already high protection that this immunized population has against tetanus. Therefore, it is recommended that routine boosters in individuals known to have had primary immunization including a reinforcing dose be given only at 10-year intervals, and that emergency boosters be given no closer than 1 year apart (335[C]). Hypersensitivity reactions may be due to hypersensitivity to the toxoid or to the proteins of *Clostridium tetani* which co-purify with toxoid during the precipitation process used in its conventional preparation (336[C]).

Neurological side effects Rutledge et al. (337[R]) have collected reports of neurological side effects following tetanus immunization published by several authors. The most common reported complication is *polyneuropathy*. In the majority of cases the onset of polyneuropathy occurred within 14 days of the last injection, and ranged in severity from a single nerve palsy to profound sensimotor involvement of the CNS, including cord and cortex. Recovery was usually complete (eight of 10 patients with onset <14 days after injection) but three patients with onset >14 days from injection had only partial recovery. The diagnosis has to be based on a temporal relationship between immunization and onset of symptoms and the exclusion of other causes of neuropathy. Quast et al. (338[C]) have reviewed *mono- and polyneuritis* following tetanus immunization during 1970 and 1977. The frequency of this side effect was 0.4 per one million distributed vaccine doses.

Individual case reports Case reports on *abscess formation* (SEDA-11, 288); *dermatomyositis*, *neuralgic amyotrophy*, *polyradiculoneuritis with paresis of the urinary bladder and bowel* (SEDA-9, 283); asymmetric *polyneuropathy*, and *demyelinating polyneuropathy*, and *Guillain-Barré syndrome* (SEDA-14, 281); *subcutaneous nodules*, and polyvinylpyrrolidone *thesaurismosis* revealed by inflammatory manifestations following tetanus booster injection (SEDA-10, 288) have been published in the Annuals.

Risk situations The only contraindication to administering tetanus toxoid is a history of severe hypersensitivity reaction or neurological reaction after a previous dose. AIDS and HIV infections are not contraindications to tetanus immunization. Data on tetanus immune response in children with AIDS showed defective responses (339[C]).

Tick-borne meningoencephalitis vaccine

This vaccine is an adsorbed formalin-inactivated virus vaccine prepared on chicken embryo tissue. The vaccine is known to be well tolerated. Mild *local reactions* (soreness, redness, swelling) have been reported in 10—25% of vaccinees; systemic reactions occur in similar rates. Fever >39°C is a rarity.

Positive *merthiolate* tests were found in eight of 30 patients with suspected adverse reactions to tetanus or tick-borne encephalitis vaccine (local inflammatory reactions at the injection site, fever, lymphadenopathy, urticarial or lichenoid exanthemas) (340[C]). A case of facial edema and pain and swelling of the left knee following the receipt of tick-borne meningoencephalitis vaccine was suspected to be caused by thiomersal sensitivity (341[C]).

Neurological complications In 1989, 172 reports on side effects following tick-borne meningoencephalitis immunization were collected in the Federal Republic of Germany, among them 72 reports on suspect neurological complications. Analyzing the 72 reports, Kappos (342[C]) has found only three *peripheral neuritis* cases to have a presumed causal link with immunization. Three cases of mild meningitis, encephalitis and convulsions were, because of incomplete diagnosis, difficult to evaluate. The database of the Swiss Drug Monitoring Center included 20 spontaneous reports (1987 to July 1992) of adverse events following the administration of tick-borne meningoencephalitis vaccine, among them 11 reports of cases with neurological symptoms (e.g., *meningism*, *polyradiculitis*, *ataxia*, *vestibulopathy*, *facialis paresis*). The majority of cases recovered completely within few days. The incompleteness of the data does not allow conclusions regarding causality of immunization (343[C]). Individual reports on *neuropathy* (SEDA-13, 290), *multifocal cerebral vasculitis and infarction* (344[C]), *cervical myelitis* (345[c]), *myelopolyradiculitis* (345[c]), and suspected *encephalitis* (SEDA-17, 363) have been provided in the Annuals.

Tuberculin

Mammalian tuberculin purified protein derivative (tuberculin PPD) is the active principle of the old tuberculin. A small test dose in a healthy individual, given intracutaneously, is likely to produce only a little local pain and pruritus. If tuberculous infection is present, the local reaction is more marked, with vesiculation, ulceration and even granuloma annulare or necrosis.

In cases of tuberculous infection receiving more than a very minimal dose, a severe and even fatal generalized *anaphylactic reaction* can develop within about 4 hours of the injection (346[C]).

Persons engaged in manufacturing of PPD may easily become sensitized to it, and severe *allergic reactions* may occur if they thereafter inhale even small quantities (347[r]).

Lymphangitis following tuberculin testing has rarely been reported (SED-11, 686). Burgoyne et al. (348[C]) have reported a case of *acute panuveitis*. The episodes developed after each of two tests carried out at intervals of 8 years and responded well to steroid therapy.

Typhoid vaccine (including typhoid-paratyphoid vaccine)

Two different typhoid vaccines are commercially available for civilian use: (a) an *oral live attenuated vaccine* based on the Ty21a strain of *Salmonellla typhi* and (b) a *parenteral heat-phenol-inactivated vaccine* containing either killed *Salmonella typhi* or killed *S. typhi* and *S. paratyphi* A, B organisms. Approaches to develop new typhoid vaccines include the *Vi* capsular *polysaccharide vaccine* and vaccines based on *auxotrophic mutants* of Vi-positive and Vi-negative *S. typhi* (SED-11, 687; SEDA-12, 278; SEDA-13, 284; SEDA-14, 281).

Oral live vaccine During volunteer studies and field trials using Ty21a vaccine, adverse reactions were rare and consisted of abdominal discomfort, nausea, vomiting, and rash or urticaria. Adverse reactions occurred with equal frequencies among groups receiving vaccine or placebo. A case report on a *typhoid-fever-like syndrome* following the receipt of Ty21a live oral vaccine has been provided (SEDA-15, 350).

Inactivated vaccine Vaccines administered parenterally are not well tolerated. Severe local pain and/or swelling occurred in 6—40% of vaccinees; systemic reactions have been reported in 9—30% (headache), and in 14—29% (fever); 13—24% of vaccinees missed work or school due to adverse effects. More severe reactions (hypotension, shock) have been reported sporadically (349[R]).

Individual case reports Reports on fatal *angioimmunoplastic lymphadenopathy*, *hemolytic uremic syndrome* (following the receipt of typhoid/paratyphoid/diphtheria vaccine), fatal *hyperpyrexia* (SED-11, 687), *transverse myelitis* (SEDA-10, 288), *erythema nodosum* (SEDA-11, 289; SEDA-14, 281) and *Reiter's syndrome* (SEDA-15, 350) have been noted in previous volumes and in the Annuals.

Varicella vaccine

A live attenuated varicella vaccine was developed in 1973 by Takahashi using the OKA strain isolated from a boy with chickenpox. Several producers are using this live vaccine strain, e.g. Biken Institute, Merck, Sharp & Dohme, and SmithKline Beecham.

Reactogenicity Many clinical trials to assess immunogenicity and safety of varicella vaccine both in healthy and immunocompromised individuals have been carried out, examples have been given in the Annuals (SEDA-12, 285; SEDA-13, 290; SEDA-14, 285; SEDA-15, 289; SEDA-17, 379). The vaccine has been found safe and immunogenic. The reports of different investigators are quite similar. Mild *local reactions* at the injection site were the most commonly reported side effects, occurring in about 10% after the first and second dose. Vaccine-associated *rashes* developing approximately 1 month after the first dose were reported in about 6%, *sore throat* in 8%, and fever >37.8°C in 2% of vaccinees. Rash and fever after the second dose of vaccine were reported by less than 1% of vaccinees.

Maculopapular or papulovesicular *rash* occurred much more often in vaccinees with suspended chemotherapy (42%) (350[C], 351[C]).

Simultaneous administration of vaccines Reaction rates were not increased if the administration of varicella vaccine was combined with the administration of other vaccines, e.g. MMR vaccine (see SEDA-15, 358).

Herpes zoster Cases of herpes zoster both in healthy and in immunosuppressed persons have been reported by Plotkin et al. (352[C]), Hammerschlag et al. (353[C]), and Magrath (354[r]).

Spread of vaccine virus Spread to siblings of immunized leukemic children has been observed: between 18 and 36 days after the receipt of varicella vaccine 2–10% of exposed children developed mild *varicella* and/or seroconversion to varicella virus. Dissemination from healthy vaccinees has not been observed (354[r]).

Individual case reports Extensive vaccine-associated *rashes* have occurred in four leukemic children; a relationship between rash and steroid treatment was discovered (355[C]). *Acute thrombocytopenic purpura* developed 3 weeks after varicella immunization (356[C]).

Complicated wild varicella in immunized individuals has been reported (357[C]); among the two cases the first reported case of varicella meningitis occurring in a child with documented immunization and seroconversion (358[C]).

Yellow fever vaccine

The vaccine contains the 17D virus strain grown in chick embryo tissue. The older (Dakar) yellow fever vaccine was prepared from more virulent material and often caused encephalitis, the risk in children being particularly high (SED-8, 712).

Side effects following yellow fever immunization These have been documented by an expert group of WHO (359[R]):

(a) *Minor postimmunization reactions* On about the 6th day after immunization, less than 5% of vaccinees develop fever, headache, and backache, lasting for 1–2 days.

(b) *Neurological complications* No more than 17 cases of encephalitis have been recorded over a period of 40 years. They all occurred in children: 12 in infants less than 4 months old, two at 4 months, one at 6 months, one at 7 months, and one at 3 years of age. The last mentioned case was the only fatal one (17D virus was isolated from the brain), all the others recovered fully. A case report on the provocation of *multiple sclerosis* was published in 1967, but this report has not been confirmed.

(c) *allergic reactions* Rash, erythema multiforme, urticaria, angioneurotic edema, and asthma occur infrequently, predominantly in persons with a history of allergy, especially to eggs.

Severe reactions of the *immediate hypersensitivity type* (*type* 1), sometimes accompanied by anaphylactic shock and circulatory collapse, have been described very rarely. Allergic reactions of the *Arthus phenomenon type*, characterized by local swelling and necrosis following less than 24 hours after immunization, have occurred in rare instances. Some of these cases have been fatal.

Two episodes have been reported from the Ivory Coast (1974) and Ghana (1982). On the Ivory Coast, 39 cases of severe reactions with eight deaths following a mass campaign, in which 730 000 persons were immunized. The clinical feature were quite uniform: a few hours after the receipt of vaccine the vaccinees developed signs of local inflammation, in severe cases, edema and inflammation extended and were followed by cardiovascular collapse. Bacterial contamination could be the cause: during the campaign, five-dose vaccine ampoules were pooled to prepare 50 and 100 doses for use in jet injectors. In Ghana, six vaccinees developed fulminant reactions 2–6 hours after immunization; there were two deaths. The clinical features resembled those in the Ivory Coast episode.

Schoub et al. (360[C]) have reported the first case of *encephalitis* following yellow fever immunization in a child older than 3 years of age and the second case over the age of 9 months: a 13-year-old boy developed the disease 1 week after receipt of vaccine. The patient recovered after one month. Recently, there have been two reports on encephalitis (in a 29-year-old man) and meningoencephalitis (in two adults) suspected to be caused by 17D yellow fever vaccine (361[c], 362[c]).

Risk situations Infants under 9 months old are not generally immunized, except if they live in rural areas with a history of yellow fever epidemics (immunization at 6 months) or in an active epidemic focus (immunization at 4 months). Persons known to be suffering from allergy, must be tested intradermally before immunization. Further contraindications are those for other live vaccines.

MISCELLANEOUS

Immunization and encephalitis disseminata (multiple sclerosis)

Aiming to investigate the possible relationship between immunization and an attack of encephalitis disseminata (ED), Quast et al. (363[C]) have analyzed reports of ED (16 confirmed cases, 24 suspected cases) in connection with the distribution of approximately 100 million doses of vaccines manufactured by Behringwerke (1980—1989). The analyzed data did not support an increased risk of initial manifestation of ED or of renewed attack in ED patients.

Jet-gun-associated infections

The first outbreak of a disease in which a jet injector has been implicated as the vehicle of transmission has been reported.

Thirty-one attendees at a weight-reduction clinic in Southern California experienced hepatitis B following daily parenteral injections of human chorionic gonadotrophin given by jet injectors. The transmission appeared to have resulted from the multiple repeated jet injections (364[C]). WHO and UNICEF have stated in their 'Guidelines for selecting injection equipment for the Expanded Programme on Immunization' that the use of jet injectors should be restricted to circumstances in which reusable or disposable equipment is not feasible because of the large number of persons to be immunized within a short period of time (365[R]).

Mixed bacterial vaccines Starting in the 1920s, dozens of mixed bacterial vaccine products (including inactivated bacteria such as *Staphylococcus aureus*, *Streptococcus* species, *Streptococcus pneumoniae*, *Moraxella catarrhalis*, *Klebsiella pneumoniae*, *Haemophilus influenzae*) were marketed worldwide. Currently, there are several products available in European countries, and one product in the US. Most vaccines have been used for treatment of recurrent and chronic infection of the respiratory tract. The efficacy of these products is doubtful. Delayed hypersensitivity to bacterial products is common. Increasingly large delayed reactions may occur after administering maintenance doses for months, associated sometimes with vague malaise or myalgia. If delayed skin reactions are accompanied by any systemic symptoms, administration of the mixed vaccine should be drastically reduced or stopped (366[R]).

Simultaneous administration of vaccines

Double-blind and placebo-controlled and other clinical trials to compare the efficacy and safety of single-component vaccines with those of combined vaccines or simultaneous administration of different vaccines have been carried out by several investigators (see SED-11, 687; SEDA-12, 285; SEDA-14, 289). In general, there were only insignificant differences both in reactogenicity and local or systemic side effects.

Vaccine adjuvants and preservatives

Edelman (367[R]) has provided an update on vaccine adjuvants in clinical trial. A vaccine adjuvant is defined as an agent that increases specific immune responses to an antigen. The only vaccine adjuvants currently licensed by the Food and Drug Administration (FDA) are aluminium salts. All other adjuvants are considered experimental and must undergo special preclinical testing. Real and theoretical risks of vaccine adjuvants are listed as follows: local acute or chronic inflammation with formation of abscess and nodules; induction of hypersensitivity to the host's own tissues, producing autoimmune arthritis, amyloidosis, anterior uveitis; cross-reactions with human antigens, such as glomerular basement membranes or neurolemma, causing glomerulonephritis or meningoencephalomyelitis; sensitization to tuberculin or to other skin test antigens; carcinogenesis; pyogenesis; teratogenesis; abortogenesis; induction of adverse pharmacological effects, such as hypoglycemia.

Reports on side effects caused by vaccines containing aluminium hydroxide (368[c]—370[C]), thimerosal (371[C], 372[C]) have been provided in the Annuals and in the vaccine-specific sections above.

Various vaccines and immunobiologicals

Reports on safety of experimental vaccines have been provided in the Annuals, e.g. *Corynebacterium parvus vaccine*, *Mycobacterium leprae vaccine*, and *Lactobacillus acidophilus vaccine* (against trichomoniasis) (SEDA-12, 286), and *malaria vaccine* (SEDA-14, 290). Case reports on side effects following the administration of *allergen extracts*, *honeybee venom*, *and biological response modifiers* (*e.g. Mycobacterium phlei vaccine*, *mixed bacterial vaccines*) have also been published in the Annuals (SEDA-13, 290; SEDA-14, 290).

REFERENCES

1. Adverse vaccine reactions workshop, cosponsored by WHO and Health and Welfare, Canada. Report on a meeting, 30—31 October 1991, Ottawa, Canada. WHO Geneva, 1992.
2. Health Council of the Netherlands. Adverse reactions to vaccines used in the national vaccination programme in 1989. Report, Gezondheidsraad, The Hague, 1991.
3. Institute of Medicine. Adverse effects of pertussis and rubella vaccines. National Academy Press: Washington, DC, 1991.
4. Centers for Disease Control, Atlanta, US. Vaccine Adverse Event Reporting System—United States. Morbid Mortal Wkly Rep 1990;39:730.
5. Bureau of Communicable Disease Epidemiology, Ottawa, Canada. Adverse events temporally associated with immunizing agents—1989 report. Can Dis Wkly Rep 1991; 17—29.
6. Dukes MNG, Swartz B. Responsibility for Drug-induced Injury. Amsterdam: Elsevier, 1988.
7. Galazka AM, Lauer BA, Henderson RA et al. Indications and contraindications for vaccines used in the Expanded Programme on Immunization. Bull WHO 1984; 62(3):357.
8. Howson CP, Howe CJ, Fineberg HV, eds. Adverse effects of pertussis and rubella vaccines. A report of the Committee to Review the Adverse Consequences of Pertussis and Rubella Vaccines. National Academy Press: Washington, DC, 1991.
9. Stratton KR, Howe CJ, Johnston RB Jr, eds. Adverse events associated with childhood vaccines. National Academy of Sciences: Washington, DC, 1994.
10. Dittmann S. Risiken von Schutzimpfungen, internationale Erfahrungen bei der Erfassung von Impfschaeden, Erfassung von Impfschaeden in Deutschland. In: Impfreaktionen—Impfkomplikationen (Hrsg. Maass G). Marburg: Kilian, 1995.
11. Grabenstein JD. A miscellany of obscure vaccines: Adenovirus, anthrax, mixed bacteria, and *Staphylococcus*. Hosp Pharm 1993;28:259—266.
12. Skegg DC. BCG vaccination and the incidence of lymphomaand leukemia. J Cancer 1978;21:18.
13. Lilienfeld AM, Pedersen E et al. Cancer epidemiology: methods of study. John Hopkins press: Baltimore, MD., 1967;72.
14. Snider DE, Comstock GW et al. Efficacy of BCG vaccination in prevention of cancer - an update, brief communication. J Nat Cancer Inst 1978;60:785.
15. Kendrick MA, Comstock GW. BCG vaccination and the subsequent developments of cancer in humans. J Nat Cancer Inst 1981;66:431.
16. Ambrosch F, Wiedermann G, Krepler, P. Studies on the influence of BCG vaccination on infantile leukemia. Dev Biol Stand 1986;58:419.
17. Härö AS. The effect of BCG vaccination and tuberculosis on the risk of leukemia. Dev Biol Stand 1986;58:433.
18. Lotte A, Le Vésinet O, Wasz-Höckert N et al. Estimates of the risks among vaccinated subjects and statistical analysis of their main characteristics. Adv Tuberc Res 1984;21:107.
19. Lotte A, Vésinet O, Wasz-Höckert N et al. A comprehensive list of the world literature since the introduction of BCG up to July 1982, supplemented by over 100 personal communications. Adv Tuberc Res 1984;21:194.
20. Lotte A, Wasz-Höckert O, Poisson N et al. Second IUATLD study on complications induced by intradermal BCG vaccination. Bull Int Union Tuberc Lung Dis 1988;63:47.
21. Gonzalez B, Morena S, Burdach R et al. Clinical presentation of BCG infections in patients with immunodeficiency syndromes. Pediatr Infect Dis J 1989;8:201.
22. Minegishi M, Tsuchiya S, Imaizuma M et al. Successful transplantation of soy bean agglutinin-fractionated, histoincompatible, maternal marrow in a patient with severe combined immunodeficiency and BCG infection. Eur J Pediatr 1985;143:291.
23. Lin CY, Hsu HC, Hsieh HC. Treatment of progressive BCG infection in an immunodeficient infant with a specific bovine thymic extract. Pediatr Infect Dis 1985;4:402.
24. Hódságy M, Uhereczky G, Király L et al. BCG dissemination in chronic granulomatous disease (CGD). Dev Biol Stand 1986;58:339.
25. Kobayashi Y, Komazawa Y, Kobayashi M. Presumed BCG infection in a boy with chronic granulomatous disease. Clin Pediatr 1984;23:586.
26. Smith PA, Wittenberg DF. Disseminated BCG infection in a child with chronic granulomatous disease. S Afr Med J 1984;65:821.
27. Trevenen CL, Pagtakhan RD. Disseminated tuberculoid lesions in infants following BCG vaccination. Can Med Assoc J 1982;127:502.
28. Baum WF, Wessel H, Exadaktylos P et al. Die BCG-Histiocytose —eine Form der generalisierten BCG-Infektion. Dtsch Gesundheitswes 1983;37:1384.
29. Künzel W, Frey G, Günther J et al. Geheilte BCG-Histiocytose bei isolierter temporärer Störung der T-Lymphocytenfunktion. Dtsch Gesundheitswes 1982;37:1384.
30. Erdös Z, Szabo I. Recovered case of BCG sepsis. Dev Biol Stand 1986;58:319.
31. Ehrengut W. BCG-itis während der Kindheit und in der Schwangerschaft. Zugleich ein Beitrag zu einer BCG-bedingten nekrotisierenden zerebralen Arteriitis. Klin Pädiatr 1990;202:303—307.
32. Heydermann RS, Morgan G, Levinsky RJ, Strobel S. Successful bone marrow transplantation and treatment of BCG infection in two patients with severe combined immunodeficiency. Eur J Pediatr 1991;150:477—480.
33. Boettiger M. Osteitis and other complications caused by generalized BCGitis. Acta Pediatr Scand 1982;71:471.
34. Boman G, Sjögren I, Dahlström G. A follow-up study of BCG-induced osteo-articular lesions in children. Bull Int Union Tuberc 1984;59:198.
35. Peltola H, Salmi I, Vahvanen V et al. BCG vaccination as a cause of osteomyelitis and subcutaneous abscesses. Arch Dis Child 1984;59:157.
36. Marik I, Kubat R, Slosarek M. BCG osteomyelitis et gonitis u batolete. Acta Chir Orthop Traum Czech 1984; 51:495.
37. Krepela K, Galliova J, Sejdova E et al. Osseous complications after BCG vaccination. Cs Pediatr 1985;40:263.
38. Krepela K, Galliová J, Kubec V, Marik J. Influence of a reduced dose of BCG vaccine on the incidence of osseous complication after BCG immunization (in Czech). Cs Pediat 1992;47:134—136.
39. Hanimann B, Morger R, Baerlocher K et al. BCG-Osteitis in der Schweiz. Schweiz Med Wochenschr 1987;117:193.

40. Aftimos S, Nicol R. BCG osteitis: a case report. NZ Med J 1986;99:271.
41. Kolandaivélu G, Manohar K, Bose JC et al. Osteitis of humerus following BCG vaccination. J Indian Med Assoc 1986;84:184.
42. Geissler W, Pumberger W, Wurnig P, Stuhr O. BCG osteomyelitis as a rare cause of mediastinal tumor in a one-year-old child. Eur J Pediatr Surg 1992;2:118—121.
43. Milstien JB, Gibson JJ. Quality control of BCG vacci-neby WHO: a review of factors that may influence vaccine effectiveness and safety. Bull WHO 1990;68:93.
44. Easton PA, Hershfield ES. Lymphadenitis as a late complication of BCG vaccination. Tubercle 1984;65:205.
45. Tshabalala. Anaphylactic reactions to BCG in Swaziland (Letter to the Editor). Lancet 1983;ii:653.
46. Tardieu M, Truffot-Pernot C, Carriere JP. Tuberculous meningitis due to BCG in two previously healthy children. Lancet 1988;i:440.
47. Morrison WL, Webb WJS, Aldred J. Meningitis after BCG vaccination. Lancet 1988;i:654.
48. Kanwar AJ, Kaur S, Bansal R et al. Lupus vulgaris following BCG vaccination. Int J Dermatol 1988;27:525.
49. Radeff B, Harms M. Acute febrile neutrophilic dermatosis (Sweet's syndrome) following BCG vaccination. Acta Dermatol-Venereol 1986;66:357.
50. Katznelson D, Gross S et al. Polyneuritis following BCG revaccination. Postgrad Med J 1982;58:496.
51. Molz, G, Hartmann HP, Griesser HR. Generalisierte BCG-Infektion bei einem 7 Wochen alten, plötzlich gestorbenen Säugling. Pathologica 1986;7:216.
52. May-Yung Yen, Jorn-Hom Liu. Bilateral optic neuritis following BCG vaccination. J Clin Neuro-Ophthalmol 1991; 11:246—249.
53. Simma B, Dietze O, Vogel W, Ellemunter H, Guggenbichler JP. Bacille Calmette-Guérin-associated neonatal hepatitis. Eur J Pediatr 1991;150:423—424.
54. Sadeghi E, Kumar PV. Eczema vaccinatum and postvaccinal BCG adenitis—case report. Tubercle 1990;71:145—146.
55. Wolff M, Dopfer R, Hassberg D, Niethammer D. Mediastinal tumor following vaccination against tuberculosis. Monatsschr Kinderheilkd 1993;141:409—411.
56. Power JT, Stewart JC, Ross JD. Erythromycin in the management of troublesome BCG lesions. Br J Dis Chest 1984;78:192.
57. Singh G, Singh M. Erythromycin for BCG cold abscess (Letter to the Editor). Lancet 1984;ii:979.
58. Akenzua GI, Sykes RM. Management of suppurative regional lymphadenitis complicating BCG vaccination in newborns. Niger J Pediatr 1986;13:65.
59. Caglayan S, Yegin O, Kayran N et al. Is medical therapy effective for regional lymphadenitis following BCG vaccination? Am J Dis Child 1987;141:1213.
60. Immunizations Practices Advisory Committee (ACIP). Recommendations on BCG vaccines. Morbid Mortal Wkly Rep 1979;28:241.
61. Global Advisory Group of the Expanded Programme on Immunization (EPI). Report on the meeting 13—17 October, 1986, New Delhi. Unedited document, WHO/EPI/Geneva/87/1, 1986.
62. Pinsky CM, Camacho FJ, Kerr D et al. Intravesical administration of BCG in patients with recurrent superficial carcinoma of the urinary bladder. Cancer Treat Rep 1985; 69:47.
63. Sawamura M, Kan-ei Lee, Kadowaki K. Experience with intravesical BCG therapy for prophylaxis of superficial cancer. Acta Urol Jpn 1985;39:125.
64. Schellhammer PF, Ladaga LE, Fillion MB. BCG for superficial transitional cell carcinoma of the bladder. J Urol 1986;135:261.
65. Droller M. BCG in the management of bladder cancer J Urol 1986;135:331.
66. Herr HW, Pinsky CM, Whitmore WF et al. Longterm effect of intravesical BCG on flat carcinoma in situ of the bladder. J Urol 1986;135:265.
67. von der Meijden APM, Steerenberg PA, de Jong WH, Debruyne FMJ. Intravesical BCG treatment for superficial bladder cancer: results after 15 years of experience. Anticancer Res 1991;11:1253—1258.
68. Kanarek A. BCG Therapeutic-treatment of urinary bladder cancer in situ. Cont Pract 1991;18:15—20.
69. Herr HW. Use of BCG vaccine. Probl Urol 1992;6:484—492.
70. Al Amin Al Khalifa M, Elfving P, Manson W, Colleen S. BCG treatment of 39 patients with superficial transitional cell carcinoma of the bladder. Scand. J Urol Nephrol 1990;25:135—139.
71. Farina LA, Laguna P, Palou J, Algaba F, Santaularia J, Vicente J. Adenoma nefrogénico en el curso del tratamiento con BCG intravesical. Arch Esp Urol 1992;45,2:153—154.
72. Modesto A, Marty L, Suc JM, Kleinknecht D, Frémont JF, Marsepoil T, Veyssier P. Renal complications of intravesical BCG therapy. Am J Nephrol 1991;11:501—504.
73. de Boisgisson Ph, Roussel F, Leclerc D, Picquenot JM. Granulomatous renal mass during endovesical BCG therapy for bladder carcinoma. Urology 1991;37:557—560.
74. Armstrong RW. Complications after intravesical instillation of BCG: rhabdomyolysis and metastatic infection. J Urol 1991;145:1264—1266.
75. Katz DS, Wogalter H, D'Esposito RF, Cunha BA. *Mycobacterium bovis* vertebral osteomyelitis and psoas abscess after intravesical BCG therapy for bladder carcinoma. Urology 1992;40:63—66.
76. Baba Y, Ishizu K, Jojima K, Joko K, Nakamura K, Takihara H, Naiti K. Multiorgan failure following intravesical BCG administration—a case report (Japanese). Acta Urol Jpn 1992;38:1063—1065.
77. Mcparland C, Cotton DJ, Gowda KS, Hoeppner VH, Martin WT, Weckworth PF. Miliary *Mycobacterium bovis* induced by intravesical BCG immunotherapy. Am Rev Respir Dis 1992;146:1330—1333.
78. Graziano DA, Jacobs D, Lozano RG, Buck RL. A case of granulomatous hepatitis after intravesical BCG administration. J Urol 1991;146:1118—1119.
79. de Gennes C, Hanslik T, Lugagne P, Sauvaget F, Le Thi Huong Du, Chatelain C, Godeau P. Polyarthrite lors d'un traitement par BCG intra-vésical: arthrie réactionelle à *Mycobacterium bovis*? Bull SNFMI 1991;12:151.
80. Truelson T, Wishnow KI, Johnson DE. Epididymo-orchitis developing as a late manifestation of intravesical BCG therapy and masquerading as a primary testicular malignancy: a report of 2 cases. J Urol 1992;148:1534—1535.
81. Miyashita H, Troncoso P, Babaian RJ. BCG-induced granulomatous prostatitis: a comparative ultrasound and pathologic study. Urology 1992;39:364—367.
82. Choi HR, Hong CK, Ro BI. A case of widespread skin tuberculosis following BCG vaccination. Ann Dermatol 1992;4:124—127.

83. Steg A, Leleu C, Debré B et al. Systemic BCG infection, 'BCGitis', in patients treated by intravesical BCG therapy for bladder cancer. Eur Urol 1989;16:161.
84. Deresiewicz RL, Stone RM, Aster JC. Fatal disseminated mycobacterial infection following intravesical BCG. J Urol 1990;144:1331–1333.
85. Rawls WH, Lamm DL, Lowe BA, Crawford ED, Sarosdy MF, Montie JE, Grossman HB, Scardino PT. Fatal sepsis following intravesical BCG administration for bladder cancer. J Urol 1990;144:1328–1330.
86. Sakamoto GD, Burden J, Fisher D. Systemic BCG infection after transurethral administration for superficial bladder carcinoma. J Urol 1989;142:1073–1075.
87. Corti-Ortiz C, Garay PR, Jasse JA, Carmona FH, MacMillan Soto G, Coc Canas LF, Delaunoy RV, de San Pedro RSS. Profilaxis del cancer vesical superficial con 1 mg de BCG endovesical: Comparacion con otras dosis. Actas Urol Esp 1993;17:239–242.
88. Rivera P, Caffarena E, Cornejo H, del Pino M, Foneron A, Haemmersli J, Sepulveda M, Ubilla A. BCG vaccine minidosesas prophylaxis for vesical cancer in stage T1. Actas Urol Esp 1993;17:243–246.
89. Lo Cigno M, Emili E, Iraci F, Soli M, Bercovich E, Rusconi R. Confronto tra BCG Berna e Pasteur F nella profilassi delle recidive neoplastiche superficiali della vescica. Acta Urol Ital 1991;6(Suppl 1):145–148.
90. Guinan P, Brosman S, Dekernion J et al. Intravesical BCG and second primary malignancies. Urology 1989;33:380.
91. Khanna OP. Intravesical BCG and second primary malignancies (Letter). Urology 1989;34:113.
92. Crispen RG. BCG and cancer. Dev Biol Stand 1986; 58:371.
93. Schult C. Nebenwirkungen der BCG-Immunotherapie bei 511 Patienten mit malignem Melanom. Hautarzt 1984;35:78.
94. Grigorovich NA, Risina DI, Nodel'son SE. Treatment of the complications occurring in BCG vaccine immunotherapy of patients with malignant neoplasma (in Russian). Vopr Onkol 1984;30:102.
95. Hoover HC, Surdyke MG, Dangel RB et al. Prospectivelyrandomized trial of adjuvant active-specific immunotherapy for human colorectal cancer. Cancer 1985;55:1236.
96. Shea CR, Imber MJ, Cropley TG. Granulomatous eruption after BCG vaccine immunotherapy for malignant melanoma. J Am Acad Dermatol 1989;21:1119.
97. Torisu M, Iwasaki K, Sakata M. Immunotherapy of cancer patients with BCG: summary of ten years experience in Japan. Dev Biol Stand 1986;58:451.
98. The Ludwig Lung Cancer Study Group (LLCSG). Immunostimulation with intrapleural BCG as adjuvant therapy in resected non-small cell lung cancer. Cancer 1986;58:2411.
99. Holmgren J, Svennerholm AM. New vaccines against bacterial enteric infections. Scand. J Infect Dis Suppl 1990;70:149–156.
100. Markman B. Symptoms of reactogenicity in field trial of oral cholera vaccine (Letter to the Editor). Lancet 1990;ii:320.
101. Cryz SJ, Levine MM, Kaper JB, Fürer E, Althaus B. Randomized double-blind placebo-controlled trial to evaluate the safety and immunogenicity of the live oral cholera vaccine strain CVD 103-HgR in Swiss adults. Vaccine 1990;8:577–580.
102. Gavrilesco CS, Constatinesco L. Tachycardie ventriculaire et fibrillation auriculaire associées après vaccination anticholériques. Acta Cardiol 1973;28:89.
103. Driehorst J, Laubenthal L. Akute Myocarditis nach Choleraschutzimpfung. Dtsch Med Wochenschr 1984; 109:197.
104. Mall T, Gyr K. Episode resembling immune complex disease after cholera vaccination. Trans R Soc Trop Med Hyg 1984;78:106.
105. Eisinger AJ, Smith JG. Acute renal failure after TAB and cholera vaccination. Br Med J 1979;1:381.
106. Gatt DT. Pancreatitis following monovalent typhoid and cholera vaccination. Br J Clin Pract 1986;40:300.
107. Van Ramshorst JD, Ehrengut W. Die Diphtherieschutzimpfung. In: Herrlich A, ed. Handbuch der Schutzimpfungen. Springer: Berlin, 1965;394.
108. Ehrengut W. Neurale Komplikationen nach Diphtherieschutzimpfung und Impfungen mit Diphtherietoxoid-Mischimpfstoffen. Dtsch Med Wochenschr 1986;111:939.
109. Onisawa S, Sekine I, Ichimura T et al. Guillain-Barré syndrome secondary to immunization with diphtheria toxoid. Dokkyo J Med Sci 1985;12:227.
110. Holliday PL, Bauer RB. Polyradiculoneuritis secondary to immunization with tetanus and diphtheria toxoids. Arch Neurol 1983;40:56.
111. Immunization Practices Advisory Committee (ACIP). Recommendations on diphtheria, tetanus, and pertussis: guidelines for vaccine prophylaxis and other preventive measures. Morbid Mortal Wkly Rep 1981;30:392.
112. Hurwitz ES, Holman RC, Nelson DB et al. National surveillance for Guillain-Barré syndrome: January 1978–March 1979. Neurology 1983;33:150.
113. Griffith RD, Miller OF. Erythema multiforme following diphtheria and tetanus toxoid vaccination. J Acad Dermatol 1988;19:758.
114. Wstepne D. Prophylactic vaccinations and seizure activity in EEG. Neurol Neurochir Pol 1981;5:553.
115. Greco D. Case-control study on encephalopathy associated with diphtheria-tetanus immunization in Campagna, Italy. WHO Bull 1985;63:919.
116. Weinberg GA, Granoff DM. Polysaccharide-protein conjugate vaccines for the prevention of *Haemophilus influenzae* type b disease. J Pediatr 1988;113:621.
117. D'Cruz OF, Shapiro ED, Spiegelman KN et al. Acute inflammatory demyelinating polyradiculoneuropathy (Guillain-Barré syndrome) after immunization with *Haemophilus influenzae* type b conjugate vaccine. J Pediatr 1989;115:743.
118. Gervaix A, Caflisch M, Suter S, Haenggeli CA. Guillain-Barré syndrome following immunisation Hib type b conjugate vaccine. Eur J Pediatr 1993;152:613–614.
119. Jakacki R, Luery N, McVerry P. *Haemophilus*-diphtheria protein conjugate immunization after therapy in splenectomized patients with Hodgkin disease. Ann Intern Med 1990;112:143.
120. Hughes PJ, Saadeh IK, Cox JPDT, Illis LS. Probable post-hepatitis A vaccination encephalopathy. Lancet 1993;342:302.
121. Francis DP, Feorino PM, McDougal S et al. The safety of the hepatitis B vaccine. J Am Med Assoc 1986;256:869.
122. Quast U, Freiburg K. Zur Verträglichkeit gentechnisch hergestellter Impfstoffe. Die gelben Hefte. Immunbiol Inform 28/1, 41, 1988
123. Shaw FE, Graham DJ, Guess HA et al. Postmarketing surveillance for neurologic adverse events reported after hepatitis B vaccination. Experience of the first three years. Am J Epidemiol 1988;127:337.

124. Safary A, André F. Clinical development of a new recombinant DNA hepatitis B vaccine. Postgrad Med J 1987;63(Suppl 2):105.
125. Wiedermann G, Ambrosch F, Kremsner P et al. Reactogenicity and immunogenicity of different lots of a yeast-derived hepatitis vaccine. Postgrad Med J 1987;63(Suppl 2):109.
126. Wahl M, Hermodsohn. Intradermal, subcutaneous or intramuscular administration of hepatitis B vaccine: side effects and antibody response. Scand J Infect Dis 1987;19:617.
127. Jilg W, Schmidt M, Deinhardt F. Immune response to hepatitis B revaccination. Med Virol 1988;24:377.
128. Hilleman MR. Yeast recombinant hepatitis B vaccine. Infection 1987;15:3.
129. Jilg W, Schmidt M, Weinel B et al. Immunogenicity of recombinant hepatitis B vaccine in dialysis patients. J Hepatol 1986;3:190.
130. Herroelen L, de Keyser J, Ebinger G. Central-nervous-system demyelination after immunization with recombinant hepatitis B vaccine. Lancet 1991;338:1174–1175.
131. Personal communication.
132. Mahassin F, Algayres JP, Valmary J, Bili H. Acutemyelitis following hepatitis B vaccination. Presse Med 1993; 22:1997–1998.
133. Trevisani F, Gattinara GC, Caraceni P. Transverse myelitis following hepatitis B vaccination. J Hepatol 1993;19:317–318.
134. Brezin AP, Lautier-Frau M, Hamedani M. Visual loss and eosinophilia after recombinant hepatitis B vaccine. Lancet 1993;342:563–564.
135. Tuohy PG. Guillain-Barré syndrome following immunization with synthetic hepatis B vaccine. NZ Med J 1989; 102:114.
136. Carmeli Y, Oren R. Hepatitis B vaccine side effect. Lancet 1993;341:250–251.
137. Hartman S. Convulsion associated with fever following hepatitis B vaccination (Letter to the Editor). J Pediatr Child Health 1990;26:65.
138. Trevisan G, Stinco G. HBV vaccination and lichen planus. G Ital Dermatol Venereol 1993;128:545–548.
139. Reutens DC, Dunne JW, Leather H. Neuralgic amyotrophy following recombinant DNA hepatitis B vaccination. Muscle Nerve 1990;13:461.
140. Biasi D, De Sandre G, Bambara LM, Carletto A. A new case of reactive arthritis after hepatitis B vaccination. Clin Exp Rheumatol 1993;11:215.
141. Tudela P, Marti S, Bonal J. Systemic lupus erythematosus and vaccination against hepatitis B (Letter to the Editor). Nephron 1992;62:236.
142. Hudson TJ, Newkirk M, Gervais F, Shuster J. Adverse reaction to the recombinant hepatitis B vaccine. J Allergy Clin Immunol 1991;88:821–822.
143. Rogerson SJ, Nye FJ. Hepatitis B vaccine associated with erythema nodosum and polyarthritis. Br Med J 1990;301:345.
144. Levy M, Koren G. Hepatitis B vaccine in pregnancy: maternal and fetal safety. Am J Perinatol 1991;8:227–232.
145. Anonymous. Alleged link between hepatitis b vaccine and chronic fatigue syndrome. Can Med Assoc J 1992; 146:37–38.
146. Giammanco G, Li Volti S, Mauro L, Giammanco Bilancia G, Salemii, Barone P, Musumeci S. Immune response to simultaneous administration of a recombinant DNA hepatitis b vaccine and multiple compulsory vaccines in infancy. Vaccine 1991;9:747–750.
147. Torres JM, Bruguera M, Vidal J, Artigas N. Immune response, efficacy and reactogenicity of hepatitis B vaccine administered simultaneously with DTP and poliomyelitis vaccine. Gastroenterol Hepatol 1993;16:470–473.
148. Rietschel RL, Adams RM. Reactions to thimerosal in hepatitis B vaccines. Dermatol Clin 1990;8:161–164.
149. Jungkunz G, Köhler P, Holbach M, Schweisfurth H. Kasuistik: Zwei Fälle mit heftiger lokaler Reaktion nach aktiver Hepatitis-B-Impfung bei Sensibilisierung auf Thiomersal. Hyg Med 1990;15:418–420.
150. Kirkland LR. Ocular sensitivity to thimerosal: A problem with hepatitis vaccine? South Med J 1990;83:497–499.
151. Cosnes A, Flechet ML, Revuz J. Inflammatory nodular reactions after hepatitis b vaccination due to aluminium sensitization. Contact Dermatitis 1990;23:65–67.
152. Hütteroth TH, Quast U. Aluminiumhydroxid-Granulome nach Hepatitis-B-Impfung (Fragen aus der Praxis). Dtsch Med Wochenschr 1990;115:476.
153. Dorozinsky A, Anderson A. Deaths in vaccine trials trigger French inquiry. Science 1991;252:501.
154. Guillaume JC, Saiag P, Wechsler J et al. Vaccinia from recombinant virus expressing HIV genes (Letter). Lancet 1991;i:1034.
155. Midthun K, Garrison L, Gershman K et al. Cellular immunity in HIV-1 rgp 160 vaccinees. In: Abstracts, V International Conference on AIDS, Montreal, 1989;544.
156. Francois A, Ninane J, Burtonboy G et al. Disseminated *Mycobacterium bovis* infection following BCG immunization in an HIV-infected infant. In: Abstracts, IV International Conference on AIDS, Stockholm, Sweden, 12–16 June, 1988.
157. Vetter N. Personal communication, 1989.
158. Clements CJ, Von Reyn CF, Mann JM. HIV infection and routine childhood immunization: a review. Bull WHO 1987;65/6:905.
159. Besnard M, Sauvion S, Offredo C, Gaudelus J, Gaillard JL, Veber F, Blanche S. BCG infection after vaccination of HIV-infected children. Pediatr Infect Dis J 1993;12:993–997.
160. Von Reyn CF, Clements CJ, Mann JM. Human immunodeficiency virus infection and routine childhood immunization. Lancet 1987;ii:669.
161. Reynes J, Perez C, Lamaury I et al. BCG adenitis 30 years after immunization in a patient with AIDS. J Infect Dis 1989;160:727.
162. Mvula M, Ryder R, Manzila T et al. Response to childhood vaccination in African children with HIV infection. In: Abstracts, IV International Conference on AIDS, Stockholm, Sweden, 12–16 June, 1988.
163. Embree J, Datta P, Braddick M et al. Vaccinations of infants of HIV-seropositive mothers. In: Abstracts, IV International Conference on AIDS, Stockholm, Sweden, 12–16 June, 1988.
164. La Force FM. Immunization of children infected with human immunodeficiency virus. WHO/EPI/GEN/86.6 Rev 1, Geneva, 1986.
165. Immunizations Practices Advisory Committee (ACIP). Recommendations on immunization of children infected with Human T-lymphotropic virus type III/lymphadenopathy-associated virus. Morbid Mortal Wkly Rep 1986;35:595.
166. McLaughlin M, Thomas P, Onorato I et al. Live virus vaccines in human immunodeficiency virus-infected children: a retrospective survey. Pediatrics 1988;82:229.
167. Gutfreund K, heatham-Speth D, Rossol S et al. The

effect of vaccination against hepatitis B on the CD4+ cell account in anti-HIV positive man. In: Abstracts, V International Conference on AIDS, Montreal, 1989;435.
168. Buchbinder SP, Hessol N, Lifson A et al. The interaction of HIV and hepatitis B vaccination in a cohort of homosexual and bisexual men. In: Abstracts, V International Conference on AIDS, Montreal, 1989;259.
169. Expanded Programme on Immunization. Immunization policy. WHO/EPI/GEN/86.7 Rev 1, Geneva, 1986.
170. Expanded Programme on Immunization. Joint WHO/UNICEF statement on immunization and AIDS. Wkly Epidemiol Rec 1987;62(9):53.
171. Committee on Immunization. Guide for adult immunization. Philadelphia: American College of Physicians, 1985; 58.
172. Immunization Practices Advisory Committee (ACIP). Recommendations on prevention and control of influenza. Morbid Mortal Wkly Rep 1987;36(24):373.
173. Stefanini M, Pionelli S, Mell R et al. Acute vascular purpura following immunization with Asiatic vaccine. N Engl J Med 1958;259:9.
174. Yar MD, Antunes JL. Relapsing encephalomyelitis following the use of influenza vaccine. Arch Neurol (Chicago) 1972;27:182.
175. Anonymous. Influenza prevention for 1985/86. Med Lett Drugs Ther 1986;27:81.
176. Retailliau HF, Curtis AC, Storr G et al. Illness after influenza vaccination reported through a nationwide surveillance system, 1976—1977. Am J Epidemiol 1980;11:270.
177. Langmuir AD, Bregman DJ, Kurland LT et al. An epidemiologic and clinical evaluation of Guillain-Barré syndrome reported in association with the administration of swine influenza vaccines. Am Epidemiol 1984;119:841.
178. Feschank R, Künzel U, Quast U. Das Guillain-Barré syndrome—eine Impfkomplikation? Z Allg Med 1986;62:71.
179. Safranek TJ, Lawrence DN, Kurland LT, Culver DH, Wiederholt WC, Hayner NS, Osterholm MT, O'Brien P, Hughes JM, and the Expert Neurology Group. Reassessment of the association between Guillain Barré syndrome and receipt of swine influenza vaccine in 1976—1977: Results of a two-state study. Am J Epidemiol 1991;133:940—951.
180. Roscelli JD, Bass JW, Pang L. Guillain Barré syndrome and influenza vaccination in the U.S. Army, 1980—1988. Am J Epidemiol 1991;133:952—955.
181. Kurland LT, Molgaard CA, Kurland EM et al. Swine flu vaccine and multiple sclerosis. J Am Med Assoc 1984; 251:2672.
182. Nagano T, Mizuguchi M, Kurihara E et al. A case of acute disseminated encephalomyelitis with convulsion, gait disturbance, facial palsy and with multifocal CT lesions. No To Hattatsu 1988;20:325.
183. Casoli P, Tumiati B. Porpora trombocitopenica idiopatica acuta dopo vaccinacione antinfluenzale. Medicina 1989; 9:417—418.
184. Ichikawa N, Takase S, Kogure K. Recurrent aseptic meningitis after influenza vaccination in a case with systemic lupus erythematosus. Clin Neurol 1983;23:570.
185. Morimoto T, Oguni H, Awaya Y. A case of rapidly progressive central nervous system disorder manifesting as a pallidal posture and ocular motor apraxia. Brain Dev 1985;7:449.
186. Beijer WEP, Sprenger MJW, Masurel N. Polymyalgia rheumatica and influenza vaccination. Dtsch Med Wochenschr 1993;118:164—165.
187. Mader R, Narendran A, Lewtas J, Bykerk V, Goodman RCJ, Dickson JR, Keystone EC. Systemic vasculitis following influenza vaccination—Report of 3 cases and literature review. J Rheumatol 1993;20:1429—1431.
188. Demmler M, Heidel G. Trigeminus-Affektion nach Influenza-Schutzimpfung. Psychiatr Neurol Med Psychol 1985; 37:428.
189. Vidal E, Gaches F, Berdah JF, Nadalon S, Lavignac C, Mitrea L, Loustaud-Ratti V, Liozon F. Vasculitis after influenza vaccination. Rev Med Intern 1993;14:1173.
190. Kobashigawa JA, Warner-Stevenson L. Influenza vaccine does not cause rejections after cardiac transplantation. Transplant Proc 1993;25:2738—2739.
191. Kramer P, McClain CJ. Depression of aminopyrine metabolism by influenza vaccination. N Engl J Med 1981;21: 1262.
192. Meredith CG, Christian CD, Johnson RF et al. Effects of influenza virus vaccine on hepatic drug metabolism. Clin Pharmacol Ther 1985;37:396.
193. Gomolin JH, Chapron DJ, Luhan PA. Lack of effect of influenza vaccine on theophylline levels and warfarin anticoagulation in the elderly. J Am Geriatr Soc 1985;33:269.
194. Grabowski N, May JJ, Pratt DS. The effect of split virus influenza vaccination on theophylline pharmacokinetics. J Am Rev Resp Dis 1985;131:934.
195. Jann MW, Fidone GS. Effect of influenza vaccine on serum anti-convulsant concentrations. Clin Pharm 1986;5: 817.
196. Gerth HG. Grippeschutzimpfung. Dtsch Med Wochenschr 1989;114:180.
197. Ducluceau R. Les accidents de la sérothérapie antitétanique. Bull Méd Lég Toxicol Méd 1971;14:26.
198. Charpin J, Louchet E, Gratecos LA. Subsiste-t-il encore des réactions allergiques de la sérothérapie? Marseille Méd 1969;106:223.
199. Bianchi R et al. Der anaphylaktische Schock des Menschen auf artfremdes Serum. Helv Chir Acta 1967; 34:257.
200. World Health Organization. The collection, fractionation, quality control, and uses of blood and blood products. Geneva: WHO, 1981.
201. Delwalde PJ et al. Deux cas de neuropathies multiples d'origine sérothérapique avec paralysie phrénique. Acta Neurol Belg 1967;67:452.
202. Czirner J, Besnyak G. Myokardinfarkt-ähnliches Bild als seltene Komplikation nach Applikation von Tetanus-Antitoxin. Z Gesamte Inn Med Grenzgeb 1969;24:119.
203. Humphrey JH, White RG, eds. Reactions due to antigen-antibody complexes (nephritis in man). In: Immunology for Students of Medicine, 3rd edn. Oxford: Blackwell Scientific Publications, 1970;458.
204. Suarez-Lopez J, Sanchez-Salorio M, Sanchez-Lado J. Uveitis exudativa de caracter sero-anafiláctico. Arch Soc Oftalmol Hisp-Am 1965;25:499.
205. Wilde H, Chomchey P, Prakongsri S et al. Adverse effect of equine rabies immune globulin. Vaccine 1989;7:10.
206. Seiffert J, Brendel W, Lob G et al. Improvement of the compatibility of ALG. Behring Inst Mitt 1972;51:255.
207. Doney KC, Weiden PL et al. Treatment of graft-versus-host disease in human allogenic marrow graft recipients: a randomized trial comparing antithymocyte globulin and corticosteroids. Am J Hematol 1981;11:1.
208. Kheirbek AO, Molnar ZV et al. Malignant lymphoma in a renal transplant recipient treated with antithymocyte globulin. Transplantation 1982;35:267.

209. Gronski P, Seiler FR, Schwick HG. Discovery of antitoxins and development of antibody preparations for clinical uses from 1890 to 1990. Mol Immunol 1991;28:1321–1332.
210. Pirofsky B, Kinzey DM. Intravenous immune globulins. Drugs 1992;43:6–14.
211. Bunnag C, Dhorranintra B, Jareoncharsri P. Effect of alleglobuline injection on serum immunoglobulin levels in ENT patients. Asian Pacific J Allergy Immunol 1991;9:45–50.
212. Oya A. Japanese encephalitis vaccine. Acta Pediatr Jpn 1988;30:175.
213. Ohtaki E, Murakami Y, Komori H, Yamashita Y, Matsuishi T. Acute disseminated encephalomyelitis after Japanese encephalitis vaccination. Pediatr Neurol 1992;8:137–139.
214. Advisory Committee on Immunization Practices (ACIP). Recommendations on Japanese Encephalitis Vaccine. Morbid Mortal Weekly Rep 1993;42(No.RR-1).
215. Amador R, Moreno A, Valero V, Murillo L, Mora AL, Rojas M, Rocha C, Salcedo M, Guzman F, Espejo F, Nunes F, Patarroyo ME. The first field trials of the chemically synthesized malaria vaccine SPf66: safety, immunogenicity and protectivity. Vaccine 1992;10:179–184.
216. Patarroyo G, Franco L, Amador R, Murillo LA, Rocha CL, Rojas M, Patarroyo ME. Study of the safety and immunogenicity of the synthetic malaria SPf66 vaccine in children aged 1–14 years. Vaccine 1992;10:175–178.
217. Immunization Practices Advisory Committee (ACIP). Recommendations on measles prevention. Morbid Mortal Wkly Rep 1982;31:217.
218. Isomura S. Measles and measles vaccine in Japan. Acta Pediatr Jpn 1988;30:154.
219. Landrigan PJ, Witte JJ. Neurologic disorders following live measles-virus vaccination. J Am Med Assoc 1973; 223:1459.
220. Bloch AB, Orenstein WA, Stetler HC. Health impact of measles vaccination in the United States. Pediatrics 1985;76:524.
221. Immunization Practices Advisory Committee. Recommendations on measles prevention. Morbid Mortal Wkly Rep 1987;36:409.
222. Pollock RM, Morris J. A seven-year survey of disorders attributed to vaccination in northwest Thames region. Lancet 1983;i:753.
223. Committee on Infectious Disease. Personal and family history of seizures and measles immunization. Pediatrics 1987;18:741.
224. Hinman AR, Orenstein WA, Bloch AB et al. Impact of measles in the United States. Rev Infect Dis 1983;5:439.
225. Zilber N, Rannon L, Alter M. Measles, measles vaccination and rate of subacute sclerosing panencephalitis (SSPE). Neurology 1983;33:1558.
226. Ueda S. SSPE-epidemiology in Japan and neurovirulence of SSPE virus. Brain Dev 1985;7:122.
227. Okuno Y, Nakao T, Ishida N et al. Incidence of subacute sclerosing panencephalitis following measles and measles vaccination in Japan. Int J Epidemiol 1989;18:684.
228. Gerike E, Dittmann S. Personal communication, 1990.
229. Cernescu C, Milea S. Epidemiology of subacute sclerosing panencephalitis (SSPE) in Romania 1976–1982. Rev Roum Med Ser Virol 1983;34:239.
230. Phadke MA, Joshi BN, Warerkar UV, Diwan MP, Panse GA, Sokhey J, Bhate SM. Toxic shock syndrome: an unforeseen complication following measles vaccination. Indian Pediatr 1991;28:663–665.
231. Milstein J, Dittmann S. Personal communication, 1995.
232. Olivares M, Walter D, Osorio M et al. Anemia of mild viral infection: the measles vaccine as a model. Pediatrics 1989;84:851.
233. Aaby B, Samb B, Simondon F, Whittle H, Coll Seck AM, Knudsen K, Bennett J, Markowitz L, Rhodes P. Child mortality after high-titre measles vaccines in Senegal: the complete data set (Letter to the Editor). Lancet 1991; 338:1518.
234. Garenne M, Leroy O, Beau J-P, Sene I. Child mortality after high-titre measles vaccines: prospective study in Senegal. Lancet 1991;338:903–907.
235. Hülsse C, Steffen W, Von Suchodeletz W. Masernausbruch in einem Heim für zerebral schwerstgeschädigte Patienten. Dtsch Gesundheitswes 1980;35:62.
236. Peltola H, Heinonen OP. True adverse reaction frequencies of MMR vaccine—a double-blind, placebo-controlled, crossover study in twins. Lancet 1986;i:939.
237. O'Brien TC, Maloney CJ, Tauraso NM. Quantitation of residual host protein in chicken empbryo-derived vaccines by radial immunodiffusion. Appl Microbiol 1971;21:780–782.
238. Fasano MB, Wood RA, Cook SK, Sampson HA. Egg hypersensitivity and adverse reactions to MMR vaccine. J Pediatr 1992;120:878–881.
239. Greenberg MA, Birx DL. Safe administration of mumps—measles—rubella vaccine in egg-allergic children. J Pediatr 1988;113:504.
240. Giampetro PG, Bruno G, Grandolfo M, Businco L. Adverse reaction to measles immunization (Letter to the Editor). Eur J Pediatr 1992;152:80.
241. Kelso JM, Jones RT, Yunginger JW. Anaphylaxis to MMR vaccine mediated by IgE to gelatin. J Allergy Clin Immunol 1993;91:867–872.
242. Kwittken PL, Rosen S, Sweinberg SK. MMR vaccine and neomycin allergy. Am J Dis Child 1993;147:128–129.
243. Juntunen-Backman K, Peltola H, Backman A et al. Safe immunization of allergic children against measles, mumps, and rubella. Am J Dis Child 1987;141:1103.
244. Adler JB, Mazzotta SA, Barkin JS. Pancreatitis caused by measles, mumps, and rubella vaccine. Pancreas 1991; 6:489.
245. Committee on Immunization. Guide for adult immunization. Philadelphia: American College of Physicians, 1985; 63.
246. Roberts JStC, Bryett KA. Incidence of reactions to meningococcal A & C vaccine among U.K. schoolchildren. Public Health 1988;102:471.
247. Hood DA, Edwards IR. Meningococcal vaccine—do some children experience side effects? NZ Med J 1989; 102:65.
248. Halvorsen S. The meningococcal serogroup B vaccine protection trial in Norway 1988–1991: trial surveillance by an independent group. Norweg Inst Publ Health Ann 1991;14:135–137.
249. Peltola H, Safary A, Kayhty H. Evaluation of two tetravalent (ACYW135) meningococcal vaccines in infants and small children: a clinical study comparing immunogenicity of *O*-acetyl-negative and *O*-acetyl-positive group C polysaccharides. Pediatrics 1985;76:91.
250. Immunization Practices Advisory Committee. Mumps prevention. Morbid Mortal Wkly Rep 1989;38:388.
251. Fujinaga T, Motegi Y, Tamura H, Kuroume T. A prefecture-wide survey of mumps meningitis associated with MMR vaccine. Pediatr Infect Dis J 1991;10:204–209.

252. Sugiura A, Yamada A. Aseptic meningitis as a complication of mumps vaccination. Pediatr. Infect Dis J 1991;10:209—213.
253. Miller E, Goldacre M, Pugh S, Colville A, Farrington P, Flower A, Nash J, MacFarlane L, Tettmar R. Risk of aseptic meningitis after measles, mumps, and rubella vaccine in UK children. Lancet 1993;341:979—982.
254. Colville A, Pugh S. Mumps meningitis and MMR vaccine (Letter to the Editor). Lancet 1992;340:786.
255. Brown EG, Furesz J, Dimock K, Yarosh W, Contreras G. Nucleotide sequence analysis of Urabe mumps vaccine strain that caused meningitis in vaccine recipients. Vaccine 1991;9:840—842.
256. Forsey T, Bentley ML, Minor N, Begg N. Mumps vaccines and meningitis (Letter to the Editor). Lancet 1992; 340:980.
257. Peltola H. Mumps vaccination and meningitis. Lancet 1993;341:994—995.
257a. Afzal MA. Personal communication, 1996.
258. Teuwen D. Personal communication, 1994.
259. Sawada H, Yano S, Oka Y, Togashi T. Transmission of Urabe mumps vaccine strain between siblings. Lancet 1993;342:371.
260. Tesovic G, Begovac J, Bace A. Aseptic meningitis after MMR vaccine (Letter to the Editor). Lancet 1993;341:1541.
261. Cizman M, Mozetic M, Radescak-Rakar R et al. Aseptic meningitis after vaccination against measles and mumps. Pediatr Infect Dis J 1989;8:302.
262. Fescharek R, Quast U, Maass G, Merkle W, Schwarz S. Measles-mumps vaccination in the FRG: an empirical analysis after 14 years of use. II. Tolerability and analysis of spontaneously reported side effects. Vaccine 1990;8:446—456.
263. Deutsche Vereinigung zur Bekämpfung der Viruskrankheiten (DVV). Mumpsschutzimpfung und Diabetes mellitus (Typ I). Bundesgesundhbl, 1989;237.
264. Baraff LJ, Manclark CR, Cherry JD. Analyses of adverse reactions to diphtheria and tetanus toxoids and pertussis vaccineby vaccine lot, endotoxin content, pertussis vaccine potency and percentage of mouse weight gain. Pediatr Infect Dis J 1989;8:502.
265. Scheifele DW, Meekison W, Arcand T et al. Local adverse reactions to DTP vaccine, adsorbed, in Surrey, BC. Can Med Assoc 1989;141:312.
266. Cody LC, Baraff LJ et al. Nature and rates of adverse reactions associated with DTP and DT immunizations in infants and children. Pediatrics 1981;68:650.
267. Centers for Disease Control. Adverse Events Following Immunization. Surveillance report No. 2, US Department of Health and Human Services, Public Health Service, CDC, Atlanta, GA, 1986.
268. Dittmann S. Atypische Impfverläufe nach Schutzimpfungen. Leipzig: Barth, 1981.
269. Pollock TM, Miller E, Mortimer JR et al. Pertussis immunization and serious acute neurological illness. Br Med J 1981;282:1595.
270. Vulginity V. Sterile abscesses after diphtheria—tetanus toxoids—pertussis vaccination. Pediatr Infect Dis J 1987; 6:497.
271. Salomon ME, Halperin R, Yee J. Evaluation of the two-needle strategy for reducing reactions to DTP vaccination. Am J Child 1987;141:796.
272. Miller DL, Madge N, Diamond J, Wadsworth J, Ross E. Pertussis immunisation and serious acute neurological illness in children. Br Med J 1993;307:1171—1176.
273. Madge N, Diamond J, Miller D, Ross E, McManus C, Wadsworth J, Yule W. The National Childhood Encephalopathy Study: A 19-year follow-up. A report of the medical, social, behavioural and educational outcomes after serious, acute, neurological illness in early childhood. Dev Med Child Neurol 1993;35(Suppl 68):1—118.
274. Institute of Medicine. Stratton KR, Howe CJ, Johnston RB Jr, eds. DPT Vaccine and Chronic Nervous System Dysfunction: A New Analysis. Washington, DC: National Academy Press, 1994.
275. Immunization Practices Advisory Committee (ACIP). Diphtheria, tetanus, pertussis: recommendations for vaccine prophylaxis and other preventive measures. Morbid Mortal Wkly Rep 1985;34:405.
276. Immunization Practices Advisory Committee (ACIP). Recommendations on pertussis immunization; family history of convulsions and use of antipyretics—Supplementary ACIP statement. Morbid Mortal Wkly Rep 1986;36:281.
277. Lewis K, Cherry JD, Sachs MH et al. The effect of prophylactic acetaminophen administration on reactions to DTP vaccination. Am J Dis Child 1988;142:62.
278. Galazka A. Update on acellular Pertussis Vaccine. WHO/EPI/GEN/88.4. Geneva: World Health Organization, 1988.
279. Aoyama T, Hagiwara S, Murase Y et al. Adverse reactions and antibody response to acellular pertussis vaccine. J Pediatr 1986;109:925.
280. Kimura M, Kuno-Sakei H. Pertussis vaccines in Japan. Acta Pediatr Jpn 1988;30:143.
281. Kimura M, Kuno-Sakei H. Reports on cases of neurological illnesses occurring after administration of acellular pertussis vaccines in Japan. Tokai J Exp Clin Med 1988; 13:165.
282. Committee on Immunization. Guide for Adult Immunization. American College of Physicians: Philadelphia, 1985;65.
283. Houston TP. mall-vessel vasculitis following simultaneous influenza and pneumococcal vaccination. NY State J Med 1983;1182.
284. Gabor EP, Seeman M. Acute febrile systemic reaction to polyvalent pneumococcal vaccine. J Am Med Assoc 1979;242:2208.
285. Maddox PR, Motley RJ. Sweet's syndrome: a severe complication of pneumococcal vaccination following emergency splenectomie. Br J Surg 1990;77:809—810.
286. Citron ML. Pneumococcal vaccine-induced thrombocytopenia, 1982. J Am Med Assoc 1982;248:1178.
287. Kelton G. Vaccination-associated relapse of immune thrombocytopenia. J Am Med Assoc 1981;245:369.
288. Bart RS, Lagin S. Keratocanthoma following pneumococcal vaccination. J Dermatol Surg Oncol 1983;9:381.
289. Immunization Practices Advisory Committee. Pneumococcal polysaccharide vaccine. Morbid Mortal Wkly Rep 1989;38:64.
290. Immunization Practices Advisory Committee. Recommendations on pneumococcal polysaccharide vaccine usage. Morbid Mortal Wkly Rep 1984;33:273.
291. Rytel MW, Dailey MP, Schiffman G et al. Pneumococcal vaccine immunization of patients with renal impairment. Proc Soc Exp Biol Med 1986;182:468.
292. Halsey, Spika JS et al. Adverse reactions to pneumococcal polysaccharide vaccine in children. Pediatr Infect Dis 1982;1:34.
293. Sutter R. Personal communication, 1995.

294. Centers for Disease Control. Adverse Events Following Immunization. Surveillance Report No.2, US Department of Health and Human Services, Public Health Service, CDC, Atlanta, GA, 1986.
295. Kinnunen E, Färkkila M, Hovi T. Incidence of Guillain-Barré syndrome during a nation-wide oral poliovirus vaccine campaign. Neurology 1989;39:1034.
296. Cockburn WC. The work of the WHO Consultative Group on Poliomyelitis Vaccine. Bull WHO 1988;66/2:143.
297. Strebel PM, Sutter RW, Cochi SL. Epidemiology of poliomyelitis in the United States. One decade after the last reported case of indigenous wild virus-associated disease. Rev Infect Dis 1992.
298. Evans DMA, Dunn G, Minor PD. Increased neurovirulence associated with a single nucleotide change in a noncoding region of the Sabin type 3 poliovaccine genome. Nature 1985;314:548.
299. Sutter RW, Patriarca PA, Suleiman AJM, Brogan S, Cochi SL, El-Bualy MS. Attributable risk of DTP injection in provoking paralytic poliomyelitis during a large outbreak in Oman. J Infect Dis 1992;165:444—449.
300. Ornoy A, Arnon J, Feingold M, Ben Ishai P. Spontaneous abortions following oral poliovirus vaccination in first trimester. Lancet 1990;i:800.
301. Harjulehto T, Hovi T, Aro T. Congenital malformations and oral poliovirus vaccination during pregnancy. Lancet 1989;ii:440.
302. Burton AE, Robinson ET, Harper WF et al. Fetal damage after accidental polio vaccination of an immune mother. J R Coll Gen Pract 1984;34:390.
303. Anonymous. Wkly Epidemiol Rec 1985;35:269.
304. Cohen J. Possible origins of AIDS. Science 1992; 256:1260—1261.
305. Global Advisory Group of the Expanded Programme on Immunization (EPI). Report on the meeting 13—17 October, 1986, New Delhi. Unedited document, WHO/EPI/Geneva/87/1, 1986.
306. Immunization Practices Advisory Committee (ACIP). Recommendation on immunization of children infected with HIV. Morbid Mortal Wkly Rep 1986;35:595.
307. Immunization Practices Advisory Committee (ACIP). Recommendations on poliomyelitis prevention. Morbid Mortal Wkly Rep 1982;31:22.
308. Department of Health and Social Security. Immunisation against infectious disease. London: Her Majesty's Stationery Office, 1988.
309 Stanislavskiy ES, Balayan SS, Sergienko AI, Makarenko TA, Edvabnaya LS, Krohina MA, Rusanov VM. Clinico-immunological trials of *Pseudomonas aeruginosa* vaccine. Vaccine 1991;9:491—494.
310. WHO. Report of the Second International Symposium on New Developments in Rabies Control, Essen, 5—7 July 1988. WHO/Rab Res/89.31, Geneva, 1988.
311. Committee on Immunization. Guide for Adult Immunization. Philadelphia: American College of Physicians, 1985;72.
312. Anonymous. Rabies vaccine. Med Lett 1991;117—118.
313. Moulignier A, Richer A, Fritzell C, Foulon D, Khoubesserian P, de Recondo J. Méningo-radiculite secondaire à une vaccination antirabique. Press Méd 1991;20:1121—1123.
314. Tornatore CS, Richert JR. CNS demyelination associated with diploid cell rabies vaccine (Letter to the Editor). Lancet 1990;i:1346—1347.
315. Anonymous. Human rabies prophylaxis, 1987. Wkly Epidemiol Rec 1988;13:357.
316. Hinman AR. Prevention of congenital rubella infection: Symposium summary. Pediatrics 1985;75:1162.
317. Peters ME, Horowitz S. Bone changes after rubella vaccination. Am J Radiol 1984;143:27.
318. Centers for Disease Control. Prospective study of persistent and recurrent arthropathy and other potential adverse events following rubella immunization of adult women (study design). Personal communication, 1991.
319. Bayer SR, Turksoy RN, Emmi AM, Reindollar RH. Rubella immunization. Fertil Steril 1992;57:229.
320. Kazarian EL, Gager WE. Optic neuritis complicating measles, mumps and rubella vaccination. Am J Ophthalmol 1978;86:544.
321. Tingle AJ, Chantler JK, Pot KH. Postpartum rubella immunization: association with development of prolonged arthritis, neurological sequelae, and chronic rubella viremia. J Infect Dis 1985;152:606.
322. Allen AD. Is RA 27/3 rubella immunization a cause of chronic fatigue? Med Hypothesis 1988;27:217.
323. Centers for Disease Control. Rubella vaccination during pregnancy: United States, 1971—1986. Morbid Mortal Wkly Rep 1987;36(28):457.
324. Centers for Disease Control. Rubella vaccination during pregnancy—United States, 1971—1988. Morbid Mortal Wkly Rep 1989;38:289.
325. Immunization Practices Advisory Committee (ACIP). Recommendation on immunization of children infected with HIV. Morbid Mortal Wkly Rep 1986;35:595.
326. Baxby D, Gaskell RM, Gaskell GC et al. Ecology of orthopox viruses and use of recombinant vaccinia vaccines. Lancet 1986;ii:850.
327. Brown F, Schild GC, Ada GL. Recombinant vaccinia viruses as vaccines. Nature 1986;319:549.
328. Dorozinsky A, Anderson A. Deaths in vaccine trials trigger French inquiry. Science 1991;252:501.
329. Guillaume JC, Saiag P, Wechsler J et al. Vaccinia from recombinant virus expressing HIV genes (Letter). Lancet 1991;i:1034.
330. Stokes SL, Atkinson WL, Becher JA, Williams WW. Vaccination against orthopoxvirus infection and adverse events among laboratory personnel, United States, 1983—1991. Personal communication, 1992.
331. Perry GF. Occupational Medicine Forum: Pro and cons of vaccinia immunization. J Occup Med 1992;34:757.
332. Collier LH. Reactions and antibody responses to reinforcing doses of adsorbed and plain tetanus vaccines. Lancet 1979;i:1364.
333. Levine L, Ipsen J, McComb JA. Adult immunization: preparation and evaluation of combined fluid tetanus and diphtheria toxoids for adult use. Am J Hyg 1961;73:20.
334. Relihan M. Reactions to tetanus toxoid. J Irish Med Assoc 1969;62:430.
335. Edsall G, Elliot MW, Peebles TC et al. Excessive use of tetanus toxoid boosters. J Am Med Assoc 1967;202:111.
336. Leen CLS, Barclay GR, McClelland DBL et al. Double-blind comparative trial of standard (commercial) and anti-body-affinity-purified tetanus toxoid vaccines. J Infect 1987;14:119.
337. Rutledge SL, Snead OC. Neurological complications of immunizations. J Pediatr 1986;109:917.
338. Quast U, Hennessen W et al. Mono- and polyneuritis after tetanus vaccination. Dev Biol Stand 1979;43:25.
339. Chen RT, Spira TJ. Tetanus prophylaxis in AIDS patients. J Am Med Assoc 1986;255:1063.

340. Lindemayr H, Drobie M, Ebner H. Impfreaktionen nach Tetanus- und Frühsommermeningoenzephalitisschutzimpfung durch Merthiolat (Thiomersal). Hautarzt 1984;35:392
341. Ackermann R. Allergische Reaktion nach FSME-Auffrischimpfung (Anfrage und Antwort). Dtsch Med Wochenschr 1990;115:1213.
342. Kappos L. Mögliche neurologische Nebenwirkungen nach FSME-Impfung. Fachpressegespräch, Frankfurter Presse Club 20 February, 1990.
343. Bohus M, Glocker FX, Jost S, Deuschl G. Myelitis after immunization against tick-borne encephalitis (Letter to the Editor). Lancet 1993;342:239—240.
344. Schabet M, Wiethoelter H, Grodd W. Neurological complications after simultaneous immunization against tick-borne encephalitis and tetanus. Lancet 1989;i:959.
345. Goerre S, Kesselring J, Hartmann K, Kuhn M. Side effects after vaccination for tick-borne encephalitis. Schweiz Med Wochenschr 1993;123:654—657.
346. DiMaio VJM, Froede RC. Allergic reactions to the tine test. J Am Med Assoc 1975;233:769.
347. Radonic M. Systemic allergic reactions due to occupational inhalation of tuberculin aerosol. Ind Med Surg 1966;35:24.
348. Burgoyne CF, Verstraeten TC, Friberg TR. Tuberculin skin-test-induced uveitis in the absence of tuberculosis. Graefe's Arch Clin Exp Ophthalmol 1991;229:232—236.
349. Immunization Practices Advisory Committee. Recommendations on typhoid immunization. Morbid Mortal Wkly Rep 1990;39:1.
350. Gershon AA, Steinberg SP, LaRussa P et al. Immunization of healthy adults with live attenuated varicella vaccine. J Infect Dis 1988;158:132.
351. Gershon AA, Steinberg SP, Gelb L et al. Live attenuated varicella vaccine use in immunocompromised children and adults. Pediatrics 1986;78:757.
352. Plotkin SA, Starr SE, Conner K et al. Zoster in normal children after varicella vaccine. J Infect Dis 1989;159:1000.
353. Hammerschlag MR, Gershon AA, Holzman R et al. Herpes zoster in an adult recipient of live attenuated varicella vaccine. J Infect Dis 1988;160:535.
354. Magrath DI. Prospective vaccines for national immunization programmes. In: Proceedings, 3rd Meeting of National Programme Managers on Expanded Programme on Immunization, St. Vincent, Italy, 22—25 May 1990. Unedited document ICP/EPI 023/31, 1990.
355. Lydick E, Kuter BJ, Zajac BA. Association of steroid therapy with vaccine-associated rashes in children with acute lymphocytic leukemia who received Oka/Merck varicella vaccine. Vaccine 1989;7:549.
356. Lee SY, Komp DM, Andiman W. Thrombocytopenic purpura following varicella-zoster vaccination. Am J Pediatr Hematol Oncol 1986;8:78.
357. Pillai JJ, Gaughan WJ, Watson B, Sivalingam JJ, Murphey SA. Renal involvement in association with postvaccination varicella (Letter to the Editor). Clin Infect Dis 1993; 17:1079—1080.
358. Naruse H, Miwata H, Ozaki T, Asano Y, Namazue J, Yamanishi K. Varicella infection complicated with meningitis after immunization. Acta Pediatr Jpn Overs Ed 1993;35:345—347.
359. WHO. Prevention and Control of Yellow Fever in Africa. WHO, Geneva, 1986.
360. Schoub BD, Dommann CJ, Johnson S, Downie C, Patel PL. Encephalitis in a 13-year-old boy following 17D yellow fever vaccine. J Infect 1990;21:105—106.
361. Merlo C, Steffen R, Landis T, Tsai T. Possible association of encephalitis and 17D yellow fever vaccination in a 29-year-old traveller. Vaccine 1993;11:691.
362. Drouet A, Chagnon A, Valance J, Carli P, Muzellec Y, Paris JF. Meningoencephalitis after immunization with 17D yellow fever virus. Rev Med Interne 1993;14:257—259.
363. Quast U, Herder C, Zwisler O. Vaccination of patients with encephalomyelitis disseminata. Vaccine 1991;9:228—235.
364. Shah RH, Mackey K, Wallace H et al. Hepatitis B associated with jet gun injection. Morbid Mortal Wkly Rep 1986;35:373.
365. Expanded Programme on Immunization. Immunization policy. WHO/EPI/GEN/86.7 Rev.1, Geneva, 1986.
366. Grabenstein JD. A miscellany of obscure vaccines: Adenovirus, anthrax, mixed bacteria, and *Staphylococcus*. Hosp Pharm 1993;28:259—266.
367. Edelman R. An update on vaccine adjuvants in clinical trial. AIDS Res Human Retrovir 1992;8:1409—1411.
368. Kaaber K, Nielsen AO, Veien NK. Vaccination granulomas and aluminium allergy: course and prognostic factors. Contact Dermatitis 1992;26:304—306.
369. Hendrick MJ, Goldschmidt MH, Shofer FS, Wang Yun-Yu, Somlyo AP. Postvaccinal sarcomas in the cat: Epidemiology and electron probe microanalytical identification of aluminium. Cancer Res 1992;52:5391—5394.
370. Cox NH, Moss C. Cutaneous reactions to aluminium in vaccines: an avoidable problem. Lancet 1988;i:43.
371. Noel I, Galloway A, Ive FA. Hypersensitivity to thiomersal in hepatitis b vaccine. Lancet 1991;338:705.
372. Aberer W. Vaccination despite thimerosal sensitivity. Contact Dermatitis 1991;24:6—10.

Meyler's Side Effects of Drugs, 13th Edition
M.N.G. Dukes, editor

SECTION EDITOR: M.N.G. DUKES

Claus Koch

33 Blood, blood components, plasma and plasma products

INTRODUCTION

Although recent years have seen major achievements in transfusion medicine to improve blood and blood product safety, the risks of transfusion reactions and transmission of infectious agents have not been eliminated. The treatment of patients with blood or blood-derived components has indeed been the subject of great public concern in recent years due mostly to the tragic outcome of human immunodeficiency virus (HIV) infection which can be transmitted by transfusion. Conditions related to the risks of transmission of infectious agents therefore play a prominent role in any discussion of the side effects of blood and blood components.

In general, the list of possible adverse effects of blood and blood components is a fairly long one. Numerous instances of morbidity and mortality mentioned in the literature may serve as evidence of this. It must however be stressed that human errors resulting in blood group mismatch remain the leading causes of transfusion-related fatalities (3). On the other hand, data on adverse reactions, including fatalities, are somewhat incomplete due to the fact that certain side effects are not manifested immediately, but may be observed only after months—perhaps even after years.

Because of the risk of serious complications in blood transfusion therapy, it has been emphasized that unnecessary transfusions should be avoided. It is clear that in most cases therapy with blood or blood components is solely a replacement therapy and should therefore be used only when deficiency of some blood component has been clearly demonstrated, and 'component blood therapy' as a more specific treatment is thus most often preferable to whole blood therapy. Also, promotion of autologous transfusions—although not always feasible—seems to be a strategy which might reduce complication rates (4).

In order to reduce risks to a minimum and at the same time secure high quality blood products, three approaches must be adopted. They relate to: (1) selection of blood donors; (2) screening of individual donations, and; (3) use of production methods specifically aimed at minimizing the risks of transmitting infectious diseases.

Blood donor selection Blood donors ought to be non-remunerated and voluntary, and their health should be checked with regular intervals. A scheme for donor selection may include permanent exclusion criteria, like previous episodes of jaundice (or laboratory tests providing evidence of acute or previous infectious hepatitis, especially hepatitis B or C), syphilis or malaria, presence of anti-HIV antibodies, a so-called risky conduct like homosexual or bisexual behaviour, or a history of treatment with non-recombinant growth factor. Time-limited exclusion criteria relate to the current health status, and may also include intake of certain kinds of medicine, recent blood transfusion, vaccination with live vaccines, recent pregnancy or travel to certain geographical areas, e.g. areas with malaria.

In most countries, donors with a history of icterus are excluded from the donor population. However, there is a substantial geographic variation in the prevalence (and in the rate of detection) of HBsAg and anti-hepatitis C in donors (296, 297). In addition, the type of donors involved influences the risk: it has been clearly shown that commercial (paid) donors carry a much higher hepatitis risk than do non-remunerated, voluntary donors (46, 298).

Laboratory screening of individual donations Donations should be tested for infectivity whenever possible. At present the following assays are performed in most countries: HIV-I/-II antibodies, antibodies to HCV, antibodies to HTLV-I/-II, hepatitis B-surface antigen (HBsAg) and syphilis. Since hepatitis C can be directly tested for, the so-called surrogate tests (hepatic enzyme ALT and antibodies to hepatitis B core antigen) are not employed in all countries, and their relevance has been questioned (310).

Serological screening of every blood or plasma donation must be performed using the most sensitive techniques. For HBsAg this screening may however be unreliable in cases with low titers of HBsAg—evidence has accumulated that HBsAg-negative but strongly positive anti-hepatitis core antigen antibody-positive blood might be infectious (299, 300). Routine screening for HBcAg antibodies is unfortunately impracticable at present. The fact must also be taken into account, that there may well be a period of time ranging from 1 to 8–10 months before antibodies appear, e.g. in HIV or hepatitis patients with viremia.

In order to further increase the sensitivity and also to minimize this so-called window period during which serological markers will not detect the infection, methods to detect nucleic acids, e.g. derived from the virus particle, have been suggested. These methods have, however, not yet been developed sufficiently to be useful; different laboratories still follow different routines, and at present both false-positive and false-negative results pose a problem. There is, however, no doubt that in the future these PCR-like methods will further increase the safety of blood and blood products.

Screening for syphilis is no longer mandatory in all countries as cost-benefit analysis demonstrates it to be of little benefit, at least when using voluntary, non-remunerated donors.

Preparation of safe plasma-derived products The risk of infectivity is eliminated—or at least reduced—by the adoption of good manufacturing practice (GMP) both in blood banks and in plasma fractionation units. The sterility of the final products is checked, and virus inactivation measures (e.g. heat treatment, chemical inactivation) are taken whenever appropriate. Up to the present, the possibility of performing inactivation procedures has been developed furthest as regards the non-cellular blood products, although recently leukodepletion procedures using filtration have seemed to offer an advantage with respect to infectious agents which are almost exclusively intracellular.

The virucidal methods currently in use (301) are based on different approaches. With heat treatment (heating in solution, heating of lyophilized product, or heating in vapor under pressure), the actual temperature, duration, and use of stabilizers vary with the individual product concerned (302, 303). Treatment of a product with a mixture of an organic solvent and a detergent (S/D treatment) has proven to be highly effective as regards lipid-enveloped viruses (295, 304). More recent virus removal or virus inactivation methods employ nano-filtration (305) or treatment with a combination of a colored photosensitizer and light (306).

COMPLICATIONS OF BLOOD DONATION

Among the various adverse effects of blood donation, *vasovagal syncope* and *convulsive reactions* are of concern to blood centers, as they may frighten potential first-time donors. First time donors have a higher frequency of these reactions (1.7%) than do repeat donors (0.2%), and donors who have experienced such reactions subsequently donate less frequently than those without reactions (5). Donors who react are generally of lower weight and have slightly lower blood pressure than those without reactions. Of the social and psychological factors which have been studied, the ingestion of caffeinated beverages and shortening of the duration between registration and the time of phlebotomy are associated with a reduced risk of reactions (5).

Bruising in the antecubital fossa is one of the commonest side effects of blood donation. The common practice of flexing the arm over a cottonwool ball or swab may aggravate bleeding, and direct compression over the puncture site with elevation of the extended arm is recommended as an alternative (6).

The only significant known drawback to whole blood donation is the potential risk of *iron deficiency*. In a study involving 948 menstruating and 141 non-menstruating female blood donors, menstruating donors had lower mean serum ferritin levels than non-menstruating donors. First-time donors had a mean ferritin level of 24 mg/l and regular donors a value of 19 mg/l. The frequency of donations was more predictive of ferritin levels than was the number of donations (7). The study concluded that female donors, especially those donating ≥3 times per year, should have their iron status checked at appropriate intervals and should receive iron supplementation.

It has commonly been thought that donation of blood by *older persons* might involve health risks for themselves, and in many countries healthy potential blood donors are therefore ineligible to donate after the age of 60. A study done of the growing demographic group beyond this age has, however, shown that when donating the standard volume of blood (450 ml), the resulting side effects were no greater than in a control group of donors aged 50–65 years (8).

Apheresis procedures when performed by experienced personnel are considered to be relatively safe. They are, however, not without their dangers, and health risks to both patients and donors undergoing apheresis may occur. Not unexpectedly, the risks are greater with therapeutic plasmapheresis on account of the underlying disease, with an estimated three deaths per 10 000 procedures (9). Frequent donations involving apheresis procedures have been reported to cause *allergic reactions*, most likely due to exposure to ethylene oxide and taking the form of urticaria, flushing, wheezing, chest pain, and in a few cases hypotension (10). Ethylene oxide is often used for sterilization of the polyvinyl chloride tubings, and similar allergic reactions in patients undergoing chronic hemodialysis have been attributed to sensitization to ethylene oxide used for sterilization of the dialyzer. One study has shown significant levels of IgE antibodies to ethylene dioxide in the sera of 78% of donors with allergic reactions and only 12% of control sera.

Although there are no important effects of *multiple blood donation*, cases of *depressed cell-mediated immunity* and *decreased lymphocyte proliferation response* have been reported in the past among such donors (11). In a group of 27 whole blood donors who had regularly donated for at least 4 years, there were no abnormalities in lymphocyte subsets, neutrophil and monocyte receptors, or in the molecules that are important in host defense, as compared with non-donor controls (12). In 25 volunteer donors undergoing regular platelet-pheresis by a discontinuous process a large number of T4 and T8 lymphocytes, a moderate number of B-lymphocytes, and a smaller number of monocytes were removed (13).

TRANSMISSION OF INFECTIOUS DISEASES BY BLOOD AND BLOOD PRODUCTS

Transmission of infectious disease with blood and blood products has remained a serious issue especially after the discovery that *HIV infection* can be transmitted with blood and/or blood products.

It is, however, important to consider two circumstances separately: on the one hand the risk of transmitting disease with whole blood or cellular blood components in situations where virus-inactivation or virus-removal methods are scarcely available, and on the other hand the risk of transmitting disease with plasma or plasma-derived products in situations where effective virus inactivation procedures can today be applied to the product.

Transmission of bacteria

Transfusion-transmitted *bacterial infection* in recipients of blood or blood components is a dreaded but rare complication when modern equipment (i.e. closed systems) is used for the collection and preparation of blood components. Since the introduction of closed systems for blood collection and of stringent regulations regarding storage of blood at 4°C, contamination of red cell products has become rare. However, platelets stored at room temperature remain a potential source of bacterial infections, and recently there has been a dramatic increase in the number of reports of septic episodes associated with both red cell and platelet concentrate transfusions (16). These reports suggest that such reactions may occur as often as in one per 4000 platelet transfusions or even more frequently (14,15). In one study, bacterial isolates from contaminated platelets included *Staphylococcus epidermidis* and *S. aureus* and *Bacillus cereus* (17). Transmission of bacterial infections through contaminated red cell concentrates have been caused mainly by *Yersinia enterocolitica*. This enteric organism is capable of efficient proliferation and even selective growth at refrigeration temperature. Of the 182 reports of transfusion-related fatalities which the United States FDA received between 1986 and 1991, 29 (16%) were due to bacterial contamination, and eight of these were caused by contamination with *Yersinia enterocolitica* (18).

Syphilis is one of the oldest recognized infectious risks of blood transfusion, and blood donors have been routinely screened for syphilis by serological tests for more than 50 years. In recent years, transfusion-transmitted syphilis has become exceptionally rare, with only very few cases reported in the literature. The general use of refrigerated blood reduces the risk of transmission as *Treponema pallidum* loses its viability within a few days in whole blood stored at 4°C.

Transmission of viruses

The occurrence of viral hepatitis (19) and acquired immune deficiency syndrome (AIDS) (20, 21) after treatment with blood or blood products underlines the importance of being aware of the risk of transmission of infections through blood products. More recently, viruses such as human T-cell lymphotropic viruses (HTLV-I and -II) and the parvoviruses have been recognized as blood borne viruses which may compromise the safety of blood products, and cytomegalovirus (CMV) may also be infective, especially in immunocompromised recipients.

HIV-1 In the late 1970s, the human immunodeficiency virus (HIV) was spreading silently and undetected. By 1981, when AIDS was first recognized, cases had already occurred in several countries, but the worldwide spread of HIV infection was only fully realized in the mid-1980s. A recent review discusses transfusion-associated AIDS in great depth and also highlights the fact that the scope of the problem has widened with recognition of other pathogenic retroviruses such as HIV-2, HTLV-I and HTLV-II (21). HIV can be transmitted by blood and blood products and since 1985 donated blood and plasma has in most countries been screened for the presence of HIV-1-antibodies and rather more recently for HIV-2 antibodies as well; HIV-positive units have been discarded. The overall level of HIV prevalence in blood donors declined from 0.035% in mid-1985 to 0.012% by mid-1987, primarily as a result of donor education and self-exclusion, and by eliminating seropositive donors from the donor pool (22). The prevalence of HIV positivity among donors now seems to be around one to two per 400 000 in countries with blood donation systems based on non-remunerated voluntary donors. Before screening of blood and plasma, and before virus inactivation procedures were applied to coagulation factor products (e.g. F-VIII and F-IX), many hemophiliacs who were treated with substitution therapy were exposed to infection with HIV. In the United States, a 1991 study noted that approximately 70% of tested persons with hemophilia A (Factor VIII-deficiency) and 35% with hemophilia B (Factor IX-deficiency) were found to be HIV seropositive (22).

Up to 1987, in 28 European countries, 4% of all reported patients with AIDS were likely to have been infected by blood transfusion. In these countries the percentage of patients with hemophilia or other coagulation disorders developing AIDS was similar up to that date (23).

Transfusion of HIV-infected blood probably still remains a public health problem, especially in parts of Africa (Central, Eastern and Southern), Asia, and parts of the Caribbean. Non-sterile needles, syringes and other skin-piercing instruments also play a role in HIV transmission.

Recently infected donors may, however, not develop detectable antibody for some weeks or months, and HIV infection in a minute number of transfusion recipients must therefore still be expected. Several recipients are reported to have seroconverted following transfusion of blood from donors who were considered anti-HIV negative at the time of donation (24). This so-called window period has been estimated to last for an average of 45 days, and in 90% of cases is probably less than 150 days (60). The HIV antibody tests currently in use have since then become more sensitive and are able to detect seroconversion 5—15 days earlier than the tests in use in the late 1980s (61). The fact that the frequency of positive tests among donors nevertheless continues to decline suggests that the actual risk of HIV infection is now significantly less than the 1990 estimate.

HIV-2 Another virus (HIV-2) closely related to HIV-1 was first reported to be associated with AIDS in 1986 in West-Africa, where the virus is believed to be endemic. Several cases of HIV-2 infection has been reported among Europeans and West-Africans residing in Europe and in the United States. The spectrum of disease and modes of transmission of HIV-2 seem to be similar to those of HIV-1 (63). However, there have been relatively few reports of HIV-2 transmission with blood. The anti-HIV-1 EIA-tests currently used for screening blood donors are estimated to detect from 42 to 92% of HIV-2 infections (62). Anti-HIV-2 assays are now available and are used routinely for blood donor screening.

HTLV-I and HTLV-II The human T-cell lymphotropic virus type I (HTLV-I) is endemic in some areas of Japan, the Caribbean and Africa and has been associated with adult T-cell leukemia. In Japan, seroconversion has been observed when anti-HTLV-I-negative patients were transfused with seropositive blood or components, and in one study the conversion rate was 62% (22). However, to date, no case of transfusion-associated adult T-cell *leukemia* has been reported (26, 27). HTLV-II was originally isolated from a patient with hairy cell leukemia, but the association has not been confirmed. For both HTLV-I and HTLV-II, the natural history, the prevalence rates in blood donors and their possible clinical consequences need to be studied further (25). In the US the current risk of post-transfusion HTLV infection appears to be approximately one in 70 000 per unit (28). For the present it is clear that risk factors for HTLV-I infection among donors are largely geographic, whereas HTLV-II infection is primarily associated with drug abuse (22). Ninety-seven percent of individuals with anti-HTLV-I show virus within their lymphocytes (24), but seroconversion has not been observed after transfusion of fresh frozen plasma or plasma-derived products from seropositive donors (22, 23).

Hepatitic viruses and viral hepatitis

Transmission of viral hepatitis continues to be a serious problem related to transfusion of whole blood, cellular blood components and whole blood, and—but to a lesser degree—related to plasma-derived products (307, 308).

It is difficult and probably impossible to obtain complete data on the true incidence of hepatitis transmitted by blood or blood products: the incubation time is long, mild anicteric cases are not recognized, and systematic follow-up studies of transfused patients are difficult and expensive (309). In addition, the epidemiology of viral-transmitted hepatitis is different in different regions.

Hepatitis transmitted by blood or blood products can be caused by several viruses. Hepatitis B virus (HBV) and hepatitis C virus (HCV) together with serologically unidentified hepatitis virus(es) causing non-A, non-B, non-C hepatitis are a major source. Less significant in the statistics are hepatitis A virus (31, 32), cytomegalovirus, Epstein-Barr virus, herpes simplex virus and other viruses that may cause liver damage.

Hepatitis A virus (HAV) Only a few reports of hepatitis A virus transmission have been published (31, 32). In 1992 an outbreak of icteric hepatitis A involving at least 83 hemophilia A patients in Italy, Belgium, Ireland and Germany who had been treated with a high purity Factor VIII concentrate produced by one manufacturer was documented (29, 30); 93% of the patients were icteric, and a diagnosis of hepatitis A was based on the presence of IgM anti-HA. The contamination source has not yet been definitively established, but it is possible that the virus did not originate from the plasma donors.

Hepatitis B virus (HBV) Following the detection of HBsAg by Blumberg and the introduction of HBsAg screening for donors of blood and plasma in all developed countries, hepatitis B virus transmission through the use of blood and blood products has been effectively prevented. Estimates based upon the sensitivities of current tests for HBsAg and for anti-HBc show that the risk is of the order of one in 200 000 per unit (33).

Passive immunization of the recipient at the time of potential exposure to hepatitis B virus is available. Prophylactic or post-exposure administration of hepatitis immunoglobulin (HBIG) has been shown to be a valuable measure in the prevention of hepatitis B. Addition of anti-hepatitis B immunoglobulin to factor concentrates appears to abolish HBV infectivity (34, 35).

Hepatitis B vaccination has been used effectively in controlled trials (36, 37). The prophylactic effectiveness of hepatitis B vaccine administered immediately after exposure to HBV has not been established (38).

Hepatitis delta (HD) Where they occur with any frequency, hepatitis delta infections raise a problem, as the hepatitis induced tends to be more severe than hepatitis B infection alone, and is more likely to progress to chronic hepatitis. Hepatitis delta virus is a defective RNA virus that can replicate only in the presence of hepatitis B virus. It has a unique hybrid structure consisting of a delta inner core encapsulated by the surface antigen of hepatitis B virus. Delta superinfection can transform asymptomatic or mild chronic hepatitis B infection to severe progressive active hepatitis and cirrhosis, and contributes substantially to fulminant hepatitis B (39, 40).

Hepatitis C virus (HCV) Hepatitis caused by hepatitis C virus was considered as belonging to the group of Non-A, Non-B hepatitis until 1989 when a test became available which specifically identified 50—70% of acute, self-limiting cases and more than 80% of chronic cases of transfusion-related Non-A, Non-B hepatitis (41). Before hepatitis C screening became available, 80—90% of post-transfusion hepatitis cases in the United States were of Non-A, Non-B type (42). Post-transfusion Non-A, Non-B hepatitis is, in general, less severe than hepatitis B and, in about 60—80% of cases, the patients are asymptomatic and anicteric. There have, however, been observations showing that Non-A, Non-B hepatitis tends to progress to chronic liver disease (43, 44).

The test for hepatitis C was originally based on a recombinant antigen selected from a cDNA-expression library prepared using DNA and RNA from plasma taken from a chimpanzee infected with Non-A, Non-B hepatitis originating with a human patient having transfusion-mediated Non-A, Non-B hepatitis (45). Although the infectious virus particle itself has not yet been isolated, the isolation of the genome of HCV, together with expression of viral proteins and synthesis of antigenic peptides of HCV have now made it possible to develop highly sensitive tests, based on multiple antigens from HCV.

The incidence of hepatitis C among donors seems to vary considerably (from 0.2 to at least 3%); recent publication demonstrated that among US blood donors, the prevalence was 0.36% among volunteer, unpaid donors, whereas it was 10.08% among commercial plasma donors (46). In another study, the per unit risk of HCV infection was 0.45% prior to any testing, falling to 0.19% after the introduction of so-called surrogate tests (ALT, anti-HBc), and to 0.03% after the additional implementation of anti-HCV tests (47). With the second- or third-generation tests now available, the risk of transmitting HCV-infection is probably as low as one in 6000 (48).

Availability of the hepatitis C antibody test has also emphasized the relationship between chronic hepatitis C, liver cirrhosis and hepatocellular carcinoma: in Japan, 58 patients with chronic hepatitis C were followed for 7 years; of them, 10 patients developed hepatocellular carcinoma and 14 developed cirrhosis; 30 continued to suffer from chronic hepatitis and in only four did the hepatitis recede (49).

Cytomegalovirus (CMV) It has been ascertained that up to about 70% of donors in Western Countries are CMV-antibody positive (50), and that about 10% have CMV-infected leukocytes. In developing countries the percentage may be greater than 95%. Transfusion from such donors, especially leukocyte transfusions and massive transfusions of fresh blood, may result in a mild illness with fever, splenomegaly, moderate elevation of ALT and AST, presence of atypical lymphoid cells in peripheral blood and perhaps additional symptoms. The syndrome usually appears about 4 weeks after transfusion and persists for 1—6 weeks. In immunocompetent individuals, infection with CMV is transient and without serious consequences, but immunocompromised subjects are at risk of serious, even fatal infections (51). Those at highest risk are premature low birthweight neonates, and bone marrow transplant recipients. CMV-Ab-screened blood and platelets are indicated in premature neonates and in CMV-Ab-negative recipients of seronegative bone marrow transplants. The use of seronegative donors has reduced significantly the risk of transfusion-induced CMV infection in newborn infants (52—54). Emergent evidence suggests that leukodepletion may be effective in preventing transmission of CMV by transfusion (55—57). This effect of leukodepletion indicates that the infective form of CMV is intracellular.

Parvoviruses The B19 parvovirus is known to be transmissible by blood and blood products. In most cases, B19 infection is of little consequence to the recipient. However, maternal infection is known to cause serious problems for the fetus, and patients with hemolytic anemias or HIV infection may suffer aplastic crises as a result of B19 infection. B19 is an essentially epidemic infection and is transmitted only during the pre-acute phase. The virus is not lipid enveloped and is thus not susceptible to solvent detergent treatment; furthermore, it is highly heat resistant. The infection risk is generally thought to be low, perhaps of the order of one in 10—50 000, although a much higher frequency has been suggested by studies based on PCR (58, 59).

Other infective agents transmitted by blood and blood products

Malaria Transfusion-induced malaria may be a life-threatening complication, especially in patients who have been repeatedly transfused, treated with immunosuppressive drugs or splenectomized (68). The disease is readily transmitted from asymptomatic donors with latent infection. The prevention and treatment of transfusion-transmitted malaria have been reviewed by DeVirgillis et al. (69). To prevent malaria transmission, donors from malaria-endemic areas are only accepted after spending 3 years in a malaria-free area; this interval may well be too short (70).

Chagas' disease In endemic areas (Central- and South America), transmission of infection caused by *Trypanosoma cruzi* occurs through transfusions. The total number of infected immigrants living in the United States has been estimated at about 50 000, and these carriers pose a risk as evidenced by reports of transfusion-associated cases.

REACTIONS TO WHOLE BLOOD AND ERYTHROCYTE TRANSFUSION *(66)*

Hemolytic post-transfusion reactions are most often caused by clerical and administrative errors involving misidentification (incorrect labelling of blood samples, faulty identification of patients) rather than due to mistakes in the laboratory (3, 64). A review of hemolytic and other transfusion reactions also stresses the importance of competent handling of whole blood and red cell suspensions (including avoidance of freezing or osmotic damage) (65). Immune-mediated hemolysis is usually avoided by routine antibody screening and cross-matching methods, and improved pre-transfusion testing has resulted in a significant decrease in the incidence of hemolytic transfusion reactions—although there are examples of transfusion reactions without detectable antibody levels both before and after transfusion (71).

Acute hemolytic post-transfusion reactions An acute hemolytic post-transfusion reaction with a measurable destruction of the donor's or recipient's erythrocytes due to incompatibility of antigens and antibodies is followed by the occurrence of hemoglobinemia. Hemoglobinemia occurs when the hemoglobin-binding capacity of haptoglobin and hemopexin in plasma is saturated. The severity of the reaction depends on the nature of the antigen and antibody, on the binding strength of the antibody, and on the volume of incompatible blood which has been transfused.

A severe acute hemolytic reaction occurring immediately or soon after the transfusion of incompatible blood is characterized by the classical incompatibility symptoms: a feeling of heat along the vein into which the blood is being transfused, a sensation of severe pain in the lumbar region, substernal tightness, dyspnea, nausea, a fall in blood pressure, tachycardia, circulatory collapse, hemoglobinemia, hemoglobinuria, and icterus. It is fatal in about 50% of cases, due to hemolytic shock, to hemorrhage from the activation of intravascular clotting or to the precipitation of acute renal failure.

Sometimes the clinical symptoms are poorly manifested with only fever (with or without chills), or they are masked by signs of the primary disease so that the reaction is not recognized. Especially in an anesthetized patient the only symptom of intravascular destruction of erythrocytes may be unexpected profuse bleeding from the operation wound and hypotension (72).

The overwhelming majority of such reactions (about 80%) are due to ABO-incompatibility.

Acute post-transfusion reactions may also occur in the presence of an irregular antibody in the recipient's plasma, directed most frequently against antigens of the Rh system, which may sometimes be difficult to detect; they cause hemolytic reactions only exceptionally. Such cases have been described in detail in the literature (73—77).

Delayed hemolytic post-transfusion reactions When the signs and symptoms of a hemolytic transfusion reaction occur later than 24 h after transfusion, the reaction is classified as a delayed reaction (78—80). It is estimated that up to 0.025% of recipients may well be at risk of delayed transfusion reactions (81); however, a recent study recorded only one occurrence among every 10 668 transfused units. The severity of this type of reaction varies widely. Many of these reactions are so mild that they remain unnoticed; only a few are severe or fatal. Almost all patients with this type of complication have a history of previous transfusion and/or pregnancy which creates the possibility of sensitization. The symptoms of the delayed hemolytic post-transfusion reactions are fever, chills, anemia, hemoglobulinemia, hemoglobinuria and reticulocytosis. Renal failure may occur, and the direct antiglobulin test is positive.

Delayed reactions are difficult to prevent. Incompatibility may not be demonstrable before transfusion by employing the currently used serological tests and, at the time of the reaction, the relevant antibodies may not be detectable. Repeated serological testing on post-transfusion blood samples is therefore necessary. The delayed reactions usually occur as a result of a secondary anamnestic response within 3—21 days after transfusion of apparently compatible blood, when the antibody concentration is high enough to bring about hemolysis of the donor's red blood cells. It would appear that a primary immune response, too, may evoke this kind of reaction (78).

New reports of delayed transfusion reactions continue to appear and they confirm the difficulty of diagnosis. In recent years, many allo-antibodies responsible for delayed reactions of various severity have been demonstrated (1, 78). Specific cases include reactions involving the usual Kidd and Rh antigens/antibodies and anti-S. Delayed reactions to the Kell antigens (e.g. $J_s^{a,b}$) have also been reported (82, 83), and anti-$F\gamma^b$ have also been reported to cause a delayed reaction (84). A possible delayed reaction due to anti-A_1 production from the group O graft and to reduction of suppressor cell activity by immunosuppressive agents has also been described (85). In sickle-cell patients a more severe delayed transfusion reaction may be misdiagnosed as a sickle-cell crisis (86, 87); this complication occurs particularly in patients with U-variants (88).

A method for examining the possibility of safe transfusion is based on the use of cells labelled with radioactive chromium (89). After administration of several ml of the labelled blood the survival of erythrocytes in the recipient's circulation is examined: poor survival in vivo indicates that transfusion with these erythrocytes will be hazardous (90, 91). A description of the pattern of survival of incompatible cells describes two types of survival curves that may be observed. A single exponential curve is seen with most potent IgG antibodies which do not bind complement, including anti-D, -C and -K. Clearance described by more than one exponential is observed with complement-binding antibodies (92). In the latter there is a slowing of red cell destruction 5—20 min after injection into the circulation, probably due to acquired resistance to complement activation.

The interpretation of delayed transfusion reactions may be difficult as the occurrence of low-grade warm acquired hemolytic anemia may resemble this form of transfusion reaction (93). Careful elution of antibody, its identification and confirmation of its relationship to the transfused red cells are all required to establish the nature of the reaction. If the indirect antiglobulin test is negative, autoimmune hemolysis is the likely pathogenesis (94).

Sensitization to HLA-antigens (95) Sensitization to HLA-antigens is undesirable in patients awaiting organ transplantation and in patients who need long-term platelet transfusion. The success of protocols which include leukocyte-depleted and frozen red cells might be limited since HLA antigens may be expressed on red cells. In a recent study the red cells of 50% of blood donors bound HLA-A, -B and -C antibodies (but not antibodies to class II-antigens or to leukocyte-specific antigens). Neither storage at 40°C for 21 days nor cryopreservation affected the expression of these antigens. The immunogenicity of HLA-antigens on red cells is unknown.

Reactions due to passive transfer of allo-antibodies Passive transfer of allo-antibodies present in donor's plasma is a further cause of hemolytic transfusion reactions. Low-titer red cell antibodies in donor blood are considered to be relatively harmless, especially when plasma-reduced or concentrated red cells are transfused to a recipient whose cells carry the relevant antigen. A complication of this type provoked by high-titer anti-E antibody has been described (96). Likewise, a hemolytic transfusion reaction occurred in a Kell-negative adult when anti-Kell contained in the plasma of a unit of whole blood reacted with Kell-positive cells transfused 4 weeks previously (97).

Transfusion-related acute lung injury This is an infrequent but life-threatening complication, clinically indistinguishable from adult respiratory distress syndrome (ARDS). It may occur after administration of whole blood, red cells, fresh-frozen plasma and cryoprecipitate, all of which contain variable amounts of plasma. In transfusion-related acute lung disease the symptoms of ACRD (pulmonary edema, severe hypoxia, fever, hypotension) occur within 1–6 hours from the start of transfusion, and usually subside within 1–4 days. There is evidence that leukoagglutinating and anti-HLA antibodies may cause the reaction. The reaction may be more frequent than reported because confounding factors may mask the symptoms (67).

Reactions to massive blood transfusions (81) Patients receiving massive transfusions in emergency situations are almost always extremely ill and suffering from prolonged shock or they are undergoing surgery, e.g. organ transplantations with heavy reliance on blood transfusions. The patient receiving massive transfusion is exposed to several risks resulting from addition of an anticoagulant, from transfusion of cold blood, and from biochemical, hematological and other changes in blood during storage. The complications lead in turn to metabolic disturbances and impaired hemostasis in proportion to the transfused volume. The main risks include:

Citrate toxicity During rapid and massive transfusion, an excess of citrate in preserved blood may result in a dangerous fall of the ionized calcium level in the recipient's plasma. The most significant warning sign of threatening citrate intoxication is an increase in peripheral or central venous pressure, and this should always be monitored during massive transfusions. An adequate intravenous dose of calcium gluconate or chloride is a reliable means of correcting dangerous hypocalcemia (98).

Hyperkalemia Hyperkalemia, sometimes associated with massive transfusion of old blood is not a common problem. Potassium intoxication threatens only patients with elevated potassium levels prior to transfusion, e.g. individuals with crush syndrome, renal failure and extensive burns.

Hyperammonemia and hyperphosphatemia Ammonia and inorganic phosphates rise significantly during blood storage, but caution is needed only when transfusions of old blood are administered to patients with liver failure.

Hypothermia Transfusion of refrigerated blood can, especially during massive transfusions or during exchange transfusions, induce hypothermia with a danger of cardiac arrest. Therefore, if several units of blood are rapidly administered, it is recommended to warm, but not overheat, the blood prior to transfusion (99).

Acidosis Since stored blood has a relatively low pH, its transfusion may lead to acidosis. Prompt and appropriate restoration of the patient's blood volume is most important to maintain sufficient tissue and organ perfusion and thereby to correct or avoid acidosis.

Circulatory overload Circulatory overload with symptoms of congestive heart failure and pulmonary edema may complicate transfusion in patients with an exhausted cardiac reserve.

Hemostatic abnormalities Hemostatic abnormalities associated with massive transfusions are regularly observed. *Thrombocytopenia* is a well-known consequence of hemodilution. A review of defects in hemostasis caused by blood transfusion also comments on thrombocytopenia, which is a more frequent clinical problem than abnormalities of coagulation (100). If the platelet count drops below 40×10^9 per liter, platelet concentrates should be transfused; 1–2 units of fresh frozen plasma are recommended after every 10 units of stored blood to correct coagulation factor deficiencies. As far as the storage lability of coagulation factors is concerned, a mild decrease of Factors V and VIII and, occasionally, of fibrinogen, occurs in the recipient. It must be emphasized, however, that significant coagulation disorders including disseminated intravascular coagulation (DIC) appear almost routinely during prolonged hypovolemia (101).

Mannucci et al. (102) studied changes in the hemostatic system in surgical patients undergoing massive transfusion. Abnormal results were observed in 93% of patients, the most frequent finding being a deranged platelet count. Well-defined hemostatic disorders, e.g. DIC, were ascertained in 48% of patients. To reduce the risk in such circumstances, careful laboratory monitoring and stringent attention to treatment of the underlying disease have been recommended.

Transport function of hemoglobin The progressively increasing oxygen affinity of stored erythrocytes caused by a fall of 2,3-diphosphoglycerate level is clinically relevant only under extreme conditions. The increasing oxygen affinity of hemoglobin is reversible in vivo within 24 hours. It is possible to restore the oxygen transport function of hemoglobin by addition of purine nucleosides to old blood (103).

Hemosiderosis Patients who have received about 100 units of erythrocytes inevitably develop siderosis of the organs and tissues as a consequence of transfusion-induced iron overload (104). Deposition of iron results in functional damage to the heart, liver, spleen and endocrine and other organs, and is often fatal. The clinical signs of iron toxicity in children are retarded growth, splenomegaly, cardiopathy and endocrinopathy. Examination of the serum ferritin level and transferrin saturation is a useful method for diagnosis of iron overload.

Subcutaneous infusion of desferrioxamine now provides effective and relatively safe treatment by increasing iron excretion. Furthermore, ascorbic acid significantly enhances urinary iron excretion (105).

Iron accumulation can be significantly reduced by transfusing young erythrocytes since the intervals between transfusions can be extended (106, 107).

Reactions to exchange transfusions (81) Exchange transfusion is the most effective therapeutic procedure in the treatment of hemolytic disease of the newborn. Bilirubin removal prevents the damage to the central nervous system caused by hyperbilirubinemia. In addition, sensitized erythrocytes are replaced by normally surviving cells and anemia is corrected. The risks of the treatment are essentially the same as described above for other massive transfusions and are dependent on the health of the newborn infant, its gestation age and weight. The transfused blood should be as fresh as possible and should not have been stored for more than 4—5 days. It must be free of antigens reacting with antibodies in the maternal plasma. Technical errors like *perforation of the umbilical vein*, *false placing of the catheter* and *air embolism* are very rare complications.

Favorable results of exchange transfusion in a variety of diseases in adults, e.g. sickle-cell disease, severe clotting disorders, hepatic failure and acute hemolytic transfusion reactions have been published. Today, however, machine apheresis procedures are available and these are more effective and safer for patients requiring exchange of cellular elements or plasma.

Transfusion reactions in oncology patients Oncology patients treated with intensive chemotherapy are usually immunosuppressed; in one report the incidence of overall reactions to blood transfusion in such patients was 0.3% of all transfused units, which is significantly lower than expected (108). Febrile non-hemolytic reactions and allergic urticarial reactions were the most frequently noted, and the number of delayed hemolytic transfusion reactions was much lower than in non-oncology patients.

This probably results from a relative inability of oncology patients to produce allo-antibodies against blood group antigens.

Allergy to contaminating drugs Allergic reactions to potentially allergenic drugs present in donated blood may explain some transfusion reactions that cannot be explained by routine tests. Although donors are in many countries asked to volunteer their history of drug intake during the previous 24 hours, common self-medication remedies may be overlooked. In an investigation among Canadian donors 6—7% of donor blood samples had detectable levels of acetylsalicylic acid and acetaminophen (109). Such drugs would be potentially capable of causing untoward reactions in the recipients. In addition the presence in donor blood of certain drugs may damage some blood components, especially platelets.

Prevention of microaggregates In preserved blood, microaggregates are formed during storage. Such microaggregates are identified as cellular material (platelet conglomerates, leukocyte ghosts, and platelet ghosts with fibrin-co-aggregates) or proteinaceous material. Blood filters with small pore sizes seem to be effective in preventing such adverse effects as febrile non-hemolytic transfusion reactions, in preventing or delaying the development of leukocyte antibodies, and in reducing the risk of respiratory distress syndrome by removing intact or disintegrating cells, debris and microaggregates (110).

REACTIONS TO LEUKOCYTES

Multi-transfused patients often develop non-hemolytic febrile transfusion reactions, caused by antibodies to allo-antigens on the leukocytes. The minimum number of leukocytes that may stimulate antibody production is unknown, but it is believed that these reactions occur when more than 0.5×10^9 leukocytes are transfused (111). The allo-antigens responsible for the reactions belong most often to either the HLA-system, or they are granulocyte-specific antigens (112). Allo-antibodies to these antigens may give rise to *neonatal neutropenia*, *febrile transfusion reactions* or to *poor response to granulocyte transfusions* (113). ABO incompatibility has been shown not to alter the in vivo fate of granulocytes (114). The *febrile reactions* are usually mild, but *pulmonary manifestations* may be more severe. Respiratory distress may develop very soon after starting the transfusion or within 24 hours. The radiologically evident pulmonary infiltrates may be associated with leukocyte aggregates and leukocyte antigen—antibody complexes. Recovery is usually uneventful.

Removal of leukocytes from blood and packed erythrocytes significantly reduces the incidence of these reactions in sensitized recipients (115—118). Numerous procedures for removing leukocytes have been described (119, 120), including filtration through cotton wool and other more sophisticated filtering devices. A decrease in leukocyte content of at least 80% must be achieved.

Centrifugal blood cell separators as well as techniques of filtration leukapheresis or reversible leukoadhesion can provide a therapeutically adequate dose of granulocytes from a single donor (121), and cells separated in this way are clinically effective.

Granulocyte transfusions

Granulocyte transfusions are indicated in severely granulocytopenic febrile patients with sepsis who are not responding to antibiotics. At least 2×10^{10} granulocytes per day are considered to comprise an adequate granulocyte transfusion, but on occasion larger numbers are probably required (122, 123). Complications after granulocyte transfusions occur in about 15—20% of the recipients (124) and are most often seen in patients given granulocytes prepared by filtration leukapheresis. The complications include predominantly severe *febrile reactions*, the transmission of *cytomegalovirus infection* and the development of *graft-versus-host disease*. Of particular importance are *respiratory reactions* with pulmonary edema, occurring mostly in allo-immunized recipients. As described above, leukocyte aggregation may be the cause, with sequestration microemboli and fluid overflow, but other causes have also been suspected. Reactions appear to be more common in patients with sepsis.

Since centrifuge-collected granulocytes are markedly contaminated with erythrocytes, the ABO-compatibility between donor and recipient will be important unless the erythrocytes can be removed before use. Some reactions, particularly allergic and febrile complications, are associated with the presence of macromolecular agents (hydroxyethyl starch, modified gelatine, dextran) used to increase the yield of centrifugal techniques.

REACTIONS TO PLATELETS

Severe *thrombocytopenia* is observed most often in connection with chemotherapy in oncology patients. The availability of platelet concentrates has improved the therapeutic possibilities.

Platelet concentrates are obtained by differential centrifugation of several fresh blood units or by plateletpheresis from single donors using a blood cell separator. The quality of platelet concentrates obtained by apheresis deteriorates rapidly after storage for more than 24 hours. Of all blood components, platelets are the most vulnerable to bacterial contamination.

The major risks associated with platelet transfusion are *allo-immunization* and *infection*. Rarely platelets cause *graft-versus-host disease* (125, 126). Allo-antibodies—especially anti-HLA antibodies—appear to be responsible for the major source of complications in patients given repeated platelet transfusions. These antibodies cause febrile reactions but they can also be responsible for partial or complete refractoriness to platelet transfusions. It has been estimated that more than 50% of recipients become allo-immunized within 4—6 weeks following repeated platelet transfusions prepared from random donors (127, 128), though other evidence indicates that this problem may well have been over-emphasized (129).

Platelet concentrates contain a considerable number of leukocytes, and it is not clear whether allo-antibody formation is caused by the platelets themselves or by these contaminating leukocytes (129). There is in fact evidence that use of leukocyte-free platelets could prevent refractoriness to platelet transfusion (130), and anti-HLA induction is also reduced when using leukocyte-free platelets (131). This report also demonstrates that the use of HLA-matched platelets almost entirely avoids allo-immunization. Severe but transient thrombocytopenia was observed after infusion of whole blood from a donor subsequently found to have a high titer platelet-specific antibody (anti-PI^{A1}) (132). This, however, has been described only in extremely rare cases.

Post-transfusion thrombocytopenic purpura Post-transfusion thrombocytopenic purpura is a rare immunological complication developing about 1 week after transfusion of blood containing platelets (133—135). Most patients have been women aged 40—80 with a history of transfusions or pregnancy. The incriminated antibody in the patient's sera reacts with the recipient's own platelets. Thrombocytopenia and purpura usually last up to 3 weeks, as the antibody disappears and the platelet count progressively rises. The responsible antibody is usually PIA1, and the patient's platelets are PI^{A1}-negative. The precise mechanism causing this platelet destruction is uncertain, but the transient presence of an autoantibody (136) or adsorption of PI^{A1}-antigen onto PI^{A1}-negative platelets (137) have been suggested. There seems to be a linkage to HLA-DR3 and DRw52 (138). Anti-PI^{A2} is only seldom implicated in post-transfusion thrombocytopenia (139, 140). This complication can be treated with plasma exchange, high-dose steroid or i.v. immunoglobulin (141).

Neonatal alloimmune thrombocytopenic purpura Neonatal alloimmune thrombocytopenic purpura is a rare, transient, severe thrombocytopenia in the newborn due to platelet destruction by maternal antibody. The mother is usually a PI^{A1}-negative person who has produced anti-PI^{A1} as a result of previous blood transfusion or pregnancy. The antibody crosses the placenta and destroys the PI^{A1}-positive platelets of the neonate. Treatment is with PI^{A1}-negative platelets (81).

GRAFT-VERSUS-HOST REACTIONS

Graft-versus-host (GvH) disease is caused by engrafted allogeneic immunocompetent T-lymphocytes (passenger lymphocytes) which are able to proliferate and to react against the recipient (142, 143). It is a serious, potentially fatal complication in allogeneic bone marrow transplantation. Development of GvH disease has been reported variously after administration of various types of blood preparations (144), whole blood used for exchange transfusion (145), packed erythrocytes, granulocytes (2, 146, 147) and platelets (142).

GvH disease is characterized by activated T-helper cells (T_H) and cytotoxic T-lymphocytes (T_C) (148). Skin lesions in GvH disease show a reduction in antigen-presenting Langerhans cells and T_H-cells and an increase in T_C/T-suppressor (T_S) cells (149); these changes parallel others elsewhere in the body. Following the transfusion of blood components containing lymphocytes, GvH disease may also develop in severely immunocompromised patients, e.g. in patients with immunodeficiency syndrome or patients undergoing massive chemotherapy. The smallest number of lymphocytes capable of inducing GvH disease is not known, but it is known that 1 unit of blood contains a sufficient number of lymphocytes to produce GvH disease in severely immunocompromised adult patients. The finding that GvH disease is encountered more often in neonates than in adults may be explained by the inadequacy of the neonatal immune defense system.

GvH disease after allogeneic bone marrow transplantation (150) gives rise to a wide range of complications, especially cutaneous, hepatic and gastrointestinal, including severe itching and persistent diarrhea. Treatment with prednisolone and—if necessary—antilymphocyte antibodies and/or ciclosporin may help. Hepatic involvement may be mild but can progress to liver failure in spite of optimal treatment (151). Oral complications may be related to GvH disease but may also be a result of intensive chemotherapy/irradiation or a result of intensive antibiotic treatment (152).

To reduce the risk of GvH disease to a minimum, one can inhibit the proliferative capacity of the donor's immunocompetent lymphocytes by irradiation of lymphocyte-containing blood products. A dose of 1500—3000 rads is used. A newer protocol using murine monoclonal antibodies to pan-T-cell antigen (e.g. CD3) to remove mature T-lymphocytes from bone marrow grafts is promising, while transplant recipients have greatly benefitted from prophylactic ciclosporin therapy (153). T-cell-depletion on the other hand does not seem to impair (and may actually enhance) functional recovery of B-cells after bone marrow transplantation (154). The post-marrow transplantation period is followed by a period of profound immunosuppression often complicated by life-threatening infections, e.g. caused by CMV (155, 156).

Bone marrow transplants are most often kept cryopreserved in dimethylsulfoxide (DMSO), and residual DMSO be responsible for toxic reactions: in one report, all 10 patients studied showed a drop in heart rate and blood pressure (157). Other factors like cell lysis or rapid infusion of large volumes may however be responsible.

Transfusion and transplantation interactions

Beneficial effects have been shown from giving blood transfusions, preferably donor-specific, prior to transplantation. The mechanism for this is not known (159—161). By contrast, pre-transplant transfusions in bone marrow recipients suffering from aplastic anemia cause major complications, and may be responsible for graft rejection and marrow transplantation failure (158). Immunosuppressed patients, e.g. with hematological malignancies, are less likely to become sensitized to histocompatibility antigens to which they are exposed by transfusions; restriction on transfusions in the pre-transplant period is not necessary.

'Passenger B-lymphocytes' may also pose problems in transplantations. Acquired hemolytic reactions due to anti-A or anti-B may be induced by group-O allografts in renal transplantation (162—165) and may be prevented by prophylactic irradiation of the kidney (166). Also cases of immune hemolytic anemia have been attributed to donor-derived red cell antibodies after allogeneic bone marrow transplantation (167, 168).

THERAPEUTIC PLASMA EXCHANGE

Intensive plasma exchange has been studied in the treatment of numerous diseases, above all in Waldenström's macroglobulinemia, thrombotic thrombocytopenic purpura, systemic lupus erythematosus, myasthenia gravis, hypercholesterolemia, hyperviscosity syndrome, hemolytic-uremic syndrome and several other autoimmune disorders (169). Its potential benefit could result from the removal of a variety of harmful substances from plasma such as antibodies, antigens, immune complexes, toxins or abnormal plasma components. If the circulating substance is a cause of the disease, plasma exchange can be effective. However, its therapeutic potential in many diseases has not so far been precisely defined.

The performance of intensive plasma exchange (removal from an adult of 2000—3000 ml of plasma with its replacement to maintain the patient's blood volume) requires cell separation, which renders possible the rapid removal of large volumes of plasma. There are two methods of plasma separation, namely centrifugal flow separation and flow filtration (170, 171).

Intensive plasma exchange is a relatively safe procedure. It is generally well tolerated, and only a few serious complications have been reported. Potential complications comprise transient hypotension, nausea, urticaria, abdominal discomfort, fever, hypothermia, air or microaggregate embolism, hypocalcemia (citrate effect) with paresthesias, tetany and cardiac depression, thrombocytopenia (frequently observed), coagulation factor depletion, as well as depletion of various intravascular proteins, visual scotomata, hepatitis, vasovagal reactions and reactions associated with phlebotomy (phlebitis, hematoma).

The fluid volume and protein removed by plasmapheresis must be replaced. Among the solutions available for replacement therapy are fresh frozen plasma and human albumin solutions.

REACTIONS TO PLASMA AND PLASMA PROTEINS

The main adverse reactions to plasma or plasma proteins can be classified as follows (78, 81, 172):

Fever Fever may result, starting 10—15 min after infusion is initiated. Fever is often seen together with headache, nausea, and shivering. These symptoms often disappear upon discontinuation of infusion.

Anaphylactoid reactions These range from mild urticaria and flushing to fatal anaphylaxis. Such reactions may occur either during the infusion or within several minutes after infusion. Mild reactions often start locally with a tendency to spreading. In more severe cases, dyspnea, arthralgia and fever appears. Stabilizers or other additives added to plasma protein preparations may be of importance. In addition, protein aggregates in the preparations may participate in anaphylactoid reactions including pulmonary abnormalities. Severe reactions have occasionally been encountered.

Hypotension Hypotension is another, sometimes severe, side effect of the administration of plasma proteins. This untoward effect may well be associated with the presence of a potent prekallikrein activator (Hageman factor—Factor XII degradation product) which is thought to stimulate the kininogen in the recipient's blood to produce kinin which causes systemic hypotension.

Development of an antibody response The development of an antibody response against a deficient or genetically different protein may be the cause of post-transfusion complications. The main problems result from formation of antibodies against antihemophilic factors—e.g. against Factor VIII or Factor IX—occurring after repeated transfusions in hemophiliacs and causing inhibition of therapeutic effect. Another situation where antibody formation may lead to side effects arises in IgA-deficient subjects who receive IgA-containing products and produce anti-IgA antibodies. Inhibitors to coagulation proteins and antibodies to IgA are described in more detail below.

WHOLE PLASMA

Fresh frozen plasma (FFP) is defined as the fluid portion of a single unit of human blood that has been individually centrifuged, separated and frozen at −188°C (or colder) within 6 hours of collection. Its use has increased considerably in most countries within the past 10—15 years (173) in spite of mounting evidence of its potential risks such as transmission of viral infections. Infrequently allo-immunization occurs, with formation of Rh antibodies from contaminating red blood cells and (as with any Intravenous administered fluid) hypervolemia and cardiac failure may occur (174). Anti-A and anti-B in plasma may hemolyze the recipient's red cells if FFP is not ABO-compatible (175).

Recently, virus-inactivated plasma is becoming an alternative where virus inactivation has been performed either using S/D treatment (NYBC method) or heat treatment.

ALBUMIN

Adverse reactions to human serum albumin are rare; usually only occasional and mild reactions are reported like itching and urticaria. Serious reactions are extremely uncommon. When they do occur, however, they tend to take the form of anaphylactoid reactions (0.011% of cases treated) and about a third of these may be life-threatening (173).

The reactions are unpredictable, and it has been known for a patient who has reacted violently to albumin on one occasion to tolerate it well on another after being given diphenhydramine (176). A newer case in which the mechanism seemed to be IgE-mediated anaphylaxis against native albumin has been reported (177).

Aggregates present in protein preparations may be the cause of some reactions. Another postulated cause may be the presence of antibodies against genetic variants of human albumin (178). Hypotensive reactions due to the presence of a prekallikrein activator in some batches of preparations may occur.

The contamination of albumin solutions with aluminium, resulting in toxicity, has been described (179). In a study measuring the aluminium content of albumin from 20 suppliers, the content varied from 1.03 to 1301 μmol/l depending on batch and manufacturer (180). Aluminium overloading may occur, especially in patients with impaired renal function who receive large volumes of albumin, leading to osteodystrophy and encephalopathy (181). The sources of contamination relate to the fractionation procedure employed and can be located to containers, filters, and final product-containers.

Albumin can be rendered virus-free through pasteurization, and treated in this way it has an unblemished safety record with regard to virus transmission; there have been no cases of HIV-transmission attributed to this type of product although many batches are known, in retrospect, to have been derived from HIV-contaminated pools (182).

IMMUNOGLOBULINS

One of the main developments in the use of plasma protein fractions in recent years has been the increase in use of immunoglobulins (183, 184).

Human immunoglobulins are prepared either for i.m./s.c. use or for i.v. administration. The preparations used for i.m./s.c. administration are mainly given to prevent or treat diseases like rhesus-disease (anti-D) or a group of infectious diseases caused by viruses, e.g. morbilli, hepatitis A, hepatitis B, rabies, CMV, etc. Preparations for i.v. use are mainly used for treatment of general immune deficiency states (primary or secondary) or for diseases like idiopathic thrombocytopenic purpura (ITP) and autoimmune disorders (184, 188).

The effect of immunoglobulin therapy is either protection against microorganisms (antibody substitution) and/or immunomodulation. The mechanism of the response to non-infectious diseases is still not clear, but in ITP, early falls in platelet-associated IgG and IgM may be a primary event due to interference with platelet—antibody binding (189). Other explanations, particularly for long-term responses, are reductions in proportion of T4-helper cells and increased immunosuppression due to transient blockade of Fc-receptor functions. Suppression of polyclonal immunoglobulin biosynthesis induced by high-dose immunoglobulin infusions has also been suggested as a possible mechanism (190).

Side effects of immunoglobulins are related to the extent to which they are foreign to the recipient, but relate also to the underlying disease for which the patient receives therapy and to the specificity of the antibodies present in the preparation in question.

IgA deficiency is one the more common genetically determined disorders and, in caucasians, the homozygote deficiency is present in 0.3—0.03% of the population. Such individuals may develop anti-IgA antibodies and develop serum sickness-like symptoms after the first administration, and sometimes more severe reactions after repeated injections (185, 311, 312). A mild reaction due to sensitization against genetic IgA variants may also be observed.

Another general—although rare—side effect to immunoglobulin is intravascular hemolysis due to presence of anti-blood group antibodies (139—141, 186, 187).

Side effects associated with i.m./s.c. immunoglobulin are extremely rare, and are most often related to IgA deficiency in the patient or to additives (e.g. antiseptics). Side effects associated with i.v. immunoglobulin are seen more often and may be either local or systemic.

Local reactions are essentially attributable to the technique used and are not specific to i.v. immunoglobulin.

Of the systemic reactions, those of an inflammatory nature are thought to be due to the presence of small complexes or microaggregates, probably leading to activation of the complement system. They are usually mild and influenza-like, and they generally respond to slowing or temporary interruption of the infusion. They take the form of headache, hypotension, sweating, chills, fever, nausea and vasomotor reactions. It has, however, been noted that the frequency of such adverse reactions decreased, probably due to improved quality of the preparations. In 1978 the frequency of adverse reactions was as high as 55% in those receiving i.v. preparations containing 10—13% polymeric immunoglobulin, whereas current i.v. immunoglobulin causes adverse reactions in only 3—4% (184). The more severe reactions are possibly also complement mediated and may be due to spontaneous activation of the complement system by the immunoglobulin preparation concerned—again immunoglobulin aggregates may possibly be involved. The symptomatology can be similar to that of inflammatory reactions though it may be more severe. Such serious effects—including the rare reactions of anaphylactic type—may occur in as few as one in 6000 cases (191).

Stroke and myocardial infarction have been reported after high-dose treatment with intravenous immunoglobulin, which causes an increase in plasma viscosity (313). High-dose immunoglobulin has also been reported to cause neutropenia, disseminated intravascular coagulation and serum sickness (314). Finally there are the occasional cases where transmission of viral disease has been suspected, e.g. non-A, non-B hepatitis (hepatitis C) (54).

Hypogammaglobulinemic patients have been reported to develop mild symptoms (10% in Ref. 192). In a study where 37 patients with primary hypogammaglobulinemia received 1235 immunoglobulin infusions, 10 patients experienced adverse reactions during 34 infusions (2.8% of all infusions), but only five were moderately severe. Symptoms were as described above. The reactions appeared to be related to the rate of administration (193); administration of 5 mg/kg per minute was tolerated well. Some reports indicate that anaphylaxis due to infusion of i.v. immunoglobulin occurs most often in this group of patients (194, 195).

Thrombocytopenic patients generally tolerate i.v. immunoglobulin well (196). In a study of 16 young patients aged from 9 months to 22 years with immune-mediated hematocytopenia (13 having childhood immune thrombocytopenic purpura) who received a total of 210 infusions, minimal side effects (transient headaches) were experienced in only four infusions, and in three of the four patients concerned later infusions were free of problems (197). Anaphylactic reactions have, however, been seen in two atopic patients with ITP, and the authors warn that children with atopic disease should not receive i.v. immunoglobulin (198). In elderly patients, thrombotic events have been described in up to 10% in patients aged over 60, some of them fatal. Thrombotic events may be related to a rapid rise in circulating platelets (199, 200). A few examples of alopecia seen when i.v. immunoglobulin was given concomitantly with steroid have been described (201, 202).

As already mentioned, i.v. immunoglobulin therapy has been used in other groups of patients (202). In a review of i.v. immunoglobulin in SLE, worsening proteinuria and/or elevation of serum creatinine was observed (203, 204)—whereas others treating similar patients could detect no deterioration (198, 205).

Due to reports of severe side effects, rheumatoid factor in patients with B-cell neoplasia might be considered a contraindication to i.v. immunoglobulin (206).

Human monoclonal antibodies *(Rodent monoclonal antibodies are described under the heading 'Non-human plasma proteins')*

The exciting potential of human monoclonal antibody (McAb) immunotherapy in clinical medicine has long been discussed, but only very few examples of successful applications of such antibodies have yet been demonstrated. One reason for this is that the production of human monoclonal antibodies of predefined specificity and with appropriate binding characteristics has proved to be a notoriously difficult task.

Treatment of neoplastic diseases with McAb is theoretically attractive. Unfortunately none of the McAbs available at present have been demonstrated to be strictly tumor specific, and binding to normal cells has been shown to be the major unknown factor for toxicity (212).

An illustration of the potential of human monoclonal antibodies is provided by the HA-1A antibody, which is a human monoclonal IgM antibody with specificity for the core/lipid A-part of endotoxin. 291 patients with gram-negative bacteremia were treated with this antibody, and a significant decrease in mortality was seen (216). Since then other patient groups have been treated, and apart from local hives, flushing and mild transient hypotension, no adverse reactions have been noted (217, 218). None of the patients have developed antibodies to HA-1A. Although the initial results seem promising, more trials are needed to substantiate the therapeutic efficacy of HA-1A.

Campath-1H is a humanized monoclonal antibody with specificity for CDw52 (present on the cell membranes of lymphocytes and monocytes). It has been used for the treatment of patients with rheumatoid arthritis and vasculitis. The major adverse effects (fever, nausea, skin rash, hypotension) might well be related not to the antibody itself but rather to cytokines, released as a consequence of lysis of the target lymphocytes (315). Out of four patients, treated with Campath-1H, three developed antibodies to Campath-1 H, but with no effect on plasma concentrations and with no obvious clinical consequences. Other side effects have included mild renal impairment and transient thrombocytopenia.

COAGULATION PROTEINS

The last 10—15 years have witnessed a more optimal treatment of patients with bleeding disorders in that more and more patients have been offered prophylactic treatment and not merely substitution therapy on demand. At the same time there has been an important new development in the respective products towards more highly purified preparations, and the time is now approaching where recombinant coagulation proteins will be available as a realistic alternative to the plasma-derived products.

By far the most serious complications to treatment with plasma-derived proteins have been transmission of viral diseases, primarily transmission of HIV. This topic and the current possibilities to prevent transmission have been dealt with already.

There are only relatively few immediate side effects from administration of coagulation proteins. They are the kind of side effects common to the infusion of plasma proteins and are described on page 973. The most important are induction of inhibitory antibodies, modulation of the immune system, and thrombotic events.

Patients suffering from bleeding disorders are at risk of developing antibodies against the factor which is absent, present in reduced amounts or present in an inactive form in their own blood. Such coagulation inhibitors render treatment very difficult. Inhibitors to F-VIII are the most common and develop in 5—15% of hemophilia A patients. Inhibitors to F-IX develop in 1—4% of hemophilia B patients (225, 226).

Patients with Factor VIII inhibitors present clinically either as 'high responders' who show a strong anamnestic response and a sharp rise in inhibitor levels after exposure to F-VIII, or 'low responders' who show little or no anamnestic response (227).

Treatment of F-VIII inhibitor patients has been attempted using many different strategies:

Regular administration of intermediate or low-dose F-VIII concentrates has been shown to lead to the rapid disappearance of F-VIII inhibitors in some high responders (227). This is thought to be due to the development of immunological tolerance.

Binding to phospholipids protects F-VIII from inactivation by inhibitors and 25—58% of F-VIII seems to be protected by this mechanism (228). This may explain the effectiveness of treating hemophiliacs who have inhibitors with *high doses of F-VIII.*

Prothrombin complex concentrate (PCC) has also been used for treating bleeding episodes in patients with F-VIII-inhibitors (229). However, thromboembolic complications related to higher doses have been described, although relatively rarely (230, 231). Thrombotic events seem to be extremely rare when highly purified F-IX is used, also when used for treatment of patients with hemophilia B. Activated PCC has also been found to be effective in the treatment of patients with F-VIII inhibitors (232). Again, serious complications are rare, but disseminated intravascular coagulation has been reported (233).

Highly purified animal material such as porcine F-VIII continues to be used to good effect in hemophiliacs with high-titer inhibitors. Adverse effects have been relatively mild, consisting of fever and rare anaphylactoid reactions (234). Platelet aggregation and progressive thrombocytopenia have also been observed (235).

Another less effective regimen which may be employed in inhibitor management is the *pharmacological elevation of F-VIII* with deamino-D-arginine vasopressin (DDAVP) which has a number of drawbacks, however, such as tachyphylaxis, flushing, headaches, myocardial ischemia, and fluid retention (236).

One of the promising strategies employed in the management of F-VIII inhibitors is the use of *activated F-VII* (F-VIIa). Plasma derived F-VIIa has been successfully used (237), and a recombinant F-VIIa is now available and it has been used with success in a number of cases (peroperatively, treatment of life-threatening hematomata). Only mild adverse effects were observed. Recently, however, a case of disseminated intravascular coagulation in a hemophiliac treated with recF-VIIa has been described (238).

There has been some concern about the possible effect of F-VIII preparations on the immune system. In vitro experiments have shown immune suppressive effects by coagulation factor concentrates (239, 240) such as impairment of Fc-receptor-mediated phagocytosis and intracellular bacterial killing (241). Also inhibition of interleukin-2 production and impaired MLR and PHA-transformation has been demonstrated (242). These phenomena could be explained as caused by the presence of immune complexes and aggregated immunoglobulin copurified with F-VIII. A decrease in T4-lymphocytes has also been found. Whether these findings reflect a functional impairment of the immune system is still unclear.

If the modulation of certain immune functions is in fact due to contaminating components in the preparations one would expect that the new generation of very high purity F-VIII would behave differently. Highly purified F-VIII with a specific activity of 100—150 units/mg protein is now available, as is F-VIII purified by immunoaffinity chromatography using mouse monoclonal antibodies.

The virus-inactivating procedures now being used (chemical inactivation and/or wet-heat treatment) should provide coagulation factors with no risk of transmitting HIV and with a very high safety for hepatitis virus. All the same, the availability of recombinant F-VIII (rF-VIII) is considered a safer alternative. rF-VIII is structurally and immunologically similar to plasma-derived F-VIII, and it has been well tolerated in patients in clinical trials. A major concern, however, is a relatively high incidence of inhibitors (20%) which might be related to the monoclonality of rF-VIII (243).

PLASMA PROTEINS OF NON-HUMAN ORIGIN

Xenogeneic polyclonal immunoglobulins

Horse antisera to diphtheria (and later to tetanus as well) were produced and used in therapy from about the turn of the century. Such products have now been replaced almost entirely by plasma fractions of human origin. There are, however, a few situations where xenogeneic antisera are still in use, despite their many and often serious side effects.

Polyclonal antilymphocyte preparations (e.g. antilymphocyte globulin (ALG) and antithymocyte globulin (ATG)) have been developed based on the evidence that T-cells are primarily responsible for rejection of transplants. Indications for treatment with, e.g. horse ALG and/or ATG are very much the same as the indications for mouse monoclonal anti-T3 (OKT3): acute rejection of transplants, but also aplastic anemia (219, 317).

Short-term toxicity has been particularly marked in patients treated with ALG/ATG preparations from immunized horses (220). Immediate adverse effects include leukopenia and thrombocytopenia, fever, arthralgia, rash, urticaria, hepatotoxicity, hyperglycemia, hypertension and diarrhea (221). A somewhat later side effect is serum sickness. Many of the effects may be due to an induced elevation of tumor necrosis factor (222).

The longer-term effects of immunosuppression and, in particular, the residual hematological and immunological abnormalities in aplastic anemia patients treated with ALG have only recently been documented: toxicity to hematopoietic cells, eventually leading to clonal marrow diseases years after treatment (223). Four to 10 years after treatment, development of paroxysmal nocturnal hemoglobinuria, refractory sideroblastic anemia, chronic myelomonocytic leukemia, or acute leukemia is seen (224).

Rodent monoclonal antibodies

The therapeutic use of rodent (mouse or rat) monoclonal antibodies in vivo as against the use of human monoclonal antibodies is disadvantageous because the foreign nature of the antibody may induce immune responses, which will abrogate the effectiveness of the McAb and/or cause adverse reactions in the recipient. One report concludes that human anti-mouse immunoglobulin responses have limited the usefulness of murine McAb in more than half the patients treated (207). Human anti-mouse antibodies have been described both when monoclonal antibodies are used as a diagnostic tool in vivo and when used therapeutically (208—211).

Common side effects of treatment with monoclonal antibodies have included fever, chills and malaise (21—23% of cases), urticaria and pruritus (15—18%) (213).

The murine monoclonal antibody OKT3 directed against the CD3-structure on T-lymphocytes has proved to be an important therapeutic agent with potent immunosuppressive actions. It is used in reversing acute rejection episodes in kidney, heart, liver or pancreas allograft-rejections, and for GvH disease in bone marrow transplant recipients, when corticosteroids have failed, or to avoid ciclosporin nephrotoxicity and the inconvenience of polyclonal antilymphocyte globulins (214). Its extensive application justifies its consideration in discussing the side effects of rodent monoclonal antibodies. Despite its efficacy in over 90% of cases, this product causes a number of problems, such as fluid retention, acute pulmonary edema (215) and intense early effects which include fever, chills, nausea, vomiting, headache, and hypotension, the last of these being attributed to systemic vasodilation.

Other monoclonal antibodies against cell membrane markers (CD molecules) have been described. The side effects of such antibody preparations can be described as general side effects due to the administration of heterologous protein, or as an effect of the cell-targeting mechanisms (e.g. cell lysis).

Bovine serum albumin (*BSA*) is often used as protein supplement in cell growth media, and residual BSA has sometimes caused side effects. Symptoms are mild, such as itching and urticaria. An anaphylactic reaction has been described in a patient undergoing bone marrow transplantation where the patient's bone marrow cells had been kept in a BSA-containing medium. As a component in sperm-processing media, BSA has caused side effects after intrauterine insemination (330).

OTHER THERAPEUTIC PROTEINS, INCLUDING RECOMBINANT PRODUCTS

Fibrin glue Fibrin glue is a tissue adhesive containing fibrinogen and thrombin. It is a two-component system that contains highly concentrated fibrinogen, Factor VIII, fibronectin and traces of other plasma proteins in one component. The other component contains thrombin, calcium chloride, and antifibrinolytic agents, such as aprotinin. Mixing of the two components promotes clotting. Fibrin glue is used for tissue sealing, hemostasis and wound healing.

Only very few side effects to fibrin glue have been reported. An anaphylactic reaction has been described after the use of fibrin glue as a sealant after mastectomy, most likely due to the presence of bovine aprotinin (319). As most preparations of fibrin glue contain bovine thrombin, its administration may result in the development of anti-bovine thrombin antibodies. In a prospective study, 13 out of 34 patients developed a thrombin inhibitor and reduced Factor-V activity (316, 321). Another study (320) reported inhibitor to Factor-V after cardiac surgery.

Antithrombin III (AT-III) AT-III is a plasma α_2-glycoprotein that accounts for the major antithrombin activity in plasma and also inhibits other enzymes. Hereditary or acquired deficiency results in thromboembolism. Treatment with AT-III is still a matter of dispute (322, 323). Apart from vasodilatation, remarkably few side effects have been noticed.

α_1-Antitrypsin (α_1-proteinase inhibitor) This inhibitor neutralizes the activity of neutrophil elastase, and is used for the treatment of patients with a homozygous deficiency of α_1-antitrypsin (318). Adverse effects occur only rarely (318).

Erythropoietin Recombinant human erythropoietin (rHUEpo) has been in clinical use for more than 10 years. It has proved to be an effective form of therapy with a very favorable risk-benefit ratio in patients with end-stage chronic renal failure in hemodialysis, and in those with progressive renal failure who are not yet being dialyzed (244). Erythropoietin also opens up new opportunities in dealing with anemia in non-uremic patients such as patients with cancer, AIDS, and rheumatoid arthritis (325). Treatment with erythropoietin results in substantial improvement in rehabilitation and in the quality of life of such patients.

Earlier fears that the renal function of pre-dialysis patients on erythropoietin might deteriorate prematurely have not been realized (245), and to date there have been no reports of specific antibody formation (246). Although the retarded growth of pediatric patients with renal failure does not improve (246, 247), well-being, energy, appetite and cardiac function are enhanced, and by obviating the need for regular blood transfusion, iron overload, allo-immunization to cellular antigens and transfusion-transmitted viral infections are avoided (248).

The main limiting factor in obtaining an optimal response to erythropoietin is adequacy of the iron stores (249, 250). Other causes for an inadequate response to erythropoietin may be concurrent infection or inflammatory disease (244), aluminium toxicity and secondary hyperparathyroidism (251).

Acute adverse effects of erythropoietin, such as pruritus, flu-like symptoms, headache, bone or abdominal pain, myalgia, nausea, have been reported. The reactions are relatively mild and appear to be dose dependent as they occur less frequently when erythropoietin is given by subcutaneous application as compared to intravenous administration (252–254). Subcutaneous injection may lead to local reactions, probably due to hypersensitivity (324).

The most prominent problem appears to be hypertension and the sequelae thereof (255). It is only seen in uremic patients. There appear to be several factors contributing to this effect. One is the loss of hypoxic vasodilation response, leading to increased peripheral vascular resistance (256), but more important is the rise in blood viscosity, which increases with the hematocrit in both normotensive and hypertensive individuals in response to therapy (257). It is still being debated whether hypertension occurs only in patients with pre-existing hypertension or in normotensive patients as well, but approximately 30% of all patients require intensified or de novo antihypertensive therapy as they respond to erythropoietin treatment (258).

Hypertensive encephalopathy is a major concern (259, 324), often in connection with sudden and extreme rises in blood pressure which occur in some cases. It is not clear why certain patients develop these problems and others do not, but particular risk situations have been defined, above all transfusion-dependent anemic patients with low hematocrit (<20%). Careful control of blood pressure during the acute phase of erythropoietin treatment, and using low doses of erythropoietin is therefore advised in patients at high risk, such as those with previous hypertension and seizures, and the severely anemic.

Other less common side effects have been thrombotic events (260, 261). As the erythrocyte volume increases under the influence of erythropoietin, the clearance achieved by the dialyzer may fall, and there can as a consequence be an increase in creatine, potassium and phosphorous (262). Treatment of patients with sickle-cell anemia has led to disastrous sickling crises (263), and there are at present no clinical data to support the use of erythropoietin in sickle-cell disease (264).

CYTOKINES

Interferon

Interferon has now been in clinical use for almost 25 years. Interferon-α now has four recognized indications: hairy cell leukemia, chronic granulocytic leukemia, Kaposi's sarcoma and condylomata acuminata. Two recent reviews outline the therapeutical potential of interferons in therapy (265, 266). The various side effects described in connection with interferon therapy are multifaceted: influenza-like symptoms with fever, myalgia, arthralgia and lethargy, starting within 1 week after treatment was initiated and lasting 1—7 days, seem to be very common (267, 268). Development of neutralizing antibodies leading to resistance of patients with hairy cell leukemia and chronic myelogenous leukemia has been described (269, 270). The route of administration is important in provoking an antibody response, and recombinant interferon-β is more likely to be immunogenic when administered subcutaneously or intramuscularly than when given intravenously (271). Finally, development of Raynaud's phenomenon has been described (272) after treatment with interferon-α, and exacerbation of multiple sclerosis has been observed after treatment with interferon-γ.

Interleukin-2 is dealt with in Chapters 37/45 of this volume.

Colony-stimulating factors

Around 10 glycoprotein myeloid hemopoietic growth factors or colony-stimulating factors (CSFs) have so far been identified and purified, their genes have been cloned and active recombinant proteins have been produced. Recombinant factors derived from yeast or mammalian cells are glycosylated, as they are in their native state, whereas those expressed in bacterial systems are not. Glycosylation may be clinically relevant with regard to efficacy and antigenicity of the molecule, although antibody formation has not been observed, even after prolonged therapy (273). Most clinical studies with CSFs have hitherto been performed with granulocyte-macrophage CSF (GM-CSF) and granulocyte-CSF (G-CSF), although clinical trials using other CSFs have also started in a number of centers. GM-CSF leads to a dose-dependent, sustained increase of peripheral neutrophils, with a delayed increase in circulating monocytes and eosinophils. The effect of G-CSF appears to be more restricted to neutrophils. Multi-CSF (IL-3) stimulates production of all types of leukocytes, as well as platelets and reticulocytes (274).

GM-CSF This is the most widely used CSF clinically and is used to reduce chemotherapy-induced myelosuppression in patients with metastatic sarcoma, breast cancer or melanoma; to facilitate harvest of peripheral blood stem cells for autologous bone marrow transplantation; in cyclic neutropenia; to aid recovery after high doses of ionizing radiation; and, less successfully, for severe aplastic anemia. It has also been applied to patients with AIDS (275).

The generalized side effects of GM-CSF are dose-related and have usually been tolerable. They include bone pain (276), fever, myalgia, headache, thrombophlebitis, nausea, facial flushing and dyspnea (326). These effects are probably due to activation of secondary cytokines (such as TNF-α and IL-1) (277). These reactions occur in 40—60% of all treated patients (274). The first dose of GM-CSF may be followed within 3 hours by flushing, hypotension, tachycardia, dyspnea, musculoskeletal pain, nausea and vomiting (326). At very high doses (generally over 16 μg/kg/day), erythroderma, weight gain and edema with pleuro-pericardial effusions and ascites have been reported (278). Renal symptoms have also been described (279, 280), and various biochemical abnormalities, possibly due to secondary hyperaldosteronism (281—283). Cutaneous reactions to GM-CSF occur in about 50% of the patients and have been reviewed (284), the authors expressing concern that autoimmune skin diseases, psoriasis and other dermatoses might be exacerbated. Earlier fears that GM-CSF might give rise to progression of preleukemic conditions have not been substantiated (285).

G-CSF G-CSF—unlike GM-CSF—stimulates the proliferation of committed myeloid precursors, rather than pluripotent stem cells (328). In all clinical studies carried out to date, this CSF, whether given subcutaneously or intravenously, has been well tolerated, with few side effects other than bone pain (which occurs in about 20% of patients), myalgia, and fever, much as with GM-CSF-therapy (328). Increased spleen size has been reported (281, 286), and a neutrophilic dermatosis (Sweet's syndrome) has been described following G-CSF therapy in a case of hairy cell leukemia (287). Transient elevation of alkaline phosphatase, lactate dehydrogenase and uric acid are considered normal physiological consequences of the rise in neutrophil count (329).

HEMIN

Hemin (hematin), an exogenous source of heme, is used for the treatment of acute intermittent porphyria and other hepatic porphyrias. It is generally well tolerated in the recommended doses, though thrombophlebitis, coagulation defects, circulatory collapse and occasional renal failure have been reported (288). Thrombophlebitis is seen in up to 36% of patients, and this effect and also the effect on coagulation (prolongation of prothrombin and thromboplastin times, increased fibrin degradation products and thrombocytopenia) may well be caused by degradation products of hemin (289). There is evidence that slowing down the rate of infusion might lower the risk of side effects (290). Heme-arginate is more stable than hemin, but it is still not established whether side effects (thrombophlebitis, anaphylaxis and psychosis (327)) are fewer and the therapeutic effect more favorable than with hematin (291).

METALLO-PORPHYRINS

Kappas et al. were the first to show that synthetic tin protoporphyrin was effective as a specific inhibitor of heme-oxygenase in causing a decrease in plasma bilirubin levels both in adults and in neonates, and thereby preventing jaundice (292, 293). The work has been reviewed (294), and although the substance is not in fact a blood product it merits brief consideration here. A variety of heme analogs, such as tin, zinc, chromium and manganese metalloporphyrins, have been shown to be effective, via a competitive inhibition of cleavage of heme to biliverdin and carbon monoxide. Stannic porphyrins seem to be the most effective. The side effects are rather limited with only occasional erythema occurring, suggesting phototoxicity of these products.

REFERENCES

1. Patten E, Reddi CR, Riglin H et al. Delayed hemolytic transfusion reaction caused by a primary immune response. Transfusion 1982;22:248.
2. Ritchey AK, Andiman W, McIntosch S et al. Mononucleosis syndrome following granulocyte transfusion in patients with leukemia. J Pediatr 1980;97:267.
3. Linden JV, Paul B, Dressler KP. A report of 104 transfusion errors in New York State. Transfusion 1992;32:601—606.
4. Qutaishat S. Autologous blood transfusion: Evaluation of an alternative strategy in reducing exposure to allogeneic blood transfusion. Immunol Invest 1995;24:435—441.
5. Kasprisin DO, Glynn SH, Taylor F. Moderate and severe reactions in blood donors. Transfusion 1992;32:23—26.
6. Blackmore M. Minimising bruising in the antecubital fossa after venepuncture. Br Med J 1987;295:332.
7. Milman N, Sondergård M, Sorensen CM. Iron stores in female blood donors evaluated by serum ferritin. Blut 1985;51:337.
8. Pindyck J, Avorn J, Kuriyan M. Blood donation by the elderly: clinical and political considerations. J Am Med Assoc 1987;257:1186.
9. Boogaerts MA. Side effects of hemapheresis. Transfus Med Rev 1987;1:186.
10. Dolovich J, Sagona M, Pearson F. Sensitization of repeat plasmapheresis donors to ethylene oxide gas. Transfusion 1987;27:90.
11. Straus RG. Apheresis donor safety: changes in humoral and cellular immunity. J Clin Apheresis 1984;2:68—80.
12. Lewis SL, van Kutvirt SG, Simon TL. Investigation of the effect of long-term whole blood donation on immunologic parameters. Transfusion 1992;32:51—56.
13. Matsui Y, Martin-Alosco S, Doenges E. Effects of frequent and sustained platelet-apheresis on peripheral blood mononuclear cell populations and lymphocyte functions of normal volunteer donors. Transfusion 1986;26:447.
14. Morrow JF, Braine JG, Kickler TS et al. J Am Med Assoc 1991;266:555—558.
15. Blajchman MA. Bacterial contamination of blood products and the value of pre-transfusion testing. Immunol Invest 1995;24:163—170.
16. Blajchman MA, Ali AM. In: Nance SJ, ed. Blood Safety: Current challenges. Bethesda, MD: AABB, 1992;213—228.
17. Hogman CF, Fritz H, Sandberg L. Transfusion 1993; 33:189—191.
18. Hoppe PA. Interim measures for detection of bacterially contaminated red cell components. Transfusion 1992; 32:199—201.
19. Conrad ME. Diseases transmissible by blood transfusion: viral hepatitis and other infectious disorders. Semin Hematol 1981;18:122.
20. AIDS—The safety of Blood and Blood Products. Chichester—New York—Brisbane—Toronto—Singapore: J Wiley and Sons, 1987.
21. Berkman SA, Groopman JE. Transfusion associated AIDS. Transfus Med Rev 1988;2:18.
22. Sullivan MT, Williams AE, Fang CT et al. Arch Intern Med 1991;151:2043—2048.
23. Bove JR, Sandler SG. HTLV-1 and blood transfusion Transfusion 1988;28:93.
24. Morishima Y, Ohya K, Ueda R et al: Detection of adult T-cell leukemia virus (ATLV) bearing lymphocytes in concentrated red blood cells derived from ATL associated antibody (ATLA-Ab) positive donors. Vox Sang 1986; 50:212.
25. Sander S. HTLV-I and -II new risks for recipients of blood transfusion? J Am Med Assoc 1986;256:16.
26. Minamoto GY, Gold JWM, Scheinberg SG. Infection with human T-cell leukemia virus type 1 in patients with leukemia. N Engl J Med 1988;318:219.
27. Editorial: HTLV-I comes of age. Lancet 1988;i:217.
28. Nelson KE, Donahue JG, Munoz A et al. Ann Intern Med 1992;117:554—559.
29. Mannucci PM. Outbreak of Hepatitis A among Italian patients with haemophilia. Lancet 1992;339:819.
30. Robinson SM, Schwinn H, Smith A. Clotting factor and hepatitis A. Lancet 1992;340:1465—1466.
31. Seeberg S, Brandberg A, Hermodsson S et al. Hospital outbreak of hepatitis A secondary to blood exchange in a baby. Lancet 1981;ii:1155.
32. Barbara JAJ, Howell DR, Briggs M et al. Post-transfusion hepatitis. Lancet 1982;i:738.
33. Dodd RY. N Engl J Med 1992;327:419—421.
34. Brummelhuis HGJ, Over J, Duiris-Vorst CC et al. Contributions to the optimal use of human blood. IX. Elimination of hepatitis B transmission by (potentially) infectious plasma derivatives. Vox Sang 1983;45:205.
35. Tabor E, Aronson DL, Gerety RJ. Removal of hepatitis-B-virus infectivity from Factor-IX complex by hepatitis-B immunoglobulin: experiments in chimpanzees. Lancet 1980; ii:68.
36. Editorial: The evolution, implications and applications of the hepatitis B vaccine. J Am Med Assoc 1982;247:2272.

37. Szmunes W, Stevens SE. Hepatitis B vaccine: demonstration of efficacy in controlled trial in high risk population in the United States. N Engl J Med 1980;303:833.
38. Szmunes W, Stevens SE. Passive-active immunization against hepatitis B. Immunogenicity studies in adult Americans. Lancet 1981;i:575.
39. Nishioka NS, Dienstag JL. Delta hepatitis: a new scourge? N Engl J Med 1985;312:1515.
40. Hatzakis A, Hadziyannis S, Maclure M et al. Infection with hepatitis delta virus. N Engl J Med 1986;318:516.
41. Alter HC, Purcell RH, Shih HJ et al. Detection of antibody to hepatitis C virus in prospectively followed transfusion recipients with acute and chronic non-A, non-B hepatitis. N Engl J Med 1989;321:1494.
42. Tremolada F, Chiapetta F, Valfre C et al. Prospective study of posttransfusion hepatitis in cardiac surgery patients receiving only blood or also blood products. Vox Sang 1983;44:25.
43. Kiyosawa K, Akahane Y, Nagata A et al. The significance of blood transfusion in non-A, non-B chronic liver disease in Japan. Vox Sang 1982;43:45.
44. Realdi G, Alberti A, Rugge M et al. Long-term follow-up of acute and chronic non-A, non-B post-transfusion hepatitis: evidence of progression to liver cirrhosis. Gut 1982;23:270.
45. Choo QL, Kuo G, Weiner AJ et al. Isolation of a cDNA clone derived from a blood borne non-A, non-B viral hepatitis genome. Science 1989;244:359.
46. Dawson GJ, Lesniewski JL, Stewart KM et al. Detection of antibodies to hepatitis C virus in U.S. blood donors. J Clin Microbiol 1991;29:551.
47. Donahue JG, Munoz A, Ness PM et al. N Engl J Med 1992;327:369—373.
48. Kleinman S, Alter H, Busch M et al. Transfusion 1992;32:805—813.
49. Kiyosawa K, Tanaka E, Sodeyama T et al. Transition of antibody to hepatitis C virus from chronic hepatitis to hepatocellular carcinoma. Jpn J Cancer Res 1990;81:1089.
50. Silvergleid AJ, Kott TJ. Impact of cytomegalovirus testing on blood collection facilities. Vox Sang 1983;44:102.
51. Barbara J, Tegtmeier GE. Cytomegalovirus and blood transfusion. Blood Rev 1987;1:207.
52. Yeagar AS, Grumel FC, Afleigh EB et al. Prevention of transfusion acquired cytomegalovirus infection in newborn infants. J Pediatr 1981;98:281.
53. Kumar A, Nankervis GA, Cooper AR et al. Acquisition of cytomegalovirus infection in infants following exchange transfusion: a prospective study. Transfusion 1980;20:327.
54. Tegtmeier GT. The use of cytomegalovirus-screened blood in neonates. Transfusion 1988;28:201.
55. Bowden RA, Slichter SJ, Sayers MH et al. Blood 1991;78:246—250.
56. Eisenfeld L, Silver H, McLaughlin J et al. Transfusion 1992;32:205—209.
57. Smith KL, Cobain T, Dunstan RA. Br J Haematol 1993;83:640—642.
58. Cohen BJ, Field AM, Gudnadottir S et al. J Virol Methods 1990;30:233—238.
59. McOmish F, Yap PL, Jordan A et al. J Clin Microbiol 1993;31:323—328.
60. Petersen LR, Satten GA, Dodd R et al. Transfusion 1994;34:283—289.
61. Busch MP. Retroviruses and blood transfusion: The lessons learned and the challenge yet ahead. In: Nance ST, ed. Blood Safety: Current Challenges. Bethesda: American Association of Blood Banks, 1992;1—44.
62. Anonymous. AIDS due to HIV-2 infection. Morbid Mortal Wkly Rep 1988;37:33.
63. Broder S. Pathogenic human retroviruses. N Engl J Med 1988;318:243.
64. Seyfried H, Walewska I. Immune hemolytic transfusion reactions. World J Surg 1987;11:25.
65. Glicher RO. Immune hemolytic transfusion reactions and pseudohemolytic transfusion reactions. Plasma Ther Transfus Technol 1985;6:7.
66. Greenwalt TJ. Pathogenesis and management of hemolytic transfusion reactions. Semin Hematol 1981;11:25.
67. Povosky MA, Chaplin HC, Moore SB. Transfusion-related acute lung injury: a neglected serious complication of hemotherapy. Transfusion 1992;32:589—591.
68. DeVirgillis S, Galanello R, Cao A. *Plasmodium malariae* transfusion malaria in splenectomized patients with thalassemia major. J Pediatr 1981;98:584.
69. Cook GC. Prevention and treatment of malaria. Lancet 1988;i:32.
70. Gilcher RO, Belcher L. Posttransfusion malaria—a new look. Transfusion 1981;21:611.
71. Harrison CR, Hayes TC, Trow LL. Intravascular hemolytic transfusion reaction without detectable antibodies: a case report and review of literature. Vox Sang 1986;51:96.
72. Isbister JP. Blood transfusion and blood component therapy. Clin Anaesthesiol 1984;2:643.
73. Molthan L. Intravascular hemolytic transfusion reaction due to anti-Vw + Mia with fatal outcome. Vox Sang 1981; 40:105.
74. Baldwin ML, Barrasso C, Gavin J. The first example of a Raddon-like antibody as a cause of a transfusion reaction. Transfusion 1980;21:86.
75. Goman MI, Glidden HM. Another example of anti-Tca. Transfusion 1981;21:579.
76. Lee EL, Bennett C. Anti-Cob which caused acute hemolytic transfusion reaction. Transfusion 1980;22:150.
77. Kurtz SR, Kuszaj Z, Quellet R et al. Survival of homozygous Coa (Colton) red cells in a patient with anti-Coa1. Vox Sang 1982;43:28.
78. Patten E, Reddi CR, Riglin H et al. Delayed hemolytic transfusion reaction caused by a primary immune response. Transfusion 1982;22:248.
79. Pineda AA, Taswell HF, Brzica SM. Delayed hemolytic transfusion reaction: an immunologic hazard of blood transfusion. Transfusion 1978;18:1.
80. Moore SB, Taswell HF, Pineda AA et al. Delayed hemolytic transfusion reactions: evidence of the need for an improved pretransfusion compatibility test. Am J Clin Pathol 1980;74:94.
81. Barton GC. Nonhemolytic, noninfectious transfusion reactions. Semin Hematol 1981;18:95.
82. Taddie SJ, Barrasso C, Ness PM. A delayed transfusion reaction caused by anti-K6. Transfusion 1982;22:68.
83. Waheed A, Kennedy MS. Delayed hemolytic transfusion reaction caused by anti-Jsb in a Js(a+b+) patient. Transfusion 1982;22:161.
84. Boyland IP, Mufti GJ, Hamblin TJ. Delayed hemolytic transfusion reaction caused by anti-Fyb in a spenectomized patient. Transfusion 1982;22:402.
85. Contreras M, Hazelhurst GR, Armitage SE. Develop-

ment of 'auto-anti-A1-antibodies' following alloimmunisation in an A2 recipient. Br J Haematol 1983;55:657.
86. Coles SM, Klein HG, Holland PV. Alloimmunization in two multitransfused patient populations. Transfusion 1981; 21:462.
87. Diamond WJ, Brown FL Jr, Bitterman P et al. Delayed hemolytic transfusion reaction presenting as sickle-cell crisis. Ann Int Med 1980;93:231.
88. Beattie KM, Sigmund KE, McGraw J et al. U-variant blood in sickle cell patients. Transfusion 1982;22:257.
89. Davey RJ, Simpkins SS. 51-Chromium survival of Yt(a+) red cells as determinant of the in vivo significance of anti-Yta. Transfusion 1981;21:702.
90. Davey RJ, Gustafson M, Holland PV. Accelerated immune red cell destruction in the absence of serologically detectable alloantibodies. Transfusion 1980;20:348.
91. Whitsett CF, Pierce JA. Red cell destruction in the absence of detectable antibody. Transfusion 1981;21:474.
92. Mollison PL. Survival curves of incompatible red cells. Transfusion 1986;26:43.
93. Rosenfield RE. Two types of delayed hemolytic transfusion reaction. Transfusion 1985;25:182.
94. Salama A, Mueller-Eckhardt C. Letter. Transfusion 1985;25:182.
95. Rivera R, Scornik JC. HLA antigens on red cells. Transfusion 1986;26:376.
96. Ballas SK, Bosch J, Miguel O. Passive transfer of anti-E antibody. Transfusion 1981;21:758.
97. West NC, Jenkins JA, Johnston BR et al. Interdonor incompatibility due to anti-Kell antibody undetectable by automated antibody screening. Vox Sang 1986;50:176.
98. Dzik WH, Kirkly SA. Citrate toxicity during massive blood transfusion. Transfus Med Rev 1988;2:176.
99. Hey E, Scopes JW. Thermoregulation in the newborn. In: Avery CB, ed. Neonatology, 3rd edn. Philadelphia: JP Lippincott, 1987;201.
100. Heinrichs C. Hämostasedefekte nach Transfusionen. Anaesthesiol Reanima 1982;7:245.
101. Harke H, Rahmann S. Hemostatic disorders in massive transfusion. Bibl Haematol 1980;46:179.
102. Manucci PM, Federici A, Sirchia G. Hemostasis testing during massive blood replacement: a study of 172 cases. Vox Sang 1982;42:113.
103. Valeri CR, Zaroulis CG, Vecchione JJ et al. Therapeutic effectiveness and safety of outdated human red cells rejuvenated to restore oxygen transport function to normal, frozen 3—4 years at −80°C, washed and stored at 4°C for 24 hours prior to rapid infusion. Transfusion 1980;20:159.
104. Halliday JW, Powell LW. Iron overload. Semin Hematol 1982;19:42.
105. Pippard MJ, Callender ST, Finch CA. Ferrioxamine excretion in iron-loaded man. Blood 1982;60:288.
106. Parry ES, Thomas MJG, Marcus RE et al. Characterization and transfusion of young erythrocytes. Br J Haematol 1982;50:701.
107. Graziano JH, Piomelli S, Seaman C et al. A simple technique for preparation of young red cells for transfusion from ordinary blood units. Blood 1982;59:865.
108. Yang O, Hugh MD, Lichtiger B. Transfusion reactions in patients with cancer. Am J Clin Pharmacol 1987;2:253.
109. Maclntyre A, Gray JD, Gorelock M et al. Salicylate and acetaminophen in donated blood. Can Med Assoc J 1986;135:215.
110. US Dept of Health and Human Services Food and Drug Administration: The Code of Federal Regulations. Title 21, Part 606. FDA, 1987.
111. Koerner K, Kubanek B. Comparison of three different methods used in the preparation of leukocyte-poor platelet concentrates. Vox Sang 1987;53:26.
112. McCullogh J, Clay M, Kline W. Granulocyte antigens and antibodies. Transfus Med Rev 1987;1:150.
113. McCullogh J. The clinical significance of granulocyte antibodies and in vivo studies of the fate of granulocytes. In: Garratty G, ed. Current Concepts in Transfusion Therapy. Arlington, VA: American Association of Blood Banks, 1985;125.
114. McCullogh J, Clay M, Loken M et al. Effect of ABO incompatibility on the fate in vivo of 111-Indium granulocytes. Transfusion 1988;28:258.
115. Ness PM, Frey E, Perkins HA. Improved blood utilization with leukocyte-poor cell masses (LPCM) prepared by cell washing. Transfusion 1981;21:124.
116. Menitove JE, McElligot MC, Aster RH. Febrile transfusion reaction: What blood component should be given next? Vox Sang 1982;42:318.
117. Liedén G, Hildén J-O. Febrile transfusion reactions reduced by of buffy-coat-poor erythrocyte concentrates. Vox Sang 1982;43:263.
118. Hughes ASB, Brozovic B. Leucocyte depleted blood: an appraisal of available techniques. Br J Haematol 1982; 50:381.
119. Goldfinger D, Lowe C. Prevention of adverse reactions to blood transfusion by the administration of saline-washed red blood cells. Transfusion 1981;21:277.
120. Sirchia G, Parravicini A, Rebulla P et al. Effectiveness of red blood cells filtered through cotton wool to prevent antileukocyte antibody production in multitransfused patients. Vox Sang 1982;42:190.
121. Arnold R, Pflieger H, Wiesneth M et al. In vitro and in vivo studies on filter collected granulocytes. Scand J Haematol 1981;26:31.
122. Highy DJ, Burnett D. Granulocyte transfusions: current status. Blood 1980;55:2.
123. Huestis DW. Leukapheresis and granulocyte transfusion. Haematologia 1982; 15:39.
124. Karp DD, Ervin TJ, Tuttle S et al. Pulmonary complication during granulocyte transfusions: incidence and clinical features. Vox Sang 1982;42:57.
125. National Institutes of Health Consensus Conference: Platelet transfusion therapy. Transfus Med Rev 1987;1:195.
126. Editorial.: Platelet transfusion therapy. Lancet 1987; ii:490.
127. Seidl S, Kilp M. The current status of platelet and granulocyte transfusions. Haematologia 1980;13:145.
128. Kutti J, Zaroulis CG, Dinsmore RE et al. A prospective study of platelet-transfusion therapy administered to patients with acute leukemia. Transfusion 1982;22:44.
129. Eernisse JG, Brand A. Prevention of platelet refractoriness due to HLA antibodies by administration of leukocyte-poor blood components. Exp Hematol 1981;9:77.
130. Sirchia G, Parravicini A, Rebulla P et al. Preparation of leukocyte-free platelets for transfusion by filtration through cotton wool. Vox Sang 1983;44:115.
131. Murphy MF, Waters AH. Immunological aspects of platelet transfusions. Br J Haematol 1985;60:409.
132. Scott EP, Moilan-Bergeland J, Dalmasso AP. Posttransfusion thrombocytopenia associated with passive transfusion of a platelet-specific antibody. Transfusion 1988;28:73.

133. Mueller-Eckhardt C, Lechner K, Heinrich D et al. Post-transfusion thrombocytopenic purpura: immunological and clinical studies in two cases and review of the literature. Blut 1980;40:249.
134. Vogelsang G, Kickler TS, Bell WR. Posttransfusion purpura. Am J Hematol 1986;21:259.
135. Mueller-Eckhardt C. Post-transfusion purpura. Br J Haematol 1986;64:419.
136. Stricker RB, Lewis BH, Corash L et al. Posttransfusion purpura associated with an autoantibody directed against a previously undefined platelet antigen. Blood 1987;69:1458.
137. Kickler TS, Ness PM, Herman JH et al. Studies of the patophysiology of posttransfusion purpura. Blood 1986; 68:347.
138. DeWaal LP, Van Dalen CM, Engelfriet CP et al. Alloimmunization against the platelet-specific Zwa antigen, resulting in neonatal alloimmune thrombocytopenia or post-transfusion purpura, is associated with the supertypic DRw52 antigen including DR3 and DRw6. Hum Immunol 1986; 17:45.
139. Ovesen H, Taaning E, Christensen BA. Post-transfusion purpura (PTP) caused by anti-Zwa (PLA2). Ugeskr Laeg 1986;148:2769.
140. Chapman JF, Murphey MF, Berney SI et al. Post-transfusion purpura associated with anti Bak[a] and anti-PL^{A2} platelet antibodies and delayed haemolytic transfusion reaction. Vox Sang 1987;52:313.
141. Slichter SJ. Post-transfusion purpura: response to steroids and association with red blood cell and lymphocytotoxic antibodies. Br J Haematol 1982;50:599.
142. Von Fliedner V, Highby DJ, Kim U. Graft-versus-host reaction following blood product transfusion. Am J Med 1982;72:951.
143. Pflieger H. Graft-versus-host disease following blood transfusions. Blut 1983;46:61.
144. Schmitz N, Kayser W, Gassmann W et al. Two cases of graft-versus-host disease following transfusion of nonirradiated blood products. Blut 1982;44:83.
145. Lauer BA, Githens JH, Hayward AR et al. Probable graft-vs-graft reaction in an infant after exchange transfusion and marrow transplantation. Pediatrics 1982;70:43.
146. Ritchey AK, Andiman W, McIntosch S et al. Mononucleosis syndrome following granulocyte transfusion in patients with leukemia. J Pediatr 1980;97:267.
147. Weiden PL, Zuckerman N, Hansen JA et al. Fatal graft-versus-host disease in a patient with lymphoblastic leukemia following normal granulocyte transfusions. Blood 1981; 57:328.
148. Schmiedmaier W, Feil W, Gebhart W et al. Fatal graft-versus-host reaction following granulocyte transfusions. Blut 1982;290:658.
149. Sloane JP, Thomas JA, Imrie SF et al. Morphological and immunohistological changes in the skin in allogeneic bone marrow recipients. J Clin Pathol 1984;37:919.
150. Slichter SJ. Transfusion and bone marrow transplantation. Transfus Med Rev 1988;2:1.
151. McDonald GB, Shulman HM, Sullivan KM et al. Intestinal and hepatic complications of human bone marrow transplantation. I. Gastroenterology 1986;90:460.
152. Carl W, Higby DJ. Oral manifestations of bone marrow transplantation. Am J Oncol 1985;8:81.
153. Filipovich AH, Krawczak CL, Kersey JH et al. Graft-versus host-disease prophylaxis with anti-T-cell monoclonal antibody OKT3, prednisone and methotrexate in allogeneic bone-marrow transplantation. Br J Haematol 1985;60:143.
154. Brenner MK, Wimperis JZ, Reittie JE et al. Recovery of immunoglobulin isotypes following T-cell depleted allogeneic bone marrow transplantation. Br J Haematol 1986; 64:125.
155. Winston DJ, Huang ES, Miller MJ et al. Molecular epidemiology of cytomegalovirus infection associated with bone marrow transplantation. Ann Intern Med 1985;1102:16.
156. Grob JP, Prentice HG, Hoffbrand AV et al. Immune donors can protect marrow-transplant recipients from severe cytomegalovirus infections. Lancet 1987;i:774.
157. Davis J, Rowley S, Braine H et al. Toxicity of bone marrow graft infusions. Transfusion 1987;27:551.
158. Storb R, Weiden PL. Transfusion problems associated with transplantation. Semin Hematol 1981;18:163.
159. Singal DP, Ludwin D, Blajchman MA. Blood transfusion and renal transplantation. Br J Haematol 1985;61:595.
160. Whelchel JD, Shaw JF, Curtis JJ et al. Effect of pretransplant stored donor-specific blood transfusions on early renal allograft survival in one-haplotype living transplant. Transplantation 1982;34:326.
161. Light JA, Metz S, Oddenino K et al. Donor-specific transfusion with diminished sensitization. Transplantation 1982;34:352.
162. Mangal AK, Sinclair M et al. Acquired hemolytic anemia due to 'auto'-anti-A or 'auto'-anti-B induced by group 0 homograft in renal transplant recipients. Transfusion 1984; 24, 201.
163. Bracey AW, Van Buren C. Immune anti-A_1 in A_2 recipients of kidneys from group O donors. Transfusion 1986; 26:282.
164. Herron R, Clark M, Tate D et al. Immune hemolysis in a renal transplant recipient due to antibodies with anti-c specificity. Vox Sang 1986:51:226.
165. Bracey AW. Anti-A of donor lymphocyte origin in three recipients of organs from the same donor. Vox Sang 1987; 53:181.
166. Mangal AK, Growe GH, Sinclair M et al. Development of 'auto'-anti-A antibodies following alloimmunisation in an A_2 recipient. Br J Haematol 1984;571:714.
167. Hows J, Beddow K, Gordon-Smith E et al. Donor-derived red blood cell antibodies and immune hemolysis after allogeneic bone marrow transplantation. Blood 1986;67:177.
168. Heim MU, Schleuning M, Eckstein R et al. Rh antibodies against the pretransplant red cells following Rh-incompatible bone marrow transplantation. Transfusion 1988; 28:272.
169. Wenz B, Barland P. Therapeutic intensive plasmapheresis. Semin Hematol 1981:18:147.
170. Heal JM, Bailey G, Helphingstine C et al. Non-centrifugal plasma collection using cross-flow membrane plasmapheresis. Vox Sang 1983;44:156.
171. Wiltbank TB, Castino F, Grapka BH et al. Filtration plasmapheresis in vivo. Transfusion 1981;21:502.
172. Braunstein AH, Oberman HA. Transfusion of plasma components. Transfusion 1984; 24, 281. Transfusion 1984; 24:281.
173. Ring J, Messmer K. Incidence and severity of anaphylactoid reactions to colloid volume substitutes. Lancet 1977; i:466.
174. National Institutes of Health Consensus Conference: Fresh frozen plasma: indications and risks. Transfus Med Rev 1987;1:201.
175. Jones J. Abuse of fresh frozen plasma. Br Med J 1987;295:287.

176. Edelman BB, Straughn MA, Getz P et al. Uneventful plasma exchange with albumin replacement in a patient with a previous reaction to albumin. Transfusion 1985;25:435.
177. Stafford CT, Lobel SA, Fruge BC et al. Anaphylaxis to human serum albumin. Ann Allerg 1988;61:85.
178. Naylor DH, Anhorn CA, Laschinger C et al. Antigenic differences between normal human albumin and a genetic variant. Transfusion 1982;22:128.
179. El Habib R, Eygonnet JP. Aluminium bone disease. Br Med J 1987;295:1415.
180. Maharaj D, Fell GS, Boyce BF et al. Aluminium bone disease in patients receiving plasma exchange with contaminated albumin. Br Med J 1987;295:693.
181. X,X.: Encephalopathy. Encephalopathy 1992;(in press).
182. Cuthbertson B, Rennie JG, Aw D. Safety of albumin preparations manufactured from plasma not tested for HIV antibody. Lancet 1987;ii:41.
183. Hassig A. Intravenous immunoglobulins: pharmacological aspects and therapeutic use. Vox Sang 1986;51:10.
184. Björkander J. Antibody deficiency syndromes. Sweden, Thesis. University of Göteborg, 1985.
185. Avoy DR. Delayed serum sickness-like transfusion reactions in a multiply transfused patient. Vox Sang 1981;41:239.
186. Lucas GS, Jobbins K, Bloom AL. Intravenous immunoglobulin and blood-group antibodies. Lancet 1987;ii:742.
187. Brox AG, Cournoyer D, Sternbach M et al. Hemolytic anemia following intravenous gamma globulin administration. Am J Med 1987;82:633.
188. Hopkins SJ. Sandoglobulin. Drugs Today 1985;21:277.
189. Ball S, Zuiable A, Roter BLT et al. Changes in platelet immunoprotein levels during therapy in adult immune thrombocytopenia. Br J Haematol 1985;60:631—633.
190. Dammacco F, Iodice G, Campobasso N. Treatment of adult patients with idiopathic thrombocytopenic purpura with intravenous immunoglobulin: effects on circulating T cell subsets and PWM-induced antibody synthesis in vitro. Br J Haematol 1986;62:125.
191. Williams PE, Yap PL, Gillon J et al. Non-A,non-B hepatitis transmission by intravenous immunoglobulin. Lancet 1988;ii:501.
192. Cunningham-Rundles C. Intravenous immune serum globulin in immunodeficiency. Vox Sang 1985;49(Suppl)1:8.
194. Hachimi-ldrissi S, de Schepper J, De Waele M et al. Type III allergic reaction after infusion of immunoglobulins. Lancet 1990;336:55.
195. McCluskey DR, Boyd NAM. Anaphylaxis with intravenous gamma globulin. Lancet 1990;ii:874.
196. Imbach P, Barandum S, D'Apuzzo V et al. High-dose intravenous gamma globulin for idiopathic thrombocytopenic purpura in childhood. Lancet 1981;i:1228.
197. Jordan SC. Intravenous gamma globulin therapy in systemic lupus erythematosus and immune complex disease. Clin Immunol Immunopathol 1989;53:S164.
198. Myer I, Andler W. Die Behandlung der idiopathischen thrombozytopenischen Purpura. Krankenhausarzt 1987; 60:105.
199. Frame WD, Crawford RJ. Thrombotic events after intravenous immunoglobulin. Lancet 1986;ii:468.
200. Mitchell AD, De Villez R. Alopecia after immunoglobulin infusion. Lancet 1987;i:1436.
201. Chan-Lam D, Fitzsimons EJ, Douglas WS. Alopecia after immunoglobulin infusion. Lancet 1987;i:1436.
202. Ballow M. Mechanisms of action of intravenous immune serum globulin therapy and potential use in auto-immune connective tissue diseases. Cancer 1991;(in press).
203. Woodruff RKe, Grigg AP, Firkin FC et al. Fatal thrombotic events during treatment of autoimmune thrombocytopenia with intravenous immunoglobulin in elderly patients. Lancet 1986;ii:217.
204. Schifferli J, Leski M, Faure H et al. High dose intravenous IgG treatment and renal function. Lancet 1991;337:457.
205. Jayne DRW, Davies MJ, Fox CJV et al. Treatment of systemic vasculitis with pooled intravenous immunoglobulin. Lancet 1991;337:1137.
206. Barton JC, Herrera GA, Galla JH et al. Acute cryoglobulinemic renal failure after intravenous infusion of gamma globulin. Am J Med 1987;82:624.
207. Larrick JW, Bourla JM. Prospects for the therapeutic use of human monoclonal antibodies. J Biol Response 1986;5:379.
208. Courtnay-Luck NS, Epenetos AA, Moore R et al. Development of primary and secondary immune responses to mouse monoclonal antibodies used in the diagnosis and therapy of malignant neoplasms. Cancer Res 1986;46:6489.
209. Scoff RW, Foon KA, Beatty SM et al. Human antimurin immunoglobulin responses in patients receiving monoclonal antibody therapy. Cancer Res 1985;45:879.
210. Shawler DL, Bartholomew RM, Smith LM et al. Human immune response to multiple injections of murine monoclonal IgG. J Immunol 1985;135:1530.
211. Reynolds JC, Vecchio SD, Sakara H et al. Antimurine antibody response to mouse monoclonal antibodies: clinical findings and implications. Nucl Med Biol 1989;16:121.
212. Lightner DJ, Vessella RL, Chiou RK et al. Immunotherapy for renal cell carcinoma: recent results. World J Urol 1986;4:222.
213. Dillman RO, Beauregard JC, Halpern SE et al. Toxicities and side effects associated with intravenous infusions of monoclonal antibodies. J Biol Response 1986;5:73.
214. Burke GW, Vercellotti GM, Simmons RL et al. Reversible pancytopenia following OKT3. Transplantation 1989; 48:403.
215. Lee CW, Logan JL, Zukoski CF. Cardiovascular collapse following orthoclone OKT3 administration: a case report. Am J Kidney Dis 1991;17:73.
216. Ziegler EJ, Fisher CJ, Spring CL et al. Treatment of gram-negative bacteraemia and septic shock with HA-1A human monoclonal antibody against endotoxin. N Engl J Med 1991;324:429—436.
217. Khazaeli MB, Wheeler R, Teng N et al. Initial evaluation of a human immunoglobulin M monoclonal antibody (HA-1A) in humans. J Biol Response Modif 1990;9:178.
218. Fisher CJ, Zimmerman J, Khazaeli MB et al. Initial evaluations of human monoclonal anti-lipid A antibody (HA-1A) in patients with sepsis syndrome. Crit Care Med 1990; 18:1311.
219. Editorial: Immunosuppression in aplastic anaemia—postponing the inevitable. N Engl J Med 1991;324:1358.
220. Kawano Y, Nissen G, Gratwohl A et al. Cytotoxic and stimulatory effects of antilymphocyte globulin (ALG) on haematopoiesis. Blut 1990;60:297.
221. Frickhofen N, Kaltwasser JP, Schrezenmeier H et al. Treatment of aplastic anaemia with antilymphocyte globulin and methyl prednisolone with or without cyclosporine. N Engl J Med 1991;324:1297.
222. Debets JM, Leunissen KML, van Hoof HF et al. Evi-

dence of involvement of tumor necrosis factor in adverse reactions during treatment of kidney allograft rejection with antilymphocyte globulin. Transplantation 1989;47:487.
223. Kawano Y, Nissen C, Grathwohl A et al. Cytotoxic and stimulatory effects of antilymphocyte globulin (ALG) on haematopoiesis. Blut 1990;60:297.
224. de Planque MH, Brand A, Kluin-Nelemans HC et al. Haematologic and immunologic abnormalities in severe aplastic anaemia patients treated with anti-thymocyte globulin. Br J Haematol 1989;71:421.
225. Hasegawa DK, Edson J. Detection of Factor VIII and IX inhibitors after first exposure to heat-treated concentrates. Lancet 1987;i:449.
226. Pasi KJ, Hamon MD, Perry DJ et al. Factor VIII and IX inhibitors after exposure to heat-treated concentrates. Lancet 1987;1:689.
227. Van Leeuwen EF, Mauser Bunschoten EP, Van Dijken PJ et al. Disappearance of factor VIII:C antibodies in patients with haemophilia A upon frequent administration of factor VIII in intermediate or low dose. Br J Haematol 1986;64:291.
228. Kemball-Cook G, Barrowcliffe TW. Factor VIII concentrates contain factor VIII procoagulant antigen bound to phospholipid. Br J Haematol 19 86;63:425.
229. Chandra S, Brummelhuis HGJ. Prothrombin complex concentrates for clinical use. Vox Sang 1981;41:257.
230. Fuerth JH, Mahrer P. Myocardial infarction after Factor IX therapy. J Am Med Assoc 1981;245:1455.
231. Small M, Lowe GDO, Douglas JT et al. Factor IX thrombogenicity: in vitro effect on coagulation activation and a case report of disseminated intravascular coagulation. Thromb Haemost 1982;48:76.
232. Abilgaard CF, Penner JA, Watson-Williams EJ. Anti-inhibitor coagulant complex (Autoplex) for treatment of Factor-VIII inhibitors in hemophilia. Blood 1980;56:978.
233. Rodeghiero F, Castronovo S, Dini E. Disseminated intravascular coagulation after infusion of FEIBA (Factor VIII Inhibitor Bypassing Activity) in a patient with acquired haemophilia. Thromb Haemost 1982;48:339.
234. Brettler DB, Forsberg AD, Levine PH et al. The use of porcine Factor VIII (Hyate:C) in the treatment of patients with inhibitor antibodies to Factor VIII. Arch Intern Med 1989;149:1381.
235. Green D, Tuite GF. Declining platelet counts and platelet aggregation during porcine VIII:C infusions. Am J Med 1989;86:222.
236. Manucci PM, Lusher JM. Desmopressin and thrombosis. Lancet 1989;ii:675.
237. Hedner U, Kisiel W. Use of human Factor VIIa in the treatment of two haemophilia A patients with high titre inhibitors. J Clin Invest 1983;71:1836.
238. Stein SF, Duncan A, Cutler D et al. Disseminated intravascular coagulation (DIC) in a haemophiliac treated with recombinant Factor VIIa. Blood 1990;76:438a.
239. Carr R, Edmund E, Prescott RJ et al. Abnormalities of circulating lymphocyte subsets in haemophiliacs in an AIDS-free population. Lancet 1984;i:1431.
240. Aledort LM. Blood products and immunological changes: impacts without AIDS infection. Semin Hematol 1988;25:14.
241. Mannhalter JW, Ahmad R, Leibl H. Comparable modulation of human monocyte functions by commercial F.VIII concentrates of varying purity. Blood 1988;71:1662.
242. Thorpe R, Dilger P, Dawson NJ et al. Inhibition of interleukin-2 secretion by Factor VIII concentrate: a possible cause of immunosuppression in haemophiliacs. Br J Haematol 1989;71:387.
243. Inhibitors after recFVIII therapy. Blood 1992.
244. Adamson JW, Eschback JW. The use of recombinant erythropoietin (rHUEpo) in humans. Cancer Surv 1990; 9:157.
245. Eschback JW, MacDougall IC. Correction of anemia in progressive renal failure with recombinant human erythropoietin. N Engl J Med 1989;321:158.
246. Watson AJ. Adverse effects of therapy for the correction of anaemia in haemodialysis patients. Semin Nephrol 1989;9:30.
247. Fischback M, Simeoni U, Mengus L et al. Le genie genetique au service de l'anemi renale. J Med Strasbourg 1990;21:433.
248. Offner G, Hoyer PF, Latta K et al. One year's experience with recombinant erythropoietin in children undergoing continuous ambulatory or cycling peritoneal dialysis. Pediatr Nephrol 1990;4:498.
249. Fischer JW, Bonner J, Eschback J et al. Statement on the clinical use of recombinant erythropoietin in anaemia of end-stage renal disease. Am J Kidney Dis 1989;14:163.
250. McMahon LP, Dawborn JK. Experience with low-dose intravenous and subcutaneous administration of recombinant human erythropoietin. Am J Nephrol 1990;10:404.
251. Eschback JW, Adamson J,W.: Anemia of end-stage renal disease (ESRD). Kidney Int 1985;28:1.
252. Winearls CHG, Oliver DO, Pippard MJ et al. Effects of human erythropoietin derived from recombinants DNA on the anemia of patients maintained by chronic haemodialysis. Lancet 1986;ii:1175.
253. Freuken LAM, Koene RPA. Recombinant human erythropoietin and the effects of different routes of administration. Nephrologia 1990;10:33.
254. McMahon LP, Dawborn K. Experience with low-dose intravenous and subcutaneous administration of recombinant human erythropoietin. Am J Nephrol 1990;10:404.
255. Frei U, Nonnast-Daniel B, Koch KM. Erythropoietin and hypertension (in German). Klin Wochenschr 1988; 66:914.
256. Raine AE. Seizures and hypertensive events. Semin Nephrol 1990;10:40.
257. Levin N. Management of blood pressure changes during recombinant human erythropoietin therapy. Semin Nephrol 1989;9:16.
258. Eschback JW, Kelly MR, Haley NR et al. Correction of anaemia in progressive renal failure with recombinant human erythropoietin (rHUEpo). N Engl J Med 1989; 321:158.
259. Tomson CRV, Venning MC, Ward MK. Blood pressure and erythropoietin. Lancet 1988;i:351.
260. Koppensteiner R, Stockenhuber F, Jahn C et al. Changes in determinants of blood rheology during treatment with haemodialysis and recombinant human erythropoietin. Br Med J 1990;300:1626.
261. MacDougall IC, Hutton RD, Cavill I et al. Treating renal anaemia with recombinant human erythropoietin: practical guidelines and a clinical algorithm. Br Med J 1990; 300:655.
262. Zehnder C. Erythropoietin treatment: Influence of hemoglobin concentration on dialyser creatinine clearance in haemodialysed patients. 1996;(in press).
263 Barber WH. Fetal hemoglobin and erythropoietin. N Engl J Med 1987;318:449.

264. Williamson PJ. Erythropoietin. Transfus Sci 1991;12:15.
265. Galvani D, Griffiths SD, Cawley JC. Interferon for treatment: the dust settles. Br Med J 1988;296:1554.
266. Merigan TC. Human interferon as a therapeutic agent. N Engl J Med 1988;318:1458.
267. Giles FJ, Gray A, Brozovic M. Alpha-interferon therapy for essential thrombocytaemia. Lancet 1988;ii:70.
268. Alexander GJM, Fagan EA, Daniels HM et al. Loss of HBsAg with interferon therapy in chronic hepatitis B virus infection. Lancet 1987;ii:66.
269. Inglada L, Porres JC, La Banda F et al. Anti-lFN-titres during interferon therapy. Lancet 1987;ii:1521.
270. Steis RG, Smith JW, Urba WJ et al. Resistance to recombinant interferon alpha-2a in a hairy cell leukemia associated with neutralizing anti-interferon antibodies. N Engl J Med 1988;318:1409.
271. Konrad MW, Childs AL, Merigan TC et al. Assessment of the antigenic response in humans to recombinant mutant interferon beta. J Clin Immunol 1987;7:365.
272. Roy V, Newland AC. Raynaud's phenomenon and cryoglobulinaemia associated with the use of recombinant human alpha-interferon. Lancet 1988;i:944.
273. Sieff CA. Haemopoietic growth factors: in vitro and in vivo studies. In: Hoffbrand AV, ed. Recent Advances in Haematology. London: Churchill Livingstone, 1988;1.
274. Klingemann HG, Shepherd JD, Eaves CJ et al. The role of erythropoietin and other growth factors in transfusion medicine. Transfus Med Rev 1991;5:33.
275. Brito-Babapule F. Therapeutic applications of the myeloid haematopoietic growth factors. Transfus Sci 1991;12:25.
276. Devereux S, Bull HA, Campos-Costa D et al. Granulocyte macrophage colony stimulating factor induced changes in cellular adhesion, molecule expression and adhesion to endothelium: in vitro and in vivo studies in man. Br J Haematol 1989;71:323.
277. Devereux S, Lynch CD. Granulocyte macrophage colony stimulating factor Biotherapy 1990;2:305.
278. Goldstone A, Khwaja A. The role of haematopoietic growth factors in bone marrow. Leuk Res 1990;14:721.
279. Brandt SJ, Peters WP, Atwater SK et al. Effect of recombinant human granulocyte-macrophage colony stimulating factor on hematopoietic reconstitution after high dose chemotherapy and autologous bone marrow transplantation. N Engl J Med 1988;318:869.
280. Herrmann F, Lindemann Mertelsmann R. Polypeptides controlling hemopoietic blood cell development and activation. Blut 1987;58:173.
281. Kojima S, Fukuda M, Miyajima Y et al. Treatment of aplastic anaemia in children with recombinant human granulocyte stimulating factor. Blood 1991;77:937.
282. Viens P, Thyss A, Garner G et al. GM-CSF treatment and hypokaliaemia. Ann Intern Med 1989;111:263.
283. Potter MN, Mott HG, Oakhill A. Granulocyte-macrophage colony stimulating factor (GM-CSF), hypocalcaemia and hypomagnesaemia. Ann Intern Med 1990;112:715.
284. Wakefield PE, James WD, Samlaska CP et al. Colony stimulating factors. J Am Acad Dermatol 1990;23:903.
285. Negri RS, Haeuber DH, Nagler A et al. Treatment of myelodysplastc syndrome with recombinant human granulocyte colony stimulating factor: a phase I-II trial. Ann Intern Med 1989;110:976.
286. Sheridan WP, Morstyn G, Wolf M et al. Granulocyte colony stimulating factor and neutrophil recovery after high-dose chemotherapy and autologous bone marrow transplantation. Lancet 1989;ii:891.
287. Glaspy JA, Baldwin GC, Robertson PA et al. Therapy for neutropenia in hairy cell leukemia with recombinant human granulocyte colony stimulating factor. Ann Intern Med 1988;109:789.
288. Khanderia Y. Circulatory collapse associated with hemin therapy for acute intermittent porphyria. Clin Pharm 1986;5:690.
289. Mustajcki P, Tenhunen R, Pierach C et al. Heme in the treatment of porphyrias and hematological disorders. Semin Hematol 1989;26:1.
290. Simionalto CS, Cabal R, Jones RL et al. Thrombophlebitis and disturbed hemostasis following administration of intravenous hematin in normal volunteers. Am J Med 1988;85:538.
291. Herrick AL, McColl KEL, Moore MR et al. Controlled trial of haem-arginate in acute hepatic porphyria. Lancet 1989;i:1295.
292. Drummond GS, Kappas A. Chemoprevention of neonatal jaundice. Potency of tin-protoporphyrin in an animal model. Science 1982;217:1250.
293. WHO. Wkly Epidemiol Rec 1990;65:390.
294. WHO. Wkly Epidemiol Rec 1991;66:33.
295. Horowitz MS, Rooks C, et al. Virus safety of solvent/detergent treated antihemophilic factor concentrate. Lancet 1988;ii:186.
296. Holland P, Golosova T, Szmuness W et al. Viral hepatitis markers in Soviet and American blood donors. Transfusion 1980;20:504.
297. Alter HJ. Transfusion-associated non-A,non-B hepatitis: the first decade. In: Zuckerman AJ, ed. Viral Hepatitis and Liver Disease. New York: Alan R. Liss, 1988;537.
298. Tabor E. Goldfield M, Black HA et al. Hepatitis Be antigen in volunteer and paid blood donors. Transfusion 1980;20:192.
299. Cossart YE, Kirsch S, Ismy SL. Post-transfusion hepatitis in Australia: report of the Australian Red Cross study. Lancet 1980;ii:192.
300. Vyas GN, Perkins HA. Non-B post-transfusion hepatitis associated with hepatitis core antibodies in donor blood. N Engl J Med 1982;306:749.
301. Suomela H. Global Blood Safety Initiative. Viral inactivation of blood and blood products. Geneva: World Health Organization, 1992.
302. Heimburger N, Karges HE. Strategies to produce virus-free blood derivatives. In: Morgenthaler JJ, ed. Virus Inactivation in Plasma Products. Berlin: Karger, 1989;23—33.
303. Piskiewicz D, Lieu MY et al. Virus inactivation by heat treatment of lyophilised coagulation factor concentrates. Curr Stud Hematol Transf 1989;56:55—69.
304. Prince AM, Brotman B. Sterilisation of Hepatitis and HTLV-III viruses by exposure to tri(*n*-butyl)phosphate and sodium cholate. Lancet 1986;ii:706—710.
305. Dideo AJ, Allegrezza AE. Validable virus removal from protein solutions. Nature 1991;351:420—421.
306. Lambrecht B, Mohr H, Knuver-Hopt J et al. Photoinactivation of viruse in human fresh plasma by phenothiazine dyes in combination with visible light. Vox Sang 1991; 60:207—213.
307. Aach RD, Kahn RA. Post-transfusion hepatitis: Current perspectives. Ann Intern Med 1980;92:539.
308. Blum HE, Vyas GN. Non-A,Non-B hepatitis: a contemporary assessment. Haematologia 1982;15:153.
309. Wenk RE, Brewer MK, Bass G et al. Surveillance for post-transfusion hepatitis by a community hospital. Transfusion 1981;21:557.

310. NIH Consensus: Infectious disease testing for blood transfusions. J Am Blood Resources Assoc 1995;4:78–87.
311. Nydegger UE. Intravenous immunoglobulin in combination with other prophylactic and therapeutic measures. Transfusion 1992;32:72–82.
312. Liblau R, Morel E, Bach JF. Autoimmune diseases, IgA deficiency and intravenous immunoglobulin treatment. Am J Med 1992;93:114.
313. Reinhart WH, Berchtold PE. Effect of high-dose intravenous immunoglobulin therapy and blood rheology. Lancet 1992;339:662–664.
314. Comenzo RL, Malachowaski ME, Meissner H et al. Immune hemolysis, disseminated intravascular coagulation and serum sickness after large doses of immune globulin given intravenously for Kawsaki's disease. J Pediatr 120; 926:928.
315. Watts RA, Isaacs JD, Hale G et al. Campath-1H in inflammatory arthritis. Clin Exp Rheumatol 1993;11(Suppl 8):S165–S167.
316. Banninger H, Hardegger T, Tobler A et al. Fibrin glue in surgery: frequent development of inhibitors of bovine thrombin and human factor V. Br J Haematol 1993;85:528–532.
317. Clark KR, Forsythe JL, Shenton BK et al. Administration of ATG according to the absolute T lymphocyte count during therapy for steroid-resistant rejection. Transplant Int 1993;6:18–21.
318. Clark JA, Gross TP. Pain and cyanosis associated with alpha 1-proteinase inhibitor. Amm J Med 1992;92:621–626.
319. Kon NF, Masumo H, Nakajima S et al. Anaphylactic reaction to aprotinin following topical use of biological tissue sealant. Masui (Japan) 1994;43:1606–1610.
320. Muntean W, Zenz W, Finding K et al. Inhibitor to factor V after exposure to fibrin sealant during cardiac surgery in a two-year-old child. Acta Paediatr 1994;83:84–87.
321. Ortel TL, Charles LA, Keller FG et al. Topical thrombin and acquired coagulation factor inhibitors: clinical spectrum and laboratory diagnosis. Am J Hematol 1994;45:128–135.
322. Lechner K, Kyrle PA. Antithrombin III concentrates—are they clinically useful? Thromb Haemost 1995;73:340–348.
323. Menache D, O'Malley JP, Schorr JB et al. Evaluation of the safety, recovery, half-life, and clinical efficacy of antithrombin III (human) in patients with hereditary antithrombin III deficiency. Blood 1990;146:137–16896.
324. McDougall IC. Adverse reactions profile 4. Erythropoietin in chronic renal failure. Journal Name Lost 1992.
325. Foa P. Erythropoietin: clinical applications. Acta Haematol 1991;86:162–168.
326. Nemunaitis J. Granulocyte-macrophage-colony-stimulating factor: a review from preclinical development to clinical application. Transfusion 1993;33:70–83.
327. Kostrzewska E, Gregor A, Tarcynska-Nosal S. Heme arginate (Normosang) in the treatment of attacks of acute hepatic porphyrias. Mat Med Pol 1991;4:259–262.
328. Lieschke G, Burgess AW. Granulocyte colony-stimulating factor (G-CSF): preclinical and clinical studies. N Engl J Med 1992;327:99–106.
329. Hermann F. G-CSF: Status quo and new indications. Infection 1992;20:183–188.
330. Sonenthal KR, McKnight T, Shaugnessi MA et al. Anaphylaxis during intrauterine insemination secondary to bovine serum albumin. Fertil Steril 1991;56:1188–1191.

Meyler's Side Effects of Drugs, 13th Edition
M.N.G. Dukes, editor

SECTION EDITOR: C.B.M. TESTER-DALDERUP

P.I. Folb

34 Intravenous infusions—solutions and emulsions

GENERAL CONSIDERATIONS

Many of the reports in the medical literature regarding adverse effects in association with intravenous fluids (including total parenteral nutrition) tend to be descriptive rather than analytical and/or investigative in nature. Nevertheless, over the years a cumulative picture has emerged that has provided much insight into the nature and pathogenesis of the bone and hepatic disorders associated with total parenteral nutrition, and the hypersensitivity reactions that characterize the occasional adverse responses to intravenous dextran. Moreover, with the greater awareness and improved understanding that have developed in recent years of the micronutrient deficiencies that may complicate prolonged total parenteral nutrition reports of these are appearing less often.

PLASMA SUBSTITUTES

Dextrans

Hypersensitivity reactions Dextran-induced allergic reactions have now been elucidated. Severe anaphylactic reactions only occur in patients with preformed dextran-reactive antibodies. Infusion of dextran causes the formation of large immune complexes that trigger activation of a cascade of enzyme systems, leukocytes and platelets. It may be possible to prevent or minimise these effects by blocking the reactive sites of the antibodies with small dextran fragments; this is hapten inhibition. The method used is to inject very low-molecular weight dextran (dextran-1, molecular weight 1000 Da) intravenously before an infusion of dextran is started; this blocks access to the antigen-combining sites by preformed circulating dextran-reactive antibodies.

There has been a reduction in the reports of severe reactions to dextran from 22 per 100 000 units of dextran administered between 1975 and 1979 to 1.2 per 100 000 units between 1983 and 1985. The number of reported fatal reactions decreased over the same period from 23 to 1. More than 600 000 units of dextran were used during each period. This represented a nearly 20-fold reduction in the reported incidence of severe dextran-induced adverse reactions in Sweden in the 3 years following the introduction of dextran-1 for the purpose of desensitization. During the same periods the incidence of grade I reactions (which are not considered to be antibody-mediated) did not change, suggesting that the decreased incidence of severe reactions after introduction of dextran-1 was not explained by a general decrease in the reporting of adverse reactions. It was emphasised that pre-injection of dextran-1 does not eliminate completely the risk of severe reactions to dextran (1[R]).

Paull studied the incidence of anaphylactoid reactions to dextran in 5745 patients over a 63-month period from January 1981 to March 1986 (2[C]). A total of 12 646 half-liter units of dextran-70 had been administered to these patients. The average number of dextran units transfused was 2.2 per patient. Fifteen (15) reactions were recorded, a rate of one reaction per 383 patients treated (0.26%). Seven of these reactions were potentially life-threatening (grade III or IV), giving a combined incidence of severe reactions of one in 821 patients treated (0.12%). The remaining eight reactions were less severe (grade I or II), and the combined incidence of the milder reactions was 1:718 patients treated (0.14%).

Ljungstrom (3C) has reported on the enhancement of the safety of dextran by hapten inhibition with dextran 1, which has been in use since 1982 for the prevention of severe dextran-induced anaphylactic reactions caused by immune complexes. Analysis of pre- and post-reaction titer of dextran-reactive antibodies was made in most Scandinavian studies (the precise number of these was not specified in the report). The incidence of severe dextran-induced anaphylactic reactions to clinical dextran after the prophylactic use of hapten inhibition was approximately 1/200 000 patients receiving dextran-1. In Sweden, where reporting of severe adverse drug reactions is mandatory, the incidence was approximately one in 70 000, indicating a 35-fold reduction. Only two fatal reactions were reported, an incidence of one per 2.5 million doses, indicating a 90-fold reduction. Both occurred in patients with extremely high titers of dextran-reactive antibodies. Side effects to dextran-1, mostly mild, were reported in approximately one case per 100 000 doses. These side effects were not antibody mediated. The author concluded that dextran with hapten inhibition has arguably become the safest plasma substitute in current clinical practice. The conclusions were reached on the basis of a postmarketing surveillance study, and were confirmed in another publication from the same center (4[C]).

It is possible for a severe dextran-induced anaphylactic/anaphylactoid reaction to develop despite prophylaxis with monovalent hapten dextran (5[c]). This has been reported in a 60-year-old patient with multiple trauma, who received a dextran infusion for prophylaxis of thrombosis due to severe thrombocytosis developing in the late postoperative period. The causal relationship to dextran was considered likely, although no serum sample was taken prior to the reaction, due to the close time relationship to the dextran-60 infusion. In addition, there were high titers of dextran-reactive antibodies in the blood drawn immediately after the reaction occurred.

Three cases of severe allergic reactions to dextran-70 (including one pregnant woman at the time of delivery) have been reported (6[C]). All three had received previous hapten prophylaxis. Although the pregnant patient recovered, the baby had evidence of serious brain damage at birth. Another patient with a very high titer of dextran-reactive antibodies died from myocardial infarction which happened at the same time. The third patient recovered without sequelae. The authors concluded that dextran-70 should be avoided in pregnancy until the baby is born, and that even in the presence of immune prophylaxis, these complications with dextran-70 may develop. Vigilant observation and resuscitation facilities are necessary in all cases.

Another case of an anaphylactoid reaction in a pregnant woman immediately after the administration of dextran 40 solution has been reported (7[cR]). The baby was delivered rapidly by cesarean section after the event, and was apparently dead at birth but successfully resuscitated. The case has prompted Barbier and colleagues to report on the safety in general of dextran administered during pregnancy (7[cR]). They have found information on 32 cases with moderate anaphylactoid reactions associated with severe fetal distress and they advised avoiding preventive fluid preload with dextran in these cases.

Acute pulmonary edema A case of pulmonary edema and coagulopathy following intrauterine instillation of 32% dextran-70 has been reported (8[c]). The volume of the agent in this case (700 ml) exceeded that recommended by the manufacturer (500 ml), and furthermore the installation time (2 hours) was in excess of that recommended (45 minutes). The authors pointed out that hyperosmolarity of the agent is such that if it enters the intravasular compartment, volume overload may result from the fact that 100 ml of intravascular dextran-70 will osmotically expand the intravascular volume by 860 ml, by drawing interstitial fluid into the central compartment. This may further aggravate the risks of pulmonary edema and dilutional coagulopathy.

Acute pulmonary edema developed in a healthy person after elective microsurgery for treatment of a malignant tumor of the forearm. It was thought to have been caused by dextran infusion (9[c]). The authors criticized the widespread use of dextran as an anticoagulant in surgery. Although thromboprophylaxis of microvascular anastomoses seems advisable theoretically, there is little clinical evidence in support of this agent for this purpose. The pulmonary edema in this case was thought to be non-cardiogenic, similar to that caused by heroin, methadone, propoxyphene and salicylates, due to a direct adverse effect on the pulmonary vasculature, rather than anaphylaxis, cardiac pump failure or volume overload. (The patient was in good physical condition before the operation, and there was no sign of volume overload perioperatively. Cardiac enzymes, electrocardiogram and echocardiogram were normal. No other medications were likely to have caused the pulmonary edema. The gradual response to diuretics suggested a non-cardiogenic cause.)

High-output left ventricular failure High output left ventricular failure has been described after hysteroscopic lysis of adhesions using dextran as a distension medium. Prolonged surgical dissection of the uterine wall, and the large volume of dextran and fluid (2 liters of 5% dextrose and an additional 800 ml dextran) that was administered, probably caused the dextran to enter into the systemic circulation, inducing a significant shift of fluid into the intravascular compartment (10[c]). (The precise duration of the operation was not stated in the report.)

Dextran deposition in tissues In biopsy and autopsy studies 32 patients treated with regular hemodialysis for 61 ± 34 months, who had also received dextran-40 as a plasma expander because of hypotension during hemodialysis, were compared with a control group of 11 hemodialyzed patients who were given other plasma expanders. In 11 of the former who had received the largest dose of dextran-40 (0.38 g/kg per week) particles were found in the cytoplasm of macrophages in various organs which were PAS-positive and diastase-resistant on light microscopy, and birefringent on polarisation. Electron microscopy revealed a fibrillar structure, but ionic analysis by electronic sampler on scanning electron microscopy excluded silicone. No intracellular inclusions were observed in the control group, or in the patients given dextran-40 in doses lower than 0.08 g/kg per week. There was a linear relationship between the number of particles and dose of dextran-40 that had been given, leading the authors to suggest that the material demonstrated in the macrophages was dextran that had been structurally modified and conglomerated by macrophage activity to a water-insoluble form (11[c]). (Infused dextran is mainly eliminated unmodified by the kidney at a rate of 50% in the first 24 hours and 20% in the following 48 hours. The remaining 30%, which is made up of the molecules having the highest molecular weight, is partly eliminated by the gastrointestinal tract, where it is thought to be hydrolyzed by coliform bacteria, and partly metabolised by splenic and hepatic dextranase (dextrano-α-1,6-glucosidase.)

Acute renal failure Of 207 patients with ischemic stroke, stages III or IV, treated with an intravenous infusion of low-molecular weight dextran (dextran-40) over 4 days, nine (4.3%) developed acute renal failure attributable to the dextran. Oliguria occurred after a mean time of 4 (3—6) days. The incidence of dextran-induced renal failure was higher in patients with pre-existing impaired kidney function (serum creatinine ⩾2.5 mg/dl). The high risk of death in the patients who developed renal failure was due to non-renal complications, notably pneumonia and pulmonary embolism (12[C]).

Acute anuric renal failure has been described following administration of dextran-40 and radiocontrast to a 59-year-old female patient. An increased risk of radiocontrast-induced renal ischemia is considered in relation to the pathogenesis of the dextran-induced renal failure. This has been demonstrated in animal studies. The mechanism of dextran-induced acute renal failure may be multifactorial, with elements of hyperoncotic acute renal failure, tubular obstruction, and direct tubular toxicity. Radiocontrast-induced acute renal failure is unusual in patients with normal baseline creatinine levels. The ischemic effect of radiocontrast seemed to be important in this case. Renal function should be carefully monitored if the simultaneous administration of dextran and radiocontrast is necessary. If renal function deteriorates and oliguria or anuria occurs, plasmapheresis may be an appropriate and effective approach for clearing dextran (13[c]).

In SED-11 (p. 726) Australian cases of acute renal failure, apparently representing a hypersensitivity reaction, were considered. Some further discussion of the problem has ensued (14[r], 15[r]).

On the basis of these observations it has been suggested that the pathogenesis of renal dysfunction during dextran-40 treatment involves mainly intraluminal hyperviscosity, decreased tubular flow, and pinocytic uptake of colloid into tubular cells (16c). Direct injury to the renal tubular epithelium cannot be ruled out (15[r]).

Abnormal liver function In a retrospective study of adverse effects of various drugs in 197 patients who underwent infertility surgery under general anesthesia and simultaneous intraperitoneal administration of 32% dextran-70, an increase in postoperative SGOT and SGPT values was noted in 86. The use of 32% dextran-70 in combination with corticosteroids or halothane (or halogenized drugs) resulted in an increased risk of temporarily disturbed liver function. Of 31 patients in whom it was possible to follow the SGOT and SGPT values after discharge from hospital, it was found that in 29 the values had returned to normal within 6 months. The authors suggested that hepatocytes may be damaged by enhanced glycogen deposition and/or lipid accumulation in patients receiving dextran. Corticosteroids potentially increase the risk of liver function disturbance (17[c]).

Acidosis The results of arterial blood gas and acid-base analyses were evaluated in 50 patients suffering from dextran-induced anaphylactic reactions. Metabolic acidosis was consistently present in severe cases, leading to cardiac arrest. Acidosis was also found in patients with less severe reactions and only slight impairment of the circulation. Bronchospastic respiratory signs were common, but it was also noted that acidosis developed in the absence of these symptoms and in patients with mild or no circulatory problems. The severity of the acidosis was often underestimated during treatment. Arterial P_{O_2} and P_{CO_2} were not significantly affected during these reactions. It was suggested from this study that the circulation is unlikely to be normalized until the metabolic acidosis is corrected, despite other therapeutic efforts that may be made (18[c]).

Intraperitoneal use of dextrans The complications of repeated postoperative intraperitoneal instillation of 6% dextran-60 (given for 5 days to 32 patients) have been monitored and compared with the outcome in 15 control patients. In the dextran-treated subjects abdominal pain and dyspnea occurred significantly more frequently than in the controls. During intraperitoneal irrigation with dextran a significant increase in body weight and in central venous pressure was noted. Bradycardia developed between the third and sixth postoperative days. Blood pressure remained unchanged. Seventy-five percent of the patients in the dextran group developed pleural effusions containing dextran by the fifth postoperative day. It was concluded that the uncertain advantages of dextran in the prevention of adhesions do not offset undesired side effects (19[c]).

After reproductive surgery 32% dextran-70 is sometimes administered intraperitoneally as adjuvant treatment for reducing adhesion formation. The high-molecular weight (70 000) dextran is thought to surround the raw peritoneal surfaces and keep them apart, in this way possibly preventing adhesion formation.

The complications of this procedure have been described in five patients (20C). In one, a right pleural effusion was detected on the third postoperative day and it had resolved 4 days later. In the remaining four cases bilateral vulvar edema developed on the first or second postoperative day, and this resolved in each case between the fifth and ninth day after surgery. Combined vulvar and leg edema in one of the patients has not been reported previously. It is thought that this edema is due to extravasation of dextran along fascial planes increasing the colloid-oncotic pressure in these spaces and promoting movement of a large amount of fluid from the vascular into the extravascular space. The right pleural effusion was thought to be due to movement of dextran through the diaphragmatic lymphatics or through small openings in the diaphragm, the majority of which are in the right hemidiaphragm.

The scientific evidence in support of the use of intraperitoneal dextran as an anti-adhesion adjuvant is scant. For this reason, it is particularly important that the safety of this therapeutic strategy should be carefully reviewed. Ricaurte and Hilgers (21[C]) found in a study of 139 consecutive patients who underwent major gynecological surgery and in whom 32% dextran-70 had been used as an anti-adhesion adjuvant (the mean amount of dextran used was 183 ml) that there was an acceptably low rate of complications.

Adverse effects involved 11 patients and included postoperative ileus (2.9%), pleural effusion (2.2%), allergic reactions (1.4%), wound infection (1.4%) and labial swelling (0.7%). There was no evidence of an increased infection rate.

Haemaccel (polygeline) *(SED-12, 866; SEDA-14, 304; SEDA-15, 379)*

Using a computer-aided model for the prediction of pseudoallergic reactions from prospective data collected from 581 patients in a controlled clinical trial with an outdated formulation of the plasma substitute Haemaccel, accurate prediction of 86% of the patients who had a systemic reaction was possible (22[C]). The data were handled by multivariate analysis using the independence-Bayes model. The predictive accuracy of other reactions was poor. A history of allergy was recorded in 26% of the patients who had systemic reactions and in 12 and 13% of the patients with no systemic or skin reactions. However, these differences were not statistically significant.

The *effects on renal function* of two modified gelatin preparations (Plasmion and Haemaccel) have been studied in 15 patients (23[C]). It was found that in both groups proteinuria appeared as soon as perfusion began, with a peak as high as 6 g/l at the third hour. At the same time, low-molecular weight proteinuria (<30 kDa) was observed. β_2-Microglobulinuria was significantly increased. The authors believed that proteinuria is either due to inhibited tubular reabsorption of filtered protein, caused by gelatin, or to the amino acids, arginine and lysine, which are released as a result of gelatin hydrolysis. The pathological significance of this finding is unexplained.

The allergic reactions that have been described in association with Haemaccel are thought to be caused by direct histamine release as a result of allergenic stimulation of mast cells. These cases raise the questions as to whether Haemaccel is appropriate for bronchoreactive patients and whether such patients should be protected by histamine receptor blockade.

Haemaccel is known to cause acute histamine release with resultant significant morbidity. Patients suffering from underlying bronchial asthma and pheochromocytoma are thought to be particularly at risk. Anaphylactoid reactions are, however, rare. Three cases of acute anaphylactoid reactions to Haemaccel have been described from Australia. The reactions were serious and the explanation for them is unclear. All three were either normovolemic or mildly hypovolemic at the time of the event (24[c]).

In a comparison of 4% human albumin solution, gelatin and dextran-40, administered as replacement fluids during plasma exchange, the gelatin solution induced two immediate allergic reactions and one delayed reaction (of 37 patients exposed). No cross-reactive allergy was observed between the two colloids. Dextran-1000 injections were well tolerated. Gelatin infusions were associated with ten times more episodes of hypovolemia (5.6 compared with 0.62%). This difference is probably explained by the faster elimination of gelatin from the vascular compartment, and it suggests that a larger volume of gelatin is required compared with dextran-40 for the same volume of plasma exchanged (25[C]).

Hydroxyethyl starch (hetastarch) *(SEDA-13, 316; SEDA-14, 304)*

Hetastarch (6%) administration to patients with septic shock (six subjects, compared with an equal number given human serum albumin) caused moderate effects on the *hemostatic coagulation profile* (prothrombin time, partial thromboplastin time, and quantitative platelet count) following 24 hours of infusion. There was no increase in bleeding as a result, and there were no statistically significant differences between these effects and those produced by human serum albumin (26[c]); however, it should be noted that the number of subjects was so small as effectively to preclude a finding of significant difference between the groups studied. The authors' conclusion that hetastarch is a safe and effective volume expander in patients with sepsis and shock needs to be considered cautiously, particularly as it is pointed out in the paper that there is an immediate decrease in Factor VIII coagulant to approximately half normal levels in patients receiving hetastarch. Furthermore, there is mention of a patient with von Willebrand's disease in whom the bleeding time was markedly prolonged and platelet adhesiveness decreased, although the patient did not suffer from overt bleeding. A comprehensive monograph summarizing the reported adverse reactions to plasma volume expanders has been published (27[R]).

There are several known mechanisms whereby synthetic macromolecular colloids such as hydroxyethyl starch disturb hemostasis. The thrombin time is shortened by a fibrinoplastic effect of the macromolecules in hydroxyethyl starch. This accelerates the conversion of fibrinogen to fibrin, resulting in a less stable thrombus which is more susceptible to lysis. The macromolecules in HES induce an acquired von Willebrand's syndrome with reduced levels of all three main Factors VIII: Factor VIII:C, vWF and von Willebrand factor antigen (vWFag). Macromolecules may coat the outer membrane of circulating platelets and cause a qualitative platelet function defect, thus prolonging bleeding time. Minor abnormalities of platelet aggregation have been observed after infusion of low volumes of hydroxyethyl starch, and platelet defects probably contribute to the hemorrhagic state.

Renal damage Hydroxyethyl starch is produced synthetically by introducing hydroxyethyl groups onto glucose units of starch molecules. This is then subjected to acid hydrolysis, which results in a product with a molecular weight of approximately 450 000 Daltons. Metabolism and elimination of the substance is complex, and it is related to the size of the particles. The smaller molecules, with a molecular weight of less than 50 000 Daltons, are excreted unchanged by glomerular filtration. Larger molecules are metabolized to smaller molecules, and distributed to various body tissues, where they may undergo hydrolysis in the reticuloendothelial system or enzymatic degradation by amylases. In a patient with normal renal function it is possible that the undamaged kidney presents a selective barrier to all but the smallest of the hetastarch molecules. The breakdown products are then eliminated by urinary excretion.

Legendre et al. (28[C]) have reported osmotic nephrosis-like lesions in kidney transplant recipients, which they attribute to hydroxyethyl starch that had been used in brainstem-dead patients before organ procurement. The incidence of these lesions was not influenced by cold ischemia time, presence and length of delayed graft function, or immunosuppressive regimen (including the use of cyclosporin). The lesions had no significant deleterious influence on the occurrence of delayed graft function and on serum creatinine at 3 and 6 months post-transplantation. Osmotic nephrosis-like lesions may be long-lasting since in three patients they were still present at 3 months post-transplantation on routine renal biopsy. In patients without osmotic nephrosis-like lesions no kidney was lost, whereas among those with such lesions, seven of 31 were lost.

Although an obvious short-term detrimental influence on renal function was not shown, these lesions might cloud the already difficult interpretation of renal transplant biopsies, especially for drug (cyclosporin) nephrotoxicity. The authors recommended avoidance of hydroxyethyl starch in potential organ donors.

There has been a recent report of hetastarch causing a discrepancy between urinary specific gravity and osmolality (29[c]). High-molecular weight molecules present in the hetastarch solution produced a disproportionate rise in urine specific gravity compared with osmolality. In two patients, the combined effects of acute tubular necrosis secondary to hypotension and abnormal glomerular permeability were thought to have allowed high-molecular weight particles of hetastarch to be excreted in the urine. The hetastarch particles elevated the urine specific gravity, but had a correspondingly lesser effect on osmolality. It was not thought that hetastarch itself was nephrotoxic. The authors concluded that in the setting of pre-existing renal disease, hetastarch may elevate the urinary specific gravity without unduly affecting the ability of the kidney to concentrate urine. They recommended that urinary osmolality, rather than specific gravity, should be regarded as the preferred method of evaluating the urine, after the administration of high-molecular weight colloid solutions.

Two cases have been reported of hemodilution therapy with hydroxyethyl starch causing acute deterioration of an already existing nephropathy (29[c]). The authors suggested, on theoretical grounds, that the deterioration in renal function in these cases was likely to have been the result of increased permeability caused by damage to the glomerular basement membrane. Hydroxyethyl starch molecules are filtered above the physiological renal threshold, and this increases the viscosity of the urine. This can be counteracted by promoting diuresis. The authors managed to avoid precipitating renal insufficiency by ensuring a fluid intake of about 3 liters a day. Without an adequate diuresis hydroxyethyl starch accumulates in patients with renal dysfunction, with consequences that include further damage to the diseased kidneys.

Cardiovascular effects In a comprehensive comparison of the pharmacokinetics and pharmacodynamics of dextran and hydroxyethyl starch (30[R]) the effects of hydroxyethyl starch on the cardiovascular system have been described. The mean arterial pressure, central venous pressure, and wedge pressure increase. The cardiac index, left ventricular stroke work index, and stroke output rise, whereas the pulmonary vascular resistance falls. Oxygen availability to the tissues is improved. The effects of hydroxyethyl starch on blood viscosity and erythrocyte aggregation, in particular, are more pronounced than with dextran.

Pruritus One of the physically uncomfortable and sometimes overlooked complications of hydroxyethyl starch is prolonged pruritus. In 481 patients treated for diseases of the microcirculation of the cochleovestibular system, 149 of them with hydroxyethyl starch, 43 (28.8%) complained of pruritus, compared with only 5.7% of another group of patients who were treated with dextran 40 (31C). In more than 40% of the patients pruritus started in normal skin 1—3 weeks after therapy and lasted between 6 weeks and 6 months; the itching was resistant to therapy with antihistamines. The problem can be socially embarrassing, particularly when hydroxyethyl starch has been given in high doses. The resistance of hydroxyethyl starch-induced pruritus to standard therapy, including antihistamines, corticosteroids, ultraviolet light, and other measures, has been described recently in a single case (32[c]).

Four patients suffering from nausea or tinnitus who received intravenous hydroxyethyl starch developed severe pruritus, especially on the trunk, without skin eruption, 1—3 weeks after the start of treatment. The pruritus was refractory to treatment, and neither oral nor topical antihistamine treatment was successful; only ultraviolet phototherapy or topical steroids gradually alleviated the pruritus after periods ranging from several weeks to 1 year (33[c]).

In a retrospective study of 491 patients treated for various cochleovestibular disorders 25 of 59 patients (42.4%) treated with hydroxyethyl starch complained of pruritus, compared with four of 35 (11.4%) treated with dextran-40 ($p<0.01$) (34[C]).

Generalized itching has been reported in 43 of 149 patients treated with hydroxyethyl starch for acute or chronic microcirculatory disease causing neuro-otological disturbances. The itching can be 'most annoying', and the authors believe that this should be taken into account when therapy is decided upon (35[C]).

In another retrospective study of 266 patients receiving hydroxyethyl starch for otological indications it was found that 32% of the patients developed pruritus, which characteristically appeared as pruritic crisis. In 55% of the patients the onset of symptoms was after the hydroxyethyl starch had been discontinued. The symptoms persisted on average for 8.8 weeks. Pruritus was generalized, but with a predilection of the trunk and genitalia. Coincidental atopic disease or higher age were not predisposing factors. The incidence of pruritus correlated well with the cumulative dosage and also depended on the type and molecular weight of the HES given (6 or 10%, molecular weight 40 or 200 kDa). Light and electron microscopic assessment showed deposits of HES, especially within dermal macrophages and endothelial cells adjacent to nerve fibers (36[c]). The authors suggested that a histamine-independent pathway is probably responsible for the induction of pruritus. Antihistamine drugs had no therapeutic effect on the patients reported.

Jurecka and others (37[c]) have made a contribution to understanding the mechanism of severe itching reported after administration of hydroxyethyl starch in hemodilution therapy. After HES treatment, vacuoles in cells of various organs in humans have been shown, predominantly affecting the mononuclear phagocyte system. These vacuoles present indirect evidence for phagocytosis of HES particles. In a study of skin biopsies of patients who had received HES and suffered subsequently from itching, it was demonstrated by light and electron microscopy, immunohistochemistry and immunoelectron microscopy using a polyclonal anti-HES antiserum, that storage of HES was present in the skin of all patients. This was mainly in dermal macrophages, endothelial cells of blood and lymph vessels, some perineural cells and endoneural macrophages of larger nerve fascicles, some keratinocytes and Langerhans cells. There were no morphological signs of histamine release from mast cells. These workers concluded that mediators other than histamine, released from HES-affected cells, must be responsible for the itching.

von Willebrand's disease Alteration of the coagulation mechanism is a recognized complication of the administration of large volumes of hydroxyethyl starch. A case has been described of a 33-year-old man who was diagnosed with von Willebrand's disease shortly after he had been given 3 liters of hetastarch over 3 days following an acute sensorineural hearing loss. The patient had a history of a prolonged activated partial thromboplastin time (APTT), although he had previously undergone bilateral hip arthroplasties with no evidence of abnormal bleeding. The patient had an episode of epistaxis and experienced weakness and pain in his leg. When hetastarch was stopped, it was noted that the patient had elevated levels of APTT, and reduced levels of Factors XII and VIIIC. Over the next few months, the von Willebrand's syndrome was reversed, although his Factor XII levels remained reduced (38[c]).

A detailed histological and immunohistochemical study of hydroxyethyl starch deposits in rat tissues has been reported (39). Thirteen days after a single intravenous injection the rats were sacrificed and liver, spleen, lymph node, lung, kidney and skin were studied. In all these organs, antihydroxyethyl starch antiserum stained cells which were mainly regarded as mononuclear phagocytes (confirmed by the use of antimacrophage monoclonal antibody ED1). These findings suggested a degree of prolonged tissue storage of either hydroxyethyl starch or of a degradation product that stains with the antibody, and this may account for persistent complications such as pruritus. However, in this histochemical study no mast cell degranulation or accumulation of inflammatory cells was observed. Immunohistochemical studies of this kind are likely to be useful in elucidating possible correlations between adverse effects and the long-term storage of hydroxyethyl starch.

General In a review of the use and value of hemodilution therapy using dextrans and hydroxyethyl starch, respectively, in ischemic brain infarction (40[R]) the authors pointed out that although this regimen has been in use for more than 20 years its value is uncertain. Studies over the past 7 years using iso- and hypervolemic hemodilution with low-molecular weight dextrans or hydroxyethyl starch have failed to show a definite beneficial effect. Thus, the adverse effects, such as anaphylaxis, volume overload, cerebral hemorrhage and acute renal failure, need to be considered in this light.

TOTAL PARENTERAL NUTRITION

Mechanisms of systemic disease caused by parenteral lipids

A theory has been proposed by, inter alia, Cooke (41[r]) and Andersson et al. (42[r]), regarding a possible mechanism by which parenteral lipid solutions injure preterm infants; namely, by free radical-induced lipid peroxidation in the lipid solution. How this happens is not explained. The result may be pulmonary damage and chronic lung disease. Premature infants are thought to be at particularly high risk.

Both Williams (43[c]) and Wilson et al. (44[c]) have suggested that Cooke's interpretation was not based on solid clinical evidence, and that the data that he derived from his observations should be tested in controlled studies before TPN is prescribed for infants of very low birthweights.

There is evidence that lipid emulsion, which is cleared by the Kupffer cells of the reticuloendothelial system (RES), may adversely affect RES function by decreasing its ability to remove blood-borne bacteria. In a study of the blood clearance and organ localisation of viable ^{35}S-radiolabelled *Escherichia coli* following slow intraperitoneal and more rapid intravenous administration of 20% fat emulsion in Sprague-Dawley rats it was found that although there was rapid bacterial blood clearance in control and test animals, there was a significant change in the organ localization of bacteria as a result of the administration of lipid emulsion. There was a slight increase in lung localization of bacteria in rats receiving intraperitoneal fat emulsion, and a significant increase in lung trapping of bacteria in rats receiving intravenous fat emulsion. Liver localization of bacteria was reduced in all groups after fat emulsion. The data are understood to indicate that intravenous fat emulsion decreases hepatic phagocytosis and increases pulmonary localization of *E. coli*, and it is thought that this may produce greater susceptibility to infection. Patients with underlying sepsis are at greatest risk. The capacity of the lungs to kill sequestered bacteria is not known. Thus, increased bacterial lung localization may result in local inflammation and other pulmonary complications, and in the re-emergence into the blood of viable *E. coli*, with systemic sepsis as a result (45[R]).

Since lipoprotein lipase activity is reduced in premature babies and babies who are small for gestational age, and since bacterial and viral infections adversely affect lipoprotein lipase activity and may precipitate fat overload, it follows that fat emulsion should be administered with great caution, or even temporarily withheld, in small infants with proven or suspected sepsis (45[R]).

Lipids have an adverse effect on carbohydrate metabolism under basal conditions. The infusion of 20% triglyceride emulsion with heparin during basal insulin and glucose turnover conditions resulted in a rise of plasma free fatty acids from 0.4 to 0.8 mM with a low rate of infusion (0.5 ml/min for 2 hours) to between 1.6 and 2.1 mM with a high rate (1.5 ml/min for 2 hours). There were similar increases in plasma concentrations of glycerol, acetoacetate, and hydroxybutyrate. The infusions resulted in significant increases in C-peptide concentrations, but had no effects on any of the other indices of carbohydrate metabolism that were examined (plasma glucose, lactate, and pyruvate concentrations), or on carbohydrate oxidation rates. By blocking the compensatory release of insulin by the intravenous administration of somatostatin and by simultaneous replacement of basal insulin and glucagon concentrations, these workers found that there was a significant increase in plasma glucose and in hepatic glucose output, and a decrease in glucose clearance. It was concluded that exogenous lipids may have adverse effects on carbohydrate metabolism under basal conditions, and that healthy individuals normally compensate for this by additional secretion of insulin (46[R]).

Critically ill patients are at greatest risk of fat overload syndrome when they are given lipid emulsions intravenously. Some of these patients already have impaired lipid metabolism and they are at risk of developing fat intolerance. These are the very patients who are likely to be given parenteral nutrition, including fat emulsions. Patients with increased serum triglyceride concentrations (for example, in hypothyroidism, with inborn errors of lipid metabolism, renal insufficiency, and severe sepsis, especially gram-negative sepsis) are at greatest risk. There is impaired metabolism of fats in advanced liver disease. Continuous heparin infusion may also lead to a decreased elimination capacity (47[R]). Lindholm (47[R]) has pointed out that drugs with a high lipid content, when given concurrently with lipid-containing parenteral nutrition, may aggravate the problems of lipid overload. The anesthetic, propofol, which is used for continuous sedation in a dose of 1—3 mg/kg/hour (an equivalent of 300—500 ml of a 10% fat emulsion), may aggravate the symptoms and pathological effects of fat overload (47[R]).

Precipitation The United States Food and Drug Administration has issued a safety alert about precipitate formation in total parenteral nutrition admixtures that can be life-threatening (48[r]). Reports have been received by the FDA of two deaths and at least two cases of respiratory distress that developed during intravenous infusion of a three-in-one (amino acids, carbohydrate, and lipids) TPN admixture. The admixture contained 10% FreAmine 111, dextrose, calcium gluconate, potassium phosphate, other minerals, and a lipid emulsion, all of which were combined. The solution may have contained a precipitate of calcium phosphate. Autopsies revealed diffuse microvascular pulmonary emboli containing calcium phosphate.

The FDA recommends that if patients on TPN develop symptoms of acute respiratory distress, pulmonary embolus, or interstitial pnemonitis, the infusion should be stopped immediately and thoroughly checked for precipitates.

Precipitates can develop in TPN admixtures because of a number of factors such as the concentration, pH, and phosphate content of the amino acid solutions, the calcium and phosphorus additives, the order of mixing, the mixing process, or the compounder.

The FDA has recommended the following steps to decrease the hazard of injury through precipitation (49[r]):

(1) The amounts of phosphorus and of calcium added to the admixture are critical. The solubility of the added calcium should be calculated from the volume at the time that the calcium is added. It should not be based on the final volume. The line should be flushed between the addition of any potentially incompatible components.

(2) A lipid emulsion in a three-in-one admixture obscures the presence of a precipitate. Therefore, if a lipid emulsion is needed, either use a two-in-one admixture with the lipid infused separately, or add the calcium before the lipid emulsion according to the recommendations in (1) above. If the amount of calcium or phosphate which must be added is likely to cause a precipitate, some or all of the calcium should be administered separately. Such separate infusions must be properly diluted and slowly infused to avoid serious adverse events related to the calcium.

(3) During the mixing process, parenteral nutrition admixtures should be periodically agitated to check for precipitates. This check should be conducted both before and during the infusion. Patients and caregivers should be trained to inspect for signs of precipitation. They should also be trained to stop the infusion and seek medical assistance if precipitates are noted.

(4) A filter should be used when infusing either central or peripheral parenteral nutrition admixtures. (Data are not available to determine which size filter is most effective in trapping precipitates.)

(5) Parenteral nutrition admixtures should be administered within the following time frames: if stored at room temperature, the infusion should be started within 24 h after mixing; if stored at refrigerated temperatures, the infusion should be started within 24 h of rewarming. Because warming parenteral nutrition admixtures may contribute to the formation of precipitates, once administration begins, care should be taken to avoid excessive warming of the admixture.

Mirtallo (50[r]) has added to the FDA guidelines for giving calcium in TPN solutions, to ensure maximum safety of the process: take care that an appropriate dose of calcium is prescribed; follow appropriate procedures when mixing TPN solutions; when using automated compounding devices, follow the device manufacturer's instructions explicitly (if deviation is necessary, apply data from research or the literature); and keep in mind that more information is needed to substantiate the usefulness of filters in preventing adverse effects caused by the infusion of particulate matter present in TPN admixtures. It has been pointed out that calcium phosphate precipitate forms more readily in warm than in cold solutions. Precipitation can occur in solution at room-temperature even if an identical cold solution is clear. A precipitate can also form when a clear solution refrigerated or at room-temperature is warmed to body temperature. Thus, visual inspection and even in-line filters - if they are distal to the side of precipitation - may be ineffective in preventing infusion of the precipitate (51[c]).

Hepatic complications The pathogenicity and management of liver injury caused by both short-term parenteral nutrition and long-term TPN have been reviewed by Baker and Rosenberg (52[R]). Progressive liver injury developing in patients needing prolonged TPN raises serious dilemmas. There is a high prevalence of hepatic complications of TPN in children. Premature or low-weight-for-age infants are at increased risk of *cholestasis*, which is the prominent abnormality both clinically and on biopsy. Infants are at high risk of developing *progressive liver injury* and *liver failure* if TPN is prolonged beyond 5 months. The outcome may be fatal. The pattern and prognosis of liver injury in children is distinct from that seen in adults, despite some overlap.

Increased hepatic lipogenesis and reduced transport function are important in the *fatty liver* associated with TPN. Providing ample quantities of essential amino acids lessens but does not prevent this. This highlights the importance of total caloric intake. If insufficient amounts of amino acids are taken together with adequate non-protein calories, a situation may develop which is analogous to kwashiorkor. Hepatic lipid accumulates, but lipoprotein synthesis is limited. Carnitine supplementation minimizes fatty infiltration of the liver in patients receiving dextrose-based TPN, which supports the idea that carnitine deficiency plays a role in the development of this complication. However, carnitine can ordinarily by synthesized from the essential amino acids, methionine and lysine, which are present in all commercially available TPN formulae. Hepatic tissue requirements may be increased under conditions of stress, contributing to the development of a fatty liver by impairment of transport and oxidation of fatty acids by mitochondria.

Several mechanisms have been proposed to explain the cholestasis that occurs during TPN, but there is little direct evidence to support any of them. Nutrient deficiencies which may be critical for hepatic uptake, biotransformation, and secretion of bile may be involved; a deficiency in taurine, which is important for bile acid conjugation, may cause cholestasis in premature infants. Certain amino acids may act as toxins. Decreased hormonal and neural stimulation of hepatic bile secretion may be a factor in patients who are not receiving nutrition enterally. Increased production of lithocholate, which is an hepatotoxic bile acid, by intestinal bacteria, or retention of lithocholate in the liver, might account for the cholestasis.

Elevated levels of lithocholate, portal bacteremia and/or endotoxemia have all been suggested as contributing to *hepatic triaditis* in patients with inflammatory bowel disease receiving TPN. Toxic amino acids or their metabolic products, excessive calorie administration and a disturbed carbohydrate/protein ratio may also influence the development of triaditis.

Steatonecrosis is also known to occur when nutritional depletion develops. Inadequate administration of a critical nutrient or combination of nutrients might be involved in the pathogenicity of this lesion.

Sixteen patients with massive bowel resection receiving long-term home TPN for periods ranging from 31 to 145 months were examined for evidence of liver disease. A small number of patients with duodenocolostomy (three cases) developed cirrhosis, but not the patients with surgically shortened small bowel (13 cases) (53[c]). There is no obvious explanation for this.

In a retrospective study of 172 neonates requiring TPN for a minimum of 1 week it was noted that the number of operations (amongst other factors) was significantly related to the development of cholestasis. This was identified as a new variable in the pathogenicity of TPN-related cholestasis, which may be related to the stress of surgery itself or to the repeated administration of anesthetic agents (54[C]). Morphine and its derivatives are known to induce cholestasis.

An animal model has been developed in young pigs which demonstrates the complications of gallbladder 'sludge' and cholestasis with TPN. Lipid was used in the solution. Weight-matched animals were used as controls. All animals in the TPN group developed 'sludge' in their gallbladders, decreased basal bile flow, decreased bile salt excretion, and a diminished response to bile salt-stimulated bile flow, compared with controls. There was no abnormality in routine liver function test or in liver histology. It was concluded from this experimental model that the gallbladder 'sludge' and cholestasis, demonstrated by bile flow studies, are the result of a decrease in both the bile salt-dependent and bile salt-independent fractions of canalicular bile flow (55[C]).

A rat model has been developed of hepatic steatosis induced by TPN administered for 3 weeks, without associated abnormal liver function tests (58). It is unclear from this experimental study whether the dissociation of TPN-induced hepatic steatosis and biochemical dysfunction is explained by the relatively short duration of the experiments, or whether the apparent difference from the human situation is due to the fact that rat livers respond differently from human livers (for example, rats do not have gallbladders). Hepatic steatosis may be an early marker of liver toxicity caused by TPN, preceding biochemical disturbance. If so, reversal of early hepatic steatosis should spare the liver from further abnormality.

Cholelithiasis King and colleagues have examined the predisposition of infants and children to cholelithiasis when treated with parenteral nutrition (56[C]). Clinically diagnosable cholelithiasis had developed in 11 patients. Six required cholecystectomy for relief of chronic abdominal pain, pancreatitis or empyema of the gallbladder. One other infant underwent cholecystectomy. Two of the remaining four patients were asymptomatic, one had episodes of abdominal colic, and one died as a result of chronic hepatic insufficiency caused by parenteral nutrition-associated cholestasis. Factors that predisposed these children to cholelithiasis included short-bowel syndrome, lack of an ileocecal valve, and an increased number of abdominal surgical procedures ($p<0.05$). Patients with biliary calculi had a longer duration of parenteral feeding and a higher incidence of both parenteral nutrition-associated cholestasis and necrotizing enterocolitis. However, intergroup differences for these characteristics did not achieve statistical significance. The authors recommend routine ultrasound examinations of the gallbladder for children maintained on parenteral nutrition for longer than 30 days, and early elective cholecystectomy for children who develop parenteral nutrition-associated cholelithiasis.

In a related study the incidence and progress of sludge, microlithiasis, and lithiasis formation in the biliary tract was studied in 12 patients who underwent total gastrectomy and postoperative TPN commencing immediately after surgery (57[C]). Serial ultrasonographic studies were carried out every 72 hours during TPN, every 7 days during the period of oral refeeding, and then once a month for a further 3 months. Sludge of the gallbladder was demonstrated in five of the 12 patients after a minimum period of 9 days after surgery, and in four of these microlithiasis of the biliary tract was subsequently revealed. In two of four patients the stone dissolved spontaneously, while in the remaining two no change occurred in dimension of the calculi after intervals of 6 and 7 months, respectively. Without exception, the sludge and microcalculi were 'silent'. This study underlines the high incidence of biliary tract sludge and microlithiasis complicating TPN, and it highlights the necessity for preventive measures and for vigilance for acute pancreatitis (57[C]).

Cholelithiasis is extremely unusual in infants and children. However, in a group of 400 children receiving TPN who were evaluated prospectively for the presence of gallstones and sludge, eight (2%) were found by ultrasonography to have developed cholelithiasis. All had received large amounts of amino acids ($\geq$1.8 g/kg/day) and relatively low amounts of fat ($\leq$1.7 g/kg/day) with a high ratio of non-protein (kcal/ml; >0.8). It was concluded that the administration of large amounts of amino acids and a high ratio of non-protein (kcal/ml) increased the risk of formation of gallstones and sludge. Conversely, these are prevented by the administration of appropriate amounts of fat (59[C]).

Histological abnormalities The histological features of liver biopsies from 20 children treated with total parenteral nutrition have been described (60[c]). All the children had received TPN for a minimum of 2 weeks. The conditions that led clinicians to use this form of treatment included prematurity, sepsis, and gastrointestinal surgical procedures. Fourteen children had a history of prematurity; in nine the birth weight was between 640 and 1300 grams. Ten of the 20 children died. The findings suggested that the morphological features observed in the liver can be correlated with the duration of TPN, the histological features beginning with cholestasis and culminating with cirrhosis.

Neonates and infants In a study of newborn infants treated with TPN for a variety of conditions, cholestasis occurred in 71% of premature infants compared with 22% of full-term babies. Infants with cholestasis had been on TPN for a longer time (37 as opposed to 27 days), but the bilirubin level did not correlate with the extent of histological injury and was frequently normal despite marked histological damage (61[C]).

A similar conclusion was reached in an evaluation of total parenteral nutrition-associated cholestasis, conducted retrospectively in 15 infants (62[C]). Two-thirds of the patients had been kept on TPN for more than 60 days. Preterm babies less than 32 weeks of age had an earlier rise of direct bilirubin and AST. The main histological findings on liver biopsy or at autopsy were cholestasis (intracellular or canalicular), periportal inflammation, fibrosis and bile ductular proliferation. Sixty percent of the patients survived; their liver function profile became normalized within a mean of 14.0—9.4 (8—34) weeks after discontinuation of TPN in the survival cases. The authors concluded that infant TPN-associated cholestasis is mostly reversible, but that younger preterm babies are susceptible to a prolonged TPN course, and that they have more marked clinical and pathological changes.

To identify the factors predictive of the development of TPN-related cholestasis, an historical cohort analysis of 62 very low-birth weight (VLBW) infants who had been treated with TPN has been conducted (63[C]). Seventeen developed cholestasis (27.4%). In the cholestatic group, the mean duration of TPN administration had been significantly longer than in those who had not developed cholestasis (25.7 compared with 8 days, $p<0.001$). The maximum daily amino acid and lipid content of the TPN infusate was greater (amino acids, 2.25 compared with 1.25 g/kg, $p<0.001$; lipid, 2.0 compared with 1.25 g/kg per day, $p<0.01$). The duration of fasting was longer (20.7 compared with 6.3 days, $p<0.001$), and the incidence of necrotizing enterocolitis was higher (58.8% compared with 15.5%, $p=0.02$). Using linear discriminant analysis with development of cholestasis as the dependent variable, the duration of TPN ($p=0.0000$) and the maximum content of amino acid in infusate each day ($p=0.0000$) were noted to be independent variables predictive of the development of cholestasis.

The high risk of hepatic injury complicating TPN in infants may be explained by factors that are specific to this age group; namely, immaturity of the enzyme systems responsible for hepatic conjugation, disturbance in the physiological patterns of enteral nutrition, and excessive secondary bile acid production and absorption from a contaminated small bowel. The bile of premature and newborn infants differs in its composition from that of adults, and this may account for the differences in solubility (64[c]).

Hematological Hematological abnormalities were associated with prolonged administration of intravenous fat emulsion in seven children on a program of long-term cyclic TPN. Each received Intralipid 20% 1—2 g/kg body weight per 24 hours during 3—18 months. Recurrent thrombocytopenia occurred in all seven children. Platelet life-span (measured with indium-111) was reduced. Sea-blue histiocytes containing granulations and hemophagocytosis were seen on bone marrow smears. There was bone marrow sequestration of radiolabelled autologous erythrocytes. The constellation of hematological abnormalities suggested an activation of the monocyte—macrophage system by the fat emulsion (66[C]).

Hematological complications of this nature pose a serious problem for children who are dependent on artificial nutrition for prolonged periods. Platelet counts should be performed on a regular basis in patients receiving prolonged TPN with Intralipid. If a low platelet count develops, reduction or termination of administration is indicated (66[C]). It was noted that secretion of plasminogen activators by monocytes was normal in one case, and increased in the other six. Circulating plasminogen levels were depressed, ranging from 4 to 10 mg/100 ml (normal range 10—70 mg/100 ml). These findings further point to hyperactivity of the macrophage in the reticuloendothelial system related to long-term treatment with Intralipid.

Sepsis In 1279 premature very low-birth weight infants the use and duration of treatment with TPN were associated with short gestational age and low birth weight. Infants treated with TPN had a higher risk of sepsis usually caused by *Staphylococcus epidermis* or *S. aureus* (65c). Thus, although the risk of sepsis in this age group appears to be significantly increased by TPN, the causative organisms were fairly benign. It was concluded that the advantages of TPN outweigh the disadvantages of sepsis in this group of infants.

Blood gas exchange The change in transcutaneous oxygen (tcP_{O_2}) and carbon dioxide (tcP_{CO_2}) tension in response to 60 minutes infusion of Intralipid (mean dose 0.16—0.07 g/kg/hour) in neonates with lung disease (hyaline membrane disease or bronchopulmonary dysplasia) has been evaluated in seven sick infants from an intensive care unit, studied on 13 different occasions. The tcP_{O_2} was 10% lower following Intralipid infusion ($p<0.05$), whereas no significant change occurred in tcP_{CO_2} measurements.

The results show that the infusion of Intralipid contributes to the hypoxia of respiratory distress in neonates. The authors recommend that Intralipid should be administered to this category of patients only in limited quantities and with extreme caution. Prolonged routine use of high-dose Intralipid is not recommended in infants with pulmonary disease, and alternative energy sources need to be considered (67[C]).

Micronutrient and enzyme deficiency Three adult cases in which *copper deficiency* developed during long-term total parenteral nutrition without copper supplementation have been described. All three patients were suffering from malabsorption when therapy was instituted, and overt symptoms of copper deficiency developed an average of 5.8 months after the start of TPN. Clinically, leukopenia with neutropenia and low plasma levels of copper and ceruloplasmin were seen in all cases (68[c]).

Low selenium levels were found in four children receiving long-term TPN who developed erythrocyte macrocytosis (three), loss of pigmentation of hair and skin (two), elevated transaminase and creatine kinase activities (two), and profound muscle weakness (one). Mean serum vitamin B_{12}, folate, and vitamin E levels were normal. Intravenous supplementation with selenium for 3–6 months resulted in an almost 3-fold elevation of serum selenium levels, with improvement of erythrocyte mean corpuscular volume in the three children with macrocytosis. After 6–12 months of supplementation hair selenium increased 3-fold, and in the two children with decreased pigmentation there was change to a darker skin and hair color. Transaminase and creatine kinase activities returned to near normal in those affected, and in the one child with severe myopathy muscle weakness improved. Erythrocyte macrocytosis and loss of skin and hair pigmentation (pseudoalbinism) have not previously been described as manifestations of selenium deficiency (69[C]).

Carnitine deficiency has been described in surgical neonates receiving TPN (70[C]). In a consecutive study of neonates who received TPN for over 2 weeks it was found that all patients had a carnitine intake far below the recommended minimal need of 11 mmol/kg per day. Although only three of the infants showed clinical symptoms suggestive of carnitine deficiency, the authors have recommended carnitine supplementation for all neonates receiving TPN for over 2 weeks. Carnitine plays a key role in the oxidation of fatty acids.

Persistent abnormalities of liver function tests developing in patients treated with home parenteral nutrition have been investigated for a possible association with diminished total and free plasma carnitine concentrations. It was suggested that a deficiency of L-carnitine may be responsible for the steatosis and steatohepatitis in these patients. Four adult women on home parenteral nutrition for a mean of 53 months (range 21–80 months) were studied before and after 1 month of intravenous L-carnitine supplementation (1 g/day). All patients had abnormalities in standard liver function tests and low total and free plasma carnitine values. The mean total and free plasma carnitine concentration and mean total hepatic carnitine concentration were reduced before supplementation and rose to normal values after treatment. However, there was no significant improvement in mean serum aspartate aminotransferase and alkaline phosphatase levels, plasma free fatty acid and triglyceride concentrations, or in the grade of hepatic steatosis on light microscopy. These results suggest that carnitine deficiency is not a major cause of steatosis and steatohepatitis in patients receiving home parenteral nutrition (72C).

The time-course for the depletion of red blood cell and plasma *glutathione peroxidase* activity has been documented in five patients receiving home parenteral nutrition (71[C]). There was a decrease in red blood cell glutathione peroxidase, general enzyme activity and protein content in these patients. Once replacement of selenium (as selenious acid) had begun, there was a rapid increase (within 6 hours) in plasma glutathione peroxidase activity. Platelet and granulocyte glutathione peroxidase activity, which was low prior to selenium treatment, normalized within a time consistent with the kinetics of platelets and polymorphonuclear production. Red blood cell glutathione peroxidase activity returned to normal within 3–4 months, which is consistent with the time-course for bone marrow red blood cell production. The authors concluded that the repletion of red blood cell glutathione peroxidase in this setting requires the presence of selenium.

Selenium in the form of selenocysteine is part of the active site of glutathione peroxidase, the enzyme which catalyzes glutathione reduction of organic hydroperoxides and hydrogen peroxide, which protects against oxidative damage. The minimum daily selenium requirement for patients receiving nutrition has not been determined.

Metabolic bone disease Parenteral nutrition-induced bone disease, which has regularly been written about in recent years in SED Annuals, has now been thoroughly reviewed (76[R]). It is difficult to identify the role of a single nutrient in the development of this bone disease. The pathogenicity may be different in patients at different ages: in growing infants increased mineral requirement may be of particular importance, whereas other factors (such as aluminium toxicity) may be common in both adults and children. Since mineral status may be critical, particularly in small preterm infants, non-nutritional factors, including chronic use of potent loop diuretics and altered acid-base status, can affect urine mineral loss, cell metabolism, and consequently bone mineralization. The author concluded, on the basis of the information and evidence that is currently available, that the cause of parenteral nutrition-related bone disease is multifactorial, and that its prevention awaits better understanding of the exact sequence of pathogenetic events.

The characteristics of bone disease associated with parenteral nutrition remain controversial. In a study aimed at elucidating the contribution of aluminium deposition to this syndrome and the spectrum of pathology in patients supported by current regimens utilizing crystalline amino acids, quantitative histomorphometry and staining for aluminium were performed on iliac crest bone biopsies from 26 long-term parenteral nutrition patients and 16 normal volunteers. Compared with normal subjects, the median trabecular bone area for a group with positive aluminium staining who were exposed to casein hydrolysate was significantly less, as was the median rate of bone formation. A variety of abnormal histological findings was present in patients without positive aluminium stains who were supported solely by regimens utilizing crystalline amino acids. Neither decreased median trabecular bone area nor decreased median rate of bone formation was uniformly characteristic of the latter patient group (73[C]).

In a study of 17 patients who first received TPN containing casein hydrolysate with high aluminium and ergocalciferol (25 μg/day) for 6—72 months followed by TPN containing amino acids with reduced aluminium and ergocalciferol (5 μg/day) for 9—58 months, and in a further cross-sectional study of 22 patients receiving casein and ergocalciferol (24μg/day) compared with 46 patients receiving amino acids and ergocalciferol (5 μg/day) for 6—58 months, the following were found: bone formation was higher and osteoid area, bone surface-stainable aluminium and total bone aluminium were lower with amino acid TPN than with casein TPN; bone formation varied inversely with both plasma aluminium and bone surface aluminium, suggesting that plasma or bone surface aluminium, acquired during TPN, reduces bone formation and leads to patchy osteomalacia. Serum levels of immunoreactive parathyroid hormone and 1,25-dihydroxyvitamin D were higher with amino acid TPN (74[C]). The data in this study demonstrate that the metabolic bone disease associated with long-term TPN improves after a change from casein to amino acids. This is associated with a reduction in the quantities of aluminium, protein and ergocalciferol in the TPN solutions.

Bone-formation rate was higher and the osteoid lower in patients who received amino acids compared with casein hydrolysate. Serum levels of 1,25-dihydroxyvitamin D were higher, and the plasma levels of aluminium and urinary excretion of aluminium and calcium were markedly lower, during the administration of amino acids compared with casein hydrolysate. The changes in the TPN solution made over the time of this study were complex, and the significance of the findings reported here is uncertain.

Nevertheless, the inverse relationships between bone-formation rate and both plasma and surface-stainable aluminium support the view that less exposure to aluminium may play a significant role in improving the bone histology in this setting.

Bone loss Bone-mass status has been studied in 10 patients aged 19—66 years who received home TPN over 0—67 months (mean 24 months), mostly for short-bowel syndrome. During a follow-up of up to 19 months a significant decrease of both cancellous and cortical bone components was found (75[C]). The authors concluded that prolonged TPN is associated with ongoing bone diminution, affecting mainly cancellous bone.

Renal impairment A profound decrease in renal function associated with long-term TPN (that is, in patients who had received home TPN for periods longer than 10 years) has been found in the majority of 33 patients. Twenty-nine of the patients had a reduction in estimated creatinine clearance of 0.6—15.4% per year. Tubular function, as determined by the tubular reabsorption of phosphate, was impaired in 52% of the subjects. Although nephrotoxic drug use, bacteremia and fungemia, age and infection rate accounted for part of the decline in renal function, most of it was unexplained (77C).

Urinary oxalate excretion Parenteral nutrition solutions contain the oxalate precursors ascorbate and glycine, and for this reason Campfield and Braden have studied the relationship between TPN administration and oxalate excretion in very low-birth weight infants (78[C]). Administration of TPN protein of approximately 0.5 g/kg per day to these infants was associated with an increased urinary oxalate/creatinine ratio, when compared with very low-birth weight infants receiving a glucose and electrolyte solution. A further rise in urinary oxalate concentration and oxalate/creatinine ratio was noted when TPN protein was increased to approximately 1.5 g/kg per day. Elevated urinary oxalate concentrations may be a factor in the pathogenesis of nephrocalcinosis in these infants.

Metabolic The problems that may result from the administration in total parenteral fluid infusions of D-fructose or sorbitol have been reviewed (79[r]). Either of these may cause life-threatening hypoglycemia, unless glucose is administered concurrently, in patients who have underlying hereditary fructose intolerance. Unless there is a clear clinical history of the condition it may not be readily identified. In some countries fructose and D-glucitol (sorbitol) have been eliminated from the pharmacopoeia for this reason.

Aluminium content Parenterally administered aluminium bypasses the gastrointestinal tract, which normally serves as a protective barrier to aluminium entry into the blood. In the past, aluminium contamination of casein hydrolysate, which was used as a source of protein in TPN solutions, was associated with low-turnover osteomalacia and with encephalopathy in uremic patients. Premature infants are still at risk of aluminium accumulation as a result of prolonged TPN (as are patients receiving plasmapheresis therapy with albumin contaminated in its preparation with aluminium). Metabolic bone disease may result (80[R]). The US Food and Drug Administration is presently considering standards for regulation of aluminium in fluids for parenteral nutrition.

Manganese toxicity When oral intake is precluded, the recommended daily parenteral supplementation of manganese is 0.15—0.8 mg. Manganese is mainly excreted in the bile; during cholestasis serum manganese levels may rise, and manganese toxicity may result. Neuropsychiatric symptoms are a prominent expression of manganese toxicity. Phenothiazine drugs may be administered, which themselves are liable to potentiate manganese toxicity. In a patient treated with TPN and supplementary manganese, together with haloperidol for anxiety and insomnia, several abnormal neurological signs developed: extrapyramidal rigidity and uncontrolled tremor, slowed speech, a mask-like face and micrographia. Once manganese and haloperidol were discontinued, all symptoms disappeared within 7 days. The parkinsonian effect of the phenothiazines may be due to free-radical formation in the presence of ionic manganese in the neuromelanin-containing regions of the brain. The neurotoxicity of manganese is thought to be due to the oxidation of excess manganese to higher valencies. Trivalent manganese promotes oxidation of phenothiazines, increasing free-radical formation. In this case, toxic levels of manganese may have increased the patient's susceptibility to haloperidol (81[c]).

Fat overload syndrome The fat overload syndrome, characterized by sudden elevation of serum triglycerides, hepatosplenomegaly, intravascular coagulopathy and end-organ dysfunction, is an uncommon complication of intravenous administration of fat emulsion. The syndrome is a consequence of fat sludging within the microvasculature in organs such as the spleen, liver, kidney, lungs, brain and retina. Necrosis in these organs suggests that emboli are responsible for the clinical symptoms and functional impairment that results. Plasma exchange has been successfully used in a patient with this syndrome who had not responded adequately to conventional medical therapy (82[c]).

Hyperammonemia Six cases of hyperammonemia which developed during TPN as a component of renal failure therapy have been described (83[c]). The hyperammonemia presented as a change in mental status in all six; this developed approximately 3 weeks after initiation of TPN therapy, and in five of the six patients the episodes were of increasing duration and paroxysmal. Serum ammonia levels were elevated in all cases, and they returned to normal when the TPN was discontinued. In three of the patients, serum amino acid analysis in the acute phase showed reduced levels of ornithine and citrulline (the substrate and product, respectively, of condensation with carbamyl phosphate at its entry into the urea cycle). Levels of arginine, the precursor to ornithine, were elevated.

Sexual function Priapism has been the subject of eight reports as a complication of TPN. A further case has been reported (84[c]) of a patient who developed persistent, painful penile erection 12 hours after the administration of a 12% fat emulsion. This was thought to have been caused by venous thrombosis in the corpora cavernosa, and the priapism was immediately relieved by bilateral corpora cavernosa spongiosa shunts, although the patient remained impotent. Three different mechanisms have been postulated for this complication of TPN: (i) an increase in blood coagulability; (ii) adverse effects on red blood cells; and (iii) fat embolism. In this case it was felt that the 20% fat emulsion had increased platelet activity, which was already increased before the start of therapy, and that this had predisposed to the development of priapism. The authors pointed out that a shunt procedure should be performed as soon as possible if erectile capacity is to be preserved.

Lymphocyte reactivity The effects of five different parenteral nutrition solutions on in vitro lymphocyte reactivity and measured lymphocyte responsiveness in patients receiving parenteral nutrition have been investigated (85[C]). Lymphocyte reactivity was measured in 15 postoperative patients allocated randomly to receive either simple electrolyte solutions or isocaloric parenteral regimens with or without fat emulsion. In vitro lymphocyte responses were significantly depressed ($p < 0.001$) by the fat emulsion at concentrations similar to those achieved in clinical practice, but were unaffected by dextrose or amino acid solutions. Lymphocyte reactivity was significantly depressed in patients during the period of infusion of the fat emulsion compared with controls ($p < 0.05$). The results indicate that careful consideration should be given before using fat emulsions in patients whose cell-mediated immunity is already impaired.

Intestinal mucosal atrophy The effects of TPN on the intestinal mucosa have been studied in a neonatal piglet model (86). In TPN-fed piglets there was a significant reduction in weight and length of the gastrointestinal tract, particularly in the proximal small bowel. The proximal small-bowel weight was reduced by 67 and 72%, respectively, compared with formula piglets and sow-fed controls. Similar, but less marked, differences were found in the distal small bowel.

It was concluded from these findings that TPN produces marked retardation of the growth and development of the entire gastrointestinal tract, but that the most prominent effects occur in the proximal small bowel, the primary site of nutrient absorption. It appears that TPN, while necessary for survival, is at least temporarily detrimental to intestinal growth and development.

Cardiovascular Intravenous nutrition by peripheral vein is associated with a high risk of thrombophlebitis. The addition of heparin (500 U/l) and hydrocortisone (5 mg/l) significantly reduced the risk of thrombophlebitis from 0.43 to 0.11 episodes per patient-day, and a reduction in osmolality of the solution resulted in a further fall in the incidence of thrombophlebitis to 0.04 episodes per patient-day, and a significant increase in the median life span of the cannula from 26 to 86 hours (87[c]). The authors suggested that the risks of peripheral thrombophlebitis with parenteral nutrition given via a peripheral vein are linked with the osmolality of the material, and that they can be reduced by lowering the osmolality and by addition of heparin and hydrocortisone. Since the risk and incidence of thrombophlebitis is directly proportional to the duration of the infusion, it is clear that peripheral intravenous nutrition should only be given in this way to patients who require nutritional support for a short period; that is, less than 10 days.

In a companion study it has been shown that the incidence of infusion phlebitis is minimized during total parenteral nutrition by cyclic infusion of nutrient solutions, and by rotation of venous access sites (88[c]).

CATHETER INFECTION

Catheter sepsis rates in TPN are variable, depending on several patient factors. These include immunosuppression or associated critical illness, multiple intravascular catheters, and bacterial transfer from another source in the body. Catheter-related sepsis may present as fever, chills, change in mental status, hypotension and leukocytosis. In patients with suspected catheter-related infection whose peripheral blood cultures do not grow the same organism as a culture drawn directly from the catheter, a guide wire exchange of the catheter may be effective. However, this is a surgical procedure which may become complicated by catheter malposition, air embolism, dislodgement of a septic thrombus, or cardiac arrhythmias (89[r]).

In a study of catheter infection in patients treated with TPN a distant septic focus was present in 165 of 244 patients (188 of 269 catheters: 69.9%). There was a colonization rate of 19.1% of the catheters of the patients with a distant septic focus, compared with 7.4% in patients without a distant septic focus ($p<0.05$). There was a high mortality rate in patients with a distant septic focus and a colonized catheter ($p<0.001$); sepsis was responsible for 33 of the 48 deaths (68.8%) in this group (90[C]).

MANNITOL

The ways in which large doses of mannitol used in treating cerebral edema may alter extracellular fluid volume, osmolality, and composition to an extent which, under some circumstances, may lead to acute renal failure, cardiac decompensation, and other complications have been reviewed by Oken (91[R]). The patient's body habitus, age, total body water content relative to body weight, pretreatment plasma sodium concentration and plasma osmolality, and the presence of edema or ascites can influence the degree of extracellular fluid change and the rate of mannitol excretion to a significant degree.

Mannitol is excreted unchanged through the kidneys, and when renal function is impaired mannitol accumulates and the movement of water into the intravascular space results in cellular dehydration. Two patients have been reported (92[c]) who suffered reversible acute oliguric renal failure following mannitol infusion given as treatment for intracranial hypertension. Both experienced nausea and vomiting, and became increasingly lethargic with the development of generalized edema. Congestive cardiac failure occurred. Laboratory tests showed severe dilutional hyponatremia with hyperosmolality.

There is still no finality in the understanding of the rebound intracranial hypertension that may develop as a result of mannitol administration in neurological situations. Kofke (93[r]) has reviewed the evidence produced by Rudehill and others (94[c]) of an increase in CSF mannitol and osmolality after intravenous administration of the agent. The review points out that the reported incidence of rebound intracranial hypertension with mannitol varies widely. There is no agreement that osmotic gradients and their reversal are the mechanisms, respectively, of intracranial pressure reduction and rebound after mannitol. Another explanation is that mannitol reduces intracranial pressure by decreasing viscosity and compensatory vasoconstriction, thus decreasing cerebral blood volume and thereby decreasing intracranial pressure. Rebound can then be explained by the delayed increase in viscosity after mannitol-induced diuresis and elimination of mannitol. It is unlikely that this provides a comprehensive explanation for the effects of mannitol. It may be that passage of mannitol across the blood—brain barrier is significantly influenced by the presence and nature of neurological disease. There may be patient subsets: one might be those with diffusely increased blood—brain barrier permeability. Another might be those with focally increased blood—brain barrier permeability but diffuse distribution of mannitol throughout the cerebrospinal fluid. Such patients might be at special risk. These observations need to be regarded as speculative for the time being, but the idea of identifying subsets of patients who are at special risk is challenging.

SODIUM CHLORIDE SOLUTIONS

Central pontine myelinolysis This subject has been reviewed in The Lancet (95[R]). Pontine and extrapontine myelinolysis are generally considered to be linked with rapid correction of severe hyponatremia. Neurological deterioration is likely to result. It is not certain what rate of sodium repletion is safe. The best data available indicate that correction should not exceed 12 mmol/l per day, although more rapid correction may be safe. The duration of treatment also seems to be important: 12 mmol/l per day may be excessive if continued for more than 2 or 3 days.

Accurate control of the serum sodium is a major difficulty in the setting of severe hyponatremia. The administration of an amount of hypertonic saline calculated to raise the sodium to mildly hyponatremic levels may result in a serum sodium in the normonatremic, or even hypernatremic, range. The serum sodium should not be allowed to rise more that 12 mmol/l over the first 24 hours, and even less over each subsequent 24-hour period. It is clear than an amount of saline calculated to raise the serum sodium by a given amount affects individuals differently. This makes frequent monitoring of serum sodium mandatory.

GLUCOSE SUBSTITUTES

Liver and urinary system Four children aged 2.5—14 years were given infusions of fructose, sorbitol and xylitol after sustaining head trauma (three patients) or after attempting suicide with carbromal (one patient). After transitory polyuria, renal failure of varying severity set in 3—6 days after initiation of the treatment. Serum osmolality fell to 265—274 mOsmol/kg, the hematocrit to 0.25—0.31, and hyponatremia developed. Serum creatinine rose to a maximum of 256—930 μmol/l. Liver damage developed in parallel with renal failure. Two of the children died of acute liver atrophy. The other patients were given symptomatic treatment with balanced equalization of the hyponatremia, administration of furosemide, and carbohydrate substitution. They were discharged after 4 and 8 weeks, respectively, with normal renal and hepatic function. Dialysis was not required. The hepatic and renal abnormalities were attributed to the high amounts of fructose, sorbitol and xylitol which had been administered to totals of 7.1—23.0 g/kg body weight on the first day, which was well above the recommended levels (96[c]).

Metabolic Severe hyperlactacidemia of 8.7, 8.6 and 7.9 ml, respectively, developed in three patients with hyperosmolar syndromes. Each had received rehydration treatment with 5% fructose in water (fructose dosage was 0.5 g/kg body weight per hour). After correction of the electrolyte disturbances the continued infusion of fructose at the same dosage elevated the plasma lactate concentration in two of the patients to 4.9 and 4.0 mmol/l, retrospectively, indicating near normalization of hepatic lactate utilization. In addition to peripheral insulin resistance and decreased muscular glucose utilization the hyperosmolar state was also associated with reduced *tolerance to fructose*. It follows that in rehydration therapy for hyperosmolar syndromes infusion solutions containing fructose should not be used. This 'functional fructose intolerance' is thought to be due to impaired gluconeogenesis. In order to administer 50 grams of fructose, infusion rates up to 1000 ml/hour are necessary to achieve a positive fluid balance and to match the osmotic diuresis that is produced. Failure to maintain proper balance may cause serious metabolic complications such as hyperlactemia, lactic acidosis and circulatory shock (97[c]).

The glucose substitutes, fructose, sorbitol and xylitol, are still widely used in parenteral nutrition in Europe. Their main advantage is the sparing of a blood-glucose-raising effect, particularly in severely ill patients with glucose intolerance. In such cases it may be possible to avoid insulin therapy since the first steps in the metabolism of these carbohydrates are insulin dependent. Keller (98[r]) has pointed out that the major objection to fructose, and to sorbitol which is metabolized via fructose, is the life-threatening *risk in patients with hereditary fructose intolerance*. This congenital disorder affects one in 21 000 persons, and there have been more than 12 severe complications caused by these solutions, several lethal. Since a prior history of fructose intolerance is often not obtained, the author feels that the use of fructose- and sorbitol-containing infusion fluids must be regarded as offering doubtful advantage but carrying definite lethal risk, and that their use should be discontinued. At least, a modified intravenous fructose tolerance test should be carried out before infusions of fructose or sorbitol are given (99[r]).

Repeated intravenous administration of fructose and sorbitol in an adult female with hereditary fructose intolerance resulted in 'hepatic and renal failure of unclear origin' (100[c]). During the course of fructose infusion in both the patient and her brother, who also suffered from hereditary fructose intolerance, the following metabolic changes were noted: hypoglycemia, elevated rise in the blood fructose concentration, hyperlactacidemia, and hyperammonemia. These metabolic changes were reversed after discontinuing the fructose infusion.

ALBUMIN AND PLASMA SUBSTITUTES

All the adverse events have been described that occurred during plasma exchange sessions in adult patients with Guillain-Barré syndrome in a study of 28 French and Swiss intensive care units. The study was based on 220 patients allocated either to plasma exchange or not. A total of 105 patients underwent 390 plasma exchanges (55 received albumin in 208 sessions as replacement fluid, and 50 patients received fresh plasma in 182 sessions). Altogether, 253 adverse incidents were recorded, and in 15 patients plasma exchange had to be discontinued because of severe intolerance which included bradycardia in three, intercurrent complications—mainly infections, and technical difficulties. Fresh frozen plasma was associated with significantly more adverse incidents than albumin. The occurrence of adverse events was related to the preplasma exchange hemoglobin level; age, sex, previous history, neurological severity and the need for mechanical ventilation did not modify the risk of adverse effects. The possibility that some of the events described in this series were attributable to the underlying disease rather than to the plasma exchange was not ruled out (101[c]).

It has been pointed out that intravenous albumin preparations contain a significant amount of ammonium (102[c]). Ammonium concentrations up to 800 μmol/l have been found. The concentration of ammonium seems to be batch dependent, and related to storage time, the highest concentration being in the oldest preparations. Ammonium is probably liberated from protein and/or amino acids during storage, and this may be enhanced in the presence of oxygen. Although this might potentially contribute to deterioration of hepatic encephalopathy in patients receiving this treatment, that was not shown in this small study.

REFERENCES

1. Ljungstrom K-G. The antithrombotic efficacy of dextran. Acta Chir Scand Suppl 1988;543:26.
2. Paull J. A prospective study of dextran-induced anaphylactoid reactions in 5745 patients. Anaesth Intensive Care 1987;15:163.
3. Ljungstrom KG. Safety of dextran in relation to other colloids—ten years experience with hapten inhibition. Infus Ther Transfusionsmed 1993;20:206—210.
4. Ljungstrom KG, Willman B, Hedin, H. Hapten inhibition of dextran anaphylaxis. Nine years of post-marketing surveillance of dextran 1. Ann Fr Anesth Reanim 1993; 12:219—222.
5. Allhoff T, Lenhart FP. Schwere dextraninduzierte anaphylactische/anaphylactoide Reaktion (DIAR) trotz Haptenprophylaxe. Infus Ther Transfusionmed 1993;20:301—306.
6. Berg EM, Fasting S, Sellevold OFM. Serious complications with dextran-70 despite hapten prophylaxis. Anaesthesia 1991;46:1033.
7. Barbier P, Jonville A-P, Autret E, Coureau C. Fetal risks with dextrans during pregnancy. Drug Safety 1992;7:71.
8. Choban MJ, Kalhan SB, Anderson RJ, Collins R. Pulmonary edema and coagulopathy following intrauterine instillation of 32% dextran-70 (Hyskon). J Clin Anesth 1991;3:317.
9. Kitziger KJ, Sanders WE, Andrews CP. Acute pulmonary edema associated with use of low-molecular weight dextran for prevention of microvascular thrombosis. J Hand Surg 1990;15A:902—905.
10. Golan A, Ron-El R, Siedner M et al. High-output left ventricular failure after dextran use in an operative hysteroscopy Fertil Steril 1990;54:939—941.
11. Bergonzi G, Paties C, Vassallo G et al. Dextran deposits

in tissues of patients undergoing hemodialysis. Nephrol Dial Transplant 1990;5:54—58.
12. Biesenbach G, Kaiser W, Zazgornik J. Häufigkeit des akuten Nierenversagens nach Infusion von niedermolekulärem Dexran bei Patienten mit ischämischen Insult Intensivmedizin 1990;27:133—137.
13. Kurnik BRC, Singer F, Groh WC. Case report: dextran-induced acute anuric renal failure. Am J Med Sci 1991; 302:28—30.
14. Stein HD. Dextran-40, acute renal failure, and elevated plasma oncotic pressure. N Engl J Med 1988;318:253.
15. Moran M, Kapsner C. Dextran-40, acute renal failure, and elevated plasma oncotic pressure. N Engl J Med 1988;318:253.
16. Druml W, Polzleitner D, Laggner AN et al. Dectran-40, acute renal failure, and elevated plasma oncotic pressure. N Engl J Med 1988;318:252.
17. Weinans MJN, Kauer FM, Klompmaker IJ, Wijma J. Transient liver function disturbances after the intraperitoneal use of 32% dextran 70 as adhesion prophylaxis in infertility surgery. Fertil Steril 1990;53:159—161.
18. Ljungstrom K-G, Renck H. Metabolic acidosis in dextran-induced anaphylactic reactions. Acta Anaesthesiol Scand 1987;31:157.
19. Gauwerky JFH, Heinrich D, Kubli F. Complications of intraperitoneal dextran application for prevention of adhesions. Biol Res Pregnancy Perinatol 1986;7:93.
20. Tulandi T. Transient edema after intraperitoneal instillation of 32% dextran 70. J Reprod Med 1987;32:472.
21. Ricaurte E, Hilgers TW. Safety of intraperitoneal 32% dextran 70 as an antiadhesion adjuvant. J Reprod Med 1989;34:535.
22. Ennis M, Ohmann C, Lorenz W et al. Prediction of risk for pseudoallergic reactions and histamine release in patients undergoing anaesthesia and surgery: a computer-aided model using independence-Bayes. Agents Actions 1988; 23:366.
23. Lazard T, Deswartes-Pipien I, Tenenhaus D et al. Protéinurie apràs perfusion de gélatine. Thérapie 1989;44:269.
24. Prevederos HP, Bradburn NT, Harrison GA. Three cases of anaphylactoid reaction to Haemaccel. Anaesth Intens Care 1990;18:409—412.
25. Bombail-Girard D, Boulechfar H, Tangre M et al. Etude comparative de l'efficacité et de la tolérance de deux substituts de plasma utilisés comme solution de remplissage au cours des échanges plasmatiques. Ann Méd Interne 1990;141:611—614.
26. Falk Jl, Rackow EC, Astiz ME et al. Effects of hetastarch and albumin on coagulation in patients with septic shock. J Clin Pharmacol 1988;28:412.
27. Fisher MMcD, Brady PW. Adverse reactions to plasma volume expanders. Drug Safety 1990;5:86.
28. Legendre Ch, Thervet E, Page B, Percheron A, Noel LH, Kreis H. Hydroxyethylstarch and osmotic-nephrosis-like lesions in kidney transplantation. Lancet 1993;342:248—249.
29. Haskell LP, Tannenberg AM. Elevated urinary specific gravity in acute oliguric renal failure due to hetastarch administration. NY State J Med 1988;July:387.
30. Schulze VH, Berlin-Buch. Plasmaersatzstoffe: Dextran und Hydroxyethylstärke im Vergleich. Krankenhauspharmazie 1991;12:551.
31. Albegger K, Schneeberger R, Franke V, Oberascher G, Miller K. Juckreiz nach Therapie mit Hydroxyathylstärke (HES) bei otoneurologischen Erkrankungen. Wiener Med Wochen 1992;i:l.
32. Vente C, Schulze H-J. Persistierender Pruritus nach niedrigmolekulärer Hydroxyethylstärke (HES)-Infusionen. Kolner Dermatol 1991;53:733.
33. Lentner A, Warmke S, Genzel I, Jansen W. Persistierender Pruritus nach Hydroxyethylstärke-Infusionen? Z Hautkr 1991;66:214—221.
34. Schneeberger R, Albegger K, Oberascher G, Miller K. Juckreiz - Eine Nebenwirkung von Hydroxyäthylstärke (HES)? HNO 1990;38:298—303.
35. Schneeberger R. Auftreten von Juckreiz als Nebenwirkung einer hochdosierten Hämodilutionstherapie mit Hydroxyathylstarke Akt Ernahr-Med 1993;18:263—265.
36. Gall H, Kaufmann R, von Ehr M, Schumann K, Sterry W. Persistierender Pruritus nach Hydroxyathylstarke-Infusionen. Hautarzt 19??;44:713—716.
37. Jurecka W, Szepfalusi Z, Parth E, Schimetta W, Gebhart W, Scheiner O, Kraft D. Hydroxyethylstarch deposits in human skin—a model for pruritus? Arch Dermatol Res 1993;285:13—19.
38. Dalrymple-Hay M, Aitchison R, Collins P, Sekhar M, Colvin B. Hydroxyethyl starch induced acquired von Willebrand's disease. Clin Lab Haematol 1992;14:209—211.
39. Parth E, Jurecka W, Szepfalusi Z, Schimetta W, Gebhart W et al. Histological and immunohistochemical investigations of hydroxyethylstarch deposits in rat tissues. Eur Surg Res 1992;24:13.
40. Lang C. Risiken und Nebenwirkungen der Hämodilutionstherapie. Nervenheilkunde 1992;11:44.
41. Cooke RWI. Factors associated with chronic lung disease in preterm infants. Arch Dis Child 1991;66:776—769.
42. Andersson S, Pitkanen O, Hallman M. Parenteral lipids and free radicals in preterm infants. Arch Dis Child 1992;67:152.
43. Williams AF. Factors associated with chronic lung disease in preterm infants. Arch Dis Childh 1992;67:351.
44. Wilson DC, McClure G, Halliday HL, Reid MMcC, Dodge JA. Nutrition and broncho-pulmonary dysplasia. Arch Dis Childh 1991;66:37—38.
45. Katz S, Plaisier BR, Folkening WJ, Grosfeld JL. Intralipid adversely affects reticuloendothelial bacterial clearance. J Pediatr Surg 1991;26:921—924.
46. Boden G, Jadali F. Effects of lipid on basal carbohydrate metabolism in normal men. Diabetes 1991;40:686—692.
47. Lindholm M. The ability of critically ill patients to eliminate fat emulsions. J Drug Dev 1991;4(Suppl 3):40—42.
48. Nightingale SL. Safety alert on hazards of precipitation associated with parenteral nutrition. J Am Med Assoc 1994;271:1472.
49. Editorial. Safety alert: Hazards of precipitation associated with parenteral nutrition. Am J Hosp Pharm 1994;51:1427—1428.
50. Mirtallo JM. The complexity of mixing calcium and phosphate. Am J Hosp Pharm 1994;51:1535—1536.
51. Hasegawa GR. Caring about stability and compatibility. Am J Hosp Pharm 1994;51:1533—1534.
52. Baker AL, Rosenberg IH. Hepatic complications of total parenteral nutrition. Am J Med 1987;82:489.
53. Ito Y, Shils ME. Liver dysfunction associated with long-term total parenteral nutrition in patients with massive bowel resection. J Parenter Enter Nutr 1991;15:271—276.

54. Drongowski RA, Coran AG. An analysis of factors contributing to the development of total parenteral nutrition induced cholestasis. J Parenter Enter Nutr 1989;13:586.
55. Truskett PG, Shi ECP, Rose M et al. Model of TPN associated hepatobiliary dysfunction in the young pig. Br J Surg 1987;74:639.
56. King DR, Ginn-Pease ME, Lloyd TV et al. Parenteral nutrition with associated cholelithiasis: another iatrogenic disease of infants and children. J Pediatr Surg 1987;22:593.
57. Gafa M, Sarli L, Miselli A et al. Sludge and microlithiasis of the biliary tract after total gastrectomy and postoperative total parenteral nutrition. Surg Gynecol Obstet 1987; 165:413.
58. Nussbaum MS, Fisher JE. Pathogenesis of hepatic steatosis during total parenteral nutrition. Surg Ann 1991;23:1–11.
59. Komura J, Yano H, Tanaka Y, Tsuru T. Increased incidence of cholestasis during total parenteral nutrition in children—factors affecting stone formation. Kurume Med J 1993;40:7–11.
60. Mullick FG, Moran CA, Ishak KG. Total parenteral nutrition: a histopathologic analysis of the liver changes in 20 children. Mod Pathol 1994;7:190–194.
61. Moss RL, Das JB, Raffensperger JG. Total parenteral nutrition-associated cholestasis: clinical and histopathologic correlation. J Paediatr Surg 1993;28:1270–1274.
62. Chou YH, Yau KI, Hsu HC, Chang MH. Total parenteral nutrition-associated cholestasis in infants: clinical and liver histologic studies. Acta Paediatr Sinica 1993;34:264–271.
63. Yip YY, Lim AKP, Joseph R, Tan KL. A multivariate analysis of factors predictive of parenteral nutrition-related cholestasis (TPN cholestasis) in VLBW infants. J Singapore Paediatr Soc 1990;32:144–148.
64. Mashako MNL, Cezard J-P, Boige N, Chayvialle JA et al. The effect of artificial feeding on cholestasis, gallbladder sludge and lithiasis in infants: correlation with plasma cholecystokinin levels. Clin Nutr 1991;10:320–327.
65. Beganovic N, Verloove-Vanhorick SP, Brand R et al. Total parenteral nutrition and sepsis. Arch Dis Child 1988;63:66.
66. Goulet O, Girot R, Maier-Redelsperger M et al. Hematologic disorders following prolonged use of intravenous fat emulsions in children. J Parenter Enter Nutr 1986;10:284.
67. Marks KH, Turner MJ, Rothberg AD. Effect of Intralipid infusion on transcutaneous oxygen and carbon dioxide tension in sick neonates. S Afr Med J 1987;72:389.
68. Fujita M, Itakura T, Takagi Y et al. Copper deficiency during total parenteral nutrition: clinical analysis of three cases. J Parenter Enter Nutr 1989;13:421.
69. Vinton NE, Dahlstrom KA, Strobel CT et al. Macrocytosis and pseudoalbinism: manifestations of selenium deficiency. J Pediatr 1987;111:711.
70. Tibboel D, Delemarre FM, Przyrembel H et al. Carnitine deficiency in surgical neonates receiving total parenteral nutrition. J Pediatr Surg 1990;25:418.
71. Cohen HJ, Brown MR, Hamilton D et al. Glutathione peroxidase and selenium deficiency in patients receiving home parenteral nutrition: time course for development of deficiency and repletion of enzyme activity in plasma and blood cells. Am J Clin Nutr 1989;49:132.
72. Bowyer BA, Miles JM, Haymond MW et al. L-Carnitine therapy in home parenteral nutrition patients with abnormal liver tests and low plasma carnitine concentrations. Gastroenterology 1988;94:434.
73. Lipkin EW, Ott SM, Klein GL. Heterogeneity of bone histology in parenteral nutrition patients. Am J Clin Nutr 1987;46:673.
74. Vargas JH, Klein GL, Ament ME et al. Metabolic bone disease of total parenteral nutrition: course after changing from casein to amino acids in parenteral solutions with reduced aluminium content. Am J Clin Nutr 1988;48:1070.
75. Foldes J, Rimon B, Muggia-Sullam M et al. Progressive bone loss during long-term home parenteral nutrition. J Parenter Enter Nutr 1990;14:139.
76. Koo WWK. Parenteral nutrition-related bone disease. J Parenter Enter Nutr 1992;16:386–395.
77. Buchman AL, Moukarzel A, Ament ME, Gornbein J, Goodson B, Carlson C, Hawkins RA. Serious renal impairment is associated with long-term parenteral nutrition. J Parenter Enter Nutr 1993;17:438–444.
78. Campfield T, Braden G. Urinary oxalate excretion by very low birth weight infants receiving parenteral nutrition. Pediatrics 1989;84:860.
79. Palyza V, Bockova M. Poruchy metabolismu fruktozy a infuze. Vnitrni Lekarstvi 1992;28:814.
80. Klein GL. The aluminum content of parenteral solutions: current status. Nutr Rev 1991;49:74–79.
81. Mehta R, Reilly JJ. Manganese levels in a jaundiced long-term total parenteral nutrition patient; potentiation of haloperidol toxicity? Case report and literature review. J Parenter Enter Nutr 1990;14:428–430.
82. Kollef MH, McCormack MT, Caras WE et al. The fat overload syndrome: sucessful treatment with plasma exchange. Ann Intern Med 1990;112:545–546.
83. Douchain F, Hode E, Paul JC et al. Priapisme aigu après une perfusion d'émulsion lipidique à 10 p. 100 chez un enfant mucoviscidosique. Presse Méd 1990;19:429.
84. Hebuterne X, Frere AM, Bayle J, Rampal P. Priapism in a patient treated with total parenteral nutrition. J Parenter Enter Nutr 1992;16:171–174.
85. Francis DMA, Shenton BK. Fat emulsion adversely affects lymphocyte reactivity. Aust NZ J Surg 1987;57:323.
86. Morgan W, Yardley J, Luk G et al. Total parenteral nutrition and intestinal development: a neonatal model. J Pediatr Surg 1987;22:541.
87. Madan M, Alexander DJ, Mellor E, Cooke J et al. A randomised study of the effects of osmolality and heparin with hydrocortisone on thrombophlebitis in peripheral intravenous nutrition. Clin Nutr 1991;10:309–314.
88. Kerin MJ, Pickford IR, Jaeger H, Couse NF et al. A prospective and randomised study comparing the incidence of infusion phlebitis during continuous and cyclic peripheral parenteral nutrition. Clin Nutr 1991;10:315.
89. Cahill SL, Benotti PN. Catheter infection control in parenteral nutrition. Nutr Clin Pract 1991;6:65–67.
90. Chuang JH, Chuang SF. Implication of a distant septic focus in parenteral nutrition catheter colonization. J Parenter Enter Nutr 1991;15:173–175.
91. Oken DE. Renal and extrarenal considerations in high-dose mannitol therapy. Renal Fail 1994;16:147–159.
92. Suzuki K, Miki M, Ono Y, Saito Y, Yamanaka H. Acute renal failure following mannitol infusion. Hinyokika Kiyo—Acta Urol Jpn 1993;39:721–724.
93. Kofke WA. Mannitol: Potential for rebound intracranial hypertension? J Neurosurg Anesthesiol 1993;5:1–3.
94. Rudehill A, Gordon E, Ohman G. Pharmacokinetics and effects of mannitol on hemodynamics, blood and cerebrospinal fluid electrolytes and osmolality during intracranial surgery. J Neurosurg Anesthesiol 1993;5:4–12.

95. Laureno R, Karp BI. Pontine and extrapontine myelinolysis following rapid correction of hyponatraemia. Lancet 1988;i:1439.
96. Galaske RG, Burdelski M, Brodehl J. Primär polyurisches Nierenversagen und akute gelbe Leberdystrophie nach Infusion von Zuckeraustauschstoffen im Kindesalter. Dtsch Med Wochenschr 1986;111:978.
97. Druml W, Kleinberger G, Lenz K et al. Fructose-induced hyperlactemia in hyperosmolar syndromes. Klin Wochenschr 1986;64:615.
98. Keller U. Zuckerersatzstoffe Fructose und Sorbit: ein unnötiges Risiko in der parenteralen Ernährung. Schweiz Med Wochenschr 1989;119:101.
99. Panning B, Piepenbrock S. Kritische Bemerkungen zu Berichten über Todesfälle durch hereditäre Fructosein-toleranz im Erwachsenenalter aus der Sicht der Neuroanästhesie. Anästh Intensivther Notfallmed 1988;23:217.
100. Sachs M, Asskali F, Forster H, Encke A. Repeated perioperative administration of fructose and sorbitol in a female patient with hereditary fructose intolerance. Z Ernahrungswiss 1993;32:56—66.
101. Bouget J, Chevret S, Chastang C, Raphael JC. Plasma exchange morbidity in Guillain-Barré syndrome: results from the French prospective, randomized, multicenter study. The French Cooperative Group. Crit Care Med 1993;21:641—643.
102. Chamuleau RAFM, Jorning GGA, Korse FG, Roos PJ. Ammonium in intravenous albumin preparations. Lancet 1993;342:1110—1111.

Meyler's Side Effects of Drugs, 13th Edition
M.N.G. Dukes, editor

SECTION EDITOR: B. VRHOVAC

J. Caron, C. Libersa and C. Thomas

35.1 Drugs affecting blood clotting, fibrinolysis, and hemostasis

HEMORRHAGE AS THE MAJOR RISK

Drugs with a proven antithrombotic action—whether by interference with the coagulation process, activation of the fibrinolytic system, or inhibition of platelet function—are known to induce a hemorrhagic diathesis, the severity of which increases with a given drug's ability to interfere with the hemostatic mechanism. The art is to adjust the dosage of the drug so that thrombus formation can no longer occur or existing thrombi will stop growing and begin to resolve, without inducing overt severe hemorrhagic complications.

For the indirectly acting anticoagulants of the *coumarin* type, satisfactory dosage adjustment can be achieved in well-instructed cooperative patients and where an INR (International Normalized Ratio) and a well-standardized prothrombin time test is used. The risk of bleeding is similar for all coumarin congeners (1, 2), although a long-acting variety such as phenprocoumon, which gives more stable hypocoagulability and hence significantly better persistence of the patient's prothrombin time within the therapeutic range, tends to lead to a slightly higher incidence of bleeding (3).

The individual adjustment of *heparin* to a clinically effective level is more difficult to accomplish, because here laboratory control is insufficiently standardized.

Even more hazardous is the control of *thrombolytic agents*; when employed in high, i.e. defibrinating dosage, these drugs are notorious for the induction of a hemorrhagic defect requiring intensive-care supervision.

Anti-platelet drugs such as aspirin and ticlopidine induce hemorrhages more strongly the more they interfere with normal platelet function, i.e. prolong the bleeding time (4, 5).

HEMORRHAGE DUE TO HEPARIN AND COUMARIN CONGENERS

Short-term gynecological, medical and surgical in-patient anticoagulation

Unfractionated heparin *Low-dose heparin prophylaxis* (5000 *IU s.c.* 2—3 *times a day*) in surgical patients is now known to be less innocuous than was originally thought (6[C]). Nevertheless, for patients without contraindications the conclusion of the Council on Thrombosis of the American Heart Association still holds good: 'low-dose heparin is well tolerated by the patient and requires no laboratory monitoring' (7). With respect to the incidence of local hematoma formation, calcium heparinate does not differ from sodium heparinate (8). The addition of dihydroergotamine (DHE) does not reduce the frequency of bleeding complications as has been demonstrated in a large, prospective, double-blind, multicenter trial of the antithrombotic potential of DHE-heparin in patients undergoing elective abdominal, pelvic and thoracic surgery (9[C]).

In a recent review of the relevant literature, *heparin, given in therapeutic dosages* (>15 000 *IU per day*) is accompanied by average daily frequencies of fatal, major, and major and minor bleeding of 0.05, 0.8 and 2.0% respectively; these frequencies are approximately twice those expected without heparin drug therapy (10[R]). The Boston collaborative Drug Surveillance Program revealed that among 2656 medical patients receiving heparin, bleeding was correlated with the intake of aspirin, with gender, and probably with age and renal function. Unfortunately, the route of heparin administration is not mentioned. The crude risk of bleeding was 9%, ranging from 4.9% for doses below 50 IU/kg per dose through 8.1% for 50—99 IU/kg per dose, up to 17.2% for doses of 100 IU/kg per dose or more. The 7-day cumulative risk for any kind of bleeding was 9.1%. Melena, hematoma, and macrohematuria were the most frequent manifestations; intracranial and pulmonary bleeding were rare. Of particular interest was the peak incidence of bleeding on the third day after initiation of heparin therapy, which points to a relatively safe initial 48-hour period in systemic heparinization. The localization of bleeding expressed in percentages and broadly classified as major/minor, was as follows: 49/11 for gastrointestinal hemorrhage, 11/8 for vaginal hemorrhage (1/3 post partum!), 11/28 for bleeding from wounds and accidental soft-tissue traumas, 6/0 for retroperitoneal bleeding, 6/35 for genitourinary bleeding other than vaginal, 5/0 for intracranial hemorrhage, 4/10 for epistaxis, and 8/8 for other forms of blood loss (11).

Fatal hemorrhage under heparin therapy occurred about once in every 1000 courses of treatment (12).

With respect to the *route of application of heparin*, prospective studies seem to confirm earlier reports stating that heparin is more safely administered by continuous drip infusion than by intermittent intravenous injection: in a pooled analysis of randomized trials comparing different methods of heparin administration, average incidences of major bleeding of 6.8% among patients given continuous infusion and of 14.2% among those given intravenous injections (odds ratio, 0.42; $p = 0.01$) have been reported (13[r]). However, it has been suggested that comparison is hazardous because of the larger 24-hour doses of heparin used in the groups receiving intermittent intravenous injections in several major studies where bleeding rate was strongly correlated to the mean total daily dose irrespective of the method of administration (14[r]). The difference in bleeding rates could thus be attributed more to the difference in the dosage than to the route of administration. In pooled analysis of randomized trials (15[r]) comparing continuous intravenous heparin infusion with subcutaneous administration, the average incidence of major bleeding was 4.4 and 4.3%, respectively (odds ratio 1.0), and no difference in bleeding risk was detected between the two groups. On the other hand, one should not forget the risk of serious bleeding when using the classical technique of 'flushing' with heparin and saline to maintain patency of venous and arterial catheters (16[C]).

Low-molecular weight heparin (LMWH) Because of its reduced activity on overall clotting, LMWH was expected to cause less bleeding than unfractionated heparin. Meta-analyses of randomized clinical trials comparing LMWH with unfractionated heparin in the prevention of post-operative deep venous thrombosis showed no difference in the incidence of major bleeding (17[R], 18[R]). However, a recent meta-analysis of randomized clinical trials comparing LMWH with unfractionated heparin in the initial curative treatment of deep venous thrombosis showed a 35% reduction in major bleeding in patients treated with LMWH; although this result is not significant, this reduction seems to indicate a reduction in bleeding rate, but larger studies in humans are still necessary (19[R]).

Oral anticoagulation With respect to *oral anticoagulation*, the risk of bleeding during the first 3 days after a loading dose is approximately twice that during the third week of treatment (12). It should be pointed out here that the prothrombin time measured before initiation of treatment has no predictive values as to either the incidence or the severity of bleeding complications (12). The *rate of bleeding per 1000 days at risk* is, as would be expected, directly related to the intensity of the drug-induced anticoagulant effect. This rate is ≤1 in patients kept at levels within the range of approximately 1.5—3 INR. It increases to 5—10 with INRs of 3—5 and exceeds 50, and thus becomes unacceptably high, when INRs >5 are instituted (12).

The overall risk of bleeding complications induced by therapeutic doses of *heparin and coumarin combined* has been well documented by authors with experience in centralized anticoagulant control, i.e. in anticoagulant units or interdepartmental groups for in-hospital patients. In a mixed medical and surgical hospital population, the incidence of clinically important bleeding was of the order of one in 20 patients. Approximately one in 50 patients required termination of therapy or blood transfusion (12, 20, 21).

Long-term outpatient anticoagulation with coumarin congeners As in short-term treatment, the intensity and stability of treatment determine, in addition to the beneficial effect of the drug, the rate and severity of bleeding complications. In a recent review of relevant literature, the average annual frequencies of fatal, major and major and minor bleeding during warfarin therapy were 0.6, 3.0 and 9.6%, respectively (10[R]). A rough approximation of the bleeding incidence, as deduced from data of authors with abundant experience, is given in Table 1 (22—28). For patients treated with an intensity of anticoagulation reflected by INRs between 2 and 5, the aim being 3—3.5, a series of well-controlled trials (see Table 2) (1, 3, 22, 23, 25, 29—34) has provided important information with respect to urogenital, gastrointestinal and cerebrovascular bleeding. Macrohematuria, taken as a parameter because of its unambiguity as a symptom of hemorrhagic diathesis, occurs with an incidence of approximately one in 40 years at risk in trials without centralized laboratory control (22, 23, 30, 32, 33) and one in 80 years at risk in trials with centralized laboratory control (1, 25, 29, 34). In an American survey, covering 978 patient years and an intensity of treatment very probably surpassing the level prevailing in most of the trials referred to in

Table 1. *Bleeding episodes related to intensity of treatment*

Conventional percentages (rough approximation)			Prolongation ratio in INR	Bleedings per 100 patient treatment years	Reference
19	P&P		2.50	13	22
20		Owren	2.60	7	23
15			1.80	0.7	26
11	TT		2.60	6	28
9			3.0	10	25
8			4.0	25*	24
15		Quick	6.0	140	27

* Results of an investigation of the bleeding complications observed for inpatients treated with coumarin or the combination coumarin/heparin and controlled by the Leiden Thrombosis Service during a 10-year period. Female patients displayed a slightly but significantly higher incidence of bleeding complications.
P&P = Owren's modification of the prothrombin time, introduced in 1951; TT = Owren's modification of the prothrombin time, introduced in 1959; INR = International Normalized Ratio.

Table 2, the incidence of hematuria was one in 22 years at risk; two patients died, one from subdural and the other from gastrointestinal bleeding (35).

Table 3 (3, 22, 25, 34) illustrates the risk of bleeding also in non-anticoagulated patients. With an intensity and stability of oral anticoagulation as applied by Dutch thrombosis centers, the risk of hemorrhagic complications increases by a factor of approximately 10. However, cerebrovascular bleeding accidents are largely compensated for by the prevention of cerebrovascular thromboembolism (see p. 1021). In the review of literature cited above (10^{R}), the average annual frequencies of bleeding were approximately 5 times those expected without warfarin therapy.

Bleeding complications observed by the centralized anticoagulant control system of the Dutch thrombosis centers (home-and outpatient treatment combined) The extensive Dutch organization for oral anticoagulant control of home patients and outpatients recommends a treatment intensity of approximately 2.5–5 INR, the mean target value being 3.5 INR (36, 37), and provides aid in ensuring therapeutic controls. In 1980, the incidence of macrohematuria amounted to between one per 20 and one per 100 years at risk, according to the intensity of treatment (Fig. 1) (3, 34, 38). This incidence is reasonably close to that calculated from the prospective studies cited in Table 2 (1, 3, 22, 23, 25, 29–34).

With respect to *lethal bleeding* complications, figures are available from three thrombosis services* achieving adequate anticoagulation. The incidence of lethal *cerebrovascular accidents* (the majority being bleeding complications) is approximately 1:300 years at risk (see also p. 1017). The second-highest drug-induced mortality is associated with *gastrointestinal bleeding*, which, as deduced from the annual reports of the large centers, has an incidence of between 1 in 1000 and 1 in 2000 years of exposure to risk.

Relation of bleeding complications to gender, age and renal failure Gender, age, and renal failure are reported to be related to the incidence of bleeding. Patients with renal failure are at risk for major bleeding during heparin or warfarin therapy, but the influence of gender or age remains controversial (10^{R}). The results of the Boston Collaborative Drug Surveillance Program for hospitalized patients treated with either heparin or coumarin, or with both, suggest that minor bleedings are independent of age, whereas for major bleedings the point estimate was 3 times higher among patients aged 60 years or older than in patients younger than 40, but this difference was not statistically significant (11). Another study dealing with bleeding complications in hospitalized elderly patients suggests that there is an even more pronounced bleeding risk for women aged 70 years or older (39). Orally anticoagulated home- and outpatients older than 65 years, controlled by one of the Dutch thrombosis centers, also displayed a higher percentage of hemorrhage than did the younger age group, the effect, as in the former study (39), being significant for female patients (28). The influence of gender, age, and renal failure is particularly clear in studies dealing with heparin treatment of elderly inpatients who appear to have a very marked susceptibility for the often rapidly lethal retroperitoneal bleeding (12, 15).

For men treated with oral anticoagulants only, the results of a multicenter prospective trial in The Netherlands (see Tables 2 and 3) suggest no increase with age in the incidence of macrohematuria, whereas gastrointestinal bleeding and cerebrovascular accidents appear

* Courtesy of Dr. A.W. Broekmans (Leiden), Dr. A. Jeletich-Bastiaanse (Amsterdam), and Dr. J. Roos (The Hague).

Table 2. *Incidence (no./years at risk) per types of bleeding, and number of lethal bleeding complications observed in long-term anticoagulation*

	Bjerkelund 1957 (22)	Borchgrevink 1960 (23)	Moschos 1964 (32)	Royston 1966 (33)	Loeliger 1967 (25)[d]	Meuwissen 1969 (31)[d]	Fekkes 1971 (1)[d]	Joly 1977 (30)[g]	Boekhout-Mussert 1981 (29)[d]	Sixty Plus Study 1982 (3, 34)[d,e]
Years at risk	418	142	60	1250	168	110	917	522	640	685
Macrohematuria	1/22	1/28	1/30	1/54	1/84	1/55	1/92	1/47	1/104	1/76
Gastrointestinal bleeding (severe)	1/46	1/71	1/20	1/83	1/168	1/110	1/152	1/47	1/213	1/69
Cerebrovascular accidents	1/105	1/179	1/168	1/229	1/40	1/62				
Lethal bleeding	4[a]	0	2[b]	7[c]	0	0	2[a]	0	2[a,h]	6[a,f]

a = cerebral; b – 2 gastrointestinal, 1 patient dying suddenly 3 days, the other of complete heart block 16 days after bleeding; c = 5 cerebral, 2 gastrointestinal; d = patients under control of Dutch Thrombosis Services; e = patients >60 years old (median 66); f = 4 proven hemorrhages; g = patients >75 years old (median 79); h = ruptured aneurysm.

Table 3. *Bleeding complications and cerebrovascular accidents (moderate to severe) observed in coumarin-treated patients and non-coumarin-treated control patients*

Years at risk	Macro-hematuria	CVA	Definite intra-cranial bleeding	Other bleeding complications+	Reference	
Coumarin	418	11	4(4)*	4(4)*	26	22
Control	360	1	5(1)*	1(1)*	4	
Coumarin	168	2	1(0)	1(0)	14	25
Placebo	138	0	1(1)*	1(1)	5	
Coumarin	685	10	12(9)*	8(6)	28** (78)***	3, 34
Placebo	667	3	20(12)*	1(1)	4** (6)***	(patients >60 years)

* Lethal cerebrovascular accidents.
** Reason for breaking the code.
*** All bleedings, including minor nose and skin bleedings.
+ None of these was lethal.

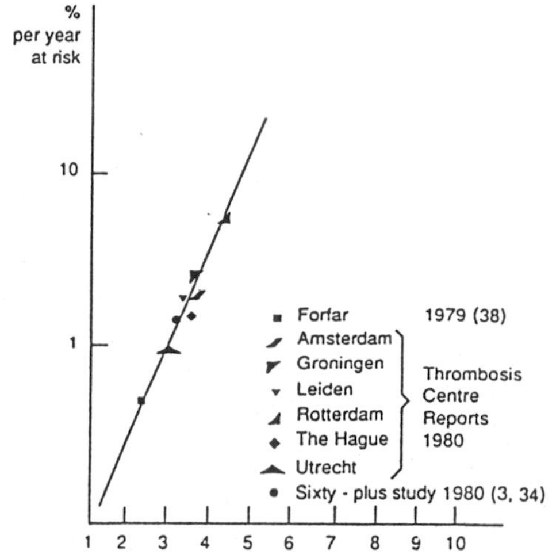

Fig. 1 *Relationship between intensity of anticoagulation (expressed by International Normalized Ratio: INR) and incidence of macrohematuria as the expression of bleeding tendency reported by the centers referred to in the figure. The percentage per year of bleeding is presented logarithmically on the y-axis. A straight line drawn through the symbols reflects the relationship reasonably well.*

to have occurred more frequently than in other studies in patients unselected with respect to age. This is in accordance with a French report on 100 patients (again mainly men) older than 75 years (median 79) on long-term treatment who were followed for 522 years at risk (30). A quarter of the major complications occurred during anticoagulation with INR values assessed at ⩾4. Blood transfusion was necessary in two cases in the French study; in the Dutch study, four patients required blood transfusion. There were no deaths due to extra-cranial bleeding in either trial. Unfortunately, there were too few female patients in both studies to permit analysis of a possible female preponderance in the incidence of a bleeding complication in the elderly. In the Sixty Plus Study, however, females tended to bleed more frequently than men (34).

Thus, data concerning female gender and advanced age remain under discussion and the *conclusion* must be that the incidence and severity of bleeding are acceptable, even in the aged, if the prothrombin times are kept within reasonable limits, but that they are perhaps greater in elderly female patients treated with heparin.

Bleeding complications and underlying organic lesions Concurrent disease is an important risk factor in patients treated with heparin. For oral anticoagulant prophylaxis, the overall percentage of bleeding patients with organic lesions exceeds 50, the majority having prothrombin times within therapeutic limits (22, 28, 33, 34). It is therefore clear that all cases of major (or recurrent mild) internal hemorrhagic complications should be investigated for possible underlying organic disease.

Interestingly, a clinical history of *gastroduodenal ulceration* (often active) is reported to be accompanied by anticoagulant-induced bleeding in only some 3% of cases. In patients with unsuspected peptic ulcerations, acute gastrointestinal bleeding during prophylaxis is as low as 0.25% of courses (12).

A report from the Mayo Clinic suggests that, in patients properly treated with antibiotics for *prosthetic-valve endocarditis*, adequate oral anticoagulation leads to a reduction in central nervous system (CNS) complications: the risk of coumarin-induced cerebral hemorrhage appeared to be lower than that of lethal thromboembolic CNS complications (40^{C}). It must be borne in mind here, however, that the therapeutic range adopted by the specialists in the Mayo Clinic (⩾1.5

times the control value of the commercially available rabbit thromboplastin, Simplastin, corresponding to approximately ≥2.5 times prolongation in terms of INR) represents moderate anticoagulation, which is rather safe. Other reports on intracranial hemorrhage in coumarin-treated patients with prosthetic heart valves corroborate the conclusion that, in patients with prosthetic-valve endocarditis, the risk of embolization is greater than the risk of hemorrhage (41[C]). The latter was relatively high, but could most probably have been reduced if the levels of anticoagulation had been those applied at the Mayo Clinic.

Relation of bleeding complications to the duration of treatment The results of a prospective study designated to quantify the bleeding risk accompanying *long-term oral anticoagulant prophylaxis* gave no indication that the incidence of bleeding depended on the duration of treatment, either with respect to the period before the patient's entry to the study (6 months to longer than 10 years, mean 6 years) or with respect to the study period itself (2 years for patients without breakage of the code) (3). This is good evidence against an important weeding-out process for patients supposed to display a special bleeding tendency.

Prevention of bleeding complications An important reduction in the risk of bleeding may be anticipated if the intensity of treatment is tailored to the indication for oral anticoagulation (42[R]). Adequate control of the level of anticoagulation in the individual patient (36) and proper selection of suitable candidates for long-term anticoagulant treatment are additional measures which can reduce the risk of bleeding (43[C]); contraindications, including severe cerebral atherosclerosis, untreated polyarteritis nodosa or septicemia, must be respected. *Uncooperative patients* must be excluded from long-term treatment with oral anticoagulants. In patients with *severe hypertension* and insufficient reaction to antihypertensive drugs, anticoagulants should be given for at most short periods and with caution. *Elderly patients*, especially those suffering from *moderate hypertension*, from *cerebral thrombosis* or from a *latent gastrointestinal ulcer*, should be supervised closely (44[C]).

Elderly patients should receive lower initial and maintenance dosages. In oral anticoagulation, optimal levels are achieved with up to 40% lower doses than with those needed by younger patients (30, 45). For heparin the difference is not known.

In oral anticoagulation, it is also of the utmost importance to adjust the dosage if the patient suffers from an *intercurrent illness* or receives another drug which might interfere with the anticoagulant (see p. 1009 and Table 4).

Drugs interfering with platelet function, as reflected by prolongation of the bleeding time, e.g. aspirin and ticlopidine, are dangerous and should be avoided in patients adequately treated with anticoagulants. Aspirin can increase the rate of gastrointestinal bleeding complications by up to 1:15 (46). Aspirin ingestion prior to heart surgery increases the incidence of operative and post-operative bleeding in patients receiving the high doses of heparin required during coronary artery bypass grafting (47[C]). However the risk of adding aspirin to a short course of regular therapeutic doses of heparin in patients with unstable angina or acute myocardial infarction seems acceptable (13[r]).

HEMORRHAGE DUE TO THROMBOLYTIC AGENTS

The major adverse effect of thrombolytic therapy in the treatment of myocardial infarction, deep venous thrombosis and pulmonary embolism is bleeding. The hemorrhagic risk induced by *urokinase*, *anistreplase* (anisoylated plasminogen streptokinase activator complex or APSAC) or *alteplase* (recombinant tissue plasminogen activator or rt-PA) is probably no different from that described for *streptokinase* (48, 49[r]).

As one might expect, *short-term thrombolytic therapy* (as applied in myocardial infarction) appears to be much safer than prolonged treatment (as applied in deep venous thrombosis and/or pulmonary embolism). So, the risk of fatal hemorrhages (almost 60% of them intracerebral) increases steadily with increasing length of treatment, with no indication of higher lethality in the first hour (50[R]).

The most obvious bleeding seen with thrombolytic agents is at the site of venepuncture or arterial catheter insertion. This, together with loss of blood due to the amount of blood taken for diagnostic procedures, largely explains the fall in hemoglobin in patients treated with thrombolytic agents, mostly occurring early (48, 51, 52[R]). The risk of bleeding is markedly increased in patients undergoing cardiac catheterization or other invasive procedures. A 1989 general review of randomized trials of thrombolytic treatments reported a 1% incidence of major bleeding in patients treated for acute myocardial infarction with streptokinase independently of the procedure (invasive or non-invasive) used (49[r]). For the purposes of this review, hemorrhage was considered to be major if it was intracranial or retroperitoneal, if it led directly to death or resulted in transfusion; in the most invasive procedure (if coronary angiography was performed during or within 12 hours

Table 4. *Interactions of drugs with coumarin congeners*

Drug (generic name)	Effect on anticoagulant response	Mechanism	Clinical comment
Acetylsalicylic acid	Potentiation (483) (at doses >1.5 g/day)	Unknown	Avoid concurrent use; may also cause thrombocytopathy and gastric erosion; ulcerogenic
Allopurinol	Potentiation (484)	Inhibition of microsomal enzymes (485)	Adjustment of dosage
Aminoglutethimide	Diminution possible (486)	Unknown	Adjustment of dosage
Aminoglycoside antibiotics	Potentiation possible (487)	Decreased availability of vitamin K (488)	Monitoring of INR
Aminosalicylic acid	Potentiation possible (489)	Unknown	Anecdotal
Amiodarone	Potentiation (490–492)	Reduced warfarin and acenocoumarol clearance (490, 493)	Adjustment of dosage
Anabolic steroids and androgens (C17-alkylated)	Potentiation (494)	Unknown	Adjustment of dosage
Antacids containing magnesium	Potentiation possible (495) (only documented for dicoumarol)	Increased absorption (495)	No practical importance
Azapropazone	Potentiation (496)	Displacement from binding sites on plasma proteins (497)	Avoid concurrent use; may also cause gastric erosion
Azathioprine	Diminution (498)	Unknown	
Barbiturates	Diminution (499)	Induction of microsomal enzymes (500)	Adjustment of dosage
Benziodarone	Potentiation (501)	Unknown	Adjustment of dosage
Bezafibrate	Potentiation (502)	Unknown	Adjustment of dosage
Carbamazepine	Diminution (503, 504)	Induction of microsomal enzymes (504)	Adjustment of dosage
Carbimazole	Diminution	Decreased catabolism of vitamin K-dependent clotting factors (505)	Adjustment of dosage
Cephalosporins	Potentiation possible (506)	Inhibition of hepatic vitamin K metabolism (507)	Monitoring of INR
Chloral hydrate	Minor potentiation during initial phase of anticoagulant therapy, not during maintenance therapy (508, 509)	Displacement from binding sites on plasma proteins (510)	No practical importance
Chloramphenicol	Potentiation (511, 512)	Unknown	Adjustment of dosage
Chlortalidone	(Pseudo)diminution (513)	Hemoconcentration (513)	No practical importance
Cholestyramine	Diminution (514)	Decreased absorption and interruption of enterohepatic circulation (514, 515)	Adjustment of dosage; separating dosage of both drugs with long time interval
Cimetidine	Potentiation (516) (not documented for phenprocoumon (517))	Stereoselective inhibition of warfarin elimination (518)	Adjustment of dosage
Cinchophen	Potentiation (519)	Unknown	Avoid concurrent use
Ciprofloxacin	Potentiation (520, 521)	Unknown	Monitoring of INR
Clofibrate	Potentiation (522)	Unknown	Adjustment of dosage
Corticosteroids	Ambiguous (523, 524)		No practical importance
Co-trimoxazole	Potentiation (525, 526)	Unknown	Adjustment of dosage
Cyclophosphamide	Diminution possible (527)	Unknown	Anecdotal
Cyclosporine	Diminution possible (528)	Unknown	Adjustment of dosage
Danazol	Potentiation (529)		
Dichloralphenazone	Diminution (530)	Induction of microsomal enzymes by phenazone (530)	Adjustment of dosage
Diflunisal	Potentiation possible (531)	Unknown	Avoid concurrent use; may also cause thrombocytopathy and gastric erosion

Table 4. *(continued)*

Drug (generic name)	Effect on anticoagulant response	Mechanism	Clinical comment
Disulfiram	Potentiation (532)	Inhibition of microsomal enzymes (532)	Adjustment of dosage
Erythromycin	Potentiation possible (533, 526)	Reduced warfarin clearance (534)	Monitoring of INR
Ethchlorvynol	Diminution (535)	Unknown	Adjustment of dosage
Ethacrynic acid	Potentiation possible (536)		Anecdotal
Feprazone	Potentiation (537)	Displacement from binding sites on plasma proteins and stereoselective metabolic changes in case of warfarin (538, 539)	Avoid concurrent use; is also ulcerogenic
Floctafenine	Minor potentiation (540)	Unknown	Monitoring of INR
Fluconazole	Potentiation possible (541–543)	Unknown	Monitoring of INR
Fluoxetine	None (544)		
Flurbiprofen	Potentiation possible (545, 546)	Unknown	Monitoring of INR
Glafenine	Minor potentiation (547)	Unknown	Monitoring of INR
Glucagon	Potentiation (548)	Unknown	Avoid concurrent use
Glutethimide	Diminution (549)	Induction of microsomal enzymes (549)	Adjustment of dosage
Griseofulvin	Diminution (550)	Unknown	Adjustment of dosage
Halofenate	Potentiation (551)	Unknown	Anecdotal
Haloperidol	Diminution possible (552)	Unknown	Anecdotal
Isoniazid	Potentiation possible (553)	Unknown	Anecdotal
Itraconazole	Potentiation possible (554)	Unknown	Monitoring of INR
Ketoconazole	Potentiation possible (555)	Unknown	Monitoring of INR
Lovastatin	Potentiation possible (556)	Unknown	Monitoring of INR
Mefenamic acid	Potentiation possible (557)		No clinical importance
Mercaptopurine	Diminution (558)	Unknown	Adjustment of dosage
Methylsalicylate	Potentiation (559) with topical methylsalicylate ointment		
Metronidazole	Potentiation (560)	Stereoselective metabolic changes in cases of warfarin (560)	Adjustment of dosage
Miconazole	Potentiation possible (561) even with topical applications (562, 563)	Unknown	Avoid concurrent use
Nafcillin	Diminution possible (564)		Anecdotal
Nalidixic acid	Potentiation possible (565)		Anecdotal
Norfloxacin	Potentiation (520)	Unknown	Monitoring of INR
Nutritional preparations	Diminution (566)	Increased avaibility of vitamin K (566)	Adjustment of dosage
Ofloxacin	Potentiation (567)	Unknown	Monitoring of INR
Omeprazole	Potentiation (568)	Unknown	Monitoring of INR
Oral contraceptives	Ambiguous (569, 570)		No practical importance
Oxametacin	Potentiation (571)		Monitoring of INR
Oxolamine	Potentiation possible (572)	Unknown	Adjustment of dosage
Oxyphenbutazone	Potentiation (573)	Displacement from binding sites on plasma proteins and stereoselective metabolic changes in case of warfarin (538, 539)	Avoid concurrent use; is also ulcerogenic
Paracetamol	Potentiation possible (574)	Unknown	No pratical importance
Phenylbutazone	Potentiation (575)	Displacement from binding sites on plasma proteins and stereoselective metabolic changes in case of warfarin (538, 539)	Avoid concurrent use; is also ulcerogenic
Phenyramidol	Potentiation (576)	Inhibition of microsomal enzymes (577)	Adjustment of dosage
Phenytoin	Diminution (578) (warfarin may give potentiation (579))	Unknown	Adjustment of dosage

Table 4. *(continued)*

Drug (generic name)	Effect on anticoagulant response	Mechanism	Clinical comment
Piracetam	Potentiation possible (580)		Anecdotal
Piroxicam	Potentiation (581)		Monitoring of INR
Quinidine	Potentiation possible (582)	Unknown	Monitoring of INR
Ranitidine	Possible potentiation for high dosage (583)	Unknown	Monitoring of INR if high dosage
Rifampicin	Diminution (584)	Induction of microsomal enzyme (585)	Adjustment of dosage
Spironolactone	(Pseudo)diminution (586)	Hemoconcentration (586)	No practical importance
Sucralfate	Diminution possible (587, 588)		Anecdotal
Sulfinpyrazone	Potentiation possible (589-592) (not documented for phenprocoumon (591))	Microsomal enzyme inhibition (593)	Adjustment of dosage
Sulfonamides	Potentiation possible (594, 595)	Unknown	Anecdotal
Sulindac	Potentiation possible (596, 597)	Unknown	Monitoring of INR
Tamoxifen	Potentiation possible (598–600)	Unknown	Adjustment of dosage
Tetracyclines	Potentiation possible (512, 525)	Decreased availability of vitamin K (488)	Monitoring of INR
Thiouracils	Diminution	Decreased catabolism of vitamin K-dependent clotting factors (505)	Adjustment of dosage
Thyroid compounds	Potentiation (601)	Increased catabolism of vitamin K-dependent clotting factors (505)	Adjustment of dosage
Tienilic acid	Potentiation (602)	Unknown	Avoid concurrent use
Ubidecarone	Reduction (603)	Unknown	Adjustment of dosage
Vitamin E	Potentiation possible (604)	Unknown	Anecdotal

of thrombolytic therapy), the incidence of major bleeding was 15% as compared to 0.8% with the non-invasive procedure. In more recent multicentric studies using a non-invasive procedure in acute myocardial infarction, the incidence of major bleedings was ≤1% in patients treated with streptokinase, anistreplase or alteplase (53[c]–58[c])

Similar increases of major bleeding have been reported in both patients undergoing invasive procedures in studies comparing streptokinase and alteplase or streptokinase and anistreplase in the treatment of acute myocardial infarction as well as in the invasive management of pulmonary emboli with streptokinase (49[r]).

Some reports of serious adverse consequences occurring in patients with aortic dissection or pericarditis (even with primary cerebrovascular accident) that mimicked clinical or ECG myocardial infarction emphasize the necessity of accurate diagnosis before thrombolytic treatment in patients with chest pain or atypical ECG alterations (59[C]–62[C]).

The incidence of hemorrhagic complications is significantly greater with *high-doses of streptokinase* in treatment of deep venous thrombosis (63[CR]). High-dosage streptokinase thrombolysis applied *for* 2–3 *days* with an initial dose of 500 000 units followed by a maintenance dose of 3 600 000 units per 24 hours led to a 10% rate of major spontaneous bleeding complications with a fatal outcome in four older subjects out of the total of 98 patients. In the majority of bleedings, residual fibrinogen levels were <1.5 g/liter (64). The fatality rate of bleeding caused by streptokinase amounts to 7% in cases treated for peripheral arterial occlusion; it is much lower, however, in young patients treated for venous thromboembolism (65, 66). The fatality rate is much higher than that known for conventional thrombosis prophylaxis with heparin and coumarin preparations (67). Thrombolysis should therefore be avoided unless there is an indisputable indication such as iliac venous thrombosis (phlegmatia alba) in young patients, in whom this treatment affords definitely better prevention of the post-thrombotic syndrome than does conventional heparin/coumarin therapy. Contraindications must be considered very carefully, especially cerebral lesions (64, 68[R]) and retinal hemorrhage (69).

It goes without saying that the combination of thrombolysis with drugs known to induce hemostatic imbalance will increase the danger of bleeding even more. The safety data on 209 US cases in the Hoechst-Roussel intracoronary streptokinase registry also underscore the danger of excessive bleeding when thrombolysis is associated with general heparinization (70[C]). In one well-controlled clinical trial, bleeding complications associated with streptokinase/ancrod treatment were significantly more severe than those seen with streptokinase/coumarin (71).

HEMORRHAGE DUE TO ANTI-PLATELET DRUGS

The most relevant information on hemorrhagic complications occurring during prophylaxis with anti-platelet drugs, whether applied singly or in combination, has been provided by well-controlled prospective trials with *aspirin* (72), *aspirin combined with dipyridamole* (73) or aspirin compared with *oral anticoagulants* (74).

With *ticlopidine*, bleeding time may be prolonged by up to 30 minutes. In well-controlled studies with ticlopidine, the overall incidence of minor bleeding can be estimated at 10% of all patients (menorrhagia, bruises and epistaxis) (75[R]). The underlying severe disturbance of the hemostatic function of platelets may be accompanied by serious per- and postoperative bleeding. As for aspirin, the disturbance of platelet function is irreversible. The bleeding time therefore will not return to normal sooner then 5—10 days after withdrawal, but can be corrected immediately by platelet transfusion. In a retrospective study comparing the post hemorrhagic risk in patients who had received platelet antiaggregants preoperatively for coronary surgery revascularization, a significant increase in postoperative hemorrhage and a higher incidence of re-operations was observed in the patients treated with ticlopidine as compared with other antiaggregants (76[C]). In a randomized trial comparing ticlopidine (500 mg daily) with aspirin (1300 mg daily) for the prevention of stroke in high risk patients, the incidences of bleeding were similar in both group, although more patients treated with aspirin developed peptic ulcerations or gastrointestinal hemorrhages (77[C]). For patients treated with ticlopidine prior to elective surgery, it is recommended that the drug be withdrawn 10 days before the operation (4). In case of emergencies, corticosteroids given intravenously may help to shorten the prolonged bleeding time (78). Thrombocytopenia, reversible on discontinuation of the drug, is another adverse reaction which can occur as early as the fifth week on ticlopidine, its probable cause being the development of antibodies against platelets.

SPECIAL BLEEDING COMPLICATIONS KNOWN TO OCCUR DURING ANTICOAGULATION AND THROMBOLYTIC TREATMENT

Unusual bleedings can occur with both anticoagulants and thrombolytic agents. Oral anticoagulants and heparin have been available for a long time, which explain why most reports of bleeding as a side effect are with these therapies. Some special case reports are specified when occurring with thrombolytic treatment.

Pineal hemorrhage One case of *pineal apoplexy* due to hemorrhage into a pineal cyst has been reported (79[C]).

Intrapituitary bleeding Two cases of intrapituitary bleeding have been reported in patients suffering from pituitary tumors, one with oral anticoagulant (80[C]), another with streptokinase, heparin and aspirin given for recent myocardial infarction (81[C]).

Bleeding into a goiter Bleeding into a cyst of a nodular colloid goiter, leading to acute respiratory distress, developed in a patient with excessive hypocoagulability in the course of long-term anticoagulation with phenprocoumon (82[C]).

Adrenal bleeding Hemorrhage into the adrenal glands—which is known to occur during heparin treatment (83[C], 84) but has also been observed in patients receiving coumarin alone (85[C], 86[C])—is rare. Under oral anticoagulation, the bleeding starts on average 1 week after the institution of the treatment; after the third week, bleeding is exceptional (87[C]). As a rule, it is seen in severely ill patients with cardiac failure. Venous congestion combined with adrenocortical stimulation (88) and cathecholamines released from the adrenal medulla and from retrograde medullary emboli in the cortex (89[C]) are thought to play an important role in the pathogenesis. The symptoms are those of acute adrenal insufficiency, in most cases combined with abdominal distress. The clinical features are pain referred to the (lower) back or abdomen, anorexia, nausea, vomiting, and sometimes diarrhea or signs of paralytic ileus, mental confusion and, finally, hypotension and shock, sometimes developing acutely during or shortly after venipuncture(s) (87[C]). The laboratory findings include leukocytosis with a persistently high number or an increase of circulating eosinophils, followed by hyperkalemia, hyponatremia, increased blood urea, and a low blood glucose level which is probably responsible for the mental confusion but the clinical picture is highly variable (87[C]). If the condition is recognized and adequately treated, the patient will recover, but normal adrenal function will not be regained.

Bleeding into a pheochromocytoma has also been described (90[C]).

Otological bleeding Otological bleeding complications are rare. A single case of otohematoma after a minor trauma (91[CR]) and cases of bleeding from the eardrum after gunshot concussion (92[C]) or even without mechanical trauma (93[c]) have been published. Otosalpingitic and labyrinthine bleeding have very occasionally been attributed to oral anticoagulation 91[CR]).

Locomotor system This system is rarely affected by hemorrhage except in cases of trauma. However, under oral anticoagulant overdosage, *hemarthrosis* may occur 'spontaneously', but this is usually preceded by some intrinsic joint pathology (94[C]). A single case was reported to have occurred during heparinization for hemodialysis (95[CR]) and three cases were reported with streptokinase in patients with or without active joint disease (96[C], 97[C]).

Recurrent hemarthrosis resembling hemophilic arthropathy has been described with warfarin (98[C]) and a case of acute hemorrhagic bursitis with alteplase (99[C]).

Carpal tunnel hemorrhage has been described (100[C]).

Massive hematomas often occur in muscles after *intramuscular injections*, but they can apparently also occur spontaneously. A hematoma of the *rectus abdominis muscle*, an uncommon but not unknown condition, is an example of the spontaneous type of bleeding which can cause severe anemia and acute anuria due to a large, deeply situated hematoma of the rectus sheath. Surgical treatment is usually indicated, and the earlier it is applied, the more favorable the result will be (101[CR]).

Ischemic compartment syndromes of the *flexor muscles of the forearm, of the thigh or of the calf* due to bleeding after puncture (102[C]) or after minor trauma (103[C]) in patients taking anticoagulants may occur. In such cases, immediate fasciotomy can prevent irreversible hemorrhagic muscle necrosis.

Respiratory system Soft-tissue bleeding in the *pharyngolaryngeal* region or *sublingual* space accompanied by upper airway obstruction with asphyxia (pseudo-Ludwig phenomenon) is extremely rare (104[C]) and often requires intubation, tracheostomy or cricothyrotomy (105[C]).

Bleeding from *lung cysts* (106[C]), from *pulmonary infarct* and from bacterial *pneumonia* lesions is rare and is most probably due to over-anticoagulation (107[C]).

Pulmonary hematoma secondary to anticoagulant therapy is a well known, though very rare, entity. It is associated with uncontrolled anticoagulation and may present with *hemothorax* (108[C]). Diffuse intrapulmonary hemorrhage has been thought to occur in cases of severe bronchopneumonia or left-sided cardiac failure, accompanied by hypoxia-hypocapnia, under strong over-anticoagulation (109[C]). Spontaneous pulmonary hemorrhage following coronary thrombolysis with alteplase and urokinase has been reported (110[C]).

Hemothorax may arise from a predisposing lesion such as those associated with postoperative adhesion, pneumonitis, and pulmonary infarction (111[C], 112[C]), but massive hemothorax can also occur spontaneously (113[C]). The mortality of these complications is approximately 50%. More than half of the reported cases occurred during heparin treatment with coumarin added (111[C]).

Cardiovascular system *Hemopericardium with tamponade*, although quite uncommon, is more frequent in cardiac patients treated with anticoagulants than in those who do not receive these drugs (114[C], 115[C]). For this reason, anticoagulants should be dosed carefully, avoiding over-anticoagulation in patients with a fresh myocardial infarction developing a pericardial friction rub (116[C]). The post-myocardial infarction syndrome (Dressler's) may also be intensified by anticoagulants (117[C]). Recurrent hemorrhagic pericardial effusion has been observed after myocardial infarction associated with a ventricular aneurysm (118[C]). The occurrence of 'spontaneous' or 'idiopathic' hemopericardium is exceptional; overdosage of the anticoagulant possibly combined with a virus infection should be considered pathogenic (119[C]—121[C]). There is one report of successful surgical treatment of a case of calcified constrictive epicardiopericarditis which had developed from hemopericardium after coumarin overdosage (122[C]). Hemopericardium is a dreaded complication of thrombolysis. Among 392 consecutive patients with acute myocardial infarction treated with intravenous thrombolysis, a hemopericardium-incidence of 1% (four patients) was reported; two patients were receiving alteplase, one anistreptlase and one streptokinase; in all cases hemopericardium evolved to cardiac tamponade within 24 hours (123[C]).

Routine anticoagulation for patients undergoing a coronary bypass operation or heart-valve replacement can, in case of over-anticoagulation, result in cardiac tamponade in spite of an open pericardium (124[C]). In patients not treated with anticoagulants or aspirin, the incidence of postoperative cardiac tamponade is about 0.5% (125[C]). The creation of a pericardial window with the insertion of a pericardial drain may be a helpful therapeutic measure (126[C]).

In a report of a well-controlled histological study of acute coronary lesions, which showed that the frequency of *hemorrhages into atheromatous plaques of the coronary arteries* does not differ between treated and untreated patients, the authors, unfortunately, did not give exact data on the intensity of anticoagulant therapy (127).

Bleeding from aortic aneurysms may well be promoted by long-term oral anticoagulation because of the inhibition of mural thrombus formation. This is suggested by the case history of a patient with an abdominal aneurysm which, on computerized tomographic analysis, showed no mural thrombosis while the patient was on long-term anticoagulant therapy. Six months after withdrawal of the anticoagulant drug, the aneurysm displayed the same circular thrombotic apposition as the aneurysms of 20 other patients who were not being treated with anticoagulants (128[C]). Systemic thrombolysis in patients with prosthetic abdominal graft may be responsible for perigraft retroperitoneal hemorrhage (129[C]).

In humans, acute myocardial infarction is generally of nonhemorrhagic (anemic) type. On the other hand, hemorrhagic infarction rarely occurs. Some clinicopathological studies have revealed the possibility of *hemorrhagic myocardial infarction* with thrombolytic agents, and the risk of extension of the hemorrhage into areas of non-infarcted myocardium in patients treated with selective coronary thrombolysis (130[C], 131[C]).

Gastrointestinal tract and intraperitoneal cavity
Hemorrhage into the *salivary gland* has been reported as an unusual complication of coumarin treatment in a patient with evidence of excessive anticoagulation (132[C]).

Bleeding complications occurring after dental extraction in patients on oral anticoagulants have been compared with those of an age-matched control group. As expected for patients with a blood coagulation disorder, there was no difference between the two groups with respect to primary (immediate) hemostasis, but there was a greater tendency for late bleeding to occur in the anticoagulated group (disturbed secondary hemostasis). After extractions, sutures were used but only to replace tissue, with no attempt to ensure primary closure (133[C]). Restorative dental procedures during mild oral anticoagulation (INR 2.0—5.0) are not accompanied by excessive bleeding (134[C]).

On the basis of the Boston Collaborative Drugs Surveillance Program, rates of 1.2 and 0.2% for *major gastrointestinal bleeding complications* were calculated for medical inpatients treated with heparin and warfarin, respectively. The group receiving both drugs before the hemorrhage showed a percentage of 0.7. These figures pertain to patients known not to suffer from any overt predisposing illness (135).

In a series of patients admitted for gastrointestinal bleeding during anticoagulant therapy, no predisposing cause for the bleeding could be detected in 20% of cases. In patients with *upper digestive tract bleeding*, ulcer disease was present in 63% of 29 cases; with *lower digestive tract bleeding*, five had a thermometer lesion (136[C]).

Several cases of *esophageal hematoma* complicating oral anticoagulation or thrombolytic treatment are known (137[C]—139[C]). The symptoms may mimic acute myocardial infarction or dissection of the aorta. Excessive hypoprothrombinemia may be present. Conservative treatments led to complete recovery.

Retroperitoneal hemorrhage is also a rare bleeding complication. It becomes manifest as pain and tenderness in the abdomen, loins and groin. A palpable mass or bruising may develop in these areas, and compression neuropathy or paralytic ileus can occur. In the majority of cases, however, the course is sudden and death rapid, the clinical picture being determined by hypovolemic shock with or without abdominal pain or paralytic ileus. Over-anticoagulation is the precondition for spontaneous retroperitoneal hematoma but, in patients with adequate prothrombin times, bleeding can occur in the first and even in the second week after a trauma such as vascular surgery, spinal, epidural and lumbar puncture, or an alcoholic sympathetic block (140[C]). Treatment should be conservative. The prognosis, however, is rather poor. An authoritative report of clinical, laboratory and postmortem findings in patients with fatal outcome, has indicated that tight clinical and laboratory control might prevent (and could possibly improve the prognosis of) this potentially lethal complication of conventional thrombosis prophylaxis (141[C]). Retroperitoneal bleeding has been reported to occur in approximately 2% of the fatalities resulting from anticoagulants (142[C], 143[C]).

Spontaneous intramural hematoma in the bowel wall and/or the visceral peritoneum is among the better-known emergencies, causing what is called 'anticoagulant ileus' (144[C]), although cases occurring during thrombolytic therapy are also known (145). In orally anticoagulated patients, the prevalence, which in a Dutch thrombosis center amounts to ≤0.1% of the patients treated, is independent of the duration of the anticoagulant treatment. The vast majority of the cases have concerned patients with a history of myocardial infarction and an undesirably severe hypocoagulability (146[CR]). The signs and symptoms are those of intestinal obstruction or, in cases of bleeding into the peritoneal cavity, of intestinal paralysis. Periumbilical pain is common, together with abdominal distension and only slight guarding and rebound tenderness. There may be leukocytosis, but little evidence of a shift to the left. Only some of the patients have tarry stools or bloody diarrhea. Fever may develop. Since surgical treatment is generally not required, the condition is known as the 'non-surgical acute abdomen'. Radiological examination performed immediately after oral ingestion of a minimal amount of barium sulfate may show typical luminal narrowing with its spiculated outline ('coiled-spring', 'spiked', 'picket-fence' pattern) (147[C]). Accurate diagnosis could be facilitated by endoscopic or ultrasonographic techniques as well as by using computed tomographic scanning (148[C]). In doubtful cases (after correction of the prothrombin time!), needle aspiration and investigation of the peritoneal fluid will confirm the diagnosis and avoid unnecessary surgery (149[C]). The treatment of choice is a combination of nasogastric suction, intravenous injection of small doses (2—5 mg) of vitamin K_1, and parenteral fluids. Laparotomy and small-bowel resection are seldom indicated (150[C], 151[C]). Non-conservative treatment seems rather dangerous: of 88 cases reported up to 1968, the 47 patients treated conservatively recovered rapidly, whereas the outcome was fatal in five of the remaining 41 patients who had undergone surgery (152[C]). It is conceivable that part of what is called *idiopathic intraperitoneal bleeding* originates (at least in men) from bleeding into the bowel wall or visceral peritoneum (153[C], 154[C]).

Ovarian follicular bleeding is another cause of hemoperitoneum, but will be treated below.

Hemobilia was reported in a patient suffering from gallstones with cholecystitis (155). Hemobilia associated with cholestatic jaundice due to obstruction of the common bile duct by a blood clot has also been reported in an elderly male suffering from gallstones (156[C]). Worth mentioning is a case of endoscopically documented massive hemobilia observed in an excessively anticoagulated 65-year-old male patient in whom laparotomy showed a gallbladder filled with clotted blood and stones, while histopathological examination of the bladder revealed a benign fundal pedunculated polyp (157[C]).

Wirsungorrhagia (bleeding originating from the pancreatic duct) (158[R]) is most likely in cases with cysts or an arterial aneurysm. Diagnosis can be made by endoscopy followed by angiography. Surgical treatment may be life-saving. In a patient treated with oral anticoagulants, simple withdrawal of the drug resulted in cessation of the pancreatic-duct bleeding (159[C]). The question of whether *hemorrhagic pancreatitis* can be caused by anticoagulants remains unanswered. Some reports suggest a causal relationship (160[C], 161[C]).

The majority of cases of *spontaneous rupture of the spleen* in patients on long-term oral anticoagulation involve over-anticoagulation (162[C], 163[C]). Some cases have been described with streptokinase (164[c]), with alteplase (165[C]) or with ticlopidine (166[C]). *Spontaneous rupture of a subcapsular hepatic or a hepatosplenic hematoma* has been described in several patients, one of them treated with a coumarin congener, the other with streptokinase or anistreplase (167[C]—171[C]).

Urogenital tract *Microhematuria* is commonly associated with adequate anticoagulant treatment. No definite correlation between the amount of erythrocyte excretion and the intensity of the treatment has been found (172[C]). During coumarin treatment, a deficiency of vitamin K-dependent glycoprotein inhibitors of calcium oxalate crystal growth might explain the propensity of the growth of microscopic kidney stones which in turn are responsible for microscopic hematuria (173[r], 174[r]).

Macrohematuria can be a valuable parameter of the hemorrhagic diathesis induced during oral anticoagulation (see p. 2), often preceding other complications; it can reflect hypertrophy of the prostate, neoplasms, or lithiasis. Occasionally, it may lead to obstruction of the ureter (175[C]). Two reports of thrombolytic therapy with *streptokinase* for deep venous thrombosis *for* 5 *days* indicate a 20—30% incidence of macrohematuria despite careful control (176, 177).

Intrarenal hematoma is extremely rare but must, in anticoagulated patients, be considered in the differential diagnosis of renal neoplasms. Very exceptionally, spontaneous unilateral kidney rupture may occur, necessitating nephrectomy (178[C]). In the case of rupture of the pyelum with intraperitoneal bleeding, death may follow (179[C]). Equally rare is hematoma of the wall of the urinary bladder (180[C]).

Menometrorrhagia is only exceptionally caused by overdosage of anticoagulants; in most instances an organic lesion, such as cervicitis, endometritis, polyposis, myoma or a malignant neoplasm, is found (181[CR]).

Ovarian follicular (*corpus luteum*) *bleeding* with hemoperitoneum is another infrequent complication of coumarin as well as heparin treatment (182[C], 183[C]). Cases of recurrent ovarian hemorrhage have also been described (184[C], 185[C]). Massive ovarian hemorrhage appears to be associated with poor anticoagulant control in the majority of cases (182[C], 183[C]). It is thought that in all probability (insufficiently controlled) anticoagulant therapy, whether long- or short-term, intensifies the natural process of corpus luteum bleeding (182[C], 184[C], 185[C]). It is important to know that prothrombin times of 2.1—2.5 times normal, as assessed with rabbit thromboplastins and considered to be optimal by some authors, usually reflect over-anticoagulation (37) and not, as is still widely believed (186[C]), adequate anticoagulation. In non-anticoagulated patients the problem of bleeding from a ruptured ovarian follicle or corpus luteum is usually self-limiting, with no major therapeutic indications for intervention (187[C]). If, in anticoagulated patients, free blood is found in the pouch of Douglas and there is clinical evidence of active bleeding, laparotomy to control intra-abdominal hemorrhage is unavoidable.

During pregnancy, both intrauterine and fetal bleeding have been ascribed to anticoagulant drugs (188[R], 189[R]). The anticoagulant level in the infant has been shown to equal the level prevailing in the mother's blood (190[C]).

Nervous system The relative risk of *intracerebral hemorrhage* during oral anticoagulant treatment was in one series more than 10 times higher for patients over 50 years of age than for similarly aged untreated individuals in the general population. Hypertension was the most important predisposing condition. The risk of bleeding rose with increasing intensity of anticoagulation (191[C]). Results of a double-blind prospective trial, performed under the same well-defined conditions of adequate treatment, corroborate the finding that the rate of intracranial bleeding is increased by about 10-fold; in patients older than 60 years anticoagulated for a transmural infarction, this rate may be as high as 1:100 years at risk (3). The prognosis of intracerebral hemorrhage during anticoagulant treatment is disastrous as has been demonstrated by a retrospective study in which 74% of fatal issues were reported (192[C]). The use of prothrombin complex concentrate would be superior to fresh frozen plasma in reversing anticoagulation and possibly preventing further bleeding in these circumstances (193).

Many iatrogenic deaths under thrombolytic therapy are the result of intracranial hemorrhage. There is a higher risk of intracranial bleeding in the elderly, in hypertensive patients, and in those with low body weight (194, 195[R]). Data from large comparative trials of thrombolytic treatment in myocardial infarction seems to indicate that streptokinase is associated with a lower incidence of intracranial bleeding than alteplase or anistreplase, although the magnitude of these differences is low (57[c], 195[R]).

Reports of fatal brain edema after early thrombolysis with alteplase in acute stroke (196[C]) make this procedure hazardous in common use. Recently, the Data Monitoring Committee for Multicentre Acute Stroke Trial-Europe (MAST-E) of streptokinase recommended to stop enrolment into the trial, because of excess mortality in the streptokinase group versus placebo group (68).

There can be no doubt that anticoagulant therapy contributes to the development and severity of a *subdural hematoma*. Whereas males predominate in the non-anticoagulated population, patients receiving oral anticoagulation show no preference for gender or for a particular age group (197). Immediate treatment with vitamin K_1 and a plasma fraction containing the coagulation factors whose synthesis is depressed by coumarin drugs, followed by surgery, may improve the prognosis considerably (198[C]). Chronic subdural hematoma had also been reported after thrombolytic therapy (199[C]).

The occurrence of *hematomyelia*, also called *ictus medullaris* or 'acute transverse myelitis' because of the acute onset of irreversible paraplegia, is highly exceptional (200[C], 201[C]).

(*Sub*)-*arachnoidal bleeding* (*hematorrhachis*) and (*sub*)-*pial spinal hematomas* are also very rare and have only been reported occasionally, after lumbar puncture (202[C]) or occurring spontaneously (203[C]). A case of spontaneous spinal epidural hematoma with cord compression requiring surgical decompression has been described after combination of heparin and streptokinase (204[C]). Of particular relevance here are the results of a well-controlled study on patients anticoagulated with heparin after a lumbar puncture. The results suggest that when a lumbar puncture is performed, postponement of anticoagulation for at least 1 hour and avoidance of aspirin may decrease the risk of developing an extraparenchymal spinal hematoma (205[C]). The occurrence of a (sub-arachnoidal) spinal cord hemorrhage—which was successfully evacuated surgically—in an orally anticoagulated patient suffering from herpes zoster has been reported. The development of bleeding near the herpes-involved ganglia was suggested (206[C]). There are also two reports—in two independent presentations, each of one case—of subarachnoidal spinal bleeding from an asymptomatic spinal neurinoma (207[C], 208[C]).

The symptomatology and prognosis of *spinal sub-(intra)-dural hematoma* (209[C]), which can also occur after lumbar puncture (210[C]), probably do not differ substantially from those of *epi-(peri)-dural hematoma* (6[C], 211[C]). Intermittent herniation of a disc may be pathogenic (212[C]). Both are recognized emergencies demanding surgical decompression to prevent irreversible paraplegia (202[C], 213[C]). However, a report published in the French literature reminds us that the prognosis of the epidural hematoma may be satisfactory even when the hematoma (L4—L5) is not evacuated until 7 days after the onset of the signs and symptoms (214[C]); a single case of spontaneous remission has been reported (215[C]). In an excellent review article, written in German, it is shown that only one-fifth of all cases of epidural hematoma are associated with anticoagulant therapy (216[CR]). Such cases may be attributable to anticoagulants in patients given peridural analgesia via an indwelling catheter (217[C]).

Peripheral facial palsy due to bleeding in the parotid gland has been reported (218[C]).

Brachial plexus paralysis, which is known to occur in hemophiliacs resorting to crutches during an episode of hemarthrosis, has been observed in one patient who was using crutches during treatment with heparin for thrombophlebitis (219[C]).

A case of *ulnar compressive neuropathy* has been reported in a patient treated with warfarin who fell on his outstretched arm (220[C]).

Palsies of the lower limb and the *quadriceps* (femoral neuropathy) (221[C]) result from bleeding in the region of the sciatic nerve root, psoas muscle, iliac muscle fascia, or in the quadriceps muscle itself. The blood compresses rather than infiltrates the (femoral) nerve (222[C]). Overdosage causing excessive hypocoagulability (221[C]) or inexpert injection leading to subfascial bleeding (223[C]), even with low-dose heparin (224[C]), may be the cause of these complications. Computerized tomography is a helpful diagnostic procedure (225[C]). Although with conservative treatment the prognosis is generally good, recovery may take more than a year (226[CR]). It is not clear whether the few reported cases of residual neurological disability occurred after spontaneous bleeding or were the consequence of femoral neuropathy caused by bleeding due to parenteral injections (227[C]). The syndrome may also be observed in cases of spurious aneurysm developing either spontaneously (228[C]) or at the site of a suture of an aorta bifurcation prosthesis (229[c]). A paradigmatic and surgically well-documented case of femoral neuropathy secondary to bleeding beneath the iliac fascia, distal to the inguinal ligament, has validated the hypothesis that compression of the femoral nerve against the iliac fascia and the inguinal ligament is one of the pathogenetic mechanisms (230[C]). This explains why surgical decompression may lead to immediate relief of the pain. However, recovery of the neurological lesion is probably no better than with immediate reversal of hypocoagulability.

Aggravation of *retinal and vitreous bleeding* associated with diabetic and hypertensive retinopathy has not been convincingly described, but Dutch experience suggests that the extent of retinal hemorrhage is related to the intensity of hypocoagulability. A single report of the occurrence of massive intraocular hemorrhage in a patient suffering from disciform macular degeneration and showing signs of gross overtreatment supports this suggestion (231[C]); similarly severe bleeding also occurs in patients not receiving oral anticoagulants (232[CR]). Thrombolytic agents have also been held responsible for severe intraocular bleeding (69[C]).

PROBLEM SITUATIONS IN ANTICOAGULATION

SKIN NECROSIS IN ORAL ANTICOAGULATION *(For heparin- and streptokinase-induced skin necrosis, see pp.* 1030 *and* 1018, *respectively)*

Skin necrosis is a rare but serious complication of oral anticoagulation, seen typically during induction of therapy and occurring in approximately 0.1% of patients. It is conceivable that the condition is more common than is generally recognized, because many *formes frustes* can occur, presenting as painful cellulitis without hemorrhagic necrosis. Severe skin necrosis in a patient on oral anticoagulation was first described in 1943. However, it was 11 years after the first description before the condition was dealt with extensively in a report on 13 patients (233[C]).

There is convincing evidence that skin necrosis occurs exclusively in patients displaying excessively severe initial coumarin-induced hypocoagulability (234[C]). This most probably obligatory precondition for the development of necrosis was overlooked by physicians monitoring the anticoagulant effect with Factor VII-insensitive thromboplastins. Authors using such thromboplastin preparations reported an incidence of skin necrosis of up to 0.7% (235[C]) and even 3.5% (236[C]). Repeated occurrence (occasionally even during prolonged treatment) when the coumarin dosage has been increased abruptly is extremely rare (237[C], 238[C] case 1).

Familiarity with the *clinical and histological pictures* is essential, because the earliest signs and symptoms must be recognized if necrosis is to be prevented. The lesion does not occur before the second day of treatment or after the second week of treatment is started, but usually develops between the third and fifth day. The lesion often appears symmetrically or at a pair of unrelated sites, with a predilection for parts in the body rich in fatty tissue such as the breasts, abdomen, buttocks, thighs and calves. Feet and toes are seldom affected, male genitalia only rarely (233[C], 239[C], 240[C]), and the vagina and uterus exceptionally seldom (241[r]). Probably due to the sites of predilection, women account for approximately 90% of the cases. The lesion begins with an evanescent, painful, slightly raised, more or less clearly demarcated erythematous patch. Histological examination at this stage reveals slight round-cell perivascular infiltration of the corium, edema, and swelling of the capillary endothelium, particularly at the cutis/subcutis boundary (the dermovascular loop), *with fibrin thrombi in the small venules*. Patches of necrotic fatty tissue, slight polymorphonuclear perivascular infiltration, and patchy interstitial edema as well as bleeding are present at this stage. Very soon, petechiae appear which become confluent within 24 hours, forming purple ecchymotic lesions surrounded by a sharply defined zone of hyperemia. During the next 24 hours, thrombotic occlusion of the veins causes infarction with necrosis of the skin, subcutaneous fat, and sometimes also of deeper anatomical structures. Hemorrhagic blisters characterize the onset of irreversible necrosis of the skin. Laboratory investigation may reveal diffuse intravascular coagulation and even hemolytic anemia (243[C]).

The *pathogenesis* is still not completely elucidated, but data suggest that transient protein C deficiency might be causative. This hypothesis is supported by the following observations:

(1) Hemorrhagic skin necrosis has been described for all coumarin congeners and indandione derivatives.

(2) During the initial phase of oral anticoagulant treatment the plasma concentration of protein C, a vitamin K-dependent protein with anticoagulant properties, decreases rapidly in parallel with Factor VII. The biological half-lives of protein C and Factor VII are much shorter than those of Factors IX, X and II so, during the initial phase of oral anticoagulation, there is a striking imbalance between procoagulant (Factors IX, X and II) and anticoagulant (protein C) vitamin K-dependent factors.

(3) Patients with hereditary (244[C], 245[C]) or acquired functional (246) protein C deficiency are particularly susceptible to the development of hemorrhagic skin necrosis.

However, skin necrosis has also been reported in patients with protein S (a cofactor for protein C) deficiency, or in patients at high thrombogenic risk linked to a constitutional antithrombin III deficit or in patients with antiphospholipid antibodies associated with disseminated erythematous lupus (247[R]-249[C]).

Prevention of coumarin necrosis can be achieved by avoiding initial overshooting of the coumarin effect. A primary precondition is the use of a Factor VII-sensitive method for laboratory control; second, cautious initial dosage is mandatory (245[C]), especially in the aged, who require up to one-third less coumarin on average than younger age groups (45); third, adequate patient surveillance is essential. The development of the full-blown picture of skin necrosis can usually be prevented by the administration, on first signs of a developing lesion, of vitamin K_1 (234[C]), vitamin K_1 plus heparin (250[C]) or vitamin K_1 plus streptokinase and heparin (251[C]). Even advanced lesions may regress partially under a vitamin K_1/heparin regimen (235[C]). Vitamin K_1/streptokinase/heparin has been recommended as the therapy of choice. A short thrombolytic course might be given by those experienced in the application of streptokinase. There is no need to suspend coumarin drugs; correction of the overshooting will suffice. Prevention of the recurrence of coumarin necrosis in patients with protein C deficiency, if treatment is necessary, could consist of transient simultaneous infusion of fresh frozen plasma (leading to a constant level of protein C) and heparin both before and at the first time of administration of an oral anticoagulant drug, associated or not with protein C concentrate (252[C], 253[C]).

PREGNANCY

Antithrombotic treatment during pregnancy carries a well-established and substantial risk for both mother and fetus. The mother has an increased chance of abortion and of perinatal bleeding complications; vitamin K antagonists, including hydroxycoumarin derivatives and indan-1,3-dione-derived drugs, may be teratogenic and can also induce bleeding in the fetus (188[C], 254[CR], 255[CR]).

The pattern of teratogenicity of congeners of the vitamin K antagonist group is generally known as *warfarin embryopathy*, also referred to as the *fetal warfarin syndrome* and *Conradi-Hünermann syndrome*, although the latter term also covers an identical hereditary disorder. The pattern is now considered to represent a specific group of malformations occurring in some of the fetuses exposed to a vitamin K antagonist during the first trimester, with a critical period during the sixth to ninth weeks of gestation. The minimal criteria for the diagnosis include either nasal hypoplasia or stippled epiphyses. In severe cases the forehead is bossed and the nose is sunken, with deep grooves between the alae nasi and the tip of the nose; other skeletal deformities may also be present. Half the affected children display upper airway obstructions, obviously secondary to underdeveloped cartilage. Radiography discloses stippling (caused by abnormal focal calcification of the epiphyseal regions), preferentially in the axial skeleton, e.g. the proximal femur, and in the calcanei. Children with milder defects may show catch-up growth and stippling may disappear after the first year of life; in severe cases, however, the nose remains small and sunken in the face. It is questionable whether mental retardation is part of the syndrome, since it has only been observed in cases of exposure for at least two trimesters.

The belief that the incidence of the overt syndrome is of the order of 5%, seemed to be confirmed by a review of 186 studies: among 1325 pregnant women who received anticoagulant drugs, 970 were allocated to warfarin treatment and the incidence of warfarin embryopathy was 4.6% (256[r]). However in a prospective survey of 72 pregnancies requiring oral anticoagulation for cardiac-valve prosthesis, the incidence of coumarin embryopathy was 25% in the 12 pregnancies in which heparin was not substituted for acenocoumarol until after the 7th week, and 29.6% in the 37 pregnancies in which acenocoumarol was given throughout pregnancy. It is of special interest to note that no signs of coumarin embryopathy were seen when acenocoumarol was discontinued from the sixth to the 12th week of gestation and the pregnant women were treated instead with heparin (257[C]).

Present knowledge of the function of vitamin K suggests that oral anticoagulation might induce changes that result in warfarin embryopathy by inhibiting post-translational carboxylation of proteins needed in the normal ossification process. Intensity of treatment appears to be of importance since no case of warfarin embryopathy was apparent in 44 consecutive children of 42 mothers exposed in the first trimester, but who were treated at levels of 40—60% prothrombin activity (258[C], 259[C]). Experiments in rats in which highly intensive long-term anticoagulants produced excessive mineralization disorders favor this causal relationship (260).

Another possible adverse reaction is *fetal central nervous system anomaly* which can occur in fetuses exposed to vitamin K antagonists at any time during pregnancy. The anomaly may be a sequela of fetal intracerebral hemorrhages with scarring. Two patterns are distinguished; one consists of *dorsal midline dysplasia*, expressed as agenesis of the corpus callosum, *Dandy-Walker malformation*, midline cerebral atrophy, or possible encephalocele; the other consists of *ventral midline dysplasia*, characterized by optic atrophy. The patients are never completely normal on follow-up, and the resulting personal and social burden is considerable. According to a review of the literature already cited above (256[r]), central nervous system anomalies were observed in 26 out of 970 pregnancies (2.7%) in which warfarin was used.

Defects other than warfarin embryopathy and central nervous anomaly occur in only approximately one in 50 pregnancies, which means that exposure to vitamin K antagonists carries no marked risk of malformation in general.

Other consequences of oral anticoagulation during pregnancy are *spontaneous abortion, stillbirth and premature birth* (261[C]). In 1980, a literature review of anticoagulant therapy during pregnancy concluded that the overall likelihood of an adverse fetal outcome is approximately one third of pregnancies for either oral anticoagulant or heparin treatment (254[CR]). It seems however, that the high rate of adverse fetal outcomes associated with heparin during pregnancy is probably a reflection of the severity of maternal diseases (262[C]). Moreover, recent studies suggest that heparin is relatively safe for the fetus and represents the anticoagulant therapy of choice during pregnancy, whereas oral anticoagulants may not be, particularly during the first trimester (263[R], 264[R]).

The risks to which a mother treated with anticoagulants is exposed should not be neglected, but the maternal rate of bleeding complications under heparin treatment is reported to amount to 2%; this rate is consistent with the reported rates of bleeding associated with heparin therapy in nonpregnant women, and in warfarin therapy when used for the treatment of venous thrombosis (263[R]).

Another hazard of long-term heparin administration is *maternal osteoporosis*, as clearly illustrated by several reports of pregnant women who developed severe osteoporosis after having received heparin, complicated by multiple vertebral fractures in some women (265[C]—267). Long-term heparin therapy during pregnancy results in changes in calcium homeostasis, for which a dose-dependent response has been suggested (268[R]). The prevalence of osteoporosis in patients treated with long-term heparin therapy is controversial, but the incidence of osteoporotic fractures was found to be 2.2% (four patients) in a series of 184 women receiving long-term subcutaneous prophylaxis with heparin twice daily during pregnancy (269[C]). Histomorphometry revealed severe osteoporosis with rarefaction of the cancellus bone; the number of osteoclasts was depressed (266[C]). Prophylaxis with 1,25- or 1α-dihydroxyvitamin D has been recommended in cases with low serum levels of the former (270).

Counseling and therapy Contraceptive counseling must be given to all women who need anticoagulants. Occurrence of pregnancy in a woman treated by oral anticoagulants should lead to the discussion of the opportunity of a therapeutic abortion. Recommendations for the use of anticoagulant therapy during pregnancy have been reassessed in recent publications (263[R], 264[R]): (1) in the case of previous venous thrombosis and/or pulmonary embolism, two reasonable approaches are possible (use low-dose heparin throughout pregnancy followed by oral anticoagulant postpartum for 4—6 weeks, or initiate clinical surveillance combined with periodic venous non-invasive tests followed by oral anticoagulant postpartum for 4—6 weeks); (2)

if venous thrombosis occurs, heparin should be administered until term, discontinued immediately before delivery, and then both heparin and oral anticoagulant can be started postpartum; (3) in the case of planning pregnancy in patients who are being treated with long-term oral anticoagulants, either replace oral anticoagulant with heparin before conception is attempted, or perform frequent pregnancy tests and substitute oral anticoagulant for heparin when pregnancy achieved; (4) in the case of mechanical heart valves, the management of patients is problematic because the efficacy of heparin is not established (two approaches have been recommended: use heparin in a therapeutic dosage throughout pregnancy or use heparin until the 13th week, followed by oral anticoagulant until the middle of the third trimester, and then by heparin until delivery).

Pregnancy is not considered to be incompatible with treatment with thrombolytic agents. No adverse reactions have been reported in the fetus (65). Septicemia occurring during treatment with streptokinase has been described (271[C]).

ANTICOAGULATION DURING THE PUERPERIUM AND LACTATION

It has long been known that the prothrombin activity in the plasma of newborns whose mothers are treated with coumarin is not significantly reduced (189[R]). Acenocoumarol-treated breast-feeding mothers may as a rule safely feed their infants (272[C]). A similar conclusion holds for phenindione (273[C]). However, in some of the work underlying these positive conclusions, the level of anticoagulation was low (274[C]). Furthermore, there are differences in the coumarin sensitivity of newborns. Some experts thus recommended weekly oral administration of 1 mg of vitamin K_1 to the child (275[C]).

A single observation of a decrease in the required dose of anticoagulant after breast-feeding was stopped may be of general importance, because the prothrombin time—which is markedly shortened in mothers during the last months of pregnancy and early in the puerperium—slowly normalizes, i.e. becomes longer, physiologically during the weeks after confinement (276). An experienced obstetrician has therefore recommended that the prothrombin time be checked twice a week in coumarin-treated mothers post partum (189[R]).

CEREBRAL EMBOLISM

Without anticoagulant treatment about 12% (range 2—22%) of patients with non-septic cerebral embolism of cardiac origin will experience a second embolic stroke within 2 weeks (277[CR]). This risk is equally distributed over the initial 14 days, with a slight predominance over the first 6 days. Cumulative data from five retrospective studies involving 80 anticoagulated and 136 non-anticoagulated patients show a beneficial effect of immediate anticoagulation (in most instances with heparin and in a minority of the patients by continuing oral anticoagulant treatment) on the early recurrence rate of cerebral embolism. Early embolism occurred in 15% of the non-anticoagulated patients, but in only 5% of the patients who received immediate anticoagulation (278[C]—282). Two prospective studies have been performed. In one non-randomized study, excluding patients with a severe neurological deficit, two patients out of 21 receiving immediate anticoagulation developed a second embolic stroke (283[C]). On the other hand, a randomized study involving 45 patients who were admitted within 48 hours after the episode and who had no evidence of hemorrhage on CT-scan, found recurrence in none of the 24 anticoagulated patients but in 10% (two of 21 patients) of the non-anticoagulated patients (284[C]).

The assessment of the risk of immediate anticoagulation in patients with cerebral embolism is difficult because many reports are anecdotal or retrospective and are often without adequate information on the degree of anticoagulation, the size of the infarct or other contributing risk factors. From the available data, it is estimated that in 3—5% of non-anticoagulated patients with cerebral embolism the initial CT-scan shows hemorrhagic infarcts (277[R]). Moreover, transition of initially pale embolic infarcts into hemorrhagic infarcts may occur not only in anticoagulated patients but also in non-anticoagulated patients (220[C], 278[C], 279[C], 284[C]). This transformation can happen within hours or be delayed for days after the initial event. Even in anticoagulated patients, original hemorrhagic infarcts may not progress and resolve under therapeutic anticoagulation (279[C], 283[C]).

In five retrospective studies comprising 151 immediately anticoagulated patients the frequency of hemorrhagic infarcts or intracerebral hemorrhage varied from 0 to 14%, suggesting differences in patient selection and/or anticoagulation practice (220, 279[C], 281, 282[C], 285[C]). Neurological deterioration associated with intracerebral hemorrhage was observed in only one retrospective study (in five of the 28 patients). Two of these five patients were over-anticoagulated prior to the clinical deterioration and another patient worsened after a loading dose of heparin (282[C]). In the non-randomized clinical study, hemorrhagic infarcts developed in two out of 21 patients, in one patient without clinical deterioration (288[C]). In the randomized prospective study the risk of intracerebral hemorrhage was shown to be low.

However, patients with hemorrhagic infarcts were excluded from the study and only a minority of patients had a large pale infarct (284[C]).

In a subsequent (mainly retrospective) study it was shown that hemorrhagic transformation associated with clinical deterioration in anticoagulated patients appears to occur predominantly in large infarcts (277[C]). Other risk factors for hemorrhage are an initial loading dose of heparin and over-anticoagulation either by heparin or oral anticoagulant treatment (277[C], 282[C]).

The Cerebral Embolism Study Group formulated the following recommendations (277[C]):

(1) Immediate anticoagulation is indicated for patients with small and moderate-sized infarcts if a CT-scan performed 24 hours from stroke does not show hemorrhage.

(2) In patients with large infarcts, postponing anticoagulation for 5–7 days may be prudent.

(3) If high-quality CT is available, cerebrospinal fluid examination is not routinely recommended prior to anticoagulation.

(4) It may be advisable to avoid bolus doses of heparin and excessive anticoagulation in patients with large infarcts and make special efforts to control hypertension.

The intensity of treatment should be monitored daily; for heparin the ellagic acid APTT (activated partial prothrombin time) should be kept between 1.5 and 2.5 times the control value; and for oral anticoagulation treatment the prothrombin time between 3.0 and 4.5 INR.

REBOUND HYPERCOAGULABILITY

Sudden discontinuation of *oral anticoagulant therapy* is not followed by either hypercoagulability of the blood or an increased incidence of thrombosis except when anticoagulant drugs are withdrawn because of severe bleeding complications (286). This has been convincingly shown by well-controlled studies, including double-blind trials in patients who were taken off long-term anticoagulants abruptly or gradually (25, 34). Thromboembolic complications after discontinuation of anticoagulant therapy occur in venous thrombosis only when treatment has been too short (286), and in patients suffering from atherothrombosis with an incidence that could be expected in patients not treated at all (287[C]). Withdrawal of anticoagulation because of hemorrhage is not necessarily associated with a greater risk of thromboembolism than is elective discontinuation (287[C]). The former conclusion that the situation may differ in patients with intermittent cerebral ischemia (288[R]) has not been confirmed.

For *heparin*, the situation is different. There is more than mere clinical evidence to indicate that neutralization of heparin with protamine sulfate or protamine chloride induces a hypercoagulable state associated with an increased risk of thromboembolism (289). In such cases, laboratory investigation reveals activation of Factor VII and/or Factor XII, which might be responsible for the hypercoagulability state, as shown by a marked shortening of Thrombotest times (290). The fibrinogen decrease described in patients undergoing a cardiopulmonary bypass (291[C]) may be the result of influences other than neutralization of heparin by protamine. It has been claimed that the presence of heparin in the patient's blood for some days reduces the level of circulating antithrombin III to such a degree that thrombosis may recur (292[C]). The finding that heparin requirements increase during the first few days of administration supports this view (293). Further sequential studies on heparin requirements, antithrombin III, Factor VIII procoagulant activity, Factor VIII-related antigen, and clinical response in patients kept on heparin for 2–3 weeks are required to assess the degree and importance of antithrombin III changes induced by heparin (294[C]). An exhaustive review article covers the main aspects as well as details relevant to this important issue and its possible relation to rebound hypercoagulability (295[R]).

Rebound hypercoagulability after a course of *thrombolytic treatment* is well known. Such treatment must therefore be continued with adequate dose of heparin/coumarin.

INTERFERENCE BY ANTICOAGULANTS IN DEFENCE AND REPAIR MECHANISMS

DELAYED HYPERSENSITIVITY

Skin-test reactivity, i.e. induration and tissue factor generation by monocytes, decreases under therapeutic levels of oral anticoagulation, but lymphocyte transformation activity does not. This constitutes the rationale for the use of oral anticoagulants in the treatment of immune diseases characterized by fibrin deposition, such as allograft rejection and lupus nephritis (296).

ANTI-TUMOR ACTION

Both a direct and an indirect anti-tumor action of anticoagulants has been postulated on the basis of experimental findings in animals (297). Warfarin given alone or in combination with cytostatic drugs appears to reduce the size of fibrosarcomas in animals (297, 298) and osteosarcoma in man (299[C]), and consequently prolongs survival times in both. The cooperative studies program of the Veterans Administration Medical Research Service suggests that, among patients with various tumors, those suffering from small-cell carcinoma of the lung had a significantly longer survival (about 4 years instead of 2) when warfarin was added to the standard treatment of this malignancy (300[C]); this is consistent with an earlier report (301[C]) and with the results of animal experiments (302). No differences in survival were observed between warfarin-treated and control groups for advanced non-small-lung, colorectal, head and neck, and prostate cancers (303[C]). The contention that cancer morbidity and/or mortality is reduced in anticoagulated patients is not, however, substantiated by the results of a retrospective study of 378 patients who had been on anticoagulants for about 10 years on average (304[C]).

It has been suggested that warfarin may have a specific effect on tumor-cell growth via the inhibition of protein synthesis (305). Another explanation of the effect of the drug is a decreasing co-adherence of tumor cells, which renders them more vulnerable to the action of the defence mechanism. The lower co-adherence is thought to be induced by an inhibitory action of anticoagulants on the fibrin network that is vital for tumor-cell growth. This hypothesis, which is supported by the dose-dependence of the inhibitory effect of both heparin and warfarin (306), has been studied in a controlled randomized trial of the use of streptokinase after surgery for tumors of the large bowel (298). Heparin is also assumed to inhibit the interstitial transmigration of tumor cells (307).

WOUND HEALING, BONE FRACTURE HEALING, AND INFECTIONS

In guinea-pigs, *wound healing* has been conclusively shown to be unaffected by heparin, heparinoids and/or dextran sulfate in doses that powerfully inhibit the coagulation process (308) though coumarin drugs seem to alter wound healing in dogs (309). In man, it has not been proven that antithrombotic treatment delays wound healing. The observation of a single case of abdominal rupture supposedly due to heparin treatment (310[C]) remains unconfirmed. Conversely, streptokinase may promote the healing of sutured arterial wounds, at least in animals (311).

The finding that *bones fractured* during oral anticoagulant therapy require more time to form adequate amounts of callus may be explained by an anticoagulant-induced increase in the size of fracture hematoma (312[C]). Another report claiming possible delayed healing of bone fractures under coumarin prophylaxis is not convincing (313[C]). However, the observation of inhibition by warfarin of calcification inside artificial hearts implanted in calves adds to the body of evidence indicating that coumarin depresses not only coagulation factors, but also other (Gla)-containing proteins, e.g. osteocalcin, a shortage of which may also delay (skeletal) calcification (260, 314). Osteocalcin is a non-collagenous bone matrix protein containing γ-carboxyglutamic acid, the synthesis of which is vitamin K-dependent. During oral anticoagulation with phenprocoumon, osteocalcin levels were found to be lower than in normal control subjects, whereas the proportion of non-carboxylated osteocalcin was significantly higher than in normal subjects (315[C]). Since osteocalcin levels reflect bone formation, but not bone resorption activity, the decreased serum total osteocalcin levels during oral anticoagulation do not necessarily imply that bone loss occurs in these patients. However, decreased bone formation and impaired γ-carboxylation of osteocalcin in patients treated with phenprocoumon may be clinically important in circumstances such as fracture healing or when there is pre-existing bone disease. It has been suggested that vitamin D regulates the synthesis of vitamin K-dependent bone protein, but no significant influence of the duration of phenprocoumon therapy on the levels of PTH and vitamin D has been observed (315[C]).

Interference with *resistance to infection* has not been substantiated so far for anticoagulants. For thrombolytic agents, interference possibly contributing to the occurrence of septicemia has occasionally been reported (271[C]).

GROSS OVERDOSAGE (ACCIDENTAL, SURREPTITIOUS AND HOMICIDAL USE)

Similarity of appearance of tablets with different contents may lead to inadvertent coumarin intoxication (316[C]). A single case of accidental overdosage in a 4.5-year-old child (80 mg acenocoumarin in 26 hours) did not produce any proven adverse reaction (317[C]). Transcutaneous uptake of warfarin contained in talcum powder for infant hygiene caused severe hypoprothrombinemia leading to death in 177 of 741 cases (318[C]). Chronic skin exposure to rat poison containing warfarin could lead to cerebral hemorrhage by percutaneous resorption (319[Cr]). Cases of possible (320[C]) or proven (321) self-intoxication with heparin have been reported, but surreptitious ingestion of coumarin congeners is quite common (322[C]-325[CR]) and criminal poisoning has been recorded (326[C]). A single case of attempted abortion with bishydroxycoumarin has been published

(327[C]). In cases of suspected intoxication, the levels of the various coumarin congeners can now be individually estimated, both qualitatively and quantitatively, either fluorometrically or by thin-layer chromatography (328–330).

Vitamin K_1 epoxide accumulation in the plasma, reaching a maximum 3–4 hours after intravenous application of 10 mg vitamin K_1, and specifically assessed by means of a gas-liquid chromatographic method, is claimed to be the best means for rapid assessment or confirmation of surreptitious or accidental ingestion/overdosage of an oral anticoagulant (331).

Patients with warfarin poisoning are generally treated with vitamin K_1. However, in cases with particularly strong indications for oral anticoagulation, e.g. patients with prosthetic heart valves, complete reversal of the anticoagulant effect by means of vitamin K_1 must be avoided. It has been shown that the prothrombin times can be adequately corrected in such cases by the use of fresh-frozen plasma, initially 500 ml given twice daily and then continued with one application of 500 ml/day until the upper limit of the therapeutic coumarin level is reached, e.g. 10 μmol/liter for warfarin-sodium (332[C]).

Large doses of oral cholestyramine may increase the elimination of warfarin (333[C]). This is in line with the usefulness of this drug in eliminating phenprocoumon taken in overdosage (334[C]).

Heparin

ADVERSE REACTION PATTERN

General and toxic reactions *Hemorrhage* is the major risk, as is discussed in the introduction to this Chapter. *Thrombocytopenia* ($\leq 100 \times 10^9$/liter) occurs in about 3–7% (335[r]) of patients, independent of the mode of administration (336, 337), the dose and the type of heparin (338[c]–340[C]). Overall incidence is probably about 5% (341[R]). Higher incidences have been described in previous reports (342) (which may be due to the presence of impurities in the heparin as a result of poor quality manufacturing techniques), some of them obviously including cases of non-heparin-induced thrombocytopenia. Two clinical types of heparin-induced thrombocytopenia have been defined: type I (mild) which occurs within the first few days of heparin administration, and type II (severe), which is less frequent, and which is generally seen after a week or more of treatment and which is often complicated by the recurrence of thromboembolic events.

Type I heparin-induced thrombocytopenia is frequent and is characterized by a mild transient thrombocytopenia (usually $>50 \times 10^9$/liter); the thrombocytopenia occurs on the first few days of heparin administration (usually 1–5 days) and requires careful monitoring but not usually the cessation of heparin therapy; type I is generally harmless and very probably results from direct heparin-induced platelet aggregation; thrombocytopenia can regress in spite of continued therapy. Type II heparin-induced thrombocytopenia is less frequent but often associated with severe thrombocytopenia (usually $<50 \times 10^9$/liter); the thrombocytopenia usually occurs with a delayed onset (a week or more) and is frequently complicated by recurrence of thromboembolic events leading to life-threatening complications (see 'Hematological' below). Type II thrombocytopenia is probably an immune-mediated phenomenon and requires immediate cessation of heparin therapy (341[R]). Withdrawal of heparin will result in remission of the thrombocytopenia within 4 days. The risk of thrombocytopenia is increased in patients with a history of previous heparin therapy (343[C]). Thrombocytopenia and/or thromboembolic complications can occur sooner in case of previous exposure to heparin, thus suggesting an anamnestic response (341[R]). Some prospective studies, including mainly transient benign thrombocypenia (type I heparin-induced thrombocytopenia), suggest that thrombocytopenia is more frequently observed in patients given the bovine lung type of heparin than in those receiving the porcine intestinal mucosa type (344–347[r]). Type II thrombocytopenia is more common in patients treated with unfractionated heparin than in those treated with low-molecular weight heparin (LMWH) (348[C]). Cross-reactions between unfractionated heparin and LMWH have been described (349[C], 350[C]). Heparin-coated catheters can sustain the thrombocytopenia in patients with heparin-associated antiplatelet antibodies (351[C], 352[c]) and therefore have to be removed from such patients. Long-term use can lead to *osteoporosis*.

Hypersensitivity reactions Hypersensitivity reactions to heparin are well known but rare. A wide range of symptoms have been described, including urticaria, conjunctivitis, rhinitis, asthma, cyanosis, tachypnea, feeling of oppression, fever, angioneurotic edema, and anaphylactic shock. Very rarely, hemorrhagic skin necrosis may develop. General vasospastic reactions have also been described, exceptionally complicated by skin necrosis (353[C]). The symptoms mentioned are pain, cyanosis, and ischemia of the affected leg or severe itching and burning, especially on the plantar surface. Cardiovascular shock may occur in parallel with disseminated intravascular coagulation (354[C], 355[C]). Heparin in these situations is considered to be the hapten of a heparin—protein complex which induces antibody production and antigen—antibody reaction associated with release of platelet and vasoactive compounds. Vasospastic reactions are probably part of the *syndrome of thrombohemorrhagic complications*. The latter and heparin-induced hemorrhagic *skin necrosis* are dealt with extensively below, under 'Hematological'. In view of the severity of the syndrome, it is recommended that heparin therapy be monitored, in addition to checking of activated partial thromboplastin time, by twice-weekly blood-platelet counts (356).

The preservatives, chlorocresol (357[C]) and chlorbutol (358[C]), have also been reported to be responsible for local and systemic anaphylactoid reactions (SED-8, 767).

Tumor-inducing effects These have not been reported. For possible tumor-reducing effects, see p. 1027.

ORGANS AND SYSTEMS

Cardiovascular and respiratory Bolus administration of heparin induces vasodilatation and a fall in arterial blood pressure of 5—10 mmHg (359). Some convincing data have been reported concerning the role in these reactions of chlorbutol which is used as a bactericidal and fungicidal ingredient of available heparin preparations (360[C]). For other cardiovascular and respiratory effects, see 'Hypersensitivity' above.

Nervous system Effects on the nervous system, other than those due to bleeding, have not been reported.

Endocrine, metabolic Heparin has been shown to have a strong *clearing action on postprandial lipidemia* (361[C]) by activating lipoprotein lipase. The latter effect has been thought to be associated with an increase in free fatty acids (362[C]) inducing arrhythmias and death in patients with myocardial infarction (363[C], 364[C]). However, during adequate intravenous application of heparin as well as a low-dose subcutaneous heparin regimen, there was neither an increase in the level of free fatty acids nor a change in the number of incidents of arrhythmia in the first 12—24 hours after myocardial infarction (365[C], 366[C]). One recent publication reported a case of substantial hypertriglyceridemia in a pregnant woman who received long-term subcutaneous heparin treatment (367[c]). Heparin-induced *hypoaldosteronism* is well documented both in patients treated with unfractionated heparin, even at low dose, as well as in patients treated with LMWH (368[R]). The most important mechanism of aldosterone inhibition appears to involve a reduction in both the number and affinity of the angiotensin-II receptors in the zona glomerulosa (368[R]). This effect is believed to be responsible for the *hyperkalemia* developing in heparin-treated patients with impaired renal function or diabetes mellitus who are not able to compensate for the reduction in aldosterone synthesis by increasing renin production by the juxtaglomerular apparatus, therefore requiring high levels of aldosterone to maintain normal potassium levels (369[C]—372[C]).

Hematological *Spontaneous arterial emboli*, which constitute a life-threatening emergency occurring 6—15 days after the institution of heparin therapy, were first described in 1958 (373[C]). Later reports authoritatively defined *the syndrome as comprising heparin-induced thrombocytopenia, thrombosis and hemorrhage* (374[C]). This thromboembolic complication usually occurs with type II heparin-induced thrombocytopenia. To distinguish this syndrome from the generally mild acute and early-onset type of thrombocytopenia (so-called type I thrombocytopenia) referred to under 'Adverse reaction pattern', the former is referred to by clinicians as *the sporadic severe type of thrombocytopenia* (375[CR]), by pathologists as the *white clot syndrome* (376[C]), and in pathogenetic terms as the *delayed-onset type of thrombocytopenia* (377). The full-blown clinical picture may be anticipated by musculoskeletal or gastrointestinal symptoms (378[CR]). Manifestations take the form of thrombotic complications, including new or recurrent arterial thromboembolism, frequently localized in the distal aorta and in a lower extremity or presenting as myocardial infarction and hemiplegia (379[C]), but also in the brachial artery (380[C]), often requiring surgical treatment. It also includes pulmonary embolism and/or progression of deep venous thrombosis (381[C], 382[Cr]). Prosthetic valve thrombosis can occur during heparin-induced thrombocytopenia (383[C]). Radiological features are reported to be suggestive or even typical of the syndrome (384[C]). The histological picture of systemic heparin-induced thrombosis is characterized by firm, pale thromboemboli composed of platelets and fibrin (380[C], 374[C]). Hemorrhagic manifestations can associate petechiae, ecchymoses, oozing from venipuncture sites, epistaxis, hemoptysis, and intracerebral hemorrhage (374[C], 385[C]). Amputation has sometimes proved necessary (376[C]). The incidence of hemorrhagic or thrombotic side effects in heparin-induced thrombocytopenia is 22.5%, with 12% mortality as reported in a series of

169 patients (386[R]). The absence of dependence between the amount of heparin and the development of the syndrome is well documented. This is confirmed by the fact that thrombocytopenia with thromboembolic complication is sometimes induced by simple heparin and saline 'flushing' to maintain the patency of venous catheters (382[Cr]). There is varying thrombocytopenia ($5-100\times10^9$/liter; mean $\pm 30\times10^9$/liter) and often moderate disseminated intravascular coagulation. After discontinuation of heparin, platelet counts return to normal within 2—3 days, i.e. much faster than in the early-onset thrombocytopenia. Rechallenge with heparin leads to an abrupt fall in the number of platelets and to reappearance of the clinical signs and symptoms (374[C]) which sometimes leads to sudden death (387[R]). The majority of cases point to an immunological etiology, i.e. platelet-bound IgG (more infrequently IgM) with, after incubation of normal donor platelets with platelet-poor patient plasma in the presence of heparin, aggregation followed by a release reaction. Heparin itself is probably not the primary antigen but, possibly through its negative charges, could induce conformational changes on the platelet membrane in certain patients, thereby exposing a neoantigen on the platelet surface resulting in the formation of antiplatelet antibodies (388[C]). Platelet factor 4 complexed to heparin has been reported to specifically bind these antibodies (389[C]). It has been suggested that the occurrence of the syndrome in patients suffering from myeloproliferative disease is more than a coincidence, since such patients are especially prone to immunization (211[C], 376[C]). It is not excluded, however, that during the acute thrombocytopenic phase there is a global activation of the coagulation cascade, as evidenced by reductions in the levels of antithrombin III, protein C and heparin cofactor II (293—295[R], 390). An immune endothelial cell injury in heparin-induced thrombocytopenia is a possible etiological factor in heparin-induced thrombosis. The heparin-dependent antibodies could interact with endothelial-linked heparin or with heparan sulfate which is synthetized by endothelial cells. This heparan sulfate exerts antithrombin III cofactor activity in intact vessels and may be accessible to circulating antibodies in heparin-induced thrombocytopenia, thereby explaining the seemingly paradoxical occurrence of thrombosis as well as the low incidence of bleeding complications in these conditions (391[R]). However preexisting pathology such as recent cardiovascular surgery, or local factors such as atherosclerosis or endothelial damage, probably localize the prothrombotic process to these sites (390). This antibody-induced platelet aggregation is probably not a passive process but an active one, which is partly linked to both prostaglandin synthesis and an ADP-dependent mechanism. This could explain the in vitro inhibition of platelet aggregation induced by aspirin and dipyridamole (392[C]), and the encouraging results described with the use of a prostacyclin analog in the treatment (393[c], 394[c]) or prevention of heparin-induced thrombocytopenia (395). Thrombolytic treatment or dermatan sulfate has been used successfully in patients with thrombosis associated with heparin-induced thrombocytopenia (383[C], 396[C]), and switching to LMWH has occasionally been successful (397[r]), although LMWH themselves can also cause thrombocytopenia and thrombosis. However, it is important to emphasize that LMHW is not indicated for the treatment of unfractionated heparin-induced thrombocytopenia, because of the extensive cross-reactivity of the two forms of heparin (254[C], 348[r], 350[C], 398[C]). Rapid reversal of immunological abnormalities due to heparin-induced thrombocytopenia was obtained in one patient undergoing emergency cardiac surgery under plasmapheresis associated with gammaglobulin infusion, thereby allowing further use of heparin (399[C]).

A local manifestation of heparin-induced thrombosis is *heparin-induced skin necrosis*, first described in 1973 (400[C]) and later observed in patients suffering from the thrombo-hemorrhagic syndrome (385[C]). The skin pathology develops on the sixth to ninth day after the initiation of subcutaneous heparin treatment and develops at the site of injection of the anticoagulant. The clinical and histological pictures of the skin necrosis are similar to those of what is called 'coumarin necrosis'. It is important to note that there is an increased risk of thrombocytopenia and thrombotic complications in patients who have had previous heparin-associated skin necrosis episodes (401[C]). This form of skin necrosis must, of course, be distinguished from vasospastic skin necrosis and from skin necrosis induced by cholesterol embolization. Ergotism should also be suspected in cases receiving prophylaxis with the combination of low-dose heparin and dihydroergotamine (402[C]). Heparin-induced skin necrosis can also be associated with local vasculitis (403[C]) which may be accompanied by fever. Laboratory examinations reveal inflammatory changes with anemia, leukocytosis, eosinophilia, raised erythrocyte sedimentation rate and a positive capillary fragility test. This vasculitis can lead to organ involvement such as glomerulonephritis (404[C]).

Systemic and localized thrombosis after heparin administration are thought to be different effects of the same kind of allergic heparin-induced platelet aggregation. This hypothesis is supported by the occurrence (after intravenous administration of heparin to patients with the localized type of thrombosis) of signs of massive systemic platelet aggregation, namely acute confusion, hemiparesis, dyspnea, and precordial or extremity pain. Platelet aggregometry seems to constitute the best method for the demonstration of suspected systemic or localized heparin-induced thrombosis. However, use of this method is not feasible until the heparin has been cleared from the circulation and the platelet count has become sufficiently high ($\geq 100 \times 10^9$/liter).

Rare cases of *hypereosinophilia* with positive rechallenge have been reported (405[c], 406[C]).

Liver The effect of heparin on *liver function* is discussed below in the section 'Interference with diagnostic routines'.

Urogenital system Heparin has been associated with *priapism* (for older literature, see SED-8, 768; 407[C]). The frequency and severity of iatrogenic priapism as a result of heparin therapy seems to be greater than with any other type of medical treatment (408[C]). The antialdosterone effect on the kidney is mentioned above under 'Endocrine, metabolic'.

Skin and appendages Besides *allergic* skin reactions and skin *necrosis* caused by heparin-induced thrombosis, vasospasm or cholesterol embolization (see above under 'Adverse reaction pattern'), *lipodystrophy* and *alopecia* have been reported (for older literature, see SED-8, 768). Lipodystrophy may be the result of lipoprotein lipase activity associated with subcutaneously injected heparin or heparinoid. Transient alopecia occurring 4—12 weeks after the administration of heparin is due to the severity of thromboembolic disease for which heparin was given rather than to heparin toxicity. Erythematous nodules or infiltrated plaques at the site of injections, common side effects of subcutaneous unfractionated heparin, which occur 3 to 21 days after starting of heparin treatment, are probably delayed-type hypersensitivity reactions and are seen with striking predominance in women (409[C], 410[C]); these local skin reactions are also seen with LMWH (411) and cross-reaction between unfractionated heparin and LMWH can occur (405[c]). Erythromelalgia has been described with enoxaparine (412[C]). Acute dermatitis at the primary site of contact can occur with heparinoid cream (413[C]).

Special senses *Conjunctivitis* due to allergy is reported above under 'Hypersensitivity reactions' (see 'Adverse reaction pattern').

Other organs and systems Patients who have received therapeutic doses of unfractionated heparin (more than 150 mg daily) for more than 4 months may display severe *osteoporosis* complicated by spontaneous bone fractures (for older literature, see SED-8, 768). Preliminary results from a prospective study which included a small number of patients suggest that a 3-month treatment with LMWH for deep venous thrombosis is associated with less reduction in bone density than a treatment of same duration with unfractionated heparin (414[c]). This osteoporosis has been ascribed to the enhancement of collagenolysis or to enzyme inhibition by heparin. Other authors stress the resemblance to hyperparathyroid osteopathy. Other possibilities include vitamin D or 1,25- or 1α-dihydroxyvitamin D (415) deficiency and ascorbic acid deprivation at the site of osteoblast activity (see also p. 1024). The report of osteoporosis in an infant treated with high-dose heparin (600 IU/kg/24 hours) over a 9-month period, accompanied by severe nephrocalcinosis (calcified granulomas) after candida septicemia adds to the evidence of heparin-induced osteolysis (416[C]). Similar evidence is given by *metastatic calcification* in patients with end-stage renal failure treated by hemodialysis, sometimes associated with calcified subcutaneous nodules (417[C]). In these patients, calcification might be promoted by the action of heparin, since the intravenous injection of 20 000 IU of heparin induced mobilization of calcium and inorganic phosphate even in patients without renal failure (418[C]).

Bacteriological discharges from osteomyelitis sinuses have been described with heparin therapy (419[C]).

Many *other effects* have been attributed to heparin (420[R]), including reduction of neomycin toxicity, protection against peptic ulcers through neutralization of histamine, an antagonistic effect on autoimmune antibodies, an anti-infectious action and the antimetastatic effect on malignant tumors referred to in the introductory section to this Chapter.

Risk situations In *paraproteinemia* a non-soluble pathogenic paraprotein—heparin complex may be formed (421[C]). Hence, patients suffering from paraproteinemia should be treated with heparin only after a test has been performed in vitro to exclude this possibility.

Withdrawal effects See 'Rebound hypercoagulability' in the introductory section to this Chapter (p. 1026).

Interference with diagnostic routines *Pseudo-hypocalcemia* can occur in hemodialysis patients, particularly in those who display chylomicronemia before administration of heparin (422). This spurious hypocalcemia is thought to be the result of lipolytic activity in vitro, sufficient to produce calcium soaps of fatty acid. The cause of hypocalcemia can therefore be detected and eliminated by the analysis of blood samples immediately after venepuncture.

Screening tests for *mucopolysacchariduria* may give strongly positive results in heparinized patients (423).

Concentrations of heparin as low as 1 IU/ml give 80% *inhibition of acid phosphatase activity in leukocytes* (424).

An asymptomatic increase in serum *aminotransferase* levels is frequent in patients receiving unfractionated heparin or LMWH given therapeutically or prophylactically (425[C]—427[R]). This elevation is more pronounced for alanine aminotransferase than for aspartate aminotransferase and occurs between days 5 and 10 of heparin treatment (427[R], 428). The source of heparin had no relation to the development of elevated aminotransferase concentrations. After discontinuation and sometimes even in spite of prolongation (425[C], 427[R]) of heparin treatment, aminotransferase levels returned to normal. The mechanism of the increase in concentrations of alanine aminotransferase and aspartate aminotransferase remains to be elucidated. A concomitant increase of γ-GT has been described in some patients (429[C], 430[C]).

In one study, the isoenzyme pattern of *lactate dehydrogenase* was studied, and all these patients showed elevated hepatic fractions. The pattern of enzyme elevations along with the increased lactate dehydrogenase isoenzyme hepatic fraction would suggest hepatocellular damage as the most likely enzyme source (425[C]).

The artefactual increases of as much as 50% in *total thyroxine*, estimated by a competitive protein-binding assay, and of as much as 30% in *triiodothyroxine* resin uptake are in all probability the results of rapid and continuing lipolytic hydrolysis of triglycerides after blood has been drawn (431). Thyroid function tests should therefore always be performed on blood samples taken before (or a sufficient time after) heparin treatment (432).

Heparin may interfere with the determination of *carcinoembryonic antigen* activity, depending on which commercial kit is used. The negative effect of heparin could be reduced by heat treatment in the presence of plasma proteins (433[C]).

Heparin may affect the *analysis of arterial blood gases* (434[C]). Addition of excess heparin, and acid mucopolysaccharide, to the syringe for blood drawing may alter the Henderson and Hasselbach equation, simulating metabolic acidosis. It is advisable to coat the syringe with heparin and remove all excess heparin prior to blood sampling.

Heparin has a dose-related inhibitory effect on the *chromogenic lysate assay for endotoxin* (435[C]). A 90% reduction in detectable endotoxin was found at concentrations of heparin as low as some 30 U/ml.

Interference with drug measurements and interaction with drugs Interference with measurement of drugs by heparin used in a blood sampling lock is well documented for *propranolol* (436).

A short communication reporting increased plasma *warfarin* binding after the administration of heparin (437) has not yet been confirmed. However, suspension of the heparin given initially in combination with warfarin may well be followed by a decrease in the patient's tolerance of the oral anticoagulant.

In normal, non-fasted subjects, 100—1000 IU of heparin given intravenously caused a rapid increase in the free fractions of *diazepam* (438, 439), *chlordiazepoxide* and *oxazepam*, but no change in the case of *lorazepam* (438). The clinical implications of this finding are not yet known.

Heparin may interfere with the determination of *aminoglycosides* using enzyme multiplied immunoassays, resulting in lower values than with the use of other assays (440[C]). In the case of gentamicin, these lower values may be due to direct binding of gentamicin to heparin, as well as a more complex interaction involving heparin, gentamicin and proteins (440[C]). Blood samples for the determination of aminoglycosides by enzyme immunoassays should not be collected in heparinized tubes or from indwelling lines.

Reduction of *digitoxin binding* to plasma proteins has been reported after administration of heparin (441[C]). In a study of 10 hemodialyzed patients on maintenance digitoxin therapy, it was demonstrated that the reduced binding was a result of heparin-induced in vitro lipolysis, and not a consequence of in vivo binding of digitoxin to plasma proteins.

Dobutamine hydrochloride and heparin should not be mixed or infused through the same intravenous line, as this causes precipitation (442[C]).

Resistance to heparin has been observed in patients hospitalized in coronary care units receiving intravenous nitroglycerin. Primarily imputed to propylene glycol in nitroglycerine preparations (443[C]), this resistance has also been described in propylene glycol-free preparations. The underlying mechanism might be a nitroglycerin-induced qualitative antithrombin III abnormality (444[CR]).

THE COUMARINS (WARFARIN AND OTHER COUMARIN CONGENERS)

The bioavailability of various oral anticoagulants can differ (445). Since in the individual patient a difference of as little as 5—10% in the warfarin dosage may result in an appreciable change in the hypocoagulability state, a small, seemingly acceptable, difference in bioavailability between different products may be clinically relevant. On the other hand, it should be kept in mind that inadequate or variable bioavailability of coumarin congener products is only a minor factor compared with the major problems which still arise when patients receive inadequate doses of anticoagulants or do not reliably follow directions (446).

The coumarins

ADVERSE REACTION PATTERN

General and toxic reactions Except for overdosage effects resulting in hemorrhage (see p. 1008) and exceptionally in hemorrhagic skin necrosis (see p. 1023) as well as potentially in embryopathy (see p. 1023), serious effects do not occur.

Hypersensitivity reactions Proven cases of allergy seem to be extremely rare (447). Maculopapular rashes with cross-sensitivity between coumarin derivates have been reported (448[C]). Nonpruritic purpuric skin eruptions, histologically presenting as vasculitis and reappearing on rechallenge with warfarin or acenocoumarol, have been incidentally described (449, 450[C]).

Tumor-inducing effects These have not been reported. For possible tumor-reducing effects, see page 1027.

ORGANS AND SYSTEMS

Cardiovascular *Vasodilatory action* on coronary arteries (451), peripheral veins, and capillaries, with purple toes as one of the most obvious consequences (452[C], 453[C]) have been reported. Sensations of cold may be due to increased loss of body heat caused by peripheral vasodilatation (454[C]). *Cholesterol embolization*, which promptly improves after the drug is discontinued (455[C]), may also well explain the purple-toe phenomenon.

Nervous system It has been suggested that gross overdosage might induce Reye's syndrome, i.e. encephalopathy with fatty degeneration of viscera (456[C]), but a cause-effect relationship has not been demonstrated.

Endocrine, metabolic An *anti-thyroid* effect of bishydroxycoumarin has been suspected (457) and a *uricosuric* effect has been reported (458, 459). In cases of hypo- or hyperthyroidism, the hypoprothrombinemic response to warfarin is abnormal (460[C]) (see also 'Risk situations' below). For pathological ossification (mineralization), see page 1026. Warfarin appears to diminish *calcium deposition* in spontaneously degenerated bioprosthetic valves (461[C]).

Hematological Blood and plasma *viscosity* has been reported to decrease by 5—10% during the administration of coumarin in healthy volunteers as well as in coronary patients (462[C]). This may also explain, at least partly, the antianginal effect of coumarin congeners. The mechanism might be related to changes in the protein composition of the plasma. A reversible increase in the white cell count has been reported with long-term use of acenocoumarol (463[C]).

Protein C, another vitamin K-dependent serine protease zymogen in plasma, has been shown to represent a regulatory protein which, when activated, limits the activity of two activated procoagulant co-factors, namely Factors V_a and VIII_a. Heterozygotes for hereditary isolated protein C deficiency tend to develop a thrombotic disease which has been successfully treated with long-term coumarin (464, 465). Apparently, the balance between the activities of the anticoagulant factor (protein C) and the procoagulant factors (II, VII, IX and X)—which is disturbed in the protein C-deficient patient—is restored under conditions of long-term treatment with coumarins.

Other possible vitamin K-dependent factors are *Factor III* (466) and the *Factor VIII-bypassing coagulant* (467), but their pathophysiological relevance is still unknown.

One case of hemolytic anemia which was thought to be related to warfarin has been described (468[C]).

Liver In 1963, a report was presented describing disturbance of several liver functions in patients on long-term treatment with phenprocoumon (469). Since then, several cases diagnosed as probable coumarin-induced *cholestatic hepatitis*, have been described; in *six* of these rechallenge caused a relapse (470[C]—474[C]).

Gastrointestinal Gastrointestinal *complications* are limited to hemorrhage (see introductory section to this Chapter, p. 1019).

Urinary tract In one case, multisystemic abnormalities including renal failure were caused by cholesterol embolization. Discontinuation of the anticoagulant resulted in dramatic improvement of renal function (455[C]).

Skin and appendages Purpura, purple toes, skin necrosis, and cholesterol embolization have been dealt with above.

Other organs and systems Preliminary results from a prospective study which included a small number of patients treated for deep venous thrombosis over a 3-

month period show identical reduction of bone density irrespective of treatment with coumarins or heparin (414[c]).

Risk situations (*See also general section of this Chapter*) Patients with *hypothyroidism* and *hyperthyroidism* should all be carefully monitored because, with the former condition, the response to the drug is greatly reduced and, with the latter, greatly enhanced (460[CR]). When treated, the susceptibility of these patients to coumarin gradually normalizes.

Other risk-enhancing factors are *inability to comply with the regimen*, severe *liver damage*, *thrombocytopenia*, endogenous *coagulation disturbances*, severe *hypertension*, *tumors*, *ulcerations* and *cerebrovascular disease*.

Patients with *impaired renal function* (475) or mild to moderate *hepatitis* (476[C]) do not appear to be subject to unusual risks.

An increased responsiveness of patients with *heart failure* (liver congestion) is assumed to be associated with a redistribution of body water and thus with accumulation of unbound anticoagulant at the site of hepatic receptors (475). In warfarin-treated patients one report suggested that *influenza vaccination* was responsible for an increase in prothrombin time (477[C]) but other reports have failed to confirm this (478[R]).

Withdrawal effects The problem of possible rebound hypercoagulability after sudden discontinuation of (oral) anticoagulation is dealt with on page 1026.

Overdosage Overdosage is discussed on page 1027.

Response to smoking and alcohol intake *Smoking* Cigarette-smoking, studied with respect to its possible influence on warfarin metabolism in volunteers, appeared to affect the clearance and apparent volume of distribution of warfarin, although the net effect on anticoagulant activity was negligible in volunteers (479) and patients (480[C]).

Alcohol Alcoholic subjects may ingest ethanol in amounts large enough (200 g) to inhibit warfarin clearance, but the daily consumption of ethanol for a period of 3 weeks in the form of wine taken with meals in moderate (28.2 g daily) or even in liberal quantities (56.4 g daily), had no effect on the hypoprothrombinemia induced by warfarin (481). A report of ethanol potentiation of aspirin-induced prolongation of bleeding time (482) is of importance in view of a putative increase, due to alcohol intake, of the hemorrhagic risk accompanying outpatient oral anticoagulation.

Table 5. *Interactions of coumarin congeners with other drugs*

Drug (generic name)	Effect	Mechanism
Phenytoin	Increased serum levels of phenytoin (605)	Unknown
Sulfonylureas	Hypoglycemia (606)	Inhibition of microsomal enzymes (606)

Interactions Commonly prescribed drugs can potentiate or antagonize the anticoagulant effect of coumarin drugs in many ways: by interfering with the resorption of the drug, the intestinal production and resorption of vitamin K_2, and the resorption of vitamin K_1 present in food; further, by affecting the binding of drugs to plasma proteins; and finally, by changing the metabolism of the drug at the microsomal level in the liver. Competition for metabolic pathways (for example of cytochrome P450 enzyme system) could lead to an increase in the anticoagulant effect, and/or in the pharmacological effects of a drug the active metabolites of which are produced by the same metabolic pathway. Hence, any patient on oral anticoagulation who has another compound added to or withdrawn from the drug regimen, must have his prothrombin times carefully monitored to avoid important changes in the level of intensity of treatment, since an excessively high intensity results in an unnecessarily high bleeding tendency, and insufficient intensity leads to recurrence of the thromboembolic disease.

The information on interactions given in Table 4 (483—604) and Table 5 (605, 606) is mainly based on well-documented prospective studies and, in a few instances, on anecdotal reports. Under the heading 'Clinical comment', an estimate is given of the extent to which interaction interferes with dosage regulation. It should be realized that a given interaction may hold for one but not for another coumarin congener.

INDANDIONE DERIVATIVES

In 0.1—0.3% of patients treated with indandione derivatives, which have the same anti-vitamin K action as the coumarins, a hypersensitivity reaction is induced and proves fatal in about 10% of the cases. Therefore, these preparations are no longer used in many countries. For further information, the interested reader is referred to earlier editions of Meyler's Side Effects of Drugs, especially SED-8 (1975).

New antithrombotic agents

Some new drugs are currently in early phases of clinical development; they especially include specific direct thrombin or factor X_a inhibitors. Clinical data are still few but we can hope that their specific pharmacological properties will decrease the incidence of certain side effects, especially bleeding. In the offing are:

Dermatane sulfate—a glycosaminoglycan—could possess pure antithrombin properties without bleeding activity.

Hirudin, the principal anticoagulant of the medicinal leech (*Hirudo medicinalis*), is now produced by recombinant DNA techniques and characterized by a high thrombin affinity, whether it is free in the plasma or absorbed on the fibrin clot. The high levels of incidence of hemorrhagic strokes occurring in patients treated with both thrombolytic and hirudin, led to suspension and redesign (with notably decrease in hirudin dose) of three major trials (GUSTO-IIA, TIMI-9A, HIT III) investigating the effect of these antithrombotic agents in myocardial infarction (607—609). Bleeding diathesis leading to life-threatening hemorrhage related to hirudin may require use of prothrombin complex concentrate (610[c]).

Thrombolytic agents

Five thrombolytic agents are now available: streptokinase, urokinase, anistreplase (anisoylated plasminogen streptokinase activator complex or APSAC), pro-urokinase (single-chain urokinase-type plasminogen activator or scu-PA), alteplase (recombinant tissue plasminogen activator or rt-PA). Although their pharmacodynamic properties do not significantly differ, some characteristics, as a result of their origin or mode of action, can explain specific side effects and pharmacokinetic differences:

Since *streptokinase* is a natural product of *Streptococcus* cultures and therefore has antigenic properties similar to those of *Streptococcus*, most of the population have anti-streptokinase antibodies. These antibodies explain both the allergic reactions and the resistance to the drug in some cases. If streptokinase has to be re-administered within 8 months of previous exposure, the neutralizing effects of plasma should be taken into account and the dose of streptokinase should be adjusted to overcome these effects (611[C]). However, the rate of fall of streptokinase antibodies after a previous exposure to streptokinase is controversial, and persistent elevation of titers can be seen in a large proportion of patients (612[C]).

Anistreplase which is a compound consisting of streptokinase and anisoylated plasminogen is also subject to allergic reactions, and possesses a longer elimination half-life, thereby allowing intravenous administration in a relatively short interval of time.

Urokinase can be extracted from human urine or from culture of fetal kidney cells and does not seem to cause allergic reactions.

Pro-urokinase and *alteplase* which are recombinant DNA products, also appear to be free of allergic reactions and possess a short elimination half-life (3—8 minutes) requiring continuous infusion administration, which may in some cases be an advantage as it allows rapid surgical intervention when necessary (613).

ADVERSE REACTION PATTERN

General and toxic reaction *Hemorrhage* is the major risk as is discussed at the beginning of this chapter (p. 1008). *Transient hypotensive reactions* are described with all thrombolytic agents. The incidence of these reactions following the infusion of streptokinase in myocardial infarction is high; despite the frequency of its occurrence, the pathophysiology of this hypotensive effect is not known and these reactions are not necessarily antibody-related, and may be due to histamine liberation or to kinin production (614[C]). They occur shortly after the initiation of infusion, may be accompanied by flushing and anxiety, and are reversible with fluid administration and temporary discontinuation of the infusion (614[C]) or vasopressive agents. The magnitude of this hypotensive reaction is directly related to the rate of infusion of streptokinase. The incidence of such reactions does not seem to be affected by premedication with steroids. Rapid injection of anistreplase can also cause transient hypotension (615[c]). The administration of alteplase (or rt-PA) appears to be associated with a lower risk of hypotensive reactions than streptokinase (56[r], 58[c]).

Hypersensitivity reactions These types of reactions are most often seen in patients who have been treated with compounds derived from *Streptococcus* cultures (streptokinase and anistreplase). See below under 'Hypersensitivity reactions'.

ORGANS AND SYSTEMS

Cardiovascular and respiratory *Embolic detachment* of components of venous or mural thrombi is sometimes involved in the development of cruoric thromboembolism or cholesterol embolization. A 10% incidence of *pulmonary embolism* occurring during thrombolysis, lethal in 0–5% (63[CR], 616, 617), points to the risk of detachment—due to the action of thrombolytic agents—of white components of the venous thrombi, especially if large veins, such as those in the pelvis, are involved (618[C]). The risk has not, however, been proven to exceed that reported in patients treated with heparin and/or coumarin. Embolic detachment coming from left ventricular thrombus seldomly occurs, but when it does, it can be responsible for renal (619[C]), cerebral (620[C]) or aortic embolism (621[C]). *Cholesterol embolization* occurring shortly after thrombolytic treatment is characterized by the development of livedo reticularis or multiple necrotic lesions of the skin of both legs (622[C]). *Acute renal failure* (623[C], 624[c]) is a dreaded and often fatal consequence (625[C]). These embolizations are thought to occur after removal of mural thrombi covering atherosclerotic plaques leading to direct exposure of free cholesterol to the arterial circulation. The most frequent *reperfusion arrhythmias* described with thrombolytic drugs when used for treatment of myocardial infarction are transient ventricular tachycardia. Apart from ventricular tachycardia, reperfusion arrhythmias include ventricular fibrillation, accelerated idioventricular rhythm, sinus bradycardia, atrio-ventricular dissociation, ventricular premature beats and supraventricular tachycardia (626[C], 627[C]). No significant differences have been observed between alteplase and streptokinase concerning the incidence of *ventricular fibrillation* (56[r]). However thrombolysis and reperfusion are much less frequently associated with tachyarrhythmias in patients than in experimental models; reperfusion of the right coronary artery might be more arrhythmogenic than reperfusion of the left coronary artery (628[r]). One report describes a *coronary arterial aneurysm* occurring in a 49-year-old man, 1 month after successful percutaneous transluminal coronary recanalization with streptokinase (629[C]). *Phlebitis* at the site of infusion of streptokinase is very frequent and troublesome (139); it is less well known for urokinase-treated patients.

Nervous system The development of *Guillain-Barré syndrome* has been reported in patients who were treated with streptokinase and anistreplase (630[C]–633[C]). As streptokinase and anistreplase are derived from *Streptococcus*, an immunological reaction is thought to induce the development of these Guillain-Barré syndromes. No other effects on the nervous system than those due to bleeding has been reported.

Hematological *Hemolysis* after intravenous streptokinase is rare (634[c]). *Platelet aggregation* due to an antibody-mediated reaction has been suggested as a cause of streptokinase-enhanced *coronary thrombosis* in patients with a specific type of antistreptokinase antibodies (635). Thrombocytopenia has been described after thrombolytic therapy but is most likely a multifactorial phenomenon since patients generally also received i.v. heparin (636[Cr]). A general side effect might be *disseminated intravascular coagulation* induced by thrombolytic agents. Urokinase may have induced a transient hypercoagulation state due to contamination with urinary thromboplastin when the drug was first introduced (637). At present, there is general agreement about the need for conventional anticoagulant treatment immediately after (and even combined with) thrombolytic treatment (51, 67, 638). Transient *lymphopenia* possibly related to immunological destruction of T-helper cells by streptokinase has been described (639[c]).

Liver See 'Interference with diagnostic routine' below. A few cases of *liver dysfunction* with or without jaundice have been reported with streptokinase and urokinase (640[C]–643[C]).

Urinary system *Haematuria* and *proteinuria* can occur without alteration of immunohistochemical features, thereby suggesting a non-immune cause such as either a direct effect on the glomeruli, or merely a reflection of the hypocoagulable state (644[C]). See also 'Cardiovascular and respiratory' above (cholesterol embolization).

Skin and appendages See 'Cardiovascular and respiratory' above (cholesterol embolization).

Special senses *Iritis and uveitis* have been reported with streptokinase (645[c], 646[c]).

Wound healing and infection This last general adverse reaction to thrombolytic agents is discussed on page 1027.

Hypersensitivity reactions The incidence of acute overall allergic reaction in streptokinase- or anistreplase-treated patients amounts to 1–5% (48, 52[R], 54[c], 56[r], 647), and prophylactic steroids do not seem to alter reports of allergic reactions (55[c]). The most common manifestation of non-anaphylactic reactions to streptokinase or anistreplase are *skin rashes* and *pyrexia*. However, *anaphylactic shock* with streptokinase is also well known, though rare, occurring in 0.1% of the patients in the GISSI trial (54[c]). Life-threatening *angioedema* has been described with streptokinase (648[C]) and with alteplase (649[C], 650[C]). *Skin rashes* are seen in about 5% of patients treated with streptokinase, but rarely, if ever, with alteplase. *Pyrexia* can occur after the initial dose of streptokinase. Concurrent administration of corticosteroids does not prevent it completely. A marked rise in body temperature with chills may be accompanied by hypotension, abdominal pain (particularly low back pain) and—very occasionally—mild psychotic reactions. In one study of patients with deep venous thrombosis, designated to compare temperature rise and loss of hemoglobin under streptokinase treatment and conventional anticoagulation with heparin, 11.8 and 85.7% of the patients displayed neither of these two side effects, whereas pyrexia ≤38°C and/or hemoglobin loss <20 g/liter occurred in 62.4 and 9.5% and pyrexia ≥38°C and/or hemoglobin >20 g/liter in 25.8 and 4.8%, respectively; pulmonary embolism was observed in 7.8 and 11.9%, respectively. The study also showed that with individually adjusted dosage of streptokinase (based on the streptokinase tolerance test), lysis can be achieved at doses lower than those generally recommended, which might reduce the severity of adverse reactions as well (48). There are two studies that have conclusively demonstrated that urokinase is non-pyrogenic, as temperature rises were identical for urokinase and heparin (48, 651). The administration of alteplase appears to be associated with a lower risk of allergic reactions than streptokinase (56[c], 58[c]). Acute *bronchospasm*, sometimes fatal (652[CR]) or *dyspnea* can occur with streptokinase. Because treatment with streptokinase and anistreplase induces the production of antibodies, repeated courses are at greater risk.

Several cases of *low back pain* associated with streptokinase or anistreplase injections for acute myocardial infarction have been described with rapid resolution once the streptokinase was stopped (653[C]—656[C]). It is presumed that the mechanism could be allergic since no such report has been published with alteplase (655[C]). Streptokinase is regularly reported to have induced an *immune complex syndrome* characterized by *plasmocytosis*, often severe, and accompanied by fever and the development of (hemolytic) anemia, occurring as early as the first week after the start of treatment; in some cases, temporary alterations in renal function are also induced (657[C]—659). *Vasculitis* has been rarely described after streptokinase or anistreplase (660[C]—663[C]) but not after urokinase or atleplase, and is characterized by lymphocyte infiltration and deposition of immune complex, fibrin and complement in the skin microvasculature. Other patients display the typical picture of serum sickness, sometimes associated with acute renal failure (664[C]-666[C]) or of Henoch-Schönlein *purpura* (667[C]) with purpuric rash, joint and abdominal pain or, in other cases, microscopic hematuria (668[C]). *Adult respiratory distress syndromes* have been reported with streptokinase and anistreptlase (669[C], 670[C]); the timing of symptom onset and the antibody profile in one case suggest an immunological response (670[C]). Stimulation of the immune system could be involved in to the development of Guillain-Barré syndrome in patients treated with streptokinase (631[C]).

Allergic reactions are uncommon with urokinase and were not observed in 172 patients given urokinase by continuous infusion for 18 hours (671). Paradigmatic is a report of successful continuation of thrombolysis with urokinase in a patient in whom streptokinase had led to severe anaphylactic shock (672[C]). A case of allergic hemorrhagic bullae has been reported (673[c]).

Bleeding, thromboembolism, fever and allergic reactions led not only to interruption of an intensive 5-day streptokinase treatment scheme intended to lyse deep venous thrombosis in a large proportion (almost half) of the cases, but also to the recommendation of strict 24-hour surveillance of the patients (674).

Risk situations See p. 1008 under 'Hemorrhage due to thrombolytic agents'.

Interactions *Combination with other antithrombotic drugs* The combination of thrombolytic agents with an anticoagulant and/or aspirin has been said to be life-threatening. An excess of major bleeding episodes with combined subcutaneous heparin and streptokinase or alteplase treatments (1.0% with heparin versus 0.5% without heparin) has been reported in the International Trial (56[r]) in patients with suspected acute myocardial infarction.

Clinical and experimental data suggested a possible increase of hemorrhage risk during thrombolytic therapy with alteplase and concomitant use of *diltiazem* (675[c]).

Interference with diagnostic routine *Interference with liver function tests* No difference was found in the course of transaminases, lactate dehydrogenase, and creatine phosphokinase in patients suffering from myocardial infarction who received an 18-hour infusion of urokinase compared with patients receiving glucose alone (671), but subacute alterations of liver function tests have been described with streptokinase and anistreplase (676[C]). Unexplained increases in alanine aminotransferase and aspartate aminotransferase activities have been reported in almost a quarter of the patients treated with streptokinase (677[C]). In view of a greater prominence of liver dysfunction with streptokinase than with alteplase it could be wiser to choose alteplase rather than streptokinase in patients with previous impaired hepatic function (678[C]).

ANTIDOTES TO ANTICOAGULANTS AND THROMBOLYTIC AGENTS

Vitamin K_1 (phytonadione) *(see also Chapter 38)*

Vitamin K_1 administered intravenously is generally tolerated well. Minute amounts (2–5 mg) of vitamin K_1 administered intravenously can be followed by severe short-lasting *cyanosis*, *dyspnea*, *tachycardia*, and *low blood pressure* in patients suffering from cardiac failure. Thirty-five cases of similar reactions have been reported, mostly from Germany, some of them severe. Fatalities have been reported in the American literature (679[C]). Re-exposure by intramuscular injection did not lead to recurrence of the reaction in two patients (679[C], 680). Avoidance of the intravenous route of administration is recommended, except in case of emergency. Vitamin K_1 should be injected intravenously preferably at an extremely slow rate, e.g. 10 min for the first milligram, followed by 1 mg per minute.

Authors who repeatedly administered large amounts of vitamin K_1, e.g. 26 doses of 100 mg each, intramuscularly to patients suffering from cirrhosis of the liver have described a remarkable cutaneous lesion which they called *localized scleroderma*, most probably an allergic skin reaction (681[C]). Scleroderma-like hypodermic induration involving both buttocks was also seen in a 7-year-old child given vitamin K_1 at birth by intramuscular injection into both buttocks; in this case the course was progressive with an exacerbation with age (682[C]). For vitamin K dermatitis, see Chapter 38.

Cerebral vein thrombosis developed after the administration of 10 mg of vitamin K_1 in two patients suffering from chronic intestinal inflammation assumed to be part of an autoimmune disease (683[C]).

Protamine sulfate and protamine chloride

Protamine, derived from salmon sperm, combines with and neutralizes heparin. The relative insolubility of protamine-insulin suspension in water slows the subcutaneous resorption of the hormone, and consequently prolongs its biological activity. In a prospective study of patients undergoing cardiopulmonary bypass, 10.7% of patients receiving protamine sulfate had adverse reactions of varying types (684).

Protamine sulfate regularly induces *hypotension* when administered too rapidly. *Hypersensitivity reactions*, characterized by flushing, urticaria, wheezing, possible angioedema and hypotension, can occur following slow intravenous use of protamine sulfate. True *anaphylaxis* with bronchospasm and or anaphylactic shock is a real, albeit very rare, adverse reaction (685[C]). Cases of anaphylactic shock after slow intravenous administration of protamine sulfate to diabetic patients suggest cross-hypersensitivity with the protamine present in protamine zinc insulin (686[C]–688[C]), especially in patients with serum antiprotamine IgE or IgG antibodies (689[C]). Insulin-dependent diabetic patients who receive protamine insulin (nowadays less often used) might be at greater risk of side effects when receiving protamine sulfate: a retrospective study of patients who received protamine sulfate to antagonize the effects of heparin during catheterization procedures or cardiac surgery, revealed a relative risk of anaphylaxis 4 times higher in diabetic patients treated with protamine insulin than in non-diabetic control subjects (690[C]). However other authors claim that protamine itself is non-antigenic and that drug hypersensitivity must be due to contaminating fish antigens. This hypothesis is supported by the fairly high frequency of allergic reactions in patients not previously treated with protamine (four out of 140 healthy donors in a leukopheresis program displayed allergic reactions) (691). Severe acute ('catastrophic') *pulmonary vasoconstriction* with cardiovascular collapse has been identified in 1983 and subsequent studies revealed that the incidence of protamine-induced pulmonary artery vasoconstriction was about 1.5% (692[R]). The protamine-induced pulmonary artery vasoconstriction is accompanied by the generation of large quantities of thromboxane A_2, which is known to be a potent vasoconstrictor (692[R]).

Intravenous administration of protamine sulfate in relatively large doses (300 mg) to neutralize heparin after a cardiopulmonary bypass operation is thought to have induced *non-cardiogenic pulmonary edema* and *peripheral vascular collapse* in four patients (693[C]). The reaction took place about 1 hour after administration; two of four patients died. No evidence of hypersensitivity was found (694[C]).

The hypothesis of a putative hypersensitivity to protamine salts in men after vasectomy has been advanced but not confirmed by clinical observation (695).

The heparin-neutralizing effect of protamine sulfate is more or less transitory (696[C]); it is antagonized by a plasma inhibitor. Better and irreversible neutralization of heparin is achieved by the use of protamine chloride (697[C]).

ANTI-PLATELET DRUGS

Three anti-platelet drugs deserve discussion here:

Ticlopidine

This thienopyridine derivative with broad antiplatelet activity, has been used in Europe since 1978. The use of ticlopidine has, however, been progressively restricted in many countries because of its serious side effects. Some reference to the risk of *hemorrhage* is made earlier in this Chapter.

The most commonly reported side effects associated with ticlopidine use are *skin rashes* and *gastrointestinal effects* including nausea, vomiting, anorexia, epigastric pain, and diarrhea. More seldom seen are *severe chronic diarrhea* with fecal incontinence and dehydration or hypokalemia which regresses with withdrawal of treatment (698[C], 699[C]).

Ticlopidine can affect the results of *liver* function tests. Several reports of hepatitis (mainly cholestatic) have been published (700[C]–702[C]) and one report of granulomatous hepatitis (703[C]).

Hematological disorders including leukopenia, agranulocytosis, thrombocytopenia and pancytopenia have been described, usually within 3 months of starting of treatment, and are reversible in most cases on discontinuation of therapy. In three well-controlled prospective studies, severe ($<0.45\times10^9$/liter) but reversible neutropenia developed respectively in 0.6, 0.9 and 0.8% ticlopidine-treated patients (77[C], 704[C], 705[C]). Thrombotic thrombocytopenic purpuras, sometimes fatal, have been reported (706[c], 707[C]).

Anagrelide

Anagrelide is a member of the imidazoquinazoline series of compounds with a powerful anti-aggregating effect. During studies in humans, anagrelide has been found to produce *thrombocytopenia*. This drawback could be an advantage in patients with thrombocytosis where the platelet reduction appears at doses far below the levels at which anti-aggregating effects are exerted (708). Other side effects include headache and nausea.

Abciximab

Abciximab is a chimeric human/murine monoclonal antibody that reacts with appropriate domains of the glycoprotein IIb/IIIa complex on the platelet surface, thereby inhibiting platelet aggregation. In addition to heparin and aspirin, abciximab reduces the incidence of acute ischemic events and restenosis in high-risk patients undergoing coronary angioplasty or/and directional atherectomy, but this beneficial effect is obtained at the cost of a significant increase in bleeding complications and transfusions (709[C], 710[C]). Thrombocytopenia can occur and human antimurine antibodies develop in a few patients.

REFERENCES

1. Fekkes N, De Jonge H, Veltkamp JJ et al. Comparative study of the clinical effects of acenocoumarol (Sintrom®) and phenprocoumon (Marcoumar®) in myocardial infarction and angina pectoris. Acta Med Scand 1971;190:535.
2. Smith R, Rodman R, Pastor BH. A comparative study of prothrombinopenic anticoagulant drugs. J Am Med Assoc 1960;174:1917.
3. Sixty Plus Reinfarction Study Research Group. Risks of long-term oral anticoagulant therapy in elderly patients after myocardial infarction. Lancet 1982;i:64.
4. Riboulot M, Dieval J, Malgouzou M et al. A propos des dangers d'un traitement anti-agrégant plaquettaire par la ticlopidine: conduite à tenir en pré, per et post-opératoire. Cah Anesthésiol 1981;29:961.
5. Stubbé LTFL, Pietersen JH, Van Heulen C. Aspirin preparations and their noxious effect on the gastrointestinal tract. Br Med J 1962;1:675.
6. Pachter HL, Riles TS. Low dose heparin: bleeding and wound complications in the surgical patient. Ann Surg 1977;186:669.
7. Council on Thrombosis of the American Heart Association. Prevention of venous thromboembolism in surgical patients by low-dose heparin. Circulation 1977;55:423A.
8. Allen JG, Arendrup H, Toftgaard C et al. Calcium-heparin or sodium-heparin in low-dose heparin prophylaxis? Thromb Haemostasis 1979;42:1064.
9. The Multicenter Trial Committee. Dihydroergotamine-heparin prophylaxis of postoperative deep vein thrombosis: a multicenter trial. J Am Med Assoc 1984;251:2960.
10. Landefeld CS, Beyth RJ. Anticoagulant-related bleeding: clinical epidemiology, prediction and prevention. Am J Med 1993;95:315.
11. Walker AM, Jick H. Predictors of bleeding during heparin therapy. J Am Med Assoc 1980;244:1209.
12. Coon WW, Willis PW. Hemorrhagic complications of anticoagulant therapy. Arch Intern Med 1974;133:386.
13. Hirsh J. Heparin. N Engl J Med 1991;324:1565.
14. Morabia A. Heparin doses and major bleedings (Letter to Editor). Lancet 1986;i:1278.
15. Levine MN, Hirsh J, Kelton JG. Heparin induced bleeding. In: Lane DA, Lindahl, eds. Heparin: chemical and biological properties, clinical applications. London: Edward Arnold, 1989:517.
16. Passannante A, Macik BG. Case report: the heparin flush syndrome—a case of iatrogenic hemorrhage. Am J Med Sci 1988;296:71.
17. Leizorovicz A, Haugh MC, Chapuis FR et al. Low molecular weight heparin in prevention of perioperative thrombosis. Br Med J 1992;305:913.
18. Nurmohamed MT, Rosendaal FR, Büller HR et al. Low-molecular weight heparin versus standard heparin in general

and orthopaedic surgery: a meta-analysis. Lancet 1992; 340:152.

19. Leizorovicz A, Simonneau G, Decousut, Boissel JP. Comparison of efficacy and safety of low molecular weight heparins and unfractionated heparin in initial treatment of deep venous thrombosis: a meta-analysis. Br Med J 1994;309:299.
20. Coon WW, Willis PW, Symons MJ. Assessment of anticoagulant treatment of venous thromboembolism. Ann Surg 1969;170:559.
21. Sevitt S, Gallagher NG. Prevention of venous thrombosis and pulmonary embolism in injured patients. Lancet 1959;ii:981.
22. Bjerkelund ChJ. The effect of long-term treatment with dicoumarol in myocardial infarction. Acta Med Scand 1957;Suppl 330:1.
23. Borchgrevink CF. Long-term anticoagulant therapy in angina pectoris and myocardial infarction. Acta Med Scand 1960;Suppl 359:1.
24. Loeliger EA. Personal experience, 1972.
25. Loeliger EA, Hensen A, Kroes F et al. A double-blind trial of long-term anticoagulant treatment after myocardial infarction. Acta Med Scand 1967;182:549.
26. Owren PA. Some perspectives of the therapeutic problem in coronary disease. Thromb Diath Haemorrh 1969; Suppl 35:1.
27. Pastor BH, Resnick ME, Rodman T. Serious hemorrhagic complications of anticoagulant therapy. J Am Med Assoc 1962;180:747.
28. Roos J, Van Joost HE. The cause of bleeding during anticoagulant treatment. Acta Med Scand 1965;178:129.
29. Boekhout-Mussert MJ, Van der Kolk-Schaap PJ, Hermans J et al. Prospective double-blind clinical trial of bovine, human and rabbit thromboplastin in the control of long-term oral anticoagulation. Am J Clin Pathol 1981;75:297.
30. Joly F, Valty J, Emar A. Traitement anticoagulant au long cours chez les sujets âgés de plus de 75 ans. Arch Mal Coeur Vaiss 1977;70:521.
31. Meuwissen OJAT, Vervoorn AC, Cohen O et al. A double-blind trial of long-term anticoagulant treatment after myocardial infarction. Acta Med Scand 1969;186:361.
32. Moschos CB, Wong PCY, Sise HS. Controlled study of the effective level of long-term anticoagulation. J Am Med Assoc 1964;190:799.
33. Royston GR. The management of adequate anticoagulant therapy and its complications. Vasc Dis 1966;3:295.
34. Sixty Plus Reinfarction Study Research Group. A double-blind trial to assess long-term oral anticoagulant therapy in elderly patients after myocardial infarction. Lancet 1980;ii:989.
35. Mosley DH, Schatz IJ, Breneman GM et al. Long-term anticoagulant therapy: complications and control in a review of 978 cases. J Am Med Assoc 1963;186:914.
36. Loeliger EA, Lewis SM. Progress in laboratory control of oral anticoagulants. Lancet 1982;ii:318.
37. Loeliger EA, Van den Besselaar AMHP, Broekmans AW. Intensity of oral anticoagulation in patients monitored with various thromboplastins. N Engl J Med 1983;308:1228.
38. Forfar JC. A 7-year analysis of haemorrhage in patients on long-term anticoagulant treatment. Br Heart J 1969;42:128.
39. Chapuy P, Philip JJ, Pasquier J. Les accidents du traitement anticoagulant chez les sujets âgés. Méd Hyg 1974; 32:954.
40. Wilson WR, Geraci JE, Danielson GK et al. Anticoagulant therapy and central nervous system complications in patients with prosthetic valve endocarditis. Circulation 1978;57:1004.
41. Lieberman A, Hass WK, Pinto R et al. Intracranial hemorrhage and infarction in anticoagulated patients with prosthetic heart valves. Stroke 1978;9:18.
42. Loeliger EA, Broekmans AW. Optimal therapeutic anticoagulation. Haemostasis 1985;15:283.
43. Von Bertrab R. Ist eine optimal Antikoagulation in der ambulanten Praxis möglich? Bericht über eine retrospektive 5-Jahres-Studie aus einer kardiologischen Praxis. Schweiz Med Wochenschr 1985;115:1092.
44. Launbjerg J, Egeblad H, Heaf J et al. Bleeding complications to oral anticoagulant therapy: multivariate analysis of 1010 treatment years in 551 outpatients. J Intern Med 1991;229:351.
45. Shepherd AMM, Hewick DS, Moreland TA et al. Age as a determinant of sensitivity to warfarin. Br J Clin Pharmacol 1977;4:315.
46. Dale J, Myhre E, Storstein O et al. Prevention of arterial thromboembolism with acetylsalicylic acid. Am Heart J 1977;94:101.
47. Sethi GK, Copeland JG, Goldman S et al. Implications of preoperative administration of aspirin in patients undergoing coronary artery bypass grafting. J Am Coll Cardiol 1990;15:15.
48. Cooperative Study. Urokinase-streptokinase embolism trial. J Am Med Assoc 1974;229:1606.
49. Fennerty AG, Levine MN, Hirsh J. Hemorrhagic complications of thrombolytic therapy in the treatment of myocardial infarction and venous thromboembolism. Chest 1989;95(Suppl):88S.
50. Straub H. Letale Komplikationen der Fibrinolyse. Münch Med Wochenschr 1982;124:57.
51. Duckert F, Müller G, Nyman D et al. Treatment of deep vein thrombosis with streptokinase. Br Med J 1975;1:479.
52. Johnson ES, Cregeen RJ. An interim report of the safety of anisoylated plasminogen streptokinase activator complex (APSAC). Drugs 1987;33(Suppl 3):298.
53. Gruppo Italiano per lo Studio della Sopravivenza nell'Infarto Miocardico. GISSI-2: a factorial randomised trial of alteplase versus streptokinase and heparin versus no heparin among 12 490 patients with acute myocardial infarction. Lancet 1990;336:65.
54. Gruppo Italiano per lo Studio della Streptochinasi nell'Infarto Miocardico (GISSI). Effectiveness of intravenous thrombolytic treatment in acute myocardial infarction. Lancet 1986;i:397.
55. ISIS-2 (Second International Study of Infarct Survival) Collaborative Group. Randomised trial of intravenous streptokinase, oral aspirin, both, or neither among 17 187 cases of suspected acute myocardial infarction: ISIS-2. Lancet 1988;ii:349.
56. The International Study Group. In-hospital mortality and clinical course of 20 891 patients with suspected acute myocardial infarction randomised between alteplase and streptokinase with or without heparin. Lancet 1990;336:71.
57. GUSTO Investigator (The). An international randomized trial comparing four thrombolytic strategies for acute myocardial infarction. N Engl J Med 1993;329:673.
58. ISIS 3 (Third International Study of Infarct Survival) Collaborative Group. A randomized comparison of streptokinase vs tissue plasminogen activator vs anistreptlase and

aspirin plus heparin vs aspirin alone among 41 229 cases of suspected acute myocardial infarction. Lancet 1992;339:753.
59. Blankenship JC, Almquist AK. Cardiovascular complications of thrombolytic therapy in patients with a mistaken diagnosis of acute myocardial infarction. J Am Coll Cardiol 1989;14:1579.
60. Butler J, Davies AH, Westaby S. Streptokinase in acute aortic dissection. Br Med J 1990;300:517.
61. Curzen NP, Clarke B, Gray HH. Intravenous thombolysis for suspected myocardial infarction: a cautionary note. Br Med J 1990;300:513.
62. Partanen HJ, Nieminen MS. Intracerebellar fatal haemorrhage after thrombolytic therapy of suspected non-Q-wave myocardial infarction (Letter to Editor). Lancet 1990;336:883.
63. Meissner AJ, Misiak A, Ziemski JM et al. Hazards of thrombolytic therapy in deep vein thrombosis. Br J Surg 1987;74:991.
64. Conard J, Samama M, Milochevitch R et al. Complications hémorragiques au cours de 98 traitements par la streptokinase. Nouv Presse Méd 1979;8:1319.
65. Brogden RN, Speight TM, Avery GS. Streptokinase: a review of its clinical pharmacology, mechanism of action and therapeutic uses. Drugs 1973;5:357.
66. Tilsner V, Greul W. Thrombolytic therapy: agents, indication, clinical performance, and side effects. Vasc Surg 1979;13:79.
67. Brinckmann W, Heinrich P, Hünemörder H. Komplikationen der Thrombolysetherapie. Zentralbl Chir 1976; 101:477.
68. Hommel M, Boissel JP, Cornu C et al. Termination of trial of streptokinase in severe acute ischaemic stroke. Lancet 1995;345:57.
69. Kohner EM, Pettit JE, Hamilton AM et al. Streptokinase in central retinal vein occlusion: a controlled clinical trial. Br Med J 1976;1:550.
70. Weinstein J. Treatment of myocardial infarction with intracoronary streptokinase: Efficacy and safety data from 209 United States cases in the Hoechst-Roussel registry. Am Heart J 1982;104:894.
71. Tibbutt DA, Chesterman CN, Williams EW et al. Controlled trial of the sequential use of streptokinase and ancrod in the treatment of deep vein thrombosis of lower limb. Thromb Haemostasis 1977;37:222.
72. Aspirin Myocardial Infarction Study Research Group. A randomized, controlled trial of aspirin in persons recovered from myocardial infarction. J Am Med Assoc 1980;243:661.
73. Persantine-Aspirin Reinfarction Study Research Group. Persantine and aspirin in coronary heart disease. Circulation 1980;62:449.
74. 'Enquête de prévention secondaire de l'infarctus du Myocarde' Research Group. A controlled comparison of aspirin and oral anticoagulants in prevention of death after myocardial infarction. N Engl J Med 1982;307:701.
75. Editorial. Ticlopidine. Lancet 1991;23:459.
76. Criado A, Juffé A, Carmona J et al. Ticlopidine as a hemorrhagic risk factor in coronary surgery. Drug Intell Clin Pharm 1985;19:673.
77. Hass WK, Easton JD, Adams HP et al., for the Ticlopidine Aspirin Stroke Study Group. A randomized trial comparing ticlopidine hydrochloride with aspirin for the prevention of stroke in high-risk patients. N Engl J Med 1989;321:501.
78. Thébault J, Blatrix C, Blanchard J et al. A possible method to control prolongations of bleeding time under antiplatelet therapy with ticlopidine. Thromb Haemostasis 1982;48:6.
79. Apuzzo MLJ, Davey LM, Manuelidis EE. Pineal apoplexy associated with anticoagulant therapy. J Neurosurg 1976;45:223.
80. Nourizadeh AR, Pitts FW. Hemorrhage into pituitary adenoma during anticoagulant therapy. J Am Med Assoc 1965;193:623.
81. Hyer SL, Soo SC, Taylor W, Nusseu SS. Spontaneous haemorrhage into a pituitary tumour after streptokinase therapy. Postgrad Med J 1993;69:244.
82. Winter J, Kantartzis M. Atemnotsyndrom als Folge einer spontanen Blutung in eine Struma. Chirurgie 1981;52: 780.
83. Delhumeau A, Houet JF, Bourrier P et al. Heparin induced thrombocytopenia with adrenal haemorrhage and acute adrenal insuffiency (in French). Ann Fr Anesth Reanim 1990;8:656.
84. Knight LL, Valentine EH. Spontaneous bilateral adrenal hemorrhage: report of a case occuring during heparin therapy. J Am Med Assoc 1962;182:1312.
85. Amador E. Adrenal hemorrhage during anticoagulant therapy: a clinical and pathological study of ten cases. Ann Intern Med 1965;63:559.
86. Geyer G, Tragl KH, Zeitlhofer J. Beidseitige tödliche Nebennierenblutung während der Antikoagulantienbehandlung. Wien Klin Wochenschr 1965;77:456.
87. Leblanc M, Michiels R, Beaufils JP et al. Les hématomes bilatéraux des glandes surrénales—complication du traitement anticoagulant: à propos d'une nouvelle observation anatomo-clinique. Sem Hôp 1968;44:302.
88. Haller RM. Experimentelle Nebennierenrindenblutungen an anticoagulierten Ratten, ausgelöst durch Stimulation der Nebennierenrinde. Virchows Arch Pathol Anat Abt A 1969;346:204.
89. Szabo S, McComb DJ, Kovacs K et al. Adrenocortical hemorrhagic necrosis. Arch Pathol Lab Med 1981;105:536.
90. Ejerblad S, Hemmingsson A. Acta Chir Scand 1981;147:497.
91. Mounier-Kuhn P, Dumolard P. Les accidents oto-rhinolaryngologiques au cours des traitements anticoagulants. J Méd Lyon 1971;52:851.
92. Sonkin N. Anticoagulation and gunshot concussion in eardrum bleeding. RI Med J 1966;49:243.
93. Feinmesser R, Gay I. An unusual adverse reaction to nicoumalone. Br J Med 1986;292:992.
94. McLaughlin GE, McCarthy DJ, Segal BL. Hemarthrosis complicating anticoagulant therapy. J Am Med Assoc 1966;196:1020.
95. Hale WB, Vishnu Moorthy A, Middleton WS. Hemarthrosis from heparin therapy. J Am Med Assoc 1980; 244:30.
96. Birnbaum Y, Stahl B, Rechavia E. Spontaneous hemarthrosis following thrombolytic therapy of acute myocardial infarction. Int J Cardiol 1993;40:289.
97. Oldroyd KG, Hornung RS, Jones AM et al. Spontaneous haemarthrosis following thrombolytic therapy for myocardial infarction. Postgrad Med J 1990;66:387.
98. Andes WA, Edmunds JO. Hemarthroses and warfarin: joint destruction with anticoagulation. Thromb Haemostasis 1983;49:187.
99. Perazella MA, Buller GK. Hemorrhagic bursitis complicating treatment with recombinant tissue plasminogen activator. Am J Med 1991;91:440.

100. Hartwell SW, Kurtay M. Carpal tunnel compression caused by hematoma associated with anticoagulant therapy. Cleveland Clin Q 1966;33:127.
101. Babb RR, Spittell JA, Bartholomew LG. Hematoma of the rectus abdominis muscle complicating anticoagulant therapy. Mayo Clin Proc 1965;40:760.
102. Neviaser RJ, Adams JP, May GI. Complications of arterial puncture in anticoagulated patients. J Bone Jt Surg 1976;58-A:218.
103. Hay SM, Allen MJ, Barnes MR. Acute compartment syndromes resulting from anticoagulant treatment. Br Med J 1992;305:1474.
104. Gooder P, Henry R. Impending asphyxia induced by anticoagulant therapy. J Laryngol Otol 1980;94:347.
105. Waldron J, Youngs RP. Respiratory arrest produced by anticoagulant-induced haemorrhage into parapharyngeal space. J Laryngol Otol 1986;100:857.
106. Kent DC. Bleeding into pulmonary cyst associated with anticoagulant therapy. Am Rev Resp Dis 1965;92:108.
107 Kaplinsky N, Thaler M, Militianu J et al. Transient pulmonary infiltrates associated with warfarin. J Am Med Assoc 1980;243:513.
108. Chakraborty AK, Dreisin RB. Pulmonary hematoma secondary to anticoagulant therapy. Ann Intern Med 1982;96:67.
109. Granthil C, Dugue P, Houvenaeghel M et al. Hemorragies occultes intrapulmonaires au cours des traitements anticoagulants. Nouv Presse Méd 1980;9:3275.
110. Nathan PE, Torres Av, Smith AJ et al. Spontaneous pulmonary hemorrhage following coronary thrombolysis. Chest 1992;101:1150.
111. Schermer MJ, Wolfson RL, Rayfield EJ et al. Hemothorax complicating pulmonary infarction and anticoagulation. Univ Mich Med Cent J 1972;38:150.
112. Simon HB, Daggett WM, DeSanctis RW. Hemothorax as a complication of anticoagulant therapy in the presence of pulmonary infarction. J Am Med Assoc 1969;208:1830.
113. Diamond MT, Fell SC. Anticoagulant-induced massive hemothorax. NY State J Med 1973;73:691.
114. Aarseth S, Lange HF. The influence of anticoagulant therapy on the occurence of cardiac rupture and hemopericardium following heart infarction. I. A study of 89 cases of hemopericardium (81 of them cardiac ruptures). Am Heart J 1958;56:250.
115. Lange HF, Aarseth S. The influence of anticoagulant therapy on the occurence of cardiac rupture and hemopericardium following heart infarction. II. A controlled study of a selected treated group based on 1044 autopsies. Am Heart J 1958;56:257.
116. Niarchos AP. Pericarditis after myocardial infarction. Br Med J 1971;3:112.
117. Stoyanov PK, Staneva MP. Postmyokard-infarkt-Syndrom und antikoagulantien-Therapie. Münch Med Wochenschr 1966;108:2042.
118. Grennfield JC, Dillon ML. Hemorrhagic pericardial effusion following myocardial infarction associated with a ventricular aneurysm. Am Heart J 1959;57:327.
119. Fell SC, Rubin IL, Enselberg CD et al. Anticoagulant induced hemopericardium with tamponade. N Engl J Med 1965;272:670.
120. Granot H, Shinar E. Spontaneous anticoagulant-induced hemopericardium with tamponade. Acta Haematol 1982;68:339.
121. Miller RL. Hemopericardium with use of oral anticoagulant therapy. J Am Med Assoc 1969;209:1362.
122. Rifle G, Viard H, Cortet P. Péricardite constrictive calcifiante à forme angineuse compliquée d'hémopéricarde et de tamponnade au décours d'un traitement anticoagulant. Acta Cardiol 1976;31:79.
123. Renkin J, De Bruyne B, Benit E et al. Cardiac tamponade early after thrombolysis after acute myocardial infarction: a rare but not reported haemorrhagic complication. J Am Coll Cardiol 1991;17:280.
124. Hochberg MS, Merrill WH, Gruber M et al. Delayed cardiac tamponade associated with prophylactic anticoagulation in patients undergoing coronary bypass grafting. J Thorac Cardiovasc Surg 1978;75:777.
125. Ofori-Krakye SK, Tyberg TI, Geha AS et al. Late cardiac tamponade after open heart surgery: incidence, role of anticoagulants in its pathogenesis and its relationship to the postpericardiotomy syndrome. Circulation 1981;63:1323.
126. Belic L, Stafford G, Allen JW et al. Cardiac tamponade during anticoagulation. J Am Med Assoc 1978;240:672.
127. Jørgensen L, Chandler AB, Borchgrevink CF. Acute lesions of coronary arteries in anticoagulant-treated and in untreated patients. Atherosclerosis 1971;13:21.
128. Brecht Th, Brecht G, Von Lilienfeld-Toal H et al. Der antithrombotische Effekt von Phenprocoumon: computertomographische Beobachtung eines abdominellen Aortenaneurysmas. Herz Kreisl 1980;12:111.
129. London NJM, Williams B, Stein A. Systemic thrombolysis causing haemorrhage around a prosthetic abdominal aortic graft. Br Med J 1993;306:1530.
130. Fujiwara H, Onodera T, Tanaka M et al. A clinicopathologic study of patients with hemorrhagic myocardial infarction treated with selective coronary thrombolysis with urokinase. Circulation 1986;73:749.
131. Waller BF, Rothbaum DA, Pinkerton CA et al. Status of the myocardium and infarct-related coronary artery in 19 necropsy patients with acute recanalization using pharmacologic (streptokinase, r-tissue plasminogen activator), mechanical (percutaneous transluminal coronary angioplasty) or combined types of reperfusion therapy. J Am Coll Cardiol 1987;9:785.
132. DeCastro CM, Hall RJ, Glasser SP. Salivary gland hemorrhage—an unusual complication of coumadin anticoagulation. Am Heart J 1970;80:675.
133. Bailey BMW, Fordyce AM. Complications of dental extractions in patients receiving warfarin anticoagulant therapy. Br Dent J 1983;155:308.
134. Rooney TP. General dentistry during continuous anticoagulation therapy. Oral Surg Oral Med Oral Pathol 1983;56:252.
135. Jick H, Porter J. Drug-induced gastrointestinal bleeding. Lancet 1978;ii:87.
136. Chaussade S, Desechalliers JP, Lerebours E et al. Les hémorragies digestives sous traitement anticoagulant: analyse rétrospective d'une série de 178 cas consécutifs. Gastroentérol Clin Biol 1984;8:152.
137. Andress M. Submucosal haematoma of the oesophagus due to anticaogulant therapy. Acta Radiol Diagn 1971; 11:216.
138. Jishi F, Sissons CE, Silverstone EJ et al. Oesophageal dissection after thrombolytic treatment for myocardial infarcton. Thorax 1992;47:835.
139. Smart RF, Stone AR. Intramural oesophageal haematoma complicating anticoagulant therapy. NZ Med J 1978;87:176.
140. Bergqvist D, Hallböök T, Hessman Y. Anticoagulation and retroperitoneal haematoma. Vasa 1976;5:329.

141. Lowe GDO, McKillop JH, Prentice AG. Fatal retroperitoneal haemorrhage complicating anticoagulant therapy. Postgrad Med J 1979;55:18.
142. Hodin E, Dass T. Spontaneous retroperitoneal hemorrhage complicating anticoagulant therapy. Ann Surg 1969;170:848.
143. Russek HI, Zohman BL. Anticoagulant therapy in acute myocardial infarction. Am J Med Sci 1953;225:8.
144. Hafner CD, Granley JJ, Krause RJ et al. Anticoagulant ileus. J Am Med Assoc 1962;182:947.
145. Delgoffe C, Régent D, Chaulieu C et al. Hématome duodénal spontané géant au cours d'un traitement fibrinolytique. J Radiol 1981;62:187.
146. Stanton PE, Wilson JP, Lamis PA et al. Acute abdominal conditions induced by anticoagulant therapy. Am Surg 1974;40:1.
147. Askey JM. Small bowel obstruction due to intramural hematoma during anticoagulant therapy. Calif Med 1966;104:449.
148. Brügger R, Walter M, Schlup P. Sonographische Diagnose eines Darmwandhämatoms bei Antikoagulation. Schweiz Med Wochenschr 1986;116:1102.
149. Jacobson BM, Fruin RC. Intestinal obstruction simulated by hemoperitoneum during anticoagulant therapy. Ann Intern Med 1966;64:401.
150. Lyon DC. Intussusception complicating anticoagulant therapy. Br Med J 1968;2:345.
151. Zer M, Chaimoff C, Dintsman M. Anticoagulant ileus with intestinal necrosis. Isr J Med Sci 1972;8:154.
152. Herbert DC. Anticoagulant therapy and the acute abdomen. Br J Surg 1968;55:353.
153. Abaza A, Rebut AM. Accidents abdominaux aigus pseudo-occlusifs de la thérapeutique anticoagulante. Presse Méd 1962;70:1622.
154. Leatherman LL. Intestinal obstruction caused by anticoagulants. Am Heart J 1968;76:534.
155. Brawner J, Trivedi H, Sataline LR. Hemocholecyst: report on a case associated with anticoagulant therapy. Ohio State Med J 1966;62:1028.
156. Baulieux J, Maillet P, Picq P. Un accident rare du traitement anticoagulant: l'hémobilie d'origine vésiculaire. Lyon Méd 1974;232:175.
157. Goldsmith JC, Drossman DA, Blatt PM. Hemobilia complicating warfarin therapy. South Med J 1979;72:748.
158. Frayssinet R, Sahel J, Sarles H. Les wirsungorragies: étude d'un cas et revue de la littérature. Gastroentérol Clin Biol 1978;2:93.
159. Couzigou P, Boisseau C, Faucher P et al. Wirsungorragie: complication d'un traitement anti-coagulant. Nouv Presse Méd 1980;9:1712.
160. Larsen RR, SawyerRB, Sawyer KC et al. Hemorrhagic pancreatitis complicating anticoagulant therapy. NY State J Med 1962;62:2397.
161. Nicora E. Pancreatite acuta emorragica in corso di terapia anticoagulante. Pathologica 1966;58:243.
162. Gernigon Y, Beaumont E, Griffe J. Rupture spontanée de la rate chez un malade traité par les anticoagulants. Arch Méd Ouest 1980;12:163.
163. Neff U, Mannhart H, Rüedi Th. Spontane Milzruptur unter Antikoagulantientherapie. Helv Chir Acta 1977; 44:503.
164. Gardner-Medwin J, Sayer J, Mahuda YR, Spiller RC. Spontaneous rupture of spleen following streptokinase therapy. Lancet 1989;ii:1398.
165. Cheung PK, Arnold JMO, McLarty TD. Splenic hemorrhage: a complication of tissue plasminogen activator treatment. Can J Cardiol 1990;6:183.
166. Loizon P, Nahon P, Founti H et al. Rupture spontanée de la rate sous ticlopidine. A propos de deux observations. J Chir Paris 1994;131:371.
167. Eklöf B, Gjöres JE, Lohi A et al. Spontaneous rupture of liver and spleen with severe intra-abdominal bleeding during streptokinase treatment of deep venous thrombosis. Vasa 1977;6:369.
168. Fox SB, Carr B, Robinson A, Wilson RM. Fatal rupture of a subcapsular liver hematoma in a patient treated with anisolylated plasminogen streptokinase activated complex. Postgrad Med 1991;5:67,699.
169. Kriesmann A, Theiss W, Lutilsky L et al. Fibrinolytische Therapie bei tiefen Venenthrombosen der oberen und unteren Extremität. Fortschr Med 1977;95:858.
170. Piper C, Remmele W, von Egidy H. Spontaneous rupture of liver under fibrinolytic therapy (in German). Münch Med Wochenschr 1990;132:412.
171. Roberts MH, Johnston FR. Hepatic rupture from anticoagulant therapy. Arch Surg 1975;110:1152.
172. Walker RL, Rost FWD. Phenindione therapy and haematuria. Med J Aust 1965;52/II:755.
173. Fowler WE, Bovarsky S. A possible cause of hematuria in patients taking warfarin. N Engl J Med 1986;315:65.
174. Nakagawa Y, Abram V, Parks JH et al. Urine glycoprotein growth inhibitors: evidence for a molecular abnormality in calcium oxalate nephrolithiasis. J Clin Invest 1985;76:1455.
175. Beirn SFO, Lavelle S. Ureteric obstruction by clot during anticoagulant treatment. Br Med J 1964;1:1162.31.
176. Schuster HP, Becker G, Prellwitz W et al. Uberwachung der Blutgerinnung und Komplikationen bei Langzeittherapie mit Streptokinase. Infusionstherapie 1980;5:260.
177. Theiss W, Hofer E, Kriessmann A et al. Tiefe Venenthrombosen: Streptokinase-Behandlung mit angepasster Erhaltungsdosis. Med Klin (Münich) 1980;75:580.
178. Luna I, Leadbetter RL, Gilbert DR. Spontaneous rupture of the kidney: a complication of anticoagulation—report of 2 cases. J Urol 1973;109:788.
179. Palaniswamy R, Singhal PC, Rao MS et al. Fatal renal haemorrhage following haemodialysis in a patient with obstructive uropathy. Postgrad Med J 1983;59:57.
180. Larrieu H, Strich M. Une complication rare du traitement anticoagulant: l'hématome de la paroi vésicale. Bull Mém Soc Chir Paris 1973;62:350.
181. Mathieu J, Dargent D, Moine C. Les méno-métrorragies chez la femme soumise à un traitement anti-coagulant au long cours. Lyon Méd 1968;26:1741.
182. Feitcher GEH, Herting W. Massive Corpus-luteum-Blutung unter Antikoagulantientherapie bei einer Dialysepatientin. Geburtshilfe Frauenheilkd 1976;36:447.
183. Waxman M, Baird GJ. Corpus luteum hemorrhage. J Am Med Assoc 1978;239:2270.
184. Peters WA, Thiagarajah S, Thornton WN. Ovarian hemorrhage in patients receiving anticoagulant therapy. J Reprod Med 1979;22:82.
185. Wong KP, Gillet PG. Recurrent hemorrhage from corpus luteum during anticoagulant therapy. Can Med Assoc J 1977;116:388.
186. Shapiro ED, Neches WH, Mathews RA. Corpus luteum hemorrhagicum: an unusual complication of anticoagulant therapy. Am J Dis Child 1980;134:523.

187. Rosenthal AH. Rupture of the corpus luteum including four cases of massive intraperitoneal hemorrhage. Am J Obstet Gynecol 1960;79:1008.
188. Hirsh J, Cade JF, Gallus AS. Anticoagulants in pregnancy: a review of indications and complications. Am Heart J 1972;83:301.
189. Ludwig H. Antikoagulantien in der Schwangerschaft und im Wochenbett. Geburtshilfe Frauenheilkd 1970;30:337.
190. Saidi P, Hoag MS, Aggeler PM. Transplacental transfer of bishydroxycoumarin in the human. J Am Med Assoc 1965;191:761.
191. Wintzen AR, De Jonge H, Loeliger EA et al. The risk of intracerebral hemorrhage during oral anticoagulant treatment: a population study. Ann Neurol 1984;16:553.
192. Peruzzi P, Rousseaux P, Bazin A et al. Hemorrhagic complications of anticoagulants seen by the neurosurgeon. Report of fifty-four cases (in French). Sem Hôp 1990;66:487.
193. Fredriksson K, Norrving B, Strömblad LG. Emergency reversal of anticoagulation after intracerebral hemorrhage. Stroke 1992;23:972.
194. Alpert JS. Intracranial hemorrhage after thrombolytic therapy: a therapeutic conflict. J Am Coll Cardiol 1992; 19:295.
195. Levine MN, Goldhaber SZ, Califf RM et al. Hemorrhagic complications of thrombolytic therapy in the treatment of myocardial infarction and venous thromboembolism. Chest 1992;102(Suppl):3645.
196. Koudstaal PJ, Stibbe J, Vermeulen M. Fatal ischaemic brain oedema after early thrombolysis with tissue plaminogen activator in acute stroke. Br Med J 1988;297:1571.
197. Wintzen AR, Tijssen JGP. Subdural hematoma and oral anticoagulant therapy. Arch Neurol 1982;39:69.
198. Snyder M, Renaudin J. Intracranial hemorrhage associated with anticoagulation therapy. Surg Neurol 1977;7:31.
199. Nathan PE, Sonenblick B, Chakote V et al. Headache, thrombolytic therapy, and chronic subdural hemorrhage. A case report. Angiology 1994;45:77.
200. Brandt M. Spontaneous intramedullary haematoma as a complication of anticoagulant therapy. Acta Neurochir 1980;52:73.
201. Constantini S, Ashkenzi E, Shoshen et al. Thoracic hematomyelia secondary to coumarin-anticoagulant therapy—a case report. Eur Neurol 1992;32:109.
202. Sadjapour K. Hazards of anticoagulation therapy shortly after lumbar puncture. J Am Med Assoc 1977; 237:1692.
203. Kohli CM, Palmer AH, Gray GH. Spontaneous intraspinal hemorrhage causing paraplegia: a complication of heparin therapy. Ann Surg 1974;179:197.
204. Mustafa MH, Galino R. Spontaneous spinal epidural haematoma causing cord compression after streptokinase therapy for acute coronary artery occlusion. South Med J 1988;81:1202.
205. Ruff RL, Dougherty JH. Complications of lumbar puncture followed by anticoagulation. Stroke 1981;12:879.
206. Friedland ML, Wittels EG. Spinal cord haemorrhage following herpes zoster: a possible complication of warfarin therapy. Postgrad Med J 1982;58:39.
207. Motomochi M, Makita Y, Nabeshima S et al. Spinal subarachnoid hemorrhage due to a thoracic neurinoma during anticoagulation therapy: a case report. Neurol Med Chir 1981;21:781.
208. Toledo E, Shalit MN, Segal R. Spinal subdural hematoma associated with anticoagulant therapy in a patient with spinal meningioma. Neurosurgery 1981;8:600.
209. Russell N, Jacob MJC. Spinal subdural hematoma in association with anticoagulant therapy. J Can Sci Neurol 1981;8:87.
210. Brandt F, Roosen K. Spinales subdurales Hämatom nach Lumbal-Punktion unter Antikoagulantien-Behandlung. Aktuel Neurol 1980;7:167.
211. Zuccarello M, Scanarini M, D'Avella D et al. Spontaneous spinal extradural hematoma during anticoagulant therapy. Surg Neurol 1980;14:411.
212. Oh S, Künzli M, Tok S. Nervwurzelsyndrom bei spontanem intraduralem Hämatom durch Antikoagulations-therapie. Schweiz Rundsch Med 1981;70:1033.
213. Strain RE. Spinal epidural hematoma in patients on anticoagulant therapy. Ann Surg 1964;159:507.
214. Pointud Ph, Uzzan B, Stilhart B. Syndrome de la queue de cheval par hématome épidural rachidien au cours d'un traitement anticoagulant. Nouv Presse Méd 1979;8:4047.
215. Harik SI, Raichle ME, Reis DJ. Spontaneously remitting spinal epidural hematoma in a patient on anticoagulants. N Engl J Med 1971;284:1355.
216. Oldenkott P, Preger R, Todorow S. Spinale epidurale Hämatome und Antikoagulantienbehandlung. Med Welt 1981;32:46.
217. Varkey GP, Brindle GF. Peridural anaesthesia and anticoagulant therapy. Can Anaesth Soc J 1974;21:106.
218. Gaillard J, Haguenauer JP, Moindrot M et al. Paralysie faciale au cours d'un traitement anticoagulant. J Fr Oto-Rhino-Laryngol 1973;22:825.
219. Salam AA. Brachial plexus paralysis: an unusual complication of anticoagulant therapy. Am Surg 1972;38:454.
220. Hoyt TE, Tiwari R, Kusske JA. Compressive neuropathy as a complication of anticoagulant therapy. Neurosurgery 1983;12:268.
221. Prill A. Ischiadikus-Lähmungen als Komplikation unter Antikoagulantienbehandlung. Med Welt 1965;1:307.
222. Zarranz JJ, Simon R, Saisachs P. Acute anticoagulant-induced compressive lumbar plexus neuropathy: a clinicopathological study. Eur Neurol 1981;20:469.
223. De Bolt WL, Jordan JC. Femoral neuropathy from heparin hematoma. Bull Los Angeles Neurol Soc 1966;31:45.
224. Kounis NG, Karatzas GE. Haemorrhagic complications of anticoagulants: heparin-induced femoral neuropathy. Practitioner 1980;224:741.
225. Uncini A, Tonali P, Falappa P et al. Femoral neuropathy from iliac muscle hematoma induced by oral anticoagulation therapy: report of three cases with CT demonstration. J Neurol 1981;226:137.
226. Castaneda LG, Goodfellow JW. The recovery of femoral nerve paralysis after iliacus haematoma in anticoagulated patients. Orthopaedics 1973;6:77.
227. Young MR, Norris JW. Femoral neuropathy during anticaogulant therapy. Neurology 1976;26:1173.
228. Razzuk MA, Linton RR, Darling RC. Femoral neuropathy secondary to ruptured abdominal aortic aneurysms with false aneurysms. J Am Med Assoc 1967;201:817.
229. Briët E. Personal communication, Thrombosis Center, Leiden, 1978.
230. Kettlekamp DB, Powers SR. Femoral compression neuropathy in hemorrhagic disorders. Arch Surg 1969;98:367.
231. Feman SS, Barlett RE, Roth AM et al. Intraocular hemorrhage and blindness associated with systemic anticoagulation. J Am Med Assoc 1972;220:1354.
232. Hogan MJ. Systemic anticoagulation and intraocular hemorrhage. J Am Med Assoc 1972;221:1516.

233. Verhagen H. Local haemorrhage and necrosis of the skin and underlying tissues, during anti-coagulant therapy with dicumarol or dicumacyl. Acta Med Scand 1954;148:453.
234. Van Amstel WJ, Boekhout-Mussert MJ, Loeliger EA. Successful prevention of coumarin-induced hemorrhagic skin necrosis by timely administration of vitamin K_1. Blut 1978;36:89.
235. Jost P. Cumarinnekrosen. Schweiz. Med. Wochenschr 1969;99:1069.
236. Leypold F, Carniel M. Nil nocere! Hautnekrosen als Komplication bei Behandlung mit Antikoagulantien. Münch Med Wochenschr 1961;103:1675.
237. Cameron ARE, Van Berkel W, Sixma JJ. Huidnecrose na drie jaar behandeling met acenocoumarine. Ned Tijdschr Geneeskd 1974;118:505.
238. Horn JR, Danziger KH, Davis RJ. Warfarin-induced skin necrosis: report of four cases. Am J Hosp Pharm 1981;38:1763.
239. Barkley C, Badalament RA, Metz EN et al. Coumarin necrosis of the penis. J Urol 1989;141:946.
240. Kandrotas RJ, Deterding J. Genital necrosis secondary to warfarin therapy. Pharmacotherapy 1988;8:351.
241. Haefeli H. Uterusnekrose bei Cumarin-Therapie. Fortschr Geburtslilfe Gynäkol 1969;39:49.
242. Koch-Weser J. Coumarin necrosis. Ann Intern Med 1968;68:1365.
243. DiCato MA, Ellman L. Coumadin-induced necrosis of breast, disseminated intravascular coagulation, and hemolytic anemia. Ann Intern Med 1975;83:233.
244. Broekmans AW, Bertina RM, Loeliger EA et al. Protein C and the development of skin necrosis during anticoagulant therapy (Letter to Editor). Thromb Haemostasis 1983;49:251.
245. Samama M, Horellou MH, Soria J et al. Successful progressive anticoagulation in a severe protein C deficiency and previous skin necrosis at the initiation of anticoagulant treatment. Thromb Haemostasis 1984;51:132.
246. Teepe RG, Broekmans AW, Vermeer BJ et al. Recurrent coumarin-induced skin necrosis in a patient with an acquired functional protein C deficiency. Arch Dermatol 1986;122:1408.
247. Comp PC, Elrod JP, Karzenski S. Warfarin-induced skin necrosis. Semin Thromb Hemostasis 1990;16:293.
248. Craig A, Taberner DA, Fischer AH et al. Type I protein S deficiency and skin necrosis. Postgrad Med J 1990;66:389.
249. Wattiaux M-J, Hervé R, Robert A et al. Coumarin-induced skin necrosis associated with acquired protein S deficiency and antiphospholipid antibody syndrom. Arthr Rheum 1994;37:1096.
250. Nalbandian RM, Mader IJ, Barrett JL et al. Petechiae, ecchymoses, and necrosis of skin induced by coumarin congeners. J Am Med Assoc 1965;192:603.
251. Leiber G, Egbring R. Zur Therapie der 'Cumarinnekrose'. Internist 1972;13:340.
252. Zauber PN, Stark MW. Successful warfarin anticoagulation despite protein C deficiency and a history of warfarin necrosis. Ann Intern Med 1986;104:659.
253. Lewandowski K, Zawilska K. Protein C concentrate in the treatment of warfarin-induced skin necrosis in the protein C deficiency. Thromb Haemostasis 1994;71:395.
254. Hall JG, Pauli RM, Wilson KM. Maternal and fetal sequelae of anticoagulation during pregnancy. Am J Med 1980;68:122.
255. Stevenson RE, Burton OM, Ferlauto GJ et al. Hazards of oral anticoagulants during pregnancy. J Am Med Assoc 1980;243:1549.
256. Ginsberg JS, Hirsh J. Use of anticoagulants during pregnancy. Chest 1989;95(Suppl):156S.
257. Iturbe-Alessio I, Fonseca MdC, Mutchinik O et al. Risks of anticoagulant therapy in pregnant women with artificial heart valves. N Engl J Med 1986;315:1390.
258. Kort HI, Cassel GA. An appraisal of warfarin therapy during pregnancy. S Afr Med J 1981;60:578.
259. Olwin JH, Koppel JL. Anticoagulant therapy during pregnancy: a new approach. Obstet Gynecol 1969;34:847.
260. Price PA, Williamson MK, Haba T et al. Excessive mineralization with growth plate closure in rats on chronic warfarin treatment. Proc Natl Acad Sci USA 1982;79:7734.
261. Chong MKB, Harvey D, DeSwiet M. Follow-up study of children whose mothers were treated with warfarin during pregnancy. Br J Obstet Gynaecol 1984;91:1070.
262. Ginsberg JS, Kowalchuk G, Hirsh J et al. Heparin therapy during pregnancy. Risks to the fetus and mother. Arch Intern Med 1989;149:2233.
263. Ginsberg JS, Hirsh J. Use of antithrombotic agents during pregnancy. Chest 1992:102(Suppl):385S.
264. Ginsberg JS, Hirsh J. Use of antithrombotic agents during pregnancy. Chest 1995:108(Suppl):305S.
265. De Swiet M, Dorrington Ward P, Fidler J et al. Prolonged heparin therapy in pregnancy causes bone demineralization. Br J Obstet Gynaecol 1983;90:1129.
266. Megard M, Cuche M, Grapeloux A et al. Ostéoporose de l'héparinothérapie: analyse histomorphométrique de la biopsie osseuse: une observation. Nouv Presse Méd 1982; 11:261.
267. Squires JW, Pinch LW. Heparin-induced spinal fractures. J Am Med Assoc 1979;241:2417.
268. Dahlman T, Sjöbery HE, Hellgren M, Bucht E. Calcium homeostasis in pregnancy during long-term heparin treatment. Br J Obst Gynaecol 1992;99:412.
269. Dahlman TC. Osteoporotic fractures and the recurrence of thromboembolism during pregnancy and the puerperium in 184 women undergoing thromboprophylaxis with heparin. Am J Obst Gynecol 1993;168:1265.
270. Aarskog D, Aksknes L, Lehmann V. Low 1,25-di-hydroxyvitamin D in heparin-induced osteopenia. Lancet 1980; ii:650.
271. Göring G. Kasuistischer Beitrag zur Streptokinase-behandlung in der Schwangerschaft. Geburtshilfe Frauenheilkd 1971;31:348.
272. Houwert-De Jong M, Gerards LJ, Tetteroo-Tempelman CAM et al. May mothers taking acenocoumarol breast feed their infants? Eur J Clin Pharmacol 1981;21:61.
273. Goguel M, Noël G, Gillet J-Y et al. Thérapeutique anticoagulante et allaitement. Rev Fr Gynécol 1970;65:409.
274. Orme MLE, Lewis PJ, De Swiet M et al. May mothers given warfarin breast-feed their infants? Br Med J 1977; 1:1564.
275. Eckstein HB, Jack B. Breast-feeding and anticoagulant therapy. Lancet 1970;i:672.
276. Gjønnaess H, Fagerhol MK, Stormorken H. Studies on coagulation and fibrinolysis in blood from puerperal women with and without oestrogen treatment. Br J Obstet Gyneacol 1975;82:151.
277. Cerebral Embolism Study Group. Immediate anticoagulation of embolic stroke: brain hemorrhage and management options. Stroke 1984;15:779.
278. Calandre L, Ortega JF, Bermejo F et al. Cerebral embolism and anticoagulation. Neurology 1983;33:1103.

279. Furlan AJ, Cavalier SJ, Hobbs RE et al. Hemorrhage and anticoagulation after nonseptic embolic brain infarction. Neurology 1982;32:280.
280. Hart RG, Coull BM, Hart D. Early recurrent embolism associated with nonvalvular atrial fibrillation: a retrospective study. Stroke 1983;14:688.
281. Koller RL. Reccurent embolic cerebral infarction and anticoagulation. Neurology 1982;32:283.
282. Shields RW, Laureno R, Lachman T et al. Anticoagulant-related hemorrhage in acute cerebral embolism. Stroke 1984;15:426.
283. Lodder J, Van der Lugt PJM. Evaluation of the risk of immediate anticoagulant treatment in patients with embolic stroke of cardiac origin. Stroke 1983;14:42.
284. Cerebral Embolism Study Group. Immediate anticoagulation of embolic stroke: a randomized trial. Stroke 1983;14:668.
285. Bass E. Anticoagulation in cerebral embolism. Can J Neurol Sci 1983;10:32.
286. Sevitt S, Innes D. Evidence against 'rebound' thrombosis after stopping oral anticoagulant drugs. Lancet 1963; ii:974.
287. Michaels L. Incidence of thromboembolism after stopping anticoagulant therapy. J Am Med Assoc 1971;215:595.
288. Editorial. Thrombotic 'rebound' after withdrawal of oral anticoagulants. Drugs Ther Bull 1966;4:92.
289. Castaneda AR, Gans H, Weber KC et al. Heparin neutralization: experimental and clinical studies. Surgery 1967;62:686.
290. Godal HC, Gjengedal G. Activation of coagulation by heparin-protamine complexes as demonstrated by Thrombotest. Scand J Haematol 1971;8:194.
291. Gans H, Castaneda AR. Problems in hemostasis during open heart surgery. VII. Changes in fibrinogen concentration during and after cardiopulmonary bypass with particular reference to the effect of heparin neutralization on fibrinogen. Ann Surg 1967;165:551.
292. Marciniak E, Gockerman JP. Heparin-induced decrease in circulating antithrombin-III. Lancet 1977;ii:581.
293. Cook MK. Heparin-induced decrease in circulating antithrombin III. Lancet 1978;i:208.
294. Woods HF, Dawson A, Ash G et al. Heparin-induced decrease in circulating antithrombin III (Letter to Editor). Lancet 1978;i:209.
295. Barrowcliffe TW, Johnson EA, Thomas D. Antithrombin III and heparin. Br Med Bull 1978;34:143.
296. Edwards RL, Rickles FR. Delayed hypersensitivity in man: effects of systemic anticoagulation. Science 1978; 200:541.
297. Hilgard P, Schulte H, Wetzig G et al. Oral anticoagulation in the treatment of a spontaneously metastasing murine tumour (3LL). Br J Cancer 1977;35:78.
298. Thornes RD. Adjuvant therapy of cancer via the cellular immune mechanism or fibrin by induced fibrinolysis and oral anticoagulants. Cancer 1975;35:91.
299. Hoover HC, Ketcham AS, Millar RC et al. Osteosarcoma: improved survival with anticoagulation and amputation. Cancer 1978;41:2475.
300. Zacharski LR, Henderson WG, Rickles FR et al. Effect of warfarin on survival in small cell carcinoma of the lung. J Am Med Assoc 1981;245:831.
301. Elias EG, Shukla SK, Mink IB. Heparin and chemotherapy in the management of inoperable lung carcinoma. Cancer 1975;36:129.
302. Williamson RCN, Lyndon PJ, Tudway AJC. Effects of anticoagulation and ileal resection on the development and spread of experimental intestinal carcinomas. Br J Cancer 1980;42:85.
303. Zacharski LR, Henderson WG, Rickles FR et al. Effect of warfarin anticoagulation on survival in carcinoma of the lung, colon, head and neck, and prostate. Cancer 1984; 53:2046.
304. Annegers JF, Zacharski LR. Cancer morbidity and mortality in previously anticoagulated patients. Thromb Res 1980;18:399.
305. Hilgard P, Maat B. Mechanism of lung tumour colony reduction caused by coumarin anticoagulation. Eur J Cancer 1979;15:183.
306. Lione A, Bosmann HB. The inhibitory effect of heparin and warfarin treatments on the intravascular survival of B16 melanoma cells in syngeneic C57 mice. Cell Biol Int Rep 1978;2:81.
307. Hilgard P, Beyerle L, Hohage R et al. The effect of heparin on the initial phase of metastasis formation. Eur J Cancer 1972;8:347.
308. Zahir M. Anticoagulants and experimental wound healing. Br J Exp Pathol 1965;46:623.
309. Deutsch E, Benda L, Zischka W. Probleme der Antikoagulantienbehandlung. Thromb Diath Haemorrh 1958; 2:510.
310. Hampton JR. The burst abdomen. Br Med J 1963; 2:1032.
311. Safar J, Gajewski J, Shedd DP et al. Effect of the streptokinase-induced fibrinolytic state on the healing of sutured arterial wounds in dogs. J Surg Res 1969;9:649.
312. Blum E. Beeinflüssung der Kallusbildung durch Antikoagulantien bei Frakturen mit thromboembolischen Komplikationen. Bruns' Beitr Klin Chir 1964;208:25.
313. Gasperini E, Parmeggiani, G. Anticoagulanti nella profilassi della malattia thromboembolica ed evoluzione del callo osseo. Clin Ortop 1969;21:394.
314. Pierce WS, Donachy JH, Rosenberg G et al. Calcification inside artificial hearts: inhibition by warfarin-sodium. Science 1980;208:601.
315. Pietschmann P, Woloszczuk W, Panzer S et al. Decreased serum osteocalcin levels in phenprocoumon-treated patients. J Clin Endocrinol Metab 1988;66:1071.
316. Breckenridge RT, Kellermeyer RW. A hemorrhagic syndrome due to dicoumarol poisoning masquerading as propylthiouracil sensitivity. Ann Intern Med 1964;60:1066.
317. Granditsch G, Pilgerstorfer HW. Vergiftung mit Acenocumarin (Sintrom®) bei einem Kind. Wien Klin Wochenschr 1971;83:62.
318. Martin-Bouyer G, Khanh NB, Linh PD et al. Epidemic of haemorrhagic disease in Vietnamese infants caused by warfarin-contaminated talcs. Lancet 1983;i:230.
319. Abell TL, Merigian KS, Lee JM et al. Cutaneous exposure to warfarine-like anticoagulant causing an intracerebral hemorrhage: a case report. J Toxicol Clin Toxicol 1994;32:69.
320. Favre-Gilly J, Thouverez JP, Tourniaire M. Diathèse hémorragique féminine avec présence dans le sang d'une antithrombine du type de l'héparine. Sang 1958;29:398.
321. Martin CM, Engstrom PF, Barrett ON Jr. Surreptitious self-administration of heparin. J Am Med Assoc 1970; 215:475.
322. Agle DP, Ratnoff OD, Spring GK. The anticoagulant malingerer: psychiatric studies of three patients. Ann Intern Med 1970;73:67.

323. Gover PA, Ingram GIC, Cork MS et al. Bleeding from self-administration of phenindione: a detailed case-study. Br J Haematol 1976;33:551.
324. Josso F, Prou-Wartelle O, Soulier JP. Intoxication volontaire itérative par phenylindane-dione (pindione). Nouv Rev Fr Hématol 1966;6:685.
325. O'Reilly RA, Aggeler PM. Surreptitious ingestion of coumarin anticoagulant drugs. Ann Intern Med 1966; 64:1034.
326. Ikkala E, Myllylä G, Nevanlinna HR et al. Haemorrhagic diathesis due to criminal poisoning with warfarin. Acta Med Scand 1964;176:201.
327. De Jager NST, Boyd NF, Ginsburg AD. Attempted abortion by the use of bishyroxycoumarin. Can Med Assoc J 1972;107:50.
328. Corn M, Berberich R. Rapid fluometric assay for plasma warfarin. Clin Chem (New York) 1967;13:740.
329. De Wolff FA, Van Kempen GMJ. Determination of phenprocoumon, an anticoagulant, in human plasma. Clin Chem (Winston-Salem) 1976;22:1575.
330. Van Kempen GMJ, Koot-Gronsveld EAM, De Wolff FA. Quantitative and qualitative analysis of the anticoagulant acenocoumarol in human plasma. J Chromatogr 1978;145:332.
331. Bechtold H, Trenk D, Jähnchen E, Meinertz T. Plasma vitamin K_1-2,3-epoxide as diagnostic aid to detect surreptitious ingestion of oral anticoagulant drugs. Lancet 1983; i:596.
332. Toolis F, Robson RH, Critchley JAJH. Warfarin poisoning in patients with prosthetic heart valves. Br Med J 1981;283:581.
333. Renowden S, Westmoreland D, Whote JP et al. Oral cholestyramine increases elimination of warfarin after overdose. Br Med J 1985;291:513.
334. Meinertz T, Gilfrich H, Bork R et al. Treatment of phenprocoumon intoxication with cholestyramine. Br Med J 1977;2:439.
335. Scott BD. Heparin-induced thrombocytopenia. A common but controllable condition. Postgrad Med 1989;86:153.
336. Ayars GH, Tikoff G. Incidence of thrombocytopenia in medical patients on 'mini dose' heparin prophylaxis. Am Heart J 1980;99:816.
337. Gallus AS, Goodall KT, Beswick W et al. Heparin-associated thrombocytopenia: case report and prospective study. Aust NZ J Med 1980;10:25.
338. Ball A, L'Huillier AM, Dreyfuss L et al. Thrombopénie à la Fraxiparine. Une observation. Presse Méd 1989;18:1254.
339. Rankin JA. Heparin-induced thrombosis (white clot syndrome) secondary to prophylactic subcutaneous administration of heparin. Can J Surg 1988;31:33.
340. Heeger PS, Backstrom JT. Heparin flushes and thrombocytopenia. Ann Intern Med 1986;105:142.
341. Kelton JG. Heparin-induced thrombocytopenia. Haemostasis 1986;16:173.
342. Bell WR, Tomasulo PA, Alving BM et al. Thrombocytopenia occuring during the administration of heparin: a prospective study in 52 patients. Ann Intern Med 1976; 85:155.
343. Kakkasseril JS, Cranley JJ, Panke T et al. Heparin-induced thrombocytopenia: a prospective study of 142 patients. J Vasc Surg 1985;2:382.
344. Bell WR, Royall RM. Heparin-associated thrombocytopenia: a comparison of three heparin preparations. N Engl J Med 1980;303:902.
345. Cipolle RJ, Rodvold KA, Seifert R et al. Heparin-associated thrombocytopenia: a prospective evaluation of 211 patients. Ther Drug Monit 1983;5:205.
346. Green D, Martin GJ, Shoichet SH et al. Thrombocytopenia in a prospective, randomized, double-blind trial of bovine and porcine heparin. Am J Med Sci 1984;288:60.
347. Rao AK, White GC, Sherman L et al. Low incidence of thrombocytopenia with porcine mucosal heparin. A prospective multicenter study. Arch Int Med 1989;149:1285.
348. Warkentin TE, Levine MN, Hirsh J et al. Heparin-induced thrombocytopenia in patients treated with low-molecular-weight heparin or unfractionated heparin. N Engl J Med 1995;332:1330.
349. Horellou MH, Conard J, Lecrubier C et al. Persistent heparin induced thrombocytopenia despite therapy with low molecular weight heparin. Thromb Haemostasis 1984; 51:134.
350. Oriot D, Wolf M. Wood C et al. Severe heparin-induced thrombocytopenia in a child with myocarditis (in French). Arch Fr Pédiatrie 1990;47:357.
351. Laster J, Silver D. Heparin-coated catheters and heparin-induced thrombocytopenia. J Vasc Surg 1988;27:667.
352. Pelouze GA, Coste B, Rassam Th, Valat JD. Thrombopénie immunoallergique déclenchée par le revêtement hépariné d'un cathéter. Presse Méd 1989;18:1481.
353. Gayer W. Seltene Beobachtungen von Heparin-Unverträglichkeit. Gynaecologia (Basel) 1968;166:25.
354. Cutcudache C, Gorun V, Brailescu G. Coagulopathie de consommation au cours d'une réaction anaphylactique à l'héparine. Coagulation 1971;4:19.
355. Schimpf K, Barth P. Heparinshock mit Verbrauchsreaktion des Blutgerinnungssystems? Klin Wochenschr 1966; 44:544.
356. Godal HC. Report of the International Committee on Thrombosis and Haemostasis: thrombocytopenia and heparin. Thromb Haemostasis 1980;43:222.
357. Ainley EJ, Mackie IG, MacArthur D. Adverse reaction to chlorocresol-preserved heparin. Lancet 1977;i:705.
358. Dux S, Pitlik S, Perry G et al. Hypersensitivity reaction to chlorbutol-preserved heparin. Lancet 1981;i:149.
359. Bjoraker DG, Ketcham TR. Hemodynamic and platelet response to the bolus intravenous administration of porcine heparin. Thromb Haemostasis 1983;49:1.
360. Bowler GMR, Galloway DW, Meiklejohn BH. Sharp fall in blood pressure after injection of heparin containing chlorbutol (Letter to Editor). Lancet 1986;i:848.
361. Woldow A, Lopez RH, Goldberg H. Effect of multiple injections of heparin on the hyperlipemia of atherosclerosis. Am J Cardiol 1964;14:64.
362. Arnesen H, Skjaeggestad Ø, Wik B. Plasma free fatty acids and the incidence of arrhythmias in acute myocardial infarction during treatment with small doses of subcutaneous heparin or warfarin. Acta Med Scand 1980;207:21.
363. Kurien VA, Yates PA, Oliver MF. Free fatty acids, heparin, and arrhythmias during experimental myocardial infarction. Lancet 1969;ii:185.
364. Rutstein DD, Castelli WP, Nickerson RJ. Heparin and human lipid metabolism. Lancet 1969;i:1003.
365. Arnesen H, Bjerkedal I, Skjaeggestad Ø et al. Plasma free-fatty-acids and small doses of subcutaneous heparin in acute myocardial infarction. Thromb Res 1979;14:541.
366. Wolf R, Beck OA, Hochrein H. Der Einfluss von Heparin auf die Häufigkeit von Rhythmusstörungen beim akuten Myokardinfarkt. Dtsch Med Wochenschr 1974;99:1549.

367. Wahs GF, Cameron J, Henderson A. Lipoprotein lipase deficiency due to long-term heparinization presenting as severe hypertriglyceridemia in pregnancy. Postgrad Med J 1991;67:1062.
368. Oster JR, Singer I, Fishman LM. Heparin-induced aldosterone suppression and hyperkaliemia. Am J Cardiol 1995;98:575.
369. Aull L, Chao H, Coy K. Heparin-induced hyperkalemia. Drug Intell Clin Pharm 1990;24:244.
370. Edes TE, Sunderrajan EV. Heparin-induced hyperkaliema. Arch Int Med 1985;145:1070.
371. Leehey D, Gannt M, Lim V. Heparin-induced hypoaldosteronism: report of a case. J Am Med Assoc 1981; 246:2189.
372. Phelps KR, Oh MS, Carroll HJ. Heparin-induced hyperkalemia: report of a case. Nephron 1980;25:254.
373. Weismann RE, Tobin RW. Arterial embolism occuring during systemic heparin therapy. Arch Surg 1958;76:219.
374. Rector TS, Cipolle RJ, Seifert RD et al. Characteristics of heparin-associated thrombocytopenia. Am J Hosp Pharm 1979;36:1561.
375. Carreras LO. Thrombosis and thrombocytopenia induced by heparin. Scand J Haematol 1980;25(Suppl):36.
376. Kitzis M, Huisse MG, Hannoun L et al. Thrombopénies induites par l'héparine: diagnostic biologique et complications. Arch Mal Coeur Vaiss 1980;73:1395.
377. Ansell J, Deykin D. Heparin-induced thrombocytopenia and recurrent thromboembolism. Am J Hematol 1980;8:325.
378. Baird RA, Convery FR. Arterial thromboembolism in patients receiving systemic heparin therapy. J Bone Jt Surg 1977;59:1061.
379. Cimo PL, Moake JL, Weinger RS et al. Heparin-induced thrombocytopenia: association with a platelet aggregating factor and arterial thromboses. Am J Hematol 1979;6:125.
380. Moore JR, Weiland AJ. Heparin-induced thromboembolism: a case report. J Hand Surg 1979;4:382.
381. Jaffray B, Welch GH, Cooke TG. Fatal venous thrombosis after heparin therapy (Letter to Editor). Lancet 1991;337:561.
382. Rizzoni WE, Miller K, Rick M. Heparin-induced thrombocytopenia and thromboembolism in the postoperative period. Surgery 1988;103:470.
383. Bernasconi F, Metivet F, Estrade G. Thrombosis of mitral valve prosthesis associated with heparin-induced thrombocytopenia: fibrinolytic treatment (in French). Presse Méd 1988;17:1366.
384. Lindsey SM, Maddison FE, Towne JB. Heparin-induced thrombo-embolism: angiographic features. Radiology 1979;131:771.
385. White PW, Sadd JR, Nensel RE. Thrombotic complications of heparin therapy. Ann Surg 1979;190:595.
386. Laster J, Cikrit D, Walker N, Silver D. The heparin-induced thrombocytopenia syndrome: an update. Surgery 1987;102:763.
387. Becker PS, Miller VT. Heparin-induced thrombocytopenia. Stroke 1989;20:1449.
388. Anderson GP. Insights into heparin-induced thrombocytopenia. Br J Haematol 1992;80:504.
389. Amiral J, Bridey F, Dreyfus M et al. Platelet factor 4 complexed to heparin is the target for antibodies generated in heparin-induced thrombocytopenia. Thromb Hemostasis 1992;67:545.
390. Boshkov LK, Warkentin TE, Hayward CPM et al. Heparin-induced thrombocytopenia and thrombosis: clinical and laboratory studies. Br J Haematol 1993;84:322.
391. Cines DB, Tomaski A, Tannenbaum S. Immune endothelial-cell injury in heparin-associated thrombocytopenia. N Engl J Med 1987;316:581.
392. Chong BH, Castaldi PA. Heparin-induced thrombocytopenia: further studies of the effects of heparin-dependent antibodies on platelets. Br J Haematol 1986;64:347.
393. Gruel Y, Lermisiaux P, Lang M et al. Usefulness of antiplatelet drugs in the management of heparin-associated thrombocytopenia and thrombosis. Ann Vasc Surg 1991;5:552.
394. Metz B, N'Guyen Ph, Chapoutot L et al. Embolie pulmonaire massive révélant une thrombopénie induite par héparine de bas poids moléculaire. Succés thérapeutique d'une prostacycline. Ann Cardiol Angéiol 1991;40:619.
395. Kappa JR, Fisher CA, Todd B. Intraoperative management of patients with heparin-induced thrombocytopenia. Ann Thorac Surg 1990;49:714.
396. Agnelli G, Ioro A, de Angelis V, Nenci GG. Dermatan sulfate in heparin-induced thrombocytopenia. Lancet 1994;344:1295.
397. Huisse MG, Huet Y, Zygelman M, Guillin MC. Thrombopénie induite par l'héparine standard. Tentative thérapeutique à l'aide d'une héparine de bas poids moléculaire. Presse Méd 1983;12:643.
398. Kikta MJ, Keller MP, Humphrey PW, Silver D. Can low molecular weight heparins and heparinoïds be safely given to patients with heparin-induced thrombocytopenic syndroms? Surgery 1993;114:705.
399. Vender JS, Matthew EB, Silverman IM et al. Heparin-associated thrombocytopenia: alternative managements. Anesth Analg 1986;65:520.
400. O'Toole RD. Heparin: adverse reaction (Letter to Editor). Ann Intern Med 1973;79:759.
401. Fowlie J, Stanton PD, Anderson JR. Heparin-associated skin necrosis. Postgrad Med J 1990;66:573.
402. Schlag G, Poigenfürst J, Gaudernak T. Risk/benefit of heparin-dihydroergotamine thromboembolic prophylaxis. Lancet 1986;ii:1456.
403. Stavorovsky M, Lichenstein D, Nissim F. Skin petechiae and ecchymoses (vasculitis) due to anticoagulant therapy. Dermatologica 1979;158:451.
404. Jones BF, Epstein MT. Cutaneous heparin necrosis associated with glomerulonephritis. Aust J Dermatol 1987;28:117.
405. Dacosta A, Mismetti P, Buchmuller A et al. Hyperéosinophilie et lésions cutanées induites par héparine de bas poids moléculaire. Presse Méd 1994;23:1540.
406. Viallard JF, Nean B, Monlun E et al. Hyperéosinophilie liée à l'héparine: une observation avec test de réintroduction. Thérapie 1994;49:513.
407. Clark SK, Tremann JA, Sennewald FR et al. Priapism: an unusual complication of heparin therapy for sudden deafness. Am J Otolaryngol 1981;2:69.
408. Adjiman S, Fava P, Bitker MO, Chatelain H. Priapisme induit par l'héparine: un pronostic plus sombre? Ann Urol 1988;22:125.
409. Klein GF, Kofler H, Wolf H, Fritsch PO. Eczema-like, erythematous, infiltrated plaques: a common side effect of subcutaneous heparin therapy. J Am Acad Dermatol 1989;21:703.
410. Tuneu A, Moreno A, de Moragas JM. Cutaneous reac-

tions secondary to heparin injections. J Am Acad Dermatol 1985;12:1072.
411. Phillips JK, Majumdar G, Hunt BJ, Savidge GF. Heparin-induced skin reaction due to two different preparations of low molecular weight heparin. Br J Haematol 1993;84:349.
412. Conri CL, Azoulai P, Constans J et al. Erythromelalgia and low molecular weight heparin (in French). Thérapie 1994;49:518.
413. Pecegueiro M, Brando M, Pinto J et al. Contact dermatitis to Hirudoid® cream. Contact Derm 1987;17:290.
414. Monreal M, Glive A, Lafoz E et al. Heparins, coumarin, and bone density. Lancet 1992;338:706.
415. Dahlman T, Lindvall N, Hellgren M. Osteopenia in pregnancy during long-term heparin treatment: a radiological study post partum. Br J Obstet Gynaecol 1990;97:221.
416. Hausdorf G, Bentele K, Hellwege HH. Nephrocalcinose nach Candida-Sepsis und Heparin-Osteoporose bei einam Säugling. Monatsschr Kinderheilkd 1982;130:168.
417. Fox JG, Walli RK, Jaffray B, Simpson HKL. Calcified subcutaneous nodules due to calcium heparin injections in a patient with chronic renal failure. Nephrol Dial Transplant 1994;9:187.
418. Korz R. Heparin-induzierte Mobilisation von Calcium und anorganischem Phosphat im Zumsammenhang mit extraossären Verkalkungen bei chronischer Hämodialyse. Klin Wochenschr 1971;49:255.
419. Argent NB, Veale D. Discharge from ostemyelitis sinus with heparin therapy (Letter to Editor). Postgrad Med J 1990;66:583.
420. Jaques LB. Heparins—Anionic polyelectrolyte drugs. Pharmacol Rev 1980;31:99.
421. Miller D. Heparin precipitability of the macroglobulin in a patient with Waldenström's macroglobulinemia. Blood 1960;16:1313.
422. Godolphin W, Cameron EC, Frohlich J et al. Spurious hypocalcemia in hemodialysis patients after heparinization. Am J Clin Pathol 1979;71:215.
423. Buist NRM, Curtis HT. Heparin and false positive tests for mucopolysacchariduria. Lancet 1972;ii:286.
424. DeChatelet LR, McCall CE, Cooper MR et al. Inhibition of leukocyte acid phosphatase by heparin. Clin Chem 1972;18:1532.
425. Dukes GE, Sanders SW, Russo J et al. Transaminase elevations in patients receiving bovine or porcine heparin. Ann Intern Med 1984;100:646.
426. Schwartz KA, Royer G, Kaufman DB et al. Complications of heparin administration in normal individuals. Am J Hematol 1985;9:355.
427. Toulemonde F, Kher A. Héparine et transaminases: une énigme sans importance en 1994? Thérapie 1994;49:355.
428. Salomon F, Schmid M. Heparin (Letter to the Editor). Lancet 1991;325:1585.
429. Lambert M, Laterre P-F, Leroy Ch et al. Modifications of liver enzymes during heparin therapy. Acta Clin Belg 1986;41:307.
430. Sonnenblick M, Oren A, Jacobsohn W. Hypertransaminasemia with heparin therapy. Br Med J 1975;3:77.
431. Thompson JE, Baird SG, Thomson JA. Effect of i.v. heparin on serum free triiodothyronine levels (Letter to Editor). Br J Clin Pharmacol 1977;4:701.
432. Wilkins TA, Midgley JEM, Giles AF. Treatment with heparin and results for free thyroxin. An in vivo or an in vitro effect? Clin Chem 1982;28:2441.
433. Wu JT. Interference of heparin in carcinoembryonic antigen radioimmunoassays. Clin Chim Acta 1983;130:47.
434. Ordog GJ, Wasserberger J, Balasubramaniam S. Effect of heparin on arterial blood gases. Ann Emerg Med 1985;14:233.
435. Mac Connell JS, Cohen J. Effect of anticaogulants on the chromogenic Limulus lysate assay for endotoxin. J Clin Pathol 1985;38:430.
436. Wood M, Shand DG, Wood AJJ. Altered drug binding due to the use of indwelling heparinized cannulas (heparin lock) for sampling. Clin Pharmacol Ther 1979;25:103.
437. Routledge PA, Bjornsson TD, Kitchell BB et al. Heparin administration increases plasma warfarin binding in man (Letter to Editor). Br J Clin Pharmacol 1979;8:281.
438. Desmond PV, Roberts RK, Wood AJJ et al. Effect of heparin administration on plasma binding of benzodiazepines. Br J Clin Pharmacol 1980;9:174.
439. Routledge PA, Kitchell BB, Bjornsson TD et al. Diazepam and *N*-desmethyldiazepam redistribution after heparin. Clin Pharmacol Ther 1980;27:528.
440. Walters MI, Roberts WH. Gentamicin/heparin interactions: effects on two immunoassays and on protein binding. Ther Drug Monit 1984;6:199.
441. Lohman JJHM, Hooymans PM, Koten MLP et al. Effect of heparin on digitoxin protein binding. Clin Pharmacol Ther 1985;37:55.
442. Hasegawa GR, Eder JF. Dobutamine-heparin mixture inadvisable. Am J Hosp Pharm 1984;41:2588.
443. Col J, Col-Debeys C, Lavenne-Pardonge et al. Propylene glycol-induced heparin resistance during nitroglycerin infusion. Am Heart J 1985;110:171.
444. Becker RC, Corrao JM, Bovill EG et al. Intravenous nitroglycerin-induced heparin resistance: A qualitative antithrombin III abnormality. Am Heart J 1990;119:1254.
445. Ruedy J, Davies RO, Gagnon MA et al. Drug bioavailability. Can Med Assoc J 1976;115:105.
446. Biron P. Dosage, compliance and bioavailability in perspective. Can Med Assoc J 1976;115:102.
447. Levi B, Süsstrunk H. Allergische Hauterscheinungen unter Antikoaguleantien. Personal communication, 1975.
448. Kruis-de Vries MH, Stricker BHC, Coenraads PJ, Nater JP. Maculopapular rash due to coumarin derivatives. Dermatologica 1989;178:109.
449. Tanay A, Yust I, Brenner S et al. Dermal vasculitis due to coumadin hypersensitivity. Dermatologica 1982;165:178.
450. Susano R, Garcia A, Altadill A, Ferro J. Hypersensitivity vasculitis related to nicoumalone. Br Med J 1993;306:973.
451. Lakin KM. Experimentelle Untersuchung der Wirkung von Antikoagulantien auf den Koronarkreislauf. Thromb Diath Haemorrh 1964;S12:115.
452. Akle CA, Joiner CL. Purple toe syndrome. J R Soc Med 1981;74:219.
453. Feder W, Auerbach R. 'Purple toes': an uncommon sequela of oral coumarin drug therapy. Ann Intern Med 1961;55:911.
454. Burton JL, Pennock P. Anticoagulants and 'feeling cold'. Lancet 1979;i:608.
455. Bruns FJ, Segel DP, Adler S. Control of cholesterol embolization by discontinuation of anticoagulant therapy. Am J Med Sci 1978;275:105.
456. Levin S, Mogilner M. Reye's syndrome (encephalopathy with fatty degeration of viscera) due to warfarin poisoning. Acta Paediatr Scand 1974;63:164.
457. Walters MB. The relationship between thyroid function and anticoagulation therapy. Am J Cardiol 1963;11:112.
458. Christensen F. Uricosuric effect of dicoumarol. Acta Med Scand 1964;175:461.

459. Thompson GR, Mikkelsen WM, Willis III PW. The uricosuric effect of certain oral anticoagulant drugs. Arthr Rheum 1959;2:383.
460. Self TH, Straughn AB, Weisburst MR. Effect of hyperthyroidism on hypoprothrombinemic response to warfarin. Am J Hosp Pharm 1976;33:387.
461. Stein PD, Riddle JM, Kemp SR et al. Effect of warfarin on calcification of spontaneously degenerated porcine bioprosthetic valves. J Thorac Cardiovasc. Surg 1985;90:119.
462. Mayer GA. Blood viscosity and oral anticoagulant therapy. Am J Clin Pathol 1976;65:402.
463. Herrmann KS, Kreuzer H. Beobachtung einer Acenocoumarol induzierten Granulocytose. Klin Wochenschr 1988;66:639.
464. Griffin JH, Evatt B, Zimmerman TS et al. Deficiency of protein C in congenital thrombotic disease. J Clin Invest 1981;68:1370.
465. Marlar RA, Kleiss AJ, Griffin JH. Mechanism of action of human activated protein C, a thrombin-dependent anticoagulant enzyme. Blood 1982;59:1067.
466. Zacharski LR, Rosenstein R, Phillips PG. Tissue factor: a vitamin K-dependent clotting factor? Ann NY Acad Sci 1981;370:311.
467. Aronson DL, Bagley J. Preliminary characterization of a 'Factor VIII bypassing coagulant'. Ann NY Acad Sci 1981;370:291.
468. Dybedal I, Lamvik J. Warfarin as a probable cause of haemolytic anaemia. Thromb Haemostasis 1990;63:143.
469. Renschler HE, Schmidt FW, Mammen EF. Untersuchungen über die Auswirkungen langdauernder Antikoagulantientherapie auf die Leber. Dtsch Arch Klin Med 1963;208:524.
470. Adler E, Benjamin SB, Zimmerman HJ. Cholestatic hepatic injury related to warfarin exposure. Arch Intern Med 1986;146:1837.
471. de Man RA, Wilson JHP, Schalm SW et al. Phenprocoumon-induced hepatitis mimicking non-A, non-B hepatitis. J Hepatol 1990;11:318.
472. Den Boer W, Loeliger EA. Phenprocoumon-induced jaundice. Lancet 1976;i:912.
473. Rehnqvist N. Intrahepatic jaundice due to warfarin therapy. Acta Med Scand 1978;204:33.
474. Slagboom G, Leoliger EA. Coumarin-associated hepatitis: report of two cases. Arch Intern Med 1980;140:1028.
475. Bachmann K, Shapiro R. Protein binding of coumarin anticoagulants in disease states. Clin Pharmacokin 1977; 2:110.
476. Williams RL, Chary WL, Blaschke TF et al. Influence of acute viral hepatitis on disposition and pharmacologic effect of warfarin. Clin Pharmacol Ther 1976;20:90.
477. Kramer P, Tsuru M, Cook CE et al. Effect of influenza vaccine on warfarin anticoagulation. Clin Pharmacol Ther 1984;35:16.
478. Bussey HI, Saklad JJ. Effect of influenza vaccine on chronic warfarin therapy. Drug Intell Clin Pharm 1988; 22:198.
479. Bachmann K, Shapiro R, Fulton R et al. Smoking and warfarin disposition. Clin Pharmacol Ther 1979;25:309.
480. Weiner B, Faraci PA, Fayad R et al. Warfarin dosage following prosthetic valve replacement: effect of smoking history. Drug Intell Clin Pharm 1984;18:904.
481. O'Reilly RA. Lack of effect of mealtime wine on the hypoprothrombinemia of oral anticoagulants. Am J Med Sci 1979;277:189.
482. Deykin D, Janson P, McMahon L. Ethanol potentiation of aspirin-induced prolongation of the bleeding time. N Engl J Med 1982;306:852.
483. Watson RM, Pierson RN. Effect of anticoagulant therapy upon aspirin-induced gastrointestinal bleeding. Circulation 1961;24:613.
484. Jähnchen E, Meinertz T, Gilfrich HJ. Interaction of allopurinol with phenprocoumon in man. Klin Wochenschr 1977;55:759.
485. Vesell ES, Passananti GT, Greene FE. Impairment of drug metabolism in man by allopurinol and nortriptyline. N Engl J Med 1970;283:1484.
486. Bruning PF. Personal communication, Antoni van Leeuwenhoekhuis, Het Nederlands Kanker Instituut, Amsterdam, 1983.
487. Udall JA. Human sources and absorption of vitamin K in relation to anticoagulation stability. J Am Med Assoc 1965;194:127.
488. O'Reilly RA, Aggeler PM. Determinants of the response to oral anticoagulant drugs in man. Pharmacol Rev 1970;22:35.
489. Self TH. Interaction of warfarin and aminosalicylic acid (Letter to Editor). J Am Med Assoc 1973;223:1285.
490. Caraco Y, Chajek-Shaul T. The incidence and clinical significance of amiodarone and acenocoumarol interaction. Thromb Haemostas 1989;62:906.
491. Hamer A, Peter T, Mandel WJ et al. The potentiation of warfarin anticoagulation by amiodarone. Circulation 1982;65:1025.
492. Martinowitz U, Rabinovici J, Goldfarb D et al. Interaction between warfarin sodium and amiodarone (Letter to Editor). N Engl J Med 1981;304:671.
493. Watt AH, Stephens MP, Buss DC et al. Amiodarone reduces plasma warfarin clearance in man. Br J Clin Pharmacol 1985;20:707.
494. Pyörälä K, Kekki M. Decreased anticoagulant tolerance during methandrostenolone therapy. Scand J Clin Lab Invest 1963;15:367.
495. Ambre JJ, Fischer LJ. Effects of coadministration of aluminum and magnesium hydroxides on absorption of anticoagulants in man. Clin Phamacol Ther 1973;14:231.
496. Grenn AE, Hort JF, Korn HET et al. Potentiation of warfarin by azapropazone. Br Med J 1977;1:1532.
497. McElnay JC, D'Arcy PF. Interaction between azapropazone and warfarin. Experientia 1978;34:1320.
498. Rivier G, Khamashta MA. Warfarin and azathioprine: a drug interaction does exist. Am J Med 1993;95:342.
499. Robinson DS, MacDonald MG. The effect of phenobarbital administration on the control of coagulation achieved during warfarin therapy in man. J Pharmacol Exp Ther 1966;153:250.
500. Levy G, O'Reilly RA, Aggeler PM et al. Pharmacokinetic analysis of the effect of barbiturate on the anticoagulant action of warfarin in man. Clin Pharmacol Ther 1970;11:372.
501. Pyörälä K, Ikkala E, Siltanen P. Benziodarone (Amplivix) and anticoagulant therapy. Acta Med Scand 1963; 173:385.
502. Blum A, Livneh A, Seligmann H, Ezra D. Severe gastrointestinal bleeding induced by a probable hydroxycoumarin-bezafibrate interaction. Isr J Med Sci 1992;28:47.
503. Denbow CE, Fraser HS. Clinically significant hemorrhage due to warfarin-carbamazepine interaction. South Med J 1990;83:981.
504. Mølholm Hansen, J, Siersbaek-Nielsen K, Skovsted L.

Carbamazepine-induced acceleration of diphenylhydantoin and warfarin metabolism in man. Clin Pharmacol Ther 1971;12:539.
505. Loeliger EA, Van der Esch B, Mattern et al. The biological disappearance rate of prothrombin, factors VII, IX and X from plasma in hypothyroidism, hyperthyroidism and during fever. Thromb Diath Haemorrh 1964;10:267.
506. Rymer W, Greenlaw CW. Hypoprothrombinemia associated with cefamandole. Drug Intell Clin Pharm 1980; 14:780.
507. Bechtold H, Andrassy K, Jähnchen E et al. Evidence for impaired heparin vitamin K_1 metabolism in patients treated with *N*-methylthiotetrazole cephalosporins. Thromb Haemostasis 1984;51:538.
508. Boston Collaborative Drug Surveillance Program. Interaction between chloral hydrate and warfarin. N Engl J Med 1972;286:53.
509. Udall JA. Warfarin interactions with chloralhydrate and glutethimide. Curr Ther Res 1975;17:67.
510. Sellers EM, Koch-Weser J. Potentiation of warfarin-induced hypoprothrombinemia by chloral hydrate. N Engl J Med 1970;283:827.
511. Korsgaard Christensen L, Skovsted L. Inhibition of drug metabolism by chloramphenicol. Lancet 1969;ii:1397.
512. Magid E. Tolerance to anticoagulants during antibiotic therapy (Letter to Editor). Scand J Clin Lab Invest 1962;14:565.
513. O'Reilly RA, Sahud MA, Aggeler PM. Impact of aspirin and chlorthalidone on the pharmacodynamics of oral anticoagulant drugs in man. Ann NY Acad Sci 1970;179:173.
514. Robinson DS, Benjamin DM, McCormack JJ. Interaction of warfarin and nonsystemic gastrointestinal drugs. Clin Pharmacol Ther 1971;12:491.
515. Meinertz T, Gilfrich H-J, Groth K et al. Interruption of the enterohepatic circulation of phenprocoumon by cholestyramine. Clin Pharmacol Ther 1977;21:731.
516. Serlin MJ, Sibeon RG, Mossman S et al. Cimetidine: interaction with oral anticoagulants in man. Lancet 1979;ii:317.
517. Harenberg J, Zimmermann R, Staiger Ch et al. Lack of effect of cimetidine on action phenprocoumon. Eur J Clin Pharmacol 1982;23:365.
518. Toon S, Hopkins KJ, Garstang FM, Rowland M. Comparative effects of ranitidine and cimetidine on warfarin in man. Br J Clin Pharmacol 1986;21:565P.
519. Jarnum S. Cinchophen and acetylsalicylic acid in anticoagulant treatment. Scand J Clin Lab Invest 1954;6:91.
520. Jolson HM, Tanner A, Green L, Grasela TH Jr. Adverse reaction reporting of interaction between warfarin and fluoroquinolones. Arch Intern Med 1991;151:1003.
521. Linville D, Emory C, Graves L. Ciprofloxacin and warfarin interaction. Am J Med 1991;90:765.
522. O'Reilly RA, Sahud MA, Robinson AJ. Studies on the interaction of warfarin and clofibrate in man. Thromb Diath Haemorrh 1972;27:309.
523. Chatterjea JB, Salomon L. Antagonistic effect of ACTH and cortisone on the anticoagulant activity of ethyl biscoumacetate. Br Med J 1954;2:790.
524. Hellem AJ, Solem JH. The inflence of ACTH on prothrombin-proconvertin values in blood during treatment with dicumarol and phenylindanedione. Acta Med Scand 1954;150:389.
525. O'Donnell D. Antibiotic-induced potentiation of oral anticoagulant agents. Med J Aust 1989;150:163.
526. O'Reilly RA, Motley CH. Racemic warfarin and trimethoprim-sulfamethoxazole interaction in humans. Ann Intern Med 1979;91:34.
527. Tashima CK. Cyclophosphamide effect on coumarin anticoagulation. South Med J 1979;72:633.
528. Snyder DS. Interaction between cyclosporin and warfarin. Ann Intern Med 1988;108:311.
529. Meeks ML, Mahaffey KW, Katz MD. Danazol increases the anticoagulant effect of warfarin. Ann Pharmacother 1992;26:641.
530. Breckenridge A, Orme ML, Throgeirsson S et al. Drug interactions with warfarin: studies with dichloralphenazone, chloral hydrate and phenazone (antipyrine). Clin Sci 1971,40:351.
531. Serlin MJ, Mossman S, Sibeon RG et al. Interaction between diflunisal and warfarin. Clin Pharmacol Ther 1980;27:493.
532. O'Reilly RA. Interaction of sodium warfarin and disulfiram (Antabuse) in man. Ann Intern Med 1973;78:73.
533. Bartle WR. Possible warfarin-erythromycin interaction (Letter to Editor). Arch Intern Med 1980;140:985.
534. Bachmann K, Schwartz JI, Forney R et al. The effect of erythromycin on the disposition kinetics of warfarin. Pharmacology 1984;28:171.
535. Johansson SA. Apparent resistance to oral anticoagulant therapy and influence of hypnotics on some coagulation factors. Acta Med Scand 1968;184:297.
536. Petrick RJ, Kronacher N, Alcena V. Interaction between warfarin and ethacrynic acid. J Am Med Assoc 1975;231:843.
537. Chierichetti S, Bianchi G, Cerri B. Comparison of feprazone and phenylbutazone interaction with warfarin in man. Curr Ther Res 1975;18:568.
538. Lewis RJ, Trager WF, Chan KK et al. Warfarin: stereochemical aspects of its metabolism and the interaction with phenylbutazone. J Clin Invest 1974;53:1607.288.
539. O'Reilly RA, Goulart DA. Comparative interaction of sulfinpyrazone and phenylbutazone with racemic warfarin: alteration in vivo of free fraction of plasma warfarin. J Pharmacol Exp Ther 1981;219:691.
540. Boeijinga JK, Van de Broeke RN, Jochemsen R et al. De invloed van floctafenine (Idalon) op antistollingsbehandeling met coumarinderivaten. Ned Tijdschr Geneeskd 1981;125:1931.
541. Seaton TL, Celum CL, Black DJ. Possible potentiation of warfarin by fluconazole. Drug Intell Clin Pharm 1990; 24:1177.
542. Bacewicz AM, Menke JJ, Bokar JA, Baud EB. Fluconazole-warfarin interaction. Ann Pharmacother 1994; 28:1111.
543. Gericke KR. Possible interaction between warfarin and fluconazole. Pharmacotherapy 1993;13:508.
544. Rowe H, Carmichael R, Lemberger L. The effect of fluoxetine on warfarin metabolism in the rat and man. Life Sci 1978;23:807.
545. Marbet GA, Ducker GF, Walter M et al. Interaction study between phenprocoumon and flurbiprofen. Curr Med Res Opin 1977;5:26.
546. Stricker BHCh, Delhez JL. Interaction between flurbiprofen and coumarins (Letter to Editor). Br Med J 1982;285:812.
547. Boeijinga JK, Van der Vijgh WJF. Double blind study of the effect of glafenine (Glifanan) on oral anticoagulant therapy with phenprocoumon (Marcoumar). Eur J Clin Pharmacol 1977;12:291.

548. Koch-Weser J. Potentiation by glucagon of the hypoprothrombinemic action of warfarin. Ann Intern Med 1970;72:331.
549. MacDonald MG, Robinson DS, Sylwester D et al. The effects of phenobarbital, chloral betaine, and glutethimide administration on warfarin plasma levels and hypoprothrombinemic responses in man. Clin Pharmacol Ther 1969;10:80.
550. Cullen SI, Catalano PM. Griseofulvin-warfarin antagonism. J Am Med Assoc 1967;199:582.
551. McMahon FG, Jain A, Ryan JR et al. Some effects of MK-185 on lipid and uric acid metabolism in man (Abstract). Univ Mich Med Cent J 1970;36:247.
552. Oakley DP, Lautch H. Haloperidol and anticoagulant treatment (Letter to Editor). Lancet 1963;ii:1231.
553. Rosenthal AR, Self TH, Baker ED et al. Interaction of isoniazid and warfarin. J Am Med Assoc 1977;238:2177.
554. Yeh J, Soo SC, Summerton C, Richardson C. Potentiation of action of warfarin by itraconazole. Br Med J 1990;301:669.
555. Smith AG. Potentiation of oral anticoagulants by ketoconazole. Br Med J 1984;288:188.
556. Ahmad S. Lovastatin warfarin interaction. Arch Intern Med 1990;150:2407.
557. Holmes EL. Pharmacology of the fenamates. IV. Toleration by normal human subjects. Ann Phys Med 1966; 9(Suppl):36.
558. Spiers ASD, Mibashan RS. Increased warfarin requirement during mercaptopurine therapy: a new drug interaction (Letter to Editor). Lancet 1974;ii:221.
559. Yip ASB, Chow WH, Tai YT, Cheung KL. Adverse effect of topical methylsalicylate ointment on warfarin anticoagulation: an unrecognized potential hazard. Postgrad Med J 1990;66:367.
560. O'Reilly RA. The stereoselective interaction of warfarin and metronidazole in man. N Engl J Med 1976;295:354.
561. Watson PG, Lochan RG, Redding VJ. Drug interaction with coumarin derivative anticoagulants (Letter to Editor). Br Med J 1982;285:1045.
562. Colquhoun MC, Daly M, Stewart P, Beeley L. Interaction between warfarin and miconazole oral gel. Lancet 1987;i:695.
563. Marotel C, Cerisay D, Vasseur P et al. Potentialisation des effets de l'acénocoumarol par le gel buccal de miconazole. Presse Méd 1986;15:1684.
564. Qureshi GD, Reinders TP, Evans HJ. Warfarin resistance with nafcillin therapy. Ann Intern Med 1984;100:527.
565. Hoffbrand BI. Interaction of nalidixic acid and warfarin (Letter to Editor). Br Med J 1974;2:66.
566. Lee M, Schwartz RN, Shafiri R. Warfarin resistance and vitamin K (Letter to Editor). Ann Intern Med 1981;94:140.
567. Baciewicz AM, Ashar BH, Locke TW. Interaction of ofloxacin and warfarin. Ann Intern Med 1993;119:1223.
568. Ahmad S. Omeprazole-warfarin interaction. South Med J 1991;84:674.
569. De Teresa E, Vera A, Ortigasa J et al. Interaction between anticoagulants and contraceptives: an unsuspected finding. Br Med J 1979;2:1260.
570. Schrogie JJ, Solomon HM, Zieve PD. Effect of oral contraceptives on vitamin-K dependent clotting activity. Clin Pharmacol Ther 1967;8:670.
571. Baele G, Rasquin K, Barbier F. Effects of oxametacin on coumarin anti-coagulation and on platelet function in humans. Arzneim-Forsch 1983;33:149.
572. Meyboom RHB. Personal communication, 1979.
573. Fox SL. Potentiation of anticoagulants caused by pyrazole compounds. J Am Med Assoc 1964;188:320.
574. Antlitz AM, Mead JA, Tolentino MA. Potentiation of oral anticoagulant therapy by acetaminophen. Curr Ther Res 1968;10:501.
575. Aggeler PM, O'Reilly RA, Leong L et al. Potentiation of anticoagulant effect of warfarin by phenylbutazone. N Engl J Med 1967;276:496.
576. Carter SA. Potentiation of the effect of orally administered anticoagulants by phenyramidol hydrochloride (Analexin). N Engl J Med 1965;273:423.
577. Solomon HM, Schrogie JJ. The effect of phenyramidol on the metabolism of bishydroxycoumarin. J Pharmacol Exp Ther 1966;154:660.
578. Mølholm Hansen, J, Siersbaek-Nielsen K, Kristensen M et al. Effect of diphenylhydantoin on the metabolism of dicoumarol in man. Acta Med Scand 1971;189:15.
579. Nappi JM. Warfarin and phenytoin interaction (Letter to Editor). Ann Intern Med 1979;90:852.
580. Pan HYM, Ng RP. the effect of nootropil in a patient on warfarin. Eur J Clin Pharmacol 1983;24:711.
581 Rhodes RS, Rhodes PJ, Klein C et al. A warfarin piroxicam drug interaction. Drug Intell Clin Pharm 1985;19:556.
582. Koch-Weser J. Quinidine-induced hypoprothrombinemic hemorrhage in patients on chronic warfarin therapy. Ann Intern Med 1968;68:511.
583. Baciewicz AM, Morgan PJ. Ranitidine-warfarin interaction (Letter to Editor). Ann Intern Med 1990;112:76.
584. Michot F, Bürgi M, Büttiger J. Rimactan (Rifampizin) und Antikoagulantientherapie. Schweiz Med Wochenschr 1970;100:583.
585. O'Reilly RA. Interaction of sodium warfarin and rifampin—studies in man. Ann Intern Med 1974;81:337.
586. O'Reilly RA. Spironolactone and warfarin interaction. Clin Pharmacol Ther 1980;27:198.
587. Braverman SE, Marino MT. Sucrafalte-warfarin interaction. Drug Intell Clin Pharm 1988;22:913.
588. Mungall D, Talbert RL, Phillips C et al. Sucralfate and warfarin. Ann Intern Med 1983;98:557.
589. Michot F, Holt NF, Fontanilles F. Über die Beeinflussung der gerinnungshemmenden Wirkung von Acenocoumarol durch Sulfinpyrazon. Schweiz Med Wochenschr 1981; 111:255.
590. Nenci GG, Agnelli G, Berrettini M. Biphasic sulfinpyrazone-warfarin interaction. Br Med J 1981;282:1361.
591. O'Reilly RA. Phenylbutazone and sulfinpyrazone interaction with oral anticoagulant phenprocoumon. Arch Intern Med 1982;142:1634.
592. Toon S, Low LK, Gibaldi M et al. The warfarin-sulfinpyrazone interaction: stereochemical considerations. Clin Pharmacol Ther 1986;39:15.
593. Walter E, Staiger Ch, De vries J et al. Induction of drug metabolizing enzymes by sulfinpyrazone. Eur J Clin Pharmacol 1981;19:353.
594. Self TH, Evans W, Ferguson T. Interaction of sulfisoxazole and warfarin (Letter to Editor). Circulation 1975; 52:528.
595. Sioris LJ, Weibert RT, Pentel PR. Potentiation of warfarin anticoagulation by sulfisoxazole. Arch Intern Med 1980;140:546.
596. Carter SA. Potential effect of sulindac on response of prothrombin-time to oral anticoagulants (Letter to Editor). Lancet 1979;ii:698.
597. Loftin JP, Vesell ES. Interaction between sulindac and

warfarin: different results in normal subjects and in an unusual patient with a potassium-losing renal tubular defect. J Clin Pharmacol 1979;19:733.
598. Lodwick R, McConkey B, Brown AM, Beeley L. Life threatening interaction between tamoxifen and warfarin (Letter to Editor). Br Med J 1987;295:1141.
599. Tenni P, Lalich DL, Byrne MJ. Life threatening interaction between tamoxifen and warfarin. Br Med J 1989;298:93.
600. Gustovic P, Baldin B, Tricoire MJ et al. Life threatening interaction between tamoxifen and acenocoumarol (in French). Thérapie 1994;49:55.
601. Owens JC, Neely WB, Owen WR. Effect of sodium dextrothyroxine in patients receiving anticoagulants. N Engl J Med 1962;266:76.
602. Detilleux M, Caquet R, Laroche C. Potentialisation de l'effet des anticoagulants coumariniques par un nouveau diurétique, l'acide tiénilique. Nouv Presse Méd 1976;5:2395.
603. Spigest O. Reduced effect of warfarin caused by ubidecarenone. Lancet 1994;344:1372.
604. Corrigan JJ, Marcus FI. Coagulopathy associated with vitamin E ingestion. J Am Med Assoc 1974;230:1300.
605. Mølholm Hansen, J, Kristensen M, Skovsted L et al. Dicoumarol-induced diphenylhydantoin intoxication. Lancet 1966;ii:265.
606. Solomon HM, Schrogie JJ. Effect of phenyramidol and bishydroxycoumarin on the metabolism of tolbutamide in human subjects. Metabolism 1967;16:1029.
607. Antmann EM. Hirudin in acute myocardial infarction. Safety report from the thrombolysis and thrombin inhibition in myocardial infarction (TIMI) 9A trial. Circulation 1994;90:1624.
608. Neuhaus KL, von Essen L, Tebbe U et al. Safety from the pilot phase of randomized r-Hirudin for improvement of thrombolysis (HIT III) study. Circulation 1994;90:1638.
609. GUSTO IIa Investigator (The). Randomized trial of intravenous heparin versus recombinant hirudin for acute coronary syndromes. Circulation 1994;90:1631.
610. Irani MS, White HJ Jr, Sexon RG. Reversal of hirudin-induced bleeding diathesis by prothrombin complex concentrate. Am J Cardiol 1995;75:422.
611. Jalihal S, Morris GK. Antistreptokinase titres after intavenous streptokinase. Lancet 1990;i:184.
612. Cross DB. Should streptokinase be readministred? Insights for recent studies of antistreptokinase antibodies. Med J Aust 1994;161:100.
613. Jolliet P, Magnin C, Unger PF. Pulmonary embolectomy after intravenous thrombolysis with alteplase (Letter to Editor). Lancet 1990;335:290.
614. Lew AS, Laramee P, Cercek B et al. The hypotensive effect of intravenous streptokinase in patients with acute myocardial infarction. Circulation 1985;72:1231.
615. Been M, de Bono DP, Muir et al. Clinical effects and kinetic properties of intravenous APSAC—anisoylated plasminogen-streptokinase activator complex (BRL26 921) in acute myocardial infarction. Int J Cardiol 1986;11:53.
616. Madar G, Duckert F, Widmer LK. Thrombolyse ou héparine dans la thrombose veineuse profonde. Gaz Méd Fr 1975;82:4113.
617. Salmon J. Les thrombolytiques dans le traitement des oblitérations artérielles aiguës. Gaz Méd Fr 1975;82:4135.
618. Grimm W, Schwieder G, Wagner T. Fatal pulmonary embolism from deep leg-pelvis veins during thrombolytic treatment (in German). Dtsch Med Wochenschr 1990; 115:1183.
619. Abassade P, Iung B, Baudouy PY et al. Embolie rénale bilatérale au cours d'une fibrinolyse par l'activateur tissulaire du plasminogène, chez un patient porteur d'un thrombus ventriculaire gauche. Arch Mal Coeur 1991;84:583.
620. Yasaka M, Yamaguchi T, Yonehara T, Moriyasu H. Recurrent embolization of tissue plasmonigen activator in acute cardioembolic stroke. Angiology 1994;45:481.
621. Zahger D, Weiss T, Anner H, Waksman R. Systemic embolization following thrombolytic therapy for acute myocardial infarction. Chest 1990;97:754.
622. Quenn M, Jay Biem H, Moe G, Sugar L. Development of cholesterol embolization syndrom after intravenous streptokinase for acute myocardial infarction. Am J Cardiol 1990;65:1042.
623. Pirson Y, Honhon B, Cosyns JP, Van Ypersele C. Cholesterol embolism in a renal graft after treatment with streptokinase. Br Med J 1988;296:394.
624. Gupta BK, Spinowitz BS, Charytan C, Wahl SJ. Cholesterol crystal embolization-associated renal failure after therapy with recombinant tissue-type plasminogen activator. Am J Kidney Dis 1993;21:659.
625. Rieben FW, Waldherr R, Oster P et al. Akutes Nierenversagen als Folge diffuser Cholesterinkristall-Embolisation unter Streptokinasetherapie. Dtsch Med Wochenschr 1979; 104:1447.
626. Been M, de Bono DP, Muir AL et al. Coronary thrombolysis with intravenous APSAC. Br Heart J 1985;53:253.
627. Jones CR, Hillis WS, Campbell BC, Fulton WFM. Coronary reperfusion following thrombolytic therapy using BRL 26 921. Haemostasis 1984;14:55.
628. Verstraete M. Thrombolytic therapy in acute myocardial infarction. Circulation 1990:82(Suppl II):II96.
629. Chen MF, Liau CS, Lee VT. Coronary arterial aneurysm after percutaneous transluminal coronary recanalization with streptokinase. Int J Cardiol 1990;28:117.
630. Ancillo P, Duarte J, Cortina JJ et al. Guillain-Barré syndrome after acute myocardial infarction treated with anistreplase. Chest 1994;105:1301.
631. Cicale MJ. Guillain-Barré syndrome after streptokinase therapy (Letter to Editor). South Med J 1987;80:1068.
632. Eden KV. Possible association of Guillain-Barré syndrome with thrombolytic therapy (Letter to Editor). J Am Med Assoc 1983;249:2020.
633. Leaf DA, MacDonald I, Kliks B et al. Streptokinase and the Guillain-Barré syndrome (Letter to Editor). Ann Intern Med 1984;100:617.
634. Mathiesen O, Grunnet N. Haemolysis after intravenous streptokinase. Lancet 1989;i:1016.
635. Vaughan DE, Krishenbaum JM, Loscalzo J. Streptokinase-induced, antibody-mediated platelet aggregation: a potential cause of clot propagation in vivo. J Am Coll Cardiol 1983;11:1343.
636. Harrington RA, Sane DC, Califf RM et al. Clinical importance of thrombocytopenia occuring in the hospital phase after administration of thrombolytic therapy for acute myocardial infarction. J Am Coll Cardiol 1994;23:891.
637. European Urokinase Study Group. Influence of various initial doses of urokinase on coagulation parameters. Thrombos Diathes Haemorrh 1971;Suppl 45:25.
638. Martin M, Schoop W, Zeitler E. Frische arterielle Verschlüsse als Komplikation der Infusionsbehandlung mit Streptokinase. Dtsch Med Wochenschr 1969;94:1240.
639. Blum A, Shohat B. CD-4 lymphopenia induced by streptokinase. Circulation 1995;91:1899.

640. Mager A, Birnbaum Y, Zlotikamien B et al. Streptokinase-induced jaundice in patients with acute myocardiol infarction. Am Heart J 1991;121:1543.
641. Phillips E, Woolfrey S, Cameron E. Streptokinase-induced jaundice. Postgrad Med J 1994;70:55.
642. Polkey MI, Olivier RM, Walker JM. Hepatic dysfunction induced by streptokinase. Am J Gastroenterol 1992; 87:1062.
643. Pavlou H, Pangiotopoulos A, Graham A, Alexoploulos G. Urokinase-induced cyto-hepatolysis in a patient with acute myocardial infarction. Eur Heart J 1995;16:291.
644. More RS, Peacock F. Haematuria and proteinuria after thrombolytic therapy (Letter to Editor). Lancet 1990; 336:1454.
645. Gary MY, Lazarus JH. Iritis after treatment with streptokinase. Br Med J 1994;309:97.
646. Kinshuck D. Bilateral hypopyon and streptokinase. Br Med J 1992;305:1332.
647. Bell WR. Thrombolytic therapy: a comparison between urokinase and streptokinase. Semin Thromb Haemost 1975;2:1.
648. Cooper JP, Quarry DP, Beale DJ, Chappell AG. Life-threatening, localized angio-oedema associated with streptokinase. Postgrad Med J 1994;70:592.
649. Francis CW, Brenner B, Liddy JP, Marder UJ. Angioedema during therapy with recombinant tissue plasminogen activator. Br J Haematol 1991;77:562.
650. Purvis JA, Booth NA, Wilson EM et al. Anaphylactoïd reaction after injection of alteplase. Lancet 1993;341:966.
651. Cooperative Study. Urokinase pulmonary embolism trial. J Am Med Assoc 1970;214:2163.
652. Shaw CED, Easthope RN. Fatal bronchospasm following streptokinase. NZ Med J 1993;106:207.
653. Dickinson RJ, Rosser A. Low back pain associated with streptokinase. Br Med J 1991;302:111.
654. Hannaford P, Kay CR. Back pain and thrombolysis. Br Med J 1992;304:915.
655. Lear J, Tajapakse R, Pohl J. Low back pain associated with streptokinase. Lancet 1992;340:851.
656. Shah M, Taylor RT. Low back pain associated with streptokinase (Letter to Editor). Br Med J 1990;301:1219.
657. Chan NS, White H, Maslowski A et al. Plasmocytosis and renal failure after readministration of streptokinase for threatened myocardial infarction. Br Med J 1988;297:717.
658. Spangen L, Liljeqvist L, Ljungdahl I et al. Temporary changes in the renal function following streptokinase therapy. Acta Med Scand 1976;199:335.
659. Straub PW, Boersma J, Rhyner K et al. Plasmozytose nach thrombolytischer Therapie mit Streptokinase. Schweiz Med Wochenschr 1974;104:1891.
660. Bucknall C, Darley C, Flax J et al. Vasculitis complicating treatment with intravenous anisoylated plasminogen streptokinase activator complex in acute myocardial infarction. Br Heart J 1988;59:9.
661. Gemmill JD, Sandler M, Hills WS et al. Vasculitis complicating treatment with intravenous anisoylated plasminogen streptokinase activator complex in acute myocardial infarction. Br Heart J 1988;60:361.
662. Ong ACM, Handler CE, Walker JM. Hypersensitivity vasculitis complicating intravenous streptokinase therapy in acute myocardial infarction. Int J Cardiol 1988;21:71.
663. Sorber WA, Herbst V. Lymphocytic angiitis following streptokinase therapy. Cutis 1988;42:57.
664. Albert F, Dubourg O, Steg G et al. Maladie sérique après fibrinoyse par streptokinase intraveineuse au cours d'un infarctus du myocarde. Arch Mal Coeur 1988;81:101.
665. Davies KA, Mathieson P, Winearls CG et al. Serum sickness and acute renal failure after streptokinase therapy for myocardial infarction. Clin Exp Immunol 1990;80:83.
666. Noel J, Rosenbaum LH, Gangaharan V et al. Serum sickness-like illness and leukocytoclastic vasculitis following intracoronary arterial streptokinase. Am Heart J 1987; 113:395.
667. Verstraete M, Vermylen J, Donati MB. The effect of streptokinase infusion on chronic arterial occlusions and stenoses. Ann Intern Med 1971;74:377.
668. Argent N, Adam PC. Proteinuria and thrombolytic agents (Letter to Editor). Lancet 1990;335:106.
669. Le SP, Chatterjee K, Wolfe CL. Adult respiratory distred syndrome following thrombolysis treatment with APSAC for acute myocardial infarction. Am Heart J 1992;123:1368.
670. Tio RA, Voorbig RHAM, Endhoven R. Adult respiratory distress syndrome after streptokinase. Am J Cardiol 1992;70:1632.
671. European Collaborative Study. Controlled trial of urokinase in myocardial infarction. Lancet 1975;ii:624.
672. Walter B, Tamm D. Thrombolyse mit Urokinase nach Streptokinase-Anaphylaxie. Med Klin (Münich) 1979; 74:239.
673. Ejaz AA, Aijaz M, Nawab ZM et al. Hemmorhagic bullae as a complication of urokinase therapy for hemodialysis catheter thrombosis. Am J Nephrol 1995;15:178.
674. Six P, Marbet GA, Walter M et al. Nebenwirkungen bei verschiedenen Thrombolysemethoden. In: Neuhaus K (Ed.), Blutgerinnung und Antikoagulation: Aktuelle Probleme für Klinik und Praxis. Stuttgart—New York: Schattauer Verlag, 1976;111.
675. Becker RC, Caputo R, Ball S et al. Hemorrhagic potential of combined diltiazem and recombinant tissue-type plasminogen activator administration. Am Heart J 1993; 126:11.
676. Sallen MK, Efrusy ME, Kniaz JL, Wolfson PM. Streptokinase-induced hepatic dysfunction. Am J Gastroenterol 1983;78:523.
677. Maclennan AC, Ahmad N, Lawrence JR. Activities of aminotransferases after treatment with streptokinase for acute myocardial infarction. Br Med J 1990;301:321.
678. Freimark D, Leor R, Hod D et al. Impaired hepatic function tests after thrombolysis for acute myocardial infarction. Am J Cardiol 1991;67:535.
679. Medical News. Doctors warned on drugs. NY State J Med 1963;63:2430.
680. Arend H. Konakion: severe reactions after i.v. injection. Paper presented at: Workshop on Clinical Toxicology, Basel, 1971.
681. Paccalin J, Texier L, Gauthier Y et al. Lésions érythémato-pigmentées pré-sclérodermiques chez un cirrhotique traité par la vitamine K1. Bull Soc Fr Dermatol Syphyligr 1973;79:490.
682. Rommel A, Saurat JH. Hypodermite fessière sclérodermiforme et injectios de vitamine K1 à la naissance. Ann Pédiatr (Paris) 1982;29:64.
683. Florholmen J, Waldum H, Nordøy A. Cerebral thrombosis in two patients with malabsorption syndrome treated with vitamin K. Br Med J 1980;281:541.
684. Weiler JM, Gellhaus MA, Carter JG et al. A prospective study of the risk of an immediate adverse reaction to protamine sulfate during cardiopulmonary bypass surgery. J Allergy Clin Immunol 1990;85:713.

685. Doolan L, McKenzie I, Krafchek J et al. Protamine sulphate hypersensitivity. Anaesth. Intensive Care 1981; 9:147.
686. Moorthy SS, Pond W, Rowland RG. Severe circulatory shock following protamine (an anaphylactic reaction). Anesth Analg 1980;59:77.
687. Gottschlich GM, Gravlee GP, Georgitis JW. Adverse reactions to protamine sulfate during cardiac surgery in diabetic and non-diabetic patients. Ann Allergy 1988;61:227.
688. Gupta SK, Veith FJ, Ascer E et al. Anaphylactoid reactions to protamine: an often lethal complication in insulin-dependent diabetic patients undergoing vascular surgery. J Vasc Surg 1989;9:342.
689. Weiss ME, Nyhan D, Peng Z et al. Association of protamine IgE and IgG antibodies with life-threatening reactions to intravenous protamine. N Engl J Med 1989;320:886.
690. Vincent GM, Janowski M, Menlove R. Protamine allergy reactions during cardiac catheterization and cardiac surgery: risk in patients taking protamin-insulin preparations. Catheter Cardio Diag 1991;23:164.
691. Caplan SN, Berkman EM. Protamine sulfate and fish allergy (Letter to Editor). N Engl J Med 1976;295:172.
692. Lowenstein D, Zapol WM. Protamine reaction, explosive mediator release, and pulmonary vasoconstriction. J Anesthesiol 1990;73:373.
693. Olinger GN, Becker RM, Bonchek LI. Noncardiogenic pulmonary edema and peripheral vascular collapse following cardiopulmonary bypass: rare protamine reaction? Ann Thor Surg 1978;29:20.
694. Nordström L, Fletcher R, Pavek K. Shock of anaphylactoid type induced by protamine: a continuous cardiorespiratory record. Acta Anaesthesiol Scand 1978;22:195.
695. Samuel T. Antibodies reacting with salmon and human protamines in serum from infertile men and from vasectomized men and monkeys. Clin Exp Immunol 1977;30:181.
696. Pifarré R, Babka R, Sullivan HJ et al. Management of postoperative heparin rebound following cardiopulmonary bypass. J Thorac Cardiovasc Surg 1981;81:378.
697. Frick PG, Brögli H. The mechanism of heparin rebound after extracorporeal circulation for open cardiac surgery. Surgery 1966;59:721.
698. Chassany O, Bacq V, Metman EH et al. Diarrhée chronique sévère au cours d'un traitement par la ticlopidine. Gastroentérol Clin Biol 1989;13:950.
699. Guedon C, Bruna T, Ducrotte P et al. Altered small bowel motility in severe chronic diarrhoea with ticlopidine (in French). Gastroentérol Clin Biol 1989;13:934.
700. Grimm IS, Litynski JJ. Severe cholestasis associated with ticlopidine. Am J Gastroenterol 1994;89:279.
701. Mamamarella A, Paoletti V, Moroni C et al. Ittero colestatico da ticlopidina. Clin Ter 1991;138:45.
702. Sinnott JA, Ligot J, Grow W Jr et al. Prolonged elevation of liver function test associated with ticlopidine induced hepatitis (Abstract). Am J Gastroenterol 1994;89:1751.
703. Ruiz-Valverde P, Zafon C, Segarra A et al. Ticlopidine-induced granulomatous hepatitis. Ann Pharmacother 1995;29:633.
704. Gent M, Blakely JA, Easton JD et al. The Canadian American Ticlopidine Study (CATS) in thromboembolic stroke. Lancet 1989;i:1215.
705. Jarzon L, Bergquist D, Boberg J et al. Prevention of myocardial infarction and strokes in patients with intermittent claudication: effects of ticlopidine. Results from STIMS, the Swedish Ticlopidine Multicentre Study. J Intern Med 1990;227:301.
706. Ellie E, Durrieu C, Besse P et al. Thrombotic thrombocytopenic purpura associated with ticlopidione. Stroke 1992;22:922.
707. Page V, Tardy B, Zeni F et al. Thrombotic thrombocytopenic purpura related to ticlopidine. Lancet 1991;337:774.
708. Silverstein MN, Petitt RM, Solberg LA Jr et al. Anagrelide: a new drug for treating thrombocytosis. N Engl J Med 1988;318:1292.
709. EPIC investigators. Use of a monoclonal antibody directed against the platelet glycoprotein IIb/IIIa receptor in high-risk coronary angioplasty. N Engl J Med 1994;300:956.
710. Topol EJ, Califf RM, Weisman HF et al. Randomised trial of coronary intervention with antibody against platelet IIb/IIIa integrin for reduction of clinical restenosis: results at six months. Lancet 1994;343:881.

Meyler's Side Effects of Drugs, 13th Edition
M.N.G. Dukes, editor

SECTION EDITOR: B. VRHOVAC

A. Castot

35.2 Hemostatic agents

In a limited number of clinical conditions, certain currently available 'hemostatic drugs' have proved to be useful, particularly aminocaproic acid, tranexamic acid, etamsylate and desmopressin. A certain number of other drugs, particularly the extracts of snake venoms, certainly promote coagulation, but in such a manner that one must, with regard to the very limited clinical evidence available, express some reserve as to the efficacy/safety ratio. Many other 'hemostatic agents' have been studied in such an unsatisfactory a manner that neither their efficacy nor their safety has been adequately delineated; some at least are apparently both harmless and useless.

For the group as a whole, one must conclude that wherever there is evidence of adverse reactions this must weigh heavily in deciding whether or not a drug with a doubtful therapeutic value will be used. In SEDA-3 (1979) both the efficacy and safety of these drugs were for this reason reviewed at some length and that discussion remains valid after 17 years. The reader of the present review is referred to that volume for a full discussion of the efficacy/safety balance in this field. In the present brief account, reference is made to mechanisms of hemostatic action only where they might be expected to result in adverse reactions, e.g. thrombosis, and without entering into a discussion of the clinical usefulness of these effects.

Tissue extracts

Numerous tissue extracts, prepared from a variety of animal tissues, including platelets, have been claimed to be hemostatic agents. Each of them has been in vogue for a period of time and only a few have survived to the present. A micellar suspension of at least six phospholipids extracted from animal brains and mixed in fixed proportions is still commercially available in some countries as a hemostatic agent (Thromboplastin, Tachostyptan). This substance accelerates in vitro coagulation, but in certain concentrations only. No adverse reactions involving circulatory or cardiac function could be observed in normal human subjects following intravenous injection of 10 ml, but a fast injection may *decrease the blood pressure* (1^c).

Aminaphthone (aminonaphthone)

This synthetic agent (2-hydroxy-3-methyl-1,4-naphthohydroquinone-2-*p*-aminobenzoate) significantly shortens the bleeding time in normal and heparinized rabbits and mice, and probably also in patients with or without a bleeding defect. No side effects were noted when patients who had initially been involved in an efficacy study of limited duration were treated with aminonaphthone for one additional year (2^c); that study was reported in 1970 and there is deplorably little recent information on the drug, though it is still sold.

Carbazochrome and carbazochrome salicylate

Adrenochrome, an oxidation product of adrenaline, becomes stable when combined with monosemicarbazone (adrenochrome monosemicarbazide). When complexed with sodium salicylate, this substance is much more soluble (carbazochrome salicylate) and is administered as a hypertonic solution which causes a brief, painful stinging sensation when injected intramuscularly. Experiments in animals demonstrate a significant reduction of normal bleeding time when adrenochrome monosemicarbazide is given (3^c). There is older evidence to show that some effects of adrenochrome are inhibited by the action of *antihistamines*.

Carbazochrome does not induce sympathetic stimulation and is remarkably non-toxic.

Etamsylate

Etamsylate is a synthetic water-soluble non-steroidal drug (diethylamine 2,5-dihydroxybenzenesulfate) which was shown many years ago to increase platelet adhesiveness to glass beads, platelet factor 3 availability and platelet factor 4 release, to increase capillary resistance and to reduce the bleeding time in animals, normal subjects and patients with a variety of bleeding disorders. This reduction in blood loss was dose related.

From a clinical point of view, two of three double-blind trials indicated that etamsylate significantly reduces blood loss in primary menorrhagia (4[c]—5[c]) and in women wearing an intrauterine device (IUD) (7[c]), and that it decreases the incidence of periventricular hemorrhage in very-low-birth-weight babies (8[c]). The latter indication was confirmed in two studies (9[c]—10[c]). The clinical benefit in patients without bleeding disorders undergoing dental extraction, adenotonsillectomy or prostatic and proctological surgery is not clearly established and carefully controlled trials are needed to substantiate the manufacturer's claims for its efficacy in these circumstances.

Minor side effects are *indigestion*, *headache* and *vertigo* (11[c]). Slight transient hypotension was occasionally observed (12[c]), and this can be more marked in the elderly after intravenous injection (12[c]). In a retrospective study, severe leucopenia was reported in children receiving etamsylate; however, the causal relationship is not clearly established (13).

5-Hydroxytryptamine creatinine sulfate

2-(5-Hydroxy-3-indolyl) ethylamine creatinine sulfate has been proposed as a hemostatic agent. Platelets are the main carriers of 5-hydroxytryptamine (5-HT), which they possibly sequester when this amine escapes from the entero-chromaffin system. Aggregating platelets release their 5-hydroxytryptamine, and this was considered to be responsible in part for the vasoconstrictor activity in platelets.

Vertigo, *tachycardia* and other *subjective symptoms* of discomfort have been reported in some patients receiving the drug by rapid intravenous injections (14[c]).

Naphthionine

It is known that Congo red can induce thrombophlebitis of the vein into which it is injected. Naphthionine (sodium 4-amino-1-naphthalene-1-sulfonate) is related to Congo red and has been reported to enhance the blood coagulation and to reduce bleeding time slightly. No side effects with naphthionin were reported (15[c], 16[c]).

Naftazone (β-naphthoquinone semicarbazone)

Naftazone is prepared by diazotization of sulfonic acid with β-naphthol and is similar to adrenochrome. Naftazone significantly reduces the normal bleeding time and blood loss in rabbits and dogs. In many ways, this drug resembles adrenochrome, but it may in addition have certain effects at the cellular level. No side effects have been reported. In a multicentric study of the efficacy and tolerance of naftazone in order to compare two dosage schemes, 4% of patients complained transient and moderate nausea and gastric pain (17).

Pectin and related substances

Pectin-like substances have an in vitro inhibitory effect on fibrinolysis. The numerous observations claiming that pectin has a hemostatic effect were based on subjective clinical judgment, which is notoriously unreliable; controlled trials are not available. Judging from the literature, the pectin preparation, Sangostop, has been administered to a large number of patients and all authors stress that the drug is completely non-toxic. Gohrbrandt (18[c]) gave it to more than 400 patients and stressed that no thrombotic complications were seen.

Natural estrogens *(see also Chapter 40.2)*

Equine estrogens A mixture of the sodium salts of sulfate esters of estrogenic substances, principally estrone and equilin, of the type excreted by pregnant mares, are the main constituents of a hemostatic agent recommended for systemic use (Premarin). It has been shown to increase the number and polymerization of acid mucopolysaccharides, which may alter the local gel-sol equilibrium of the ground substance in favour of the gel phase (19[c]). There is no consistent or major change in blood coagulation or fibrinolysis in patients given this substance. Conjugated estrogens have been reported to reduce bleeding in uremic patients (20[c]).

Headache and *nausea* have been recorded after intravenous injections (81[c]) and slow injection is advised to avoid flushing. The evidence of side effects occurring in long-term use (which may include venous thrombosis and endometrial carcinoma) is mainly derived from studies of long-term hormonal therapy and is reviewed in Chapter 40.2.

Estriol disodium succinate This is an ester of a weak natural estrogen. Its mechanism of action is likely to be similar to that of conjugated equine estrogens. The doses given for hemostatic purposes (up to 40 mg daily i.m.) are many times greater than those used for estrogen replacement therapy (2 mg daily or less), and might be expected to result in endometrial stimulation if given for some time. No side effects have been reported during short-term use of this drug.

Extracts of snake venoms

For many years, extracts of snake venoms have been prepared for their coagulatory properties and used as hemostatic agents.

Botropase Botropase (*Bothrops jararaca*) splits only fibrinopeptide A from fibrinogen (des-A-fibrin) and in vivo produces low-grade disseminated intravascular coagulation associated with the formation of soluble fibrin monomer complexes. Moreover, the drug has a thromboplastin-like activity, but the thrombin generated is rapidly neutralized by the efficient antithrombin system present in plasma (22[c]).

Botropase shortens the coagulation time and induces low-grade intravascular coagulation, which may have harmful consequences. Since the benefits and disadvantages of the drug are not known, Botropase cannot be recommended as a general hemostatic agent before appropriate and stringent clinical trials are performed.

Reptilase Reptilase (*Bothrops atrox*) also has a thrombin-like activity and a thromboplastin-like moiety. The effect of reptilase on patients with a bleeding disorder or menorrhagia/metrorrhagia is conjectural until more valid clinical data are assembled.

No major side effects attributable to the drug have been reported in the literature. However, the report of a high mortality rate amongst post-prostatectomy patients with cardiovascular complications who had received Reptilase must be noted (23[c]).

Inhibitors of fibrinolysis

Some of these can be used in adapted doses as an antidote to thrombolytic agents, or as hemostatic agents.

Aminocaproic acid (EACA, 6-aminohexanoic acid) EACA is an inhibitor of plasminogen activation and of plasmin and other proteolytic enzymes. The hemostatic properties of aminocaproic acid are thought to be related to its ability to inhibit plasminogen activators and so preserve fibrin in hemostatic plugs threatened by normal fibrinolytic activity. There are also other possible activities such as inhibition of kinin and C_1-esterase release.

Well-controlled studies on aminocaproic acid performed in a limited number of patients revealed no serious toxicity. Minor unwanted, probably partially allergic, effects include nasal congestion, conjunctival suffusion, nausea, vomiting, diarrhea, maculopapular or morbilliform rashes, and transient hypotension (24[c]).

Rather exceptional side effects have been reported: purpuric rash (25[c]), bullous eruption (26[c]), psychotic reactions (27[c]); and convulsions: a grand mal seizure was reported immediately after intravenous administration of aminocaproic acid (28[c]) in a 60-year-old man treated for bleeding esophageal varices.

That aminocaproic acid can counteract the rare primary and also secondary hyperfibrinolysis could be anticipated; its hemostatic value in bleeding conditions, in which there is no evidence for an increase in systemic fibrinolysis, is surprising but striking. In some instances, local fibrinolysis may be enhanced in some tissues, e.g. endometrium and colon, but this is often difficult to study. *Prolongation of template bleeding time* has been convincingly demonstrated in connection with serious intra- or postoperative bleeding complications (29). The prolongation was shown to be dose-dependent. All 13 patients given doses ≥36 g/day had prolonged bleeding times, which in seven of them exceeded 20 minutes. Seven patients on smaller doses showed no prolongation. In vitro, a dose-dependent inhibition of ADP and collagen-induced platelet aggregation was demonstrated. The abnormalities disappeared within 24—48 hours after discontinuation of the drug.

In low doses, EACA is an important inhibitor of fibrinolysis and it seems effective in patients with hereditary hemorrhagic telangiectasia with epistaxis, gastrointestinal bleeding and moderate anemia (30[c]).

EACA significantly reduces bleeding in patients undergoing cardiopulmonary bypass; a retrospective study shows that prophylactic treatment with EACA decreased blood replacement therapy, and minimized the number of patients who required re-explorations for bleeding after cardiopulmonary bypass surgery (31[R]).

Obstruction of urine flow after aminocaproic acid treatment in hemophiliacs (32—33) and non-hemophiliacs (34[C]) is a warning against its use in urinary tract bleeding, especially when heavy bleeding occurs in the upper part of the tract.

Intrapleural clot formation (35[C]) has also been reported. In patients suffering from a malignant disease in all probability associated with disseminated intravascular coagulation, the development of acute right heart failure (36[C]) and renal failure due to glomerular capillary thrombosis (37[C], 38[C]) during treatment with aminocaproic acid have been reported. Such a coincidence strongly suggests aggravation by the drug or even induction of *thrombotic angiopathy* and caution should therefore be exercised in the administration of antifibrinolytic agents in disseminated intravascular coagulation. Equally suggestive of a thrombogenic effect is the observation of increased mortality due to massive pulmonary embolism in patients with ruptured intracranial aneurisms given aminocaproic acid as part of preoperative management (39[C]). Extracranial thrombotic complications have also been described repeatedly in patients treated conservatively with aminocaproic acid for subarachnoid hemorrhage (40[C], 41[C]). A case of symptomatic subclavian vein thrombosis with rapid resolution after discontinuation of aminocaproic acid has been reported in a patient with promyelocytic leukemia, while heparin treatment was continued (42[C]). However, in a double-blind multicenter study of 515 patients after prostatectomy, the mortality due to pulmonary embolism and myocardial infarction was comparable in the control and the aminocaproic acid-treated groups (43[C]). The risk of thrombosis may be increased in women taking oral contraceptives. In other subjects, there is no firm evidence that aminocaproic acid predisposes to thrombosis, but it certainly maintains existing fibrin deposits. Hypotension and ST-T wave ECG changes were described in a 81-year-old woman with traumatic hyphema, after 3 days of oral treatment with aminocaproic acid, 4 grams every day (44[c]).

Painful *muscle necrosis* with *myoglobinuria* probably due to microvascular thrombosis, incidentally leading to acute renal failure (45[c]), may develop up to several weeks after the institution of high-dose (30 g/day) aminocaproic acid treatment which suggests a cumulative dose-related or time-related effect (46[c]–50[c]).

More recently, myonecrosis developed in a 22-year-old man who presented dark smoky urine, calf tenderness with progressive weakness and difficulty in walking, after 5 weeks of aminocaproic acid treatment for traumatic hematuria: recovery ensued over the next 3 weeks after discontinuing treatment (51[c]).

In a single case, cardiac and hepatic necrosis was seen, but it is uncertain whether the drug was responsible (52[c]).

Aminomethylbenzoic acid The antifibrinolytic properties of aminomethylbenzoic acid (PAMBA) are well known; it is about 3 times more active than ϵ-aminocaproic acid in inhibiting plasminogen activators. A paper from 1966 noted that since aminomethylbenzoic acid has a low toxicity, enough can be administered to maintain the required plasma level needed to give 80% inhibition (53). Again there is a lack of recent reliable data.

Tranexamic acid This is a synthetic amino acid (4-amino-methyl cyclohexane carboxylic acid). It is known that primarily high-affinity lysine-binding sites of plasminogen are involved in its binding to fibrin. Saturation of these binding sites with tranexamic acid displaces plasminogen from the fibrin surface and results in a retardation of fibrinolysis if tissue plasminogen activator is used for activation (54[r], 55[c]). This and other properties are similar to those of ϵ-aminocaproic acid, but tranexamic acid is about 10 times more potent. Its use is indicated in conditions involving increased fibrinolysis with bleeding or an augmented risk of bleeding (56[r]).

The clinical efficacy of tranexamic acid has been convincingly demonstrated in primary or IUD-induced menorrhagia, urinary tract bleeding, bleeding in the lower intestinal tract, prevention of rebleeding during the first 10 days in ruptured intracranial aneurysms, and recurrent epistaxis. The value of fibrinolysis inhibitors in the prevention of bleeding after tooth extraction in patients with hemophilia is now amply documented and routinely used in hemophiliac treatment centers. Excessive bleeding can also be prevented after prostatectomy and adenotonsillectomy (56[r]). Several clinical trials confirmed the efficacy in patients with upper gastrointestinal tract bleeding (57[c], 58[c]) or undergoing coronary revascularization (59): tranexamic acid reduces blood loss and blood transfusion requirement. There is considerable uncertainty as to whether a fibrinolytic inhibitor is helpful in patients with recurrent abruptio placentae or amegakaryocytic thrombocytopenia. Tranexamic acid was found to be effective in the treatment of traumatic hyphema (56[r]). Patients with acute promyelocytic leukemia often develop a bleeding diathesis during cytostatic treatment which can be predicted by a decrease of α_2 antiplasmin to below 30% of normal. Treatment with tranexamic acid was shown to be effective in an open study and also in a double-blind trial (60, 61).

Side effects of tranexamic acid are rare and mainly limited to nausea, diarrhea or abdominal pain (56[r], 62[c], 63[c]–67[c]) and an occasional orthostatic reaction. It is likely that the better safety of tranexamic acid as compared with EACA is due to the lower daily dose required of the former (3–6 grams) than of the latter (18–30 grams). Psychiatric disturbances and restlessness may occur (68[c]). More recently tranexamic acid has been associated with fixed drug eruption (69[c]), and with bullous eruption (70[c]).

However, tranexamic acid appears to have the same thrombogenic effect as aminocaproic acid (71) and may increase the risk of thrombosis and infarction. It has been demonstrated that it may cause or aggravate cerebral ischemia complications when administered for prevention of rebleeding in patients with subarachnoid hemorrhage (72[c], 73[c]); systemic thromboembolic complications have been reported, including mesenteric thrombosis (74[c]), retinal artery occlusion (75[c]), deep vein thrombosis (76[c]), intracranial arterial thrombosis (77[c]–79[c]); a massive pulmonary thromboembolism was reported in a 62-year-old Chinese woman 7 days after treatment with high doses for subarachnoid haemorrhage (80[c]). Central venous stasis retinopathy was observed in two young women after oral treatment for menorrhagia (81[c]).

Although all these reports of thrombotic complications are anecdotal, they warrant prophylactic anticoagulation in patients suffering from angio-edema who have been given surgical treatment (82).

It is well known that extravascular blood clots formed when the inhibitor is in the circulation may be resistant to physiological fibrinolysis, e.g. thrombi in the renal pelvis or bladder in patients with hematuria (83[c]). Acute renal failure has also been described in two patients: in one case the transient episode was observed in a patient treated for diffuse intravascular coagulation (84[c]); the second patient was anuric for 15 days with clots and fibrin deposits in the bladder and ureter after receiving traxenamic acid for severe thrombocytopenia. (85[c]).

Overall, the association between tranexamic acid and thrombosis may be fortuitous and the risk of this potential hazard very rare. Indeed, the adverse reaction follow-up data of the Swedish National Board of Health and Welfare did not find an increase in thromboembolic complications in women with menorrhagia treated with tranexamic acid. During a 9-year period, corresponding to 238 000 women years, 11 thromboembolic complications were reported. This corresponds to an annual incidence of 0.005% which is not higher than the spontaneous incidence of thrombosis in fertile women (see SEDA-14, 312). A retrospective study of 256 patients treated with tranexamic acid for abruptio placentae and bleeding during pregnancy found no evidence for any thrombogenic effect of the drug (86). Moreover a recent clinical study in patients undergoing cardiac surgery does not show any potential increased thrombotic complications (59).

Pregnancy Aminocaproic acid, aminomethylbenzoic acid and tranexamic acid should not be given in the early stages of pregnancy since a teratogenic effect in animals has been reported (87).

Aprotinin This is a well-defined serine protease inhibitor, isolated from bovine lung, and is identical to the basic pancreatic trypsin inhibitor. Its chemical structure is precisely known and its inhibitory effect on plasmin has been extensively studied.

The administration of aprotinin at the start of cardiovascular bypass surgery appears to reduce blood loss and to protect against global myocardial ischemia (88[c], 89[c], 90[r]). When a very high dose, 700 mg, was given intravenously from the start of anesthesia to the end of the operation in patients undergoing repeat open heart surgery through a previous sternotomy, a significant reduction of blood loss was obtained. The patients mean drainage blood loss was reduced by an average of 81%, from 1509 ml in the controls to 286 ml in the patients receiving aprotinin ($p<0.001$). The mean hemoglobin losses were 78 and 8.3 grams, respectively, a reduction of 89% ($p<0.001$). Blood transfusion requirements were 8-fold higher in the control group than in the aprotinin group, seven of whom received only the single unit of their own blood taken before cardiopulmonary bypass (91[c], 92[c]). The mode of action is unclear: it is postulated that this beneficial effect of aprotinin is related to the preservation of two platelet receptors that are removed by plasmin: the von Willebrand glycoprotein Ib receptor required for platelet adhesion and the fibrinogen receptor on platelets required for aggregation (93[r]). Nevertheless, in a retrospective study in patients undergoing deep hypothermic perfusion, with or without circulatory arrest, a greater incidence of bleeding was recorded for the aprotinin-treated patients (94). A combination of aprotinin with tranexamic acid may be effective in preventing or delaying rebleeding after rupture of an intracerebral aneurism; the addition of aprotinin seems to decrease the incidence of delayed cerebral vasospasm and ischemic complications which are sometimes noted when tranexamic acid is used alone (95[c]).

As could be expected, allergic reactions may occur and repeated use carries the risk of anaphylactic reactions (96[c]). The reported incidence of anaphylactic reactions ranged from 0.3 to 0.6%, and approached 5% with prior aprotinin exposure. In some cases, the reaction was IgE mediated (97[c]).

Up to 1980, 32 cases of shock attributed to aprotinin had been reported to the Japanese Ministry of Health and Welfare, the majority concerning patients treated for pancreatitis. Ten case histories of major shock are presented in detail; all of the patients recovered. The risk seems to be higher in patients intermittently treated after a rest period of several days up to 2 months (98). Well documented cases of lethal anaphylaxis have been reported (99).

The incidence of allergic reactions is low. Adverse effects such as erythema, urticaria, bronchospasm, nausea and vomiting, diarrhea, muscle pains, and blood pressure changes, have been reported (100[c], 101[c]). One article describes an allergic pancreatitis caused by the drug (102[c]).

Rare cases of psychotic reactions, delirium, hallucinations and confusion have been reported (103[c]). Delirium, hallucination and disorientation in time and space can, however, also be symptoms of severe pancreatitis, which in the cases in question was the indication for the administration of aprotinin.

Disseminated intravascular coagulation especially in elderly patients may be developed or aggravated (104[c], 105[c]).

Aprotinin has remarkably few recorded side effects when used as a hemostatic agent; three cardiac arrests were recorded in some 2000 patients receiving the drug intravenously following surgery (106[c]). Recently a case of profound hypotension and marked flushing of the skin, in a 3.5-year-old child who underwent cardiac surgery was described, a few minutes after a rapid and high-dose infusion of aprotinin: the mechanism of this adverse hemodynamic effect is unclear (107[c]).

Some anecdotal cases of thrombotic events could indicate that there is some evidence for a potential risk of thrombosis with aprotinin administration but, in all cases, the role of the drug remains unclear (108[c], 109[cr], 110[c]).

Some studies show that aprotinin might be associated with an increased risk of thrombotic graft occlusion and myocardial infarction (111).

In a prospective randomized double-blind study, in patients undergoing cardiac surgery, the use of high-dose aprotinin induces hypercoagulability with elevated thrombin—antithrombin-III complexes, d-dimers and plasminogen, and a decrease of plasminogen activitor inhibitor (112[r]).

However, the use of aprotinin appears to be safe in a recent multicenter placebo-controlled study in a US population of patients undergoing coronary artery bypass grafting (113[r]). Further and larger studies are needed to define more adequately the risk of thromboembolism with aprotinin (114).

Desmopressin

Desmopressin (1-deamino-8-D-arginine vasopressin, desmopressin acetate) is a synthetic analog of the neurohypophyseal nonapeptide arginine vasopressin. It has enhanced antidiuretic potency, markedly diminished pressor activity and a prolonged half-life and duration of action compared to the natural hormone (115[r]). This compound has become the most effective agent available for treatment of central diabetes insipidus. Desmopressin acetate also has significant hematological effects and can raise circulating levels of Factor VIII and Von Willebrand's factor. It is used for non-transfusional treatment of mild and moderate hemophilia (congenital or acquired) Von Willebrand's disease, and in patients with coagulation disorders due to ticlopidine treatment (116[c]—120[c]). Intravenous injection is the most common route. However, nasal spray administration has been proved to be efficient for home treatment of patients with bleeding episodes and can be used prophylactically for minor surgical procedures in patients with mild hemophilia A (121). It also shortens the prolonged skin bleeding time in patients with renal failure (122[c], 123[c]), liver cirrhosis (124, 125), congenital or acquired platelet function defects (126[c]—129[c]), and intake of aspirin (130[c]). The use of desmopressin seems to be of no benefit in patients with adequate hemostasis whose bleeding is not excessive after surgery, but its administration may be a helpful ancillary measure when hemorrhage is a problem in such patients undergoing cardiac surgery (131[c]). Recently, a review of 18 published double-blind, placebo-controlled, randomized clinical trials of desmopressin and blood loss after cardiac surgery showed a significant reduction of blood loss in desmopressin-treated patients, in studies where the blood loss in the placebo groups was equal or over 1180 ml (132).

The side effects of desmopressin include rare instances of headache, abdominal pain and sweating (115[r]), facial flushing after intravenous administration (116[c]—126[c]), and changes in blood pressure: desmopressin acetate is known to lower the mean blood pressure and increase the pulse rate in normal subjects. Two cases of hypotension following cardiovascular bypass have also been reported (133[c]). A first case of marked cyanosis and dyspnea requiring resuscitation was reported in a 23-month-old boy with tetralogy of Fallot who received desmopressin prior to surgery (134[c]). Thrombocytopenia after desmopressin is usually observed in patients with type II-B Von Willebrand disease; a case has been recently reported in a patient with type I platelet discordant Von Willebrand disease (135[c])

Allergic reactions have been described after intranasal administration: these reactions could also be due to the preservative chlorobutanol. Decreased activity can occur in relation to changes in nasal absorption, such as during coryza, or during swimming (nasal washout), or when using oral hypoglycemic agents (115[r]).

A drawback is that desmopressin acetate may induce arterial thrombosis in patients with coronary or cerebral atherosclerosis (136[c]—139[c]), or with vascular risk factors.

Close surveillance of the drug is warranted especially in elderly patients and those with clinical or laboratory evidence of atherosclerosis (140). The mechanism is unclear: Desmopressin acetate stimulates the release of all the multimeric forms of Von Willebrand factor found in normal plasma, and of large forms not normally present in the circulation (141[r]). These abnormal multimers can aggregate platelets during conditions of artificially raised fluid shear stress that resemble those found in partly obstructed atherosclerotic arteries. Concomitant use of antifibrinolytic agents should be avoided (142[r]).

Nine trials evaluating the hemostatic efficacy of desmopressin in reducing blood and transfusion requirements in 763 patients, showed no significant differences between the frequencies of thromboembolism in desmopressin recipients and controls (143[c]). An analysis of 31 clinical trials of desmopressin in patients undergoing cardiac, vascular, orthopedic or other major surgery indicates that desmopressin does not increase the incidence of thrombosis (144[r]). However, a case of myocardial infarction was reported in a blood donor in excellent health, with no risk factors and no signs of vascular disease (145[c]). Recently a case of cerebral infarction, following surgery has been reported in a 7-month-old girl who had congenital nephrotic syndrome (146[c]).

Another potential risk is that of water intoxication with resultant hyponatremia. Fluid intake should be monitored closely to prevent water intoxication with resultant hyponatremia, particularly in children and elderly patients. Rapid decreases in serum sodium concentration may result in seizures. Development of seizures in association with hyponatremia after intravenous administration of desmopressin to promote hemostasis during surgery were described in a 8.5-year-old girl with Von Willebrand disease and in a 13-month-old boy with moderate hemophilia A (147[c]). Although it is a potent antidiuretic, water retention is not a prominent clinical problem; however, a case of pulmonary edema has been reported in a 27-year-old man, following the administration of desmopressin to reduce blood loss during surgery. Fluid balance should be monitored closely during intra- and postoperative periods (148[c]).

REFERENCES

1. Reichel HH, Martini F, Bleichert A. Untersuchungen über die Kreislaufwirkung eines neuen Haemostypticums. Arzneim-Forsch 1953;3:252.
2. Jurgens J. Clinical practice in the bleeding prophylaxis of thrombocytogenic haemorrhagic diatheses using the haemostatic preparation ‘aminophaton’. Quad Coagul 1970;14:1.
3. Klemm WR, Bolton GR. Comparative evaluation of systemic anticoagulants in dogs. Arzneim-Forsch 1967;17:1573.
4. Jaffe G, Wickham A. A double-blind pilot study of Dicynene in the control of menorrhagia. J Int Med Res 1973;1:127.
5. Harrison R, Campbell S. A double-blind trial of ethamsylate (Dicynene) in the treatment of excessive menstrual bleeding in patients with and without intrauterine contraceptive devices. Lancet 1976;ii:283.
6. Kasonde JM, Bonnar J. Effect of ethamsylate and aminocaproic acid on menstrual blood loss in women using intrauterine devices. Br Med J 1975;4:21.
7. Kovács J, Annus J. Effectiveness of ethamsylate in intrauterine-device menorrhagia. Gynecol Obstet Invest 1978;9:161.
8. Morgan MEI, Benson JWT, Cooke RWI. Ethamsylate reduces the incidence of periventricular haemorrhage in very low birth-weight babies. Lancet 1981;ii:830.
9. Harrison RF, Matthews T. Intrapartum ethamsylate. Lancet 1984;ii:296.
10. Benson JW, Drayton MR, Hayward C et al. Multicentre trial of ethamsylate for prevention of periventricular haemorrhage in very low birth weight infants. Lancet 1986;ii:1297.
11. Sevin R, Cuindet JF. Capillary resistance and diabetic retinopathy: the effect of etamsylate (cyclonamine or Dicynone). Ophtalmologica 1968;155:186.
12. Watson B. Transient hypotension following intravenous ethamsylate (Dicynene) (Letter to Editor). Br Med J 1977;1:1472.
13. Ritter L, Schlosser H, Boos J, Heyen P. Einfluss von Etamsylat auf die Blutungsneigung von Kindern mit onkologischen Erkrankungen—Retrospektive Matched-pair-Analyse von 64 Patienten bei Untersuchung von 100 Patienten der Universitätskinderklinik Münster (Effect of etamsylate on hemorrhagic diathesis of children with oncologic diseases—Retrospective matched-pair analysis of 64 patients in a study of 100 patients of the Münster University Pediatric Clinic). Klin Pädiatr 1991;203:296—301.
14. Greco AS. Impiego del solfato dopio di 5-ossitriptamina e creatinina (Antemovis) in soggetti con emostasi normale operati di tonsillectomia. Minerva Otorinolaringol 1957;7:3.
15. Poller L. A study of Naphtionin, a new haemostatic drug. J Clin Pathol 1955;8:331.
16. Poller L, More JRS. A study of Naphtionin in the management of the bleeding defect in patients with thrombocytopenia. J Clin Pathol 1964;17:680.
17. Zicot M. Etude multicentrique de l’efficacité et de la tolérance de la naftazone (Mediaven 10 mg). Comparaison de deux schémas posologiques. Rev Med Liàge 1993;48:224.
18. Gohrbrandt E. The action of pectin as a blood coagulant. Dtsch Med Wochenschr 1936;62:1625.
19. Schiff M, Burn HF. The effect of intravenous oestrogens on ground substance. Arch Otolaryngol 1961;73:44.
20. Lin YK, Kosfeld RE, Marcum SG. Treatment of uraemic bleeding with conjugated oestrogens. Lancet 1984;ii:887.
21. Jacobson P. Spontaneous hemorrhage. Arch Otolaryngol 1954;59:523.
22. De Nicola P, Guccione G, Manara G, Cipolli PL. Manifestazioni emorragiche in pazienti con reperti normali dell’emocoagulazione e dell’emostasi. Minerva Otorinolaryngol 1969;17:183.
23. Durante LJ, Moutsos A, Ambrose RB et al. Prostatectomy bleeding. Ann Surg 1962;156:781.
24. McNicol GP, Fletcher AP, Alkjaersig N et al. The use

of ε-aminocaproic acid, a potent inhibitor of fibrinolytic activity, in the management of postoperative hematuria. J Urol 1961;86:829.
25. Chakrabarti A, Collett KA. Purpuric rash due to ε-aminocaproic acid. Br Med J 1980;2:197.
26. Brooke CP, Spiers EM, Omura EF. Noninflammatory bullae associated with ε-aminocaproic acid infusion. J Am Acad Dermatol 1992;27:880.
27. Wysenbeek AJ, Sell AA, Vardi M et al. Acute delirious state after ε-aminocaproic acid. Lancet 1978;i:221.
28. Rabinovici R, Heyman A, Kluger Y et al. Convulsions induced by aminocaproic acid infusion. Ann Pharmacother 1989;23:780.
29. Glick R, Green D, Ts'ao C et al. High dose epsilon-aminocaproic acid prolongs the bleeding time and increases rebleeding and intraoperative hemorrhage in patients with subarachnoid hemorrhage. Neurosurgery 1981;9:398.
30. Saba HI, Morelli GA, Logrono LA. Brief report: treatment of bleeding in hereditary hemorrhagic telangiectasia with aminocaproic acid. N Engl J Med 1994;330:1789.
31. Jordan D, Delphin E, Rose E. Prophylactic ε-aminocaproic acid (EACA) administration minimizes blood replacement therapy during cardiac surgery. Anesth Analg 1995;80:827.
32. Van Itterbeek H, Vermylen J, Verstraete M. High obstruction of urine flow as complication of treatment with fibrinolysis inhibitors of haematuria. Acta Haematol 1968;39:237.
33. Stark SN, White JG, Langer L et al. ε-Aminocaproic acid therapy as a cause of intrarenal obstruction in haematuria of haemophiliacs. Scand J Haematol 1965;2:99.
34. Goggins JT, Allen TD. Insobluble fibrin clots within the urinary tract as a consequence of ε-aminocaproic acid therapy. J Urol 1972;107:647.
35. McNicol GP. Disordered fibrinolytic activity and its control. Scott Med J 1962;7:266.
36. Johansson SA. Acute right heart failure during treatment with epsilon amino-caproic acid (E-ACA). Acta Med Scand 1967;182:331.
37. Charytan C, Purtilo D. Glomerular capillary thrombosis and acute renal failure after epsilon-amino-caproic acid therapy. N Engl J Med 1969;280:1102.
38. Gralnick HR, Greipp P. Thrombosis with epsilon aminocaproic acid therapy. Am J Clin Pathol 1971;56:151.
39. Jotkowitz S. Epsilon aminocaproic acid and possible pulmornary emboli (Letter to Editor). N Engl J Med 1974;290:861.
40. Tahmouresie A. Venous thrombosis (Letter to Editor). J Neurosurg 1979;51:266.
41. Tubbs RR, Benjamin SP, Dohn DE. Recurrent subarachnoid hemorrhage associated with aminocaproic acid therapy and acute renal artery thrombosis. J Neurosurg 1979;51:94.
42. Schwartz BS, Williams EC, Conlan MG, Mosher DF. Epsilon-amino-caproic acid in the treatment of patients with acute promyelocytic leukemia and acquired alpha-2-plasmin inhibitor deficiency. Ann Int Med 1986;105:873.
43. Vinnicombe J, Shuttleworth KED. Aminocaproic acid in the control of haemorrhage after prostatectomy: safety of aminocaproic acid: a controlled trial. Lancet 1966;i:232.
44. Jennings T, Safran M. Coronary artery disease as a contraindication to the administration of aminocaproic acid. Arch Ophthamol 1987;105:895.
45. Biswas CK, Reid Milligan DA, Agte SD et al. Acute renal failure and myopathy after treatment with aminocaproic acid. Br Med J 1980;2:115.
46. Brodkin HM. Myoglobulinuria following epsilon-aminocaproic acid (EACA) therapy. J Neurosurg 1980;53:690.
47. Frank MM, Sergent JS, Kane MA et al. Epsilon-aminocaproic acid therapy of heditary angioneurotic edema. N Engl J Med 1972;286:808.
48. Korsan-Bengtsen K, Ysander L, Blohme G et al. Extensive muscle necrosis after long-terrn treatment with aminocaproic acid (EACA) in a case of hereditary periodic edema. Acta Med Scand 1969;185:341.
49. Rizza RA, Sclonick S, Conley CL. Myoglobinuria following aminocaproic acid administration. J Am Med Assoc 1976;236:1845.
50. Kennard C, Swash M, Henson RA. Myopathy due to aminocaproic acid. Muscle Nerv 1980;3:202.
51. Johnstone BR, Syme RRA. Myonecrosis complicating epsilon aminocaproic acid treatment of traumatic haematuria. Br J Urol 1987;60:81.
52. Sweeney WM. Aminocaproic acid, an inhibitor of fibrinolysis. Am J Med Sci 1965;249:576.
53. Vogel G. Klinische Erfahrungen mit *p*-Aminomethylbenzoesäure. Z Gesamte Inn Med 1966;21/2:1.
54. Astedt B. Clinical pharmacology of tranexamic acid. Scand J Gastroenterol 1987;137:22.
55. Hoylaerts M, Lijnen HR, Collen D. Studies on the mechanism of the antifibrinolytic action of tranexamic acid. Biochim Biophys Acta 1981;673:75.
56. Verstraete M. Clinical application of inhibitors of fibrinolysis. Drugs 1985;29:236.
57. Staël Von Holstein C, Eriksson SBS, Källén R. Tranexamic acid as an aid to reducing blood transfusion requirements in gastric and duodenal bleeding. Br Med J 1987;294:7.
58. Henry DA, O'Connell DL. Effects of fibrinolytic inhibitors on mortality from upper gastrointestinal haemorrhage. Br Med J 1989;298:1142.
59. Rousou JA, Engelman RM, Flack JE et al. Tranexamic acid significantly reduces blood loss associated with coronary revascularization. Ann Thorac Surg 1995;59:671.
60. Schwartz BS, Williams EC, Conlan MG, Mosher DF. Epsilon aminocaproic acid in the treatment of patients with acute promyelocytic leukemia and acquired alpha 2 plasmin inhibitor deficiency. Ann Int Med 1986;105:873.
61. Avvisati G, Buller HR, Ten Cate JW, Mandelli F. Tranexamic acid for control of haemorrhage in acute promyelocytic leukemia. Lancet 1989;ii:122.
62. Munch EP, Weeke B. Non hereditary angioedema treated with tranexamic acid: a 6-month placebo controlled trial with follow-up 4 years later. Allergy 1985;40:92.
63. Nilsson L, Rybo G. Treatment of menorrhagia with an antifibrinolytic agent, tranexamic acid (AMCA): a double-blind investigation. Acta Obstet Gynecol Scand 1967;46:572.
64. Hedlung PO. Antifibrinolytic therapy with cyklokapron in connection with prostatectomy: a double-blind study. Scand J Urol Nephrol 1969;3:177.
65. Sheffer AL, Austen KF, Rosen FS. Tranexamic acid therapy in hereditary angioneurotic edema. N Engl J Med 1972;287:452.
66. Vermylen J, Verhaegen-Declercq ML, Verstraete M et al. A double blind study of the effect of tranexamic acid in

essential menorrhagia. Thromb Diath Haemorrh 1968;20:583.
67. Weström L, Bengtsson LP. Effect of tranexamic acid (AMCA) in menorrhagia with intrauterine contraceptive devices: a double-blind study. J Reprod Med 1970;5:154.
68. Adams MP, Nibbelink DW, Torner JC, Sahs AL. Antifibrinolytic therapy in patients with aneurysmal subarachnoid hemorrhage. Arch Neurol 1982;38:25.
69. Kavanagh GM, Sansom JE, Harrison P et al. Tranexamic acid (Cyklokapron Rm)-induced fixed-drug eruption. Br J Dermatol 128:229.
70. Carrion-Carrion C, Del Pozzo-Losada J, Gutierrez-Ramos R et al. Bullous eruption induced by tranexamic acid. Ann Pharmacother 1994;28:1305.
71. Swedish Adsverse Drug Reaction Committee. Tranexamic acid—thromboembolism and visual disturbances. Läkartidningen 1980;77:4974.
72. Vermeylen H, Lindsay KW, Murray GD et al. Antifibrinolytic treatment in subarachnoid hemorrhage. N Eng J Med 1984;311:432.
73. Tsementzis SA, Hitchcock ER, Meyer CH. Benefits and risks of antifibrinolytic therapy in the management of ruptured intracranial aneurysms. A double blind placebo controlled study. Acta Neurochir 1990;102:1.
74. Razis PA, Coulson IH, Gould TR, Findley IL. Acquired C1-esterase inhibitor deficiency. Anaesthesia 1986;41:838.
75. Parsons MR, Merritt DR, Ramsay RC. Retinal artery occlusion associated with tranexamic acid therapy. Am J Ophthalmol 1988;105:688.
76. Endo Y, Nishimura S, Miura A. Deep vein thrombosis induced by tranexamic acid in idiopathic thrombocytopenic purpura. J Am Med Assoc 1988;259:3561.
77. Davies D, Howell DA. Tranexamic acid and arterial thrombosis. Lancet 1977;i:49.
78. Agnelli G, Gresele P, Decunto M et al. Tranexamic and intrauterine contraceptive devices, and fatal cerebral arterial thrombosis. Br J Obstet Gynaecol 1982;89:681.
79. Humbert P, Gutknecht J, Mallet H et al. Acide tranexamique et thrombose du sinus londitudinal supérieur. Thérapie 1987;42:65.
80. Woo KS, Tse LKK, Woo LFJ, Vallance-Owen J. Massive pulmonary thromboembolism after tranexamic acid antifibrinolytic therapy. Br J Clin Pract 1989;43:465.
81. Snir M, Axer-Siegel R, Buckman G, Yassur Y. Central venous stasis retinopathy following the use of tranexamic acid. Retina 1990;10:181.
82. McNicol GP, Douglas AS. Epsilon-aminocaproic acid and other inhibitors of fibrinolysis. Br Med Bull 1964;20:233.
83. Gebauer D, Heigel K. Therapeutische Beeinflussung der Hamophilie durch AMCHA. Med Klin 1969;64,:378.
84. Albronda T, Gökemeyer JDM, van Haeften TW. Transient acute renal failure due to tranexamic acid therapy for diffuse intravascular coagulation. Neth J Med 1991;39:127.
85. Fernández Lucas M, Liaño F, Navarro JF et al. Acute renal failure secondary to antifibrinolytic therapy. Nephron 1995;69:478.
86. Lindoff C, Rybo G, Åstedt B. Treatment with tranexamic acid during pregnancy, and the risk of thrombo-embolic complications. Thromb Haemost 1993;70:238.
87. Johnson AJ, Skoza L, Claus E. Observation on epsilon aminocaproic acid. Thromb Diath Haemorrh 1962;7:203.
88. Popov-Cenic S, Urban AE, Noe G. Studies on the cause of bleeding during and after surgery with a heart lung machine in children with cyanotic and acyanotic cardiac defects and their prophylactic treatment. In: McConn, ed. Role of Chemical Mediators in the Pathophysiology of Acute Illness and Injury. New York: Raven Press, 1982;229.
89. Hack G, Kirchhoff PG, Popov-Cenic S et al. Aprotinin bei Operationen am offenen Herzen. Med Welt 1983;34:726.
90. Davis R, Whittington R. Aprotinin: a review of its pharrnacology and therapeutic efficacy in reducing blood loss associated with cardiac surgery. Drugs 1995;49:954.
91. Bidstrup BP, Royston D, Sapsford RN, Taylor KM. Reduction in blood loss and blood use after cardiopulmonary bypass with high dose aprotinin (Trasylol). J Thor Cardiov Surg 1989;97:364.
92. Royston D, Bisdtrup BP, Taylor KM, Sapsford RN. Effect of aprotinin on need for blood tranfusion after repeat open-heart surgery. Lancet 1987;ii:1289.
93. Van Oeveren W, Eijsman L, Roozendaal KJ, Wildevuur CHR. Platelet preservation by aprotinin during cardiopulmonary bypass. Lancet 1989;i:644.
94. Westaby S, Fomi A, Dunning J et al. Aprotinin and bleeding in profoundly hypotherrnic perfusion. Eur J Cardiothorac Surg 1994;8:82.
95. Guidetti B, Spallone A. The role of antifibrinolytic therapy in the preoperative management of recently ruptured intracranial aneurysm. Surg Neurol 1981;15:239.
96. Gregori P. Allergic shock after treatment with protease inhibitors. Med Klin (Munich) 1967;62:1868.
97. Wüthrich B, Schmid P, Schmid ER, Tornic M, Johansson SGO. IgE-mediated anaphylactic reaction to aprotinin during anaesthesia. Lancet 1992;340:173.
98. Japanese Ministry of health and Welfare. Information on adverse reaction to drugs. Jpn Med Gaz 1980;April 20:10.
99. Proud G, Chamberlain J. Anaphylactic reaction to aprotinin. Lancet 1976;ii:48.
100. Editorial. Today's Drugs: Trasylol. Br Med J 1966;2:1580.
101. Körtge P. Die thrombolystische Therapie. Dtsch Med J 1967;18:255.
102. Siegel M, Werner M. Allergische Pankreatitis bei einer Sensibilisierung gegen den Kallikrein-Trypsin-Inaktivator. Dtsch Med Wochenschr 1965;90:1712.
103. Vonk J. Ervaringen met Trasylol bij de behandeling van acute pancreatitis. Ned Tijdschr Geneeskd 1965;109:1510.
104. Saffitz JE, Stahl DJ, Sundt TM, Wareing TH, Kouchoukos NT. Disseminated intravascular coagulation after administration of aprotinin in combination with deep hypothermic circulatory arrest. Am J Cardiol 1993;72:1080.
105. Loeliger EA. Personal Experience, 1972.
106. Matis P. Effect of Trasylol on blood clotting and wound healing. In: Marx R, Imdahl H, Haberland GL, eds. New Aspecls of Trasylol Therapy. Reports on Symposia in Bad Godesberg and in Munich. Stuttgart: Schattauer Verlag, 1967;21.
107. Söhrer H, Bach A, Fleischer F, Lang J. Adverse haemodynamic effects of high-dose aprotinin in a paediatric cardiac surgical patient. Anaesthesia 1990;45:853.
108. Baubillier E, Cherqui D, Dominique C et al. A fatal thrombotic complication during liver transplantation after aprotinin administration. Transplantation 1994;57:1664.
109. Thorpe CM, Murphy WG, Logan M. Use of aprotinin in knee replacement surgery. Br J Anaesth 1994;73:408.
110. Umbrain V, Christiaens F, Camu F. Intraoperative coronary thrombosis: can aprotinin and protamine be incriminated? J Cardiothor Vasc Anaesth 1994;8:198.
111. Van Der Meer J, Hillege HL, Ascoop CAPL et al. Risk

benefit ratio of aprotinin therapy in coronary artery by pass surgery. Circulation 1994;90:1–640.
112. Feindt P, Seyfert V, Volkmer I et al. Is there a phase of hypercoagulability when aprotinin is used in cardiac surgery. Eur J Cardiothorac Surg 1994;8:308.
113. Lemmer JH, Stanford W, Bonney SL et al. Aprotinin by coronary bypass operations. Efficacy, safety and influence on early saphenous vein graft patency. A multicenter randomized, double blind placebo controlled study. J Thorac Cardiovasc Surg 1994;107:543.
114. Underwood HJ, Cooper GJ. Aprotinin and vein graft occlusion after coronary artery bypass. J Thorac Cardiovas Surg 1995;109:1022.
115. Richardson DW, Robinson AG. Desmopressin. Ann lnt Med 1985;103:228.
116. Ockelford PA, Menon NC, Berry EW. Clinical experience with arginine vasopressin (desmopressin acetate) in Von Villebrand's disease and mild haemophilia. NZ Med J 1980;92:375.
117. Gralnick HR, Williams SB, MC Keown LP et al. Desmopressin acetate in type II a Von Villebrand's disease. Blood 1986;67:465.
118. De La Fuente B, Kasper CK, Rickles FR, Hoyer LW. Response of patients with mild and moderate hemophilia A and Von Villebrand's disease to treatment with desmopressin. Ann Intern Med 1985;103:6.
119. Naorose-Abadi SM, Bond LR, Chitolie A, Beavan DH. Desmopressin therapy in patients with acquired factor VIII inhibitors. Lancet 1988;i:366.
120. Calenda E, Papion H, Borg JY et al. Normalisation du temps de saignement, apres administration de desmopressine, chez une femme traitee par ticlopidine. Presse Méd 1988;17:2143.
121. Lethagen S, Ragnarson-Tenvall G. Self treatment with desmopressin intranasal spray in patients with bleeding disorders: effect on bleeding symptoms and socioeconomic factors. Ann Hematol 1993;66:257.
122. Mannucci PM, Remuzzi G, Pusineri F et al. Deamino-8-D-arginine vasopressin shortens the bleeding time in uremia. N Engl J Med 1983;308:8.
123. Watson AJ, Keogh JAB. 1-Deamino-8-D-arginine vasopressin as a therapy for the bleeding diathesis of renal failure. Am J Nephrol 1984;4.
124. Burroughs A, Matthews K, Qadiri M et al. Desmopressin and bleeding time in patients with cirrhosis. Br Med J 1985;291:1377.
125. Mannucci PM, Vicente V, Vianello L et al. Controlled trial of desmopressin (desmopressin acetate) in liver cirrhosis and other conditions associated with a prolonged bleeding time. Blood 1986;67:1148.
126. Kobrinsky N, Gerrard JM, Watson CM et al. Shortening of bleeding time by 1-deamino-8-D-arginine desmopressin in various bleeding disorders. Lancet 1984;ii:1145.
127. Schulman S, Johnsson H, Egberg N, Blomback M. Desmopressin acetate-induced correction of prolonged bleeding time in patients with congenital platelet function defects. Thromb Res 1987;45:165.
128. Mannucci PM. Desmopressin: a non transfusional form of treatment for congenital and acquired bleeding disorders. Blood 1988;72:1449.
129. Di Michele DM, Hathaway WE. Use of Desmopressin acetate in inherited and acquired platelet dysfunction. Am J Hematol 1990;33:39.
130. Chard RB, Kam CA, Nunn GR, Jonhson DC, Meldrum-Hanna W. Use of desmopressin in the management of aspirin-related and intractable haemorrhage after cardiopulmonary bypass. Aust NZ J Surg 1990;60:125.
131. Salzman EW, Weinstein MJ, Weintraub RM et al. Treatment with desmopressin acetate to reduce blood loss after cardiac surgery: a double blind randomized trial. N Eng J Med 1986;314:1402.
132. Cattaneo M, Mannucci PM. Desmopressin and blood loss after cardiac surgery. Lancet 1993;342:812.
133. D'alaumo FS, Johns RA. Hypotension related to desmopressin administration following cardiopulmonary bypass. Anesthesiology 1988;69:962.
134. Israels SJ, Kobrinsky NL. Serious reaction to desmopressin in a child with cyanotic heart disease. N Engl J Med 1989;320:1563.
135. Castaman G, Rodeghiero F, Lattuada A, Mannuci PM. Desmopressin induced thrombocytopenia in type I platelet discordant Von Willebrand disease. Am J Hematol 1993;43:5.
136. Salzman EW, Weinstein M, Weintraub RM et al. Myocardial infarction in a patient with hemophilia treated with Desmopressin acetate. N Engl J Med 1988;318:121.
137. Bond L, Bevan D. Myocardial infarction in a patient with hemophilia treated with desmopressin acetate. N Engl J Med 1988;318:121.
138. O'Brien JR, Green JP, Salmon G et al. Desmopressin and myocardial infarction. Lancet 1989;i:664.
139. Van Dantzig JM, Duren DR, Ten Cate JW. Desmopressin and myocardial infarction. Lancet 1989;i:664.
140. Editorial. Desmopressin and arterial thrombosis. Lancet 1989;i:938.
141. Ruggeri ZM, Mannucci PM, Lombardi R, Federici AD, Zimmerman TS. Multimetric composition of Factor WIII/Von Villebrand Factor following administration of desmopressin acetate: implication for pathophysiology and therapy of Von Villebrand's disease subtypes. Blood 1982;59:1272.
142. Moake JL, Turner NA, Stathopoulos NA et al. Involvement of large plasma Von Villebrand factor (VWF) mullimers and unusually large (UWF) forms derived from endothelial cells in shear stress induced plateled aggregation. J Clin Invest 1986;78:1456.
143. Mannucci PM, Lusher JM. Desmopressin and thrombosis. Lancet 1989;ii:675.
144. Mannuci PM, Carlsson S, Harris AS. Desmopressin, surgery and thrombosis. Thromb Haemost 1994;71:154.
145. McLeod B. Myocardial infarction in a blood donor after administration of desmopressin Lancet 1990;ii:137.
146. Grunwald Z, Cook Sather SD. Intraoperative cerebral infarction after desmopressin administration in infant with end-stage renal disease. Lancet 1995;345:1364.
147. Sheperd LL, Hutchinson RJ, Worden EK, Koopmann CF, Coran A. Hyponatremia and seizures after intravenous administration of desmopressin acetate for surgical hemostasis. J Pediat 1989:144:470.
148. Cone A, Riley R. DDAVP and pulmonary oedema. Anaesth. Intensive Care 1994;22:502.

Meyler's Side Effects of Drugs, 13th Edition
M.N.G. Dukes, editor

SECTION EDITOR: M.N.G. DUKES

M.N.G. Dukes

36 Gastrointestinal drugs

Antacids *(SEDA-16, 417; SEDA-17, 413; SEDA-18, 370)*

ADVERSE REACTION PATTERN (1^R)

General and toxic reactions When given in conventional doses for symptomatic relief, antacids are safe, and adverse effects seldom limit the choice of preparation, except when troublesome diarrhea occurs. Change of bowel habit, usually in the form of mild diarrhea, is common. Other adverse effects usually arise as a direct consequence of ion absorption. They include alkalosis (particularly with large doses of soluble antacids), milk alkali syndrome when calcium is included, and the consequences of absorbing individual ions, particularly sodium but also bismuth and aluminium. Antacids can also interfere with the absorption of other drugs to a clinically important extent.

Hypersensitivity reactions These have not been described.

Tumor-inducing effects These have not been described.

ORGANS AND SYSTEMS

Cardiovascular *Circulatory collapse* could occur as a symptom of severe hypermagnesemia if magnesium-containing products are taken in large amounts in high-risk patients; heart failure can be precipitated in susceptible patients by antacids with a high sodium content (see below).

Respiratory *Respiratory paralysis* is a terminal event in severe hypermagnesemia (see below).

Nervous system Aluminium and bismuth can cause *encephalopathies*; these are dealt with primarily in Chapter 22.

Endocrine, metabolic Some antacids contain enough sugar to derange diabetic control. Since the sugar is not an active component, it will not be declared on the packaging in many countries.

Mineral and fluid balance *Milk alkali syndrome and alkalosis* These can occur. Simple alkalosis as a consequence of antacid ingestion is seldom important clinically except where a source of calcium is included, and in the presence of renal insufficiency when milk alkali syndrome can be induced. This presents acutely with headache, nausea, irritability, and weakness, or chronically with azotemia, alkalosis and hypercalcemia.

Absorption of individual ions For certain problems relating to the absorption of metallic ions, the reader is referred to Chapter 22 (Metals).

Aluminium Aluminium *encephalopathy*, and sometimes death, can be associated with high blood aluminium levels and has been well documented in patients with renal insufficiency taking large amounts of phosphate-binding aluminium gels. Aluminium absorption resulting in raised blood levels has been detected in babies given 'Infant Gaviscon' (which is based on aluminium alginate and is not in fact recommended by the manufacturer in the very young) and in adults given aluminium sucrose sulfate, though without apparent ill-effect. Aluminium absorbed into the system is excreted in the bile, with no obvious consequences (SEDA-12, 316).

The ability of aluminium gels to bind phosphate can result in clinical significant hypophosphatemia, which usually presents as *myalgia*, *weakness* and *bone pain*, but can have more extreme consequences; one report described *rickets* with *hypercalciuria* after prolonged use, though the subject was an immobilized boy with spastic quadriplegia which can itself have affected the skeleton (2^C).

Bismuth Bismuth encephalopathy, discussed in Chapter 22, is characterized by ataxia, confusion, speech disorder and myoclonus. The subgallate and oxychloride have been implicated, as has the subcitrate when used in a patient with impaired bismuth clearance. The chelate tripotassium dicitratobismuthate, which contains very small amounts of bismuth, appears for the present to be safe in this respect for normal use, as does the occasional use of more traditional bismuth products for conditions such as travellers' diarrhea. Use of bismuth subnitrate ('Roter' tablets) does not seem to lead to metal absorption (3^C), but such absorption does occur from bismuth salicylate (4^C).

Calcium Even small amounts raise serum calcium levels. Calcium ions stimulate antral gastrin release, and hence gastric acid secretion, rendering calcium salts an illogical treatment for acid-peptic disorders (5[C]). Sustained high dosage and/or concurrent renal disease are the classical antecedents of the milk-alkali syndrome (see above). In a pregnant woman, calcium-containing antacids raised the calcium level to a point where hemodialysis was required (SEDA-17, 413).

Sodium The sodium content of antacids varies greatly; a daily dose of some products may contain sodium equivalent to more than 1 gram of salt. As in the case of sugar, this may not be clear from the labeling, and it may not even be obvious from the name of the preparation (e.g. 'Mist mag trisil BPC') yet the amount can be sufficient to *precipitate heart failure* in predisposed individuals. *Absence seizures* have been described during sodium bicarbonate treatment.

Copper deficiency Severe copper deficiency has followed the taking of a gel containing bismuth, aluminium, magnesium and sodium in a patient with pyloric stenosis (6[C]).

Gastrointestinal Magnesium salts, given alone or in combination with other antacids, commonly induce *diarrhea* of osmotic origin; this is often not realized by those who use products such as 'milk of magnesia' long-term in the belief that they are innocuous, and physicians faced with unexplained instances of diarrhea should enquire as to magnesium intake. Aluminium and bismuth can on the other hand *constipate*, and impacted tablets of this type have in some cases even caused *obstruction* (see SEDA-16, 417, also Chapter 22). The belief that calcium salts cause constipation is almost certainly ill-founded.

With sodium bicarbonate, *gastric rupture* due to massive carbon dioxide release has been described, though it is very rare (7[C])

With calcium hydrogen phosphate, *neonatal gastrointestinal obstruction and inspissation* are on record. Alginic acid preparations can cause gastric *bezoars*, as can tube-feed thickening when antacids are added (8[C]).

In low-birthweight infants, use of magnesium-containing antacids has caused *hypermagnesemia* and *intestinal perforation* (SEDA-16, 417).

Bismuth can *darken the feces*, even to the extent of giving a melena-like appearance.

Urinary system Some reviewers have claimed that bismuth can cause reversible *acute renal failure*, but if this indeed occurs it must be excessively rare; it might be part of a nephrotic syndrome. A Japanese patient treated with magnesium silicate developed *urolithiasis*, the stone consisting of 98% silicate (9[Cr]); some 15 cases of silica stones have been reported in Japan but it is not clear how many of these patients had used magnesium silicate. A similar case from Australasia concerned an individual who grossly overused an aluminium and magnesium antacid and presented with *nephrolithiasis* and bilateral *ureteric obstruction* as well as a symptomless hypophosphatemia (SEDA-16, 417).

Skin and appendages A single case of *fixed drug eruption* during magnesium trisilicate treatment has been reported (SEDA-11, 321).

Musculoskeletal *Myalgia* is a common sign of aluminium-induced hypophosphatemia. *Osteomalacia* due to prolonged use of aluminium salts is similarly well described in association with phosphate-binding treatment for renal failure (SEDA-16, 417). It has, however, also been seen with sufficiently high doses of mixed magnesium and aluminium antacids in individuals with normal renal function (10[C]). *Soft tissue calcification* has been reported.

Risk situations For reasons given in the preceding sections, special risks are attached to the use of certain (but not all) antacids in neonates (especially those with a low-birthweight), tube-fed patients, patients with cardiac failure, diabetics and cases of renal disease.

Second-generation effects There appears to be no known adverse effect of antacids on fertility, conception or pregnancy. It would however seem advisable to be cautious with their use during lactation since they could affect the pH of the milk and it would seem unwise to expose the neonate to the trivalent metals with their ability to cause encephalopathy.

Interactions Concurrent antacid intake can reduce the rate of absorption of many other drugs or the peak level obtained, and/or reduce general drug bioavailability. Effects are not always of clinical importance (Table 1).

ANTIEMETICS AND DRUGS AFFECTING GASTROINTESTINAL MOTILITY *(SEDA-16, 418; SEDA-17, 413; SEDA-18, 370)*

The antiemetic drugs form a heterogeneous group and its members have to be viewed individually. The only general warning is that the prescriber should realize how many of these drugs, derived from the metoclopramide example, are in fact members of the neuroleptic family, and therefore capable of producing such effects as parkinsonism and tardive dyskinesias; any antiemetic of that type is likely to be capable of producing any of the effects of antipsychotic drugs, as reviewed

Table 1. *Effects of aluminium-containing antacids on the absorption of other drugs*

Drug	Effect
Of probable or known clinical significance	
Diflunisal	
Digoxin	
Ferrous iron	reduced absorption
Ketoconazole	
Tetracycline	
^{99m}TcPYP	altered distribution*
Quinolone antibiotics	reduced circulating levels (11[r])
Of dubious or unlikely clinical significance	
Aminophylline	absorption retarded
Oral antidiabetic agents	partly adsorbed on antacids
Cimetidine	reduced peak level
Diazepam	absorption retarded but complete
Indomethacin	reduced absorption
Isoniazid	reduced peak level
Levodopa	reduced absorption
Phenothiazines	adsorbed in vitro
Phenytoin	absorption retarded

* Accumulation of the radiopharmaceutical in the liver and reticuloendothelial system (12[c]).

in Chapter 6. The range of antiemetics has now been extended by the $5HT_3$ antagonists.

Alizapride

This is a substituted benzamide and thus neuroleptic related. In one study it was found that in doses which were less effective than normal doses of metoclopramide, alizapride was equally prone to cause *extrapyramidal effects* and indeed more prone to cause *hypotension* (SED-12, 939; SEDA-17, 413). Doses of 5 mg/kg (but not less) were found in another study to cause *diarrhea* as well as orthostatic hypotension (SEDA-9, 311); the incidence of diarrhea may well be higher than with metoclopramide (11[c]). The drug has been found to increase the absorption rate of concurrently administered diazepam (12[C]). Other recorded effects include a sensation of bodily heat and trismus (SEDA-10, 323).

Batanopride

This is again a substituted benzamide; it has 5-HT_3 receptor antagonist activity and is claimed to be free of dopaminergic properties. Clinical studies have concentrated on its use in patients suffering severe vomiting as a result of cytostatic therapy, but have run into problems because of poor tolerance at effective dose levels. The most important dose-limiting side effect has seemed to date to be severe *hypotension* (13[C]) but diarrhea and ECG changes also occur.

Bendectin (Debendox) *(see also Chapter 13)*

This mixture of doxylamine succinate and pyridoxine (at one time combined with dicyclomine) was withdrawn after a campaign had incriminated it of teratogenicity. Used mainly in some Anglo-Saxon countries, it was employed primarily to treat nausea and vomiting during pregnancy in situations in which, in other countries, dietary measures and/or low doses of antihistamines are more customary. No consistent picture of the congenital defects which it was alleged to produce (e.g. pyloric stenosis) ever emerged and reviews in these volumes have never concluded otherwise than that it was at most a low-grade teratogen (SEDA-9, 311) or entirely innocent.

Cannabinoids *(see also Chapter 4)*

Adverse effects appear to be more common with the cannabinoids than with the benzamide antiemetics of the metoclopramide type. *Sedation*, *dry mouth*, *dysphoria*, *incoordination*, and *hypotension* have all been noted. It is unclear if there are material differences in the frequency of such effects as between nabilone, tetrahydrocannabinol or levonantradol. Other effects suggested include *hyperalgesia* at injection sites, and in the case of tetrahydrocannabinol *diminished mixed-function oxidase activity* (SEDA-8, 336).

One member of the group (δ^9-tetrahydrocannabinol, also known as THC or generically as dronabinol) has been officially accepted as an antiemetic drug for use in cancer chemotherapy. With the doses needed for this purpose it seems to be better tolerated in younger patients; older patients are more prone to develop *drowsiness*, *autonomic changes*, *disorientation*, *anxiety*, *depression*, *paranoia*, *visual hallucinations* or even *manic psychosis* (SEDA-11, 32). The adverse effects are usually mild and resolve rapidly on withdrawal of treatment (SEDA-17, 413).

Cisapride

Cisapride is structurally similar to metoclopramide (qv) but has no dopamine receptor blocking activity and hence no central antiemetic effect; since, however, it stimulates the release of acetylcholine in the gastrointestinal tract it is effective in conditions such as reflux esophagitis and gastroparesis. During clinical trials of this compound, suspected adverse effects were limited to *transient gastric pain*, *borborygmi* or *diarrhea*, which are found to occur in some 5% of patients. There can also be mild *headache* or *dizziness*; overviews of field use on a large scale in Germany noted the absence of serious complications, but there was diarrhea in about 2% of cases and headache in 1% (SEDA-18, 370). All the same, there are pointers to a number of organic complications which might easily be overlooked in this type of overview.

Over a 3-year period, the WHO programme for International Drug Monitoring received seven notifications of cases in which *disturbances of cardiac rhythm* (palpitations or extra beats) had occurred; in some cases there was tremor or chest pain. The symptoms resolved on drug withdrawal and there was a positive rechallenge in three of the cases. It is postulated that cisapride may cause tachycardia through a procainamide-like effect (14[CR]).

In some 16% of a series of children treated with cisapride for intestinal pseudo-obstruction, treatment was followed by mild *irritability* and *hyperactivity* (SEDA-18, 370). In one adult, *aggressive behaviour* seemed to be a direct complication of treatment (15[c]).

In one elderly man receiving cisapride, *hepatitis* was seen; it resolved rapidly on drug withdrawal and there was no detectable cause other than the use of cisapride (16[C])

It now seems possible that cisapride can cause functional changes in the *urinary tract* because of increased pressure in the bladder; this may be a problem in individuals with hyperactive bladders. Carone et al. treated a series of individuals who had complete traumatic spinal cord injury, and the increase in reflex bladder contractions was sufficient to reduce compliance markedly (17[c]).

Like other prokinetic agents cisapride can alter the pattern of absorption of *other drugs*; this is seldom important except perhaps where dosage is extremely critical. *Cimetidine* impairs the metabolism of cisapride, but to date this has not been found to be of clinical significance.

Clebopride

Like alizapride, clebopride has *extrapyramidal effects* which were initially overlooked; a warning was issued in 1988 (18[r]). The problem has continued to be reported, the incidence in effective doses probably being as high as 25%; relevant reports include one of a respiratory dyskinesia, which can easily be mistaken for psychogenic hyperventilation (SEDA-17, 414).

At the time of writing the overall efficacy/safety balance of this drug gives rise to concern. In a 1991 report on a crossover trial, a third of the participants had to withdraw because of adverse effects, among which *drowsiness*, *dizziness*, *tremors* and *anxiety* were prominent (19[C]).

Domperidone

This neuroleptic antiemetic has the expected range of *dystonic and extrapyramidal adverse effects* (20[r]) which seem, as with metoclopramide, to be more prone to occur in childhood (21[C]). It is difficult to accept that claims for lower frequencies than with metoclopramide are justified, particularly when one reads a recent report of the drug having induced a *neuroleptic malignant syndrome* (22[C]) Like its congeners, domperidone has repeatedly been shown to induce symptoms attributable to *hyperprolactinemia* (galactorrhea, amenorrhea and breast tenderness) despite claims that there is a lower incidence of effects on prolactin levels.

The intravenous infusion of domperidone, withdrawn some years ago, has caused *convulsions* and *cardiac arrest*.

Metoclopramide

Although this compound has lost some ground to newer congeners, it has been the most widely used of the neuroleptic-type antiemetics and therefore the one with which the clearest picture of adverse effects has emerged, with neuroleptic and endocrine effects occupying the first place. Reactions are generally short-lived provided treatment is stopped; the duration of reactions does not always seem to be explained by simple pharmacokinetic considerations.

The long-term use of metoclopramide should be avoided; it is unfortunate that in many old people with vague gastrointestinal complaints the drug is so readily prescribed over long periods because of failure to appreciate its risks.

Cardiovascular Complete *heart block* (SED-12, 939; 23[c]) and *supraventricular tachycardia* (24[C]), presumably a vagolytic effect, have been described and if there are predisposing conditions heart failure can be precipitated (SEDA-16, 418). *Hypertensive crisis* has been precipitated in patients with pheochromocytoma. *Depressed renal plasma flow* has been noted.

Nervous system *Dyskinesias* of various types (see Chapter 6) are classic; in adult use, *tardive dyskinesia* and *myoclonus* have been described (SEDA-9, 312; SEDA-17, 414); dyskinesias tend to occur after some months of use. As with the classic neuroleptics, *neuroleptic malignant syndrome* can occur with this drug and its congeners (25[Cr]). The '*blue tongue*' sign, in which the tongue is blue, swollen and obstructs the upper airway, is an unusual but dangerous manifestation of the same group of adverse effects (SED-12, 940). Dystonic reactions seem to be particular problems in the very young and the very old, but the frequency is disputed (26[CR]); one overview concluded that acute movement disorders occurred in about one in 80 young adults (SEDA-17, 414). When the drug is used by intravenous injection, e.g. as an aid to gastric emptying imaging, *akathisia* seems to occur mainly in females or young males, and more frequently if the injection is more rapid.

The fact that the neurological reactions can be difficult or impossible to distinguish from spontaneous Parkinsonism perhaps explains those reports which claim that the effects are sometimes irreversible; almost certainly in such cases the disorders were not exclusively due to the drug.

A lengthy *withdrawal reaction* has also been described after 6 months of treatment, characterized by an alternation of an akinesian (rigid) state and a akathisian condition reminiscent of the restlessness seen in parkinsonism (27[C]); even after a year of symptomatic treatment the effects had not fully subsided.

Liver Complex pictures of liver disorders are very occasionally seem, e.g. with *cholestasis* and opening of arteriovenous shunts in the liver (SEDA-16, 419); in two cases a condition resembling *Reye's syndrome* has been seen (28[Cr]).

Respiratory Two cases of acute bronchospasm have been reported after intravenous use, one in a patient with pre-existing asthma (SEDA-16, 419). In view of the drug's pharmacology, this is not unexpected.

Endocrine, metabolic Hyperprolactinemia and galactorrhea, sometimes with gynecomastia, are classic complications (SEDA-9, 312). Vasopressin release has been claimed to be enhanced, while aldosterone release is impaired (SED-12, 940).

Hematological Effects on the blood are very uncommon, but *neutropenia* has been reported in circumstances suggesting that a causal link is likely (SEDA-13, 329). *Methemoglobinemia* has been reported following gross accidental overdosage to an infant (SEDA-15, 392).

Interactions *Anticholinergic drugs* and *narcotic analgesics* can be expected to counter the effects of metoclopramide.

Risk situations Drugs of this type are clearly contraindicated in situations where stimulation of gastrointestinal motility could be dangerous, e.g. where there is hemorrhage, obstruction or a risk of perforation. For obvious reasons, patient with existing dyskinesias should not receive such drugs, and both the very young and the very old have a greater risk of adverse reactions, as do patients with cardiac disorders or asthma. If there is impaired liver function the drug may accumulate.

Withdrawal reactions See above under 'Nervous system'.

Ondansetron (GR-38O32F)
Granisetron
Tropisetron *(SEDA-16, 419; SEDA-17, 415; SEDA-18, 370; 29[R])*

These $5HT_3$-antagonists are effective antiemetics used in treating cytotoxic-induced vomiting. They have gained ground rapidly but long-term experience is still limited. In the doses recommended, ondansetron appears much more effective than the benzamide antiemetics; at those doses, adverse reactions which are being reported—with provisional estimates of incidence—include mild *elevation of the transaminases* (up to 17%), slight *headache* (8—42%), transient *diarrhea* (2—5%, which may be followed in longer-term therapy by *constipation*), *dizziness* (5%) and *dry mouth* (5—17%); the incidence of xerostomia seems to be rather higher than with metoclopramide. There is also incidental reference to *anorexia*, *paresthesias*, *constipation* or *abdominal discomfort*, *changes in blood pressure*, *fever*, *facial edema*, *leg cramps*, *hot flushes* and *enlargement of the spleen* (29[C]). One recent trial noted a patient with *syncope*, presumably because of blood pressure changes (SEDA-18, 370).

Both neurological and cardiological complications could in principle occur and monitoring for both is advisable. With ondansetron, several cases of *extrapyramidal reactions* (30[c]) have been noted in recent reviews; in two cases the reaction did not recur after reduction in dosage or a change in the infusion time. Some patients have experienced *electrocardiographic changes* (mainly prolongation of the QT-interval) and episodes of *angina*. *Thrombocytopenia* has been observed but could have been coincidental.

Some data from a single trial suggest that ondansetron might enhance the nephrotoxicity of the cytostatic drug zenoplatin (SEDA-17, 415); this possibility demands further study.

To date, granisetron appears to have the same safety profile as ondansetron (31[R]); too little is known of tropisetron to draw firm conclusions (SEDA-17, 416; SEDA-18, 371).

INTERACTIONS OF ANTIEMETIC DRUGS

Drugs which affect the rate of gastric emptying are known to affect the absorption of other drugs from the stomach or intestine. Metoclopramide (and no doubt all related drugs) can, by accelerating gastric emptying, cause more rapid absorption of *alcohol* and *paracetamol*. It has been suggested that it raises the bioavailability of *ciclosporin* (SED-12, 940). On the other hand, it has been found to lower the blood levels attained after giving *theophylline*.

Concern about interference with absorption is clearly justified where a drug with a narrow efficacy/toxicity margin is given concurrently. When *digoxin* is given in a slowly dissolving form, the blood levels attained may be reduced by a third if metoclopramide is given at the same time (32[C]); liquid or readily dissoluble solid forms of digoxin (which are currently most commonly used) are unlikely to be affected. Also potentially important in cardiac patients is the ability of metoclopramide to raise the serum levels of *quinidine* by up to 20% (33[C]).

Depressed renal plasma flow has been noted, suggesting that concurrent metoclopramide use could increase the nephrotoxicity of *cisplatin* (34[C]), an important observation in view of the specific usefulness of these antiemetics during cisplatin treatment.

Alongside such effects one should bear in mind that if one of the neuroleptic-type antiemetics is given to a patient who is also being treated with a *neuroleptic* for antipsychotic purposes, there could well be an additive adverse effect, notably as regards induction of dyskinesias.

ANTI-ULCER AGENTS

HISTAMINE H_2-ANTAGONISTS *(SEDA-16, 420; SEDA-17, 371)*

The overall safety record of the currently marketed agents, particularly cimetidine and ranitidine, which have extensive world-wide use, is excellent, and in clinical practice safety issues seldom affect drug choice (35[R]), except perhaps where it is necessary to avoid interactions with phenytoin, theophylline and warfarin. Surveillance studies which have been going on for a quarter of a century (including 10-year studies in many patients, mainly involving cimetidine and ranitidine), have failed to detect any serious adverse effects other than those recognized by 1980 or any adverse effect on mortality (36[C]).

Cimetidine *(SEDA-16, 422; SEDA-17, 417; SEDA-18, 371)*

ADVERSE REACTION PATTERN

General and toxic reactions The main varieties of side effects described relate to the anti-androgenic properties of cimetidine and its action in sufficient concentrations on the central nervous system. There is also a spectrum of drug interactions, mainly attributable to inhibition of hepatic mixed-function oxidase, but they only have clinical consequences under special circumstances.

Occasional, generally minor, effects include bradycardia and conduction defects, thrombocytopenia, neutropenia, interstitial nephritis, mild hepatic dysfunction, and headache. Intestinal infection due to loss of the gastric acid barrier also occurs, and myalgia, fever, monoamine oxidase-like interaction and neuropathies have been well documented occasionally.

Hypersensitivity reactions Hypersensitivity reactions such as bronchospasm have rarely been described. Anaphylaxis (with recurrence on rechallenge) is on record, as are asthma and skin effects.

Tumor-inducing effects have been much discussed ever since the introduction of these drugs but their existence has not been established. The discussion was seeded by: (a) findings of 'intestinal metaplasia' of the gastric epithelium in rats used for chronic toxicity studies, though only at extraordinarily high dose levels, followed by the appearance of intramucosal carcinomas in the pyloric region after 11 months of study. (b) Reports to adverse reaction monitoring agencies (and incidentally in the literature) of patients on cimetidine in whom gastric carcinoma was diagnosed. However, the drug has been widely (and sometimes without careful prior diagnosis) used in patients with a range of gastric disorders, and some of these are believed to have had early carcinomas at the time when cimetidine was started (37[C]). (c) The fact that cimetidine can undergo nitrosation to form a mutagen. (d) The structural resemblance of cimetidine to tiotidine, which in animals can induce gastric carcinoma. It is always unwise to conclude categorically that a drug used long-term will *not* prove to be carcinogenic. There is still, in 1996, no valid reason for considering cimetidine, as used in humans, to be tumorigenic, and indeed where cohort studies have detected some excess incidence of gastric cancer in long-term users of cimetidine this seems attributable to selection bias (38[C]). All the same, watchfulness remains necessary; a case discussed in the ranitidine section below suggests that the concerns are not purely theoretical. The fact that drugs of this type have in many countries now been released for self-medication seems very likely to lead to an increase in the incidence of cases in which an H_2-blocker is used without prior exclusion pre-malignant or malignant change, thus confusing the situation further.

ORGANS AND SYSTEMS

Cardiovascular (39[R]) Rapid infusions of cimetidine cause an increase in plasma histamine and this could be one reason for the cardiac effects. A marked degree of *bradycardia* (e.g. a 30% reduction in heart rate) is uncommon though well recognized (SEDA-17, 417); *sinoatrial* and *atrioventricular conduction effects* and *arrhythmias* of every possible type have occasionally been noted, particularly following infusions but also with oral therapy. It has been suggested that if a patient is particularly at risk (e.g. because of poor renal function) the EGG should be monitored (SEDA-15, 394).

Respiratory *Bronchospasm* is occasionally reported, reflecting the possibility of allergy to the drug, and the need for some caution with its initial use in any asthmatic patient (SEDA- 15, 394); in pre-existing atopic asthma, H_2-antagonists may enhance bronchial reactivity (SEDA-16, 421). Central nervous effects can lead to *respiratory depression* (see below), although this is rare.

As noted below, loss of the gastric acid barrier can predispose to intestinal infection, and pulmonary aspiration of infected gastrointestinal secretions can very occasionally cause *pneumonia* after anesthesia or during intensive care (40[C]). *Interstitial lung disease* can occur under these conditions.

Nervous system Cimetidine crosses the blood—brain barrier and can cause *confusion*, particularly in those elderly or sick individuals with compromised hepatic or renal systems, and especially after intravenous treatment; very rarely, an acute confusional psychosis has been seen in a younger person (41[C]). *Delirium* has been thought to be a particular problem with intravenous use, but this is more likely to be a reflection of patient selection. Other postulated, but less well proven, adverse events include central *respiratory depression* (see above), and *extrapyramidal* and *cerebellar disturbances*; isolated reports of *choreiform movements* appear well founded. *Depression* rarely occurs.

Severe central neurological problems are not common; one intensive survey of nearly 10 000 patients followed for 3 months noted only five cases of confusion, though there were 34 with sensations of dizziness, 23 with headache and 74 with other milder central nervous effects (33[C]). The overall incidence of adverse neurological effects reported to the US public health authorities (which naturally represent only a small proportion of those which actually occur) was 8.6 per million prescriptions for cimetidine and virtually the same for ranitidine. Healthy elderly people are probably not at particular risk.

Occasionally, *neuropathies* have been documented (42[C]). The fear that cimetidine or ranitidine might increase the incidence of motor neurone disease was raised in the light of case-control work but seems to have been allayed by data from the Oxford Record Linkage Study published in 1993 (43).

Endocrine, metabolic *Fever* is occasionally noted (44[C]). Mild anti-androgenic properties, which are dose-related, are associated with binding to androgen receptors; *reduced sperm counts* have been reported, as have modestly *raised serum prolactin* levels after intravenous treatment (SEDA-9, 313). Some slight degree of *male breast enlargement* is not uncommon (e.g. in one series of 25 men, five experienced it) (45[Cr]), but it can regress with continued treatment; very rarely can it be massive and unilateral; there is no strict parallel between the effects on the breast and the blood prolactin levels. *Impotence* has been suggested in the light of some case experiences; this type of effect is always difficult to prove but it has been described repeatedly with various H_2-blockers. One well-documented case suggested that in an infant girl reversible *premature puberty* was induced, but it must be noted that domperidone was also being given (SEDA-15, 394); in another instance an 18-month-old infant showed marked enlargement of one breast (SEDA-16, 421—422), but this is probably similar to the effect sometimes seen in adult men (see above) rather than a true endocrine effect. In the earlier years of cimetidine use there were scattered (though well-documented) reports of the drug having destabilized severe *diabetes*, resulting in impaired control; most diabetics are unlikely to be affected.

Modest *increases in serum high-density lipoproteins* have occasionally been noted (SED-12, 942).

Hematological *Thrombocytopenia* has been reported with recurrence on rechallenge, and *neutropenia* has also been documented as an occasional adverse effect, possibly related to experimental inhibition of granulocyte colony growth (SEDA-10, 325); the effects appear to occur with all H_2-antagonists in an incidence roughly proportional to their sales. Exceptionally, thrombocytopenia and leukopenia have occurred together (SEDA-17, 417). There was concern during the first years of cimetidine therapy that the drug might produce severe blood dyscrasias, but most of those that have been described have occurred in patients who were already severely ill or exposed to other toxic influences (SED-12, 942; SEDA-15, 394). In one case of pancytopenia a cimetidine dose-dependent inhibition of normal human CFU-GM colon formation was observed (SEDA-16, 422).

Liver For a drug of this importance it should be noted that no real suspicion of hepatotoxicity has ever been put upon cimetidine. The reports received by large national monitoring centers make occasional references to hepatitis, jaundice, or changes in liver function tests, but these could be coincidental and systematic surveillance appears to point to an absence of risk.

Gastrointestinal An older concern here was the possibility that H_2-blockers could predispose to gastric carcinogenesis (see general section on tumor-inducing effects above); this seems to have been allayed, as was the fear once expressed that ulcers might be more liable to perforate after cimetidine had been given and withdrawn.

Removal of the acid barrier to infection increases the chances of bacterial or *parasitic colonization of the upper gut* and thereby the chances of pulmonary infection from aspirated gastric contents (see ‘Respiratory’ above).

Pancreatitis has several times been suggested as a complication of treatment, but this thesis has remained unconfirmed. *Parotitis* with positive rechallenge has been documented in one case (46^C).

Urinary system Minor rises in serum creatinine levels reflect interference with tubular function; this seems to be clinically unimportant and fully reversible. There were two early reports of reversible acute *renal failure*, one of them with a positive rechallenge and with a biopsy finding of interstitial infiltrates of inflammatory cells (47^C).

Skin and appendages *Xerosis* and *asteatotic dermatitis* are among the rare cutaneous effects which can occur; they may be of anti-androgenic origin (see above). Allergic skin reactions can comprise *urticaria*, *dermatitis*, *erythema multiforme* and various forms of *rash*. A possibly unique case of *alopecia* affecting the entire body was described in 1981; in that case the temporal association was convincing and there was a correlation with an anti-androgenic effect on hormone levels (48). Several cases of *psoriasis* have been precipitated or aggravated by cimetidine; ranitidine has the same rare effect (49^C).

Musculoskeletal A small proportion of patients develop troublesome *myalgia* when treated with cimetidine (50^C). There have been incidental reports of *polymyositis* and a form of *myopathy* probably of motor neuron origin. Myalgia may also be associated with *arthritis* and *joint effusion*, but this is extremely unusual (SED-12, 942).

Interactions The large number of drug interactions described with cimetidine are largely attributable to the binding of the drug to hepatic mixed-function oxidase (and hence to inhibition of drug metabolism) or to cimetidine-induced interference with hepatic or renal clearance of drugs. Cimetidine-induced reduction of hepatic blood flow can, for example, reduce the clearance of *lidocaine* while at the renal level cimetidine interferes slightly with the tubular excretion of *procainamide* and *quinidine*. Both effects are of a modest degree, and the long list of drugs for which interference is demonstrable (Table 2) is out of all proportion to the number for which interference is of clinical significance. In most cases the slowing of the metabolism of other drugs, by a third at most, is only likely to be troublesome for drugs with a narrow margin between the therapeutic and toxic dose, such as *theophylline*, *phenytoin* and *warfarin*; clearance of theophylline may be reduced by up to 22% and the half-life increased by 50% (SEDA-16, 421).

Cimetidine has proven to reduce slightly the rate of metabolism of *alcohol* and to alter its absorption but it is doubtful if these effects are clinically significant. More important is that H_2-antagonists cause a significant reduction in the absorption of *vitamin* B_{12} from food because of the decrease in gastric acid secretion; this can be sufficient to cause vitamin deficiency, notably in

Table 2. *Groups of drugs interacting with cimetidine*

Drug	Effect
Antiarrhythmic agents	
Lidocaine	Toxic levels in normal volunteers
Procainamide	Increased plasma levels
Quinidine	Increased plasma levels
Anticoagulants	
Warfarin	Enhanced activity*
Antidiabetic drugs	
Gliclazide	Increased levels
Anticonvulsants	
Phenytoin	Raised steady-state levels*
Valproate	Toxic levels reached*
Antidepressants	
Imipramine	Retarded metabolism
Anti-inflammatory agents	
Indomethacin	Retarded metabolism
Antimitotic agents	
Fluorouracil	Increased levels
Benzodiazepines	
Diazepam	Increased plasma levels
Nitrazepam	Increased plasma levels
Cardiovascular drugs	
Propranolol	Enhanced activity
Nifedipine	Increased plasma levels
Diltiazem	Increased plasma levels
Verapamil	Increased plasma levels
Diuretics	
Furosemide	Increased area under plasma curve
Immunosuppressant	
Ciclosporin	Increased plasma levels*
Muscle relaxants	
Succinylcholine	Delayed recovery*
Respiratory agents	
Theophylline	Toxic levels reached*

* Effects likely to be of clinical importance are marked by an asterisk.

patients who have low body stores of vitamin B_{12} and are taking an H_2-antagonist over a long period (51[R]).

In some patients MAOI-like interactions (e.g. with tyramine) have been described.

Risk situations The principal situation of increased risk exists in *old age*, since neurological adverse effects are more likely to occur in those elderly persons having *impairment of hepatic or renal function*. It has been suggested that women with *spinal cord injuries* may be at increased risk of the galactorrhea induced by H_2-antagonists, since such injuries themselves can lead to galactorrhea (SEDA-17, 417).

Withdrawal reactions A complex neurobehavioral and gastroenteric withdrawal syndrome has been seen with both cimetidine and ranitidine; characteristics included anxiety, sleeplessness, anorexia with loss of weight, irritability, tachycardia, diarrhea, nausea and vomiting, abdominal pain, headache and vertigo. The syndrome virtually disappeared when the drugs were given again, but reappeared when they were withdrawn once more. The syndrome may be related to a fall in prolactin levels; it reacted well to domperidone (52[C]).

Famotidine

This drug seems to be free of effects upon drug metabolism and it has been claimed to be free of the antiandrogenic effect of cimetidine; however in one woman who accidentally took double doses of the drug for some months it did induce hyperprolactinemia and breast engorgement (SEDA-18, 372). In other ways it bears a very close resemblance to cimetidine, e.g. *headache* and *confusion* with intravenous use are reported; *thrombocytopenia* and *pancytopenia* are also described (SEDA-15, 395). One case of *vasculitis* in a patient who tolerated cimetidine well is on record. A case of acute *rhabdomyolysis* has been documented and might reflect the immunomodulating effect of the drug (SEDA-17, 418). An unusual case of *hyperpyrexia* is on record, but the patient had a pre-existing cerebral trauma as a facilitating factor (SEDA-16, 422).

Although it is impossible to make a direct comparison between famotidine and cimetidine since the former has been used on a much smaller scale, it seems possible at present that the hematological problems occur more frequently with famotidine; one repeatedly encounters well-documented reports of both thrombocytopenia and neutropenia, sometimes severe (SEDA-17, 417).

Nizatidine

Experience with this less widely used drug is still too limited to make valid comparisons with its earlier congeners. Data sheet warnings of possible adverse effects refer to *skin rash*, *urticaria*, *somnolence* and *thrombocytopenia*. The drug is said not to give problems with interactions or to affect the androgen status.

Ranitidine *(SEDA-16, 422; SEDA-17, 418; SEDA-18, 372; 53[R])*

Compared with cimetidine, this drug inhibits hepatic

metabolism of other substances only to a very slight extent and it is not anti-androgenic. In most other respects there are very close similarities to cimetidine; with respect to the central nervous system, occasional *confusion*, *behavioral disturbance* and *chorea* are reliably reported, as is *headache*; *lethargy* has been described in a neonate (SEDA-18, 372); *depression* has been estimated to occur in 1—5% of patients treated (SEDA-17, 418; 54[C]). Where the cardiovascular system is concerned *atrioventricular block* is on record as well as a case of *bradycardia* in an neonate receiving the drug intravenously. *Skin rash* and *vasculitis* can occur and both *pancytopenia* and *agranulocytosis* have been documented. In one case where *pancreatitis* occurred without identifiable cause other than ranitidine, it was confirmed by rechallenge on two occasions (SEDA-16, 422). As with cimetidine, *acute interstitial nephritis* has been documented in a few cases (55[C]). The fact that a fair number of cases of *impotence* have been described strongly suggests that this is an effect which all H_2-blockers can on occasion exert.

There seem to be individuals with a metabolic idiosyncrasy who develop serious but probably fully reversible *liver injury* when exposed to ranitidine; the Netherlands Centre for Monitoring of Adverse Reactions has published data on six cases, in most of which other causal factors could be excluded (56[CR]), and a fatal case of liver injury has been reported from France (SEDA-16, 422).

The prolonged discussion regarding the possibility that H_2-antagonists might induce gastric tumours (see under 'Cimetidine' above) was extended by a 1993 report on a case in which a *gastric carcinoid tumor* was found in a man of 62 taking ranitidine; in this instance the dosage was unusually high and there was pre-existing chronic renal failure as well as diabetes, but the tumor was similar in type to that seen in animals; it was successfully removed by partial gastrectomy and did not recur (57[c]).

The ability of H_2-antagonists to induce respiratory infections has been explained in the above monograph on cimetidine, but the possible significance of this effect has been studied most concretely with ranitidine; there seems to be no reason for concern in most patients, but the risk might be considerable in some older patients with pre-existing health problems rendering them unduly susceptible to infection (SEDA-18, 372).

A clearly identified risk situation is renal impairment, which at least in the case of intravenous use can double the frequency of adverse reactions (SEDA-18, 371). A significant effect on the absorption or metabolism of alcohol has been both boldly claimed and equally firmly denied.

PROTON PUMP INHIBITORS

Omeprazole *(SEDA-16, 422; SEDA-17, 418; SEDA-18, 373)*

Omeprazole is still the only proton pump inhibitor with which widespread experience has been gained; others such as lansoprazole, have followed. This class of compounds is currently being exposed to the same doubts and concerns as those raised with the H_2-blockers when they were first introduced, namely as regards their safety in long-term use. Not surprisingly, there have been controversies between the manufacturers of this type of drug and the H_2-blockers as regards the relative safety of the two types of product. Certainly in shorter-term use omeprazole has a good safety record; no substantial problems have come to the fore as a result of monitoring its side effects since introduction.

ADVERSE REACTION PATTERN

General and toxic reactions Headache, skin rash and diarrhea have all been recorded by adverse event registries sufficiently often to suggest causal relationships (58[R]).

Hypersensitivity reactions Hypersensitivity might underlie the thrombocytopenia which has been incidentally documented.

Tumor-inducing effects (*SEDA*-16, 423) In part repeating the debate on the alleged carcinogenicity of cimetidine is the argument that, with omeprazole, gastric neoplasia may be more prone to occur. In this case, the argument derives in the first instance from studies in rats where carcinoid nodules were detected in the stomach of animals given large doses over prolonged periods. A variety of evidence, however, suggests that these findings were neither specific to the drug nor likely to indicate material risks to man (59[R]), and that other arguments for a tumor-inducing effect are equally unconvincing. Firstly, similar carcinoid change has been detected with other drugs, notably secretory antagonists, and with the fibrates which are antisecretory in rats. Secondly carcinoidogenesis can be inhibited by antrectomy, presumably by removing an antral gastrin drive and it can be enhanced by partial fundectomy, when relative anacidity increases antral gastrin release. Thirdly, although omeprazole treatment can raise serum gastrin levels quite markedly in man, they do so by a level of magnitude less than in pernicious anemia, in which carcinoid tumors are recorded, albeit rarely.

Fourthly, despite close searching, carcinoids have not been detected complicating ordinary ulcer treatment in man. Others have claimed on the basis of tissue work in vitro that omeprazole may itself be a mitogen or mutagen; it has been counter-claimed that the technique used in the studies concerned is inherently unreliable and that other standard techniques have failed to reveal mutagenic potential (SED-12, 943–449). Finally, selective and important actions on a cytochrome which would activate carcinogens have been claimed, but seem unlikely experimentally. This is one of the situations in which there is inherent difficulty in disproving a postulate relationship. Currently, however, it seems very unlikely that appreciable risk exists.

ORGANS AND SYSTEMS

Gastrointestinal Moderate *nausea*, *diarrhea* or *abdominal pain* can occur. There is an increased incidence of the severe interstitial and atrophic forms of *gastritis*, associated with moderate hypergastrinemia and hyperplasia of the argyrophil cells (60[C]). This is not necessarily a side effect—it could represent the natural history of chronic gastritis associated with peptic ulcer disease.

Gastric *polyps* have been observed in a number of patients, but they disappear spontaneously during follow-up (SEDA-18, 373). It may be noted that most or all patients taking omeprazole exhibit a non-pathological 'pseudohypertrophy' of the parietal cells.

The possibility that, as with H_2-blockers, the achlorhydria resulting from use of this drug will raise the risk of gastrointestinal infection (leading perhaps to respiratory infection) has been advanced both on theoretical grounds and in the light of a number of cases, including one of esophageal candidiasis (SED-12, 944; 61[c], 62[c]).

Endocrine, metabolic There have been occasional reports of *gynecomastia*, regressing after drug withdrawal, and a single report of *painful erections* after each dose in an elderly man (SEDA-17, 419). In patients with Zollinger-Ellison syndrome, omeprazole causes significant weight gain, perhaps because of shifts in the hormonal balance (SEDA-17, 419; 63[Cr]).

Mineral and fluid balance *Hyponatremia* has been described in an elderly alcoholic patient taking omeprazole (SEDA-17, 419).

Hematological There is a documented case of *thrombocytopenia* in a male adult with a history of chronic alcoholism; the blood disorder appeared on the fourth day of treatment and receded after drug withdrawal (64[c]). To date there is also a single report of severe hemolytic anemia, with recovery following withdrawal of omeprazole (SEDA-17, 419).

Skin and appendages A case of *angio-edema* and *urticaria* triggered by omeprazole, but not by the enteric granules devoid of the capsule shell, has been described (SEDA-18, 373).

Interactions Omeprazole is a modest inhibitor of mixed-function oxidase. Interactions, however, are less likely than with cimetidine and probably of no practical importance even when drugs like phenytoin are co-administered. One effect claimed has been that, in the acid-free stomach, a differing and shorter-acting pattern of metabolites of *digoxin* is produced, which could clinically change that drug's duration of action (65[C]).

Omeprazole appears to increase the blood level of *ciclosporin* substantially (SEDA-17, 420). However it will reduce the absorption of those drugs demanding a low gastric pH (*ketoconazole*, *iron salts*, *ampicillin*) and may decrease the hepatic clearance of drugs (*diazepam*, *warfarin*, *phenytoin*)

Risk situations In the light of one case of a *Yersinia entercolitica* septicemia it seems just possible that in a patient on *heavy oral iron supplementation* the intraluminal iron together with the raised intestinal pH resulting from the use of omeprazole may contribute to the enhanced proliferation and dissemination of this organism (66[C])

Lansoprazole

One of the first papers to provide an overview of the safety profile of this drug is based on the pre-marketing clinical work, and has to be regarded with the reservations appropriate to this type of material. In a total of 4749 patients the most frequent adverse effects reported were headache (4.7%), diarrhea (3.2%), abdominal pain (2.2%), pharyngitis (1.8%) and nausea (1.4%); some patients had upper respiratory complaints or suffered anxiety or depression, or myalgia (67[R]). For the moment it would be wise to assume that in the field the adverse reaction profile will be closer to that of omeprazole.

ANTIMUSCARINICS

Pirenzepine *(SEDA-16, 423)*

It was claimed, when this anticholinergic agent was introduced, that in the doses necessary to affect gastric secretion it would be almost entirely free of other atropine-like effects. The dissociation has not in fact gone as far as one would wish; though such atropine-type side effects as dry mouth and difficulty of accommodation are less common with pirenzepine than with atropine itself, they can still occur in a frequency related to dose and are likely to be present in about half the patients using the drug (68[C]). Cardiac conduction effects resulting in sinus tachycardia, atrial fibrillation and nodal tachycardia can also occur.

Idiosyncratic adverse effects seem limited, but granulocytopenia and thrombocytopenia are on record (SED-12, 944).

Scopolamine *(see also Chapter 13)*

Scopolamine regained some popularity with its introduction in the form of transdermal patches, for use as an antinauseant and antisecretory agent. Use of these forms, however, does not lessen the chance of unwanted atropine-type effects. Serious effects on the nervous system, i.e. confusion, delirium and psychosis are well documented.

Telenzepine *(SEDA-13, 335)*

On a weight-for-weight basis this drug is 25—50 times more potent than pirenzepine, but after a dosage adjustment is made it seems, if anything, to be more likely to have undesired anticholinergic effects.

OTHER ULCER-HEALING AGENTS

Bismuth compounds *(see also under 'Antacids' above and in Chapter 23)*

Since 1990, bismuth has tended to come into vogue again as a component in a combined therapy to eliminate *Helicobacter pylori*; it is given here together with metronidazole and either amoxycillin or tetracycline; the incidence of adverse effects (particularly gastrointestinal) demanding drug withdrawal is high, but it is not entirely clear which component(s) of this triple therapy should be blamed.

Carbenoxolone
Liquorice
Deglycyrrhizinated liquorice

Liquorice owes its ulcer-healing properties to glycyrrhizin and glycyrrhizic acid; carbenoxolone is related to the latter. All these substances have unwanted mineralocorticoid-like effects. Deglycyrrhizinated liquorice and lauryl glycyrrhetinic acid, which are also used in some countries for their ulcer-healing effects, do not have mineralocorticoid-like effects. It should be noted that liquorice is sometimes present in laxatives, e.g. prepared by herbalists, and that hyperaldosteronism can appear unexpectedly in such cases where the intake of liquorice has gone unrecognized (SEDA-16, 425).

The mineralocorticoid properties are probably exerted by displacing aldosterone from non-specific receptor sites within cells, thus making it more available to affect mineral metabolism. What this in practice means is that in normal doses carbenoxolone can cause *salt and water retention* with occasional *hypokalemia*. The effects are common but usually mild; they are detected more often during treatment if patients are weighed, their blood pressure measured and serum potassium levels checked. Those given prolonged courses, the elderly and those with hepatic, cardiac and renal impairment are at special risk; severe effects with serious hypertension, heart failure and hypokalemia of sufficient degree to induce myopathy and tubular necrosis can usually be ascribed to ill-advised treatment of persons in whom carbenoxolone is contraindicated, to its use in the elderly, or to prolonged intake without supervision.

Hyperprolactinemia has been noted in a woman with secondary amenorrhea and hypertension who was ingesting large amounts of liquorice; all abnormalities reversed on stopping treatment (69[c]). This effect could reflect some involvement of prolactin in adrenal steroidogenesis or salt and water homeostasis.

Because of the mineralocorticoid properties, these preparations counter the therapeutic effects of most diuretics and other drugs used to treat hypertension, their effects being counteracted by carbenoxolone. Conversely, both spironolactone and amiloride inhibit the healing action of carbenoxolone (SEDA-6, 317).

Emprostil *(SEDA-17, 420)*

Even in doses insufficient to control ulcer symptoms this drug has a higher incidence of adverse effects than do the H_2-blockers, though they amount to little more than *abdominal pain* and *diarrhea*.

Misoprostol *(SEDA-16, 424; SEDA-17, 420; SED-18, 374)*

This compound is dealt with in the section of this volume reviewing the prostaglandins.

Sucralfate *(SEDA-16, 424; SEDA-17, 420; SEDA-18, 374)*

Sucralfate, a basic aluminium salt of sucrose octasulfate, probably acts by binding to inflamed surfaces; it is possible, however, that its binding properties are more generalized, and it has indeed been used as an intra-alimentary phosphate-binding agent in uremic patients.

Plasma aluminium levels rise in patients with renal failure and one might expect aluminium to accumulate with long-term drug use (70[C]); it would seem unwise to use the drug in such patients.

Bezoar formation has more than once been recorded with esophageal obstruction by inspissated drug (SEDA-17, 421; SEDA-18, 374; 71[C]), and a gastric bezoar can be formed when tube feeds include sucralfate; the formation of bezoars reflects the binding of sucralfate to protein in the food.

As to possible interactions, concurrent sucralfate treatment has been claimed to reduce *warfarin* bioavailability (SED-12, 945), and in view of the mode of action it may be expected to do the same with other drugs, including the H_2-blockers which may be used concurrently. Even anecdotal reports of such effects (including those relating to phenytoin, tetracycline or digoxin) therefore need to be taken seriously, particularly where the drugs concerned have a narrow therapeutic index or are being used to treat serious conditions.

OTHER DRUGS FOR THE TREATMENT OF GASTRIC DISORDERS

Dimeticone

Although no adverse toxic effects have been attributed to this antiflatulent agent, commonly compounded with antacids, its use has been associated with elevated hydrogen levels in the breath.

Since dimeticone is a surfactant, one might expect it to enhance the absorption of drugs, and there are some reports showing that this happens with warfarin and (in animal studies) digoxin. Again the rule applies that in a patient taking such a drug where the dose is crucial a careful watch for such interference should be kept.

Tritiozine

Tritiozine is presented as a non-anticholinergic, antisecretory agent. Its use has been associated with drowsiness and with occasional slight increases in transaminase levels (72[c]). A series of cases of predominantly sensory neuropathies with wallerian degeneration of the myelinated fibers has been published (61[C]).

EMETICS

Ipecacuanha *(SEDA-16, 424; SEDA-17, 421)*

Ipecacuanha, with emetine as its main active component, has often been used as a home remedy for various purposes, and not only as an emetic. Use in infancy generally seems safe, but reversible *myopathy* secondary to abuse by individuals with eating disorders has been noted (SED-12, 945; SEDA-17, 421); the active alkaloid may have been responsible. The question is discussed further in Chapter 49. There is some suggestion of *cardiac impairment* with such overdosage, presumably also myopathic. Forced emesis can lead to *esophageal damage* or even complete rupture; *pneumomediastinum* and *pneumoperitoneum* have therefore sometimes complicated induced emesis (SEDA-10, 326). A bizarre case of *neonatal vomiting, irritability and hypothermia* was attributed to the mother having added ipecacuanha surreptitiously to her baby's feed; at any age, however, emetine in excess can be very irritant to the gastrointestinal tract, resulting for example in bloody *diarrhea*. *Asthma* can occasionally be induced by ipecacuanha; when the compound was more widely used in medicine this was a familiar problem for those compounding medicines (73[cR])

Saline

Gastric and upper small bowel necrosis have been described after ingestion of massive amounts of concentrated saline (1 kg salt in 660 ml of water) as an emetic.

ANTIDIARRHEAL AGENTS *(SEDA-16, 424; SEDA-17, 421)*

Fluid replacement is more important than the use of any of these agents in simple diarrhea. Oral rehydration salts or fluids (ORS, ORF) promoted by the World Health Organization and other bodies fortunately largely displaced the dangerous use of antidiarrheals in children in developing countries; ORS are now being displaced in turn by the simple advice to continue feeding the child normally, with use of adequate fluids.

Halogenated quinolines

Since a major epidemic of subacute myelo-opticoneuropathy (SMON) in Japan among users of clioquinol (peaking during the period 1966—1970) led to the withdrawal of that drug in Japan itself and subsequently elsewhere, the halogenated quinolines have been used on a much smaller scale than formerly. Once regarded as a prophylactic and remedy for simple diarrhea, some of them remain in limited use for special purposes, notably for the treatment of amebiasis where no alternative is available.

The events in Japan have been fully documented in earlier volumes from 1968 onwards (see, e.g. SEDA-4, 253) and are now largely of historical interest. However, the condition continues to be reported very sporadically (SEDA-10, 326). The main abdominal symptoms are diarrhea and abdominal pain, sometimes accompanied by nausea, vomiting, constipation, a bloated feeling in the abdomen, and meteorism. The neurological symptoms are acute or subacute in nature, and sensory disturbances are characteristic and spread gradually from the feet up to the navel. Some 20—40% of cases have visual disturbances ranging from blurred vision to atrophy of the optic nerve and blindness. A wide range of mental symptoms is seen. The clearest proof of the cause/effect relationship in Japan was the finding of clioquinol chelates in the green furring of the tongue and the greenish urine. There has been no clear explanation for the much higher incidence of cases in Japan than elsewhere, but a number of hypotheses have been raised (74[R]).

There is every reason to believe that the adverse effects seen with clioquinol can occur with the other hydroxyquinolines, yet a number of them are still sold freely in various parts of the world (75[R]).

Kaolin

Kaolin, commonly given together with pectin, is generally regarded as safe, but its absorbent properties could result in the binding of other drugs which are given at about the same time. Kaolin has, for example been shown to adsorb mefenamic acid and flufenamic acid, phenylbutazone and indomethacin, so one should not be surprised if it reduces the effect of any non-steroidal anti-inflammatory agent, requiring an increase in dosage by 50— 100% to maintain efficacy. The reduction of lincomycin absorption is quite drastic, perhaps amounting to 90% of the dose given.

Lomotil (diphenoxylate + atropine)

Diphenoxylate is a synthetic compound intended to possess the antidiarrheal effects of the opiates, but it also retains some less desirable opiate effects. Atropine, added to the formulation many years ago in the hope of preventing misuse, can itself cause problems, especially if the drug is intentionally or accidentally used to excess; in one instance *keratoconjunctivitis* occurred, confirmed by rechallenge but not with diphenoxylate alone (SEDA-16, 425). Adverse effects are rare during ordinary use in adults, but children can be particularly sensitive to the adverse effects of both components, and in cases of poisoning complex and prompt measures may be needed, particularly since the respiratory depression may be delayed until a day after ingestion and may recur even after a good response to narcotic antagonists.

This and other drugs which reduce intestinal motility can interact with other drugs by affecting their absorption, e.g. the absorption of nitrofurantoin can be doubled.

Even more strongly than in the case of loperamide (see below) one must advise against any use of this drug in childhood diarrhea.

Loperamide

As compared with Lomotil, a further degree of dissociation of unwanted opiate effects has been attained with this compound, which acts mainly peripherally; recognition of its safety if appropriately used has led to its being released in many countries for sale without prescription. It does nevertheless retain some central activity, and *nausea*, *dizziness*, *dry mouth*, *abdominal pain*, *ileus* and *lethargy* all occur in a minority of users, with occasional reports of more serious central reactions such as a possible association with *delirium* in a child (76[C]). Some cases of *necrotizing enterocolitis* have been reported in infants developing paralytic ileus after treatment for mild diarrhea (77[C]); this is only one of the good reasons to avoid the drug in young children—the most important is that diarrhea in infants should not be suppressed pharmacologically (78[R]).

Oral rehydration fluids (ORF) *(SEDA-17, 422)*

Oral hydration fluids, as long recommended for example by WHO, should cause no problems. Not all available mixtures are however ideal, and some home-made versions have caused more problems than they relieved; solutions of appropriate salt content should be used to avoid hyponatremia, and the sugar content should not be such as to cause osmotic diarrhea. As noted above, it is now realized that continuation of normal feeding and fluid intake is as effective as the use of ORF.

LAXATIVES *(SEDA-16, 425; SEDA-17, 422; SEDA-18, 374)*

Side effects of laxatives as such If laxatives of any type are heavily used, not necessarily to the point of abuse, *diarrhea* will be common, as well as a tendency to *nausea* and to *fluid and electrolyte imbalance*. The possibility of laxative-induced *colonic injury*, with damage to the autonomic nervous innervation of the large intestine, was formerly much discussed; in fact it was probably a problem with the violent cathartics formerly used (podophyllin, aloes) and might still occur with cascara, but is not on record with the laxatives normally used today.

Laxative abuse Habitual, usually secretive, abuse of laxatives is much more common in women than in men and there is overlap with the anorectic/bulemic syndrome. Abuse of irritant agents such as senna and cascara have been the commonest varieties (SED-10, 704), but in recent years reports show that a range of proprietary laxatives have been abused. Abuse can lead to a condition characterized by chronic diarrhea, hypokalemia and fluid depletion. Features also include hypomagnesemia, hypocalcemia and hypoalbuminemia with thirst, lassitude, weight loss, edema, and occasionally osteomalacic bone pain and clubbing. In one small series of cases of laxative abusers, *pseudo-Bartter's syndrome* was induced; complications included confusion, convulsions, muscle weakness (with or without paralysis or rhabdomyolysis) and bone changes; hypokalemia and hypophosphatemia were common, and when the laxatives were withdrawn some patients suffered prolonged edema (79[CR]).

Interactions Any laxative could in principle derange drug absorption from the intestine (e.g. of quinidine).

Anthraquinones

All anthraquinones, of which cascara and senna are the best known, can cause *cramping* and *abdominal discomfort*. Chronic use can be associated with *melanosis coli*. The urine can be colored red. The possibility of colonic injury has been discussed (see general section above). There is a fairly recent case of *hepatitis* on record, confirmed by rechallenge, and possibly due to re-absorption of rhein anthron produced in the intestine (SEDA-16, 425).

Senna is widely used in fairly low doses without serious problems; it is also employed in a very high dosage form (X-Prep) to clear the colon before radiological examination. In this form it is generally well tolerated but it should certainly not be used if there is any predisposition to colonic rupture. An unusual antabuse-type reaction reported on one occasion seems to have been due to an interaction of metronidazole with the alcohol present in X-Prep (SEDA-15, 398).

Dantron Dantron is a synthetic analog of the anthraquinones, others being aloe-emodin, chrysophanic acid, emodin, physicon, and rhein. All seem to be bacterial mutagens: dantron itself, in addition to being genotoxic as assessed by DNA repair testing, seems to be capable of inducing intestinal tumors in animals (SED-11, 788). Because of these properties the drug has already been withdrawn in some countries, except for concurrent use with morphine in terminal cancer patients.

Bisacodyl This synthetic agent increased peristalsis by a direct effect on the small intestine. The only specific adverse effect described is *abdominal cramping* which a minority of patients find troublesome. As with other laxatives however, heavy or chronic use can derange the system in various ways, e.g. inducing hypokalemia with rhabdomyolysis (SEDA-16, 425).

Liquid paraffin

It has been recommended for many years that the use of liquid paraffin should be discontinued because of its propensity to cause *malabsorption of fat-soluble vitamins*, to leak and soil the perineal skin, and to cause *lipid pneumonia* if aspirated; at the very least the drug should be avoided in young children (80[r]).

Oxyphenisatin (oxyfenisatin)

This laxative, once very widely used, was withdrawn prior to 1980 in most countries because of the occurrence of chronic persistent/active *hepatitis*; a full account will be found in volumes in this series from 1971.

Phenolphthalein

This remains a widely employed laxative for self-treatment, often camouflaged in chocolate and thus liable to abuse or accidental use. Skin *rashes* of various types are reported repeatedly, sometimes with *pruritus*. *Pigmentation defects* have been described. The most serious (but rare) effect to have been reliably documented is *toxic epidermal necrolysis*. A *fixed drug eruption* with bullous *erythema multiforme* has been shown to be associated with auto-sensitization, and direct intracellular immunofluorescence is found (81).

Sodium picosulfate *(SEDA-16, 425; SEDA-17, 422)*

A 1992 report described two cases of *generalized urticarial skin reactions* after a first dose of sodium picosulfate. This may have represented an interaction with aminosalicylic acid derivatives which were being administered at the same time, or a simple adverse effect to one of the agents. A dubious case of status epilepticus has been published (SEDA-16, 425).

BULKING AGENTS AND OSMOTIC LAXATIVES

The bulking agents include vegetable fiber products (such as bran), paraffin and methylcellulose (which absorbs water into the intestinal), agar (which similarly expands to form a gel) and psyllium seeds or other mucilaginous plant products. The osmotic laxatives include inorganic salts and the synthetic disaccharide, lactulose as well as magnesium salts and sodium phosphate.

Bulking and osmotic agents are largely free of adverse effects, but any non-absorbable agent can aggravate symptoms associated with pre-existent intestinal stricture. Abdominal bloating due to bacterial fermentation of unabsorbed carbohydrate is a common sequel to excessive intake. The sugar content of some bulk laxatives may be sufficient to impair diabetic control; the vegetable matter in other preparations can cause bezoars to form and is potentially allergenic. Various of these laxatives are discussed individually below.

Glycerol (glycerin)

Glycerol is used as a laxative given orally, as an enema, or in the form of suppositories. Large oral doses can cause *nausea* or *headache*, as well as severe *derangements of water balance* which may be dangerous in patients in poor physical condition. The substance can also *raise plasma insulin levels* and thereby derange diabetes; in debilitated (and young) diabetic patients it is a particularly risky form of treatment which should be avoided since it has even led to fatalities. Rectal administration can cause *mucosal erosion*.

Lactulose
Lactilol

No significant adverse effects of lactulose solutions have been described, but *non-toxic megacolon* has been seen in some elderly patients and, as with other laxatives, there is always a possibility of *dependence* (SEDA-11, 374).

Lactilol is another disaccharide similar to lactulose. It has been claimed to be more palatable and to have fewer adverse effects but these are no more than first impressions (SEDA-18, 374).

Magnesium salts

Enema treatment with these salts can cause severe *hypermagnesemia* (82[C]). Absorbed magnesium ions can cause *focal cerebral signs*, *coma*, *apnea*, *muscular paralysis*, and *cardiac arrhythmias*.

Mannitol

Oral use can raise intracolonic hydrogen concentrations sufficiently high to cause *explosions* at diathermy.

Psyllium

The bulk laxative Perdiem, which is based largely on psyllium with senna, has been found to cause several cases of *esophageal impaction*, one of which also had a gastric bezoar (SEDA-15, 398).

Occupational exposure of a nurse to a psyllium-based laxative has been found to give rise to *allergy*. This problem arises in a more serious form among the personnel of pharmaceutical factories processing psyllium (SEDA-16, 426), and *eosinophilia* has also been recorded in these situations. The allergen appears to reside in the endosperm or embryonic seed components and not in the husk which is the component with laxative effect; in principle therefore it should be feasible to supply a non-antigenic form of purified psyllium husk (SEDA-17, 423).

Sodium phosphate

Absorption of large amounts of phosphate from enemas can cause *hyperphosphatemia*, *hypocalcemia*, and *cardiac arrest*. Adults with normal excretory functions should not be at risk, but infants and those with renal failure are likely to experience complications (SEDA-17, 425; SEDA-18, 374).

Salazosulfapyridine (sulfasalazine) *(SEDA-16, 426; SEDA-17, 423; SEDA-18, 375)*

Sulfasalazine is a compound comprising both a sulfonamide moiety and 5-aminosalicylic acid. When the drug was introduced for the treatment of ulcerative colitis it was believed that both elements would contribute to the therapeutic effect, but in fact the sulfonamide merely serves as a carrier from which the 5-aminosalicylic acid is progressively released; at the same time the sulfonamide exerts the adverse effects of its own class (see Chapter 29.1). Adverse reactions are frequent and the withdrawal rate for this reason can be as high as 30% (SEDA-16, 426).

ADVERSE REACTION PATTERN

General and toxic reactions Dose-related nausea and vomiting are common and minor hematological changes and skin rash are often seen; a substantial minority of patients withdraw from treatment themselves. Severe hematological abnormalities, lung complications and liver disease with severe sensitization are rare; reversible male infertility with oligospermia is well documented. Hemolysis can occur to a minor degree in many ordinary patients. Heinz bodies may be detected in peripheral blood samples. A Kawasaki-like syndrome has once been reported (SEDA-16, 427) in a patient who later reacted in the same manner to mesalazine.

Hypersensitivity reactions Skin reactions are common and general sensitization can occur, as with other sulfa derivatives. The clinical features, besides skin rash, include granulomatous liver disease, positive lupus phenomenon, hypocomplementemia and fever (83[CR]). More serious skin conditions can also occur (see below). In the case of mild reactions, patients can often be desensitized by giving small (and then progressively increasing) doses of the drug. Various complex auto-immune syndromes can occur (SEDA-17, 423); in long-term studies of the use of the drug in rheumatoid arthritis, 12—20% of evaluable patients developed antinuclear antibodies during treatment (SEDA-16, 426; SEDA-18, 375).

Tumor-inducing effects These have not been described.

ORGANS AND SYSTEMS

Cardiovascular *Raynaud's phenomenon* has been described.

Respiratory *'Sulfasalazine lung'*, *fibrosing alveolitis* and *eosinophilic pleurisy* are variants on a well-recognized though unusual lung complication. Most commonly it presents with fever, eosinophilia, dyspnea and pulmonary infiltrates (SEDA-15, 309; 84[cR]). The disease usually develops 1—9 months after the start of treatment and the fibrosing alveolitis can be fatal (85[C]). Whether the salicylate or the sulfa moiety is responsible is unclear; both can cause pulmonary eosinophilia. Differentiation from lung disease simply associated with ulcerative colitis can be difficult, particularly because the drug-induced state sometimes itself takes the form of an interstitial pneumonitis without evidence of a hypersensitivity reaction (86[C]) and rechallenge can be dangerous (SEDA-16, 427).

Nervous system *Vivid dreams* and daytime *hallucinations* have been noted on one occasion. On another an *aseptic meningitis* appeared in a patient with a pre-existing Sjögren's syndrome; and the drug link was confirmed by a positive rechallenge (87[C]). In a slow-acetylator, drug toxicity may have underlain an *axonal sensorimotor neuropathy* (SEDA-17, 424); an unusual but not unique case of *transverse myelitis* was reported in 1991, and other published case reports suggest links with *chorea* and *ataxia* (SEDA-16, 427).

Hematological Minor changes with Heinz body formation and minor degrees of hemolysis are common. *Agranulocytosis* is very unusual but well described, and can occur suddenly and very early in treatment (88[Cr]); a degree of *granulocytopenia* may be more common in rheumatoid patients taking the drug than in those with inflammatory bowel disease, and one study showed an incidence of neutropenia in 10% of cases (SEDA-16, 426). Folic acid absorption is reduced but rarely to a clinically significant extent, though *megaloblastic anemia* has been documented as a rare complication. *Methemoglobinemia* can occur in patients with a particular pattern of hepatic metabolism of sulfapyridine (89[C]).

Liver See also 'Hypersensitivity reactions' above. Exceptionally, fulminant *hepatic failure with massive necrosis* has been seen; two cases were reported in 1992 and both failed to survive (SEDA-17, 424).

Gastrointestinal *Nausea* and *vomiting*, as well as *taste disturbances* (SEDA-17, 424), *anorexia* and *abdominal discomfort* can occur. They are particularly common in slow acetylators, but symptoms remit with dose reduction. *Pancreatitis* has several times been ascribed to the drug and may well be the expression of a hypersensitivity reaction; cases with positive rechallenge are on record. Exacerbation of existing *colitis* is rare but well-recognized; more recently it has appeared that sulfasalazine can induce a colitis de novo; *pseudomembranous colitis* with *Clostridium difficile* was reported in 1991, as was a fatal neutropenic colitis with no evidence of *C. difficile* growth (SEDA-17, 424).

The finding of *E. coli* antibiotic resistance on rectal swabs with a range of resistance extending beyond the sulfa drugs, is difficult to evaluate. The clinical relevance is doubtful.

Skin and appendages Simple rashes are not uncommon. *Raynaud's phenomenon* and *toxic epidermal necrolysis* associated with *erythroid hypoplasia* and agranulocytosis (see above) have occurred; in one case of toxic epidermal necrolysis very marked immunosuppression was found (SEDA-18, 375). A rare case of skin *hyperpigmentation* (apparently a phototoxic reaction) has been associated with sulfasalazine lung (see above) (90[C]). Hair loss seems to be a possible but rare effect (SEDA-16, 427).

Urinary system Two cases have been reported of patients with long-standing ulcerative colitis who after several years of treatment with sulfasalzine developed what seemed to be a drug-induced *chronic interstitial nephritis* with no other detectable cause (91[C]); it may be noted that the same problem has arisen with mesalazine (see below). *Nephrotic syndrome* with minimal change nephropathy has been described both with this drug and with mesalazine (SEDA-16, 427).

Genital system *Oligospermia*, with reduced motility and a high frequency of abnormal forms, and male *infertility* are well documented. Oral and rectal treatment have the same effects, which reverse when treatment ceases. *Impotence* has been described on many occasions, sometimes with positive rechallenge (92[Cr])

Risk situations As noted above, gastrointestinal adverse reactions occur more commonly in *slow acetylators*, and they should receive lower doses. *Glucose-6-phosphate dehydrogenase deficiency* may be associated with a tendency to hemolysis. Finally, where chronic inflammatory bowel disease coexists with *acute intermittent porphyria*, the bowel condition itself has been proven to bring with it an increased risk of acute porphyric attacks; salazosulfapyridine can trigger such an attack in this condition (SEDA-17, 425).

Second-generation effects Pregnant colitic patients have generally fared better if they continued to take the drug. Though salazosulfapyridine crosses the placenta, competes for albumin-binding sites with bilirubin and can be detected in breast milk, no adverse effects on the offspring have been detected.

Interactions *Ferrous sulfate* interferes with salazosulfapyridine absorption, possibly by chelation; the significance of this phenomenon is doubtful, given that the beneficial effect of salazosulfapyridine depends on 5-aminosalicylate release in the large intestine from sulfapyridine which apparently only serves as a carrier and therefore does not need to be absorbed. *Oral antimicrobial agents* will, however, inhibit the splitting reaction. *Digoxin* blood levels may be reduced by salazosulfapyridine treatment.

5-Aminosalicylic acid (mesalazine) *(SEDA-16, 427; SEDA-17, 425; SEDA-18, 375; 93[R])*

Mesalazine, as pointed out above, is the active principle of salazosulfapyridine in chronic inflammatory bowel disease and it can be equally well administered using carriers other than salazosulfapyridine (thereby hoping to avoid those adverse reactions due to the sulfonamide moiety) or administered without a carrier at all in the form of a slow- or controlled-release preparation. Since the desired action takes place in the gut lumen and wall, one or the other of these approaches must be adopted; the substance should not be administered in its simple form; if it is, absorption will be greater (and systemic side effects are likely to be perhaps more common) and the local efficacy may be less. Olsalazine (diazo-5-aminosalicylic acid) is a newer example of the carrier approach.

With both these newer preparations some adverse reactions persist; in the light of recent evidence and a major meta-analysis it seems increasingly doubtful whether their profile is substantially more favourable than that of sulfasalazine, despite the elimination of the sulfonamide moiety (94[R]).

Hypersensitivity The possibility of hypersensitivity reactions has been suggested, but they may be rather less of a problem than with sulfasalazine. A *lupus-like syndrome* has been described on several occasions (SEDA-15, 400; 95[c]).

Cardiovascular There is a single Scandinavian case report reliably attributing a fatal *myocarditis* to mesalazine (96[C]).

Hematological Heinz body formation occurs but has not been a clinical problem. A case of *thrombocytopenia* has been published but the causal link is doubtful; *leukopenia* has however been seen in a patient who had earlier reacted to salazosulfapyridine in the same way (SEDA-17, 425).

Respiratory A symptomatic bilateral *lung reaction* with interstitial infiltrates and impaired function has been observed in a patient treated with mesalazine for

2 years; the condition had developed insidiously but recovered within 8 months following drug withdrawal (97[C]). The condition is not necessarily identical to the lung reaction seen with sulfasalazine.

Gastrointestinal *Pancreatitis* has been noted often enough to be taken seriously (98[Cr]); it has occurred in children as well as adults and has sometimes been confirmed by rechallenge (SEDA-18, 375). *Nausea*, *vomiting* and *stomatitis* can occur. *Diarrhea* seems rather more common with olsalazine than with sulfasalazine.

Skin and appendages See also 'Genital system' below. Rashes have not generally proved an important problem, but two cases of oral and cutaneous *lichen planus* which had developed during salazosulfapyridine treatment recurred when the patients later received mesalazine (SEDA-17, 425).

Urinary system Interstitial nephritis has been well documented (SEDA-17, 425; 99[R]). The adverse effect was predictable from animal toxicology.

Sexual organs Inflammation of external genitalia has been described but may be due to the stabilizer content. Male infertility caused by salazosulfapyridine can be reversed by switching to mesalazine.

Second-generation effects Even during high dosing, only very small amounts of mesalazine enter the breast milk; toxic effects are unlikely but allergic effects might be exerted (SEDA-18, 376).

Olsalazine *(SEDA-16, 427; SEDA-17, 425; SEDA-18, 376)*

Olsalazine consists of two molecules of 5-aminosalicylate linked by an azo-bond which is lysed in the gut to yield the active molecules at the point where they are required to act. Side effects would be expected to be those of 5-aminosalicylate, and this is largely the case. However *diarrhea* has been sufficiently common to suggest that it may be a particular problem with olsalazine, with an incidence of some 13%; it is probably a small-intestinal secretory diarrhea (SEDA-17, 425; 100[C]). Similarly, a case of *cholestatic hepatitis* has been described which was confirmed on rechallenge yet did not recur with mesalazine in similar doses (SEDA-16, 428). In one case there was a marked hypersensitivity reaction in a man previously intolerant of sulfasalazine, but the circumstances suggested a reaction to 5-aminosalicylate rather than to the double molecule (SEDA-18, 376).

Para-aminosalicylate (4-aminosalicylate)

The adverse reactions to this long-established antituberculous drug, which has also been developed as a treatment for ulcerative colitis, are considered in Chapter 30.

ANTISPASMODIC AGENTS

Mebeverine *(See also Chapter 13)*

This agent is claimed to act directly on the colonic muscle and is virtually free of systemic adverse reactions, but its therapeutic effect is weak. Surprisingly. a case of *colonic perforation* was described in 1990, but the patient concerned was suffering from the distal intestinal syndrome of cystic fibrosis and may have been at particular risk (SEDA-16, 428).

Peppermint oil

Peppermint oil seems generally free of adverse effects.

SECRETORY STIMULANTS

Ceruletide

This decapeptide can cause *sweating*, *dizziness* and *vomiting* (see Chapter 48).

Histamine and betazole (ametazole)

Unwanted vasomotor effects of histamine injections can be partially blocked by H_1-antihistamines, while incorporation of benzyl alcohol in the injection prevents pain at the injection site. Betazole has a more selective gastric effect but is not entirely free of systemic histamine-like reactions.

Pentagastrin

Nausea, *abdominal cramp*, *headache*, *drowsiness* and *giddiness* can occur, but the gastric effect is largely dissociated from these unwanted effects.

Secretin and pancreozymin (cholecystokinin)

Allergic reactions may accompany use of these hormones which are only partially purified.

RECTAL PREPARATIONS

Bisacodyl suppositories

These can make the rectal mucosa appear inflamed, but the effect is transient; the effect can be mistaken for idiopathic proctitis. As noted above, cramping is a problem for some patients with this laxative.

Corticosteroid and salazosulfapyridine mixtures

Steroid absorption from these suppositories or enemas does occur but is seldom a clinical problem.

Soap enemas

Local inflammation may occur. *High pressure injection* can perforate the bowel; the treatment is obsolete.

Sodium phosphate enemas

As noted above, infants and patients with renal failure are particularly prone to develop hyperphosphatemia and associated hypocalcemia when these enemas are administered.

CHOLELITHOLYTIC AGENTS

BILE ACIDS

Chenodeoxycholic acid *(SEDA-16, 428; SEDA-17, 426; SEDA-18, 376)*

ADVERSE REACTION PATTERN

General and toxic reactions Mild diarrhea and slightly elevated serum transaminase levels are very common.

Hypersensitivity reactions These have not been reported.

Tumor-inducing effects These have not been described.

ORGANS AND SYSTEMS

Endocrine, metabolic Although most studies have shown no consistent effects on *serum cholesterol* concentrations, in the National Cooperative Gallstone Study a 10% increase was noted over a 2-year period in treated people as against a 5% rise in controls. Low-density lipoprotein levels rose in association; other varieties were unaffected.

Liver *Serum transaminase levels* tend to double or triple in the early weeks of treatment in about a third of cases treated. There is a hypothesis that this is due to the mechanisms of lithocholate sulfation. Lithocholic acid is formed by the 7-dehydroxylation of chenodeoxycholic acid; this potentially toxic substance is ordinarily inactivated by sulfation. Hypertransaminasemia has been detected in nearly 75% of persons with a low sulfation capacity (this capacity being bimodally distributed) and in less than one in ten of those with high capacities. All the same, chenodeoxycholic acid is substantially, if not totally, devoid of serious hepatotoxic actions. Liver biopsy has shown no significant changes; minor changes can include fatty change and lipofuscin accumulation.

Gastrointestinal About half of all patients given the usual dose of 15 mg/kg per day will develop diarrhea. Unabsorbed bile acid causes water to be secreted into the large bowel. Symptoms remit with dose reduction and may not recur if the dose is then slowly raised again.

Skin and appendages *Lichen planus* developed in one patient taking a combination of chenodeoxycholic and ursodeoxycholic acid (SEDA-17, 428).

Risk situations Because of the hepatic effects the drug should not be used where there is a liver disorder. Because of its effect on the intestine it is best avoided in inflammatory bowel disease.

Second-generation effects These have not been reported, though it is generally considered wise to avoid the drug in pregnancy.

Interactions No effects upon the clearance of other drugs have been found.

Ursodeoxycholic acid *(SEDA-16, 428; SEDA-17, 426; SEDA-18, 376)*

Ursodeoxycholic acid, the 7β-epimer of chenodeoxycholic acid, seldom causes significant diarrhea or induces hypertransaminasemia. The lack of transaminasemia is puzzling since ursodeoxycholic acid, like chenodeoxycholate, is metabolized to lithocholate, and some if not all animal studies have revealed evidence of hepatotoxicity. One undesirable property of ursodeoxycholic acid is that occasionally treatment is followed by the development of *resistant* (*and radio-opaque*) *coatings to gallstones*, thus retarding or preventing further dissolution.

Tauroursodeoxycholic acid *(SEDA-18, 376)*

Experience with this agent is limited; in a comparative trial it seemed to be less effective than ursodeoxycholic acid and to produce more side effects. Recently, two patients were described who took the drug for primary biliary cirrhosis; both developed severe right upper quadrant pain, and rechallenge with tauroursodeoxycholic acid was positive (101[c]).

INTRADUCTAL INFUSIONS *(SEDA-18, 376)*

Methyl-*tert*-butylether
Mono-octanoin

Fever, *abdominal pain*, *nausea*, *vomiting* and *diarrhea* all occur frequently with these substances, as can mildly *raised levels of serum amylase or liver enzymes generally*; *stone impaction* has been described; cholecystitis can be induced, at least when methyl-*tert*-butylether is used alongside ethylene diaminetetra-acetic acid (SEDA-16, 428). Most such effects are probably attributable to over-rapid infusion. *Necrotizing choledochomalacia* has also been described with mono-octanoin, as has non-cardiogenic *pulmonary edema* after appropriate intra-biliary use (102[Cr]); if mono-octanoin is in error injected intravenously, fatal respiratory and cardiac arrest can occur (103[C]).

OTHER GASTROINTESTINAL DRUGS

Activated charcoal *(SEDA-17, 426; SEDA-18, 376)*

Though usually innocuous, activated charcoal can in large or multiple doses, such as may be needed in severe poisoning, repeatedly cause genuine *intestinal obstruction*; a pseudo-obstruction can also occur if drugs inhibiting intestinal motility are given at the same time, and sometimes it is not clear which process has occurred (SED-12, 951; SEDA-17, 426; 104[C]). *Hyponatremic dehydration* has been described when charcoal was combined with sorbitol to treat theophylline overdose in a child (SED-12, 951). *Pulmonary aspiration* is an ever-present risk when using charcoal, especially in the semiconscious patient, to treat poisoning; a particular problem in that situation arises from pneumonitis caused by povidone (used as a suspending agent) which can lead to respiratory failure and death.

Choleretics

Little is known of any of the properties of the wide range of proprietary choleretics available. Many are ancient polypharmaceuticals.

Ion-exchange resins *(See also Chapter 44)*

Cholestyramine and colestipol are discussed elsewhere in this volume since their intended effect is not actually on the gastrointestinal system. *Sequestration* of orally administered drugs, as well as of bile acids, can occur; the interactions are most likely to cause problems with *digoxin* and *warfarin* because of their narrow therapeutic index. The drugs are not pleasant to take, so compliance is often poor.

Cysteamine

Nausea, *flushing*, *vomiting* and *drowsiness* are reported.

Pancreatic enzymes

When held in the mouth, these can cause *oral ulceration*. Tissue extracts may be bacterially contaminated.

Percutaneous hepatic tumour ablation with alcohol

This treatment commonly induces *severe pain*, *fever* and *hepatic dysfunction*; there can also be *pleural effusion*, *pneumothorax*, *ascites*, *vasovagal reaction*, *transient hypotension*, *myoglobinuria* and *portal thrombosis*. A fatal case of massive *hepatic necrosis* distant from the injection site has also been attributed to this treatment (SEDA-18, 377).

Sclerosant injections

Following the use of sclerosants, such as ethanolamine oleate 5%, to treat esophageal varices, patients commonly experience early *dysphagia* and *retrosternal pain*, as might be expected. More serious complications can arise later if the *fibrosis* which is a natural consequence of the treatment extends too far, or if the sclerosant escapes from the veins which are being treated. Complications can include fibrosis (leading for example to *esophageal stricture*) as well as *perforation*, *sepsis* and *respiratory problems*. *Mediastinal pain* can be precipitated by excessively deep or large injections. *Mesenteric thrombosis* has been claimed to occur as a complication and would not be unexpected; *chylothorax* and *cerebral embolism* have also been described.

A number of case reports suggest that sclerosant therapy could be *carcinogenic* (SEDA-15, 401).

Current impressions are that local use of propranolol is safer, but that neither this nor the use of sclerosing agents, with all their attendant risks, is particularly effective (SEDA-18, 377).

REFERENCES

1. Sewing KF. Tolerance of antacids. J Physiol Pharmacol 1993;44(Suppl 1):75–77.
2. Foldes J, Balena R, Parfitt AM et al. Hypophosphatemic rickets with hypocalcuria following long-term treatment with aluminium-containing antacid. Bone 1991;12:67–71.
3. Nwokolo CU, Prewett EJ, Sawyer AA et al. Lack of bismuth absorption from bismuth subnitrate (Roter) tablets. Eur J Gastroenterol Hepatol 1989;5:433.
4. Nwokolo CU, Mistry P, Pounder RE. The absorption of bismuth and salicylate from oral doses of Pepto-Bismol (bismuth salicylate). Aliment Pharmacol Ther 1990;4:163.
5. Levant JA, Walsh JH, Isenberg JI. Stimulation of gastric secretion and gastrin release by single oral doses of calcium carbonate in man. N Engl J Med 1973;239:555.
6. Kalmthoot PMV, Engels LGJ, Baker HH et al. Severe copper deficiency, due to excessive use of an antacid combined with pyloric stenosis. Dig Dis Sci 1982;57:859.
7. Brismar B, Standberg A, Wiklund B. Stomach rupture following ingestion of sodium bicarbonate. Acta Chir Scand Suppl 1986;530:97.
8. Schulthess HK, Valli C, Escher F et al. Ösophagusobstruktion während Sondenernährung: Folge von Eiweissfallung durch Antazida? Schweiz Med Wochenschr 1986; 118:960.
9. Mihara S, Kawamura H, Nemoto R et al. Silicate urolithiasis; a case report. Nishiniton J Urol 1992;54:875–877.
10. Neumann A, Jensen BG. Osteomalacia from Al and Mg antacids. Acta Orthop Scand 1989;60:361.
11. Moreno I, Rosell R, Abad A et al. Randomized trial for the control of acute vomiting in cisplatin-treated patients: high dose metoclopramide with dexamethasone and lorazepam as adjuncts versus high dose alizapride plus dexamethasone and lorazepam. Oncology 1991;48:397–402.
12. McGeown MG. Renal disease associated with drugs. In: D'Arcy PF, Griffin JP, eds. Iatrogenic Diseases, 3rd edn. Oxford–New York–Tokyo: Oxford University Press, 1986; 790.
13. Herrstedt J, Jeppesen BH, Dombenowsky P. Dose-limiting hypotension with the 5-HT3-antagonist batanopride (BMY-25801). Ann. Oncol 1991;2:154–155.
14. Olsson S, Edwards IR. Tachycardia during cisapride treatment. Br Med J 1992;305:748–749.
15. Anon. Cisapride–aggressive behaviour. Bull Swed Adverse Drug React Advisory Comm 1991;57:1.
16. Denie C, Gohy P. Hepatite cytolytique attributable au cisapride. Gastroenterol Clin Biol 1992;16:368–376.
17. Carone R, Vercelli D, Bertapelle P. Effects of cisapride on anorectal and vesicourethral function in spinal cord injured patients. Paraplegia 1993;31:125–127.
18. Anon. Clebopride: warning on extrapyramidal symptoms. WHO Drug Inform 1988;2(2):69.
19. Bleiberg H, Piccart M, Lips S et al. A phase I trial of a new aniemetic drug–clebopride maleate–in cisplatin-treated patients. Ann Oncol 1992;3:141–143.
20. Anon. Clebopride: warning on extrapyrimidal symptoms. WHO Drug Inform 1988;3:141–143.
21. Pellegrino M, Sacco M, Lotti F. Sindrome extrapiramidale da moderato hiperdosaggio di domperidone. Ped Med Chir 1990;12:205–206.
22. Spirt MJ, Chan W, Thieberg W et al. Neuroleptic malignant syndrome induced by domperidone. Dig Dis Sci 1992; 37:946–948.
23. Vidal A, Rodriguez A, Barrio A et al. Bloqueo A-V por intoxicación con metoclopramida. An Esp Pediatr 1991; 34:313–314.
24. Bevacqua BK. Supraventricular tachycardia associated with postpartum metoclopramide administration. Anesthesiology 1988;68:124.
25. Brower RD, Dreyer CF, Kent TA. Neuroleptic malignant syndrome in a child treated with metoclopramide for chemotherapy-related nausea. J Child Neurol 1989;4:230.
26. Bateman DN, Darling WM, Boys R et al. Extrapyramidal reactions to metoclopramide and prochlorperazine. Q J Med 1989;71:307.
27. Noll AM, Pinsky D. Withdrawal effects of metoclopramide. West J Med 1991;154:726–728.
28. Casteels-van Daele M. Reye syndrome or effects of antiemetics? Eur J Pediatr 1991;150:456–459.
29. Finn AL. Toxicity and side effects of ondansetron. Semin Oncol 1992;19:53–60.
30. Halperin JR, Murphy B. Extrapyramidal reaction to ondansetron. Cancer 1992;69:1275.
31. Del Favero A, Roila F, Tonato M. Reducing chemotherapy-induced nausea and vomiting. Current perspectives and future possibilities. Drug Safety 1993;9:410–428.
32. Manninen V, Apajalahti A, Melin J et al. Altered absorption of digoxin in patients given propantheline and metoclopramide. Lancet 1973;i:398.
33. Guckenbieh W, Gilfrich HJ, Just H. Einfluss von Laxantien und Metoclopramid auf die Chinidin-Plasmakonzentration während Langzeittherapie bei Patienten mit Herzrhythmusstörungen. Med Welt 1976;57:1273.
34. Israel R, O'Mara V, Austin B et al. Metoclopramide decreases renal plasma flow. Clin Pharmacol Ther 1986; 39:261.
35. Feldman M, Burton ME. Histamine H_2-receptor antagonists. Standard therapy for acid-peptic disease. N Engl J Med 1990;353:1672.
36. Colin-Jones DG, Langman MJS, Lawson DH et al. Postmarketing surveillance of the safety of cimetidine: 10 year mortality report. Gut 1992;33:1280–1284.
37. Colin-Jones DC, Langman MJS, Lawson DH et al. Cime-

tidine and gastric cancer: preliminary report from postmarketing surveillance study. Br Med J 1983;285:1311.
38. Møller H, Nissen A, Mosbech J. Use of cimetidine and other ulcer drugs in Denmark 1977—1990 with analysis of the risk of cancer among cimetidine users. Gut 1992; 33:1166—1169.
39. Hinrichsen H, Halabi A, Kirch W. Haemodynamic effects of H_2-antagonists. Eur J Clin Invest 1992;22:9—18.
40. Höltmann BJ, Schött D, Ulmer WT. Diffuse interstitielle Lungerkrankung nach Anwendung von Cimetidin bei einem Patienten mit schwerer Refluxkrankheit der Speiseröhre. Med Klin 1989;84:405.
41. Bhatia MS, Agrawal P, Khastgir U et al. Cimetidine induced psychosis. Indian Pediatr 1989;26:1061—1062.
42. Pouget J, Pellissier JF, Jean P et al. Neuropathie périphérique au cours d'un traitement par la cimétidine. Rev Neurol 1986;142:34.
43. Vssey MP, Goldacre MJ, Seagroatt V et al. Peptic ulcer, cimetidine, and motor neurone disease—a record linkage study. Gut 1993;34:1660—1661.
44. Potter H, Byrne EB, Levobitz S. Fever after cimetidine and ranitidine. J Clin Gastroenterol 1986;5:275.
45. Spence RW, Celestin LE. Gynaecomastia associated with cimetidine. Gut 1979;20:154.
46. Trechot PF, De Romemont E, De Romemont M et al. Parotidite récidivante avec un antihistaminique H_2. J Fr Oto-Rhino-Laryngol 1991;40:173—174.
47. Payne CR, Ackrill P, Ralston AJ. Acute renal failure and rise in alkaline phosphatase activity caused by cimetidine. Br Med J 1982;285:100.
48. Vircburger MI, Prelevic GM, Burkie S et al. Transitory alopecia and hypergonadotrophic hypogonadism during cimetidine treatment. Lancet 1981;i:1160.
49. Andersen M. Forværring af psoriasis under behandling med H_2-antagonister. Ugeskr Læg 1991;153:132.
50. Labeeuw M, Cabanne JE, Dubot P. Recurrent myalgias associated with cimetidine. Int J Clin Pharmacol Ther Toxicol 1986;24:349.
51. Force RW, Nahata NC. Effect of histamine H_2-receptor antagonists on vitamin B_{12} absorption. Ann Pharmacother 1992;26:1283—1286.
52. Rampello L, Nicoletti G. Sindrome da sospension della terapia con H_2-antagonisti. Med Riv EMI 1990;10:294—296.
53. Wormsley KG. Safety profile of ranitidine. Drugs 1993; 46:976—985.
54. Stocky A. Ranitidine and depression. Aust NZ J Psychiatry 1991;25:415—418.
55. Gaughan WJ, Shet VR, Francos GC et al. Ranitidine-induced acute interstitial nephritis with epithelial cell foot process fusion. Am J Kidney Dis 1993;22:337—340.
56. Van Bommel EFH, Meyboom RHG. Leverbeschadiging door ranitidine. Ned Tijdschr Geneeskd 1992;136:435—437.
57. Rao SSC, Nayak KS, Swarnalata G et al. Gastric carcinoid associated with ranitidine in a patient with renal failure. Am J Gastroenterol 1993;88:1273—1274.
58. UK Committee on Safety of Medicines. Diarrhoea, skin reactions and headache following omeprazole therapy. Curr Probl 1991;31.
59. Langman MJS. Omeprazole. Br Med J 1991;303:481.
60. Lamberts R, Creutzfeldt W, Strüber HS et al. Long-term omeprazole therapy in peptic ulcer disease; gastrin, endocrine cell growth, and gastritis. Gastroenterology 1993;104:1356—1370.
61. Littman A. Potent acid reduction and risk of enteric infection. Lancet 1990;335:222.
62. Lesur G, Paupard T, Turner L et al. Mycose oesophagienne au décours d'un traitment par l'oprémazole. Gastroenterol Clin Biol 1993;17:598.
63. Raoul JL, Bretagne JF, Ropert A et al. Zollinger-Ellison syndrome, antisecretory treatment and body weight. Dig Dis Sci 1992;37:1308—1309.
64. Rudelli A, Leduc I, Traulle C et al. Thrombopénie survenue après traitement par oméprazole. Press Méd 1993; 20:966.
65. Cohen AF, Kroon R, Schoemaker HC et al. Effect of gastric acidity on the bioavailability of digoxin. Evidence for a new mechanism for interactions with omeprazole. Br J Clin Pharmacol 1991;31:565P.
66. Fakir M, Saison C, Wong T et al. Septicemia due to Yersinia enterocolitica in a hemodialyzed iron-depleted patient receiving omeprazole and oral iron supplementation. Am J Kidney Dis 1992;19:282—284.
67. Colin-Jones DG. Safety of lansoprazole. Aliment Pharmacol Ther 1993;7(Suppl 1):56—60.
68. Londong W, Londong V, Federle C. Pharmacokinetic and pharmacodynamic studies in man simulating acute and chronic treatment with oral pirenzepine. Eur J Clin Pharmacol 1989;36:369.
69. Werner S, Brismar K, Olsson S. Hyperprolactinemia and liquorice. Lancet 1979;i:319.
70. Leung MCT, Henderson IS, Halls DJ et al. Aluminium hydroxide versus sucralfate as a phosphate binder in uraemia. Br Med J 1989;286:1379.
71. Anderson W, Weatherston C, Veal C. Esophageal medication bezoar in a patient receiving enteral feedings and sucralfate. Am J Gastroenterol 1989;84:205.
72. Pellegrini R. Clinical effects of trithiozine, a newer gastric antisecretory agent. J Int Med Res 1979;7:452.
73. Persson CGA. Ipecacuanha asthma: more lessons. Thorax 1991;46:467—468.
74. Dukes MNG. The paradox of clioquinol and SMON. In: D'Arcy PF, Griffin JP, eds. Iatrogenic Diseases, Update 1981. Oxford—New York—Toronto: Oxford University Press, 1981;105.
75. Chetley A. Problem Drugs. London and Atlantic Highlands: Zed Books, 1995;62—68.
76. Schwart RH, Rodriguez WJ. Toxic delirium possibly caused by loperamide. J Pediatr 1991;118:656—657.
77. Chow CB, Li SH, Leung NK. Loperamide associated necrotising enterocolitis. Arch Paediatr Scand 1986;75:1034.
78. Chetley A. Not for children. In: Chetley A, ed. Problem Drugs. London and Atlantic Highlands: Zed Books, 1995.
79. Meyers AM, Feldman C, Sonnekus MI et al. Chronic laxative abusers with pseudo-idiopathic oedema and autonomous pseudo-Bartter's syndrome. South Afr Med J 1990;78:631—636.
80. Anon. Liquid paraffin—restricted indications and availability. Int Pharm J 1990;4:205.
81. Shelley WB, Schlappner OLA, Heis HB. Demonstration of intercellular immunofluorescence and epidermal hysteresis in bullous fixed drug eruption due to phenolphthalein. Br J Dermatol 1972;86:118.
82. Collinson PO, Burroughs AK. Severe hypermagnesemia due to magnesium sulphate enemas in patients with hepatic coma. Br Med J 1986;293:1013.
83. Pettersson T, Gripenberg M, Molander G et al. Severe immunological reaction induced by sulfasalazine. Br J Rheumatol 1990;59:239.
84. Armentia L, Mar A, Ramos Dias F. Toxicidad pulmonar inducida por salazosulfapiridina. Farm Clin 1989;6:275.

85. Leino R, Liipo K, Ekfors T. Sulphasalazine-induced reversible hypersensitivity pneumonitis and fatal fibrosing alveolitis; report of two cases. J Intern Med 1991;229:553–556.
86. Hamadeh MA, Atkinson J, Smith LJ. Sulfasalazine-induced pulmonary disease. Chest 1992;101:1033–1037.
87. Merrin P, Williams IA. Meningitis associated with sulphasalazine in a patient with Sjögren's syndrome and polyarthritis. Ann Rheum Dos 1991;50:645–646.
88. Guilleman F, Aussebat R, Guerci A et al. Fatal agranulocytosis in sulfasalazine treated rheumatoid arthritis. J Rheumatol 1989;16:1166.
89. Pirmohamed M, Coleman MD, Hussain F et al. Direct and metabolism dependent toxicity of sulphasalazine and its principal metabolites towards human erythrocytes and leucocytes. Br J Clin Pharmacol 1991;32:303.
90. Gabazza EC, Taguchi O, Yamakami T et al. Pulmonary infiltrates and skin pigmentation associated with sulfasalazine. Am J Gastroenterol 1992;87:1654–1657.
91. Dwarakanath AD, Michael J, Allan RD. Sulphasalazine induced renal failure. Gut 1992;33:1006–1007.
92. Ireland A, Jewell DP. Sulfasalazine-induced impotence: a beneficial resolution with olsalazine. J Clin Gastroenterol 1989;11:711.
93. Anon. Asacol: mesalazine for ulcerative colitis. Drug Ther Bull 1986;24:38.
94. De Franchis R, Vecchi M, Carpinelli L et al. Comparison of the efficacy and safety of sulphasalazine and mesalazine in the maintenance treatment of ulcerative colitis; a meta-analysis. Eur J Gastroenterol Hepatol 1993;5:505–510.
95. Dent MT, Ganapathy S, Holdsworth CD et al. Mesalazine induced lupus-like syndrome. Br Med J 1992;305:159.
96. Kristensen KS, Hoegholm A, Bohr L et al. Fatal myocarditis associated with mesalazine. Lancet 1991;335:605.
97. Reinoso MA, Schroeder KW, Pisani RJ. Lung disease associated with orally administered mesalazine for ulcerative colitis. Chest 1992;101:1469–1471.
98. Sachedina B, Saihil F Cohen LB et al. Acute pancreatitis due to 5-aminosalicylate. Ann Intern Med 1989;110:490.
99. UK Committee on Safety of Medicines. Nephrotoxicity associated with mesalazine (Asacol). Curr Probl 1990;30.
100. Meyers S, Sachar DB, Present DH et al. Olsalazine sodium in the treatment of ulcerative colitis among patients intolerant of sulfasalazine. A prospective, randomised, placebo-controlled double blind dose ranging clinical trial. Gastroenterology 1987;93:1255.
101. Pratt DS, Kaplan MM. Abdominal pain after taking ursodiol. New Engl J Med 1993;328:1502.
102. Shustak A, Noseworth TW, Johnson RG. Noncardiogenic pulmonary edema during intrabiliary infusion of monooctanoin. Crit Care Med 1986;214:659.
103. Hejka AG, Poquette M, Wiebe DA et al. Fatal intravenous injection of monoctanoin. Am J Forensic Med Pathol 1990;11:165–170.
104. Atkinson SW, Young Y, Trotter GA. Treatment with activated charcoal complicated by gastrointestinal obstruction requiring surgery. Br Med J 1992;305:563.

Meyler's Side Effects of Drugs, 13th Edition
M.N.G. Dukes, editor

SECTION EDITOR: C.B.M. TESTER-DALDERUP

Thierry Vial and Jacques Descotes

37 Drugs acting on the immune system

THERAPEUTIC CYTOKINES

Cytokines and growth factors are proteins produced in minute quantities by various cells to regulate a variety of physiological processes, particularly in the immune system and hematopoietic system (1[R]). Cytokines and growth factors are also involved in the pathophysiology of many human diseases, and their potential use as therapeutic agents is being actively investigated for the treatment of cancer, immunodepression and infectious diseases (2[R], 3[R]). Recombinant technology has been successfully used to produce sufficient quantities of cytokines and growth factors to conduct clinical trials (4[R], 5[R]).

Because of their pleiotropic effects and because doses far greater than the amount naturally released in man are administered to patients, a wide spectrum of side-effects have been described. Some of these side-effects are expected, in that they are related to the biological activities of cytokines and growth factors, but several side-effects are unexpected. With the rapidly progressing field of cytokine therapy, new side-effects are described nearly each day and this Chapter is an attempt to provide an updated review of recognized or potential side-effects associated with cytokine and growth factor therapy.

INTERFERONS (IFNs)

Three types of naturally occurring IFNs, which differ both structurally and antigenically, are used in the clinic. IFN-α and IFN-β share 30—40% of sequence homology. They exert antiviral and antiproliferative activities. IFN-γ, produced by activated T cells and natural killer cells, is recognized by a different receptor and acts primarily as an immunoregulatory cytokine. Although IFNs have been approved in a limited number of indications (6[R]), a wide range of viral diseases or cancers are candidates for IFN therapy (7[r]).

Interferon-α (IFN-α)

IFN-α is used as purified natural leukocyte or lymphoblastoid human IFN, or as recombinant preparations, via subcutaneous, intramuscular, or intravenous routes. Trade name and approved indications are indicated in Table 1. Several other antitumoral and antiviral uses of IFN-α, as well as their combination with cytotoxic agents and other cytokines, are still under investigation (8—10[R]). Relatively low doses (1—10 MU/day) are now used in most indications, except in Kaposi's sarcoma which requires high doses (≥20 MU/m^2/day) for antitumoral efficacy. Although the half-life is only 4—5 hours, biological activities extend for 2—3 days after administration. Toxicities of IFN-α have mostly been reported via systemic administration, and intranasal use has not been associated with more frequent adverse effects compared to placebo (11[c]). The pharmacokinetics, pharmacological activities and therapeutic use of IFN-α have recently been reviewed (12[R]).

GENERAL TOXICITY

Whatever the dose, virtually all patients experience a flu-like syndrome, namely fever, tachycardia, chills, headache, arthralgias and myalgias (13[R]). Although the severity increases with the dose, the flu-like syndrome is rarely dose-limiting. Tachyphylaxis usually occurs after 1 week of treatment, but isolated cases have involved IFN-α in late febrile reactions (14[c], 15[c]).

ORGANS AND SYSTEMS

Cardiovascular Dose-dependent cardiovascular effects, namely hypotension or hypertension, benign sinusal tachycardia or supraventricular tachycardia, and distal cyanosis, have been experienced by 5—15% of patients within the first days of treatment (13[R], 16[R]).

Severe cardiotoxicity was rarely described and included atrioventricular block, life-threatening ventricular arrhythmias, asymptomatic or symptomatic myocardial ischemia or even infarction and sudden death (17—19[R]). No clear relationship with the dose or the age

Table 1 *Type of interferons and indications*

Generic name and trade name	Indications
IFN-α	
Human natural leucocyte (IFN-$\alpha n3$: Alferon N®) or lymphoblastoid IFN-α (IFN-$\alpha n1$: Wellferon®)	*Malignant diseases*: hairy cell leukemia, Kaposi's sarcoma, diffuse melanoma, renal cell carcinoma, chronic myelogenous leukemia
Recombinant preparations (rIFN-α_{2a}: Roferon®, rIFN-α_{2b}: Intron A®, rIFN-α_{2c}: Berofor®)	*Viral diseases*: condylomata acuminata, chronic active hepatitis B and C
IFN-β	
Natural fibroblast (Fiblaferon®)	*Multiple sclerosis*
Recombinant preparation (INF-β_{1b}: Betaseron®)	
INF-γ	
Recombinant preparation (IFN-γ_{1b}: Actimmune ®)	*Chronic granulomatous disease*

could be found, but most cases were observed in patients with pre-existing heart disease or previous doxorubicin exposure. Anecdotal reports of severe but reversible dilated cardiomyopathy have been described after high-dose IFN-α treatment in patients without prior evidence of cardiac disease (20—24[C]). Irreversible congestive cardiomyopathy was however reported in a patient with previous doxorubicin treatment (25[C]). The possible role of IFN-α and IFN-γ in the development of progressive right ventricular heart failure with confirmed pulmonary hypertension has also been discussed (26[C]).

Patients with a previous history of arrhythmias, coronary disease or cardiac dysfunction, should be considered at high risk of developing cardiac toxicity. Careful cardiac assessment is thus mandated before treatment and this was recently highlighted in a prospective study of 11 patients receiving low-dose IFN-α (27[C]). Forty-five percent of the patients experienced a reversible reduction in left ventricular ejection of more than 10%, which might be critical in patients with existing cardiac dysfunction. Finally, the combination of high-dose interleukin-2 (IL-2) with IFN-α was found to enhance cardiovascular complications, namely cardiac ischemia and ventricular dysfunction (28—30[C]).

Respiratory The occurrence of interstitial pneumonia associated with IFN-α was recently described in patients with chronic hepatitis (31—34[C]), chronic myeloid leukemia (35, 36[C]) or renal cell carcinoma (37[C]). One patient experienced interstitial pneumonia, hemolytic anemia and cholestatic liver dysfunction (38[C]). IFN-α was also suspected to be involved in one case of biopsy-proven bronchiolitis obliterans organizing pneumonia (39[C]). Overall, clinical symptoms appeared 3—12 weeks after the onset of IFN-α therapy. In all reported cases, except one (31[C]), symptoms completely resolved after IFN-α discontinuation, spontaneously or after a short corticosteroid treatment. Diffuse pulmonary interstitial fibrosis was also attributed to the combination of IFN-α with piroxicam in one patient (40[C]). Most reported cases were described in Japanese patients who also commonly use herbal remedies, so that the causal relationship between interstitial pneumonia and IFN-α treatment awaits further confirmation from Western countries. Although most patients have received at least 18 MU/week, an immune-mediated pulmonary toxicity involving activation of T-cell immune functions is possible.

Nervous system Reports describing the clinical relevance of neuropsychiatric effects associated with IFN-α have been increasing over the years.

The most frequently reported symptoms, namely headache, fatigue and weakness, malaise, drowsiness and memory disorders were observed concomitantly with the flu-like syndrome and usually disappeared after the first injections (41[R]). Severe symptoms including significant weight loss, marked somnolence or lethargy, frank encephalopathy with visual hallucinations, dementia, delirium, ataxia and sometimes coma, have been reported only in patients receiving very high doses (42[C]). Other neurological side-effects included vertigo, cramps, apraxia, tremor and dizziness (43, 44[C]).

Neurobehavioral symptoms were among the most frequent treatment-limiting toxicities and appeared either subacutely in patients receiving high doses or more insidiously during the first 3 months of treatment in those receiving low doses (45[C], 46[R], 47[c], 48[C]). Behavioral and emotional changes included psychomotor slowing, hypersomnia, loss of interest, lack of spontaneity, affective disorders, depression or mania, irritability, agitation and aggressiveness (47, 48). Cognitive impairment included visuospatial disorientation, attentional deficits and lack of concentration, abnormalities in immediate memory recall, slurred speech, difficulties in reading and changes in handwriting. Cerebral changes on EEG have confirmed the organic nature of the psychiatric disturbances, with slowing of dominant α rhythm in the frontal lobes and occasional appearance of diffuse δ or intermittent θ activity (43, 49[C]). This pattern of psychometric changes is identical whatever the dose, but the severity of symptoms is typically dose- and schedule-related (41). Neuropsychiatric symptoms usually resolved following discontinuation of treatment or lowering of the dose, but a retrospective evaluation has suggested the presence of a protracted neurotoxicity, namely impaired memory, deficits in motor coordination and frontal lobe executive functions, parkinson-like tremor and mild dementia (50[C]).

Depressive disorders and confusion has recently appeared as a major reason for treatment discontinuation. The incidence of depression increased with the duration of treatment from 14% of patients during the first weeks up to 39% after 12—28 weeks of treatment (47[c]). Suicidal ideation or suicidal attempt has been reported (47[c], 51[C]) but its incidence or the excess risk related to IFN-α treatment has not yet been carefully determined. Fluoxetine and nortriptyline were both suggested to alleviate depressive symptoms (52, 53[C]). Controlled trials are required to clarify these effects.

The frequency of neuropsychiatric symptoms varied from 7 to 17% and up to 35% when minor or subclinical manifestations detected only by neuropsychological tests are also included (47[c], 48[C]). Although intraventricular IFN-α, chemo-immunotherapy, previous or concomitant cranial irradiation, asymptomatic brain metastases, pre-existing intracerebral arteriosclerosis, cerebral atrophy, previous organic brain injury, or drug and alcohol abuse, have all been suggested as risk factors to develop neuropsychiatric symptoms (48[C], 54[C], 55[C], 56[c], 57[C], 58[C]), no specific predictive medical profile has yet been identified. A recent non-controlled study performed in patients with active psychiatric disease has shown that most patients tolerated IFN-α under strict psychiatric surveillance and maintenance of psychotropic drugs (59[C]). The mechanisms underlying neurotoxicity were supposedly the result of an IFN-α effect on fronto-subcortical functions (45, 50). IFN-α induced a direct vascular effect, alterations of neuroendocrine hormone production, modifications of the dopaminergic pathways, or an effect mediated by secondary cytokine release (IL-1, IL-2, TNF), were all suggested to be involved (41, 46).

Other severe neurological symptoms have only been recorded as single case reports. Seizures were described during clinical trials using high doses of IFN-α, but generalized tonic clonic convulsions and status epilepticus have also appeared in several patients receiving intermediate or low doses (60—62[C]). Dose-related distal paresthesias occurred in as much as 7% of patients (13). Acute and reversible peripheral neuropathy was however documented in only very few patients receiving low doses for chronic myeloid leukemia (63—65[C]). The role of IFN-α was confirmed by prompt recurrence after re-administration, but dose reduction was sometimes sufficient to alleviate symptoms (65). Reversible acute axonal polyneuropathy after IFN-α for chronic hepatitis C has also been reported (66[C]). Other isolated and non-confirmed neurological side effects included trigeminal sensory neuropathy (67[c]), bilateral neuralgic amyotrophy (68[C]), permanent mild spastic diplegia (69[C]), and symptoms suggestive of leuko-encephalopathy (70[C]).

Endocrine, metabolic Since the first reports of thyroid disorders in patients receiving long-term therapy with leukocyte-derived IFN-α (71[C]), numerous investigators have reported thyroid disorders induced by different IFN sources in patients treated for chronic viral hepatitis (72—83[C]), solid tumours (84, 85[C]) or hematological malignancies (86, 87[C]). Hyperthyroidism, hypothyroidism and biphasic thyroiditis were reported to occur after 2—6 months of treatment, and occasionally after the cessation of treatment (78). Antithyroid hormone antibodies have also been found in one patient and this could be the cause of erroneously elevated thyroid hormone levels (88[C]). Although, not enough data are available on the long-term consequences of IFN-α-induced thyroid dysfunction, all affected patients recovered normal thyroid function within 1.5 years after IFN-α withdrawal in a study involving 68 patients (73). However, long-term substitutive treatment was needed in some patients with severe and sustained hypothyroidism despite IFN-α discontinuation (74, 78, 79, 82, 89[C]). The management of clinical thyroid dysfunction still needs to be clarified. Discontinuation of IFN-α was not always required in patients with hypothyroidism and thyroxine replacement was often sufficient (85). By contrast, hyperthyroidism would probably require the prompt withdrawal of IFN-α.

The estimated incidence of thyroiditis varied largely because the follow-up duration, the nature of the study (prospective or retrospective), and the biological monitoring, differed from one study to another (90[R]). Furthermore, the underlying disease may also play a role, as recently illustrated in two Italian prospective studies to evaluate the incidence of thyroid disorders. Only 5% of patients treated for hematological malignancies during a mean time of 15.9 months, developed autoantibodies, and none had clinical thyroid disorders (91[C]). By contrast, a 34.3% incidence of hypo- or hyperthyroidism was found in patients treated during 12 months for chronic active hepatitis C, as compared to 3.7% in patients treated for chronic active hepatitis B (92[C]). Overall, investigators found that the incidence was 1—2% in patients treated for chronic hepatitis B, ranged from 5 to 10% in patients treated for chronic hepatitis

C, and was 10—45% in cancer patients (90[R]). Hypothyroidism was found to be more frequent in cancer patients, while hyperthyroidism and hypothyroidism were both equally observed in patients treated for chronic hepatitis. Even more impressive was the escalating incidence of thyroid disorders in patients receiving both IFN-α and IL-2 (see 'Interleukin-2').

Gender is not a significant risk factor for developing thyroid disorders (82). The duration of IFN-α therapy has been suggested as a risk factor while no clear relation has been found with dose regimen (73, 78, 86). Finally, the incidence of thyroid disease was not different between natural or recombinant IFN-α (76[c], 85, 90). The most relevant risk factor in developing thyroid disorders was the presence of thyroid peroxidase antibodies before IFN-α treatment (82). De novo occurrence of thyroid autoantibodies during treatment was also frequently noted in patients who further developed thyroid dysfunction. In any case, most authors now agree that the assay of thyroid antibodies before treatment, and a regular assessment of TSH levels in treated patients, are useful to predict the risk of thyroid disorders.

The mechanism of IFN-α-induced thyroid disorders is not fully established. The presence of thyroid antibodies at the time of diagnosis strongly supports an autoimmune cause. However, in some cases, thyroid antibodies were not detected (85, 86), and a direct influence of IFN-α on TSH release, a direct IFN-α- or a secondary cytokine-mediated cytotoxicity on thyrocytes (86) were suggested to be involved. Studies in healthy volunteers have shown that a single IFN-α injection significantly decreases TSH level (50% suppression) and slightly decreases thyroid hormone levels (93[C]). In vitro studies also argue for a direct inhibitory effect of IFN-α on human thyrocyte functions at clinically observable levels (94[C]).

The development of insulin-dependent diabetes mellitus (IDDM) has been reported in cancer or chronic hepatitis patients after IFN-α treatment (95—100[C]). That IDDM improved or resolved after IFN-α discontinuation in several patients is in keeping with the role of IFN-α (97—99). Again, an autoimmune mechanism has been suggested as several patients had HLA-DR4 haplotype and islet cell antibodies (ICA) at the time of diagnosis (96, 98, 100). However, the induction of ICA antibodies in IFN-α-treated patients has never been otherwise demonstrated (77, 101, 102[C]). It has also been suggested that IFN-α may accelerate the destruction of stimulated β-cells via the induction of insulin resistance (103), and that it was a possible mechanism in patients with diabetes without islet cell antibodies (95, 97). This is also in keeping with the induction or exacerbation of type 2 diabetes mellitus in two patients (104, 105[C]). More recently, the occurrence of IgE and IgG insulin antibodies associated with signs of insulin allergy was reported in an IDDM patient after 6 weeks of treatment (106[C]).

Isolated reports have suggested that IFN-α may be the cause of biological hypoparathyroidism (107[C]) and reversible hypopituitarism with pituitary antibody for GH_3 cells, suggesting an autoimmune mechanism (108[C]).

That IFNs affected lipid metabolism has been known for a long time, and a reversible decreases in plasma cholesterol or increases in triglyceride levels have consistently been found (109, 110[C], 111[cR]). Further studies identified hypertriglyceridemia as the major metabolic consequence of IFN-α in the setting of cancer or chronic hepatitis treatment (112—114[C]). Very severe, but reversible hypertriglyceridemia upon treatment discontinuation were sometimes observed, with plasma levels over 10 g/l (114—117[C]) and even 19.8 g/l in one case (118[C]). An IFN-α-mediated suppression of hepatic triglyceride lipase has been suggested (117). Diet and lipid-lowering drugs have been proposed to maintain acceptable triglyceride levels during long-term IFN-α therapy (115, 118). No clinical consequences of hypertriglyceridemia has been reported to date, but a risk of acute pancreatitis should be borne in mind.

Neuroendocrine effects observed in patients treated with IFN-α included a reversible stimulation of the hypothalamic-pituitary adrenal axis with a marked increase in cortisol and adrenocorticotrophic hormone secretion (119, 120[C]). Prolactin and growth hormone secretion were not significantly affected following acute or subacute administration of IFN-α (120, 121[C]). However, the rate of growth was significantly lower than predicted in 35% of pediatric patients receiving long-term treatment for recurrent respiratory papillomatosis (122[c]), and growth retardation was also recently reported in a female patient during a 3-year treatment (123[C]).

Mineral and fluid balance Several hydroelectrolytic disturbances and a syndrome resembling inappropriate antidiuretic hormone secretion was described following high-dose IFN-α (124[C]). Severe hyponatremia attributed to an inappropriate secretion of antidiuretic hormone was recently reported (125[C]).

Hematological Hematological toxicity commonly included dose-related leukopenia, neutropenia and thrombopenia, while anemia has been rarely observed (126[C]). In a recent trial in patients with chronic hepatitis C, severe neutropenia (<900 leukocytes/mm^3) and thrombopenia (<49 000/mm^3) were observed in 20 and 10% of patients, respectively, and was sometimes treatment limiting (127[c]). In a survey of 11 241 patients treated for chronic viral hepatitis, life-threatening neutropenia or thrombopenia were reported in six patients only (128[c]). Possible risk factors for severe hematological toxicity include cirrhosis and hypersplenism. Pancytopenia or aplasia, sometimes fatal, have been reported only in patients who had received previous chemotherapy (129—132[C]). Severe and even fatal erythrocytosis during low-dose IFN-α therapy for hairy cell leukemia has been described in several patients (133[C]).

Immune-mediated thrombocytopenia resembling idiopathic thrombocytopenic purpura has been observed (134—136[C]) as well as reversible cases of positive direct Coombs' test with or without clinical hemolysis (137—139[C]). A mechanism close to that observed with α-methyldopa was suggested to be involved in IFN-α-induced autoimmune hemolytic anemia (138), but Coomb's-negative hemolytic anemias were also reported (140—141). Although sometimes used in the treatment of idiopathic thrombocytopenic purpura (ITP), a dramatic worsening of thrombopenia and severe or even fatal bleeding has been described in several patients (142—144[C]).

IFN-α treatment might also induce multiple antibody formation to transfused blood cell antigens with subsequent massive hemolysis (145[C]). The development of an anti-factor VIII autoantibody in one hemophiliac (146[C]) and in one non-hemophiliac patient diagnosed as acquired hemophilia with subsequent fatal hemorrhage (147[C]) was also considered as a possible consequence of IFN-α therapy.

Isolated cases of venous thrombosis have been observed (148[C]). Recently, Becker et al. reported the development of antiphospholipid antibodies (APA) in 40% of patients treated with IFN-α alone or IFN-α plus IL-2 (149[C]). Prolongation of the partial thromboplastin time and venous thrombosis were observed in 80% of APA-positive patients. The causative role of IFN-α was suggested by the absence of APA in similar patients treated with IL-2 alone or not receiving immunotherapy. This is also in keeping with previous reports of reversible coagulation abnormalities in patients receiving high-dose continuous IFN-α (150[C]).

Liver An asymptomatic and reversible rise in liver transaminases has been reported in 25—30% of patients receiving high-dose IFN-α (151[cR]). In the treatment of chronic hepatitis B, HBe seroconversion is sometimes preceded by a moderate worsening of serum aminotransferase levels (152[c]), but unusually severe exacerbation of chronic hepatitis B infection and fatal liver failure occurred (153—155[C]). Such fatalities were reported in nine patients among 2490 treated for chronic viral hepatitis (156[c]).

More disturbing are the reports of acute revelation or exacerbation of latent chronic autoimmune hepatitis in IFN-α-treated patients (157—162[C]). Further analysis has demonstrated that these patients were initially misdiagnosed as having seronegative chronic viral hepatitis and reversible autoimmune hepatitis was later proven to be the correct diagnosis. The reversibility of acute liver injury after corticosteroid treatment further support an exacerbation of a latent autoimmune process. IFN-α-induced exacerbation of autoimmune chronic active hepatitis was also reported in patients with unequivocal chronic hepatitis C (164, 165[C]) and this has posed the question of how to recognize at-risk patients (166[r]). Only the sudden increase in alanine aminotransferase levels appeared to be a marker of this event, while the systematic detection of autoantibodies failed to predict the risk of autoimmune hepatitis (164). In patients presenting with both hepatitis C virus positivity and autoantibodies, corticosteroid therapy has been considered as first line treatment. Among six patients with LKM-1 antibody and hepatitis C virus RNA-positive serum, IFN-α was beneficial in three, while the three other patients developed prompt increase in transaminase levels (163[C]). Interestingly, a HLA-B51, DR2 and DQ1 haplotype was found in the three latter patients. The possibility of a de novo induction rather than exacerbation of autoimmune hepatitis has only been suggested in isolated reports, including three patients with chronic hepatitis B or C (167—169[C]) and in one patient with chronic myeloid leukemia (170[C]). Such a rare event is in keeping with the lack of autoantibodies linked to autoimmune liver disease among IFN-α-treated patients (101, 102, 171[C]). IFN-α induced unexplained acute exacerbation of liver disease in one chronic hepatitis C patient (172[C]) and severe liver failure in two leukaemia patients (173, 174[C]) also suggested a direct hepatotoxicity.

Gastrointestinal Gastrointestinal disorders, namely nausea, vomiting, diarrhea or anorexia were observed in 30—40% of patients and their severity is typically dose-dependent (16[R], 150[c]). Transient taste or smell alterations, and dryness or inflammation of oropharynx, were also sometimes reported (16, 43). The occurrence or exacerbation of ulcerative colitis has been described in isolated cases (83[C], 175, 176[C]) as has a severe case of painful oral ulcerations recurring after IFN-α re-administration (177[C]). Asymptomatic elevation of the pancreatic enzymes (178[C]) and acute pancreatitis (179[C]), both of which reversed after IFN-α withdrawal, were reported in one patient with no mention of hypertriglyceridemia.

Urinary system Mild and usually clinically not significant proteinuria, leukocyturia, hematuria or moderate increases in serum creatinine levels were observed in 15—25% of patients (151[R]). In patients with multiple myeloma receiving high-dose IFN-α, severe proteinuria and nephrotic syndrome were sometimes noted (180[C]). A deterioration of glomerular and tubular renal function was found in most IFN-α-treated patients assessed prospectively with a number of renal function markers (181[C]).

Acute renal insufficiency has been rarely described and was mostly reported in patients with underlying renal disease (182, 183[C]), in those receiving high-dose IFN-α (184—186[C]) or patients treated either for multiple myeloma (187—189[C]) or chronic myelogenous leukemia (190—192[C]). Pathological findings in IFN-α-induced renal disorders included nephrotic syndrome with minimal change nephropathy and acute tubulointerstitial nephritis (184, 186), nephrotic syndrome with severe glomerular changes (190—192), membrano-proliferative glomerulonephritis (185), extracapillary glomerulonephritis with crescents (191), and acute tubular necrosis (187). Although renal dysfunction usually resolved after IFN-α withdrawal, irreversible alteration or incomplete resolution of renal function were occasionally noted (182, 183, 186, 188, 190). In several cases, the role of concomitant NSAIDs therapy could not be completely excluded. According to several investigators, the mechanism of nephrotoxicity may have involved a direct nephrotoxic effect (187, 191), a T-cell-mediated immune effect (184, 186), an immune-complex renal disease (185) or an autoimmune etiology (190).

Reports of acute renal insufficiency have also recently been attributed to the consequence of IFN-α induced hemolytic-uremic syndrome (193, 194[C]) or renal thrombotic microangiopathy (195[C]).

Skin and appendages A wide range of skin lesions, namely skin dryness, rash, diffuse erythema or urticaria has been reported in 5—12% of patients (13[R]). Reversible alopecia secondary to telogen effluvium appeared as a frequent complication. It was noted in 7% (196[c]) up to 23—30% of patients (197[C]) receiving various types of IFN-α, and sometimes reversed despite continuation of treatment. Excessive growth of eyelashes has also been reported (198, 199[C]).

Subcutaneous IFN-α administration sometimes induced local erythema or skin induration, but isolated reports have described the occurrence of more severe reactions, ranging from inflammatory painful nodules (200[C]) to local ulcerations and frank necrosis at sites of IFN-α injections (201—204[C]). Regular change in the area of injection is thus strongly recommended. A localized intradermic bullous eruption which recurred following each IFN-α injection was also reported (205[C]).

Leukocytoclastic vasculitis was rarely noted (85[c], 206[C]). Digital vasculitis (207[C]) and angiographic confirmed digital artery occlusion (208[C]) have appeared as isolated reports and could have been related to a paradoxal angiogenic effect of IFN-α (209[C]).

Since the first report of induction or exacerbation of psoriasis in cancer patients treated with high-dose IFN-α (210[C]), which was followed by a controversial debate (211, 212), several investigators have confirmed that IFN-α may either induce clinically and histologically typical psoriasis or worsen preexisting psoriasis (213—220[C]). This was particularly exemplified by the reversibility of the lesions after the cessation of treatment and the prompt recurrence of symptoms following IFN-α re-administration (214—217). While symptoms usually developed within the first month in patients with previous psoriasis, lesions were observed after a minimum of 2—3 months of treatment in patients without psoriasis history. Psoriatic lesions at the sites of injection was suggested as a potential indication for further generalization of psoriasis (213, 214, 216). More disturbing cases involved the concomitant development of mono- or polyarticular joint symptoms (214—218). Pustular psoriasis with balanitis and erosive monoarthritis in one HLA-B27 patient suggesting an incomplete Reiter's syndrome was reported also (221[C]).

More recently, numerous reports described the occurrence or the exacerbation of lichen planus in IFN-α-treated patients (222—230[C]). Although most patients had received IFN-α for chronic hepatitis C, suggesting a possible causal role of hepatitis C virus infection, the association of this disease with a high incidence of lichen planus remains debated (231[c]). Furthermore, recurrence of the lesions following IFN-α re-administration (230) or cases of lichen planus in cancer patients (232[C], 233[CR]) strongly argue for a direct causal link with IFN-α treatment. Local treatment and PUVA-therapy were sometimes sufficient to alleviate symptoms (222, 230), but the discontinuation of IFN-α was required in most severe cases (223, 227, 228).

Other dermatological immune or autoimmune diseases included single cases of bullous pemphigus and pemphigoid with circulating pemphigus-like autoantibodies (234[C]), pemphigus foliaceus with anti-intercellular IgG antibodies (235[C]) and paraneoplastic pemphigus (236[C]). Although not previously reported in malignant melanoma patients receiving IFN-α alone, the occurrence of vitiligo was recently attributed to the combination of IFN-α with piroxicam in one responder (40[c]).

Special senses Recent reports highlighted the risk of neurosensorial manifestations. Ten cases of reversible retinal disorders have been reported and consisted of cotton-wool spots in all cases, retinal capillary non-perfusion, arteriolar occlusions, retinal edema and hemorrhages in several other patients (237[C]). Visual loss was observed in one patient only. Further prospective ophthalmological investigations have confirmed these findings and revealed asymptomatic and reversible retinopathy and subconjunctival hemorrhage in 38% of non-diabetic patients (238[C]). It was suggested that retinal hemorrhage could be predicted on the basis of high C5a levels (239[C]). Other reports described the occurrence of transient bilateral decrease of vision without ocular vascular disorders (240[C]) or sudden onset of severe ocular pain with exophthalmos and irreversible visual loss (241[C]). Optic tract neuropathy with blurring of vision (242[C]), cortical blindness and fatal encephalopathy (243[C]), mononeural abducent nerve paralysis (244[C]) and complete reversible bilateral oculomotor nerve paralysis (245[C]) were also described.

A recent prospective study assessed auditory functions in 49 patients treated with IFN-α or IFN-β for chronic viral hepatitis and found tinnitus, hearing loss or both disorders in 8, 16 and 20% of patients, respectively (246[C]). These disorders tended to occur more frequently in patients on high cumulative doses, but led to treatment discontinuation in only two patients, and completely reversed after discontinuation of treatment.

Musculoskeletal system Musculoskeletal toxicity has already been noted and included mostly severe muscle pains. A recent report of symptomatic myopathy developing in a patient treated for chronic hepatitis C suggested that a possible exacerbation of latent muscular disorders may occur as a consequence of IFN-α treatment because of persistent biological myopathic abnormalities (247[C]). One case of polymyositis reversible upon IFN-α discontinuation has also been described (248[C]), as well as the occurrence of severe necrotic myopathy shortly after IFN-α was instituted (249[C]). In the latter case, the myopathy was associated with severe bullous lesions and the patient died. Finally, a direct muscular toxicity of IFN-α was suggested by the report of acute rhabdomyolysis after IFN-α dose was increased (250[C]).

Sexual function Decreased libido, usually observed together with various neuropsychiatric symptoms, and reversible cases of impotence have been reported anecdotally (128[c], 251[C]). Interestingly, gonadal toxicity or sexual dysfunction have not been found in a clinical and biological prospective monitoring in 43 male patients treated for hairy cell leukemia compared to 33 patients receiving no systemic therapy (252). Although a decrease in serum progesterone and estradiol levels has also been noted in women (253), a decrease in fertility was not observed.

Miscellaneous The development of autoimmune disorders during IFN-α treatment has been the scope of an increasing number of papers and the spectrum of interferon-induced immune diseases is expanding year after year, including thyroiditis, diabetes, hematological disorders, systemic lupus erythematosus (SLE), rheumatoid arthritis, dermatological disease, myasthenia gravis, etc. Several of them have been previously discussed in the corresponding 'Organs and systems' section. Moreover, there is some evidence for a link between hepatitis C and several immune-mediated disease (254[R]), so that the exact role of IFN-α is often difficult to ascertain.

A number of studies in patients with malignant tumors or chronic hepatitis have investigated the presence before treatment, and the occurrence during treatment, of a wide range of autoantibodies (72—75, 77, 79—83, 101, 102, 171). Several antibodies (mostly antinuclear antibodies, parietal cell antibodies, rheumatoid factor, liver/kidney microsome antibody and smooth muscle antibodies) have been detected before any IFN-α treatment in 24.5—32% of patients and titers increased during therapy. Overall, the new occurrence of autoantibodies was observed in 4—30% of previously autoantibody-negative patients (90). They were mostly antinuclear antibodies, rheumatoid factors, smooth muscle antibodies, parietal cell antibodies, and antithyroid antibodies. A clear correlation between the development of autoantibodies and the response to IFN-α treatment has not been shown (85, 102).

The occurrence of systemic lupus erythematosus (SLE) has been described in several IFN-α-treated patients (255—261[C]), including one case with recurrence of symptoms following IFN-α re-administration (257[C]). All but one affected patient were young and had never suffered from lupus symptoms before treatment. In several cases, renal or dermatological involvement, the presence of antibodies to dsDNA or a short onset after starting treatment, the predominance of female gender, and the persistence of symptoms after IFN-α withdrawal, are more in keeping with a naturally occurring SLE unmasked in patients receiving IFN-α (258, 260, 261) than a newly interferon-caused illness. An association between HLA-A2, B7 and DR2 and interferon-related SLE suggested a genetic predisposition (257). Scleroderma and vitiligo with high levels of IL-2 and IL-6 were also described in one woman receiving both IFN-α and IL-2 (262[C]).

The reactivation or appearance of inflammatory rheumatological disorders were also consistently reported (263—266[C]) and sometimes required antimalarials or immunosuppressive drugs (263[C]). The clinical or serological features were consistent with rheumatoid arthritis or lupus-like polyarthritis, and most patients had pre-existing clinical or biological abnormalities before treatment. Other reports included seronegative polyarthritis (263[C]), acute seronegative monoarthritis of the hip (267[C]) and seropositive monoarthritis of the metatarsophalangeal of the right foot (268[C]). Wandl et al. found an unexpectedly high incidence of rheumatoid and lupus-like symptoms, namely arthralgia, arthritis, myalgia, Raynaud's phenomenon, in 19.8% of patients treated with IFN-α alone or in combination with IFN-γ (266[C]). Only a minority of affected patients fulfilled the criteria of SLE.

Reversible cases of Raynaud's phenomenon, sometimes associated with cryoglobulinemia, were reported (269, 270[C]). Although a strong correlation between cryoglobulinemia and hepatitis C has been consistently reported with a beneficial effect of IFN-α in such cases (254[R], 271[C]), several isolated reports suggested that an exacerbation of cryoglobulinemia may also be the result of IFN-α treatment (272–274[C]).

Since one brief mention of exacerbation of sarcoidosis in 1992 (266[c]), several authors have reported the occurrence of subcutaneous sarcoid nodules (277–277[C]) or generalized sarcoidosis following IFN-α (278[C]). Reversible outcome following treatment discontinuation suggests the causal involvement of IFN-α.

The occurrence of clinically and biologically confirmed myasthenia gravis after 3–5 months of IFN-α was recently described (279, 280[C]). Although long-term follow-up was not available, both pyridostigmine maintenance or persistence of anti-acetylcholine receptor antibodies were compatible with the exacerbation of an underlying disease.

IFNs exert various effects on the immune system, and both immunostimulating or immunosuppressive effects, which probably depend on the IFN dosage, can be observed. Recent reports highlighted several unexpected immunosuppressive effects of IFN-α in humans. This has been exemplified by the occurrence of severe *Candida* esophagitis in immunocompetent patients treated with IFN-α (281, 282[c]), or the development of Kaposi's sarcoma together with a decrease in CD4+ cells in a patient treated for T-cell lymphoma (283[C]). An abrupt decrease in CD4+ cells with the occurrence of opportunistic infections was also observed after IFN-α in several HIV-infected patients negative for the serum p24 antigen (284, 285[c]). An autoimmune destruction of CD4+ cells in several subjects with a particular HLA haplotype has been suggested (285[c]). Soriano et al. found such a CD4+ cell drop in four of 72 HIV-infected patients several days after beginning IFN-α for hepatitis C infection (286[c]). These potential immunosuppressive effects of IFN-α are based on limited data and no conclusion can be drawn on the presently reported association between CD4+ cell decline and IFN-α therapy.

The increased incidence of viral infections in transplant recipients has led to the consideration of use of IFN-α therapy in such patients, but the experience is still limited. In one placebo-controlled trial of prophylactic IFN-α in renal transplant recipients, a significantly higher incidence of irreversible rejection was found in IFN-α-treated patients (287[C]). Deterioration of renal function and acute rejection were later found in five of 15 patients treated for chronic viral hepatitis, while IFN-α was found to be beneficial in other patients (288[c]). In another study, IFN-α was poorly tolerated by renal transplant recipient, 20% of whom had to stop treatment and one third experienced rapid or progressive deterioration in renal function (289[c]). Finally, IFN-α for recurrent hepatitis C virus infection in liver transplant recipients is under investigation, but preliminary results have suggested an increased risk of acute rejection with histological findings of acute vanishing bile duct syndrome (290[c]).

Isolated case reports have suggested that IFN-α might enhance the incidence or severity of graft-versus-host disease (GVHD) (291, 292[c]) but conflicting results have emerged. Three of 11 patients receiving IFN-α after allogeneic transplantation developed acute GVHD (293[c]), while no difference in the likelihood or severity of GVHD was found in a randomized trial involving 40 controls and 39 patients treated with IFN-α after transplantation (294[c]). Late allograft rejection was also anecdotally observed (295[C]).

The appearance of IFN-antibodies in treated patients is a critical issue as regards the clinical application of IFN-α, and a considerable amount of investigators have reported on the characteristics, incidence and clinical significance of these antibodies (13[R], 296[R]). Both non-neutralizing antibodies, the most frequent, and neutralizing antibodies have been detected in IFN-treated patients. Titers usually increased during treatment, but a dramatic fall was mostly observed after treatment discontinuation and was sometimes even noted despite prolonged continuous treatment (297[R]). No correlation between the occurrence of autoantibodies and anti-IFN-α antibodies has so far been reported (298[R]). While antibodies to a recombinant form are able to cross-react with other recombinant IFN-α, their ability to neutralize natural species has not or seldom been documented (297[R], 299–301[C]). Furthermore, a change to natural IFN-α in patients losing therapeutic responses after rIFN-α antibody formation was successfully used in some patients (302[R], 303[R], 304[C], 305[C]), and it was suggested that neutralizing antibodies resulted from a specific immune response to the recombinant preparations (306[R]). Indeed, although a loss of therapeutic response was not found in earlier studies (307[R]), a lack of response or the reversal of clinical response were later reported in patients treated for malignancies or chronic viral hepatitis (303[R], 304[C], 305[C], 308[c], 309[C]). A large-scale study in 251 chronic hepatitis C patients recently confirmed that the clinical response to rIFN-α is significantly less in patients with neutralizing antibodies (302[R]), and it has been suggested that neutralizing antibodies in chronic hepatitis C (309, 310[C]) or chronic myelogenous leukemia (311[C]) patients mostly accounted for relapse or secondary resistance of the disease before completion of treatment. Additionally, patients showing a clinical response despite IFN-α antibody formation presented either with transient low titers or a late occurrence of neutralizing antibodies. On the other hand, neutralizing antibodies were not associated with immune complex-associated diseases or hypersensitivity reactions, and exerted no influence on IFN-α-associated side effects (312[cR]). An improvement of the flu-like syndrome was even suggested (313[c]). The clinical significance of binding antibodies is yet unknown although changes in pharmacokinetic IFN-α parameters might be expected. The rate of antibody formation differed greatly between studies, from none to more than 50% of patients, probably because of several features (i.e. the population studied and the race, the type of IFNs, the route of administration, dose regimen, duration of treatment and method of assay) have not been always taken into account when interpreting these results. IFN antibody formation has been reported to be higher in patients receiving long-term, instead of short-term, treatment, in patients receiving subcutaneous rather than intravenous IFN, and in patients receiving low rather than high doses (13[R]). A higher frequency of antibodies to rIFN-α_{2a} has repeatedly been reported as compared to other recombinant or natural IFN preparations. This difference has been nicely illustrated in a population of 296 chronic hepatitis patients receiving various preparations of IFN-α (299[C], 314[C]). Binding antibodies and neutralizing antibodies were found in 44.6 and 20.2%, respectively, of patients receiving rIFN-α_{2a} as compared to 14.6 and 6.9% of those receiving rIFN-α_{2b}, and 9.4 and 1.2% of those receiving IFN-α_{N1}. Similar significant differences in the immunogenic potential of these two recombinant IFN-α preparations were also demonstrated in 159 patients treated for chronic myelogenous leukemia (311[R]).

Hypersensitivity reactions Type I reactions have never been clearly documented in IFN-α-treated patients. One single case of contact dermatitis suggested that IFN-α_{2c} may induce a cell-mediated delayed hypersensitivity (315[C]). A recurrent anaphylactoid reaction possibly due to mast cell degranulation has been described in a patient treated for mastocytosis (316[c]).

Tumour-inducing effects The occurrence of lymphoid or myeloid malignancies has recently appeared as a possible late complication of IFN-α treatment. At the moment, isolated reports included cases of: lymphoblastic leukemia or non-Hodgkin's B-cell lymphoma in two children (317[C]), the triggering of aggressive plasma cell leukemia in two multiple myeloma patients (318, 319[C]), an early lymphoid blastic transformation in a patient treated for chronic myeloid leukemia (320[C]), one case of acute myeloid leukemia (321[C]), and the occurrence of pseudolymphoma of the liver in a patient with chronic hepatitis B infection (322[C]). A tumor-enhancing effect of IFN-α was also suspected in the development of late metastases of latent melanoma (323[C]). The causative role of IFN-α remains speculative. Similarly, the mechanisms are unclear although an effect mediated by secondary cytokine secretion, such as IL-6, or an IFN-induced cytogenetic abnormality might have been involved (324[c]).

Second-generation effects Experimental models were unable to find mutagenic or teratogenic effects of IFN-α. Clinical experience in humans is still scarce. A recent study using ex vivo placental perfusion suggested that IFN-α_{2a} does not cross the human placenta (325). Uncomplicated and successful pregnancy has been detailed in 10 patients treated for chronic myelogenous leukemia or essential thrombocythemia and have included exposure during the first 2 months in two cases and the whole pregnancy in three, while the treatment was started during the late first trimester in five (326–332[C]). Healthy babies were delivered at full-term in seven cases, premature delivery was observed at 34 weeks in one case and moderate intrauterine growth retardation occurred in two cases. Further examination of six babies up to 2 and 3 years after delivery showed normal growth or development (326–330). Although IFN-α does not seem to interfere with embryo-fetal development, safety during pregnancy still awaits to be further documented and delayed therapy of non-life-threatening disease is advisable, especially in the first trimester of pregnancy.

Interactions Because increased physiological production of IFN and experimental in vitro and in vivo data in experimental animals or human liver tissue have shown reduced activity of hepatic microsomal cytochrome P450s (333[R], 334–337), several workers have investigated the effect of IFN on probes or drugs metabolized by hepatic microsomal cytochrome P450. However, drug interaction studies in humans are still very scarce.

Single dose of IFN-α was reported to induce a mean 16% fall in antipyrine clearance and a 51% decrease in theophylline clearance in healthy volunteers or patients with chronic active hepatitis B (338–339[C]). A 3-day treatment was found to decrease the plasma clearance of theophylline in 11 healthy volunteers (340[C]). Long-term treatment produced conflicting results with significant and reversible decrease in aminopyrine breath test value during the second and fourth month of treatment (341[C]), and no change in salivary antipyrine clearance following a 2-week regimen (342[C]). A significant decrease in theophylline clearance has also been found in cancer patients on low-dose maintenance IFN-α treatment (343[C]).

One recent report also suggested that IFN-α can significantly increase serum warfarin concentration and prothrombin time (344[C]).

Reduced efficacy of human erythropoietin has been clearly documented in several patients receiving IFN-α (345, 346[C]), an effect probably mediated by IFN-α-induced suppression of erythropoiesis.

Although synergistic hematotoxicity resulted from the combination of IFN-α and zidovudine in AIDS-related Kaposi's sarcoma, this regimen has been considered relatively safe (347[R], 348[c]).

Even though IFN are increasingly used in association with other cytokines or cytotoxic drugs, no specific and unexpected adverse effects have been reported, but acute toxicity was sometimes enhanced (349[R], 350[R]). That was the case for a 5-fluorouracil (5-FU) and IFN-α combination which produced increased 5-FU serum concentrations and significantly enhanced gastrointestinal and myelosuppressive toxicities (351–353[C]). The pharmacokinetic interaction was not reproduced when folic acid was added to the regimen (351, 352), and less toxicity was found with continuous infusions of 5-FU plus folic acid and IFN-α (354[C]).

Finally, interferon-induced fever may have also increased the rate of elimination of melphalan (355[C]).

Interferon-β (IFN-β)

IFN-β, used as natural fibroblast or recombinant preparation (IFN-β_{1b}) by systemic or local administration, share similar antiviral and antiproliferative properties to IFN-α and has been approved in the treatment of multiple sclerosis (356[R], 357[R]). Other potential antiviral and antiproliferative indications are yet under investigation.

General toxicity of IFN-β is very similar to that of IFN-α (358[c]). Toxicities are dose-related and tachyphylaxis to fever and chills usually developed after several doses. On the other hand, IFN-β is considered as markedly less toxic for the central nervous system (46[R]), a suggestion which was mostly based on a prospective study assessing electrophysiological and neuropsychological functions in 22 patients receiving intravenous infusion (359[C]). However, central nervous system toxicity was sometimes reported (360[c], 361[C]) and one case of suicide was noted (358[c]).

Unexpected immune consequences of IFN-β treatment have been scarcely evaluated. Thyroid dysfunction and antithyroid antibodies were not observed in 20 patients receiving IFN-β during 24 weeks for hematological malignancies (362[C]). The possible involvement of IFN-β in asymptomatic and regressive pulmonary sarcoidosis has been discussed (363[C]). Finally, only one report described allergic contact dermatitis with positive epicutaneous patch tests in a patient using eyedrops containing IFN-β (364[C]).

Local and benign inflammatory reactions were commonly observed after subcutaneous injections. In the reference multicenter placebo-controlled trial, 65% of patients receiving IFN-β had reactions at the injection site compared to 6% in the placebo group (358). Skin necrosis appeared in eight of 38 patients receiving high-dose IFN-β, with an inverse relation between the dose and the delay of onset (365[C]); recent reports have emphasized the possibility that severe skin necrosis with focal thrombosis of deep dermal vessels after several weeks of self-injections of lower dose recombinant IFN-β_{1b} may occur (366, 367[C]). Interestingly, skin necrosis did not recur after IFN-α use. Induction of psoriatic lesions at the injection site has also been associated with subcutaneous injections of IFN-β (368[C]).

Still limited information is available on antibodies to IFN-β. The incidence of neutralizing antibodies to rIFN-β was found to be only 3.4% among 428 patients (369[C]) and reached 56% in patients receiving natural IFN-β for malignant melanoma (370[C]). Possible differences in the immunogenic potential of recombinant and natural IFN-β preparations were found in a small study (371[c]), but the clinical significance of these antibodies has not yet been clearly assessed.

Drug interactions with IFN-β have been poorly investigated and only one study reported a mean decrease of 27% in theophylline clearance in seven patients with chronic hepatitis C (372[C]).

Interferon-γ (IFN-γ)

IFN-γ is available only as recombinant (IFN-γ_{1b}) and has been approved in the treatment of chronic granulomatous disease (373[R]). Other potential immunoregulatory indications, namely rheumatoid arthritis, Behçet's disease, infectious disease or combination with other cytokines in cancer treatment are still under investigation.

Relevant information on the clinical toxicity of long-term IFN-γ treatment has been obtained from the ICGDSCG trial which revealed a mild toxicity profile with transient and tolerable side effects (374[c]). At the dose currently recommended (1.5 μg/kg or 50 $\mu g/m^2$), only mild fever and flu-like symptoms, headache and erythema at the injection site were significantly more frequent with IFN-γ_{1b} compared to placebo, the incidence of which increased with age. Although confusional episodes have sometimes been described, symptoms of neurotoxicity were usually not observed despite EEG monitoring and psychometric tests in treated patients (375[c]). However, careful examinations led to suggest that IFN-γ can induce similar neurophysiological changes to IFN-α (376[C]).

Other forms of toxicity have been reported as isolated cases or in patients receiving higher doses. Most have been reported to the manufacturer and causal evaluation is lacking (373[R]). Dose-related benign and asymptomatic proteinuria was sometimes observed (377[c]) and severe proteinuria and nephrotic syndrome was reported once after low-dose IFN-γ (378[C]). Reversible acute renal failure was attributed to IFN-γ-induced focal segmental glomerulosclerosis and acute tubular necrosis (379[C]). High-dose IFN-γ has been reported to induce several cardiovascular side-effects, namely hypotension and arrhythmia which were mostly observed in patients with previous cardiovascular disorders (19[cR], 375[c]). Heart failure and myocardial infarction have also been cited as a possible cardiac toxicity (373[R]). However, heart rate, frequency of ventricular or supraventricular ectopic beats and asymptomatic cardiac events were not significantly different during treatment compared to baseline tests in a prospective trial performed in 20 patients on IFN-γ (380[C]).

Only minimal effects of IFN-γ on the white blood cell counts have been observed (381). Asymptomatic and recurring acute hemolytic anemia without evidence of immune hemolysis was attributed to IFN-γ in one patient receiving both IL-2 and IFN-γ (382[C]). Metabolic, mineral and hormonal disturbances during treatment are limited to increased cortisol levels (383[c]) and reversible dose-dependent hypertriglyceridemia (384[c]).

Induction of psoriatic lesions at the injection site has been observed in 10 of 42 patients treated with IFN-γ for psoriatic arthritis, while joint symptoms were improved (385[c]). Single or multiple erythema nodosum leprosum was observed in 60% of patients treated for lepromatous leprosy with intradermal IFN-γ; severe systemic symptoms required thalidomide treatment in two patients (386[C]). Anaphylactoid reaction and severe bronchospasm was reported following the first injection of IFN-γ (375[c]).

Although IFN-γ is mainly used for immunoregulatory properties, the clinical immune adverse consequences of IFN-γ treatment in humans has been addressed in a limited number of studies. All eleven patients included in a 6-month study with IFN-γ were shown to develop new autoantibodies which sometimes persisted over several months after the end of treatment (387[C]). The development of autoantibodies or an increase in titers of previously positive antinuclear antibodies or smooth muscle antibodies have been reported after 16 weeks of treatment (388[C]). None of the patients studied developed clinical evidence of autoimmune disease. However, disturbing reports suggested that IFN-γ can both improve and deteriorate immune or inflammatory conditions. Although no change in antinuclear antibodies was reported in a trial of 54 patients with rheumatoid arthritis (389[c]), increased or newly developed antinuclear antibodies were observed in three of six rheumatoid arthritis patients receiving IFN-γ for 2–8 months, including two patients who experienced clinical exacerbation of the disease (390[c]). In addition, isolated cases of development (391[C]) or life-threatening exacerbation (392[C]), of systemic lupus erythematosus have been reported in patients receiving IFN-γ for rheumatoid arthritis. Rheumatoid or lupus-like symptoms associated with elevated antinuclear antibodies titers were noted in 17% of patients receiving IFN-γ and IFN-α for myeloproliferative disorders, while only 8.3% of patients treated with IFN-α alone experienced similar symptoms (266[c]). IFN-γ treatment was also involved in the induction or reactivation of sero-negative arthritis in patients treated for cutaneous psoriasis (393[C]) and the unexpected exacerbation of multiple sclerosis in 39% of patients (394[C]). Other possible deleterious effects of IFN-γ on the immune system may also include the rapid exacerbation and occurrence of multiple Kaposi's sarcoma lesions in a patient with AIDS treated for visceral leishmaniasis (395[C]).

Finally, neutralizing antibodies were not found in 334 patients receiving rIFN-γ (396[C]).

INTERLEUKINS

Interleukin-1 (IL-1)

Although IL-1α and IL-1β are produced by two distinct genes with only 25% homology, they act through the same receptor and share similar in vitro biological properties. IL-1 also acts synergistically with TNF-α to mediate sepsis and inflammation and with other colony-stimulating factors (e.g. GM-CSF, G-CSF, IL-3 or IL-6) to promote colony formation, exert direct antiproliferative activity, and stimulate hematopoietic recovery in patients undergoing autologous bone marrow transplantation or receiving cytotoxic anticancer treatment (397[R]). Both forms of IL-1 are currently under investigation.

Very similar toxicities are observed with IL-1α and IL-1β. Fever and chills, within hours after intravenous infusion (398—400[C]) or subcutaneous administration (401[c]), are quite universal, but only occasionally treatment-limiting. Tachyphylaxis may develop during prolonged administration (398). Although intensity can increase with dose escalation, fever and chills were observed at all dose levels. Other frequent, but moderate side-effects included transient fatigue, myalgia, arthralgia, headache, nausea, vomiting, diarrhea, and abdominal pain. Only headache appeared to be increased in intensity in patients receiving the highest doses (400[c]). Few patients receiving IL-1α complained of somnolence, agitation, delusional ideation, photophobia or subjective blurred vision (402); seizures or severe somnolence appeared in a single phase II trial of IL-1β (403). Local phlebitis was observed with both cytokines and required the use of a central venous catheter, while subcutaneous injection of IL-1β induced pain and erythema at the injection sites (401[c]). IL-1α treatment was also involved in mucositis and xerostomia (402[c])

Self-limited, but significant hypertension usually occurring within minutes after starting the infusion, precedes the occurrence of chills and rigor, and is probably caused by venoconstriction induced by adrenergic stimulation (404[C]). The most significant adverse effect of IL-1 is a dose-limiting hypotension resulting from the secondary decrease in systemic vascular resistance. Usually, tachyphylaxis is not observed. Saline infusion or low-dose dopamine was sometimes required. In IL-1α trials, hypotension requiring blood pressure support was observed in 60% of patients receiving 0.3 μg/kg/day (398). In IL-1β trials, hypotension requiring treatment developed in 29% of patients (400). The most probably involved mechanism is an IL-1-induced increase in nitric oxide production by vascular smooth muscles (405). Although mild weight gain, pulmonary infiltrates and dyspnea have been observed in about 20—40% of IL-1α treated patients (402), none exhibited a severe capillary leak syndrome. Shortness of breath requiring oxygen was also noted in a few patients receiving IL-1β (400) and benign supraventricular arrhythmias occurred sometimes (398, 406).

Biological side-effects in IL-1α-treated patients included a transient and moderate increase in bilirubin, aspartate aminotransferase and serum creatinine levels (399, 402). IL-1β was sometimes associated with transient hypoglycemia within hours of administration (406) Overall, the maximum tolerated doses of IL-1 was 0.3 μg/kg/day for IL-1α (402) and 0.068 μg/kg/day for IL-1β in patients with intensive support (406). Higher doses of IL-1 are probably tolerable providing that patients are closely monitored and receive careful intensive blood support. Indomethacin may lower the maximum tolerated dose of IL-1 (397[R], 402). The mechanism of IL-1-associated toxicities is unclear and may be the result of a direct or indirect cytokine-mediated effect.

Interleukin-2 (IL-2)

Interleukin-2, produced by activated T-lymphocytes, has pleiotropic immunological effects mediated by specific receptors. Non-glycosylated recombinant IL-2 (aldesleukin, teceleukin) has been approved for the treatment of metastatic renal cell carcinoma. The current recommended dose is 600 000 UI/kg by intermittent bolus intravenous infusion. The pharmacological properties, pharmacokinetics and therapeutic use of IL-2 have been extensively reviewed elsewhere (407—412[R]). IL-2 alone or in combination has been used in patients with advanced cancer refractory to conventional treatment. Overall, the addition of LAK cells does not significantly potentiate IL-2 toxicity, but neither does it improve the therapeutic response in renal cell carcinoma (411[R]).

Considerable efforts have been made to limit IL-2-associated toxicities which are dose- and schedule-dependent (412, 413[R]). Low dose IL-2, continuous infusion and/or subcutaneous administration are preferred by various investigators because of their reluctance to use conventional high-dose or bolus administration; such regimens were considered as effective and safe for outpatients (414—417[R]). A complete analysis of 255 patients included in seven phase II trials during a 5-year period and treated with the currently recommended high dose of IL-2 for metastatic renal cell carcinoma has recently been reported (418).

Table 2. *Severe clinical toxicities (grade 3 or 4 of the National Cancer Institute) associated with high-dose IL_2 (from 418)*

General symptoms	
Fever and chills	24%
Asthenia	4%
Edema	2%
Sepsis	6%
Cardiovascular complications	
Hypotension	74%
Supraventricular arrhythmias	3%
Myocardial injury (angina, infarction)	4%
Hematological abnormalities	
Thrombocytopenia	21%
Anemia	18%
Renal complications	
Oliguria or anuria	46%
Elevated blood urea nitrogen	16%
Elevated serum creatinine	14%
Acidosis	6%
Neuropsychiatric complications	
Coma, seizures	4%
Behavorial changes	28%
Dermatological findings	
Pruritus and erythema	4%
Pulmonary complications	
Dyspnea	17%
Adult respiratory distress	<1%
Respiratory failure	2%
Hepatic abnormalities	
Hyperbilirubinemia	21%
Elevated transaminase level	10%
Elevated alkaline phosphatase level	8%
Gastrointestinal disorders	
Nausea and vomiting	25%
Diarrhea	22%
Stomatitis	4%
Gastrointestinal bleeding	4%
Intestinal perforation	<1%
Other findings	
Arthralgia	1%
Myalgia	1%
Death	4%

Although severe toxicities generally attributable to the capillary leak syndrome were found in most patients (Tables 2 and 3), they reversed promptly after treatment discontinuation. Death related to IL-2-induced toxicity was, however, reported in 4% of patients, and followed myocardial infarction and respiratory failure associated with the capillary leak syndrome, gastrointestinal toxicity or sepsis. Toxicities associated with IL-2 can be caused by the release of secondary cytokines such as TNF-α, IFN-γ, IL-1, IL-6 and IL-8 (409).

Table 3. *Most frequent reasons (one or more) for discontinuation of high-dose intravenous IL-2 treatment*

Constitutional symptoms	17%
Hypotension	19%
Atrial arrhythymias	10%
Oliguria	9%
Elevated creatinine level	13%
Disorientation	10%
Pulmonary toxicity	12%
Nausea or vomiting	4%
Diarrhea	6%
Thrombocytopenia	7%
Hyperbilirubinemia	5%

GENERAL TOXICITY

Constitutional symptoms (generalized malaise, fever and chills, or asthenia) are universal in patients treated with high-dose IL-2. Although usually suppressed by acetaminophen, indomethacin and meperidine administration, they were one of the major reasons for stopping treatment (413[R]). Myalgias and arthralgias are sometimes associated with flu-like symptoms.

ORGANS AND SYSTEMS

Cardiovascular Hemodynamic and cardiac complications are among the most serious complications of IL-2 therapy. A significant hypotension with a consecutive increase in heart rate was noted in almost all patients (419[C]). These findings are frequently dose-limiting and clinically very similar to the hemodynamic pattern seen in early septic shock. IL-2-induced synthesis of nitrous oxide has been proposed as the underlying mechanism (409[r]).

In previous reports, hypotension requiring fluids and vasopressor support was observed in the majority of patients receiving high-dose IL-2 (413[R]). Cardiac arrhythmias were experienced by 6—10% of patients, angina pectoris or documented myocardial infarction was reported in 3—4% of patients and mortality due to myocardial infarction in 1—2%. New guidelines have considerably improved the cardiac tolerance of IL-2. These included prudent maintenance intravenous fluid (100—125 ml/hour) or saline boluses, low-dose dopamine or phenylephrine as required. White et al. (420[C]) have recently reported their 5-year experience on the cardiopulmonary toxicity of high-dose intravenous bolus IL-2 in metastatic melanoma or renal cell carcinoma patients without underlying cardiac disease. Hypotension was the most frequent adverse effect, in up to 53% of treatment courses, and it resolved promptly with vasopressor treatment. Unexpectedly, response to treatment was significantly higher in melanoma patients who experienced hypotension. Although 11.1% of all patients had elevated creatine phosphokinase (CPK) serum level before or during treatment, only 2.5% had elevated CPK associated with a documented elevation in their MB isoenzyme fraction. CPK elevations were mostly asymptomatic with only one patient who experienced symptoms. Cardiac arrhythmias were observed in 9% of patients (6% of treatment courses) and mostly consisted of limited atrial fibrillation or supraventricular tachycardia which responded well to conventional treatment such as digoxin. Further courses of IL-2 in 11 of these patients produced recurrent arrhythmias in only two, and long-term treatment of arrhythmias was never required. Third-degree atrioventricular block and repetitive episodes of ventricular tachycardia in a patient with myocarditis were each observed once. High-degree atrioventricular block was also documented in isolated reports (421[C]). Cardiovascular events occurred within hours after starting infusion, persisted throughout IL-2 therapy, and normalized within 1—3 days after treatment cessation. Only isolated reports have indeed documented chronic cardiac impairment after myocardial infarction (422[C]), or the persistence of left ventricular dysfunction beyond 4 weeks after treatment withdrawal (423[C]).

At-risk patients include those with known or suspected coronary disease. Owing to the high risk of ischemic myocardial injury, it is reasonable to monitor cardiac function and CPK levels closely in all patients, or to exclude those with significant underlying coronary or cardiorespiratory diseases. Pretreatment cardiac screening has indeed greatly decreased the incidence of myocardial infarction, ischemia and related arrhythmias. The concomitant use of L-carnitine has also been proposed to reduce IL-2-related cardiac complications in metastatic cancer patients with heart disease (424[c]), but the relevance of these results will need more extensive evaluation. Age, performance status and gender were not significantly associated with cardiopulmonary toxicity (420).

A decrease in systemic vascular resistance, stroke work index and left ventricular ejection fraction are usually involved in the pathophysiology of cardiac dysfunction and, although as yet unproven, the production of TNF-α may be a key factor in the cardiovascular toxicity of IL-2 (413[r]). Clinical, electrocardiographic and radionuclide ventriculography monitoring in 22 patients undergoing a 5-day continuous intravenous infusion of IL-2 for various cancers clearly demonstrated that reversible left ventricular dysfunction accounted for most of the hemodynamic changes observed (425[C]). Indeed, significant coronary disease was usually not observed in patients undergoing cardiac catheterization which argues for a direct myocardial damage (420). Additionally, clinical and histological findings of eosinophilic or mixed lymphocytic-eosinophilic myocarditis have sometimes been observed, and also suggested a drug hypersensitivity reaction (426, 427[C]).

The capillary leak syndrome is characterized by damage to endothelial cells with a subsequent leakage of fluid into the extravascular space (428) and a third-space clinical syndrome with generalized or peripheral edema, weight gain, cardiovascular complications, hypotension, pulmonary congestion and pleural effusions, ascites, oliguria and prerenal azotemia (431[R]). Symptoms resolve in a few days following IL-2 discontinuation. Studies on the mechanism of increased vascular permeability have raised a number of hypotheses. LAK cells are likely to play a major role. Suppression of endothelin-1 secretion by endothelial cells, activation of the complement cascade, IL-8 and TNF release with subsequent activation of polymorphonuclear neutrophils have all been suggested to be involved (409, 410, 429, 430).

Respiratory In their series, White et al. (420[C]) noted severe respiratory distress in 3.2% of treatment courses, but intubation was required in only one patient. This is far less than reported in a previous study where 10—30% of patients developed respiratory distress, severe enough to warrant mechanical ventilation in 5—20% of cases (413[R]). This discrepancy may be related to the strict selection criteria now used for the evaluation of pulmonary function, limited fluid management strategy, prophylactic antibiotics and prompt withdrawal of treatment in patients presenting with shortness of breath, rales or persistent hypoxemia.

Previously described pulmonary features consisted of lung opacities, diffuse pulmonary interstitial edema, pleural effusions, alveolar edema and hypoxemia with full recovery within one day after treatment cessation (431, 432[C]). This, together with a slight increase in central venous pressure suggested an IL-2-induced increase in lung capillary permeability or direct cardiac dysfunction. LAK cells infused in combination with IL-2 exerted an additional toxic effect on the lung (433[C]). No significant association was found between previous clinical dysfunction and radiological interstitial edema (432). Very severe adult respiratory distress syndrome requiring double lung transplantation was recently reported in a young woman treated with 18 MU/day for acute myeloid leukemia (434[C]).

Nervous system Neuropsychiatric effects of IL-2 given alone or in combination with LAK cells have been carefully studied in a longitudinal survey of 44 patients (435[C]). Overall, 66% of patients showed severe behavioral to moderate cognitive changes, several of whom required transient neuroleptic administration or emergency psychiatric therapy. Half of the patients also had cognitive impairment with disorientation and confusion. Other infrequent side-effects included paranoid delusions, hallucinations, loss of interest, sleep disturbances or drowsiness, decreased energy, fatigue, anorexia and malaise. Coma and seizures were exceptionally observed. Symptoms usually occurred within 1 week of treatment and most patients recovered completely within 4 days after cessation of treatment. No predictive or predisposing factors could be clearly identified. Clinically relevant neuropsychiatric symptoms were less frequent with subcutaneous IL-2. Although observed in 14% of treatment courses in 61 patients (436[c]) and in 40% of patients receiving IL-2 plus IFN-α (437[c]), treatment-limiting psychiatric symptoms occurred in two and <6% of patients in these studies, respectively.

Even though perivascular foci demyelination was found in the brain of a patient dead from acute leukoencephalopathy (438[C]), and delayed progressive cognitive dysfunction was observed after intraventricular IL-2 treatment (439[C]), long-term neurological damage has not been so far explored. In a small study of seven metastatic melanoma patients, cognitive impairment was identified at the end of each intravenous IL-2 course using clinical evaluation and neuropsychological tests (440[C]). Furthermore, increased latency and a decrease amplitude in event-related evoked potentials were noted. All patients recovered baseline values within 1 week after the last IL-2 administration. Similar findings were found in patients receiving subcutaneous IL-2 (441[C]). The mechanisms of IL-2 neurotoxicity remain to be more clearly established (46).

Other neurological side effects, such as bilateral carpal tunnel syndrome (442[C]) have been reported as single case reports. Brachial plexopathy in two patients (443[C]), which recurred upon rechallenge in one, is in keeping with a possible side effect of IL-2 treatment.

Endocrine, metabolic Since the first report of hypothyroidism described after IL-2 plus LAK cell treatment (444[C]), a number of studies have reported the occurrence of thyroid dysfunction in patients receiving IL-2 alone (445, 446[C]), or in association with LAK cells (445, 447, 448[C]), IFN-α or IFN-γ (445, 446, 449—454[C]) or TNF (446, 453[C]).

Features of hypothyroidism were the most frequent in patients receiving IL-2 alone or with LAK cells (89% of affected patients), and were usually observed after 2—4 months of treatment (445, 446). By contrast, patients receiving IL-2 plus IFN developed either biphasic thyroiditis with subsequent hypothyroidism or hyperthyroidism (449—454). Most patients recovered after immunotherapy withdrawal or thyroxin treatment (446, 452). Female gender and the presence of antithyroid antibodies also correlated significantly with the development of thyroid disease (446).

In prospective clinical studies, the incidence of IL-2-induced or -aggravated thyroid disorders ranged from 9 to 16.4% in patients receiving IL-2 alone (446) to 47% in patients receiving IL-2 plus LAK cells (448). Thyroid abnormalities tended to correlate with cumulative IL-2 dose and were strongly correlated with treatment duration (445). IL-2 plus IFN-α produced a greater incidence of thyroid dysfunction affecting 20—91% of patients (449—452, 454). In addition, the incidence of laboratory thyroid dysfunction increased by up to 100% in patients given five or six cycles of both cytokines (449). IL-2 plus IFN-γ also tended to be a risk factor for the development of biphasic thyroiditis (446).

The presence of antithyroid antibodies and the findings of strong expression of HLA-DR antigens on thyrocytes make an autoimmune process likely, especially in patients receiving IL-2 plus IFNs (446, 450). However, several investigators also suggested a possible effect of immunotherapy on thyroid hormonal function because thyroid disorders were sometimes observed without any thyroid antibodies (447, 449, 452, 453). A significant decrease in TSH level and elevated thyroid hormones was indeed observed in most patients treated with IL-2 and IFN-α, while thyroid autoantibodies were not significantly elevated (454).

Adrenal hemorrhage leading to acute adrenal insufficiency has been reported in one patient (455[C]). Various hormonal and metabolic effects of IL-2 treatment have been reported and were temporally related to hypotension (456[C]). Elevated plasma concentrations of ACTH, cortisol, β-endorphin, epinephrine and norepinephrine have also been found (456, 457[C], 458[C]). No significant changes in the plasma levels of several other hormones were detected (410[r]).

Recurrent and marked hypocholesterolemia with decreased high- and low-density lipoproteins have been described following high-dose IL-2 (459[C]). Slight increases in plasma triglycerides were also observed. Severe but completely reversible hypovitaminosis C was also noted in patients on high-dose IL-2 plus LAK cells (460[C]).

Hematological Hematological side effects of IL-2 typically included transient anemia, thrombocytopenia, eosinophilia, neutropenia, extreme lymphopenia and rebound lymphocytosis (381[R], 413[C]). Transient suppression of hematopoiesis by secondary cytokines, peripheral platelet destruction and increased endothelium margination of lymphocytes are possible mechanisms.

The hematological toxicity in 199 carefully managed patients treated for metastatic melanoma or renal cell carcinoma with currently used high-dose intravenous bolus IL-2 regimen was recently analyzed retrospectively (461[CR]). Anemia requiring transfusions was noted in 14% of all treatment courses and severe thrombocytopenia occurred in 2.2%, with three patients suffering from serious hemorrhages. Most patients had coagulation disorders with elevated partial thromboplastin time as the most frequent effect. Severe leukopenia was rarely observed and was not associated with infectious episodes. Early transient lymphopenia (93% decrease) was followed by rebound lymphocytosis of up to 198% of baseline values. Except for severe thrombopenia, treatment cessation was not required. Intravenous polyvalent immunoglobulins have been successfully used in one patient to reduce IL-2-induced thrombopenia (462[c]). The severity of hematological disorders was not affected by previous chemotherapy and no correlation with response to treatment was found (461). However, other investigators have found that moderate to severe dose-related thrombocytopenia was observed particularly in those patients previously treated with cytotoxic agents (463[C]). Life-threatening thrombopenia was also suggested to be partly due to LAK cell administration (464[C]). Finally, decreases in platelet count correlated with significant ex vivo platelet functional activity and were not associated with clinical hemostatic consequences (465[C]). Sustained eosinophilia, possibly mediated by IL-5 or GM-CSF, was sometimes observed during IL-2 treatment but was not associated with clinical evidence of hypersensitivity (466[C]). Subcutaneous low-dose IL-2 therapy has been shown to improve dramatically the frequency and intensity of hematological toxicity, and the combination of IL-2 and IFN-α produced either moderate additional toxicity or no significant enhancement (467[cR]).

Decreased levels of several clotting factors and a significant fall in prothrombin time have been reported in IL-2-treated patients (468, 469[C]). In a prospective evaluation of coagulation disorders performed within 6 hours after the last IL-2 dose, a significant prolongation of the partial thromboplastin time and a decrease in the functional levels of factors II, IX, X, XI and XII were noted (470[C]). Complete normalization was observed in the following 2 or 3 days, and no clear mechanism of IL-2-induced coagulopathy was found.The efficacy of prophylactic vitamin K use (468) has recently been disputed (470[C]). Other data suggested that IL-2 may activate the coagulation and fibrinolytic system (463, 471). Except for one patient who experienced mesenteric thrombosis, no clinical relevance was observed.

Liver About 20% of patients developed mild-to-severe intrahepatic cholestasis (413) with reversible and dose-dependent elevation of bilirubin and alkaline phosphatase levels while liver transaminases were only slightly elevated (472[C]). Recurrence of cholestasis following IL-2 rechallenge was not always observed (473[C]). The mechanism of IL-2-induced intrahepatic cholestasis remains unknown but it may be mediated by the release of cytokines known to affect liver function (474[R]). Focal fatty infiltrates of the liver that mimicked metastasis were also reported in a patient receiving both IL-2 and a short course of IFN-α (475[C]).

Cholecystopathy was recently described in cancer patients (476[c], 477[c]) and was fully investigated in seven of 29 HIV-infected patients receiving IL-2 infusion (478[CR]). Right upper quadrant abdominal pain and gallbladder wall thickening at sonography developed after 4—5 days of treatment and spontaneously resolved after treatment cessation or dosage reduction. Similar symptoms re-occurred after IL-2 re-administration. Although suggestive of acalculous cholecystitis, surgery is not required because this disorder is usually benign.

Gastrointestinal Minor and reversible gastrointestinal side-effects, i.e. anorexia, nausea, vomiting and diarrhea, were noted in more than 80% of IL-2 treatments, but ileus or ascites were far less common (413). Mucositis, glossitis, spontaneously reversible oral dryness, and various oral signs or complaints were also reported (479[C]). An increase (24—65%) in spleen size was initially observed in five of nine patients (480[c]). A mean splenic index increase of 64% was recently found on computed tomography after a mean of 66.2 days of IL-2 treatment for non-hematological malignancies (480[C]). Splenomegaly persisted after an average of 215 days following the completion of IL-2 treatment and was not associated with tumor progression.

Severe and sometimes fatal intestinal complications including intestinal ischemia, necrosis or perforation, and diffuse bowel ulceration requiring surgery have been described in 1.3—7% of patients receiving IL-2 alone or in combination with LAK cells or IFN-α (482—484[C]). Severe diarrhea was suggested as a potential indicator for subsequent colonic ischemia (484). A symptomatic exacerbation of Crohn's disease occurred in two patients (485[C]) and the rapid onset of acute pancreatitis secondary to high-dose bolus IL-2 therapy has been reported in two patients (486[C]).

Urinary system Oliguria or anuria, azotemia and increased serum creatinine levels have been encountered in more than 90% of patients receiving high-dose IL-2 (413[R]). Proteinuria, ranging in degree from mere traces (487[C]) to a frank but reversible nephrotic syndrome (488[C]), was sometimes observed, and a possible role of contaminants has been discussed (489).

Renal function in 199 carefully managed patients treated for metastatic melanoma or renal cell carcinoma with high-dose intravenous bolus IL-2 was recently analyzed retrospectively (490[CR]). Severe oliguria, hypotension and weight gain were encountered in most treatment courses, and elevated serum creatinine levels (mean peak at 2.7 mg/dl) were the cause of treatment discontinuation in 13% of cycles. Proteinuria, and various urinalyses modifications were also observed. The higher peaks of creatinine values were found in patients with renal carcinoma, older patients, males and nephrectomized patients. No evidence of long-term renal defect was observed and renal dysfunction is not considered as a treatment-limiting factor providing that patients are carefully managed for hypotension or oliguria. Again, low-to-intermediate doses of IL-2 alone or associated with IFN-α have been suggested to be safe and effective in the setting of outpatient regimens (416).

Previously elevated serum creatinine levels, especially in patients over 60, have been claimed to predict the severity and duration of renal impairment, but neither previous nephrectomy nor the interval between nephrectomy and initiation of IL-2 therapy were associated with a higher risk of renal failure (413). A typical prerenal mechanism secondary to the vascular leak syndrome is commonly involved in the pathophysiology of acute renal failure. In addition, a direct intrinsic intrarenal effect of IL-2 with a higher than expected decrease in glomerular filtration rate (487) or tubular dysfunction (491[C]) have been suggested to be involved. Several isolated cases of acute interstitial or tubulointerstitial nephritis with a predominant T lymphocyte infiltration of the kidneys (492—494[C]) and exacerbation of a subclinical IgA glomerulonephritis (495[C]) suggested altered cell-mediated immunity.

Skin and appendages A wide spectrum of reversible cutaneous reactions have been observed, generally comprising pruritus, flushing, mild-to-moderate desquamative macular erythematous rash while generalized erythroderma or photosensitivity were rarely observed (496[R]). The severity of cutaneous complications was not dose-dependent and did not correlate with other systemic reactions. Histological and immunopathological examination of the skin showed mild infiltrates of activated T helper lymphocytes and an increased expression of HLA-DR and intercellular adhesion molecule-1 on keratinocytes and endothelial cells, and a possible role for IFN-γ was suggested (497—499). Other side-effects included erosions in surgical scars, multiple superficial cutaneous ulcerations and telogen effluvium (496).

IL-2 treatment has also been involved in the clinical exacerbation or the occurrence of severe cutaneous reactions associated with altered cell-mediated immunity or an autoimmune process, namely the recurrence of quiescent pemphigus vulgaris (500[C]), fatal dermatitis exfoliativa compatible with the diagnosis of pemphigus vulgaris (501[C]), the exacerbation of localized or widespread psoriasis (496[r]), and the rapid progression of scleroderma with myositis (502[C]). Immunostimulation due to IL-2 may have also played a role in the occurrence or unmasking of erythema nodosum (503[C]), linear IgA bullous dermatosis (504[C]), and life-threatening extensive bullous skin eruption with the possible additive role of concomitant antibiotic use (505[C]). One possible case of toxic epidermal necrolysis, which is thought to result from antibody-dependent cellular cytotoxicity, was also described (506[C]). A high incidence of de novo vitiligo has been reported in patients undergoing chemotherapy followed by IL-2 and IFN-α for metastatic melanoma (507[C]), and was more recently reported in several similar patients receiving IL-2 (508[c]) or IL-2 plus IFN-α without antineoplastic therapy (509[C]). A correlation between IL-2-induced vitiligo and a favorable tumor response was found (507) but was recently disputed (508). The association of scleroderma and vitiligo was also reported in a single patient (510[C]). Finally, lobular panniculitis occurred after subcutaneous injections and was further exacerbated by intravenous IL-2 (511[C]).

Special senses Transient episodes of amaurosis or scotoma in the right superior quadrant of vision, both of which recurred after IL-2 rechallenge, have been described (512[C]). Three other patients experienced visual phenomena including diplopia, scotoma and palinopsia during treatment, and resolved upon IL-2 discontinuation (513[C]).

Musculoskeletal system Joint or muscle pains have sometimes been reported (413) as well as shoulder arthralgias with normal radiographs and scintigraphic imaging consistent with bilateral synovitis (514[C]). Several reports also suggested that IL-2 can reactivate or induce rheumatoid arthritis (515[C]).

Sexual Reversible decrease in testosterone levels has been observed in male patients (410).

Miscellaneous *Infectious complications* An increased incidence of clinically relevant infectious complications has now been largely documented following intravenous IL-2 with an incidence of 10—40% (516, 517[C]). A recent retrospective study reported a 13% incidence of documented bacterial infections during 935 treatment courses of high-dose IL-2 and also noted that opportunistic infections were not more frequent (518[C]). The most commonly isolated pathogens were *Staphylococcus aureus*, *S. epidermidis* and *Escherichia coli*. Documented infections affected mostly the catheter site or the urinary tract. Infections were usually noted during the first (68%) or the second (21.3%) course of IL-2 therapy, i.e. 4—9 days and 13—18 days after the start of treatment. Bacterial sepsis was mostly related to the use of central venous catheters and fatal septic shock was rarely recorded. However, an elevated incidence of infectious complications has also been noted in patients receiving subcutaneous IL-2 and IFN-α (519[c]) but these findings were disputed by other investigators who did not find any increased incidence of infections in patients receiving subcutaneous IL-2 alone (520[c], 521[c]). The prophylactic use of antibiotics and systematic screening led to a significant decrease in the frequency of infections, from 21.8 to 7% of patients over a 3-year surveillance (518).

Risk factors of bacterial infection are many-fold (518). Previous colonization of the skin with *S. aureus* and skin desquamation increased the risk of nosocomial bacteremia. Age, underlying tumor, source, dose and duration of intravenous IL-2 or the concomitant use of LAK cells, were not associated factors. Finally, severe neutropenia was not associated with bacteremia (413, 461). The mechanism of these complications is not fully understood (413). A decrease in circulating neutrophil chemotaxis, superoxide production and/or neutrophil Fc receptor expression have been suggested to be involved. Impaired cell-mediated or humoral immune responses have also been shown following high-dose IL-2 but the clinical consequences of these findings remain unknown.

IL-2 antibodies In a recent investigation of 205 patients with metastatic cancer, rIL-2 binding antibodies were detected in 50% and neutralizing antibodies in only 7% (522[C]). No significant difference in incidence was found between subcutaneous and continuous intravenous administration. Another study was unable to detect neutralizing antibodies in patients receiving IL-2 alone, but identified 18% of patients who developed neutralizing activity when receiving IL-2 in combination with IFN-α_{2b} (523[C]). Anti-IL-2 antibodies have been shown to recognize both the recombinant and the natural cytokine (524[C]), and patients developing neutralizing anti-IL-2 antibodies had a significantly lower serum-soluble IL-2 receptor level than patients without antibodies (523). The clinical relevance of rIL-2-neutralizing antibodies has not been accurately evaluated but a loss of response was apparently documented in one single patient (524).

Hypersensitivity reactions The report of angioneurotic edema and urticaria in two patients receiving IL-2 questioned the role of IL-2 in hypersensitivity reactions (525[C]). No hypersensitivity reactions or anaphylaxis directly related to IL-2 have seemingly been described so far.

Interestingly, more frequent, but delayed, severe atypical acute hypersensitivity reactions to iodinated and non-ionic contrast media injection have been observed after 2—6 weeks following IL-2 discontinuation in patients who had previously well tolerated contrast media (526—530[C]). Symptoms appeared within 1—4 hours after contrast media injection and consisted of diarrhea, vomiting, malaise, fever and chills, skin rash, facial edema and sometimes itching, hypotension, dyspnea and oliguria. They resolved rapidly, recurred after each injection (526), but the patients could further receive IL-2 without adverse effects. The incidence of these reactions after contrast media injection in IL-2-treated patients ranged from 5 to 15% (526, 527, 529), and was up to 28% of patients receiving IL-2 via arterial infusion (530). Prior therapy with IL-2 seemed to be a prerequisite. 'Recall' reactions to IL-2 have been proposed as these complications more closely resembled IL-2-induced immediate side effects than typical contrast media reactions. The mechanism remains largely unknown, but prior exposure to IL-2 may have sensitized a proportion of patients. A putative enhancement of the immune response against iodine-containing contrast media following IL-2 has been suggested (530), but was not substantiated (527). More recently, an unexpected high incidence of similar type I hypersensitivity reactions to cisplatin and dacarbazine was also found within several hours after administration in patients on a combination of IL-2 and IFN-α (531[C]). The reactions occurred at least after the first cycle and increased in incidence thereafter, suggesting again that immunotherapy can sensitize patients to several chemotherapeutic agents.

Tumor-inducing effects Few data are available on the possibility that IL-2 can promote leukemic cell growth or stimulate B lymphocytes in vivo. Only isolated case reports have described relapses of acute myeloid leukemia (532[C]) or the proliferation of leukemic blasts cells with phenotypic changes in a patient treated for acute myelocytic leukemia (533[C]). Interestingly, a high percentage of blasts expressed the CD25 antigen in both reports. Reversible increase of peripheral monoclonal B cell lymphocytosis in a patient with B cell lymphocytic lymphoma (534[C]) or the development of Hodgkin's disease in a woman receiving IL-2 for metastatic melanoma (535[C]) were also documented as single reports.

Interactions Since IL-2 may cause fluid retention, edema and renal failure, the potential for significant pharmacokinetic drug interactions does exist. However, very few relevant data are available (348[R]). Acute encephalopathy with typical signs of morphine intoxication was recently attributed to IL-2-induced renal failure or a toxic central nervous system synergy of both treatments (536[C]).

On the other hand, non-steroidal anti-inflammatory agents used to reduce fever and other IL-2 adverse effects may theoretically potentiate IL-2 nephrotoxicity through the inhibition of prostaglandin synthesis. However their role was deemed unlikely by several authors (487).

Interleukin-3 (IL-3)

IL-3, which is produced by activated T lymphocytes, stimulates the proliferation and differentiation of the granulocyte, macrophage, eosinophil, basophil, erythroid, megakaryocyte and mast cell lineages (537[R]). Subcutaneous recombinant IL-3 is under clinical investigation in patients with chemotherapy-induced myelotoxicity, in the setting of autologous bone marrow transplantation or peripheral stem cell harvesting, or in patients with myelodysplastic syndrome, aplastic anemia and Diamond-Blackfan anemia (537, 538[R]).

Subcutaneous doses of 5—10 μg/kg/day have been suggested to be acceptable by most patients for further studies. Overall, treatment discontinuation because of side effects ranged from 17 to 50% of patients on doses of 10 μg/kg/day (539, 540[C]), and the incidence or severity of constitutional symptoms, generalized skin reaction and facial edema, were the most frequent dose-limiting adverse events. In autologous bone marrow transplantation, the maximum tolerated dose was only 2 μg/kg/day (541[C]). Intravenous administrations were suggested to be less well tolerated than subcutaneous injections (542[c]). Although no comparative study has yet been performed, the side effects of yeast or *E. coli*-derived IL-3 do not appear to be different (543[c], 544[c]). No antibodies to IL3 have so far been detected in human sera (544[c]).

The specific toxicity of *E. coli*-derived rhIL-3 was recently studied in healthy volunteers after a 4-day regimen of once-daily subcutaneous IL-3 at 2.5, 5 and 7.5 μg/kg/day (545[C]). All subjects experienced at least one mild-to-moderate symptom and the most frequently reported were flu-like symptoms with fever, chills, headache, conjunctival congestion, myalgia and diffuse aching. Minor erythematous reactions at the injection site and facial flushing were also consistently described. Malaise, eye pain, nasal congestion, asthenia or lethargy, tachycardia and gastrointestinal disorders, all occurred in less than 16% of patients. None of these effects were clearly related to the dose, and discontinuation of treatment was not required. A similar safety profile was reported in treated patients with flu-like symptoms, flushing and headache as the most frequent adverse events; tachyphylaxis usually developed during treatment (546[R]). IL-3-associated fever was supposedly the result of a dose-dependent increase in IL-6 and acute phase protein production. Mild-to-severe skin rash or urticaria were sometimes observed. Although they were not easily attributable to IL-3 because patients received many other drugs and/or presented with severe underlying disease, other significant adverse events possibly related to IL-3 in phase I/II trials included bullae and hemorrhagic necrosis of the skin (544[c]), exacerbation or new onset of atrial fibrillation (539[c], 544[c]), dyspnea (540[c]), exacerbation of arthralgia in a seronegative patient (544[c]), and transient thrombocytopenia in myelodysplastic syndrome or aplastic anemia patients (547[c]). Signs of meningismus with neck rigidity were sometimes found (543[c]). Although weight gain and peripheral edema may develop, no convincing report of capillary leak syndrome has so far been described.

Whereas hypotension was rarely observed in clinical trials, severe hypotension within hours after IL-3 injection was observed in three of 26 patients treated with angiotensin-converting enzyme (ACE) inhibitors (548[c]). An indirect synergism of ACE and IL-3 on nitric oxide production was suggested to be involved. Thrombophlebitis was observed in 45% of patients treated for advanced ovarian cancer who also received intravenous IL-3 (542[c]), and deep venous thromboses were reported in children treated with maintenance IL-3 for Diamond-Blackfan anemia (549[c]). In addition, one smoking breast cancer patient developed severe hypotension and acute thrombosis of the cerebellar and superior mesenteric arteries after subcutaneous IL-3 administration (550[C]). Although an increased risk of thrombosis with IL-3 remains to be demonstrated, these case reports suggest that IL-3 may contribute to the development of thrombosis.

Similarly to G-CSF or GM-CSF, the presence of IL-3 receptors on leukemia cells indicated a theoretical risk for disease acceleration. No accelerated tumor growth was noted in patients with non-hematopoietic tumors (551[c]), or newly diagnosed non-Hodgkin's lymphoma (552[c]). Overall, some types of disease progression were observed in 11 of 86 patients with myelodysplastic syndrome (544, 547, 553—555[c]), but no clear relation between IL-3 and disease acceleration can be assessed at the moment. Other long-term consequences of IL-3 have included a transient rise in circulating atypical B lymphocytes with enlargement of the spleen and lymph nodes in two patients with large cell lymphoma (551[c]), and the development of a clonally-related transient plasmocytosis with paraproteinemia in one patient with relapsing follicular non-Hodgkin's lymphoma (556[C]). Finally, one single case of bone marrow histocytosis was described in a patient treated with IL-3 for refractory aplastic anemia (557[C]).

Interactions Although clinical trials of combined sequential administration of IL-3 plus GM-CSF did not reveal additional significant toxicity (558[R]), recent data in patients treated for myelodysplastic syndrome suggested unacceptable toxicity (559[C]).

In ovarian cancer patients, the combination of IL-3 with high-dose carboplatin was poorly tolerated with severe fever, malaise, protracted nausea, vomiting, severe hypotension and nephrotoxicity, requiring IL-3 discontinuation in 60% of patients when IL-3 was administered only 24 hours after high-dose carboplatin (560[C]).

No evidence has emerged from clinical studies that the incidence or severity of side-effects are increased in patients receiving other chemotherapy (539).

Interleukin-4 (IL-4)

IL-4 is a pleiotropic cytokine, mostly produced by activated T cells, which acts on the proliferation and differentiation of B and T lymphocytes, and enhances the function of natural killer cells, eosinophils and mast cells (561[R]). The potential anti-tumoral and hematopoietic activities of yeast or *E. coli*-derived IL-4 are under investigation (562—565[C]).

Moderate-grade fever with flu-like symptoms, arthralgia, fatigue, anorexia, nausea or vomiting, headache and nasal congestion, was observed in most patients at all doses and by all routes of administration (562—565). Mild and transient hypotension was also noted. These side effects were suggested to be dose related with the more severe and protracted symptoms at high dose levels (563, 564). Periorbital, facial and peripheral edema were also noted and discomfort caused by severe and resistant nasal congestion, supposedly due to edema and vascular engorgement from histamine stimulation, was sometimes dose limiting (562, 563). Other adverse events, as yet not clearly related to IL-4, included reversible Coomb's-positive hemolytic anemia (565), transient partial blindness, photophobia and visual hallucinations (563, 564).

The vascular leak syndrome, a dose-limiting side effect, was observed at the dose level of 15 μg/kg by bolus or continuous intravenous administration (562, 565). A moderate capillary leak syndrome was also noted at a lower subcutaneous doses (564). Mild and asymptomatic elevations in liver enzymes and minimal changes in serum creatinine levels were sometimes noted, and isolated coagulation abnormalities with minor prolongation of prothrombin time were also consistently observed particularly in patients with pre-existing liver disease (563).

Several recent reports focused on severe and unexpected IL-4 side effects. Cardiac toxicity, clinically consistent with myocardial infarction, was observed in three of seven metastatic cancer patients receiving intravenous bolus IL-4 to a daily total of 800 $\mu g/m^2$ (566[C]). A unique pattern of myocarditis with predominant polymorphonuclear, eosinophil and mast cells infiltrate was found to be the possible cause of death in one fatal case and suggested an allergic inflammatory myocardial process.

Significant gastrointestinal toxicity was described in patients receiving IL-4 alone or in combination with IL-2 for advanced malignancy (567[C]). Antral or prepyloric ulcers, and erosive gastritis were identified at endoscopy following 12 of 84 courses of IL-4 in 72 patients, of whom three suffered from life-threatening bleeding. No treatment-related death was observed and no clear correlation with the dose of IL-4 could be demonstrated. A possible protective effect of IL-2 on the gastrointestinal mucosa was suggested. Although all but one of these patients also received indomethacin, no recurrence of symptoms was found in several patients who developed ulcers during IL-4 treatment, and further received IL-2 and indomethacin. The ability of IL-4 to affect prostaglandin E_2 synthesis strongly suggests that IL-4 alone can contribute to the development of digestive mucosal injury.

A papular eruption on the forearms was noticed in one of nine patients in a phase I trial (563[c]). Pruritic papulovesicular eruption and histological findings consistent with transient acantholytic dermatosis were recently described in detail in three patients receiving IL-4 for the treatment of melanoma or renal cancer (568[C]). The eruption reappeared soon after an additional course of IL-4 in two patients.

Interleukin-6 (IL-6)

IL-6 is produced by T cells, monocytes, fibroblasts, endothelial cells and keratinocytes, and regulates pleiotropic biological functions (546[R]).

Recombinant IL-6 was investigated for its thrombopoietic and potential antitumoral effects and very few trials have evaluated the safety of intravenous and subcutaneous IL-6 administration (569, 570[C]). Moderate fever and flu-like symptoms were observed in all patients, and mild nausea sometimes occurred. No clear relationship between the dose of IL-6 and constitutional symptoms has been demonstrated. Moderate reactions at the site of injection usually followed subcutaneous IL-6 administration (569). In contrast to several other cytokines, IL-6 has not been associated with signs of vascular leak syndrome or hypotension.

Dose-dependent and reversible normocytic anemia was consistently noted within several days after starting IL-6, and required blood transfusion at the highest dose level (570). Other biochemical changes included asymptomatic increases in liver function tests, transient proteinuria, increased serum creatinine and blood glucose levels and a dose-dependent decrease in serum albumin and cholesterol levels (570).

Overall, no major toxicities appeared at daily doses up to 20 μg/kg when IL-6 was used alone in patients with malignant disease, and constitutional symptoms or anemia are the main dose-limiting events (569). By contrast, the maximum tolerated dose of subcutaneous IL-6 was only 1 μg/kg/day in autologous bone marrow transplantation, because of severe maculopapular rash or hyperbilirubinemia with microvesicular steatosis (571[c]). In patients with myelodysplasia or thrombocytopenia, a dose-limiting toxicity was observed at 5 μg/kg/day IL-6 (572[c]). Preliminary results showed that combination of IL-6 with G-CSF or GM-CSF was not associated with significant synergism or new forms of toxicity (573, 574[c]).

Isolated reports documented decreased visual acuity and bilateral uveitis in a patient receiving a 2-week regimen of IL-3 and IL-6 for secondary myelodysplastic syndrome (575[C]). One case of diffuse maculopapular erythema with histological features consisting of epidermal spongiosis and interstitial mixed inflammatory cell infiltrate was reported after IL-6, the causative role of which was suggested by the recurrence of symptoms after re-administration (576[C]). Finally, the possibility that IL-6-induced acceleration of tumor growth was recently suggested in two patients with solid tumors (577[c]).

Tumor necrosis factor-α (TNF-α)

TNF-α, naturally produced by activated macrophages and monocytes, is recognized to exert pleiotropic effects on normal and malignant cells (578[R]). Numerous phase I or II trials of recombinant TNF-α as a single agent or in combination were conducted using intravenous bolus or infusion, and subcutaneous and intramuscular administration. The main results of trials up to 1992 were recently reviewed (579[R]).

Overall, the systemic administration of TNF-α as a single agent gave disappointing results with no significant clinical antitumor effect. In this setting, the maximum tolerated dose ranged from 160 to 200 $\mu g/m^2$ (578, 579). Severe hypotension, thought to be nitrous oxide-mediated and requiring fluid replacement or vasopressors, was the main dose-limiting toxicity in most studies, and was observed at all dose levels. Other frequent and sometimes dose-limiting toxicities included fever, chills and rigors, myalgia, diarrhea, nausea or vomiting, as well as local reactions at the injection site (SEDA-17, 433; 579, 580).

TNF-α has also been considered as a major neurotoxic agent (46[R]), and the great majority of patients treated with this agent have developed central nervous system symptoms, with headache, lethargy, fatigue, confusion, disorientation and decreased performance status being the most frequently observed (580). Meyers et al. (581[C]) recently evaluated the cognitive function of patients receiving TNF-α alone or combined with IL-2, and reported documented reversible attentional deficits, memory disorders, deficits in motor coordination and frontal lobe executive functions. Seizures, transient amnesia, aphasia, hallucinations and diplopia have sometimes occurred. Reversible hypoperfusion in the frontal lobes was found using single photon emission computerized tomography. Epidoses of tremor, resembling essential tremor and myoclonus, were also reported in a young patient with Ehler-Danlos syndrome after each TNF-α intravenous administration over 4 months (582[C]).

Hemorrhagic gastritis has appeared in three of 27 phase I patients with cancer (583). Significant pulmonary injury evidenced by a reversible decline in pulmonary diffusing capacity was found in most TNF-α-treated patients (584), and dyspnea or acute bronchospasm were sometimes noted, especially in patients with extensive metastatic pulmonary disease (580, 583). One case of reversible pulmonary hemorrhage (585[C]) and one case of permanent decrease in myocardial contractility with subsequent congestive cardiomyopathy (586[C]) have been described.

Transient liver dysfunction affecting transaminases and bilirubin, oliguria and elevated creatinine levels were commonly reported. Dose-related thrombopenia, granulocytopenia, decreased monocyte and lymphocyte counts were frequent, whereas anemia was rarely observed (580, 587). Septic episodes were sometimes associated with leukopenia (580). Coagulation disorders, with laboratory evidence of disseminated intravascular coagulopathy, were observed in 30% of patients and were sometimes associated with thromboembolic events (588). Modifications in prothrombin time and partial thromboplastin time were noted (579), and a rise in the plasma levels of von Willebrand factor was also found in healthy volunteers (589). Metabolic disorders included a decrease in cholesterol and high-density lipoproteins, an increase in triglycerides and very-low-density lipoproteins, and hyperglycemia (579, 588). One single case report described the exacerbation of hypothyroidism after TNF-α treatment in a patient with chronic thyroiditis (590[C]).

The systemic administration of TNF-α in combination with IFN-γ, IL-2 or cytotoxic drugs produced positive clinical results, but such combinations reduce the maximum tolerated dose of TNF-α 2—4-fold, with hyperbilirubinemia, neurotoxicity, severe febrile reaction and hypotension as the main dose-limiting toxicities (578, 579, 591, 592). Anaphylactic-like reactions, bronchospasm and adult respiratory distress syndrome were also found in patients with extensive pulmonary metastases receiving both TNF-α and IL-2 (593[c]). In a recent pilot study of TNF-α combined with the monoclonal anti-disialoganglioside GD3 antibody in eight patients with metastatic melanoma, one patient with steroid-treated adrenal insufficiency experienced an acute and multivisceral massive tumour lysis syndrome within hours after starting treatment and the reasons for this response to treatment were unexplained (594).

Local (intralesional, intra-arterial or intraperitoneal) administration was suggested to be a more promising route of administration for TNF-α, with milder toxicities (579). Severe metabolic disorders were however reported, such as hypophosphatemia with clinically significant myocardial dysfunction in patients with liver metastases receiving TNF-α by continuous hepatic arterial infusion (SEDA-17, 433). A recent trial of TNF-α administered by the intratumoral route showed adverse effects similar to those reported after intravenous administration, namely fever, hypotension and fatigue, but coagulation disorders, pulmonary, central nervous system, liver and renal toxicities were not observed (595).

Isolated perfusion of the limbs with high-dose TNF-α has also been proposed as a regional therapy for melanoma (596). In a recent trial using high-dose TNF-α, melphalan and IFN-γ under hyperthermic conditions in patients with advanced melanoma and malignant soft tissue tumors, severe hemodynamic changes were observed in all patients and consisted of a pure distributive or a mixed distributive cardiogenic shock, mimicking septic shock and requiring vasopressive or inotropic agents in 94% of patients (597). Other frequently observed effects included altered delivery and uptake of oxygen, radiologically visible lung infiltrates, fever, granulocytopenia and infections, thrombopenia, coagulation disorders, elevated transaminase levels and hyperbilirubinemia.

Granulocyte-macrophage colony-stimulating factor (GM-CSF)

GM-CSF primarily increases production and functions of neutrophils, and also stimulates the proliferation of monocytes and eosinophils and the production of cytokines (e.g. IL-1, IL-6, M-CSF, TNF). *Escherichia coli*-derived recombinant GM-CSF (molgramostim) is not glycosylated, whereas yeast-derived rGM-CSF (sargramostim) is heavily glycosylated. The relevance of these differences as regards efficacy, safety or antigenicity is unknown. Based on a retrospective review and a historical comparison, the tolerance of molgramostim was suggested to be poorer than that of sargramostim (598[c]), but no controlled trials have been conducted to compare adequately their respective safety. GM-CSF was approved to reduce neutropenic states following myelotoxic chemotherapy or myeloablative treatment with autologous bone marrow transplantation at doses of 1—6 μg/kg. In several countries, it was also approved in ganciclovir-induced neutropenia of AIDS patients. The pharmacodynamics, pharmacokinetics and clinical applications of GM-CSF have been reviewed comprehensively (599—602[R]).

At usually recommended doses, systemic side effects occur in 25—30% of patients, but are rarely treatment-limiting. Doses greater than 250 $\mu g/m^2$ and/or the intravenous route are associated with more frequent adverse effects. Flu-like symptoms with myalgia and chills, erythematous eruptions at the injection site, facial flushing and gastrointestinal disorders with anorexia and weight loss were commonly reported (600, 603[R]). Severe fatigue and asthenia are rare. Fever was observed in up to 50% of patients at doses $\geqslant$3 μg/kg (603[R]). Peak of fever at a constant time after GM-CSF injection, the lack of clinical and biological signs of infection and a prompt response to paracetamol have been proposed as criteria to recognize GM-CSF-induced iatrogenic fever (604[r]), a concept disputed by others (605). Finally, a rapidly reversible first-dose syndrome (dyspnea with hypoxia, tachycardia and hypotension) within the first hour after the first continuous infusion was reported in 15—30% of patients (600[R]).

ORGANS AND SYSTEMS

Cardiovascular Mild local phlebitis sometimes occur at intravenous sites of administration (606[c]). Central venous catheter site thrombosis, inferior vena cava thrombosis and possible pulmonary embolism have been observed only in patients receiving very high doses of GM-CSF (607, 608[c]). Continuous infusion via the inferior vena cava for peripheral stem cell (PSC) collection before autologous transplant has been associated with significantly more frequent catheter thrombotic occlusions during apheresis than in an historical control group of patients receiving aspirin prophylaxis only (54 vs 3%) (609[C]).

Although chemotherapy for breast cancer is associated with a higher risk to develop vascular thrombosis, the previously not described occurrence of iliac artery thrombosis in two patients receiving high-dose chemotherapy was attributed to GM-CSF (610[C]). Raynaud's phenomenon has also been reported in patients on high-dose chemotherapy (611[c]).

A dose-limiting vascular leak syndrome was consistently described in patients receiving 30 μg/kg/day GM-CSF or more (600[R]). Lower doses were also reported to induce a clinically relevant capillary leak syndrome (598[c], 612[C], 613[C]). Continuation of GM-CSF treatment, using the same or a lowered dose, proved to be possible in some patients given corticosteroids and oxygen (598[c]). An increase in the transcapillary escape rate of albumin, supposedly due to endothelial cell damage, was observed in patients receiving 10 μg/kg/day GM-CSF intravenously (614[C]), and a possible role of IL-1 and TNF production by GM-CSF-activated monocytes was also suggested (613).

Respiratory It has recently been suggested that GM-CSF may increase the pulmonary toxicity of bleomycin (615[C]) and to facilitate the development of the adult respiratory distress syndrome (ARDS) (616[C]). An increased neutrophil expression of surface proteins with enhanced neutrophil adhesion to endothelium cells was suggested to be involved (616). Life-threatening pulmonary toxicity together with massive hyperleukocytosis has also been observed in one patient which supports the role of increased neutrophil count in ARDS (617[C]). Reversible interstitial pulmonary edema with pulmonary failure may also have resulted from a first-dose reaction syndrome following the first low-dose administration of GM-CSF (618[C]).

Endocrine, metabolic Reversible hypothyroidism or biphasic thyroiditis developed in two of 25 cancer patients with previously normal thyroid function receiving intermittent cycles of GM-CSF with doxorubicin plus cyclophosphamide (619[c]). Both patients had thyroid peroxidase (TPO) antibodies prior to treatment, and no similar thyroid dysfunction was observed in patients without pre-existing thyroid antibodies. The possible exacerbation of an underlying autoimmune thyroiditis was later exemplified in a TPO-positive patient who developed hypothyroidism and a transient rise in antibody titers following 3 weeks of GM-CSF treatment (620[C]).

Mineral and fluid balance A transient and moderate reversible rise in leukocyte alkaline phosphatase, lactate dehydrogenase (LDH) and uric acid serum levels is usually observed concomitantly with increased neutrophil production (600, 603[R]). Increase in serum LDH should thus not be interpreted as an absolute sign of disease progression. Severe and symptomatic hypokalemia was thought to result from an increased intracellular potassium uptake linked to massive leukocytosis after GM-CSF treatment (621[C]). Decreases in serum cholesterol levels have also been reported (603[R]). Marked hypoalbuminemia lower than 25 g/l, eventually associated with edema and ascites, developed after 3—10 μg/kg/day GM-CSF in four of nine patients treated for myelodysplastic syndrome or aplastic anemia (622[C]).

Hematological Expectedly, dose-related and sometimes marked hypereosinophilia was described after GM-CSF treatment (623[C]). Although usually not associated with toxic symptoms, excessive eosinophilia with fatal necrotizing pneumonia and Loeffler's endocarditis has been described (624[C]).

Patients with previous autoimmune blood disorders could be at an increased risk of hematological GM-CSF toxicity. Acute exacerbation of autoimmune thrombocytopenia (625[c]) or hemolytic anemia (626[C]) may be linked to macrophage activation. A marked decrease in vitamin K-dependent coagulation factors over several days was reported in an open randomized trial involving patients treated with GM-CSF for acute myeloid leukemia (614[C]). Prophylactic intravenous vitamin K prevented these disorders in further patients and a transient decrease in hepatic factor synthesis was supposedly involved. Typical vaso-occlusive crisis with increased hemolysis occurred within minutes after intracutaneous injections of GM-CSF at the site of a leg ulcer in a stable patient with sickle cell disease (627[C]). Topical applications of GM-CSF were later uneventful in this patient.

Although GM-CSF acts primarily on the myeloid lineage, splenomegaly with histologically documented splenic extramedullary hematopoiesis of all three lineages has been described (628[C]).

Liver A moderate increase in serum aminotransferases was sometimes noted in GM-CSF-treated patients and severe hepatotoxicity following GM-CSF in the setting of autologous bone marrow transplantation for advanced Hodgkin's disease was briefly reported (629[c]). The prompt occurrence of hyperbilirubinemia was later found in 8% of bone marrow transplant patients and considered as possible grounds for molgramostim discontinuation (598[c]).

Urinary system No evidence of nephrotoxicity secondary to GM-CSF was been identified during clinical trials, but the possible occurrence of transient renal insufficiency has sometimes been discussed (598[c]).

Skin and appendages GM-CSF frequently induced erythema and itching at the site of subcutaneous injections (600[R]). A particularly high incidence of relapsing macular pruritic infiltrates at the site of injection was noted in patients with inflammatory breast cancer (630[c]). Based on a retrospective review, molgramostim-induced rash was found to be the most common adverse event leading to the discontinuation of treatment in bone marrow transplant patients, but further administration of sargramostim was sometimes well tolerated (598).

Cutaneous reactions have been carefully described in 57 cancer patients and included localized immediate angioedematous reactions (8%), generalized cutaneous reactions (21%) or both (16%) (631[C]). Generalized reactions consisted mostly of maculopapular, exfoliative and urticarial eruptions, which resolved following topical treatments, dose reduction or treatment discontinuation. Hyperkeratosis, mild spongiosis, lymphocytic exocytosis and a perivascular infiltration by lymphocytes, neutrophils and eosinophil, was usually found. Eosinophil activation was probably involved in the pathogenesis of these lesions. However, the exact mechanism remains speculative and may also involve other cytokines or inflammatory mediators. GM-CSF was also involved in atopic dermatitis-like eruptions in two of five bone marrow transplant patients (632[c]).

Several reports suggested that GM-CSF may induce (633[C]) or exacerbate (606[c], 634[C]) cutaneous leukocytoclastic vasculitis, a side effect which was substantiated by a prompt recurrence of vasculitis after drug re-administration (606, 634). Renal or pulmonary involvement was sometimes noted (633, 634). Relapsing necrotizing vasculitis at all GM-CSF injection sites has also been described and an immune-mediated mechanism suggested to be involved (635[C]). Single cases of neutrophilic dermatoses have been reported following GM-CSF and included the acute exacerbation of previous pyoderma gangrenosum (636[C]) or the occurrence of subcorneal pustular dermatosis around injection sites with linear subcorneal IgA deposits (637[C]). GM-CSF was involved in a reversible acute bullous eruption further diagnosed as epidermolysis bullosa acquisita (638[C]). An acute revelation of this autoimmune bullous disease in a previously asymptomatic patient cannot be ruled out. More recently, Stasi et al. (639[C]) reported a reversible erythema multiforme after 2 weeks of GM-CSF, and an immunological hypersensitivity response with inappropriate cytokine secretion was suggested to be involved. Acute and generalized exacerbation of pre-existing moderate psoriasis has been reported following GM-CSF administration (640[C]) and is in keeping with the finding that GM-CSF is sometimes elevated in patients with psoriasis.

Musculoskeletal system Mild-to-moderate transient bone pains were commonly observed (603[R]). Reactivation or worsening of rheumatoid symptoms associated with a prompt increase in acute phase proteins has sometimes been observed shortly after starting GM-CSF for Felty's syndrome (641[C]). Reversible flare-up of rheumatoid symptoms in a seropositive rheumatoid arthritic patient has also been reported (642[C]). GM-CSF induced acute IL-6 release from synovial cells was thought perhaps to be involved.

Miscellaneous The stimulating effects of GM-CSF on the myeloid lineage and other cells of the immune system were sometimes associated with deleterious consequences. Histiocytic bone marrow proliferation following several days of GM-CSF administration (643, 644[C]) and reactive hematophagic histiocytosis resulting in persistent and fatal pancytopenia were possible consequences of overstimulation of the host immune system (645[C]). This adverse outcome may be explained by the effects of GM-CSF on the proliferation and activation of mononuclear phagocytes. Because the production of cytokines (mostly IL-1 or TNF-α) involved in the stimulation of cells responsible for graft-versus-host disease (GvHD) can be enhanced by hematopoietic growth factors, their use after allogeneic transplantation is theoretically risky. Reviews of clinical trials using G-CSF or GM-CSF in the setting of allogeneic bone marrow transplantation were however unable to identify any possible increase in the risk of late engraftment failure, relapse rate, or exacerbation of GvHD (601, 602[R]).

Although they were not clearly observed in clinical

trials (646[R]), other theoretical effects of growth factors may also include enhanced HIV replication in myeloid cells and acceleration of HIV-associated diseases (603[R]). At the moment, only one AIDS patient with ultrasonographic confirmation of enhanced Kaposi's sarcoma lesions temporally related to GM-CSF used for interferon- and zidovudine-related severe neutropenia has been reported (647[C]).

Antibodies to GM-CSF, cross-reacting with *E. coli*-derived GM-CSF but not with mammalian-derived GM-CSF were initially described in four of 13 patients treated with yeast-derived rhGM-CSF (648[C]). The immunogenic potential of rGM-CSF was further confirmed in patients receiving molgramostim, of whom 95% developed neutralizing antibodies against the exogenous cytokine after the second cycle (649[C]). Although the clinical relevance remains to be more clearly established, a significant modification of exogenous GM-CSF pharmacokinetics, a reduction in the rise of leukocyte count, and a reduction of GM-CSF-associated adverse effects were suggested as possible consequences. The subcutaneous route and repeated schedule of administration in this study can be expected to increase the likelihood of antibody occurrence. That most patients receiving growth factors are likely to be immunocompromised as a result of chemotherapy, might also account for discrepancies observed between the wide use of growth factors and the paucity of reports on antibodies against growth factors. Importantly, only one patient with very low anti-GM-CSF antibody titers was found among eight multiple myeloma patients receiving intensive chemotherapy. Again, antibodies to GM-CSF were not found after prolonged use in AIDS patients (650[C]).

Hypersensitivity reactions GM-CSF has exceptionally been associated with anaphylaxis, and a recurrent immediate local reaction followed by systemic hypersensitivity reaction was reported once after a 7-month regimen of sargramostim (651[C]). Prick skin tests to GM-CSF were positive and the patient further tolerated G-CSF uneventfully. Anaphylactic-type reactions without documented immune-mediated mechanism have been reported in approximately 8% of GM-CSF treatments in advanced testicular cancer (652[c]).

Tumour-inducing effects The possibility that growth factors may stimulate the growth of malignant and leukemic cells, or accelerate the progression of a myelodysplastic syndrome to acute myeloid leukemia was pointed out by Schriber and Negrin (603[R]), and is further discussed in the G-CSF section.

At the moment, there is no indication from clinical trials that GM-CSF actually does increase the risk of tumor growth or raise the relapse rate in patients treated for various malignancies (600, 602, 603). No increased risk of graft failure, leukemogenesis, relapse or death was indeed found after a median follow-up of 36 months in 128 patients (653[c]). De novo occurrence of diffuse oligoclonal plasmocytosis following a 10-month treatment with multiple chemotherapy and both GM-CSF and G-CSF in a young patient with high-grade glioma was recently reported (654[C]).

In addition, although reversible increases in circulating blasts during GM-CSF treatment has sometimes been noted in patients with myelodysplastic syndrome or myeloid leukemia, no evidence of significant leukemic cell proliferation has been found in controlled trials of patients treated for acute myeloid leukemia (600, 602, 603, 655[R]). More recently, a placebo-controlled, randomized trial in elderly patients with acute myelogenous leukemia did not show a significant difference in the regrowth of leukemia in the GM-CSF-treated versus control groups (656[C]). One single case report recently described a B cell non-Hodgkin's lymphoma 4.5 years after short-duration GM-CSF treatment for aplastic anemia (657[C]). An abrupt rise in peripheral blasts with diffuse infiltration of the spleen and subsequent fatal hemorrhagic spleen rupture shortly after GM-CSF was also attributed to splenic proliferation of leukemic blast cells in a patient primed for acute monocytic leukemia (658[C]).

Granulocyte colony-stimulating factor (G-CSF)

G-CSF primarily increases neutrophil production and function. *Escherichia coli*-derived recombinant G-CSF (filgrastim) is not glycosylated while Chinese hamster ovary cells-derived recombinant G-CSF (lenograstim) is partly glycosylated. Although the in vitro potency of lenograstim is higher than filgrastim, no comparative study evaluated the therapeutic and safety relevance of these differences.

Filgrastim was approved for chemotherapy-induced neutropenia and in patients receiving high-dose chemotherapy followed by bone marrow transplantation at daily doses ranging from 5 to 10 μg/kg. In several countries, G-CSF was also approved for use in severe chronic neutropenic diseases (United Kingdom), aplastic anemia, myelodysplastic syndrome or acute leukemia (Japan). The pharmacodynamics, pharmacokinetics and clinical applications of lenograstim or filgrastim were recently reviewed (601, 602, 659, 660).

At the recommended doses, G-CSF is usually well-tolerated with generalized musculoskeletal and transient bone pains, headache, and mild rash as the commonest adverse effects (603[R]). Fever is less common than with GM-CSF. Limited experience in 10 children treated with higher doses (400–2000 $\mu g/m^2$/day) for aplastic anemia showed no major toxicity (661[c]). Adverse events were infrequent and led to the discontinuation or temporary withdrawal of treatment in only seven of 44 patients with severe congenital neutropenia treated for 4–6 years (662[C]).

ORGANS AND SYSTEMS

Cardiovascular A possible excess in cardiovascular events and unexpected death was recently suggested (663[c]) and was also found in a randomized controlled trial (664[c]), but further evaluation of the actual risk is needed. Acute popliteal arterial thrombosis has been described during antineoplastic and G-CSF therapy in a single patient (665[C]). Hypercoagulability associated with extreme leukocytosis and a G-CSF-induced increase in ADP-induced platelet aggregation could have both played a role (666). Nevertheless, caution is warranted in patients predisposed to thromboembolic events.

Although it was not described during clinical trials, a typical capillary leak syndrome associated with central intravenous G-CSF administration has been reported in two patients with malignant lymphoma treated with high-dose chemotherapy (667[C]).

Respiratory Several isolated reports and small case series of patients recently focused on the possibility that G-CSF can increase the pulmonary toxicity of bleomycin (668–670[C]) and cyclophosphamide (671[C]). Interestingly, pulmonary failure was observed while the neutrophil count was significantly increased. Non-infectious interstitial pneumonia, sometimes fatal, was reported in eight of 40 patients receiving antineoplastic drugs (mostly methotrexate and bleomycin) and G-CSF for malignant lymphoma, while no such cases had appeared prior to G-CSF use among 35 historical controls (672[c]). Another retrospective study found severe pulmonary complications (fatal in three) in four of 12 patients with non-Hodgkin's lymphoma treated with the BACOP (bleomycin, doxorubicin, cyclophosphamide, vincristine and prednisone) regimen plus G-CSF in comparison to one of 24 historical control patients treated with the same regimen without G-CSF (673[c]). However, French authors strongly disagreed with these results as they found no difference in the incidence of pulmonary complications in their randomized trials of 278 G-CSF vs placebo patients who received a bleomycin-containing regimen for non-Hodgkin's lymphoma (674[c]). In a recent randomized trial, finger-pulse oximetry was used to monitor pulmonary function in 35 consecutive admissions (675[C]). Transient slight hypoxia with a median reduction in O_2 saturation from 5 to 16% was found 12 times, and corresponded to G-CSF use in 83% of these cases. However, no relation with a specific cytotoxic treatment or previous radiotherapy was found.

The abrupt increase in neutrophil counts and functions induced by exogenous growth factors may also play an additional role in the development of the adult respiratory distress syndrome (ARDS). ARDS has been described during the neutrophil recovery in three of nine patients receiving G-CSF for drug-induced agranulocytosis (676[C]). Although worsening of an underlying illness (i.e. previous pulmonary failure and severe sepsis) is possible, the contributing role of G-CSF cannot be ruled out. The worsening of underlying ARDS with impaired gas exchange in one patient treated with G-CSF for antibiotic-induced neutropenia emphasizes again the need to evaluate carefully the use of growth factors in drug-induced agranulocytosis (677[C]).

Although the mechanism of G-CSF pulmonary toxicity has not been established, endothelial damage subsequent to increased neutrophil functions (i.e enhancement of superoxide release, increase in adhesion molecule expression and adherence) or the release of cytokines (IL-1, IL-6, TNF) have been advanced as possibilities (669, 672, 673, 676).

Endocrine, metabolic No influence on thyroid function, thyroid peroxidase antibody and thyroglobulin antibody titers was observed in 20 breast cancer patients receiving subcutaneous G-CSF, including two patients with positive thyroid antibodies prior to treatment (678). Minor biological abnormalities, namely transiently elevated leukocyte alkaline phosphatase and uric acid serum levels, are considered to be physiological consequences of the rise in neutrophil count observed after G-CSF treatment (SEDA-17, 396). The frequent occurrence of moderate increase in serum lactate dehydrogenase (LDH) and alkaline phosphatase (ALP) should not be interpreted as disease progression, but rather as enzyme release following leukocyte recovery (679–681). Decreases in serum cholesterol levels have also been observed (659[r]).

Hematological Eosinophilia was sometimes observed in patients on long-term G-CSF for congenital neutropenia (662[c]). Patients treated with G-CSF for congenital neutropenia or Felty's syndrome could also be predisposed to develop anemia and/or thrombocytopenia (662[c], 682[C]). Emperipolesis of neutrophils within megakaryocytes, an unusual feature of thrombocytopenia, was found in one patient on high-dose G-CSF (683[C]).

Asymptomatic increase in spleen volume (from 2 to 148%) concomitant with neutrophilia has been reported in about 25% of patients treated with G-CSF for severe chronic neutropenia (659, 662, 684[c]) and splenomegaly with documented extramedullary hematopoiesis attributable to the mobilization of early hematopoietic progenitors from the marrow to the spleen was also described (685[C]).

Coagulation disorders have not appeared during clinical trials. However, the occurrence and subsequent worsening of a disseminated intravascular coagulopathy was noted in a young HIV-infected boy treated with zidovudine and increasing G-CSF doses (686[C]). Thrombopenia was retrospectively found in nine of 28 similar patients after a median of 11 weeks of subcutaneous G-CSF with various antiretroviral drugs and five had various coagulation abnormalities (686[C]). The relevance of such findings and the role of G-CSF is unknown.

Liver Clinical trials did not suggest G-CSF-induced hepatotoxicity. A reversible increase in transaminase and γ-glutamyl transpeptidase levels was observed in two patients (687, 688[C]). Although this hepatic reaction may have been coincidental, a further increase in liver tests after G-CSF re-administration is in keeping with drug-induced hepatotoxicity (688). One case of fatal fulminant hepatitis after a short G-CSF treatment could have be due to alcohol abuse and several concomitant drugs (687[R]). Acute hepatitis and pancreatitis in an HIV-infected patient with previously normal hepatic and pancreatic functions were described, and both abnormalities promptly recurred after G-CSF re-administration (689[C]).

Urinary system No evidence of nephrotoxicity emerged from clinical trials, but transient and isolated hematuria was sometimes observed in long-term G-CSF treatments of congenital neutropenias (662[c]).

Skin and appendages Skin disorders were mostly minor with skin rash or itching reported in approximately 8% of G-CSF-treated patients (659[R]). In addition, widespread vesiculopustular lesions developing after each subcutaneous G-CSF injection (690[C]), localized cutaneous reactions similar to those described with GM-CSF (691[C]) and the occurrence of subcutaneous nodules infiltrated by leukemic blast cells at the injection sites for acute myelomonocytic leukemia (692[C]) were described in isolated reports. Atypical leukemic cells were also found in erythematous eruptions after each G-CSF administration in two patients with acute myelogenous leukemia (693[C]).

Leukocytoclastic vasculitis is a well-recognized side effect of G-CSF (694–698), and the literature includes cases with positive rechallenge (696–698). Jain recently analyzed 18 cases reported in the literature or to the manufacturer (699[cR]). Among 16 assessable cases, vasculitis was identified in 6% of patients treated for chronic benign neutropenia, and in only six of approximately 200 000 patients treated for malignant disease. This author noted also that vasculitis developed usually when the neutrophil count was above 800/μl, thus suggesting that an increase in neutrophil counts may play a role in necrotic vasculitis. Although most cases were confined to the skin, renal failure with hematuria and proteinuria was sometimes observed (696). The occurrence of vasculitis is not treatment-limiting and does not preclude further G-CSF administration providing that the absolute neutrophil count is maintained below 1000/μl (699).

Reports of induction or exacerbation of neutrophilic dermatitis is in keeping with the stimulating effects of G-CSF on the production and functions of neutrophils. Although initially debated (SEDA-17, 396), recent reports of biopsy-proven Sweet's syndrome (acute febrile neutrophilic dermatosis) (700–703[C]) are convincing due to the close temporal relationship between treatment onset and the neutrophil count increase, to the spontaneous regression following G-CSF withdrawal and the white blood cell decrease (703), or the recurrence of the lesions after G-CSF re-administration (700–702). Bullous pyoderma gangrenosum, which disappeared after G-CSF discontinuation and topical or systemic corticosteroid treatment, was also reported in two cancer patients (704, 705[C]).

Lenograstim was reportedly involved in a case of corticosensitive erythema nodosum which recurred after filgrastim (706[C]). Finally, several reports involved G-CSF treatment in the exacerbation of pre-existing psoriasis (694[C], 707[c]).

Musculoskeletal system Transient bone pain within 2–3 days before myeloid recovery were the commonest side-effects of G-CSF as compared to GM-CSF. They occurred in up to 20–25% of patients receiving intravenous or subcutaneous injections (603, 659). Bone pain used to disappear despite continuation of treatment.

Worsening of rheumatoid symptoms was sometimes reported in patients treated for neutropenia of Felty's syndrome (708–710[C]). In one typical case, a flare of rheumatoid symptoms recurred after G-CSF rechallenge (710). The mechanisms involved are unclear and G-CSF-induced neutrophil activation in the joint, or G-CSF-mediated increase in local neutrophil response to TNF-α have both been suggested to be involved (708, 710).

A possible exacerbation of osteoporosis was recently reported in patients on long-term G-CSF for severe congenital neutropenia (662), but improvement or stabilization during treatment was also noted in other patients. Furthermore, no apparent effect on height, head circumference and weight was found in patients under 18 years of age. Severe osteoporosis was extensively investigated in a child (711[C]) who experienced osteoporotic vertebral collapse, reduced bone mineral content, decreased levels of osteocalcin and features of osteoporosis on bone biopsy. Only prospective monitoring of growth and bone mineral content in chronically G-CSF-treated patients would be useful to further assess this potential complication.

Miscellaneous The clinical consequences of stimulation of immune cells have been illustrated by the development of a rapid and generalized lymph node enlargement with a decrease in peripheral blood lymphocytes 1 week after G-CSF administration (712[C]). Interestingly, lymphadenopathy reappeared following a further course of G-CSF.

Antibodies to rG-CSF have not so far been reported (659, 660), even in patients on long-term treatment (662).

Hypersensitivity reactions Anaphylaxis after subcutaneous filgrastim was reported in a patient receiving multiple other medications (713[C]). Severe systemic reactions were suggested to be type-I immune reactions because of positive intradermal tests and elevated IgE level in two patients treated with filgrastim and lenograstim, respectively (714[C]). Cross-reactions between the two recombinant products were not found, and one patient who presented with hypersensitivity reactions to GM-CSF further tolerated G-CSF administration (651). However, anaphylaxis to G-CSF is supposedly extremely rare and the manufacturer is aware of only two cases of anaphylactoid reactions among 20 000 filgrastim-treated patients (715).

Tumor-inducing effects As with GM-CSF, there was some concern that G-CSF may stimulate the growth of leukemic cells, promote myeloid malignancies, or accelerate the progression of myelodysplastic syndromes to acute myeloid leukemias. However, although receptors to growth factors have been demonstrated on leukemic blasts and several carcinoma or melanoma lines, no clear clinical evidence of disease acceleration was found in G-CSF-treated patients (603[R]). Published reports were essentially based on temporal relationships between the start of G-CSF administration and the development or acceleration of malignancies in single patients treated for gastric cancer (717[C]) or Hodgkin's disease (718, 719[C]). G-CSF has been involved in blast mobilizations with a phenotype change from common acute lymphoblastic leukemia to biphenotypic leukemia (719[C]). Pseudoleukemia features on bone-marrow biopsy was also observed after only a 2-day administration of G-CSF in a pancytopenic lymphoma patient (720[C]). Available clinical data or results of several randomized controlled trials in patients with various malignancies provide no evidence for increased relapse rates (603, 659, 660[R]).

There was also some reluctance in the use of G-CSF in acute myeloid leukemia. No clear evidence of disease acceleration was found in several recent reviews (602, 659, 660). In addition, a double-blind, placebo-controlled, randomized clinical trial in elderly patients receiving chemotherapy for acute myelogenous leukemia did not find a significant difference in the regrowth of leukemia in the G-CSF versus control groups (721).

The progression of myelodysplastic syndromes to acute myeloid leukemia is of greater concern as several investigators noted reversible increases in circulating blasts during G-CSF treatment in this setting (603[R]). However, no increased incidence of the confirmed progression to acute myeloblastic leukemia was found in G-CSF patients compared to controls (659[R]). In any case, myelodysplastic syndrome patients with more than 20% of blast cells in the bone marrow should be considered to be at a higher risk of leukemic transformation.

Isolated reports suggested a shortened delay in the occurrence of myelodysplasia and/or acute myeloid leukemia in patients on G-CSF maintenance therapy for aplastic anemia or severe congenital neutropenia (722–725[C]), but a previous history of immunosuppressive therapy may also play a role. In most cases, acquired monosomy 7 was observed and in vitro proliferation of myeloblasts by G-CSF was obtained in one patient (723[C]). The long-term outcome (median follow-up of 43 months) of 123 pediatric patients treated with G-CSF did not show a difference in the incidence of secondary myelodysplasia or acute myeloid leukemia in aplastic anemia patients surviving longer than 2 years as compared to the expected rate calculated prior to G-CSF use (726). Similarly, no evidence for an increased risk of myelodysplasia or acute myeloid leukemia was found in 54 patients treated with G-CSF during 4–6 years for severe congenital neutropenia (662). Although aplastic anemia might be a preleukemic disorder, a possible increased rate of myelodysplastic syndrome or acute myeloid leukemia after G-CSF should be borne in mind.

The safety of growth factors in myeloma patients is also of concern as they can stimulate the proliferation of myeloma cells through IL-6 expression, but few clinical data are available. The mobilization of clonal myeloma cells into the peripheral circulation in one patient receiving G-CSF to mobilize peripheral stem cells for autologous rescue (727[C]), the rapid progression of a multiple myeloma shortly after G-CSF treatment to mobilize hematopoietic stem cells (728[C]), and the onset of a monoclonal gammopathy only 3 days after G-CSF administration in one patient with acute myelogenous leukemia (729[C]), directly or indirectly support the view that caution should be exercised in patients with multiple myeloma.

Macrophage colony-stimulating factor (M-CSF)

M-CSF stimulates the growth and differentiation of the monocyte lineage, and promotes the survival, proliferation and functions of mature monocyte/macrophage. M-CSF also enhances myelopoiesis through the amplified production of G-CSF and GM-CSF by monocytes, and exerts antitumoral activity. Both purified human urinary M-CSF (hM-CSF) and recombinant human M-CSF have been investigated in humans.

Recombinant M-CSF (RhM-CSF)

The most significant side effect of glycosylated mammalian-derived rhM-CSF in a phase I trial was a dose- and schedule-related severe thrombopenia which typically occurred after 7—10 days of treatment (730[C]). By contrast, a 7-day regimen produced a significant, but not treatment-limiting thrombopenia. Thrombopenia correlated with monocytosis and reversed within 2—3 days after cessation of treatment, and was the only significant toxicity in most other trials. In severe cases, a 50% reduction in rhM-CSF dose was sufficient to decrease the severity of thrombopenia and to permit continued treatment (731). The mechanism of rhM-CSF-induced thrombopenia is unknown, but splenomegaly and a possible splenic sequestration might account for this effect.

Other significant toxicities observed with high-dose rhM-CSF consisted of subclinical conjunctival injection in 50% of patients undergoing ophthalmological examination, and was associated with moderate but symptomatic episcleritis and blurred vision in one patient (730[c]). Asymptomatic retinal or perilimbal hemorrhages were also sometimes noted and no clear correlation with platelet counts was found. Subjective ophthalmological symptoms, ocular inflammation, iridocyclitis or malaise also appeared as dose- or treatment-limiting toxicities in other trials (732, 733[c]). Constitutional symptoms consisting of malaise, fatigue, insomnia, headache, nausea, fever, chills were sometimes noted (732—734), as was local toxicity after subcutaneous injection (732[c]). In addition, the development of multiple subcutaneous nodules which recurred after each administration, and were consistent with a panniculitis on skin biopsy, was recently described (735[C]). No further toxicities were observed in the long-term follow-up of patients receiving rhM-CSF after allogeneic bone marrow transplantation (731).

Human urinary M-CSF

The safety of hM-CSF in allogeneic and syngeneic bone marrow transplantation was evaluated in a randomized double-blind placebo-controlled phase III trial involving 119 patients (736). Only transient mild fever was noted in 6.7% of patients and there were no significant adverse effects on platelet count. The incidence of graft-versus-host disease, engraftment failure and the leukemic relapse rate were not affected as compared to the placebo group. Similarly, a 21-day intravenous infusion regimen of hM-CSF was not associated with significant toxicity in autologous bone marrow transplant patients compared to a control group (737). However, severe erythrodermia after high-dose hM-CSF was recently described (738[C]), and a dramatic proliferation of blast cells with mobilization in peripheral blood was also noted after each hM-CSF dose in a patient with acute myeloblastic leukemia and karyotypic 5q anomaly (739[C]).

IMMUNOSUPPRESSIVE DRUGS

GENERAL CONSIDERATIONS

Malignancies and infectious diseases These represent the two major causes of morbidity and/or mortality after the fifth year of transplantation.

Updating data from the Cincinnati Transplant Tumor Registry, published in 1993, has rendered possible a comprehensive description of the characteristics of several neoplasms observed in organ transplant recipients (740). Skin and lip cancers are the most common, aggressive squamous cell carcinoma being most frequently observed as compared to the general population. Non-Hodgkin's lymphomas represented the majority of lymphoproliferative disorders, and the incidence was 30—50-fold higher than in controls (741). An excess of Kaposi's sarcomas, carcinomas of the vulva and perineum, hepatobiliary tumors and various sarcomas, is also reported in transplant patients. By contrast, the incidence of common neoplasms encountered in the general population is not increased after transplantation. In renal transplant patients, the actuarial cumulative risk of cancer is 18% at 10 years, 33% at 15 years and 50% at 20 years, and men are more frequently affected by skin cancer than are women (742). In addition, the relative risk of skin tumors tends to increase with time, whereas it remains similar for non-skin tumors. Very similar figures have been found by other investigators (743). The longer survival of transplant recipients clearly underlies the extent of this problem and the need for close monitoring of patients.

Whilst there is no doubt that the incidence of malignancies is increased in the transplant population, there are still some controversies as to which factor, namely treatment duration, total dosage, the degree of immunosuppression or the type of immunosuppressive regimens, is the most relevant. Partial or complete regression of lymphoproliferative disorders and Kaposi's sarcomas after reduction of immunosuppressive therapy strongly argues for the role of the degree of immunosuppression (740). The incidence of cancer was significantly higher in renal transplant patients receiving triple therapy regimens as compared to double therapy (744). Similarly, aggressive immunosuppressive therapy may account for the higher incidence of lymphomas in cardiac versus renal allograft patients. In a large multicenter study involving more than 52 000 kidney and heart transplant patients between 1983 and 1991, the rate of non-Hodgkin's lymphomas in the first post-transplantation year was 0.2% in kidney and 1.2% in heart recipients, and decreased substantially thereafter (745). Initial immunosuppression with both azathioprine and ciclosporin, and prophylactic treatment with antilymphocyte antibodies was associated with a significantly increased incidence of non-Hodgkin's lymphomas as compared to other immunosuppressive regimens, which confirmed the major role of the initial degree of immunosuppression. No increased incidence of lymphoma was observed in patients receiving ciclosporin without azathioprine. Other authors were also unable to find evidence that ciclosporin specifically increases the risk of tumors as compared to previously used immunosuppressive regimens (742, 746), and some even suggested a possibly lower incidence in ciclosporin-treated patients (747, 748). Patients with rheumatoid arthritis receiving ciclosporin had an increased relative risk of malignancies as compared to those given corticosteroids, but it was similar to the risk in patients treated with disease-modifying antirheumatic drugs (749). The spontaneous occurrence of cancers unrelated to the treatment cannot be excluded, and an increased risk of lymphomas has been repeatedly found in patients with rheumatoid arthritis (750). Among 3700 patients treated with ciclosporin for autoimmune disease, the overall incidence of lymphoma was 0.14% (751). Finally, the most striking difference between conventional and modern immunosuppressive regimens, including ciclosporin, was the average time to the appearance of tumors, in particular skin cancers and lymphomas, which was shorter in ciclosporin-treated patients (747, 748).

Multiple factors with complex interactions are obviously involved in the observed pattern and increased incidence of neoplasms in transplant patients. They include severely depressed immunity with an impaired immune surveillance against various carcinogens, the activation of several oncogenic viruses in immunosuppressed patients, as suggested by the early of occurrence of several tumors, and a possible mutagenic effect of the drugs. Viruses, such as papillomavirus, cytomegalovirus and Epstein-Barr virus are believed to play an important role in the development of several post-transplant cancers. From a theoretical point of view, the use of antiviral drugs active against herpes viruses which are commonly implicated as cofactors, can be expected to produce a reduction in the incidence of post-transplant lymphoproliferative disorders. Future studies designed to evaluate the incidence of neoplasms in transplant patients should take into account the use of these drugs.

Infections, in particular bacterial and viral pathogens (cytomegalovirus, herpes simplex virus, Epstein-Barr virus), and also protozoal and fungal infections, are also a cause of morbidity and mortality in the post-transplantation period, whatever the immunosuppressive regimen used (752—756).

Teratogenesis A number of reports have described the outcome of pregnancies following organ transplantation (757). Drugs commonly used in transplant patients do not appear to increase the risk of congenital malformations, and no difference in the rate of malformations was found when comparing ciclosporin to other immunosuppressive regimens (758, 759). Similarly, no birth defects were observed among 10 children from tacrolimus-treated women (760). However, very high tacrolimus cord levels were found in one child who presented with neonatal anuria.

The National Transplantation Pregnancy Registry has recently analyzed 197 pregnancies in women treated with ciclosporin (761). Hypertension, pre-eclampsia and infections were frequently noted. Ectopic pregnancies and miscarriages seemed to occur at a similar rate as compared to the general population. Pregnancies resulted in liveborn infants in 68%, and half of the newborns were premature while the other half were low-birthweight. A decreased renal graft function during pregnancy was associated with a greater risk of lower birthweight newborns and graft loss. Another study of 133 pregnancies confirmed that intrauterine growth retardation, premature birth, low birthweight and increased perinatal mortality rate, are critical complications (759). Ciclosporin was associated with more frequent miscarriage, pre-term birth and intrauterine growth retardation, but the comparison was based on a small number of patients. Other risk factors associated with adverse outcomes are many-fold and include a short time interval between transplantation and pregnancy, impaired renal function prior to pregnancy, and hypertension (759, 762).

Long-term effects of in utero exposure to immunosuppressive agents have been studied in a limited number of children. Reduced renal function was not found in children prenatally exposed to ciclosporin (763). No adverse effects on the immune system were found in a 2-year-old girl exposed in utero to ciclosporin (764). Similarly, while changes in T-lymphocytes subsets were found in seven children born to azathioprine- or ciclosporin-treated mothers, immune function assays were normal (765).

Azathioprine

Azathioprine, a pro-drug converted to 6-mercaptopurine (6-MP), is widely used as a post-transplant thiopurine immunosuppressant or in various autoimmune or inflammatory disorders, such as rheumatoid arthritis, dermatomyositis, systemic lupus erythematosus, chronic skin and inflammatory bowel diseases. In a recent meta-analysis of nine randomized, placebo-controlled trials of azathioprine or 6-MP in Crohn's disease, adverse events requiring drug withdrawal, namely allergy, leukopenia, pancreatitis and nausea, were 5 times more frequent in the purine analog group (766).

ORGAN AND SYSTEMS

Hematological Dose-dependent hematological toxicity, namely pancytopenia or predominant leukopenia and thrombopenia, remains the most commonly reported adverse effect in patients receiving azathioprine. In a 27-year survey of 739 patients treated with 2 mg/kg azathioprine for inflammatory bowel disease, dose reduction or discontinuation of the drug because of bone marrow toxicity was necessary in 37 patients (5%) (767). Moderate or severe leukopenia was the most frequent (3.8%) and was associated with pancytopenia resulting in death or severe sepsis in three patients. Isolated thrombopenia without severe clinical consequences was also sometimes observed. Macrocytic anemia has been previously reported in several patients. Reversible pure red cell aplasia has been rarely reported and may occur late after starting the treatment (768). Hematotoxicity usually occurs in the first 4 weeks of treatment, but strict and continuous surveillance of blood cell counts is required as delayed occurrence has also been observed (769).

Abnormalities in purine enzyme activities with resulting increases in the levels of cytotoxic thionucleotides and enhancement of bone marrow toxicity has been thought to be involved. Several recent papers strongly argue for a pharmacogenetic basis to explain myelotoxicity in transplant recipients (770, 771), or in patients with rheumatoid arthritis (772) or autoimmune hepatitis (773). Compared to rheumatoid arthritis subjects without azathioprine-associated bone marrow toxicity, erythrocyte thiopurine methyltransferase (TPMT) and/or lymphocyte 5′-nucleotidase (5-NT) activities were low or even completely absent in the three patients who presented with severe bone marrow toxicity (772). Again, TPMT deficiency was associated with very high levels of red blood cell 6-thioguanine metabolites in heart transplanted patients with severe leukopenia following azathioprine (771). TPMT deficiency in a pancytopenic patient receiving azathioprine was also found in several members of his family and this resulted in higher 6-MP plasma levels (774). Very low TPMT activity is not sufficient to account for azathioprine-induced bone marrow toxicity (775), and low activity of 5-NT was found as another major cause in patients without TPMT deficiency (776). Finally, xanthine oxidase deficiency might also contribute to azathioprine hematotoxicity (777). At the moment, the screening for purine enzyme activities, i.e. TPMT and/or 5-NT, is not routinely used but deficiency in purine enzymes should be suspected in patients presenting with bone-marrow toxicity shortly after the beginning of treatment.

Liver Hepatotoxicity is an infrequent, but well-known side effect of azathioprine (SED-8, 1118) requiring careful and regular monitoring of liver test functions (769, 778). Reversible cholestatic hepatitis is the most frequent side effect, and bile duct injury has been suggested as a possible cause (779). Hepatocellular injury was rarely found. Other histological features included lesions of the liver venous system, namely peliosis hepatitis, sinusoidal dilatation, perivenous fibrosis and nodular regenerative hyperplasia (780, 781), and were associated with portal hypertension (SEDA-16, 520; 778).

Interestingly, in 29 cardiac transplant recipients who had experienced liver dysfunction, probably related to azathioprine, cyclophosphamide was safely substituted and liver enzyme levels improved without an increased incidence of rejection episodes or a significant change in corticosteroid and/or ciclosporin doses (782).

Severe and potentially fatal veno-occlusive liver diseases have been reported in renal and allogeneic bone marrow transplanted patients receiving chronic administration of azathioprine (SED-8, 1118). Similar complications have been described shortly after liver transplantation (783, 784). A previous episode of acute liver rejection affecting mostly the hepatic veins was supposedly a contributing factor and the presence of non-inflammatory small hepatic vein lesions was considered as a possible early indicator of azathioprine hepatotoxicity following hepatic transplantation (783). In any case, liver biopsy should be considered in azathioprine-treated patients with elevated serum transaminase activity or cholestasis, so that discontinuation of the treatment can be carried out rapidly if necessary (784).

Gastrointestinal Pancreatitis has sometimes been reported as part of the azathioprine or 6-MP hypersensitivity reaction (SEDA-16, 520), and required withdrawal of treatment in 1.3% of patients with Crohn's disease (766). Pancreatitis or hyperamylasemia were not found to be significantly different in renal transplant patients randomly assigned to receive azathioprine or ciclosporin, and other causative factors were found in most patients with pancreatitis (785).

Musculoskeletal system Severe myalgia and symmetrical polyarthritis have been reported. Eight cases of azathioprine-associated arthritis were identified in the WHO drug monitoring database including six cases with a typical hypersensitivity syndrome and two cases in whom joint involvement was the only reported symptom (786).

Miscellaneous The risk of infectious complications linked to azathioprine immunosuppressive activity has never been carefully assessed. A fatal case of Epstein-Barr virus-associated hemophagocytic syndrome was reported in a young male patient receiving azathioprine and prednisone for Crohn's disease (787). Donor-specific blood transfusion in the preparation for transplantation was found to be complicated by a higher incidence of cytomegalovirus infection in patients receiving azathioprine (788).

Hypersensitivity reactions Azathioprine-associated systemic hypersensitivity is well known, with various symptoms occurring separately or concomitantly, namely fever and rigors, arthralgias, myalgias, leukocytosis, cutaneous reactions, gastrointestinal disturbances, hypotension, cholestasis or hepatocellular injury, pancreatitis, interstitial nephritis or pneumonitis (789). There is no evidence to suggest that the incidence of azathioprine hypersensitivity is different depending on the underlying treated disease. Allergic reactions were found in 2% of patients with Crohn's disease (766). Symptoms usually occurred within the first 6 weeks of treatment and sometimes mimicked sepsis (790). The more rapid recurrence and/or severe symptoms following azathioprine rechallenge were in keeping with a putative immune-mediated reaction (791, 792), but no immunological mechanism has yet been clearly evidenced. On the basis of rapidly recurring pneumonitis with pulmonary hemorrhage and the positivity of leukocyte migration inhibition test, a cell-mediated immune mechanism has been suggested to be involved (793). A genetic predisposition is also suspected, with a possible association between the hypersensitivity syndrome and the Bw4 and Bw6 phenotypes (791, 792). Interestingly, 6-MP was re-administered safely in two patients who had previously experienced a severe systemic hypersensitivity mimicking gastroenteritis (794) or Goodpasture's syndrome (795) following azathioprine, suggesting a major role for the imidazole moiety of azathioprine.

Anaphylactic shock has also been reported occasionally (796). Moreover, delayed contact hypersensitivity with positive patch test was found in a pharmaceutical handler of azathioprine (797).

Drug interactions Allopurinol inhibits xanthine oxidase, an enzyme involved in the inactivation of azathioprine and 6-MP, and several cases of bone marrow suppression have appeared following the concomitant use of allopurinol and azathioprine (SEDA-16, 114; 798). A reduction of at least 25% in azathioprine or 6-MP dosage, and careful hematological monitoring have been proposed if their combined use is required (769).

Tumour-inducing effects An increased incidence of secondary tumors specifically related to azathioprine immunosuppressive treatments remains difficult to demonstrate. Squamous cell carcinomas of the skin are the most frequently reported effects after transplantation. In renal transplant recipients, premalignant dysplastic keratotic lesions were shown to increase linearly by 6.8% per year after 3.5 years following transplantation, and were finally observed in all 167 patients within 16 years of transplantation (799). Interestingly, no relation with sun exposure or skin type was found in this study. The great majority of these patients were on prednisolone and azathioprine, but azathioprine was considered as the main causative factor, possibly due to a carcinogenic effect rather than to immunosuppression itself.

Few studies addressed the risk of cancer in non-transplant patients treated with azathioprine. Although an increased risk of non-Hodgkin's lymphomas, possibly related to treatment duration, has been found in rheumatoid arthritis patients (800), several other studies were unable to find evidence that azathioprine increased the incidence of cancer. Overall, no increased incidence of cancer was noted after a median of 9 years of follow-up in 755 patients who had received less than 2 mg/kg/day azathioprine during a median of 12.5 years for inflammatory bowel disease (801). Only colorectal cancers (mostly adenocarcinoma) were more frequent, but their incidence is also increased in chronic inflammatory bowel diseases. More specifically, there was no excess of non-Hodgkin's lymphoma, but the power of the study to detect an increased risk of this disorder was low. However, promptly reversible EBV-associated lymphomas are still reported as single case reports in azathioprine-treated patients (802), and two cases of acute myeloid leukemia with 7q deletion have been recently described following treatment for polymyositis (803) or rheumatoid arthritis (804). Severe and rapidly aggressive squamous-cell carcinomas developed in three patients with a moderate-to-excessive sun exposure who had received long-term azathioprine treatment for dermatological conditions (805).

Cyclophosphamide

INTRODUCTION

Cyclophosphamide is a alkylating nitrogen mustard derivative mainly used in oncological patients. Comprehensive reviews of cyclophosphamide toxicity and its management in oncological patients and in the setting of bone marrow transplantation, can be found elsewhere (778, 806).

The use of cyclophosphamide as an immunosuppressant in solid organ transplantation is now limited. However, it has been successfully used in patients with various inflammatory disorders or autoimmune diseases. Cyclophosphamide-induced side effects at low immunosuppressive doses, are similar but less frequent as compared to those observed in oncological patients. For example, in 25 patients receiving intravenous (15 mg/kg) cyclophosphamide alone, or followed by oral cyclophosphamide (5 mg/kg) pulse therapy for various inflammatory rheumatic diseases, mild-to-moderate nausea was the most common side effect and was significantly more frequent in those who had received the higher total intravenous dose (807). Other side effects included alopecia (two cases), leukopenia (two cases), thrombocytopenia (one case). Infectious complications were noted in 52% of patients and hemorrhagic cystitis was not observed.

ORGANS AND SYSTEMS

Respiratory (*SED*-8, 1112; *SEDA*-17, 518) Interstitial pneumonitis and pulmonary fibrosis have rarely been reported and did not clearly correlate with dosage (806). Indeed, interstitial pulmonary inflammation with rapid progression to fatal lung fibrosis has recently been associated with low-dose cyclophosphamide in two patients treated for polyarteritis nodosa (808) and renal transplantation (809), respectively.

Nervous system Although progressive multifocal leukoencephalopathy is sometimes associated with Wegener's granulomatosis, one case occurred upon low-dose cyclophosphamide with subsequent significant improvement after treatment discontinuation (810).

Endocrine, metabolic Treatment of inflammatory disorders or autoimmune diseases with cyclophosphamide can induce ovarian dysfunction (807). Only minor side effects were observed on the menstrual cycles and fertility in women under 40 years (811), In a recent study involving 92 women treated with oral cyclophosphamide for systemic lupus erythematosus, patients who started treatment after 30 years of age and received high cumulative doses of cyclophosphamide, had a greater prevalence of menstrual disturbances, namely amenorrhea or oligomenorrhea (812). Permanent amenorrhea was found in 27.2% of patients and premature menopause was suggested in two patients who had previously regained menstruation after treatment.

Mineral and fluid balance Low-dose intravenous cyclophosphamide has recently been associated with reversible hyponatremia and water intoxication (813), an effect which was supposedly due to a direct effect of cyclophosphamide on the kidney.

Liver Cyclophosphamide-associated hepatic injury was previously thought to be dose-related, presenting as an asymptomatic rise in serum aminotransferase levels in patients with neoplasia (SED-8, 1119). However, several convincing reports described reversible acute hepatitis within 10 weeks of low-dose cyclophosphamide as an immunosuppressant in patients with Wegener's granulomatosis (814, 815), systemic lupus erythematosus (816), or nephrotic syndrome (817). Although corticosteroids were given concomitantly in most of these patients, no data are available to indicate a possible increase in the hepatotoxic potential of this drug combination. This side-effect is very rare anyway. Low-dose cyclophosphamide has also been involved in the occurrence of hepatic veno-occlusive disease (818), and in four separate episodes of recurrent serum transaminase level fluctuations in a patient with hepatitis C virus infection treated for Wegener's granulomatosis (819).

Miscellaneous Infectious complications associated with cyclophosphamide have been initially reported in patients treated for vasculitis and also receiving corticosteroids (820). Subsequently, infections were found as the most prevalent complications in cyclophosphamide-treated patients (807). Older age and disease rather than treatment duration, and the total dose, seemed to predispose to severe infectious episodes (807). More specifically, an increased risk of severe, life-threatening *Pneumocystis carinii* pneumonia has been identified in patients with connective tissue disease treated with cyclophosphamide plus corticosteroids, particularly in those with lymphocytopenia (821—823). Fatal aspergillosis infection has also been reported (824).

Hypersensitivity reactions (*SED*-8, 1126; *SEDA*-17, 522) Anaphylactic reactions have been reported following intravenous cyclophosphamide, and positive skin tests to the parent drug and/or 4-OH cyclophosphamide were found in several well-documented case reports (825, 826). Although other mechanisms are to be considered, the possible contribution of IgE antibody was further suggested by the positivity of immediate skin tests to cyclophosphamide metabolites in five patients, and the recurrence of symptoms following intravenous or oral rechallenge in several of them (827).

Tumour-inducing effects Whether the increased incidence of malignancies after cyclophosphamide treatment is a consequence of mutagenicity/carcinogenicity, rather than immunosuppression is still a matter of debate. In a cohort of non-Hodgkin's lymphoma patients, bladder cancer was significantly increased in survivors who had received cyclophosphamide and the excess risk was dependent on the total cumulative dose, i.e more than 20 grams (828). Although these results are not readily transposable to patients receiving long-term low-dose cyclophosphamide, this potential risk should be kept in mind when considering long-term cyclophosphamide treatment for non-neoplastic conditions. Indeed, an increased incidence of cancers, mostly bladder and skin cancers, was found in a 20-year follow-up study involving 119 patients with rheumatoid arthritis, with a high total dose of cyclophosphamide, i.e. 80 grams, again as the main risk factor (829). Isolated cases of squamous cell carcinomas of the bladder in patients treated for Wegener's granulomatosis with cumulative cyclophosphamide doses of 80 and 120 grams have also been reported (830). By contrast, previous exposure to cyclophosphamide did not appear as a risk factor of cancer in patients with systemic lupus erythematosus, but the number of cases was again very low (831).

Ciclosporin

A major breakthrough in the management of organ-transplanted patients, use of ciclosporin has also been proposed for the treatment of various inflammatory or autoimmune diseases (751), including rheumatoid arthritis (832), psoriasis (833), inflammatory bowel disease (834), idiopathic nephrotic syndrome, and uveitis.

Considerable efforts have been paid in the last years to define the optimal ciclosporin dose to reduce toxicity while retaining efficacy. Based on the analysis of several studies, an approximate ciclosporin dose of 4 mg/kg/day was proposed for long-term maintenance (835). Although a correlation between early post-transplantation ciclosporin whole blood levels and the occurrence of ciclosporin-induced toxicity was suggested, most of the patients remained in the therapeutic range, so that the identification of susceptible patients has yet to be achieved (836). In an attempt to overcome the poor and unpredictable absorption of the standard oral formulation, a microemulsion-based formulation Neoral has been evaluated, with no significant difference in the nature, severity and incidence of side effects (837).

ORGANS AND SYSTEMS

Cardiovascular Hypertension is a common side-effect with the highest incidence of 95% in heart transplant recipients and the lowest incidence in renal transplant recipients. Compared to azathioprine, hypertension requiring treatment was considered to be one of the main risks in ciclosporin-treated patients (838). In addition, about 10% of patients treated for psoriasis experienced hypertension (833), indicating that ciclosporin is specifically involved in hypertension observed in organ transplant patients.

The pathophysiology of ciclosporin-induced hypertension has been suggested to be related to renal vasoconstriction with subsequent sodium—water retention and/or an increased activity of the sympathetic nervous system, while no role was found for the renin angiotensin system (778). However, hypertension often occurs, whereas minimal reductions in the glomerular filtration rate are observed (839), or even more in healthy volunteers, before any change in renal function (840). Numerous studies have evaluated several antihypertensive agents in this setting (778). Because nifedipine has no effect on ciclosporin blood levels, it is usually the drug of choice. However, a possible increased prevalence of gingival overgrowth should be borne in mind (see Interactions). Other calcium channel blockers have been considered, but careful monitoring of ciclosporin blood levels is recommended because several of them inhibit ciclosporin metabolism.

A possible role of ciclosporin in the exacerbation or the development of Raynaud's disease has been suggested, and may involve endothelial damage or changes in platelet functions (841).

Nervous system A wide variety of neurological symptoms, ranging from mild and common toxicity such as headaches, tremor, paresthesias, confusion and visual hallucinations, to severe and rare toxicity, including psychosis, cerebellar disorders, cortical blindness, spinal motor dysfunction, seizures and coma, have been described in organ-transplanted patients treated with ciclosporin (SED-8, 1115; SEDA-17, 520; SEDA-16, 516). Mild-to-moderate symptoms were observed in up to 25% of liver-transplant patients (842), but severe neurotoxicity, such as seizures, was encountered in only a minority of patients (843). Neurological symptoms usually appeared within the first month of treatment, but a delayed occurrence proven by positive rechallenge was sometimes observed (844). Infrequently reported symptoms included catatonia (845), recurrent migraine-like headaches (846), and the abrupt onset of chorea in a patient with previous asymptomatic lesions of the putamen (847).

Although the role of many other factors, including combined therapy, should be considered, reports of neurotoxicity in non-transplanted patients are in keeping with the causal role of ciclosporin (848, 849). Elevated serum ciclosporin level are a possible contributive factor, but severe neurological symptoms have been observed despite normal ciclosporin levels. Possible risk factors, such as hypocholesterolemia (842), hypomagnesemia (845), high-dose steroid therapy, systemic hypertension, or the presence of microangiopathic hemolytic anemia, were suggested to correlate with the development of ciclosporin neurotoxicity (850—852). According to Schwartz et al. (851), clinical symptoms as well as computerized tomography and/or magnetic resonance imaging features were very similar to those observed in hypertensive encephalopathy, with predominant white matter reversible occipital lesions. Complete neurological recovery was subsequently noted in most patients after blood pressure normalized. Fatality due to intracranial hemorrhage was reported exceptionally (851).

Endocrine, metabolic *Hyperlipidemia* Hyperlipidemia, encountered in a large number of transplant recipients, is a possible, but yet unproven, additional risk factor for cardiovascular diseases (853, 854). Although hyperlipidemia in the transplant patient is obviously multifactorial, ciclosporin has been considered as a possible independent risk factor (854). The fact that hyperlipidemia has also been reported in nontransplant patients receiving ciclosporin alone and the transient decrease in hyperlipidemia after ciclosporin discontinuation provide indirect evidence for a causal role of ciclosporin (SED-8, 1131; SEDA-17, 524; 854). The possible impact of ciclosporin on lipid parameters included an increase in cholesterol, LDL cholesterol and apolipoprotein B levels. A significant correlation between ciclosporin blood levels and LDL cholesterol and apolipoprotein B levels, and the cholesterol/HDL cholesterol ratio was found (855). The treatment of hyperlipidemia in transplanted patients is a major dilemma because of several drug interactions and an increased risk of myopathy and rhabdomyolysis has been shown with the concomitant use of ciclosporin and several lipid-lowering drugs (see Drug interactions).

Diabetes mellitus A possible association between ciclosporin treatment and glucose abnormalities has been previously discussed. Interestingly, all cases of post-transplantation diabetes mellitus or abnormal glucose tolerance have been noted in patients receiving corticosteroids, and no abnormal glucose metabolism was found in those treated with ciclosporin and azathioprine (856).

Mineral and fluid balance *Hyperuricemia* Significant hyperuricemia has been observed in as many as 80% of ciclosporin-treated patients, and resulted from a decrease in renal urate clearance (857). Episodes of gout developed mostly in male patients receiving diuretics, but the incidence was suggested to be lower than in the general hyperuricemic population (778). In nine studies performed in renal transplant patients, the incidence of gout was found to range from 5 to 24% (858) and the rapid development of tophi after the onset of gout was sometimes noted (859).

Hyperkalemia Mild and uncomplicated hyperkalemia is also commonly observed in patients on ciclosporin and is generally prevented by a low-potassium diet (778). An inappropriate renal response to hyperkalemia with tubular insensitivity to exogenous mineralocorticoid has been found, and a beneficial effect of acetazolamide was suggested (860). Other electrolytic disturbances included hypomagnesemia (861) and hypercalcemia without increased parathormone serum levels (862).

Hematological Very few cases of ciclosporin-induced immune hemolytic anemia have been reported (863, 864). A direct causal relationship with ciclosporin remains difficult to establish.

Liver (*SED*-18, 1118) Abnormalities in liver function tests, which consisted of hyperbilirubinemia and moderate increases in transaminase and alkaline phosphatase levels, were observed in up to 49% of patients taking ciclosporin, but improvement was usually observed upon decreased dose (SED-18, 1118). Experiments on isolated human hepatocytes showed that ciclosporin competitively inhibits the uptake of cholate and glycocholate bile acids (865). In accordance, the biological features of ciclosporin-associated hepatotoxicity are mostly those of cholestasis with decreased bile excretion (866, 867). In addition, cholestasis from other causes can also increase the accumulation of ciclosporin or its metabolites, which in turn can worsen hepatic dysfunction (866). This mechanism has been suggested in a patient with Crohn's disease who presented with an aggravation of hyperbilirubinemia from total parenteral nutrition following the addition of ciclosporin (868). At the moment, long-term hepatotoxicity resulting from ciclosporin treatment has not been reported.

Gastrointestinal Gastrointestinal symptoms are usually mild and transient. Gastrointestinal intolerance has been reported in 50% of rheumatoid arthritis patients, and that was the main cause for ciclosporin discontinuation in 8% of patients (832). Whereas no cases of worsening colitis have occurred in patients treated for inflammatory bowel diseases, in isolated cases ciclosporin treatment was involved in the development of acute colitis with recurrence of symptoms upon ciclosporin rechallenge (869, 870).

Nephrotoxicity Among the many ciclosporin-associated side effects, much attention has been focused on nephrotoxicity and two main distinct patterns are recognized (871). Acute functional nephrotoxicity consisting of decreased renal function is the most frequently observed. It develops within the first month, and includes a dose-related rise in serum creatinine levels sometimes associated with hyperkalemia. Although clinically often difficult to differentiate from acute allograft rejection in renal transplant patients, the alteration in renal function promptly resolves upon ciclosporin discontinuation or decreased dosage. Several conditions, such as pre-existing hypovolemia, concomitant diuretic treatment or renal artery stenosis, are known risk factors (778). Hypothyroidism was also thought to increase acute ciclosporin nephrotoxicity through an impaired hepatic ciclosporin metabolism (872). Another instance of very severe acute nephrotoxicity is the hemolytic uremic syndrome with histological findings of thrombotic microangiopathy, and a possible evolution to graft rejection or death (873). The clinical distinction with acute rejection is also often very difficult, and no reliable mechanism has been established. In addition, two patients with a history of reversible thrombotic microangiopathy, were successfully retreated several months later with lower ciclosporin doses (874).

In contrast, chronic impairment of the renal function, as first reported by Myers et al. (875) in cardiac transplant patients, is considered to be a major consequence of ciclosporin treatment because of possible irreversible end-stage renal disease. Since then, a considerable amount of work has accumulated on the development of progressive renal dysfunction in patients receiving long-term ciclosporin. This remains a major concern and a change to a ciclosporin-free regimen was considered in 40% of patients because of the progressive renal deterioration with histological signs of nephrotoxicity (838). Following the initial assumption that ciclosporin can cause irreversible chronic nephropathy leading to end-stage renal disease, the clinical relevance of chronic nephrotoxicity following long-term use of ciclosporin in renal transplant patients remains strongly debated, as no clear increase in the incidence of graft losses has been demonstrated since the introduction of ciclosporin (876). Several investigators showed that despite an initial decrease in the renal function, serum creatinine levels stabilized after several years of surveillance. No evidence of progressive nephropathy has been found retrospectively among 347 ciclosporin-treated patients with a follow-up as long as 10 years after renal transplantation (877). From a recent retrospective multicenter analysis of 1663 renal-transplant recipients who had received long-term ciclosporin treatment (mean follow-up: 36 months), it was also suggested that graft failure was mostly due to chronic rejection rather than to ciclosporin-induced progressive nephropathy (878). Mihatsch et al. (879) found that severe ciclosporin arteriopathy was the cause of renal transplant failure in less than 1% of patients. Several prospective studies involving a few patients argued against a strong effect of ciclosporin, as compared to azathioprine, on renal allograft function (880) and a chronic immune injury was suggested to account for the renal dysfunction (881).

There is also much concern in other organ-transplanted patients, and progressive renal failure secondary to ciclosporin nephrotoxicity has been consistently reported in heart- (882, 883), liver- (884) and lung-transplant recipients (885). However, in most patients followed for a long period of time, renal function stabilized after an initial decline (884, 886), and ciclosporin nephropathy-associated end-stage renal disease which required dialysis or renal transplantation rarely developed (882, 884). Among 430 cardiac transplants, end-stage renal disease developed in 14 (3.3%) of patients after a mean of 82 months and was supposedly consecutive to ciclosporin nephrotoxicity in 13 patients (887).

Obviously, the current use of lower ciclosporin doses can account for these results suggesting that end-stage renal failure should not be regarded as a major limitation to ciclosporin treatment in organ-transplant patients. In addition, once-daily morning ciclosporin dosing was suggested to improve the glomerular filtration rate and the renal blood flow when compared to half the dose taken twice daily in stable heart-transplant patients (888).

Ciclosporin nephrotoxicity is also an important issue for patients treated for autoimmune diseases, because the risk can outweigh the benefit in these patients. An increase of greater than 30% in serum creatinine levels has been reported within the first 3 months of treatment in 50% of rheumatoid arthritis patients, persisting thereafter (832). Although renal dysfunction is reversible when large rises in serum creatinine levels are avoided or after short-term ciclosporin treatment (889), clinical and morphological evidence of sustained or progressive ciclosporin nephropathy in patients with autoimmune diseases treated with low-doses for long-term maintenance is accumulating (890—894).

The histopathological features in patients with chronic nephropathy consist mostly of non-specific tubular atrophy and interstitial fibrosis (895). The presence of arteriolar lesions is considered as very suggestive of ciclosporin nephrotoxicity, but the prevalence has strongly decreased with the use of lower doses. Interestingly, arteriolopathy sometimes improved after reducing or discontinuing ciclosporin. Morphological features in patients treated for autoimmune diseases were again non-specific and included a wide range of lesions which mostly consisted of tubulointerstitial changes and arteriolopathy (893, 895). No significant correlation between histological findings and ciclosporin doses was found (891). Moreover, severe histological lesions were identified in patients with normal renal function, and the severity of tubulointerstitial lesions was considered to be a better index than the glomerular filtration rate, to predict the occurrence of chronic nephropathy.

Although a large number of studies investigated the pathogenesis of ciclosporin nephrotoxicity in humans and animal models, the exact mechanisms remain ill-understood (778, 871, 896). A sustained vasoconstriction of the afferent arterioles associated with a decrease in the renal blood flow and the glomerular filtration rate, is the main finding in reversible acute renal dysfunctions. Possible mechanisms include an imbalance between vasodilator prostaglandins and thromboxane, endothelin-1 release from damaged endothelium, increased sensitivity to vasoactive peptides, and the stimulation of the sympathetic nervous system, whereas the role of the renin—angiotensin—aldosterone system has never been clearly demonstrated in humans (839, 881, 896). However, it is unclear whether a continuous elevation in renal vascular resistance can account for the chronic progressive obliterative vasculopathic renal dysfunction observed in patients on long-term ciclosporin maintenance.

Factors putatively associated with ciclosporin nephrotoxicity are many-fold. Although several studies found that the high initial doses of ciclosporin increased the risk of chronic nephrotoxicity (877, 890), others suggested that patients maintained on high ciclosporin concentrations had no more chance of toxic nephropathy (878). Several investigators found that neither the mean daily dose or ciclosporin blood levels nor the duration of ciclosporin treatment, appear to be significant risk factors (883, 891). Initial acute renal insufficiency was not clearly associated with the development of ultimate renal dysfunction (882, 883), whereas a higher risk for progressive renal failure was identified in patients with decreased glomerular filtration rate at 6 months post-transplantation (883). Age, sustained hypertension, hypertriglyceridemia or low HDL cholesterols can also contribute to chronic renal failure (883). In patients treated for autoimmune diseases, age, large initial ciclosporin daily dose, and maximum percentage increase in serum creatinine levels were possible risk factors (890). Recurrent episodes of severe acute nephrotoxicity also increased the likelihood of subsequent chronic nephropathy (893).

The prevention and management of ciclosporin-associated nephrotoxicity has been reviewed elsewhere (778). Low-dose ciclosporin in association with other immunosuppressive agents or the delayed introduction of ciclosporin after renal function has returned to normal, are the currently recommended measures to decrease nephrotoxicity. An increase in serum creatinine levels greater than 30% above baseline levels indicates the need for ciclosporin dose adjustment (751). Attempts to reduce ciclosporin doses or even to withdraw ciclosporin after several months of treatment, especially within the first year following transplantation, should be regarded with caution and balanced with the risk of acute rejection (835, 897—899). Based on retrospective investigations, ciclosporin withdrawal after a

1-year rejection-free period has been successful in carefully selected patients (900) and older white patients with preserved renal function and a well-matched graft, were suggested to be possible candidates for elective ciclosporin withdrawal (901). However, a retrospective analysis in more than 12 000 renal transplant patients over a 5-year period showed that long-term maintenance with a steroid-free ciclosporin regimen (ciclosporin alone or in association with azathioprine) significantly increased graft and patient survival compared to patients on other immunosuppressive regimens, and this allowed use of higher doses of ciclosporin without increasing nephrotoxicity (902). The use of several drugs to prevent ciclosporin nephrotoxicity has been investigated in numerous studies (778). Calcium channel blockers have repeatedly been suggested to reduce the incidence of ciclosporin-associated nephrotoxicity. Based on randomized prospective trials, nifedipine has been proposed as a reliable adjunctive treatment to minimize the long-term nephrotoxic effects of ciclosporin in renal transplant patients (903, 904).

Skin and appendages Widespread hypertrichosis is the most common complication. Changes in facial features have been reported in children (SED-8, 1125), as well as a possibly more frequent occurrence of acne vulgaris and keratosis pilaris (905). Several nail changes, such as excess granulation tissue (906) and ingrowing toenails (907), have been reported.

Special senses Ciclosporin-associated gingival overgrowth was noted in the early 1980s, and subsequent studies have investigated the prevalence and pathophysiology of this side effect. Clinically significant gingival overgrowth, that is to say requiring treatment or surgical excision, affected approximately 30% of patients within the first 6 months of treatment (908). In multiple sclerosis, a 35%-incidence of gingival overgrowth was found in patients treated for at least 1 year versus 14% in controls (909).

The duration of ciclosporin treatment appeared to be the significant risk factor (910), and the cumulative ciclosporin dose administered during the first 6 months following transplantation significantly correlated with the development on gingival overgrowth in renal transplant children (911). Accordingly, reduction of the ciclosporin dose has been suggested to improve gingival overgrowth (908), and the use of lower ciclosporin dose in recent years supposedly decreased the prevalence of gingival overgrowth (911). Although ciclosporin is preferentially secreted in the saliva, a clear relationship between saliva and blood ciclosporin concentrations has not been found (909). Conflicting results regarding the incidence of gingival overgrowth have also emerged on the effect of ciclosporin daily doses and plasma blood levels (909–911). Young age and male sex were significantly correlated to the presence of gingival overgrowth (909, 910). This latter finding is further supported by the report of an increased androgen metabolism in gingival hyperplasia induced by ciclosporin (912). The combination of ciclosporin and nifedipine was additive, and the resulting increased prevalence and/or severity of gingival overgrowth has been confirmed in recent studies in both children (913) and adults (910–914). An inhibitory effect of these drugs on the calcium-dependent collagenase production was suggested. As most calcium channel blockers can produce gingival overgrowth, more frequent gingival hyperplasias should be expected, at least theoretically, when these drugs are combined with ciclosporin.

The relationship between either bacterial plaque, gingival bleeding index or inflammation in the development of gingival overgrowth remains a matter of debate, and it is not yet clearly established whether these problems are the cause or the result of gingival overgrowth (908–911). In any case, poor oral health with subsequent local inflammation appears to be a contributing factor (915).

Various studies have shown that the clinical and histological features of gingival overgrowth in ciclosporin-treated patients is very similar to that associated with phenytoin or nifedipine (908). Compared to control specimens, ultrastructural gingival examinations in ciclosporin-treated patients showed many fibroblasts, abundant amorphous substance and marked plasma cell infiltration (916). Although an imbalance between the production and the removal of collagen is supposed to account for gingival hyperplasia, the mechanism of ciclosporin-induced gingival overgrowth has not yet been clearly established. A possible local lymphocyte resistance to ciclosporin resulting in an increasing number of several inflammatory cells in the gingival lamina propria has also been suggested (915). There has been speculation concerning genetic differences in the susceptibility to develop gingival overgrowth (908).

Based on single case reports, it has been suggested that azithromycin (917) or metronidazole (918) dramatically improve ciclosporin-associated symptomatic gingival hyperplasia in renal transplant patients, but these findings await confirmation.

Musculoskeletal system In an analysis of published or spontaneous case reports, the manufacturer found 29 cases of muscular disorders in ciclosporin-treated patients, the complications falling into two categories (919). Myopathic symptoms, i.e. myalgias and muscle weakness without rhabdomyolysis, were reported in 0.17% of patients and receded after dose reductions or treatment withdrawal. Rhabdomyolysis occurred in less than 0.05% of patients and was mostly observed in patients taking concomitant drugs, such as lovastatin or colchicine.

Several reports have described the possible association of bone pain with the addition of ciclosporin to immunosuppressive regimens. Acute and bilateral deep bone pains, mostly involving the knees and ankles, have been retrospectively identified in 19.1% of patients receiving ciclosporin, with the highest prevalence in renal transplant recipients (920). In addition, about half of the patients presenting images of osteonecrosis had a history of episodic bone pains. Interestingly, calcium channel blockers dramatically improved bone pains in prospectively evaluated transplant patients, suggesting a possible vascular etiology.

Osteopenia is a potential side-effect in patients on long-term treatment after renal transplantation and the impact of ciclosporin on bone metabolism is controversial. No effects of ciclosporin have been found on bone mineral metabolism and bone remodeling in normocalcemic renal transplant patients with normal renal function while on long-term treatment (921). Measurement of forearm bone density in a few patients showed that significant bone loss was observed less frequently in patients treated with ciclosporin alone as compared to those treated with azathioprine/prednisone regimens (922). Moreover, ciclosporin did not appear to have a negative influence on post-transplantation growth in prepubertal children (923).

Hypersensitivity reactions Anaphylactoid reactions, sometimes after the first administration, have been reported with the intravenous formulation only. Pruritic rash, respiratory symptoms, chest pain (924) and, rarely, cardiopulmonary arrest (925) have been observed. The presence of cremophor EL, the polyoxyethylated castor oil base pharmaceutical solvent, is likely to account for this life-threatening reaction.

Overdosage Ciclosporin overdose has been reviewed by the manufacturer using published data or cases communicated to the Sandoz Drug Monitoring Centre (926). Accidental overdose was the most common and doses ranged from 20 to 400 mg/kg. In adults, no clinical consequences were observed for doses up to 100 mg/kg, and only minor clinical or biological manifestations, namely transient hypertension, tachycardia, headache, gastrointestinal symptoms or slight increase in serum creatinine levels, were observed. Life-threatening reactions occurred in three neonates, of whom one died after severe metabolic acidosis and renal insufficiency. Sub-chronic ciclosporin overdose over 8 days did not appear to cause any additional risk (927). Taken together, the available data suggests that acute ciclosporin toxicity is low in adults, while more severe intoxication should be expected in neonates.

Interactions Ciclosporin is variably absorbed by the gastrointestinal tract and almost completely metabolized in both the liver and small intestine by cytochrome P4503A which is known to metabolize a large number of drugs. Inducers, inhibitors or substrates of cytochrome P4503A have thus the potential to interact with ciclosporin. In addition, ciclosporin has a wide inter- and intrapatient pharmacokinetic variability and a narrow therapeutic index (928). Indeed, numerous significant pharmacokinetic drug interactions have been described in patients on ciclosporin. Experimental models using human hepatocytes can be used to screen for potential inducers or inhibitors of ciclosporin metabolism (929). On the other hand, pharmacodynamic interactions resulting from additive or synergistic toxicities, such as nephrotoxicity or neurotoxicity, can be encountered. Drug interactions with ciclosporin have been reviewed (930—933). The clinical relevance of the interaction of NSAIDs and ciclosporin is still uncertain (SEDA-17, 107). Table 4 presents the most common interactions as well as possible new drug interactions.

Whereas erythromycin—ciclosporin interactions leading to a significant increase in ciclosporin blood levels and serum creatinine levels have been consistently demonstrated, only isolated reports indicated a possible interaction with josamycin or pristinamycin (950). A 2-fold increase in ciclosporin concentrations has been reported in patients receiving miocamycin (950), and several case reports suggested a potential interaction between ciclosporin and newer macrolides, such as azithromycin (951), clarithromycin (952) or midecamycin (953). By contrast, spiramycin or roxithromycin did not significantly change ciclosporin concentrations (950).

In the light of case reports, ciprofloxacin was initially thought to increase ciclosporin blood levels and to enhance ciclosporin nephrotoxicity. Hoey et al. (954) were unable to find evidence to support this interaction, and suggested that the recommended dose of ciprofloxacin can be safely used in ciclosporin-treated patients. Only one case of norfloxacin-induced increase in ciclosporin blood levels has been reported (933), while ofloxacin did not appear to alter ciclosporin metabolism (955).

Nafcillin has been thought to increase ciclosporin hepatic metabolism. However, a recent retrospective study found an increased risk of ciclosporin-associated early nephrotoxicity in nafcillin-treated patients, despite the fact that ciclosporin concentrations were not different from controls (956). A possible interference

Table 4. *Drug interactions affecting ciclosporin (CsA) pharmacokinetics and toxicity (updated from 930–933)*

Pharmacokinetic interactions		Pharmacodynamic interactions
Drugs which increase CsA blood levels	Drugs which decrease CsA blood levels	Drugs which increase CsA toxicity
Anti-infectives		
Macrolides or related drugs (see text)		
Azithromycin	*Bile acid resin*	**Increased nephrotoxicity**
Clarithromycin	*Carbamazepine*	*ACE inhibitors*
Erythromycin	*Griseofulvin* (944)	*Aciclovir (see text)*
Josamycin	*Phenobarbital*	*Aminoglycosides*
Midecamycin	*Phenytoin*	*Amphotericin B*
Miocamycin	*Probucol* (945)	*Cotrimoxazole*
Pristinamycin	*Pyrazinamide* (946)	*Melphalan*
Ciprofloxacin (unproven, see text)	*Rifampicin*	*Foscarnet (see text)*
Antifungals	*Sulfadiazine* (947)	*Nafcillin (see text)*
Ketoconazole		*NSAIDs*
Fluconazole		
Itraconazole		**Increased muscular toxicity** (see text)
Metronidazole (934)		*Lovastatin*
Cardiovascular drugs		*Simvastatin*
Amiodarone (935,936)		*Fibric acid derivatives*
Clonidine (937)		
Calcium channel blockers		**Increased gingival hyperplasia**
Nicardipine		*Nifedipine*
Diltiazem		
Verapamil		**Increased neurotoxicity**
Miscellaneous		*Imipenem/cilastatin*
Allopurinol (938)		
Chloroquine (939)		**Increased risk of hepatotoxicity**
Corticosteroids		*Androgens* (948, 949)
Danazol (940)		
Grapefruit juice (941-943)		
Oral contraceptives		
Tacrolimus		

of nafcillin with ciclosporin assay, giving rise to falsely low levels, is a possible explanation.

Although a possible enhancement of nephrotoxicity has been suggested in patients receiving aciclovir and ciclosporin (957), no such findings were found in a retrospective analysis of a double-blind study (958). Foscarnet (959), but not ganciclovir (960), has also been involved in reversible renal failure after concomitant use with ciclosporin.

Conflicting data have emerged on the omeprazole—ciclosporin association, with isolated case reports suggesting that omeprazole can increase (961) or decrease (962) ciclosporin concentrations, whereas no effect of omeprazole was demonstrated in a randomized blind cross-over placebo trial (963).

The deliberate use of several enzymatic inhibitors to reduce the required dose of ciclosporin resulting in marked cost saving and potential minimization of ciclosporin-associated adverse effects, is under extensive investigation, with ketoconazole (964—966), diltiazem or verapamil (903, 967, 968). Co-administration of calcium channel blockers is probably valuable in the treatment of ciclosporin-induced hypertension, or to prevent ciclosporin nephrotoxicity. By contrast, nicardipine, diltiazem and verapamil (but not nifedipine (967), isradipine (969), amlodipine (970) or felodipine (971)) significantly affected ciclosporin pharmacokinetics.

The treatment of ciclosporin-induced hypercholesterolemia in transplant recipients has been the matter of numerous recent trials to assess the efficacy and safety of lipid-lowering drugs. A possibly increased risk of muscular disorders should be considered with fibric acid agents and HMG-CoA reductase inhibitors (853). Rhabdomyolysis involving the concomitant use of ciclosporin and simvastatin (972), or more frequently lovastatin (973), have been seen. However, lower doses of these drugs have been safely administered in a small number of transplant recipients receiving ciclosporin (974—976). Fluvastatin (977, 978) and pravastatin (979, 980) were also suggested to be safe and effective to reduce cholesterol levels and/or to decrease the incidence of coronary vasculopathy.

Ciclosporin-induced impairment of the hepatic metabolism of other drugs has seldom been evaluated (981). High-dose ciclosporin was however shown to increase the area-under-the-curve for doxorubicin and doxorubicinol, and to produce greater doxorubicin-related myelotoxicity (982).

Mycophenolate mofetil

Mycophenolate mofetil, the morpholinoethyl ester of mycophenolic acid, is an antimetabolite which interferes with the synthesis of nucleic acids and selectively inhibits the proliferation of T and B lymphocytes. It has been used in the treatment of psoriasis. Clinical trials assessing the safety and efficacy of mycophenolate mofetil in kidney (983, 984) or heart (985) transplant recipients reported symptoms in accordance with the known antiproliferative effect of this drug. Compared to placebo, the combination of mycophenolate mofetil with ciclosporin and corticosteroids induced more frequent gastrointestinal disorders, leukopenia and opportunistic infections (983). A similar profile of side effects was found in a randomized, double-blind study which compared mycophenolate mofetil (2 and 3 grams) and azathioprine as part of a quadruple sequential induction protocol after renal transplantation (984). More frequent symptoms in the mycophenolate group included dose-dependent diarrhea, esophagitis, gastritis, gastrointestinal hemorrhage, neutropenia and CMV-tissue invasive disease. Three cases of lymphoproliferative disorders occurred in the first 6-months of follow-up, and all were observed in the mycophenolate group. Interestingly, nephrotoxicity or hepatotoxicity were not observed in clinical trials reported so far.

Tacrolimus

Tacrolimus (FK506), a macrolide immunosuppressive agent, approximately 100 times more potent than ciclosporin on a weight basis, has become recently available for use in liver transplantation, and appeared as a relevant alternative to ciclosporin for baseline immunosuppression (986, 987).

Two large open, randomized multicenter 1-year trials have compared the efficacy and safety of tacrolimus-based and ciclosporin-based immunosuppressive regimens in liver transplant recipients (988, 989). Both trials found a similar incidence of patient and graft survival, whereas tacrolimus significantly reduced acute and refractory acute rejection episodes. Overall, side effects were similar whatever the regimen used, but their incidence, including those which required withdrawal from the study, was higher in tacrolimus-treated patients. Neurological symptoms, nephrotoxicity and hyperglycemia were more commonly reported in the tacrolimus group, but severe neurological or renal complications seemed to be as frequently reported in both groups. In addition, both studies noted a decreased incidence of side effects after the starting tacrolimus dose was reduced. This is in accordance with early trials showing that the initially proposed dose of tacrolimus was too high (990). When dose reduction failed, severe or persistent tacrolimus-related side effects usually reversed after replacement by ciclosporin (991).

ORGANS AND SYSTEMS

Cardiovascular Rare, but troublesome, severe and recurrent hypertrophic cardiomyopathies developing within 3 months have been reported, both in children (992) and adults (993).

Nervous system Insomnia, tremor and headaches are more frequently reported as compared to ciclosporin, whereas more severe neurological side-effects such as psychosis, neuropathy, convulsions, coma and paralysis were observed with a similar incidence (988, 989). In addition to a possible, but yet unproven specific tacrolimus neurotoxicity, various other factors contribute to the development of severe neurological symptoms. The higher incidence of moderate or severe late neurotoxicity in tacrolimus- versus ciclosporin-treated patients, was indeed strongly associated with severe post-operative infections, multiple-organ failure and fatal outcome, and an increase in several biological parameters (bilirubin, creatinine, transaminases) (994). Similar conclusions were reached by others (995) who also failed to find any relationship between tacrolimus blood levels and the occurrence of major neurotoxicity. All the same, patients experiencing neurological complications significantly improved after dose reduction (996) or conversion to ciclosporin treatment (997, 998).

Endocrine, metabolic Whilst glucose tolerance tended to improve over time in steroid-free tacrolimus- or ciclosporin-treated patients, glucose intolerance remained more frequent in the tacrolimus group after a median of 23 months (999). However, post-transplant diabetes mellitus requiring permanent insulin treatment after 1-year follow-up was as frequent in ciclosporin as in tacrolimus-treated liver graft recipients (1000). Compared to ciclosporin-based immunosuppressive regimens, total cholesterol and LDL cholesterol serum levels were found to be lower in patients receiving tacrolimus for 1 year (1001). Both findings were considered to result from a significant steroid-sparing effect of tacrolimus.

Hematological Although multiple factors are involved in the development of immune hemolysis in transplant recipients, in vitro experiments argued for a possible triggering role of tacrolimus in a few patients (1002). In a single case report, tacrolimus has been thought to cause isolated anemia due to a selective hypoplasia of erythropoiesis (1003).

Liver Mild-to-moderate liver function test abnormalities have been observed. The normalization of liver function tests, namely moderate or frank alanine aminotransferase and alkaline phosphatase elevations, upon tacrolimus reduction or discontinuation, was suggestive of a possible dose-related hepatotoxicity (1004). In addition, liver biopsy showed a centrilobular hepatocellular dropout with sinusoidal dilatation and congestion, and no features of cellular rejection or acute hepatitis.

Urinary system Tacrolimus nephrotoxicity has clinical and morphological features similar to those of ciclosporin (1005, 1006). Late nephrotoxicity evaluated by the mean serum creatinine concentration and/or glomerular filtration rate at 1 year was similar in ciclosporin- and tacrolimus-treated patients (1007, 1008). Interestingly, a significantly lower prevalence of antihypertensive treatment was noted in tacrolimus-treated patients (1008), confirming earlier results which suggested that the incidence of de novo hypertension is lower under tacrolimus regimen. The possible association between tacrolimus and the occurrence of hemolytic uremic syndrome is based upon isolated cases (1009—1011). By contrast, tacrolimus has successfully been used in patients suffering from hemolytic uremic syndrome related to ciclosporin (1012).

Reversible but severe hyperuricemia and acute renal failure was also thought to be related to high-dose tacrolimus rescue therapy in a patient who had previous gouty arthritis under ciclosporin (1013).

Miscellaneous Several other mild-to-moderate side effects, such as alopecia, pruritus, anemia, and hyperkalemia, have been more frequently observed in patients receiving tacrolimus (988, 989). Severe gastrointestinal toxicity and weight loss requiring drug discontinuation can also occur (991). Finally, and in contrast to ciclosporin, hirsutism and gingival hyperplasia have not been described.

Another interesting difference in tacrolimus-based immunosuppression is the possibly lower incidence of major infectious complications, namely CMV and pneumonia (989, 1014). However, a retrospective study found an increased incidence of symptomatic Epstein-Barr virus infections and lymphoproliferative disorders in children under 5 years of age, who received tacrolimus as compared to ciclosporin (1015); this was considered to be the consequence of over-immunosuppression which requires careful screening for EBV infections and dosage monitoring.

Tumour-inducing effects Based on a first evaluation of 936 patients, mostly liver and renal transplant recipients, who had received tacrolimus as the primary immunosuppressive therapy for a mean of 10 months, 1.6% of patients developed post-transplant lymphoproliferative disorders after a median of 70 days (1016). This incidence as well as the described pathological features, are similar to those previously described in relation to ciclosporin treatment. Additional data including larger studies and longer period of follow-up are not yet available.

Overdosage Minimal side effects, or none, were observed in four patients after an acute tacrolimus overdose (1017). Continuous veno-venous hemofiltration was found to dramatically increase the elimination rate of tacrolimus in two other patients who experienced acute renal and liver failure with elevated plasma tacrolimus blood levels (1018).

Drug interactions The hepatic metabolism of tacrolimus is primarily mediated by the cytochrome P4503A enzyme subfamily, and experimental evidence suggested a potential for interactions with drugs known to induce or inhibit cytochrome P4503A (1019, 1020). However, the clinical experience is still limited. Isolated reports have described increases in tacrolimus blood concentrations of patients receiving erythromycin (1021—1023), clarithromycin (1024), fluconazole (1025), or ketoconazole (1026) clotrimazole (1027) or danazol (1028) while rifampicin was shown to decrease tacrolimus blood concentrations (1021). Acute renal failure in association with the use of ibuprofen has also been described in liver transplant recipients (1029), and the relevance of this interaction is probably similar to that reported with ciclosporin (SEDA-17, 107).

MONOCLONAL ANTIBODIES

Orthoclone OKT3

Muromonab CD3 (orthoclone OKT3) is a murine monoclonal antibody targeted against the human CD3-receptor—T cell complex. It is a powerful immunosuppressive agent for the treatment of acute allograft transplant rejection which has also been successfully used for the prevention of acute rejection in the post-transplant period (1028). However, the effectiveness of OKT3 prophylaxis remains subject to debate. It has recently been reported that renal transplant patients with a high risk of rejection are probably the best candidates for OKT3 prophylaxis (1029).

Excessive immunosuppression and unexpected overactivation of the immune system are the main consequences of OKT3 treatment (1030).

GENERAL REACTIONS

Acute systemic symptoms have been described after the initial doses of OKT3, used either for induction or anti-rejection therapy, and this reaction is now referred to as the 'cytokine-release syndrome' (755). A flu-like reaction is the key component of this syndrome, typically occurring within 1 hour after the first two or three OKT3 infusions, and with decreased incidence and severity following subsequent doses (1031). Symptoms included fever, chills, headache, myalgias, tachycardia and gastrointestinal symptoms which lasted for several hours. The OKT3-induced cytokine-release syndrome was more frequent after conventional than low doses of OKT3 (1032) and it was also thought to be more severe and of longer duration in patients treated for moderate-to-severe graft rejections (1033). Other systemic manifestations of the cytokine-release syndrome included acute pulmonary edema, neurological, renal and hematological symptoms (see below).

Considerable efforts have been paid to prevent or control the cytokine-release syndrome, including careful patient management and pharmacological interventions (755, 1034). Whilst high-dose steroids given prior to OKT3 administration remained the basis of treatment (1035), it was recently proposed that two separate 250-mg methylprednisolone doses given prior to OKT3, are more effective in reducing OKT3 induced side-effects, than a single 500-mg dose of methylprednisolone (1036). Indomethacin, even at low doses, has been successfully used to minimize the incidence or the severity of the cytokine-releasing syndrome, without impairing rejection reversal or renal function (1037, 1038). Low-dose OKT3 induction therapy also significantly improved OKT3 tolerance without impairing efficacy (1039, 1040).

Although the production of a wide range of cytokines has been found to be increased after OKT3 administration, TNF-α and IL-6 were suggested to play a pivotal role in this acute activation syndrome. Monoclonal anti-TNF-α antibody administration has indeed successfully reduced acute clinical symptoms (1041). A role for the activation of complement and neutrophils was more recently suggested (1032, 1042).

ORGANS AND SYSTEMS

Cardiovascular Cardiovascular manifestations are usually associated with the febrile reaction which is observed during the cytokine-release syndrome. These mostly include transient and benign hypertension, hypotension or tachycardia (755, 1031). Fluid overload or volume depletion may also play a role. Chest pain or severe arrhythmia are infrequent (1043).

Several retrospective studies have focused on a possibly increased risk of graft thrombosis affecting renal arteries, veins or glomerular capillaries, and leading to a higher incidence of rejection episodes (1044, 1045). These clinical findings were not substantiated by others (1046, 1047). A triggering of systemic procoagulant activity and activation of fibrinolysis has been found in OKT3-treated patients and may be the result of TNF-α and/or release of other cytokines, and cellular adhesion to the vascular endothelium (1044, 1047). In spite of these results, only very few cases of intragraft thrombosis putatively related to OKT3 have been reported. In a retrospective review of 231 kidney transplant recipients who received OKT3 prophylaxis, intragraft thromboses were found in 13 (5.6%), and high-dose methylprednisolone (30 mg/kg) was suggested to be a major risk factor (1048).

Respiratory Dyspnea and pulmonary edema have sometimes developed after the first OKT3 injections. Initially, pulmonary toxicity was mostly observed in patients who had fluid retention and weight gain before OKT3, and the incidence has been markedly reduced following the new guidelines for management (755, 1031). Cytokine release and complement activation with further neutrophil activation and pulmonary vascular endothelium damage were suggested to be involved (1042).

Nervous system Self-limited and benign central nervous system manifestations resembling those of aseptic meningitis, i.e. fever, headache, nuchal rigidity, cognitive disorders and photophobia, were observed in 3—10% of patients (755). Symptoms were delayed for 2—3 days, resolved spontaneously and did not require treatment discontinuation. More severe neurological disorders included slowly reversible diffuse encephalopathy with mental-status changes, neurosensorial hallucinations, generalized seizures, cortical blindness, psychotic symptoms, obtundation and coma; this was found in 7% of renal transplant patients undergoing OKT3 treatment, usually requiring treatment withdrawal (1049—1051). Focal neurological dysfunctions, namely cerebritis with focal seizures (1052) and transient hemiparesis (1053), including in one case a CT scan-proven cerebral infarction (1054), have been described. Neurotoxic symptoms were supposedly mediated by cytokine release and/or potentiated by uremic toxins. Elevated TNF-α levels in the cerebrospinal fluid were suggested to play a major role in OKT3-induced aseptic meningitis and encephalopathy (1054). Diabetes patients and severely impaired renal function with serum creatinine above 500 μM/l, were suggested to be significant risk factors for OKT3-associated neurotoxicity (1051, 1055).

Urinary system A spontaneously reversible acute increase in serum creatinine levels has been noted within 2—5 days in 8—18% of OKT3-treated patients, and was thought to result from the inhibition of renal prostaglandin synthesis and the release of cytokines (1056, 1057). No adverse consequences on short-term graft survival or graft function have been shown (1056). Isolated cases of recurrence of hemolytic uremic syndromes have been reported (1058, 1059).

Special senses Spontaneously reversible mild conjunctivitis and episcleritis have been found in 75 and 10%, respectively, of patients receiving OKT3. Diffuse anterior scleritis responding to an increased prednisone dosage was noted in a single patient only (1060). Severe and repeated isolated visual loss without any obvious cause developed in two female patients shortly after OKT3 administration (1061).

Miscellaneous An antibody response directed against the murine monoclonal OKT3 has been detected in the majority of patients within the first 3 weeks of treatment. Using a 14-day induction regimen of 5 mg OKT3 daily, anti-OKT3 antibody developed in 40.3% of patients (1034). However, sensitization was not relevant in most patients. Only elevated IgG anti-idiotypic antibody levels, i.e. higher than 1:1000, were able to significantly neutralize the binding of OKT3 to CD3 receptor and to reduce clinical efficacy, thus precluding further OKT3 administration.

Immediate IgE-mediated anaphylactic reactions, namely anaphylactic shock, bronchospasm, urticaria, remained very exceptionally reported (1062, 1063). Late-onset reactions occurring after the first week of treatment and including cutaneous erythema, a fall in blood pressure, or serum sickness-like reactions have been infrequently observed (1064).

Tumor-inducing effects As expected from its pronounced immunosuppressive activity, it was felt at the start that OKT3 was a significant risk factor in the development of post-transplant lymphoproliferative disorders, especially when high doses or sequential courses were used (1065). Whether OKT3 specifically increases the incidence of cancer or it reflects a severely immunocompromised status is still a matter of debate (755), and conflicting results have emerged from the literature. Several retrospective or controlled studies were unable to show more frequent post-transplantation malignancies in patients receiving OKT3, as compared to those receiving other immunosuppressive regimens and/or polyclonal antibodies (1066—1068). Others found some evidence that the rate of non-Hodgkin's lymphomas is higher in kidney and heart transplant recipients receiving OKT3 prophylaxis versus antithymocyte/antilymphocyte globulin (745). Although several authors suggested that even high cumulative doses or repeated courses do not increase the risk of lymphoproliferative disorders (1066, 1067), others recommended that OKT3 treatment should not exceed 14 days with a cumulative dose of less than 70 mg (755).

Risk of infectious diseases In a review of OKT3-associated side effects, Kreis (755) discussed multiple possible biases in studies of the incidence of OKT3-associated infections and was unable to find differences among patients receiving OKT3 when compared to those receiving other immunosuppressive regimens. Actually, the incidence and the severity of infections are mostly correlated with the degree of immunosuppression (1069) as was illustrated by several studies.

In a randomized, prospective study, the overall incidence of infections, mostly urinary tract and cytomegalovirus infections, during the first three post-transplantation months, was found to be significantly higher in renal transplant patients receiving prophylactic OKT3 versus ciclosporin (1070), whereas no significant difference in the severity of infections was noted in a similar multicenter trial (1028). Both studies failed to identify any adverse impact of infectious episodes on patient survival. In a randomized prospective trial of prophylactic ATG-Fresenius versus OKT3 in renal transplant patients, only minor infections (e.g. cutaneous mycosis, herpes simplex virus infections) were more common in OKT-3 treated patients while the incidence of life-threatening or severe infections was similar in both groups and generally observed after retreatment with either drug (1071). In contrast to these findings, a large retrospective study found a significantly higher incidence of infection-related deaths among patients receiving OKT3 for induction therapy as compared to those not receiving OKT3 (1072). However, renal graft survival was significantly improved in OKT-3-treated patients and no viral death was subsequently observed after the routine use of appropriate prophylaxis and treatment with cotrimoxazole, aciclovir and ganciclovir was instituted.

Several retrospective studies performed in liver- (1014, 1073) or heart-transplant recipients (1074) have found that OKT3 treatment is an additional or independent risk factor for symptomatic CMV infections in CMV-seropositive patients or in recipients of CMV-seropositive donors, suggesting that CMV prophylaxis should be implemented in this group of patients. Early OKT3 administration in the post-transplant period was also suggested to increase the likelihood of invasive CMV disease after liver transplantation (1075). By contrast, other investigators failed to show an increased incidence of CMV infections after OKT3 versus triple drug therapy in heart transplant patients (1076). Based on a small number of patients, OKT-3 administration was also suggested as a risk factor for the development of *Pneumocystis carinii* pneumonia following liver transplantation (1077).

Other monoclonal antibodies

Numerous investigators have reported and reviewed the clinical application of monoclonal antibodies (Mab) in various areas, including organ transplantation, neoplastic diseases, severe sepsis and inflammatory diseases (1078—1083). Overall, the rapid development of human anti-murine antibodies appears to be one of the most important clinical limitations to their therapeutic use. These antibodies can abrogate the effectiveness of Mab and/or cause adverse reactions following a second treatment. The development of humanized Mab is expected to improve the safety of currently available Mab (1084). At the moment, no Mabs, except OKT3, are routinely used as immunosuppressive agents in the clinic and it is beyond the scope of this Chapter to review the very limited information available from clinical trials on what may be specific side effects of Mabs under current investigation.

Although pan-T cell reactive Mab were not found to be more effective than OKT3 in immunosuppressive post-transplantation regimens (1078), several anti-T cell receptor Mabs, such as BMA031 (1085) or T10B9.1A-31 (1086), have produced only minimal side effects as compared to OKT-3. Other Mabs directed against lymphocyte subsets have been evaluated in the setting of organ transplantation. Mild-to-moderate first dose symptoms, such as fever and rigors, nausea and vomiting, bone pain, dyspnea and headache have been observed following the administration of CAMPATH-1H, a humanized Mab reactive against the CDw52 antigen present on all peripheral blood lymphocytes (1087). Interestingly, similar adverse effects were noted in rheumatoid arthritis patients treated with CAMPATH-1H (1088). Humanized anti-CD4 (1089) or anti-CD7 (1090), murine anti-ICAM-1 (CD54) (1091) or murine anti-IL2 receptor antibody (1092) were devoid of or produced only minimal and transient side-effects.

CD-4 Mabs have been extensively used in rheumatoid arthritis and significant immunomodulation has been obtained in several patients with only transient and self-limited side effects, such as flu-like symptoms, gastrointestinal disturbances, hypotension and tachycardia (1093). Anti-CD5 plus immunoconjugate administration produced common, but transient adverse effects, namely constitutional symptoms, fluid retention, skin rash and myalgias. Anaphylactoid reactions were sometimes reported (1094). Similarly, cA2, a chimeric Mab to TNF-α was found beneficial and well-tolerated with only one case of pneumonia possibly related to treatment (1095). No side effects were noted after anti-IL6 Mab administration in patients with rheumatoid arthritis (1096).

In a review of available unconjugated Mabs in the treatment of cancer, Dillman (1079) suggested that toxicity was not a major problem, but he was unable to detect significant therapeutic benefit with these agents. Potentiation and selective delivery of Mab to tumors can be obtained when drugs, isotopes and toxins are conjugated with monoclonal antibodies (1081). Immunoconjugates comprising a ricin A chain conjugated with murine Mab directed against various neoplastic antigens have thus been developed, but fluid retention with a vascular leak syndrome was found to be the main dose-limiting toxicity (1097—1099).

Finally, anti-endotoxin Mabs (e.g. nebacumab and edobacomab) have so far not been found useful in the treatment of severe sepsis (1100). Similarly, no significant reduction in the overall 28-day mortality was found when anti-TNF-α monoclonal antibody was compared with placebo in a large multicenter clinical trial (1101).

IMMUNOENHANCING DRUGS

Immunomodulating agents can be defined as chemically defined drugs with the capacity to enhance or restore the immune competence. Despite extensive research in the past years (1102), very few agents of this class are still in use today. Actually, the field of immunostimulation has dramatically shifted to the therapeutic use of cytokines so that limited new information has been published recently on the side effects of older immunomodulating agents. Interestingly however, the clinical experience gained with recombinant cytokines (see elsewhere in this Chapter), which are potent inducers of immune activation, has largely confirmed initial findings and case reports.

UNTOWARD CONSEQUENCES OF IMMUNOMODULATION

It has been known for the last decade at least, that agents capable of enhancing or restoring the immune competence of patients with a variety of immunopathological disorders, induced several types of untoward consequences directly related to their immunopharmacological activity (SED-12).

Fever Fever is the most common side-effect. In contrast to recombinant cytokines, fever associated with chemically defined immunomodulating agents is often mild, with pyrexia up to 39—40°C, chills, malaise and hypotension, inconsistent, and easily prevented or reversed by the administration of antipyretics, such as paracetamol. The mechanism likely to account for this 'flu-like reactions' involves the activation of macrophages and leukocytes, which release TNF-α and interleukin-1.

Exacerbation of the primary underlying disease This has initially been reported with levamisole. Similarly, exacerbation or reappearance of psoriatic lesions have been described. Although extremely few case reports have been published, it is known that exacerbation of asthma or eczema can occur in some patients treated with immunomodulating agents. Interestingly, exacerbation of the primary underlying disease has been reported with various recombinant cytokines.

Hypersensitivity reactions Immune complex-mediated hypersensitivity (type III) reactions have been shown to be associated with levamisole therapy.

Drug interactions Inhibition of microsomal drug-metabolizing activity has been shown with many immunomodulating agents as well as with some vaccines, either at therapeutic or at suprapharmacological dose levels. No simple mechanism is likely to account for these findings, even though the release of interleukin-1 by activated macrophages, resulting in the further release of interleukin-6 is an attractive hypothesis.

EFFECTS RELATED TO INDIVIDUAL COMPOUNDS

As indicated above, few immunomodulating agents remain in use today.

Bacillus Calmette-Guérin (BCG)

Intravesical administration for the treatment of bladder cancer is currently the main therapeutic use of BCG as an immunostimulating agent. In their review of 1278 bladder cancer patients, Lamm et al. (1103) noted cystitis in 91% of patients. Other side-effects included fever (1.3%), hepatitis (0.9%), arthritis or arthralgias (0.5%), hematuria (0.5%), skin rash (0.4%), epididymo-orchitis (0.2%), bladder contracture (0.2%), hypotension (0.1%) and cytopenia (0.1%). Lowering the BCG dose did not decrease the incidence of side effects, and even increased the incidence of pollakiuria, hematuria, fever and headache (1104).

Local reactions with redness and itching have been very commonly reported. Arthritis and Reiter's syndrome have been described recently (1105—1109). Mycobacterial infection is another possible complication. Systemic (1110) or localized, often granulomatous, infections to the lung (1111—1113), the bone (1114) and the liver (1115) have been described. Treatment with antituberculous drugs is usually effective.

Bucillamine

Renal complications have been noted with this drug, which bears a resemblance to penicillamine, when it has been used in the treatment of rheumatoid arthritis. At least 14 cases of nephrotic syndrome have been reported in Japan (1116). The first case of pulmonary eosinophilia in a 60-year-old woman with rheumatoid arthritis has been published recently (1117). A few cases of autoimmune diseases associated with bucillamine, including pemphigus (1118) and myasthenia gravis (1119) have also been described. Finally, a yellowish discoloration of the nails has been suggested to be a possible complication of bucillamine treatment (1120).

Isoprinosine

Neither therapeutic efficacy or side-effects were evidenced in two recent clinical trials of isoprinosine for the treatment of HIV infection (1121) and multiple sclerosis (1122).

Levamisole

Apart from side-effects possibly related to immunomodulation as discussed above, e.g. flu-like reaction or exacerbation of primary underlying disease, levamisole may induce specific complications which are reviewed elsewhere in this volume (see Chapter 31). Multifocal inflammatory leukoencephalopathy has been described in cancer patients treated with levamisole alone (1123) or in association with 5-fluorouracil (1124). One case of inappropriate antidiuretic hormone syndrome has been reported in a patient with sigmoid-colon carcinoma treated with levamisole and with 5-fluorouracil (1125). Finally, seizures (1126) have been noted in two children receiving levamisole for the treatment of nephrotic syndrome.

OK-432 (Picibanil)

Fever, nausea and vomiting, and pain at injection site were commonly reported following OK-432 administration, whereas joint pain, mild liver dysfunction, and anemia were seldom described.

Thymostimulin

One case of anaphylactic shock has been reported immediately after the injection of thymostimulin (1127).

REFERENCES

1. Arazi KI, Lee F, Miyajima A et al. Cytokines: coordinators of immune and inflammatory responses. Annu Rev Biochem 1990;59:783—836.
2. Takaku F. Clinical applications of cytokines for cancer treatment. Oncology 1994;51:123—128.
3. Talmadge JE, Dean JH. Immunopharmacology of recombinant cytokines. In: Dean JH, Luster MI, Munson AE, Kimber I, eds. Immunotoxicology and Immunopharmacology, 2nd edn. New York: Raven Press, 1994;227—247.
4. Evens RP, Witcher M. Biotechnology: an introduction to recombinant DNA technology and product availability. Ther Drug Monitor 1993;15:514—520.
5. Thomas JA, Thomas MJ. New biologics: their development, safety and efficacy. In: Thomas JA, Myers LA, eds. Biotechnology and Safety Assessment. New York: Raven Press, 1993;1—22.
6. Weinstock-Guttman B, Kinkel RT, Rudick RA. The interferons: biological effects, mechanism of actions and use in multiple sclerosis. Ann Neurol 1995;37:7—20.
7. Volz MA, Kirkpatrick CH. Interferons 1992. How much of the promise has been realised? Drugs 1992;43:285—294.
8. Agarwala SS, Kirkwood JM. Interferons in the therapy of solid tumors. Oncology 1994;51:129—136.
9. Baron S, Dianzani F. The interferons: a biological system with therapeutic potential in viral infections. Antiviral Res 1994;24:97—110.
10. Urabe A. Interferons for the treatment of hematological malignancies. Oncology 1994;51:137—141.
11. Wiselka MJ, Nicholson KG, Kent J et al. Prophylactic intranasal α_2 interferon and viral exacerbations of chronic respiratory disease. Thorax 1991;46:706—711.
12. Dorr RT. Interferon-α in malignant and viral diseases. Drugs 1993;45:177—211.
13. Vial T, Descotes J. Clinical toxicity of the interferons. Drug Safety 1994;10:115—150.
14. Chowhan NM, Zarrabi MH. Late febrile reaction to interferon. Am J Hematol 1992;41:144.
15. Gaudin JL, Dumortier J, Souquet JC, Bel A. Fièvre tardive sous interféron alpha recombinant. Presse Med 1994;23:1041.
16. Spiegel RJ. The alpha interferons: clinical overview. Sem Oncol 1987;14(Suppl 2):1—12.
17. Kubota T, Kaseda S, Yoshida M et al. Two cases of second-degree atrioventricular block associated with interferon therapy for chronic hepatitis C. Kokyu to Junkan 1994;42:983—987.
18. Mansat-Krzyzanowska E, Dréno B, Chiffoleau A, Litoux P. Manifestations cardio-vasculaires associées à l'interféron α-2a. Ann Med Int 1991;142:576—581.
19. Sonnenblick M, Rosin A. Cardiotoxicity of interferon: a review of 44 cases. Chest 1991;99:557—561.
20. Chapelon-Abric C, Chemlal K, Leblond V et al. Insuffisance ventriculaire gauche aiguë réversible induite par l'interféron. Rev Med Int 1994;15:857.
21. Cohen MC, Huberman MS, Nesto RW. Recombinant alpha2 interferon-related cardiomyopathy. Am J Med 1988;85:549—551.
22. Deyton LR, Walker RE, Kovacs JA et al. Reversible cardiac dysfunction associated with interferon alpha therapy in AIDS patients with Kaposi's sarcoma. N Engl J Med 1989;321:1246—1249.
23. Guillot P, Barbuat C, Richard B, Jourdan J. Myocardiopathie réversible induite par l'interféron. Thérapie 1993; 48:65—66.
24. Sonnenblick M, Rosenmann D, Rosin A. Reversible cardiomyopathy induced by interferon. Br Med J 1990; 300:1174—1175.
25. Zimmerman S, Adkins D, Graham M et al. Case report: irreversible, severe congestive cardiomyopathy occurring in association with interferon alpha therapy. Cancer Biother 1994;9:291—299.
26. Kramers C, de Mulder PHM, Barth JD et al. Acute right ventricular heart failure in a patient with renal cell carcinoma after interferon therapy. Neth J Med 1993;42:65—68.
27. Sartori M, Andorno S, La Terra G et al. Assessment of interferon cardiotoxicity with quantitative radionuclide angiocardiography. Eur J Clin Invest 1995;25:68—70.
28. Azar JJ, Theriault RL. Acute cardiomyopathy as a consequence of treatment with interleukin-2 and interferon-alpha in a patient with metastatic carcinoma of the breast. Am J Clin Oncol 1991;14:530—533.
29. Kruit WM, Punt KJ, Goey SH et al. Cardiotoxicity as a dose-limiting factor in a schedule of high dose bolus therapy with interleukin-2 and alpha-interferon. Cancer 1994; 74:2850—2856.
30. Schechter D, Nagler A, Ackerstein A et al. Recombinant interleukin-2 and interferon alpha immunotherapy following

autologous bone marrow transplantation. Cardiology 1992;80:168–171.
31. Chin K, Tabata C, Satake N et al. Pneumonitis associated with natural and recombinant interferon alfa therapy for chronic hepatitis C. Chest 1994;105:939–941.
32. Kamisako T, Adachi Y, Chihara J, Yamamoto T. Intersitial pneumonitis and interferon-alfa. Br Med J 1993;306:896.
33. Matsui M, Sawada K, Ohta M. Acute interstitial pneumonia which developed during interferon-therapy for type C chronic hepatitis. Nippon Kyobu Rinsho 1993;52:884–890.
34. Moriya K, Yasuda K, Koike K et al. Induction of interstitial pneumonitis during interferon treatment for chronic hepatitis C. J Gastroenterol 1994;29:514–517.
35. Murata M, Nagai M, Bando S et al. Emergence of acute interstitial pneumonia following high dose interferon alpha treatment in a case of chronic myelogenous leukemia. Intern Med 1993;32:716–718.
36. Yufu Y, Yamashita S, Nishimura J, Nawata H. Interstitial pneumonia caused by interferon-α in chronic myelogenous leukemia. Am J Hematol 1994;47:253.
37. Watanabe N, Miura S, Yamaguchi E et al. A case of interferon-alpha-induced pneumonitis. Nippon Kyobu Shikkan Gakkai Zasshi 1993;31:1308–1312.
38. Hizawa N, Kojima J, Kojima T et al. A patient with chronic hepatitis C who simultaneously developed interstitial pneumonia, hemolytic anemia and cholestatic liver dysfunction after alpha-interferon administration. Intern Med 1994;33:337–341.
39. Ogata K, Koga T, Yagawa K. Interferon-related bronchiolitis obliterans organizing pneumonia. Chest 1994; 106:612–613.
40. Harris J, Bines S, Das Gupta T. Therapy of disseminated malignant melanoma with recombinant α 2b-interferon and piroxicam: clinical results with a report of an unusual response-associated feature (vitiligo) and unusual toxicity (diffuse pulmonary interstitial fibrosis). Med Pediatr Oncol 1994;22:103–106.
41. Bocci V. Central nervous system toxicity of interferons and other cytokines. J Biol Regul Homeostat Agents 1988;2:107–118.
42. Smedley H, Katrak M, Sikora K, Wheeler T. Neurological effects of recombinant human interferon. Br Med J 1983;286:262–264.
43. Iaffaioli RV, Fiorenza L, D'Avino M et al. Neurotoxic effects of long-term treatment with low-dose alpha 2B interferon. Curr Ther Res 1990;48:403–408.
44. Merimsky O, Reider-Groswasser I, Inbar M, Chaitchik S. Interferon-related mental deterioration and behavioural changes in patients with renal cell carcinoma. Eur J Cancer (1990)26, 596–600.
45. Adams F, Quesada JR, Gutterman JU. Neuropsychiatric manifestations of human leukocyte interferon therapy in patients with cancer. J Am Med Assoc 1984;252:938–941.
46. Meyers CA, Valentine AD. Neurological and psychiatric adverse effects of immunological therapy. CNS Drugs 1995;3:56–68.
47. Prasad S, Waters B, Hill PB et al. Psychiatric side effects of interferon alfa-2b in patients treated for hepatitis C. Clin Res 1992;40:840A.
48. Renault PF, Hoofnagle JH, Park Y et al. Psychiatric complications of long-term interferon alfa therapy. Arch Intern Med 1987;147:1577–1580.
49. Mattson K, Niiranen A, Iivanainen M et al. Neurotoxicity of interferon. Cancer Treat Rep 1983;67:958–961.
50. Meyers CA, Scheibel RS, Forman AD. Persistent neurotoxicity of systemically administered interferon-alpha. Neurology 1991;41:672–676.
51. Janssen HLA, Brouwer JT, van der Mast RC, Schalm SW. Suicide associated with alfa-interferon therapy for chronic viral hepatitis. J Hepatol 1994;21:241–243.
52. Goldman LS. Successful treatment of interferon alfa-induced mood disorder with nortriptyline. Psychosomatics 1994;35:412–413.
53. Levenson JL, Fallon HJ. Fluoxetine treatment of depression caused by interferon-alpha. Am J Gastroenterol 1993;88:760–761.
54. Adams F, Fernandez F, Mavligit G. Interferon-induced organic mental disorders associated with unsuspected pre-existing neurologic abnormalities. J Neuro-Oncol 1988; 6:355–359.
55. Meyers CA, Obbens EA, Scheibel RS, Moser RP. Neurotoxicity of intraventricularly administered alpha-interferon for leptomeningeal disease. Cancer 1991;68:88–92.
56. Hagberg H, Blomkvist E, Ponten U et al. Does alpha-interferon in conjunction with radiotherapy increase the risk of complications in the central nervous system. Ann Oncol 1990;1:449.
57. Laaksonen R, Niiranen A, Iivanainen M et al. Dementia-like, largely reversible syndrome after cranial irradiation and prolonged interferon treatment. Ann Clin Res 1988;20:201–203.
58. Mitsuyama Y, Hashiguchi H, Murayama T et al. An autopsied case of interferon encephalopathy. Jpn J Psychiatr Neurol 1992;46:741–748.
59. Van Thiel DH, Friedlander L, Molloy PJ et al. Interferon-alpha can be used successfully in patients with hepatitis C virus-positive chronic hepatitis who have a psychiatric illness. Eur J Gastroenterol Hepatol 1995;7:165–168.
60. Hibi H, Itoh K, Kamiya T et al. Grand mal like attack by interferon injection in case of renal cell carcinoma. Hinyokika Kiyo 1991;37:69–72.
61. Janssen HLA, Berk L, Vermeulen M, Schalm SW. Seizures associated with low-dose alpha-interferon. Lancet 1990;336:1580.
62. Miller VS, Zwiener RJ, Fielman BA. Interferon-associated refractory status epilepticus. Pediatrics 1994;93:511–512.
63. Cudillo L, Cantonetti M, Venditti A et al. Peripheral polyneuropathy during treatment with alpha-2 interferon. Haematologica 1990;75:485–486.
64. Gastineau DA, Habermann TM, Hermann RC. Severe neuropathy associated with low-dose recombinant interferon-alpha. Am J Med 1989;87:116.
65. Jaubert D, Hauteville D, Pelissier JF, Muzellec Y. Neuropathie périphérique au cours d'un traitement par interféron alpha. Presse Med 1991;20:221–222.
66. Negoro K, Fukusako T, Morimatsu M, Liao CM. Acute axonal polyneuropathy during interferon α-2a therapy for chronic hepatitis C. Muscle Nerve 1994;17:1351–1352.
67. Read SJ, Crawford DHG, Pender MP. Trigeminal sensory neuropathy induced by interferon-alpha therapy. Austr NZ J Med 1995;25:54.
68. Bernsen P, Wong Chung RE, Vingerhoets HM, Janssen JTP. Bilateral neuralgic amyotrophy induced by interferon treatment. Arch Neurol 1988;45:449–451.

69. Vesikari T, Nuutila A, Cantel K. Neurologic sequelae following interferon therapy of juvenile laryngeal papilloma. Acta Paediatr Scand 1988;77:619–622.
70. Merimsky O, Reider I, Merimsky E, Chaitchik S. Interferon-related leukoencephalopathy in a patient with renal cell carcinoma. Tumori 1991;77:361–362.
71. Fentiman IS, Balkwill FR, Thomas BS et al. An autoimmune aetiology for hypothyroidism following interferon therapy for breast cancer. Eur J Cancer Clin Oncol 1988; 24:1299–1303.
72. Barreca T, Picciotto A, Franceschini R et al. Long term therapy with recombinant interferon alpha 2b in patients with chronic hepatitis C: effect on thyroid function and autoantibodies. J Biol Regul Homeost Agents 1993;7:58–62.
73. Baudin E, Marcellin P, Pouteau M et al. Reversibility of thyroid dysfunction induced by recombinant alpha interferon in chronic hepatitis C. Clin Endocrinol 1993;39:657–661.
74. Chung YH, Shong YK. Development of thyroid autoimmunity after administration of recombinant human interferon-α2b for chronic viral hepatitis. Am J Gastroenterol 1993;88:244–247.
75. Fonseca V, Thomas M, Dusheiko G. Thyrotropin receptor antibodies following treatment with recombinant alpha-interferon in patients with hepatitis. Acta Endocrinol 1991;125:491–493.
76. Graus J, Barcena R, Urena V et al. Thyroid disease during therapy of chronic hepatitis C with IFN. J Hepatol 1993;18(Suppl 1):126.
77. Imagawa A, Itoh N, Hanafusa T et al. Autoimmune endocrine disease induced by recombinant interferon-α therapy for chronic active type C hepatitis. J Clin Endocrinol Metabol 1995;80:922–926.
78. Lisker-Melman M, Di Bisceglie AM, Usala SJ et al. Development of thyroid disease during therapy of chronic viral hepatitis with interferon alfa. Gastroenterology 1992;102:2155–2160.
79. Nagayama Y, Ohta K, Tsuruta M et al. Exacerbation of thyroid autoimmunity by interferon a treatment in patients with chronic viral hepatitis, our studies and review of the literature. Endocrine J 1994;41:565–572.
80. Schultz M, Müller R, von zur Mühlen A, Brabant G. Induction of hyperthyroidism by interferon-α-2b. Lancet 1989;i:1452.
81. Tsianos EV, Dalekos GN, Merkouropoulos MH et al. Frequency of thyroid dysfunction after recombinant alpha-interferon therapy in Greek patients with chronic active hepatitis. Eur. J Gastroenterol Hepatol 1994;6:547–551.
82. Watanabe U, Hashimoto E, Hishamitsu T et al. The risk factors for develoment of thyroid disease during interferon-α therapy for chronic hepatitis C. Am J Gastroenterol 1994;89:399–403.
83. Yoshikawa M, Sakamoto T, Mitoro A et al. Autoimmunity during alpha-interferon therapy for chronic hepatitis C Gastroenterol Jpn 1993;28(Suppl 5):109–114.
84. Burman P, Tötterman TH, Berg K, Karlsson FA. Thyroid autoimmunity in patients on long term therapy with leukocyte-derived interferon. J Clin Endocrinol Metabol 1986;63:1086–1090.
85. Rönnblom LE, Alm GV, Oberg KE. Autoimmunity after alpha-interferon therapy for malignant carcinoid tumors. Ann Intern Med 1991;115:178–183.
86. Gisslinger H, Gilly B, Woloszczuk W et al. Thyroid autoimmunity and hypothyroidism during long-term treatment with recombinant interferon-alpha. Clin Exp Immunol 1992;90:363–367.
87. Kalkner M, Hagberg H, Karlsson-Parra A. Autoantibody occurrence in hairy-cell leukemia during prolonged interferon treatment. Eur J Haematol 1990;45:233–234.
88. Papo T, Oksenhendler E, Izembart M et al. Antithyroid hormone antibodies induced by interferon-α. J Clin Endocrinol Metabol 1992;75:1484–1486.
89. Marcellin P, Pouteau M, Renard P et al. Sustained hypothyroidism induced by recombinant alpha interferon in patients with chronic hepatitis C. Gut 1992;33:855–856.
90. Vial T, Descotes J. Immune-mediated side-effects of cytokines in humans. Toxicology 1995;105:31–57.
91. Vallisa D, Cavanna L, Berté R et al. Autoimmune thyroid dysfunctions in hematologic malignancies treated with alpha-interferon. Acta Haematol 1995;93:31–35.
92. Preziati D, La Rosa L, Covini G et al. Autoimmunity and thyroid dysfunction in patients with chronic active hepatitis treated with recombinant interferon alpha-2a. Eur J Endocrinol 1995;132:587–593.
93. Wiedermann CJ, Vogel W, Tilg H et al. Suppression of thyroid function by interferon-alpha2 in man. Naunyn-Schmiedeberg's Arch Pharmacol 1991;343:665–668.
94. Yamazaki K, Kanaji Y, Shizume K et al. Reversible inhibition by interferons alpha and beta of ^{125}I incorporation and thyroid hormone release by human thyroid follicules in vitro. J Clin Endocrinol Metab 1993;77:1439–1441.
95. Bibas M, Andriani A, Rinaldi PL. Diabetic ketoacidosis with coma after interferon therapy for a metastatic melanoma: a case report. Br J Haematol 1994;87(Suppl 1):204.
96. Fabris P, Betterle C, Floreani A et al. Development of type 1 diabetes mellitus during interferon alpha therapy for chronic HCV hepatitis. Lancet 1992;340:548.
97. Gori A, Caredda F, Franzetti F et al. Reversible diabetes in patient with AIDS-related Kaposi's sarcoma treated with interferon α-2a. Lancet 1995;345:1438–1439.
98. Guerci AP, Guerci B, Lévy-Marchal C et al. Onset of insulin-dependent diabetes mellitus after interferon-alfa therapy for hairy cell leukaemia. Lancet 1994;343:1167–1168.
99. Mathieu E, Fain O, Sitbon M, Thomas M. Diabète autoimmun après traitement par interféron alpha. Presse Med 1995;24:238.
100. Waguri M, Hanafusa T, Itoh N et al. Occurrence of IDDM during interferon therapy for chronic viral hepatitis. Diabetes Res Clin Pract 1994;23:33–36.
101. Fattovitch G, Betterle C, Brollo L et al. Induction of autoantibodies during alpha interferon treatment in chronic hepatitis B. Arch Virol 1992;4(Suppl):291–293.
102. Mayet WJ, Hess G, Gerken G et al. Treatment of chronic type B hepatitis with recombinant α-interferon induces autoantibodies not specific for autoimmune chronic hepatitis. Hepatology 1989;10:24–28.
103. Koivisto VA, Pelkonen R, Cantell K. Effects of interferon on glucose tolerance and insulin sensitivity. Diabetes 1989;38:641–647.
104. Khan BA, Gordon SC. Development of diabetes during interferon alpha therapy for chronic HCV hepatitis. Am J Gastroenterol 1994;89:1736.
105. Lopes EPA, Oliveira PM, Silva AE et al. Exacerbation of type 2 diabetes mellitus during interferon-alfa therapy for chronic hepatitis B. Lancet 1994;343:244.
106. Krug J, Fritzsch J, Aust G. Induction of insulin antibodies and insulin allergy under alfa-interferon treatment of renal cell carcinoma in a patient with insulin-treated diabetes mellitus: a case report. Int Arch Allerg Immunol 1995; 106:169–172.

107. Ueki K, Tsuchida A, Murakami H et al. Hypoparathyroidism during alpha-INF therapy in a patient with multiple myeloma J Med 1989;20:391–397.
108. Sakane N, Yoshida T, Yoshioka K et al. Reversible hypopituitarism after interferon-alfa therapy. Lancet 1995;345:1305.
109. Massaro ER, Borden EC, Hawkins MJ et al. Effects of recombinant interferon-α2 treatment upon lipid concentrations and lipoprotein composition. J Interfer Res 1986; 6:665–662.
110. Schectman G, Kaul S, Mueller RA et al. The effect of interferon on the metabolism of LDLs. Arteriosclerosis Thromb 1992;12:1053–1062.
111. Oberg K, Eriksson B. Medical treatment of neuroendocrine gut and pancreatic tumors. Acta Oncol 1989;28:425–431.
112. Ruiz-Moreno M, Carreno V, Rua MJ et al. Increase in triglycerides during α-interferon treatment of chronic viral hepatitis. J Hepatol 1992;16:384–388.
113. Jaubert D, Galzin M, de Jaureguiberry JP, Hadjali Y. Hypertriglycéridémies au cours des traitements par interféron alpha. Rev Med Interne 1994;15(Suppl 3):422s.
114. Penarrubia MJ, Steegmann JL, Lavilla E et al. Hypertriglyceridemia may be severe in CML patients treated with interferon-α. Am J Hematol 1995;49:240–241.
115. Berruti A, Gorzegno G, Vitetta G et al. Hypertriglyceridemia during long-term interferon-alpha therapy: efficacy of diet and gemfibrosil treatment. A case report. Tumori 1992;78:353–355.
116. Sunderkötter C, Luger T, Kolde G. Severe hypertriglyceridaemia and interferon-alpha. Lancet 1993;342:1111–1112.
117. Yamagishi SI, Abe T, Sawada T. Human recombinant interferon alpha-2a (rIRFN alpha-2a) therapy suppresses hepatic triglyceride lipase, leading to severe hypertriglyceridemia in a diabetic patient. Am J Gastroenterol 1994;89:2280.
118. Graessle P, Bonacini M, Chen S. Alpha-interferon and reversible hypertriglyceridemia. Ann Intern Med 1993; 118:316–317.
119. Gisslinger H, Svoboda T, Clodi M et al. Interferon-α stimulates the hypothalamic-pituitary-adrenal axis in vivo and in vitro. Neuroendocrinology 1993;57:489–495.
120. Müller H, Hiemke C, Hammes E, Hess G. Sub-acute effects of interferon-α2 on adrenocorticotrophic hormone, cortisol, growth hormone and prolactin in humans. Psychoneuroendocrinology 1992;17:459–465.
121. Barreca T, Picciotto A, Franceschini R et al. Effects of acute administration of recombinant interferon alpha 2b on pituitary hormone secretion in patients with chronic active hepatitis. Curr Ther Res 1992;52:695–701.
122. Crockett DM, Lusk RP, McCabe BF, Mixon JH. Side effects and toxicity of interferon in the treatment of recurrent respiratory papillomatosis. Ann Otol Rhinol Laryngol 1987;96:601–607.
123. Kikawa K, Nishida K, Tanizawa A et al. Growth retardation as a long-term side-effect of alpha-interferon therapy. Eur J Pediatr 1995;154:591–592.
124. Färkkilä AM, Iivanainen MV, Färkkilä MA. Disturbance of the water and electrolyte balance during high-dose interferon treatment. J Interfer Res 1990;10:221–227.
125. Lei KIK, Wickham NWR, Johnson PJ. Severe hyponatremia due to syndrome of inappropriate secretion of antidiuretic hormone in a patient receiving interferon-α for chronic myeloid leukemia. Am J Hematol 1995;48:100.
126. Ernstoff MS, Kirkwood JM. Changes in the bone marrow of cancer patients treated with recombinant interferon alpha-2. Am J Med 1984;76:593–596.
127. Poynard T, Bedossa P, Chevallier M et al. A comparison of three interferon alfa-2b regimens for the long-term treatment of chronic non-A, non-B hepatitis. N Engl J Med 1995;332:1457–1462.
128. Giustina G, Favarato S, Ruol A, Fattovitch G. A survey of clinical toxicity of alfa interferon in 11,241 patients with chronic viral hepatitis. Ital J Gastroenterol 1994;26:203–204.
129. Harousseau JL, Milpied N, Bourhis JH et al. Aplasie fatale après traitement par interféron alpha d'une leucémie myéloïde chronique en rechute après greffe de moelle osseuse allogénique. Presse Med 1988;17:80–81.
130. Hoffmann A, Kirn E, Krueger GRF, Fischer R. Bone marrow hypoplasia and fibrosis following interferon treatment. In Vivo 1994;8:605–612.
131. Shepherd PCA, Richards S, Allan NC. Severe cytopenias associated with the sequential use of busulphan and interferon-alpha in chronic myeloid leukaemia. Br J Haematol 1994;86:92–96.
132. Talpaz M, Kantarjian H, Zurzrock R, Gutterman JU. Bone marrow hypoplasia and aplasia complicating interferon therapy for chronic myelogenous leukaemia. Cancer 1992;69:410–412.
133. Steis RG, VanderMolen LA, Lawrence J et al. Erythrocytosis in hairy cell leukaemia following therapy with interferon-alpha. Br J Haematol 1990;75:133–135.
134. Abdi EA, Brien W, Venner PM. Auto-immune thrombocytopenia related to interferon therapy. Scand J Haematol 1986;36:515–519.
135. Lopez Morante AJ, Saez-Royuela F, Casanova Valero F et al. Immune thrombocytopenia after alpha-interferon therapy in a patient with chronic hepatitis C. Am J Gastroenterol 1992;87:809–810.
136. Shrestha R, McKinley C, Bilir BM et al. Possible idiopathic thrombocytopenic purpura associated with natural alpha interferon therapy for chronic hepatitis C infection. Am J Gastroenterol 1995;90:1146–1147.
137. Akard LP, Hoffman R, Elias L, Saiers JH. Alpha-interferon and immune hemolytic anemia. Ann Intern Med 1986;105:306.
138. Barbolla L, Paniagua C, Outeirino J et al. Haemolytic anaemia to the alpha-interferon treatment: a proposed mechanism. Vox Sanguinis 1993;65:156–157.
139. Braathen LR, Stavem P. Autoimmune haemolytic anaemia associated with interferon alpha-2a in patients with mycosis fungoides. Br Med J 1989;298:1713.
140. Fornaciari G, Bassi C, Beltrami M et al. Hemolytic anemia secondary to interferon treatment for chronic B hepatitis. J Clin Gastroenterol 1991;13:596–597.
141. Hirashima N, Mizokami M, Orito E et al. Chronic hepatitis C complicated by Coombs-negative hemolytic anemia during interferon treatment. Intern Med 1994;33:300–302.
142. Benjamin S, Bain BJ, Dodsworth H. Severe bleeding associated with worsening thrombocytopenia following alpha-interferon therapy for autoimmune thrombocytopenic purpura. Clin Lab Haematol 1991;13:315–317.
143. Matthey F, Ardeman S, Jones L, Newland AC. Bleeding in immune thrombocytopenic purpura after alpha-interferon. Lancet 1990;335:471–472.
144. Stern SCM, Asagba GO, Hedge UM. Prolonged thrombocytopenia following alpha-interferon for refractory im-

mune thrombocytopenic purpura. Clin Lab Haematol 1994;16:183–185.
145. McNair ANB, Jacyna MR, Thomas HC. Severe haemolytic transfusion reaction occurring during alpha-interferon therapy for chronic hepatitis. Eur J Gastroenterol Hepatol 1991;3:193–194.
146. Castenskiold EC, Colvin BT, Kelsey SM. Acquired factor VIII inhibitor associated with chronic interferon-alpha therapy in a patient with haemophilia A. Br J Haematol 1994;87:434–436.
147. Stricker RB, Barlogie B, Kiprov DD. Acquired factor VIII inhibitor associated with chronic interferon-α therapy. J Rheumatol 1994;21:350–352.
148. Durand JM, Quiles N, Kaplanski G, Soubeyrand J. Thrombosis and recombinant interferon-α. Am J Med 1993;95:115.
149. Becker JC, Winkler B, Klingert S, Bröcker EB. Antiphospholipid syndrome associated with immunotherapy for patients with melanoma. Cancer 1994;73:1621–1624.
150. Mirro J, Kalwinsky D, Whisnant J et al. Coagulopathy induced by continuous infusion of high doses of human lymphoblastoid interferon. Cancer Treat Rep 1985;69:315–317.
151. Quesada JR, Talpaz M, Rios A, et al. Clinical toxicity of interferons in cancer patients: a review. J Clin Oncol 1986;4:234–243.
152. Davis GL, Balart LA, Schiff ER et al. Treatment of chronic hepatitis C with recombinant α-interferon: a multicentre randomized controlled trial J Hepatol 1990;11(Suppl 1):S31–S35.
153. Laskus T, Radkowski M, Slusarczyk J, Cianciara J. Severe exacerbation of chronic active hepatitis B during interferon alpha therapy. Digestion 1992;52:61–64.
154. Marcellin P, Colin JF, Boyer N et al. Fatal exacerbation of chronic hepatitis B induced by recombinant alpha-interferon. Lancet 1991;338:828.
155. Rossetti F, Pontini F, Crivellaro C et al. Interferon therapy of chronic delta-hepatitis in a patient cured of pediatric malignancies: possible harmful effect. Liver 1991; 11:255–259.
156. Janssen HLA, Brouwer JT, Nevens F et al. Fatal hepatic decompensation associated with interferon alfa. Lancet 1993;306:107–108.
157. Farhat BA, Johnson PJ, Williams R. Hazards of interferon treatment in patients with autoimmune chronic active hepatitis. J Hepatol 1994;20:560–561.
158. Papo T, Marcellin P, Bernuau J et al. Autoimmune chronic hepatitis exacerbated by alpha-interferon. Ann Intern Med 1992;116:51–53.
159. Payen JL, Rabbia I, Combis JM et al. Révélation d'une hépatite auto-immune par l'interféron. Gastroenterol Clin Biol 1993;17:404–405.
160. Ruiz-Moreno M, Rua MJ, Carreno V et al. Autoimmune chronic hepatitis type 2 manifested during interferon therapy in children. J Hepatol 1991;12:265–266.
161. Tran A, Beusnel C, Montoya ML et al. Hépatite autoimmune de type 1 révélée par un traitement par interféron. Gastroenterol Clin Biol 1992;16:722–723.
162. Vento S, Di Perri G, Garofano T et al. Hazards of interferon therapy for HBV-seronegative chronic hepatitis. Lancet 1989;ii:926.
163. Muratori L, Lenzi M, Cataleta F et al. Interferon therapy in liver/kidney microsomal antibody type-1 positive patients with chronic hepatitis C. J Hepatol 1994;21:199–203.
164. Garcia-Buey L, Garcia-Monzon C, Rodriguez S et al. Latent autoimmune hepatitis triggered during interferon therapy in patients with chronic hepatitis C. Gastroenterology 1995;108:1770–1777.
165. Maeda T, Onishi S, Miura T et al. Exacerbation of primary biliary cirrhosis during interferon α-2b therapy for chronic active hepatitis C. Dig Dis Sci 1995;40:1226–1230.
166. Heathcote EJ. Autoimmune hepatitis and chronic hepatitis C: latent or initiated by interferon therapy. Gastroenterology 1995;108:1942–1944.
167. Muratori L, Zauli D, Giostra F et al. LKM1 appearance in a HLA-DR3+ patient with chronic hepatitis C during interferon treatment. J Hepatol 1993;18:259–260.
168. Shindo M, Di Bisceglie AM, Hoofnagle JH. Acute exacerbation of liver disease during interferon alfa therapy for chronic hepatitis C. Gastroenterology 1992;102:1406–1408.
169. Silva MO, Reddy KR, Jeffers LJ et al. Interferon-induced chronic active hepatitis? Gastroenterology 1991; 101:840–842.
170. Ariad S, Song E, Cohen R, Bezwoda WR. Interferon-alpha induced autoimmune hepatitis in a patient with Philadelphia chromosome-positive chronic myeloid leukemia with cytogenetically normal T lymphocytes. Mol Biother 1992;4:139–142.
171. Sarraco G, Touscoz A, Durazzo M et al. Autoantibodies and response to α-interferon in patients with chronic viral hepatitis. J Hepatol 1990;11:339–343.
172. Shimizu Y, Joho S, Watanabe A. Hepatic injury after interferon-alpha therapy for chronic hepatitis C. Ann Intern Med 1994;121:723.
173. Durand JM, Kaplanski G, Portal I et al. Liver failure due to recombinant alpha interferon. Lancet 1991; 338:1268–1269.
174. Wandl UB, Kloke O, Niederle N. Liver failure due to recombinant alpha interferon for chronic myelogenous leukaemia. Lancet 1992;339:123–124.
175. Pecorari P. Colite ulcerosa in corso di leucemia a cellule capellute: descrizione di un caso. Rec Prog Med 1991; 82:269–271.
176. Mitoro A, Yoshikawa M, Yamamoto K et al. Exacerbation of ulcerative colitis during alpha-interferon therapy for chronic hepatitis C. Intern Med 1993;32:327–331.
177. Qaseem T, Jafri W, Abid S et al. A case report of painful oral ulcerations associated with the use of alpha interferon in a patient with chronic hepatitis due to Non-A Non-B Non-C virus. Military Med 1993;158:126–127.
178. Motoo Y, Watanabe H, Okai T, Sawabu N. Interferon-induced pancreatic injury. J Clin Gastroenterol 1994; 19:268–269.
179. Sotomatsu M, Shimoda M, Ogawa C, Morikawa A. Acute pancreatitis associated with interferon-α therapy for chronic myelogenous leukemia. Am J Hematol 1995; 48:211–212.
180. Selby P, Kohn J, Raymond J et al. Nephrotic syndrome during treatment with interferon. Br Med J 1985;290:1180.
181. Kurschel E, Metz-Kurschel U, Niederle N, Aulbert E. Investigations on the subclinical and clinical nephrotoxicity of interferon alpha-2B in patients with myeloproliferative syndromes. Renal Failure 1991;13:87–93.
182. Ayub A, Zafar M, Al-Harbi A et al. Acute renal failure with α-interferon therapy: a case report. Med Science Res 1993;21:123–124.
183. Nair S, Ernstoff MS, Bahnson RR et al. Interferon-induced reversible acute renal failure with nephrotic syndrome. Urology 1992;39:169–172.

184. Averbuch SD, Austin HA, Sherwin SA et al. Acute interstitial nephritis with the nephrotic syndrome following recombinant leukocyte A interferon therapy for mycosis fungoides. N Engl J Med 1984;310:32—35.
185. Kimmel OL, Abraham AA, Phillips TM. Membranoproliferative glomerulonephritis in a patient treated with interferon-α for human immunodeficiency virus infection. Am J Kidney Dis 1994;24:858—863.
186. Traynor A, Kuzel T, Samuelson E, Kanwar Y. Minimal-change glomerulopathy and glomerular visceral epithelial hyperplasia associated with alpha-interferon therapy for cutaneous T-cell lymphoma. Nephron 1994;67:94—100.
187. Fahal IH, Murry N, Chu P, Bell GM. Acute renal failure during interferon treatment. Br Med J 1993;306:973.
188. Noël C, Vrtovsnik F, Facon T et al. Acute and definitive renal failure in progressive multiple myeloma treated with recombinant interferon alpha-2a: report on two patients. Am J Hematol 1992;41:298—299.
189. Sawamura M, Matsushima T, Tamura J et al. Renal toxicity in long-term alpha-interferon treatment in a patient with myeloma. Am J Hematol 1992;41:146.
190. Lederer E, Truong L. Unusual glomerular lesion in a patient receiving long-term interferon alpha. Am J Kidney Dis 1992;20:516—518.
191. Durand JM, Retornaz F, Cretel E et al. Glomérulonéphrite extracapillaire au cours d'un traitement par interféron alpha. Rev Med Interne 1993;14:1138.
192. Viallard JF, Pommereau A, Punthous M et al. Glomérulopathie inhabituelle au cours d'un traitement par interféron alpha. Rev Med Interne 1994;15(Suppl 3):421s.
193. Schlaifer D, Dumazer P, Spenatto N et al. Hemolytic-uremic syndrome in a patient with chronic myelogenous leukemia treated with interferon alpha. Am J Hematol 1994;47:254—255.
194. Stratta P, Canavese C, Dogliani M et al. Hemolytic uremic syndrome during recombinant alpha-interferon treatment for hairy cell leukemia. Renal Failure 1993;15:559—561.
195. Jadoul M, Piessevaux H, Ferrant A et al. Renal thrombotic microangiopathy in patients with chronic myelogenous leukaemia treated with interferon-alpha-2b. Nephrol Dial Transplant 1995;10:111—113.
196. Demelia L, Vallebona E, Poma R et al. Adverse effects of alpha-interferon therapy in chronic hepatitis. Gastroenterology, 10th World Congress of Gastroenterology 1994; Abstract II:2638P.
197. Tosti A, Misciali C, Bardazzi F et al. Telogen effluvium due to recombinant interferon alpha-2b. Dermatology 1992;184:124—125.
198. Berglund EF, Burton GV, Mills GM, Nichols GM. Hypertrichosis of the eyelashes associated with interferon-alpha therapy for chronic granulocytic leukemia. South Med J 1990;83:363.
199. Foon KA, Dougher G. Increased growth of eyelashes in a patient given leukocyte A interferon. N Engl J Med 1984;311:1259.
200. Klapholz L, Ackerstein A, Goldenhersh MA et al. Local cutaneous reaction induced by subcutaneous interleukin-2 and interferon alpha-2a immunotherapy following ABMT. Bone Marrow Transplant 1993;11:443—446.
201. Christian B, Derriennic X, Aymard JP. Nécrose cutanée locale après injection d'interféron alpha. Presse Med 1993;22:783.
202. Cnudde F, Gharakhanian S, Luboinski J et al. Cutaneous local necrosis following interferon injections. Int J Dermatol 1991;30:147.
203. Oeda E, Shinohara K. Cutaneous necrosis caused by injection of α-interferon in a patient with chronic myelogeneous leukemia. Am J Hematol 1993:44:213—214.
204. Orlow SJ, Friedman-Kein AE. Cutaneous ulcerations secondary to interferon alfa therapy of Kaposi's sarcoma, Arch Dermatol 1992;128:566.
205. Andry P, Weber Buisset MJ, Fraitag S et al. Toxidermie bulleuse à l'Introna. Ann Dermatol Venereol 1993;120:843—845.
206. Liet JM, Casasnovas RO, Terraz A et al. Vascularite aiguë leucocytoclastique à dépôts d'IgA au cours d'un traitement par interféron alpha. Rev Med Interne 1992;13(Suppl 6):169.
207. Sangster G, Kaye SB, Calman KC, Toy JL. Cutaneous vasculitis associated with interferon. Eur J Cancer Clin Oncol 1983;19:1647—1649.
208. Reid IT, Lombardo FA, Redmond IJ et al. Digital vasculitis associated with interferon therapy. Am J Med 1992;92:702—703.
209. Dreno B, Huart A, Billaud E et al. Alpha-interferon therapy and cutaneous vascular lesions. Ann Intern Med 1989;111:95—96.
210. Quesada JR, Gutterman JU. Psoriasis and alpha-interferon. Lancet 1986;i:1465—1468.
211. Hartmann F, von Wussow P, Deicher H. Psoriasis-Exazerbation bei Therapie mit α-Interferon. Deutsche Med Wochenschr 1989;114:96—98.
212. Harrison PV, Peat MJ. Effect of interferon on psoriasis. Lancet 1986;ii:457—458.
213. Cervoni JP, Serfaty L, Picard O et al. Le traitement des hépatites B et C par interféron alpha peut induire ou aggraver un psoriasis. Gastroenterol Clin Biol 1995;19:324—325.
214. Funk J, Langeland T, Schrumpf E, Hanssen LE. Psoriasis induced by interferon-alpha. Br J Dermatol 1991; 125:463—465.
215. Georgetson MJ, Yarze JC, Lalos AT et al. Exacerbation of psoriasis due to interferon-α treatment of chronic active hepatitis. Am J Gastroenterol 1993;88:1756—1758.
216. Jucgla A, Marcoval J, Curco N, Servitje O. Psoriasis with articular involvement induced by interferon alfa. Arch Dermatol 1991;127:910—911.
217. Kusec R, Ostoji S, Planinc-Peraica A et al. Exacerbation of psoriasis after treatment with alpha-interferon. Dermatologica 1990;181:170.
218. Makino Y, Tanaka H, Nakamura K et al. Arthritis in a patient with psoriasis after alpha-interferon therapy for chronic hepatitis C. J Rheumatol 1994;21:1771—1772.
219. Pauluzzi P, Kokelj F, Perkan V et al. Psoriasis exacerbation induced by interferon-α: report of two cases. Acta Dermatol Venereol 1993;73:395.
220. Wolfe JT, Singh A, Lessin SR et al. De novo development of psoriatic plaques in patients receiving interferon alfa for treatment of erythrodermic cutaneous T-cell lymphoma. J Am Acad Dermatol 1995;32:887—893.
221. Cleveland MG, Mallory SB. Incomplete Reiter's syndrome induced by systemic interferon α treatment. J Am Acad Dermatol 1993;29:788—789.
222. Barreca T, Corsini G, Franceschini R et al. Lichen planus induced by interferon-alpha-2a therapy for chronic active hepatitis C. Eur J Gastroenterol Hepatol 1995;7:367—368.

223. d'Agay-Abensour L, Benamouzig R, de Belilovsky C et al. Lichen plan au cours d'une hépatite virale chronique C traitée par interféron alpha. Gastroenterol Clin Biol 1992;16:610–611.
224. Dupin N, Chosidow O, Francés C et al. Lichen planus after alpha-interferon therapy for chronic hepatitis C. Eur J Dermatol 1994;4:535–536.
225. Heintges T, Frieling T, Goerz G, Niederau C. Exacerbation of lichen ruber planus but not of acute intermittent porphyria during interferon therapy in a patient with hepatitis C J Hepatol 1993;18(Suppl 1):129.
226. Papini M, Bruni PL, Bettacchi A, Liberati F. Sudden onset of oral ulcerative lichen in a patient with chronic hepatitis C on treatment with alpha-interferon. Int J Dermat 1994;33:221–222.
227. Perreard M, Constant T, Monges D et al. Lichen plan cutanéo-muqueux induit par une deuxième cure d'interféron alpha à forte dose chez un malade atteint d'une hépatite virale C chronique. Gastroenterol Clin Biol 1994;18:1051.
228. Protzer U, Ochsendorf FR, Leopolder-Ochsendorf A, Holtermüller KH. Exacerbation of lichen planus during interferon alfa-2a therapy for chronic active hepatitis C. Gastroenterology 1993;104:903–905.
229. Sassigneux P, Michel P, Joly P, Colin R. Lichen plan cutanéo-muqueux éruptif au cours du traitement d'une hépatite C chronique par interféron alpha. Gastroenterol Clin Biol 1993;17:764.
230. Strumia R, Venturini D, Boccia S et al. UVA and interferon-alfa therapy in a patient with lichen planus and chronic hepatitis C. Int J Dermat 1993;32:386.
231. Cribier B, Garnier C, Laustriat D, Heid E. Lichen planus and hepatitis C virus infection: an epidemiologic study. J Am Acad Dermatol 1994;31:1070–1072.
232. Rodrigues B, Oliveira M, Inock A. Lichen plan induit par l'interféron alpha 2b chez un malade avec un myélome à IgG. Nouv Dermatol 1989;8:29–31.
233. Aubin F, Bourezane Y, Blanc D et al. Severe lichen planus-like eruption induced by interferon-alpha therapy. Eur J Dermatol 1995;5:296–299.
234. Parodi A, Semino M, Gallo R, Rebora A. Bullous eruption with circulating pemphigus-like antibodies following interferon-alpha therapy. Dermatology 1993;186:155–157.
235. Niizeki H, Inamoto N, Nakamura K et al. A case of pemphigus foliaceus after interferon alpha-2a therapy. Dermatology 1994;189(Suppl 1):129–130.
236. Kirsner RS, Anhalt GJ, Kerdel FA. Treatment with alpha interferon associated with the development of paraneoplastic pemphigus. Br J Dermatol 1995;132:474–478.
237. Guyer DR, Tiedeman J, Yannuzzi LA et al. Interferon-associated retinopathy. Arch Ophtalmol 1993;111:350–356.
238. Hayasaka S, Fujii M, Yamamoto Y et al. Retinopathy and subconjonctival haemorrhage in patients with chronic viral hepatitis receiving interferon alfa. Br J Ophthalmol 1995;79:150–152.
239. Sugano S, Yanagimoto M, Suzuki T et al. Retinal complications with elevated circulating plasma C5a associated with interferon-alpha therapy for chronic active hepatitis C. Am J Gastroenterol 1994;89:2054–2056.
240. Ene L, Géhénot M, Horsmans Y et al. Transient blurred vision after interferon for chronic hepatitis C. Lancet 1994;344:827–828.
241. Yamada H, Mizobuchi K, Isogai Y. Acute onset of ocular complications with interferon. Lancet 1994;343:914.
242. Manesis EK, Petrou C, Brouzas D, Hadziyannis S. Optic tract neuropathy complicating low-dose interferon treatment. J Hepatol 1994;21:474–477.
243. Merimsky O, Nisipeanu P, Loewenstein A et al. Interferon-related cortical blindness. Cancer Chemother Pharmacol 1992;29:329–330.
244. Fukumoto Y, Shigemitsu T, Kajii N et al. Abducent nerve paralysis during interferon alpha-2a-therapy in a case of chronic active hepatitis C. Intern Med 1994;22:637–640.
245. Bauherz G, Soeur M, Lustman F. Oculomotor nerve paralysis induced by alpha II-interferon. Acta Neurol Belgica 1990;90:111–114.
246. Kanda Y, Shigeno K, Kinoshita N et al. Sudden hearing loss associated with interferon. Lancet 1994;343:1134–1135.
247. Arai H, Tanaka M, Ohta K et al. Symptomatic myopathy associated with interferon therapy for chronic hepatitis C. Lancet 1995;345:582.
248. Matsuya M, Abe T, Tosaka M et al. The first case of polymyositis associated with interferon therapy. Intern Med 1994;33:806–808.
249. Miglino M, Pierri I, Canepa L et al. An unusual reaction to alpha interferon in a case of non Hodgkin's lympoma. Haematologica 1993;78:411–413.
250. Greenfield SM, Harvey RS, Thompson RPH. Rhabdomyolysis after treatment with interferon alfa. Br Med J 1994;309:20–27.
251. Alvarez JS, Sacristan JA, Alsar MJ. Interferon alfa-2a-induced impotence. Ann Pharmacother 1991;25:1397.
252. Schilsky RL, Davidson HS, Magid D et al. Gonadal and sexual function in male patients with hairy cell leukemia: lack of adverse effects of recombinant alpha 2-interferon treatment. Cancer Treat Rep 1987;71:179–181.
253. Kauppila A, Cantell K, Janne O et al. Serum sex steroid and peptide hormone concentrations, and endometrial estrogen and progestin receptors levels during administration of human leukocyte interferon. Int J Cancer 1982;29:291–294.
254. Lunel F. Hépatites C et anomalies immunologiques. Gastroenterol Clin Biol 1994;18:829–838.
255. Flores A, Oliv A, Feliu E, Tena X. Systemic lupus erythematosus following interferon therapy. Br J Rheumatol 1994;33:787.
256. Mehta ND, Hooberman AL, Vokes EE et al. 35-year-old patient with chronic myelogenous leukemia developing systemic lupus erythematosus after alpha-interferon therapy. Am J Hematol 1992;41:141.
257. Rönnblom LE, Alm GV, Oberg KE. Possible induction of systemic lupus erythematosus by interferon-alpha treatment in a patient with a malignant carcinoid tumour. J Intern Med 1990;227:207–210.
258. Sanchez Roman J, Castillon Palma MJ, Garcia Diaz E, Ferrer Ordinez JA. Systemic lupus erythematosus induced by recombinant alpha interferon treatment. Med Clin 1994;102:198.
259. Schilling PJ, Kurzrock R, Kantarjian H et al. Development of systemic lupus erythematosus after interferon therapy for chronic myelogenous leukemia. Cancer 1991; 68:1536–1537.
260. Tolaymat A, Leventhal B, Sakarcan A et al. Systemic lupus erythematosus in a child receiving long-term interferon therapy. J Pediatr 1992;120:429–432.
261. Yoshida A, Takeda A, Koyama K et al. Systemic lupus erythematosus with nephropathy after interferon alpha 2A therapy Clin Rheumatol 1994;13:382.
262. Böni R, Dummer R, Burg G. Scleroderma and vitiligo following treatment with interferon-alpha and interleukin-2

in a patient with metastatic melanoma. Dermatology 1994;189:330.
263. Chazerain P, Meyer O, Ribard P et al. Trois cas de polyarthrite survenant au cours d'un traitement par interféron-alpha recombinant. Rev Rhum Mal Osteoart 1992;59:303—309.
264. Conlon KC, Urba WJ, Smith JW et al. Exacerbation of symptoms of autoimmune disease in patients receiving alpha-interferon therapy. Cancer 1990;65:2237—2242.
265. Maccari S, Bassi C, Giovannini AG, Plancher AC. A case of arthropathy and hypothyroidism during recombinant alpha-interferon therapy. Clin Rheumatol 1991;10 452—454.
266. Wandl UB, Nagel-Hiemke M, May D et al. Lupus-like autoimmune disease induced by interferon therapy for myeloproliferative disorders. Clin Immunol Immunopathol 1992;65:70—74.
267. Kiely PD, Bruckner FE. Acute arthritis following interferon-α therapy. Br J Rheumatol 1994;33:502—503.
268. Chan GCB, Lee SS, Yeoh EK. Mono-arthritis in a chronic hepatitis B patient after alpha-interferon treatment. J Gastroenterol Hepatol 1992;7:432—433.
269. Arslan M, Ozyilkan E, Kayhan B, Telatar H. Raynaud's phenomenon associated with alpha-interferon therapy. J Intern Med 1994;235:503.
270. Roy V, Newland AC. Raynaud's phenomenon and cryoglobulinaemia associated with the use of recombinant human alpha-interferon. Lancet 1988;i:944—945.
271. Schirren CA, Zachoval R, Schirren CG et al. A role for chronic hepatitis C virus infection in a patient with cutaneous vasculitis, cryoglobulinemia, and chronic liver disease. Effective therapy with interferon-α. Dig Dig Sci 1995; 40:1221—1225.
272. Bojic I, Lilic D, Radojcic C, Mijuskovic P. Deterioration of mixed cryoglobulinemia during treatment with interferon-alpha-2a. J Gastroenterol 1994;29:369—371.
273. Harlé JR, Disdier J, Pelletier J et al. Dramatic worsening of hepatitis C virus-related cryoglobulinaemia subsequent with treatment with interferon alfa. J Am Med Assoc 1995;274:126.
274. Zimmermann R, Konig V, Banditz J, Hopf U. Interferon alpha in leucocytoclastic vasculitis, mixed cryoglobulinemia, and chronic hepatitis C. Lancet 1993;341:561—562.
275. Blum L, Serfaty L, Wattiaux MJ et al. Nodules hypodermiques sarcoïdosiques au cours d'une hépatite virale C traitée par interféron alpha 2b. Rev Med Interne 1993; 14:1161.
276. Christian B, Derriennic X, Guilhot F. Sarcoïdose au cours d'une leucémie myéloïde chronique traitée par interféron alpha 2b. Rev Med Interne 1992;13;S462.
277. Ohhata I, Ochi T, Kurebayashi S et al. A case of subcutaneous sarcoid nodules induced by interferon alpha. Nippon Kyobu Shikkan Gakkai Zasshi 1994;32:996—1000.
278. Liozon E, Cransac M, Remenieras L et al. La sarcoïdose: une nouvelle complication de traitement par l'interféron alpha. Rev Med Interne 1993;14:1160.
279. Batocchi AP, Evoli A, Servidei S et al. Myasthenia gravis during interferon alfa therapy. Neurology 1995; 45:382—383.
280. Quilichini R, Mazzerbo F, Amiel O et al. Myasthénie au cours d'un traitement par interféron alpha. Rev Med Interne 1994;15(Suppl 3):421s.
281. Hassanein T, Schade R, Lasky S, Van Thiel D. Is interferon an immunosuppressant? Gastroenterology 1994; 106(Suppl):905.
282. Prignet JM, Galzin M, Demarquay F et al. Candidose oesophagienne au cours d'un traitement par l'interféron d'une hépatite chronique à virus C. Gastroenterol Clin Biol 1994;18:796—797.
283. Ariad S, Lewis D, Bezwoda WR. Kaposi's sarcoma after alpha-interferon treatment for HIV-negative T-cell lymphoma. S Afr Med J 1993;83:430—431.
284. Pesce A, Taillan B, Rosenthal E et al. Opportunistic infections and CD4 lymphocytopenia with interferon treatment in HIV-1 infected patients. Lancet 1993;341:1597.
285. Vento S, Di Perri G, Cruciani M et al. Rapid decline of CD4+ cells after IFNα treatment in HIV-1 infection. Lancet 1993;341:958—959.
286. Soriano V, Bravo R, Samaniego JG et al. CD4+ T-lymphocytopenia in HIV-infected patients receiving interferon therapy for chronic hepatitis C. AIDS 1994;8:1621—1622.
287. Kovarik J, Mayer G, Pohanka E et al. Adverse effect of low-dose prophylactic human recombinant leucocyte interferon-alpha treatment in renal transplant patients. Transplantation 1988;45:402—405.
288. Durlik M, Gaciong Z, Rancewicz Z et al. Renal allograft function in patients with chronic viral hepatitis B and C treated with interferon alpha. Transplant Proc 1995;27:958—959.
289. Rostaing L, Izopet J, Baron E et al. Treatment of chronic hepatitis C with recombinant alpha 2b interferon in kidney transplant recipients: preliminary results and side effects. Transplant Proc 1995;27:948—950.
290. Dousset B, Conti F, Houssin D, Calmus Y. Acute vanishing bile duct syndrome after interferon therapy for recurrent HCV infection in liver-transplant recipients. N Engl J Med 1994;330:1160—1161.
291. Browett PJ, Nelson J, Tiwari S et al. Graft-versus-host disease following interferon therapy for relapsed chronic myeloid leukaemia post-allogeneic bone marrow transplantation. Bone Marrow Transplant 1994;14:641—644.
292. Pavord S, Sivakumaran M, Durrant S, Chapman C. The role of alpha interferon in the pathogenesis of GVHD. Bone Marrow Transplant 1992;10:477.
293. Klingemann HG, Grigg AP, Wilkie-Boyd K et al. Treatment with recombinant interferon (α-2b) early after bone marrow transplantation in patients at high risk for relpase. Blood 1991;78:3306—3311.
294. Meyers JD, Flournoy N, Sanders JE et al. Prophylactic use of human leucocyte interferon after allogeneic bone marrow transplantation. Ann Intern Med 1987;107:809—816.
295. Ornellas de Souza MH, Abdelhay E, Silva MLM et al. Late marrow allograft rejection following alpha-interferon therapy for hepatitis in a patient with paroxysmal nocturnal hemoglobinuria. Bone Marrow Transplant 1992;9:495—497.
296. Antonelli G. Development of neutralizing and binding antibodies to interferon (IFN) in patients undergoing IFN therapy. Antiviral Res 1994;24:235—244.
297. Prümmer O. Interferon-alpha antibodies in patients with renal cell carcinoma treated with recombinant interferon-alpha-2A in an adjuvant multicenter trial. Cancer 1993;71:1828—1834.
298. Figlin RA, Itri LM. Anti-interferon antibodies: a perspective. Sem Hematol 1988;25(Suppl 3):9—15.
299. Antonelli G, Currenti M, Turriziani O, Dianzani F. Neutralizing antibodies to interferon-α: relative frequency in patients treated with different interferon preparations. J Infect Dis 1991;163:882—885.

300. Bekisz JB, Zur Nedden DL, Enterline JC, Zoon KC. Antibodies to interferon-alpha 2 for hairy cell leukemia. J Interfer Res 1989;9(Suppl 1):S1–S7.
301. Brand CM, Leadbeater L, Bellati G et al. Antibodies developing against a single recombinant interferon protein may neutralize many other interferon-alpha subtypes. J Interfer Res 1993;13:121–125.
302. Antonelli G, Giannelli G, Pistello M et al. Clinical signifiance of recombinant interferon-α2 neutralizing antibodies in hepatitis patients. J Interfer Res 1994;14:211–213.
303. Steis RG, Longo DL. Clinical relevance of recombinant interferon-α2a antibodies in patients with hairy cell leukemia. J Interfer Res 1994;14:207–209.
304. von Wussow P, Jakschies D, Freund M et al. Treatment of anti-recombinant interferon-alpha 2 antibody positive CML patients with natural interferon-alpha. Br J Haematol 1991;78:210–216.
305. von Wussow P, Pralle H, Hochkeppel HK et al. Effective natural interferon-α therapy in recombinant interferon-α-resistant patients with hairy cell leukemia. Blood 1991;78:38–43.
306. Nolte KU, Jakschies D, Pestka S, von Wussow P. Different specificities of SLE-derived and therapy-induced interferon-α antibodies. J Interfer Res 1994;14:197–199.
307. Spiegel RJ, Jacobs SL, Treuhaft MW. Anti-interferon antibodies to interferon-alpha 2b: results of comparative assays and clinical perspective. J Interfer Res 1989;9(Suppl 1):S17–S24.
308. Casato M, Lagana B, Antonelli G et al. Long-term results of therapy with interferon-α for type II essential mixed cryoglobulinemia. Blood 1991;78:3142–3147.
309. Milella M, Antonelli G, Sanantonio T et al. Neutralizing antibodies to recombinant alpha-interferon and response to therapy in chronic hepatitis C virus infection. Liver 1993;13:146–150.
310. Diodati G, Bonetti P, Noventa F et al. Treatment of chronic hepatitis C with recombinant human interferon-α2a: results of a randomized controlled clinical trial. Hepatology 1994;19:1–5.
311. von Wussow P, Hehlmann R, Hochhaus T et al. Roferon (rIFN-α2a) is more immunogenic than Intron A (r-IFN-α2b) in patients with chronic myelogenous leukemia. J Interfer Res 1994;14:217–219.
312. Spiegel RJ, Spicehandler JR, Jacobs SL, Oden E. Low incidence of serum neutralizing factors in patients receiving recombinant alfa-2b interferon (Intron A). Am J Med 1986;80:223–228.
313. Lok ASF, Lai CL, Leung EKY. Interferon antibodies may negate the antiviral effects of recombinant α-interferon treatment in patients with chronic hepatitis B virus infection. Hepatology 1990;12:1266–1270.
314. Antonelli G, Currenti M, Turriziani O et al. Relative frequency of nonneutralizing antibodies to interferon in hepatitis patients treated with different IFN-alpha preparations. J Infect Dis 1992;165:593–594.
315. Detmar U, Agathos M, Nerl C. Allergy of delayed type to recombinant interferon α-2c. Contact Dermatitis 1989; 20:149–150.
316. Pardini S, Bosincu L, Bonfilgi S et al. Anaphylactic-like syndrom in systemic mastocytosis treated with alpha-2-interferon. Acta Haematol 1991;85:220.
317. Arico M, Maggiore G, De Stefano P et al. Acute-B lineage lymphoid malignancy after interferon therapy for chronic viral hepatitis. Blood 1994;83:869–870.
318. Blade J, Lopez-Guillermo A, Tassies D et al. Development of aggressive plasma cell leukaemia under interferon-alpha therapy. Br J Haematol 1991;79:523–525.
319. Sawamura M, Murayama K, Ui G et al. Plasma cell leukaemia with alpha-interferon therapy in myeloma. Br J Haematol 1992;82:631.
320. Ambrosetti A, Krampera M, Veneri D et al. Early lymphoid blastic crisis following major karyotypic conversion in a chronic myeloid leukemia patient treated with interferon-α. Int J Clin Lab Res 1994;24:58–59.
321. Spielberger RT, Dickstein JI, Le Beau MM et al. Acute myeloid leukaemia following interferon-alfa treatment of hairy cell leukaemia. Br J Haematol 1993;83:519–520.
322. Ohtsu T, Sasaki Y, Tanizaki H et al. Development of pseudolymphoma of liver following interferon-alpha therapy for chronic hepatitis B. Intern Med 1994;33:18–22.
323. Bork K, Braüninger W, Röhrborn W. Metastases of malignant melanoma due to interferon alpha-2a? Dermatologica 1988;177:249–250.
324. Hild F, Freund M, Fonatsch C. Chromosomal aberrations during interferon therapy for chronic myelogenous leukemia. N Engl J Med 1991;325:132.
325. Waysbort A, Giroux M, Mansat V et al. Experimental study of transplacental passage of alpha interferon by two assay techniques. Antimicrob Agents Chemother 1993; 37:1232–1237.
326. Baer MR, Ozer H, Foon KA. Interferon-α therapy during pregnancy in chronic myelogenous leukaemia and hairy cell leukaemia. Br J Haematol 1992;81:167–169.
327. Crump M, Wang XH, Sermer M, Keating A. Successful pregnancy and delivery during α-interferon therapy for chronic myeloid leukemia. Am J Hematol 1992;40:238–239.
328. Pardini S, Dore F, Murineddu M et al. α2b-Interferon therapy and pregnancy: report of a case of essential thrombocythemia. Am J Hematol 1993;43:78.
329. Petit JJ, Callis M, Fernandez de Sevilla A. Normal pregnancy in a patient with essential thrombocythemia treated with interferon-α2b. Am J Hematol 1992;40:80.
330. Reichel RP, Linkesch W, Schetitska D. Therapy with recombinant interferon alpha-2c during unexpected pregnancy in a patient with chronic myeloid leukaemia. Br J Haematol 1992;82:472–473.
331. Thornley S, Manoharan A. Successful treatment of essential thrombocythemia with alpha interferon during pregnancy. Eur J Haematol 1994;52:63–64.
332. Vianelli N, Gugliotta L, Tura S et al. Interferon-α2a treatment in a pregnant woman with essential thrombocythemia. Blood 1994;83:874–875.
333. Mannering GJ, Deloria LB. The pharmacology and toxicology of the interferons: an overview. Ann Rev Pharmacol Toxicol 1986;26:455–515.
334. Craig PI, Mehta I, Murray M et al. Interferon down regulates the male-specific cytochrome P450IIIA2 in rat liver. Mol Pharmacol 1990;38:313–318.
335. Cribb AE, Delaporte E, Kim SG et al. Regulation of cytochrome P-4501A and cytochrome P-4502E induction in the rat during the production of interferon α/β. J Pharmacol Exp Ther 1994;268:487–494.
336. Okuno H, Kitao Y, Takasu M et al. Depression of drug-metabolizing activity in the human liver by interferon-α. Eur. J Clin Pharmacol 1990;39:365–367.
337. Donato MT, Herrero E, Gomez-Lechon MJ, Castell JV. Inhibition of monooxygenase activities in human hepatocytes by interferons. Toxicol In Vitro 1993;7:481–485.

338. Williams SJ, Farrell GC. Inhibition of antipyrine metabolism by interferon. Br J Clin Pharmacol 1986;22:610–612.
339. Williams SJ, Baird-Lambert JA, Farrell GC. Inhibition of theophylline metabolism by interferon. Lancet 1987; ii:939–941.
340. Jonkman JHG, Nicholson KG, Farrow PR et al. Effects of α-interferon on theophylline pharmacokinetics and metabolism. Br. J Clin Pharmacol 1989;27:795–802.
341. Horsmans Y, Brenard R, Geubel AP. Short report: interferon-α decreases ^{14}C-aminopyrine breath test values in patients with chronic hepatitis C. Aliment Pharmacol Ther 1994;8:353–355.
342. Echizen H, Ohta Y, Shirataki H et al. Effects of subchronic treatment with natural interferons on antipyrine clearance and liver function in patients with chronic hepatitis. Gastroenterology 1990;30:562–567.
343. Israel BC, Blouin RA, McIntyre W, Shedlofsky SI. Effect of interferon-α monotherapy on hepatic drug metabolism in cancer patients. Br J Clin Pharmacol 1993;36:229–235.
344. Adachi Y, Yokoyama Y, Nanno T, Yamamoto T. Potentiation of warfarin by interferon. Br Med J 1995;311:292.
345. Desai RG. Drug interaction between alpha interferon and erythropoietin. J Clin Oncol 1991;9:893.
346. Nordio M, Guarda L, Lorenzi S et al. Interaction between alpha-interferon and erythropoietin in antiviral and antineoplastic therapy in uraemic patients on haemodialysis. Nephrol Dial Transplant 1993;8:1308.
347. Burger DM, Meehorst PL, Koks CHW, Beijnen JH. Drug interactions with zidovudine. AIDS 1993;7:445–460.
348. Krown SE, Gold JWM, Niedzwiecki D et al. Interferon-α with zidovudine: safety, tolerance, and clinical and virologic effects in patients with Kaposi sarcoma associated with the acquired immunodeficiency syndrome (AIDS). Ann Intern Med 1990;112:812–821.
349. Sznol M, Longo DL. Chemotherapy drug interactions with biological agents. Sem Oncol 1993;20:80–93.
350. Meadows LM, Walther P, Ozer H. α-Interferon and 5-fluorouracil: possible mechanisms of antitumor action. Sem Oncol 1991;18(Suppl 7):71–76.
351. Czejka MJ, Schüller J, Jäger W et al. Influence of different doses of interferon-α-2b on the blood plasma levels of 5-fluorouracil. Eur J Drug Metabol Pharmacokinet 1993; 18:247–250.
352. Schüller J, Czejka MJ, Schernthaner G et al. Influence of interferon alfa-2b with or without folinic acid on pharmacokinetics of fluorouracil. Sem Oncol 1992;19(Suppl 3):93–97.
353. Sinnige HAM, Buter J, de Vries EGE et al. Phase I–II study of the addition of α-2a interferon to 5-fluorouracil/leuvovorin. Pharmacokinetic interaction of α-2a interferon and leucovorin. Eur J Cancer 1993;29A:1715–1720.
354. Punt CJA, Burghouts JTM, Croles JJ et al. Continuous infusion of high-dose 5-fluorouracil in combination with leucovorin and recombinant interferon-alpha-2b in patients with advanced colorectal cancer. A multicenter phase II study. Cancer 1993;72:2107–2111.
355. Ehrsson H, Eksborg S, Wallin I et al. Oral melphalan pharmacokinetics: influence of interferon-induced fever. Clin Pharmacol Ther 1990;47:86–90.
356. Connelly JF. Interferon beta for multiple sclerosis. Ann Pharmacother 1994;28:610–616.
357. Panitch HS. Interferons in multiple sclerosis. A review of the evidence. Drugs 1992;44:946–962.
358. The IFNB Multiple Sclerosis Study Group. Interferon beta-1b is effective in relapsing-remitting multiple sclerosis. I. Clinical results of a multicenter, randomized, double-blind, placebo-controlled trial. Neurology 1993;43:655–661.
359. Liberati AM, Biagini S, Perticoni G et al. Electrophysiological and neuropsychological functions in patients treated with interferon-β. J Interfer Res 1990;10:613–619.
360. Ettinger DS, Harwood K. Phase II study of recombinant beta interferon in patients with advanced non-small-cell lung carcinoma. Med Pediatr Oncol 1988;16:30–32.
361. Matsumura S, Takamatsu H, Ara S. Central nervous system toxicity of local interferon-β therapy. Neurol Med Chir 1988;28:265–270.
362. Pagliacci MC, Pelicci G, Schippa M et al. Does interferon-beta therapy induce thyroid autoimmune phenomena. Horm Metabol Res 1991;23:196–197.
363. Abdi EA, Nguyen GK, Ludwig RN, Dickout WJ. Pulmonary sarcoidosis following interferon therapy for advanced renal cell carcinoma. Cancer 1987;59:896–900.
364. Pigatto PD, Bigardi A, Legori A et al. Allergic contact dermatitis from beta-interferon in eyedrops. Contact Dermatitis 1991;25:199–200.
365. Miles SA, Wang H, Cortes E et al. Beta interferon therapy in patients with poor prognosis Kaposi sarcoma related to the acquired immunodeficiency syndrome (AIDS). Ann Intern Med 1990;112:582–589.
366. Bérard F, Canillot S, Balme B, Perrot H. Nécrose cutanée locale après injections d'interféron bêta. Ann Dermatol Venereol 1995;122:105–107.
367. Sheremata WA, Taylor JR, Elgart GW. Severe necroziting cutaneous lesions complicating treatment with interferon beta-1b. N Engl J Med 1995;332:1584.
368. Kowalzick L, Meyer U. Psoriasis induced at the injection site of recombinant interferons. Arch Dermatol 1990;126:1515–1516.
369. Larocca AP, Leung SC, Marcus SG et al. Evaluation of neutralizing antibodies in patients treated with recombinant interferon-βser. J Interfer Res 1989;9(Suppl 1):S51–S60.
370. Dummer R, Müller W, Nestle F et al. Formation of neutralizing antibodies against natural interferon-β, but not against recombinant interferon-γ during adjuvant treatment therapy for high-risk malignant melanoma patients. Cancer 1991;67:2300–2304.
371. Fierlbeck G, Schreiner T. Incidence and clinical signifiance of therapy-induced neutralizing antibodies against interferon-β. J Interfer Res 1994;14:205–206.
372. Okuno H, Takasu M, Kano H et al. Depression of drug-metabolizing activity in the human liver by interferon-beta. Hepatology 1993;17:65–69.
373. Todd PA, Goa KL. Interferon gamma-1b: a review of its pharmacology and therapeutic potential in chronic granulomatous diseases. Drugs 1992;43:111–122.
374. International Chronic Granulomatous Disease Cooperative Study Group (ICGDCSG). A controlled trial of interferon gamma to prevent infection in chronic granulomatous disease. New Engl J Med 1991;324:509–516.
375. Mattson K, Niiranen A, Pyrhonen S et al. Recombinant interferon gamma treatment in non-small cell lung cancer. Antitumour effect and cardiotoxicity. Acta Oncol 1991; 30:607–610.
376. Born J, Späth-Schwalbe E, Pietrowsky R et al. Neurophysiological effects of recombinant interferon-gamma and -alpha in man. Clin Physiol Biochem 1989;7:119–127.
377. Sriskandan K, Tee DE, Pettingale KW. Nephrotic syn-

drome during treatment with interferon. Br Med J 1985;290:1590–1591.
378. Weiss KS. Nephrotic range of proteinuria and interferon therapy. Ann Intern Med 1992;116:347.
379. Ault BH, Stapleton FB, Gaber L et al. Acute renal failure during therapy with recombinant human gamma interferon. N Engl J Med 1988;319:1397–1400.
380. Friess GG, Brown TD, Wrenn RC. Cardiovascular rhythm effects of gamma recombinant DNA interferon. Invest. New Drugs 1989;7:275–280.
381. Aulitzky W, Tilg H, Vogel W et al. Acute hematologic effects of interferon alpha, interferon gamma, tumor necrosis factor alpha and interleukin 2. Ann Hematol 1991;62:25–31.
382. Rabinowitz AP, Hu E, Watkins K, Mazumder A. Hemolytic anemia in a cancer patient treated with recombinant interferon-gamma. J Biol Response Modif 1990;9:256–259.
383. Krishnan R, Ellinwood EH, Laszlo J et al. Effect of gamma interferon on the hypothalamic-pituitary-adrenal system. Biol Psychiatry 1987;22:1163–1166.
384. Kurzrock R, Rohde MF, Quesada JR et al. Recombinant γ interferon induces hypertriglyceridemia and inhibits post-heparin lipase activity in cancer patients. J Exp Med 1986;164:1093–1101.
385. Fierlbeck G, Rassner G, Muller C. Psoriasis induced at the injection site of recombinant interferon gamma. Results of immunohistologic investigations. Arch Dermatol 1990; 126:351–355.
386. Sampaio EP, Moreira AL, Sarno EN et al. Prolonged treatment with recombinant interferon-γ induces erythema nodosum leprosum in lepromatous leprosy patients. J Exp Med 1992;175:1729–1737.
387. Weber P, Wiedmann KH, Klein R et al. Induction of autoimmune phenomena in patients with chronic hepatitis B treated with gamma-interferon. J Hepatol 1994;20:321–328.
388. Kung AWC, Jones BM, Lai CL. Effects of interferon-gamma therapy on thyroid function, T-lymphocytes subpopulation and induction of autoantobodies. J Clin Endocrinol Metabol 1990;71:1230–1234.
389. Cannon GW, Emkey RD, Denes A et al. Prospective 5-year follow up of recombinant interferon-γ in rheumatoid arthritis. J Rheumatol 1993;20:1867–1873.
390. Seitz M, Kranke M, Kirchner H. Induction of antinuclear antibodies in patients with rheumatoid arthritis receiving treatment with recombinant human gamma interferon. Ann Rheum Dis 1988;47:642–644.
391. Graninger WB, Hassfeld W, Pesau BB et al. Induction of systemic lupus erythematosus by interferon-gamma in a patient with rheumatoid arthritis. J Rheumatol 1991; 18:1621–1622.
392. Machold KP, Smolen JS. Interferon-gamma induced exacerbation of systemic lupus erythematosus. J Rheumatol 1990;17:831–832.
393. O'Connell PG, Gerber LH, DiGiovanna JJ, Peck GL. Arthritis in patients with psoriasis treated with gamma-interferon. J Rheumatol 1992;19:80–82.
394. Panitch HS, Hirsch RL, Schindler J, Johnson KP. Treatment of multiple sclerosis with gamma interferon: exacerbations associated with activation of the immune system. Neurology 1987;37:1097–1102.
395. Albrecht H, Stellbrink HJ, Gross G et al. Treatment of atypical leishmaniasis with interferon gamma resulting in progression of Kaposi's sarcoma in an AIDS patient. Clin Invest 1994;72:1041–1047.
396. Jaffe HS, Chen AB, Kramer S, Sherwin SA. The absence of interferon antibody formation in patients receiving recombinant human interferon-gamma. J Biol Response Modif 1987;6:576–580.
397. Curti BD, Smith JW. Interleukin-1 in the treatment of cancer. Pharmac Ther 1995;65:291–302.
398. Smith JW II, Longo DL, Alvord G et al. The effects of treatment with interleukin-1α on platelet recovery after high-dose carboplatin. N Engl J Med 1993;328:756–761.
399. Weisdorf D, Katsanis E, Verfaillie C et al. Interleukin-1α administered after autologous transplantation: a phase I/II clinical trial. Blood 1994;84:2044–2049.
400. Nemunaitis J, Appelbaum FR, Lilleby K et al. Phase I study of recombinant interleukin-1β in patients undergoing autologous bone marrow transplant for acute myelogenous leukemia. Blood 1994;83:3473–3479.
401. Kanz L, Birken R, Brugger W et al. Biological activities of subcutaneous rhIL-1β in cancer patients. Blood 1992; 80(Suppl 1):92a.
402. Smith JW II, Urba WJ, Curti BD et al. The toxic and hematologic effects of interleukin-1 alpha administered in a phase I trial to patients with advanced malignancies. J Clin Oncol 1992;10:1141–1152.
403. Redman BG, Abubakr Y, Chou T et al. Phase II trial of recombinant interleukin-1 beta in patients with metastatic renal cell carcinoma. J Immunother Emphasis Tumor Immunol 1994;16:211–215.
404. Haefeli WE, Bargetzi MJ, Starnes HF et al. Evidence for activation of the sympathetic nervous system by recombinant human interleukin-1β in humans. J Immunother 1993;13:136–140.
405. Kilbourn RG, Gross SS, Lodato RF et al. Inhibition of interleukin-1-α induced nitric oxide synthase in vascular smooth muscle and full reversal of interleukin-1-α induced hypotension by $N\omega$-amino-L-arginine. J Natl Cancer Inst 1992;84:1008–1016.
406. Crown J, Jakubowski A, Kemeny N et al. A phase I trial of recombinant human interleukin-1β alone and in combination with myelosuppressive doses of 5-fluorouracil in patients with gastrointestinal cancer. Blood 1991;78:1420–1427.
407. Anderson PM, Sorenson MA. Effects of route and formulation on clinical pharmacokinetics of interleukin-2. Clin Pharmacokinet 1994;27:19–31.
408. Parkinson DR, Sznol M. High-dose interleukin-2 in the therapy of metastatic renal-cell carcinoma. Sem Oncol 1995;22:61–66.
409. Wagstaff J, Baars JW, Wolbink GJ et al. Renal cell carcinoma and interleukin-2: a review. Eur J Cancer 1995;31A:401–408.
410. Whittington R, Faulds D. Interleukin-2: a review of its pharmacological properties and therapeutic use in patients with cancer. Drugs 1993;46:446–514.
411. Bruton JK, Koeller JM. Recombinant interleukin-2. Pharmacotherapy 1994;14:635–656.
412. Oppenheim MH, Lotze MT. Interleukin-2: solid-tumor therapy. Oncology 1994;51:154–169.
413. Vial T, Descotes J. Clinical toxicity of interleukin-2. Drug Safety 1992;7:417–433.
414. Caligiuri MA. Low-dose recombinant interleukin-2 therapy: rationale and potential clinical applications. Sem Oncol 1993;20(Suppl 9):3–10.
415. Maas RA, Dullens HFJ, Den Otter W. Interleukin-2 in cancer treatment: disappointing or (still) promising: a review. Cancer Immunol Immunother 1993;36:141–148.

416. Schomburg A, Kirchner H, Atzpodien J. Renal, metabolic and hemodynamic side-effects of interleukin-2 and/or interferon α: evidence of a risk/benefit advantage of subcutaneous therapy. J Cancer Res Clin Oncol 1993;119:745—755.
417. Stadler WM, Vogelzang NJ. Low-dose interleukin-2 in the treatment of metastatic renal-cell carcinoma. Sem Oncol 1995;22:67—73.
418. Fyfe G, Fisher RI, Rosenberg SA et al. Results of treatment of 255 patients with metastatic renal cell carcinoma who received high-dose recombinant interleukin-2 therapy. J Clin Oncol 1995;13:688—696.
419. Groeger JS, Bajorin D, Reichman B et al. Haemodynamic effects of recombinant interleukin-2 administered by constant infusion. Eur J Cancer 1991;27:1613—1616.
420. White RL, Schwartzentruber DJ, Guleria A et al. Cardiopulmonary toxicity of treatment with high dose interleukin-2 in 199 consecutive patients with metastatic melanoma or renal cell carcinoma. Cancer 1994;74:3212—3222.
421. Landiono G, Granata LG, Baiocchi C. Atrioventricular block following therapy with recombinant interleukin-2. G Ital Cardiol 1991;21:691.
422. Ravaud A, Lakdja F, Delaunay M et al. Cardiomyopathy after acute myocardial infarction after therapy with interleukin-2 and tumour infiltrating lymphocytes. Eur J Cancer 1992;28A:1772.
423. Goel M, Flaherty L, Lavine S, Redman BG. Reversible cardiomyopathy after high-dose interleukin-2 therapy. J Immunother 1992;11:225—229.
424. Lissoni P, Galli MA, Tancini G, Barni S. Prevention by L-carnitine of interleukin-2-related cardiac toxicity during cancer immunotherapy. Tumori 1993;79:202—204.
425. Fragasso G, Tresoldi M, Benti R et al. Impaired left ventricular filling rate induced by treatment with recombinant interleukin-2 for advanced cancer. Br Heart J 1994;71:166—169.
426. Samlowski WE, Ward JH, Craven CM, Freedman RA. Severe myocarditis following high-dose interleukin-2 administration. Arch Pathol Lab Med 1989;113:838—841.
427. Schuchter LM, Hendricks CB, Holland KH et al. Eosinophilic myocarditis associated with high-dose interleukin-2 therapy. Am J Med 1990;88:439—440.
428. Ballmer-Weber BK, Dummer R, Küng E et al. Interleukin 2-induced increase of vascular permeability without decrease of the intravascular albumin pool. Br J Cancer 1995;71:78—82.
429. Baars JW, Hack CE, Wagstaff J et al. The activation of polymorphonuclear neutrophils and the complement system during immunotherapy with recombinant interleukin-2. Br J Cancer 1992;65:96—101.
430. Hack KE, Ogilvie AC, Eisele B et al. C1-inhibitor substitution therapy in septic shock and in the vascular leak syndrome induced by high doses of interleukin-2. Intensive Care Med 1993;19(Suppl 1):S19—S28.
431. Davis SD, Berkmen YM, Wang JCL. Interleukin-2 therapy for advanced renal cell carcinoma: radiographic evaluation of response and complications. Radiology 1990;177:127—131.
432. Saxon RR, Klein JS, Bar MH et al. Pathogenesis of pulmonary edema during interleukin-2 therapy: correlation of chest radiographic and clinical findings in 54 patients. Am J Roentgenol 1991;156:281—285.
433. Villani F, Galimberti M, Rizzi M, Manzi R. Pulmonary toxicity of recombinant interleukin-2 plus lymphokine-activated killer cell therapy. Eur Respir J 1993;6:828—833.
434. Brichon PY, Barnoud D, Pison C et al. Double lung transplantation for adult respiratory distress syndrome after recombinant interleukin-2. Chest 1993;104:609—610.
435. Denicoff KD, Rubinow DR, Papa MZ et al. The neuropsychiatric effects of treatment with interleukin-2 and lymphokine-activated killer cells. Ann Intern Med 1987;107:293—300.
436. Buter J, de Vries EGE, Sleijfer DT et al. Neuropsychiatric symptoms during treatment with interleukin-2. Lancet 1993:341:628.
437. Fenner MH, Hänninen EL, Kirchner HH et al. Neuropsychiatric symptoms during treatment with interleukin-2 and interferon-α. Lancet 1993;341:372.
438. Vecht CJ, Keohane C, Menon RS et al. Acute fatal leukoencephalopathy after interleukin-2 therapy. N Engl J Med 1990;323:1146—1147.
439. Meyers CA, Yung WKA. Delayed neurotoxicity of intraventricular interleukin-2: a case report. J Neuro Oncol 1993;15:265—267.
440. Caraceni A, Martini C, Belli F et al. Neuropsychological and neuro-physiological assessment of the central effects of interleukin-2 administration. Eur J Cancer 1992;29A:1266—1269.
441. Pace A, Pietrangeli A, Bove L et al. Neurotoxicity of antitumoral IL-2 therapy: evoked cognitive potentials and brain mapping. Ital J Neurol Sci 1994;15:341—346.
442. Heys SD, Mills KLG, Eremin O. Bilateral carpal tunnel syndrome associated with interleukin-2 therapy. Postgraduate Med J 1992;68:587—588.
443. Loh FL, Herskovitz S, Berger AR, Swerdlow ML. Brachial plexopathy associated with interleukin-2 therapy. Neurology 1992;42:462—463.
444. Atkins MB, Mier JW, Parkinson DR et al. Hypothyroidism after treatment with interleukin-2 and lymphokine-activated killer cells. N Engl J Med 1988;318:1557—1563.
445. Kruit WHJ, Bolhuis RLH, Goey SH et al. Interleukin-2-induced thyroid dysfunction is correlated with treatment duration but not with tumor response. J Clin Oncol 1993;11:921—924.
446. Vialettes B, Guillerand MA, Viens P et al. Incidence rate and risk factors for thyroid dysfunction during recombinant interleukin-2 therapy in advanced malignancies. Acta Endocrinol 1993;129:31—38.
447. Kung AWC, Lai CL, Wong KL, Tam CF. Thyroid functions in patients treated with interleukin-2 and lymphokine-activated killer cells. Q J Med 1992;297:33—42.
448. Weijl NI, Van Der Harst D, Brand A et al. Hypothyroidism during immunotherapy with interleukin-2 is associated with antithyroid antibodies and response to treatment. J Clin Oncol 1993;11:1376—1383.
449. Jacobs EL, Clare-Salzer MJ, Chopra IJ, Figlin RA. Thyroid function abnormalities associated with the chronic outpatient administration of recombinant interleukin-2 and recombinant interferon-alpha. J Immunother 1991;10:448—455.
450. Pichert G, Jost LM, Zobeli L et al. Thyroiditis after treatment with interleukin-2 and interferon-α2a. Br J Cancer 1990;64:915—918.
451. Reid I, Sharpe I, McDevitt J et al. Thyroid dysfunction can predict response to immunotherapy with interleukin-2 and interferon-α2. Br J Cancer 1991;64:915—918.
452. Schwartzentruber DJ, White DE, Zweig MH et al. Thyroid dysfunction associated with immunotherapy for patients with cancer. Cancer 1991;68:2384—2390.

453. Vassilopoulou-Sellin R, Sella A, Dexeus FH et al. Acute thyroid dysfunction (thyroiditis) after therapy with interkeukin-2. Horm Metabol Res 1992;24:434–438.
454. Mönig H, Hauschild A, Lange S, Fölsch UR. Suppressed thyroid-stimulating hormone secretion in patients treated with interleukin-2 and interferon-α2b for metastatic melanoma. Clin Invest 1994;72:975–978.
455. Van der Molen LA, Smith JW, Longo DL et al. Adrenal insufficiency and interleukin-2 therapy. Ann Intern Med 1989;111:185.
456. Chambrier C, Mercatello A, Tognet E et al. Hormonal and metabolic effects of chronic interleukin-2 infusion on cancer patients. J Biol Response Modif 1990;9:251–255.
457. Denicoff KD, Durkin TM, Lotze MT et al. The neuroendocrine effects of interleukin-2 treatment. J Clin Endocrinol Metabol 1989;69:402–410.
458. Spinazze S, Viviani S, Bidoli P et al. Effect of prolonged subcutaneous administration of interleukin-2 on the circadian rhythms of cortisol and beta-endorphin in advanced small cell lung cancer patients. Tumori 1991;77:496–499.
459. Lissoni P, Brivio F, Pittalis S et al. Decrease in cholesterol levels during the immunotherapy of cancer with interleukin-2. Br J Cancer 1991;64:956–958.
460. Marcus SL, Dutcher JP, Paietta E et al. Severe hypovitaminosis C occuring as the result of immunotherapy with high-dose interleukin-2 and lymphokine-activated killer cells. Cancer Res 1987;47:4208–4212.
461. MacFarlane MP, Yang JC, Guleria AS et al. The hematologic toxicity of interleukin-2 in patients with metastatic melanoma and renal cell carcinoma. Cancer 1995;75:1030–1037.
462. Cottin V, Nègrier S, Ranchère JY et al. Treatment of interleukin-2-induced thrombocytopenia by intravenous immunoglobulin. Eur J Cancer 1994;30A:2187.
463. Fleischmann JD, Shingleton WB, Gallagher C et al. Fibrinolysis, thrombocytopenia, and coagulation abnormalities complicating high-dose interleukin-2 immunotherapy. J Lab Clin Med 1991;117:76–82.
464. Guarini A, Sanavio F, Novarino A et al. Thrombocytopenia in acute leukaemia patients treated with IL-2: cytolytic effect of LAK cells on megakaryocytic progenitors. Br J Haematol 1991;79:451–456.
465. Oleksowicz L, Zuckerman D, Mrowiec Z et al. Effects of interleukin-2 administration on platelet function in cancer patients. Am J Hematol 1994;45:224–231.
466. MacDonald D, Gordon AA, Kajitani H et al. Interleukin-2 treatment-associated eosinophilia is mediated by interleukin-5 production. Br J Haematol 1990;76:168–173.
467. Schomburg A, Kirchner H, Atzpodien J. Hematotoxicity of interleukin-2 in man: clinical effects and comparison of various treatment regimens. Acta Haematol 1993; 89:119–131.
468. Birchfield GR, Rodgers GM, Girodias KW et al. Hypoprothrombinemia associated with interleukin-2 therapy: correction with vitamin K. J Immunother 1992;11:71–75.
469. Richard V, Bernier M, Themelin L et al. Blood coagulation abnormalities during adoptive immunotherapy with interleukin-2. Ann Oncol 1991;2:67–68.
470. Oleksowicz L, Strack M, Dutcher JP et al. A distinct coagulopathy associated with interleukin-2 therapy. Br J Haematol 1994;88:892–894.
471. Baars JW, De Boer JP, Wagstaff J et al. Interleukin-2 induces activation of coagulation and fibrinolysis: resemblance to the changes seen during experimental entotoxaemia. Br J Haematol 1992;82:295–301.
472. Fisher B, Keenan AM, Garra BS et al. Interleukin-2 induces profound reversible cholestasis: a detailed analysis in treated cancer patients. J Clin Oncol 1989;7:1852–1862.
473. Punt CJA, Henzen-Logmans SC, Bolhuis RLH, Stoter G. Hyperbilirubinaemia in patients treated with recombinant human interleukin-2. Br J Cancer 1990;61:491.
474. Andus T, Bauer J, Gerok W. Effects of cytokines on the liver. Hepatology 1991;13:364–371.
475. Lilenbaum RC, Lilenbaum AM, Hyrniuk WM. Interleukin-2-induced focal infiltrate of the liver that mimic metastases. J Natl Cancer Inst 1995;87:609–610.
476. Dickey KW, Barth RA, Stewart JA. Recurrent transient gallbladder wall thickening associated with interleukin-2 chemotherapy. J Clin Ultrasound 1993;21:58–61.
477. Levy R, Cargill M, Le Maignan C et al. Cholécystites aiguës alithiasiques sous interleukine-2. Presse Med 1994; 23:1583.
478. Powell FC, Spooner KM, Shawker TH et al. Symptomatic interleukin-2-induced cholecystopathy in patients with HIV infection. Am J Roentgenol 1994;163:117–121.
479. Marmary Y, Shiloni E, Katz J. Oral changes in interleukin-2 treated patients: a preliminary report. J Oral Pathol Med 1992;21:230–231.
480. Pozniak MA, Christy PS, Albertini MR et al. Interleukin-2-induced splenic enlargement. Cancer 1995;75:2737–2741.
481. Ratcliffe MA, Roditi G, Adamson DJA. Interleukin-2 and splenic enlargement. J Natl Cancer Inst 1992;84:810–811.
482. Post AB, Falk GW, Bukowski RM. Acute colonic pseudo-obstruction associated with interleukin-2 therapy. Am J Gastroenterol 1991;86:1539–1541.
483. Rahman R, Benrstein Z, Vaickus L et al. Unusual gastrointestinal complications of interleukin-2 therapy. J Immunother 1991;10:221–225.
484. Sparano JA, Dutcher JP, Kaleya R et al. Colonic ischemia complicating immunotherapy with interleukin-2 and interferon-alpha. Cancer 1991;68:1538–1544.
485. Sparano JA, Brandt LJ, Dutcher JP et al. Symptomatic exacerbation of Crohn disease after treatment with high-dose interleukin-2. Ann Intern Med 1993;118:617–618.
486. Birchfield GR, Ward JH, Redman BG et al. Acute pancreatitis associated with high-dose interleukin-2 immunotherapy for malignant melanoma. West J Med 1990; 152:714–716.
487. Shalmi CL, Dutcher JP, Feinfeld DA et al. Acute renal dysfunction during interleukin-2 treatment: suggestion of an intrinsic renal lesion. J Clin Oncol 1990;8:1839–1846.
488. Hisanaga S, Kawagoe H, Yamamoto Y et al. Nephrotic syndrome associated with recombinant interleukin-2. Nephron 1990;54:277–278.
489. Heslan JMJ, Branellec AI, Lang P, Lagrue G. Recombinant interleukin-2-induced proteinuria: fact or artifact. Nephron 1991;57:373–374.
490. Guleria AS, Yang JC, Topalian SL et al. Renal dysfunction associated with the administration of high-dose interleukin-2 in 199 consecutive patients with metastatic melanoma or renal carcinoma. J Clin Oncol 1994;12:2714–2722.
491. Heys SD, Eremin O, Franks CR et al. Lithium clearance measurements during recombinant interleukin 2 treatment: tubular dysfunction in man. Renal Failure 1993;15:195–201.
492. Diekman MJM, Vlasveld LT, Krediet RT et al. Acute interstitial nephritis during continuous intravenous administration of low-dose interleukin-2. Nephron 1992;60:122–123.

493. Feinfeld DA, D'Agati V, Dutcher JP et al. Interstitial nephritis in a patient receiving adoptive immunotherapy with recombinant interleukin-2 and lymphokine-activated killer cells. Am J Nephrol 1991;11:489–492.
494. Vlasveld LT, van de Wiel-van Kemenade E, de Boer AJ et al. Possible role for cytotoxic lymphocytes in the pathogenesis of acute interstitial nephritis after recombinant interleukin-2 treatment for renal cell cancer. Cancer Immunol Immunother 1993;36:210–213.
495. Chan TM, Cheng IKP, Wong KL et al. Crescentic IgA glomerulonephritis following interleukin-2 therapy for hepatocellular carcinoma of the liver. Am J Nephrol 1991; 11:493–496.
496. Asnis LA, Gaspari AA. Cutaneous reactions to recombinant cytokine therapy. J Am Acad Dermatol 1995; 33:393–410.
497. Blessing K, Park KG, Heys SD et al. Immunopathological changes in the skin following recombinant interleukin-2 treatment. J Pathol 1992;167:313–319.
498. Dummer R, Miller K, Eilles C, Burg G. The skin: an immunoreactive target organ during interleukin-2 administration. Dermatologica 1991;183:95–99.
499. Wolkenstein P, Chosidow O, Wechsler J et al. Cutaneous side effects associated with interleukin-2 administration for metastatic melanoma. J Am Acad Dermatol 1993;28:66–70.
500. Prussick R, Plott RT, Stanley JR. Recurrence of pemphigus vulgaris associated with interleukin 2 therapy. Arch Dermatol 1994;130:890–893.
501. Ramseur WL, Richard IF, Duggan DB. A case of fatal pemphigus vulgaris in association with beta interferon and interleukin-2. Cancer 1989;63:2005–2007.
502. Puett DW, Fuchs HA. Rapid exacerbation of scleroderma in a patient treated with interleukin 2 and lymphokine activated killer cells for renal cell carcinoma. J Rheumatol 1994;21:752–753.
503. Weinstein A, Bujak D, Mittelman A, Davidian M. Erythema nodosum in a patient with renal cell carcinoma treated with interleukin-2 and lymphokine-activated killer cells. J Am Med Assoc 1987;258:3120–3121.
504. Guillaume JC, Escudier B, Espagne E et al. Dermatose bulleuse avec dépots linéaires d'IgA le long de la membrane basale au cours d'un traitement par l'interferon gamma et l'interleukine-2. Ann Dermatol Venereol 1990;117:899–902.
505. Staunton M, Scully MC, Le Boit PE, Aronson FR. Life-threatening bullous skin eruptions during interleukin-2 therapy. J Natl Cancer Inst 1991;83:56–57.
506. Wiener JS, Tucker JA, Walther PJ. Interleukin-2-induced dermatotoxicity resembling toxic epidermal necrolysis. South Med J 1992;85:656–659.
507. Richards JM, Gilewski TA, Ramming K et al. Effective chemotherapy for melanoma after treatment with interleukin-2. Cancer 1992;69:427–429.
508. Wolkenstein P, Revuz J, Guillaume JC et al. Autoimmune disorders and interleukin-2 therapy: a step toward 'unanswered questions'. Arch Dermatol 1995;131:615–616.
509. Scheibenbogen C, Hunstein W, Keilholz U. Vitiligo-like lesions following immunotherapy with IFN-α and IL-2 in melanoma patients. Eur J Cancer 1994;30A:1209–1211.
510. Böni R, Dummer R, Burg G. Scleroderma and vitiligo following treatment with interferon-alpha and interleukin-2 in a patient with metastatic melanoma. Dermatology 1994;189:330.
511. Baars JW, Coenen J, Wagstaff J et al. Lobular panniculitis after subcutaneous administration of interleukin-2 (IL-2), and its exacerbation during intravenous therapy with IL-2. Br J Cancer 1992;66:698–699.
512. Bernard JT, Ameriso S, Kempf RA et al. Transient focal neurologic deficits complicating interleukin-2 therapy. Neurology 1990;40:154–155.
513. Friedman DI, Hu EH, Sadun AA. Neuro-ophtalmic complications of interleukin-2 therapy. Arch Ophthalmol 1991;109:1679–1680.
514. Baron NW, Davis LP, Flaherty LE et al. Scintigraphic findings in patients with shoulder pain caused by interleukin-2. Am J Roentgenol 1990;154:327–330.
515. Massarotti E, Liu NY, Mier J, Atkins MB. Chronic inflammatory arthritis after treatment with high-dose interleukin-2 for malignancy. Am J Med 1992;92:693–697.
516. Blaise D, Stoppa AM, Viens P et al. Intensive immunotherapy with recombinant IL-2 after autologous bone marrow transplantation is associated with a high incidence of bacterial infections. Bone Marrow Transplant 1992;10:193–194.
517. Morère JF, Darras C, Boaziz C et al. Complications infectieuses au cours des traitements par l'interleukine-2. Presse Med 1993;22:413–416.
518. Pockaj BA, Topalian SL, Steinberg SM et al. Infectious complications associated with interleukin-2 administration: a retrospective review of 935 treatment courses. J Clin Oncol 1993;11:136–147.
519. Jones AL, Cropley I, O'Brien MER et al. Infectious complications of subcutaneous interleukin-2 and interferon-alpha. Lancet 1992;339:181–182.
520. Buter J, de Vries EGE, Sleijfer DT et al. Infection after subcutaneous interleukin-2. Lancet 1992;339:552.
521. Schomburg AG, Kirchner HH, Atzpodien J. Cytokines and infection in cancer patients. Lancet 1992;339:1061.
522. Scharenberg JGM, Stam AGM, von Blomberg BME et al. The development of anti-interleukin-2 (IL-2) antibodies in patient treated with recombinant IL-2 does not interfere with clinical responsiveness. Proc Am Assoc Cancer Res 1993;34:464.
523. Atzpodien J, Hänninen EL, Kirchner H et al. Human antibodies to recombinant interleukin-2 in patients with hypernephroma. J Interfer Res 1994;14:177–178.
524. Kirchner H, Körfer A, Evers P et al. The development of neutralizing antibodies in a patient receiving subcutaneous recombinant and natural IL-2. Cancer 1991;67:1862–1864.
525. Baars JW, Wagstaff J, Hack CE et al. Angioneurotic oedema and urticaria during therapy with interleukin-2. Ann Oncol 1992;3:243–244.
526. Abi-Aad AS, Figlin RA, Belldegrun A, de Kernion JB. Metastatic renal cell cancer: interleukin-2 toxicity induced by contrast agent injection. J Immunother 1991;10:292–295.
527. Choyke PL, Miller DL, Lotze MT et al. Delayed reactions to contrast media after interleukin-2 immunotherapy. Radiology 1992;183:111–114.
528. Heinzer H, Huland E, Huland H. Adverse reaction to contrast material in a patient treated with local interleukin-2. Am J Roentgenol 1992;158:1407.
529. Shulman KL, Thompson JA, Benyunes MC et al. Adverse reactions to intravenous contrast media in patients treated with interleukin-2. J Immunother 1993;13:208–212.
530. Zukiwski AA, David CL, Coan J et al. Increased incidence of hypersensitivity to iodine-containing radiographic

contrast media after interleukin-2 administration. Cancer 1990;65:1521–1524.
531. Heywood GR, Rosenberg SA, Weber JS. Hypersensitivity reactions to chemotherapy agents in patients receiving chemoimmunotherapy with high-dose interleukin 2. J Natl Cancer Inst 1995;87:915–922.
532. MacDonald D, Jiang YZ, Swirsky D et al. Acute myeloid leukemia relapsing following interleukin 2D2 treatment expresses the alpha chain of the interleukin 2D2 receptor. Br J Haematol 1991;77:43–49.
533. Spiekermann K, O'Brien S, Estey E. Relapse of acute myelogenous leukemia during low dose interleukin-2 (IL-2) therapy: phenotypic evolution associated with strong expression of the IL-2 receptor alpha chain. Cancer 1995;75:1594–1597.
534. Tiberghien P, Racadot E, Deschaseaux ML et al. Interleukin-2-induced increase of a monoclonal B-cell lymphocytosis. Cancer 1992;69:2583–2588.
535. Flaherty LE, Schwert R, Redman BG. Development of Hodgkin's disease in patient receiving long-term administration of dacarbazine and interleukin-2 for metastatic melanoma. J Natl Cancer Inst 1990;82:1360.
536. Bortolussi R, Fabiani F, Savron F et al. Acute morphine intoxication during high-dose recombinant interleukin-2 treatment for metastatic renal cell cancer. Eur J Cancer 1994;30A:1905–1907.
537. Gianella-Borradori A. Present and future clinical relevance of interleukin-3. Stem Cells 1994;12(Suppl 1):241–248.
538. de Vries EGE, van Gameren MM, Willemse PHB. Recombinant human interleukin-3 in clinical oncology. Stem Cells 1993;11:72–80.
539. Tepler I, Elias A, Kalish L et al. Effect of recombinant human interleukin-3 on haematological recovery from chemotherapy-induced myelosuppression. Br J Haematol 1994;87:678–686.
540. Veldhuis GJ, Willemse PHB, van Gameren MM et al. Recombinant human interleukin-3 to dose-intensify carboplatin and cyclophosphamide chemotherapy in epithelial ovarian cancer: a phase I trial. J Clin Oncol 1995;13:733–740.
541. Nemunaitis J, Appelbaum FR, Singer JW et al. Phase I trial with recombinant interleukin-3 in patients with lymphoma undergoing autologous bone marrow transplantation. Blood 1993;82:3273–3278.
542. Biesma B, Willemse PHB, Mulder NH et al. Effects of interleukin-3 after chemotherapy for advanced ovarian cancer. Blood 1992;80:1141–1148.
543. Ganser A, Lindemann A, Seipelt G et al. Effects of recombinant human interleukin-3 in aplastic anemia. Blood 1990;76:1287–1292.
544. Nimer SD, Paquette RL, Ireland P et al. A phase I/II study of interleukin-3 in patients with aplastic anemia and myelodysplasia. Exp Hematol 1994;22:875–880.
545. Huhn RD, Yurkow EJ, Kuhn JG et al. Pharmacodynamics of daily subcutaneous recombinant human interleukin-3 in normal volunteers. Clin Pharmacol Ther 1995;57:32–41.
546. Aulitzky WE, Schuler M, Peschel C, Huber C. Interleukins. Clinical pharmacology and therapeutic use. Drugs 1994;48:667–677.
547. Ganser A, Seipelt G, Lindemann A et al. Effects of recombinant human interleukin-3 in patients with myelodysplastic syndromes. Blood 1990;76:455–462.
548. Dercksen MW, Hoekman K, Visser JJ et al. Hypotension induced by interleukin-3 in patients on angiotensin-converting enzyme inhibitors. Lancet 1995;345:448.
549. Gillio AP, Failkner LB, Alter BP et al. Treatment of Diamond-Blackfan anemia with recombinant human interleukin-3. Blood 1993;82:744–751.
550. Theodossiou C, Kroog G, Ettinghaussen S et al. Acute arterial thrombosis in a patient with breast cancer after chemotherapy with fluorouracil, doxorubicin, leucovorin, cyclosphosphamide, and interleukin-3. Cancer 1994;74:2808–2810.
551. Ganser A, Lindemann A, Seipelt G et al. Effects of recombinant human interleukin-3 in patients with normal hematopoiesis and in patients with bone marrow failure. Blood 1990;76:666–676.
552. Hovgaard DJ, Nissen NI. Effects of interleukin-3 following chemotherapy on non-Hodgkin's lymphoma: A prospective, controlled phase I/II study. Eur J Haematol 1995;54:78–84.
553. Kurzrock R, Talpaz M, Estrov Z et al. Phase I study of recombinant human interleukin-3 in patients with bone marrow failure. J Clin Oncol 1991;9:1241–1250.
554. Ganser A, Ottman OG, Seipelt G et al. Effect of long-term treatment with recombinant human interleukin-3 in patients with myelodysplastic syndromes. Leukemia 1993;7:696–701.
555. Willemze R, Fenaux P, Gerhartz H et al. A randomized phase I/II multicenter study (EORTC 06891) of rhIL-3 in patients with myelodysplastic syndroms at relatively low risk of developing leukemia. Blood 1992;80(Suppl 1):86a.
556. Kramer MHH, Kluin PM, Wijburg ER et al. Differentiation of follicular lymphoma cells after autologous bone marrow transplantation and haematopoietic growth factor treatment. Lancet 1995;345:488–490.
557. Herrmann F, Lindemann A, Lange W et al. Medullary histiocytosis following treatment of severe aplastic anemia with recombinant human interleukin-3 in combination with antilymphocyte globulin, cyclosporin-A, and methylprednisolone. Ann Hematol 1991;63:229–231.
558. Ganser A, Ottman OG, Hoelzer D. Interleukin-3 and interleukin 3/GM-CSF combination therapy: clinical implications. Stem Cells 1993;11:465–473.
559. Nand S, Sosman J, Godwin JE, Fisher RI. A phase I/II study of sequential interleukin-3 and granulocyte-macrophage colony-stimulating factor in myelodysplastic syndromes. Blood 1994;83:357–360.
560. Dercksen MW, Hoekman K, ten Bokkel Huinink WW et al. Effects of interleukin-3 on myelosuppression induced by chemotherapy for ovarian cancer and small cell undifferentiated tumours. Br J Cancer 1993;68:996–1003.
561. Peyron E, Banchereau J. Interleukin-4: structure, function and clinical aspects. Eur J Dermatol 1994;4:181–188.
562. Atkins MB, Vachino G, Tilg HJ et al. Phase I evaluation of thrice-daily intravenous bolus interleukin-4 in patients with refractory malignancy. J Clin Oncol 1992;10:1802–1809.
563. Gilleece MH, Scarffe JH, Ghosh A et al. Recombinant human interleukin 4 (IL-4) given as daily subcutaneous injections: a phase I dose toxicity trial. Br J Cancer 1992;66:204–210.
564. Prendiville J, Thatcher N, Lind M et al. Recombinant human interleukin-4 (rhu IL-4) administered by the intravenous and subcutaneous routes in patients with advanced

cancer: a phase I toxicity study and pharmacokinetic analysis. Eur J Cancer 1993;29A:1700–1707.
565. Sosman JA, Fisher SG, Kefer C et al. A phase I trial of continuous infusion interleukin-4 (IL-4) alone and following interleukin-2 (IL-2) in cancer patients. Ann Oncol 1994; 5:447–452.
566. Trehu EG, Isner JM, Mier JW et al. Possible myocardial toxicity associated with interleukin-4 therapy. J Immunother 1993;14:348–351.
567. Rubin JT, Lotze MT. Acute gastric mucosal injury associated with the systemic administration of interleukin-4. Surgery 1992;111:274–280.
568. Mahler SJ, de Villez RL, Pulitzer DR. Transient acantholytic dermatosis induced by recombinant human interleukin 4. J Am Acad Dermatol 1993;29:206–209.
569. van Gameren MM, Willemse PH, Mulder NH et al. Effects of recombinant human interleukin-6 in cancer patients: a phase I-II study. Blood 1994;84:1434–1441.
570. Weber J, Yang JC, Topalian SL et al. Phase I trial of subcutaneous interleukin-6 in patients with advanced malignancies. J Clin Oncol 1993;11:499–506.
571. Lazarus HM, Winton EF, Williams SF et al. Phase I study of recombinant human interleukin-6 (rhIL-6, *E. coli*) after autologous bone marrow transplant (ABMT) in patients with poor-prognosis breast cancer. Blood 1993; 82(Suppl 1):676.
572. Gordon MS, Nemunaitis J, Hoffman R et al. Phase I trial of subcutaneous recombinant human interleukin-6 in patients with myelodysplasia and thrombocytopenia. Blood 1992;80(Suppl 1):249a.
573. Crawford J, Figlin R, Chang A et al. Phase I/II trial of recombinant human interleukin-6 (rhIL-6) and granulocyte colony-stimulating factor (rhG-CSF) following ifosphamide, carboplatin and etoposide (ICE) chemotherapy in patients with advanced non-small cell lung carcinoma. Blood 1993;82(Suppl 1):367a.
574. Fay JW, Collins R, Pineiro L et al. Concomitant administration of interleukin-6 and Leucomax (rhGM-CSF) following autologous bone marrow transplantation: a phase I trial. Blood 1993;82(Suppl 1):431a.
575. Wu WCS, Magnnion B, Stone RM. Uveitis associated with interleukin-3 and interleukin-6 therapy. Arch Ophthalmol 1995;113:408–409.
576. Fleming TE, Mirando WS, Soohoo LF et al. An inflammatory eruption associated with recombinant human IL-6. Br J Dermatol 1994;130:534–536.
577. Ravoet C, De Greve J, Vandewoude K et al. Tumour stimulating effects of recombinant human interleukin-6. Lancet 1994;344:1576–1577.
578. Sidhu RS, Bollon AP. Tumor necrosis factor activities and cancer therapy—A perspective. Pharmacol Ther 1993;57:79–128.
579. Hieber U, Heim ME. Tumor necrosis factor for the treatment of malignancies. Oncology 1994;51:142–153.
580. Mittelman A, Puccio C, Gafney E et al. A phase I pharmacokinetic study of recombinant human tumor necrosis factor administered by a 5-day continuous infusion. Invest New Drugs 1992;10:183–190.
581. Meyers CA, Valentine AD, Wong FL et al. Reversible neurotoxicity of IL-2 and TNF: correlation of SPECT with neuropsychological testing. J Neuropsychiatry Clin Neurosci 1994;6:285–288.
582. Ferbert A, Biniek R, Kindler J, Maurin N. Myoclonus and tremor induced acutely by administration of tumor necrosis factor in a patient with Ehlers-Danlos syndrome. Movement Disorders 1993;8:232–233.
583. Krigel RL, Padavic-Shaller KA, Rudolph AA et al. Hemorrhagic gastritis as a new dose-limiting toxicity of recombinant tumour necrosis factor. J Natl Cancer Inst 1991;83:129–131.
584. Kuei JH, Tashkin DP, Figlin RA. Pulmonary toxicity of recombinant human tumor necrosis factor. Chest 1989;96:334–338.
585. Schilling PJ, Murray JL, Markowitz AB. Novel tumor necrosis factor toxic effects. Cancer 1992;69:256–260.
586. Hegewisch S, Weh HJ, Hossfeld DK. TNF-induced cardiomyopathy. Lancet 1990;335:294–295.
587. Logan TF, Kaplan SS, Bryant JL et al. Granulocytopenia in cancer patients treated in a phase I trial with recombinant human tumor necrosis factor. J Immunother 1991; 10:84–95.
588. Muggia FM, Brown TD, Goodman PJ et al. High incidence of coagulopathy in phase II studies of recombinant tumor necrosis factor in advanced pancreatic and gastric cancers. Anti-Cancer Drugs 1992;3:211–217.
589. van der Poll T, van Deventer SJH, Pasterkamp G et al. Tumor necrosis factor induces von Willebrand factor release in healthy humans. Thromb Haemost 1992;67:623–626.
590. Miyakoshi H, Ohsawa K, Yokoyama H et al. Exacerbation of hypothyroidism following tumor necrosis factor-alpha infusion. Intern Med 1992;31:200–203.
591. Schiller JH, Witt P, Storer B et al. Clinical and biological effects of combination therapy with gamma-interferon and tumor necrosis factor. Cancer 1992;69:562–571.
592. Smith JW II, Urba WJ, Clark JW et al. Phase I evaluation of recombinant tumor necrosis factor given in combination with recombinant interferon-gamma. J Immunother 1991;10:355–362.
593. Negrier MS, Pourreau CN, Palmer PA et al. Phase I-trial of recombinant interleukin-2 followed by recombinant tumor necrosis factor in patients with metastatic cancer. J Immunother 1992;11:93–102.
594. Minasian LM, Szatrowski TP, Rosemblum M et al. Hemorrhagic tumor necrosis during a pilot trial of tumor necrosis factor-α and anti-GD3 ganglioside monoclonal antibody in patients with metastasic melanoma. Blood 1994;83:56–64.
595. Watanabe N, Yamauchi N, Maeda M et al. Recombinant human tumor necrosis factor causes regression in patients with advanced malignancies. Oncology 1994;51:360–365.
596. Lejeune F, Liénard D, Eggermont A et al. Clinical experience with high-dose tumor necrosis factor alpha in regional therapy of advanced melanoma. Circ Shock 1994;43:191–197.
597. Eggimann P, Chiolero R, Chassot PG et al. Systemic and hemodynamic effects of recombinant tumor necrosis factor alpha in isolation perfusion of the limbs. Chest 1995;107:1074–1082.
598. Ippoliti C, Przepiorka D, Smith T et al. Adverse effects of molgramostim in marrow transplant recipients. Clin Pharm 1993;12:520–525.
599. Cebon JS, Lieschke GJ. Granulocyte-macrophage colony-stimulating factor for cancer treatment. Oncology 1994;51:177–188.
600. Grant SM, Heel RC. Recombinant granulocyte-macrophage colony-stimulating factor (rGM-CSF) A review of its pharmacological properties and propective role in the management of myelosuppression. Drugs 1992;43:516–560.

601. Lazarus HM, Rowe JM. Clinical use of hematopoietic growth factors in allogeneic bone marrow transplantation. Blood Rev 1994;169–178.
602. Vose JM, Armitage JO. Clinical applications of hematopoietic growth factors. J Clin Oncol 1995;13:1023–1035.
603. Schriber JR, Negrin RS. Use and toxicity of the colony-stimulating factors. Drug Safety 1993;8:457–468.
604. Gluck S, Gagnon A. Neutropenic fever in patients after high-dose chemotherapy followed by autologous haematopoietic progenitor cell transplantation and human recombinant granulocyte-macrophage colony-stimulating factor. Bone Marrow Transplant 1994;14:989–990.
605. Khwaja A, Chopra R, Goldstone AH, Linch DC. Acute-phase response in patients given rhIL-3 after chemotherapy. Lancet 1992;339:1617.
606. Welte K, Zeidler C, Reiter A et al. Differential effects of granulocyte-macrophage colony-stimulating factor and granulocyte colony-stimulating factor in children with severe congenital neutropenia. Blood 1990;75:1056–1063.
607. Antman KS, Griffin JD, Elias A et al. Effect of recombinant human granulocyte-macrophage colony-stimulating factor on chemotherapy-induced myelosuppression. N Engl J Med 1988;319:593–598.
608. Nissen C, Tichelli A, Gratwohl A et al. Failure of recombinant human granulocyte-macrophage colony-stimulating factor therapy in aplastic anemia patients with very severe neutropenia. Blood 1988;72:2045–2047.
609. Stephens LC, Haire WD, Schmit-Pokorny K et al. Granulocyte macrophage colony stimulating factor: high incidence of apheresis catheter thrombosis during peripheral stem cell collection. Bone Marrow Transplant 1993;11:51–54.
610. Tolcher AW, Giusti RM, O'Shaughnessy JA, Cowan KH. Arterial thrombosis associated with granulocyte-macrophage colony-stimulating factor (GM-CSF) administration in breast cancer patients treated with dose-intensive chemotherapy: a report of two cases. Cancer Invest 1995;13:188–192.
611. Gianni AM, Bregni M, Siena S et al. Recombinant human granulocyte-macrophage colony-stimulating factor reduces haematologic toxicity and widens clinical applicability of high-dose cyclophosphamide treatment in breast cancer and non-Hodgkin's lymphoma. J Clin Oncol 1990;8:768–778.
612. Arning M, Kliche KO, Schneider W. GM-CSF therapy and capillary-leak syndrome. Ann Hematol 1991;62:83.
613. Emminger W, Emminger-Schmidmeier W, Peters C et al. Capillary leak syndrome during low dose granulocyte-macrophage colony-stimulating factor (rh GM-CSF) treatment of a patient in a continuous febrile state. Blut 1990;61:219–221.
614. Hansen PB, Johnsen HE, Lund JO et al. Unexpected hepatotoxicity after priming and treatment with molgramostim (rhGM-CSF) in acute myeloid leukemia during induction chemotherapy. Am J Hematol 1995;48:48–51.
615. Philippe B, Couderc LJ, Balloul-Delclaux E et al. Pulmonary toxicity of chemotherapy and GM-CSF. Resp Med 1994;88:715.
616. Verhoef G, Boogaerts M. Treatment with granulocyte-macrophage colony stimulating factor and the adult respiratory distress syndrome. Am J Hematol 1991;36:285–287.
617. Einzig AI, Dutcher JP, Wiernik PH. Life-threatening hyperleukocytosis and pulmonary compromise after priming with recombinant human granulocyte-macrophage colony-stimulating factor in a patient with acute myelomonocytic leukemia. J Clin Oncol 1995;13:304–305.
618. Miniero R, Madon E, Artesani L et al. Acute pulmonary failure after the first administration of recombinant human granulocyte-macrophage colony-stimulating factor. Leukemia 1992;6:352–353.
619. Hoekman K, von Blomberg-van der Flier BME, Wagstaff J et al. Reversible thyroid dysfunction during treatment with GM-CSF. Lancet 1991;338:541–542.
620. Hansen PB, Johnsen HE, Hippe E. Autoimmune hypothyroidism and granulocyte-macrophage colony-stimulating factor. Eur J Haematol 1993;50:183–184.
621. Viens P, Thyss A, Garnier G et al. GM-CSF treatment and hypokaliemia. Ann Intern Med 1989;111:263.
622. Kaczmarski RS, Mufti GJ. Hypoalbuminaemia after prolonged treatment with recombinant granulocyte-macrophage colony-stimulating factor. Br Med J 1990;301:1312–1313.
623. Gonzales-Chambers R, Rosenfeld C, Winkelstein A, Dameshek L. Eosinophilia resulting from administration of recombinant granulocyte-macrophage colony-stimulating factor (rhGM-CSF) in a patient with T-γ lymphoproliferative disease. Am J Hematol 1991;36:157–159.
624. Donhuijsen K, Haedicke C, Hattenberger S et al. Granulocyte-macrophage colony-stimulating factor-related eosinophilia and Loeffler's endocarditis. Blood 1992;79:2798.
625. Lieschke GJ, Maher D, Cebon J et al. Effects of bacterially synthetized recombinant human granulocyte-macrophage colony-stimulating factor in pateints with advanced malignancy. Ann Intern Med 1989;110:357–364.
626. Nathan FE, Besa EC. GM-CSF and accelerated hemolysis. N Engl J Med 1992;326:417.
627. Pieters RC, Rojer RA, Saleh AW et al. Molgramostim to treat SS-sickle cell leg ulcers. Lancet 1995;345:528.
628. Lindemann A, Hermann F, Mertelsmann R et al. Splenic haematopoiesis following GM-CSF therapy in a patient with hairy cell leukaemia. Leukemia 1990;4:606–607.
629. Haferlach T, Schmitz N, Suttorp M et al. Hepatotoxicity of GM-CSF in patients with advanced Hodgkin's disease given autologous bone marrow transplants? Bone Marrow Transplant 1990;5(Suppl 2):83.
630. Steger GG, Locker G, Rainer H et al. Cutaneous reactions to GM-CSF in inflammatory breast cancer. N Engl J Med 1992;327:286.
631. Mehregan DR, Fransway AF, Edmonson JH, Leiferman KM. Cutaneous reactions to granulocyte-monocyte colony-stimulating factor. Arch Dermatol 1992;128:1055–1059.
632. Yamada H, Tubaki K, Ashida T et al. Does recombinant granulocyte-macrophage colony-stimulating factor (GM-CSF) play a crucial role in the pathogenesis of atopic dermatitis after bone marrow transplantation (BMT). Med Science Res 1991;19:395.
633. Kluin-Nelemans JC, Hollander AAMJ, Fibbe WE et al. Leucocytoclastic vasculitis during GM-CSF therapy. Br J Haematol 1989;73:419–420.
634. Dreicer R, Schiller JH, Carbone PP. Granulocyte-macrophage colony-stimulating factor and vasculitis. Ann Intern Med 1989;111:91–92.
635. Steichen Kabalin CA, Kanwar Y, Roholt N et al. Cutaneous reaction to granulocyte-macrophage colony stimulating factor (GM-CSF): a case report. J Allerg Clin Immunol 1994;94(part 2):242.
636. Perrot JL, Benoit F, Segault D et al. Pyoderma gangrenosum aggravé par administration de GM-CSF. Ann Dermatol Venerol 1992;119:846–848.

637. Lauthenschlager S, Itin PH, Hirsbrunner P, Büchner SA. Subcorneal pustular dermatosis at the injection site of recombinant human granulocyte-macrophage colony-stimulating factor in a patient with IgA myeloma. J Am Acad Dermatol 1994;30:787–789.
638. Ward JC, Gitlin JB, Garry DJ et al. Epidermolysis bullosa acquisita induced by GM-CSF: a role for eosinophils in treatment-related toxicity. Br J Haematol 1992;81:27–32.
639. Stasi R, Gatti S, Perrotti A et al. Erythema multiforme during GM-CSF therapy. Acta Dermatol Venereol 1994; 74:132–134.
640. Kelly R, Marsden RA, Bevan D. Exacerbation of psoriasis with GM-CSF therapy. Br J Dermatol 1993;128:468–469.
641. Hazenberg BPC, van Leeuwen MA, van Rijswijk MH et al. Correction of granulocytopenia in Felty's syndrome by granulocyte-macrophage colony-stimulating factor. Simultaneous induction of interleukin-6 release and flare-up of the arthritis. Blood (1989)74, 2769–2770.
642. De Vries EGE, Willemse PHB, Biesma B et al. Flare-up of rheumatoid arthritis during GM-CSF treatment after chemotherapy. Lancet 1991;338:517–518.
643. Lang E, Cibull ML, Gallicchio VS et al. Proliferation of abnormal bone marrow histiocytes and undesired effect of granulocyte macrophage-colony-stimulating factor therapy in a patient with Hurler's syndrome undergoing bone marrow transplantation. Am J Hematol 1992;41:280–284.
644. Wilson PA, Ayscue LH, Jones GR, Beentley SA. Bone marrow histiocytic proliferation in association with colony-stimulating factor therapy. Am J Clin Pathol 1993;99:311–313.
645. Risti B, Flury RF, Schaffner A. Fatal hematophagic histiocytosis after granulocyte-macrophage colony-stimulating factor and chemotherapy for high-grade malignant lymphoma. Clin Invest 1994;72:457–461.
646. Groopman JE. Granulocyte-macrophage colony-stimulating factor in human immunodeficiency virus disease. Sem Hematol 1990;27(Suppl 3):8–14.
647. Hermans P, Gori A, Lemone M et al. Possible role of granulocyte-macrophage colony stimulating factor (GM-CSF) on the rapid progression of AIDS-related Kaposi's sarcoma lesions in vivo. Br J Haematol 1994;87:413–414.
648. Gribben JG, Devereux S, Thomas NSB et al. Development of antibodies to unprotected glycosylation sites of recombinant human GM-CSF. Lancet 1990;335:434–437.
649. Ragnhammar P, Friesen HJ, Frodin JE et al. Induction of anti-recombinant human granulocyte-macrophage colony-stimulating factor (*Escherichia coli*-derived) antibodies and clinical effects in nonimmunocompromised patients. Blood 1994;84:4078–4087.
650. Scadden DT, Agosti J. No antibodies to granulocyte macrophage colony-stimulating factor with prolonged use in AIDS. AIDS 1993;7:438.
651. Engler RJM, Weiss RB. Recombinant human granulocyte-macrophage-colony stimulating factor (GM-CSF) as a cause of anaphylaxis. J Allerg Clin Immunol 1995;95(part 2):283.
652. Bokemeyer C, Schmoll HJ, Harstrick A. Side-effects of GM-CSF treatment in advanced testicular cancer. Eur. J. Cancer 1993;29A:924.
653. Rabinowe SN, Neuberg D, Bierman PJ et al. Long-term follow-up of a phase III study of recombinant human granulocyte-macrophage colony-stimulating factor after autologous bone marrow transplantation for lymphoid malignancies. Blood 1993;81:1903–1908.
654. Csaki C, Ferencz T, Sipos L et al. Multifocal oligoclonal plasmocytosis in a child with high-grade glioma following high-dose chemotherapy with intensive cytokine support. Med Pediatr Oncol 1994;23:273.
655. Estey EH. Use of colony-stimulating factor in the treatment of acute myeloid leukemia. Blood 1994;83:2015–2019.
656. Stone RM, Berg DT, George SL et al. Granulocyte-macrophage colony-stimulating factor after initial chemotherapy for elderly patients with primary acute myelogenous leukemia. N Engl J Med 1995;332:1671–1677.
657. Foot ABM, Potter MN, Mott MG, Oakhill A. Effects of haemopoietic growth factors for aplastic anaemia. Lancet 1994;344:757.
658. Zimmer BM, Berdel WE, Ludwig WD et al. Fatal spleen rupture during induction chemotherpay with rh GM-CSF priming for acute monocytic leukemia. Clinical case report and in vitro studies. Leuk Res 1993;17:277–283.
659. Frampton JE, Lee C R, Faulds D. Filgrastim: a review of its pharmacological properties and therapeutic efficacy in neutropenia. Drugs 1994;48:731–760.
660. Frampton JE, Yarker YE, Goa KL. Lenograstim. A review of its pharmacological properties and therapeutic efficacy in neutropenia and related clinical settings. Drugs 1995;49:767–793.
661. Kojima S, Matsuyama T. Stimulation of granulopoiesis by high-dose recombinant human granulocyte colony-stimulating factor in children with aplastic anemia and very severe neutropenia. Blood 1994;83:1474–1478.
662. Bonilla MA, Dale D, Zeidler C et al. Long-term safety of treatment with recombinant human granulocyte colony-stimulating factor (r-metHuG-CSF) in patients with severe congenital neutropenias. Br J Haematol 1994;88:723–730.
663. Lindemann A, Rumberger B. Vascular complications in patients treated with granulocyte colony-stimulating factor (G-CSF). Eur J Cancer 1993;29A:2338–2339.
664. Pettengell R, Gurney H, Radford JA et al. Granulocyte colony-stimulating factor to prevent dose-limiting neutropenia in non-Hodgkin's lymphoma: a randomized controlled trial. Blood 1992;80:1430–1436.
665. Conti JA, Scher HL. Acute arterial thrombosis after esclated-dose methotrexate, vinblastine, doxorubicin and cisplatin chemotherapy with recombinant granulocyte colony-stimulating factor. A possible new recombinant granulocyte colony-stimulating factor toxicity. Cancer 1992;70:2699–2702.
666. Shimoda K, Okamura S, Inaba S et al. Granulocyte colony-stimulating factor and platelet aggregation. Lancet 1993;341:633–634.
667. Oeda E, Shinohara K, Kamei S et al. Capillary leak syndrome likely the result of granulocyte colony-stimulating factor after high-dose chemotherapy. Intern Med 1994; 33:115–119.
668. Dirix LY, Schrijvers D, Druw P et al. Pulmonary toxicity and bleomycin. Lancet 1994;344:56.
669. Katoh M, Shikoshi K, Takada M et al. Development of interstitial pneumonitis during treatment with granulocytes colony-stimulating factor. Ann Hematol 1993;67:201–202.
670. Matthews JH. Pulmonary toxicity of ABVD chemotherapy and G-CSF in Hodgkin's disease: possible synergy. Lancet 1993;342:988.
671. Van Woensel JBM, Knoester H, Leeuw JA, Van Aalderen WMC. Acute respiratory insufficiency during doxorubicin, cyclophosphamide, and G-CSF therapy. Lancet 1994;344:759–760.

672. Iki S, Yoshinaga K, Ohbayashi Y, Urabe A. Cytotoxic drug-induced pneumonia and possible augmentation by G-CSF: clinical attention. Ann Hematol 1993;66:217–218.
673. Lei KIK, Leung WT, Johnson PJ. Serious pulmonary complications in patients receiving recombinant granulocyte colony-stimulating factor during BACOP chemotherapy for aggressive non-Hodgkin's lymphoma. Br J Cancer 1994; 70:1009–1013.
674. Bastion Y, Reyes F, Bosly A et al. Possible toxicity with the association of G-CSF and bleomycin. Lancet 1994;343:1221–1222.
675. White K, Cebon J. Transient hypoxaemia during neutrophil recovery in febrile patients. Lancet 1995;345:1022–1024.
676. Demuynck H, Zachée P, Verhoef GEG et al. Risks of rhG-CSF treatment in drug-induced agranulocytosis. Ann Hematol 1995;70:143–147.
677. Schilero GJ, Oropello J, Benjamin E. Impairment in gas exchange after granulocyte colony stimulating factor (G-CSF) in a patient with the adult respiratory distress syndrome. Chest 1995;107:276–278.
678. Van Hoef MEHM, Howell A. Risk of thyroid dysfunction during treatment with G-CSF. Lancet 1992;340:1169–1170.
679. Fossa SD, Poulsen JP, Aaserud A. Alkaline phosphatase and lactate dehydrogenase changes during leucocytosis induced by G-CSF in testicular cancer. Lancet 1992; 340:1544.
680. Higa GM. Significance of granulocyte colony-stimulating factor (G-CSF)-induced increase in LDH. Ann Pharmacother 1994;28:118.
681. Sarris AH, Majlis A, Dimopoulos MA et al. Rising serum lactate dehydrogenase often caused by granulocyte-or granulocyte-macrophage colony stimulating factor and not tumor progression in patients with lymphoma and myeloma. Leuk Lymph 1995;17:473–477.
682. Wun T. The Felty syndrome and G-CSF-associated thrombocytopenia and severe anemia. Ann Intern Med 1993;118:318–319.
683. Migita M, Fukunaga Y, Watanabe A et al. Emperipolesis of neutrophils by megakaryocytes and thrombocytopenia observed in a case of Kostmann's syndrome during intravenous administration of high-dose rhG-CSF. Br J Haematol 1992;80:413–415.
684. Dale DC, Bonilla MA, Davis MW et al. A randomized controlled phase III trial of recombinant human granulocyte colony-stimulating factor (filgrastim) for treatment of severe chronic neutropenia. Blood 1993;81:2496–2502.
685. Litam PP, Friedman HD, Loughran TP. Splenic extramedullary hematopoiesis in a patient receiving intermittently administered granulocyte colony-stimulating factor. Ann Intern Med 1993;118:954–955.
686. Mueller BU, Burt R, Gulick L et al. Disseminated intravascular coagulation associated with granulocyte colony-stimulating factor therapy in a child with human immunodeficiency virus infection. J Pediatr 1995;126:749–752.
687. Buntzel J, Küttner K. Hepatic injury due to G-CSF. Onkologie 1995;18:54–56.
688. Günther G, Mauz-Körholz C, KörholzD, Burdach S. G-CSF and liver toxicity in a patient with neuroblastoma. Lancet 1992; 340:1352.
689. Zylberberg H, Zylberberg L, Hagege H et al. Probable G-CSF-induced hepatitis and pancreatitis in an HIV-seropositive patient. J Hepatol 1995;22:596–597.
690. Ostlere LS, Harris D, Prentice HG, Rustin MHA. Widespread folliculitis induced by human granulocyte-colony-stimulating factor therapy. Br J Dermatol 1992; 127:193–194.
691. Samlaska CP, Noyes DK. Localized cutaneous reactions to granulocyte colony-stimulating factor. Arch Dermatol 1993;129:645–646.
692. Duhrsen U, Renges HH, Mayer U, Hossfeld DK. Leukemic nodules at the site of G-CSF injection in acute myelomonocytic leukemia. Eur J Haematol 1995;54:51–52.
693. Yamashita N, Natsuaki M, Morita H et al. Cutaneous eruptions induced by granulocyte colony-stimulating factor in two cases of acute myelogenous leukemia. J Dermatol 1993;20:473–477.
694. Couderc LJ, Philippe B, Franck N et al. Necroziting vasculitis and exacerbation of psoriasis after granulocyte colony-stimulating factor for small cell lung carcinoma. Resp Med 1995;89:237–238.
695. Mulligan SP, Wegman A, Cooke B. Leukocytoclastic vasculitis occuring with the second dose of granulocyte-colony stimulating factor for severe chronic neutropenia. Aust NZ J Med 1995;25:75.
696. Schliesser G, Pralle H, Lohmeyer J. Leukocytoclastic vasculitis complicating granulocyte colony-stimulating factor (G-CSF) induced neutrophil recovery in T-γ lymphocytosis with severe neutropenia. Ann Hematol 1992;65:151–152.
697. Wodzinski MA, Hampton KK, Reilly JT. Differential effect of G-CSF and GM-CSF in acquired chronic neutropenia. Br J Haematol 1991;77:249–250.
698. Yang YM, Mankad VM, Manci E. Granulocyte colony-stimulating factor associated leukocytoclastic vascultitis mimicking Henoch-Schönlein purpura. Pediatr Hematol Oncol 1993;10:193–195.
699. Jain KK. Cutaneous vasculitis associated with granulocyte colony-stimulating factor. J Am Acad Dermatol 1994;31(Part 1)213–215.
700. Fukutoku M, Shimizu S, Ogawa Y et al. Sweet's syndrome during therapy with granulocyte colony-stimulating factor in a patient with aplastic anaemia. Br J Haematol 1994;86:645–648.
701. Park JW, Mehrotra B, Barnett BO et al. The Sweet syndrome during therapy with granulocyte colony-stimulating factor. Ann Intern Med 1992;116:996–998.
702. Paydas S, Sahin B, Seyrek E et al. Sweet's syndrome associated with G-CSF. Br J Haematol 1993;85:191–192.
703. van Kamp H, van den Berg E, Timens W et al. Sweet's syndrome in myeloid malignancy: a report of two cases. Br J Haematol 1994;86:415–417.
704. Johnson MML, Grimwood CRE. Leukocyte colony-stimulating factors. A review of associated neutrophilic dermatoses and vasculitides. Arch Dermatol 1994;130:77–81.
705. Ross HJ, Moy LA, Kaplan R, Figlin RA. Bullous pyoderma gangrenosum after granulocyte colony-stimulating factor treatment. Cancer 1991;68:441–443.
706. Nomiyama J, Shinohara K, Inoue H. Erythema nodosum caused by the administration of granulocyte colony stimulating factor in a patient with refractory anemia. Am J Hematol 1994;47:333.
707. Negrin RS, Haeuber DH, Nagler A et al. Treatment of myelodysplastic syndrome with recombinant human granulocyte colony-stimulating factor. A phase I–II trial. Ann Intern Med 1989;110:976–984.
708. Hayat SQ, Hearth-Holmes M, Wolf RE. Flare of ar-

thritis with successful treatment of Felty's syndrome with granulocyte colony stimulating factor (GCSF). Clin Rheumatol 1995;14:211–212.
709. Vidarsson B, Geirsson AJ, Onundarson PT. Reactivation of rheumatoid arthritis and development of leukocytoclastic vasculitis in a patient receiving granulocyte colony-stimulating factor for Felty's syndrome. Am J Med 1995; 98:589–591.
710. Yasuda M, Kihara T, Wada T et al. Granulocyte colony-stimuling factor induction of improved leukocytopenia with inflammatory flare in a Felty's syndrome patient. Arthr Rheum 1994;37:145–146.
711. Bishop NJ, Williams DM, Compston JC et al. Osteoporosis in severe congenital neutropenia treated with granulocyte colony-stimulating factor. Br J Haematol 1995; 89:927–928.
712. Kawachi Y, Ozaki S, Sakamoto Y et al. Richter's syndrome showing pronounced lymphadenopathy in reponse to administration of granulocyte colony-stimulating factor. Leuk Lymph 1994;13:509–514.
713. Jaiyesimi I, Giralt SS, Wood J. Subcutaneous granulocyte colony-stimulating factor and acute anaphylaxis. N Engl J Med 1991;325:587.
714. Sasaki O, Yokoyama A, Uemura S et al. Drug eruption caused by recombinant human G-CSF. Intern Med 1994;22:641–643.
715. Brown SL, Hill E. Subcutaneous granulocyte colony-stimulating factor and acute anaphylaxis. N Engl J Med 1991;325:587.
716. Cannell PK, Davies JM, Jackson JM. Sideroblastic anemia following autotransplantation for Hodgkin's disease using rHu-G-CSF. Bone Marrow Transplant 1992;9:301–302.
717. Soutar RL. Acute myeloblastic leukaemia and recombinant granulocyte colony stimulating factor. Br Med J 1991;303:123–124.
718. Stathopoulos GP, Moschopoulos N, Apostolopoulou E et al. Acute non-lymphocytic leukaemia complicating gastric cancer treated with epidophyllotoxin containing chemotherapy and G-CSF. Acta Oncol 1994;33:713–714.
719. Matsuzaki A, Ohga S, Ueda K et al. Induction of CD33-positive blasts by granulocyte colony-stimulating factor in a child with common acute lymphoblastic leukemia. Int J Ped Hematol Oncol 1994;1:339–341.
720. Reale MA, Yen Y, Strair RK et al. Pseudoleukemia after granulocyte colony-stimulating factor therapy. South Med 1995;J88:462–464.
721. Dombret H, Chastang G, Fenaux P et al. A controlled study of recombinant human granulocyte colony-stimulating factor in elderly patients after treatment for acute myelogenous leukemia. N Engl J Med 1995;332:1678–1683.
722. Imashuku S, Hibi S, Katahoka-Morimoto Y et al. Myelodysplasia and acute myeloid leukaemia in cases of aplastic anaemia and congenital neutropenia following G-CSF administration. Br J Haematol 1995;89:188–190.
723. Izumi T, Muroi K, Takatoku M et al. Development of acute myeloblastic leukaemia in a case of aplastic anaemia treated with granulocyte colony-stimulating factor. Br J Haematol 1994;87:666–668.
724. Kojima S, Tsuchida M, Matsuyama T. Myelodysplasia and leukemia after treatment of aplastic anemia with G-CSF. N Engl J Med 1992;326:1294–1295.
725. Weinblatt ME, Scimeca P, James-Herry A et al. Transformation of congential neutropenia into monosomy 7 and acute nonlymphoblastic leukemia in a child treated with granulocyte colony-stimulating factor. J Pediatr 1995; 126:263–265.
726. Imashuku S, Hibi S, Nakajima F et al. A review of 125 cases to determinate the risk of myelodysplasia and leukemia in pediatric neutropenic patients after treatment with recombinant human granulocyte colony-stimulating factor. Blood 1994;84:2380–2381.
727. Vora AJ, Toh CH, Peel J, Greaves M. Use of granulocyte colony-stimulating factor (G-CSF) for mobilizing peripheral blood stem cells: risk of mobilizing clonal myeloma cells in patients with bone marrow infiltration. Br J Haematol 1994;86:180–182.
728. De la Rubia J, Bonanad S, Palau J et al. Rapid progression of multiple myeloma following G-CSF mobilization. Bone Marrow Transplant 1994;14:475–476.
729. Sawamura T, Sakura T, Miyawaki S. Exacerbation of monoclonal gammopathy in a patient treated with G-CSF. Ann Intern Med 1993;118:318.
730. Cole DJ, Sanda MG, Yang JC et al. Phase I trial of recombinant human macrophage colony-stimulating factor administered by continuous intravenous infusion in patients with metastatic cancer. J Natl Cancer Inst 1994;86:39–45.
731. Nemunaitis J, Shannon-Dorcy K, Appelbaum FR et al. Long-term follow-up of patients with invasive fungal disease who received adjunctive therapy with recombinant human macrophage colony-stimulating factor. Blood 1993;82:1422–1427.
732. Bukowski RM, Budd GT, Gibbons JA et al. Phase I trial of subcutaneous recombinant macrophage colony-stimulating factor: clinical and immunomodulatory effects. J Clin Oncol 1994;12:97–106.
733. Sanda MG, Yang JC, Topalian SL et al. Intravenous administration of recombinant human macrophage colony-stimulating factor to patients with metastatic cancer: a phase I study. J Clin Oncol 1992;10:1643–1649.
734. Zamkoff KW, Hudson J, Groves ES et al. A phase I trial of recombinant human macrophage colony-stimulating factor by rapid intravenous infusion in patients with refractory malignancy. J Immunother 1992;11:103–110.
735. Dutcher JP, Benchabbat A, Jones JG, Wiernik PH. Unique dermatological complication of rhM-CSF treatment. Leuk Lymph 1994;15:347–349.
736. Masaoka T, Shibata H, Ohno R et al. Double-blind test of human urinary macrophage colony-stimulating factor for allogeneic and syngeneic bone marrow transplantation: effectiveness of treatment and 2-year follow-up for relapse of leukaemia. Br J Haematol 1990;76:501–505.
737. Khwaja A, Yong K, Jones M et al. The effect of macrophage colony-stimulating factor on haematopoietic recovery after autologous bone marrow transplantation. Br J Haematol 1992;81:288–295.
738. Masumoto A, Kawada H, Fukuda R et al. Severe erythrodermia caused by M-CSF. Am J Hematol 1994; 47:147–148.
739. Yasuda N, Ohmori S, Usui T. Mobilization of myeloblasts with 5q-anomaly during treatment with macrophage-colony stimulating factor (M-CSF). Am J Hematol 1995; 48:60.
740. Penn I. Tumors after renal and cardiac transplantation. Hematol. Oncol Clin North Am 1993;7:431–445.
741. Penn I. The changing pattern of posttransplant malignancies. Transplant Proc 1991;23:1101–1103.
743. London N, Farmery S, Will E et al. Risk of neoplasia in renal transplant patients. Lancet 1995;346:403–406.

744. Kehinde E, Petermann A, Morgan J et al. Triple therapy and incidence of de novo cancer in renal transplant recipients. Br J Surg 1994;81:985–986.
745. Opelz G, Henderson R. Incidence of non-Hodgkin lymphoma in kidney and heart transplant recipients. Lancet 1993;342:1514–1516.
746. Sheil A, Disney A, Mathew T et al. Cancer development in cadaveric donor renal allograft recipients treated with azathioprine (AZA) or cyclosporine (CyA) or AZA/-CyA. Transplant Proc 1991;23:1111–1112.
747. Gruber SA, Gillingham K, Sothern RB et al. De novo cancer in cyclosporine-treated and non-cyclosporine-treated adult primary renal allograft recipients. Clin Transplant 1994;8:388–395.
748. Hiesse C, Kriaa F, Rieu P et al. Incidence and type of malignancies occurring after renal transplantation in conventionally and cyclosporine-treated recipients: analysis of a 20-year period in 1600 patients. Transplant Proc 1995;27:972–974.
749. Arellano F, Krupp P. Malignancies in rheumatoid arthritis patients treated with cyclosporin A. Br J Rheumatol 1993;32(Suppl 1):72–75.
750. Gridley G, McLaughlin J, Ekbom A et al. Incidence of cancer among patients with rheumatoid arthritis. J Natl Cancer Inst 1993;85:307–311.
751. Feutren G. The optimal use of cyclosporin A in autoimmune diseases. J Autoimmun 1992;5(Suppl A):183–195.
752. Garcia V, Keitel E, Almeida P et al. Morbidity after renal transplantation: role of bacterial infection. Transplant Proc 1995;27:1825–1826.
753. Grossi P, Minoli L, Percivalle E et al. Clinical and virological monitoring of human cytomegelovirus infection in 294 heart transplant recipients. Transplantation 1995; 59:847–851.
754. Kekec Y, Tavli S, Tokyay R, Haberal M. Infections after kidney transplantation. Transplant Proc 1992;24:1932–1933.
755. Kreis H. Adverse events associated with OKT3 immunosuppression in the prevention or treatment of allograft rejection. Clin Transplant 1993;7:431–446.
756. Wade J, Rolando N, Hayllar K et al. Bacterial and fungal infections after liver transplantation: an analysis of 284 patients. Hepatology 1995;21:1328–1336.
757. Huynh L, Min D. Outcomes of pregnancy and the management of immunosuppressive agents to minimize fetal risks in organ transplant patients. Ann Pharmacother 1994; 28:1355–1357.
758. Armenti V, Ahlswede K, Ahlswede B et al. National Transplantation Pregnancy Registry: outcomes of 154 pregnancies in cyclosporine-treated female kidney transplant recipients. Transplantation 1994;57:502–506.
759. Cararach V, Carmona F, Monleon F, Andreu J. Pregnancy after renal transplantation: 25 years experience in Spain. Br J Obstet Gynaecol 1993;100:122–125.
760. Jain A, Venkataramanan R, Lever J et al. FK506 and pregnancy in liver transplant recipients. Transplant Proc 1993;56:751.
761. Armenti V, Ahlswede K, Ahlswede B et al. Variables affecting birthweight and graft survival in 197 pregnancies in cyclosporine-treated female kidney transplant recipients. Transplantation 1995;59:476–479.
762. Armenti V, Ahlswede B, Morits M, Jarrell B. National Transplantation Pregnancy Registry: analysis of pregnancy outcomes of female kidney recipients with relation to time interval from transplant to conception. Transplant Proc 1993;25:1036–1037.
763. Shaheen F, Al-Sulaiman M, Al-Khader A. Long-term nephrotoxicity after exposure to cyclosporine in utero. Transplantation 1993;56:224–225.
764. Baarsma R, Kamps W. Immunological responses in an infant after cyclosporine A exposure during pregnancy. Eur J Pediatr 1993;152:476–477.
765. Pilarski L, Yacyshyn B, Lazarovits A. Analysis of peripheral blood lymphocyte populations and immune function from children exposed to cyclosporine or to azathioprine in utero. Transplantation 1994;57:133–144.
766. Pearson D, May G, Fick G, Sutherland L. Azathioprine and 6-mercaptopurine in Crohn disease. A meta-analysis. Ann Intern Med 1995;123:132–142.
767. Connell W, Kamm M, Ritchie J, Lennard-Jones J. Bone marrow toxicity caused by azathioprine in inflammatory bowel disease: 27 years experience. Gut 1993;34:1081–1085.
768. Creemers G, van Boven W, Lowenberg B, van der Heul C. Azathioprine-associated pure red cell aplasia. J Intern Med 1993;233:85–87.
769. Wijnands MJH, van Riel PLCM. Management of adverse effects of disease-modifying antirheumatic drugs. Drug Safety 1995;13:219–227.
770. Escousse A, Rifle G, Sgro C et al. Azathioprine toxicity, 6-mercaptopurine accumulation and the 'poor' 6-thiopurine methylator phenotype. Eur J Clin Pharmacol 1995;48:309–310.
771. Schütz E, Gummert J, Mohr F et al. Azathioprine myelotoxicity related to elevated 6-thioguanine nucleotides in heart transplantation. Transplant Proc 1995;27:1298–1300.
772. Kerstens P, Stolk J, Abreu R et al. Azathioprine-related bone marrow toxicity and low activities of purine enzymes in patients with rheumatoid arthritis. Arthr Rheum 1995;38:142–145.
773. Ari Z, Mehta A, Lennard L, Burroughs A. Azathioprine-induced myelosuppression due to thiopurine methyltransferase deficiency in a patient with autoimmune hepatitis. J Hepatol 1995;23:351–354.
774. Escousse A, Mousson C, Santona L et al. Azathioprine-induced pancytopenia in homozygous thiopurine methyltransferase-deficient renal transplant recipients: a family study. Transplant Proc 1995;27:1739–1742.
775. Soria-Royer C, Legendre C, Mircheva J et al. Thiopurine methyltransferase activity to assess azathioprine myelotoxicity in renal transplant patients. Lancet 1993;341:1593–1594.
776. Kerstens P, Stolk J, Hilbrands L et al. 5-Nucleotidase and azathioprine-related bone-marrow toxicity. Lancet 1993;342:1245–1246.
777. Serre-Debeauvais F, Bayle F, Amirou M et al. Hématotoxicité de l'azathioprine à déterminisme génétique aggravé par un déficit en xanthine oxyase chez une transplantée rénale. Presse Med 1995;24:987–988.
778. Rossi S, Schroeder T, Hariharan S, First M. Prevention and management of the adverse effects associated with immunosuppressive therapy. Drug Safety 1993;9:104–131.
779. Horsmans Y, Rahier J, Geubel A. Reversible cholestasis with bile duct injury following azathioprine therapy: a case report. Liver 1991;11:89–93.
780. Duvoux C, Kracht M, Lang P et al. Hyperplasie nodulaire régénérative du foie associée à la prise d'azathioprine. Gastroenterol Clin Biol 1991;15:968–973.
781. Mion F, Napoleon B, Berger F et al. Azathioprine in-

duced liver disease: nodular regenerative hyperplasia of the liver and perivenous fibrosis in a patient treated for multiple sclerosis. Gut 1991;32:715–717.
782. Wagoner L, Olsen S, Bristow M et al. Cyclophosphamide as an alternative to azathioprine in cardiac transplant recipients with suspected azathioprine-induced hepatotoxicity. Transplantation 1993;56:1415–1418.
783. Mion F, Cloix P, Boillot O, et al. Maladie veino-occlusive après transplantation hépatique. Association d'un rejet aiguë cellulaire et de la toxicité de l'azathioprine. Gastroenterol Clin Biol 1993;17:863–867.
784. Sterneck M, Wiesner R, Ascher N et al. Azathioprine hepatotoxicity after liver transplantation. Hepatology, 1991;14:806–810.
785. Frick T, Fryd D, Goodale R et al. Lack of association between azathioprine and acute pancreatitis in renal transplantation patients. Lancet 1991;337:251.
786. Pillans P, Tooke A, Bateman E, Ainslie G. Acute polyarthritis associated with azathioprine for interstitial lung disease. Resp Med 1995;89:63–64.
787. Posthuma E, Westendorp R, van der Sluys Veer A et al. Fatal infectious mononucleosis: a severe complication in the treatment of Crohn's disease with azathioprine. Gut 1995;36:311–313.
788. Suassuna J, Machado R, Sampaio J et al. Active cytomegalovirus infection in hemodialysis patients receiving donor-specific blood transfusions under azathioprine coverage. Transplantation 1993;56:1552–1554.
789. Saway P, Heck L, Bonner J, Kirklin J. Azathioprine hypersensitivity. Case report and review of the literature. Am J Med 1988;84:960–964.
790. Wilson B, Parsonnet J. Azathioprine hypersensitivity mimicking sepsis in a patient with Crohn's disease. Clin Infect Dis 1993;17:940–941.
791. Jeurissen M, Boerbooms A, van de Putte L, Kruijsen M. Azathioprine induced fever, chills, rash, and hepatotoxicity in rheumatoid arthritis. Ann Rheum Dis 1990;49:25–27.
792. Meys E, Devogelaer J, Geubel A et al. Fever, hepatitis and acute interstitial nephritis in a patient with rheumatoid arthritis. Concurrent manifestations of azathioprine hypersensitivity. J Rheumatol 1992;19:807–809.
793. Refabert L, Sinnassamy P, Leroy B et al. Azathioprine-induced pulmonary haemorrhage in a child after renal transplantation. Pediatr Nephrol 1995;9:470–473.
794. Godeau B, Paul M, Autegarden J et al. Hypersensitivity to azathioprine mimicking gastroenteritis. Absence of recurrence with 6-mercaptopurine. Gastroenterol Clin Biol 1995; 19:117–119.
795. Stetter M, Schmidli M, Krapf R. Azathioprine hypersensitivity mimicking Goodpasture's syndrome. Am J Kidney Dis 1994;23:874–877.
796. Jones J, Ashworth J. Azathioprine-induced shock in dermatology patients. J Am Acad Dermatol 1993;29(Part 1):795–796.
797. Burden A, Beck M. Contact hypersensitivity to azathioprine. Contact Dermatitis 1992;27:329–330.
798. Garcia-Ortiz R, De Los Angeles Rodriguez M. Pancytopenia associated with the interaction of allopurinol and azathioprine. J Pharm Technol 1992;7:224–226.
799. Taylor A, Shuster S. Skin cancer after renal transplantation: the causal role of azathioprine. Acta Dermatol Venereol 1992;72:115–119.
800. Silman A, Petrie J, Hazleman B, Evans S. Lymphoproliferative cancer and other malignancy in patients with rheumatoid arthritis treated with azathioprine: a 20 year follow up study. Ann Rheum Dis 1988;47:988–992.
801. Connell W, Kamm M, Dickson M et al. Long-term neoplasia risk after azathioprine treatment in inflammatory bowel disease. Lancet 1994;343:1249–1252.
802. Larvol L, Soule J, Le Tourneau A. Reversible lymphoma in the setting of azathioprine therapy for Crohn's disease. N Engl J Med 1994;331:883–884.
803. Krishnan K, Adams P, Silveira S et al. Therapy-related acute myeloid leukaemia following immunosuppression with azathioprine for polymyositis. Clin Lab Haematol 1994; 16:285–289.
804. Mok C, Kwong Y, Lau C. Secondary acute myeloid leukaemia with 7q-complicating azathioprine treatment for rheumatoid arthritis. Ann Rheum Dis 1995;54:155–156.
805. Bottomley W, Ford G, Cunliffe W, Cotterill J. Aggressive squamous cell carcinomas developing in patients receiving long-term azathioprine. Br J Dermatol 1995;133:460–462.
806. Fraiser LH, Kanekal S, Kehrer JP. Cyclophosphamide toxicity. Characterising and avoiding the problem. Drugs 1991;42:781–795.
807. Omdal R, Husby G, Koldingsnes W. Intravenous and oral cyclophosphamide pulse therapy in rheumatic diseases: side effects and complications. Clin Exp Rheumatol 1993; 11:283–288.
808. Diaz-Gonzalez F, Castaneda-Sanz S, Lopez-Robledillo J, Garcia-Vicuna R. Lung fibrosis in a patient with polyarteritis nodosa receiving cyclophosphamide therapy. J Rheumatol 1992;19:325–327.
809. Queffeulou G, Ducloux D, Faucher C et al. Fatal cyclophosphamide-induced interstitial pneumonitis in a renal transplant patient. Nephrol Dial Transplant 1994;9:1655–1657.
810. Morgenstren L, Pardo C. Progressive multifocal leukoencephalopathy complicating treatment for Wegener's granulomatosis. J Rheumatol 1995;22:1593–1595.
811. Langevitz P, Klein L, Pras M, Many A. The effect of cyclophosphamide pulses on fertility in patients with lupus nephritis. Am J Reprod Immunol 1992;28:157–158.
812. Wang CL, Wang F, Bosco JJ. Ovarian failure in oral cyclophosphamide treatment for systemic erythematosus. Lupus 1995;4:11–14
813. McCarron M, Wright G, Roberts S. Water intoxication after low dose cyclophosphamide. Br Med J 1995;311:292.
814. Du L, Rigaud D, Papo T. Cyclophosphamide-induced hepatitis in Wegener's granulomatosis. Mayo Clin Proc 1994;69:912–913.
815. Snyder L, Heigh R, Anderson M. Cyclophosphamide-induced hepatotoxicity in a patient with Wegener's granulomatosis. Mayo Clin Proc 1993;68:1203–1204.
816. Cleland B, Pokorny C. Cyclophosphamide related hepatotoxicity. Aust NZ J Med 1993;23:408.
817. Milford D, Butler N, Clarke R et al. Reversible hepatic dysfunction in association with cyclophosphamide therapy. Eur J Pediatr 1995;154:411–412.
818. Modzelewski JR, Daeschner C, Joshi VV et al. Veno-occlusive disease of the liver induced by low-dose cyclophosphamide. Mod Pathol 1994;7:967–972.
819. Arend S, Hagen E, Kroes A et al. Activation of chronic hepatitis C virus infection by cyclophosphamide in a patient with cANCA-positive vasculitis. Nephrol Dial Transplant 1995;10:884–887.
820. Bradley JD, Brandt KD, Katz BP. Infectious complica-

tions of cyclophosphamide treatment for vasculitis. Arthr Rheum 1989;32:45–53.
821. Godeau B, Coutant-Perronne V, Le Thi Huong D et al. *Pneumocystis carinii* pneumonia in the course of connective tissue disease: report of 34 cases. J Rheumatol 1994;21:246–251.
822. Jarrousse B, Guillevin L, Bindi P et al. Increased risk of Pneumocystis carinii pneumonia in patients with Wegener's granulomatosis. Clin Exp Rhumatol 1993;11:615–621.
823. Porges AJ, Beattie SL, Ritchlin C et al. Patients with systemic lupus erythematosus at risk for *Pneumocystis carinii* pneumonia. J Rheumatol 1992;19:1191–1194.
824. Kattwinkel N, Cook L, Agnello V. Overwhelming fatal infection in a young woman after intravenous cyclophosphamide therapy for lupus nephritis. J Rheumatol 1991;18:79–81.
825. Cromar B, Colvin M, Casale T. Validity of skin tests to cyclophosphamide and metabolites. J Allerg Clin Immunol 1991;88:965–967.
826. Knysak D, McLean J, Solomon W et al. Immediate hypersensitivity reaction to cyclophosphamide. Arthr Rheum 1994;37:1101–1104.
827. Popescu N, Sheehan M, Kouides P et al. Allergic reactions to cyclophosphamide: delayed clinical expression associated with positive immediate skin tests to drug metabolites in five patients. J Allerg Clin Immunol 1995;95:288.
828. Travis L, Curtis R, Glimelius B et al. Bladder and kidney cancer following cyclophosphamide therapy for non-Hodgkin's lymphoma. J Natl Cancer Inst 1995;87:524–530.
829. Radis C, Kwoh C, Morgan M et al. Risk of malignancy in cyclophosphamide treated patients with rheumatoid arthritis: a 20-year follow-up study. Arthr Rheum 1993; 36(Suppl):R19.
830. Stein J, Skinner E, Boyd S, Skinner D. Squamous cell carcinoma of the bladder associated with cyclophosphamide therapy for Wegener's granulomatosis: a report of two cases. J Urol 1993;149:588–589.
831. Petterson T, Pukkala E, Teppo L, Friman C. Increased risk of cancer in patients with systemic lupus erythematosus. Ann Rheum Dis 1992;51:437–439.
832. Landewe R, Goei H, van Rijthoven A et al. Cyclosporine in common clinical practice: an estimation of the benefit/risk ratio in patients with rheumatoid arthritis. J Rheumatol 1994;21:1631–1636.
833. Zachariae H, Olsen T. Efficacy of cyclosporin A (CyA) in psoriasis: an overview of dose/response, indications, contraindications and side-effects. Clin Nephrol 1995;43:154–158.
834. Brazier F, Finet L, Duchmann J, Dupas J. Ciclosporine A et maladies inflammatoires chroniques du tube digestif. Gastroenterol Clin Biol 1995;19:494–504.
835. Helderman J, van Buren D, Amend W, Pirsch J. Chronic immunosuppression of the renal transplant patient. J Am Soc Nephrol 1994;4(Suppl 8):S2–S9.
836. Azoulay D, Lemoine A, Dennison A et al. Incidence of adverse reations to cyclosporine after liver transplantation is predicted by the first blood level. Hepatology 1993;18:1123–1126.
837. Noble S, Markham A. Cyclosporin. A review of the pharmacokietic properties, clinical efficacy and tolerability of a microemulsion-based formulation (Neoral®). Drugs 1995;50:924–941.
838. Thiel G, Bock A, Spöndlin M et al. Long-term benefits and risks of cyclosporin A (Sandimmun). An analysis at 10 years. Transplant Proc 1994;26:2493–2498.
839. Graham R. Cyclosporine: mechanisms of action and toxicity. Clev Clin J Med 1994;61:308–313.
840. Sturrock N, Lang C, Struthers A. Cyclosporin-induced hypertension precedes renal dysfunction and sodium retention in man. J Hypertension 1993;11:1209–1216.
841. Davenport A. The effect of renal transplantation and treatment with cyclosporin A on the prevalence of Raynaud's phenomenon. Clin Transplant 1993;7:4–8.
842. de Groen P, Aksamit A, Rakela J et al. Central nervous system toxicity after liver transplantation. The role of cyclosporin and cholesterol. N Engl J Med 1987;317:861–866.
843. Cilio M, Danhaive O, Gadisseux J et al. Unusual cyclosporin related neurological complications in recipients of liver transplants. Arch Dis Child 1993;68:405–407.
844. Welge-Lussen U, Gerhartz H. Late onset of neurotoxicity with cyclosporin. Lancet 1994;343:293.
845. Bernstein L, Levin R. Catatonia responsive to intravenous lorazepam in a patient with cyclosporine neurotoxicity and hypomagnesemia. Psychosomatics 1993;34:102–103.
846. Steiger M, Farrah T, Rolles K et al. Cyclosporin associated headache. J Neurol Neurosurg Psychiatry 1994; 57:1258–1259.
847. Combarros O, Fabrega E, Polo J, Berciano J. Cyclosporine-induced chorea after liver transplantation for Wilson's disease. Ann Neurol 1993;33:108–109.
848. Monteiro L, Almeida-Pinto J, Rocha N et al. Case report: cyclosporin A-induced neurotoxicity. Br J Radiol 1993;66:271–272.
849. Shimizu C, Kimura S, Yoshida Y et al. Acute leucoencephalopathy during cyclosporin A therapy in a patient with nephrotic syndrome. Pediatr Nephrol 1994;8:483–485.
850. Reece D, Frei-Lahr D, Sheperd J et al. Neurologic complications in allogeneic bone marrow transplant patients receiving cyclosporin. Bone Marrow Transplant 1991; 8:393–401.
851. Schwartz R, Bravo S, Klufas R et al. Cyclosporine neurotoxicity and its relationship to hypertensive encephalopathy: CT and MR findings in 16 cases. Am J Roentgenol 1995;165:627–631.
852. Ghany A, Tutschka P, McGhee R et al. Cyclosporine-associated seizures in bone marrow transplant recipients given busulfan and cyclophosphamide preparative therapy. Transplantation 1991;52:310–315.
853. Kirk J, Dupuis R. Approaches to the treatment of hyperlipidemia in the solid organ transplant recipient. Ann Pharmacother 1995;29:879–891.
854. Hricik D. Posttransplant hyperlipidemia: the treatment dilema. Am J Kidney Dis 1994;23:766–771.
855. Kuster G, Drexel H, Bleisch J et al. Relation of cyclosporine blood levels to adverse effects on lipoproteins. Transplantation 1994;57:1479–1483.
856. Isoniemi H, Ahonen J, Tikkanen M et al. Long-term consequences of different immunosuppressive regimens for renal allografts. Transplantation 1993;55:494–499.
857. Lin H, Rocher L, McQuillan M et al. Cyclosporine-induced hyperuricemia and gout. N Engl J Med 1989; 321:287–292.
858. Ben Hmida M, Hachicha J, Bahloul Z et al. Cyclosporine-induced hyperuricemia and gout in renal transplants. Transplant Proc 1995;27:2722–2724.
859. Baethge B, Work J, Landreneau M, McDonald J. Tophaceous gout in patients with renal transplants treated with cyclosporine. J Rheumatol 1993;20:718–720.
860. Kamel K, Ethier J, Quaggin S et al. Studies to

determine the basis for hyperkalemia in recipients of a renal transplant who are treated with cyclosporine. J Am Soc Nephrol 1992;2:1279–1284.
861. Nozue T, Kobayashi A, Kodama T et al. Pathogenesis of cyclosporine-induced hypomagnesemia. J Pediatr 1992;120:638–640.
862. Thomas M, Hannoun L, Loria A. Hypercalcémie liée au traitement par ciclosporine A chez un transplanté hépatique. Presse Med 1994;23:51.
863. Faure J, Causse X, Bergeret A et al. Cyclosporine induced hemolytic anemia in a liver transplant patient. Transplant Proc 1989;21:2242–2243.
864. Rougier J, Viron B, Ronco P et al. Autoimmune haemolytic anaemia after ABO-match, ABDR full match kidney transplantation. Nephrol Dial Transplant 1994; 9:693–697.
865. Azer S, Stacey N. Cyclosporine-induced interference with uptake of bile acids by human hepatocytes. Transplant Proc 1993;25:2892–2893.
866. Bluhm R, Rodgers W, Black D et al. Cholestasis in transplant patients. What is the role of cyclosporin? Aliment Pharmacol Ther 1992;6:207–219.
867. Cadranel J, Erlinger S, Desruenne M et al. Chronic administration of cyclosporin A induces a decrease in hepatic excretory function in man. Dig Dis Sci 1992;37:1473–1476.
868. Moore R, Greenberg E, Tangen L. Cyclosporine-induced worsening of hepatic dysfunction in a patient with Crohn's disease and enterocutaneous fistula. South Med J 1995;88:843–844.
869. Murphy E, Morris A, Walker E et al. Cyclosporine A induced colitis and acquired selective IgA deficiency in a patient with juvenile chronic arthritis. J Rheumatol 1993;20:1397–1398.
870. Bowen J, Sahi S. Cyclosporin induced colitis. Br Med J 1993;307:484.
871. Bennett W. The nephrotoxicity of immunosuppressive drugs. Clin Nephrol 1995;43(Suppl 1):S3–S7.
872. Leong S, Lye W, Tan C, Lee E. Acute cyclosporine A nephrotoxicity in a renal allograft recipient with hypothyroidism. Am J Kidney Dis 1995;25:503–505.
873. Hochstetler L, Flanigan M, Lager D. Transplant-associated thrombotic microangiopathy: the role of IgG administration as initial therapy. Am J Kidney Dis 1994;23:444–450.
874. Dhib M, Moulin B, Abderrahim E et al. Cyclosporine-associated thrombotic microangiopathy: report of two cases with good outcome and successful subsequent reuse. Transplant Proc 1993;25:2294–2296.
875. Myers R, Ross J, Newton L et al. Cyclosporine-associated chronic nephropathy. N Engl J Med 1984;311:699–705.
876. Ben-Maimon C, Burke J, Besarab A et al Evidence against chronic progressive cyclosporine nephrotoxicity. Transplant Proc 1991;23:1260–1262.
877. Almond P, Gillingham K, Sibley R et al. Renal transplant function after ten years of cyclosporine. Transplantation 1992;53:316–323.
878. Burke J, Pirsch J, Ramos E et al. Long-term efficacy and safety of cyclosporine in renal-transplant recipients. N Engl J Med 1994;331:358–363.
879. Mihatsch M, Morozumi K, Strom E et al. Renal transplant morphology after long-term therapy with cyclosporine. Transplant Proc 1995;27:39–42.
880. Beveridge T, Calne R. Cyclosporine (Sandimmun) in cadaveric renal transplantation. Ten-year follow-up of a multicenter trial. Transplantation 1995;59:1568–1570.
881. Van Buren D, Burke J, Lewis R. Renal function in patients receiving long-term cyclosporine therapy. J Am Soc Nephrol (1994) 4, S17-S22.
882. Greenberg A, Thompson M, Griffith B et al. Cyclosporine nephrotoxicity in cardiac allograft patients—A seven-year follow-up. Transplantation 1990;50:589–593.
883. Sehgal V, Radhakrishnan J, Appel G et al. Progressive renal insuffisiency following cardiac transplantation: cyclosporine, lipids, and hypertension. Am J Kidney Dis 1995;26:193–201.
884. Gonwa T, Klintmalm G, Levy M et al. Impact of pretransplant renal function on survival after liver transplantation. Transplantation 1995;59:361–365.
885. Zaltzman J, Pei Y, Maurer J et al. Cyclosporin nephrotoxicity in lung transplant recipients. Transplantation 1992;54:875–878.
886. Ruggenenti P, Perico N, Amuchastegui S et al. Following an initial decline, glomerular filtration rate stabilizes in heart transplant patients on chronic cyclosporine. Am J Kidney Dis 1994;24:549–553.
887. Kuo P, Luikart H, Busse-Henry S et al. Clinical outcome of interval cadaveric renal transplantation in cardiac allograft recipients. Clin Transplant 1995;9:92–97.
888. Bunke M, Sloan R, Brier M, Ganzel B. An improved glomerular filtration rate in cardiac transplant recipients with once-a-day cyclosporine dosing. Transplantation 1995; 59:537–540.
889. Brown A, Wilkinson R, Thomas T et al. The effect of short-term low-dose cyclosporine on renal function and blood pressure in patients with psoriasis. Br J Dermatol 1993;128:550–555.
890. Feutren G, Mihatsch MJ. Risk factors of cyclosporine-induced nephropathy in patients with autoimmune diseases. N Engl J Med 1992;326:1654–1660.
891. Habib R, Niaudet P. Comparison between pre- and posttreatment renal biopsies in children receiving ciclosporine for idiopathic nephrosis. Clin Nephrol 1994;42:141–146.
892. Korstanje M, Bilo H, Stoof T. Sustained renal function loss in psoriasis patients after withdrawal of low-dose cyclosporin therapy. Br J Dermatol 1992;127:501–504.
893. Pei Y, Scholey J, Katz A et al. Chronic nephrotoxicity in psoriatic patients treated with low-dose cyclosporine. Am J Kidney Dis 1994;23:528–536.
894. Young E, Ellis C, Messana J et al. A prospective study of renal structure and function in psoriasis patients treated with cyclosporin. Kidney Int 1994;45:1216–1222.
895. Mihatsch M, Antonovych T, Bohman S et al. Cyclosporin A nephropathy: standardization of the evaluation of kidney biopsies. Clin Nephrol 1994;41:23–32.
896. Niaudet P. La néphrotoxicité de la ciclosporine est-elle inéluctable? Presse Med 1994;23:1061–1063.
897. Delmonico F, Tolkoff-Rubin N, Auchincloss H et al. Management of the renal allograft recipient: immunosuppressive protocols for long-term sucess. Clin Transplant 1994;8:34–39.
898. Kasiske B, Heim-Duthoy K, Ma J. Elective cyclosporine withdrawal after renal transplantation: a meta-analysis. J Am Med Assoc 1993;269:395–400.
899. Sanders C, Curtis J, Julian B et al. Tapering or discontinuing of cyclosporine for financial reasons: a single center experience. Am J Kidney Dis 1993;21:9–15.
900. Heim-Duthoy K, Chitwood K, Tortorice K et al. Elec-

tive cyclosporine withdrawal 1 year after renal transplantation. Am J Kidney Dis 1994;24:846–853.
901. Smith S, Minda S, Samsa G et al. Late withdrawal of cyclosporine in stable renal transplant recipients. Am J Kidney Dis 1995;26:487–494.
902. Opelz G. Effect of the maintenance immunosuppressive drug regimen on kidney transplant outcome. Transplantation 1994;58:443–446.
903. McCulloch T, Harper S, Donnelly P et al. Influence of nifedipine on interstitial fibrosis in renal transplant allograft treated with cyclosporin A. J Clin Pathol 1994;47:839–842.
904. Wilkie M, Beer J, Evans S et al. A double-blind, randomized, placebo-controlled study of nifedipine on early renal allograft function. Nephrol Dial Transplant 1994; 9:800–804.
905. Halpert E, Tunnessen W, Fivush B, Case B. Cutaneous lesions associated with cyclosporine therapy in pediatric renal transplant recipients. J Pediatr 1991;119:489–491.
906. Wakelin S, Emmerson R. Excess granulation tissue development during treatment with cyclosporin. Br J Dermatol 1994;131:147–148.
907. Olujohungbe A, Cox J, Hammon MD, Prentice HG. Ingrowing toenails and cyclosporin. Lancet 1993;342:1111.
908. Seymour R. Drug-induced gingival overgrowth. Adverse Drug React Toxicol Rev 1993;12:215–232.
909. Hefti A, Eshenaur A, Hassell T, Stone C. Gingival overgrowth in cyclosporin A treated multiple sclerosis patients. J Periodontol 1994;65:744–749.
910. Thomason J, Seymour R, Ellis J et al. Iatrogenic gingival overgrowth in cardiac transplantation. J Periodontol 1995;66:742–746.
911. Wondimu B, Dahllöf G, Berg U, Modéer T. Cyclosporin-A-induced gingival overgrowth in renal transplant children. Scand J Dental Res 1993;101:282–286.
912. Sooriyamoorthy M, Gower D, Eley B. Androgen metabolism in gingival hyperplasia induced by nifedipine and cyclosporin. J Periodontol Res 1990;25:25–30.
913. Bökenkamp A, Bohnhorst B, Beier C et al. Nifedipine aggravates cyclosporine A-induced gingival hyperplasia. Pediatr Nephrol 1994;8:181–185.
914. Thomason J, Seymour R, Rice N. The prevalence and severity of cyclosporin and nifedipine-induced gingival overgrowth. J Clin Periodontol 1993;20:37–40.
915. O'Valle F, Mesa F, Gomez-Morales M et al. Immunohistochemical study of 30 cases of cyclosporin A-induced gingival overgrowth. J Periodontol 1994;65:724–730.
916. Mariani G, Calastrini C, Carinci F et al. Ultrastructural features of cyclosporin A-induced gingival hyperplasia. J Periodontol 1993;64:1092–1097.
917. Wahlstrom E, Zamora J, Teichman S. Improvement in cyclosporine-associated gingival hyperplasia with azithromycin therapy. N Engl J Med 1995;332:753–754.
918. Wong W, Hodge M, Lewis A et al. Resolution of cyclosporin-induced gingival hypertrophy with metronidazole. Lancet 1994;343:986.
919. Arellano F, Krupp P. Muscular disorders associated with cyclosporin. Lancet 1991;337:45.
920. Barbosa L, Gauthier V, Davis C. Bone pain that responds to calcium channel blockers. A retrospective and prospective study of transplant recipients. Transplantation 1995;59:541–544.
921. Dumoulin G, Hory B, Nguyen N et al. Lack of evidence that cyclosporine treatment impairs calcium-phosphorus homeostasis and bone remodelling in normocalcemic long-term renal transplant recipients. Transplantation 1995;59:1690–1694.
922. McIntyre H, Menzies B, Rigby R et al. Long-term bone loss after renal transplantation: comparison of immunosuppressive regimens. Clin Transplant 1995;9:20–24.
923. Hokken-Koelega A, van Zaal M, de Ridder M et al. Growth after renal transplantation in prepubertal children: impact of various treatment modalities. Pediatr Res 1994; 35:367–371.
924. Howrie D, Ptachcinski R, Griffith B et al. Anaphylactoid reactions associated with parenteral cyclosporin use: possible role of cremophor EL. Drug Intell Clin Pharm 1985;19:425–427.
925. Friedman L, Dienstag J, PWN et al. Anaphylactic reaction and cardiopulmonary arrest following intravenous cyclosporine. Am J Med 1985;78:343–345.
926. Arellano F, Monka C, Krupp P. Acute cyclosporin overdose. A review of present clinical experience. Drug Safety 1991;6:226–276.
927. Sketris I, Onorato L, Yatscoff R et al. Eight day of cyclopsorin overdose: a case report. Pharmacotherapy 1993;13:658–660.
928. Fahr A. Cyclosporin clinical pharmacokinetics. Clin Pharmacokinet 1993;24:472–495.
929. Pichard L, Fabre I, Fabre G et al. Cyclosporin A drug interactions. Screening for inducers and inhibitors of cytochrome P-450 (cyclosporin A oxidase) in primary culture of human hepatocytes and in liver microsomes. Drug Metabol Disp 1990;18:595–606.
930. Billaud E, Ropers J, Fortineau N et al. Analyse critique des interactions médicamenteuses de la ciclosporine. Therapie 1992;47:335–342.
931. Chan G, Sinnott J, Emmanuel P et al. Drug interactions with cyclosporine: focus on antimicrobials. Clin Transplant 1992;6:141–153.
932. Yee G, McGuire T. Pharmacokinetic drugs interaction with cyclosporin (Part I). Clin Pharmacokinet 1990;19:319–332.
933. Yew G, McGuire T. Pharmacokinetic drug interactions with cyclosporin (Part II). Clin Pharmacokinet 1990;19:400–415.
934. Vincent F, Glotz D, Kreft-Jais C et al. Insuffisance rénale aiguë chez un transplanté rénal traité par cyclosporine A et métronidazole. Therapie 1994;49:155.
935. Chitwood K, Abdul-Haqq A, Heim-Duthoy K. Cyclosporine-amiodarone interaction. Ann Pharmacother 1993; 27:569–571.
936. Mamprin F, Mullins P, Graham T et al. Amiodarone-cyclosporine interaction in cardiac transplantation. Am Heart J 1992;123:1725–1726.
937. Gilbert R, Kahn D, Cassidy M. Interaction between clonidine and cyclosporine A. Nephron 1995;71:105.
938. Gorrie M, Beaman M, Nicholls A, Backwell P. Allopurinol interaction with cyclosporin. Br Med J 1994;308:113.
939. Nampoory M, Nessim J, Gupta R, Johny K. Drug interaction of chloroquine with ciclosporin. Nephron 1992; 62:108–109.
940. Passfall J, Schuller I, Keller F. Pharmacokinetics of cyclosporin during administration of danazol. Nephrol Dial Transplant 1994;9:1807–1808.
941. Ducharme M, Warbasse L, Edwards D. Disposition of intravenous and oral cyclosporine after administration with grapefruit juice. Clin Pharmacol Ther 1995;57:485–491.
942. Proppe D, Hoch O, McLean A, Visser K. Influence of

chronic ingestion of grapefruit juice on steady-state blood concentrations of cyclosporine A in renal transplant patients with stable graft function. Br J Clin Pharmacol 1995;39:337–338.
943. Yee G, Stanley D, Pessa L et al. Effect of grapefruit juice on blood cyclosporin concentration. Lancet 1995; 345:955–956.
944. Abu-Romeh S, Rashed A. Ciclosporin A and griseofulvin: another drug interaction. Nephron 1991;58:237.
945. Gallego C, Sanchez P, Planells C et al. Interaction between probucol and cyclosporine in renal transplant patients. Ann Pharmacother 1994;28:940–943.
946. Jimenez del Corro L, Hernandez F. Effect of pyrazinamide on ciclosporin levels. Nephron 1992;62:113.
947. Spes C, Angermann C, Stempfle H et al. Sulfadiazine therapy for toxoplasmosis in heart transplant recipients decreases cyclosporine concentration. Clin Invest 1992; 70:752–754.
948. Vinot O, Cochat P, Dubourg-Derain L et al. Jaundice associated with concomitant use of norethandrolone and cyclosporine. Transplantation 1993;56:470–471.
949. Wood P, Liu Y, JA. Oxymetholone hepatotoxicity enhanced by concomitant use of cyclosporin A in a bone marrow transplant patient. Clin Lab Haematol 1994;16:201–204.
950. Amsden G. Macrolides versus azalides: a drug interaction update. Ann Pharmacother 1995;29:906–917.
951. Ljuti D, Rumboldt Z. Possible interaction between azithromycin and cyclosporin. Nephron 1995;70:130.
952. Ferrari S, Goffin E, Mourad M et al. The interaction between clarithromycin and cyclosporine in kidney transplant recipients. Transplantation 1994;58:725–727.
953. Finielz P, Mondon J, Chuet C, Guisereix J. Drug interaction between midecamycin and cyclosporin. Nephron 1995;70:136.
954. Hoey L, Lake K. Does ciprofloxacin interact with cyclosporine? Ann Pharmacother 1994;28:93–96.
955. Wynckel A, Toupance O, Melin J et al. Traitement des légionelloses par ofloxacine chez le transplanté rénal. Absence d'interférence avec la ciclosporine A. Presse Med 1991;20:291–293.
956. Jahansouz F, Kriett J, Smith C, Jamieson S. Potentiation of cyclosporine nephrotoxicity by nafcillin in lung transplant recipients. Transplantation 1993;55:1045–1048.
957. Ahmed T, Fenton T, McGraw M. Reversible renal failure in renal transplant patients receiving acyclovir. Pediatr Nephrol (1993) 7, C58.
958. Duganzic R, Sketris I, Belitsky P et al. Effect of coadministration of acyclovir and cyclosporine on kidney function and cyclosporine concentrations in renal transplant patients. Ann Pharmacother 1991;25:316–317.
959. Morales J, Munoz M, Fernandez Zatarain G et al. Reversible acute renal failure caused by the combined use of foscarnet and cyclosporin in organ transplanted patients. Nephrol Dial Transplant 1995;10:882–883.
960. Cantarovich M, Latter D. Effect of prophylactic ganciclovir on renal function and cyclosporine levels after heart transplantation. Transplant Proc 1994;26:2747–2748.
961. Schouler L, Dumas F, Couzigou P et al. Omeprazole-cyclosporin interaction. Am J Gastroenterol 1991;86:1097.
962. Arranz R, Yanez E, Franceschi J, Fernandez-Ranada J. More about omeprazole-cyclosporine interaction. Am J Gastroenterol 1993;88:154–155.
963. Blohmé I, Idström J, Andersson T. A study of the interaction betwwen omeprazole and cyclosporine in renal transplant patients. Br J Clin Pharmacol 1993;35:156–160.
964. Albengres E, Tillement J. Cyclosporin and ketoconazole, drug interaction or therapeutic association. Int J Clin Pharmacol Ther Toxicol 1992;30:555–570.
965. First M, Schroeder T, Michael A et al. Cyclosporine-ketoconazole interaction. Long-term follow-up and preliminary results of a randomized trial. Transplantation 1993; 55:1000–1004.
966. Keogh A, Spratt P, McCosker C et al. Ketoconazole to reduce the need for cyclosporine after cardiac transplantation. N Engl J Med 1995;333:628–633.
967. Sketris I, Methot M, Nicol D et al. Effect of calcium-channel blockers on cyclosporine clearance and use in renal transplant patients. Ann Pharmacother 1994;28:1227–1331.
968. Smith C, Hampton E, Pederson J et al. Clinical and medicoeconomic impact of the cyclosporine-diltiazem interaction in renal transplant recipients. Pharmacotherapy 1994;14:471–481.
969. Vernillet L, Bourbigot B, Codet J et al. Lack of effect of isradipine on cyclosporin pharmacokinetics. Fund Clin Pharmacol 1992:6:367–374.
970. Toupance O, Lavaud S, Canivet E et al. Antihypertensive effect of amlodipine and lack of interference with cyclosporine metabolism in renal transplant recipients. Hypertension 1994;24:297–300.
971. Pedersen E, Sorensen S, Eiskjaer H et al. Interaction between cyclosporine and felodipine in renal transplant recipients. Kidney Int 1992;41(Suppl 36):S82–S86.
972. Blaison G, Weber J, Sachs D et al. Rhabdomyolyse causée par la simvastatine chez un transplanté cardiaque sous ciclosporine. Rev Med Interne 1992;13:61–63.
973. Corpier C, Jones P, Suki W et al. Rhabdomyolysis and renal injury with lovastatin use. Report of two cases in cardiac transplant recipients. J Am Med Assoc 1988;260:239–241.
974. Cheung A, DeVault G, Gregory M. A prospective study on treatment of hypercholesterolemia with lovastatin in renal transplant patients receiving cyclosporine. J Am Soc Nephrol 1993;3:1884–1891.
975. Kandus A, Kovac D, Koselj M et al. Lovastatin treatment of hyperlipidemia in kidney transplant recipients on cyclosporine immunosuppression. Transplant Proc 1994; 26:2642–2643.
976. Vanhaecke J, Cleemput J, Lierde J et al. Safety and efficacy of low dose simvastatin in cardiac transplant recipients treated with cyclosporine. Transplantation 1994; 58:42–45.
977. Goldberg R, Roth D. A preliminary report of the safety and effiacy of fluvastatin for hypercholesterolemia in renal transplant patients receiving cyclosporine. Am J Cardiol 1995;76:107A–109A.
978. Li P, Mak T, Wang A et al. The interaction of fluvastatin and cyclosporin A in renal transplant patients. Int J Clin Pharmacol Ther 1995;33:246–248.
979. Kobashigawa J, Katznelson S, Laks H et al. Effect of pravastatin on outcomes after cardiac transplantation. N Engl J Med 1995;333:621–627.
980. Yoshimura N, Ohmori Y, Tsuji T, Oka T. Effect of pravastatin on renal transplant recipients treated with cyclosporine—4-year follow-up. Transplant Proc 1994;26:2632–2633.
981. Isogai M, Shimida N, Kamataki T et al. Changes in the amounts of cytochromes P450 in rat hepatic microsomes produced by cyclosporin A. Xenobiotica 1993;23:799–807.

982. Rushing D, Raber S, Rodvold K et al. The effects of cyclosporine on the pharmacokinetics of doxorubicin in patients with small cell lung cancer. Cancer 1994;74:834–841.
983. European Mycophenolate Mofetil Cooperative Study Group. Placebo-controlled study of mycophenolate mofetil combined with cyclosporin and corticosteroids for prevention of acute rejection. Lancet 1995;345:1321–1325.
984. Sollinger HW. Mycophenolate mofetil for the prevention of acute rejection in primary cadaveric renal allograft recipients. Transplantation 1995;60:225–232.
985. Ensley R, Bristow M, Olsen S et al. The use of mycophenolate mofetil (RS-61443) in human heart transplant recipients. Transplantation 1993;56:75–82.
986. Hooks M. Tacrolimus, a new immunosuppressant. A review of the literature. Ann Pharmacother 1994;28:501–511.
987. Winkler M, Christians U. A risk-benefit assessment of tacrolimus in transplantation. Drug Safety 1995;12:348–357.
988. The US Multicenter FK506 Liver Study Group. A comparison of tacrolimus (FK506) and cyclosporine for immunosuppression in liver transplantation. N Engl J Med 1994;331:1110–1115.
989. European FK506 Multicentre Liver Study Group. Randomised trial comparing tacrolimus (FK506) and cyclosporin in prevention of liver allograft rejection. Lancet 1994; 344:423–428.
990. Alessiani M, Cillo U, Fung J et al. Adverse effects of FK506 overdosage after liver transplantation. Transplant Proc 1993;25:628–634.
991. Mor E, Sheiner P, Schwartz M et al. Reversal of severe FK506 side effects by conversion to cyclosporine-based immunosuppresion. Transplantation 1994;58:380–382.
992. Atkinson P, Joubert G, Barron A et al. Hypertrophic cardiomyopathy associated with tacrolimus in paediatric transplant patients. Lancet 1995;345:894–896.
993. Natazuka T, Ogawa R, Kizaki T et al. Immunosuppressive drugs and hypertrophic cardiomyopathy. Lancet 1995; 345:1644.
994. Mueller A, Platz K, Bechstein W et al. Neurotoxicity after orthotopic liver transplantation. A comparison between cyclosporin and FK506. Transplantation 1994;58:155–170.
995. Burkhalter E, Starzl T, Van Thiel D. Severe neurological complications following orthotopic liver transplantation in patients receiving FK 506 and prednisone. J Hepatol 1994;21:572–577.
996. Wijdicks E, Wiesner R, Dahlke L, Krom R. FK 506-induced neurotoxicity in liver transplantation. Ann Neurol 1994;35:498–501.
997. Ayres R, Dousset B, Wixon S et al. Peripheral neurotoxicity with tacrolimus. Lancet 1994;343:862–863.
998. Bronster D, Yonover P, Stein J et al. Demyelinating sensorimotor polyneuropathy after administration of FK 506. Transplantation 1995;59:1066–1068.
999. Krentz A, Dmitrewski J, Mayer D et al. Postoperative glucose metabolism in liver transplant recipients. A two-year prospective randomized study of cyclosporine versus FK506. Transplantation 1994;57:1666–1669.
1000. Jindal R, Popescu I, Schwartz M et al. Diabetogenicity of FK506 versus cyclosporine in liver tranplant recipients. Transplantation 1994;58:370–372.
1001. Abouljoud MS, Levy MF, Klintmalm GB. Hyperlipidemia after liver transplantation: long term results of the FK506/cyclosporine US multicenter trial. Transplant Proc 1995;27:1121–1123.
1002. Abu-Elmagd K, Bronsther O, Kobayashi M et al. Acute hemolytic anemia in liver and bone marrow transplant patients under FK 506 therapy. Transplant Proc 1991; 23:3190–3192.
1003. Winkler M, Schulze F, Jost U et al. Anaemia associated with FK 506 immunosuppression. Lancet 1993; 341:1035–1036.
1004. Fisher A, Mor E, Hytiroglou P et al. FK506 hepatotoxicity in liver allograft recipients. Transplantation 1995;59: 1631–1632.
1005. Bäckman L, Nicar M, Levy M et al. Chronic nephrotoxicity of FK 506 after liver transplantation. Transplant Proc 1994;26:1803.
1006. Connolly J, Gane E, Higgins R. Renal arteriopathy associated with FK 506 therapy following liver transplantation. Nephrol Dial Transplant 1994;9:834–836.
1007. Platz K, Mueller A, Blumhardt G et al. Nephrotoxicity following orthotopic liver transplantation. A comparison between cyclosporine and FK506. Transplantation 1994; 58:170–178.
1008. Porayko M, Gonwa T, Klintmalm G, Wiesner R. Comparing nephrotoxicity of FK506 and cyclosporine regimens after liver transplantation: preliminary results from US multicenter trial. Transplant Proc 1995;27:1114–1116.
1009. Holman M, Gonwa T, Cooper B et al. FK506-associated thrombotic thrombocytopenic purpura. Transplantation 1993;55:205–206.
1010. Ichihashi T, Naoe T, Yoshida H et al. Haemolytic uraemic syndrome during FK506 therapy. Lancet 1992; 340:60–61.
1011. Schmidt R, Venkat K, Dumler F. Hemolytic-uremic syndrome in a renal transplant recipient on FK 506 immunosuppression. Transplant Proc 1991;23:3156–3157.
1012. Kaufman D, Kaplan B, Kanwar Y et al. The successful use of tacrolimus (FK506) in a pancreas/kidney transplant recipient with recurrent cyclosporine-associated hemolytic uremic syndrome. Transplantation 1995;59:1737–1739.
1013. Williams M, Lewis D. Hyperuricemic acute renal failure associated with FK506 nephrotoxicity. Clin Transplant 1992;6:194–195.
1014. Hadley S, Samore M, Lewis W et al. Major infectious complications after orthotopic liver transplantation and comparison of outcomes in patients receiving cyclosporine or FK506 as primary immunosuppression. Transplantation 1995;59:851–859.
1015. Cox K, Lawrence-Miyasaki L, Garcia-Kennedy R et al. An increased incidence of Epstein-barr virus infection and lymphoproliferative disorder in young children on FK506 after liver transplantation. Transplantation 1995;59:524–529.
1016. Reyes J, Tzakis A, Green M et al. Posttransplant lyphoproliferative disorders occurring under primary FK506 immunosuppression. Transplant Proc 1991;23:3044–3046.
1017. Mrvos R, Hodgman M, Dean B et al. FK506 overdose: a report of four cases. J Toxicol Clin Toxicol 1995;33:487.
1018. Hopp L, Lobardozzi S, Gilboa N et al. Removal of FK 506 by continuous hemofiltration: report of two allograft recipients with renal and liver failures. Clin Transplant 1993;7:546–551.
1019. Iwasaki K, Matsuda H, Nagase K et al. Effects of twenty-three drugs on the metabolism of FK506 by human liver microsomes. Res Commun Chem Pathol Pharmacol 1993;82:209–216.
1020. Prasad T, Stiff D, Subbotina N et al. FK506 (tacroli-

mus) metabolism by rat liver microsomes and its inhibition by other drugs. Res Commun Chem Pathol Pharmacol 1994;84:35—46.
1021. Furlan V, Perello L, Jacquemin E et al. Interactions between FK506 and rifampicin or erythromycin in pediatric liver recipients. Transplantation 1995;59:1217—1218.
1022. Jensen C, Jordan M, Shapiro R et al. Interaction between tacrolimus and erythromycin. Lancet 1994;344:825.
1023. Shaeffer M, Collier D, Sorrell M. Interaction between FK506 and erythromycin. Ann Pharmacother 1994;28:280—281.
1024. Wolter K, Wagner K, Philipp T, Fritschka E. Interaction between FK506 and clarithomycin in a renal transplant patient. Eur. J Clin Pharmacol 1994;47:207—208.
1025. Braun F, Schutz E, Grupp C et al. Interaction of tacrolimus (FK-506) and fluconazole. Ther Drug Monit 1995; 17:397.
1026. Assan R, Fredj G, Larger E et al. FK506/fluconazole interaction enhances FK506 nephrotoxicity. Diabetes Metab 1994;20:49—52.
1027. Sheiner, PA, Mor E, Chodoff L et al. Acute renal failure associated with the use of ibuprofen in two liver transplant recipients on FK506. Transplantation 1994; 57:1132—1133.
1028. Norman D, Kahana L, Stuart F et al. A randomized clinical trial of induction therapy with OKT3 in kidney transplantation. Transplantation 1993;55:44—50.
1029. Abramowicz D, Norman D, Goldman M et al. OKT3 prophylaxis improves long-term renal graft survival in high-risk patients as compared to cyclosporine: combined results from the prospective, randomized Belgian and US studies. Transplant Proc 1995;27:852—853.
1030. Sgro C. Side-effects of a monoclonal antibody, muromonab CD3: orthoclone OKT3. Toxicology 1995;105:23—29.
1031. Jeyarajah D, Thistlethwaite J. General aspects of cytokine-release syndrome: timing and incidence of symptoms. Transplant Proc 1993;25(Suppl 1):16—20.
1032. Parlevliet K, Bemelman F, Yong S et al. Toxicity of OKT3 increases with dosage: a controlled study in renal transplant recipients. Transplant Int 1995;8:141—146.
1033. Vasquez E, Fabrega A, Pollak R. OKT3-induced cytokine-release syndrome: occurence beyond the second dose and association with rejection severity. Transplant Proc 1995;27:873—874.
1034. Norman D, Chatenoud L, Cohen D et al. Consensus statement regarding OKT3-induced cytokine-release syndrome and human antimouse antibodies. Transplant Proc 1993;25(Suppl 1):89—92.
1035. Peces R, Urra J, Escalada P et al. High-dose methylprednisolone inhibits the OKT3-induced cytokine-related syndrome. Nephron 1993;63:118.
1036. Bemelman F, Buysmann S, Wilmink J et al. Effects of divided doses of steroids on side effects, cytokines, and activation of complement and granulocytes, coagulation and fibrinolysis after OKT3. Transplant Proc 1994;26:3096—3097.
1037. First M, Schroeder T, Hariharan S, Weiskittel P. Reduction of the initial febrile response to OKT3 with indomethacin. Transplant Proc 1993;25(Suppl 1):52—54.
1038. Gaughan W, Francos B, Dunn S et al. A retrospective analysis of the effect of indomethacin on adverse reactions to orthoclone OKT3 in the therapy of acute renal allograft rejection. Am J Kidney Dis 1994;24:486—490.
1039. Brown M, Korb S, Light J et al. Low-dose OKT3 induction therapy following renal transplantation leads to improved graft function and decreased adverse effects. Transplant Proc 1993;25:553—555.
1040. Norman D, Kimball J, Bennett W et al. A prospective, double blind, randomized study of high-versus low-dose OKT3 induction immunosuppression in cadaveric renal transplantation. Transplant Int 1994;7:356—361.
1041. Chatenoud L. OKT3-induced cytokine-release syndrome: preventive effect of anti-tumour necrosis factor monoclonal antibody. Transplant Proc 1993;25(Suppl 1):47—51.
1042. Raasveld M, Bemelman F, Schellekens P et al. Complement activation during OKT3 treatment: a possible explanation for respiratory side effects. Kidney Int 1993; 43:1140—1149.
1043. Hall K, Dole E, Hunter G et al. Hyperpyrexia-related ventricular tachycardia during OKT3 induction therapy. Transplantation 1992;54:1112—1113.
1044. Abramowicz D, Pradier O, Marchant A et al. Induction of thromboses within renal grafts by high-dose prophylactic OKT3. Lancet 1992;339:777—778.
1045. Gomez E, Aguado S, Gaco E et al. Main graft vessels thromboses du to conventional-dose OKT3 in renal transplantation. Lancet 1992;339:1612—1613.
1046. Hollenbeck M, Westhoff A, Bach D, Grabensee B. Doppler sonography and renal graft thromboses after OKT3 treatment. Lancet 1992;340:619—620.
1047. Raasveld M, Hack C, ten Berge I. Activation of coagulation and fibrinolysis following OKT3 administration to renal transplant recipients: association with distinct mediators. Thromb Haemost 1992;68:264—267.
1048. Abramowicz D, Pradier O, de Pauw L et al. High-dose glucocorticosteroids increase the procoagulant effects of OKT3. Kidney Int 1994;46:1596—1602.
1049. Marks W, Perkal M, Bia M, Lorber M. Aseptic encephalitis and blindness complicating OKT3 therapy. Clin Transplant 1991;5:435—438.
1050. Min D, Fallo S. Encephalopathy associated with muromonab-CD3. Clin Pharm 1993;12:610—612.
1051. Shihab F, Barry J, Bennett W et al. Cytokine-related encephalopathy induced by OKT3: incidence and predisposing factors (Part 1). Transplant Proc 1993;25:564—565.
1052. Capone P, Cohen M. Seizures and cerebritis associated with administration of OKT3. Pediatr Neurol 1991;7:299—301.
1053. Osterman J, Trauner D, Reznik V, Lemire J. Transient hemiparesis associated with monoclonal CD3 antibody (OKT3) therapy. Pediatr Neurol 1993;9:482—484.
1054. Reiss R, Makoff D, Rodriguez H et al. Encephalopathy and cerebral infarction in OKT3-treated patients with concomitant elevation of cerebrospinal fluid tumour necrosis factor alpha. Nephrol Dial Transplant 1993;8:464—468.
1055. Kehinde E, Scriven S, Feehally J et al. Adverse effects of OKT3 therapy: increased risk with impaired renal function. Transplant Proc 1994;26:1945—1947.
1056. Batiuk T, Bennett W, Norman D. Cytokine nephropathy during antilymphocyte therapy. Transplant Proc 1993;25(Suppl 1):27—30.
1057. First M, Schroeder T, Hariharan S. OKT3-induced cytokine-release syndrome: renal effects (cytokine nephropathy). Transplant Proc 1993;25(Suppl 1):25—26.
1058. Doutrelpont J, Abramowicz D, Florquin S et al. Early recurrence of hemolytic uremic syndrome in a renal transplant recipient during OKT3 therapy. Transplantation 1992;53:1378—1379.

1059. Goodman D, Walker R, Birchall I et al. Reccurent haemolytic uraemic syndrome in a transplant recipient on orthoclone (OKT3). Pediatr Nephrol 1991;5:240–241.
1060. McCarthy J, Sullivan K, Keow P, Rollins D. Diffuse anterior scleritis during OKT3 monoclonal antibody therapy for renal transplant rejection. Can J Ophthalmol 1992; 27:22–24.
1061. Dukar O, Barr C. Visual loss complicating OKT3 monoclonal antibody therapy. Am J Ophthalmol 1993;115:781–785.
1062. Abramowicz D, Crusiaux A, Goldman M. Anaphylactic shock after retreatment with OKT3 monoclonal antibody. N Engl J Med 1992;327:736.
1063. Georgitis J, Browning M, Steiner D, Lorentz W. Anaphylaxis and desensitization to the murine monoclonal antibody used for renal graft rejection. Ann Allergy 1991; 66:343–347.
1064. Turner M, Holman J. Late reactions during initial OKT3-treatment. Clin Transplant 1993;7:1–3.
1065. Swinnen LJ, Costanzo-Nordin MR, Fisher SG et al. Increased incidence of lymphoproliferative disorders after immunosuppression with the monoclonal antibody OKT3 in cardiac-transplant recipients. N Engl J Med 1990;323:1723–1728.
1066. Anderson P, Schroeder T, Hariharan S, First M. Incidence of posttransplant lymphoproliferative disease in OKT-3 treated renal transplant recipients. Clin Transplant 1993;7:582–585.
1067. Batiuk T, Barry J, Bennett W et al. Incidence and type of cancer following the use of OKT3: a single center experience with 557 organ transplants. Transplant Proc 1993;25:1391.
1068. McAlister V, Grant D, Roy A et al. Posttransplant lymphoproliferative disorders in liver recipients treated with OKT3 or ALG induction immunosuppression. Transplant Proc 1993;25:1400–1401.
1069. Costanzo-Nordin M, Swinnen L, Fisher S et al. Cytomegalovirus infections in heart transplant recipients. Relationship to immunosuppression. J Heart Lung Transplant 1992;11:837–846.
1070. Abramowicz D, Goldman M, de Pauw L et al. The long-term effects of prophylactic OKT3 monoclonal antibody in cadaver kidney transplantation. A single-center, prospective, randomized study. Transplantation 1992;54:433–437.
1071. Bock H, Gallati H, Zürcher R et al. A randomized prospective trial of prophylactic immunosuppression with ATG-Fresenius versus OKT3 after renal transplantation. Transplantation 1995;59:830–840.
1072. Petrie J, Rigby R, Hawley C et al. Effect of OKT3 in steroid-resistant renal transplant rejection. Transplantation 1995;59:347–352.
1073. Portela D, Patel R, Larson-Keller J et al. OKT3 treatment for allofraft rejection is a risk factor for cytomegalovirus disease in liver transplantation. J Infect Dis 1995; 171:1014–1018.
1074. Wechsler M, Giardina E, Sciacca R et al. Increased early mortality in women undergoing cardiac transplantation. Circulation 1995;91:1029–1035.
1075. Hooks M, Perlino C, Henderson J et al. Prevalence of invasive cytomegalovirus disease with administration of muromonab CD-3 in patients undergoing orthotopic liver transplantation. Ann Pharmacother 1992;26:617–620.
1076. Lake K, Anderson D, Milfred S et al. The incidence of cytomegalovirus disease is not increased after OKT3 induction therapy. J Heart Lung Transplant 1993;12:537–538.
1077. Hayes M, Torzillo P, Sheil A, McCaughan G. *Pneumocystis carinii* pneumonia after liver transplantation in adults. Clin Transplant 1994;8:499–503.
1078. Cosimi A. Future of monoclonal antibodies in solid organ transplantation. Dig Dis Sci 1995;40:65–72.
1079. Dillman R. Antibodies as cytotoxic therapy. J Clin Oncol 1994;12:1497–1515.
1080. Panayi G. The pathogenesis of rheumatoid arthritis and the development of therapeutic strategies for the clinical investigation of biologics. Agents Actions 1995; 47(Suppl):1–21.
1081. Pietersz G, Krauer K. Antibody-targeted drugs for the therapy of cancer. J Drug Target 1994;2:183–215.
1082. Revillard J, Robinet E, Goldman M et al. In vitro correlates of the acute toxic syndrome induced by some monoclonal antibodies: a rationale for the design of predictive tests. Toxicology 1995;96:51–58.
1083. Schroeder T, First M. Monoclonal antibodies in organ transplantation. Am J Kidney Dis 1994;23:138–147.
1084. Mountain A, Adair J. Engineering antibodies for therapy. Biotechnol Genet Eng Rev 1992;10:1–142.
1085. Chatenoud L, Legendre C, Kurrle L et al. Absence of clinical symptoms following the forst injection of anti-T cell receptor monoclonal antibody (BMA031) despite isolated TNF release. Transplantation 1993;55:443–445.
1086. Waid T, Lucas B, Thompson J et al. Treatment of acute cellular rejection with T10B9.1A-31 or OKT3 in renal allograft recipients. Transplantation 1992;53:80–86.
1087. Friend P, Rebello P, Oliveira D et al. Successful treatment of renal allograft rejection with a humanized antilymphocyte monoclonal antibody. Transplant Proc 1995; 27:869–870.
1088. Watts R, Isaacs J, Hale G et al. CAMPATH-1H in inflammatory arthritis. Clin Exp Rheumatol 1993;11(Suppl 8):S165–S167.
1089. Meiser B, Reiter C, Reichenspurner H et al. Chimeric monoclonal CD4-antibody: a novel immunosuppressant for clinical heart transplantation. Transplantation 1994;58:419–423.
1090. Lazarovits A, Rochon J, Banks L et al. Human mouse chimeric CD7 monoclonal antibody (SDZCHH380) for the prophylaxis of kidney transplant rejection. Transplant Proc 1993;25:820–822.
1091. Haug C, Colvin R, Delmonico F et al. A phase I trial of immunosuppression with anti-ICAM-1 (CD54) mAb in renal allograft recipients. Transplantation 1993;55:766–772.
1092. van Gelder T, Zietse R, Mulder A et al. A double-blind, placebo-controlled study of monoclonal anti-interleukin-2 receptor antibody (BT563) administration to prevent acute rejection after kidney transplantation. Transplantation 1995;60:248–252.
1093. Moreland L, Pratt P, Sanders M, Koopman W. Experience with a chimeric monoclonal anti-CD4 antibody in the treatment of refractory rheumatoid arthritis. Clin Exp Rheumatol 1993;11(Suppl 8):S153–S159.
1094. Strand V, Lipsky P, Cannon G et al. Effects of administration of anti-CD5 plus immunoconjugate in rheumatoid arthritis. Arthr Rheum 1993;36:620–630.
1095. Elliot M, Maini R, Feldmann M et al. Randomised double-blind comparison of chimeric monoclonal antibody to tumor necrosis factor alpha (cA2) versus placebo in rheumatoid arthritis. Lancet 1994;344:1105–1110.
1096. Wendling D, Racadot E, Wijdenes J. Treatment of severe rheumatoid arthritis by anti-interleukin 6 monoclonal antibody. J Rheumatol 1993;20:259–262.

1097. Amlot P, Stone M, Cunningham D et al. A phase I study of an anti-CD22-deglycosylated ricin A chain immunotoxin in the treatment of B-cell lymphomas resistant to conventional therapy. Blood 1993;82:2624—2633.
1098. Selvaggi K, Saria EA, Schwartz R et al. Phase I/II study of murine monoclonal antibody-ricin A chain (Xomazyme-Mel) immunoconjugate plus cyclosporine A in patients with metastatic melanoma. J Immunother 1993;13:201—207.
1099. LoRusso PM, Lomen PL, Redman et al. Phase I study of monoclonal antibody-ricin A chain immunoconjugate Xomazyme-791 in patients with metastatic colon cancer. Am J Clin Oncol 1995;18:307—312.
1100. Susla G, Dew R. Antiendotoxin monoclonal antibodies. What future now? Drug Safety 1994;11:215—222.
1101. Abraham E, Wunderink R, Silverman H et al. Efficacy and safety of monoclonal antibody to human tumor necrosis factor alpha in patients with sepsis syndrome. A randomized controlled, double-blind, multicenter clinical trial. TNF-alpha Mab Sepsis Study Group. J Am Med Assoc 1995;273:934—941.
1102. Hadden JW. Immunostimulants. Immunol Today 1993;14:275—280.
1103. Lamm DL, Stogdill VD, Stogdill BJ, Crispen RG. Complications of Bacillus Calmette-Guerin immunotherapy in 1,278 patients with bladder cancer. J Urol 1986;135:272—274.
1104. Galvan L, Ayani I, Arrizabalaga MJ et al. Intravesical BCG therapy of superficial bladder cancer: study of adverse effects. J Clin Pharm Ther 1994;19:101—104.
1105. Chazerain P, Desplaces N, Ziza JM et al. BCG osteoarthritis on kness arthroplasty after bacillus Calmette-Guérin (BCG) for bladder cancer. Rev Rhum Mal Osteoart 1992;59:836—838.
1106. Goupille P, Soutif D, Valat JP. Arthritis after Calmette-Guérin Bacillus immunotherapy for bladder cancer. J Rheumatol 1992;19:1825—1826.
1107. Faus S, Martinez Montauti J, Puig L. Reiter's syndrome after administration of intravesical bacille Calmette-Guérin. Clin Infect Dis 1993;17:526—527.
1108. Nesher G. Reiter's syndrome following intravesical therapy with Bacillus Calmette-Guérin (BCG). Rev Rhum 1993;60:814.
1109. Price GE. Arthritis and iritis after BCG therapy for bladder cancer. J Rheumatol 1994;21:564—565.
1110. Geffray L, Duche A, Cevallos R et al. Generalized BCGitis after intra-ureteral BCG therapy. Presse Med 1994;23:544.
1111. Gonzalez JA, Marcol BR, Wolf MC. Complications of intravesical bacillus Calmette-Guérin: a case report. J Urol 1992;148:1892—1893.
1112. LeMense GP, Strange G. Granulomatous penumonitis following intravesical BCG. What therapy is needed? Chest 1994;106:1624—1626.
1113. Reinert KU, Sybrecht GW. T helper cell alveolitis after bacillus Calmette-Guérin immunotherapy for superficial bladder tumor. J Urol 1994;151:1634—1635.
1114. Fishman JR, Walton DT, Flynn NM et al. Tuberculous spondylitis as a complication of intravesical bacillus Calmette-Guérin therapy. J Urol 1993;149:584—587.
1115. Proctor DD, Chopra S, Rubenstein SC et al. Mycobacteremia and granulomatous hepatitis following intravesical bacillus Calmette-Guérin instillation for bladder carcinoma. Am J Gastroenterol (1993)88, 1112—1115.
1116. Isozaki T, Kimura M, Ikegaya N et al. Bucillamine (a new therapeutic agent for rheumatoid arthritis) induced nephrotic syndrome: a report of two cases and review of the literature. Clin Invest 1992;70:1036—1042.
1117. Ogawa H, Fujimura M, Heki U et al. Eosinophilic bronchitis presenting with only severe dry cough due to bucillamine. Resp Med 1995;89:219—221.
1118. Amasaki Y, Sagawa A, Atsumi T et al. A case of rheumatoid arthritis developing pemphigus-like skin lesion during treatment with bucillamine. Jpn J Rheumatol 1992;4:66.
1119. Fujiyama J, Tokimura Y, Ijichi S, Arimura K. Bucillamine may induce myasthenia gravis. Jpn J Med 1991; 30:101—102.
1120. Ishizaki C, Sueki H, Kohsokabe S, Nishida H. Yellow nail induced by bucillamine. Int J Dermatol 1995;34:493—494.
1121. Thorsen S, Pedersen C, Sandström E et al. One-year follow-up on the safety and efficacy of isoprinosine for human immunodeficiency virus infection. J Intern Med 1992;231:607—615.
1122. Milligan NM, Miller DH, Compston DAS. A placebo-controlled trial of isoprinosine in patients with multiple sclerosis. J Neurol Neurosurg Psychiatr 1994;57:164—168.
1123. Kimmel DW, Wijdicks EFM, Rodriguez M. Multifocal inflammatory leukoencephalopathy associated with levamisole therapy. Neurology 1995;45:374—376.
1124. Ferroir JP, Fenelon G, Beaugerie L, Avenin Recoing D. inflammatory leucoencephalopathy caused by adjuvant therapy with 5 fluorouracil and levamisole for colon carcinoma. Rev Neurol 1994;150:471—474.
1125. Tweedy CR, Silverberg DA, Scott L. Levamisole-induced syndrome of inappropriate antidiuretic hormone. N Engl J Med 1992;326:1164.
1126. Palcoux JB, Niaudet P, Goumy P. Side effects of levamisole in children with nephrosis. Pediatr Nephrol 1994; 8:263—264.
1127. Mieles L, Venkataramanan R, Yokoyama I et al. Interaction between FK506 and clotrimazole in a liver transplant recipient. Transplantation 1991;52:1086—1087.
1028. Shapiro R, Venkataramanan R, Warty VS et al. FK506 interaction with danazol. Lancet 1993;341:1344—1345.
1129. Marcos C, Quirce S, Compaired JA et al. Severe anaphylactic reaction to thymostimulin. Allergy 1991;46:235—237.

Meyler's Side Effects of Drugs, 13th Edition
M.N.G. Dukes, editor

SECTION EDITOR: M.N.G. DUKES

Elisabet Helsing

38 Vitamins

Vitamins are essential organic substances, the usual source of which is food. They are required by humans in amounts ranging from micrograms to milligrams per day. There are four fat-soluble vitamins (A, D, E and K) and nine water-soluble vitamins (thiamin, riboflavin, niacin, pantothenic acid, folic acid, biotin and vitamins B_6, B_{12} and C) are chemically heterogeneous, but all are essential for normal growth, development and maintenance of the human organism (1). They cannot be synthesized by the organism itself, but have to be supplied externally. The main indications for vitamin supplementation are threatening or manifest deficiency states.

The name 'vitamin' itself is a misnomer, created by one of the early nutrition researchers, C. Funk (1920) who knew that the substances they were trying to identify were not necessarily 'amines', but he felt he needed 'a name that would sound well and serve as a 'catch word'' (2). Funk proved to be far-sighted indeed; the name 'vitamins' has proved to have extraordinary selling power.

A typical example of the creation of fallacious beliefs in the positive effects of vitamin supplements was an article published in 1988 about increased intelligence in a group of supplemented schoolchildren (3[c]). Although later studies were unable to reproduce the results and the study methodology has been criticized, this has not hindered the sales of 'intelligence pills' to zealous parents (4[R]).

Vitamins are not infrequently used by medical workers as placebos against poorly defined general malaise, without consideration of the patient's actual vitamin status (5[R]). Self-medication with vitamin supplements is very common in most countries, and commonly the users are not objectively deficient of the vitamin in question (6[r]). In general, physicians in an industrialized society can expect that approximately half of their adult patients will currently use vitamin supplements (7[R]); among athletes 75% have been found to use supplements (8[R]).

As micronutrient deficiencies more or less ceased to be a large public health problem in western countries, the attention of scientists and manufacturers was turned towards the many other functions these substances have in human metabolism. For the last decade or so, pharmacological doses of most of the vitamins have been claimed to be of therapeutic value in a wide variety of conditions which have only a superficial resemblance to the classic vitamin-deficiency syndromes. The literature on which many of these claims are based unfortunately often consists of poorly conducted clinical trials or anecdotal reports. Only recently have properly designed studies been performed. Evidence from such studies suggests a beneficial therapeutic effect of vitamin E in intermittent claudication and fibrocystic breast disease, and of vitamin C in pressure sores. The use of vitamin A in acne vulgaris, vitamin E in angina pectoris or hyperlipidemia or for enhancement of athletic capacity, of vitamin C in advanced cancer, and of niacin in schizophrenia have been rejected.

The possible prophylactic effect of relatively high intakes of vitamins with antioxidant properties (in doses several times higher than the average requirements, but not as large as the 'mega'-doses described above) are the subject of intense investigation by several research teams; the results are not equivocal (9), and no authoritative body has proposed quantitative recommendations or reference values for public health policy. Food fortification and 'designer foods' specially formulated to prevent chronic diseases are enthusiastically advocated by the vitamin industry and its proponents (10[C]). Unrestrained fortification has now reached levels in some countries where concern about potential harmful effects of oversupply of some micronutrients have been raised (11[r], 12).

According to some authors, the increased accessibility and use of high-dose vitamin preparations has been encouraged by the multi-million-dollar health food industry, increased emphasis placed by physicians on more 'natural' approaches to disease treatment, a population of consumers interested in 'holistic medicine' and, in the USA, a court decision that vitamins are not drugs and may be marketed without control by the health authorities. In therapeutic usage, the physician has to keep in mind the cost-benefit of use of high-dose vitamin supplementation for disorders where proof of efficacy is lacking (13[R]).

There is widespread and easy availability of high-dose vitamin preparations, often wrongly presented as food supplements. This situation has a dangerous potential for abuse of high doses of vitamins and the occurrence of unanticipated side effects (14^R, 15^r) and, indeed, a growing number of cases of various forms of vitamin intoxication are being reported in the literature. These cases often involve children, who may be specially vulnerable to the effects of accidental overdosage by well-meaning parents. The Canadian Paediatric Society's Nutrition Committee in 1990 issued a warning to physicians based on an estimation that as many as 10% of healthy Canadian children were exposed to vitamin polypharmacy and a substantial risk of accidental overdose (16^C).

Since vitamin overdosage can produce unexpected signs and symptoms, physicians should ask patients presenting with vague symptoms, including those described below, about their use of unusual or unapproved therapies, including the use of vitamins in mega-doses (17^R). It has indeed been suggested that a medical history is not complete without vitamin-mineral supplement information (8^R). A summary of notable symptoms reported with vitamin overdosage is given in Table 1.

Reference values for vitamins Nutritionists have in the early 1990s, based on an increased body of evidence, changed the nomenclature with regard to what used to be called 'Recommended Dietary Allowance' (RDA), 'Recommended Daily Intakes' (RDI) or Nutrient Reference Values (18^R). When in 1993 the Scientific Committee for Food of the European Communities published 'Nutrient and Energy Intakes for the European Community' (19^R), a new approach was introduced allowing for more flexibility with regard to quantitative values. Based on what is known about the 'average requirement' (AR) for a nutrient in a population, and assuming a normal distribution of requirements, a value two standard deviations above the AR will indicate the Population Reference Intake (PRI)—a level at which deficiency of the micronutrient is probable in less than 2.5% of any population. A value two standard deviations below the AR, the Lowest Threshold of Intake (LTI), will denote a level where the probability of deficiency in a population is almost 97.5%. In the monographs which follow, these three values, as suggested by the EC Report, are given for individuals in an adult population.

Table 1. *Notable symptoms reported with vitamin overdosage*

Vitamin A	Hypercarotenosis
	Dry skin, fissures, depigmentation and pruritus
	Bone tenderness
	Chronic liver disease
	Increased intracranial pressure
	Hair loss
	Diarrhea
	Vomiting
	Nausea
	Headache
	Sleep disturbances
	Teratogenesis (renal and nervous system)
Vitamin D	Bone demineralization
	Renal calcinosis and kidney failure
	Hypercalcemia
	Metastatic calcification
	Hypertension
Vitamin K	Hemolytic anemia
	Neonatal jaundice
Vitamin B_6	Peripheral sensory neuropathy
	Ataxia
Niacin	Skin flushing
	Hypotension
	Arrhythmias
	Hyperuricemia, gout
	Pruritus
	Hyperglycemia
	Hepatotoxicity
	Headaches
	Alopecia
	Peptic ulcer
Vitamin E	Increased action of warfarin
Vitamin C	Gastrointestinal symptoms
	Oxalate stones in predisposed persons
	Possible teratogenesis and carcinogenesis in very high doses
	Impairment of work at high altitudes

Source: SEDA-13, 345, Dukes MNG, Editor. Data supplied by Evans and Lacey (17), supplemented by Fike (8).

Vitamin A (retinol)*

Average Requirement (AR) for vitamin A is set to 500 μg RE for adult men and 400 μg for women. Population Reference Intake (PRI) are 700 and 600 μg RE, respectively, while Lowest Threshold Intake (LTI) is set at 300 and 250 μg RE for adult men and women, respectively. While slightly higher PRI are advised for

* Vitamin A activity may be expressed either as international units IU (1 IU equalling 0.3 μg of all-*trans*-retinol or 0.6 μg of all-*trans*-β-carotene), or more correctly, in retinol equivalents (RE) where 1 RE equals 1 μg of all-*trans*-retinol, 6 μg of all-*trans*-β-carotene or 12 μg of other provitamin A carotenoids.

pregnancy and lactation (700 and 950 μg RE, respectively), concern about the possible teratogenic effect of vitamin A has led health authorities to advise pregnant women against taking vitamin A supplements (18[R]). Much higher doses—over 200 000 IU—are, however, routinely distributed as half yearly doses to children in populations deemed to be suffering from vitamin A deficiency, mainly in developing countries. Toxicity is occasionally observed during these massive dose prophylactic programs (20[r]), and their effect has sometimes been called into question (21[C], 22[C]). Supplements that contain 25 000 IU or more of vitamin A per capsule are available as over-the-counter (OTC) preparations in many countries (23). The 'Nutrient and Energy Intakes for the European Community' advises against single doses >120 000 μg, and regular intakes >9000 μg/day in men and 7500 μg in women.

Normal serum levels of vitamin A are within the range of 30—150 IU/100 ml.

ADVERSE REACTION PATTERN

General and toxic reactions Acute intoxication has been observed following ingestion of vitamin A-rich liver from the polar bear, halibut or shark, or, lately, fish oil supplements used to lower plasma lipids (24[c], 25[c]). In adults, toxic doses have been in the range of one or more million units of vitamin A, but in children as low as 30 000 IU, or even in a few children <2000 IU/kg/day (26[R]). Symptoms occur from 6—24 hours after ingestion and comprise acute onset of drowsiness, irritability, vertigo, headache, delirium and convulsions, intolerance to food, and diarrhea (SEDA-8, 344).

Long-term administration of 10 000 IU daily may cause chronic hypervitaminosis A, and at greatest risk in this regard are persons with impaired liver function (26[R], 27[c]). Because of the multisystemic manifestations of hypervitaminosis A, symptoms are often misjudged and diagnosis delayed. Main symptoms of chronic intoxication include malaise, headache, vertigo, intracranial hypertension, nystagmus, photophobia, hyperkeratosis, gastrointestinal complaints, changes in the skin and mucous membranes, tenderness and pain in the bone and joints and fever.

Long-term treatment with high doses of vitamin A seems to be a doubtful procedure, since in some patients side effects, especially disturbed liver function, become evident only when irreversible damage, e.g. liver cirrhosis or fibrosis with portal hypertension, is already present. It seems that the total cumulative intake of vitamin A, rather than the size of any dosage, may be the critical factor for damage to the liver (28[C]); this might hold also true for other side effects.

Hypersensitivity reactions These do not seem to occur, although increased serum IgM values were reported in an analysis of patients with severe liver disease after prolonged administration of vitamin A (29[C]).

Tumor-inducing effects These have so far been indicated only with regard to prostatic cancer especially in those 70 years of age and over (SEDA-13, 346).

ORGANS AND SYSTEMS

Cardiovascular Persons with severe hypertriglyceridemia associated with Type V hyperlipoproteinemia may be at increased risk for hypervitaminosis A, even with moderate levels of vitamin A supplementation (30[C]). Long-term vitamin A administration is associated with an increase in serum cholesterol and serum triglyceride concentrations (31[c]) and consequently might be linked with atherosclerosis (SEDA-1, 274; SEDA-8, 345; 32[R]).

Nervous system *Acute poisoning* produces symptoms such as drowsiness, sluggishness, irritability, an irresistible desire to sleep, severe headache and papilledema. In young children, raised intracranial pressure with bulging of the fontanelle, papilledema and diplopia have been observed (SED-8, 799, 801; SEDA-15, 411; 33[C]).

In 50% of *chronic* vitamin A intoxications intracranial hypertension occurs, sometimes together with skin and hair changes, pain in the musculoskeletal system and fatigue (34[CR]). Benign intracranial hypertension (pseudotumor cerebri), vertigo and papilledema have appeared following the daily intake of 10 000—20 000 IU vitamin A for 2 years; in young children even a few months of treatment may suffice (35[R]) and symptoms may occur at low doses (even in a few children as low as <2000 IU/kg/day (26[R]). The precise cause of increased intracranial pressure in hypervitaminosis A is controversial and remains unclear (29[C]). Daily doses of 3 000 000 IU of vitamin A have induced central nervous symptoms such as acute symptomatic psychosis with striking disturbances in the electroencephalogram and pathological changes in the cerebrospinal fluid (36[C]). After cessation of medication with vitamin A and administration of low doses of neuroleptics the psychotic symptoms disappeared within a week.

Neuropsychiatric changes were reported to be the

earliest dose-limiting symptomatic toxicity in cancer patients on high doses of retinol (37[C]).

Endocrine, metabolic Chronic intoxication with vitamin A has been reported to cause hypercalcemia, hyperglycemia, increased alkaline phosphatase, hypoproteinemia, hypoprothrombinemia, increased sulfobromphthalein retention, elevated serum transaminases, low serum ascorbic acid, decreased protein content of the cerebrospinal fluid, elevated urinary hydroxyproline and hypercalciuria (SED-8, 800; SEDA-1, 274; 38[c]).

Mineral and fluid balance Edema and ascites are sometimes seen in chronic intoxication (SED-8, 799).

Hematological High doses of vitamin A reduce the stability of the lipoprotein boundary layer of the erythrocytes, which can lead to hemolysis and anemia (39[C]). Neutropenia, leukocytosis, thrombocytopenia, aplastic anemia and increased sedimentation rate have also been reported after high doses of vitamin A (40[r], 41[C]).

Liver Enlargement of the liver, spleen and lymph nodes have been reported in adults (39[C], 40[r], 41[C]).

Liver biopsies have been performed in some patients with chronic vitamin A intoxication. Perisinusoidal fibrosis and massive accumulation of lipid-storing cells were found. Impairment of blood flow by perisinusoidal fibrosis probably resulted in the secondary alterations in hepatocytes which included cellular atrophy and formation of cytoplasmic bullae. Histological examination also revealed central vein sclerosis and focal congestion associated with perisinusoidal storage. The vitamin A concentration of the liver was found to be increased (42[c], 43[C], 44[c]).

For the diagnosis of hypervitaminosis A, plasma levels and retinol-binding protein (RBP) may be misleading. Four cases were reported of hepatic fibrosis in siblings, secondary to chronic ingestion of massive doses of vitamin A, but plasma levels of vitamin A and RBP at the time of diagnosis were in the normal range (45[C]).

A long-term observation of 41 patients with varying forms of liver disease, all caused by prolonged vitamin A consumption has given further insight into the range of histological lesions and the prognosis of liver disease related to hypervitaminosis A (40[C]). Clinical examination revealed hepatomegaly in 18 of the patients, splenomegaly in 13, signs of chronic hepatic disease in 12, ascites in nine and icterus in eight. Repeat liver biopsies in three patients 3—6 years after diagnosis showed progression from steatosis or fibrosis to fully developed micronodular cirrhosis in all cases, demonstrating that the liver damage may be irreversible. Nine patients died during follow-up, six of terminal liver failure. Plasma retinol concentrations were, however, above the reference range in only about 40%. The damage is not always irreversible; one patient, after prolonged intake of excessive amounts of vitamin A for treatment of psoriasis (270 000 IU) showed not only reversible chronic intoxication, but a reversible portal hypertension and deranged liver function tests without any histological signs of cirrhosis (46[C]). In a similar case, portal hypertension disappeared after a 6-month low vitamin A diet. The fact that no decrease in Ito cells either in size or number could be seen suggests that lipid venous obstruction is unlikely to be the only mechanism responsible for portal hypertension in vitamin A-induced liver disease 47[C].

Even moderate intakes of vitamin A, when taken over a prolonged period of time, can cause significant hepatocellular injury, as seen in three family members with symptoms and biochemical evidence of hepatitis, who were found to have been ingesting 20 000—45 000 IU per day for 7—10 years (48[c]). A similar case involved a 45-year-old woman who had taken an OTC supplement over 6 years, who developed severe and fatal liver damage (49).

Gastrointestinal Nausea, vomiting and anorexia are common symptoms of acute vitamin A intoxication, as are dryness and scaling of the lips, gingivitis and bleeding from the gums. Polydipsia has been described (SED-8, 799, 800).

Urinary system In chronic intoxication polyuria, increased frequency of micturition, urinary incontinence, enuresis and acute renal failure due to tubular necrosis may occur (39[C], 40[C]).

Patients with renal dysfunction are known to have elevated circulating vitamin A levels. In chronic dialysis patients, the level may rise steadily. The significantly increased osmotic fragility of erythrocytes observed in hemodialyzed patients also seems to be related to high vitamin A levels. The similarity between uremic symptoms and those of vitamin A excess may, however, explain why hypervitaminosis A in uremic patients is rarely associated with clinical toxicity (SEDA-12, 327).

Skin and appendages In acute intoxication, peeling of the entire skin can occur as a delayed symptom (50[C]). Among the early and most commonly reported symptoms of chronic vitamin A intoxication are erythema, pruritus, hyperkeratosis, dryness and hemorrhages and fissures of the lips. A yellow to yellow-orange discoloration of the skin, decreased tolerance to sunlight, changes in pigmentation, hair loss and brittle nails have been observed as well as spider angiomas and palmar erythema in patients with serious hepatic damage due to chronic use of vitamin A (SED-8, 800).

Special senses Nystagmus, diplopia, photophobia, palsy of the ocular muscle, retinal hemorrhage and protrusio bulbi (SED-8, 801; 51[c]) have all been reported and are an effect of the raised intracranial pressure. Intoxication can also lead to papilledema, which in some cases may be the only symptom (SEDA-11, 333; 52[C], 53[C]).

Musculoskeletal Excessive intake of vitamin A leads to accelerated resorption of trabecular and cortical bone due to increased osteoclastic activity. The elevated alkaline phosphatase, increased urinary hydroxyproline levels and hypercalciuria mentioned above correlate with these findings (54[C]).

Pain in the bones and joints is a common symptom. Bone tenderness often occurs without other bone symptoms, but possible complications include elevation of the periosteum, hyperostosis and, in children, premature closure of the epiphyses of the long bones causing growth arrest (54[C], 55).

Skeletal deformities involving the lower limbs and the spine were seen in a 15-month-old girl who during the previous few months had received a total dose of 10.5 million IU of vitamin A (56[c]). Skeletal signs were also seen in a nursing infant who was given 35 drops of a vitamin preparation 5 times a day for the first month of life, corresponding to daily dosages of 25 000 IU vitamin A, 5000 IU vitamin D, 15 mg vitamin E and 250 mg vitamin C. Other symptoms included hydrocephalus, cutaneous and hepatic signs (57[c]).

Another fatal case of hypervitaminosis A involved a premature neonate who died after having ingested 60 times the suggested dose of vitamin A per day (90 000 IU) for 11 days. On autopsy the skeleton showed marked alterations of endochondral bone formation. There was also evidence of accelerated resorption of bone, hypercalcemia and metastatic calcification of the skin, soft tissues and organs (58[c]). The above three cases also point to the dangerous misunderstanding with regard to vitamins common among lay people and professionals alike: vitamins are believed to be innocuous substances - and if a little of them is good for you, much must be better. Table 2 puts this statement into perspective (59[R]).

Risk situations In view of the above data, young children would seem to be particularly at risk. Symptoms of chronic intoxication are seen with intakes from about 2500 to 50 000 IU/kg body weight (35[R]).

At special risk are persons whose liver function is compromised by drugs, viral hepatitis or protein-energy malnutrition (26[R]). Children with restricted protein intake may have reduced tolerance to vitamin A; one case is reported where about 20 000 IU vitamin A daily given to a 6-year-old child over a long period led to hypervitaminosis, possibly because the liver's normal role in vitamin A metabolism in this case was circumvented (60[C]).

In alcoholics, vitamin A supplementation might have been a useful measure but is complicated by the fact that large amounts of this vitamin may be hepatotoxic and that chronic alcohol consumption results in an enhanced susceptibility to this effect (61[R]).

Second-generation effects In animals both deficiency and massive overdose with vitamin A can be teratogenic. In humans only a few cases of teratogenicity associated with vitamin A have been observed (62[C], 63[C], 64[R]), although a high incidence of spontaneous abortions and of birth defects have been observed in women ingesting therapeutic doses of isotretinoin (13-*cis*-retinoic acid) during the first trimester of pregnancy (see Chapter 14). Recommendations concerning dosage of vitamin A in pregnant women have been issued by several institutions (18[R]), including the Teratology Society (65), the American College of Obstetricians and Gynecologists (66). The Health Protection Branch of Health and Welfare Canada accepted the recommendation that the use of retinoic acid for acne be regarded as contraindicated in women during pregnancy and in those of childbearing age (67). A study in Hungary of 1203 births to women who had received a supplement containing 6000 IU/day, compared with 1510 receiving placebo, did not show any evidence of teratogenic effect (68). The lower limit of supplementation recommended varies between 5000 and 10 000 IU of vitamin A per day (SEDA-14, 330). Manufacturers have been urged to lower the doses in OTC preparations correspondingly and include warnings on labels (65). A summary of some cases of birth defects associated with high maternal intake of vitamin A is found in Table 3 (from Hathcock, 26[R]).

Interactions Vitamin A added to *infusions* can be absorbed by the plastic containers often used (see Chapter 36). Liquid paraffin used as a *laxative* can prevent absorption of Vitamin A and other fat-soluble vitamins. *Oral contraceptives* can lead to an increase in plasma levels of vitamin A. Since increased vitamin A levels may have a negative effect on conception, this might provide an explanation for the reduced fertility sometimes seen during the period immediately following withdrawal of contraceptive steroids.

Administration of large doses of vitamin A to children in poor socioeconomic conditions has often for logistic reasons been combined with other health care interventions, such as immunization. A randomized

Table 2. *Toxic doses of vitamin A*

Population	Sex	Age (years)	Country or region	Retinol equivalents (μg)
Toxic concentrations (28[c])				
Adults			Nordic	7 500
			Australia	20 000
Pregnant women	F		Australia	10 000
			U.S.A.	5 000–10 000
*Chronic intoxication**				
Children				758/kg
Adults				15 000–30 000
*Acute intoxication*** (35[c])				
Children				22 500–30 000
Adults				300 000–600 000

Table 3. *Some cases of birth defects associated with high material intake of vitamin A*

Maternal intake	Duration	Symptoms	Other conditions
Reports of individual cases			
~500 000 IU	Single dose, second month	Preauricular appendices, epibulbar dermatoid (eye malformations similar to Goldenhar's syndrome)	Dose caused acute toxicity in the pregnant women
150 000 IU	Periconceptual −2 to +3 mo	Facial dysmorphism, pterygium colli, distended abdomen, absence of external genitalia and of anal and urethral openings, polycystic kidneys, dysmorphism of lumbar spine	Fetus aborted at 20 wk because of spinal abnormality and polycystic kidney
25 000 IU 50 000 IU	0–13 wk 14 wk to term	Unilateral ureteral duplication with one ureter ending in the vagina, hydronephrosis, hydroureters	
Reports of multiple cases 18 000–100 000 IU	Before and throughout pregnancy	Abnormalities of the head, face, ears, eyes, mouth, lips, jaws, heart and urinary system; other defects	Cases reported by physicians to FDA; cases reported to State Birth Defects Registry

Source: Hathcock et al. 1990 (15[r]).

case-control study of 336 infants receiving either 100 000 IU of vitamin A or placebo simultaneously with measles vaccine, showed a lower seroconversion to measles in the vitamin A group. At the moment of writing, the discussion of whether this observation is valid or not, is still ongoing (69[C]).

Interference with diagnostic routines See above under 'Organs and systems'.

RETINOIDS

Retinoids are dealt with exclusively in Chapter 14.

VITAMINS OF THE B GROUP

Thiamine (vitamin B_1)

The requirement for thiamine depends on the utilization of energy-yielding substrates, and increases with the energy expenditure, and is therefore expressed relative to energy intake. The AR is 72 μg/MJ, the PRI is 100 μg/MJ, and the LTI is 50 μg/MJ. Expressed for average energy expenditure, this would mean an AR of 0.8 mg/day for males and 0.6 for females; a PRI of 1.1 and 0.9 mg/day, and an LTI of 0.6 and 0.4 mg/day, respectively, have been suggested. Excess thiamine is normally easily cleared by the kidneys. The adverse reactions which one has to take into account are usually associated with parenteral feeding with doses much larger than the RDA and over long periods of time. One such case involved fatty degeneration of the liver, possibly caused by thiamine overloading, resulting in hyaline necrosis and ascites (70[c]).

More common are hypersensitivity reactions, which also have been observed mainly after parenteral administration. The clinical symptoms are weakness, precordial pain, palpitation, dyspnea, epigastric pain, vomiting, itching, erythema, scaling of the facial skin, severe rash, tachycardia, hypotension, purpura, a semicomatose state and even fatal anaphylactic shock. Respiratory failure has been reported after parenteral administration of high doses. Although not very common, several cases are reported in the literature.

Anaphylactic reactions have mainly been observed after parenteral administration, occasionally also after muscular injections. In some cases an oral challenge did not produce any reaction (71[R], 72[c]). Thiamine hydrochloride and possibly its intermediates, such as thiothiamide, may constitute a risk of allergic contact dermatitis (73[c], 74[c]).

A prospective study of the toxicity of parenteral thiamine hydrochloride in a large group of patients showed adverse reactions in only 1.1% of the cases, mainly in the form of local irritation. Only one out of the 11 adverse reaction cases was of a serious nature (75[C]). Adverse effects of thiamine may possibly be confined to patients with an allergic disposition, and intradermal test doses of such patients may be warranted prior to high dose thiamine administration.

Riboflavin

The AR is 1.3 mg/day for males and 1.1 mg/day for females, the PRI 1.6 and 1.3 mg/day, respectively, and the LTI 0.6 mg/day for both sexes.

Riboflavin may cause discoloration of the urine; the vitamin is poorly absorbed and adverse reactions are almost unknown.

Nicotinic acid
Nicotinyl alcohol

High-dose niacin is of recognized value in the treatment of elevated blood cholesterol. Its use can be complicated by side effects: skin reactions due to the vasodilator effect, changes in glucose tolerance and liver function. A sustained-release form of nicotinic acid may decrease the vasodilator effect, but there have been several case reports of hepatotoxicity with this form of the drug (SEDA-16, 438). It has been questioned whether the sustained-release form of the drug, which is available over the counter in some countries, ought to continue to be available for self medication (76[C], 77[r]) given its serious side effects.

Skin problems may be persistent in a proportion of patients, variously estimated at 10—59%, and can severely limit medication compliance. The skin reaction may be ameliorated by concomitant use of non-steroidal anti-inflammatory agents such as aspirin and indomethacin (SEDA-15, 412). Transient exanthema, pruritus and sometimes wheals are seen, as well as uniform dryness and scaling of the epidermis, brown pigmentation and even on occasion an acanthosis nigricans-like dermatosis. Persistent rashes can also occur. Doses in excess of 5 grams per day are routinely associated with skin manifestations and can on occasion cause liver damage, gout and ulcer formation. These reactions may be associated with nicotinic acid rather than nicotinamide, which is sometimes recommended as an alternative (78[c]). Increased hair loss has been described. Tingling of the fingertips, faintness and dizziness have been observed. Intravenous administration of nicotinic acid or nicotinyl alcohol tartrate can induce short-lived fibrinolytic activity. Symptoms observed after high doses of nicotinic acid (such as giddiness, faintness and vasovagal attacks) result from drug-induced dilatation of the small arteries and arterioles, resulting in decreased peripheral resistance and blood pressure, and anaphylactic shock can occur. Some cases of EEG abnormalities associated with vitamin B therapy have been reported (SEDA-15, 412; 79[c]).

General gastrointestinal symptoms include heartburn, vomiting, nausea, meteorism and hunger pains. With nicotinyl alcohol, mild stomach complaints and diarrhea may occur. Late adverse effects may comprise hepatic dysfunction, with deranged liver function tests and hyperbilirubinemia.

After prolonged use of nicotinic acid and nicotinyl alcohol, histological changes, e.g. parenchymal cell injury, portal fibrosis, cholangitis, cholestasis, biliary casts and lymphocytic infiltrations around the bile duets, have occasionally been seen.

Prolonged administration of nicotinic acid may indeed have a diabetogenic effect and decompensation of previously stable diabetes may be induced. A case has been described of severe hyperglycemia, precipitated by niacin treatment of high serum lipids (80[c]). During long-term treatment, uric acid levels tend to rise slightly. Some cases of myopathy, with nocturnal leg aching and cramps have been reported. These symptoms may be exacerbated by simultaneous use of other

Table 4. *Peripheral sensory neuropathy during vitamin B_6 megatherapy*

Authors	Cases	Daily dose	Duration of treatment
Schaumburg et al. (1983)	7	2—6 g	2—40 months
Berger and Schaumburg (1974)	1	500 mg	1 year
Vasile et al. (1984)	1	3 g	6 months
De Zegher et al. (1985)	1	1 g	no specification
Dalton (1985)	23	50—300 mg	no specification
Parry and Bredesen (1985)	16	200—5000 mg	1—36 months
Podell (1985)	1	500 mg	8 years
Baer and Stillman (1984)	1	4 g	4 years (dermatosis)
Friedman et al. (1986)	1	2 g	1 year (dermatosis)

From Camarasa et al. (15).

lipid lowering drugs associated with similar side effects, or alcohol which also has myopathic effects (SEDA-15, 413; 81[C]). Apparent interaction between niacin and alcohol has been seen to cause toxic delirium and lactic acidosis (82[c]). Interaction between niacin and nicotine transdermal patches has been observed, causing flushing and dizziness (83).

Some cases of niacin maculopathy have also been observed but the incidence is low, reportedly 0.67% of patients treated with niacin for hyperlipidemia (SEDA-14, 331).

Pyridoxine (vitamin B_6)

Requirements for vitamin B_6 vary with protein intake, and the AR is set at 13 μg/g protein intake, the PRI at 15 μg/g protein intake. In adults this translates into an AR of 1.3 mg/day for males and 1.0 mg/day for females, and a PRI of 1.5 and 1.1 mg/day for males and females, respectively.

Pyridoxine mega-doses are commonly used therapeutically in homocysteinuria, cystathionuria and primary oxalosis type I. In some diseases it is used empirically; they include rheumatic diseases, degenerative joint diseases, carpal tunnel syndrome, Chinese restaurant syndrome and premenstrual syndrome. Several reports have accumulated over the last years demonstrating that neurotoxicity may be associated with pyridoxine megavitamin therapy (84[C]).

Extremely high doses, even up to 6000 mg/day, have sometimes been used therapeutically. Many patients have been self-medicating, with more than 2000 mg/day, for long periods of time (SEDA-10, 334; 85[C], 86[C]). The main symptom of pyridoxine toxicity is peripheral sensory neuropathy (see Table 4; SEDA-16; 87[R]).

While generally no problems arise from controlled application of high doses of pyridoxine under medical supervision, self-medication in doses exceeding 300—500 mg/day can lead to adverse effects, especially when continued over a long period of time.

Sensory neuropathy was reported as an adverse effect in eight patients with homocysteinuria treated with 600—1200 mg/day of pyridoxine for 4—22 years. Nerve conduction studies of the sural nerve showed abnormalities in four of five affected patients (88[C]). Neuropathies have been observed in women on doses as low as 50—500 mg/day taken for one to several months (89[C], 90[R]). Reviews of sensory neuropathies and pyridoxine toxicity have been published (91[R], 92[R]). Pyridoxine (given alone or in combination with vitamin B_{12}) may induce deterioration of acne vulgaris or eruption of an acneiform exanthema (93[C]). Excessive doses of pyridoxine appear to cause a metabolic defect that impairs the structural integrity of the skin, especially during the summer months (94[c]). Vesicular skin lesions on the hands and feet have also been reported, possibly as a symptom secondary to the neurological disturbances (95[c]).

Vitamin B_6 appears to possess both dopamine-enhancing and dopamine-blocking properties: on the one hand pyridoxine (like dopamine) depresses the release of prolactin from the pituitary gland; on the other hand, the vitamin in oral doses of 10—20 mg rapidly reverses the therapeutic effect of dopamine (96[r]). This should be borne in mind if pyridoxine is prescribed for nursing mothers or for patients treated with levodopa for Parkinson's disease or syndrome, although the problem does not seem to arise when using the combination of levodopa with decarboxylase inhibitors.

Decreased serum folate levels have been demonstrated in patients with homocysteinuria while receiving pyridoxine. The mechanism of this effect may depend upon removal of substrate inhibition of the enzyme, N^5-methyltetrahydrofolate homocysteine methyltransferase, due to pyridoxine-induced lowering of the substrate, homocysteine (97[C]).

One case has been reported of a malformed infant

whose mother had taken daily doses of pyridoxine during pregnancy (50 mg for the first 7 months as well as unknown doses of lecithin and vitamin B_{12}). The girl was born with near-total amelia of her left leg at the knee (98[C]). As a precaution, high doses of pyridoxine during pregnancy should be avoided.

The pyridoxine RDA for infants is set at a rather high level in many countries. Consequently, infant formulae are commonly enriched with pyridoxine in relatively high amounts. A recent study found that in comparison with breastfed infants, those fed formula had very high biochemical measures of vitamin B_6 status, which appeared to be dose dependent. During the first 6 months the vitamin B_6 status of the formula-fed infants was above the 95th percentile for the breastfed infants. The authors conclude that reducing the B_6 content of formulas would ensure a more physiological vitamin B_6 status in formula-fed infants (99).

High-dose (300 mg/day) pyridoxine treatment of patients with severe, steroid-requiring asthma was studied in a 9-week double-blind placebo-controlled trial, where no significant differences between the treatment and the control group was found. One patient developed neurological symptoms which may have been due to vitamin B_6 toxicity (100).

Pantothenic acid (vitamin B_5)

Pantothenic acid has no known therapeutic use or adverse reactions. The related racemic alcohol (pantenol) has been claimed to have a parasympathicomimetic effect and hence to interact with other cholinergic drugs and suxamethonium.

RELATED SUBSTANCES

Hopantenate

Hopantenate (calcium D-(+)-4-(2,4-dihydroxy-3,3-dimethylbutyramido) butyrate hemihydrate), or calcium hopantenate, is a homoanalog of L-pantothenate and has been used in Japan for the treatment of mental retardation with behavioural abnormalities. It represents one of the many attempts which have been made—so far unsuccessfully—to develop derivatives of substances belonging to the vitamin B group as agents for the treatment of brain or nervous disorders (SEDA-12, 328; SEDA-13, 347).

Side effects have been reported, sometimes fatal, in patients receiving calcium hopantenate, notably encephalopathy with metabolic acidosis and semicoma (101[c]) and Reye-like syndrome (102[c]), possibly due to the induction of pantothenic acid deficiency, as hopantenate is a pantothenic acid antagonist. In elderly people, liver dysfunction and gastrointestinal upsets have been reported (103[C], 104[C]). As a pantothenic acid analog, hopantenate may affect lactate generation, glucose metabolism and ammonia disposal. Two fatal cases in elderly people presenting with this syndrome have been reported (105). In Japan, where the product was introduced in 1978, the control authorities issued a series of warnings with respect to problems induced by hopantenate in 1988 (106[CR]).

Folic acid

For folic acid (pteroyl glutamic acid) the ADR in adults has been set at 140 μg/day for adults, while the PRI is 200 μg/day. Neural tube defects have been shown to be prevented in offspring by periconceptual ingestion of 400 μg folic acid per day in the form of supplements. Red cell folate values above 150 μg per liter are an indication of sufficiency (107).

High levels of folic acid—commonly 4—5 mg have been used in pregnancy without apparent ill effects.

An interaction of anticonvulsant drugs with the metabolism of folate has been described (SEDA-13, 348). Rare but serious cases of sensitivity to this epileptogenic effect of folic acid have been reported (108[c]); however, it is well tolerated by many other epileptics requiring folic acid. Further investigations are needed concerning folate metabolism in a wide range of clinical disorders now being treated with *antifolate medications* such as cancer, leukemia, psoriasis, rheumatoid arthritis, bronchial asthma, bacterial infections, malaria, hypertension, Crohn's disease, gout, epilepsy and AIDS (SEDA-15, 414).

The intake of high doses of folic acid as well as vitamin B_{12} increases the reticulocyte counts. Thus, use of one of these vitamins might mask the deficiency of the other (SEDA 17, 440). On suspicion of anemia due to deficiency of one of these nutrients, serum levels of both vitamin B_{12} and folic acid should be assessed (109).

A recommendation to supplement all pregnant women with 5 mg folic acid daily in order to prevent neural tube defects (NTD) was issued by health authorities in England in 1991 (110). In 1992 the US Public Health authorities recommended a considerably lower daily intake, 0.4 mg/day (111). This is what a woman would consume if she followed the US Dietary Guidelines and Dietary Pyramid (112). The etiology of neural tube defects is not entirely clear, the condition may have several different causes, only some of which may be responsive to folate (113). Rates of NTD vary considerably between countries; in the US, rates of NTD isolated from other birth anomalies declined over the period 1968–1989 (114). The justification for a recommendation for general high-dose supplementation is still under discussion.

RELATED SUBSTANCES

Folinic acid

Reduced folates are co-factors for the 5-fluorodeoxyuridine monophosphate-thymidylate synthetase reaction. Leucovorin (calcium folinate) therefore potentiates the toxicity of 5-fluorouracil, and fatal side effects have been reported in patients over 65 years of age receiving high-dose treatment with leucovorin simultaneously with fluorouracil. This has led some groups to recommend that initial use of fluorouracil should be lowered by 20% and that therapy be stopped temporarily at the first sign of distal gastrointestinal side effects (SEDA-15, 414).

Cyanocobalamin (vitamin B_{12})

The AR for adults is 1.0 μg/day, PRI is 1.4 μg/day and LTI is 0.6 μg/day.

Side effects of high intakes have been described: urticaria, eczematous and exanthematous skin lesions, and anaphylactic reactions (SEDA-4, 265), but it is not clear whether the reactions are caused by the drug itself, a preservative or possibly by contaminants. High oral or parenteral doses of vitamin B_6 and especially hydroxocobalamin are also on rare occasions suspected to induce acne which is always benign (SEDA-5, 347; 115[C]). Several cases of vitamin B_{12}-induced folliculitis and acneiform eruptions have been described in the literature, recently in connection with a patient on total parenteral nutrition (TPN) (116[C]). Nutritional support teams managing TPN should be aware of this potential adverse effect.

A mild form of polycythemia as well as peripheral vascular thrombosis has been described in patients with pernicious anemia treated with high doses of vitamin B_{12} (117[C]).

RELATED SUBSTANCES

Hydroxocobalamin
Mecobalamin

Hydroxocobalamin (vitamin B_{12a}) has the same pattern of adverse reactions as cyanocobalamin; the same appears to apply to the methyl derivative, mecobalamin.

Vitamin C (ascorbic acid)

The AR of vitamin C is set at 30 mg/day; the PRI is set at 45 mg/day for adults; the LTI, for which considerable evidence exists, is 12 mg/day.

ADVERSE REACTION PATTERN

In spite of lack of unequivocal evidence of a beneficial effect of large doses of vitamin C for the common cold, the use of vitamin C for this indication is widespread. Vitamin C in daily doses of some grams can generally be ingested without any serious ill effects, but occasionally problems do occur.

General and toxic reactions Hot flushes, headache, fatigue, insomnia, nausea, vomiting and diarrhea have been observed with large doses, but it is difficult to tell to what extent these are real or placebo effects. The best evidence of problems caused by high doses in fact relates to stone formation, mainly in patients with chronic renal failure and certain hematological and metabolic effects, mainly in premature infants. Lately, several cases of hemolysis have been reported.

Hypersensitivity reactions Four cases of respiratory and cutaneous allergies to ascorbic acid have been described (118[C]).

Tumor-inducing effects These have not been reported.

ORGANS AND SYSTEMS

Cardiovascular Patients with idiopathic (genetic) hemochromatosis constitute a risk group, since ingestion of large doses of vitamin C may lead to deterioration in cardiac function (119[R]).

Respiratory A trial in 868 children showed that in those with high plasma ascorbic acid concentrations, the duration of upper respiratory infection was greater than in those with low levels (120[C]), but this finding (contrasting with the optimistic expectations of other workers) requires confirmation.

Endocrine, metabolic Data have been presented indicating a diabetogenic effect of dehydroascorbic acid and an increased excretion of glucose after giving ascorbic acid. A recent double-blind, placebo-controlled study demonstrated that plasma insulin response to an oral glucose tolerance test in normoglycemic, ascorbic-acid-'saturated' (2 grams/day) adults was significantly depressed 0.5 hours postprandially, and significantly elevated 2 hours postprandially in comparison with controls, thus indicating that elevated ascorbic acid levels may delay the insulin response to a glucose challenge and prolong postprandial hyperglycemia (121[C]).

An increase in serum cholesterol has been seen in atherosclerotic patients taking high doses of vitamin C (122[CR]).

Daily doses of 3 grams of ascorbic acid for 6 days have been found to induce a significant loss of high altitude resistance, persisting for 2 weeks after withdrawal of the treatment. The ingestion of large doses may therefore constitute a risk in persons taking them under conditions where the oxygen supply may suddenly become impaired, and would also seem to be undesirable in persons with pathological hypoxia, e.g. due to respiratory diseases (123[C]).

Doses of 4 grams have been shown to raise uric acid clearance in volunteers (124[C]), although the vitamin does not seem to reduce protein-bound uric acid in blood.

Daily doses of 4—12 grams do result in acidification of the urine, which may induce precipitation of urate and cystine and consequently formation of urate stones or cysteinuria. Vitamin C is apparently excreted largely as oxalate; hyperoxaluria results when large doses are taken. In patients with pre-existing oxalosis, gram doses of ascorbic acid further increase oxalate excretion (122[R], 125[C]).

Controlled trials to verify a cause-and-effect relationship between ascorbic acid ingestion, calcium oxalate and urinary stone formation have not yet been conducted, but a relationship can be assumed in individuals who have a proclivity to stone formation (126[R]).

Hematological Under experimental conditions, daily 5-gram doses of ascorbic acid have been found to raise the lytic sensitivity of erythrocytes to hydrogen peroxide (127[C]). Similar doses, given with mandelamine or antibiotics, lower urinary pH and have a slight effect on blood pH: in patients with sickle-cell anemia, such doses can induce a crisis (122[R]). Studies indicate that the erythrocytes of premature infants may be damaged by vitamin C (SEDA-14, 332); reduced glutathione levels and increased Heinz-body formation have been seen (128[C]). Possible explanations may be a higher glucose consumption and an increase in glycolytic enzyme activities as compared with erythrocytes from adults, accompanied by increased sensitivity to hemolysis (129[r]). Also at risk are patients with glucose-6-phosphate dehydrogenase (G6PD) deficiency, in whom vitamin C may denature hemoglobin and reduce the erythrocyte glutathione level; one such case has proved fatal (130[CR]). This is further demonstrated by recent case reports of hemolytic effects (131[c]) in two young erythrocyte G6PD-deficient subjects, induced by excessive intake of 'fizzy drinks' fortified with ascorbic acid in 132[c].

Gastrointestinal Nausea, abdominal cramps and diarrhea are not uncommon (122[R]). In runners taking daily doses of 1 gram of vitamin C for reduction of musculoskeletal symptoms, mild diarrhea is frequently observed (133[c]). Ascorbic acid stones have been found to obstruct the ileocecal valve (134[C]).

Urinary system The provision of ascorbic acid to patients with *renal failure* should be carefully monitored to avoid accelerated development of secondary oxalosis; hyperoxalemia has been reported to be aggravated by vitamin C supplementation in regular hemodialysis patients (135[C]). The pharmacological mechanism has been clarified in animal experiments (SEDA-15, 414—415; 136[C]). See also: 'Endocrine, metabolic'.

Skin As pointed out above, cutaneous allergy has been described.

Bone In animal experiments, it has been shown that high doses of ascorbic acid adversely influenced skeleton stability. In chicks, supplementary ascorbic acid at levels of 220 mg/kg in the food increased mobilization of calcium and phosphate from the skeleton, as demonstrated by ^{45}Ca studies and determination of acid phosphatase activity in plasma. Increased ascorbic acid also resulted in increased oxygen consumption and decreased lactic acid production by cultured chick tibiae; in growing swine, large doses (about 1 g/day for 32 days) led to a significant increase in the excretion rate of hydroxyproline, indicating an increased rate of collagen breakdown (SED-8, 803).

Risk situations See above under 'Cardiovascular', 'Urinary system' and 'Hematological', and below under 'Interactions'.

Ascorbic acid has been thought to precipitate widespread tumor hemorrhage and necrosis with disastrous consequences in patients with very rapidly proliferating and widely disseminating tumors. These observations suggest that ascorbic acid should be prescribed with extreme caution to persons with advanced cancer (126[R]).

Ascorbic acid-induced esophageal stricture has been reported in one *elderly patient* who had taken the drug for 2 months. Surgical pathology revealed ulceration, inflammation and fibrosis (137[C]). A 500-mg tablet of ascorbic acid dissolves only slowly and is associated in vitro with a shift in saliva pH from 6.2 to 2.8. Since elderly individuals usually have less frequent esophageal contractions, it is not uncommon for this group to have a capsule lodged for a time in the esophagus (SEDA-13, 348), and it is entirely possible that cases like the above are more frequent than previously thought.

Second-generation effects Earlier evidence that ascorbic acid in gram doses might reduce fertility was disputed; recently, however, a further case of sterility apparently due to this treatment has been described (122[R]).

Animal teratological evidence is not entirely uniform, but very high doses in rats and mice have been given without deleterious effects on the fetus (64[R]).

Interactions Binding of zinc and copper has been reported (122[R]). Ascorbic acid is well known for its ability to promote the absorption of iron, a reason for caution in giving high doses of vitamin to patients with iron overload conditions (SEDA-9, 324). Especially patients with hemochromatosis, polycythemia and leukemia who present with marked iron overload should keep their intake of vitamin C to a minimum (138[R]). However, ascorbic acid can also interfere with the distribution of iron in the body in patients suffering from these conditions. One consequence is that in patients with iron overload who are at the same time suffering from scurvy, iron tends to be deposited in the reticuloendothelial system rather than the parenchymal cells, a situation which may lessen the risks for the liver, the heart or the endocrine glands. It has conversely been noted that in cases of β-thalassemia major with iron overload, administration of ascorbic acid can be associated with a deterioration of cardiac function (139[r]).

Because ascorbic acid in the gastrointestinal tract can reduce much of the vitamin B_{12} content of food, patients with vitamin B_{12} deficiency should always be questioned about their intake of vitamin C (126[R]).

The effect of ascorbate on prothrombin time during *oral anticoagulation* is potentially dangerous. In a patient receiving dicoumarol the prothrombin time fell from 19 seconds to normal values after intake of vitamin C. A similar effect was noted in a patient with thrombophlebitis given 16 grams of ascorbic acid daily (122[R]). Earlier data have suggested that even doses of 200 mg may have resulted in a slight increase in mortality from thromboembolism in the population of a geriatric unit. Impaired response to the anticoagulant warfarin, enhanced drug crystalluria with aspirin, and decreased renal tubular reabsorption of amphetamines and tricyclic antidepressants can be caused by simultaneously ingested vitamin C (126[R]). In one patient an interaction between ascorbic acid and the neuroleptic *fluphenazine* has been described; ascorbic acid may lower the serum fluphenazine levels not only by liver enzyme induction, but also by interference with absorption (140[CR]).

Vitamin C in large doses (5 grams daily) decreases the chronotropic effect of concomitantly administered *isoprenaline* in man (141[C]).

Interference with diagnostic routines The presence of high concentrations of ascorbic acid in the urine may interfere with tests for *urinary glucose*. With concentrations as low as 20 mg/100 ml, tests performed with glucose-oxidase paper may be inhibited, thus giving a false-negative result (142[C]).

Ascorbic acid can, however, also result in false-positive tests for glucose in urine (Benedict's test, Clinitest®) and blood. Any reports of glycosuria or hyperglycemia in patients on vitamin C therapy must therefore be regarded with suspicion unless a specific (e.g. chromatographic) test for glucose has been performed (122[R]).

Plasma *ethinylestradiol* concentrations increase when it is administered with ascorbic acid. This interaction is of some significance in women taking oral contraceptives (SEDA-6, 328).

Vitamin C also interferes with the auto-analyzer determination of *serum transaminases* and *lactic dehydrogenase* (122[R]). Serum *bilirubin* concentrations may be reduced by ascorbic acid, so that the presence of liver disease may be masked (122[R]).

False-negative results of tests for occult blood were found after ingestion of high doses of vitamin C. Daily doses of as much as 500 mg can be absorbed in the intestine, but quantities in excess of this are excreted and may influence the test for occult blood (143[C]). Lack of ascorbic acid can, because of its effect on iron distribution, derange the laboratory indices for iron overload, causing the plasma iron or ferritin levels (or the degree of iron excretion after a challenge with deferoxamine) to be considerably less than the degree of severity of the iron overload would normally lead one to expect (144[c]).

Vitamin D (calciferol) and analogs (calcitriol)

Dietary intake and synthesis of vitamin D in the skin under the influence of ultraviolet light complement one another. In practice, the PRI for adults varies between

5 and 10 μg/day, and for infants and children between 10–25 μg/day*.

Fortification of margarine and dairy products with vitamin D is mandatory in some countries, and permitted in others. Infant formulae and liquid milk are commonly fortified with vitamin D, and two recent studies demonstrated fortification vastly in excess of what was stated on the label (145[C], 146). In one of the cases this was detected when hypervitaminosis was detected in the population. One case of hypercalcemia after prolonged feeding with premature formula which is higher than normal in vitamin D, was also reported (147[c]).

ADVERSE REACTION PATTERN

General and toxic reactions Vitamin D intoxication is characterized by hypercalcemia and hypercalciuria as a result both of excessive gastrointestinal calcium absorption and of enhanced mobilization of calcium from bone (SED-9, 637). Unintentional intoxication may result from addition of vitamin D to food, especially to milk and milk products for prevention of vitamin D deficiency. The established dosage for prophylaxis of vitamin D-deficient rickets, 400 IU (10 μg), is commonly regarded as safe. The large vitamin D doses used in hypoparathyroidism, renal osteodystrophy, vitamin D-resistant rickets and osteomalacia may predispose patients to become intoxicated. Close clinical and biochemical monitoring of patients receiving vitamin D or vitamin D analogs is necessary since intoxication may occur independent of dose and period over which the drug has been given. There are indications that early high-dosage prophylaxis or treatment may induce later nephrocalcinosis and hypercalciuria in children (148[C], 149[C]).

Initial symptoms of hypervitaminosis D comprise weakness, fatigue, lassitude, headache, nausea, vomiting, and diarrhea. Renal function can be impaired at an early stage with polyuria, polydipsia, nocturia, decreased urinary concentrating ability, and proteinuria.

The characteristic features of chronic intoxication are deposition of calcium salts in various tissues. A follow-up study of 24 children with vitamin D intoxications (13 900–200 000 IU/day) for up to 13 years found that 22.7% of the patients remained with permanent damage. The severity of renal, neurological and digestive symptoms was related to the daily dose administered, but the final consequences were dependent on the duration of overdosage (150[C]). Vitamin D-intoxication has also been seen after so-called 'Stoss'-prophylaxis in children, i.e. the use of single very high doses of vitamin D, and it has therefore been suggested that this procedure should be avoided (151[C]).

It has been suggested that it is the 25-hydroxyvitamin D metabolite which is the main factor involved in vitamin D intoxication (152[c]). The level of this metabolite in serum may remain high for several months after ingestion of excessive amounts, at least in infants (SEDA-12, 329; 153[c]).

In elderly people, it should be remembered that the amount of body fat is usually increased and total body fluid is decreased. These changes affect drug distribution, and should be considered when administering lipophilic substances such as vitamin D, which may have a higher relative distribution volume, increased accumulation and a prolongation of their pharmacological effect. Reduced dosages of vitamin D should therefore be given to older patients (154[r]).

Hypersensitivity reactions Hypersensitivity reactions of allergic type are very rare (see 'Risk situations').

Tumor-inducing effects These are not known.

ORGANS AND SYSTEMS

Cardiovascular Some individuals develop hypertension, which may be directly related to hypercalcemia in some cases and which may be reversible when renal function is normalized (155[C]). Metastatic calcification is observed in various tissues, but arterial calcifications are the most usual (SED-8, 805). In some patients undergoing dialysis, calcification of the blood vessels was so extensive that cannulation could not be performed.

Respiratory Calcification of the lung is a rare occurrence, but has been reported in an infant following ingestion of toxic doses (156[c]).

Nervous system There have been very occasional reports of mental disturbances, cerebellar ataxia, peripheral facial paresis, apathy, lack of interest and (in the event of acute poisoning) even stupor. Mental changes may occur prior to the appearance of any somatic symptom (SED-8, 804).

There may be a correlation between the seriousness of hypervitaminosis D and the extent of electroencephalographic change.

* As cholecalciferol: 10 μg cholecalciferol=400 IU of vitamin D.

Endocrine, metabolic In patients with pancreatitis associated with hypercalcemia of unclear origin, vitamin D poisoning may be responsible, especially when episodes are recurrent (157[C]).

Mineral and fluid balance Earlier, a somewhat arbitrary cut-off point for the presence of hypercalciuria led to the conclusion that treatment of postmenopausal osteoporosis with $1{,}25(OH)_2D_3$ would easily generate hypercalciuria. More accurate studies have led to revision of previous standards; it is now proposed that 7.5 mmol/100 ml in women and 10 mmol/100 ml in men, which is based on serum values of normal elderly subjects, be a more realistic cut-off reference value (158[R]).

A single high dose of vitamin D can usually be given without ill effects, even though some workers have described subsequent characteristic changes in the level of phosphorus and calcium in the blood (SED-8, 804, 805). With continued dosage, hypophosphatemia can occur which is more persistent than the hypercalcemia. Hypercalcemia can last for several months after discontinuing the drug. Examination of the urine in cases of overdosage has demonstrated proteinuria, cylindruria and increased excretion of calcium and phosphate. Studies of serum are likely to show increased calcium, increased urea nitrogen, decreased phosphate, decreased cholesterol and sometimes secondary disturbances of other electrolytes (e.g. increased Na^+ and decreased K^+) with acidosis. Due to changes in electrolyte balance, electrocardiographic changes may occur (SEDA-6, 328).

Hypervitaminosis D may easily occur during the treatment of renal rickets since, on the one hand, there is a greatly increased requirement for vitamin D and, on the other, impaired renal function. The renal ability to excrete calcium is so limited that hypercalciuria does not develop as a warning of imminent vitamin D intoxication. Careful monitoring of the plasma biochemistry is therefore essential when treating these cases, and vitamin D must be withdrawn if the serum calcium reaches 10 mg/100 ml or the alkaline phosphatase level falls to normal (159[C]).

Gastrointestinal Besides the general gastrointestinal symptoms mentioned above, acute pancreatitis can develop, possibly due to metastatic calcification of the pancreatic ducts (see also 'Endocrine, metabolic' above). High doses of vitamin D can also affect dental enamel. In one published case, dental hypoplasia was observed many years after an episode of hypervitaminosis D (SED-8, 804).

Urinary system Daily doses of more than 40 μg of vitamin D can cause calcium deposition in the kidneys. Renal damage is largely due to this deposition of calcium. Tubular function is impaired first, glomerular function later (SED-8, 804, 805). Medullary nephrocalcinosis can develop as a result of therapy with high doses of vitamin D combined with calcium, mainly seen in infants and school children. Ultrasound screening of children treated with high doses of vitamin D and calcium is therefore recommended (160[C]) (see also 'Mineral and fluid balance' above).

Special senses Band dystrophia of the cornea has been reported in the past, as have been calcium deposits in the cornea and the conjunctiva. Tympanic membrane calcification may lead to severe, irreversible conductive deafness.

Bone In severe hypervitaminosis D signs of hypo- and demineralisation of the long bones as well as calcification of the soft tissues can be observed radiologically. Patients with osteoporosis or osteomalacia have been treated with pharmacological doses of vitamin D for extended periods of time. Some cases of hypervitaminosis D with hypercalcemia and acute renal failure have been reported, and suggest that such therapy should be avoided. Published data on the use of vitamin D for prophylaxis or treatment of osteoporosis fail to document benefits superior to those of calcium alone or calcium with estrogens and fluoride (SEDA-14, 332; 161[CR]).

Risk situations Deposition, inactivation and catabolism of vitamin D apparently differ quite markedly from one individual to another, since adverse effects have been observed in some cases after administration of doses as low as 0.1 mg. Plasma activity of vitamin D in these cases remained high for an unusually long period of time.

During treatment of hypoparathyroidism, hypercalcemia may occur, probably due to an increased sensitivity to vitamin D (SED-8, 805). Hypercalcemia developing in the course of vitamin D therapy for hyperparathyroidism is often correlated with gastroduodenal ulcer. An increased sensitivity to vitamin D is also observed in sarcoidosis and in patients undergoing renal dialysis and having an abnormal calcium/phosphorus ratio. The risks in renal rickets have been noted above. Patients on continuous ambulatory peritoneal dialysis (CAPD) who develop secondary hyperparathyroidism may already have low bone turnover or adynamic bone lesions, and if treated indiscriminately with calcitriol their low bone turnover may get worse (162[R]).

It has also been suggested that newborn infants with subcutaneous fat necrosis may exhibit transient hypersensitivity to vitamin D (163[C]). There seems indeed to be a relationship between the syndrome known as *infantile idiopathic hypercalcemia* and vitamin D intake and/or vitamin D metabolism (164[C]).

Second-generation effects High doses of vitamin D during pregnancy, possibly together with genetic factors, may induce spontaneous abortion or a severe form of idiopathic hypercalcemia, and a clinical entity in the offspring comprising valvular stenosis of the aorta, peculiar facies, mental retardation and abnormal tooth formation (SED-8, 805). However, such abnormalities can also occur in the absence of hypervitaminosis D, and the doses needed to treat hypoparathyroidism in pregnancy, e.g. 100 000 IU daily, have been well tolerated (64[R]).

A female with hereditary insensitivity to 1,25-dihydroxyvitamin D had an extraordinarily high serum concentration of 1,25-dihydroxyvitamin D throughout the course of gestation, but bore a normal child. This case demonstrates that high serum concentrations need not be teratogenic, although the maternal metabolite may enter the fetal circulation (165[C]).

Interactions *Anticonvulsants* (barbiturate, phenytoin) and other drugs inducing liver enzymes (such as rifampicin) are capable of inducing an accelerated hepatic catabolism of vitamin D; they can lead to reductions in serum 25-hydroxyvitamin D levels and osteomalacia (166[r]). Prophylactic vitamin D treatment of patients receiving long-term treatment with such drugs can therefore be meaningful and should be given at least in case of anticonvulsant drug-induced osteomalacia (167[r], 168[C]).

Symptomatic and reversible hypercalcemia was seen in two elderly patients on apparently safe amounts of vitamin D and thiazide diuretics. The 'hypersensitivity' resulted from an interaction with *calcium carbonate* which had been ingested simultaneously. In the presence of other predisposing factors, hypercalcemia may develop in patients taking 5—10 grams of calcium carbonate daily (169[c], 170[c]).

The combined effects of vitamin D, calcium and *anabolic steroids* in the treatment of senile osteoporosis has been investigated (171[C]). Neither methandienone nor vitamin D_3 alone, but only the two together, seemed to increase coronary morbidity and mortality and possibly in women only. Simultaneous use of these two drugs should thus apparently be avoided.

SPECIFIC NOTE ON VITAMIN D ANALOGS

The vitamin D analogs, 1 α-hydroxycholecalciferol (1 α-OHD_3) and 1,25-dihydroxycholecalciferol (1,25$(OH)_2D_3$), have some advantages over vitamin D (calciferol), but their high potency involves the risk of hypercalcemia developing even after small dose increments, due to increased intestinal calcium absorption. The induction of hypercalcemia concomitant with such clinical symptoms as anorexia, vomiting, (persistent) renal damage and tissue calcification has been described (SEDA-7, 371, 372). Due to the cumulative effect of vitamin D analogs, constant vigilance is required to prevent hypercalcemia, especially in patients with chronic renal failure and associated renal osteodystrophy (SED-9, 639; SEDA-7, 371—372).

Hypercalcemia is not necessarily accompanied by clinical symptoms and disappears within 48 hours when administration of the drug is discontinued. In patients with hypoparathyroidism or chronic renal failure, the rate of reversal of hypercalcemia after stopping treatment with the vitamin D analogs is lower than in normal subjects. In these diseases, frequent control of blood biochemistry is recommended during treatment with vitamin D analogs (SEDA-2, 307; SEDA-9, 325; 172).

Of 19 chronic hemodialysis patients receiving a combination of 1-OHD_3 and 1,25$(OH)_2D_3$ for 12 months, six showed increased bone resorption. Another six showed decreased bone resorption, and seven no change. Histologically documented aggravation of hyperparathyroidism was associated with a statistically significant increase in plasma concentrations of phosphate and parathyroid hormone. The administration of vitamin D analogs may therefore be either beneficial or noxious depending on whether or not the induced hyperphosphatemia is adequately prevented (173[c]).

A child suffering from X-linked hypophosphatemic rickets developed vitamin D intoxication during treatment with 1α-OHD_3 and phosphorus. Besides the usual findings in this condition he showed precocious synostosis of the skull with signs of raised intracranial pressure. In view of earlier reports of coincidence of craniostenosis and X-linked hypophosphatemic rickets the authors conclude that the possibility exists that intoxication with 1α-OHD_3 was the precipitating factor. In addition, hypersensitivity to 1α-OHD_3 was found 2 months after cessation of treatment, with normal levels of calcitriol (1,25$(OH)_2D_3$) (174[C]).

Renal function There is controversy in the literature as to whether the long-term use of C_1-hydroxylated vitamin D analogs in non-dialyzed patients with chronic renal insufficiency is associated with an impairment of glomerular filtration rate (SED-9, 639; SEDA-3, 300; SEDA-4, 267; SEDA-5, 349). At present the question remains unresolved. Nevertheless, the following suggestions are valid ones. Treatment with these drugs should be restricted to patients with severe renal osteodystrophy. A proper dose should be administered in order to avoid a deleterious effect on renal function. Serum calcium and creatinine levels should be monitored carefully. The treatment should be discontinued as hypercalcemia develops.

In a comparative study the efficacy and side effects of calcitriol and ergocalciferol were investigated in 18 children with chronic renal failure and histological evidence of renal osteodystrophy. Whereas therapeutic effects were similar with cholecalciferol and calcitriol, hypercalcemia was more common in the calcitriol-treated patients (11 episodes following calcitriol therapy and three episodes following ergocalciferol therapy) (175[c]).

VITAMIN E (TOCOPHEROL)

Since vitamin E requirement depends on the dietary intake of polyunsaturated fatty acids which varies considerably between individuals, it has not been seen as expedient to establish a single PRI value.

ADVERSE REACTION PATTERN

Several reviews on side effects of vitamin E have been undertaken in the course of the last decade (176[CR], 177[R]), especially of those related to premature infants (178[R]), where high doses have been associated with infectious complications and fatal hepatic failure. In adults, thrombophlebitis, thromboembolism, pulmonary embolism, hypertension, fatigue, gynecomastia and breast tumors have been described as particularly serious complications of vitamin E ingestion, but there is little evidence as to their frequency. Diarrhea and abdominal pain may occur. For some of these effects there seems to be a dose relationship: 800 mg daily for 30 days was recently shown to have no reported side effects in healthy elderly subjects (179). Table 5 shows reported side effects related to dosage in a review of about 50 publications on vitamin E (180[R]).

ORGANS AND SYSTEMS

Cardiovascular Daily administration of 300 mg of vitamin E may lead to an increase in serum cholesterol by an average of 74 mg/100 ml (180[R]). It is therefore advisable to use vitamin E with caution in patients with a family history of heart disease, particularly in view of the doubts about its therapeutic value.

Hematological A significant depression of the bactericidal activity of leukocytes and mitogen-induced lymphocyte transformation occurred after administration of 300 mg of DL-tocopherol, given daily for 3 weeks (181[C]). A reduction of platelet adhesion to collagen has been described (182[C]), and experimentally confirmed (182[C]) and has been seen in doses from 400 mg/day (184[C]).

Skin Although the topical use of vitamin E lacks proof of any beneficial effects, it continues to be popular. Allergic contact dermatitis has been reported rarely; when used in baths, vitamin E is known to cause a follicular eruption.

Risk situations Premature neonates are reported to have a relative deficiency of vitamin E at birth, which has been associated with hemolytic anemia. As increased incidence of necrotizing enterocolitis was reported when oral tocopherol was given to such infants (185[C], 186[C]), parenteral tocopherol was for a while recommended for use in very ill neonates (180[C], 187[c], 188[C]).

However, an increasing number of commonly fatal cases of the 'E-Ferol syndrome' was reported in the course of the 1980s (SEDA-12, 329; 178[R]). This was characterized by progressive clinical deterioration with unexplained thrombocytopenia, renal dysfunction, cholestasis and ascites (189[C]). Persistent liver dysfunction indicated irreversible intrahepatic injury in the neonates and, in 1986, Alade et al. presented evidence of a plausible mechanism for this damage (190[C]). They suggested that E-Ferol suppresses the response of human lymphocytes to phytohemagglutinin and that the factor responsible for this suppression was polysorbate 80, used as an emulsifier in E-Ferol. The authors considered that polysorbate-induced alteration of membrane fluidity in cells of vessel walls might lead to changes in structure and function. Large doses of polysorbate 80 and polysorbate 20 were unavoidably administered when E-Ferol was used and, indeed, a high level of polysorbate 89 (100 μg/ml) was found in ascitic fluid obtained from an affected infant long after discontinuance of E-Ferol. This explanation has been complemented by animal studies (191[C]). A report from the Office of Epidemiology and Biostatistics (Center for Drug Evaluation and research) of the US Food and Drug Administration presented the results of a survey of neonatal intensive care units in which E-Ferol had been used. The analysis clearly indicated that exposure to E-Ferol was associated with increased morbidity and mortality among the infants. Again high levels of polysorbate in body fluids were observed (192[C]). While in adults excretion of polysorbate after hydrolysis of the

Table 5. *Side effects of high doses of vitamin E**

Dosage	Symptoms of changes
	Clinical symptoms
≥300 mg	Gastrointestinal irritation, nausea, vomiting, headache, muscular weakness, dizziness, stomatitis, visual complaints
400 mg	Thrombophlebitis, urticaria, vaginal bleeding
800 mg	Faintness, fatigue, creatinuria
1200 mg	Ecchymosis
1600 mg	Deterioration of angina pectoris
unknown	Deterioration of diabetes melitus
unknown	Transient hypertension
unknown	Allergic contact dermatitis
unknown	Gynecomastia, breast cancer
	Laboratory findings
≥300 mg	Decreased incorporation of thymidine in PHA-stimulated lymphocytes, decreased bactericidal activity of leukocytes and decreased blood glucose levels
600 mg	Decreased concentrations of T3 and T4 in serum
300 mg	Increased concentrations of lipids, cholesterol, carotenoids and blood coagulation factors
600 mg	Increased levels of free cholesterol in LDL- and VLDL-fractions
800 mg	Increased serum creatinine kinase, creatinuria
1000 mg	Increased excretion of steroids in urine
1200 mg	Increased warfarin activity
unknown	Increased dehydroepiandrosterone levels in blood
unknown	Increased gonadotrophin levels

Source: (ref. 180[R]).

fatty acid chain is very fast, the neonate excretes only the polyoxyethylated metabolite (193[R]).

Pre-term infants receiving <25 mg/kg/day tocopherol acetate supplement intravenously had highly variable serum tocopherol concentrations. High serum concentrations were correlated with the occurrence of necrotizing enterocolitis (194[C]).

It appears that another side effect to mega-dose vitamin E therapy in the very low-birthweight infant, first reported in Japan in 1986, may be an increased incidence of infection, even sepsis, after intramuscular injection (SEDA-12, 330). A review of the literature in 1992 concluded that pharmacological serum concentrations of vitamin E might predispose premature infants to infectious complications, possibly caused by an inhibitory effect of vitamin E on the formation of superoxide anion in leukocytes (195).

A statistically significant increase in retinal hemorrhage with parenteral vitamin E was found in premature infants (196[C]). This has led some researchers to conclude that tocopherol should not be recommended for the prevention of retinopathy in prematurity (197[C]), particularly in infants with birth weights of less than 1 kg.

Interactions Vitamin E therapy in vitamin K-deficient subjects and subjects on anticoagulant therapy decreases active plasma prothrombin levels (198[C]).

VITAMIN K* (PHYLLOQUINONE (K_1), MENAQUINONE (MK-*n*)) (*See also Chapter* 35.1)

Vitamin K is in many countries routinely administered to newborn babies in varying doses and by various routes, most commonly either orally or by intramuscular injection, to prevent hemorrhagic disease in the newborn (HDN) (see Table 6).

Side effects of vitamin K are rare, and apparently more common with parenteral administration than with oral (199[R]), and may in a few cases be related to solubilizers, such as polyethoxylated castor oil, added to the fat-soluble vitamin K (SEDA-13, 350; 200[R]).

The most important side effects are jaundice and kernicterus, which may occur in the small and premature baby even after small doses, probably because of immature liver function (SED-8, 806). Hemolytic anemia may occasionally be induced by high doses of vitamin K; severe hemolysis due to this vitamin has also been reported in glucose-6-phosphate dehydrogenase deficiency, particularly if infection is present. In severe

* Vitamin K is the name for a group of compounds, all of which contain the 2-methyl-1,4-naphthoquinone moiety. Common nomenclature is: Vitamin K_1 (phytomenadione), vitamin K_2 (phytonadione), vitamin K_3 (menadione).

Table 6. *Classification of hemorrhagic disease of the newborn (HDN)*

Syndrome	Time of presentation	Common bleeding sites	Comments
Early HDN	0–24 hours	Cephalohematoma, intracranial, intrathoracic, intra-abdominal	Maternal drugs a frequent cause (e.g. warfarin, anticonvulsants)
Classic HDN	1–7 days	Gastrointestinal, skin, nasal, circumcision	Mainly idiopathic, maternal drugs
Late HDN	2–12 weeks	Intracranial, skin, gastrointestinal	Mainly idiopathic, may be presenting feature of underlying disease (e.g. cystic fibrosis, α1-antitrypsin deficiency, biliary atresia. Some degree of cholestasis often present.

Source: Shearer MJ. Vitamin K. Lancet 1995;i(345):229–234.

hepatocellular disease the prothrombin concentration may be further depressed by high doses of vitamin K (SED-8, 806). High doses of vitamin K administered to patients with thrombosis and myocardial infarction treated with dicoumarol may induce relapses (SED-8, 806).

A case-control study in 1990 suggested a causal relation between intramuscular administration of vitamin K to newborns and the subsequent development of leukemia in the babies (201[C]). Later studies have not been able to confirm this finding (202[C], 203[C], 204[r]), but several ongoing studies are expected to shed further light on this problem.

Rapid intravenous administration of the vitamin may cause facial flushing, sweating, fever, rise in blood pressure, a feeling of constriction of the chest, and cyanosis. Cases of cardiovascular collapse after intravenous injection of vitamin K_1 and phytonadione have been reported (205[C]). Intravenous injection of vitamin K_1 is recommended to be performed slowly at a rate not exceeding 5 mg/min. The benefits of intravenous administration of K_1 and phytonadione have to be weighed against the serious, although rare, adverse effects of this drug.

Skin reactions These have been observed after intramuscular injection of vitamin K_1. These lesions appear 4–16 days and even weeks after intramuscular injection, and persist for up to 2 months (SEDA-4, 268; 94[R], 206[C]). The condition is rare; up to now only about 40 cases have been reported in the literature. As a rule, only a rash occurs, generally after high doses of the oil-soluble analog. However, intramuscular injection of vitamin K_1 may also induce lumbar scleroderma around the injection site. The scleroderma is reported to develop in four stages; erythematous, erythematopigmented, established scleroderma and resolvent scleroderma. A case of localized pseudoscleroderma (Texier's syndrome) has also been reported (207[c]). This particular adverse reaction has occurred mainly in patients with hepatic insufficiency (SED-8, 806; SEDA-12, 330), but skin reactions have also been seen in patients with a normal hepatic condition (208[cR]). Brown pigmentation in the trochanteric region has been reported in a cirrhotic patient (SEDA-3, 301).

Allergic reactions have been attributed to vitamin K_1, K_3 and K_4. In mice, vitamin K_3 induced marked hypodynamia and hypothermia. This effect was potentiated by vitamin B_2 (SED-8, 806). Allergic reactions to the systemic administration of vitamin K are immunologically mediated, and generally arise in patients with coagulation or liver problems.

Intradermal tests with vitamin K_1 and K_3 in 145 normal subjects induced an allergic skin reaction 7–22 days after injection in 13 of them. The results indicate that the index of cutaneous sensitivity lies somewhere between 5.5 and 8.9%. The absence of side effects with oral phytomenadione supports the theory that oral administration of the molecule responsible for the dermatitis promotes tolerance rather than inducing or aggravating dermatitis. Continuation of treatment orally can in some cases prevent dermatitis (209[C]). No cross-sensitivity has been seen between vitamin K_1 and K_3 (210[C]). Anaphylactoid reactions to vitamin K_1 have been reported (SEDA-15, 416), especially with intravenous use, some of these even fatal (211[R]).

REFERENCES

1. AMA Council on Scientific Affairs, American Medical Association Vitamin preparations as dietary supplements and as therapeutic agents. J Am Med Assoc 1987;257(14):1929–1936.
2. Combs GF. The Vitamins. Fundamental Aspects in Nutrition and Health. New York: Academic Press, 1992;22.
3. Benton D and Roberts G. Effect of vitamin and mineral supplementation on intelligence of a sample of schoolchildren. Lancet 1988;i:140–143.
4. Whitehead RG. Vitamins, minerals, schoolchildren, and IQ. Br Med J (1990) 302, 548.
5. Schrijver J, Dukes MNG, Helsing E, Bruce Å. Use and Regulation of Vitamin and Mineral Supplements. A Study with Policy Recommendations. Published for the WHO Regional Office for Europe by STYX Publications, Groningen.
6. Koplan JP, Annest JL, Layde DM et al. Nutrient intake and supplementation in the United States. Am J Publ Health (1986) 76, 287–289.
7. Muncie HL, Sobal J. The vitamin-mineral supplement history. J Family Pract (1987) 24, 365.
8. Fike S. Vitamin preparations: recommendations for use. Natl Strength Condition Assoc J (1987) 9, 32.
9. Steinberg, D. Antioxidant vitamins and coronary heart disease (Editorial). New Engl J Med 1993;328(20):1487–1489.
10. Gey KF, Stähelin HB, Eichholzer M. Poor plasma status of carotene and vitamin C is associated with higher mortality from ischemic heart disease and stroke: Basel Protective Study. Clin Invest 1993;71(1):3–6.
11. Heiskanen K, Salmenperä L, Perheentupa J, Siimes MA. Infant vitamin B-6 status changes with age and with formula feeding. Am J Clin Nutrition 1994;60(6):907–910.
12. American Dietetic Association. Positions of the American Dietetic Associsation: enrichment and fortification of foods and dietary supplements. J Am Dietetic Assoc 1994;94(6):661–663.
13. Ovesen L. Vitamin A therapy in the absence of obvious deficiency: What is the evidence? Drugs (1984) 27, 148.
14. Anonymous. Vitamin intoxication is new abuse. Am Pharm (1981) 821, 91.
15. Philen RM et al. Survey of advertising for Nutritional Supplements in Health and Bodybuilding Magazines. J Am Med Assoc 1992;268(8):1008–1011.
16. Nutrition Committee, Canadian Paediatric Society. Megavitamin and megamineral therapy in childhood. Can Med Assoc J (1990) 143, 1009–1013.
17. Evans CD, Lacey JH. Toxicity of vitamins: complications of a health movement. Br Med J (1986) 292, 509.
18. Committee On Medical Aspects of Food Policy. Dietary Reference Values for Food Energy and Nutrients for the United Kingdom. Report of the Panel on Dietary Reference Values. Report on Health and Social Subjects No 41, Department of Health. London: Her Majesty's Stationery Office, 1991.
19. Scientific Committee for Food. Nutrient and energy intakes for the European Community. Luxembourg: Directorate-General Industry Commission of the European Communities, 1993.
20. McLaren DS. Vitamin A deficiency and toxicity. In: Present Knowledge In Nutrition, 5th edn. Washington, DC: Nutrition Review, 1984;203.
21. Abdeljaber MH et al. The impact of Vitamin A supplementation on morbidity: a randomized community intervention trial. Am J Public Health 1991;(81)12:1654–1656.
22. Herrera G et al. Vitamin A supplementation and child survival. Lancet 1992;340(8814):267–271.
23. Guest Editorial. Position Paper by the Teratology Society: vitamin A during pregnancy. Teratology (1987) 35, 269–275.
24. Yetiz JZ. Clinical applications of fish oils. J Am Med Assoc (1985) 260, 665.
25. Grubb BP. Hypervitaminosis A following long-term use of high dose fish oil supplements. Chest (1990) 97, 1260.
26. Hathcock JN, Hattan DG, Jenkins MY et al. Evaluation of vitamin A toxicity. Am J Clin Nutr (1990) 52, 183–202.
27. Theiler R, Wirth, HP, Flury R, Hanck A, Michel BA. Chronic vitamin A intoxication with musculoskeletal symptoms and morphologic hepatic alterations: description of a case. Schweiz Med Wochenschr (1993) 123, 2405–2412.
28. Geubel AP, DeGalocsy C, Alves N, Rahier J. Liver damage caused by therapeutic vitamin A administration: estimate of dose-related toxicity in 41 cases. Farm Tijdschr Belg (1993) 790, 17–26.
29. Marti TJ, Rusinol E, Santana JM et al. Papiledema per ingesta excessiva de vitamina A: a proposit d'un cas. Bull Soc Catalana Pediatr (1985) 45, 193.
30. Ellis JK, Russell RM, Markrauer FL, Schaefer EJ. Increased risk for vitamin A toxicity in severe hypertriglyceridemia. Ann Intern Med (1986) 105, 877.
31. Pastorino U, Chiesa G, Infante M, Soresi E, Clerici M, Valente M, Belloni PA, Ravasi G. Safety of high-dose vitamin A: randomized trial on lung cancer chemoprevention. Oncology (1991) 48, 131–137.
32. Gerber LE, Erdman JW. Changes in lipid metabolism during retinoid administration. J Am Acad Dermatol (1982) 6, 664.
33. De Francisco A, Chakraborty J, Chowdhury HR, Yunus M, Baqui AH, Siddique AK, Sack RB. Acute toxicity of vitamin A given with vaccines in infancy. Lancet (1993) 342, 526–527.
34. Lombaert A, Carton H. Benign intracranial hypertension due to A-hypervitaminosis in adults and adolescents. Eur Neurol (1976) 14, 340.
35. Bauernfeind JC. Vitamin A—Application Technology: A Report of the International Vitamin A Consultative Group. Washington, DC: The Nutrition Foundation, 1980.
36. Haupt R. Akute symptomatische Psychose bei Vitamin A-Intoxikation. Nervenarzt (1977) 48, 91.
37. Goodman GE, Alberts DS, Meyskens FL. Phase I trial of retinol in cancer patients. J Clin Oncol (1983) 1, 394.
38. Muntaner P, Rodriguez C, Arnau JM. Molecular lesion in patients with medium chain acyl-CoA dehydrogenase deficiency. Lancet (1990) 335, 1588–1589.
39. Leicht E, Strunz J, Von Seebach HB et al. Akute Vitamin-A-Intoxikation mit hämolytischer Anämie, Hyperkalzämie und toxischer Hepatose. Med Klin (1973) 68, 54.
40. Muenter MD, Perry HO, Ludwig J. Chronic vitamin A intoxication in adults. Am J Med (1971) 50, 129.
41. Goeckenjan G, Goerz G, Pöttgen W et al. Lebensbedrohliche Komplikationen der hochdosierten Vitamin-A-Behandlung bei Psoriasis. Dtsch Med Wochenschr (1972) 97, 1424.

42. Reuter H. Vitamine: Chemie und Klinik. Stuttgart: Hippokrates Verlag. 1970.
43. Fleischmann R, Schlote W, Schomerus H et al. Kleinknotige Leberzirrhose mit ausgeprägter portaler Hypertension als Folge einer Vitamin A-Intoxikation bei Psoriasisbehandlung. Dtsch Med Wochenschr (1977) 102, 1637.
44. Frøkiær E, Hertel L. Langvarig A-vitaminindtagelse og levercirrhose. Ugeskr Læg (1981) 143, 2038.
45. Sarles J, Scheiner C, Sarran M, Giraud F. Hepatic hypervitaminosis A: a familial observation. J Pediatr Gastroenterol Nutr (1990) 10, 71.
46. Kistler HJ, Plüer S, Dickenmann W, Pirozynski W. Portale Hypertonie ohne Leberzirrhose bei chronischer Vitamin-A-Intoxikation. Schweiz Med Wochenschr (1977) 107, 825.
47. Noseda A, Adler M, Ketelbant P et al. Massive vitamin A intoxication with ascites and pleural effusion. J Clin Gastroenterol (1985) 7, 344.
48. Minuk GY, Kelly JK, Hwang W-S. Vitamin A hepatotoxicity in multiple family members. Hepatology (1988) 8, 272.
49. Kowalski TE, Falestiny M, Furth E and Malet PF. Vitamin A Hepatotoxicity: A Cautionary Note Regarding 25 000 IU Supplements. Am J Med 1994;97(6):523–528.
50. Nater JP, Doeglas HMG. Halibut liver poisoning in 11 fishermen. Acta Dermatol-Venereol (Stockholm) (1970) 50, 109.
51. Morrice G, Havener WH, Kapetansky F. Vitamin A intoxication as a cause of pseudotumor cerebri. J Am Med Assoc (1960) 173, 1802.
52. Marcus DF, Turgeon P, Aaberg TM et al. Optic disk findings in hypervitaminosis A. Ann Ophthalmol (1985) 17, 397.
53. Hawkins TE, Burlon DT. Vitamin A intoxication. J Am Osteopath Assoc (1974) 73, 371.
54. Frame B, Jackson CE, Reynolds WA, Umphrey JE. Hypercalcemia and skeletal effects in chronic hypervitaminosis A. Ann Intern Med (1974) 80, 44.
55. Bartolozzi G, Bernini G. Chronic hypervitaminosis A. Helv Paediatr Acta (1979) 25, 301.
56. Ruby L, Mital MA. Skeletal deformities following chronic hypervitaminosis A: a case report. J Bone Jt Surg (1974) 56, 1283.
57. Gottrand F, Leclerc F, Chenaud M et al. Une cause rare d'hydrocéphalie du nourrison: l'intoxication chronique par la vitamine A. Arch Fr Pédiatr (1986) 43, 501.
58. Bush ME, Dahms BB. Fatal hypervitaminosis A in a neonate. Arch Pathol Lab Med (1984) 108, 838.
59. Noirfalise A. (1991) La vitamin A est-elle dangereuse? Rev Med Liege 16, 461–464.
60. Silverman SH, Lecks HI. Protein calorie deficiency and vitamin indiscretion in an atopic child who developed hypervitaminosis A. Clin Pediatr (1982) 21, 172.
61. Lieber CS. Interaction of ethanol with drugs and vitamin therapy. Pharmacol Phys (1985) 19, 1.
62. Rosa FW, Wilk AL, Kelsey FO. Teratogen update: vitamin A congeners. Teratology (1986) 33, 355.
63. Stange L, Carlström K, Eriksson M. Hypervitaminosis A in early human pregnancy and malformations of the central nervous system. Acta Obstet Gynaecol Scand (1978) 57, 298.
64. Nishimura H, Tanimura T. Clinical Aspects of the Teratogenicity of Drugs. Amsterdam—Oxford: Excerpta Medica, 1976;251.
65. Teratology Society. Teratology Society Position Paper: Recommendations for vitamin A use during pregnancy. Teratology (1987) 35, 269–275.
66. ACOG Committee Opinion: Committee on Obstetrics. Maternal and fetal medicine, vitamin A supplementation during pregnancy. Int J Gynecol Obstet 1993;40(2):175.
67. Danby FW. Retinoic acid in acne therapy. Can Med Assoc J (1978) 119, 854.
68. Dudas I, Czeizel AE. Use of 6000 IU vitamin A during early pregnancy without teratogenic effect. Teratology 1992;45(4):335–336.
69. Semba RD, Munasir Z, Beeler J, Akib A, Muhilal, Audet, S, Sommer A. Reduced seroconversion to measles in infants given vitamin A with measles vaccination. Lancet (1995) 345, 1330–1332.
70. Buligescu I Mileu B, Serbanescu M et al. Un caz de steatoza hepatoica masiva secundara abuzului de tiamina. Med Interna (1986) 38, 183.
71. Kolz R, Lonsdorf G, Burg G. Unverträglichkeitsreaktionen nach parenteraler gabe von Vitamin B_1. Hautarzt (1980) 31, 657.
72. Leung R, Puy R, Czarny D. Thiamine anaphylaxis. Med J Aust (1993) 159, 355.
73. Larsen IA, Jepsen JR, Thulin H. Allergic contact dermatitis from thiamine. Contact Dermatitis (1989) 20, 387.
74. Villas Martinez F, Joral A, Garmendia Goitia JF. Anaphylactic reaction by vitamin B_1. Med Clin (1993) 100, 316.
75. Wrenn, KD, Murphy F, Slovis CM. A toxicity study of parenteral thiamine hydrocloride. Ann Emergency Med (1989) 18, 867.
76. McKenney JM, Proctor JD, Harris S, Vernon M, Chinchili A. A Comparison of the efficacy and toxic effects of sustained- vs immediate-release niacine in hypercholesterolemic patients. J Am Med Assoc 1994;271(9):672–677.
77. Lasagna L. Over-the-counter Niacin (Editorial). J Am Med Assoc 1994;271(9):709–710.
78. Warady B, Kriley M, Alon U, Hallerstein S. Nicotinic acid-induced flush. Periton Dial (1989) 9, 81.
79. Santanelli F, Cobbi G, Albani F, Gastaut H. Apparition d'anomalies EEG chez deux patients en traitement chronique par des vitamines B. Neurophysiol Clin (1988) 18, 549.
80. Schwartz ML. Severe reversible hyperglycemia as a consequence of niacin therapy. Arch Intern Med (1993) 153, 2050–2052.
81. Litin SC, Anderson CF. Nicotinic acid-associated myopathy. Am J Med (1989) 86, 481.
82. Schwab RA, Bachhuber BH. Delirium and lactic acidosis caused by ethanol and niacin coingestion. Am J Emerg Med (1991) 9, 363–365.
83. Rockwell KA. Potential interaction between niacin and transdermal nicotine. Ann Pharmacother (1993) 27, 1283–1284.
84. Schaumburg H, Kaplan J, Windebank A et al. Sensory neuropathy from pyridoxine abuse: a new megavitamin syndrome. N Engl J Med (1983) 309, 445.
85. Dalton K. Pyridoxine overdose in premenstrual syndrome. Lancet 1985;i:1168.
86. Parry GJ, Bredesen DE. Sensory neuropathy with low-dose pyridoxine. Neurology (1985) 35, 1466.
87. Bässler KH. Nutzen und Gefahren einer Megavitamintherapie mit Vitamin B_6. Dtsch Apoth Ztg (1990) 130, 1964–1966.
88. Ludolph AC, Masur H, Oberwittler C, Koch HG, Ullrich

K. Sensory neuropathy and vitamin B_6 treatment in homocysteinuria. Eur J Pediatr (1993) 152, 271.
89. Dalton K. Toxicity of vitamins. Br Med J (1986) 292, 903.
90. Heinrich HC. Neuro- und embryotoxische Nebenwirkungen von Vitamin B_6. Med Monatsschr Pharm (1989) 12, 392.
91. Bendich A, Cohen M. Vitamin B_6 safety issues. Ann NY Acad Sci (1990) 585, 321–330.
92. Bernstein AL. Vitamin B_6 in clinical neurology. Ann NY Acad Sci (1990) 585, 250–260.
93. Braun-Falco, Lincke H. Zur Frage der Vitamin B_6/B_{12}-Akne: ein Beitrag zur Acne medicamentosa. Münch Med Wochenschr (1976) 118, 155.
94. Baer RL. Cutaneous skin changes probably due to pyridoxine abuse. J Am Acad Dermatol (1983) 10, 527.
95. Freidman MA, Resnick JS, Baer RL. Subepidermal vesicular dermatosis and sensory peripheral neuropathy caused by pyridoxine abuse. J Am Acad Dermatol (1986) 14, 915.
96. Greentree LB. Dangers of vitamin B_6 in nursing mothers. N Engl J Med (1979) 300, 141.
97. Wilcken B, Turner B. Homocystinuria: reduced folate levels during pyridoxine treatment. Arch Dis Child (1973) 48, 58.
98. Garner LIG, Welsh-Sloan J, Cady RB. Phocomelia in an infant whose mother took large doses of pyridoxine during pregnancy. Lancet 1985;i:636.
99. Heiskanen K, Salmenperä L, Perheentupa J et al. Infant vitamin B_6 status changes with age and with formula feeding. Am J Clin Nutrition 1994;60(6):907–910.
100. Sur S et al. Double-blind trial of pyridoxine (vitamin B_6) in the treatment of steroid-dependent asthma. Ann Allergy 1993;70(2):147–152.
101. Kimura A, Yoshida I, Ono E et al. Acute encephalopathy with hyperammonemia and dicarboxylic aciduria during calcium hopantenate therapy: a patient report. Brain Dev (1986) 8, 601.
102. Togashi K, Miura Y, Ishiyama S et al. Two autopsied cases of sudden death associated with calcium hopantenate. Brain Dev (1984) 6, 230.
103. Noda, A, Umezaki H, Yamamoto K, Araki T, Murakami T, Ishii N. Reye-like syndrome following treatment with the pantothenic acid antagonist, calcium hopantenate. J Neurol Neurosurg Psychiatry (1988) 51, 582–585.
104. Ohsuga S, Ohsuga T, Takeoka T et al. Metabolic acidosis and hypoglycemia during calcium hopantenate administration. Report on 5 patients. Clin Neurol (1989) 29, 741.
105. Otsuka M, Akiba T, Okita Y et al. Lactic acidosis with hypoglycemia and hyperammonemia observed in two uremic patients during calcium hopantenate treatment. Jpn J Med (1990) 29, 324–328.
106. Anonymous. Calcium hopantenate. Information on Adverse Reactions to Drugs, No. 85. Tokyo: Ministry of Health and Welfare, 1988.
107. Chanarin I. The Megaloblastic Anaemias, 2nd edn. Oxford: Blackwell Scientific Publications, 1979.
108. Bramanti P, Ricci RM, Bagala S et al. Does folic acid exert a provocative action on the EEG of epileptic patients? A preliminary report. Acta Neurol (1987) 42, 250.
109. Wald NJ, Bower C. Folic acid and the prevention of neural tube defects (Editorial). Br Med J 1995; 310(6986):1019–1020.
110. Acheson D, Poole AAB. Folic acid in the prevention of neural tube defect: Circular letter to all doctors in England. Issued by the Department of Health, London, 1991.
111. United States Public Health Service. US Public Health Says B Vitamin Can Cut Birth Defects Risk (Press release). 14 September 1992.
112. Scott JM et al. Folic acid to prevent neural tube defects (Letter). Lancet 1991;338(8765):505.
113. Holmes LB. Prevention of neural tube defects (Editorial). J Pediatr 120(6):918–919.
114. Yen IH et al. The changing epidemiology of neural tube defects. Am J Dis Child 1992;146(7):857–861.
115. Dupre A, Albarel N, Bonafe JL et al. Acnes induites par la vitamine B_{12}. Rev Med Toulouse (1975) 11, 391.
116. Gallastegui C, Cardona D, Pujol R et al. Vitamin B_{12}-induced folliculitis. Drug Intell Clin Pharm Ann Pharmacother (1989) 23, 1033–1034.
117 Klemetti L. Is the vitamin B_{12} treatment of pernicious anaemia a predisposing factor for thrombosis in aged patients? Acta Med Scand (1964) 176, 121.
118. Vasal P. A propos de trois allergies respiratoires et cutanes d l'acide ascorbique. Rev Fr Allergol (1976) 16, 103.
119. Van der Weyden MB. Vitamin C, desferrioxamine and iron loading anemias. Aust NZ J Med (1984) 14, 593.
120. Coulchan JL, Eberhard S, Kapner L et al. Vitamin C and acute illness in Navajo schoolchildren. New Engl J Med (1976) 295, 973.
121. Johnston CS, Yen M-F. Megadose of vitamin C delays insulin response to a glucose challenge in normoglycemic adults. Am J Clin Nutr (1994) 60, 735–738.
122. Barness LA. Safety considerations with high ascorbic acid dosage. Ann NY Acad Sci (1975) 258, 523.
123. Schrauzer GN, Ishmael D, Kiefer GW. Some aspects of current vitamin C usage: diminished high-altitude resistance following overdosage. Ann NY Acad Sci (1975) 258, 377.
124. Stein HB, Hasan A, Fox IH. Ascorbic acid-induced uricosuria: a consequence of megavitamin therapy. Ann Intern Med (1976) 84, 385.
125. Roth DA, Brettenfield RV. Vitamin C and oxalate stones. J Am Med Assoc (1977) 237, 768.
126. Sestili MA. Possible adverse effects of vitamin C and ascorbic acid. Semin Oncol (1983) 10, 299.
127. Mengel CE, Greene HL. Ascorbic acid effects on erythrocytes. Ann Intern Med (1976) 84, 490.
128. Ballin A, Brown EF, Koren G, Zipursky A. Vitamin C-induced erythrocyte damage in premature infants. J Pediatr (1988) 113, 114.
129. Petrich C, Goebel U. Vitamin C-induced damage of erythrocytes in neonates. J Pediatr (1989) 114, 341.
130. Campbell GD, Steinberg MH, Dower JD. Ascorbic acid-induced hemolysis in G6PD deficiency. Ann Intern Med (1975) 82, 810.
131. Rees DC, Kelsey H, Richards JDM. Acute haemolysis induced by high dose ascorbic acid in glucose-6-phosphate dehydrogenase deficiency. Br Med J, 1993;306(6881):841–842.
132. Mehta JB, Singhal SV, Meutch BC. Ascorbic acid-induced hemolysis in G-6-PD deficiency. Lancet (1990) 336, 944.
133. Hoyt CJ. Diarrhea from vitamin C. J Am Med Assoc (1980) 244, 1674.
134. Vickery RE. Unusual complication of excessive ingestion of vitamin C tablets. Int Surg (Chicago) (1973) 55, 422.
135. Ono K. Secondary hyperoxalemia caused by vitamin C supplementation in regular hemodialysis patients. Clin Nephrol, 1986;239.

136. Ono K, Ono H, Ono T et al. Effect of vitamin C supplementation on renal oxalate deposits in five-sixths nephrectomized rats. Nephron (1989) 51, 536.
137. Bonavina L, DeMeester TR, McChesney L et al. Drug-induced esophageal strictures. Ann Surg (1987) 206, 173.
138. Hallberg L. Effect of vitamin C on the bioavailability of iron from food. In: Counsell JN, Hornig DH, eds. Vitamin C (Ascorbic Acid). New Jersey: Applied Science Publishers, 1981;49.
139. Cohen A, Cohen IJ, Schwartz E. Scurvy and altered iron stores in thalassemia major. N Engl J Med (1981) 304, 158.
140. Dysken MW, Cumming RJ, Channon RA, Davis JM. Drug interaction between ascorbic acid and fluphenazine. J Am Med Assoc (1979) 241, 2008.
141. Hajdu E, Jrnyi B, Matos L. The effect of large oral doses of vitamin C on the chronotropic action of isoprenaline in man. Br J Pharmacol (1979) 66, 4607.
142. Mayson JS, Schumaker 0, Nakamura RM. False negative test for urinary glucose in the presence of ascorbic acid. Am J Clin Pathol (1972) 58, 297.
143. Anonymous. Vitamin C verfälscht Bluttests. Klinikarzt (1976) 5, 515.
144. Nienhuis AW. Vitamin C and iron. N Engl J Med (1981) 304, 170.
145. Jacobus CH et al. Hypervitaminosis D associated with drinking milk. New Engl J Med 1992;326(18):1173—1177.
146. Holick MF et al. The vitamin D content of fortified milk and infant formula. New Engl J Med 1992;326(18):1178—1181.
147. Nako Y, Fukushima N, Tomomasa T et al. Hypervitaminosis D after prolonged feeding with a premature formula. Pediatrics 1993;92(6):862—864.
148. Misselwitz J, Hesse V, Markestad T. Nephrocalcinosis, hypercalciuria and elevated serum levels of 1,25-dihydroxyvitamin D in children. Acta Paediat Scand (1990) 79, 637—643.
149. Weber G, Cazzuffi MA, Frisone F et al. Nephrocalcinosis in children and adolescents: sonographic evaluation during long-term treatment with 1,25-dihydroxycholecalciferol. Child Nephrol Urol 1988/1989;9:273—276.
150. Navarro M, Espinosa L, Pena A, Picazo ML, Larrauri M. Intoxicación por vitamina D_3 y secuelas irreversibles. An Esp Pediatr (1984) 22, 99.
151. Hoppe B, Genhm HE, Wopmann M et al. Vitamin-D-intoxikation beim Säugling: eine vermeidbare Ursache von Hypercalciurie und Nephrocalcinose. Schweiz Med Wschr (1992) 122, 257—262.
152. Saggese G, Baroncelli GI, Bertelloni S. Intossicazione da vitamina D. Minerva Pediatr (1986) 38, 1057.
153. Misselwitz, J. Hesse V. Hypercalzämie nach Vitamin-D Stossprophylaxe. Kinderärztl Prax (1986) 54, 431.
154. Schütz R-M. Aspekte der Pharmakotherapie im Alter. Dtsch Med Wochenschr (1993) 118, 1652—1654.
155. Blum M, Kirsten M, Worth MH. Reversible hypertension: caused by the hypercalcemia of hyperparathyroidism, vitamin D toxicity, and calcium infusion. J Am Med Assoc (1977) 237, 262.
156. Bartolozzi G, Calzolari C, Pela I et al. Pulmonary calcification in vitamin D poisoning in an infant. Pediatr Med Chir (1988) 10, 541.
157. Waele BD, Smitz, J, Willems G. Recurrent pancreatitis secondary to hypercalcemia following vitamin D poisoning. Pancreas (1989) 4, 378.
158. Gallagher JC, Goldgar D. Treatment of postmenopausal osteoporosis with high doses of synthetic calcitriol. A randomized controlled study. Ann Intern Med (1990) 113, 649—655.
159. Stanbury SW. The treatment of renal osteodystrophy. Ann Intern Med (1966) 65, 1133.
160. Gückel C, Benz-Bohm G. Roth B. Die Nephrokalzinose in Kindesalter: Sonographische Befunde und Differentialdiagnostik. Fortschr Röntgenstr (1989) 3, 301.
161. Schwartzmann MS, Franck WA. Vitamin D toxicity complicating the treatment of senile, postmenopausal, and glucocorticoid-induced osteoporosis: four case reports and a critical commentary on the use of vitamin D in these disorders. Am J Med (1987) 82, 224.
162. Delmez JA. Calcitriol and secondary hyperparathyroidism in continuous ambulatory peritoneal dialysis patients. Peritoneal Dial Int (1993) 13, 122—125.
163. Wehinger H. Spätrachitis nach Vitamin-D-Überempfindlichkeit bei Adiponekrosis subcutanea in der Neugeborenenperiode. Z Kinderheilk (1969) 107, 42.
164. Fraser D. The relation between infantile hypercalcemia and vitamin D—public health implications in North America. Pediatrics (1976) 40, 1050.
165. Marx SJ, Swart EG, Hamstra AJ, Deluca HF. Normal intrauterine development of the fetus of a woman receiving extraordinarily high doses of 1,25-dihydroxyvitamin D. J Clin Endocrinol Metab (1980) 51, 1138.
166. Hahn TJ. Drug-induced disorders of vitamin D and mineral metabolism. Clin Endocrinol Metab (1980) 9, 107.
167. Hahn TJ. Drug-induced disorders of vitamin D and mineral metabolism. Clin Endocrinol Metab (1980) 9, 107.
168. Krause KH, Bohn T, Schmidt-Gayk H et al. Zur prophylaktischen Gabe von Vitamin D_2 und D_3 bei Anfallskranken. Nervenarzt (1978) 49, 174.
169. Crowe M, Wollner L, Griffiths RA. Hypercalcemia following vitamin D and thiazide therapy in the elderly. Practitioner (1984) 228, 312.
170. Drinka PJ, Nolten WE. Hazards of treating osteoporosis and hypertension concurrently with calcium, vitamin D, and distal diuretics. J Am Geriatr Soc (1984) 32, 405.
171. Inkovaara J, Gothoni G, Halttula R et al. Calcium, vitamin A and anabolic steroid in treatment of aged bones: double-blind placebo-controlled long-term clinical trial. Age Ageing (1983) 12, 124.
172. Chan JCM, Young RB, Alon U, Mamunes P. Hypercalcemia in children with disorders of calcium and phosphate metabolism during long-term treatent with 1,25-dihydroxyvitamin-D_3. Pediatrics (1983) 72, 225.
173. Coevoet B, Sebert J L, DeGueris J et al. Adverse effect of vitamin D metabolites on osteitis fibrosa in patients on chronic hemodialysis: critical role of induced hyperphosphatemia. Miner Electrolyte Metab (1979) 2, 217.
174. Carlsen NLT, Krasilnikoff PA, Eiken M. Premature cranial synostosis in X-linked hypophosphatemic rickets: possible precipitation by 1-alpha-OH-cholecalciferol intoxication. Acta Paediatr Scand (1984) 73, 149.
175. Hodson EM, Evans RA, Dunstan CR et al. Treatment of childhood renal osteodystrophy with calcitriol or ergocalciferol. Clin Nephrol (1985) 24, 192.
176. Roberts HJ. Perspective on vitamin E as therapy. J Am Med Assoc (1981) 246, 129.
177. Hale WE, Perkins LL, May FE et al. Vitamin E effect on symptoms and laboratory values in the elderly. J Am Diet Assoc (1986) 114, 625.

178. Balistreri WF, Farrell MK, Bove KE. Lessons from the E-Ferol tragedy. Pediatrics (1986) 78, 503.
179. Meydani SN, Meydani M, Rall LC et al. Assessment of the safety of high-dose, short-term supplementation with vitamin E in healthy older adults. Am J Clin Nutr (1994) 60, 704–709.
180. Elmadfa IE. Nutzen und Gefahren hochdosierter Vitamin E-Präparate. Fette Seifen Anstrichmittel (1985) 87, 571.
181. Prasad JS. Effect of vitamin E supplementation on leucocyte function. Am J Clin Nutr (1980) 33, 606.
182. Steiner M. Effect of alpha tocopherol administration on platelet function in man. Thromb Haemost (1983) 49, 73.
183. Jandok J, Steiner M. An effective inhibitor of platelet adhesion. Blood (1986) 68, 1153.
184. Srivastave KC. Vitamin E exerts antiaggregatory effects without inhibiting the enzymes of the arachidonic acid cascade in platelets. Prostaglandins Leukotrienes Med (1986) 21, 177.
185. Finer NN, Peters KL, Hayek Z et al. Vitamin E and necrotizing enterocolitis. Pediatrics (1984) 73, 387.
186. Johnson L, Bowen P, Herman N et al. The relationship of prolonged elevation of serum vitamin E levels to neonatal bacterial sepsis (SEP) and necrotizing enterocolitis (NAC) (Abstract). Pediatr Res 1983;17:Abstr 319.
187. Pantoja A, Ukrainski C, Belendy D et al. Vitamin E kinetics in children 1500 grams: intramuscular vs oral administration (Abstract). Pediatr Res 1984;18:Abstr 371.
188. Phelps DL, Pool W, Bauernfeld JC et al. Safety of intravascular tocopherol in a randomized double-blind trial in premature infants. Pediatr Res (1984) 18, 158A.
189. Bove KE, Kosmetatos N, Wedig KE et al. Vasculopathic hepatoxicity associated with E-Ferol. J Am Med Assoc (1985) 254, 2422.
190. Alade SL, Brown RE, Paquet A. Polysorbate 80 and E-Ferol toxicity. Pediatrics (1986) 77, 593.
191. Varma RD, Kraushal R, Junnarkar AY et al. Polysorbate 80: a pharmacological study. Arzneim Forsch (1985) 35, 804.
192. Arrowsmith JB, Faich GA, Tomita DK et al. Morbidity and mortality among low birth weight infants exposed to an intravenous vitamin E product, E-Ferol. Pediatrics (1989) 83, 244.
193. Pesce AJ, McKean DL. Toxic susceptibilities in the newborn with special consideration of polysorbate toxicity. Ann Clin Lab Sci (1989) 19, 70.
194. Friedman CA, Wender DF, Temple DM et al. Serum alpha-tocopherol concentrations in pre-term infants receiving less than 25 mg/kg/day alpha-tocopherol acetate supplements. Dev Pharmacol Ther (1988) 11, 273.
195. Mino M. Clinical uses and abuses of vitamin E in children. Proc Soc Exp Biol Med (1992) 200, 266–270.
196. Rosenbaum AL, Phelps DL, Isenberg SJ et al. Retinal hemorrhage in retinopathy of prematurity associated with tocopherol treatment. Ophthalmology (1985) 92, 1012.
197. Phelps DL, Rosenbaum AL, Isenberg SJ et al. Tocopherol efficacy and safety for preventing retinopathy of prematurity: a randomized, controlled, double-masked trial. Pediatrics (1987) 79, 489.
198. Helson L. The effect of intravenous vitamin E and nenadiol sodium diphosphate on vitamin K-dependent clotting factors. Thrombos Res (1984) 35, 11.
199. Mosser C, Janin-Mercier A, Souteyrand P. Les réactions cutanées après administration parentérale de vitamine K. Ann Dermatol Vénéréol (1987) 114, 243.
200. Havel M, Graninger W, Lindemayr H. Tolerability of a new vitamin K_1 preparation for parenteral administration to adults: one case of anaphylactoid reaction. Clin Ther (1987) 9, 373.
201. Golding J, Paterson M, Kinlen JL. Factors associated with childhood cancer in a national cohort study. Br J Cancer (1990) 62, 304–308.
202. Klebanoff MA, Read JS, Mills JL et al. The risk of childhood cancer after neonatal exposure to vitamin K. New Engl J Med (1993) 329, 905–908.
203. Ekelund H, Finnström O, Gunnarskog J et al. Administration of vitamin K to newborn infants and childhood cancer. Br Med J (1993) 307, 89–91.
204. McWirther WR. Vitamin K and childhood cancer. Med J Aust (1993) 159, 499.
205. Pelletier G, Attali P, Ink O. Arrêt cardiorespiratoire après injection intraveineuse de vitamine K_1. Gastroentérol Clin Biol (1986) 10, 615.
206. Earnes HM, Sarkany I. Adverse skin reaction from vitamin K. Br J Dermatol (1976) 95, 653.
207. Brunskill NJ, Beth-Jones J, Graham-Brown RAC. Pseudosclerodermatous reaction to phytomenadione injection (Texier's syndrome). Clin Exp Dermatol (1988) 13, 276.
208. Sanders MN, Winkelmann RK. Cutaneous reactions to vitamin K. J Am Acad Dermatol (1988) 19, 699.
209. Pigatto PD, Bigardi A, Fumugali M et al. Allergic dermatitis from parenteral vitamin K. Contact Dermatitis (1990) 22, 307–308.
210. Hwang SW, Kim YP, Chung BS, Kim HK. Vitamin K_1 dermatitis. Korean J Dermatol (1983) 21, 91.
211. ADRAC. Slow down on parenteral vitamin K. Aust Adverse Drug React Bull (1991) 10, 3.

Meyler's Side Effects of Drugs, 13th Edition
M.N.G. Dukes, editor

SECTION EDITOR: M.N.G. DUKES

M.N.G. Dukes

39 Corticotrophins and corticosteroids

Editorial note *Corticosteroids used on the skin are reviewed in Chapter 14; corticosteroids used in the eye are discussed in Chapter 47.*

GENERAL

The main human anti-inflammatory corticosteroid—the glucocorticoid cortisol (hydrocortisone) as secreted by the adrenal—has, for therapeutic purposes, generally been replaced by related steroids of synthetic origin. These Δ^1-dehydrated glucocorticoids are designed to imitate the physiological hormone, possessing marked glucocorticoid potency but having only minor effects on sodium retention and potassium excretion; the relative glucocorticoid and mineralocorticoid potencies of the best known compounds, in so far as these potencies are agreed, are compared in Table 2.

In the course of the years a great deal of research has been devoted to producing better steroids for therapeutic use. It would be fair to say that those endeavors have only in part succeeded; from the start the mineralocorticoid effects were sufficiently minor to be without problems; the fact that successive synthetic steroids had an increasing potency in terms of weight was not of direct therapeutic significance; and the most hoped-for aim, that of dissociating wanted from unwanted glucocorticosteroid effects was hardly achieved at all (1[R]). Most untoward effects, such as those due to the catabolic and gluconeogenic activities of the glucocorticoid family, probably cannot be dissociated entirely from the anti-inflammatory activity (2[R]); it is possible that myopathy and muscle wasting are actually more common when triamcinolone or dexamethasone are used, but this may merely reflect overdosage of these potent substances. Some progress in achieving a dissociation of effects has however been made. Beclamethasone does prove to have a relatively greater local than systemic effect, though the latter remains clinically significant. Deflazacort, one of the few new glucocorticoids to have been developed in recent years, bears some promise of a reduced intensity of side effects, e.g. on bone mineral density, but the work available so far does not provide a firm basis for conclusions (SEDA-18, 389). Cloprednol seems to affect much less the hypothalamic-pituitary-adrenal axis function, and to cause less excretion of nitrogen and calcium than older steroids (3[C]).

When considering the adverse reactions to corticosteroids, one has to take into account the fact that the great majority of patients who are therapeutically treated with glucocorticoids do not have a deficiency of these hormones. The adverse reactions to corticosteroids depend very largely upon the way in which (and the purpose for which) they are used. There are essentially four groups of indications:

(1) *Substitution therapy* is employed in cases of primary and secondary adrenocortical insufficiency; the aim is to provide glucocorticoids and mineralocorticoids in physiological quantities, and the better the dosage regime is adapted to the individual's needs the less chance of side effects.

(2) *Antiphlogistic therapy* is used mainly to exploit the immunosuppressive, anti-allergic, anti-inflammatory, anti-exudative and anti-proliferative effects of the glucocorticoids. The desired pharmacodynamic effects reflect a general influence of these substances on the mesenchyme, where they suppress those mesenchymal reactions that result in the symptoms of inflammation, exudation and proliferation; the non-specific effects of corticosteroids on mesenchyme are part of their physiological activity but they can only be obtained to a clinically useful extent by using dosage levels at which the more specific (and in this situation unwanted) physiological effects also become manifest to an inconvenient degree.

(3) *Suppression therapy* can be used, e.g. to inhibit the adrenogenital syndrome. Again higher doses are employed. The treatment of the adrenogenital syndrome is only partly substitutive and has to be adapted to the individual case, but dose levels are needed at which various hormonal effects of the mineralo- and glucocorticoids are likely to become troublesome. High doses sufficient to *suppress immune reactions* are used in patients who have undergone organ transplants.

(4) *Massive doses*, far exceeding physiological levels, can be used in occasional situations, notably to treat shock and sometimes to obtain an antiemetic effect in an emergency. At such levels of dosage, both the desired and the undesired effects reflect overdosage; the corticosteroid is no longer acting as nature intended; the treatment is however usually of brief duration and the resultant problems are therefore few.

Any physician prescribing corticosteroids long term should have a check-list in mind of the undesired effects which they can exert both during treatment and on withdrawal, so that any harm which occurs cam be promptly detected and countered.

Many of the adverse effects to corticotrophin (ACTH) and glucocorticoids became known well over a generation ago. Earlier evidence on those effects which are well quantified and beyond dispute, will be found in the older volumes in this series, and original sources will be indicated only where certain matters, e.g. the quantification of an effect, are still unsettled or knowledge is still accumulating.

Nomenclature The two main classes of adrenal corticosteroids (including the substances sythesized to emulate their effects) are properly known as the *glucocorticosteroids* and the *mineralocorticosteroids*. Particularly the former are often known by shorter names; they are commonly referred to as 'glucocorticoids', 'corticosteroids', 'corticoids' or even simply 'steroids'. Shorter names will for the sake of convenience be used at various points in this Chapter in so far as there is no risk of confusion with the mineralocorticosterioids.

ACTH (corticotrophin) and tetracosactide

(SEDA-16, 453; SEDA-17, 451; SEDA-18, 386)

ACTH stimulates the adrenal cortex to secrete hydrocortisone (cortisol), corticosterone, aldosterone and a number of weakly androgenic substances as well as a small amount of testosterone. Aldosterone synthesis is also regulated by renin and angiotensin. Fluctuations in the rates of secretion from the adrenal cortex are determined by variations in the rate of release of ACTH from the anterior pituitary, and this in turn is controlled by the hypothalamic corticotrophin-releasing hormone (CRH). Since release of the latter is affected by circulating corticosteroid levels, a negative-feedback control operates to keep the system in balance. It follows from the above that if corticosteroids are administered exogenously they will operate through this feedback to suppress adrenal function; ACTH, on the other hand, will promote adrenal cortical function, which explains the fact that there are some differences between the effects of the two.

In patients with functionally normal adrenals the indications for corticosteroids and ACTH are the same, but if the adrenal needs to be stimulated (as it may where its function has been suppressed by prolonged corticosteroid treatment) there can a sufficient reason for a course of ACTH. The only proven practical advantage of ACTH treatment over that with glucocorticosteroids lies in the avoidance of secondary adrenal insufficiency, whilst hypophyseal production of ACTH also appears to be hardly suppressed; against these relative benefits one must set the disadvantages of sodium and water retention and of increased androgen secretion from the adrenal. The main indications for corticotrophin and tetracosactide are thus in the diagnostic rather than the therapeutic field, in which they are being replaced increasingly by CRH.

ACTH (corticotrophin) is a polypeptide consisting of 39 amino acids. Its hormonal activity is related to the first 24 amino acids in a sequence to be found both in preparations of animal origin and in the human pituitary. The differing sequence of the remaining 15 amino acids in animal products may lead to antibody formation and hence to allergic reactions when these animal hormones are injected into human subjects. Even the highly purified ACTH preparations of animal origin were, therefore, from 1970 onwards largely displaced by the so-called 'synthetic ACTH' or 'synthetic corticotrophin'—better known by its generic name of tetracosactide, since it in fact contains only the first 24 amino acids, hence avoiding much of the antigenicity of the complete molecule.

The mode of inactivation and excretion of ACTH is still almost completely unknown; its biological half-life has been variously assessed as several minutes or several hours.

The following monograph should be consulted alongside that on glucocorticosteroids later in this chapter: it is not always clear which adverse effects are actually specific to ACTH/tetracosactide and which simply result from the secretion of corticosteroids which they induce; conversely, almost any adverse effect associated with corticosteroids can in principle also occur with ACTH.

ADVERSE REACTION PATTERN

General and toxic reactions Corticotrophins share all the adverse effects of corticosteroids, including reduction of the body's defenses against infection and infestation, but they do not depress adrenocortical function. For the effects of the glucocorticoids and mineralocorticoids which are secreted in response to ACTH (or tetracosactide) administration the reader is referred to the later sections on these substances themselves. In addition, the melanocyte-stimulating hormone (MSH) sequence in the ACTH molecule can result in hyperpigmentation, and the induction of androgen secretion can lead to virilization. Corticotrophins may also have additional unwanted effects of their own, such as myoclonic encephalopathy and adrenal hemorrhage.

Hypersensitivity reactions Although the incidence of severe allergic reactions to natural ACTH of animal origin fell in the course of the years as progressively purer products were introduced, the problem for a small minority of patients remained. Exact figures are difficult to cite, but hypersensitivity reactions were sometimes described even in patients with no known history of ACTH treatment, presumably sensitized by other animal material. Hypersensitivity to ACTH may cause only dizziness, nausea and vomiting or cutaneous hypersensitivity reactions, but in several instances shock with circulatory failure has been observed (4[C]). In a number of patients allergic to porcine ACTH, no such problems were observed when synthetic corticotrophin was given, i.e. the absence of most of the antigenic part of the original molecule reduces the risk of sensitivity reactions. The smaller synthetic molecule is, however, still capable of inducing the formation of antibodies in some individuals (SEDA-12, 979; 5[C]); allergic reactions and anaphylactic shock have been observed during treatment with tetracosactide and the condition has even proved fatal. Local reactions have even been seen after the administration of small doses for intracutaneous testing. In the early years of tetracosactide use, the frequency of local and general reactions to a long-acting acetylated synthetic corticotrophin was estimated at as little as one in 30 000 (SED-12, 979), but it is doubtful whether this figure can be supported today, unless one interprets it as referring only to major calamities. Indeed, subclinical immune reactions to both natural and synthetic ACTH appear to be fairly common during long-term treatment of asthmatic patients, with an incidence of intradermal reactions of about 50%, a prevalence of IgE antibodies which is significantly higher than in controls, and a high incidence of low-titered agglutinating antibodies to ACTH. The antibodies can result in a gradual loss of effect of the product.

Tumor-inducing effects These have not been observed; see, however, the monograph on glucocorticosteroids.

ORGANS AND SYSTEMS

Cardiovascular The cardiovascular system can be involved in severe *anaphylactic reactions* (see above). There is also clearly a risk of *myocardial hypertrophy* in children on prolonged treatment, an effect which could reflect increased androgen secretion and thus be more likely to occur than with steroids. *Hypertension*, with or without simultaneous hypertrophic myopathy, is a common feature of adrenal stimulation which seems to be common when using depot tetracosactide but not simple tetracosactide (SEDA-18, 386; 6[c]).

Respiratory ACTH and in lesser measure tetracosactide can induce *asthma* in sensitive subjects (7[R]). The question as to whether synthetic ACTH or corticoids should be preferred for the treatment of chronic asthmatic bronchitis has been discussed in the literature mainly with respect to the side effects (see 'Endocrine' and 'Bone and growth' below); an earlier belief that ACTH might be more effective in children has not been confirmed.

Nervous system *Psychic disturbances* may be induced by corticotrophin treatment. Mood changes continue to be reported in association with ACTH treatment (8[C]). Emotional instability or psychotic tendencies may be aggravated, whilst euphoria, insomnia, personality changes such as hypomania and depression may be precipitated, sometimes even with psychotic manifestations. Although it seems reasonable to assume that one is dealing here mainly with an effect of the corticoids secreted in response to ACTH treatment, it should be recalled that segments of the ACTH molecule themselves have effects on brain function and could conceivably play a role.

Myoclonic encephalopathy appears to be a specific though rare complication of ACTH, not seen with the corticosteroids (9[c]).

Brain shrinkage has been described as a possible adverse effect of ACTH treatment of infantile spasms, and using magnetic resonance imaging in five Japanese children so treated this seems to have been confirmed (10[C]). Ventricular dilatation and cortical atrophy were found, and while loss of water is the most likely explanation it should be realized that in animal experiments evidence was obtained of inhibition of brain growth by ACTH.

Endocrine, metabolic ACTH can promote the development of a more or less pronounced *Cushingoid state*. ACTH treatment also results in an *increased meta-*

bolic clearance rate of cortisol, aldosterone and desoxycorticosterone (SEDA-1, 282).

Prolonged stimulation by adrenocorticotrophin leads to *adrenocortical cell hyperplasia* and an increase in the size and weight of the adrenal glands; massive enlargement can today be demonstrated by computerized tomography as well as clinical examination (11[c]). Acute *adrenal hemorrhage*, either unilateral (12[c]) or bilateral (13[C]) following ACTH administration has been observed repeatedly, and results in an acute abdominal crisis; though usually seen in children, hemorrhage can also occur in adults (SEDA-17, 451).

Even a single dose of ACTH may cause *inhibition of thyrotrophic hormone secretion*, although the effect is brief. Conversely, hyperthyroidism increases the sensitivity to corticotrophin treatment.

Suppression of the growth hormone response to hypoglycemia by ACTH has been reported (see also below). Androgen secretion may cause symptoms of *virilization* in women.

Mineral and fluid balance The mineral and fluid balance is affected in varying degrees, as would be expected from the effect on mineralocorticoid secretion (see 'Mineralocorticoids' later in this Chapter).

Development of renal calcinosis as a result of *hypercalciuria* is a major concern in the treatment of infantile spasms with ACTH. A study in 16 infants (14[C]) showed that this form of treatment, often associated with anticonvulsants, results in an increased urinary excretion of calcium and phosphate, with increased parathormone serum levels and generalized aminoaciduria in some cases. This makes it imperative that the dose of ACTH and the duration of this treatment be kept to the minimum required to ensure efficacy. In one case reported in 1992, in which the calcified stones were removed surgically, recurrence was apparently prevented, despite the presence of a Cushingoid state, by chlorthiazide maintenance treatment (15[cr]).

Hematological Marked *leukocytosis* has incidentally been described, despite the absence of infection, in a patient treated with tetracosactide (SED-12, 980); the effect may well be due to corticoid secretion rather than to ACTH itself (see monograph on 'Glucocorticosteroids').

Gastrointestinal A relative indication for ACTH treatment is the occasional gastrointestinal intolerance to glucocorticoids given orally. In these cases, however, only the locally exerted effects of the steroids can be avoided, and not their systemic effects on the gastrointestinal tract (16[r]).

Urinary system The problem of *renal calcinosis* is dealt with under 'Mineral and fluid balance' above.

Skin and appendages The possibility of allergic skin reactions, e.g. *urticaria*, has been discussed above. Since the first 13 amino acids in the ACTH peptide are the same as in the MSH molecule, treatment with ACTH can thus occasionally result in *hyperpigmentation*. The shorter peptide chain in the synthetic ACTH molecule may perhaps even cause rather more pronounced melanocyte-stimulating effects; long-term treatment with depot synthetic ACTH has, however, itself caused melanoderma (SED-12, 980) and, in one series of 41 patients, hyperpigmentation was observed in three of them (SEDA-1, 281).

Special senses The appearance of *bilateral subcapsular cataracts* and *glaucoma* have been mentioned in the literature as possible risks (17[Cr]), but they presumably reflect corticosteroid effects. Bilateral *macular degeneration* has been described with tetracosactide (ibid).

Bone and growth Although it has been stated in reviews that treatment with ACTH *inhibits growth* much less than does glucocorticoid treatment, the growth hormone response to stimuli is reduced, and since growth hormone secretion is impaired during ACTH treatment claims for the greater safety of this therapy in asthmatic children must be regarded with much reserve.

Risk situations These are as for glucocorticoids: in addition, patients with a known allergic tendency should preferably not receive these substances unless sufficient supervision is possible to cope with unexpected allergic reactions, at least until tolerance has been demonstrated.

Withdrawal effects Relative adrenocortical insufficiency can follow termination of ACTH treatment (presumably because the cortex has adapted itself to a constant high level of stimulation) and may persist for some months; steroid substitution has to be provided during this period. The risk of this effect can be reduced by keeping the dose of ACTH at the lowest possible level.

Second-generation effects There are no firm data on the use of ACTH in pregnancy; both corticosteroid and androgenic effects might affect the fetus.

Interactions The principal interactions of ACTH are those interfering with the *glucocorticoids*; the reader is referred to that section. In addition, *thyroxine* treatment may increase sensitivity to ACTH treatment.

Other modifications to the ACTH molecule

Since the development of tetracosactide, other modifications to the ACTH molecule have been made, and some clinical work has been done with products containing less than 24 amino acids, e.g. 1—18, but none has proved more usable than tetracosactide; the replacement of some naturally occurring amino acids by others may intensify or prolong the effect of the polypeptide.

Corticotrophin releasing hormone (CRH)

For complete functional evaluation of the hypothalamic-hypophyseal-adrenal axis one can use CRH which is today available both in human (hCRH) and the ovine (oCRH) forms. Single bolus injections in standard doses (e.g. 200 μg hCRH or oCRH), whether given on a single occasion or at fixed intervals, have a very low rate of complications. Continuous infusions of several hours using hCRH or oCRH have also been well tolerated but side effects (see above) appeared when cumulated doses of 200—300 μg/hour were given and these 'nonstandard' doses should at present only be used in experimental work with well-designed safety precautions.

The *cardiovascular system* is predominantly affected (e.g. tachycardia, hypotension, flushing); other symptoms are only seen sporadically (e.g. *dizziness*). It has been found that standard doses of hCRH and oCRH are as a rule well tolerated even in severely ill patients. However, the higher doses may provoke marked side effects in persons with neurological disorders, in subjects with coronary heart disease and in patients with endocrinological disorders of the pituitary-adrenal axis, especially if the blood—brain barrier has been damaged (e.g. by a head injury or during intracranial surgery).

Glucocorticosteroids *(SEDA-16, 447; SEDA-17, 445; SEDA-18, 386)*

The incidence and severity of adverse reactions to glucocorticosteroids depend upon the dose level, but to an even greater degree upon the duration of treatment; even the vast doses of glucocorticosteroids sometimes used in shock are without serious adverse effects since they are given so briefly.

The main groups of risks arising from longer treatment with glucocorticosteroids are summarized in Table 1. The comparative potency of the corticoids in common system use is summarized in Table 2.

ADVERSE REACTION PATTERN

General and toxic reactions The two classic risks of long-term corticosteroid therapy are adrenal suppression and the induction of Cushing-like changes. During prolonged treatment with anti-inflammatory doses one is likely to encounter glucose intolerance, osteoporosis, acne vulgaris and a greater or lesser degree of mineralocorticoid-induced change. In children growth can be retarded, and adults given high doses can experience mental changes. There may be a risk of peptic ulceration, though this is much less certain than previously thought. Infections and abdominal crises can be masked. Some of the above effects reflect the 'catabolic' properties of the glucocorticosteroids, i.e. their ability to accelerate the breakdown of tissue and in some situations to impair its build-up.

Hypersensitivity reactions Since the glucocorticoids have immunosuppressive and anti-phlogistic properties one would not expect allergic reactions to constitute a problem, except where the excipients act as allergens. Nevertheless, allergenic reactions to those steroids themselves have been reported. Urticaria after corticoid treatment has been explained as a reaction of the mesenchyme. Also an increase of eosinophilic leukocytes (which normally are diminished by glucocorticoids) has been reported as a first reaction to treatment with such a steroid. Anaphylactic shock has been described after intranasal hydrocortisone acetate application. A life-threatening anaphylactic-like reaction to intravenous hydrocortisone has been described in patients with asthma (see also under 'Respiratory'). There is some reason to believe that sodium succinate esters are more prone to cause hypersensitivity reactions (SEDA-17, 449), but unconjugated steroids can definitely produce allergy in some cases (SEDA-16, 452).

Tumor-inducing effects Direct tumor-inducing effects of the glucocorticosteroids are not known, but the particular risk that malignancies in patients undergoing immunosuppression with these or other drugs will spread more rapidly is a well-recognized problem. A case of progressive endometrial carcinoma associated with azathioprine and prednisone therapy has for example been reported. Rapid progression of Kaposi's sarcoma 10 weeks after combined treatment with corticosteroids and cyclophosphamide has been described; marked im-

Table 1. *Risks of glucocorticosteroid therapy (I)*

I. Exogenous hypercorticism with 'Cushing's syndrome'	*II. Endogenous hypocortisolism (atrophy of the adrenal cortex)*
Moon face (facial rounding)	Insufficient or absent stress reaction. Withdrawal effects
Central obesity	Relapse of the disease being treated
Striae	
Hirsutism	*III. Unwanted results accompanying the desired effects*
Acne	Increased risk of infection
Ecchymosis	Disturbed wound healing
Hypertension	Peptic ulcer risks such as bleeding and perforation
Osteoporosis	Retardation of growth
Myopathy (atrophy of hip muscles)	
Disorders of sexual function	*IV. Untoward side effects with unknown correlations*
Diabetes mellitus	Mental disturbance
Hyperlipidemia	Encephalopathy
Disorders of mineral and fluid balance	Increased risk of thrombosis
(depending on the type of corticosteroid)	Cataract
	Increased intraocular pressure and glaucoma
	Aseptic necrosis of bone
	Corticoid dependence (with long-term therapy)

Table 2. *Relative potencies of systemic glucocorticosteroids*

Compound (or its esters)	Glucocorticoid potency as compared to hydrocortisone (mg for mg basis)	Mineralocorticoid potency	Equivalent doses (mg)
Hydrocortisone	1.0	++	20.0
Betamethasone	30	0	0.6
Cortisone	0.8	++	25.0
Dexamethasone	30	0	0.75
Fluprednisolone	10	0	1.5
Meprednisone	5	0	4.0
Methylprednisolone	5	0	4.0
Paramethasone	10	0	2.0
Prednisolone	4	+	5.0
Prednisone	4	+	5.0
Triamcinolone	5	0	4.0

Note: A number of experimental or recently developed corticosteroids are omitted from this table since their potency has not yet been fully agreed; early work with such compound often proves to have been conducted with inappopriate doses.

provement of the skin lesions was noted after discontinuation of prednisone therapy (18[Cr]). A study of seven patients with an accelerated growth of Kaposi's sarcoma lesions during corticosteroid therapy suggests that these steroid hormones may alter the biological behavior of this malignant disease (19[Cr]). Hydrocortisone accelerates the growth of cell lines derived from AIDS-Kaposi's sarcoma cultured in vitro and this may partially explain the findings cited above. Reports continue to point to the reversibility of the condition when steroids are withdrawn (20[c]).

There have been repeated reports of an acute tumor lysis syndrome when corticosteroids are administered in patients with pre-existing tumors.

ORGANS AND SYSTEMS

Cardiovascular The secondary mineralocorticoid activity of a glucocorticoid may lead to salt and water retention (see below) which also can result in *hypertension*. Cortisone-induced *cardiac lesions* are sometimes reported and *ECG changes* have been seen in corticosteroid-treated patients (21[C]). Whereas abnormal *myocardial hypertrophy* in children has perhaps been associated more readily with ACTH treatment, it has been seen on occasion during high dosage of steroids with normalization after dose reduction and discontinuation. The heart is also almost certainly a site for *myopathic changes* analogous to those affecting other muscles. These findings point to the need to monitor myocardial form and function, particularly during intensive or prolonged treatment or in high-risk cases (see below) (SEDA-10, 343).

Hypokalemia (see below) can naturally lead to *arrhythmias* and *cardiac arrest*.

Long-term treatment with corticosteroids may be accompanied by the occurrence of *arteritis*, but rheumatic patients have a special disposition to vascular reactions, and cases of occurrence of periarteritis nodosa after discontinuation of long-term corticosteroid treatment have been reported; *acute myocardial infarction* in an old man with coronary insufficiency and giant cell arteritis following treatment with prednisolone has been described (SEDA-10, 343) but could well have been coincidental.

Respiratory In recent years corticosteroids have been given locally in the form of aerosols for allergic rhinitis and for asthma. *Atrophic changes, fungal and other infections* may alter the nasal mucosa after aerosol treatment (22[C]), and since most systematic published documentation on these intranasal products is limited to 1—2 years of experience (though they have been in use for a far longer period) some reserve is warranted with respect to their long-term safety and the wisdom of continual use.

The inhalation aerosols used for asthma have proved valuable, and whilst a rarely symptomatic oral candidiasis is seen in some 5—10% of cases, particularly where oral hygiene is poor, no reports documenting an increased frequency of lower respiratory tract infections have emerged. *These products for inhalation are reviewed fully in Chapter* 16 *of this volume.*

Patients with aspiration of gastric material who were treated with corticosteroids did not exhibit improved survival but showed a higher incidence of *pneumonia* (SED-12, 982).

As pointed out elsewhere, allergic reactions to corticosteroids (or their excipients) are possible, and serious or even fatal *anaphylactic reactions* involving respiratory impairment have been seen in a few patients given intravenous hydrocortisone (23[Cr]).

In cases of pneumothorax with closed thoracotomy tube drainage, chronic corticosteroid treatment has been reported to *delay and impede re-expansion of the lung* (SED-8, 820).

Hiccup is a rare complication of steroid therapy; five cases have been published at various times (24[cr]).

Nervous system *Mental disturbances* The psychostimulant effects of the corticosteroids are well known (25[cR]), and their dose dependency is recognized (SED-11, 817); they may amount to little more than euphoria or comprise severe mental derangement, e.g. mania in an adult with no previous psychiatric history (SEDA-17, 446) or catatonic stupor demanding electroconvulsive therapy (26[cr]). In their mildest form, and especially in children, the mental changes may be detectable only by specific tests of mental function (27[R]).

Mental effects can even occur in patients treated with fairly low doses; they can also appear following withdrawal or omission of treatment apparently because of adrenal suppression (28[Cr], 29[c]). Obviously, there must be factors related to the personality of the patient or to the underlying disease that make some patients more prone than others to this adverse reaction. A report of two cases of prednisolone-induced psychosis, which improved upon giving the drug in three divided daily doses, and in whom recurrence was avoided by switching to enteric-coated tablets, suggests that in susceptible patients the margin of safety may be quite narrow (SED-12, 982). It is possible that reduced absorption accounted for the improvement, but attention should perhaps be focused on peak concentrations in plasma rather than on average levels. Interestingly, the association between low serum albumin levels and psychiatric as well as other complications of prednisone has been recognized for years and it is an elementary pharmacokinetic notion that peak levels of the free drug in plasma—the fraction that can reach the CNS—will be increased when binding of a drug to serum albumin is decreased (30[C]).

Large doses are clearly most likely to cause the more serious behavioral and personality changes, ranging from extreme nervousness, severe insomnia or mood swings to psychotic episodes which can include both manic and depressive states, paranoid states and acute toxic psychoses. A history of emotional disorders does not necessarily preclude corticosteroid treatment, but existing emotional instability or psychotic tendencies may be aggravated by these steroids. Such patients as these should be carefully and continuously observed for signs of mental changes, including alterations in the sleep pattern. Such an aggravation of psychic alterations may occur not only during high-dose oral treatment but also following any increase in dosage in long-term maintenance therapy; it may possibly also occur with inhalation of a corticosteroid (31[C]). The psychomotor stimulant effect is said to be most pronounced with dexamethasone and to be much less with 6-methylprednisolone, but this concept of a differential psychotropic effect still has to be confirmed. The management of a psychotic reaction in an Addisonian patient on corticosteroid treatment needs special care (SED-8, 820). Psychotic reactions which do not recede promptly when corticosteroid dosage is reduced to the lowest effective level (or withdrawn) may need to be treated with antipsychotic drugs; occasionally these fail and antidepressants are needed (SEDA-18, 387), but in other cases antidepressants appear to aggravate the symptoms.

Organic changes Long-term treatment with corticosteroids may result in CAT-scan evidence of cerebral atrophy (32[C]; see also ACTH above). The development of a severe organic brain syndrome has been observed in six patients undergoing prolonged treatment with corticosteroids (SEDA-3, 304). The manifestations included confusion, disorientation, apathy, confabulation, irrelevant speech and slow mentation, with abrupt onset of these symptoms.

Pseudotumor cerebri Some few patients receiving these drugs for a range of indications develop the *pseudotumor cerebri* syndrome, i.e. benign intracranial hypertension. In one Japanese case it was found that warfarin prevented recurrence of the syndrome after a break in corticoid therapy (33[Cr]).

Neurological phenomena Latent *epilepsy* can be rendered manifest by corticosteroid treatment. Long-term treatment may result in *papilledema* and *increased intracranial pressure*, particularly in children; benign intracranial hypertension in a 7-month-old child has been seen after withdrawal of topically applied betamethasone ointment (see Chapter 14) and in a 7-year-old boy treated with a 1% cortisol ointment in large amounts. The symptoms may simulate those of an intracranial tumor. Paradoxically, cerebral edema occurring during a surgical procedure can be partly prevented by corticosteroid treatment. An *encephalopathy* can occur at any age (SEDA-18, 387), not necessarily in association with intracranial hypertension, and there are repeated reports of *epidural lipomatosis*, which can lead to spinal cord compression (34[cR], 35[Cr]); in one instance, the excised lipomata contained brown fat, a phenomenon which may prove to be not unusual in steroid lipomata (SEDA-16, 451).

In the past there has been some reason to think that corticosteroids could precipitate *multiple sclerosis*, but this has not been confirmed and there is currently evidence that a special corticosteroid regime may actually be capable of retarding deterioration in the latter condition (SEDA-18, 387). A *Guillain-Barré* syndrome was described in 1991 in a patient on high-dose intravenous therapy (SEDA-16, 449).

Effects of intrathecal administration are discussed in a later section of this chapter

Endocrine, metabolic The endocrine effects of the glucocorticoids involve variously the pituitary-adrenal axis, the genitals, the parathyroid and the thyroid; there are also metabolic effects, primarily involving carbohydrates.

Pituitary-adrenal axis Elevated glucocorticoid plasma levels usually result, after 2 weeks, in the first signs of iatrogenic Cushing's syndrome. The characteristic symptoms may occur individually or in combination. Whereas in spontaneous Cushing's syndrome or the ACTH-induced syndrome, the predominant symptoms are in part determined by hyperandrogenicity and tend to comprise hypertension, acne, impaired sight, disorders of sexual function, hirsutism or virilism, striae of the skin and plethora, Cushing's syndrome due to glucocorticosteroid therapy is likely to cause benign intracranial hypertension, glaucoma, subcapsular cataract, pancreatitis, aseptic necrosis of the bones and panniculitis. Obesity, facial rounding, psychiatric symptoms, edema and delayed wound healing are common to these different forms of Cushing's syndrome. It has been said that Cushing-like effects are to be expected if the function of the adrenal cortex is suppressed by daily doses of more than 50 mg hydrocortisone or its equivalent. However, pituitary-adrenal suppression has been described at lower dosage equivalents, e.g. during prolonged intermittent therapy with dexamethasone (36[C]). Tolerance to the glucocorticosteroids in this, as in some other respects, varies from individual to individual; some patients tolerate 30 mg of prednisone for a long time without developing Cushing's syndrome, while others show distinct symptoms at 7.5 mg; the doses recommended today to avoid the appearance of Cushing's syndrome in the majority of patients are usually equivalent to 20 mg hydrocortisone. It must always be recalled that Cushing's syndrome is induced not only by oral application and injections of the steroids; it can also result from topical treatment and intranasal (37[C]) or intrapulmonary application (see below and in Chapters 14 and 16).

The *secondary adrenal insufficiency* caused by therapeutically effective doses can be observed even after giving 5 mg prednisone 3 times daily for only 1 week; after discontinuation the adrenal suppression lasts in that case for some days. If one continues this treatment for about 20 weeks, then maximal atrophy of the adrenal cortex results, and lasts for some months. This effect, which is dose- and time-dependent, begins with an inhibition of the hypothalamus, and culminates in true atrophy of the adrenal cortex. It can occur even with steroids given by inhalation (38[c]). Patients with liver disease may experience adrenal suppression with lower doses of corticosteroids (39[C]). Many physicians consider it advisable to use alternate day therapy (reviewed below) to avoid a complete suppression of the ACTH secretion; in most indications this appears to produce the same therapeutic effect as daily dosage. Intercurrent application of ACTH has been tried but it does not inhibit atrophy of the adrenal cortex and extends the phase of restitution of the hypothalamo-pituitary-adrenal system; the role of ACTH comes later as an instrument for reviving a suppressed adrenal system when steroid therapy has been completed. It can be helpful to measure the degree of suppression of ACTH secretion during long-term steroid treatment of asthmatic children, as a means of optimizing therapy and avoiding excessive dosage (40[C]).

The adrenal suppression caused by these compounds

results in withdrawal problems (see 'Withdrawal reactions' below). In addition, corticosteroid-treated patients with inadequate adrenal function who are due to undergo surgery will have an inadequate reaction to the resulting stress and need to be temporarily protected by additional steroid dosage (41^R). A comparable situation, requiring additional steroids, may be provoked by an accident or sickness with fever.

Menstrual cycle Since amenorrhea is a symptom of Cushing's syndrome, disorders of menstruation are a common complaint in fertile women receiving higher doses of corticosteroids (SEDA-3, 305). On the other hand it is known that plasma cortisol levels in normally menstruating women exhibit marked circadian variation; the extent of this variation may reach 200% or more (42^R), with the peak of the cortisol plasma levels at the mid-cycle and near its end. Inhibition of ovulation by 25 mg triamcinolone has been reported when the drug is given on days 1 or 2 of the cycle. How corticosteroids interfere with the hormonal control of the menstrual cycle is still unknown (43^R).

Testicular function Reduced sperm count and motility and inhibition of the secretory function of the testicle during glucocorticosteroid treatment have been reported and discussed in relation to the suppression of adrenal androgen production. These reports still await confirmation.

Parathyroid function The antagonism between the parathyroids and hypercorticism is well known. Latent hyperparathyroidism may be unmasked by administration of corticosteroids.

Thyroid function Even a single dose of ACTH briefly inhibits the secretion of thyrotrophic hormone. The uptake of radioactive iodine is also suppressed by ACTH and by glucocorticosteroids, but this is without clinical relevance. Pathological degrees of change in thyroid function induced by corticosteroid treatment are reported to be rare.

Carbohydrate metabolism All glucocorticoids increase gluconeogenesis. The turnover of glucose is increased, more being metabolized to fat, and blood glucose is increased 10—20%. Glucose tolerance and sensitivity to insulin are decreased, but provided pancreatic islet function is normal carbohydrate metabolism will not be noticeably deranged. The so-called 'steroid diabetes', a benign diabetes without a tendency to ketosis, but with a low sensitivity to insulin and a low renal threshold to glucose, only develops in one-fifth of the patients treated with high glucocorticosteroid dosage. Even in patients with diabetes, ketosis is not to be expected since the glucocorticosteroids have antiketotic activity, presumably due to suppression of growth hormone secretion. Corticosteroid treatment of known diabetics normally leads to deregulation but this can be compensated for by adjusting the dose of insulin. The increased gluconeogenesis induced by glucocorticosteroid treatment mainly takes place in the liver, but corticosteroid treatment is especially prone to disturb carbohydrate metabolism in liver disease. When hyperglycemic coma occurs it is almost always of the hyperosmolar non-ketotic type. After termination of corticosteroid treatment steroid diabetes normally disappears. An apparent exception to these optimistic findings is provided by the 1992 case of a patient in whom corticosteroid treatment was followed by severe diabetes with diabetic nephropathy, but this was a seriously ill individual who had already undergone renal transplantation (SEDA-17, 449).

The effect of steroids on carbohydrate mechanisms is probably exerted in more than one way. An increase in fasting glucagon levels has been observed in volunteers given 40 mg prednisolone daily for 4 days, and this effect may be involved, alongside gluconeogenesis, in corticoid-induced hyperglycemia. Some newer steroids have been claimed to cause less derangement of blood glucose (as well as less salt and water retention) but further studies are needed to confirm whether this interesting therapeutic approach has indeed been successful (SEDA-13, 353).

Lipid metabolism (*SEDA*-15, 421; *SEDA*-16, 450) High-dose corticoid therapy may induce marked hypertriglyceridemia with milky plasma. It has been suggested that this is caused by abnormal accumulation of dietary fat, decreased post-heparin lipolytic activity and glucose intolerance (44^{CR}). An association between corticoid exposure and hypercholesterolemia has been found in several studies (45^C) and may contribute to an increased risk of atherosclerotic vascular disease.

Derangements of fat deposition is repeatedly recorded; epidural lipomatosis has been referred to above, but fat can be deposited at other sites instead; *adiposis dolora*, involving the symmetrical appearance of multiple painful fat deposits in the subcutaneous tissue, has on one occasion been attributed to steroids (SEDA-16, 451).

Mineral and fluid balance Hydrocortisone has only one thousandth of the mineralocorticoid activity of aldosterone; whether mineralocorticoid effects, notably *salt and water retention*, appear during glucocorticoid treatment depends on the compound selected and the dosage and duration of therapy (cf. Table 2); there are reports of *pseudohyperaldosteronism* even after intranasal application of 9α-fluoroprednisolone (SEDA-11, 340). There can be an increase in *calcium and phosphorus loss* because of effects both on the kidney and the bowel, with increased excretion and decreased resorption; tetanic states which have been observed in patients on high-dose long-term intravenous treatment with corticosteroids have been explained as being due to hypocalcemia and there are also effects on bone (see below). The severity of the potassium loss depends partly on the amount of sodium in the diet; the most widely used synthetic corticosteroids cause less potassium excretion than does natural hydrocortisone. Prednisone and prednisolone have a glucocorticoid activity 4—5 times that of hydrocortisone, yet their mineralocorticoid activity is less (see Table 1); even at high dosage they do not cause noteworthy sodium and water retention. Of the major synthetic steroids, dexamethasone has the strongest antiphlogistic, hyperglycemic and ACTH-inhibitory activity; sodium retention is completely absent; the degree of corticosteroid-induced metabolic alkalemia may also be less with dexamethasone than with hydrocortisone or methylprednisolone (SEDA-10, 343).

The administration of large doses of corticosteroids to patients with major burns presenting with a low cardiac output syndrome has been reported to produce a reversible drop in serum *zinc* which might lead to impairment of tissue repair (SED-8, 824), but it is not clear that this manifests itself clinically.

Hematological Not all the various classes of leukocytes are affected by glucocorticoid treatment in the same way. The total *leukocyte count is increased*, but the number of *eosinophilic leukocytes* decreases, as does the *lymphocyte* count (see below). The number of *monocytes* and their capacity to perform phagocytosis is reduced. The *thrombocyte count* increases. *Polycythemia* is a symptom of Cushing's syndrome and *anemia* is correlated to Addison's disease, but polycythemia is not generally encountered as a consequence of treatment with glucocorticoids, perhaps because there is no increased secretion of androgens; an increase in hemoglobin correlated to a *polyglobular reaction of the hematopoietic system* was nevertheless the most frequent side effect observed in a study over 8 years of 77 patients treated for hyperergic-allergic reactions. At the beginning of treatment more than 40% (and during continuous therapy more than 70%) of the patients showed this change in erythrocytes (46[C]). Leukocytosis was in the early phases observed in more than 60% and later in more than 40%. This leukocyte reaction was dose dependent, as was the less frequent thrombocytosis (5—10% during continuous treatment). This report agrees fairly well with some older publications, but it has been noted in the past that, in the long run, very high-dose corticoid treatment can result in suppression of the activity of the bone marrow with fatty infiltration replacing hematopoietic tissue (ibid.).

In children a *leukemoid reaction* has been induced by betamethasone treatment (90[c]); this possibility must always be borne in mind since corticosteroids can actually be used to treat leukemia or its complications. A case of very high white blood cell counts and neutrophilia in a pre-term infant whose mother had received two doses of betamethasone prenatally, to enhance fetal lung maturation, is one of a short list of leukemoid reactions possibly attributable to antenatal steroid treatment (47[c]).

It is possible that in children with *acute lymphoblastic leukemia* corticosteroid therapy adversely affects the duration of remissions, and it has therefore been suggested that leukemia should be ruled out in children before starting long-term therapy with corticosteroids (SEDA-11, 340). A *depression of the lymphocyte count* seems to be a general and direct action of the corticosteroids on the lymphatic tissue (48[C]), but the mechanism of this action is still incompletely known; certainly, *lymphocytolysis* seems to be increased by glucocorticosteroids. Studies of lymphocyte subpopulations show a preferential decrease in T-cells while B-cells are constant or slightly decreased. B-lymphocyte function (measured as immunoglobulin synthesis) decreases, suppressor T-lymphocyte activity is suppressed, and helper T-lymphocyte function is unaffected by corticosteroids (SEDA-3, 308; 49[cr]).

The influence of glucocorticosteroids in promoting *blood coagulation* is a known effect which seems to be less frequent than the reaction of the lymphatic tissue and the bone marrow, but may cause thrombosis (SED-12, 985) and has to be looked for during long-term treatment. In many diseases in which corticosteroids are likely to be used, the disease itself and the application of other drugs may of course themselves alter coagulation parameters, and the continuous control of hematological parameters should therefore not be restricted to cell counts and measurement of hemoglobin. An increased incidence of *subcutaneous ecchymosis* in older women has been observed during treatment with triamcinolone acetate. *Purpura* has been observed during corticosteroid treatment and an increased fragility of the capillaries is thought to occur in about 60% of these patients.

One recent report described repeated occurrence in a single patient of the *blue toe syndrome* when treated with steroids to increase the platelet count (SEDA-16, 451).

Liver The process of gluconeogenesis, which is promoted by glucocorticosteroids, takes place mainly in the liver. The glycolytic enzymes of the liver are also activated by these steroids. The synthesis of ribonucleic acid and of enzymes involved in protein catabolism is increased but the process of protein catabolism takes place outside the liver as well, e.g. in the muscles. There is experimental evidence for a corticosteroid-induced enhancement of hepatic lipid synthesis (SEDA-3, 308), but the main effect of corticosteroids in this connection is lipid mobilization from adipose tissue. The influence of long-term corticosteroid treatment on liver function is still unknown. If pathological changes are diagnosed, the possible influence of the disease which is being treated has to be borne in mind.

The risks and benefits of corticosteroid treatment in hepatitis are still being discussed (SEDA-3, 308); there may be risks—a transition to chronic active hepatitis has been seen after corticosteroid treatment of the early phase of acute viral hepatitis (SEDA-3, 308).

Gastrointestinal *Peptic ulceration* (*SEDA*-12, 335; *SEDA*-13, 354; *SEDA*-15, 421) There is today no longer a serious belief in a markedly increased risk of peptic ulcer during corticosteroid treatment of adults (50[R]), though the symptoms of existing peptic ulcer can certainly be masked and complications (such as perforation) can probably be induced; there may also be a genuine risk of induction of ulcerative disorders in premature children (discussed later in this Chapter). The issue has often been complicated by the simultaneous (sometimes unrecorded) use of ulcerogenic non-steroidal anti-inflammatory agents. Data on 3064 patients participating in 71 clinical trials showed, however, a significantly higher incidence of peptic disease in the steroid-treated patients (1.8%) versus controls (0.8%), and this incidence varied directly with the dosage of steroids (51[C]). Gastrointestinal hemorrhage also occurred more frequently in steroid-treated patients (2.25%) than in controls (1.6%). The risk of a fatal outcome due to ulcer complications was in an Australian case-control study found to be elevated roughly four-fold (52[Cr]). The frequency of gastrointestinal bleeding in these studies complies well with earlier observations in the Boston Collaborative Surveillance Program's 1978 report, according to which 0.5% of a large series of medical in-patients on corticosteroids had a gastrointestinal bleeding sufficiently severe to require transfusions and 28% had minor bleeding (SED-12, 986).

The mechanism of whatever harm corticosteroids may do to the stomach is not entirely clear; cortisol neither consistently increases acid nor pepsinogen secretion but is considered to diminish the protective production of mucin by the gastric mucosa. Serum gastrin concentrations have been found elevated in patients on prolonged corticosteroid treatment and in Cushing's syndrome. Some reports suggest that cases with hepatic cirrhosis or nephrotic syndrome are particularly at risk. Whatever the degree of risk, patients on long-term treatment with corticosteroids the patients should be regularly checked to detect peptic ulcers which may develop, bleed and even perforate without producing pain during such treatment. No differences in gastric tolerance between the various synthetic glucocorticosteroids seem to exist, and the extent of benefit of prophylactic treatment with various agents (antacids, misoprostol, H_2-antagonists) has still to be evaluated.

Pancreatitis A series of case reports over a long period show that pancreatitis and derangements of pancreatic secretion can appear at any time during long-term corticosteroid treatment (SED-12, 986; SEDA-14, 339; 53[c]). Necrosis of the pancreas during corticosteroid treatment has been described and can be lethal. Impairment of pancreatic function may predispose to steroid-induced metabolic pancreatitis. Although the literature suggests a causal relationship between corticosteroid therapy and these various pancreatic complications there is still no certainty; corticosteroid treatment is, after all, often given simultaneously with other forms of therapy which may produce pancreatitis (SED-11, 82). The strongest evidence that there is a causal relationship is provided by a Japanese report on 52 autopsies which showed marked changes in pancreatic histology in steroid-treated patients as compared with controls (SEDA-17, 449).

Regional ileitis While corticosteroids may have a beneficial effect on regional ileitis, it is a fact that, following such treatment, perforation of the ileum, lymphatic dilatation and microscopic fistulae have been observed.

Ulcerative colitis A possible risk of corticosteroid treatment of ulcerative colitis is thought to lie in an increased chance that toxic megacolon will develop or that perforation of the colon will occur.

Perforation of existing diverticula can probably be promoted; a series of cases point in this direction (SEDA-18, 387).

Urinary system There is an increased possibility of formation of urinary *calculi* during corticosteroid treatment because of the raised excretion of calcium and phosphate referred to above. An increase in the incidence of *proteinuria* during corticosteroid treatment of children has also been reported but confirmation of the causal relationship is still awaited. Changes resembling *diabetic nodular glomerular sclerosis* have been seen in corticoid-treated nephrosis. Treatment with corticoids can result in minor *increases in the urinary content of leukocytes and erythrocytes* without clear renal injury. The use of high doses of glucocorticoids to counter rejection of renal transplants is still a matter of intensive study; the optimal dose to ensure an effect without undue risk of complications has yet to be agreed on (54[R]). *Nocturia* is fairly common during glucocorticoid treatment (55[R]).

Skin and appendages (*for topical corticosteroid treatment, see Chapter* 14) Besides *hirsutism* and *striae* (see 'Endocrine') the corticosteroids can induce atrophic changes in the skin. *Subcutaneous atrophy* after intramuscular and after intra-articular injection has often been reported; the corticosteroids have been shown to reduce subcutaneous collagen. *Ecchymosis* and *paper-thin skin folds* recalling those seen in old people are typical symptoms. *Acne* frequently occurs during treatment; the effect, which has mainly been seen after topical application, is said to be correlated with the use of those compounds having a particularly strong local effect (56[C]), but this is not proven. *Depigmentation* can also occur at the site of injection of steroids. Three cases of severe *lipoatrophy*, one also with leukoderma, occurring within the same family after intramuscular injection of triamcinolone, suggest a genetic susceptibility to this adverse effect (SEDA-3, 303). *Leukoderma* can appear, accompanied by normal melanocyte function but a diminished phagocytic activity of the keratinocytes to eliminate the melanosomes (57[C]). An inhibition of the function of the *sebaceous glands* in the skin is caused by corticosteroids whilst androgens stimulate their function.

The appearance of erythematous, firm, warm subcutaneous nodules within 2 weeks of discontinuation of large doses of steroids is recognized as *post-steroid panniculitis*; this is an infrequently reported complication of steroid therapy but case reports confirm that restitution without scarring is the rule, and that re-institution of corticosteroids is not necessary for improvement of this condition (58[C]).

Infections of the skin are often caused by suppression of the immune system as a result of corticosteroid treatment (see below).

Special senses The eye can be involved in generalized adverse reactions to systemically administered corticosteroids, e.g. *conjunctivitis* can occur as part of an allergic reaction and *infections of the eye* may be masked as a result of the anti-inflammatory and analgesic effect of these drugs. *Ophthalmoplegia* can appear as one of the consequences of steroid myopathy (SEDA-16, 450). Two complications requiring special discussion are cataract and glaucoma.

Cataract The incidence of posterior subcapsular cataract in patients undergoing prolonged treatment with corticosteroids often seems to be about 10%, but a 1993 study by Kaye et al. in children on low-dose prednisone found cataract in seven of 23 cases (59[C]). Some studies show a clear correlation with the duration of treatment and total dosage, others do not (SEDA-17, 449). It has been suggested that the risk of cataract is higher in patients with rheumatoid arthritis than in patients with bronchial asthma, and it is also higher in children. The reversibility of the lenticular changes has often been discussed (60[R], 61[R]), but even without corticoid withdrawal regression has been found in children on long-term treatment (62[cr]). Nevertheless, some 7% of the patients who develop cataract caused by steroid treatment have to be operated on. A change in permeability of the capsule followed by an alteration in electrolyte concentration in the lens as well as a change of the mucopolysaccharides of the lens have been advanced as reasons for the development of the cataract.

Increased intraocular pressure and glaucoma (*SEDA*-17, 449) The pathogenesis of corticosteroid-induced glaucoma is still unknown, but there is decreased outflow, and excessive accumulation of mucopolysaccharides may be a major factor. An association with cataract and papilledema has often been observed. The rise in intraocular pressure is variable: the pediatric study of low doses by Kaye cited above found some (reversible) effect in only two of 23 subjects as compared with controls, but other papers record serious increases in pressure which may lead to blindness. There is almost certainly a genetic predisposition to steroid-induced glaucoma, as there is to glaucoma in general.

Papilledema A case of papilledema as a manifestation of raised intracranial pressure has been reported following withdrawal of topical steroids (SEDA-3, 305).

Toxic optic neuropathy This can occur and may underlie the various reports of *sudden blindness*; in one case transient visual loss occurred on several occasions, each time following administration of a corticosteroid (SEDA-17, 447). In another, blindness occurred suddenly and paradoxically after corticosteroid injections into the nasal turbinates (63[C]). It may be noted that, although corticosteroids are sometimes used successfully to relieve pre-existing optic neuritis, a number of such patients react adversely with increased episodes of visual loss.

Exophthalmos This has been described incidentally as a complication, a 1989 report presenting a series of 21 cases; it seems to occur only after very long-term administration.

Complications of topical administration of corticoids in the eye are dealt with in Chapter 47.

Bones and joints (*SEDA*-16, 448) Of the effects of corticosteroids on the skeleton, *osteoporosis* is the most important clinically; manifestations can include vertebral compression fractures, scoliosis resulting in respiratory embarrassment, and fractures of the long bones. Provided no fractures have occurred, the effects seem to be reversible when treatment is withdrawn (SEDA-18, 389).

Several mechanisms seem to underlie the effect of corticosteroids on bone. As noted earlier, treatment with glucocorticoids can result in a deficit of calcium and phosphate; glucocorticosteroids increase the excretion of calcium into the bowel and inhibit its absorption; they also inhibit the tubular re-absorption in the kidney and promote the mobilization of calcium from the skeleton; when calcium homeostasis cannot be maintained, the resulting hypocalcemia may have serious consequences (SEDA-18, 388; 64[R], 65[R]). This so-called 'steroid hyperparathyroidism' was the explanation traditionally most prominently advanced for steroid osteoporosis, but it is not the only one and may not be the most central. In addition the catabolic effect of these substances on protein metabolism causes a reduction of the bone matrix. Vitamin D metabolism can also be altered; the levels of vitamin D_3 metabolites in plasma are also reduced in children receiving either daily or intermittent long-term glucocorticoid therapy for various disorders (66[C]). Finally, a dose-dependent fall of serum osteocalcin, a bone matrix protein that appears to correlate with bone formation, has been found and its measurement is now regarded as a useful marker for steroid-induced osteoporosis; it can be used alongside other measures noted below.

The overall effect of corticoids on the bone mineral content differs between patients on comparable treatment, which suggests that some patients are more predisposed than others (SEDA-3, 306), and probably also that the standards of evaluation employed by different clinics are not comparable. This variability and the wide range of products and dosage schemes employed means that one does not have a clear impression of what constitutes a safe regimen as far as the skeleton is concerned (SEDA-18, 388), or whether indeed any regimen is safe in this respect. Certainly in a series of men with rheumatoid arthritis even a very low dose of corticosteroids (e.g. 10 mg/day or less of prednisolone daily) has proved to have a significant effect on bone mineral density (67[C]); other recent work has provided similar results (SEDA-18, 388—389). Post-menopausal women seem to be particularly susceptible. The fluorinated glucocorticosteroids are said to have relatively more catabolic activity than others and might have a greater effect on the skeleton but, as noted elsewhere, such impressions may merely reflect the general potency of some newer steroids and a tendency to use them in inappropriate doses.

Infusion of ionic calcium has sometimes been used to counteract the malabsorption of calcium in patients on long-term glucocorticoid treatment, particularly in patients who develop secondary hypoparathyroidism (SEDA-3, 306). There is also promising evidence that in amenorrheic or menopausal women requiring corticosteroids the adverse effects on the vertebrae can be countered by hormonal replacement therapy with estrogen and progesterone (68[C]); progestagens similarly seem to have a promising effect in the male, and while they cause a decline in serum testosterone they apparently do not undermine the desired effects of the corticosteroid (SEDA-16, 449). There is also hopeful experience with the use of salmon calcitonin (SEDA-17, 447) and tamoxifen (ibid, 448).

The diagnostic routines to detect steroid-induced osteoporosis now often include measurement of bone mineral mass content by photon absorptiometry and by quantitative computed tomography, and these methods can be valuable in the monitoring of patients on long-term corticoids. Other methods such as the fasting urinary hydroxyproline/creatinine ratio, the alkaline phosphatase level, dual-absorption photometry of the hip and serum osteocalcin measurements can also be used, depending on an individual clinic's equipment and experience (SEDA-17, 447).

Avascular aseptic necrosis of bone has often been described (SEDA-16, 449; 69[C], 70[C]); it occurs in a wide range of patients suffering from many different disorders and is particularly likely to involve the femoral and the humeral head. The first lesions are often localized small osteolytic areas in the subchondral bone, where they can be diagnosed early with X-rays; magnetic resonance imaging has been suggested as a way of identifying necrosis of the femoral head before other radiological studies become abnormal. Normal hips are rarely involved in avascular osteonecrosis; aseptic osteonecrosis of the femoral head is, however, often seen in young patients; the lunate, capitate and patella are their locations. Usually only one joint is involved, though it seems possible that the lesions can be multiple. Whether intra-articular injections of corticosteroids may cause necrosis of bone is still uncertain (see below).

Effects on muscle and tendons (*SEDA*-15, 419) The presence of physiological amounts of corticosteroids in necessary for the normal functioning of the muscular system. Excessive corticoid levels, by contrast, result in protein catabolism and apparently also in a reduced rate of muscle protein synthesis (71[C]), and hence in *muscular atrophy* and *fibrosis*. Muscular symptoms (weakness) can of course also result from steroid-induced hypokalemia. In naturally occurring Cushing's syndrome, muscle involvement can be observed in some 50% of cases (72[R]); among relevant case reports on corticosteroid treatment, descriptions and studies of myopathy involving the respiratory muscles are prominent (73[C], 74[C]), possibly because this is particularly likely to have clinical consequences. Patients on mechanically assisted ventilation may be particularly at risk of developing myopathy (SEDA-18, 390). However any musculature can be affected; one often sees weakness and atrophy of the hip muscles and (in about half the cases) the shoulder muscles and the proximal musculature of the limbs. The myopathy usually develops gradually, without pain and symmetrically. There is a suggestion that the incidence of myopathy is greatest during treatment with a compound fluorinated at the 9α-position such as triamcinolone but once again this may simply reflect its general potency. In children, the risk of muscular effects is relatively high. After termination of treatment the myopathy normally improves over a period of several months.

Biopsy is not justified as a routine, but it is useful as a diagnostic tool in distinguishing suspected corticoid myopathy from those diseases of the muscles or vascular system with inflammation which may have been the indication for giving corticosteroids in the first place; electromyographic measurements cannot confirm the diagnosis.

Tendons may be injured by corticosteroid treatment and can rupture (75[C]); a recent report describes 10 cases of Achilles tendon rupture seen in a single clinic over a 10-year period (SEDA-17, 448). The risk seems to be greater if local (e.g. intra-articular) injections are used.

Effects on immune defence mechanisms and incidence of infection Corticoids inhibit the formation of antibodies; they thereby also inhibit immune responses. With long-term treatment IgG subclass deficiencies can become marked (76[C]). There is suppression of the antigen—antibody reaction, and since this reaction itself normally results in a liberation of kinines, the latter is also suppressed. Failure of kinine liberation leads in turn to inhibition of invasion of sensitized leukocytes and reduced production and maturation of phagocytes. Undoubtedly it is true that using minimal effective doses will avoid the most serious consequences, but the problem cannot be fully circumvented since the antiphlogistic effects themselves involve some inhibition of the migration of leukocytes and phagocytosis.

The consequence of this interference with the immune reaction can be multiplication of bacteria and an increased risk of bacterial intoxication when infection does occur; the frequency and severity of clinical infections hence tend to increase during glucocorticoid therapy. Aggravation of existing tuberculosis and reactivation of completely quiescent cases of this infection are classic consequences demanding prophylactic measures; atypical mycobacteria have also caused tissue infections (SEDA-17, 449). Other bacterial infections, some severe and proceeding to sepsis, have followed glucocorticosteroid treatment. A particularly difficult situation arises when very high doses of corticosteroids have to be used to treat septic shock, since under these circumstances an adverse effect on the immune situation could be disastrous; the corticosteroid treatment should be backed up with appropriate antibiotic cover. There are clearly other situations as well in which a combination of corticosteroids with antibiotics is needed because of the presence or risk of grave infection, whether acute or chronic.

Fungal and candidial infections (including cases of fulminant fungal pericarditis and one of mucomycosis) may similarly be aggravated by corticosteroid treatment (SEDA-17, 449; SEDA-18, 390; 77[C]). Virus infections bear the same risk; smallpox vaccination, now obsolete, has in the past resulted in vaccinia gangrenosum in patients receiving corticosteroids, and the current type of varicella vaccine proves much more likely to produce rashes in children already receiving steroids than in controls (SEDA-16, 452). In renal transplantation two cases of death from herpes simplex as a result of steroid treatment are on record (SED-8, 827; SEDA-17, 449). Strongyloidiasis, listeriosis, amebic dysentery and toxoplasmosis have all on some occasion been precipitated or aggravated by corticosteroids.

Effects on growth The growth-inhibiting effects of corticosteroids in children have long been recognized; they are not only related to the inhibition of growth hormone secretion, but also to the sensitivity of the peripheral tissue to the hormone's effects. By means of overnight profile analysis it was shown that steroid treatment reduces the amplitude but not the number of pulses of the physiological growth hormone secretion (SEDA-14, 335; 78[C]).

Effects on growth appear early in treatment: with sensitive testing methods they can be detected in growing children within a few weeks of starting therapy. The effects can be produced by any route of administration, including even inhalation therapy (at least when using dexamethasone) (SEDA-18, 391). It is generally agreed that use of single doses of prednisone on alternate mornings minimizes growth retardation but does not avoid it; in children it has been shown that biochemical markers of growth are lower in patients receiving daily corticosteroid therapy than in patients treated with an alternate-day regimen or not receiving corticosteroids (SED-12, 988; 79[C]).

It has long been thought by some physicians that the impairment of growth caused by corticosteroids can be lessened by switching to ACTH but, as pointed out in the monograph on corticotrophin, this is uncertain. Compensatory treatment with 'anabolic' hormones is definitely not recommended today, since they do not stimulate growth but actually impede it by promoting closure of the epiphyses. Growth hormone has been tried (80[C]) but this approach must be regarded as experimental. Provided steroid treatment is terminated before the end of puberty, total growth may catch up with the physiological norm (SEDA-17, 448). Concern has been expressed that fear of growth retardation may result in unjustifiable denial of corticosteroid therapy; it does however seem highly advisable to keep doses as low as possible, and to switch to a therapeutic regimen that excludes steroids, as children approach the expected onset of puberty (SEDA-14, 335).

Serum osteocalcin determinations (see above in connection with osteoporosis) appear to be a helpful marker to evaluate the effects of steroids on growth in children.

Risk situations In patients with acute hepatitis and active hepatitis, protein binding of the glucocorticoids will be reduced, peak levels of administered corticoids increased, and half-lives somewhat prolonged. Cases of *hepatic disease* suffer adrenal suppression more readily. However, a diseased liver may not be capable of transforming prednisone efficiently into active prednisolone.

In patients due to undergo *surgery* who are already on long-term oral corticosteroid therapy, parenteral therapy should be temporarily substituted.

Children are considered to be particularly at risk as regards raised intracranial pressure or interference with growth. Facial plethora has been found in *workers manufacturing synthetic glucocorticoids*, some of them having grossly abnormal responses to tetracosactide. It has been recommended that all workers manufacturing potent steroids should be screened regularly for corticosteroid overdosage and should be moved regularly to units processing other drugs (81[C]).

Withdrawal effects As discussed above, suppression of adrenal cortical function is one of the consequences of repeated administration of glucocorticoids; after termination of treatment a withdrawal syndrome may be experienced. In many cases this is unpleasant rather than acutely dangerous; in such instances the patients may experience headache, nausea, dizziness, anorexia, weakness, emotional changes, lethargy and perhaps fever; in some cases severe *mental disorders* occur (see above) and there are repeated reports of *benign intracranial hypertension* (82[c]). The steroid withdrawal syndrome also seems to underlie the '*steroid pseudorheumatism*' which can occur when the drugs are withdrawn in rheumatic patients. Withdrawal symptoms disappear if the corticosteroid is resumed, but as a rule they will in any case vanish spontaneously within a few days. More serious consequences can ensue, however, in certain types of cases and if adrenal cortical atrophy is severe. In patients treated with corticoids for the nephrotic syndrome and apparently cured, the syndrome is particularly likely to *relapse* on withdrawal of therapy if the adrenal cortex is atrophic (SEDA-3, 305). In some cases acute adrenocortical insufficiency after glucocorticoid treatment has actually proved *fatal*.

It is advisable to withdraw long-term corticosteroid therapy gradually so that the cortex has sufficient opportunity to recover. If this is done, there is no need for other measures (such as ACTH therapy) to ensure cortical recovery.

Second-generation effects *Teratogenic effects* of glucocorticosteroids, which have been demonstrated in animal experiments since 1950, have not been confirmed in man. The question whether a disease which has had to be treated with corticosteroids in pregnancy or the steroid treatment itself may have caused congenital anomalies reported anecdotally usually cannot be answered in any individual case. Dexamethasone, for instance, given in suppressive dosage, seems to have been therapeutically effective in endocrine abnormal pregnancy with congenital adrenogenital syndrome (83[R]); how is one to distinguish cause and effect here? The cleft lip and palate seen in animal studies have not been encountered more frequently in the offspring of corticoid-treated women than in those of non-treated women. In several small series of cases in whom corticosteroids were used before and during pregnancy no congenital abnormalities were seen on follow-up, but material on which to base a firm judgement is lacking. Certainly, the evidence to date does not suggest that on teratological grounds one should hesitate to administer corticosteroids for therapeutic reasons during pregnancy (SEDA-3, 306).

Effects when steroids are given very late in pregnancy are discussed below in connection with the treatment of lung immaturity in premature infants

Retardation of intrauterine growth by glucocorticosteroids has been reported not only in animals but also in man. In a 1990 case from France, dwarfism (as well as *Cushing's syndrome*) was recorded in a child whose mother had received high-dose steroids during pregnancy.

The possibility has been advanced that the *risk of*

stillbirth may be increased by glucocorticoid treatment; the figures are suggestive, but the possibility that the disorder which led to the use of the corticoid was itself responsible for the less favorable outcome cannot be excluded (84[C]).

Use in premature infants is discussed below.

Prevention of the respiratory distress syndrome (RDS) in anticipated prematurity This has become a widely accepted (though not uncontroversial) indication for corticoids in late pregnancy, the compound most often used being dexamethasone. The timing of such treatment in late pregnancy seems to be of crucial importance (SEDA-3, 306); the possible side effects for the mother and the child are still being discussed. The issue was extensively reviewed in SEDA-17 (1994).

In the mother, *labor may be advanced* by such glucocorticosteroid therapy (SEDA-3, 306); the combination of this treatment with sympathomimetic drugs may bear a risk for the mother of *fluid retention with pulmonary edema* (SED-12, 990), though it is not clear whether this problem indeed only occurs when both drugs are used.

As far as the child is concerned, one may well find only moderate *adrenal suppression* (85[c]), though in some cases substitution treatment with corticosteroids can be necessary in such babies; this short-term treatment with betamethasone shortly before birth has generally been found not to inhibit the infant's adrenal capacity to react to ACTH (86[C]). A single case of *leukemoid reaction* in a pre-term infant has been observed, after the mother was given betamethasone shortly before delivery (SEDA-3, 306).

On the other hand there are many reports of *hypertension* (87[Cr]), and ECG and other studies often confirm the presence of a disproportionately serious and bilateral *hypertrophic obstructive cardiomyopathy*, which unless it proves fatal is in general reversible once the corticosteroids are withdrawn (SEDA-18, 386). Although the issue is confounded by the possibility that infants with bronchopulmonary dysplasia may be innately hypertensive, there seems no doubt as to the effect. Most babies treated with steroids for lung dysplasia also show an appreciable *rise in blood urea nitrogen*, due almost entirely to an increase in structural protein catabolism (88[Cr]). Serious *gastrointestinal complications* can occur; in one typical series of premature neonates treated in this way there were three such instances (perforated duodenal ulcer, perforated gastric ulcer and upper gastrointestinal hemorrhage, the last two proving fatal) (89[cR]); the symptoms are apparently not masked by the glucocorticoid as one would expect to be the case in adults. These treated infants also tend to show a low pH, which is unusual in premature babies (SEDA-18, 445).

Clearly the duration of such treatment after delivery should be kept as brief as possible, but there is no reason for such concern as would lead to the withholding of therapy; one Dutch study with a 10-year follow-up of the children detected no problems with their intellectual, motor or social functioning as compared with controls (90[C]).

Interactions Glucocorticosteroids may alter the response to *anticoagulants*. A raised tolerance to heparin has been reported while a fall in fibrinolytic activity has been seen during glucocorticoid treatment (SED-8, 816). For such reasons, the entire clotting mechanism and particularly the prothrombin time should be checked periodically in patients receiving these steroids concomitantly with anticoagulants, particularly if the steroid dose is changed. In addition the possibility of an increased risk of gastric bleeding in patients receiving both corticoids and anticoagulants should be borne in mind.

Diphenylhydantoin and *phenobarbital* increase the metabolism of glucocorticoids, reducing the plasma half-life by some 50%. *Rifampicin* and other drugs inducing liver enzymes may be expected to have a similar effect, sufficient to impede the effects of corticosteroid maintenance treatment, e.g. in asthma.

Glucocorticoids reduce the plasma level of *salicylates* and if they are given alongside aspirin or other anti-inflammatory drugs there may well be an additive effect on the gastric wall leading to ulceration. The undesirability of using fixed combinations of corticosteroids with *non-steroidal anti-inflammatory agents* has been stressed above.

Glucocorticoids potentiate potassium loss when they are given alongside potassium-losing *diuretics*.

SPECIAL FORMS AND PATTERNS OF ADMINISTRATION OF GLUCOCORTICOIDS

Most knowledge of the adverse effects of corticosteroids has been acquired with their use as oral products. Various other routes of administration have however been developed, sometimes specifically in the hope of securing a local therapeutic effect while avoiding systemic adverse reactions. Although experience has shown that the latter cannot be eliminated in this way, they can be diminished in some cases. In other cases, new problems arise. In addition, attempts have been made to reduce the adverse effects of oral treatment by special dosage schemes.

Daily or alternate-day administration The unwanted effects of the glucocorticoids can apparently be prevented to some extent by alterations in the dosage routine, e.g. giving them on alternative days or administering the total daily dose every morning. The latter is logical in view of the circadian rhythm of endogenous corticoid production; giving a therapeutic dose of a corticosteroid in the evening may inhibit the normal increase in the endogenous corticosteroid level the following morning.

Use in fixed combinations Fixed combinations of oral corticosteroids with non-steroidal anti-inflammatory analgesic or broncholytic drugs which have to be given repeatedly during the day are undesirable, since their pattern of administration is determined in part by the demands of the other components; the corticoid is thus likely to be given in such a way that it deranges the circadian rhythm of the endogenous glucocorticoids.

Inhalation therapy with corticosteroid aerosols (*See also above and Chapter* 16) To some extent, the side effects of these hormones can be reduced in asthma patients by the use of an aerosol, but the dose required to affect the bronchi depends on the size of the particles; if sufficient amounts of the hormone can reach the bronchioles or are deposited elsewhere and absorbed, the treatment will obviously produce systemic effects. Beclomethasone dipropionate or flunisolide are the most common active ingredients of aerosols, their systemic effects are said to be relatively mild, although some suppression of the hypothalamo-hypophyseal-adrenal system may occur (SEDA-6, 332). Oral candidiasis is a frequent but usually minor local complication. In some patients the propellant used in certain aerosols may produce acute bronchoconstriction (SEDA-6, 332). Systemic corticosteroid reactions to inhalation therapy are mentioned at various points in the above review and in Chapter 16: it is important to realize that they can extend to adrenal suppression and psychiatric syndromes.

Nasal sprays The local application of glucocorticosteroids for the treatment of seasonal or perennial rhinitis often results in systemic side effects, and various of these have been mentioned in the present review. The use of nasal sprays containing a corticosteroid which has specific topical activity (such as beclomethasone dipropionate or flunisolide) seems to reduce the systemic side effects, but these can nevertheless occur, even to the extent of suppression of basal adrenal function in children (91[c]). Local side effects include *candida infection*, *nasal stinging*, *epistaxis*, *throat irritation* (92[cR]) and exceptionally *anosmia* (93[c]).

Pulse or megadose therapy Extremely large intravenous doses of glucocorticosteroids given at longer intervals may sometimes be effective when a patient does not respond to conventional high doses. Systemic lupus erythematosus, various rheumatic diseases and the treatment of renal graft rejection are indications for this type of application (SEDA-6, 331). As mentioned above, no side effects need be expected after a single injection of a high dose, but some serious complications have been observed with repeated use, comprising both infections and the known direct side effects of glucocorticosteroids. Cases of dysrhythmia and atrial fibrillation have been reported (SEDA-18, 391). With pulse therapy the nature of the injected glucocorticosteroids seems to be important, e.g. the more rapidly metabolized hydrocortisone seems to be better tolerated than dexamethasone (SEDA-6, 331).

Intraspinal injections The question as to whether oral glucocorticosteroid therapy should be preferred to intrathecal injections is raised by the harmful effects which have sometimes occurred after the latter, though some of these may have been caused by irritative substances in the injection fluid (SEDA-6, 331—332). The same local steroid concentrations can probably be attained with fewer problems when oral administration is used. Epidural injection of corticosteroids seems to be safer than intrathecal injection, but injection of high doses can cause the same systemic side effects as seen with oral treatment.

The effects of *intrathecal* administration, both wanted and unwanted, are still much debated (94[R]). Corticosteroids given intrathecally can cause *elevation of cerebrospinal fluid protein* and carry the risk of *arachnoiditis* (SED-8, 820). Also *chemical meningitis* has been reported after two intrathecal injections of methylprednisolone acetate (95[C]) and after lumbar facet joint block (SEDA-17, 450). *Intraspinal* injections of hydrocortisone for multiple sclerosis apparently led in one case to a *cauda equina syndrome* with subsequent ulceromutilating acropathy (SEDA-17, 450). *Intra-discal* injections of triamcinolone acetonide led in a number of French cases to disk or epidural *calcification*, sometimes symptomless (SEDA-17, 450).

Table 3. *Approximate potency of various mineralocorticoids compared to cortisone*

Compound	Route of administration	Glucocorticoid effect	Mineralocorticoid effect
Cortisone	Oral	1	1
Desoxycorticosterone	Sublingual	Negligible	50
Fludrocortisone	Oral	10–20	150
Aldosterone	Injected	None	500

Intra-articular and periarticular administration Local injections of steroids into and around the joints can have a dramatic therapeutic effect but the catabolic effect can have serious consequences, including adverse effects on the joint structure (96[Cr]) and on local tendons (see above), subcutaneous atrophy and possibly induction of osteonecrosis. Provided the state of the joint is carefully inspected before any new injection is given, and the interval between the injections is not less than 4 weeks, the risk seems to be small enough to justify treatment in invalidating cases (SEDA-3, 307).

Inadvertent intra-arterial injection Particularly when injecting corticoids locally, e.g. to relieve an arthritis of the wrist, accidental injection into an artery is possible. Severe local ischemia can result (SEDA-17, 450).

Use of high doses as antiemetics in cancer patients

High doses of glucocorticoids which show an antiemetic effect in cancer patients can increase the risk of metastases, e.g. in breast cancer. Therefore these hormones should only be used in those types of tumors for which they are known to improve the efficacy of the cancer treatment already used. A curious reaction after intravenous high-dose dexamethasone, used as an antiemetic agent in cancer chemotherapy or for other purposes, is the appearance of a sudden and severe itching, burning sensation and constrictive *pain in the perineal region*. This has been described in several published reports (SEDA-11, 336; 97[C]).

Mineralocorticoids

Aldosterone is the principal physiological salt-retaining corticoid, but it is unsuitable for routine medical use since it is rapidly inactivated when given orally. Desoxycorticosterone (DCA, DOCA, desoxycortone) was used for a long period but had to be taken sublingually (or implanted or injected) to avoid inactivation during liver passage. Overdosage of desoxycorticosterone leading to hypertensive encephalopathy and permanent brain damage has been described (SED-8, 820). Fludrocortisone is the compound most often used at present for long-term mineralocorticoid treatment.

The approximate potency of various mineralocorticoids as compared to cortisone is shown in Table 3.

Fludrocortisone acetate

The dose of fludrocortisone needed in chronic adrenocortical insufficiency varies very widely, from 0.05 to 1.0 mg daily, and in salt-losing forms of the congenital adrenogenital syndrome up to 0.2 mg daily may be needed. In doses appropriate to the individual's needs, adverse reactions to the glucocorticoid effects rarely prove problematical; the main problem is to adjust the dosage (as well as the intake of salt) to these needs, since the adverse effects which can be experienced mainly reflect relative overdosage, and if high doses are to be used meticulous monitoring is required. *Edema*, *hypertension*, *hypokalemia* and *cardiac hypertrophy* can occur. *Hypertension* is the most common reason to reduce dosage. The hypokalemia can lead to *muscular weakness* (98[C]) requiring KCl supplementation.

REFERENCES

1. Kaiser H. Cortisonederivate in Klinik und Praxis. Stuttgart—New York: Thieme, 1987.
2. Labhart A. Adrenal cortex. In: Labhart A, ed. Clinical Endocrinology, Ch. VII. Berlin—Heidelberg—New York: Springer, 1985;373.
3. Medici TC, Rüegsegger P. Does alternate-day cloprednol therapy prevent bone loss? A longitudinal double-blind controlled clinical study. Clin Pharmacol Ther 1990;48:455-466.
4. Rukonen R, Simell O, Dunkel L et al. Hormonal backgroud of the hypertension and fluid derangements associated with adrenocorticotrophic hormone treatment of infants. Eur J Pediatr 1989;148:737.
5. Glass D, Nuki G, Daly JR. Development of antibodies during long-term therapy with corticotrophin in rheumatoid arthritis. Ann Rheum Dis 1971;30:593.
6. Kusse MC, van Nieuwenhuizen O, van Huffelen AC et al. The effect of non-depot $ACTH_{(1-24)}$ on infantile spasms. Dev Med Child Neurol 1993;35:1067-1073.
7. Grabner W. Zur induzierten NNR-lnsuffizienz. Fortschr Med 1977;95:1866.
8. Minden SL, Orav J, Schildkraut JJ. Hypomaniac reactions to ACTH and prednisone treatment for multiple sclerosis. Neurology 1988;38:1631.
9. Rutgers, AWF, Links OP, Coultre R et al. Behavioural disturbances after effective ACTH-treatment of the dancing-eyes syndrome. Dev Med Child Neurol 1988;30:407.
10. Konishi Y, Yasujima M, Kuriyama M et al. Magnetic resonance imaging in infantile spasms: effects of hormonal therapy. Epilepsia 1992;33:304-309.
11. Liebling MS, Stare TJ, McAlister WH et al. ACTH induced adrenal enlargement in infants treated for infantile spasms and acute cerebellar encephalography. Pediatr Radiol 1993;23:454-456.
12. Levin TL, Morton E. Adrenal hemorrage complicating ACTH therapy in Crohn's disease. Pediatr Radiol 1993; 23:457-458.
13. Dunlap SK, Meiselman MS, Breuer Rl et al. Bilateral adrenal hemorrhage as a complication of intravenous ACTH infusion in two patients with inflammatory bowel disease. Am J Castroenterol 1989;84:1310.
14. Rukonen R, Simell I, Jaaskelainen J et al. Disturbed calcium and phosphate homeostasis during treatment with ACTH of infantile spasms. Arch Dis Child 1986;61:671.
15. Katzir Z, Shvil Y, Landau EH et al. Thiazide therapy for ACTH-induced hypercalciuria and nephrolithiasis. Acta Paediatr 1992;81:277-279.
16. Mathies H. Probleme der symptomatischen Therapie rheumatischer Erkrankungen mit Glukokortikoiden und nichtsteroidalen Antirheumatika. Internist 1979:20:414.
17. Williamson J. Posterior subcapsular cataracts and macular lesions after long term corticotrophin therapy. Br J Ophthalmol 1967;51:839.
18. Erban SB, Sokas RK. Kaposi's sarcoma in an elderly man with Wegener's granulomatosis treated with cyclophosphamide and corticosteroids. Arch Intern Med 1988; 148:1201
19. Gill PS, Loureiro C, Bernstein-Singer M et al. Clinical effect of glucocorticoids on Kaposi sarcoma related to the acquired immunodeficiency syndrome (AIDS). Ann Intern Med 1989;110:937.
20. Tebbe B, Mayer-da-Silva A, Garbe C et al. Genetically determined coincidence of Kaposi sarcoma an psoriasis in an HIV-negative patient after prednisolone treatment. Spontaneous regression 8 months after discontinuing therapy. Int J Dermatol 1991;30:114—120.
21. Stewart IM, Marks JS. E.C.G. abnormalities in steroid-treated rheumatoid patients. Lancet 1977;ii:1237.
22. Poynter D. Beclomethasone dipropionate aerosol and nasal mucosa. Br J Clin Pharmacol 1977;4(Suppl 3):295S.
23. Hayhurst M, Braude A, Benatar SR. Anaphylactic-like reaction to hydrocortisone. S Afr Med J 1978;53:259.
24. Lim BS, Choi WY, Choi JW. A case of steroid-induced intractable hiccup. Tuberc Respir Dis 1991;38:304—307.
25. Klein JF. Adverse psychiatric effects of systemic glucocorticoid therapy. Am Fam Phys 1992:46:1469—1474.
26. Doherty M, Garstin I, McClelland RG et al. A steroid stupor in a surgical ward. Br J Psychiatry 1991;158:125—127.
27. Satel SL. Mental status in children receiving glucocorticoids. Clin Pediatr 1990;29:382—388.
28. Alpert E, Seigerman C. Steroid withdrawal psychosis in a patient with closed head injury. Arch Phys Med Rehabil 1986;67:766.
29. Hasanyeh F, Murray RB, Rodgers H. Adrenocortical suppression presenting with agitated depression, morbid jealousy, and a dementia-like state. Br J Psychiatry 1991; 159:870-872.
30. Lewis GP, Jusko W, Burke CW et al. Prednisone side effects and serum protein levels. Lancet 1971;ii:778
31. Kaiser H. Psychische Storungen nach Beclomethasondipropionat-lnhalation? Med Klin 1978;73:1334.
32. Bentson J, Reza M, Winter J, Wilson G. Steroids and apparent cerebral atrophy on computed tomography. J Comput Assist Tomogr 1978;2:16.
33. Sakamaki Y, Nakamura R, Uchida M et al. A case of pseudotumor cerebri following glucocorticoid therapy in which warfarin prevented recurrence. Jpn J Med 1990; 29:566—570.
34. Laroche F, Chemouilli R, Carlier P. Efficacy of conservative treatment in a patient with spinal cord compression due to corticosteroid-induced epidural lipomatosis. Rev Rheum (English Edn), 1993;30:729—731.
35. Roy-Camille R, Mazel CH, Husson JL et al. Symptomatic spinal epidural lipomatosis induced by a long-term steroid treatment. Spine 1991;16:1365—1371.
36. Rabhan NB. Pituitary-adrenal suppression and Cushing's syndrome after intermittent dexamethasone therapy. Ann Intern Med 1968;69:1141.
37. Reiner M, Galeazzi RL, Studer H. Cushing-Syndrom und Nebennierenrinden-Suppression durch intranasale Anwendung von Dexamethasonpraparaten. Schweiz Med Wochenschr 1977;107:1836.
38. Zwaan CM. Odink RJH, Delemarre-van de Waal HA. Acute adrenal insufficiency after discontinuation of inhaled corticosteroid therapy. Lancet 1992;340:1289—1290.
39. Marazzi MG, Agnese G, Gremmo M et al. Problemi relativi alla funzionalita surrenalica in corso di terapia cortisonica protratta in soggetti con epatite cronica: nota preliminare. Minerva Pediatr 1978;30:937.
40. Dutau G, Rochiccioli P. Exploration corticotrope au cours des traitements prolongés par le dipropionate de béclométhasone chez l'enfant. Poumon Coeur 1978;34:247.
41. Grabner W. Zur induzierten NNR-lnsuffizienz bei chirurgischen Eingriffen. Fortschr Med 1977;95:1866.

42. Diczfalusy E, Landgren BM. Hormonal changes in the menstrual cycle. In: Diczfalusy D, ed. Regulation of Human Fertility. Copenhagen: Scriptor, 1977;21.
43. Cunningham GR, Goldzieher JW, De la Pena A et al. The mechanism of ovulation inhibition by triamcinolone acetonide. J Clin Endocrinol 1978;46:8.
44. Bagdade J, Porte D Jr, Bierman EC. Steroid induced lipemia. Arch Intern Med 1970;125:129.
45. Ettinger WH, Hazzard WR. Elevated apolipoprotein-B levels in corticosteroid-treated patients with systemic lupus erythematosus. J Clin Endocrinol Metab 1988;67:425.
46. Schneider J, Burmeister H, Riuz-Torres A. Langzeitstudien uber die Wirksamkeit der Dauertherapie bei hyperergisch-allergischen Erkrankungen mit Prednisolon. Verh Dtsch Ces Inn Med 1977;83:1785.
47. Bielawski D, Kiati IM, Hegyi T. Betamethasone induced leukaemoid reaction in pre-term infant. Lancet 1978;i:218.
48. Craddock CG. Corticosteroid-induced Iymphopenia, immunosuppression, and body defense. Ann Intern Med 1978;88:564.
49. Saxon AS, Stevens RH, Ramer SJ et al. Glucocorticoids administered in vivo inhibit suppressor T Iymphocyte function and diminish B Iymphocyte responsiveness in in vitro immunoglobulin synthesis. J Clin Invest 1978;61:922.
50. Spiro HM. Is the steroid ulcer a myth? N Engl J Med 1983;309:21.
51. Messer J, Reitman D, Sachs HS et al. Association of adrenocorticosteroid therapy and peptic ulcer disease. N Engl J Med 1983;309:21.
52. Henry DA, Johnston N, Dobson A, Duggan J. Fatal peptic ulcer complications and the use of non-steroidal anti-inflammatory drugs, aspirin, and corticosteroids. Br Med J 1987;295:1227.
53. Hamed I, Lindemann RD, Czerwinski AW. Case report: acute pancreatitis following corticosteroid and azathioprine therapy. Am J Med Sci 1978;276:211.
54. Gray S, Daar A, Shepherd H, Oliver DO. Oral versus intravenous high-dose steroid treatment of renal allograft rejection. The big shot or not? Lancet 1978;i:117.
55. Editorial. Nocturia during steroid therapy. Br J Med J 1970;4:193.
56. Wendt H. Klinisch-pharmakologische Untersuchungen zur akneinduzierenden Wirkung von Fluorcortinbutylester. Arzneim-Forsch 1977;27:2245.
57. Bioulac P, Beylot C. Etude ultrastructurale d'une leucodermie secondaire à une injection intraarticulaire de corticoides. Ann Dermatol Venereol 1977;104:883.
58. Silverman RA, Newman AJ, LeVine MJ et al. Poststeroid panniculitis: a case report. Pediatr Dermatol 1988;5:92.
59. Kaye LD, Kalenak JW, Price RL et al. Ocular implications of long-term prednisone therapy in children. J Pediatr Ophthal Strabismus 1993;30:142—144.
60. Abramson HA. May corticosteroid cataracts be reversible? (Editorial). J Asthma Res 1977;14:7.
61. Lubkin VL. Steroid cataract—a review and a conclusion. J Asthma Res 1977;14:55.
62. Forman AR, Loreto JA, Tina LU. Reversibility of corticosteroid-associated cataracts in children with nephrotic syndrome. Am J Ophthalmol 1977;84:75.
63. Byers B. Blindness secondary to steroid injections into the nasal turbinates. Arch Ophthalmol 1979;97:79.
64. Lukert BP, Adams JS. Calcium and phosphorus homeostasis in man. Arch Intern Med 1976;136:1249.
65. Hahn TJ. Corticosteroid induced osteopenia. Arch Intern Med 1978;138:882.
66. Chesney RW, Mazess RB, Hamstra AJ et al. Reduction of serum 1,25-dihydroxyvitamin-D3 in children receiving glucocorticoids. Lancet 1979;ii:1123.
67. Garton MJ, Reid DM. Bone mineral density of the hip and of the anteroposterior and lateral dimensions of the spine in men with rheumatoid arthritis. Arthr Rheum 1993;36:222—228.
68. Lukert BP, Johnson BE, Robinson RG. Estrogen and progesterone replacement therapy reduces glucocorticoid-induced bone loss. J Bone Miner Res 1992;7:1063—1069.
69. Herve J, De Gouyon F, Bonnet-Gajdos M et al. Ostéonecrose ischémique des têtes fémorales et des têtes humerales par corticotherapie chez l'enfant. Arch Fr Pediatr 1978; 35:420.
70. Abeles M, Urman JD, Rothfield NF. Aseptic necrosis of bone in systemic lupus erythematosus: relationship to corticosteroid therapy. Arch Intern Med 1978;138:750.
71. Gibson JNA, Poyser NL, Morrison WL. Muscle protein synthesis in patients with rheumatoid arthritis: effect of chronic corticosteroid therapy on prostaglandin $F_2\alpha$ availability. Eur J Clin Invest 1991;21:406-412.
72. Anon. Corticosteroid myopathy. Lancet 1970;ii:1118.
73. Janssens S, Decramer M. Corticosteroid-induced myopathy and the respiratory muscles. Report of two cases. Chest 1989;95:1160.
74. Weiner P, Azgad Y, Weiner M. The effect of corticosteroids on inspiratory muscle performance in humans. Chest 1993;104:1788—1791.
75. Halpern AA, Horowitz BT, Nagel DA. Tendon ruptures associated wiht corticosteroid therapy. West J Med 1977; 127:378.
76. Klaustermeyer WB, Gianos ME, Kurohara ML et al. IgG subclass deficiency associated with corticoteroids in obstructive lung disease. Chest 1992;102:1137-1142.
77. Pingleton WW, Bone RC, Kerby GR et al. Oropharyngeal candidiasis in patients treated with triamcinolone acetonide aerosol. J Allergy Clin Immunol 1977;60:254.
78. Daly JR. The effect of short- and long-term corticosteroid treatment on sleep-associated growth hormone secretion. Clin Endocrinol 1978;8:315.
79. Travis LB, Chesney R, McNery P et al. Growth and glucocorticoids in children with kidney disease. Kidney Int 1978;14:365.
80. Allen DB, Goldberg BD. Stimulation of collagen synthesis and linear growth by growth hormone in glucocorticoid-treated children. Pediatrics 1992;89:416-421.
81. Newton RW, Browning MCK, Iqbal J et al. Adrenocortical suppression in workers manufacturing synthetic glucocorticoids. Br Med J 1978;1:73.
82. Lucas A, Coll J, Salinas I et al. Hipertensión arterial begigna tras suspensión de corticoterapia en una paciente previaments intervenida por enfermedad de Cushing. Med Clin 1991;97:473.
83. Stöckli A, Keller M. Kongenitales adrenogenitales Syndrom und Schwangerschaft. Schweiz Med Wochenschr 1969; 99:126.
84. Warrell DW, Taylor R. Outcome for the foetus of mothers receiving prednisolone during pregnancy. Lancet 1968;i:117.
85. Kairalla AB. Hypothalamic-pituitary-adrenal axis function in premature neonates after extensive prenatal treatment with betamethasone: a case history. Am J Perinatol 1992;9:428—430.
86. Ohrlander S, Gennser G, Nilsson KO, Eneroth P. ACTH

test to neonates after administration of corticosteroids during gestation. Obstet Cynecol 1977;49:691.
87. Ohlsson A, Calvert SA, Hosking M et al. Radomized controlled trial of dexamethasone treatment in very-low-birth-weight infants with ventilator-dependent chronic lung disease. Acta Paediatr 1992;81:751–756.
88. Brownless KG, Ng Pc, Henderson MJ et al. Catabolic effect of dexamethasone in the preterm baby. Arch Dis Child 1992;67:1–4.
89. O'Neil EA, Chwals WJ, O'Shea MD et al. Dexamethasone treatment during ventilator dependency: possible life threatening gastrointestinal complications. Arch Dis Child 1992;67:10–11.
90. Schmand B, Neuvel J, Smolders-de Haas et al. Psychological development of children who were treated antenatally with corticosteroids to prevent respiratory distress syndrome. Pediatrics 1990;86:58–64.
91. Priftis K, Everard ML, Milner AD. Unexpected side-effects of inhaled steroids: a case report. Eur J Pediatr 1991;150:448-449.
92. Stead RJ, Cooke NJ. Adverse effects of inhaled corticosteroids. Not serious if care is taken. Br Med J 1988;298:403.
93. Whittet HB, Shinkwin C, Freeland AP. Anosmia due to nasal administration of corticosteroid. Br Med J 1991; 303:651.
94. Wilkinson HA. Intrathecal Depo-medrol: a literature review. Clin J Pain 1992;8:49–56.
95. Plumb VJ, Dismukes WE. Chemical meningitis related to intrathecal corticosteroid therapy. South Med J 1977; 70:1241.
96. Sparling M, Malleson P, Wood B et al. Radiographic followup of joints injected with triamcinolone hexacetonide for the management of childhood arthritis. Arthr Rheum 1990;33:821–825.
97. Klygis LM. Dexamethasone-induced perineal irritation in head injury. Am J Emerg Med 1992;10:268.
98. Rivera VM. Fludrocortisone acetate and muscular weakness. J Am Med Assoc 1973;225:993.

Meyler's Side Effects of Drugs, 13th Edition
M.N.G. Dukes, editor

SECTION EDITOR: B. VRHOVAC

P. Senanayake and M.F. McCann

40.1 Hormonal contraceptives

Editorial note *The present chapter deals specifically with acute adverse reactions to hormonal contraceptives. Tumorigenic effects and most of the possible second-generation effects are discussed in Chapter 40.2.*

GENERAL

Oral contraceptives (OCs) have been in use for more than 30 years. The pattern of immediate adverse reactions is by now well known, but late effects can be difficult to study, especially if they are rare and the condition also occurs spontaneously. The influence of geographical variation and of progressive changes in formulation, which is very marked in some of the relevant studies, must always be borne in mind. Retrospective case-control studies are now difficult to perform, since the proportion of women who have never been exposed to oral contraceptives is decreasing rapidly; in 1992 there were probably some 20–40 million current users. Information on the duration and time of treatment is crucial, but it is usually difficult to obtain retrospectively. It is thus important to continue to follow the large cohorts of women included in the prospective studies currently being conducted in various countries or sponsored by the World Health Organization.

Hormonal contraceptives are among the most effective forms of contraception. During typical use, 3% of women using combined oral contraceptives become pregnant in the first year (1[R]). The pregnancy rate for progestogen-only pills (POPs) is somewhat higher, about 5% (2[R]). As compared to the original high-dose combination products, the lower dosages now in current use offer a lesser margin for error if tablets are missed (as they undoubtedly are); the efficacy of POPs is even more dependent on correct use. The accidental pregnancy rates for injectable and implanted hormonal contraceptives are lower than for the oral products and are not dependent on daily pill-taking. The 1-year rate for depot medroxyprogesterone acetate (injectable) is 0.3% and for levonorgestrel implants is 0.09% (1[R]).

Hormonal contraceptives offer many health benefits (3[r], 4[R]), in addition to being a highly effective method of pregnancy prevention. Combined oral contraceptives (COCs) greatly reduce the risk of epithelial ovarian cancer and endometrial adenocarcinoma. COCs also prevent benign breast disease (fibroadenoma and cystic changes), pelvic inflammatory disease, and ectopic pregnancy. They have beneficial effects on menstrual patterns, including reduction in amount of menstrual flow and thus lower prevalence of iron deficiency anemia, as well as reduction in the prevalence and severity of dysmenorrhea. Finally, there is some evidence that they also prevent functional ovarian cysts, uterine fibroids and rheumatoid arthritis and that their use may lead to increased bone mineral density.

The classic oral contraceptives are those based on both estrogen and progestogen, which together inhibit gonadotropin secretion and thus prevent ovulation (1[R], 4[R]). Estrogen also stabilizes the endometrium and potentiates the action of the progestogen. In addition, the progestogen exerts contraceptive effects on the cervical mucus (thickening the mucus to make it hostile to sperm penetration), the endometrium (interfering with implantation), and the Fallopian tubes (altering ovum transport). The original fixed combinations have given way to others employing lower doses, as well as to variants on the principle. The estrogen dosage today normally lies in the range of 30–50 μg ethinylestradiol, since lower levels result in an unsatisfactory bleeding pattern. To calculate the dose of progestogen which offers the highest benefit/risk ratio is not as easy, particularly since their relative potency can be expressed in various ways (e.g. in terms of their effect on the human endometrium, their androgenic or corticosteroid potency on their ability to inhibit ovulation), and it is not at all clear which of these activities are relevant to long-term safety issues (2[R]).

Oral contraceptives

ADVERSE REACTION PATTERN

General and toxic reactions The incidence of common adverse reactions to oral contraceptives varies with population and product. Common side effects of combined OCs include intermenstrual bleeding, nausea or vomiting, breast tenderness and headaches. Occasionally OC users report depression or decreased libido, acne or weight gain. Women taking COCs are also at greater risk of chlamydia infection and of modest impairment in glucose and lipid metabolism. The most serious complications attributable to OC use are cardiovascular diseases, but these are extremely rare and are even less common now, with lower dose formulations, than in earlier decades.

Hypersensitivity reactions These have been observed, but only very rarely.

Tumor-inducing effects (see also Chapter 40.2) The risk of epithelial ovarian and endometrial cancer is reduced by combined OCs. It is unclear whether breast or cervical cancer rates are affected by COCs; any possible increase in risk appears to be quite small.

Second-generation effects (see also Chapter 40.2) Inadvertent use of OCs during pregnancy does not increase the risk of congenital anomalies. Women using combined OCs are much less likely to have ectopic pregnancies than either women using other contraceptive methods or non-contracepting women; users of progestogen-only contraception have an ectopic pregnancy incidence similar to non-contraceptors. After OC discontinuation, there is sometimes a 1–2 month delay in return to fertility. Use of hormonal contraceptives during lactation is associated with a modest reduction in milk quantity for combined OCs but no effect for progestogens alone.

ORGANS AND SYSTEMS

Cardiovascular (*For thromboembolism, see special section below. Also, see 'Endocrine, metabolic' section*) The association between COCs and *hypertension* has been explored in a pair of reports from a multicenter clinical trial carried out by WHO (5[Cr], 6[Cr]). When women were randomly assigned to take COCs containing either 30 or 50 μg ethinylestradiol, both with 250 μg levonorgestrel, there were no significant differences in either blood pressure measurements or life-table probability of developing hypertension. However, a parallel cohort of women with nonhormonal IUDs had significantly lower systolic and diastolic blood pressure and rate of hypertension incidence compared to the 50-μg estrogen COC group. Thus, there appears to be an adverse effect of COCs which is unrelated to estrogen dose. Most, but not all, studies of progestagen dose in COCs also find no dose-response relationship (2[R]).

Hypertension in connection with oral contraception was first reported in 1961 and proved by rechallenge. It is still not clear why certain women develop hypertension when using oral contraceptives. It has been shown that the drugs have an effect on the renin–angiotensin system, but there actually seems to be some decrease in responsiveness to plasma renin activity. Possible pathophysiological mechanisms discussed so far include: (a) insufficient adaptation to increased production of angiotensin and aldosterone, (b) an increase in cardiac output, and (c) changes in the metabolism of catecholamines. The estrogenic component of oral contraceptives appears to be the more important factor in producing abnormalities in the renin system, but the progestogen may also play a role. In a 1977 analysis of data from the large prospective study by the Royal College of General Practitioners (RCGP) it was found that with oral contraceptives containing ethinylestradiol 50 μg and 1, 3 or 4 mg of norethisterone acetate the rate of hypertension increased with an increasing progestogen dose (7[C]). Recent evidence implicates progestogens as well (8[R]). Other studies have not shown a dose-response effect for either norethisterone acetate or D-norgestrel, even with the higher doses used in the past (2[R]).

By 1978, by which time fairly low-dosed products had become more widely used, it seemed clear (9[R]) that many users of oral contraceptives react at some time with a rise in blood pressure, although it cannot always be regarded as hypertension; clinical hypertension may not occur with current products in more than 1–5% of women (10[R]). The rise in blood pressure can appear at any time during treatment and persists for at least as long as the drug is taken; sometimes it lasts several months longer, but even then it generally returns to normal values. Severe or malignant hypertension is rare, but 4% of users are found to have a diastolic blood pressure of 90 mmHg or more. This prevalence is about twice as high as in women of the same age who are not using oral contraceptives. Even current low-dose products have this effect; it is not clear whether the frequency was in fact higher with the older drugs. Thus, blood pressure measurements should be an integral part of the follow-up care of all women taking oral contraceptives (1[R]).

As might be expected, women with hypertension who take oral contraceptives run a somewhat greater risk of *acute secondary complications due to hypertension*, such as subarachnoid hemorrhage (11[C]); if the hypertension is severe and persistent one might anticipate long-term effects on the cardiovascular system and kidneys. Nested case-control studies utilizing data from the RCGP study found that hypertension was an independent risk factor for both stroke (12[C]) and myocardial infarction (13[C]); after controlling for other variables, including OC use, the odds ratios (or estimated relative risks) associated with hypertension were 2.8 for stroke and 2.4 for myocardial infarction. OC use did not further increase the risk associated with either hypertension or history of toxemia of pregnancy. Nonetheless, hypertensive women who take OCs should be monitored carefully.

No confirmation has been obtained of early beliefs that hypertension during oral contraception was more prone to occur in Black American women, or in women with a history of hypertension during pregnancy (4[R], 14[C]). Lehtovirta et al. (15[Cr]) have however advanced clinical evidence that the women involved may have a defect in dopaminergic transmission affecting blood pressure and prolactin secretion; pre-existent abnormalities of platelet function and fibrinolysis have also been linked with this complication (SEDA-6, 348).

Thromboembolism An international Consensus Development Meeting in 1990 issued the following statement regarding the relationship between oral contraceptive use and *cardiovascular disease* (16[R]):

> 'The majority of epidemiological studies strongly suggest an association between current OC use and certain cardiovascular deaths. Although the relative risk is increased, the absolute risk is small .... Because the risk of myocardial infarction is apparent in current users, disappears on cessation of use, and is not associated with duration of use, there is no *epidemiologic* support for the hypothesis that risk of cardiovascular diseases is of atherogenic origin .... Whether particular formulations or progestogens have qualitative advantages or disadvantages merits further study. Estrogens and progestogens interact at many levels, and in epidemiologic studies of users of combined OCs it is difficult to assign a risk to either component separately. Moreover, it is physiologically unsound to do so .... Alterations in plasma lipid, carbohydrate, and hemostasis variables are of major importance for the development of cardiovascular diseases, and their level can be influenced by sex steroids, including artificial steroids contained in OCs. The pharmacodynamic responses ... are dependent on not only the type and dosage of sex steroids, but also on intra- and interindividual variability in pharmacokinetics.'

Evidence is now accumulating regarding the low cardiovascular risk associated with use of OCs containing low estrogen dose (<50 μg ethinylestradiol) (17[R]). These recent epidemiological studies have found that current users of low dose pills have small, and often statistically non-significant, elevations in risk of *myocardial infarction* (SEDA-16, 465; 18[Cr]; 19[C]), *thrombotic stroke* (12[C], 20[Cr], 21[Cr]), *venous thromboembolism* (22[C]), and *subarachnoid hemorrhage* (12[C], 21[CR], 23[C]). Several of these studies compared the risk for pills with low dose compared to higher dose ($\geq$50 μg ethinylestradiol) and found somewhat lower rates among women currently using the lower dose preparations (12[C], 18[Cr], 20[Cr], 24[C]). Even with the low dose oral contraceptives, *cigarette smoking* further elevates the risk for myocardial infarction (19[C]) and thrombotic stroke (12[C], 20[Cr]).

A recent review of the safety of OCs notes that early epidemiological studies of high-dose oral contraceptives are not relevant to the clinical situation today, for several reasons (25[R]). COCs prescribed initially had 3–4 times the estrogen dose and 10 times the progestogen dose compared to those commonly used in the 1990s. Secondly, early studies did not consider the potentially confounding effects of other risk factors, most notably cigarette smoking. Finally, women desiring OCs are evaluated more carefully now for these other risk factors and are advised not to use this contraceptive method if they have serious underlying medical conditions or if they are older women who smoke.

Cause and effect relationships The consensus statement noted above includes the following comment on *coagulation* parameters (16[R]):

> 'Oral contraceptives induce alterations in hemostasis variables. There are changes in the concentrations of a large number of specific plasma components of the coagulation and fibrinolytic systems, although usually within the normal range . . . It is conceivable that these effects are estrogen mediated because they have not been demonstrated in progestogen-only preparations. There is a dose-dependent relationship in the case of estrogen, although in combination pills, the progestogens might exert a modifying effect .... Further attention should be given to changes in factor VIIc and fibrinogen induced by OCs and also to the association between carbohydrate metabolism and fibrinolysis.'

Beller (26[R]) has recently noted that quantification of coagulation factors is notoriously difficult because of the interrelationships among the various components of the coagulation cascade, the broad range of normal values, and the considerable inter-laboratory variability. This variability is illustrated by a WHO study of COC users, conducted on several continents, which found statistically significant differences among clinical centers in prothrombin time, fibrin plate lysis, plasminogen, and activated partial thromboplastin time (SEDA-16, 464).

Several problems confuse the discussion of oral contraception and the risk of thrombosis. The term 'hypercoagulability' has been used to describe a supposed prethrombotic state, identifiable by certain changes in the hemostatic system, yet to date no laboratory test can in fact assess the risk of thrombosis occurring in a given individual; similarly, coagulation changes in vitro have sometimes been regarded as proof of an existent thrombotic state. Further, laboratory data from patients with existing thrombosis have been interpreted as demonstrating the cause of the thrombosis, whereas they may simply be a consequence. Studies of effects on clotting mechanisms have been obtained on different populations, using different contraceptives, with different methods and at different periods of the medication cycle (27[C]—31[C]).

There are numerous methodological issues inherent in most epidemiological studies of OCs and cardiovascular disease, as well. Bias in the ascertainment of drug exposure is an unresolved issue for most of the case-control studies on actual incidence of thrombosis. Because of the multiplicity of cardiovascular disease risk factors (some of which are interrelated), proper control of confounding is not possible. Epidemiological data on thrombosis can at best demonstrate an association between two events, but not establish a causal relationship.

It is today clear that oral contraceptives do have thrombogenic activity, the proof emerging from an accumulation of epidemiological and biochemical evidence. That has not however been a smooth process; as soon as the risk of thromboembolism came to light around 1961, the evidence was contested and the conflict was prolonged. The first major evidence of thromboembolism as a risk came in 1967 from Britain's Medical Research Council (32[CR]). This and other large studies (32[CR]—37[CR]) concluded that women using oral contraceptives ran a greater risk than non-users of developing deep venous thrombosis, pulmonary embolism, cerebral thrombosis, myocardial infarction and retinal thrombosis. Later papers and case reports described deep venous thrombosis, portal venous thrombosis and pulmonary embolism (38[c]—40[c]). The Boston Collaborative Drug Surveillance Program follow-up study of more than 65 000 healthy women from 1980 through 1982 found a positive association between current oral contraceptive use and venous thromboembolism (rate ratio 2.8); there was also a positive association between current oral contraceptive use and stroke or myocardial infarction (41[c]). A British study using data from 1978, by which time lower-dose products were increasing in use, pointed to an approximate doubling of the risk of thromboembolism when compared with controls (SEDA-7, 387). The early 1980s were nevertheless marked by a series of critical papers which sought to question the entire concept of there being a link.

A landmark paper to resolve the issue, co-authored by Realini and Goldzieher in 1985 (42[R]), provides a thorough critique of the methodological strengths and weaknesses of the epidemiological evidence. The authors concluded that an association between current oral contraceptive use and the incidence of venous thromboembolism in subjects without predisposition had been consistently observed in case-control and cohort studies. The evidence regarding myocardial infarction, various types of stroke, and cardiovascular mortality was less consistent. Among the numerous methodological shortcomings, particularly in the earlier studies, is lack of control for the confounding effects of smoking and the likelihood of detection bias (particularly for venous thromboembolism). It is important to note that venous thromboembolism is much more common in young women than myocardial infarction or stroke; although venous thromboembolism is less often fatal, the greater incidence implies that it has a greater public health impact.

Incidental case reports of severe cardiovascular events continue to appear, including incidents of cerebral venous thrombosis and subarachnoid hemorrhage (43[c], 44[c]), fatal central angiitis (45[c]), sinus thrombosis (SEDA-16, 465) and cerebral ischemia (46[c]). In one series of 22 cases of cerebral infarction concerning either arteries or veins, all oral contraceptives involved contained a low dosage of ethinylestradiol (47[c]). Basilar artery occlusion secondary to thrombosis (48[c]), occlusion of cerebral arteries (49[c]), retinal vascular complications (50[c]) as well as encephalopathy with renovascular hypertension (51[c]) and acute myocardial infarction (52[c]) have all been reported in more recent papers. Thromboembolism with other localizations, such as in the mesenteric vessels and the hepatic vein, i.e. Budd-Chiari syndrome, has been occasionally reported (53[c]); the first 10 such cases were reported as long ago as 1972 and the increasing number since then has begun to give rise to some concern (SEDA-6, 344; SEDA-7, 386). Forty-one cases of intestinal ischemia and infarction in oral contraceptive users have been published, the latter being associated with a high mortality rate (54[c]). A case of renal vein thrombosis has also occurred (55[c]).

Degree of risk It is extremely important in all these matters to distinguish between effects on morbidity and on mortality (which are far from running parallel) and to maintain a sense of proportion as regards the importance of the risk in the community at large.

West German data over the period 1955—1980, for example, showed no community-wide increase in the incidence of ischemic heart disease, cerebral vascular embolism or pulmonary embolism, despite the rapid growth in oral contraceptive use during that period (56[CR]).

The Oxford Family Planning Association's cohort study which followed up more than 17 000 women for an average of nearly 16 years found no significant overall effect of oral contraceptive use on mortality, with a relative risk of 0.9 (57[C]). Mortality from diseases of the circulatory system had slightly increased; the relative risk of death from ischemic heart disease in current or past oral contraceptive users was 3.3 (95% confidence interval 0.9—17.9), while data on fatal cerebrovascular disease were too few to be interpreted. Pills containing 50 μg estrogen accounted for about 70% of the woman-years of pill use, with most of the remainder being lower dosages.

A massive Finnish mortality study, covering 1 585 000 women-years of oral contraceptive use and 1 975 000 women-years of copper-bearing intrauterine device use found no increase in relative risk among oral contraceptive users for myocardial infarction or cerebral hemorrhage deaths; there might however have been an increased risk of death from pulmonary embolism among oral contraceptive users (58[C]). The authors stress that the low incidence rates of death from cardiovascular diseases could, at least in part, be explained by the influence of risk factors, such as a history of ischemic heart disease or its predisposing factors, or hypertension and age, on the contraceptive choice, owing to the exclusion of oral contraceptives in high-risk women.

A recent analysis by Schwingl and colleagues has modeled the cardiovascular disease mortality risk associated with low dose (<50 μg ethinylestradiol) OCs in the United States (17[R]). For non-smokers and light smokers (<25 cigarettes per day) of all ages, the results indicate that the mortality among current OC users is likely to be lower than the mortality due to pregnancy. Only among heavier smokers who are over age 30 would the risk of OC use exceed the risk of pregnancy. The researchers note that in countries with higher maternal mortality than the US, even older women who are both heavy smokers and OC-users would have lower mortality risk than that associated with pregnancy.

Mechanisms The risk of thrombosis is almost certainly associated with the *estrogen component* (59[R]) for both arterial and venous events and to the progestogen for arterial events. Estrogen alone has been incriminated as a cause of thromboembolism when given to men (60[Cr]); the risk of puerperal thromboembolism following estrogen inhibition of lactation has been demonstrated in several studies (e.g. 61[CR]); non-contraceptive estrogens clearly increase the risk of acute myocardial infarction in women younger than 46 years of age (62[CR]). The changes in coagulation factors (see below) appear to be related to the estrogen dose, and the thrombogenic effect is generally regarded as dose related (63[CR]—65[CR]).

Oral contraceptives cause an increase of the *coagulation factors* I (fibrinogen), II, VII, IX, X, and XII, as well as a decrease in antithrombin III levels, which would be expected to predispose to venous thromboembolism, especially if not counterbalanced by an increase either in fibrinolytic activity or of other inhibitory proteins of the coagulation, such as protein C (66[r]). The overall impression is one of some imbalance of the hemostatic mechanism towards hypercoagulability. Progestogen-only preparations have not been shown to have any significant effect on the coagulation system. Numerous studies have shown that lower estrogen dosages (30 μg) have less effect on coagulation parameters than higher dosages (50 μg) (67[C], 68[R]). Ernst (69[R]) has reviewed the evidence regarding fibrinogen and OC use, concluding that there is a significant rise in fibrinogen levels during the early months of OC use, with levels returning to baseline after cessation of use.

Prolonged use of oral contraception seems to lower levels of anti-aggregatory *prostacyclin* (70[C]).

There is also fairly strong evidence that *immunological mechanisms* play a role in thrombotic episodes associated with oral contraceptives, especially when they occur in the absence of risk factors for vascular disease (71[C]), though this has been contested (72[C]). In one series of reports on cerebral infarction, circulating immune complexes and/or specific antihormone antibodies were found in 15 of 20 patients assessed (47[c]). In a recent large series of women with venous or arterial thrombosis, Beaumont has reported that anti-ethinylestradiol antibodies (anti-EEAb) were absent in non-OC users but present in 72% of users; they were also present in 33% of OC users without thrombosis (SEDA-16, 465). Anti-EEAb plus smoking were found jointly in half of the cases.

Other risk factors For a long time it has been considered on strong grounds that smoking, obesity, and age in excess of 35 years are exogenous risk factors which raise the risk of thromboembolic changes.

The role of *smoking* is generally regarded as clear (73[CR], 74[R]); it increases the risk of myocardial infarction as well as of subarachnoid hemorrhage, and it can double or treble mortality (75[C]—80[R]). There is a definite dose-response effect, with light smokers having twice the risk of coronary heart disease and heavier smokers having up to four times the risk, compared to non-smokers (74[R]). Cessation of smoking is accompanied by a reduction in risk of coronary heart disease to that of nonsmokers within 3–5 years (74[R]). The mechanism for smoking's effect on cardiovascular disease is less clear. Smoking may contribute to effects on the pro-coagulation process in young women smokers (81[c]). Oral contraceptive users who were smokers have been found to have significantly lower values for fibrinolytic activity than those who were non-smokers (82[c]), but not consistently (31[c]). A recent study by Fruzzetti et al. (67[C]) has shown that the effects of OCs on the coagulation system are much greater in smokers than non-smokers.

The 1989 case-control analysis of the RCGP cohort study found that current oral contraception did increase the risk of acute myocardial infarction, but only among smokers (13[C]). The estimated relative risk for current OC use was 0.9 for non-smokers, 3.5 for women smoking <15 cigarettes per day, and increasing to 20.8 for ≥15 cigarettes per day, suggesting a synergistic effect of OCs and smoking. There was no relationship with previous OC use. Results from the other large British cohort study, conducted by the Oxford Family Planning Association (OFPA) indicate no significantly increased risk of myocardial infarction or angina pectoris for either current or former use of OCs, but a strong dose-response effect of current smoking (83[C]).

Numerous studies have shown that the risk of coronary heart disease increases directly with *body weight* (74[R]). For example, the OFPA data confirm that the risk of myocardial infarction or angina increases significantly with weight (83[C]). The underlying risk of cardiovascular disease is very low among reproductive-age women, but there is a gradual increase in risk with *age* during this period (84[R]). However, because the risks associated with pregnancy also increase markedly with age, the US Food and Drug Administration has concluded that the benefits may outweigh the possible risks for healthy nonsmoking women over age 40.

As far as endogenous risk factors are concerned, early epidemiological data on the recurrence of thrombosis (85[CR]) indicated something of an inherited predisposition, and others found a *low content of fibrinolytic activators* in the vessel wall of women who 6–12 months earlier had experienced a thrombotic complication while using oral contraceptives (86[CR]); high doses of estrogen affected the levels of such activators (87[CR]). However, such lesions are apparently not exclusive to users of oral contraceptives (SEDA-8, 360) and examination of the vessel wall is not of predictive value in determining risk. It was shown at an early stage that women belonging to blood group Type O run rather less risk of thromboembolism (88[CR]). French authors have advanced a hypothesis that an *allergic arteritis* is involved in the complication, which again would suggest the presence of endogenous predilection. The risk of thromboembolic complications may be greater where there is a history of *diabetes*, *hypertension* and *pre-eclamptic toxemia*. In some studies there has been an association with *Type II hyperlipoproteinemia*, *hypercholesterolemia and atheromatosis* (33[CR], 75[CR], 89[c]–91[c]). *Hypertension* may be an additional risk factor when considered in relation to oral contraceptive use (*see above*).

Early work suggested a greater risk following *major surgery* (92[CR]–94[CR]). However, epidemiological studies of *postoperative venous thromboembolism* are limited and subject to divergent interpretations (95[R]). There is no documented excess risk of postoperative thrombosis associated with low-dose combined OCs among women without other risk factors (3[r], 26[R]). A recent study examined changes in hemostasis after cessation of COCs (30 μg ethinylestradiol plus either desogestrel or gestodene) (96[Cr]). Several weeks elapsed before plasma concentrations of fibrinogen, factor X and antithrombin III returned to baseline; the authors therefore conclude that even low dose COCs should be stopped at least 4 weeks before major surgery. A 1991 journal editorial makes this same recommendation, but notes that one of the reasons for this advice is concern about litigation (95[R]). From a practical point of view, any decision regarding possible discontinuation of COCs prior to surgery should take into consideration the possibility of conception occurring during the interim period. If the woman chooses to suspend use of combined OCs, progestogen-only preparations (as well as barrier methods) are deemed suitable (95[R]). A recommended alternative to COC discontinuation is low-dose prophylactic heparin (26[R]).

Product-related risk factors relate to the selection of an oral contraceptive. Mestranol was the estrogen almost universally used in early COC formulations; ethinylestradiol is much more common today. Ethinylestradiol has greater estrogenic potency and therefore can be used at a somewhat lower dose, though it has never been clear whether this means that the risk of thromboembolic complications is also reduced. Though as late as 1985 the relevance of the estrogen dose was incidentally challenged (SEDA-11, 349), there has been a universal effort to develop products employing the lowest possible effective doses of estrogens and progestogens. Whether the risk is different for dose levels of 30, 40 or 50 μg of estrogen is still not known; the primary evidence of risk was obtained at higher levels. In the individual woman, the preparation of choice is the lowest-dosed one which suits her needs. In some cases low-dosed progestogen-only products can be used, despite their often poor control of endometrial bleeding. The choice of estrogen might still be relevant to the extent that (physiological) 17β-estradiol in microcrystalline form later became available for oral use and in theory might prove safer in some respects than synthetic estrogens since it seems to have less effect on the fibrinolytic system; it is discussed in a later section.

Persistence of risk Most, but not all, studies find no effect of prior OC use on cardiovascular disease risk (97[C]—104[C]). It is now generally acknowledged that the increased risk of cardiovascular disease associated with current use virtually disappears upon cessation of COC use (25[R], 74[R], 84[R]). This conclusion is supported most strongly by a 1990 meta-analysis of published studies on the relationship between past use of OCs and myocardial infarction, which produced an adjusted relative risk estimate of 1.01, indicating no association (105[CR]). The authors note, however, that there have been only a few studies of stroke in relation to previous OC use, and that those studies have produced inconsistent results; thus, meta-analysis of stroke data are precluded.

The Nurses' Health Study found no differences in either incidence of or mortality from various cardiovascular diseases between never- and past-users, regardless of the duration of use, or time since last use (105[CR]). A recent analysis of mortality data from this study reports that death rates due to coronary heart disease, stroke, and other cardiovascular conditions are similar for ever-users (including current users) and never-users of OCs (106[Cr]). The nested case-control analysis of the RCGP study determined that, although stroke risk was elevated among current OC users regardless of smoking status, former users had an increased risk only if they were current smokers (12[C]). Thorogood et al. (18[Cr]) found that the risk of fatal myocardial infarction was similar for current and past users, whereas Lidegaard and colleagues (20[Cr]) reported a lower risk of cerebral thromboembolic attack for former users compared to never-users.

This lack of an association between previous OC use and cardiovascular disease further supports the above discussion on biological mechanisms. There does not appear to be a long-term mechanism at work, such as atherosclerosis, but rather an effect confined to current use, such as thrombosis (25[R], 74[R], 105[CR]).

Conclusions As techniques become more refined, errors in earlier work will continue to be detected, but it is clear that oral contraception does carry a risk of thromboembolic complications. The degree of risk is small, except where ancillary risk factors are present. There seems however to be no doubt that under the influence of all these studies of risk, the formulation of oral contraceptives has been changed for the better, resulting in a decrease in thromboembolic morbidity and mortality (25[R], 84[R]).

Respiratory system No known effects.

Nervous system *Headache* is sometimes reported as a side effect of OC use (1[R], 4[R]). However, in a placebo-controlled trial, headache was not found to be associated with use of COCs containing either 50 or 100 μg mestranol (107[C]). In many other studies of OC side effects, it is not possible to ascertain whether the prevalence of specific complaints such as headache is actually elevated, because there is no appropriate comparison group.

Because *migraine headaches* are of vascular origin, it is pertinent to consider whether hormonal contraception is appropriate (108[R]). No association of migraine headache and stroke has been demonstrated. However, some women with migraine experience an increase in severity and frequency of headache when taking COCs. As a precaution, women who have migraine headaches with focal neurological symptoms should not take COCs (1[R], 4[R]).

Despite initial concern (SEDA-6, 349), COCs do not appear to worsen seizure control in most women with *epilepsy*, although seizure frequency should nonetheless be carefully monitored (108[R]). The primary consideration regarding contraceptive method selection for epileptic women is the importance of high effectiveness, yet those antiepileptic agents that are enzyme inducers reduce the effectiveness of hormonal contraceptives. Women who wish to take COCs but for whom enzyme-inducing medication provides the best seizure control should be prescribed COCs with 50 μg ethinylestradiol. Reversible electroencephalographic changes probably due to progestational action (109[r]) have been observed in 25—60% of oral contraceptive users. It has been demonstrated that fewer seizures occur during the luteal phase (low estrogen) of the menstrual cycle, opening the possibility that estrogens (or oral contraceptives) may be epileptogenic.

There are various reports of *chorea* (110[c], 111[c]), *hemichorea* (112[c]) and *paraballism* (113[c]). In one case, chorea was the first sign of lupus erythematosus (114[c]).

Psychiatric symptoms have been described in single case reports (115[c], 116[c]), probably reflecting a nonspecific derangement of balance in susceptible individuals. As to psychological effects, many physicians have found that certain women react to oral contraceptives by becoming morose or unhappy, but this does not necessarily mean that they meet the clinical criteria of a true depression (117[C]), the incidence of which has not been found to be increased (118[CR]). Several possible biological mechanisms for pill-induced depression have been hypothesized (1[R]). However, when nervousness and depression among COC users are carefully evaluated over time, the prevalence has been found to be highest during the pretreatment control cycle and to be similar for women taking the placebo and the COCs (107[C]), thus indicating no physiological relationship.

Many OC users find greater *sexual satisfaction* (1[R], 118[CR]) because of relief from worry about pregnancy. Occasionally women report decreased libido, which may have a hormonal basis. One study found that users of oral contraceptives had no rise in female-initiated sexual activity at the time when ovulation should have occurred, whereas non-users did show such an increase in sexual activity (119[CR]).

Endocrine, metabolic The report of the Consensus Development Meeting stated the following regarding the effects of oral contraceptives on *carbohydrate and lipid metabolism* (16[R]):

'All currently used OCs can cause deterioration in glucose tolerance accompanied by hyperinsulinemia. There is no evidence that the use of combined OCs is accompanied by overt symptoms of diabetes.... The progestogen component is mainly responsible for the effects of OCs on carbohydrate metabolism, but the estrogen component may modulate the influence. The magnitude of the impact on glucose metabolism depends on the type of progestogen and also on the doses of a given steroid.

Oral contraceptives induce changes in lipid and lipoprotein metabolism and these changes are dose dependent and can be related to both estrogens and progestogens. The effects of oral contraceptives on lipids may change with time—rendering short-term studies, that is, shorter than 6 months, difficult to interpret.... Although the lipid changes are quite definite, there is no evidence that they are related to atherogenesis in OC users.

The insulin resistance syndrome has recently been described by Godsland and Crook (120[R]) as a set of metabolic risk factors for cardiovascular disease (specifically, coronary heart disease/arterial disease). These interrelated risk factors include hyperinsulinemia and impaired glucose tolerance, hypertriglyceridemia, reduced high-density lipoprotein (HDL) concentrations, and hypertension, with insulin resistance as a potential underlying factor. Hormonal contraceptives may variously affect these metabolic conditions, with the effect dependent in part on steroid type and dose. Newer formulations do not change HDL levels or increase blood pressure, but insulin resistance and hypertriglyceridemia still occur. These latter changes are caused primarily by the estrogen component of combined OCs, but the progestogen component may also modify these effects. The preparations with the more favorable metabolic effects are those containing norethindrone or the newer, more selective progestogens (desogestrel or norgestimate).

These metabolic disturbances attributable to estrogen must be weighed against the direct beneficial effects of estrogens on the artery wall that have recently been demonstrated. Collins and colleagues (121[R]) suggest that estrogen has a calcium antagonist effect that relaxes the vessel walls, thus increasing blood flow. Williams et al (122[Cr]) have documented in cynomolgus monkeys that estrogen administration leads to dilation of the coronary arteries and that these vascular responses were not related to plasma lipid concentrations, blood pressure or heart rate. It has also been shown by this same group of researchers that estrogen-progestogen administration to hypercholesterolemic cynomolgous monkeys reduces both their HDL cholesterol levels and their arterial lesions (123[C]).

A recent review of the relationship of hormonal contraception to carbohydrate metabolism by Elkind-Hirsch and Goldzieher (124[R]) reports that low-dose COCs are associated with only a small elevation in risk of impaired glucose tolerance. They note that there is no difference in incidence of diabetes mellitus for ever-users compared to never-users and conclude that the minor changes in glucose metabolism are not of clinical importance.

Findings as to effects on *carbohydrate* metabolism are not fully consistent (125[R]). A diabetogenic action has been claimed, but various prospective studies in England (126[CR]–128[CR]) showed no increased risk of diabetes in oral contraceptives users compared with controls or ex-users. All the same, effects on carbohydrate metabolism do occur. A mild to moderate degree of insulin resistance has been found in some investigations (129[C]–133[C]). The clear impression persists that oral contraceptives can in some individuals cause deterioration in glucose tolerance (134[r]) and that patients with serious or brittle diabetes should not use them (135[c]). Because of the increased risk of pregnancy complications in diabetic women, a highly effective contraceptive method such as COCs is often desirable. A clinical study of young women with insulin-dependent diabetes mellitus has recently documented no significant differences between women using various COCs (≤0.05 mg ethinylestradiol) and non-users in hemoglobin A_{1c} values, albumin excretion rates, and diabetic retinopathy (136[C]). Whether OC use by women with a history of *gestational diabetes* further increases their underlying propensity for developing diabetes when not pregnant is uncertain (4[R]).

Arteriosclerotic vascular diseases have been extensively discussed as a possible complication of oral contraceptives related to *lipid* changes (137[R]). Early studies mostly showed an increase of both triglycerides and cholesterol, involving very low-density lipoproteins (VLDL), low-density lipoproteins (LDL) and high-density lipoproteins (HDL) (138[CR]). The lower-dose products now in use have less marked effects, but the combined effects of oral contraceptives and lifestyle have to be considered here as well (137[R]). In one investigation (139[CR]) in which three low-estrogen dose combinations were studied, the HDL fraction (which is thought to have a protective effect against arteriosclerosis) was lowered. However, not all products behave in the same way (140[C]). The changes appear to be dose-related (141[c]) as regards both components; in a Kaiser-Permanente study (142[Cr]) in some 5000 women, it was found that estrogen administration increased the HDL-cholesterol by 0.18—0.39 mmol/l while progestogen lowered the HDL-cholesterol by 0.41 mmol/l. With combined therapy an intermediate result was obtained. A retrospective Belgian study of treatment up to 12 years found that pure progestogen contraceptives caused a moderate decrease in triglycerides, HDL-cholesterol and apoprotein A1, whereas mainly estrogen oral contraceptives increased the same parameters; long- and short-term use had the same effects (143[C]). Some studies however suggest an early effect on certain lipid/lipoprotein changes followed by a leveling off for some groups of patients (139[c], 144[c]).

In the light of these and other findings (145[C]—147[C]) it has been argued that the progestogen component is capable of increasing the risk of arteriosclerosis (137[R]), but not all progestogens have the same effect. Certain combinations using desogestrel, chlormadinone or low-dose norgestrel have been found to have little or no deleterious effect on lipid levels (147[C]—149[C]), while pure progestogen preparations seem to have no effect on lipids (149[C]). Smoking has been found not to affect the lipid and lipoprotein changes observed in oral contraceptive users (150[c]).

Whether there is an increased risk of developing atherosclerotic disease is still controversial but the consensus view has indicated that the risk is slightly increased. Various findings make it impossible to draw direct conclusions from the biochemical data. HDL-cholesterol, for example, may be divided into subfractions, of which HDL_2 seems to be more responsive to estrogens and progestogens; HDL_2 concentration has been thought to correlate better with a reduced risk of cardiovascular disease than does total HDL-cholesterol (151[R]). The picture is further complicated by the fact that when estrogens are used in post-menopausal women they can raise HDL, i.e. have a favorable effect (152[C]—155[C]); it may be that they raise the risk in the short term, as suggested above, but lower it in the long term. Again, whether the higher HDL_2 level induced by some oral contraceptives could offer some protection against the development of cardiovascular disease is uncertain since the disease is determined by several factors and not by lipids alone (148[C]). Risks may differ in certain subgroups of users (156[c]). The only general rules emerging from what is now known are that one should—for this and other reasons—use the lowest possible dose of active components in an oral contraceptive, and that, other things being equal, preference might be given to combinations having little effect on LDL- and HDL_2-cholesterol concentrations (157[R]).

There are certain *thyroid* effects. Oral contraceptives raise plasma protein-bound iodine and thyroxine (158[C]) whilst the resin triiodothyronine uptake decreases. The uptake of radioactive iodine in the thyroid is normal as a rule; total uptake of radioactive iodine may be lowered (159[Cr]). The effect of the progestogen on thyroxine-binding globulin may possibly counteract the estrogenic action. The net result will be a rise in protein-bound iodine and a fall in resin triiodothyronine uptake (160[C]). It has been suggested that oral contraceptives may actually exert some protective effect against thyroid disease.

Alterations of plasma *vitamin* levels have been observed in oral contraceptive users due to changes in plasma protein-binding capacity, and partly also because of impairment of absorption (161[R]). While most vitamin levels in the blood decrease (134[r]), vitamin A levels are increased, though carotene levels fall. Curiously, an isolated case-report of hypercarotenemia has been recently reported (162[c]). Ascorbic acid levels are lower in the leukocytes and platelets of 'pill' users. It seems that the conversion of vitamin D_3 to 25-hydroxy-D_3 is inhibited. Both sequential and non-sequential types of oral contraceptives impair the absorption of polyglutamic folate but not that of monoglutamic folate; the change can result in megaloblastic anemia in predisposed subjects, e.g. those with celiac disease or a deficient diet. Vitamin B_{12} deficiency has also been seen in healthy 'pill' users in whom serum vitamin B_{12}-binding proteins were not altered. Alterations in vitamin B_6 metabolism have been discussed, particularly in connection with the suspicion that the 'pill' might cause depression. An additional daily intake of pyridoxine has been suggested to correct the complex changes observed during 'pill' intake (163[C], 164[C]); there are no firm data proving that such medication has any useful effect in most women, but the approach may be tried empirically where the mood changes are a problem (1[R], 165[R]). All in all, one must doubt whether the effects of these products on vitamin metabolism are of any significance, except possibly in severely undernourished populations.

Both long- and short-term progestational therapy can suppress pituitary *ACTH* production to some extent, as studied with the metyrapone test. Medroxyprogesterone and chlormadinone have been shown to suppress the reaction to metyrapone almost completely. Recovery was rapid after discontinuation of therapy; no conclusion was drawn as to the relative effect of the ethinylestradiol that was also given. The cortisol secretion rate is depressed in women receiving norethindrone and mestranol, and the suggestion has been made that the gluconeogenic effect of corticosteroids is markedly potentiated in subjects receiving estrogens or estrogen-like substances. Adrenal cortical insufficiency has been related to the use of ethinylestradiol and dimethisterone taken during 1 year. The ascorbic acid content of the anterior pituitary is diminished in the presence of estrogen-induced adenohypophyseal hypertophy.

Fasting *growth hormone* levels are higher in women using a contraceptive agent than in controls.

The *body weight* tends to increase in some women without a clear explanation, although it could be attributable in some individuals to improved appetite, water retention or conceivably the anabolic effect of an 'androgenic' progestogen. The increase is usually less than 2 kilograms and occurs during the first 6 months of use (134[r]). This physiological increase in weight associated with OCs occurs only rarely. Studies that record weight change over time have generally found similar fluctuations in OC users and non-users (4[R], 107[C]). Cyclic weight gain due to fluid retention may also occur (1[R]).

The effects of oral contraceptives on *lactation* have been examined carefully (166[R], 167[R]), since estrogens are well-known inhibitors of ovulation in large doses, and even products containing 30 μg ethinylestradiol will reduce the milk volume (168[C]); the composition of the milk is also slightly altered (134[r]), but again one has the impression that the effect is not important except in a very poorly nourished population. Both progestogens and estrogens are excreted in the milk, their proportions being correlated with those in plasma but lower. The plasma/milk ratio varies from compound to compound, probably due to variations in the degree of protein binding and (for progestogens) also with the amount of fat in the milk. The amount of steroid transferred in 600 ml of milk is estimated at 0.1% or less, of the daily dose taken. Although newborn infants might be relatively sensitive to these hormonal substances because of the immaturity of detoxification systems, no adverse effects have been found when they were looked for systematically; nevertheless, isolated cases of gynecomastia have been noted in babies when their mothers were taking oral contraceptives during lactation. Eight-year follow-up of Swedish children whose mothers used COCs while breastfeeding indicates no negative effects on health, growth or development (169[Cr]). It should be realized that the hormonal content of natural human and cows' milk is not negligible. If hormonal contraception is to be used during lactation, it would seem sensible to prefer low-dose progestogens rather than combinations with estrogens; they are not the most effective contraceptives, but probably sufficient to supplement the contraceptive effect of lactation itself and they are unlikely to inhibit lactation (2[R]).

Mineral and fluid balance (*Also, see 'Musculoskeletal system' below*) Both lowering and elevation of plasma *zinc* have been reported following the use of sex hormones. Serum *copper* has been shown to rise, but serum *magnesium* has been found to remain unchanged. The clinical importance of these effects is not known. Users of oral contraceptives have been shown to excrete significantly less *calcium* than non-users (170[C]) and estrogen treatment has been shown to prevent bone loss in postmenopausal women (171[CR]); it is thus likely that the diminished urinary calcium excretion observed in women using oral contraceptives results from suppression of bone resorption by exogenous estrogens. Long-term use of oral contraceptives may therefore affect skeletal bone stores and prevent the development of osteoporosis. In line with these findings is an investigation showing an increase in radio-opacities in the mandibles of women using oral contraceptives (172[C]).

Hematological *Iron status* is improved in most OC users because of decreased menstrual blood loss; thus, an important benefit of OC use is the reduction in prevalence of *iron deficiency anemia* (161[R]). As with so many other issues, much of the research on iron status has been with higher hormone dosages than are currently used. A recent study of a low-dose COC (ethinylestradiol 30 μg plus desogestrel 0.15 mg) documented a significantly lower menstrual blood loss during pill administration than at baseline (173[C]). Most women had normal values for hemoglobin, hematocrit, erythrocyte index, and serum ferritin both before and during OC administration, with no significant changes. However, two women who had menorrhagia (defined as menstrual blood loss greater than 80 ml) and low serum ferritin prior to OC use experienced improvement in both of these parameters while taking OCs. The cyclic variation of serum iron during the menstrual cycle has also been found to be less pronounced during the use of anovulatory agents (174).

Although *sickle cell disease* is sometimes listed as a contraindication to OC use, a recent review concludes that this may not be justified (175[R]). Women with this condition need highly effective contraception because pregnancy is associated with increased morbidity and mortality to both mother and fetus, as well as the increased likelihood that the infant would have sickle cell disease. Theoretically, combined OCs should be given with caution because of the increased risk of thrombosis associated with both sickle cell disease and COCs, but the limited available evidence indicates no change in hematological parameters among women using hormonal contraceptives (2[R]). Progestogen-only preparations may be preferred, not only to avoid potential risk of thrombosis but also because studies suggest that sickle cell crises may be inhibited.

The *binding capacity of serum proteins* is altered by oral contraceptives (176[R]) and leads to alterations in the serum levels of various substances including thyroxine, cortisol and serum iron (177[C]) and in *serum iron binding capacity*, which are all increased. Erythrocyte enzymopathies have been observed during pregnancy and oral contraceptive treatment (178[CR]) and in these cases a cause—effect relationship seems likely. The reaction, however, appears to be observed very rarely (*see also Chapter* 40.2). A hemolytic and uremic syndrome seen in one very long-term user may have been due to antisteroid hormone antibodies (179[c]).

Liver (*Tumorigenic effects are discussed in Chapter* 40.2) Hepatobiliary complications of OCs have been thoroughly reviewed by Lindberg (53[CR]). While most women experience no adverse effects, occasionally hepatic changes may occur, including intrahepatic cholestasis, cholelithiasis, hepatic adenomas, hepatocellular carcinoma, and vascular complications of the liver. Lindberg specifies that women with a history of liver disease whose liver function tests have returned to normal can take OCs, with careful monitoring. However, women with the following conditions should not be given OCs: history of cholestatic jaundice of pregnancy; past or current benign or malignant hepatic tumors; active hepatitis; and familial defects of biliary excretion.

Oral contraceptives have been shown to cause mild hepatocellular damage manifested by a transient rise in serum transaminases (180). Long-term use has been shown to lead to changes in the hepatic ultrastructure with involvement of the mitochondria, which develop crystalline inclusions. Furthermore, hypertrophy of the smooth endoplasmic reticulum and changes in the biliary canaliculi have been demonstrated (181, 182). These changes are not usually accompanied by any clinical symptoms. The Budd-Chiari syndrome is discussed in connection with thromboembolism (above).

Benign liver tumors (hepatocellular adenoma and focal nodular hyperplasia) are extremely rare conditions which appear to be related to OC use (183[R]).

Jaundice as a result of oral contraceptive treatment has been repeatedly described (53[R]). The overall incidence has been estimated at about 1:10 000 (184), but in the Swedish population figures between 1:100 and 1:4000 were published when high-dose preparations were still in use (185[CR]). When hepatic symptoms appear, they usually do so within the first month of medication (186), and comprise anorexia, malaise, pruritus and jaundice. Very few cases are seen after the third month of medication and those reported are regarded by some as unlikely to be due to oral contraceptives. Elevation in serum alkaline phosphatase is usual, while serum transaminases can be normal to highly elevated (187). Microscopic examination of the liver shows intrahepatic cholestasis. When medication is stopped, symptoms usually disappear rapidly and the reaction does not seem to leave any sequelae (188[CR]). Genetic components seem to be important for the development of the reaction; women who have experienced jaundice or severe pruritus in late pregnancy seem to be especially susceptible to develop jaundice or gallbladder disease when using oral contraceptives (189[CR]). Discussion of mechanisms has related mostly to estrogens (190), but cases have been described in individuals receiving progestogens only (185[CR]); the explanation might be the conversion of the latter to estrogens in vivo (191). The cause of cholestasis is unknown, but animal data indicate that there is an inhibition of bile flow and of the biliary excretion of bilirubin and bile salts.

Peliosis hepatis has been described in association with contraceptive-induced hepatic tumors (see Chapter 40.2) and has sometimes developed in isolation, perhaps as a herald of more serious changes to follow, e.g. cirrhosis and portal hypertension developed (53[R]); one such case ultimately required an orthotopic liver transplant (192[c]).

Sinusoidal dilatations in the liver have been reported rarely (53[R]). For example, a 23-year-old woman developed an acute painful syndrome with cytolysis after 7 years of oral contraceptive use; she recovered promptly after oral contraceptive withdrawal (193[c]).

A recent meta-analysis of the relationship between COCs and *gallbladder disease* has yielded a small increased risk for women who had ever used OCs (pooled estimated relative risk ratio=1.38) (194[R]). A dose-response effect was noted, indicating that, although the risk is less with lower dose COCs, a weak relationship may still remain. The increased risk appears to be concentrated in the early years of OC use, suggesting that OCs accelerate the development of the disease.

The association between oral contraceptive use and gallbladder disease has long been disputed. Recently, the Nurses' Health Study II showed no substantial increase in risk associated with ever-use of OCs, but relative risks of 1.6 for long-term use and for current use, after adjusting for body mass index and several other confounding variables (195[C]). A 1994 report from the Oxford FPA study similarly indicates no relationship with ever-use of OCs (196[C]). The Boston Collaborative Drug Surveillance Program (197[CR]) found that of a large series of 212 patients with gallbladder disease 31% were using oral contraceptives, as compared with only 20% of controls. Stolley et al. (198[CR]) found that the risk of gallbladder surgery was twice as high for oral contraceptive users as for non-users. A 1982 RCGP Study (199[C]) report concluded, however, that no overall increased risk of gallbladder disease occurred in the long term and that the previously demonstrated short-term increase in risk is due to an acceleration of the onset of gallbladder disease in women already susceptible to it. The risk may also be age dependent, the relative risk of gallstone disease being higher in young women using OCs than in older users (195[C], 200[C], 201[c]).

The finding that oral contraceptive use causes an increase in the cholesterol concentration of hepatic bile and a shift in the chenodeoxycholic/cholic acid ratio suggests a biochemical basis for the increase in gallbladder disease among oral contraceptive users (195[C], 202[C], 203[CR]). Effects on gallstone formation may well be due to the estrogen content, e.g. since estrogens seem to raise the risk of gallbladder disease in men (204[CR]), and in women can raise the cholesterol saturation of bile and hence the lithogenic index (203[C], 205[C]).

Results from the Boston Collaborative Drug Surveillance Program suggest that oral contraceptive users are more often diagnosed as having *acute hepatitis* than are non-users (206[CR]). There was no similar finding in the study by the British RCGP (126[CR]).

Gastrointestinal Mild gastrointestinal complaints such as *nausea*, *vomiting* and vague *abdominal pain* were seen in 10–30% of patients in earlier studies, but are less common with the low doses used today. *Nausea* is associated with the estrogen component of COCs. Frequency and severity generally decline over time (1[R], 3[r]). A placebo-controlled clinical trial by Goldzieher and colleagues (107[C]) documented a higher prevalence of nausea and vomiting among COC users than among women taking either a placebo or a progestogen-only oral contraceptive; the prevalence was also higher for the combined OC containing 100 μg mestranol than for the combination product containing 50 μg mestranol.

Gingivitis, of varying degrees of severity, is sometimes associated with OC use, apparently because the steroids alter the microbial flora in the mouth (207[R]). *Gingival hypertrophy* has incidentally been described. Even a low-dose combination has been found to have an effect on the *composition of saliva* (208[CR]); although large individual variations were noted, protein, sialic acid, hexosamine, fucose, hydrogen ion concentration and total electrolyte concentration decreased, while the secretion rates increased. The sodium and hydrogen ion concentrations increased in parotid gland secretion and sodium in submandibular gland secretion. To what extent these changes might affect the dental status of the patient is not known.

Oral *pyogenic granuloma* has been reported both in pregnant patients and in patients using oral contraceptives (209[CR]). Progestogens, alone or together with estrogen, cause an increase in the width and tortuosity of peripheral blood vessels in the oral mucosa, which become more susceptible to local irritants and show increased permeability.

Acute pancreatitis has been reported during oral contraceptive treatment (210[CR]) as well as serum amylase increases (211[C]).

The relationship between OC use and *inflammatory bowel disease* has been analyzed in two case-control studies published in the 1990s (212[C], 213[C]). Both found a significant elevation in risk among current users compared to never-users for Crohn's disease, but only one (212[C]) detected an increased risk for ulcerative colitis. A dose-response effect was suggested for Crohn's disease, but not for ulcerative colitis (212[C]). When the data were stratified by smoking status in one of these analyses (213[C]), the increased risk was found only among current smokers.

Diarrhea has been mentioned as an occasional individual reaction.

Urinary system A few reports point to a higher incidence of urinary infections in users of oral contraceptives (134[r]), but this could reflect differing or altered patterns of sexual behavior.

Skin and appendages Various types of *skin reactions* can certainly occur during oral contraceptive treatment, but bearing in mind the vast number of women using the 'pill', major skin reactions due to oral contraceptive treatment seem to be rare. The incidence, even including all minor complications, has been estimated at 5% (214). The figure includes *chloasma*, *acne*, *seborrhea*, *hirsutism*, *pruritus*, *herpes gestationis*, *porphyria cutanea tarda* and allergic reactions such as *urticaria*. Low-dose COC use generally results in improvement of acne, although occasionally a user experiences a worsening of acne due to the androgenic potency of the progestin (1[R], 4[R]).

There is a possible association with *erythema nodosum* which has been linked to the use of either estrogens or progestogens or the combination of the two; probably, however, neither hormone directly causes the condition but merely creates a fertile background for its generation by other antigens (214). *Alopecia* during treatment and following withdrawal has been seen, but the association may be coincidental. *Condyloma acuminata* has been stated to increase during oral contraception, with regression after withdrawal (215). Increased *pigmentation* of areas exposed to sunlight as well as photosensitivity have been observed in some users. One case of *pityriasis lichenoides* disappearing after withdrawal of oral contraceptives has been described (216[c]).

Special senses An aggravation of existing *otosclerosis* has been observed several times; in one series of five cases, withdrawal of the medication stabilized four cases while the fifth was improved (217[C]).

In a study of 7046 American women, hearing was generally better among current oral contraceptive users than in never-users, and intermediate for past users (218[C]). There is no reason to expect a decline in hearing except in cases of otosclerosis (see above). A long-term study of chronic OC users, which included otological, audiological and vestibular examinations, found no impairment of the function of the healthy internal ear (219[c]).

It is still difficult to judge whether a correlation exists between *ocular pathology* and the use of oral contraceptives (1[R], 2[R], 4[R]), with the exception of thromboembolic incidents affecting the retinal venous flow. Oral contraceptives have several times been reported to decrease the tolerability to contact lenses, but in any case this declines in some people as the years pass. However, pregnancy itself may result in loss of contact-lens tolerance both for scleral and corneal lenses, lenses often having to be refitted after pregnancy; a similar effect of oral contraceptives is thus not entirely unlikely (220[C]), even though other workers have failed to detect any such effect (221[C]). Similar doubts relate to the induction of macular hole with retinal detachment, but in one study 20 out of 24 women with this complication were found to be using oral contraceptives (SEDA-6, 348). Finally, there is one case report of retinal migraine linked to the end of oral contraceptive treatment cycles (222).

Musculoskeletal system Although some studies have shown that COCs increase bone mineral density, the available evidence suggests that any beneficial effect is rather small (25[R], 223[Cr]), and presumably is related to the dosage of estrogen (224[CR]). The effects may depend in part on the age of women being studied, as normally bone mass density continues to increase until it peaks in women in their 20s and 30s, and then remains constant until the premenopausal period when it begins to decline. For example, a recent study of young women (age 19—22) found that those taking very low-dose (20 μg ethinylestradiol) COCs had no change in bone density over 5 years, whereas non-users had a significant increase (224[CR]).

Genital system (*Tumorigenic effects are dealt with in Chapter* 40.2) *Breast tenderness or pain* can appear in some women, especially with estrogen-dominant preparations, although it is notable that other women with a history of breast discomfort experience improvement when they begin to take oral contraceptives (134[r]).

Women currently taking OCs are less likely than non-users to have *functional ovarian cysts* (3[r]). This protective effect appears to be more modest with lower dose monophasic formulations than with those containing >35 μg estrogen (225[C], 226[C]). Multiphasic preparations neither increase nor decrease the risk.

Women taking combined OCs experience improvement in several parameters of *menstrual function* (3[r], 173[C], 227[C]). Menses generally become more regular and predictable, and dysmenorrhea is less common and less severe. The number of days of each menstrual period is reduced, as is the amount of menstrual flow (173[C]); thus women who previously experienced iron deficiency anemia associated with menorrhagia have increased iron stores (see 'Hematological' section above). An analytic comparison of women who kept menstrual diary records as part of WHO clinical trials has demonstrated that users of COCs have more regular menstrual cycles than users of other hormonal methods (228[C]). None of the COC users in these studies had amenorrhea (defined as absence of bleeding throughout a 90-day reference period), although shorter periods of amenorrhea have occasionally been reported in other studies, particularly with very low-dosage formulations and with longer-term use (1[R], 4[R]).

Intermenstrual bleeding (also called *breakthrough bleeding* or *spotting*) often occurs, especially during the first few cycles of treatment, and is frequently the reason that women choose to discontinue OC use (228[R], 229[R]). Prospective OC users should be advised to expect this problem. A recent review urges more rigorous study of this important side effect (229[R]). The authors state that available evidence suggests that better cycle control is offered by preparations containing gestodene than desogestrel and by levonorgestrel compared to norethindrone, but the absence of standardized methodology makes these conclusions tentative. Research on triphasic preparations is too sparse to permit even tentative conclusions. A recent analysis has shown that intermenstrual bleeding rates vary inversely with both estrogen and progestogen dose (230[C]). However, there is no evidence that breakthrough bleeding is an indication of reduced contraceptive efficacy (4[R]), despite speculation regarding a possible relationship.

Dysmenorrhea is less common and less severe among women using oral contraceptives. A prospective study in Sweden has demonstrated that, both at study entry and 5 years later, dysmenorrhea was less severe among women using OCs than among women using neither OCs nor IUDs (227[C]). There were no significant differences among the three groups of OCs (monophasic, low gestogen activity; monophasic, progestogen-dominated; triphasic).

Since *post-'pill' amenorrhea* of more than 6 months duration was first suggested as an adverse reaction around 1965, much work has been devoted to delineating the risk and prognosis. It is now recognized that amenorrhea following pill discontinuation occurs in 0.7–0.8% of former users, which is no different than the background rate of spontaneous secondary amenorrhea (4[R]). No cause and effect relationship between OC use and subsequent amenorrhea has been documented. Hull et al. (231[C]) in London found that in 48 patients classified as having post-'pill' amenorrhea the subsequent conception rate was no lower than in a control group not suffering from this condition.

Although there may be a delay of 1–2 months in *return of fertility* after COC discontinuation, within a few months conception rates are similar to those of women discontinuing nonhormonal contraception (4[R], 25[R], 232[C], 233[C]). There appears to be a shorter delay with low-dose pills compared to high-dose pills (234[C]). Delay in the return of ovulation has on occasion led to the erroneous conclusion that the first post-'pill' pregnancy might be unduly prolonged (SEDA-6, 351).

Another post-contraceptive change reported primarily during the period when highly dosed products were in use was a *condensation of the superficial cortical layers of the ovary* (SEDA-8, 863). Severe *atrophy of the endometrium* following a period of oral contraception has been described (235), but the incidence is not known since the endometrium is not usually examined. To what extent such changes are associated with OC use and affect subsequent fertility is again not known.

Pelvic inflammatory disease (PID), often resulting in infertility, ectopic pregnancy or chronic pelvic pain, occurs at a somewhat lower incidence in OC users and also tends to be less severe in OC users, compared to non-contraceptors (236[R]–238[R]). The biological mechanism for this protective effect may be the changes in cervical mucus or decreased menstrual bleeding (and thus decreased retrograde menstrual blood in the uterus).

In contrast, COCs provide no protection against *lower reproductive tract infection* (particularly cervical chlamydial and gonococcal infection) and may even have an adverse effect (236[R]–238[R]). This possible increased risk appears to be the result of the expanded area of cervical ectropion associated with the estrogen in COCs. *Candidiasis* of the vagina in oral contraceptive users without evidence of diabetes mellitus has been frequently reported.

Data on the risk of *human immunodeficiency virus* infection with COCs are sparse, with some studies indicating an adverse effect and others showing no association (236[R], 238[R], 239[R]).

Benign breast disease (including fibroadenoma and cystic changes) is less common among COC users (183[R]).

Epidemiological studies of the relationship between OC use and *pelvic endometriosis* have variously shown an increased risk, a decreased risk, and no effect (240[R]). For example, an Italian study recently found an elevated risk among ever-users of OCs, but this elevation occurred only among former users, not current users (241[C]). Furthermore, the authors note that a similar pattern has been shown in several large cohort studies (OFPA, RCGP, and Walnut Creek). There was no association in the Italian study with recency, latency, or duration of use, suggesting that any relationship with OC use is not a true biological relationship but instead the result of selection and other biases.

There are conflicting reports of the association between OC use and *uterine leiomyomas* (*fibroids*), but the data suggest a modest protective effect of current use (183[R]).

Immunological A recent review of the immunological effects of estrogens and progestogens concludes that, although understanding of any relationship is incomplete, it is not likely that the low doses used in OCs would have negative effects on the immune system (242[R]). A sex difference in immune responsiveness has been known to exist for a long time, but little attention has been paid to the possible role played by sex hormones in its regulation. In the study by the British Royal College of General Practitioners (126[CR]) oral contraceptive users showed a higher incidence of certain *infectious diseases*. Support for the concept that oral contraceptives might raise risks of infection has been presented in other studies, and workers from the tropics have remarked that pregnant women appear to be unduly sensitive to malarial infestation (WHO, unpublished data). The antibody response to tetanus toxoid in women has been shown to be considerably lower in oral contraceptive users than in controls (243[CR]). A depressed lymphocyte response to phytohemagglutinin (PHA) has been observed in a series of women taking oral contraceptives (244[R]); the reduction in PHA response reflects impaired T-cell function, and this finding is of interest in view of the concept that a deficiency of T-cell function is important in certain autoimmune diseases. Another consequence of prolonged impairment of T-cell function would be an increased susceptibility to infectious diseases.

During recent years, several studies of the effect of sex hormones on serum immunoglobulin titers have been published. Klinger et al. (245[Cr]) studied the effect of four different oral contraceptives on the serum concentration of IgA, IgC and IgM and found that the concentration of all three immunoglobulins decreased during the first course of treatment and returned to normal during the subsequent cycles. There was some evidence that the steroid-induced reduction of immunoglobulins was predominantly caused by the estrogenic component. More recently, a study has been conducted in which plasma from women currently taking combined oral contraceptives, past users of the pill, women who have never used the pill, and non-users with a history of venous thrombosis was examined for the presence of immunoglobulin G (IgG) that showed specific binding of ethinylestradiol (246[C]). No increase in 'specific' IgG and no evidence of ethinylestradiol binding was observed in oral contraceptive users in comparison to non-users. This study therefore provides no support for the hypothesis that a significant percentage of oral contraceptive users develops a specific IgC showing a high binding affinity to ethinylestradiol, which might be causally linked to the development of thrombotic phenomena in oral contraceptive users (see above).

It appears that OC use reduces the prevalence of severe disabling *rheumatoid arthritis*. Although studies of this issue have produced discrepant results, a meta-analysis of studies that met specific methodological criteria produced an overall adjusted pooled odds ratio of 0.73 (247[R]). The authors suggest that OCs do not actually prevent rheumatoid arthritis, but modify the disease process to prevent progression to severe disease. Pregnancy has similar effects. It is unclear whether it is the estrogen or the progestogen component of OCs that is responsible (242[R]).

Numerous case reports have suggested that COCs can induce *systemic lupus erythematosus* (114[c], 242[R], 248[c]). However, examination of this issue systematically, in a 1994 case-control study, has shown no association with OC use (249[C]).

Results from the Oxford FPA study indicate no relationship between OC use and *multiple sclerosis* incidence (250[C]). Conversely, multiple sclerosis is no longer considered to be a contraindication for hormonal contraceptive use.

Other organs and systems There were some early reports of localized *mandibular osteitis* in women using oral contraceptives subsequent to surgery of the mandibular molar teeth (SEDA-2, 316). The possibility has been put forward that changes in the hemostatic mechanism (see above) could be the cause.

Hypersensitivity reactions Aggravation of *bronchial asthma, eczema, rashes, angioneurotic edema and vasomotor rhinitis* have been incidentally observed and *cold urticaria* has been reported (251[c]). It is not know whether in any particular individual the hypersensitivity reaction is due to the hormonal substances themselves or to other ingredients in the tablet. Nasal provocation tests with suspensions of contraceptive steroids (252[c]), in patients suffering from allergic rhinitis or pollinosis who had been taking these products, showed a positive response in one third of cases; the same patients also reacted to topical estrogens. Life-threatening *anaphylaxis* with rechallenge has occurred in a young woman using oral contraceptives (253).

Tumor-inducing effects (see also Chapter 40.2) Combined oral contraceptives have a strong, well-documented protective effect on both epithelial ovarian and endometrial cancer (183[R]). A recent meta-analysis of epidemiological studies of *ovarian cancer* found a summary estimated relative risk of 0.64 for ever-use of combined OCs, indicating a 36% reduction in ovarian cancer risk (254[R]). This protective effect increased with increasing duration of OC use and continued for at least 10 years after discontinuation. Although most of the OCs reported in these studies were older, higher-dose formulations, the Cancer and Steroid Hormone (CASH) study included users of pills containing 35 μg or less of ethinylestradiol, and this subgroup of women was found to have a reduced risk of ovarian cancer (255[C]). Because ovarian cancer causes more deaths than any other gynecological malignancy, at least in developed countries, prevention of ovarian cancer is a particularly important non-contraceptive benefit of OCs (25[R]).

Numerous studies have also shown a duration-related protective effect of COCs on *endometrial cancer*, with risk before age 60 reduced by 38% for 2 years of use and up to a 70% reduction for 12 years (256[R]). This beneficial effect continued for at least 15 years after cessation of use. As with ovarian cancer, the CASH study results indicate that the lower dose COCs have a protective effect that is similar to that of the higher dose pills (257[C]).

Research on the association with *breast cancer* generally finds no effect on overall risk (183[R]). The exception is for breast cancer diagnosed at young ages (a very small percentage of breast cancer cases), for which OCs have been shown to have a modest adverse effect. The hormonal composition of COCs does not appear to alter breast cancer risk.

Although studies indicate that OCs increase the risk of *cervical squamous cell carcinoma* and *carcinoma in situ*, there are numerous methodological problems inherent in examination of this relationship (183[R]). Thus it is unclear whether the data reflect a true biological relationship.

The incidence of reproductive cancers attributable to OC use has been estimated in a modeling analysis by Coker and colleagues (258[R]). The authors assumed a 50% reduction in ovarian and endometrial cancers associated with 5 or more years of pill use, and utilized two alternative scenarios for breast and cervical cancer effects. If OC use produces a 20% increase in breast cancer before age 50 and in cervical cancer, then for every 100 000 pill users there would be 44 fewer reproductive cancers and these users would gain one more day free of cancer. If instead the elevation in risk of early breast cancer and of cervical cancer is 50%, then OC users would have 11 fewer cancer-free days.

In developed countries, where *liver cancer* is quite rare, OCs are associated with an increased risk (183[R]). In contrast, in developing countries, where liver cancer is more common, OC use does not appear to affect the risk.

The available evidence does not demonstrate any relationship of OC use with *malignant melanoma of the skin*, *colorectal cancer*, *gallbladder cancer*, or *pituitary tumors* (183[R]).

Second-generation effects (*See also Chapter* 40.2) *Use in pregnancy*: see Chapter 40.2. *Use in lactation*: see 'Endocrine, metabolic'. *Effects on fertility*: see 'Genital system'. *Genetic effects*: see Chapter 40.2.

The likelihood of *ectopic pregnancy* depends on both the pregnancy rate and the proportion of those pregnancies that are ectopic (259[R]). The proportion of pregnancies that implant at an extrauterine site is 0.005 for both COC users and women using no contraception but, because OC users are much less likely to conceive, their rate of ectopic pregnancy is much lower (0.005 per 1000 woman years, compared to 2.6 per 1000 woman years for women using no contraception). The incidence of ectopic pregnancies is also somewhat lower for COCs than for other contraceptive methods. The proportion of ectopic implantations seems to be increased when low-dose progestogens are used either as oral contraceptives or in intrauterine devices (SEDA-1, 303; 2[R], 134[r]), although the incidence is no higher than for non-contraceptors (259[R]). In the past there was some concern about a possible increased risk of ectopic gestation after oral contraceptives have been discontinued (260), but this is no longer considered to be an issue.

The American College of Obstetrics and Gynecology (ACOG) has recently issued a statement concluding that oral contraceptives have not been shown to be causally related to *congenital anomalies* (261[R]). OCs are neither teratogens nor mutagens. Detailed literature reviews by Bracken (262[R]) and by Simpson and Phillips (263[R]) have come to the same conclusion.

Risk situations and contraindications There are no hard and fast rules about prescribing oral contraceptives; the degree of risk resulting from a particular factor has to be looked at from case to case. Specific risk factors for cardiovascular complications have been considered above. The following classification, based in part on data which will be considered in Chapter 40.2, is therefore merely a guideline.

Combined oral contraceptives should not be provided to women with the following *absolute contraindications*:
(a) thrombophlebitis or thromboembolic disorders (current or past);
(b) cerebrovascular disease (current or past);
(c) coronary artery or ischemic heart disease (current or past);
(d) breast cancer (current or past);
(e) endometrial cancer or other estrogen-dependent neoplasia (current or past);
(f) hepatic adenoma or carcinoma (current or past);
(g) impaired liver function (current);
(h) less than 2 weeks postpartum;
(i) breastfeeding and less than 6 weeks postpartum;
(j) known or suspected pregnancy;
(k) use of enzyme-inducing drugs, specifically the antibiotics rifampicin and griseofulvin and most anticonvulsants.

Combined OCs should be provided only with caution and careful monitoring to women with the following *relative contraindications*:
(a) over age 35 and currently smoking ≥15 cigarettes per day;
(b) migraine headaches, particularly with focal neurological symptoms;
(c) hypertension (current, controlled);
(d) diabetes, particularly with retinopathy, neuropathy or vascular disease;

(e) familial hyperlipidemia or current treatment for hyperlipidemia;
(f) gallbladder disease (current);
(g) cholestatic jaundice of pregnancy or with prior OC use;
(h) unexplained abnormal vaginal bleeding;
(i) breastfeeding, particularly if less than 6 months postpartum;
(j) major surgery, with prolonged immobility.

Withdrawal effects (*See 'Genital system'*) Although it was originally believed that women discontinuing OCs were more likely to have *amenorrhea*, careful analysis reveals that this is not the case. The likelihood of *conception* is reduced for the first 1—2 months after discontinuation, but cumulative conception rates after several months are not affected.

Overdosage Children below the age of 6 years who have accidentally ingested oral contraceptives have experienced nausea and vomiting during 10—15 hours after ingestion (SEDA-1, 306). Occasionally apathy, drowsiness and a slight increase in transaminase level have been reported.

Interactions Two categories of drug interactions (264[R], 265[R]) have been reported:
(a) Those where other drugs impair the effect of oral contraceptives, leading to breakthrough bleeding and pregnancy. The interaction is due primarily (but not exclusively) to enzyme induction, resulting in accelerated breakdown of the contraceptive. This is a greater problem today than it was when higher-dose contraceptives with a greater reserve of contraceptive potency were in use. In a few cases the activity of oral contraceptives is enhanced. This is of some concern, because of the suggestion that high ethinylestradiol blood levels will correlate to adverse effects (266[R]).

(b) Situations in which oral contraceptives may interfere with the metabolism of other drugs, resulting in an increase in their efficacy and/or impaired tolerance, or in decreased efficacy. These interactions are rarely of clinical significance.

Effect of other drugs on oral contraceptives **(a) Drugs that can impair contraceptive efficacy** Many of the reports in the literature are single cases and care must be taken to establish that, in fact, 'pill failure' was not due to poor compliance, diarrhea or vomiting (266[R]). However, with at least two types of drugs, anticonvulsants and rifampicin, there are well-established interactions.

Anticonvulsant drugs Failure of contraceptive therapy and breakthrough bleeding have been noted repeatedly in patients concurrently taking various enzyme-inducing anticonvulsant drugs (264[R], 265[R], 267[CR]). The latter include phenytoin, primidone, ethosuximide, phenobarbital and carbamazepine. In contrast, valproic acid, which has not be shown to be an enzyme inducer, has no detectable effect on the pharmacokinetics of progestogens and estrogens (264[R], 266[R]).

The specific isozyme responsible for metabolic 2-hydroxylation of ethinylestradiol is $P450_{Nf}$ (subfamily IIIA); some studies seem to confirm that anticonvulsants can induce this isozyme (264[R]). However, in addition to enzyme induction, the anticonvulsants may increase the binding of sex hormone-binding globulin (SHBG). Since sex steroids bind with high affinity to SHBG and since phenobarbital is able to increase SHBG capacity, 'free' active steroid concentrations will tend to decrease during treatment with phenobarbital (266[R], 268[CR]—271). In addition, it has been shown that phenobarbital is able to increase steroid metabolism in both the gut wall and liver (272[C]).

The use of an alternative contraceptive method has long been advised in women taking antiepileptic drugs unless they can be treated with the traditional high-dose oral products, e.g. containing between 80 and 100 μg estradiol (266[R], 267[R]); for effective protection they may also need a shortened 'pill'-free interval. A fair test is to see whether a woman taking oral contraceptives alongside anticonvulsants has adequate cycle control; if not, this is a sign of interference and an alternative method will certainly be advisable.

Antituberculosis drugs (*rifampicin*) Increased intermenstrual or breakthrough bleeding and pregnancy have been reported in women taking rifampicin in conjunction with contraceptive steroids (265[R], 268[CR], 273, 274[r]). Evidence has been produced that rifampicin increases the rate of metabolism of both the estrogenic and progestrogenic components of oral contraceptives through hepatic microsomal enzyme induction (264[R], 275[C]) involving the same isozyme as that induced by anticonvulsants ($P450_{Nf}$ P450-IIIA3). A 4-fold increase in the rate of steroid metabolism has been demonstrated; hence, it would appear unwise for women on rifampicin to rely on steroid contraception.

Griseofulvin has been shown to modify hepatic enzyme activity in mice. Though there is no good evidence of a major enzyme-inducing effect in humans, several case reports of pregnancies occurring in women receiving both oral contraceptives and griseofulvin suggest an interaction (264[R]—266[R]).

Other antibiotics There are sporadic, but well documented, reports of women using oral contraceptive steroids who became pregnant while taking a variety of other antibiotics (264[R], 266[R], 276). However, there is much inter-individual variation (268[CR], 277[R], 278[c]). Suspicion focuses primarily on the broad-spectrum antibiotics and tetracycline. The purported mechanism here is apparently not enzyme induction but interference with the entero-hepatic circulation of ethinylestradiol. Ethinylestradiol can be conjugated with both sulphate and glucuronic acid; sulphation occurs primarily in the small intestinal mucosa, while glucuronidation occurs mainly in the liver. These conjugates are excreted in the bile and then reach the colon where they may be hydrolyzed by the gut bacteria to liberate unchanged ethinylestradiol, which can be reabsorbed into the portal circulation (264[R]). The antibiotics may suppress this bacterial effect, resulting in reduced plasma hormone concentration (264[R], 266[R]). The antibiotics doxycycline and tetracycline have recently been shown to have no effect on serum levels of exogenous estrogens and progestogens among women taking COCs with 35 μg ethinylestradiol (279[C], 280[C]). One of these studies also assessed endogenous progesterone and found no mid-cycle elevation of progesterone suggestive of ovulation (279[C]). Several other studies have also found no overall interaction between antibiotics and OCs, but it is possible that, because of the large interindividual differences in pharmacodynamic responses, a small percentage of women would experience this problem (265[R]).

Antacids These apparently do not affect the bioavailability of oral contraceptives (266[R]), but since a magnesium-containing antacid preparation can induce diarrhea the latter might reduce absorption of the oral contraceptive (264[R]).

Other drugs Phenacetin or pyrazolone-containing-analgesics, meprobamate and chlordiazepoxide have been used by women who became pregnant, although they were regularly taking oral contraceptives. *Clomethiazole* has been shown to be a potent enzyme inducer in animals and is a drug commonly used for the treatment of mycosis in man; it might, in theory, interfere with oral contraception.

Smoking The polycyclic hydrocarbons in cigarette smoke are potent inducers of certain cytochrome P450 isozymes. There is a marked increase in the 2-hydroxylation of natural estradiol in smokers, but not of ethinylestradiol, suggesting that the two estrogens are metabolized by different P450 enzymes (264[R]). There is thus probably no pharmacokinetic interaction between smoking and oral contraceptives, but women on the 'pill' should be encouraged to stop smoking because of the risks involving the cardiovascular system (see above, Cardiovascular section).

(b) Drugs that can increase oral contraceptive levels Several drugs increase the circulating levels of oral contraceptive steroids, and in some instances an increase in their potency and hence their adverse effects may result:

Ascorbic acid This (vitamin C) is extensively sulphated in the gastrointestinal mucosa and competes with ethinylestradiol, which is also extensively sulphated. Although plasma ethinylestradiol concentration has been shown to be increased by ascorbic acid in women, both in studies with single dose of ethinylestradiol or during long-term oral contraceptive use (264[R]), a recent study showed no such effect (265[R]).

Paracetamol Paracetamol might have a similar effect to ascorbic acid, i.e. competing with ethinylestradiol for sulphation capacity in the gut. There is a significant decrease in the area under the curve of ethinylestradiol sulphate after taking paracetamol, but no effect on plasma levonorgestrel concentrations. This interaction could be of clinical significance in women on the 'pill' who take paracetamol regularly or suddenly stop taking it (264[R], 266[R]).

Troleandomycin Several reports of hepatic cholestasis in women taking both troleandomycin and oral contraceptives have been published. Oxidation of troleandomycin by a P450 isozyme produces a derivative (probably a nitroso-derivative) which binds itself tightly to the enzyme and thereby causes inactivation. This inhibition is highly selective for $P450_{Nf}$ (see above, 'anticonvulsants') and hepatic accumulation of ethinylestradiol is possible (264[R], 281[c]).

Roxithromycin This has been shown in a small specific study not to interfere with oral contraceptives (282[c]).

Effect of oral contraceptives on other drugs Studies in animals and more recently in vitro studies with human liver microsomes have shown that oral contraceptives can inhibit the metabolism of other drugs undergoing various forms of oxidative metabolism. In contrast, oral contraceptives seem to induce glucuronidation (264[R]). It has been suggested that the estrogenic component of oral contraceptives is necessary for the inhibition of drug oxidation, since women receiving progestogens alone had a normal clearance of antipyrine, whereas those receiving a combination tablet had impaired antipyrine elimination (283[C]).

(a) Oral contraceptives increasing the effect of other drugs *Benzodiazepines* Oral contraceptives influence in humans the metabolism of some benzodiazepines undergoing oxidation (*chlordiazepoxide, alprazolam, diazepam*) or nitro-reduction (*nitrazepam*). For these drugs, oral contraceptives inhibit enzyme activity and reduce clearance. There is nevertheless little evidence that this interaction is of clinical importance. It should be noted that for other benzodiazepines undergoing oxidative metabolism, such as bromazepam or clotiazepam, no change was found in oral contraceptive users (264[R], 266[R], 284[c]).

Corticosteroids In oral contraceptive users there is a 30—50% reduction in the clearance of *prednisolone* and a prolonged elimination half-life. These alterations result from changes in both protein binding, which is increased, presumably due to increased corticosteroid binding globulin levels, and unbound drug clearance, which is decreased, presumably due to the inhibition of metabolism. It has therefore been suggested that lower doses of prednisolone should yield clinical efficacy in oral contraceptive users (264[R], 266[R], 285[c]).

Antidepressants Oral contraceptives decrease clearance of *imipramine* (probably by reducing hepatic oxidation) and thus increase elimination half-life. Hydroxylation of *amitriptyline* is also inhibited by contraceptive steroids. The clinical significance is uncertain, but caution should probably be exercised when tricyclic antidepressants are used in women taking oral contraceptives (264[R], 286[R]).

Methylxanthines The clearance of both *theophylline* and *caffeine* is reduced in oral contraceptive users and half-lives are increased, probably because of inhibition of hepatic metabolism by cytochrome P450. Again, caution in dosage is advisable (264[R], 266[R], 287[C]).

β-Blockers Oral contraceptives increase the area under the curve and the plasma concentrations of metoprolol, oxprenolol and propranolol, but statistical significance is reached only with metoprolol. The changes are consistent with inhibition of hydroxylating enzymes, but are unlikely to be of clinical relevance (264[R], 288[c]).

Ciclosporin Several case reports have suggested that ciclosporin elimination may be impaired by oral contraceptives, resulting in increased plasma ciclosporin concentrations. Ciclosporin undergoes hydroxylation and N-demethylation for which cytochrome P450 is involved ($P450_{Nf}$), so enzyme competition probably explains the interaction. Since ciclosporin is toxic, dosage should be reviewed carefully (264[R], 266[R], 289[C]).

Neuroleptics A single case of neuroleptic malignant syndrome has been described in a woman treated with haloperidol and thioridazine, 12 hours after starting an oral contraceptive. The authors suggested that this could be a pharmacodynamic interaction involving dopaminergic neurotransmission (290[c]).

(b) Oral contraceptives reducing the effect of other drugs Pharmacokinetic interactions have been described with drugs metabolized mainly by glucuronidation, which is induced by oral contraceptives, but other mechanisms can also produce problems.

Anticoagulants Oral contraceptives have been reported to reduce the effect of anticoagulants, probably due to the fact that oral contraceptives have an antagonistic effect on certain clotting factors (see above, also Chapter 37a), although they have incidentally been stated to potentiate the action of acenocoumarol (SEDA-5, 371). One study showed a significant increase in the clearance of phenprocoumon, due to an accelerated glucuronidation. As phenprocoumon is metabolized by hydroxylation as well as by direct glucuronidation, the increased clearance may mean that induction of the latter process overrides inhibition of the former (291).

Benzodiazepines Some benzodiazepines are metabolized by glucuronic acid conjugation. Of these, temazepam showed increased clearance when oral contraceptives were concomitantly administered, but lorazepam and oxazepam did not (292[C]). It is unlikely that this is an interaction of clinical importance (264[R], 266[R]).

Analgesics *Paracetamol* is metabolized essentially in the liver by glucuronidation and sulphation; oral contraceptives increase only glucuronidation. *Salicylic acid* clearance is also higher in users of oral contraceptives, due to increase in both the glycine and glucuronic acid conjugation pathways. Increased glucuronidation may also explain the fact that oral contraceptives enhance *morphine* clearance. These changes could have some significance for short- or long-term pain relief (264[R], 266[R]).

There is also considerable evidence that the elimination of a number of drugs metabolized by the hepatic mixed-function oxidation system is impaired in women receiving oral contraceptives. These drugs, for example, reduce the clearance of *aminopyrine* (293[C]), *antipyrine* (294[C], 295[C]), and *pethidine* (296[C]). This effect on antipyrine clearance has recently been documented even with low-dose COCs (265[R]).

Clofibric acid Oral contraceptives increase plasma clearance of clofibric acid, a drug mainly metabolized by glucuronidation (264[R], 266[R]).

Alcohol Women on oral contraceptives showed a significant decrease in the absolute elimination rate of ethanol (105 mg/kg/hour) as compared to controls (121 mg/kg/hour; $P<0.005$). The percentage ethanol elimination rate was also significantly decreased in women taking oral contraceptives (0.015% per hour) as compared to control subjects (0.019% per hour; $P<0.001$). These results were consistent during the three phases of the menstrual cycle and when body leanness was taken into consideration (297[C]).

Overall benefit-risk evaluation A comprehensive

analysis by The Alan Guttmacher Institute in the US has evaluated the health risks of various contraceptive methods, as well as no method, using simulation analysis models (84[R]). Because combined oral contraceptives are highly effective, they prevent pregnancy-related deaths, particularly those associated with ectopic pregnancy. This factor more than offsets the small increased risk of cardiovascular disease related to current use, resulting in averted deaths at all ages (ranging from 3.9 per 100 000 current users at ages 15—19 up to 18.7 per 100 000 at ages 40—44 in the US). They also prevent future deaths from ovarian and endometrial cancers (from 23 per 100 000 at ages 15—19 to 10 per 100 000 at ages 40—44). Current pill use also prevents 1614 hospitalizations per 100 000 users annually. Most of these avoided hospitalizations are because of prevention of pregnancy complications, but they also include a reduced rate of hospitalizations due to ovarian cysts, benign breast disease, upper genital tract infection, urinary tract infection, and invasive cancers of the ovary and endometrium. The conditions for which hospitalization rates may be slightly increased among COC users include: myocardial infarction; stroke; venous thrombosis and embolism; invasive cancers of the breast, cervix and liver; cervical intraepithelial neoplasia; and gallbladder disease.

Data from the Nurses' Health Study indicate no difference in all-cause mortality between women who had ever used OCs and those who had never used them (106[Cr]). There was also no increase in mortality associated with duration of use, and no relationship with time since first use or time since last use. Similarly, in the OFPA study, the overall 20-year mortality risk for OC users compared to women using diaphragms or IUDs was 0.9, indicating no effect (57[C]). Although the number of deaths from each cause was small, the pattern is consistent with the risks shown in other studies. OC users had somewhat higher death rates for ischemic heart disease and cervical cancer, but lower rates of ovarian cancer mortality. Breast cancer mortality was similar for OC users and non-users.

In developing countries (184[CR]) it has been found, as one would expect, that wherever high maternal mortality prevails, the risk of oral contraception is low in comparison. For all women in developing countries below the age of 40, oral contraceptive use is substantially safer than no method at all or traditional methods, about as safe as IUDs, but not as safe as sterilization or as traditional methods backed by legal abortion performed by trained physicians.

Some of the risks have only become evaluable with much longer experience, e.g. those relating to effects on development of malignancies. Data on these matters too seem reassuring (see Chapter 40.2); any cancer-promoting effect is counterbalanced by the halving (at least a 40% reduction) of the risk of endometrial and ovarian cancers. In addition, any consideration of major risk/benefit issues should be supplemented by a consideration of minor ones, e.g. the decrease in disorders of the menstrual cycle (such as dysmenorrhea, menorrhagia, and the premenstrual syndrome) and the decreased risks of iron deficiency anemia, functional ovarian cysts, uterine fibroids, benign breast disease, pelvic inflammatory disease and ectopic pregnancy (298[R], 299[R]).

Since much of the work on overall risk/benefit equations is old, relating to high-dose products, it is important to note that more recent work confirms the even greater relative safety of the products today in use (298[R], 299[R]). Even at an earlier phase, such authoritative workers as Vessey and Doll (300[CR]) stressed that the medical and social benefits of oral contraceptive use considerably outweighed the risks, while emphasizing the need to contain such risks as there are, i.e. by careful patient selection and supervision and by use of oral contraceptives with the lowest possible dosage.

ALTERNATIVE ORAL PRODUCTS

ALTERNATIVE COMBINATIONS OF ESTROGEN AND PROGESTOGEN

As pointed out earlier, the doses of progestogen and estrogen used in combined oral contraceptives have been progressively reduced, most recently with the wide acceptance of products containing only 30 μg ethinylestradiol. At present, preparations with estrogen levels as low as 20 μg are on trial and attempts continue to find more satisfactory progestogen-only products.

The *estrogen* component in oral contraceptives is usually ethinylestradiol. A few newer preparations contain the 'natural' steroid 17β-estradiol in micronized form. In acute studies, this has been shown not to depress fibrinolysis and to have less effect on liver function and lipid metabolism. Whether it will prove safer when used on a large scale is still uncertain.

The oral *progestogens* used today are all 19-nortestosterone derivatives. The difficulty in deciding which measure of progestogen potency is most relevant to oral contraception has been alluded to above; if one relies on the 'menstrual delay test' D-norgestrel is more potent than norethindrone. D-Norgestrel also has an anti-estrogen effect and drugs containing D-norgestrel are therefore regarded as progestogen-dominated. There is no means to determine beforehand which women should preferably receive a progestogen- or an estrogen-dominated oral contraceptive. Furthermore, because D-norgestrel is more potent than norethindrone, it is usually given at a lower dose, so the actual progestogenic (as well as androgenic and antiestrogenic) activity of COCs containing these two progestogens may actually be similar (2[R]).

Three new progestogens have been synthesized, all derivatives of levonorgestrel: desogestrel, gestogene and norgestimate. These new progestogens are described as more 'selective' because their relative binding affinity for the progesterone receptor is greater than for the androgen receptor, and thus they would be expected to have less of an androgenic effect than levonorgestrel or norethindrone. This expectation is born out in clinical studies which show HDL cholesterol levels to generally be increased (or unchanged) with gestodene and desogestrel preparations, according to a recent review by Fotherby and Caldwell (301[R]); data on norgestimate formulations are sparse. This is in contrast to levonorgestrel studies, which often show a decrease in HDL cholesterol (or no change) and of norethindrone, which usually show no change. Differences among the progestogens in other serum lipid effects are less obvious. Whether the HDL differences have any important ramifications on cardiovascular disease has not been demonstrated. This review also comes to the following conclusions about other aspects of these new progestogens. Efficacy is similar for both the older and newer progestogens, in combination with ethinylestradiol 30—35 μg. Cycle control and minor side effects also appear to be similar, although differences in analytic methodology make it difficult to compare study results. A review by Kaunitz (302[R]) echoes this assessment of satisfactory cycle control with low dose COCs containing desogestrel (the most commonly used of the three new progestogens), adding that the desogestrel combination appears to be particularly suitable for women prone to androgen-excess conditions such as acne and hirsutism.

Pharmacokinetic studies (303[c]—309[c]) suggest that replacement of one progestogen by another can have *unexpected consequences on the total effect*, and they also demonstrate the need to re-examine kinetics at various phases during long-term use of a combined product. Ethinylestradiol levels were in some studies higher in women receiving an oral contraceptive containing gestodene than in those receiving an oral contraceptive with desogestrel (303[c]—305[c]), though not all workers could confirm this (309[c]) and inter-individual variations are considerable. A progressive rise in ethinylestradiol levels was observed during each oral contraceptive cycle (299[c]—305[c]). As ethinylestradiol is metabolized by oxidation by human liver cytochrome P450 (310[c]), this was interpreted as a reduction in oxidative metabolism by ethinylestradiol itself and possibly by the progestogen. This could be of major concern as elevated ethinylestradiol levels have been described in women who developed hypertension during oral contraceptive use (306[c]). Dibbelt et al. (309[c]) suggest that there could be possible correlations between the high ethinylestradiol serum levels and irregularities in the pretreatment hormone status; Stadel (307[c]) thinks this could be mainly due to genetic disposition.

In cases where withdrawal bleeding is small or does not occur, oral contraceptives of the *normophasic* type can be tried. In these drugs the seven first tablets contain only estrogen and the following 14 tablets both estrogen and progestogen, which give an endometrium of a more normal secretion phase type; this in turn leads to a more pronounced withdrawal bleeding. A further development of this principle, the *triphasic* type of product, involves administering a 3-step regimen in which the change from estrogenic to progestogenic dominance is more gradual. The recent review of the new progestogens also examines the triphasic preparations, concluding that their greatest advantage is a reduction in inter-menstrual bleeding (301[R]). The authors state that the levonorgestrel triphasics are also less likely to cause a decrease in HDL cholesterol than are the monophasics containing the same progestogen. One cannot generalize about the properties of these variants; it is good that they are available as alternatives to widen the choice of approaches, but there is again no way of determining in advance which type of product will best suit the individual woman, and theoretical arguments that they are more 'physiological' than earlier products have yet to be proven to be of practical significance.

PROGESTOGEN-ONLY ORAL CONTRACEPTIVES

Progestogen-only oral contraceptives not only lack the estrogen component of COCs but also have a lower dose of progestogen than even the current low-dose combined OCs. Progestogen-only pills (POPs) are therefore indicated for women who desire oral contraception but who have contraindications to the estrogen in COCs, are breastfeeding, are older (especially smokers), or simply wish to minimize their exogenous hormone intake (2[R], 299). The drawbacks of POPs are that *menstrual irregularity* is common and that careful compliance is necessary in order to achieve high *efficacy*.

The *pharmacokinetics* of progestogens in POPs are

somewhat different than in COCs, because of the interaction of estrogen and progestogen in the combination products (2[R]). One of the major differences is that the plasma levels of progestogen rise over time in COC users but not in women taking POPs. This is due in part to estrogen stimulation of *serum hormone-binding globulin* (*SHBG*) production, increased binding of progestogen to SHBG, and reduced progestogen clearance with COCs. In contrast, SHBG levels decline with POP use and administration of POPs results in modest declines in progestogen levels over time.

Pregnancy rates during the first year of use are estimated to be 0.5%, if the pills are taken precisely on schedule (1[R]). However, POPs are less 'forgiving' of incorrect use than are COCs, with pregnancy risk increased by a delay in pill-taking of as little as 3 hours (2[R]). Up to 10% of pregnancies among POP users implant outside the uterus; the actual incidence of *ectopic pregnancy* is similar to that of non-contracepting women, but higher than for women using other methods (2[R], 259[R]). The reason for the high percentage of pregnancies that are ectopic may be related to changes in tubal motility and delay in ovum transport.

There does not appear to be any clinically significant delay in *return of fertility* following POP discontinuation (2[R]). Although there have been no large studies, data from several small studies indicate no effect. Furthermore, because POPs prevent ovulation in only about half of cycles, and because the pregnancy prevention effects decline rapidly if a pill is taken late, the normal reproductive physiology presumably returns quickly after pill discontinuation.

Evidence continues to accumulate that progestin-only contraceptives (including pills, injectables and implants) have no adverse effects on *lactation* (311[Cr], 312[Cr]) and thus are preferred to COCs. Not only is there no inhibition of milk production by POPs (whereas there is a modest inhibition by COCs), but the steroid dose transmitted to the infant is less with POPs than with COCs (2[R]). Although these progestin-only methods can be initiated early in the postpartum period, there is no reason to begin use of any contraceptive method if the mother is still amenorrheic and not yet giving the infant supplementary foods (313[R]).

Changes in *lipid metabolism* among POP users are minimal (2[R]). Some studies find very small decreases in HDL and HDL_2 cholesterol, but no effect on other parameters of lipid metabolism. The androgenicity of progestogens parallels their effect on lipoprotein metabolism, but dosage must also be taken into account. For example, although levonorgestrel is more androgenic than norethindrone, its progestational potency is also greater and so levonorgestrel is given at a much lower dose for contraceptive purposes; the net result is that there is no clinical difference in lipid effects, as was demonstrated most conclusively in a clinical trial by Ball et al. (314[C]) in England.

Most studies of *carbohydrate metabolism* have found little effect of POPs, but there is a suggestion of slight deterioration in glucose tolerance and elevated plasma insulin concentrations (2[R]). Women with diabetes mellitus can generally take POPs without a change in their insulin requirements.

Coagulation factors in POP users have not been studied extensively using current laboratory methods, but there appears to be little effect (2[R]). Perhaps the most informative study is the randomized clinical trial of two POPs (norethindrone 0.35 mg and levonorgestrel 0.03 mg) by Ball et al. (314[C]), which found a decrease in several coagulation factors among women who switched from a COC but no change among women who had not previously been using a hormonal contraceptive. Thus POPs appear to be particularly suitable for women who desire oral contraception but who are at increased risk of thrombosis, including older women who are smokers (2[R]).

Considerable research has found no overall increase in *blood pressure* measurements or in prevalence of *hypertension* associated with POP use (2[R]).

Epidemiological data on risk of *cardiovascular disease* among POP users are sparse, but the limited available information indicates no association (2[R]). Because progestogens have no clinically significant effect on coagulation parameters, POPs are unlikely to cause thrombogenesis, which is the primary causal pathway for the small elevated risk of cardiovascular disease among COC users.

Similarly, there is little information available regarding *cancer* risk, because both POP use and most cancers are rare (2[R]). Studies that have categorized POPs separately have found very few cancer cases among these women. Based on data regarding COCs and post-menopausal hormone replacement therapy, POPs may have a modest protective effect on *endometrial cancer*. They may also have a beneficial relationship with *ovarian cancer*, although to a lesser degree than COCs, based on the hypothetical mechanisms for the protective effect of COCs. Whether there is an association with *cervical or breast cancer* is even less well understood for POPs than for COCs, but there is no reason to suspect a greater effect of POPs.

While the ovaries are inactivated by high-dose progestogen preparations, low-dose preparations quite often cause endogenous *hyperestrogenemia* as a result of their mild suppression of gonadotropins—by altering the follicle-stimulating hormone (FSH)/luteinizing hormone

(LH) ratio. This may be responsible for some of the clinical symptoms including not only menstrual disturbances such as breakthrough bleeding, but also *breast pain* and *cystic ovaries* (315[R], 316). *Functional ovarian cysts* (or persistent ovarian follicles) occur more frequently in POP users than in COC users or in women using no hormonal contraceptive method (2[R]). Follicular development is delayed and the follicle continues to grow for a period of time, but these enlarged follicles usually regress spontaneously and are not of clinical significance.

Because POPs exert some of the same effects that may explain the protection against *pelvic inflammatory disease* among COC users, notably decreased penetrability of cervical mucus, POPs may also provide a small degree of protection (2[R]). On the other hand, the expanded cervical ectropion that may be responsible for the possible increased risk of *lower genital tract infection* among COC users is not present in POP users, and thus POPs are unlikely to have any effect.

Menstrual irregularities are common among women taking POPs and are often the reason a user chooses to discontinue the method (2[R], 315, 317). POP users are more likely than users of other hormonal contraceptive methods to have frequent bleeding (228[R]). Infrequent bleeding, amenorrhea and irregular bleeding among POP users are more likely than among COC users, but less likely than among women using levonorgestrel-releasing vaginal rings or DMPA. Women deciding to discontinue taking POPs often do so because of menstrual irregularities, but informing prospective users that this is a common side effect often alleviates their concern.

Other side effects are generally less prevalent with POPs than with COCs because of the absence of estrogen and lower dose of progestogen (2[R]). *Headache, breast tenderness*, and, less commonly, *nausea* and *dizziness* have been reported by POP users, but it is not clear whether POPs actually play a causal role. Androgenic side effects, such as *acne*, *hirsutism* and *weight gain* occur, but rarely.

Most recently in the field of oral contraceptives interesting discussions took place which must be mentioned in this Chapter. In December 1995 and January 1996 three independently conducted epidemiological studies (383—385) with oral contraceptives of the third generation containing either gestodene or norgestrel have been published. Compared with second generation OCs the risk of thromboembolism associated with desogestrel and gestoden was found to be 1.5 (385), 2.3 (384) or 2.6 (383) times greater. The reaction of the CPMP (Committee on Safety of Medicine of the European Community) was moderate. Its position statement indicated that the risk of venous thromboembolism is higher in users of desogestrel and gestodene containing OC than in levonorgestrel containing OC. It mentioned that the impact of biases and confounders on the difference cannot be fully evaluated (386). The UK Committee on Safety of Medicines (CSM) recommended very early in October 1995 "that women taking third generation progestagen should be advised to switch to another brand (387) not containing either of progestagens". Germany prolonged instructions for prescribing these drugs until January 1997. As previously, women younger than 30 years and first time users should not receive third generation progestagens.

The different evaluation of the same data is interesting. One should conclude that despite the fact that studies showed an approximately 2-fold increased risk of venous thromboembolism associated with desogestrel and norgestrel, the actual risk associated with these products is still low. Excess risk is about 11—20 cases per 100 000 woman-years. These figures for progestagens of earlier generation is about five to ten per 100 000 woman years.

INJECTABLE HORMONAL CONTRACEPTIVES

Injectable hormonal contraceptives, normally composed of long-acting esters of a progestogen, have obvious practical advantages over oral products where user compliance is poor, e.g. in the illiterate or mentally subnormal woman or in some populations in developing countries. It is however precisely the fact that they are used in this type of patient which has led to some social protest against their use and this may in turn explain some unbalanced criticism of them in terms of efficacy and safety. However they can be considered as an effective, reversible, and relatively safe method of contraception, which could be used in some women who smoke or when estrogen is contraindicated (298[R], 299[R]).

Depot medroxyprogesterone acetate

Depot medroxyprogesterone acetate (DMPA) is by far the most widely used preparation of this type; the assessment of it produced by the World Health Organization in 1983 (318[C]) remains valid (319[C]—323[R]). It is estimated that the drug has been used by 30 million women in more than 90 countries (323[R]). Peak levels in the blood are reached around the 10th day after injection, but the drug is still detectable in the blood at the 90th day; there is wide inter-individual variation. It acts primarily by inhibiting ovulation but, as with the oral contraceptives, there seem to be secondary mechanisms. The product is extremely *effective*, with less than one pregnancy per 100 woman-years. Currently, it is used as a 3-monthly injectable contraceptive given generally in a dose of 150 μg.

DMPA is derived from 17α-hydroxy-progesterone, whereas the progestogens used in oral contraceptives and the NORPLANT implant are structurally related to 19-nortestosterone. One of the metabolic differences is that these 19-nortestosterone derivatives form strong bonds with SHBG, but DMPA does not (2[R]). Another difference is that, unlike most other progestogen-only methods, ovulation is usually suppressed (4[R]).

The majority of women using the product unfortunately experience either *irregular bleeding* and *spotting* or *amenorrhea* linked to endometrial atrophy (324[CR]); only one in 1000 women, however, bleed sufficiently to warrant an aggressive therapy such as curettage. As the duration of use increases, amenorrhea becomes more common. DMPA is associated with greater variability in *menstrual patterns* than other hormonal contraception (228[C], 325[Cr]). Bleeding/spotting episodes are infrequent but prolonged, and the prevalence of amenorrhea increases over time to more than half of users after the first year. Fewer than 10% of users have bleeding patterns defined as 'acceptable', compared to 85—90% of non-contracepting women (325[Cr]). However, with appropriate patient selection and counseling, many users view amenorrhea positively.

Because DMPA users are often amenorrheic, they may experience improvements in such menstrual cycle conditions as *menorrhagia and dysmenorrhea* and in *iron deficiency anemia*. Other potential benefits include reduction in the risk of *pelvic inflammatory disease*, improvement in *sickle cell disease* parameters, and lessened seizure frequency in women with *epilepsy* (3[r]).

Other reported side effects include *headache*, *bloating of the abdomen or breasts*, *mood changes and weight gain* (3[r], 4[R], 324[R]). Weight gain appears to be more common among women using DMPA than among those using other progestogen-only methods.

Like other progestogens, DMPA has some slight *metabolic effects* (324[R]), but they do not seem to be serious. A multicenter study of *lipid metabolism* conducted by WHO found considerable difference in serum lipids and apolipoproteins among the centers, with overall small decreases in HDL cholesterol and increases in LDL levels (326[Cr]). There is a disputed effect on *carbohydrate metabolism* but certainly no precipitation of diabetes in healthy women. Carbohydrate metabolism has been shown to be unaffected by DMPA use in a study that simultaneously did find modest impairment in glucose tolerance among users of levonorgestrel-containing low dose COCs and progestogen-only pills (327[Cr]).

Researchers have found little or no effect of medroxyprogesterone acetate, administered either orally or by injection, on *blood coagulation*, as recently reviewed by Beller (26[R]). No increased risk of thrombosis has been noted (4[R]).

The only study of DMPA and *HIV infection*, conducted among Thai prostitutes, showed an increased risk for women using DMPA, after adjustment for other variables (328[C]).

For women with *epilepsy*, DMPA is a particularly useful contraceptive method because it has been shown to reduce seizure frequency (108[R]). The dosage is sufficiently high that reduced efficacy due to enzyme-inducing antiepileptic medication is not an issue.

The suitability of DMPA for women with *sickle cell disease* has been evaluated in a controlled crossover trial, which found that both hematological and clinical parameters were improved during DMPA administration (329[C]).

Three cases of *clitoral hypertrophy* have been described in infants exposed to DPMA in utero. In view of the hormonal spectrum of DPMA, this is a conceivable side effect, but there is no confirmation, nor is it clear whether the drug harms the fetus in any other way (319[r]).

Return of fertility may be delayed for several months following DMPA discontinuation (3[r], 4[R]). The length of the delay is not related to duration of use. There is no evidence of any permanent impairment of fertility (323[R], 330[c]).

Numerous studies have shown that *lactation* is not adversely affected by DMPA use and that breast milk production may even be increased (167[R]). Because of the low binding affinity of DMPA to SHBG, the concentration of steroids in the milk is close to that in the maternal plasma, unlike the 19-nortestosterone derivatives. Children whose mothers used DMPA while breastfeeding have been followed-up in Thailand for 17 years and in Chile for 4.5 years, with no documented effect on growth or development (2[R]). In undernourished lactating women the metabolic effects seem to be more pronounced than among healthy users (331[c]). Serum cholesterol levels tended to be higher during the first 6 months of lactation, but there was no alteration in glucose tolerance, serum triglycerides or total protein levels during 1 year of treatment.

Effects of DMPA on *reproductive cancers* appear to be similar to COCs (3[r]) (See Chapter 40.2). Most notably, despite initial concerns about *breast cancer* in beagle dogs who were administered large doses of DMPA, a recent pooled analysis of epidemiological studies documented that women using DMPA are not at increased overall risk of breast cancer (332[R]). Furthermore, risk did not increase with increasing duration of use. However, women who had begun use within the past 5 years had a significantly elevated risk, perhaps because of accelerated growth of pre-existing tumors or increased surveillance. Another recent review concludes that DMPA has a protective effect against *endometrial cancer* that is at least as strong as for COCs, but that, based on the limited available evidence, there is no association with *ovarian cancer* (333[R]). Regarding *cervical neoplasia*, studies of DMPA do not show a strong adverse effect, but as with COCs it is uncertain whether there is no association or a slight increased risk (334[R]).

The very high *contraceptive efficacy* of DMPA does not appear to be affected by *interaction with other drugs* (1[R], 3[r]).

Bone mineral density has been found in one cross-sectional study to be lower among current DMPA users, with cessation of use being accompanied by almost complete recovery of bone density (335[C]).

Anaphylactic reaction to DMPA injection occurs very rarely (1[R]).

No consistent effects have been found with respect to *liver function*, and indeed primary biliary cirrhosis and chronic active hepatitis have appeared to improve during treatment (319[r]).

When used in the *treatment of breast and endometrial cancer*, DMPA side effects regarded as corticoid-like occur (336[C]—339[C]). Although adrenal suppression has been observed when using high doses of DMPA for cancer chemotherapy or precocious puberty, this is not found to occur when the drug is used in contraceptive doses (134[r]).

Taken as a whole, one can say that DMPA is a product which has some inconvenient side effects on the menstrual pattern. Containing no estrogen, it does not embody the thromboembolic risks of the oral contraceptives. There is no evidence that it causes cancer, and on theoretical grounds one would anticipate that it would be at least as safe in this respect as the oral contraceptives, perhaps safer in the long run. It should not be used in cases of breast cancer, genital cancer, undiagnosed uterine bleeding or suspected pregnancy (320[r]), but these are merely logical precautions.

Norethisterone enantate

The side effects of norethisterone enantate when used as a 2-monthly injectable contraceptive have been compared to those of DMPA (340[c], 341[c]). The largest single trial conducted, covering some 9000 women-months of use, provides a fair picture of its adverse effects. *Menstrual irregularity* was the main complaint (prolonged bleeding, spotting or amenorrhea). Other side effects were periodic *abdominal bloating* and the complaint of *tender breasts*, both of which were thought to be due to water retention and could be relieved by diuretics. No associated weight gain was observed. The injections given to over 50 women who had mild *hypertension* did not significantly affect blood pressure which generally remained below 140/90 mmHg, nor was *blood clotting* affected. *High-density lipoprotein-cholesterol* values in the women treated were significantly lower than those of the control group. The results of *glucose tolerance tests* did not differ significantly between both groups (342[C]).

Three studies carried out in Bangladesh (343[c]), Pakistan (344[c]) and China (345[c]) showed similar adverse reaction patterns. In the Bangladesh study nine out of 254 women showed a rise in both systolic and diastolic *blood pressure*, while five had a reduction of the same magnitude. In the Chinese women no significant changes in blood pressure were seen, but five showed *abnormal liver function* tests and three of these women had liver enlargement following treatment for more than 2 years.

Other compounds

Other progestin-only injectables are being developed but to date appear to have similar properties to those already available (346[C]).

Combined estrogen-progestogen injectables

Combined estrogen-progestogen injectables, to be administered monthly, have been developed in an effort to produce more regular vaginal bleeding patterns (325[Cr]). Numerous formulations have been evaluated and two of these have undergone Phase III clinical trials by WHO: (1) DMPA 25 mg plus estradiol cypionate 5 mg and (2) norethisterone enanthate 50 mg plus estradiol valerate 5 mg. Analysis of daily menstrual diary record cards for women using these methods, compared to several other contraceptive methods and no method, reveals that bleeding patterns for women receiving monthly injections are more regular, but not entirely normal (325[Cr]). Although the median experience is similar to that of non-contracepting women, the range of menstrual patterns is much wider. Women not using hormonal contraceptives were found to have an 'acceptable' menstrual pattern in 85—90% of cycles, compared to about 70% of cycles by the end of the first year of use of monthly injectables. Fewer than 10% of women discontinued use during the first year because of bleeding irregularities or amenorrhea, a rate that is presumably related in part to thorough counseling in these carefully conducted clinical trials.

IMPLANTED HORMONAL CONTRACEPTIVES

Levonorgestrel implants (nonbiodegradable)

Subdermal implanted silastic rods containing levonorgestrel (NORPLANT®; this is the registered trademark of The Population Council for subdermal levonorgestrel implants) have also been used for long-term, reversible contraception. Six nonbiodegradable silicone rubber capsules, each containing 35 mg levonorgestrel, are inserted in the woman's arm. This system provides effective contraception for approximately 5 years. The contraceptive effect of the implants does not seem to be caused by ovulation inhibition, since the hormone levels are low in the majority of women (347[c], 348[c]).

The most frequent side effect is *irregular menstrual bleeding* (349[R], 350[C]). Although most users of levonorgestrel implants have irregular menstrual cycles during the first year of use, menstrual patterns tend to become more regular over time (351[R], 352[Cr], 353[C]). Amenorrhea is uncommon. Menstrual irregularity does not appear to be correlated with body mass index (352[Cr]). Total *menstrual blood loss* is not increased, nor are *hemoglobin* or *serum ferritin* levels reduced (351[R], 354[C]). One NORPLANT study seemed to show that monthly bleedings were more commonly reduced than increased (355[c]).

Headache is the most common side effect (349[R], 354[C]). Just as with progestogen administered continuously by mouth, *functional ovarian cysts* (or persistent ovarian follicles) are common in NORPLANT users. Some women also experience *acne*, because of the androgenic activity of levonorgestrel (4[R]), and others report breast discharge. Two cases of *major depression and panic disorder*, developing soon after NORPLANT insertion and resolving after removal, have been reported, but a causal association has not been proven (356[c]).

Numerous studies of various *metabolic laboratory tests* have generally found no marked deviation from normal values (4[R], 351[R]). A recent laboratory report from Singapore indicates that, both during NORPLANT use and after implant removal, *lipid metabolism* parameters and *liver function* tests are similar to baseline measurements, although there were some minor fluctuations, particularly during the early period of use (357[C]). Two recent studies of *carbohydrate metabolism* in NORPLANT users have found small changes, within normal limits, and only during the first 1–2 years of use (358[C], 359[C]).

Research on *blood coagulation* has produced inconsistent results, usually showing little effect (2[R]). Notably, a study that compared women using NORPLANT with those using low-dose COCs found that the coagulation system was affected less by the progestin-only implant (360[C]). NORPLANT use is not accompanied by any significant changes in *blood pressure* (354[C]).

A study that documented *weight* over time showed no change in body mass index among NORPLANT users (352[C]). Earlier studies indicated a similar lack of effect on weight (354[C]).

Pregnancy rates among NORPLANT users are the lowest among all contraceptive methods (0.09% during the first year) (1[R]). With the original Silastic tubing, heavier women had higher pregnancy rates, but this is not usually true with the newer tubing (except for slightly higher failure rates toward the end of the 5-year life span) (1[R], 4[R]). Women with regular menstrual cycles during NORPLANT use are somewhat more likely to have an accidental pregnancy than those with irregular cycles or amenorrhea (353[C]). Because the pregnancy rate among NORPLANT users is quite low, the rate of *ectopic pregnancy* is also very low (351[R], 354[R]). There is no evidence that infants conceived during NORPLANT use are at higher risk of *birth defects* (351[R], 354[C]).

As with other hormonal contraceptives, there is considerable variation in *menstrual irregularity* and other effects, which may be mediated in part by inter-individual differences in steroid levels associated with differences in SHBG (354[R]).

Several insertion-related complications can occur, including *infection*, *hematoma formation*, *local irritation*, *implant expulsions*, and *allergic reaction* to the dressing (4[R]). The rods can usually be *removed* in less than 1 hour under local anesthesia, but removal may be more difficult if the clinician is inexperienced in their removal, if the rods were not positioned properly at insertion, or if fibrous tissue has grown around the rods (4[R]).

A pooled analysis of *insertion site complications* in multi-country studies found that 0.8% of women develop infection after NORPLANT insertion, generally within the first week, but sometimes several months later (361[R]). Implant expulsion occurred in 0.4% of users, often because of infection but sometimes because of improper placement. Contrary to expectations, one-third of infections and two-thirds of expulsions were reported more than 2 months after insertion. Notably, the rates of infection, expulsion, and local reaction varied widely among countries and among clinics within countries.

A paper has recently been published describing serious adverse events among NORPLANT users reported to the US Food and Drug Administration from 1991 through 1993 (362[C]). Although true incidence rates cannot be computed because these voluntary reports are presumably an undercounting of the actual number of events, it should be noted that supplies for 891 000 implants were distributed during this time period; assuming a continuation rate of 80%, the authors calculate reported event rates using a denominator of 713 000. The FDA received reports of 24 women hospitalized for *infection* at the insertion site and 14 who were either hospitalized or disabled because of *difficulties associated with capsule removal*. Fourteen women (2.0 per 100 000) were reportedly hospitalized due to *stroke*. There were also three women who developed *thrombotic thrombocytopenia purpura* and six who developed *thrombocytopenia*. Finally, 39 NORPLANT users developed *pseudotumor cerebri* (benign intracranial hypertension), for a reported incidence rate of 5.5 per 100 000; this condition is known to be associated with obesity or recent weight gain, conditions which were present for the majority of these cases for whom such data were given. Although the rates of stroke and pseudotumor cerebri were less than the expected rates in the general population of reproductive-age women, they were sufficiently close to the expected rates to suggest that, because these rates are presumably underreported, NORPLANT users may actually be at increased risk.

A very large series (10 718 women) has recently been reported from China, in conjunction with The Population Council (363[C]). The annual pregnancy rate averaged 0.3 per 100 woman-years over the course of the 5 years of use. Pregnancy rates increased significantly with weight, but even in the heaviest group the annual rates were less than one per 100. Only 3.1 per 100 pregnancies were ectopic, higher than for the general population in Beijing but much lower than in US studies of NORPLANT (presumably because of lower rates of pelvic inflammatory disease in China). There were no deaths attributable to NORPLANT use and no cardiovascular/cerebrovascular deaths. The 5-year continuation rate was 72.1 per 100 acceptors. Menstrual cycle disruption was the primary side effect and the most common reason for implant removal. Hemoglobin levels increased during the first year of use and remained elevated. Early in the study low platelet counts led to removal in 17 women, including one with primary thrombocytopenia and another with chronic thrombocytopenia. Therefore, during the second phase of the study, platelet counts were recorded before insertion, as well as annually during use; admission values were found to be well below normal, with very little change after insertion. Supervised training in insertion and removal was emphasized; insertion-related complications necessitated removal for only 21 users.

Complications in the removal of NORPLANT capsules have been evaluated in a series of 3416 cases from 11 countries (364[Cr]). Complications were reported in 4.5% of removals, usually attributable to implants being broken during removal (1.7%) or being embedded below the subdermal plane (1.2%). Logistic regression analysis revealed the most important risk factors for complicated removals to be complications at insertion and an infection at the implant site (before or at the time or removal). For women without complications, the mean removal time was 11.5 minutes, but for those with complications the mean increased to 29.7 minutes. These results illustrate the necessity of proper insertion technique, under aseptic conditions. Capsules are known to be surrounded by a fibrous sheath within 3 months after implantation; beyond a few months, there was no difference in complication rate by duration of use. As with insertion-related complications, the rate of complications varies considerably.

Several studies of NORPLANT use by *lactating mothers* have shown that there are no negative effects on infant growth or health and that the rate of steroid transfer is quite low (2[R]). There are no data on insertion earlier in the postpartum period.

There have not yet been any studies of NORPLANT and *cancer* risk.

Return of fertility is rapid (3[r], 4[R]). Serum levonorgestrel levels are undetectable within a week after implant removal, and normal ovulatory cycles usually resume during the first month.

The *NORPLANT-2 system*, which requires only two capsules, is undergoing clinical trials. This system is effective for 3 years.

Levonorgestrel implants (biodegradable)

Also long-acting is the biodegradable subdermal capsular implant Capronor, that releases levonorgestrel over a 12—18-month period; the small study available to date compared a 12- and a 21.6-mg dose in capsules of differing size. Ovulation occurred in all cycles at the lower dose and in a quarter of cycles at the higher dose, so it is likely that the contraceptive effect results essentially from changes in the cervical mucus and the endometrium. Several patients experienced local swelling or itching of the skin at the capsule insertion site, relieved by topical corticosteroids (365[c]).

Other compounds

The active components used in such implants have varied. In one early study (366[R]) implants filled with *megestrol acetate* gave an unexpectedly high incidence of tubal pregnancies and the absolute number of ectopic pregnancies was clearly greater than that expected for the general population; this finding has also from time to time been described with oral progestogen-only products. One delivery system of this type employs subcutaneous implants of fused pellets made from *norethisterone and pure cholesterol* (367[c]).

Clinical trials of *desogestrel implants* have recently been carried out (368[C]). These were found to be effective, with *bleeding irregularities* and *ovarian cysts* as the primary side effects.

INTRAVAGINAL HORMONAL CONTRACEPTIVES

As early as 1978, the vaginal administration of steroids for contraceptive purposes was attempted, at that time using vaginal rings containing *medroxyprogesterone acetate* or both *norgestrel and estradiol*. More recently, complete inhibition of ovulation has been attained in women by the daily intravaginal application of a product containing 1 mg *noresthisterone* and 0.05 mg *mestranol* (369[C]).

A low-dose *levonorgestrel* vaginal ring has also been studied. Women using vaginal rings releasing 20 μg levonorgestrel daily have more bleeding/spotting days than women using other hormonal contraceptives, with *menstrual patterns* similar to those of progestogen-only pill users (228[C]). Irregular and infrequent bleeding was also recorded by some women. Recent analysis of menstrual calendar data from WHO Phase III clinical trials finds that the percentage of women who experience bleeding patterns defined as 'acceptable' increases steadily from 39.4% in the first 3 months to 55.8% during months 10—12 (325[Cr]). Frequent and irregular bleeding were the most common problems. In another study, among 108 women there were four pregnancies during 1 year of investigation with a discontinuation rate of 71.2%. Menstrual disturbances were the main adverse effects and also the most common reason for discontinuation, occurring in 45% of cycles during the first month (370[c]).

INTRACERVICAL HORMONAL CONTRACEPTIVES

When an intracervical device (ICD) releasing 20 μg levonorgestrel per day was studied in 198 women for 2 years of its use, a total of seven pregnancies occurred, all of them during the first year and six of them occurred after the unnoticed expulsion of the device. One pregnancy occurred in an epileptic woman taking carbamazepine, with the ICD remaining in situ. In three cases the ICD was removed due to infection, all three occurring during the first year of use; in one case, *Neisseria gonorrhoeae* and, in another, *Chlamydia trachomatis*, were found. During the study the mean body weight increased, but remarkably there was a statistically significant decrease in both the mean diastolic and systolic blood pressures after 1 and 2 years of ICD use compared to the pre-insertion values (371[c]).

POSTCOITAL 'CONTRACEPTION'

Diethylstilbestrol has been widely used as a postcoital contraceptive. However it is no longer in use in many countries as a postcoital contraceptive, because of the possible effect on the surviving fetus (see Chapter 40.2). *Ethinylestradiol* has also been used in the past, with a daily dose of 5 mg/day for 5 days. This method has a high incidence of adverse reactions, nausea, vomiting and tender breast being the most frequent (372[c]).

The most common method today is *four tablets of ethinylestradiol* 50 μg and norgestrel 500 μg: two tablets are to be taken immediately and the other two 12 hours later. This treatment must begin within 72 hours of unprotected intercourse. It seems to be as effective as ethinylestradiol alone and with less nausea and vomiting (373[cr]). Overall failure rates are about 2—3%, with perhaps twice this failure rate when taken at mid-cycle. It should not be used when absolute contraindications to estrogen are present. These include pregnancy, unstable angina, transient ischemic attacks, liver disease, undiagnosed genital bleeding or a history of thromboembolism. Some absolute contraindications to long-term use, such as breast cancer and arterial disease, are not contraindications for short-term use (374).

Use of *lower dose COCs*, in a larger quantity, are also presumed to be effective for postcoital contraception (375[R]). *Progestin-only pills* can be used, at a single dose of 0.6 mg levonorgestrel taken within 12 hours (1[R]). One study found that levonorgestrel alone had a low failure rate but that intermenstrual bleeding, nausea and dizziness were common side effects (SEDA-16,

466). Danazol, a synthetic *androgen*, has been evaluated, but with inconsistent research results (1[R], 375[R]).

The antiprogesterone *mifepristone* (RU486), almost exclusively used as an abortifacient, has also been tried as a postcoital contraceptive (376). A randomized trial of a single dose of mifepristone 600 mg, compared to the standard treatment described above, demonstrated that mifepristone is at least as effective as the usual regimen (377[Cr]). Women receiving mifepristone had lower rates of side effects, particularly nausea and vomiting, but their next menstrual period was more likely to be delayed. Another randomized trial, comparing the standard treatment, danazol, and RU486, found that all methods were equally effective (SEDA-16, 466). The standard treatment had a higher total incidence of side effects, but RU486 was associated with the greatest cycle disruption.

A non-hormonal approach to emergency contraception is insertion of an *IUD*, up to 7 days after ovulation in a cycle during which unprotected intercourse has occurred (1[R]).

HORMONE-RELEASING INTRAUTERINE DEVICES *(see also Chapter 49)*

One of the main disadvantages of conventional intrauterine devices (IUDs) is the increased *menstrual blood loss* associated with their use. In an attempt to ameliorate this problem, various IUDs have been designed to release either progesterone or synthetic progestogen (e.g. levonorgestrel) (4[R], 378[R]).

IUDs releasing levonorgestrel are somewhat more *effective* than copper-containing devices, while those releasing progesterone are least effective (379[R]). The proportion of pregnancies that are *ectopic* is higher for both levonorgestrel- and progesterone-releasing devices, compared to copper IUDs. Thus, both types of hormonal devices have higher overall rates of ectopic pregnancy per 1000 woman years than do copper devices, but rates vary inversely with hormone dose. At the most common dosage levels, the ectopic pregnancy rate for levonorgestrel-containing IUDs (20 μg/day) was less than that of non-contraceptors, but for progesterone IUDs (65 μg/day) the risk was elevated.

Because the greatest risk of microbacterial contamination of the endometrium is at IUD insertion, progesterone-releasing devices that must be re-inserted annually may increase the likelihood of *pelvic inflammatory disease* (PID) (1[R]). In contrast, a randomized clinical trial of an IUD that releases 20 μg levonorgestrel daily, for a period of several years, suggests a protective effect against PID (380[Cr]). The 36-month rate of PID was significantly lower for the levonorgestrel device (0.5 per 100 woman-years) than for a copper-releasing IUD (2.0). The *pregnancy rate* was also significantly lower (0.3 for the progestogen-devices, compared to 3.7), as was the rate of *ectopic pregnancies* (0.03 compared to 0.25). The rate of *expulsion* was similar, while the rates of removal because of *amenorrhea* and the *hormonally-related side effects* were significantly higher for the levonorgestrel-releasing device.

The administration of progesterone-only contraception via IUDs in this way is clearly associated with some of the problems seen when other routes are used. The effect is apparently largely at the uterine level, but the partial and variable effects on ovulation seem to cause a greater risk of *functional ovarian cysts* (381[C], 382[C]).

REFERENCES

1. Hatcher RA, Guest F, Stewart F et al. Contraceptive Technology. 16th revised edition. New York: Irvington Publishers, 1994.
2. McCann MF, Potter LS. Progestin-only oral contraception: a comprehensive review. Contraception 1994; 50(Suppl):1.
3. American College of Obstetricians and Gynecologists (ACOG). Hormonal Contraception. ACOG Technical Bulletin No. 198, Washington, DC, 1994.
4. Speroff L, Darney PD. A Clinical Guide for Contraception. Baltimore, Maryland: Williams & Wilkins, 1992.
5. WHO Task Force on Oral Contraceptives. The WHO multicentre trial of the vasopressor effects of combined oral contraceptives: 1. Comparisons with IUD. Contraception 1989;40:129.
6. WHO Task Force on Oral Contraceptives. The WHO multicentre trial of the vasopressor effects of combined oral contraceptives: 2. Lack of effect of estrogen. Contraception 1989;40:147.
7. Royal College of General Practitioners' Oral Contraception Study. Effect of hypertension and benign breast disease of progestagen component in combined oral contraceptives. Lancet 1977;i:624.
8. Woods JW. Oral contraceptives and hypertension. Hypertension 1988;11(Suppl II):11.
9. Editorial. Hypertension and oral contraceptives. Br Med J 1978;2:1570.
10. Connell EB. Oral contraceptives: the current risk-benefit ratio. J Reprod Med 1984;29(Suppl):513.
11. Thorogood M, Adam SA, Mann JI. Fatal subarachnoid haemorrhage in young women: role of oral contraceptives. Br Med J 1981;293:762.
12. Hannaford PC, Croft PR, Kay CR. Oral contraception and stroke. Evidence from the Royal College of General Practitioners' oral contraception study. Stroke 1994;121: 168.
13. Croft P, Hannaford PC. Risk factors for acute myocardial infarction in women: evidence from the Royal College of

General Practitioners' oral contraception study. Br Med J 1989;298:165.
14. Pritchard JA, Pritchard SA. Blood-pressure response to estrogen-progestin oral contraceptive after pregnancy-induced hypertension. Am J Obstet Gynecol 1977;129: 733.
15. Lehtovirta P, Ranta T, Seppala M. Elevated prolactin levels in oral contraceptive pill-related hypertension. Fertil Steril 1981;36:403.
16. Skouby SO (Committee Chairman) et al. Consensus Development Meeting: Metabolic aspects of oral contraceptives of relevance for cardiovascular diseases. Am J Obstet Gynecol 1990;162:1335.
17. Schwingl PJ, Ory HW, King TDN. Modeled estimates of cardiovascular mortality risks in the U.S. associated with low dose oral contraceptives, 1995-draft. Unpublished.
18. Thorogood M, Mann J, Murphy M et al. Is oral contraceptive use still associated with an increased risk of fatal myocardial infarction? Report of a case-control study. Br J Obstet Gynecol 1991;98:1245.
19. Rosenberg L, Palmer JR, Shapiro S. Use of lower dose oral contraceptives and risk of myocardial infarction (abstract). Circulation 1991;83:723.
20. Lidegaard O. Oral contraception and risk of a cerebral thromboembolic attack: results of a case-control study. Br Med J 1993;306:956.
21. Thorogood M, Mann J, Murphy M et al. Fatal stroke and use of oral contraceptives: findings from a case-control study. Am J Epidemiol 1992;136:35.
22. Thorogood M, Mann J, Murphy M et al. Risk factors for fatal venous thromboembolism in young women; a case-control study. Int J Epidemiol 1992;21:48.
23. Longstreth WT, Nelson LM, Koepsell TD et al. Subarachnoid hemorrhage and hormonal factors in women: a population based case-control study. Ann Intern Med 1994;121:168.
24. Gerstman BB, Piper JM, Tomita DK et al. Oral contraceptive estrogen dose and the risk of deep venous thromboembolic disease. Am J Epidemiol 1991;133:32.
25. Grimes DA. The safety of oral contraceptives: Epidemiologic insights from the first 30 years. Am J Obstet Gynecol 1992;166:1950.
26. Beller FK. Cardiovascular system: coagulation, thrombosis, and contraceptive steroids—Is there a link? In: Goldzieher JW, Fotherby K, eds. Pharmacology of the Contraceptive Steroids. New York: Raven Press, 1994:309.
27. Gevers Leuven JA, Kluft C, Bertina RM et al. Effects of two low-dose oral contraceptives on circulating components of the coagulation and fibrinolytic systems. J Lab Clin Med 1987;109:631.
28. Cohen C, Mackie IJ, Walshe K et al. A comparison of the effects of two triphasic oral contraceptives on haemostasis. Br J Haematol 1988;69:259.
29. Ernst E, Schmölzl CH, Matrai A et al. Hemorheological effects of oral contraceptives. Contraception 1989;40:571.
30. Farag A, Bottoms SF, Mammen EF et al. Haemostasis and oral contraceptives. Folia Haematol 1988;115:340.
31. Von Hugo R, Briel RC, Schindler AE. Wirkung oraler Kontrazeptiva auf die Blutgerinnung bei rauchenden und nichtrauchenden Probandinnen. Aktuel Endokrinol Stoffwechsel 1989;10:6.
32. Medical Research Council. Risk of thromboembolism in women taking oral contraceptives. Br Med J 1967;2:355.
33. Inman WHW, Vessey MP. Investigation of deaths from pulmonary, coronary and cerebral thrombosis and embolism in women of childbearing age. Br Med J 1968;2:193.
34. Vessey MP, Doll R. Investigation of relation between use of oral contraceptives and thromboembolic disease. Br Med J 1968;2:199.
35. Sartwell PE, Masi AT, Arthes FG et al. Thromboembolism and oral contraceptives: an epidemiological case-control study. Am J Epidemiol 1969;90:365.
36. Seigel DG, Markush RE. Oral contraceptives and relative risk of death from venous and pulmonary thromboembolism in the United States. Am J Epidemiol 1969; 90:11.
37. Vessey MP. The Walnut Creek Contraceptive Drug Study. Br J Fam Plann 1981;7:83.
38. Miwa LJ, Edmunds AL, Shaefer MS et al. Idiopathic thromboembolism associated with triphasic oral contraceptives. DICP Ann Pharmacother 1989;23:773.
39. Lamy L, Roy PH, Morissette JJ et al. Intimal hyperplasia and thrombosis of the visceral arteries in a young woman: possible relation with oral contraceptives and smoking. Surgery 1988;103:706.
40. Scolding NJ, Gibby OM. Fatal pulmonary embolism in a patient treated with Marvelon. J R Coll Gen Pract 1988;38:568.
41. Porter JB, Hunter JR, Jick H et al. Oral contraceptives and nonfatal vascular disease. Obstet Gynecol 1985;66:1.
42. Realini JP, Goldzieher JW. Oral contraceptives and cardiovascular disease: a critique of epidemiologic studies. Am J Obstet Gynecol 1985;152:729.
43. Chilvers E, Rudge P. Cerebral venous thrombosis and subarachnoid haemorrhage in users of oral contraceptives. Br Med J 1986;292:524.
44. Granato DB, Archer CR, Awwad EE. Magnetic resonance imaging of cerebral venous thrombosis secondary to 'low-dose' birth control pills. Clin Imag 1989;13:220.
45. Nagaratman N, James WE. Isolated angiitis of the brain in a young female on the contraceptive pill. Postgrad Med J 1987;63:1085.
46. Xnereb M, Pullicino P. Oral contraceptive use and risk of stroke. Stroke 1988;19:22.
47. Chopard JL, Moulin T, Bourrin JC et al. Contraception orale et accident vasculaire cérébral ischémique. Semin Hôp (Paris) 1988;64:2075.
48. Biller J, Haberland C, Toffel Gl et al. Basilar artery occlusion in an adolescent girl: a risk of oral contraceptives? J Child Neurol 1986;1:347.
49. Iuliano G, Di Domenico G, Masullo C et al. Terapia contracettiva trifasica et ictus cerebri. Riv Neurobiol 1985; 85:231.
50. Lalive d'Epinai SP, Trüb P. Retinale vaskuläre Komplikationen bei oralen Kontrazeptiva. Klin Mbl Augenheilkd 1985;188:394.
51. Bradley IR, Reynolds J, Williams PF et al. Encephalopathy in renovascular hypertension associated with the use of oral contraceptives. Postgrad Med J 1986;62:1031.
52. Landau E, Lessing JB, Weintraub M et al. Acute myocardial infarction in a young woman taking oral contraceptives. J Reprod Med 1986;31:1008.
53. Lindberg MC. Hepatobiliary complications of oral contraceptives. J Gen Intern Med 1992;7:199.
54. Schneiderman DJ, Cello JP. Intestinal ischemia and infarction associated with oral contraceptives. West J Med 1986;145:350.

55. Böhler J, Hauenstein KH, Hasler K et al. Renal vein thrombosis in a dehydrated patient on oral contraceptive. Nephrol Dial Transplant 1989;4:993.
56. Detering K, Kallischnig G. The cardiovascular risk of oral contraception with special reference to German mortality statistics. N Trends Gynecol Obstet 1985;1:360.
57. Vessey MP, Villard-Mackintosh L, McPherson K et al. Mortality among oral contraceptive users: 20 year follow up of women in a cohort study. Br Med J 1989;299:1487.
58. Hirvonen E, Indänpään-Heikkilä J. Cardiovascular death among women under 40 years of age using low-estrogen oral contraceptives and intrauterine devices in Finland from 1975 to 1984. Am J Obstet Gynecol 1990;163:281.
59. Porter JB, Hunter JR, Danielson S et al. Oral contraceptives and nonfatal vascular disease—recent experience. Obstet Gynecol 1982;59:299.
60. Bailar JC, Byar DP. Oestrogen treatment for cancer of the prostate. Cancer 1970;26:257.
61. Badaracco MB, Vessey MP. Recurrence of venous thromboembolism disease and use of oral contraceptives. Br Med J 1974;1:215.
62. Jick H, Dinan B, Herman R et al. Myocardial infarction and other vascular diseases in young women. J Am Med Assoc 1978;240:2548.
63. Stadel BV. Oral contraceptives and cardiovascular disease. I. N Engl J Med 1981;305:612.
64. Stadel BV. Oral contraceptives and cardiovascular disease. II. N Engl J Med 1981;305:627.
65. Böttiger LE, Boman G, Eklund G et al. Oral contraceptives and thromboembolic disease: effect of lowering oestrogen content. Lancet 1980;i:1097.
66. Poller L. Oral contraceptives, blood clotting and thrombosis. Med Bull 1978;34:151.
67. Fruzzetti F, Ricci C, Fioretti P. Haemostasis profile in smoking and nonsmoking women taking low-dose oral contraceptives. Contraception 1994;49:579.
68. Thorogood M, Villard-Mackintosh L. Combined oral contraceptives: risks and benefits. Br Med Bull 1993;49:124.
69. Ernst E. Oral contraceptives, fibrinogen and cardiovascular risk. Atherosclerosis 1992;93:1.
70. Ylikokkala O, Pnolakka J, Viinakka L. Estrogen containing oral contraceptives decrease prostacyclin production. Lancet 1981;i:42.
71. Plowright D, Adam SA, Thorogood M et al. Immunogenicity and the vascular risk of oral contraceptives. Br Heart J 1985;53:556.
72. Syner FN, Moghissi KS, Agronow SJ. Study of the presence of abnormal proteins in the serum of oral contraceptive users. Fertil Steril 1983;40:202.
73. Frederiksen H, Ravenholt RT. Oral contraceptives, cigarette smoking. Public Health Rep 1970;85:197.
74. Rich-Edwards JW, Manson JE, Hennekens CH et al. The primary prevention of coronary heart disease in women. New Eng J Med 1995;332:1758.
75. Arthes FG, Masi AT. Myocardial infarction in younger women. Chest 1976;70:594.
76. Jain AK. Cigarette smoking, use of oral contraceptives and myocardial infarction. Am J Obstet Gynecol 1977; 126:301.
77. Beral V, Kay R. Mortality among oral-contraceptive users: Royal College of General Practitioners' Oral Contraception Study. Lancet 1977;ii:727.
78. Petiti DP, Wingerd J. Use of oral contraceptives, cigarette smoking, and risk of subarachnoid haemorrhage. Lancet 1978;ii:234.
79. Vessey MP, Doll R, Peto R et al. A long-term follow-up study of women using different methods of contraception—an interim report. J Biosoc Sci 1976;8:373.
80. Royal College of General Practitioners' Oral Contraception Study. Incidence of arterial disease among oral contraceptive users. J R Coll Gen Pract 1983;33:75.
81. Bruni V, Rosati D, Bucciantini S et al. Platelet and coagulation functions during triphasic oestrogen-progestogen treatment. Contraception 1986;33:39.
82. Kjaeldgaard A, Larsson B. Long-term treatment with combined oral contraceptives and cigarette smoking associated with impaired activity of tissue plasminogen activator. Acta Obstet Cynaecol Scand 1986;65:219.
83. Mant D, Villard-Mackintosh L, Vessey MP et al. Myocardial infarction and angina pectoris in young women. J Epidemiol Commun Heatlh 1987;41:215.
84. Harlap S, Kost K, Forrest JD. Preventing Pregnancy, Protecting Health: A New Look at Birth Control Choices in the United States. The Alan Guttmacher Institute, New York, 1991.
85. Cirkel U, Schweppe KW. Fettstoffwechsel und orale Kontrazeptiva. Äztl Kosmetol 1985;15:253.
86. Astedt B, Isacson S, Nilsson HM et al. Thrombosis and oral contraceptives: possible predisposition. Br Med J 1973;4:631.
87. Astedt B. Low fibrinolytic activity of veins during treatment with ethinyloestradiol. Acta Obstet Gynaecol Scand 1971;50:279.
88. Jick H, Slone D, Westerholm B et al. Venous thromboembolic disease and ABO blood type. Lancet 1969;i:539.
89. Koenig W, Gehring J, Mathes P. Orale Kontrazeptiva und Myokardinfarkt bei jungen Frauen. HerzKreisl 1984; 16:508.
90. Zatti M. Contraccettivi orali: alterazioni delle variabili fisiologiche. C Ital Chim Clin 1983;8:249.
91. Leone A, Lopez M. Rôle du tabac et de la contraception orale dans l'infarctus du myocarde de la femme: description d'un cas. Pathologica 1984;76:493.
92. Vessey MP. Postoperative thromboembolism. Br Med J 1970;3:123.
93. Green GR, Sartwell PE. Oral contraceptive use in patients with thromboembolism following surgery trauma or infection. Am J Publ Health 1972;63:680.
94. Ratnoff OD, Kaufman R. Arterial thrombosis in oral contraceptives users. Ann Intern Med 1982;142:447.
95. Whitehead EM, Whitehead MJ. The pill, HRT, and postoperative thrombosis: cause for concern? (editorial) Anaesthesia 1991;46:521.
96. Robinson GE, Burren T, Mackie IJ et al. Changes in haemostasis after stopping the combined contraceptive pill: implications for major surgery. Br Med J 1991;302:269.
97. Ananijevic-Pandey I, Vlajinac H. Myocardial infarction in young women with reference to oral contraceptive use. Int J Epidemiol 1989;18:585.
98. Vessey MP, Lawless M, Yeates D. Oral contraceptives and stroke: findings in a large prospective study. Br Med J 1984;289:530.
99. Collaborative Group for the Study of Stroke in Young Women. Oral contraception and increased risk of cerebral ischemia or thrombosis. N Engl J Med 1973;288:871.
100. Inman WHW. Oral contraceptives and fatal subarachnoid haemorrhage. Br Med J 1979;2:1468.
101. Pettiti DB, Wingerd J, Pellegrin F et al. Risk of vascular disease in women. J Am Med Assoc 1979;242:1150.

102. Thorogood M, Adam SA, Mann J I. Fatal subarachnoid haemorrhage in young women: role of oral contraceptives. Br Med J 1981;283:762.
103. Helmich S, Rosenberg L, Kaufman DW et al. Venous thromboembolism in relation to oral contraceptive use. Obstet Gynecol 1987;69:91.
104. Rosenberg L, Palmer JR, Lesko SM et al. Oral contraceptive use and the risk of myocardial infarction. Am J Epidemiol 1990;131:1009.
105. Stampfer MJ, Willett WC, Colditz GA et al. Past use of oral contraceptives and cardiovascular disease: a meta-analysis in the context of the Nurses' Health Study. Am J Obstet Gynecol 1990;163:285.
106. Colditz GA (for The Nurses' Health Study Research Group). Oral contraceptive use and mortality during 12 years of follow-up: The Nurses' Health Study. Ann Intern Med 1994;120:821.
107. Goldzieher JW, Moses LE, Averkin E et al. A placebo-controlled double-blind crossover investigation of the side effects attributed to oral contraceptives. Fertil Steril 1971;22:609.
108. Mattson RH, Rebar RW. Contraceptive methods for women with neurologic disorders. Am J Obstet Gynecol 1993;168:2027.
109. Lobo RA, Gibbons WE. The role of progestin therapy in breast disease and central nervous system function. J Reprod Med 1982;(Suppl 8):515.
110. Asherson RA, Harris NE, Gharavi AE et al. Systemic lupus erythematosus, antiphospholipid antibodies, chorea, and oral contraceptives. Arthr Rheum 1986;29:1535.
111. Leys D, Destée A, Petit H et al. Chorea associated with oral contraception. J Neurol 1987;235:46.
112. Buge A, Rancurel DV, Chéron F. Hémichorée et contraceptifs oraux. Rev Neurol 1985;141:663.
113. Driesen JJM, Walters ECh. Oral contraceptive induced paraballism. Clin Neurosurg 1987;89:49.
114. Mathor AK, Gatter RA. Chorea as the initial presentation of oral contraceptive-induced systemic lupus erythematosus. J Rheumatol 1988;15:1042.
115. Calanchini C. Die Auslösung eines Zwangssyndroms durch Ovulationshemmer. Schweiz. Arch Neurol Psychiatr 1986;137:25.
116. Van Winter JT, Miller KA. Breakthrough bleeding in a bulimic adolescent receiving oral contraceptives. Pediat Adolesc Gynecol 1986;4:39.
117. Chang AMZ, Chick P, Milburn S. Mood changes as reported by women taking the oral contraceptive pill. Aust NZ J Obstet Gynecol 1982;22:78.
118. Fleming O, Seager CP. Incidence of depressive symptoms in users of oral contraceptives. Br J Psychiatry 1978; 132:431.
119. Adams DB, RossGold A, Burt AD. Rise in female-initiated sexual activity at ovulation and its suppression by oral contraceptives. N Engl J Med 1978;299:1146.
120. Godsland IF, Crook D. Update on the metabolic effects of steroidal contraceptives and their relationship to cardiovascular disease risk. Am J Obstet Gynecol 1994;170:1528.
121. Collins P, Rosano GMC, Jiang C et al. Cardiovascular protection by oestrogen—a calcium antagonist effect? Lancet 1993;341:1264.
122. Williams JK, Adams M, Herrington DM et al. Short-term administration of estrogen and vascular responses of atherosclerotic coronary arteries. J Am Coll Cardiol 1992; 20:452.
123. Clarkson TB, Shively CA, Morgan TM et al. Oral contraceptives and coronary artery atherosclerosis of cynomolgus monkeys. Obstet Gynecol 1990;75:217.
124. Elkind-Hirsch K, Goldzieher JW. Metabolism: carbohydrate metabolism. In: Goldzieher JW, Fotherby K, eds. Pharmacology of the Contraceptive Steroids. New York: Raven Press, 1994:345.
125. Spellacy WN. Carbohydrate metabolism during treatment with estrogen, progestogen and low-dose oral contraceptives. Am J Obstet Gynecol 1982;142:732.
126. Royal College of General Practitioners. Oral Contraceptives and Health. An Interim Report from the Oral Contraceptive Study of the Royal College of Practitioners. London: Pitman Medical, 1974.
127. Wingrave ST, Kay CR, Vessey MP. Oral contraceptives and diabetes mellitus. Br Med J 1979;1:23.
128. Hannaford PC, Kay CR. Oral contraceptives and diabetes mellitus. Br Med J 1989;299:1315.
129. Ramamoorthy R, Saraswathi TP, Kanaka TS. Carbohydrate metabolic studies during twelve months of treatment with a low-dose combination oral contraceptive. Contraception 1989;40:563.
130. Eschwége E, Fontbonne A, Simon D et al. Oral contraceptives, insulin resistance and ischemic vascular disease. Int J Gynecol Obstet 1990;31:263.
131. Miccolo R, Orlandi MC, Fruzetti F et al. Effeti dei contracettivi orali a basse dosi sul metabolismo glucidico. Minerva Ginecol 1989;41:44.
132. Godsland IF, Crook D, Simpson R et al. The effects of different formulations of oral contraceptive agents on lipid and carbohydrate metabolism. N Engl J Med 1990;323:1375.
133. Simon D, Senan C, Garnier P et al. Effects of oral contraceptives on carbohydrate and lipid metabolism in a healthy population: the Telecom study. Am J Obstet Gynecol 1990;163:382.
134. World Health Organization. Oral Contraceptives: Technical and Safety Aspects. WHO Offset Publications, 64. World Health Organization, Geneva, 1982.
135. Gaspard U. Contraception orale, métabolisme glucidique et critéres de surveillance. Contracept Fertil Sex 1988;16:113.
136. Garg SK, Chase HP, Marshall G et al. Oral contraceptives and renal and retinal complications in young women with insulin-dependent diabetes mellitus. J Am Med Assoc 1994;271:1099.
137. Knopp RH. Arteriosclerosis risk: the role of oral contraceptives and postmenopausal estrogens. J Reprod Med 1986;31(Suppl 9):913.
138. Rössner S, Larsson-Cohn U, Carlsson LA et al. Effects of an oral contraceptive agent on plasma lipids, plasma lipoproteins, the intravenous fat tolerance and the post-lipoproteins, the intravenous fat tolerance and the post-heparin lipoprotein lipase activity. Acta Med Scand 1971;190:301.
139. Burkman RT, Zacur HA, Kimball AW et al. Oral contraceptives and lipids and lipoproteins. I. Variations in mean levels by oral contraceptive type. Contraception 1989;40:553.
140. Wallace RB, Hoover J, Barret-Connor E et al. Altered plasma lipid and lipoprotein levels associated with oral contraceptives and oestrogen use. Lancet 1979;ii:111.
141. Frankman O, Marsk L, Rössner S. P-piller och HDL-kolestrol. Läkartidningen 1979;76:15.
142. Bradley DD, Wingerd J, Petiti DB et al. Serum high-density-lipoprotein cholesterol in women using oral contraceptives, oestrogens and progestin. N Engl J Med 1978; 299:17.

143. Deslypere JP, Thiery M, Vermeulen A. Effect of long-term hormonal contraception on plasma lipids. Contraception 1985;31:633.
144. Lussierl-Cacan S, Davignon J, Nestruck AC et al. Influence of a triphasic oral contraceptive preparation on plasma lipids and lipoproteins. Fertil Steril 1990;58:28.
145. Lipson A, Stoy DB, LaRosa JC et al. Progestins and oral contraceptive-induced lipoprotein changes: a prospective study. Contraception 1986;34:121.
146. Klosterboer HJ, Van Wayjen RGA, Van den Ende A. Comparative effects of monophasic desogestrel plus ethinyloestradiol and triphasic levonorgestrel plus ethinyloestradiol on lipid metabolism. Contraception 1986;34:135.
147. Notelovitz M, Feldman EB, Gillespy M et al. Lipid and lipoprotein changes in women taking low-dose, triphasic oral contraceptives: a controlled, comparative, 12-month clinical trial. Am J Obstet Gynecol 1989;160:1269.
148. Van der Vange N, Kloosterboer HJ, Haspels AA. Effects of seven low-dose combined oral contraceptives on high density lipoprotein subfractions. Br J Obstet Gynaecol 1987;94:559.
149. Ball MJ, Ashwell E, Jackson MC et al. Which Pill? The effect of various modern preparations on lipoproteins and glucose metabolism. Br J Fam Plann 1989;14:110.
150. Leuven JAG, Drijkoningen GJA, Alers J et al. The effect of low dose contraceptives on lipoprotein lipid and apolipoprotein levels in smoking and non-smoking women. J Drug Ther Res 1988;13:355.
151. Fotherby K. Oral contraceptives and lipids. Br Med J 1989;289:1049.
152. Holt LH, Herbst AL. DES-related female genital changes. Semin Oncol 1982;9:341.
153. Burch JC, Byrd EF Jr, Vaughn WK. The effects of long-term estrogen on hysterectomized women. Am J Obstet Gynecol 1974;118:778.
154. Gordon T, Kannel WB, Hjortland MC et al. Menopause and coronary heart disease. Ann Intern Med 1978;89:157.
155. Hammond CB, Jelovsek RR, Lee K et al. Effect of long-term estrogen replacement therapy. Am J Obstet Gynecol 1979;133:525.
156. Burkman RT. Oral contraceptives, lipid and lipoprotein changes, and risk of coronary heart disease. Semin Reprod Endocrinol 1989;7:224.
157. Knopp RH. Cardiovascular effects of endogenous and exogenous sex hormones over a woman's lifetime. Am J Obstet Gynecol 1988;158:1630.
158. Walden CE, Knopp RH, Johnson JL et al. Effect of estrogen/progestin potency on clinical chemistry measures: the Lipid Research Clinics Program prevalence study. Am J Epidemiol 1986;123:517.
159. Bersivala V, Virka K, Kulkarni RD. Thyroid function of women taking oral contraceptives. Contraception 1974; 9:305.
160. WHO Task Force on Oral Contraceptives. Oral and injectable hormonal contraceptive and signs and symptoms of vitamin deficiency and goitre: prevalence studies in five centres in the developing and developed world. WHO Bull, 1983.
161. Amatayakul K. Metabolism: vitamins and trace elements. In: Goldzieher JW, Fotherby K, eds. Pharmacology of the Contraceptive Steroids. New York: Raven Press, 1994:363.
162. Malnick SDH, Halperin M, Geltner D. Hypercarotenemia associated with an oral contraceptive. DICP Ann Pharmacother 1989;23:811.
163. Rose DP. The influence of oestrogens on tryptophan metabolism in man. Clin Sci 1966;31:265.
164. Price SA, Toseland PA. Oral contraceptives and depression. Lancet 1969;ii:158.
165. Anonymous. Depression and oral contraceptives: the role of pyridoxine. Drug Ther Bull 1978;16:85.
166. Nilsson S, Nygren KG. Transfer of contraceptive steroids to human milk. Res Reprod 1979;11:1.
167. McCann MF, Liskin LS, Piotrow PT et al. Breast-feeding, fertility, and family planning. Population Reports, Series J, No. 24. Baltimore, Maryland, Population Information Program, 1984.
168. WHO Task Force on Oral Contraceptives. Effects of hormonal contraceptives on breast milk composition and infant growth. Stud Fam Plann 1988;19:361.
169. Nilsson S, Mellbin T, Hofvander Y et al. Long-term follow-up of children breast-fed by mothers using oral contraceptives. Contraception 1986;34:443.
170. Goulding A, McChesney R. Diminished urinary calcium excretion by women using oral contraceptives. Aust NZ J Med 1976;6:251.
171. Recker RR, Saville PD, Heaney RP. Effect of oestrogens and calcium carbonate on bone loss in postmenopausal women. Ann Intern Med 1977;87:649.
172. Darzenta NC, Giunta JL. Radiographic changes of the mandible related to oral contraceptives. Oral Surg 1977; 43:478.
173. Larsson G, Milsom I, Lindstedt G et al. The influence of a low-dose combined oral contraceptive on menstrual blood loss and iron status. Contraception 1992;46:327.
174. Mardell M, Silva JF. Effect of oral contraceptives on the variations in serum iron during the menstrual cycle. Lancet 1967;ii:1323.
175. Howard RJ, Tuck SM. Haematological disorders and reproductive health. Br J Fam Plann 1993;19:147.
176. Lucis OJ, Lucis R. Oral contraceptives and endocrine changes. Bull WHO 1972;46:443.
177. Rahman HA et al. A report on the effect of oral contraceptives on blood picture, serum iron and TIBC in twenty cases of healthy Egyptian women. Bull Alexandr Fac Med 1982.
178. Kendall AG, Charlow GF. Red cell pyruvate kinase deficiency: adverse effect of oral contraceptives. Acta Haematol 1977;57:116.
179. Schillinger F, Montagnac R, Birembaut P et al. Syndrome hémolytique et urémique au décours d'une contraception orale. Rev Fr Gynécol Obstet 1986;81:721.
180. Hargreaves T. Oral contraceptives and liver function. J Clin Pathol 1970;23(Suppl):3.
181. Larsson-Cohn U, Stenram U. Liver ultrastructure and function in icteric and non-icteric women using oral contraceptive agents. Acta Med Scand 1967;181:257.
182. Perez V, Gorodisch S, De Martire J et al. Oral contraceptives: long-term use produce fine structural changes in liver mitochondria. Science 1969;165:1805.
183. WHO Scientific Group. Oral Contraceptives and Neoplasia. WHO Technical Report Series No. 817, Geneva, 1992.
184. Population Information Program. Update on usage, safety and side effects. Population Reports, Oral Contraceptives, Ser. A, No. 5. Johns Hopkins University, Baltimore, MD, 1979.
185. Westerholm B. Oral contraceptives and jaundice. In: Baker SB de C, Tripot T, eds. Proceedings, European So-

ciety for the Study of Drug Toxicity, Oxford, 1969. Amsterdam: Excerpta Medica, 1968:158.
186. Ockner RK, Davidson CS. Hepatic side-effects of oral contraceptives. N Engl J Med 1976;276:331.
187. Stoll BA, Andrews JT, Mofferam R. Liver damage from oral contraceptives. Br Med J 1966;1:960.
188. Briggs MH, Briggs M. Metabolic effects of hormonal contraceptives. In: Chang Chai Fen et al. eds. Recent Advances in Fertility Regulation, Beijing, 1980, 1981:83.
189. Dalén E, Westerholm B. Occurrence of hepatic impairment of women jaundiced by oral contraceptives and in their mothers and sisters. Acta Med Scand 1974;195:459.
190. Adlercreutz H, Tenhunen R. Some aspects of the interaction between natural and synthetic female sex hormones and the liver. Am J Med 1970;49:630.
191. Brown JB, Blair H-AF. Urinary oestrogen metabolites of 17-norethisterone and esters. Proc R Soc Med 1960; 53:433.
192. Van Erpecum KJ, Janssens AR, Kreuning J et al. Generalized peliosis hepatis and cirrhosis after long-term use of oral contraceptives. Am J Gastroenterol 1988;83:572.
193. Heresbach D, Deugnier Y, Brissot P et al. Dilatations sinusoïdales et prise de contraceptifs oraux. Ann Gastroentérol 1988;24:189.
194. Thijs C, Knipschild P. Oral contraceptives and the risk of gallbladder disease: a meta-analysis. Am J Pub Health 1993;83:1113.
195. Grodstein F, Colditz GA, Hunter DJ et al. A prospective study of symptomatic gallstones in women: relation with oral contraceptives and other risk factors. Obstet Gynecol 1994;84:207.
196. Vessey M, Painter R. Oral contraceptive use and benign gallbladder disease; revisited. Contraception 1994;50:167.
197. Boston Collaborative Drug Surveillance Programme. Oral contraceptives and venous thromboembolic disease, surgically confirmed gall bladder disease, and breast tumours. Lancet 1973;i:1399.
198. Stolley PD, Tonascia JA, Tockman MS et al. Thrombosis with low-oestrogen oral contraceptives. Am J Epidemiol 1975;102:197.
199. Royal College of General Practitioners' Oral Contraception Study. Oral contraceptives and gallbladder disease. Lancet 1982;ii:957.
200. Scragg RKR, McMichael AJ, Seamark RF. Oral contraceptives, pregnancy, and endogenous estrogen in gallstone disease: a case-control study. Br Med J 1984;288:1795.
201. Strom BL, Ravikiran MPH, Tamragouri N et al. Oral contraceptives and other risk factors for gallbladder disease. Clin Pharmacol Ther 1986;39:335.
202. Bennion LJ, Ginsberg RL, Garnich MB et al. Effects of oral contraceptives on the gallbladder bile of normal women. N Engl J Med 1976;294:189.
203. Tritapepe R, Padova C, Bellomi M et al. Lithogenic bile after conjugated oestrogen. N Engl J Med 1976;295:960.
204. Coronary Drug Project Research Group. Gallbladder disease as a side-effect of drugs influencing lipid metabolism. N Engl J Med 1977;296:1185.
205. Kern F, Everson GT, DeMark B et al. Biliary lipids, bile acids, and gallbladder function in the human female: effects of contraceptive steroids. J Lab Clin Med 1982; 99:798.
206. Morrisson AS, Jick H, Ory HW. Oral contraceptives and hepatitis: a report from the Boston Collaborative Drug Surveillance Program, Boston University Medical Center. Lancet 1977;i:1142.
207. Zachariasen RD. Ovarian hormones and gingivitis. J Dental Hygiene 1991;65:150.
208. Magnusson I, Ericson T, Hugoson A. The effect of oral contraceptives on the concentration of some salivary substances in women. Arch Oral Biol 1975;20:119.
209. Musalli NG, Hopps RM, Johnson NW. Oral pyogenic granuloma as a complication of pregnancy and the use of hormonal contraceptives. Int J Gynaecol Obstet 1976;14:187.
210. Mungall IPF, Hague RV. Pancreatitis and the pill. Postgrad Med J 1975;51:855.
211. Burk M. Pregnancy, pancreatitis and the pill. Br Med J 1972;4:551.
212. Boyko EJ, Theis MK, Vaughan TL et al. Increased risk of inflammatory bowel disease associated with oral contraceptive use. Am J Epidemiol 1994;140:268.
213. Sandler RS, Wurzelmann JI, Lyles CM. Oral contraceptive use and the risk of inflammatory bowel disease. Epidemiology 1992;3:374.
214. Barriére H, Roubeix Y. Dermatoses et oestroprogestatifs. Gaz Med Fr 1977;84:1485.
215. Mariotti F, Ruocco V. Oral contraceptives and sharpened condylomas. Riforma Med 1971;85:429.
216. Hollander A, Crots IA. Mucha-Haberman disease following oestrogen-progestogen therapy. Arch Dermatol 1973;107:465.
217. Jorge A, Schwartzman Y. Efectos de los anticonceptivos sobre la otosclerosis. Rev Bras Oto-Rino-Laringol 1975; 41:46.
218. Loveland DB. Auditory levels according to use of oral contraceptives in 5449 women. J Am Aud Soc 1975;1:28.
219. Zanker K, Kessler L. Innenohrstörung durch orale hormonale Kontrazeptive? Z Klin Med 1985;40:1897.
220. Soni PS. Effects of oral contraceptives steroids on the thickness of human cornea. Am J Optom Physiol Opt 1980;57:825.
221. De Vries-Reilingh A, Reiners H, Van Bijsterveld OP. Contact lens tolerance and oral contraceptives. Ann Ophtalmol 1978;10:947.
222. Byrne E. Retinal migraine and the pill. Med J Aust 1979;66:659.
223. Fortney JA, Feldblum PJ, Talmage RV et al. Bone mineral density and history of oral contraceptive use. J Reprod Med 1994;39:105.
224. Polatti F, Perotti F, Filippa N et al. Bone mass and long-term monophasic oral contraceptive treatment in young women. Contraception 1995;51:221.
225. Holt VL, Daling JR, McKnight B et al. Functional ovarian cysts in relation to the use of monophasic and triphasic oral contraceptives. Obstet Gynecol 1992;79:529.
226. Lanes SF, Birmann B, Walker AM et al. Oral contraceptive type and functional ovarian cysts. Am J Obstet Gynecol 1992;166:956.
227. Milsom I, Sundell G, Andersch B. The influence of different combined oral contraceptives on the prevalence and severity of dysmenorrhea. Contraception 1990;42:497.
228. Belsey EM, WHO Task Force on Long-Acting Systemic Agents for Fertility Regulation. Vaginal bleeding patterns among women using one natural and eight hormonal methods of contraception. Contraception 1988;38:181.
229. Rosenberg MJ, Long SC. Oral contraceptives and cycle control: a critical review of the literature. Adv Contraception 1992;8(Suppl 1):35.
230. Saleh WA, Burkman RT, Zacur HA et al. A randomized trial of three oral contraceptives: comparison of bleeding

patterns by contraceptive types and steroid levels. Am J Obstet Gynecol 1993;168:1740.
231. Hull MGR, Bromhan DR, Savage PE et al. Normal fertility in women with post-pill amenorrhoea. Lancet 1981;i:1329.
232. Vessey MP, Wright NH, McPherson K et al. Fertility after stopping different methods of contraception. Br Med J 1978;1:265.
233. Harlap S, Davies AM. The Pill and Births: The Jerusalem Study, Final Report. US Department of Health, Education and Welfare, National Institute of Child Health and Development, Center for Population Research, Bethesda, MD, 1978:219.
234. Bracken MB, Hellenbrand KG, Holford TR. Conception delay after oral contraceptive use: the effect of estrogen dose. Fertil Steril 1990;53:21.
235. Toth F, Kerenyin T. Changes of endometrium during contraceptive treatment. Acta Morphol Acad Sci Hung 1973;14:114.
236. Cates W Jr, Stone KM. Family planning, sexually transmitted diseases and contraceptive choice: a literature update—Part II. Fam Plann Perspect 1992;24:122.
237. National Institutes of Health (NIH) Expert Committee on Pelvic Inflammatory Disease. Pelvic inflammatory disease. Research directions in the 1990s. Sex Transm Dis 1991;18:46.
238. McGregor JA, Hammill HA. Contraception and sexually transmitted diseases: interactions and opportunities. Am J Obstet Gynecol 1993;168:2033.
239. Howe JE, Minkoff HL, Duerr AC. Contraceptives and HIV. AIDS 1994;8:861.
240. Vercellini P, Ragni G, Trespidi L et al. Does contraception modify the risk of endometriosis? Hum Reprod 1993;8:547.
241. Parazzinni F, Ferraroni M, Bocciolone L et al. Contraceptive methods and risk of pelvic endometriosis. Contraception 1994;49:47.
242. Schuurs AHWM, Geurts TBP, Goorissen EM et al. Immunologic effects of estrogens, progestins, and estrogen-progestin combinations. In: Goldzieher JW, Fotherby K, eds. Pharmacology of the Contraceptive Steroids. New York: Raven Press, 1994:379.
243. Joshi UM, Rao SS, Kora SJ et al. Effect of steroidal contraceptives on antibody formation in the human female. Contraception 1971;3:327.
244. Hagen C, Froland A. Depressed lymphocyte response to PHA in women taking oral contraceptives. Lancet 1972;ii:1185.
245. Klinger G, Schubert H, Stelzner A et al. Zum Verhalten der Serumimmunoglobulin-Titer von IgA, IgG und IgM bei Kurz- und Langzeitapplikation verschiedener hormonaler Kontrazeptiva. Dtsch Gesundheitswes 1978;33:1057.
246. Huang NH. Absence of antibodies to ethinyloestradiol in users of oral contraceptive steroids. Fertil Steril 1984;41:587.
247. Spector TD, Hochberg MC. The protective effect of the oral contraceptive pill on rheumatoid arthritis: an overview of the analytic epidemiological studies using meta-analysis. J Clin Epidemiol 1990;43:1221.
248. Bojarski JK, De la Serna AR, Gols AR et al. Migraña acompañada como manifestación del lupus eritematoso sislemicon: presentación de 2 casos. Med Clín (Barcelona) 1986;87:112.
249. Strom BL, Reidenberg MM, West S et al. Shingles, allergies, family medical history, oral contraceptives, and other potential risk factors for systemic lupus erythematosus. Am J Epidemiol 1994;140:632.
250. Villard-Mackintosh L, Vessey MP. Oral contraceptives and reproductive factors in multiple sclerosis incidence. Contraception 1993;47:161.
251. Burns MP, Schoch DR, Grayzel AI. Gold urticaria and an oral contraceptive. Ann Intern Med 1983;98:1025.
252. Pelikan Z. Possible immediate hypersensitivity reaction of the nasal mucosa to oral contraceptives. Ann Allergy 1978;40:211.
253. Scinto J, Enrione M, Bernstein D et al. In vitro leukocyte histamine release to progesterone and pregnanediol in a patient with recurrent anaphylaxis associated with exogenous administration of progesterone. J Allergy Clin Immunol 1990;85:228.
254. Hankinson SE, Colditz GA, Hunter DJ et al. A quantitative assessment of oral contraceptive use and risk of ovarian cancer. Obstet Gynecol 1992;80:708.
255. Cancer and Steroid Hormone Study (CASH) of the Centers for Disease Control and the National Institute of Child Health and Human Development. The reduction in risk of ovarian cancer associated with oral-contraceptive use. N Engl J Med 1987;316:650.
256. Schlesselman JJ. Oral contraceptives and neoplasia of the uterine corpus. Contraception 1991;43:557.
257. Cancer and Steroid Hormone Study (CASH) of the Centers for Disease Control and the National Institute of Child Health and Human Development. Combination oral contraceptive use and the risk of endometrial cancer. J Am Med Assoc 1987;257:796.
258. Coker AL, Harlap S, Fortney JA. Oral contraceptives and reproductive cancers: weighing the risks and benefits. Fam Plann Perspect 1993;25:17.
259. Franks AL, Beral V, Cates W Jr et al. Conception and ectopic pregnancy risk. Am J Obstet Gynecol 1990;163:1120.
260. Weiss DB, Aboulafia Y, Kilewidsky A. Ectopic pregnancy and the pill. Lancet 1976;ii:196.
261. American College of Obstetricians and Gynecologists (ACOG). Contraceptives and congenital anomalies. ACOG Committee Opinion: Committee on Gynecologic Practice, No. 124. Int J Gynecol Obstet 1993;42:316.
262. Bracken MB. Oral contraception and congenital malformations in offspring: a review and meta-analysis of the prospective studies. Obstet Gynecol 1990;76:552.
263. Simpson JL, Phillips OP. Spermicides, hormonal contraception and congenital malformations. Adv Contracept 1990;6:141.
264. Back DJ, Orme ME. Pharmacokinetic drug interactions with oral contraceptives. Clin Pharmacokinet 1990;18:472.
265. Back DJ, Orme MLE. Drug interactions. In: Goldzieher JW, Fotherby K, eds. Pharmacology of the Contraceptive Steroids. New York: Raven Press, 1994:407.
266. Shenfield GM, Griffin JM. Clinical pharmacokinetics of contraceptive steroids. An update. Clin Pharmacokinet 1991;20:15.
267. Crawford P, Chadwick DJ, Martin C et al. The interaction of phenytoin and carbamazepine with combined oral contraceptive steroids. Br J Clin Pharmacol 1990;30:892.
268. Bach AM, Breckenridge AM, Crawford FE et al. Interindividual variation and drug interactions with hormonal steroid contraceptives. Drugs 1981;21:46.
269. Conney AH. Pharmacological implications of microsomal enzyme induction. Pharmacol Rev 1967;19:317.

270. Breckenridge AM. Clinical implications of enzyme induction. In: Parke ed. Enzyme Induction. London: Plenum, 1975:273.
271. Nilsson S, Victor A, Nygren KG. Plasma levels of D-norgestrel and sex hormone binding globulin during oral D-norgestrel medication immediately after delivery and legal abortion. Contraception 1977;15:87.
272. Back DJ, Breckenridge AM, Crawford FE et al. Phenobarbitone interaction with oral contraceptive steroids in the rabbit and rat. Br J Pharmacol 1980;69:441.
273. Skolnick JI, Stoler BS, Kotz DG et al. Rifampicin, oral contraceptives and pregnancy. J Am Med Assoc 1976; 236:1382.
274. Plosker GL, Hawes EM. Oral contraceptive drug interaction. J Gynaecol Endocrinol 1986;11:17.
275. Bolt HM, Kappus H, Bolt M. The effect of rifampicin treatment on the metabolism of oestradiol and 17α-ethinylestradiol by human liver microsomes. Eur J Clin Pharmacol 1975;8:301.
276. Hughes BR, Cunliffe WJ. Interactions between the oral contraceptive pill and antibiotics. Br J Dermatol 1990; 122:717.
277. Helton ED, Goldzieher JW. The pharmacokinetics of the ethinyl estrogens: a review. Contraception 1977;15:255.
278. Friedman CI, Hunek AL, Kim MH et al. The effect of ampicilin on oral contraceptive effectiveness. Obstet Gynecol 1980;55:33.
279. Neely JL, Abate M, Swinker M et al. The effect of doxycycline on serum levels of ethinyl estradiol, norethindrone, and endogenous progesterones. Obstet Gynecol 1991;77:416.
280. Murphy AA, Zacur HA, Charache P et al. The effect of tetracycline on levels of oral contraceptives. Am J Obstet Gynecol 1991;164:28.
281. Miguet JP, Vuitton D, Pessayre D et al. Jaundice from troleandomycin and oral contraceptives. Ann Intern Med 1980;92:434.
282. Meyer B, Müller F, Wessels P et al. A model to detect interactions between roxithromycin and oral contraceptives. Clin Pharmacol Ther 1990;47:671.
283. Chambers DM, Jefferson GC, Chambers M et al. Antipyrine elimination in saliva after low-dose combined or progestogen-only oral contraceptive steroids. Br J Clin Pharamacol 1982;13:229.
284. Jochemsen R, Van der Graaf M, Boeijinga JK et al. Influence of sex, menstrual cycle and oral contraception on the disposition of nitrazepam. Br J Clin Pharmacol 1982;13:319.
285. Legler UF, Benet LZ. Marked alterations in dose-dependent prednisolone kinetics in women taking oral contraceptives. Clin Pharmacol Ther 1986;39:425.
286. Krishnan KRR, France RD, Ellinwood EH. Tricyclic-induced akathisia in patients taking conjugated estrogens. Am J Pscyhiatry 1984;141:696.
287. Patwardhan RV, Desmond PV, Johnson RF et al. Impaired elimination of caffeine by oral contraceptive steroids. J Lab Clin Med 1980;95:603.
288. Kendall MJ, Quarterman CP, Jack DB et al. Metoprolol pharmacokinetics and the oral contraceptive pill. Br J Clin Pharmacol 1982;14:120.
289. Deray G, Le Hoang P, Cacoub P et al. Oral contraceptive interaction with cyclosporin. Lancet 1987;i:158.
290. Rivera JM, Iriarte LM, Lozano F et al. Possible estrogen-induced NMS. DICP Ann Pharmacother 1989;23:811.
291. Mönig H, Baese C, Heidemann HT et al. Effect of oral contraceptive steroids on the pharmacokinetics of phenprocoumon. Br J Clin Pharmacol 1990;30:115.
292. Patwardhan RV, Mitchell MC, Johnson RF et al. Differential effects of oral contraceptive steroids on the metabolism of benzodiazepines. Hepatology 1983;3:248.
293. Sonnenberg A, Koelz HR, Herz R et al. Limited usefulness of the breast test in evaluation of drug metabolism: a study in human oral contraceptive users treated with dimethylamino-antipyrine and diazepam. Hepatogastroenterology 1980;27:104.
294. Homeida M, Haliwell M, Branch RA. Effects of an oral contraceptive on hepatic size and antipyrine metabolism in premenopausal women. Clin Pharmacol Ther 1978;24:228.
295. Teunissen MWE, Srcvastava AK, Breimer DD. Influence of sex and oral contraceptives on antipyrine metabolite formation. Clin Pharmacol Ther 1982;32:240.
296. Rudolfsky S, Crawford JS. Some alterations in pattern of drug metabolism associated with pregnancy, oral contraceptives and the newly-born. Br J Anaesth 1966;38:446.
297. Jones M, Morgan Jones B. Ethanol metabolism in women taking oral contraceptives. J Am Med Soc Alcohol Res Soc Alcohol 1984;8:24.
298. Da Vanzo J, Parnell AM, Foege WH. Health consequences of contraceptive use and reproductive patterns. Summary of a report from the US National Research Council. J Am Med Assoc 1991:265:2692.
299. Szarewski A, Guillebaud J. Contraception. Current state of the art. Br Med J 1991;302:1224.
300. Vessey MP, Doll R. Evaluation of existing techniques: is 'the pill' safe enough to continue using? Proc R Soc Med 1976;195:69.
301. Fotherby K, Caldwell ADS. New progestogens in oral contraception. Contraception 1994;49:1.
302 Kaunitz AM. Combined oral contraception with desogestrel/ethinyl estradiol: tolerability profile. Am J Obstet Gynecol 1993;168:1028.
303. Kuhl H, Jung-Hoffmann C, Heidt F. Alterations in the serum levels of gestodene and SHBG during 12 cycles of treatment with 30 μg ethinylestradiol and 75 μg gestodene. Contraception 1988:38:477.
304. Kuhl H, Jung-Hoffmann C, Heidt F. Serum levels of 3-keto-desogestrel and SHBG during 12 cycles of treatment with 30 μg ethinylestradiol and 150 μg desogestrel. Contraception 1988;38:381.
305. Jung-Hoffmann C, Kuhl H. Interaction with the pharmacokinetics of ethinylestradiol and progestogens contained in oral contraceptives. Contraception 1989;40:299.
306. Kaul L, Curry CL, Ahluwalia BS. Blood levels of ethinylestradiol, caffeine, aldosterone and desoxycorticosterone in hypertensive oral contraceptive users. Contraception 1981;23:643.
307. Stadel BC, Sternthal PM, Schlesselman JJ et al. Variation of ethinylestradiol blood levels among healthy women using oral contraceptives. Fertil Steril 1980;33:257.
308. Jung-Hoffmann C, Kuhl H. Pharmacokinetic cross-over studies with low dosed oral contraceptives. Acta Endocrinol 1991;124(Suppl 1):78.
309. Dibbelt L, Knuppen R, Jütting G. Group comparison of serum ethinylestradiol, CBG and SHBG concentrations in 83 women using two low-dose combination oral contraceptive for three months. Acta Endocrinol 1991;124(Suppl 1):79.
310. Guengerich FP. Oxidation of 17-ethinylestradiol by

human liver cytochrome P-450. Mol Pharmacol 1988; 33:500.

311. WHO Task Force for Epidemiological Research on Reproductive Health. Progestogen-only contraceptives during lactation: I. Infant growth. Contraception 1994;50:35.

312. WHO Task Force for Epidemiological Research on Reproductive Health. Progestogen-only contraceptives during lactation: II. Infant development. Contraception 1994;50:55.

313. Kennedy KI, Rivera R, McNeilly AS. Consensus statement on the use of breastfeeding as a family planning method. Contraception 1989;39:478.

314. Ball MJ, Ashwell E, Gillmer MDG. Progestagen-only oral contraceptives: comparison of the metabolic effects of levonorgestrel and norethisterone. Contraception 1991; 44:223.

315. Mall-Haefeli M. Was bringt die Micropille? Ther Umschau 1986;43:365.

316. Fraser IS. Menstrual changes associated with progestogen-only contraception. Acta Obstet Gynaecol Scand 1986; (Suppl 134):21.

317. Deteuf M, Kuttenn F. Hyperestrogénie sous contraception par micropilule progestative. Contracept Fertil Sex 1982;10:377.

318. World Health Organization. Injectable Hormonal Contraceptives. Technical and Safety Aspects. WHO Publication No. 65, Geneva, 1982.

319. World Health Organization. Multinational comparative clinical trial of long-acting injectable contraceptives: norethisterone enanthate given in two dosage regimens and depot-medroxyprogesterone acetate: final report. Contraception 1983;28:1.

320. Fraser I, Holck SE. Depot-medroxyprogesterone acetate. In: Mishell D, ed. Advances in Contraceptive Technology, 1982.

321. Holck SE. Safety and effectiveness of long-acting injectable contraceptives. In: Proceedings, International Symposium on Hormonal Contraception, Basle, 1983.

322. Nash HA. Depo Provera: a review. Contraception 1975;12:377.

323. Kaunitz AM. Long-acting injectable contraception with depot medroxyprogesterone acetate. Am J Obstet Gynecol 1994;170:1543.

324. Hyazi Y, Maes E, Hurlet A et al. Acétate de médroxyprogestérone-dépôt: effets cliniques et métaboliques (lipides, glucose, hémostase). J Gynecol Obstet Biol Reprod 1985; 14:93.

325. Fraser IS. Vaginal bleeding patterns in women using once-a-month injectable contraceptives. Contraception 1994;49:399.

326. WHO Task Force on Long-Acting Systemic Agents for Fertility Regulation. A multicentre comparative study of serum lipids and apolipoproteins in long-term users of DMPA and a control group of IUD users. Contraception 1993;47:177.

327. Kamau RK, Maina FW, Kigondu C et al. The effect of low-oestrogen combined pill, progestogen-only pill and medroxyprogesterone acetate on oral glucose tolerance test. East Afr Med J 1990;67:550.

328. Rehle T, Brinkmann UK, Siraprapasiri T et al. Risk factors of HIV-1 infection among female prostitutes in Khon Kaen, Northeast Thailand. Infection 1992;20:328.

329. deCeulaer K, Gruber C, Hayes R et al. Medroxyprogesterone acetate and homozygous sickle-cell disease. Lancet 1982:229.

330. Fotherby K, Howard G. Return of fertility in women discontinuing injectable contraceptives. J Obstet Gynaecol 1986;6(Suppl 2):110.

331. Joshi UM, Virkar KD, Amatayakul K et al. Metabolic side effects of injectable depot-medroxyprogesterone acetate, 150 mg three-monthly, in undernourished lactating women. Bull WHO 1986;64:587.

332. Skegg DC et al. Depot medroxyprogesterone acetate and breast cancer: a pooled analysis of the World Health Organization and New Zealand studies. J Am Med Assoc 1995;273:799.

333. Pisake L. Depot-medroxyprogesterone acetate (DMPA) and cancer of the endometrium and ovary. Contraception 1994;49:203.

334. LaVecchia CL. Depot-medroxyprogesterone acetate, other injectable contraceptives, and cervical neoplasia. Contraception 1994;49:223.

335. Cundy T, Cornish J, Evans MC et al. Recovery of bone density in women who stop using medroxyprogesterone acetate. Br Med J 1994;308:247.

336. Cavalli F, Goldhirsch A, Jungi F et al. Randomized trial of low- versus high-dose medroxyprogesterone acetate in the induction treatment of postmenopausal patients with advanced breast cancer. J Clin Oncol 1984;2:414.

337. Hedley D, Tattersall MHN, Dalgleish A. Advanced breast cancer: response to high dose oral medroxyprogesterone acetate. Aust NZ J Med 1984;14:251.

338. Johansson J-E, Lingardh G. High-dose medroxyprogesterone in the treatment of advanced therapy resistant prostatic carcinoma. Eur Urol 1985;11:9.

339. Mahlke M, Grill H-J, Knapstein P et al. Oral high-dose medroxyprogesterone acetate (MPA) treatment: cortisol/MPA serum profiles in relation to breast cancer regression. Oncology 1985;42:144.

340. Salem HT, Salah M, Aly MY et al. Acceptability of injectable contraceptives in Assiut, Egypt. Contraception 1988;38:697.

341. Kazi AI. Comparative evaluation of two once-a-month contraceptive injections. J Pale Med Assoc 1989;39:98.

342. Howard G, Blair M, Fotherby K et al. Seven years clinical experience of the injectable contraceptive, noresthisterone oenanthate. Br J Fam Plann 1985;11:9.

343. Chowdhury TA. A clinical study of injectable contraceptive Noristerat. Bangladesh Med J 1985;14:28.

344. Kazi A, Holck S, Diethelm P. Phase IV study of the injection Norigest in Pakistan. Contraception 1985;32:395.

345. Han Ziyan, Xiao Ruiqui. A follow-up study of the efficacy and safety ofinjectable microencapsulated megestrol acetate and a discussion on its contraceptive mechanism. Int J Gynecol Obstet 1985;23:207.

346. Hall PE. Clinical trial of the monthly injectable contraceptives, cycloprovera and HRP 102. In: Zatuchni GI et al, eds. Long-acting Contraceptive Delivery Systems. Philadelphia: Harper and Row, 1984.

347. Alvarez F, Brache V, Tejeda AS et al. Abnormal endocrine profile among women with confirmed or presumed ovulation during long-term Norplant® use. Contraception 1986;33:111.

348. Hingorani V, Jalinawala SF, Kochhar M. Phase II randomized comparative clinical trial of Norplant® (six capsules) with Norplant® (two covered rods) subdermal implants for long term contraception: report of a 24-month study. Contraception 1986;33:233.

349. Shoupe D, Mishell DR. Norplant: subdermal implant

system for long-term contraception. Am J Obstet Gynecol 1989;160:1266.
350. Singh K, Viegas OAC, Liew D et al. The effects of Norplant-2 rods: one year experience in Singapore. Contraception 1988;38:429.
351. Croxatto HB. NORPLANT: Levonorgestrel-releasing contraceptive implant. Ann Med 1993;25:155.
352. Pasquale SA, Knuppel RA, Owens AG et al. Irregular bleeding, body mass index and coital frequency in Norplant contraceptive users. Contraception 1994;50:109.
353. Shoupe D, Mishell DR, Bopp BL et al. The significance of bleeding patterns in Norplant implant users. Obstet Gynecol 1991;77:256.
354. Davies GC, Newton JR. Subdermal contraceptive implants—a review: with special reference to Norplant. Br J Fam Plann 1991;17:4.
355. Balogh SA, Klavon SL, Basnayake S et al. Bleeding pattern and acceptability among Norplant users in two Asian countries. Contraception 1989;39:541.
356 Wagner KD, Berenson AB. Norplant-associated major depression and panic disorder. J Clin Psychiatry 1994;55:478.
357. Singh K, Viegas OAC, Loke DFM et al. Evaluation of liver function and lipid metabolism following Norplant-2 rods removal. Adv Contracept 1993;9:233.
358. Konje JC, Otolorin EO, Odukoya OA et al. Return of ovulation after removal of Norplant subdermal implants. Br J Fam Plann 1992;18:44.
359. Singh K, Viegas OAC, Loke D et al. Effect of Norplant-2 rods on liver, lipid and carbohydrate metabolism. Contraception 1992;45:463.
360. Shaaban MM, Elwan SI, El-Kabsh MY et al. Effect of levonorgestrel contraceptive implants, Norplant, on blood coagulation. Contraception 1984;30:421.
361. Klavon SL, Grubb GS. Insertion site complications during the first year of NORPLANT use. Contraception 1990;41:27.
362. Wysowski DK, Green L. Serious adverse events in Norplant users reported to the Food and Drug Administration's MedWatch spontaneous reporting system. Obstet Gynecol 1995;85:538.
363. Gu SJ, Du MK, Zhang LD et al. A 5-year evaluation of NORPLANT contraceptive implants in China. Obstet Gynecol 1994;83:673.
364. Dunson TR, Amaty RM, Krueger SL. Complications and risk factors associated with the removal of Norplant Implants. Obstet Gynecol 1995;85:543.
365. Darney PD, Monroe SC, Klaisle CM et al. Clinical evaluation of the Capronor contraceptive implant: preliminary report. Am J Obstet Gynecol 1989;160:1292.
366. Croxatto HD, Diaz S, Rosati S et al. Adnexal complications in women under treatment with progestogen implants. Contraception 1976;12:629.
367. Gupta G, Saxena BB, Landesman R et al. Preparation, properties, and release rate of norethindrone (NET) from subcutaneous implants. In: Zatuchni GI, Goldsmith A, Shelton JD et al, eds. Long-Acting Contraceptive Delivery Systems. Harper and Row, Philadelphia, 1984:425.
368. Diaz S, Pavez M, Moo-Young AJ et al. Clinical trials with 3-keto-desogestrel subdermal implants. Contraception 1991;44:393.
369. Coutinho EM, Silva AR, Carreira C et al. Ovulation inhibition following vaginal administration of pills containing norethindrone and mestranol. Contraception 1984;29:197.
370. Ji G, Hong-zhu S, Gui-ying S. Clinical investigation of a low-dose levonorgestrel releasing vaginal ring. Fertil Steril 1986;46:626.
371. Ratsula K. Clinical performance of a levonorgestrel-releasing intracervical contraceptive device during the first two years of use. Contraception 1989;39:187.
372. Haspels AA, Van Santen MR. Post coital contraception. J Gynaecol Endocrinol 1986;11:17.
373. Haspels AA, Van Santen MR. Postcoital contraception. Pediatr Adolesc Gynecol 1984;2:63.
374. Reader FC. Emergency contraception. Br Med J 1991;302:801.
375. Trussell J, Stewart F, Guest F et al. Emergency contraceptive pills: a simple proposal to reduce unintended pregnancies. Fam Plann Perspect 1992;24:269.
376. Glasier A, Thong KJ, Dewar M et al. Postcoital contraception with mifepristone. Lancet 1991;337:1414.
377. Glasier A, Thong KJ, Dewar M et al. Mifepristone (RU 486) compared with high-dose estrogen and progestogen for emergency postcoital contraception. N Engl J Med 1992;327:1041.
378. Odlind V. Review: New methods for fertility regulation in women. Clin Reprod Fertil 1987;3:221.
379. Sivin I. Dose- and age-dependent ectopic pregnancy risks with intrauterine contraception. Obstet Gynecol 1991;78:291.
380. Toivonen J, Luukkainen T, Allonen H. Protective effect of intrauterine release of levonorgestrel on pelvic infection: three years' comparative experience of levonorgestrel- and copper-releasing intrauterine devices. Obstet Gynecol 1991; 77:261.
381. Robinson GE, Bounds W, Kubba AA et al. Functional ovarian cysts associated with the levonorgestrel releasing intrauterine device. J Fam Plann 1989;14:131.
382. Barbosa I, Bakos O, Olsson S-E et al. Ovarian function during use of a levonorgestrel-releasing IUD. Contraception 1990;42:51.
383. World Health Organization. Effect of different progestagens in low oestrogen oral contraceptives on venous thromboembolic disease. Lancet 1995:346:1582—1588.
384. Jick H, Jick SS, Gurewich V et al. Risk of idiopathic cardiovascular death and nonfatal venous thromboembolism in women using oral contraceptives with differing progestagen components. Lancet 1995; 346:1589—1592.
385. Spitzer WO, Lewis MA, Heinemann LAJ et al. Third generation oral contraceptives and risk of venous thromboembolic disorders: an international case-control study. Br Med J 1996:312:83—87.
386. WHO Collaborating Centre for International Drug Monitoring. Oral contraceptives. Adverse Reaction Newsletter 1996, No 2:8—11.
387. Committee on Safety of Medicines. Combined oral contraceptives and thromboembolism (letter). London, 18 October 1995.

Meyler's Side Effects of Drugs, 13th Edition
M.N.G. Dukes, editor

SECTION EDITOR: B. VRHOVAC

M.N.G. Dukes

40.2 Sex hormones

Editorial note *It is not possible to separate the discussion of adverse reactions to hormonal contraceptives (Chapter* 40.1) *strictly from the present review of adverse reactions to estrogens, progestogens and related sex hormones used for other indications. The more immediate effects, such as thromboembolism, are mainly dealt with under oral contraceptives, while later effects, such as tumorigenicity and second-generation effects, will for this entire series of compounds be discussed in this Chapter.*

SECOND-GENERATION EFFECTS OF FEMALE SEX HORMONES *(see also Chapter 40.1)*

In 1980, an authoritative Scientific Group of the World Health Organization (WHO) surveyed the entire question of the effects of female sex hormones on fetal development and infant health (1^R) and after 16 years one can conclude that later reports in the literature have almost entirely supported its conclusions. They are still reflected at many points in the review which follows.

Chromosomal abnormalities The fear that oral contraceptives might induce chromosomal abnormalities was expressed when they were relatively new, but largely laid to rest. When aborted fetuses from women who used oral contraceptives were compared with those from non-users, no difference could be demonstrated in the frequency of abnormal karyotypes or in the sex ratio between the two groups. Certainly, data have been presented showing a slightly raised frequency of minor chromosomal changes in children whose mothers had been exposed to oral contraceptives before pregnancy, but from a genetic point of view, these scattered findings are not alarming.

Sex of offspring Slight evidence has been put forward in the past that the use of oral contraceptives might result in a predominance of female births. Later evidence on the issue has been indecisive; if there is any effect at all it must be extremely slight. Interestingly enough, the same type of evidence is now coming to the fore as regards the outcome of pregnancy in women successfully treated for sterility (see later).

Congenital abnormalities A number of American studies reviewed in previous editions of this volume appeared to show that children exposed in utero to oral contraceptives ran a slightly increased risk of being born with certain types of birth defects; in particular a 'syndrome' was identified comprising multiple malformations involving the vertebrae, anus, cardiac structures, trachea, esophagus, renal structures and limbs (abbreviated to 'VACTERL'). The entire VACTERL syndrome was in fact seldom or never encountered; clusters of defects falling within this group were seen, but the associations were very variable. Furthermore, virilization of the female fetus and some of the other elements in the VACTERL group have been described following exposure to certain progestogens, hormonal pregnancy tests or (rarely) to oral contraceptives taken in error in early pregnancy.

McCredie et al. (2^C) published in 1983 a retrospective study on 155 children with congenital limb reductions: 18 mothers (12%) were found to have taken oral contraceptives inadvertently during early pregnancy compared with only one mother in a control group, pointing to a relative risk of 23.9; adjustment for smoking hardly altered the figure. Other work has however indicated that smoking carries a higher risk of malformations than the use of oral contraceptives (SED-12, 1022).

The results of such studies have led some reviewers to conclude that oral contraceptives are slightly teratogenic, but caution is needed; the conclusion of the 1980 WHO report cited above that such an effect is slight or absent probably remains valid for all widely used oral contraceptives: naturally, newer products might have other effects.

Congenital malformations may well occur after the use of hormonal (estrogen/progestogen) pregnancy tests, now obsolete, since these high doses of a hormonal combination represented an aggressive interference with any early pregnancy which might exist. A 1967 report suggested some association with meningomyelocele or hydrocephalus, and later retrospective studies provided some evidence of cardiac defects or limb reduction anomalies. Such studies always raise methodological doubts, but it is not unthinkable that these tests were harmful, since they sometimes induced bleeding even in early pregnancy; they could thus derange embryonic nutrition.

With regard to progestogens given alone to prevent threatened or habitual abortion, there is no good evidence of beneficial effects, and much evidence to the contrary; effects on the sexual development of the fetus cannot however be excluded (3[R]; see also section on progestogens later in this Chapter).

Late effects: the diethylstilbestrol (DES) story DES, a non-steroidal estrogen, was used extensively in pregnancies between 1940 and about 1975 in the belief that it could protect pregnancy and counter the risk of spontaneous abortion. So far, DES is the only estrogen known to have an effect on the fetus which leads to an adverse reaction which does not become apparent until puberty or adulthood, and perhaps extends even to third-generation injury. It is naturally not excluded that some structurally related non-steroidal estrogens might have the same effect, but these have never been used in the same way in pregnancy.

The causal relationship is here well established and has been reviewed in the literature and repeatedly in these volumes; unfortunately, despite the abandonment of DES treatment in pregnancy for habitual or threatened abortion, the late effects continue to be reported. It was indeed not until some 12—15 years after the peak of its use had passed that it was found that female children of these pregnancies tended to develop vaginal changes (adenosis, with cervical ectropion) when reaching adolescence or adulthood and that these could give rise to a clear-cell adenocarcinoma. Whereas carcinomas are a late and infrequent event, even in exposed subjects, cervical vaginal adenosis is common, the incidence probably being some 30% (4[r]). The estimated tumor risk is only 0.14—1.4 per 1000 DES-exposed subjects, but since up to 6 million persons were exposed in utero to DES between 1940 and 1970 the total number of victims may be very high indeed. There is also a high incidence of fertility disturbances among these daughters, and their own pregnancies apparently stand a high chance of not going normally to term (SED-12, 1023; 5[CR]). Analogous changes were found in the male offspring (6[c]). As in the thalidomide case, an important element in determining cause and effect was the characteristic nature of the defect: the vaginal pathology does occur spontaneously but is highly unusual. A major problem has been the fact that the defect is as a rule only recognizable many years after birth, at which time the history of the original treatment may be difficult or impossible to reconstruct. Even today the material is not homogeneous and strict statistical analysis of some of the epidemiological data has been claimed to point to a series of shortcomings. This does not undermine the clear conclusion that the drug is indeed responsible for the effects described (7[R]).

Epidemiological studies on the complications of DES use in pregnancy will certainly produce new data as time goes on: most of the data will probably continue to come from the United States and The Netherlands, where DES was much more widely used to treat habitual or threatened abortion than elsewhere. In France 150 000—200 000 pregnancies were involved; in The Netherlands, with a much smaller population, 180 000—380 000 pregnant women were treated with DES up to 1976.

Second- (and possible third-) generation effects of DES continue to be reported yearly and are reviewed in the *Side Effects of Drugs Annuals* and elsewhere (8[R], 9[R]). Typical is a 1987 update analyzing 519 cases of clear-cell carcinoma of the vagina and cervix identified by the Registry for Research on Hormonal Transplacental Carcinogenesis of the University of Chicago (10[C]); in 60% of all cases the patient's mother had received DES during pregnancy. The median age at diagnosis was 19.0 years. The authors argue that in view of the relative rarity of the tumors, even in exposed women, one could consider that DES is not a complete carcinogen and that some other factor is also involved in the pathogenesis of this carcinoma.

During the last decade, various additional aspects of this problem have given rise to concern. One emerged in 1988 from a large multicenter epidemiological cohort study established by the US National Cancer Institute (DESAD Project): it was found here that the women exposed in utero to DES had a 50% increased incidence of *autoimmune disease* (11[C]). Another worrying finding appears to be emerging from the current case-reports and discussions in litigation strongly suggesting that some of the changes induced by DES indeed continue to appear in the *third generation* (see above).

Baseline exposure to estrogens (*SEDA*-18, 394) In 1993, Sharpe and Skakkebaek published a theory that environmental and other forms of exposure to estrogens, particularly during fetal life, might explain the increasing incidence of reduced sperm counts and developmental disorders of the male genital system (12). Such exposure could be in part due, for example, to dietary changes in mothers: a low-fiber diet results in a great reabsorption of endogenous estrogens, and there is an increasing use in the diet of soya, which is a rich source of phytoestrogens. The topic goes beyond the scope of this volume, but it is not impossible that baseline exposure to estrogens in the diet or environment could increase the sensitivity of individuals to estrogens which are administered therapeutically or for purposes of contraception.

SEX STEROIDS AND TUMOR INDUCTION

Knowledge of tumor induction by sex steroids is largely based on interpretation of epidemiological data, with careful exclusion of possible confounding elements.

Liver tumors In dealing with liver tumors, it is essential to consider all the various types of sex steroids in a single review since they seem to resemble one another closely in their long-term effects on this organ. The nomenclature used in the literature is unfortunately confusing: most reports differentiate between 'hepatic adenoma' and 'focal nodular hyperplasia', but the latter term is also sometimes employed to cover the whole range. Other terms, which have been used are 'focal cirrhosis', 'regenerative hyperplasia', 'hamartoma', 'mixed adenoma' and 'benign hepatoma'.

Androgens and anabolics As will be pointed out later in this Chapter, there is no essential difference between androgens and 'anabolics'. High doses of either, such as maybe used in refractory anemias, have been associated with the induction of benign liver tumors as well as primary hepatocellular carcinoma.

The fact that primary hepatoma, liver adenoma and peliosis are uncommon conditions and that only a tiny fraction of the population is receiving high-dose androgens strongly suggests that the association of both events is more than a coincidence (13[C]): some animal studies and in vitro studies also indeed point to a hepatocarcinogenic effect of 'anabolic' compounds. No cases seem to have been described in sportsmen who have used high-dose androgens or in girls suffering from precocious puberty but the former, at least, often use these drugs for a relatively short period; longer-term use is likely to be surreptitious and thus poorly documented. Most of the widely used compounds in this class, including methyltestosterone, have been reported to induce liver tumors. The apparent exceptions are the nortestosterone derivatives without 17α-substitution. Whether these drugs are indeed safer or whether they have merely been employed less frequently for high-dose therapy is not known.

The incidence of liver tumors following the use of androgens and anabolic steroids (see also later in this Chapter) still cannot be calculated. What is clear is that if these products are indeed to be used in high doses or over periods of time—and there is now much doubt as to whether they are effective in such indications as osteoporosis and aplastic anemia—techniques such as computed tomographic scanning and ultrasonographic examination should be employed for early detection of any liver lesions which appear.

Oral contraceptives, estrogens and benign liver tumors The effects of oral contraceptives on the liver comprise not only benign liver tumors (focal nodular hyperplasia, hepatic adenoma and hemangioma) (14[c]) and hepatocellular carcinoma but also peliosis hepatitis (15[CR]), sinusoid dilatations (16[r]), and such probably unrelated complications as jaundice and gallstones (see Chapter 40.1).

The causal association between oral contraceptive use and *benign tumors* can be considered well documented in humans, and the same problem clearly arises with conjugated estrogens (17[CR]), diethylstilbestrol and probably antiestrogens. The evidence for the link is based on very numerous case reports from the field, reviewed in the *Annuals* in this series, but also on some case-control studies. Studies of the latter type first appeared in 1976 and 1981, and both pointed to a correlation (SED-12, 1024). The relative risk of benign liver tumours in users of conjugated estrogens or oral contraceptives as compared to non-users may be about 40:1, although the figure is still low in absolute terms. Animal studies indicate that estrogens alone or in combination with progestogens can increase the size of pre-existing liver tumors, but do not initiate tumor formation themselves; whether these preparations are actually inducing tumors or promoting a latent tendency to tumor development is not of essential importance. Although there is some evidence that liver cell adenoma can regress after oral contraceptives are withdrawn (SEDA-15, 347; 18[C]) they do not always do so (19[C]). It is clear that any woman with 'pill'-associated liver lesions should avoid all further use of hormonal contraceptives and related products.

Oral contraceptives and malignant liver cancer Malignant cancer of the liver is still a very rare disease in young women, but case-control studies can be carried out. Evidence from both sides of the Atlantic suggested from 1987 onwards that a significant relationship might exist between oral contraceptives and hepatocellular carcinoma (20[r], 21[r], 22[C]). Even the best of these studies however had some limitations, e.g., incomplete data as regards a past history of hepatitis or the extent of contraceptive use. One authoritative attempt to estimate the degree of risk was made by WHO in 1989, matching 122 newly diagnosed cases of primary liver cancer to 802 controls; the relative risk of liver cancer in women who had ever used combined oral contraceptives was estimated to be 0.71; no consistent link with months of use or time since first or last use was observed (23[C]). A major examination of the issue by Hsing et al. appeared in 1992, and used both material from the US National Mortality Followback Survey and the group's own work; it was concluded that the relative risk for sometime users of OCs was 1.6, rising to 2.0 in those using the products for more than 10 years (24[CR]).

The issue is by no means simple to resolve and the ultimate answer may not be a simple one. Prentice and Thomas, who reviewed the earliest studies on hepatocellular carcinoma, concluded that oral contraceptives may not interact with other hepatic carcinogens, and may not be found to enhance measurably the risk of liver cancer in parts of the world where hepatitis B virus (HBV) is endemic and hepatocellular carcinoma is common (25[R]). Others have since then suggested a positive association between parity or gravidity and hepatocellular carcinoma, which needs to be further explored (SEDA-17, 458).

Tumors of the genital system *Hormonal replacement therapy and endometrial carcinoma* In untreated women, the main risk factors for endometrial carcinoma are age, obesity, nulliparity, late menopause (and possibly early menarche), the Stein-Leventhal syndrome, certain systemic diseases including diabetes mellitus, hypertension, hypothyroidism and arthritis, radiation, and exposure to exogenous estrogens (SED-12, 1024; 26[C]). Certain of these risk factors indicate that an altered endocrine state with increased estrogen stimulation is a predisposing cause, and one might thus in theory expect estrogen treatment (and notably hormonal replacement therapy) to increase the risk.

Two epidemiological studies published in 1975 first indicated that estrogen use during and after the menopause did indeed increase the risk of endometrial cancer, and in 1986 an authoritative review (27[R]) endorsed these findings, concluding that there was a 4—9-fold increase in risk among users, relative to non-users; the risk increased with both the strength of the medication and the duration of use. A 1990 review of data up to that time indicated that estrogen replacement therapy for over 2 years without concurrent progesterone therapy was associated with an approximately three-fold increase in risk for both localized and extra-uterine cancer; this risk was found to increase with duration of use and to persist for over 6 years after discontinuation of therapy (28[R]). These studies have been criticized from a methodological point of view, particularly since, as Horwitz and Feinstein had noted earlier (29[CR]), there is evidence of a detection bias that arises from the increased diagnostic attention received by women with uterine bleeding after estrogen exposure and perhaps also from a greater tendency of women to bleed from a pre-existing tumor when estrogens are given. It could be that the magnitude of the association between estrogens and endometrial cancer has been greatly overestimated for such reasons and that the real odds ratio is less than estimated, but it seems unlikely that the risk can be disproved. There is, for example, some older evidence that even where the above-mentioned bias has largely been eliminated, there is still a correlation between estrogen use and endometrial carcinoma, the evidence being strongest for the 'first-generation' oral contraceptive products containing large amounts of estrogen. One such study (30[CR]) still found a six-fold risk among estrogen users compared with non-users; long-term users (over 5 years) had a 15-fold risk; excess risk was present for both diethylstilbestrol and conjugated estrogens. Another well-controlled study, from 1986, similarly found increased risk with conjugated estrogens, the greatest increases in risk being associated with a dosage of 0.625 mg or greater, and duration of use of 10 years or more (31[C]). Although according to this study the risk remained elevated even among women who had stopped using conjugated estrogens 5 or more years previously, one may not ignore an earlier finding by Jick et al. (32[CR]) from evidence in a large group practice that a sharp downward trend in the incidence of endometrial cancer did occur parallel with a substantial reduction in prescriptions for replacement estrogens.

Among the many papers which have since then incriminated estrogens, particularly the conjugated estrogens so widely used in North America, there are some which present more subtle conclusions. One paper specifically incriminates estrone (33[C]), but this is of course a major component of conjugated estrogens. A case-control study from Buffalo, NY, found that while histories of menopausal estrogen use did not differ between endometrium cancer patients and healthy controls, estrogen users had a significantly higher frequency of low-grade tumors with a correspondingly better survival rate (34[C]).

Menopausal estrogens became popular much later in Europe, and relatively little evidence has emerged to complement the US findings. In 1983, however, when Persson in Sweden completed a very large cohort study, he found that while among women treated with estrogens there was no significant increase in endometrial cancer compared with the control population, there was indeed a significantly increased incidence of premalignant lesions among women using estrogens alone for more than 3 years (35[CR]). A long and continuing case-control study in a Swiss population points in the same direction; use of HRT for 5 years or more creates a mean relative risk of 1.9, use for 5 years or more creates a relative risk of 5.1 (CI 2.7–9.8) (36[CR]). This, as well as existing evidence that progestogens have some protective effect on the endometrium (37[R]), emphasizes the need for prospective studies in different sub-populations using different types of replacement therapy. Such studies may also help to clarify further the risk factors; there is for example an impression that the risk is greater in lean than in overweight women, while the risk may be less in women who have a history of having used oral contraceptives as well.

In summary Although our knowledge is still incomplete and needs to be extended, it is highly likely that estrogen replacement therapy given without progestagens does indeed considerably increase the risk of endometrial cancer both during and after treatment. Because of the evidence that progestogens provide partial protection of the endometrium (and might, if one knew how to employ them optimally, provide substantial protection) they are today correctly incorporated in many regimens of estrogen therapy in postmenopausal women.

Oral contraceptives and endometrial cancer Here too, suggestive case histories raised, at an early phase, the notion of a possible correlation. As noted above, among cases of endometrial cancer there indeed seemed to be an excess of users of oral contraceptives, particularly of the early high-estrogen type. With the virtual demise of these early products, the situation seems to have reversed itself: a 1983 study from the CDC in Atlanta (38[C]) found that women who had used fixed combinations for oral contraception at some time in their lives had a relative risk of endometrial cancer of only 0.5 as compared with never-users. The protective effect occurred only in women who had used oral contraception for at least 12 months, and lasted for at least 10 years after cessation. A further population-based case-control study 4 years later came to a similar conclusion, and found that the protection persisted for at least 15 years after discontinuation (SED-12, 1043). WHO adopted the same view in 1988 in the light of multinational data (39[C]). As in the case of hormonal replacement therapy, the protective effect seems to be due to the progestogen component.

Oral contraceptives, cervical neoplasms and adenosis A 1988 statistical analysis of data from the Royal College of General Practitioners study in Britain pointed clearly to an association between oral contraceptive use and cervical neoplasms (40[C]); of 47 000 women followed since 1965, those who had at some time used oral contraceptives ('ever-users') had a significantly higher incidence rate of cervical cancer than 'never-users' after standardization of other variables including a history of sexually transmitted disease. The incidence increased with increasing duration of use, attaining four-fold control values after 10 years of use. Other studies (41[C], 42[cr]) similarly found an increased risk with increased duration of use but also with the use of 'pills' containing a higher proportion of estrogen or in users having a history of genital infections or abnormal Pap smears. Benign cervical *adenosis* and adenomatous *polyps* have been seen in oral contraceptive users and were prominent in some early reports (SED-11, 857). They often (but do not always) disappear when medication is stopped.

By the mid 1980s it was fair to conclude that: (a) oral contraceptive use did not appear to increase the subsequent incidence of abnormal cytology among women who had normal smears at the time they began to use the products; (b) extended oral contraceptive use (over 6 years) appeared to increase by several times the rate of conversion of pre-existing cervical dysplasia to carcinoma in situ. Generally speaking, subsequent data have tended to be compatible with those conclusions, e.g. pointing to an increased incidence of micro-invasive cervical carcinoma and again stressing the changes in cytology and the extent to which the effect may differ with the strength and composition of the product. The average risk figures which emerge are generally in line with those found in a northern Norwegian study published in 1992 where, after correcting for other risk factors, relative rates were found of 1.5 for current users and 1.4 for past users as compared with 'never users' (SEDA-17, 456). Clearly, confounding factors such as differences in sexual activity, age at first coitus and the number of sexual partners can confuse the issue and render study more complex (43[CR]). In addition, any discussion of the issue must today take into account the current view of the human papilloma virus (HPV) as a sexually transmitted agent which is now accepted as the main cause of cervical cancer (44[C]), and the possible influence of herpes simplex virus type 2, smoking and other known or emergent risk factors.

The most authoritative view on cervical cancer at present is that expressed by WHO in 1992:

> 'Recent studies suggest that use of oral contraceptives for more than 5 years is associated with a modest increase in relative risk (ranging from 1.3 to 1.8). The extent to which this reflects a biological relationship is uncertain, particularly given the absence of reliable information on the role of possible infectious agents, such as the human papilloma viruses . . .' (45[R]).

To summarize In the present state of knowledge, all

women taking oral contraceptives over long periods should undergo regular routine screening by cervical cytology to ensure early detection of premalignant and malignant processes.

Uterine fibroids In a long-term follow-up study in Scandinavia published in 1986 the risk of fibroids was found to *decrease* consistently with increasing duration of oral contraceptive use (SEDA-12, 340). A decade earlier, the British Royal College of Physicians study had similarly suggested a protective effect, while an Oxford study had not, but once more the issue is confused by the change in composition of oral contraceptives over the years, and more recent papers thus carry the most weight. On the other hand a causal relationship between apoplectic leiomyomas and oral contraceptive usage was strongly suggested by Myles and Hart in the light of their 1985 study of five histologically distinctive uterine smooth muscle neoplasms with multifocal hemorrhages (46[C]). The effects of hormonal steroids on the blood vessels in pre-existing leiomyomas may in their view be responsible for intimal hyperplasia with or without accompanying thrombi.

Oral contraceptives, estrogens and ovarian tumors Two major British prospective studies of 1974 and 1976 (47[CR], 48[R]) indicated that *oral contraceptive treatment* was unrelated to the development of benign ovarian tumors; these and other studies also indicated that follicular and lutein cysts are suppressed in women using oral contraceptives. With regard to ovarian cancer, somewhat later data indicated a decreased risk in oral contraceptive users; impressive case-control work from the US in 1981 (49[C]) seemed to show this protective effect when oral contraceptives had been taken for 4 years or more, the risk of ovarian cancer then being decreased by a mean of some 40%; the effect was even greater when the contraceptives had been used for a longer period. Very similarly, in 1988, a multi-country study backed by WHO indicated that ever-users of combined oral contraceptives had a risk rate which was only 71% of that in non-users, while women who had used oral contraceptives for 5 or more years had about a 50% reduction in risk (SEDA-12, 1026). It should be added, however, that not all reviewers find these trends significant.

With *conjugated estrogens* the risk of ovarian cancer was stated in 1977 to *increase* two- to three-fold (SED-12, 1026), but this was based primarily on findings in women who had also taken diethylstilbestrol, and the conclusion was therefore not generally accepted. A 1982 paper which found an apparent slight increase in ovarian epithelial carcinoma among American women taking estrogens is similarly open to challenge (SEDA-7, 385) and the link cannot be regarded as established (50[r]).

Breast neoplasms (51[R]) Shortly after the first oral contraceptives were introduced, around 1959, the fact that some women noticed acute effects on the breast led to fears that the ultimate consequence might be the induction of mammary disorders, particularly tumors; the same concerns were raised about replacement therapy. The debate on this issue has now continued for more than 30 years and it is characterized by contradictions, discrepancies in scientific findings, qualified statements and controversies and, all in all, a massive output of data and opinions. The present review will necessarily be confined to some of the highlights of the discussion (presented in Table 1), leading up to a summary of the present situation and the questions which still remain open.

It is clear from Table 1 that there is obviously no simple relationship between treatment with hormonal oral contraceptives (or other products containing estrogens) and the incidence of breast cancer. As in the case of other neoplasms, studies are confounded by the influence of many factors including age, parity, age at first delivery, family history, pre-existent fibrocystic disease, geographical or environmental influences, the age at which the menarche and menopause occurred as well as by the progressive change in the spectrum of contraceptives in use. Information bias can easily mislead researchers. The possible influence on findings of the long latency likely to be involved in any effect has been heavily contested; breast tumors may have been present for many years by the time they become clinically detectable; hence many tumors induced by oral contraceptives may have so far been missed, but conversely oral contraceptives must often have been prescribed to women who unknowingly were already suffering from breast cancer. One must also bear in mind the apparently spontaneous increase in the incidence of breast cancer over the last 40 years. Finally, where cancers are found, there is little or nothing to distinguish them histologically from tumours arising spontaneously (SEDA-17, 456).

All in all, it would seem clear that there is no overall, measurable risk of inducing breast cancer by taking *oral contraceptives* for a number of years, but there are some possible risk situations which it is prudent to avoid, or in which frequent control of the state of the breasts is essential. These would be:

(a) Very long-term use before the first full pregnancy;
(b) Prolonged use of high-dose preparations;
(c) Uninterrupted use in women with a family history

Table 1. *Oral contraceptives (OC), hormone replacement therapy (HRT) and estrogens (E) and possible associations with breast neoplasms; selected literature*

WHO, 1978 (52[R])	Review of nine major studies of OC; decreased risk of breast cancer found in eight of them. Greater effect with higher doses; clinically significant with 2 years of use.
Herbst, 1978 (53[CR])	25-year follow up of women receiving DES in pregnancy; very slightly more breast tumors, significantly more cancer deaths.
Jick et al., 1979 (54[C])	HRT: positive link to breast cancer provided menopause was natural.
RCGP (UK), 1981 (55[C])	OC breast cancer link, but only in 30–34 age group; coincidental?
Pike et al., 1981 (56[C])	OC breast cancer link if used before first full-term pregnancy; high doses = more risk.
Vessey et al., 1981 (57[C])	Case control: no link between OC and breast cancer.
Hulka et al., 1982 (58[C])	History of breast cancer cases shows four-fold risk increase with injectable estrogens.
Ory et al., 1982 (59[C])	Case control: no link between OC and breast cancer.
Brinton et al., 1982 (60[C])	Case control: ever-users of OC had 1.1 risk as compared with never-users (N.S.); higher doses = slightly higher risk. Duration of use irrelevant. Family history: higher risk. Use after age 40: risk raised 50%.
Drife, 1983 (61[R])	Editorial: greater risk if OC used long term in early life?
Vessey et al., 1983 (62[C])	Pike's results not confirmed; may be some protective effect of OC?
CDC (US), 1983 (63[C])	Case control: ever-users of OC had 0.9 0.8–1.2) risk compared with never users; N.S. Family history and use of OC before first pregnancy irrelevant.
Pike et al., 1983 (64[C])	Enlarged study: OC breast cancer link if used before first full-term pregnancy: high doses = more risk.
Jannerich et al., 1983 (65[C])	Case control: no link with OC.
Rosenberg et al., 1984 (66[C])	Case control: no link with OC except for 30% increase if taken before first full pregnancy.
Stadel et al., 1985 (67[C])	Epidemiological study: no OC link even in sub-populations.
CDC (US), 1986 (68[C])	Epidemiological study: no OC link even in sub-populations.
Ellery et al., 1986 (69[C])	Case-control: evidence of risk if duration and dosage considered.
Meirik et al., 1986 (70[C])	Risk doubled by 12-year OC use; risk raised by duration of use; risk raised by use before first pregnancy; results may only be valid for Swedish women under 40. Not seen in older or Norwegian women.
CASH (US), 1986 (71[C])	No link with OC detected.
Shapiro, 1986 (72[R])	Authoritative review: no risk.
Stadel et. al., 1986 (73[R])	Greater risk with OC in women having history of fibroadenoma.
Lee et al., 1987 (74[C])	Case control: Significantly more breast cancer if (injected) depot-medroxyprogesterone used. No link with OC found.
Stadel et al., 1988 (75[C])	11.8-fold risk increase when young women use OC 12 years or more.
Bergkvist, 1989 (76[C])	Cohort study following up long-term HRT users: slight increase in breast cancer, possibly accentuated by progestagen. Study criticized methodologically (SED-12, 1027)
WHO, 1990 (77[R])	Analysis: Most studies have found no link to OC; no reason for serious concern; possibly slightly higher frequency in industrialized countries.
MacLennan, 1991 (78[R])	HRT: Risk increase up to 30%.
WHO, 1992 (79[R])	No increased risk from past OC use in women aged over 45 years; weak link in younger women with long-term use.
Gambrell, 1993 (80[R])	Link between HRT and breast cancer uncertain, but Nurse's Health Study suggested relative risk of 1.36. Adding progestogens reduces risk.
Colditz et al., 1993 (81[R])	17 relevant studies of HRT reviewed; risk raised 20% by use for >10 years, 50% by use for >20 years.
Stewart, 1993 (82[R])	Review: at least ten acceptable epidemiological papers point to link between long-term HRT and breast cancer.

of breast cancer or with a personal history of fibroadenoma.

As far as *hormonal replacement therapy* is concerned one must provisionally conclude, with the authors of a major Canadian study published in 1992, that long-term past use of estrogens is not related to risk, but that current estrogen use increases the risk of breast cancer to a modest degree, and that the addition of progestagens probably does not remove the increased risk resulting from the use of unopposed estrogen (83[C]).

Finally, it is clear that the increase in the use of estrogen-used contraceptives during the last quarter of a century cannot be held responsible for the current population-wide increase in breast cancer; as the International Committee for Research in Reproduction pointed out in 1989, the overwhelming proportion of the current rise in cases of breast cancer is among women who are too old to have taken OCs when they were younger. In addition, calculations suggest that even if an adverse effect among younger users of OCs were proved, it would still only account for a few percent of all breast cancers occurring in Western countries.

Malignant melanoma Mortality and incidence rates

of malignant melanoma and skin cancer have increased in most western countries during the last 15 years, obviously for reasons unconnected with oral contraception. However, endocrinological factors can affect the melanocytes and the spread of malignant melanoma, estrogen receptors have been noted in malignant melanoma cells and estrogens are known to stimulate melanogenesis, an effect which is enhanced by simultaneous administration of progestogens. Oral contraceptives might therefore have an effect; the fact that chloasma has long been known to occur in some oral contraceptive users is perhaps relevant (84[Cr]).

One large epidemiological study from California indeed found that women taking oral contraceptives, particularly long-term users, had a relatively high incidence of malignant melanoma (85[CR]). In Australia, a significant association with melanoma was seen in women who had used oral contraceptives for at least 10 years prior to diagnosis (86[C]). In a Canadian study on the other hand no association was found between the risk of superficially spreading melanoma or nodular melanoma and the use of either oral contraceptives or menopausal estrogens (SED-12, 1029); it was suggested that there might, however, be a risk in some subpopulations. One must be alert for confounding factors: e.g. contraceptive users may be more prone to expose themselves to sunlight. A recent case control study in Philadelphia on intra-ocular malignant melanoma concluded that hormonal factors played only a limited role in the causation of this condition (SEDA-12, 1029).

Other neoplasms The 1978 WHO report cited above quoted an unpublished study by March in which *pituitary adenomas* were found in 26% of women with secondary amenorrhea following the use of oral contraceptives, yet in only 13% of cases who had not used these products. The difference is significant, but selection bias might explain the results.

Estrogens

ESTROGEN REPLACEMENT THERAPY (ERT) HORMONAL REPLACEMENT THERAPY (HRT)

Hormonal replacement therapy consists primarily of the administration of low doses of oral estrogens to women, either in cycles or continuously. The drugs mainly used are conjugated estrogens, estriol (1—2 mg) and estrone. They may be given for a brief period at the time of the climacteric to relieve acute symptoms, such as hot flushes, or long-term in the hope of slowing or arresting certain involutional changes, such as osteoporosis. Their efficacy for some of these purposes is still disputed; the effects on osteoporosis are the best documented. In some regimens, progestogens are also used (see below) and cyclical patterns of administration are adopted.

Many of the adverse reactions listed below have actually been observed when estrogens were used in adults for other purposes. Quantification of risk is rarely possible since preparations, doses and patient populations differ so much; in addition, the placebo effect in estrogen replacement therapy is very marked, and some of these products have been administered at doses which are only marginally active.

ADVERSE REACTION PATTERN

General and toxic reactions Water and salt retention may result in weight gain and some rise in blood pressure. Changes in liver function tests can occur and jaundice is sometimes seen. Mild gastrointestinal upsets are not unusual. Unwanted endocrine effects can include painful stimulation of the breast and endometrial bleeding.

Hypersensitivity reactions These are rare but not impossible, e.g. urticaria, edema and slight dyspnea have been described as an allergic reaction to quinestrol (SEDA-12, 1030; see also Chapter 40.1).

Tumor-inducing effects The risk of endometrial carcinoma was long disputed, but current evidence points to a strong association, especially after prolonged use. Higher doses of estrogens can probably induce various forms of liver tumors. Both questions are dealt with in the general sections at the beginning of this Chapter.

ORGANS AND SYSTEMS *(see also Chapter 40.1)*

Cardiovascular There are contradictory data on the relationship between cardiovascular disease and postmenopausal estrogen use and only randomized clinical trials would resolve some of the doubts which persist.

Even weak estrogens in effective doses tend to *increase the blood pressure* in sensitive subjects (87[Cr]) and regular monitoring is desirable (see also Chapter 40.1). This may in part explain the trend to a higher incidence of *cardiac disorders*. In the 1985 Framingham Heart Study on 1234 postmenopausal women (88[CR]) it was shown that women reporting postmenopausal estrogen use at one or more biennial examinations had over a 50% elevation in the risk of cardiovascular morbidity and a more than two-fold risk of cerebrovascular disease after the index examination. Increased rates for myocardial infarction were observed particularly among estrogen users who smoked cigarettes. Among nonsmokers estrogen use was associated with an increased incidence of stroke. A further case-control study published in the United Kingdom in 1989 examined the possible association between the use of HRT and the risk of stroke and myocardial infarction (89[C]). No link, positive or negative, was found, but the subjects examined had on average used estrogens for only 15 months some 9 years before. One must set against this the results of a much larger prospective study in more than 120 000 women aged 30–55 years, designed to clarify the possible role of postmenopausal estrogen use in coronary heart disease. The age-adjusted relative risk of coronary disease in those who had at some time used hormone replacement therapy was here 0.5 as compared with controls, and the risk in current users was 0.7. The relative risks were similar for fatal and nonfatal disease and were unaltered after adjustment for a long list of confounding factors (90[C]). Jaffe found, on the electrocardiogram, a degree of ST-depression consistent with ischemia, which might indicate that these preparations induce *coronary spasm* (91[C]), but neither small- nor large-scale studies suggest any increase in the incidence of cardiovascular disease as a whole in women on such therapy; there may in some respects be a decrease, reflecting the favorable effect of estrogens in increasing high-density lipoprotein cholesterol.

Respiratory Allergic *bronchospasm* very rarely occurs but has been reported several times in the past decade, apparently in women with an existing allergic tendency or history of asthmatic disease; it may be noted that some asthmatic women are known to show an increase in their symptoms during the luteal phase of the menstrual cycle. In affected cases, the link with HRT is likely to be demonstrable by rechallenge (SEDA-12, 1030; 61[cr]).

Nervous system *Headache* can occur; in a series of patients with a latent or known tendency to *migraine*, attacks clearly have been precipitated, usually with prominent visual phenomena (92[cr]). In a woman with history of *chorea* in the distant past, a vaginal cream containing estrogens precipitated a renewed attack.

Endocrine, metabolic A significant decrease in *glucose tolerance* in women on HRT replacement therapy has been shown, although a sequential-type product with mestranol and norethisterone was being used (94[C]). Conflicting data concerning the effects of oral contraceptives on *carbohydrate metabolism* have been presented (see Chapter 40.1); the effects are probably insignificant. Effects on lipids are discussed primarily in Chapter 40.1.

In postmenopausal women on long-term treatment with mestranol a decrease in the serum-free *thyroxine* concentration has been demonstrated, but it was not associated with any degree of hypothyroidism. The serum concentrations of thyroid-stimulating hormone remained unchanged.

In one comparative study, ethinylestradiol was found to have an unfavorable effect on *liver protein synthesis* (SED-12, 1030). When a Canadian group administered conjugated estrogens or medroxyprogesterone acetate for 1 year, however (95[C]), all the various treatment regimes had favorable effects on lipid metabolism in a dose-related manner: after 1 year of treatment high-density lipoprotein levels increased and the high-density lipoprotein/low-density lipoprotein ratios, an anti-atherogenic index, also increased in all groups compared with pre-treatment values.

Mineral and fluid balance *Retention of water and salt* and *weight gain* are common during estrogen therapy. *Protein-bound iodine* and serum *copper* increase (SED-12, 1030). Effects on serum *calcium* are dealt with in Chapter 40.1; it should be recalled that hypercalcemia can occur during estrogen treatment of patients with metastasized mammary carcinoma.

Hematological There is clearly a thrombotic risk with estrogens, reviewed in full in Chapter 40.1. The mechanisms may be multiple. *Fibrinolytic activity* decreases in postmenopausal women when a high dose (250 μg) of ethinylestradiol is given daily for 10 days in preparation for prolapse operation (96[c]). On the other hand, long-term administration of 80 μg mestranol to postmenopausal women for 1 year or longer increased the concentration of fibrinogen and L-trypsin inhibitor while plasminogen decreased (SED-12, 1030–1031). There is also evidence that even low doses of oral estrogens frequently increase the *amount of thrombin generated* in vivo. It has been suggested on the basis of a case history of multiple systemic arterial thrombi in a patient with a prosthetic heart valve that, if estrogens are needed in such individuals, they should be combined with anticoagulants. One would be inclined to extend the warning; any women with a pre-existing thrombosis risk should be examined very carefully before deciding to give estrogens at all.

Liver *Changes in liver function tests, cholestasis and jaundice* are well known (see Chapter 40.1). The possibility of tumor induction is discussed above.

Gastrointestinal Dose-dependent *nausea* can occur; it is not lessened by using coated tablets. *Ischemic colitis* has been described (97[Cr]).

Pancreas There is a small but significant risk of *acute pancreatitis* starting 2–78 weeks after beginning of treatment; pain usually ceases within 10 days of HRT withdrawal (98[r]).

Urinary system In the distant past, hypernephroma was thought to be a result of estrogen treatment. There is, in fact, no clear evidence that this is so. However, there is some work suggesting that older women with intact uteri can be rendered more susceptible to urinary tract infections by taking estrogens (99[c]). The notion is surprising since some other studies, admittedly in selected material, have shown a decrease in such infections when HRT is used, and further work is needed (SEDA-17, 463).

Skin and appendages In susceptible subjects, *chloasma and* skin *nevi* can be induced by active doses of estrogen. *Porphyria* can be precipitated and familial *porphyria cutanea tarda* can become manifest (100[C]) (see also Chapter 40.1).

Special senses Apart from retinal thrombosis, *optic neuritis* has been described. In older women, estrogens cause a slight *rise in intra-ocular pressure* (SED-12, 1031).

Genital system All estrogens, even the weaker ones, can induce endometrial bleeding after the menopause. In therapeutically active doses, *bleeding* and *endometrial hyperplasia* are common. The risk of endometrial and cervical carcinoma is discussed above.

Breast Active doses of estrogens can result in *painful tingling and swelling* of the breast, sometimes requiring withdrawal of treatment. Frank *gynecomastia* can be induced by exposure to estrogen in a factory environment and it has even been described in an elderly man whose wife used an estrogen-containing vaginal lubricant (SEDA-6, 350). The risk of breast cancer is discussed earlier in this Chapter.

Effects on the immune system Recently reported laboratory data indicate that estrogens may have adverse immunological effects which could predispose to symptomatic infections (101[R]). See also 'Urinary system' above.

Risk situations For reasons discussed in extenso elsewhere in this Chapter and in Chapter 40.1, special risks are attached to the administration of active doses of estrogens in patients with a history of *jaundice in pregnancy*, *hepatic disease*, *thromboembolism* or *porphyria*, or where the presence of an *estrogen-dependent tumor* cannot be entirely excluded. Many of the risk situations and contraindications listed in Chapter 40.1 for hormonal contraceptives are clearly relevant to estrogen therapy as well.

Second-generation effects HRT is generally given at a time when pregnancy can be excluded, but in principle some of the risks discussed in connection with oral contraceptives would arise if a women receiving HRT were to become pregnant (see introduction to this Chapter).

Interactions The effects of *anticoagulants* may be somewhat antagonized by active doses of estrogens.

Other interactions are largely the same as those described for the oral contraceptives except for the fact that the dosage in HRT is not so critical as to render acceleration of metabolism a problem (see Chapter 40.1).

The question has been raised, but not so far entirely answered, whether the addition of progestogens to HRT might not cancel out the desired protective effect of estrogens against cardiac disorders; at present there seems to be no evidence from the field that this happens (SEDA-16, 459)

COMBINED ESTROGEN–PROGESTOGEN REPLACEMENT THERAPY

Because of the fear of certain risks (particularly malignancy) which might result from unilateral estrogen therapy in postmenopausal women over a long period, the use of combined estrogen–progestogen regimens with a monthly interruption to allow for withdrawal bleeding has, as pointed out earlier in this Chapter, been propagated as an alternative, it has been suggested that long-term therapy with estrogens alone should be periodically interrupted by a cycle of such combined treatment. These approaches have not been tested on a large scale and are unlikely to be; few women welcome the prospect of regular 'menstrual' bleeding persisting for many years after the menopause, and it might introduce new and unforeseen risks, particularly to the aging uterus. On theoretical and practical grounds, however, such combinations have been developed and used for relatively short periods of treatment during the climacteric itself to regularize bleeding and to relieve menopausal symptoms. The pattern of short-term adverse effects of these products is very similar to that of the combined oral contraceptives (see SEDA-12, Chapter 40.1).

Jensen and colleagues studied the effect on lipids of norethisterone acetate (1 mg/day given in the second half of the cycle) added to estrogen hormone replacement therapy (17α-estradiol, 1 mg or more orally/day) in the treatment of healthy postmenopausal women. The mixture as a whole produced no adverse effects on serum lipids or lipoproteins (102[C]).

TRANSDERMAL ESTROGENS

These have been used, mostly on an experimental basis to date, as a convenient means of giving estrogen supplementation, for example to women with established postmenopausal osteoporosis. Typical patches contain 50 μg estradiol, which appears to be sufficient to have an effect on bone if the pharmaceutical formulation is optimal. The wash-out period of transdermally applied estradiol seems to be about 6 weeks. In effective doses all the familiar adverse effects of estrogens can occur, including endometrial hyperplasia and bleeding *per vaginam*. Some local irritation can occur, with erythema and itching (103[C]).

ADMINISTRATION OF ESTROGENS TO MALES

Males receiving estrogens generally do so in the course of palliative treatment for malignancies (prostatic carcinoma) for which high doses may be given. Many of the effects described elsewhere in this Chapter may occur under these conditions, including thromboembolic complications.

Cardiovascular In one study, treated men with coronary heart disease were found to have higher serum estradiol concentrations and serum cholesterol, while high-density lipoprotein cholesterol was lower (104[C]). These data confirm the results of the Coronary Drug Project in which men treated with different doses of estrogens showed a dose-dependent increase in *myocardial infarction* and *thromboembolic diseases*. The effects of estrogens on lipid metabolism are considered to be the cause of the coronary heart disease.

Two other small studies in Europe have also concluded that a high risk of cardiovascular complications is associated with estrogens during long-term estrogen therapy (SED-12, 1032); in one of these, male patients treated with estrogens were found to have increased levels of Factor VII, Factor VIII and fibrinogen, pointing to a hypercoagulable state and platelet activation (105[C]). Two cases of mesenteric venous thrombosis in men taking estrogen therapy for carcinoma of the prostate have been reported (SED-12, 1032).

Swedish workers have sought to develop a test system to define patients who are at a higher risk of cardiovascular complications when treated with estrogens for cancer of the prostate (106[C]). An investigational battery using exercise stress testing, evaluation of the peripheral circulation, blood volume estimation, chest X-ray, blood tests including hormonal status, lipoproteins, antithrombin III, and a physical examination and history taken by a cardiologist is claimed to render it possible to classify 84% of estrogen-treated patients as individuals with or without particular risk of a cardiovascular complication and to identify an extremely high-risk sub-group.

A combination of diethylstilbestrol with cyproterone acetate and medroxyprogesterone acetate in patients with previously untreated prostatic cancer was tested in a randomized European trial (107[C]). It was concluded that patients treated with medroxyprogesterone acetate had a less favorable course with a shorter duration of survival and time to progression than those treated with the other two drugs. Cardiovascular side effects were reported more often in patients treated with diethylstilbestrol than in those treated with cyproterone acetate. The risk of developing severe cardiovascular complications was the highest during the first 6 months of treatment.

Hematological *Thrombocytopenia* was observed on two occasions in a patient treated with high doses of synthetic estrogens for prostatic carcinoma (SED-12, 1032). In another series, treatment with a non-steroid estrogen compound consistently *lowered hemoglobin levels* in patients with prostatic carcinoma, but also in healthy eunuchs (108[C]).

Endocrine, metabolic A case of profound *hypocalcemia* in a patient with osteoblastic metastatic carcinoma of the prostate has been reported, occurring after treatment with 15 mg diethylstilbestrol per day for 7 days (SED-12, 1032).

Genital system and breasts Administration of estrogens results in *pigmentation of the male areola* followed by *gynecomastia*, both during oral treatment and local application (109[c]). Estrogen-induced gynecomastia can be prevented in patients with prostatic carcinoma by irradiating the breast region before starting therapy.

Decrease in libido and sexual activity are to be expected in men treated with estrogens.

ADMINISTRATION OF ESTROGENS TO CHILDREN

Precocious puberty has been observed in young girls after contact with hair lotions and other products containing estrogens (SED-12, 1032). Contamination of isoniazid tablets with stilbestrol was the cause of an 'epidemic' of precocious puberty in a children's tuberculosis ward.

In boys as in men, estrogens can produce gynecomastia.

INDIVIDUAL ESTROGENS

17β-Estradiol
Ethinylestradiol
Mestranol

Ethinylestradiol has been discussed in Chapter 40.1. 17β-Estradiol might in theory be better tolerated, e.g. by the liver, than the synthetic derivatives (ethinylestradiol and mestranol). Of the above three estrogens, only ethinylestradiol itself has been extensively employed for specifically estrogenic purposes, often in very small doses.

Diethylstilbestrol
Chlorotrianisene

Diethylstilbestrol and other non-steroidal estrogens came into vogue at a time when the cost of producing steroidal estrogens, whether synthetic or of natural origin, was still prohibitive.

Diethylstilbestrol (DES, stilbestrol) and other non-steroidal estrogens such as chlorotrianisene (TACE) have largely lost favor in view of the association between DES in pregnancy and second-generation injury (see Introductory Section of this Chapter). There seems to be no reason for believing that the acute adverse reactions to these non-steroidal compounds differ from those of steroids. DES has been shown to induce hepatocellular carcinoma in males (SEDA-6, 341) and although it has become accepted by long tradition for the treatment of prostatic carcinoma, it could probably equally well be replaced (and often has indeed been replaced) by a steroid estrogen.

Estriol
Estrone
Conjugated equine estrogens

For estrogen replacement therapy, North America became accustomed to using conjugated estrogens (apparently since their original mode of production from mares' urine gave them a 'natural' connotation) while Europe has tended to use estriol or estrone.

Estriol is a very weak estrogen, usually given in oral doses of 1—2 mg, which has effects similar to those of ethinylestradiol at about 1/100th of this dosage: i.e. the vulva and vagina respond, but there is little effect on the endometrium. Similar considerations apply to estrone and to conjugated equine estrogens; most of the activity in the latter is in fact due to the presence of sodium estrone which appears to be added to most preparations in view of the limited supply of genuine equine estrogens.

Conjugate estrogens are also available as intravenous preparations for the treatment of severe uterine bleeding which is unresponsive to oral therapy. A severe anaphylactic reaction has been described in one case (SED-12, 1033), which might be anticipated since conjugated estrogens contain foreign (equine) material.

Most other relevant data on the adverse effects of the above products will be found in the monograph on 'Hormonal replacement therapy' earlier in this Chapter.

Quinestrol

Quinestrol is an ether of ethinylestradiol which is stored in the body fat and hence acts for weeks or months after a single oral dose; in the event of adverse reactions, this storage renders impossible the prompt termination of exposure.

GONADOTROPHINS AND OVULATION-INDUCING DRUGS

Gonadotrophins

Human chorionic gonadotrophin (HCG) has mainly luteinizing hormone (LH) activity; human menopausal gonadotrophin (HMG) contains both follicle-stimulating hormone (FSH) and LH in approximately equal amounts. The relative content of the pituitary gonadotrophin preparations in FSH and LH varies with the extraction procedure used. Treatment schedules for the induction of ovulation have been described in a number of papers, but the individual sensitivity of the ovaries varies greatly. Complications presumably occur primarily where the dose is excessive as compared with individual need; their incidence varies greatly from clinic to clinic. Problems include super-ovulation, multiple pregnancy and the hyper-stimulation syndrome (110[CR]) consisting of rapid ovarian enlargement with intraperitoneal effusion. Ascites and hydrothorax (111[c]) are occasionally seen, probably due to an increase in vascular permeability at high estrogen levels. Vascular accidents have also been reported, namely thrombophlebitis (112[c]) and obstruction of the basilar artery (SED-12, 1033). Gonadotrophins have also been reported, though with much less certainty, to cause cardiomyopathy and behavioral and intellectual disturbances (SED-12, 1033).

Treatment with FSH of porcine origin has resulted in an allergic reaction; it may be recalled that formation of antigens to the pregnant mare serum gonadotrophins (PMS) formerly in use was by no means uncommon. One subfertile man treated with HMG/HCG developed a malignant teratoma of the testis; in view of his history the causal relationship is dubious (113[C]).

Clomiphene

Clomiphene is a very weak non-steroidal estrogen; like some other weak hormonal substances it can block feedback mechanisms (and thereby impede the secretion of an endogenous hormone) while exerting little effect itself; the net result is that clomiphene can act as an antiestrogen.

The primary use of clomiphene is in the induction of ovulation. In one large study, some adverse reactions in treated women were found to result from its ovulatory effects, and others to be direct reactions to the substance itself (114[C]). The most common problem was ovarian enlargement (13.8%), followed by hot flushes (10.6%), abdominal and pelvic discomfort (7.0%), and nausea and vomiting (2.1%). Incidental symptoms were breast discomfort, vaginal changes, psychological symptoms, headache, heavier menses and increased urinary frequency. Sporadic case-reports on clomiphene in the literature relate to fetal ovarian dysplasia or maternal psychosis (SEDA-7, 391), either of which may have been coincidental. However, it must be borne in mind that the substance is related structurally to triparanol.

Suspicions that clomiphene treatment might adversely affect the fetus developing as a result of successful ovulation induction are difficult to confirm or allay, since the condition for which clomiphene is being used, i.e. subfertility, might itself carry some risk of malformation. The fear originally arose after 18 cases of trisomy had been reported to the authorities in the United States; later data on a large series of clomiphene-induced pregnancies (115[CR]) indicated that if there was indeed such risk it must be very small; a study of 200 instances of Down's syndrome showed that none of them had been exposed to the drug) (SEDA-6, 357). Another older report concerned a case of congenital retinopathy (SEDA-7, 391). The principal current concern is that there may be a risk of neural tube defects in the offspring; Cornel and colleagues concluded that there was a relative risk of at least 2 of an association between disturbed fertility and neural tube defects (116[C]), but others found no evidence for an association between maternal clomiphene use and such defects (117[C]).

One unusual possibility is a change in the sex ratio; when James examined the number of males per 100 females among infants conceived after induction of ovulation with clomiphene he found it to be 85 and significantly different from the normal human sex ratio at birth, which is about 106 (118[R]).

Mammary cancer in the mother has been suspected as a risk, but specific investigation into the matter does not support this suspicion (SED-12, 1034).

A case of testicular seminoma in a man receiving both clomiphene and mesterolone for 15 months for oligospermia has been described (119[C]), but it would hardly seem likely that the drug was responsible. In a multi-center study by WHO of the possible use of clomiphene in male infertility, two patients withdrew because of visual disturbances, dizziness and headaches (SEDA-17, 466).

Tamoxifen

Tamixofen is another weak estrogen which binds to receptors and therefore. Where adverse effects are concerned however, one needs to be cautious with this simple view of the mechanism of action. It is perfectly likely that in some organs and tissues it is the drug's estrogenic activity which is dominant and provides the best explanation for its effects.

Tamoxifen is used for the treatment of tumors with estrogen receptors and of endometrial carcinoma. It is also available in a number of countries for the induction of ovulation in patients with anovulatory infertility and has also been used in men with oligospermia.

The overall rates published for adverse effects vary enormously, between 1 and 60% (120[R], 121[R]). The acute side effects reported with this preparation when used for the treatment of mammary cancer are largely those which one would expect to be associated with a decrease in estrogenic activity, i.e. *hot flushes* (which can be severe), *dry skin*, *mental or CNS effects* (such as mild depression, headache, fatigue, nervousness and tremor), *oligomenorrhea and amenorrhea*, *loss of libido*, and rare events such as *pruritus*, *migraine* and *edema* (SED-12, 1034; 122[C]). Nausea and vomiting are not uncommon. There are also references in the literature to cases of hirsutism, weight gain, rashes, thrombocytopenia, and leukopenia (SED-12, 1034); the hirsutism could reflect a relative dominance of endogenous androgen activity as the level of estrogenic activity declines.

Thrombosis and *pulmonary embolism* have been described (123[R], 124[C]); the number of cases is still small, but the association would not be unexpected in view of what is known about the effects of other sex hormones. The primary condition might be responsible, at least in part, for the occurrence of such complications. The drug does reduce antithrombin III but not to a level at which a major risk would be expected (SEDA-18, 402), and other measurable effects on the coagulation process seem to be slight (SEDA-17, 465).

Liver dysfunction and *peliosis hepatis* have been are other reactions incidentally reported, and either of these seems credible on theoretical grounds and observations advanced elsewhere in this Chapter for related compounds. The possibility of tamoxifen raising the incidence of *liver cancer* has been discussed but no conclusion is possible; in rats given doses equivalent to 20 mg in humans there was indeed an 11.5% incidence of hepatic carcinoma.

Cases of *uterine fibroids* and *endometrial polyps* (sometimes with bleeding) have been reported in menopausal women who were treated with tamoxifen for periods of months or years (SEDA-16, 466; 125[R], 126[C]). In view of this, the question as to whether the action of tamoxifen on the endometrium may increase the risk of *endometrial cancer* has been discussed for more than a decade. A 1993 paper, which reviews the outcome of six major trials, tends strongly to the conclusion that tamoxifen can induce both endometrial hyperplasia and endometrial cancer to an extent which is proportional to the total dose administered (127[r]); the figures point to an overall incidence of endometrial cancer of 0.5% in tamoxifen users and 0.1% in controls. Another major review up to 1992 concluded that in the world literature there were 70 cases of uterine malignancies with tamoxifen, including 61 cases of adenocarcinoma of the endometrium and four cases of *uterine sarcoma* (128[R]).

The most specific and dangerous complication is *hypercalcemia*, a known direct consequence of the successful treatment of mammary carcinoma having bony metastases: again, the figures for its incidence vary greatly, but one will continuously have to be prepared for this potentially life-threatening complication. In principal an anti-estrogen might also precipitate osteoporosis, but tamoxifen has not been shown to do so—indeed there is good reason to believe that it protects the skeleton against steroid-induced bone loss (129[r]), and in some work performed to examine the state of the bones during treatment with tamoxifen there was actually a higher bone density than in controls.

An unusual case of rapidly fatal *renal failure* reported in 1993 could reflect an interaction between tamoxifen and one or more *cytostatic agents*, with mitomycin C a prime suspect; in a series of breast cancer patients some 10% of those treated both with tamoxifen and a cytostatic agent developed abnormal renal function, progressing towards various stages of hemolytic uremic syndrome (130[cr]).

There have been repeated reports of *ophthalmic complications*, including irreversible retinopathy with seriously decreased visual acuity, refractile opacities, cystoid macular edema, retinal yellow-white dots and keratopathy (SEDA-6, 356; SEDA-7, 391; SEDA-16, 466); one other report deals with bilateral optic neuritis developing in a woman with breast cancer who was treated for 6 months with tamoxifen (131[C]), and in 1992 Pavlidis et al. published a prospective study of the entire question of the drug's ocular toxicity (132[cR]). Their clear conclusion was that even in low doses (e.g. 10 mg or lower) tamoxifen can induce ocular toxicity if it is given for a sufficiently long period; most of the changes are reversible but they justify very close monitoring. Again it may be recalled that the related compound, MER-29 (triparanol), caused cataract and had various other adverse reactions in common with tamoxifen as well. but the considerable value of tamoxifen in treating mammary carcinoma must be borne in mind when reviewing these problems.

In premenopausal women, tamoxifen seems to have complex effects upon *ovarian function*, compatible with the accelerated development of multiple follicles (133[CR]): this might be expected in view of the product's similarity to clomiphene.

Second-generation effects These do not appear to have been documented in human subjects, but since animal studies suggested the possibility of fetal and neonatal malformations it has for a long time been customary to exclude pregnancy before administering tamoxifen.

Interactions It is not clear how tamoxifen might interact with a drug the efficacy of which is based on its estrogenic activity; the question is important since in excluding pregnancy before prescribing tamoxifen a physician may rely on the use of *hormonal contraceptives* and, in theory, their efficacy might be undermined by an anti-estrogen. A possible interaction with *cytostatics* is discussed above under 'Urinary system'.

Droloxifene

Droloxifene is 3-OH-tamoxifen citrate, but it was found in the laboratory to have a higher affinity for estrogen receptors than tamoxifen itself and (presumably for that reason) a lower ratio of estrogenic to anti-estrogenic activity. The pattern of adverse reactions nevertheless seems very similar, with up to a third of patients affected by menopausal-type sensations, e.g. hot flushes (25—33%) and lassitude (21—24%). Incidental patients in a multi-center controlled study of 369 users suffered from pulmonary embolism, thrombosis, erythema, a transient rise in serum γ-glutamyltransferase levels and fatal aggravation of hypercalcemia (134[C]).

Toremifene

This triphenyl derivative is structurally related to tamoxifen, but in animal studies it was relatively less estrogenic. From the limited experience published to date, the adverse reaction pattern appears to be closely similar to that of droloxifene (135[C]).

OTHER COMPOUNDS

Cyclofenil

Cyclofenil is another weak non-steroidal estrogen related to stilbestrol which was in use for a number of years but has largely lost favor. Up to 2% of patients taking this drug complain of nausea, vomiting, hot flushes, or headache: slight abdominal pain has been reported in up to 18%, ovarian enlargement without cysts in 3%, and galactorrhea in 4%. There have been a few case reports of hemolytic anemia (SED-12, 1034). Some cases of reversible mild cholestatic jaundice have been observed. The symptoms regressed rapidly following cessation of therapy.

Olsson and colleagues, reviewing 30 patients with hepatic reactions to cyclofenil (136[cR]), conclude that the liver derangement is probably related to metabolic idiosyncrasy rather than to a direct toxic effect. There is a surprising lack of such reports from countries where cyclofenil was widely used: in France, at least, the number of cases of hepatitis occurring is known to have been much greater than that reported in print; the drug was abandoned in France in 1988.

Epimestrol

The adverse effects of epimestrol (3-methoxy-17-epiestriol), also a very weak estrogen with some ovulation-inducing effects, are largely as one would expect. In one series hot flushes, insomnia, anorexia, nausea and vomiting were reported in 1.5%, headache in 3%, and uterine bleeding in 38% (137[Cr]). Ovarian hyperstimulation is rare but not unknown. As is usual with such treatment, the incidence of the adverse effects reported varies greatly, no doubt related to the motivation of the patients and the schemes of administration employed.

PROGESTOGENS

Most aspects of progestogens have been dealt with in Chapter 40.1. While the progestogens do have certain characteristic effects of their own, notably on the female menstrual cycle, the spectrum of adverse effects of any particular progestogen (particularly when given in high doses) is likely to be heavily dependent on the extent to which it also possesses glucocorticoid, mineralocorticoid or estrogenic or androgenic properties. Some individuals receiving progestogens for the treatment of breast cancer will thus for example experience painful swelling of the breast and prolonged amenorrhea (which are progestogenic) but also weight gain and hypercalcemia (which are likely to be corticosteroidal). Patients treated with progestogens during pregnancy are said to be prone to prolonged post-partum bleeding, but this probably reflects the pregnancy disorder for which these drugs were given, e.g. threatened abortion. Virilization of the female fetus has been described following administration of various progestogens in early pregnancy and is presumably an androgenic effect.

Progestogens given alone as oral contraceptives can induce a number of side effects (see Chapter 40.1), some of which may reflect their other hormonal properties while others are non-specific. Headache, nausea and vomiting, breast tenderness and pain in the back or abdomen can occur.

Animal studies cannot be regarded as providing a reliable indicator of the spectrum of activity of individual compounds; suggestions that derivatives of 17α-hydroxyprogesterone (such as megestrol acetate, chlormadinone acetate, medroxyprogesterone acetate) are more 'natural' because of their progesterone-like structure than derivatives of 19-nortestosterone (such as norgestrel, lynestrenol, ethynodiol acetate, norethisterone and allylestrenol) are not based on biological evidence. Experience, too, can be misleading; there is some suggestion that hydroxyprogesterone caproate can have adverse reactions on the fetus when used in pregnancy whilst similar reports on allylestrenol (used for the same purpose) are lacking, but one must bear in mind the anecdotal nature of such evidence and especially the fact that hydroxyprogesterone caproate appears to be a more widely used compound than allylestrenol and hence one on which adverse reaction reports are more likely to appear.

Progestogens belonging to the ethisterone family (norethisterone, levonorgestrel, desogestrel) have some androgenic activity; those in the hydroxyprogesterone family (hydroxyprogesterone caproate, chlormadinone, cyproterone acetate) tend to be antiandrogenic, while norgestimate, mentioned in Chapter 40.1, seems to be somewhat estrogenic. Water retention occasionally occurs and may reflect a degree of desoxycortone acetate (DOCA)-like activity; virilization of a female fetus is more likely to occur with a product possessing some androgenic activity, and breast tenderness with a product possessing estrogenic activity.

Cardiovascular system Medroxyprogesterone has been variously reported to induc a fall in blood pressure in some initially hypertensive patients while rapidly raising diastolic pressure in some other women or to have no effect on blood pressure at all.

Liver Administration of some progestogens may result in elevation of non-conjugated bilirubin (138[R]). Norethisterone acetate has been implicated (139[c]).

Endocrine, metabolic Medroxyprogesterone, while suppressing spermatogenesis, also depresses insulin- or arginine-induced growth hormone release (140[C]). Basal growth hormone levels have been reported to become elevated (SED-12, 1035).

INDIVIDUAL PROGESTOGENS

Desogestrel

Desogestrel is one of the newer progestogenic steroids intended for use in oral contraceptives, and is mentioned in Chapter 40.1. It was developed and introduced because of its relatively favorable effect on blood lipids in experimental work; this led to the hope that it might, in the long run, have a relatively favorable effect on the risk of atherogenesis. In the short term, its effects are very similar to those of other progestogens.

Gestonorone caproate

Gestonorone (17α-hydroxy-19-norprogesterone) has been found useful in doses of 200 mg i.m. weekly for benign prostatic hypertrophy. Mild side effects, in two trials discussed earlier in these volumes (SED-12, 1035—1036), included loss of appetite and mild fever, but more remarkable was a significant *decrease in erythrocyte count, hemoglobin and hematocrit*, normalizing after drug withdrawal.

Hydroxyprogesterone caproate

High doses of this compound and the related norderivative have been used to treat benign prostatic hyperplasia. Very striking is the high incidence of *impotence* recorded in these studies; it may affect two-thirds of patients and seems to persist in some patients after withdrawal of the drug (141[C]).

Lynestrenol

Lynestrenol is one of the older progestagens used in oral contraceptives and has been very widely and successfully employed; as monotherapy it has been used to regulate the menstrual cycle.

A Finnish study was conducted to analyze the association between the prolonged use of lynestrenol (to suppress menstruation in mentally retarded women) and arterial disease detected at autopsy. The conclusion was that such treatment—here given for a mean of more than 6 years—indeed raises the risk of arterial disease and that such treatment must be very carefully considered (142[C]).

Medroxyprogesterone acetate

High doses of medroxyprogesterone acetate are widely used for the treatment of hormone-dependent carcinomas (notably of the breast) and the side effects occurring under these conditions have received primary attention (SEDA-12, 343). Its combination with cytostatic drugs may induce additional side effects. In doses effective in breast cancer, e.g. 800 mg/day, toxic effects are likely to include excessive *weight gain* (in 40—90% of eases), *cushingoid facies* (10—20%), *worsening of diabetes mellitus* (up to 8%), *edema* (10—20%) and other effects suggestive of hypercorticism. The changes are especially marked in women treated for more than 5 weeks; effects are less severe at a dosage of 400 mg/day. Smaller groups of patients may develop *rash*, *thromboembolism*, *dysuria*, *nervousness*, *headache*, or *nausea and vomiting*.

Treatment with low-dose medroxyprogesterone acetate (50 and 150 mg/day) for endometriosis resulted in a *decrease in HDL-cholesterol* (143[C]) confined to the HDL_2 subfraction which was decreased by as much as 58% after 24 weeks of treatment; the effect was clearly dose dependent.

The pharmaceutical formulation of oral medroxyprogesterone acetate preparations may be of importance for their efficacy because of its marked effect on bioavailability, and variations in the latter can also explain inconsistencies in side-effect data. Well-formulated oral products have an excellent bioavailability, rendering parenteral treatment for most therapeutic purposes unnecessary.

Mental or personality changes, a typical corticosteroid effect, have been reported to be more severe and more frequent with combined aminoglutethimide plus medroxyprogesterone acetate treatment than with monotherapy in patients with bone metastases from breast cancer. The increased frequency of depressive syndromes on the two-drug therapy could not be attributed to the physical side effects of the combination, since the mental disorders appeared only during the first weeks of treatment, whereas the cushingoid features did not become apparent until some 6–8 weeks of treatment had been given (144[C]).

Megestrol acetate

Megestrol acetate, like medroxyprogesterone acetate, is regarded as a reasonably effective hormonal treatment for metastatic breast cancer in postmenopausal women. The commonest side effects are typical for the progestagens as a group, but corticosteroid-like effects seem less prominent than with medroxyprogesterone acetate. Typical effects and incidence figures for effective doses in cancer patients (SED-12, 1036; SEDA-17, 467; 145[C]) have been cited as *weight gain* (81–88%), mild *edema* reversible with diuretics (7–34%), *hypertension* (17–25%), *constipation* (13–17%), *dyspnea* (6.5–21%), *pyrosis* (6.5%) *chest tightness* (4–8%), *hyperglycemia* (8–13%), *heart failure* (4%), *urinary frequency* (4–11%), *diarrhea* (6%), *gastrointestinal upset* (6%) and *phlebitis or thrombosis* (4%). Isolated cases of *blood pressure increase*, *headache*, *dyspnea*, *vaginal bleeding*, *nervousness*, *sweating*, *vertigo*, *gastrointestinal symptoms*, *skin rash*, *pruritus* and *thrombocytopenia* have also been reported.

Megestrol acetate has also proved of value in patients with metastatic prostatic cancer, epithelial ovarian cancer or malignant melanoma. In one clinical study of 43 men with recurrent and metastatic cancer of the prostate given megestrol acetate 160 mg/day orally, side effects comprised *thromboembolic phenomena* (two patients), *peripheral edema* (two), increasing *cardiomegaly* (one), nausea and vomiting (four). In five patients, an asymptomatic *rise in liver enzyme levels* was noted but it resolved during further treatment. In three patients, increasing *bone pain* occurred, no doubt relating to changes in bony metastases and requiring analgesia. Another patient developed *hypercalcemia* and one patient developed *convulsive epilepsy* (146[C]).

Several other trials in other forms of cancer provide a picture of side effects similar to the above, with the risks of thrombosis and hypertension demanding particular attention, since they are serious though not common; as a rule, patients with a history of thromboembolic disease or heart failure are excluded. *Loss of libido and potency* has been seen in some men. The gain in body weight when it occurs is often linked to an evident improvement in appetite (147[C]), which can be a positive advantage in cachectic patients with advanced cancers.

When used alongside diethylstilbestrol or ethinylestradiol in men with previously untreated metastatic carcinoma of the prostate, a high incidence of feminizing side effects (70–74%, no doubt attributable to the estrogens) was seen; a higher than expected rate of cardiovascular complications (18%) and an unexpected need for cortisone replacement (13%) were also observed (148[C]).

Norethisterone

A curious survival of an obsolete practice was to be found in Melbourne, Australia, up to 1991, where a practitioner had continued for 20 years to prescribe norethisterone routinely to pregnant women with a history of habitual abortion or interuterine death in previous pregnancies. When the results were examined it was found that in five of 39 females exposed in utero there was hypertrophy of the clitoris, a sign of masculinization (SEDA-17, 466–467).

Progesterone

This natural progestogen is unsuitable for oral use (unless given in a special micronized form), but it is employed by other routes.

Intra-articular use When 1 mg/kg body weight of progesterone was injected intra-articularly in 12 patients with rheumatoid arthritis no important side effects were observed during the 2 months of follow-up (SED-12, 1037).

Systemic use Among the variants on estrogen replacement therapy which have been tried is the combination of the estrogen with either tamoxifen or with injections of progesterone to inhibit estrogenic development of the postmenopausal endometrium. In a study where both regimens were compared, a minority of women on each regimen complained of short-lasting dizziness following the progesterone injections (200 mg/day for 10 days); these also proved less effective than tamoxifen in suppressing endometrial development.

Intranasal use Preparations of progesterone in a polyethylene glycol base ointment have been tested, using single doses of 20, 30 and 40 mg intranasally. The side effects were mainly a transient unpleasant taste in the mouth or a slight feeling of nasal congestion after administration (SED-12, 1037).

TRANSDERMAL PROGESTOGENS

An older 19-*nor*-progesterone (ST 1435, Merck Darmstadt) has been used experimentally in a transdermal form as a possible hormonal contraceptive. A daily application of 0.8–1 mg was needed to inhibit ovulation in all subjects. There was some irregularity of bleeding, and some subjects experienced breast tenderness (SEDA-17, 468).

PROGESTERONE ANTAGONISTS

Mifepristone

Mifepristone (RU-486) binds with high affinity to receptors for progesterone and glucocorticoids, blocking the actions of these hormones on their target tissues. The anti-fertility effects of mifepristone during early pregnancy have been attributed to the blockade of endometrial progesterone receptors. Mifepristone also impedes the production of human chorionic gonadotrophin and progesterone in the placenta. When given in a single dose of 10 mg/kg body weight by mouth to induce menses, heavy bleeding was reported in some cases (149[C]).

The most widely discussed use of RU-486 has been as an abortifacient. When a single dose of 600 mg p.o. was used in a clinical study on 150 healthy pregnant women, 131 attained a complete abortion. Three women reported bleeding over 2 weeks after abortion: 16 women had a reduced hemoglobin level of less that 11 g/100 ml, justifying iron therapy. Other side effects were uterine contractions and pelvic pain (four patients), transient asthenia (three patients) and nausea (two patients) (150[C]). These findings seem to be typical, even though dosage schemes have varied, as little as 100 mg p.o. having been used successfully with similar adverse effects (SED-12, 1037).

COMPARATIVE EFFECTS OF SEX HORMONE ON PLASMA VALUES

A large number of plasma values are affected by sex hormones; the information is to be found at the appropriate points in this as well as the previous Chapter.

ANDROGENIC AND ANABOLIC STEROIDS

The classic androgen is natural testosterone, which today can be given orally in a special pharmaceutical form, but has more often been used as the orally active 17-methyl derivative or an injectable ester. From about 1955 onwards, however, a number of 'anabolic steroids' were developed for which it was claimed, on the basis of animal experiments, that the virilizing effects had been reduced compared with testosterone, whereas the effects on tissue build-up and nitrogen retention had been maintained. These compounds were therefore promoted for such purposes as the promotion of appetite and weight increase in children and the advancement of convalescence. In fact, it has never been at all clear that these compounds are anything other than weak and expensive androgens. Even in these 'tonic' doses, they can cause virilization in women and precocious development of secondary characteristics in children. In the much higher doses later developed for use in such conditions as aplastic anemia, mammary carcinoma and terminal uremia, their androgenic effects are very pronounced indeed. It may be noted that one formerly well-known 'anabolic' steroid, metandienone (Dianabol), was withdrawn in 1982 and other withdrawals have followed.

A fair amount of use of 'anabolic' steroids is still made surreptitiously among sportsmen and body builders and undoubtedly injury is being done.

Cardiovascular 'Anabolic' steroids used by body builders, often apparently in grossly excessive amounts, appear to lead cardiac disorders, including cardiomegaly and heart failure (SEDA-15, 440). It is difficult to distinguish the effects of the drug from those of overexertion and perhaps also other forms of 'tonic' therapy used by this group.

Liver The high milligram doses of 'anabolic' steroids in use seem to carry a considerable risk of liver dysfunction. perhaps attributed to the alkylation of the steroid. Whereas the liver damage induced by methyltestosterone has been shown to be reversible (151[C]), that resulting from use of other 'anabolics' may not be. It is impossible, however, to make valid comparisons in view of the irregularity with which reports appear; cases of severe *cholestasis* were, for example, only reported in patients treated daily with stanozol after it had been in clinical use for more than 20 years; in that instance the patients recovered biochemically over 3–6 months after withdrawal of the drug (152[c]).

The effects of these compounds on the liver may vary somewhat with their structure: even when misused in athletes, nandrolone decanoate (which has no 17-substitution) did not appear to adversely affect liver function, but other agents readily cause *jaundice*.

Both pre-cancerous and cancerous changes in the liver have repeatedly been recorded; *peliosis hepatis* is probably a precancerous condition. Large hepatocellular carcinomas have been described (153[C]; see also 'Sex steroids and tumor induction' earlier in this Chapter). A case of a *liver cell adenoma* in a child (154[c]) and two cases of *nodular hepatocellular carcinoma* (155[c]) have been reported in patients treated with oxymetholone, metenolone acetate or other 'anabolic' steroids for 5–15 years.

Liver complications may make it necessary to interrupt the use of 'anabolics' in such conditions as aplastic anemia: one patient, for example, receiving no less than 2 mg/kg oxymetholone daily with oral prednisone, showed hematological improvement but developed HBsAg-negative cholestatic hepatitis; the drugs were discontinued and the condition relapsed (156[C]). When an 8-year-old child was treated with as little as 0.3 mg/kg oxymetholon daily for 5 years; a hepatic adenoma of the left lobe of the liver developed and required surgical removal (SED-12, 1038).

The use of fluoxymesterone, ethylestrenol, metandienone, oxandrolone, oxymetholone and stanozolol by athletes has often been reported (as pointed out in the discussion of malignancies earlier in this Chapter) and is a well-known problem in professional sport (157[r]). Even if adverse reactions such as hepatocellular carcinoma are rare, it seems doubtful whether one can justify the treatment of healthy persons for non-medical reasons with a drug which has even a limited potential for liver damage.

Skin The skin commonly shows acne and hirsutism, the latter again often being irreversible: in women, loss of scalp hair can occur. Multiple halo nevi have been described in a case treated with oxymetholone (SED-12, 1038). When the effect of testosterone and anabolic steroids on the size of sebaceous glands was studied in a series of male athletes, high doses of all the products tested were found to enlarge the glands (158[C]).

Other systems Other adverse effects of androgens (and hence of 'anabolics') are largely those which would be expected from their properties as male sex hormones. The effect on the *voice* in women and children may initially be reversible, but soon becomes permanent: *polyps of the larynx* have also been observed (159[R]). *Menstrual derangement* is likely. Like other hormones, androgens have certain effects on *plasma levels* of enzymes, minerals and vitamins and cause decreased levels of HDL-cholesterol in athletes using them (160[C]). An unusual complication reported in 1981 was the induction of a *toxic confusional state* and *choreiform movements* by an anabolic steroid (SED-12, 1038), but here one is probably dealing with the non-specific results of endocrine stress in a susceptible individual (see Chapter 39). Other unusual complications on record are an *obstructive sleep apnea syndrome* induced by testosterone (161[c]) and *superior sagittal sinus thrombosis*.

The 'anabolic' steroid oxandrolone, used for some years in boys to promote growth, proved to induce *gynecomastia* in a high proportion of subjects treated; 23 of the 33 patients affected subsequently required mastectomy (SEDA-17, 469–470).

Treatment of hypogonadism The approved indications for androgen therapy concern their substitution in male hypogonadism. Testosterone enanthate (TE) or transdermal testosterone have commonly been used.

Severe *priapism* is occasionally experienced; such a complication occurred in a 20-year-old man with idiopathic hypogonadotrophic hypogonadism receiving TE 250 mg i.m. every 2 weeks (162[cr]).

Acne is a common complaint with testosterone enanthate, but it has been claimed to be largely eliminated by using testosterone implants in equivalent doses; it is not clear why this might be expected.

A clinical study of transdermal testosterone using doses of 315 ± 69 mg/day reported no local reactions to patch application (163[C]); however, when *serum dehydrotestosterone* (DHT) was determined it was found to be significantly higher than in normal men who had similar testosterone levels. The possible effects of such raised DHT concentrations on the prostate and other tissues have yet to be systematically studied.

Interactions (*See also Chapter* 40.1) Many androgens and anabolic steroids have been shown to reduce the dose of *anticoagulants* which a patient requires, sometimes by as much as 25% (164[R]), and hemorrhages have sometimes resulted from their use. This is in part due to their own effect on clotting factors (see also above); stanazol, fluomesterone, metandienone, methyltestosterone, oxymesterone and oxymetholone have been reported to decrease the synthesis or increase the degradation of clotting factors; however, other mechanisms may also be involved. A study with stanozolol in which it reduced the warfarin requirement led the investigators to conclude that the drug increased fibrinolysis, reduced the production of vitamin K-dependent clotting factors and increased the amount of the natural anticoagulant, antithrombin III (165[c]).

Older data pointed to some reduction in *insulin* requirements when diabetics received androgenic 'anabolics', but today it would seem wise to avoid these drugs in the diabetic patient altogether.

NEWER ANDROGEN-LIKE SUBSTANCES

Testolactone
Drostanolone
Calusterone

During the last three decades several papers have appeared on newer androgen-like substances used in treatment of advanced mammary carcinoma. The ratio between their desired and unwanted effects is still uncertain. Of these substances, *testolactone* showed no masculinizing or feminizing activity at a recommended dosage of 100 mg/day; in 8% of all cases, vomiting, nausea and diarrhea were observed (166[C]).

The androgenic effect of *drostanolone* was only slight when a dose of 100—200 mg per week was given, but higher doses did cause virilization (167[C]); hypercalcemia has been observed (168[c]).

Calusterone, found to be a weak androgen, caused facial flush and increased sulfobromphthalein retention; vomiting occurred in 5% of cases (169[c]).

Danazol

Danazol, an inhibitor of pituitary gonadotrophin and a very weak androgen, is used for the treatment of endometriosis and fibrocystic mastopathy. Common adverse effects are primarily androgenic and comprise hirsutism, edema, weight gain, voice change, oiliness of the skin or hair, depression, anxiety, fatigue, sedation and dizziness, gastrointestinal tract symptoms, muscle cramps, skin rash and vasomotor symptoms (170[C], 171[C]). Enlargement of the clitoris and deepening of the voice in girls have occasionally been noted, while women become amenorrheic (172[C]); the amenorrhea can persist for a considerable period.

Mild hypertension can occur and blood pressure should therefore be monitored during treatment. Although danazol has a specific effect on gonadotrophin secretion, it does not lead to any change in basal levels of thyroid-stimulating hormone, prolactin or cortisol (173[C]); however, a decrease in serum thyroxine-binding protein may lead to an erroneous diagnosis of hypothyroidism.

Other reactions incidentally but clearly documented with danazol are reversible lipid changes (decrease in mean HDL-cholesterol and increase in LDL-cholesterol, amenorrhea, a rise in serum transaminase levels, cholestasis or jaundice, hearing loss, hypercalcemia, reduced bone density and benign intracranial hypertension (SED-12, 1039). The reduction in bone density appears to be considerably less than that seen with equieffective doses of the gonadotrophin releaser inhibitor leuprolide (see later), but the lipid changes could in the longer term prove serious (SEDA-18, 399—400).

Danazol can cause a mild impairment of glucose tolerance (174[CR]) associated with elevated plasma insulin levels and this may represent a risk in diabetics. A case report of apparent danazol-induced primary hepatocellular carcinoma has been described (175[C]). No significant changes have been found in the total blood picture, platelet count, bleeding or coagulation time (176[C]).

Effects on the fetus Because danazol is capable of causing amenorrhea, a pregnancy occurring while taking the medication may not be diagnosed until considerable fetal exposure has occurred. Evidence is accumulating that danazol has an androgenic effect on the fetus leading to fetal genital malformations (177[R]). It has therefore been urged that therapy with danazol should begin after several days of a normal menstrual flow and at a dose greater than 200 mg/day, since lower doses may not effectively inhibit hormonal output, folliculogenesis and ovulation.

Interactions A metabolic interaction between danazol and *carbamazepine* was detected in patients with both epilepsy and fibrocystic breast disease; carbamazepine serum levels increased almost two-fold in the presence of danazol (178[R]). Another study showed that the plasma clearance of carbamazepine decreased substantially and that its half-life increased from 11 to 24 hours: danazol inhibits the epoxide-*trans*-diol pathway of carbamazepine metabolism (179).

ANTIANDROGENS

Cyproterone and cyproterone acetate

Cyproterone is a strong antiandrogen. Its 17α-acetoxy derivative cyproterone acetate possesses, in addition to its intrinsic antiandrogenic activity, strong progestational and antigonadotrophic properties. The excretion of the steroid is slow due to storage in adipose tissue (180, 181). The acetate is used for the treatment of female hirsutism, for prostatic cancer, for undesirable hypersexual activity in the male, for precocious puberty and for severe acne in both sexes. A low-dosage preparation of cyproterone acetate (2 mg) combined with 50 mg of ethinylestradiol has been available in a few countries as an oral contraceptive for women with mild symptoms of virilization.

Frequency of adverse effects Cyproterone acetate as monotherapy in prostatic cancer seems to produce fewer side effects than estrogen therapy. A dosage of 100 mg given daily by mouth to 39 patients resulted in a 10% incidence of side effects, comprising phlebitis (3%), pulmonary embolism (3%) and gynecomastia (5%), as well as edema, mental aberration and fairly frequent gastrointestinal disorders (182[C]). When other workers used a higher (400 mg daily) dose of cyproterone acetate in 20 patients with breast cancer, eight patients themselves stopped treatment because of adverse effects after an average of 17 weeks; further treatment was withheld in two patients because of a cerebrovascular accident and a pulmonary embolism, respectively. Problematical side effects in this series were nausea (seven patients), severe nausea and weight loss exceeding 10% of body weight (three), necrotizing hepatitis recovering after drug withdrawal (two) and depression (two) (183[C]).

Endocrine, metabolic Cyproterone acetate probably has some glucocorticoid effects, as judged clinically from its apparent ability to substitute for cortisol in adrenocortical-suppressed children. Not surprisingly, therefore, endocrine side effects of cyproterone acetate include the inhibition of pituitary ACTH (corticotrophin) secretion and interference with the biogenesis and metabolism of steroid hormones in the adrenal cortex, gonads, liver, kidney and peripheral tissues. The acetate also influences the properties of steroid-binding globulins, and steroid conjugation in the liver and the kidney, thereby playing a role in the inactivation and excretion of steroid hormones. Cyproterone acetate has in addition considerable progestational activity; the appropriate dosage for a secretory transformation of the human endometrium is 20—30 mg. Amenorrhea and irregular uterine bleeding are therefore common side effects of treatment with cyproterone acetate alone.

Liver Reversible necrotizing hepatitis has been noted above. Various other case reports have described severe hepatitis with hepatic failure, e.g. after 3 weeks of high-dose treatment in an elderly man, but recovering after drug withdrawal (184[C]); fulminant hepatitis has also been recorded (SED-12, 1040). In one series of cases of advanced breast cancer receiving 200—400 mg/day for a mean of 24 weeks, five of 20 patients showed liver function disturbances during cyproterone acetate therapy that could not be attributed to non-drug causes; biopsies performed in two other patients showed hepatitis with bridging and confluent necrosis and evidence of early post-hepatitic scarring which in the long run could lead to cirrhosis (185[C]).

Thromboembolism Thrombosis and embolism have been noted in trials summarized above but also by others, sometimes even with low doses. A case of deep vein thrombosis in a 19-year-old woman with no risk factors other than oral contraception using cyproterone acetate 2 mg with ethinylestradiol 35 μg has been published: the circumstances suggested that the drug was responsible, and it is now known that in such cases antibodies to the drug may be demonstrable (186[C]).

Respiratory Three cases of breathlessness in patients with prostatic carcinoma treated with 300 mg daily of cyproterone acetate have been described (187[C]). In the absence of any other cause for the breathlessness, it was suggested that it was due to the progestogenic effect of cyproterone acetate, increasing ventilation in patients with a pre-existing mild to moderate degree of abnormal pulmonary function.

Effects in men (*See also 'Second-generation effects' above*) Most effects in men partly resemble those in women taking comparable doses and include tiredness, drowsiness, vertigo, headache, weakness and depression in about 30% of the patients, particularly in the second to the sixth week of treatment. Gynecomastia (ca. 20%), reduction of body hair (ca. 10%), genital pain (2—3%), galactorrhea (0.3%) and gain or loss of weight have also been reported (SED-12, 1040; 188[CR]).

Effects in children One must expect cyproterone acetate, when used in high doses in children for precocious puberty, to inhibit the pituitary-adrenal axis: signs of adrenal suppression are sometimes indeed observed (189[C]). This is in accordance with earlier observations in the rat but appears not to occur in human adults (190[C]). It has been recommended that steroid cover be considered for these children during intermittent illness and prior to surgery.

Miscellaneous Reference has been made above to antibody formation. One report described two male patients treated for hypogonadism and four women taking cyproterone acetate as a contraceptive who developed recurrent *angioedema*. It was suggested that these cases point to an androgen deficit due to either hypogonadism or to prior androgen treatment (191[C]).

Second-generation effects Since sexual differentiation in the male in early embryonic life is androgen dependent, antiandrogenic treatment of pregnant animals may cause feminization of the male fetus. Although this serious side effect has not yet been reported in the human, pregnancy has to be excluded before the onset of therapy. During treatment, inhibition of ovulation is virtually certain but in cases of drug interaction, pregnancy can occasionally occur during treatment (*unpublished notifications*).

Reversible impairment of spermatogenesis occurs and data sheets provide warnings (presumably based on unpublished data) that abnormal spermatozoa may be found.

Combination products

To overcome the problem of amenorrhea and menstrual disturbances with cyproterone acetate when treating such conditions as acne and hirsutism in women, a combination with ethinylestradiol in acyclical 'reversed sequential regime' has been developed. A 2 mg dose of cyproterone acetate was originally combined with 0.05 mg ethinylestradiol, later with 0.035 mg ethinylestradiol. With the latter dose, tolerance is improved, but adverse effects have included weight loss (13%), varicose veins (3.2%) and breast enlargement (20%) (192[c]).

In the literature as a whole, most of the adverse effects attributable to the reversed sequential regimen and of the low-dose contraceptive (193[C]) are closely similar to those recorded with orthodox oral contraceptives, although breast pain and tenderness seem to be more common (10%). The only late adverse effect, which may appear even after 1 year of treatment, is mastopathy.

Flutamide

The non-steroidal antiandrogen, flutamide, is described as being equipotent to the steroidal antiandrogen, cyproterone acetate, as shown in laboratory studies; it has been used in prostatic carcinoma. Side effects seen in clinical studies comprise particularly gynecomastia and breast tenderness (34% in one study of 243 patients), nausea and vomiting (occasional), and rare (less than 3%) thromboembolic-cardiovascular complications (194[R]). The thromboembolic complications may in some cases have a correlation to prior estrogen treatment. Elevation of liver function tests has also been reported.

GONADOTROPHIN-RELEASING HORMONE ANTAGONISTS

Leuprolide

A discussion of leuprolide belongs primarily in the section of the volume dealing with miscellaneous hormones, but a brief mention is warranted here in view of the drug's current interest as an alternative to danazol in the treatment of endometriosis.

Administered as a suspension of the acetate (Lupron Depot), leuprolide exerts an effect for 4 weeks following intramuscular injection, e.g. of 3.75 mg. The side effects are a consequence of its induction of a prolonged hypoestrogenic state. As might be expected, they include bone loss as well as menopausal-like symptoms (irritability, nervousness, anxiety insomnia, hot flushes). In a 4-week multi-center clinical trial by Wheeler et al. comparing leuprolide with danazol in 270 patients, the drugs proved to have similar efficacy. Seven patients out of total of 101 taking leuprolide dropped out during treatment, the reasons being severe menopausal symptoms in five cases, eye pain, nausea and vomiting and hypertonia in one and (probably coincidental) enlargement of the clitoris in one case. Leuprolide was much less prone than danazol to alter blood fats or clotting factors. Patients became amenorrheic during treatment but menstruation returned in all but two patients. With leuprolide there was a significant decrease in bone density during treatment and this effect was more marked than with danazol; after completion of the treatment, the bone density parameters showed considerable recovery over a period of years; longer follow-up would be desirable (195[Cr]).

REFERENCES

1. World Health Organization Scientific Group. Effect of female sex hormones on fetal development and infant health. WHO Techn Rep Ser 1980;657.
2. McCredie J, Kricker A, Elliott J et al. Congenital limb defects and the pill. Lancet 1983;ii:623.
3. World Health Organization. Treatment of threatened or habitual abortion. In: Drugs in Pregnancy and Delivery. 11th European Symposium on Clinical Pharmacological Evaluation in Drug Control. Copenhagen: WHO Regional Office for Europe, 1984;6.
4. Sopena-Bonnet B. L'adénose cervico-vaginale: l'une des conséquences possibles de l'exposition in utero au DES. Contracept Fertil Sex 1989;17:461.
5. Senenekjian EK, Potkul RK, Frey K et al. Infertility among daughters either exposed or not exposed to diethylstilbestrol. Am J Obstet Gynecol 1988;158:493.
6. Hembree WC, Nagler HM, Fang JS et al. Infertility in a patient with abnormal spermatogenesis and in utero DES exposure. Int J Fertil 1988;33:173.
7. Buitendijk S. Diethylstilbestrol and the next generation—a challenge to the evidence? In: Dukes MNG, ed. Side Effects of Drugs, Annual 12. Amsterdam: Elsevier, 1988;346.
8. Lynch HT, Quinn T, Severin MJ. Diethylstilbestrol, teratogenesis and carcinogenesis: medical/legal implications of its long-term sequelae, including third-generation effects. Int J Risk Safety Med 1990;1:171.
9. Curran WJ. The DES product liability story in America:

The third generation litigation. Int J Risk Safety Med 1992;3:229.
10. Melnick S, Cole P, Anderson D et al. Rates and risks of diethylstilbestrol-related clear cell adenocarcinoma of the vagina and cervix. N Engl J Med 1987;316:514.
11. Noller KL, Blair PB, O'Brien PC et al. Increased occurrence of autoimmune disease among women exposed in utero to diethylstilbestrol. Fertil Steril 1988;49:1080.
12. Sharpe RM, Skakkebaek NE. Are oestrogens involved in falling sperm counts and disorders of the male reproductive tract? Lancet 1993;341:1392.
13. Oda K, Oguma N, Kawano M et al. Hepatocellular carcinoma associated with long-term anabolic steroid therapy in two patients with aplastic anemia. Acta Haematol Jpn 1987;50:29.
14. Greer T. Hepatic adenoma and oral contraceptive use. J Fam Pract 1989;28:322.
15. Brooks JJ. Hepatoma associated with diethylstilbestrol therapy for prostatic carcinoma. J Urol 1982;128:1044.
16. Heresbach D, Deugnier Y, Brissot P et al. Dilatations sinusoidales et prise de contraceptifs oraux. Ann Gastroentérol 1988;24:189.
17. Christopherson WM. Liver tumours and the pill. Br Med J 1975;4:756.
18. Firovino M, Akovblantz A et al. Regression of liver cell adenoma. Gastroenterology 1982;55:775.
19. Marks WH, Thompson N, Appleman H. Failure of hepatic adenomas (HCA) to regress after discontinuance of oral contraceptives. Ann Surg 1988;208:190.
20. Ross RK, Bernstein L, Garabrant D et al. Avoidable nondietary risk factors for cancer. Am Fam Physician 1988;38:153.
21. La Vecchia C, Negri E, Parazzini F. Oral contraceptives and primary liver cancer. Br J Cancer 1989;59:460.
22. Neuberger J, Forman D, Doll R, Williams R. Oral contraceptives and hepatocellular carcinoma. Br Med J 1986; 292:1355.
23. World Health Organization. Combined oral contraceptives and liver cancer. The WHO Collaborative Study of Neoplasia and Steroid Contraceptives. Int J Cancer 1989; 43:254.
24. Hsing AW, Hoover RN, McLaughlin JK et al. Oral contraceptives and primary liver cancer among young women. Cancer Causes Control 1992;3:43.
25. Prentice RL, Thomas DB. On the epidemiology of oral contraceptives and disease. Adv Cancer Res 1987;49:285.
26. Parazzini F, Negri E, Vecchia C et al. Population attributable risk for endometrial cancer in Northern Italy. Eur J Cancer Clin Oncol 1989;25:1451.
27. Brosens I, Johannisson E, Baulieu E-E et al. Oral contraceptives and hepatocellular carcinoma. Br Med J 1986; 292:1667.
28. Rubin GL, Peterson HB, Lee NC et al. Estrogen replacement therapy and the risk of endometrial cancer: remaining controversies. Am J Obstet Gynecol 1990;162:149.
29. Horwitz RI, Feinstein AR. Alternative analytic methods for case-control studies of estrogens and endometrial cancer. N Engl J Med 1978;299:1089.
30. Antunes CMF, Stolley PD, Rosenhein NB et al. Endometrial cancer and estrogen use: report of a large case-control study. N Engl J Med 1979;300:9.
31. Buring JE, Bain CJ, Ehrmann RL. Conjugated estrogen use and risk of endometrial cancer. Am J Epidemiol 1986;124:434.
32. Jick H, Watkins RN, Hunter JR et al. Replacement estrogens and endometrial cancer. N Engl J Med 1979; 300:218.
33. Ziel HK, Finkle WD. Association of estrone with the development of endometrial carcinoma. Am J Obstet Gynecol 1976;124:735.
34. Spengler KF, Clarke EA, Woolever AM et al. Exogenous estrogens and endometrial cancer: a case-control study and assessment of potential biases. Am J Epidemiol 1981;114:497.
35. Persson I. Climacteric Treatment with Estrogens und Estrogen - Progestogen Combinations: The Risk of Endometrial Neoplasia. Results of a Cohort Study. Thesis, University of Uppsala. Stockholm: Almqvist and Wiksell, 1983.
36. Levi F, La Vecchia C, Gulie C et al. Oestrogen replacement treatment and the risk of endometrial cancer; an assessment of the role of covariates. Eur J Cancer 1993;29A:445.
37. Jacobs HS, Loeffler FE. Postmenopausal hormone replacement therapy. Br Med J 1992;305:1403.
38. Centers for Disease Control: Cancer and Steroid Hormone Study. Oral contraceptive use and the risk of endometrial cancer. J Am Med Assoc 1983;249:1600.
39. World Health Organization. The WHO Collaborative Study of Neoplasia and Steroid Contraceptives. Epithelial ovarian cancer and combined oral contraCeptives. Int J Epidemiol 1988;18:538.
40. Beral V, Hannaford P, Kay C. Oral contraceptive use and malignancies of the genital tract. Lancet 1988;ii:1331.
41. Brinton LA, Huggins GR, Lehman HF et al. Long term use of oral contraceptives and risk of invasive cervical cancer. Int J Cancer 1986;38:339.
42. Slattery ML. Overall JC, Abbott TM et al. Sexual activity. contraception, genital infections, and cervical cancer: support for a sexually transmitted disease hypothesis. Am J Epidemiol 1989;130:248.
43. Bosch FX, Munoz N, De Sanjosé et al. Risk factors for cervical cancer in Colombia and Spain. Int J Cancer 1992;52:750.
44. McNab JCM, Walkinshaw SA, Cordiner JW et al. Human papillomavirus in clinically and histologically normal tissue of patients with genital cancer. New Engl J Med 1986;315:1052.
45. World Health Organization. Oral contraceptives and neoplasia: report of a WHO Scientific Group. WHO Tech Rep Ser 1992;817.
46. Myles JL, Hart WR. Apoplectic leiomyomas of the uterus. Am J Surg Pathol 1985;9:798.
47. Royal College of General Practitioners. Oral Contraceptives and Health. London: RCGP 1974.
48. Vessey MP, Doll R, Peto R et al. A long-term follow-up study of women using different methods of contraception—an interim report. J Biosoc Sci 1976;8:373.
49. Weiss S, Lyon L, Liff M et al. Incidence of ovarian cancer in relation to the use of oral contraceptives. Int J Cancer 1981;28:669.
50. Mack TM. Hormone replacement therapy and cancer. Baillière's Clin Endocrinol 1993;7:113.
51. Nisker JA, Siiteri PK. Estrogens and breast cancer. Clin Obstet Gynecol 1981;24:301.
52. World Health Organization. Steroid contraception and the risk of neoplasia. WHO Techn Rep Ser 1978;619.
53. Herbst AL, ed. Intrauterine exposure to diethylstilbestrol in the human. In: Proceedings, 'Symposium on DES',

1977. Chicago: American College of Obstetricians and Gynecologists, 1978.

54. Jick H, Watkins RN, Hunter JR et al. Replacement estrogens and endometrial cancer. N Engl J Med 1979; 300:218.

55. Royal College of General Practitioners. Oral Contraceptive Study. London: RCGP, 1981.

56. Pike MC, Henderson BE, Casagrand JT et al. Oral contraceptive use and early abortion as risk factors for breast cancer in young women. Br J Cancer 1981;43:72.

57. Vessey MP, McPherson K, Doll R. Breast cancer and oral contraceptives: findings in Oxford Family Planning Association Contraceptive Study. Br Med J 1981;282:2093.

58. Hulka B, Chambless L, Deubner D et al. Breast cancer and estrogen replacement therapy. Am J Obstet Gynecol 1982;143:638.

59. Ory GW, Layde OM et al. Long term oral contraceptive use and the risk of breast cancer. Paper presented at 31st Annual Epidemic Service Conference. Georgia: Atlanta, 1982.

60. Brinton LA, Hoover R, Szklo M et al. Oral contraceptives and breast cancer. Int J Epidemiol 1982;11:4.

61. Drife J. Which Pill? (Editorial) Br Med J 1983;287:1397.

62. Vessey MP, McPherson K, Yeates D et al. Oral contraceptive use and abortion before first term pregnancy in relation to breast cancer risk. Br J Cancer 1983;45:327.

63. Centers for Disease Control Cancer and Steroid Hormone Study. Long-term oral contraceptive use and the risk of breast cancer. J Am Med Assoc 1983;249:1591.

64. Pike MC, Henderson BE, Krailo MD et al. Breast cancer in young women and use of oral contraceptives: possible modifying effects of formulation and age at use. Lancet 1983;ii:926.

65. Janerich D, Polednak A et al. Breast cancer and oral contraceptive use: a case-control study. J Chronic Dis 1983;36:639.

66. Rosenberg A, Miller D, Kaufman D et al. Oral contraceptives and breast cancer. Am J Epidemiol 1984;119:167.

67. Stadel BC, Rubin GL, Webster LA et al. Oral contraceptives and breast cancer in young women. Lancet 1985;ii:970.

68. The Cancer and Steroid Hormone Study of the Centers for Disease Control and the National Institute of Child Health and Human Development. Oral contraceptive use and the risk of breast cancer. N Engl J Med 1986;105:405.

69. Ellery C, MacLennan R, Berry G et al. A case control study of breast cancer in relation to the use of steroid contraceptive agents. Med J Aust 1986;144:173.

70. Meirik O, Lund E, Adam H-O et al. Oral contraceptive use and breast cancer in young women. Lancet 1986;ii:922.

71. The Cancer and Steroid Hormone Study of the Centers for Disease Control and the National Institute of Child Health and Human Development. Oral contraceptive use and the risk of breast cancer. N Engl J Med 1986;105:405.

72. Shapiro S. Oral contraceptives—time to take stock. N Engl J Med 1986;315:450.

73. Stadel BV, Schlesselman JJ. Oral contraceptive use and the risk of breast cancer in women with a 'prior' history of benign breast disease. Am J Epidemiol 1986;123:373.

74. Lee NC, Rosero-Bixby L, Oberle MW et al. A case control study of breast cancer and hormonal contraception in Costa Rica. J Natl Cancer Inst 1987;79:1247.

75. Stadel BV, Lai S, Schlesselman JJ et al. Oral contraceptives and premenopausal breast cancer in nulliparous women. Contraception 1988;35:287.

76. Bergkvist L, Adami HO, Persson I et al. The risk of breast cancer after estrogen and estrogen-progestin replacement. N Engl J Med 1989;321:293.

77. The WHO Collaborative Study of Neoplasia and Steroid Contraceptives. Breast cancer and combined oral contraceptives: result from a multinational study. Br J Cancer 1990;61:110.

78. MacLennan A. Hormone replacement therapy and the menopause. A consensus statement of the Australian Menopause Society. Med J Aust 1991;155:43.

79. World Health Organization. Oral contraceptives and neoplasia: report of a WHO Scientific Group. WHO Tech Rep Ser 1992;817.

80. Gambrell RD. Estrogen replacement therapy and breast cancer risk. A new look at the data. Female Patient 1993;18:55.

81. Golditz GA, Egan KM, Stampfer MJ. Hormone replacemen therapy and risk of breast cancer. Results from epidemiologic studies. Am J Obstet Gynecol 1993;168:1473.

82. Stewart GR. Hormone replacement therapy and breast cancer. Med J Aust 1993;158:436.

83. Colditz GA, Stammfer MJ, Willett WC et al. Type of postmenopausal hormone use and risk of breast cancer. 12-year follow-up from the Nurses' Health Study. Cancer Causes Control 1992;3:475.

84. Carruthers R. Chloasma and oral contraceptives. Med J Aust 1966;2:17.

85. Beral V, Ramcharan S, Faris R. Malignant melanoma and oral contraceptive use among women in California. Br J Cancer 1977;36:804.

86. Beral V, Shaw H, Milton G. Oral contraceptive use and malignant melanoma in Australia. Br J Cancer 1984;50:681.

87. Notclovttz M. Effect of natural oestrogens on blood pressure and weight in postmenopausal women. South Afr Med J 1975;49:2551.

88. Wilson PWF, Garrison RJ, Castelli WP. Postmenopausal estrogen use, cigarette smoking, and cardiovascular morbidity in women over 50: The Framingham Study. N Engl J Med 1985;313:1038.

89. Thompson SG, Meade TW, Greenberg G. The use of hormonal replacement therapy and the risk of stroke and myocardial infarction in women. J Epidemiol Community Health 1989;43:173.

90. Stampfer MJ, Willett WC, Colditz GA et al. A prospective study of postmenopausal estrogen therapy and coronary heart disease. N Engl J Med 1985;313:1044.

91. Jaffe MD. Effect of oestrogens on post exercise electrocardiogram. Br Heart J 1977;39:1299.

92. Collins LC, Peiris A. Bronchospasm secondary to replacement estrogen therapy. Chest 1993;104:1300.

93. Kise HJ, Meienberg O. Deterioration or onset of migraine under estrogen replacement in the menopause. J Neurol 1993;240:195.

94. Sturdee DW, Gustafson RC, Moore B. Glucose tolerance and hormone replacement therapy: a preliminary study. Postgrad Med J 1976;55(Suppl 6):52.

95. Sherwin BB, Gelfland MM. A prospective one-year study of estrogen and progestin in post-menopausal women: effects on clinical symptoms and lipoprotein lipids. Obstet Gynecol 1989;73:759.

96. Astedt B. Low fibrinolytic activity of veins during treatment with ethinyloestradiol. Acta 0bstet Gynaecol Scand 1971;50:279.

97. McClennan BL. Ischemic colitis secondary to Premarin: report of a case. Dis Colon Rectum 1976;19:618.

98. Underwood TW, Frye CB. Drug-induced pancreatitis. Clin Pharm 1993;12:440.
99. Orlander JD, Jicks S, Dean AD et al. Urinary tract infections and estrogen use in older women. J Am Geriatr Soc 1992;40:817.
100. Malina L, Chlumsky J. Oestrogen-induced familial porphyria cutanea tarda. Br J Dermatol 1975;92:707.
101. Styrt B, Sugarman B. Estrogens and infection. Rev Infect Dis 1991;13:1139.
102. Jensen J, Christiansen C. Dose-response effects on serum lipids and lipoproteins following combined oestrogen—progestogen therapy in post-menopausal women. Maturitas 1987;9:259.
103. Selby PL, Reacock M. The effect of transdermal estrogen on bone, calcium regulating hormones and liver in postmenopausal women. Clin Endocrinol 1986;25:543.
104. Kainz W, Aldor E, Titscher G et al. Hyperöstrogenismus als möglicher Risikofaktor bei Männern mit koronarer Herzkrankheit. Herz Kreisl 1985;17:21.
105. Henrikson P, Blomback M, Bratt G et al. Effects of estrogen therapy and orchidectomy on coagulation and prostanoid synthesis in patients with prostatic cancer. Med Oncol Tumor Pharmacother 1989;6:219.
106. Henriksson P, Johansson SE. Prediction of cardiovascular complications in patients with prostatic cancer treated with oestrogen. Am J Epidemiol 1987;125:970.
107. Pavone-Macaluso M, De Voogt HJ, Viggiano G et al. Comparison of diethylstilbestrol, cyproterone acetate and medroxyprogesterone acetate in the treatment of advanced prostatic cancer: final analysis of a randomized phase III trial of the European Organization for Research on Treatment of Cancer Urological Group. J Urol 1986;136:624.
108. Feustel A, Nietzsschmann U. Der Einfluss gegenschlechtlicher Hormonbehandlung und Kastration auf Hb und Blutkörperchensenkunggeschwindigkeit beim Prostatkarzinom. Urol Int 1974;29:1.
109. Bazex A, Salvader R, Dupré A et al. Gynécomastie et hyperpigmentation aréolaire après oestrogénothérapie locale anti-séborrhéique. Bull Soc Fr Dermatol Syphiligr 1967; 74:466.
110. Engel T, Jewelewicz R, Dyrenfurth I et al. Ovarian hyperstimulation syndrome. Am J Obstet Gynccol 1972; 112:1052.
111. Mrouch A, Kase N. Acute ascites and hydrothorax after gonadotropin therapy. Obstet Gynecol 1976;30:346.
112. Nwosu OF, Corson L, Bolognese RJ. Hyperstimulation and multiple side-effects of menotropin therapy: a case report. J Reprod Med 1974;12:117.
113. Rubin SO. Malignant teratoma of testis in a subfertile man treated with HCG and HMG. Scand J Urol Nephrol 1973;7:81.
114. Kistner RW. The use of clomiphene citrate in the treatment of anovulation. Semin Drug Treat 1973;3:159.
115. Gysler M, March M et al. A decade's experience with individualized clomiphene treatment regimen. Fertil Steril 1982;37:161.
116. Cornel MC, Ten Kate LP, Dukes MNG et al. Ovulation induction and neural tube defects. Lancet 1989;i:1386.
117. Gluckle H, Wald N. Clomifene and neural tube defects. Lancet 1991;337:853.
118. James WH. The sex ratio of infants born after hormonal induction of ovulation. Br J Obstet Gynaecol 1985;92:299.
119. Neoptolemos JP, Locke TJ et al. Testicular tumour associated with hormonal treatment for oligospermia. Lancet 1981;ii:754.
120. Insler V, Lunenfeld B. Anovulation. Contrib Gynecol Obstet 1978;4:6.
121. De Muylder X, Neven P. Tamoxifen and potential adverse effects. Cancer J 1993;6:111.
122. Sawka CA, Pritchard Kl, Paterson AHG et al. Role and mechanism of action of tamoxifen in premenopausal women with metastatic breast carcinoma. Cancer Res 1986;46:3152.
123. Ferrazzi E, Cartel G, De Besi P et al. Tamoxifen in disseminated breast cancer. Tumori 1977;63:463.
124. Millward MJ, Cantwell BMJ, Lien EA et al. Intermittent high-dose tamoxifen as a potential modifier of multidrug resistance. Eur J Cancer 1992;28A:805.
125. Boudouris O, Ferrand S, Guillet JL. Efféts paradoxaux du tamoxifène sur l'utérus de la femme. J Gynecol Obstet Biol Reprod 1989;18:372.
126. Nuovo MA, Nuovo GJ, McCaffrey RM et al. Endometrial polyps in postmenopausal patients receiving tamoxifen. Int J Gynecol Pathol 1989;8:125.
127. Rutqvist LE, Mattson A. Cardiac and thromboembolic morbidity among post-menopausal women with early-stage breast cancer in randomized trial of adjuvant tamoxifen. J Natl Cancer Inst 1993;85:1398.
128. Seoud MAF, Jonson J, Weed JC. Gynecologic tumours in tamoxifen-treated women with breast cancer. Obstet Gynec 1993;82:165.
129. Fentiman IS, Fogelman I. Breast cancer and osteoporosis—a bridge at last. Eur J Cancer 1993;29A:485.
130. Montes A, Powles TJ, O'Brien MER. A toxic interaction between mitomycin C and tamoxifen causing the haemolytic uraemic syndrome. Eur J Cancer 1993;29A:1854.
131. Pugesgaard T, Von Eyben F. Bilateral optic neuritis evolved during tamoxifen treatment. Cancer 1956;58:383.
132. Pavlidis NA, Petris C, Briassoulis E et al. Clear evidence that long-term, low-dose tamoxifen treatment can induce ocular toxicity. Cancer 1992;69:2961.
133. Sherman BM, Chapler FK, Crickard K et al. Endocrine consequences of continuous antiestrogen therapy with tamoxifen in premenopausal women. J Clin Invest 1978;64: 398.
134. Bruning PF. Drolixifene, a new antiestrogen in postmenopausal advanced breast cancer: preliminary results of a double-blind dose-finding phase II trial. Eur. J. Cancer 1992;28A:1404.
135. Hamm JT, Tormey DC, Kohler PC et al. Phase I study of toremifene in patients with advanced cancer. J Clin Oncol 1991;9:2036.
136. Olsson R, Tyllström J, Zettergren L. Hepatic reactions to cyclophenil. Gut 1983;24:260.
137. Schmidt-Elmendorff H, Kämmerling R. Vergleicehende klinsche Untersuchungen von Clomiphen. Cyclofenil und Epimestrol. Geburtsh Frauenheilkd 1977;37:531.
138. Boyer JL, Preisig R, Zbinden G et al. Guidelines for assessment of potential hepatotoxic effects of synthetic androgens, anabolic agents and progestogens in their use in males as antifertility agents. Contraception 1976;13:461.
139. Werner T. Ikterus mit Worschluss-syndrom nach Behandlung mit Noresthisteronazetat. Z Gastroenterol 1969; 7:186.
140. Simon E, Schiffer M, Glick SM et al. Effect of medroxyprogesterone acetate upon stimulated release of growth hormone in men. J Clin Endocrinol 1967;57:1633.
141. Palanca E. Juco W. Conservative treatment of benign prostatic hyperplasia. Curr Med Res Opin 1977;4:513.

142. Huovinen K, Autio S, Kaprio J. Peroral lynestrenol and arterial disease in mentally retarded women. Acta Obstet Gynaecol Scand 1988;67:211.

143. Teichmann AT, Cremer P, Wieland H et al. Lipid metabolic changes during hormonal treatment Of endometriosis. Maturitas 1988;10:27.

144. Wander HE, Nagel GA, Blossey HC et al. Aminoglutethimide and medroxyprogesterone acetate in the treatment of patients with advanced breast cancer. Cancer 1986; 58:1985.

145. Tschekmedyian NS, Tait N, Aisner J. High-dose megestrol acetate in the treatment of postmenopausal women with advanced breast cancer. Semin Oncol 1986;13:20.

146. Crombie D, Raghaven D, Page J et al. Phase II study of megestrol acetate for metastatic carcinoma of the prostate. Br J Urol 1987;59:443.

147. Löffler TM, Weber FW, Hausamen TU. Einfluss von mittelhoch dosiertem Megestrolacetat auf Appetitstimulation und gewichtszunahme bei gleichzeitiger zytostatische therapie. Tumordiagn Ther 1992;13:72.

148. Johnson DE, Babaian RJ, Swanson DA et al. Medical castration using megestrol acetate and minidose estrogen. Urology 1988;31:371.

149. Nieman LK, Choute TM, Chrousos GP et al. The progesterone antagonist RU 486: a potential new contraceptive agent. N Engl J Med 1987;316:187.

150. Maria B, Stampf F, Foepp A, Ulmann A. Termination of early pregnancy by a single dose of mifepristone (RU 486), a progesterone antagonist. Eur J Obstet Gynecol Reprod Biol 1988;28:249.

151. Lowdell CP, Murray-Lyon IM. Reversal liver damage due to long-term methyltestosterone and safety of non-17α-alkylated androgens. Br Med J 1985;291:637.

152. Evely RS, Triger DR, Milnes JP et al. Severe cholestasis associated with stanazolol. Br Med J 1987;294:612.

153. McGaugham GW, Bilous MJ, Gallagher ND. Long-term survival with tumor regression in androgen-induced liver tumors. Cancer 1985;56:2622.

154. Sanchez JMC, Becerra EP, Martin AA et al. Adenoma hepatico después del tratamiento con oximetolona. Rev Esp Pediatr 1988;44:195.

155. Oda K, Oguma N, Kawano M et al. Hepatocellular carcinoma associated with longterm anabolic steroid therapy in two patients with aplastic anemia. Acta Haematol Jpn 1987;50:29.

156. Pandita R, Quadri MI. Constitutional aplastic anemia. Indian Pediatr 1988;25:469.

157. Perlmutter C, Löwenthal D. Use of anabolic steroids by athletes. Aust Fam Physician 1985;32:208.

158. Kiraly CL, Collan Y, Alein M. Effect of testosterone and anabolic steroids on the size of sebaceous glands in power athletes. Am J Dermatopathol 1987;9:515.

159. Keul J, Deus B, Kindermann W. Anabole Hormone: Schädigung, Leistungsfähigkeit und Stoffwechsel. Med Klin 1976;71:497.

160. Costill DL, Pearson DR, Fink WJ. Anabolic steroids use among athletes: changes in HDL-C levels. Phys Sportsmed 1984;12:113.

161. Sandblom RE, Matsumoto AM, Schoene RB et al. Obstructive sleep apnea syndrome induced by testosterone administration. N Engl J Med 1983;9:508.

162. Zelissen PMJ, Stricker BHC. Severe priapism as a complication of testosterone therapy. Am J Med 1988;85:273.

163. Ahmed SR, Boucher AE, Manni A et al. Transdermal testosterone therapy in the treatment of male hypogonadism. J Clin Endocrinol Metab 1988;66:546.

164. Koch-Weser J, Sellers EM. Drug interactions with coumarin anticoagulants. N Engl J Med 1971;285:547.

165. Acomb D, Shaw PW. A significant interaction between warfarin and stanozolol. Pharm J 1985;234:73.

166. Volk H, Deupree RH, Goldenberg IS et al. A dose-response evaluation of delta-1-testolactone in advanced breast cancer. Cancer 1974;33:9.

167. Seay DG, Bradshaw JD, Nicol NL. Clinical experience with dromostanolone-propionate (CNSC-12198) in breast carcinoma. Cancer Chemother Rep 1972;56:89.

168. Gorins A. Le traitement du cancer du sein en phase avancée par le drostanolone propionate. CR Soc Fr Gynécol 1970:40:553.

169. Gordan GS, Halden A, Horn Y et al. Improved treatment for metastatic breast cancer. Clin Res 1971;19:573.

170. Buttram VC, Reiter RC, Ward S. Treatment of endometriosis with danazol: report of a 6-year prospective study. Fertil Steril 1985;43:353.

171. Gorins A, Perret F, Tournant B et al. A French double-blind crossover study (danazol versus placebo) in the treatment of severe fibrocystic breast disease. Eur J Gynaecol Oncol 1984;2:85.

172. Peress MR. Persistent amenorrhea following discontinuation of danazol therapy. Fertil Steril 1984;41:322.

173. Franchimont P, Cramilion CI. The effect of danazol on anterior pituitary function. Fertil Steril 1977;28:814.

174. Wynn V. Metabolic effects of danazol. J Int Med Res 1977;5(Suppl 3):25.

175. Middleton C, McCaughan GW, Painter DM et al. Danazol and hepatic neoplasia: a case report. Aust NZ J Med 1989;19:733.

176. Rakoff AE. Side-effects of danazol therapy. In: Greenblatt RB, ed. Recent Advances in Endometriosis. Proceedings of a Symposium, Augusta, GA, 1975. Amsterdam: Excerpta Medica, 1976;108.

177. Wentz AC. Adverse effects of danazol in pregnancy. Ann Intern Med 1982;96:672.

178. Nelson MV. Interaction of danazol and carbamazepine. Int J Psychiatry 1988;145:768.

179. Krämer G, Theison M, Von Unruh GE et al. Carbamazepine—danazol drug interaction: its mechanism examined by a stable isotope technique. Ther Drug Monit 1986;8:387.

180. Kolb KH. Zur Pharmacokinetik des Cyproteronacetat: biologisch-experimentelle Studien. Adv Biosci 1969;1:71.

181. Röpke H. Simulierung der Pharmakokinetik des Cyproteronacetat mit dem Analogcomputer. Adv Biosc 1969;1:61.

182. Beurton D Grall J, Davody Ph et al. Treatment of prostatic cancer with cyproterone acetate as monotherapy. Prog Clin Biol Res 1987;243A:369.

183. Willemse PHB, Dikkeschei LD, Mulder NH et al. Clinical and endocrine effects of cyproterone acetate in postmenopausal patients with advanced breast cancer. Eur J Cancer Clin Oncol 1988;24:417.

184. Blake JC, Sawyer AM, Dooley JS et al. Severe hepatitis caused by cyproterone acetate. Gut 1990;31:556.

185. Meijers WH, Willemse PHB, Sleijfer DT et al. Hepatocellular damage by cyproterone acetate. Eur J Cancer Clin Oncol 1986;22:1121.

186. Leroy O, Beuscart C, Senneville E. Deep venous thrombosis and antibodies to cyproterone acetate. Lancet 1990;336:509.

187. Green NA, Harrison BWD. Breathlessness in patients

with prostatic carcinoma treated with cyproterone acetate. Br Med J 1989;298:1524.
188. Micheroli R, Battegay R. Ambulante Behandlung von Sexualdelinquenten mit Cyproteronacetat (Androcur). Schw Arch Neurol Neurochir Psychiatr 1985;136:37.
189. Stanhope R. Huen KF, Buzi F et al. The effect of cyproterone acetate on the growth of children with central precocious puberty Eur J Pediatr 1987;46:500.
190. Laschet U. Eine Möglichkeit zur Behandlung von sexuellen Deviationen und Perversionen beim Mann. Med Mitt 1973;2:11.
191. Pichler WK, Lehner R, Spath PJ. Recurrent angioedema associated with hypogonadism or antiandrogen therapy. Ann Allergy 1989;63:301.
192. Keil TU. Behandlung androgenabhängiger Harterkrankungen. Fortschr Med 1985;103:51.
193. Hammerstein J, Meckies J, Leo-Rossberg I et al. Use of cyproterone acetate (CPA) in the treatment of acne, hirsutism and virilism. J Steroid Biochem 1975;6:827.
194. Koch H. Flutamide—a new non-steroidal anti-androgen. Drugs Today 1984;20:561.
195. Wheeler JM, Knittle JD, Miller JD. Depot leuprolide acetate versus danazol in the treatment of women with symptomatic endometriosis: A multicenter,double-blind randomized clinical trial. Am J Obstet Gynecol 1993;169:26.

Meyler's Side Effects of Drugs, 13th Edition
M.N.G. Dukes, editor

SECTION EDITOR: M.N.G. DUKES

J. Weeke

41 Thyroid and antithyroid drugs

Drugs affecting thyroid function can be divided into those which mimic the effects of endogenous hormones (thyroid hormones) and those interfering with their synthesis and/or secretion ('antithyroid drugs'). A third group of drugs—the 'iodine preparations'—may interfere with the natural physiological function of the thyroid because of their excessive iodine content. Also, the destructive properties of radioactive iodides can be used in the treatment of thyroid diseases. Before, during and occasionally after treatment with thyroid and/or antithyroid drugs, control of serum concentrations of thyroid-stimulating hormone and thyroid hormones should be performed to monitor their effect and adjust the dosage.

The normal adult thyroid gland secretes about 90 μg of thyroxine (T4) and less than 10 μg of triiodothyronine (T3) per day. Somewhat less than half of the T4 is converted to T3 by several tissues (especially the liver). Most of the daily production of T3 thus comes from peripheral 5-deiodination of T4 and not by direct glandular secretion. The thyroid hormones are tightly bound (T4 even more than T3) to plasma transport proteins, thus explaining their prolonged half-life (about 8 days for T4 and about 1 day for T3). Nuclear receptors for thyroid hormones bind T3 much more efficiently than T4, thereby explaining the more rapid onset of action and greater biological potency of T3. The intestinal absorption and hepatic clearance of orally ingested thyroid hormones also differ. T3 is much better absorbed and in earlier studies was found to have a higher bioavailability than T4, only about 60% of which appears in the peripheral circulation after oral intake (1[R]). More recent studies, however, have found a higher intestinal absorption of T4 (±80%), at least when administered in the form of new pharmaceutical preparations designed to optimize its absorption, and when its content was validated by high-pressure liquid chromatography (2). These basic data form the background of optimal thyroid substitution. Thyroid hormones are used either to replace the failing function of the thyroid gland (spontaneous or drug-induced) or to suppress the endocrine function of abnormal thyroid tissues (especially non-toxic struma, goiter or after thyroidectomy for thyroid neoplasms). Although abnormalities of the peripheral metabolism of thyroid hormones are known to be present in some forms of under- or overnutrition, thyroid drug therapy cannot be considered a safe means of treating obesity.

Treatment with thyroid hormones therefore poses only a few essential questions: which dosage should be used, which preparation chosen and how can therapy best be monitored so as to avoid short- and long-term risks?

THYROID HORMONES

L-Thyroxine (T4), triiodothyronine (T3) and thyroid extract

For a long period, the cheapest preparations of thyroid hormone (and at one time the only ones available) were simple *extracts of animal thyroid glands*. Although these products have been used for many decades with remarkably few side effects, such crude extracts also have some important disadvantages. Animal thyroid glands contain different ratios of T4/T3 (range 2—5:1 by weight) and therefore differ widely from the most common human ratio of 10:1. The absolute quantity of thyroid hormone may also vary independently of the total iodine content. One grain (60 mg) of a thyroid preparation was found to vary by as much as 15—110% in its T4 content and by 53—120% in its T3 content (3[CR]). The problem of the absolute amount of thyroid hormones can probably be overcome by (bio)assaying the true thyroid hormone content, but the inappropriate T4/T3 ratio results in abnormally high serum T3 concentrations, especially in the postabsorptive phase. This seems to be a sufficient argument to discontinue the use of thyroid extracts whenever T4 is available and certainly when full substitution rather than partial suppression is necessary (SEDA-3, 340).

Triiodothyronine (*T*3) can be used for thyroid substitution, but it has the disadvantage of being short-lived and its intestinal absorption may give rise to unusually high post-absorption peaks inducing symptoms of tachycardia. Moreover, the dosage necessary to obtain euthyroidism is more difficult to evaluate due to fluctuations in serum T3: measurements of thyroid-stimulating hormone (TSH) are also probably less reliable since its secretion is more dependent on the extracellular T4 than on T3 concentration. The therapeutic use of T3 is therefore generally only recommended when a more rapid onset of action is necessary, e.g. when thyroid therapy needs to be interrupted for the administration of ^{131}I in treatment of thyroid cancer. In myxedema coma it is controversial if the therapeutic choice should be T3 or T4 or a combination (95[R]). Moreover, long-term therapy with T3 is more likely to cause secondary osteoporosis than T4 (see below).

The drug of choice for thyroid replacement therapy is therefore *L-thyroxine* (T4) since it is the natural secretory product of the thyroid, has a long half-life and will be metabolized in the peripheral tissues according to the general body requirements. The optimal dosage of T4 is more difficult to determine and should be based on repeated measurements of both T4 and TSH serum concentrations. Prior to the 1980s when these measurements were unavailable, 300 μg daily was frequently advised. Today, the daily recommended dose is more usually 100—200 μg, a level which is designed to restore a normal T4 and TSH concentration.

The daily recommended dose depends on the aim of the therapy. Thyroid replacement therapy for control of spontaneous or iatrogenic hypothyroidism should aim at a dosage of T4 which maintains TSH concentrations within the normal range (certainly not undetectably low using sensitive immunoradiometric TSH assays). This will usually be associated with a high-normal range for free T4 and a T3 concentration within the low-normal range. The mean requirement for such patients has been found to be 112 ± 19 μg/day (2[CR]) and 1.57 μg/kg per day (4[CR]). This dose is lower than that recommended previously because of a better knowledge of the real T4 production rate, availability of better pharmaceutical preparations allowing greater bioavailability and especially because of better methods for drug monitoring (SEDA-12, 353; SEDA-15, 444; 5[CR]—7[CR]). A confusing factor has been the presence of incorrect amounts of thyroxine in some older branded preparations of T4 (SEDA-10, 366). Even in 1987 some thyroid preparations still contained much less hormone than stated (2[CR]). High-pressure liquid chromatographic evaluation of the T4 content of thyroxine tablets is now a standard routine in the United States (8[CR]) and should be adopted everywhere. During pregnancy the replacement dose should be increased at least according to recent data obtained from a retrospective analysis of pregnant hypothyroid patients. The mean increase in T4 dosage was 40% (9[CR]).

When thyroid therapy is used not only in replacement of a failing gland but also to prevent growth of remnants of a differentiated thyroid carcinoma, a suppressive thyroid dosage is used aiming at high-normal T4 concentrations and TSH in the undetectable or at least lower than normal range, as measured by two-sided assays. Such therapy is warranted because of its long-term safety, efficacy and tolerance, but some additional therapy for osteoporosis prevention should be considered (see below).

As with all forms of long-term therapy, compliance with the prescribed dosage of T4 is not always optimal and an unwarranted fear of thyroid-induced osteoporosis or breast cancer may add to this lack of compliance. Inadequacy of thyroxine replacement therapy is not always easily recognized. Several patients were reported with clearly inadequate or excessive T4 consumption despite a correct prescription. All patients suffered from depression. Depression could indeed be an additional risk factor by promoting lack of compliance, and the resulting hypo- or hyperthyroidism could further aggravate the depression (10[C]).

In contrast to other protein-bound drugs for which a loading dose is given to achieve rapid steady-state concentrations, a slow and stepwise increase in thyroid hormone replacement therapy is advisable. This is preferred mainly to avoid sudden cardiac side effects, especially in older patients with long-standing myxedema. Moreover, since thyroid hormone substitution may change the metabolic clearance of this drug, steady-state concentrations are obtained only after several months (SEDA-6, 363).

ADVERSE REACTION PATTERN

General and toxic reactions The main adverse effects of thyroid hormones are those which would be expected to result from overdosage. These can largely be avoided by adjusting the dosage according to the appropriately selected laboratory tests. The adverse effects essentially comprise the symptoms of hyperthyroidism and include weight loss despite a normal or increased appetite, increased nervousness, tachycardia or arrhythmia of various types, increased general metabolism and its symptoms (sweating, thermophobia, etc.).

Hypersensitivity reactions Allergy to pure thyroid preparations was first reported as late as 1986. Fever, liver dysfunction and eosinophilia appeared during T3 or T4 treatment of a hypothyroid patient disappearing after discontinuation of the therapy

(12). In vitro lymphocyte testing confirmed sensitization for thyroid hormones. Progressive re-institution of T3 subsequently proved possible in this patient without recurrence of hypersensitivity. T3 was considered preferable because of the shorter biological half-life.

Tumor-inducing effects A possible link between breast cancer in women and thyroid hormone therapy was suggested on the basis of a retrospective study of patients with breast cancer (SEDA-3, 340). A subsequent statistical re-analysis of the original data failed, as have other more recent studies, to confirm such a relationship (SEDA-3, 340; SEDA-4, 294; 11[R]).

ORGANS AND SYSTEMS

Cardiovascular Overdosage of thyroid hormones induces *tachycardia or palpitations* but may also result in several types of *arrhythmia*, e.g. auricular fibrillation. Pre-existing cardiac disease, always to be suspected in the elderly or after long-standing hypothyroidism, may be severely aggravated by sudden thyroid substitution, resulting in severe angina pectoris. myocardial infarction or sudden cardiac death (SEDA-13, 375). In such patients, the initial dosage should be low and the stepwise increase should be spaced out over a prolonged period and with careful clinical and ECG control. In some circumstances, e.g. three-vessel disease, substitution should be postponed until after coronary bypass surgery (SEDA-6, 363). Cardiac decompensation may also result from the increased circulatory demand induced by thyroid hormone substitution or overtreatment. However, patients receiving long-term treatment with T4 had no change in morbidity, mortality and quality of life, including cardiovascular manifestations (96[C]).

Nervous system *Insomnia*, *psychic stimulation*, *general nervousness* and *tremor* are among the hyperthyroid symptoms resulting from relative overdosage. *Pseudotumor cerebri* has incidentally been observed shortly after T4 was given for juvenile hypothyroidism. The headache and bilateral papilledema without focal neurological defects subsequently disappeared even when T4 treatment was continued (13[C]). Several cases of mania have also been reported even after the intake of what is usually considered as safe doses of T4 (14[c]).

Metabolic With overdosage, increased metabolism results in *increased heat production*, with increased perspiration and thermophobia and possible weight loss despite normal or even increased appetite.

Skeletal The occurrence of a *slipped capital femoral epiphysis* has been described during the treatment of hypothyroidism (SEDA-3, 340). Since it is known that slipping occurs more frequently during the pubertal growth spurt, it is advisable to check for the occurrence of this complication during the pubertal period in children receiving thyroid treatment. Prolonged overtreatment may result in osteopenia.

Thyroid hormones have a direct effect on bone cells, thereby increasing both bone resorption and formation with subsequent mild adaptation of the systemic calciotrophic hormones (15[CR]). Increased bone turnover can result in a small deficit during each cycle and therefore finally result in mild *osteoporosis*. No good data regarding fracture incidence are available, but the bone mineral content of several areas known to be at risk for fractures (lumbar spine, forearm, femur) has been measured, mainly in cross-section, but also in a few prospective studies. During replacement therapy for hypothyroidism a small bone deficit was associated with a prior history of Graves' disease and/or later therapy with T3 or T4 dosages which suppress TSH concentrations (SEDA-16, 471). Since overt hyperthyroidism is well recognized to be associated with bone loss, it is possible that the reduction in bone density reported in some studies of T4 treatment reflect an adverse effect of previous thyrotoxicosis rather than T4 therapy itself (SEDA-17, 473). The best idea about the effects of prolonged T4 therapy can probably be obtained from bone mineral content measurements in patients with suppressive T4 dosage for thyroid carcinoma (Table 1). Therefore postmenopausal women with intact parathyroid glands on prolonged suppressive T4 therapy may have an increased risk for osteoporosis and should have their BMC measured and/or receive preventive osteoporosis therapy. Cautious use of T4, avoiding overdosage and unnecessary use, is probably safe for bone.

After-effects Prolonged adrenocortical insufficiency is well known after prolonged steroid therapy. Thyroid function usually recovers within 4 weeks after withdrawal of thyroid hormone therapy. Hypothalamic secretion of thyrotrophin-releasing hormone (TRH) is the last part of the thyroid-hypophyseal axis to recover.

Risk situations *Pre-existing cardiac disease* and *long-standing hypothyroidism* carry serious risks (see above). *Adrenal insufficiency* may be associated with hypothyroidism (either by autoimmune destruction or due to hypophyseal disease) and carries the risk of an acute Addison's crisis if thyroid substitution precedes corticosteroid therapy. The diagnostic problem presented by the fact that a few patients with central hypothyroidism have a moderately increased serum TSH should be kept in mind (98[C]). Some goitrous patients have an auto-

Table 1. *Bone mineral content and thyroid replacement therapy: longitudinal studies*

Author (Ref.)	*n*/Sex (Age)	Disease	FU	Results BMC		
				Femur	Spine	Radius
Krolner et al. (16a[C])	7 F/1 M (57 yr)	Primary hypothyroidism 125 μg T4	1 yr	—	−9%/yr	
Ribot et al. (16b[C])	6 F/4 M (50 yr)	Hypothyroidism R/135 μg T4	1 yr −7%	−5%	—	
Toh et al. (17[C])	24 M (50 yr)	Primary hypothyroidism (8) post-^{131}I (16)	3 yr	N.S.	N.S.	N.S.
Stall et al. (18[C])	18 F postm. (60 yr)	Hypothyroidism treated for 14 yr	2 yr			
		(a) low TSH (T4 dose 170)		−1.4%/yr	−2.9%/yr	−1.2%/yr
		(b) normal TSH		−0.3%/yr	−1.1%/yr	−0.13%/yr

FU = duration of follow-up

nomous thyroid hormone secretion which quantitatively is still within the normal limits, but they become hyperthyroid even with relatively small amounts of exogenous thyroid hormones since the latter accumulate with the endogenous autonomous thyroid secretion.

Second-generation effects Thyroid hormones virtually do not cross the placental barrier except for small amounts during early fetal development. The fetus is therefore dependent on its own thyroid hormone secretion. Thyroid hypo- or hyperfunction of the mother may, however, in itself unfavorably influence the fetal outcome or well-being. Thyroid therapy should therefore be carefully adjusted during or before pregnancy.

Thyroid hormone secretion is not markedly increased during pregnancy and it has generally been considered that thyroid replacement therapy should therefore not generally be increased during pregnancy. Recent experience, however, with the use of a minimal replacement dosage outside pregnancy casts doubt on this belief, experience pointing to the need for a mean increase of 40% increase in such thyroid replacement dosage during pregnancy (9[CR]).

Interactions T4 increases the toxicity of *cardiac glycosides* and enhances the effect of *coumarin anticoagulants*. *Oral antidiabetic drugs* and *clofibrate* may enhance the effect of T4. *Cholestyramine* reduces its absorption. *Estrogens*, e.g. in oral contraceptives, increase the thyroxine-binding globulin concentration, leading to diagnostic and therapeutic errors. Several drugs (*androgens*, *corticosteroids*, *diphenylhydantoin*, *salicylates*) and diseases (*liver or kidney disease*, *malnutrition*) may interfere with the transport or metabolism of thyroid hormones and thereby profoundly influence thyroid function tests.

OTHER THYROID HORMONES

Dextrothyroxine

Dextrothyroxine (D-T4) is used as a lipid-lowering agent. It significantly lowers the serum cholesterol (19a[R]) as does levothyroxine (L-T4). However, the D-form has a much smaller hormonal effect on body tissues than the L-isomeric form. The literature is confusing since older preparations of D-T4 contained considerable amounts of L-T4. For example, in the US Coronary Drug Project (19b[R]) a D-T4 preparation was used with a so-called low L-T4 content. It was necessary to terminate the study because of an excessive number of cardiac deaths and non-fatal infarcts.

Overdosage Inadvertent excessive use of thyroid hormones (by eating ground beef contaminated with thyroid hormones), the incorrect use of these drugs for the treatment of obesity, excessive thyroid substitution therapy and factitious use of thyroid hormones for psychiatric reasons result in mild hyperthyroidism, but serious short-term side effects are rare. Accidental or suicidal injection of large amounts of thyroid hormones is exceptional (20[R]). Clinical symptoms do not necessarily correlate well with plasma T4 levels and range from anxiety, confusion or coma to tachycardia, atrial fibrillation and angina. At least three lethal cases have been reported previously (SEDA-8, 371). Treatment of thyroid overdosage is not well standardized and may include gastric lavage, sedatives, β-blockers, hydrocortisone or specific antiarrhythmic drugs. Plasmapheresis and exchange transfusion have been used successfully to treat life-threatening cases. More recent studies have found beneficial effects of iodine-containing organic radiographic agents (ipodate) since they are potent inhibitors of the peripheral conversion of T4 to T3, but rebound effects are not impossible (20[R]).

PITUITARY HORMONES AND RELEASERS

Thyrotrophin (thyroid-stimulating hormone; TSH)

Since antibodies to TSH can develop, it is used only as a diagnostic and not as a therapeutic agent. *Allergy* to commercial bovine TSH has been reported as an immediate Type I hypersensitivity reaction directed towards the bovine albumin and gammaglobulin of the preparation. The recent cloning of human TSH will probably allow the safer use of biosynthetic hTSH for clinical in vitro and in vivo diagnosis.

Thyrotrophin-releasing hormone (TRH)

TRH, a synthetic tripeptide which stimulates the hypophyseal secretion of TSH, is also used mainly for diagnostic purposes although some experiments have been performed to evaluate its effects in mental disorders. Its side effects are discussed in Chapter 43.1.

ANTITHYROID DRUGS

Several natural or synthetic substances interfere with the synthesis and/or secretion of the thyroid hormones. For the treatment of hyperthyroidism, only thioamines are used (containing the thiourea structure) which are either derivatives of thiouracil (especially propylthiouracil) or of thioimidazole (especially methimazole or Strumazol and its carbethoxy-derivative, carbimazole or Neo-mercazole, which is converted in the body to methimazole) (21[R], 22[R]). All these drugs interfere with the thyroid peroxidase system and inhibit the synthesis of the thyroid hormones and are thus effective in reducing their overproduction in cases of hyperthyroidism. However, if these drugs are used in too high dosages, they can induce hypothyroidism and hypersecretion of thyroid-stimulating hormone (TSH) which in turn will stimulate thyroid growth and goiter development. To avoid these problems, regular adjustment of dosage or combination with synthetic thyroid hormones is necessary as soon as the euthyroid state is obtained.

The favorable effect of antithyroid drugs may also be due to their suppressive effect on lymphocytic infiltration into the thyroid and thereby they directly modulate the basic disorder of autoimmune hyperthyroidism (SEDA-6, 364; SEDA-9, 344). Propylthiouracil, but not the thioimidazoles, inhibits the conversion of L-thyroxine to its more active derivative triidothyronine. This effect is significant during high-dose treatment and propylthiouracil may therefore be preferred if a more rapid onset of action is desired, e.g. thyrotoxic crisis, although clear experimental proof of the advantageous effect is still lacking (1[R]). The antithyroid drugs are well absorbed from the intestinal tract, but the half-life of propylthiouracil is much shorter (±2 hours) than that of the thioimidazoles (±6 hours). The in vivo half-life may however be longer due to a clear accumulation and retention of the drug in the thyroid gland (23[R]).

Dosage and timing Two general patterns of use of antithyroid drugs exist. The first uses monotherapy with progressive reduction in dosage during recovery from hyperthyroidism. The second maintains a higher dosage of antithyroid drugs but associates a thyroid replacement therapy to avoid hypothyroidism. No convincing evidence for a better short- or long-term control of Graves' disease with either form of therapy exists, but combination therapy followed by monotherapy with L-T4 increased the remission rate substantially. The administration of thyroxine during antithyroid drug treatment decreases both the production of antibodies to TSH receptors and the frequency of recurrence of hyperthyroidism (93[C]). During combination therapy with propylthiouracil and L-thyroxine in normal therapeutic doses the inhibition of the conversion of T4 to T3 is of no importance. A single dose of antithyroid drugs per day cannot completely block iodine organification but can nevertheless control most cases of hyperthyroidism. Such therapy can therefore be used in some patients to improve compliance. The duration of therapy is also controversial, but a more prolonged duration of therapy is usually associated with a higher remission rate (SEDA-12, 354).

The thiouracils

ADVERSE REACTION PATTERN

General and toxic reactions Both the thiouracils and the thioimidazoles can produce hypothyroidism and goiter (see above). Most of their other side effects are allergic rather than toxic. The overall percentage of untoward reactions is between 2 and 14%, but severe reactions occur in less than 1% of the patients. Some data indicate that thioimidazoles have a lower incidence of side effects than thiouracils (24[R]). An association between the dosage of thionamide and the development of untoward reactions has been found in several studies (99[C]). It has therefore been proposed that the initial dose of carbimazole should not exceed 30 mg/day and that of propylthiouracil 300 mg/day (SEDA-17, 474).

Hypersensitivity reactions These can comprise drug fever, lymphadenopathy, arthralgia, agranulocytosis, thrombocytopenia, leukopenia or skin reactions (21[R], 25[R]). In view of the in vivo conversion of carbimazole to methimazole, cross-allergy between the two compounds can be expected and has indeed been observed. Cross-allergy between thiouracil and thioimidazoles is rare, but a few cases have been reported.

Tumor-inducing effects These have not been reported.

ORGANS AND SYSTEMS

Cardiovascular *Changes in cardiac activity* consistent with hypothyroidism are only to be expected if the thiouracils are given in relative overdosage. An *allergic vasculitis* can occur (see 'Skin and appendages' below).

Nervous system *Neuritis* and some cases of *taste disturbance* have been incidentally described (SEDA-7, 398; SEDA-11, 357).

Endocrine, metabolic *Sexual precocity* associated with hypothyroidism has been reported after long-term treatment of children with propylthiouracil, and may reflect relative overdosage. The occurrence of *hypothyroidism* and of *goiter* has been referred to above.

Hematological *Agranulocytosis*, *thrombocytopenia* and *leukopenia* are the most important adverse reactions to antithyroid drugs. A distinction may also be made between a slight dose-dependent reduction in leukocyte count and a true allergic agranulocytosis (SEDA-10, 368). Such a severe agranulocytosis (or more rarely pancytopenia), however, occurs in less than 1% of cases and is usually only observed during the first few months of therapy. Since such agranulocytosis can develop very rapidly, periodic leukocyte counts are usually considered to be of little help, but recent studies have revealed that weekly leukocyte counts can detect presymptomatic cases and allow more rapid intervention (94[R]). Patients should therefore be warned to seek immediate medical help if fever or sore throat develop during antithyroid drug treatment. If the drug is discontinued immediately recovery is the rule, but fatal cases have also been reported.

The risk of agranulocytosis has been estimated during several surveys. A large European-Israeli study (26[CR]) revealed a risk of about three per 10 000 users. The mortality in this survey was however small (one in 45 cases) (SEDA-13, 376). In two hospital surveys of agranulocytosis (27[CR], 28[CR]) an increased risk was observed in women over 40 years and when more than 40 mg of methimazole (thiamazole) was taken per day. In vitro lymphocyte testing can confirm the sensitization of the immune system to the antithyroid drugs and may occasionally indicate cross-sensitivity between methimazole and propylthiouracil (SEDA-8, 372; SEDA-9, 344).

Liver *Hepatitis* with lymphocyte sensitization has been reported and both *cholestatic jaundice* (especially with methimazole) and *toxic necrosis* (especially when using propylthiouracil) have been reported (SEDA-14, 367). Some lethal cases of hepatic necrosis have been observed (25[R]).

Skin and appendages The most common reaction to antithyroid drugs is a benign skin *rash or pruritus* without rash. Although such a reaction is usually not serious and may even disappear during continuous treatment, it nevertheless indicates an allergic reaction and requires discontinuation of therapy. Thiouracil may then be replaced by thioimidazoles, but allergy to both products may occasionally be observed. Several cases of 'collagen-like' or 'lupus-like' disease have been reported (joint pain, skin rash and positive antinuclear antibodies) both during treatment with propylthiouracil and with methimazole (SEDA-8, 372; SEDA-10, 368). Some cases of general vasculitis can be fatal, although high-dose glucocorticoid therapy may be helpful (29).

Special senses *Exophthalmos* can occur; although this is probably due to the autoimmune thyroid disease itself it is frequently aggravated by overtreatment with antithyroid drugs. *Ototoxicity* has been suggested but is poorly documented.

Musculoskeletal system Symptoms of *arthritis* and signs of a *'collagen disease'-like state* (including lupus, polymyositis or vasculitis-like symptoms) (SEDA-13, 377) probably reflect allergic reactions to the thiouracils.

Risk situations The antithyroid drugs should not be used in patients with a large intrathoracic *goiter*, which may further increase in size. In severe *hepatic disease*, the dosage should be very cautiously determined.

Second-generation effects *Use in pregnancy and during lactation* Both the thiouracils and thioimidazoles readily cross the placenta and can induce fetal hypothyroidism, resulting in a slight delay in neurological or bone maturation. Various degrees of goiter have also been observed, even to the extent of severe tracheal compression and death. Antithyroid drug dosage should therefore be reduced to the minimum required to maintain a euthyroid state without supplementation of T4 (101[R]). Methimazole has also been associated with a small scalp defect, but no other congenital malformations have been observed. The reported association between thiouracil intake and scalp defects of the fetus has been questioned (SEDA-13, 377; 30[C], 31[C]), but a further case was nevertheless reported later (SEDA-14, 367).

Since propylthiouracil does not cross the placenta quite so easily as the thiouracils, and has not been associated with scalp defects, it could be the preferred drug to treat maternal hyperthyroidism (32[R], 33[CR]). When used cautiously in minimal amounts and with frequent dose adjustments, it probably remains the safest form of treatment of hyperthyroidism during pregnancy (SEDA-8, 373; SEDA-11, 357). The antithyroid drugs also appear in human milk, and breast feeding has therefore been considered contraindicated during such treatment. More recent work, however (34[CR], 35[CR]), found that the level of drug transfer in human milk was too low to affect thyroid function in the breast-fed infant.

Overdosage An acute overload with 13 grams of propylthiouracil remained without serious side effects, except for a temporary decrease in serum triiodothyronine (SEDA-5, 382).

Interactions Treatment with antithyroid drugs induces changes in the metabolism of *other drugs*, the dosage of which may need adjusting. The antithyroid drugs also interfere with the incorporation of *iodine* into thyroglobulin and should therefore be interrupted before and shortly after the administration of therapeutic doses of radioactive iodine.

OTHER ANTITHYROID DRUGS

Several other drugs interfere in some way with thyroid physiology. Propranolol or other β-adrenergic antagonist drugs have become an integral part of the management of hyperthyroidism providing a symptomatic treatment of hyperadrenergic-like symptoms. Some of the β-adrenergic antagonist drugs reduce the conversion of thyroxine to triiodothyronine, but the clinical efficacy of drugs that reduce T3 is similar to drugs without this effect (102[R]). Propranolol has been used without other antithyroid drugs in preparation for thyroid surgery (SEDA-7, 398) (see Chapter 19).

Potassium perchlorate

This thyrostatic drug is still used (in a dose of 1000 mg/day or more) as an alternative to the thionamides, especially in cases of allergy. Compared with the thionamides, it has two disadvantages: (a) treatment cannot be directly changed to radioiodine therapy since perchlorate elimination lasts for some weeks; (b) brief high-dose iodine therapy cannot be used as a preoperative thyrostatic measure.

Potassium perchlorate produces goiter, as do the thionamides, but its effects on the hematological system are the main reason for using it sparingly. Fatal aplastic anemias following potassium perchlorate treatment have been reported (36[C], 37[C]). Agranulocytosis and pancytopenia have also been described (SED-8, 897).

A new indication for potassium perchlorate may be the iodine-induced form of thyrotoxicosis, since low-dose perchlorate (<1 g/day) combined with methimazole was found to be superior to all other forms of treatment in amiodarone-induced hyperthyroidism (38).

Erythema nodosum associated with lupus erythematosus cells has been described as an adverse effect (SED-8, 897).

Lithium salts *(see also Chapter 3)*

Lithium salts are used at a dosage of 900—1500 mg/day for the treatment of hyperthyroidism. In contrast to the thionamides, lithium does not inhibit the uptake of radioiodine by the thyroid gland (see Refs. 75—77). The blood levels have to be checked every 2—3 days initially and thereafter weekly. Lithium has a small safety margin and is therefore not used in long-term treatment of thyroid diseases (39[R]).

IODINE AND THE IODIDES

Iodine must be present in the normal diet to prevent iodine-deficiency goiter or cretinism and iodine deficiency-related disorders are still a world-wide (although preventable) group of diseases that affect about 150 million people in at least 40 countries. The WHO is sponsoring a program to control these disorders by the year 2000 (40[R], 41[R]). Scepticism to the introduction of programs to prevent iodine-deficiency disorders is occasionally encountered in regions of mild iodine deficiency, especially in Europe (103[r]). The main arguments against introduction of iodized salt are a temporary rise in the incidence of hyperthyroidism (48[R]), a possible increase in the incidence of Graves' disease, and the fact that the remission rates with antithyroid drug therapy will decrease (104[c]). Prevention of mild iodine deficiency is supported by a longitudinal study from Switzerland; 109 000 persons in a defined catchment area were studied before and for 9 years after correction of mild iodine deficiency. The incidence of toxic nodular goiter increased the first year by 27%, but thereafter a steady decrease in the incidence of both toxic nodular goiter (−73%) and of Graves' disease (−33%) was observed (105[r]). The controversy is however not settled, and further carefully controlled studies are needed.

Pharmacological amounts of iodine either in its inorganic form or as an element of several organic drugs may however have specific thyroid effects (induction of hypo- or hyperthyroidism or goiter) and general adverse reactions.

Potassium iodide

Potassium iodide is the inorganic iodide most commonly used in high dosage for acute thyrotoxicosis. Indeed, large amounts of iodine induce a temporary block of thyroid hormone secretion (Wolff-Charkoff effect) and therefore result in a more rapid thyrostatic effect than synthesis inhibitors. Potassium iodine is also used for preoperative treatment of goiter, especially to reduce preoperative bleeding. It can be employed in combination with thyrostatic drugs but should never be prescribed in combination with perchlorate since each abolishes the other's effects. The thyrostatic effects of iodide are evident even at a dose of 6 mg/day, but doses between 50 and 100 mg/day are usually recommended. In some cases of intolerance to higher doses, perchlorate may be used, e.g. for preoperative treatment.

The term '*iodism*' covers a group of adverse effects which include irritation of the skin, the mucous membranes and the conjunctiva. *Allergic reactions* seem to be rare and are mainly observed as exanthema, pruritus, fever, eosinophilia and allergic vasculitis (42[R], 43[R], 44[CR], 45[C]). *Leukocytosis*, *swelling of the salivary glands*, *iodine coryza* and *gastric upsets* have also been reported. *Headache* may accompany the other reactions. In rare cases, *jaundice*, *bleeding* from the mucous membranes and *bronchospasm* may occur. *Inflammatory states* may be aggravated by these adverse reactions.

Effects on thyroid function Iodine excess may induce hyper- or hypothyroidism (SEDA-12, 355; SEDA-13, 378). Pharmacological amounts of iodine induce only a temporary inhibition of thyroid hormone secretion since, even during continuous administration of iodine, normal thyroid function reappears ('escape from inhibition'), at least in most normal subjects. For some unknown reasons, thyroid function may remain suppressed, resulting in hypothyroidism, secondary hypersecretion of TSH and development of goiter (46[R]). Patients with autoimmune thyroiditis, partial thyroid resection and very young infants (or fetuses) are especially prone to develop such iodine-induced hypothyroidism. That therapeutic doses of iodine could induce hyperthyroidism was already known in the nineteenth century shortly after its introduction for the prevention and treatment of iodine deficiency (47[C], 48[R]). Thereafter, similar observations were made in several other parts of the world when iodine supplementation was introduced in iodine-deficient areas. Such iodine-induced hyperthyroidism or 'Iod-Basedow' can also occur in patients with other thyroid diseases (especially multinodular goiter), even when the diet was sufficient in iodine prior to the excess intake of iodine. This may even be found in patients with apparently normal thyroid glands. Iod-Basedow is usually associated with a slight goiter increase, high concentration of both free L-thyroxine (T4) and triiodothyronine (T3) and a very low uptake of radioactive iodine. The disease disappears spontaneously weeks or months after interruption of the excess iodine (49[R]—51[R]). Such a disorder should be differentiated from the temporary increase in T4 and a reciprocal decrease in T3 which can occur 1—2 weeks after the administration of iodine or iodine-containing drugs and which is not associated with clinical symptoms of thyroid dysfunction (52[CR]).

Iodine-containing drugs *(see also Chapter 17)*

Many drugs contain iodine in amounts considerably exceeding the optimum daily intake of inorganic iodine. Such drugs include most radiographic contrast media, amiodarone (Cordarone), iodoquinoline (Mexaform) and benziodarone (Amplivix), but also iodine-containing antiseptics (e.g. povidone iodine or betadine). Some 'natural' foods such as seaweed may also contain substantial amounts of iodine and result in thyroid dysfunction. Shortly after the administration of such iodine-containing drugs, a self-limited increase in serum T4 which sometimes exceeds the normal range and a reciprocal decrease in serum T3 is observed. This situation usually disappears but may persist during further treatment (so-called isolated hyperthyroxinemia). In some patients, true hyperthyroidism (increase in both T4 and T3 with clinical symptoms) occurs, e.g. in about 5% of patients on long-term treatment with amiodarone, whereas evolution to iodine-induced hypothyroidism is less frequent (53[CR], 54[C], 55[R]). On the other hand, the frequency of iodine-induced hyperthyroidism can comprise about half of all cases of hyperthyroidism, at least in elderly patients taking several drugs (SEDA-7, 399). It is therefore logical to omit iodine from all pharmaceutical preparations whenever possible, and at least require the clear labeling of its presence when it is inherently necessary. The more generous use of iodine has also been held responsible for the increasing frequency of relapse of Graves' disease in the United States. Treatment of more severe cases of iodine-induced hyperthyroidism may be difficult, as thyroid synthesis inhibitors are not immediately active and ^{131}I cannot be used because of a low thyroid uptake. The carefully supervised combination of perchlorate and methimazole has been found to be effective (56[CR]), but surgery has also been occasionally advocated.

Second-generation effects Iodine readily crosses the placenta and the fetal concentration usually exceeds the maternal concentration. The placenta does not seem to have a regulating transfer mechanism, implying that excess maternal intake of iodine will also expose the fetus to iodine intoxication. This usually results in hypothyroidism and development of goiter. Such goiters may become very large and even create obstetrical problems during delivery or mechanical compression during early postnatal life (SEDA-4, 295; SEDA-5, 328). A similar warning against the use of iodine or iodine-containing drugs applies during lactation since iodine is actively secreted in milk.

Stable iodine in radiation protection of the thyroid *(SEDA-11, 358)*

Accidents with nuclear reactors or nuclear bombs could expose large numbers of people to several decay products of uranium, and iodine isotopes are among the most abundant compounds released in such reactions. It is therefore logical to use stable isotopes of iodine to prevent the accumulation of radioiodine in a person or population at risk of such exposure. The accidents in Windscale (UK), Three Mile Island (USA) and particularly Chernobyl (Ukraine) have drawn much attention to such problems. The major question is therefore whether the potential side effects of stable iodine when given indiscriminately to large groups of people might not outweigh the risk of radioiodine exposure. One also needs to find ways of making stable iodine available rapidly when disasters occur since, in order to be effective, iodine has to be given in sufficient amounts (± 100 mg) within a short time before or after (-12 to $+3$ hours) radioiodine exposure. KIO_3 has a better stability than KI tablets since KI may easily evaporate during prolonged storage. The main toxic side effects of stable iodine are shown in Table 2. Extensive discussion and reports (57[R]–62[R]) lead one to conclude that iodine should be administered to the general population if the risk of radioiodine exposure is sufficient (>15–100 rem), but excluding people with increased risk of adverse effects to iodine (previous thyroid disease or known serious allergy). In the elderly the benefit of stable iodine probably does not outweigh its potential side effects, while in pregnant women and infants the risk/benefit ratio is not established, so that rapid evacuation of such persons from fallout zones should be given the highest priority (SEDA-11, 358).

Table 2. *Side effects of iodine given for radioprotection*

Effects on the thyroid gland
Iodine-induced goiter
Iodine-induced hypothyroidism
Special risk groups: fetus and neonate
Iodine-induced hyperthyroidism
Special risk groups
People living in iodine-deficient areas
People with a history of hyperthyroidism
Extrathyroidal side effects
Gastrointestinal complaints (nausea, pain)
Sialoadenitis and taste abnormalities
Cutaneous and mucous membranes; irritation, rash, edema (including face and glottis)
Allergic-like reactions: iodine fever, eosinophilia, serum-sickness-like symptoms, vasculitis
Special risk groups: patients with hypocomplementic vasculitis

RADIOACTIVE IODINE COMPOUNDS

Two radioactive isotopes of ^{127}I are used in clinical medicine: ^{131}I ($t_{1/2}$ of 8 days and a high-energy emitter) used mainly for therapy of hyperthyroidism and thyroid cancer and replaced by ^{123}I ($t_{1/2}$ 13 hours) for diagnostic purposes. ^{125}I ($t_{1/2}$ of 60 days and a low energy emitter) is now hardly ever used for the treatment of hyperthyroidism and ^{132}I has too short a half-life to be used diagnostically. Radioactive isotopes of iodide are handled by the thyroid as stable iodide and thus actively concentrated, incorporated into thyroglobulin, stored, metabolized and secreted as thyroid hormones. Small amounts of radioactive iodine are therefore ideal probes to analyze the uptake of iodine, the distribution of iodine in the gland, and possibly even its turnover and incorporation into thyroid hormones. Larger amounts of radioactive iodine selectively radiate the thyroid gland and therefore selectively impair the function of the follicular thyroid cells and eventually destroy them.

Three dosage ranges for radioactive iodines are used: for diagnostic purposes usually much less than 1 mCi is given with thyroid radiation doses of a few rads (^{123}I) up to 50–200 rads (^{131}I). For treatment of hyperthyroidism the amount of ^{131}I is usually a few millicuries and *is either roughly estimated or calculated according to the size of the thyroid gland, the uptake of a tracer dose of iodine and the type of thyroid disorder (diffuse or nodular) with doses ranging from* 80 *to* 150 μCi per gram of thyroid tissue (63[c], 64[c]). In thyroid cancer, ^{131}I can also be used to eliminate tumoral tissue which cannot be removed surgically but still captures iodine. In such circumstances, amounts of 100 mCi of ^{131}I or more are not unusual. With such high amounts, other tissues besides the thyroid gland can also receive substantial amounts of radiation.

Iodine-131

ADVERSE REACTION PATTERN

General and toxic reactions *Radiation thyroiditis* is an infrequent complication resulting in swelling and localized pain over the thyroid gland which subsides spontaneously or with anti-inflammatory or corticosteroid therapy (SEDA-1, 314).

Acute exacerbation of hyperthyroidism, resulting particularly in cardiac complications (arrhythmias or decompensation) or even 'thyroid storm', has been reported several times (SEDA-1, 314) and should be avoided by treating very severely hyperthyroid patients with antithyroid drugs prior to the administration of ^{131}I. A temporary increase in serum triiodothyronine and L-thyroxine without clinical symptoms of exacerbation of hyperthyroidism, however, occurs much more frequently (SEDA-1, 314).

Hypothyroidism All patients with autoimmune hyperthyroidism seem to have an increased incidence of late hypothyroidism, but the risk increases markedly after extensive thyroid surgery and especially after ^{131}I treatment. Analysis of the cumulative incidence of hypothyroidism reveals two phases: an early phase of radiation death of thyroid cells, dependent on the ^{131}I dosage and occurring during the first 1—2 years after treatment: a second period of a lower (±3% per year) (Table 3) (65[CR]—67[CR]) but life-long risk of developing hypothyroidism for a variety of reasons (natural history of the disease, autoimmune processes). The total incidence of hypothyroidism may therefore be reduced by lowering the therapeutic dose but at the expense of a higher incidence of more prolonged or recurrent hyperthyroidism. Calculation of the therapeutic dose according to thyroid gland size, iodine uptake or biological half-life and type of thyroid disorder may help to reduce the total incidence of hypothyroidism, although this is less well documented than many believe (68[R], 69[C]). Moreover, the occurrence of post-^{131}I-hypothyroidism should not be dramatized since treatment is much simpler than abandoning the patient first to the prolonged risk of recurrent hyperthyroidism and thereafter to life-long follow-up for occurrence of hypothyroidism. Hypothyroidism after ^{131}I can also be temporary and replacement therapy should not be started too early (70[C]).

Graves' ophthalmopathy Several papers have reported that radioiodine therapy may lead to worsening of ophthalmopathy, possibly because of the release of thyroid antigens during the inflammatory reaction after ^{131}I therapy. The worsening could be prevented by glucocorticoid therapy (106[C]).

Hypersensitivity reactions These do not occur.

Tumor-inducing effects The association between radiation and induction of tumors is so well known that radioactive iodine therapy is under constant surveillance to detect any increased incidence of malignant tumors in patients thus treated. Moreover, external radiation of the neck is definitely a risk factor in thyroid cancer, but the radiation dose is usually much smaller than for the treatment of hyperthyroidism and is moreover given to children instead of adults.

The total number of case-reports of thyroid cancer after ^{131}I is however very small (±26 cases) (71[CR]) in relation to the estimated number of patients treated with ^{131}I since 1941 (≥1 000 000 patients). Moreover, systematic follow-up or retrospective studies were unable to reveal an increased risk of thyroid carcinoma in patients treated with ^{131}I for hyperthyroidism. Results of two such studies are shown in more detail in Tables 4 and 5. In another follow-up study of 1005 women treated with ^{131}I no increase in total morbidity or in the incidence of thyroid cancer could be observed (72[CR]).

In a recent study cancer mortality was investigated in 10 552 Swedish patients (mean age: 57 years) who received ^{131}I therapy for hyperthyroidism (mean follow-up 15 years). There were increases in overall cancer mortality and deaths due to carcinoma of the stomach, lung and kidney, and while the findings for stomach cancer may be of significance because of an association with time after ^{131}I treatment (58 cases at 10 years or more of follow-up against the expected 44 cases) the lack of a relation between cancer mortality and either

Table 3. *Hypothyroidism after* ^{131}I

No. of cases	^{131}I dose (mCi)	Total follow-up period (yr)	% Hypothyroidism						Total annual cumulative incidence (%)	Ref. no.
			One-year follow-up			End of follow-up				
			Diffuse goiter	Nodular goiter	Total	Diffuse goiter	Nodular goiter	Total		
4473	8–20	26 (1951–75)	8	3	6	77	64	72	3	65[CR]
1369	9	17 (1959–76)	6	3	6	26	14	—	3.5	66[CR]
248	6–10	10	38	11	—	70	18	—	0.5/4	67[CR]

Table 4. ^{131}I *treatment and thyroid cancer: Cooperative Thyrotoxicosis Therapy Follow-Up Study (62[CR])**

Incidence of thyroid cancer	Thyroidectomy (n = 11 732)	^{131}I (n = 21 714)	Antithyroid drugs (n = 1238)
Within 1 year of treatment	50	9	0
After 1 year of treatment	4	19	4
Total	54 (4.6‰)	28 (1.3‰)	4 (3.2‰)
No. of deaths from thyroid cancer	4	6	0

* Maximum follow-up time: 22 years.

Table 5. ^{131}I *treatment and thyroid cancer (74[CR])*

No. of patients treated with ^{131}I	3000
Mean age	57 yr
Mean dose of ^{131}I	13.3 mCi
Mean observation period	13 yr
Thyroid cancer	
Observed incidence	4
Expected incidence*	3.2
Thyroid cancer occurring more than 5 yr after ^{131}I treatment	
Observed incidence	2.1
Expected incidence	3

* According to the (Compulsatory) Swedish Cancer Registry.

the time from radioiodine treatment or the dose administered, for tumors at other sites, argues against a carcinogenic effect of radioiodine (SEDA-17, 475; 108[C]).

The use of ^{131}I in children is however quite different from its use in adults. Experience worldwide is much more limited as regards both the number of children treated and the total number of years of observation. Concern about possible second-generation effects is difficult to allay but has not been substantiated, since there is an absence of obvious birth defects or genetic changes in the offspring of patients treated with ^{131}I (71[CR]–75[CR]). Moreover, the radiation dose to the ovaries in ^{131}I therapy for hyperthyroidism is usually below 3 roentgens and thus comparable to the radiation due to common radiographic abdominal examinations. If ^{131}I is given during pregnancy, fetal hypothyroidism and chromosomal aberrations may occur (76[C]). The risk of eventual tumor-inducing effects in the thyroid or other tissues remains real. The young thyroid is indeed very sensitive to external radiation or to nuclear fall-out: 66% of young adults developed thyroid lesions 25 years after such exposure (77[CR]). One report on a high prevalence of post-^{131}I hypothyroidism found no cases of thyroid or other malignancy after a mean follow-up period of almost 15 years (78[CR]). Others, however, found an increased frequency of thyroid nodules: among case-reports on thyroid cancer after ^{131}I in the world literature the younger age group is largely overrepresented due to the frequency of ^{131}I use in this age group (71[CR]). In view of the small number of long-term results (±400 cases reported up to 1979) (95[R]) in a young population with probably higher susceptibility for thyroid tumors it seems unwise to use ^{131}I as preferred treatment for adolescents or young adults with hyperthyroidism. Much longer follow-up periods will be necessary, preferably with central registration to allow a definite conclusion about treatment (79[R], 80[R]). Many experts, however, already consider the present follow-up period sufficiently long to extend the use of ^{131}I to all patients with Graves' disease above the age of 25 (SEDA-14, 368; 81). There are, however, large discrepancies in the treatment strategies globally (109[r]).

The use of very high amounts of ^{131}I for thyroid cancer imposes special care and risks: the frequency of radiation thyroiditis is much higher (more than 20%) and similar symptoms of pain and swelling can also be observed in the salivary glands. Nausea and vomiting may also occur. The incidence of leukemia is increased: 15 cases being reported in 5000 patients treated with ^{131}I for thyroid cancer (80^R); it therefore seems wise to limit the total dose of ^{131}I in a single patient to 500 mCi unless the thyroid disease activity permits higher long-term risks. It is also important to keep such patients well hydrated to allow rapid elimination of ^{131}I not retained by thyroid tissue. The radiation dose to the ovaries is not negligible, being approximately 200 roentgens after 500 mCi of ^{131}I, a dose sufficient to increase slightly the subsequent risk of miscarriage or congenital abnormalities. However, no apparent increase in the rate of abnormalities has been observed in the outcome of pregnancies among women previously treated for thyroid cancer.

ORGANS AND SYSTEMS

Cardiovascular In a study of a series of thyrocardiac patients it was found that of those dying primarily from thyrotoxicosis more than 21% did so within 3 weeks of ^{131}I treatment (82^R), presumably reflecting too sudden a change in metabolic activity for patients with existing cardiac complications.

Respiratory Acute respiratory embarrassment due to thyroid swelling or subsequently due to cicatrization occurs only rarely.

Nervous system Although cases of aseptic meningitis have been associated with the use of radioactive iodine, the products used were albumin complexes (^{131}I-RISA); this complication is almost certainly attributable to the protein content or to pyrogens rather than to the radioactive iodine (82^R).

Endocrine Both hyperfunction (83^c) and hypofunction of the parathyroid glands have been described, but a causal relationship is doubtful (84^C). The calcitonin-producing cells of the thyroid are usually also destroyed by ^{131}I and this calcitonin deficiency may contribute to later *osteoporosis* (SEDA-14, 369).

Hematological *Leukemia* does not occur more frequently in patients treated with ^{131}I for hyperthyroidism than in similar patients treated by surgery. After the high doses used in the treatment of thyroid cancer a definite increase in the incidence of leukemia is observed (80^R).

Genital system Large amounts of ^{131}I, as used in thyroid cancer therapy, may produce testicular damage as documented from hormonal and sperm analysis (85^c), but long-term results are nevertheless reassuringly normal (72^R).

Second-generation effects *Use in pregnancy* Radioactive iodine passes the placenta and accumulates in the fetal thyroid where the concentration probably exceeds that in the maternal thyroid. Detailed studies demonstrate that the fetal dose of iodine is virtually nil before the 90th day of gestation but sharply increases thereafter (86^R). This alone is sufficient reason to avoid the use of ^{131}I in pregnancy, but there is also some controversial evidence that various congenital deformities have been produced by the isotope (87^R).

Use in lactation For similar reasons, ^{131}I, which is transferred in the milk, should not be given during lactation. Even the diagnostic use of radioisotopes of iodine should be avoided (88^c).

Genetic effects Mutagenic effects on the sexual organs are difficult to determine in clinical practice. However, while the radiation dose to the ovary and testes is rather small after ^{131}I treatment for hyperthyroidism (maximum ±5 roentgens) it may be substantial after the higher amounts of ^{131}I used for thyroid cancer (see above). In any case, children born to mothers previously treated with ^{131}I did not have an increased incidence of congenital malformations. The number of such observations is too small, however, to allow definite conclusions about its safety (79^R).

Interference with diagnostic routines Injections of ^{131}I given to detect pulmonary embolism may result in false-negative results in the ^{125}I-labeled fibrinogen test for venous thrombosis.

OTHER RADIOACTIVE IODINES

Iodine-125

This isotope was introduced for the treatment of thyrotoxicosis in the hope that it would have less effect on the nuclei of the thyroid cells. The therapeutic results have been disappointing (89^R, 90^R). The problems are generally similar to those discussed in connection with ^{131}I.

RADIOPROTECTION

The administration of ^{131}I to patients also requires safety measurements to reduce to a minimum the irradiation of medical personnel treating such patients and to avoid contamination of rooms and family members of patients. ^{131}I capsules are therefore to be preferred to the administration of liquid iodide. With doses above 25 mCi (555 MBq), usually intended only for treatment of patients with thyroid cancer, isolation in a specially constructed room of a service for nuclear medicine is necessary. Waste disposal should also be carefully handled so as to avoid overall contamination (91[R], 92[R]).

REFERENCES

1. Chopra IJ, Cody V. Triiodothyronines in health and disease. In: Gross F, ed. Monographs on Endocrinology, Vol 18. Berlin—Heidelberg—New York: Springer-Verlag, 1981:1.
2. Fish LH, Schwartz LH, Cavanaugh J et al. Replacement dose, metabolism, and bioavailability of levothyroxine in the treatment of hypothyroidism. N Engl J Med 1987;316:764.
3. Rees-Jones RW, Rolla AR, Larsen PR. Hormonal content of thyroid replacement preparations. J Am Med Assoc 1980;243:549.
4. Carr D, McLeod DT, Parry G, Thornes HM. Fine adjustment of thyroxine replacement dosage: comparison of the thyrotrophin releasing hormone test using a sensitive thyrotrophin assay with measurement of free thyroid hormones and clinical assessment. Clin Endocrinol 1988;28:325.
5. Paul TL, Kerrigan J, Kelly AM et al. Long-term L-thyroxine therapy is associated with decreased hip bone density in premenopausal women. J Am Med Assoc 1988;259:3137.
6. Hiasa Y, Ishida T, Aihara T et al. Acute myocardial infarction due to coronary spasm associated with L-thyroxine therapy. Clin Cardiol 1989;12:161.
7. Kologlu S, Baskal N, Kologlu LB et al. Hirsutism due to the treatment with L-thyroxine in patients with thyroid pathology. Rev Roum Med Sér Endocrinol 1988;26:179.
8. Iranmanesh A, Lizarralde G, Johnson ML, Veldhuis JD. Dynamics of 24-hour endogenous cortisol secretion and clearance in primary hypothyroidism assessed before and after partial thyroid hormone replacement. J Clin Endocrinol Metab 1989;70:155.
9. Mandel SJ, Larsen PR, Seely EW, Brent GA. Increased need for thyroxine during pregnancy in women with primary hypothyroidism. N Engl J Med 1990;323:91.
10. Exley A, O'Malley BP. Depression in primary hypothyroidism masquerading as inadequate or excessive L-thyroxine consumption. Q J Med New Ser 1989;72/269:867.
11. Gorman CA, Becker DV, Greenspan et al. Breast cancer and thyroid therapy statement by the American Thyroid Association. J Am Med Assoc 1977;237:1459.
12. Shibata H, Hayakawa H, Hirukawa M et al. Hypersensitivity caused by synthetic thyroid hormone in a hypothyroid patient with Hashimoto's thyroiditis. Arch Intern Med 1986;146:1624.
13. Van Dop C, Conte FA, Koch TK et al. Pseudotumor cerebri associated with initiation of levothyroxine therapy for juvenile hypothyroidism. N Engl J Med 1983:308:1076.
14. Evans DL, Strawn SK, Haggerty JJ et al. Appearance of mania in drug-resistant bipolar depressed patients after treatment with L-triiodothyronine. J Clin Psychiatry 1986;47:521.
15. Auwerx J, Bouillon R. Mineral and bone metabolism in thyroid disease: a review. Q J Med 1986;232:737.
16a. Krolner B, Versterdal Jørgensen J, Pors Nielsen S. Spinal bone mineral content in myxoedema and thyrotoxicosis: effect of thyroid hormones and antithyroid treatment. Clin Endocrinol 1983;18:439.
16b. Ribot C, Tremollières F, Pouilles JM, Louvet JP. Bone mineral density and thyroid hormone therapy. Clin Endocrinol 1990;33:143.
17. Toh SH, Brown PH. Bone mineral content in hypothyroid male patients with hormone replacement: a 3-year study. J Bone Miner Res 1990;5:463.
18. Stall GM, Harris S, Sokoll LJ, Dawson-Hughes B. Accelerated bone loss in hypothyroid patients overtreated with L-thyroxine. Ann Antern Med 1990;113:265.
19a. Pristanz H, Leb C, Raber J et al. Beeinflussung laborchemischer und nuklearmedizinischer Schilddrüsenparameter unter der Behandlung mit einem hochgereinigten D-Thyroxin-Präparat. Münch Med Wochenschr 1980;122:199.
19b. Coronary Drug Project Research Groups. Coronary Drug Project: Findings leading to further modifications of its protocol with respect to dextrothyroxine. J Am Med Assoc 1972;220:996.
20. Cohen JH, Ingbar SH, Braverman LE. Thyrotoxicosis due to ingestion of excess thyroid hormone. Endocr Rev 1989;10:113.
21. Kampmann JP, Hansen JM. Clinical pharmacokinetics of antithyroid drugs. Clin Pharmacokinet 1981;6:401.
22. Langer P, Greer MA, eds. In: Antithyroid Substances and Naturally Occurring Coitrogens. Basel—München—Paris—London—New York—Sidney: Karger, 1977:54.
23. Jansson R, Dahlberg PA, Johansson H, Lindström B. Intrathyroidal concentrations of methimazone in patients with Graves' disease. J Clin Endocrinol Metab 1983;57:129.
24. Marchant B, Lees JF, Alexander WD. Antithyroid drugs. Pharmacol Ther (B) 1978;3:305.
25. Cooper DS. Antithyroid drugs. N Engl J Med 1984;311:1353.
26. Retsagi G, Kelly JP, Kaufman DW. Risk of agranulocytosis and aplastic anaemia in relation to use of antithyroid drugs. Br Med J 1988;297:262.
27. Cooper DS, Goldminz D, Levin AA et al. Agranulocytosis associated with antithyroid drugs. Ann Intern Med 1983;98:26.
28. Kaaja R, Ebeling P, Lamberg BA. Tyreostaathioidon aiheuttama agranulosystocs. I Duodecim 1986;102:872.
29. Wing SS, Fantus IG. Adverse immunologic effects of antithyroid drugs. Can Med Assoc J 1987;136:121.
30. Momotoani N, Ito K, Hamada N et al. Maternal hyperthyroidism and congenital malformation in the offspring. Clin Endocrinol 1984;20:695.
31. Van Dijke CP, Heyendael RJ, De Kleine MJ. Methimazole, carbimazole and congenital skin defects. Ann Intern Med 1987;106:60.
32. Burrow GN. Current concepts: the management of thyrotoxicosis in pregnancy. N Engl J Med 1985;313:562.
33. Momotani N, Noh J, Oyanagi H et al. Antithyroid drug therapy for Graves' disease during pregnancy: optimal regimen for fetal thyroid status. N Engl J Med 1986;315:24.
34. Johansen K, Kampmann JP, Mølholm Hansen J et al. Udskillelsen af antityreoide stoffer i modermælk. Ugeskr Læg 1982;144:1635.
35. Cooper DS, Bode HH, Nath B et al. Methimazole phar-

macology in man: studies using a newly developed radioimmunoassay for methimazole. J Clin Endocrinol 1984;58:473.
36. Johnson RS, Moore GW. Fatal aplastic anemia after treatment of thyreotoxicosis with potassium perchlorate. Br Med J 1961;1:1369.
37. Krevans JR, Asper Jr SP, Rienhoff WF Jr. Fatal aplastic anemia following use of potassium perchlorate in thyreotoxicosis. J Am Med Assoc 1962;181:162.
38. Martino E, Aghini-Lombardi F, Mariotti S et al. Amiodarone: a common source of iodine-induced thyrotoxicosis. Hormone Res 1987;26:158.
39. Baldessarini RJ, Lipinski JF. Lithium salts. Ann Intern Med 1975;83:527.
40. Anonymous. Prevention and control of iodine deficiency disorders. Lancet 1986;ii:433.
41. Hetzel BS. The Prevention and Control of Iodine Deficiency Disorders. Nutrition policy discussion paper no. 3, United Nations ACC/SCN, Rome, 1988.
42. Friend DG. Iodide therapy. N Engl J Med 1960;263:1358.
43. Utiger RD. The diverse effects of iodide on thyroid function. N Engl J Med 1972;287:562.
44. Hoorn B, Kabins SA. Iodide fever. Am J Med Sci 1972;264:467.
45. Eeckhout E, Willemsen M, Deconinck A, Somers G. Granulomatous vasculitis as a complication of potassium iodide treatment for Sweet's syndrome. Acta Dermatol-Venereol 1987;67:362.
46. Vagenakis AG, Braverman LE. Drug induced hypothyroidism. Pharmacol Ther (C) 1976;1:149.
47. Coindet J-F. Découverte d'une remàde contre le goitre. Bibl Univ Sci BL Arts 1820;14:90.
48. Kohn LA. A look at iodine-induced hyperthyroidism: recognition. Bull NY Acad Med 1975;51:959.
49. Ingbar SH. Autoregulation of the thyroid: the effects of thyroid iodine enrichment and depletion. In: Hall R, Köbberling J, eds. Thyroid Disorders Associated with Iodine Deficiency and Excess. Serono Symposia Publications, Vol. 22. New York: Raven Press, 1985:153.
50. Savoie J-C, Massin P, Thomopoulos P et al. Hyperthyroïde induite par l'iode: une variété mal connue de pathologie iatrogàne. Concours Med 1977;99-20:3227.
51. Evered D, Yeo PPB. Drug-induced endocrine disorders. Drugs 1977;13:353.
52. Burger A, Dinichert D, Nicod P et al. Effect of amiodarone on serum triiodothyronine, reverse triiodothyronine, thyroxin and thyrotropin: a drug influencing peripheral metabolism of thyroid hormones. J Clin Invest 1976;58:255.
53. Jonckheer MH. Amiodarone and the thyroid gland: a review. Acta Cardiol 1981;36:199.
54. Andersen ED. Long-term antiarrhythmic therapy with amiodarone: high prevalence of thyrotoxicosis (11%). Eur Heart J 1981;2:199.
55. Karpman BA, Rapoport B, Filetti S, Fisher DA. Treatment of neonatal hyperthyroidism due to Graves' disease with sodium ipodate. J Clin Endocrinol Metab 1987;64:119.
56. Martino E, Aghini-Lombardi F, Mariotti S et al. Amiodarone: a common source of iodine-induced thyrotoxicosis. Hormone Res 1987;26:158.
57. Yalow RS. Risks in mass distribution of potassium iodide. Bull NY Acad Med 1983;59:1020.
58. Robbins J. Indications for using potassium iodide to protect the thyroid from low level internal irradiation. Bull NY Acad Med 1983;59:1028.
59. Schleien B, Halperin JA, Bilstad JM et al. Recommendations on the use of potassium iodide as a thyroid-blocking agent in radiation accidents: an FDA update. Bull NY Acad Med 1983;59:1009.
60. Crocker DG. Nuclear reactor accidents: the use of KI as a blocking agent against radioiodine uptake in the thyroid: a review. Health Phys 1984;46:1265.
61. Helsing E, Dukes MNG. The Safety of Stable Iodine When Used to Provide Protection against Nuclear Fallout. Internal advisory report. Copenhagen: WHO Regional Office for Europe, 1986.
62. Wolff J. Risks for stable and radioactive iodine in radiation protection of the thyroid. In: Hall R, Köbberling J, eds. Thyroid Disorders Associated with Iodine Deficiency and Excess. Serono Symposia Publications, Vol. 22. New York: Raven Press, 1985:111.
63. Holm LE, Lundell G, Dahlqvist I, Israelsson A. Cure rate after ^{131}I therapy for hyperthyroidism. Acta Radiol 1981;20:161.
64. Bliddal H, Hansen JM, Rogowski P et al. ^{131}I treatment of diffuse and nodular toxic goiter with or without antithyroid agents. Acta Endocrinol 1982;99:517.
65. Holm LE, Lundell C, Israelsson A, Dahlqvist I. Incidence of hypothyroidism occurring long after iodine-131 therapy for hyperthyroidism. J Nucl Med 1982;23:103.
66. Best JD, Chan V, Khoo R et al. Incidence of hypothyroidism after radioactive iodine therapy for thyrotoxicosis in Hong-Kong Chinese. Clin Radiol 1981;32:57.
67. Kamphuis JJ. Behandeling van hyperthyreoïdie met ^{131}I: een retrospectief onderzoek. Ned T Geneeskd 1980; 124:1045.
68. Hays MT. Hypothyroidism following iodine-131 therapy. J Nucl Med 1982;23:176.
69. Watson AB, Brownlie BEW, Frampton CM et al. Outcome following standardized 185 MBq dose ^{131}I therapy for Graves' disease. Clin Endocrinol 1988;28:487.
70. MacFarlane, IA, Shalet SM, Beardwell CG, Khara JK. Transient hypothyroidism after iodine-131 treatment for hyperthyroidism. Br Med J 1979;2:421.
71. McDougall I, Nelsen TS, Kempson RL. Papillary carcinoma of the thyroid seven years after I-131 therapy for Graves' disease. Clin Nucl Med 1981;6:368.
72. Hoffman DA, McConahey WM, Diamond EL, Kurland LT. Mortality in women treated for hyperthyroidism. Am J Epidemiol 1982;115:243.
73. Dobyns BM, Sheline GE, Workman JB. Malignant and benign neoplasms of the thyroid in patients treated for hyperthyroidism: a report of the Cooperative Thyrotoxicosis Therapy Follow-up Study. J Clin Endocrinol Metab 1974;38:976.
74. Holm LE, Dahlqvist I, Israelsson A, Lundell G. Malignant thyroid tumors after iodine-131 therapy: a retrospective cohort study. N Engl J Med 1980;303:188.
75. Sakar SD, Beierwaltes WH, Gill SP, Cowley BJ. Subsequent fertility and birth histories of children and adolescents treated with ^{131}I for thyroid cancer. J Nucl Med 1976;17:460.
76. Goh K. Radioiodine treatment during pregnancy: chromosomal aberrations and cretinism associated with maternal iodine-131 treatment. J Am Med Assoc 1981;36:262.
77. Larsen PR, Conard RA, Knudsen K. Thyroid hypofunction appearing as a delayed manifestation of accidental exposure to radioactive fallout in a Marshallese population. In: Biological Effects of Ionizing Radiation, Vol. 1. Vienna: International Atomic Energy Agency, 1978:101.
78. Freitas JE, Swanson PD, Gross MD, Sisson JC. Iodine-131: optimal therapy for hyperthyroidism in children and adolescents? J Nucl Med 1979;20:847.

79. Maxon HR, Thomas SR, Chen I-W. The role of nuclear medicine in the treatment of hyperthyroidism and well-differentiated thyroid adenocarcinoma. Clin Nucl Med 1981; 6:P87.
80. Blahd WH. Treatment of malignant thyroid disease. Semin Nucl Med 1979;19:95.
81. Graham GD, Burman KD. Radioiodine treatment of Graves' disease. Ann Intern Med 1986;105:900.
82. Shani J, Atkins HL, Wolf W. Adverse reactions to radiopharmaceuticals. Semin Nucl Med 1976;6:305.
83. Triggs SM, Williams ED. Irradiation of the thyroid as a cause of parathyroid adenoma. Lancet 1977;i:593.
84. Jialal I, Pillay NL, Asmal AC. Radio-iodine-induced hypoparathyroidism. S Afr Med J 1980;58:939.
85. Handelsman DJ, Conway AJ, Donnelly PE, Turtle JR. Azoospermia after iodine-131-treatment for thyroid carcinoma. Br Med J 1980;281:1527.
86. Johnson JR. Fetal thyroid dose from intakes of radioiodine by the mother. Health Phys 1982;43:573.
87. Nishimura H, Tanimura T. Clinical Aspects of Teratogenicity of Drugs. Amsterdam: Excerpta Medica, 1976.
88. Dydek GJ, Blue PW. Human breast milk excretion of iodine-131 following diagnostic and therapeutic administration to a lactating patient with Graves' disease. J Nucl Med 1988;29:470.
89. Glanzmann Ch, Kaestner F, Horst W. Therapie der Hyperthyreose mit Radioisotopen des Jods: Erfahrungen bei über 2000 Patienten. Klin Wochenschr 1975;88:669.
90. Glanzmann Ch, Horst W. Iodine-125 and iodine-131 in the treatment of hyperthyroidism. Clin Nucl Med 1980;5:325.
91. Thomas SR, Maxon HR, Fritz KM. A comparison of methods for assessing patient body burden following ^{131}I therapy for thyroid cancer. Radiology 1980;137:839.
92. Radioprotection Committee. Radioprotection in radioactive iodine therapy. Belg Tijdschr Radiol 1980;63:39.
93. Hashizume K, Ichikawa K, Sakurai A et al. Administration of thyroxine in treated Graves' disease. Effects on the level of antibodies to thyroid-stimulating hormone receptors and on the risk of recurrence of hyperthyroidism. N Engl J Med 1991;324:947.
94. Tajiri J, Noguchi S, Murakami I, Murakami N. Antithyroid drug-induced agranulocytosis. The usefulness of routine blood cell count monitoring. Arch Intern Med 1990;150:621.
95. Wartofsky L. Myxedema Coma. In: Braverman LE, Utiger RD, JB eds. Werner and Ingbar's The Thyroid, 6th edn. Philadelphia: J.B. Lippincott, 1991:1089.
96. Petersen K, Bengtsson C, Lapidus L et al. Morbidity, mortality and quality of life for patients treated with levothyroxine. Arch Intern Med 1990;150:2077.
97. Reference deleted.
98. Martino E, Bambini G, Bartalena L et al. Human serum thyrotrophin measurement by ultrasensitive immunoradiometric assay as a first-line test in the evaluation of thyroid function. Clin Endocrinol (Oxford) 1986;24:141.
99. Reinwein D, Benker G, Lazarus JH, Alexander WD, and the European Multicenter Study Group on Antithyroid Drug Treatment. A prospective randomized trial of antithyroid drug dose in Graves' disease therapy. J Clin Endocrinol Metab 1993;76:1516.
100. Reference deleted.
101. Hamburger JI. Diagnosis and management of Graves' Disease in Pregnancy. Thyroid 1992;2:219.
102. Feely J, Peden N. Use of β-adrenoceptor blocking drugs in hyperthyroidism. Drugs 1984;27:425.
103. Laurberg P. Editorial: iodine intake. What are we aiming at? J Clin Endocrinol Metab 1994;79:17.
104. Solomon BL, Evaul JE, Burman KD, Wartofsky L. Remission rates with antithyroid drug therapy: continuing influence of iodine intake? Ann Intern Med 1987;107:510.
105. Delange F. Correction of iodine deficiency: benefits and possible side effects. Eur J Endocrinol 1995;132:542.
106. Bartalena L, Marcocci C, Bogazzi F et al. Use of corticosteroids to prevent progression of Graves' ophthalmopathy after radioiodine therapy for hyperthyroidism. N Engl J Med 1989;321:1349
107. Reference deleted.
108. Holm L-E, Hall P, Wiklund K et al. Cancer risk after iodine-131 therapy for hyperthyroidism. J Natl Cancer Inst 1991;83:1072.

Meyler's Side Effects of Drugs, 13th Edition
M.N.G. Dukes, editor

SECTION EDITOR: M.N.G. DUKES

H.M.J. Krans

42 Insulin, glucagon and oral hypoglycemic drugs

INSULIN *(SEDA-16, 480; SEDA-17, 477; SEDA-18, 409)*

Insulin is an essential life saving drug for many persons with diabetes. Its major side effect is hypoglycemia. This is specifically dangerous when patient's awareness of hypoglycemia is reduced or when long-acting preparations are used. Allergic reactions, although less common with newer preparations, are regularly seen. Insulin has to be given by injection, with pumps or specific devices for intensive therapy, which all generate specific problems. Rare complications are lipo-atrophy or -hypertrophy and edema.

Insulin is used for substitution therapy in patients with an absolute or relative deficiency of insulin. It differs from many drugs used in medicine in that it is a synthetic human product or, when of animal origin, closely related to human insulin. However, the manner and the site of administration and the variation in duration of action of the various insulin preparations, the grade of purification and differences in concentration elicit specific problems. Most of the insulins now prescribed are either synthetic human or highly purified insulins of animal origin. The use of insulin of lesser purity is declining, but it is still used in considerable quantities in Eastern and Central Europe and in less developed countries. In some countries both highly purified insulins of Western origin in concentrations of 100 U/ml and locally produced less pure insulins in concentrations of 20, 40 or 80 U/ml are available at the same moment, creating confusion. Patients have to realize that the syringe used for injection has to be concordant with the specific strength of insulin for which it has been made. The major adverse effects originate from overdosage or from allergic reactions. Additives introduced as preservatives or to change the duration of action of insulin may also induce side effects.

All insulins may generate side effects in man. The effects of insulin are modified by various factors. The absorption of insulin depends, for example, on the site of injection (1) (abdominal wall, over or under the umbilica, buttock, upper arm or upper leg), depth of the subcutaneous injection, skin temperature (2), presence of lipodystrophy, variation in inactivation of injected insulin, etc. The disposal of insulin depends on many factors. The half-life of intravenously injected insulin is about 5 minutes. Exercise and hard labor lower the blood glucose and thereby increase the effect of insulin. Infections and obesity decrease the effect. The timing of food intake and the composition of meals is also related to the action of insulin.

A useful overview of major factors influencing the fate of injected insulin (and thereby also its risks) has been provided by Binder et al. (3[r]); Table 1 is reprinted from this paper.

The duration of action of various forms of insulin is indicated in Table 2.

HYPOGLYCEMIA

The most frequent complication of insulin therapy is inadvertent hypoglycemia (4[R], 5[R]). Over 5% of death in diabetes may be attributed to hypoglycemia. The frequency increases with the current trend towards rigorous maintenance of normoglycemia (6[r]). In the DCCT trial (7[R]) the frequency of serious hypoglycemia was more than three times increased in the intensively treated group and the frequency of the attacks was related to the value of HbA_{1c} (8[r]). The reasons for hypoglycemia may be inaccurate or excessive insulin injections, heavy physical exercise, or omission of meals. Often, hypoglycemic attacks are preceded by smaller attacks, which are unnoticed or not reported to the family or physician. Attacks can be caused by decreased resistance to insulin or switch to a type of insulin with a different duration of action. The action of highly purified insulins, even when in long-acting form, is somewhat faster and shorter compared with less pure preparations. Errors in injection techniques

Table 1. *Summary of factors of major importance for the fate of injected insulin*

Variable	Present knowledge indicates that:
Insulin preparation	Regular insulin $T_{50\%}$ ~2—4 h Intermediate-acting insulin $T_{50\%}$ ~16—20 h Prolonged-acting insulin $T_{50\%} \geqq 36$ h Intraindividual variation in absorption up to 50% Interindividual variation from day to day up to 25%
Insulin species	Of minimal importance
Fortuitous injection technique	Contributes to variance
Injected region	Absorption faster from abdominal region than from femoral and gluteal region; exercising injected limb speeds up absorption; applies especially to regular insulin
Subcutaneous blood flow	Major determinant for absorption rate and clinically significant for regular insulin (influenced by smoking, ambient temperature, exercise, local massage etc.)
Subcutaneous degradation of insulin	Usually of no clinical significance; in rare cases after insulin need exceeds 120 IU it might explain brittleness
Insulin antibodies	Increase unpredictably the circulating part of insulin and prolong its half-life; rare cause of insulin resistance

Reprinted from Binder et al. (3[R]) with permission from the American Diabetes Association, Inc.

such as superficial subcutaneous injections forming nodules or bleeding may cause variation in the daily uptake of insulin, resulting in an increase in the mean administered dose and in inadvertent hypoglycemic attacks. They are often not immediately seen after the transfer, but after 2—3 weeks. Somogyi phenomena, unnoticed hypoglycemic instances during sleep, induce a rise in blood glucose with accompanying glucosuria. When long-acting insulin is increased in the evening, the hypoglycemias during the night increase as well. Blood glucose monitoring late at night helps to establish the diagnosis. Hypoglycemic periods may also be induced by concomitantly developing diseases, e.g. renal disease, hepatic disease (cirrhosis), hypopituitarism, hypoadrenocorticism, hypoglucagonism, hypothyroidism, malnutrition, anorexia nervosa, pregnancy, termination of pregnancy, recovery from infections, operations or stress states.

Some drugs may increase the hypoglycemic action of insulin, e.g. β-blockers (propranolol), or β-stimulating agents, anesthesia, excessive use of alcohol (SEDA-5, 386), salicylate, oxytetracycline, EDTA, mebanazine and manganese (5[r]). The decrease of a prescribed dose of prednisone may induce hypoglycemia as well. In poorly controlled diabetics hypoglycemic symptoms may be mild, absent or unnoticed (9).

The *symptoms* of hypoglycemia vary from patient to patient and may vary in the same patient. The principal symptoms are a feeling of hunger, restlessness, profuse sweating, tachycardia, palpitations and paleness. Most of these symptoms are induced by excessive release of noradrenaline or adrenaline as a consequence of the hypoglycemia (adrenergic symptoms). The patient may also experience headache, confusion, drowsiness, fatigue, difficulties in finding words, frequent yawning, anxiety, blurred vision, diplopia and numbness of the nose, lip and fingers (neuroglycopenic symptoms). This indicates that the nervous system is affected by hypoglycemia. When hypoglycemia does not recede spontaneously or is not terminated, cerebral dysfunction becomes manifest as confusion or reduction of consciousness. Lethargy and depression or obstructive behavior develop and are accompanied by loss of consciousness, snoring, deep respiration and facial paralysis. Neurological involvement may appear as cramps, paralysis, hemiplegia or paraplegia. Epileptic seizures may accompany hypoglycemic attacks. In deep coma the pupils are dilated, but they may react to light. Coma may develop very rapidly.

Some patients do not experience the noradrenergic symptoms of hypoglycemia. They are taken by surprise, may lose consciousness and have hypoglycemic blood glucose values without any preceding symptom. This may be more frequent when human insulin is used or after frequent preceding hypoglycemic instances (9[R], 10[R], 11[R]). It is difficult to substantiate altered awareness of hypoglycemia. Repeated hypoglycemic periods reduce the awareness of hypoglycemic symptoms. Indications are given that this is accompanied by lowering of the blood glucose levels, which elicit the response of contraregulatory hormones (12[r]).

It has been stated that decreased 'awareness' has been noted as an accompanying event with the increased use of human insulin (SEDA-15, 452). Double-blind studies providing human or animal insulin to persons complaining of increased unawareness when using human insulin could not substantiate the claims (SEDA-17, 480; 13[r]). This has not, however, ended the discussion. Training seems to be a possible means of increasing awareness. If the problem is experienced β-blockers, sometimes used for the treatment of hypertension, also suppress the prodromal symptoms.

Every patient treated with insulin (or with hypoglycemic agents) who develops a neurological or psychia-

Table 2. *Insulin preparations: type and duration of action*

Type	Onset of action	Maximum action (hours after subcutaneous injection)	Duration of action
Short-acting			
Regular insulin**	20–30	1–3	5–8
Crystalline	20–40	1–3	5–8
MC insulin*	15–30	1–3	4–8
Human insulin*	15–30	1–3	4–8
Intermediate-acting			
Zinc	1–2	6–10	12–16
Isophane	1–2	4–6	11–20
Globin	1–2	6–10	10–18
Lente	2–4	3–12	14–24
NPH**	1–2	8–12	14–24
MC Lente*	2–3	3–12	14–24
Depot	1–2	3–12	14–24
Long-acting			
Protamine zinc	4–6	16–24	24–36
Ultralente**	4–6	16–24	24–36
Ultratard	4–6	16–24	24–36
Insulinetard	4–6	16–12	24–36
Combined preparations			
Mixtard	$\frac{1}{2}$–1	3–18	12–24

* Highly purified.
** Also available highly purified or as human insulin.

tric disorder has to be considered to be hypoglycemic until proven otherwise. With modern methods (blood glucose strips) instant information about the blood glucose level is available. A rapid fall in blood glucose in a diabetic patient may elicit hypoglycemic symptoms even when blood glucose values are still normal or above normal. Experience with pumps has shown that many patients continue to feel hypoglycemic for a long time after normoglycemia has been attained.

Differentiation from hyperglycemic coma is usually not difficult. The development of hyperglycemic coma takes a longer time and blood glucose is high. However, urine testing during suspected hypoglycemic attacks may show positive glucosuria, if urine produced before the hypoglycemic period is still in the bladder. Even ketonuria may be present if a patient has been fasting for a long period. True epilepsy or cerebrovascular accidents may cause comparable symptoms or accompany hypoglycemia. When a patient does not react rapidly to sufficient therapy (see below), other diagnoses have to be considered. Vascular episodes in older diabetics may mimic hypoglycemic attacks. In hypoglycemic attacks the symptoms disappear rapidly after sugar intake. After a hypoglycemic attack patients often felt less well for a period of up to 48 hours. Headache, tiredness and lack of initiative may disappear only gradually. These symptoms in the morning may indicate unnoticed hypoglycemic periods during sleep. Wet pyjamas or sheets may also indicate unnoticed hypoglycemia. During anesthesia, profuse sweating may indicate hypoglycemia. Alcohol may confuse the diagnosis of hypoglycemia (for review, see SEDA-5, 386). Alcohol inhibits gluconeogenesis. It makes the patient more susceptible to hypoglycemia and can even cause hypoglycemia in normal persons. The symptoms of alcohol abuse and hypoglycemia are almost identical. If hypoglycemia is predominant, glucose administration will help.

Hypoglycemia is an important problem in children (14[r]). Children do not always establish the connection between the symptoms of threatening hypoglycemia and the danger involved. Overdosage of insulin is relatively common (SEDA-7, 406).

Older patients are particularly susceptible to hypoglycemia. Factors such as cerebral blood flow, blood P_{O_2} and P_{CO_2}, permeability of the blood-brain barrier or the presence of underlying neurological defects influence the hypoglycemic effects. Hypoglycemic symptoms have to be expected when the blood glucose level is lower than 2.6 mmol/l. This value depends on the method of estimation of blood glucose. Cardiovascular effects of hypoglycemia including angina pectoris, arrhythmia, premature ventricular contractions, electrocardiographic changes and coronary thrombosis have been reported. Raised levels of catecholamines and decreased levels of potassium seem to be a reason for cardiac damage during hypoglycemia.

Hypoglycemic periods are often seen in 'brittle diabetics', many of whom are overtreated with insulin. Changes in the insulin regimen (decreased use of long-acting insulin, frequent small injections of short-acting insulin) or the use of continuous infusion pumps can often lead to better results, but not every brittle diabetes can be corrected in that way (SEDA-7, 405). Errors in injection techniques such as superficial subcutaneous injections forming nodules or bleeding may cause variation in the daily uptake of insulin, resulting in an increase in the mean administered dose and in inadvertent hypoglycemic attacks.

Long periods of (deep) hypoglycemia may induce permanent brain damage. There is concern that frequent attacks of hypoglycemia impair brain function but there are few hard data. If it is absolutely impossible to stabilize brittle diabetes factitious hypoglycemia, Von Münchhausen syndrome by proxy (SEDA-18, 413), or manipulation of the prescribed doses may be suspected.

The emergence of hypoglycemic attacks depends upon the times and amounts of food eaten and the duration of action of the insulin used (see Table 2). Where only one type of insulin is employed the hypoglycemic symptoms are mostly seen at the end of the period of maximal activity of insulin (i.e. for short-acting insulins at the end of the morning or in the evening, for long-acting insulins, when they are given in the evening, during the night or early in the morning). Modern insulin therapy involves using a combination of long- and short-acting insulins. Long-acting insulins are given once or twice a day in combination with and/or in addition to short-acting insulins, which are administered 2—4 times a day. Hypoglycemia can then develop at moments when the combined effects are most prominent. Hypoglycemia in the midmorning may be a consequence of the action of the long-acting insulin of the previous day and the short-acting insulin given earlier in the same morning. Repeated hypoglycemic symptoms at the same time of the day indicate that the timing of the insulin injection or the proportion long-acting/short-acting insulin has to be changed. If the interval between insulin injection and the subsequent meal is very short, the effective insulin concentration in the blood is still low, when glucose is taken out of the gut. This induces very high post-meal glucose levels. Increase of insulin dosage induces hypoglycemia at a later moment. It is than advisable to try first to increase the interval between injection and start of the meal. New synthetic insulins like Lys-Pro-insulin are supposed to give a more rapid increase and fall of insulin levels than regular insulin, but this product is still in the phase of testing.

In factitious hypoglycemia (in which hypoglycemic periods are caused by surreptitious self-injection (of excessive) amounts of insulin) low blood glucose values are accompanied by high insulin levels but by low C-peptide levels (15[cr]). Suicide attempts with insulin in diabetic patients or non-diabetic patients may be less uncommon than is often thought.

Treatment of hypoglycemia Patients have to be instructed to have sugar available at all times and to use it when the first symptoms of hypoglycemia are felt. Often they fail to do so (16). If patients are used to self-monitoring, it is advisable that they monitor blood glucose first. When they feel hypoglycemic, a rapid drop in blood glucose without reaching hypoglycemic values may suffice to elicit a hypoglycemic reaction. Hypoglycemic reactions are sometimes difficult to discriminate from other feelings of malaise. Sugar will always give instantaneous relief.

The conscious patient should take glucose orally at once. If this does not suffice, he should receive a glucose infusion to keep the blood glucose level at 7—12 mmol/l (SED-9, 707). The treatment of choice in hypoglycemic coma is immediate intravenous injection of 20—50 grams of glucose. The patient may try to resist the injection, and help with the immobilization of the arm may therefore be needed. Injection of concentrated glucose solution outside a blood vessel leads to inflammatory and necrotic reactions. If intravenous injection of glucose is impossible 1 mg of glucagon can be injected subcutaneously. Where the patient has received high doses of long-acting insulin, hypoglycemia may relapse after a single dose of sugar has provided temporary relief, and monitoring should continue for a longer period. After hypoglycemic reactions elicited by long-acting insulins or oral hypoglycemic drugs the patient should be observed for possible recurrences during the next few days (17[r]). The longer the duration of the coma, the poorer the prognosis. Persistent posthypoglycemic coma is probably due to cerebral edema. Fever may accompany this severe form of coma, which demands treatment with intravenous mannitol and glucocorticoid injections. Such a severe coma may last for several days and demand intensive clinical treatment. Encephalopathy with various neurological symptoms may be the consequence.

ALLERGIC REACTIONS TO INSULIN

Insulin allergy remains a frequent side effect (SEDA-7, 403; 18[R]—20[R]) though serious systematic reactions are rare. Local reactions at the site of injection are not infrequent. They appear as reddening, swelling, heat, burning and itching and may be with or without frankly painful sensations. They may set in immediately or after some hours. The patch may extend gradually and remain for increasingly long periods. Some immediate reactions are related to IgE (or IgE/IgG) levels (21[R]). Other reactions are of the tuberculin granulomatous type or of the local vasculitis Arthus type. The local reactions may be accompanied, preceded or followed by a generalized reaction, such as urticaria, nausea, vomiting, diarrhea, angioneurotoxic edema, wheezing or anaphylactic shock. The latter complication is rare, but sometimes fatal. A direct relation between allergic reactions and a specific IgG fraction cannot be established (22[r]).

The allergic reactions were originally thought to be caused by impurities present in the insulin preparation used. After the introduction of monocomponent insulin these reactions continued to be seen in patients during treatment with monocomponent insulin or human synthetic insulin, even without a previous history of treatment with other insulins (23[C]). Transferring a patient from animal to human insulin may, paradoxically, induce allergic reactions, which subside when treatment with animal insulin is re-instituted (24[C]). In 20-year-old sera of patients who were never treated with human insulin, antibodies against human insulin could be demonstrated (25[r]).

Allergic reactions may also be elicited by Surfen (aminoquinuride) (26[C]) (a constituent of various insulin preparations, which delays the uptake of insulin), by zinc (29[C]) or by zinc and/or protamine (NPH) (28[C], 29[C]). Remnants of fluids used for cleansing the skin may be co-injected in micro-amounts and elicit allergic reactions (30[c]).

Intermittent insulin administration seems to favor the development of allergic reactions (SEDA-6, 369). General edema (SEDA-11, 364) or abscesses (SEDA-7, 406) generated by insulin injections are extremely rare. Insulin may induce local, painful lumps on injection sites. Sclerosing granuloma is occasionally seen (31[C]) and could be induced by zinc (32[C]). Such reactions are most commonly a consequence of an incorrect injection technique, generally the use of too short a needle or too superficial an injection.

In excised (infected) lumps, amyloid fibrils, proteins containing intact insulin, could be demonstrated (33[C]). Plastic syringes may release silicone particles; these may diminish the effect of insulin (34[C]), or themselves induce granulomatous reactions (35[C]).

Lipodystrophy, lipoatrophy or lipohypertrophy may be a consequence of chronic local insulin reactions which can be elicited by less pure as well as by highly purified preparations (36[C]), but such reactions can also develop at sites distant to the injection. Circulating insulin-binding antibodies may increase insulin resistance (37[C], 38[R]) and extend insulin action by slowing release. The mean levels of antibodies decrease when purified insulins or human insulin are used, but they can be demonstrated even when modern insulins of high purity have been used exclusively. Anti-receptor antibodies are seldom seen.

Treatment In 95% of cases the local reactions disappear spontaneously. A switch to less immunogenic, highly purified insulins is necessary if the reactions persist. For local allergic reactions, antihistamines or the addition of hydrocortisone (2 mg) along with the insulin preparation are seldom needed. For generalized reactions, skin testing is often necessary to establish allergic desensitization. One should start with low intradermal doses and, if necessary, add hydrocortisone.

For therapy of local lumps, extravasation, etc., one should first seek to improve the injection technique. Substitution with highly purified insulin is recommended. Injection with purified insulin in the affected area may speed up resorption of the lumps. *Lipodystrophy* or *lipoatrophy* improve after transfer to human or highly purified insulin. *Lipohypertrophy* in the other hand often fails to respond to changes in the insulin regimen (39[C]). Variation in injection site may help, but differences in absorption rate then have to be taken into account.

Insulin resistance is said to be present when more than 200 units per day have to be injected; it is generally due to the antibodies discussed above. In general, antibody titers decrease when highly purified insulins are used, but they sometimes remain elevated after the switch-over. Some diseases, such as infections, endocrine hyperfunctional states (acromegaly, Cushing's syndrome, thyrotoxicosis), leukemia or stress may contribute to a seemingly higher resistance to insulin.

Insulin edema Insulin edema is a rare complication more frequently seen in the earlier years of insulin therapy (for review see SEDA-11, 364). It is mostly seen when disregulated patients with progressive weight loss are treated with relatively high amounts of insulin. Decreased sodium excretion (40[C]), sodium reabsorption and water retention by a possible direct action of insulin on the kidney may be involved (41[R]). The role of aldosterone or of inhibition of the renin-angiotensin-aldosterone system in insulin edema is unclear. Insulin edema is a specific side effect, but it may aggravate pulmonary edema, congestive heart failure and hypertension. The treatment consists of reduction of the insulin dose, than the edema subsidizes in 3—4 days. A specific complication of high amounts of insulin during hyperosmolar diabetic coma is *rhabdomyolysis* (42[C]). Low intra-muscular phosphate and potassium, often masked by relatively high blood glucose values, may be an important contributing factor.

SECOND-GENERATION EFFECTS

In animals, teratogenicity of insulin during pregnancy has been observed (SED-8, 908). No proof has been given that this also holds good for man.

NEW INSULINS

Pushed by industrial developments, the use of synthetic human insulin, produced by recombinant DNA techniques, has increased strongly (43). The clinical value or clinical significance of the differences in antigenicity between human and animal insulins is not clear. Even in patients never treated with other types of insulin, allergic reactions can be seen and anti-insulin antibodies can be demonstrated when human insulin is used (SEDA-8, 379; 44[r]). They generally tend to act more rapidly, but for shorter periods than the comparable, unpurified counterparts. Human ultra-lente (45) and human NPH insulin (46) are more rapidly absorbed.

Reports about increased unawareness of hypoglycemia after transfer from animal insulin to human insulin preparation induced by disappearance of adrenergic (warning) symptoms of hypoglycemia (47) have been extensively debated (SEDA-15, 452; SEDA-17, 478).

Human insulins may be the treatment of choice in new diabetic patients, provided that there are no important differences in price between both insulin types. For short periods of insulin therapy (operations, pregnancy, etc.) they are the first choice, because allergies seem to develop more frequently in interrupted insulin treatment. They must also be tried when insulin allergy, insulin resistance or lipoatrophy emerge.

Chemically modified insulins (with one or more amino acid substituted) and other ways of absorption (nasal insulin, encapsulated insulins) are still in an experimental phase. These newer formulations may induce more rapid and constant release of insulin from the injection site, since they consist of pockets with monomeric insulin. Natural insulin in high concentrations tends to aggregate and to form dimers or hexamers, which are less active and more slowly resorbed. The change of one or more amino acids in the insulin molecule by recombinant DNA technology may inhibit insulin to form dimers or hexamers. More rapid resorption, rapid availability and rapid inactivation makes the action better comparable with the action of endogenously secreted insulin. In recent years, new attention has been given to the role of zinc in insulin. The pharmacokinetics and the pharmacodynamics of lente/regular mixtures seem to be less reliable (48) and more negatively influenced by refrigerated storage (49). Granuloma with furunculated lesions, containing rhomboid insulin crystals and leukocytes appeared to be induced by zinc present in insulin preparations (32).

Product variation The formulation of insulin differs in various countries. One hundred U/ml insulin is increasingly used in many countries, but in other countries 20, 40 or 80 U/ml are still in use. The increased frequency of travelling and tourism has increased the importance of the problem. In some countries in various parts of the world, both U40 insulin of variable purity and highly purified U100 insulin are available at the same time. U100 insulin in U40 syringes causes severe unexpected hypoglycemia and the reverse induces apparent insulin resistance (SEDA-6, 367).

Intranasal administration of insulin is still experimental. Nasal irritations, sometimes with congestion, are seen. A problem in nasal administration is still how to get a daily reproducible identical dose (50[R]). Delivering by aerosol inhalation is another experimental method. No lung obstruction was reported, but the uptake varied considerably (51[c]).

NEW DEVICES FOR INSULIN ADMINISTRATIONS

Insulin pumps The usefulness of devices for constant subcutaneous, intravenous or intraperitoneal insulin administration is now well established. To establish feed-back systems reliable, constantly functioning insulin sensors are essential but they have been in a developmental phase for more than 20 years, and still no long-acting glucose sensors for non-experimental use are available (52[R]). Experience with pumps in large groups of patients has been reported (53, 54[CR], 55[r]). When starting intensive therapy, temporary worsening of secondary complications, mostly retinopathy but sometimes nephropathy, have been reported (SEDA-14, 374). Weight gain is also a 'complication' (7). Type I diabetics, pregnant patients, some types of brittle diabetics, patients wanting to become pregnant and children are major candidates for insulin pump therapy. Most of the pumps deliver insulin subcutaneously. Implantable pumps delivering insulin intraperitoneally with remote control devices are also used (for a recent review, see Ref. 56[R]). Pumps delivering insulin intravenously are almost out of use. The pump provides signals to alert the user to malfunction, but leakage of connections often does not activate the alarm. Since the patient has no natural reserve of insulin, breakdown of the pump, leakage or intercurrent infection without adjustment of the dose leads to very rapid development of ketoacidosis. The sudden release of insulin from a 'runaway' pump is an exceptional event. Hypoglycemic deaths, infections, local allergic reactions and infections, thrombosis in intravenous systems, nickel allergy for needles (57[C]), dermal infections (58[r]), needle breakage (SEDA-13, 382), problems with bad batteries, breakdown of the pump, leakage in delivery systems or wrong insertion of the needle have all been described (SEDA-7, 405; 59). Pumps with sealed reservoirs (waterproof) can expel more insulin when used at high altitudes (skiing, mountaineering, pressured cabins in airplanes) inducing serious hypoglycemia (60[C], SEDA-16, 486).

The tendency of insulin to conglomerate in concentrated solutions requires sometimes specific insulin for pumps. There is still a difference of opinion whether insulin resorption kinetics changes (improves) during the placement of the catheter (SEDA-16, 488; SEDA-18, 412). Change-over of the injection site and the renewal of the infusion system every 2—4 days is important for prevention of clogging, local allergy, and infection at the insertion site. In the implanted pumps, catheters for continuous intraperitoneal insulin infusion can be obstructed by deposits of fibrin on the catheter tip. They mostly reappear after the plug is blown out, necessitating replacement (61[r]). A hematoma with a fulminant *Streptococcus* infection in the pump pocket has been reported (62[C]). During the start of pump therapy, some patients feel as if they are constantly hypoglycemic, even though low blood glucose values cannot be objectified. In the intravenous pumps, thrombosis, vasculitis and septicemia may emerge.

Other devices Other devices, like long-term subcutaneous (63) or intraperitoneal (64) catheters for children or intraperitoneal catheters (65) for pumps, meet the same type of problems as subcutaneous catheters for pumps, except that the catheters are indwelling for longer periods. Other devices, like the jet-stream injector, propagated as an alternative for persons afraid for injections, have given problems with delayed pain and bleeding. The advantages of the methods are questionable.

The insulin pen is increasingly used for intensive insulin therapy. In general, intensive therapy induces lower blood glucose levels and decreased HbA_{1c}. This may induce worsening of proliferative retinopathy (66[c]), which is often temporary, or weight gain (7). Pens may develop inaccuracies in rare instances, which may be unnoticed by the patient (67). Clogging of the system is often the cause. The result is diabetic coma or keto-acidosis, but this is not more frequent than with other systems. When needles are not regularly renewed, infections may emerge.

A thin fat layer may result in intramuscular injections, leading to faster absorption of long-acting insulins. This may reduce the absorption time to a half (68). Disposable syringes may release silicon particles into the insulin vials, reducing the effectiveness of insulin (69[C]). This may happen when insulin is reversed into the bottle, during correction for the desired dose. This is specifically seen when low doses are used for long periods. Flocculation of insulin, found before the expiry date, may be related to this problem (SEDA-12, 360). Flocculated insulin may also block the jet-holes.

Frequent self control by pricking the finger-tips may induce anemia (70[C]) or pyoderma gangrenosum and finger-tip ulceration (71[C]).

GLUCAGON *(SEDA-17, 484; SEDA 18, 413)*

Glucagon is used subcutaneously (1 mg, repeated once or twice) in hypoglycemic coma, when glucose cannot be given intravenously. In some countries it is frequently used by personnel (family members), who are not medically qualified, as the first action when the patient cannot take sugar orally. The anti-hypoglycemic effect of an intramuscular injection is longer lasting and more potent than that of intravenous glucagon (72). It is used as a stimulatory test in C-peptide testing, pheochromocytoma, hyperinsulinism and Zollinger-Ellison syndrome or as an additive in upper gastrointestinal X-ray investigations (0.5—1 mg). It has been used in myocardial infarction, although its inotropic effects may present a risk. Glucagon induces nausea and vomiting and it may induce erythema multiforme even after the injection of a small amount (73[C]). Hand eczema has been found when glucagon was used as an adjuvant during X-rays of the gastrointestinal tract.

ORAL HYPOGLYCEMIC DRUGS

Four groups of glucose lowering drugs can be distinguished: sulfonylureas, biguanides, α-glucosidase inhibitors and, still in development, the quidinidilones. Moreover, drugs are primarily developed to prevent or postpone secondary complications (aldose reductase inhibitors).

SULFONYLUREAS AND SULFAPYRIMIDINES *(SEDA-16, 479; SEDA-17, 489; SEDA-18, 413)*

The most frequent complication is hypoglycemia, specifically when normalization of blood glucose is the goal of the treatment. Incidental side effects are presented under the various headings. When a side effect is not mentioned under a specific drug it does not mean that it cannot develop with this drug (for a recent review, see Ref. 74[R]).

Sulfonylureas and sulfapyrimidines have the same mode of action. They act by increasing the amount of insulin released from the β-cells; this effect is supported by the increased glucose levels. The β-cells of patients treated with these drugs are chronically stimulated. It has not been established whether this benefits the patient in the long run.

A rise in insulin receptors (binding sites), amelioration of the post-binding defect and inhibition of the (increased) glucose output from the liver have been described (SEDA-5, 391). Most of the in vitro or animal experiments in which these findings were obtained were of short duration, however. The data are difficult to translate into data relevant to the extensive pathophysiological changes present in diabetes mellitus. In diabetes mellitus Type II, changes in (the) insulin secretion (pattern) and increased peripheral resistance to insulin, both resulting in an increased output of glucose from the liver are found. The primary defect in NIDDM is still not known.

Sulfonylureas are mainly used in Type II diabetes mellitus. The extra amount of insulin released results in a decrease in blood glucose and glucosuria and contributes to a decrease in energy loss (and may thereby contribute to an increased storage of body fat when more is eaten than is necessary to meet daily energy needs); it will also provoke feelings of hunger. They should therefore not be prescribed to overweight diabetics, who primarily need to lose weight. The decrease in adipose tissue contributes to a greater effectiveness of the available insulin. Nowadays, as supported by the DCCT results (7[R]), we know that a sustained increase in the blood glucose level may accelerate the development of secondary complications of diabetes mellitus. Being overweight may be the price to be paid for normalization of blood levels. However, not all secondary changes, like macroangiopathy, seem to be directly dependent on blood glucose levels. It is beyond the scope of this book to discuss the matter in more detail.

The experiences of 30 years of treatment with oral drugs were reviewed by Nabarro (75[R]).

General side effects

Hypoglycemia Hypoglycemia remains the most frequent complication in diabetes treated with tablets (4[r], 13[r], 76[R], 77[r]). These drugs are mostly used by elderly people, and the characteristic warning symptoms of hypoglycemia (dizziness, transpiration, a feeling of hunger) are often absent or not well-interpreted. The hypoglycemic situation takes the patient and the environment by surprise. Confusion with neurological symptoms of other origin (transient ischemic attack, cerebrovascular accidents, etc.) is not uncommon. Hypoglycemia may be the result of an overdose of sulfonylureas. Decreased intake of food or of alcohol may also play a role (5[r]). Most sulfonylureas are metabolized in the liver (SED-9, 709), hence *liver insufficiency*, liver disease, and liver enzyme inhibition (alcohol) or induction (drugs) may influence the half-life of the drug and its duration of action. *Renal dysfunction* is another cause of hypoglycemia. Some sulfonylureas such as chlorpropamide (for 30%) or tolbutamide (50%) are excreted by the kidney. With other drugs, such as acetohexamide, glibenclamide, glibornuride, glyburide or glymidine, the metabolites which sometimes also have a hypoglycemic effect, are excreted. The decrease in insulin metabolism in diseased kidneys may contribute to the hypoglycemia since it increases the half-life of insulin. A third cause of hypoglycemia is the simultaneous use of drugs which have glucose-lowering effects or which inhibit the expression of the first warning signs, e.g. β-blockers.

The potency and the duration of action of oral hypoglycemic drugs vary (see Table 3). The duration of action is determined by the biological half-life, the velocity of metabolism in the liver, binding to plasma proteins, the hypoglycemic effect of their metabolic products, and the speed of excretion. Blood levels of the drugs do not always determine the duration of action. When blood levels are falling, stimulation of insulin secretion may continue for some time. Oral drugs may make the cell more sensitive to insulin, and it is difficult to predict how long the hypoglycemic effect will last. For some drugs (e.g. glibenclamide), two compartments have been postulated (78), i.e. a first (rapidly equilibrating) and a second (slowly equilibrating) compartment. The latter may act as a 'granary' which continues to release the drug even during prolonged hypoglycemic attacks.

In general, hypoglycemia caused by oral hypoglycemic drugs is more dangerous and of longer duration than hypoglycemia caused by insulin (13[r]). The warning symptoms (dizziness, transpiration, a feeling of hunger) may not be present or are not well-interpreted as danger

Table 3. *Principal oral hypoglycemic drugs (sulfonylureas)*

Generic name	Dose (mg)		Duration of action (h)	Half-life (h) Renal function	
	Mean/day	Maximum/day		Normal	Anuric
Acetohexamide	250–1000	1500	12–24	16	48
Carbutamide	500–1500	2500			
Chlorpropamide	100–500	1000	20–60	35	200
Glibenclamide (glyburide)	2.5–10	20	12–18	5–8	11–14
Glibornuride	12.5–100		10–15		
Gliclazide	40–240	240	12–18	8–11	
Glipizide	2.5–20	30	6–12	3–5	unchanged*
Gliquidone	15–90	120	6–12	6–10	unchanged*
Glisoxepide	2–12	15	5–10		
Glymidine (= glycodiazine)	500–1500	3000	6–12		
Tolazamide	100–500	1000	12–16	8–10	?
Tolbutamide	500–2000	3000	6–12	3–5	48

* Hypoglycemia is seen in spite of the unchanged half-life.

signs by the patient. The factors described above contribute to the prolongation of the hypoglycemic effect.

Most dangerous are hypoglycemic attacks produced by long-acting preparations such as chlorpropamide and by so-called second-generation drugs such as glibenclamide (SEDA-4, 303). Increases in the maximum attainable effect of second-generation drugs could result in deeper hypoglycemia after overdosage. Frequent occurrence of hypoglycemic episodes has occasionally resulted in encephalopathy and after discontinuation of the hypoglycemic drug the cerebral injury has proved to be persistent. It is not exceptional for a prolonged hypoglycemic coma to end fatally (4[r], 77[r]). In 494 cases of severe hypoglycemia, 10% of the patients died and 9% had permanent sequelae (79[c]). Hypoglycemia factitia induced by tablets is difficult to diagnose since C-peptide levels will be high and not suppressed. Treatment of hypoglycemia (80[R]) and of overdose with sulfonylureas has been reviewed recently. Somatostatin (octreotide (81[CR]) but not diazoxide is recommended.

Resistance to diuretic treatment in patients treated with oral hypoglycemics may be caused by water containing agents like chlorpropamide or, to a lesser extent, tolbutamide. Changing to a sulfonylurea without an antidiuretic effect (glibenclamide) or to one which enhances water excretion (acetohexamide, tolazamide) may be advisable (SED-8, 913). Slight hyponatremia was seen, predominantly with chlorpropamide, but also with glybornuride, carbutamide, gliclazide and glibenclamide. Extreme hyponatremia was only seen with chlorpropamide and, in one case, with glibenclamide (82[r]).

Hematological The most dangerous adverse reaction is *agranulocytosis*. *Aplastic anemia* (83[c], 84[C]), *pure white cell aplasia* (85[C]), *bone marrow aplasia* and *hemolytic anemia* have been described during chlorpropamide (86[C]), glibenclamide (87[C], 88[C]) or tolbutamide treatment. *Hemorrhagic thrombocytopenic purpura* has been described with chlorpropamide (89[r]), tolbutamide (90[C]), glibenclamide (91[C], 92[C]), acetohexamide and tolazamide, and *hypersensitive vasculitis* (93[c]) has been described with glibenclamide (SED-9, 712).

Liver The risk of *hepatotoxicity* with the sulfonylureas varies both with the drug which is used and the dosage. It has been described for chlorpropamide (94[cr]), tolbutamide (95[C]), glipizide and glibenclamide (96[C]). *Anicteric, cytolytic hepatitis* has been described after glibenclamide (97[C]). *Cholestatic jaundice* is probably of allergic origin (SED-8, 911); it is rare and has been described with glibenclamide (98[C]), acetohexamide (99[c]), chlorpropamide (100[CR]) and tolazamide (101[C]). *Hepatitis* has been described with glibenclamide (102[C]). An Antabuse-like effect after use of alcohol has been described with chlorpropamide, but also with gliclazide, glipizide and acetohexamide. *Jaundice* during treatment with sulfonylureas is difficult to distinguish from viral hepatitis.

Gastrointestinal Gastrointestinal tract disturbances are frequent. The are described for all sulfonylureas. They comprise *nausea*, *vomiting*, *heartburn*, *dyspepsia*, a *metallic taste* and *abdominal pain*. They are less troublesome when the drugs are taken after meals.

Pancreas A possible relationship between 2 years of treatment with sulfonylurea and damage to the islets of Langerhans has been reported (103). A fatal case of pancreatitis induced by glyburide has been described (104[C]).

Urinary system *Nephrotic syndrome* and immune complex *glomerulonephritis* have been induced by chlorpropamide (105[C]).

Skin *Photosensitization* has been described for tolbutamide (106[C]), chlorpropamide (107[C]) and glibenclamide (108[r]), sometimes combined with *porphyrinuria* (SED-8, 911). *Allergic reactions* have been described for all sulfonylureas. They include pruritic rashes, erythema nodosum, urticaria, blisters (97[c]), erythema multiforme, exfoliative dermatitis, Quincke's edema, erythrodermia and itching, while lichenoid drug reactions with ulcerations have occurred after chlorpropamide and tolazamide (109[C]). More generalized hypersensitivity reactions may actually prove fatal, but they are rare.

Special senses A change in *taste* sensations has been reported with glipizide (110).

Miscellaneous effects *Eosinophilic infiltrations* have been described for tolbutamide (SED-8, 917) and (chronic) eosinophilic pneumonia has been described during chlorpropamide (111[C], 112[C]) and tolazamide (113[C]) treatment.

Risk situations *Hypopituitarism*, *hypoadrenalism*, *hypothyroidism*, *insulinoma*, *malnutrition* and *old age* all increase sensitivity to sulfonylureas. The delay or omission of a meal or other reasons for a *smaller caloric intake*, as well as unexpected *hard exercise*, may increase the hypoglycemic effects of sulfonylureas. Excessive use of *alcohol*, sometimes found in older persons living alone, may also contribute to changes in sensitivity to oral drugs. Hypoglycemia has been reported in a worker, not wearing a mask, working with a machine preparing ultrafine sulfonylurea powder (114[C]).

Second-generation effects The possible teratogenicity of sulfonylureas in man naturally cannot be judged from animal data. Because of anecdotal evidence of risk and on theoretical grounds it is however inadvisable to give sulfonylurea therapy to women of fertile age (115[c]). In women using self administered hypoglycemic drugs during pregnancy, chlorpropamide, glyburide and tolbutamide induced serious malformations like microtia, deafness, facial deformities, ventricular septum defect (with or without aortic rotation), atrial septum defect and single umbilical artery (116[C]). An effect of high blood glucose could not be excluded. The choice for pregnant diabetics is between insulin given frequently in a short-acting form to avoid overdosage, or a continuous insulin infusion system, since overdosage of insulin may be harmful to the developing fetus. *Chromosomal damage* is described with chlorpropamide (117[c]). The same drug may have contributed to the development of a cleft palate (118[C]). Transient diabetes insipidus was seen in a child born to a mother treated with chlorpropamide in pregnancy (119[C]).

Interactions (*see also Table* 4) Drug mechanisms which result in potentiation of the hypoglycemic effects of the sulfonylureas comprise: (1) prolongation of the half-life by inhibition of metabolism or excretion (*phenylbutazone*, *coumarins*, *chloramphenicol*, *doxycycline*, *probenecid*, *sulfaphenazole*, *fenyramidol*); (2) competition with plasma protein binding sites (*phenylbutazone*, *salicylates* and *sulfonamides*); (3) potentiation of their hypoglycemic action by inhibition of gluconeogenesis, enhancement of oxidation of glucose or stimulation of insulin secretion (β-adrenergic receptor blockers, mono-amine-oxidase inhibitors, salicylates, tranylcypromine).

The hepatic effects of sulfonylureas include the inhibition of enzymatic degradation of *ethanol*. This effect is only partly comparable with the action of disulfiram, which blocks the aldehyde degradation but not that of the ethanol molecule itself. It results in a vasomotor reaction with giddiness, tachycardia, headache, angina pectoris and skin reactions. The most prominent drug to elicit these effects seems to be chlorpropamide, but it has also been described for tolbutamide and other drugs. The specific effect of alcohol and chlorpropamide has been propagated to be of use as a genetic marker, but this has not been confirmed (for review, see SEDA-7, 407). ACE-inhibitors may contribute to the hyponatremia seen during chlorpropamide (120[r]).

Recently, a number of reports on confusion around hypoglycemic prescriptions have been published (SEDA-16, 490; SEDA-17, 495; SEDA-18, 414) like chlorpropamide instead of chlorpromazine or chloroquine and diabinese (chlorpropamide) or acetohexamide instead of diamox (acetazolamide).

INDIVIDUAL SULFONYLUREAS *(see SED-11, 898)*

First- and second-generation sulfonylureas

Sometimes distinctions are made between hypoglycemic drugs of the first and second generation. One of the distinctions is that the first-generation drugs are prescribed in gram doses and the second-generation drugs (glibenclamide, glipizide) in milligram doses. However, toxic effects are not likely to be primarily dependent on the actual weight of the drug administered; they are more likely to relate to the potency of

Table 4. *Drug interactions involving oral hypoglycemic agents*

Interactions	Mechanisms	Notes
Enhanced hypoglycemic effect		
Salicylates	(2) (6)	
Probenecid	(1) or (2)	
Allopurinol	(1)	
Pyrazoles	(1) or (2)	
β-Adrenergic blockers	(3)	
Levodopa	(3)	
Perhexiline	(3)	
Chloramphenicol	(1)	
Sulfonamides	(1) (2)	(6)
Isoniazid	(5)	
Coumarin-type anticoagulants	(6)	
Azopropazan	(2)	
Ace inhibitors	(5)	
Impaired hypoglycemic effect		
Barbiturates	(4)	
Phenothiazines	(5)	Involves only sulfonylurea
Thiazide diuretics	(6)	Involves only sulfonylurea
Furosemide	(5)	
Sulfamethoxydiazine	(5)	
Corticosteroids	(6)	
Oral contraceptives	(6)	
Acetazolamide	(5)	
Other effects		
Tetracyclines		Increased risk of lactic acidosis when biguanides are given
Alcohol		Lowers blood glucose; impairs gluconeogenesis
Diuretics		With biguanides, increased risk of lactic acidosis

(1) Inhibition of drug-metabolizing enzymes.
(2) Displacement of drug from protein-binding site.
(3) Impairment of glucose homeostatic mechanism.
(4) Induction of metabolizing enzymes.
(5) Unknown.
(6) Other mechanisms.

the dose used. The frequency of side effects reported (which is difficult to measure when compared with the frequency of the administrations of the drug) does not seem to differ greatly as between the two 'generations'. The seriousness and the type of the side effects are the same. The supposedly greater success of the second generation drugs in secondary failures is difficult to support when the body weight is included in the observation (122[R]). A high percentage of the second-generation drugs are often bound to serum proteins, resulting in an effect of longer duration. In this Chapter no further distinctions will be made between first- and second-generation drugs.

Acetohexamide

This drug is readily absorbed; the maximum hypoglycemic effect occurs after 3—5 hours. However, its main metabolite (hydroxyhexamide) also has hypoglycemic activity; it has a longer half-life and a duration of action of 12—24 hours.

Carbutamide

This sulfonamide with bacteriostatic properties is no longer permitted in many countries. It is one of the most toxic oral hypoglycemic drugs with many and severe side effects.

Chlorpropamide

Chlorpropamide, according to many authors, is now the most toxic of the sulfonylureas in general use. Various combinations of adverse effects have been described. The frequency with which problems arise seems to reflect the fact that the drug is both potent and long-acting, and that elimination from the body may take several weeks. Hypoglycemic attacks are therefore often of prolonged duration, and they may be lethal (4[C]). Chlorpropamide must not be given when clear contraindications, such as impaired liver or renal function, alcoholism or insufficient food intake, are present. Its antidiuretic actions are specific and may lead in 2% (122[r]) to a syndrome of appropriate antidiuretic hormone secretion (SEDA-4, 303) or to low sodium levels with impairment of mental function (123[r]). It has also caused a disulfiram-like syndrome when combined with alcohol and, in another patient, a similar reaction seems to have been triggered by concomitant treatment with gold (124).

Gliclazide

Gliclazide is a slow-acting sulfonylurea which is not used in many countries. Gliclazide is 85—97% bound to plasma proteins; 20% is excreted in the urine. The metabolites have no hypoglycemic effect. The side effects and interactions of gliclazide have been extensively reviewed (125[R]).

Glibenclamide (glyburide)

The dosage of glibenclamide can (and often must) be lowered after some weeks of treatment. A slowly equilibrating 'deep compartment' for this drug which is gradually filled during prolonged glibenclamide therapy may be present (76). A major metabolite with hypoglycemic properties may accumulate during renal failure (78). More than 99% of glibenclamide is bound to plasma proteins.

Hypoglycemia is not infrequent (77[R]); because of the drug's kinetics it often runs an extended course and can be lethal.

Since the glibenclamide patent expired in some countries, new formulations have been marketed, and one can of course not exclude changes in effect as a result of differing bioavailability or excipients (e.g. skin reactions have occurred with one such new formulation (126) and a fatal case of cholestatic hepatitis (127[CR])).

Glibornuride

About 95—97% of glibornuride is bound to plasma proteins; 65% of the drug and its metabolites is eliminated by the kidney. Kidney disease may prolong its half-life some 3.7-fold.

Glipizide

Glipizide (128[R]) is nearly as potent as glibenclamide; 95—97% is bound to plasma proteins. The half-life is shorter than that of glibenclamide.

Glisoxepide

Glisoxepide is the most potent hypoglycemic drug, being on a weight basis about 500 times more potent than tolbutamide.

BIGUANIDES *(SEDA-16, 492; SEDA-17, 488; SEDA-18, 415)*

Of the three biguanides, buformin and phenformin have been withdrawn in many countries (SEDA-4, 306) because of dangerous side effects, but they are still available in a few countries. Metformin (129[R]) is the only biguanide commonly used. The major reason for restrictions, imposed in various countries, is the risk of lactic acidosis (130[R]), which is fatal in 50% of the cases (131[R]). The relative risk of metformin treatment is significantly lower than that of phenformin or buformin (132), but lactic acidosis, caused by metformin, has been repeatedly reported (SEDA-6, 371; 133[C], 134[R]), even in cases in the absence of known contraindications (135[C]).

The biguanides have a special affinity for the mitochondrial membrane, which causes an alteration in electron transport and results in a decrease in oxygen consumption. Inhibition of the active transport of glucose in the intestinal mucosa, absent activation of glucose transporters, inhibition of gluconeogenesis, inhibition of fatty acid oxidation and of lipid synthesis are the effects which are considered to cause lowering of the blood glucose and an increase in blood lipids in the diabetic.

All biguanides have plasma half-lives of 2—3 hours. Peak levels are reached after 1.5—4 hours; 70—90% of the drugs are eliminated via the kidneys. Biguanides have been reviewed recently (136[R]).

Adverse reactions *Hypoglycemia* can occur. Early symptoms of *lactic acidosis* are nausea, vomiting and diarrhea; since these are common adverse reactions to biguanides as such, a careful watch should be kept for their sudden onset or aggravation, which might point to lactic acidosis (129).

Gastrointestinal discomfort is frequent (15—25%), but dose-dependent. *Vomiting* and *diarrhea* (without lactic acidosis) occur. *Anorexia* and *weight loss* are common. Weight loss is often seen at the beginning of treatment by interference with intestinal absorption. *Metformin* and *phenformin* (137) interfere with the absorption of vitamin B_{12}. *Urticaria* and *rash* are seen occasionally. Phenformin induced *pancreatitis* (138[C]) and *hemorrhagic gastritis* (139[C]), and metformin induced *hepatitis* (140[C]). *Leukocytoblastic vasculitis* and *pneumonitis*, induced by metformin, have been reported (141[C]).

No clear information is available as to the effect of metformin in pregnancy.

Risk situations Contraindications for the treatment with biguanides are: (1) impaired renal function (serum creatinine may not be a sufficient indicator; creatinine clearance has to be estimated); (2) elevated risk of impaired renal function in intercurrent diseases with fever, congestive heart failure or infections of the urinary tract, during treatment with diuretic drugs, intravenous pyelographic studies or severe dieting; (3) states with tissue hypoxia (respiratory insufficiency, heart insufficiency, anemia and peripheral vascular deficiencies); (4) hepatitis and hepatic cirrhosis; (5) excessive use of alcohol; (6) wasting diseases; (7) pre- and postoperative states. In general they should not be used in persons over 75 years.

Interactions The action of *insulin* is enhanced by biguanides just as by the sulfonylureas. Potentiation of the anti-coagulant action of *warfarin* or *phenprocoumon* by metformin (and phenformin) has been reported (142). Decreased serum levels of metformin were reported when it was combined with insulin or acarbose (143). The reader is further referred to Table 4.

ENZYME INHIBITORS

α-GLUCOSIDASE INHIBITORS *(SEDA-16, 493; SEDA-17, 489; SEDA-18, 416)*

The two α-glucosidase inhibitors (polyhexose mimickers) in use are acarbose and miglitol. They delay absorption of glucose and fat. In diabetes, the extended resorption lowers peak blood glucose levels after the meals and makes it effective to inhibit states of reactive hypoglycemia, as can be seen after gastric operation, in idiopathic forms and in dumping syndrome. In many studies a decrease of HbA_{1c} of 0.3—0.8% is seen. When combined with insulin most effects are seen in regimens with only once or twice a day administration. They seem to be less effective when combined with intensive insulin therapy (144[R]). In combination with insulin or oral hypoglycemic drugs the frequency of hypoglycemic episodes may increase; sucrose or higher carbohydrates are reported to be less effective, which can be understood from its mechanism of action. Frequent side effects are flatulence and meteorism, sometimes preventing further use. In prospective studies this amounts to 6—10% of the participants on 50 mg t.i.d.; the frequency increases when higher doses are used. Abdominal pain and (malabsorption) diarrhea have been described. Miglitol gave the same results (145[r]). Acarbose is not absorbed and excreted with the feces. Miglitol is resorbed from the gut and is almost completely absorbed and excreted unchanged in the urine (146[R]).

OTHER ORAL DRUGS *(SEDA-16, 493; SEDA-17, 488)*

THIAZOLIDINEDIONES

A new type of drugs, upregulating the insulin inducible glucose transporter Glut 4. It should reduce insulin resistance in muscle, fat and liver. They may be registered in some countries in the coming years. Side effects are nausea, vomiting, abdominal fullness and diarrhea. Small decreases in Hb, Ht and blood cell counts and increases in LDH and BUN were described (147[r]).

ALDOSE REDUCTASE INHIBITORS *(SEDA-16, 493; SEDA-17, 489; SEDA-18, 417)*

Aldose reductase inhibitors are used for the treatment of secondary complications in diabetes (for recent reviews see Refs. 148[R], 149[R]). They inhibit or reduce secondary complications induced by diabetes, specifically in tissues in which glucose uptake is not insulin dependent (probably neural tissue, the lens and glomeruli). A study on the effectiveness in neuropathy has been published (150[Cr]). The long-term effect on neuropathy, retinopathy and nephropathy has still to be established, awaiting the results of current 5-year studies. Increased blood glucose concentrations increase the levels of glucose in non-insulin-dependent tissues. At normal blood glucose concentrations the intracellular glucose is metabolized to myoinositol. When the intracellular glucose levels are increased, more glucose is metabolized to sorbitol. This results in a decrease of ATP-levels and of myoinositol, a substrate for the membrane phospholipid, phosphatidylinositol.

The key enzyme in this process, aldose reductase, exerts little activity when intracellular glucose levels are normal, but high glucose levels activate the enzyme.

Most aldose reductase inhibitors (alrestatin, sorbinil, ponalrestat, imirestat and ONO-554) have been used in clinical trials, but have been withdrawn because of side effects or lack of effect (149[R]). Sorbinil, which resembles phenytoin (151), showed toxic reactions in about 10% of the patients. They comprise rash, often with fever, nausea, diarrhea, marked thrombocytopenia, mild neutropenia and decreased hematocrit, lymphadenopathy and splenomegaly. Adult respiratory distress syndromes have been reported. Epidermal necrolysis and Stevens-Johnson syndrome have been observed.

At this moment only tolrestat and epalrestat are in clinical use. They have been registered in some countries. Both less, and less severe, side effects are reported, like dizziness, increases in hepatic enzymes, slight increase in creatinine and blisters.

GUAR GUM

Guar gum is sometimes recommended as it results in slower uptake of glucose in the gut. The effectiveness is lower than acarbose, and side effects like regurgitation, obstipation, abdominal cramps, diarrhea and itching are more frequently reported (152[Cr]).

REFERENCES

1. Koivisto VA, Felig P. Alterations in insulin absorption and in blood glucose control associated with varying insulin injection sites in diabetic patients. Ann Intern Med 1980;92:59—61.
2. Sindelka G, Neinemann L, Berger M, Frenck W, Chantelau E. Effect of insulin concentration, subcutaneous fat thickness and skin temperature on subcutaneous insulin absorption in healthy subjects. Diabetologia 1994;37:377—380.
3. Binder C, Lauritzen T, Faber O, Pramming S. Insulin pharmacokinetics. Diabetes Care 1984;7:188—199.
4. Auzepy Ph, Caquet R. Severe hypoglycemia due to insulin: adverse side-effects of antidiabetic drugs. Semin Hop 1983;59:697—705.
5. Seltzer HS. Severe drug-induced hypoglycemia: a review (official publication, American Society of Contemporary Medicine and Surgery). Compr Ther 1979;5:21—29.
6. Gold AE, Deary IJ, Frier BM. Recurrent severe hypoglycaemia and cognitive function in type I diabetes. Diabetic Med 1993;10:503—508.
7. DCCT research group. The effect of intensive treatment of diabetes in the development of long-term complications in insulin-dependent diabetes mellitus. N Engl J Med 1993;329:977—986.
8. Crofford OB. Diabetes Control and Complications. Annu Rev Med 1995;46:267—279.
9. Gale EAM, Tattersall RD. Unrecognised nocturnal hypoglycaemia in insulin-treated diabetics. Lancet 1979;i: 1049—1052.
10. Gerich JE, Mokam M, Veneman T Korytkowski M, Mitrakou A. Hypoglycemic unawareness. Endocrine Rev 1991;12:356—371.
11. Cryer PE. Hypoglycemic Unawareness in IDDM. Diabetes Care 1993;16(Suppl 3):40—47.
12. Hepburn DA, MacLeod KM, Frier BM. Physiological, symptomatic and hormonal responses to acute hypoglycaemia in type 1 diabetic patients with autonomic neuropathy. Diabetic Med 1993;10:940—949.
13. Colagiuri S, Miller JJ, Petocz P. Double-blind crossover comparison of human and porcine insulins in patients reporting lack of hypoglycaemia awareness. Lancet 1992;339:1432—1435.
14. Daneman D, Frank M, Perlman K, Tamm J, Ehrlich R. Severe hypoglycemia in children with insulin-dependent diabetes mellitus: frequency and predisposing factors. J Pediatr 1989;115:681—685.
15. Arem R, Zoghbi W. Insulin overdose in eight patients: insulin pharmacokinetics and review of the literature. Medicine 1985;64:323—332.
16. Clarke B, Ward JD, Enoch BA. Hypoglycaemia in insulin-dependent diabetic drivers. Br Med J 1980;281:586.
17. Torres Marti A, Font J, Cano F, Rodriguez de Castro L, Camp J, Borras A, Milla J. Epidemiologic study of hypoglycemic syndrome in an emergency unit: study of 71 cases. Med Clin 1981;77:405—409.
18. Kahn CR, Rosenthal AS. Immunologic reactions to insulin: insulin allergy, insulin resistance, and the autoimmune insulin syndrome. Diabetes Care 1979;2:283—295.
19. DeShazo RD, Boehm TM, Kumar D, Galloway JA, Dvorak HF. Dermal hypersensitivity reactions to insulin: correlations of three patterns to their histopathology. J Allergy Clin Immunol 1981;69:229—237.
20. Ross JM. Allergy to insulin. Pediatr Clin North Am 1984;31:675—687.
21. Kumar D. Insulin allergy: differences in the binding of porcine, bovine, and human insulins with anti-insulin IgE. Diabetes Care 1981;4:104—107.
22. Soto-Aguilar MC, deShazo RD, Morgan JE, Mather P, Ibrahim G, Frentz JM, Lauritano AA. Total IgG and IgG subclass specific antibody responses to insulin in diabetic patients. Ann Allergy 1991;67:499—503.
23. Jones GR, Statham B, Owens DR et al. Lipoatrophy and monocomponent porcine insulin. Br Med J 1981;282:190.
24. Silverstone P. Generalised allergic reaction to human insulin. Br Med J 1986;292:933—934.
25. Patterson R, Roberts M, Grammer LC. Insulin allergy: re-evaluation after two decades. Ann Allergy 1990;64:459—462.
26. Goerz G, Ruzicka T, Hofmann N, Drost H, Gruneklee D. Granulomatöse allergische Reaktion vom verzögerten Typ auf Surfen. Hautarzt 1981;32:187—190.
27. Feinglos MN, Jegasothy BV. 'Insulin' allergy due to zinc. Lancet 1979;i:122—124.

28. Bruni B, Barolo P, Gamba S, Grassig G, Blatto A. Case of generalized allergy due to zinc and protamine in insulin preparation. Diabetes Care 1986;9:552.
29. Gin H, Aubertin J. Generalized allergy due to zinc and protamine in insulin preparation treated with insulin pump. Diabetes Care 1987;10:789–790.
30. Diem P. Allergy to insulin. Br Med J 1980;281:1068–1069.
31. Elte JWF, Van der Schroeff JG, Van Leeuwen AWFM, Radder JK. Sclerosing granuloma after short-term administration of depot-insulin Hoechst. Klin Wochenschr 1982; 60:1461–1464.
32. Jordaan HF, Sandler M. Zinc-induced granuloma—a unique complication of insulin therapy. Clin Exp Dermatol 1989;14:227–229.
33. Dische FE, Wernstedt C, Westermark GT, Westermark P, Pepys MB, Rennie JA, Gilbey SG, Watkins PJ. Insulin as an amyloid-fibril protein at sites of repeated insulin injections in a diabetic patient. Diabetologia 1988;31:158–161.
34. Chantelau EA, Berger M. Pollution of insulin with silicone oil, a hazard of disposable plastic syringes. Lancet 1985;i:1459.
35. Lapière CM, Pierard GE, Hermanns JF, Lefebvre P. Unusual extensive granulomatosis after long-term use of plastic syringes for insulin injections. Dermatologica 1982;165:580–590.
36. Young RL, Steel JM, Frier BM, Duncan LJP. Insulin injection sites in diabetes—a neglected area? Br Med J 1981;283:349.
37. Shinozuka M, Hirose K, Guji M et al. Diabetic coma due to insulin resistance associated with insulin allergy: a case report. J Jpn Diabet Soc 1981;24:755.
38. Kurtz AB, Nabarro JDN. Circulating insulin-binding antibodies. Diabetologia 1980;19:329–334.
39. Valenta LJ, Elias AN. Insulin-induced lipodystrophy in diabetic patients resolved by treatment with human insulin. Ann Intern Med 1985;102:790–791.
40. Saule H. Insulin-induzierte ödeme bei Adoleszenten mit Diabetes mellitus Typ I. Dtsch Med Wochenschr 1991;116:1191–1194.
41. DeFronzo RA. The effect of insulin on renal sodium metabolism: a review with clinical implications. Diabetologia 1981;21:165–171.
42. Singhal PC, Abramovici M, Venkatesan J. Rhabdomyolysis in the Hyperosmolal State. Am J Med 1990;88:9–12.
43. Brogden RN, Heel RC. Human insulin, a review of its biological activity. Pharmacokinetics and therapeutic use. Drugs 1987;43:350.
44. Ganz MA, Unterman T, Roberts M, Uy R, Sahgal S, Samter M, Gammer LC. Resistance and allergy to recombinant human insulin. J Allergy Clin Immunol 1990;86:45–51.
45. Hildebrandt P, Berger A, Volund AA and Kühl C. The subcutaneous absorption of human and bovine ultra-lente insulin formulations. Diabetic Med 1985;2:355–359.
46. Benzi L, Marchetti P, Carriero PL et al. Long term therapy with biosynthetic human insulin: importance of short acting/intermediate acting insulin ratio on determining efficacy of treatment. Clin Drugs Exp 1987;13:321.
47. Teuscher A, Berger WG. Hypoglycaemia unawareness in diabetics transferred from beef/porcine insulin to human insulin. Lancet 1987;ii:382–385.
48. Klauser R, Schernthaner G, Prager R. Mixtures of human intermediate and human regular insulin in type I diabetic patients. Diabetes Res Clin Pract 1988;5:185–190.
49. Perriello G, Torlone E, Di Santo S, Fanelli C, DeFeo P, Santeusanio F, Brunetti P, Bolli GB. Effect of storage temperature of insulin on pharmacokinetics and pharmacodynamics of insulin mixtures injected subcutaneously in subjects with type I (insulin-dependent) diabetes mellitus. Diabetologia 1988;31:811–815.
50. Gizurarson S, Bechgaard E. Intranasal administration of insulin to humans. Diabetes Res Clin Pract 1991;12:71–84.
51. Laube BL, Georgopoulos A, Adams GK. Preliminary study of the efficacy of insulin aerosol delivered by oral inhalation in diabetic patients. J Am Med Assoc 1993; 269:2106–2109.
52. Fischer U. Fundamentals of glucose sensors. Diabetic Med 1991;8:309–321.
53. Mecklenburg RS, Benson EA, Benson JW Jr, Blumenstein BA, Fredlund PN, Guinn TS, Metz RJ, Nielsen RL. Long-term metabolic control with insulin pump therapy: report of experience with 127 patients. N Engl J Med 1985;313:465–468.
54. Mecklenburg RS, Guinn TS, Sannar CA, Blumenstein BA. Malfunction of continuous subcutaneous insulin infusion systems: a one-year prospective study of 127 patients. Diabetes Care 1986;9:351–355.
55. Chantelau E, Spraul M, Mühlhauser I, Gause R, Berger M. Long-term safety, efficacy and side-effects of continuous subcutaneous insulin infusion treatment for Type 1 (insulin-dependent) diabetes mellitus: a one centre experience. Diabetologia 1989;32:421–426.
56. Saudek CD. Implantable insulin pumps: a current look. Diabetes Res Clin Pract 1990;10:109–114.
57. Morton C. Nickel allergy: a complication of CSII. Pract Diabetes 1990;7:179.
58. Chantelau E, Lange G, Sonnenberg GE, Berger M. Acute cutaneous complications and catheter needle colonization during insulin-pump treatment. Diabetes Care 1987; 10:478–482.
59. Fishman V, Fishman M. Practical problems with insulin pumps. N Engl J Med 1982;306:1369–1370.
60. Wredling R, Lin PE, Adamson U. Pump 'run-away' causing severe hypoglycaemia. Lancet 1989;ii:273.
61. Bousquet-Rouaud R, Castex F, Gostalat G, Bastide M, Hedon B, Bouanani M, Jouvert S, Mirouze J. Factors involved in catheter obstruction during long-term peritoneal insulin infusion. Diabetes Care 1993;16:801–805.
62. Levy RP, Borchelt MD, Kremer RM, Francis SJ, O'Connor CA. *Hemophilus influenzae* infection of an implantable insulin-pump pocket. Diabetes Care 1992; 15:1449–1450.
63. Hanas R, Ludvigsson J. Side effects and indwelling times of subcutaneous catheters for insulin injections. A new device for injecting insulin with a minimum of pain in the treatment of insulin-dependent diabetes mellitus. Diabetes Res Clin Pract 1990;10:73–83.
64. Käär MJ, Mälenpää J, Knip M. Insulin administration via a subcutaneous catheter, effects on absorption. Diabetes Care 1993;16:1412–1413.
65. Wredling R, Adamson U, Lins PE, Backman L, Lundgren D. Experience of long-term intraperitoneal insulin treatment using a new percutaneous acces device. Diabetic Med 1991;8:597–600.
66. Rosenlund EF, Haakens K, Brinchmann-Hansen O, Dahl-Jorgensen K, Hanssen KF. Transient proliferative diabetic retinopathy during intensified insulin treatment. Am J Ophthalmol 1988;105:618–625.

67. Hardy K, Gill G. Bubble ketoacidosis. Lancet 1988; i:1336—1337.
68. Vaag A, Handberg A, Lauritzen M, Hendriksen JE, Pedersen KD, Beck-Nielsen H. Variation on absorption of NPH insulin due to intramuscular injection. Diabetes Care 1990;13:74—76.
69. Chantelau E, Berger M, Böhlken B. Silicone oil released from disposable insulin syringes. Diabetes Care 1986;9:672—673.
70. Cordray JP, Merceron RE, Guillerd X, Nys P. Baisse du fer sérique due à l'auto-surveillance glycémique chez le diabétique. Presse Med 1991;20:310.
71. Cox NH, Dufton Pa. Pyoderma gangrenosum and fingertip ulceration in a diabetic patient. Pract Diabetes 1987; 4:236.
72. Namba M, Hanafusa T, Kono N, Tarui S and the GL-G Hypoglycemia Study Group. Clinical evaluation of biosynthetic glucagon treatment for recovery from hypoglycemia developed in diabetic patients. Diabetes Res Clin Pract 1993;19:133—138.
73. Edell SL. Erythema multiforme secondary to intravenous glucagon. Am J Roentgenol 1980;134:385—386.
74. Sulfonylurea Drugs: Basic and Clinical Considerations. Lebovitz HE, Melander A, eds. Diabetes Care 1990; 13(Suppl 3):1—59.
75. Nabarro JDN. Oral hypoglycaemic agents: the first thirty years. J R Coll Phys London 1992;26:50—55.
76. Berger W, Caduff F, Pasquel M, Rump A. Die relative Häufigkeit der schweren Sulfonylharnstoff-Hypoglykämie in den letzten 25 Jahren in der Schweiz. Schweiz Med Wochenschr 1986;116:145—151.
77. Asplund K, Wiholm B-E, Lithner F. Glibenclamide-associated hypoglycaemia: a report on 57 cases. Diabetologia 1983;24:412—417.
78. Samimi H, Loutan L, Balant L, Tilloles M, Fabre J. Métabolites des sulfonylurées hypoglycéniantes; intérêt clinique: expériences avec le glibenclamide chez le rat. Schweiz Med Wochenschr 1977;107:1291—1296.
79. Kennedy TD, Keat AC, Chester M et al. Predisposing factors in fatal glibenclamide induced hypoglycaemia. Pract Diabetes 1988;5:217.
80. Moore DF, Wood DF, Volans GN. Features, prevention and management of acute overdose due to antidiabetic drugs. Drug Safety 1993;9:218—229.
81. Boyle PJ, Justice K, Krentz AJ, Nagy RJ, Schade DS. Octreotide reverses hyperinsulinemia and prevents hypoglycemia induced by sulfonylurea overdoses. J Clin Endocrinol Metab 1993;76:752—756.
82. Gin H, Lars I, Morlat Ph, Beauvieux JM, Aubertin J. Hyponatrémie induite par les sulfamides hypoglycémiants. Ann Med Interne 1989;139:455—459.
83. Planas AT, Kranwinkel RN, Soletsky HB, Pezzimenti JF. Chlorpropamide-induced pure RBC aplasia. Arch Intern Med 1980;140:707—708.
84. Gill MJ, Ratliff DA, Harding LK. Hypoglycemic coma, jaundice, and pure RBC aplasia following chlorpropamide therapy. Arch Intern Med 1980;140:714—715.
85. Levitt LJ. Chlorpropamide-induced pure white cell aplasia. Blood J Am Soc Hematol 1987;69:394—400.
86. Saffouri B, Cho JH, Felber N. Chlorpropamide-induced haemolytic anaemia. Postgrad Med 1981;57:44—45.
87. Nataas OB, Nesthus I. Immune haemolytic anaemia induced by glibenclamide in selective IgA deficiency. Br Med J 1987;295:366—367.
88. Abbate S, Hoogwerf BJ. Hemolytic anemia associated with sulfonylurea use. Diabetes Care 1990;13:904—905.
89. Augustyniak W, Giermaziak H, Gebicki L. Haemorrhagic drug-induced thrombocytopenic purpura of allergic origin. Wiad Lek 1980;33:487—490.
90. Raisp J. Thrombocytopenic purpura in combined oral therapy of diabetes. Diab Croat 1974;3:41.
91. Gundersen K, Molony BA, Crim JA et al. Micronase (glyburide): clinical overview. In: Rifkin H, ed. Micronase: Pharmacological and Clinical Evaluation. Amsterdam: Excerpta Medica, 1975:254.
92. Väätainen N, Fräki JE, Hyvönen M, Neittaanmaki H. Purpura with a linear epidermo-dermal deposition of IgA. Acta Dermatol-Venereol 1983;63:169—170.
93. Ingelmo M, Vivancos J, Bruguera M, Sierra J, Balcells A. Hypersensitivity vasculitis and granulomatous hepatitis induced by glybenclamide: a case report. Med Clin (Barcelona) 1980;75:306—308.
94. Schneider HL, Hornback KD, Kniaz JL, Efrusy ME. Chlorpropamide hepatotoxicity: report of a case and review of the literature. Am J Gastroenterol 1984;79:721—724.
95. Rumboldt Z, Bota B. Favorable effects of glibenclamide in patient exhibiting idiosyncratic hepatotoxic reactions to both chlorpropamide and tolbutamide. Acta Diabetol Lat 1984;21:387—391.
96. De Rosa G, Corsello SM, Pizzi C et al. Epatopatia citolitica amitterica da glibenclamide. Epatologia 1980;26:73.
97. Wongpaitoon V, Mills PR, Russell RI, Patrick RS. Intrahepatic cholestatic and cutaneous bullae associated with glibenclamide therapy. Postgrad Med J 1981;57:244—246.
98. Lambert M, Geubel A, Rahier J, Branquinho F. Cholestatic hepatitis associated with glibenclamide therapy. Eur J Gastroenterol Hepatol 1990;2:389—391.
99. Rank JM, Olson RC. Reversible cholestatic hepatitis caused by acetohexamide. Gastroenterology 1988;96:1607—1608.
100. Frier BM, Steward WK. Cholestatic jaundice following chlorpropamide selfpoisoning. Clin Toxicol 1977;11:13—17.
101. Nakao NL, Gelb AM, Stenger RJ, Siegel JH. A case of chronic liver disease due to tolazamide. Gastroenterology 1985;89:192—195.
102. Goodman RC, Dean PJ, Radparvar A, Kitabchi AE. Glyburide-induced hepatitis. Ann Intern Med 1987; 106:837—839.
103. Tavani E, Giardini R. Alterazione istopatologiche delle isole di Langerhans in un caso di diabete trattato con sulfaniluree. Pathologica 1978;70:105—108.
104. Roblin X, Abnader Y, Baziz A. Pancréatite aigue sous gliclazide. Gastroenterol Clin Biol 1992;16:96.
105. Appel GB, D'Agati V, Bergman M, Pirani CL. Nephrotic syndrome and immune complex glomerulonephritis associated with chlorpropamide therapy. Am J Med 1983;74:337—342.
106. Kar PK, Das Gupta SK, Das KD. Tolbutamide photosensitivity. J Indian Med Assoc 1984;82:289—291.
107. Kang JS, Kim TH. A case of Chlorpropamide induced photo sensitivity. Korean J Dermatol 1993;31:788—791.
108. Salazar JJ, León-Quintero GI, Arenas R. Dermatosis por medicamentos. Relación de 169 casos revisados en 3 años. Dermatol Rev Mex 1993;37:240—242.
109. Barnett JH, Barnett SM. Lichenoid drug reactions to chlorpropamide and tolazamide. Cutis 1984;34:542—544.
110. Feinglos MN, Lebovitz HE. Long-term safety and efficacy of glipizide. Am J Med 1983;75:60—66.

111. Ahmad S. Pulmonary infiltration eosinophilia with chlorpropamide therapy. South Med J 1984;77:1615.
112. Bell RJM. Pulmonary infiltration with eosinophils caused by chlorpropamide. Lancet 1964;i:1249.
113. Bondi E, Slater S. Tolazamide-induced chronic eosinophilic pneumonia. Chest 1981;86:652.
114. Ludwig A. Akzidentelle Hypoglykämie durch Inhalation von Sulfonylharnstoffstaub. Arbeitsmed Sozialmed Praventivmed 1991;26:31–32.
115. Watson WAF, Petrie JC, Galloway DB, Bullock I, Gilbert JC. In vivo cytogenetic activity of sulphonylurea drugs in man. Mutat Res 1976;38:71–80.
116. Piacquadio K, Hollingsworth DR, Murphy H. Effects of in-utero exposure to oral hypoglycaemic drugs. Lancet 1991;338:866–869.
117. Berger W. Orale Antidiabetika: eine Standort-Bestimmung. Z Allg Med 1978;54:513–524.
118. Ansaldi E, Gilardi GB. Chlorpropamide and cleft palate. J Foetal Med 1984;4:50.
119. Uhrig JD, Hurley RM. Chlorpropamide in pregnancy and transient neonatal diabetes insipidus. Can Med Assoc J 1983;128:368, 370–371.
120. Hirokawa CA, Gray DR. Chlorpropamide-induced hyponatremia in the veteran population. Ann Pharmacother 1992;26:1243–1244.
121. Schöffling K. Möglichkeiten un Risiken der Behandlung des Zuckerkranken mit oralen Antidiabetika. Therapiewoche 1979;29:5024.
122. Hirokawa CA, Gray DR. Chlorpropamide-induced hyponatremia in the veteran population. Ann Pharmacother 1992;26:1243–1244.
123. Sloan RW, Kreider RM, Luderer JR. The effect of chlorpropamide hyponatremia on mental status in a nursing home population. J Fam Pract 1983;16:937–942.
124. Wolfsthal SD, Wiser TH. Chlorpropamide and an antabuse-like reaction. Ann Intern Med 1985;103:158.
125. Palmer KJ, Brogden RN. Gliclazide. An update of its pharmacological properties and therapeutic efficacy in non-insulin-dependent diabetes mellitus. Drugs 1993;46:92–125.
126. Tabatabai S, Grossmann D. Diabetestherapie mit Glibenclamid. Med Welt 1985;36:123.
127. Van Basten JP, Van Hoek B, Zeijen R, Stockbrugger R. Glyburide-induced cholestatic hepatitis and liver failure. Case-report and review of the literature. Neth J Med 1992;40:305–307.
128. Lebovitz HE. Glipizide: a second-generation sulfonylurea hypoglycemic agent. Pharmacotherapy 1985;5:63–77.
129. Vigneri R, Goldfine ID. Role of metformin in treatment of diabetes mellitus. Diabetes Care 1987;10:118–122.
130. Seufert CD. Lactacidose. Med Klin 1979;74:850–857.
131. Cohen RD, Woods HF. Lactic acidosis revisited. Diabetes 1983;32:181–191.
132. Berger W. Zur Problematik der Biguanidbehandlung. Pharma-Kritik (Bern) 1979;1:9.
133. Hermann LS, Magnusson S, Möller B, Casey C, Tucker GT, Woods HF. Lactic acidosis during metformin treatment in an elderly diabetic patient with impaired renal function. Acta Med Scand 1981;209:519–520.
134. Hermann LS. Metformin: a review of its pharmacological properties and therapeutic use. Diabete Metabol 1979; 5:233–245.
135. Tymms DJ, Leatherdale PA. Lactic acidosis due to metformin therapy in a low risk patient. Postgrad Med J 1988;64:230–231.
136. Bailey CJ. Biguanides and NIDDM. Diabetes Care 1992;15:755–772.
137. Adams JF, Clark JS, Ireland JT, Kesson CM, Watson WS. Malabsorption of vitamin B_{12} and intrinsic factor secretion during biguanide therapy. Diabetologia 1983;24:16–18.
138. Graeber GM, Marmor BM, Hendel RC, Gregg RO. Pancreatic and severe metabolic abnormalities due to phenformin therapy. Arch Surg 1976;111:1014–1016.
139. Florianello F, Gatti C, Marinoni M, Bagni CM. Gastrite emorragica da antidiabetici. Acta Chir Ital 1978;34:597.
140. Çubukçu A, Yilmaz MT, Satman I et al. Metformin kullanimina bağli bir akut hepatit vakasi (metformin-induced hepatitis). Tip Fak Mecm 1991;54:447–452.
141. Klapholz L, Leitersdorf E, Weinrauch L. Leucocytoclastic vasculitis and pneumonitis induced by metformin. Br Med J 1986;293:483.
142. Ohnhaus EE, Berger W, Duckert F, Oesch F. The influence of dimethylbiguanide on phenprocoumon elimination and its mode of action. Klin Wochenschr 1983;61:851–858.
143. Gregorio F, Santeusanio F. Le biguanidi: aspetti farmacologici ed impiego clinico. G Ital Diabetol 1993;13:43–60.
144. Liebl A, Renner R, Hepp KD. Acarbose bei insulinbehandelten Diabetikern. Ein kritischer Überblick Akt Endokr 1993;14:42–47.
145. Johnston PS, Coniff RF, Hoogwerf BJ, Santiago JV, Pi-Sunyer FX, Krol A. Effects of the carbohydrase inhibitor miglitol in sulfonylurea-treated NIDDM patients. Diabetes Care 1994;17:20–29.
146. Clissold WR, Edwards C. Acarbose. A preliminary review of its pharmacodynamic and its pharmacokinetic properties and its therapeutic potential. Drugs 1988;35:214–243.
147. Kuzuya T, Iwamoto Y, Kosaka K, Takebe K, Yamanouchi T, Kasuga M, Kajinuma H, Akanuma Y, Yoshida S, Shigeta Y et al. A pilot clinical trial of a new oral hypoglycemic agent, CS-045, in patients with non-insulin dependent diabetes mellitus. Diabetes Res Clin Pract 1991;11:147–154.
148. Tsai SC, Burnakis TG. Aldose reductase inhibitors: an update. Ann pharmacother 1993;27:751–754.
149. Krans HMJ. Recent clinical experience with aldose reductase inhibitors. Diabetic Med 1993;10(Suppl 2):44S-48S.
150. MacLeod AF, Boulton AJM, Owens DR, Van Rooy P, Van Gerven JM, Macrury S, Scarpello JH, Segers O, Heller SR, Van der Veen EA. A multicentre trial of the aldose reductase inhibitor tolrestat in patients with symptomatic diabetic peripheral neuropathy. Diabetes Metab 1992; 18:14–20.
151. Pitts NE, Gundersen K, Mehta DJ, Vreeland F, Shaw GL, Peterson MJ, Collier J. Aldose reductase inhibitors in clinical practice: preliminary studies on diabetic neuropathy and retinopathy. Drugs 1986;32(Suppl 2):30–35.
152. Chuang L-M, Jou T-S, Yang W-S, Wu HP, Huang SH, Tai TY, Lin BJ. Therapeutic effect of guar gum in patients with non-insulin-dependent diabetes mellitus. J Formosan Med Assoc 1992;91:15–19.

Meyler's Side Effects of Drugs, 13th Edition
M.N.G. Dukes, editor

SECTION EDITOR: C.B.M. TESTER-DALDERUP

L.G. Cleland and P. Coates

43.1 Miscellaneous hormones

Calcitonin

Calcitonin inhibits osteoclastic bone resorption, increases the urinary excretion of calcium and phosphate and decreases serum calcium. It is used in the treatment of disorders with increased bone turnover, in particular Paget's disease when this is associated with bone pain, osteolytic lesions or neural compression (1[CR]). Calcitonin is less effective than other therapeutic measures in the treatment of acute hypercalcemia (2[R]). Long-term administration of calcitonin may be beneficial in cases of osteogenesis imperfecta (3[C]) and algoneurodystrophy. Pharmacological doses of calcitonin have also been used to prevent bone loss in high turnover osteoporosis. When used continuously at high doses, its therapeutic effect is sustained for only a few months; this may be due to down-regulation of osteoclast receptors, and the duration of the response to calcitonin can be extended by periodically interrupting the treatment. A number of different regimes, ranging from cycles of a few days to several months, have been found to be effective in both normal postmenopausal women and in established osteoporosis (4[R], 5[C]). However, there has been no reduction in fracture risk with this treatment (6[R]). No information appears to be available about any possible relationship between calcitonin treatment, physical activity and the fracture risk. Calcitonin also has a potent analgesic effect independent of its effect on bone, possibly mediated through the endogenous opioid system (7[R]). It appears to be more effective when given intranasally than parenterally for this indication.

Salmon and eel calcitonin are the most potent varieties, but human and pork calcitonins are also used. Both the parenteral (subcutaneous) and intranasal routes of administration may be used, although the latter requires an increased dose. Antibodies against calcitonin are frequently found after prolonged treatment, more commonly with salmon (30–69%) or eel calcitonin than with the human hormone. These do not usually affect the clinical activity of calcitonin, and have not been reported to cause any harmful effect to the patient. Antibody-mediated resistance is exceptional. However, neutralizing antisalmon calcitonin antibodies have been found after previous exposure to subcutaneous or intramuscular calcitonin.

The side effects of calcitonin, although common, are usually mild, and their incidence can be reduced by using the nasal or the subcutaneous rather than the intramuscular route. There are no studies which compare the incidence of side effects in calcitonin from different species. Side effects primarily comprise vascular, gastrointestinal, local and allergic reactions. *Flushing* occurs shortly after administration in up to 20% of all patients, and lasts from a few minutes to up to an hour. Nausea is also common, but vomiting or diarrhea are rare. These effects usually subside if the drug is continued. Other less common effects, which tend to be unpleasant rather than serious are included in the overview in Table 1.

Parathyroid hormone and analogs

Synthetic human PTH has been used in diagnostic testing for hyperparathyroidism and pseudohypoparathyroidism: no adverse reactions have been reported with infusions of up to 60 mg (8[c], 9[c]). Although bone resorption increases if the hormone is given continuously or in high doses, it has an anabolic effect on bone when given intermittently (10[CR]). Synthetic parathyroid hormone fragments have therefore been used in the treatment of slow turnover osteoporosis. However, trabecular bone volume increases at the expense of cortical bone and the anabolic effect last for less than 12 months (11[C]). In a recent 12-month study of PTH(1–34) in osteoporotic patients when combined with estrogen cortical bone was protected and a short-term anabolic effect was evident (12[c]). Evaluation of PTH in osteoporosis continues (4[R]) and its use should still be considered experimental.

Human growth hormone (somatotrophin; hGH)

Deficiency of growth hormone is responsible for short stature in up to one in 5000 children. Growth hormone (hGH) extracted from human pituitaries was used to

Table 1. *Side effects of calcitonin*

Cardiovascular reactions
Vascular flushing
Sensation of warmth in the face or hands
Tingling in the extremities
Gastrointestinal
Nausea vomiting
Abdominal pain
Diarrhea
Metallic taste in the mouth
Urinary system
Increased frequency of micturition
Polyuria
Skin and appendages
Rash

treat hormone-deficient patients until several cases of the fatal neurological disorder *Creutzfeldt-Jakob disease* were reported, notably where the selection and extraction procedures had devoted insufficient attention to the elimination of possible slow viruses in the starting material. The infectious agent, a virus-like particle (prion) had probably contaminated several batches of hGH. The natural human product was therefore withdrawn from the market in most countries, but was rapidly replaced by biosynthetic hGH preparations. Mean growth velocity rates achieved using these agents are equal to those obtained earlier with the native hormone, even with early formulations which induced antibodies in up to 75% of patients. Antibody-induced resistance may be overcome by increasing the dosage or changing the formulation.

The usage, optimal timing and dosage of hGH therapy have been extensively studied (SEDA-14, 379; 13[R]). Continuous intravenous infusion and small frequent intravenous bolus injections are equally effective in raising the serum IGF-1 concentration in GH-deficient subjects. However, the same amount given in two divided doses produces a much smaller response. The duration of effective GH concentration may thus be more important than its pulsatility for biological activity. An evening injection of growth hormone is more effective, or at least associated with a more physiological profile, than the same injection given in the morning.

Additional indications include Turner's syndrome: in this condition, GH therapy increases the pretreatment growth rate by more than 2 cm per year in 50% of patients given 0.5 U/kg/week and in more than 80% receiving 1.0 U/kg/week. This occurs without accelerating bone age and a real height increase may therefore be expected. Addition of low dose ethinylestradiol does not further accelerate growth in these girls. Growth hormone is also used in children with chronic renal failure (14[C]) and in Noonan's syndrome (15[C]). It has not been adopted for routine use in children with constitutional short stature.

Growth hormone replacement therapy in GH-deficient adults remains experimental. There is a small increase in muscle and bone mass, with a similar reduction in fat mass and normalization of blood lipids. Patients also report an improvement in general well-being (16[R]). Growth hormone treatment has also been given to critically ill patients in the intensive care setting. To date, although there is a measurable reduction in nitrogen turnover, no fall in mortality and no improvement in recovery rate has been detected in patients so treated, and the therapy should still be considered experimental (17[R]).

Long-term treatment is associated with a low incidence of adverse effects (18[C]). *Thyroid dysfunction* is common, due to enhanced T4 to T3 conversion (19[C]). There is no increase in the incidence of diabetes mellitus (20[C]). 23 cases of *benign intracranial hypertension* (*pseudotumor cerebri*) have been reported since 1986. All were symptomatic and over half presented within 8 weeks of starting treatment. The condition resolved in all cases when the hormone was withdrawn (21[R]). A *slipped femoral capital epiphysis* has been reported, but this may have been related to the growth spurt itself rather than a direct toxic effect. In a recent study of 100 critically ill patients receiving hGH, 43 became hypercalcemic; in 10 subjects total calcium was higher than 3.12 mmol/l. Patients with poor renal function were at higher risk of hypercalcemia, probably due to reduced calcium clearance (22[c]).

Local irritation or *lipodystrophy* at the injection site have been described.

Systemic allergic reactions are rare, but may be overcome by desensitization (23[c]).

Eleven cases of *leukemia* were reported between 1959 and 1987 in children treated with growth hormone (SEDA-13, 388), although several of those in whom a causal link was possible had undergone cranial irradiation for a brain tumour. In a recent study, six cases of leukemia were identified in extended follow-up of 6284 hGH recipients (24[CR]). This represented a relative risk of 1.8 compared to a matched population. The greatest incidence was in patients with craniopharyngioma and in those patients who received radiotherapy (four patients in each group). It therefore remains unclear how much of the increased risk is due to growth hormone itself.

Growth hormone-releasing hormone (GHRH)

The hypothalamic peptide GHRH has been used to test hypophyseal growth hormone secretion in cases of suspected growth hormone deficiency or excess, and can be used in combination with other releasing factors. An intravenous bolus of 1 mg/kg synthetic GHRH increases growth hormone concentration above 5 mmol/l in most healthy subjects. Higher doses are no more effective. When using the intranasal or subcutaneous route, however, an increased dose is necessary. The response to GHRH also decreases markedly with age in both sexes. This test is not able to detect GH deficiency in a single procedure, and full endocrinological evaluation is necessary to substantiate the diagnosis. In prepubertal children, a single intravenous injection of 2 mg/kg was well tolerated, and peak growth hormone concentration at 120 min correlated well with area under the curve. A greater response may be obtained by priming patients with testosterone. GHRH at a dose of 5 mg/kg/day for 6 days beforehand also increased the predictive value of the test (25[c]), as did priming with octreotide 5 hours before GHRH testing (26[C]).

Prolonged pulsatile GHRH treatment (e.g. 1 mg/kg every 3 hours s.c. for 6 months followed by 2 mg/kg for a further 6 months) has been found to be well tolerated in a series of GH-deficient children. The acute growth hormone response to GHRH is usually a poor predictor of growth response in response to such treatment, but a marked improvement in mean growth rate can occur without serious adverse effects. This increase is no greater than with growth hormone therapy when given in this fashion.

Adverse effects are frequent but mild. Transient *facial skin flushing* was reported in 81 of 574 children undergoing GHRH testing, whereas a *sensation of thoracic constriction, pallor, transient taste sensations, headache, nausea, bradycardia or tachycardia and transient hypotension or hypertension* occurred in less than 2% of the patients. No alteration in either hepatic or renal function was observed in subjects after prolonged administration. Pre-existing *thyroid failure worsened* in one of these children.

Anti-GHRH antibodies may develop with prolonged treatment. These may be associated with a decreased growth rate, which is still correctable with GH therapy.

Growth hormone release-inhibiting hormone (somatostatin) and analogs

Somatostatin was first isolated from the hypothalamus, and was shown to inhibit growth hormone release. It has since been found in neuroendocrine cells in the gastrointestinal tract, particularly within the gastric antrum and the myenteric plexus as well as the D cells of the pancreatic islets. It is the major inhibitory peptide in the gut. The native hormone must be given as a continuous infusion, due to its very short half-life. Somatostatin has been studied in many syndromes of hormone excess, as has a synthetic analog with a prolonged duration of action of up to 12 hours (SMS-201-985, octreotide) and has been found to be effective and well tolerated. Other long-acting analogs are currently being developed. Octreotide is more potent than the native hormone. It is also more selective in its inhibition of growth hormone relative to insulin, when compared to somatostatin.

In acromegalic patients treated with octreotide, suppression of the growth hormone level to less than 5 mmol/l occurred in 42—80%. This was associated with improvement in clinical symptoms (soft tissue swelling, paresthesia, headache, weakness and excessive sweating). Shrinkage of the pituitary adenoma was observed in 19—37% overall and was dose related, as was the incidence of adverse reactions (27[CR]). Octreotide is usually given subcutaneously in three divided doses per day. Continuous subcutaneous infusion has been shown to give similar results with one third of the total daily dose, and may therefore lead to fewer side effects (28[CR]). Depot formulations of somatostatin analogs are currently under investigation.

The use of somatostatin and its analogs is well established in the management of gastroentero-pancreatic tumours, with a large series reporting benefit in up to 90% of patients with carcinoid syndrome, and up to 50% of patients with VIPoma, glucagonoma, gastrinoma or insulinoma (29[CR]). Experience with the rarer peptide-secreting tumours is limited.

Other indications include treatment of bleeding esophageal varices, for which octreotide is equipotent with vasopressin analogs (30[C]), and in the treatment of postvagotomy and postgastrectomy syndromes (31[C]). It has also been used in the management of TSH-secreting pituitary adenomas (32[C]), in countering the hypoglycemia of severe malaria (33[C]), and to reduce stool volume in intractable AIDS diarrhea (34[C], 35[R]). The side-effect profile does not appear to be affected by the immunosuppression of this last group. A growing application is in pancreatic surgery, where octreotide has been reported to reduce the incidence of postoperative pancreatic fistula (36[C]) and pancreatitis (37[R]).

Octreotide and related somatostatin analogs under development have been used as labeled probes for the identification of endocrine tumours (38[R], 39[R]) and in the investigation of Graves' ophthalmopathy (40[C]).

Transient gastrointestinal symptoms (*nausea, diarrhea, abdominal discomfort, loose stools*) are common during the first few days of treatment. The frequency (30—50%) is dose related and is similar in healthy volunteers, acromegalic patients and patients with gastrointestinal tumours (27[R]). Of more significance is the increased risk of cholelithiasis (6–18% in the long term), related to *decreased gall bladder contraction* (41[C]). Postprandial insulin secretion is reduced by both somatostatin and its analogs, and results in *impaired glucose tolerance* or in *diabetes mellitus* in some patients. In a recent study of 90 treated acromegalic subjects, glucose intolerance was demonstrated in 20% and diabetes in 28%. Conversely, however, 18% of this group who were diabetic at baseline became normoglycemic with treatment (42[C]). Fecal fat excretion is frequently increased, although *steatorrhea* develops only occasionally.

Rebound gallbladder hypermotility can occur on withdrawal of octreotide and can be associated with *biliary colic* or *pancreatitis* (43[C], 44[c]).

Vasopressin and analogs

Vasopressin is a hypothalamic octapeptide secreted from the neurohypophysis, with both antidiuretic and vasoconstrictor properties (45[R]). It has a very short blood half-time (about 10 min), necessitating continuous intravenous infusion or frequent nasal application. Its vasoconstrictive effects limit the use of the native hormone. Dose-related adverse effects reported include *cutaneous pallor*, *hypertension*, *arrhythmias*, *myocardial ischemia* or *infarction*. *Intestinal and peripheral vasoconstriction* may follow prolonged infusion, resulting in *gangrene of intestinal segments or of skin, fingers or limbs*. This has been fatal in several cases, and vasopressin infusion should be ceased if skin necrosis occurs (46[C]). Profound *hyponatremia* due to reduced free water clearance is a further predictable dose-related effect. This is a particular risk in patients who are unconscious, or who have disturbed thirst sensation. *Uterine and abdominal cramps*, *nausea* and an *urge to defecate* have also been reported. *Antibodies* to vasopressin have been documented by several authors. These were more commonly seen with crude 'pituitary snuff' preparations, and led mostly to *nasal irritation*.

The difficulties of administration and frequent adverse effects of vasopressin led to its replacement by DDAVP (1-amino-8-D-arginine vasopressin or desmopressin), a synthetic analog with a prolonged duration of action and antidiuretic properties, but little vasoconstrictor effect (47[R]). Complete cranial diabetes insipidus can usually be controlled with twice daily intranasal applications of 5–10 mg. It has also been used successfully in the treatment of enuresis due to a variety of causes, either alone or in combination with imipramine. *Hyponatremia* and *convulsions* have both been reported in this setting (48[c], 49[C], 50[R]).

Desmopressin also has hemostatic properties. It increases plasma concentrations of von Willebrand factor antigen, factor VIII and tissue plasminogen activator by 2–6-fold. There is a similar increase in platelet adhesiveness. DDAVP can therefore replace cryoprecipitate treatment in some patients with factor IX deficiency. It can also be used in the management of bleeding diatheses due to platelet dysfunction, for example in uremia or following aspirin treatment (51[R]). Triglycinelysine vasopressin (terlipressin), a precursor of vasopressin, is used in the treatment of bleeding esophageal varices. Although rebleeding is reduced, mortality does not fall with treatment (30[C]). *Hyponatremia*, *hypertension* and *headache* are increasingly reported with desmopressin. Other effects such as *flushing*, *sweating* and *abdominal* pain have been reported very infrequently. Careful control of water intake is usually sufficient to control problems due to overhydration (47[R]).

Hypersensitivity reactions can occur: *tachyphylaxis* (52[c]) and *thrombocytopenia* (53[c]) have developed in a few patients treated with DDAVP for hemophilia and von Willebrand disease. Increased platelet aggregation is the likely cause.

Oxytocin

Oxytocin is a hypothalamic nanopeptide which selectively stimulates the smooth muscle of the uterus and mammary glands. It is used in the induction or augmentation of labor. It is well tolerated and effective in a wide range of infusion rates and concentrations, although a higher dose is generally necessary for labor induction. Contraindications to its use include placenta or vasa previa, previous classical uterine incision, pelvic structural deformities and abnormal fetal lie. Large fetal size and high maternal parity may also be relative contraindications. Uterine contractions and fetal heart rate should be monitored during oxytocin administration (54[R], 55[R]). Prior non-classical cesarean delivery is not currently considered to preclude oxytocin therapy. A number of recent investigations found no significant increase in uterine complications or in fetal morbidity or mortality in women with a previous cesarean, although oxytocin-treated patients had a higher rate of failed trial of labor for reasons which are still unclear (56[R], 57[C], 58[C]). Oxytocin is structurally quite similar to vasopressin, and like the latter has water-retaining properties when used in pharmacological doses.

Severe *hyponatremia* and *convulsions* have been observed in newborns after administration of oxytocin and salt-poor fluids to the mother. Oxytocin-induced hemodilution of fetal blood may promote *hemolysis*, increasing the frequency of *neonatal physiological jaundice*.

The effect is not large, and its mechanism has not been determined (59[R]).

Acute water intoxication has produced maternal *cerebral edema* and *convulsions* in fewer than 50 cases in the literature. This effect was most frequent in women given high doses of the drug, in combination with salt-poor intravenous fluids. In rare cases this has been fatal. *Transient hypotension*, due to a direct effect of oxytocin on the vascular smooth muscle, has also been observed with large doses. *Uterine hyperstimulation*, with associated *fetal distress*, can occur, and oxytocin infusion should be halted in affected patients (54[R]). *Anaphylaxis* is also rare. A single case of oxytocin-induced *rupture of an unscarred uterus* during the second trimester has been reported.

Table 2. *Current and proposed applications of GnRH and its analogs*

Gonadotrophin-stimulating effects:

1. Diagnostic testing of pituitary-gonadal function
2. Induction or timing of ovulation (66[CR], 67[R], 68[R])
3. Induction of ovulation in polycystic ovarian syndrome (69[R])
4. Treatment of hypothalamic hypogonadal male infertility (70[R], 71[R])
5. Treatment of undescended testis (72[CR])

Gonadotrophin-inhibiting effects

1. Treatment of idiosexual precocious puberty (73[C])
2. Reversible female contraception
3. Reversible male contraception (74[c], 75[R])
4. Treatment of hormone-dependent cancers
   (a) Prostatic (77[R])
   (b) Breast (77[CR], 78[c])
5. Benign prostatic hyperplasia (SED-12, 1086)
6. Female hirsutism (79[R])
7. Endometriosis (80[R])
8. Premenstrual syndrome (81[R])
9. Uterine leiomyoma (82[R])
10. Catamenial epilepsy (83[C])

Thyrotrophin-releasing hormone (protirelin; TRH)

Thyrotrophin-releasing hormone is a widely distributed tripeptide. Prolactin and TSH release are stimulated by high local hypothalamic concentrations of TRH. TRH is also believed to have a role as a neurotransmitter in several other tissues, including other areas of the central nervous system, retina, pancreas and gastrointestinal tract. The synthetic peptide is principally used in dynamic tests of pituitary and hypothalamic function. Its use in the assessment of hyperthyroidism has been superseded by the advent of sensitive TSH assays (60[R]). It is generally given intravenously (200 mg bolus) as oral and intranasal absorption is erratic. However, the frequency of side effects is much reduced when these alternative routes are employed.

TRH and analogs have occasionally been used in the management of a variety of neurodegenerative disorders, including motor neuron disease, without evidence of sustained improvement. It has also been given in combination with antenatal glucocorticoid treatment, in an attempt to reduce the incidence of infant respiratory distress syndrome. However, the infants in the treated group had increased ventilation requirements and their mothers experienced increased nausea, lightheadedness and hypertension (61[C]). It should not, therefore, be given to pregnant patients.

The side effects of TRH are usually mild. These include *facial flushing*, *urinary urgency*, *vaginal sensations*, *nausea*, *chest pain* and *altered taste sensation* (62[c]). A transient *rise or fall in blood pressure* without serious outcome has been observed (63[c]). In very rare cases, transient *amaurosis* and *bronchospasm* have been reported. These were thought to be due to either vasopressor syncope or cardiac arrhythmia. *Orthostatic hypotension* may be more pronounced in the elderly; *loss of consciousness* or *convulsions* were seen in a few patients who received high doses (400 mg) of TRH intravenously. The most serious adverse event reported is *pituitary apoplexy* (pituitary hemorrhage or infarction, characterised by *severe headache*, *visual loss*, and often by *pituitary failure*, *hypotension* and *coma*). This complication has been described in 15 cases in the literature following pituitary function testing with TRH. Pituitary macroadenoma was present in all cases. Although insulin and GnRH were also used in these patients, TRH was considered to be the most likely agent responsible due to its vasoactive properties (64[cR]).

Gonadotrophin-releasing hormone (GnRH) and analogs

The hypothalamic releasing factor for both luteinizing hormone and follicle-stimulating hormone is a decapeptide, commonly used in tests of hypothalamic-pituitary-gonadal function. Several superagonist analogs have been synthesized, with varying durations of action, and these have recently been reviewed (65[R]). GnRH and its analogs initially stimulate the secretion of gonadotrophins. When given continuously by nasal or depot administration, down-regulation of hypophyseal receptors occurs, with a resultant antigonadotrophic effect. The number of therapeutic indications claimed for GnRH and analogs continues to increase (Table 2); not all have proved equally successful.

In females, the most frequent adverse effects are symptoms of *hypoestrogenism*, with *hot flushes* in almost all patients and, less frequently, *vaginal dryness*, *reduced libido*, *mood disturbance or depression*, *breast discomfort*, *initial headache* and *bleeding*. Severe flushing may be treated effectively with either clonidine (84[c]) or the dopamine receptor antagonist veralipride (85[c]). Ovarian hyperstimulation is less common than with gonadotrophin treatment in amenorrheic women (86[CR]). *Osteoporosis*, with trabecular bone being most affected, has been regularly observed in both sexes with chronic GnRH agonist treatment (87[c], 88[c]). Female patients, however, tend to be younger, and to have a longer period of treatment. They also have a lower average initial bone mass than males, and their fracture risk is therefore higher. Osteoporosis is reversible in premenopausal patients within 6 months of GnRH withdrawal, and is not considered to be an absolute contraindication (89[R]). Treatment for endometriosis should, however, be limited to 6 months because of the lack of proven preventive treatment for bone loss. Norethisterone (90[c]), etidronate (91[c]) and parathyroid hormone (92[c]) have been used in short-term trials to prevent osteoporosis in patients treated with GnRH. Estrogens had no protective effect (93[c]).

Pelvic pain has been reported in patients treated with gonadorelins for leiomyoma, and is associated with tumour shrinkage (94[c]). One hundred and four women treated with leuprorelin for 12 months showed an *increase in both total cholesterol and HDL cholesterol*, with no increase in the LDL:HDL ratio (95[C], 96[C]). *Fatigue*, *headache* and *depression* were reported in one study to be more common in patients taking an intranasal rather than a subcutaneous formulation (97[C]): this has yet to be confirmed.

Males also experience hypogonadal symptoms with prolonged GnRH administration, including hot flushes and *reduced libido*, although this is a therapeutic effect rather than a side effect. When used in the treatment of prostate cancer, an initial *tumor flare* occurs, unless an anti-androgen is given concurrently. This does not alter the overall prognosis, but is useful if neurological compression is threatened. *Acne* has developed in some men receiving GnRH treatment, when it is used for either its stimulating or inhibitory effects. When given as an infusion for treatment of male hypogonadism, mild *gynecomastia* occasionally occurs.

Corticotrophin-releasing hormone (CRH)

Synthetic human and ovine CRH are commonly used in provocation tests of the function of the hypothalamic-pituitary-adrenal axis. The CRH test is useful in the evaluation of patients with Cushing's disease, both as an intravenous bolus injection of 1–2 mg/kg (98[R]) and in petrosal sinus sampling (99[CR]), in which it improves the predictive value. CRH may also be used to assess patients with adrenal insufficiency (100[R]).

Side effects occur in almost 40% of patients (101[R]). They mainly comprise *flushing* or a feeling of warmth (30%), a sensation of *discomfort* (5%), *palpitations* (3%) and *dyspnea* (1%), with a dose of 1 mg/kg body weight. Higher doses (more than 200 mg) may cause *hypotension* or *coronary ischemia*. Patients with brain injury may be more prone to adverse reactions (101[R]). No serious allergic reactions have been reported.

REFERENCES

1. Singer FR. Clinical efficacy of salmon calcitonin in Paget's disease of bone. Calcif. Tissue Int 1991;9(Suppl 2):S7.
2. Hall TG, Schaiff RAB. Update on the medical treatment of hypercalcemia of malignancy. Clin Pharm 1993;12:117.
3. Nishi Y, Hamamoto K, Kajiyama M et al. Effect of long-term calcitonin therapy by injection and nasal spray on the incidence of fractures in osteogenesis imperfecta. J Pediatr 1992;121:477.
4. Gennari C, Nuti R, Agnusdei D, Camporeale A, Martini G. Management of osteoporosis and Paget's disease. An appraisal of the risks and benefits of drug treatment. Drug Safety 1994;11:179.
5. Reginster JY, Meurmans L, Deroisy R et al. A 5-year controlled randomized study of prevention of postmenopausal trabecular bone loss with nasal salmon calcitonin and calcium. Eur J Clin Invest 1994;24:565.
6. Wallach S. Calcitonin treatment in osteoporosis. Drug Ther 1993;23:61.
7. Gennari C, Agnusdei D, Camporeale A. Use of calcitonin in the treatment of bone pain associated with osteoporosis. Calcif Tissue Int 1991;49(Suppl 2):S9.
8. Mallette LE. Synthetic human parathyroid 1–34 fragment for diagnostic testing. Ann Intern Med 1988;109:800.
9. Mallette LE, Kirland JL, Gagel RF, Law WM Jr. Synthetic human parathyroid hormone (1–34) for the study of pseudohypoparathroidism. J Clin Endocrinol Metab 1988; 67:964.
10. Dempster DW, Cosman F, Parisien W et al. Anabolic actions of parathyroid hormone on bone. Endocrine Rev 1993;14:690.
11. Neer R, Slovik D, Daly M et al. Treatment of postmenopausal osteoporosis with daily parathyroid hormone plus calcitriol. Osteoporosis Int 1990;Suppl 1:S204.
12. Reeve J, Arlot ME, Bradbeer et al. Human parathyroid peptide treatment of vertebral osteoporosis. Osteoporosis Int 1993;Suppl 3:S199.
13. Laron Z, Butenandt O. Optimum use of growth hormone in children. Drugs 1991;42:1.
14. Fine RN, Kohaut EC, Brown D, Perlman A. Growth after recombinant growth hormone treatment in children with chronic renal failure: report of a multicenter randomized double-blind placebo-cotrolled study. J Pediatr 1994;124:374.

15. Thomas BC, Stanhope R. Long-term treatment with growth hormone in Noonan's syndrome. Acta Pediatr 1993; 82:853.
16. Rosen T, Johansson G, Johansson JO, Bengtsson BA. Consequences of growth hormone deficiency in adults and the benefits and risks of recombinant human growth hormone treatment. A review paper. Horm Res 1995;43:93.
17. Riedel M, Brabant G, Riegen K, von zur Muhlen A. Growth hormone therapy in adults: rationales, results and perspectives. Exp Clin Endocrinol 1994;102:273.
18. Price DA, Clayton PE, Crowne EH, Roberts CR. Safety and efficacy of human growth hormone in girls with Turner Syndrome. Horm Res 1993;39(Suppl 2):44.
19. Grunfeld C, Sherman BM, Cavalieri RR. The acute effects of human growth hormone administration on thyroid function in normal men. J Clin Endocrinol Metab 1988; 67:1111.
20. Czernichow P, Albertsson-Wikland K, Tuvemo T, Gunnarsson R. Growth hormone treatment and diabetes: survey of the Kabi Pharmacia Internaional Growth Study. Acta Pediatr Scand 1991;37(Suppl):104.
21. Malozowski S, Tanner LA, Wysowski D, Fleming GA. Growth hormone, insulin-like growth factor 1, and benign intracranial hypertension. New Engl J Med 1993;329:665.
22. Knox JB, Demling RH, Wilmore DW et al. Hypercalcemia associated with the use of human growth hormone in an adult surgical intensive care unit. Arch Surg 1995;130:442.
23. Walker SB, Weiss ME, Tattoni DS. Systemic reaction to human growth hormone treated with acute desensitization. Pediatrics 1992;90:108.
24. Fradkin JE, Mills JL, Schonberger LB et al. Risk of leukemia after treatment with pituitary growth hormone. J Am Med Assoc 1993;270:2829.
25. Bueno G, Bueno M, Garagoni JM et al. Priming with GHRH (1—29) NH2: an aid in differential diagnosis between hypothalamic and pituitary deficiencies. J Pediatr Endocrinol 1994;7:309.
26. Dickerman Z, Guyda H, Tannenbaum GS. Pretreatment with somatostatin analog SMS 201-995 potentiates growth hormone (GH) responsiveness to GH-releasing factor in short children. J Clin Endocrinol Metab 1993;77:652.
27. Ezzat S, Snyder PJ, Young WF et al. Octreotide treatment of acromegaly. A randomized, multicenter study. Ann Intern Med 1992;117:711.
28. Christensen SE, Weeke J, Orskov A et al. Long-term efficacy and tolerability of octreotide treatment in acromegaly. Metabolism 1992;41:44.
29. Trautmann ME, Neuhaus CH, Lenze H et al. The role of somatostatin analogs in the treatment of endocrine gastrointestinal tumours. Horm Metab Res 1993;27(Suppl):24.
30. Walker S, Kreichgauer HP, Bode JC. Terlipressin vs somatostatin in bleeding esophageal varices: a controlled, double-blind study. Hepatology 1992;15:1023.
31. Mackie CR, Jenkins SA, Hartley MN. Treatment of severe postvagotomy/postgastrectomy symptoms with the somatostatin analod octreotide. Br J Surg 1991;78:1338.
32. Chanson P, Warnet A. Treatment of thyroid-stimulating hormone-secreting adenomas with octreotide. Metabolism 1992;41:62.
33. Phillips RE, Looareesuwan S, Molyneux ME et al. Hypoglycaemia and couterregulatory hormone responses in severe falciparum malaria: treatment with Sandostatin. Q J Med 1993;86:233.
34. Garcia-Compean D, Ramos-Jiminez J, Guzman de la Garza F et al. Octreotide therapy in AIDS-related, refractory diarrhea: results of a multicentre Canadian-European study. AIDS 1994;8:1563.
35. Farthing MJ. Octreotide in the treatment of refractory diarrhoea and intestinal fistulae. Gut 1994;35(Suppl 3):S5.
36. Montorsi M, Zago M, Mosca F et al. Efficacy of octreotide in the prevention of pancreatic fistula after elective pancreatic resections: a prospective, controlled, randomized clinical trial. Surgery 1995;117:26.
37. Maton PM. Expanding uses of octreotide. Baillieres Clin Gastroenterol 1994;8:321.
38. Lamberts SWJ, Hofland LJ, De Herder WW et al. Octreotide and related somatostatin analogs in the diagnosis and treatment of pituitary disease and somatostatin scintigraphy. Front Neuroendocrinol 1993;14:27.
39. Fahlbusch R, Giovanelli M, Buchfelder M, Losa M. Advances in the medical and surgical treatment of pituitary adenomas: the role of long-acting somatostatin analogs. J Endocrinol Invest 1993;16:449.
40. Kahaly G, Diaz M, Hahn K et al. Indium-111 pentetreotide scintigraphy in Graves' ophthalmopathy. J Nucl Med 1995;36:550.
41. Eastman RC, Arakaki RF, Shawker T et al. A prospective examination of octreotide-induced gall-bladder changes in acromegaly. Clin Endocrinol 1992;36:265.
42. Koop BL, Harris AG, Ezzat S. Effect of octreotide on glucose tolerance in acromegaly. Eur J Endocrinol 1994; 130:58.
43. Rhodes M, James RA, Bird M et al. Gallbladder function in acromegalic patients taking long-term octreotide: evidence of rebound hypermotility on cessation of treatment. Scand J Gastroenterol 1992;27:115.
44. Sadoul JL, Benchimol D, Thyss A et al. Acute pancreatitis following octreotide withdrawal. Am J Med 1991;90:763.
45. Cross BA, Leng G. The neurohypophysis: Structure, function and control. Prog Brain Res 1983;60:1.
46. Moreno-Sanchez D, Casis B, Martin A et al. Rhabdomyolysis and cutaneous necrosis following intravenous vasopressin infusion. Gastroenterology 1991;101:529.
47. Seckl JR, Dunger DB. Diabetes insipidus. Current treatment recommendations. Drugs 1992;44:216.
48. Hamed M, Mitchell H, Clow DJ. Hyponatremic convulsion associated with desmopressin and imipramine treatment. Br Med J 1993;306:1169.
49. Eckford SD, Swami KS, Jackson SR, Abrams PH. Desmopressin in the treatment of nocturia and enuresis in patients with multiple sclerosis. Br J Urol 1994;74:733.
50. Robson WL, Leung AK. Side effects and complications of treatment with desmopressin for enuresis. J Natl Med Assoc 1994;86:775.
51. Lethagen S. Desmopressin (DDAVP) and hemostasis. Ann Hematol 1994;69:173.
52. Mannucci PM, Bettega D, Cattaneo M. Patterns of development of tachyphylaxis in patients with haemophilia and von Willebrand disease after repeated doses of desmopressin (DDAVP). Br J Haematol 1992;82:87.
53. Castaman G, Rodeghiero F, Lattuada A, Mannucci PM. Desmopressin-induced thrombocytopenia in type I platelet discordant von Willebrand disease. Am J Hematol 1993;43:5.
54. Owen J, Hauth JC. Oxytocin for the induction or augmentation of labour. Clin Obstet Gynaecol 1992;35:464.

55. ACOG Technical Bulletin Number 157. Int J Obstet (July) 1991;39:139.
56. Rosen MG, Dickinson JC, Weshoff CL. Vaginal birth after cesarean: A meta-analysis of morbidity and mortality. Obstet Gynecol 1991;77:465.
57. Chelmow D, Laros RK Jr. Maternal and neonatal outcomes after oxytocin augmentation in patients undergoing a trial of labor after prior cesarean delivery. Obstet Gynecol 1992;80:966.
58. Sakala EP, Kaye S, Murray RD, Munson LJ. Oxytocin use after previous cesarean: why a higher rate of failed labor trial? Obstet Gynecol 1990;75:356.
59. Friedman L, Lewis PJ, Clifton P, Bulpitt CJ. Factors influencing the incidence of neonatal jaundice. Br Med J 1978;1:1235.
60. Surks MI et al. American Thyroid Association guidelines for use of laboratory tests in thyroid disorders. J Am Med Assoc 1990;263:1529.
61. Australian collaborative trial of antenatal thyrotropin-releasing hormone (ACTOBAT) for prevention of neonatal respiratory disease. Lancet 1995;345:877.
62. Dolva LO, Riddervold F, Thorsen RK. Side effects of thyrotropin releasing hormone. Br Med J 1983;287:532.
63. Aikibi M, Shirakawa Y, Komatsu H et al. Hypotensive and bradycardic responses to thyrotropin-releasing hormone in a comatose patient. Clin Neuropharmacol 1992;15:236.
64. Masago A, Ueda Y, Kanai H et al. Pituitary apoplexy after pituitary function test: a report of two cases and review of the literature. Surg Neurol 1995;43:158.
65. Filicori M. Gonadotrophin-releasing hormone agonists. A guide to use and selection. Drugs 1994;48:41.
66. Filicori M, Flamigni C, Dellai P et al. Treatment of anovulation with pulsatile gonadotropin-releasing hormone: prognostic factors and clinical results in 600 cycles. J Cln Endocrinol Metab 1994;79:1215.
67. Martin K, Santoro N, Hall J et al. Management of ovulatory disorders with pulsatile gonadotropin-releasing hormone. J Cln Endocrinol Metab 1990;71:1081A.
68. Carr JS, Reid RL. Ovulation induction with gonadotropin-releasing hormone (GnRH). Semin Reprod Endocrinol 1990;8:174.
69. Barnes RB, Rosenfield RL, Burstein S et al. Pituitary-ovarian responses to nafarelin testing in the polycystic ovary syndrome. New Engl J Med 1989;320:559.
70. Clayton RN. Gonadotropin releasing hormone: from physiology to pharmacology. Clin Endocrinol 1987;26:361.
71. Matsumoto AM. Hormonal therapy of male hypogonadism. Endocrinol Metab Clin North Am 1994;23:857.
72. Olsen LH, Genster HG, Mosegaard A et al. Management of the non-descended testis: doubtful value of lutenizing-hormone-releasing hormone (LHRH). A double-blind placebo-controlled multicentre study. Int J Androl 1992; 15:135.
73. Swaenepoel C, Chaussin JL, Roger M. Long-term results of long-acting lutenizing-hormone-releasing hormone agonist in central precocious puberty. Horm Res 1991;36:126.
74. Tom L, Bhasin S, Salameh W et al. Induction of azoospermia in normal men with combined Nal-Glu gonadotropin-releasing hormone agonist and testosterone enanthate. J Clin Endocrinol Metab 1992;75:476.
75. Cummings DE, Bremner WJ. Prospects for new male hormonal contraceptives. Endocrinol Metab Clin North Am 1994;23:857.
76. Plosker GL, Brogden RN. Leuprorelin. A review of its pharmacology and therapeutic use in prostatic cancer, endometriosis and other sex hormone-related disorders. Drugs 1994;48:930.
77. Blamey RW, Jonat W, Kaufman M et al. Goserelin depot in the treatment of premenopausal advanced breast cancer. Eur J Cancer 1992;28A:810.
78. Lopez M, Natali M, Di Lauro L et al. Combined treatment with buserelin and cyproterone acetate in metastatic male breast cancer. Cancer 1993;72:502.
79. Andreyko JL, Monroe SE, Jaffe RB. Treatment of hirsutism with a gonadotropin-releasing hormone agonist (nafarelin). J Cln Endocrinol Metab 1986;63:854.
80. Barbieri RL. Gonadotropin releasing hormone agonists: treatment of endometriosis. Clin Obstet Gynaecol 1993; 36:636.
81. Mortola JF. Applications of gonadotropin releasing hormone in the treatment of premenstrual syndrome. Clin Obstet Gynaecol 1993;36:753.
82. Nakamura Y, Yoshimura Y. Treatment of uterine leiomyomas in perimenopausal women with gonadotropin-releasing hormone agonists. Clin Obstet Gynaecol 1993; 36:660.
83. Bauer J, Wildt L, Flugel D, Stefan H. The effect of a synthetic GnRH analogue on catamenial epilepsy: a study in ten patients. J Neurol 1992;239:284.
84. Bressler LR, Murphy CM, Shevrin DH, Warren RF. Use of clonidine to treat hot flushes secondary to leuprolide or goserelin. Ann Pharmacother 1993;27:182.
85. Vercellini P, Vendola N, Colombo A et al. Veralipride for hot flushes during gonadotropin releasing hormone agonist treatment. Gynaecol Obstet Invest 1992;34:102.
86. Rizk B, Smitz J. Ovarian hyperstimulation syndrome after superovulation using GnRH agonists for IVF and related procedures. Hum Reprod 1992;7:320.
87. Goldray D, Weisman Y, Jaccard N, Merdler C. Decreased bone density in elderly men treated with the gonadotropin-releasing hormone agonist decapeptyl (D-Trp6-GnRH). J Clin Endocrinol Metab 1993;76:288.
88. Whitehouse RW, Adams JE, Bancroft K et al. The effects of nafarelin and danazol on vertebral trabecular bone mass in patients with endometriosis. Horm Res 1990;32:161.
89. Fogelman I. Gonadotropin releasing hormone agonists and the skeleton. Fertil Steril 1992;57:715.
90. Riis BJ, Christiansen C, Johansen JS, Jacobson J. Is it possible to prevent bone loss in youg women treated with lutenizing hormone-releasing agonists? J Clin Endocrinol Metab 1990;70:920.
91. Surrey ES, Fournet N, Voigt B, Judd HL. Effects of sodium etidronate in combination with low-dose norethindrone in patients administered a long-acting GnRH agonist: a preliminary report. Obstet Gynecol 1993;81:581.
92. Finkelstein JS, Klibanski A, Schaefer EH et al. Parathyroid hormone for the prevention of bone loss induced by estrogen deficiency. N Engl J Med 1994;331:1618.
93. Leather AT, Studd JWW, Watson NR, Holland EFN. The prevention of bone loss in young women treated with GnRH analogues with 'add-back' estrogen therapy. Obstet Gynecol 1993;81:104.
94. Chipato T, Healy DL, Vollenhoven B, Buckler HM. Pelvic pain complicating LHRH analogue treatment of fibroids. Aust New Zealand J Obstet Gynecol 1991;31:383.
95. Gerhard I, Schindler AE, Buhler K et al. Treatment of endometriosis with leuprorelin acetate depot: a German multicentre study. Clin Ther 1992;14(Suppl A):3.

96. Buhler K, Winkler U, Schindler AE. Influence on hormone levels, lipid metabolism and reversibility of endocrinological changes after leuprorelin acetate depot therapy. Clin Ther 1992;14(Suppl A):104.
97. Tapanaien J, Hovatta O, Juntunen K. Subcutaneous goserelin versus intranasal buserelin for pituitary down-regulation in patients undergoing IVF: A randomized comparative study. Hum Reprod 1993;8:2052.
98. Chrousos GP, Schulte HM, Oldfield EH et al. The corticotropin-releasing factor stimulation test: An aid in the evaluation of patients with Cushing's syndrome. N Engl J Med 1984;310:622.
99. Oldfield EH, Doppman JL, Nieman LK et al. Petrosal sinus sampling with and without corticotropin-releasing hormone for the differential diagnosis of Cushing's syndrome. N Engl J Med 1991;325:897.
100. Schlaghecke R, Kornley E, Santen RT, Ridderskamp P. The effect of long-term glucocorticoid therapy on pituitary-adrenal responsiveness to exogenous corticotropin-releasing hormone. N Engl J Med 1992;326:226.
101. Nink M, Krause U, Lehnert H, Beyer J. Safety and side effects of human and ovine corticotropin-releasing hormone administration in man. Klin Wochenschr 1991;69:185.

Meyler's Side Effects of Drugs, 13th Edition
M.N.G. Dukes, editor

SECTION EDITOR: C.B.M. TESTER-DALDERUP

C.L. Hill and L.G. Cleland

43.2 Prostaglandins

Prostaglandin E_2, prostaglandin $F_{2\alpha}$, prostaglandin I_2 and analogs

INTRODUCTION

Eicosanoids are the oxygenated metabolites of 20-carbon unsaturated fatty acids found in the phospholipids of cell membranes (Greek eicosa=20). The eicosanoids include the prostaglandins, thromboxanes and leukotrienes. Precursor fatty acids include arachidonic acid C20:4*n*-6 (for 2-series prostaglandins and thromboxane and 4-series leukotrienes), dihomogammalinolenic acid C20:3*n*-6 (for PGE_1) and eicosapentaenoic acid, C20:5*n*-3 (for 3-series prostaglandins and 5-series leukotrienes). Naturally occurring eicosanoids are predominantly metabolites of the arachadonic acid reflecting the dominance of *n*-6 fatty acids in the terrestrial food chain.

The principal biologically active, naturally occurring prostaglandins are prostaglandin E_2 (PGE_2), prostaglandin $F_{2\alpha}$ ($PGF_{2\alpha}$), prostacyclin (PGI_2) and thromboxane (TXA_2). These agents have various—sometimes opposed—biological actions ([1R]). Their half-life is short due to their rapid breakdown (a few minutes for PGE_2 and $PGF_{2\alpha}$, a few seconds for PGI_2) ([2R]). Prostaglandins thus have principally local biological actions. Analogs (mostly methyl derivatives) have been synthesized which are more slowly inactivated. The adverse reactions encountered when prostaglandins are used therapeutically will depend on the background indications (see Table 1), since these will determine the dose, route of administration and hence the type of reaction likely to occur. Many of the problems experienced are attributable to their main pharmacological effects (Table 2).

PROSTAGLANDINS IN OBSTETRICS

Prostaglandins of the E- and F-type are widely used in obstetrics for ripening the uterine cervix and stimulating uterine contraction at any stage of pregnancy. They are used in first- and second- trimester abortions, cervical priming, the induction and augmentation of labor, and postpartum hemorrhage ([3C], [4C], [5CR], [6CR], [7C]–[9C]). The route of administration can be vaginal, cervical, extra-amniotic, intra-amniotic, per-oral, intramuscular or intravenous, and varies according to indication.

A less established application involves intratubal injection of $PGF_{2\alpha}$ for ectopic pregnancy ([10CR], [11c]). Oral PGE_2 can be used to suppress lactation for which it is as effective as bromocriptine with less breast tenderness ([12c]).

ADVERSE REACTION PATTERN

General and toxic reactions The most prominent and frequent adverse effects of prostaglandins are those on the gastrointestinal tract. However, the most dangerous are likely to be the cardiovascular effects which in predisposed patients can sometimes cause life-threatening collapse and heart failure. Hyperthermia and headache are frequent CNS effects. Epileptiform convulsions rarely occur. When used for pregnancy termination, cases of uterine hyperstimulation and less frequently uterine rupture have been reported.

Hypersensitivity reactions Allergy to prostaglandins can cause skin reactions, bronchospasm (also seen as a direct pharmacological effect) and occasionally anaphylaxis.

Tumor-inducing effects These have not been reported.

Second-generation effects There are small number of infants reported with limb deformities with and without Möbius sequence when exposed to misoprostol (PGE analog) in the first trimester.

Table 1. *Possible indications for prostaglandin therapy*

In Obstetrics	
First- and second-trimester abortion	
Cervical reopening	
Induction of labor	
Augmentation of labor	
Postpartum hemorrhage	
Ectopic pregnancy	
Lactation suppression	
In cardiovascular disease	
Congenital cardiac malformation	
Raynaud's syndrome	
Chronic obstructive pulmonary disease	
Adult respiratory distress syndrome	
Pulmonary hypertension	
Arterial occlusion disease	
Extracorporeal circulation	
In gastrointestinal disease	
Peptic ulceration	
Liver transplantation	
Chemotherapy-induced mucosal lesions	
Other applications	
Urology	Peyronie's disease
	Erectile dysfunction
	Post-chemotherapy/radiation cystitis
Ophthalmology	Glaucoma

Table 2. *Pattern of action of prostaglandins*

Prostaglandin E-type predominant factors
Increase in hormone secretion
Growth hormone, adrenocorticotrophin, thyrotrophin, luteinizing hormone, thyroid hormone, insulin, glucocorticoids, progesterone, erythropoiten, renin
Increase in body temperature
Sensitization of pain-mediating nerve fibers
Increase in force of myocardial contraction
Increase in blood flow in gastric mucosa, liver, kidney and placenta
Increase in renal secretion of sodium, potassium and water
Antagonistic action against antidiuretic hormone
Increase in intraocular pressure
Increase in permeability of blood capillaries
Increase in gastrointestinal motility
Decrease in gastrointestinal secretion
Decrease in blood pressure
Bronchial dilatation
Inhibition of bronchial secretion
Sedation
Contraction of non-pregnant human uterus
Induction of abortion and labor
Prostaglandin F-type predominant effects
Bronchial constriction, especially in asthma patients
Decrease in pulmonary blood flow and increase in pulmonary blood pressure
Increase in erythropoietin secretion
Increase in neural transmission at sympathetic nerve endings
Increase in gastrointestinal motility
Decrease in blood pressure
Sedation (effects on the central nervous system)
Luteolytic effects in mammalian species (except in man)
Induction of abortion and labor
Prostaglandin I-type predominant effects
Decrease in platelet aggregation
Decrease in mean arterial pressure
Decrease in total peripheral and pulmonary resistance
Increase in heart rate
Increase in renal secretion of sodium (tubular effect)

ORGANS AND SYSTEMS

Cardiovascular Both PGE_2 and $PGF_{2\alpha}$ commonly cause a *fall in blood pressure* and a degree of *bradycardia* (1[R], 13[R]). PGE_2 can cause *vasodilatation* of small vessels whilst $PGF_{2\alpha}$ may cause *vasoconstriction* (14[R]). These changes are common but often mild. However, angina pectoris and myocardial infarction are increasingly being reported with prostaglandins of all types, particularly after inadvertent intramyometrial injection (15[C], 16[c]–18[c]). A single case of pulmonary edema after the infusion of PGE_1 has been reported (19[c]). In patients with pre-existing cardiovascular disease the risk of serious aggravation is very real, and both pre-existing hypertension and states of shock will be worsened. A severe *rise in blood pressure* occurred in a few cases in which fetal death was associated with unresolved pre-eclampsia.

Respiratory Asthmatics are more sensitive than normal subjects to *bronchoconstriction* induced by $PGF_{2\alpha}$ (20[CR], 21[C]).

Nervous system An *increase in body temperature*, *pyrexia* (both intra- and post-partum) and *chills* are thought to result from central stimulation of temperature regulatory centres (22[r], 23[c]). Headache and migraine are the most common side effects affecting the central nervous system (24[c], 25[r]). Prostaglandin can cause *EEG abnormalities* (26[C]). *Convulsions*, which occur occasionally, are a particular risk for epileptic patients (24[c], 25[r], 26[Cr]). The combination of prostaglandins and oxytocin can be complicated by grand mal-like seizures (27[C]). Enhancement of the pain sensation may reflect a direct effect on nerve fibers. The presence of pain correlates well with efficacy.

Gastrointestinal Gingivitis has been associated with obstetric prostaglandin use (25[r]). *Nausea*, *vomiting*, *diarrhea* and *abdominal pain* (28[R]) occur in about 90% of all patients when given prostaglandins systemically. The frequency and duration of these adverse effects depend on the mode of application, the dosage and the molecule used, and are very variable (29[R]).

Special senses An increase of *intraocular pressure* and *miosis* has been reported (24[r], 25[r]).

Effects on the fetus Prostaglandins have, like oxytocin, been responsible rarely for fetal distress and even fetal death (30[C], 31[C]). The risk of fetal fatalities underlines the importance of cardiotocography during prostaglandin (pre)induction. Prostaglandins should be used with extreme caution if there is a risk of placental insufficiency (31[C]). The incidence of neonatal jaundice was not increased after induction of labor with prostaglandins (32[C]).

Gonzalez et al. have described seven Brazilian infants with limb deficiency both with and without Möbius sequence who were exposed to misoprostol in the first trimester during unsuccessful abortion attempts (33[C]). There did not appear to be any particular time of relative vulnerability within the first trimester. A case of hydrocephalus and abnormal digits was reported earlier (SED-12, 1092). There is a paucity of reports on this subject.

Reproductive system Uterine hypertonia and hyperstimulation are well-recognized side-effects of induction of abortion and labor with prostaglandins. Cervical and uterine rupture have been reported with every prostaglandin and analog, even in previous unscarred uteri (25[R], 34[C]—39[C], 40[c], 41[c]). The risks can be minimized by using lower doses (0.5 mg intracervically or 3 mg intravaginally), allowing longer intervals between reapplications, and by avoiding combination with oxytocin, which has a potentiating effect. However, there is a single case report of uterine rupture in a multiparous woman with unscarred uterus following low-dose (1.5 mg) intravaginal PGE_2 application (42[c]). In the event of uterine hyperstimulation, β_2-adrenoceptor agonists may reduce uterine contractility. Intensive monitoring of uterine activity and fetal condition is mandatory since the rate of absorption of PGE_2 after intravaginal or cervical administration is unpredictable.

Methods of application in relation to side effects Intrauterine infusion (intra- or extra-amniotic) has been reported to be associated with fewer gastrointestinal symptoms and less fever than parenteral or intravaginal administration (43[C]). In intra-amniotic application the puncture must be guided by echography and before injection a control aspiration of some amniotic fluid is essential in order to minimize intrauterine or intravascular injection. Occurrence of uterine rupture has been described with intra-amniotic treatment.

Inflammation and pain are common at the site of injection when prostaglandins are given intramuscularly or intradermally (44[R], 45[R]). Prostaglandins have been used intravenously, both for induction mid-trimester abortion and for induction of labor in cases of intrauterine death. The same side effects as described above are found, and are usually very pronounced. Routine premedication with an antiemetic and an antidiarrheal agent significantly reduces gastrointestinal side effects.

Risk situations When PGE_2 and $PGF_{2\alpha}$ are used for the induction of labor and abortion, contraindications have to be respected which (until proven otherwise) also apply to the methyl analogs of these two prostaglandins.

Contraindications to the induction of labor are: *previous cesarean section* or *hysterotomy* (because of the risk of rupture) (35[CR]), *previous major abdominal surgery*, *prior abnormal delivery*, *a history of severe abdominal inflammation* and/or *infection*; pelvic deformities with obstruction of the birth canal; predisposition to *uterine cramps* or *tetanus uteri*. However uneventful vaginal deliveries have been reported in patients with two previous cesarean sections with labor induced with vaginal PGE_2 (46[c]). Women with a *history of six or more deliveries* and *anomalies of the fetus* (e.g. hydrocephalus causing cephalopelvic disproportion) must also be excluded.

Predispositions to *glaucoma*, *epilepsy*, *pre-eclampsia*, *hypertension*, *asthma* and *ischemic heart disease* are relative contraindications.

SYNTHETIC ANALOGS OF PGE_2 AND $PGF_{2\alpha}$

The use of synthetic analogs allows reduction of dosage and adverse effects. Sulprostone (16-phenoxy-ω-17,18,19,20-tetra-nor-PGE_2-methylsulfonylamide), gemeprost (16,16-dimethyl-*trans*^{2}-PGE_2-methylester), and (15*S*)-15-methyl-$PGF_{2\alpha}$ have been tested clinically and typically display fewer adverse effects than their naturally occurring counterparts, although this depends on the method of administration.

Seizures have been described during pregnancy termination induced by sulprostone (47[C]). Sulprostone has been associated with minor abnormalities of liver and kidney function (48[C]). Two myocardial infarctions (one fatal) have been reported in patients receiving sulprostone with mifepristone (49[c], 50[c]).

Vomiting was experienced by more than 90% of patients given (15*S*)-15-methyl-$PGF_{2\alpha}$ intramuscularly.

Vaginally applied gemeprost is effective in inducing first and second trimester abortion and in cervical priming before vacuum aspiration. Pyrexia, vomiting and diarrhea were experienced in 20% of patients (6[CR]).

Vaginally applied misoprostol (PGE_1 analog) is more effective and better tolerated than oral misoprostol for the induction of first trimester abortion following the administration of mifepristone (51[CR]). It appears more effective than both gemeprost or sulprostone combined with mifepristone for induction of first trimester abortion.

PROSTAGLANDINS IN CARDIOVASCULAR DISEASE

Maintenance of the ductus arteriosis

PGE_1 and PGE_2 are effective in maintaining the patency of the ductus arteriosus in the initial management of congenital cardiac malformations (52[CR], 53[CR]). The most frequent adverse effects during prolonged treatment are diarrhea, necrotizing enterocolitis, cortical hyperostosis (54[CR], 55[Cr]), fever, respiratory depression and apnea and seizure-like activity (56[CR]). The frequency of adverse effects may not necessarily be reduced with low dose intravenous or oral administration (57[CR]). Maternal/fetal hyperglycemia due to reduced insulin secretion is rare, except in the infants of diabetic mothers (58[c]). Less common side effects include gastric outlet obstruction due to antral hyperplasia (59[CR]).

Raynaud's phenomenon and digital ischemia

Studies of PGE_1 infusion for treatment of Raynaud's syndrome have had contradictory effects on frequency of attacks and of healing ischemic digital ulcers (60[Cr], 61[C]–63[C]). Prostacyclin infusion (using PGI_2 or its synthetic analog, iloprost) appear to have beneficial effects in both reducing the severity and frequency of attacks and healing of ischemic digital ulcers. Adverse effects are common and include headache, flushing, jaw pain, nausea, vomiting, diarrhea and inflammation and pain at the injection site (64[C], 65[C]). Iloprost has also been used effectively in the treatment of local gangrene secondary to chemotherapy (66[c]). Dermal application of PGE_2 analog results in both subjective and objective improvement in patients with Raynaud's syndrome and produced only minor self-limiting side effects of headache, flushing and diarrhea (67[C]).

Primary pulmonary hypertension

Initial studies of continuous intravenous prostacyclin infusion in patients with primary pulmonary hypertension have showed sustained improvement in pulmonary artery pressure, exercise capacity and survival compared with historical controls (68[CR], 69[C]). Minor complications (diarrhea, jaw pain, flushing, photosensitivity, headaches) were dose-related. Serious complications were related to problems with the drug delivery system including catheter thrombosis, sepsis and temporary interruption of infusion resulting in abrupt deterioration (68[CR]).

Regulation of pulmonary vascular perfusion in advanced respiratory disease

PGE_1 significantly reduces right ventricular pulmonary afterload in patients with pulmonary hypertension due to chronic obstructive airway disease (70[C]). It may also have utility in the treatment of adult respiratory distress syndrome (71[C]). Preliminary studies using aerosolized prostacyclin show a reduction of pulmonary artery pressure and improved arterial oxygenation with reduction in intrapulmonary shunt in ventilated patients with adult respiratory distress syndrome (72[c]) and severe community acquired pneumonia (73[C]). However, ventilated patients with severe community acquired pneumonia and pre-existing fibrosis required much higher doses with reduction in systemic vascular resistance and increase in intrapulmonary shunt (73[C]). A single report described improved oxygenation, mainly due to reduction of intrapulmonary shunting in two neonates with pulmonary hypertension treated with aerosolized prostacyclin (74[C]).

Miscellaneous applications of PGI_2

Prostacyclin infusions (using PGI_2 or its synthetic analog, iloprost) have been administered during extracorporeal circulation to prevent blood clotting in the dialyzer coil (75[CR]). The risk of severe hypotension can be avoided by carefully controlling the infusion rate.

Synthetic PGI_2 has been used in arterial occlusive disease as an anti-aggregatory drug (76[C]–80[C]). Side effects are common. Fever, nausea, anorexia, diarrhea, pain at the infusion site and arthralgia are the most prominent. A single study has suggested an increased risk of thromboembolism after the use of iloprost in peripheral vascular disease (81[c]).

New uses of PGI_2 include a suggested reduction of restenosis rate during transluminal coronary angioplasty (82[C]). Newer analogs (83[R]) and oral forms (84[c]) are in development.

PROSTAGLANDINS IN GASTROINTESTINAL DISEASE

Peptic ulceration and NSAID-induced gastropathy

Prostaglandins of the E-type (misoprostol, enprostil) have anti-ulcer activity in the upper gastrointestinal tract (85[CR]). They inhibit gastric acid secretion at modest doses, provide mucosal protection against noxious agents including non-steroidal anti-inflammatory drugs, smoking, alcohol and chemotherapy. They are the only agents proven to prevent NSAID-induced gastroduodenal lesions (86[CR], 87[C]). They may also be effective in prevention of NSAID-induced renal impairment (88[c]).

The cure rate for gastric and duodenal ulcers is comparable to the results with H_2-receptor antagonists (89—91). Relapses appear to be fewer with prostaglandin therapy. Healing of duodenal ulcers refractory to H_2-receptor antagonists has been described.

Diarrhea (between 4 and 38%), abdominal pain or cramp, flatulence and nausea or vomiting account for most of the side effects reported. No biochemical or hematological side effects have been noted.

These agents are contraindicated in women of childbearing age unless they are using adequate contraceptive measures due to uncertain abortifacient effects. They have been used as illegal abortifacients in some countries (33).

Liver failure and transplant dysfunction

Prostaglandins of the E-series (both intravenous and oral forms) have been used in treatment of fulminant hepatic failure, primary non-function following orthotopic liver transplantation and recurrent hepatitis B infection following orthotopic liver transplantation in open trials (92[C], 93[c], 94[Cr]). Adverse effects are almost universal. They include gastrointestinal symptoms (abdominal pain and cramping, watery diarrhea) affecting 33—100% which appear more common with oral formulations and possibly amongst those with elevated serum glucose. Cardiovascular effects which affect about 33% include migraine, hypotension, peripheral edema, and myocardial infarction (in those with preexisting risk factors). Painful clubbing and cortical hyperostosis (92—100%) developed 10—60 days after initiating intravenous or oral therapy. Arthritis/arthralgia developed in 8% of those receiving intravenous and 92% of those receiving oral PGE_1 or PGE_2. All adverse reactions appear to be dose-related and resolve with reduction in dose. Two patients also developed calcium oxalate stones after 1 year of oral therapy (95[CR]).

OTHER INVESTIGATED APPLICATIONS

Urology Prostacyclin infusion in men with persistent pain associated with Peyronie's disease was of little value but produced marked side effects (bradycardia, hypotension, nausea, flushing) (96[CR]).

A single dose of intracorporeally applied PGE_1 is most effective in inducing artificial penile erection in cases of erectile dysfunction. The reported side effects include pain and a burning sensation (75%) (97[CR]) and prolonged penile erection (12%) (98[C]). Burning and pain can be reduced by using a lower initial dose with incremental increases until a satisfactory erection is produced (99[C]). Prolonged erections induced by PGE_1 usually require drainage and phenylephrine irrigation, although a small percentage can be managed with oral terbutaline or oral pseudoephedrine if treated within 3 hours of PGE_1 injection (98[C]). A single case of Peyronie-like plaque and penile curvature deformity has been reported following repeated intracorporeal PGE_1 use (100[c]).

Massive diffuse hemorrhage due to cyclophosphamide-induced or radiation cystitis has been treated successfully with PGE_1, PGE_2, (15*S*)-15-methyl-$PGF_{2\alpha}$ and carboprost intravesically. Febrile reactions and severe bladder spasm are dose-dependent (101[C], 102[C], 103[Cr]).

Ophthalmology Topical PGE_2 and $PGF_{2\alpha}$ significantly reduce intraocular pressure for at least 24 hours and are useful for the treatment of glaucoma. The $PGF_{2\alpha}$-isopropyl ester ($PGF_{2\alpha}$-IE) derivatives appear to be most effective. Transient ocular adverse effects include conjuctival hyperemia, local irritation, intermittent photophobia and pain in the eye (104[C], 105[C]). Newer $PGF_{2\alpha}$-IE derivatives appear to be better tolerated with less severe and less frequent adverse effects (106[R]). The ocular pressure lowering effect of latanoprost appears to be additive with timolol, with mild transient hyperemia noted in 50% of those treated with latanoprost alone (107[C]).

REFERENCES

1. Dusting GJ, Moncada S, Vane JR. Prostaglandins, their intermediates and precursors: cardiovascular actions and regulatory roles in normal and abnormal circulatory systems. Prog Cardiovasc Dis 1979;21:405—430.
2. Nakano J. General pharmacology of prostaglandins. In: Cuthbert MF, ed. The Prostaglandins: Pharmacological and Therapeutic Advances. Philadelphia: JB Lippincott Co, 1973:23—124.
3. Hayashi RH, Castillo MS, Noah ML. Management of severe postpartum hemorrhage due to uterine atony using an analogue of prostaglandin F_2 Obstet Gynecol 1981;58:426.
4. Pulkkinen MO, Kajanoja P, Kivikoski A et al. Abortion with sulprostone, a prostaglandin E_2 derivative. Int J Gynaecol Obst 1980;18:40.
5. Robins J, Surrago E. Alternatives in midtrimester abortion induction. Obstet Gynecol 1980;56:716.

6. Thong KJ, Robertson AJ, Baird DT. A retrospective study of 932 second trimester terminations using gemeprost (16,16-dimethyl-*trans*-δ_2 PGE_1 methyl ester). Prostaglandins 1992;44:65—74.
7. Hill NCW, Selinger M, Ferguson J, MacKenzie IZ. Management of intra-uterine fetal death with vaginal administration of gemeprost or prostaglandin E_2: a random allocation controlled trial. J Obstet Gynaecol 1991;11:422—426.
8. Poulsen HK, Moller LK, Westergaard JG, Thomsen SG, Giersson RT, Armgrimsson R. Open randomized comparison of prostaglandin E_2 given by intracervical gel or vaginatory for preinduction cervical ripening and induction of labor. Acta Obstet Gynecol Scand 1991;70:549—553.
9. Jaschevatzky OE, Dascalu S, Noy Y, Rosenberg RP, Anderman S, Ballas S. Intrauterine $PGF_{2\alpha}$ infusion for termination of pregnancies with second trimester rupture of membranes. Obstet Gynaecol 1992;79:32—34.
10. Egarter CH, Husslein P. Treatment of tubal pregnancy by prostaglandins. Lancet 1988;i:1104.
11. Eckford S, Fox R. Intratubal injection of prostaglandin in ectopic pregnancy. Lancet 1993;342:803.
12. England MJ, Tjallinks A, Hofmeyr J et al. Suppression of lactation: a comparison of bromocriptine and prostaglandin E_2. J Reprod Med 1988;33:630.
13. Lee JB. Cardiovascular-renal effects of prostaglandins. Arch Intern Med 1974;133:56.
14. Olsson AG, Carlson LA. Clinical, haemodynamic and metabolic effects of intra-arterial infusions of prostaglandin E_2 in patients with peripheral vascular disease. In: Samuelsson B, Paoletti R, eds. Advances in Prostaglandin and Thromboxane Research. New York: Raven Press, 1976.
15. Bugiardini R, Galvani M, Ferrini D et al. Myocardial ischemia induced by prostacyclin and iloprost. Clin Pharmacol Ther 1985;38:101.
16. Fliers E, Duren DR, van Zwieten PA. A prostaglandin analogue as a probable cause of myocardial infarction in a young woman. Br Med J 1991;302:416.
17. Lennox CE, Martin J. Cardiac arrest following intramyometrial prostaglandin E_2. J Obstet Gynaecol 1991;11: 263—264.
18. Meyer WJ, Benton SL, Hoon TJ, Gauthier DW, Whiteman VE. Acute myocardial infarction associated with prostaglandin E_2. Am J Obstet Gynecol 1991;165:359—360.
19. White JL, Fleming NW, Burke TA, Katz NM, Moront MG, Kim YD. Pulmonary edema after PGE_1 infusion. J Cardiothor Anesth 1990;4:744—747.
20. Smith AP, Cuthbert MF. The response of normal and asthmatic subjects to prostaglandin E_2 and $F_{2\alpha}$ by different routes and their significance in asthma. In: Samuelsson ES, Paoletti R, eds. Advances in Prostaglandin and Thromboxane Research. New York: Raven Press, 1976:449.
21. Fishburne JI Jr, Brenner WE, Braaksma JT et al. Bronchospasm complicating intravenous prostaglandin $F_{2\alpha}$ for therapeutic abortion. Obstet Gynecol 1972;39:892.
22. Milton AS. Modern views on the pathogenesis of fever and the mode of action of antipyretic drugs. J Pharm Pharmacol 1976;28:393.
23. Callen PJ, De Louvois J, Hurley R, Trudinger BJ. Intrapartum and postpartum pyrexia and infection after induction with extra-amniotic prostaglandin E_2 in tylose. Br J Obstet Gynaecol 1980;87:513.
24. Haller U, Kubli R. Klinische Nebenwirkungen und Komplikationen der Prostaglandine bei Abortinduktion. Gynekologie 1978;11:39.
25. Karim SMM. Prostaglandin-physiological basis of practical applications. In: Proceedings, 6th Asia and Oceania Congress in Endocrinology, 1978.
26. Lyneham RC, McLeod JG, Low PA et al. Convulsions and EEG abnormalities after intra-amniotic prostaglandin $F_{2\alpha}$. Lancet 1973;ii:425.
27. Sedeberg-Olsen J, Olsen CE. Prostaglandin-oxytocin induction of mid-trimester abortion complicated by grand mal-like seizures. Acta Obstet Gynaecol Sand 1983;62:79.
28. Rachmilewitz D. Prostaglandins and diarrhoea. Dig Dis Sci 1980;25:897.
29. Kirton KT, Kimball FA, Porteus SE. Reproduction physiology:prostaglandin associated events. In: Samuelsson B, Paoletti R, eds. Advances in Prostaglandin and Thromboxane Research. New York: Raven Press, 1976.
30. Quinn MA, Murphy AJ. Fetal death following extra-amniotic prostaglandin gel. Br J Obstet Gynaecol 1981,88:650.
31. Beck I, Clayton JK. Hazards of prostaglandin pessaries in postmaturity. Lancet 1982;ii:161.
32. Lange PK, Sestergaard G, Secher J, Skogaard I. Neonatal jaundice after labour induced or stimulated by prostaglandin E_2 or oxytocin. Lancet 1982;i:992.
33. Gonzalez CH, Vargas FR, Perez ABA, Kim CA, Brunoni D, Marques-Dias MJ, Leone CR, Neto JC, Llerena JC, de Almeida JCC. Limb deficiency with or without Möbius Sequence in seven Brazilian children associated with misoprostol use in the first trimester of pregnancy. Am J Med Genetics 1993;47:59—64.
34. Cederqvist L, Birnbaum J. Rupture of the uterus after midtrimester prostaglandin abortion. J Reprod Med 1980; 3:136.
35. Bromham DR, Anderson RS. Uterine scar rupture in labour induced with vaginal prostaglandin E_2. Lancet 1980;ii:485.
36. El-Etriby EK. Rupture of the cervix during prostaglandin termination of pregnancy. Postgrad Med J 1981;57:265.
37. Sawyer MM, Lipshitz J, Anderson GD, Dilts PV. Third trimester uterine rupture associated with vaginal prostaglandin E_2. Am J Obstet Gynecol 1981;140:710.
38. Geirsson RT. Uterine rupture following induction of labour with prostaglandin E_2 pessaries, an oxytocin infusion and epidural analgesia. J Obstet Gynecol 1981;2:76.
39. Thavarasah AS, Siva Achanna K. Uterine rupture with the use of Cervagem (prostaglandin E_1) for induction of labour on account of intra-uterine death. Singapore Med J 1988;29:351.
40. Maymon R, Schulman A, Pomeranz M, Holtzinger M, Haimovich L, Bahary C. Uterine rupture at term pregnancy with the use of intracervical prostaglandin E_2 gel for induction of labor. Am J Obstet Gynecol 1991;165:368—370.
41. Maymon R, Haimovich L, Schulman A, Pomeranz M, Holtzinger M, Bahary C. Third-trimester uterine rupture after prostaglandin E_2 use for labor induction. J Reprod Med 1992;37:449—452.
42. Azem F, Jaffa A, Lessing JB, Peyser MR. Uterine rupture with the use of a low-dose vaginal PGE_2 tablet. Acta Obstet Gynecol Scand 1993;72:316—317.
43. Quinn MA, Shekleton PA, Wein R, Kloss M. Single dose extra-amniotic prostaglandin gel for midtrimester termination of pregnancy. Aust NZ J Obstet Gynaecol 1980;20:77.

44. Moncada S, Ferreira SH, Vane JR. Sensitization of pain receptors of dog knee joint by prostaglandins. In: Robinson HJ, Vane JR, eds. Prostaglandin Synthetase Inhibitors. New York: Raven Press, 1974:189.
45. Ferreira SH, Moncada S, Vane JR. Prostaglandins and signs and symptoms of inflammation. In: Robinson HJ, Vane JR, eds. Prostaglandin Synthetase Inhibitors. New York: Raven Press, 1974:175.
46. Chattopadhyay SK, Sherbeeni MM, Anokute CC. Planned vaginal delivery after two previous caesarean sections. Br J Obstet Gynaecol 1994;101:498–500.
47. Brandenburg H, Jahoda MGJ, Wladimiro H et al. Convulsions in epileptic women after administration of prostaglandin E_2 derivative. Lancet 1990;311:1138.
48. Ranjan V, Hingorani V, Kinra G. Evaluation of sulprostone for second trimester abortions and its effects on liver and kidney functions. Contraception 1982;25:175.
49. A death associated with mifeprostone/sulprostone. Lancet 1991;337:969–970.
50. Ulmann A, Silvestre L, Chemama L, Rezvani Y, Renault M, Aguillaume CJ, Baulieu E. Medical termination of early pregnancy with mifepristone (RU486) followed by a prostaglandin analogue. Acta Obstet Gynecol Scand 1992;71:278–283.
51. el Refaey H, Rajasekar D, Abdalla M, Calder L, Templeton A. Induction of abortion with mifepristone (RU486) and oral or vaginal misoprostol. N Engl J Med 1995;332:983–987.
52. Momma K, Takao A, Sone K, Tashiro M. Prostaglandin E_1 treatment of ductus-dependent infants with congenital heart disease. Int Angiol 1984;3:33.
53. Van der Sijp JRM, Rohmer J. Prostaglandinetherapie bij pasgeborenen met een ductus Botalli-afhankeliijke circulatie. Tijdschr Kindergeneeskd 1985;53:20.
54. Woo K, Emery J, Peabody J. Cortical Hyperostosis: A compication of prolonged prostaglandin infusion in infants awaiting cardiac transplantation. Pediatrics 1994;93:417–420.
55. Letts M, Pang E, Simons J. Prostaglandin-induced neonatal periostitis. J Pediat Orthop 1994;14:809–813.
56. Lewis AB, Freed MD, Heymans MA, Roehl SL, Kensey RC. Side effects of therapy with prostaglandin E_1 in infants with critical congenital heart disease. Circulation 1981; 64:893–898.
57. Singh GK, Fong LV, Salmon AP, Keeton BR. Study of low dosage prostaglandin—usages and complications Eur Heart J 1994;15:377–381.
58. Cohen MH, Nihill MR. Postoperative ketotic hyperglycemia during prostaglanding E_1 infusion in infancy. Pediatrics 1983;71:842.
59. Peled N, Dagan O, Babyn P, Silver MM, Barker G, Hellmann J, Scolnik D, Koren G. Gastric-outlet obstruction induced by prostaglandin therapy in neonates. New Engl J Med 1992;327:505–513.
60. Gryglewski RJ. Prostacyclin: pharmacology and clinical trials. Int Angiol 1984;3:89.
61. Kato K, Kawai T, Narita M, Uemura J, Tani K, Okubo T. Use of prostaglandin E_1 (lipo-PGE1) to treat Raynaud's phenomenon associated with connective tissue disease: thermographic and subjective assessment. J Pharm Pharmacol 1992;44:442–444.
62. Langevitz P, Buskila D, Lee P, Urowitz MB. Treatment of refractory ischaemic skin ulcers in patients with Raynaud's phenomenon with PGE_1 infusion. J Rheumatol 1989; 16:1433–1435.
63. Mohrland JS, Porter JM, Smith FA, Belch J, Simms MH. A multiclinic, placebo-controlled, double-blind study of prostaglandin E_1 in Raynaud's syndrome. Ann Rheum Dis 1985;44:754–760.
64. Wigley FM, Wise RA, Seibold JR, McCloskey DA, Kujala G, Medsger TA, Steen VD, Varga J, Jimenez S, Mayes M, Clements PJ, Weiner SR, Porter J, Ellman M, Wise C, Kaufman LD, Williams J, Dole W. Intravenous iloprost infusion in patients with Raynaud phenomenon secondary to systemic sclerosis. Ann Intern Med 1994;120:199–206.
65. Belch JJF, Drury JK, Capell H, Forbes CD, Newman P, McKenzie F, Leiberman P, Prentice CRM. Intermittent epoprostenol (prostacyclin) infusion in patients with Raynaud's syndrome Lancet 1983;i:313–315.
66. Vowden P, Wilkinson D, Kester RC. Treatment of digital ischaemia associated with chemotherapy using the prostacyclin analogue iloprost. Eur J Vasc Surg 1991;5:593–595.
67. Belch JJF, Shaw B, Sturrock RD, Madhok R, Leiberman P, Forbes CD. Double-blind trial of Cl115,347, a transdermally absorbed prostaglandin E_2 analogue, in treatment of Raynaud's phenomenon. Lancet 1985;i:1180–1183.
68. Barst RJ, Rubin LJ, McGoon MD, Caldwell EJ, Long WA, Levy PS. Survival in primary pulmonary hypertension with long-term continuous intravenous prostacyclin infusion. Ann Intern Med 1994;121:409–415.
69. Higenbottam TW, Spiegelhalter D, Scott JP, Fuster V, Dinh-Xuan AT, Caine N, Wallwork J. Prostacyclin (epoprostenol) and heart-lung transplantation as treatments for pulmonary hypertension. Br Heart J 1993;70:366–370.
70. Gassner A, Sommer G, Fridrich L et al. Der Einfluss von Proastalandin E_1 (Alprostadil) auf die pulmonale Hypertonie bei Patienten mit chronisch obstructiven Atemwegserkrankungen (COPD). Prax Klin Pneumol 1988;42:521.
71. Sinzinger H, Fitscha P. Leberfunktionsparameter und Fibrinogen bei i.a. und i.v. PGE_1-infusion. Wien Klin Wochenschr 1988;14:488.
72. Walmrath D, Schneider T, Pilch J, Grimminger F, Seeger W. Aerosolised prostacyclin in adult respiratory distress syndrome. Lancet 1993;342:961–962.
73. Walmrath D, Schneider T, Pilch J, Schermuly R, Grimminger F, Seeger W. Effects of aerosolized prostacyclin in severe pneumonia Am J Respir Crit Care Med 1995; 151:724–730.
74. Bindl L, Fahnenstich H, Peukert U. Aerosolised prostacyclin for pulmonary hypertension in neonates. Arch Dis Child 1994;71:F214-FF216.
75. Zusman MR, Rubin RH, Cata AE et al. Hemodialysis using prostacyclin instead of heparin as the sole antithrombotic agent. N Engl J Med 1981;304:934.
76. Gruss JD, Vargas-Montano H, Bartels D et al. Use of prostaglandins in arterial occlusion diseases. Int Angiol 1984;3:7.
77. Shionoya S. Clinical experience with prostaglandin E_1 in occlusive arterial disease. Int Angiol 1984;3:99.
78. Tanabe T, Mishima Y, Shionoya Y et al. Effect of intravenous drip infusion of prostaglandin E_1 on peripheral vascular reconstruction. Int Angiol 1984;3:63.
79. Nizankowski R, Krolikowski W, Bielatowicz J, Szczelklik A. Prostacyclin for ischemic ulcers in peripheral arterial disease: a random assignment placebo controlled study. Thromb Res 1985;37:21.
80. Telles GS, Campbell WB, Wood RFM et al. Prostaglandin E_1 in severe lower limb ischaemia: a double-blind controlled trial. Br J Surg 1984;71:506.

81. Kovacs IB, Mayou SC, Kirby JD. Infusion of a stable prostacyclin analogue, iloprost, to patients with peripheral vascular disease; lack of antiplatelet effect but risk of thromboembolism. Am J Med 1991;90:41—46.
82. Darius H, Nixdorff U, Zander J, Rupprecht HJ, Erbel R, Meyer. Effects of ciprostene on restenosis rate during therapeutic transluminal coronary angioplasty. Agents Actions 1992;37(Suppl):305—311.
83. Hattori R, Yui Y, Shirotani M, Kawai C. A stable prostacyclin analogue, 9B methylcarbacyclin (U-61, 431F). Cardiovasc Drug Rev 1992;10:233—242.
84. Hildebrand M, Pfeffer M, Mahler M, Staks T, Windt-Hanke F, Schutt A. Oral iloprost in healthy volunteers. Eiconasoids 1991;4:149—154.
85. Okeefe SJD, Spitaels JM, Mannion G, Naiker N. Misoprostol, a synthetic prostaglandin E_1 analogue, in the treatment of duodenal ulcers. A double-blind, cimetidine-controlled trial. South Afr Med J 1985;67:321.
86. Graham DY, White RH, Moreland LW, Schubert TT, Katz R, Jaszewski R, Tindall E, Triadafilopoulos G, Stromatt SC, Teoh LS and the Misoprostol Study Group. Duodenal and gastric ulcer prevention in arthritis patients taking NSAIDs. Ann Intern Med 1993;119:257—262.
87. Grazioli I, Avossa M, Bogliolo A, Broggini M, Carcassi A et al. Multicenter stucy of the safety/efficacy of misoprostol in the prevention and treatment of NSAID-induced gastroduodenal lesions. Clin Exp Rheumatol 1993;11:289—294.
88. Wilkie ME, Davies GR, Marsh FP, Rampton DS. Effect of indomethacin and misoprostol on renal function in healthy volunteers. Clin Nephrol 1992;38:334—337.
89. Goldin E, Fich A, Eliakim R et al. Comparison of misoprostol and ranitidine in the treatment of duodenal ulcer. Isr J Med Sci 1988;24:282.
90. Wilson DE. Misoprostol and gastroduodenal mucosal protection (cytoprotection). Postgrad Med J 1988;64(Suppl 1):7.
91. Watkinson G, Hopkins A, Abkar FA. The therapeutic efficacy of misoprostol in peptic ulcer disease. Postgrad Med J 1988;64(Suppl 1):60.
92. Greig PD, Woolf GM, Sinclair SB, Abecassis M, Strasberg SM, Taylor BR, Blendis LM, Superina RA, Glynn MFX, Langer B, Levy GA. Treatment of primary liver graft nonfunction with prostaglandin E_1 Transplantation 1989; 48:447—453.
93. Flowers M, Sherker A, Sinclair SB, Greig PD, Cameron R, Phillips MJ, Blendis L, Chung SW, Levy GA. Prostaglandin E in the treatment of recurrent hepatitis B infection after orthotopic liver transplantation. Transplantation 1994; 58:183—191.
94. Tancharoen S, Jones RM, Angus PW, Michell ID, McNicol L, Hardy KJ. Prostaglandin E_1 therapy in orthotopic liver transplantation recipients: Indications and outcomes. Transplant Proc 1992:24:2248—2249.
95. Cattral MS, Altraif I, Greig PD, Blendis L, Levy GA. Toxic effects of intravenous and oral prostaglandin E therapy in patients with liver disease. Am J Med 1994;97:369—373.
96. Strachan JR, Pryor JP. Prostacyclin in the treatment of painful Peyronies disease. Br J Urol 1988;61:516.
97. Waldhauser M, Schramek P. Efficiency and side effects of prostaglandin E_1 in the treatment of erectile dysfunction. J Urol 1988;140 525.
98. Lowe FC, Jarow JP. Placebo-controlled study of oral terbutaline and pseudoephedrine in management of prostaglandin E_1-induced prolonged erections. Urology 1993; 42:51—54.
99. Chen J, Godschalk M, Katz PG, Mulligan T. The lowest effective dose of prostaglandin E_1 as treatment for erectile dysfunction. J Urology 1995;153:80—81.
100. Chen J, Godschalk M, Katz PG, Mulligan T. Peyronie's-like plaque after penile injection of prostaglandin E_1. J Urol 1994;152:961—962.
101. Hemal AK, Vaidyanathan S, Sankaranarayanan et al. Control of massive vesical hemorrhage due to radiation cystitis with intravesicalinstillation of (15*S*)-15-methylprostaglandin $F_{2\alpha}$. Int J Clin Pharmacol 1988;26:477.
102. Levine LA, Jarrard DF. Treatment of cyclophosphamide-induced hemorrhagic cystitis with intravesical carboprost tromethamine. J Urol 1993;149:719—723.
103. Trigg ME, O'Reilly J, Rumelhart S, Morgan D, Holida M, de Alarcon P. Prostaglandin E_1 bladder installations to control severe hemorrhagic cystitis. J Urol 1990;143:92—94.
104. Flach AJ, Eliason JA. Topical prostaglandin E_2 effects on normal human intraocular pressure. J Ocul Pharmacol 1988;4:13.
105. Lee PY, Shao H, Xu L et al. The effect of prostaglandin $F_{2\alpha}$ on intraocular pressure in normotensive human subjects. Invest Ophthalmol 1988;29:1474.
106. Serle JB. Pharmacological advances in the treatment of glaucoma. Drugs Aging 1994;5:156—170.
107. Rulo AH, Greve EL, Hoymg PF. Additive effect of latanoprost, a prostaglandin $F_{2\alpha}$ analogue, and timolol in patients with elevated intaocular pressure. Br J Ophthalmol 1994;78:899—902.

Meyler's Side Effects of Drugs, 13th Edition
M.N.G. Dukes, editor

SECTION EDITOR: M.N.G. DUKES

I. Aursnes

44 Drugs affecting lipid metabolism

GENERAL

The effectiveness of lipid-lowering drugs in reducing or retarding human atherosclerosis is well documented, most recently also as regards their effect on total mortality 1[C]. It has been suspected that low levels of serum cholesterol would be associated with increased cancer or all-cause mortality. In a more recent epidemiological study these risks are reduced to become almost nonexistent by adjusting for confounding factors, the only remaining risk being higher mortality due to hemorrhagic stroke (2[C]).

Fibrates *(SED-12, 1097)*

Adverse events are essentially the same with all fibrates, generally being mild or absent during short-term treatment.

ADVERSE REACTION PATTERN

General and toxic reactions These are usually mild or not present. Reactions from various organs have been reported; slight increases in liver and muscle enzymes in blood are frequent. Gastrointestinal upset is experienced by some patients.

Hypersensitivity reactions These reactions, especially from the skin, are rare, the incidence being reported with slightly different frequencies with the various drugs.

Tumor-inducing effects These have not been demonstrated in animal studies. There have been suspicions in man, especially from studies with clofibrate.

Second-generation effects These cannot be ruled out, and fibrates are therefore not recommended during pregnancy.

ORGANS AND SYSTEMS

Cardiovascular Earlier suspicions of cardiovascular adverse effects have not been supported by more recent observations.

Respiratory Acute respiratory complications due directly to the drug are unknown.

Nervous system Gemfibrozil-induced *headache* has been reported (3[C]) and occurred in one patient after 24 hours on bezafibrate (4[C]). One patient with myositis taking bezafibrate also had *conduction blocks* in the tibial nerves, indicating demyelinating neuropathic changes (5[C]). *Peripheral neuropathy* has been observed with bezafibrate (6[r]).

Endocrine, metabolic A consistent picture has not emerged; but one must be prepared for unexpected *changes in carbohydrate tolerance* in either normal subjects or diabetics.

Mineral and fluid balance Clofibrate has a mild *antidiuretic effect*, and animal studies seem to indicate that this is due to its inducing release of antidiuretic hormone (ADH). In patients with diabetes insipidus the effect is sufficient to result in measurable *water retention*, but in the clofibrate-using population as a whole it is not of great consequence and no problems of 'inappropriate ADH secretion' arise.

Hematological *Leukopenia* is mentioned as an important side effect with gemfibrozil and is also seen with fenofibrate (7[R]).

Liver Documentation of good renal and hepatic function is mandatory before beginning treatment with the fibrates (8[R]). *Serum transaminase changes* are regularly seen and *hepatitis* does occur (7[R]). One case of *liver failure* probably due to beclobrate has been reported (9[c]). Several cases of *hepatitis* due to fenofibrate have been reviewed (10[R]).

Gastrointestinal *Abdominal discomfort* is seen in 5–10% of all patients. *Epigastric fullness*, *nausea*, *meteorism and mild diarrhea* have been repeatedly described, and *stomatitis* has been incidentally mentioned. There are wide discrepancies in the figures given for such complications, ranging as they do from 2 to 20%; the truth appears to be that during the first few days and weeks of treatment *mild discomfort of one sort or another* is quite commonly experienced, although some of it is due merely to a placebo effect; serious symptoms are most unusual. Bezafibrate is seemingly better tolerated than gemfibrozil (11[C]). In a double-blind trial with fenofibrate the incidence of *gastrointestinal side effects* was not different from that seen with placebo (12[R]).

Diarrhea was complained of by five out of 1213 individuals receiving beclobrate (13[R]).

Fibrates produce bile that is supersaturated with cholesterol. Although gallstones are frequently seen with clofibrate, no excess frequency has been observed with fenofibrate (7[R]). In the WHO study, 59 patients in the clofibrate group had to be operated on for gallstones, compared with 24 and 25, respectively, in the two placebo groups. The Coronary Drug Project produced similar findings, the incidence of *cholelithiasis* and *cholecystitis* being increased from 2.6 to 4.0% over a 6-year period (14C).

Skin *Non-specific rash* has been reported. With fenofibrate it is reported significantly more often than with placebo (15[R]), and occurs in some 0.6% of patients in several studies taken together (7[R]). In a double-blind trial the incidence of *cutaneous adverse effects* was 11% with fenofibrate and less than 1% with placebo; they included hives and urticaria (12[R]). In another report the difference was 6% (16[R]). *Photosensitivity* is also seen (17[C]). *Psoriasis* was exacerbated in one case during treatment with gemfibrozil (18[C]). *Serious skin disorders* are rarely associated with clofibrate and a clofibrate-induced *Steven-Johnson syndrome* has been reported (19[C]).

Cancer A trend towards *increased frequency of cancer* was found in the World Health Organization Study (14[C]), but follow-up of these patients did not support this notion. No increased cancer incidence has been found in other studies, except for an increased frequency of basal cell carcinomas in the Helsinki Heart Study, approaching statistical significance (7[R]), but this is most probably due to chance, in view of the later reversal of the trend after the study (20[C]).

Musculoskeletal system *Creatine kinase increased* in 0.8% of patients receiving fenofibrate compared with 0.6% of controls (9[R]), and in five out of 1213 patients receiving beclobrate (13[R]). A case of *myopathy* occurring during treatment with gemfibrozil alone has been reported (21[C]), and is also seen with ciprofibrate (22[r], 23[c]). Acute *rhabdomyolysis* and *hemoglobin reduction* occurred after bezafibrate overdose in hyperlipidemic patients on hemodialysis (24[C]).

Hypothyroidism seemingly enhances the tendency towards muscle toxicity (25[C], 26[C]). The muscular syndrome appears to be a special risk in nephrotic patients, in whom up to 18% of the circulating fibrate may be unbound because of low serum albumin levels; in one classic report four out of six nephrotic individuals developed the syndrome within 3 days of starting to take clofibrate (27[Cr]). *Severe reversible renal failure* has been observed with bezafibrate (28[C]). *Acute compartment syndrome* has been reported as an unusual presentation of gemfibrozil-induced myositis in a patient with chronic renal failure (29[C]).

Sexual function Gemfibrozil has been suspected to *reduce libido* in two cases (30[c], 31[c]), an effect which is well known with clofibrate. *Loss of libido and impotence* have been associated with use of fibrates, altogether four such cases involving gemfibrozil being reported from Spain (32[Cr]).

Risk situations In view of data presented elsewhere in this monograph, it would seem fair to regard certain groups of patients as running greater risks than normal when taking fibrates. Individuals with *nephrosis* or *renal failure* stand to develop the muscular syndrome perhaps because there is less protein to bind the drug and excretion is impaired. *Hypothyroidism* may be another factor predisposing to the muscular syndrome. Individuals with *liver disease* of any type should probably not be taking fibrates. If there is *biliary cirrhosis* or if *gallstones* are present, *biliary complications* are more prone to occur.

Withdrawal effects No problems appear to *arise* when fibrates are withdrawn, even if treatment has been prolonged and the withdrawal is sudden.

Second-generation effects There has been no systematic study of the use of fibrates in pregnancy. In animals, no teratogenic potential has been demonstrated, but in the rabbit the drug is found *to cumulate in the fetal serum*. The significance of this, if any, is unknown. No data are on record of possible effects of fibrates during lactation or on fertility.

Immunological and hypersensitivity reactions *Arthritis* is not unheard of with fibrates, and one case of *vasculitis, Raynaud's phenomenon and polyarthritis* has been reported (33[Cr]).

Interactions Rhabdomyolysis when used with *statins* is well known, and has been seen when bezafibrate was combined with *furosemide* (33[C]). In 80 patients with primary mixed hyperlipidemia, gemfibrozil used together with *lovastatin* resulted in 3% discontinuation because of myositis, but none attributable to rhabdomyolysis or myoglobinuria (35[C]). In one patient, the same combination caused severe proximal muscle weakness and a biopsy showed multiple foci of mononuclear cell infiltration (36[C]). Rhabdomyolysis in a patient taking ciprofibrate has been attributed to an interaction with the antifungal drug miconazole which was thought to have caused reduced metabolism of ciprofibrate (37[C]).

Hypoglycemia in a diabetic patient was the result of *glyburide* combined with gemfibrozil (38[C]). Since fibrates are strongly bound to albumin, they will displace other similarly bound drugs. In practice, this has been shown to have important repercussions for simultaneous treatment with the *oral anticoagulants*, *furosemide and the sulfonylureas*, and other interactions of this type should be watched for.

Ion-exchange resins

The incidence of adverse effects with ion-exchange resins varies markedly with the selection of patients.

ADVERSE REACTION PATTERN

General and toxic reactions Ion-exchange resins exert their effects within the gastrointestinal tract; their adverse reactions are therefore generally the result of local intolerance or of interference with the absorption of drugs or fat-soluble vitamins.

Hypersensitivity reactions These can occur.

Tumor-inducing effects These are unknown.

Second-generation effects Due to their interference with absorption of fat-soluble vitamins it would seem unwise to give resins during pregnancy.

Cholestyramine *(SED-12, 1099)*

Gastrointestinal *Constipation* is often experienced, but foods rich in fiber can reduce the problem. Other effects are *upper abdominal pain, gas, heartburn and nausea*. About half the patients taking this drug complain of *mild or moderate constipation* and even *fecal impaction* may occur; particularly in the elderly a mild laxative may be needed. Many other patients complain of *anorexia, nausea, meteorism, heartburn and cramp*; occasionally there is *diarrhea*. A fatality has been described in a small child where the *impacted resin obstructed the colon* (SED-8, 935). Doses higher than the 10–16 grams normally used can cause *steatorrhea*.

Metabolic Levels of *triglycerides* tend to increase, especially in patients with hypertriglyceridemia.

Mineral and fluid balance In young children with renal insufficiency, *hypochloremic acidosis* can occur (39[C]).

Hematological *Vitamin K* deficiency may in theory lead to hypoprothrombinemia and hence to bleeding.

Skin *Pruritus and rash* have occurred.

Bone A degree of *osteoporosis or osteomalacia* can occur because of *deranged vitamin D absorption*; the risk should be borne in mind in the elderly.

Second-generation effects It would seem unwise to give cholestyramine in pregnancy in view of the effects which it can have on absorption of vitamin K, calcium and other vitamins and nutrients.

Interactions Binding of substances present in the gastrointestinal tract explains all the interactions of cholestyramine; the process has been studied in vitro, in animals and in man. There is reason to anticipate problems if the resin is given along with acidic and some other drugs having a narrow safety margin such as *anticoagulants* (coumarins), *cardiac glycosides* and *thyroid hormones* (thyroxine, triiodothyronine). It has been pointed out, in the context of a patient taking warfarin and cholestyramine in whom the prothrombin time was extremely prolonged, that cholestyramine on its own has been reported to cause hypoprothrombinemic hemorrhage in the absence of anticoagulants (40[C]). Interference with the absorption of other acidic drugs, including the *barbiturates*, *naproxen*, *phenylbutazone* and its congeners and the thiazide diuretics can almost certainly occur, but it is of little or no clinical importance since the dose of these substances can easily be adjusted as time goes on to allow for any decrease in absorption, or alternative drugs can be sought. Interference with *anticoagulants* and *cardiac glycosides* presents the most acute problem because of the need for exact dosage of these drugs. It has often been said that problems can be avoided provided the drugs are not given simultaneously; however, this is not true where the drug in question undergoes enterohepatic circulation, as is the case with *digitoxin* and *phenprocoumon*, as a result of which these substances are present in the gastrointestinal tract for a long period. The interval principle for other drugs is indeed useful, but the interval should be at least 1 hour and in the case of *thyroxine* 4–5 hours, the drug in question being given prior to the resin.

Interference with absorption is also of importance as regards: (a) *vitamin K*, quantities of which sequestrated in the gastrointestinal tract can be so great that bleeding ensues (so far, no increased bleeding tendency has been reported); (b) *vitamin D*, lack of which can lead to osteomalacia or osteoporosis (the fact that high doses of the resin can cause an increase in alkaline phosphatase levels in young people suggests a subclinical effect of the same type); (c) *iron*, at least in patients particularly susceptible to iron deficiency.

Malabsorption of *folic acid* with decreased erythrocyte folate levels has been reported, more commonly in children (41[r]). There is apparently no recorded case of clinical deficiency of vitamin A among patients taking cholestyramine, but it is advisable to give both vitamins A and D in water-soluble form to patients on this resin.

Colestipol *(SEDA-2, 360; SEDA-3, 358)*

Like cholestyramine, colestipol is a basic anion-exchange resin. It is of more recent origin and there has been correspondingly less clinical experience, but the *gastrointestinal side effects* are similar. One might also anticipate a similarity to cholestyramine as regards other adverse reactions and interactions, provided equally effective doses are used, which has not always been the case.

The commonest reported side effect has been *constipation* (30%). In the first months of therapy *nausea and bloating* can occur. A disappointingly low compliance is found with young patients (42[C]). The encapsulated form of the drug is better tolerated (43[C]).

Interactions The binding capacity of colestipol includes concurrently administered *anionic drugs* and it also reduces the enterohepatic recirculation of *digitoxin, thyroxine, tetracycline and hydrochlorothiazide*. No interference was reported with the absorption of fat-soluble vitamins, but at high doses in children supplemental folic acid may need to be provided (44[r]).

Polidexide (DEAE-Sephadex)

Although structurally different from the other products in use, polidexide appears in practice to cause the same patterns of adverse reactions and interactions as cholestyramine.

HMG coenzyme-A reductase inhibitors

(SEDA-13, 404; SEDA-14, 395; SEDA-15, 478)

ADVERSE REACTION PATTERN

General and toxic reactions These are mostly limited to slight increases in liver and muscle enzymes in the blood, thus bearing a striking resemblance to the effects of the fibrates.

Hypersensitivity reactions These do occur.

Tumor-inducing effects These cannot be ruled out, but no indications of such have been observed so far.

Second-generation effects These are suspected. The drugs should not be used during pregnancy.

ORGANS AND SYSTEMS

Nervous system In type II diabetics, two cases of etiologically obscure *eye muscle palsies* have been reported (45[c]). In the EXCEL-study, which was a double-blind, placebo-controlled study for 48 weeks in 8245 individuals, the prevalence of adverse events was similar during placebo and active treatment. Notably, *depression* was reported in 1.7% of those receiving placebo versus 1.4% of all those given lovastatin (46[C]). Accordingly, in an analysis of two large Finnish cohorts monitored for 10 and 15 years, the risk of *accidents, suicides*, and other *violent deaths* was not related to serum cholesterol concentration (9[C]). In the 4S-study there were five *suicides* in the simvastatin group and four in controls (1[C]).

Statins interfere with the *production of isoprene* which is somehow connected with sleep. Lovastatin-associated *sleep* and *mood disturbances* were concluded from observations in two patients in whom discontinuation of lovastatin resulted in prompt abatement of sleep disturbance and anxiety (47[C]). Parallel experiences have been reported with simvastatin and pravastatin (48[r], 49[C]). An analysis of sleep EEG measures relevant to *insomnia* provided no evidence of significant differences between pravastatin, simvastatin, and placebo (50[C]). In another study comparing pravastatin and lovastatin, neither drug affected *nocturnal sleep*, but lovastatin significantly affected *daytime performance*. In subjects who took lovastatin there was more *divided attention* and *less vigilance* (51[C]). In a group of male patients with primary hypercholesterolemia, neither lovastatin nor pravastatin caused any substantial or objective change in the quality of *sleep* (52[C]).

Endocrine, metabolic *Diabetes mellitus* was diagnosed in a 63-year-old woman 5 months after she began pravastatin 20 mg/day. Insulin could be withdrawn soon after she stopped taking pravastatin (53[C]). *Vascular collapse* can possibly be related to low production of corticosteroids (54[C]).

Liver Judged from the enzyme increases seen with statins one suspects liver toxicity, although a return to normal or only slightly increased values is often seen after a short period. Rarely frank *hepatitis* is observed. A *cholestatic picture* has also been reported (55[C], 56[C]). The mechanisms behind these reactions are not known.

In one series the frequency of *liver toxicity* was similar in patients treated with pravastatin or simvastatin (57[C]), while in another study there was a difference 6 months after the start of the study. At that time liver enzymes showed a statistically significant but transient increase in the simvastatin group (58[C]).

Pancreas *Pancreatitis* has been observed during

treatment with statins (59[C]). HMG CoA reductase inhibitors could increase the risk of *acute pancreatitis in hemodialysis patients*. The records of 56 patients were reviewed over an 8-year period in one hospital. After lipid lowering with drugs was started, five of them experienced an episode of *acute pancreatitis* (60[C]). Three cases of *pancreatitis* have been reported with simvastatin (61[C], 62[C]).

Skin A case of simvastatin-induced *lichenoid eruption* with skin and mucosal involvement has been reported (63[C]). Similar reactions have been reported previously (SEDA-18, 427).

Vision One should be aware of any appearance of color blindness (64[c]). *Conjunctivitis* (65[c]) has also been observed. Due to the high cholesterol content of the human lens, *ocular changes* have been looked for during trials with statins. It has been concluded that *cataract* does not occur. Although the degree of *lens opacities* increases during treatment, the incidence does not differ from that seen in an untreated control population (66[C]).

Altogether 150 patients suffering from primary hypercholesterolemia, were studied for 2 years with lovastatin or simvastatin, fenofibrate serving as control. Increases or decreases in the *visual acuity* were distributed very similarly in the three groups (67[C]).

Sexual function Cholesterol is necessary for the *production of steroid hormones*, and a case of *hypospermia* has been reported (68[C]).

Musculoskeletal system The *serum coenzyme-Q level* is regularly reduced by about 30% during statin treatment, because the enzyme is carried by low-density lipoprotein particles, although the concentrations during long-term treatment are equal to those in healthy controls (69[C], 70[C]). Ubiquinone (coenzyme-Q) is part of the oxidative respiratory pathway generating ATP, and shortage of supply could impede the function of myocytes leading to increase in serum creatine phosphokinase and even cell destruction with release of myoglobin which in its turn can block kidney tubuli and thereby produce *anuria*. One in 1000 patients receiving both placebo and 20 mg lovastatin daily experienced transaminase elevations 3 times the upper normal level, increasing to 1.5% in those receiving 80 mg daily. *Myopathy*, which was defined as muscle symptoms with a *creatine kinase elevation* greater than 10 times the upper limit of normal, was found in only one patient receiving 40 mg once daily and in four patients receiving 80 mg/day. The number of patients with *rhabdomyolysis* was, according to post-marketing reporting from the first million individuals taking lovastatin, 24 cases altogether. Seventeen of those had taken other medications which are known to increase this risk (71[R]). There is some evidence that patients with complicated medical histories may be at somewhat greater risk of developing *myopathy* than would be anticipated from experience in controlled trials.

Immunological reactions A *lupus-like syndrome* (72[r]) and also a *lichenoid reaction* (63[c]) can occur. *Arthralgia* has been recorded and has been associated with rapid lowering of cholesterol concentrations (51[C]).

Miscellaneous Although *fever* is well known, the first report of *severe hyperthermia* has been published. A 55-year-old woman with Parkinson's disease, rheumatoid arthritis and hyperthyroidism, experienced hyperthermia following therapy with lovastatin for hypercholesterolemia. She responded equally strongly to repeated challenges suggesting a cause-and-effect relationship (73[C]).

Hypersensitivity reactions There were 25 serious hypersensitivity reactions (such as *arthralgia* and *thrombocytopenia*) among the first million patients taking lovastatin. At least some of these are considered to be due to the drug (74[R]).

Interactions In a compiled series, four (5%) out of 80 subjects receiving lovastatin and *gemfibrozil* developed myopathy. Based on this and on reports to US Food and Drug Administration the combined use of the two drugs is discouraged, especially in patients with compromised renal and/or hepatic function (75[C]). Elderly women might be a group at special risk (76[c], 77[C]). In addition, discontinuation of lovastatin should be considered during acute illness due to alterations in drug metabolism and frequent use of *multiple medications* including *erythromycin* (78[C]). In view of the higher risk of severe myopathy with combined treatment, it is noteworthy that patients with mixed hyperlipidemia can be well treated with a statin only (79[C]). Ten cases of interaction with *warfarin* resulting in an increased bleeding tendency have been reported (71[R]).

Estrogen-replacement therapy appeared to have no effect on either the efficacy or safety profile of lovastatin (80[C]).

Second-generation effects Based on a general consideration of risk, these drugs should not be administrated during pregnancy and only in very exceptional circumstances to any woman of child-bearing age.

INDIVIDUAL HMG COENZYME-A REDUCTASE INHIBITORS

The frequency of *discontinuation of treatment* because of adverse effects was similar for the statins in one series (81[C]) but a slight difference in the benefit:risk ratio could be of importance.

Fluvastatin

It has been suggested that the pharmacokinetics of fluvastatin, including extensive biliary excretion and absence of circulating active metabolites, might be associated with a low incidence of systemic adverse effects compared with other statins. Common adverse effects associated with fluvastatin in clinical trials have been *fatigue, headache, nausea, diarrhea, dyspepsia, abdominal pain and rash* (82[r]).

Clinical experience with fluvastatin in >1800 patients treated for an average of 61 weeks has shown it to be safe and tolerable. Although *dyspepsia* was observed more commonly in fluvastatin patients, the incidence, along with that of other adverse events (e.g. *headache*), and the number of *treatment discontinuations* proved statistically indistinguishable from those of placebo controls (83[R]). Notably, drug-related *myositis* or *rhabdomyolysis* have not been observed with fluvastatin.

Lovastatin *(SED-11, 924)*

The adverse event profile in 8245 patients with moderate hypercholesterolemia has been evaluated in a double-blind, diet- and placebo-controlled trial (84[C]). The difference between lovastatin and placebo in the incidence *of clinical adverse experiences* requiring discontinuation was small, ranging from 1.2% at 20 mg twice daily to 1.9% at 80 mg/day. Among a variety of clinical symptoms registered in the study, only *constipation* differed significantly between drug and placebo with a slight increase in frequency in the treated group. It was also noted that the treated patients gained on the average 0.4 kg *more weight* than controls. *Deaths* were few (36), and none of these was due to accidental causes. Lovastatin-induced rhabdomyolysis can occur in the absence of other drug therapy (SED-12, 1101). *Severe rhabdomyolysis* with *hepatopathy* was observed during low-dose lovastatin treatment. There were no drug interactions, nor were other causes of rhabdomyolysis present (85[C]).

Pravastatin

A series of 1142 hypercholesterolemic patients treated with pravastatin has been followed with a placebo-controlled design during the first 8—16-week period (86[R]). The numbers of '*adverse drug experiences*' were similar in treated and untreated individuals. *Rash* was the only single adverse clinical event that was different (4.0 vs 1.1%). In the same patients *discontinuation of therapy* during follow-up was found to be necessary in 3.2% of those given pravastatin alone. *Myopathy* was observed in one instance only, whereas increases in creatine kinase in the treated group did not differ significantly from controls. Marked, *persistent increases in transaminases* occurred in 1.1% with no cases of *symptomatic hepatitis*. Because of the hydrophilic property of the drug, it might have limited entry into peripheral cells and thereby produce few adverse effects (87[R]). It is believed to have a particularly low potential for *CNS-related adverse effects*, as it has not been shown to enter the cerebrospinal fluid (88[C]). Clinical experience so far suggests that *muscle toxicity* occurs less often with pravastatin than with lovastatin (89[r]).

Interactions Pravastatin has not been tried together with drugs that are known to increase the risk of myopathy such as *fibrates*. Prothrombin time was not affected with the concurrent administration of *warfarin* (90[R]). *Cholestyramine* significantly reduces the systemic availability of pravastatin (91[c]).

Simvastatin

Long-term follow up of 2423 patients receiving simvastatin has shown that it is well tolerated with no reports of *new or unexpected adverse effects* (92[C]). Episodes of *gout* occurred in three out of nine patients with chronic renal failure who were treated with simvastatin (93[c]). According to authors who reported a case of *protein-losing enteropathy, diarrhea* during simvastatin treatment may be a fairly harmful adverse effect (94[C]).

Rhabdomyolysis has been reported (95[C], 96[C]). In a series of 66 patients during a 1-year study two experienced *myalgia* and *weakness* with creatine kinase values above 3000 (normally <100) (97[C]).

Two cases of *cholestatic hepatitis* have been reported (98[C], 99[C]). It has been claimed that physicians should bear in mind the *nephrotoxic potential* of this drug (100[C]), but there is no definite evidence that simvastatin is associated with the development of *proteinuria* (101[C]).

Nicotinic acid derivatives *(SED-11, 923; SEDA-13, 405; SEDA-14, 395; SEDA-15, 480)*

It is not entirely clear to what extent the incidence of adverse reactions of nicotinic acid (niacin) is the same as that encountered with its various derivatives. The monograph below applies primarily to nicotinic acid itself; its congeners are discussed briefly later.

ADVERSE REACTION PATTERN

General and toxic reactions With the doses used for lipid lowering, reactions are rather severe due to the vasodilating effect, but not associated as a rule with any great danger. Hepatotoxicity is infrequently seen.

Hypersensitivity reactions These do not seem to occur, but the itching and flush can easily be mistaken for evidence of allergic reactions.

Tumor-inducing effects These have not been reported.

ORGANS AND SYSTEMS

Cardiovascular *Coronary steal* with worsening of myocardial ischemia related to niacin's vasodilating property is a possible side effect suggested from a case report (102[C]). The drug should therefore perhaps be withheld in patients with unstable angina. *Flushing of the skin* is a normal reaction to high doses of nicotinic acid until tolerance to it develops. Some patients experience a much more *severe vascular reaction* with sensations of *heat*, *throbbing of the head*, *vertigo*, *faintness* and sometimes a marked *fall in blood pressure*.

Nervous system *Tingling* in the orofacial region has been attributed to a *neuropathic effect*, but this could have been due to the *vascular reaction*.

Liver Particular concern is connected with the drug's *hepatotoxicity*, and the slow release form of the drug is suspected to increase this danger (103[R], 104[C]). Rechallenge with crystalline preparations has been tolerated (105[C]). A case of *fulminant hepatic failure* following low-dose modified-release niacin therapy has been reported (106[R]). The causal association is supported by previous reports and it has been stated that awareness of possible toxicity associated with high dosages of time-release niacin formulations is important (107[C]). More common is an *asymptomatic increase in liver enzymes* during niacin therapy.

Endocrine, metabolic Of special concern is niacin's *hyperglycemic action* and it is therefore not recommended as a first-line hypolipidemic drug in patients with non-insulin-dependent diabetes mellitus (108[C]). Life-threatening *hyperglycemia* has been observed in a normoglycemic individual who had no evidence of glucose intolerance after withdrawal of niacin therapy (109[C]. Long-acting forms of niacin have also been linked with the development of *lactic acidosis* (110[C]).

Skin and appendages *Flushing* occurs transiently in all patients and persists in 10–15% of cases. When starting with a high dose, *hypotension* may occur (111[R]). *Itching*, *dry skin*, and *gastrointestinal distress* are other common adverse effects of nicotinic acid. The *flushing of the skin with pruritus* is a transitory reaction, but *urticaria* can occur at any time and dryness of the skin, mild *exfoliation*, an *acanthosis nigricans*-like state and *loss of hair* have all been described in prolonged treatment. *Brown pigmentation of the skin* can be observed in about a quarter of all patients on long-term therapy. *Sebum secretion* tends to increase. In a few cases *acanthosis nigricans* may develop (111[R]).

Vision Reversible *blurring of vision* due to cystoid macular edema is a rare but recognized complication. *Retinal edema*, when it happens, will subside on stopping administration of niacin (111[R]).

Musculoskeletal system Niacin has also been connected with the development of *myopathy* (112[C]). Together with lovastatin it can produce *rhabdomyolysis* (113[C]). Myopathy was reported in two patients taking niacin without predisposing factors. Moreover, it occurred both with crystalline and sustained-release niacin (114[C]).

Interference with diagnostic routines The high blood levels of nicotinic acid attained when it is given as a hypolipidemic agent are sufficient to give false-positive reactions to tests for blood *bilirubin* and to interfere with tests for *catecholamines*.

EFFECTS SPECIFIC TO PARTICULAR NICOTINIC ACID DERIVATIVES

Niacin

Adverse effects are common with niacin, especially in children (115[C]). A general warning against indiscriminate use of niacin as a vitamin supplement has been given (116[R]). In a comparison between sustained-release and immediate-release niacin, many patients withdrew from the study because of adverse drug reactions or *abnormal laboratory results*. Only 22% of the patients on sustained-release niacin and 61% of the immediate-release group completed the study (117[C]). It has been pointed out that because controlled-release niacin seems to be more potent than crystalline niacin, product substitution without dose adjustment should be avoided (118[C]). It has been hypothesized that retained clinical effects on long-term survival after recovery from myocardial infarction could be obtained with only 1 gram of niacin daily (119[R]). If this holds true, a dramatic reduction in side effects from this drug will occur. Possibly an important HDL-increasing effect related to this drug is operative also at this low dose level.

Acipimox

Acipimox (*S*-methylpyrazine-2-carboxylic acid 4-oxide) is structurally related to nicotinic acid. The recommended dosage of 750 mg/day was not in one study associated with significant alterations in lipids (120[C]), in contrast to the results of another recent study (121[C]).

Flush and *gastrointestinal disturbances*, but no elevating effect on *blood glucose* and *uric acid* was observed in a study with 7137 patients, of whom 15% stopped taking the drug because of side effects (122[c]). In another open study blood glucose was on average slightly lowered in 3009 type II diabetics given acipimox for at least 2 months (123[C]).

Aluminium nicotinate
Nicotinyl alcohol

The adverse reactions to these compounds appear to be identical to those experienced with nicotinic acid. Aluminium nicotinate perhaps causes slightly less *gastrointestinal distress*, but the same can be achieved by buffering the acid, and neither approach in fact solves the problem, which is probably not primarily one of acidity.

Xanthinol nicotinate

A severe *toxicoderma* has been reported with this compound and confirmed by a provocation test (SEDA-1, 333). *Flushing* is claimed to be less frequent than with nicotinic acid, but has nevertheless been repeatedly observed, and the *other adverse reactions* are likely to be those of nicotinic acid.

MISCELLANEOUS DRUGS

Eicospentaenoic acid
Docosahexaenoic acid

These long-chain, polyunsaturated fatty acids from fish oil are in use as triglyceride lowering agents. Few adverse effects have been reported. Belching or eructation with fishy taste or smell, vomiting, flatulence, diarrhea or obstipation are relatively common. No episodes of spontaneous or severe bleeding have been seen, although potentiation of bleeding time has been suspected from one study using a combination with aspirin (124[C]) and was reported in some patients on warfarin (125[C]).

Probucol *(SED-11, 924; SEDA-14, 395; SEDA-15, 480)*

Probucol, which is also an antioxidant, reduces both low-density lipoprotein and high-density lipoprotein cholesterol concentrations, in one study by 11 and 26%, respectively (126[c]). The side effects of probucol have been reviewed (127[R]) and extensively dealt with in previous editions of this book.

Cardiovascular Probucol *prolongs the QT-interval* in electrocardiograms, but it does not regularly produce *arrhythmia*. *Torsades de pointes* has occurred in one patient with the Romano-Ward syndrome (128[C]), and in one patient with no particular risk factors, in whom the dysrhythmia was nevertheless life threatening (129[C]).

However, a retrospective analysis of 89 patients has shown that ECG monitoring may be necessary, especially in women, as well as in those with hypoalbuminemia or with ischemic heart disease (130[C]).

Gastrointestinal According to long-term studies covering 7—9 years, probucol seems to be well tolerated with a reasonably low incidence of side effects. All the documented side effects were concentrated in the gastrointestinal tract. The incidence of *diarrhea* fell from 19% in the first year to 5% in the following year. Only in some 3% of cases do symptoms such as *diarrhea* or *abdominal pain* lead to discontinuation of treatment. Diarrhea and *flatulence* which resolve after a few months are often seen.

Triparanol (Mer-29)

Although the gravity of its adverse effects led to the withdrawal of triparanol in 1961—1962, the data must remain on record as a basis for comparison when preliminary findings on new lipid-lowering drugs are examined.

Triparanol is closely related to various non-steroidal estrogens and antiestrogens and inhibits the reduction of the 24,25 double-bond in the side chain during cholesterol synthesis, hence leading to accumulation of desmosterol. Major complications included *cataract formation*, disorders of the *skin and hair (including discoloration and alopecia)*, *liver function disturbances*, *proteinuria and malabsorption syndrome*. *Loss of libido* was noted, as with some other lipid-lowering drugs. Triparanol was *teratogenic* in mice. The problems have been reviewed in earlier editions of this book (SED-5, 462).

REFERENCES

1. Scandinavian Simvastatin Survival Study Group. Randomised trial of cholesterol lowering in 4444 patients with coronary heart disease. the Scandinavian Simvastatin Survival Study (4S). Lancet 1994;344:1383—1389.
2. Iribarren C, Reed DM, Burchfiel CM, Dwyer JH. Serum toral cholesterol and mortality. Confounding factors and risk modification in Japanes-American men. J Am Med Assoc 1995;273:1926—1932.
3. Sabin JA, Codina A, Rodriguez C, Laporte JR. Gemfibrozil-induced headache. Lancet 1988;ii:1246.
4. Hodgetts TJ, Tunnicliffe C. Bezafibrate-induced headache. Lancet 1989;i:163.
5. Ismail HM, Al-Indrisi HY, Al-KalafJ. Combined myoneuro-toxicity by bezafibrate. Saudi Med J 1993;14(1):86—87.
6. Ellis CJ, Wallis WE, Caruana M. Peripheral neuropathy with bezafibrate. Br Med J 1994;309:929.
7. Roberts WC. Safety of fenofibrate—US and worldwide experience. Cardiology 1989;76:169—179.
8. Brown WV. Fibric acid derivatives. J Drug Dev 1990; 3:211—216.
9. Vartiainen E, Puska P, Pekkanen J, Tuomilehto J, Lönnquist J, Ehnholm C. Serum cholesterol concentration and mortality from accidents, suicide, and other violent causes. Br Med J 1994;309:445—447.
10. Rigal J, Furet Y, Autret E, Breteau M. Hépatite mixte sévère au fénofibrate? Revue de la littérature à propos d'un cas. Rev Med Interne 1989;10:65—67.
11. Kremer P, Marowski C, Jones C, Acacia E. Therapeutic effects of bezafibrate and gemfibrozil in hyperlipoproteinaemia type IIa and IIb. Curr Med Res Opin 1989;11:293—303.
12. Brown WV. Treatment of hypercholesterolaemia with fenofibrate. a review. Curr Med Res Opin 1989;11:321—330.
13. Capurso A. Drugs affecting triglycerides. Cardiology 1991;78:218—225.
14. Committee of Principal Investigators. A cooperative trial in the primary prevention of ischaemic heart disease using clofibrate. Br Heart J 1978;40:1069.
15. Zimetbaum P, Frishman WH, Shoshonah K. Effects of gemfibrozil and other fibric acid derivatives on blood lipids and lipoproteins. J Clin Pharmacol 1991;31:25—37.
16. Knopp RH. Review of the effects of fenofibrate on lipoproteins, apoproteins, and bile saturation. US studies. Cardiology 1989;76:14—22.
17. Leroy D, Dompmartin A, Lorier E, Leport Y, Audebert C. Photosensitivity induced by fenofibrate. Photodermatol Photoimmunol Photomed 1990;7:136—138.
18. Fisher DA, Elias PM, LeBoit PL. Exacerbation of psoriasis by the hypolipidemic agent, gemfibrozil. Arch Dermatol 1988;124:854—855.
19. Wong SS. Steven-Johnson syndrome induced by clofibrate. Acta Dermatol-Venereol 1994;74:475.
20. Huttunen JK, Heinonen OP, Manninen , Koskinen P, Hakulinen T, Teppo L, Manttari M, Frick MH. The Helsinki Heart Study. an 8.5-year safety and mortality follow-up. J Intern Med 1994;235:31—39.
21. Magarian GJ, Lucas LM, Colley C. Gemfibrozil-induced myopathy. Arch Intern Med 1991;151:1873—1874.
22. Harvengt C. Drugs recently released in Belgium. Acta Clin Belgica 1991;46:117—119.
23. Delangre T, Vernier L, Moore N, Mihout. Rhabdomyolyse aiguë au cours d'un traitement par le ciprofibrate. Presse Méd 1990;19:1811—1812.
24. Bedani PL, Perini L, Gilli P. Acute rhabdomyolysis and hemoglobin reduction after bezafibrate overdose in hyperlipidemic patients on hemodialysis. Nephron 1994;68:512—513.
25. Tregouet B. L'hypothyroïdie favorise-t-elle la toxicité musculaire des fibrates? Rev Med Interne 1991;12:159.
26. Hattori N, Shimatsu A, Murabe H, Nishimura M, Nakamura H, Imura H. Clofibrate-induced myopathy in a patient with primary hypothyroidism. Jpn J Med 1990;29:545—547.
27. Bridgman CJF, Rosen SM, Thorp JM. Complications during clofibrate treatment of nepfrotic-syndrome hyperlipoproteinaemia. Lancet 1972;ii:506.
28. Lipkin, GW, Tomson CR. Severe reversible renal failure with bezafibrate. Lancet 1993;341:371.
29. Chow LT, Chow W. Acute compartment syndrome. an unusual presentation of gemfibrozil induced myositis. Med J Aust 1993;158(1):48—49.
30. Bain SC, Lemon M, Jones AF. Gemfibrozil-induced impotence. Lancet 1990;336:1389.
31. Pizarro S, Bargay J, D'Agosto P. Gemfibrozil-induced imptence. Lancet 1990;336:1135.
32. Figueras A, Castel JM, Laporte JR, Capella D. Gemfibrozil-induced impotence. Ann Pharmacother 1993;27(7—8):982.
33. Smith GW, Hurst NP. Vasculitis, Raynaud's phenomenon and polyarthritis associated with gemfibrozil therapy. Br J Rheumatol 1993;32(1):84—85.
34. Venzano C, Cordi GC, Corsi L, Dapelo M, De Micheli A, Grimaldi GP. Un caso di rabdomiolisi acuta con insufficienza renale acuta da assunzione contemporanea di furosemide e bezafibrato. Minerva Med 1990;81:909—911 .
35. Glueck, CJ, Oakes N, Speirs J, Tracy T, Lang J. Gemfibrozil- lovastatin therapy for primary hyperlipoproteinemias. Am J Cardiol 1992;70:1—9.
36. Chucrallah A, De Girolami U, Freeman R, Federman M. Lovastatin/gemfibrozil myopathy. a clinical, histochemical, and ultrastructural study. Eur Neurol 1992;32:293—296.
37. Ory JP, Cleau D, Jobard JM, Bourscheid D. Interaction miconazole—cipofibrate responsable d'une rhabdomyolyse. A propos d'un cas. Ann Med Nancy Est 1993;32:305.
38. Ahmad S. Gemfibrozil. Interaction with glyburide. Southern Med J 1991;84:102.
39. Blom HJ, Monasch E. Metabole acidose bij een patient met gestoorde nierfunctie na cholestyramine toediening. Ned Tijdschr Geneeskd 1983;127:1446.
40. Lawlor DP, Hyers TM. Extreme prolongation of the prothrombin time in a patient receiving warfarin and cholestyramine. Cardiovasc Rev Rep 1993;14(4):72—74.
41. Kane JP, Malloy MJ. Treatment of hypercholesterolemia. Med Clin North Am 1982;66:537.
42. Kruse W, Kohlmeier M, Nikolaus T, Vogel G, Schlierf G. Langzeitbehandlung mit colestipol. Münch Med Wschr 1989;131:407—409.
43. Linet OI, Grzegorczyk CR, Demke DM. The effect of encapsulated, low-dose colestipol in patients with hyperlipidemia. J Clin Pharmacol 1988;28:804—806.
44. Glueck CJ. Colestipol and Probucol. Treatment of pri-

mary and familial hypercholesterolemia and amelioration of atherosclerosis. Ann Intern Med 1982;96:475.
45. Baldermann H, Schweighart C, Rett K, Scholz B, Fabricius E-M, Wicklmayr M et al. Wirksamheit und verträglichkeit von lovastatin (mevinacor) bei typ-II-diabetikern mit hyperlipoproteinämie. Akt Endokrinol 1992;13:94—98.
46. Lines, C. Hazards of reducing cholesterol. Br Med J 1994;309:541.
47. Rosenson RS, Goranson NL. Lovastatin-associated sleep and mood disturbances. Am J Med 1993;95(5):548—549.
48. Duits N, Bos FM. Depressive symptoms and cholesterol-lowering drugs. Lancet 1993;341(8837):114.
49. Duits N, Bos FM. Psychiatric complications with the use of simvastatin. Ned Tijdschr Geneeskd 1993;137(26):1312—1315.
50. Eckernas SA, Roos BE, Kvidal P, Eriksson LO. The effects of objective and subjective measures of nocturnal sleep. A comparison of two structurally different HMG CoA reductase inhibitors in patients with primary moderate hypercholesterolaeia. Br J Clin Pharmacol 1993;35(3):284—289.
51. McDonagh J, Winocour P, Walker DJ. Musculoskeletal manifestations during simvastatin therapy. Br J Rheumatol 1993;32(7):647—648.
52. Partinen M, Phil S, Strandberg T, Vanhanen H, Murtomaki E, Block G, Neafus R, Haigh J, Miettinen T, Reines S. Comparison of effects on sleep of lovastatin and pravastatin in hypercholesterolemia. Am J Cardiol 1994;73:876—880.
53. Jonville-Bera AP, Zakian A, Bera FJ, Carré P, Autret E. Possible pravastatin and diuretics-induced diabetes mellitus. Reactions. Ann Pharmacother 1994;28:964—965.
54. French J, White H. Transient symptomatic hypotension in patients on simvastatin. Lancet 1989;2:807—808.
55. McQueen MJ. Cholestatic jaundice associated with lovastatin (mevacor) therapy. Can Med Assoc J 1990;142:841—842.
56. Spreckelsen U, Kirchoff R, Haacke H. Cholestatischer ikterus während lovastatin-einnahme. Dtsch Med Wschr 1991;116:739—740.
57. Ballare M, Campanini M, Airoldi G, Zaccala G, Bertoncelli MC, Cornaglia G and others. Hepatotoxicity of hydroxy-methyl-glutaryl-coenzyme A reductase inhibitors. Min Gastroenterol Dietol 1992;38:41—44.
58. Muggeo M, Travia D, Querena M, Zenti MG, Bagnani M, Branzi P others. Long term treatment with pravastatin, simvastatin and gemfibrozil in patients with primary hypercholesterolaemia. a controlled study. Drug Invest 1992;4:376—385.
59. Lons T, Chousterman M. La simvastatine. Une nouvelle molécule responsable de pancréatite aiguë? Gastroenterol Clin Biol 1991;15:93—94.
60. Lozano L, Tornero F, Usón J, Rincón B, Garzón A et al. HMG CoA reductase inhibitors in haemodialysis patients. A risk factor for acute pancreatitis? Nephrol Dialysis Transplant 1994;9:992.
61. Ramdani M, Schmitt, A-M, Liautard J, Duhamel 0, Legroux P, Gislon J et al. Pancréatite aiguë à la simvastatine. Deux cas. Gastroenterol Clin Biol 1991;15:986.
62. Couderc M, Blanc P, Rouillon J-M, Bauret P, Larrey D, Michel H. Un nouveau cas de pancréatite aiguë après la prise de simvastatine. Gastroenterol Clin Biol 1991;15:986—987.
63. Roger D, Rolle F, Labrousse F, Brosset A, Bonnetblanc JM. Simvastatin-induced lichenoid drug eruption. Clin Exp Dermatol 1994;19:88—89.
64. Lintott CJ, Scott RS, Nye ER, Robertson MC, Sutherland WHF. Simvastatin (mk 733). An effective treatment for hypercholesterolemia. Aust NZ J Med 1989;19:317—320.
65. Steyn K, Weich HFH, Vermaak WJH, Marais AD, Omar MAK, Van Gelder AL et al. A 6-month trial of simvastatin (HMG-CoA reductase inhibitor) in the treatment of hypercholesterolaemia. S Afr Med J 1991;79:639—645.
66. Laties AM, Shear CL, Lippa EA, Gould AL, Taylor HR, Hurley DP, Stephenson WP, Keates EU, Tupy-Visich MA, Chremos AN. Expanded clinical evaluation of lovastatin (EXCEL) study results. II. Assessment of the human lens after 48 weeks of treatment with lovastatin. Am J Cardiol 1991;67:447—453.
67. Schmidt J, Schmitt C, Hockwin O, Paulus U, Bergmann K. Ocular drug safety and HMG-CoA-reductase inhibitors. Ophthalmic Res 1994;26:352—360.
68. Hildebrand RD, Hepperlen TW. Lovastatin and hypospermia. Ann Intern Med 1990;112:549—550.
69. Laaksonen R, Ojala JP, Tikkanen MJ, Himberg JJ. Serum ubiquinone concentrations after short- and long-term treatment with HMG-CoA reductase inhibitors. Eur J Clin Pharmacol 1994;46:313—317.
70. Laaksonen R, Jokelainen K, Sahi T, Tikkanen MJ, Himberg J-J. Decreases in serum ubiquinone concentrations do not result in reduced levels in muscle tissue during short-term simvastatin treatment in humans. Clin Pharmacol Ther 1995;57:62—66.
71. Mantell G, Burke MT, Staggers J. Extended clinical safety profile of lovastatin. Am J Cardiol 1990;66:11—15.
72. Ahmad S. Side effects of HMG CoA reductase inhibitors. Heart Dis Stroke 1993;2:262.
73. Von Pohle WR. Recurrent hyperthermia due to lovastatin. Western J Med 1994;161:427—428.
74. Tobert JA, Shear CL, Chremos AN, Mantell GE. Clinical experience with lovastatin. Am J Cardiol 1990;65:23—26.
75. Pierce LR, Wysowski DK, Gross TP. Myopathy and rhabdomyolysis associated with lovastatin-gemfibrozil combination therapy. J Am Med Assoc 1990;264:71—75.
76. Goldstein MR. Myopathy and rhabdomyolysis with lovastatin taken with gemfibrozil. J Am Med Assoc 1990; 264:2991.
77. Kogan AD, Orenstein S. Lovastatin-induced acute rhabdomyolysis. Postgrad Med J 1990;66:294—296.
78. Spach DH, Bauwens JE, Clark CD, Burke WG. Rhabdomyolysis associated with lovastatin and erythromycin use. Western J Med 1991;154:213—215.
79. Vega GL, Grundy SM. Management of primary mixed hyperlipidemia with lovastatin. Arch Intern Med 1990; 150:1313—1319.
80. Bradford RH, Downton M, Chremos AN, Langendorfer A, Stinnett S, Nash DT, Mantell G, Shear CL. Efficacy and tolerabiliy of lovastatin in 3390 women with moderate hypercholesterolemia. Ann Intern Med 1993;118:850—855.
81. Kostner GM. Statine verringern cholesterin am besten. Therapiewoche 1992;10:634—641.
82. Anonymous. Sandoz' fluvastatin for hypercholesterolaemia. SCRIP 1994;1886/7:29.
83. Jokubaitis LA. Updated clinical safety experience with fluvastatin. Am J Cardiol 1994;73:18D—24D.
84. Bradford RH, Shear CL, Chremos AN, Dujovne C,

Downton M, Franklin FA, Gould AL, Hesney M, Higgins J, Hurley DP, Langendorfer A, Nash DT, Pool JL, Schnaper H. Expanded clinical evaluation of lovastatin (EXCEL) study results. Arch Intern Med 1991;151:43–49.
85. Fernández Zataraín G, Navarro ?, García H, Villatoro J, Calvo C. Rhabdomyolysis and acute renal failure associated with lovastatin. Nephron 1994;66:483–484.
86. Newman TJ, Kassler-Taub KB, Gelarden RT, Korzin EG, DeVault AR, McGovern ME, Pan HY. Safety of pravastatin in long-term clinical trials conducted in the united states. J Drug Dev 1990;3:275–280.
87. Betteridge DJ. Clinical efficacy and tolerability of pravastatin. J Drug Dev 1992;4:9–14.
88. Botti RE, Triscari J, Pan HY, Zayat J. Concentrations of pravastatin and lovastatin in cerebrospinal fluid in healthy subjects. Clin Neuropharmacol 1991;14:256–61.
89. Jungnickel PW, Cantral KA, Maloley PA. Pravastatin. A new drug for the treatment of hypercholesterolemia. Clin Pharm 1992;11:677– 89.
90. Catalano P. Pravastatin safety. an overview. Round Table Ser 1990;16:26–31.
91. Broisman L, Engster P, Chow MSS. Focus on pravastatin. An HMG-coA reductase inhibitor for the treatment of hypercholesterolemia. Hosp Formul 1991;26:552–563.
92. Boccuzzi SJ, Keegan ME, Hirsch LJ, Shapiro DR, Plotkin DJ, Mitchel YB. Long term experience with simvastatin. Drug Invest 1993;5:135–140.
93. Harris DCH, Simons LA, Mitchell P, Stewart JH. Management of non-nephrotic hyperlipidaemia of chronic renal failure with simvastatin. Med J Australia 1991;155:573.
94. Chagnon JP, Cerf M. Simvastatin-induced protein-losing enteropathy. Am J Gastroenterol 1992;87:257.
95. Deslypere JP, Vermeulen A. Rhabdomyolysis and simvastatin. Ann Intern Med 1991;114:342.
96. Berland Y, Vacher Coponat H, Durand C, Baz M, Laugier R, Musso JL. Rhabdomyolysis with simvastatin use. Nephron 1991;57:365–366.
97. Emmerich J, Aubert I, Bauduceau B, Dachet C, Chanu B, Erlich D, Gautier D, Jacotot B, Rouffy J. Efficacy and safety of simvastatin (alone or in association with cholestyramine). A 1-year study in 66 patients with type II hyperlipoproteinaemia. Eur Heart J 1990;11:149–155.
98. Feydy P, Bogomoletz WV. Un cas d'hépatite à la simvastatine. Gastroenterol Clin Biol 1991;15:94–95.
99. Ballaré M, Campanini M, Catania E, Bordin G, Zaccala G, Monteverde A. Acute cholestatic hepatitis during simvastatin administration. Rec Prog Med 1991;82:233–235.
100. Deslypere JP, Delanghe J, Vermeulen A. Proteinuria as complication of simvastatin treatment. Lancet 1990; 336:1453.
101. La Belle P, Mantel G. Simvastatin and proteinuria. Lancet 1991;337:864.
102. Pasternak RC, Kolman BS. Unstable myocardial ischemia after the initiation of niacin therapy. Am J Cardiol 1991;67:904–906.
103. Gibaldi M. Adverse drug effects. Perspect Clin Pharm 1991;9:3–8.
104. Etchason JA, Miller TD, Squires RW, Allison TG, Gau GT, Marttila JK, Kottke BA. Niacin-induced hepatitis. a potential side effect with low-dose time-release niacin. Mayo Clin Proc 1991;66:23–28.
105. Henkin Y, Johnson KC, Segrest JP. Rechallenge with crystalline niacin after drug-induced hepatitis from sustained-release niacin. J Am Med Assoc 1990;264:241–243.
106. Fischer DJ, Knight LL, Vestal RE. Fulminant hepatic failure following low-dose sustained-release niacin therapy in hospital. West J Med 1991;155:410–412.
107. Rader JI, Calvert RJ, Hathcock JN. Hepatic toxicity of unmodified and time-release preparations of niacin. Am J Med 1992;92:77–81.
108. Garg A, Grundy SM. Nicotinic acid as therapy for dyslipidemia in non-insulin-dependent diabetes mellitus. J Am Med Assoc 1990;264:723–726.
109. Schwartz ML. Severe reversible hyperglycemia as a consequence of niacin therapy. Arch Intern Med 1993; 153(17):2050–2052.
110. Earthman TP, Odom L, Mullins CA. Lactic acidosis associated with high-dose niacin therapy. Southern Med J 1991;84:496–497.
111. Carlson LA. The broad spectrum hypolipidaemic drug nicotinic acid. J Drug Dev 1990;3:223–226.
112. Litin SC, Anderson CF. Nicotinic acid-associated myopathy. A report of three cases. Am J Med 1989;86:481.
113. Reaven P, Witztum JL. Lovastatin, nicotinic acid, and rhabdomyolysis. Ann Intern Med 1988;109:597–598.
114. Gharavi AG, Diamond JA, Smith DA, Phillips RA. Niacin-induced myopathy. Am J Cardiol 1994;74:841–842.
115. Currie R. Side effects of acipimox (Olbetam). NZ Med J 1993;106(956):211.
116. Miller SM. Potential perils of niacin therapy. Clin Lab Sci 1991;4:156–158.
117. McKenney JM, Proctor JD, Harris S, Chinchili M. A comparison of the efficacy and toxic effects of sustained- vs immediate-release niacin in hypercholesterolemic patients. J Am Med Assoc 1994;271:672–677.
118. Gray DR, Morgan T, Chretien SD, Kashyap ML. Efficacy and safety of controlled-release niacin in dyslipoproteinemic veterans. Ann Intern Med 1994;121:252–258.
119. Luria MH. Atherosclerosis. the importance of HDL cholesterol and prostacyclin. a role for niacin therapy. Med Hypotheses 1990;32:21–28.
120. O'Kane MJ, Trinick TR, Tynan MB, Trimble ER, Nicholls DP. A comparison of acipimox and nicotinic acid in type 2b hyperlipidaemia. Br J Clin Pharmacol 1992;33:451–453.
121. Tornvall P, Walldius G. A comparison between nicotinic acid and acipimox in hypertriglyceridaemia—effects on serum lipids, lipoproteins, glucose tolerance and tolerability. J Intern Med 1991;230:415–21.
122. Ganzer BM. Langzeitstudie zu acipimox. Pharmazie 1990;135:31.
123. Laverzzari M, Milanesi G, Oggioni E, Pamparana F. Results of a phase IV study carried out with acipimox in type II diabetic patients with concomitant hyperlipoproteinaemia. J Int Med Res 1989;17:373–380.
124. Eritsland J, Arnesen H, Smith P, Seljeflot I, Dahl K. Effects of highly concentrated omega-3 polyunsaturated fatty acids and acetylsalicylic acid, alone and combined, on bleeding time and serum lipid profile. J Oslo City Hosp 1989; 39:97.
125. Smith P, Arnesen H, Opstad T, Dahl K, Eritsland J. Influence of highly concentrated n-3 fatty acids on serum lipids and hemostatic variables in survivors of myocardial infarction receiving either oral anticoagulants or matching placebo. Thromb Res 1989;53:467.
126. Davidson MH, Gwynne JT, Khachadurian AK, LaRosa JC, Miller ?, Lindner M et al. Combination of pravastatin and probucol in the treatment of primary hypercholesterolemia. Coronary Artery Dis 1991;2:1061–8.

127. Zimetbaum P, Eder H, Frishman W. Probucol. Pharmacology and clinical application. J Clin Pharmacol 1990;30:3–9.
128. Matsuhashi H, Onodera S, Kawamura Y, Hasebe N, Kohmura Y, Yamashita H, Tobise K. Probucol-induced QT prolongation and torsades de pointes. Jpn J Med 1989; 28:612–615.
129. Gohn DC, Simmons TW. Polymorphic ventricular tachycardia (torsade de pointes) associated with the use of probucol. N Engl J Med 1992;326:1435–1436.
130. Ohya Y, Kumamoto K, Abe I, Tsubota Y, Fujishima M. Factors related to QT interval prolongation during probucol treatment. Eur J Clin Pharmacol 1993;45(1):47–52.

Meyler's Side Effects of Drugs, 13th Edition
M.N.G. Dukes, editor

SECTION EDITOR: P.I. FOLB

P.I. Folb

45 Cytostatics and immunosuppressive drugs

CARDIOVASCULAR TOXICITY

Anthracyclines

Doxorubicin (adriamycin) This anthracycline has been documented to cause cardiotoxicity acutely in the form of arrhythmias (1^{R}) and in the long term as a dose-related cardiomyopathy. Several studies have shown cardiotoxicity early in treatment by electrocardiography, echocardiography (2^{C}, 3^{C}) or by serial radionuclide angiography (4^{R}). Endomyocardial sampling (5^{cr}) is probably most reliable, but its invasive nature precludes general use.

Anesthesia is difficult in patients with cumulative anthracycline-induced cardiotoxicity, and it has proved fatal on occasions (6^{cr}). Heart transplantation has been successful in patients with late, progressive cardiomyopathy without recurrence of the underlying malignant disease (7^{c}).

The development of cumulative dose-related cardiotoxicity limits the total dose of doxorubicin that can safely be administered, and the search continues for drugs which are as effective but lack this side effect. Although several anthracycline and anthraquinone derivatives appear to be less cardiotoxic than doxorubicin, patients nevertheless require careful monitoring for the development of cardiac symptoms and signs (7^{R}, 9^{C}—29^{C}).

Severe doxorubicin cardiotoxicity is generally considered irreversible, and it is associated with a poor prognosis and high mortality. However, four cases have been reported in which the advanced cardiac dysfunction associated with doxorubicin recovered completely (30^{C}).

Mortensen et al. (31^{c}) have studied 11 patients with anthracycline cardiotoxicity by heart catheterization and endomyocardial biopsy. Myocytic damage correlated linearly with cumulative dose. There was a non-linear relationship between electron microscopic changes and the extent of hemodynamic impairment. There was pronounced fibrous thickening of the endocardium in most patients, especially in the left ventricle. Endocardial fibrosis may be the first morphological sign of cardiotoxicity.

Chronic toxicity of the anthracyclines, particularly when used in children, has been addressed by Lipshultz et al. who conclude that doxorubicin in childhood impairs mycocardial growth in a dose-related manner resulting in progressive increase in left ventricular afterload, sometimes associated with impaired myocardial contractility (32^{Cr}).

Viniegra et al. (33^{Cr}) have shown that a significant number of patients receiving anthracycline therapy develop cardiac autonomic dysfunction.

Lahtinen et al. have performed a randomized double-blind study to compare the cardiotoxicity of epirubicin and doxorubicin. They found a significant decrease in left ventricle ejection fraction with doxorubicin but not with epirubicin (34^{c}).

An 11% incidence of ECG changes was attributed to aclarubicin used in the treatment of acute leukemia in adults. The author stated that aclarubicin does not necessarily share the toxic effects of either doxorubicin or daunorubicin, but does not comment on whether the cardiotoxicity of the different drugs given sequentially is additive (35^{CR}).

Abnormalities of right ventricular wall motion are added to the list of conduction defects documented as being due to doxorubicin (36^{c}).

The subtle chronic abnormalities in myocardial function that occur in children 10—20 years after anthracycline exposure are best detected by exercise echocardiography, since these patients may have normal resting cardiac function (37).

Further information regarding the pathogenesis of chronic anthracycline cardiotoxicity is provided in a report of 201 pediatric patients who received 200—1275 mg/m^{2} of doxorubicin and/or daunorubicin. Of these, 23% had abnormal cardiac function 4—20 years afterwards. In the group of patients followed-up for more than 10 years, 38% had abnormal cardiac function compared with 18% in the group followed up for less than 10 years (38, 39).

In another study, more than one-half of the children studied by serial echocardiogram, following doxorubicin therapy for acute lymphoblastic leukemia, developed increased left ventricular wall stress due to decreased wall thickness. This stress progressed with time (40[R]).

Casper et al. conducted a prospective randomized trial of adjuvant chemotherapy with bolus against continuous intravenous infusion of doxorubicin 60 mg/m^2 either as a bolus over a few minutes or by infusion over 72 hours. They defined cardiotoxicity as a 10% or greater decrease in left ventricular ejection fraction. They concluded that cardiotoxicity was seen in 61% of patients on bolus median dose equal to 420 mg/m^2 compared with 42% on the continuous infusion schedule median dose of 540 mg/m^2. Also, the rate of cardiotoxicity as a function of the cumulative dose of doxorubicin was significantly higher in the bolus treatment arm (41[C]). Thus, total dose, method of administration and source of the anthracycline all have an impact on the cardiotoxic profile of this group of drugs. All eventually have a cardiotoxic ceiling.

Moreb and Oblon concluded that 63% (n=19; all diagnosed with anthracycline-induced congestive cardiac failure) of patients recover from clinical anthracycline-induced congestive heart failure, although reversal of the cardiac problem may be modest and unpredictable (42[c]).

Corrected QT interval prolongation as a measure of myocardial repolarization may offer an easy, non-invasive test to predict those patients at special risk of late cardiac decompensation following anthracycline treatment for childhood cancer (43[c]).

Epirubicin Epirubicin is considered to cause less cardiotoxicity than doxorubicin (44[R]). This is possibly due to its more rapid clearance rather than a different action (45[r]).

Epirubicin is an epimer of doxorubicin with similar anticancer activity. Torti et al. (46[C]) have studied 29 patients treated with epirubicin in cumulative doses ranging from 147 to 888 mg/m^2. The ultrastructural myocardial lesions produced by epirubicin were similar to those produced by doxorubicin (partial and total myofibrillar loss in individual myocytes). With both drugs severe lesions were associated with replacement fibrosis. None of the patients who received epirubicin in the study developed congestive cardiac failure.

Idarubicin This anthracycline appears to have a profile of cardiotoxicity similar to that of older members of the series. It has been reported to cause short-term cardiac toxicity when used in high doses in leukemia, and there is no doubt a cumulative dose-related toxicity as well (47[R]).

Amsacrine (m-AMSA) Cardiac arrhythmias have been reported after amsacrine therapy in association with hypokalemia. Pre-existing supraventricular arrhythmias or ventricular ectopic beats are not absolute contraindications to its use (48[c]).

An estimation of the incidence of cardiotoxic reactions with m-AMSA has been made by Weiss et al. (49[R]). Of 5430 patients treated with m-AMSA, 65 developed cardiotoxicity, including prolongation of the QT interval, non-specific ST-T wave changes, ventricular tachycardia and ventricular fibrillation. Thirty-one patients had serious ventricular arrhythmias resulting in cardiopulmonary arrest; 14 died as a result. The arrhythmias occurred within minutes to several hours after drug administration. The manifestation of cardiotoxicity was not related to total cumulative dose, and hypokalemia was possibly a risk factor for the arrhythmias.

Cisplatin/5-fluorouracil There is reason to believe that these drugs exert synergistic cardiotoxicity. This is supported by evidence from Coninx et al. who have described patients with anginal pain and ischemic changes on ECG following combined administration of cisplatin 100 mg/m^2 and 5-fluorouracil 1000 mg/m^2 for 7 days (50[C]).

Coronary vascular spasm leading to myocardial infarction has been reported following 5-fluorouracil given in a total dose of 3000 mg/m^2 over 2 days (51[C]). This is the mechanism thought to underlie the cardiotoxicity of the drug (52[r]). There is a report of acute myocardial infarction, rather than generalized cardiomyopathy, occurring during cisplatin therapy (53[c]).

Evidence is mounting for a direct association between cisplatin and major cardiovascular events, including myocardial infarction (54[C]), angina pectoris, coronary heart disease and arterial occlusive events (55[cr]).

5-Fluorouracil (5-FU) The number of reports of 5-FU-induced cardiac toxicity manifesting as constrictive anginal chest pain during infusion is increasing. Non-specific ST-T electrocardiographic changes are seen. This is sporadic, and the outcome is favourable if the drug is stopped. Re-introduction of the drug has been associated with occasional fatal outcome and is not recommended (56[c]). Sudden deaths, presumed to be caused by ventricular fibrillation, have been reported (57[c], 58[c]). Acute dilated cardiomyopathy with left ventricular dysfunction related temporally to 5-FU and cisplatin infusion, with subsequent complete recovery, has been tentatively linked to 5-FU (59[c]). Other similar events have been reported (60[c], 61[c]).

The precise mechanisms of 5-FU cardiotoxicity are not known. Those that have been suggested include: (i) direct uncoupling of electromechanical myocardial function at the level of ATP generation (62[c]); (ii) an immunoallergic reaction following sensitization by a complex of 5-FU and cardiac cells; (iii) vasospasm secondary either to 5-FU or to released products; (iv) a direct toxic effect of the drug on the myocardium. Most reports have attributed chest pain to vasospasm (63[c]).

Keefe et al. have described the cardiotoxicity of 5-fluorouracil in a series of 910 patients; they found life-threatening toxicity in 0.55% (64[c]). Robben et al. reported on the cardiotoxicity of 5-FU in a review of 135 cases from the literature (65[CR]). Lynch et al. (66[c]) studied the cardiotoxicity of a combination of cisplatin, 5-FU and etoposide given for advanced non-small cell cancer of the lung. Whilst the combination caused only the expected amount of hematological toxicity, it was associated with a higher than expected incidence of cardiac, pulmonary and cerebrovascular toxicity, including two myocardial infarcts, two cases of congestive heart failure, one pulmonary embolus, and one cerebrovascular accident in a study of 35 patients.

Cisplatin Cardiotoxicity of cisplatin has been reported in a few cases, most of them heavily pretreated with other potentially cardiotoxic drugs. Fassio et al. (67[C]) have observed an untreated patient who developed paroxysmal supraventricular tachycardia during administration of cisplatin given in a dose of 20 mg/m^2 together with etoposide 75 mg/m^2. The arrhythmia appeared to be related to cisplatin since normal rhythm was restored after cisplatin was withdrawn.

Cisplatin/bleomycin/vinblastine Twenty-one cases have been reported of life-threatening disease affecting large arteries in patients treated with cisplatin, bleomycin and vinblastine in combination for germ cell tumors (68[CR], 69[CR]). Five patients died during or after therapy, three from acute myocardial infarction, one from rectal infarction, and one from cerebral infarction. Other patients who developed major vascular disease, including coronary artery and cerebrovascular disease, have been reported. Symptoms occurred acutely in some (within 48 hours of starting therapy) and after months or years had elapsed in others.

Gamelin et al. (70[C]) report a 5% incidence of cardiotoxicity complicating high-dose infusion of 5-FU (1000 mg/m^2/day for 4 days), and they correlated its development with plasma levels of the drug in excess of 450 mg/ml. Thyss et al. have shown significant elevation of endothelin plasma levels in patients with 5-FU cardiotoxicity (71[C]).

Cyclophosphamide High-dose cyclophosphamide (120—200 mg/kg) is often used in immunosuppression of patients for bone marrow transplantation. This dose may cause lethal cardiotoxicty with severe congestive heart failure developing 1—10 days after the first dose. Severe congestive heart failure is accompanied by ECG findings of diffuse voltage loss, cardiomegaly, pulmonary vascular congestion, and pleural and pericardial effusion. Pathological findings include hemorrhagic myocardial necrosis, thickening of the left ventricular wall and fibrinous pericarditis.

Goldberg et al. (72[C]) have studied 80 patients who received cyclophosphamide 50 mg/kg/day for 4 days in preparation for bone marrow grafting. Seventeen percent of patients had symptoms consistent with cyclophosphamide cardiotoxicity. Six died from congestive heart failure. Older patients were at greatest risk of developing cardiotoxicity.

Mitoxantrone Anthracyclines have the ability inherent in their quinone structure to form free-radical semiquinones which directly interact with oxygen causing peroxidation of the lipid membranes of the heart. However, this reaction has not been demonstrated with mitoxantrone, and the mechanism of its cardiotoxicity is unknown. The South West Oncology Group (73[CR]) reported on 801 patients treated with mitoxantrone; 1.5% developed congestive cardiac failure, an additional 1.5% had a reduced left ventricular ejection fraction (LVEF), and 0.25% developed acute myocardial infarction. Predisposing factors to mitoxantrone cardiotoxicity include increasing age, prior anthracycline therapy, previous cardiovascular disease, mediastinal radiotherapy, and a cumulative dose of the drug exceeding 120 mg/m^2.

Abnormalities in left ventricular ejection fraction have been described in 46% of patients (n=14) treated with mitotoxantrone (14 mg/m^2) and with vincristine and prednisolone (74[C]). Pre-existing history of cardiac disease or previous anthracycline exposure was excluded. Only one patient developed clinically overt congestive cardiac failure. Other reports have described less cardiotoxicity compared with the parent compound, doxorubicin (75[r], 76[r]).

In 801 patients treated with mitoxantrone prior treatment with doxorubicin and mitoxantrone was significantly associated with risk of cardiotoxicity, but age, sex and prior mediastinal radiotherapy were not useful predictors (77[c]).

Hypokinetic heart wall motion abnormalities and

early signs of chronic cardiomyopathy have been identified as a significant toxic effect of mitoxantrone in patients who received cumulative doses of 32—174 mg mitoxantrone (78[C]). Electrocardiographic T wave inversion and cardiac complications have been described in intensive therapy with mitoxantrone 40 mg/m^2 over 5 days and cyclophosphamide 1550 mg/m^2 for 4 days, given prior to bone marrow transplantation for metastatic breast cancer. All patients had had previous exposure to doxorubicin in cumulative doses that did not exceed 442 mg/m^2 (79[C]).

PULMONARY TOXICITY

Bleomycin *(SEDA-11, 937)* Diffuse interstitial pneumonitis with significant mortality is a well-recognized complication of bleomycin therapy. The mechanism of the toxicity is not known. Lipid peroxidation of cell membranes has been suggested, but recent work does not support this hypothesis (80[r]). Others have suggested a role for angiotensin-converting enzyme in production of the lung damage (81[r]), but the data are unconvincing. Lung toxicity may occur at low cumulative bleomycin doses during concurrent treatment with cyclophosphamide (which independently causes pulmonary toxicity). In a series of 19 patients (82[C]) there was a high (26%) incidence of fatal pulmonary toxicity in patients receiving the combination of these two drugs, which warrants special caution.

Estimates of the incidence of bleomycin pulmonary toxicity range from 11 to 23% (83[R]). Of 99 patients previously treated with bleomycin together with other cytostatic drugs for testicular tumors, 16 developed abnormal lung function tests; amongst those who received more than 500 mg bleomycin cumulatively, 75% had abnormal lung function tests, Raynaud's phenomenon or both (84[C]). Rapid progression to fatal pulmonary fibrosis has been documented previously and, in all but one instance, there had been previous or concurrent chest radiotherapy. Two cases have been reported of rapidly progressive fatal pulmonary fibrosis in patients receiving bleomycin who had had no previous lung disease, and who had not undergone radiotherapy to the chest (85[C]).

Bleomycin is also associated with a hypersensitivity pneumonitis. This should be considered when interpreting cytological swab preparations in patients treated with the drug, since the acute cytological changes may be misinterpreted (86[C]).

A syndrome of acute chest pain occurring during bleomycin infusion has been described in 10 patients with features which cannot be ascribed to pulmonary fibrosis, hypersensitivity pneumonitis or cardiovascular toxicity (87[C]). The pain was sudden in onset, occurring during the first or second course, usually on the second or third day. Retrosternal pressure or pleuritic in nature, in some cases it was severe enough to require narcotic analgesics. Stopping or slowing the infusion produced a marked improvement. In two of seven patients who received a subsequent course, the pain recurred. One patient experienced dyspnea and two developed an erythematous rash. On examination, one had a pleural friction rub, one a pericardial friction rub, and fever was noted during five episodes. There were no other physical abnormalities. ECG changes suggestive of pericarditis were noted in two patients; one patient developed transient blunting of a costophrenic angle on X-ray of the chest, and another a transient and small retrocardiac pulmonary infiltrate. The pain resolved spontaneously on analgesics, and there were no long-term pulmonary or cardiac sequelae. Possible underlying mechanisms include pleuropericarditis due to serosal inflammation or vascular pathology.

Busulfan Vergnon described three cases of busulfan-induced interstitial pneumonitis (88[c]). Each had circulating immune complexes and alveolitis, and histology demonstrated consistent abnormalities of type I pneumocytes and depletion of type II pneumocytes.

Ciclosporin (cyclosporine) Adult respiratory distress syndrome has been described after intravenous ciclosporin. It was thought that a high concentration of the drug in the pulmonary vasculature due to administration through a central vein was responsible for capillary leakage, but a patient has been reported in whom the pulmonary capillary leak resolved rapidly when the intravenous route of administration was changed to oral (89[c]). This suggested that cremaphor, the solvent for parenteral ciclosporin, was responsible. However, an adult patient has been described who developed respiratory distress syndrome in association with oral ciclosporin given after renal transplantation (90[C]).

Cyclophosphamide Twenty-nine cases of cyclophosphamide-induced pneumonitis have been described (91[c]). Considering the widespread use of this drug over many years, this is a rare adverse effect.

Mitomycin (mitomycin C) Biopsy-proven mitomycin pneumonitis occurred in five of 44 patients treated with the drug in conjunction with weekly low-dose doxorubicin (20 mg) (92[c]). The picture was of pulmonary infiltrates clinically and radiologically, progressive dyspnea and hypoxia, and improvement on steroids. The mean total dose of mitomycin that had been given in the five patients was 89 mg.

Verweij and co-workers have published the results of a prospective study of 44 patients treated with mitomycin (93[CR]). Combining their data with a review of the world literature, they conclude that the incidence of mitomycin-induced interstitial pneumonitis is less than 10%. This side effect is dose dependent, occurring at cumulative dose levels of 20 mg/m^2 or greater, although doses up to 30 mg/m^2 have been safe.

Linette et al. (94[R]) have concluded that mitomycin C causes pulmonary toxicity in between 2 and 38% of cases. It is characteristically of slow-onset, at cumulative doses greater than 79 mg/m^2 (94[C]).

Methotrexate In a review of the respiratory complications of methotrexate, the authors concluded that methotrexate pneumonitis occurs in 7% of patients, of which 25% are fatal as a result of respiratory failure (95[R]). This can occur with any dose of methotrexate, given via any route; it has occurred following 12 mg given intrathecally for central nervous system prophylaxis (96[c]).

Cisplatin and bleomycin Seven patients died from irreversible respiratory failure following combined cisplatin and bleomycin chemotherapy. Five had raised serum creatinine and all received cisplatin before the bleomycin. The authors recommended extreme caution with this combination, and suggested that bleomycin should precede the cisplatin infusion (97[CR]).

Carmustine Carmustine pulmonary toxicity is well documented. Hasleton et al. (98[C]) have described eight patients who developed interstitial pulmonary fibrosis 12—17 years after exposure to carmustine in a total dose of carmustine of 770—1410 mg/m^2. Lung fibrosis has been described in a long-term follow up 13—17 years after treatment of 31 children treated for brain tumours; six died, and of eight still available for study, six had upper zone fibrotic changes of their lungs on X-ray (99[C]).

Procarbazine The permanent and acute reversible forms of lung disease attributed to procarbazine have been reviewed (100[CR]).

Actinomycin Actinomycin increases the pulmonary toxic effects of radiation by an estimated 30%, and it reduces the radiation tolerance of the lung by at least 20% (101[CR]).

NEUROTOXICITY

Neurological symptoms occurring in patients with cancer are common; more than 20% of cancer patients develop this disability. Cytostatic therapy may increase the frequency of neurotoxicity in cancer patients. Acute and late neurotoxic syndromes involve a number of cytostatic agents (Table 1).

Acivicin Acivicin is a potent inhibitor of L-asparagine synthetase and other L-glutamine amidotransferases, and it kills the cell by blocking nucleotide biosynthesis. Besides myelotoxicity, acivicin has other neurological toxicity, manifesting in lethargy and auditory as well as visual hallucinations. Some patients experience nystagmus, incontinence and severe depression (102[c], 103[c]).

L-Asparaginase Thrombosis and hemorrhage are well recognized complications of L-asparaginase therapy in 1—2% of patients receiving the drug. This is due to the coagulopathy which has been variously attributed to decreased levels of fibrinogen, Factor IX, Factor XI, Factor VIII complex, antithrombin III and plasminogen (104[cr]). In a review of 28 central nervous system thrombotic or hemorrhagic events and eight peripheral thromboses related to L-asparaginase, the median time from initial treatment to adverse reaction was 16—17 days (105[r]). Most patients recovered completely, although five cases had residual neurological deficits and one died from superior sagittal sinus thrombosis.

Carmustine (BCNU) and nimustine (ACNU) Eye pain and blindness due to retinal and optic nerve damage are recognized hazards of intracarotid BCNU therapy. They are thought to be due, at least in part, to the ethanol content of the diluent. ACNU is water-soluble and ethanol-free. In a study of 30 patients with malignant gliomas, 123 infusions of ACNU and 53 BCNU were administered (106[c]). Eye pain was experienced during all BCNU infusions but not with ACNU, and one patient developed unilateral blindness after BCNU. In another study, BCNU was administered in solution with 5% dextrose in water (107[c]). All the patients experienced ipsilateral orbital pain and scleral erythema, suggesting that BCNU itself contributes to the toxicity. Seven additional patients were treated wearing an ocular compression device to decrease blood flow and had not experienced any ocular complications.

Cisplatin Infusions of cisplatin into the axillary artery have led to a bronchial plexopathy rather than the more

Table 1. *Cystostatic agents that may be toxic to the nervous system*

Drug	Neurotoxic effects
Alkylating agents	
Mechlorethamine	Rare encephalopathy following high doses
Chlorambucil	Disorientation, cognitive dysfunction
Ifosfamide	Mild memory disturbance
Nitrosoureas	
Carmustine	Brain damage in conventional doses when combined with radiation
Antimetabolites	
Methotrexate	Inthrathecal: acute meningitis; acute fatal cerebral dysfunction; chronic leukoencephalopathy
Fluorouracil	Cerebellar ataxia in high doses
Vidarabine	Generalized rigidity, myoclonic jerks
Cytarabine	Cerebellar ataxia in high doses
Vinca alkaloids	
Vincristine	Peripheral neuropathy, abdominal pain, constipation
Vinblastine	Jaw pain, myopathy, inappropriate ADH secretion
Vindesine	Overdose or accidental intrathecal injection is usually fatal
Cisplatin	Peripheral neuropathy, deafness, cerebral cortical blindness, epileptic seizures
Ciclosporin	Loss of visual acuity, visual hallucinations, seizures, tremor and depression
L-Asparaginase	Acute encephalopathy
Sparfosic acid (PALA)	Encephalopathy, seizures
2′-Deoxycoformycin	Lethargy, somnolence, coma
Nitroimidazole radiosensitisers	Peripheral neuropathy
Spirogermanium	Dizziness, somnolence, altered mental status, seizures in overdose

commonly described lumbosacral nerve plexus lesion (108[c]).

Cisplatin causes a well-recognized reversible sensory peripheral neuropathy, commencing with depressed deep tendon reflexes and loss of vibration sense, progressing to a sensory ataxia (109[c]). This may be age-related, as the use of high-dose cisplatin in children with neuroblastoma has not been associated with peripheral neuropathy (110[c]). Motor nerves are spared (111[r]).

Walker et al. have reported five cases of cerebral herniation following cisplatin therapy (112[C]). However, all had evidence of intracerebral tumour with mass effect and the herniation of the brain was thought to be multifactorial rather than directly attributable to cisplatin treatment.

Hypomagnesemia secondary to cisplatin administration may be severe enough to present as generalized seizures (113[R]). It more commonly presents with muscular weakness, tremulousness, peripheral paresthesias, tetany and personality changes. It is dose- and schedule-dependent. Loss of magnesium may be prevented by prophylactic magnesium infusion prior to and during cisplatin administration (114[c]), but this is not universally recommended because of the risk of acute uremia (115[r]).

Further evidence of paresthesias in the extremities developing 5 years after adjuvant cisplatin-based treatment for stages I and II testicular cancer has been reported; no acute cardiovascular complications were observed (116[c]). Four of eight children developed acute neurological toxicity. Three had seizures and one transient blindness following high-dose cisplatin (200 mg/m^2) administered by continuous infusion over 5 days, followed 10 days later by a further 2 days with 40 mg/m^2/day. These children showed the greatest deterioration in renal function, and they may have had impaired clearance of and increased exposure to cisplatin (117[c]). Sghirlanzoni et al., using a clinical model, demonstrated that peripheral neuropathy with clinical signs and/or symptoms was found in 80% of patients who had received a cumulative dose of 576 mg/m^2 of cisplatin. They demonstrated a dose-related decrease in sensory action potential amplitudes (118[C]). The clinical and neurophysiological time progression of the severity of cisplatin polyneuropathy during and after treatment with cisplatin up to a cumulative dose of 600 mg/m^2 has been described (119[C]). The paraneoplastic neuropathy experienced by women with epithelial ovarian cancer receiving cisplatin has been attributed in certain cases to the drug (120[C]). When three different schedules of cisplatin were evaluated with regard to the drug's neurotoxicity, using the same dose of 450 mg/m^2 for each of the schedules, it was found that cisplatin-induced peripheral neuropathy depended on both total-dose and single-dose intensity (121[C]).

Pratt et al. (122[C]) showed that neurotoxicity in 22 adolescents was related to the prior cumulative dose of cisplatin that had been received; the relative risk increased 3.2-fold up to a dose of 600 mg/m^2, and 4.1-fold up to a dose of 1340 mg/m^2. Persistent Lhermitte's signs suggestive of irreversible spinal cord toxicity have been reported (123[cr]). By comparing 50 mg/m^2 weekly with 75 mg/m^2 3 times weekly, using detailed neurological and neurophysiological examination, it has been concluded that cisplatin neuropathy is either of sensory or axonal type, and that both are related to total and single doses (124[C]). However, Pollera et al. believe that cisplatin-induced peripheral neurotoxicity is related to dose intensity rather than to the total dose received (125[cr]). A 47% incidence of peripheral neuropathy of all grades has been reported with cisplatin (126[Cr]), and a 31% 'off' therapy deterioration of peripheral neuropathy presenting as muscle cramps and demyelination syndromes has been described (127[Cr]).

High-dose cisplatin (CDDP) The use of aggressive hydration using hypertonic saline and sodium thiosulfate, with dose-scheduling, reduces the risks of dose-limiting nephrotoxicity of cisplatin, and this has made possible the use of high-dose cisplatin (defined as >200 mg/m^2/course). At such doses there are severe chronic peripheral neuropathy, ototoxicity and myelosuppression. There is evidence that these effects can be reduced by lengthening the infusion time of cisplatin (128[Cr]). Peripheral neuropathy is the commonest manifestation of cisplatin neurotoxicity; with high-dose administration the incidence and severity increase with the total dose, and it appears to be age-related. It was not seen in 47 children treated with high-dose cisplatin (40 mg/m^2/day for 5 days) for neuroblastoma (129[C]). Autonomic neuropathy, motor neuropathy and denervation changes in muscles are occasionally encountered. In a clinical and electrophysiological study of eight patients treated with high-dose cisplatin (800—1400 mg), in conjunction with etoposide and bleomycin, all developed a peripheral sensory neuropathy (130[C]). A reduction in vibratory sensation was the earliest manifestation of the neuropathy and the findings were compatible with primary damage to the dorsal root ganglia with a central-distal axonopathy. No motor nerve abnormalities were detected apart from one patient with carpal tunnel syndrome, but two patients had prolonged brainstem auditory-evoked potentials, indicating a central transmission defect. In another clinical and electrophysiological study of seven patients treated with cisplatin, the sensory neuropathy was also found to be of axonal type, with considerable involvement of proprioception (131[C]). Postmortem study of one case showed degeneration of the posterior columns of the spinal cord and evidence of neuronal loss in the lumbar spinal ganglion.

There have been several reports of local neurotoxicity after intra-arterial cisplatin. In 63 patients pretreated with low-dose cisplatin given by arterial infusion for head and neck cancer (up to 25 mg/day for 1—10 days), before definitive local treatment, cranial nerve palsies developed on the same side as the cannulated artery in four cases (132[C]). Ipsilateral involvement of the 9th, 10th, 11th and 12th cranial nerves occurred in two patients, and the 12th and 7th nerves alone were affected in the other two patients. The palsies appeared at the end of treatment or up to 10 days later and only the 12th nerve palsy in one of the patients with multiple cranial nerve involvement recovered completely. In each patient, no other cause for paresis was found and CT scans showed that the nerves were not infiltrated by tumour. The cumulative dose of cisplatin administered to these four patients was less than that received by the unaffected 59 patients (median 200 mg, range 160—250; compared with 250 mg, range 160—400 mg).

Eleven patients referred for neurological evaluation after cisplatin infusion into the internal or external iliac arteries for pelvic or lower limb tumours all developed symptoms within 48 hours of nerve or plexus dysfunction within the territory supplied by the cannulated artery (133[C]). The lumbosacral plexus was affected in nine patients, the femoral nerve in one, and the peroneal nerve in one. The doses of cisplatin ranged from 50 to 160 mg/m^2 and they did not correlate with the severity or course of the neuropathy. Small-vessel injury and infarction or a direct toxic effect seem likely explanations.

A correlation has been shown between the total dose of cisplatin and the vibratory perception threshold of the hand (134[c]).

Ciclosporin (cyclosporine) Various neurological syndromes have been reported with ciclosporin, including loss of visual acuity and visual hallucinations, and acute cerebral cortical blindness complicating ciclosporin therapy in a 5-year-old girl (135[C]).

Neurotoxicity is a serious side effect of ciclosporin treatment. Three patients who developed neurotoxicity following treatment with ciclosporin manifested with grand mal seizures and dysarthria. The plasma concentration of ciclosporin in these patients increased as the neurological signs appeared, and the signs resolved quickly after dose reduction (136[C]).

Prolonged confusion, where non-convulsive status epilepticus seemed to be the underlying cause, is a recognized complication of ciclosporin (137[CR]). A 19% incidence of central nervous system toxicity with ciclosporin has been reported in pediatric renal transplantation patients. The symptoms included seizures, drowsiness, confusion, hallucinations, visual disturbances and mental changes (138[CR]).

Cytarabine (ara-C, cytosine arabinoside) Central nervous system disturbance, especially impaired cerebellar function, is the dose-limiting toxicity for cytarabine, and age is known to be an important predictive factor. Of 418 patients who received 36—48 g/m^2 only 35 (8%) experienced severe cerebellar toxicity, which was irreversible or fatal in four (1%) (139[C]). Patients over 50 years of age are significantly more likely to develop cerebellar problems than younger patients (26/137, 19%, compared with 9/281, 3%); a second course did not increase the incidence, implying that it is the individual rather than the cumulative dose which is important. The cerebellar syndrome is the most common complication of high-dose cytarabine therapy.

In another study of the cerebellar syndrome caused by cytarabine (140[C]), in which it was found in seven of 30 patients (23%) treated, clinical symptoms of toxicity appeared between the third and seventh days of starting chemotherapy, manifesting first as lethargy and confusion (140[C]). Within the next 24 hours signs of cerebellar dysfunction were observed. These included dysarthria, ataxia, tremor, nystagmus and dysmetria. In most patients in whom neurotoxicity developed, liver function worsened during chemotherapy. Abnormal liver function at the start of therapy and development of neurotoxicity appear to be linked. The symptoms of neurotoxicity resolved within 4—49 days.

Signs of cerebellar dysfunction following administration of a lower dose of cytarabine (24 g/m^2), in association with aseptic meningitis, have been reported (141[c]). Aseptic meningitis may be observed in patients given intrathecal cytarabine. This may be the first case of aseptic meningitis following intravenous cytarabine.

Doxifluridine (5′-deoxy-5-fluorouridine) Doxifluridine is a compound of 5-fluorouracil. In a neurological evaluation of 17 patients treated with the drug 10 patients developed symptoms of central nervous system toxicity while receiving the drug in doses of 3 or 5 g/m^2/h/day for 5 days every 4 weeks for 3 months. The neurological symptoms, cerebellar and encephalopathic, developed simultaneously and were commonly first noted by the patients during the second week of the first cycle. The neurotoxicity was dose-related and it worsened during subsequent treatment. The symptoms of cerebellar disease ranged from a subjective feeling of unsteady gait to disability, while encephalopathy manifested by difficulties in concentration and with memory. Patients with marked weight loss and with a generalized dysrhythmia on ECG are at greatest risk of developing neurotoxicity with doxifluridine (142[C]).

Etoposide (VP-16-23) Acute neurological dysfunction with exacerbation of pre-existing neurological disorders has been reported following treatment with high-dose (>800 mg/m^2/day ×3 days) etoposide given with autologous bone marrow transplantation (143[C]). This happened 9—10 days after the start of treatment, and it abated without sequelae after prompt steroid therapy. Changes in intracranial pressure may explain this acute disturbance.

Fludarabine phosphate Fludarabine phosphate is a purine nucleoside antitumor agent, with ability to inhibit DNA synthesis. Dose-limiting myelotoxicity, nausea and vomiting, and elevation of liver enzymes were observed during early clinical studies. Fludarabine phosphate causes severe central nervous system toxicity (144[c]). A total of 70 patients with acute leukemia received 95 courses of the drug in daily doses ranging from 20 to 220 mg/m^2 for 5—7 days. Neurotoxicity was noted in 36% of patients who received doses greater than 96 mg/m^2/day, but in only 0.2% of patients treated with lower doses. The onset of neurological symptoms was delayed, appearing 21—60 days after the last course of fludarabine phosphate. Visual symptoms were the most common. Progressive deterioration of mental status or encephalopathy leading to a vegetative state developed in 11 patients. Clinicopathological findings showed a progressive demyelination in the central nervous system to be the main factor causing the neurotoxic symptoms.

Ifosfamide The development of convulsions, severe facial spasms and trismus 7 hours after an infusion of ifosfamide in a dose of 7 g/m^2, which had not occurred at a dose of 5 g/m^2, was reported during a phase II study of the drug used as a single agent ifosfamide in pediatric solid tumors (145[C]). A higher incidence of ifosfamide encephalopathy is associated with the oral form compared with the intravenous; this has been attributed to metabolic differences between the two (146[CR]).

Severe encephalopathy has been noted in children treated with ifosfamide (1.8 g/m^2) alone. No predisposing risk factors such as impaired renal function or lowered albumin were present. Electroencephalographic abnormalities and seizures were reversible, despite prolonged coma (147[c]).

Ifosfamide is associated with moderate toxicity and peripheral neuropathy when administered in combination with cisplatin (148[C]). These symptoms improved within a few days after treatment with haloperidol.

In an evaluation of ifosfamide in 57 pediatric patients with malignant solid tumors, all patients received 1.6 g/m^2/day for 5 days followed by mesna 400 mg/m^2 at 0.25, 4, and 6 hours after ifosfamide (149[C]). Neurological toxicity occurred in 13 patients. The usual symptoms were somnolence and general weakness followed by confusion, tremors, ataxia, aphasia, urinary incontinence and cranial nerve paralysis. The symptoms of neurotoxicity disappeared spontaneously within 72 hours of completion of the 5-day course. Some patients had a recurrence of neurotoxicity on rechallenge. In an analysis of the incidence and features of electroencephalographic changes associated with ifosfamide + mesna therapy there was no significant association between the EEG record before and during treatment; EEG changes developed 12—24 hours before clinical toxicity. Discriminant analysis identified low serum albumin, high serum creatinine levels, and pelvic involvement by the underlying malignant disease as factors predisposing to the development of severe encephalopathy (150[C]).

Methotrexate Reports of necrotizing leukoencephalopathy in association with methotrexate have been verified by biopsy or autopsy (151[c], 152[c]). Serial electroencephalography may predict this, with slow-wave activity developing with administration of high-dose methotrexate. Autopsy has shown widespread necrosis and spongiosis in the cerebral and cerebellar white matter in such cases (151[c]). Chronic brain edema, multifocal white matter necrosis and deep brain atrophy have been reported in patients who received high-dose methotrexate therapy, with an incidence of 4% (153[c]). All patients received 8—9 g/m^2 methotrexate intravenously over 4 hours. The encephalopathy began abruptly, an average of 6 days after the second or third weekly treatment, presenting with behavioural abnormalities. These ranged from laughter to lethargy or unresponsiveness. In some patients, there were focal sensorimotor or reflex signs and generalized seizures. The disorder lasted from 15 minutes to 72 hours, and it disappeared as abruptly as it began, without specific treatment.

Vinca alkaloids Neurotoxicity is dose-limiting with the vinca alkaloids. In a study of cindesine (154[C]), administered in a dose of 2 mg/m^2 on 2 consecutive days weekly, peripheral neuropathy with paresthesias was noted in four of 22 patients, and muscle weakness with loss of deep tendon reflexes in five patients. Neuropathies were pronounced at sites of pre-existing nerve damage. If a tumour had previously damaged peripheral nerves, or if a chordotomy had been performed, the paresthesias that developed at that site were often painful. Neurotoxicity was reversible, and the longest interval to full recovery was 3 months.

The vinca alkaloids may have a synergistic toxic effect on the nervous system. Amongst 17 patients with metastatic breast cancer given the four-drug combination, vincristine + vinblastine + doxorubicin + cyclosphosphamide, there was a high incidence of acute neurotoxicity observed at half the usual therapeutic dose of vincristine and vinblastine (155[c]).

Vincristine Pre-existing neurological disease may predispose to severe vincristine neuropathy (156[R], 157[R]); a diagnosis of Charcot-Marie-Tooth (CMT) disease is regarded as a contraindication to the use of the drug (158[C]). Four cases have been described of vincristine-induced neuropathy in CMT disease; one was fatal, and in the other three there was severe quadriplegia which recovered. A predisposition to development of vincristine neuropathy has been described in a patient with pre-existing Friedreich's ataxia (159[r]).

Scheduling of vincristine by 5-day infusion may reduce the risk of dose-related neurotoxicity manifesting as marked paresthesias, paralytic ileus and grand mal seizures (160[r]). In a study of seven patients (median age 7 years), limb and jaw muscle pain starting at days 3—5 of the infusion requiring opiate analgesia was the most pronounced toxic effect (161[c]).

In a prospective double-blind placebo-controlled study, concurrent oral administration of 500 mg glutamic acid three times daily with vincristine reduced the incidence of subjective and objective signs of vincristine neurotoxicity (162[C]). There were no differences in constipation, weakness or loss of knee reflexes. Severe gastrointestinal side effects were not noted.

Platinum and vinca alkaloid regimens Decreased peripheral circulation, Raynaud's phenomenon, and polyneuropathy has been described following the combined use of cisplatin, bleomycin and vinblastine for testicular tumors. Of eight cases with polyneuropathy that were investigated, it was not possible to confirm an causative association between Raynaud's phenomenon and the chemotherapy (163[c]).

Cranial nerve toxicity of the vinca alkaloids is less well documented. Three cases have been reported of vincristine-induced laryngeal nerve paralysis (164[C]). Forty patients have been described with orofacial pain developing as a manifestation of neuropathy about 3 days after vincristine administration, lasting for a mean duration of 2 days. One-half of the patients were affected in the first week, and the occurrence of pain was commonest in young patients and in smokers; it was dose-related (165[c]).

Busulfan High concentrations of busulfan in the cerebrospinal fluid have been correlated with development of myoclonic epilepsy and/or other electroencephalographic changes, following high-dose busulfan conditioning regimens for acute leukemia (166[c]).

Methotrexate A rare case of a reversible neurological disturbance associated with focal subcortical white matter pathology has been described after administration of 3 g/m^2 methotrexate. In patients receiving 8–12.5 g/m^2 methotrexate the incidence of neurological abnormality was 4%. All of these patients were also receiving methotrexate intrathecally as well, but the relevance of this is not known (167[c]).

HEPATOTOXICITY

Azathioprine Four cases have been reported of hepatotoxicity characterized by severe jaundice and intrahepatic cholestasis, presenting in patients receiving azathioprine (168[c]).

Cholestatic hepatitis is an uncommon adverse effect of azathioprine. Veno-occlusive disease (SEDA-12), and an unusual diffuse liver disease with sinusoidal dilatation (SEDA-11) have been described. An association with hepatocellular necrosis is less clear. A patient has been reported in whom hypersensitivity to azathioprine was associated with biochemical hepatitis and a normal liver biopsy appearance besides marked lipofuscin deposition (169[C]). These findings, combined with patchy isotope uptake on technetium scintigraphy, are suggestive of focal hepatocellular necrosis which has not previously been described as a manifestation of azathioprine hypersensitivity.

Four patients with renal transplants developed hepatic veno-occlusive disease after immunosuppression with azathioprine. The diagnosis of was based on typical histopathological findings: perivenular fibrosis, trilobular sinusoidal dilatation and congestion, and perisinusoidal fibrosis. The patient presented with severe progressive portal hypertension followed by fulminant liver failure and death. The disease was associated with cytomegalovirus infection, and it was not related to the dose of azathioprine that had been administered (170[c]).

Ciclosporin (cyclosporine) At least one episode of hepatotoxicity occurred in 228 of 466 patients (49%) with renal transplants who were treated with ciclosporin. Laboratory analysis of the patients experiencing hepatotoxicity indicated that 110 (48%) had hyperalbuminemia, 108 (47%) an elevated SGOT, and 167 (59%) an elevated AP. Ciclosporin dose reduction resulted in resolution of hepatotoxicity in 185 patients (81%), while 32 (14%) experienced recurrent or persistent liver function abnormalities. Eleven (2.4%) of the patients developed biliary calculous disease. The concentration of ciclosporin in the serum was high among the patients with hepatotoxicity (171[C]). Pharmacokinetic studies showed an increased area under curve of the drug, probably accounted for by decreased drug clearance in the hepatotoxic patients.

A causal association has been shown between the hepatotoxicity of ciclosporin and cold ischemic liver damage occurring during preservation prior to liver transplantation (172[C]). This presents a problem when ciclosporin is used following liver transplantation. In a study of more than 1000 patients, an incidence of mild reversible hepatoxicity of 40% was found in patients receiving 5-fluorouracil and levamisole as adjuvants for more than 1 year. The toxicity was predominantly elevated alkaline phosphatase, associated with elevation of transaminase or serum bilirubin. The incidence of mild hepatotoxicity in the group receiving levamisole alone, and amongst those receiving no treatment at all, was the same—a little more than above 16% (173[C]).

Cyclophosphamide Cyclophosphamide-induced, dose-dependent hepatic injury is probably caused as a result of impaired clearance of the metabolite, acrolein (174[r]). This presents clinically as raised serum aminotransferase levels (175[c]), and it may be aggravated by prior exposure to azathioprine.

Dacarbazine (DTIC) Hepatotoxicity has been reported with single-dose dactinomycin (176[C]) and DTIC (177[c], 178[c]), presenting as acute liver necrosis with hepatic venous thrombosis which may be fatal.

Fatal hepatotoxicity has been associated with dacarbazine following 500 mg/day for 5 days (179[c]). The cause of this reaction is unclear; an allergic hepatic vasculitis with thrombosis is possible.

Dactinomycin (actinomycin D) Severe hepatotoxicity, not found with standard treatment schedules, has been noted in children treated with a pulsed, intensive regimen actinomycin D for Stages I and II Wilm's tumors of favorable histology (180[C]). The treatment regimen included 15 μg/kg/day actinomycin D for 5 days in weeks 1, 5 and 13, together with vincristine. Five of 40 patients who received the pulsed regimen of 60 μg/kg actinomycin D every 3 weeks up to and including week

15, developed severe hepatotoxicity, manifesting with sharp rises in liver function test values, ascites and liver enlargement. One child with complicating factors died, the others recovered. All five had possible contributing factors, such as repeated anesthesia.

Floxuridine (5′-fluoro-5′-deoxyuridine; FUDR) Floxuridine is used in regional arterial chemotherapy for primary and metastatic malignancies, delivered using an implantable pump. The principle of hepatic arterial infusion is based on the fact that hepatic tumours derive much of their blood supply from the hepatic artery, whereas the liver parenchyma receives its supply from the portal venous circulation.

Acute and chronic cholecystitis has been reported, secondary to floxuridine hepatic artery infusion (181[c]). Chemotherapy in this patient was associated with persistent epigastric pain with radiation to the back which was not accompanied by any fever or white blood cell elevation. Cholescystectomy revealed a shrunken, thickened fibrotic gallbladder that was filled with thick, pasty, hemorrhagic material. There were no gallstones.

Methotrexate Elevation of the plasma phenylalanine/tyrosine ratio in pediatric and adolescent patients may provide clinical evidence of liver damage prior to the appearance of clinical symptoms in patients who have been treated with high doses of methotrexate (182[c]).

Elevated AST levels are common in patients receiving methotrexate for prolonged periods. These may indicate cirrhosis. Measurement of the serum aminoterminal propeptide of Type III procollagen (PIII PI) has been used as an alternative to liver biopsy; high levels correlate with fibrosis on liver biopsy (183[r]). No patient with a normal serum PIII NP level had an abnormal biopsy.

Hepatotoxicity due to long-term administration of low-dose methotrexate is a serious side effect of treatment in patients with chronic non-neoplastic disorders such as psoriasis or rheumatoid arthritis. Since routine liver function tests are not a reliable indicator of liver damage, and they may become abnormal when there is already considerable liver damage, it is common practice to monitor patients by conducting annual liver biopsies. Folate depletion may be a factor in the pathogenesis of methotrexate-induced liver disease. In a study of 30 patients on long-term methotrexate therapy, aimed at determining whether erythrocyte levels of folate and methotrexate might provide an indication for liver biopsy, no difference was found between red cell levels of folate in patients with cirrhosis or progressive liver fibrosis, and patients without fibrosis or with non-progressive hepatic fibrosis. Erythrocyte methotrexate levels were higher in patients with progressive hepatic disease, but cumulative dose and length of treatment were stronger predictors. In individual cases, erythrocyte folate and methotrexate levels were not a reliable guide (184[C]).

In 22 of 29 patients (76%) who were treated with low-pulse doses of methotrexate for rheumatoid arthritis, liver biopsy specimens showed variability in liver cell nuclear size, glycogenated nuclei, and fatty change. A mild portal infiltration with lymphocytes was found occasionally. There were no significant differences in age, duration of treatment or cumulative dose amongst the cases. Serial elevation of serum aminotransferase and/or alkaline phosphatase levels and development of hypoalbuminemia during treatment were indicators of development of liver disease (185[C]).

In a meta-analysis of 636 patients from 15 studies who received low-dose chronic methotrexate therapy it was concluded that the risk of liver toxicity is substantial and that it increased with cumulative dose and heavy alcohol intake (186[C]). At cumulative doses of 1500 mg, methotrexate has a consistent effect on a number of liver parameters (187[C]).

Thiopurines The thiopurines (azathioprine, 6-mercaptopurine and 6-thiouracil) are implicated in peliosis hepatitis (a liver vascular disorder) (188[c]) and hepatic veno-occlusive disease. Azathioprine has been associated with development of nodular regenerative hyperplasia of the liver (189[c]). It is possible that this precedes the veno-occlusive disease.

Actinomycin D Four cases of hepatotoxicity occurred when actinomycin D was studied in a United Kingdom trial of the treatment of Wilm's tumor; there was a steep dose-toxicity relationship (190[CR], 191[r]). There is evidence from other studies of Wilm's tumour that hepatotoxicity of actinomycin D is dose- and schedule-dependent; mild hepatotoxicity is described in up to 12% of patients (192[R]).

Thioguanine The United Kingdom Medical Research Council chronic myeloid leukemia group reported 18 cases of thioguanine-induced non-cirrhotic portal hypertension. This was commonly associated with deterioration in liver function (193[C]).

NEPHROTOXICITY

Cisplatin (*cis*-dichlorodiammine platinum; CDDP) Cisplatin is nephrotoxic, and the nephrotoxicity is often dose-limiting (194[R]). This is mainly due to proximal tubular dysfunction (195[r]), and the risk is lessened by adequate hydration which reduces drug concentration in the renal tubules. Impaired renal function may continue for at least 6 months after treatment has been discontinued.

Sodium thiosulfate protects against cisplatin-induced nephrotoxicity by reacting covalently with cisplatin in the renal tubules. Other protectors include probenecid, orgotein, fosfomycin (196[c]), amifostine (WR-2721) and anthiol. The beneficial role of furosemide is uncertain.

Cisplatin-induced nephrotoxicity may be detected by a rise in blood urea or creatinine clearance. Tubular dysfunction may manifest in a fall in serum levels of sodium (197[r]), potassium, magnesium (198[r]), and phosphorus.

Hyponatremia has been reported secondary to renal sodium loss (199[R]), and inappropriate ADH secretion may be partly responsible (200[r]).

Renal magnesium wasting is the main mechanism responsible for the hypomagnesemia associated with cisplatin (201[r]), and it may be associated with enhanced tubular reabsorption of calcium and consequent hypocalciuria (202[r]). This dissociation in the renal handling of calcium and magnesium is similar to what is found in Bartter's syndrome. The site of the renal tubular defect in these conditions is not known, but there is evidence that the active renal tubular transport systems are disrupted.

The nephrotoxicity of cisplatin is primarily tubular, although changes in renal blood flow and glomerular filtration also occur, and hypomagnesemia is common (SEDA-12; 203[R], 204[R]). Proximal tubular damage is well recognized, and fragments of distal tubular cells have been demonstrated in the urine of patients receiving chemotherapy that included cisplatin (205[c]). Although the use of hydration and saline diuresis has improved the situation, it remains an important clinical problem and research continues into ways of reducing the nephrotoxicity of cisplatin and into seeking less toxic analogs.

In experiments in mice the trace element selenium, which interacts with heavy metals, reduces the renal, intestinal, hepatic and hematological toxicity of cisplatin without affecting its antitumour activity (206).

WR-2721, an organic thiosulfate compound which has been shown in animal studies to protect normal tissues against toxicity of radiation, cisplatin and alkylating agents, has been used in pretreatment of patients with metastatic melanoma before administration of cisplatin 60—150 mg/m^2 in an uncontrolled trial of 36 patients (207[C]). There was a response rate of 53% and a low incidence of nephrotoxicity; transient nephrotoxicity occurred in 4% of 82 courses of WR-2721 given with 120 mg/m^2 cisplatin.

A number of case reports describe hypomagnesemia and renal magnesium wasting following administration of cisplatin. In a prospective study of 28 patients who received a total of 82 doses of cisplatin hypomagnesemia occurred in all patients and it was associated with significant and prolonged dose-related magnesium wasting. Serum magnesium was 1.8 ± 0.1 mg/100 ml after the fourth dose. Examination of the urine sediment 2—4 days after each dose of cisplatin revealed renal tubular epithelial cells, suggesting that the drug directly injures the tubules, leading to decreased tubular reabsorption of magnesium, renal magnesium wasting and hypomagnesemia (208[C]). In another study, patients receiving cisplatin and concomitant magnesium supplementation developed significantly less renal tubular damage as assessed by urine *N*-acetyl-β-D-glucosaminidase (209[c]). No patient developed clinical signs of hypomagnesemia when intravenous or oral supplementation of magnesium was given as soon as the serum magnesium fell to or below 0.45 mmol/l. In patients receiving intracavitary cisplatin in high doses (100—200 mg/m^2) together with intravenous thiosulphate there was a lower incidence of hypomagnesemia as a result of the thiosulfate; thiosulfate probably inactivated cisplatin before it reached the kidney, by complex formation (210[c]).

Carboplatin Carboplatin is a second-generation platinum analog with dose-limiting myelosuppression. When used at doses causing similar hematological toxicity to cisplatin, it has negligible renal, neurological and auditory toxicity (211[r]—214[r]). In combination with other cytotoxic agents the maximum tolerated dose is less than normal because of the risk of myelosuppression (215[r]). However, if the dose is increased, as happens in treatment of acute non-lymphocytic leukemia when 200—300 mg/m^2 daily for 5 days are given, high-tone hearing loss and renal impairment may develop (216[C]). In this study, all but one patient developing these side effects had also received aminoglycoside antibiotics.

Mild to moderate reduction in creatinine clearance with elevation in serum urea and creatinine were reported in 14.3% of patients receiving carboplatin in a dose of 400 mg/m^2 for gynecological malignancies. Of the patients who received carboplatin 400 mg/m^2 with vincristine but without hydration for lung cancer, 19% developed renal changes. Hyperzincuria and hypozincemia can occur concurrently in patients treated with cisplatin, due to variable excretion of zinc in these cases (217[C]).

Cisplatin, in combination The effect of age on nephrotoxicity after treatment with ifosfamide or cisplatin has been studied (218[C]). Children aged 5 years or less had more severe proximal tubular toxicity associated with ifosfamide than older patients. They also had significantly lower plasma phosphate levels and a higher fractional excretion of glucose. There was no evidence of glomerular or distal renal tubular damage after ifosfamide, and no difference was found between the older and younger children in any other aspect of renal function. In general, patients' age predicts independently for the likelihood and severity of genitourinary toxicity caused by cisplatin in combination chemotherapy (219[C]).

Ciclosporin The renal toxicity of ciclosporin has been described as being an adverse effect of the drug on the compensatory mechanisms of the kidney, without proximal tubular function (urea and sodium reabsorption) being affected (220[CR]). A rise in serum creatinine level may be adequate to identify acute-onset ciclosporin nephrotoxicity, but it is not suitable for identification of chronic, late-onset ciclosporin nephrotoxicity (221[r]).

Intrarenal vasoconstriction may play an important part in the nephrotoxicity of ciclosporin, particularly the acute nephrotoxicity (222[R]). A marked reduction in renal blood flow associated with an increase in renal vascular resistance, probably due to post-glomerular vasoconstriction, has been demonstrated in acute ciclosporin toxicity (223[C], 224[C]). The explanations that have been proposed include activation of the renin-angiotensin system, prostaglandin inhibition and sympathetic nervous system activation (225[r]).

It is less clear whether hemodynamic alterations are important in chronic ciclosporin nephrotoxicity. The main morphological abnormality that has been demonstrated in the kidneys of patients receiving ciclosporin long-term is interstitial fibrosis. Vascular lesions, predominantly arteriolar, with arterial intimal fibrosis have been noted in renal biopsies from patients with chronic ciclosporin nephrotoxicity (226[C]).

The long-term effects of ciclosporin on renal function in 11 liver transplant recipients were evaluated over a follow-up period of 6–26 months (227[C]). Immediately post-operatively, glomerular filtration rate (GFR) and effective renal plasma flow (ERPF) fell by 60%, subsequently settling at 45–60% of normal. There were additional toxic effects on renal tubular function. Histopathological findings were mild to moderate; notably, arterial and arteriolar nephrosclerosis. Renal function improved as the dose of ciclosporin was reduced, despite continued administration of the drug. This suggests a persistent, potentially reversible, functional component to chronic ciclosporin nephrotoxicity. Whether this is in the main vascular or tubular is unclear.

The respective roles of organ preservation and ciclosporin in the pathogenesis of post-transplant renal damage have been studied in an in vitro model that simulates the hypothermic kidney preserved before surgery in Collins' solution and exposed after transplantation to ciclosporin (228). The results showed that preservation sensitizes the kidney to ciclosporin injury, which is consistent with clinical experience (229[R]). If the preserved kidney cells were given a period of repair before administration of ciclosporin, further injury did not happen. In animal experiments prolonged cold preservation causes progressive deterioration in the renal cortical microcirculation; concentration of ciclosporin in the renal cortex of hypoperfused kidneys markedly potentiates the vascular damage caused by cold preservation (230). In animal studies the calcium blocker, nifedipine, moderates the toxic effects of long-term exposure to ciclopsorin.

In a retrospective study of 106 patients following renal transplantation who had been treated with ciclosporin, 85% were hypertensive compared with 54% of patients taking azathioprine becoming hypertensive (231[C]). Renal function was significantly better in hypertensive patients treated with nifedipine than with other antihypertensive medication (β-blockers and vasodilators), and it was similar to that of normotensive patients treated with ciclosporin.

It is important to monitor plasma levels in order to minimize the risk of ciclosporin nephrotoxicity. Ciclosporin pharmacokinetics vary considerably between patients, and even in an individual patient from time to time, with changes in the clinical condition and treatment, particularly with administration of other drugs (232[C]). In a study of ciclosporin use in 53 bone marrow transplant recipients in which the drug was used to suppress graft-versus-host disease, 63% developed acute nephrotoxicity (233[C]). These patients had significantly higher plasma ciclosporin levels during the first month post-transplant than those patients who did not develop acute nephrotoxicity, even though they received the same cumulative dose. Children received a higher cumulative dose, but their plasma levels did not differ significantly from the adults, and they suffered less nephrotoxicity.

Ciclosporin and ketoconazole used together (the latter elevates the serum concentration of the former) are liable to cause severe nephrotoxicity. Plasma levels of ciclosporin may become excessively high in patients receiving the two drugs concomitantly (234[c]).

Renal morphology has been studied in 17 patients who received ciclosporin for sight-threatening uveitis. Most had not received other potentially nephrotoxic drugs. Variable interstitial fibrosis, frequently associated with tubular atrophy, was noted in all 17. The extent of the pathological changes did not correlate with the age, treatment period or average cumulative dose (235[C]). Ciclosporin nephrotoxicity mimics the histological features of acute allograft rejection and tubular necrosis. It is important to be able to distinguish clinically between ciclosporin toxicity on the one hand (necessitating a reduction in dose) and rejection (requiring an increase in dose) on the other.

Ciclosporin nephrotoxicity is aggravated when the drug is given together with other nephrotoxic agents. Severe nephrotoxicity has been reported in three renal transplant patients who received ciclosporin and gentamicin, and in others receiving both drugs before surgical procedures, even though toxic serum levels of either drug were not reached (236[c]).

Cyclophosphamide and ifosfamide Each of these drugs causes a hemorrhagic cystitis in a high proportion of patients, with an occasionally fatal outcome. The damage to urinary bladder epithelium is caused by acrolein, a metabolite of each that is excreted in the urine. In bone marrow transplant recipients, prior administration of busulfan which itself causes hemorrhagic cystitis may increase this risk of cyclophosphamide (237[C]). Mesna (2-mercaptoethane sodium sulfonate) is used to prevent this toxicity. It is excreted by the kidney, and it binds and detoxifies acrolein which is then excreted in the urine; mesna also prevents the breakdown of acrolein precursors. Intravesical prostaglandin E_2 has been suggested for treating this toxic cystitis (238[c]).

Renal toxicity of ifosfamide in children appears to be temporary. Children and adolescents given cumulative doses of 32—112 g/m^2 showed only transient disturbances in renal function (250[Cr]). In a series of five children with renal tubular Fanconi syndrome caused by the drug, all went on to develop rickets in the face of declining renal function. None had had pre-existing tubular damage and the syndrome developed at cumulative doses of ifosfamide of 39—99 g/m^2. Typical low serum bicarbonate and phosphate levels were noted, and supplementation of these resulted in bone healing but not renal recovery (251[c]).

High-dose methotrexate Renal toxicity is seen with high-dose methotrexate. This is more likely to occur with concomitant administration of other nephrotoxic agents such as aminoglycosides, cephalosporins, non-steroidal anti-inflammatory agents and diuretics (239[R]).

The pathogenesis of methotrexate-induced nephrotoxicity is not understood, but it is thought to be the result of crystallization of methotrexate in the renal tubules. Adequate hydration and urinary alkalinization are necessary to minimize this effect (240[r]). Urinary β_2-microglobulin may be a useful marker of methotrexate nephrotoxicity (241[r]).

When the serum levels of the drug are high, leucovorin rescue may protect against renal failure. Methotrexate levels are only transiently lowered by hemoperfusion, and they are unaffected by peritoneal dialysis once there is acute renal failure. Sustained reduction in drug levels and recovery of renal function have been reported following charcoal hemoperfusion followed by hemodialysis (242[c], 243[c]).

Coadministration of methotrexate and procarbazine in the treatment of medulloblastomas increases the risk of methotrexate nephrotoxicity. Delayed administration of methotrexate until 72 hours after procarbazine therapy has been given may decrease this risk (244[c]).

Mitomycin (mitomycin C) Hemolytic uremic syndrome has previously been described in more than 50 patients treated with mitomycin (245[R]). It presents as Coombs-negative microangiopathic hemolytic anemia, thrombocytopenia and renal failure, and the outcome is often fatal. The underlying pathology is thought to be drug-induced vascular endothelial damage. It occurs 4—7 months after the start of chemotherapy. Blood transfusion may cause clinical deterioration in those affected (246[r]). Treatment with hemodialysis and immunosuppressive drugs is not always successful.

Histology of the kidney in the hemolytic uremic syndrome caused by mitomycin shows mesangial proliferative glomerulonephritis with partial thickening and/or splitting of the basement membrane. On electron microscopy there is accumulation of non-homogeneous material in the subendothelial spaces. Neither immunoglobulin nor complement deposition is found (247[r]).

Other clinical reports have also brought attention to the association of hemolytic uremic syndrome with mitomycin (248[c], 249[C]).

Interferon-α The nephrotoxicity of interferon-α_{2B} has been studied at clinical and subclinical levels. Using a number of markers of renal function, all patients receiving interferon showed up to 20% deterioration in renal glomerular and tubular function (252[c]).

GASTROINTESTINAL TOXICITY

A retrospective analysis over 13 years of cytotoxic therapy for various conditions revealed 12 cases in which chemotherapy had induced gastrointestinal perforation (253[CR]). Six doses of etoposide each of 250 mg/m^2 induced an advanced stage (grade 4) of mucositis. Fifty percent of patients receiving epirubicin 120 mg/m^2 developed grade 2 or 3 mucositis. Severe stomatitis complicated epirubicin 1250 mg/m^2 (254[C]). Increased intestinal permeability has been shown in children receiving low-dose methotrexate therapy (255[CR]).

Oral cyclophosphamide in combination therapy A case of toxic megacolon following five cycles of epirubicin 70 mg/m^2, 5-FU 500 mg/m^2 and oral cyclophosphamide 75 mg/m^2 for 14 days has been reported. The clinical presentation includes an elevated erythrocyte sedimentation rate and a colonic diameter of greater than 9 cm; the outcome may be fatal (256[c]). Two-thirds of patients treated with cyclophosphamide orally for 4 months and intravenous 5-FU and methotrexate (CMF) for breast cancer developed Barrett's epithelium, presumably as a result of CMF-induced esophagitis (257[C]). An esophagitic mechanism, rather than one of mucosal re-epithelialization by undifferentiated stem cells has been proposed (258[r]).

Other drugs In an endoscopic study of the acute gastroduodenal toxicity of intravenous cisplatin 10 mg/m^2 and etoposide 107 mg/m^2 (mean dose) given for three doses, a significant number of patients developed gastroduodenal lesions several of which progressed (259[c]).

SKIN TOXICITY

Ciclosporin (cyclosporine) Changes in facial appearance have been described in 19 children treated with ciclosporin and prednisone after renal transplantion (260[C]). There was coarsening of facial features with thickening of the nares, lips and ears, puffiness of the cheeks, prominence of the supraorbital ridges, and mandibular prognathism. This was found in all the children who had been treated for 6 months.

Hypertrichosis was noted in 95% of 56 diabetics receiving ciclosporin long-term (261[C]). Ninety-five percent of the patients developed hypertrichosis due to an increase in the number of hairs and conversion of vellous to terminal hair. This appears to be a direct effect of ciclosporin rather than androgen-mediated, and with cessation of therapy it reverted to normal telogen effluvium.

Cyclophosphamide High doses of cyclophosphamide can induce the erythrodysesthesia syndrome, that is, a plantar-palmar erythema of the hands and feet (262[C]).

Cytosine arabinoside/5-fluorouracil (5-FU) Acute, painful, swollen and self-limiting erythema of the hands and soles has been reported following induction therapy for acute myeloid leukemia (263[Cr]). Histology was not specific. This has been attributed to cytosine, and it has also been documented in association with protracted (5-FU) infusion (264[c]). 5-FU commonly causes other mucocutaneous complications such as hyperpigmentation and multiple pigmented macules (265[c]).

Mitomycin C There have been several reports of erythematous blistering skin eruption of the palms and soles affecting patients treated with intravesical mitomycin. This has been attributed to a contact dermatitis, but more widespread skin involvement and an association with eosinophilic interstitial cystitis suggest that it may be a more generalized allergic reaction (266[C], 267[C], 268[c]—270[c]).

Extravasation of mitomycin causes inflammation and ulceration starting within 7—10 days, lasting several weeks. Four cases have been reported in whom the onset of tissue necrosis was delayed several weeks or months after exposure (271[C], 272[C]). In one case ulceration seemed to have been precipitated by drinking ethanol, and in another by exposure to the sun.

Mitoxantrone (mitozantrone) Mitoxantrone can cause the urine and sclera to turn blue or blue-green (273[c], 274[c]). There has been a single report of hidradenitis associated with mitoxantrone (275[c]). Painful onycholysis, blue discoloration of the nails (276[c]), and reversible loss of fingernails (277[c]) have been described.

Teniposide Dose-related, non-IgE-mediated hypersensitivity has been reported in 16 children receiving teniposide (278[C]). Other published reports of hypersensitivity or anaphylactoid reactions to teniposide include degranulation of basophils (279[c], 280[Cr]), and eight anaphylactic reactions in pediatric patients, all associated with the use of intravenous teniposide in a dose of 150 mg/m^2 (281[C]).

Other drugs Hypersensitivity reactions have been ascribed to a variety of drugs: cytarabine, azathioprine, methotrexate, and asparaginase (282[C]—284[C], 285[c], 286[Cr]).

Platinum compounds Six cases of type 1 anaphylactic reactions to platinum compounds (cisplatinum or carboplatin) have been reported (287[c]). In another series, 16 patients of more than 200 experienced allergic reactions to carboplatin (288[C]). The authors warn about the risk of immediate anaphylactoid reactions, especially with multiple courses of therapy, given the common use of carboplatin in out-patients.

Mitomycin C Three cases of allergic dermatitis have been described following intravesical mitomycin C (289[c]). A type IV hypersensitivity reaction was demonstrated on patch testing. Six cases of purpuric allergic drug eruption from intravesicular mitomycin C have been reported which the authors believe may be the first such reports, despite the frequency (9%) of allergic cutaneous reactions to mitomycin C (290[c]).

Other drugs in combination Five of 32 patients treated with the alternating drug regimen CAMBO-VIP (cyclophosphamide, doxorubicin, methotrexate, bleomycin, vincristine, etoposide, ifosfamide and prednisolone) for non-Hodgkin's lymphoma have been reported to have developed blisters under the thickened skin of the palms and/or soles, followed by desquamation (291[c]). Two cases of discrete cutaneous hyperpigmentation following high-dose chemotherapy with cyclophosphamide, etoposide and carboplatin are recorded (292[c]). A case of Beu's lines (transverse ridging of the nails) has been reported following multiple drug therapy for Hodgkin's disease (293[c]); other possible causes were considered.

Other drugs Hypersensitivity to the epipodophyllotoxins etoposide and tenoposide has been reported in an incidence of 46% in one series of 108 patients receiving one of these drugs. The risk is related to the cumulative dose, reaching a maximum at 1500—2000 mg/m^2 in the case of tenoposide and 2000—3000 mg/m^2 for etoposide (294[C]). Acute hypersensitivity reactions characterized by hypotension, bronchospasm and facial flushing has been associated with etoposide (295[c], 296[c]). Rechallenge (with appropriate prophylactic cover) supported the association. Similar anaphylactoid reactions have also been linked with intravenous cyclophosphamide (297[cr]).

Four cases of hyperkeratotic seborrheic warts appearing over a 2-year period, 25 years after the patients had been started on 2.5 mg/kg doses of azathioprine, have been reported (298[c]).

OCULAR TOXICITY

Doxorubicin A review of ocular adverse reactions to doxorubicin refers to conjunctivitis, periorbital edema, lacrimation, blepharospasm, keratitis and decreased visual acuity (299[R]). Two cases of persistent photophobia and chronic inflammation of the eye following accidental topical exposure to doxorubicin have been reported (300[c]).

Interferon In a report of 57 patients treated with interferon for renal cell carcinoma, two developed multiple retinal exudates associated with visual disturbance. This association has previously been unreported. Both patients received vinblastine concurrently. The precise role of interferon in this reaction is unknown (301[cr]).

Vinca alkaloids Peripheral neuropathy and cranial nerve palsies are common with the vinca alkaloids. Optic neuropathy following a single small dose of vincristine has been reported in a single case (302[cr]). The dose of vincristine was small (1.275 mg), and the latent period before onset of visual loss was brief (6—8 weeks). Previously reported cases have had multiple injections of vincristine and the latent period was longer than 3 months.

Studies on monkeys have demonstrated visual loss and optic atrophy with intravitreous injection of vincristine. Clinical reports of post-vincristine optic atrophy are rare. Most are irreversible, progressing to permanent blindness. There is commonly coexistent peripheral or cranial neuropathy (303). It is possible that certain patients are predisposed to vincristine-induced optic atrophy.

Other drugs A 2.7% ocular complication rate in 112 patients treated with a cumulative dose of BCNU 370 mg/m^2 for intracranial tumors has been recorded (304[C]).

Transient cortical blindness and occipital seizures with visual impairment have been reported in association with ciclosporin (305[c], 306[c]). Cyclophosphamide-induced anemia has led to retinopathy presenting as striated hemorrhage of the retina (307[C]).

Keratoconjunctivitis is a well-recognized complication of cytarabine therapy with a reported incidence of 30—100%; it is commonly associated with high doses (3 g/m^2). Corneal and conjunctival toxicity have been described following 4 days' therapy, 235 mg (100 mg/m^2) daily (308[c]).

Ciclosporin Eight cases of optic disc edema have been reported in bone marrow transplant patients treated with ciclosporin. In two of the patients there were other possible explanations, but in all cases discontinuation of ciclosporin resulted in resolution of the papilledema (309[C]).

5-Fluorouracil Striate melanokeratosis of the retina

has been associated with 5-fluorouracil in reports from a number of centers; there has been no consistent explanation of the pathogenesis of this side effect (310[c]—312[c]). 5-Fluorouracil-containing regimens have been linked with several ocular side effects, including marked lacrimation, ocular pruritus and a burning sensation in the eyes (313[CR]).

OTOXICITY

Cisplatin (CDDP) Sudden bilateral deafness without tinnitus has been described after a single course of cisplatin at a dose of 120 mg/m^2; the patients showed only slight improvement after 4 weeks (314[c]).

High-tone hearing loss is consistently present in patients receiving cisplatin. Progressive hearing loss develops as a result of repeated administration of the drug, until a threshold plateau is reached at 3000—8000 Hz (315[c]). This is the result of damage to the organ of Corti. The ototoxicity is bilateral, symmetrical, progressive and irreversible. Following one course of cisplatin (150—225 mg/m^2) the mean hearing loss recorded was 27 dB at 8000 Hz, 21 dB at 6000 Hz, and 11 dB at 4000 Hz. Development of hearing loss is independent of pre-treatment hearing function (316[c]).

Otoxicity is a common and prominent side effect of cisplatin treatment. The two main symptoms reported, independently or together, are tinnitus and hearing loss. There is considerable individual variation in susceptibility, and both peak plasma levels and cumulative dose are important. Transient reversible tinnitus occurs commonly, even after low doses, but hearing impairment is more dose-dependent and affected by age, renal function, pre-existing inner ear damage and concomitant loop diuretic and/or aminoglycoside treatment. In in vitro studies selective damage to hair cells in the cochlea and in the supporting cells in the cochlear and vestibular parts of the labyrinth have been shown, with arrest of morphogenesis and cytodifferentiation. Morphological changes in the stria vascularis have been noted (317[R]).

One hundred and eighty-six women receiving treatment with cisplatin 50 mg/m^2, 4-weekly, for gynecological cancers underwent audiological testing before and after treatment (318[C]). Forty developed significant hearing loss of at least 15 dB, but there was no significant loss in the speech frequency range. Prior hearing acuity did not influence the incidence or extent of the deterioration.

Animal experiments indicate that cisplatin is only weakly vestibulotoxic (319), and clinical vestibular toxicity is found less frequently than hearing loss. Of 10 patients who received 80— 550 mg cisplatin, clinical features of vestibulotoxicity were analyzed in addition to hearing, and patients underwent audiometry, body sway, caloric, optokinetic and pendular rotation testing (320[C]). Four patients sustained significant hearing loss, five had tinnitus, and three complained of dizziness, giddiness and/or unsteadiness rather than vertigo. These symptoms were transient, and they occurred usually after several weeks of administration; they were not consistently dose-related. Spontaneous nystagmus was observed in seven, positional nystagmus in six, and caloric and body sway tests were abnormal in the early stages in several patients. The findings were suggestive of a cumulative toxic effect.

It was previously reported (SEDA-11, 394) that hearing loss with ciclosporin depends on the total cumulative dose, and that the first changes are observed at frequencies exceeding 8000 Hz. The nature of the drug injury caused by cisplatin is not clear.

In an in vitro study of the toxicity of cisplatin on hair cells and other inner ear structures, aimed at determining whether selective damage occurs in inner ear hair cells and whether morphogenesis and cytodifferentiation are influenced by low cisplatin concentrations, it was found that even at low cisplatin concentrations (0.1 μg/ml) selective damage to hair cells occurs. Incubation at a cisplatin concentration of 1 μg/ml caused morphological damage in the supporting cochlear and vestibular cells, and 10 μg/ml caused total collapse of the membranous labyrinth. Drug exposure arrested morphogenesis as well as cytodifferentiation (321).

Difluoromethylornithine (DFMO) Hearing loss appears to be the dose-limiting toxic effect for DFMO in patients receiving 4×2 g/day (SEDA-11, 394). In one study, it was found in 48% of patients treated with DFMO (3×2 g/day). In some cases the hearing loss was characterized audiographically as bilateral, sensorineural, primarily high frequency, with a median loss of 25—30 dB. All patients recovered within 1—3 months of cessation of therapy. There was no clear association between total dose of DFMO and the degree of hearing loss (322[C]).

Cisplatin It has been suggested that otoxicity caused by cisplatin may be more closely related to single dose rather than to the cumulative total dose of drug, as hearing disorders were detected in all patients who had received a single dose in excess of 150 mg, but there were no hearing disorders in patients who received less than 100 mg in a single dose (323[C]). An attempt has been made to quantify the ototoxic effects of cisplatin in children by cumulative platinum dose and decibel hearing loss at certain predetermined frequencies. The findings provide useful insight into this toxicity (324[C]). In a study of cisplatin otoxicity in children (325[C]) it was concluded that 77% experienced ototoxicity with a median cumulative dose of 360 mg/m^2; younger patients, and patients who had undergone prior cranial irradiation, are more particularly susceptible to audiological changes which progress in severity with increasing dose (326[C]).

In a series of 154 audiograms it has been shown that ototoxicity increases with cumulative dosage of cisplatin and that low-dose or monthly regimens cause the lowest toxicity. Those patients who were given high doses over short periods of time, or who developed tinnitus and hearing loss in the speech frequencies, were at the highest risk (327[C]). In a small series of patients it was confirmed that pre-treatment hearing loss does not increase the risk of cisplatin ototoxicity (328[cr]). It has been postulated that cisplatin ototoxicity is inversely related to the patient's age (329[Cr]). A 600-mg/m^2 'plateau' dose of cisplatin, beyond which hearing loss shows no apparent further deterioration in children and adolescents, is described (330[CR]). A hearing loss greater than 20 dB with frequency as 5% at 1000 Hz, 31% at 2000 Hz, 59% at 4000 Hz and 95% at 8000 Hz is described (330[CR]).

Carboplatin The ototoxicity of carboplatin is not well documented; however, an incidence of 27% has been reported in a series of closely monitored patients (327[C]).

It has been estimated that 19% of patients receiving carboplatin have significant hearing loss greater than 30 dB; the hearing loss is cumulative and maximum at 8000 Hz; the authors reported two of these patients with hearing loss greater than 10 dB at 1000 Hz. The overall conclusion is that with low-dose, short-schedule, carboplatin therapy routine audiometry is not justified (331[CR]).

In another study, carboplatin-induced ototoxicity was reported in 32% of exposed patients. This was similar to cisplatin otoxicity, although occurring at a lower frequency (4000–8000 Hz), compared to the often quoted 6000–8000 Hz for cisplatin. The extent of otic damage was proportional to the dose of carboplatin (332[C]). In serial audiometric testing in 66 patients receiving cisplatin 100 mg/m^2 per course, of 39 evaluable patients, 54% had no or mild hearing loss, 36% developed early hearing loss and 10% had late loss. If early hearing loss occurred and treatment was nevertheless continued, the speech frequencies were eventually affected in 71% of patients (333[C]).

REPRODUCTIVE, GENETIC AND SEXUAL TOXICITY *(SEDA-11, 489)*

In men receiving chemotherapy the sperm count will return to normal within 2 years of discontinuing chemotherapy in 78% of cases; however, intensive treatment, such as with doses of cisplatin in excess of 500 mg/m^2, reduces the chances of recovery of normal spermatogenesis (334[CR]).

When cytostatic drugs are used in children an effect on sexual development can be expected. Cyclophosphamide, or testicular and cranial irradiation, in the treatment of childhood malignancies can lead to small testicular size and decreased sperm production in adulthood (335[CR]). A cumulative dose-response toxic effect of cisplatin affects gonadal function when the drug is used in children around puberty; this damage is reversible in girls, but not in boys (336[CR]).

Gynecomastia is frequent in men with testicular tumours producing large amounts of human chorionic gonadotrophin (HCG), and its appearance after completion of chemotherapy may indicate residual or recurrent disease. However, not uncommonly, gynecomastia is a harmless, although troubling late side effect of chemotherapy. Sixteen patients who developed gynecomastia 2–9 months after treatment, and who were in complete remission, were found to have significantly elevated levels of estradiol. Follicle-stimulating hormone (FSH) had a higher estradiol/testosterone ratio than similarly treated patients without gynecomastia (337[C]). It is likely that this was due to increased secretion of testicular estrogen in response to a compensatory increase in pituitary gonadotrophins after cytotoxic damage to Leydig cells and spermatogenesis.

Primary ovarian failure has previously been recognized in adults after intermittent low-dose melphalan, and it has now been reported in three adolescents after high-dose melphalan (338[C]).

An increased incidence of gene aberration is to be expected in the offspring of a male patient being treated at the time of conception with chemotherapy for testicular tumours (339[CR]). Various drug regimens for Hodgkin's disease and high grade non-Hodgkin's lymphoma produce different patterns of changes in sister chromatid exchange frequency, and the changes may reflect the potential of the drugs concerned to induce second malignancies (340[CR]).

Cyclophosphamide Following treatment with cyclophosphamide after bone marrow transplantation, ovarian function may occasionally recover resulting in a successful pregnancy up to 7 years after treatment

(341[R]). No specific factors were found to correlate with recovery of normal ovarian function. However, recovery was rare if the patient had undergone concurrent total body irradiation (342[R]).

Of 23 men treated with either cyclophosphamide or non-alkylating agent combinations, there was a dose-related disturbance in gonadotrophin secretion in the cyclophosphamide group (343[C]). The chances of maintaining normal gonadal function following combined modality treatment of Hodgkin's disease are significantly greater among girls than boys at 9-year follow-up (344[Cr]). Pre- and post-pubescent boys were affected by six cycles of MOPP, whether or not pelvic radiation was administered; on the other hand, in girls similarly treated, ovarian function was directly affected by the number of courses of chemotherapy and the ovarian radiation dose (345[CR]). In a study of male gonadal function at 9 years follow-up after regimens containing cyclophosphamide, mechlorethamine, vincristine or procarbazine, azoospermia was found, whereas regimens containing dactinomycin and vinblastine did not have a toxic effect on spermatogenesis (346[Cr]). Testicular volume and sperm count in 18 patients, 1—13 years after chemotherapy, showed that all those who had received chemotherapy which did not include cisplatin had normal testicular size and sperm counts, whereas of seven who had received cisplatin, six had small testes and azoospermia and one was oligozoospermic with normal-sized testes (347[c]).

Nitrosoureas In a study of boys treated with carmustine (BCNU) or lomustine (CCNU) alone or in combination with procarbazine and vincristine for brain tumors, there were 20 cases of persistent testicular damage of the 21 cases studied (348[c]). From assessment of testicular size it was thought that the majority of those affected would remain infertile. This supports the idea that germinal epithelium is more susceptible than Leydig cells to cytotoxic-induced damage.

PVB (cisplatin/vinblastine/bleomycin) Sexual function may be compromised in men following treatment with PVB chemotherapy. In a study of 54 patients, 54% experienced disorders of sexual function 2 years after completion of treatment (349[R]). Ejaculatory dysfunction was tentatively linked to chemotherapy in 30% of those affected. Diminished libido, usually reversible, was found in 75% at the time of receiving chemotherapy.

ABVD, COPP, MOPP, MVPP The gonadal effects of MOPP and MVPP in patients with Hodgkin's disease have been described in SEDA-11 (pp. 397, 403). Similar studies have been conducted in patients treated with ABVD (adriamycin / bleomycin / vinblastine / dacarbazine) and COPP (cyclophosphamide/vincristine/procarbazine/prednisone) chemotherapy (350[C]). The results suggest that all men experience irreversible sterility with preservation of normal Leydig cell function after COPP, which is more spermatotoxic than MOPP and much more so than ABVD. Ovarian failure was age-related after COPP, occurring in 86% of those over 24 years of age at the time of therapy, compared with 28% in women patients less than 24 years old. In contrast to male patients, sterility in women was always associated with ovarian endocrine failure requiring estrogen replacement. Pregnancies and normal births did occur: 14 women became pregnant and five healthy children were born.

Buserelin The possibility of preventing sterility caused by treatment of Hodgkin's disease, by 'down-regulating' the gonad during chemotherapy, has been investigated using buserelin, a gonadotrophin-releasing hormone (GnRH agonist analog) (351[C]). Twenty men and 10 women received buserelin, the men at two different dosage schedules, which suppressed luteinizing hormone (LH) responses to GnRH throughout treatment. Follicle-stimulating hormone (FSH) responses were suppressed initially. At follow-up assessments up to 3 years after completion of therapy, all the buserelin-treated and untreated men were profoundly oligospermic; four of the eight treated women and six of nine untreated female controls were amenorrheic.

PPMB/ACE Gonadal function was evaluated in 59 men and 31 women after successful treatment of germ-cell tumors with the POMB/ACE (cisplatin/vincristine / methotrexate / bleomycin / dactinomycin / cyclophosphamide/etoposide) regimen (352[C]). The majority of patients recovered fertility; 81% of men who did not receive para-aortic radiotherapy, whose original tumor bulk was less than 5 cm in diameter, and whose duration of chemotherapy was less than 6 months recovered compared with 32% who had larger tumours or who received longer courses of chemotherapy, or both. Fertility and pregnancies were undisturbed in 24 female patients treated for invasive trophoblastic tumours with methotrexate alone, with methotrexate and dactinomycin in combination, or with other combination chemotherapy (353[C]). There were nine subsequent pregnancies, with the birth of eight healthy babies, and one woman requested a termination of pregnancy.

The endocrine effects of cisplatin-based chemotherapy were studied in 22 male patients 9—24 or more months after completion of treatment for germ-cell tumors (354[C]). Mean basal FSH and stimulated LH and FSH levels were elevated but serum testosterone levels were similar to untreated controls. Younger patients (under 25 years old) appeared more resistant to these effects of chemotherapy, and the hormonal abnormalities recovered with time.

The long-term prognosis for sperm counts after chemotherapy with and without radiation in 71 males treated for non-Hodgkin's lymphoma on the CHOP-Bleomycin combination has been studied (355[C]). Pelvic radiotherapy and cumulative cyclophosphamide dosages of greater than 9.5 g/m^2 are associated independently and in combination with a greater risk of permanent sterility.

Cisplatin A Danish study group has reported a fertility problem of 53% in patients with unilateral germ cell tumours, but there was no significant difference between orchiectomy and cisplatin-based chemotherapy or subdiaphragmatic irradiation. Eight patients remained infertile despite evident recovery of spermatogenesis, and all 22 children conceived post-treatment were born normal and without malformations (356[C]).

Intensive multi-drug regimens A decreased chance of paternity has been reported in 67% of patients who had been treated with MOPP/ABVD for Hodgkin's disease. This included oligospermia, asthenozoospermia and/or teratozoospermia. The recovery of spermatogenesis was documented in only 40% (357[C]).

Gynecomastia severe enough to necessitate discontinuation of therapy was the main side effect of estramustine therapy following its use at 560 mg/day for more than 1 year in prostatic carcinoma (358[c]). Breast pain with vaginal bleeding and diarrhea were dose-limiting when estramustine 840 mg/day was given for breast cancer (359[CR]).

HEMATOLOGICAL TOXICITY *(SEDA-15, 487)*

L-Asparaginase The use of L-asparaginase in patients with leukemia is associated with thrombotic and hemorrhagic coagulation disorders. Five patients with cerebral thrombosis complicating asparaginase/prednisone/vincristine induction therapy for acute lymphoblastic leukemia were found to have a decreased platelet count following the event and, in three of them, sequential changes in von Willebrand factor multimer pattern (360[C]). The other two patients were only studied at presentation and their multimer pattern was not appreciably different to pooled plasma from seven controls without thromboses. The findings were consistent with thrombotic complications caused by platelet agglutination by plasma Von Willebrand factor.

In another study, 12 children in complete remission treated with L-asparaginase alone daily were investigated for platelet and clotting abnormalities (361[C]). Changes in prothrombin time, partial thromboplastin time and fibrinogen remained close to the normal range, and platelet function was normal. Decreased levels of physiological inhibitors of coagulation (protein C and antithrombin III) were found. Clinical thrombosis was uncommon. These results are consistent with another study of L-asparaginase therapy as a single agent in 14 children with acute lymphoblastic leukemia (362[C]). A severe deficit of antithrombin III and protein C was observed with a coexisting hypocoagulable state; an equilibrium between the two partly explained the lack of thromboembolic phenomena. The hypocoagulability was due to hypofibrinogenemia and reduced levels of vitamin K-dependent factors.

Three patients with bilateral venous sinus thrombosis have been described following L-asparaginase treatment; the diagnosis and follow-up of this complication have been succinctly reviewed (365[cR]). In another patient who developed central nervous system thrombosis whilst receiving L-asparaginase it was shown that this was associated with a transient acquired type II pattern of von Willebrand's disease (368[c]).

Combination drug therapy Forty patients with lung cancer, treated with a combination of cisplatin, mitomycin C, vinblastine, doxorubicin, cyclosphosphamide and methotrexate, showed a significant post-treatment increase in fibrinopeptide A and a decrease in fibrinolytic activity, reflected by a fall in functional tissue activator; this appeared to be cumulative, depending upon the extent of drug exposure (363[CR]).

Mitomycin C Eighty-five cases of cancer-associated hemolytic uremic syndrome were reported up to 1990 to the United States National Cancer Registry; 84 had received a cumulative dose of 60 mg mitomycin C or more in their treatment as part of their treatment (364[C]).

Amsacrine Prolongation of prothrombin time following amsacrine in dose of 1200 mg/m^2 for acute myeloid leukemia was found to be related to transient deficiency of Factor X (366[c]).

Interleukin-2 Suppression of bone marrow function by interleukin-2, an endogenous glycoprotein lymphokine with immune modulating properties and indirect antitumour activity in vitro and in vivo, has a different etiology to the myelosuppression associated with other chemotherapeutic agents. In a detailed study of 42 patients with advanced cancer treated with interleukin-2 and lymphokine-activated killer (LAK) cells from autologous lymphocytes, there were reduced numbers of circulating erythroid and granulocyte/macrophage progenitors which rebounded after discontinuation of therapy (367[C]). Patients developed severe significant anemia (partly due to phlebotomy, cytopheresis and hemodilution), thrombocytopenia, lymphopenia and eosinophilia with mild neutropenia and rebound lymphocytosis after treatment was stopped. The pathogenesis of the hematopoietic suppression was not clear, but it was thought to involve complex interaction of several regulatory lymphokines.

Cisplatin Cisplatin causes an elevation of erythropoeitin, but anemias associated with platinum therapy are independent of this mechanism (369[c]).

BIOCHEMICAL AND HORMONAL CHANGES

Ciclosporin (cyclosporine) Ciclosporin is potentially more toxic in patients with altered LDL levels or a low total serum cholesterol (370[Cr]). Ciclosporin therapy itself significantly raises plasma lipoprotein levels by increasing the total serum cholesterol; this is due to an increase in LDL cholesterol, demonstrated in a prospective double-blind randomized placebo-controlled trial in 36 male patients with amyotrophic lateral sclerosis (371[CR]). Twenty-two patients have been described who developed significant elevation of mean serum triglycerides and cholesterol, 2 weeks after starting low-dose ciclosporin therapy; this may be a risk factor for cardiovascular disease (372[C]). Seven cases of hypertriglyceridemia were reported in patients receiving ciclosporin 2.0—7.5 mg/kg/day for psoriasis. This developed during the first month of therapy; the values were greater than the upper limit for age- and sex-matched controls (376[C]).

Another study has provided evidence that ciclosporin-induced immunosuppression in patients undergoing renal transplants may induce (or be associated with) diabetes mellitus (428[cr]). Renal magnesium wasting occurred in 24% of a series of renal transplant patients treated with ciclosporin; other renal function indicators remained normal (373[Cr], 374[R]).

Hyperuricemia occurred in 72% of male and 82% of female patients receiving ciclosporin post heart transplant; there was also an increased incidence of gouty arthritis in these patients (375[C]).

Cisplatin Magnesium wasting is a common adverse effect of cisplatin therapy. Hyponatremia is rare, and persistent hyponatremia very rare (377[c]). In a detailed description of the biochemical abnormalities that may result from renal tubular dysfunction following cisplatin therapy it was noted that hypocalciuria is more common than hypomagnesemia, and that there tends to be a state of reduced serum bicarbonate. The most severe renal tubular damage caused by cisplatin is characterized by hypocalciuria, total body magnesium deficiency and hypokalemic metabolic alkalosis (378[cr]).

Methotrexate Of patients receiving high-dose methotrexate (5—8 g/m^2) 95% developed a significant increase in serum phenylalanine levels, probably due to inhibition of dihydropteridine reductase enzymes (381[C]). The clinical significance of this is not obvious, although it is possible that it may contribute to the transient neurological disturbance observed in some patients receiving high-dose treatment.

Mitotane Mitotane given in dose of 1—5 grams daily for 4 weeks was associated with the development of hypercholesterolemia in three cases. The effect had not reverted to normal 3 months later (379[c]).

Combined cytotoxic drug therapy Combined cytotoxic drug therapy for Hodgkin's disease in childhood often results in abnormal endocrine function; this appears particularly to be an increase in follicle-stimulating hormone, prolactin and thyroid-stimulating hormone (380[CR]).

SECONDARY CANCERS

Malignant tumours have been documented with increasing frequency over the last 30 years as a long-term complication of cytotoxic therapy.

Thirty-one patients developed new malignancies among 949 renal allograft recipients (3.3%); an increased risk of malignant tumour developing in patients receiving ciclosporin was noted (381[C]). The actuarial risks of developing secondary malignancy and/or myelodysplastic syndrome at 5, 10 and 15 years post-treatment for Hodgkin's disease have been calculated (382[c]). A case of lymphoblastic leukemia has been described following treatment of a malignant germ cell tumour;

it was suggested that this was related to the etoposide component of the treatment, and that development of secondary leukemia after etoposide may not be confined to the myeloid cell lineage (383[c]).

Three cases of malignant neoplasm have been described in patients receiving a prolonged course of methotrexate in doses of 7.5—15 mg weekly (384[c]).

Alkylating agents Alkylating agents have been implicated in the causation of secondary tumours, including acute myeloid leukemia, myelodysplastic syndromes (385[R]), solid tumours (386[c], 387[c]), Hodgkin's disease (388[c], 389[CR]), ovarian cancer (390[c], 391[c]), and gastric cancer (392[R]). Survival from the time of diagnosis of secondary malignancies is usually very short (393[R]).

In a multicenter case-controlled study the incidence of acute myeloid leukemia in treated Hodgkin's disease was 64 times higher than in the general population, the risk being higher in males. It was also shown that there was a significant association between the use of extensive radiotherapy, vincristine/procarbazine, splenectomy and the dose of mechlorethamine and the development of acute myeloid leukemia in those patients (394[CR]). The problem is thought to be the result of chromosomal aberrations developing in patients treated with alkylating agents (395[r]), although there is no general agreement about this (396[cr]).

Azathioprine It has not been possible to demonstrate a consistent increase in the incidence of secondary tumours as a result of long-term azathioprine treatment, over and above that in matched controls, yet sporadic reports are published. Skin (predominantly squamous-cell carcinoma), cancer of the lip, Kaposi's sarcoma, and carcinoma of the cervix and anus are reported to be more common following azathioprine than in the general population (397[r]).

Ciclosporin (cyclosporine) There is a disproportionately high incidence of lymphomas, Kaposi's sarcoma (398[c]), and renal cell carcinoma in ciclosporin-treated patients (399[c]—401[c]). Of interest is a report of complete regression of Kaposi's sarcoma following discontinuation of ciclosporin treatment (402[c]). An increase in chromosomal abnormalities has been correlated with serum ciclosporin levels in one study (403[c]).

Other case reports and reviews A large international collaborative study by cancer registries has published the incidence of second malignancies following testicular cancer, ovarian cancer and Hodgkin's disease (404[C]): 3157 second cancers were observed among 133 411 patients diagnosed between 1945 and 1984. Patients with Hodgkin's disease were at particular risk, having an 80% excess of cancer. It confirms the high incidence of this complication noted in other reports involving smaller numbers of patients (405[C]—408[c]).

Other conclusions deriving from the international collaborative study (404[C]) include the following:
(i) patients with testicular cancer had a 30% greater chance of developing cancer than the general population, and those with ovarian cancer 20%;
(ii) leukemia, previously linked to alkylating agents, occurred in excess after testicular cancer, ovarian cancer and Hodgkin's disease (relative risk 6.1), as did non-Hodgkin's lymphoma (relative risk 1.8) (the latter particularly after Hodgkin's disease);
(iii) other cancers with significant excesses were lung cancer following Hodgkin's disease (relative risk 1.9), breast cancer following Hodgkin's disease (relative risk 1.4), and bladder cancer following ovarian cancer and Hodgkin's disease (relative risks 1.7 and 2.2 in women, respectively);
(iv) a marked excess in incidence of secondary malignancies was found in the salivary gland, thyroid, bone, and connective tissue (there was a smaller excess for colorectal cancers following ovarian cancer).

In general, a casual relationship between treatment of the first malignancy and development of the second seems likely. Alkylating agents are strongly implicated in the pathogenesis of the leukemias. Non-Hodgkin's lymphoma occurred after a 10-year latency in patients with ovarian cancer, suggesting a possible radiation effect, but early in patients with testicular tumours or Hodgkin's disease possibly related to the immunosuppressive effect of the cytotoxic therapy. The excess of bladder cancers in patients with Hodgkin's disease and ovarian cancer may be related to radiotherapy (subdiaphragmatic in the former), and/or cyclophosphamide which is widely used in the treatment of both and is a known human bladder carcinogen.

The increased incidence of breast cancer after Hodgkin's disease may be related to supradiaphragmatic irradiation, but the risk was higher for patients with ovarian cancer, which is consistent with a common predisposition to breast and ovarian cancer. However, cytotoxic drugs may have contributed to the risk.

Organ transplant recipients Renal transplant recipients are known to be at increased risk of developing malignant disease, the risk increasing with time after the transplant. The commonest cancers in this setting are squamous carcinoma of the skin and lip, in situ carcinoma of the cervix, and non-Hodgkin's lymphoma. An increased incidence of hepatocellular carcinoma has been reported (409[CR]). In Australia and New Zealand tumours of the urogenital tract, especially of the kidney and bladder, are the commonest non-cutaneous tumours encountered in renal transplant recipients (410[r]). Severe metaplastic and dysplastic changes, suggestive of premalignancy, have been found in the lining epithelium of collecting ducts and tubules of cadaveric renal transplants in two patients receiving azathioprine and prednisolone (411[c]).

Rheumatoid disease An increased incidence of non-Hodgkin's lymphomas has been noted in patients receiving long-term immunosuppression with azathioprine and prednisolone for rheumatoid disease, although the latent period appears to be longer than in other situations, perhaps reflecting a different pathogenesis (412[C]).

Epipodophyllotoxins Etoposide and teniposide are prominent causes of secondary malignancies, particularly secondary myeloid and lymphoid leukemias. The risk appears to be related to both the schedule and the cumulative dose, and it may be aggravated by addition of alkylating agents and/or radiotherapy (413—418). There are differences between the chromosomal abnormalities and the subsequent acute myeloid leukemia associated with the alkylating agents and those following topoisomerase inhibition by epipodophyllotoxin therapy (419[cR]). The alkylating agents cause abnormalities of chromosomes 5 and 7, singly or together, and the epipodophyllotoxins damage the 11q23 chromosome locus (420[R]).

MISCELLANEOUS *(See Tables 2 and 3)*

Fever In a report from Japan of fever higher than 38°C in nine of 31 children receiving maintenance vincristine chemotherapy for either leukemia or lymphoma, an allergic mechanism has been proposed. Concurrent corticosteroids as part of the regimen appeared to be protective. Younger children are at greater risk. Peak temperatures occur within 24 hours of vincristine administration. The pyrexia may last from 6 hours to 4 days, and the condition is self-limiting (421[C]).

Sixty milligrams of bleomycin administered intrapleurally caused a fever greater than 39°C in two of 21 patients treated for malignant pleural effusion (422[c]). This settled without treatment and was not associated with local discomfort.

Mitomycin C Ten cases of bladder wall calcification have been reported following intravesicular administration of mitomycin C. These lesions can resemble tumour recurrence in the bladder, and biopsy is advocated to distinguish between the two (423[c]).

ORAL TOXICITY

Mucositis is a well documented toxic effect of anthracyclines; it has been reported in 8% of combination chemotherapeutic courses including epirubicin in a dose of 180 mg/m^2 (424[C]). Gingival overgrowth during ciclosporin treatment is well recognized, with incidence of between 8 and 70% (425[c]). There may be an additive effect (incidence and severity) when patients receive more than one drug with a gingival proliferative effect, such as nifedipine.

OLFACTORY TOXICITY

Thirty percent of patients treated with cisplatin have been reported to have some degree of anosmia, which in 1% is severe or complete; the sense of smell returns to normal within 3—4 months of completing cisplatin therapy (426[C]).

BIOLOGICAL RESPONSE MODERATORS

Recombinant interleukin-2 (rIL-2) The toxicity of IL-2 is well documented and the effects are consistent and common. They include fever, chills, malaise, skin rash, nausea, vomiting (often resistant to antiemetics), diarrhea, fluid retention, myalgia, insomnia, disorientation, life-threatening hypotension and the capillary leak syndrome (which may be preceded by weight gain) (SEDA-15, 491; 427[C]).

The renal toxicity and hypotension associated with IL-2 is dose-related. It manifests as uremia, oliguria, fluid retention and pronounced renal tubular sodium reabsorption (428[C]). No evidence of tubular dysfunction has been found. Anemia, eosinophilia, and neutropenia, and an increased SGOT, alkaline phosphatase and transaminase are described. Mild liver dysfunction, hypophosphatemia and hypomagnesmia are the most common laboratory abnormalities (429[c], 430[c]). The development of pulmonary edema may be part of a capillary leak syndrome. Occasional signs of cardiac toxicity such as atrial fibrillation are described. These effects are dose- and schedule-related, and they are similar for adults (431[c], 432[c]) and children (433[c]).

Table 2. *Recent articles on toxic effects of cytostatic drugs, immunomodulators and cytoprotective agents*

Drug/topic	Nature of report	Ref.
Filgrastim (G-CSF)	Musculoskeletal pain 8–18% of patients, severe in 3%; possible toxicity to other blood cell lines not established; leukocytosis exceeding 100 000/mm^3 in fewer than 5% of patients	452[R]
	Myelodysplasia and acute myeloid Leukemia	524[c]
	Sweet's syndrome	533[c]
	Fatal heart disorders	540[c]
	Capillary leak syndrome	550[c]
Buserelin	Thrombocytopenia (aggravation in SLE)	576[c]
Buserelin implant (LH-RH agonist)	Hot flushes (64%), loss of libido (30%), impotence (25%); voiding difficulties or urinary retention (2.5%)	453[R]
Lenograstim (glycosylated G-CSF)	Bone pain (13%), reaction or pain at injection site (13%), headache (7%)	454[R]
Interferon	Autoimmune thyroid disease (three forms: hypothyroidism, hyperthyroidism, biphasic thyroiditis); lupus-like syndrome; polyarthropathy	455[R]
	Autoimmune chronic active hepatitis (exacerbation)	551[c]
Interferon-α	Autoimmune hepatitis	546[c]
	Skin eruptions	646[c]
	Neuropsychiatric disturbances	645[c]
	Retinal hemorrhage (with elevated plasma C5a levels)	513[c]
	Membranoproliferative glomerulonephritis	515[c]
	Glomerulonephritis	525[c]
	Sarcoid nodules, subcutaneous	513[c]
	Hyperthyroidism (?autoimmune)	523[c]
	Autoimmune thyroid disorders	528[c] 539[c]
	Myelofibrosis	526[c]
	acute vanishing bile duct syndrome	527[c]
	Diabetes mellitus, insulin dependent	532[c]
	Acquired factor VIII inhibitor	554[c]
	Necrotic myopathy	563[c]
	Pneumonia, hemolytic anemia and liver dysfunction	596[c]
	Arthritis (aggravation in)	598[c]
	psoriasis	646[c]
	Raynaud's disease	599[c]
	Lichen planus, oral ulcerative	600[c]
	Lichen planus, mucocutaneous	604[c]
	Blindness in elderly patient	601[c]
	Optic neuritis	610[c]
	Thrombocytopenia	613[c]
	Pancreatitis	614[c]
	Hemolytic uremic syndrome	603[c]
	Rhabdomyolysis	605[c]
	Transient blurred vision	606[c]
	Pseudolymphoma of liver	607[c]
	Bone marrow disorders	609[c]
	CD4 lymphopenia	608[c]
	Hemolytic anemia	615[c]

Table 2. *(continued)*

Drug/topic	Nature of report	Ref.
Ciclosporin	Hirsutism in women when used to treat Behçet's disease	456[R]
	Epithelial dysplasia	522[c]
	Nail disorders	616[c]
	Reflex sympathetic dystrophy	536[c]
	Acute leukoencephalopathy (with prednisolone)	537[c]
	Thrombotic microangiopathy	547[c]
	Hypertension (in lung transplant recipients)	561[c]
	Hypertension (in liver transplant recipients)	586[c]
	Spastic paraparesis	565[c]
	Encephalopathy	570[c]
	Late onset CNS disorders	572[c]
	Recurrent migraine-like headaches	573[c]
	Gingival hyperplasia	583[c]
	Gingival hypertrophy	584[c]
Ciclosporin + tacrolimus	Glucose intolerance	585[C]
Paclitaxel (taxol)	Myelosuppression	655[c]
	Optic nerve disturbances	652[c]
	Sensory neuropathy	653[c]
	Myocardial damage	650[c]
	Radiation recall dermatitis	651[c]
	Neuropathy and hypotension	595[c]
	Recall reaction	654[c]
Molgramostim (GM-CSF)	Reactions at injection site (45%), skin rash (36%); fever, bone and muscle pain; acute reaction after first dose: dyspnea with hypoxia, flushing, tachycardia, hypotension, nausea, vomiting, musculoskeletal pain;	458[R]
	Aggravation of Kaposi's sarcoma in AIDS patient	656[c]
	Erythema multiforme	648[c]
	Subcorneal pustular dermatosis	649[c]
Interferon-α_{2b}	Lichen planus exacerbation	520[c]
Methotrexate	Malignant lymphoma (rare)	459[R]
	Hyperthermia	518[c]
	Cutaneous pseudolymphoma	519[c]
	Non-Hodgkin's lymphoma	558[c]
	Megaloblastic anemia and pneumonitis	589[c]
	Pneumonitis	590[c]
	Blood dyscrasias	591[c]
	Pleural and pericardial effusion	592[c]
	Cirrhosis	593[c]
	Proteinuria in children	594[c]
Pentostatin	Linked with (but not proven) neutropenia; fall in CD4+ lymphocytes; both effects were reversible; herpes zoster infections; neurological disorders (drowsiness, headache, fatigue); nephrotoxicity	460[R]
Fotemustine (nitrosourea)	Toxic for hematopoietic stem cells (leukopenia and/or thrombocytopenia after lag time of several weeks) (25%)	461[R]
Interferon-α_{2a}	Influenza-like symptoms (69%), skin dryness (60%), nausea, diarrhea, depressive symptoms (30%)	462[R]
	Hemolytic uremic syndrome	597[c]
Tamoxifen	Hot flushes, vaginal dryness, depressive tendency; more rarely, possible increased risk of endometrial cancer, thrombo-embolism, hepatitis, retinopathy	463[R]
	Hepatocellular carcinoma (lack of association with)	644[C]
	Fatal neutropenia	643[c]
	Ocular toxicity	642[c]
	Eye disorders	626[c]
	Endometriosis	639[c]
	Endometriosis	625[c]

Table 2. *(continued)*

Drug/topic	Nature of report	Ref.
	Uterine proliferation	640[c]
	Endometrial proliferation	621[R]
	Endometrial cancer	622[R]
	Endometrial cancer	623[C]
	Depression	624[C]
	Tamoxifen flare	641[c]
	Ovarian cysts	638[c]
	Ovarian cysts	637[c]
	Granulosa cell tumour	627[c]
	Fallopian tube adenocarcinoma	628[c]
	Thrombocytopenia, immune mediated	629[c]
	Fatal neutropenia	630[c]
Bleomycin	Flagellate dermatitis	464[cR]
	Fatal pulmonary fibrosis (in conjunction with G-CSF)	557[c]
Vincristine	Neurological consequences of accidental intrathecal vincristine (lower motor neuron neuropathic bladder)	465[c]
	Visual hallucinations	512[c]
	Anaphylaxis (in child with acute basophilic leukemia)	517[c]
	Myocardial ischemia	631[c]
	Acute neuropathy	634[c]
Carmustine + mitomycin	Ocular toxicity: qualitative and quantitative changes in tear films, with corneal and conjunctival epithelial damage	466[c]
Mitomycin	Alveolitis	612[c]
Carmustine (BCNU)	Acute interstitial pneumonitis (fatal outcome)	467[c]
Procarbazine	Prolonged thrombocytopenia;	468[c]
	hypersensitivity reactions, including various pulmonary toxic effects	469[c]
Hydroxyurea	Acute leukemia (following treatment for polycythemia vera); severe thromboembolism	470[C]
Ifosfamide	Fanconi syndrome; renal failure	471[c]
	Cerebral atrophy (fatal outcome)	531[c]
	Ventricular arrhythmias	545[c]
	CNS disorders	553[c]
	Hallucinations	617[c]
	Pancreatitis	618[c]
	Peripheral nerve disorders	620[c]
	Progressive renal failure	619[c]
Azothioprine + prednisolone	Progression of enterovirus-induced myocarditis to dilated cardiomyopathy	473[c]
Methotrexate	Gynecomastia	474[c]
	Acute urticaria and hepatitis	475[c]
	Neuropsychological effects of cranial irradiation, intrathecal methotrexate and systemic methotrexate	476[c]
Azathioprine	Long-term neoplasia risk (no substantial increased risk when given for inflammatory bowel disease);	477[R]
	Hypersensitivity resembling Goodpasture's syndrome	478[R]
	Drug fever	564[c]
	Epstein-Barr virus-related lymphoma	574[c]
Cytosine	Pulmonary insufficiency;	479[C]
Arabinoside	Granulocytopenia, drug fever, thrombocytopenia	480[c]
Busulphan + cyclophosphamide	Severe mucositis, hemorrhagic cystitis, interstitial pneumonia, liver toxicity, hyperpigmentation of the skin	481[c]
Busulphan + cyclosporin	Retinopathy	578[c]
Busulphan	Renal cancer	577[c]

Table 2. *(continued)*

Drug/topic	Nature of report	Ref.
Cisplatin	Delayed emesis renal toxicity and toxicity-modulating strategies	635[C]
	Hyperbilirubinemia	549[c]
	Ototoxicity	568[R]
	Severe exfoliative dermatitis	569[c]
	Optic neuritis	581[c]
Etoposide	Acute myelomonocytic leukemia	483[c]
	Acute promyelocytic leukemia	484[c]
	Hypersensitivity reactions	485[c]
	Secondary infantile leukemia	486[c]
	Peripheral neuropathy	487[c]
	Acral erythema	488[c]
	Secondary leukemias	489[R]
	Hypersensitivity reactions	542[cR]
Carboplatin + etoposide	Recurrent salt wasting	490[c]
Ciclosporin	Antidiuretic effect	491[c]
	Myopathy	492[c]
	Hypertrichosis (hair growth)	559[c]
	Autoimmune hemolytic anemia	588[c]
Carboplatin	Hypersensitivity reactions	493[c]
	Hyponatremia	555[c]
	Renal salt wasting, recurrent	560[c]
	Fatal anaphylaxis	566[c]
Doxorubicin + cyclophosphamide	Therapy-related leukemia	494[R]
Farmorubicin	Photoprovoked erythematobullous skin eruption	495[c]
Floxuridine	Gastric mucosal injury	496[C]
Interleukin-2	Cardiopulmonary toxicity:	497[C]
	Respiratory distress, arrhythmias, hypotension, atrial fibrillation (recurrent), ventricular tachycardia; hepatotoxicity	498[C]
	Cholecystopathy	499[C]
	Cholecystitis	602[c]
	Antiphospholipid syndrome	500[C]
	Left ventricular dysfunction	501[C]
	Renal dysfunction (transient)	647[c]
	Coagulation disorders	516[C]
DAB486 inter-leukin 2	Adrenal hemorrhage and insufficiency	538[c]
Cyclophosphamide	Facial discomfort: burning of face and scalp; oropharyngeal tingling; nasal congestion; rhinorrhea; sneezing; lacrimation	502[C]
Cyclophosphamide + thiotepa	Episodic complete heart block	503[c]
Cyclophosphamide + filgrastim	Fatal respiratory insufficiency	582[c]
Melphalan	Long-term neuropathy after regional isolated perfusion	504[C]
Aminoglutehimide	Primary hypothyroidism	505[C]
Vindesine	Transient neutropenia	506[C]
L-Asparaginase	Hyperglycemia, ketoacidosis	507[C]
	Cerebrovascular disorders	556[c]
Actinomycin D	Hepatic veno-occlusive disease	508[c]
Menogaril (semisynthetic anthracycline)	Leukopenia	509[c]
TNF-α + monoclonal antibody R24	Hemorrhagic tumour necrosis	510[c]
Cyclophosphamide	Hemorrhagic cystitis	511[C]
	Hemorrhagic colitis	571[c]
	Hepatitis	587[c]

Table 2. *(continued)*

Drug/topic	Nature of report	Ref.
Fludarabine	Progressive multifocal leukoencephalopathy	514[c]
	Tumour lysis syndrome ('lysis pneumonopathy')	521[c]
	CNS disorders	541[c]
	Autoimmune thrombocytopenia	543[c]
Mercaptopurine	Myelosuppression	529[c]
Fluorouracil	Fatal myocarditis	530[c]
	Toxic myocarditis	535[c]
	Cardiotoxicity, life-threatening	544[c]
	coronary artery spasm	552[c]
Fluorouracil + interferon-α	Cytomegalovirus colitis	580[c]
Flutamide	Fulminant hepatitis	548[c]
Busulfan	Cataract	562[c]
Chlorambucil	Pneumonitis	575[c]
	Interstitial pneumonitis	636[c]
Aminoglutethimide	Purpura simplex	579[c]
Lomustine	Aplastic anemia	611[c]
Vinorelbine	Cardiotoxicity	632[c]
	acute pain at tumour site	633[c]

Table 3. *Other recent reports on toxic effects of cytostatic drugs*

Drug/topic	Nature of report	Ref.
Antiandrogens	Gynecomastia: LH-RH agonists (triptorelin, leuprorelin, buserelin, goserelin)	614[R]
Azathioprine	Lack of carcinogenesis: incidence study	663[C]
Chemotherapy	Secondary leukemia following antineoplastic therapy	664[C]
Cisplatin	Nephrotoxicity	661[C]
Cyclophosphamide	Hyponatremia	668[r]
Ciclosporin	Carcinogenesis incidence	660[C]
Immunosuppressants	Adverse effects in renal transplant recipients during pregnancy	662[C]
Immunosuppressants	Carcinogenesis in children and infants after heart transplantation	671[C]
Interferon	Clinical toxicity	658[C]
Interferon-α	Adverse effects incidence	665[C]
LH-RH agonists	Gynecomastia (triptorelin, leuprorelin, buserelin, goserelin)	667[R]
Methotrexate	Adverse effects incidence	659[C]
Tamoxifen	Adverse effects incidence	657[C]
Tamoxifen	Carcinogenicity (uterus, ovaries)	670[C]
Tamoxifen	Endometrial cancer	669[r]
Teniposide	Risk of acute myeloid leukemia	666[C]
Vincristine	Hyponatremia	613[R]

The nephrotoxic effect of IL-2 infusion is associated with a rise in creatinine clearance and a reduction in renal plasma flow; this is associated with reduced renal prostaglandin synthesis and increased plasma renin activity, which may explain the mechanism of this effect (434[c]).

Interferons Neuropsychiatric complications have been described in association with interferon in adults but not previously in children. Two children treated with interferon experienced confusion, somnolence and syncope associated with transient EEG abnormalities. The symptoms abated and the EEG findings improved once treatment was discontinued, and there was no recurrence when it was resumed at a lower dose (435[c]).

Eleven adults undergoing interferon treatment with various preparations and for various indications experienced unexpected severe organic mental disorders. These included delirium, extrapyramidal symptoms, mania and neuresthenia with catatonic episodes. Computerized tomographic (CT) scans of the brain disclosed unsuspected pre-existing neurological abnormalities in all the patients (436[C]). Fever, fatigue, anorexia, weight loss and malaise are non-specific and common 'flu-like' symptoms associated with interferon therapy (437[C]—439[C]). Myelosuppression (which is usually not of clinical significance) (440[C]), gastrointestinal adverse effects and elevation of liver enzymes are reported (441[C]). Most of these effects are dose-related, tachyphylaxis occurs (442[C]), and control of adverse effects is easy with dose manipulation (549[C]). However, these effects may seriously impair quality of life and lead to patients abandoning therapy (450[C]).

Clinical hypothyroidism preceded by appearance in the blood of thyroid autoantibodies has been reported in patients receiving daily long-term interferon. This has been explained as being related to aberrant induction of Class II HLA expression, and it is suggested that autoimmune response may be related to contaminants in the interferon preparation (451[r]). Agreement on this has not been reached.

REFERENCES

1. Okuma K, Ariyoshi Y, Ota K. Clinical study of acute cardiotoxicity of anti-cancer agents—analysis using Holter ECG monitoring. Jpn J Cancer Chemother 1988;15:1893.
2. Solymar L, Marky I, Mellander L, Sabel K. Echocardiographic findings in children treated for malignancy with chemotherapy including adriamycin. Pediatr Hematol Oncol 1988;5:209.
3. Nakamura K, Miyake T, Kawamura T, Maekawa I. Prospective monitoring of adriamycin cardiotoxicity with systolic time intervals. J Jpn Soc Cancer Ther 1988;23:1633.
4. Dey HM, Kassamali H. Radionuclide evaluation of doxorubicin cardiothoxicity: the need for cautious interpretation. Clin Nuclear Med 1988;13:565.
5. Rowan R, Masek M, Billingham M. Ultrastructural morphometric analysis of endomyocardial biopsies. Am J Cardiol Pathol 1988;2:137.
6. McQuillan P, Morgan B, Ramwell J. Adriamycin cardiomyopathy. Anaesthesia 1988;43:301.
7. Goenen M, Baele P, Lintermans J et al. Orthotopic heart transplantation eleven years after left pneumonectomy. J Heart Transplant 1988;7:309.
8. Henderson C, Hayes DF, Corne S et al. New agents and new medical treatments for advanced breast cancer. Semin Oncol 1987;14:34.
9. Ando K, Hirai K, Kubo Y et al. Intra-arterial administration of epirubicin in the treatment of nonresectable hepatocellular carcinoma. Cancer Chemother Pharmacol 1987; 19:183.
10. Sampi K, Masaoka T, Shirakawa S et al. Phase II study of epirubicin in acute leukaemia: a cooperative group study. Anticancer Res 1987;7:29.
11. Zittoun R, Eghbali H, Audebert A et al. Association d'epirubicin bleomycine, vinblastine et predisone (EBVP) avant radiotherapie dans les stades localises de la maladie de Hodgkin. Bull Cancer 1987;74:151.
12. Becouarn Y, Bui BN, Kerbrat et al. Traitement des sarcomes des tissues moux de l'adulte par une association de vindesine et de cisplatine avec doxorubicine ou epirubicin: une etude pilote. Bull Cancer 1987;74:109.
13. Hakes B, Raymond V. Phase II study of idarubicin in advanced endometrial carcinoma. Cancer Treat Rep 1987;71:535.
14. Bastholt L, Dalmark M. Phase II study of idarubicin given orally in the treatment of anthracycline-naive advanced breast cancer patients. Cancer Treat Rep 1987;71:451.
15. Kolaric K, Mechl Z, Potrebica V et al. Phase II study of oral 4-demethoxydaunorubicin in previously treated (except anthracyclines) metastatic breast cancer patients. Oncology 1987;44:82.
16. Echardt S, Szanto J, Cerar O et al. Activity of epirubicin in combination chemotherapy of advanced ovarian cancer. Oncology 1987;44:69.
17. Deliliers GL, Maiolo AT, Annaloro C et al. Idarubicin in sequential combination with cytosine arabinoside in the treatment of relapsed and refractory patients with acute non-lymphoblastic leukaemia. Eur J Cancer Clin Oncol 1987;23:1041.
18. Mittleman A, Magill GB, Raymond V et al. Idarubicin in patients with pancreatic cancer. Cancer Treat Rep 1987;71:657.
19. Tan CTC, Hancock C, Steinherz P et al. Phase I and clinical pharmacological study of 4-demethoxydaunorubicin (idarubicin) in children with advanced cancer. Cancer Res 1987;47:2990.
20. Frustaci S, Gasparini G, Veronesi A et al.. Phase II study of esorubicin (4'-deoxydoxorubicin) in locally advanced or metastatic head and neck carcinoma. Invest. New Drugs 1987;5:307.
21. Carison RW, Billingham ME, Kohler M et al. Esorubicin in refractory carcinoma of the breast: a Northern California Oncology Group Study. Cancer Treat Rep 1987;4:427.
22. Follezou JY, Palangie T, Feuilhade F. Essai randomise comparant la mitotoxantrone a l'adriamycine dans les cancers du sein evolues. Press Med 1987;16:765.
23. Pazdur R, Samson MK, Baker LH. Aclacinomycin A: Phase II evaluation in bronchogenic squamous cell carcinoma. Eur J Clin Oncol 1987;10:234.
24. Pazdur R, Samson MK, Baker LH. Aclacinomycin A: Phase II evaluation in advanced soft tissue carcinoma. Eur J Clin Oncol 1987;10:237.

25. Kerpel-Fronius S, Gyergyay F, Hindy I et al. Phase I-II trial of aclacinomycin A given in four-consecutive day schedule to patients with solid tumours. Oncology 1987;44:159.
26. Rosell R, Abad-Esteve A, Morera J et al. A randomised study comparing platinum doxorubicin and VP-16 with platinum 4′-epidoxorubicin and VP-6 in patients with non-small cell lung cancer. Eur J Clin Oncol 1987;10:245.
27. Yamada K, Shirakawa S, Ohno R et al. A phase II study of 2″R)-4′-*O*-tetrahydroxy-randyladriamycin (THP) in hematological malignancies. Invest New Drugs 1987;5:299.
28. Mathe G, Umezawa H, Oka S et al. An oriented phase II trial of THP-adriamycin in breast carcinoma. Biomed Pharmacother 1986;40:376.
29. Bardakji Z, Jolivet J, Lnagelier Y et al. 5-Fluorouracil-metronidazole combination therapy in metastatic colorectal cancer. Cancer Chemother Pharmcol 1986;18:140.
30. Saini J, Rich MW, Lyss AP. Reversibility of severe left ventricular dysfunction due to doxorubicin. Ann Intern Med 1987;106:814.
31. Mortensen SA, Olsen HS, Baandrup U. Chronic anthracycline cardiotoxicity: haemodynamic and histopathological manifestations suggesting a restrictive endomyocardial disease. Br Heart 1986;55:274.
32. Lipshultz SE, Colan SD, Gelber RD, Perez-Atayde AR, Sallan SE, Sanders SP. Late cardiac effects of doxorubicin therapy for acute lymphoblastic leukemia in childhood. N Engl J Med 1991;324:808—815.
33. Viniegra M, Marchetti M, Losso M, Navigante A, Litovska S, Senderowicz A. Cardiovascular autonomic function in anthracycline-treated breast cancer patients. Cancer Chemother Pharmacol 1990;26:227—231.
34. Lahtinen R, Kuikka J, Nousiainen T, Uusitupa M, Lansimies E. Cardiotoxicity of epirubicin and doxorubicin: a double-blind randomized study. Eur J Haematol 1991; 46:301—305.
35. Cohen IJ, Loven D, Schoenfeld T, Sandbank J, Kaplinsky C, Yaniv Y, Jaber L, Zaizov R. Dactinomycin potentiation of radiation pneumonitis: a forgotten interaction. Pediatr Hematol Oncol 1991;8:187—192.
36. Barendswaard E, Prpic H, Van Der Wall E, Camps J, Keizer H, Pauwels E. Right ventricular wall motion abnormalities in patients treated with chemotherapy. Clin Nucl Med 1991;July:513—516.
37. Weesner K, Bledsoe M, Chauvenet A, Wofford M. Exercise echocardiography in the detection of anthracycline cardiotoxicity. Cancer 1991;68:435—438.
38. Steinherz L, Steinherz P, Tan C, Heller G, Murphy L. Cardiac toxicity 4 to 20 years after complete anthracycline therapy. J Am Med Assoc 1991;266:1672—1677.
39. Drug news. Anthracycline cardiotoxicity uncovered. Drug Ther Dec 1991:57.
40. Fahey J. Cardiovascular function in children with acquired and congenital heart disease. Curr Opin Cardiol 1992;7:111—115.
41. Casper E, Gaynor J, Hajdu S, Magil G, Tan C, Friedrich C, Brennan M. A prospective randomised trial of adjuvant chemotherapy with bolus versus continuous infusion of doxorubicin in patients with high-grade extremity soft tissue sarcoma and an analysis of prognostic factors. Cancer 1991;68:1211—1229.
42. Moreb J, Oblon D. Outcome of clinical congestive heart failure induced by anthracycline chemotherapy. Cancer 1992;70:2637—2641.
43. Rubin AM, Kang H,. Cerebral blindness and encephalopathy with cyclosporin A toxicity. Neurology 1987;37:1072.
44. Okuma K, Ariyoshi Y, Ota K. Clinical study of acute cardiotoxicity of anti-cancer agents—analysis using Holter ECG monitoring. Jpn J Cancer Chemother 1988;15:1893.
45. Camaggi C, Comparsi R, Strocchi E et al. Epirubicin and doxorubicin comparative metabolism and pharmacokinetics. Cancer Chemother Pharmacol 1988;21:221.
46. Torti FM, Bristow MM, Lum BI. Cardiotoxicity of epirubicin and doxorubicin: assessment by endomyocardial biopsy. Cancer Res 1986;46:3722.
47. Concetta Petti M, Mandelli F. Idarubicin in acute leukaemias: experience of the Italian Cooperative Group GIMEMA. Semin Oncol 1989;16(Suppl 2):10.
48. Puccio C, Feldman E, Arlin Z. Amasacrine is safe in pateints with ventricular ectopy. Am J Hematol 1988;28:197.
49. Weiss RB, Grillo-Lopez AJ, Marsoni S et al. Amsacrine-associated cardiotoxicity: an analysis of 82 cases. J Clin Oncol 1986;4:918.
50. Coninx P, Nasca S, Lebrun D et al. Sequential trial of initial chemotherapy for advanced cancer of the head and neck DDP versus DDP+5-fluorouracil. Cancer 1988; 62:1888.
51. Murin J, Kasper J, Danko J et al. Development of myocardial infarction in a patient treated with 5-fluorouracil. Vnitrni Lekarstvi 1989;35:1020.
52. Mazoyer G, Assouline D, Fourchard V et al. Cardiotoxicity of 5-fluorouracil. A case report. Rev Mal Respir 1989;6:551.
53. Sasaki M, Suzuki A, Ishhara T. A case of acute myocardial infarction after treatment with cisplatin. Jpn J Cancer Chemother 1989;16:2289.
54. Steven MAJ, Gouge F, David MAJ, Tietjen P, Jack Moore LTC. Irreversible renal failure after intraperitoneal cisplatin administration. J Reprod Med 1989;34:931—933.
55. Stefenelli T, Kuzmits R, Ulrich W, Glogar D. Acute vascular toxicity after combination chemotherapy with cisplatin, vinblastine and bleomycin for testicular cancer. Eur Soc Cardiol 1988;9:552.
56. Clavel M, Simeone P, Grivet B. Toxicite cardiaque du 5-fluorouracile. Presse Med 1988;17:1675.
57. Eskilsson J, Albertsson M, Mercke C. Adverse cardiac effects during induction chemotherapy treatment with cisplatin and 5-fluorouracil. Radiother Oncol 1988;13:41.
58. Mortimer J, Higano C. Continuous infusion 5-fluorouracil and folinic acid in disseminated colorectal cancer. Cancer Invest 1988;6:129.
59. Coronel B, Madonna D, Mercatello A et al. Myocardiotoxicity of 5-fluorouracil. Intensive Care Med 1988;14:429.
60. Chaudary S, Thomas Song S, Jaski B. Profound, yet reversible heart failure secondary to 5-fluorouracil. Am Med 1988;85:454.
61. Jakubowski A, Kemeny N. Hypotension as a manifestation of cardiotoxicity in three patients receiving cisplatin and 5-fluorouracil. Cancer 1988;62:266.
62. Chaudary S, Thomas Song S, Jaski B. Profound, yet reversible heart failure secondary to 5-fluorouracil. Am Med 1988;85:454.
63. Kleiman N, Lehane D, Geyer C et al. Prinzmetal's angina during 5-fluorouracil chemotherapy. Am J Med 1987;82:566.
64. Keefe D, Roistacher N, Pierri M. Clinical cardiotoxicity of 5-fluorouracil. J Clin Pharmacol 1993;33:1060—1070.
65. Robben N, Pippas A, Moore J. The syndrome of 5-

fluorouracil cardotoxicity. An elusive cardiopathy. Cancer 1993;71:493–509.
66. Lynch T, Kass F, Kalish L, Elias A, Strauss G, Shulman L et al. Cisplatin, 5-fluorouracil and etoposide for advanced non-small cell lung cancer. Cancer 1993;71:2953–2957.
67. Fassio T, Canobbio L, Gasparini G et al. Paroxysmal supraventricular tachycardia during treatment with cisplatin and etoposide combination. Oncology 1986;43:219.
68. Samuels BL, Vogelzange NJ, Kennedy BJ. Vascular toxicity associated with vinblastine, bleomycin and cisplatin chemotherapy. Int J Androl 1987;10:363.
69. Samuels BL, Vogelzange NJ, Kennedy BJ. Severe vascular toxicity associated with vinblastine, bleomycin and cisplatin chemotherapy. Cancer Chemother Pharmacol 1987; 19:253.
70. Gamelin E, Gamelin L, Larra F, Turcant A, Alain P, Maillart P, Allain Y. Acute cardiac toxicity of 5-fluorouracil: pharmacokinetic correlation. Cancer Bull 1991;78:1147–1153.
71. Thyss A, Gaspard M, Marsault R, Milano G, Frelin C, Schneider M. Very high endothelin plasma levels in patients with 5-FU cardiotoxicity. Reference incomplete.
72. Goldberg MA, Antin JH, Guinan EC et al. Cyclophosphamide cardiotoxicity: an analysis of dosing and risk factor. Blood 1986;68:1114.
73. South West Oncology Group. Cancer Treat Rep 1987;71:609.
74. Cassidy J, Merrick M. Cardiotoxicity of mitoxantrone assessed by stress and resting nuclear ventriculography. Eur J Clin Oncol 1988;24:935.
75. Okuma K, Ariyoshi Y, Ota K. Clinical study of acute cardiotoxicity of anti-cancer agents—analysis using Holter ECG monitoring. Jpn J Cancer Chemother 1988;15:1893.
76. Brusamolino E, Bertini M, Guidi S et al. CHOP vs CNOP (N = mitoxantrone) in non-Hodgkin's lymphoma: an interim report comparing efficacy and toxicity. Haemotologica 1988;73:217.
77. Mather FJ, Simon RM, Clark GM et al. Cardiotoxicity in patients treated with mitoxantrone: Southwest Oncology Group Studies. Cancer Treat Rep 1987;71:609.
78. Kwok-Hung L, Yang-Te T, Shou-Dong L et al. Phase 2 study of mitoxantrone in unresectable primary hepatocellular carcinoma following hepatitis B infection. Cancer Chemother Pharmacol 1989;23:54.
79. South West Oncology Group. Cancer Treat Rep 1987;71:609.
80. Jenkinson S, Duncan C, Lawrence R, Collins J. Lack of enhancement of bleomycin lung injury in vitamin E-deficient rats. J Crit Care 1987;2:264.
81. Nussinovitch N, Peleg E, Yaron A et al. Angiotensin converting enzyme in bleomycin-treated patients. Clin Pharmacol Ther Toxicol 1988;26:310.
82. Quigley M, Brada M, Heron C, Horwich A. Severe lung toxicity with a weekly low-dose chemotherapy regimen in patients with non-Hodgkin's lymphoma. Haematol Oncol 1988;6:319.
83. Potash RJ. Acute dyspnoea in a chemotherapy recipient. Respir Care 1987;32:279.
84. Creutzig A, Polking W, Schmoll HJ et al. Raynaud's syndrome and alteration of pulmonary function following cytostatic therapy of testicular cancer. Med Klin 1987;4:131.
85. Dee GJ, Austin JHM, Mutter GL. Bleomycin-associated pulmonary fibrosis: rapidly fatal progression without chest radiotherapy. J Surg Oncol 1987;35:135.
86. Hartmann CA, Weisse I, Voigt D et al. Gefahr zytologischer Fehlinterpretation bei Zytostatikapneumopathie. Prax Klin Pneumol 1987;41:223.
87. White DA, Schwartzberg LS, Kris MG et al. Acute chest pain syndrome during bleomycin infusion. Cancer 1987; 59:1582.
88. Vergnon J, Boucheron S, Riffat J et al. Pneumopathies interstitielles au busulfan: analyse histologigue, evolutive et par lavage broncho-alveolaire de trois observations. Rev Med Intern 1988;9:377.
89. Blaauw AAM, Leunissen KML, Cheriex EC et al. Disappearance of pulmonary capillary leak syndrome when intravenous cyclosporine is replaced by oral cyclosporine. Transplantation 1987;43:758.
90. Powel-Jackson PR, Carmichael FJL, Calne RY et al. Adult respiratory distress syndrome associated with oral cyclosporine. Transplantation 1987;43:767.
91. Glatt V, Henke M, Sigmund G, Costable U. Cyclophosphamid-induzierte Pneumonitis. Fortschr Rontgenschr 1988;148:545.
92. Colozza M, Tonato M, Grignani F, Davis S. Low-dose mitomycin and weekly low-dose doxorubicin combination chemotherapy for patients with metastatic breast carcinoma previously treated with cyclophosphamide, methotrexate, and 5-fluorouracil. Cancer 1988;62:262.
93. Verweij J, Zanten T, Souren T et al. Prospective study on the dose relationship of mitomycin C-induced interstitial pneumonitis. Cancer 1987;60:756.
94. Linette D, McGee K, McFarland J. Mitomycin-induced pulmonary toxicity: case report. Ann Pharmacother 19?? ;26:481–484.
95. Massin F, Coudert B, Marot JP, Foucher P, Camus PH, Jeannin L. Methotrexate pneumonitis. Rev Mal Respir 1990;7:5–15.
96. Martins da Canha AC, Bartsch CH, Gadner H. Acute respiratory failure after intrathecal methotrexate administration. Pediatr Hematol Oncol 1990;7:189–192.
97. Rabinowits M, Souhami L, Gil RA, Andrade CAV, Paiva HC. Increased pulmonary toxicity with bleomycin and cisplatin chemotherapy combinations. Am J Clin Oncol 1990;13:132–138.
98. Hasleton PS, O'Driscoll BR, Lynch P, Webster A, Kalra SJ, Gattamaneni HR, Woodcock AA, Poulter LW. Late BCNU lung: A light and ultrastructural study on the delayed effect of BCNU on the lung parenchyma. J Pathol 1991;164:31–36.
99. O'Driscoll BR, Hasleton PS, Taylor PM, Poulter LW, Gattamaneni HR, Woodcock AA. Active lung fibrosis up to 17 years after chemotherapy with carmustine (BCNU) in childhood. N Eng J Med 1990;82:378–382.
100. Millward MJ, Cohney SJ. Pulmonary toxicity following MOPP chemotherapy. Aust NZ J Med 1990;20:245–248.
101. Cohen IJ, Loven D, Schoenfeld T, Sandbank J, Kaplinsky C, Yaniv Y, Jaber L, Zaizov R. Dactinomycin potentiation of radiation pneumonitis: a forgotten interaction. Pediatr Hematol Oncol 1991;8:187–192.
102. Wilson JKV, Knulman MV, Skeel RT et al. Phase II clinical trial of acivicin in advanced breast cancer: an Eastern Cooperative Oncology Group Study. Cancer Treat Rep 1986;70:1237.
103. Booth BW, Korzun AH, Weiss RB et al. Phase II trial of acivicin in advanced breast carcinoma: a Cancer and Leukemia Group B study. Cancer Treat Rep 1986;70:1247.
104. O'Meara A, Daly M, Hallinan F. Increased antithrom-

bin III concentration in children with acute lymphatic leukaemia receiving L-asparaginase therapy. Med Pediatr Oncol 1988;16:169.
105. Ott N, Ramsay N, Priest J et al. Sequelae of thrombotic of hemorrhagic complications following L-asparaginase therapy for childhood lymphoblastic leukemia. Am J Pediatr Hematol Oncol 1988;10:191.
106. Papavero L, Loew F, Jaksche H. Intracarotid infusion of ACNU and BCNU as adjuvant therapy of malignant gliomas. Acta Neurochir 1987;85:128.
107. Johnson DW, Parkinson D, Wolpert SM et al. Intracarotid chemotherapy with 1,3-bis-(2-chloroethyl)-l-nitrosourea (BCNU) in 5% dextrose in water in the treatment of malignant glioma. Neurosurgery 1987;20/4.
108. Kahn CE, Messersmith RN, Samuels BL. Bronchial plexopathy as a complication of intraarterial cisplatin chemotherapy. Cardiovasc Intervent Radiol 1989;12:47.
109. Gessini L, Jandolo B, Pollera C et al. Neuropatia da cisplatino: un nuovo tipo di polineuropatia assonale ascendente progressiva. Riv Neurobiol 1987;33:75.
110. Holleran W, De Gregorio M. Evolution of high-dose cisplatin. Invest New Drugs 1988;6:135.
111. Riggs J, Ashaf M, Snyder R, Gutmann L. Prospective nerve conduction studies in cisplatin therapy. Ann Neurol 1988;23:92.
112. Walker R, Cairncross J, Posner J. Cerebral herniation in patients receiving cisplatin. J Neuro-Oncol 1988;6:61.
113. Bellin S, Selim M. Cisplatin-induced hypomagnesemia with seizures: a case report and review of the literature. Gynecol Oncol 1988;30:104.
114. Kibirige M, Morris-Jones P, Addison G. Prevention of cisplatin-induced hypomagnesemia. Pediatr Hematol Oncol 1988;5:1.
115. Bauer F, Westhofen M. Vestibular disorders in patients with head and neck tumors receiving carboplatin. HNO 1992;40:19–24.
116. Nichols C, Roth B, Williams S, Gill I, Muggia F, Stablein D, Weiss R. No evidence of acute cardiovascular complications of chemotherapy for testicular cancer. J Clin Oncol 1992;10:760–765.
117. Highley M, Meller S, Pinkerton C. Seizures and cortical dysfunction following high dose cisplatin administration in children. Med Paediatr Oncol 1992;20:143–148.
118. Sghirlanzoni A, Silvani A, Scaioli V, Pareyson D, Marchesan R, Boiardi A. Cisplatin neuropathy in brain tumor chemotherapy. Ital J Neurol Sci 1992;13:311–315.
119. LoMonaco M, Milone M, Batocchi A, Padua L, Restuccia D, Tinali P. Cisplatin neuropathy: clinical and neurophysiological findings. J Neurol 1992;239:199–204.
120. Cavaletti G, Bogliun G, Marzorati L, Marzola M, Pittelli M, Tredici G. The incidence and course of paraneoplastic neuropathy in women with epithelial ovarian cancer. J Neurol 1991;238:371–374.
121. Cavaletti G, Marzorati L, Bogliun G, Colombo N, Marzola M, Pittelli M, Tredici G. Cisplatin-induced peripheral neurotoxicity is dependent on total-dose intensity and single-dose intensity. Cancer 1992;69:203–207.
122. Pratt CB, Goren MP, Meyer WH, Singh B, Dodge RK. Ifosfamide neurotoxicity is related to previous cisplatin treatment for pediatric solid tumors. J Clin Oncol 1990;8:1399–1401.
123. List AF, Kummet TD. Spinal cord toxicity complicating treatment with cisplatin and etoposide. Am J Clin Oncol/CTT 1990;13:256–258.
124. Marzorati L, Bogluin G, Cavaletti G, Tredici G, Pittelli MR. Neurotoxicity of two different cisplatin treatments. Rev Neurobiol 1990 26:459–464.
125. Pollera CF, Pietrangeli A, Giannarelli D. Cisplatin induced peripheral neurotoxicity: relationship to dose intensity. Ann Oncol 1991;2:212.
126. Gerritsen R, Van der Burg MEL, ten Bokkel Huinink WW, van Houwelingen JC, Neijt JP. Incidence of neuropathy in 395 patients with ovarian cancer treated with or without cisplatin. Cancer 1990;66:1697–1702.
127. Siegal T, Haim N. Cisplatin induced peripheral neuropathy. Cancer 1990;66:1117–1123.
128. Holleran W, De Gregorio M. Evolution of high-dose cisplatin. Invest New Drugs 1988;6:135.
129. Philip T, Ghalie R, Pinkerton R et al. A phase II study of high-dose cisplatin and VP-16 in neuroblastoma. J Clin Oncol 1987;5:941.
130. Daugaard GK, Petrera J, Trojaborg W. Electrophysiological study of the peripheral and central neurotoxic effect of cisplatin. Acta Neurol Scand 1987;76:86.
131. Amiel H, Gherardi R, Giroux C et al. Neuropathie au cisplatine. Ann Med Interne 1987;138:101.
132. Frustaci S, Barzan L, Comoretto R et al. Local neurotoxicity after intra-arterial cisplatin in head and neck cancer. Cancer Treat Rep 1987;71:3.
133. Castellanos AM, Glass P, Yung WKA. Regional nerve injury after intra-arterial chemotherapy. Neurology 1987; 37:834.
134. Oshita F, Saijo N, Shinkai T, Eguchi K, Sasaki Y et al. Correlation between total dose of cisplatin and vibratory perception threshold in chemotherapy-induced peripheral neuropathy of cancer patients. Cancer J 1992;5:165–169.
135. Rubin AM, Kang H. Cerebral blindness and encephalopathy with cyclosporin A toxicity. Neurology 1987;37:1072.
136. Labar B, Bogdanic V, Plasvic F et al. Cyclosporin neurotoxicity in patients treated with allogenic bone marrow transplantation. Biomed Pharmacother 1986;40:148.
137. Delpont E, Thomas P, Gugenheim J, Chichmanian, Mahagne MH, Suisse G. Prolonged confusion with cyclosporine: non convulsive status epilepticus. Neurophysiol Clin 1990;20:207–215.
138. Bohlin AB, Berg U, Englund M, Malm G, Persson A, Tibell A. Central nervous system complications in children treated with cyclosporin after renal transplantation. Child Nephrol Urol 1990;10:225–230.
139. Herzig RH, Hines JD, Herzig GP et al. Cerebellar toxicity with high-dose cytosine arabinoside. J Clin Oncol 1987;5:927.
140. Nand S, Messmore HL, Patel R et al. Neurotoxicity associated with systemic high-dose cytosine arabinoside. J Clin Oncol 1986;4:571.
141. Thordarson H, Talstad I. Acute meningitis and cerebellar dysfunction complicating high-dose cytosine arabinoside therapy. Acta Med Scand 1986;220:493.
142. Heier MS, Fossa SD. Wernicke-Korsakoff-like syndrome in patients with colorectal carcinoma treated with high-dose doxifluridine. Acta Neurol Scand 1986;73:449.
143. Leff R, Thompson J, Daly M et al. Acute neurologic dysfunction after high-dose etoposide therapy for malignant glioma. Cancer 1988;62:32.
144. Chun HG, Leyland-Jones BR, Caryk S et al. Central nervous system toxixicity of fludarabine phosphate. Cancer Treat Rep 1986,70:1225.
145. Pinkerton CR, Pritchard J. A phase 2 study of ifosfam-

ide in paediatric solid tumours. Cancer Chemother Pharmacol 1989;24(Suppl):S13.
146. Lind MJ, Margison JM, Cerny T et al. Comparative pharmacokinetics and alkylating activity of fractionated intravenous and oral ifosfamide in patients with bronchogenic carcinoma. Cancer Res 1989;49:735.
147. Gieron M, Barak L, Estrada J. Severe encephalopathy associated with ifosfamide administration in two children with metastatic tumours. J Neuro-Oncol 1988;6:29.
148. Drings P, Abel U, Bulzebruck H et al. Experience with ifosfamide combinations (etoposide or DDP) in non-small cell lung carcinoma. Cancer Chemother Pharmacol 1986;18(Suppl 2):S34.
149. Pratt CB, Horowitz ME, Meyer WH et al. Phase II trial of ifosfamide in children with malignant solid tumors. Cancer Treat Rep 1987;71:131.
150. Meanwell CA, Blake AE, Kelly KA et al. Prediction of ifosfamide/mesna associated encephalopathy. Eur J Cancer Clin Oncol 1986;22:815.
151. Fujii Y, Mizuno Y, Hongo T et al. Serial spectral EEG analysis in a patient with non-Hodgkin's lymphoma complicated by leukoencephalopathy induced by high-dose methotrexate. Jpn J Cancer Chemother 1988;15:713.
152. Postkitt K, Steinbok P, Flodmark O. Methotrexate leukoencephalopathy mimicking cerebral abcess on CT brain scan. Child Nerv Syst 1988;4:119.
153. Ebner F, Ranner G, Slave J et al. MR findings in methotrexate induced CNS abnormalities. Am J Neuroradiol 1989;10:959.
154. Rhomberg WU. Vindesine for recurrent and metastatic cancer of the uterine cervix: a phase II study. Cancer Treat Rep 1986;70:1455.
155. Stewart DJ, Maroun JA, Lefebre B et al. Neurotoxicity and efficacy of combined Vinca alkaloids in breast cancer. Cancer Treat Rep 1986;70:591.
156. Dickerhoff R, Lindner W, Scheiber W. Severe emboli in patients receiving chemotherapy for non-Hodgkin's lymphoma. Chest 1988;94:589.
157. Thoumie P, Diverrez JR, Guidet B. Polynevrite aigue a la vincristine prescrite pour un cancer du sein chez une patiente atteinte de maladie de Friedreich. Sem Hop Paris 1989;65:30.
158. Dickerhoff R, Lindner W, Scheiber W. Severe emboli in patients receiving chemotherapy for non-Hodgkin's lymphoma. Chest 1988;94:589.
159. Thoumie P, Diverrez JR, Guidet B. Polynevrite aigue a la vincristine prescrite pour un cancer du sein chez une patiente atteinte de maladie de Friedreich. Sem Hop Paris 1989;65:30.
160. Hurwitz R, Mahoney D, Armstrong D, Browder T. Reversible encephalopathy and seizures as a result of conventional vincristine administration. Med Pediatr Oncol 1983;16:216.
161. Pinkerton C, McDermott B, Philip T, Biron P. Continuous vincristine infusion as part of a high dose chemoradiotherapy regimen: drug kinetics and toxicity. Cancer Chemother Pharmacol 1988;22:271.
162. Jackson D, Wells H, Atkins J. Amelioration of vincristine neurotoxicity by glutamic acid. Am J Med 1988;84:1016.
163. Heier MS, Nilsen T, Graver V, Aass N, Fossa SD. Raynaud's phenomenon after combination chemotherapy of testicular cancer, measured by laser Doppler flowmetry. A pilot study. Br J Cancer 1991;63:550—552.
164. Annino D, MacArthur C, Friedman E. Vincristine-induced recurrent laryngeal nerve paralysis. Laryngoscope 1992;102:1260—1262.
165. McCarthy G, Skillings J. Jaw and other orofacial pain in patients receiving vincristine for the treatment of cancer. Oral Surg Oral Med Oral Pathol 1992;74:299—304.
166. Meloni G, Raucci U, Pinto R, Spalice A, Vignetti M, Iannetti P. Pretransplant conditioning with busulphan and cyclophosphamide in acute luekemia patients. Ann Oncol 1992;3:145—148.
167. Borgna-Pignatti C, Battisti L, Marradi P, Balter R, Caudoma R. Transient neurologic disturbances in a child treated with moderate-dose methotrexate. 1992.
168. Ramalho HJ, Terra EG, Cartapatti E et al. Hepatoxicity of azathioprine in renal transplant recipients. Transplant Proc 1989;21:1716.
169. Cooper C, Cotton DWK, Minihane N et al. Azathioprine hypersensitivity manifesting as acute + focal hepatocellular necrosis. J R Soc Med 1986;79:171.
170. Read AE, Wiesner RH, LaBrecque DR et al. Hepatic veno-occlusive disease associated with renal transplantation and azathioprine therapy. Ann Intern Med 1986;104:651.
171. Lorber MI, Van Buren CT, Flechner SM et al. Hepatobiliary and pancreatic complications of cyclosporine therapy in 466 renal transplant recipients. Transplantation 1987; 43:35.
172. Harihara Y, Sanjo K, Idezuki Y. Cyclosporine hepatotoxicity and cold ischemia liver damage. Transplant Proceed 1992;24:1984.
173. Moertel C, Fleming T, MacDonald J, Haller D, Laurie J. Hepatic toxicity associated with fluorouracil plus levamisole adjuvant therapy. J Clin Oncol 1993;11:2386—2390.
174. Honjo I, Suou T, Hirayama C. Hepatotoxicity of cyclophosphamide in man: pharmacokinetic analysis. Res Commun Chem Pathol Pharmacol 1988;61:149.
175. Shaunak S, Munro J, Weinbren K et al. Cyclophosphamide-induced liver necrosis: a possible interaction with azathioprine. Q J Med 1988;67:309.
176. Green D, Finklestein J, Norkool P, D'Angio GJ. Severe hepatic toxicity after treatment with single-dose dactinomycin and vincristine. Cancer 1988;62:270.
177. Ceci G, Bella M, Melissari M et al. Fatal hepatic vascular toxicity of DTIC. Cancer 1988;61:1988.
178. Lejeune F, Macher E, Kleeberg U et al. Assessment of DTIC vs levamisole or placebo in treatment of high risk stage I patients after surgical removal of a primary melanoma of the skin: a Phase III adjuvant study. Eur J Cancer Clin Oncol 1988;24:81.
179. McClay E, Lusch MJ, Manstrangelo MJ. Allergy-induced hepatic toxicity associated with decarbazine. Cancer Treat Rep 1987;71:219.
180. D'Angio GJ. Hepatoxicity with actinomycin D. Lancet 1987;ii:104.
181. Pietrafitta JJ, Anderson BG, O'Brien MJ et al. Cholecystitis secondary to infusion chemotherapy. J Surg Oncol 1986;31:287.
182. Hilton MA, Bertolone S, Patal CC. Daily profiles of plasma phenylalanine and tyrosine in patients with osteogenic sarcoma during treatment with high dose methotrexate citrovorum rescue. Med Paediatr Oncol 1989;17:265.
183. Risteli J, Sogaard H, Oikarinen A et al. Aminoterminal propeptide of type III procollagen in methotrexate-induced liver fibrosis and cirrhosis. Br J Dermatol 1988;119:321.
184. Zachariae H, Schroder H, Foged E et al. Methotrexate hepatotoxicity and concentrations of methotrexate and folate

in erythocytes—relation to liver fibrosis and cirrhosis. Acta Dermatol Venereol 1987;67:336.
185. Tolman KG, Glegg DO, Lee DG et al. Methotrexate and the liver. J. Rheumatol 1985;12(Suppl):29.
186. Whiting-O'Keefe Q, Fye K, Sack K. Methotrexate and histologic hepatic abnormalities: a meta-analysis. Am J Med 1991;90:711—716.
187. Lin Y, Huang Y, Lee S, Wu J, Chang C, Chen C, Hwang S. Clinical study of methotrexate-induced hepatic injury in patients with psoriasis. Chin J Gastroenterol 1991;8:277—281 (in Chinese).
188. Larrey D, Freneaux E, Berson A et al. Peliosis hepatis induced by 6-thioguanine administration. Gut 1988;29:1265.
189. Jones M, Best P, Catto G. Is nodular regenerative hyperplasia of the liver associated with azathioprine therapy after renal tansplantation? Nephrol Dialysis Transplant 1988;3:331.
190. Pritchard J, Raine J, Wallendszus K. Hepatoxicity of actinomycin-D. Lancet 1989;i:168.
191. White L, Tobias V, O'Gorman-Hughes DW. Actinomycin-D induced hepatoxicity. Pediatr Hematol Oncol 1989;6:53.
192. D'Angio GJ. Hepatotoxicity and actinomycin. Lancet 1990;335:1290.
193. Shepherd P, Fooks J, Gray R, Allan N. Thioguanine used in maintenance therapy of chronic myeloid leukaemia causes non-cirrhotic portal hypertension. Br J Haematol 1991;79:185—192.
194. Bergevin P. Nephrotoxicity of cisplatin (*cis*-diamminedichloroplatinum (II). Drug Today 1988;24:403.
195. Daugaard G, Abildgaard U, Holstein Rathlou N et al. Renal tubular function in patients treated with high-dose cisplatin. Clin Pharmacol Ther 1988;44:164.
196. Saito M, Masaki T, Kato H. A clinical evaluation of the protective effect of fosfomycin (FOM) against the *cis*-diamminedichloroplatinum (CDDP)-induced nephrotoxicity. Acta Urol Jpn 1988;34:782.
197. Mariette X, Paule B, Bennet P et al. Cisplatin and hyponatremia. Ann Intern Med 1988;108:770.
198. Mavichak V, Coppin C, Wong N et al. Renal magnesium wasting and hypocalciuria in chronic *cis*-platinum nephropathy in man. Clin Sci 1988;75:203.
199. Mariette X, Paule B, Bennet P et al. Cisplatin and hyponatremia. Ann Intern Med 1988;108:770.
200. Daugaard G, Abildgaard U, Holstein Rathlou N et al. Renal tubular function in patients treated with high-dose cisplatin. Clin Pharmacol Ther 1988;44:164.
201. Bellin S, Selim M. Cisplatin-induced hypomagnesemia with seizures: a case report and review of the literature. Gynecol Oncol 1988;30:104.
202. Mavichak V, Coppin C, Wong N et al. Renal magnesium wasting and hypocalciuria in chronic *cis*-platinum nephropathy in man. Clin Sci 1988;75:203.
203. Safirstein R, Wiston J. Cisplatin nephrotoxicity. J QUEH 1987;9(Suppl):216.
204. Safirstein R, Winston J, Moel D et al. Cisplatin nephrotoxicity: insights into mechanism. Int J Androl 1987;10:325.
205. Falkenberg FW, Mondorf U, Pierard E et al. Identification of fragments of proximal and distal tubular cells in the urine of patients under cytostatic treatment by immunoelectron microscopy with monoclonal antibodies. Am J Kidney Dis 1987;9:129.
206. Imura N, Naganuma A, Satoh M et al. Depression of toxic effects of anticancer agents by selenium or pretreatment with metallothionein inducers. J QUEH 1987;9(Suppl):223.
207. Glover D, Glick JH, Weiler C et al. WR-2721 and high-dose cisplatin: an active combination in the treatment of metastatic melanoma. J Clin Oncol 1987;5:574.
208. Lam M, Adelstein DJ. Hypomagnesemia and renal magnesium wasting in patients treated with cisplatin. Am J Kidney Dis 1986;8:164.
209. Willox JC, McAllistar EJ, Sangster G et al. Effects of magnesium in testicular cancer patients receiving cisplatin. Br J Cancer 1986;54:19.
210. Markman M, Cleary S, Howell SB. Hypomagnesemia following high-dose intracavitary cisplatin with systemically administered sodium thiosulfate. Am J Clin Oncol Cancer Clin Trials 1986 9:440.
211. Ten Bokke Huinink W, Van der Burg M, Van Oosterom A et al. Carboplatin in combination therapy for ovarian cancer. Cancer Treat Rev 1988;15(Suppl B):9.
212. Calvert A, Horwich A, Newlands E et al. Carboplatin or cisplatin? Lancet 1988;ii:577.
213. Conte P, Bruzzone M, Chiara S et al. Carboplatin (JM8), adriamycin and cyclophosphamide (JAC) in advanced ovarian carcinoma: a pilot study. Tumori 1988; 74:217.
214. Anderson H, Wagstaff J, Crowther D et al. Comparative toxicity of cisplatin, carboplatin (CBDCA) and iproplatin (CHIP) in combination with cyclophosphamide in patients with advanced epithelial ovarian cancer. Eur J Cancer Clin Oncol 1988;24:1471.
215. Calvert A, Horwich A, Newlands E et al. Carboplatin or cisplatin? Lancet 1988;ii 577.
216. Lee E, Egorin M, van Echo D et al. Phase I and pharmacokinetic trial of carboplatin in refractory adult leukaemia. J Natl Cancer Inst 1988;80:131.
217. Sweeney J, Ziegler P, Pruet C et al. Hyperzincuria and hypozincemia in patients treated with cisplatin. Cancer 1989;63:2093.
218. Skinner R, Peearson A, Price L, Courtland M, Craft A. The influence of age on nephrotoxicity following chemotherapy in children. Br J Cancer 1992;66(Suppl XVIII):S30—S35.
219. Hargis J, Anderson J, Porpert K, Green M, VAn Echo D, Weiss R. Predicting genitourinary toxicity in patients receiving cisplatin-based combination chemotherapy: a Cancer and Leukemia Group B Study. Cancer Chemother Pharmacol 1992;30:291—296.
220. Laskow DA, Curtis JJ, Luke RG, Jullian BA, Jones P, Deierhoi MH. Cyclosporine induced changes in glomerular filtration rate and urea excretion. Am J Med 1990;88:497—502.
221. Mobb GE, Veitch PS, Bell PRF. Are serum creatinine levels adequate to identify the onset of chronic cyclosporine A nephrotoxicity? Transplant Proc 1990;22:1708—1710.
222. Tindall RSA, Rollins JA, Phillips JT et al. Preliminary results of a double-blind randomized, placebo-controlled trial of cyclosporin in myasthenia gravis. N Engl J Med 1987;316:719.
223. Hadj-Aissa A, Labeeuw M, Lareal MC et al. Effets de la cyclosporine (CyA) sur le rein isole:comparaison avec l'excipient (Exc). Nephrologie 1987;8:73.
224. Hoyer PF, Krohn HP, Offner G et al. Renal function after kidney transplantation in children. Transplantation 1987;43:489.
225. Wheatley HC, Datzman M, Williams JW et al. Long-term effects of cyclosporine on renal function in liver transplant recipients. Transplantation 1987;43:641.

226. Mihatsch MJ, Thiel G, Ryffel B. Brief review of the morphology of cyclosporin A nephropathy. Nephrologie 1987;8:143.
227. Wheatley HC, Datzman M, Williams JW et al. Long-term effects of cyclosporine on renal function in liver transplant recipients. Transplantation 1987;43:641.
228. Raphael L, Fish JC. An in vitro model for analyzing the nephrotoxicity of cyclosporine and preservation injury. Transplantation 1987;43:703.
229. Anaise D, Waltzer WC, Arnold AN et al. Adverse effects of cyclosporine A on the microcirculation of the cold preserved kidney. NY State J Med 1987;87:141.
230. Feehally J, Walls J, Mistry N et al. Does nifedipine ameliorate cyclosporin A nephrotoxicity? Br Med J 1987;295:310.
231. Feehally J, Walls J, Mistry N et al. Does nifedipine ameliorate cyclosporin A nephrotoxicity? Br Med J 1987;295:310.
232. Le Bigot JF, Lavene D, Kiechel JR. Pharmacocinetique et metabolisme di la cyclosporine: interaction medicamenteuse. Nephrologie 1987;8:135.
233. Lindholm A, Ringden O, Lonnqvist B. The role of cyclosporine dosage and plasma levels in efficacy and toxicity in bone marrow transplant recipients. Transplantation 1987;43:680.
234. Schroeder TJ, Melvin DB, Clardy CW et al. Use of cyclosporine and ketoconazole without nephrotoxicity in two heart transplant recipients. J Heart Transplant 1987;6:84.
235. Palestine AG, Austin HA, Balow JE et al. Renal histopathologic alterations in patients treated with cyclosporine for uveitis. N Engl J Med 1986;314:1293.
236. Termeer A, Hoistma AJ, Koene RAP. Severe nephrotoxicity caused by the combined use of gentamicin and cyclosporine in renal allograft recipients. Transplantation 1986;42:220.
237. Thomas AE, Patterson J, Prentice HG et al. Haemorrhagic cystitis in bone marrow transplantation patients: possible increased risk associated with prior busulphan therapy. Bone Marrow Transplant 1987;1:347.
238. Thomas AE, Patterson J, Prentice HG et al. Haemorrhagic cystitis in bone marrow transplantation patients: possible increased risk associated with prior busulphan therapy. Bone Marrow Transplant 1987;1:347.
239. Maiche A, Lappalainen K, Teerenhovi L. Renal insufficiency in patients treated with high dose methotrexate. Acta Oncol 1988;27:73.
240. Christensen M, Rivera G, Crom W et al. Effect of hydration on methotrexate plasma concentrations in children with acute lymphocytic leukema. J Clin Oncol 1988;6:797.
241. Amino K, Kawaguchi N, Matsumoto S et al. Urinary β_2-microglobulin as an indicator of impaired excretion of methotrexate. Jpn J Cancer Chemother 1988;15:3103.
242. Molina R, Fabian C, Cowley B. Use of charcoal hemoperfusion with sequential hemodialysis to reduce serum methotrexate levels in a patient with acute renal insufficiency. Am J Med 1987;82:350.
243. Relling M, Bruder Stapleton F, Ochs J et al. Removal of methotrexate, leucovorin and their metabolites by combined hemodialysis and hemoperfusion. Cancer 1988;62:884.
244. Price P, Thompson H, Bessell E, Bloom H. Renal impairment following the combined use of high-dose methotrexate and procarbazine. Cancer Chemother Pharmacol 1988;21:265.
245. Mackintosh J, Tattersal M. Mitomycin-C induced hemolytic-uraemic syndrome. Aust NZ J Med 1988;18:182.
246. Ries F. Nephrotoxicity of chemotherapy. Eur J Cancer Clin Oncol 1988;21:951.
247. Hayano K, Fukui H, Otsuka Y, Hattori S. Three cases of renal failure associated with microangiopathic hemolytic anemia after mitomycin-C therapy (in Japanese). Jpn J Nephrol 1988;7:835.
248. Vervey J, De Vries J, Pinedo HM. Mitomycin C-induced renal toxicity, a dose dependent side effect? Eur J Cancer Clin Oncol 1987;23:195.
249. Sheldon R. Slaughter D. A syndrome of microangiopathic hemolytic anemia, renal impairment, and pulmonary edema in chemotherapy-treated patients with adenocarcinoma. Cancer 1986;58:1428.
250. Goren MP, Pratt CB, Viar MJ. Tubular nephrotoxicity during long term ifosfamide and mesna therapy. Cancer Chemother Pharmacol 1989;25:70—72.
251. Burk CD, Restaino I, Kaplan BS, Meadows AT. Ifosfamide induced renal tubular dysfunction and rickets in children with Wilms tumor. J Pediatr 1990;117:331—335.
252. Kurschel E, Metz-Kurschel U, Niederie N, Aulbert E. Investigations on the sub-clinical nephrotoxicity of interferon alpha-2B in patients with myeloproliferative syndromes. Renal Failure 1991;13:87—93.
253. Ricci JL, Turnbull ADM. Spontaneous gastroduodenal perforation in cancer patients receiving cytotoxic therapy. J Surg Oncol 1989;41:219.
254. Vorobiof DA, Falkson G. Phase 2 study of high dose 4′-epidoxorubicin in the treatment of advanced gastrointestinal cancer. Eut J Cancer Clin Oncol 1989;25:563.
255. Vorobiof DA,FAlskon G. Phase 2 study of high dose 4′-epidoxorubicin in the treatment of advanced gastrointestinal cancer. Eut J Cancer Clin Oncol 1989;25:563.
256. De Gara C, Gagic N, Arnold A, Seaton T. Toxic megacolon associated with anticancer chemotherapy. CJS 1991;34:339—341.
257. Spechler S. Columnar-lined (Barret's) esophagus. Curr Opin Gastroenterol 1991;7:557—561.
258. Mullai N, Sivarajan K, Shiomoto G. Barrett esophagus. Ann Intern Med 1991;114:913.
259. Sartori S, Neilson I, Maestri A, Beltrami D, Trevisani L, Pazzi P. Acute gastroduodenal mucosal injury after cisplatin plus etoposide chemotherapy. Oncology 1991;48:356—361.
260. Reznik VM, Durham BL, Lyons-Jones et al. Changes in facial appearance during cyclosporin treatment. Lancet 1987;i:1405.
261. Wysocki GP, Daley TD. Hypertrichosis in patients receiving cyclosporine therapy. Clin Exp Dermatol 1987; 12:191.
262. Matsuyama JR, Kwok KK. A variant of the chemotherapy associated erythrodysesthesia syndrome related to high dose cyclophosphamide. DCIP Ann Pharmacother 1989;23:776.
263. Shall L, Lucas G, Whittaker J, Holt P. Painful red hands: a side effect of leukaemia therapy. Br J Dermatol 1988;119:249.
264. Bellmunt J, Navarro M, Hidalgo R, Sole L. Palmar-plantar erythrodysesthesia syndrome associated with short-term continuous infusion (5 days) of 5-fluorouracil. Tumori 1988;74:329.
265. Cho K, Chung J, Lee A et al. Pigmented macules in patients treated with systemic 5-fluorouracil. J Dermatol 1988;15:342.
266. Inglis JA, Tolley DA, Grigor KM. Allergy to mitomycin

C complicating topical administration for urothelial cancer. Br J Urol 1987;59:547.
267. Sala F, Crosti C, Bencini PL et al. Esantema tossiallergico da instillazione endovesicale di mitomicina C. G Ital Dermatol Vernereol 1987;122:265.
268. Mobley WC, Loening SA, Narayana AS et al. Use of intravesical cisplatin and mitomycin-C for recurrent transitional cell carcinoma of bladder refractory to thiotepa. Urology 1986;4:335.
269. Beer RAM, Muhlethaler JP, Bartlome F et al. Adjuvant intravesicle chemotherapy of superficial bladder cancer with monthly doxoribicin or intensive mitomycin. Eur Urol 1987;13:10.
270. Hetherington JW, Newling DWW, Robinson MRG et al. Intravesical mitomycin C for the treatment of recurrent superficial bladder tumours. Br J Urol 1987;59:239.
271. Aizawa H, Tagami H. Delayed tissue necrosis due to mitomycin C. Acta Dermatol Venereol 1987;67:364.
272. Bikkers THA, Verweij J, Stoter AN. Ernstige weefselnecrose ten gevolge van extravasatie van mitomycine. Ned Tijdschr Geneeskd 1987;131:588.
273. Koppensteiner R, Minar E. Survival following an extremely high-dose of mitoxantrone in a 73 year old female with small-cell bronchial carcinoma (Letter to Editor). J Cancer Res Clin Oncol 1988;114:324.
274. Anonymous. Mitoxantrone. Med Lett 1988:68.
275. Burg G, Bieber T, Langecker P. Lokalisierte neutrophile ekkrine Hidradenitis unter Mitroxantron: eine typische Zytostatikanebenwirkung. Hautarzt 1988;39:233.
276. Speechly-Dick ME, Owen ERTC. Mitozantrone induced onycholysis. Lancet 1988;i:113.
277. Werner Hansen S, Nissen N, Mork Hansen M et al. High activity of mitoxantrone in previously untreated lowgrade lymphomas. Cancer Chemother Pharmacol 1988;22:77.
278. Carstensen H, Nolte H, Hertz H. Teniposide induced hypersensitivity reactions in children. Lancet 1989;ii:55.
279. Nolte H, Carstensen H, Hertz H. VM-26 (teniposide) induced hypersensitivity and degranulation of basophils in children. Am J Pediatr Hematol/Oncol 1988;10:308.
280. Van de Kerkhof PCP, de Vaan GAM, Holland R. Pyoderma gangrenosum in acute myeloid leukaemia during immunosuppression. Eur J Pediatr 1988;148:34.
281. Siddall SJ, Martin J, Nunn AJ. Anaphylactic reactions to teniposide. Lancet 1989;i:394.
282. Fondevila CG, Milone GA, Pavlovsky S. Cutaneous vasculitis after intermediate dose of methotrexate (IDMTX). Br J Haematol 1989;72:591.
283. Huber A. Anaphylactoid-type reaction to methotrexate. Allergologie 1990;13:S33.
284. Williams SF, Larson RA. Hypersensitivity reaction to high dose cytarabine. Br J Haematol 1989;73:274.
285. Korholz D, Wahn U, Jurgens H et al. Allergic reactions during treatment with L-asparaginase: role of specific IgE antibodies. Monatsschr Kinderheilkd 1990;138:23.
286. Riedel RR, Schmitt A, de Jonge JPA et al. Gastrointestinal type I hypersensitivity to azathioprine. Klin Wochenschr 1990;68:50.
287. Saunders M, Denton C, O'Brien M, Blake P, Gore M, Wiltshore E. Hypersensitivity reactions to cisplatin and carboplatin. Ann Oncol 1992;3:574–576.
288. Hendrick A, Simmons D, Cantwell B. Allergic reactions to carboplatin. Ann Oncol 1992;3:239–240.
289. Vidal C, de la Fuente R, Gonzalez Quintela A. Three cases of allergic dermatitis due to intravesicle mitomycin. Dermatology 1992;184:208–209.
290. De Groot A, van der Meyden A. Purpuric allergic drug eruption from intravesicle instillation of the antitumor antibiotic mitomycin C. Dermatosen 1991;39:84–86.
291. Hirano M, Okamoto M, Maruyama F, Ezaki K, Shimizu K, Ino T, Matsui T. Alternating non-cr chemotherapy for non-Hodgkin's lymphoma of intermediate-grade and high grade malignancy. Cancer 1992;69:772–777.
292. Singal R, Tunnessen W, Wiley J, Hood A. Discrete pigmentation after chemotherapy. Pediatr Dermatol 1991; 8:231–235.
293. Requena L. Chemotherapy-induced transverse ridging of the nails. Cutis 1991;48:129–130.
294. Kellie S, Crist W, Pui C, Crone M, Fairclough D, Rodman J, Rivera G. Hypersensitivity reactions to epidophyllotoxins in children with acute lymphoblastic leukemia. Cancer 1991;67:1070–1075.
295. Cersosimo R, Calarese P, Karp D. Acute hypotensive reaction to etoposide with successful rechallenge: case report and review of the literature. DICP Ann Pharmacother 1989;23:876–877.
296. Tester W, Cohn J, Fleekop P, Rabinowitz M. Successful rechallenge to etoposide after acute vasomotor response. J Clin Oncol 1990;8:1660–1661.
297. Salles G, Vial T, Archimbaud E. Anaphylactoid reaction with bronchospasm following intravenous cyclophosphamide administration. Ann Hematol 1991;62:74–75.
298. Moens Ch, Moens Ph, Philippart G. Azathioprine and warts. Ann Rheum Dis 1990;49:269.
299. Curran CF, Luce JK. Ocular adverse reactions associated with adriamycin (doxorubicin). Am J Ophthalmol 1989;108:709.
300. Curran CF, Luce JK. Accidental acute exposure to doxorubicin. Cancer Nurs 1989;12:329.
301. Fossa SD. Is interferon with or without vinblastine the 'treatment of choice' in metastatic renal cell carcinoma? The Norwegian Radium Hospital's experience. Semin Surg Oncol 1988;4:178.
302. Teichmann K, Dabbagh N. Severe visual loss after a single dose of vincristine in a patient with spinal cord astrocytoma. J Ocul Pharm 1988;4:117.
303. Pinkerton C, McDermott B, Philip T, Biron P. Continuous vincristine infusion as part of a high dose chemoradiotherapy regimen: drug kinetics and toxicity. Cancer Chemother Pharmacol 1988;22:271.
304. Elsa T, Watne K, Fostad K et al. Ocular complications after intracarotid BCNU for intracranial tumors. Acta Ophthalmol 1989;67:83.
305. Rubin AM. Transient cortical blindness and occipital seizures with cyclosporine toxicity. Transplantation 1989; 47:572.
306. Wilson SE, de Groen PC, Aksamit AJ et al. Cyclosporin A induced reversible cortical blindness. J Clin Neuro-Ophthalmol 1988;8:215.
307. Kadoya K, Suda Y, Tonaki M et al. Two cases of anemic retinopathy. Folia Ophthalmol Jpn 1989;40:148.
308. Barletta J, Fanous M, Margo C. Corneal and conjuctival toxicity with low-dose cytosine arabinoside. Am J Ophthalmol 1992;113:587–588.
309. Avery R, Jabs D, Wingard J, Vogelsang G, Saral R, Santos G. Optic disc edema after bone marrow transplantation—possible role of cyclosporine toxicity. Ophthalmology 1991;98:1294–1301.

310. Rajeev B, Thomas R. Striate melanokeratosis following trabeculectomy with 5-fluorouracil. Arch Ophthalmol 1990;108:1216–1217.
311. Stank T, Krupin T, Feitl M. Subconjuctival 5-fluorouracil induced transient striate melanokeratosis. Arch Ophthalmol 1990;108:1210.
312. Lemp M. Striate melanokeratosis. Arch Ophthalmol 1991;109:917.
313. Loprinz C, Love R, Garrity J, Ames M. Cyclophosphamide, methotrexate and 5-fluorouracil (CMF) induced ocular toxicity. Cancer Invest 1990;8:459–465.
314. Domenech J, Santabarbara P, Carulla M et al. Sudden hearing loss in an adolescent following a single dose of cisplatin. Otorhinolaryngology 1988;50:405.
315. Kopelman J, Budnick A, Sessions RB, Wong GY. Ototoxicity of high-dose cisplatin by bolus administration in patients with advanced cancers and normal hearing. Laryngoscope 1988;98:858.
316. Laurell G, Borg E. Ototoxicity of cisplatin in gynaecological cancer patients. Scand Audiol 1988;17:241.
317. Laurell G, Engstrom B, Hirsch A et al. Ototoxicity of cisplatin. Int J Androl 1987;10:359.
318. Laurell G, Engstrom B, Hirsch A et al. Ototoxicity of cisplatin. Int J Androl 1987;10:359.
319. Caston J, Doinel L. Comparative vestibular toxicity of dibekacin, habekacin and cisplatin. Acta Otolaryngol 1987;104:315.
320. Kobayashi H, Ohashi N, Watanabe Y et al. Clinical features of cisplatin vestibulotoxicity and hearing loss. Otorhinolaryngology 1987;49:67.
321. Annilo M, Sobin A. Cisplatin: evaluation of its ototoxic potential. Am J Otolaryngol 1986;7:276.
322. Meyskens FL, Kingsley EM, Glattke T et al. A phase II study of difluoromethylornithine (DFMO) for the treatment of metastatic melanoma. Invest New Drugs 1986;4:257.
323. Liren T, Aoyagi M, Fuse T, Yokota M, Suzuki T, Kim Y, Koike Y. (1991).
324. Cohen B, Zweidler P, Goldwein J, Molloy J, Packer R. Ototoxic effect of cisplatin in children with brain tumours. Pediatr Neurosurg 1990/91;16:92–296.
325. Pasic T, Dobie R. *Cis*-platinum ototoxicity in children. Laryngoscope 1991;101:985–991.
326. Weatherly R, Owens J, Catlin F, Mahoney D. *Cis*-platinum ototoxicity in children. Laryngoscope 1991; 101:917–924.
327. Bauer F, Westhofen M. Vestibular disorders in patients with head and neck tumours receiving carboplatin: HNO 1992;40:19–24.
327. Waters G, Ahmed M, Katsarkas A, McKay J. Ototoxicity due to *cis*-diamminedichloroplatinum in the treatment of ovarian cancer: influence of dosage and schedule of administration. Ear Hear 1991;12:91–102.
328. Durrant J, Rodgers D, Myers E, Johnson J. Hearing loss—risk factors for cisplatin ototoxicity? Observations. Am J Otol 1990;11:375–377.
329. Vantrappen G, Rector E, Debruyne F. The ototoxicity of cisplatin: clinical study. Acta Otorhinolaryngol Belg 1990;44:415–422.
330. Skinner R, Pearson A, Amineddine H, Mathias D, Craft A. Ototoxocity of cisplatinum in children and adolescents. Br J Cancer 1990;61:927–931.
331. Kennedy I, Fitzharris B, Colls B, Atkinson C. Carboplatin is ototoxic. Cancer Chemother Pharmacol 1990;26:232–234.
332. Bauer F, Westhofen M, Kehrl W. Carboplatin ototoxicity in head and neck cancer patients. Laryngo-Rhino-Otol 1992:412–415.
333. Blakley B, Myers S. Patterns in hearing loss resulting from *cis*-platinum therapy. Otolaryngol. Head Neck Surg 1993;109:385–391.
334. Meistrich ML, Chawla SP, da Cunha MF et al. Recovery of sperm production after chemotherapy for osteosarcoma. Cancer 1989;63:2115.
335. Siimes MA, Rautonen J. Small testicles with impaired production of sperm in adult male survivors of childhood malignancies. Cancer 1990;65:1303.
336. Wallace WHB, Shalet SM, Crowne EC et al. Gonadal dysfunction due to *cis*-platinum. Med Pediatr Oncol 1989; 17:409.
337. Saeter G, Fossa SD et al. Gynaecomastia following cytotoxic therapy for testicular cancer. Br J Urol 1987;59:348.
338. Kellie SJ, Kingston JE. Ovarian failure after high-dose melphalan in adolescents. Lancet 1987;i:1425.
339. Schubert J, Tolkendorf E, Held HJ et al. Can the genetic risk be evaluated for offspring of testicular cancer patients exposed to chemotherapy treatment? Aktuel Urol 1989;20:199.
340. Brown T, Dawson AA, Bennett B et al. The effects of four drug regimens on sister chromatid exchange frequency in patients with lymphomas. Cancer Genet Cytogenet 1988;36:89.
341. Sanders J, Buckner C, Amos D et al. Ovarian function following marrow transplantation for aplastic anemia or leukemia. J Clin Oncol 1988;6:813.
342. Gradishar W, Schilsky R. Effects of cancer treatment on the reproductive system. CRC Crt. Rev Oncol Hematol 1988;8:153.
343. Hoorweg-Nijman J, Delemarre-van de Waal H, de Waal F, Behrendt H. Cyclophosphamide-induced disturbance of gonadotropin secretion manifesting testicular damage. Acta Endocrinol 1992;26:143–148.
344. Jackson D, Craig J, Spurr C, White D, Muss H, Cruz J. Vincristine infusion with CHOP-CCNU in diffuse large cell lymphoma. Cancer Invest 1990;8:7–12.
345. Sy-Ortin T, Shostak C, Donaldson S. Gonadal status and reproductive function following treatment for Hodgkin's disease in childhood; the Stanford experience. Int J Radiat Oncol Biol Phys 1990;19:873–880.
346. Aubier F, Flamant F, Brauner R, Caillaud J, Chaussain J, Lemerle J. Male gonadal function after chemotherapy for solid tumours in childhood. J Clin Oncol 1989;7:304–309.
347. Siimes M, Elomaa I, Koskimies A. Testicular function after chemotherapy for osteosarcoma. Eur J Cancer 1990;26:973–975.
348. Clayton P, Shalet S, Price D, Campbell R. Testicular damage after chemotherapy for childhood brain tumors. J Pediatr 1988;112:922.
349. Nijman J, Koops H, Oldhoff J et al. Sexual function after surgery and combination chemotherapy in men with disseminated nonseminomatous testicular cancer. J Surg Oncol 1988;38:182.
350. Kreuser ED, Xiros N, Hetzel WD et al. Reproduction and endocrine gonadal capacity in patients treated with COPP chemotherapy for Hodgkin's disease. J Cancer Res Clin Oncol 1987;113:260.
351. Waxman JH, Ahmed E, Smith D et al. Failure to preserve fertility in patients with Hodgkin's disease. Cancer Chemother Pharmacol 1987;19:159.

352. Rustin GJS, Pektasides D, Bagshaw KD et al. Fertility after chemotherapy for male and female germ cell tumours. Int J Androl 1987;10:389.
353. Richter VOP, Bucholz K et al. Course of pregnancy and delivery afte cytostatic treatment of trophoblastic tumours. Zentralbl Gynakol 1987;109:586.
354. Bosl GJ, Bajorunas D. Pituitary and testicular hormonal function after treatment for germ cell tumours. Int J Androl 1987;10:381.
355. Pryzant R, Meistrich M, Wilson G, Brown B, McLaughlin P. Long-term reduction in sperm count after chemotherapy with and without radiation therapy for non Hodgkin's lymphomas. J Clin Oncol 1993;11:239—247.
356. Hansen P, Glavind K, Panduro J, Pedersen M. Paternity in patients with testicular germ-cell cancer: pretreatment and post-treatment findings. Eur J Cancer 1991;27:1385—1389.
357. Viniani S, Ragni G, Santoro A, Perotti L, Caccamo E, Negretti E, Valagussa P. Testicular dysfunction in Hodgkin's disease before and after treatment. Eur J Cancer 1991;27:1389—1392.
358. Kawakita J, Horii A, Hayahara N, Morikawa Y, Umeda M, Yamamoto K. Clinical study of estramustine phosphate disodium (estracyt) on prostatic cancer—results of long term therapy for 38 patients with prostatic cancer. Acta Urol Jpn 1990;36:1361—1369.
359. Wada T, Morikawa E, Houjou T, Kadota K, Mori N, Matsunami N. Clinical evaluation of estramustine phosphate for a treatment of patients with advanced breast cancer. Jpn J Cancer Chemother 1990;17:1901—1904.
360. Pui CH, Jackson CW, Chesney CM et al. Involvement of von Willebrand factor in thrombosis following asparaginase, prednisolone, vincristine therapy for leukemia. Am J Haematol 1987;25:291.
361. Homans AC, Rybak ME, Baglini RL et al. Effect of L-asparaginase administration on coagulation and platelet function in children with leukaemia. J Clin Oncol 1987;5:811.
362. Mielot F, Danel P, Boyer C et al. Deficits acquis en antithrombine III et en proteine C au cours due traitement par la L-asparaginase. Arch Fr Pediatr 1987;44:161.
363. Ruiz MA, Marugan I, Estelles A et al. The influence of chemotherapy on plasma coagulation and fibrinolytic systems in lung cancer patients. Cancer 1989;63:643.
364. Lesene JB, Rothschild N, Erickson B et al. Cancer associated hemolytic uremic syndrome: analysis of 85 cases from a national registry. J Clin Oncol 1989;7:781.
365. Schick RM, Jolesz F, Barnes PD et al. M.R. diagnosis of dual venous sinus thrombosis complicating L-asparaginase therapy. Comput Med Imaging Graph 1989;13:319.
366. Carter C, Winfield DA. Factor X deficiency during treatment of relapsed acute myeloid leukeamia with amsacrine. Clin Lab Haematol 1988;10:225.
367. Ettinghausen SE, Moore JG, White De et al. Haematologic effects of immunotherapy with lymphokineactivated killer cells and recombinant interleukin-2 cancer patients. Blood 1987;69:1654.
368. Shapiro A. Clarke S, Christain J, Odom L, Hathaway W. Thrombosis in children receiving L-asparaginase. Am J Pediatr Hematol Oncol 1993;15:400—405.
369. Hasegawa I, Tanaka K. Serum erythropoietin levels in gynecologic cancer patients during cisplatin combination chemotherapy. Gyn Oncol 1992;46:65—68.
370. Raine AEG, Carter R, Mann JI et al. Adverse effect of cyclosporin on plasma cholesterol in renal transplant recipients. Nephrol Dial Transplant 1988;3:458.
371. Ballantyne CM, Podet EJ, Patsch WP et al. Effect of cyclosporine therapy on plasma lipoprotein levels. J Am Med Assoc 1989;262:53.
372. Stiller M, Pak G, Kenny C, Jondreau L, Davis I, Wachsman S, Shupack J. Elevation of fasting serum lipids in patients treated with low dose cyclosporine for severe plaque-type psoriasis. J Am Acad Dermatol 1992;27:434—438.
373. Scoble J, Freestone A, Varghese Z, Fernando O, Sweny P, Moorhead J. Cyclosporin induced renal magnesium leak in renal transplant patients. Nephrol Dial Transplant 1990;5:812—815.
374. Nozue T, Kobayashi A, Kodama T, Uemasu F, Endoh H, Sako A, Takayagi Y. Pathogenesis of cyclosporine-induced hypomagnesemia. J Pediatr 1992;120:638—640.
375. Burack D, Griffith B, Thompson M, Kahl L. Hyperuricemia and gout among heart transplant recipients receiving cyclosporine. Am J Med 1992;92:141—146.
376. Grossman R, Delaney R, Brinton E, Carter D, Gottlieb A. Hypertriglyceridemia in patients with psoriasis treated with cyclosporine. J Am Acad Dermatol 1991;25:648—651.
377. Orbo A, Simonson E. Cisplatin-induced sodium anbd magnesium wastage. Eur J Cancer 1992;28 A:1294.
378. Bianchetti M, Kanaka C, Ridolfi-Luthy A, Hirt A, Wagner H, Oetliker O. Persisting renotubular sequelae after cisplatin in children and adolescents. Am J Nephrol 1991;11:127—130.
379. Vassilopoulou-Sellin R, Samaan N. Mitotane administration: an unusual cause of hypercholesterolemia. Horm Metab Res 1991;23:619—620.
380. Perrone L, Sinisi AA, Tullio M et al. Endocrine function in subjects treated for childhood Hodgkin's disease. J Pediatr Endocrinol 1989;3:175.
381. Dhondt J, Farriaux J, Millot F, Taret S, Hayte J, Mazingue F. Hyperphenylalninemia during high dose methotrexate therapy. Arch Fr Pediatr 1991;48:249—251.
382. Hoppe RT. Secondary leukemia and myelodysplastic syndrome after treatment for Hodgkin's disease. Leukemia 1992;6(Suppl 4):155—157.
383. Bokemeyer C, Freund M, Schmoll HJ, Rieder H, Fonatsch C. Secondary lymphoblastic leukemia following treatment of a malignant germ cell tumour. Ann Oncol 1992; 3:771.
384. Trenkwalder P, Eisenlohr H, Prechtel K, Lydtin H. Three cases of malignant neoplasm, pneumonitis, and pancytopenia during treatment with low-dose methotrexate. Clin Invest 1992:70:951—955.
385. Bennett J, Moloney W, Green M, Boice J. Acute myeloid leukemia and other myelopathic disorders following treatment with alkylating agents. Hematol Pathol 1987;1:99.
386. Pedersen-Bjergaard J, Ersbal J, Hansen V et al. Blasenkarzinom nach Cyclophosphamid-Langzeittherapie. Aktuel Urol 1988;19:275.
387. O'Keane J. Carcinoma of the urinary bladder after treatment with cyclophosphamide (Letter to Editor). N Engl J Med 1988;319 871.
388. Mahe M, Raffi F, Rojouan J et al. Cancers secondaires apres maladie de Hodgkin. Semin Hop Paris 1988;64:3013.
389. Van der Velden J, Van Putten W, Guinee V et al. Subsequent development of acute non-lymphocytic leukemia in patients treated for Hodgkin's disease. Int J Cancer 1988;42:252.
390. Gyotat D, Coiffier B, Camos L et al. Acute leukaemia following high-dose chemoradiotherapy with bone marrow rescue for ovarian teratoma. Acta Haematol 1988;80:52.

391. Einhorn N, Eklund G, Lambert B. Solid tumours and chromosome aberrations as late side effects of melphalan therapy in ovarian carcinoma. Acta Oncol 1988;27:215.
392. Bennett J, Moloney W, Greene M, Boice J. Acute myeloid leukemia and other myelopathic disorders following treatment with alkylating agents. Hematol Pathol 1987;1:99.
393. Bennett J, Moloney W, Greene M, Boice J. Acute myeloid leukemia and other myelopathic disorders following treatment with alkylating agents. Hematol Pathol 1987;1:99.
394. Van der Velden J, Van Putten W, Guinee V et al. Subsequent development of acute non-lymphocytic leukemia in patients treated for Hodgkin's disease. Int J Cancer 1988;42:252.
395. Genuardi M, Zollino M, Serra A et al. Long-term cytogenetic effects of antineoplastic treatment in relation to secondary leukemia. Cancer Genet Cytogenet 1988;33:201.
396. Einhorn N, Eklund G, Lambert B. Solid tumours and chromosome aberrations as late side effects of melphalan therapy in ovarian carcinoma. Acta Oncol 1988;27:215.
397. Penn I. Immunosuppression and neoplasia cancers after cyclosporine therapy. Transplant Proc 1988;20:276.
398. Qunibi W, Akhtar M, Ginn E, Smith P. Kaposi's sarcoma in cyclosporine-induced gingival hyperplasia. Am J Kidney Dis 1988;11:349.
399. Penn I. Immunosuppression and neoplasia cancers after cyclosporine therapy. Transplant Proc 1988;20:276.
400. Penn I. Posttransplant malignancies. World J Urol 1988;6:125.
401. Penn I, Brunson M. Cancers after cyclosporine therapy. Transplant Proc 1988;20:885.
402. Pilgrim M. Spontane Manifestation und Regression eines Kaposi-Sarkoms unter Cyclosporin A. Hautarzt 1988;39:368.
403. Fukuda M, Ohmori Y, Aikawa I et al. Mutagenicity of cyclosporine in vivo. Transplant Proc 1988;20:929.
404. Kaldor JM, Day NE, Band P et al. Second malignancies following testicular cancer, ovarian cancer and Hodgkin's disease: an international collaborative study among cancer registries. Int J Cancer 1987;39:571.
405. Bjergaard JP, Larsen SO, Stuck J et al. Risk of therapy-related leukaemia and preleukaemia after Hodgkin's disease: relation to age, cumulative dose of alkylating agents, and time from chemotherapy. Lancet 1987;ii:83.
406. Donaldson SS, Link MP. Combined modality treatment with low-dose radiation and MOPP chemotherapy for children with Hodgkin's disease. J Clin Oncol 1987;5:742.
407. Wijlhuizen TJ, Breed WPM,. Secundaire maligniteiten na behandeling van de ziekte van Hodgkin. Ned Tijdschr Geneeskd 1987;131:1342.
408. Blayney DW, Longo DL, Young RC et al. Decreasing risk of leukaemia with prolonged follow-up after chemotherapy and radiotherapy for Hodgkin's disease. N Engl J Med 1987;316:710.
409. Gruber S, Dehner LP, Simmons RL. De novo hepatocellular carcinoma without chronic liver disease but with 17 years of azathioprine immunosuppression. Transplantation 1987;43:597.
410. Mittal BV, Cotton RE. Severely atypical changes in renal epithelium in biopsy and graft nephrectomy specimens in two cases of cadaver renal transplantation. Histopathology 1987;11:833.
411. Kelly G, Scheibner A, Murray E et al. T6+ and HLA-DR+ cell numbers in epidermis of immunosuppressed renal transplant recipients. J Cutaneous Pathol 1987;14:202.
412. Pitt PI, Sultan AH, Malone M et al. Association between azathioprine therapy and lymphoma in rheumatoid disease. J R Soc Med 1987;80:428.
413. Pui C, Ribeiro R, Hancock M, Rivera G, Evans W, Raimondi S, Head D. Acute myeloid leukemia in children treated with epipodophyllotoxins for acute lymphoblastic leukemias. New Engl J Med 1991;325:1682—1687.
414. Pui C. Epipodophyllotoxin-related acute myeloid leukemia. Lancet 1991;338:1468.
415. Hawkins M. Secondary leukaemia after epipodophyllotoxins. Lancet 1991;338:1408.
416. Whitlock J, Greer J, Lukens J. Epipodophyllotoxin-related leukaemia. Cancer 1991;68:600—604.
417. Ratain M, Rowley J. Therapy-related acute myeloid leukemia secondary to inhibitors of topoisomerase II. Ann Oncol 1992;3:107—111.
418. Hawkins M, Wilson L, Stovall M, Marsden H, Potok M, Kingston J, Chessells J. Epipodophyllotoxins, alkylating agents, and radiation and risk of secondary leukaemia after childhood cancer. Br Med J 1992;304:951—958.
419. Pedersen-Bjergaard J, Philip P. Two difference cases of therapy-related and de-novo acute myeloid leukemia.
420. Rubin C, Arthur D, Woods W, Lange B, Nowell P, Rowley J, Nachman J. Therapy-related myeloid syndrome and acute myeloid leukemia in children. Blood 1991;78:2982—2988.
421. Ishii E, Hara T, Mizuno Y, Ueda K. Vincristine-induced fever in children with leukaemia and lymphoma (in Japanese). Saishin Igaku 1988;6:1341.
422. Hsu NY, Chen C. Intrapleural bleomycin in the management of malignant pleural effusion. J Surg Assoc ROC 1988;21:302.
423. Garrigos J, Auladell A, Perez P, Garcia J, Matoses M, Marcos M, Linares A. Lesions/calcification secondary to mitomycin C instillation. Arch Esp Urol 1991;44:1060 (in Spanish).
424. Zuckerman K, Case D, Gams R, Prasthofer E. Chemotherapy of intermediate and high grade non-Hodgkin's lymphomas with an intensive epirubicin containing regimen. Blood 1993;82:3564—3573.
425. Pan W, Chan C, Huang C, Lai M. Cyclosporine-induced gingival overgrowth. Transplant Proc 1992;24:1393—1394.
426. Soni N, Bajaj B. Toxic effects of cisplatin on olfaction. Pak J Otolaryngol 1991;7:23—25.
427. Javadpour N, Lalehzarian M. A Phase I-II study of high dose recombinant human interleukin-2 in disseminated renal-cell carcinoma. Semin Surg Oncol 1988;4:207.
428. Webb D, Austin H, Belldegrun A et al. Metabolic and renal effects of interleukin-2 immunotherapy for metastatic cancer. Clin Nephrol 1988;30:141.
429. Sondel P, Kohler P, Hank J et al. Clinical and immunological effects of recombinant interleukin-2 given by repetitive weekly cycles to patients with cancer. Cancer Res 1988; 48:2561.
430. Webb D, Austin H, Belldegrun A et al. Metabolic and renal effects of interleukin-2 immunotherapy for metastatic cancer. Clin Nephrol 1988;30:141.
431. Sosman JA, Kohler PC, Hank JA et al. Repetitive weekly cycles of interleukin 2. Clinical and immunologic effects of dose, schedule, and addition of indomethacin. J Natl Cancer Inst 1988;80:1451.
432. Richards JM, Barker E, Latta J et al. Phase I study of weekly 24 hour infusions of recombinant human interleukin 2. J Natl Cancer Inst 1988;80:1325.

433. Nasr S, McKolanis J, Pais R et al. A phase I study of interleukin 2 in children with cancer and evaluation of clinical and immunologic status during therapy. Cancer 1989;64:783.
434. Christiansen NP, Skubitz KM, Nath K et al. Nephrotoxicity of continuous intravenous infusion of recombinant interleukin 2. Am J Med 1988;84:1072.
435. Katz JA, Mahoney DH, Steuber CP et al. Human leukocyte alpha interferon induced transient neurotoxicity in children. Invest New Drugs 1988;6:115.
436. Adams F, Fernandez F, Mavligit G. Interferon induced organic mental disorders associated with unsuspected preexisting neurologic abnormalities. J Neuro-Oncol 1988; 6:355.
438. Kogawa T, Togashi S, Yanagiya H et al. The treatment of renal cell carcinoma with interferon. J Jpn Soc Cancer Ther 1988;23:649.
439. Aderka D, Michalevicz R, Daniel Y et al. Recombinant interferon alpha C for advanced hairy cell leukemia. Cancer 1988;61:2207.
440. Ahre A, Bjorkholm M, Osterborg A et al. High doses of natural α-interferon [α-IFN] in the treatment of multiple myeloma—a pilot study from the Myeloma Group of Central Sweden (MGCS). Eur J Haematol 1988;41:123.
441. Cetto G, Franceschi T, Turrina G et al. Recombinant alpha-interferon and vinblastine in metastatic renal cell carcinoma: efficacy of low doses. Semin Surg Oncol 1988;4:184.
442. Borden E, Hawkins M, Sielaff K et al. Clinical and biological effects of recombinant interferon-β administered intravenously daily in Phase I trial. J Interferon Res 1988;8:357.
443. McLeod G. Alpha-interferons in malignant melanoma. Br J Clin Pract 1988;(Suppl):62.
450. Levens W, Fischer N, Ingehag W, Rubben H. Adverse reactions in long-term interferon treatment. Semin Surg Oncol 1988;4:204.
451. Fentiman I, Balkwill F, Thomas B et al. An autoimmune aetiology for hypothyroidism following interferon therapy for breast cancer. Eur J Cancer Clin Oncol 1988;24:1299.
452. Editorial. Filgrastin (G-CSF). Prescrire Int 1995;4:45.
453. Editorial. Buserelin (LH-RH agonist). Prescrire Int 1995;4:36.
454. Editorial. Lenograstim (glycosylated G-CSF). Prescrire Int 1995;4:34.
455. Editorial. Autoimmune diseases as an adverse event of interferon: thyroid disease is by far the most frequent. Prescrire Int 1994;14(143):471—473.
456. Editorial. Cyclosporin. Prescrire Int 1994;14(143):462—465.
457. Editorial. Pacilitaxel. Prescrire Int 1994;14(141):332—333.
458. Editorial. Molgramostim (GM-CSF). Prescrire Int 1994;14(140):271—274.
459. Editorial. Malignant lymphoma during low-dose methotrexate therapy. Prescrire Int 1994;14(138):154.
460. Editorial. Pentostatin. Prescrire Int 1994;14(139):205—206.
461. Editorial. Fotemustine. Prescrire Int 1994;14(137):69—70.
462. Editorial. Interferon alpha-2a. Prescrire Int 1994; 14(137):80—82.
463. Editorial. Tamoxifen prophylaxis: warning. Prescrire Int 1994;3:62.
464. Mowad CM, Nguyen TV, Elenitsas R, Leyden JJ. Bleomycin-induced flagellate dermatitis: a clinical and histopathological review. Br J Dermatol 1994;131(5):700—702.
465. Zaragoza MR, Ritchey ML, Walter A. Neurourologic consequences of accidental intrathecal vincristine: a case report. Med Pediatr Oncol 1995;24(1):61—62.
466. Cruciani F, Tamanti N, Abdolrahimzadeh S, Franchi F, Gabrieli CB. Ocular toxicity of systemic chemotherapy with megadoses of carmustine and mitomycin. Ann Ophthalmol 1994;26(3):97—100.
467. Lena H, Desrues B, Le Coz, Quinquenel ML, Delaval P. Severe diffuse interstitial pneumonitis induced by carmustine (BCNU). Chest 1994;105(5):1602—1603.
468. Hadjiyanni M, Valianatou K, Tsilianos M, Seitanidis B. Prolonged thrombocytopenia after procarbazine 'overdose' (Letter). Eur J Cancer 1992;28A(6—7):1299.
469. Coyle T, Bushunow P, Winfield J, Wright J, Graziano S. Hypersensitivity reactions to procarbazine with mechlorethamine, vincristine, and procarbazine chemotherapy in the treatment of glioma (Review). Cancer 1992;69 (10):2532—2540.
470. Weinfeld A, Swolin B, Westin J. Acute leukaemia after hydroxyurea therapy in polycythaemia vera and allied disorders: prospective study of efficacy and leukaemogenecity with therapeutic implications. Eur J Haematol 1994; 52(3):134—139.
471. Hanquinet S, Wouters M, Devalck C, Perlmutter N, Sariban E. Inreased renal parenchymal echogenicity in ifosfamide-induced renal Fanconi syndrome. Med Pediatr Oncol 1995;24(2):116—118.
472. Kramer A, Goldschmidt H, Hahn U, Andrassy K. Progressive renal failure in two breast cancer patients after high-dose ifosfamide (Letter). Lancet 1994;344:1569.
473. Heim A, Stille-Siegener M, Kandolf R, Kreuzer H, Figulla HR. Enterovirus-induced myocarditis: hemodynamic deterioration with immunosuppressive therapy and successful application of interferon-alpha. Clin Cardiol 1994; 17(10):563—565.
474. Thomas E, Leroux JL, Blotman F. Gynecomastia in patients with rheumatoid arthritis treated with methotrexate (Letter). J Rheumatol 1994;21(9):1777—1778.
475. Al-Lamki Z, Thomas E, el-Banna N, Jaffe N. Acute urticaria and hepatitis complicating high-dose methotrexate therapy. Med Pediatr Oncol 1995;24(2):137—40.
476. Butler RW, Hill JM, Steinherz PG, Meyers PA, Finlay JL. Neuropsychologic effects of cranial irradiation, intrathecal methotrexate, and systemic methotrexate in childhood cancer. J Clin Oncol 1994;12(12):2621—2629.
477. Connell WR, Kamm MA, Dickson M, Balkwill AM, Ritchie JK, Lennard-Jones JE. Long-term neoplasia risk after azathioprine treatment in inflammatory bowel disease. Lancet 1994;343:1249—1252.
478. Stetter M, Schmidl M, Krapf R. Azathioprine hypersensitivity mimicking Goodpasture's syndrome. Am J Kidney Dis 1994;23(6):874—877.
479. Shearer P, Katz J, Bozeman P, Jenkins J, Laver J, Krance R, Hurwitz C, Mahmoud H, Mirro J. Pulmonary insufficiency complicating therapy with high dose cytosine arabinoside in five pediatric patients with relapsed acute myelogenous leukemia. Cancer 1994;74(7):1953—1958.
480. Wysocki M, Kurylak A, Pilecki O, Balcar-Boron A. Preliminary evaluation of adverse effects after administration of arabinoside cytosine (Ara-C) in high doses to children with acute myelogenous leukemia (Polish). Acta Haematol Pol 1994;25(1):37—42.
481. Bandini G, Belardinelli A, Rosti G, Calori E, Motta MR, Rizzi S, Benini C, Tura S. Toxicity of high-dose busul-

phan and cyclophosphamide as conditioning therapy for allogeneic bone marrow transplantation in adults with haematological malignancies. Bone Marrow Transplant 1994; 13(5):577–581.
482. Anonymous. Cisplatin-induced delayed emesis: pattern and prognostic factors during three subsequent cycles. Italian Group for Antiemetic Research. Ann Oncol 1994;5(7):585–589.
483. Goto H, Shimazaki C, Tatsumi T, Yamagata N, Inaba T, Fujita N, Moriguchi T, Yamamoto K, Seto M, Ueda R. et al. Acute myelomonocytic leukemia after treatment with chronic oral etoposide: are MLL and LTG9 genes targets for etoposide? Int J Hematol 1994;60(2):145–149.
484. Matsuzaki A, Inamitsu T, Watanabe T, Ohga S, Ishii E, Nagotoshi Y, Tasaka H, Suda M, Ueda K. Acute promyelocytic leukaemia in a patient treated with etoposide for Langerhans cell histiocytosis. Br J Haematol 1994; 86(4):887–889.
485. de Souza P, Friedlander M, Wilde C, Kirsten F, Ryan M. Hypersensitivity reactions to etoposide. A report of three cases and review of the literature. Am J Clin Oncol 1994;17(7):387–389.
486. Iida H, Taji H, Iida M, Suzuki R, Sugihara T, Minami S, Kodera Y, Yamamoto K, Seto M, Ueda R. Secondary leukemia after etoposide treatment involved MLL gene rearrangement (Japanese). Rinsho Ketsueki 1994;35(6):569–575.
487. Imrie KR, Couture F, Turner CC, Sutcliffe SB, Keating A. Peripheral neuropathy following high-dose etoposide and autologous bone marrow transplantation. Bone Marrow Transplant 1994;13(1):77–79.
488. Portal I, Cardenal F, Garcia-del-Muro X. Etoposide-related acral erythema (Letter). Cancer Chemother Pharmacol 1994;34(2):181.
489. Bokemeyer C, Schmoll HJ, Poliwoda H. Secondary leukemias after etoposide chemotherapy (German). Dtsch Med Wochenschr 1994;119(19):707–713.
490. Tscherning C, Rubie H, Chancholle A, Claeyssens S, Robert A, Fabre J, Bouissou F. Recurrent renal salt wasting in a child treated with carboplatin and etoposide. Cancer 1994;73(6):1761–1763.
491. Sturrock ND, Lang CC, Clark G, Struthers AD. Acute haemodynamic and renal effects of cyclosporin and indomethacin in man. Nephrol Dial Transplant 1994;9(8):1149–1156.
492. Larner AJ, Sturman SG, Hawkins JB, Anderson M. Myopathy with ragged red fibres following renal transplantation: possible role of cyclosporin-induced hypomagnesaemia. Acta Neuropathol (Berlin) 1994;88(2):189–192.
493. Weidmann B, Mulleneisen N, Bojko P, Niederle N. Hypersensitivity reactions to carboplatin. Report of two patients, review of the literature, and discussion of diagnostic procedures and management. Cancer 1994;73(8):2218–2222.
494. Shepherd L, Ottaway J, Myles J, Levine M. Therapy-related leukemia associated with high-dose 4-epi-doxorubucin and cyclophosphamide used as adjuvant chemotherapy for breast cancer (Letter). J Clin Oncol 1994;12(11):2514–2515.
495. Balabanova MB. Photoprovoked erythmatolbullous eruption from farmorubicin. Contact Dermatitis 1994; 30(5):303–304.
496. Doria MI Jr, Doria LK, Faintuch J, Levin B. Gastric mucosal injury after hepatic arterial infusion chemotherapy with floxuridine. A clinical and pathologic study. Cancer 1994;73(8):2042–2047.
497. White RL Jr, Schwartzentruber DJ, Guleria A, MacFarlane MP, White DE, Tucker E, Rosenberg SA. Cardiopulmonary toxicity of treatment with high dose interleukin-2 in 199 consecutive patients with metastatic melanoma or renal cell carcinoma. Cancer 1994;74(12):3212–3222.
498. Schomburg A, Kirchner H, Lopez-Hanninen E, Menzel T, Rudolph P, Korfer A, Fenner M, Poliwoda H, Atzpodien J. Hepatic and serologic toxicity of systemic interleukin-2 and/or interferon-alpha. Evidence of risk-benefit advantage of subcutaneous therapy. Am J Clin Oncol 1994;17(3):199–209.
499. Powell FC, Spooner KM, Shawker TH, Premkumar A, Thakore KN, Vogel SE, Kovacs JA, Masur H, Feuerstein IM. Symptomatic interleukin-2-induced cholecystopathy in patients with HIV infection. Am J Roentgenol 1994; 163(1):117–121.
500. Becker JC, Winkler B, Klingert S, Brocker EB. Antiphospholipid syndrome associated with immunotherapy for patients with melanoma. Cancer 1994;73(6):1621–1624.
501. Fragasso G, Tresoldi M, Benti R, Vidal M, Marcatti M, Borri A, Besana C, Gerundini PP, Rugarli C, Chierchia S. Impaired left ventricular filling rate induced by treatment with recombinant interleukin 2 for advanced cancer. Br Heart J 1994;71(2):166–169.
502. Kosirog-Glowacki JL, Bressler LR. Cyclophosphamide-induced facial discomfort. Ann Pharmacother 1994; 28(2):197–199.
503. Ramireddy K, Kane KM, Adhar GC. Acquired episodic complete heart block after high-dose chemotherapy with cyclophosphamide and thiotepa. Am Heart J 1994; 127(3): 701–704.
504. Vrouenraets BC, Eggermont AM, Klaase JM, Van Geel BN, Van Dongen JA, Kroon BB. Long-term neuropathy after regional isolated perfusion with melphalan for melanoma of the limbs. Eur J Surg Oncol 1994;20(6):681–685.
505. Figg WD, Thibault A, Sartor AO, Mays D, Headlee D, Calis KA, Cooper MR. Hypothyroidism associated with aminoglutethimide in patients with prostate cancer. Arch Intern Med 1994;154(9):1023–1025.
506. Aoshiba K, Nagai A, Ueno H, Konno K. Transient neutropenia after intravenous injection of vindesine in patients with lung cancer. Eur J Clin Pharmacol 1994; 47(1):25–32.
507. Cetin M, Yetgin S, Kara A, Tuncer AM, Gunay M, Gumrak F, Gurgey A. Hyperglycemia, ketoacidosis and other complications of L-asparaginase in children with acute lymphoblastic leukemia. J Med 1994;25(3–4):219–229.
508. Barclay KL, Yeong ML. Actinomycin D associated hepatic veno-occlusive disease—a report of 2 cases. Pathology 1994;26(3):257–260.
509. Taylor SA, Blumenstein BA, Stephens RL, Crawford ED, Pistone B, Hill JB. Phase II trial of menogaril in metastatic adenocarcinoma of the prostate. A Southwest Oncology Group study. Invest New Drugs 1994;12(1):67–70.
510. Minasian LM, Szatrowski TP, Rosenblum M, Steffens T, Morrison ME, Chapman PB, Williams L, Nathan CF, Houghton AN. Hemorrhagic tumor necrosis during a pilot trial of tumor necrosis factor-alpha and anti-GD3 ganglioside monoclonal antibody in patients with metastatic melanoma. Blood 1994;83(1):56–64.
511. Meisenberg B, Lassiter M, Hussein A, Ross M, Vredenburgh JJ, Peters WP. Prevention of hemorrhagic cystitis after

high-dose alkylating agent chemotherapy and autologous bone marrow support. Bone Marrow Transplant 1994; 14(2):287—291.
512. Ghosh K, Sivakumaran M, Murphy P, Chapman CS, Wood JK et al. Visual hallucinations following treatment with vincristine. Clin Lab Haematol 1994;16:355—357.
513. Sugano S, Yanagimoto M, Suzuki T, Sato M, Onmura H et. al. Retinal complications with elevated circulating plasma C5a associated with interferon-alpha therapy of chronic active hepatitis C. Am J Gastroenterol 1994;89:2054—2056.
513. Ohhata I, Ochi T, Kurebayashi S, Kikui M, et al. A case of subcutaneous sarcoid nodules induced by interferon-alpha (Japanese). Nippon Kyobu Shikkan Gakkai Zasshi 1994;32:996—1000.
514. Zabernigg A, Maier H, Thaler J, Gattringer C. Late-onset fatal neurological toxicity of fludarabine. Lancet 1994;344:1780.
515. Kimmel OL, Abraham AA, Phillips TM. Membranoproliferative glomerulonephritis in a patient treated with interferon-alpha for human immunodeficiency virus infection. Am J Kidney Dis 1994;24:858—863.
516. Oleksowicz L, Strack M, Dutcher JP, Sussman I, Caliendo G et al. A distinct coagulopathy associated with interleukin-2 therapy. Br J Haematol 1994;88:892—894.
517. Bernini JC, Timmons CF, Sandler ES. Acute basophilic leukemia in a child: anaphylactoid reaction and coagulopathy secondary to vincristine-mediated degranulation. Cancer 1994;75:110—114.
518. Maillot F, Machet L, Mommeja-Marin H. Vaillant L. Hyperthermia associated with methotrexate in Still's disease (French). Therapie 1994;49:520—521.
519. Cardon T, Heuschling C, Delaporte E, Cotten H, Catteau B et al. Cutaneous pseudolymphoma occurring during methotrextae therapy for rheumatoid arthritis. Rev Rhum 1994;61:651.
520. Heintges T, Frieling T, Goerz G, Niederau C. Exacerbation of lichen planus but not of acute intermittent hepatic porphyria during interferon therapy in a patient with chronic hepatitis C. J Hepatol 1994;21:1152—1153.
521. Crowley JJ, Knight L, Charan N. Lysis pneumonopathy associated with the use of fludarabine phosphate. Western J Med 1994;161:597—599.
522. Bulengo-Ransby SM, Sahn EE, Metcalf JS, Maize JC. Bowenoid change in association with graft-versus-host disease: a cyclosporine toxicity? J Am Acad Dermatol 1994;31:1052—1054.
523. Ching DWT. Severe disseminated, life threatening herpes zoster infection in a patient with rheumatoid arthritis treated with methotrexate. Ann Rheum Dis 1995;54:155.
524. Imashuku S, Hibi S, Kataoka-Morimoto Y, Yoshihara T, Ikushima S et al. Myeloodysplasia and acute myeloid leukaemia in cases of aplastic anaemia and congenital neutropenia following G-CSF administration. Br J Haematol 1995;89:188—190.
525. Traynor A, Kuzel T, Samuelson E, Kanwar Y. Minimal-change glomerulopathy and glomerular visceral epithelial hyperplasia associated with alpha-interferon therapy for cutaneous T-cell lymphoma. Nephron 1994;67:94—100.
526. Hoffman A, Kirn E, Krueger GRF, Fischer R et al. Bone marrow hypoplasia and fibrosis following interferon treatment. In Vivo 1994;8:605—612.
527. Dousset B, Conti F, Houssin D, Calmus Y. Acute vanishing bile duct syndrome after interferon therapy for recurrent HCV infection in liver-transplant recipients. New Engl J Med 1994;330:1160—1161.
528. Eugene C, Tennenbaum R, Anciaux ML et al. Autoimmune thyroid disorders induced by alpha-interferon in 2 females with chronic non-A hepatitis, non-B hepatitis (French). Gastroenterol Clin Biol 1993;17:594—597.
529. Lennard L, Gibson BES, Nicole T, Lilleyman JS. Congenital thiopurine methyltransferase deficiency and 6-mercaptopurine toxicity during treatment for acute lymphoblastic leukaemia. Arch Dis Child 1993;69:577—579.
530. Kaufmann O, Meyer R, Matthias M. Fatal myocarditis induced by regionary appplication of 5-fluorouracil (German). Tumor Diagnost Ther 1994;15:159.
531. Bruggers CS, Friedman HS, Tien R, Delong R. Cerebral atrophy in an infant following treatment with ifosfamide. Med Pediatr Oncol 1994;23:380—383.
532. Bibas M, Andriani A, Rinaldi PL. Diabetic ketoacidosis with coma after interferon therapy for a metastatic melanoma. A case report. Br J Haematology 1994;87(Suppl 1):204.
533. Fakutoku M, Shimizu S, Ogawa Y, Takeshita S, Masaki Y et al. Sweet's syndrome during therapy with granulocyte colony-stimulating factor in a patient with aplastic anaemia. Br J Haematol 1994;86:645—648.
534. Lautenschlager S, Itin PH, Hirsbrunner P, Buchner SA et al. Subcorneal pustular dermatosis at the injection site of recombinant human granulocyte-macrophage colony-stimulating factor in a patient with IgA myeloma. J Am Acad Dermatol 1994;30:787—789.
535. Sasson Z, Morgan CD, Wang B, Thomas G, MacKenzie B et al. 5-Fluorouracil related toxic myocarditis: case reports and pathological confirmation. Can J Cardiol 1994;10:861—864.
536. Petit H, Schaeverbeke T, Malavialle P, Marce S, Antoine JF et al. Reflex sympathetic dystrophy syndrome of the foot in liver transplant patient treated with ciclosporin A. Rev Rhum (English Edition; Joint, Bone, Spine Dis) 1993;60:616.
537. Shimizu C, Kimura S, Yoshida Y, Nezu A, Kazuyo S et al. Acute leucoencephalopathy during cyclosporin A therapy in a patient with nephrotic syndrome. Pediatr Nephrol 1994;8:483—485.
538. Cohen R, Jaffe ES, Stetler-Stevenson M-A, Sausville EA, DeNigris EC et al. Bilateral adrenal hemorrhage and adrenal insufficiency in a patient with lymphomatous adrenal infiltration following administration of a fusion toxin (DAB486 interleukin-2). J Immunother 1994;16:229—233.
539. Eugene C, Tennenbaum R, Anciaux ML et al. Autoimmune thyroid disorders induced by alpha-interferon in 2 females with chronic non-A hepatitis, non-B hepatitis (French). Gastroenterol Clin Biol 1993:594—597.
540. Lindemann A, Rumberger B. Vascular complications in patients treated with granulocyte colony-stimulating factor (G-CSF). Eur J Cancer (Part A) 1993;29A:2338—2339.
541. Johnson PWM, Fearnley J, Domizio P, Goldin J, Nagendran K et al. Neurological illness following treatment with fludarabine. Br J Cancer 1994;70:966—968.
542. De Souza P, Friedlander M, Wilde C, Kirsten F, Ryan M et al. Hypersensitivity reactions to etoposide: a report of three cases and review of the literature. Am J Clin Oncol Cancer Clin Trials 1994;17:387—389.
543. Montillo M, Tedeschi A, Leoni P. Recurrence of autoimmune thrombocytopenia after treatment with fludarabine in a patient with chronic lymphocytic leukemia. Leukemia Lymphoma 1994;15:187—188.

544. Weidmann B, Jansen W, Bojko P, Hanseler Th, Tauchert M et al. Life-threatening cardiotoxicity of 5-fluorouracil (German). Intensivmed Notfallmed 1993;30:153–158.
545. Takahashi J, Kawashima R, Abe Y et al. Ventricular premature contraction observed after anti-cancer chemotherapy with ifosfamide (Japanese). Gan to Kagaku Ryoho 1994;21:1681–1684.
546. Eisenburg J. Interferon- or virus-C-induced autoimmune chronic hepatitis? Report on observations and review of the literature (German). Fortschr Med 1994;112:317–321.
547. Hochstetler LA, Flanigan MJ, Lager DJ. Transplant-associated thrombotic microangiopathy: the role of IgG administration as initial therapy. Am J Kidney Dis 1994; 23:444–450.
548. Dourakis SP, Alexopoulou AA, Hadziyannis SJ. Fulminant hepatitis after flutamide treatment. J Hepatol 1994;20:350–353.
549. Onishi Y, Hatae M, Nakamura T et al. Case report: severe hyperbilirubinemia after cisplatin-based chemotherapy (Japanese). Nippon Gan Chiryo Gakkai Shi 1994;29:552.
550. Oeda E, Shinohara K, Kamei S, Nomiyama J, Inoue H et al. Capillary leak syndrome likely the result of granulocyte colony-stimulating factor after high-dose chemotherapy. Intern Med 1994;33:115–119.
551. Farhat BA, Johnson PJ, Williams R. Hazards of interferon treatment in patients with autoimmune chronic active hepatitis. J Hepatol 1994;20:560–561.
552. Keefe DL, Roistacher N, Pierri MK. Clinical cardiotoxicity of 5-fluorouracil. J Clin Pharm 1993;33:1060–1070.
553. Kupfer A, Aeschliman C, Wermuth B, Cerny T et al. Prophylaxis and reversal of ifosfamide encephalopathy with methylene-blue. Lancet 1994;343:763–764.
554. Castenskiold EC, Colvin BT, Kelsey SM. Acquired factor VIII inhibitor associated with chronic interferon-alpha therapy in a patient with haemophilia A. Br J Haematol 1994;87:434–436.
555. Tscherning C, Rubie H, Chancholle A, Claeyssens S, Robert A et al. Recurrent renal salt wasting in a child treated with carboplatin and etoposide. Cancer 1994;73:1761–1763.
556. Kingma A, Tamminga RYJ, Kamps WA et al. Cerebrovascular complications of L-asparaginase therapy in children with leukemia—asphasia and other neuropsychological deficits. Pediatr Heamatol Oncol 1993;10:303–309.
557. Dirix LY, Schrijvers D, Druwe P, Van Den Brande J, Verhoeven D et al. Pulmonary toxicity and bleomycin. Lancet 1994;344:56.
558. Zimmer-Galler I, Lie JT. Choroidal infiltrates as the initial manifestation of lymphoma in rheumatoid arthritis after treatment with low-dose methotrexate. Mayo Clin Proc 1994;69:258–261.
559. Tosti A, Misciali C, Piraccinin BM, Peluso AM, Bardazzi F et al. Drug-induced hair loss and hair growth: incidence, management and avoidance. Drug Safety 1994;10:310–317.
560. Tscherning C, Rubie H, Chancholle A, Claeyssens S, Robert A et al. Recurrent renal salt wasting in a child treated with carboplatin and etoposide. Cancer 19??;73:1761–1763.
561. Morrison RJ, Short HD, Noon GP, Frost AE. Hypertension after lung transplantation. J Heart Lung Transplant 1993;12:928–931.
562. Soysal T, Bavunoglu I, Baslar Z, Aktuglu G. Cataract after prolonged busulphan therapy. Acta Haematol 1993;90(4):213.
563. Miglino M, Pierri I, Canepa L, Carrara P, Celesti L et al. An unusual reaction to alpha interferon in a case of non-Hodgkin's lymphoma. Haematologica 1993;78:411–413.
564. Pandhi RK, Gupta LK, Girdhar M. Azathioprine-induced drug fever. Int J Dermatol 1994;33:198.
565. Jalan R, Plevris JN, MacGilchrist A, Hayes PC et al. Reversible spastic paraparesis due to cyclosporin toxicity. Am J Gastroenterol 1994;89:645–646.
566. Zweizig S, Roman LD, Muderspach LI. Death from anaphylaxis to cisplatin: a case report. Gynecol Oncol 1994;53:121–122.
567. Shenkier T, Gelmon K. Paclitaxel and radiation-recall dermatitis. J Clin Oncol 1994;12:439.
568. Blakly BW, Gupta AK, Myers SF, Schwan S. Risk factors for ototoxicity due to cisplatin. Arch Otolaryngol Head Neck Surg 1994;120:541–546.
569. Lee TC, Hook CC, Long HJ. Severe exfoliative dermatitis associated with hand ischemia during cisplatin therapy. Mayo Clin Proc 1994;69:80–82.
570. Mabin D, Fourquet I, Richard P et al. Reversible leucoencephalopathy related with high dose cyclosporine A (French). Rev Neurol 1993;149:576–578.
571. Yudis M, Gronich J, Sirota R et al. Hemorrhagic ileocolitis after pulse cyclophosphamide therapy in lupus nephritis. Am J Kidney Dis 1993;22:A11.
572. Welge-L Ussen UC, Gerhartz HH. Late onset of neurotoxicity with cyclosporin. Lancet 1994;343:293.
573. Steiger MJ, Farrah T, Rolles K, Harvey P, Burroughs AK et al. Cyclosporin associated headache. J Neurol Nuerosurg Psychiatry 1994;57:1258–1259.
574. Larvol L, Soule J-C, Le Tourneau A. Reversible lymphoma in the setting of azathioprine therapy for Crohn's disease. New Engl J Med 1994;331:883–884.
575. Crestani B, Jaccard A, Israel-Biet D, Couderc L-J, Frija J et al. Chlorambucil-associated pneumonitis. Chest 1994;105:634–636.
576. Miyagawa S, Shirai T, Shimamoto I, Ichijo M, Ueki H, et al. Worsening of systemic lupus erythmatosus-associated thrombocytopenia after administration of gonadotropin-releasing hormone analog. Arthr Rheum 1994;37:1708–1709.
577. Iurlo A, Foa P, Sala M, Maiolo AT. Renal cancer after busulphan treatment for chronic myeloid leukemia. A case report. Tumori 1993;79:278–279.
578. O'Riordan JM, FitzSimon S, O'Connor M, McCann SR. Retinal microvascular changes following bone marrow transplantation: the role of cyclosporine. Bone Marrow Transplant 1994;13:101–104.
579. Stratakis CA, Chrousos GP. Capillaritis (purpura simplex) associated with use of aminoglutethimide in Cushing's syndrome. Am J Hosp Pharm 1994;51:2589–2591.
580. Baker JL, Gosland MP, Herrington JD, Record KE. Cytomegalovirus colitis after 5-fluorouracil and interferon-alpha therapy. Pharmacotherapy 1994;14:246–249.
581. Mansfield SH, Castillo M. MR of *cis*-platinum induced optic neuritis. Am J Neuroradiol 1994;15:1178–1180.
582. Van Woensel JBM, Knoester H, Leeuw JA, van Aalderen WMC. Acute respiratory insufficiency during doxorubin, cyclophosphamide, and G-CSF therapy. Lancet 1994;344:759–760.
583. Wondimu B, Dahllof G, Berg U, Modeer T. Cyclosporin-A-induced gingival overgrowth in renal transplant children. Scand J Dent Res 1993;101:282–286.
584. Wong W, Hodge MG, Lewis A, Sharpstone P, Kingswood JC et al. Resolution of cyclosporin-induced gingival hypertrophy with metronidazole. Lancet 1994;343:986.

585. Krentz AJ, Dmitrewski J, Mayer D, McMaster P, Buckels J et al. Postoperative glucose metabolism in liver transplant recipients: a two-year prospective randomized study of cyclosporine versus FK506. Transplantation 1994;57: 1666–1669.
586. Winkler M, Brinkmann C, Jost U, Oldhafer K, Ringe B et al. Long-term side effects of cyclosporin-based immunosuppression in patients after liver transplantation. Transplant Proc 1994;26:2679–2682.
587. Du LTH, Rigaud D, Papo T. Cyclophosphamide-induced hepatitis in Wegener's granulomatosis. Mayo Clin Proc 1994;69:912–913.
588. Rougier JP, Viron B, Ronco P, Khayat R, Michel C et al. Autoimmune haemolytic anaemia after ABO-match, ABDR full match kidney transplantation. Nephrol Dialysis Transplant 1994;9:693–697.
589. Bolla G, Disdier P, Harle JR, Verrot D, Weiller PJ. Concurrent acute megaloblastic anaemia and pneumonitis: a severe side-effect of low-dose methotrexate therapy during rheumatoid arthritis. Clin Rheumatol 1993;12:535–537.
590. Leduc D, De Vuyst P, Lheureux P et al. Pneumonitis complicating low-dose methotrexate therapy for rheumatoid arthritis. Discrepancies between lung biopsy and bronchcalveolar lavage findings. Chest 1993;104:1620–1623.
591. Adverse Drug Reaction Advisory Committee. Low dose methotrexate therapy—toxic if not taken correctly. Med J Australia 1994;161:152.
592. Abu-Shakra M, Nicol P, Urowitz MB. Accelerated nodulosis, pleural effusion, and pericardial tamponade during methotrexate therapy. J Rheumatol 1994;21:934–937.
593. Chandran G, Ahern MJ, de la M. Hall P, Geddes R, Smith M et al. Cirrhosis in patients with rheumatoid arthritis receiving low dose methotrexate. Br J Rheumatol 1994;33:981–984.
594. Kovacs GT, Paal Ch, Somlo P, Koos R, Schuler D et al. Proteinuria due to suboptimal hydration with high-dose methotrexate therapy. Cancer Chemother Pharmacol 1993;33:262–263.
595. Jerian SM, Sarosy GA, Link CJ Jr, Fingert HJ, Reed E et al. Incapacitating autonomic neuropathy precipitated by taxol. Gynecol Oncol 1993;51:277–280.
596. Hizawa N, Kojima J, Kojima T, Sukoh N, Yamaguchi E et al. A patient with chronic hepatitis C who simultaneously developed interstitial pneumonia, hemolytic anemia and cholestatic liver dysfunction after alpha-interferon administration. Intern Med 1994;33:337–341.
597. Stratta P, Canavese C, Dogliani M, Thea A, Degani G et al. Hemolytic uremic syndrome during recombinant alpha-interferon treatment for hairy cell leukemia. Renal Failure 1993;15:559–561.
598. Makino Y, Tanaka H, Nakamura K, Fujita M, Akiyama K et al. Arthritis in a patient with psoriasis after interferon-alpha therapy for chronic hepatitis C. J Rheumatol 1994;21:1771–1772.
599. Arslan M, Ozyilkan E, Kayhan B, Telatar H. Raynaud's phenomenon associated twith alpha-interferon therapy. J Intern Med 1994;235:503.
600. Papini M, Bruni PL, Bettacchi A, Liberati F et al. Sudden onset of oral ulcerative lichen in a patient with chronic hepatitis C on treatment of alfa-interferon. Int J Dermatol 1994;33:221–222.
601. Yamada H, Mizobuchi K, Isogal Y. Acute onset of ocular complications with interferon. Lancet 1994;343:914.
602. Levy R, Cargill M, Le Maignan C et al. Acute alithiasic cholecystitis in patients given interleukin-2. Presse Med 1994;23:1583.
603. Stratta P, Canavese C, Dogliani M, Thea A, Degani G, et al. Hemolytic uremic syndrome during recombinant alpha-interferon treatment for hairy cell leukemia. Renal Failure 1993;15:559–561.
604. Sassigneux P, Michel P, Joly P, Colin R et al. Lichen planus during interferon alpha-2a therapy for chronic hepatitis-C. Gastroenterol Clin Biol 1993;17:764.
605. Greenfield SM, Harvey RS, Thompson RPH. Rhabdomyolysis after treatment with interferon alfa. Br Med J 1994;309:20–27.
606. Ene L, Gehenot M, Horsmans Y, Detry-Morel M, Geubel AP et al. Transient blurred vision after interferon for chronic hepatitis C. Lancet 1994;344:827–828.
607. Ohtsu T, Sasaki Y, Tanizaki H, Kawano N, Ryu M et al. Development of pseudolymphoma of liver following interferon-alpha therapy for chronic hepatitis B. Intern Med 1994;33:18–22.
608. Soriano V, Bravo R, Samaniego JG, Gonzalez J, Odriozola PM et al. CD4− T-lymphocytopenia in HIV-infected patients receiving interferon therapy for chronic hepatitis C. AIDS 1994;8:1521–1622.
609. Hoffmann A, Kirn E, Krueger GRF, Fischer R et al. Bone marrow hypoplasia and fibrosis following interferon treatment. In Vivo 1994;8:605–612.
610. Manesis EK, Petrou C, Brouzas D, Hadziyannis S. Optic tract neuropathy complicating low-dose interferon treatment. J Hepatol 1994;21:474–477.
611. Elis A, Lishner M, Savin H, Ravid M. Aplastic anemia induced by cyclohexylchloroethylnitrosurea. Anti-Cancer Drugs 1994;5:105–107.
612. Lenci G, Muller-Quernheim J, Lorenz J, Schweden F, Ferlinz R. Toxic lung damage by mitomycin C (German). Pneumologie 1994;48:197–201.
613. Stern SCM, Asagba GO, Hegde UM. Prolonged thrombocytopenia following alpha-interferon for refractory immune thrombocytopenic purpura. Clin Lab Haematol 1994;16:183–185.
614. Motoo Y, Watanabe H, Okai T, Sawabu N. Interferon-induced pancreatic injury. J Clin Gastroenterol 1994; 19:268–269.
615. Hirashima N, Mizokami M, Orito E, Yamauchi M, Narita M et al. Chronic hepatitis C complicated by Coombs-negative hemolytic anemia during interferon treatment. Intern Med 1994;33:300–302.
616. Wakelin SH, Emmerson RW. Excess granulation tissue development during treatment with cyclosporin. Br J Dermatol 1994;131:147–148.
617. DiMaggio JR, Brown R, Baile WF, Schapira D. Hallucinations and ifosfamide-induced neurotoxicity. Cancer 1994;73:1509–1514.
618. Izraeli S, Adamson PC, Blaney SM, Balis FM. Acute pancreatitis after ifosfamide therapy. Cancer 1994;74:1627–1628.
619. Kramer A, Goldschmidt H, Hahn U, Andrassy K. Progressive renal failure in two breast cancer patients after high-dose ifosfamide. Lancet 1994;344:1569.
620. Patel SR, Forman AD, Benjamin RS. High-dose ifosfamide-induced exacerbation of peripheral neuropathy. J Natl Cancer Inst 1994;86:305–306.
621. Uziely B, Lewin A, Brufman G et al. The effect of tamoxifen on the endometrium. Breast Cancer Res Treat 1993;26:101–105.

622. Van Leeuwen FE, Benraadt J, Coebergh JWW, Kiemeney LALM, Gimbrere CHF et al. Risk of endometrial cancer after tamoxifen treatment of breast cancer. Lancet 1994;343:448—452.
623. Fisher B, Costantino JP, Redmond CK, Fisher ER, Wickerham DL et al. Endometrial cancer in tamoxifen-treated breast cancer patients: findings from the National Surgical Adjuvant Breast and Bowel Project (NSABP) B-14. J Natl Cancer Inst 1994;86:527—537.
624. Cathcart CK, Jones SE, Pumroy CS, Peters GN, Knox SM et al. Clinical recognition and management of depression in node negative breast cancer patients treated with tamoxifen. Breast Cancer Res Treat 1993;27:277—281.
625. Morgan MA, Gincherman Y, Mikuta JJ. Endometriosis and tamoxifen therapy. Int J Gynecol Obstet 1994;45:55—57.
626. Heier JS, Dragoo RA, Enzenauer RW, Waterhouse WJ et al. Screening for ocular toxicity in asymptomatic patients treated with tamoxifen. Am J Ophthalmol 1994;117:772—775.
627. Gherman RB, Parker MF, Macri CI. Granulosa cell tumor of the ovary associated with antecedent tamoxifen use. Obstet Gynecol 1994;84:717—719.
628. Sonnendecker HEM, Cooper K, Kalian KN. Primary fallopian tube adenocarcinoma in situ associated with adjuvant tamoxifen therapy for breast carcinoma. Gynecol Oncol 1994;52:402—407.
629. Candido A, Bussa S, Tartaglione R, Mancini R, Rumi C et al. Tamoxifen-induced immune-mediated platelet destruction. A case report. Tumori 1993;79:231—234.
630. Mike V, Currie VE, Gee TS. Fatal neutropenia associated with long-term tamoxifen therapy. Lancet 1994;344:541—542.
631. Cargill RI, Boyter AC, Lipworth BJ. Reversible myocardial ischaemia following vincristine containing chemotherapy. Respir Med 1994;88:709—710.
632. Raymond E, Espie M, Extra JM, Marty M et al. Cardiotoxicity of vinorelbine (Navelbine Rm) (French). Therapie 1994;49:63.
633. Gebbia V, Testa A, Valenza R, Cannata G, Verderame F et al. Acute pain syndrome at tumour site in neoplastic patients treated with vinorelbine: report of unusual toxicity. Eur J Cancer (Part A) 1994;30A:889.
634. Dubois A, Reynaud D, Yeche S et al. Acute vincristine neurotoxicity: a new case. Therapie 1993;48:515.
635. Pinzani V, Bressolle F, Haug IJ, Galtier M, Blayac JP, Balmes P. Cisplatin-induced renal txocity and toxicity-modulating strategies: a review. Cancer Chemother Pharmacol 1994;35(1):1—9.
636. Crestani B, Jaccard A, Israel-Biet D, Couderc LJ, Frija J, Clauvel JP. Chlorambucil-associated pneumonitis. Chest 1994;105(2):634—636.
637. Shulman A, Cohen I, Altaras MM, Maymon R, Ben-Nun I, Tepper R, Beyth Y. Ovarian cyst formation in two premenopausal patients treated with tamoxifen for breast cancer. Hum Reprod 1994;9(8):1427—1429.
638. Re A, Wierdis T, Tessarolo M, Leo L, Bellino R, Lauricella A, Lanza A. Two cases of ovarian cysts in postmenopausal patients under antiestrogen treatment. Clin Exp Obstet Gynecol 1994;21(4):221—224.
639. Morgan MA, Gincherman Y, Mikuta JJ. Endometriosis and tamoxifen therapy. Int J Gynaecol Obstet 1994; 45(1):55—57.
640. Ugwumadu AH, Harding K. Uterine leiomyomata and endometrial proliferation in postmenopausal women treated with the anti-oestrogen tamoxifen. Eur J Obstet Gynecol Reprod Biol 1994;54(2):153—156.
641. Gorlich M. Tamoxifen flare. Zentralbl Gynakol 1994;116(4):239—241.
642. Mihm LM, Barton TL. Tamoxifen-induced ocular toxicity. Ann Pharmacother 1994;28(6):740—742.
643. Mike V, Currie VE, Gee TS. Fatal neutropenia associated with long-term tamoxifen therapy. Lancet 1994; 344:541—542.
644. Muhlemann K, Cook LS, Weiss NS. The incidence of hepatocellular carcinoma in US white women with breast cancer after the introduction of tamoxifen in 1977. Breast Cancer Res Treat 1994;30(2):201—204.
645. Janssen HL, Brouwer JT, van der Mast RC, Schalm SW. Suicide associated with alfa-interferon therapy for chronic viral hepatitis. J Hepatol 1994;21(2):241—243.
646. Makino Y, Tanaka H, Fujita M, Akiyama K, Makino I. Arthritis in a patient with psoriasis after interferon-alpha therapy for chronic hepatitis C. J Rheumatol 1994; 21(9):1171—1772.
647. Guleria AS, Yang JC, Topalian SL, Weber JS, Parkinson DR, MacFarlane MP, White RL, Steinberg SM, White DE, Einhorn JH et al. Renal dysfunction associated with the administration of high-dose interleukin-2 in 199 consecutive patients with metastatic melanoma or renal carcinoma. J Clin Oncol 1994;12(12):2714—2722.
648. Stasi R, Gatti S, Perrotti A, Orlandi A, Spagnoli LG, Papa G. Erythema multiforme during GM-CSF therapy. Acta Dermatol-Venereol 1994;74(2):132—134.
649. Lautenschlager S, Itin PH, Hirsbrunner P, Buchner SA. Subcorneal pustular dermatosis at the injection site of recombinant human granulocyte-macrophage colony-stimulating factor in a patient with IgA myeloma. J Am Acad Dermatol 1994;30:787—789.
650. Jekunen A, Heikkila P, Maiche A, Pyrhonen S. Paclitaxel-induced myocardial damage detected by electron microscopy (Letter). Lancet 1994;343:727—728.
651. Shenkier T, Gelmon K. Paclitaxel and radiation-recall dermatitis (Letter). J Clin Oncol 1994;12(2):439.
652. Capri G, Munzone E, Tarenzi E, Fulfaro F, Gianni L, Caraceni A, Martini C, Scaioli V. Optic nerve disturbances: a new form of paclitaxel neurotoxicity (Letter). J Natl Cancer Inst 1994;86(14):1099—1101.
653. Sahenk Z, Barohn R, New P, Mendell JR. Taxol neuropathy. Electrodiagnostic and sural nerve biopsy findings. Arch Neurol 1994;51(7):726—729.
654. Meehan JL, Sporn JR. Case report of Taxol administration via central vein producing a recall reaction at a site of prior Taxol extravasation (Letter). J Natl Cancer Inst 1994;86(16):1250—1251.
655. Greco FA, Hainsworth JD. Paclitaxel (Taxol): phase I/II trial comparing 1-hour infusion schedules. Semin Oncol 1994;21(5 Suppl 8):3—8.
656. Hermans P, Gori A, Lemone M, Franchioly P, Clumeck N. Possible role of granulocyte-macrophage colony stimulating factor (GM-CSF) on the rapid progression of AIDS-related Kaposi's sarcoma lesions in vivo. Br J Haematol 1994;87(2):413—414.
657. Moredo Anelli TF, Anelli A, Tran KN, Lebwohl DE, Borgen PI et al. Tamoxifen administration is associated with a high rate of treatment-limiting symptoms in male breast cancer patients. Cancer 1994;74:74—77.
658. Vial T, Descotes J. Clinical toxicity of the interferons. Drug Safety 1994;10:115—150.

659. Halla JT, Hardin JG. Underrecognised postdosing reactions to methotrexate in patients with rheumatoid arthritis. J Rheumatol 1994;21:1224–1226.
660. Gruber SA, Gillingham K, Sothern RB, Stephanian E, Matas AJ et al. De novo cancer in cyclosporine-treated and non-cyclosporine-treated adult primary renal allograft recipients. Clin Transplant 1994;8:388–395.
661. Anand AJ, Bashey B. Newer insights into cisplatin nephrotoxicity. Ann Pharmacother 1993;27:1519–1525.
662. Talaat KM, Tyden G, Bjorkman U, Groth CGI. Thirty successful pregnancies in organ transplant recipients: a single-center experience. Transplant Proc 1994;26:1773.
663. Connel WR, Kinlen LJ, Ritchie JK, Blakwill A, Lennard-Jones JE et al. Cancer risk from azathioprine in inflammatory bowel disease. Gastroenterology 1994; 106(Suppl):667.
664. Chasen MR, Falkson G. Leukemia after chemotherapy for cancer. Cancer Biother 1993;8:115–122.
665. Giustina G, Favarato S, Ruol A, Fattovich G. A survey of clinical toxicity of alfa interferon in 11 241 patients with chronic viral hepatitis. Ital J Gastroenterol 1994;26:203–204
666. Smith MA, Rubinstein L, Ungerleider RS. Therapy-related acute myeloid leukemia following treatment with epipodophyllotoxins: estimating the risks. Med Pediatr Oncol 1994;23:86–98
667. Editorial. Drug-induced gynaecomastia. Rev Prescr 1994;14(136):21–22.
668. Editorial. Drug-induced hyponatraemia. Rev Presc 1993;13(134):587–588.
669. Friedl A, Jordan VC. What do we know and what don't we know about tamoxifen in the human uterus (Review). Breast Cancer Res Treat 1994;31(1):27–39.
670. Kedar RP, Bourne TH, Powles TJ, Collins WP, Ashley SE et al. Effects of tamoxifen on uterus and ovaries of postmenopausal women in a randomised breast cancer prevention trial. Lancet 1994;343:1318–1321.
671. Bernstein D, Baum D, Berry G, Dahl G, Weiss L et al. Neoplastic disorders after pediatric heart transplant. Circulation 1993;88:230–237.

Meyler's Side Effects of Drugs, 13th Edition
M.N.G. Dukes, editor

SECTION EDITOR: M.N.G. DUKES

M.N.G. Dukes*

46 Radiological contrast media and radiopharmaceuticals

GENERAL

In examining the adverse effects of contrast media several complementary approaches have to be adopted. Firstly, as in other drug fields, one has to consider the adverse effects, be they toxic, idiosyncratic or allergic, associated with a *particular compound or class of compounds*. Secondly, one must look at those reactions which are associated with the *type of investigation performed* (e.g. myelographic, gastrointestinal, angiographic) rather than with particular media. Thirdly, one needs to consider those adverse events which result from *technical errors or failings* in the administration or removal of a contrast medium. In some circumstances it may not be at all clear which of these issues underlies a particular reaction.

In using this chapter to determine whether a particular type of reaction has been described in the past it can thus be helpful to consult the sections dealing with the use of other contrast media in the same situation, or experience with the same contrast media for other situations. Clearly, however, not all these things can be extrapolated, since the reactions to a particular contrast medium do differ with the purpose for which it is used; apparent discrepancies in the figures for the incidence of side effects with a given contrast medium often simply reflect the fact that for one purpose it may be given in a higher dosage, at a higher rate, or into a more sensitive tissue than where another application is concerned.

During the last two decades there has been a marked shift in the types of contrast media in general use in industrialized countries. Some older media must nevertheless be considered since they remain in use for special purposes or in certain countries, and a number of obsolete media still deserve attention because residues can persist in the body and elicit adverse reactions many years after they have been administered.

THE NATURE OF CONTRAST MEDIA

The radio-opacity of contrast media is dependent upon the fact that they contain substances having a high atomic number, which absorb X-rays. *Bismuth*, now largely obsolete (except for gastrointestinal examination) has an atomic number of 83, barium of 56. Since the soluble salts of barium are poisonous, the insoluble salt, barium sulfate, is used as a suspension.

Soluble contrast media are based on *iodine*, which has an atomic number of 53. This means that in principle they could exert the various adverse effects of other iodine compounds as reviewed in Chapter 41.

The *ionic compounds* for a long time dominated the field; they include diatrizoate, iothalamate, iodamide and metrizoate; all these are triiodobenzoic acid derivatives and are similar in terms of toxicity; modifications of the cations (using various ratios of sodium, methylglucamine and calcium) can however affect the toxicity in specific circumstances. Particularly for the many types of radiological examination which involve intravascular injection, the ionic compounds present disadvantages. Members of the class are relatively toxic, and the older compounds have a high osmolarity. Since intolerance to such contrast media (including reactions such as pain on injection and thrombosis) is in part due to their hypertonicity, lower-osmolar media have recently been introduced and have rapidly replaced them for most purposes (1^R); sodium methylglucamine ioxaglate is itself an ionic medium but, being a monoacid dimer, it has approximately one-half the osmolarity of the older compounds.

The other main development among the field of iodine-based media has been the introduction of the *non-*

* This Chapter owes much to the extensive reviews prepared by Dr George Ansell for previous editions of *Meyler's Side Effects of Drugs* and eighteen successive *Side Effects of Drugs Annuals*. I would also like to acknowledge the expert advice which I have received from Dr Ole Jonsen.

-ionic contrast media which in most (but not all) fields are better tolerated as substances (2[R]) and which also avoid the problem of high osmolarity. The first was metrizamide, which has now essentially been superseded by newer non-ionic compound media such as iopamidol, iohexol, iopramide and ioversol. There was early acceptance of the need to use such media in weak patients and children (3[R]). Initially, the non-ionic media were used more restrictively in other individuals because of their higher price, but this problem is progressively being overcome, particularly in those areas where it has been shown that the higher costs are outweighed by a substantial reduction in the costs of managing adverse reactions (4[CR]).

The choice of contrast media for particular purposes depends primarily on their suitability for reaching a particular organ and/or the sensitivity of the tissues with which they will come into contact:

- For many types of investigation, contrast media have to be given by the intravascular route. Intravascular iodine-based contrast media are used for *angiography* and *computed tomography*, but since they are excreted mainly by the kidney they are also used for *excretory urography*. Here, for the reasons explained above, there has been a strong shift to the non- ionic and low-osmolar media (SEDA-18, 441).
- For *cholecystography* one will need those which are excreted primarily by the liver; in this field, iodipamide and ioglycamide were long preferred, but the newer iodoxamate and iotroxate are more efficiently excreted via this route.
- The media used to *outline cavities* may be either water-soluble, water-insoluble, or oily in nature.
- In the *gastrointestinal tract* the insoluble barium sulfate is still most commonly used, but water-soluble iodinated media may be used in special circumstances.
- For *retrograde urography*, many different media can be used provided they are diluted sufficiently.
- For *arthrography*, *ductography* and *sinography* one similarly has a wide choice provided the media are diluted.
- For *lymphography and ductography*, iodized oil is used.
- *Hysterosalpingography* is at most centers now performed with water-soluble media.
- *Bronchography* can be performed with an aqueous or oily suspension.
- *Myelography* represents a special challenge because of the sensitivity of nervous tissue to direct toxic effects; for this purpose the ionic media (which are neurotoxic) and the oily medium iophendylate have now been superseded by non- ionic media; two recently developed members of this class, iotrolan and iodixanol, were selected since they are approximately isotonic with cerebrospinal fluid.

GENERAL AND IDIOSYNCRATIC REACTIONS TO CONTRAST MEDIA *(5[R])*

Although some systemic reactions reflect the present of iodine in the contrast medium, or a frankly toxic effect of a particular compound, there is a family of 'idiosyncratic' reactions to soluble contrast media which affect a range of systems, occur in susceptible individuals and represent the main problems with these media; they occur more particularly with media of the ionic type and when contrast media are given by the intravascular route, but they can occur in any situation. Idiosyncratic reactions may be slightly less common following arteriography than after urography. The main types of reactions encountered are listed in Table 1 and their nature and mechanism are discussed in more detail below; Table 2 indicates the type of reactions which are more prone to come to the fore with intravenous urography.

In various earlier surveys relating to conventional ionic contrast media, the *incidence* of minor reactions was one in 13—30 cases, that of intermediate reactions was one in 57—130 cases, and that of severe reactions to one in 1000—4000 applications. The figures for the non-ionic media are much more favorable. The Japanese Committee on the Safety of Contrast Media (6[CR]) surveyed in 1990 169 284 cases receiving ionic media and 168 363 receiving non-ionic contrast media. In patients with a previous history of reactions to contrast media, the incidence of severe reactions was 0.73% with ionic media and only 0.18% with non-ionic media. Among patients with asthma, severe and very severe reactions developed in 1.88% with ionic media and 0.23% with non- ionic media. In a Canadian survey of 1992, the overall incidence of adverse effects to contrast media was 3.9% for ionic media and only 0.9% for non-ionic media, despite the fact that the proportion of patients with heart disease as a pre-existing risk factor was much higher in the non-ionic group (7[CR]).

As to the *time sequence*, most such reactions occur within 5—10 minutes of injection, but they may be delayed; it is advisable for patients to be under close observation for approximately 20 minutes after injection. In a series comprising part of the survey by Shehadi cited below, 80% of reactions commenced in the first 5 minutes after injection, and the remaining 20% of reactions commenced between 5 and 15 minutes after injection. There are also a series of late but mild

Table 1. *Idiosyncratic reactions to soluble contrast media*

Minor	Intermediate	Severe
Nausea, retching	Faintness	Collapse
Slight vomiting	Severe vomiting	Loss of consciousness
Feeling of heat	Extensive urticaria	Bronchospasm
Limited urticaria	Edema of face or glottis	Edema of the glottis
Mild pallor or sweating	Bronchospasm	Pulmonary edema
Itchy skin rashes	Dyspnea	Cardiac arrest
Arm pain	Rigors	Myocardial infarction syndrome
	Chest pain	Cardiac arrhythmias
	Abdominal pain	
	Headache	
	Tetany	

Table 2. *Intravenous urograms: risk ratios related to clinical history*

History	Minor reactions	Intermediate reactions	Severe reactions	Death
Allergy (all types)	1.6	2.6	3.9	
Hay fever	1.7	1.8	2.3	
Urticaria	1.5	4.8	2	
Asthma	1.2	2.7	5.1	
Previous reaction to contrast medium	6.9	8.7	10.9	
Previous reaction to other drugs	1.8	2	3.2	
Heart disease	1.1	0.9	4.5	8.5

reactions, notably those reflecting 'iodism' (SEDA-11, 411).

PATTERN OF IDIOSYNCRATIC REACTIONS

Cardiovascular The majority of severe reactions are associated with cardiovascular manifestations causing *hypotensive shock* and in some cases *ventricular fibrillation* and *cardiac arrest*; these events are reversible in most cases receiving prompt treatment. In a case of hypotensive collapse reported in 1977, and followed by a small number of others, *disseminated intravascular coagulation* was found (8[C]). In milder cases there is only hypertension which may be transient and symptomless; in certain cases of hypotension there is bradycardia (due apparently to vagal over-activity) rather than tachycardia (SEDA-2, 373).

Routine ECG monitoring during intravenous urography shows that significant *ECG abnormalities* occur in patients with heart disease and that the incidence of these abnormalities appears to be related to the dose of contrast medium and the speed of injection (9[C]).

It should be noted that certain contrast media, notably the sodium methylglucamine-based high osmolar products Renografin-76 and MD- 76, have calcium-binding properties and cause more hemodynamic changes and a higher risk of ventricular fibrillation (e.g. in cardiography) than do the calcium-enriched media Angiovist and Hypaque-76 (10[CR]).

Non-ionic contrast media are almost sodium free; they have little tendency to induce ventricular fibrillation or depress cardiac motility, and this small risk might (if studies on animal material in vitro are a dependable guide) be further reduced by the addition of a very small amount of sodium (11[r]).

Respiratory *Bronchospasm* may be severe, particularly in asthmatic patients, and may cause cardiac arrest (12[CR]). Subclinical bronchospasm may occur after bolus injections of ionic contrast medium; the incidence is lower with non-ionic media (SEDA-8,427).

In patients with incipient cardiac failure, there is a particular risk of precipitating *pulmonary edema* when large doses of contrast medium are used. Occasionally non-cardiogenic pulmonary edema can occur though it is notable that it has several times been seen in patients with a prior history of myocardial infarct (SEDA- 16, 531); it can also be a component of anaphylactic shock (SEDA-5, 420).

Adult respiratory distress syndrome has been seen in one case, accompanied by *disseminated intravascular coagulation* (SEDA-16, 531).

Nervous system *Loss of consciousness* may occur if there is hypotensive collapse; rarely there may be prolonged coma.

Convulsions, seen as part of an idiosyncratic reaction, tend to occur in patients with an existing tendency to epilepsy, or to appear as consequences of hypotensive collapse, cardiac arrest or overdose (see also section on Computed Tomography below).

Endocrine, metabolic *Enzymes* inhibited to some extent by these contrast media include cholinesterase, glucose-6- phosphate dehydrogenase and alcohol dehydrogenase (13[R]).

Transient *hyperthyroid changes* may occur (SEDA-6, 408); however, when an excessive dose of diluted ioxaglate was used to opacify and render visible the catheters in infants on parenteral nutrition, three of 28 patients developed transitory *hypothyroidism* (14[C]).

Contrast media caused release of *vasoactive intestinal polypeptide* in a patient with a vipoma of the pancreas and hepatic secondaries (SEDA-11, 411).

Mineral and fluid balance It has been known for a generation that contrast media may cause some depression of the *calcium* and *magnesium* levels in the blood (15[c]), an effect which might be relevant to the occasional occurrence of *tetany* (see also SEDA-7, 452).

Hematological A single case of severe but reversible *hypoplastic anemia* has been attributed to sodium diatrizoate (16[C]). *Acute thrombocytopenic purpura* has also been reported in three patients (SEDA-11, 413). Ionic contrast media have a *disaggregating effect* on erythrocytes, and hypertonic media reduce their *elasticity* (SEDA-4, 335). There is some (disputed) evidence that use of the generally safer non-ionic media actually increases the risk of *thromboembolic complications* as compared with the ionic products, possibly because the non-ionic products lack the anticoagulant effect of the ionic media; the risk has been described in some contested studies as being 4—10 times higher (SEDA-17, 537; SEDA-18, 444; 17[CR]); certainly the non- ionic substances do produce profound degranulation of platelets in vitro, but this proves to be unrelated to thrombin generation (18[R]). Some workers do however currently prefer to heparinize when giving the non-ionic media.

Gastrointestinal *Nausea* and *vomiting* in idiosyncratic reactions have been mentioned above. *Diarrhea* is less common but has been repeatedly reported, sometimes with *angio-edema of the bowel* (19[CR]).

Swelling of the *parotid glands* has been recognized as an occasional effect for very many years (20[C]), occurring particularly in cases where there is renal failure (see below); the swelling usually occurs 2—4 days after the procedure and may last for several days, but evanescent salivary gland enlargement may also occur within a few minutes of injection and last for a number of hours. In one published case, the complication was associated with *paralysis of the facial nerve*, which largely subsided over the next 9 weeks (SED-8, 1033). Transitory enlargement of the *pancreas* may also occur (SEDA-11, 411).

Urinary system Not surprisingly, complications affecting the kidneys are more likely to occur when one is performing urographic investigations in cases of suspected renal disease, i.e., in high risk situations. However, the kidneys can be adversely affected by other intravenous techniques as well.

A number of cases of *renal failure* have occurred, but most particularly in patients with myelomatosis; in most of these, diodone or acetrizoate had been used, and these older media cause precipitation of Bence-Jones protein, whereas more recent agents such as diatrizoate do not. Nevertheless, renal failure has incidentally been described following the use of diatrizoate (SED- 8, 1032); dehydration or oliguria may have been contributing factors. However, urography may precipitate renal failure in myelomatosis even if the patient is well hydrated (SEDA-2, 374).

Dehydration predisposes to renal failure. It is not generally accepted that there is an increased risk of causing renal failure by contrast media examinations in diabetic patients with renal disease and particularly in juvenile-onset diabetes. Pre-existing renal disease with azotemia is an important factor. Other possible predisposing factors include cardiac disease, diuretics, multiple examinations within a short period, and multiple myeloma.

There are conflicting opinions concerning the relevance of the dose and choice of contrast medium used. One analysis certainly shows a significant correlation of contrast nephropathy with higher doses (21[CR]). Although under clinical experimental conditions the non-ionic media iohexol and iopamidol appear to be less nephrotoxic than diatrizoate (22[C]), contrast nephropathy has occurred with these non-ionic media as well (SEDA-13, 434) and, in an earlier randomized trial comparing iopamidol and diatrizoate, no significant difference in nephrotoxicity was demonstrated. However, less than 5% of patients in the second study had advanced renal impairment (23[CR]). Low osmolar media as a whole appear to be less nephrotoxic than high osmolar media but this only appears to be of clinical importance in patients with existing renal disorders (24[CR]). The new non-ionic agent iodixanol may be less toxic than its congeners but further work is needed to verify this (SEDA-18, 444).

As to *risk situations*: urate nephropathy and increased oxalate excretion may be factors in causing renal failure (SEDA-7, 452). In hyperuricemic children with Burkitt's lymphoma, urography caused urate nephropathy in three of four untreated patients (SEDA- 10, 423). Although there have been many cases of myelomatosis where urography has been undertaken without incident, the examination should only be performed in this condition if absolutely imperative.

Diagnosis Kidney *biopsy* in cases of renal complications may show changes resembling an osmotic nephrosis, but these can also be found in some cases with no evidence of impaired renal activity.

The presence of an *abnormally prolonged or increasingly dense nephrogram* can provide a clue to incipient acute renal failure. In addition, if the kidney is not capable of excreting an intravenous contrast medium adequately, blood levels will be elevated for some days and under these circumstances part of the medium is excreted in the bile, resulting in X-ray *visualization of the gallbladder and bowel*. However, one should bear in mind that ioxaglate is actively secreted into the bile and when using this contrast medium gallbladder opacification may occur in the absence of renal failure (25[C]).

Prevention of contrast nephropathy rests largely on the exclusion of high-risk cases, such as very ill patients with diabetic renal failure, severe cardiovascular disease with diminished renal blood flow, jaundice, pre-existing azotemia and multiple myeloma. Where the investigation is nevertheless needed in these conditions, the physiological state should be corrected as a far as possible: adequate hydration should be assured and sufficient volume expansion ensured to induce a gentle diuresis (e.g. 75 ml/hour), before and for several hours after the administration the contrast medium. Concomitant use of other potentially nephrotoxic agents should be avoided. Finally, since the small amounts of contrast medium that remain in the body after a radiographic examination may potentiate renal damage resulting from subsequent events, there should be a delay of at least 12 hours after the examination before any surgery is undertaken which could adversely effect the kidney, e.g. procedures requiring temporary renal clamping or percutaneous balloon dilatation of the renal artery. A similar delay is advised between cerebral angiography and renal harvesting for transplantation. If renal glomerular filtration is reduced by 50% or more, a delay of 24 hours or more may be advisable after aortofemoral angiography (SEDA-15, 502). There is currently some disputed evidence that calcium channel blockers might reduce the nephrotoxicity of contrast media, but other work has suggested that they could have a deleterious effect, particularly in patients receiving high osmolar media or in diabetics (SEDA-18, 444).

Skin and appendages The skin may be involved in idiosyncratic reactions (see above) or more rarely in typical *iododerma*, sometimes alongside other dermal and systemic complications (26[CR]). Delayed skin *rashes* have been noted in 5% of patients undergoing urography. Rarely *acute vasculitis*, *Stevens-Johnson syndrome* and *bullous lichen planus* have been reported (SEDA-11, 411; SEDA-14, 422). Other rarities reported sporadically (but all in more than one case) include the *Köbnor phenomenon* (27[Cr]), fixed drug eruptions (e.g. with iothalamate (28[CR])) and delayed reactions of various types. Reports of severe drug eruptions have become more frequent since the introduction of the non-ionic contrast media, but this may well be due simply to the fact that there has in recent years been a greater awareness of such reactions (SEDA-16, 538).

Chromosomal changes An increased frequency of *chromosomal aberrations* and sister chromatid exchanges has been found in lymphocytes up to a week after intravenous urography; diatrizoate produced more changes than ioxaglate (29). Earlier it was reported that the incidence of chromosomal aberrations in the lymphocytes of seven infants who underwent angiocardiography had been found to be higher than expected (SEDA-3, 379). Whether this means that contrast media produce significant cytogenetic damage is not at all clear (SEDA-3, 379).

Miscellaneous (*SED*-12, 1172) A transitory case of *myopathy* has been reported after iopamidol and a fatal case of *malignant hyperthermia* after 100 ml of diatrizoate. A fatal reaction has been reported in a case of *Waldenström's IgM paraproteinemia*.

Risk situations (30[CR]) Certain individual factors may increase the risk of reaction and have been outlined above. In *infants*, the low glomerular filtration rate may result in delayed excretion; reactions in the *elderly* are often severe. In patients with *myasthenia gravis*, crises may be precipitated (31[CR]). Patients with pre-existent *thyrotoxicosis* present a problem since the condition may be aggravated, even to the point of precipitating a thyroid storm (32[CR]). Patients with a history of *previous reactions* to contrast media have a 35—40% chance of reacting again if re-examined. Sufferers from *asthma* or *heart disease* have a higher risk of developing a severe reaction. There also appears to be an *ethnic* element: Indian and, to a lesser extent, patients of Mediterranean origin have a significantly increased risk of reactions. A relation was also shown between the size of the *dose* of contrast medium used and the incidence of severe reactions.

Interactions *Drugs which increase uric acid excretion* may precipitate nephropathy (SEDA-7, 452). *Non- steroidal anti-inflammatory drugs* may possibly also increase the risk (SEDA-15, 502). If *metformin* is being taken, there is a greater risk of it producing lactic acidosis (33[CR]). Field experience, backed by a case-control study of 1991, strongly indicates that patients taking β- blockers have an increased risk ratio of 2.7

as regards adverse reactions to contrast media, tending in particular to become hypotensive, sometimes dangerously so, even with non-ionic media (SEDA-11, 411; SEDA-17, 536; 34[Cr]). Contrast media should not be mixed with *antihistamines* in a syringe since precipitation can result (SED-8, 1034). Diatrizoate and *strophanthin K* may have a synergistic toxic effect (SEDA-4, 334). Prior *Interleukin*-2 therapy can clearly induce atypical contrast medium hypersensitivity in the form of toxic recall reactions of various types (SEDA-17, 537–538), and these cannot be prevented by steroid premedication (35[CR]). *Hydralazine* seems to increase the risk of acute cutaneous vasculitis (36[C]).

Interference with diagnostic routines Urinalysis after intravenous urography may give misleading results. Increased specific gravity, false-positive tests for protein (with the sulfosalicylic acid and nitric acid ring methods, but not the bromophenyl dye test) and the presence of needle-like crystals have been reported. A positive result in the black copper reduction test, suggesting alcaptonuria, may follow the use of diatrizoate, iothalamate or iodipamide (37[c]). Methylglucamine-based contrast media interfere with the estimation of urinary catecholamines in pheochromocytoma (SEDA-10, 423). Diatrizoate may interfere with PAH extraction studies (SEDA-15, 502; 38[CR]).

Overdosage Fatal cases of accidental overdosage in infants have been reported; the complications leading to death were either pulmonary edema or convulsions (SED-8, 1035). The latter can be due to the hyperosmolar state (leading to hypertonic dehydration) or to the chemical toxicity of the contrast medium.

Cause of fatalities Shehadi (39[cr]) reviewed in 1985 the available findings in 449 fatal reactions to ionic media. Deaths occurred in all age groups, but the incidence peaked in the 50–70 year age group; in this older group, cardiovascular collapse, cardiac arrest and pulmonary edema were the most common features, but pulmonary edema appeared to be the commonest autopsy finding in all age groups. Lalli (40[CR]) examined the causes of 53 deaths due to urography or computed tomography; 35 were of cardiac origin and eight were attributed to pulmonary edema. The presenting features in eight cases were nausea and vomiting, whilst seven cases presented with shock or hypotension.

Prediction of risk Intravenous pre-testing is unreliable in determining susceptibility; in one survey of 33 400 patients, the great majority of reactions were not predicted by pre-testing, though a positive pretest did indicate an increased risk of a reaction occurring (41[CR]). The value of the lymphoblast transformation test is very limited, though it certainly provides interesting evidence that contrast media can sometimes act as antigens (SEDA-16, 531; 42[C]).

Mechanisms The mechanisms underlying idiosyncratic adverse reactions are far from clear. Although many resemble allergic or anaphylactic events, the evidence does not suggest that they are as a whole induced immunologically, though some certainly are, and there is no doubt that in some situations contrast media can act as antigens (see above). Lalli believes that all contrast media reactions are explicable on a neurological basis; the hypothesis is not generally accepted, but most would agree that anxiety can be an important predisposing factor, e.g. to cardiac arrhythmias. It has been suggested that contrast media may act as histamine liberators, and there is animal experimental evidence that this is the case, the methylglucamine media being more potent in this respect than the corresponding sodium salts (though ioxaglate may apparently also elicit histaminoid reactions (43[CR])); the antihistamine diphenhydramine has been recommended both for preventing and treating reactions (see below) and may have some efficacy. A further theory is that bradykinin is an essential mediator in systemic contrast media reactions (44[R]). There is also older experimental evidence that contrast media can activate serum complement by the 'alternative pathway' and it is postulated that this may be one of the factors in systemic adverse reactions, possibly by liberation of anaphylatoxin and with a risk of disseminated intravascular coagulation (SEDA-2, 374).

Treatment of reactions Treatment of idiosyncratic reactions goes beyond the scope of this volume. In severe reactions, intravenous steroids are usually given on an empirical basis with oxygen administration as required. Non-cardiogenic hypotensive shock usually responds best to fluid replacement, but vasopressors may occasionally be required. Adrenaline is primarily indicated for bronchospasm and other allergic-type reactions, but caution is required to avoid cardiac arrhythmias. Intravenous antihistamines are useful in angioneurotic edema, but may aggravate hypotensive reactions. Chemotoxic convulsions require intravenous diazepam and oxygenation.

Prevention of idiosyncratic reactions In high-risk patients, and more particularly those with a history of poor tolerance of contrast media, measures will need to be taken to contain risks of hypersensitivity reactions. Quite apart from using non-ionic and low osmolar media, and diluting media for certain purposes, one can consider prophylactic premedication. Steroid premedication alone has often been advocated, particularly in asthmatic patients; although it has been condemned as unnecessary with the present generation of contrast media (SEDA-18, 442) it seems to be well founded in experience, reducing both the frequency and severity of reactions, but it certainly does not eliminate risk (45[R]). A double regimen based on prednisolone and the antihistamine diphenhydramine has been advocated in various centres (46[CR], 47[R]; SEDA-16, 531; SEDA-18, 442). To be effective, steroids should be given sufficiently far in advance; an intravenous injection of dexamethasone given immediately before an infusion of contrast media has failed to prevent an anaphylactic reaction (48[CR]).

Prophylactic use of H_1 and H_2 antagonists, aminocaproic acid and hyposensitization have all been proposed as means of reducing risk. ϵ-Aminocaproic acid was formerly used prophylactically in France, but introduced a particular risk of massive intravascular coagulation (SEDA-17, 536).

The prevention of renal risks is dealt with separately above.

LOCAL TOXICITY OF CONTRAST MEDIA

Intravenous injection With highly concentrated sodium media, such as sodium iothalamate 420, severe *arm pain* may occur and a number of cases of late *thrombosis* have developed (49[cR]). In a comparison of the sodium and methylglucamine salts of diatrizoate, even with lower concentrations, the incidence of arm pain was higher with the sodium salt (SED-8, 1033). Extravasation of ionic contrast medium in the soft tissues may cause a *chemical cellulitis* leading to skin necrosis particularly if the circulation is compromised (SEDA-10, 424); tissue damage is less severe with the non-ionic media. The risk of extravasation is greatest with the rapid injection of large doses needed in computer tomography (see below). In rare cases, gangrene has followed, particularly in venography. Arterial insufficiency probably results in slower removal of the agent and hence more prolonged exposure to it.

As in many other areas, the non-ionic media are in this respect less noxious; this is shown in animal studies (SEDA-16, 530) and in a number of clinical cases where extravasation of medium to large volumes of iopamidol responded to palliative measures and had no lasting ill-effects (50[CR]). Among the ionic media, the methylglucamine media seem to have more local toxicity than their sodium equivalents.

Subcutaneous or intramuscular injection In the past, when intravascular injection proved difficult, contrast media were sometimes given by the subcutaneous or intramuscular route. On occasion, severe sloughing of tissue resulted. Addition of hyaluronidase in order to alleviate this problem only aggravated it, and dilution with water, saline or procaine solution also proved useless (SED-8, 1021). If, in exceptional circumstances, these routes have to be used, the medium should be injected in small quantities at multiple sites (see also section on 'Amniography').

Intra-articular injection Minor reversible edematous changes have been noted in the synovial membrane following arthrography, and a chemical synovitis may occur (SEDA-10, 425).

EFFECTS OF ADDITIVES

Several additives used in proprietary contrast media could have adverse effects; they include surfactants (e.g. Thesat), dextran (used as a thickening agent), local anesthetics (which in animal experiments seem to be more toxic to the tissues when combined with a surfactant) and antibiotics; others are mentioned elsewhere in this chapter, e.g. parabens. Neomycin, present in 2.5% concentration in one such product, has on occasion caused precipitation when mixed with sodium alginate contained in a catheter lubricant, resulting in a congealed mass in the bladder. Neomycin in this product has also caused temporary paralysis due to neuromuscular blockade in an infant following retroperitoneal extravasation of the contrast medium.

RADIOLOGY OF THE ALIMENTARY TRACT

Barium sulfate

Oral barium sulfate is theoretically non-toxic, but constipation and abdominal pain are not uncommon after barium meals or barium enemas (51[CR]). The main risk is that *accumulations* of barium will remain in the colon; they may persist for 6 weeks or longer in elderly patients or cases of colonic obstruction; barium fecoliths may even have to be removed surgically. Prolonged stasis of barium may occur following a barium enema into the distal loop of a colostomy. Residues in the appendix have caused appendicitis. Toxic dilatation of the colon may be aggravated by barium enema.

Perforation into the peritoneal cavity Following barium enema, perforation occurs rarely in children and debilitated adults or where the colon is already weakened by inflammatory, malignant or parasitic disease; the perforation may be triggered by manipulations involved in giving the barium enema or result from hydrostatic pressure. In one recorded case, perforation followed air contrast insufflation for barium enema in a patient in whom the sigmoid colon became trapped in an inguinal hernia (SEDA-2, 373).

At least 12 cases of perforation of the colon by barium enema, with four deaths resulting, were reported in a series of publications (SED-12, 1165). The incidence of perforation was approximately one in 6000 examinations. Even sterile barium sulfate can cause marked peritoneal irritation with considerable fluid loss into the peritoneal cavity, but in practice it is usually a mixture of barium and feces which escapes and this not surprisingly produces severe peritonitis and dense adhesions. The mortality has been reported to be 58% with conservative treatment, and still as high as 47% with surgical intervention (52[C]). Early operation is indicated and large volumes of intravenous fluids improve the prognosis. Patients who recover may develop fibrogranulomatous reactions and adhesions which can lead to bowel obstruction or ureteric occlusion.

Perforation may not only occur in the colon; in one reported case a duodenal ulcer appeared to perforate. In both this and another case of perforation (of a sigmoid diverticulum) the complication was not immediately recognized, the duodenal perforation only being detected 5 days after the administration of the barium meal (SEDA- 17, 535).

Finally, it may be noted that in air-contrast examinations colonic perforation may actually precede the giving of the barium enema itself, being attributable to the preparatory insufflation of air if this is conducted with excessive enthusiasm in a high-risk case (e.g. an elderly patient with a hitherto unrecognized epigastric hernia) (53[cr]).

Extraperitoneal perforation and leakage of barium may cause few immediate symptoms, but delayed endotoxic shock can develop some 12 hours later, frequently causing death. Bowel infarction may also result. Barium granulomata may occur, causing painful masses, rectal strictures or ulcers. On proctoscopy, the presence of an ulcer with a whitish base may mimic a carcinoma. In one rare case where a barium enema perforated into a sigmoid abscess, this was followed by intravasation into the portal venous system (54[CR]).

Accidental venous intravasation of barium during administration of a barium enema usually has a high immediate mortality due to barium embolism in the lungs, but occasionally it causes few symptoms (SEDA-1, 352). In one intermediate case there was hypotension and evidence of disseminated intravascular coagulation (SEDA-9, 407); this patient recovered after intensive treatment.

ECG changes have been recorded in older patients during administration of barium enemas and could represent a hazard in cases of cardiac disease.

Transient bacteremia was recorded in 11.4% of a series of 175 patients who had undergone barium enema examination; it appeared almost at once and lasted up to 15 minutes (55[CR]). Although a second study elsewhere failed to confirm these findings (SEDA-2, 373), a subsequent fatal case of staphylococcal septicemia in an elderly patient with an immune deficiency suggests that the risks are not merely theoretical (56[CR]).

Allergy Hypersensitivity reactions to barium itself are not known, but reactions to other constituents of barium sulfate enemas, formerly believed to be rare, are now being recognized with increasing frequency (SED-18, 441) and could be as common as one in 1000. They vary from urticarial rashes to severe anaphylactic collapse, and can be particularly severe in patients with asthma (57[CR]). Hypersensitivity to the latex balloon catheter used in double contrast barium enemas appears to be a common mechanism (58[CR]), but hypersensitivity to glucagon, to the preservative methylparabens or to other additives seems to be responsible in some cases. Insofar as the latex balloon is concerned, it seems that thorough washing will remove the allergen responsible for the reaction (59[R]).

Poisoning A fatal case of poisoning resulted from the use of barium sulfide which had been mistaken for barium sulfate (SED- 8, 1022). Isolated cases of barium encephalopathy (see Chapter 23) have been attributed to absorption of barium following the use of barium sulfate (SEDA-15, 498).

Technical errors Accidental administration of a barium enema into the vagina instead of the rectum may occur and can be very hazardous: in a number of these patients there has been fatal rupture of the vagina with venous intravasation of barium (SEDA-1, 352). Barium given orally may be inhaled, and if there is incoordination of swallowing, inhalation of thick paste may cause fatal asphyxiation (60[C]); aspiration of barium may also cause fatal pneumonia (61[CR]).

Tannic acid

Tannic acid (up to 1.5%) was at one time added to barium enemas to improve the quality of the radiological picture. Tannic acid is hepatotoxic and fulminant liver disease very occasionally resulted from this practice. Although it was perhaps avoidable, being apparently associated mainly with higher tannic acid concentrations, mucosal damage or a prior tannic acid washout of the bowel, the risks involved have rendered this technique virtually obsolete (SED-8, 1023).

Water-soluble media

The high osmolar media diatrizoate and iothalamate were formerly recommended for oral use in preference to barium where there was a risk of perforation, but the osmotic effect of such material can lead to diarrhea and fluid loss which may be dangerous in weak patients. Diatrizoate, despite its cathartic action, may occasionally induce ileus when given postoperatively (62[C]); it can also can be precipitated as a solid mass in the stomach when gastric acidity is high, but also in an achlorhydric gastric stump following partial gastrectomy if stomal obstruction is present (SEDA-1, 352). On one occasion when diatrizoate was used to fill the gastric balloon of a Sengstaken- Blakemore tube, hydrogen ions from the gastric content apparently penetrated into the balloon, precipitating the contrast medium and preventing the balloon's removal (SED-8, 1024). Accidental inhalation of hypertonic contrast media during oral administration may cause fatal pulmonary edema (63[C]).

Low-osmolar media such as iohexol are now preferred for oral use; they can still often cause some diarrhea, e.g. in 18 out of 40 cases in one series (SEDA-16, 529). Absorption can be increased if there is mucosal damage in the bowel, such as in Crohn's disease, resulting in delayed excretion but not apparently involving risk (SEDA-18, 441).

Diatrizoate enemas are still sometimes used to treat meconium ileus or constipation and it is important to give intravenous fluids so as to avoid dehydration. Hypomagnesemia may also occur (64[CR]). Osmotic effects lower in the gastrointestinal tract have even led to distension and cecal perforation (65[CR]). Stasis of diatrizoate in dilated loops of bowel may cause inflammatory changes or necrosis (66, 67[CR]).

Severe systemic reactions to enterally administered water-soluble contrast media are rare but they do occur, e.g. with oral iohexol (68[CR]).

SIALOGRAPHY

A randomized study of sialography in 60 patients compared Lipiodol ultrafluid (ethiodized oil) with meglumine diatrizoate 290. Pain and swelling of the parotid gland was more frequent after Lipiodol UF (69[CR]).

ORAL CHOLECYSTOGRAPHY

Contrast media used for oral cholecystography are weak iodinated organic acids which are absorbed, then largely conjugated with glucuronic acid. The most widely used agents are iopanoic acid and sodium or calcium ipodate; also used are tyropanoate and iocetamic acid. Bunamiodyl sodium, which proved toxic to the kidneys, has been withdrawn.

Allergy As in other situations, patients allergic to additives, such as parabens in sodium ipodate, can react to them, e.g. with rash (70[C]).

Cardiovascular A hypotensive reaction associated with a vasovagal reaction probably explains four deaths from acute coronary insufficiency (two each with iodoalphionic acid and iopanoic acid) reported in patients with ischemic heart disease.

Endocrine, metabolic Iopanoic acid is as potent a uricosuric agent as probenecid and this effect might explain some renal complications which have been seen (see below); aspirin diminishes the uricosuric effect but may also impair X-ray visualization due to competition at plasma protein-binding sites. Fluctuations of serum urate after oral cholecystography can *interfere with diagnostic tests* and even precipitate an attack of *gout* (71[C]).

Most oral cholecystographic agents raise serum protein-bound iodine (*PBI*) levels for a period varying from 1 week to 2 years. With iophenoxic acid (now obsolete), PBI levels up to 14 000 μg/ml were found after a single dose; in this case it was estimated that it would take 30 years for the level to fall to the physiological norm (72[C]).

Liberation of iodine from these agents may produce some *thyroid inhibition* in normal subjects for up to 3 months, but can also increase hormonal synthesis in a thyroid adenoma, and cases of frank *thyrotoxicosis* have been attributed to these media, the effect starting within a few days (73[C]).

Hematological Severe *thrombocytopenia* has rarely been reported after both iopanoic acid (74[CR]), iocetamic acid (75[CR]) and sodium ipodate; in the last case there was evidence that the patient had developed platelet antibodies of the type associated with other drug-induced thrombocytopenias (76[C]).

Liver Sulfobromphthalein (*BSP*) retention is increased by sodium ipodate or iopanoic acid, probably by competition in the hepatic excretory pathway. The mechanism is not clear. Serum bilirubin concentration may rise, and there can be a slight increase in serum enzymes, persisting for a few days.

Gastrointestinal *Nausea*, *vomiting*, *colicky abdominal pains* and *diarrhea* are common and occasionally severe. Iopanoic acid seems particularly prone to cause diarrhea.

Urinary system A slight transitory increase in *serum creatinine* commonly occurs and there may be *dysuria*. Acute *renal insufficiency* is uncommon with the agents currently in use, but some 100 fatalities were reported with bunamiodyl sodium. The clinical course is that of acute renal failure with oliguria or anuria and raised blood urea beginning a few hours to several days after cholecystography; most patients recover without sequelae in a few days, but fatalities can still occur. The mechanism is not clear; a diffuse acute tubular necrosis, sometimes with crystals of calcium salts, is found at biopsy or autopsy (77[C]). A decrease in creatinine clearance within the normal range is common. The possibility that these agents might simply block the renal tubules has been advanced, but they are only present in the urine in small amounts in their non-conjugated, i.e. relatively insoluble, form. The effect on uric acid excretion (see 'Endocrine, metabolic') might be involved. In any event, sufficient fluid should be given to ensure an adequate flow of urine.

The risk of renal failure is greater in the presence of existing hepatic insufficiency, apparently because under these conditions both blood levels and renal excretion of the contrast medium are greater (SEDA-10, 422).

Skin and appendages Urticarial or erythematous rashes may occur and persist for a few days. Iocetamic acid seems more prone than other agents to cause skin reactions (SEDA-1, 352). A persistent urticaria has been seen in cases where iophendylate was used in myelography and the residue remained in situ (SED-12, 1180, SEDA-16, 536); similar cases are referred to elsewhere in this Chapter.

Risk situations These contrast media should not be given if there is hypersensitivity. Patients with ischemic heart disease may also be at increased risk. Oral cholecystography is contraindicated in jaundice and in renal failure. Excretion occurs in breast milk and cholecystography should therefore also be avoided in lactation (SEDA-6, 404).

Second-generation effects It has been realised for a generation that iophenoxic acid passes the placental barrier. In 1961 a series of mothers and their children were found to have abnormal elevation of PBI 7 years after ingestion of iophenoxic acid for cholecystography (see 'Endocrine, metabolic') (78[C]). A little later the first case was reported of a child with congenital hypothyroidism born 5 years after the mother had undergone cholecystography; at the age of 2 the PBI in the child was still 469 μg/100 ml (79[C]); in a similar case the mother had been given iophenoxic acid 8 years prior to pregnancy (SED-12, 1167). iophenoxic acid is, as pointed out above, now obsolete.

Overdosage In a case where 30 grams of iopanoic acid was given, instead of 3 grams, the patient experienced severe nausea with vomiting and diarrhea but no more serious effects (SED-12, 1167).

Interactions Oral media may partially block the excretion of intravenously administered methylglucamine iodipamide into the biliary tract, and when they are given just before the latter may increase the incidence of toxic reactions; an interval of some days between oral and intravenous examination is therefore advisable.

Interference with diagnostic routines Errors in evaluating liver function are likely if BSP tests are carried out within 2 days after cholecystography. There may be an increase in serum T3 and a decrease in TSH after injection of iodinated radiological compounds (SEDA-6, 408). Measurements of serum butanol-extractable iodine are less affected by contrast media than those of PBI. As pointed out above, fluctuations of serum urate may occur after oral cholecystography. Pseudo-albuminuria may occur with a false- positive sulfosalicylic acid test (80).

Ceruletide *(See also Chapter* 36)

Ceruletide, a synthetic compound resembling cholecystokinin, causes contraction of the gallbladder and is sometimes used instead of the traditional 'fatty meal' in cholecystography. With intramuscular injection, *nausea*, *vomiting*, *diarrhea* and *cramps* have been reported; intravenous injections can cause spasm of the gallbladder neck and severe *pain* with tingling sensations, sweating and mild hypotension (81[C]).

INTRAVENOUS CHOLECYSTOGRAPHY AND CHOLANGIOGRAPHY

Note *Many of the adverse effects of contrast media given intravenously for this or other purposes will be found in the section on general and idiosyncratic reactions earlier in this Chapter.*

While the classic literature concerning adverse reactions to intravenous cholangiography is mainly based on experience with iodipamide and ioglycamide, work with two newer media, iodoxamate and iotroxate, is now coming to the fore. They are excreted more efficiently and can be used in lower doses. They are also believed to be less toxic but there are even today insufficient data for this to be fully evaluated.

In a national survey conducted in Britain in 1970, when these drugs were generally given in a single injected dose, intermediate reactions to iodipamide occurred once in every 700 cases, severe reactions once in every 1600, and deaths once in every 5000 (SED- 12, 1168). The introduction of infusion cholangiography (in which the contrast medium is given over a 15—30-minute period) has decreased the incidence of minor reactions; it allows the liver to excrete the contrast medium more efficiently so that doses as low as 3—5 ml of ioglycamide or 10 ml of 50% iodipamide can be used. According to a 1975 report from France, serious reactions nevertheless occurred once in every 310 infusion cholangiographies (82[CR]; see also SEDA-10, 422).

Idiosyncratic reactions The major immediate reactions are *hypotensive collapse* and *bronchospasm*, but other reactions include nausea, abdominal pain, diarrhea, tetany and skin rashes. The picture is broadly similar to that encountered with the urographic media.

Cardiovascular Hypotension has been referred to above; it is more marked if injection is rapid (see also 'Gastrointestinal'). *Prinzmetal angina* with ECG changes has been seen 10 minutes after giving iodipamide (SEDA-2, 373).

Endocrine, metabolic Iodipamide has a uricosuric action similar to that of the oral cholecystographic media (see also 'Interference with diagnostic routines' above).

Gastrointestinal Idiosyncratic reactions can involve the gastrointestinal system (see above). When pethidine is given with iodipamide, a myocardial infarction-like syndrome may occur due to *spasm of the sphincter of Oddi* (SED-8, 1026). Oral and intravenous cholangiography have in the past very rarely been reported to precipitate acute pancreatitis (83[c]).

Liver There have been several incidents pointing to the *hepatotoxicity* of iodipamide, variously characterized by epigastric pain, nausea and vomiting, jaundice, pyrexia and tenderness over the liver; the liver function tests are deranged and biopsy where performed has shown centrilobular necrosis (84[C]). The incidence of abnormal liver function tests may be as high as 18% after a 40-ml dose, and the quantity given should be as small as possible since the complication seems to be dose related.

Prior administration of corticosteroids or sulfonylureas impairs hepatic excretion of ioglycamide (SEDA-1, 353). Both of the newer contrast media may also affect liver function tests; in a small series of cases, the degree of intrahepatic cholestasis appeared to be relatively more marked after iodoxamate than after iotroxate (SED-12, 1168).

Urinary system *Renal failure* may occur after iodipamide and ioglycamide, particularly with large doses (SED-8, 1027).

Miscellaneous Ioglycamide produced fatal *gel precipitation of the plasma* in a case of Waldenström's IgM monoclonal paraproteinemia (SEDA-7, 451). *Malarial relapse* followed administration of iodipamide in two cases (SED-8, 1028).

PERCUTANEOUS TRANSHEPATIC CHOLANGIOGRAPHY

Using a fine needle with sodium diatrizoate as the contrast medium, this is a relatively safe technique for use in cases of obstructive jaundice in which the high serum bilirubin precludes oral or intravenous techniques. The complications of *bile peritonitis* and *internal hemorrhage* are best avoided by decompression of dilated ducts. Bile blood fistula can lead to fatal *endotoxic shock* due to bacteria escaping from the obstructed biliary tract (85[C]). The rapid appearance of a pyelographic shadow may be a useful diagnostic sign calling for immediate antibiotic therapy. However, it is now usual to give a broad-spectrum antibiotic immediately before commencing the examination. Acute renal failure has been reported following transhepatic cholangiography (SEDA-10, 423).

T-TUBE AND OPERATIVE CHOLANGIOGRAPHY

Pyrexial reactions occurred in 5.3% of cases following postoperative cholangiography through the T-tube. In two patients, there was endotoxic shock (SEDA-5, 420).

A fatal reaction occurred when diatrizoate was used for operative cholangiography and contrast medium entered the bloodstream (86[CR]).

ENDOSCOPIC RETROGRADE CHOLANGIOPANCREATOGRAPHY (ERCP)

Although a severe *contrast medium reaction* with shock has been observed, this was the only contrast medium reaction in a series of 2000 ERCP examinations reported on in 1977 (87[CR]). In some other reports, milder degrees of allergic reactions have been noted (88[cr]) In a series of 10 000 cases reported on in the United States in 1976 (89[CR]) the most serious side effects were *cholangitic sepsis* (0.8%, fatal in 0.08%) and *pancreatic sepsis* (0.3%, fatal in 0.06%) but there was a 1% incidence of *injection pancreatitis* and other cases of drug interactions (diazepam, spasmolytic agents), instrumental injury and aspiration pneumonia. Pancreatitis can result from over- filling of the pancreatic duct. Significant quantities of contrast medium may be absorbed after ERCP and even after duodenal instillation of diatrizoate. Endoscopists must therefore be prepared to treat contrast medium reactions.

Transient asymptomatic *hypermylasemia* may occur (SEDA-14, 422), and a recent report showed a 15% incidence of *mild renal dysfunction* only detected by prospective study (90[cR]).

EXCRETION UROGRAPHY

Note *Many of the adverse effects of contrast media given intravenously for this or other purposes will be found in the section on general and idiosyncratic reactions earlier in this Chapter.*

The water-soluble products used for excretion urography are largely the same as those used for angiography, and in checking for data on adverse reactions the reader should consult the angiographic section as well as the present one. The products are based variously on diatrizoate, metrizoate, iothalamate and iodamide; both sodium and meglumine salts are used. Acetrizoate has largely been abandoned. The products generally contain some sodium citrate as a buffer and salts of ethylenediaminetetra-acetic acid to stabilize the solutions. This might theoretically lead to sensitization.

The contrast media used in this field exhibit protein-binding properties and inhibit various enzyme systems to a differing extent; these properties seem to correlate to the relative toxicity of the different substances in use as judged by the LD_{50}; they are most marked with iopanoate, iodipamide and acetrizoate and less so with diatrizoate and iothalamate. Protein binding might perhaps alter the function of the proteins in the cell membranes or blood vessel endothelium, but the significance of protein binding in causing adverse effects is uncertain.

The overall pattern of general and idiosyncratic reactions is as discussed in an earlier section of this Chapter for soluble contrast media as a whole, the frequency of problems apparently being somewhat greater than when performing angiography, with a particular tendency towards renal reactions.

RETROGRADE AND ANTEGRADE UROGRAPHY

For this purpose, the salts of diatrizoate or iothalamate are generally used. Barium sulfate has been employed for cystography, but is inadvisable for reasons given below.

Effects on urethra and bladder Retrograde urography is often followed by *irritation and edema of the urethral and bladder mucosa*. In experimental animals this effect was found to be maximal at 48 hours and to persist for at least a week. Factors which lessened the inflammatory response in the bladder were dilution of the medium and the use of smaller volumes instilled at lower pressure. In clinical use, diatrizoate has seemed to be less irritant than acetrizoate (91[R]).

Renal effects Retrograde pyelography may rarely cause deterioration of renal function with acute renal failure, particularly if there has been marked pyelorenal back flow; exceptionally the complication can be fatal (92[C]). Retrograde pyelography with potassium bromide has caused renal failure (SEDA-11, 413).

Barium sulfate has in the past been used for cystography, but if ureteric reflux occurs the barium may become inspissated in the calyceal system of the kidney; in view of experimental findings, this might be expected to cause granulomatous reactions with fibrosis.

Systemic effects Retrograde pyelography would seem safer than intravenous urography in patients who are highly sensitive to contrast media, but small amounts of contrast medium can be absorbed, mainly via the calyces. In one reported case of pyelorenal back flow dating back to 1968, 12.5% of the contrast medium was absorbed (93[C]). A severe generalized reaction has been reported following cystography with diatrizoate (SED-12, 1174) and another in a patient with ureteric reflux treated with meglumine iothalamate; in the latter case there was circulatory collapse but it responded to simple change in posture and epinephrine was not required (SEDA-18, 445). Miliary dissemination of tubercle bacilli from an infected urinary system following retrograde pyelography with pyelovenous back flow is a very rare complication (SED-8, 1036).

Severe and prolonged hypotensive collapse has also been seen following antegrade pyelography through a nephrostomy tube under general anesthesia, but the patient in question had a previous history of an acute reaction (SEDA-18, 445).

CYSTOURETHROGRAPHY

Bladder rupture is a risk here. In two children with myelomengingoceles and ventriculoperitoneal shunts, bladder rupture had particularly serious consequences; the diatrizoate which was being used passed into the peritoneal cavity and then via the shunt into the cerebral ventricles and subarachnoid space, causing tonic convulsions (SEDA-17, 538).

COMPUTED TOMOGRAPHY

Large intravenous doses of contrast media may be used during computed tomography (CT). Side effects are broadly similar to those of excretion urography, but the incidence of serious reactions and deaths may possibly be higher due to greater difficulty in treating reactions when the patient is in a scanner (SEDA-7, 451). *Renal failure* may occur in diabetics with pre-existing renal disease or as a particular result of multiple examinations. In herpes simplex encephalitis, *prolonged retention* of contrast medium may occur in the brain. In patients with spinal tumors, stimulus-sensitive *extensor spasms* may occur in the trunk and limbs (SEDA-7, 453).

In a randomized trial, *seizures* occurred in 14 (16%) of 86 patients with gliomas undergoing contrast CT examinations; however, in 83 other patients with gliomas receiving diazepam prophylaxis, seizures occurred in only two patients (2.2%). There was an increased risk of seizure in patients with a previous history of seizures and in association with antineoplastic therapy (94[CR]). Patients with thrombotic thrombocytopenic purpura (TTP) also appear to be at greater risk of developing seizures during contrast examination. Fatal status epilepticus can occur during CT (113[cr]). The non-ionic medium, iopamidol, appears to be less likely to cause seizures (114[CR]).

An *acute myasthenic crisis* with apnea was induced by contrast CT with diatrizoate in two patients with myasthenia gravis and this was followed by prolonged aggravation of the myasthenia (95[CR]). This has also occurred with iopamidol (SEDA-12, 396).

For computed tomography, large volumes of contrast medium have to be injected under pressure and this can lead to several problems. Subclinical *air embolism* may occur (SEDA-14, 422) as may serious *extravasation*; in one series of 20 950 CT scans using non-ionic media there was extravasation ranging from an estimated 3 ml to 100 ml in 28 cases, the degree of extravasation depending on the pressure applied. Where extravasation occurs, the extent of tissue damage depends primarily on the osmolarity of the contrast medium but it is clear that with ionic media the methylglucamine salts cause more damage than do the sodium salts (96[R]).

ANGIOGRAPHY, DIGITAL SUBTRACTION ANGIOGRAPHY AND CARDIOGRAPHY

Note *Many of the adverse effects of contrast media given intravenously for this or other purposes will be found in the section on general and idiosyncratic reactions earlier in this Chapter.*

NATURE AND INCIDENCE OF SIDE EFFECTS

If ionic media are to be used for investigations of the vascular system, it is preferable to employ methylglucamine salts for cerebral arteriography, whereas for cardiography mixtures of sodium and methylglucamine salts are required. However, low-osmolar contrast media (in particular the non-ionic media) are increasingly being used in vascular radiology because of their lower risk rate. An analysis of more than 90 000 cardiac angiographies performed in American hospitals during 1991 showed that for diagnostic catheterization non-ionic media were now being used in some 72% of cases; the overall rate of complications here was 1.5%, including idiosyncratic reactions in 0.25%, vascular complications in 0.44%, neurological complications in 0.05%, arrhythmias in 0.31% and myocardial infarction in 0.06%; the death rate was 0.11%. In percutaneous coronary angioplasty major complications, generally of the same type, occurred in 5% of cases (97[Cr]). In one large series of DSA examinations using iopamidol the overall incidence of reactions was 2.5%; some occurred with a delay of an hour or more (98[C]).

Idiosyncratic reactions seem to be less common following arteriography than after urography (see above), perhaps because the medium here does not pass directly through the lungs, but the data are limited. Mild 'allergic' reactions were noted in six out of 167 patients who underwent arteriography with iodamide (SED-12, 1175). Two severe delayed generalized cutaneous reactions with blistering have occurred following lumbar aortography with iopamidol and iohexol (SED-12, 1174). In two published cases, injection of diatrizoate during arteriography under general anesthesia caused severe hypotensive collapse (SEDA-7, 452). In another patient with two previous reactions to contrast media, a severe reaction occurred after the injection of only 2 ml meglumine iothalamate into the abdominal aorta (SEDA-4, 333).

When large volumes of contrast media are injected for angiographic examinations, a number of factors influence toxicity. With rapid injections, as in angiocardiography or digital subtraction angiography (DSA), the toxicity is much greater than when it is possible to use a slow drip; many unwanted effects reported in the course of the years are predominantly due to the hypertonicity of the older media, but even the newer products have some chemotoxicity. In critical areas, such as the myocardium, brain spinal cord or kidney, tolerance may be low.

Special precautions should be taken in performing DSA in patients with cardiac disease; a patient with a history of angina may develop ischemic ECG changes with or without chest pain following the injection of a contrast medium bolus into the superior vena cava for DSA and one such patient developed ventricular fibrillation (99[CR]).

Not all untoward events in vascular radiology are due to the contrast medium. On more than one occasion, a petechial rash has developed in the distribution of the injected vessel, and has been found to be due to glove-powder or cotton fiber embolism as a result of contamination of saline used for irrigating syringes or from wiping needles or Seldinger wires with gauze swabs (SED-8, 1037). Again, disruption of an atheromatous plaque during angiography may cause cholesterol embolism which is often fatal (SEDA-14, 423).

CARDIAC ANGIOGRAPHY *(See also 'Selective coronary angiography' below)*

Incidence of complications (*see also above*) In one US study of cardiac angiography published in 1993 the incidence of adverse events was 31.6% for diatrizoate and only 10.2% for iohexol; it should be noted however that the diatrizoate used in that study (Renografin 76[TM]) causes calcium binding and may have elevated the rate of cardiac complications (100[CR]). Progress appears to continue: the new non-ionic agent Iodixanol 320, which is virtually iso-osmolar, has been tested in cardiac angiography against iohexol and seemed to be even better tolerated (101[CR]).

Hemodynamic effects *Blood pressure changes*, *cardiac arrhythmias* and *cardiac arrest* have been described. *Tachycardia* is probably compensatory, as are the concomitant *increases in venous pressure and pulmonary arterial pressure*. However, the site and rate of administration are relevant in determining the exact nature and pattern of these reactions.

Rapid peripheral intravenous injection of concentrated ionic contrast media produces a brief rise in systemic arterial pressure followed by a prolonged fall; the diastolic pressure decreases more than the systolic pressure and the heart slows; the pulse contour changes, and the venous pressure rises. The electrocardiogram may show flattening, splitting, or inversion of the T-waves.

Injection into the right side of the heart or pulmonary artery may be followed, especially if the older media are employed, by transient pulmonary hypertension but systemic hypotension. The pulmonary hypertension is partially due to an increase in the pulmonary vascular resistance from capillary blockage by the altered erythrocytes, which have a reduced elasticity due to the effect of a hypertonic contrast medium (SEDA- 4, 335). Decreased cardiac output accompanied by cardiac slowing and diminished force of contraction seem to explain the initial systemic hypotension; persistence of hypotension thereafter is probably due to the vasodilator effect of the contrast medium on the systemic vessels. Pulmonary angiography is particularly dangerous when the right ventricular end-diastolic pressure exceeds 20 mmHg (SEDA-6, 407). Iohexol appears to be a safer medium for pulmonary angiography (SEDA-14, 423).

Injection into the left ventricle or the proximal aorta is likely to produce more marked effects. Cardiac rate, stroke volume and output increase. There is elevation of the right and left atrial pressures and of the left ventricular end-diastolic pressure. The pulmonary arterial pressure is also increased. The blood volume expands and the peripheral blood flow increases and then falls as the systemic resistance is lowered. The hematocrit falls and venous pressure gradually rises. As the systemic arterial pressure declines, the heart rate increases. These responses are largely due to the injection of strongly hypertonic solutions, which promote a rapid expansion of the plasma volume; water shifts from the extravascular fluid spaces to the blood and moves out of the erythrocytes which shrink and become crenated. Blood viscosity rises, but plasma viscosity does not increase significantly. The erythrocytes give up potassium to the plasma and this might contribute to the observed decrease in peripheral vascular resistance.

Hematological Ionic contrast media may, as noted elsewhere in this Chapter, exert an *anticoagulant* effect (SED-8, 1038), particularly marked in large doses. In vitro experiments with normal plasma showed that contrast media potentiate the anticoagulant action of heparin; the effect is particularly strong with plasma from patients with liver disease or coagulation diseases. Clotting time measured in a patient shortly after administration of contrast media may show abnormally elevated levels and may cause problems in monitoring (102[r]). Non- ionic contrast media, as discussed in this chapter in connection with the question of thrombogenesis, do not have a similar anticoagulant action. If blood is allowed to mix with a non-ionic medium in the syringe or catheter, thrombus formation may occur and this could be a potential cause of thromboembolic phenomena (SEDA- 15, 502; 103[r]).

When blood is diluted with 90% sodium diatrizoate in vitro, there is initially a decrease in erythrocyte diameter due to the hypertonic environment, but as more contrast medium is added, the erythrocytes show an increase in diameter because of damage to the cell wall; this tallies with the fact that cases of hemolysis and hemoglobinuria have in the past been reported with diatrizoate (104[C]).

In patients with sickle-cell disease, a high local concentration of contrast medium in the blood during arteriography may cause sickling with resulting thrombosis (SED-8, 1053). One patient with hemoglobin sickle-cell disease developed severe intravascular hemolysis, thrombocytopenia, leukocytosis and pulmonary infiltrates following left ventriculography and coronary angiography with meglumine diatrizoate (105[CR]). In vitro studies indicate that the non-ionic medium, iopamidol, causes significantly less sickling than a conventional ionic contrast medium, and iopamidol would therefore be preferable for arteriography in patients with this disorder (SEDA-7, 453).

Urinary system Infants receiving large doses of ionic contrast media during cardioangiography may suffer renal damage. Fatal cases, occurring after doses of more than 3 ml/kg, showed *renal medullary necrosis* or severe *proximal tubular vacuolation*. Such doses have in other infants produced *microscopic hematuria*. *Renal necrosis* has occurred in infants following intravenous administration of 1—3 ml/kg of sodium diatrizoate, but these children were in very poor general condition (SED-8, 1038). In high risk adults, cardioangiography may similarly cause contrast nephropathy (SEDA- 15, 501).

Miscellaneous Following a difficult cardiac angiography in the supine position in an elderly man with arteriosclerosis *transient cortical blindness* occurred, and on CT there was contrast enhancement of the occipital lobes; the best explanation seems to be that a large amount of contrast medium may have entered the vertebral artery and passed upwards, passing a defective blood- -brain barrier (106[Cr]). Similar complications have been described in other patients, sometimes with amnesia, following cardiac catheterization and angiography (SEDA-18, 444).

SELECTIVE CORONARY ARTERIOGRAPHY

Contrast medium entering the coronary arteries following injection into the ascending aorta is usually partially diluted, unless the catheter is misplaced at the opening of the coronary artery. With selective coronary arteriography, the injection is made directly into the right and left coronary arteries.

Contrast media entering the coronary circulation may cause *decreased myocardial contractility*, *transient EGG changes*, *dysrhythmias* and even *ventricular fibrillation*. The latter is most likely to occur following injection into the right coronary artery. Provided the expert radiologist can rely upon a contrast medium having consistent properties such as these, even if they are inconvenient, he can adapt to them, but serious problems can arise if a product is suddenly and unexpectedly modified:

> Following studies in dogs in which methylglucamine salts of diatrizoate or iothalamate produced only temporary T-wave changes whilst sodium salts of these same media produced more marked changes with a fall in blood pressure and increase in coronary flow, the US manufacturers of a sodium methylglucamine diatrizoate product removed virtually all of its sodium content, but without announcing the change. Radiologists using the altered contrast medium noticed an unexpected increase in the incidence of ventricular fibrillation following coronary arteriography. Subsequent animal experiments confirmed that the new medium caused this effect, apparently by prolonging the time of depolarization. The addition of small quantities of sodium to the medium lessened this prolongation of the depolarization phase (107).

It should be noted that non-ionic media cause fewer EGG changes than ionic media, and they are therefore increasingly preferred for coronary arteriography (SEDA-10, 424; SEDA-11, 412).

In a series of nine patients undergoing coronary arteriography, plasma measurements from the coronary sinus showed a significant *depression of ionized calcium levels* immediately following injection of Renografin 76 (sodium methylglucamine diatrizoate) into the coronary arteries. The depression was most marked and lasted longer in patients with arteriosclerosis. The depression of ionized calcium was attributed to the chelating agents (disodium EDTA and sodium citrate) present in some contrast media. This may be a factor in causing electromechanical dissociation in the cardiac muscle (SEDA-1, 356; SEDA-11, 412). The hypocalcemic effect of ionic contrast media may potentiate the effect of a calcium blocker such as verapamil (SEDA-8, 429; SEDA-9, 410).

Obeid and co-workers reported two cases of severe hypotensive collapse with generalized itching which followed left ventricular angiography with 76% sodium methylglucamine diatrizoate; the hypotension failed to respond to vasoconstrictors, and measurements of right auricular and right ventricular pressures showed marked reduction in 'filling pressures'. Rapid intravenous infusion of isotonic saline caused prompt improvement in the blood pressure. A similar case of hypotension with a beneficial response to plasma expanders has been reported in a case of prolonged shock after intravenous urography (SEDA-1, 356).

An anaphylactoid reaction occurring after left ventriculography was associated with EGG changes apparently due to coronary artery spasm (108[CR]).

Coronary arteriography is usually carried out in association with left ventriculography. Increase of left ventricular end-diastolic pressure may occur after either of these procedures. Since the coronary injections are the more dangerous part of the investigation, they should be performed first, before myocardial function has been compromised. If the left ventricular end- diastolic pressure then rises above 40 mmHg, left ventriculography should be delayed.

Technical complications Major catheter hazards are *dissection of the coronary artery* or *clot embolism* in the coronary arteries due to transfer of clots from the Seldinger wire to a second catheter (109[R]).

AORTOGRAPHY AND PERIPHERAL ARTERIOGRAPHY

Hemodynamic effects Intra-arterial injection of conventional ionic contrast media results in *vasodilatation*; this is due mainly to hypertonicity of the medium, but toxicity is also a factor; the vasodilatation may in addition be partly due to an anti-cholinesterase action, since it is partially blocked by atropine. In clinical practice, aortography and peripheral arteriography are usually associated with a slight fall in blood pressure, tachycardia and discomfort in the limbs, such as heat or pain.

Acetrizoate has a more marked effect in this respect than an equi- osmolar solution of diatrizoate. Methylglucamine salts appear to be relatively less vasoactive in the peripheral vessels. All these changes are considerably less marked with low-osmolar media such as ioxaglate, iopamidol or iohexol, but not necessarily absent. Abdominal aortography with iohexol has been found to produce both a decrease in the systemic blood pressure and an increase in the plasma concentration of atrial natriuretic peptide; this may be due to increased intravascular volume (SEDA-16, 533).

Five cases of *pulmonary edema* have been reported following retrograde aortic injection of sodium iothalamate (Conray 325 or 420) in a series of 65 patients being investigated for intermittent claudication under general anesthesia. Three of the five cases had a history of myocardial disease and another had received 200 ml Conray 420. Pre-angiographic cardiological assessment is important, as is limitation of contrast medium dose, and control of the volume of saline used for flushing the Seldinger catheter (SEDA-3, 379).

Gastrointestinal Selective angiography of the gastrointestinal tract is widely practised and with a correct technique it is a relatively safe procedure.

Infarction of the bowel was formerly a very occasional complication of abdominal aortography and was due to injection of contrast medium into the mesenteric arteries. Most of these cases were due to the older media such as acetrizoate; however, small bowel injury has occurred following the injection of a concentrated bolus of sodium iothalamate (110[C]). *Ileus* has been reported following mesenteric angiography in a patient with renal failure (SEDA-12, 1177).

Intra-arterial injection of lipiodol (iodized oil) has been used to enhance the accuracy of computed tomography in hepatic tumors. This may cause transient *bowel ischemia* with nausea, vomiting and diarrhea. Embolization of the cystic artery may cause *acute acalculous cholecystitis* (SEDA-15, 505).

Urinary system In abdominal aortography, the contrast medium reaching the renal parenchyma is relatively undiluted, so that factors of concentration and volume are more important, particularly if a bolus of high concentration is accidentally injected directly into the renal artery. In the early days of abdominal aortography, *renal damage* was a significant hazard, mainly because the media then in use were relatively toxic, but at high-dose levels or high concentrations the media now used may also cause renal injury. In one series of 400 patients undergoing angiography with high doses of ionic contrast medium, the overall incidence of acute renal dysfunction was 11.3%, but in those patients with pre-existing renal disease the incidence was 41.7%. Injections close to the renal arteries are more likely to cause renal changes than a similar dose of contrast medium injected intravenously for digital vascular imaging (SEDA-9, 408). In one case reported by Stark and Coburn in 1966, the patient had renal artery stenosis and there had been an intra-aortic injection of 30 ml of 50% methylglucamine diatrizoate at the level of the renal arteries; here oliguria with pyrexia occurred within a few hours, and the urine output only gradually recovered over a period of some 2 months (111[C]). Diabetes was a predisposing factor in another case (SED-12, 1177). In two further cases, renal failure was followed by nephrogenic diabetes insipidus and nephrotic syndrome, respectively (SED-8, 1042).

Transient *proteinuria* commonly occurs after aortography and selective nephro-angiography due to an increase in glomerular permeability. Ioxaglate, iopamidol and iohexol cause only negligible proteinuria (SEDA-8, 428; SEDA-11, 413).

Effects on the spinal cord *Paraplegia* is a rare complication of angiography. Mishkin et al. (112[CR]) suggested in 1973 that the relative rarity of published reports did not reflect the true incidence of these complications, quoting five cases notified to their group during a 3-month period. There were four cases of tetraplegia (three being due to parathyroid arteriography and one following angiography of the posterior fossa); in their fifth case, paraplegia followed attempted renal angiography. When these neurological complications occur following angiography, the iodine content of the cerebrospinal fluid is raised.

There are various explanations, backed by animal studies, for this complication. Where there is an obstruction to the normal outflow of blood from the aorta, there is an increased risk of the contrast medium being diverted into the spinal circulation. This effect may be aided by a gravitational factor if the examination is performed in the supine position (SED-8, 1042).

The risk may not be the same for all media in current use; the relationship between the compound used and the neurotoxic effects is discussed below in connection with cerebral angiography.

Cerebral effects These may complicate thoracic aortography when excessive doses of concentrated medium are injected, particularly if the catheter is sited so that the major dose of contrast medium is directed into the cerebral circulation. In one published case, 10 ml of sodium iothalamate 70% was injected into the carotid artery, being mistaken for methylglucamine iothalamate 60%; this was followed by an immediate *convulsion* with *loss of consciousness* for 2 minutes. The patient at first appeared to recover completely, but *hemiparesis* followed and persisted for some 24 hours. Such changes are presumably due to cerebral edema following transient damage to the blood—brain barrier. In a fatal case, a massive overdose of 340 ml Renigrafin 76 was injected in a 7-year-old child with coarctation of the aorta and computed tomography showed persistence of contrast medium in the brain (113[CR]).

CEREBRAL ANGIOGRAPHY

Animal experiments with the *ionic media* have shown that these damage the blood-brain barrier, thereby creating a degree of risk to brain tissue when they are employed in cerebral angiography—though one must stress that they have often been used safely. Other work indicates that the sodium cation increases the neurotoxicity of the contrast medium, possibly by increasing its diffusibility into the brain substance. Methylglucamine, on the other hand, decreases the neurotoxicity. The addition of a small quantity of calcium also appeared to reduce toxicity, at least when added to the sodium preparations. There are only marginal differences in neurotoxicity as measured in animal experiments between the diatrizoate, iothalamate and metrizoate anions. Calcium methylglucamine metrizoate has probably the lowest neurotoxicity of the ionic media, followed closely by methylglucamine iothalamate. In clinical use, however, the calcium preparations appear to cause a greater degree of discomfort due to their inducing a sensation of heat (SED-8, 1042).

Although the *non-ionic media* produced less injury to the blood—brain barrier in animal studies, clinical work has not generally shown them to be better tolerated when used for cerebral angiography and it has been argued that these expensive media should now only be used where the blood—brain barrier is thought to be defective (114[CR]).

It is not entirely simple to consider separately the cardiovascular and neurological complications of cerebral angiography since they seem to be in part interdependent.

Cardiovascular events can be followed by polygraphic recordings during cerebral angiography; they indicate that both with the ionic and non-ionic media *hypotension*, *bradycardia* and even transient *asystole* may occur, though there may also be reflex tachycardia (115[C]) which can proceed to produce hypertension. These changes are more marked during vertebral angiography when the posterior cerebral arteries have been filled, suggesting that they are due to involvement of centers in the hypothalamus or brain stem. *Visual disturbances* may also occur due to involvement of the occipital cortex (116[C]). The reflex cardiovascular changes may be more serious in patients with coronary artery disease and may give rise to left ventricular failure. Both ECG and EEG involvement are less common when methylglucamine salts are used. Premedication with atropine has been found to decrease the incidence of the cardiovascular changes, but not that of focal EEG effects. Their incidence has also been reduced by use of very small doses of contrast media, and premedication with hypertonic mannitol in those patients with raised intracranial pressure.

Many of the *psychic* complications of cerebral angiography may be due to arterial trauma rather than to the toxic effect of the contrast medium. If the investigation is undertaken under general anesthesia, the use of a volatile anesthetic may in itself cause an increase in intracranial pressure and thereby constitute an aggravating factor (117[C]). *Focal EEG changes* may occur on the side of the injection and if these are prolonged they may be followed by evidence of neurological involvement. Transient *global amnesia* and *confusional states* have been reported following cerebral angiography, even with nonionic media (SEDA-8, 429; SEDA-9, 410; 118[CR]). There appears to be an increased risk of *seizures* due to vasospasm if cerebral angiography is performed during or shortly after an attack of migraine (SEDA-11, 412).

In a series of 308 cerebral angiograms where metrizamide and meglumine metrizoate were compared on a randomized double-blind basis, metrizamide caused a lower incidence of EEG changes, but the incidence of clinical complications showed no significant difference in the two groups, suggesting that these were mainly caused by other factors such as thromboembolism (SEDA-5, 422); thromboembolism has indeed been suspected after cerebral angiography, even with iohexol (SEDA-13, 435).

MISCELLANEOUS COMPLICATIONS OF ANGIOGRAPHY

Technical complications of angiography (*SED*-8, 1039, 1043) Problems arising as a result of *mechanical injury* rather than from the presence of contrast media will not be reviewed in detail in this volume, since they can hardly be considered as adverse reactions to the products in question. Local *vascular complications* associated with angiography include intramural injection of contrast medium (leading to dissection of the arterial wall), arterial thrombosis, phlebitis, venous thrombosis, embolic phenomena and damage to atheromatous plaques in the aorta leading to cholesterol embolism (SEDA-14, 423; 119[C]). Any vascular injury can naturally have serious consequences for the organ or limb served by the affected vessel.

Hemorrhage into the *neurovascular sheath* at the site of an axillary artery puncture can lead to nerve compression and damage (120[C]). Some retroperitoneal bleeding commonly accompanies translumbar aortography and this may rarely be complicated by retroperitoneal or perinephric infections (121[C]). Injection of contrast material into an intervertebral disc during this same procedure may produce lumbar pain associated with disc necrosis. *Acute pancreatitis* has been reported after aortography with sodium acetrizoate 70% w/v which was accidentally injected into the *celiac axis*. A report from 1958 described a fatal case of bilateral *adrenal necrosis* following lumbar aortography (SED-12, 1178). Aortography in cases of pheochromocytoma can produce *adrenal hemorrhage* into and around the tumor, though it is not clear whether a technical fault was involved; adrenal insufficiency followed bilateral adrenal venography in another case.

Air embolism has been reported as a complication of injections of contrast media. A rare but serious complication of translumbar aortography is *chylothorax* due to injury of the thoracic duct. Intra-osseous venography may be followed by *fat embolism*.

Diatrizoate is extremely neurotoxic if it enters the *subarachnoid space*. This has sometimes occurred as a result of misplacement of the needle in arteriographic investigations (see section on 'Myelography' below).

Particulate contamination of contrast media Contrast media used for arteriography contain a variety of microscopic particles. When glass ampoules are opened they contain a larger number of particles than rubber-capped vials due to the vacuum effect on glass particles during the opening of the ampoule (122). This may theoretically cause microembolism. Angiographic catheters and guide wires also contain a very large number of particles derived from the manufacturing process and the release of these particles is increased some 6-fold after the insertion of the guide-wire into the catheter (SED-12, 1179). Vials should be opened by removing the cap and not by puncture of the membrane, since the needle usually pushes large rubber particles into the solution. Ideally, contrast media should be filtered before injection, but this will often not be practicable.

In the case of glass ampoules, if the ampoule is allowed to stand for 30—60 seconds after opening, most of the larger particles will have sedimented to the bottom of the ampoule. These can then be avoided by leaving the lower 2—3 mm of contrast medium in the ampoule.

Interactions *Protamine sulfate* has a pH of 3—4 and causes precipitation of diatrizoic acid; if injected into a catheter containing diatrizoate in heparinized patients, it could cause a precipitate which in theory might result in an embolus (SEDA-1, 356). Ioxaglate has been reported to be precipitated by *papaverine* which is frequently used in penile cavernosography (SEDA-11, 413), but some cases may have been due to an interaction between heparin and papaverine, perhaps not involving the contrast medium (SEDA-18, 444); in one case, use of iopamidol 370 immediately after an injection of papaverine was followed by extensive intra-arterial thrombosis (SEDA-17, 537). Ionic contrast media cause temporary prolongation of clotting time in patients treated with *heparin*; this effect may last for 6 hours and may interfere with laboratory assays (123). As noted elsewhere in this Chapter, non-ionic media do not have this anticoagulant effect, and if blood is allowed to mix with a non- ionic medium in the syringe or catheter, thrombus formation may occur, which could be a potential cause of thromboembolism (SEDA- 15, 502).

VENOGRAPHY

Phlebography of the legs This technique sometimes causes a superficial *thrombophlebitis* of the injected vein. In a follow-up of 61 previously normal patients who had undergone phlebography, four showed clear evidence of subsequent *deep vein thrombosis* and in two of these there were signs of non- fatal *pulmonary embolism*. The incidence of thrombosis may indeed have been higher since an abnormal fibrinogen uptake test developed in 20 individuals, though the result could have been non- specific (124[CR]). The risk of thrombophlebitis is significantly less when low-osmolar media are used (SEDA-9, 410; SEDA-11, 414).

Necrosis of the skin was described many years ago following peripheral venography (125[C]); in these cases there had been some extravenous injection, and the presence of impaired circulation probably resulted in slower removal of the agent and hence more prolonged exposure to it. *Gangrene* of the toes has also occurred (SEDA-8, 430).

Polyarthropathy, occurring in a severe and acute form, has been described as a rare complication of venography in patients with end-stage renal failure (SEDA-18, 445).

Intraosseous phlebography *Fat embolism* is a rare complication of intra-osseous phlebography (SEDA-1, 356).

Orbital venography Orbital venography has been largely superseded by computed tomography and magnetic resonance imaging. This technique was usually safe, but individual cases have been reported of *hemorrhage in a lymphangioma* of the orbit and of transitory *retinal artery spasm* or *retinal hemorrhage*, the latter two involving diabetic subjects (SED- 12, 1179).

Cavernosography *Priapism* due to venous thrombosis has been reported after penile cavernosography with ioxaglate and diluted iothalamate (126[C]). Contrast media may cause endothelial damage in the corpus cavernosum. Prior injection of 1000—2000 units of heparin into the corpus cavernosum and use of diluted non-ionic media have therefore been advocated for this procedure (127[r]).

MYELOGRAPHY AND VENTRICULOGRAPHY

Myelography and ventriculography are techniques which of themselves, irrespective of the medium employed, have some unpleasant effects: e.g., *headache*, *nausea* and *dizziness* are frequent problems; they are possibly more frequent in women (SEDA-1, 357), in cases of multiple sclerosis (SEDA-2, 375) and in investigations at the higher levels of the central nervous system. Nevertheless, the nature and incidence of the adverse reactions do depend on the contrast medium employed, and it is more convenient to consider these in three main classes: the oily media, the ionic water-soluble media and the non-ionic water-soluble media.

OILY MEDIA

Iofendylate was formerly widely used for myelography and to some extent for ventriculography. In the United States, where myelography was generally performed with large volumes of contrast medium, it has been the custom to aspirate the iofendylate at the end of the investigation, whereas in some other countries smaller volumes have been used and it had been assumed that these would be gradually absorbed. In patients with multiple sclerosis, myelography with iofendylate may cause particularly severe reactions (SEDA-2, 375).

Aseptic meningitis has occurred 3—67 days after myelography, and in one case it was associated with evidence of *cerebral vasospasm* and *infarction* (SED-8, 1044). An unusual *ophthalmic complication* in another patient followed the passage of iofendylate into the region of the clivus and along the course of the optic nerve during a cervical myelogram; the patient experienced transient pain and flashes of light in the eye, followed by 2 days of periorbital pain. A month later, severe visual impairment with renewed pain occurred; the condition responded to systemic steroids (128[C]).

Venous intravasation may rarely occur during lumbar myelography and *pulmonary oil embolization* has resulted. The latter has also been described following ventriculography with iofendylate in a hydrocephalic child with a ventriculovenous shunt. In that case the symptoms were mild, but the compound can obstruct the valve and in any patient the medium should therefore be removed at the completion of the procedure.

Arachnoiditis is a recognized problem and much-discussed problem, which has given rise to group litigation. Extensive adhesions due to iofendylate have been described, leading to neurological complications and death; there are two cases on record with clinical changes resembling Sudeck's atrophy (SED-8, 1045). Animal experiments have shown that the ability of iofendylate to cause arachnoiditis is especially pronounced if it is mixed with blood; the compound should thus be avoided if there is the possibility of bleeding having occurred into the cerebrospinal fluid.

As noted earlier, it is common to see evidence of iofendylate *residues* for many years after myelography, and one consequence of this is that the *serum protein-bound iodine* may remain elevated, e.g. for as long as 12 years (SED-8, 1045). The residue problem also extends to the skull and it is common to find symptomless deposits of iofendylate there following myelography; in several patients however such residues in the skull have apparently caused *convulsions* (SEDA-6, 407; SEDA-14, 424). They may also be associated with persistent *headache* (SEDA-8, 430) and perhaps with the development of vestibular disturbances many years later (SEDA-17, 538).

In two reported cases, ventriculography with iofendylate resulted in *adhesions* with obstructions to the outflow of cerebrospinal fluid (in one case at the level of the third ventricle, in the other at the level of the fourth) producing an obstructive *hydrocephalus* (SED-12, 1180; 129[CR]).

A case of recurrent febrile *nodular non-suppurative panniculitis* (Weber-Christian syndrome) has been described which occurred a month after myelography with iofendylate; the causal link is uncertain (SEDA-1, 357).

Persistent symptoms due to residues of iofendylate following myelography have been noted elsewhere in this Chapter; *allergy with urticaria and anaphylactic episodes* recurring for 17 years was described in one such patient who was hypersensitive to iofendylate; after removal of most of the residue, the symptoms improved (130[C]). In one unusual case of anaphylactic collapse, marked *bilateral parotid enlargement* was the presenting sign (SEDA-18, 442; see also 'General and idiosyncratic reactions' above).

IONIC WATER-SOLUBLE MEDIA

The earliest water-soluble medium used for lumbar myelography or radiculography, sodium methiodal, had an irritant effect and required spinal anesthesia which sometimes caused hypotension. Methylglycamine iothalamate proved to be less irritant, whilst methylglucamine iocarmate had a still lower neurotoxicity. However, even these two media could cause convulsions or muscle spasms if the contrast medium came into contact with the conus medullaris. For this reason the patient was postured with the head elevated for several hours after the examination to prevent the contrast medium passing above the L-l vertebral level. Diazepam might also be given prophylactically. When convulsions did occur they could be severe, even resulting in fractures or dislocation of a hip. Convulsive pattern have also been seen on the EEG in some patients without actual convulsions.

Methylglucamine iocarmate and methylglucamine iothalamate have both caused persistent *arachnoiditis*, leading to obliteration of nerve roots and constriction of the dural sac; operative treatment after myelography has been found to increase the risk of arachnoiditis. The risk of arachnoiditis was dose-dependent and varied with the contrast medium used (131[cR], 132[C]).

Four cases of *cauda equina syndrome* have been described with methylglucamine iocarmate used for radiculography, although in two cases faulty technique was perhaps contributory (SEDA-2, 375).

Diatrizoate is extremely neurotoxic if *injected into the subarachnoid space*. This has occurred accidentally as a result of misplacement of the needle in arteriographic investigations, in discography or from inadvertent use in myelography or injection of a myelocele. Severe *convulsions* with extensor spasms occur and may result in death, particularly if the medium comes into contact with the brain; onset of convulsions may be rapid, but they can also be delayed for several hours. Two patients developed *renal failure* as an additional complication (SEDA-8, 1046). After the use of iohexol, convulsions are rare (SEDA-16, 536).

Accidental misuse of diatrizoate for myelography, with fatal consequences, continues to be a serious problem. Lavage of the subarachnoid space with saline in such cases has been effective in reducing toxicity (SEDA-15, 504).

It is at the present day regarded as extremely dangerous to use ionic media intrathecally and stern warnings against such use have been issued, e.g. by the American FDA (SEDA-18, 445). Where they have accidentally been used, fatalities have resulted (SEDA-18, 445; 133[CR]).

NON-IONIC WATER-SOLUBLE MEDIA

Metrizamide

Nature and incidence of adverse reactions Metrizamide was the first non-ionic contrast medium and became widely used for myelography and also for ventriculography. It was much less neurotoxic than iocarmate, though EEG changes lasting up to 3 days were found in some 16% of cases in early studies (SED-8, 1047).

Gelmers (134[CR]) analyzed a series of 439 myelo-

Table 3. *Lumbar myelography: frequency of side effects in 4568 myelographies (SEDA-4, 335)*

Side effects	Percentage	No. of patients
Headache	32	
Nauseat	11	
Vomiting	7	
Dizziness	7	
Increased pain	7	
Hypotension	<1	
Numbness, paresthesia		4
Muscular fibrillations		16 (9 from 1 center)
Micturition problems		52 (42 from 3 centers)
Vasovagal collapse		3
Temperature rise		12
Neck stiffness		5
Meningism		3
Allergic reactions		6

graphies with metrizamide. The most frequent side effect was *headache*, which could be differentiated as early-onset headache (related to hydrodynamic modifications in the spinal fluid following lumbar puncture) and late-onset headache reflecting a metrizamide effect. The frequency of late-onset headache was at least 27%, but altogether 46% of the patients had headache at one time or another. In this series, *meningeal irritation* was seen in 5%, sometimes in a severe form, mimicking a septic complication. *Spinal irritation* and *epileptic fits* were encountered in two cases and one case, respectively. Striking was the occurrence of an *acute psychotic organic syndrome*, frequently observed after cervical myelography with high doses of medium. A severe *anaphylactic reaction* occurred in one patient. The results of the above study have generally been confirmed by others; seizures are clearly very rare with these non-ionic media, though they have occurred, even with iohexol (135[Cr]), as have *involuntary movements and facial twitching* (136[cr]) and *nystagmus* (137[c]). Meningeal irritation and paraplegia have both been seen with iohexol (SEDA-16, 536) and a case of aseptic meningitis when using the newer non-ionic dimer iotrolan (ibid).

The incidence of side effects is somewhat higher when metrizamide is used for cervical myelography and appears to be related to the frequency with which the contrast medium enters the cranial cavity. The incidence of symptoms in lumbar myelography and cervical myelography is shown in Tables 3 and 4.

Psychic effects An early (1977) report by the manufacturer on experience in 2500 cervical myelograms with metrizamide throws light on the psychic complications with this first of the non-ionic media (138[C]). There were transient mental reactions in 25 of these instances, including 13 cases of *confusion* or *disorientation*, four of *depression*, two of *hallucinations*, two of *psychosis*, and one each of *anxiety*, *drowsiness*, *dysphasia* and *nightmares*.

Among 18 German study patients (139[CR]) undergoing lumbar myelography with metrizamide in 1979, an *organic psychosyndrome* was found in six of them, characterized by impaired memory and depression, but it could be demonstrated only by psychometric tests and it had disappeared within 5 days. In four of the 18 patients there was *hypo- or areflexia* and in three there were *EEG changes*; there was no correlation between these various types of effect.

Electroencephalographic changes Lundervold and Sortland monitored the EEG in 292 patients undergoing examinations with metrizamide. In 13% there were minor non-specific EEG changes which occurred 24 hours after the injection. In 4% there were more marked abnormalities such as spikes, spikes and waves, or paroxysms of bilateral synchronous high voltage rhythmic δ-waves, apparently due to a direct toxic action of metrizamide on the cerebral cortex. They occurred shortly after the injection, and in the patients involved a large amount of the contrast medium had flowed intracranially. Diazepam did not appear to have any significant effect on the EEG changes (reviewed in SEDA-4, 337; see also SEDA-15, 504).

Convulsions Up to 1979 it was estimated that some 360 000 myelographies had been performed with metrizamide and that there had been 40 cases of epileptic attacks after its use (140[R]); although they tended to relate to investigations in the upper part of the spine, three related to cases of lumbar myelography; a further case was later described. In some of these instances the use of other drugs may have played a role, including chlorpromazine, antihypertensive agents, diphenhydramine and pethidine (SED-12, 1182). The role of chlorpromazine in facilitating metrizamide-induced convulsions has been confirmed in animal studies; it was formerly recommended that phenothiazines should be withdrawn at least 48 hours before intrathecal use of metrizamide (see below). Some, but by no means all, of the patients experiencing convulsions with metrizamide have a history of epilepsy.

Neurological changes Transient neurological changes may occur (see also under 'Psychic effects' above). They include *asterixis* (flapping tremor), *aphasia* and reversible *visual defects*. In one patient, asterixis and head bobbing were still present 3 months after myelography with metrizamide (SEDA-7, 453). An isolated case of persistent *cervical myelopathy* has also been reported after lumbar myelography with metrizamide (SEDA-5, 423).

A variety of other neurological complications have also been recorded. These include *Guillain-Barré syn-*

Table 4. *Cervical myelography: side effects other than grand mal (1232 examinations) (SEDA-4, 33)*

Symptoms or signs	No. of patients	Incidence (%)	Range
Headache	457	37	10–53
Nausea	245	20	2–45
Vomiting	173	14	0–43
Dizziness	61	5	
Mental changes	25	2	
Pain	88		
Numbness, paresthesia	8		
Myoclonia	4		
Weakness in arms or legs	6		
Micturition disturbances	8		
Neck stiffness	2		
Allergic reaction	2		
Hematemesis	1		
Eye flickering	1		

drome (SEDA-6, 407), *auditory or visual disturbance*, *motor aphasia*, *VI nerve palsy* (SEDA-8, 431), *manic syndrome*, *organic brain syndrome* (SEDA-10, 425), *confusional changes* and *absence status*. Absence status responds rapidly to intravenous diazepam (SEDA-14, 415).

In The Netherlands around 1979 there were several reports of *aseptic meningitis* after the use of metrizamide (SED-12, 1183) and the complication has been reported since with iopamidol (141[Cr]). *Streptococcal meningitis* has also been reported (142[CR]).

Death has occurred following deterioration of neurological status. There has been a higher incidence of such complications in diabetics (SEDA-11, 415). Aspiration of 20–25 ml of cerebrospinal fluid after metrizamide myelography appears to reduce the incidence of neurological adverse effects (143[CR]).

Skin A few *urticarial* and *anaphylactic* reactions have been noted (SEDA-8, 431; SEDA-10, 425).

Use in cisternography When metrizamide was used to outline the basal cisterns in association with computed tomography of the skull, *headache* occurred in some 50% of patients and *vomiting* in 26–56%, depending on the dose used; the symptoms occurred 2–6 hours after injection and cleared within 12 hours. *Convulsions* have occurred with this procedure (144[C]).

Miscellaneous Transient *exacerbation of systemic lupus erythematosus* has occurred after metrizamide myelography (SEDA-9, 411). Several patients have developed *hyperthermia* (SEDA-10, 425) and one patient with metrizamide encephalopathy developed severe *hypertension* (SEDA-11, 415; SED-12, 1182).

Mechanism of effects on the brain Examination by computed tomography following metrizamide cisternography shows that metrizamide penetrates the superficial parts of the cerebrum and cerebellum adjacent to the subarachnoid surface. This penetration is maximal between 6 and 12 hours after the injection and coincides with the main incidence of acute adverse (SEDA-4, 337). It has been suggested that the position of the head may be important in determining the localization of metrizamide toxicity on the brain. Aphasia without a confusional state was noted in some 12% patients who were placed in the left lateral decubitus position for tomography of the spine. In one of these cases computed tomography showed accumulation of metrizamide over the left hemisphere. In 34 patients who were placed on their right side for tomography, there were no speech disturbances.

Reduction in the size of the cerebral ventricles has been detected in some cases following myelography with metrizamide. It was suggested that this may indicate cerebral swelling and that this may be harmful in patients with raised intracranial pressure.

Metrizamide causes inhibition of the enzyme hexokinase, through competition with substrate glucose, and it has been suggested that it may therefore interfere with the glucose metabolism of the brain.

Intraventricular metrizamide may cause perivascular mononuclear infiltration in the walls of the ventricles. This histological appearance may be mistaken for an encephalitis if previous exposure to metrizamide is not considered (SEDA-7, 454).

Adhesive arachnoiditis Adhesive arachnoiditis does not appear to occur clinically with metrizamide, but it has been seen in high-dose animal studies (SEDA-2, 375).

Iopamidol and iohexol

The second-generation non-ionic water-soluble media—iopamidol and iohexol—are cheaper than metrizamide and more convenient to use. Using these newer contrast media for the purpose, and with appropriate selection of patients and supervision at home, myelography has become acceptable as an outpatient procedure. There does not appear to be any contraindication to phenothiazines with iopamidol or iohexol. In comparative trials, iopamidol and iohexol produced fewer side effects than metrizamide and they do not so far appear to have given rise to the psychosyndrome, but slight *EEG changes* may occur even with the newer media. *Seizures and clonic jerks* have been reported when relatively large doses of iopamidol have been used in myelography (SEDA-7, 455; SEDA-13, 436).

More minor side effects such as *headache*, *nausea* and *vomiting* were more frequent in women than in men, particularly in women between the age of 26 and 50 years. Early ambulation has been found to increase the incidence of headaches. In one study, there was a higher incidence of delayed headaches after iopamidol in comparison with iohexol. Long-distance travel also appeared to increase the incidence of post-myelogram headaches (SEDA-15, 503). *Dizziness* was more frequent in patients over the age of 50 years. In a meta-analysis of 25 published studies, the incidence of post-myelographic symptoms was significantly higher when needles larger than 22G were used.

Myelography with either iopamidol or metrizamide may cause transitory *deterioration in memory operations* as determined by psychological tests, but the effect is less with iopamidol (145[Cr]). Measurement of the visual evoked response 20 hours after myelography may show a delayed response. This appears to show a correlation with the severity of post- myelogram headaches; the delay in the visual-evoked response is less marked with iopamidol than with metrizamide. It is suggested that this technique may be useful in the assessment of myelographic contrast media toxicity (146[Cr]).

Hydration is usually recommended after myelography but it can be excessive and cause problems greater than those due to the contrast medium. One patient who had been given 2 liters of water to drink prior to iohexol myelography developed an *encephalopathy* with confusion and disorientation. There was evidence of a dilution hyponatremia, possibly with water intoxication. With restriction of fluids and use of dexamethasone the condition was largely resolved within 48 hours and recovery was complete (147[Cr]); the case is not unique (148[CR]) and it is clearly essential to give patients clear instructions as to their water intake.

A few cases of severe purulent *meningeal reactions* to iopamidol have been briefly described in the course of the years (149[CR]). In one exceptional case-report, a *hemorrhagic meningeal reaction* and *thrombosis of the superior longitudinal sinus* followed sacroradiculography with iopamidol (150[CR]). A case of *transitory abducent nerve palsy* has been reported after myelography with iopamidol (SED-12, 1183).

Table 5. *Incidence of serious complications in 32 000 lymphographies (175[C])*

Event	No. of cases	Incidence
Death	18	0.0006
Pulmonary infarcts	81	0.0025
Pulmonary edema	10	0.0003
Pneumonia	13	0.0004
Hypertensive crisis	6	0.0002
Prolonged fever	24	0.0008
Hypersensitivity reactions		
Oily contrast medium	40	0.0012
Vital blue dye	57	0.0017
Cerebral disorders	9	0.0003

DISCOGRAPHY

A case of subdural *empyema* with residual quadriparesis has been reported as a rare complication of discography (151[CR]). Accidental injection of diatrizoate into the subarachnoid space causes *convulsions*, as noted above.

LYMPHOGRAPHY

Iodized oils are usually used as contrast media for lymphography; they can cause *iodism*. Reactions may also occur to the dye 'patent blue violet' which is injected subcutaneously prior to the lymphogram to enable the lymphatics to be visualized; it *colors the skin and urine* blue. The incidence of serious reactions to lymphography in 32 000 cases is indicated in Table 5.

Hypersensitivity Allergic or even anaphylactic reactions can occur either to the iodized oil or to the dye; in hypersensitive patients, prior use of steroids and antihistamines may fail to prevent a severe reaction (152[C]).

Skin and appendages The skin may be involved in allergic reactions. *Dermatitis* has also been described in the past occurring some days after lymphography and apparently due to extravasation of the iodized oil into the tissues (SED-12, 1184). Since lymphography requires an incision, wound infections may occur and, rarely, lymphangitis.

In 17 out of 53 cases with obstructive lymphedema

there was an *increase in limb volume* following lymphangiography with Lipiodol ultrafluid (iodinated poppy seed oil) and 10 cases had features resembling *lymphangitis*. In one patient there was an *allergic reaction* with rapid development of edema and increase of limb volume by 2000 ml. Whereas contrast medium virtually disappears from normal lymphatics within 8 hours, in cases of obstructive lymphedema Lipiodol remains in the lymphatics for several days and it appears to cause a low grade *chemical inflammation* with obliteration of the lymphatics (SEDA-7, 454).

A woman with inoperable carcinoma of the cervix developed multi- centric *reticulohistiocytosis* with arthritis and skin papules following lymphography with Lipiodol ultrafluid. Two later examinations with diatrizoate caused exacerbation of the disease within 24 hours. The condition receded spontaneously after 12 months and subsequent examinations with metrizamide and iodamide were symptom-free (153[CR]).

Pulmonary embolism Some of the injected contrast medium inevitably reaches the lungs; tracer studies 30 years ago showed that some degree of pulmonary oil embolism occurred in every patient (154[C]); pulmonary function studies have shown abnormalities, in particular a decrease in pulmonary diffusing capacity and pulmonary capillary blood volume, even in the absence of clinical signs or symptoms (155[C]). Most cases are indeed symptomless, though there can be mild pyrexia, whilst X-rays show stippling or an arborization pattern. If hypotension, cyanosis, dyspnea and pleuritic pain appear, infarction should be suspected. The risk that the blockage of the lung capillaries by oil will endanger the patient is naturally greater if pulmonary function is already compromised, e.g. by neoplastic or fibrotic disease, or by radiotherapy.

In some patients this phase of mechanical obstruction is followed after some days or 3—4 weeks by a chemical reaction, presumably as the oil breaks down to irritant fatty acids, which cause exudation and hemorrhage. Interference with the production of lung surfactant may also occur and a marked intravascular cellular reaction has been described (156[C]). The chemical irritative phase is marked by fever, cough with sputum (often blood) and a variable degree of respiratory distress; there may even be tachycardia and hypotension.

Lymphatic obstruction is also an important factor in the etiology of oil embolism during lymphography causing shunting via distal lymphovenous communications.

Operations or anesthesia may be poorly tolerated in the immediate post-lymphography period when lung diffusion is diminished.

A case of pulmonary fibrosis and microlithiasis has been reported as a late complication of lymphography with iodized oil, but a causative relation is uncertain (SEDA-12, 397).

Cerebral oil embolism Cerebral oil embolism has been described in nine patients in one series of 3500 lymphograms (157[R]) and in eight patients in another series of 16 501 investigations (158[Cr]). All nine patients in the former series developed neurological signs, usually within 48 hours, reaching a peak in 4—7 days; the symptoms variously comprised motor dysfunction, paraplegia and deep coma lasting for some weeks; three of the nine died. The EEG findings in these patients pointed to diffuse brain emboli.

Retinal fat embolism may be useful in confirming the diagnosis; computed tomography may also show collections of ethiodol in the brain. In the early phase after radiotherapy to the lungs, the vasculature is damaged so that contrast medium is less effectively retained in the lungs. If lymphography is performed at this stage, there is an increased risk of cerebral embolism (SED-8, 1048).

Hepatic oil embolism This has been described but appears to be virtually symptomless.

Effects on the lymph nodes Within a few hours after lymphography, the lymph nodes show dilatation of the marginal and intermediate sinuses and a giant-cell reaction, the foreign body reaction consisting of diffuse reticulocytosis and sinus histiocytosis. Diffuse plasmacytosis and an increase in the eosinophil count may also be seen. The response is maximal after 10—14 days, but the changes in the lymph nodes may not be eliminated for as long as 15 months (SED-12, 1184).

Facilitation of metastasis There has been some suggestion from individual cases that the passage of contrast media through malignant lymph nodes may facilitate metastases; one relevant case relates to Hodgkin's disease (159[C]), another to melanoma (160[C]). There is also a little animal evidence in this direction. Generally, it has been considered that lymphography is unlikely to be a significant factor promoting malignant dissemination and that its diagnostic value in planning treatment far outweighed any theoretical risk. Computed tomography and magnetic resonance imaging have now largely replaced lymphography for the demonstration of malignant lymph nodes.

Endocrine system Mild *hypothyroidism* with a goiter developed in a 15-year-old boy 6 weeks after lymphangiography with Lipiodol ultrafluid. The goiter disappeared after 3 months treatment with L-thyroxine (SEDA-7, 454).

BRONCHOGRAPHY

Computed tomography of the lungs has decreased the requirement for bronchography, but the latter is still of value in selected cases. The currently used preparation for bronchography is propyliodone (either in aqueous suspension with carboxymethylcellulose or in an oily suspension), but the newer non-ionic dimer iotrolan has attained some popularity. Of the two propyliodone preparations, the aqueous version is reputed to be more irritant, though some work found no difference between the two. The oily medium has tended to cause more peripheral filling and to be associated with a higher incidence of pyrexial reactions and pneumonic change.

Of the earlier products used in the field, Hytrast (a mixture of iopydol and iopydone in aqueous suspension with carboxymethylcellulose) was generally withdrawn because it gave rise to a foreign body reaction. Iodized oil was formerly popular, but iodism was not uncommon and sometimes even fatal; sulfonilamide was added to one particular preparation of iodized oil to increase its viscosity and on occasion produced methemoglobinemia and cyanosis. Late granulomatous reactions in the lungs followed by long-term fibrosis were also described with iodized oil, as were early allergic granulomatous reactions as well as other types of allergic reaction, such as pneumonitis and urticaria.

Approximately one-third of patients undergoing bronchography appear to have experienced some type of reaction. The most common symptoms are *headache*, *nausea and vomiting*, *fever*, *'iodism'* and *dyspnea*. Less frequent reactions are *wheezing*, *diarrhea*, *dizziness*, *cyanosis*, *chest pain* and *pneumonia*. Aqueous propyliodone has produced rather more reactions than the oily form, but as a rule the product producing most reactions has also produced the best visualization. Symptoms are also related to the volume of medium used and the degree of alveolarization (161[CR]).

In a survey of 100 000 bronchograms published in 1967, 18 *deaths* were attributed to the technique. Half the fatalities were however due to the local anesthetic, generally used in excessive amounts. Fatalities tended to occur in children, patients with limited respiratory reserves, or subjects experiencing severe hypersensitivity reactions (SED-12, 1185).

Transitory *changes in lung function* may occur after bronchography due to retention of the contrast medium in the bronchi; normal diffusing capacity may not return for 3 days and it is better to avoid thoracic surgery during this period (162[C]). When bronchography is performed during fiber optic bronchoscopy, there may be marked arterial oxygen desaturation. Iotrolan is more fluid than propyliodone and appears to cause less arterial oxygen desaturation (SEDA-15, 504).

In pediatric bronchography, *segmental collapse* occurs in half the cases, but is particularly common with the aqueous media. Collapse also seems to be more common when halothane and oxygen are used as the anesthetic agents (SEDA-15, 504); this has been attributed to the rapid absorption of the anesthetic gases combined with the partial bronchial block caused by the contrast medium.

If the cricothyroid route is used for bronchography, contrast medium may be accidentally injected into the *soft tissues of the neck*; propyliodone has under these conditions produced an inflammatory reaction leading to dysphagia, pain on movement of the neck, and mediastinal spread, rarely with EGG changes suggesting pericarditis. Oral steroids with antibiotic cover usually produce dramatic relief of symptoms.

Heating lowers the viscosity of propyliodone and should be avoided. Death from progressive acute respiratory failure resulted from bilateral bronchography under general anesthesia using propyliodone which had been heated in an autoclave.

HYSTEROSALPINGOGRAPHY

Water-soluble media are now generally preferred for hysterosalpingography, the urographic media such as diatrizoate or iothalamate being most commonly selected. It has sometimes been suggested that low-osmolar contrast media should be preferred; however, a double-blind comparison of the low-osmolar medium Hexabrix 320 (ioxaglate) with Conray 280 (methylglucamine diatrizoate) in 100 patients showed no difference in the incidence of early or late side effects between the two media (163[Cr]).

There is no justification for using specialized preparations based on the more toxic molecules of acetrizoate or iodipamide; these cause more severe pain and may also cause hypotension and shock.

Iodized oil, at one time widely used, causes less pain but was suspected of causing adhesions and there was certainly some risk of oil embolism following intravasation, e.g. a case of retinal embolism occurred with visual impairment lasting for some months (SED-8, 1050) and several cases of pulmonary oil embolism were described (SEDA-16, 537). Skin testing with iodized oil on occasion resulted in both local and generalized reactions (SEDA-1, 357). Like later agents, lipiodol could also cause salpingitis.

The main remaining disadvantage of the currently used water-soluble media is their tendency to cause *lower abdominal pain*, which may be severe, during or shortly after the injection; it can last for 24 hours or longer. *Vaginal bleeding* may occur and the next menstrual period may be deranged. With all contrast media there is a possibility of *hypersensitivity reactions* occurring, and dextran as an additive has on occasion produced anaphylactic symptoms (SEDA-15, 505). *Salpingitis* can occur with any of these contrast media.

AMNIOGRAPHY (SED-8, 1051)

Ultrasound has now generally superseded the use of amniography, a procedure in which contrast media can be injected into the amniotic sac during pregnancy to determine fetal normality. Diatrizoate, iothalamate and earlier iodized oil were employed. There is a theoretical risk of the hypertonic medium causing premature labor (particularly if sodium media were used). Accidental injection of contrast medium into the fetal subcutaneous tissue could cause sloughing of the skin or subcutaneous necrosis. Cases of thyroid hyperplasia or hypothyroidism were also described, with presence of oily contrast medium in the soft tissues.

ARTHROGRAPHY

Following the injection of contrast medium into a joint, the synovium becomes edematous and hemorrhagic within 2 hours. At 24 hours there is tissue eosinophilia and vascular congestion. Eosinophilia of the synovial fluid may also occur. The complications reported in a survey of 126 000 examinations are shown in Table 6.

Table 6. *Complications of arthrography in 126 000 examinations (164[CR])*

Complications	Number
Death	0
Severe reactions	
Hypotension	4
Vasomotor collapse and laryngeal edema	1
Air embolism	1
Vagal reactions	83
Subsequent seizures	6
Apnea	1
Hives	61
Cellulitis	1
Sepsis	3
Massive effusion	1
Severe pain	5
Sterile chemical synovitis	150

HEPATIC ENHANCEMENT

Perfluoro-octylbromide

Preliminary assessment of an intravenous infusion of an emulsion of perfluoro-octylbromide as a hepatic and splenic enhancement agent caused lower back pain and transitory fever (SEDA-15, 505). This problem appeared to be due to the lipid emulsion and seems to have been overcome with more recent preparations.

MAGNETIC RESONANCE IMAGING (MRI)

Gadolinium pentate dimeglumine (*GdDTPA*) is used as a contrast agent in magnetic resonance imaging. In a manufacturer's survey, adverse reactions were reported in 19.9% of patients, but these were predominantly minor (SEDA-15, 505). Several severe anaphylactoid reactions and of angioneurotic edema have however also been reported (SED-12, 1187; SEDA-16, 537; SEDA-17, 538; 165[cr]).

Gadoteridol is a newer non-ionic agent used for MRI. A moderately severe anaphylactic reaction has been described in a patient with known drug allergies, and milder reactions in a series of other patients (SEDA-18, 446).

RADIOPHARMACEUTICALS *(166[R]) (For radioactive iodine, see also Chapter 41)*

Radioactive substances may be used in medicine as tracers—the quantities used in this case being merely sufficient to enable them to be detected—or as therapeutic agents, in which case the quantities employed and the amount of radiation emitted may be considerable. Risks resulting from the radiation itself fall outside the scope of this volume.

Adverse reactions to isotope scanning have from time to time been reported. Reactions vary from mild symptoms such as flushing, headache, tachycardia or nausea to collapse, cardiac arrest and death.

A few cases of cardiovascular collapse and death have formerly occurred after injection of *radioactive mac-*

ro-aggregated albumin particles (MAA) for lung perfusion scanning in patients with advanced pulmonary disease. These all occurred prior to 1975 when high doses were in use and quality standards lower. A recent study in 12 patients confirms that lung scanning with MAA does not significantly impair lung function as measured by carbon monoxide diffusion (167[CR]).

A case of anaphylaxis occurred after the injection of a leukocyte suspension labeled with ^{99m}Tc-hexamethyl propylene amine oxime (168[CR]).

^{99m}Tc-labeled serum albumin microspheres have in one case caused collapse, apparently because the patient in question had earlier been sensitized by blood transfusions (SEDA-2, 376).

A severe anaphylactic reaction occurred 7 minutes after injection of *orthoiodohippurate* for renography in a patient who had previously had a severe reaction following intravenous urography with Conray 400. It was estimated that the dose of radiopharmaceutical contained approximately 11 μg of iodine (169[CR]).

Inhalation of *Technigas* (an ultrafine suspension of ^{99m}Tc-labeled carbon particles) for ventilation scintigraphy in a series of patients led to a temporary decrease in oxygenation in 87% of cases, often in sufficient degree to cause some discomfort (SEDA-17, 539; 170[C]). Injection of ^{99m}Tc-MAA for perfusion scintigraphy similarly tended to cause a decrease in oxygenation, but insufficient to cause symptoms (ibid).

In bone scanning, a severe systemic reaction due to *diphosphonate* sensitivity has been described (171[Cr]). Vasculitis and erythema multiforme have also occurred (SEDA-14, 425).

Aseptic meningitis has been reported following isotope cysternography with *serum albumin labeled with radioactive iodine* (172[C], 173[C]), but also after giving the (non-protein) *indium diethylenetriaminopentaacetic acid* (SEDA-2, 376).

Dipyridamole-thallium-201 imaging is being increasingly used to assess cases of suspected coronary disease (SEDA-15, 506; SEDA-16, 537; SEDA-17, 539); the substance can be given either orally or intravenously. Dipyramidole can cause *bronchospasm*, which may demand treatment with aminophylline. In one series of 400 examinations, severe chest pain due to *myocardial ischemia* occurred in 9% of cases, milder chest pain (probably not associated with cardiac events) in 21%; there was severe hypotension in 2.5% of cases (174[CR]). Others have reported instances of cardiovascular collapse (SEDA-15, 506).

The Society of Nuclear Medicine has maintained a register of adverse reactions to radiopharmaceuticals occurring in the United States since 1976. The incidence rates of reactions appear to be declining due to improved quality control of radiopharmaceuticals. Many of the earlier adverse reactions were attributed to iron-containing preparations, gelatin-stabilized preparations, materials such as albumin contaminated with pyrogens and other products no longer in use. The overall incidence of reactions for the year 1978 was estimated to lie between one and six per 100 000 examinations. Reactions reported during 1978 are shown in Table 7 and the estimated range of incidence per 100 000 examinations is shown in Table 8.

When Keeling and Sampson (176[R]) reviewed UK reports of adverse reactions to radiopharmaceuticals from 1977 to 1983, they found a changing distribution pattern (Table 9). This is partly due to elimination of some of the earlier, more toxic preparations and partly due to changing usage, more particularly the increased use of phosphonate preparations. The authors estimated that only 10% of reactions were reported and that the probable incidence rate was between one in 1000 and one in 10 000. There was one death associated with a hypotensive reaction to colloid in a severely ill patient. One elderly patient had a cardiac arrest after injection of macro-aggregated albumin but was resuscitated.

RADIOPHARMACEUTICALS IN LACTATION

Many radiopharmaceuticals are excreted in breast milk and a review has discussed the implications of nuclear medicine examinations in the nursing mother (177[R]). Iodides are excreted in high concentrations in breast milk.

The use of the short half-life ^{123}I in preference to ^{131}I partly overcomes this problem, but iodide or perchlorate which is used to block thyroid uptake in the mother may be excreted in the milk. Likewise, furosemide or cholecystokinin, which may be used to alter the distribution of radiopharmaceuticals, may be excreted in breast milk. Technetium compounds are now the most widely used radiopharmaceuticals; the highest excretion in breast milk occurs with sodium pertechnetate and the lowest with technetium diethylenetriaminepenta-acetic acid which is rapidly excreted by the kidneys. Depending on the type of examination and the dose of radiopharmaceutical the mother may be advised to withhold breastfeeding for 12—24 hours. Advice may also be required concerning external radiation when the mother holds the child. Before deciding to perform nuclear medicine tests in young women, it is important to consider the possibility of future lactation. Only essential investigations should be performed: the most appropriate radiopharmaceutical should be selected,

Table 7. *Reactions to radiopharmaceuticals in the United States in 1978 (175[CR])*

Radiopharmaceutical	Reported symptoms in order of decreasing frequency of observation, with time of onset (summary of 1978 data only)
^{99m}Tc-HSA	Up to 1 hour: flushing, respiratory difficulty; rapid pulse; rash; high temperature
^{99m}Tc-HAM	1 hour: flushing, respiratory distress; cyanosis; itching, rash; pyrogen; bronchospasm; anaphylactic shock
^{99m}Tc-Sulfur-colloid	1 hour: hives, rash, itching; redness/swelling; nausea, vomiting, dizziness, loss of consciousness; respiratory difficulty, flushing, cyanosis; pain at injection site; bronchospasm. After 1 hour: rash; pyrogen reaction
^{99m}-Glucoheptonate	Rash, hives; nausea, dizziness, chills
^{99m}-DTPA (Fe)	Seizure; dizziness, hypotension; swelling, redness, itching
^{99m}-DTPA (SSn)	Hives, itching; flushing, hypertension
^{99m}Tc-MAA	Up to 1 hour: hives; itching, redness; respiratory difficulty; cardiac arrest; metallic taste
Nal(^{131})I	Several hours: nausea, vomiting, chest pain; tachycardia; itching skin; rash, hives
Orthoiodohippurate (^{131})I	Immediate: anaphylactic shock After one hour: pyrogen reaction. Several hours: meningitis

Table 8. *Estimated range for incidence of adverse reactions to radiopharmaceuticals in the United States in 1978*

Radiopharmaceutical	Estimated range for incidence per 100 000
^{99m}Tc-HSA	18–89
^{99m}Tc-HAM	13–65
^{99m}Tc-Sulfur-colloid	2–8
^{99m}Tc-Glucoheptonate	2–8
NaI(^{131})	1–7
^{99m}Tc-pyrophosphate	1–5
^{99m}Tc-MAA	1–3
^{99m}Tc-Tc0_4	0.01–0.4

Table 9. *Major groupings of adverse reactions to radiopharmaceuticals reported in the United Kingdom from January 1977 to December 1983 (176[R])*

	Colloids	Phosphonates	Albumin particulates	Others
1977 to mid-1980	12(12)	2(2)	5(4)	8(7)
	48%	8%	16%	28%
Mid-1980 to 1983	8(6)	15(13)	3(3)	8(7)
	21%	45%	10%	24%
Total	20(18)	17(15)	8(7)	16(14)
	33%	28%	13%	26%

Figures in brackets are totals *less* those considered as 'unlikely to be due to the radiopharmaceutical'.

and the dose reduced to the minimum compatible with obtaining a diagnostic result.

RADIOACTIVE SUBSTANCES OF HISTORICAL INTEREST

Thorotrast

Thorotrast (thorium dioxide) was at one time a widely used contrast medium; introduced in 1928, it had by 1933 been shown to induce malignancy in rats. It was prohibited in various countries from 1936 onwards, though it continued to be used in some parts of the world for another three decades. The late effects of this radioactive material continue to be reported. Thorotrast deposits are predominantly localized in the liver and reticuloendothelial system, the major late effects have been those of portal fibrosis, malignant liver tumors and myeloproliferative disorders, but granulomatous, fibrotic and malignant changes of many organ systems have been described. Thorotrast is the most potent human leukemogen yet identified. The risk of developing a fatal blood dyscrasia after Thorotrast is very much greater than after external radiotherapy, but the latent period (20 years) is very much longer than that after external irradiation (5–7 years).

A 1993 follow-up study in Denmark of mortality among 999 patients who had received Thorotrast between 1935 and 1947 showed that excess mortality could only be explained in part by diseases known to be induced by thorotrast such as cirrhosis and cancer of the liver, leukemia and other hematological disorders; it was suggested that non-specific effects induced by the α-radiation emitted by Thorotrast may have contributed to this excess mortality (178[CR]).

For full reviews of this topic the reader is referred to

earlier volumes in this series (SED-8, 1051 and SED Annuals 1–19).

Radium

In a follow-up of 5058 persons with therapeutic or occupational exposure to radium, there were 21 patients with a carcinoma of the mastoid and 11 patients with malignant tumours of the nasal sinuses (SEDA-4, 337).

During the period 1944–1952, a large number of German patients were injected with 'Peteosthor', a solution containing radium-224. In high doses, this has resulted in an increased frequency of bone sarcoma, leukemia and other tumors. Benign exostoses, growth retardation, tooth breakage, kidney disease, liver disease and cataracts have also occurred (SEDA-11, 417)

REFERENCES

1. Thomsen HS, Dorph S. High osmolar and low osmolar contrast media. An update on frequency of adverse drug reactions. Acta Radiol 1993;34:205–209.
2. Siegle RL. Rates of idiosyncratic reactions. Ionic versus nonionic media. Invest Radiol 1993;28(Suppl 5):595–598.
3. Cohen MD. A review of the toxicity of nonionic contrast agents in children. Invest Radiol 1993;28(Suppl 5):587–593.
4. Powe NR, Davidoff AJ, Moore RD et al. Net costs from three perspectives of using low versus high osmolarity contrast medium in diagnostic angiocardiography. J Am Coll Cardiol 1993;21:1701–1709.
5. Bush WH, Swanson DP. Acute reactions to intravenous contrast media: types, risk factors, recognition and specific treatment. Am J Roentgenol 1991;157:1153–1161.
6. Katayama H, Yamaguchi K, Kozuka T et al. Adverse reactions to ionic contrast media. A report from the Japanese Committee on the Safety of Contrast Media. Radiology 1990;175:621.
7. Barrett BJ, Parfrey PS, McDonald JR et al. Nonionic low- osmolality versus ionic high-osmolality contrast media for intravenous use in patients perceived to be at high risk: randomized trial. Radiology 1992;183:105–110.
8. Zeeman RK. Disseminated intravascular coagulation following intravenous pyelography. Invest Radiol 1977;12:203.
9. Pfister RC, Hutter AM. Cardiac alterations during intravenous urography. Invest Radiol 1980;15:S239.
10. Matthai WM, Hirshfeld JW. Choice of contrast agents for cardiac angiography: review and recommendations based on clinically important distinctions. Cathet Cardiovasc Diagn 1991;22:278–289.
11. Bääth L, Almén T, Öksendal A. Cardiac effects from addition of sodium ions to nonionic contrast media for coronary arteriography. An investigation in the isolated rabbit heart. Invest Radiol 1990;25:5137–5140.
12. Ansell G. Adverse reactions to contrast agents: scope of problem. Invest Radiol 1970;5:374.
13. Lasser EC. Metabolic basis of contrast material toxicity: status 1971. Am J Roentgenol 1971;113:415.
14. Girouk JD, Sizun J, Rubio S et al. Hypothyroïdie transitoire après opacification iodées des cathéters epicutanéocaves au réanimation néonatale. Arch Fr Pediatr 1993; 50:273.
15. Kutt H, Milhorat TH, McDowall F. The effect of iodinated contrast media upon blood proteins, electrolytes and red cells. Neurology 1963;13:492.
16. Stemerman M, Goldstein ML, Schulman PL. Pancytopenia associated with diatrizoate. NY State J Med 1971;71:19.
17. Esplugas E, Cequier MD, Burwell LR et al. Influence of contrast media on thrombus formation during coronary angioplasty. J Am Coll Cardiol 1991;18:443–450.
18. Chronos NAF, Goodall AH, Wilson DJ et al. Profound platelet degranulation is an important side effect of some types of contrast media used in interventional cardiology. Circulation 1993;88:2035–2044.
19. Polgen M, Kuhlmen JE, Hansen FC et al. Case report. Computed tomography of angiooedema of small bowel due to reaction to radiographic contrast medium. J Comput Assist Tomogr 1988;12:1044.
20. Navani S, Taylor CE, Kaufman SA et al. Evanescent enlargement of salivary glands following triiodinated contrast media. Br J Radiol 1972;45:19.
21. Taliercio CP, Vlietstra RE, Fisher LD et al. Risks for renal dysfunction with cardiac angiography. Ann Intern Med 1986;104:501.
22. Waxler L, Cohen B, Rudnick MR et al. Multicentre trial of ionic and nonionic contrast media. Radiology 1991; 292(Abstr 1159, RSNA Annual Meeting, Chicago).
23. Schwab SJ, Hiatky MA, Pieper KS et al. Contrast nephrotoxicity, a randomized controlled trial of a nonionic and an ionic radiographic contrast agent. N Engl J Med 1989;320:149.
24. Barrett BJ, Carlisle EJ. Meta-analysis of the relative nephrotoxicity of high and low osmolarity iodinated contrast media. Radiology 1993;188:171–178.
25. Bellamy P, Patrick D. Biliary opacification following intravenous Hexabrix: a normal phenomenon detected by computed tomography. Br J Radiol 1986;59:79.
26. Vaillant L, Pengloan J, Blanchier D et al. Iododerma and acute respiratory distress with leucocytic vasculitis following the intravenous injection of contrast medium. Clin Exp Dermatol 1990;15:232–233.
27. Shah AM, Hutchison SJ. Case report: The Koebnor phenomenon—an unusual localization of a contrast reaction. Clin Radiol 1990;42:136–137.
28. Benson PM, Giblin WJ, Douglas DM. Transient nonpigmenting fixed drug eruption caused by radiopaque contrast media. J Am Acad Dermatol 1990;23:379–381.
29. Nuñez ME, Sinués B. Cytogenic effects of diatrizoate and inaglate on patients undergoing excretory urography. Invest Radiol 1990;25:692–697.
30. Katayama H, Yamaguchi K, Kozuka T et al. Full-scale investigation into adverse reactions in Japan. Risk factor analysis. Invest Radiol 1991;26:S33–S36.
31. Eliashiv S, Wirguin I, Brenner T et al. Aggravation of

human and experimental myasthenia gravis by contrast media. Neurology 1990;40:1623–1625.
32. Shimura H, Takazawa K, Endo T et al. T_4-thyroid storm after CT scan with iodinated contrast medium. J Endocrinol Invest 1990;13:73–76.
33. Jamet P, Lebas de Lacour JCI, Christoforov B et al. Acidose lactique mortelle après urographie intraveineuse chez une diabétique recevant de la metformine. Sem Hôp 1980;56:9.
34. Pozzato C, Marozzi F, Brenna F. et al. Un caso di morte consequente all somministrazione endevenoza di mezzo di contrasto organiodato a basa osmolalita. Radiol Med 1990; 80:107–108.
35. Shulman KL, Benyunes MC, Winter TC et al. Adverse reactions to intravenous contrast media in patients treated with Interleukin-2. J Immunother 1993;13:208–212.
36. Reynolds NJ, Wallington TB, Burton JL. Hydralazine predisposes to acute cutaneous vasculitis following urography with iopamidol. Brit J Dermatol 1993;129:82–85.
37. Lee S, Shoen I. Black copper reduction reaction stimulating alcaptonuria—occurrence after intravenous urography. N Engl J Med 1966;275:266.
38. Tidgren B, Golman K. Effect of diatrizoate on renal extraction of PAH in man. Acta Radiol 1989;30:521.
39. Shehadi WH. Death following intravascular administration of contrast media. Acta Radiol Diagn 1985;26:457.
40. Lalli AF. Contrast media deaths. Australas Radiol 1984;28:133.
41. Katayama H, Tanaka T. Clinical survey of adverse reactions to ionic contrast media. Invest Radiol 1988;23(Suppl 1):S88.
42. Stejskal V, Nillson R, Grepe A. Immunologic basis for adverse reactions to radiographic contrast media. Acta Radiol 1990;31:605– 610.
43. Spataro RF, Katzberg RW, Fischer HW et al. High-dose clinical urography with the low-osmolality contrast agent Hexabrix: comparison with a conventional contrast agent. Radiology 1987;162:9.
44. Lasser EC, Lyon SG. Inhibition of angiotensin-converting enzyme by contrast media. 1. In vitro findings. Invest Radiol 1990;25:698- -702.
45. Dunnick NR, Cohan RH. Cost, corticosteroids and contrast media. Am J Roentgenol 1994;162:523–526.
46. Greenberger PA, Patterson R. The prevention of immediate generalised reactions to radiocontrast media in high-risk patients. J Allergy Clin Immunol 1991;87:867–872.
47. Bush WH, McClennan BL, Swanson DP. Contrast media reactions: prediction, prevention and treatment. Postgrad Radiol 1993;13:137– 147.
48. Melki PH, Mugel TL, Cléro B et al. Parotidite aiguë bilatérale. Prodrome isolé d'un choc anaphylactoide après injection de produit de contraste iodé. J Radiol 1993;74:51–54.
49. National Radiographic Survey (United Kingdom): unpublished reports up to 1990 made available by Dr G. Ansell.
50. Cohan RH, Dunnick NR, Leder RA et al. Extravasation of nonionic radiologic contrast media: efficacy of conservative treatment. Radiology 1990;176:65–67.
51. Smith HJ, Jones K, Hunter TB. What happens to patients after upper and lower gastrointestinal studies? Invest Radiol 1988;23:822.
52. Zheutlin N, Lasser EC, Rigler LG. Clinical studies on the effect of barium in the peritoneal cavity following rupture of the colon. Surgery 1952;32:967.
53. Rai AM, Johnson E. Epigastric hernia during air-contrast barium examination. Am J Roentgenol 1990;155:420.
54. Wheatley MJ, Eckhauser FE. Portal venous barium intravasation complicating barium enema examination. Surgery 1991;109:788–791.
55. LeFrock J, Ellis CA, Klainer AS et al. Transient bacteraemia associated with barium enemas. Arch Intern Med 1975;135:835.
56. Hammer JL. Septicaemia following barium enema. South Med J 1977;70:1361.
57. Stringer DA, Hassal E, Ferguson AC et al. Hypersensitivity reaction to single contrast barium meal studies in children. Paediatr Radiol 1993;23:587–588.
58. Ownby DR, Tomlanovich M, Sammons N et al. Anaphylaxis associated with latex allergy during barium enema examinations. Am J Roentgenol 1991;156:903–908.
59. Literature Review: Allergic reactions to barium procedures and latex rubber. E-Z-EM Ltd., London.
60. Lareau DG, Berta JW. Fatal aspiration of thick barium. Radiology 1976;120:317.
61. Gray C, Sivaloganathan S, Simkins KC. Aspiration of high- density barium contrast medium causing acute pulmonary inflammation—report of two fatal cases in elderly women with disordered swallowing. Clin Radiol 1989;40:397.
62. Davies NP, Williams JA. Tubeless vagotomy and pyloroplasty and the "Gastrografin test". Am J Surg 1971;122:368.
63. Chiu CL, Gambach RR. Hypaque pulmonary edema: a case report. Radiology 1974;111:91.
64. Godson C, Ryan MP, Brady HR et al. Acute hypomagnesaemia complicating the treatment of meconium ileus equivalent in cystic fibrosis. Scand J Gastroenterol 1988;23(Suppl 143):148.
65. Seltzer SE, Jones B. Cecal perforation associated with Gastrografin enema. Am J Roentgenol 1978;130:997.
66. Creteur V, Douglas D, Galante M et al. Inflammatory colonic changes produced by contrast material. Radiology 1983;147:77.
67. Leonidas JC, Burry F, Fellows RA et al. Possible adverse effect of methylglucamine diatrizoate compounds in the bowel of newborn infants with meconium ileus. Radiology 1975;121:693.
68. Glover JR, Thomas BM. Severe adverse reaction to oral iohexol. Clin Radiol 1991;44:137.
69. Nicholson DA. Contrast media in sialography: a comparison of lipiodol ultra fluid and Urografin 290. Clin Radiol 1990;42:423– 426.
70. Kuwano A, Sugai T, Mochida K. Systemic contact dermatitis induced by oral contrast media or the gallbladder. Skin Res 1993;35(Suppl 16):114–120.
71. Kelly WN. Uricosuria and X-ray contrast agents. N Engl J Med 1971;248:975.
72. Astwood EB. Occurrence in the serum of certain patients of large amounts of a newly isolated iodine compound. Trans Assoc Am Physicians 1957;70:183.
73. Fairhurst BJ, Naqvi N. Hyperthyroidism after cholecystography. Br Med J 1975;3:630.
74. Hysell LK, Hysell JW, Gray JM. Thrombocytopenic purpura following iopanoic acid ingestion. J Am Med Assoc 1977;237:361.
75. Insauti CLG, Lechin F, Van der Digs B. Severe thrombo-

cytopenia following oral cholecystography with iocetamic acid. Am J Hematol 1983;14:285.
76. Stacher A. Schwerste Thrombopenie durch ein perorales trijodiertes Gallenkontrastmittel. Wien Klin Wochenschr 1966;78:286.
77. Schreiner GE. Nephrotoxicity and diagnostic agents. J Am Med Assoc 1966;196:413.
78. Shapiro R. The effect of maternal ingestion of iophenoxic acid with serum protein bound iodine of the progeny. N Engl J Med 1961;264:378.
79. De Jonge GA. Vruchtbeschadiging door farmaca. Folia Med Neerl 1965;8:65.
80. Sanen FJ. Consideration of cholecystographic media. Am J Roentgenol 1962;88:797.
81. Sargent EN, Boswell W, Hubsher J. Cholecystokinetic cholecystography: efficacy and tolerance studies of ceruletide. Am J Roentgenol 1978;130:1051.
82. Nahum H, Desbleds M, Marsault C. Les accidents de la cholangiographie intraveineuse: résultats de l'enquête de la Société Française de Radiologie. J Radiol Electrol 1975;56:595.
83. Müller K, Jorge A. Rezidive akuter Pankreatitis nach Cholezystographie. Med Klin 1965;60:1693.
84. Sutherland LR, Edwards LA, Medline A et al. Meglumine iodipamide (Cholegrafin) hepatotoxicity. Ann Intern Med 1977;86:437.
85. Keighley MRB, Wilson G, Kelly JP. Fatal endotoxic shock of biliary tract origin complicating transhepatic cholangiography. Br Med J 1973;3:147.
86. Sakahira K, Ebata T, Tsunoday Y et al. Serum diatrizoate level during intraoperative cholangiography without choledochal obstruction. Dig Dis Sci 1990;35:1085—1088.
87. Gmelin E, Kramann B, Weiss H-D. Kontrastmittelzwischenfall bei einer endoskopischen retrograden Cholangiopancreatikographie. Münch Med Wochenschr 1977;119: 1439.
88. Lorenz R. Allergic reaction to contrast medium after endoscopic retrograde pancreatography. Endoscopy 1990;22:196.
89. Bilbao MK, Dotter CT, Lee TG et al. Complications of endoscopic retrograde cholangiopancreatography (ERCP): a study of 10,000 cases. Gastroenterology 1976;70:314.
90. Seibert DG, Al-Kawas FH, Graves J et al. Prospective evaluation of renal function following ERCP. Endoscopy 1991;23:355—356.
91. Shopner CE. Clinical evaluation of cystourethrographic contrast media. Radiology 1967;88:491.
92. Mihalecz K. Wölfer E, Czâszár J, Pintér J. Akute Niereninsuffizienz nach unilateraler retrograder Pyelographie. Z Urol Nephrol 1967;60:783.
93. Lytton B, Brooks MB, Spencer RP. Absorption of contrast material from urinary tract during retrograde pyelography. J Urol 1968;100:779.
94. Pagani JG, Hayman LA, Bigelow RH et al. Prophylactic diazepam in prevention of contrast media-induced seizures in glioma patients undergoing cerebral computed tomography. Cancer 1984;54:2200.
95. Chagnac Y, Hadani M, Goldhammer Y. Myasthenic crisis after intravenous administration of iodinated contrast agent. Neurology 1985;35:1219.
96. Kim SH, Park KH, Kim YI et al. Experimental tissue damage after subcutaneous injection of water soluble contrast media. Invest Radiol 1990;26:678—685.
97. Johnson LW, Krone R. Cardiac catheterization 1991: a report of the registry of the Society for Cardiac Angiography and Intervention Catheter. Cardiovascul Diagn 1993; 28:219—220.
98. Gross-Fengels W, Beyer D, Fischbach R. Akute Nebenwirkungen und Komplikationen der zentralvenösen DSA. Ergebnisse bei 2600 Untersuchungen. Med Klin 1991; 86:561—565.
99. Hesselink JR, Hayman LA, Chung JG et al. Myocardial ischaemia during intravenous DSA in patients with cardiac disease. Radiology 1984;153:577.
100. Hill JA, Winniford N, Cohen MB et al. Multi centre trial of ionic versus nonionic contrast media for cardiac angiography. Am J Cardiol 1993;72:770—775.
101. Kløw NE, Levorstad K, Berg KJ et al. Iodixanol in cardioangiography in patients with coronary artery disease. Tolerability, cardiac and renal effects. Acta Radiol 1993; 34:72— 77.
102. Parvez A, Moncada R, Messmore HL et al. Ionic and non-ionic contrast media interaction with anticoagulant drugs. Acta Radiol Diagn 1982;23:401.
103. Robertson HJE. Blood clot formation in angiographic syringes containing non-ionic media. Radiology 1927; 162:621.
104. Cohen AG, Kokko JP, Williams WH. Hemolysis and hemoglobinuria following angiography. Radiology 1969; 92:329.
105. Rao AK, Thompson R, Durlacher L et al. Angiographic contrast agent-induced acute hemolysis in a patient with hemoglobin SC disease. Arch Intern Med 1985;145:759.
106. Parry P, Rees JR, Wilde P. Transient cortical blindness after coronary angiography. Br Heart J 1993;70:563—564.
107. Snyder CF, Formanek A, Frech RS et al. The role of sodium in promoting ventricular arrhythmia during selective coronary arteriography. Am J Roentgenol 1971;113:567.
108. Druck MN, Johnstone DE, Staniloff H et al. Coronary artery spasm as a manifestation of anaphylactoid reaction to iodinated contrast material. Can Med Assoc J 1981;125:1133.
109. Editorial. Transfemoral cardiac catheterisation can cause fatal blood clots. J Am Med Assoc 1972;221:547.
110. Sewell R, Killen DA, Foster JH. Small bowel injury by angiographic contrast medium. Surgery 1968;64:459.
111. Stark FR, Coburn JW. Renal failure following methylglucamine diatrizoate (Renografin) aortography: report of a case with unilateral renal artery stenosis. J Urol 1966;96:848.
112. Mishkin MM, Baum S, Di Chiro G. Emergency treatment of angiography induced paraplegia and tetraplegia. N Engl J Med 1973;288:1184.
113. Junck L, Marshall WH. Fatal brain edema after contrast agent overdose. Am J Neuroradiol 1986;7:522.
114. Latchaw RE. The use of nonionic contrast agents in neuroangiography. A review of the literature and recommendations for clinical use. Invest Radiol 1993;(Suppl 5):555—561.
115. Mitsumori M, Hayakawa K, Abe M. E.C.G. changes during cerebral angiography: a comparison of low osmolarity contrast media. Eur J Radiol 1991;13:55—58.
116. Wishart DL. Complications in vertebral angiography in 447 studies. Am J Roentgenol 1971;113:527.
117. Jennett WB, Barker J, Fitch W et al. Effect of anaesthesia on intracranial pressure in patients with space-occupying lesions. Lancet 1969;i:61.
118. Brady AP, Hough DM, Lo R et al. Transient global amnesia after cerebral angiography with iohexol. Can Assoc Radiol J 1993;44:450— 452.

119. Harrington D, Amplatz K. Cholesterol embolism and spinal infarction following aortic catheterisation. Am J Roentgenol 1972;115:171.
120. Carroll SE, Wilkins WW. Two cases of brachial plexus injury following percutaneous arteriograms. Can Med Assoc J 1970;102:861.
121. Viville C, Gillet M, Reins R. Les complications de l'aortographie lombaire (ou aortographie directe) et leur prévention. J Radiol Electrol 1966;47:289.
122. Winding O. Intrinsic particles in angiographic contrast media. Radiology 1920;134:317.
123. Parvez A, Moncada R, Messmore HL et al. Ionic and non-ionic contrast media interaction with anticoagulant drugs. Acta Radiol Diagn 1982;23:401.
124. Albrechtsson U, Olison C-G. Thrombotic side-effects of lower- limb phlebography. Lancet 1976;i:723.
125. Gothlin J, Hallbrook T. Skin necrosis following extravasal injection of contrast medium at phlebography. Radiologe 1971;11:161.
126. Sellam R, Economou C, Amer M et al. Priapisme après cavernographie. Raport d'un cas original. Ann Urol 1988; 22:145.
127. Bookstein JS. Comment. Radiology 1990;174:286.
128. Tabbador K. Unusual complication of iophendylate injection myelography. Arch Neurol 1973;29:435.
129. Gupta SR, Naheedy MH, O'Hara RJ et al. Hydrocephalus following iophendylate injection myelography with spontaneous resolution: case report and review. Comput Radiol 1986;9:359.
130. Lieberman P, Siegle RL, Caplan RJ et al. Chronic urticaria and intermittent anaphylaxis: reactions to iophendylate. J Am Med Assoc 1976;236:1495.
131. Ahlgren P. Long term side effects after myelography with water soluble contrast media: Conturax, Conray meglumin 282 and Dimer-X. Neuroradiology 1973;6:206.
132. Hansen EB, Fahrenjrug A, Praestholm J. Late meningeal effects of myelographic contrast media with special reference to metrizamide. Br J Radiol 1978;51:321.
133. Rosati G, Leto DI, Priolo S et al. Serious fatal complications after inadvertent administration of ionic water-soluble contrast media in myelography. Eur J Radiol 1992;15:95—100.
134. Gelmers HJ. Adverse effects of metrizamide in myelography. Neuroradiology 1979;18:119.
135. Altschuler EM, Segal R. Generalised seizures following myelography with iohexol (Omnipaque). J Spinal Disord 1990;3:59—61.
136. Dalen K, Kerr HH, Wang A-M et al. Seizure activity after iohexol myelography. Spine 1991;16:84.
137. Belanger JG, Blair IG, Elder AM et al. Adult myelography with iohexol. J Can Assoc Radiol 1990;41:191—194.
138. Nyegaard & Co. Summarising notes from the Amipaque Symposium, 1977.
139. Richart S, Sartor K, Holl B. Subclinical organic psychosyndromes on intrathecal injection of metrizamide for lumbar myelography. Neuroradiology 1979;18:177.
140. Mejlhede A. Et tilfaelde med universelle krampeanfald efter lumbal myelografi med metrizamid (Amipaque). Ugeskr Læg 1979;141:2761.
141. Mallat Z, Vassal T, Naiuri JF et al. Aseptic meningitis after myelography. Lancet 1991;338:252.
142. Schlesinger JJ, Salit IE, McCormack G. Streptococcal meningitis after myelography. Arch Neurol 1982;39:576.
143. Numaguchy Y, Weems AM, Mizushima A et al. Myelography with metrizamide: effect of contrast removal on side-effects. Am J Neuroradiol 1986;7:683.
144. Robertson CH, Taveras JM, Tadmor R et al. Computed tomography in metrizamide cisternography: importance of coronal and axial views. J Comput Assisted Tomogr 1977; 1:241.
145. Hammeke TA, Haughton VM, Grogan JP et al. A preliminary study of cognitive and affective alterations following intrathecal administration of iopamidol or metrizamide. Invest Radiol 1984;19(Suppl):S268.
146. Broadbridge AT, Bayless SG, Firth R et al. Visual evoked response changes following intrathecal injection of water-soluble contrast media: a possible method of assessing neurotoxicity and a comparison of metrizamide and iopamidol. Clin Radiol 1984;35:371.
147. Muxi M, Pérez-Soler J, Alcon S et al. Presentación de dos casos di hiperplasia del tiroides, posiblemente desencadenada por la administractión de productos yodados en la aminografia previo a la T.l.U. Toko-Ginecol Práct 1972;31:79.
148. Soriano-Soriano C, Jiminez-Jiminez FJ, Egido-Herero JA et al. Acute encephalopathy following lumbar myelography with iohexol. Acta Neurol 1992;14:127—129.
149. Wallers K, Chaudhuri AKR et al. Severe meningeal irritation after intrathecal injection of iopamidol. Br Med J 1985;291:1688.
150. Glowinski J, Breuillard Ph, Delafolie A et al. Thrombose du sinus longitudinal superieur après sacroradiculographie au iopamidol. Rev Rhum 1986;53:183.
151. Lowrie SP, Ferguson GG. Spinal subdural empyema complicating cervical discography. Spine 1989;14:1415.
152. Lossef SV, Barth KH. Severe delayed hypotensive reaction after ethiodol lymphangiography despite premedication. Am J Roentgenol 1993;161:417—418.
153. Bork K, Hoede N. Paraneoplastische multizentrische Reticulohistiozytose: durch jodhaltige Röntgen-Kontrastmittel ausgelöst und provozierbar. Z Hautkr 1985;60:729.
154. Richardson P, Crosby EH, Bean HA et al. Pulmonary oil deposition in patients subjected to lymphography: detection by thoracic photoscan and sputum examination. Can Med Assoc J 1966;94:1086.
155. Fraimow W, Wallace S, Greening RR et al. Pulmonary function studies. Cancer Chemother Rep 1968;52:99.
156. Hallgrimson J, Clouse ME. Pulmonary oil emboli after lymphography. Arch Pathol 1965;80:426.
157. Koehler PR. Complications of lymphography. Lymphology 1968;1:116.
158. Rasmussen KE. Retinal and cerebral fat emboli following lymphography with oily contrast media. Acta Radiol Diagn 1970;10:199.
159. Engeset A. Dissemination of tumor cells by lymphangiography. In: Ruttmann E, ed. Proceedings, International Symposium on Lymphology, Zurich, 1966. Stuttgart: Georg Thieme Verlag, 1967;308.
160. Desmons M, Ramioul H. Perilymphatic spread of a melanoma of the foot after lymphography. J Radiol Electrol 1964;45:703.
161. Rayl JE. Clinical reactions following bronchography. Ann Otol Rhinol Laryngol 1965;74:1120.
162. Suprenant E, Wilson, A, Bennett L et al. Changes in regional pulmonary function following bronchography. Radiology 1968;91:736.
163. Davies AC, Keightley A, Borthwick-Clarke A et al. The use of a low-osmolality contrast medium in hysterosal-

pingography: comparison with a conventional contrast medium. Clin Radiol 1985;36:533.
164. Newberg AH, Munn CS, Robbins AH. Complications of arthrography. Radiology 1985;155:605.
165. Takebayashi S, Sugiyama M, Nagase M et al. Severe adverse reaction to I.V. gadopentate dimeglumine. Radiology 1993;160:659.
166. Sampson CB. Adverse drug reactions and drug interactions with radiopharmaceuticals. Drug Safety 1993;8:280–294.
167. Oldham R, Staab EV. Aseptic meningitis following the intrathecal injection of radio-iodinated serum albumen. Radiology 1970;97:317.
168. Giaffer MH. Tindale WB, Senior S et al. Anaphylactoid reaction associated with the use of ^{99m}Tc hexamethyl propylene amine oxime as a leukocyte labeling agent. Br J Radiol 1991;64:625- -626.
169. Støckel M, Ennow K, Kristensen K et al. Anaphylactic reactions to orthoiodohippurate. Eur J Nucl Med 1983;8:89.
170. James JM, Lloyd JJ, Leahy BC et al. The incidence and severity of hypoxia associated with 99Tcm Technigas ventilation scintigraphy and 99Tcm MAA perfusion scintigraphy. Br J Radiol 1992;65:403–408.
171. Ramos-Gabatin A, Orzel JA, Moloney TR et al. Severe systemic reaction to diphosphonate bone imaging agents: skin testing to predict allergic response and a safe alternative agent. J Nucl Med 1986;27:1432.
172. Oldham R, Staab EV. Aseptic meningitis following the intrathecal injection of radio-iodinated serum albumen. Radiology 1970;97:317.
173. Earnes B, Fish M. Chemical meningitis as a complication of isotope cisternography. Neurology 1971;21:426.
174. Perper EJ, Segall GM. Safety of dipyramidole-thallium in high risk patients with known or suspected coronary artery disease. J. Nuclear Med 1991;32:2107–2114.
175. Rhodes BA, Cordova MM. Adverse reactions to radiopharmaceuticals: incidence in 1978 and associated symptoms (Report of the Adverse Reactions Subcommittee of the Society of Nuclear Medicine). J Nucl Med 1980;21:1107.
176. Keeling DH, Sampson CB. Adverse reactions to radiopharmaceuticals: United Kingdom 1977–1983. Br J Radiol 1984;57:1091.
177. Coakley AJ, Mountford PJ. Nuclear medicine and the nursing mother. Br Med J 1985;291:159.
178. Andersson M, Juel K, Storm HH. Pattern of mortality among Danish Thorotrast patients. J Clin Epidemiol 1993; 46:637–644.

Meyler's Side Effects of Drugs, 13th Edition
M.N.G. Dukes, editor

SECTION EDITOR: P.I. FOLB

B.C.P. Polak

47 Drugs used in ocular treatment

GENERAL CONSIDERATIONS

The nature of risks Ophthalmic drugs may give problems of local tolerance, but with variable frequencies. They can induce pain on instillation, allergic reactions, delayed healing, punctate keratitis, disturbances of lacrimal secretion and disturbances of accommodation. These local problems may be responsible for poor patient compliance.

Eye drops are a specialized pharmaceutical formulation allowing concentration of the active drug in ocular structures; administration of a lower dose than would be necessary to obtain the same effect by systemic administration is needed. Eighty percent of the drug present in an eye drop however diffuses into the general circulation and by this way it may exert systemic effects, even at low concentrations (1[R]). The lacrimal pump is the essential route of diffusion from an eye drop into the systemic circulation, through active cellular absorption in the lacrimal secretory pathways. The active ingredient avoids the first-pass effect and reaches its site of action directly, resulting in an increased bioavailability. All the same, this form of treatment is generally very well tolerated, when one bears in mind the immense volume of eye drops prescribed by ophthalmologists each day.

The systemic effects exerted by eye drops are most pronounced in the case of agonists and antagonists of the autonomic nervous system. β-Blockers in eye drops can cause bronchospasm, heart failure, syncope and psychiatric disorders, especially at high doses and with non-selective β-blockers, though these adverse reactions are usually related to failure to comply with the prescribing precautions. α-Adrenergic agonists, which exert dose-dependent effects, can induce hypertensive crises or angina attacks. Except in patients at special risk (children under the age of 30 months and the elderly) *parasympathicomimetics* cause few systemic adverse effects (SEDA-16). *Anticholinesterases* which have curare-like properties are contraindicated for 6 weeks before general anesthesia. In the very young and the very old patient *atropinic* eye drops carry a risk of cardiovascular collapse and neuropsychiatric disturbances. Problems may also develop with *anti-infectives*, *antiseptics* and *contact lens products*.

Risk factors and risk reduction The *elderly* are particularly likely to make errors in the administration of ophthalmic medications, resulting in overdoses and adverse toxic effects or underdosage with inadequately controlled glaucoma (2[R]). This may be the result of impaired memory, mental confusion, impaired vision, hearing and mobility or a combination of these factors. It would be wise practice to assess both compliance and the administration technique of elderly patients to ensure the safe and effective use of ophthalmic preparations (SEDA-16).

A few simple rules can reduce the incidence of adverse effects and improve compliance:
(1) comply with the contraindications and precautions applicable to the drug;
(2) start with lower doses, especially in children and the elderly;
(3) never administer more than 30 μl of an eye drop at any time, and give it only into the superolateral corner of the eye;
(4) close the medial canthus with the finger after instillation of the eye drop.

CLASSIFICATION

Ophthalmic drugs are often classified broadly into diagnostic and therapeutic agents, but many such drugs are in fact used for both diagnostic and therapeutic purposes, and they will therefore be considered together in this chapter, broadly by pharmacological groups. Most of the drugs dealt with in this Chapter are actually applied to the eye; where the same drugs are also used by other routes of administration for other purposes, the adverse effects of such uses are dealt with in other chapters of this book.

In the latter part of this chapter, attention is devoted to a number of agents important as additives in ophthalmic preparations.

DIAGNOSTIC AND THERAPEUTIC OPHTHALMIC DRUGS

ANTIALLERGIC AGENTS

The common features of allergic conjunctivitis include pronounced itching, a mild conjunctival appearance, a stringy or ropey discharge and papillary hypertrophy of the tarsal conjunctiva in severe cases. There may be a family history of allergy. An IgE-mediated immediate hypersensitivity mechanism is associated with most types of allergic conjunctivitis, most frequently the result of exposure to airborne allergens.

Contact allergy is mediated by lymphocytes rather than antibodies. Seen with increasing frequency are external eye diseases related to contact lenses or prolonged use of ophthalmic medications. Treatment of allergic conjunctivitis is based on the diagnosis and severity of signs and symptoms. *Cromoglycate* (*cromolyn*), *Nedocromil and Levocabastine* (*levocab*) are available for topical ocular application, and the regimen of choice should be based on the response to milder forms of therapy and a consideration of adverse effects (see SEDA-18).

Sodium cromoglycate inhibits the release of pharmacologically active chemical mediators from sensitized cells and is effective when applied topically to mucous membranes in asthma and other atopic disorders. When applied topically to the eye it is effective in the treatment of vernal keratoconjunctivitis (vernal catarrh, spring catarrh), allergic conjunctivitis and hay fever. While no systemic or severe adverse reactions have been attributed to ocular sodium cromoglycate even after as such as 8 months of therapy, transient local stinging and burning have been reported in 13—77% of patients receiving the original formulation of this drug which contained 2-phenylethyl alcohol as a preservative. These effects regressed during continued treatment and may vary greatly depending on both the individual and the underlying disease. Ocular sodium cromoglycate without 2-phenylethyl alcohol has been reported to be more effective than preparations containing this preservative; stinging, leading to increased lacrimation, dilutes the drug and reduces the time it is retained in the conjunctival sac. Thus, the topical effects of sodium cromoglycate will be less if it is formulated with 2-phenylethyl alcohol.

Unpreserved 2% *nedocromil* sodium eye drops and placebo were used for 6 weeks in a double-masked comparative study of 45 patients with contact lens-associated papillary conjunctivitis. There was significantly less itching in the nedocromil sodium group compared with placebo, and biomicroscopic assessment showed a significant difference in the amount of mucus on the upper tarsal surface in favor of nedocromil sodium by the end of the study. In the nedocromil group, however, 21 patients had adverse effects, especially taste changes and/or stinging on application of the drops (16^C).

ANTISEPTIC AND ANTI-INFECTIVE DRUGS

Antibiotics and sulfonamides *(see also Chapters 25.1—5, 26, 27, 30 and 'Antiviral agents' and 'Preservatives' below)*

Various antibiotic eye drops and ointments are available including *aminoglycosides*, *chloramphenicol*, *fusidic acid*, *ofloxacin*, *oxytetracycline*, *polymyxin* and *rifamycin*.

Local adverse effects *Allergic* reactions may occur, but the incidence is low compared with the volume of prescriptions; these reactions consist of conjunctivitis, keratitis, palpebral and periocular eczema. Aminoglycosides are considered to be highly sensitizing. Modifications of the saprophytic flora by antibiotic treatment and selection of resistant strains may occur.

Local *irritation* occurs with all antibiotics, particularly sulfonamides and aminoglycosides.

Systemic effects Systemic chloramphenicol is hematotoxic, but this toxicity can also occur via the ocular route (see 'Individual drugs' below).

Individual drugs The hematological risks with *chloramphenicol* have long been recognized; the first death resulting from bone marrow aplasia induced by chloramphenicol eye drops was described in 1955 (11^c). In 1993 the American National Register of Drug Induced Ocular Side Effects had received reports of 23 patients with blood dyscrasias which might have been related to topical ocular administration of chloramphenicol (12^R).

Chloramphenicol causes two types of bone marrow toxicity: the first is a dose-related, reversible depression generally affecting erythroid cells and the second is an idiosyncratic reaction which affects all three cell lines and is generally fatal. Ocular chloramphenicol may cause this idiosyncratic reaction only in genetically predisposed patients. The overall risk of developing aplastic anemia after oral administration of chloramphenicol is 1:30 000 to 1:50 000, which is 13 times greater than the risk of idiopathic aplastic anemia in the population as a whole. Since topical administration achieves systemic effects by absorption through the conjunctival membrane or through drainage down the lacrimal duct with eventual absorption from the gastrointestinal tract, the risk may be similar to that after oral administration of the antibiotic.

It is difficult to justify subjecting patients to this potential risk in view of the availability of other antibiotics for use in the eye. In the United States the Physician Desk Reference emphasizes with repeated warnings the importance of not using ocular chloramphenicol unless there is no alternative, and this warning should be supported on both sides of the Atlantic (13^r).

Aminoglycosides, frequently used in ophthalmology to treat or to prevent bacterial infections, may be toxic for retinal structures if high concentrations are administered in the vitreous. Retinal ultrastructure was examined at various intervals following a single intravitreal injection of 100—4000 μg of gentamicin in rabbit eyes. Three days after injection of 100-500 μg, numerous abnormal lamellar lysosomal inclusions were observed in the retinal pigment epithelium (RPE) and in macrophages in the subretinal space. These changes were typical of drug-induced lipid storage and were comparable to inclusions reported in kidney and other tissues as manifestations of gentamicin toxicity. One week after similar injections focal areas of RPE necrosis and hyperplasia with disruption of outer segments appeared, but the inner segments and inner retina were intact. Doses of 800-4000 μg produced a combined picture of RPE/macrophage lipidosis within the first 3 days, with increasing superimposed inner retinal necrosis (20).

Sulfacetamide sodium (*Albucid*) in solutions stronger than 5% can cause burning and stinging, but this brief discomfort is usually tolerated without serious complaints. Sulfacetamide still compares favorably with the newer antibiotics since it is effective against superficial ocular infections caused by a variety of micro-organisms. Serious allergic reactions may develop after ocular treatment (2^R).

The *sulfonamides* have a bacteriostatic rather than a bactericidal action. Many local anesthetics used in the eye are esters of *p*-aminobenzoic acid and such drugs will interfere with the action of sulfonamides. To obtain the maximum effect from instillation of sulfonamide eye drops, these drugs should therefore not be used until the effect of the local anesthesia disappears.

Antiviral drugs *(Certain drugs listed below are also discussed in Chapter 14 or Chapter 29.2)*

Antiviral drugs for topical ocular use are *aciclovir* (*Zovirax*), *idoxuridine* (*IDU*) and *trifluorothymidine* (*TFT*).

Aciclovir can also be given systemically, especially to treat stromal disease, uveitis anterior and posterior and to eradicate the virus from the trigeminal ganglion and other reservoirs. There is also evidence that it may be effective against herpes zoster. Various local adverse effects have been reported, including pruritus, burning sensations and irritative or allergic conjunctivitis. Superficial punctate keratitis, delayed epithelial healing and epithelial dysplasia may develop. TFT is twice as potent as IDU and gives excellent results in herpetic ulcers previously treated with topical steroids and in IDU-unresponsive ulcers (SED-12, 1203).

Idoxuridine (*iododeovuridine*, *IDU*) can be used to treat superficial keratitis; the poor results in deep stromal diseases are due to the poor solubility of the drug. Idoxuridine is unstable, cannot eliminate the virus from the eye, is locally toxic, especially in dry-eye patients due to its increased concentration (or decreased tear solution), and is topically sensitizing. Drug allergy and toxicity may have an incidence as high as 5—8%. Lacrimal punctum stenosis, lacrimation, follicular conjunctivitis, narrowing of meibomian gland orifices, inhibition of keratocyte mitosis and corneal stromal repair, and a decrease in the strength of healing corneal wounds and in the rate of epithelial regeneration are observed (21). After prolonged administration many changes in the conjunctival and corneal epithelium may occur, such as conjunctival cicatrization, punctate keratitis, subepithelial and intra-epithelial edema and corneal opacities. Idoxuridine may also induce the emergence of resistant virus strains (22^C).

Trifluridine (*trifluorothymidine*, *TFT*, *F3-TDR*) is twice as potent as (and 10 times more soluble than) idoxuridine in 1% solution. Trifluridine has been reported to heal dendritic keratitis faster than idoxuridine, to be as effective as vidarabine when used five times a day, to have no cross-toxicity with idoxuridine or vidarabine, to heal stromal corneal defects more effectively than idoxuridine, and to produce topical allergy, punctal narrowing and punctal keratitis only rarely. Furthermore, trifluridine gives excellent results in herpetic ulcers previously treated with topical steroids and in idoxuridine-unresponsive ulcers. Allergic reactions, however, may occur.

Vidarabine (*ara-A*, *adenine arabinoside*) is oncogenic and mutagenic in animals, whilst its rapid inactivation and poor solubility are practical disadvantages. Vidarabine has proved effective in the treatment of kerato-uveitis in animals and man, and may be used intravenously to treat herpetic kerato-uveitis in man. It is effective in herpetic keratitis unresponsive to idoxuridine, has a low toxicity and no cross-allergenicity.

Other anti-infective and antiseptic drugs

All antiseptics can cause local irritation and allergy, and may cause the emergence of resistant bacteria. Treatment with nitrates and phenylmercuryl acetate may cause band-shaped corneal opacities ([1]R). The case of a severe iodine-induced thyrotoxicosis in a patient who had been using iodine-containing eye drops for more than 10 years has been reported (14[c]).

Argyrosis has occurred in many patients treated with *silver nitrate*. Several cases of chemical burns of the eyes in newborn babies have been reported, but most of these complications followed incorrect administration of the preparation.

β-ADRENERGIC BLOCKERS

β-Adrenergic receptor blockers are successfully used as ocular tension-lowering drugs without notable effects on pupillary size or refraction. Systemic effects are greater than one would expect since there is no first-pass effect with ocular administration and the plasma concentration can therefore attain therapeutic levels. *Timolol* (*Timoptol*, *Timoptic*), *metipranolol and levobunolol* (*Betagan*) are non-selective β_1- and β_2-adrenoreceptor blockers. *Betaxolol hydrochloride* (*Betoptic*) is a relatively cardioselective β_1-adrenoreceptor blocking agent; Selective β-blockers block β_1-adrenoreceptors at concentrations below those required to block β_2-adrenoreceptors in the bronchi; in low doses, therefore, they may be less likely to precipitate bronchospasm. This and other systemic effects can nevertheless occur (SED-12, 1201).

β-Blockers are generally well tolerated following topical application to the eye, but adverse systemic reactions may occasionally be severe enough to require discontinuation of the drug.

Local adverse effects *Dry eyes* have been reported after the systemic or ocular use of timolol. Usually transitory sensations of dry eyes develop, and a reduction in the Schirmer test and tear film break-up time may occur. Symptomatic superficial punctate keratitis in association with complete corneal anesthesia has been observed.

Systemic effects Of the possible adverse reactions attributable to β-blockers, 50—70% are systemic side effects, which may be idiosyncratic and non-dose-related and the same as those seen with any oral β-adrenergic receptor blocking agent.

Cardiovascular effects can be prominent. Hemodynamic changes after the topical ocular use of β-blocking agents sometimes include only small decreases in heart rate and resting pulse rate, and insignificant reduction in blood pressure. However, patients with cardiovascular disorders, especially those with an irregular heart rate and dysrhythmias, are certainly at risk. Bradycardia, cardiac arrest, heart block, hypotension, palpitations, syncope, cerebral ischemia and cerebrovascular accidents may occur.

The *pulmonary system* can be susceptible: these drugs can aggravate or precipitate bronchospasms and potentially life-threatening respiratory failure may occur.

It is not surprising to find the *nervous system* being involved in adverse reactions to ophthalmic β-blockers, since central nervous system effects are well recognized complications of β-blockers in general. Lightheadedness, mental depression, weakness, fatigue, acute anxiety, dissociative behaviour, disorientation and memory loss may develop a few days to some months after initiating timolol therapy. Central nervous system complaints are more common in patients with the greatest reduction in intraocular pressure. Patients may be unaware of the symptoms until the medication is stopped.

Endocrine effects can occur: one should be aware of the possibility of hypoglycemia in insulin-dependent diabetics with masking of the tachycardia that otherwise provides a warning. Conversely, in diabetic patients treated with oral antidiabetics hyperglycemia may develop due to an enhanced decrease of the insulin secretion.

Of *miscellaneous* systemic effects which have been described, sexual impotence is a recognized but rare complication of β-blockers given systemically, which also may be experienced with ophthalmic treatment. Aggravation of myasthenia gravis has been observed during ophthalmic timolol therapy. Bilateral pigmentation of the finger- and toe-nails, marked hyperkalemia and arthralgia following ocular timolol have all been reported (SED-12; 6[c]).

Interactions Any of the interactions associated with systemically administered β-blockers can in principle occur when eyedrops are used. Administration of β-blockers in eyedrops should clearly be avoided in patients receiving systemically administered β-adrenergic receptor antagonists.

Risk factors Because their long-term effects are unknown β-adrenergic receptor blockers should be used with caution in infants and, if possible, avoided during pregnancy and lactation. If topical β-blockers have to be used in asthmatic patients or in patients with a past history of bronchial asthma, careful monitoring is essential. To exclude the risk of precipitating glaucoma in a susceptible individual, gonioscopy is recommended before starting local β-adrenergic receptor blocking therapy. Eyes with potential angle closure require a miotic and should not be treated with β-blocking agents alone. Tachyphylaxis may develop after a short period of treatment.

It has been shown that a genetic fault in the oxidative

metabolism of β-blockers may be detected in some patients, and there are significantly higher plasma levels in these poor metabolizers, who are at greater risk of developing systemic effects (23^R).

Individual drugs In 165 patients treated with *timolol* in a 0.5% concentration, adverse effects were reported in 23% of cases, including psychiatric effects (39.5%), cardiovascular effects (18.6%), respiratory effects (7%) and local effects (25.6%) (5^R). A 'rebound' tachycardia has been reported after withdrawal of ophthalmic timolol therapy (24). Amaurosis fugax has been reported in association with topical timolol, as has severe hyperkalemia, confirmed by rechallenge. With *Betaxalolol*, the relative absence of β_2-adrenergic inhibition reduces the incidence of some systemic effects; in particular it has been found to be better tolerated in patients with compromised pulmonary systems, in whom timolol and levobunolol have been shown to reduce pulmonary function by 25—30%.

CORTICOSTEROIDS *(see also SEDA-18, 169, 190)*

Corticosteroids administered alone

Since corticosteroids reduce the immunological defenses of the body to most types of infection, their use in the eye should be monitored carefully. It should be stressed that excessive use of corticosteroids may result in corneal herpes infection and mycosis.

The ophthalmological follow-up of patients using topical corticosteroids should include at least twice a year repeated tonometry, careful slit-lamp examination for early signs of herpetic or fungal keratitis and for changes in the equatorial and posterior subcapsular portions of the lens, examination of pupillary size and lid position, and staining of the cornea for possible punctate keratitis. Blood glucose concentrations should be checked if there are symptoms which suggest hyperglycemia.

Local adverse effects The ocular effects which may develop after local or systemic administration of steroids include *cataracts*, *glaucoma*, *papilledema*, *pseudotumor cerebri*, *activation of corneal infections*, *superficial keratitis*, *ptosis*, *pupillary dilatation*, *conjunctival palpebral petechiae*, *uveitis and scleromalacia*. Topical ocular application, but also facial application, may give rise to high corticosteroid concentrations in the anterior compartment of the eye. Serious *visual loss* may occur owing to the development of cataract in patients using corticosteroid creams.

It may be noted here that steroid creams applied topically to the skin are routinely used in the treatment of many skin disorders, and their use on the face in severe atopic eczema is relatively common. Three patients developed advanced *glaucoma* while using topical facial steroids. Two other patients have been described with ocular hypertension secondary to topical facial steroids (17^c).

Systemic effects Precautions should be taken in administering systemic corticosteroids to patients with diabetes, congestive heart failure, peptic ulcers, systemic hypertension, glaucoma and tuberculosis. Systemic adverse effects do not generally occur with limited topical administration to the eye.

Individual drugs *Medrysone*, *fluorometholone* and *tetrahydroxytriamcinolone* have been shown to have a topical inflammatory effect with a reduced propensity to crease intraocular pressure. Methylprednisolone acetate provides a source of steroid that lasts for up to 2 weeks.

Clobetasone butyrate eye drops with or without neomycin have been found to be as effective as betamethasone with or without neomycin, respectively. Clobetasone butyrate has been reported to be less prone to raise intraocular pressure.

Corticosteroid and antibiotic combinations

The use of steroid + antibacterial combinations is illogical and should generally be avoided because of the possibility of resistant bacterial strains emerging. It would be highly advisable if prescriptions for these drugs were issued by ophthalmologists only, at least in those parts of the world where adequate medical services are available.

CYCLOPLEGICS AND MYDRIATRICS

Anticholinergic agents *(see also Chapter 13)*

By counteracting the effects of the parasympathetic nervous system these drugs induce passive pupillary dilatation by paralysis of the iridial sphincter, suppress accommodation by paralysis of the ciliary muscle and increase the vascular permeability of the iris and ciliary bodies. Anticholinergics are used for diagnostic and refractive purposes, and in combination with other drugs as part of the treatment of several serious ocular conditions, including inflammatory states.

The main agents are *atropine*, *homatropine and hyoscine* (*scopolamine*) as well as synthetic molecules, such as *cyclopentolate* (*Cyclogyl*) *and tropicamide* (*Mydriaticum*).

Local adverse effects All anticholinergic agents can induce acute *closed angle glaucoma* in patients with an anatomical predisposition. They also cause *photophobia* and *disturbances of accommodation* leading to difficulties in reading and driving.

Systemic effects The occurrence of peripheral as well as central unwanted reactions is mainly dose-dependent. The unwanted peripheral effects of all atropine-like drugs include *flushing of the skin, dryness of the mucous membranes with fever, tachycardia, decreased salivary secretion and dryness of the mouth, drying up of the gastrointestinal secretions and decreased gastric acidity, decreased muscle tone in the gut and constipation*. Bladder tone and frequency of micturition are decreased and acute *urinary retention* is a risk, especially in older men. Nasal, bronchial and lacrimal *secretions* are decreased.

Central nervous system effects include confusion, excitement, hallucinations, sedation and tachypnea. The state of excitement is followed by increasing drowsiness, stupor and general central depression. When the drug is not stopped there is a risk of coma with cardiovascular collapse or even death (SED-12; 1[R]). These complications essentially occur in children and in the elderly; they are dose-dependent, but there is a certain degree of individual susceptibility. Serious effects may be countered using physostigmine.

Individual drugs When using *atropine*, systemic toxicity may be decreased by using 0.5% rather than 1% solutions; the lower concentration should always be used in children. Hypersensitivity reactions can occur, usually in the form of contact dermatitis and conjunctival redness. *Cyclopentolate* is a short-acting cycloplegic with a rapid onset (and considerable intensity) of action, which particularly in children has been reported to cause hallucinations and psychotic episodes (25). It has been suggested that a partial structural affinity of the side-chain to some hallucinogens aggravates the problems associated with this drug. *Eucatropine*, being a relatively weak cycloplegic, may be better tolerated in the elderly and patients with glaucoma. With *hyoscine*, bradycardia is more likely than tachycardia, and central stimulation only rarely precedes depression. Idiosyncratic reactions are more common than with atropine, but contact dermatitis is less likely to occur (21). *Tropicamide* tends to have a greater mydriatic than cycloplegic effect. Allergic reactions can occur (21).

ENZYMES *(see also Chapter 33)*

Chymotrypsin

Chymotrypsin has been used for enzymatic zonulolysis during operations for cataract. The possible role of this enzyme in precipitating postoperative intraocular hypertension has been studied, but the use of enzymatic zonulolysis does not seem to increase significantly the risk of glaucoma.

Chrondroitin sulfate-hyaluronate sodium (Viscoat)

Sodium chondroitin sulfate and other viscoelastic substances have been shown to protect the corneal endothelium during intraocular surgery (see also 'Hyaluronic acid'). Viscoat itself is currently used in corneal transplant preservation media. One of the major complications noted with the use of viscoelastic substances during cataract surgery is the potential for increased intraocular pressure following the operation. Chondroitin sulfate has been reported to be relatively less likely to precipitate such extreme elevations in intraocular pressure because it is cleared rapidly from the trabecular meshwork. However, with any new technique or chemical used in surgery there is always the potential for an unexpected side effect, and recent publications suggest that Viscoat is no exception, the risks perhaps including subepithelial calcium deposits and keratopathies (26[r]).

Hyaluronic acid (hyaluronate sodium, Healon)

Hyaluronate sodium is a high-molecular weight substance originally developed as a vitreous replacement. Although 98% of the product consists of water, it is very viscoelastic. The drug is considered to have low inflammatory and antigenic potential, and has been employed in various intraocular procedures. In addition to filtration bleb formation, it has been used to protect the corneal endothelium during intraocular lens implantation and keratoplasty, to reform the anterior chamber, to push back a bulging vitreous face, and in retinal detachment surgery as a vitreous replacement.

Certain mechanical problems may occur with its use, although these are not true side effects. The major side effect associated with the use of hyaluronate sodium has been a transient rise in intraocular pressure in the immediate postoperative period, attributed to its viscoelastic nature, resulting in coating and plugging of the trabecular meshwork. For this reason, it is advisable to dilute hyaluronate sodium at the end of the surgical procedure with a balanced salt solution.

LOCAL ANESTHETICS *(see SEDA-17, 542)*

The anesthetics applied topically to the eye for diagnostic or surgical purposes are *oxybuprocaine* (*benoxinate, Novesin, Dorsacaine, ambucaine*), *cocaine*, *tetracaine*

(*Pontocaine*), *and Proparacaine* (*Ophthaine*, *proxymetacaine*).

Use of local anesthetics creates the risk of dual toxicity of both the agent itself and the added preservative. Non-preserved anesthetics should be used when examining an eye in which a penetrating or perforating injury is suspected and during intraocular procedures if surface anesthesia is required.

Abuse of topical ocular anesthetics is a serious disorder, causing persistent epithelial defects. It is generally accepted that frequent use of topically applied ocular anesthetics causes poor healing of epithelial defects, leading to corneal stromal infiltration. Loss of the epithelial barrier may set the stage for infection and permanent corneal scarring. Increased pain in the otherwise anesthetic cornea may induce the patient to apply anesthetic drops more and more frequently, rendering the withdrawal of the anesthetic in some patients impossible without administration of large doses of analgesics. The patient who abuses ocular anesthetics may appear with a corneal abrasion, recurrent erosion, or similar surface disease. Careful questioning will generally yield a diagnosis. Sometimes hospitalization or even tarsorrhaphy may be required for diagnostic purpose after withdrawal of all topical medication (9[c], 10[c]).

Local adverse effects Topical anesthetics may *alter lacrimation and tear film stability* and cause *direct epithelial toxicity*. *Endothelial toxicity* may occur in the case of penetrating or perforating injuries. Furthermore, the agent and its vehicle may both serve as a reservoir of *microbial contamination*, with the potential for infection. Especially benoxinate in combination with sodium fluorescein (Fluocaine; Fluress) may be easily contaminated, particularly with *Pseudomonas aeruginosa* (SEDA-17, 543).

Interactions Topical anesthetics cause loosening of the desmosomal area of cell—cell adhesion, resulting in a more permeable epithelial cell layer. When this occurs other pharmaceutical agents are more able to penetrate this normally poorly permeable layer.

Anesthetics also reduce the reflex secretion of tears, causing an increase in the length of time required for tear washout. This allows topically applied agents to be in contact with the epithelial surface for a prolonged period of time.

Systemic effects Both idiosyncratic and allergic reactions may occur. Stevens-Johnson syndrome may be caused or exacerbated by topical anesthetics.

Individual drugs With *cocaine*, poisoning can occur with doses as small as 20 mg (10 drops of cocaine 4%). Victims generally collapse and die after associated cardiovascular abnormalities, dysrhythmias and respiratory failure. Signs and symptoms of intoxication include excitement, restlessness, headache, nausea, vomiting, abdominal pain, convulsions and delirium. *Oxybuprocaine* (*benoxinate*, *Novesin*, *Dorsacaine*, *ambucaine*) causes little punctate epithelial staining and is therefore useful during applanation tonometry; this popular topical anesthetic has an additional advantage in that it possesses bactericidal properties. Serious loss of vision due to keratitis following abuse of benoxinate has been described (14[C]). Its usage and prescription should be subject to strict guidelines.

Instillation of *tetracaine*, a popular topical anesthetic used in ophthalmology, may cause a burning sensation; the initial discomfort is less severe if the eyes are closed after instillation. The transitory presence of tiny superficial corneal epithelial lesions is commonly noted after tetracaine anesthesia. Although local allergy to tetracaine may develop because of repeated use, such reactions are extremely uncommon (15[C]).

Instillation of *proparacaine* is considerably more comfortable than the use of tetracaine. Proparacaine causes much less stinging and squeezing of the lids and is often completely painless. Patients allergic to tetracaine are not necessarily allergic to proparacaine and vice versa.

For discussion of the side effects of *lidocaine* and *procaine*, see Chapter 11.

PARASYMPATHICOMIMETIC DRUGS

Traditional 'direct-acting' cholinergic drugs used for many years in antiglaucomatous therapy are *acetylcholine* (used for its brief effect during ophthalmic surgery) and *carbachol* (having a strong and longer-lasting effect since it is not destroyed by cholinesterases). The modern direct parasympathicomimetics include *aceclidine*, which again has a short duration of action. Cholinesterase inhibitors act indirectly by inhibiting the enzyme; they have included *pilocarpine*, *ecothiophate iodide*, *prostigmine*, *eserine and DFP* (*dyfios*); they are naturally only effective in the presence of acetylcholine and they have a longer duration of action.

The ocular action of the direct and indirect parasympathicomimetics is identical: they increase the flow rate of aqueous humor across the trabeculum, decrease the resistance to its flow and consequently lower the intraocular pressure.

Local adverse effects The expected and inevitable effects of parasympathicomimetic eye drops are more intense in myopic and young patients, *causing aggravation of the myopia*, *blurred vision and periorbital pain* due to congestion of the iris and ciliary body. Anterior and posterior synecchiae may develop. *Allergic reac-*

tions have also been reported as well as epithelial toxicity. The anticholinesterases have caused pseudopemphigoid reactions in the eyelids and occlusion of the lacrimal puncta (SED-12, 1198; 7[r]). The danger of a miotic agent inducing *retinal detachment* is directly proportional to the capacity of the drug to produce spasm of the ciliary body. Retinal detachments have been reported after the use of cholinergic agents, but they may also be coincidental.

Systemic effects The commonest effects are headache and periorbital pain. Signs of vagal stimulation may be observed with nausea, vomiting, sweating, hypersalivation, lacrimation, hypotension, bradycardia, bronchial constriction, respiratory failure and nightmares. These reactions essentially occur during intensive treatment for acute closed angle glaucoma, requiring frequent instillations of pilocarpine. The elderly and young children are at particular risk.

Interactions During induction of general anesthesia the presence of anticholinesterase activity in the serum may potentiate the effect of curare-like drugs such as suxamethonium, used as muscle relaxants, with prolonged apnea after intubation and death. Such eye drops should be stopped 6 weeks before the operation (8[c]).

The importance of inquiring about the use of drugs cannot be overemphasized. Patients often do not regard antiglaucomatous eye drops as 'medication' and omit this information from their medical history. Complaints of excessive sweating, intermittent diarrhea, muscle weakness and fatigue over a long period may be due to the usage of echothiopate eye drops (phospholine iodide 0.25%) for glaucoma and may disappear when the eye drops are withdrawn (27[C]). Topically applied anticholinesterase eye drops or exposure to organophosphate insecticides can reduce the amount of plasma cholinesterase and pseudocholinesterase, creating a potentially fatal hazard for surgical patients receiving succinylcholine.

SYMPATHICOMIMETIC DRUGS

Sympathicomimetics are used to produce mydriasis for ophthalmoscopic evaluation. Mydriasis is not maximal as with the anticholinergic mydriatics, but especially in younger patients sympathicomimetic mydriasis is quite effective and causes little or no disturbance of accommodation. Sympathicomimetic agents are also used as vasoconstrictors in surgical procedures, for symptomatic relief of allergic reactions and hyperemia of the conjunctiva, and to lower intraocular pressure in open angle glaucoma. *Epinephrine* (*adrenaline*), *phenylephrine*, *dipivefrin*, *naphazoline and tetrahydrozoline* are the drugs available. *Clonidine and p-aminoclonidine* eye drops have been introduced more recently.

Local adverse effects *Allergic* reactions can occur with all adrenergic agonists.
Melanic conjunctivocorneal *pigmentation* has been reported with an incidence of 30% with epinephrine, but not with dipivefrin.

Conjunctival *irritation* and a feeling of ocular burning can occur, as well as reactive conjunctival *vasodilatation* following the initial vasoconstriction (1[R]).

Acute closed-angle *glaucoma* during mydriasis is an uncommon event with sympathicomimetics.

Retinopathy (cystoid macular edema) has been reported to occur in 2.8% of the patients receiving epinephrine and exceptionally with dipivefrin, especially in aphakic or pseudophakic eyes (3[R]).

Systemic effects Systemic toxicity can result from topical application: *headache*, *blood pressure elevation*, *extrasystoles*, *tachycardia*, *faintness* and *cerebrovascular accidents* have been reported. The incidence of adverse effects is high with 10% phenylephrine, but is less with lower concentrations; this applies to all drugs of this class. It should be noted that phenylephrine is in some countries available in a non-prescription concentration of 0.12% for use as an ocular decongestant. Patients with contraindications to phenylephrine should be instructed to consult their physician before using these preparations. Phenylephrine should be used cautiously in the elderly and in patients with hypertension, coronary heart disease, aneurysms and diabetic autonomic neuropathy. There is also a clear *interaction* problem: patients on medications with pressor effects, such as monoamine oxidase inhibitors, tricyclic antidepressants and anticholinergic agents should be monitored closely if phenylephrine is to be used (SEDA-16, 542).

Individual drugs With *para-aminoclonidine*, headaches, attributable to ocular vasoconstriction, as well as anxiety, vomiting, dry mouth, tremor and pallor have been reported (4[c]). With *phenylephrine*, several cases of allergic blepharoconjunctivitis have been seen, even at low concentrations; the reaction begins 3–4 hours after drug application, persists for 12 hours, and regresses gradually within 72 hours (28). Biopsy of the conjunctiva reveals marked infiltration with cells of various types; there is some evidence that a sensitization mechanism is involved. The 10% solution has sometimes caused extremely severe cardiovascular complications, even including myocardial infarction. In newborn infants the benefit of accurate assessment of gestational age by examination of the anterior vascular capsule of the lens and the value of funduscopic examination in ill premature babies must be weighed against the possible risks of the associated increase in blood pressure produced by the pupillary dilators. Since there is no increase in mydriatic effect with repeated instillation or increasing concentration, and their small body mass places premature neonates at increased risk of phenylephrine overdose, it seems prudent to use the lowest possible concentration, as well as the most effective combination of mydriatics for indirect ophthalmoscopy in premature infants where such examination is absolutely necessary. Again with phenylephrine it should be noted that the hypertensive effect is likely to be maximal at some time within the first 20 minutes, and wherever possible (or where risk factors are present) the blood pressure should be monitored.

Potential advantages of *dipivefrine* (dipivalylepinephrine; DPE; Propine), which is an adrenaline prodrug include greater duration of action, increased bioavailability, greater potency, greater stability and reduced incidence of side effects, compared with standard preparations. The effect on pupil size is insignificant, no objective sight threatening effects are observed, and central visual acuity and visual fields are not affected after application of a 0.1% solution of dipivefrine into the eye. However, minor sporadic and transient burning or stinging sensations may be experienced.

As noted above, cystoid macular edema of the retina has been seen after the use of dipiveprin, but it may be noted that in the classic case described in 1982 (29[C]) pretreatment with timolol maleate might have predisposed the eye to this complication.

Tetryzoline (tetrahydrozolin), an α-adrenergic agent with vasoconstrictor and decongestant properties, is widely available without prescription for symptomatic relief of 'pink eye' and is found in various products in a 0.05% concentration.

Tetryzoline eye drops are considered safe when used appropriately in the eye. However, relatively small amounts can produce profound central nervous depression and can lead to serious toxicity, especially in children under 2 years of age. A Poison Center reported 64 cases of tetryzoline poisoning over a period of 3 years; ingestions accounted for 59 cases, but three were attributable to administration into the eye, ear or nose. It is important that these products be kept safety out of reach of children.

Similar reactions in young children have been reported with other sympathicomimetics sometimes on free sale, such as *naphazoline*, commonly known by such trade names as Privine, Clear Eyes, Naphcon and Vaso Clear, and *oxymetazoline*, commonly present in Afrin, Duration, and Neo-Synephrine 12 hour.

MISCELLANEOUS ANTIGLAUCOMATOUS DRUGS

In addition to various drugs already reviewed above which are used in glaucoma a number of others are or have been employed in this condition.

Guanethidine (*see also Chapter 20*)

Guanethidine, an adrenergic neuron-blocking agent, is useful in cases of glaucoma, chemical sympathectomy, ptosis and eyelid retraction. The reduction in intraocular pressure is small. In general, tissues treated topically with guanethidine become sensitized to sympathicomimetic acting drugs. This is useful in glaucoma therapy where adrenaline may be administered in low dosage in combination with guanethidine. After instillation of guanethidine-containing eye drops, conjunctival hyperemia and stinging have been described.

Carbonic-anhydrase inhibitors (*see also Chapter 20*)

Carbonic-anhydrase inhibitors cause a reduction in aqueous formation and may therefore be useful in certain cases of glaucoma. These drugs should be used with caution in the long-term control of glaucoma because of their serious systemic side effects.

The incidence and severity of many adverse reactions to carbonic-anhydrase inhibitors are dose-related and usually respond to lowering of the dosage or withdrawal of the drug. Symptoms of depression, confusion, fatigue, impotence, irritability, malaise, nervousness and weight loss are often present to some extent in patients on long-term acetazolamide or methazolamide therapy (Table 1). These symptoms may be related to systemic metabolic acidosis (due to renal excretion of bicarbonate) which is often accompanied by a decrease in serum potassium levels (30[R]). Gastrointestinal intolerance, manifested as abdominal cramping, dyspepsia and nausea with or without diarrhea, is another common problem. Carbonic-anhydrase inhibitors decrease the urinary excretion of citrate and uric acid, which may lead to renal calculi and gouty arthritis. Pulmonary edema, taste disorders and alopecia have also been associated with carbonic-anhydrase inhibitors.

The most serious side effect of carbonic-anhydrase inhibitors is bone marrow depression. Complete blood cell counts should be performed prior to initiation of carbonic-anhydrase inhibitor therapy, at least once during the first 6 months and at intervals of every 6 months thereafter.

Risk factors Carbonic-anhydrase inhibitors should

be used with caution in patients with respiratory acidosis or those with severe loss of respiratory capacity, and in patients with diabetes mellitus. Carbonic-anhydrase inhibitors are contraindicated in patients with hepatic disease or insufficiency, depressed serum concentrations of sodium or potassium, and in those with adrenocortical insufficiency, hyperchloremic acidosis, or severe renal disease or dysfunction. These drugs should also not be administered to patients receiving salicylates or to pregnant women, especially in the first trimester.

Osmotic agents

The commonly recognized complications of osmotic agents used in patients with acute closed-angle glaucoma are mild headache, neck pain, nausea and vomiting; the intravenous agents urea, mannitol and sodium ascorbate present the added risk of thrombophlebitis. The postgastrectomy patient should be treated cautiously with oral glycerol, as should patients with heart failure or advanced liver disease.

MISCELLANEOUS THERAPEUTIC AND DIAGNOSTIC AGENTS

Artificial tears

Allergic reactions may occur. Tear-film break-up time may be increased 4-fold.

Indomethacin

Indomethacin in eye-drop form may cause burning sensations, pruritus, local congestion and irritation, corneal epithelial changes and edema of the eyelids (18[c]).

Silicone oil

The use of silicone oil injection in the treatment of retinal detachment with massive periretinal proliferation has been found to induce macular attachment in a high percentage of treated patients. There is no difference in the success rate between phakic and aphakic eyes. The filling of the vitreous cavity with silicone oil, however, may cause *changes in refraction*. Complications attributed to intraocular silicone oil include *cataract*, *keratopathy* and *glaucoma*. Of 103 phakic eyes, 73% developed lens opacities after 1—3 years, 87% after 3—5 years, and 90% after 5 years or longer. Few of these cataracts were however sufficiently dense to require surgery, and those that did were managed with intra- or extracapsular lens extraction without difficulty.

Keratopathy developed in nine eyes, and in two of these penetrating keratoplasty was undertaken successfully. In 16 eyes persistently raised intraocular pressure (greater than 25 mmHg) occurred; although silicone oil was found to be present in the chamber angle on gonioscopy in 33% of the cases, in only six eyes was raised intraocular pressure associated with oil in the anterior chamber.

ADDITIVES, EXCIPIENTS AND STAINING AGENTS

PRESERVATIVES USED IN EYE DROPS AND CONTACT LENS SOLUTIONS

The ocular risk related to the use of contact lenses is not only due to the lenses themselves, but also to the toxic or allergic effects of cleaning solutions (19[r]) and the preservatives which they contain. The latter are also found in various eyedrops. Preservatives are known to exert toxic side effects on the corneal epithelium and endothelium. Preservative-containing eye drops should not be used in patients with ocular surface disease, in cases of perforating injury or during surgery.

Cases of allergic conjunctivitis and blepharitis have been reported with the preservatives *benzalkonium chloride* and *mercurial salts*, though benzalkonium at the commonly used concentration of 0.01% produces no evident damage. These adverse reactions can be prevented by rinsing hard lenses in clean water before insertion in the eye and by boiling soft lenses in normal saline after cleaning.

The use of mercurials on the eye may lead to a bluish gray deposit of mercuric oxide on the eyelids, conjunctivae and Descemet's layer. Phenylmercuric nitrate used in a 0.004% concentration may lead to mercuria lentis. Mercurial compounds have been found in the aqueous humor, having penetrated the eye from hydrophilic-gel contact lenses preserved with thiomersal. Although it remains to be established whether deposition of mercury in the eye is clinically important, the concentrations found are similar to those reported with systemic poisoning by organic mercurials (31[r]).

Thiomersal is more soluble and stable than the older mercurials. It does not influence tear-film wetting of cornea or contact lenses, or the stability of the tear film itself. Thiomersal has been known to cause both a blepharoconjunctivitis and a punctate keratitis in contact lens wearers which may be attributed incorrectly to allergies.

Allergic reactions caused by thiomersal preservative have also been reported.

Chlorhexidine digluconate is a biguanide surfactant with low toxicity, but it is a strong contact sensitizer. Its mucus-binding capacity limits its use: it binds to hydrophilic (soft) contact lenses. Build-up of proteinaceous debris in lenses may greatly increase the binding of chlorhexidine to the lens.

Use of *chlorobutanol* is limited to pH levels below 6. It is subject to thermal degradation and may be adsorbed on to the walls of containers. It is however without major toxic effects. Chlorobutanol has no effect on wetting of cornea or contact lenses, as do surface-active agents. When tested with soft lenses, chlorobutanol, concentrated in the lenses, causes mild conjunctivitis.

STAINING AGENTS

Fluorescein *(See also Chapter 49)*

Local use Contamination of fluorescein eye drops is a very serious risk. *Pseudomonas aeruginosa* is an especially dangerous pathogenic micro-organism liable to invade fluorescein eye drops. Fluorescein is most safely dispensed in sterile single-dose units or as sterile fluorescein-impregnated paper strips.

Fluorescein transiently stains the skin and mucous membranes yellow.

Systemic use The majority of the systemic reactions following intravenous fluorescein in fluorescein angiography are allergic, but some may be due to contamination with dimethylformamide, an industrial solvent (32[C]). The most frequent side effect is nausea; urticaria, hypersalivation, rhinorrhea and chills have been seen in a few cases.

It is difficult to predict side effects to fluorescein by intracutaneous testing of the drug. Reactions once experienced tend to recur following subsequent intravenous injection. Serious or fatal accidents during fluorescein angiography were assessed by an international survey involving 594 687 angiographies. The incidence of fatal accidents was one case per 49 557 angiographies, and of non-fatal but serious accidents one case per 18 020 angiographies. The total number of accidents reported was 45 cases, equal to one per 13 215 angiographies. Age, general health of the patients and the experience of the different clinics which perform this examination may influence the frequency and the severity of these accidents (33[R]).

Indocyanine green

Indocyanine green, successfully used for infrared angiography of the choroidal vessels, is well tolerated intravenously and the side effects are less pronounced than those following intravenous fluorescein.

Methylene blue

Methylene blue is somewhat irritant, and topical anesthesia is recommended before its use. Prolonged systemic exposure to methylene blue may cause the fundus to turn visibly blue (34[C]).

Rose bengal

Discomfort and irritation are more pronounced with rose bengal than with fluorescein. Discoloration of the skin of the patient's eyelids and the examiner's fingers as well as ocular staining are more persistent than when fluorescein is used (21[R]).

VEHICLES USED IN FORMULATIONS

The vehicles included in modern ophthalmic medicines increase the viscosity of the agent, help to maintain the drug in solution or suspension, and are thought to stay longer on the exterior of the eye, leading to a longer contact time and possibly greater absorption of the drug than is the case with a simple aqueous solution (2[R]).

Methylcellulose

Methylcellulose is a useful vehicle in eye drops and contact lens solutions; it is non-irritating and has a good refractive index. A 1% solution is well retained in the conjunctival sac. Corneal cultures have been stimulated by methylcellulose, resulting in increased growth of cells. Tear-film break-up time was increased 4-fold with 2% methylcellulose.

Petrolatum-mineral oil

Petrolatum-mineral oil ointment is retained longer on the eye than other vehicles. The large molecules of the petrolatum-mineral oil-base ointment are not easily removed by blinking, and a component of the corneal tear film is a non-polar oil. The fact that ointments are oil bases and non-polar explains why they are readily absorbed by the pre-corneal and conjunctival tear films. To maintain drug contact with the eye, patching is recommended (2[R]).

Polyvinyl alcohol

Polyvinyl alcohol (PVA), a synthetic long-chain alcohol, has been used as a component of various ophthalmic drug vehicles. If one wishes to retain clear vision and retain longer drug contact with the eye, PVA is superior to saline. PVA has good drug compatibility and it acts as a wetting agent, lowering surface tension; at a concentration of 1.4% it does not interfere with corneal wound healing (2[R]).

REFERENCES

1. Hugues FC, le Jeunne C. Systemic and local tolerability of ophthalmic drug formulations. Drug Safety 1995;8:365—380.
2. Anand KB, Beizer JL. Extraocular effects of ophthalmic drugs in the geriatric patient. Geriatr Med Today 1990; 9:15—23.
3. Larricart P. Les affections retiniennes. In Raspiller et al, eds. Les effets indesirables de medicaments en ophtalmologie. Bulletin des Societes d'Ophtalmologie de France, rapport annuel, 1985;193—211.
4. Abraham D, Robin A, Pollack I, de Faller J, de Santis L. The safety and efficacy of topical 1% ALO 2145 (*p*-aminoclonidine hydrochloride) in normal volunteers. Arch Ophthalmol 1987;105:1205—1207.
5. McMahon D, Shaffer RN, Hoskins HD, Hetherington J. Adverse effects experienced by patients taking timolol. Am J Ophthalmol 1979;88:736—738.
6. Diggory, P, Cassels-Brown A, Vail A, Abbey LM, Hillman JS. Avoiding unsuspected respiratory side-effects of topical timolol with cardioselective or sympathicomimetic agents. Lancet 1995;345:1604—1606.
7. Fellman RL, Starita RJ. Ocular and systemic side effects of topical cholinergic and anticholinesterase drugs. In: Sherwood and Spaeth, eds. Complications of Glaucoma Therapy. Thorofare: Slack Inc., 1990;6—18.
8. Everitt DE, Avorn J. Systemic effects of medications used to treat glaucoma. Ann Intern Med 1990;112:120—125.
9. Rosenwasser GOD, Holland S, Pflugfelder SC. Topical anesthetic abuse. Ophthalmology 1990;97:967—972.
10. Henkes HE, Waubke TN. Keratitis from abuse of corneal anaesthetics. Br J Ophthalmol 1978;62:62.
11 Rosenthal RL, Blackman A. Bone marrow hypoplasia following the use of chloramphenicol eye drops. J Am Med Assoc 1955;191:36—37.
12 Fraunfelder FT, Morgan RL, Yunis AA. Blood dyscrasias and topical ophthalmic chloramphenicol. Am J Ophthal 1993;115:812-813.
13. Doona M, Walsh JB. Use of chloramphenicol as topical eye medication: time to cry halt? Br Med J 1995;310:1217—1218.
14. Andre F, Bielefeld P, Besancenot JF, Belleville I, Sgro C. Fausse inocuite des collyres: a propos d'une observation de thyrotoxicose induite par l'iode, Therapie 1988;43:431—432.
15. Bernstein JA, Bernstein IL. Cromolyn and nedocromil, novel anti-allergic drugs. Immunol Allergy Clin North Am 1993;13:891—902.
16. Bailey CS, Buckley RJ. Nedocromil sodium in contact lens-associated papillary conjunctivitis. Eye 1993;7(Suppl): 29—33.
17. Aggarwal RK, Potamitis T, Chong NHV, Guarro M, Shah P, Kheterpal S. Extensive visual loss with topical facial steroids. Eye 1993;7:664—666.
18. Pichon P, Moreau G. Complications corneennes par usage de collyre a l'indometacine. Bull Soc Ophtalmol France 1990;90:449—451.
19. Polak BCP, Beekhuis WH. Risk and safety of contact lenses. Int J Risk Safety Med 1990;1:219—223.
20. D'Amico DJ, Libert J, Kenyon KR. Retinal toxicity of intravtireal gentamycin. Invest Ophthalmol Visual Sci 1984;25:564.
21. Havener WH. Ocular Pharmacology, 4th edn. St Louis: C.V. Mosby, 1978.
22. Lass JH, Thoft RA, Dohlman Ch. Idoxuridine-induced conjunctival cicatrization. Arch Ophthalmol 1983;101:747.
23. Fraunfelder FT. Ocular beta-blockers and systemic effects. Arch Intern Med 1986;146:1073.
24. Nelson WL, Fraunfelder FT, Sills JM, Arrowsmith JB Kuritsky JN. Adverse respiratory and cardiovascular events attributed to timolol ophthalmic solution, 1978—1985. Am J Ophthalmol 1986;102:606.
25. Khurana AK, Ahluwalia BK, Rajan C, Vohra AK. Acute psychosis associated with topical cyclopentolate hydrochloride. Am J Ophthalmol 1988;105:91.
26. Coffman MR, Mann PM. Corneal subepithelial deposits after use of sodium chondroitin. Am J Ophthalmol 1986;102:279.
27. Alexander WD. Systemic side effects with eye drops. Br Med J 1981;282:1359.
28. Geyer O, Yust I, Lazar M. Allergic blepharoconjunctivitis due to phenylephrine. J Ocul Pharmacol 1988;4:123.
29. Mehelas TJ, Kollarits CR, Martin WG. Cystoid macular edema presumably induced by dipivefrin hydrochloride (Propine). Am J Ophthalmol 1982;94:682.
30. Fraunfelder FT, Meyer SM. Systemic adverse reactions to glaucoma medications. Int Ophthalmol 1989;29:143.
31. Burstein NL. Corneal cytotoxicity of topically applied drugs, vehicles and preservatives. Surv Ophthalmol 1980; 25:15.
32. Jacob JSH, Rosen ES, Young E. Report on the presence of a toxic substance, dimethyl formamide, in sodium fluorescein for fluorescein angiography. Br J Ophthalmol 1982;66:567.
33. Zografos L. Enquête internationale sur l'incidence des accidents graves ou fatals pouvant survenir lor d'une angiographie fluorescéinique. J Fr Ophthalmol 1983;6:495.
34. Flewellen EH. Hazards of intravenous indigo carmine, fluorescein and methylose blue. Tex Med 1980;76(10):49.

Meyler's Side Effects of Drugs, 13th Edition
M.N.G. Dukes, editor

E. Ernst and P.A.G.M. De Smet

48 Risks associated with complementary therapies

INTRODUCTION

In most industrialized countries the prevalence of complementary (the frequently-used term 'alternative' is inappropriate and should be abandoned) medicine (CM) is high and still growing. In the US every third individual uses some form of CM (1) and in Europe the prevalence ranges from 24% in The Netherlands to 49% in France (2). The reasons for this popularity are diverse but to a large extent they represent a criticism of the content and style of modern mainstream medicine.

The effectiveness of CM is largely unknown and more definitive evidence is urgently needed (3). For responsible therapeutic decision making such information has to be complemented by safety data. One of the foremost claims of the proponents of CM is that it is natural and hence harmless; this, of course, is *not* true and dangerously misleading. Like other types of medicine, CM can be *directly* harmful (i.e. through adverse effects of a herbal drug) or *indirectly* harmful (i.e. through being applied incompetently) or harmful through causing needless expense (4). Some would also argue that injudicious use of ineffective CM leads to injury because the application of appropriate treatment is delayed, but this naturally applies in the case of some orthodox medical treatments as well.

The potential health risks (i.e. not the financial risks) will be discussed below and the following therapies will be considered: (a) phytomedicines; (b) homeopathy; (c) other unconventional drugs; (d) acupuncture; (e) manipulation.

INDIRECT RISKS

Even a perfectly safe remedy (mainstream or unorthodox) can become unsafe when applied incompetently. Medical competence can be defined as doing everything in the best interest of the patient. There are numerous situations, both in orthodox and complementary medicine where competence is jeopardized (Table 1). The only way to minimize incompetence is proper education and training combined with responsible regulatory control. While training and control are self-evident features of mainstream medicine they are often not fully incorporated in CM. Thus the issue of indirect health risk is particularly pertinent to CM. Whenever complementary practitioners take full responsibility for a patient, this should be matched with full medical competence; if on the other hand, competence is not demonstrably complete, the healer in question should not assume full responsibility (5).

The indirect risks of CM are grossly under-researched, and at present we can but guess the size of the problem (6). There is, however, one particular aspect where some data does exist: the *attitude of practitioners towards immunization*. The majority of homeopaths (7–9) and chiropractors (10) are unconvinced of the benefit of immunization. They claim that it causes more illness than it prevents disease and advise, in many instances successfully, their patients against it (11).

This attitude not only exposes individual patients to unjustifiable risks but also jeopardizes herd immunity which develop into a threat to the health of the population at large. A homeopathic remedy might be totally safe, but the homeopath might not be (12)! Further data in related areas are urgently required (6).

DIRECT RISKS

There are several possibilities of direct risks through complementary drug therapies (Table 2). While we have at least some data on certain of these aspects, others (like drug interactions) represent almost a white spot on the map of medical science (4, 13).

Table 1. *Indirect risks of complementary medicine*

Missed diagnoses
Misdiagnoses
Disregarding contraindications
Preventing/delaying more effective therapy
Clinical deterioration not diagnosed
Adverse reaction to therapy not diagnosed
Discontinuation of prescribed drugs
Self-medication

Table 2. *Direct risks associated with drugs used in complementary medicine*

Allergic reactions
Toxic effects
Interactions with concomitant medications
Contamination
False authentication
Lack of quality control

PHYTOMEDICINES

In principle, drugs derived from plants can elicit the same types of adverse reactions as synthetic drugs (Table 3)—the body has no way of distinguishing between 'natural' and man-made compounds. Usually phytomedicines are more complex, containing more than one potentially active molecule. Herbalists therefore claim that a 'synergy' can exist between several active constituents leading to a desired effect. Although there are examples of synergy (14), little evidence exists for this actually happening. Theoretically the synergy could, of course, also apply to adverse effects, rendering herbal preparation potentially more hazardous than single compound drugs.

Type A reactions are usually readily recognisable but type C, B and D reactions will often be missed. Contrary to the belief of most herbalists, long-standing experience is therefore by no means a reliable yardstick when it comes to judging the risk of adverse reactions.

Table 3. *Types of adverse reactions to herbal remedies*

Type	Characteristic	Example
A	Pharmacologically predictable, usually dose dependent	Drowsiness after administration of kava-kava
B	Idiosyncratic, not pharmacologically predictable, not dose dependent	Hypersensitivity
C	Pharmacologically predictable, develop gradually during long-term use	Slowed bowel function after prolonged use of herbal laxatives
D	Effects with a latency period of months or years	Carcinogenic effects of the *Aristolochia* species

The following is not an exhaustive compilation of the literature on adverse effects of herbal remedies. Instead, the more pertinent and newer data have been collected, primarily on the basis of information already published in previous editions of this handbook and the corresponding Annuals. Plants with well-known toxicity (e.g. herbs with anticholinergic belladonna alkaloids) have not generally been excluded, but only concise information is given in such cases. Priority has been given to adverse reactions to remedies which are not readily found in pharmacological handbooks.

***Achillea millefolium* (yarrow)**

This material can produce contact dermatitis; a generalized eruption following the drinking of yarrow tea has also been reported.

***Aconitum* species (aconite)**

Aconite roots can produce serious heart failure due to the presence of toxic alkaloids, such as aconitine. Among the other symptoms of aconite poisoning are numbing of mouth and tongue, gastrointestinal disturbances, muscular weakness, incoordination and vertigo (15). A recent review from Hong Kong reports 17 cases of aconite poisoning after the administration of Chinese herbal mixtures (SEDA-18, 1). The toxicity of raw aconite can be decreased substantially by decoction, as this process leads to a change in alkaloid composition (16).

***Acorus calamus* (sweet flag)**

Commercial calamus preparations have yielded mutagenic effects in bacteria, while calamus oil (Jammu variety) has been shown to be carcinogenic in rats; as studies on the calamus constituent, β-asarone in calamus rhizomes and their volatile oils varies considerably with the botanical variety: high levels in triploid calamus from Eastern Europe and no detectable level in the diploid North American variety (SEDA-12, 408).

***Adonis vernalis* (pheasant's eye)**

Due to the presence of cardioactive glycosides, digitalis-like effects and potentiation of digitalis toxicity are possible.

Aescin

This complex mixture of triterpene saponins is prepared from the seeds of *Aesculus hippocastanum* (horse chestnut) and consists of a water-soluble fraction (α-aescin) and a water-insoluble fraction (β-aescin). The latter has been repeatedly associated with acute renal failure, when given intravenously in massive doses. Whether such effects can also occur after oral administration is unclear, as animal studies have shown a poor absorption of β-aescin from the gastrointestinal tract.

***Allium sativum* (garlic)** *(SED-12, 1214; SEDA-16, 546)*

Topical exposure can lead to allergic contact dermatitis or burn-like skin lesions (17), and occupational inhalation of garlic powder can lead to asthma (18). A case of spontaneous spinal epidural hematoma resulting in paraplegia in an 87-year-old patient was attributed to the chronic, excessive intake of garlic cloves (19).

Allyl isothiocyanate

This is the major component of the volatile oils of *Armoracia rusticana* and *Brassica nigra* seeds (see separate entries). This compound is a potent irritant and shows mutagenic activity in bacterial testing, as well as fetotoxic and carcinogenic potential in rats. However, as allyl isothiocyanate also occurs in ordinary mustard, it would not be realistic to ban all botanical drugs containing this compound, which commonly provide no more than a normal daily dose of mustard (e.g. 5 mg allyl isothiocyanate per 5 grams of mustard).

***Aloe* species**

These contain laxative anthranoid derivatives (see separate entry). Large doses are claimed to cause nephritis and use during pregnancy is discouraged, since intestinal irritation might lead to pelvic congestion. Aloe is thought to aggravate hemorrhoids.

***Ammi majus* (greater ammi)**

Injudicious use of the fruit in combination with skin exposure to the sun can cause severe phototoxic dermatitis due to the presence of psoralens (20).

***Ammi visnaga* (toothpick ammi)**

Prolonged use or overdosing of the fruit may produce nausea, dizziness, constipation, loss of appetite, headache, pruritus and sleeping disorders.

***Anisodus tanguticus* (Zangqie)**

This traditional Chinese herbal medicine contains hyoscyamine and related toxic tropane alkaloids (4).

***Anthemis* species**

See entry on 'chamomile'.

***Anthoxanthum odoratum* (sweet vernal grass)**

Rich in coumarin (see separate entry).

Anthranoid derivatives *(SEDA-13, 453)*

These occur primarily in various laxative herbs (such as aloe, cascara sagrada, medicinal rhubarb and senna) in the form of free anthraquinones, anthrones, dianthrones and/or *O*- and *C*-glycosides derived from these substances. They produce harmless discoloration of the urine. Depending on intrinsic activity and dose, they can also produce abdominal discomfort and cramps, nausea, violent purgation, and dehydration. They can be distributed into breast milk, but not always in sufficient amounts to affect the suckling infant. Long-term use may result in electrolyte disturbances and in atony and dilation of the colon.

Several anthranoid derivatives (notably the aglycones aloe-emodin, chrysophanol, emodin, and physcion) show genotoxic potential in bacterial and/or mammalian test systems (e.g. SEDA-12, 409), and two anthranoid compounds (the synthetic laxative danthrone and the naturally occurring 1-hydroxyanthraquinone) have shown carcinogenic activity in rodents [Drug Saf]. In a recent epidemiological study, chronic abusers of anthranoid laxatives (identified by the detection of pseudomelanosis coli) showed an increased relative risk of 3.04 (95% confidence interval of 1.18—4.90) for colorectal cancer (21). More studies are still needed to clarify this issue, if only to exclude the possibility that chronic constipation per se might increase the risk for colorectal cancer and would thus act as a confounding factor. Pending the results of such studies, the German health authorities have restricted the indication of herbal anthranoid laxatives to constipation which has not responded to bulk-forming therapy (which rules out their inclusion in slimming aids). In addition, the German authorities have imposed restrictions to the laxative use of anthranoid-containing herbs (e.g. not to be used for more than 1—2 weeks without medical advice, not to be used in children under 12 years of age, and not to be used during pregnancy and lactation) (21, 22).

See also the entries on *Cassia* species and on *Rubia tinctorum*.

***Arctostaphylos uva-ursi* (bearberry)**

The reputed antibacterial activity of bearberry is ascribed to the urinary metabolite hydroquinone, which is excreted in the form of inactive conjugates and needs an alkaline urine to be liberated. As the urine of people on a Western non-vegetarian diet is usually acidic, it is sometimes suggested that one should alkalinize the urine of bearberry users with sodium bicarbonate. However, as the dosage recommended for this purpose is usually high, this carries well-known risks such as a high sodium load and interference with the renal clearance of certain other drugs.

The urine of patients taking bearberry may darken on standing. Toxic reactions to bearberry have not been reported, except for an anomalous case of dyspnea, cyanosis, and skin reactions following the intake of an aqueous decoction (23). However, recent reports of carcinogenicity of hydroquinone following prolonged administration of high doses to rats or mice raise a question about the long-term safety of *Arctostaphylos uva-ursi* and other medicinal herbs containing substantial amounts of arbutin (4).

***Areca catechu* (areca, betel)**

A substantial part of the world's population chews betel nut quid, a combination of areca nut, betel pepper leaf (from *Piper betle*), lime paste and tobacco leaf. The major alkaloid of the areca nut, arecoline, can produce cholinergic side effects (such as bronchoconstriction) (24) as well as antagonism of anticholinergic agents (25). Under the influence of the lime in the betel quid, arecoline hydrolyzes into arecaidine, a central nervous system stimulant which accounts, together with the essential oil of the betel pepper, for the euphoric effects of betel quid chewing. The use of the areca nut is widely implicated in the development of oral cancers, and it has been documented that the saliva of betel nut chewers contains nitrosamines derived from areca nut alkaloids (26).

***Aristolochia* species**

Plants belonging to the genus of *Aristolochia* are rich in aristolochic acids and aristolactams. Aristolochic acid I and aristolochic acid II are mutagenic in several test systems. A mixture of these two compounds was found to be so highly carcinogenic in rats that even homeopathic *Aristolochia* dilutions have been banned from the German market. The closely related aristolactam I and aristolactam II have not been submitted to carcinogenicity testing, but these compounds show mutagenic activity in bacteria as well. Aristolochic acids have been demonstrated to pass into human breast milk. Massive intravenous doses of aristolochic acids result in renal toxicity, sometimes even in fatal nephrosis.

In Belgium, an outbreak of nephropathy in 70 individuals has been attributed to a slimming preparation that supposedly included the Chinese herbs *Stephania tetrandra* and *Magnolia officinalis*. Analysis showed that the root of *Stephania tetrandra* (Chinese name 'Fangji') was in all probability substituted or contaminated with the root of *Aristolochia fangchi* (Chinese name 'Guang fangji') (27, 28). The nephropathy was characterized by extensive interstitial fibrosis with atrophy and loss of the tubules (29). At least one patient showed evidence suggestive of urothelial malignancies (30).

***Armoracia rusticana* (horseradish)**

This contains 0.05—0.2% of essential oil consisting for 85% of allyl isothiocyanate (see separate entry). Abdominal discomfort and convulsive syncope were observed following the ingestion of raw horseradish which had not been properly aired before use (31).

***Arnica montana* (mountain arnica)**

The flowers contain skin-sensitizing sesquiterpene lactones, which can cross-react with related allergens in other medicinal plants. Ingestion of tea prepared from *Arnica* flowers can result in gastroenteritis. Large oral doses of undiluted *Arnica* tincture are said to produce various serious symptoms.

***Artemisia absinthium* (wormwood)**

The volatile oil is used to flavor the alcoholic liqueur absinthe, which can damage the nervous system and cause mental deterioration. This toxicity is attributed to thujone (a mixture of α- and β-thujone), which constitutes 3—12% of the oil, which in its turn attains concentrations of 0.25—1.32% in the whole herb. Alcoholic extracts and the essential oil are forbidden in most countries.

***Artemisia cina* (wormseed)**

This contains the toxic lactone, santonin, which was formerly used as an anthelminthic, but has now been superseded by other less toxic anthelminthics.

***Artemisia vulgaris* (common wormwood)**

The herb contains 0.03—0.3% essential oil with variable composition. Depending on origin, 1,8-cineole, camphor, linalool and thujone may all be major components. Allergic skin reactions (32) and abortive activity have been described.

***Asclepias tuberosa* (pleurisy root)**

Due to the presence of cardioactive glycosides, digitalis-like effects and potentiation of digitalis toxicity may occur. Interference with assays of the plasma digoxin level is also possible (33).

***Asperula odorata* (sweet woodruff)**

Rich in coumarin (see separate entry).

***Atropa belladonna* (deadly nightshade)**

This contains toxic tropane alkaloids (see separate entry).

***Azadirachta indica* (neem tree)**

Margosa oil, which is extracted from the seeds, has been implicated as a potential cause of Reye's syndrome.

Barberry

'Barberry' is a vernacular name for *Berberis vulgaris* (European barberry), but may also refer to the *Berberis* species, *M. Mahonia aquifolium* and *nervosa*. In the United States, only the latter species have had official status as a source of barberry, but *B. vulgaris* is said to serve similar medicinal purposes and to contain similar principles. Its root bark yields the quaternary isoquinoline alkaloid, berberine (see separate entry), and several other tertiary and quaternary alkaloids. The literature sometimes cautions that barberry alkaloids may cause arterial hypotension.

Berberine

'Berberine' is a major alkaloid in the root bark of *Berberis vulgaris*, the bark of *Mahonia aquifolium* and *M. nervosa*, and the root of *Hydrastis canadensis*. Secondary sources claim that berberine has produced toxic effects in a medical setting, but fail to provide details about the administered dose and route of administration. This is unfortunate since berberine is a quaternary base and may thus be poorly absorbed from the gastrointestinal tract. In a trial on the effect of berberine in acute watery diarrhea, oral doses of 400 mg were well tolerated, except for complaints about the bitter taste and a few instances of transient nausea and abdominal discomfort. However, patients with cholera given tetracycline plus berberine, were more ill, suffered longer from diarrhea and required larger volumes of intravenous fluid than those given tetracycline alone (34).

Berberis vulgaris

See entry on 'barberry' above

***Blighia sapida* (akee)**

The unripe fruit of this tree has a high level of a potent hypoglycemic amino acid, known as 'hypoglycin A'. Animal experiments have shown that this compound is teratogenic.

***Brassica nigra* (black mustard)**

External application of preparations from black mustard has declined because of skin irritation. The mustard oil derived from the seeds consists largely of allyl isothiocyanate (see separate entry).

***Bryonia alba* (white bryony)**

This is a drastic laxative and emetic, which contains toxic cucurbitacins.

***Callilepis laureola* (impila)**

Callilepis contains the toxic compound atractyloside and related compounds. The plant is responsible for the deaths of many Zulu people in Natal, who use its roots as a herbal medicine. Post-mortem analysis has revealed hepatic and renal tubular necrosis (SEDA-13, 454).

Canthaxanthin *(SED-12, 1216; SEDA-16, 546)*

Canthaxanthin is an orange carotenoid which naturally occurs in fruits and vegetables, mushrooms, shellfish, algae and other forms of marine life. It has been approved by the US Food and Drug Administration as a food coloring agent. It is also being promoted as a skin-tanning agent in oral doses supplying larger amounts than would be normally consumed as a food additive. Unlike certain other carotenoids, canthaxanthin is not a precursor of vitamin A, and therefore does not carry the risk of hypervitaminosis A. Retinopathy due to deposition of the substance in the retina, which is seen as gold-yellow deposits around the macula, and one case of canthaxanthin-associated aplastic anemia has been reported (35).

***Capparis spinosa* (caper plant)**

The leaf and fruit of *Capparis spinosa* both contain isothiocyanates. Allergic contact dermatitis following their application in the form of wet compresses has been reported (36).

***Capsicum annuum* (chili pepper)**

Capsaicinoids, such as capsaicin, produce an intense burning sensation when they come in contact with the eyes or the skin.

***Cassia* species (senna)**

The leaves and fruits of *Cassia angustifolia* and *Cassia senna* contain laxative anthranoid derivatives (see separate entry). Mutagenicity testing of sennosides has produced negative results in several bacterial and mammalian systems, except for a weak effect in *Salmonella typhimurium* strain TA102 (37, 38). No evidence of reproductive toxicity of sennosides has been found in rats and rabbits (39). When a standardized preparation containing senna pods (providing 15 mg of sennosides per day) was given to breast-feeding mothers, the suckling infants were only exposed to a non-laxative amount of rhein, which remained a factor 10^{-3} below the maternal intake of this active metabolite (40). A well-defined purified senna extract was not carcinogenic, when administered orally to rats in daily doses up to 25 mg/kg for 2 years (41).

Exceptional complications of senna abuse include hepatitis as well as finger clubbing and hypertrophic osteopathy.

***Catha edulis* (khat)**

The chewing of khat leaves results in subjective mental stimulation, physical endurance, increase of self-esteem and social interaction. Until recently, this habit was confined to Arabian and East African countries, because only fresh leaves are active, but due to increased possibilities of air transportation, khat is now also chewed in other parts of the world. Tachycardia and increased blood pressure, irritability, psychosis and psychic dependence have been described as adverse effects. Although cathine (=norpseudoephedrine) is quantitatively the main alkaloid, the amphetamine-like euphorigenic and sympathicomimetic cardiovascular effects of khat are primarily attributed to cathinone (42). Khat chewing by a breast-feeding mother can lead to the presence of cathine in the urine of the suckling child (SEDA-13).

***Cephaelis acuminata* (ipecac)**

Ipecac syrup contains the toxic alkaloids, cephaeline and emetine. When it is used as an emetic or in accidental poisoning, serious adverse effects are usually absent. However, misuse by anorectic and bulimic patients has resulted in severe myopathy, lethargy, erythema, dysphagia, cardiotoxicity and even death (SEDA-11, 422).

Chamomile

This is the vernacular name of *Chamomilla recutita* and *Anthemis* spp. The latter are more potent skin sensitizers (delayed-type) than the former, presumably because they can contain a higher level of the sesquiterpene lactone, anthecotullid. This allergic compound is present, at low levels, in only one of four chemotypes of *C. recutita*. Cross-sensitivity with related allergenic sesquiterpene lactones in other plants is possible.

Internal use of chamomile tea preparations has been associated with rare cases of anaphylactic reactions (43) and their applications as an eye-wash can cause allergic conjunctivitis (44).

Chamomilla recutita

See entry on 'Chamomile'

***Chelidonium majus* (celandine)**

A number of alkaloids have been detected in the herb and root, including chelidonine, chelerythrine, sanguinarine and berberine (see separate entry). Some authors caution that its use in children should be discouraged because of an early fatal colitis in an almost 4-year-old boy has been observed (45); however, this report does not provide convincing evidence that the victim had indeed taken *C. majus*. One case of hemolytic anemia following the oral use of a celandine extract was reported (46).

***Chenopodium ambrosioides* (American wormseed)**

Chenopodium oil contains the toxic principle, ascaridole, which was formerly used as an anthelminthic, but has now been superseded.

***Chrysanthemum vulgaris* (common tansy)**

This contains essential oil with neurotoxic thujone in such amounts that even normal doses may be toxic.

***Citrullus colocynthis* (colocynth)**

The dried pulp of the fruit is a drastic laxative, which contains toxic cucurbitacins. Pseudomembranous colitis secondary to ingestion of colocynth has been reported.

***Conium maculatum* (poison hemlock)**

Hemlock contains the poisonous piperidine alkaloid, coniine, and related alkaloids. It has well-established teratogenic activity in certain animal species.

***Convallaria majalis* (lily of the valley)**

As cardioactive glycosides are present in this herb, digitalis-like effects and potentiation of digitalis toxicity are believed to be possible.

***Convolvulus scammonia* (Mexican scammony)**

The resin is a drastic purgative with irritant properties, which has now been superseded.

***Coriaria arborea* (tutu)**

The tutu plant is a traditional Maori medicine. Ingestion of portions or concoctions of the plant can result in grand mal convulsions, respiratory arrest, and death. The responsible toxin, tutin, is allied to the picrotoxin group (47).

Coumarin

The plant lactone coumarin (not to be confused with coumarin anticoagulants) is a major constituent of tonka beans (the seeds of *Dipteryx odorata* and *Dipteryx oppositofolia*) and the dried herb of sweet clover (*Melilotus officinalis*). It is devoid of anticoagulant activity, but the molding of sweet clover can increase the hemorrhagic potential of this herb by transforming coumarin to the anticoagulant dicoumarol. This transformation could explain a case of abnormal clotting function and mild bleeding after the drinking of a herbal tea prepared from tonka beans, sweet clover and several other ingredients. Unfortunately, this possibility was not investigated, as the reporting physician was not aware of the exact phytochemistry and pharmacology of coumarin-yielding plants.

Coumarin has hepatotoxic potential in man, when taken in daily doses of 25—100 mg (48). Bile-duct carcinomas have been reported to occur in rats fed coumarin, but the correctness of this diagnosis has been seriously criticized.

***Crataegus* species (hawthorn)**

Although *Crataegus* extracts do not contain digitalis-like glycosides, potentiation of digitalis activity has been reported to occur in guinea-pigs. This study has been challenged, however, and further investigations are needed to establish whether *Crataegus* preparations can enhance digitalis toxicity.

***Crocus sativus* (saffron)**

The stamens have been used primarily as a coloring and flavoring agent. No risks have been documented for daily doses up to 1.5 grams, but 5 grams are toxic, 10 grams are abortive and 20 grams are a lethal dose.

***Crotalaria* species**

These plants have hepatotoxic potential due to the presence of pyrrolizidine alkaloids (see separate entry).

Croton tiglium

Croton oil has a violent purgative action and contains tumor-promoting phorbol diesters.

***Cyamopsis tetragonolobus* (cluster bean)**

Guar gum, which comes from the endosperm of the seeds, has been repeatedly associated with esophageal obstruction (SEDA-14, 445). Interference with the absorption of other drugs has also been reported.

***Cycas circinalis* (false sago palm)**

The seeds contain the non-protein amino acid α-*N*-methylamino-L-alanine. Monkeys fed on this amino acid have been shown to develop a syndrome closely resembling amyotrophic lateral sclerosis (ALS) and parkinsonism dementia (PD). There is some preliminary evidence to suggest that the use of poultices prepared from cycad seeds as a topical cure for skin lesions could be related to the occurrence of ALS/PD in Eastern Irian Jaya (SEDA-13, 453).

***Cynoglossum officinale* (hound's tongue)**

This contains alkaloids with curare-like activity as well as hepatotoxic and carcinogenic pyrrolizidine alkaloids (see separate entry).

***Cytisus scoparius* (Scotch broom)**

This contains the toxic alkaloid sparteine and related quinolizidine alkaloids, such as isosparteine and cytisine. Inexpert self-medication with a broom tea has resulted in fatal poisoning with clinical symptoms of ileus, heart failure and circulatory weakness. It would be prudent to avoid broom preparations during pregnancy, not only because sparteine (see separate entry) has abortifacient potential but also because of preliminary information that the plant produced malformed lambs in feeding trials.

***Datura* species**

Datura contains toxic tropane alkaloids (see separate entry). Intoxications with *Datura stramonium* (jimson weed) and related species continue to pose a problem (49—51).

***Delphinium consolida* (larkspur)**

Delphinium spp. contain complex diterpenoid alkaloids that cause acute intoxication and death from respiratory paralysis in cattle. Alkaloids and their concentrations vary with the species and plant part involved, which causes variability in toxicity. With respect to *D. consolida*, toxic alkaloids are found in non-medicinal plant parts (root, seed, herb), but they are purportedly absent in the medicinal plant part (flower).

***Dictamnus* species**

The root bark of *Dictamnus dasycarpus* shows mutagenic activity in bacteria, which is not due to dietary flavonoids, but to the furoquinoline alkaloids dictamnine and γ-fagarine. The clinical relevance of this finding remains to be established. *D. albus* can induce bullous phototoxic contact dermatitis.

Dictamnus dasycarpus is a common ingredient of the complex traditional Chinese herbal medicines that have been associated with liver damage; however, a causative role remains to be established (52—55).

Dionaea muscipula

The expressed sap of this fly-catching plant has been available in Germany as a herbal oncolytic in the form of ampoules and oral drops. However, when it became apparent that intramuscular administration could produce shivers, fever and anaphylactic shock, the health authorities banned the ampoules. They also ruled that the product information on the oral drops should warn against use in pregnancy and should list reddening of the face, headache, dyspnea, nausea and vomiting as adverse effects (SEDA-11, 424).

***Dipteryx* species**
The seeds of *Dipteryx odorata* (Dutch tonka bean) and *D. oppositofolia* (English tonka bean) are said to yield 1—3% of coumarin (see separate entry).

***Dryopteris filix-mas* (male fern)**
The rhizome was formerly used as an anthelminthic, but it is highly toxic and has been superseded by other, less dangerous agents. In spite of poor absorption, serious poisoning may occur: e.g. when absorption is increased by the presence of fatty foods.

***Dysosma pleianthum* (bajiaolian)**
This traditional Chinese herbal medicine is rich in toxic podophyllotoxin (56).

***Ecbalium elaterium* (squirting cucumber)**
The fruit juice of the squirting cucumber is a violent purgative due to the presence of toxic cucurbitacins. Intranasal use has been associated with Quincke's edema (57) and with fatal cardiac and renal failure (58).

***Echinacea* species**
Intravenous administration has been associated with anaphylactic reactions. An allegation that oral ingestion can also lead to allergic symptoms (59) requires further substantiation.

Eleutherococcus senticosus
See entry on 'Ginseng'.

***Ephedra* species**
These contain the tertiary alkaloid ephedrine and can therefore produce central and peripheral adrenergic effects such as stimulation, insomnia and tachycardia. Interference with conventional antihypertensive therapy is possible.

***Erythroxylum* species (coca)**
The leaves contain cocaine as principal alkaloid and a variety of minor alkaloids. Only decocainized coca products are legal in the United States, but some commercially available tea products were found to have a cocaine level normally found in coca leaves (about 5 mg of cocaine per 1 gram tea bag). This level results only in mild symptoms when package directions to drink a few cups per day are followed, but massive overdosing can result in severe agitation, tachycardia, perspiration and elevated blood pressure (SEDA-11, 425).

***Euonymus* species**
The fruit of *Euonymus europaeus* (European spindle tree) and the bark of *E. atropurpureus* (Wahoo bark) are said to have cathartic and emetic activity.

***Eupatorium* species**
Several *Eupatorium* species, such as *E. cannabinum* (hemp agrimony) and *E. purpureum* (gravel root), have hepatotoxic potential due to the presence of pyrrolizidine alkaloids (see separate entry). There is no evidence of pyrrolizidine alkaloids in *Eupatorium rugosum* (white snakeroot) but this plant also has poisonous properties, which are attributed to an unstable toxin called tremetol. Transfer in cow's milk to humans can produce a condition known as milk sickness, including trembles, weakness, nausea and vomiting, prostration, delirium, and even death.

***Exogonium purga* (jalap)**
The resin is a drastic cathartic with irritant action, which has been superseded by less toxic laxatives.

***Ferula assa-foetida* (asafetida)**
A case of methemoglobinemia in a 5-week-old infant treated with a gum asafetida preparation has been recorded.

***Gaultheria procumbens* (wintergreen)**
The volatile oil of wintergreen leaves consists largely of methyl salicylate (see separate entry).

***Genista tinctoria* (dyer's broom)**
Contains 0.3—0.8% of toxic quinolizidine alkaloids, such as anagyrin, cytisine and *N*-methylcytisine. The latter two constituents have peripheral effects similar to those of nicotine, whereas their central activity may be different. Anagyrine is a suspected animal teratogen and cytisine has been shown to have teratogenic activity in rabbits.

***Gentiana* species**
Gentian root shows mutagenic activity in bacteria, which is not due to dietary flavonoids, but to the xanthone derivatives, gentisin and isogentisin. The clinical relevance of this finding remains to be established.

Ginseng *(see also Chapter 49, SED-12, 1219; SEDA-16, 547)*
Ginseng is an ambiguous vernacular term, which may refer to *Panax* species such as *P. ginseng* (Asian ginseng) and *P. quinquefolius* (American ginseng), *Eleutherococcus senticosus* (Siberian ginseng), *Pfaffia paniculata* (Brazilian ginseng) or unidentified material (e.g. Rumanian ginseng). Of all these sources, only the *Panax* species contain ginsenosides. Among the variety

of adverse effects, which have been attributed in the literature to ginseng preparations, are hypertension, pressure headaches, dizziness, estrogen-like effects, vaginal bleeding and mastalgia. Prolonged use has been associated with a 'ginseng abuse syndrome' including symptoms like hypertension, edema, morning diarrhea, skin eruptions, insomnia, depression, and amenorrhea. Most reports are difficult to interpret, however, because of the absence of a control group, the simultaneous use of other agents, insufficient information about dosage and, last but not least, the lack of botanical authentication. The botanical quality of ginseng preparations continues to be a problem (60). For instance, when a case of neonatal androgenization was associated with maternal use of Siberian ginseng tablets during pregnancy, botanical analysis showed that the incriminated material almost certainly came from *Periploca sepium* (Chinese silk vine) (61).

Glycyrrhiza glabra **(liquorice)**

Prolonged use and/or high doses may produce mineralocorticoid adverse effects and drug interactions due to the saponin glycoside glycyrrhizin, which is naturally present in liquorice root in the form of calcium and potassium salts of glycyrrhizinic acid. Most individuals can consume 400 mg of glycyrrhizin daily without adverse effects, but some individuals will develop adverse effects following regular daily intake of as little as 100 mg of glycyrrhizin (62).

Gossypol *(SED-11, 1019; SEDA-13, 456)*

Gossypol occurs in certain *Gossypium* species (cotton), mostly in the seeds and root bark. Clinical studies have confirmed its efficacy as a male contraceptive agent. Reported side effects include fatigue, changes in appetite, transient elevation of SGPT levels, and hypokalemia. Hypokalemic paralysis may occur with muscular weakness and severe fatigue as prodromal signs. To what extent gossypol entails the risk of irreversible sterility would seem to require further assessment.

Gossypol is a racemic mixture of (+)- and (−)-gossypol. When tested separately in male rats at a dosage of 30 mg/kg orally for 14 days, only the latter enantiomer had a clear anti-fertility effect. It was also found that (+)-gossypol has lower acute toxicity than (−)-gossypol following intraperitoneal administration to mice. In a human study, the enantiomers showed remarkable pharmacokinetic differences in the mean elimination half-life; less than 5 hours for (−)-gossypol as compared to 133 hours for the (+)-enantiomer.

Guar gum *(SEDA-17, 547)*

Guar gum is promoted, amongst others, as a slimming aid. It can lead to the obstruction of the gastrointestinal tract, particularly when there is pre-existing pathology.

Harpagophytum procumbens **(devil's claw)**

It is sometimes stated that this plant should be avoided during pregnancy because of its supposed abortifacient capacity, but the oxytoxic properties of the plant remain to be verified.

Hedeoma pulegiolides

See the entry on 'Pennyroyal oil'.

Heliotropium **species**

These have a well-established hepatotoxic potential due to the presence of pyrrolizidine alkaloids (see separate entry).

Hintonia latiflora **(copalchi)**

Copalchi bark has been advocated primarily as an antidiabetic agent. Its use has been associated with liver toxicity but a causal relationship could not be established (63).

Hydrastis canadensis **(golden seal)**

The root contains isoquinoline alkaloids, including the quarternary base berberine (see separate entry) and the tertiary base hydrastine. As the latter may stimulate uterine contractions, it would be prudent to avoid golden seal root preparations during pregnancy, even though the actual risk of premature labor still has to be verified.

Hyoscyamus niger **(henbane)**

This contains toxic tropane alkaloids (see separate entry).

Hypericum perforatum **(St John's wort)**

It is well-established that ingestion of this herb by grazing animals can cause photosenitization. These effects are generally ascribed to the red-colored pigment, hypericin.

Juglans regia *(English walnut)*

The fresh fruit-shell contains the naphthoquinone constituent juglone, which is mutagenic and possibly carcinogenic. The juglone content of dried shells has not yet been studied adequately.

Juniperus communis *(juniper)*

The volatile oil distilled from the berries can act as

a gastrointestinal irritant. It is said that excessive doses may result in renal damage, and use during pregnancy is discouraged because of a fear that this might also stimulate the uterus.

Inula helenium *(elecampane)*

Higher doses of the root can produce vomiting, diarrhea, cramps and paralytic symptoms.

Iphigenia indica *(shancigu)*

This traditional Chinese herbal medicine contains the toxic alkaloid colchicine (4).

Kelp *(SED-12, 1220; SEDA-16, 547; SEDA-17, 547)*

Kelp is a general name for seaweed preparations obtained from different botanical species (such as *Fucus vesiculosus*, *Fucus serratus*, *Ascophyllum nodosum* and *Macrocystis pyrifera*). As kelp contains iodine, it occasionally produces hyperthryroidism (64), hypothyroidism or extrathyroidal reactions, such as skin eruptions. It can also contain contaminants like arsenic, and bone marrow depression and autoimmune thrombocytopenia have been described in consequence (65).

Krameria triandra **(rhatany)**

Contact dermatitis has been reported.

Laminaria **species**

As the stalks contain iodine, their use can be associated with intrathyroidal and extrathyroidal adverse reactions (cf. the entry on 'kelp').

Larrea tridentata **(chaparral)**

There are a number of case reports of hepatotoxicity attributed to herbal medicines containing chaparral leaves (66, 67). The major phenolic component of chaparral (a catechol lignan called nordihydroguaiaretic acid) was found to produce lymphatic and renal lesions, when given chronically in high doses to rodents. The first case of cystic renal cell carcinoma and acquired renal cystic disease associated with consumption of chaparral tea has been recently reported (68).

Laurus nobilis **(laurel)**

Laurel oil obtained from the berries is a potent skin sensitizer due to the presence of allergenic sesquiterpene lactones (SEDA-11, 427).

Ledum palustre **(marsh tea)**

The essential oil is a potent irritant of the gastrointestinal tract, kidneys and urinary tract; other toxic effects include abortion.

Lentinus edodes **(shiitake)**

The use of this edible mushroom is occasionally associated with skin reactions (69, 70).

Lobelia inflata **(Indian tobacco)**

This herb contains lobeline and other pyridine alkaloids. Lobeline has peripheral effects similar to those of nicotine, whereas its central activity may be different. Its use has been associated with nausea, vomiting, headache, tremors and dizziness. Symptoms caused by overdosage include profuse diaphoresis, paresis, tachycardia, hypertension, Cheyne-Stokes respiration, hypothermia, coma and death. Large doses are convulsant.

Mahonia **species**

See the entry on 'Barberry' above.

Mandragora officinarum **(European mandrake)**

This contains toxic tropane alkaloids (see separate entry).

Medicago sativa **(alfalfa)**

Prolonged ingestion of alfalfa seeds or alfalfa tablets has been associated with the induction of a lupus-like syndrome in humans. Dermatitis following the ingestion of alfalfa seed infusions has also been recorded.

Melaleuca alternifolia **(tea tree)**

The undiluted essential oil from the leaves of *Melaleuca alternifolia* is increasingly used as a topical natural cure for bacterial and fungal skin infections. Several patients have been described in whom such use resulted in an allergic contact eczema which was most commonly caused by the constituent *d*-limonene (71). Internal use of half a teaspoonful of the oil may result in a dramatic rash (72), whereas half a tea cup may induce a coma followed by a semi-conscious state with hallucinations (73). Less than 10 ml is sufficient to produce serious signs of toxicity in small children.

Melilotus officinalis **(sweet clover)**

The herb contains coumarin, 3,4-dihydrocoumarin (=melilotine), *o*-coumaric acid, *o*-hydroxycoumaric acid and the *o*-glucoside of *o*-coumaric acid (=melilotoside). As withering leads to enzymatic glycoside hydrolysis and since the resulting *o*-coumaric acid is spontaneously transformed to coumarin, the dried herb smells strongly of coumarin (see separate entry).

Mentha pulegium

See the entry on 'Pennyroyal oil'.

Methyl salicylate

This compound constitutes more than 95% of oil of wintergreen. It has been responsible for rare cases of allergic skin reactions, and accidental ingestion in young children has resulted in fatal salicylate poisoning.

Methylsalicylate is also an important constituent of the Red Flower Oil preparations which belong to the popular herbal analgesics for topical application in Southeast Asia. Some users take small amounts of the oil orally to enhance its analgesic effects. There are many different brands, which provide variable amounts of declared or undeclared methylsalicylate (up to 0.78 g/ml of oil). A suicide attempt by deliberate ingestion of approximately 100 ml has resulted in severe salicylate poisoning (74).

Mistletoe

This is an ambiguous vernacular term, as it may refer to *Phoradendron* species such as *P. flavescens* (American mistletoe) and to *Viscum album* (European mistletoe). The stems and leaves of the latter plant have been reported to contain alkaloids, viscotoxins and lectins. While the toxicity of the alkaloids remains to be assessed, the viscotoxins and lectins have been found to be very poisonous in animals, when given parenterally. However, the literature consulted does not provide experimental data on their oral toxicology profile. The phytochemistry of the genus *Phoradendron* is less well known but the presence of so-called phoratoxins (related to the viscotoxins) has been demonstrated. Teas prepared from unspecified plant parts or berries of *Phoradendron* are said to have caused fatal intoxications, but there seem to be no similar data on *Viscum album*.

Parenteral administration of a *Viscum album* preparation can result in a serious allergic reaction (75).

Mistletoe is sometimes assumed to have hepatotoxic potential, based on a case-report of hepatitis due to a herbal combination product claimed to have had mistletoe as one of its ingredients (76). However, the allegation that mistletoe was the probable cause of the illness has been rightly criticized, inter alia because the botanical material was not authenticated. As the incriminated product also contained skullcap, it should be noted that herbal combination therapies providing skullcap have also been associated with hepatotoxicity on other occasions (see the entry on Skullcap).

***Momordica charantia* (karela)**

It is well-established that oral preparations of the karela fruit have hypoglycemic activity in a majority of maturity-onset diabetic patients (77), and interference with conventional treatment by diet and chlorpropamide has been observed (78). It has also been reported that subcutaneous injection of a principle obtained from the fruit may lower blood glucose levels in juvenile diabetes. The agent(s) responsible for the hypoglycemic effects of karela and the mechanism(s) of action require further study.

***Myristica fragrans* (nutmeg)**

Large doses of the seed can cause nausea, vomiting, flushing, dry mouth, tachycardia, CNS stimulation possibly with epileptiform convulsions, miosis, mydriasis, euphoria and hallucinations. Nutmeg is sometimes abused for its hallucinogenic potential; ingestion of less than one tablespoon can be enough to produce severe symptoms similar to those seen in anticholinergic poisoning (79). The essential oil contains the mutagenic and animal carcinogenic compound, safrole (see separate entry).

***Nerium oleander* (oleander)**

Due to the presence of cardioactive glycosides, digitalis-like effects and potentiation of digitalis toxicity are possible. A fatality due to drinking a herbal tea prepared from oleander leaves, erroneously believed to be eucalyptus leaves, has been reported.

***Nicotiana tabacum* (tobacco)**

The leaves contain the toxic alkaloid, nicotine, as major constituent, and several other pyridine alkaloids as minor constituents. Although tobacco enemas have been abandoned in official medicine because of their life-threatening toxicity, unorthodox self-medication with this agent has not completely died out. A case-report in the 1970s described nausea and confusion, followed by hypotension and bradycardia, due to an enema apparently prepared from 5—10 cigarettes.

***Oenothera biennis* (evening primrose)**

The seeds yield evening primrose oil, which is used in various disorders, such as atopic eczema, premenstrual syndrome, and benign breast pain. When used as directed, only minor side effects, such as nausea, diarrhea and headache, or none are encountered. Allegations that evening primrose oil may trigger hitherto undiagnosed temporal lobe epilepsy in patients receiving known epileptogenic drugs (e.g. phenothiazines) still need to be substantiated.

Panax ginseng

See the entry on 'Ginseng'.

***Papaver somniferum* (opium poppy)** *(see Chapter 8)*

Opium, which is the dried latex obtained from the unripe capsules, contains morphine and other toxic narcotic alkaloids. Among its commonest side effects are nausea, vomiting, sedation, drowsiness and confusion. It entails risks such as respiratory depression, physical dependence and interactions with other central depressants.

Poppy dependence due to the frequent sucking of poppy seeds (80) or to the regular drinking of a tea infusion from poppy heads (81) is rare but has been documented. The ingestion of poppy seeds can result in detectable urinary levels of morphine and codeine (82).

Pausinystalia yohimbe **(yohimbe)**

The bark contains the toxic alkaloid, yohimbine (see separate entry), and other alkaloids.

Pennyroyal oil

This volatile oil can be obtained from *Hedeoma pulegioides* and from *Mentha pulegium*. A major constituent is pulegone, which may even constitute 80% or more of samples from the latter source. The oil has a long history as a folk medicine for the induction of menses and abortion. Ingestion of large doses for these purposes has resulted in serious symptoms including vomiting, abortion, seizures, hallucinations, renal damage, hepatotoxicity, shock and death. The hepatotoxic potential of pulegone has been confirmed in animal experiments.

Petasites **species**

These have hepatotoxic potential due to the presence of pyrrolizidine alkaloids (see separate entry).

Pfaffia paniculata

See the entry on 'Ginseng'.

Phoradendron **species**

See the entry on 'Mistletoe'.

Phytolacca americana **(pokeweed)**

Severe emesis and diarrhea, accompanied by tachycardia, have been observed after ingestion of raw leaves and after drinking tea prepared from the powdered root.

Pilocarpus pennatifolius **(jaborandi)**

The leaves contain pilocarpine as the major alkaloid as well as a variety of minor alkaloids. Pilocarpine is a potent cholinergic drug, which enhances salivary flow, sweating and gastrointestinal motility when doses of 2.5—7.5 mg are taken orally. It may interfere with asthma therapy and the effect of anticholinergic drugs.

Piper methysticum **(kava-kava)**

South Pacific natives prepare a ceremonial beverage from the rhizome. The major constituents are non-alkaloidal pyrone derivatives, which produce sedation and centrally induced muscle relaxation in laboratory animals. Case-reports have described erythema, rashes, yellow discoloration of the skin, sensory disturbances, sleepiness and ataxia.

Heavy chronic consumption of kava-kava can lead to a pellagroid dermopathy that appears to be unrelated to niacin deficiency (83).

Pithecellobium jiringa **(jering fruit)**

Jering fruit is valued in Malaysia and Indonesia as a delicacy and for its antidiabetic properties. Acute renal failure is a rare complication. Among the presenting symptoms are dysuria, hematuria, vomiting, abdominal pain and blue urine (84).

Plantago **species**

Plantago seeds are widely used as bulk laxatives under the names of 'psyllium' (from *P. psyllium* or *P. indica*) and 'ispaghula' (from *P. ovata*). Occupational exposure to the powered drug has resulted in sensitization with symptoms ranging from rhinitis and lacrimation to more severe respiratory compromise (SEDA-9, 424). Ingestion has been associated with rare cases of generalized urticarial rash and anaphylactic shock (85). The possibility that the intestinal absorption of lithium and other drugs may be inhibited should also be considered (86).

Podophyllum peltatum **(American mandrake)**

The resin prepared from the dried rhizome and roots contains podophyllotoxin, α-peltatin and β-peltatin. When applied topically, it is a strong irritant to the skin and mucous membranes and may lead to poisoning because of systemic absorption. When taken by mouth, it has a drastic laxative action and produces violent peristalsis. Ingestion of large doses can result in severe neuropathic toxicity (SEDA-11, 426). The oral and local use of the resin should be avoided during pregnancy, as this has been associated with teratogenicity and fetal death.

Prunus **species**

The raw pits or kernels of various *Prunus* species (such as apricot, bitter almond, choke cherry and peach) are promoted as health foods. When ingested in sufficient quantity, however, they are poisonous due to the cyanogenic glycoside, amygdalin, which yields hydrogen cyanide after ingestion. For instance, a total consumption of approximately 48 apricot kernels produced forceful vomiting, headache, flushing, heavy perspiration, dizziness, and faintness before vomiting was induced in the emergency room, whereafter the symptoms rapidly subsided. Besides the risk that a large dose can lead to acute cyanide poisoning, there is also the question whether continued ingestion of cyanogenic pits or kernels might induce chronic intoxication.

An outbreak of congenital malformations in swine has been associated retrospectively with the eating of cherries, leaves and bark of wild black cherries (*Prunus serotina*). Prospective experimental evidence of teratogenicity was not available at that time, but amygdalin was later reported to be teratogenic in hamsters.

Psoralea corylifolia

Infusions prepared from the seed can result in photosensitivity due to the presence of psoralens (87).

***Pulsatilla vulgaris* (meadow windflower)**

Higher doses may irritate the kidneys and urinary tract; pregnancy is considered a contraindication.

Pyrrolizidine alkaloids *(SED-11, 1016)*

Pyrrolizidine alkaloids occur in a large number of plants, notably in the genera *Crotalaria*, *Cynoglossum*, *Eupatorium*, *Heliotropium*, *Petasites*, *Senecio* and *Symphytum*. It is well-established that certain representatives of this class and the plants in which they occur are hepatotoxic as well as mutagenic and hepatocarcinogenic. They can produce veno-occlusive disease of the liver with clinical features like abdominal pain with ascites, hepatomegaly and splenomegaly, anorexia with nausea, vomiting, and diarrhea. Sometimes there is also damage to the pulmonary region (SEDA-13, 449).

It would be prudent to avoid any exposure of the unborn or suckling child to herbal remedies containing pyrrolizidine alkaloids. Animal studies have shown that transplacental passage and transfer to breast milk are possible, and there is a human case of fatal neonatal liver injury, in which the mother had used a herbal cough tea containing pyrrolizidine alkaloids throughout her pregnancy (SEDA-13, 452).

The German Federal Health Office has restricted the availability of botanical medicines containing unsaturated pyrrolizidine alkaloids as follows (88, 89): herbal medicines providing >1 mg internally or >100 mg externally per day, when used as directed, are not permitted; herbal medicines providing 0.1—1 mg internally or 10—100 mg externally per day, when used as directed, may be applied only for a maximum of 6 weeks per year, and they should not be used during pregnancy or lactation.

***Raphanus sativus* var. *niger* (black radish)**

The root contains 0.0025% of essential oil with glycosides yielding allyl isothiocyanate (see separate entry) and butyl isothiocyanate. According to secondary literature, consumption of several roots may produce miosis, pain, vomiting, slowed respiration, stupor and albuminuria. It is also claimed that poisoning secondary to the use of black radish sap for bile-stones has occurred.

***Rauwolfia serpentina* (rauwolfia)**

The root contains numerous alkaloids, of which reserpine and rescinnamine are said to be the most active as hypotensive agents. Inexpert use can lead to serious toxicity including symptoms such as hypotension, sedation, depression and potentiation of other central depressants.

***Rhamnus purshianus* (cascara sagrada)**

The bark contains laxative anthranoid derivatives (see separate entry).

***Rheum palmatum* (rhubarb)**

The rhizome contains laxative anthranoid derivatives (see separate entry).

***Ricinus communis* (castor bean)**

Castor oil is the fixed oil obtained from the seeds by cold expression. When taken by mouth, especially in large doses, it may produce violent purgation with nausea, vomiting, colic, and a risk of miscarriage. One study suggests that maternal self-medication with castor oil may be associated with an increased incidence of fetal meconium passage (SEDA-13, 455).

***Rubia tinctorum* (madder)**

The use of herbal medicines prepared from madder root is no longer permitted in Germany. Root extracts have shown genotoxic effects in several test systems, which are attributed to the presence of the anthraquinone derivative lucidin. One of the other main components, alizarin primeveroside, is transformed into 1-hydroxyanthraquinone, when given orally to the rat, and this metabolite shows carcinogenic activity in rats (90).

***Ruscus aculeatus* (butcher's broan)**

Topical use of *Ruscus aculeatus* as vasocontrictive treatment of varices and hemorrhoids may lead to allergic contact dermatitis (91).

***Ruta graveolens* (rue)**

The essential oil not only can produce contact dermatitis and phototoxic reactions, but also can induce severe hepatic and renal toxicity. Use as an abortive agent has resulted in fatal intoxications. Therapeutic doses can lead to melancholia, sleep disorders, fatigue, dizziness and cramps. The sap of the fresh leaf can produce painful gastrointestinal irritation, fainting, sleepiness, weak pulse, abortion, swollen tongue and a cool skin.

Safrole

Safrole is the major component (e.g. 80%) of oil of sassafras, and lesser quantities occur in essential oils from nutmeg, star anise, mace, and cinnamon leaf. Some of its known or possible metabolites show mutagenic activity in bacterial testing and it has been proven to have weak hepatocarcinogenic effects in rodents. Experiments in mice have suggested the possibility of transplacental and lactational carcinogenesis.

Whether the metabolism of safrole in rodents is similar to that in man remains to be determined.

***Salix* species (willow)**

The bark of various *Salix* species contains glycosides of saligenin (=salicylalcohol), namely the simple *O*-glycoside salicin and more complex glycosides like salicortin. When taken orally, these glycosides may undergo intestinal transformation to saligenin, which in turn may be rapidly absorbed and then converted by the liver to salicylic acid. When willow bark preparations are used according to current dosage recommendations, they will not provide sufficient salicylic acid, to produce acute salicylate poisoning. However, the risk of an idiosyncratic response (skin reactions, bronchospasm) in sensitive individuals cannot be excluded.

***Salvia miltiorrhiza* (danshen)**

In China, the root of *Salvia miltiorrhiza* has been used traditionally for the treatment of coronary diseases. A pharmacodynamic and pharmacokinetic study in rats suggests that this traditional agent may enhance the anticoagulant activity of warfarin, when both drugs are taken together. This animal study was initiated because of observations in Hong Kong that patients on routine warfarin therapy experienced an adverse drug interaction when they self-medicated with a freely available Danshen preparation (92).

***Salvia officinalis* (sage)**

The leaf contains 1—2.5% of essential oil consisting of 35—60% of thujone. This compound may produce toxicity when the herb is taken in overdose (more than 15 grams per dose) or for a prolonged period. Pregnancy is listed as a contraindication to the use of the essential oil or alcoholic extracts.

***Sassafras albidum* (sassafras)**

The wood of sassafras root contains 1—2% of volatile oil, which in turn consists largely of safrole. This constituent is a weakly hepatocarcinogenic agent in laboratory animals (see separate entry).

In Germany, the health authorities have recently proposed the withdrawal of *Sassafras*-containing medicines, including homeopathic products up to D3, from the market (93).

Of particular concern is the uncontrolled availability of sassafras oil because of its use in so-called 'aromatherapy'. Internal use of this oil in recommended doses up to 12 drops per day this can lead to a daily intake up to 0.2 grams of safrole (94).

Scopalia carniolica

This contains toxic tropane alkaloids (see separate entry).

***Scutellaria* species**

See the entry on 'Skullcap'.

***Sechium edule* (chayote)**

The tuber is valued as a potent diuretic by Latin American populations. Its use as a decoction by a pregnant woman suffering from pedal edema may have been the cause of a severe case of hypokalemia (SEDA-13, 453).

***Senecio* species**

Many *Senecio* species, such as *S. jacobaea* (ragwort) and *S. longilobus* (thread leaf groundsel) contain a hepatotoxic level of pyrrolizidine alkaloids (see separate entry).

***Silybum marianum* (St. Mary's thistle)**

A case of anaphylactic shock following the use of a herbal tea containing an extract of the fruit has been reported (95).

Skullcap

Herbal therapies comprising skullcap as one of their ingredients have been repeatedly associated with hepatotoxic reactions. One of these cases was originally attributed to mistletoe, even though there were insufficient grounds for this allusion (cf. the entry on mistletoe). Although Western skullcap preparations are supposed to come from *Scutellaria lateriflora*, it remains unclear whether this plant is responsible. In the United Kingdom, the American germander (*Teucrium canadense*) has been widely used to replace *Scutellaria lateriflora* in commercial skullcap materials and products. In one UK case of skullcap-associated hepatotoxicity, the material was found to come from *Teucrium canadense*. This raises the possibility that other cases of skullcap toxicity may also have involved *Teucrium* rather than *Scutellaria* (4).

Sparteine *(SEDA-17, 548)*

This is a major quinolizidine alkaloid in *Cytisus scoparius*. Among its reported effects are a lessening of cardiac conductivity, stimulation of uterine motility, circulatory collapse and respiratory arrest. Pharmacokinetic studies have shown that its metabolic oxidation exhibits genetic polymorphism and that about 6—9% of the Caucasian population are poor metabolizers. Sparteine was contained in a slimming aid ('Herbal Slimming Aid', UK). It was formerly used to induce labour; at the very least it should be contraindicated during pregnancy.

Quinidine, haloperidol and moclobemide are all potent inhibitors of the oxidative metabolism of sparteine (4).

***Spirulina* species**

Promotional claims that *Spirulina* is a good source of vitamin B_{12} for vegetarians are inappropriate (4).

***Strophantus* species**

The seeds contain toxic cardiac glycosides.

Strychnos nux-vomica

The dried ripe seeds contain the alkaloids strychnine and brucine, together with traces of other alkaloids. Strychnine is a well-known powerful convulsant, which may readily produce serious and even lethal poisoning.

Swertia japonica

This shows mutagenic activity in bacteria, which is due not to dietary flavonoids, but to several xanthone derivatives. The clinical relevance of these findings remains to be established.

***Symphytum officinale* (comfrey)** *(SEDA-13, 450; SEDA-17, 547)*

This plant has hepatotoxic potential due to the presence of pyrrolizidine alkaloids (see separate entry) and their *N*-oxides. The percutaneous absorption of the *N*-oxides in an alcoholic extract of comfrey root has been investigated in rats: about 0.1—4% of the dermal dose could be recovered from the urine in 48 hours.

***Tanacetum parthenium* (feverfew)**

As this herb is rich in allergenic sesquiterpene lactones, such as parthenolide, it is not surprising that contact dermatitis has been observed. The most common adverse effect of oral feverfew products is mouth ulceration. A more widespread inflammation of the oral mucosa and tongue, swelling of the lips and loss of taste have been reported as well (SEDA-11, 426).

Taxus celebica

This plant, which contains the flavonoid sciadopitysin, is traditionally used in China as a herbal treatment of diabetes mellitus. There have been two instances in which the ingestion of a massive dose was followed by acute renal failure. Both patients initially presented with gastrointestinal upset and fever (96).

Tetrahydropalmatine (Jin Bu Huan)

l-Tetrahydropalmatine has been identified as the active constituent in Chinese 'Jin Bu Huan Anodyne' tablets on the Western market. The package insert suggested *Polygala chinensis* as source plant, but in reality this alkaloid comes from a *Stephania* species. Both *l*-tetrahydropalmatine and its racemic *dl*-form are used in Chinese medicine as analgesic and hypnotic agents. Reported side effects include vertigo, fatigue, nausea, and drowsiness, which effects could make users unfit for driving. Recent case reports have documented life-threatening bradycardia and respiratory depression in small children following unintentional overdosing (97) and acute hepatitis in adult users (98).

***Teucrium canadense* (American germander)**

See the entry on 'Skullcap'.

***Teucrium chamaedrys* (wall germander)**

In France, numerous cases of hepatitis have been associated with the normal use of this herb. The frequency of this adverse effect has been estimated at one case in about 4000 months of treatment (99). Although most cases were not very serious, fatal outcome has been reported (100), and progression to liver cirrhosis has also been described (101). An animal study suggests that the hepatotoxicity resides in one or more reactive metabolites of its furanoditerpenoids (102).

***Tripterygium wilfordii* (Leigongteng)**

Extracts from the root of *Tripterygium wilfordii* are used in China for the treatment of various disorders, such as rheumatoid arthritis, ankylosing spondylitis, systemic lupus erythematosus and glomerulonephritis. The potential benefits in such serious diseases should be carefully weighed against a substantial risk of adverse reactions, including gastrointestinal disturbances, skin rashes, amenorrhea, leukopenia, and thrombocytopenia. In male users, prolonged use can induce oligospermia and azoospermia, and a decrease in the size of the testis (103–105). In addition, the immunosuppressive properties of Leigongteng may promote the development of infectious diseases (106).

Tropane alkaloids

The occurrence of tropane alkaloids, such as hyoscyamine and/or scopolamine, in the solanaceous plants *Atropa belladonna*, *Datura stramonium*, *Hyoscyamus niger* and *Mandragora officinarum* is well established. These alkaloids are powerful anticholinergic agents and can elicit peripheral symptoms (e.g. blurred vision, dry mouth) as well as central effects (e.g. drowsiness, delirium). They can potentiate the effects of synthetic drugs with similar pharmacological activity.

***Tussilago farfara* (coltsfoot)**

This may have hepatotoxic potential due to the presence of pyrrolizidine alkaloids (see separate entry) in low concentrations (SEDA-13, 452).

***Urginea maritima* (squill)**

As the bulb contains cardioactive glycosides, it may produce digitalis-like effects and potentiation of digitalis toxicity. In a recent Turkish case, the ingestion of two bulbs as a folk remedy for arthritic pains was sufficient to result in fatal poisoning (107).

***Urtica* species (stinging nettle)**

The blister-raising properties of locally applied stinging nettle extracts are well known. They are said to be reduced by drying or heat-treatment. A secondary source states that tea prepared from stinging nettle leaves may occasionally give rise to gastric irritation, skin reactions, edema and oliguria, but primary references are not provided. A positive patch test reaction to *Urtica dioica* has been obtained in a patient who had developed edematous gingivostomatitis following the regular use of stinging nettle tea as a tonic. The patient also showed positive reactions to chamomile (*Anthemis nobilis*) and its allergens (sesquiterpene lactones) (108).

***Valeriana* species (valerian)**

The valepotriates which occur in valerian roots have alkylating properties. Valtrate/isovaltrate and dihydrovaltrate are mutagenic in bacterial test systems in the presence of a metabolic activator, and their degradation products baldrinal (from valtrate) and homobaldrinal (from isovaltrate) are already mutagenic without metabolic activation. These latter compounds also show direct genotoxic activity in SOS-chromotesting. As far as is known, decomposition of dihydrovaltrate does not yield baldrinals.

The levels of valepotriates and baldrinals in valerian extracts depend on the botanical species: root extracts of *V. officinalis* contain up to 0.9% of valepotriates, compared to 2–4 and 5–7% of valepotriates in root extracts of *V. wallichii* and *V. mexicana*, respectively. Another relevant parameter is the dosage form:

- When a *herbal tea* is prepared by hot extraction from valerian root, up to 60% of the valepotriates remains behind in the root material and only 0.1% can be recovered from the tea.
- A freshly prepared *tincture* contains 11% of the valepotriates originally found in the root material. Storage at room temperature rapidly reduces this level to 3.7% after 1 week and 0% after 3 weeks. In view of this rapid degradation, it is not surprising that commercially available tincture samples yield baldrinals when analyzed.
- Valerian-containing *tablets and capsules* may provide up to 1 mg of baldrinals per piece.

Valepotriates show poor gastrointestinal absorption, but 2% is degraded in vivo to baldrinals following the oral application of valtrate/isovaltrate to mice. In other words, a tablet with 50 mg of valepotriates may add 1 mg of baldrinals to the amount of baldrinals, which are already present before ingestion (see above). In contrast to the valepotriates, the degradation product homobaldrinal is absorbed fairly well following oral application to mice. As much as 71% of the administered dose can be recovered from the urine in the form of baldrinal glucuronide. Since no unchanged homobaldrinal can be demonstrated in body fluids or liver samples following oral administration, the compound appears to undergo substantial first-pass metabolism. As this glucuronidation leads to loss of the mutagenic properties, the primary target organs which may be at risk from valepotriates and baldrinals are the gastrointestinal tract and the liver (109). The toxicological significance of all these data is still unclear, however, since the carcinogenic potential of valerian preparations and their constituents has not yet been evaluated.

***Veratrum* species**

The rhizome and root of *Veratrum album* (white hellebore) and the rhizome of *V. viride* (green hellebore) contain many alkaloidal constituents, including hypotensive ester alkaloids. Among the major toxic symptoms are hypotension and bradycardia. The related species *V. californicum* has well-established teratogenic activity in livestock, due to the presence of the alkaloids, cyclopamine, cycloposine and jervine. The latter alkaloid is also found in white and green hellebore.

Viscum album
See the entry on 'Mistletoe'.

***Vitex-agnus castus* (chaste tree)**
Vitex-agnus castus is a plant with estrogen-like activities, used for a variety of gynecological problems, particularly on the European continent. One case report describes a woman who, while undergoing in vitro fertilization, took this remedy during an unstimulated cycle (110). She was closely monitored for hormone levels and showed considerable derangement of gonadotrophin and ovarian hormone levels. *Vitex-agnus castus* may therefore lead to ovarian hyperstimulation and may increase the risk of miscarriage.

Xysmalobium undulatum
The root contains toxic cardiac glycosides.

***Yohimbine** (SED-11, 1024; SEDA-13, 457)*
Yohimbine is a major alkaloid in the bark of *Pausinystalia yohimbe*. It has α_{-2}-adrenoreceptor antagonistic properties and can thereby counteract the effects of antihypertensives. A dose of 15—20 mg p.o. can increase blood pressure and induce anxiety in healthy volunteers. In patients on tricyclic antidepressants, hypertension may already occur at 4 mg t.i.d. The toxicity of yohimbine can also be enhanced by other drugs, such as phenothiazines. A dose of 5 mg is sufficient to produce adverse effects in patients with autonomic failure, and 10 mg can elicit manic-like symptoms in patients with bipolar depression. Bronchospasm and a lupus-like syndrome have also been reported (111).

***Ziziphus jujuba* (Dazao)**
The fruit of *Ziziphus jujuba* is often consumed in Eastern Asia as food or as a tonic and sedative. A case of angioneurotic edema following the oral ingestion of dazao preparations has been described (112).

HOMEOPATHY

Most *but not all* homeopathic remedies are too diluted to bring about toxic effects. Potentially toxic concentrations of arsenic (113) and cadmium (114) in homeopathic remedies have been described. Concern has also been voiced about potentially carcinogenic effects of low potencies of *Aristolochia* (115). One case of acute pancreatitis has been reported following the medication of a complex homeopathic drug containing 19 different ingredients (116). Low potencies can also cause allergic reactions (117, 118). Recently, three cases of severe allergic and anaphylactic reactions have been reported (SEDA-16, 547). In cases of concomitant drug treatments, interactions are conceivable, even though there is no published evidence on this matter.

Generally speaking, ADRs to homeopathic medications are *probably* rare. Yet the fact is that we cannot, at present, tell their true incidence as no definitive study of this has ever been carried out.

For some of the potential indirect risks associated with homeopathy, see above.

OTHER UNCONVENTIONAL DRUGS

Animal drugs

Drug substances of animal origin can produce anaphylactic or anaphylactoid reactions, particularly after parenteral administration (119). It is also possible that the animal drug may transmit an infectious disease because of the presence of a pathogenic microbe.

Arumalon *(SEDA-14, 440)*
Arumalon is a 'chondroprotective' agent containing an extract of cartilage and an extract of the red bone marrow of calves. Parenteral use has been associated with local reactions at the site of the injection and with allergic symptoms (such as fever, malaise, symptoms of pronounced inflammation, nephrotic syndrome). Polymyositis and fatal dermatomyositis are also alleged to be possible.

Arteparon *(SEDA-14, 441)*
This 'chondroprotective' agent is prepared from bovine lung and tracheal cartilage. Mucopolysaccharide polysulfuric acid ester (also known as glycosaminoglycan polysulfate) is declared as its major principle. This substance resembles heparin in its molecular structure and can have the same dose-dependent effect on platelet aggregation. Cross-reactivity with heparin is possible. The use of Arteparon has been associated with life-threatening thromboembolic complications (myocardial infarction, pulmonary embolus, hemiplegic apoplexia, cerebral hemorrhage, death).

Other reported side effects include local reactions at the site of the injection, serious allergic symptoms, arthropathy, subcutaneous fat necrosis, and reversible alopecia.

Carp bile
In Asia, the raw bile of the grass carp (*Ctenopharyngodom idellus*) is believed by some to be health promoting. However, eating this substance can result in hepatic dysfunction and nephrotoxicity (120). The former reaction may resolve within a few days, but the latter is more serious, culminating in acute renal failure within

2—3 days after ingestion (121). Experiments in rats have shown that the bile of the grass carp loses its lethality when treated with cholestyramine, a drug known to form insoluble complexes with bile acids (122).

Cell therapy *(SED-11, 1026; SED-12, 1226; SEDA-13, 457; SEDA-16, 546) (see also Chapter 49)*

Cell therapy consists of the parenteral or enteral administration of cells or cell parts obtained from animal organs and/or tissues of bovine donors, sheep, pigs or rabbits. Two different types of cell preparations are in use: fresh cells, which are administered in fresh form, and dried cells or so-called sicca cells, which are worked up for later use. The most prevailing risk of cell therapy seems to be local and generalized allergic reactions (fever, nausea, vomiting, urticaria, and anaphylactic shock). Other untoward consequences include fatal and non-fatal encephalomyelitis (SEDA-11, 429), polyneuritis, Laundry-Guillain-Barré syndrome, fatal serum sickness, perivenous leukoencephalitis, and immune-complex vasculitis.

Copper

A patient has been described who developed acute liver failure and cirrhosis resembling Wilson's disease due to chronic overdosing of a dietary copper supplement (10—20 times the maximum recommended dose of 3 mg per day for years) (123).

Fish oil *(SEDA-13, 460; SEDA-18, 3)*

Fish oil supplements rich in long-chain polyunsaturated omega-3 fatty acids (eicosapentaenoic acid, docosahexaenoic acid) can reduce plasma levels of triglycerides and VLDL, decrease platelet aggregation, prolong bleeding time, reduce blood pressure, increase the fluidity of blood and affect leukotriene production. Reported side effects include fullness and epigastric discomfort, diarrhea, and a fishy taste after belching. In addition to these mild symptoms, certain areas have been identified in which problems of a more serious nature could arise, such as:
(a) a potential risk that the favourable changes in plasma lipids could be offset by a deleterious increase in LDL cholesterol or LDL apoprotein B;
(b) the possible adverse consequence of the capacity to increase bleeding time and to reduce platelet aggregation, especially in patients with pre-existing bleeding and platelet abnormalities and in those taking other anti-thrombotic agents;
(c) some preliminary evidence that a detrimental effect on patients with aspirin-sensitive asthma is possible;
(d) an adverse effect on the metabolic control of patients with non-insulin-dependent diabetes mellitus, when these patients are not being treated with a sulfonylurea derivative (124);
(e) pro-thrombotic effects through changes on clotting factor concentration (125);
(f) possible contamination.

Gangliosides (Cronassial®, Sygen®

Gangliosides extracted from bovine brain tissue have been widely used in Western Europe and South America for several neurological disorders. Reported side effects (other than discomfort at the injection site) included motoneuron disease-like illness, cutaneous erythema (with or without fever and nausea) and anaphylaxis. After the evaluation of reported associations between the use of gangliosides and Guillain-Barré syndrome (126, 127), the Committee for Proprietary Medicinal Products (CPMP) of the European Commission recommended in September 1994 that the marketing authorizations for Cronassial® (a mixture of gangliosides for treating peripheral neuropathies) should be withdrawn. At the same time, the CPMP recommended that marketing authorizations for Sygen® (a monosialoganglioside known as GM-1 for treatment of cerebral vascular insufficiency) should be suspended for 1 year, pending the completion of ongoing trials.

Ghee

Ghee is the clarified butter from the milk of water buffaloes or cows. Although the butter is heated enough to eliminate non-sporulating organisms, the process is unlikely to kill *Clostridium tetani* spores. This may explain why a case-control study in rural areas of Pakistan identified its traditional use as an umbilical cord dressing as a risk factor for the development of neonatal tetanus (128).

Green-lipped mussel *(SED-11, 1021)*

An extract of the New Zealand green-lipped mussel (*Perna canaliculus*) is advocated for the treatment of arthritic symptoms. Reported adverse effects include flare-up of the disease, epigastric discomfort, flatulence and nausea. A case of jaundice appearing some weeks after starting treatment has been reported.

Imedeen

Imedeen is the trade name of an oral health food product containing freeze-dried proteins from the cartilage of deep-sea fish, which is advocated as an antiwrinkling agent. Its use has been associated with generalized skin reaction and extensive Quincke's edema (129).

Oyster extract

A food supplement consisting of oyster extract, ginseng, taurine and zinc (Ostrin plus GTZ 611® has been associated with a case of Quincke's facial edema. The reaction developed immediately after intake of the food supplement and the oyster extract was considered to be its most likely cause (130).

Propolis *(SEDA-12, 410; SEDA-13, 459; SEDA-18, 4)*

Propolis or bee-glue is a resinous material used by bees to seal hive walls and to strengthen the borders of the combs as well as the hive entrance. It is increasingly associated with cases of allergy following use of the substance in bio-cosmetics and in self-treatment of various diseases. Although most cases involve allergic contact dermatitis arising from topical application, a few reports describe an allergic reaction to oral ingestion (78[R]). Contamination of propolis capsules with an excessive level of lead has been recently reported from New Zealand (131).

Rattlesnake meat *(SEDA-14, 442; SEDA-18, 2)*

Dried rattlesnake meat is a well-known Mexican folk remedy, which can be purchased without prescription in Mexico, El Salvador, and the southwestern part of the United States. It is available as such and in the form of powder, capsules or pills, which may be labeled in Hispanic as *víbora de cascabel*, *pulvo de víbora* or *carne de vḑbora*. As the rattlesnake is a well-established reservoir for *Salmonella arizona*, such products can cause serious systemic infections. Typically, victims are Hispanic patients with a medical illness undermining their immunological integrity (e.g. SLE, AIDS). Although most patients respond well to intravenous therapy with ampicillin or co-trimoxazole, fatalities have been observed. Recently one case of *Salmonella arizonae* peritonitis was reported from Texas.

Royal jelly

Royal jelly is a viscous secretion produced by the pharyngeal glands of the worker bee, *Apis mellifera*, which is widely used in alternative medicine as a health tonic. Its internal use by atopic individuals can induce severe, sometimes even fatal, asthma and anaphylaxis (132, 133). Topical application can lead to contact dermatitis.

Spanish fly *(SED-11, 1023)*

Spanish fly (also known as cantharides) is the dried blistering beetle (*Cantharis vesicatoria* and related spp.), which contains cantharidin as major active constituent. A related drug, which serves as an alternative cantharidin source in the East, is the Chinese blistering beetle (*Mylabris* spp.). Spanish fly has gained a considerable reputation as an aphrodisiac agent following observations that nearly toxic doses could cause priapism in men, and pelvic congestion, occasionally with uterine bleeding, in women. These effects are due to an irritant effect on the genitourinary tract, which could be misinterpreted as increased sensuality. Cantharidin was formerly used medicinally as a counter-irritant and vesicant, but this use has been abandoned because of its high toxicity. Manifestations of cantharidin poisoning range from local vesicobullous formation to gross hematuria, hepatotoxicity, myocardial damage, denudation of the gastrointestinal tract, and occasionally death. The lethal dose is not well established, however, with one patient dying after the ingestion of only 10 mg, and another patient surviving the intake of 50 mg. A recent report from Hong Kong described a fatal case due to ingesting a decoction of more than 200 dried *Mylabris* beetles as an abortifacient (134).

Squalene

Squalene is a popular over-the-counter Asian folk remedy derived from shark liver oil. Oral capsules are readily available in Asian health food stores and the substance is also widely used in cosmetics. Ingestion of squalene capsules has been associated with a case of severe lipoid pneumonia due to aspiration; the patient also had abnormal liver function which raises the possibility of hepatotoxicity (135).

Thyroid hormones *(see also Chapter 37)*

Over the years, thyroid hormones have been repeatedly incorporated in non-orthodox drug programs for weight reduction. Although it is well recognized that these hormones can help to reduce weight, primarily by increasing the metabolic rate, they have no place in the therapy of obese euthyroid patients. When dietary intake of protein and calcium is inadequate, they may induce worrying catabolic losses of these muscular and skeletal components, and the weight loss is not sustained after termination of therapy. Furthermore, the large doses needed for weight reduction may suppress endogenous thyroid function and have potentially dangerous effects of the heart, such as tachyarrhythmias and cardiomegaly (136).

Toad venom

The dried venom of the Chinese toad (*Bufo bufo gargarizans*) is one of the ingredients of the traditional Chinese medicine 'kyushin'. It contains bufalin and cinobufaginal, which are structurally related to digoxin antibodies, they create the false impression of high plasma digoxin levels (137). Deliberate overdosing of 'kyushin' in an attempt to commit suicide resulted in nausea, vomiting, general malaise, and ECG changes (e.g. atrioventricular block) (138).

Mineral drugs

Non-orthodox preparations may contain all kinds of minerals in a wide range of dosages. Most often these ingredients will provide nutritional electrolytes and/or trace elements. One should bear in mind that adverse reactions are certainly possible when excessive doses are taken (139).

Germanium *(SED-12, 1227; SEDA-13, 459; SEDA-16, 545; SEDA-17, 545)*

The daily intake of germanium through foodstuffs is estimated to be in the range of 0.4—3.5 mg. In recent years, germanium preparations supplying much larger amounts have hit the health food markets. Various case-reports have shown that a daily intake of 30—700 mg germanium for months or years (corresponding to a cumulative dose varying from 8.5 to more than 324 grams germanium) can lead to serious renal failure, which is not always reversible. Neuropathy, myopathy and hepatic damage may also occur. Biopsies of the kidney or liver have verified germanium concentrations up to 70 and 140 times the normal levels. Some patients ultimately died from gastrointestinal bleeding, cardiogenic shock or multiple organ failure. The majority of cases involved the use of inorganic germanium dioxide or an unidentified germanium compound, but carboxyethylgermanium sesquixide and germanium lactate-citrate have also been incriminated (140).

Exotic remedies and cosmetics *(SEDA-18, 4)*

In various parts of the world, toxic metal salts or oxides are deliberately included in traditional medicines and cosmetics (see Table 4), even though such preparations may be associated with a risk of serious poisoning (136). For instance, Ayurvedic medicines have repeatedly been associated with arsenic poisoning including hyperpigmentation and hyperkeratosis (141).

There is a recent practice among urbanized South African blacks to replace traditional herbal ingredients of purgative enemas with sodium or potassium dichromate. This switch can result in serious toxicity, characterized by acute renal failure, gastrointestinal hemorrhage, and hepatocellular dysfunction (142, 143).

Miscellaneous drugs

Vitamins can cause all kinds of serious adverse reactions, when taken in massive doses for non-orthodox purposes, but these problems are discussed elsewhere in this volume (see Chapter 38). The adverse effects of some other non-orthodox medicines are reviewed below.

Table 4. *Potential contaminants that should be taken into account in the quality control of herbal medicines (14^R)*

Type of contaminant	Examples
Botanicals	*Atropa belladonna*, *Digitalis*, *Colchicum*, *Rauwolfia serpentina*, pyrrolizidine-containing plants
Micro-organisms	*Staphylococcus aureus*, *Escherichia coli* (certain strains), *Salmonella*, *Shigella*, *Pseudomonas aeruginosa*
Microbial toxins	Bacterial endotoxins, aflatoxins
Pesticides	Chlorinated pesticides (e.g. DDT, DDE, HCH-isomers, HCB, aldrin, dieldrin, heptachlor), organic phosphates, carbamate insecticides and herbicides, dithiocarbamate fungicides, triazin herbicides
Fumigation agents	Ethylene oxide, methyl bromide, phosphine
Radioactivity	^{134}Cs, ^{137}Cs, ^{103}Ru, ^{131}I, ^{90}Sr
Metals	Lead, cadmium, mercury, arsenic
Synthetic drugs	Analgesic and anti-inflammatory agents (e.g. aminophenazone, phenylbutazone, indomethacin), corticosteroids, hydrochlorothiazide, diazepam
Animal drugs	Thyroid hormones

Carnitine

The natural amino acid L-carnitine functions in the body in the transport of fatty acids into mitochondria, and its therapeutic value in the treatment of primary carnitine deficiencies and some secondary deficiencies is well-established. Its direct toxicity seems negligible, and only minor adverse effects (e.g. gastrointestinal discomfort) have been observed in its consumers.

According to a recent case report, however, the addition of L-carnitine (1 gram orally per day) to long-term acenocoumarol therapy may result in marked potentiation of this anticoagulant.

DL-Carnitine may be advocated in health food stores as a means to improve athletic performance. It competitively inhibits L-carnitine and can thus cause symptoms of carnitine deficiency. An exemplary case involved an athlete who took 500 mg of DL-carnitine for 2 days before running a long-distance race. No problems were encountered during the race, but later he developed muscle weakness and urinary discoloration suggestive of myoglobinuria.

Fumaric acid and derivatives *(SEDA-13, 458)*

Monoethyl fumarate and dimethyl fumarate are being used in some countries for psoriasis. The major risk is nephrotoxicity, which can take the form of an acute renal failure that is only partially reversible. Other side effects include gastrointestinal disturbances, skin reactions, flushing, reversible elevation of transaminases, reversible lymphopenia, and eosinophilia. Osteomalacia due to renal tubular toxicity has also been reported (144). As a consequence, the use of fumaric acid esters requires regular hematological control as well as periodic renal and hepatic function determinations.

A recent randomized double-blind trial in patients with severe psoriasis has confirmed the antipsoriatic efficacy of a mixture of dimethylfumarate and monoethylhydrogenfumarate, whereafter this mixture was licensed as a medicine in Germany. However, a renewed assessment of the benefit/risk ratio was subsequently announced (145).

γ-Hydroxybutyrate

γ-Hydroxybutyrate (GHB or sodium oxybate) has been illicitly promoted in the United States for body building, weight control, as a sleeping aid, and as a replacement for L-tryptophan after this amino acid had been recalled from the market. Ingestion of 0.5 to 3 teaspoons can produce vomiting, drowsiness, hypotonia and/or vertigo, and loss of consciousness, irregular respiration, tremors, or myoclonus may follow. Seizure-like activity, bradycardia, hypotension and/or respiratory arrest have also been reported. Severity and duration of symptoms depend on the dose of GHB and on the presence of other CNS depressants, such as alcohol.

D-Glucosamine *(SEDA-14, 440)*

Parenteral administration of this chondroprotective agent may produce a local reaction at the site of the injection as well as serious allergic reactions. Among the other reported side effects are nausea, vomiting, stupor, and isolated cases of blood disorders. It is likely that such reactions are partly due to the presence of lidocaine in the injection fluid.

Hydrogen peroxide

Intravenous injection of hydrogen peroxide as an unconventional therapy for cancer or AIDS has resulted in acute hemolytic anemia, which can be followed by fatal complications such as cardiopulmonary arrest (146) or progressive renal impairment (147).

Lorenzo's oil *(SEDA-18, 453)*

This preparation of 20% erucic acid and 80% oleic acid has been advocated as a miracle cure for adrenoleukodystrophy but it has failed to live up to this popular image. Prolonged treatment has been associated with thrombocytopenia.

L-Tryptophan *(SEDA-15, 514)*

L-Tryptophan (LT) is a naturally occurring essential amino acid, which has been advocated as an innocuous health food for the treatment of depression, insomnia, stress, behavioral disorders, premenstrual syndrome, and so on. At the end of 1989, LT-containing health food products were associated in the United States with an epidemic of the so-called eosinophilia-myalgia syndrome (EMS). This syndrome was characterized by an eosinophil count of $\geqslant 10^9$/liter and intense generalized myalgia. Other relatively frequent signs and symptoms were complaints of fatigue, arthralgia, skin rash, cough and dyspnea, edema of the extremities, fever, scleroderma-like skin abnormalities, increased hair loss, xerostomia, pneumonia or pneumonitis with or without pulmonary vasculitis, and neuropathy. About one third of the cases required hospitalization, and a substantial number of patients died. Although there is good evidence that the epidemic was triggered by a contaminant, the responsible substance has not yet been identified.

In 1994, LT was reintroduced on the UK market under the strict condition that it should only be prescribed by hospital specialists for patients with long-standing resistant depression (148).

Ubidecarenone

Ubidecarenone (coenzyme Q10) is not only an investigational cardiovascular drug but is also widely available as a non-orthodox over-the-counter product. Several patients have been described in whom a reduced effect of warfarin was observed following the addition of non-orthodox ubidecarenone to their warfarin regimens. Ubidecarenone is chemically closely related to menaquinone (vitamin K_2) but the exact mechanism of this interaction remains to be identified (149, 150).

ACUPUNCTURE

Acupuncture is used predominantly to alleviate pain, but numerous other indications have been proposed. While the question of *efficacy* of this treatment is still unresolved, it is often assumed that the therapy is essentially free of risks. This is clearly not entirely true (151).

Peacher (152) mentions various minor adverse reactions. In addition there have been numerous reports

Table 5. *The most frequently reported complications of acupuncture*

Condition	Number of cases in the world literature
Cardiac trauma	4
Contact dermatitis	5
Drowsiness	79
Endocarditis	3
Erythema	4
Hepatitis	126
Perichondritis	12
Peripheral nerve injury	3
Pneumothorax	32
Renal injury	17
Retained needle	12
Septicemia	3
Spinal cord injury	19
Syncope	53

Modified from Ref. 125.

about serious complications (Table 5). Acupuncture needles must be handled adequately to guarantee sterility of the needle on insertion. If such safety rules are not strictly adhered to, there is a high risk of transmitting infectious diseases. In at least three published case-reports, acupuncture was the only plausible explanation for infections with the HIV virus (153, 154). Similarly hepatitis infections may be transmitted in this way (155—157).

Furthermore, osteomyelitis (158), endocarditis (159, 160) or generalized *Staphylococcus aureus* infections (161) have been associated with acupuncture. In principle one can assume that any blood-borne infection is transmittable through the (mis)-use of acupuncture needles.

By definition, acupuncture entails tissue trauma. If the technique is performed properly and on the correct acupuncture points, trauma will affect only the skin and the connective tissue below. If, however, acupuncture needles are inserted at the wrong site or penetrate too deeply, other tissues or organs can be affected.

One recent review identified 32 cases of pneumothorax and two of hemothorax (162). Damage to the middle ear (following auriculoacupuncture), injury to the spinal cord (152), cardiac tamponade have been other serious traumatic complication (163, 164). Needles may also break while in situ, and parts of acupuncture needles have been found in patients' kidney (165), carpal tunnel (166), cervical spine (167), spinal cord (168) and heart (169). Petechiae and other forms of bleeding have also been reported (162). If a nerve is punctured the patient might experience (unnecessary) pain and even sustain minor, in extreme cases persistent nerve damage.

Cases of allergies to the various metals used in acupuncture needles have been described (170); Chiu warned that acupuncture in pregnant women might carry a risk for the foetus; it is postulated that acupuncture can increase oxytocin release in the mother which subsequently might induce harmful effects on the unborn (171). Convulsions, inadvertent anesthesia, loss of co-ordination and tinnitus have also been reported (172). Aggravation of pre-existing symptoms, abortion, miscarriage (152) skin malignoma, (172) and Koebner phenomenon (173) have also been associated with acupuncture.

MANIPULATION

Manipulative therapies (chiropractic and osteopathy) are amongst the most prevalent of complementary treatments. Particularly when involving the cervical spine, they are associated with serious complications.

The Stroke Council of the AHA registered 359 cases of vascular accidents until 1981 (174). In Switzerland 1255 such incidents were recorded in 1 535 000 manipulations (175). Others estimated the incidence of *reported* vascular accidents to be one to four per million treatments (176—178). The mortality/severe long-term impairment rate of these is 28% (179).

The incidence rate is, of course, higher if minor symptoms are included and specifically searched for: out of a total of 75 500 procedures applied, 25 such cases were reported (180). The reported incidence rates are probably a gross under-estimation of the true figures; in a series of 13 cases of clinically and radiologically verified vertebral artery dissection, eight were spontaneous, two occurred after manipulation and three after minor injury (181).

The mechanisms of vascular complications of cervical manipulations involve vertebral artery dissection, intramural bleeding or pseudo-aneurysm leading to thrombosis or embolism (179) as well as transient cerebral ischemia through mechanical artery compression during cervical rotation (182) and vasospasm (183). The vertebral artery at the C_1/C_2 segment is most often affected. Combined rotation, extension and traction movements apparently create the highest risk, particularly when executed forcefully (184). The most frequent clinical findings are Wallenberg's (28%), other brain stem (49%), cerebellar (8%), occipital lobe (5%) and unclassified syndromes (179). They occur usually during or promptly after the intervention, but delays of hours, or days have also been observed (178, 185, 186). Symptoms may start as headache and neck pain which are frequent reasons for applying manipulative therapies in the first place. At least one case has been described where neck pain was the first sign of dissection, which

Table 6. *Patch testing results for five commercial herbal ointments in 1032 dermatological patients seen for patch testing*

Trade name (Supplier)	Herbal ingredient	Patients with positive reaction (11 in total)
Arniflor (VSM)	*Arnica* tinct. 10%	no. 1[a] 2[a] 3
Kamillosan (Homburg)	Chamomile extr. 4%	no. 1[a] 2[a] 4[b] 5[b] 6[c]
Echinacea (VSM)	*Echinacea* tinct. 10%	no. 7 8
Hamametum (VSM)	*Hamamelis* extr. 25%	no. 1[a] 2[a] 9 10
Calendula (VSM)	*Calendula* tinct. 10%	no. 1[a] 11

[a]Also positive to woolfat.
[b]Also positive to *Matricaria* leaf.
[c]Also positive to colophony.

in turn was treated by manipulation which resulted in a fatal stroke (187).

Dislocations and fractures of vertebra have also been reported and are not confined to the upper spine (188, 189). Patients with osteoporosis are at high risk; manipulation is therefore contra-indicated in these individuals. Nerval lesions range from plexus paralysis and ophthalmoplegia to tetraplegia, disk herniation and phrenic nerve palsy (188, 190). A recent review reported 89 neurological complications following manipulation, in the English language literature; the number of unreported cases could well be considerably higher.

INCIDENCE

Most data on adverse effects following complementary treatments are anecdotal and tell us little about the true size of the problem; unfortunately there are few systematic attempts to identify the incidence of adverse reactions to unorthodox remedies. One group studied the incidence of contact dermatitis (191). These researchers evaluated the contact sensitization potential of five commercial herbal ointments in 1032 consecutive or randomly selected patients visiting their patch test clinics. Eleven patients reacted positively to one or more ointments. Two of these patients were sensitized by wool fat, a non-herbal constituent of the ointments, but the reactions in the nine remaining patients (8.7%) could very well have been herb-induced (Table 6). In two of the patients reacting positive to the chamomile ointment, this was verified by additional testing with the plant material itself (*Matricaria* leaf).

Another group retrospectively studied all 2695 patients admitted to a Taiwan department of medicine during a period of 10 months. Four percent of these patients were admitted because of drug-related problems, and herbal remedies ranked third amongst the categories of medicines responsible (192). One case control study on nasopharyngeal carcinoma from the Philippines (193) identified herbal medicine use as one of the risk factors for this condition. A study of 1701 patients admitted to two general wards of a Hong Kong hospital revealed that only 0.2% of these cases were due to adverse reactions to Chinese herbal drugs—sadly though, two of the three cases were serious (194).

The London based National Poisons Unit surveyed retrospectively the time span between January 1983 and March 1989 and prospectively the entire year 1991 (133). 1070 enquiries were made in relation to herbal and other traditional drugs. Of these patients, 25.2% suffered from symptoms. Most adverse reactions were associated with herbal sedatives. In several cases a causal relationship between herbal medication and adverse effects were rated as highly probable: one case of hepatitis after an Ayurvedic remedy, one case of fatal liver failure after a Chinese herbal tea for eczema, one case of atropine poisoning following ingestion of a belladonna tea, one case of abdominal pain after taking a herbal tonic containing capsicum, one case of liver damage after a combined herbal sedative of valerian, hops, gentian and skullcap, one case of photodermatitis after ingestion of rue, one case of jaundice after skullcap and broom.

Vis-à-vis the high and growing popularity of complementary therapies, it would be unethical not to study their potential hazards systematically and in more detail than has been done so far.

REFERENCES

1. Eisenberg DM, Kessler RC, Foster C, Norlock FE, Calkins DR, Delbanco TL. Unconventional medicine in the United States. N Engl J Med 1993;328:246–52.
2. Fisher P, Ward A. Complementary Medicine in Europe. Br Med J 1994;309:107–111.
3. Ernst E. Phytomedicine research. Br Med J 1994; 308:673–674.
4. De Smet PAGM. Health risks of herbal remedies. Drug Safety 1995;13:81–93.
5. Ernst E. Competence in complementary medicine. Comp Ther Med 1995;3:6–8.
6. Boström H, Rössner S. Quality of alternative medicine—complications and avoidable deaths. Quality Assurance Health Care 1990;2:111–117.
7. Sulfaro F, Fasher B, Burgess MA. Homoeopathic vaccination, what does it mean? Med J Austr 1994;161:305–307.
8. Rasky E, Freidl W, Haidvogl M, Stronegger WJ. Arbeits-und Lebensweise von homöopathisch tätigen Arztinnen und Arzten in Österreich. Wien Med Wschr 1994;144:419–424.
9. Ernst E, White A. Homoeopathy and immunization. Br J Gen Pract 1995;48:629–630.
10. Colley F, Haas M. Attitudes on immunization: a survey of American chiropractors. J Manipul Physiol Ther 1994; 17:584–590.
11. Simpson N, Lenton S, Randall R. Potential refusal to have children immunized: extent and reasons. Br Med J 1995;310:227.
12. Ernst E. The safety of homoeopathy. Br Homoeopathy J 1995;84:193–194.
13. De Smet PAGM, D'Arcy PF. Drug interactions with herbal and other non-orthodox drugs. In: D'Arcy PF, McElnay JC, Welling PG, eds. Mechanisms of Drug Interactions. Heidelberg: Springer Verlag, in press.
14. Phillipson JD. Traditional medicine treatment for eczema: experience as a basis for scientific acceptance. Eur Phytotelegram 1994;6:33–40.
15. Kelly SP. Aconite poisoning. Med J Aust 1990;153:499.
16. Hikino H, Yamada C, Nakamura K et al. Change of alkaloid composition and acute toxicity of Aconitum roots during processing. Yakugaku Zasshi 1977;97:359.
17. Lee TY, Lam TH. Contact dermatitis due to topical treatment with garlic in Hong Kong. Contact Dermatitis 1991;24:193–196.
18. Canduela V, Mongil J, Carrascosa M, Docio S, Cagigas P. Br J Dermatol 1995;132:161–162.
19. Rose KD, Croissant PD, Parliament CF, Levin MB. Spontaneous spinal epidural hematoma with associated platelet dysfunction from excessive garlic ingestion: a case report. Neurosurgery 1990;26:880–882.
20. Ossenkoppele PM, Van der Sluis WG, Van Vloten WA. Fototoxische dermatitis door het gebruik van de Ammi majus-vrucht bij vitiligo. Ned Tijdschr Geneeskd 1991;135:478–480.
21. Siegers CP, Von Hertzberg-Lottin E, Otte M. Antranoid laxative abuse—a risk for colorectal cancer? Gut 1993; 34:1099–1001.
22. Kommission E. Aufbereitungsmonographien. Dtsch Apoth Ztg 1993;133:2791–2794.
23. Meijers FS. Idio-synkrasie voor folia uvae ursi. Ned Tijdschr Geneeskd 1902;46:1226–1228.
24. Taylor RFH, Al-Jarad N, John LME. Betel-nut chewing and asthma. Lancet 1992;339:577–578
25. Deahl M. Betel nut-induced extrapyramidal syndrome: an unusual drug interaction. Movement Disorders 1989; 4:330–333.
26. Pickwell SM, Schimelpfening S, Palinkas LA. 'Betelmania'. Betel quid chewing by Cambodian women in the United States and its potential health effects. West J Med 1994;160:326–330
27. Vanherweghem JL, Depierreux M, Tielemans C, Abramowicz D, Dratwa M, Jadoul M, Richard C, Vandervelde D, Verbeelen D, Vanhaelen-Fastre R et al. Rapidly progressive interstitial renal fibrosis in young women: association with slimming regimen including Chinese herbs. Lancet 1993; 341:387–391
28. Vanhaelen M, Vanhaelen-Fastre R, But P, Vanherweghem JL. Identification of aristolochic acid in Chinese herbs. Lancet 1994;343:174.
29. Depierreux M, Van Damme B, Vanden Houte K, Vanherweghem JL. Pathologic aspects of a newly described nephropathy related to the prolonged used of Chinese herbs. Am J Kidney Dis 1994;24:172–180.
30. Cosyns J-P, Jadoul M, Squifflet J-P, Van Cangh P-J, Van Ypersele De Strihou C. Urothelial malignancy in nephropathy due to Chinese herbs. Lancet 1994;344:188.
31. Rubin HR, WuAW. The bitter herbs of Seder: more on horseradish horrors. J Am Med Assoc 1988;259:1943.
32. Kurz G, Rapaport MJ. External/internal allergy to plants (Artemisia). Contact Dermatitis 1979;5:407–408.
33. Longerich L, Johnson E, Gault MH. Digoxin-like factors in herbal teas. Clin Invest Med 1993;16:210–218.
34. Khin-Maung-U, Myo-Khin, Nyunt-Nyunt-Wai, Aye-Kyaw, Tin-U. Clinical trial of berberine in acute watery diarrhoea. Br Med J 1985;291:1601–1605.
35. Bluhm R, Branch R, Johnston P, Stein R. Aplastic anemia associated with canthaxanthin ingested for 'tanning' purposes. J Am Med Assoc 1990;264:1141–1142.
36. Angelini G, Vena GA, Filotico R, Foti C, Grandolfo M. Allergic contact dermatitis from Capparis spinosa L. applied as wet compresses. Contact Dermatitis 1991;24:382–383.
37. Mengs U. Toxic effects of sennosides in laboratory animals and in vitro. Pharmacology 1988;36(Suppl 1):180–187.
38. Sandnes D, Johansen T, Teien G, Ulsaker G. Mutagenicity of crude senna and senna glycosides in *Salmonella typhimurium*. Pharmacol Toxicol 1992;71:165–172.
39. Mengs U. Reproductive toxicological investigations with sennosides. Arzneim Forsch 1986;36:1355–1358.
40. Faber P, Strenge-Hesse A. Relevance of rhein excretion into breast milk. Pharmacology 1988;36(Suppl 1):212–220.
41. Lydén-Sokolowski A, Nilsson A, Sjöberg P. Two-year carcinogenicity study with sennosides in the rat: emphasis on gastro-intestinal alterations. Pharmacology 1993;47(Suppl 1):209–215.
42. Widler P, Mathys K, Brenneisen R, Kalix P, Fisch HU. Pharmacodynamics and pharmacokinetics of khat: a controlled study. Clin Pharmacol Ther 1994;55:556–562.
43. Subiza J, Subiza JL, Hinojosa M et al. Anaphylactic reaction after the ingestion of chamomile tea: a study of cross-reactivity with other composite pollens. J Allergy Clin Immunol 1989;84:353–358.

44. Subiza J, Subiza JL, Alonso M et al. Allergic conjunctivitis to chamomile tea. Ann Allergy 1990;65:127—132.
45. Koopman H. Tödliche Schöllkraut-Vergiftung (*Chelidonium majus*). Vergiftungsfälle 1937;8:93—98.
46. Pinto Garcia V, Vicente PR, Barez A, Soto I et al. Anemia hemolitica inducida por *Chelidonium majus*. Observ Cl2n Sangre 1990;35:401—403.
47. Anonymous. Twenty-fifth Annual Report of the National Toxicoloy Group. Dunedin: New Zealand National Poisons and Hazardous Chemicals Information Centre, 1990;4.
48. Cox D, O'Kennedy R, Thornes RD. The rarity of liver toxicity in patients treated with coumarin (1,2-benzopyrone). Hum Toxicol 1989;8:501—506.
49. Guharoy SR, Barajas M. Atropine intoxication from the ingestion and smoking of jimson weed (*Datura stramonium*). Vet Hum Toxicol 1991;33:588—589.
50. Coremans P, Lambrecht G, Schepens P, Vanwelden J, Verhaegen H. Anticholinergic intoxication with commercially available thorn apple tea. Clin Toxicol 1994;32:589—592.
51. Anonymous. Jimson weed poisoning—Texas, New York, and California. MMWR 1995;44:41—44.
52. Pillans P, Eade MN, Massey RJ. Herbal medicine and toxic hepatitis. New Zealand Med J 1994;107:432—433.
53. Kane JA, Kane SP, Jain S. Hepatitis induced by traditional Chinese herbs; possible toxic components. Gut 1995;36:146—147.
54. Vautier G, Spiller RC. Safety of complementary medicines should be monitored. Br Med J 1995;311:633.
55. Perharic L, Shaw D, Leon C, De Smet PAGM, Murray VSG. Liver damage associated with certain types of traditional Chinese medicines used for skin diseases. Hum Exp Toxicol (in press).
56. Kao W-F, Hung D-Z, Lin K-P, Deng J-F. Podophyllotoxin intoxication: toxic effect of Bajiaolian in herbal therapeutics. Hum Exp Toxicol 1992;11:480—487.
57. Plouvier B, Trotin F, Deram R, De Coninck P, Baclet JL. Concombre d'ane (*Ecbalium elaterium*) une cause peu banale d'oedème de Quincke. Nouv Press Méd 1981;10:2590.
58. Vlachos P, Kanitsakis NN. Fatal cardiac and renal failure due to *Ecbalium elaterium* (squirting cucumber). Clin Toxicol 1994;32:737—738.
59. Anonymous. Immunallergische Reaktionen nach Echinacea-Extrakten (Echinacin, Esberitox N u.a.). Arznei-Telegramm 1991;4:39.
60. Cui J, Garle M, Eneroth P, Björkhem I. What do commercial ginseng preparations contain? Lancet 1994;344:134.
61. Awang DVC. Maternal use of ginseng and neonatal androgenization. J Am Med Assoc 1991;266:363.
62. Stormer FC, Reistad R, Alexander J. Glycyrrhizic acid in liquorice—evaluation of health hazard. Food Chem Toxicol 1993;31:303—312.
63. Hänsel R, Keller K, Rimpler H, Schneider G, eds. Hagers Handbuch der Pharmazeutischen Praxis. 5th edn. Band 5. Drogen E-O. Berlin: Springer-Verlag, 1993.
64. De Smet PAGM, Stricker BHC, Wilderink F, Wiersinga WM. Hyperthyreoïdie tijdens het gebruik van kelptabletten. Ned Tijdschr Geneeskd 1990;134:1058—1059.
65. Pye KG, Kelsey SM, House IM, Newland AC. Severe dyserythropoiesis and autoimmune thrombocytopenia associated with ingestion of kelp supplements. Lancet 1992; 339:1540.
66. Gordon DW, Rosenthal G, Hart J, Sirota R, Baker AL. Chaparral ingestion. The broadening spectrum of liver injury caused by herbal medications. J Am Med Assoc 1995; 273:489—490.
67. Batchelor WB, Heathcote J, Wanless IR. Chaparral-induced hepatic injury. Am J Gastroenterol 1995;90:831—833.
68. Smith AY, Feddersen RM, Gardner KD Jr, Davis CJ Jr. Cystic renal cell carcinoma and acquired renal cystic disease associated with consumption of chaparral tea: a case report. J Urol 1994;152:2089—2091.
69. Nakamura T, Kobayashi A. Toxikodermie durch den Speisepilz Shiitake (*Lentinus edodes*). Hautarzt 1985;36: 591—593.
70. Nakamura T. Shiitake (*Lentinus edodes*) dermatitis. Contact Dermatitis 1992;27:65—70.
71. Knight TE, Hausen BM. Melaleuca oil (tea tree oil) dermatitis. J Am Acad Dermatol 1994;30:423—427.
72. Elliott C. Tea tree oil poisoning. Med J Aust 1993; 159:830—831.
73. Seawright A. Tea tree oil poisoning. Med J Aust 1993; 159:831.
74. Chan TH, Wong KC, Chan JCN. Severe salicylate poisoning associated with the intake of Chinese medicinal oil (Red Flower Oil). Aust NZ J Med 1995;25:57.
75. Pichler WJ, Angeli R. Allergie auf Mistelextrakt. Dtsch Med Wschr 1991;116:1333—1334.
76. Harvey J, Colin-Jones DG. Mistletoe hepatitis. Br Med J 1981;282:186.
77. Leatherdale BA, Panesar RK, Singh G et al. Improvement In glucose tolerance due to *Momordica charantia* (karela). Br Med J 1981;282:1823—1824.
78. Aslam M, Stockley IH. Interactions between curry ingredient (karela) and drug (chlorpropamide). Lancet 1979;i:607.
79. Abernethy MK, Becker LB. Acute nutmeg intoxication. Am J Emerg Med 1992;10:429—430.
80. Kaplan R. Poppy seed dependence. Med J Aust 1994;161:176.
81. Unnithan S, Strang J. Poppy tea dependence. Br J Psychiatry 1993;163:813—814
82. ElSohly HN, ElSohly MA, Stanford DF. Poppy seed ingestion and opiates urinalysis. A closer look. J Anal Toxicol 1990;14:308—310.
83. Ruze P. Kava-induced dermopathy: a niacin deficiency? Lancet 1990;335:1442—1445.
84. Yong M, Cheong I. Jering-induced acute renal failure with blue urine. Trop Doctor 1995;25:31.
85. Lantner RR, Espiritu BR, Zumerchik P, Tobin MC. Anaphylaxis following ingestion of a psyllium-containing cereal. J Am Med Assoc 1990;264:2534 -2536.
86. Perlman BB. Interaction between lithium salts and ispaghula husk. Lancet 1990:335:416.
87. Maurice PDL, Cream JJ. The dangers of herbalism. Br Med J 1989;299:1204.
88. Anonymous. Vorinformation Pyrrolizidinalkaloidhaltige Human arzneimittel. Pharm Ztg 1990;135:2532—2533 and 2623—2624.
89. Anonymous. Aufbereitungsmonographien Kommission E. Pharm Ztg 1990;135:2081—2082.
90. De Smet PAGM, Stricker BHC. Meekrapwortel in Duitsland niet langer toegestaan. Pharm Weekbl 1993;128:503.
91. Landa N, Aguirre A, Goday J, Ratón JA, Diaz-Pérez JL. Allergic contact dermatitis from a vasoconstrictor cream. Contact Dermatitis 1990;22:290—291
92. Lo ACT, Chan Km Yeung JHK, Woo KS. The effects

of Danshen (*Salvia miltiorrhiza*) on pharmacokinetics and pharmacodynamics of warfarin in rats. Eur J Drug Metab Pharmacokin 1992;17:257–262.

93. Arzneimittelkommission der Deutschen Apotheker. Vorinformation Sassafras-haltige Arzneimittel. Dtsch Apoth Ztg 1995;135:366–368.

94. De Smet PAGM. Een alternatieve olie met een luchtje. Pharm Weekbl 1994;129:258.

95. Geier J, Fuchs T, Wahl R. Anaphylaktischer Schock durch einen Mariendistel-Extrakt bei Soforttyp-Allergie auf Kiwi. Allergologie 1990;13:387–388.

96. Lin JL, Ho YS. Flavonoid-induced acute nephropathy. Am J Kidney Dis 1994;23:433–440.

97. Horowitz RS, Gomez H, Moore LL, Fulton B, Feldhaus K, Brent J, Stermitz FR, Beck JJ, Alessi JR, De Smet PAGM. Jin Bu Huan toxicity in children—Colorado 1993. Morb Mortal Weekly Rep 1993;42:633–636.

98. Woolf GM, Petrovic LM, Rojter SE, Wainwright S, Villamil FG, Katkov WN, Michieletti P, Wanless IR, Stermitz FR, Beck JJ, Vierling JM. Acute hepatitis associated with the Chinese herbal product Jin Bu Huan. Ann Intern Med 1994;121:729–735.

99. Castot A, Larrey D. Hépatites observées au cours d'un traitement par un médicament ou une tisane contenant de la germandrée petit-chêne. Bilan des 26 cas rapportés aux Centres Régionaux de Pharmacovigilance. Gastroenterol Clin Biol 1992;16:916–922.

100. Mostefa-Kara N, Pauwels A, Pines E, Biour M, Levy VG. Fatal hepatitis after herbal tea. Lancet 1992;340:674.

101. Dao T, Peytier A, Galateau F, Valla A. Hépatite chronique cirrhogène à la germandrée petit-chêne. Gastroenterol Clin Biol 1993;17:609–610.

102. Loeper J, Descatoire V, Letteron P, Moulis C, Degott C, Dansette P, Fau D, Pessayre D. Hepatotoxicity of germander in mice. Gastroenterology 1994;106:464–472.

103. Yu D-Y. Clinical observation of 144 cases of rheumatoid arthritis treated with glycoside of Radix *Tripterygium wilfordii*. J Tradit Chin Med 1983;3:125–129.

104. Tao X-L, Sun Y, Dong Y et al. A prospective, controlled, double-blind, cross-over study of *Tripterygium wilfordii* Hook f in treatment of rheumatoid arthritis. Chin Med J 1989;102:327–332.

105. Qian SZ. *Tripterygium wilfordii*, a Chinese herb effective in male fertility regulation. Contraception 1987; 36:335–345.

106. Guo J-L, Yuan S-X, Wang X-C, Xu S-X, Li D-D. *Tripterygium wilfordii* Hook in rheumatoid arthritis and ankylosing spondylitis. Preliminary report. Chin Med J 1981;94:405–412.

107. Tuncok Y, Kozan O, Cavdar C, Guven H, Fowler J. *Urginea maritima* (squill) toxicity. Clin Toxicol 1995;33:83–86.

108. Bossuyt L, Dooms-Goossens A. Contact sensitivity to nettles and camomile in 'alternative' remedies. Contact Dermatitis 1994;31:131–132.

109. Dieckmann H. Untersuchungen zur Pharmakokinetik, Metabolismus und Toxikologie von Baldrinalen. Inaugural Dissertation, Free University, Berlin, 1988.

110. Cahill DJ, Fox R, Wardle PG, Harlow CR. Multiple follicular development associated with herbal medicine. Hum Reprod 1994;9:1469–1470

111. De Smet PAGM, Smeets OSNM. Potential risks of health food products containing yohimbe extracts. B Med J 1994;309:958.

112. Chan TYK, Chan AY, Critchley JA. Hospital admissions due to adverse reactions to Chinese herbal medicines. J Trop Med Hyg 1992;95:296–298.

113. Kerr HD, Saryan LA. Arsenic content of homoeopathic medicines. Clin Toxicol 1986;24:451–459.

114. De Smet PAGM. Giftige metalen in homeopathische preparaten Pharm Weekbl 1992;127:125–126.

115. Oepen I. Kritische Argumente zur Homöopathie. Dtsch Apoth Ztg 1983;123:1105.

116. Pancreatitis following ingestion of a homeopathic preparation. N. Engl J Med 1986;414:1642.

117. Van Ulsen J, Stolz E, Joost T. Chromate dermatitis from a homoeopathic drug. Contact Dermatitis 1988;18:56–57.

118. Forsman S. Homeopati kan vara farling vid hudsjukdomar och allergier. Läkartidningen 1991;88:1672.

119. De Smet PAGM, Pegt GWM, Meyboom RHB. Acute circulatoire shock na toepassing van het niet-reguliere enzympreparaat Wobe-Mogus. Ned Tijdschr Geneesk 1991; 135:2341–2344.

120. Anonymous. Acute hepatitis and renal failure following ingestion of raw carp gallbladders—Maryland and Pennsylvania 1991 and 1994. MMWR 1995;44:566–569.

121. Chan DWS, Yeung CK, Chan MK. Acute renal failure after eating raw fish gall bladder. Br Med J 1985;290:897.

122. Chen CF, Lin MC, Liu HM. Plasma electrolyte changes after ingestion of bile extract of the grass carp (*Ctenopharyngodon idellus*) in rats. Toxicol Lett 1990;50:221–228.

123. O'Donohue JW, Reid MA, Varghese A, Portmann B, Williams R. Micronodular cirrhosis and acute liver failure due to chronic copper self-intoxication. Eur J Gastroenterol Hepatol 1993;5:561–562

124. Sorisky A, Robbins DC. Fish oil and diabetes. The net effect. Diabetes Care 1989;12:302–304.

125. Haines AP, Sanders TAB, Imerson JD. Effects of fish oil supplement on platelet function, homeostatic variables and albuminuria in insulin dependent diabetics. Thromb Res 1986;43:643–655.

126. Anonymous. Ganglioside (Cronassial u.a.) und neurologische Erkrankungen. Arznei-Telegramm 1992;12:126.

127. Nobile-Orazio E, Carpo M, Scarlato G. Gangliosides: their role in clinical neurology. Drugs 1994;47:576–585.

128. Traverso HP, Bennett JV, Kahn AJ et al. Ghee applications to the umbilical cord: a risk factor for neonatal tetanus. Lancet 1989;i:486–488.

129. Anonymous. Imedeen®, bron der eeuwige jeugd? Gebu Prikbord 1993;27:68.

130. Anonymous. Quincke's oedeem bij gebruik van oesterextract in Ostrin plus GTZ 611®. Gebu Prikbord 1994;28:67.

131. Anonymous. Propolis—recalled because of lead contamination. WHO Pharmac Newslett 1995;1:3.

132. Bullock RJ, Rohan A, Straatmans JA. Fatal royal jelly-induced asthma. Med J Aust 1994;160:44.

133. Perharic L, Shaw D, Colbridge M, House I, Leon C, Murray V. Toxicological problems resulting from exposure to traditional remedies and food supplements. Drug Safety 1994;11:284–294.

134. Kok-Choi C, Hee-Ming L, Bobby SSF, David YCP. A fatality due to the use of cantharides from *Mylabris phalerata*, an aboritfacient. Med Sci Law 1990;30:336–340.

135. Asnis DS, Saltzman HP, Melchert A. Shark oil pneumonia. An overlooked entity. Chest 1993;103:976–977

136. De Smet PAGM. Toxicological outlook on the quality assurance of herbal remedies. In: De Smet PAGM, Keller

K, Hänsel R, Chandler RF, eds. Adverse Effects of Herbal Drugs, Vol 1. Heidelberg: Springer-Verlag, 1992;1–72.
137. Fushimi R, Tachi J, Amino N, Miyai K. Chinese medicine interfering with digoxin immunoassays. Lancet 1989; i:339.
138. Lin CS, Lin MC, Chen KS et al. A digoxin-like immunoreative substance and atrioventricular block induced by a Chinese medicine 'Kyushin'. Jpn Circ J 1989;53:1077–1080.
139. Dreosti IE, Wahlqvist ML. Prescribing trace elements in clinical practice. Aust Prescr 1989;12:39–44.
140. Van der Spoel JI, Stricker BHC, Schipper MEI et al. Toxische beschadigung van nier, lever en spier toegeschreven aan het gebruik van germanium-lactaat-citraat. Ned Tijdschr Geneeskd 1991;135:1134–1137.
141. Treleaven J, Meller S, Farmer P, Birchall D, Goldman J, Piller G. Arsenic and Ayurveda. Leukaemia Lymphoma 1993;10:343–345
142. Wood R, Mills PB, Knobel GJ et al. Acute dichromate poisoning after use of traditonal prugatives. A report of 7 cases. S Afr Med (1990) J 77, 640–642.
143. Dunn JP, Krige JE, Wood R et al. Colonic complications after tozic tribal enemas. Br J Surg 1991;78:545–548.
144. Spiegel P, Fliegner L, Delling G. Osteomalazie infolge Fumarsäure-induzierten Tubulus-Defektes (sekundäres De-Toni-Debré-Fanconi-Syndrom). Nieren Hochdruckkrankh 1991;20:280–288.
145. Thesen R. Fumarsäureester bei Psoriasis. Pharm Ztg 1994;139:4122–4123.
146. Hirschtick RE, Dyrda SE, Peterson LC. Death from an unconventional therapy for AIDS. Ann Intern Med 1994; 120:694.
147. Jordan KS, Mackey D, Garvey E. A 39-year-old man with acute hemolutic crisis secondary to intravenous injection of hydrogen peroxide. J Emerg Nurs 1991;17:8–10.
148. D'Arcy PF. L-Tryptophan (Optimax): limited availability for resistant depression. Int Pharm J 1994;8:56.
149. Spigset O. Reduced effect of warfarin caused by ubidecarenone. Lancet 1994;344:1372–1373.
150. Anonymous. Coenzym Q10 (Qumin Q10 u.a.) stört orale Antikoagulation. Arznei-Telegramm 1994;12:120.
151. Ernst E. The risks of acupuncture. Int J Risk Safety Med 1995;6:179–186.
152. Peacher WC. Adverse reactions, contraindications and complications of acupuncture and moxibustion. Am J Chin Med 1975;3:35–46.
153. Castro KG, Lifson AR, White CR, Bush TJ, Chamberland ME, Lekatsas AM, Jaffe HW. Investigations of AIDS patients with no previously identified risk factors. J Am Med Assoc 1988;259:1338–1342.
154. Vittecoq D, Mettetal JF, Rouzioux C, Bach JF, Bouchon JP. Acute HIV infection after acupuncture treatments. New Engl J Med 1988;320:250–251.
155. Kent GP, Brondum J, Keenlyside RA, Lafazia LM, Scott HD. A large outbreak of acupuncture-associated hepatitis B. Am J Epidemiol 1988;127:591–598.
156. Mitchitaka K, Horiike N, Ohta Y. An epidemiological study of hepatitis C virus infection in a local district in Japan. Rinsho Bvori 1991;39:586–591.
157. Boxall EH. Acupuncture hepatitis in the west midlands. J Med Virol 1978;2:377–379.
158. Jones RD, Cross G III. Suspected chronic osteomyelitis secondary to acupuncture treatment. J Am Pociatry Assoc 1980;70:149–151.
159. Scheel O, Sundsfjord A, Lunde P. Bacterial endocarditis after treatment by a natural healer. Tidsskr Nor Laegeforen 1991;111:2741–2742.
160. Scheel, Sundsfjord A, Lunde P, Anderson BM. Endocarditis after acupuncture and injection-treatment by a natural healer. J Am Med Assoc 1992;267:56.
161. Baltimore RS, Moloy PJ. Perichondritis of the ear as a complication of acupuncture. Arch Otolarvngol 1976; 102:572–573.
162. Rampes H, James R. Complications of acupuncture. Acupunct Med 1995;13:26–33.
163. Schiff AF. A fatality due to acupuncture. Med Times 1965;93:630–631.
164. Cheng TO. Pericardial effusion from self-inserted needle in the heart. Eur Heart J 1991;12:958.
165. Keller WJ, Palmer SG, Garvin JP. Possible renal complications of acupuncture. J Am Med Assoc 1972;222:1559.
166. Southworth SR, Hartwig RH. J Hand Surg 1990; 15:111–112.
167. Murata K, Nishio A, Nishikawa M, Ohinata Y, Sakaguchi M, Nishimura S. Subarachnoid haemorrhage and spinal root injury caused by acupuncture needle-case report. Neurol Med Chir 1990;30:956–959.
168. Shiraishi S, Kuroiwa Y, Nishio S, Kinoshita. Spinal cord injury as a complication of acupuncture. Neurology 1979;29:1188–1190.
169. Hasegawa J, Noguchi N, Yamasaki J, Kotake H, Mashiba H, Sasaki S, Mori T. Delayed cardiac tamponade and hemothorax induced by an acupuncture needle. Cardiology 1991;78:58–63.
170. Tanii T, Kono T, Katoh J, Mizuno N, Fukuda M, Hamada T. A case of prurigo pigmentosa considered to be contact allergy to chromium in an acupuncture needle. Acta Dermatol Venereol 1991;71:66–67.
171. Chiu DT. The use of acupuncture during pregnancy. Intern J Med 1984;1:19–21.
172. Tsukerman IM. A rare case of carcinoma of the skin arising after acupuncture. Voprosy Onkol 1970;16:88.
173. Kirschbaum JO. Koebner Phenomenon following acupuncture. Arch Dermatol 1972;106:767.
174. Robertson JF. Neck manipulation as a cause of stroke. Stroke 1981;12:1.
175. Dvorakj J. Manuelle Medizin. Stuttgart: Thieme, 1983.
176. Hosek RS, Schram SB, Silverman H, Myers JB, Williams SE. Cervical manipulation. J Am Med Assoc 1981;245:922–925.
177. Gutmann G. Injuries to the vertebral artery caused by manual therapy. Mannuelle Ther 1983;21:2–14.
178. Hamann G, Felber S, Haass A, Strittmatter M, Kujat C, Schimrigk K, Piepgras U. Cervicocephalic artery dissection due to chiropractic manipulations. Lancet 1993; 341:764–765.
179. Frisoni GB, Anzola GP. Vertebrobasilar ischemia after neck motion. Stroke 1991;22:1452–1460.
180. Michaeli A. Dizziness testing of the cervical spine: can complications of manipulations be prevented? Physiother Theory Pract 1991;7:243–250.
181. Mas JL, Bousser MG, Hasboun D, Laplane D. Extracranial vertebral artery dissections—a review of 13 cases. Stroke 1987;18:1037–1047.
182. Green D, Joynt RJ. Vascular accidents to the brain stem with neck manipulation. J Am Med Assoc 1959; 170:522–524.
183. Smith RA, Estridge MN. Neurologic complications of head and neck manipulations. J Am Med Assoc 1962; 182:528–531.

184. Stevens AJJE. Zur Dopplersonographie der A. vertebralis bei Rotation des Kopfes. In: Gutman G. ed. Arteria Vertebrals. Traumatologie und Funktionelle Pathologie. Berlin: Springer, 1985;90–99.

185. Okawara S, Nibbelink D. Vertebral artery occlusion following hyperextension and rotation of the head. Stroke 1974;5:640–642.

186. Frumkin LR, Baloh RW. Wallenberg's syndrome following neck manipulation. Neurology 1990;40:611–615.

187. Mas JL, Henin D, Bousser MG Chain F, Haw JJ. Dissecting aneurysm of the vertebral artery and cervical manipulation: a case report with autopsy. Neurology 1989;39:512–515.

188. Schmitt HP. Risiken und Komplikationen der Manualtherapie der Wirbelsäule aus neurologischer Sicht. Nervenarzt 1988;59:32–35.

189. Halderman S, Rubinstein SM. Compression fractures in patients undergoing spinal manipulative therapy. J Manipulative Physiol Ther 1992;15:45–54.

190. Tolge C, Iyer V, McConnell J. Phrenic nerve palsy accompanying chiropractic manipulation of the neck. South Med J 1993;86:688–690.

191. Bruynzeel DP, Van Ketel WG, Young E, Van Joost Th., Smeenk G. Contact sensitization by alternative topical medicaments containing plant extracts. Contact Dermatitis 1992;27:278–279.

192. Lin SH, Lin MS. A survey on drug related hospitalisation in a community teaching hospital. Int J Clin Pharmacol Ther Toxicol 1993;31:66–99.

193. West S, Hildesheim A, Dosemeci M. Non-viral risk factors for nasopharyngeal carcinoma in the Philippines. Int J Cancer 1993;55:722–727.

194. Chan TYK, Chan AYW, Critchley JAJH. Hospital admissions due to adverse reactions to Chinese herbal medicines. J Trop Med Hyg 1992;95:296–298.

Meyler's Side Effects of Drugs, 13th Edition
M.N.G. Dukes, editor

SECTION EDITOR: P.I. FOLB

H. Haak

49 Miscellaneous drugs and materials

Many drugs, agents and devices which do not strictly fall within the scope of the previous chapters (some of which lie at the fringe of medicinal drug therapy) can cause adverse reactions, some serious. In this chapter priority is given to new information. For additional and older information the reader is referred to previous volumes and to the Annuals (see Table 1 at the end of the chapter). Toxicological and safety issues pertaining to foods are not considered in this Chapter.

SURGICAL, OPHTHALMIC AND DENTAL MATERIALS AND APPLIANCES

Acrylic bone cement

Local biocompatibility Although polymerized polymethylmethacrylate is a biocompatible material, it is not so during the brief period of setting. During that stage it releases 130 calories per gram and a rise in temperature up to 120°C is possible. This temperature rise can be reduced by various techniques, although the thermal tolerance of the tissues affected is low (56 and 72°C for coagulation of body proteins and bone collagen, respectively). This is the main factor responsible for bone necrosis associated with acrylic bone cement. To avoid this, sucrose crystals have been added to acrylic cement. The mixture has a lower polymerization temperature and greater porosity, allowing for better ingrowth of bone into the cement pores (1[r]); however, the resultant lower mechanical resistance limits its use (2[c], 3[c]). The same can be achieved by adding tricalcium phosphate which lowers the reaction temperature. The non-polymerized monomer is cytotoxic (4[c]), which can cause histopathological changes in soft tissues and bones.

Methylmethacrylate is essentially an immunologically inert implant material, but it induces an inflammatory mononuclear cell migration (5[r], 6[R]). Both cemented and cementless prostheses cause a foreign body-type host response. A new connective tissue capsule is formed around the artificial joint, which is coarser than normal. The reaction is partly granulomatous, with a tendency to necrosis and loosening of the prosthesis. After an initial necrotic phase of 2—3 weeks repair follows, leading to stabilization within 2 years.

Addition of materials (e.g. antibiotics or radiopaque contrast material) to acrylic bone cement may cause mechanical weakness due to loss of homogeneity and greater water resorption. Antibiotics have been added to combat the problem of microbial adherence. However, they may lead to a considerable dead biofilm mass on the polymethylmethacrylate surface, promoting late infections by providing a surface attractive to other strains of bacteria (7[c]).

General toxicity Since side effects in humans develop within 2—5 minutes of fixation, with features of pulmonary insufficiency, direct pulmonary damage has been postulated with the cardiovascular effects a consequence of hypoxemia (8[c], 9[c], 10[r]). This has been demonstrated by lactase dehydrogenase isomer determinations, fractions 3 and 4 being significantly elevated. These isoenzymes are released as a result of pulmonary mitochondrial injury caused by hypoxia. Methylmethacrylate monomer vapor may irritate the respiratory tract, eyes, and skin.

Regional damage This is generally the result of poor surgical technique, whereby the cement inadvertently reaches other tissues and structures. For example, leaking methylmethacrylate cement during fixation of the acetabular cup in a total hip replacement may cause sciatic nerve compression and result in severe lasting leg pain (11[C]).

Allergy Sensitization may occur in patients, surgeons and dentists, and it is reported occasionally in the literature (12[c]). As most surgical gloves do not provide a reliable barrier, additional gloves are recommended. Contact dermatitis, dizziness, nausea and vomiting occur. Ethylene oxide present in acrylic bone cement may induce acute allergic reactions in sensitized patients (13[c]).

Neoplastic effects So far, no malignancies have been described as a consequence of orthopedic use of acrylic bone cement. However, one should keep in mind that the latent period for carcinogenicity in humans is long

(20–30 years), and that the first of such cases may only start to appear now. Moreover, acrylic bone cement tends to be used most often in individuals who do not have such a long period left to live.

Cardiovascular effects Cardiovascular reactions to acrylic bone cement are a common complication in bone surgery. It is believed that cementation activates an adrenocortical response, elevating the blood pressure during general anesthesia (14[C], 15[c]); during spinal anesthesia this response is suppressed and blood pressure drops. The mechanism is thought to be by direct influence on blood pressure through the kallikrein-kinin system, since aprotinin (Trasylol), an inhibitor of kallikrein, prevents the fall in arterial pressure if it is given during acrylic bone-application (16[c]). Some investigators suggested that implantation of acrylic bone cement into the femur may increase plasma histamine which, specially in elderly patients with pre-existing cardiac diseases or/and hypovolemia, may cause serious, sometimes fatal cardiovascular complications (17[R]).

Collagen

Purified solubilized bovine collagen (Zyderm) is used as biomaterial for the treatment of soft tissue defects. Injected material precipitates at body temperature, forming a matrix allowing fibroblastic infiltration and formation of new tissue. It has been used for cosmetic purposes by injection in the dermis to correct scars and other contour deformities of the skin.

Despite its low antigenicity, the preparation is contraindicated in patients with immunological disorders. Patients should be tested with 0.1 ml Zyderm and reassessed at 4 weeks. Approximately 3% of the patients tested in this way developed *hypersensitivity reactions to collagen*, whereas 1% of treated patients have symptoms of hypersensitivity at treatment sites (18[c]). In this series, *erythema* was the sole symptom in 24%, and erythema and induration occurred in an additional 42%. Of the patients with complications, 45% reported an onset of symptoms within 10 days, while in 22% the onset was more than 30 days following treatment with collagen. *Abscesses* as a manifestation of hypersensitivity to bovine collagen occur rarely (four in 10 000 cases), but the possibility of contamination should always be considered. Local *tissue necrosis* occurs rarely after implantation (nine reported in 10 000 cases) and this is thought to be the result of local vascular interruption rather than a hypersensitivity reaction. The incidence varies widely according to the site of implantation, but more than one-half of the cases involve the glabellar region, probably because of its special vascular distribution (19[r]). Despite pretreatment collagen testing, anaphylactic shock has been reported in one patient, necessitating adrenergic agents and corticosteroids, and an allergic rash has been described after collagen injection (20[c]). These reports underline the need for adequate follow-up when collagen implants are used.

Contact lenses

Ulcerative keratitis is considered the most serious adverse effect of the use of soft contact lenses. However, it is known that this risk can be greatly reduced by avoiding overnight wear of the lenses (21[R], 22[C]). One study determined that extended wear was associated with a 5–6 times higher risk of keratitis than daily wear (23[R]). Soft contact lenses, especially extended-wear lenses, carry a significantly higher risk than do hard lenses for this disease. In a case-control study, it was found that the relative risk for overnight wear soft lenses was 21, for daily-wear soft lenses 3.6, and for polymethylmethacrylate hard lenses 1.3, as compared with gas-permeable hard lenses (24[c]).

Micro-organisms may infiltrate into soft hydrophillic lenses, causing *infection* and possibly corneal ulcers. *Acanthamoeba* is the most common cause. A recent case-control study determined that an increased risk of *Acanthamoeba* infection could be largely attributed to lack of disinfection or the use of chlorine based disinfection (the latter having little protective effect against the organism). Around 80% of cases of *Acanthamoeba* keratitis could have been avoided by the use of lens disinfection systems that are effective against this organism (25[R]). *Pseudomonas aeruginosa* adherence to corneal epithelial cells was also found to be enhanced in those who use extended-wear soft contact lenses (26[c]).

Oxygen deficiency may occur under the lens. The dimension of the lens, duration of wear and hygiene are determining factors. Tolerance is individual, and less hydrophillic materials produce a higher degree of corneal hypoxia. This is manifested by edema, and sometimes by vascularization and even limbus hyperemia and pannus corneae (27[C], 28[C]). Tear-film disruption may be a contributing factor.

Dental materials

Composite epoxy resins may cause a generalized *allergic skin rash*. Formation of *lichenoid lesions* associated with resin restoration has been described in 17 cases (SEDA-14, 456).

Fibrin glue

Fibrin glue is a physiological epoxy substance used in a variety of clinical situations including bleeding, organ injury (29[c]), cardiac surgery (30[c]), and dural defects (31[c]). *Severe hypotension* has been reported after the use of fibrin glue for hemostasis in hepatic injuries (32[c]). In one there was cardiac arrest and death. These effects may be the result of an *anaphylactic reaction* to one or more components of the glue. Of the three ingredients used to prepare fibrin glue, cryoprecipitate and bovine thrombin are antigenic and potentially the most likely causes of anaphylaxis.

One report gives case histories of three patients who underwent cardiovascular surgery (33[c]). Subsequent *abnormalities in hemostasis*, characterized by increased activated partial thromboplastin time, prothrombin time, bovine thrombin time, and by a markedly reduced factor V level, developed between the seventh and eighth postoperative days after exposure to fibrin glue containing bovine thrombin. It was suggested that the glue also contains small amounts of factor V and that this may have caused the abnormalities.

Fluorescein

A *thrombocytopenic reaction* resulting in transient purpura may occur when fluorescein is used in ocular angiography (SED-11, 1039). Severe anaphylaxis has been reported after oral administration of fluorescein (34). Allergic and inflammatory reactions to fluorescein are discussed in Chapter 47.

Glycine

Glycine solution is frequently used during transurethral prostatectomy for bladder irrigation, sometimes continuously for 24 hours after surgery. This may have an adverse effect on renal function in about 1% of cases, although it is rarely severe. Absorption of glycine may occur, with the development of *hyperoxaluria*. High initial values of urine oxalate decrease progressively over 2 weeks. This is long enough for calcium oxalate deposition to occur, if urine output is low. It has been recommended that glycine irrigation should be confined to the time of operation, and an adequate diuresis should be ensured postoperatively (35[Cr]). Rapid and massive fluid absorption due to *leakage of fluid into the peritoneal cavity* has also been reported during percutaneous nephrolithotomy (36[r]).

Glycine can act as an inhibitory neurotransmitter, which may explain why absorption of glycine—containing irrigating fluid from the pelvic cavity or directly into the blood during transurethral prostate resection has been linked to *loss of sight* and vivid *postoperative hallucinations* (37[c]). *Ammonia production* due to accumulation of glycine in tissues, and the mentioned neuroinhibitory effects of glycine should be considered risk factors when deciding on glycine as an irrigating fluid (38[c]).

Histoacryl (histocyl, enbucrilate)

Histoacryl is a tissue adhesive used in duraplasty. The sites at which it is used should be carefully chosen. Infection may develop in the frontal area and at the lateral base of the skull, even after a symptom-free interval of several years; the lesions may be characterized by infected *granular nodules*, *chronic sinusitis* or *otogenic meningitis* (39[r]).

Intrauterine contraceptive devices An intrauterine contraceptive device (IUD) may break the protective barrier of cervical mucus because of the vaginal thread attached to it. This creates a locus minoris resistentiae for various infections, although this may be explained more by poor hygiene than by the device itself. The incidence of *salpingitis* and other pelvic inflammation is believed to be higher in IUD users. A study of cervical smears in women using IUD contraception compared with others using other methods of contraception showed the incidence of *cervical inflammation* to be higher in the former (40[C]).

Genital tract *actinomycosis* has come increasingly to the fore (41[c], 42[c]). In one study in Britain, the pelvic smears of nearly one-third of women using plastic devices were positive for *Actinomyces*-like organisms, compared with two of 165 women using copper-loaded IUDs and none in a series of oral contraceptive users. There was a highly significant correlation between the presence of these organisms on smear and pain or other symptoms of pelvic inflammatory disease.

Current users of IUDs suffer more frequently from *acute rather than chronic pelvic inflammatory disease* (1.51 compared with 0.54 times per 1000 woman-years). In ex-users the situation was reversed, chronic pelvic inflammatory disease being more common (0.95 compared with 0.48 times per 1000 woman-years) (43[C]).

Whether the risk of *ectopic pregnancy* is increased in women using an IUD is a question to which there is not yet a final answer (44[R], 45[C]). The proportion of these pregnancies has been reported as 6–8%, or higher. Primary *ovarian pregnancies* develop in IUD users, suggesting that ovarian implantation is not fully prevented (46[Cr]).

Two pregnancies (with normal outcome) have been described in renal transplant patients using an IUD. It seems that an *intact immune system* is needed for effective contraception by IUD, and that immunosuppressive therapy may render an IUD ineffective. Immunosuppressed patients should be advised to use another means of contraception (47[Cr]).

The tissue effects of copper-containing IUDs have been evaluated (48[cr]). Abnormal cells were observed on the surface of the device as well as in the copper ions escaping to the surface of the device may be responsible for *local endometrial damage*.

The *fibrinolytic activity* of menstrual blood in Lippes loop wearers exceeds that of menorrhagic patients, while the values in Cu-T (200) users are in the same range as normally menstruating and untreated women. In Lippes loop users no fibrin was found in endometrial stroma. This may explain the increased blood loss associated with the use of the Lippes loop, which may be severe enough to cause anemia (49[C]).

Polytetrafluoroethylene (teflon, polytef)

Polytetrafluoroethylene (Polytef) is widely used in industry. 'Teflon' is used in household appliances, to avoid sticking of food. Polytef paste is used for a variety of medical purposes, including replacement grafts in vascular surgery, vocal cord or fold augmentation, and correction of vesicoureteric reflux and urinary incontinence.

Refluxing ureters can be treated endoscopically with subureteric injection of polytetrafluoroethylene paste (Polytef), the 'STING' procedure. However, *ureteric obstruction* has been described as a complication (50[C]). Urinary incontinence has been treated by periurethral or submucosal injections of Polytef, but reports of urinary obstruction (51[c]) and poor long-term success (52[C], 53[C]) have limited the range of indications for this treatment. Other reported complications of teflon injection for stress urinary incontinence include *periurethral abscess*, *urethral diverticulum*, *teflon granuloma* with urethral wall prolapse (54[C]), and *microembolization* (55[r]). Teflon injected in a young woman for urinary incontinence migrated to the pulmonary vascular system (56[c]).

Particles of Teflon may detach from a cardiac valve prosthesis, producing *embolic complications* (57[c]). Postoperative failure after Teflon sling repair of a rectal prolapse is probably due to poor technique (58[c]). Interposition of Teflon-Proplast implants for internal derangement of the temperomandibular joint has been used, although cases of *osseous destructive changes* have been reported (59[r]).

Polyurethane

Polyurethane is commonly used in implants. Complications are not uncommon, mainly due to a *foreign-body reaction* to the material (60[R]) such as with the microporous polyurethane (Mitrathane) cardiac patch implant and with breast implants.

Silicone

Injectable silicone, used in cosmetic surgery, for example for breast enlargement, may produce various complications. These include *formation of cysts* and *granulomas*, both soon after injection, and later (61[r], 62[R]). Thorough examination to exclude breast cancer may be necessary. Silicone implants sometimes provoke systemic adverse effects. More than 20 women developed *muscle pain*, *joint pain and swelling*, *pulmonary disease* including pleural effusions, pulmonary infiltrates, and reduced pulmonary diffusing capacity, *dry eyes*, *dysphagia*, *bladder dysfunction*, *neurological abnormalities*, and *skin disease* (including localized and diffuse *scleroderma-like changes*) (63[c]). The authors assumed that *rupture of the gel-filled prosthesis* was the most likely cause of these symptoms. The prosthesis was intact in some patients, but amorphous silicone-like material was identified by light microscopy in surgically removed fibrous tissue. In another study (64[c]), similar granulomatous inflammatory reactions developed when silicone elastomers were used as skin expanders. This was attributed to leakage of particles of the plastic material through the expander wall.

Silicone implants (especially joint prostheses) carry the risk of migration of silicone, causing *lymphadenitis* and *destructive synovitis* (65[c], 66[C]). Removal of silicone implants was the only way to cure pain due to implants in some cases (67[R]). *Foreign-body reaction* to silicone may complicate silicone elastomer joint prostheses, manifesting as *synovitis* and/or *lymphadenopathy*, sometimes at remote locations (68[C]).

Use of silicone in dialysis tubing has led to *dissemination of silicone* causing splenomegaly and deposits in liver, bone marrow, skin and visceral lymph nodes. Exposure for less than 53 months did not elicit these complications (69[Cr], 70[C]). Pneumonitis and pulmonary edema following subcutaneous injection of silicone have been reported (71[C], 72[r], 73[r]).

Spermicides

These are widely used for contraception. Use in the year before pregnancy or during pregnancy has been associated with adverse reproductive outcomes, including *spontaneous abortion* and *Down syndrome*. In a preliminary analysis an association was found between spermicide use at conception and tetraploid and hypertriploid conceptions (74[CR]). An association between the use of vaginal spermicides and birth defects has been suggested (75[R]).

Spermicide use for more than a year at any time prior to conception was more common in cases aborting a trisomic conception than in controls. The association varied with maternal age, and was confined to women aged 30 years or older (76[c]).

Talc

Talc is principally used as inert filler material in medicinal tablets or as a drying ingredient in baby powders. Inappropriate use can lead to severe pulmonary toxicological responses.

Intravenous injection of 'solubilized' psychoactive pills containing talc can produce microemboli in small pulmonary vessels, leading to *talc granulomatosis*, a common finding in drug abusers. Medications intended for oral use may be injected or sniffed, together with talc particles. Pulmonary hypertension due to talc microemboli is a well—known cause of respiratory failure in heroin addicts. A case has been described in which a heroin addicted patient, who had been followed-up for 6 months for increasing dyspnea due to chronic cor pulmonale, was admitted to an intensive care unit. She died shortly after. Postmortem lung biopsies revealed talc particles within alveolar walls and alveolar macrophages, as well as alterations in blood vessels (77[c]). A case of talc granulomatosis has been ascribed to sniffing cocaine (78[c]).

Overzealous application of baby powder may cause *severe pulmonary complications* if the infant inhales the powder (79[R]). Formation of *umbilical granulomas* has been described as an adverse effect of talc in a newborn infant (80[c]).

An experimental animal study undertaken to determine whether cornstarch powder suspended in physiological saline causes *intraperitoneal adhesions* after laparotomy showed a significantly higher incidence of adhesions than in the control group 2 weeks after surgery. It was recommended that powder—free surgical gloves should be used to prevent adhesion formation after abdominal surgery (81[C]).

Twenty-two to 35 years after they were treated for idiopathic spontaneous pneumothorax with talc poudrage, or by simple drainage, a group of patients underwent lung function testing. The former showed mild *restrictive impairment of lung function* with a mean total lung capacity 89% of predicted, compared with a mean total lung capacity of 96% in subjects who had been treated by simple drainage. None of the subjects had developed a mesothelioma (82[r]).

Although described in association with conglomerate masses and bullous disease in end—stage talc granulomatosis, *spontaneous pneumothorax* can also occur earlier in the course of talc-induced lung disease (83[c]).

Ovarian cancer has been increasing in frequency over the past 40 years, and a role for environmental factors in its etiology has been inferred from its higher incidence in industrialized countries. Cosmetic talc, deposited in the vagina following direct application to the perineum or to undergarments, sanitary napkins, or diaphragms, or through use of a talc-dusted condom during intercourse may play an important role. One recent case-control study sought to determine whether the use of talc in genital hygiene increases the risk of epithelial ovarian cancer (84[C]). The risk of ovarian cancer was significantly elevated in women who applied talc directly as a body powder, on a daily basis, for more than 10 years. The greatest risk for ovarian cancer risk was found in the subgroup of women estimated to have made more than 10 000 talc applications during years when they were ovulating. However, this exposure was found in only 14% of women with ovarian cancer. The report concluded that a life—time pattern of perineal talc use may increase the risk for epithelial ovarian cancer, but that it is unlikely to be the cause of the majority of epithelial ovarian cancers.

Vaginal tampons

Although *toxic shock syndrome* (TSS) is generally associated with the use by women of internal vaginal tampons, it is not confined to this situation.

Two large clinical epidemiological studies (85[C], 86[C]) have contributed to an understanding of the conditions leading to TSS. Of all patients with TSS, 95% were women; in 98% of cases it began during the menstrual period, and in 98% *Staphylococcus aureus phage group* 1 was isolated from the vaginal swab. In no case was the organism isolated from the blood. It is clear that shock was caused not by bacteremia but by an epidermal toxin. Only some 8% of healthy controls harbored *St. aureus* vaginally. The mortality rate of TSS is estimated to be 10—15% (87[R], 88[R]). Since *Staphylococcus* contamination, vaginal and extravaginal, usually occurs without any clinical consequences, special attention has focused on the association with vaginal tampons. A particular brand (Rely) has been withdrawn from the market, but other brands have also been linked with the syndrome.

A number of surviving patients had several recurrences during subsequent menstrual periods (up to five), these events each being progressively less severe in their clinical course (89[C], 90[C]). Insertion of a contraceptive diaphragm may trigger the TSS, even at times other than during menstruation.

The pathogenesis of TSS is not well understood. The tampons were not contaminated, and they cannot be regarded as the direct cause of TSS; they are rather a trigger for the events leading to the syndrome. A plausible explanation is that the toxin produced by *St. aureus* accumulates in the tampon and is absorbed either directly from the vagina or after reflux of menstrual blood through the fallopian tubes into the peritoneal cavity. In support of this, a number of cases have occurred in women leaving the tampon in situ for a long period, up to 3 days. It is unclear why the incidence of TSS has increased since 1978. Highly absorbent tampons may partly explain this, but it is not the only explanation. The TSS is likely to be the result of the coincidence of virulent *Staphylococcus* in the vagina and conditions favoring their growth or colonization, such as a tampon saturated with menstrual blood.

The risk of TSS in association with vaginal tampons is nevertheless small: 10—15 per 100 000 menstruating women per year. Poor hygiene (leaving tampons in situ for several days) is not the only cause; TSS has been described in women changing their tampons regularly. Women who have previously had febrile episodes during menstruation should use tampons with utmost restraint or abandon them in favor of external tampons.

Toxic shock syndrome has also been described in association with use of a vaginal contraceptive sponge (91[c]). Vaginal cultures grew *St. aureus*.

Women using contraception, either oral contraceptive pills or topical spermicides, appear to be at lower risk of developing TSS. A study analyzing patients suffering from TSS found only six spermicide users and eight oral contraception users, against 60 not using a contraceptive method (92[Cr]). It has been suggested that an antibacterial effect of spermicidal ingredients prevents the intravaginal growth of *St. aureus*. The postulated protective action of oral contraceptives has been explained by reduced menstrual flow and duration, and an alteration in cervical mucus.

Variceal sclerotherapy

In sclerotherapy an irritant is introduced in varicose veins and esophageal varices, causing a local inflammatory reaction and obliteration of the veins concerned. Sclerosing agents include ethanolamine oleate, sodium tetradecylsulfate, and sodium morrhuate.

Bleeding esophageal varices are treated by inserting a needle-tipped catheter through an endoscope to the site of the varices, and injecting a sclerosing agent directly into the bleeding varix. Side effects are common, occurring in 10—15% of patients. These include severe *local edema and necrosis* at the site of sclerosis (93[c]), *bacterial peritonitis* (94[c]), and *pneumococcal bacteremia* (95[c]). *Fever*, *chest pain*, and *odynophagia* are common after esophageal sclerotherapy, but they tend to be of short duration (96[r]). Local complications at the site of injection, such as *esophageal perforation* (1%) and *abscess formation* (0.3%), are infrequent but they are associated with substantial mortality. A patient who received endoscopic sclerotherapy for a bleeding duodenal ulcer (not a recognized indication) had a fatal outcome (97[c]).

Sclerotherapy has been used in the extremities for treating varicose and telangiectatic leg veins (98[c], 99[c]). *Telangiectatic matting* may develop—bluish areas due to post-treatment neovascularization, in which new blood vessels, less than 0.2 mm in diameter, appear distally to the treated site, most commonly on the thigh. The incidence of this has been reported to be between 5 and 35%. Resolution often occurs spontaneously over 3—12 months, although in some patients it may be permanent or require further sclerotherapy to which it may be resistant (100[c]).

DIETARY PREPARATIONS AND SWEETENERS

Acesulfame

Acesulfame is an artificial sweetener derived from acetoacetic acid, and it is used in a wide range of non-medicinal products (101[R]). The studies on the basis of which acesulfame gained approval showed no evidence in animals of mutagenicity, teratogenicity or adverse reproductive effects; a 2-year toxicology study in beagles showed no untoward adverse effects. The incidence of lymphocytic leukemia was slightly increased in high-dosed female mice, but not beyond the spontaneous variation with this strain. No other evidence of potential carcinogenicity was obtained, and it has been concluded that at the estimated level of exposure acesulfame and its metabolites are not a health hazard (102[R]).

Aspartame

Despite numerous studies of its safety during the past two decades, aspartame has proven to be a safe sweetener and the incidence of serious side effects has been difficult to determine in controlled studies. Since one of the metabolic products of aspartame is phenylalanine, excessive use of aspartame should be avoided by patients with phenylketonuria (103[r], 104[r]). Toxicity of another metabolic product, methanol, is unlikely, even when aspartame is used in extraordinary amounts (105[r], 106[R]).

Aspartame may cause *urticaria*, *angioedema*, and *granulomatous septal panniculitis* (107[c]). *Lobular panniculitis* has been described in a 57-year-old diabetic man who ingested large amounts of aspartame as a sweetener, in soft drinks and other products. After stopping aspartame intake the tender subcutaneous nodules disappeared (108[r]). The role of aspartame in sensitivity reactions is controversial. In a multicenter, randomized, double—blind, placebo—controlled, crossover study aspartame was more likely than placebo to cause urticaria or angioedema (109[R]).

Headaches may follow aspartame ingestion. In a double—blind crossover study using volunteers with self—identified headaches after aspartame, some were found to be particularly susceptible, and their headaches were attributed to aspartame (110[R]). Individuals with mood disorders are thought to be particularly sensitive to aspartame, and it has been suggested that its use in such patients should be discouraged (111[C]).

Butylated hydroxytoluene

Butylated hydroxytoluene (BHT) is an additive used as an antioxidant in foods, such as packet cake mixes, potato crisps, salted peanuts and dehydrated mashed potatoes. Its safety has been critically reviewed in a Danish study, together with a number of other food additives (112[R]). Although it has been suggested that BHT induces tumors in rats, others have suggested that it may protect tissues against the carcinogenic effects of many different substances. It is impossible to decide from experimental findings in animals what the result will be of prolonged human exposure to low concentrations of such substances. BHT causes various allergies; symptoms of hay fever and asthma have been reported.

Chewing gum should be considered as a possible cause of unexplained food allergy. BHT in chewing gum caused disseminated *urticarial eruption* in a young female (113[c]). An adverse drug reaction was ruled out, and the only recent dietary change had been regular use of chewing-gum containing BHT. The skin lesions revealed signs of *vasculitis* with a perivascular cellular infiltrate, intra-endothelial deposits of IgM, C′9, C3 and C9, and heavy extravascular deposition of fibrinogen. Within a week of stopping use of the gum the eruption had subsided. Oral provocation test confirmed that BHT was responsible, the cutaneous signs returning within several hours of BHT rechallenge.

Cyclamate

Sodium cyclamate is a potent sweetening agent which is widely used. It has been subjected to numerous safety and carcinogenicity studies. Animal data led to warning against excessive and indiscriminate use a long time ago, causing the World Health Organization in 1967 to adopt a safety limit of 50 mg/kg. However, in 1982 a joint FAO/WHO expert committee on food additives revised this recommendation to allow for a maximum daily intake of up to 11 mg of sodium or calcium cyclamate (as cyclamic acid) per kg body-weight (114[R]). Nonetheless, since in certain climates and populations the amount of cyclamate in soft drinks and other beverages may exceed these limits, more epidemiological data are needed to evaluate, for example, a possible association with *cancer of the uropoietic system* (115[CR]), and with *histological and radiological abnormalities of the small intestine* and *malabsorption* (116[c]).

Ginseng *(See also Chapter 48)*

In previous volumes of Meyler it has been pointed out that ginseng preparations vary, and some apparently contain no ginseng at all. Ginseng, which is taken in the belief that it will improve stamina, may in fact have the opposite effect. In a study of the influence of ginseng on the performance of runners it was suggested that it had a superior effect to placebo on achievement (117[c]). On re-analysis of the results it was concluded that there had been a miscalculation, and that six of the nine runners performed better on placebo (118[r]). Serum creatine kinase and SGOT levels the day after the run were more than twice as high when ginseng had been used as placebo. It may be that ginseng aggravates the muscular injury of extreme exercise (119[r]).

Saccharin

As with sodium cyclamate, saccharin has been considered to be a possible human carcinogen on the basis of animal experiments. This suspicion has now been disregarded. There is no evidence that diabetics known to consume larger quantities of saccharin than nondiabetics are at greater risk of developing bladder cancer (120[R]), or other malignancies. In the United States saccharin-containing medicines are required to carry the following warning: "Use of this product may be hazardous to your health. This product contains saccharin which has been determined to cause cancer in laboratory animals" (121[r]).

Sorbitol

Sorbitol, a polyhydric alcohol, is used as a sweetening agent in many oral medicinal liquids. In addition to enhancing the palatability of these liquids, it improves solution stability and reduces crystallization of syrup vehicles (122[r]). It is used as a sweetener in many sugar-free food products and confectioneries. Sorbitol-containing food products are often recommended for diabetic patients, because the sweetener does not raise blood glucose concentrations or require insulin for its metabolism (123[r]).

Sorbitol is slowly absorbed by passive diffusion in the small intestine. After oral administration, it increases osmotic pressure in the bowel by drawing in water, and is thus an effective osmotic laxative, sometimes leading to *diarrhea* (124[c]). Bacterial fermentation of sorbitol in the large bowel is associated with increased *flatulence* and *abdominal cramping*. Ten grams of sorbitol may cause flatulence and *bloating*, and 20 grams abdominal cramps and diarrhea.

Many healthy individuals are intolerant of sorbitol, and develop abdominal cramping and diarrhea with less than the normal laxative dose (125[r]). It has been suggested that more than 30% of healthy adults, irrespective of ethnic origin, cannot tolerate 10 grams of sorbitol (126[R]).

Certain patients may be especially sensitive to the gastrointestinal effects of sorbitol; for example, diabetics may be prone to sorbitol intolerance, because of altered gastrointestinal transit time and motility. They may also have a higher consumption of sorbitol-containing dietary foods. Patients on chronic hemodialysis may be predisposed to sorbitol intolerance as a result of carbohydrate malabsorption (127[r]).

Colonic necrosis has been reported after Kayexalate (sodium polystyrene sufonate suspension) in sorbitol retention enemas before and immediately after renal transplantation. Although the cause was not proven, it was recommended that sorbitol should not be included in Kayexalate enemas given for hyperkalemia in renal transplant recipients (128[c]).

DYES AND COLORANTS

Methylene blue

Significant neonatal morbidity may occur after transabdominal infusion of methylene blue to diagnose premature rupture of fetal membranes, to stain the amniotic fluid in twin pregnancies, or following postpartum administration of methylene blue. Toxic manifestations include *hyperbilirubinemia*, *Heinz body hemolytic anemia*, and possible *desquamation of the skin*. In most cases it appears that toxicity was the result of an overdose of methylene blue (129[C], 130[r], 131[r], 132[r]).

Multiple ileal occlusions have been reported in babies born to mothers who had twin pregnancies and who had received methylene blue administered during amniocentesis (133[r], 134[r], 135[c]). In a number of cases it was found that methylene blue had been injected into the amniotic sac of the affected twins.

Methylene blue is sometimes administered intrathecally for tracking the source of a cerebrospinal fluid leak. This procedure involves considerable risk of *spinal cord damage*, and the attendant neurological consequences.

When methylene blue is used prophylactically to prevent urinary stone formation, it may cause *dysuria*, *diarrhea* and *gastric discomfort*.

Overdosage of methylene blue given intravenously, which may happen inadvertently during urinary tract surgery, may cause shock and pseudocyanosis. The latter is due to the blue tinge of methylene blue, and it may create confusion as to the patient's circulatory status. Patients receiving methylene blue should be examined for unstable hemoglobins or an abnormal hexose-monophosphate pathway if the risk of *methemoglobinemia* is to be minimized; this has been described with a normal dose (136[C]).

Synthetic food coloring

In a study of 220 children referred for suspected *hyperactivity*, 55 were subjected to a 6-week trial of the Feingold diet, which is free of artificial colorants. The behavior of 40 improved, of whom 26 remained improved after relaxation of the diet. The children's parents believed that a particular pattern of behavior was associated with the ingestion of foods containing synthetic colorants. A double-blind cross-over study of eight of the children was conducted. Subjects were maintained on a diet free of synthetic additives and they were challenged daily for 18 weeks with either placebo or 50 mg of either tartrazine or carmoisine, each for two separate weeks. The two agents were significantly associated with extreme *irritability*, *restlessness*, and *sleep disturbance* (137[CR]). The findings raise the issue as to whether the strict inclusion criteria set for studies of hyperactivity based on 'attention deficit disorders' may miss children whose behavioral abnormalities are associated with ingestion of food additives.

Sulfite food additives have been linked to several *hyperreactive conditions* (SEDA-15, 537; 138[c]) (see section on metabisulfites).

MEDICAL DEVICES

Apnea monitors

In 1985, the United States FDA alerted hospitals and home users to the risks of *electrocution* and *burns* with apnea monitors. The alert resulted from reports of electrocution or burns when older children plugged the connector pins of the electrode leads from an infant's apnea monitor system into either AC power cords or a wall socket.

Recently, the FDA again alerted health-care workers to risk of electrocution of infants on apnea monitors when inappropriate lead wires and cables are used, and certain precautions have been recommended (139[r]). A safety alert was issued in 1993 after a baby on a hospital apnea monitor was electrocuted when inappropriate lead wires were substituted and connected to an electrical power source instead of to the monitor.

Dialysis membranes

Anaphylaxis as a side-effect of hemodialysis has been analyzed from records of approximately 260 000 courses of dialysis treatment, at three centers. There were 21 severe reactions over the 10.5-year period of the survey, all highly suggestive of anaphylaxis (140[CR]). Reactions appeared within minutes of initiating dialysis and were characterized by cardiopulmonary, mucocutaneous and/or gastrointestinal tract symptoms. Four respiratory arrests occurred and there was one death. When the individual histories and treatments were analyzed, there was strong evidence that hollow-fiber dialyzers made of cuprammonium cellulose (CC) were responsible. No obvious factors could be found to identify predisposed patients; sub-optimal rinsing of the CC hollow-fiber dialysis prior to use may have been responsible for some, but not all, reactions. Repeated dialysis anaphylaxis in one patient has been reported (141[c]).

Glass capillary tubes The United States FDA has recommended that health professionals should consider using safer alternatives to glass capillary tubes for collecting small quantities of blood (142[r]). The slender fragile tubes may break when they are sealed with putty or shatter during centrifugation (143[r]). If they break, health professionals are at risk of injury and infection from blood-borne pathogens, including HIV. In one case, a tube broke while it was being sealed manually with putty, resulting in the *transmission of HIV* to a physician (144[c]).

Safer blood collecting devices include products that are not made of glass, or are glass coated with shatter-resistant film. Another product uses a method of sealing that does not require pushing one end of the tube into putty to form a plug. Other devices allow the hematocrit to be measured without centrifugation.

Latex

Because of reports of severe allergic reactions to medical devices containing latex (natural rubber), the United States FDA currently advises health-care professionals to identify latex-sensitive patients and to be prepared to treat allergic reactions promptly. Reports of *allergic reactions* to latex-containing medical devices have included a recall of latex-cuffed enema tips after several patients died as a result of *anaphylactoid reactions* during barium enema. Condoms do not appear to cause serious latex reactions, but repeated exposure to latex both in medical devices and in consumer products (including condoms) may partly explain the rising prevalence of latex sensitivity. It has been reported that 6–7% of surgical personnel and 18–40% of spina bifida patients are latex-sensitive. Proteins in the latex itself appear to be the principal source of allergic reactions. Although it is not now known how much protein is likely to cause severe reactions, the FDA is working with manufacturers of latex-containing medical devices to set the protein levels in their products as low as possible (145[R]).

Latex is present in many medical devices, including surgical and examination gloves, catheters, intubation tubes, anesthesia masks, and dental fillers. Patient reactions to latex range from *contact urticaria* to *anaphylaxis* (146[c]). *Urethritis* may develop in patients managed with latex catheters (147[R]). In a study of 100 male patients, the incidence of urethritis with latex catheters was 22% compared with 2% in patients managed with silicone catheters. In all cases, symptoms developed within 12 hours of use and urine specimens were sterile.

Polyacrylonitrile dialyzers

The FDA has issued a safety alert about *life-threatening anaphylactoid reactions* associated with the concurrent use of angiotensin-converting enzyme (ACE) inhibitors and polyacrylonitrile (PAN) dialyzers (148[c]). The warning was followed by increased reports in the literature and to the FDA—to the latter of severe, sudden and sometimes fatal reactions. Symptoms include nausea, abdominal cramps, burning, angioedema, and shortness of breath, leading rapidly to severe hypotension. When these symptoms are recognized, dialysis should be stopped immediately and aggressive treatment for anaphylactoid reactions begun. Antihistamines do not relieve the symptoms. This does not constitute a warning to stop prescribing ACE inhibitors when patients are dialyzed with PAN membranes. The mechanism of the interaction between ACE inhibitors and PAN membrane dialyzers has not been established, and the incidence and scope of the problem remain unknown.

Volume ventilators

The FDA has alerted physicians and other health-care workers to several reports of deaths and injuries resulting from malfunctioning volume ventilators and/or heated humidifiers (149[R]). The reports link hospital fires, overheating and electric injuries to ventilators of the Puritan-Bennett series. There are also reports of overheating of humidifiers and volume ventilators from other firms. To prevent further deaths and injuries, the FDA has recommended that precautions should be taken with all volume ventilators and heated humidifiers used in either a health-care facility or at home.

MISCELLANEOUS ORGANIC COMPOUNDS

Aluminium hydroxide

Aluminium hydroxide is astringent and may cause *constipation*, or even *intestinal obstruction*. In addition, aluminium hydroxide may interfere with the absorption of other drugs from the gastrointestinal tract, if administered concomitantly.

When aluminium is used as a phosphate binder, often in renal dialysis patients, absorption and accumulation may occur. Phosphate depletion accompanied by increased bone resorption and hypercalciuria (with a risk of osteomalacia) may result. Low phosphate diets exacerbate this risk. Concurrent use of oral citrate solutions may increase absorption of aluminium from aluminium hydroxide, resulting in high blood levels, especially when renal function is impaired (150[c]). Citrate—containing preparations are included in many effervescent or dispersible tablets and increased absorption of aluminium from the gastrointestinal tract has been reported (151[r], 152[c], 153[r]).

Encephalopathy due to high serum aluminium levels has been reported in acute renal failure (154[c]).

Hyperaluminemia has been described in premature infants receiving prolonged intravenous alimentation, and in recipients of plasmapheresis receiving large volumes of replacement albumin solutions which contain high concentrations of aluminium (155[r]—157[r]).

Aminohydroxypropylidene biphosphonate (APD)

The aminohydroxypropylidene biphosphonates (APD), which include pamidronate, are commonly used to control blood calcium levels in hypercalcemic states in malignancy, primary hyperparathyroidism and Paget's disease. Side effects include low—grade transient fever and headache; other effects are asymptomatic hypocalcemia, hypophosphatemia and hypomagnesemia (158[c]—160[c]). Mineralization defects and impaired bone turnover have been reported during pamidronate therapy for Paget's disease, occasionally leading to osteomalacia. Pamidronate has a narrow therapeutic range between inhibition of bone resorption and development of mineralization defects. Short courses given to achieve biochemical remission should be administered with caution.

Serious side-effects of APD were reported after its use in otospongiosis. Of two patients with stapedial otosclerosis and sensorineural hearing loss, one developed total bilateral deafness and the other retained minimal auditory function in the low frequencies (161[cr]). It was recommended that sensorineural deafness in selected patients with otosclerosis should be treated with sodium fluoride, and that patients with Paget's disease treated with APD should be closely monitored and the drug discontinued immediately if hearing deteriorates.

Catergen (cianidanol)

In one report (162[r]) nine cases of acute *intravascular hemolysis*, severe enough to cause death in one and to necessitate hemodialysis in two others, were attributed to cianidanol on the basis of a close temporal relationship and serological tests. Cianidanol has been used in chronic active hepatitis (163[R]). Twenty-two patients received 3 grams daily, and 18 others placebo. Side-effects of cianidanol were *fever* (four patients), *hemolysis* (one) and *urticaria* (one).

Serious side effects were not observed when cianidanol was used to treat HBe antigen-positive chronic hepatitis in 338 patients (164[c]). The only side effect of note which appeared to be drug related was a *transient pyrexia* in 13, necessitating cessation of therapy in eight. Four patients also had a *skin eruption*.

Cyanamide

Cyanamide has been used in the same way as disulfiram to treat alcoholism (SED-11, 1041). It has been linked to *liver cell alterations* (SED-12, 1244), but caution is needed in attributing hepatic damage in alcoholic patients to drugs.

Dimethylsulfoxide (DMSO)

The efficacy and safety of DMSO are still relatively unclear; few studies have been performed in such a way as to permit reliable conclusions. DMSO penetrates quickly through the tissues, and there are no great differences between its effects with different administration forms. Adverse reactions to DMSO are common, but usually minor and related to the concentration of DMSO in the medication solution. The most frequent side effects can be avoided in large part by employing more dilute solutions (165[R]). Although DMSO's systemic toxicity is considered to be low, it may *potentiate the effect of simultaneously administered drugs*. Combinations of DMSO with other toxic agents probably constitute its greatest toxic potential (166[c]).

In topical use on the skin in high concentrations (90—100%) DMSO causes *irritation*, although this effect can be reduced by using lower concentrations (70%). Besides topical use on the skin and eyes, DMSO is used as an excipient to aid penetration of another substance.

Intravenous use of DMSO poses the greatest problems. Intravenous administration causes transient systemic *hemolysis with hemoglobinuria*, but without gross hematuria. The hemolysis is dose dependent and appears within several minutes after 20—40% infusions (167[c]). No evidence has been found of kidney damage because of handling higher amounts of hemoglobin after hemolysis.

DMSO caused gastrointestinal discomfort in volunteers being subjected to topical application of an 80% solution (1 g/kg/day). Nausea developed in 32%, vomiting in 6%, diarrhea in 5%, constipation in 3% and anorexia in 2% (168[R]). A *garlic-like breath* occurs in almost all patients using topical DMSO (169[c]) and probably by any other route of administration.

DMSO is currently used in cryopreservation of bone marrow concentrate, in concentrations of 10%. Severe reversible encephalopathy was experienced by two patients following infusion of peripheral blood stem cells cryopreserved in 10% dimethylsulfoxide (DMSO). In one patient, reduction of DMSO level with plasmapheresis resulted in marked improvement in encephalopathy (170[c]). Other cases of DMSO induced *encephalopathy* have been described (171[c], 172[c]).

A new presentation of dimethylsulfoxide (RIMSO 100) has introduced a problem since, when it is diluted with water, a strong *exothermic reaction* results. This caused thermal injury on intracystic instillation unless one waits until the mixture cools (173[c]).

Animal studies have documented a characteristic *change in the ocular lens, resulting in myopia* which becomes more severe with long—term administration or high concentrations of DMSO. However, studies and clinical experience have not shown similar effects in humans (174[c], 175[c]).

Disulfiram

ADVERSE REACTION PATTERN

General and toxic reactions Adverse drug reactions to disulfiram (one per 200—2000 treatment years) consist mainly of hepatic, neurological, skin, and psychiatric reactions, in decreasing order of frequency. Deaths occur at the very low frequency of one per 25 000 treatment years (176[R]).

Hypersensitivity Mild allergic reactions can occur.

Tumor-inducing effects These have not been described.

ORGANS AND SYSTEMS

Hypersensitivity reactions *Allergic reactions* to disulfiram implants are reported, but are limited in degree. The possibility of hypersensitivity developing should be borne in mind in patients who have experienced allergic reactions in the past, regardless of the allergen concerned.

Cardiovascular system A dose of 250—300 mg/day does not affect pulse rate, blood pressure or plasma noradrenaline levels, whereas 500 mg/day causes an increase in plasma noradrenaline, increased systolic blood pressure in recumbent and standing positions, and an increased pulse rate in the erect position. The *elevated blood pressure* does not reach hypertensive levels, but the results suggest increased sympathetic nervous system activity in patients receiving disulfiram. Caution should be exercised in using disulfiram in hypertensive patients. Close monitoring of blood pressure is advised, and the dose of disulfiram preferably reduced to 250 mg/day (177[C]).

Nervous system *Polyneuritis*, occasionally fulminant, is a recognized side effect of disulfiram; this includes retrobulbar neuritis, with dramatic reduction in visual acuity and impaired color perception (SEDA-10, 349; 178[R]). This complication is rare but serious. Tobacco abuse is thought to be a predisposing factor. The complication is seen with doses of 500 mg/day, and there is a latent period before onset of 2–36 months. Disulfiram may cause optic neuropathy (179[c], 180[c]).

Disulfiram may cause distressing adverse *neuropsychiatric effects* by a mechanism that is not properly understood. Side effects develop more frequently in subjects with low plasma dopamine β-hydroxylase (DBH) levels than in those with high levels. A research subject having a low level of DBH developed a schizophrenic reaction to disulfiram; it would be useful to know whether determining blood DBH levels predicts the risk of adverse reactions to disulfiram (181[C]).

Mechanism of disulfiram toxicity The neurotoxic effects of disulfiram have been compared with those of carbon disulfide, a disulfiram metabolite (182[R]). The results suggest that carbon disulfide may be responsible for the behavioral and neurological adverse effects of disulfiram. If so, other toxic effects of carbon disulfide might follow administration of high doses of disulfiram, such as parkinsonism, psychotic behavior and encephalopathy.

Liver Approximately 25 cases of disulfiram-induced *liver damage* (apparently as a result of an immunological mechanism) have been reported, some fatal. There has been uncertainty as to causality, since many alcoholic patients who use the drug have pre-existing liver damage. Nevertheless, it is believed that the drug does sometimes trigger a serious liver reaction (SEDA-10, 438); severe hepatitis, sometimes fatal, has been reported (183[c], 184[c], 185[r]). Liver function should be checked before giving the drug, especially since there may be a long history of alcohol abuse (186[C]).

Malodor In a colostomy patient the smell of the colostomy was present only so long as disulfiram exposure continued (187[c]). The explanation for this was obscure. Bad breath has been reported in patients receiving disulfiram concurrently with warfarin (188[C]).

Second-generation effects Disulfiram should not be used in women who may become pregnant while receiving therapy (189[cr]).

Interaction The interaction of disulfiram with *alcohol*, the metabolism of which is interfered with at the aldehyde stage, is the basis for its therapeutic use; disulfiram renders alcohol intake unpleasant, and dangerous if much alcohol is taken.

Disulfiram inhibits other hepatic drug metabolism and it may prolong the effects of substances normally metabolized in the liver. This has been studied for various *benzodiazepines*. The $t_{1/2}$ of chlordiazepoxide and diazepam increases significantly after disulfiram, while the clearance is decreased, with accumulation of these drugs in the body. No change in $t_{1/2}$ or clearance has been noted for oxazepam (which is not metabolized in the liver) (190[C]). The benzodiazepines are effective in reducing the disulfiram reaction to alcohol. *Amitriptyline* potentiates the disulfiram reaction. Close observation of any patient taking both drugs is essential.

Dextran-70 *(See also Chapter 34)*

Dextran-70 is a high-molecular weight dextran, widely used as a distending medium for hysteroscopy. Administration of large volumes of dextran during this procedure has been associated with *adult respiratory distress syndrome*, *pulmonary edema*, *coagulopathy and anaphylactic reactions* (191[r], 192). Severe anaphylactic reactions after hysteroscopy due to dextran have been described, within 10 minutes of exposure to dextran (193[c]). Anaphylactic reactions to dextran have been reported when used as a plasma expander. The incidence of severe dextran-induced anaphylactic reactions fell 35-fold over the period 1982–1992 in Sweden, after introduction of prophylactic hapten inhibition with dextran 1 (194[R]).

Dipyridamole

Dipyridamole, a potent coronary arteriolar vasodilator, is used with 201-thallium imaging for the detection of coronary artery disease. In a prospective study of 435 patients, followed up after infusion of dipyridamole, adverse events were noted in 40%. Three patients experienced major events necessitating hospitalization (*myocardial infarction*, *chest pain*, and a *partial seizure*). Moderately severe adverse events occurred in 9%, requiring intravenous aminophylline. These were electrocardiographic *ST segment abnormalities* (26), *nausea* (seven), *headache* (three), *chest pain* (two), *bronchospasm* (one), *protracted vomiting* (one) and *diarrhea* (one). Minor adverse events not requiring aminophylline were experienced in 30% of patients (195[CR]).

The incidence of life-threatening adverse reactions to dipyridamole is negligible (196[R]). *Fatal respiratory insufficiency* following dipyridamole—thallium imaging has been described in a patient with a history of chronic obstructive lung disease (197[c]). The authors concluded that patients with a history of chronic obstructive lung disease may have an increased risk of bronchospasm after dipyridamole infusion, and caution is advised in such patients. A patient with aortoiliac occlusive vascular disease and hypertension suffered a *stroke* 6.5 min after administration of intravenous dipyridamole during a 201-thallium myocardial study (198[c]). Aminophylline administration did not reverse its progression.

Fructose

Attention has been drawn to the dangers of fructose and sorbitol solutions in patients with hereditary fructose intolerance following the death of a 16-year-old girl who died after an uncomplicated appendicectomy (199[c]). She had undiagnosed hereditary fructose intolerance and was given sorbitol and fructose postoperatively.

Hereditary fructose intolerance is an autosomal recessive disorder with reduced activity of aldolase B in the liver, kidney, and small intestine. Ingestion of only a few grams of fructose, sorbitol, or sucrose causes *abdominal pain and vomiting* (SEDA-13, 479). Affected individuals develop an aversion to sugary foods and drinks, and in severe cases exposure during infancy may result in progressive *liver damage* and death. Exclusion of fructose from the diet allows them to develop and grow normally.

Gallium nitrate

The pathophysiology and treatment of hypercalcemia of malignancy has been reviewed and the role of gallium nitrate considered (200[r], 201[r]). The main adverse effect is nephrotoxicity, and it should be avoided in renal dysfunction and in patients taking nephrotoxic drugs. In a comparative study of gallium nitrate and etidronate in acute control of cancer-related hypercalcemia, a significantly higher proportion of the patients treated with gallium nitrate developed *asymptomatic hypophosphatemia* (202[R]).

Glycerol

In 122 patients with trigeminal neuralgia who underwent percutaneous retrogasserian glycerol injection (203[R]) complications associated with the treatment were significant: 63% had marked *hyperesthesia* of the face and 29% unpleasant *dysesthesias*, including two cases of anesthesia dolorosa. *Sensory disturbances* were most frequent in patients who had previously undergone an alcohol block procedure. Because of the high rates of recurrence and sensory disturbances, the authors prefer microvascular decompression for the management of trigeminal neuralgia.

In another study of glycerol injection in trigeminal neuralgia the only immediate complications were *herpes simplex* and *keratitis*, both disappearing in a few days. *Paresthesia* and *dysesthesia* were also reported (204[r]).

Intravascular hemolysis occurred during intravenous glycerol therapy in patients with acute stroke (205[r]).

Iodinated glycerol

Iodinated glycerol is used as a mucolytic agent in respiratory disorders. Organically-bound iodine is changed to unbound iodide after absorption. Iodide inhibits the binding of iodine to the tyrosine residue of the thyroglobulin molecule, inhibiting the synthesis of thyroxine and triiodothyronine. In patients with iodide-induced goiter, there is increased iodine transport, further reducing thyroid hormone synthesis and causing *thyroid hyperplasia* (206[r]).

Reversible *hypothyroidism* has been reported in nursing-home residents without a history of thyroid disease, who had been taking iodinated glycerol as an expectorant (207[c]). Hypothyroidism has been reported after long-term treatment with iodinated glycerol (208[c]).

L-Tryptophan

L-Tryptophan, an amino acid which has been used as an antidepressant and hypnotic, has been linked with an epidemic of the eosinophilic myalgia syndrome (209[r]). In a case of *interstitial pneumonitis* and *pulmonary vasculitis* ascribed to L-tryptophan, unintended rechallenge supported a causal relation (210[c]). The syndrome appears to be only part of a spectrum of adverse effects associated with tryptophan (211[R]).

Metabisulfite

Sulfiting agents are antioxidants widely used in the pharmaceutical and food industries. As an additive agent in various pharmaceutical products, metabisulfite can cause unpleasant adverse reactions. Metabisulfite-induced anaphylaxis through an IgE-mediated mechanism has been described in a patient who developed *urticaria*, *angioedema* and *nasal congestion* following provocative challenge with sodium metabisulfite (212[cR]).

Preservatives in subconjunctival gentamicin were identified as the cause of *conjunctival chemosis* and *capillary closure* in a recent study (213[C]). Patients undergoing cataract surgery were divided into three groups: one was given a subconjunctival injection of a preservative-free solution of gentamicin at the end of the cataract procedure, another received a subconjunctival injection of gentamicin containing sodium metabisulfite and disodium edetate as preservatives, and the third was the control group not given a subconjunctival injection. There was a significant difference in the severity of conjunctival chemosis between patients who received gentamicin with and without preservatives, respectively (214[C]).

The presence of sodium metabisulfite as an antioxidant in commercial lignocaine with adrenaline significantly increased *discomfort during injection* (215[C]). *Anaphylactoid shock* occurring during epidural anesthesia for cesarean section has been attributed to metabisulfite (216[c]). *Status asthmaticus* and *acute bronchospasm* have been linked with the use of metabisulfites (217[R]).

Nicotine replacement agents

The use of nicotine chewing-gum by people trying to give up smoking continues to provide evidence of side effects. *Atrial fibrillation* is described in association with normal or large doses (218[r], 219[c]), suggesting that accumulation may occur when nicotine gum is taken daily, causing *chronic nicotine intoxication*.

The safety and efficacy of nicotine transdermal patches, used to stop smoking, has been reviewed (220[R]). Study subjects experienced *headache* (4%), *nausea* (4%) and *vertigo* (4%) slightly more frequently than the placebo group. Skin reactions such as *mild itching* under the patch, lasting for 15—30 minutes, and *erythema* and *acute eczema*, persisting for several days after removal, also occurred. Skin reactions necessitating discontinuation of the patches occurred in 10% of a study group (221[c]); in the same report *sleep disturbances* of varying severity was a common side effect.

Perfluorochemicals, Fluosol-DA

Emulsions of perfluorochemicals are used to absorb, transport, and release oxygen and carbon dioxide. They may replace gaseous transport in red blood cells (222, 223). There are now several reports of side effects.

Mild allergic reactions have been reported following the administration of Fluosol-DA, one of the first commercially available perfluorochemicals, which is used to deliver oxygen to ischemic myocardium during percutaneous transluminal coronary angioplasty (SEDA-13, 479). *Ventricular arrhythmias*, *pruritus*, *bradycardia*, *chest pain*, *dyspnea* and *increased respiratory rate* are described (224[R]). In another study, transient leukopenia, pulmonary distress, and death were noted after administration of perfluorochemicals (225[R]).

Fluorocarbons are also used as propellants for inhalers. There have been reports of hallucinations linked to fluorocarbons after use of such inhalers (226[c], 227[r]). Earlier suggestions that fluorocarbon inhalation (often in polluted work environments) may cause cardiac arrhythmias and even death, have been difficult to prove (228[c], 229[r]).

Phenol

Phenol is a toxic substance, and side effects may occur through absorption from intact skin or wounds, ingestion, or absorption of vapor through the skin or via the lungs. Phenol is cardiotoxic, and various *cardiac dysrhythmias* have been noted after application to the skin, or less commonly when used for neurolysis. Life-threatening premature ventricular complexes were noted during topical application of phenol and croton oil in hexachlorophene soap and water for chemical peeling of a giant hairy nevus (230[c]). Three of 16 children treated with motor point blocks for cerebral palsy with a phenolic solution under halothane anesthesia developed cardiac dysrhythmias (231[c]). Severe cardiac dysrhythmia followed by circulatory arrest occurred in an elderly patient with pancreatic cancer, injected with a phenolic solution to produce splanchnic neurolysis (232[c]). The authors recommended that ethanol should replace phenol for this purpose.

Acute life-threatening *epiglottitis* developed in a patient after the use of a throat spray containing the equivalent of 1.4% phenol. The reaction may have been anaphylactic, or a direct toxic effect (233[c]).

Polyvinylpyrrolidone (Povidone)

Polyvinylpyrrolidone, a variable-weight polymer of the monomer *N*-vinylpyrrolidone, has been used for industrial, cosmetic, and medical purposes. When it enters the body it causes histologically characteristic reactions in tissues with which it comes into contact (234[r], 235[r]). It is used as a component of hair sprays, as a retardant for subcutaneous injections, and intravenously as a plasma expander. The latter results in deposition of polyvinylpyrrolidone in the reticuloendothelial system and other mesenchymal cells, including osteocytes. *Pathological fractures* of several bones and additional destructive lesions seen radiologically in other bones, were reported in a patient who had received repeated intravenous injections of polyvinylpyrrolidone for 10 years (236[c]). Biopsies of the fracture sites showed both intracellular deposits of polyvinylpyrrolidone and mucoid changes in the affected cells. If of sufficient severity, this may cause a virtual 'melt down' of osseous tissue.

Some products intended for parenteral administration contain povidone as an excipient. Adverse effects (deposition of povidone in tissues with consequent lesions and pain) have been associated with these. There have been reports of liver involvement (237[R]).

Propylene glycol

Propylene glycol is widely used as a solvent in topical steroids, other medicines, foodstuffs and cosmetics. It may be used in allergic individuals, although propylene glycol itself can cause *allergic skin reactions*. The incidence of propylene glycol allergy among patients with eczema is thought to be greater than 2% (238[r]). Used in dermatological preparations, propylene glycol may occasionally perpetuate eczema in hypersensitive patients (239[Cr]).

Propylene glycol causes *acute hemolysis* with elevated lactic dehydrogenase, bilirubin and plasma hemoglobin after use of a stock solution during intravenous nitroglycerin therapy (240[R]). *Lactic acidosis* and *convulsions* have been associated with the use of propylene glycol (SEDA-15, 537).

Sodium morrhuate

Sodium morrhuate is a fatty acid extract of cod liver oil; its sclerosant effect was discovered with the use of the agent in treating leprosy (241[R]). It is cytotoxic, as demonstrated by autopsy studies in 10 patients (242[c]).

Vascular thrombosis is thought to be secondary to tissue damage. Other sclerosant agents in current use, ethanolamine oleate, sodium tetradecylsulfate and polydocanol, cause effects similar to sodium morrhuate. It has been concluded that these drugs cause *phlebosclerosis* not through induction of plasma coagulation, but directly by damaging vascular endothelium and red cells, triggering platelets, and aggregating granulocytes at the venous wall endothelium. These effects probably derive from the surfactant properties of sodium morrhuate and from its high arachidonate content (243[c]).

Fever and *pneumonia* have been reported after the use of sodium morrhuate sclerosant solution (SEDA-14, 456).

MISCELLANEOUS INORGANIC COMPOUNDS

Calcium salts

In general, there is an increased risk of *nephrolithiasis* with prolonged high calcium intake. In one report on calcium carbonate used in chronic hemodialysis as a phosphate binder there was a low incidence of hypercalcemia with daily doses less than 6 grams (244[c]), whereas in another report on 26 dialysis patients using calcium carbonate for 3 years 42% developed new *calcification* (245[C]). In studies aimed at determining whether high calcium intake increases the risk of *nephrolithiasis*, it was found that in patients at risk of developing nephrolithiasis or with a history of nephrolithiasis, calcium can be safely given for treatment of osteoporosis, provided there is careful monitoring (246[r], 247[c]).

Calcium edetate may cause mild *transient hypercalcemia* (248[CR]).

Excipients

Previous volumes in this series have drawn attention to adverse reactions to excipients, notably hypersensitivity reactions.

An asthmatic patient whose salbutamol preparation was replaced by another containing *benzalkonium chloride* as excipient developed bronchospasm as a result (249[c]). The Federal German health authorities have issued a warning that patients who cannot tolerate *sulfite* should take care to avoid medicines and other products to which it has been added (250[r]).

To reduce the risk of hypersensitivity reactions to excipients it is necessary that the names of both active and inactive components are indicated on the package of pharmaceutical products. The Swedish authorities took the initiative a decade ago of publicising the colorants used in medicines on sale, and Norway eliminated them. There has been some opposition from manufacturers who regard the nature of the additives they use as a commercial secret. In 1988 the Japanese health authorities ruled on the listing of all inactive components of medicines, the identity and quantities of which have to be indicated in package inserts and similar materials, for the information of health professionals. Separate lists are provided for all components to be listed with drugs for oral use, injection, and use on skin and mucosal surfaces (251[r]).

Table 1. *Miscellaneous drugs, agents and materials*

Drug/agent/material	Side effects	SED/SEDA	Page no.
Acamprosate	Erythema multiforme	SEDA-17	556
Acetate dialysate	Hypersensitivity reaction	SEDA-17	556
Acrylic cranioplasties	Infection	SEDA-16	556
Activated charcoal	Pulmonary aspiration	SEDA-17	556
Adenosine	Chest pain	SEDA-16	556
Amino-oxyacetic acid	Nausea, disequilibrium	SEDA-16	556
Bucrylate embolization	Serious hemorrhage, ischemic complications	SEDA-16	556
Butel hip plate	Pseudoarthrosis, femoral head necrosis, sepsis	SED-12	1234
Chloral hydrate	Toxicity in children	SEDA-18	464
Chlorocresol	Anaphylactic shock	SEDA-18	464
Chondroprotective agents (Dona-200-SR)	Abscesses, pruritic rash, hematological changes	SED-12	1237
Clodronate	Mild diarrhoea	SEDA-16	556
Colorants	Urticaria	SEDA-17	556
Cyanoacrylate injection	Pancreatoduodenal necrosis	SEDA-16	556
Dexon-mesh sling	Intestinal complications	SEDA-16	556
Dichloroacetate	Congenital lactic acidosis	SEDA-16	556
Disodium clodronate	Gastrointestinal effects	SEDA-17	556
Endothelin-l	Edema formation	SEDA-16	556
Ethanol	Testicular infarction	SED-12	1242
	Microhematuria, proteinuria	SEDA-16	551
	Systemic hypertension	SEDA-18	459
Etidronate	Pseudogout	SEDA-17	556
Etomidate	Pain on i.v. injection	SEDA-18	464
Flucytosine, oral	Myelotoxicity	SEDA-18	464
Fluoride	Rheumatoid arthritis, extremity pain, stress fractures	SEDA-17	553
Flunitrazepam, i.v.	Respiratory depression	SEDA-18	464
Galactosoaminoglucuronoglycan sulfate	Gastrointestinal diseases	SEDA-17	556
Gelatin	Acute renal failure	SEDA-16	556
γ-Hydroxybutyrate	Coma, tonic-clonic seizure-like activity	SEDA-17	553
Gelfoam	Meningeal inflammation	SEDA-16	556
Gentian violet	Tissue discoloration	SEDA-17	556
Glutamate	Facial pressure and burning sensations	SEDA-17	556
Hepatic arterial embolization	Pain, nausea, pyrexia, hepatic enzyme disturbances	SEDA-16	556
Hypertonic saline amnioinfusion	Hemorrhagic complications	SEDA-17	556
Indigo carmine	Diencephalic dysregulation	SEDA-16	556
Isaxonine	Allergic hepatitis	SEDA-16	556
Ivalon	Mimicking of peritoneal malignancy	SEDA-18	461
Lorenzo's oil	Thrombocytopenia	SEDA-18	453
Lumbotrain (back support)	Discomfort, skin irritation	SEDA-17	556
Matrix	Nausea	SEDA-17	556
Menthol	Shaking chills, allergic contact dermatitis	SED-12	1242
Monosulfiram	Flushing, sweating, tachycardia	SEDA-16	556
Nonoxynal-9 contraceptive sponge	Genital ulcers and vulvitis	SEDA-17	556
Oxidized cellulose	Paraplegia	SEDA-16	556
Phosphorus	Nephrocalcinosis	SEDA-16	556
Polychlorinated biphenyls	Malignant melanoma	SEDA-18	
Polyethylene glycol	Renal failure, CNS depression	SEDA-17	556
Potassium chloride	Nausea, diarrhea, stomach irritation	SEDA-17	556
Rifamycin, intra-articular	Intense local pain after injection	SEDA-18	464
Silicone	Facial swelling and erythema, facial granulomas, respiratory symptoms	SEDA-18	462
^{153}Sm-EDTMP	Myelosuppression	SEDA-18	464
Sodium bicarbonate	Proteinuria	SEDA-16	555
Sodium lactate	Panic disorders	SEDA-17	556
Sodium phosphate	Hypernatremia	SEDA-17	556
Sodium polystyrene sulfonate	Intestinal necrosis	SEDA-17	556

Table 1. *Continued*

Drug/agent/material	Side effects	SED/SEDA	Page no.
Sodium tetradecylsulfate, intravariceal	Pyrexia after injection	SEDA-18	464
Sulfur dioxide	Bronchoconstriction	SEDA-17	556
Thermal waters	Epidemic of pneumonitis and meningitis	SED-12	1247
Throat lozenge	Anaphylactic shock	SEDA-16	556
Today-Sponge	Irritation, vaginal itching	SEDA-18	464
Trichosanthin	Eever, headache, sore throat, eruption	SEDA-16	556
Vascular grafts	Aneurysm formation, thrombosis	SED-12	1234
Xylit infusion (calcium oxalate)	Cerebrorenal oxalosis	SEDA-17	556

Fluoride

The main pharmacological importance of fluoride is its effect on dental enamel and bone. Fluoride binds to the calcium ion, stimulating trabecular bone formation. Sodium fluoride is used to treat osteoporosis. However, there is a risk of stress fractures in treatment of osteoporosis with fluorides (252[r], 253[c]—255[c]). *Perimalleolar pain with swelling* (SED-12, 1243) and *extremity pain* after fluoride treatment in postmenopausal osteoporosis (256[cr]) have been reported.

Fluoride poisoning may occur: after chronic ingestion of excessive amounts of fluoride, causing *osteosclerosis* and *dental fluorosis* (mottled enamel), due to accidental ingestion of fluoride mixtures during dental treatment (257[R], 258[R]), or after ingestion of insecticides or rodenticides containing fluoride salts.

Although 5—10 grams fluoride is considered to be the acute lethal dose, a *fatality* has been reported in a patient who took less than 50 mg, suggesting a wide variation in the lethal dose. Other toxic effects of fluoride in therapeutic doses are *gastrointestinal bleeding* and *atopic dermatitis* (259[C]). In a pediatric patient there were *tetanic spasms* and a *convulsion* more than 12 hours after fluoride ingestion, with a normal serum calcium. It is advisable that cases of intoxication should remain under surveillance for at least 24 hours, after the usual acute symptoms such as vomiting and diarrhea have settled (SEDA-10, 439).

In a study of the adverse effects of fluorinated drinking water (260[Cr]) a small number of patients suffered *non-specific ailments* of varying duration, involving different systems. Severe headache, loss of strength and abdominal cramps were noted, sometimes with polydipsia and polyuria. The symptoms disappeared promptly when fluorinated water was withdrawn, and reappeared immediately after rechallenge.

In a United States study designed to determine whether fluoride affects human birth rate (261[R]) the annual total fertility rate (TFR) in women aged 10—49 years was calculated for 1970—1988 in counties with water fluoride levels of at least 3 parts per million (ppm). For each region separately, the annual TFR was tested by regression against the water fluoride content and sociodemographic covariables. In most regions there was an *association between increasing fluoride levels in drinking water and decreasing TFR*, and the combined result was a negative TFR/fluoride association. The study was based on population means rather than individual data, but there was no indication that the result was influenced by selection bias, inaccurate data, or inappropriate analytical methods. It does not necessarily follow that the fluoride effect on fertility rate also applies to individual women, and this is a matter for further research.

Magnesium salts

Magnesium-containing urological irrigation solutions, used for dissolution of urinary calculi, may cause slight elevation of serum magnesium. However, this may be sufficient to cause *respiratory depression or muscle paralysis*.

Iatrogenic *hypermagnesemia with respiratory depression* has been reported in patients who received hemiacidrin, a magnesium-containing irrigation fluid, through an ureteric catheter, together with magnesium citrate orally (262[c]). The renal pelvis is able to absorb magnesium, at least when it is inflamed (263[C]), and it is suggested that absorption of magnesium through inflamed pelvic mucosa results in hypermagnesemia. With impaired renal function there may be reduced magnesium excretion and cumulation, with parathyroid inhibition and consequent calcium and phosphorus abnormalities. Intravenous calcium directly antagonises respiratory depression due to magnesium, possibly by displacement by calcium of magnesium from cell membranes.

Severe hyperkalemia has been reported in pregnant intravenous drug abusers during prolonged parenteral magnesium sulfate therapy for treatment of toxemia (264[R]). Hypermagnesemia was thought to be responsible. In patients with suspected myocardial infarction who received magnesium infusions there was an increased incidence of *atrioventricular conduction distur-*

bances (265[c]). A 3-week-old girl who was treated with magnesium oxide as a laxative developed severe *hypermagnesemia* as a result. Treatment was with a combination of hyperhydration, forced diuresis and natriuresis and administration of intravenous calcium and insulin (266[c]).

Phosphate enemas, Fleet Enema®

Phosphate enemas in children under 5 years may carry risks of significant morbidity due to *hyperphosphatemia, hypocalcemia, hypokalemia and dehydration* (267[c]). *Hypocalcemic tetany* developed in a child following two phosphate enemas administered for fecal retention (268[cR]). The authors advised against the use of phosphate enemas in children under 2 years, and they recommend use only with extreme caution in children 2–5 years, especially when there is underlying bowel disease or renal dysfunction. Rectal necrosis has been described in a child after phosphate enemas (269[r]).

In elderly patients phosphate enemas (Fleet Enema®) have caused serious side effects. A 77-year-old patient with diverticulitis, who received phosphate enemas in preparation for a barium enema, developed *hyperphosphatemia* and *hypocalcemic coma* (270[c]). This case suggests that caution is required in administering phosphate enemas to patients with abnormal colonic mucosa. In a fatal case, a Fleet Enema® was given to a 91-year-old patient who lapsed into coma and died a few hours afterwards, despite treatment with phosphate binders and calcium (271[c]).

Potassium

Oral potassium chloride is used to prevent or correct hypokalemia due to diuretic use or other conditions, and it is irritating to the gastrointestinal tract, even to the extent of causing perforation.

Potassium chloride tablets are available not only for medicinal purposes but also as a food supplement or salt substitute. This wide availability may contribute to accidental fatal *hyperkalemia*. Hyperkalemia has been reported following ingestion of salt substitutes (272[c], 273[r]), and over-the-counter potassium supplements (274[c]).

The problems surrounding enteric-coated potassium chloride tablets are unresolved. Despite recommendations that they be withdrawn, some are still available. The risks seem to be less with slow-release potassium chloride tablets. Simple dietary measures provide adequate potassium intake, and it is questionable whether for most patients potassium supplementation in any pharmaceutical form is necessary (Chapter 21).

MISCELLANEOUS REPORTS

Older reports of side effects of miscellaneous drugs and materials included in SED-12, and additional new information included in SEDA 16–18, are listed in Table 1.

REFERENCES

1. Rijke AM, Rieger MR, McLaughlin RE, McCoy S. Porous acrylic cement. J Biomed Mater Res 1977;11(3):373–394.
2. Feith R. Arcrylement. Ned Tijdschr Geneeskd 1978; 122:64.
3. Rijke AM. Bijwerkingen van methylmethacrylaat-botcement. Ned Tijdschr Geneeskd 1980;124:180.
4. Fediukovich LV, Egorova AB. Genotoksicheskii effekt akrilatov (Genotoxic effect of acrylates). Gig Sanit (USSR) 1991;12:62–64.
5. Santavirta S, Konttinen YT, Bergroth V, Gronblad M. Lack of immune response to methyl methacrylate in lymphocyte cultures. Acta Orthop Scand 1991;62(1):29–32.
6. Santavirta S, Gristina A, Konttinen YT. Cemented versus cementless hip arthroplasty. A review of prosthetic biocompatibility. Acta Orthop Scand 1992;63(2):225–232.
7. Chang CC, Merritt K. Microbial adherence on polymethyl methacrylate (PMMA) surfaces. J Biomed Mater Res 1992;26(2):197–207.
8. Saint-Maurice C, Migne J, Maurin JP, Lmas JP. Accidents consécutifs au scellement des prothèses articulaires. Ann Anesthésiol Fr 1977;18:647.
9. Shirai K. The hazard for the respiratory system of acrylic bone cement during anesthesia. Jpn J Anesthesiol 1975; 24:886.
10. Pickering CAC, Bainbridge B, Birtwistle IH. Occupational asthma due to methylmethacrylate in an orthopedic theater sister. Br Med J 1986;292:1362.
11. Oleksak M, Edge AJ. Compression of the sciatic nerve by methylmethacrylate cement after total hip replacement. J Bone Joint Surg 1992;74(5):729–730.
12. Donaghy M, Rushworth G, Jacobs JM. Generalized peripheral neuropathy in a dental technician exposed to methyl methacrylate monomer. Neurology 1991;41(7):1112–1116.
13. Rumpf KW, Rieger J, Jansen J, Scherer M, Seubert S, Seubert A, Sellin HJ. Quincke's edema in a dialysis patient after administration of acrylic bone cement: possible role of ethylene oxide allergy. Arch Orthop Trauma Surg 1986; 105(4):250–252.
14. Svartling N, Lehtinen AM, Tarkkanen L. The effects of

anaesthesia in changes in blood pressure and plasma cortisol levels induced by cementation with methylmethacrylate. Acta Anaesthesiol Scand 1986;30:247.
15. Esemenli T, Toker K, Lawrence R. Hypotension associated with methylmethacrylate in partial hip arthroplasties. Orthoped Rev 1991;XX:619–623.
16. Arac SS, Ercan ZS, Turker RK. Prevention by aprotinin of the hypotension due to acrylic cement implantation into the bone. Curr Ther Res 1980;28:554.
17. Tryba M, Linde I, Voshage G, Zenz M. Histaminfreisetzung und kardiovaskulare Reaktionen nach Implantation von Knochenzement bei totalem Huftgelenkersatz. Anaesthesist 1991;40(1):25–32.
18. De Lustro F, Smith ST, Sundsmo J et al. Reaction to injectable collagen: results in animal models and clinical use. Plast Reconstr Surg 1986;79:581.
19. Hanke CW, Higley HR, Jolivette DM, Swanson NA, Stegman SJ. Abscess formation and local necrosis after treatment with Zyderm or Zyplast collagen implant. J Am Acad Dermatol 1991;25:319–326.
20. Lipsky H. Endoscopic treatment of vesicoureteral reflux with collagen. Pediatr Surg Int 1991;6:301–303.
21. Schein OD, Glynn RJ, Poggio EC, Seddon JM, Kenyon KR. The relative risk of ulcerative keratitis among users of daily-wear and extended-wear soft contact lenses. A case-control study. N Engl J Med 1989;321(12):773–778.
22. Schein OD, Buehler PO, Stamler JF, Verdier DD, Katz J. The impact of overnight wear on the risk of contact lens-associated ulcerative keratitis. Arch Ophthalmol 1994; 112(2):186–190.
23. Nilsson SE, Montan PG. The annualized incidence of contact lens induced keratitis in Sweden and its relation to lens type and wear schedule: results of a 3-month prospective study. CLAO J 1994;20(4):225–230.
24. Dart JK, Stapleton F, Minassian D. Contact lenses and other risk factors in microbial keratitis. Lancet 1991; 338(8768):650–653.
25. Radford CF, Bacon AS, Dart JK, Minassian DC. Risk factors for acanthamoeba keratitis in contact lens users: a case-control study. Br Med J 1995;310(6994):1567–1570.
26. Fleiszig SM, Efron N, Pier GB. Extended contact lens wear enhances Pseudomonas aeruginosa adherence to human corneal epithelium. Invest Ophthalmol Vis Sci 1992;33(10):2908–2916.
27. Marechal-Coutois CH, Delcourt JC. Klinische Resultate einer Untersuchung mit einer 70%ig hydratisierten Linse: die Linse Tp 70 (Yumecon). Contactologie 1981;3D:89.
28. Pickering CAC, Bainbridge B, Birtwistle IH. Occupational asthma due to methylmethacrylate in an orthopedic theater sister. Br Med J 1986;292:1362.
29. Kram HB, Reuben BI, Fleming AW. Using of fibrin glue in hepatic trauma. J Trauma 1988;28:1195–1201.
30. Spotnitz WD, Dalton S, Baker JW. Reduction of perioperative hemorrhage by anterior mediastinal spray application of fibrin glue during cardiac operations. Am Thorac Surg 1987;44:529–531.
31. Jessen C, Sharma P. Use of fibrin glue in thoracic surgery. Ann Thorac Surg 1985;39:522–524.
32. Berguer R, Staerkel RL, Moore EE, Moore FA, Galloway WB, Mockus MB. Warning: Fatal reaction due to the use of fibrin glue in deep hepatic wounds. Case reports. J Trauma 1991;31:408–411.
33. Berruyer M, Amiral J, French P, Belleville J, Bastien O, Clerc J, Kassir A, Estanove S, Dechavanne M. Immunization by bovine thrombin used with fibrin glue during cardiovascular operations. Development of thrombin and factor V inhibitors. J Thorac Cardiovasc Surg 1993;105(5):892–897.
34. Gomez-Ulla F, Gutierrez C, Seoane I. Severe anaphylactic reactions to orally administered fluorescein. Am J Ophthalmol 1991;109:94.
35. Fitzpatrick JM, Kasidas GP, Rose GA. Hyperoxaluria following glycine irrigation for transurethral prostatectomy. Br J Urol 1981;53:250.
36. Rao PN. Absorption of irrigating fluid during transcervical resection of endometrium. Br Med J 1990;300:748–749.
37. Hahn RG. Hallucinations and visual disturbances in transurethral prostatic resection. Intensive Care Med 1988; 14:668–671.
38. Norlen H, Dimberg M, Algen LG, Vinnars E. Water and electrolytes in muscle tissue and free amino acids in muscle and plasma in connection with transurethral resection of the prostate. II. Scand J Urol Nephrol 1990;24:95–101.
39. Chilla R. Histoacryl-induced late complications after duraplasty of the base of the skull. HNO 1987;35:250.
40. Burgaresi P, Confortini M, Galanti L, Gargano D. Inflammatory changes and cervical intra-epithelial neoplasia in IUD users. Cervix 1989;7:207–212.
41. Duguid HLD, Parratt D, Traynor R. *Actinomyces*-like organisms in cervical smears from women using intrauterine contraceptive devices. Br Med J 1980,2:534.
42. Leeton J. Female genital actinomycosis and the intrauterine device. Med J Aust 1980;1:518.
43. Vessey MP, Yeates D, Flavel R, McPherson K. Pelvic inflammatory disease and the intrauterine device: findings in a large cohort study. Br Med J 1981;282:855.
44. Editorial. Unanswered question on ectopic pregnancy. Br Med J 1980;1:1127.
45. Vessey MP, Yeates D, Flavel R. Risk of ectopic pregnancy and duration of use of intrauterine device, Lancet 1979;ii:501.
46. Shamai A, Peretz BA, Kerner H, Paldi E. Four cases of primary ovarian pregnancy and two of them associated with an intrauterine device. Infertility 1979;2:233.
47. Zerner J, Doil LK, Drewry J, Leeber D. Intrauterine contraceptive device failures in renal transplant patients. J Reprod Med 1981;26:99.
48. Patai K, Balogh I. Clinicopathological problems of tissue effects caused by IUDs containing copper. Mag Noorv Lapja 1988;51:240.
49. Hefnawi F, Salek A, Kandil O et al. Fibrinolytic activity of menstrual blood in normal and menorrhagic women and in women wearing the Lippes loop and the Cu-T (200). Int J Gynaecol Obstet 1979;16:400.
50. Davies N, Atwell JD. Primary vesicoureteric reflux: treatment with subureteric injection of Polytef paste. Br J Urol 1991;67(5):536–540.
51. Boykin W, Rodriguez RF, Brizzolara JP, Thompson IM, Zeidman EJ. Complete urinary obstruction following periurethral polytetrafluoroethylene injection for urinary incontinence. J Urol 1989,141:1199–1200.
52. Kiilholma P, Makinen J. Disappointing effect of endoscopic Teflon injection for female stress incontinence. Eur Urol 1991;20(3):197–199.
53. Beckingham IJ, Wemyss-Holden G, Lawrence WT. Long-term follow-up of women treated with periurethral Te-

flon injections for stress incontinence. Br J Urol 1992; 69(6):580–583.
54. Kiilholma PJ, Chancellor MB, Makinen J, Hirsch IH, Klemi PJ. Complications of Teflon injection for stress urinary incontinence. Neurourol Urodyn 1993;12(2):131–137.
55. Smart RF. Polytef paste for urinary incontinence. Aust NZ J Surg 1991;61:663–666.
56. Claes H, Stroobants D, van Meerbeek J, Verbeken E, Knockaert D. Pulmonary migration following periurethral polytetrafluoroethylene injection for urinary incontinence. J Urol 1991;145:839–840.
57. Weingarten J, Kaufman SL. Teflon embolisation to pulmonary arteries. Ann Thorac Surg 1977;23:371.
58. Lescher J, Gorman L, Coller A, Veidenheimer MC. A management of late complications of Teflon sling repair for rectal prolapse. Dis Colon Rect 1979;22:445.
59. Kaplan PA, Ruskin JD, Tu HK et al. Erosive arthritis of the temporomandibular joint caused by Teflon-Proplast implants. Plain film features. Am J Radiol 1988;151:337.
60. Mastres CA, Cugat E, Ninot S et al. Severe fibrous epicarditis after microporous polyurethane cardiac patch implantation. Thorac Cardiovasc Surg 1986;34:137.
61. Ellenbogen R et al. Injectable fluid silicone therapy: human morbidity and mortality. J Am Med Assoc 1975; 234:308–309.
62. Savrin RA, Martin EW Jr, Ruberg RL. Mass lesion of the breast after augmentation mammoplasty. Arch Surg 1979;114:1423–1424.
63. Vasey FB, Espinoza LR, Osuna PM, Seleznick MJ, Brozena SJ, Penske NA. Silicone and rheumatic disease: replace implant or not. Arch Dermatol 1991;127:907.
64. Maturri L, Azzolini A, Campiglio GL, Tardito E. Are synthetic prostheses really inert? Preliminary results of a study on the biocompatibility of dacron vascular prostheses and silicone skin expanders. Int Surg 1991;76:115–118.
65. Atkinson RE, Smith RJ. Silicone synovitis following silicone implant arthroplasty. Hand Clin 1986;2:291.
66. Nalbandian RM et al. Long-term silicone implant arthroplasty: implications of animal and human autopsy findings. J Am Med Assoc 1983;250:1195–1198.
67. Christie AJ, Pierret G, Levitan JA. Silicone synovitis. Semin Arthr Rheum 1989;19:166–171.
68. Kircher T. Silicone lymphadenopathy: a complication of silicone elastomer finger joint prostheses. Hum Pathol 1980;11:240.
69. Bommer J, Ritz E, Waldherr R. Silicone-induced splenomegaly: treatment of pancytopenia by splenectomy in a patient on hemodialysis. N Engl J Med 1981;308:1077.
70. Bommer J, Waldherr R, Gastner M. Iatrogenic multiorgan silicone inclusions in dialysis patients. Klin Wochenschr 1981;59:1149.
71. Chastre J et al. Acute pneumonitis after subcutaneous injections of silicone in transsexual men. N Engl J Med 1983;308:764–767.
72. Celli BR, Kovnat DM. Acute pneumonitis after subcutaneous injections of silicone. N Engl J Med 1983;309:856–857.
73. Manresa JM, Manresa F. Silicone pneumonitis. Lancet 1983;ii:1373.
74. Strobino B, Kline J, Stein Z et al. Exposure to contraceptive creams, jellies and douches and their effect on the zygote. Am J Epidemiol 1980;223:434.
75. Manjuck JE. Relationship of vaginal spermicides to birth defects. J Fl Med Assoc 1989;75:316–321.
76. Strobino B, Kline J, Stein Z et al. Vaginal spermicides and spontaneous abortion of known karyotype. Am J Epidemiol 1986;123:431.
77. Magnan A, Ottomani A, Garbe L, Arnaud A, Manelli JC. Detresse respiratoire chez une heroinomane seropositive pour le virus de l'immunodeficience humaine. Ann Fr Anesth Reanim 1991;10(1):74–76.
78. Oubeid M, Bickel JT, Ingram EA, Scott GC. Pulmonary talc granulomatosis in a cocaine sniffer. Chest 1990; 98(1):237–239.
79. Hollinger MA. Pulmonary toxicity of inhaled and intravenous talc. Toxicol Lett 1990;52(2):121–127.
80. Sparrow SA, Hallam LA. Talc granulomas. Br Med J 1991;18(302):1200–1201.
81. Kamffer WJ, Jooste EV, Nel JT, de Wet JI. Surgical glove powder and intraperitoneal adhesion formation. An appeal for the use of powder-free surgical gloves. S Afr Med J 1992;81(3):158–159.
82. Lange P, Mortensen J, Groth S. Lung function 22 to 35 years after treatment of idiopathic spontaneous pneumothorax with talc poudrage or simple drainage. Thorax 1988; 43:559.
83. Rhodes RE, Chiles C, Vick WW. Talc granulomatosis presenting as spontaneous pneumothorax. South Med J 1991;84(7):929–930.
84. Harlow BL, Cramer DW, Bell DA, Welch WR. Perineal exposure to talc and ovarian cancer risk. Obstet Gynecol 1992;80(1):19–26.
85. Davis JP, Chesney PJ, Wand PJ, La Venture M. Toxic shock syndrome. N Engl J Med 1980;303:1429.
86. Shands KN, Schmid GP, Dan BB et al. Toxic shock syndrome in menstruating women. N Engl J Med 1980; 303:1436.
87. Glasgow LA. Staphylococcal infection in the toxic-shock syndrome. N Engl J Med 1980;303:1473.
88. Editorial. Toxic shock and tampons. Br Med J 1980; 281:1161.
89. Medical student. Toxic shock and tampons. Br Med J 1980;281:1426.
90. Lea S, Ellis-Pegler RB. Toxic shock and tampons. Br Med J 1980;281:1639.
91. Faich G, Pearson K, Fleming D et al. Toxic shock syndrome and the vaginal contraceptive sponge. J Am Med Assoc 1986;255:216.
92. Shelton JD, Higgins JE. Contraception and toxic shock syndrome: a re-analysis. Contraception 1981;24:631.
93. Chait S, Adler OB, Rosenberger A. Intramural dissection of the oesophagus after sclerotherapy. Value of CT. Fortschr Rontgenstr 1990;152:107–108.
94. Tam F, Chow H, Prindiville T, Cornish D, Haulk T, Trudeau W, Hoeprich P. Bacterial peritonitis following oesophageal injection sclerotherapy for variceal hemorrhage. Gastrointest Endosc 1990;36:131–133.
95. Low DE, Shoenut JP, Kennedy JK, Harding GKM, Den Boer B, Micflikier AB. Infectious complications of endoscopic injection sclerotherapy. Arch Intern Med 1986; 146:569–571.
96. Zeller FA, Cannan CA, Prakash UBS. Thoracic manifestations after esophageal variceal sclerotherapy. Mayo Clin Proc 1991;66:727–732.
97. Dell Abate P, Spaggiari L, Carboynani P, Soliani P, Karake E. An unusual complication of sclerotherapy. Endoscopy 1991;23:352–353.
98. Davis LT, Duffy DM. Determination of incidence and

risk factors for postsclerotherapy telangiectatic matting of the lower extremity: a retrospective analysis. J Dermatol Surg Oncol 1990;16:327—330.

99. Weiss RA, Weiss MA. Resolution of pain associated with varicose and telangiectatic leg veins after compression sclerotherapy. J Dermatol Surg Oncol 1990;16:333—336.

100. Duffy DM. Small vessel sclerotherapy: an overview. Adv Dermatol 1988;3:221—242.

101. Anonymous. Acesulfame. Fed Regist 1988;53(145): 28379.

102. FAO/WHO. Evaluation of certain food additives and contaminants: thirty-seventh report of the joint FAO/WHO expert committee on food additives. WHO Tech Rep Ser 806, 1991.

103. Council on Scientific Affairs. Aspartame: review of safety issues. J Am Med Assoc 1985;254:400—402.

104. Stegink LD, Koch R, Blaskovics ME et al. Plasma phenylalanine levels in phenylketonuric heterozygous and normal adults administered aspartame at 34 mg/kg body weight. Toxicology 1981;20:81.

105. Stegink LD, Filer LJ, Baker GL et al. Aspartame metabolism in human subjects. In: Health and Sugar Substitutes. Proceedings of ERGOB Conference, Geneva, 1978;160—165.

106. Shahangian S, Ash KE, Rollins DE. Aspartame not a source of formate toxicity. Clin Chem 1984;30:1254—1265.

107. Kulczycki A. Aspartame-induced urticaria. Ann Intern Med 1986;104:207—208.

108. McCauliffe DP, Poitras K. Aspartame-induced lobular panniculitis. J Am Acad Dermatol 1991;24:298—300.

109. Geha R, Buckley CE, Greenberger P, Patterson R, Polmar S, Saxon A, Rohr A, Yang W, Drouin MTI. Aspartame is no more likely than placebo to cause urticaria/angioedema: results of a multicenter, randomized, double-blind, placebo-controlled, crossover study. J Allergy Clin Immunol 1993;92(4):513—20.

110. Van den Eeden SK, Koepsell TD, Longstreth-WT Jr, van Belle G, Daling JR, McKnight B. Aspartame ingestion and headaches: a randomized crossover trial. Neurology 1994;44(10):1787—1793.

111. Walton RG, Hudak R, Green-Waite RJ. Adverse reactions to aspartame: double-blind challenge in patients from a vulnerable population. Biol Psychiatry 1993;34(1—2):13—17.

112. Zinck O, Hallas-Møller. E-nummer Bogen. Forlaget komma, Copenhagen, 1986.

113. Moneret-Vautrin DA, Bene MC, Faure G. She should not have chewed. Lancet 1986;i:617.

114. FAO/WHO. Evaluation of certain food additives and contaminants: twenty-sixth report of the joint FAO/WHO expert committee on food additives. WHO Technical Reports Series 683, 1982.

115. Lark H, Comisarow RH, Taranger LA, Canada A. Three cases of human bladder cancer following high dose cyclamate ingestion. J Urol 1977;118:258.

116. Derfler K, Siegfried M, Herold C et al. Reversible malabsorption caused by high doses of cyclamate. Am J Med 1988;85:446.

117. Le Faou M. The effect of geriatric pharmacon versus placebo on physical fatigue and recovery. Sport Méd Spec Issue 1985;41:34.

118. Ekblom B. Ginsengs effect på fysisk uthålighet ej bevisad. Läkartidningen 1988;85:1409.

119. Anonymous. Ginseng—muskelskada? Inf Socialstyr Läkemedelsavd 1988;4:114.

120. Walker AM, Dreyer NA, Friedlander E et al. An independent analysis of the national cancer institute study on non-nutritive sweeteners and bladder cancer. Am J Publ Health 1982;72:376.

121. US Food and Drug Administration. Saccharin. FDA Talk Paper T87-38, 1 September, 1987.

122. Lutomski DM, Gora ML, Wright SM, Martin JE. Sorbitol content of selected oral liquids. Ann Pharmacother 1993;27:269—274.

123. Dills WL. Sugar alcohols as bulk sweeteners. Ann Rev Nutr 1989;9:161—186.

124. Gatto-Smith AG, Scott RB, Machida HM, Gall DG. Sorbitol as a cryptic cause of diarrhea. Can J Gastroenterol 1988;2:140—142.

125. Badiga MS, Jain NR, Casanova C, Pitchumoni CS. Diarrhoea in diabetics: the role of sorbitol. J Am Coll Nutr 1990;9:578—582.

126. Jain JK, Patel VP, Pitchumoni CS. Sorbitol intolerance in adults. J Clin Gastroenterol 1987;9:317—319.

127. Coyne MJ, Rodriguez H. Carbohydrate malabsorption in black and Hispanic dialysis patients. Am J Gastroenterol 1986;81:662—665.

128. Wootton FT, Rhodes DF, Lee WM, Fitts CT. Colonic necrosis with Kayexalate-sorbitol enemas after renal transplantation. Ann Intern Med 1989;111:947—949.

129. Sills MR, Zinkham WH. Methylene blue induced Heinz body hemolytic anemia. Arch Pediatr Adolesc Med 1994;148(3):306—310.

130. Elias S, Gerbie AB, Simpson JL et al. Genetic amniocentesis in twin gestations. Am J Obstet Gynecol 1980; 138:169.

131. Kirsch IR, Cohen HJ. Heinz-body hemolytic anemia from the use of methylene blue in neonates. J Pediatr 1980;96:276.

132. Serota FT, Bernbaum JC, Schwartz E. The methylene blue baby. Lancet 1979;ii:1142.

133. Nicolini V, Monni G. Intestinal obstruction in babies exposed in utero to methylene blue. Lancet 1990;336:1258—1259.

134. Dolk H. Methylene blue and atresia or stenosis of ileum and jejunum. Lancet 1991;338:1021—1022.

135. Cragan JD, Martin ML, Khoury MJ, Fernhoff PM. Dye use during amniocentesis and birth defects. Lancet 1993; 341:1352.

136. Whitwam JG, Taylor AR, White JM. Potential hazards of methylene blue. Anaesthesia 1979;34:181.

137. Rowe KS. Synthetic food colouring and hyperactivity: a double-blind cross-over study. Aust Paediatr J 1988;24:143.

138. Frick WE, Lemanske RF. Oral sulfite sensitivity and provocative challenge in a 2-year-old. J Asthma 1991; 28:221—224.

139. Anonymous. Medical devices safety alerts. Unsafe apnea monitors lead wires. FDA Med Bull 1993;23:7.

140. Daugiras JT, Ing TS et al. Severe anaphylactoid reactions to cuprammonium cellulose hemodialyzers. Arch Intern Med 1985;145:489.

141. Wenzel-Seifert K, Sharma AM, Keller F. Repeated dialysis anaphylaxis. Nephrol Dial Transplant 1990;5:821—824.

142. Anonymous. Glass capillary tubes pose risk to healthcare workers. FDA Med Bull 1993;23:6.

143. Jagger J, Hunt EH, Pearson RD. Sharp object injuries in the hospital: causes and strategies for prevention. Am J Infect Control 1990;18:227—231.

144. Aoun H. When a house officer gets AIDS. New Engl J Med 1989;321:693–696.
145. Anon. Allergic reactions to Latex-containing medical devices. FDA Med Bull 1991;91:2–3.
146. Gaignon I, Veyckemans F, Gribomont BF. Latex allergy in a child: report of a case. Acta Anaesth Belgica 1991;42:219–223.
147. Nacey JN, Tulloch AGS, Ferguson AF. Catheter-induced urethritis: a comparison between latex and silicone catheters in a prospective clinical trial. Br J Urol 1985; 57:325.
148. Anon. Severe allergic reactions associated with dialysis and ACE inhibitors. FDA Med Bull 1992;22(1):4.
149. Anon. Medical devices safety alerts. Volume ventilator hazards. FDA Med Bull 1993;23:6.
150. Kirschbaum BB, Schoolwerth AC. Hyperaluminaemia associated with oral citrate and aluminium. Hum Toxicol 1989;45–47.
151. Mees EJD, Basci A. Citric acid in calcium effervescent tablets may favour aluminium intoxication. Nephron 1991; 59:322.
152. Main J, Ward MK. Potentiation of aluminium absorption by effervescent analgesic tablets in a haemodialysis patient. Br Med J 1992;304:1686.
153. Domingo JL et al. Effect of ascorbic acid on gastrointestinal aluminium absorption. Lancet 1992;338:1467.
154. Moreno A, Domingnez P, Domingnez C, Balabriga A. High serum aluminium levels and acute reversible encephalopathy in a 4-year-old boy with acute renal failure. Eur J Paediatr 1991;150:513–514.
155. Sedman AB, Klein GL, Merrit AR. Evidence of aluminium loading in infants receiving intravenous therapy. N Engl J Med 1985;312:1337–1343.
156. Milliner DS, Shinoberger JH, Shuman P, Coburn JW. Inadvertent aluminum administration during plasma exchange due to aluminum contamination of albumin replacement solutions. N Engl J Med 1985;312:165–167.
157. Monteagudo F, Wood L, Jacobs P, Folb P, Cassidy M. Aluminum loading during therapeutic plasma exchange. J Clin Apheresis 1987;3:161–163.
158. Nussbaum SR, Younger J, Vandepol CJ, Gagel RF, Zubler MA, Chapman R, Henderson IC, Mallette LE. Single-dose intravenous therapy with pamidronate for the treatment of hypercalcemia of malignancy: comparison of 30-, 60-, and 90-mg dosages. Am J Med 1993;95(3):297–304.
159. Redalieu E, Coleman JM, Chan K, Seaman J, Degen PH, Flesch G, Brox A, Batiste G. Urinary excretion of aminohydroxypropylidene bisphosphonate in cancer patients after single intravenous infusions J Pharm Sci 82(6):665–667.
160. Daragon A, Peyron R, Serrurier D, Deshayes P. Treatment of hypercalcemia of malignancy with intravenous APD. Cur Ther Res 1991;50:10–21.
161. Boumans LJJM, Poublon RML. The detrimental effect of aminohydroxypropylidene biphosphonate (APD) in otospongiosis. Eur Arch Otorhinol 1991;248:218–221.
162. Rotoli B, Giglio F, Bile M et al. Immune mediated acute intravascular hemolysis caused by catergen (cyanidanol). Haematologica 1985;70:495.
163. Bar-Meir S, Halpern Z, Gutman M. Effect of (+)-cyanidanol-3 on chronic active hepatitis: a double blind controlled trial. Gut 1985;26:975.
164. Suzuki H, Yamamoto S, Hirayama C et al. Cianidanol therapy for HBe-antigen positive chronic hepatitis. Liver 1986;6:35.
165. Swanson BN. Medical use of dimethyl sulfoxide (DMSO). Rev Clin Basic Pharm 1985;5(1–2):1–33.
166. Brayton CF. Dimethyl sulfoxide (DMSO): a review. Cornell Vet 1986;76(1):61–90.
167. Muther RS, Bennett WM. Effects of dimethyl sulfoxide on renal function in man. J Am Med Assoc 1980;244:2081–2083.
168. Brobyn RD. The human toxicology of dimethyl sulfoxide. Ann NY Acad Sci 1975;243:497–505.
169. John H, Laudahn G. Clinical experiences with the topical application of DMSO in orthopedic diseases. Evaluation of 4180 cases. Ann NY Acad Sci 1967;141:506.
170. Dhodapkar M, Goldberg SL, Tefferi A, Gertz MA. Reversible encephalopathy after cryopreserved peripheral blood stem cell infusion. Am J Hematol 1994;45(2):187–188.
171. Bond GR, Curry SC. Dimethylsulfoxide-induced encephalopathy. Lancet 1989;335:1134–1135.
172. Yellowlees P, Greenfield C, McIntyre N. Dimethylsulphoxide induced toxicity. Lancet 1980;ii:1004–1006.
173. Albert NE. Exothermal reaction with RIMSO 100. Urology 1982;20:662.
174. Rubin LF. Toxicity of dimethyl sulfoxide, alone and in combination. Ann NY Acad Sci 1975;243:298.
175. Olson RJ. Dimethylsulfoxide and ocular involvement. J Toxicol Cut Ocul Toxicol 1982;1:147–152.
176. Enghusen-Poulsen H, Loft S, Andersen JR, Andersen M. Disulfiram therapy: adverse drug reactions and interactions. Acta Psychiatr Scand Suppl 1992;369:59–65.
177. Lake CR, Major LF, Ziegler MG, Kopin IG. Increased sympathetic nervous system activity in alcoholic patients treated with disulfiram. Am J Psychiatr 1977;134:1411.
178. Frisoni GB, Dimonda V. Disulfiram neuropathy: a review. (1971–1988) and report of a case. Alcohol Alcoholism 1989;24:449–458.
179. Piliyath S, Schwartz BD. Disulfiram neuropathy: electrophysiological study. Electromyogr Clin Neurophysiol 1988;28:245.
180. Acheson JF, Howard RS. Reversible optic neuropathy associated with disulfiram. Neuroophthalmology 1988;8:175.
181. Ewing JA, Rouse BA, Mueller RA, Silver D. Can dopamine beta-hydroxylase levels predict adverse reactions to disulfiram? Alcohol Clin Exp Res 1978;2:93.
182. Rainey JM. Disulfiram toxicity and carbon disulfide poisoning. Am J Psychiatry 1977;134:371.
183. Knudsen TE, Nielsen-Kudsk JE. Letalt forlobende hepatitis efter disulfiram. Ugeskr Laeg 1990;152:1457–1458.
184. Vanjak D, Samuel D, Gosset F, Derrida S, Moreau R, Soupison T, Soulie A, Bismuth H, Sicot C. Disulfiram-induced fulminant hepatitis in a patient with alcoholic cirrhosis. Favourable outcome after liver transplantation. Gastroenterol Clin Biol 1989;13:1075–1078.
185. Mason NA. Disulfiram-induced hepatitis: a case report and review of the literature. Ann Pharmacother 1989; 23:872–874.
186. Bartle WR, Fisher MM, Kerenyl N. Disulfiram induced hepatitis. Dig Dis Sci 1985;30:1834.
187. Miller SI. Disulfiram: an unusual side effect. J Am Med Assoc 1977;237:2602.
188. Reilley RA, Mothley CH. Breath odor after disulfiram. J Am Med Assoc 1977;238:2600.
189. Nora AH, Nora JJ, Blu J. Limb reduction anomalies in infants born to disulfiram-treated mothers. Lancet 1977; ii:664.

190. MacLeod SM, Sellers EM, Giles HG et al. Interaction of disulfiram with benzodiazepines. Clin Pharmacol Ther 1978;24:583.
191. Manager D, Gerson J, Constantine RM, Lenzi V. Pulmonary edema and coagulopathy due to Hyskon (32% dextran 70) administration. Anesth Analg 1989;68:686—689.
192. Jediekin R, Olsfanger D, Kessler I. Disseminated intravascular coagulopathy and adult respiratory distress syndrome: life threatening complications of hysteroscopy. Am J Obstet Gynecol 1990;44:142—146.
193. Ahmed N, Falcone T, Tulandi T, Houle G. Anaphylactic reaction because of intrauterine 32% dextran-70 instillation. Fertil Steril 1991;55:1014—1016.
194. Ljungstrom KG. Safety of dextran in relation to other colloids—ten years experience with hapten inhibition. Infusionsther Transfusionsmed 1993;20(5):206—210.
195. Dubrey SW, Bomanji JB, Noble MI, Jewkes RF. Safety of intravenous dipyridamole thallium myocardial perfusion imaging: experience in 435 patients. Nucl Med Commun 1993;14(4):303—309.
196. Beller GA. Pharmacologic stress imaging. J Am Med Assoc 1991;265:633—638.
197. Ottervanger JP, Haan D, Gans SJ, Hoorntje JC, Stricker BH. Bronchospasme, apnoe en hartstilstand na een dipyridamol-perfusiescintigrafie. Ned Tijdschr Geneeskd 1993;137(3):142—143.
198. Whiting JH Jr, Datz FL, Gabor FV, Jones SR, Morton KA. Cerebrovascular accident associated with dipyridamole thallium-201 myocardial imaging. J Nucl Med 1993; 34(1):128—130.
199. Collins J. Metabolic diseases. Time for fructose solutions to go. Lancet 1993;341:600.
200. Schaiff RAB, Hall TG, Bar RS. Medical treatment of hypercalcemia. Clin Pharm 1989;8:108—121.
201. Hall TG, Schaiff RAB. Update on the medical treatment of hypercalcemia of malignancy. Clin Pharm 1993;12:117—125.
202. Warrell RP Jr, Murphy WK, Schulman P, O'Dwyer PJ, Heller G. A randomized double-blind study of gallium nitrate compared with etidronate for acute control of cancer-related hypercalcemia. J Clin Oncol 1991;9(8):1467—75.
203. Fujimaki T, Fukushima T, Miyazaki S. Percutaneous retrogasserian glycerol injection in the management of trigeminal neuralgia: long-term follow-up results. J Neurosurg 1990;73:212—216.
204. Orlandini G, Pareti A. Trattamento della neuragia del trigemino con glicerolizzazione retrogasseriana. Acta Anaesthesiol Ital 1990;41:617--624.
205. Kumana CR, Chan GTC, Yu YL, Lauder IJ, Chau TKP, Kou M. Investigation of intravascular hemolysis during treatment of acute stroke with intravenous glycerol. Br J Clin Pharmacol 1990;29:347—353.
206. Kalant H, Roschlan W. Organically bound iodine. In: Principles of Medical Pharmacology, 5th edn. Washington, DC: Decker, 1989;484—485.
207. Drinka PJ, Nolten WE. Effects of iodinated glycerol on thyroid function studies in elderly nursing home residents. J Am Geriatr Soc 1988;36:911—913.
208. Mather JL, Baycliff CD, Paterson NAM. Hypothyroidism secondary to iodinated glycerol. Can J Hosp Pharm 1993;46:177—178.
209. Kilbourne EM, Swygert LA, Philen RM, Sun RK, Anerbach RB, Miller L, Nelson DE, Falk H. Interstitial pneumonitis and pulmonary vasculitis in a patient taking an L-tryptophan preparation. Eur Respir J 1991;4:1033—1036.
210. Bogaerst Y, Van Renterghem D, Vanvughelen J, Praet M, Michielssen P, Blaton V, Willemot JP. Interstitial pneumonitis and pulmonary vasculitis in a patient taking an L-tryptophan preparation. Eur Resp J 1991;4:1033—1036.
211. Varga J et al. The cause and pathogenesis of the eosinophilia-myalgia syndrome. Ann Intern Med 1992;116:140—147.
212. Sokol WN, Hydick IB. Nasal congestion, urticaria, and angioedema caused by an IgE-mediated reaction to sodium metabisulfite. Ann. Allergy 1990;65(3):233—238.
213. Pande M, Ghanchi F. The role of preservatives in the conjunctival toxicity of subconjunctival gentamicin injection. Br J Ophthalmol 1992;76(4):235—237.
214. Pande M, Ghanchi F. The role of preservatives in the conjunctival toxicity of subconjunctival gentamicin injection. Br J Ophthalmol 1992;76(4):235—237.
215. Long CC, Motley RJ, Holt PJ. Taking the 'sting' out of local anaesthetics. Br J Dermatol 1991;125(5):452—455.
216. Soulat JM, Bouju P, Oxeda C, Amiot JF. Choc anaphylactoide aux metabisulfites au cours d'une cesarienne sous anesthesie peridurale Cah Anesthesiol 1991;39(4):257—259.
217. Maria Y, Vaillant P, Delorme N, Moneret-Vautrin DA. Les accidents graves liés aux metabisulfites. Rev Méd Interne Janvier-Février 1989:36—40.
218. Stewart PM, Catterall JR. Chronic nicotine ingestion and atrial fibrillation. Br Heart J 1985;54:222.
219. Ottervanger JP, Stricker BHC, Klomps HC. Transdermal nicotine. J Am Med Assoc 1993;269:1939—1941.
220. Tonnesen P, Norregaard J, Simonsen K, Sawe U. A double-blind trial of a 16-hour transdermal nicotine patch in smoking cessation. New Engl J Med 1991;325:311—315.
221. Mant D, Fowler G. Effectiveness of a nicotine patch in helping people stop smoking: results of a randomised trial in general practice. Br Med J 1993;306:1304—1308.
222. Maugh TH II. Blood substitutes passes its first test. Science 1979;206:205.
223. Urbaniak SJ. Artificial blood. Br Med J 1991; 303:1348—50.
224. Garrelts JC. Fluosol: an oxygen-delivery fluid for use in percutaneous transluminal coronary angioplasty. Ann Pharmacother 1990;24:1105—1112.
225. Nyberg SL, Cerra FB. Treatment of severe anemia with perfluorocarbon blood substitutes: a clinical overview. Clin Intensive Care 1991;2:226—232.
226. Schnapf BM, Santeiro ML. Beta-agonist inhaler causing hallucinations. Pediatr Emerg Care 1994;10:87—88.
227. Adinoff A, Tellez P, Lanier R. Fluorocarbon propellants and central nervous system stimulation in asthma. Pediatrics 1983;72:438—439.
228. Antti-Poika M, Heikkila J, Saarinen L. Cardiac arrhythmias during occupational exposure to fluorinated hydrocarbons. Br J Indust Med 1990;47:138—140.
229. Edling C, Ohlson CG, Ljungkvist G, Oliv A, Soderholm B. Cardiac arrhythmia in refrigerator repairmen exposed to flucrocarbons. Br J Indust Med 1990;47:207—212.
230. Warner MA, Harper JV. Cardiac dysrhythmias associated with chemical peeling with phenol. Anesthesiology 1985;62:366—367.
231. Morrison JE, Matthews D, Washington R, Fennesey PV, Harrison LM. Phenol motor point blocks in children: plasma concentrations and cardiac dysrhythmias. Anaesthesiology 1991;73:359—362.
232. Gandy JH, Tricot C, Sezeur A. Troubles du rythme cardiaque graves apres phenolisation splanchnique peroperatoire. Can J Anaesth 1993;40:357—359.

233. Ho SL, Hollinrake K. Acute epiglottitis and Chloraseptic. Br Med J 1989;298:1584.
234. Bergman M, Flance IJ, Blumenthal HT. Thesaurosis following inhalation of hair therapy. A clinical and experimental study. New Engl J Med 1958;258:471–476.
235. Bergman M, Flance IJ, Cruz PT, Klam N, Aronson PR, Joshi RA, Blumenthal HT. Thesaurosis due to inhalation of hair therapy. Report of twelve new cases including three autopsies. New Engl J Med 1962;266:750–755.
236. Kepes JJ, Chen WYK, Yick FJ. Mucoid dissolution of bones and multiple pathologic fractures in a patient with past history of intravenous administration of polyvinylpyrrolidone (PVP). A case report. Bone Miner 1993;22:33–41.
237. Golightly LK et al. Pharmaceutical excipients: adverse effects associated with 'inactive ingredients' in drug products (part II). Med Toxicol 1988;3:209–240.
238. Catanzaro JM, Smith JG. Propylene glycol dermatitis. J Am Acad Dermatol 1991;24:90–95.
239. Andersen KE. Hudreaktioner fremkaldt af propylenglykol. Ugeskr Laeg 1980;142:2478.
240. Demey HE, Daelemans RA, Verpooten GA et al. Propylene glycol-induced side effects during intravenous nitroglycerin therapy. Intensive Care Med 1988;14:221.
241. Rogers L. Intravenous sclerosing solutions. Br Med J 1930;1:59.
242. Hammerschmidt DE, Craddock PR, McCullough JJ et al. Complement activation and pulmonary leukostasis during nylon-fiber filtration leukapheresis. Blood 1978;51:721.
243. Stoncek DF, Hutton SW, Silvis SE. Sodium morrhuate stimulates granulocytes and damages erythrocytes and endothelial cells: probable mechanism of an adverse reaction during sclerotherapy. J Lab Clin Med 1985;106:498.
244. Malberti F, Surian M, Poggio F, Minoia C, Salvadeo A. Efficacy and safety of long-term treatment with calcium carbonate as a phosphate binder. Am J Kidney Dis 1988;12:487–491.
245. Von Sperschneider H, Gunther K, Stein G, Marzoll I, Kirchner E. Untersuchungen zum Einsatz von Calciumcarbonat als Phosphatbinder bei Dialysepatienten im Langzeitverlauf uber 3 Jahre. Z Urol Nephrol 1990;83:449–458.
246. Pak CYC, Sakhaee K. Nephrolithiasis from calcium supplementation. J Urol 1987;137:1212–1213.
247. Ringe JD. The risk of nephrolithiasis with oral calcium supplementation. Calcif Tissue Int 1991;48:69–73.
248. Emmett M, Sirmon MD, Kirkpatrick WG, Nolan CR, Schmitt GW, Cleveland MB. Calcium acetate control of serum phosphorus in hemodialysis patients. Am J Kidney Dis 1991;XVII:544–550.
249. Ontario Medical Association. Preservatives: bronchospasm. Ontario Medical Association's Committee on Drugs and Pharmacotherapy. The Drug Report, No. 24, December, 1987.
250. Bundesgesundheitsamt. Gegenanzeigen bei Arzneimitteln beachten Probleme mit Sulfithaltigen Arzneimitteln. BGA-Presse-Dienst, 20 January, 1989.
251. Japanese Ministry of Health and Welfare. Notice on the indication of the inactive ingredients in prescription drugs. Notification No. 853. Pharmaceutical Affairs Bureau, Ministry of Health and Welfare, 1 October, 1988.
252. Harrison JE. Fluoride treatment of osteoporosis. Calcif Tissue Int 1990;46:287–288.
253. Schnitzler CM, Wing JR, Mesquita JM, Gear AK, Robson HJ, Smyth AE. Risk factors for the development of stress fractures during fluoride therapy for osteoporosis. J Bone Miner Res 1990;5:S195–S200.
254. Bayley TA, Harrison JE, Murray TM, Josse RG, Sturtridge W, Spitzker KP, Strauss A, Vieth R, Goodwin S. Fluoride induced fractures: relation to osteogenic effect. J Bone Miner Res 1990;5:S217–S222.
255. Orcel PH, de Vernejoul MC, Prier A, Miravet L, Kuntz D, Caplan G. Stress fractures of the lower limbs in osteoporotic patients treated with fluoride. J Bone Miner Res 1990;5:S191–S194.
256. Weingrad TR, Eymontt MJ, Martin JH. Periostitis due to low dose fluoride intoxication demonstrated by bone scanning. Clin Nucl Med 1991;16:59–60.
257. Stadtler P. Fluorides. Int J Clin Pharmacol Ther Toxicol 1990;28:20–26.
258. Spak CJ, Sjostedt S, Eleborg L, Veress B, Perbeck L, Ekstrand J. Studies of human gastric mucosa after application of 0.42% fluoride gel. J Dent Res 1990;62:426–429.
259. Editorial. Another fluoride fatality: a physician's dilemma. Fluoride 1979;12:55.
260. Waldbott GL. Fluoridation: a clinician's experience. South Med J 1980;73:301.
261. Freni SC. Exposure to high fluoride concentrations in drinking water is associated with decreased birth rates. J Toxicol Environ Health 1994;42(1):109–121.
262. Fassler CA, Rodriguez MR, Badesch DB et al. Magnesium toxicity as a cause of hypotension and hypoventilation. Arch Intern Med 1985;145:1604.
263. Jenny DB, Goris GB, Urrvilley RD, Brian AB. Hypermagnesemia following irrigation of renal pelvis. J Am Med Assoc 1978;240:1378.
264. Spital A, Greenwell R. Severe hyperkalemia during magnesium sulfate therapy in two pregnant drug abusers. South Med J 1991;84:919–921.
265. Feldstedt M, Boesgaard S, Bouchelouche P, Svenningsen A, Brooks L, Lech Y, Skagen K. Magnesium substitution in acute ischemic heart syndromes. Eur Heart J 1991;12:1215–1218.
266. Versteegh FGA, Van Vught AS, Van de Walle JGS, Rademaker CMA. Magnesiumintoxicatie bij een zuigeling. Ned Tijdschr Geneesk 1991;135:1186–1188.
267. Hunter MF, Ashton MR, Griffiths DM et al. Hyperphosphataemia after enemas in childhood prevention and treatment. Arch Dis Child 1993;68:233–234.
268. Craig JC, Hodson EM, Martin HC. Phosphate enema poisoning in children. Med J Aust 1994;21, 160(6):347–51.
269. Goldman M. Phosphate enemas in childhood. Br Med J 1991;302:1273–1274.
270. Rohack JJ, Mehta BR, Subramanyam K. Hyperphosphatemia and hypocalcemic coma associated with phosphate enema. South Med J 1985;78:1241–1242.
271. Spinrad S, Sztern M, Grosskopf Y et al. Treating constipation with phosphate enema: an unnecessary risk. Israel J Med Sci 1989;25:237–238.
272. Van der Loeff HJS, Strack van Schijndel RJM, Thijs LG. Cardiac arrest due to oral potassium intake. Intensive Care Med 1988;15:58–59.
273. McCaughan D. Hazards of non-prescription potassium supplements. Lancet 1984;i:513–514.
274. Browning JJ, Channer KS. Hyperkalaemic cardiac arrhythmia caused by potassium citrate mixture. Br Med J 1981;283:1366.

International drug monitoring*

For nearly 30 years an international collaboration in monitoring adverse drug reactions, under the auspices of the World Health Organization, has been in operation. The program started in 1968 as a pilot project with the participation of 10 countries. The intent was to develop international collaboration to make it easier to detect adverse drug reactions (ADR) not revealed during clinical trials. Some years later, the Swedish government assumed operational and financial responsibility for technical aspects of the program and a WHO Collaborating Centre for International Drug Monitoring was created in Uppsala (the Uppsala Monitoring Centre (UMC)).

Now the system is based on interchange of adverse reactions information between national drug monitoring centres in 45 countries (listed on pp. 1484-1492). Collectively these centres annually provide more than 150 000-200 000 individual reports of reactions suspected of being drug-induced. The cumulative database that has been constructed from these reports now comprises over 1.4 million records (Fig. 1). In addition to the full members of the Program, there are contacts with drug safety professionals in other countries who are active in developing drug monitoring facilities. About 10 of these collaborators are close to being recognised as 'national centres' by their own governments, and consequently by WHO when a formal application has been made and they can comply with the basic technical requirements.

In each country it is the national centre which processes and evaluates adverse reaction reports, sent to them either directly from health professionals and/or, in some countries, from pharmaceutical manufacturers. Information obtained from these reports is passed back to the medical profession on a national basis, but also contributes to drug experience at the international level.

The summarized case material is collected in the WHO database, which is updated in a weekly routine. It is screened using agreed output routines 4 times a year for new and serious reactions, as well as the reporting frequencies of associations of particular interest chosen by national centres or by Uppsala Monitoring Centre Staff. In addition, the national centres receive an annual reference document containing summary data on all suspected reactions reported to the WHO program.

The main aim of the international program, i.e. the early identification of new adverse reactions, has been re-emphasized during the last few years. At the start of the program it was hoped that by applying carefully designed statistical analysis to the large amount of data available, it would be possible to identify new, unexpected reactions of medical significance. In spite of a good deal of effort, with the state of knowledge at that time, it was impossible to realise the goal of automated signal generation. It was thought that the heterogeneous nature of the data collected, and the frequency of missing data would not allow such an approach. Recently, a pilot study, in collaboration with a research unit at Stockholm's Royal Institute of Technology, has shown that the use of a Bayesian neural network may be successful in automated support for signal generation. In principle, the neural network can generate *a priori* probabilities and correlations for the relationships between any data elements (or combinations thereof) in the total data base reports or selected parts of the data base. It is possible to compare any selected data against such backgrounds. For example, the probabilities and strengths of correlation for new drugs, their reported doses, the type of ADR and patient characteristics and concomitant medication can be compared with all drugs in the data base or drugs in the same therapeutic or other class. Apart from using state-of-the-art technology, the routine comparison of different aspects of reported drug risk with the background of reports is a novel approach, essentially answering the question 'Are the ADRs reported with the selected drug (or patient group etc.) significantly different from our background reporting experience?' The neural network approach is robust from the point of view of incomplete and heterogeneous data. Work is proceding to automate the process for routine use.

The review of adverse reaction signals has been intensified during the last 10 years by the appointment of reviewers in national centres to analyze reactions pertaining to particular body systems. Short summaries of their findings are circulated to participating national centres in a memorandum called 'Signal'. In order not to miss important signals, reports of adverse drug reaction associations that are new adverse reactions are reviewed by Centre staff every 3 months for critical adverse reaction terms. Any signal based on 3 or more good quality reports that are not already in the readily available

*Contributed by Prof. I.R. Edwards, Director, on behalf of the WHO Collaborating Centre for International Drug Monitoring, Uppsala, Sweden (Uppsala Monitoring Centre).

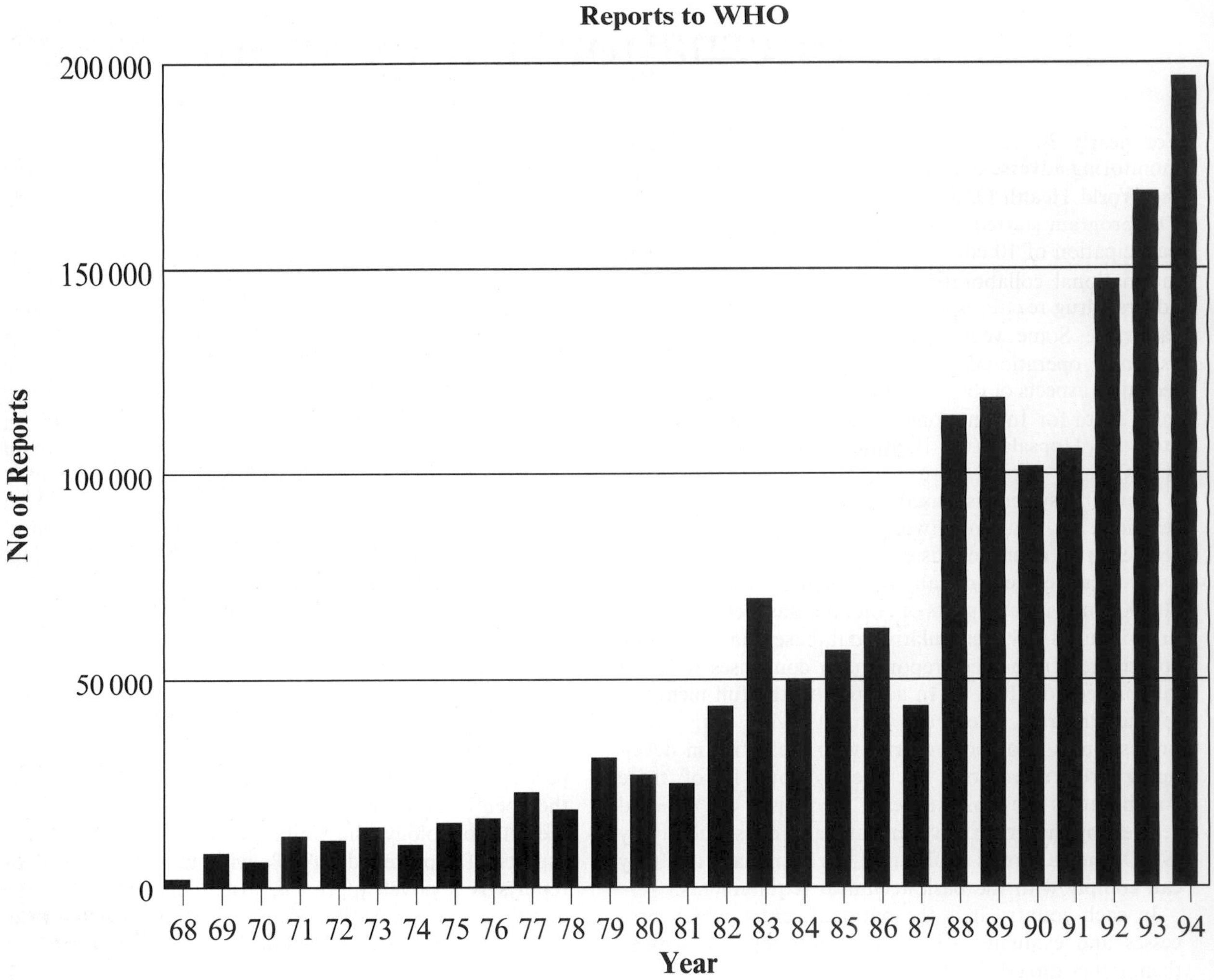

Fig. 1. *Number of individual case reports submitted regularly from national drug monitoring centres to the WHO Collaborating Centre located in Uppsala, Sweden. 1 437 052 reports (10 April 1995) are stored in the database INTDIS (International Drug Information System).*

international literature are also reported to participating centres in 'Signal'. This provides a back-up for the reviews performed by national centres' experts. The success of the signalling function is also dependent on a speedy input of reports from national centres to the UMC. One of the main objectives at the moment is to reduce delay in this input as much as possible. Whilst few centres take advantage of the facility at the moment it is possible for any national centre to use file transfer of cases via computer networks to the WHO data base.

Apart from rapidity of transfer, capture of more information is possible using automated systems. The UMC has a working data model, based on the CIOMS 1a report (obtainable from the Council for International Organisations of Medical Sciences, WHO, Geneva), which allows for much more data to be stored at the same time being compatible with the current WHO data-base and that being proposed by ICH (see below). The UMC will encourage industry to use this facility, parallel to, and not in place of, the national centres' data bases. This will ensure that all spontaneous reports are in the international arena, though users will need to be aware that duplications will occur between the two sets of data.

Increased communication between national centres during the past few years has resulted in a number of publications in medical journals. The focal point of the analyses behind many of these publications is the WHO database. There are always opportunities to intensify research activities on the basis of the WHO register. There are opportunities for researchers to stay at the UMC for short periods to study specific drug-related problems, though funding issues need to be discussed with each situation.

There is a general need to quantify adverse drug reactions information. Under-reporting of adverse drug reactions in routine monitoring is the norm. There is, however, a considerable difference in the degree from time-to-time, place-to-place and between drugs. Publicity and the novelty of the drug or reaction are but two of the reasons for changes in reporting rate. The UMC is working jointly with IMS International, who have a variety of drug use data from most of the countries that are also in the WHO Program. This allows national differences in reporting rates to be further analyzed for reasons that may be due to differences in indications for use, medical practice and demographics, amongst many others. The EU's BIOMED Program is funding a research project in this area, and already the data have been useful in dealing with a drug safety signal, as well as raising a new issue for consideration. This project was termed the ADR Signals Analysis Project (ASAP). It is now clear that it bridges the gap between having raw numbers of spontaneous reports, as the earliest signal of a problem with a drug, and the expensive and time consuming efforts that are entailed by observational and, certainly, interventional studies.

The aim was to provide more definition to an ADR signal as quickly as possible (thus the acronym ASAP: as soon as possible). Speed is important, since, if a signal is of a serious nature, an early decision must be made on whether a formal study is needed and what features in its design are necessary to give the best result. It is also necessary to provide as much information as quickly as possible to all the players in the drug safety field.

Two questions which the ASAP may be able to answer for any given signal are:

1. is there an urgent public health concern or not? e.g. is the reporting rate high or low? is there a consistant international picture? are there obvious confounding variables which provide alternative explanations for the signal other than the drug in question?

2. if there could be a problem, what type of further investigation is needed? e.g., does the reporting rate and type of reaction suggest a problem that can be studied by a case control or cohort method or other? What kind of investigation should be done of an at risk group? is a mechanistic study indicated?

In short, the objective of ASAP is to focus the gaze of pharmacovigilance on the more important issues for follow up.

An important part of the Centre's activities is also to act in other ways as a communication centre – a clearing house for information on drug safety at the service of drug regulatory agencies. In view of the current trends in pharmacoepidemiology, the Centre is also trying to increase its collaboration with groups involved with databases which may be useful in pharmacovigilance. The EU has supported an important initiative in the creation of a European Pharmacovigilance Working Group. This has allowed regulators and drug safety specialists from a variety of European countries to come together to plan co-ordinated drug safety exercises. This approach may pave the way for a much more logical development and investigation of drug safety signals world wide.

Requests for special database searches and investigations are also accepted by the Centre from participating national centres. Through searches in the WHO register, direct communication can be established between centres with a similar drug problem. The fastest way for a national centre to gain access to international experience is through an on-line connection to the WHO Centre computer.

There is also a continuous flow of external enquiries from parties outside the Collaborative Program concerning the pooled international data, and flexible search programs are available to allow for the most complex of these enquiries. On-line access, within confidentiality limits agreed by the Program members, also allows a range of do-it-yourself searches. Some countries maintain the right to refuse release of their own information if they so wish. Use of the information released is subject to a caveat document as to its proper use. At present 130–140 queries from parties outside the programme are processed annually. In addition about 15 external users subscribe to on-line access to information from the approximately 30 countries that agree to general release of data without prior consultation.

Since 1982, the UMC has been distributing an *Adverse Reactions Newsletter* to participating centres, with reviews of national adverse reaction bulletins and news of drug problems being investigated in the various countries, supplemented with figures from the WHO register.

The WHO program has assumed responsibility for

developing a standardized adverse reaction terminology (WHO-ART) and a comprehensive index of reported drugs (WHO-DD), both of which have a utility beyond their importance to the monitoring system. These tools are used in the pre-marketing safety area, as well as for post-marketing studies, by many pharmaceutical companies. WHO-ART has also been adopted by the International Program on Chemical Safety as the medical terminology used to describe poisoning incidents. The WHO-ART has been continuously developed over the 25 years of the Program and is in need of some renovation. Discussions are being undertaken with the International Committee on Harmonisation (ICH), comprising regulators and industry representatives from Japan, the EU and the USA on the development of a new terminology. This will be a difficult task, raising as it does, complicated problems of definition and hierarchical relationships that must be acceptable to Program member states with differing kinds of medical practice and language. Throughout the world, there has been concern over the introduction of a new medical terminology. The UMC is committed to maintain the WHO-ART for as long as it is required and to try to work with the managers of the new terminology to ensure as much compatability as possible. Now, there is an arrangement whereby updates of terms in the two terminologies are exchanged. The WHO-DD is unique in its coverage of drugs marketed throughout the world, but the Centre is trying to develop it further with the co-operation of industry users. There is now a working data model of a new Drug Dictionary which will allow the entry of many more details about drugs e.g. dosage forms, strengths and licence holders.

The Collaborating Centre is developing new tools for drug safety use on a continuous basis. New logic systems are under preparation for the examination of the data-base for new types of signal, and new output documents will enhance the ability of experts to evaluate the data.

There are new challenges in the drug safety arena. One is the increasing use of herbal preparations in western countries. In other countries the dangers of the use of the wrong or badly prepared herbs are better known; in western countries, 'herbal' or 'natural' remedies are synonymous with safety. The Collaborating Centre has over 5000 adverse reaction reports involving herbals, but the vast majority are impossible to interpret because of uncertainty over the contents of what are frequently multiple-ingredient, unregistered products. The Centre is discussing, with a variety of authorities throughout the world, better ways of collecting and classifying information. It is clear that international co-operation is vital, since these drugs are marketed with little control throughout the world. Much work has been done to improve the recording of herbal products in the data-base consistantly. A new joint project is proposed with the Royal Botanical Gardens, Kew, London, and the Department of Complementary Health Studies, University of Exeter, England and Dr. Peter de Smet in The Netherlands. This will also link with known projects in S. Africa, Kenya and Zimbabwe. Other countries are actively being contacted and the project is also linked with the International Programme on Chemical Safety project on poisonous plants.

Poisoning from drugs (and other chemicals) has not fallen within the scope of 'adverse drug reactions'. Indeed, the widely used WHO definition of an ADR specifically excludes doses outside the normal therapeutic range: 'A response to a drug which is noxious and unintended, and which occurs at doses normally used in man for the prophylaxis, diagnosis, or therapy of disease, or for the modification of physiological function' (WHO Technical Report No. 498 (1972). This definition has always begged the question of what is 'normal', particularly for a new drug, but it has also meant that useful information on drug safety from overdose situations may not have been collected. Many overdose patients are treated by poison control centres, or, with their advice, by general physicians and intensive care experts. Their records are not usually sent to national ADR centres. The Collaborating Centre has been involved in a pilot exercise with several poison control centres throughout the world to capture information on poisoned patients. This has been a successful study and has included much physiological data from the most severely affected patients, which will improve the understanding of dose-related ADRs and aid in the treatment of overdose patients.

The UMC is particularly conscious of the need to consider the benefit to risk balance in relationship to drug safety. This requires, amongst other things, the ability to balance the risk of the disease being treated together with the likely benefit of the drug against the risks of the drug, using similar measures. The merits of the use of a particular drug (or other therapy) are context dependant. Different indications for use, individuals with varieties of concurrent diseases are just two examples of such different contexts. Some overall public health view of a drug's merits seems desirable and this is another very different situation. Some of these issues have been aired in a joint publication and are the subject of new work with CIOMS.

Both this activity, and others that have broader implications in the general area of pharmacovigilance, are being pursued in collaboration with other interested parties. It is likely that co-operation with groups interested in developing early signals of significance will broaden within the scope of this important WHO program. Development of pharmacoepidemiology is one area where this can occur, and also in the area of risk-benefit assessment. The role of CIOMS (Council for International Organizations of Medical Sciences) is pivotal in bringing interested parties together to mount various collaborative projects, as is that of the ISPE (International Society for Pharmacoepidemiology). These organizations are specifically interested in the science of pharmacovigilance, whereas many others, such as HAI (Health Action International), INRUD (International Network for the Rational Use of Drugs), the IFPMA (International Federation of Pharmaceutical Manufacturers Associations), and the DIA (Drug Information Association), have a broader interest in the area of drug use.

These possibilities for co-operation are exciting since they have in prospect a more rational, cost-effective, and safe drug therapy, but the negative potential for duplication of both effort and dialog must be avoided, since patient safety is at stake.

In order to foster education and communication in pharmacovigilance in general, the Centre now offers an annual course, which is increasingly popular. The course is in 3 consecutive modules. The first offers some insight into the clinical aspects and diagnosis of adverse drug reactions; the second is about the Collaborating Program and also gives 'hands on' experience in using the Collaborating Centre's database; and the final module is an introduction to wider issues in pharmacoepidemiology.

There has also been an increasing trend towards both local and regional meetings in pharmacovigilance. Attendance by Centre staff at such meetings is increasingly requested, but it is to those meetings in developing countries that the Centre gives its priority. Regional meetings have been particularly useful in showing the links between pharmacovigilance, toxicovigilance, drug information, and drug regulation. In many countries developing these kind of activities, it has been possible to suggest considerable savings using shared staff and resources.

Finally, the needs of the general public must not be forgotten. It is clear from some publications, and many discussions with consumer groups, that issues of drug safety and risk and benefit in clinical care are not well understood. This is not surprising, since they are complex and often not considered by an individual until illness supervenes and they change from person to patient. The threat of illness must make it difficult to objectively contemplate different therapeutic management proposals, even if they are offered to the patient by the physician. Thus, the empowerment of patients to be involved in decisions that affect their lives seems to be a nearly impossible task, given the variety of intelligence, knowledge, and attitudes displayed by patients. One effort that has met with success, if sales are anything to judge by, is the provision of a 'Patient Pharmacopoeia'. This is the most widely selling publication in Sweden. A meeting in Verona, Italy, was recently organised by the UMC, the Department of Clinical Pharmacology, University of Verona and Equus Training, Marketing and Business Services (UK). Both the World Health Organisation (Division of Drug Management and Policy) and the Council for International Organisations of Medical Sciences (CIOMS) were sponsors.

The meeting was of professionals reflecting the major groups of players concerned with drug safety issues: consumers, health professionals, the pharmaceutical industry, drug regulators, health professional teachers, clinical pharmacology researchers, the professional media, the legal profession as well as the organisations mentioned above. It was thought essential to involve all the players in a dialogue in order to achieve greater maturity and effectiveness through greater understanding of themselves and others. A general communications model was proposed for examination which should be used to test communications traffic between the players.

The focus of communication in drug safety should be towards the empowerment of consumers and patients to make realistic decisions on their therapy.

Further meetings are being planned, under the CIOMS umbrella, to discuss several issues in more detail. A larger, more global meeting is proposed, under the WHO umbrella, to ensure that pharmacovigilance communications principles and practices can be developed which will benefit all cultures and countries.

Address list national centres participating in the WHO drug monitoring programme

Argentina (ARG)	Dr Mabel Teresa Foppiano Tel +54-1-345 7135 Fax +54-1-345 7135	Administración Nacional de Medicamentos, Alimentos y Tecnologia Medica (ANMAT) Departamento de Farmacovigilancia Avenida de Mayo 869, piso 11o (1084) BUENOS AIRES Argentina
Australia (AUS)	Dr Ian Boyd Tel +61-6-289 8671 Fax +61-6-289 7694 E-mail ian.boyd @tga.ausgovhhcs.telememo.au	Therapeutic Goods Administration Department of Community Services and Health P.O. Box 100 WODEN, A.C.T. 2606 Australia
Austria (AUT)	Ms Eva Hofbauer Tel +43-1-711 72, ext 4641 Fax +43-1-712 0823 E-mail Eva.Hofbauer@BMGSK.ADA.AT	Federal Ministry of Health and Consumer Protection Pharmacovigilance Department II/A/3 Radetzkystraße 2 A-1030 VIENNA Austria
Belgium (BEL)	Mr Thierry Roisin Tel +32-2-210 4909 Fax +32-2-210 4909	Ministry of Health Pharmacy General Inspectorate Centre National de Pharmacovigilance Vesale Building, 20 rue Montagne de l'Oratoire B-1010 BRUSSELS Belgium
Bulgaria (BUL)	Dr Jasmina Mircheva Director Tel +359-2-434 71 Fax +359-2-442 697	National Drug Institute Committee on Adverse Drug Reactions 26, Yanko Sakazov Boulevard BG-1504 SOFIA Bulgaria
Canada (CAN)	Dr Philippe Duclos Tel +1-613-957 0325 Fax +1-613-998 6413 E-mail PDUCLOS@HPB.HWC.CA	Health Canada Division of Immunization Laboratory Centre for Disease Control OTTAWA, ONTARIO K1A 0L2 Canada

Canada (CAN)	Dr L Bruce Rowsell Director Tel +1-613-957 0337, 954 6522 Fax +1-613-957 0335, 952 7738 Telex 0533679	Health Canada Bureau of Drug Surveillance ADR Monitoring Division OTTAWA, ONTARIO K1A 1B9 Canada
Chile (CHL)	Dr Q F Cecilia Morgado-Cadiz Tel +56-2-239 1105 Fax +56-2-239 6960	Ministerio de Salud Instituto de Salud Publica de Chile National Drug Information Center Avenida Marathon 1000 Casilla 48 SANTIAGO Chile
Costa Rica (COR)	Dr Albin Chaves Matamoros Tel +506-222 1878 Fax +506-257 7004	Caja Costarricense de Seguro Social Departamento de Farmacoterapia Apartado 10105 SAN JOSÉ 1000 Costa Rica
Croatia (CRO)	Prof Bozidar Vrhovac Tel +385-1-213 861 Fax +385-1-213 861 Telex 221252	National ADR Monitoring Centre Section of Clinical Pharmacology Department of Medicine University Hospital Centre 12 Kispaticeva 41000 ZAGREB Croatia
Cuba (CUB)	Dr Carlos Dotres Martinez Fax +53-7-333 299	Ministerio de Salud Publica Calle 23 esq. N. Vedado C.P. 10 400 CIUDAD DE LA HABANA Cuba
Czech Republic (CZE)	MUDr Dana Stolbová Tel +42-2-670 828 17 Fax +42-2-744 944 E-mail sukl@sukl.anet.cz Telex 122662 ihec	State Institute for Drug Control Státni ústav pro Kontrolu Léciv Committee on Adverse Drug Reactions Srobárova 48, post. prihr. 87 100 41 PRAHA 10 Czech Republic
Denmark (DEN)	Mrs Kirsten G Astrup Head Tel +45-4-488 9111 Fax +45-4-284 7077 Telex 35333 ipharm dk	National Board of Health Sundhedsstyrelsen Pharmacotherapeutic secretariat Medicines Division, Lægemiddelafdelingen 378, Frederikssundsvej DK-2700 BRONSHØJ Denmark

Finland (FIN)	Dr Erkki Palva Research Director Tel +358-9-396 725 18 (396 7250) Fax +358-9-396 725 11	National Agency for Medicines (NAM) Lääkelaitos Drug Information Centre P.O. Box 278 Siltasaarenkatu 18 A SF-00531 HELSINKI Finland
France (FRA)	Dr Anne Castot Tel +33-1-481 322 85 Fax +33-1-481 322 83 Telex 250011	Agence du Médicament Unité de Pharmacovigilance 143-145, boulevard Anatole France F-93285 SAINT-DENIS Cedex France
France (FRA)	Dr Claude Larousse Tel +33-40-084 096 Fax +33-40-084 097	CHR Institut de Biologie Centre Regional Pharmacovigilance BP 1005 F-44035 NANTES Cedex France
Germany (GFR)	Dr Jürgen Beckmann Tel +49-30-454 830 00, 454 833 11 Fax +49-30-454 832 07 Telex 17308062	Federal Institute for Drugs and Medical Devices Bundesinstitut für Arzneimittel und Medizinprodukte Seestraße 10 D-13353 BERLIN Germany
Germany (GFR)	Dr Karl-Heinz Munter Secretary-General Tel +49-221-400 4525 Fax +49-221-400 4539 Telex 8882161	Arzneimittelkommission der Deutschen Ärzteschaft P.O. Box 41 01 25, Aachener Straße 233-237 D-50931 KÖLN Germany
Greece (GRC)	Ms Antonia Pandouvaki Tel +30-1-654 9585 Fax +30-1-654 5535	National Drug Organization (EOF) Adverse Drug Reactions Section 284 Messogion Av. GR-155 62 HOLARGOS Greece
Hungary (HUN)	Dr János Borvendég Tel +36-1-215 8977 Fax +36-1-215 8977 Telex 224656 ogyih	National Institute of Pharmacy Adverse Drug Reactions Monitoring Centre Zrínyi u. 3, Box 450 H-1372 BUDAPEST Hungary

Iceland (ICE)	Dr Olafur Olafsson Director Tel +354-5-627 555 Fax +354-5-623 716 Telex 2050 extern is, 2225 extern is	Director General of Public Health Landlæknir Laugavegi 116 IS-150 REYKJAVIK Iceland
Indonesia (INO)	Dra Andajaningsih Chairman Tel +62-21-424 5459 Fax +62-21-424 3605 Telex 46142	Ministry of Health Directorate General of Drug & Food Control National Centre for Monitoring of Adverse Drug Reactions Jalan Percetakan Negara No. 23 JAKARTA 10560 Indonesia
Ireland (IRE)	Ms Niamh Arthur Senior Adverse Reactions Officer Tel +353-1-676 4971 Fax +353-1-676 7836 Telex 90542	Irish Medicines Board Adverse Reactions Section Earlsfort Centre Earlsfort Terrace DUBLIN 2 Ireland
Israel (ISR)	Dr Dina Hemo Msc Pharm Tel +972-2-782 508, 705 744 Fax +972-2-672 58 20 Telex 25206	Ministry of Health Clinical Pharmacology Department Drug Monitoring Center Horkania 3a street, P.O. Box 1176 JERUSALEM, 91010 Israel
Italy (ITA)	Dr Dina De Stefano Tel +39-6-5994 32 12 Fax +39-6-5994 33 65	National Pharmacovigilance Center Pharmacovigilance Department Ministry of Health Via Civiltà Romana 7 I-00144 ROMA Italy
Japan (JPN)	Dr T Kurokawa Tel +81-3-350 145 07 Fax +81-3-350 843 64 Telex 02225132	Ministry of Health and Welfare Pharmaceutical Affairs Bureau Safety Division Office of Appropriate Use of Drugs 2-2, 1-Chome, Kasumigaseki, Chiyoda-ku TOKYO 100-45 Japan
Korea, Rep of (KOR)	Mr Byung-Woo Moon Director Tel +82-2-503 7585 Fax +82-2-503 7591 E-mail bokji12@nownuri.newcom.co.kr	Ministry of Health & Welfare Pharmaceutical Affairs Bureau Pharmaceutical Development Division 1, Chung-ang Dong KWACHON CITY, Kyungkido, 427-760 Korea, Rep of

Malaysia (MAL)	Dr Anis bin Ahmad Tel +60-3-757 3611 Fax +60-3-756 2924	Ministry of Health Malaysia National Pharmaceutical Control Bureau National ADR Monitoring Center Jalan Universiti, P.O. Box 319 MA-46730 PETALING JAYA Malaysia
Morocco (MOR)	Dr Rachida Soulaymani-Bencheikh Tel +212-7-770 137 Fax +212-7-772 067	Institut National d'Hygiène Centre Anti Poisons et de Pharmacovigilance Avenue Ibn Batouta 27 B.P. 769, Agdal M-11400 RABAT Morocco
Netherlands (NET)	Dr Arthur P Meiners Tel +31-70-340 7487, 340 7152 Fax +31-70-340 5155 E-mail ameiners@pi.net	Medicines Evaluation Board P.O. Box 5811 Sir Winston Churchilllaan 362 2280 HV RIJSWIJK The Netherlands
New Zealand (NEZ)	Dr Peter Pillans Medical Assessor Tel +64-3-479 7248, extension 8345 Fax +64-3-477 0509 E-mail peter.pillans@stonebow.otago.ac.nz Telex 5706	University of Otago Medical School National Toxicology Group P.O. Box 913 DUNEDIN New Zealand
Norway (NOR)	Mrs Krystyna Hviding Tel +47-22-897 700 Fax +47-22-897 799	Norwegian Medicines Control Authority Statens Legemiddelkontroll (SLK) Adverse Drug Reaction Section Sven Oftedals vei 6 N-0950 OSLO 9 Norway
Oman (OMN)	Dr Ph Sawsan Ahmad Jaffar Tel +968-600 016, 601 044 Fax +968-602 287, 604 684 Telex 5465	Ministry of Health Directorate General of Pharmaceutical Affairs and Drug Control P.O. Box 393 113 MUSCAT Oman
Philippines (PHL)	Mrs Nazarita T Lanuza Tel +63-2-842 5606, 807 0731 Fax +63-2-842 4603	Bureau of Food and Drugs Department of Health Compound Alabang 1702, Muntinlupa METRO MANILA Philippines

Poland (POL)	Prof Andrzej Czarnecki Head Tel +48-22-410 652 Fax +48-22-410 652 E-mail anczarn@il.waw.pl	Institute for Drug Research and Control Centre for Monitoring of Adverse Effects to Drugs 30/34 Chelmska Street PL-00725 WARSAW Poland
Portugal (POR)	Dr Ana Maria Corrêa Nunes Head Tel +351-1-790 8500, 795 7836 Fax +351-1-795 9116, 795 9069 E-mail infarmed@mail.telepac.pt	Centro Nacional de Farmacovigilancia Instituto Nacional da Farmácia e do Medicamento (INFARMED) Parque de Saúde de Lisboa Avenida do Brasil, no. 53 P-1700 LISBOA Portugal
Romania (ROM)	Dr Rodica Badescu Tel +40-1-666 6035 Fax +40-1-312 9783 Telex 11595	State Institute for Drug Control and Pharmaceutical Research Str Aviator Sanatescu no 48, Sector 1 R-71 324 BUCURESTI Romania
Singapore (SIN)	Ms Amy Lim Tel +65-325 5629 Fax +65-224 2352 E-mail kbtoh@cs.gov.sg	Adverse Drug Reaction Monitoring Unit Drug Administration Division (DAD) No. 2 Jalan Bukit Merah SINGAPORE 0316 Singapore
Slovakia (SVK)	Dr Pavol Gibala Tel +42-7-566 5075, 211 860, 211 952 Fax +42-7-566 4127, 566 40	National Centre for Monitoring Adverse Reactions to Drugs State Institute for the Control of Drugs Kvetná 11 825 08 BRATISLAVA Slovakia
South Africa (SOA)	Ms Ushma Mehta Tel +27-21-471 618 Fax +27-21-448 6181 E-mail umehta@uctgsh1.uct.ac.za	National ADE Monitoring Centre c/o Department of Pharmacology Faculty of Medicine University of Cape Town OBSERVATORY 7925 South Africa
Spain (SPA)	Dr Fransisco José de Abajo Tel +34-1-509 7947 Fax +34-1-509 7948 Telex 47209 insan e	Centro Coordinador del Sistema Español de Farmacovigilancia Instituto de Salud 'Carlos III' Centro Nacional de Farmacobiología Carretera a Pozuelo, Km 2 E-28220 MAJADAHONDA (MADRID) Spain

Sweden (SWE)	Dr Bengt-Erik Wiholm Tel +46-18-17 46 00 Fax +46-18-54 85 66 Telex 76059	Medical Products Agency Division of Drug Epidemiology, Information & Inspection Adverse Drug Reaction Section P.O. Box 26, Husargatan 8 S-751 03 UPPSALA Sweden
Switzerland (SCH)	Dr Rudolf Stoller Tel +41-31-302 3651 Fax +41-31-302 0654, 302 8789	Interkantonale Kontrollstelle für Heilmittel Pharmacovigilance Centre Erlachstraße 8 CH-3000 BERN Switzerland
Tanzania (TAN)	Mr Henry Irunde Tel +255-51-262 11, ext 2571 Fax +255-51-462 29 Telex 41505 muhmed tz	Tanzania Drug and Toxicology Information Service P.O. Box 65088 DAR ES SALAAM Tanzania
Thailand (THA)	Mrs Suboonya Hutangkabodee Tel +66-2-591 8449, 591 8458, 591 8459 Fax +66-2-591 8457 E-mail suboonya@health.moph.go.th Telex 82573	Drug Info Center and NADRM, Techn. Div. National ADR Monitoring Centre Ministry of Public Health Food and Drug Administration Ti-wa-nondh Rd NONTHABUREE 11000 Thailand
Tunisia (TUN)	Prof Chelbi Belkahia Tel +216-1-264 763 Fax +216-1-571 390	Centre National de Pharmacovigilance Sis Höpital Charles Nicolle TUNIS 1006 Tunisia
Turkey (TUR)	Ms Sevgi Öksüz Chemist Tel +90-312-431 1446 Fax +90-312-434 4518 E-mail saglik@servis.net.tr Telex 42770	Turkish ADR Monitoring Center (TADMER) Türk Ilac Advers Etkilerini Izleme ve Skolas str 28 Saglik Bakanligi Ilac ve Eczacilic Genel Müdürlügü 06434 Sihhiye ANKARA Turkey
United Kingdom (UNK)	Dr Susan Wood Head Tel +44-171-273 0400 Fax +44-171-273 0282, 273 0675 Telex 883669	Medicines Control Agency Pharmacovigilance, Department of Health Market Towers, 1 Nine Elms Lane Vauxhall LONDON SW8 5NQ United Kingdom

United States of America (USA)	Dr Richard M Kapit Tel +1-301-594 5682 Fax +1-301-827 3529 E-mail kapit@a1.cber.fda.gov	Food and Drug Administration Center for Biologics Evaluation and Research Adverse Event Section, HFM-225 1401 Rockville Pike ROCKVILLE, MARYLAND 20852 United States of America
United States of America (USA)	Dr Robert O'Neill Tel +1-301-443 4227 Fax +1-301-443 5161 Telex 898488	Food and Drug Administration Center for Drug Evaluation and Research Office of Epidemiology and Biostatics Room 15B-31 (HFD-730) 5600 Fishers Lane ROCKVILLE, MARYLAND 20857 United States of America
Venezuela (VEN)	Dra Evelyn Uzcátegui Tel +58-2-662 4797 Fax +58-2-662 5074, 662 509	Instituto Nacional de Higiene 'Rafael Rangel' Sección de Farmacología Sanitaria Centro Nacional de Vigilancia Farmacológia Ciudad Universitaria Apartado Postal 60.412 - Oficina del Este CARACAS Venezuela
(EU)	Mr Philippe Meyer Principal Administrator Tel +32-2-295 1891, 295 6650 Fax +32-2-296 1520 Telex COMEU B 21877	European Commission Pharmaceuticals NERV 2/11, CEE, DG III C 3 Rue de la Loi 200 B-1049 BRUSSELS Belgium
(WHO)	Dr Martijn ten Ham Chief Tel +41-22-791 2111, 791 3638 Fax +41-22-791 0746 E-mail tenhamm@who.ch Telex 415416	World Health Organization Drug Safety Unit 10 Avenue Appia CH-1211 GENEVA 27 Switzerland

ASSOCIATE MEMBERS

China, People's Republic of	Prof Zhu Yonghong Tel +86-10-701 7755, extension 339 Fax +86-10-701 3755	National Centre for ADR Monitoring c/o National Institute for Drug Control Temple of Heaven BEIJING, P R C 100050 China, People's Republic of

Cyprus	Dr Eftychios Kkolos Director Tel +357-2-302 001 Fax +357-2-302 721	Ministry of Health Pharmaceutical Services 44 Kimonos Street NICOSIA 138 Cyprus
Egypt	Dr Gamila Mohamed Moussa Tel +20-2-354 9802 Fax +20-2-354 2627	Ministry of Health Directorate General of Drug Control CAIRO Egypt
Iran	Dr S Haghighi Tel +98-21-640 6174, 640 0081 Telex 212500 fdcl ir Fax +98-21-640 4330	Ministry of Health and Medical Education Food & Drug Control Laboratories (FDCL) No 31, Emam Khomeini Ave P.O. Box 9385 11136 TEHERAN Iran
Pakistan	Prof M Sultan Farooqui President Tel +92-21-588 2997, 589 2801 Fax +92-21-589 3062, 588 7513 E-mail whocpsp%paknetbbs @sdnpk.undp.org	College of Physicians & Surgeons Pakistan (CPSP) Department of Clinical Pharmacology 7th Central Street Phase II, Defence Housing Authority KARACHI - 75500 Pakistan
Sri Lanka	Dr U Ajith Mendis Director Tel +94-1-695 173 Fax +94-1-695 173	Ministry of Health Medical Technology and Supplies Division No. 120, Norris Canal Road COLOMBO 10 Sri Lanka
Yugoslavia, Fed. Rep. of	Prof Vaso Antunovic	Clinical Centre of Serbia National Centre for Adverse Drug Effects Visegradska 26 11000 BELGRADE Yugoslavia, Fed. Rep. of
Zimbabwe	Registrar Tel +263-4-792 165 Fax +263-4-736 980	Drugs Control Council P.O. Box UA 599, 106 Baines Avenue Union Avenue HARARE Zimbabwe

Index of drugs

When a drug is not listed individually, it is advisable to look for relevant information under the group name since closely related products with very similar side effects have in some cases been reviewed and indexed as a group. Page numbers in **bold** indicate where the given drug is discussed in detail.

Index of side effects